Textbook of Family Practice

ROBERT E. RAKEL, M.D.
Chairman, Department of Family Medicine
Associate Dean for Academic and Clinical Affairs
Baylor College of Medicine
Houston, Texas

Textbook of Family Practice

4th edition

W.B. SAUNDERS COMPANY
Harcourt Brace Jovanovich, Inc.
Philadelphia
London Toronto Montreal Sydney Tokyo

W. B. SAUNDERS COMPANY
Harcourt Brace Jovanovich, Inc.

The Curtis Center
Independence Square West
Philadelphia, PA 19106–3399

Library of Congress Cataloging in Publication Data

Textbook of family practice / [edited by] Robert E. Rakel.—4th ed. p. cm.

Includes bibliographical references.

Includes index.

1. Family medicine. I. Rakel, Robert E.

[DNLM: 1. Comprehensive Health Care. 2. Family Practice. WB110 T355]

RC46.T327 1990 610–dc20

ISBN 0-7216-3115-0

DNLM/DLC 90-8566
for Library of Congress CIP

Editor: John Dyson
Developmental Editor: Kathleen McCullough
Designer: Karen O'Keefe
Production Manager: Bill Preston
Manuscript Editor: Carol DeBerardino
Illustration Coordinator: Walt Verbitski
Indexer: Angela Holt
Cover Designer: Ellen Bodner

Listed here is the latest translated edition of this book together with the language of the translation and the publisher.

Spanish (1st edition) NEISA (McGraw-Hill/Interamericana de Mexico) Cedro 512, 06450 Mexico D.F., Mexico

Japanese (3rd edition) Igaku Shoin Ltd., 5-24-3 Hongo, Bunkyo-ku, Tokyo 113-91, Japan

Textbook of Family Practice ISBN 0–7216–3115–0

Last digit is the print number: 9 8 7 6 5 4 3 2

This edition is dedicated to the memory of
NICHOLAS J. PISACANO, M.D.,
1924–1990,
who contributed so much to our discipline
through the creation and development of the
American Board of Family Practice.

Contributors

Allan V. Abbott, M.D.
Associate Professor of Clinical Family Medicine, University of Southern California School of Medicine; University of Southern California Medical Center, Los Angeles, California
Cardiovascular Disease: Preventive Cardiology; Cardiovascular Disease: Rehabilitation After Myocardial Infarction

Abdulla M. Abdulla, M.D., F.A.C.P., F.A.C.C.
Clinical Professor, Medical College of Georgia School of Medicine; Active Staff, University Hospital, St. Joseph Hospital, Humana Hospital, Augusta, Georgia
The Use of Personal Computers in Medicine

Lois A. Addison, M.A., M.L.T.
Office Laboratory Consultant, Dunrobin, Ontario, Canada
Interpreting Laboratory Tests

John E. Arradondo, M.D., M.P.H.
Adjunct Professor, School of Public Health, University of Texas Medical School at Houston; Director, Houston Department of Health and Human Services, Houston, Texas
Utilization of Community Resources

Donald S. Asp, M.D.
Associate Professor, Department of Family Practice and Community Health, University of Minnesota Medical School—Minneapolis; St. Joseph's Division, St. John's Eastside Hospital, St. Paul, Minnesota
Sociocultural Influences on Medicine and Health

Sanford Auerbach, M.D.
Assistant Professor of Neurology, Boston University School of Medicine; Director, Sleep Laboratory, University Hospital, Boston, Massachusetts
Neurology: Behavioral Disturbances

Robert F. Avant, M.D.
Professor of Family Medicine; Chairman, Department of Family Medicine; Parker-Sanders Professor of Primary Care, Mayo Medical School; Department of Family Medicine, Methodist Hospital, Mayo Clinic and Mayo Foundation, Rochester, Minnesota
Obstetrics

Viken Babikian, M.D.
Assistant Professor of Neurology, Boston University School of Medicine; Chief, Neurovascular Intensive Care Unit, Veterans Administration Medical Center, Boston, Massachusetts
Neurology: Coma and Altered States of Consciousness

John W. Bachman, M.D.
Assistant Professor of Family Medicine, Mayo Medical School; Consultant, Department of Family Medicine, Mayo Clinic and Mayo Foundation, Rochester, Minnesota
Statistical Methods

Byron J. Bailey, M.D.
Wiess Professor and Chairman, Department of Otolaryngology, University of Texas Medical School at Galveston, Galveston, Texas
Otolaryngology

Macaran A. Baird, M.D.
Professor and Chairman, Department of Family Medicine, State University of New York Health Science Center at Syracuse College of Medicine; Director of Medical Education, St. Joseph's Hospital Health Center; Staff, Crouse-Irving Memorial Hospital; Staff, Community General Hospital, Syracuse, New York
Marriage and Family Counseling

Collin Baker, M.D.
Professor Emeritus, Department of Family Medicine, University of South Carolina School of Medicine, Columbia, South Carolina
Endocrinology

Bonnie Baldwin, M.D.
Resident, Division of Plastic Surgery, Baylor College of Medicine, Houston, Texas
Plastic and Reconstructive Surgery

Andrew M. Barclay, M.B., Ch.B.
Associate Professor and Chairman, Department of Family and Community Medicine, University of Kansas Medical Center School of Medicine—Wichita; Medical Staff, Wesley Medical Center; St. Francis Regional Medical Center; St. Joseph Medical Center, Wichita, Kansas
Genetic Problems

Renaldo N. Battista, M.D., Sc.D.
Associate Professor, Departments of Epidemiology and Biostatistics, Family Medicine, and Medicine, McGill University Faculty of Medicine; Director, Division of Clinical

Epidemiology, Department of Medicine, Montreal General Hospital, Montreal, Quebec, Canada
The Periodic Health Examination

Alexander Berger, M.D.
Professor, Department of Family and Community Medicine, Eastern Virginia Medical School of the Medical College of Hampton Roads, Norfolk; Director, Portsmouth Family Medicine Residency, Portsmouth General Hospital; Maryview Hospital, Portsmouth, Virginia
Ophthalmology

Kent D. Bergh, M.D.
Assistant Professor, Department of Family Medicine and Community Health, University of Minnesota Medical School—Minneapolis; North Memorial Medical Center, Robbinsdale, Minnesota
Sociocultural Influences on Medicine and Health

Lawrence H. Bernstein, M.D.
Assistant Clinical Professor of Medicine, University of Connecticut School of Medicine, Farmington; Attending Physician, Windham Community Memorial Hospital, Willimantic, Connecticut
Home Care

Paul A. Bilodeau, M.D.
Staff Physician, University Hospital; Humana Hospital-Augusta; St. Joseph Hospital, Augusta, Georgia
Hematology

F. Marian Bishop, Ph.D., M.S.P.H.
Professor and Chairman, Department of Family and Preventive Medicine, University of Utah School of Medicine, Salt Lake City, Utah
Interviewing Techniques

David H. Blankenhorn, M.D.
Professor of Medicine and Director of the Atherosclerosis Research Institute, University of Southern California School of Medicine, Los Angeles, California
Cardiovascular Disease: Preventive Cardiology

Alan Blum, M.D.
Assistant Professor, Department of Family Medicine, Baylor College of Medicine, Houston, Texas
Substance Abuse: Nicotine Addiction

Philip J. Bohnert, M.D.
Assistant Professor, Department of Family Medicine, Department of Psychiatry, Baylor College of Medicine, Houston, Texas
Psychiatric Emergencies

Donald A. Bosshart, Ed.D.
Associate Professor of Medical Education, Associate Professor of Educational Psychology in Family Medicine, Northeastern Ohio Universities College of Medicine, Rootstown, Ohio
Patient Education

James H. Bray, Ph.D.
Associate Professor, Department of Family Medicine, Baylor College of Medicine, Houston, Texas
Impact of Divorce on the Family

Baruch A. Brody, Ph.D.
Leon Jaworski Professor of Biomedical Ethics, Baylor College of Medicine, Houston, Texas
Ethics in Primary Care Medicine

Thomas R. Browne III, M.D.
Professor of Neurology (Vice Chairman), Associate Professor of Pharmacology and Experimental Therapeutics, Boston University School of Medicine; Associate Chief, Neurology Services, Veterans Administration Medical Center, Boston, Massachusetts
Neurology: Epilepsy

Leonard H. Brubaker, M.D.
Professor of Medicine, Medical College of Georgia School of Medicine; Medical College of Georgia Hospital Clinics, Augusta, Georgia
Hematology

Paul C. Brucker, M.D.
Alumni Professor and Chairman, Department of Family Medicine, Jefferson Medical College of Thomas Jefferson University; Attending Physician-in-Chief and Chairman, Department of Family Medicine, Thomas Jefferson University Hospital, Philadelphia, Pennsylvania
Childhood and Adolescence

Erich E. Brueschke, M.D.
Professor and Chairman, Department of Family Practice; Professor of Physiology, Rush Medical College of Rush University, Chicago; Senior Attending Physician, Rush-Presbyterian-St. Luke's Medical Center, Chicago; Active Attending Physician, Christ Hospital and Medical Center, Oak Lawn, Illinois
The Somatic Patient

Jon M. Burch, M.D.
Associate Professor of Surgery, Baylor College of Medicine; Attending Surgeon, Ben Taub General Hospital, Houston, Texas
General Surgery

David E. Burdette, M.D.
Teaching Fellow in Neurology, Boston University School of Medicine; Chief Resident, Neurology Department, University Hospital, Boston, Massachusetts
Neurology: Epilepsy

Sandra K. Burge, Ph.D.
Assistant Professor, Department of Family Practice, University of Texas Health Science Center at San Antonio, San Antonio, Texas
Spouse and Elder Abuse

John C. Camp, M.D.
Clinical Assistant Professor of Medicine (Cardiology), University of Southern California School of Medicine, Los Angeles; Active Medical Staff, Presbyterian Intercommunity Hospital, Whittier; Los Angeles County–USC Medical Center, Los Angeles; Rancho Los Amigos Medical Center, Downey, California
Cardiovascular Disease: Rehabilitation After Myocardial Infarction

David C. Campbell, M.D., M.Ed.
Clinical Associate Professor, Saint Louis University School of Medicine; Residency Program Director, Chief of Family Medicine, Deaconess Hospital, St. Louis, Missouri
Sports Medicine

Thomas L. Campbell, M.D.
Assistant Professor of Family Medicine and Psychiatry, University of Rochester School of Medicine and Dentistry; Attending Physician, Highland Hospital of Rochester, Rochester, New York
The Family's Influence on Health

Hilmon Castle, M.D.
Professor, Family and Preventive Medicine and Internal Medicine, University of Utah School of Medicine; Active Staff, Cardiology, University Hospital, Holy Cross Hospital, Salt Lake City, Utah
Cardiovascular Disease: Hypertension; Cardiovascular Disease: Chest Pain; Cardiovascular Disease: Heart Sounds and Murmurs; Cardiovascular Disease: Valvular Heart Disease

E. Bruce Challis, M.D.
Professor and Head, Department of Family Medicine; Medical Director, University Health Services, University of Calgary Faculty of Medicine; Director, Department of Family Medicine; Active Staff, Foothills Hospital; Courtesy Staff, Alberta Childrens Hospital; Calgary General Hospital; Calgary District Hospital Group; Tom Baker Cancer Centre, Calgary, Alberta, Canada
Oncology

Christopher V. Chambers, M.D.
Clinical Assistant Professor, Department of Family Medicine, Jefferson Medical College of Thomas Jefferson University, Philadelphia, Pennsylvania
Childhood and Adolescence

Jeannette Chirico-Post, M.D.
Associate Professor of Neurology, Boston University School of Medicine; Assistant Chief of Staff, Veterans Administration Medical Center, Boston, Massachusetts
Neurology: Disturbance of Motor Function

Rex B. Conn, M.D.
Professor and Vice Chairman, Department of Pathology and Cell Biology, Jefferson Medical College of Thomas Jefferson University; Active Staff, Director of Clinical Laboratories, Thomas Jefferson University Hospital, Philadelphia, Pennsylvania
Laboratory Values of Clinical Importance

John F. Connolly, M.D.
Professor and Chairman, Department of Orthopaedic Surgery, University of Nebraska College of Medicine; Professor, Section of Orthopaedics, Creighton University School of Medicine; Staff, University of Nebraska Hospital; Veterans Administration Medical Center; Childrens Memorial Hospital; Methodist Hospital; Bishop Clarkson Memorial Hospital; Immanuel Medical Center; AMI Saint Joseph Hospital, Omaha, Nebraska
Orthopedics

James C. Coyne, Ph.D.
Associate Professor of Family Practice and Psychiatry, University of Michigan Medical School; Attending Psychologist, University of Michigan Hospitals, Ann Arbor, Michigan
Depression

Michael H. Crawford, M.D.
Robert S. Flinn Professor, Chief, Division of Cardiology, University of New Mexico School of Medicine, Albuquerque, New Mexico
Cardiovascular Disease: Myocardial Diseases; Cardiovascular Disease: Heart Failure; Cardiovascular Disease: Acute Pericarditis; Cardiovascular Disease: Peripheral Arterial Disease; Cardiovascular Disease: Surgery for Patients with Heart Disease

Sydney H. Croog, M.D.
Professor of Behavioral Sciences and Community Health, University of Connecticut Health Center, Farmington, Connecticut
Assessment of Functional Health Status

Earl R. Crouch, Jr., M.D.
Professor and Chairman, Department of Ophthalmology, Associate Professor of Pediatrics, Eastern Virginia Medical School of the Medical College of Hampton Roads, Member, Professional Information Committee, American Academy of Ophthalmology; Norfolk General Hospital; Leigh Memorial Hospital; Children's Hospital of the King's Daughters; DePaul Hospital, Norfolk; Virginia Beach General Hospital, Virginia Beach, Virginia
Ophthalmology

Kathleen A. Culhane-Pera, M.D.
Post-Doctoral Fellow, Institute for Health Policy Studies, University of California, San Francisco, School of Medicine, San Francisco, California
Sociocultural Influences on Medicine and Health

Larry Culpepper, M.D., M.P.H.
Associate Professor of Family Medicine, Brown University Program in Medicine, Providence; Director of Research, Memorial Hospital, Pawtucket, Rhode Island
Interpreting the Medical Journal Literature

Marvin Derezin, M.D.
Clinical Professor of Medicine, Division of Gastroenterology, University of California, Los Angeles School of Medicine, Los Angeles, California
Gastroenterology

William J. Doherty, Ph.D.
Associate Professor, Family Social Science Department; Lecturer, Department of Family Practice and Community Health, University of Minnesota Medical School—Minneapolis, Minneapolis, Minnesota
Marriage and Family Counseling

Charles E. Driscoll, M.D.
Professor and Head, Department of Family Practice, University of Iowa College of Medicine; University of Iowa Hospitals and Clinics; Mercy Hospital, Iowa City, Iowa
Sexual Health Care: A Life Cycle Approach

Robert Eidus, M.D.
Clinical Associate Professor, Department of Family Medicine, University of Medicine and Dentistry of New Jersey Robert Wood Johnson Medical School, New Brunswick; Medical Director, U.S. Healthcare, Paramus, New Jersey
Managed Health Care

David V. Espino, M.D.
Assistant Professor and Director, Division of Geriatrics, Department of Family Practice, University of Texas Health Science Center at San Antonio; Active Staff, Medical Center Hospital; Provisional Staff, Lutheran General Hospital, San Antonio, Texas
Spouse and Elder Abuse

C. Edward Evans, M.B.
Professor of Family Medicine, Faculty of Health Sciences, McMaster University School of Medicine; Active Staff, McMaster University Medical Centre, Hamilton, Ontario, Canada
Patient Compliance

W. E. Fabb, A.M.
National Director of Education, Family Medicine Program, The Royal Australian College of General Practitioners, Jolimont, Victoria, Australia
Family Practice Around the World: Australia

Patrick J. Fahey, M.D.
Assistant Professor, Department of Family Medicine, The Ohio State University College of Medicine; Attending Physician, Ohio State University Hospitals, Columbus, Ohio
Nutrition

Donna R. Falvo, R.N., Ph.D.
Associate Professor, Rehabilitation Institute and School of Medicine, Southern Illinois University School of Medicine at Carbondale, Carbondale, Illinois
Patient Education

Jan A. Fawcett, M.D.
Professor and Chairman, Department of Psychiatry, Rush-Presbyterian-St. Luke's Medical Center, Chicago, Illinois
Substance Abuse: Controlled Substances

Lorraine Fay, M.D.
Assistant Professor, Department of Pediatrics, Medical College of Ohio at Toledo; Medical College of Ohio Hospital; Toledo Hospital, Toledo, Ohio
Growth and Development

Robert G. Feldman, M.D.
Professor of Neurology (Chairman), Professor of Pharmacology, Boston University School of Medicine; Professor of Public Health (Environmental Health), Boston University School of Public Health; Chief, Neurology Services, Veterans Administration Medical Center; University Hospital, Boston, Massachusetts
Neurology: Epilepsy

David V. Feliciano, M.D.
Professor of Surgery, University of Rochester School of Medicine and Dentistry; Director, Surgical Intensive Care Unit; Director, Section of Trauma, Department of Surgery, Strong Memorial Hospital of the University of Rochester, Rochester, New York
General Surgery

Richard E. Finlayson, M.D.
Associate Professor of Psychiatry, Mayo Medical School; Consultant, Section of Psychiatry and Consultant, Department of Family Medicine, Mayo Clinic and Mayo Foundation, Rochester, Minnesota
Dementia

Paul M. Fischer, M.D.
Associate Professor, Department of Family Medicine, Medical College of Georgia School of Medicine, Augusta, Georgia
Interpreting Laboratory Tests

Jules Friedman, M.D.
Assistant Professor of Neurology, Boston University School of Medicine, Boston; Chief, Neurology Service, Braintree Hospital, Braintree, Massachusetts
Neurology: Dizziness

Robert E. Froelich, M.D.
Professor, Department of Psychiatry, University of Utah School of Medicine; Chief, Mental Health Treatment Services, Department of Veterans' Affairs, Veterans Administration Medical Center, Salt Lake City, Utah
Interviewing Techniques

John Fry, C.B.E., M.D.
Family Physician, Beckenham, Kent, England
Family Practice Around the World: Britain

Charlette R. Gallagher-Allred, Ph.D.
Clinical Assistant Professor, Department of Family Medicine, Ohio State University College of Medicine; Nutrition Consultant, Ross Laboratories, Columbus, Ohio
Nutrition

John Geyman, M.D.
Professor and Chairman, Department of Family Practice, University of Washington Medical School, Seattle, Washington
Anxiety

Roland A. Goertz, M.D.
Clinical Assistant Professor, Department of Family Practice, University of Texas Health Science Center at San Antonio, San Antonio; Director, Corpus Christi Family Practice Residency Program; Active Staff, Memorial Medical Center, Corpus Christi, Texas
Cardiovascular Disease: Myocardial Diseases; Cardiovascular Disease: Heart Failure; Cardiovascular Disease: Acute Pericarditis; Cardiovascular Disease: Peripheral Arterial Disease; Cardiovascular Disease: Surgery for Patients with Heart Disease

Larry A. Green, M.D.
Woodward-Chisholm Chairman of Family Medicine, University of Colorado Health Sciences Center School of Medicine; Rose Medical Center; University Hospital, Denver, Colorado
Community-Oriented Primary Care

Troy H. Guthrie, M.D.
Associate Professor, Department of Medicine, Medical College of Georgia School of Medicine; Medical College of Georgia Hospital and Clinics, Augusta, Georgia
Hematology

Jean Haggerty, M.Sc.
Faculty Lecturer, Departments of Family Medicine and Epidemiology and Biostatistics, McGill University Faculty of Medicine; Research Associate, Division of Clinical Epidemiology, Department of Medicine, Montreal General Hospital, Montreal, Quebec, Canada
The Periodic Health Examination

James W. Hanson, M.D.
Professor of Pediatrics, University of Iowa College of Medicine; Director, Division of Medical Genetics, University of Iowa Hospitals and Clinics, Iowa City, Iowa
Genetic Problems

R. Brian Haynes, M.D., Ph.D.
Professor of Clinical Epidemiology and Medicine, Faculty of Health Sciences, McMaster University School of Medicine; Attending Staff, Section of Internal Medicine, Chedoke-McMaster Hospitals, Hamilton, Ontario, Canada
Patient Compliance

Warren A. Heffron, M.D.
Professor and Chairman, Department of Family, Community and Emergency Medicine, University of New Mexico School of Medicine; Chief of Service, Family Medicine, University of New Mexico Hospital-Bernalillo County Medical Center, Albuquerque, New Mexico
Preventive Health Care in Family Medicine

John S. Henke
Technical Editor, *Physician and Computer*, Chicago, Illinois
The Use of Personal Computers in Medicine

William Leon Heth, M.D.
Urology Chief Resident, Medical College of Ohio at Toledo, Toledo, Ohio; Midelfort Clinic, Eau Claire, Wisconsin
Urinary Tract Disorders: Urology

Robert W. Higgins, M.D.
Deputy Surgeon-General of the Navy, Deputy Chief of the Navy Bureau of Medicine and Surgery, Chief of the Navy Medical Corps
Behavioral Problems in Children and Adolescents

Joseph Hobbs, M.D.
Associate Professor, Department of Family Medicine, Medical College of Georgia School of Medicine; Medical College of Georgia Hospital and Clinics, Augusta, Georgia
Hematology; Urinary Tract Disorders: Acid-Base, Fluid, and Electrolyte Disorders; Urinary Tract Disorders: Renal Failure

Georgianna S. Hoffmann, R.N., M.A.
The Center for Marital and Sexual Counseling, Iowa City, Iowa
Sexual Health Care: A Life Cycle Approach

Warren L. Holleman, Ph.D.
Assistant Professor, Department of Family Medicine and Center for Ethics, Medicine, and Public Issues, Baylor College of Medicine, Houston, Texas
Ethics in Primary Care Medicine

Leo E. Hollister, M.D.
Professor of Psychiatry and Pharmacology, University of Texas Medical School at Houston; Medical Director, Harris County Psychiatric Center, Houston, Texas
Psychotherapeutic Drugs

Richard L. Holloway, Ph.D.
Associate Professor and Research Director, Department of Family Medicine, Baylor College of Medicine, Houston, Texas
Research Methodology

Rebecca Jackson, M.D.
Assistant Professor, University of New Mexico School of Medicine; Staff Physician, University of New Mexico Hospital-Bernalillo County Medical Center, Albuquerque, New Mexico
Sexual Assault: Rape

O. Max Jardon, M.D.
Associate Professor, Department of Orthopaedic Surgery, University of Nebraska College of Medicine; Staff, University of Nebraska Hospital; Childrens Memorial Hospital; Bishop Clarkson Memorial Hospital; Veterans Administration Medical Center; Ehrling Bergquist U.S. Air Force Regional Hospital; Immanuel Medical Center, Omaha, Nebraska
Orthopedics

L. Martin Jerry, M.D., Ph.D.
Clinical Professor of Medicine, University of Calgary Faculty of Medicine; Director, Tom Baker Cancer Centre; Attending Staff, Foothills Hospital; Calgary General Hospital, Calgary, Alberta, Canada
Oncology

Duane M. Johnson, Ph.D.
President, Productivity, Inc., Atlanta, Georgia
Personnel and Time Management

Jerry E. Jones, M.D., M.S.
Chairman, Department of Family Medicine, University of Alabama School of Medicine, Tuscaloosa Program, Tuscaloosa, Alabama
Parasitology

Marc Kamin, M.D.
Assistant Professor of Neurology, Boston University School of Medicine; Staff Neurologist, Boston City Hospital, Boston, Massachusetts
Neurology: Headache

Wayne Katon, M.D.
Associate Professor of Psychiatry and Behavioral Sciences, Chief of Division of Consultation Liaison Psychiatry, Adjunct Associate Professor of Family Medicine, University of Washington School of Medicine, Seattle, Washington
Anxiety

Sanford R. Kimmel, M.D.
Assistant Professor, Department of Family Medicine, Medical College of Ohio at Toledo; Medical College of Ohio Hospital; St. Vincent Hospital and Medical Center; Toledo Hospital, Toledo, Ohio
Growth and Development

Jan Kucera, M.D.
Professor of Neurology, Boston University School of Medicine; Staff Neurologist, Veterans Administration Medical Center, Boston, Massachusetts
Neurology: Disturbance of Motor Function

Walker A. Lea, Jr., M.D.
Active Staff, Hillcrest Baptist Medical Center; Providence Hospital; Consultant, Veterans Administration Medical Center, Waco, Texas
Dermatology

Greg L. Ledgerwood, M.D.
Clinical Associate Professor of Family Medicine, University of Washington School of Medicine, Seattle, Washington; Attending Physician, Mid-Valley Hospital, Omak, Washington
Allergy

Simmons Lessel, M.D.
Professor of Ophthalmology, Harvard Medical School; Director, Neuro-ophthalmology, Massachusetts Eye and Ear Infirmary, Boston, Massachusetts
Neurology: Visual Disturbances

John H. Leversee, M.D.
Associate Professor, Department of Family Medicine, University of Washington School of Medicine; Active Staff, University Hospital; Courtesy Staff, Children's Orthopedic Hospital and Medical Center; Providence Medical Center, Seattle, Washington
Contraception

Jerry M. Lewis, M.D.
Clinical Professor of Psychiatry, Family Practice, and Community Medicine, Southwestern Medical School; Senior Research Psychiatrist, Timberlawn Psychiatric Research Foundation; Director of Research, Timberlawn Psychiatric Hospital, Dallas, Texas
Family Structure and Functioning

Bruce S. Liese, Ph.D.
Assistant Professor, Department of Family Practice, University of Kansas Medical Center School of Medicine; University of Kansas Medical Center, Kansas City, Kansas
The Family Life Cycle

Carolyn C. Lopez, M.D.
Assistant Professor, Rush Medical College of Rush University; Associate Attending Physician, Rush-Presbyterian-St. Luke's Medical Center, Chicago, Illinois
Occupational Medicine

Christine C. Matson, M.D.
Assistant Professor of Family Medicine, Baylor College of Medicine; Active Staff, St. Luke's Episcopal Hospital; Courtesy Staff, Texas Children's Hospital, Houston, Texas
General Surgery; Plastic and Reconstructive Surgery

Harry E. Mayhew, M.D.
Professor and Chairman, Department of Family Medicine, Medical College of Ohio at Toledo; Chairman, Division of Family Medicine, Medical College of Ohio Hospital, Toledo, Ohio
Urinary Tract Disorders: Urology

John W. McCall III, Ph.D.
Assistant Professor; Director of Research, Department of Family Medicine, University of Tennessee, Memphis, College of Medicine, Memphis, Tennessee
Interpreting the Medical Journal Literature

Kay F. McFarland, M.D.
Professor of Medicine, Associate Dean of Continuing Medical Education, University of South Carolina, Columbia, South Carolina
Endocrinology

I. R. McWhinney, M.D.
Professor, Department of Family Medicine, University of Western Ontario Faculty of Medicine; Medical Director, Palliative Care Unit, Parkwood Hospital, London, Ontario, Canada
Clinical Problem-Solving in Family Practice

Clifford Michaelson, M.D.
Assistant Professor of Neurology, Boston University School of Medicine; Staff Neuro-ophthalmologist, University Hospital, Boston, Massachusetts
Neurology: Visual Disturbances

Cathi Chambley Miller
Contributor, *Physician and Computer,* Chicago, Illinois
The Use of Personal Computers in Medicine

Susan M. Miller, M.D.
Assistant Professor, Departments of Family and Internal Medicine, Baylor College of Medicine; Staff, St. Luke's Episcopal Hospital; Harris County Hospital District, Houston, Texas
Ambulatory Management of AIDS; Primary Care of the Homosexual Patient

R. Michael Morse, M.D.
Associate Professor, Department of Family Medicine, University of Virginia School of Medicine; Medical Director, Department of Family Medicine, University of Virginia Hospitals; Director, University of Virginia Wellness and Fitness Center, Charlottesville, Virginia
Preventive Health Care in Family Medicine

Steven D. Morse, M.D.
Attending Physician, Department of Emergency Medicine, Montgomery Hospital, Norristown, Pennsylvania
Emergency Medicine

Herbert L. Muncie, Jr., M.D.
Associate Professor, Department of Family Medicine, University of Maryland School of Medicine; University Hospital, Baltimore, Maryland
Obesity

Harold C. Neu, M.D.
Professor of Medicine and Pharmacology, Columbia University College of Physicians and Surgeons; Hospital Epidemiologist, Presbyterian Hospital in the City of New York, New York, New York
Infectious Diseases

Victoria Nichols-Johnson, M.D.
Associate Professor; Chief, General Division, OB/GYN, Southern Illinois University School of Medicine; St. John's Hospital; Memorial Medical Center, Springfield, Illinois
Office Gynecology

Michael L. Noel, M.D.
Assistant Professor and Director, Residency Program, Department of Family Medicine; Clinical Instructor, Department of Community Medicine, Baylor College of Medicine; Attending Physician, St. Luke's Episcopal Hospital; Texas Children's Hospital, Houston, Texas
Systemic Family Medicine: An Evolving Concept

Kenneth L. Noller, M.D.
Professor and Chair, Department of Obstetrics and Gynecology, University of Massachusetts Medical School; Chair, Department of Obstetrics and Gynecology, The Medical Center of Central Massachusetts—Hahnemann; Medical Center of Central Massachusetts—Memorial, Worcester, Massachusetts
Obstetrics

Paul A. Nutting, M.D.
Director of Research, Indian Health Service; Sells Indian Hospital, U.S. Public Health Service, Tucson, Arizona
Community-Oriented Primary Care

Peter C. O'Brien, Ph.D.
Professor of Biostatistics, Mayo Medical School; Consultant, Section of Biostatistics, Mayo Clinic and Mayo Foundation; Rochester, Minnesota
Statistical Methods

Patrick J. O'Connor, M.D., M.P.H.
Assistant Professor of Family Medicine, University of Connecticut School of Medicine and Saint Francis Hospital and Medical Center; Assistant Attending Physician, Saint Francis Hospital and Medical Center, Hartford, Connecticut
Assessment of Functional Health Status

Michael F. Parry, M.D.
Associate Clinical Professor of Medicine, Columbia University College of Physicians and Surgeons, New York, New York; Director of Infectious Diseases and Microbiology, Stamford, Connecticut
Infectious Diseases

Reg L. Perkin, M.D.
Professor (Retired), Department of Family and Community Medicine, University of Toronto Faculty of Medicine, Toronto; Executive Director, College of Family Physicians of Canada, Willowdale, Ontario, Canada
Family Practice Around the World: Canada

Charles M. Plotz, M.D., Med.Sc.D.
Professor and Chairman, Department of Family Practice, State University of New York Health Science Center at Brooklyn College of Medicine, Brooklyn, New York
Rheumatic Disease

Max R. Polliack, M.B., Ch.B., M.P.H.
Professor and Chairman, Department of Family Medicine, Sackler School of Medicine, Tel Aviv University, Tel Aviv; Director and Head Physician, Kupat Holim Clinic, Herzlia, Israel
Family Practice Around the World: Israel

James G. Price, M.D.
Professor and Chairman, Department of Family Practice, University of Kansas Medical Center School of Medicine, Kansas City, Kansas
The Family Life Cycle

John G. Prichard, M.D., M.HS.
Clinical Associate Professor of Family Medicine, University of California, Los Angeles, UCLA School of Medicine, Los Angeles; Chief, Medical Services, Ventura County Medical Center, Ventura, California
Pulmonary Medicine

Peter Pritchard, M.D.
General Practitioner, Oxfordshire, England
Patient Advisory Councils

Robert E. Rakel, M.D.
Richard M. Kleberg Senior Professor and Chairman, Department of Family Medicine, Baylor College of Medicine; Associate Dean for Academic and Clinical Affairs, Baylor College of Medicine; Attending Physician, St. Luke's Episcopal Hospital and the Methodist Hospital, Houston, Texas
The Family Physician; Care of the Dying Patient; Use of Consultants; Establishing Rapport; Substance Abuse: Nicotine Addiction; The Problem-Oriented Medical Record; The Family Genogram: Standard Genogram Structure

Christian N. Ramsey, Jr., M.D.
Professor and Chairman, Department of Family Medicine, University of Oklahoma College of Medicine; Active Staff, Oklahoma Medical Center; Courtesy Staff, Presbyterian Hospital; Consulting Staff, St. Anthony Hospital, Oklahoma City, Oklahoma
Family Structure and Functioning

Janet P. Realini, M.D.
Associate Professor, Department of Family Practice, University of Texas Health Science Center at San Antonio; Active Medical Staff, Medical Center Hospital, San Antonio, Texas
Contraception

William Y. Rial, M.D.
Visiting Lecturer, Northwestern University Medical School, Chicago, Illinois; Former Clinical Professor of Medicine (General Practice), Medical College of Pennsylvania, Philadelphia; Honorary Staff, Crozier-Chester Medical Center,

Chester; Emeritus Staff, Delaware County Memorial Hospital, Drexel Hill; Riddle Memorial Hospital, Media; Taylor Hospital, Ridley Park, Pennsylvania
Emergency Medicine

John Richards, M.B.Ch.B.
Associate Professor of General Practice, School of Medicine, University of Auckland, Auckland, New Zealand
Family Practice Around the World: New Zealand

Shelley Roaten, Jr., M.D.
Associate Professor of Clinical Family Medicine, Baylor College of Medicine; Active Staff, Hillcrest Baptist Medical Center; and Providence Hospital, Waco, Texas
Dermatology

Richard G. Roberts, M.D., J.D.
Assistant Professor, Department of Family Medicine and Practice, University of Wisconsin School of Medicine; Active Staff, St. Mark's Hospital Medical Center; Courtesy Staff, Meriter Hospital, Madison, Wisconsin
Risk Management

Wm. MacMillan Rodney, M.D.
Professor and Chairman, University of Tennessee, Memphis, College of Medicine, Memphis, Tennessee
Gastroenterology

Alex R. Rodriguez, M.D.
Lecturer, Yale University School of Medicine, New Haven; Naval Hospital, Groton, Connecticut
Behavioral Problems in Children and Adolescents

John C. Rogers, M.D., M.P.H.
Associate Professor, Department of Family Medicine; Director, Predoctoral Programs, Baylor College of Medicine; Staff, St. Luke's Episcopal Hospital; Texas Children's Hospital, Houston, Texas
The Family Genogram: The Self-Administered Genogram; Research Methodology

John S. Rolland, M.D.
Assistant Clinical Professor, Department of Psychiatry, Yale University School of Medicine; Medical Director, Center for Illness in Families; Attending Physician, Yale-New Haven Hospital, New Haven, Connecticut
The Impact of Illness on the Family

Marie Saint-Hilaire, M.D.
Assistant Professor of Neurology, Boston University School of Medicine; Staff Neurologist, University Hospital, Boston, Massachusetts
Neurology: Disturbance of Motor Function

Susan Schooley, M.D.
Assistant Professor, Department of Family Medicine, University of North Carolina at Chapel Hill School of Medicine; North Carolina Memorial Hospital, Chapel Hill, North Carolina
Child Abuse

Marc A. Schuckit, M.D.
Professor of Psychiatry, University of California, San Diego, School of Medicine; Veterans Administration Medical Center, San Diego, California
Substance Abuse: Alcohol

Thomas L. Schwenk, M.D.
Associate Professor and Chairman, Department of Family Practice, University of Michigan Medical School; Attending Physician, University of Michigan Hospitals, Ann Arbor, Michigan
Depression

Steven H. Selman, M.D.
Professor of Surgery (Urology), Medical College of Ohio at Toledo; Attending Urologist, Medical College of Ohio Hospital, Toledo, Ohio
Urinary Tract Disorders: Urology

Marc A. Shampo, Ph.D.
Instructor in Biomedical Communications, Mayo Medical School; Editor, Section of Publications, Mayo Clinic and Mayo Foundation, Rochester, Minnesota
Statistical Methods

Kevin M. Sherin, M.D., M.P.H.
Assistant Professor, Department of Family Practice, Rush Medical College of Rush University; Visiting Attending Physician, Department of Family Practice, Rush-Presbyterian-St. Luke's Medical Center, Chicago, Illinois; Courtesy Attending Staff, Walker Memorial Hospital, Avon Park, Florida
Occupational Medicine; Substance Abuse: Controlled Substances

Gabriel Smilkstein, M.D.
William Ray Moore Professor, Department of Family Practice, University of Louisville School of Medicine; Staff, Humana Hospital-University, Louisville, Kentucky
Psychosocial Influences on Health

Charles W. Smith, Jr., M.D.
Professor of Family and Community Medicine, University of Arkansas for Medical Sciences; Executive Associate Dean for Clinical Affairs and Medical Director, University Hospital of Arkansas, Little Rock, Arkansas
Otolaryngology

Jeffery Sobal, Ph.D., M.P.H.
Associate Professor, Division of Nutritional Sciences, Cornell University, Ithaca, New York
Obesity

Walter O. Spitzer, M.D., M.H.A., M.P.H.
Chairman, Department of Epidemiology and Biostatistics, McGill University Faculty of Medicine; Senior Physician, Department of Medicine, Montreal General Hospital; Senior Medical Scientist, Department of Medicine, Royal Victoria Hospital, Montreal, Quebec, Canada
The Periodic Health Examination

R. H. Sprinkle, M.D., Ph.D.
Clinical Assistant Professor of Pediatrics and Family Medicine, Robert Wood Johnson Medical School, The University of Medicine and Dentistry of New Jersey, New Brunswick, New Jersey
Care of the Newborn

Samuel Stal, M.D.
Associate Professor, Baylor College of Medicine; Chief of Plastic Surgery, Texas Children's Hospital; The Methodist Hospital; St. Luke's Episcopal Hospital, Houston, Texas
Plastic and Reconstructive Surgery

Michael A. Stocker, M.D., M.P.H.
Executive Vice President, U.S. Healthcare, Paramus, New Jersey
Managed Health Care

Porter Storey, M.D.
Clinical Assistant Professor, Department of Medicine, Baylor College of Medicine; Adjunct Assistant Professor of Medicine, Division of Medicine, University of Texas, M.D. Anderson Cancer Center; Medical Director, The Hospice at the Texas Medical Center, Houston, Texas
Care of the Dying Patient

Chester L. Strunk, M.D.
Assistant Professor, Department of Otolaryngology, University of Texas Medical School at Galveston, Galveston, Texas
Otolaryngology

David N. Sundwall, M.D.
Clinical Professor of Family Medicine, Uniformed Services University of the Health Sciences F. Edward Hébert School of Medicine, Bethesda, Maryland; Clinical Associate Professor of Medicine, Georgetown University School of Medicine and Health Sciences, Washington, D.C.
Family Practice Around the World: United States

John E. Sutherland, M.D.
Professor, Department of Family Practice, Southern Illinois University School of Medicine; St. John's Hospital; Memorial Medical Center, Springfield, Illinois
Office Gynecology

E. Lee Taylor, M.D.
Professor and Chairman, Department of Family and Community Medicine; Assistant Dean for Off-Campus, Family Practice Programs, University of Alabama School of Medicine; Chief of Family Medicine Service, University of Alabama Hospital; The Children's Hospital of Alabama, Birmingham, Alabama
The Economics of Family Practice

Mason P. Thompson, M.D.
Associate Professor, Medical College of Georgia School of Medicine; Medical College of Georgia Hospital and Clinics, Augusta, Georgia
Caring for the Elderly

Lawrence M. Tierney, Jr., M.D.
Professor of Medicine, University of California, San Francisco, School of Medicine; Assistant Chief, University of California, San Francisco Medical Center; Veterans Administration Medical Center, San Francisco, California
Pulmonary Medicine

Joseph W. Tollison, M.D.
Professor and Chairman, Department of Family Medicine, Medical College of Georgia School of Medicine; Active Staff, Medical College of Georgia Hospital and Clinics; Consulting Staff, University Hospital, Augusta, Georgia
Caring for the Elderly

Donald F. Treat, M.D.
Associate Professor of Family Medicine, University of Rochester, School of Medicine and Dentistry; Courtesy Physician, Highland Hospital of Rochester, Rochester, New York
The Family's Influence on Health

Jack Valancy, M.B.A.
Principal, Jack Valancy Consulting, Management for Health Care, Cleveland Heights; Clinical Instructor, Department of Family Medicine, Case Western Reserve University School of Medicine, Cleveland, Ohio
Accounting Systems

Carlos Vallbona, M.D.
Professor and Chairman, Department of Community Medicine, Baylor College of Medicine; Chief, Community Medicine Service, Harris County Hospital District; Active Staff, General Medicine Service, Texas Children's Hospital; Active Staff, Family Medicine Service, St. Luke's Episcopal Hospital; Active Staff, Institute for Rehabilitation and Research; Consultant, Cardiac Rehabilitation, Veterans Administration Medical Center, Houston, Texas
Interpretation of the Electrocardiogram; Cardiovascular Disease: Arrhythmias

Paul P. VanArsdel, Jr., M.D.
Professor of Medicine, Head, Section of Allergy, University of Washington School of Medicine, Seattle; Attending Physician, University Hospital, Seattle, Washington
Allergy

Donald S. Williamson, Ph.D.
Associate Professor and Director of Family Psychology Section, Department of Family Medicine, Baylor College of Medicine, Houston, Texas
Systemic Family Medicine: An Evolving Concept; Primary Care of the Homosexual Patient

Philip A. Wolf, M.D.
Professor of Neurology, Research Professor of Medicine (Preventive Medicine and Epidemiology), Boston University School of Medicine; Staff Neurologist, University Hospital, Boston, Massachusetts
Neurology: Cerebrovascular Disease

John T. Yetter, M.D.
Faculty, Family Medicine Residency; Director, Division of Sports Medicine, Deaconess Hospital, St. Louis, Missouri
Sports Medicine

Robert E. Zitter, Ph.D.
Assistant Professor, Departments of Family Practice and Psychology, Rush Medical College of Rush University, Chicago; Christ Hospital and Medical Center, Oak Lawn, Illinois
The Somatic Patient

Preface

The public's increasing awareness of the vital role that continuing comprehensive primary care plays in a quality health care delivery system makes this new decade an exciting time for the field of family practice. The goal of this text is to help physicians in family practice develop new skills and remain current with recent advances in their specialty; it also seeks to provide a reliable source of the knowledge essential to effective practice.

The fourth edition differs significantly from the first, which was published in 1973. It contains 83 chapters: 11 more than in the third edition, which was published in 1984. There are a total of 142 contributors, most of whom are family physicians. As in past editions, we have often paired a qualified subspecialist with an experienced family physician to maintain practical relevance.

More than half the chapters of this edition are entirely new: the most important change of all. There are 33 new chapter titles; 19 chapters from the third edition have been rewritten by new authors. The remaining material has been thoroughly revised and updated.

The family physician has many resources that offer fresh clinical knowledge. Our text pays close attention to the many social issues that affect health care. It is in this area that we have added a number of new chapters. Significant among these are: Family Life Cycle; Systemic Family Medicine; The Family's Impact on Health; Impact of Divorce on the Family; Ethics in Primary Care; Psychosocial Influences on Health; Community-Oriented Primary Care; Home Care; Patient Advisory Councils; and two chapters on abuse in the family. These new materials offer a wealth of practical information to prepare the family physician to deal with the issues of great concern to patients.

Every attempt has been made to keep the information in this text as current as possible, especially in those rapidly changing areas of great importance to practicing physicians. For example, recent recommendations for a second measles immunization have been added, and there are new chapters on Care of the Newborn, Growth and Development, and Childhood and Adolescence. Other new chapters include: Ambulatory Management of AIDS; Care of the Homosexual Patient; Nutrition; Obesity; Hematology; The Somatic Patient; Psychiatric Emergencies; and Dementia.

The chapter entitled Interpreting the Electrocardiogram contains many useful illustrations, as do other chapters focusing on clinical concerns such as Plastic Surgery, Gastroenterology, Dermatology, and Orthopedics. Five hundred and twenty tables and five hundred and fifty illustrations (figures, plates, and tracings) are included in this new edition.

Other newly added chapters are: Managed Health Care; Risk Management; Research Methodology; and Interpreting the Medical Literature. Recent recommendations of the U.S. Preventive Services Task Force have been added to the extensive appendices that again contain both laboratory values and conversion tables. Added to this edition in response to many requests is a chapter on Interpreting Laboratory Tests. This chapter lists conditions that should be considered when a test is abnormal, and the actions that can be taken either to confirm the diagnosis or to correct the problem.

It is our desire to make the knowledge contained here available to a broad audience. For the first time, a companion review book will be published containing questions based on this text. It is being compiled by Edward Bope, M.D., Alvah Cass, M.D., and Michael Hagen, M.D. Also, a shorter version of this text, *Essentials of Family Practice,* is being planned to meet the needs of undergraduate medical students.

Producing a text of this size is a complex task that requires many months of effort. I want to extend my special thanks to my editorial assistant, Roxy Cuddy, for her help in preparing this book; to John Dyson and the staff at W. B. Saunders for their high standards; and to my wife, Peggy, who continues to support my penchant for publishing despite the tremendous demands it makes on my time.

ROBERT E. RAKEL, M.D.

Contents

Part I Principles of Family Practice, 1

Part II Community Medicine, 207

Part VI Research in Family Medicine, 1797

Textbook of Family Practice

Part I

Principles of Family Practice

1

The Family Physician

Robert E. Rakel

The family physician provides continuing, comprehensive care in a personalized manner to patients of all ages and to their families, regardless of the presence of disease or the nature of the presenting complaint. Family physicians accept responsibility for managing an individual's total health needs while maintaining an intimate, confidential relationship with the patient. The family physician personally takes care of most of the patient's health needs; for the remainder of the patient's problems, the physician selects appropriate consulting physicians or other health professionals to assist in care. The efforts of all health professionals are coordinated by the family physician, who has ongoing responsibility for the patient's care.

Family medicine is the body of knowledge and the skills that constitute the medical discipline; when applied to the care of patients and their families, that discipline becomes the specialty of family practice. Family medicine emphasizes responsibility for total health care—from the first contact and initial assessment through the ongoing care of chronic problems (from prevention through rehabilitation). Coordination and integration of all necessary health services with the least amount of fragmentation are important features of the discipline.

Family practice is a specialty that shares many areas of content with other clinical disciplines, incorporating this shared knowledge and using it uniquely to deliver primary medical care. Similarly, other medical specialties have incorporated components from a variety of disciplines to create new disciplines that function effectively and uniquely. Thus, ophthalmology includes components of anatomy, surgery, medicine, and physics; anesthesiology involves physiology, pharmacology, biochemistry, and clinical medicine. In addition to sharing content with other medical specialties, family practice emphasizes knowledge from areas such as family dynamics, interpersonal relations, counseling, and psychotherapy. The specialty's foundation, however, remains clinical, with the primary focus on the medical care of people who are ill.

Devotion to continuing, comprehensive, personalized care; to early detection and management of illness; to the prevention of disease and maintenance of health; and to the ongoing management of patients in a community setting uniquely qualify the family physician to deliver primary care.

Development of the Specialty

About 1923, Francis Peabody commented that the swing of the pendulum toward specialization had reached its apex and that modern medicine had fragmented the health care delivery system to too great a degree. He called for a rapid return of the generalist physician who would give comprehensive, personalized care.

Dr. Peabody's declaration proved premature; society and the medical establishment were not ready for such a proclamation. The trend toward specialization gained momentum through the 1950's, and fewer physicians entered general practice. In the early 1960's, leaders in the field of general practice began advocating a seemingly paradoxical solution to reverse the trend and correct the scarcity of general practitioners—the creation of still another specialty. However, the physicians envisioned a specialty that embodied the knowledge, skills, and ideals they knew as primary care. In 1966, the concept of a new specialty in primary care received official recognition in two separate reports published 1 month apart. The first of these was the "Report of the Citizens' Commission on Graduate Medical Education of the American Medical Association," also known as the Millis Commission Report. The second report came from the Ad Hoc Committee on Education for Family Practice of the Council of Medical Education of the American Medical Association, also called the Willard Committee. Three years later, the American Board of Family Practice (ABFP) came into being as the 20th medical specialty board, thus giving birth to the specialty of family practice.

Much of the impetus for the Millis and Willard reports came from the American Academy of General Practice, which was renamed the American Academy of Family Physicians (AAFP) in 1971. The name change reflected a desire to increase emphasis on family-oriented health care and to gain academic acceptance for the new specialty of family practice.

The ABFP has distinguished itself by being the first specialty board to require recertification (every 6 years) to ensure the ongoing competence of its members. Among basic requirements for certification and recertification, the ABFP has included continuing education—the foundation on which the American Academy of General Practice had been built when organized in 1947. A member of the ABFP must participate in 50 hours of acceptable continuing education activity each year to be eligible for recertification. Once eligible, a candidate's competence is examined by cognitive testing and performance evaluation. The ABFP's emphasis on quality of education, knowledge, and performance has facilitated the rapid increase in prestige for the family physician in our health care system. The obvious logic of the ABFP's emphasis on continuing education to maintain required knowledge and skills has been adopted by other specialties and state medical societies.

Definitions

Family Practice. The AAFP and ABFP have defined family practice as

> *. . . the medical specialty which provides continuing and comprehensive health care for the individual and the family. It is the specialty in breadth which integrates the biological, clinical and behavioral sciences. The scope of family practice encompasses all ages.*
>
> *Family practice is the continuing and current expression of the historical medical practitioner and is uniquely defined within the family context.*

Any definition of family practice must be built on a base of data that is appropriate to the activities of physicians practicing the specialty. For this reason, a sincere attempt is being made to design the curriculum for training family physicians so as to represent realistically the skills and body of knowledge they will require in practice. This curriculum definition relies heavily on an accurate analysis of the problems seen and the skills used by family physicians in their practices. Unfortunately, the content of residency training programs for the primary care specialties has not always been appropriately directed toward solving the problems most commonly encountered by physicians practicing in these specialties. The situation is changing rapidly, however, and in the near future training programs should be more appropriately designed to meet the needs of the practicing physician. The almost randomly educated primary physician of previous years is being replaced by one specifically prepared to address the kinds of problems likely to be encountered in practice. For this reason, the "model office" is an essential component of all family practice residency programs.

Primary Care. The specialty of family practice is designed specifically to deliver primary care, which was defined in 1975 by the AAFP as

> *. . . a form of medical care delivery that emphasizes first-contact care and assumes ongoing responsibility for the patient in both health maintenance and therapy of illness. It is personal care involving a unique interaction and communication between the patient and the physician. It is comprehensive in scope and includes the overall coordination of the care of the patient's health problems, be they biological, behavioral or social. The appropriate use of consultants and community resources is an important part of effective primary care.*
>
> (AAFP REPORTER, JUNE 1975)

Because many physicians deliver primary care in different ways and with varying degrees of preparation, the staff of the ABFP further clarified the definition:

> *Primary care is a form of delivery of medical care which encompasses the following functions:*
>
> *1. It is "first-contact" care, serving as a point-of-entry for the patient into the health care system;*
>
> *2. It includes continuity by virtue of caring for patients over a period of time, both in sickness and in health;*
>
> *3. It is comprehensive care, drawing from all the traditional major disciplines for its functional content;*
>
> *4. It serves a coordinative function for all the health-care needs of the patient;*
>
> *5. It assumes continuing responsibility for individual patient follow-up and community health problems; and*
>
> *6. It is a highly personalized type of care.*

Primary Physician. The Millis Commission defined the "primary physician" as one who

> *. . . should usually be primary in the first contact sense. He will serve as the primary medical resource and counselor to an individual or family. When a patient needs hospitali-*

zation, the service of other medical specialists, or other medical or paramedical assistance, the primary physician will see that the necessary arrangements are made, giving such responsibility to others as is appropriate and retaining his own continuing and comprehensive responsibility.

Few hospitals and few existing specialists consider comprehensive and continuing medical care to be their responsibility and within their range of competence.

Personalized Care

It is much more important to know what sort of patient has a disease than what sort of disease a patient has.

SIR WILLIAM OSLER

Family physicians do not just treat patients, they care for people. This caring function of family medicine emphasizes the personalized approach to understanding the patient as a person, respecting the person as an individual, and showing compassion for his or her discomfort. Compassion means co-suffering and reflects the physician's willingness somehow to share the patient's anguish and understand what the sickness means to that person. Compassion is an attempt to "feel" along with the patient. Pellegrino (1979) states that "we can never *feel* with another person when we pass judgment as a superior, only when we see our own frailties as well as his." Pellegrino goes on to comment that a compassionate authority figure is effective only when others can receive the "orders" without being humiliated. The physician must not "put down" the patients but must be ever ready, in Galileo's words,

to pronounce that wise, ingenuous, and modest statement—'I don't know'.

Compassion, practiced in these terms in each patient encounter, is the irreducible base for mitigating the inherent dehumanizing tendencies of today's highly institutionalized and technologically oriented patterns of patient care.

Physicians engaged primarily in hospital-based medicine must make a stronger effort to maintain personalized care because of the added exposure to and the necessary use of devices and techniques directed toward specific diseases. The physician should guard against thinking in terms of diseases and instead think in terms of patients who have problems needing attention. The whole-person approach to patient care is hampered by focusing primarily on the disease; specific diseases require specific treatments and tend to direct the physician's attention away from other needs of the whole patient.

Peabody (1930) noted that "The treatment of a disease may be entirely impersonal; the care of a patient must be completely personal." If an intimate relationship with patients remains our primary concern as physicians, high-quality medical care will persist, regardless of the way it is organized and financed. For this reason, family practice emphasizes consideration of the individual patient in the full context of his or her life rather than the episodic care of a presenting complaint. The Millis Commission Report stresses that the family physician

. . . focuses not upon individual organs and systems but upon the whole man who lives in a complex social setting; and knows that diagnosis or treatment of a part often overlooks major causative factors and therapeutic opportunities.

It is generally recognized that medicine has become depersonalized owing to the rapid rise of superspecialization and technology. In 1956, L. W. Batten in *The Lancet* lamented the loss of personalized care, once the hallmark of private practice:

Personal continuous care was the very substance of that unfashionable institution—private practice. . . . If it ceases to be personal, then practice, as I have experienced and understood it, will have altogether ceased to be.

In a lighter, but more poignant fashion, Theodore F. Fox, as editor of *The Lancet* (April 2, 1960), wrote:

I know, too, that we must get used to a world in which ices no longer taste of cream, nor new potatoes of new potatoes; and . . . ghastly plastic flowers seem to be commoner than real ones. But nobody is going to persuade me that a nice receptionist, some good notes, and an internist keeping office hours adds up to a personal doctor who knows me and my home. Even if you throw in a psychiatric social worker, I still feel that I am being put off with a plastic substitute for the real thing. And I am supported in this belief by the knowledge that when personal medical care is abolished, it is sooner or later re-invented.

Indeed, as Fox predicted, personalized care is returning to medicine, largely because of the advent of the specialty that provides family physicians who know patients in their home environment and who assess the psychosocial factors that exist within the family setting as well as the individual's problems.

Family physicians assess the illnesses and complaints presented to them, dealing personally with the majority and arranging special assistance for a few. The family physician serves as the patients' advocate, explaining the causes and implications of illness to the patients and their families, and serves as an advisor and confidant to the family—both individually and collectively. The family physician receives many intellectual satisfactions from this practice, but the greatest reward arises from the depth of human understanding and personal satisfaction inherent in family practice.

Patients have adjusted somewhat to a more impersonal form of health care delivery and frequently look to institutions rather than to individuals for their health care; yet, their need for personalized concern and compassion remains. Tumulty (1970) found that patients consider a good physician one who (1) shows genuine interest in them; (2) thoroughly evaluates their problem; (3) demonstrates compassion, understanding, and warmth; and (4) provides clear insight into what is wrong and what must be done to correct it.

The family physician's relationship with each patient should reflect compassion, understanding, and patience, combined with a high degree of intellectual honesty. The physician must be thorough in approaching problems but also possess a keen sense of humor. He must be capable of encouraging in each patient optimism, courage, insight, and the self-discipline necessary for recovery. Sometimes, if the physician is unable to cure, he must nevertheless *always* comfort and give "the gentle relief of another's care."

Characteristics and Functions of the Family Physician

ATTRIBUTES OF THE FAMILY PHYSICIAN

The following characteristics are certainly desirable for all physicians, but they are of greatest importance for the physician in family practice.

1. A strong sense of responsibility for the total, ongoing care of the individual and the family during health, illness, and rehabilitation.
2. Compassion and empathy, with a sincere interest in the patient and the family.
3. A curious and constantly inquisitive attitude.
4. Enthusiasm for the undifferentiated medical problem and its resolution.
5. An interest in the broad spectrum of clinical medicine.
6. The ability to deal comfortably with multiple problems occurring simultaneously in one patient.
7. A desire for frequent and varied intellectual and technical challenges.
8. The ability to support children during growth and development and during their adjustment to family and society.
9. The ability to assist patients in coping with everyday problems and in maintaining stability in the family and community.
10. The capacity to act as coordinator of all health resources needed in the care of a patient.
11. A continuing enthusiasm for learning and for the satisfaction that comes from maintaining current medical knowledge through continuing medical education.
12. The ability to maintain composure in times of stress and to respond quickly with logic, effectiveness, and compassion.
13. A desire to identify problems at the earliest possible stage (or to prevent disease entirely).
14. A strong wish to maintain maximum patient satisfaction, recognizing the need for continuing patient rapport.
15. The skills necessary to manage chronic illness and to ensure maximal rehabilitation following acute illness.
16. An appreciation for the complex mix of physical, emotional, and social elements in holistic and personalized patient care.
17. A feeling of personal satisfaction derived from intimate relationships with patients that naturally develop over long periods of continuous care, as opposed to the short-term pleasures gained from treating episodic illnesses.
18. A skill for and commitment to educating patients and families about disease processes and the principles of good health.

The ideal family physician is an explorer, driven by a persistent curiosity and the desire to know more. He is part theologian, as was Paracelsus; part politician, as was Benjamin Rush; and part humorist, as was Oliver Wendell Holmes. At all times, however, he or she holds the care of the patient—the whole patient—as a primary goal.

CONTINUING RESPONSIBILITY

One of the essential functions of the family physician is the willingness to accept ongoing responsibility for managing a patient's medical care. Once a patient or a family has been accepted into the physician's practice, responsibility for care is both total and continuing. The Millis Commission chose the word "primary physician" to emphasize the concept of primary responsibility for the patient's welfare; however, the term "primary care physician" is more popular and refers to any physician who provides first-contact care.

The family physician's commitment to patients does not cease at the end of illness but is a continuing responsibility, regardless of the patient's state of health or the disease process. There is no need to identify the beginning or end-point of treatment, since care of a problem can be reopened at any time—even though a later visit may be primarily for another problem. This prevents the family physician from focusing too narrowly on one problem and helps maintain a perspective on the total patient in his or her environment. Peabody (1930) felt that much patient dissatisfaction results from the physician's neglecting to assume personal responsibility for supervision of the patient's care:

> *For some reason or other, no one physician has seen the case through from beginning to end, and the patient may be suffering from the very multitude of his counselors.*

The physician who is well acquainted with the patient not only provides more personal and humane medical care but does so more economically than the physician involved only in episodic care. The physician who knows his or her patients well can assess the nature of their problems more rapidly and accurately. Because of the intimate, ongoing relationship, the family physician is under less pressure to exclude diagnostic possibilities by use of expensive laboratory and radiologic procedures than is the physician who is unfamiliar with the patient.

The greater the degree of continuing involvement with a patient, the more capable the physician is in detecting early signs and symptoms of organic disease and functional problems. Patients with problems arising from emotional and social conflicts can be managed most effectively by a physician who has intimate knowledge of the individual and of his or her family and community background. This knowledge comes only from insight gained by observing the patient's long-term patterns of behavior and responses to changing stressful situations. This longitudinal view is particularly useful in the care of children and allows the physician to be more effective in assisting children to reach their full potential. The closeness that develops between physicians and young patients increases a physician's ability to aid the patient with problems that occur during later periods in life—such as adjustment to puberty, problems with marriage or employment, and changing social pressures. As the family physician maintains this continuing involvement with successive generations within a family, the ability to manage intercurrent problems increases with knowledge of the total family background.

By virtue of this ongoing involvement and intimate association with the family, the family physician develops a perceptive awareness of a family's nature and style of operation. This ability to observe families over time allows valuable insight that improves the quality of medical care provided to an individual patient. One of the greatest challenges in family medicine is the need to be alert to the changing stresses, transitions, and expectations of family members over time and to the effect that these and other family interactions have on the health of individuals.

Although the family is the family physician's primary concern, his or her skills are equally applicable to the individual living alone or to people in other varieties of family living. Individuals with alternative forms of family living interact with others who have significant effects on their lives. The principles of group dynamics and interpersonal relationships that affect health are equally applicable to everyone.

The family physician needs to assess an individual's personality so that presenting symptoms can be appropriately evaluated and given the proper degree of attention and emphasis. A complaint of abdominal pain may be treated lightly in one patient who frequently presents with minor problems, but the same complaint would be investigated immediately and in depth in another individual who has a more stoic personality. The decision regarding which studies to perform and when is influenced by knowledge of the patient's life style, personality, and previous response pattern. The greater the degree of knowledge and insight into the patient's background, which is gained through years of previous contact, the more capable the physician is in making an appropriate early and rapid assessment of the presenting complaint. The less background information the physician has to rely on, the greater is the need to depend upon costly laboratory studies and the more likely is overreaction to the presenting symptom. Families receiving continuing comprehensive care have fewer incidences of hospitalization, fewer operations, and fewer physician visits for illnesses compared with those who have no regular physician. This is due, at least in part, to the physician's knowledge of the patients; seeing them earlier for acute problems and thus preventing complications that would require hospitalization; being available by telephone; and seeing them more frequently in the office for health supervision. Care is also less expensive, since there is less need to rely on x-ray and laboratory procedures and visits to emergency rooms.

The United States has the most expensive health care system in the world, with 12 per cent of the gross national product devoted to health care. Schroeder (1984) believes that this situation will continue as long as the system accepts a high concentration of specialists, fee-for-service payment, patient self-referral directly to specialists, practice of specialties by physicians who have not gone through the specialty certification process, and a high dependency on specialists for primary care.

Clearly, the increasing complexity of our health care system multiplies expense and wastefulness when a patient self-diagnoses his or her problems or selects his or her own specialist rather than developing a firm and ongoing relationship with a family physician. The most efficient and cost-effective system involves a single personal physician who ensures the most logical and economical management of a problem. Medical care should be available to patients in the precise degree needed—neither too extensive nor too limited. This ensures that simple problems will not be magnified out of proportion. The more complex and involved a diagnostic process is, the more costly it becomes, and the greater is the potential for error.

The quality of our health care system is being eroded by physicians' being extensively trained at great expense to practice in one area and instead practicing in another, such as anesthesiologists practicing in emergency rooms and surgeons practicing as generalists.

Primary care, to be done well, requires extensive training specifically tailored to problems frequently seen in primary care. These include the early detection, diagnosis, and treatment of depression; the early diagnosis of cancer (especially of the breast and the colon); the management of gynecologic problems; and the care of those with chronic and terminal illnesses.

The need for a primary physician who accepts continuing responsibility for patient care is emphasized by Michael Balint (1965) in his concept of "collusion of anonymity." In this situation, the patient is seen by a variety of physicians, not one of whom is willing to accept total management of the problem. Important decisions are made—some good, some bad—but without anyone's feeling fully responsible for them.

Francis Peabody (1930) examined the futility of a patient's making the rounds from one specialist to another without finding relief because he

> *. . . lacked the guidance of a sound general practitioner who understood his physical condition, his nervous temperament and knew the details of his daily life. Many a patient who on his own initiative had sought out specialists has had minor defects extenuated so that they assume a needless importance and has even undergone operations that might well have been avoided. These are often pathetically tragic figures as they veer from one course of treatment to another—like ships that lack a guiding hand upon the helm, they swing from tack to tack with each new gust of wind but get no nearer to Port of Health because there is no pilot to set the general direction of their course.*

The family physician must also be committed to managing the common chronic illnesses that have no known cure but for which continuing management by a personal physician is all the more necessary to maintain an optimal state of health for the patient. It is a difficult and often trying job to manage these continuing, unresolvable, and progressively crippling problems, control of which requires a remolding of the life style of the entire family.

COMPREHENSIVE CARE

The term "comprehensive medical care" spans the entire spectrum of medicine. The effectiveness with which a physician delivers primary care depends upon the degree of involvement attained during training and practice. The family physician must be comprehensively trained to acquire all the medical skills necessary to care for the majority of patient problems. The greater the number of disciplines omitted from the family physician's training and practice, the more frequent is the need to refer minor problems to another physician. A truly comprehensive primary physician adequately manages acute infections, biopsies skin and other lesions, repairs lacerations, treats musculoskeletal sprains and minor fractures, removes foreign bodies, treats vaginitis, provides obstetric care and care for the newborn infant, gives supportive psychotherapy, and supervises diagnostic procedures. The needs of a family physician's patient will range from a routine physical examination, when the patient feels well and wishes to identify potential risk factors, to a problem that calls for referral to one or more narrowly specialized physicians with highly developed technical skills. The family physician must be aware of the variety and complexity of skills and facilities available to help manage patients and must match these to the individual's specific needs, giving full consideration to the patient's personality and expectations.

Management of an illness involves much more than a diagnosis and an outline for treatment. It also requires an awareness of all the factors that may aid or hinder an individual's recovery from illness. This requires consideration of religious beliefs; social, economic, or cultural problems; personal expectations; and heredity. The outstanding clinician recognizes the effects that spiritual, intellectual, emotional, social, and economic factors have on a patient's illness.

Family Practice is a comprehensive specialty involving varying depths of knowledge in many disciplines. A primary physician requires knowledge and skills of varying degrees in each specialty area, depending upon the prevalence of problems encountered in everyday practice and the degree of skills needed to become an excellent diagnostician. A physician specializing in only one discipline, however, will have a much shallower base in comprehensive medicine and a much greater depth in the chosen discipline. The subspecialist is an excellent consultant, but is not trained and cannot function effectively as a primary generalist. The distribution of his or her knowledge and skills is no more appropriate to that task than is the comprehensive physician's competence in the esoteric nuances of a limited discipline. The family physician's ability to confront relatively large numbers of unselected patients with undifferentiated conditions and carry on a therapeutic relationship over time is a unique primary care skill. The skilled family physician will have a higher level of tolerance for the uncertain than will his or her consultant colleague.

Society will benefit more from a surgeon who has a sufficient volume of surgery to maintain proficiency through frequent use of well-honed skills than from one who has a low volume and serves also as a primary care physician. The early identification of disease while it is in its undifferentiated stage requires specific training and is not a skill that can automatically be assumed by someone whose training has been mostly in hospital intensive care units. It is unfortunate that when the number of procedures is inadequate to fully occupy specialists skilled in complex technical procedures, their remaining time is spent providing care (frequently primary care) in areas where training was limited and often deficient. John Fry (1977) has said that

> *. . . working in general practice broadens the mind and humbles the soul. It is very different from the sheltered world of hospital practice. It is as though we, in general practice, work in the natural habitat of the jungle, seeking and stalking our prey in its own environment, whereas our hospital colleagues have to function behind the bars of a zoo, dealing with patients and diseases in highly artificial situations.*

Gonnella and Veloski (1982) studied the impact that one year of graduate training in different specialties has on performance in Part III of the National Board Examination, which is designed to measure general clinical knowledge. After just 1 year of a 3- or 4-year residency, the performance of physicians in all specialties *except family practice* deteriorated when compared to scores on Part II taken 1 year earlier. Only physicians in family practice training programs improved, increasing an average of eight points. The most dramatic change was among physicians in pathology training programs, in which the mean score was 95 points *lower* than on Part II. Since Part III is designed to measure the essential diagnostic and therapeutic skills that the medical profession and society expect all physicians to have, academic medicine is being asked whether or not it is appropriately preparing physicians. Many physicians eventually enter a type of practice different from what their residency prepared them for; the question remains whether many, especially those entering primary care, will undergo the difficult and costly retraining necessary to do the job well.

The World Health Organization, United Nations, and other organizations sponsored a World Conference on Medical Education in Edinburgh, Scotland, in 1988, addressing the need for reform in medical education. The meeting made a number of recommendations to medical schools in its "Edinburgh Declaration":

1. Enlarge the range of settings in which educational programs are conducted, to include all health resources of the community, not hospitals alone.
2. Ensure that curriculum content reflects national health priorities and the availability of affordable resources.
3. Ensure continuity of learning throughout life, shifting emphasis from the passive methods so widespread now to more active learning, including self-directed and independent study as well as tutorial methods.
4. Build both curriculum and examination systems to ensure the achievement of professional competence and social values, not merely the retention and recall of information.
5. Train teachers as educators, not solely as experts in content, and reward education excellence as fully as excellence in biomedical research or clinical practice.
6. Complement instruction about the management of patients with increased emphasis on promotion of health and prevention of diseases.
7. Pursue integration of education in science and education in practice, also using problem-solving in clinical and community settings as a base for learning.
8. Employ selection methods for medical students that go beyond intellectual ability and academic achievement to include evaluation of personal qualities.
9. Encourage and facilitate cooperation between the Ministries of Health, Ministries of Education, community health services and other relevant bodies in joint policy development, program planning, implementation, and review.
10. Ensure admission policies that match the numbers of students trained with national needs for doctors.
11. Increase the opportunity for joint learning, research, and service with other health and health-related professions as part of the training for teamwork.
12. Clarify responsibility and allocate resources for continuing medical education.

INTERPERSONAL SKILLS

One of the foremost skills of the family physician is the ability to effectively utilize the knowledge of interpersonal relations in the management of patients. This powerful element of clinical medicine is perhaps the specialty's most useful tool. Modern society considers the medical care system inadequate in those situations in which understanding and compassion are important to the patient's comfort and recovery from illness. Physicians are too often seen as lacking this personal concern and as being unskilled in understanding personal anxiety and feelings. There is an obvious need to nourish the seed of compassion and concern for sick people with which students enter medical school.

Family practice emphasizes the integration of compassion, empathy, and personalized concern to a greater degree than does a more technical or task-oriented specialty. Some of the earnest solicitude of the old country doctor and his untiring compassion for people must be incorporated as the effective yet impersonal modern medical procedures are applied. The patient should be viewed compassionately as a person in distress who needs to be treated with concern, dignity, and personal consideration. He or she has a right to be given some insight into his or her problems; a reasonable appraisal of the potential outcome; and a realistic picture of the emotional, financial, and occupational expenses involved in his or her care. To relate well to patients, a physician must develop compassion and courtesy, the ability to establish rapport and to communicate effectively, the ability to gather information rapidly and to organize it logically, the skills required to identify all significant patient problems and to manage these problems appropriately, the ability to listen, the skills necessary to motivate people, and the ability to observe and detect nonverbal clues.

Much of the family physician's effectiveness in interpersonal relationships depends upon his or her charisma. Charisma is a personal magic of leadership, a magnetic charm or appeal that arouses special loyalty or enthusiasm. The charismatic physician is most likely to engender maximal patient compliance and satisfaction. The physician must be aware of his or her own feelings, however, and their effect upon the patient. Charisma can be a useful therapeutic tool, but one must learn how and when to use it effectively because it can also rebound with unfavorable consequences. The physician should be aware that the patient's needs are paramount. The temptation to take an "ego-trip" is frequent and hazardous.

ACCESSIBILITY

Just as charisma is therapeutic, so too is the mere *availability* of the physician. The feeling of security that the patient gains just by knowing he can "touch" the physician, either in person or by phone, is in itself therapeutic and has a comforting and calming influence. Accessibility is an essential feature of primary care. Services must be available when needed and should be within geographic proximity. When primary care is not available, many individuals turn to hospital emergency departments. Emergency room care is, of course, fine for emergencies, but it is no substitute for the personalized, long-term, comprehensive care a family physician can provide.

DIAGNOSTIC SKILLS—UNDIFFERENTIATED PROBLEMS

The family physician, above all, must be an outstanding diagnostician. Skills in this area must be honed to perfection, since problems are usually seen in their early, undifferentiated state and without the degree of resolution that usually is present by the time patients are referred to consulting specialists. This is a unique feature of family practice, because symptoms seen at this stage are often vague and nondescript, with signs being either minimal or absent. Unlike the consulting specialist, the family physician does not evaluate the case after it has been preselected by another physician, and the diagnostic procedures used by the family physician must be selected from the entire spectrum of medicine.

At this stage of disease, there are often only subtle differences between the early symptoms of serious disease and those of self-limiting, minor ailments. To the inexperienced person, the clinical pictures may appear identical, but to the astute and experienced family physician, one symptom will be more suspicious than another because of the greater probability that it signals a potentially serious illness. Diagnoses are frequently made on the basis of probability, and the likelihood that a specific disease is present frequently depends upon the incidence of the disease relative to the symptom seen in the physician's community during a given time of year. Approximately one fourth of all patients seen will never be assigned a final, definitive diagnosis, since the resolution of a presenting symptom or a complaint will come before a specific diagnosis can be made. Pragmatically, this is an efficient method that is less costly and achieves high patient satisfaction—even though it may be disquieting to the purist physician who feels a thorough work-up and specific diagnosis should always be obtained.

The family physician is an expert in the rapid assessment of a problem presented for the first time. He or she evaluates its potential significance, often making a diagnosis by exclusion rather than by inclusion, after making certain the symptoms are not those of a serious problem. Once assured, he allows some time to elapse, using time as one of his most efficient diagnostic aids. Follow-up visits are scheduled at appropriate intervals to watch for subtle changes in the presenting symptoms. The physician usually identifies the symptom that has the greatest discriminatory value and watches it more closely than other symptoms. The most significant clue to the true nature of the illness may depend upon subtle changes in this key symptom. The family physician's effectiveness is often determined by his or her knack for perceiving the hidden or subtle dimensions of illness and following them closely.

The maxim that an accurate history is the most important factor in arriving at an accurate diagnosis is especially appropriate in family medicine, since symptoms may be the only obvious feature of an illness at the time it is presented to the family physician. Further inquiry into the nature of the symptoms, time of onset, extenuating factors, and other unique subjective features may provide the only diagnostic clues available at such an early stage. Above all, the family physician must be a skilled clinician with the ability to evaluate symptoms, verbal and nonverbal communication, and early signs of illness in order to choose those diagnostic tests that are of greatest value in diagnosing a problem early.

The family physician attempts to minimize the degree of morbidity resulting from illness. For example, he or she pays close attention to the complete eradication of a urinary tract infection in an effort to prevent permanent damage that could result in renal failure, requiring expensive and incapacitating renal dialysis or a kidney transplant. Similar examples include the early identification of carcinoma in situ of the cervix to prevent the lethal spread of uterine carcinoma as well as the early identification of a dysplastic hip, which, if undetected could result in a permanent deformity.

The family physician must be a perceptive humanist, alert to early identification of new problems. Arriving at an early diagnosis may, in fact, be of less importance than determining the real reason the patient came to the physician. The symptoms may be due to a self-limiting or acute problem, but anxiety or fear may be the true precipitating factor. Although the symptom may be hoarseness that has resulted from postnasal drainage accompanying an upper respiratory tract infection, the patient may fear it is caused by a laryngeal carcinoma similar to that recently found in a friend or celebrity. Clinical evaluation must rule out the possibility of laryngeal carcinoma, but the patient's fears and apprehension regarding this possibility must also be allayed. Similarly, a 42-year-old man with influenza and pleuritic chest pain may be anxious and apprehensive because his father died at age 45 of an acute myocardial infarction. (In fact, a frequent reason for a patient's requesting a complete check-up and electrocardiogram is the recent heart attack of an acquaintance at work.) Mild thrombophlebitis in a 35-year-old woman could bring her to the physician in a more anxious state than is warranted because her mother died from a pulmonary embolus, or a housewife's anxiety about breast cancer may well stem from a friend's recent radical mastectomy.

Every physical problem has an emotional component, and although this factor is usually minimal, it can be extremely significant. A patient's personality, fears, and anxieties all play a role in every illness and are important factors to consider in all primary care.

THE FAMILY PHYSICIAN AS COORDINATOR

Francis Peabody, Professor of Medicine at Harvard Medical School from 1921 to 1927, was a man ahead of his time; his comments remain appropriate today:

> *Never was the public in need of wise, broadly trained advisors so much as it needs them today to guide them through the complicated maze of modern medicine. The extraordinary development of medical science with its consequent diversity of medical specialists and the increasing limitations in the extent of special fields, the very factors indeed which are creating specialists, in themselves create a new demand. Not for men who are experts along narrow lines but for men who are in touch with many lines.*

The family physician, by virtue of his or her breadth of training in a wide variety of medical disciplines, has unique insights into the skills possessed by physicians in the more limited specialties. The family physician is best prepared to select specialists whose skills can be applied most appropriately to a given case as well as to coordinate the activities of each so that they are not counterproductive. The AAFP (1982) has described this role of the family physician:

> *As long as there is a need for health care services, there will be a need for a physician who assumes continuing responsibility for the health care of the patient as an individual, and for the family as the basic social unit of society. Such a physician must possess a basic core of knowledge current through constant use. This physician must be proficient in basic techniques and must know when patients require more sophisticated skills.*

As medicine becomes more specialized and complex, the family physician's role as the integrator of health services becomes increasingly important. The family physician not only facilitates the patient's access to the whole health care system but also interprets the activities of this system to the patient, explaining the nature of the illness, the implication of the treatment, and the effect of both on the patient's way of life. The following statement from the Millis Commission Report concerning expectations of the patient is especially appropriate:

> *The patient wants someone of high competence and good judgment to take charge of the total situation, someone who can serve as coordinator of all the medical resources that can help solve his problem. He wants a company president who will make proper use of his skills and knowledge of more specialized members of the firm. He wants a quarterback who will diagnose the constantly changing situation, coordinate the whole team, and call on each member for the particular contributions that he is best able to make to the team effort.*

Such breadth of vision is important for a coordinating physician. He or she must have a realistic overview of the problem and an awareness of the many alternative routes in order to select the most appropriate one. Consider, for example, three different patients with peptic ulcers. One may benefit most by medical management and another by psychiatric care, whereas the third may require surgery. The physician familiar with one form of treatment tends to rely on it excessively, whereas the family physician can select the best approach from all possible alternatives. As Pellegrino (1966) has stated:

> *It should be clear, too, that no simple addition of specialties can equal the generalist function. To build a wall one needs more than the aimless piling up of bricks, one needs an architect. Every operation which analyzes some part of the human mechanism requires to be balanced by another which synthesizes and coordinates.*

The complexity of modern medicine frequently involves a variety of health professionals, each with highly developed skills in a particular area. In planning the patient's care, the family physician, having established rapport with a patient and family and having knowledge of the patient's background, personality, fears, and expectations, is best able to select and coordinate the activities of appropriate individuals from the large variety of medical disciplines. He or she can maintain effective communication among those involved, as well as function as the patient's advocate and interpret to the patient and family the many unfamiliar and complicated procedures being used. This prevents any one consulting physician, unfamiliar with the concepts or actions of all others involved, from ordering a test or medication that would conflict with other treatment. J. E. Dunphy (1964a) has described the value of the surgeon and the family physician working closely as a team:

> *It is impossible to provide high quality surgical care without that knowledge of the whole patient which only a family physician can supply. When their mutual decisions . . . bring hope, comfort and ultimately, health to a gravely ill human being, the total experience is the essence and the joy of medicine.*

The ability to orchestrate the knowledge and skills of diverse professionals is a skill to be learned during training and cultivated in practice. It is not an automatic attribute of all physicians or merely the result of exposure to a large number of professionals. These coordinator skills extend beyond the traditional medical disciplines into the many community agencies and allied health professions as well. For the family physician to be an effective coordinator, it is essential that all pertinent health information be channeled through him or her—regardless of what institution, agency, or individual renders the service. The family physician helps remove barriers to health care, whether they be economic, emotional, social, or occupational. Because of his or her close involvement with the community, the family physician is ideally suited to being the integrator of the patient's care, coordinating the skills of consultants when appropriate and involving community nurses, social agencies, the clergy, or other family members when needed. A knowledge of community health resources and a personal involvement with the community can be used to maximum benefit not only for diagnostic and therapeutic purposes but also to achieve the best possible level of rehabilitation.

The family physician synthesizes the opinions and skills of a multitude of medical consultants with the individual patient's personal needs and the community agencies available. These must be matched to the patient's expectations and to his or her ability to respond to appropriate changes in life style. The recommended changes in life style, however, must be realistic and based on consideration of the patient's ability to comply. For example, treatment of a newly diagnosed diabetic patient recovering from ketoacidosis and who is married to a woman whose main satisfaction in life is cooking for her family requires a significant amount of tact and skill by the family physician to help both the patient and his wife readjust their life styles.

The Family Physician in Practice

The advent of family medicine not only heralds a renaissance in medical education but also involves a reassessment of the traditional medical education environment in a referral hospital. It is now considered more realistic to train a physician in a community atmosphere, providing exposure to the diseases and problems most closely approximating those he or she will encounter during practice. The ambulatory care skills and knowledge that most medical graduates need cannot be taught totally within the tertiary medical center. The specialty of family practice emphasizes training in ambulatory care skills in an appropriately realistic environment, using patients representing a cross section of a community and incorporating those problems most frequently encountered by physicians practicing primary care.

The lack of relevance in the referral medical center also applies to the hospitalized patient. Figure 1–1, which is derived from data accumulated in the United States and Great Britain, places the health problems of an average community in perspective. In an adult population of 1000 people aged 16 years or older, 750 will experience at least one illness or injury during an average month. Most of these people will be managed by self-treatment, but 250 patients will consult a physician. Of these, five patients will be referred for consultation to another physician, and nine will be hospitalized—eight of them in a community hospital and one in a university medical center. It is obvious that patients seen in the medical center (frequently the majority of cases used for teaching) represent atypical samples of illness occurring within the community. Students exposed only in this manner develop an unrealistic concept of the kinds of medical problems prevalent in society. It focuses their training on knowledge and skills of limited usefulness in later practice.

In a typical family practice that cares for 1500 to 3000 individuals, two thirds will be seen at least once each year. Many practicing family physicians and most family practice residency programs are recording the type and frequency of problems seen. Undergraduate and graduate curricula are now being revised upon information from these studies.

PRACTICE CONTENT

The first major system for classifying disease was the International Classification of Disease, which was modified for use in the United States and became the International Classification of Diseases Adapted for Use in the United States. This was further modified by hospitals into the Hospital International Classification of Diseases Adapted for Use in the United States, which included perinatal mortality and psychiatric problems and contained more than 4000 items. This classification system had major deficiencies when applied to the problems most frequently encountered by practicing family physicians, so the Royal College of General Practitioners developed a classification system pertinent to its members' needs in the administration of ambulatory care. That system served as a nucleus for an international classification of problems seen by practicing family physicians throughout the world. The sponsoring organization is the World Organization of National Colleges, Academies, and Academic Associations of General Practitioners/Family Physicians. The classification was developed by an international working party, which gave it the name International Classification of Health Problems in Primary Care, also called Ich-Pic and Pri-Care. The working party conducted a large-scale international trial that isolated the 371 items most commonly encountered by family physicians. In this manner, a large number of problems included in the International Classification of Disease but infre-

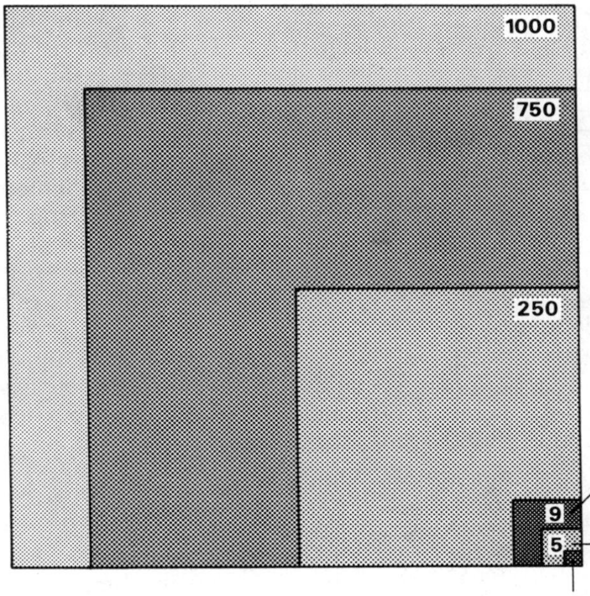

Figure 1–1. Number of persons experiencing illness or injury during an average month, per 1000 adult population. (From White, K.L., Williams, F., and Greenberg, B.: Ecology of medical care. N. Engl. J. Med., *265:*885, 1961.)

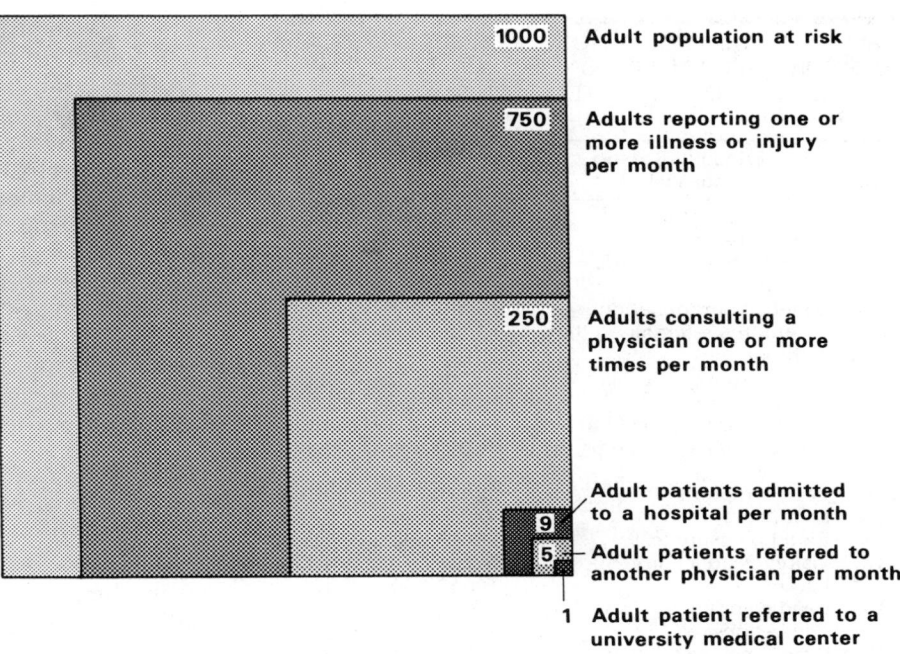

quently encountered in family practice have been eliminated. The International Classification of Health Problems in Primary Care is compatible with the larger International Classification of Disease, however, and can be used interchangeably or expanded at will.

The need for such a classification arose when it was realized that as many as 25 per cent of the problems seen by family physicians were not classifiable according to the International Classification of Disease. Many of these are undifferentiated, indefinite symptoms that resolve either spontaneously or with empiric treatment before progressing to a definitive diagnosis. It is no surprise to family physicians that respiratory tract infections, emotionally based symptoms and syndromes, skin disorders, gastrointestinal problems, and musculoskeletal and cardiovascular diseases are the most frequently encountered disorders. This classification system has permitted family physicians to institute investigative projects that are pertinent to the needs of those supplying primary care yet impossible to conduct using the research methodologies of the tertiary medical center.

Marsland and associates (1976) used the International Classification of Health Problems in Primary Care to document the problems encountered by family physicians practicing in Virginia. They showed what family practice residents in the United States could expect to see in their practices. The Virginia Study, the first of its kind, has had enormous impact on the development of family practice curricula throughout the country. The content of family practice, however, varies significantly from region to region within the United States, so it is difficult to extrapolate from a regional study.

The ABFP has defined the "content validity" of family practice by using a survey scientifically designed to obtain information about the content of family practice as performed. The results have been shared with the Medical Education for Requirements in Training Committee of the AAFP, and together the two organizations have set forth a graduate curriculum based on firm data about practice.

The National Ambulatory Medical Care Survey conducted by the National Center for Health Statistics of the United States Department of Health and Human Services has, since 1975, annually reported the problems seen by office-based physicians (in all specialties) in the United States. A symptom classification was developed to document the complaints presented by patients to physicians in their offices. The National Ambulatory Medical Care Survey reverses the previous trend of evaluating the prevalence of disease after the fact (measuring causes of death or diagnosis upon discharge from a hospital) by evaluating the presenting complaints or symptoms at the onset of the illness. This change in approach is a formidable and difficult task but one that is yielding a large amount of new and valuable information. The 20 most common symptoms or reasons prompting office visits in 1985 are shown in Table 1–1. The principal diagnoses resulting from these visits are also documented by the participating physicians. Table 1–2 lists the 50 most common patient problems diagnosed by office-based physicians in 1985.

As interest in primary care continues to grow and data continue to be collected, increasing information will be available as to what problems are being seen in practices throughout the country. Data from studies such as these, combined with ABFP

Table 1–1. THE TWENTY MOST COMMON PRINCIPAL REASONS FOR OFFICE VISITS IN THE UNITED STATES, 1985*

Rank	Principal Reason for Visit	Number of Visits	Per Cent
1	General medical examination	38,224,561	5.7
2	Prenatal examination, routine	25,746,790	4.0
3	Well-baby examination	16,447,086	2.6
4	Symptoms referable to the throat	16,370,903	2.6
5	Postoperative visit	16,303,152	2.6
6	Cough	16,133,598	2.5
7	Earache or ear infection	11,402,494	1.8
8	Abdominal pain, cramps, spasms	11,391,938	1.8
9	Back symptoms	11,310,845	1.8
10	Skin rash	10,350,091	1.6
11	Blood pressure test	9,445,594	1.5
12	Vision dysfunctions	9,266,316	1.5
13	Fever	9,049,800	1.4
14	Head cold, upper respiratory infections	8,902,340	1.4
15	Hypertension	8,813,973	1.4
16	Headache, pain in head	8,683,502	1.4
17	Chest pain and related symptoms	8,099,162	1.3
18	Knee symptoms	7,407,293	1.2
19	Eye examination	7,170,285	1.1
20	Neck symptoms	5,889,486	0.9
	All other reasons	379,976,412	59.9

*From the National Ambulatory Medical Care Survey, 1985.

surveys and audits of office records, will enable family practice training programs to revise their curricula according to the realities of everyday practice.

OFFICE VISITS

Available data concerning primary care indicate that more people use this type of medical service than any other kind, and that, contrary to popular opinion, sophisticated medical technology is not normally either required or overused in basic primary care encounters (Gold and Azevedo, 1982). Indeed, most primary care visits arise from patients requesting care for relatively uncomplicated problems, many of which are self-limiting but which cause them concern or discomfort. Treatment is often symptomatic, consisting of pain relief or anxiety reduction rather than a "cure." The greatest level of cost efficiency results when these patients' needs are satisfied while the self-limiting course of the disease is recognized without incurring unnecessary costs for additional tests.

In 1981, 37 per cent of the complaints treated by U.S. physicians were acute and 37.2 per cent were chronic, with "chronic" defined as having an onset 3 months or more before the visit (unpublished data from the Ambulatory Medical Care survey, 1981). Only 1.6 per cent of all physician visits made during 1985 ended in hospital admission, and only 3.2 per cent were referred to other physicians (Advance Data, Jan. 23, 1987).

Each year 75 per cent of people in the United States make at least one visit to a physician (Current Estimates, 1977). In 1985, the average was 2.7 office visits per person (Advance Data, Jan. 23, 1987). Females accounted for 60.9 per cent of all visits (3.2 visits per person per year), and males had 2.2 visits per person per year. The annual visit rate ranged from 1.9 visits per person per year for young adults 15 to 24 years of age to more than twice that (4.8 visits per person per year) for those 65 years of age and older. Approximately 30 per cent of all visits were made to physicians in general and family practice, and 51 per cent were made to solo practitioners.

HOUSE CALLS

At one time, house calls were a routine feature of medical practice in the United States. As general practice declined, so did the number and frequency of house calls. However, the house call continues to be a valuable tool used by family physicians to develop a thorough understanding of patients and their environment, and family practice residencies are encouraged to include house calls in their training programs.

The cost containment pressures that arose in the 1980's with the advent of Diagnostic Related Groups and Professional Review Organizations have led to a resurgence in home care. More patients with acute as well as chronic illnesses are being managed at home, and the home care industry has grown at a rate of 20 per cent a year, whereas the availability of nursing home beds has increased only 2 per cent annually (Kavesh, 1986).

Elderly patients, especially the frail elderly, often have considerable difficulty getting to and from the physician's office. The patient is more comfortable and under less stress at home and more problems can be identified, leading to improved care. Ramsdell and coworkers (1989) have shown that home visit assessments reveal two new problems and up to eight new treatment recommendations when home visits follow physician office-based assessments. Home visits may be the only way to identify some environmental hazards and to accurately evaluate the patient's functional status.

Home visits are more considerate of patients who have impaired mobility, and these patients respond better and may improve more rapidly when cared for at home by health professionals and family members (Kavesh, 1986). Only 15 per cent of patients who need long-term supportive care in the home turn to available community resources; 85 per cent receive care entirely from family and friends.

Cauthen (1981) has described eight different types of house calls: the emergency house call; the acute illness house call; the chronic illness house call;

Table 1–2. RANK ORDER OF OFFICE VISITS BY DIAGNOSIS (1985)*

Rank	Diagnosis	Per Cent	Cumulative Per Cent
1	Essential hypertension	4.1	4.1
2	Normal pregnancy	3.8	7.9
3	Health supervision: infant, child	2.7	10.6
4	Otitis media, suppurative	2.5	13.1
5	General medical examination	2.3	15.4
6	Acute upper respiratory infection	2.3	17.7
7	Diabetes mellitus	1.9	19.6
8	Neurotic disorders	1.5	21.1
9	Acute pharyngitis	1.5	22.6
10	Disorders of refraction and accommodation	1.3	23.9
11	Diseases of sebaceous glands	1.3	25.2
12	Allergic rhinitis	1.2	26.4
13	Bronchitis, not specified	1.2	27.6
14	Chronic ischemic heart disease	1.1	28.7
15	Asthma	1.0	29.7
16	Cataract	1.0	30.7
17	Certain adverse effects (allergic reactions)	0.9	31.6
18	Special investigations and examinations (e.g., gynecologic examination)	0.9	32.5
19	Contact dermatitis and other eczema	0.9	33.4
20	Disorders of urethra and urinary tract	0.9	34.3
21	Chronic sinusitis	0.9	35.2
22	Osteoarthrosis and allied disorders	0.9	36.1
23	Sprains and strains, unspecified	0.8	36.9
24	Unspecified disorders of the back	0.8	37.7
25	General symptoms (e.g., syncope, dizziness)	0.8	38.5
26	Diseases due to viruses and *Chlamydiae*	0.7	39.2
27	Noninfectious gastroenteritis and colitis	0.7	39.9
28	Peripheral enthesopathies and allied syndromes (e.g., tenosynovitis)	0.7	40.6
29	Disorders of conjunctiva (e.g., conjunctivitis)	0.7	41.3
30	Disorders of external ear (e.g., otitis externa)	0.7	42.0
31	Glaucoma	0.7	42.7
32	Acute tonsillitis	0.7	43.4
33	Inflammatory disease of the cervix and vagina (e.g., vaginitis)	0.6	44.0
34	Observation and evaluation	0.6	44.6
35	Other disorders of soft tissues	0.6	45.2
36	Contraceptive management	0.6	45.8
37	Unspecified arthropathies	0.6	46.4
38	Other disorders of synovium, tendon, and bursa	0.5	46.9
39	Affective psychoses	0.5	47.4
40	Obesity, other hyperalimentation	0.5	47.9
41	Other dermatoses	0.5	48.4
42	Disorders of menstruation and other abnormal bleeding from female genital tract	0.5	48.9
43	Otitis media, nonsuppurative	0.5	49.4
44	Sprains and strains of sacroiliac region	0.5	49.9
45	Viral infection	0.5	50.4
46	Menopausal and postmenopausal disorders	0.5	50.9
47	Symptoms involving respiratory system and other chest symptoms (e.g., cough)	0.5	51.4
48	Rheumatoid arthritis and other inflammatory polyarthropathies	0.5	51.9
49	Streptococcal sore throat and scarlet fever	0.5	52.4
50	Acute bronchitis and bronchiolitis	0.5	52.9

*Constructed from information from the 1985 National Ambulatory Medical Care Survey.

the dying patient house call; the house call to pronounce death; the grief house call; home management–versus–hospitalization house call; and the home visit house call. Although the chronic illness house call is by far the most common type, the home visit can be especially rewarding in family practice. Some family physicians routinely visit patients in the home after a mother returns from the hospital with her new baby or after a patient is discharged following a serious illness.

Dr. Nicholas T. Grace, a family physician in California, makes a home visit whenever he enrolls a new family into his practice (Family Practice News, Aug. 15, 1977) because a personal visit to the family's home is an excellent way to begin a long-term relationship and is valuable in establishing good relations, not to mention the insight gained by the physician.

GROUP OR SOLO PRACTICE

Approximately half of graduating family practice residents enter a partnership or a group practice. Twenty-eight per cent enter family practice groups, 9 per cent join multispecialty groups, and 14.8 per cent form two-person practices (partnerships). Although

Table 1–3. DISTRIBUTION OF 1989 GRADUATING RESIDENTS BY COMMUNITY SIZE*

Character and Population of Community	Number of Reporting Graduates	Percentage of Total Reporting Graduates	Cumulative Percentage of Total Reporting Graduates
Rural area or town (less than 2500) not within 25 miles of a large city	68	4.8%	4.8%
Rural area or town (less than 2500) within 25 miles of a large city	46	3.3%	8.1%
Small town (2500 to 25,000) not within 25 miles of a large city	253	17.9%	26.0%
Small town (2500 to 25,000) within 25 miles of a large city	222	15.7%	41.7%
Small city (25,000 to 100,000)	263	18.6%	60.3%
Suburb of small metropolitan area	55	3.9%	64.2%
Small metropolitan area (100,000 to 500,000)	144	10.2%	74.4%
Suburb of large metropolitan area	197	13.9%	88.3%
Large metropolitan area (500,000 or more)	113	7.9%	96.2%
Inner city/low income area (500,000 or more)	54	3.8%	100.0%
	1,415	100.0%	

*From the American Academy of Family Physicians Reprint No. 1550.

only 9.8 per cent of graduates now enter solo practice, in 1975, 74 per cent of all family physicians in the United States were in solo practice (American Academy of Family Physicians Survey, 1989).

Many graduates are attracted to group practice because of the opportunity to share calls. Such an arrangement allows physicians more time with their families and time to remain current with medical advances through continuing education. Many physicians also select group practice because of the professional stimulation of working with colleagues. Group practices allow for overhead to be shared and the cost of expensive equipment for x-ray studies and cryotherapy can be spread over a wider financial base. Employment of paramedical personnel such as a nutritionist, clinical pharmacist, or marriage and family counselor is another luxury more easily borne by groups.

Group practice does, however, involve sacrificing some privacy and individuality, since each physician must adhere to the will of the majority. Solo practice, with the individual freedom it provides, is still alive and well in the United States. Solo physicians sacrifice the financial advantage of shared office space and more elaborate equipment for the privilege of being their own boss and making decisions unencumbered by the hassles and delays of group decision-making.

Group practices are more likely to draw physicians into rural and inner-city areas, where solo physicians are unlikely to want to practice "in isolation." Approximately 42 per cent of the 1989 graduates of family practice residencies were located in towns of 25,000 population or less. Table 1–3 shows the size of community selected by 1988 residency graduates, 1667 of whom responded to an AAFP survey (out of 2257 total graduates).

Physician Supply

The 1988 report of the American Medical Association's Council on Long Range Planning and Devel-

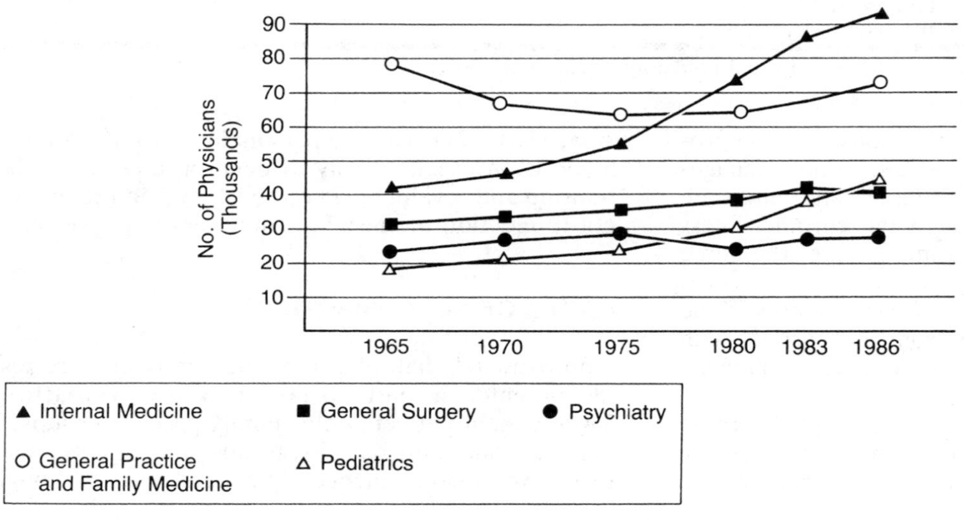

Figure 1–2. Trends in distribution of federal and nonfederal physicians by specialty for selected years. (From Roback, G., Mead, L., and Randolph, L.: Physician Characteristics and Distribution in the U.S. Chicago, American Medical Association, 1987.)

opment notes that although the number of family physicians will increase by 9 per cent by the year 2000, the U.S. population will increase by 12.3 per cent. Also, managed care systems will place increased demands on the need for family physicians, thus decreasing even further the number available in some rural areas.

The Graduate Medical Education National Advisory Committee in 1980 projected a surplus of 150,000 physicians in the United States by the year 2020, with the greatest need in primary care. Mulhausen and McGee (1989) project an even greater demand for primary care physicians than was estimated by the Graduate Medical Education National Advisory Committee.

Another federally convened group, the Council on Graduate Medical Education and the American Medical Association Center for Health Policy Research have issued reports (1988) indicating more conservative estimates of physician surplus, but emphasizing that whatever the numbers, there will be a significant shortage of family physicians and psychiatrists and a significant excess of pediatricians, internal medicine subspecialists, and obstetricians and gynecologists.

If the growth in physician supply continues, American Medical Association analysts warn that "soon some physicians might not have enough work to stay proficient, and the status of the profession might decline." Similarly, the quality of primary care will decline as physicians trained in a surplus subspecialty practice primary care without retraining. Rhee and associates (1981) showed that when physicians practice outside their specialty areas, the relative quality of their performance declines.

Figure 1–2 shows the changing distribution of physicians in selected specialties in the United States. Although there has been a sharp increase in the number of internists, 60 per cent are in subspecialties. This leaves family practice as the largest primary care discipline and the only one whose goal is to produce primary care physicians.

As much-needed changes in the American medical system are implemented, it would be wise to keep some perspective on the situation regarding physician distribution. Paul Beeson (1974) has commented,

> *I have no doubt at all that a good family doctor can deal with the great majority of medical episodes quickly and competently. A specialist, on the other hand, feels that he must be thorough, not only because of his training but also because he has a reputation to protect. He, therefore, spends more time with each patient and orders more laboratory work. The result is a waste of doctors' time and patients' money. This not only inflates the national health bill, but also creates an illusion of doctor shortage when the only real need is to have the existing doctors doing the right things.*

References

Ad Hoc Committee on Education for Family Practice of the Council on Medical Education of the American Medical Association (Willard Committee): Meeting the Challenge of Family Practice (report), September 1966. *Known best as the Willard Report, this document outlines the basic principles of education in family practice and the essential components of a residency program. It supported the recognition of family practice as a specialty and provided much of the impetus for the establishment of the American Board of Family Practice.*

American Academy of Family Physicians: Official definition of family practice and family physician. AAFP publication No. 303.

American Academy of Family Physicians: Official AAFP Definition of Primary Care. AAFP Reporter, *2*(6):1, 1975.

American Medical Association: Council on Long Range Planning and Development. The Future of Family Practice. Chicago, American Medical Association, 1988.

Balint, M.: The Doctor, His Patient and the Illness. New York, Pitman Publishing Corp., 1965. *Balint's approach to physician-patient relations remains a classic in this all-important aspect of primary care.*

Batten, L. W.: The essence of general practice. Lancet *2:*365, 1956.

Beeson, P. B.: Some good features of the British National Health Service. J. Med. Educ., *49:*43, 1974.

Cauthen, D. B.: The house call in current medical practice. J. Fam. Pract., *13:*209, 1981.

Citizens' Commission on Graduate Medical Education of the American Medical Association (Millis Commission): The Graduate Education of Physicians (report), August 1966. *Known as the Millis Commission Report, this article popularized the term primary physician and outlined the teaching of comprehensive health care in undergraduate and graduate programs. It emphasized the need for medical schools to play an active role in comprehensive care and was a stimulus for developing departments of family practice.*

Current Estimates from the Health Interview Study: United States, 1977, Department of Health, Education, and Welfare. Washington, D.C., U.S. Government Printing Office, 1978 (DHEW pub. no. [PHS] 78-1544).

Darley, W.: We need a new specialty: Family practice. New Medical Materia, *4*(3):29, 1962.

Dunphy, J. E.: Responsibility and authority in American surgery. Bull. Am. Coll. Surg., *49:*9, 1964a.

Dunphy, J. E.: Role of the family physician in the medical care of the future. New Physician, *13:*331, 1964b.

End—or beginning? Lancet, *2:*165, 1965.

Family practice, a concept or a reality? J.A.M.A., *185:*208, 1963.

Fox, T. F.: The personal doctor and his relation to the hospital. Lancet, *1:*743, 1960.

Fry, J.: Common sense and uncommon sensibility. J. R. Coll. Gen. Pract., *27:*9, 1977.

Geyman, J. P.: Family Practice: Foundation of Changing Health Care. New York, Appleton-Century-Crofts, 1980. *Geyman provides a comprehensive overview of family practice after 10 years as a recognized specialty. He describes its progress from clinical research and organizational perspectives, and suggests new issues that will face the specialty in its next stage of development. It contains useful appendices, including the Virginia Study and the WONCA-ICHPPA classification system.*

Gold, M., and Azevedo, D.: The content of adult primary care episodes. Public Health Rep *97:*48, 1982.

Gonnella, J. S., and Veloski, J. J.: The impact of early specialization on the clinical competence of residents. N. Engl. J. Med., *306:*275, 1982.

Graduate Medical Education National Advisory Committee (GMENAC): Final Report, v. 1. Hyattsville, Md., Health Resources Administration, September 1980 (DHHS pub. no. [HRA] 81-651). *This committee consisting of 22 representatives from the medical profession and the federal government projected physician needs in the United States by 1990. Emphasis was upon those disciplines that will have an excess of physicians and the impact this will have on the health care system. Recommendations were made for correcting the maldistribution.*

Halsted, J. A.: Personal care in medicine of the future. N. Engl. J. Med., *267:*1233, 1962.

James, G.: The general practitioner of the future. N. Engl. J. Med., *270:*1286, 1964.

Kavesh, W. N.: Home care: Process, outcome, cost. Ann Rev Gerontol. Geriatr. *6:*135–195, 1986.

Marsland, D. W., Wood, M., and Mayo, F.: Content of family practice. *In* Geyman, J.P. (Ed.): A Statewide Study in Virginia with Its Clinical, Educational, and Research Implications. New York, Appleton-Century-Crofts, 1976. *Known as the Virginia Study, this was the earliest report of an in-depth analysis of family physicians' practices. The study, conducted over a 2-year period, documented the problems seen by 36 family physicians and 92 family practice residents in the state of Virginia.*

McWhinney, I. R.: An Introduction to Family Medicine. New York, Oxford University Press, 1981. *A well-written discussion of the fundamentals of family medicine intended for senior medical students and residents. It begins with a chapter on the origins of family medicine and includes chapters on practice management, preventive medicine, and problem-solving.*

Mulhausen, R. and McGee, J.: Physician Need: An alternative projection from a study of large, prepaid group practices. J.A.M.A., *261*(13):1930–1934, 1989.

National Center for Health Statistics. National Ambulatory Medical Care Survey: U.S. 1975–1981 and 1985 Trends. Vital and Health Statistics, Series 13, No. 93. DHHS pub. no. (PHS)88-1754. Public Health Service, Washington, D.C. *The NAMCS is the most comprehensive study of ambulatory care conducted in the United States. This ongoing study, begun in 1975, documents the problems presenting to physicians in office practices and lists both the patient's presenting complaint and the physician's diagnosis. Physicians in all specialties with an office practice are included.*

National Center for Health Statistics. (McLemore, T. and DeLozier, J.) 1985 Summary: National Ambulatory Medical Care Survey. Advance Data from Vital and Health Statistics, No 128. DHHS pub. no. (PHS) 87-1250. Public Health Service. Hyattsville, M.D. Jan. 23, 1987.

Osler, W.: Aequanimitas, with Other Addresses. 3rd ed. Philadelphia, The Blakiston Co., 1932.

Peabody, F. W.: Doctor and Patient. New York, The Macmillan Co., 1930. *Since this book is out of print, the student is encouraged to review the original paper on the care of the patient published in J.A.M.A. 88:877, 1927.*

Pellegrino, E. D.: The generalist function in medicine. J.A.M.A., *198:*541, 1966.

Pellegrino, E. D.: Humanism and the Physician. Knoxville, University of Tennessee Press, 1979. *These previously published or delivered essays by one of medicine's most eloquent and learned representatives provide a convenient collection of both theoretical and practical thoughts on medicine and the humanities as interrelated intellectual disciplines, as the bases for significant moral and ethical decisions, and as interacting forces in medical education.*

Ramsdell, J. W., Swart, J. A., Jackson, J. E., and Renvall, M.: The yield of a home visit in the assessment of geriatric patients. J. Am. Geriatr. Soc., *37*(1):17–24, 1989.

Rhee, S., Luke, R., Lyons, T., and Payne, B.: Domain of Practice and the Quality of Physician Performance. Med. Care, *19*(1):14–23, 1981.

Schroeder, S. A.: Western European Responses to Physician Oversupply. J.A.M.A., 252(3):373–384, 1984.

Steinwachs, D. M., Levine, D. M., Elzinga, J., et al: Changing patterns of graduate medical education. N. Engl. J. Med., *306:*10, 1982. *A planning model of graduate medical education is developed based on changes in postgraduate medical education in the 1970's. Projections suggest that the increase in primary care recommended by Graduate Medical Education National Advisory Committee will probably not occur spontaneously.*

Surgeon-General's Consultant Group on Medical Education: Physicians for a Growing America (Bane Report). Washington, D.C., U.S. Government Printing Office, 1959 (PHS pub. no. 709).

Tumulty, P. A.: What is a clinician and what does he do? N. Engl. J. Med. *283*(1):20–24, 1970.

Tumulty, P. A.: The Effective Clinician: His Methods and Approach to Diagnosis and Care. Philadelphia, W. B. Saunders Co., 1973. *A well-written book describing the communication and clinical skills of a good primary care physician.*

White, K. L., Williams, F., and Greenberg, B.: Ecology of medical care. N. Engl. J. Med., *265:*885, 1961.

2

Family Structure and Functioning

Christian N. Ramsey, Jr.
Jerry M. Lewis

From the first cry at birth to the last words at death, the family surrounds us and finds a place for all ages, roles and relationships for both sexes. Our needs for physical, emotional and intellectual exchange, and for nurturance, control, communication and genital sexuality can all exist side by side and find satisfaction in harmonious relationship to one another. It exists to make itself unnecessary, to release its members into the wider community as separate, autonomous beings, only to recreate there images of itself anew. It has enormous creative potential, including that of life itself, and it is not surprising that, when it becomes disordered, it possesses an equal potential for terrible destruction.

A. C. ROBIN SKYNNER, SYSTEMS OF FAMILY AND MARITAL PSYCHOTHERAPY

Whether in solo, group, or team practice, the family physician is increasingly concerned with the family as the basic unit that is treated. Family physicians are concerned with the relationship of life in small groups to health, illness, and medical care. Diagnosis and intervention often occur at the level of interaction between members of families or between the family and its environment. In this chapter, we examine the rationale for the family as the unit of care in family medicine, the definition(s) of family, some characteristics of a healthy family, theories of family functioning and their relationships to illness in the family system, methods for the study of families, and the role of the family physician in caring for the family.

The Family as The Unit of Care in Family Medicine

Several major themes lend support to the concept of the family as the basic unit of care in family medicine: (1) the necessity of groups for the survival of humanity and the power of the family as an emotional force, (2) the roots of the specialty of family practice, (3) the relationship of the family unit to health and illness, and (4) improved health outcomes when the family is treated as a unit of care.

The Family in Society

Survival in groups is an inherent and basic element of the human condition, and the family is the most enduring social form of small group. Humans have survived in all societies by belonging to aggregates that vary in different cultures in their level of organization and differentiation. Primitive cultures rely on large groupings with relatively stable distributions of functions among subgroups. In more complex societies requiring new survival skills, the social structures and groupings are more widely differentiated. Throughout history, the family has undergone changes that parallel changes in society and has given up or taken over many of the functions of protecting and socializing its members' responses to society's needs. Today, many people are wondering what is happening to the family. People are troubled about many aspects of current family life, including the divorce rate, reports of widespread child abuse, accounts of violence between spouses, and the abundance of couples in nontraditional living and social arrangements—contract marriages, people living in communes, and mothers who are voluntarily without husbands. Urban industrial society intruded forcefully on the family of the early 20th century, taking over many of the functions that were previously the family's duties. The old now live apart in nursing homes, housing developments, or other arrangements, and economic support to members of society is provided through social security and welfare more often than it has been in the past.

As society changes, the family—which must adapt to society—changes with it. Despite the disturbing aspects of current family life, a number of observers believe that the family has demonstrated an enormous capacity for innovation and endurance throughout the ages, that the family is in the process of a transition reflecting the changes in society, and that it will survive because it is the optimal human unit. The more flexibility and adaptability society requires of its members, the more significant the family becomes as the matrix of psychosocial development.

Research on the stressful effects of life events illustrates the powerful impact of family in our lives. Holmes and Rahe (1967) developed a system for quantifying the effects of various stresses on an individual, and they found that the most stressful events are family disruptions (divorce, death, or birth of a family member). Almost all medical students in interviews for residency, when asked to rank their goals in life, say: "Family is first."

The Roots of the Specialty of Family Practice

The general practitioner of the past usually treated all members of the family and participated in the milestone events of family life: birth, illness, and death of family members. Furthermore, the general practitioner usually saw patients in the family's home and observed the repeated interactions of family members over the course of many years. The general practitioner did not have sophisticated diagnostic and therapeutic equipment such as x-ray machines, electrocardiogram machines, or computerized axial tomography scanners. Instead, the practitioner used scientific knowledge and a "data base" about the family that was gathered over years of diagnosing and treating family members. This "data base" would often involve several generations of the family.

An interesting and humorous situation involving a general practitioner and a family comes from Dr. W. L. Crosthwait's (1956) account of his early practice in Texas.

There was an old couple, the Beermans, who lived on a ranch a few miles from town. She was the whining kind. One cold night she wanted her husband to call the doctor; she thought she was going to die. The doctor went out and examined her and told her there was nothing wrong with her. The husband said, "I told you so." She ordered both the husband and doctor out of her room and said, "Don't you ever come back."

The couple lived on for 20 years, but never spoke to each other directly. They had one of those old-fashioned double houses; that is, there were two sections with a breezeway hall in between. They lived there separately and communicated with each other by note or through the hired help or the children. The husband was the whimsical type; otherwise he would have found a way to soften her up and resume normal marital relations.

Another night there came the familiar "Hello!" at my front gate. A 15-year-old boy, mounted on a work mule, said: "Doctor, you are wanted at once."

"What's the trouble?"

"Mr. Beerman's wife is dying. I am the neighbor's boy. My mammy is over there and she said for you to come quick."

I saddled up my pony and loped out there.

I got there just before the husband arrived; he had been in town all day and was pretty well loaded with his favorite beverage. He viewed the situation in silence. His wife was flat on the bed with four neighbor women rubbing her hands and feet. Her jaws were locked, lips closed tight and eyes shut, but her breathing and pulse were normal. She had been that way since noon. That was about the time she had expected her husband to return from town.

I looked the situation over and decided she was "throwing a hissy" for the benefit of the neighbors and to punish her husband.

So I said, in a loud voice, "She's in bad shape, liable to die any minute." (Moans and groans from the other women.) "But I have a remedy here that either will finish her off or bring her to; more often it kills."

I called for some hot water. I began to prepare a sterile water hypo and got her arm ready for the injection. She jerked the other arm free, slapped the hypodermic needle out of my hand, and jumped up yelling, "Get out of here, all of you!" That meant me, too. She spied her husband cowering over in one corner of the room, and she bolted into the kitchen after a skillet, a rolling pin or some other weapon. We didn't wait to see. The husband was right on my heels going out. After he got a safe distance he said to me, "Damn that woman, I'll fix her."

I don't know what he ever did, if anything, but I was glad to get out, and I was never called out there again.

The process of medical care—involving house calls and home visits—assisted the physician in using knowledge of family problems, past family behavior, and family relationships in treating problems such as the Beermans'. The physician was also able to enlist the aid of family members in the care of the patient.

Relationship of Family Functioning to Illness

There is growing appreciation that what goes on in the family may influence a family member's illness.

Disturbances in family structure and function can predispose, precipitate, or sustain illness in a family member. Many years ago, for example, Richardson (1945) studied the families of patients and noted that certain types of family structure were frequently associated with either chronic illnesses or acute, repetitive illnesses in family members. Kellner (1963) and Peachey (1963) presented evidence regarding the temporal patterns of illnesses within families and emphasized the tendency for illnesses to cluster in time in some families. These studies suggest that there may be something about the structure of the family that predisposes family members to illness.

Other studies focus on family events that precipitate illness. In particular, the loss of a loved one has been noted by Rees and Lutkins (1967), Livsey (1972), and Parkes and Brown (1972) to lead to increased rates of illness, hospitalization, and death for surviving family members. Kraus and Lilienfield's review (1959) of the mortality of widowed people in the United States emphasizes an increased mortality rate for young persons who have lost a spouse. Table 2–1 shows that, for all causes of death, the mortality rate for widowed persons was greater than that for married persons.

Recent studies, such as the work of Blotcky (1981), underscore the role that family factors may play in sustaining the illness of a family member. Meyer and Haggerty (1962) studied the various ways in which family stress can influence the incidence of streptococcal infections in family members, the carrier state of the individual, and family members' immune responses.

It seems clear that family factors can play a role in the course of illnesses of family members. However, it is necessary to emphasize that illness in a family member may also change the structure and function of the family. This is particularly true if the illness is severe or life-threatening and if its presence overwhelms the adaptive capacity of the family. Under such circumstances, a previously well-functioning family may change to a rigidly controlled system and, if the illness persists, disintegration of the family may follow. Anthony's (1970) study of families facing a potentially fatal illness in a family member is an illustrative example.

Treatment of the Family Unit Yields Improved Health Care Outcomes

The works of several investigators lend credence to the hypothesis that treatment of the family as a unit yields important benefits with regard to prevention, more complete diagnoses, and better outcomes of medical care. Medalie and coworkers (1973) studied 10,000 Israeli men and found that family dysfunction was equal in magnitude to hypertension and elevated cholesterol levels as risk factors in the incidence of angina and was a greater risk factor than cigarette smoking. As shown in Table 2–2, there was a threefold increase (from 31/1000 to 88/1000) in the incidence of angina in men from families with severe problems as compared with those with no problems.

There is evidence that health behavior is influenced by family behavior. For instance, smoking patterns are strongly influenced by families. A study done by the U. S. Department of Health, Education, and Welfare in 1971 showed that in families in which both parents smoked, 23 per cent of the 15- to 16-year-old boys smoked; in families in which neither parent smoked, only 9 per cent of boys in this age group smoked.

The family also has a major influence on the nutritional and dietary practices of its members. An obvious factor is that most persons' diets are highly dependent on the food provided from the family kitchen. Litman (1964), in a study of the dietary practices of schoolchildren in Minnesota, found that sanctioning of food behavior is a family-centered activity.

Attempting to understand patients' concerns about family members and their problems can lead to more complete diagnoses. In a family practice training program in New Jersey, Goldstein and asso-

Table 2–1. AVERAGE ANNUAL DEATH RATES FOR SELECTED CASES IN THE MARRIED AND THE WIDOWED, FOR THE 25- TO 35-YEAR-OLD GROUP, BY SEX, UNITED STATES 1949–1951*

Cause	Sex	Married	Widowed	Widowed-Married
Tuberculosis	M	11.2	141.8	12.7
	F	15.4	76.1	4.9
Vascular lesions of the central nervous system	M	3.6	29.3	8.1
	F	4.1	17.4	4.2
Hypertension with heart disease	M	1.7	18.3	10.8
	F	2.3	10.9	4.7
Influenza and pneumonia	M	2.6	20.1	7.7
	F	2.7	13.4	5.0
Arteriosclerotic heart disease	M	8.6	42.1	4.9
	F	2.8	16.5	5.9

*Death rates per 100,000 population in each specified group. (Adapted from Kraus, A. S., and Lilienfield, A. M.: J. Chronic Dis., *10*:207, 1959.)

Table 2–2. ANGINA PECTORIS INCIDENCE (1963–1968) AS RELATED TO FAMILY PROBLEMS IN 1963

Severity Score of Family Problems*	Number of Subjects	Number of Cases	Age-Area Adjusted Rate/1000
0 (least)	1636	50	31
1	3972	125	33
2	1836	68	38
3	865	41	49
4 (most)	219	16	88

*The severity score indicates the number of times a subject reported serious or very serious problems with respect to questions within the psychosocial area (e.g., 0 = no serious problems, 3 = a serious problem in each of the three questions related to relevant problem area). (Adapted from Medalie, J. H., et al.: Am. J. Med., 55:583, 1973.)

ciates (1981) studied patients' concerns about their families. They administered a questionnaire to assess patient concerns with regard to the developmental, psychologic, and social functioning of their families. Sixty-four per cent of the patients perceived one or more areas of concern in their families. Half of the patients had concerns about themselves, whereas concerns about the well-being of spouses, children, and parents' emotional health followed in rank order. Although 64 per cent of the patients expressed concern about family problems, only 26 per cent of these patients' charts contained indications acknowledging psychosocial problems during the patient visits.

Widmer and Cadoret (1979) report changes in patient behaviors during specific time periods before episodes of depression. The depressed patients showed an increased number of office visits, an increased incidence of hospitalizations, an increased number of functional complaints, an increased number of pain complaints, and increased feelings of tension compared with controls during the 7 months prior to diagnosis. Meyer and Haggerty (1962) found that families overutilized health services during periods of stress. They found that mothers tend to overutilize services for their children during stress but tend to underutilize these services for themselves.

Treatment of the family as a unit has yielded improved outcomes in a number of illnesses. Studies of diabetic children by Minuchin and coworkers (1975) at the Philadelphia Child Guidance Center showed a significant decrease in the number of admissions for ketoacidosis after family therapy. Of 13 diabetic children who were hospitalized an average of 12 times per year for severe ketoacidosis, three had only one admission per year after family therapy, whereas 10 children had none. Minuchin (1978) has also treated the families of patients with anorexia nervosa. As illustrated in Table 2–3, his research data show a recovery rate of 86 per cent.

Litman (1966) studied 100 patients with severe orthopedic disabilities. Their response to rehabilitation was graded by several groups including physicians, occupational therapists, and physical therapists. Seventy-three per cent of those with a good response to rehabilitation received positive reinforcement from their families. Seventy-seven per cent of those with a poor response did not obtain encouragement from their families. Hoebel and coworkers (1976) studied a group of men with cardiovascular disease and demonstrated that high-risk cardiac behavior could be altered by counseling sessions with the spouses, even though efforts with the patients themselves toward improving compliance were ineffective.

In summary, there is considerable evidence that treating the family as a unit may have significant impact on the prevention, diagnosis, and treatment of disease. Moreover, a number of family-centered health demonstrations, including those at Denver (Comen and Sarbara, 1972) and New Haven (Beloff et al., 1969), have shown that patients benefited from family-centered health care. The Montefiore Family Health Demonstration (Silver, 1974) showed improved health status for the families included in the study as compared with that of control families.

Family: Definition and Purpose

The family can be defined from a sociologic viewpoint as the enduring social form in which a person is incorporated. From a biologic standpoint, the family can be defined as a genetic transmission unit. From a psychologic perspective, the family is the matrix of personality development and is the most intimate emotional unit of society. A few examples of the differing definitions of family illustrate the many perspectives from which people view the family.

Rogers' (1973) sociologic definition is:

The family is a semi-closed system of actors occupying inter-related positions defined by the society of which the family system is a part as unique to that system with respect to the role content of the positions and to the ideas of kinship relatedness. The definitions of positional role content change over the history of the group.

Murdock (1965) provides a classic sociologic definition of the family:

The family is a social group characterized by common residence, economic cooperation, and reproduction. It includes adults of both sexes at least two of whom maintain a socially approved sexual relationship and one or more children, own or adopted, of the sexually cohabiting adults. The family is to be distinguished from marriage, which is a

Table 2–3. MEDICAL AND PSYCHOSOCIAL ASSESSMENT OF 50 ANORECTIC PATIENTS FOLLOWING FAMILY THERAPY*

Rating	Characteristic	Number of Cases	Percentage of Total
	Medical Assessment		
Recovered	Eating patterns normal, body weight stabilized within normal limits for height and age	43	86
Fair	Weight gain but continuing effects of illness (borderline weight, obesity, occasional vomiting)	2	4
Unimproved	Little or no change	3	6
Relapsed	Reappearance of symptoms of anorexia after apparently successful treatment	2	4
	Psychologic Assessment		
Good	Satisfactory adjustment in family, in school or work, and in social and peer relationships	43	86
Fair	Adjustment in one or another of these areas unsatisfactory	2	4
Unimproved	Inability to function even at borderline levels; disturbances of behavior, thought, and affect	3	6
Relapsed	Reappearance of symptoms of anorexia after apparently successful treatment	2	4

*Adapted from Minuchin, S.: Psychosomatic Families. Cambridge, Mass., Harvard University Press, 1978. Reprinted by permission.

complex of customs centered upon the relationship between a sexually associating pair of adults within the family.

Other definitions of the family are based on the relationships of family members. For instance, Ransom and Vandervoort (1973) define the family as a significant group of intimates with a history and a future. Gordon's (1978) definition is based more on the concept of kinship as a form of relationship: "The family is the unit made up of individuals a person is related to by blood or marriage and to whom he/she feels ties of social obligation." Gordon believes that this definition avoids the problems of attempting to specify composition or family functions. Smilkstein (1975) defines the family, with emphasis on the environment and relationships among family members, as "adult partners with and without children and single parents with children who function in a setting where there is a sense of home, and who have an agreement to establish nurturing relationships."

Some workers emphasize growth and development as a major factor in defining the family. Berman (1978) has defined the family as "a small social system made up of individuals related to each other by reason of strong reciprocal affections and loyalties and comprising a permanent household (or cluster of households) that persists over years and decades. Members enter through birth, adoption, or marriage and leave only by death." Parsons and Bales (1955) define the family as being that social unit whose primary tasks are the socialization of children and the stabilization of adult personalities.

Each of these definitions defines the family in terms of membership, relationships, functions, or developmental tasks. The authors have developed a definition that comprises many of these elements of the family and can be useful to the family physician working with families from a clinical, teaching, or research perspective:

The family is a small social system made up of individuals related to each other, biologically or by reason of strong affections and loyalty, that comprises a permanent household (or cluster of households) and persists over decades. Members enter through birth, adoption, or marriage and leave by death; therefore, the roles of members change over time and through the history of the groups. The operative, emotional field of the family at any given moment may include three generations. For the purposes of this chapter, family may refer to subdivisions (subsystems) of the small social system that possess the attributes of affection, loyalty, and permanent membership. In this context, a married couple with several children, units of a single parent and several children, three-generation units, and units evolved by remarriage from parts of previously existing groups are families. Such terms as couple, nuclear family, single-parent family, and extended family specify or define certain attributes of membership, but the family groups so designated are neither more nor less families.

Terkelsen and coworkers (1980) conclude that the basic purpose of the family is to help members satisfy their needs and that this is done by evoking sequences of interactions between members. Such interactions are sustained over a lifetime, support survival, and stimulate the development of all members. They suggest that all family units promote member-to-member interactions that are suffused with attachment behavior. In healthy families, the ambience should be nurturing and the relationships filled with loving, caring, affection, and loyalty. In dysfunctional families, relationships take on the qualities of hate, guilt, retribution, and punishment, and the ambience is pathogenic. In both healthy and dysfunctional families, the emotional attachments are intense, pervading the whole life of the family, and the outcome of these interactions is survival and personal development of the members.

At least two unique characteristics of families as a group distinguish them from other social systems. First, in contrast to other social organizations, membership in the family unit is virtually permanent. Members are not expelled because of decreased ability to function or because of a change in priorities of the family as an organization. Second, relationships are principally affectional in nature, since the family places a higher value on caring, loving, and affection than other social groups. When loyalty comes before competence in task-oriented organizations such as businesses or professional societies, there may be trouble in achieving the group's objectives.

The fundamental needs that are uniquely addressed in the family unit are those pertinent to survival and to development. The family unit must be committed to providing for physical security and development of its members: food and shelter, and intellectual, emotional, and spiritual resources. As Terkelsen (1980) points out, the condition by which a family unit is able to address the developmental needs of its members is through meeting the survival needs of the members. In other words, a family cannot adequately address the intellectual development of its members if there are not provisions for adequate food and shelter. This suggests that meaningful attention to developmental issues begins when the family is able to meet the survival needs of its members.

The way in which a family is organized corresponds to the requirements of fulfilling the combined and interacting needs of its members. In other words, there may be specific patterns of family organization, communication, and functioning that are determined by the requirements of the family members at that time in the history of the family. Family structure evolves in the service of satisfying basic needs. Haley (1973) defines family structure as the patterned sequence of behaviors that are the observable interactions between two or more members. A sequence of behavior is patterned when there is consistency in the behaviors and in their temporal relationship to each other. Thus, the family's structure is made up of a set of patterned sequences of behaviors that respond to the combined and interacting needs of family members.

Healthy Families

In this section we examine the mechanisms by which healthy families function. It is unfortunate that the study of family pathology has been done without a more thorough investigation of family health. One approach to the study of physical health was made by Pratt (1976), who studied the health practices of families in New Jersey in the late 1960's.

Her study population was a representative sample of families (N = 273) of a community of 150,000 people. Each family had a husband and wife in residence and at least one child aged 9 to 13. Her study methods involved separate interviews with each of three members during which fixed questions with structured response categories were asked. The interviews with husband and wife each lasted approximately 1½ hours, and the child's interview lasted about 45 minutes. Pratt's basic finding was that a combination of structural elements enables families to function effectively in support of their members' health. Pratt defines these as energized families:

Some families are highly energized in the sense that all members interact with each other regularly in a variety of contexts—tasks and leisure, or conversation and activity, both inside and outside the home. Energized families maintain varied and active contacts with other groups and organizations—the whole range of medical, educational, political, recreational, and business resources of the community that can be utilized to advance family members' interests. These families actively attempt to cope and master their lives, for example, by grasping the opportunity to join a sports team, seeking out information on how to improve their diet, and weighing the advantages and disadvantages of various schools or hospitals.

The energized family tends to be fluid in the internal organization. Role relationships are flexible; for example, house cleaning may be shared and everyone may take a turn at sick care. Power is shared, each person participating in decisions that affect him or her. Relationships among members tend to support personal growth and to be responsive and tolerant. Members have a high degree of autonomy within the family.

In Pratt's conceptualization, the term "energized" refers to the exchange that occurs between family members in interactions, the stimulation that comes from outside groups, and problem-solving efforts that result from the number of family interactions. She found that energized families promote their members' capacities to function fully as persons and develop the family members' capability for taking care of themselves. Specifically, five aspects of the concept of family structure were reviewed in her study: (1) interaction among family members, (2) family links to other social systems, (3) active coping efforts by family members, (4) freedom and responsiveness to individual members of the family, and (5) flexibility-rigidity of family role relationships. Several indices used to represent each of these areas are displayed in Table 2–4.

Pratt assessed health and behavior by measuring the level of (1) health and illness, (2) the quality of personal health practices, and (3) the appropriateness of professional medical services. The indices used to represent the health concepts are shown in Table 2–5.

Pratt found that an energized pattern of family structure worked more effectively than a nonenergized pattern in fostering members' efforts to protect and care for their health. She found that the form of family functioning that fosters members' health practices may be characterized as follows:

All members are actively engaged in varied, regular interaction with each other. The family has ties to the broader community through active participation of its members; a high degree of autonomy and a tendency to encourage individuality; the family is engaged in creative problem-

Table 2–4. ASPECTS OF FAMILY STRUCTURE AND THEIR INDICES*

Structural Elements	Index
Interaction Among Family Members	1. Husband-wife interaction (frequency and variety) 2. Mother-child interaction 3. Father-child interaction 4. Man's emphasis on father role versus job role 5. Combined family interaction
Links to Other Social Systems	1. Extent of community participation (membership and attendance in clubs and organizations) 2. Number of towns used (for recreation, health, church) 3. Extent of cultural participation (lessons, performance, attendance) 4. Variety of child's activities 5. Combined family extramural participation
Active Coping Efforts	1. Health training efforts by parents 2. Household health facilities 3. Child's health care equipment 4. Child's exercise equipment
Freedom and Responsiveness to Individual Members	1. Low aversive control of child by parents 2. Little obstructive conflict between husband and wife 3. Supportiveness of child by parents 4. Child's autonomy 5. Autonomy of members
Flexibility-Rigidity of Family Role Relationships	1. Conjugal division of tasks (segregation of flexibility in major task areas) 2. Conjugal division of task of child health care 3. Conjugal division of task of spouse health care 4. Conjugal power (shared or unilateral decision-making)

*Adapted from Pratt, L.: Family Structure and Effective Health Behavior: The Energized Family. Boston, Houghton Mifflin Company, 1976. Copyright © 1976 by Houghton Mifflin Company. Used with permission.

solving and active coping. It is the men's deep involvement in internal family functioning, rather than the more traditional deep involvement of women and children, that contributes most significantly to health practices of the whole family.

With regard to the use of professional medical services, Pratt's research showed that the energized pattern of family structure provides the family with advantages over the nonenergized form. With regard to use of medical services, the most important aspect of family structure was the extent of family links with organizations, activities, and resources of the broader community. The energized family achieved its advantages in the use of professional medical services by having women and children actively engaged in community activities and groups. With regard to health and illness, the dimensions of family structure that had the strongest relationship to good health were low levels of aversive control and obstructive conflict and high levels of autonomy, support, encouragement, and interaction among members. The level of health in the family as a whole was related significantly to good health of the individuals. A combined pattern of supportive family relationships and a supportive family health climate accounted for a third of the variance in the extent of health problems among family members. Since both personal health practices and the use of professional medical services are forms of task performance requiring competent and dedicated coping activity, those aspects of family structure that tended to facilitate effective coping behavior were critical ones for these two forms of health behavior, but were less crucial for health itself. On the other hand, family freedom and support that enable family members to develop and use their full physical faculties were crucial aspects of family structure for health but were of less significance for health care behavior.

Lewis and coworkers (1976, 1980) at the Timberlawn Psychiatric Research Foundation in Dallas spent 7 years performing an in-depth interactional study of families. They proposed measures of "family

Table 2–5. ASPECTS OF HEALTH AND HEALTH BEHAVIOR AND INDICES*

Health/Health Behavior	Index
Level of Health and Illness	1. Extent of health problems (self-rating) 2. Level of present health (self-rating)
Use of Professional Medical Services	1. Use of preventive medical services (tests, examinations, immunizations) 2. Use of specialized medical services 3. Use of medical services for illness 4. Total use of professional medical services (preventive, specialized, restorative)
Personal Health Practices	1. Personal health practices (sleep, exercise, elimination, dental, smoking, alcohol, and nutrition) 2. Sleep (regularity and effectiveness) 3. Exercise (regularity and amount) 4. Elimination (successful functioning) 5. Dental hygiene (regularity and appropriateness of timing) 6. Smoking (quantity) 7. Alcohol (frequency and quantity) 8. Nutrition (regularity and adequacy)

*Adapted from Pratt, L.: Family Structure and Effective Health Behavior. The Energized Family. Boston, Houghton Mifflin Company, 1976. Copyright © 1976 by Houghton Mifflin Company. Used with permission.

competence" and suggested that at any given level of competence there may be specific patterns of family organization, communication, and conflict that predispose the members either to health or to psychologic dysfunction. The model assumes that there are certain basic tasks facing all families and that families vary in their competence to promote the children's development into autonomous adults and to stabilize the parents' personalities.

Lewis's research with psychologically healthy families was done with a group of upper middle-class families in suburban Dallas, each of whom had an adolescent child. The basic hypothesis was that the competence of the family is determined by the extent to which a family accomplished the tasks of maturation and stabilization of parental personalities and the production of autonomous children. Family structure and other variables were measured by the use of 5-point rating scales. The families were videotaped performing a series of five tasks. Trained evaluators reviewed 10- to 50-minute segments of videotaped family testing. The five tasks were: (1) Main Problems—adapted from Strodbeck (1951), (2) Plan Something Together—following the method developed by Riskin and Faunce (1970), (3) Marital Relationship—the parents' relationship with each other, (4) Family Closeness—discussion stimulated by a board-type game depicting the closeness of family members to each other, and (5) Family Strengths—a discussion of what is strong about the family.

The scales used assess 14 interactional areas on continua in the areas of structure, mythology, negotiation, autonomy, and affect. These scales are shown in Table 2–6.

The study involved 33 families containing an adolescent. Significant correlations between the interactional scales and the independent ratings of global family competence were found in evaluating these families. Subsequently, a scheme of variable levels of competence among families was proposed: (1) optimal families, (2) competent, but pained, families, (3) dysfunctional families, and (4) severely dysfunctional families. The following description of families at each of these levels is derived from observations using the Family Evaluation Scales:

Optimal Families. These families vary widely in style. The parents have evolved a relationship in which power is shared. Each sees the other as competent, and leadership in the family is shared. The parents have achieved high levels of psychologic intimacy, and there seems to be an unusually affectionate bond, high levels of sexual satisfaction, and highly evolved individuality.

There are no competing coalitions. Relationships with their own parents or friends are warm and satisfying, but they do not have the intensity of the marital relationship. There is an absence of emotionally charged coalitions that compete with the marital relationship.

These families rely on negotiation as an approach to problems, and they are efficient in its use. They

Table 2–6. FAMILY EVALUATION SCALES*

Overt Power. Measures patterns of leadership, authority, control, and interpersonal influence. Scale ranges from chaos, to degrees of dominance, to a leadership pattern, to shared leadership

Parenteral Coalition. Assesses the nature of the parental relationship

Closeness. Based on the concept that one must be separate to be close. Scale ranges from families with distinct boundaries and high levels of closeness, to those families with distinct boundaries and great interpersonal distance, to those families with vague and indistinct boundaries among members

Mythology. Measures congruence between family members' image of how it functions and the rater's appraisal. Reflects the observable level of validation or the shared denial within the family

Goal-Directed Negotiation. Measures how a family solves problems. Efficient negotiation involves the exploration of each member's opinions and feelings and search for a consensus, or the ability to compromise

Clarity of Expression. Measures communications that range from those that are very clear to those in which hardly anything is ever clear

Responsibility. Measures the degree to which the family system encourages members to accept the responsibility for individual actions, feelings, and thoughts

Invasiveness. Measures invasions, or "mind reading"; that is, one person's telling (not asking) another family member what that other member thinks or feels

Permeability. Measures the degree to which the family acknowledges the messages from family members. Such acknowledgements may be verbal or nonverbal, and families range from those that are very open and responsive to such communications to those in which communications are ineffective.

Range of Feelings. Measures aspects of the breadth of a family's affective system, that is, the degree to which the family encourages or tolerates the expression of feelings of all kinds

Mood and Tone. Measures the quality of what can be called the family's basic mood. Unless a family is under stress, it has a characteristic affective tone. This may range from warm, affectionate, and optimistic to polite, hostile, depressed, pessimistic, or hopeless

Unresolvable Conflict. Measures the impact of conflict on the problem-solving capacity of the family, that is, the observer's judgment about whether or not—or to what degree—the family appears unable to resolve conflict

Empathy. Measures the degree to which the family responds to family members' feelings with understanding. ("I know what it's like to be angry, to be sad, or to be happy.") Rates the degree to which the family system is sensitive to communication of feelings

Global Health-Pathology. Measures the family's overall level of competence or, in earlier language, health or pathology

*Adapted from Lewis, J. M., Beavers, W. R., Gossett, J. T., and Phillips, V. A.: No Single Thread: Psychological Health in Family Systems. New York, Brunner/Mazel, 1976.

are clear in their communication, despite high levels of spontaneity. Family members take responsibility for thoughts and actions, and the system as a whole has high levels of permeability. Optimal families express a wide range of feelings. There are high levels of empathy and nothing to suggest unresolvable conflict. The basic family mood is warm, affectionate, humorous, and optimistic.

The studies of the individuals who make up these families strongly suggest high levels of psychological maturity. The fathers are successful in their vocations, indicate that major satisfactions come from being mentors to younger people, and work hard and for long hours. They have, however, some time left over for their families. The mothers in these families find major satisfactions within their marriages and families, but many have extensive extracurricular interests and many have jobs outside the home. The children are accomplishing age-appropriate developmental tasks in cognitive, social, and intrapsychic realms. As a group, they are friendly, open, active, often athletic, and in both interviews and testing are seen as healthy. Younger children, regardless of gender, are more apt to be less self-disciplined but more expressive and openly affectionate. This finding is in contrast with that in less well-functioning families in which these characteristics are more closely related to gender than to birth order.

Competent, but Pained, Families. These families are characterized by the failure of the parental marriage to meet the wife's emotional needs. The woman in the competent, but pained, family experiences herself as emotionally deprived as a result of her husband's affective unavailability. To observers, these women appear sour and angry. As a group they tend to be obese, have frequent physical complaints, see their physicians often, and are apt to be receiving anti-anxiety agents. Often, they form an intense coalition with a child, parent, or friend who appears to function as an ally.

The husbands appear much as described by these unhappy women. Although they are as successful vocationally as husbands in optimal families, they are more detached, less open with feelings, and tend to see interpersonal relationships as less rewarding than instrumental accomplishments. They recognize their wives' unhappiness, but do not accept responsibility for much, if any, of it. Rather, they focus on how difficult it is to be with their wives. Despite this flaw in their marriages, these couples have high levels of involvement with their children and are committed to the importance of the family. In most of these families, one parent tends to be moderately dominant, and there is no clear pattern of shared leadership.

These families often have good negotiating skills and are efficient problem-solvers if the problems are external and do not impinge too directly on the marital pain. They encourage autonomy by high levels of expressive clarity, reasonable permeability to each other, and general acceptance of responsibility for individual behavior.

In the family affective system, there is some restriction in the range of feelings expressed. It is as if the family gingerly skirts some intense affects—perhaps to avoid touching on the pain of the parents' relationship. Although warmth and caring (particularly of the children) are obvious, there is less humor and joy. Empathy is present to a moderate degree. Parental conflict is subdued, but its impact on the family is obvious. The children appear healthy. They achieve appropriate developmental milestones and function well socially and educationally. None of the children is symptomatic. In fact, raters cannot distinguish them from the children from optimal families.

Dysfunctional Families. These families demonstrate two patterns of family organization: dominant-submissive and conflicted. Both patterns are characterized by rigidity in the sense that each type of family responds to any stressful event with but one stereotyped reaction. In the dominant-submissive family, the reaction is overcontrol; in the chronically conflicted family, the reaction is increased conflict.

The *dominant-submissive pattern* is one in which one parent dominates and controls every aspect of family life. His or her dominance may be accepted fairly passively, or it may be circumvented by acting-out behavior—most often outside the home. Although both parents demonstrate clear individual ego boundaries, the parental coalitions are strained by the gross inequality in parental power. There is little closeness or intimacy, and family members are distant with each other.

Often these families see their situation as normal, and they explain any difficulty by blaming a person or condition outside the family or scapegoating one family member who is blamed for everything that is wrong with life in the family. These families do not negotiate. The dominant parent makes every decision, paying little, if any, attention to the opinions and feelings of others. The expression of feelings is often masked (particularly in the presence of the dominant parent). The pervasive family mood is either hostile or sad. There is little to suggest that empathy is valued or used. The conflict, however muted, is omnipresent.

The second type of dysfunctional family is the chronically *conflicted* one. In this pattern of family organization, the parents constantly war with each other. Each parent seeks to dominate the other; neither will share power, and neither is willing to accept a submissive role. They maintain the struggle by any technique, device, or manipulation. The children are drawn into the conflict, sometimes in stable coalitions with one parent but often in brief, transient coalitions, first with one parent, then the other. Although individual boundaries are clear, there is neither closeness nor trust.

Despite the endless conflict, many such families deny difficulty—often relying on both internal and external scapegoating. They cannot negotiate because each problem precipitates another round of conflict.

The parents, having never worked out an acceptable answer to the question "Who has the right to decide what?," cannot work together, and children do not learn to solve problems.

It is tempting to generalize and suggest that in dysfunctional families, the parents' attempts to solve the issue of their power or influence lead to relinquishing any hope of closeness or intimacy. As a consequence, regardless of whether or not family members experience a diagnosable psychiatric disorder, many are limited in their capacities for relating. Thus, they fail to achieve the emotional strength available to those more fortunate individuals who spend their lives in families sustained by closeness and intimacy.

Severely Dysfunctional Families. These families neither support maturation and growth for the parents nor encourage autonomy in the children. Families at this level of dysfunction reveal one of two patterns. The first is a pattern dominated by the influence of one parent and in which that parent's view of the world is idiosyncratic. The dominant parent is often psychotic or borderline. As a consequence, there is considerable clouding of meaning and high levels of invasiveness. Such families, however, show many of the characteristics of the dominant-submissive dysfunctional family. This pattern of severely dysfunctional families is much like the families described by Lidz and coworkers (1957) as "skewed."

The second pattern is the chaotic family. No member has enough influence to provide leadership. The family demonstrates amorphous or vague and indistinct boundaries between members, much as Bowen's (1966) "amorphous ego mass." As a consequence, it is often difficult for family members to know the meaning of family communication. When presented with problems, the family avoids, denies, and only rarely comes to closure and solves problems. Expressive clarity is low, invasions are common, and members are frequently unreceptive to each other. There is a cynical or hopeless family mood, feelings are avoided, and fusion of individual members obscures conflict.

These chaotic families often appear strange and bizarre to others. They do not relate to the surrounding world, and often the only real connections are with the parents' families of origin. Clumped together, they drift in a world of meaning all their own. Obtaining an individual sense of selfhood is terribly difficult in such a system.

Pratt's work was concerned with physical health in the family and Lewis's with psychological health, yet there are many similarities between Lewis's *optimal* families and Pratt's *energized* families. From these studies, certain fundamental characteristics of healthy families are noted: (1) shared power, (2) flexible organization, (3) adaptive problem-solving abilities capable of seeking different solutions, (4) active coping mechanisms, (5) high levels of interaction, (6) multiple and varied contacts within and without the family system, (7) support for personal growth, and (8) encouragement of a high degree of autonomy. As a group, these families tell us what is healthy and possible in family life under the best circumstances.

Theories of Family Functioning

In this section, the authors outline three major theoretical approaches explaining the functioning of families. The development of theory has been undertaken primarily from the study of families with an identified patient (mostly in the area of mental illness) rather than from the study of healthy families. Psychodynamic theories, systems theories, and developmental theories of family functioning are discussed.

Psychodynamic theories attempt to explain family functioning in terms of individual psychologic development of family members. A basic premise of psychodynamic theories is that human beings' perceptions of self and others are strongly influenced by the quality of their emotional dependency and family relationships.

Systems theories describe human or family systems in terms of General Systems Theory. A system is a set of different parts that meets the requirements of being directly or indirectly related through a network of reciprocal causal effects, and each part is related to one or more of the other parts in a reasonably stable way during any particular period of time. Family systems theory is principally concerned with relationships and information processing.

Developmental theories address family functioning as related to evolutionary passage of the family through a series of predictable stages. Each stage is characterized by a major emotional transition, and the development of the family is governed by the family's success in making the transition from stage to stage. We want to emphasize that among these different schools there is no right or wrong theory. The different theoretical explanations of family functioning simply represent different perspectives from which to view the family, and each has some validity.

PSYCHODYNAMIC THEORY

The *Bowen Family Theory* is a classic example of the psychodynamic theory of family development. Murray Bowen (1966) has been developing his theory of family functioning for more than 25 years. His early research (1960b) at the National Institute of Mental Health focused on mother-child relationships in families with a schizophrenic child. Bowen articulated a concept of the family as an emotional system and schizophrenia as a family problem in order to understand and work more effectively with these families. His theory postulates certain processes that apply in all families rather than only in those families in his clinical studies.

Bowen's initial conceptualization of the family as an "undifferentiated family ego mass" has been superseded by a theory that includes eight interlocking concepts that together describe the emotional systems within all families: (1) differentiation of self, (2) triangles, (3) nuclear family emotional system, (4) family projection process, (5) emotional cutoff, (6) multigenerational transmission process, (7) sibling position profile, and (8) emotional process in society.

Differentiation of Self. This term is used to describe degrees of human functioning—a kind of emotional maturity. When the self is differentiated, behavior is goal-directed with clear awareness of distinctions between thinking and feeling activities. When the self is less differentiated, behavior is largely emotionally responsive, or reactive, and shows less indication of being thought-directed.

Triangles. Bowen defines the triangle, or three-person system, as the basis for understanding the functioning of all emotional systems. This relationship unit can be found in any family. When sufficient stress occurs in a two-person relationship, the most uncomfortable participant in this system draws a third person into the twosome. This process creates a triangle. When triangles in a family are not readily apparent, they remain dormant and can be activated at any time, particularly in periods of stress.

Nuclear Family Emotional System. The level of intensity of the process is in inverse ratio to the level of differentiation of the spouses. Bowen postulates that mechanisms used by families to deal with the overload of anxiety that amasses in the nuclear system are marital conflict, dysfunction of a spouse, or projection of anxiety to a child. He further postulates that most families use a combination of the three mechanisms to dilute the intensity resulting from an overload of anxiety.

Family Projection Process. Parents stabilize their relationship with each other by viewing a child as their shared problem. This overinvestment of feeling in a child may impair the child's ability to function effectively. A family projection can be a scapegoating process in which one person is singled out as a family problem (i.e., the patient). The child so selected ends up with a lower level of differentiation than the parents.

Emotional Cutoff. Family members may distance themselves from each other and become emotionally divorced in an attempt to deal with fusion or lack of differentiation in their intimate relationships. Cutoffs are frequent between parent and grandparent generations in families. A direct consequence of cutoff is the burdening of the nuclear system with an equivalent overinvestment and expectation.

Multigenerational Transmission Process. This concept describes the pattern that develops over multiple generations as children emerge from the parental family with higher, equal, or lower basic levels of differentiation than the parents. Bowen believes that the successive repetition of impaired patterns of emotional behavior culminates in lowered levels of differentiation of self for certain members of the younger generations.

Sibling Position Profile. This concept is based on the work of Toman (1961), who described the expected behavior from different sibling positions. Seniority and sex distribution are strong influences on behavior.

Emotional Process in Society. The emotional forces in society may make differentiation difficult or impossible. When togetherness forces in society are strong, anxiety is high and problem behavior is pervasive. Extreme behavior sequences such as violence and destructive political leadership are much more likely to occur when the intensity of the emotional process is high than when less anxiety exists in society.

The Bowen Theory can be summarized as a general theory of emotional processes in human relationship systems with an emphasis on biologic variables. An important difference between the Bowen Theory and other family theories that are applied clinically is the goal of Bowen family therapists to operate as much as possible outside the emotional field of a patient or family. Whereas conventional family theorists and psychotherapists try to work within the emotional field, the Bowen Theory hypothesizes that therapists achieve effective clinical results to the extent that they remain outside the emotional field of the family in the clinical setting. Hall (1981) has reviewed the clinical application of the Bowen Theory.

SYSTEMS THEORY

Systems theory is a cybernetic-like interpretation of family functioning and processes. It is drawn from General Systems Theory (Buckley, 1967; von Bertalanffy, 1968). Systems theory of families is also based on concepts from communication theory, information theory, computer theory, and thermodynamics. Family systems theory attempts to relate the family to other social, environmental, and biologic systems in which it is included and with which it interacts. It is broad and offers a conceptual context in which all of the factors relative to a particular family or part of a family can be interrelated and analyzed. Our description of family systems theory is drawn from the works of Miller (1969), Beavers (1977), Kantor and Lehr (1975), and Fogarty (1976, 1978).

A system is a set of units with interrelationships. The state of each unit is constrained by the state of other units. The system is larger than the sum of all of the individual units. For instance, the characteristics of a family as a unit are different from the sum of its individual members. Knowing the attributes of all of the individuals in a family is not the same as understanding the family as an entity. The family unit has a history and has functions of its own, the specifics of which differ from those of its individual members. Marriages and families need to be thought of as interacting milieus in which transactions between component parts are continually taking place. Thus, the action of any one member affects the entire family. A ripple set up anywhere—internally or externally—that impinges on the family will reverberate throughout the family.

In his paper, "Evolution of a Systems Thinker in the Family," Fogarty (1978) gives a clinical example of the systems concept as applied to the family:

Rose is an 18-year-old girl who complains of feeling lonely and being easily rejected by people. She has occasional dates, but feels empty and does not know what she wants out of life. In treatment, she talks a little about herself but does nothing to narrow the distance between herself and her father. Her mother, toward whom she always felt close, remains her confidant. Where is the problem? In the lonely Rose, the overclose mother, or the distant father?

After some time, she meets a boy and they get rather serious. She is unsure of her relationship with him and brings him into the office with her. She tends to be possessive of him and yet yearns to be close to him. He genuinely cares about her but also wants to preserve his network with his friends. He wants some independence. Where is the problem? In Rose, or in Jim, her boyfriend, or between the two of them?

Rose and Jim get married. For the first year, things go on. He is busy with work, friends, and Rose. She feels somewhat lonely, complains mildly about his going out with the boys but is also busy with her job and housework. Where is the problem? In Rose, in Jim, in the marriage? Is there a problem?

After 2 years, Rose has a child—a son named Phil. She stops working because Phil demands much care. There is a burden to some extent, but she also finds out that she is not so lonely when she is with her son. She can talk and coo to him. Jim's responsibilities are now larger. He finds himself spending more time at work and feeling somewhat neglected—as if there were not enough time and caring about being delivered to him. At home, he is critical of Rose but she seems preoccupied with her son. Rose's mother visits often and sometimes Rose and her mother fight over the proper way to raise Phil. Jim finds himself sitting in the living room with his father-in-law. They watch TV together, get along "well," but have little to say to each other. Whenever there is an excuse, he manages to leave to do some work, to play golf, or to socialize outside the house. Phil, the son, is a little forward and naughty, but seems to be thriving. Where is the problem? In grandma or grandpa? In husband or wife? In son or in father's peer group? Is there a problem?

Time passes. Phil is now 16 years old. The phone rings in the office. It is Jim and Rose and they have a problem with their son. Ever since he turned 13, Phil has been keeping late hours, doing poorly in school and hanging out with the "wrong kids." Father and mother, who had been so distant, are now sincerely united in their efforts to change Phil. A common bond has been established between the parents—indeed a common problem. Phil is silent, wants to be left alone, and when he does speak is very critical of his parents. The parents reassure me that they have no major difficulties. Ask yourself again. Where is the problem? In whom? Between whom? In what generation? The grandparents, the parents, or the child? In the peer group, the school or the family?

With the threesome in the room, the heat is taken off of Phil by asking him what he thinks of his parents. The parents are interested because the speaker is Phil—the "problem." Phil warms up because the focus is on his parents. He talks about feeling close to mother in earlier years and then being cramped by her possessiveness in later years. He talks about not knowing his father at all. Mother agrees about father's distance and father agrees about mother's possessiveness. Phil's function improves but now the parents are bickering and fighting. They feel that things are getting worse. Where is the problem? In son, in mother, in father, or between whom? Are they all problems? Do we need three therapists, six, or ten? Who should go where about what?

Time passes again and changes begin to occur. "Therapy" is so directed that distant relationships are narrowed and overclose relationships are distanced. Father and son are put together by giving father control and responsibility over what son is doing or not doing. Mother is left out. In the past she always had someone, or did she? She had her mother, her husband, her son, and again her husband. There was always someone to be with and someone to be against. Where is grandfather? He is dead, but is he? Is he somewhere in the room? Now there is no one to be with.

Mother expresses her intense loneliness, feelings of being empty, and that no one cares about her. Not even herself. As father approaches son, he feels awkward, foolish, impatient, and intolerant. It is difficult but he must learn to control himself and to express his tenderness. Son tends to be self-righteous, to say, "See, I was right, you are the problem." He, too, has trouble with giving. If one has been the center, either of adoration or of a problem, it is difficult to give up that position. In time each one plunges inside himself but opens up to others. The despair, the tenderness, the bitterness, and anger, the impatience, the unsureness pop to the surface. As things improve, one scratches his head. Who had the problem? When did it start? How did it happen? What went into the creation of it? Where did it occur?

Kantor and Lehr (1975) describe four concepts of family systems that are based on Buckley's General Systems Theory. These workers suggest that family systems are organizationally complex, open, adaptive, information-processing systems.

Family Systems Are Organizationally Complex. This is a concept fundamental to systems orientation. Families evolve networks of interdependent causal relations that are governed primarily by mechanisms of feedback control. The component parts of a family system are neither fixed and unchanging nor chaotic, but the relations among component parts are reciprocally influencing.

Family Systems Are Open Systems. The use of the word open means that a system must have interchange with the environment as an essential factor underlying the system's viability, its reproductive ability or continuity, and its ability to change. Open systems exhibit a great deal of two-directional traffic with the larger environment. A system's openness suggests that what is inside and what is outside the system can be redefined depending on which part of the system is in focus.

Family Systems Are Adaptive. The heavy stress of the environment may dissolve a closed mechanical system. An open system's growth and development occur as a consequence of the interchange of the system with the environment. Strain and tension do not cause the open system to dissolve but instead cause it to respond productively (or destructively) to the stress.

Family Systems Are Information-Processing Systems. The information-processing capacity of the family system is responsible for the open system's ability to adapt its structure in response to environmental stimuli. Informational interchange is selectively mapped and coded in families. Kantor and Lehr believe that a fundamental principle of systems analysis is that as one moves from mechanical systems to more complex open systems, emphasis shifts away from the flow of energy required by parts of the system to the interrelationship of the parts to the transmission of information. The significance of this shift from energy flow to information flow is that a small amount of energy from one component of the system can set off a large amount of activity or behavior in other components. The researchers believe that the information processed by the family system is primarily distance-regulating.

Christie-Seely (1981) observed that teaching family systems concepts to physicians is difficult because such teaching entails a new way of thinking that is different from the familiar linear medical model that focuses on the individual patient. Figure 2–1 shows three causality schemes for illness.

In the linear medical model, A leads to illness X. The multiple causality scheme no longer views illness as solely caused by A, but caused also by B, C, and D as well. Christie-Seely suggests that a familiar model should be used to teach a new concept and points out that the endocrine system illustrates four concepts of General Systems Theory and is applicable to the family as a system: (1) the whole system must be understood in order to understand the diseased organ—the whole is greater than the sum of its parts; (2) homeostasis is essential to well-being, operates in sickness as well as in health, and is maintained by complex positive and negative feedback mechanisms; (3) the emphasis is not only on the organs themselves but on the hormones or interrelationships that are also means to assess the system's function (information-processing); and (4) changes may occur in many areas remote from original pathologic focus—all organs may be affected by a change in one organ. The endocrine system depends on constant interaction with other systems for survival and effective functioning.

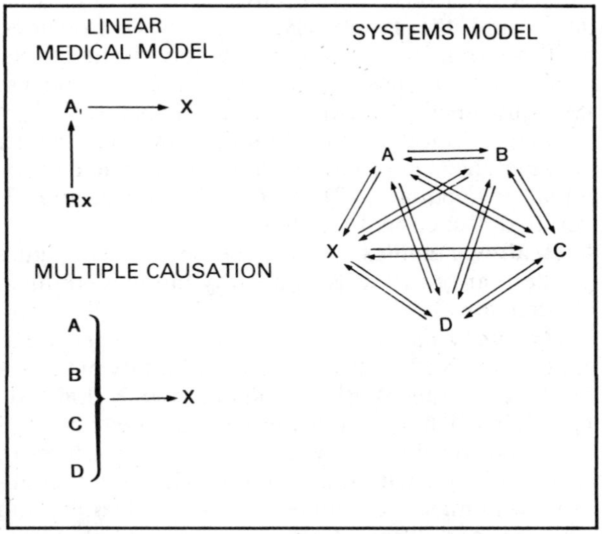

Figure 2–1. Three causality schemes. (From Christie-Seely, J.: Teaching the family system concept in family medicine. J. Fam. Pract., *13:*391, 1981, by permission of Appleton-Century-Crofts.)

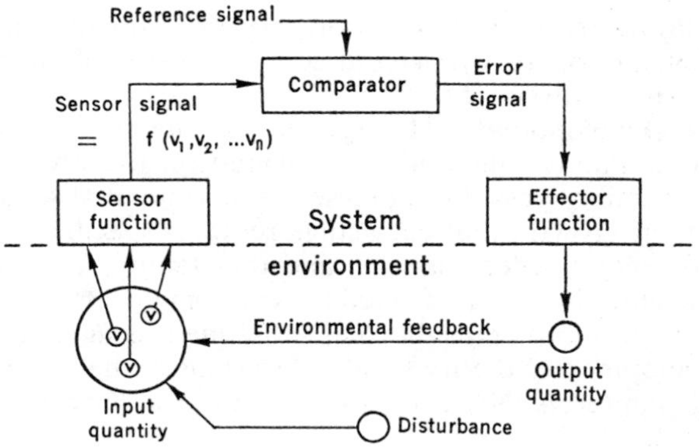

Figure 2–2. A basic control-system unit of behavioral organization. (From Powers, W. T.: Feedback: beyond behaviorism. Science, *179:*351, 1973. Copyright 1973 by the AAAS.)

The key systems concept to which the preceding four concepts point is the feedback loop. Figure 2–2 shows a basic control system unit of behavioral organization.

This diagram is a version of a prototypic feedback loop as proposed by Powers (1973). Feedback begins when a stimulus or disturbance occurs in the social field, which generates an input signal. A sensor function receives the input signal and transmits its own sensor signal to the system as a whole, alerting it to the quantity of the input signal. The sensor signal is then compared with a reference signal that states the desired level of regulation for the system. The system comparator makes an error signal based on the discrepancy between the sensor signal and reference signal. This error signal actuates the system's effector function to produce the system's response to the original stimulus. The outcome provides a feedback link to the input stimulus.

Kantor and Lehr (1975) have developed a distance-regulation model of the family based on systems concepts and particularly that of the feedback loop. They believe that the principal activity of family process is distance-regulation. The distance-regulation process can be understood by understanding the subsystems, the access and target dimensions, the mechanisms, the typal design, and the interactional player parts of family structure. Discussion of the many variables of this model is beyond our scope.

Family systems theory is a descriptive approach for explaining and predicting interpersonal and family processes. More and more research is being done today by case studies, laboratory experiments, and clinical trials to advance our comprehension of family systems analysis.

Developmental Theory. The developmental theory of family function is predicated on the premise that families pass through a series of sequential stages in their growth, that each stage requires specific first- and second-order changes, and that failure to make a specific change is reflected in symptom development or family problems at the subsequent stage. The developmental theory is fully discussed in the following chapter as the basis of the Family Life Cycle.

Clinical Models for the Study of Families

As we have seen, research on families and the development of theories about family functioning have been evolving with a number of different approaches. Because of the expanding rate at which theories about families have been developing, a number of workers have found it helpful to develop specific models that depict the functioning of families in a variety of settings. The value of such models lies in their presenting conceptual and often schematic diagrams that provide simple structures analogous to other biologic or behavioral systems. In addition, models provide a common language and a means of organizing information to show relationships. Models may suggest mechanisms for directing therapeutic intervention into family systems. In this section, we review four models that have been used to aid in the clinical understanding of family function. Two of these models, the *Systems Model of Family* and the *Circumplex Model,* are based principally on family systems theory, whereas the *Cycle of Family Function* is based on the developmental theory of families. The *Family Epidemiologic Model* is based on epidemiologic principles.

THE SYSTEMS MODEL OF FAMILY

This model, developed by Beavers (1981), integrates family systems research in healthy and disturbed families at Timberlawn and Beaver's clinical practice covering a period of nearly 20 years. The model provides a tool for a cross-sectional, process-oriented assessment of family competence, task performance, and operating style. The model is shown in Figure 2–3.

As can be seen, there are two dimensions of family structure and function depicted in this model: adaptability and style.

Adaptability is depicted on the horizontal axis and reflects structure, flexibility, and types of interaction within the family unit. Specifically, the model covers five areas of family behavior: (1) structure, (2) mythology, (3) goal-directed negotiation, (4) system encouragement of individual autonomy, and (5) expression of feeling. The structure of the family is reflected in three variables: (1) the distribution of overt power, or how power is used and shared, (2) the quality of the parental coalition, and (3) the degree of family closeness, or clarity of individual boundaries and the amount of sharing and intimacy. Mythology is defined as the shared view of themselves held by family members as compared with what an outsider sees. Goal-directed negotiation refers to the efficiency of the family in making decisions and acting on them and the encouragement of participation by all family members. System encouragement of individual autonomy is a broad aspect of family functioning covering the clarity of communication, the assumption of personal responsibility, the receptiveness of the members to each other, and the level of evasiveness or mind-reading statements (see Table 2–6). Affect is evaluated by observing expressiveness, mood and feeling tone, unresolvable conflict, and empathy. Beavers and his colleagues at Timberlawn developed *Family Evaluation Scales* that were used to measure specific aspects of family interaction and together to assess the level of family competence.

The vertical axis relates to the family's interactional *style* and is derived from Stierlin (1972). The stylistic dimension divides families into three groups—centripetal, mixed, and centrifugal—on the basis of their emotional investment.

The *centripetal* family is inner-oriented; members find it difficult to leave or to develop emotional investment outside of family. The family itself is the most trustworthy source of satisfaction, and members must put up a front to the outside world to hide family trouble or pain.

In contrast, the *centrifugal* family is outer-oriented; independence is encouraged, and satisfaction is sought from the external environment rather than from within the family. Between these extremes, which are seen most easily in severely dysfunctional families, are families designated as *mixed,* who use both centrifugal and centripetal mechanisms.

Beavers' model depicts families in three ranges of competence: (1) healthy families, which may be optimal or adequate, (2) midrange families, and (3) severely dysfunctional families.

Healthy Families. As can be seen from Figure 2–3, there are two levels of healthy families, optimal and adequate.

Optimal Families. These families are the paradigm of effective family functioning. Family members are aware of the multiple influences they have on each other's behavior and the circular movement of causes and results. They try many approaches to solving problems within the family. The family members seek intimacy, parents share power flexibly, and boundaries and differentiation between members are clear and respected.

Adequate Families. These families are more control-oriented. The parents strive more for overt power

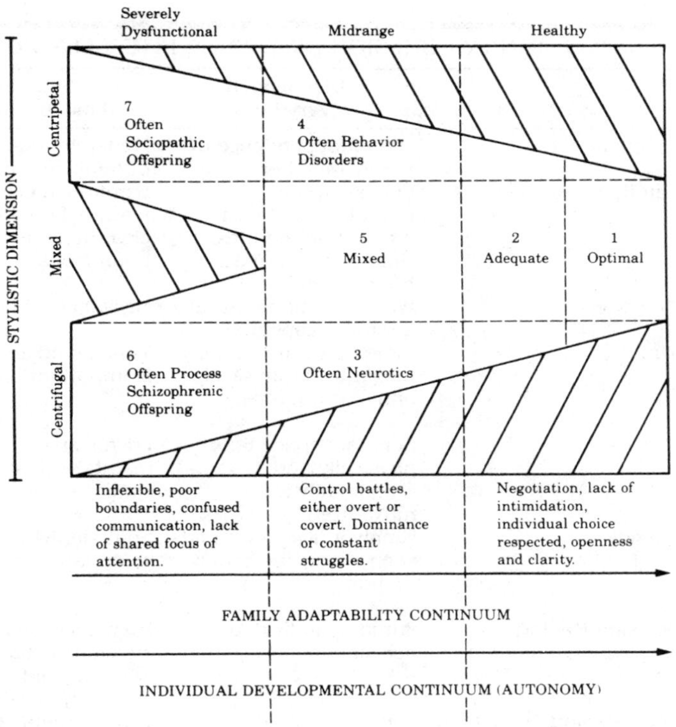

Figure 2–3. A systems model of family structure and function. (From Beavers, W. R.: A systems model of the family for family therapists. J. Mar. Fam. Ther., 7:299, 1981.)

and find themselves correspondingly less able to feel intimate and trusting. Sex-role stereotyping is more apparent: the males are unemotive and the females are more emotive. Children in these families appear to be as capable as those from optimal families, probably the result of the parents' strong belief in the importance of parenting and family life.

Midrange Families. The first group of dysfunctional families are termed midrange. Their members are sane but limited and susceptible to emotional illness. Midrange families are oriented to control and characterized by overt struggles for power. They assume that people are basically antisocial and depraved and must be controlled.

Midrange Centripetal Families. These families use direct control and expect to be successful in doing so. Hostility is repressed, rules and authority are emphasized, and spontaneity is diminished. A family member who is an identified patient is likely to be considered neurotic.

Midrange Centrifugal Families. These families use indirect control and manipulation or intimidation, but seldom expect to succeed. They are openly hostile, constantly blame and attack others, and seldom express warmth. Parents spend little time at home. Children play in neighborhood streets much earlier than the norm. Members battle for control, ending with difficulty and contempt for authority inside and outside the home. A family member who becomes an identified patient is likely to have a behavior disorder.

Midrange Mixed Families. Some midrange families have alternating and conflicting centripetal and centrifugal behavior. In this group, the parental coalition varies in one interview from dominant-submissive to bickerings and blaming the children. The children alternate between accepting and resisting parental control.

Severely Dysfunctional Families. At the low end of the continuum of family competence are those whose most serious deficiencies are in the area of coherence. They lack a shared focus of attention and sense of engagement. Members have difficulty choosing goals and resolving ambivalence. No one is clearly in charge, so power is exercised covertly and indirectly. Family interaction is chaotic. The members are pathetically limited in ability to negotiate; boundaries between members are poor, and individuals frequently speak for the feelings and motives of others.

Severely Disabled Centripetal Families. These families have nearly impermeable boundaries to the outside world. The members are seen as strange or queer. Family rules are forever blurred and static. Ambivalence is denied. Children are seriously handicapped in their struggle to grow up and to function apart from the family. A schizophrenic break is one way of expressing and trying to solve this dilemma.

Severely Dysfunctional Centrifugal Families. These families have a tenuous perimeter, sometimes with uncertainty about who constitutes the family. Family interaction is characterized by open hostility and contempt. Ambivalence is denied, with negative feelings expected. Warm, tender feelings are expressed indirectly or by behavior. Children from these families are as handicapped in developmental evolu-

Table 2–7. FAMILY COHESION DIMENSION: INTERRELATED CONCEPTS*

	Disengaged (Very Low)	Separated (Low to Moderate)	Connected (Moderate to High)	Enmeshed (Very High)
Independence	High independence of family members	Moderate independence of family members	Moderate depedence of family members	High dependence of family members
Family Boundaries	Open external boundaries, closed internal boundaries, rigid generational boundaries	Semi-open external and internal boundaries, clear generational boundaries	Semi-open external boundaries, open internal boundaries, clear generational boundaries	Closed external boundaries, blurred internal boundaries, blurred generational boundaries
Coalitions	Weak coalitions, usually a family scapegoat	Marital coalition clear	Marital coalition strong	Parent-child coalitions
Time	Time apart from family maximized (physically and/or emotionally)	Time alone and together is important	Time together is important, time alone permitted for approved reasons	Time together maximized, little time alone permitted
Space	Separate space both physically and emotionally is maximized	Private space maintained, some family space	Family space maximized, private space minimized	Little or no private space at home
Friends	Mainly individual friends seen alone, few family friends	Some individual friends, some family friends	Some individual friends, scheduled activities with couple and family friends	Limited individual friends, mainly couple or family friends seen together
Decision-Making	Primarily individual decisions	Most decisions are individually based, able to make joint decisions on family issues	Individual decisions are shared, most decisions made with family in mind	All decisions, both personal and relationship, must be made by family
Interests and Recreation	Primarily individual activities done without family, family not involved	Some spontaneous family activities, individual activities supported	Some scheduled family activities, family involved in individual interests	Most or all activities and interests must be shared with family

*From Olson, D. H., Sprenkle, D. H., and Russell, C. S.: Circumplex model of marital and family systems: I. Cohesion and adaptability dimensions, family types, and clinical applications. Fam. Process, *18*:3, 1979.

tion as those from the severely dysfunctional centripetal families. The more usual result is an antisocial personality resulting from deficiencies in nurturing, warmth, and tenderness. Child abuse, sexual deviance, and drug abuse are common in these families.

A central feature of the Beavers Family Systems Model is the concept that movement from the incoherent, unsatisfying encounters toward shared transactions is typical of progress toward competence and health within family systems. Regression in a system reverses this sequence. The overall goal of analysis and intervention in family functioning is to help the family move from a dysfunctional to a more functional level.

Family assessment can be performed quickly and efficiently by giving the family a task such as discussing "What would you like to change about your family?" and then leaving them alone for 15 minutes. A videotape recording is made and subsequently analyzed according to the variables used in the two dimensions of this model. Using this approach, it is possible to conceptualize the family's style and level of adaptability and to outline the movement to a more competent and healthy system.

CIRCUMPLEX MODEL

The Circumplex Model is a two-dimensional model developed by Olson and coworkers (1979) to address the psychosocial interior and internal milieu of the family. The authors of this Circumplex Model believe that the clustering of numerous concepts from family therapy and other social science fields reveals that adaptability and cohesion are two significant dimensions of family behavior. The model proposes that a balanced level of cohesion and adaptability is most functional to marital and family development. In the cohesion dimension, it postulates the need for a balance between too much closeness, which leads to enmeshed systems, and too little closeness, which leads to disengaged systems. There also needs to be a balance in the adaptability dimension between too much change, which leads to chaotic systems, and too little change, which leads to rigid systems. The model was developed as a tool for clinical diagnosis and for the planning of treatment goals in working with families.

The cohesion dimension describes two fundamental aspects of family functioning: (1) the emotional bonding between family members and (2) the degree of individual autonomy of family members. In developing the cohesion dimension, the theoretical concepts of Bowen (1960a), Hess and Handel (1959), Kantor and Lehr (1975), Lidz and coworkers (1957), Minuchin (1974), Reiss (1971), Stierlin (1972), Vogel and Bell (1960), and Wynne and coworkers (1958) were related with reference to extremely low cohesion, balanced cohesion, or extremely high cohesion.

Extremely high family cohesion (enmeshment or overidentification with the family) results in extreme amounts of bonding and limited individual autonomy. An extremely low amount of cohesion (disengagement) is characterized by a low degree of bonding and a high degree of autonomy from the family. A balanced degree of cohesion is the most conducive to effective family functioning and to optimal individual development. A number of specific variables are used to assess the degree of family cohesion, including emotional bonding, independence, boundaries, coalitions, time, space, friends, decision-making, interests, and recreation. These are shown in Table 2–7.

The adaptability dimension deals with the ability of the marital/family system to change its power structure, role relationships, relationship rules, and responses to cope with situational or developmental stresses. In other words, an adaptive system requires balancing between growth *(morphogenesis)* and stability *(morphostasis)*. Adaptability implies that families are capable of change and of reordering their structure. For instance, the family development approach postulates continuing shifts in family composition and the consequent need for reidentification of rules and roles in families. A family locked into a rigid morphostatic pattern is in trouble. A family must be able to adapt to normal crises of transition (parenthood, placement of children in school, adolescence, launching of children, and adjustment to retirement) in order to negotiate successfully the transitions of the family life cycle. Specific variables involved in overall adaptability include family power structure, negotiation styles, role relationships, relation rules, and feedback. Table 2–8 shows how these variables are rated under four levels of adaptability.

The authors of the Circumplex Model list eight objectives for the development of the model:

1. To identify and describe the central dimensions of family cohesion and family adaptability in our culture.
2. To demonstrate the utility of these dimensions in conceptually reducing the diversity of family process concepts.
3. To indicate how relationships can deal with the dynamic balance between constancy and change (adaptability dimension) and between enmeshment and disengagement (cohesion dimension).
4. To demonstrate how these dimensions can provide a more concrete and useful understanding of the application of General Systems Theory to the family.
5. To describe more directly and clearly group properties of families rather than only dyadic properties or individual characteristics.
6. To provide a way of integrating concepts of the individual as a system with concepts of the marital and family systems.
7. To create a dynamic model that can describe how marital and family systems can adapt to situational stresses (crises) and developmental changes that occur over the family life cycle.
8. To provide a framework that can be applied to clinical intervention and education programs for couples and families.

Figure 2–4 identifies the 16 family types in the Circumplex Model. The four types in the central area of the model reflect balanced levels of both adaptability and cohesion and are seen as most functional to the individual and family development. The four extreme types reflect very high or very low levels of adaptability and cohesion and are seen as most dysfunctional to individual and family development. Based on the design of the model and the scaling of its dimensions, the four types of families in the center circle—flexible separateness, flexible connectedness, structured connectedness, and structured separate-

Table 2–8. FAMILY ADAPTABILITY DIMENSIONS: INTERRELATED CONCEPTS*

	Chaotic (Very High)	Flexible	Structure	Rigid (Very Low)
Assertiveness	Passive and aggressive styles	Generally assertive	Generally assertive	Passive or aggressive styles
Control	No leadership	Egalitarian with fluid changes	Democratic with stable leader	Authoritarian leadership
Discipline	Laissez-faire, very lenient	Democratic, unpredictable consequences	Democratic, predictable consequences	Autocratic, overly strict
Negotiation	Endless negotiation, poor problem-solving	Good negotiation, good problem-solving	Structured negotiations, good problem-solving	Limited negotiations, poor problem-solving
Roles	Dramatic role shifts	Role-making and sharing, fluid change of roles	Some role-sharing	Role rigidity, stereotyped roles
Rules	Dramatic rule shifts, many implicit rules, few explicit rules, arbitrarily enforced rules	Some rule changes, more implicit rules, rules often enforced	Few rule changes, more explicit than implicit rules, rules usually enforced	Rigid rules, many explicit rules, few implicit rules, strictly enforced rules
System Feedback	Primarily positive loops, few negative loops	More positive than negative loops	More negative than positive loops	Primarily negative loops, few positive loops

*Adapted from Olson, D. H., Sprenkle, D. H., and Russell, C. S.: Circumplex model of marital and family systems: I. Cohesion and adaptability dimensions, family types, and clinical applications. Fam. Process, *18*:22, 1979.

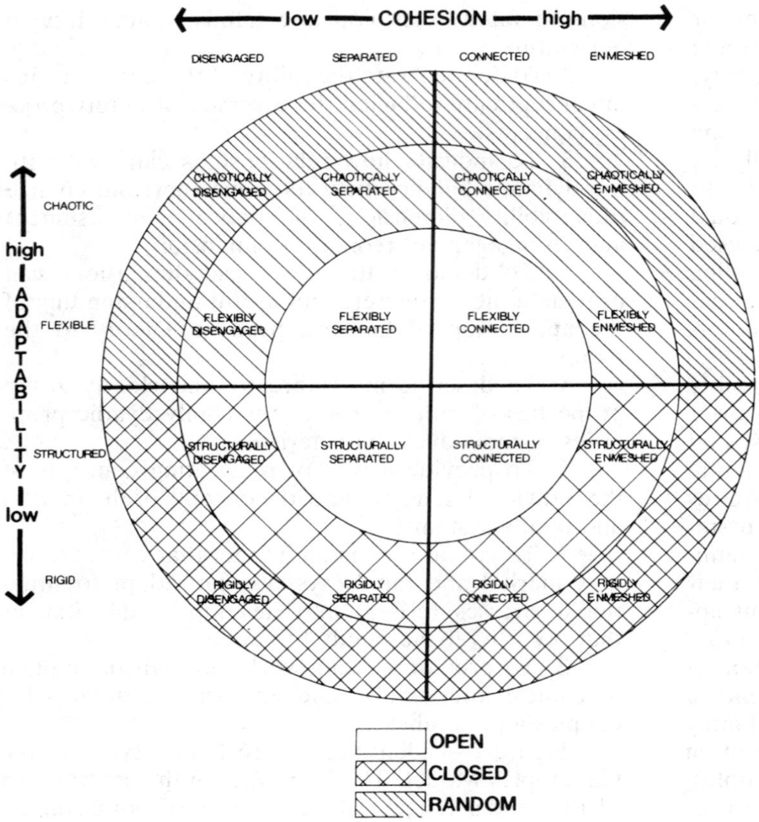

Figure 2–4. Sixteen possible types of marital and family systems derived from the circumplex model. (From Olson, D. H., Sprenkle, D. H., and Russell, C. S.: Circumplex model of marital and family systems: I. Cohesion and adaptability dimensions, family types, and clinical applications. Fam. Process, *18:3*, 1979.)

ness—represent more functional marital and family systems. An open system is distinguished by the ability of the individuals to experience and balance extremes of being independent from and connected to their families.

The four extreme types in the outer circle—chaotically disengaged, chaotically enmeshed, rigidly enmeshed, and rigidly disengaged—are the least functional to individual and family development. Families in these categories are described by the extremes of family cohesion and adaptability. The creators of the Circumplex Model believe that these behaviors are continuous with functional behavior but represent exaggerated versions of functional behavior. For instance, a chaotically disengaged family is an exaggerated form of the flexibly separated type of family.

One of the major goals in developing the Circumplex Model was to provide a framework to be used by clinicians to make more systematic diagnoses and establish more specific intervention strategies. It is possible, using the Circumplex Model, to determine clinically the degree of cohesion of a marital or family unit. It is also possible operationally to define and assess adaptability with regard to the variables of assertiveness and control, discipline, negotiation, role relationships, rules, and system feedback. Family Adaptability and Cohesion Evolution Scales (FACES) (Olson et al., 1978) is a self-administered questionnaire for the evaluation of family adaptability and cohesiveness. Once an assessment has been made of the cohesion and adaptability of a couple or family, it is possible to place the couple into one of the 16 cells of the model and then to formulate intervention or treatment goals.

THE FAMILY EPIDEMIOLOGIC MODEL

The family epidemiologic model was developed to aid in practice and research in family medicine by Medalie and his colleagues (1981). Medalie's model is based on epidemiology being defined as a study of distribution, determinants, and control of factors and processes involved in a continuum of health and disease in groups of people. Epidemiology, according to Medalie, uses a scientific method and accumulates a body of knowledge.

A Venn-type diagram of the family epidemiologic model (Fig. 2–5) is made up of three interacting and overlapping circles designating the three elements of the model: the host, the agents, and the environment. The host for this model is the family system. When the three circles of the Venn diagram overlap, there are three areas common to two of the larger circles and one area common to all three. For example, when the environment and the family system interact, the resistance of the family system can be decreased or increased. As shown in the diagram, the area common to the family and the environment is

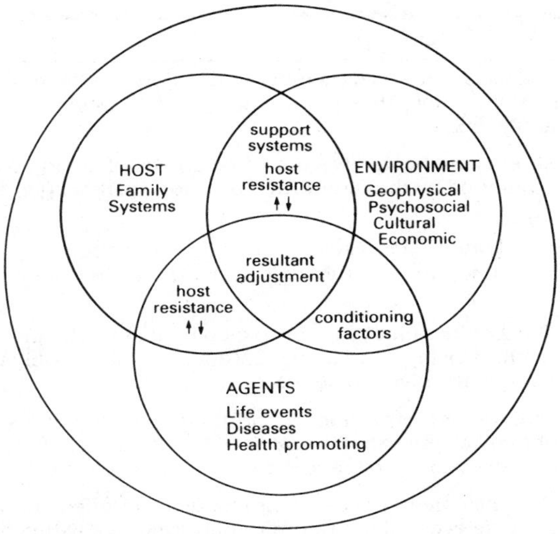

Figure 2–5. Family epidemiologic model. (From Medalie, J. H., Kitson, G. C., and Zyzanski, S. J.: A family epidemiologic model: A practice and research concept for family medicine. J. Fam. Pract. *12*:79, 1981, by permission of Appleton-Century-Crofts.)

designated as support systems. This implies that the support can be part of the family system only, it can be supplied by environmental agencies alone, or it is a combination of activities within as well as outside the family. The interacting environmental and agent variables result in a series of conditioning factors. According to Medalie's concepts, agents or stressors such as life events or diseases can cause the increase or decrease in host resistance, depending on the circumstances. The middle area, which is the result of the overlapping of all three circles, is termed resultant adjustment and implies that adjustment of a family at all times is a result of multiple interacting factors. The position and size of the large circles in the figure imply that family environment and agent are of equal importance. Although this is sometimes the case, another situation may be that the family system is of major importance with factors from the environment and agent acting as background influences. Further description of the environment and the agents is useful in understanding the family epidemiologic model.

Environment. The environment is made up of a number of subsystems that interact with each other to form the environmental system. These subsystems can be classified as follows:

1. *Economic.* Economic status is determined by ability to purchase goods and services and is vital for each family. When family income does not meet the most basic needs, the effect pervades all other aspects of living and is a severe and debilitating handicap.

2. *Social.* Social environment includes all associations, for instance, political, racial, occupational, educational, recreational, and medical care systems as well as informal social contacts.

3. *Cultural.* Cultural environment includes values and behavior of people of similar beliefs. Cultural environment can be enormously important in determining the health behavior of families or groups of people.

4. *Geophysical.* Geophysical subsystems include geologic, geographic, climatic, seasonal, and soil conditions, as well as composition of air, water, and soil. All of these variables have influences on health.

5. *Biologic.* Biologic environment is the universe of living things that surround human beings.

Agents. The agent is one or more elements, substances, forces, or processes that act as stressors of the human system that, if not countered, can lead to disequilibrium, maladjustment, or other symptoms or disease syndromes. Agents or stressors can be grouped into biologic and psychosocial categories. Biologic agents include microbiologic, chemical, physical, mechanical (floods and earthquakes), and nutritional stressors. Psychosocial stressors include life events, transitions, unexpected crises, war, revolution, terrorism, and riots. The effect of the agent system obviously depends on the resistance of the host and the interaction between other systems. Medalie regards each of the three large circles as a type of system with units and subunits being interdependent and interacting. Each of these systems has within it many variables and parameters so that the family epidemiologic model can be seen as an interactive, multisystem, multivariant model. Medalie believes that this model offers a framework for thinking, organizing data, and planning research of families and their relationships to illness and health.

THE CYCLE OF FAMILY FUNCTION

Smilkstein (1980) conceptualized a model that includes components that have been identified as basic

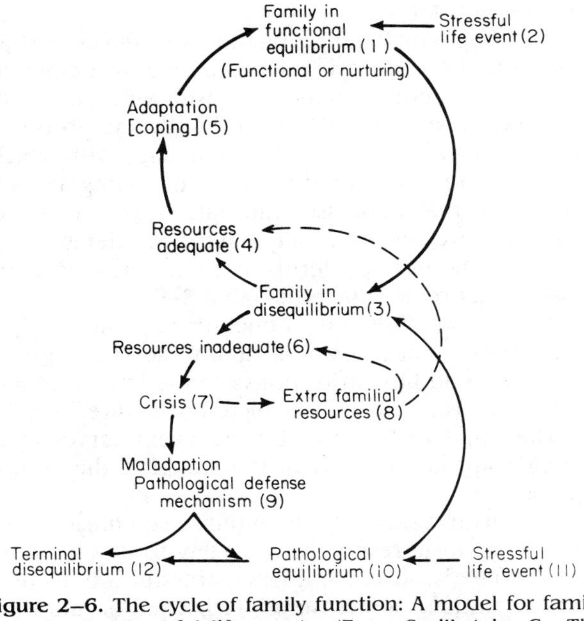

Figure 2–6. The cycle of family function: A model for family response to stressful life events. (From Smilkstein, G.: The cycle of family function: A conceptual model for family medicine. J. Fam. Pract. *11*:223, 1980, by permission of Appleton-Century-Crofts.)

Table 2–9. DEFINITION OF TERMS USED IN THE CYCLE OF FAMILY FUNCTION*

Equilibrium	A state of family homeostasis in which member interaction results in emotional and physical nurturing, thus promoting growth of family members and the family unit
Stressful Life Event	A life experience that requires the family's use of resources of coping or adapting not usually required by the family members for the management of daily activities
Crisis	A state of family disequilibrium that results from failure to identify resources adequate to allow family members to cope with a stressful life event
Disequilibrum	A state of impaired functioning, nurturing, or role-complementarity in which a family, for the time being, can neither escape nor solve problems with their customary problem-solving resoures
Resources	Those assets that serve the process of family nurturing and fall in the general categories of familial and extrafamilial social, cultural, religious, economic, educational, environmental, and medical support systems
Adaptation	The process by which family members use their resources to effect a resolution of a stressful life event and a return to nurturing family function or equilibrium
Maladaptation	The process by which a family in crisis or disequilibrium chooses abnormal defense mechanisms to achieve some measure of equilibrium in family function
Pathologic Equilibrium	A state of impaired interaction or nurturing within a family that follows the use of abnormal defense mechanisms to escape from anxiety of unresolved family crisis. Families in pathologic equilibrium may have members who are so isolated from their fellow members that they cannot receive help, or individuals who are so adhesive to their family members that independent function is paralyzed

*From Smilkstein, G.: The cycle of family function: A conceptual model for family medicine. J. Fam. Pract., *11*:226, 1980.

to the recognition and understanding of the family in trouble. He believes that the knowledge of family function as represented by the model will help the family physician assess and manage problems presented by patients who are victims of stress related to family problems.

The Cycle of Family Function was developed as a conceptual framework for presenting an empirical view of the responses that may result when a family experiences a stressful life event. Smilkstein proposes that the model offers a common language with which to discuss and understand family functioning as well as a format that addresses the data base needed to assess and care for the family having problems.

The definition of terms used in the Cycle of Family Function is shown in Table 2–9.

The Cycle of Family Function is a model that reflects the manner in which family members' interactions ebb and flow in response to the impact of life events. This is graphically depicted in Figure 2–6.

The impact of a stressful life event serves as a starting point in the study of the model of the family function.

A nurturing family maintains equilibrium by using its intrinsic resources on a day-to-day basis to meet the needs of its members. Stressful life events, however, induce a measure of disequilibrium that requires a special coping response on the part of family members. At these times, family resources are put to the test. The major extra-family resources are found in the social, cultural, religious, economic, educational, environmental, and technological (e.g., medical) phases of family life.

When the family lacks adequate resources, the consequences of a stressful life event may be a crisis. In order to relieve the stress and pain of the feelings that result from a family crisis, family members, unable to find resources with which to cope appropriately, adopt some form of ego defense such as avoidance, conversion, denial, projection, somatization, or transference (Freud, 1946).

Pathologic equilibrium exists in families that have accumulated a series of unresolved crises and have incorporated into their family system pathologic defense mechanisms that allow some measure of family nurturing to continue even though normal function is markedly impaired. Smilkstein believes that families in pathologic equilibrium not only are marginal in their nurturing, but are also symptomatic. The physician may recognize members from families in pathologic equilibrium since they will report symptoms such as depression, fighting, scapegoating, criticizing, and arguing. For some families, the cycle of functioning is ever downward. Failure to resolve crises results in discomfort of living with pathologic defense mechanisms, poor nurturing environment, and pathologic equilibrium, leading families to terminal disequilibrium. In this state, nurturing functions are not discernible, and dissolution of the family frequently occurs.

Summary. We have presented four models for the clinical study of families. Each has utility in conceptualizing issues in family functioning in differing circumstances. Both the Beavers Family Systems Model and the Circumplex Model describe overall family status as a resultant of dimensions of adaptability and cohesion or style. These models have a number of similarities in structure but are quite different in interpretation and use in that within the Circumplex Model, chaos and rigidity are at opposite ends of the spectrum and are separated by the normal zone of flexibility and structure, whereas in the Family Systems Model, chaos and rigidity are on a scaled continuum. These models have similarities on the cohesion or stylistic dimension in that disengagement and centrifugality are similar terms, and enmeshment and centripetality are similar. Therefore, a fundamental difference between these models is related to a difference in the construction of the adaptability scale. The scale is continuous in the Family Systems Model and discontinuous in the Circumplex Model.

The Family Epidemiologic Model is oriented more toward understanding the contextual issues about family, such as the nature of stressors, the effects of environment, and the relationship of these subsystems to the family system. The Cycle of Family Function is a model that aids in the understanding of the family's reaction to stress such as life cycle transitions. This model demonstrates how the family outcomes are influenced by family resources, coping behavior, extrafamilial resources, and defense mechanisms.

References

Anthony, J. E.: The impact of mental and physical illness on family life. Am. J. Psychiatry, *127:*138, 1970.

Beavers, W. R.: Systems theory, family systems and the self. *In* Beavers, W. R.: Psychotherapy and Growth: A Family Systems Perspective. New York, Brunner/Mazel, 1977. *A noted clinician and researcher presents a unifying conceptual framework for the kind of significant therapeutic interaction that promotes healthy growth. The author combines systems concepts with analysis of behavior patterns seen in competent and incompetent families in order to describe a total growth-oriented approach to psychotherapy that draws on varied clinical techniques. The basis of the therapeutic approach presented is knowledge of family systems variables that help determine why some people develop into sane, well-functioning adults whereas others exhibit madness.*

Beavers, W. R.: A systems model of the family for family therapists. J. Marital Fam. Ther., *7:*299, 1981.

Beloff, J. S., Snobe, P. S., and Weinerman, E. R.: Yale studies in family health care. Part 2. Organization of a comprehensive family health care program. J. A. M. A., *204:*355, 1969.

Berman, E. M.: Adult developmental stages and marital interaction. Audio-Digest (Psychiatry), *7:*1, 1978.

Bertalanffy, L. von: General Systems Theory. New York, George Braziller, 1968.

Blotcky, A. D.: Family functioning and physical health: an exploratory study with practical implications. Family Therapy, *8:*197, 1981.

Bowen, M.: The family as the unit of study and treatment. Am. J. Orthopsychiatry, *31:*40, 1960a.

Bowen, M.: A family concept of schizophrenia. *In* Jackson, D. (Ed.): The Etiology of Schizophrenia. New York, Basic Books, Inc., Publishers, 1960b, p. 346.

Bowen, M.: Use of family theory in clinical practice. Compr. Psychiatry, *7:*345, 1966.

Buckley, W.: Sociology and Modern Systems Theory. Englewood Cliffs, N. J., Prentice-Hill, Inc., 1967.

Christie-Seely, J.: Teaching the family system concept in family medicine. J. Fam. Pract., *13:*391, 1981.

Comen, D. L., and Sarbara, J. A.: Family-centered health care: a viable reality? Med. Care, *10:*164, 1972.

Crosthwait, W. L., and Fischer, E. G.: The Last Stitch. New York, J. B. Lippincott Co., 1956. *The poignant chronicle of the development of general practice in Texas around the turn of the century. This work is enriched with anecdotes and the philosophy of life of the early frontier physician.*

Fogarty, T. F.: Systems concepts and the dimensions of self. *In* Guerin, P. J. (Ed.): Family Therapy: Theory and Practice. New York, Gardner Press, 1976.

Fogarty, T. F.: Evolution of a Systems Thinker in the Family. New York, The Center for Family Learning, 1978.

Freud, A.: The Ego and the Mechanisms of Defense. New York, International Universities Press, Inc., 1946.

Goldstein, H. S., Snope, F. C., and McGreeham, D. M.: Family emotional health: a survey of family practice patients. J. Fam. Pract., *10:*85, 1981.

Gordon, M.: The American Family. New York, Random House, 1978. *A text in family sociology that concentrates on how our present concepts of family sociology relate to the history of the family in society. Applies the newer techniques of social sciences to the study of historical phenomena about the American family.*

Haley, J.: Uncommon Therapy. New York, W. W. Norton and Co., Inc., 1973. *A case book of an innovative psychiatrist's work in short-term therapy that is based on the psychiatric techniques of Milton Erickson. This book provides a comprehensive look at Dr. Erickson's theories, strategic therapy, and practice through a series of case studies covering kinds of problems that are likely to occur at various stages of the human life cycle.*

Hall, C. M.: The Bowen Family Theory and Its Uses. New York, Jason Aronson, Inc., 1981. *This book is an exploration in a series of applications of the pioneering Family Theory of Murray Bowen. The first section of the book provides a detailed description of the Bowen Family Theory, including the theoretical prospectus of the family process and the concepts that form the theory. The second section deals with the applications of the theory to one's own family of origin. The healing processes and other family issues in the third section explore the issues and implications involving the Bowen Family Theory and its uses.*

Hess, R., and Handel, G.: Family Worlds: A Psychosocial Approach to Family Life. Chicago, The University of Chicago Press, 1959.

Hoebel, F. C.: Family-Interactional therapy in the management of cardiac-related high-risk behaviors. J. Fam. Pract., *3:*613, 1976.

Holmes, T. H., and Rahe, R. H.: The social readjustment rating scale. J. Psychosom. Res., *11:*213, 1967. *This is the classic article with regard to the development and application of the social readjustment rating scale as a method for scaling the life-event and life-style items that were derived from psychophysics. The scale is used to investigate the similarities and differences among cultures to study recall of life events and to evaluate the relationship of life changes to the occurrence of disease.*

Kantor, D., and Lehr, W.: Inside the Family: Toward a Theory of Family Process. New York, Harper Colophon Books, 1975. *Trained observers actually lived with families of various ethnic, religious, education, and class backgrounds, recording and interviewing them in their own houses. From the data collected, Kantor extracts the fundamental processes common to all families and describes how different families run their lives, how families arrange living space, time, and effort according to particular demands.*

Kellner, R.: Family Ill Health. Springfield, Ill., Charles C Thomas, 1963.

Kraus, A. S., and Lilienfield, A. M.: Some epidemiologic aspects of the high mortality rate in the young widowed group. J. Chronic Dis., *10:*207, 1959.

Lewis, J. M.: The family matrix in health and disease. *In* Hofling, C. K., and Lewis, J. M. (Eds.): The Family: Evaluation and Treatment. New York, Brunner/Mazel, 1980. *This volume is published by the American College of Psychiatrists to bring together outstanding leaders in the fields of family research and therapy. The focus is on the family as an interacting system that promotes or inhibits the growth of its members. Procedures and techniques for evaluating the healthy and dysfunctional characteristics of families from different perspectives are presented.*

Lewis, J. M., Beavers, W. R., Gossett, J. T., et al.: No Single Thread: Psychological Health in Family Systems. New York, Brunner/Mazel, 1976. *The authors present the results of a long-term pioneering study of how healthy families function based on the concept of family systems as an outgrowth of general systems theory. This study searches out characteristics of optimally functioning families, focusing on family variables that are interactional rather than on individual observations.*

Lidz, T., Cornelison, A. R., Fleck, S., et al.: The intrafamilial environment of schizophrenic patients. Am. J. Psychiatry, *114:*241, 1957.

Litman, T. J.: The views of Minnesota school children on food. J. Am. Diet. Assoc., *45:*438, 1964.

Litman, T. J.: The family and physical rehabilitation. J. Chronic Dis., *19:*21, 1966.

Livsey, G. G.: Physical illness and family dynamics. Adv. Psychosom. Med., *8:*237, 1972.

Medalie, J. H., Kitson, G. C., and Zyzanski, S. J.: A family epidemiological model: a practice and research concept for family medicine. J. Fam. Pract., *12:*79, 1981.

Medalie, J. H., Snyder, M., Groen, J. J., et al.: Angina pectoris among 10,000 men. 5 year incidence and univariate analysis. Am. J. Med., *55:*583, 1973.

Meyer, R. J., and Haggerty, R. J.: Streptococcal infections in families. Factors altering individual susceptibility. Pediatrics, *29:*539, 1962.

Miller, J. G.: Living systems: basic concepts. *In* Grey, W., Duhl, F. J., and Rizzo, N. D. (Eds.): General Systems Theory and Psychiatry. Boston, Little, Brown and Company, 1969.

Minuchin, S.: Families and Family Therapy. Cambridge, Mass., Harvard University Press, 1974. *Reviews and strategies of a master clinician are presented here in a clear and concise form so that readers can proceed directly from the book to compare and modify their own styles and working situations. Minuchin presents six chapter-length transcripts of actual family sessions: two devoted to ordinary families who are meeting problems with success, four to families seeking help. Accompanying each transcript is the author's running interpretation of what is taking place, laying particular emphasis on the therapist's tactics and maneuvers.*

Minuchin, S.: Psychosomatic Families. Cambridge, Mass., Harvard University Press, 1978. *This book gives a detailed exploration of the application of theories of family structure and family therapy to an illness that has long resisted treatment—anorexia nervosa. The book presents a new theory of psychosomatic disease and data to confirm the theory and contains actual therapeutic situations with anorectic patients. A classic work on the relationship of the psychosomatic illness and family structure and functioning.*

Minuchin, S., Baker, L., Rosman, B. L., et al.: A conceptual model of psychosomatic illness in children: family organization and family therapy. Arch. Gen. Psychiatry, *32:*1031, 1975.

Murdock, G. P.: Social Structure. 2nd ed. New York, The Free Press, 1965.

Olson, D. H., Bell, R., and Portner, J.: FACES: Family Adaptability and Cohesion Evolution Scales. Department of Family of Social Science, St. Paul University, 1978.

Olson, D. H., Sprenkle, D. H., and Russell, C. S.: Circumplex model of marital and family systems: I. Cohesion and adaptability dimensions, family types, and clinical applications. Fam. Process, *18:*3, 1979. *The authors review the work of a number of leading experts in the field of family therapy and family systems to derive the critical components of the circumplex model in its adaptability and cohesiveness dimensions. A vast number of elements of different works are synthesized into this concept of family functioning.*

Parkes, C. M., and Brown, J., Jr.: Health after bereavement. Psychosom. Med., *34:*5, 1972.

Parsons, T., and Bales, R.: Family Socialization and Interaction Process. Glencoe, Ill., The Free Press of Glencoe, 1955.

Peachey, R.: Family patterns of stress. Gen. Pract., *27:*82, 1963.

Powers, W. T.: Feedback: beyond behaviorism. Science, *179:*351, 1973.

Pratt, L.: Family Structure and Effective Health Behavior: The Energized Family. Boston, Houghton Mifflin Company, 1976. *This book explores the types of structure a family needs in order to function effectively in contemporary society. It assesses the effectiveness of alternative forms of family structure and the family's performance of one of its major functions—personal health care. This is a report of an in-depth study conducted in the State of New Jersey over a period of several years.*

Ransom, D. C., and Vandervoort, H. E.: The development of family medicine: problematic trends. J. A. M. A., *225:*1098, 1973.

Rees, W. D., and Lutkins, S. G.: Mortality of bereavement. Br. Med. J., *40:*13, 1967.

Reiss, D.: Varieties of consensual experience. I. A theory for relating family thinking to individual thinking. Fam. Process, *10:*1, 1971.

Richardson, H. B.: Patients Have Families. New York, Commonwealth Fund, 1945.

Riskin, J., and Faunce, E. E.: Family interaction scales. Arch. Gen. Psychiatry, *22:*504, 1970.

Rogers, R. H.: Family Interaction and Transaction: The Developmental Approach. Englewood Cliffs, N.J., Prentice-Hall, Inc., 1973.

Silver, G. A.: Family Medical Care: A Design for Health Maintenance. Cambridge, Mass., Ballinger Publishing Company, 1974.

Smilkstein, G.: The family in trouble—how to tell. J. Fam. Pract., *2:*19, 1975.

Smilkstein, G.: The family APGAR: a proposal for a family function test and its use by physicians. J. Fam. Pract., *6:*1231, 1978.

Smilkstein, G.: The cycle of family function: a conceptual model for family medicine. J. Fam. Pract., *2:*223, 1980.

Stierlin, H.: Separating Parents and Adolescents. New York, Quadrangle, 1972.

Strodbeck, F. L.: Husband-wife interaction over revealed differences. Am. Sociological Rev., *16:*468, 1951.

Terkelsen, K. G.: Toward a theory of the family life cycle. *In* Carter, E. A., and McGoldrick, M. (Eds.): The Family Life Cycle: A Framework for Family Therapy. New York, Gardner Press, 1980.

Toman, W.: Family Constellation. New York, Springer Publishing Company, 1961. *The first part is devoted to the psychosocial understanding of the modern family in health and illness, whereas the second part provides a broad background from more specific family studies including presentation of general living systems theory. The final part is concerned with the treatment of families and their members. This book describes how sibling position influences personality and shapes the course of an individual's relationships outside the family. More than 60 prevailing types of relationships between siblings, spouses, and children are presented, which are based on the research in clinical psychology of a study of more than 3000 families.*

U.S. Department of Health, Education, and Welfare: Teenage Smoking: National Patterns of Cigarette Smoking, Age 12 Through 18 in 1968 and 1970. Public Health Service, Washington, D. C., 1971.

Vogel, E. F., and Bell, N. W.: The emotionally disturbed child as a family scapegoat. *In* Bell, N. W., and Vogel, E. F. (Eds.): The Family. Glencoe, Ill., The Free Press of Glencoe, 1960.

Widmer, R. B., and Cadoret, R. J.: Depression in family practice: changes in pattern of patient visits and complaints during subsequent developing depression. J. Fam. Pract., *9:*1017, 1979.

Wynne, L. C., Ryckoff, I. M., Day, J., and Hirsch, S. I.: Pseudomutuality in the family relations of schizophrenics. Psychiatry, *21:*205, 1958.

3

The Family Life Cycle

Bruce S. Liese
James G. Price

People undergo many psychologic changes over the life span that have important implications for their health. These developmental changes occur in stages (e.g., childhood, adolescence, young adulthood, middle age, old age) that are predictable and observable. Similarly, over the family life cycle, the family system undergoes important psychosocial changes. These changes also occur in predictable, observable stages (e.g., the newlywed couple, families with young children, families with adolescents, the launching years, families in later life). Since the family physician cares for families and for individuals from birth to death, an awareness of individual and family life cycle changes and the skills needed for dealing with problems they can create may enhance patient care. Thus, this chapter reviews and discusses the development of individuals and families from a family life cycle perspective.

The typical family physician is accustomed to organizing most areas of medical knowledge in a compartmentalized fashion (e.g., the three trimesters of pregnancy, the hormonal differences between the 5-year-old and the 15-year-old, the various types of cardiovascular diseases). It is equally possible to view the varied behaviors of people at different ages and life stages in an organized fashion. For example, consider the case of Barry, a 15-year-old insulin-dependent diabetic teenager:

Barry has been relatively problem-free and compliant with his treatment since his diabetes was diagnosed 4 years ago. Recently, however, Barry's parents have become upset with him because they perceive him as not eating properly, not monitoring his blood sugar levels, and not taking his insulin reliably. These problems are compounded by Barry's frustration with his parents who suddenly seem to him to be terribly strict and critical of his behaviors.

Barry's behavior is understandable when considered in the context of normal adolescent development. He has entered a stage in his life in which popularity is very important. In fact, dating and popularity seem far more important to Barry right now than his diabetes. Barry has become self-conscious about his disease and he is afraid that his friends won't like him because of his unusual eating habits and his need for daily injections. Thus, Barry neglects monitoring, dieting, and insulin for the pursuit of seemingly more important social interests.

This example illustrates that an awareness of psychologic developmental processes may be relevant to the practice of family medicine. The family physician who understands normal stage-related behaviors will be better prepared to treat patients and families with difficulties in these stages than the physician who is unaware of these processes.

This example also illustrates that some medical problems are best managed from the family systems perspective, which is central to the family life cycle model. According to the family systems perspective, the actions of each family member affect other family members as well as the family as a whole. Barry's diabetes was under control until he reached the developmental stage of adolescence. As an adolescent, Barry changed his usual behaviors (i.e., compliance) to unusual behaviors (i.e., noncompliance) as a result of the changing goals in his life. These changes caused anxiety in Barry's parents, since they are an important and responsible part of his family system. Their distress and subsequent criticism regarding his adolescent behaviors resulted in Barry's rebelliousness, which further troubled his parents. Thus, a disruption in Barry's entire family system was triggered by his individual developmental process.

The purpose of this chapter is to present the family life cycle as it relates to individual development and health. It is assumed that the typical physician may not choose to diagnose and treat problems in the life cycle of the family, since such problems do not lend themselves to direct or simple cures. It is believed, however, that the family physician who addresses individual and family life cycle development will be more helpful to patients who struggle with family life cycle issues (e.g., pregnancy, the death of a family member) than physicians who do not address them.

The Impact of Family Processes and the Family Life Cycle on Health

In their now classic work, Holmes and Rahe (1967) found that the death of a spouse or child, divorce, marriage, and other stressful life cycle events may all have significant negative effects on health. These authors, through their development of the Social Readjustment Rating Scale, have created a standardized method for assessing the impact of stressful life span events on health. Ten of the first 15 items on the Social Readjustment Rating Scale are stressful events that occur in the context of the family (see Table 3–1). Of these 10 items, five are normal family life cycle events: marriage, pregnancy, gain of a new family member, retirement, and the death of a spouse. This scale has stimulated at least two decades of research on the effects of stressful events (including family life cycle events) on health.

More recently, Campbell (1986) conducted a comprehensive review of research on the impact of the family on health (see also chapter 6 of this text). He looked critically at studies of demographic and family structure variables, stressful family life events, and family interaction and functioning in terms of how these variables affect disease severity, symptoms, compliance, and mortality. The medical problems that were studied included cardiovascular disease, hypertension, diabetes, asthma, pregnancy, schizophrenia, depression, substance abuse, anorexia nervosa, and others. Campbell drew multiple conclusions from his review, including the following:

1. Family support and marital status influence the incidence of cardiovascular disease as well as overall mortality, with spouse support offering protection against disease processes. As an extension of this finding, bereavement is associated with an increased risk of death in widowers.

2. Simple family interventions (with hypertensive patients, for example) and family support (with obese patients) can have a major impact on improving compliance and, therefore, lowering overall mortality.

3. Poor diabetic control and chronic family conflict tend to coexist.

4. Dysfunctional family communication is commonly found in schizophrenic families.

5. Personal criticism and marital discord are both associated with depression in family members.

Thus, there is an empirical basis for the assump-

Table 3–1. SOCIAL READJUSTMENT RATING SCALE*

Rank	Life Event	Mean Value
1	Death of spouse	100
2	Divorce	73
3	Marital separation	65
4	Jail term	63
5	Death of close family member	63
6	Personal injury or illness	53
7	Marriage	50
8	Fired at work	47
9	Marital reconciliation	45
10	Retirement	45
11	Change in health of family member	44
12	Pregnancy	40
13	Sexual difficulties	39
14	Gain of new family member	39
15	Business readjustment	39
16	Change in financial state	38
17	Death of close friend	37
18	Change to different line of work	36
19	Change in number of arguments with spouse	35
20	Mortgage over $52,300†	31
21	Foreclosure of mortgage or loan	30
22	Change in responsibilities at work	29
23	Son or daughter leaving home	29
24	Trouble with in-laws	29
25	Outstanding personal achievement	28
26	Wife begin or stop work	26
27	Begin or end school	26
28	Change in living conditions	25
29	Revision of personal habits	24
30	Trouble with boss	23
31	Change in work hours or conditions	20
32	Change in residence	20
33	Change in schools	20
34	Change in recreation	19
35	Change in church activities	19
36	Change in social activities	18
37	Mortgage or loan less than $10,000	17
38	Change in sleeping habits	16
39	Change in number of family get-togethers	15
40	Change in eating habits	15
41	Vacation	13
42	Christmas	12
43	Minor violations of the law	11

*From Holmes, T. H., and Rahe, R. H.: The social readjustment rating scale. J. Psychosom. Res., *11*:213–218, 1967.
†This figure was $10,000 in the original Holmes and Rahe scale. The updated amount of $52,300 is based on average mortgage rate increase from $15,000 in 1967 to $78,500 in 1989.

tion that family processes and family life cycle events are related to health and wellness. Returning to the above example, Barry's family physician suspected that Barry's noncompliance was related to his need to "fit in" with his friends as well as being related to recent family conflicts. As a result of this awareness, Barry's physician discussed friendship and dating with him and helped Barry see that he could both be popular and take care of his diabetes. His family physician also helped Barry's parents to understand the problem, and he convinced them that Barry would benefit from their understanding and support of his personal life changes. This family systems–oriented intervention resulted in Barry's return to his earlier high level of compliance. It also helped improve relationships within Barry's family system.

According to family life cycle models, patients' problems can be best understood and treated in the context of their stage of family life cycle development. In order to understand family life cycle development, however, an understanding of individual life span psychosocial development is necessary. This is true because families are collections of individuals who are at various stages of their own development. Thus, in the next section, individual psychosocial life span development is reviewed.

Individual Life Span Development

Most physicians are familiar with developmental processes in infants and children (e.g., physical, language, motor, and cognitive growth), but development in adulthood is often overlooked where it is also important. It is probably overlooked because (1) it is less dramatic and apparent than childhood development and (2) less information (i.e., research) exists on adulthood development.

Many investigators and theorists have studied the psychologic development of adults. Some of this work has been general (e.g., Baltes, 1979; Birren and Schaie, 1985; Colarusso and Nemiroff, 1981; Erikson, 1963; Gould, 1978; Kegan, 1982; Levinson, 1986; Neugarten, 1976, 1979; Sheehy, 1976; Stevens-Long, 1988), whereas others have focused on such specific topics as moral development (Kohlberg, 1981), women's development (Gilligan, 1982), men's development (Levinson et al., 1978; Vaillant, 1977), and career development (Super, 1957; Super et al., 1957; Super and Hall, 1978).

Eric Erikson (1963) was the first to systematically examine the psychosocial development of individuals across the entire life span. In his model, Erikson proposed the following eight stages of life span development:

1. Basic trust versus mistrust (birth to 18 months)
2. Autonomy versus shame and doubt (18 months to 3 years)
3. Initiative versus guilt (3 to 6 years)
4. Industry versus inferiority (6 to 12 years)
5. Identity versus role confusion (puberty and adolescence)
6. Intimacy versus isolation (young adulthood)
7. Generativity versus stagnation (middle adulthood)
8. Ego integrity versus despair (late adulthood)

According to Erikson, individuals develop as a result of the interaction between internal (i.e., psychologic) and external (i.e., social) processes. As individuals encounter critical developmental issues over the course of the life span, they experience normal, predictable crises. By confronting these crises, they proceed through the stages of psychosocial development. When crises are resolved in a satisfactory manner, individuals develop healthy personality characteristics and they move to the next stage of development. When individuals do not resolve crises effectively, they may either develop psychopathology or be stunted in further psychologic development during later stages.

Each stage of development is organized around a specific developmental issue. This section provides a brief summary of the developmental processes and issues across the eight stages of individual development, according to Erikson. Later in this chapter these stages are related to family life cycle development. For example, we examine the effects of adolescent development on the family and vice versa.

In the first stage of life, infants learn *basic trust* or *mistrust* of themselves and others, depending on the treatment they receive from their parents. In particular, infants who are comforted by consistently loving and nurturing parents are more trusting than those whose parents do not behave in this manner.

In the second developmental stage, toddlers learn either *autonomy* or *shame and doubt,* depending on how parents handle their failure experiences (e.g., during toilet training). Autonomy is defined as independence, or the separation of self from others, including parents. During this period, toddlers begin to experiment with self-control and self-determination and such experimentation is often expressed as stubbornness, refusal (i.e., shouting "NO!"), temper tantrums, and so on. (The "terrible two's" may occur during this stage.) Parents who support and encourage appropriate self-determined behaviors during this stage teach their children to become autonomous. On the other hand, parents who are excessively critical, restrictive, and punishing towards their children during this stage teach their children to feel ashamed, self-doubtful, and self-critical.

In the third stage, young children begin to internalize their parents' rules and to take initiative. This is the stage during which a high level of activity (i.e., play) takes place, and language develops rapidly. *Initiative* (versus *guilt*) develops to the extent that the child is supported emotionally during initiative-taking activities. Children who are discouraged from exploring and experimenting during this stage may lack initiative and instead be overly dependent on others.

In the fourth stage, the school-aged child is

focused on productivity and social skills. During this stage, a sense of *industry* (versus *inadequacy*) can develop in children who are productive in the school setting and get along with other children. Parents contribute positively to this process by actively listening to their children and helping them understand their experiences in school. Furthermore, parents support a sense of industry by actively sharing in the learning process at home (by reading, helping with homework and so on).

In the fifth stage, the adolescent is faced with the task of developing a *personal identity*. A personal identity is defined as a consistent, continuous personality and self-concept (i.e., a sense of self). Such an identity does not develop automatically; instead the adolescent must actively pursue such growth. Those who do not develop a personal identity during this period experience *role diffusion* and *identity confusion*.

Adolescence can be a period of turmoil for both the child and the family. As a natural part of the development process, the adolescent becomes increasingly concerned (sometimes to the point of preoccupation) about the opinions of peers regarding clothing, music, friends, language, and behaviors. During this stage, social experimentation is necessary for the adolescent to examine the various roles and identities available to him or her. In this context, it is understandable that Barry, described earlier, would neglect his health to pursue social approval. The effects of the adolescent on the family and vice versa are discussed in greater detail later in this chapter.

In the sixth stage of development, the young adult must develop a sense of *intimacy* (versus *isolation*) in relationships. Intimacy is defined as the ability to develop and maintain close, enduring relationships. Such relationships typically require significant compromises and sacrifices. During this stage, the young adult's peer group should become less important as intimacy becomes more important. It is usually during this stage that serious dating and marriage take place.

As a prerequisite for a sense of intimacy, an individual must first acquire a personal identity in the adolescent stage of development. Problems may occur in intimate relationships (especially in marriages) when one partner continues to be preoccupied, after adolescence, with others' opinions of him or her. Furthermore, the unattached single person who has not developed an identity during adolescence may avoid commitment to intimate relationships, instead seeking superficial sexual or unstable relationships.

In the seventh stage, adults are faced with the challenge of achieving *generativity* versus *stagnation*. Generativity is defined as productivity and creativity, especially as these qualities contribute to the growth of other people. Healthy individuals in this stage nurture others and become invested in their growth rather than selfishly pursuing personal gain. Such persons typically have a family to love and nurture, while also contributing to the personal and professional growth of nonfamily members (e.g., peers, friends, coworkers, and subordinates). It is common for psychologically healthy individuals at this stage to serve as mentors to others. Those who do not accomplish generativity at this stage of life face stagnation (i.e., termination of further psychosocial development).

In the eighth and final stage of life, the older adult achieves either *ego integrity* or *disgust and despair*. Ego integrity is defined as the successful integration and appreciation of one's own life experiences as well as acceptance of the inevitability of death. Arrival at this stage requires the successful culmination of all preceding stages; positive growth in this stage (i.e., ego integrity) is characterized by wisdom, maturity, independence, spirituality, and leadership. Those who do not satisfactorily achieve ego integrity face old age and death with feelings of disgust, despair, fear, bitterness, and regret.

Since the publication of Erikson's classic work, Levinson and his colleagues (Levinson, 1986; Levinson et al., 1978) have further studied adult psychosocial development. Levinson's first study of 40 men has been considered by some to be the most comprehensive modern study of adulthood development (Colarusso and Nemiroff, 1981).

From his research, Levinson (1986) has divided the life cycle into four discrete periods: (1) preadulthood (0 to 22 years); (2) early adulthood (17 to 45 years); (3) middle adulthood (40 to 65 years); and (4) late adulthood (60+ years). Each of these periods is further divided into "structure-building" periods and "structure-changing" (transitional) periods. Structure-building periods, which last between 5 and 10 years, are separated by transitional periods lasting approximately 5 years. During structure-building periods, individuals form a life structure based on their relationships, vocational commitments, and so on. From this structure, individuals pursue personal values and goals.

Transitional periods are characterized by the termination of an existing life structure and the beginning of a new life structure. Such transitional periods have been referred to as "predictable life crises" by Sheehy (1976). One example of a critical transitional period is the time between early and middle adulthood. This period has been referred to as the time of "midlife crisis" (i.e., a time of asking oneself "what does it all mean?") In Erikson's terms, this should be the time of movement into the stage of generativity. Those who have not adequately developed a sense of identity or intimacy might have a more severe midlife crisis as a result of being unprepared to begin the next phase of development.

Thus it is seen that different investigators have noted the developmental and psychologic changes that take place in individuals during different times of life. Although these investigators have arrived at varying labels for the stages and the tasks therein, they share the common theme of the need for each individual's successful passage through each stage to achieve healthy psychologic growth.

As mentioned earlier, an understanding of individual psychosocial development is essential to an understanding of family life cycle development. This is true because families consist of persons whose individual stages of development affect their family systems and vice versa. In the following sections, development is examined in the context of family life cycle stages and family life cycle events. An attempt is made to integrate individual and family life cycle development and to relate these factors to the practice of family medicine.

The Family Life Cycle

Marriage, birth, illness, and death are family life cycle events that may have a profound impact on the family as a system as well as on the psychologic development of its individual members. As mentioned previously, these events may also have significant influence on individuals' health.

Models of family life cycle development grew from individual adult life span developmental models (e.g., Erikson, 1963; Levinson, 1986). According to family life cycle developmental models, certain life cycle events, or "turning points" (e.g., marriage, becoming parents, retirement) may delineate stages in a family's life, although more often there is no single specific triggering event that initiates a new family life cycle stage.

Many different models of family life cycle development have been proposed (e.g., Barnhill and Longo, 1978; Breunlin, 1989; Carter and McGoldrick, 1980; Duvall, 1977; Haley, 1973; Rhodes, 1977; Solomon, 1973; Weeks and Wright, 1979; Wynne, 1984). All of these models have certain elements in common. For example, all models assume a family systems perspective. That is, the family as an entity is assumed to be more complex than the sum of its parts. Furthermore, when one family member enters a new stage of psychosocial development (e.g., adolescence), all family members are assumed to be affected and can be expected to react to the individual's changes. (For a more detailed discussion of family systems theory, see chapter 4 of this text.)

In most family life cycle models, it is believed that families fulfill important emotional needs for their family members, and these needs vary from stage to stage of the family life cycle. Similar to individual models of development, the transitions between stages of the family life cycle are considered important and potentially stressful times. When the tasks of a stage are not successfully completed, development may be stunted at transition points (i.e., the transition may be interrupted) or symptoms may emerge, resulting in problems in further family development.

Recently, Breunlin (1989) has proposed a revised view of the family development process. He suggests that families continuously change across the family life cycle rather than changing specifically at transition points. He describes a recursive relationship between the development of individual family members and the family: "As each family member develops, he or she increases the potential to possess additional competence that can be used in the service of increasing the flexibility and complexity of the family." Thus, in most families, individuals change continuously, resulting in challenges to the family system. To the extent that the family system accommodates to these changes, it increases its flexibility and complexity. These changes, however, occur in an oscillating rather than in a smooth (i.e., linear) or stepwise fashion. Each oscillation has the potential to result in an increment of growth for the individual and family.

In this chapter, we follow the model proposed by Carter and McGoldrick (1980), which divides the family life cycle into six stages (see Table 3–2).

STAGE 1: BETWEEN FAMILIES: THE UNATTACHED YOUNG ADULT

Mark is a 23-year-old single male who is about to enter medical school. He has lived with his family throughout his undergraduate school years, and he will soon move away from his parents' home for the first time to go to medical school. Although he has dated throughout college, none of Mark's relationships have become "serious." While visiting his family physician for a required school physical he expresses excitement and some concern about his ability to succeed in medical school. He also expresses the hope that he will soon "meet some nice girl" so he can "settle down and start a family."

Even as an unmarried young adult without a spouse or children, Mark is still in Stage 1 of the family life cycle. Stage 1 is defined as the time period between leaving one's parents' home and entering into a long-term intimate relationship (typically marriage) to begin a new family. During this stage, Mark will develop behaviors, values, attitudes, and skills that will impact on his later role as a family member (i.e., husband and father). This is a time of separating and differentiating himself from his family of origin (i.e., his parents and siblings) and forming substantial intimate relationships. This should also be a time for developing and actively pursuing his career goals and dreams.

Intimacy and Love

In the process of separating and differentiating from one's parents, the young adult must develop intimate relationships with others outside his or her family of origin. Intimacy, as defined earlier, is the ability to develop and maintain close, enduring relationships. Intimacy includes the elements of commitment, reciprocity, similarity, compatibility, attachment, and dependency (Stevens-Long, 1988). In order for two people to be intimate, they must engage in self-disclosure (i.e., they must discuss personal matters). The young adult's success at achieving intimacy will therefore depend, to a large extent, on the degree to which he or she has developed an

Table 3–2. THE STAGES OF THE FAMILY LIFE CYCLE*

Family Life Cycle Stage	Emotional Proces of Transition: Key Principles	Second Order Changes in Family Status Required to Proceed Developmentally
1. Between Families: The Unattached Young Adult	Accepting parent-offspring separation	a. Differentiation of self in relation to family of origin b. Development of intimate peer relationships c. Establishment of self in work
2. The Joining of Families Through Marriage: The Newly Married Couple	Commitment to new system	a. Formation of marital system b. Realignment of relationships with extended families and friends to include spouse
3. The Family with Young Children	Accepting new members into the system	a. Adjusting marital system to make space for child(ren) b. Taking on parenting roles c. Realignment of relationships with extended family to include parenting and grandparenting roles
4. The Family with Adolescents	Increasing flexibility of family boundaries to include children's independence	a. Shifting of parent-child relationships to permit adolescent to move in and out of system b. Refocus on midlife marital and career issues c. Beginning shift toward concerns for older generation
5. Launching Children and Moving On	Accepting a multitude of exits from and entries into the family system	a. Renegotiation of marital system as a dyad b. Development of adult to adult relationships between grown children and their parents c. Realignment of relationships to include in-laws and grandchildren d. Dealing with disabilities and death of parents (grandparents)
6. The Family in Later Life	Accepting the shifting of generational roles	a. Maintaining own and/or couple functioning and interests in face of physiologic decline; exploration of new familial and social role options b. Support for a more central role for middle generation c. Making room in the system for the wisdom and experience of the elderly; supporting the older generation without overfunctioning for them d. Dealing with loss of spouse, siblings, and other peers and preparation for own death. Life review and integration.

*From Carter, E., and McGoldrick, M.: The Family Life Cycle: A Framework for Family Therapy, New York, Gardner Press, Inc., 1980.

identity during the previous developmental stage of adolescence. This is true, according to Stevens-Long (1988), because "Meaningful self-disclosure requires a strong sense of self." She poses the question, "How can you tell someone else about who you are if you don't really know yourself?" (p. 111).

Love, which is related to intimacy, is an important issue for the unattached young adult. Mature love (versus romantic love) is defined as an unselfish commitment to another person's growth and development or the willingness to care about another person as much as one cares about one's self. Romantic love, on the other hand, is associated with physiologic (and often sexual) arousal and excitement. Tennov (1979) has coined the term "limerance" to refer to the concept of romantic love. Limerance is the intense feeling occurring at the beginning of an intimate relationship that may include intrusive thoughts, acute longing, fear of rejection, dependency, and acute sensitivity to another person (i.e., the limerant object). People in romantic love tend to idealize each other, seeing their partners as they wish them to be rather than for their actual qualities and characteristics. According to Tennov, limerance lasts approximately 2 years before it fades. She explains that fading occurs because the novelty of the relationship usually ends by that time.

Many individuals confuse romantic love with mature love. By doing so, they may experience confusion, disappointment, and disillusionment when they no longer feel the intense feelings of romantic love for their partner. During the unattached young adult stage of the family life cycle, it is important that individuals learn to distinguish between mature and romantic love in order to enter the next stage of family life cycle development (i.e., marriage) with realistic expectations for love. Individuals who are unable to develop mature loving bonds with others during this stage may become "retarded" in their abilities to enter satisfying, enduring marital relationships.

Sexuality

Sexuality is an area of concern for most unmarried young people, since a substantial number of single people engage in premarital sex. In particular, contraception is important to many young adults who visit the family physician for advice and recommendations. At different stages of the family life cycle, individuals may have different contraceptive needs and different reasons for selecting various contraceptive methods. For example, unmarried young adults are likely to be more concerned about safety against sexually transmitted diseases than married persons. Thus, an unmarried young adult may be more interested in the use of condoms for contraception than birth control pills. A married couple with adolescent children might be more concerned about contraceptive efficacy, and therefore they might be more likely to choose tubal ligation or vasectomy over condoms. In addition to helping the patient choose the most appropriate method for contraception, an office visit for contraception provides the family physician with an opportunity to explore issues of sexuality.

Sexual beliefs and attitudes, to a large extent, determine sexual behaviors and satisfaction levels. As unmarried young adults, individuals typically explore and test the sexual beliefs and attitudes they began to develop in childhood. Unfortunately, some acquired sexual beliefs are inaccurate, irrational, and dysfunctional. Such beliefs, known as "sexual myths," may contribute to sexual problems in all stages of the family life cycle. Sexual myths include the following (Zilbergeld, 1978):

1. Men shouldn't express certain feelings.
2. Sex is a performance.
3. A man must orchestrate sex.
4. A man always wants and is ready to have sex.
5. All physical contact must lead to sex.
6. Sex equals intercourse.
7. Sex requires an erection.
8. Good sex is increasing excitement terminated only by orgasm.
9. Sex should be natural and spontaneous.
10. In this enlightened age, the preceding myths no longer have an influence on us.

Sexual myths tend to result in sexual problems because they lead individuals to have unrealistic expectations about their sexuality and sexual functioning. When sexual myths do not become reality, individuals may experience "performance anxiety" (i.e., feelings of disappointment or self-consciousness, resulting in difficulties achieving or maintaining sexual arousal.) In contrast, satisfying sexual relations tend to be characterized by spontaneous intimacy and a feeling of comfort with one's body and sexual expression. The act of sexual intercourse, per se, is only part of a person's broader sexuality. Too much emphasis on intercourse and orgasm (i.e., performance) can interfere with the full expression of individuals' sexuality.

The physician helping patients with sexual problems should inquire about the sexual myths believed by patients. Through an educational process, the family physician can then begin to dispel these myths, replacing them with more accurate and functional thoughts and knowledge. The family physician can also encourage patients to engage in effective communication toward improving their sexual functioning. High-quality communication between sexual partners is the key to healthy sexual growth, adjustment, and satisfaction. Most individuals find it difficult to communicate emotions (especially sensitive, intimate emotions) in words because they fear they are vulnerable. (Sexual functioning and dysfunction are discussed in more detail in a later section on The Newly Married Couple).

Career Development

In order for young unattached adults to separate from their families of origin, they must develop careers that facilitate financial as well as psychologic independence. Career development progresses through five stages over the life span (Super et al., 1957). These stages, which are presented in Table 3–3, include the following: (1) growth (birth to 14 years old); (2) exploration (15 to 24 years old); (3) establishment (25 to 44 years old); (4) maintenance (45 to 64 years old); and (5) decline (over 65 years old). Thus, during the stage of unattached young adulthood, individuals should explore and begin to establish their careers. Such exploration requires an examination of interests and aptitudes by experimentation and risk-taking behaviors at work or in educational programs.

Mark, from the example given earlier, has been thinking about becoming a physician since high school, where he discovered his strong interest in the natural sciences and helping others. During this time of exploration he was advised by his biology teacher to volunteer at a local hospital where he actually observed the activities of physicians and other medical professionals. Mark's experiences at the hospital convinced him of his desire to become a physician. His entry into medical school at the present time is, therefore, an important part of his long-standing career dream. Career development is not always this linear or straightforward, however. Many young adults, even after completing college, are still undecided in their career goal. Such individuals are at risk for difficulties in their family life cycle development, since they may feel unsettled and insecure about their careers, resulting in floundering at a time when they need to be settled.

Health Issues in the Unattached Young Adult

Medically, the unattached young person must begin to take responsibility for his or her own body. Prior to this stage in life, most young people have had their nutritional, medical, and even recreational activities mediated by their parents and school. The family physician can educate individuals at this stage of life in the areas of health maintenance, the role of the family physician, and so on.

To summarize, successful development of the unattached young adult requires physical and psychologic separation from one's family of origin, as well as the development of intimacy with others outside of the family. In order to accomplish these tasks, it is necessary for the individual to gain self-knowledge and experience regarding intimacy, sex, and career. This process can be facilitated by the motivated family

Table 3–3. VOCATIONAL LIFE STAGES*

1. **Growth Stage (Birth to 14)**
   Self-concept develops through identification with key figures in family and in school; needs and fantasy are dominant early in this stage; interest and capacity become more important in this stage with increasing social participation and reality-testing. Substages of the growth stage are:
   Fantasy (4 to 10). Needs are dominant; role-playing in fantasy is important.
   Interest (11 to 12). Likes are the major determinant of aspirations and activities.
   Capacity (13 to 14). Abilities are given more weight, and job requirements (including training) are considered.

2. **Exploration Stage (Age 15 to 24)**
   Self-examination, role tryouts, and occupational exploration take place in school, leisure activities, and part-time work. Substages of the exploration stage are:
   Tentative (15 to 17). Needs, interests, capacities, values, and opportunities are all considered. Tentative choices are made and tried out in fantasy, discussion, courses, work, and so on.
   Transition (18 to 21). Reality considerations are given more weight as the youth enters labor market or professional training and attempts to implement a self-concept.
   Trial (22 to 24). A seemingly appropriate field having been located, a beginning job in it is found and is tried out as a life work.

3. **Establishment Stage (Age 25 to 44)**
   Having found an appropriate field, effort is put forth to make a permanent place in it. There may be some trial early in this stage, with consequent shifting, but establishment may begin without trial, especially in the professions. Substages of the establishment stage are:
   Trial (25 to 30). The field of work presumed to be suitable may prove unsatisfactory, resulting in one or two changes before the life work is found or before it becomes clear that the life work will be a succession of unrelated jobs.
   Stabilization (31 to 44). As the career pattern becomes clear, effort is put forth to stabilize, to make a secure place, in the world of work. For most persons these are the creative years.

4. **Maintenance Stage (Age 45–64)**
   Having made a place in the world of work, the concern is now to hold it. Little new ground is broken, but there is continuation along established lines.

5. **Decline Stage (Age 65 on)**
   As physical and mental powers decline, work activity changes and in due course ceases. New roles must be developed; first that of selective participant and then that of observer rather than participant. Substages of this stage are:
   Deceleration (65 to 70). Sometimes at the time of official retirement, sometimes later in the maintenance stage, the pace of work slackens, duties are shifted, or the nature of the work is changed to suit declining capacities. Many men find part-time jobs to replace their full-time occupations.
   Retirement (71 on). As with all the specified age limits, there are great variations from person to person. But, complete cessation of occupation comes for all in due course, to some easily and pleasantly, to others with difficulty and disappointment, and to some only with death.

*Reprinted by permission of the publisher from Super, Donald E. et al.: Vocational Development: A Framework for Research. New York: Teachers College Press, © 1957 by Teachers College, Columbia University. All rights reserved, pp. 40–41.

physician who addresses these issues with patients. When these tasks are accomplished, the individual is prepared for marriage and the joining of families together.

STAGE 2: THE JOINING OF FAMILIES THROUGH MARRIAGE: THE NEWLY MARRIED COUPLE

Marsha is a 28-year-old recently married woman, without children, who visits her family physician requesting assistance with birth control. She has been married to her husband, Phil, for 6 months and she explains that "marriage isn't exactly what I expected it to be." She admits that their interaction is not as "easy" as it was when they were dating, Phil is critical of her close relationships with her parents, and sexually, the couple just does not seem "terribly compatible."

Stage 2 of the family life cycle is defined as the time of "joining families through marriage." The newly married couple has formed a new family system that is both part of, and separate from, the couple's families of origin. The key process of this stage, according to Carter and McGoldrick (1980), is commitment to the newly formed family system. Such commitment requires that each member of a couple be willing to compromise self-centered beliefs and behaviors for more collaborative attitudes and actions.

When a couple decides to marry they have many hopes, dreams, and expectations for themselves and their new relationship. Some of these dreams are realistic and achievable, whereas others are unrealistic, potentially resulting in marital dissatisfaction. In this stage of the family life cycle, the couple must make many adjustments, both psychologic and behavioral, in order to have a rich and rewarding marriage. These adjustments may relate to such issues as friendships, finances, in-laws, recreation, life style, sexuality, and so forth.

When Marsha and Phil agreed to be married they expected each other to be completely supportive, attentive, and noncritical. Furthermore, each expected the other to know exactly what he or she was thinking and feeling without direct communication. (They thought "Can't he/she read my mind?") The couple also expected that there would be few, if any, conflicts between them. (They thought "We should never fight!"). And finally, they expected that they would automatically be sexually compatible. Such expectations are common in new marriages, although most of these are unrealistic. When such expectations are not met, substantial resentment may develop between the couple, which must be resolved through effective communication and conflict resolution skills.

Marital Satisfaction

Marital satisfaction has been widely researched over the past decade. Some studies have focused on marital satisfaction as it varies over the family life cycle (e.g., Reedy et al., 1981; Schram, 1979), whereas other research has focused on the ingredients that contribute to marital satisfaction, such as effective communication and skills to resolve conflict (e.g., Doherty and Jacobson, 1982; Jacobson and Holtzworth-Munroe, 1986; Jacobson & Margolin, 1979).

Research conducted to date suggests that marital satisfaction varies in its nature and intensity over the family life cycle. In general, self-reported feelings of marital satisfaction are greatest in the newly married couple without children, whereas almost all studies show an initial decrease in marital satisfaction after the first child is born (Schram, 1979). Some studies have suggested that marital satisfaction again increases after the launching years; however, this finding has been questioned by Schram (1979).

Reedy et al. (1981) studied the nature of love relationships across the adult life span. These authors found that passion and sexual intimacy are important in early adulthood, whereas tender feelings of affection and loyalty are more important in later stages of the family life cycle. They also found that "over time, satisfying love relationships are less likely to be based on intense companionship and communication and more likely to be based on the history of the relationship, traditions, commitment and loyalty" (p. 61). Finally, these investigators found that communication and self-disclosure are most important to love early in relationships, whereas a sense of loyalty, security, and commitment are "primary bonding forces in satisfying relationships which have weathered many years" (p. 61).

According to the research on the ingredients contributing to marital satisfaction (Doherty and Jacobson, 1982; Jacobson and Holtzworth-Munroe, 1986; Jacobson and Margolin, 1979), satisfying marriages are characterized by a high proportion of rewards to punishments. Rewards in a relationship can be either practical (e.g., washing the car, shopping, taking out the garbage) or they can be romantic (e.g., physical intimacy, playfulness, praise). Punishments can be verbal, nonverbal, or physical behaviors that are intended to inflict discomfort and induce behavior change in an individual's partner. Punishments in an unsatisfying marriage may include verbal abuse (e.g., name-calling), withdrawal (e.g., silence), or physical abuse.

In an unsatisfying marriage, partners may regularly punish each other when they do not get what they want from their relationship. For example, Marsha punishes Phil by angrily criticizing him when he does not do household chores or when he does not initiate romance. Phil, in turn, punishes Marsha by becoming silent and withdrawn when she criticizes him. In an unhealthy relationship such negative reciprocal behaviors are common, resulting in an escalation of marital conflicts. In healthy relationships members of a couple try to influence each other by nonpunishing behaviors (e.g., honest, direct communication and active listening), rather than by coercion (e.g., blaming, name-calling).

Some unsatisfying marriages are characterized by boredom. Boredom occurs either as a result of insufficient rewards or the "erosion" of existent rewards in the relationship. Erosion is defined as habituation to (i.e., becoming accustomed to) rewards that have existed for some time. To illustrate the effects of reward erosion, again consider the example of Phil and Marsha. Early in their relationship Phil regularly gave flowers and candy to Marsha. At first Marsha received Phil's gifts with appreciation and enthusiasm. Later, however, Marsha did not seem excited about Phil's gifts. As a result, Phil felt frustrated and inadequate about his abilities to satisfy Marsha. He, in turn, stopped giving gifts to Marsha. As a result of this and other decreases in rewards in the relationship, the couple became bored with each other and with the marriage. Boredom also occurred in their sexual relationship when they became habituated to "the same old routine." To avoid boredom, Phil and Marsha needed to be creative and innovative in their responses to each other. In other words, they needed to regularly introduce novelty into their relationship.

Sexual Intimacy in Marriage

Sexual intimacy is an important part of most couples' marital relationship. Although premarital sex is common, most couples only begin to address sexual issues after they are married. It is important that the family physician be comfortable with patients' sexual concerns. In a classic study by Frank, Anderson, and Rubenstein (1978), it was found that at least 50 per cent of happily married couples had some concerns about sexual functioning. Specifically, women reported problems achieving and maintaining sexual excitement and reaching orgasm, whereas men were most commonly concerned about ejaculating too quickly. Both sexes reported difficulties with too little foreplay before sex, partners choosing inconvenient times to initiate sex, difficulty relaxing, and disinterest in sex.

Despite the high prevalence of sexual problems in the general public, some studies (e.g., Moore and Goldstein, 1980) have found that physicians tend to underdiagnose sexual problems. Nease and Liese (1987) found that attention to sexual problems in the medical setting may be related to perceptions of physicians' willingness and abilities to address sexual problems. It is important that the family physician deal directly with patients' sexual concerns since they occur as a normal part of family life cycle development.

Returning to the example above, in order for Marsha's physician to help her with her sexual problems with Phil, he must be willing to ask about their sexual needs, the importance of sexuality in their lives, their methods for communicating about intimacy and sexuality, and so on. Their physician must also be willing to elicit very personal and specific information about such sexual issues as masturbation, sexual preference, and foreplay. With this information, the physician can diagnose sexual problems, provide sex education (including dispelling sexual myths), and make referrals to sex therapists, where indicated. (Chapter 62 of this text provides a more elaborate discussion of sexual health care.)

Family Planning and Pregnancy

At some time in their relationship, the married couple must make a decision (either explicit or implicit) about having children. This decision is critical to their identity as a family, to their individual development, and to their marital relationship. The decision to become parents varies in terms of the degree to which it is planned. Some couples plan methodically to have children at very specific times in their lives, whereas others do not plan at all for children. The family physician can assist with family planning early in the marital relationship simply by encouraging the couple to articulate their plans for having children prior to pregnancy.

The first pregnancy is an event of unparalleled importance in the individual and family life cycles. It typically results in major alterations in the couple's roles; it represents a pivotal point in their relationship; it has implications for the woman's long-term life plans (i.e., career and marriage); and it holds major existential importance for the couple. (These factors hold less importance in later pregnancies.)

According to Gloger-Tippelt (1983), the woman's emotional experience of pregnancy can best be understood as affecting three domains: biologic, psychologic, and social. The biologic domain includes embryonic and fetal growth, along with physical changes in the woman (alterations in hormones, organs, abdominal cavity). The psychologic domain includes perceptions and emotions. The social domain includes relationships with partner, family, friends, career, and health care setting. Gloger-Tippelt further explains that the psychosocial processes of the 40-week pregnancy can usefully be divided into four phases: Disruption, Adaptation, Centering, and Anticipation.

The Disruption Phase (conception to week 12) is a period of radical change on all levels: biologic, psychologic, and social. On the biologic level, the pregnant woman experiences hormonal and physiologic changes that include amenorrhea, increased estrogen and progesterone production, growth of the uterus, increased sensitivity of the breasts, and so forth. Psychologically, the woman must face alterations in her personal, social, and professional identities, while socially she may experience changes in the way she is perceived by family, friends, employer, and spouse. The woman in this phase may experience a wide range of emotions, including excitement, ecstasy, curiosity, impatience, depression, and fear of miscarriage (Gloger-Tippelt, 1983).

The Adaptation Phase (weeks 12 to 20) is a period of adjustment to the initial disruptions. The pregnant woman in this phase becomes familiar with the feelings and changes associated with being pregnant, and the emotional distress of the previous phase is reduced to a relative calm. Morning sickness, vomiting, and fatigue should have subsided by this phase, typically resulting in feelings of relief and satisfaction.

The Centering Phase (weeks 20 to 32) is dominated by the central task of producing a healthy child. During this phase, the pregnant woman begins to experience physical evidence (e.g., the child's movement) that the child is developing. In response to this evidence, the woman should feel increased responsibility for the health of the fetus and this can be a time of delight, joy, and excitement for the couple.

The Anticipation Phase (weeks 32 to birth) is the final period during which active preparation is made for the birth of the child. During this phase, as birth becomes imminent, the mother begins to look to the future and preparations are made for the child's arrival. (This preparation has sometimes been referred to as "nesting.") In addition to the positive feelings associated with this phase, the woman may experience some normal physical discomfort (e.g., constipation, indigestion, insomnia, and abdominal discomfort), resulting in the feeling: "I can't wait to get this over with!" As childbirth approaches, the pregnant woman may also experience fear of pain, loss of self-control, helplessness, and more.

The father-to-be may undergo significant stress during his wife's pregnancy. Shapiro (1987) conducted a series of interviews with 227 expectant and recent fathers. From these interviews, he found that fathers-to-be experience seven major areas of fear and concern about their wife's pregnancy, the birth process, and fatherhood. These areas include the following: queasiness, increased responsibility, obstetric-gynecologic matters, uncertain paternity, loss of spouse or child, being replaced, and their own life and death. Shapiro further explained that fathers seldom express these concerns to spouse, family, or friends.

Thus, the emotions experienced by a couple during pregnancy can be strongly positive or negative, depending on the phase and course of the pregnancy as well as conditions preceding the pregnancy (Gloger-Tippelt, 1983). Both the pregnant woman and the father-to-be might benefit from the family physician who is willing to discuss the psychosocial aspects of the pregnancy. In fact, such discussions will assist the couple in moving into the next stage of the family life cycle: the family with young children.

STAGE 3: THE FAMILY WITH YOUNG CHILDREN

Michael and Linda, a couple in their early thirties, have been married for the past 7 years. They visit their family physician with their 18-month-old daughter, Jessica, for a well-child exam. During the exam they explain that "things have changed" in their marriage. They feel "out of control" of Jessica's behaviors and their lives in general. They turn to their family physician for guidance.

Stage 3 of the family life cycle begins with the birth of a couple's first child. Baker and Ramsey (1984) point out that "the entry of the first child into a family system is one of the most dramatic changes a family experiences" (p. 56). Michael and Linda, like most couples with young children, face profound challenges and role changes in their lives as a result of becoming new parents. They find that they must accept a new family member into their family system. Their time alone together is much more limited than in the past, which diminishes their overall marital satisfaction. They discover that the responsibilities of parenting itself (e.g., discipline) can be awesome, and this may be complicated by extended family members who volunteer to become involved in the parenting process.

The Effects of Children on the Marital Relationship

The entry of a child into the marital relationship can have a significant effect on the couple's levels of physical and emotional intimacy. As mentioned earlier, marital satisfaction generally decreases after the birth of the first child (Schram, 1979). In fact, it is not uncommon for divorces and extramarital affairs to occur during this time in the couple's relationship.

Since the couple has less time together, intimate communication may decrease, including such nonverbal communication as touching, hugging, and kissing. Sexual relations may also decrease, related to the woman's body-image changes or the man's discomfort with these changes. Specifically, the husband may feel less attracted to his wife as a result of these changes, or the wife may feel self-conscious about her body, believing that her husband sees her as less attractive. In addition to these factors, intimacy may decrease simply due to the physical demands of the new family member. Infants and children require a great deal of attention, resulting in altered parental eating, sleeping, and work patterns. The entry of children into the family will also result in a decrease in privacy between the couple as they discover that children make demands on their time with little regard for their parents' needs or activities.

Michael and Linda were very excited when they first learned that Linda was pregnant with Jessica. In fact, they had planned for Jessica, and becoming parents had always been very important to them. As Linda progressed in her pregnancy, however, the couple became less sexually active, since both she and Michael felt self-consciousness about sex during pregnancy. When Jessica was first born, the couple was physically exhausted most of the time as a result of her awakening throughout the night. Even when she finally began to sleep through the night, the couple found themselves exhausted from the increased demands of parenting. Linda and Michael both found that they were paying more attention to Jessica than they were paying to their own relationship. In fact, the couple had not gone out alone together since she was born, explaining that they "could not trust a babysitter."

The couple's family physician, on hearing about their concerns, arranged for an extended discussion about their relationship and parenting. During this discussion, he helped them to explore their thoughts and feelings about these issues. He assured them that conflict during this period is normal. He advised them not to misinterpret their difficulties as "fatal flaws" in the relationship. He also recommended that they increase "quality communication" between themselves, especially active listening. And finally, he recommended that they spend more time alone together, engaging in activities they enjoyed prior to the pregnancy (e.g., intimate dinners or movies.) The couple followed this advice, which resulted in some immediate improvements in the relationship.

Effective Parenting

During this stage of the family life cycle, certain conditions in the home climate are necessary for effective parenting. These conditions fall into two broad categories, according to Jensen and Kingston (1986): love and organization. A loving home climate is characterized as having emotional expressiveness, freedom of choice, encouragement of individuality, affection, and a sense of belonging. A well-organized home climate is characterized as safe and nourishing, meaningful (regarding values and beliefs), awareness-oriented (regarding self and the world), balanced between work and play, and relatively structured. Parents are responsible for establishing loving and well-organized homes for their children's healthy development.

Michael and Linda will provide a loving home climate for Jessica by encouraging her to experience a wide range of emotions, while at the same time helping her to cope with difficult emotions. For example, at times she might experience rejection by her friends, and feel lonely, sad, and disappointed. In response, Michael and Linda can help her to cope with these feelings by having her discuss them in an open, honest, supportive, expressive environment. They may also demonstrate their love for her by allowing her the freedom to make independent choices and to learn from her mistakes. If she is to develop in a healthy fashion, Jessica must be encouraged to be unique and individualistic while also seeing herself as part of a collective, collaborative group (i.e., the family). Much of Jessica's sense of belonging to her family will result from her parents' demonstrated physical and verbal affection towards her.

Michael and Linda provide an organized home by offering Jessica a sense of structure, including "rules, expectations, limits, standards, encouragement, guidelines, and laws" (Jensen and Kingston, 1986, p. 149). Although playtime is strongly encouraged, work must also be encouraged to teach Jessica a sense of responsibility. Values are taught in order to give her a sense of the meaning of life as well as a desire for knowledge and truth about herself and the world. Another component of organization is safety and protection from danger. Jessica will grow up feeling competent and confident about herself to the extent that her parents, Linda and Michael, provide a home with these qualities.

STAGE 4: THE FAMILY WITH ADOLESCENTS

Denise Doe is a 38-year-old married woman with two adolescent children, a 16-year-old son (Danny) and a 14-year-old daughter (Dana). Her husband, Dan, is an engineer and Denise is a homemaker. Denise is visiting her family physician because she has been having difficulty sleeping. She also reports that she feels sad, helpless, and irritable lately, and she relates her feelings to concerns about her children.

The time of adolescence (approximately 12- to 18-years-old) can be turbulent for both adolescents and their families. In order to cope effectively with the changes associated with this period, the family must increase its flexibility and "soften" its boundaries to allow for the adolescent's need for autonomy and independence. This "easing up on the reins" may be very difficult for parents, but it is necessary for the healthy emotional development of the child and family.

According to Muuss (1975) adolescence is "a period of social, personal, sexual, religious, political, and vocational adjustments as well as a period of striving for increasing emotional and financial independence from parents" (p. 10). These adjustments occur as the adolescent experiments with new styles of thinking, feeling, and behaving, which are influenced by peers, the media, and popular public figures (especially in music, television, sports, and so on). Thus, it is no surprise to find that this period can affect the entire family and create parent-child and parent-parent conflicts.

In a healthy, stable family, the adolescent's development will be integrated into the family system and the changes will lead to further growth for the entire family. However, in a disorganized and unstable family these changes will lead to disruption and disharmony, and the family may feel alienated, threatened, and confused, rejecting the adolescent. The family's health and stability at this stage will be a function of their successful progression through the previous stages of family life cycle development. Specifically, by young adulthood, the adolescent's parents should have developed a secure sense of their own identity and self-confidence. If this has not occurred, the adolescent's changes will be especially threatening to parents. As a newly married couple, parents should have established strong and secure bonds between themselves as a result of effective communication, mutual support, and trust. Such bonds are important when the adolescent challenges the integrity or stability of the marital relationship. As a couple with young children, the family should have developed a loving and organized home atmosphere. Such an atmosphere will provide the adolescent with a sense of support and emotional safety as well as a place to test new thoughts, feelings, and behaviors.

If the developmental tasks listed earlier are not achieved, the adolescent and family will stagnate or pathologic symptoms will appear in one or more family members. Consider, for example, the case of the Doe family mentioned earlier. Denise has developed depressive symptoms in response to her family's difficulties with adolescence. Specifically, Danny has begun to listen to "punk rock" music and he wears his hair "spiked" when he goes out with his friends. He recently began to drive and he wishes to borrow the family car frequently; this worries his mother who now seriously doubts Danny's level of responsibility. When Danny's mother confronts him, he becomes argumentative, exclaiming "You just don't understand me!" Dana, on the other hand, has been a "perfect child," though recently her grades have dropped from mostly A's to B's and C's. To her mother, Dana seems preoccupied with boys, clothing, and makeup. Her mother fears that she, like Danny, is changing and that "she will not amount to anything if she doesn't get her grades up." To make matters worse, Dan denies that there is a problem in the family. In response, Denise becomes quite frustrated with Dan as she perceives him as a "passive, disinterested father."

In terms of family life cycle development, Denise's emotional distress can be explained as follows. First, she has been reluctant to allow her children to move in and out of the family system and experiment with new behaviors and beliefs. In other words, she has been overprotective towards her children by trying to keep them within family boundaries and away from external controversial phenomena. Second, Denise has not adequately focused on her own career and personal development, and therefore she has extra time and energy on her hands. Unfortunately, she uses this time to worry about the children. And third, she and Dan have not adequately developed their level of intimacy as evidenced by Dan's inability to listen to Denise's fears without rejecting them as irrational.

In response to Denise's depressive symptoms, her family physician prescribed antidepressants. However, he also met with Denise and Dan to discuss the predictable crises and challenges of adolescence, including experimentation, the shifting of values, and so forth. He assured the couple that their adolescents' behaviors are normal and important for their growth, as well as the family's growth. He emphasized the importance of Denise's career and he recommended that she pursue this area of growth. And finally, he observed that the couple does not communicate well regarding controversial issues. He emphasized the importance of listening and recommended that they discuss the children on a regular basis, using their best listening skills. As a result of this intervention, the Doe family has become more willing to accept each others' differences, and they tend to be more satisfied with their interrelationships. In addition to these improvements, Denise's depressive symptoms have begun to subside and the family environment is less stressful because Denise is no longer symptomatic.

STAGE 5: LAUNCHING THE CHILDREN AND MOVING ON

Steve is a 53-year-old married man with a history of hypertension and heart disease. He visits his family physician because recently he has been feeling "tightness" in his chest. Steve's physical examination, ECG, and laboratory work are all within normal limits, and he admits that "things are strained at home since the kids went to college." Steve explains that his wife, Alice, has been "pressuring" him for more time together, and for more intimacy in the relationship. He is also preoccupied with his job as an engineer and his decreased sex drive, "compared with a few years ago."

The launching stage of the family life cycle begins with the first child becoming a young adult and leaving home. It ends with the "empty nest," as the last child of a family leaves his or her family of origin. Duvall (1977) describes seven family developmental tasks at this stage:

1. Rearranging the physical facilities and resources
2. Meeting the expenses of a launching-center family
3. Reallocating responsibilities among grown and growing children
4. Coming to terms with themselves as husband and wife
5. Maintaining open systems of communication within the family and between the family and others
6. Widening the family circle through release of young adult children and recruitment of new members by marriage
7. Reconciling conflicting loyalties and philosophies of life

Thus, in this stage the family must begin to accept the departures of their own children as well as the entrances of their children's new families into their own lives. These departures and entrances may result in changes in the nature and quality of the married couple's relationship.

As the children of a family leave their parents' home during this stage, there are typically positive and negative consequences. To the extent that the family has developed appropriately through the family life cycle, the children will be prepared to leave home. Their departure will allow for further growth of the marital relationship as well as the children's personal growth. Failure to develop appropriately as a family will likely result in children who are poorly equipped to face the social and psychologic demands of life outside the immediate family circle. Furthermore, a married couple who has not grown together over the family life span may be less inclined to feel compatible with each other at this time in their relationship.

In the case of Steve and Alice, the exit of their children from home left Alice feeling somewhat lonely and empty. She had served the family as their homemaker for the past 27 years. When the children departed, she no longer had clearly defined full-time responsibilities. In response to her loneliness and emptiness she began to exert pressure on Steve to be "more of a husband and father." In particular, she wanted him to spend more time at home and she felt the desire to be more involved in close relationships with their children and grandchildren. Steve, at the same time, had just begun to feel increasingly vulnerable at his job, since younger employees were taking the jobs of older employees. As a result of these new demands of the launching stage, Steve felt nervous and inadequate about his abilities to live up to the new standards of his family relationships. In fact, he began developing the symptoms described above when his youngest son and daughter-in-law had their first child.

Steve's problems during this launching stage actually began at an earlier time in his life. Specifically, he has had difficulties at this stage because of his inadequate development through the previous stages of the family life cycle. As a young unmarried person he never established himself in a career; instead he accepted positions that allowed little room for advancement or security. This made him more vulnerable to job threats as a married adult with children. As a newly married man, Steve never adequately developed the skills and self-confidence necessary for the development of a healthy intimate relationship with Alice. Specifically, he did not feel comfortable discussing "deep, personal" matters with his wife or children, and as a result he felt out of place when called upon for his family's personal and emotional support. And finally, Steve never took an active parenting role as a result of his long hours at work and his belief that parenting was Alice's responsibility. This example well illustrates the potential effects of the launching years as well as the need for individuals' adequate development prior to this stage. In the next section the final stage of family development is presented: the family in later life.

STAGE 6: THE FAMILY IN LATER LIFE

Martha, a 66-year-old woman, has a history of arthritis that causes her significant pain and severely limits her mobility. She visits her family physician regularly for "checkups" and during one particular visit she expresses concern that her 67-year-old husband, Joseph, has not visited a doctor in years. In addition to her concern about his physical health, she admits to being worried about his mental status: his memory apparently has been failing and his judgment has been questionable since his retirement 2 years ago.

During this, the final stage of the family life

cycle, elderly persons must accept the shifting of generational roles. In other words, they must accept the fact that their children will create families of their own, be responsible for their own life decisions, and play a less active role in the family circle in which they grew up. They may also note a gradual reversal in dependency roles as their children assume advice-giving and "looking out" for their parents.

The quality of later life will be dependent upon the aging person's adjustment to psychosocial changes (e.g., departure of children from the home, retirement, grandparenthood, widowhood), as well as adjustment to physical changes and illness (Walsh, 1980).

Adjustment to Psychosocial Changes

Couples who are able to let go of their children and become independent during the previous launching stage will experience a sense of freedom that may enhance their intimate relationship. Retirement can also result in increased freedom and an enhanced marital relationship, depending on the couple's financial status, their desire for retirement, their support networks, and their preretirement relationship. Couples who have had difficulties with separation from their children, as well as those who are financially unstable or without adequate support systems, will have a more difficult time in their later years of life.

The death of a spouse is another important concern of families in their later years. According to Walsh (1980), women are four times more likely than men to suffer the spouses' death. They are also "more likely to be widowed at an earlier age with many years of life ahead" (p. 202). She explains that the death of a spouse may produce an initial sense of loss, disorientation, and loneliness, contributing to an increase in death and suicide rates in the first year after it occurs.

Grandparenthood is an important experience that characterizes this stage of the family life cycle for most older adults. Becoming a grandparent can be an exciting and meaningful experience that provides a variety of challenges and joys to all three generations, including the grandparent, parent, and grandchild. The grandparent-grandchild relationship offers a "special bond which is not complicated by the responsibilities, obligations, and conflicts inherent in the parent-child relationship" (Walsh, 1980, p. 204). In fact, Walsh suggests that perhaps "grandparents and grandchildren get along so well because they have a common enemy" (p. 204). She further warns that problems can occur in the interrelationships between the three generations if a grandchild is "triangulated in a conflict between parent and grandparent."

Adjustment to Physical Changes and Illness

Although aging is not synonymous with disease, illness is a reality to most families in later life. LaRue and Jarvik (1982) review epidemiologic data that demonstrate that the frequency of illness increases with age. For example, 86 per cent of elderly Americans have chronic health problems, while between 15 and 25 per cent of older persons living in the community are affected with mental illnesses.

Aging affects most of the body's systems in an adverse fashion (Stevens-Long, 1988). The skin and bones lose their resilience over time, resulting in increased vulnerability to wrinkles, age spots, bone loss, fractures, osteoporosis, generalized aches and pains, and so on. Most internal organ systems, including the heart, lungs, kidneys, and intestines are also affected by aging. Examples of changes that occur in the older patient are coronary atherosclerosis, which may produce angina pectoris; diminished pulmonary vital capacity; decreased production of digestive juices, which may result in impaired ability to tolerate favorite foods; prostatic hypertrophy, which may produce bothersome nocturia; and reduced exercise tolerance.

The central nervous system is also affected by aging. In the later years, the weight of the brain declines and it contains less water and protein, with more fatty tissue and inorganic salt. Blood circulation to the brain also declines, and as much as 40 per cent of the cells in some cortical areas are lost by the age of 80 or 90 years. Despite these neurologic changes, however, there is no evidence that the normal aging process causes mental illness or senility in the elderly (Stevens-Long, 1988). Nonetheless, mental illnesses do affect the elderly. For example, many elderly persons (i.e., between 10 and 20 per cent of people over 65 years old) suffer from cognitive impairment related to neurologic changes. Of these persons, 22 to 57 per cent are believed to have Alzheimer's disease. It is important that the physician distinguish these problems from the benign forgetfulness sometimes related to aging. Among older persons living in the community, 25 per cent show significant depressive symptoms, while up to 70 per cent experience one depressive episode. Sometimes depression can result in memory impairment (i.e., pseudodementia), which can be mistaken for Alzheimer's disease.

These physical changes and the deterioration of their health can result in serious concerns for the elderly and their families. In fact, these changes are primarily responsible for the family's need to become caretakers of their parents. As elderly individuals become less physically strong and healthy, they become more dependent upon others, especially family members, to take care of them. The results of these new demands on some family members depends, to a large extent, on the family's development prior to this stage of the family life cycle. For example, if the family has developed healthy, supportive relationships over the years, there will be a greater likelihood that the transition to this new dependency role will be smooth.

Martha and Joseph, from the example, face most of the issues described above, including retirement, illness, and the potential death of a spouse. In fact their problems seemed relatively minor to them until 2 years ago when Joe was forced into retirement by his company. In an extended discussion arranged by the couple's family physician, it became apparent that Joe had become increasingly depressed over his job loss and the sudden resulting changes in his personal identity, self-esteem, and life style. His depression probably accounted for his cognitive problems (since they improved substantially after he later received counseling for depression.) In response to Joe's changes, Martha began to feel concerned and depressed. In fact, she admitted to her family physician that she was afraid of "losing Joe to widowhood." Furthermore, the couple felt "guilty" about "leaning on their children," who were "happily married with their own families now." Their family physician encouraged them to discuss their concerns with their children, who responded with concern, love, and support for Martha and Joe.

DISRUPTIONS IN THE LIFE CYCLE: DIVORCE, REMARRIAGE, ILLNESS, AND DEATH

Bill and Sally have been married for 20 years. The couple has three children who are aged 14, 16, and 18 years old. Bill is seeing his family physician because recently he decided that he no longer wishes to be married to Sally. He explains that the marriage is "dull and boring" and he feels that he is "stagnating."

The family life cycle model assumes that families experience certain predictable and observable changes over the course of the family's life. However, it is also assumed that this cycle may be disrupted by events that are unexpected or unplanned. Such events include divorce, remarriage, serious illness, and death. In this section, these events are examined in terms of how they affect families across the family life cycle.

Divorce

Between one third and one half of all marriages end in divorce. Divorce is a complex process, consisting of multiple stages (Kaslow and Schwartz, 1987). Each stage has its own unique challenges and emotions that affect the entire family. (For a general discussion of the impact of divorce, see chapter 7 of this text.)

Carter and McGoldrick (1980) examine divorce as it relates to family life cycle development (see Table 3–4). These authors divide the process into four phases: the decision to divorce, planning the breakup of the system, separation, and the divorce itself (including single-parenthood: custodial and noncustodial). In each phase, they present attitudes necessary for emotional transition into the next phase. They also present developmental issues that must be resolved for healthy coping with each phase of the divorce process.

According to the model proposed by Carter and McGoldrick (1980), in the first phase of a divorce individuals must accept that they cannot resolve their problems sufficiently for the relationship to continue. They must also accept their own contributions to the marital problems and failure. In the second phase, the couple must make viable arrangements for the breakup of the system. This includes working cooperatively on resolving issues of custody, visitation, and finances. They must also deal with their extended family about the divorce. In the separation phase of divorce, individuals must be willing to cooperate in their coparental relationship (assuming that they have children), while also resolving their feelings of attachment to their spouse. This process entails mourning the loss of their intact nuclear family, adapting to living apart, and realigning relationships with the extended family. During the divorce itself, the couple must work on overcoming their emotional pain, including hurt, anger, and guilt. This is accomplished by giving up fantasies of reunion; retrieving hopes, dreams, and expectations from the marriage; and staying connected with extended families.

In the post-divorce family, parents must be willing to maintain constructive contact with their ex-spouse in order to maximize parenting relationships with children. They must also minimize conflicts with their ex-spouse in order to avoid emotional trauma to children. As part of coping after a divorce, individuals are also encouraged to develop social networks outside of the context of their ex-marriage.

Bill, from the example above, is in the first phase of the divorce process; he does not believe that his marital problems can be solved and he is willing to consider termination of the relationship. For his healthy development in this phase Bill needs to recognize his contributions to the marital problems. However, he is unwilling to do so; instead he blames the problems on Sally. For example, he reports that his marriage has been dull and boring; yet he does not admit that he could have stimulated more excitement and growth in the relationship. As long as Bill continues to engage in such denial, he is likely to experience similar difficulties in future relationships.

During this disruption of the family life cycle it is extremely important that the family physician offer unconditional support to both patients, since this period is quite painful. It is also important that the physician challenge divorcing couples to discover and change problematic relationship behaviors. For example, Bill and Sally's family physician should gently and tactfully challenge both to consider their contributions to the dullness and boredom in the relationship. Perhaps Bill stopped listening to Sally, assuming that he knew everything she had to say. Or perhaps Bill became so preoccupied with work that he became disinterested in his family. In addition, Sally might have become stagnant in her personal life, resulting in marital boredom for herself and her partner. In

Table 3–4. DISLOCATIONS OF THE FAMILY LIFE CYCLE REQUIRING ADDITIONAL STEPS TO RESTABILIZE AND PROCEED DEVELOPMENTALLY*

Phase	Emotional Process of Transition—Prerequisite Attitude	Developmental Issues
Divorce		
1. The decision to divorce	Acceptance of inability to resolve marital tensions sufficiently to continue relationship	Acceptance of one's own part in the failure of the marriage
2. Planning the breakup of the system	Supporting viable arrangements for all parts of the system	a. Working cooperatively on problems of custody, visitation, finances b. Dealing with extended family about the divorce
3. Separation	a. Willingness to continue cooperative coparental relationship b. Work on resolution of attachment to spouse	a. Mourning loss of intact family b. Restructuring marital and parent-child relationships; adaptation to living apart c. Realignment of relationships with extended family; staying connected with spouse's extended family
4. The divorce	More work on emotional divorce: Overcoming hurt, anger, guilt, etc.	a. Mourning loss of intact family: giving up fantasies of reunion b. Retrieval of hopes, dreams, expectations from the marriage c. Staying connected with extended families
Post-Divorce Family		
A. Single-parent family	Willingness to maintain parental contact with ex-spouse and support contact of children with ex-spouse and his family	a. Making flexible visitation arrangements with ex-spouse and his or her family
B. Single-parent (Noncustodial)	Willingness to maintain parental contact with ex-spouse and support custodial parent's relationship with children	a. Finding ways to continue effective parenting relationship with children b. Rebuilding own social network

*From Carter, E., and McGoldrick, M.: The Family Life Cycle: A Framework for Family Therapy. New York, Gardner Press, Inc., 1980.

any event, a family physician can help a couple like Bill and Sally by understanding and discussing their particular stage of the family life cycle. If they are not experiencing the appropriate developmental milestones for their stage in the process (e.g., acceptance of fault in the relationship), they might be encouraged to do so by the family physician.

Beal (1980) relates the effects of divorce to the couple's stage in the family life cycle. For example, he explains that divorce in a marriage without children has the fewest immediate consequences. He reports that the highest incidence of divorce occurs in families with young children. Much of the stress of divorce is felt by children and parents in the first year after divorce; however, parental conflict tends to prolong the healing process in children. Thus, family physicians seeing divorcing parents should encourage them to minimize conflict "for the sake of the children." Beal further explains that adolescents, when their parents are divorced, "have a capacity to establish more emotional distance than younger children." Divorce in later life can be especially difficult if one member is "cut off" from extended families. Furthermore, dating may be difficult for older divorced individuals who have not dated for between 20 and 50 years.

Remarriage

Remarriage is a life cycle event that involves complicated and substantial adjustments for family members. According to McGoldrick and Carter (1980), a second marriage involves the interweaving of three, four, or more families whose previous family life cycle course has been disrupted by death or divorce" (p. 265). They further elaborate on the process of remarriage, emphasizing the difficulties involved: "new relationships are . . . harder to negotiate because they do not develop slowly as intact families do but must begin midstream, after another family's life cycle has been dislocated. Naturally, second families carry the scars of first families" (p. 266).

McGoldrick & Carter (1980) offer a developmental model of the remarried family (see Table 3–5, based on a developmental schema presented by Ransom, Schlesinger, and Dendeyer, 1979).

Serious Illness and Death

Serious illnesses (chronic or acute) and death have the potential to disrupt the family life cycle as well as the individual lives of most family members. To some degree, the effects of illness and death will depend on the age of the ill or deceased person as well as the stage of the family life cycle in which the death has occurred. For example, the sudden death of a healthy young child will result in overwhelming shock and despair. Herz (1980) explains: "The death of a child is viewed by most people as life's greatest tragedy. This view derives from the fact that a child's

Table 3–5. REMARRIED FAMILY FORMATION: A DEVELOPMENTAL OUTLINE*†

Steps	Prerequisite Attitude	Developmental Issues
1. Entering the new Relationship	Recovery from loss of first marriage (adequate "emotional divorce")	Recommitment to marriage and to forming a family with readiness to deal with the complexity and ambiguity
2. Conceptualizing and planning new marriage and family	Accepting one's own fears and those of new spouse and children about remarriage and forming a stepfamily Accepting need for time and patience for adjustment to complexity and ambigutiy of: 1. Multiple new roles 2. Boundaries: space, time, membership and authority 3. Affective Issues: guilt, loyalty conflicts, desire for mutuality, unresolvable past hurts	a. Work on openness in the new relationships to avoid pseudomutuality b. Plan for maintenance of cooperative co-parental relationships with ex-spouses c. Plan to help children deal with fears, loyalty conflicts, and membership in two systems d. Realignment of relationships with extended family to include new spouse and children e. Plan maintenance of connections for children with extended family of ex-spouses(s)
3. Remarriage and reconstitution of family	Final resolution of attachment to previous spouse and ideal of "intact" family; Acceptance of a different model of family with permeable boundaries	a. Restructuring family boundaries to allow for inclusion of new spouse–stepparent b. Realignment of relationships throughout subsystems to permit interweaving of several systems c. Making room for relationships of all children with biologic (noncustodial) parents, grandparents, and other extended family members d. Sharing memories and histories to enhance stepfamily integration

*From Carter, E., and McGoldrick, M.: The Family Life Cycle: A Framework for Family Therapy. New York, Gardner Press, Inc., 1980.
†Variation on a developmental schema presented by Ransom *et al.* (1979)

death appears so egregiously out of place in the life cycle" (p. 227).

The death of a sick elderly patient, on the other hand, might be a relief to a family if the patient is very old, debilitated, or in pain. Streim and Marshall (1988) discuss the importance of the physician's role in helping a family to cope with the death of an elderly patient. These authors point out that the physician commonly regards the care of a dying elderly patient as a "hopeless endeavor." Alternatively, they explain that the physician might help the patient and family to face death, diminish fears, and reduce the patient's suffering, isolation, and loss of autonomy.

After the death of a family member the developmental task to be accomplished is to "grieve over the loss and then to reinvest in future functioning" (Walsh, 1980, p. 203). For many widows, especially young widows, remarriage is a desirable way to reinvest in future functioning. To some extent, remarriage for the older adult will be "successful" to the degree that the children, including adult children, are integrated into the new family.

Applying Family Life Cycle Concepts to Family Practice

Thus far we have presented a model for understanding individual behavior and development in the context of the family life cycle. It has been shown that most individuals function in the context of a larger family system that they impact on and that impacts on them. In this section, we present some direct implications of the family life cycle, as well as applications of various techniques to the treatment of family life cycle issues.

According to Doherty and Baird (1987), physicians vary in their levels of involvement in family issues (see Table 61–1). A physician may become involved in family issues at five levels, ranging from minimal to extreme involvement (i.e., family therapy). The level to which a physician intervenes with a family will be dependent on the physician, the patient, and the illness.

Some physicians have the motivation and skills to engage patients in family interventions, regardless of the type of the presenting complaint, whereas other physicians lack the motivation or skills to do so. Patients also vary in their levels of interest in family interventions, with some patients desiring minimal involvement and others wishing to have their physician fully involved in almost all medical and many nonmedical problems. And finally, patients' illnesses will likely determine the level of physician intervention. In acute nondebilitating injuries (e.g., sprained ankles), the physician would be less likely to become deeply involved with family dynamics. On the other hand, the patient with a terminal illness would require much more attention to family issues.

Attentiveness to family developmental processes

Table 3–6. HEALTH MAINTENANCE SCHEDULE AS RELATED TO STAGES OF THE FAMILY LIFE CYCLE*

Stage (Length of Time)	Adults—Age at End of Each Stage M	Adults—Age at End of Each Stage F	Type of Health Encounter	Number of Visits for Parents M	Number of Visits for Parents F	Number of Visits for Children	Issues in M.D.'s Assessment of Family Development
Between families (0–2 years)	20	20	Employment Physical	1	1		a. Relationship to family of origin b. Motivation and readiness for marriage
Newly married (2 years)	22	22	Premarital Contraception Health maintenance	1 1	1 1 1		a. Knowledge of sexuality b. Awareness of contraceptive methodology c. Patient understanding of marriage, marital commitment d. Planning for family medical services
Young children (13 years)	35	35	Prenatal care Parent education	 5	9 5		a. Understanding of importance of prenatal care b. Knowledge of parenting and child health care (may be spaced over many years)
			Child care 1st year 2nd year Age 3 to 14 Health maintenance M—q 5 yr F—q yr	 2	 13	 6 3 3	c. Parents' assessment of child's psychologic and emotional development d. Parents' reaction to adjustment to children, participation in child-related activities
Adolescents (7 years)	44	44	School/camp physical Health maintenance M—1 at 40 to q 2 yr F—q yr	 3	 9	3	a. Work history and progress b. Child's relationship to parents c. Parents' understanding and preparedness for adolescence
Moving on (15 years)	59	59	M—q 2 yr till 50th q yr F—q yr	13	15		a. Assessment of adjustment to life as a couple b. Work plans and retirement plans c. Assessment of frequency of visits d. Reaction to physiologic changes of middle age e. Relationship to children vis-à-vis acceptance of parent-offspring separation
Later life (15 years)	70	70		11	11		a. Nutritional assessment b. Relationship with children and their spouses c. Relationship with grandchildren
Total Visits by Family Members				37	66	15	= 118 family visits

*From Ramsey, C. N. Jr.: Developmental theory of families: The family life cycle. *In* Rakel, R. (Ed.): Textbook of Family Practice. 3rd ed. Philadelphia, W. B. Saunders Co., 1984.

can be facilitated by the physician's use of the genogram (see Chapter 74). The genogram, or family tree, is a diagram that maps out family structure and organization across at least three generations. This diagram provides an efficient means of constructing a visual clinical summary of family members' names, ages, life experiences, family relational patterns and other information important to life cycle development. The genogram can be constructed relatively quickly by the physician and patient, and the genogram can be revised as new information becomes available.

Health maintenance schedules that include family process interventions can provide appropriate methods for applying family life cycle concepts. Ramsey (1984) has constructed a schedule for providing health maintenance across the family life cycle (see Table 3–6). The farthest right hand column of this table outlines issues to be addressed by the family physician, according to the family's stage of family life cycle development. Ramsey demonstrates, by this schedule, that a family of three members (mother, father, and child) can be seen for health maintenance for 118 visits over 50 years. He further points out that most (41) of the family visits take place during the early marriage and childbearing years, with 15 visits for child health maintenance. Sixty-two visits are for health maintenance in adults over 44 years old.

References

Baker, L., and Ramsey, C. N.: The birth of the first child. *In* Rakel, R. E. (Ed.): Textbook of Family Medicine. 3rd ed. Philadelphia, W. B. Saunders Co., 1984.

Baltes, P. B.: Life-span developmental psychology: Some converging observations on history and theory. *In* Baltes, P. B., and Brim, O. G., Jr. (Eds.): Lifespan Development and Behavior. Vol. 2. New York, Academic Press, 1979.

Barnhill, L., and Longo, D.: Fixation and regression in the family life cycle. Fam. Process, *17*(4):469–478, 1978.

Beal, E. W.: Separation, divorce, and single-parent families. *In* Carter, E. A., and McGoldrick M. (Eds): The Family Life Cycle: A Framework for Family Therapy. New York, Gardner Press, Inc., 1980.

Berman, E. M., and Lief, H. I.: Marital therapy from a psychiatric perspective: An overview. Am. J. Psychiatry, *132*(6):583–592, 1975.

Birren, J. E., and Schaie, K. W. (Eds.): Handbook of the Psychology of Aging. 2nd ed. New York, Van Nostrand Reinhold, 1985.

Breunlin, D. C.: Clinical implications of oscillation theory: Family development and the process of change. *In* Ramsey, C. N., Jr. (Ed.): Family Systems in Medicine. New York, Guilford Press, 1989.

Campbell, T. L.: Family's impact on health: A critical review. Fam. Sys. Med., *4*(2 and 3):135–328, 1986. *Campbell provides a comprehensive critical review of the research on the family's impact on health, including cardiovascular disease, hypertension, diabetes, asthma, pregnancy, obesity, mental illness, and others. He reviews epidemiologic and family systems studies, and he draws conclusions that have important implications for research and practice.*

Carter, E., and McGoldrick, M. (Eds.): The Family Life Cycle: A Framework for Family Therapy. New York, Gardner Press, Inc., 1980. *These authors offer an excellent overview of family life cycle development (in six stages), special issues in families and in family therapy, and major variations in the family life cycle. Their edited text is written primarily for family therapists; however, others with strong interests in family systems theory and the family life cycle will certainly find it interesting, comprehensive, and useful. The present chapter has been organized according to the model presented in this book.*

Colarusso, C. A., and Nemiroff, R. A.: Adult Development: A New Dimension in Psychodynamic Theory and Practice. New York, Norton, 1981. *The authors of this three-part book review past theories of adult development; they develop a current psychodynamic theory of adult development; and they describe the relevance of these theories to clinical work. Their review of past theories is brief but inclusive, from "antiquity to the present." Their psychodynamic section, which includes seven hypotheses about adult development is interesting and insightful. And their final section offers diagnostic and treatment applications of value to individual and family psychotherapists.*

Doherty, W. J., and Baird, M.: Family-Centered Medical Care: A Clinical Casebook. New York, Guilford Press, 1987. *The authors of this book provide a structure for evaluating levels of physician involvement with families, ranging from "minimal emphasis on family" to "family therapy." They then organize 71 actual case studies submitted by family physicians according to the level of involvement of the physician caring for the patient. This is an interesting and sensitive book written for family physicians and others involved in family-centered medical care.*

Doherty, W. J., and Jacobson, N. S.: Marriage and the family. *In* Wolman, B. B. (Ed.): Handbook of Developmental Psychology. Englewood Cliffs, Prentice Hall, 1982.

Duvall, E.: Marriage and Family Development. 5th ed. Philadelphia, J. B. Lippincott Co., 1977. *This is Duvall's fifth edition of her comprehensive and important text on marriage and family development. The author was among the first researchers to introduce the concept of family life cycle development, and this text provides valuable theoretical, conceptual, and statistical information about marriage and family development.*

Erikson, E. H.: Childhood and Society. 2nd ed. New York, W. W. Norton, 1963.

Frank, E., Anderson, C., and Rubenstein, D.: Frequency of sexual dysfunction in "normal" couples. N. Engl. J. Med., *299*(3):111–115, 1978.

Gilligan, C.: In a Different Voice. Cambridge, Howard Press, 1982. *Much research on individual lifespan development has been based on studies of men. Alternatively, this important text presents a view of the development of women as contrasted with the development of men.*

Gloger-Tippelt, G.: A process model of the pregnancy course. Hum. Dev., *26*:134–148, 1983.

Gould, R. L.: Transformations: Growth and Change in Adult Life. New York, Simon and Schuster, 1978.

Haley, J.: Uncommon Therapy: The Psychiatric Techniques of Milton Erikson. New York, W. W. Norton, 1973. *The author of this book presents the work of the clinical hypnotist, Milton Erickson, as it relates to family life cycle development. Most of Haley's presentation is accomplished through case studies of his and Erickson's patients during the stages of courtship, marriage, childbirth and families with young children, weaning parents from children, and old age.*

Hall, D. T.: Careers in Organizations. Santa Monica, Goodyear, 1976.

Herz, F.: The impact of death and serious illness on the family life cycle. *In* Carter, E. A., and McGoldrick, M. (Eds.): The Family Life Cycle: A Framework for Family Therapy. New York, Gardner Press, Inc., 1980.

Holmes, T. H., and Rahe, R. H.: The social readjustment rating scale. J. Psychosom. Res. *11*:213–218, 1967. *This is the original presentation of the important Social Readjustment Rating Scale (i.e., the "Holmes and Rahe Scale"). This scale provides weighted values for 43 stressful events according to the effects of these events on health. The Holmes and Rahe Scale is one of the most frequently used psychosocial instruments in medicine.*

Jacobson, N. S., and Holtzworth-Munroe, A.: Marital therapy: A social learning-cognitive perspective. *In* Jacobson, N. S., and Gurman, A. S. (Eds.): Clinical Handbook of Marital Therapy. New York, Guilford Press, 1986.

Jacobson, N. S., and Margolin, G.: Marital Therapy: Strategies Based on Social Learning and Behavior Exchange Principles. New York, Brunner/Mazel, 1979.

Jensen, L. C., and Kingston, M.: Parenting. New York, Holt, Rinehart and Winston, 1986. *This textbook provides a thorough review of research and theories of parenting, and the authors propose their "Home Climate Theory" of effective parenting, which is a thoughtful integration of previous work in the area. They also review theories of discipline, and they address issues of special parenting situations (e.g., handicapped children, single parenting).*

Kaslow, F. W., and Schwartz, L. L.: The Dynamics of Divorce: A Life Cycle Perspective. New York, Brunner/Mazel, 1987. *This book provides an excellent overview of divorce from family systems and life cycle perspectives. The authors present information regarding legal, financial, economic, psychologic, and social aspects of divorce, as well as the effects of divorce on children and parents.*

Kegan, R.: The Evolving Self. Cambridge, Howard Press, 1982.

Kohlberg, L.: The Philosophy of Moral Development. San Francisco, Harper & Row, 1981.

La Rue, A., and Jarvik, L. F.: Old age and biobehavioral changes. *In* Wolman, B. B. (Ed.): Handbook of Developmental Psychology. Englewood Cliffs, Prentice Hall, 1982.

Levinson, D. J.: A conception of adult development. Am. Psychol., *41*(1):3–13, 1986.

Levinson, D. J., Darrow, C. N., Klein, E. B., et al.: The Seasons of a Man's Life. New York, Knopf, 1978. *This book reports Levinson's classic study of the development of 40 adult men, including biologists, novelists, business executives, and blue collar workers. Some have called Levinson's research "the most comprehensive and heuristic modern study of adult development." This book is quite readable and it is recommended to anyone interested in individual adulthood development.*

Liese, B. S., Larson, M. W., Johnson, C. A., and Hourigan, R. J.: An experimental study of two methods for teaching sexual history taking skills. Fam. Med., *21*(1), 1989.

Like, R. C., Rogers, J., and McGoldrick, M.: Reading and interpreting genograms: A systematic approach. J. Fam. Pract., *26*(4):407–412, 1988.

McGoldrick, M., and Carter, E. A.: Forming a remarried family. *In* Carter E. A., and McGoldrick, M. (Eds.): The Family Life Cycle: A Framework for Family Therapy. New York, Gardner Press, 1980.

McGoldrick, M., and Gerson, R.: Genograms in Family Assessment. New York, W. W. Norton, 1985. *This book outlines one approach to constructing genograms for collecting family diagnostic information. The authors describe genogram applications in clinical practice as well as the future of computerized genograms for family research. This book is made particularly interesting by the authors' use of well-known family genograms for illustrative purposes (e.g., the families of Freud, Churchill, Gandhi, Einstein, and Roosevelt).*

Moore, J. T., and Goldstein, Y.: Sexual problems among family practice patients. J. Fam. Pract., *10*(2):243–247, 1980.

Muuss, R. E.: Theories of Adolescence. 3rd ed. New York, Random House, 1975.

Nease, D. F., and Liese, B. S.: Perceptions and treatment of sexual problems. Fam. Med., *19*(6):468–470, 1987.

Neugarten, B.: Adaptation and the life cycle. The Counseling Psychologist, *6*(1):16–20, 1976.

Neugarten, B.: Time, age, and the life cycle. Am. J. Psychiatry, *136*(7):887–894, 1979.

Ramsey, C. N. Jr.: Developmental theory of families: The family life cycle. *In* Rakel, R.: Principles of Family Practice. 3rd ed. Philadelphia, W. B. Saunders Co., 1984.

Ransom, J. W., Schlesinger, S., and Dendeyer, A.: A step family in formation. Am. J. Orthopsychiatry, *49*:1, 1979.

Reedy, M. N., Birren, J. E., and Schaie, K. W.: Age and sex differences in satisfying love relationships across the adult life span. Hum. Dev. *24*:52–66, 1981.

Rhodes, S. L.: A developmental approach to the life cycle of the family. Social Casework, *58*:301–311, 1977.

Schram, R. W.: Marital satisfaction over the family life cycle: A critique and proposal. J. Marriage Fam., *41*:7–12, 1979.

Shapiro, J. L.: The expectant father. Psychology Today, *21*(1):36–42, 1987.

Sheehy, G.: Passages: Predictable Crises of Adult Life. New York, Dutton and Co., 1976. *This popular paperback, written for the lay public, presents a lively and entertaining discussion of individual adult development. The author places emphasis on the predictable crises, or "marker events," which relate to the developmental processes in men and women. This book is highly recommended for those who wish to gain a basic understanding of individual adulthood development.*

Solomon, M.: A developmental conceptual premise for family therapy. Fam. Process, *12*:179–188, 1973.

Stevens-Long, J.: Adult Life. (3rd ed.) Mountain View, CA, Mayfield Publishing Co., 1988. *This recently revised textbook, written for college life span development courses, presents a current overview of research on adult development and aging. It is divided into four parts, including The Foundations of Adult Development; Young Adulthood; Middle Age; and Later Life. Each of the latter three parts is further divided into sections on the biologic, interpersonal, and social aspects of aging.*

Streim, J. E., and Marshall, J. R.: The dying elderly patient. Am. Fam. Physician, 38(5):175–183, 1988.

Super, D. E.: The Psychology of Careers. New York, Harper and Row, 1957. *This classic book on career development over the life span is just as relevant and interesting as it was over 30 years ago when it was first published. The author has made tremendous contributions to the literature on vocational psychology, and this text is recommended to anyone wishing to examine their own or others' career development.*

Super, D. E., Crites, J. O., Hummel, R. C., et al.: Vocational Development: A Framework for Research. New York, Teachers College Press, 1957.

Super, D. E., and Hall, D. T.: Career development: Exploration and planning. Annu Rev. Psychol., *29*:333–372, 1978.

Tennov, D.: *Love and Limerence.* New York, Stein and Day, 1979. *This interesting book presents a study of, and conclusions about, the "limerence" phenomenon. Limerence, a term coined by the author, is defined as the ecstatic, hopeful, and intrusive feelings associated with being in love. Included in this text are sections on the social effects of limerence, the opinions of experts on limerence, limerence among the sexes, limerence and biology, and the control of limerence.*

Vaillant, G. E.: Adaptation to Life. Boston, Little Brown, 1977.

Walsh, F.: The family in later life. *In* Carter, E., and McGoldrick, M. (Eds.): The Family Life Cycle: A Framework for Family Therapy. New York, Gardner Press, 1980.

Weeks, G. R., and Wright, L.: Dialectics of the family life cycle. Am. J. Fam. Ther., *7*:85–91, 1979.

Wynne, L. C.: The epigenesis of relational systems: A model for understanding family development. Fam. Process, *23*(3), 297–318, 1984.

Zilbergeld, B.: Male Sexuality. New York, Bantam, 1978. *This paperback is one of the best available resources on sexual functioning and dysfunction. In common sense, straightforward language it describes and explains most male sexual problems (e.g., impotence and premature ejaculation) and it describes methods for resolving these problems. This sensitive and insightful book is highly recommended for both physicians and lay persons who wish to learn about sexual problems and their treatments.*

4

Systemic Family Medicine: An Evolving Concept

Donald S. Williamson
Michael L. Noel

The Rationale for Systemic Thinking

This chapter offers a perspective and recommends a direction toward understanding the concepts of the practice of family medicine, its evolution as a specialty, and its maturation (Doherty et al., 1987).

The World Health Organization (Callahan, 1973) defines health as ". . . a state of complete physical, mental and social well-being and not merely the absence of disease or infirmity." This definition clearly points toward the understanding of health as an interactional pattern. In a recent survey, an epidemiologist (Sagan, 1987) concludes:

> *The history of rapid health gains in the United States is not unique; the rate at which death rates have fallen is even more rapid in more recently modernizing countries. The usual explanations for this dramatic improvement—better medical care, nutrition, or clean water—provide only partial answers. More important in explaining the decline in death worldwide is the rise of hope and the decline in despair and hopelessness.*

From the beginning, family medicine has intuitively connected medicine with the family and both elements with human values. This philosophy offers a way of understanding the practice of medicine in general. Medicine is seen as fundamentally a *healing art* grounded in science, particularly when it provides direct personal contact with patients and patients' families. This concept is valid regardless whether care is offered on an outpatient basis or in the hospital, or whether care is primary or secondary. All medical practice represents an interface between the medical arts, human consciousness, and human values. This philosophy or ethic can guide every patient encounter. This interface is systemic in character and, therefore, encourages a systemic understanding of the practice of medicine. Consequently, both health and illness are most richly understood when viewed from an ecologic-systemic perspective.

However, "thinking systemically" does not necessarily mean focusing on the family as *a unit of care*. Such a notion is limited in its usefulness because it overlooks the fundamental importance of the boundary of the skin. Rather, thinking systemically is a way of understanding human behaviors in general as they are observed in the individual and in the group. At the same time, thinking systemically within family medicine does imply acknowledging the family as a crucial dimension of primary health care. Even though only one person is seen routinely by the family physician, that person is viewed within the broader social and emotional context of how the patient relates to other persons who make up the patient's ongoing family life.

An ecologic-systemic perspective assumes that the fundamental elements of the human experience, whether they are biologic-physiologic or psychologic-social or epistemologic-spiritual, are all welded into circular and recursive networks of experience and behavior. These patterns develop within and between individuals, between individuals and social groups, and between individuals and the environment. This, then, is a core understanding about the essential nature of the human organism. And it places human consciousness at the very center of human experience. Consequently, family medicine (like family therapy) seeks to counter the prevailing cultural temptation to move through life in an autohypnotic or semiconscious state, which results in minimizing personal responsibility for behavior, especially responsibility for personal well-being. Family medicine (like family therapy) calls the individual patient (and the patient's family) to consciousness, to awareness, to attentiveness, and, consequently, to accountability. It is, therefore, incumbent on the physician to be attentive to all aspects of the patient's social context.

Family medicine also recognizes that social support is a crucial buffer to social stress. It is a primary guarantor of good health, including physical health. Measuring the stress-support ratio is a quick way to evaluate the emotional quality of the patient's present life situation. This ratio acknowledges the importance of love in relationships and the importance of relationships in human life. For the majority of people, the most important relationships are within the family, since it represents the most powerful biologic bond. This sphere, then, is the arena for *family* medicine.

Different aspects of human experience have traditionally been distinguished conceptually into physical, psychologic, and spiritual spheres. But these spheres are separable only at the level of conceptualization. Furthermore, what can be distinguished into parts conceptually can also be seen in terms of *patterns*. Some of these patterns of health behavior persist over time, whereas some are endlessly changing, like the patterns of color within the kaleidoscope. Learning to see the patterns as well as the parts and learning to see changing patterns so as to be able to create responsive *patterns of intervention* constitute the essence of the systemic approach to family medicine. It is not that the family physician exercises this option on every occasion. Rather, he or she carries the awareness of these patterns of intervention and knows both when and how to use them.

As Bloch (1987) has pointed out, usually the essential features of medical practice are:

> *(1) The restriction of contextual information; (2) the ordering of relational (causal) sequences in linear fashion over short time periods, with the arrow of time pointing in one direction only; (3) the elimination of the observer or the observing system from the field of inquiry.*

Family medicine calls this "specialist" philosophy into question as it moves slowly toward a contextual understanding of both family and health and therefore toward a systemic understanding of medical practice. This shift could be as revolutionary for primary care medicine as it has been for psychotherapy. Huygen (1982) suggests that the greatest challenge facing family medicine today is "to make use of the family." The question facing the discipline is, "How does one do that?"

Systemic understanding does not deny the usefulness and appropriateness of linear thinking when called for. It can be held as a "both . . . and" posture, the more useful perspective being selected by the context and the task of the moment. In that sense, linear thinking is a subset of systemic thinking. It is analogous to the dual theory in physics, in which it is sometimes more useful to view matter as mass and at other times as energy. As Hawkins (1988) has explained, Heisenberg's "uncertainty principle" states that as the exactness of the position of a particle increases, so the uncertainty regarding its velocity increases, and vice versa. Likewise, too much "linear understanding" and too much "systemic understanding" increase our uncertainty. The question is can one look into a microscope with one eye and through a wide-angle lens with the other simultaneously? Another appropriate metaphor is found in the world of television. One camera may be taking a wide-angle picture of the entire field, whereas another is simultaneously shooting an isolated close-up of a particular play or player. This composite picture can indeed be viewed at one time, but there are always two cameras and two camera operators. This offers a compelling argument for an intimate and interdependent collaboration between family physician and family therapist.

We believe that these two perspectives are better handled sequentially than simultaneously, at least in the context of the medical examination room. It will also be proposed here that these dual perspectives, if brought together through a systemic and interdisciplinary approach, can provide an effective intellectual basis for family practice.

From the Biomedical to the Bio-Psycho-Social Model

In a watershed article (and in an important step toward systemic understanding), Engel (1977) developed what he named the bio-psycho-social model of practice in medicine. He analyzed the existing prevalent biomedical model and its shortcomings as follows:

> *It (the biomedical model) assumes disease to be fully accounted for by deviations from the norm of measurable biological (somatic) variables. It leaves no room within its framework for the social, psychological, and behavioral dimensions of illness. The biomedical model not only requires that disease be dealt with as an entity independent of social behavior, it also demands that behavioral aberrations be explained on the basis of disordered somatic (biochemical*

or neurophysiological) processes. Thus the biomedical model embraces both reductionism, the philosophic view that complex phenomena are ultimately derived from a single primary principle, and mind-body dualism, the doctrine that separates the mental from the somatic.

Engel goes on to suggest that in modern western society, the perspective of biomedicine has not simply been the foundation for the scientific study of disease but has also become the folk model, indeed a "dominant folk model of disease in the western world." He suggests that it has even acquired the status of dogma, defining dogma as a point of view that "requires that discrepant data be forced to fit the model or be excluded." In speculating why a reductionistic and dualistic biomedical model should have evolved and prevailed in this way in the west, Engel quotes Rasmussen (1975), who has offered a fascinating explanation. He points out that approximately 5 centuries ago, the church finally permitted dissection of the human body. However it did so with

. . . a tacit interdiction against a corresponding scientific investigation of man's mind and behavior. . . . this compact may be considered largely responsible for the anatomical and structural base upon which scientific western medicine eventually was to be built. . . . entities to be investigated (must) be resolved into isolable causal chains or units, from which it was assumed that the whole could be understood, both materially and conceptually, by reconstituting the parts. . . . classical science readily fostered the notion of the body as a machine, of disease as the consequence of breakdown of the machine, and of the doctor's task as repair of the machine (Engel, 1977).

Understandably, it follows that the biomedical model would place less importance on the patient's subjective account of his or her illness experience and would instead place great emphasis on objective procedures and laboratory tests.

In contrast, Engel argues that the most necessary and the most complex skills of the physician are the ability to elicit an accurate verbal account of the patient's illness experience and then to analyze it properly. He believes that it takes a careful discipline to develop reliable skills in the interviewing process and to understand "the meaning of the patient's report in psychological, social and cultural as well as anatomical, physiological, or biochemical terms" (Engel, 1977). He believes that a bio-psycho-social approach would do justice to all of these various elements, which together constitute the medical interview.

Further support for this point of view comes from a recent survey of the literature on the etiology of illness by Justice (1987). He writes

No one factor determines who gets sick . . . we are talking about . . . co-factors—not single causes.

These cofactors can be anything in one's thinking, behavior, body, or environment.

And a key co-factor, now intensely researched as part of the new science of biological and molecular psychology, is the cognitive—how our heads affect our health. Since it is now known that the brain has power to regulate all bodily functions, disregulation of the central nervous system is increasingly being implicated as a contributing factor in disease.

It should be clear by now that the bio-psychosocial model does represent something of an epistemologic shift in the ways in which physicians can conceptualize disease and illness behaviors. Engel points out that this conceptualization will determine

what are considered the proper boundaries of professional responsibility and how they influence attitudes towards and behavior with patients.

He concludes that

some medical outcomes are inadequate not because appropriate technical interventions are lacking, but because our conceptual thinking is inadequate. (Engel, 1977).

More recently, Baird and coworkers (1987), in assessing the current state of the field, create a distinction between what they call the split bio-psycho-social model and the bio-psycho-social model. The latter overcomes the usual dichotomy between mind and body by

. . . viewing diagnosis and treatment in terms of the interplay of biological, psychological, and social factors. Each domain serves as a context *for the others, and all function in* relation *to one another. . . . the physician will always be open to the presence of multiple interacting elements in diagnosing patients' health problems. . . . in the most basic form of integration, the physician's relationship with the patient is always a potentially healing dimension of medicine. . . .*

In a book with the suggestive title, *The Second Medical Revolution,* Foss and Rothenberg (1987) present an alternative concept to biomedicine, which they label infomedicine. They write

The biomedical model recognizes the internalization of unconscious (autonomic) self-regulating processes like the regulation of blood sugar levels in the body. But it does not formally recognize the internalization of self-regulating processes that initially require conscious decision-making, like the . . . regulation of "autonomic" nervous system functions . . . in clinical biofeedback therapy.

Through this more precise formulation of the bio-psycho-social model, it progresses little further forward. It is then our thesis that the concept of *systemic family medicine* takes yet another half step forward toward the completion of the epistemologic shift begun by Engel. The goal is to understand in a more *patterned way* the etiology and course of health and illness experiences and their relationship to medical theory and practice.

The Transition to Systems Thinking

Stein (1987) has suggested that Whitehead in philosophy, Weiner in cybernetics, Von Bertalanffy in biology, and Bateson in the principles behind family systems theory "all argue for the primacy of the ideas of *context* and *relations* in understanding nature and our position in it." He then quotes Doherty (1987) who concludes

> *. . . the central scientific theme of the 20th century are the ideas of context and relations as central principles in scientific study.*

The reference here is to the central tenet of systems theory that all levels of organization are connected in a hierarchical way, so that change in any part of the system will bring about change that reverberates throughout the entire system.

Recently, Kerr and Bowen (1988) have offered a fascinating perspective on the historical development of systems thinking, suggesting that while the applications may be new, systems thinking is itself quite old. They define systems thinking as the ability to observe the *process* as opposed to the *content* of nature. In distinguishing the process from the content of nature, these authors propose that

> *. . . it is analogous to a movie being equivalent to a* process *and an individual frame of the movie being equivalent to* content *(Kerr and Bowen, 1988).*

So defined, they suggest that this kind of thinking originated at least 2500 years ago with the Greeks living in Ionia in the 6th century, B.C. However, subsequent to that, systems thinking was largely ignored for 2000 years, and they suggest, for understandable reasons

> *It certainly must have seemed that everything did revolve around us. . . . it did appear that we were stationary and that everything else was moving. We ascribed individual characteristics to the planets to explain their movements. Since we did not comprehend the interrelationship of the planets, it was natural to explain their journeys through the night sky by the character we projected onto each one. Mars was the god of war, Venus was the goddess of love and beauty, Mercury was the messenger, Saturn oversaw agriculture, and Jupiter was in charge (Kerr and Bowen, 1988).*

Kerr and Bowen credit Copernicus in the mid-16th century for reintroducing systemic thinking in modern times. He did so through his revolutionary proposition that the sun is at the center of the solar system, with the planets moving in circular orbits around it. They suggest that this discovery would forever dramatically change humanity's thinking about its place in the universe. Subsequently, Johannes Kepler created a mathematical model to describe the actions of all the planets.

> *Kepler was certain that the precise planetary motions he had described were based on some sort of force that held it all together. [He] sensed that their individual parts were somehow related to one another, but he did not know the basis for this suspected interrelationship.*

Kerr and Bowen suggest that Newton solved Kepler's problem in the mid-17th century through his theory of universal gravitation. They quote Carl Sagan's summary of Newton's theory:

> *Things had been falling down since the beginning of time. That the Moon went around the Earth had been believed for all of human history. Newton was the first person ever to figure out that these phenomena were due to the same force. This is the meaning of the word "universal" as applied to Newtonian gravitation. The same law of gravity applied everywhere in the universe (Sagan, 1980).*

These authors continue with a graphic description of Newton's achievement.

> *Like all great scientists, Newton saw simplicity where others saw clutter and detail. He saw a* process *where others had seen only* content. *Gravity is what accounts for the motions of the planets. Each planet does not have a mind of its own, but each, by virtue of its mass, contributes to a gravitational field, and it is this "field" that regulates the velocity and path of each planet. It is a beautifully balanced system. . . . Copernicus, Kepler and Newton had brought us back into the realm of systems thinking, at least in the physical world (Kerr and Bowen, 1988).*

Since Newton's time, the physical sciences have continued to evolve systems perspectives, with Einstein making a quantum leap in this type of thinking in the modern era. But these authors question whether or not in theoretical development the life sciences have kept pace with the physical sciences. Certainly, when it comes to human behavior, psychology in general and theories of motivation in particular have focused heavily upon the individual. Von Bertalanffy (1968), the pioneer of general systems theory, has written

> *American psychology in the first half of the 20th century was dominated by the concept of the reactive organism or, more dramatically, by the model of man as a robot.*

Freud created dynamic psychiatry and offered the first and perhaps still the only depth theory of human behavior. His thinking was systemic at the very least in the sense that

> *he proposed that disturbances in brain* function *rather than brain* structure *were the basis of most neurotic and psychotic symptoms (Kerr and Bowen, 1988).*

Kerr and Bowen point out that Freudian theory differs from family systems theory in at least two ways. First, it was based on observations of individual patients, whereas family systems theory evolved out of the study of whole families and the relational patterns that characterize whole family behavior. Second, psychoanalysis has emphasized the uniqueness of humans as a form of life. In contrast, Bowen's family systems theory assumes that human behavior, for better or for worse, expresses that part of humanity that is shared with the lower animals. They write

. . . to say that the human is part of all life is to imply that man is fortunate to be part of a smoothly orchestrated system that guides all living things.

Bowen had declared that families behave in ways that indicate that they are natural systems. Therefore, they are to be understood in terms of systems principles, and these systems principles are "rooted in nature."

Unlike many other family theorists, Bowen did not try to apply the developing concepts of general systems theory to the understanding of the human family. Instead he assumed that the family is itself a naturally occurring system. As defined by Bowen, the word natural refers to ". . . something formed by nature without human intervention." Consequently, the concept of a "natural system" implies that systems exist in nature itself and, therefore, are not created by human theories. (This raises an interesting epistemologic question, since the very notion of a system is itself a human theory.) However, the argument that the human family system is analogous to the rest of systems behaviors in nature is compelling. Kerr and Bowen (1988) conclude

The solar system, the ant colony, the tides, the snail, the family of Homo erectus *are all natural systems. The family systems sprung from the evolutionary process and not from the human brain.*

In Bowen's view, the human family as a natural system can be identified and characterized as an *emotional system.* He believes that this emotional system is the outcome of an evolutionary process that eventually led to Homo sapiens. This view of the human family as essentially an emotional system is at the heart of Bowen's theory and continues to be a core principle of family systems theory in general. In this theory, each individual, when born into a family, fully participates in and becomes an integral part of that family's emotional system. Consequently, the challenge in growing up psychologically is to "differentiate a self," i.e., an emotional self with clear and distinct boundaries, within the family of origin. This differentiation, in turn, means to discover and declare the emotional boundaries of the self in the context of and in relationships with the other members of one's own family, especially the father and the mother (Williamson, 1981, 1982). This understanding of the family system as an emotional system in which all members participate is being emphasized here because it is one of the basic principles on which the understanding and practice of systemic family medicine can be built.

Systems Theory and Systems Thinking

The dictionary (Random House, 1987) in part defines "system" as

a regularly interacting or interdependent group of items forming a unified whole; an organized set of doctrines, ideas or principles usually intended to explain the arrangement or working of a systematic whole; a harmonious arrangement or pattern.

Other definitions include,

a set of objects together with the relationships between the objects (parts) and between their attributes (the properties of objects or parts)" Glenn (1984); and, "the most general definition of system (Greek word systema, a composite thing) is the ordered composition of (material or mental) elements into a unified whole (Simon et al., 1987).

In attempting to develop a premise for general systems theory, Von Bertalanffy (1968) tried to identify underlying principles that would apply to all systems. The purpose was to try to discover an organizational pattern rather than yield to the urge toward reductionism as the guiding principle in scientific inquiry. When applied to human behavior, this process results in principles relevant to human experience. Therefore, although Bowen's family systems theory developed independently of general systems theory, both shared the underlying assumption that social organization among human beings has "an underlying and unifying structure or pattern" (Von Bertalanffy, 1968). It has been suggested that Levi-Strauss in anthropology, Chomsky in linguistics, and Piaget in developmental psychology have all offered theories about organizing patterns in human behavior. Seeing things as patterns creates a new reality. In their book of definitions, Simon and associates (1987) note that

the premises of systems theory are based on the insight that a system as a whole is qualitatively different and "behaves" differently from the sum of the system's individual elements. . . . natural systems are always parts of larger systems and, therefore, are not fully predictable.

They go on to point out that

In the framework of family therapy, the application of the term "system" is identical to its application in the field of cybernetics. The foundations of cybernetic theory lie in control theory, in which rules were found to have validity outside the realm of mechanical systems where the theory originated. The field of biology in particular proved to exhibit a number of controlling structures (Simon et al., 1987).

Since every unit can be perceived as a system, the outcome is a "hierarchy of systems, depending on what is viewed as a whole and what is regarded as a part."

As noted earlier, traditional psychology has perceived the individual as a whole or a unit, whereas family systems theory sees the individual as one part of the larger (emotional) system of the family, with the family seen as the whole. So individual behavior is to be understood in the context of the behavior of the family as a whole. This in turn is believed to be

> *determined by the rules of communication and interaction applicable in the family system, as well as by the structure of the family itself; in other words, by the type of reciprocal relations that exist between the members of the family (Simon et al., 1987).*

In dealing with the complex issue of systems within systems and the matter of where to place the boundary to a given system, Bloch (1987) writes

> *How should systems be demarcated from each other? And how should they be connected to each other? This, in fact, constitutes a single question that acknowledges two kinds of distinctions: between what is within a system and outside of it, and between the components that make up a system. "Environment," "context," and "surround," are expressions of a particular location from which a scene is viewed . . . the disease in the body-as-context reflects our viewing stance: a virus-eyed view would be quite different.*

As to health care systems in interaction, he notes that

> *Within a particular language system, such as that of physiology and biomedicine, it is necessary to be able to demonstrate the neural-endocrine–mediating links connecting psychosocial systems to organ systems . . . the entire entity with which we are concerned . . . includes at a minimum, the biology, psychology, and physiology of the patient, the relational structure of the multigenerational family, and the relevant aspects of the health-care system . . . (Bloch, 1987).*

And so each system or subsystem is always part of a larger system, whether it begins with the cardiovascular system, the whole body system, the whole person system, or the whole family system. Each of these systems, or subsystems, is in constant interaction with all other smaller subsystems that are within it, as well as in constant interaction with the larger supra-system of the environment that is around it. And so, all living organisms are made up of smaller subsystems and simultaneously are parts in a sequence of larger systems.

In family medicine, the systems approach can therefore be used to extend the systemic model already being applied to the biologic study of the individual. This can include (1) the mind and the emotionality (that is, the emotional or feeling system) of the individual patient; (2) the patient's intergenerational family emotional system; (3) the work (family) system; and (4) any other crucial and idiosyncratic elements of the local community. Finally, the physician system and the health care system must also be considered.

The individual life experience is constructed out of various subsystems, ranging from an organ system within an individual all the way up to the ecosystem of the environment. Complex natural and social systems range all the way from the smallest cellular level to the largest populations of peoples on earth. However, most of these relationships are experienced and interpreted by the individual through the small social unit of the family. Consequently, the family emotional system is the most dominating and emotionally compelling system or subsystem in human experience. Therefore the significant *conceptual boundary* (or boundary of understanding) for systemic family medicine is moved from the boundary of the individual as a single entity to the boundary of the individual in the intergenerational family.

Systems are usually defined in light of certain universal characteristics, such as (1) the whole is greater than the sum of the parts (for example a person is more than the sum of different organ systems); (2) whatever affects the system as a whole will affect each part (consider the multiple potential side effects from particular medications); and (3) a change in any one part will affect all the other parts and will affect the system as a whole (an example of this is the way in which any disease problem focused in a particular part of the body will affect the life of the individual patient as a whole, and illness in any one family member will affect the life of the family as a whole).

It should now be evident how family systems theory has already influenced the thinking and philosophy of family medicine.

From Family Systems Medicine to Systemic Family Medicine

Family systems theory has in recent years influenced family medicine theory and practice in the direction of systems thinking. Several writers have shown the usefulness of family systems perspectives, family assessment, and family therapy initiatives in family practice (Doherty and Baird, 1983; Christie-Seeley, 1984; Sawa, 1985; Crouch, 1987; Glenn, 1987). However, the authors believe that it will not serve the discipline of family medicine well to try to incorporate routinely the treatment modalities and practices of family therapy. Such a practice encourages identity confusion and is impeded by incompatibilities of professional structure, style, and temperament. The point of connection between the disciplines is rather at the level of theoretical understandings and ethical commitments as a shared basis for practice more than it is at the point of similar clinical and treatment behaviors. It is therefore timely to now acknowledge that the concept of systemic family medicine does not come about through an *integration* of behavioral science (or family psychology) with family practice.

Rather, systemic family medicine is being presented here as another higher level of conceptualization within family medicine theory (with clear implications for practice), which draws from both traditional family medicine theory and family systems theory.

The meaning of the term family has evolved significantly within the field of family medicine over recent years. Obviously, general practitioners and the early family physicians routinely knew all the members of families who were being treated and knew them over significant periods of time. Furthermore, in an earlier time, the term family in family medicine may have been a political slogan as much as it was an intellectual or professional concept. Over the years, things have progressed rapidly to the point where Stein (1987) has suggested that what was initially a "naturalistic approach" to the medical care of families, developed in the early 1980's into "an ideological solution to the problem of family medicine's chronic identity conflict." In a telling comment he writes

> *Just as cardiologists have the cardiovascular organ system as a unit of research and clinical competence . . . so now many family physicians can stake their claim to biomedical specialness, legitimacy and respectability, by demonstrating that their unit "the family" is itself something of a bounded organ-system that can be assessed, measured, diagnosed, and intervened with, in a way that utilizes the high status cultural model of biomedicine with a new organ system. . . . family studies researchers and family therapists . . . are recruited to . . . rationalize and implement this ideology. . . . at its extreme, family medicine could come to treat its own ideological artifact.*

It would indeed be ironic if family medicine used the idea of "family" to create its own "organ system," and thereby to seek to achieve status as a medical specialty or subspecialty in the usual sense. The more attractive alternative is for systems thinking, which has spawned and permeated the culture of the family therapy movement, to continue to influence thinking within the culture of family medicine. Consequently, through interdisciplinary efforts, there might emerge a comprehensive model of family-centered health care practice, the dominant characteristic of which would be *systemic family thinking*. Since ideologic thinking is by definition nonsystemic, maintaining the open mind that systemic thinking encourages will bode well for the future of the field. Obviously, the principles of general systems theory, together with the principles of family systems theory as developed by Bowen and others, have worked to expand the limitation of human consciousness. Also, family medicine has already incorporated several fundamental principles from the general field of psychotherapy, especially family psychotherapy.

Fundamental Principles Subsumed from the Field of Psychotherapy

I. The first principle is the idea *that the relationship is the medium of healing*. This is an acknowledgment of the power of empathy in changing human behavior. It is now better understood by physicians that responses like listening, acknowledging, clarifying, reassuring, validating, and empowering do at times constitute significant *treatment interventions,* and are not simply polite or kind conversation. They can be effective, for example, to create a healing context, and to encourage commitment to well-being on the part of a patient or to encourage compliance. They frequently have a significant emotional impact on patient expectations and, therefore, often a physical effect as well. A systemic perspective helps the physician understand why his or her person and presence are key elements in the equation.

II. There is an awareness in family medicine of *the importance of language,* since language is the medium of the relationship and the treatment. Language creates a reality in the patient's mind (as well as in the physician's). And the language of each one co-creates the reality of the other. Given the universal human tendency to move in the direction of our expectations, the physician's prognostications often take on a prophetic character. Therefore, it is valuable to learn to use language to craft positive suggestions and to find ways to create positive expectations in the patient's mind. Even in cases with more dire circumstances, it is possible to create an awareness of the most optimistic outcome possible and to presume that the patient will view the problem in that way. Family psychotherapy can help here, for it has already developed the language skills of reframing (that is, creating a new context or frame of meaning around an event or a sequence of events) and "positive connotation" to a high art (Erickson and Rossi, 1979; Selvini-Palazzoli et al., 1980; Haley, 1973; Watzlawick et al., 1974).

However, frequently the language used by physicians, even with the best intentions, can be experienced by the patient as a powerful negative suggestion. The tendency to use negative suggestion unwittingly is a consequence of medical education. It is illustrated by the fact that being symptom free is described as a negative condition, or is at least a matter of achieving negative test results. And frequently, the presumption is that it is just a matter of time until positive findings (that is, a pathology) will appear. The implication is that everyone should stay alert, which is interpreted by the patient as meaning expectant of health problems. The physician's intent is good but the effect is often discouraging for the patient. The ability to use positive language and positive suggestion is part of the art to be mastered in systemic family practice.

III. As indicated, *the belief systems of the patient and the patient's family* (and consequently their expectations) *are important influences* on the future health of the patient and other family members. The belief system expresses the family's mythology about its health. Often this includes decisions about who is to be healthy and who is to be sick and when and with what outcome and to serve what purpose in family emotionality. It also includes beliefs about the sources of and reasons for illnesses as well as their meaning in the life of the patient and the patient's family. Therefore, as is appropriate and timely, the systemically oriented physician will explore the patient's beliefs about, understanding of, and expectations for his or her own present and future health and illness experiences. Therapeutic interventions in the offices of both family physicians and family therapists are likely to be more effective if the patient's and family's belief system is taken into consideration when these interventions are administered. This simply means that the physician must make an attempt to understand what is going on in the patient's mind and be attentive and responsive to it. However, this explanation may be misleadingly simple, since such a practice requires considerable empathy and self-discipline.

IV. Family physicians already realize that a systems approach *does not mean that there must always be more than one person* in the examination room at the same time. In fact, this occurs infrequently. Rather, a systems approach is directed toward the physician's thought processes, namely the ways in which he or she thinks and perceives, constructs reality and creates meaning, and so delimits and interprets data. It requires an awareness and an attitude whereby the physician is cognizant of the interrelatedness and interconnectedness of the patient's body with the mind and the meanings constructed in the mind, and that the patient is part of a greater whole, namely, the family. All of these elements constitute both the context for and the process within which the patient is evaluated. With this orientation, the physician can both think systemically and make systemically oriented treatment interventions with only one person in the room. Systemic practice allows the physician to work with an individual so as to penetrate the boundary of a family but to do so compassionately and also without being recruited into membership in the family.

V. A systems perspective acknowledges that *there is no fully objective position outside the system* from which to observe or influence the (system) patient. To observe is to join. The presence of the physician includes not only his or her belief and value systems with regard to health and illness and indeed life itself but also includes his or her own family, both nuclear family and family of origin. A systemic understanding brings a vivid awareness that there are many "unseen guests" in the examination room who contribute to the physician-patient interaction.

Doherty and Baird (1987) have pointed out that the physician is part of a triad involving himself, the patient, and the patient's family. Again, the patient's family may be represented by their physical presence, or simply through their contribution to the patient's emotionality. In any event, there is always the possibility that the physician will get caught between the patient and the patient's family, and occasionally that the patient will get caught between the physician and the family. As Doherty and Baird (1987) write, "The worst mistake the physician can make is not coming late to diagnoses for unusual diseases (the nemesis of family practice), but rather neglecting the family and then becoming the family villain."

Systemic Family Medicine—Preliminary Presuppositions

The notion of systemic family medicine has certain presuppositions embedded within it.

I. The first presupposition is that *biologic processes including illnesses are rarely functionally autonomous from psychosocial processes, i.e., consciousness.* It is assumed that all human behavior, including health and illness behavior, is motivated at some level and, therefore, purposeful. It is not necessarily or even usually purposive in the sense that, clearly, the patient does not choose the experience of illness, its symptoms, or its outcome. The patient has no voluntary control over any of it. Rather, illness behavior is purposive in the sense that, like all human behavior, it is intended to be instrumental, i.e., to solve some problem, however ineffective that solution may be. And so it is inappropriate to create axiomatic splits between the biologic self and the mental (and moral) self.

II. There are *two different and sometimes confusing hierarchies of systems involved in everyday family practice.* Each one of these systems is more useful and appropriate than the other at different times and with different purposes. First is the chronologic hierarchy, wherein when a patient initially presents with physical symptoms, then the physician directs his or her attention toward the biomedical presenting problem and the biomedical clinical differential diagnosis. From the perspective of a more comprehensive understanding of health and illness, the psychologic and epistemologic (or "meaning") levels of consciousness are presumed to be where the deeper and more significant long-term decisions are made, e.g., with regard to health and illness experiences and outcomes over time.

III. The *individual and not the family is the unit of care;* this refers of course to "family practice" care. The physical boundary of the skin defines the patient completely from the biomedical point of view, and the family physician is first and foremost a "medical doctor." It is important to learn to think systemically about the individual self, since the individual self is itself a complex "system of systems" (Fig. 4–1). First there is the biologic system, including the various body systems; second is the emotional system; and third is what might be called the spiritual system, which includes beliefs, values, and ethics. All three factors are the basis for the construction of personal reality in life. The patient's conscious mind functions at all three levels of awareness and of being. Also,

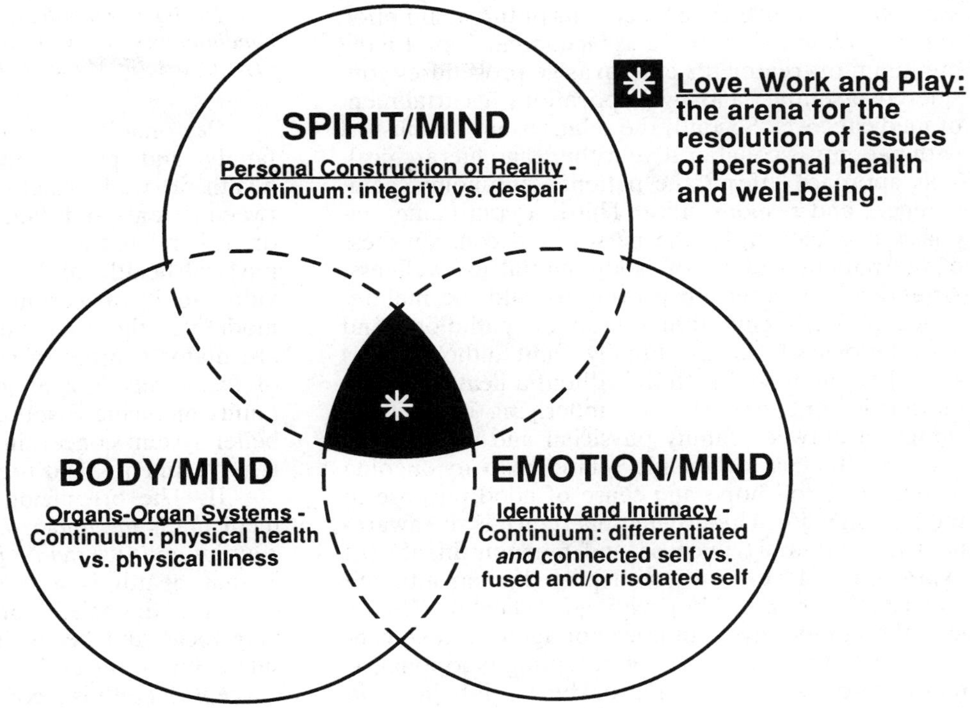

Figure 4–1. The self system (of subsystems).

the interface between these levels creates an overlapping pattern of consciousness, meanings, and decisions. This interface constitutes a personal epistemology and is a fundamental stance toward "being alive." A quick evaluation of this consciousness measures the integrity and good hope present in the patient's thoughts and feelings and, metaphorically, in his or her body as well at any given moment in time. However, having first acknowledged the primacy of the self system, nonetheless a systemic understanding of family is essential for effective continuous medical care for the individual family member. Also, on those occasions when the patient's symptoms, whether physical or psychosocial in nature, are clearly either a sign or a source of family distress, then the family itself becomes the unit of care.

IV. *The context for systemic practice is the family life cycle.* First and foremost, this is so because the human experience is embedded in a social context and the major structure of that context is the three-generational family. Many people have had important relationships with their grandparents and sometimes with grandchildren as well. But the fundamental relationships are those grounded in direct biologic connections, e.g., with one's own parents and one's own children. For most people, the life experience is set within these boundaries. Second, and as noted earlier, the transgenerational family develops and transmits a pattern of family emotionality in which all members participate. Finally, the family experience (and family emotionality) occurs over a series of family life-cycle stages and via developmental tasks. Health problems consequently occur during one or other of these stages. (This aspect will be addressed in more detail later.) Therefore, although it may be inappropriate to designate the family as the unit of care from a biomedical standpoint, nonetheless the family certainly is the major continuing influence on individual health and well-being. Therefore, it is the primary reference point for contextual understanding.

V. A systemic family approach *adds a new dimension to the notion of "continuity of care."* The essence of continuity of care resides in the fact that the family physician, over time, comes to know all members of the family and also something of the personal history of each member. He or she then has some grasp of family emotionality. (It is presumed that the family physician understands the individual and family life cycle developmental sequences and can discern where the individual patient fits within these cycles.)

Attaining this kind of family information makes it much easier and safer to formulate diagnoses in complex, undifferentiated, and unfamiliar situations and to do so quickly. The clear advantage is that it gives many additional contextual clues about how to understand the quality, severity, meaning, and likely outcome of the presenting medical problem of a given family member. This understanding is available because of information about the patient's illness history as well as personal and family emotional history. Contextual understanding and systemic evaluation of health patterns leading to comprehensive but discriminating feedback to the patient over time, are essential to the art of good "family doctoring."

VI. The final assumption is that systemic family medicine constitutes *an implicit ethical stance toward medical care*. Some of the elements of this assumption are as follows: first there is a commitment to the minimum of treatments and invasive procedures considered essential, and by implication, a curtailment of medical costs. Second, the relationship established with patients is collaborative rather than hierarchical. This approach affirms the patient's autonomy, competence, and responsibility. Third, a continuing emphasis is placed upon the person and consciousness of the patient and his or her potential for wellness. Attention is focused on prevention and the maintenance of well-being rather than on pathology and expectations of illness. Finally, and although this should be discussed tactfully without a heavy hand or moralistic tone, there is an underlying implicit assumption between family physician and patient that good health has a dynamic relationship to ongoing feelings of good hope and sense of good purpose in the patient's life. Underlying this stance is the awareness that attaining purpose and meaning in life, as expressed in love, work, and play, has an intimate and circular relationship with good health. This is why the family physician does not agree to take care of the patient in the sense of accepting emotional or moral responsibility for his or her well-being. He encourages the patient to be attentive to his or her body, to listen to its messages, and to respond accordingly. This approach is similar to that of the family therapist who encourages family members to listen to and acknowledge their feelings. The physician does not regard the patient as helpless or incompetent or as a dependent and passive observer of his or her own experience. This nonjudgmental, nonblaming, and empathic "call to consciousness" and, therefore, to accountability, flows from a systemic understanding of health and leads us toward a definition of systemic family medicine.

Systemic Family Medicine: Toward a Definition

I. Systemic family medicine is fundamentally *an epistemology about human health and illness behaviors.* It is an epistemology in the classic sense of that term. That is, it is a point of view about what data are relevant to the understanding of health and illness, along with a point of view about the way or ways in which we can come to know the information that we believe to be both important and accessible. Systemic family medicine declares that there are a variety of different ways of gathering information about a patient. On a continuum, these information-gathering methods range from the empirically verifiable at one end to the physician's intuitive awareness and both rational conclusions and not fully rational hunches at the other. Somewhere in the middle is the patient's subjective description of the experience of his or her illness. From one perspective the body can be regarded as a vehicle of communication.

> *The body is not the source of its own health. The body's condition lies solely in your interpretation of its function (The Course in Miracles, 1975).*

Personal health is influenced by a complex set of family and psychosocial factors. Better parental health, as well as better quality of relationships between parents and their adult children and grandchildren, is related to less anxiety and depression, better physical health, and less life stress. Stress enhances vulnerability to certain diseases, and social support moderates the effects of stress. Family relationships are major sources of social support, and disruption of the family is a major source of stress. Systemic family medicine is subsequently and by implication a belief system concerning the causes of illness, effective treatments, and preventive measures.

II. The organizing principle in systemic family medicine is *the understanding of health as a systemic concept and a systemic pattern.* The core proposition is that health is a total holistic or an experience involving the whole organism, although symptoms may focus and be exhibited through one particular subsystem of the self. Health is, therefore, a systemic concept. Health is a concept about patterns in human behavior and experience. Health encompasses ever-changing patterns of empirically measurable biologic and physiologic processes, along with nonmeasurable subjective experience. These aspects of health occur simultaneously and are present at different levels of awareness.

Individual health occurs in an influential social and cultural context. Not all of these variables are empirically measurable, but all are in compelling dynamic and circular interaction with each other at all times. Also, the whole is greater than the sum of the parts. Therefore, outcome is never fully predictable. This fact has considerable significance for the language used in both diagnosis and prognosis, since it creates a reality and, therefore, an expectation (matching or otherwise) in the minds of both the physician and the patient. The challenge to the family physician is to be flexible enough to see the broad picture of systemic relationships and patterns, while at the same time being able to narrow his or her focus to make the required differential diagnosis at a clinical biomedical level.

III. Systemic family medicine as an epistemology, *is a way of perceiving patients in the context of other systems.* The system of self-systems (see Fig. 4–1) constitutes the internal sphere of the individual. This system is simultaneously external in that it includes the patient-physician system, the patient's family system, the physician's family system, and the larger health care system (Fig. 4–2). Consequently, the patient is seen in the context of multiple important social interactional processes.

IV. Systemic family medicine assumes that *health patterns maintain a circular and recursive interaction with individual and family emotionality.* The clear implication of this is the importance of being able to

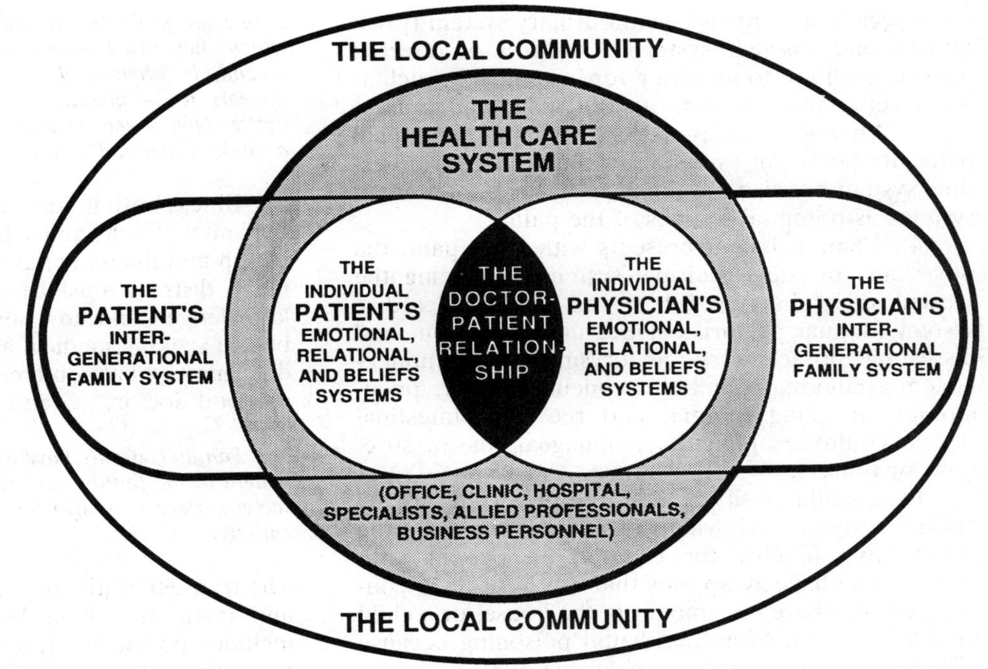

Figure 4–2. Contextual family medicine. The supra system (or system of systems).

think systemically, including being able to think in terms of the family. Although the individual is the unit of treatment, the family is the unit of understanding. Family dynamics and family emotionality, as understood in family systems theory, constitute a rich theoretical framework within which to understand the health and illness behaviors of individual family members.

V. At the same time, everything that the systemically oriented family physician does in his or her practice is, by definition, *systemic family medicine and not family therapy*. Many of the behaviors of the family physician are psychotherapeutic in nature. However, they are nonetheless always expressive of and within the province of his or her practice as a family physician. As in psychoanalysis, from which certain fundamental notions about unconscious processes, the sexuality of the child, and the importance of brain function have seeped into the culture, so the principles of family systems theory are useful for structuring family practice and indeed family life in general. However, the family physician does not seek to practice family therapy per se any more than he or she would want to practice psychoanalysis. Psychoanalysis as a way of understanding individual human behavior has served a very useful purpose historically. However, as an intervention used to resolve human problems, psychoanalysis has a more limited value and certainly has minimal relevance to family practice.

Likewise, family systems theory is most valuable as an intellectual source or a theoretical framework, but family therapy as a technique has limited usefulness in the everyday practice of family medicine. The family physician who thinks systemically and can view the individual patient within the context of his or her family can use systemic family medicine interventions to induce change in the family system by working with the individual patient. This method is similar to that of the family therapist who intervenes in a family's behavior by working alone with one family member, if he or she works within a family systems framework. As noted earlier, if a sub-system changes at any point, then the whole system changes. The general assumption is that systemic thinking and practice transcend the dichotomies usually associated with the biologic and the psychosocial, the body and the mind, the individual and the family, and the physician and the patient.

Characteristics of the Systemically Oriented Family Physician

I. First and foremost the family physician has *a systemic understanding of the body and body systems*. So he or she initially focuses on the body systems that are causing the patient's symptoms. This understanding arises from medical training, which has been thoroughly internalized. For example:

1. When a patient presents with swelling of the lower extremities, the physician assesses the cardiac system (for congestive heart failure), the renal system (for renal failure), and the gastrointestinal system (for hepatic failure).

2. When a patient presents with low back pain, the physician considers the gastrointestinal system

(retrocecal appendicitis), genitourinary system (prostatitis), and vascular system as sources of referred pain, in addition to assessing for local factors such as disc disease and osteoarthritis of the lumbar spine.

3. When a patient presents with upper abdominal pain, the physician assesses not only the gastrointestinal system but also the renal cardiac and pulmonary systems as potential sources of the pain.

4. When a patient presents with chest pain, the physician considers multiple systems, including the musculoskeletal system (chest wall pain), the cardiac system (angina pectoris, myocardial infarction, and dissecting thoracic aortic aneurysm), the pulmonary system (pulmonary embolus, pneumothorax, pneumonia, and lung tumor), and the gastrointestinal system (reflux esophagitis, esophageal spasm, stricture, or tumor).

In a similar fashion, a family physician already "thinks systemically" when considering aspects of the home environment; for example, a patient with asthma may have symptoms that are difficult to control because there is a smoker in the house, or a child may be a victim of an accidental poisoning because of improper safety precautions in the home.

Clearly, the family physician is already accustomed to thinking systemically at one level. But he or she is also accustomed to setting a limiting boundary around the kinds of information he or she will normally solicit and evaluate before making a differential diagnosis and offering treatment. Consequently, the next step is to add to the systems checklist the individual and the family emotional systems. The thrust of the argument in this chapter is to widen the boundary and enlarge the context of assessment so that this principle of systemic thinking can be applied more radially and encompass more systems at different levels.

II. Family physicians are known to be *enthusiastic problem solvers, frequently doing so by enlarging the context of inquiry.* Enlarging the context will contribute to the solving of many complex presenting situations. The question then becomes one of the timeliness and appropriateness of *enlarging the context.* The assumption is that the family physician who has learned to think systemically about the body systems can also learn to think systemically about the body system in relation to all the other systems, such as the emotional systems that comprise a given family. Huygen (1982) has suggested several situations in which direct contact with and knowledge about the family is essential

> *A first is when the family appears to be harboring, generating, or promoting the illness of one of its members. A second is when an illness intrudes so suddenly, so cataclysmically, upon a family that it needs help in orienting itself to the stress and coping with it. A third is when chronic illness appears to be relapsing uncontrollably. A fourth is when compliance seems to be an issue defying the physician's control. A fifth is when an illness appears to be psychosomatic or stress related, but the index patient admits of no problem or concern. A sixth is when the family members phone the physician repeatedly to offer secret information which they insist cannot be relayed on to the patient. A seventh is when a child or other member of the family appears to be getting ill in the context of severe conflict between two other members. An eighth is when death touches a family (Glenn, 1984).*

Illness both influences and is influenced by family dynamics. Each family has its own mythology about health and illness behaviors. These rules include how much distress must be experienced before it is acknowledged and how serious the symptoms must be before seeking medical attention. Family culture also determines what good medical care is and what makes a "good doctor." Glenn (1984) points out that,

> *Families usually have a sense of which member(s) is the patient in the family, and which member(s) are caretakers, secret sufferers, or will be hidden from the medical system entirely.*

The transgenerational transmission of beliefs, values, and mandates about health and illness sometimes includes powerful suggestions as to who should get sick, with what kind of sickness, what kind of outcome, and in the service of what transgenerational family goals. Consequently, an individual patient may think of himself or herself as a potential candidate to suffer the same medical problems as other members of the family. Obviously, evidence exists of biologic predisposition and genetic vulnerability. But social learning also transmits expectations, mandates, and loyalties from generation to generation at both conscious and unconscious levels of awareness (Bowen, 1978, Boszormenyi-Nagy and Spark, 1973). To be a good problem solver is to know that the interrelationships between health and illness behaviors of family members and the family as a whole apply to all human experience and continue through all stages of the individual and family life cycles.

III. The systemically oriented family physician is *an expert in differential diagnosis in a more comprehensive sense of that term,* that is, a differential diagnosis of the health status of the whole person and not simply the person's body. Rakel and Pisacano (1984) have noted that, "the ideal family physician" is "part theologian . . . part politician . . . part humorist." They go on to note that decisions with regard to diagnostic possibilities are influenced by

> *knowledge of the patient's lifestyle, personality and previous response pattern. . . . the less background information the physician has to rely on, the greater will be his need to depend upon costly laboratory studies and the more likely he is to overreact to the presenting symptom. . . . The skilled family physician will have a higher level of tolerance for the uncertain than his consultant colleague. . . . [He] is an expert in the rapid assessment of a problem presented for the first time. . . . he uses time as one of his most effective diagnostic aids.*

The role of the family physician as an expert "in the rapid assessment of a problem presented for the first time" will be greatly facilitated by his or her understanding of the principles of family systems theory in general and knowledge about a given patient in the context of his or her family. As has been argued earlier, a given patient and family are best understood in light of family emotionality patterns and the present life cycle stages of the patient and the family. Certain physical and emotional issues tend to correlate with particular life cycle stages. The following examples are presented not to suggest interventions but to illustrate the complexity of both presenting problems and the subsequent challenge to multifaceted differential diagnosis.

The Unattached Young Adult. Presenting medical issues are sexually transmitted diseases, for example AIDS and issues involving contraception. The related psychologic issues may be in the area of human sexuality, identity, and fear of intimacy. Clinical examples follow:

1. A 20-year-old female presented with a 1-month history of abdominal pain. The pain was nondescript, intermittent, and not related to meals. The pain was initially in the epigastrium but later localized to the pelvis. No associated symptoms or exacerbating or alleviating factors were present. At first, the patient said she was not sexually active and, therefore, had no desire for contraception. After reviewing current sources of stress in her life, she acknowledged that she was in fact sexually active and did in fact desire contraception. She was obviously embarrassed and felt guilty.

2. A 19-year-old male college student presented complaining of hand tremors. Neurologic examination proved negative. He was concerned about this because he wanted to play football. He indicated that this was his first year in college and first time away from his mother, with whom he had lived alone for the previous 10 years subsequent to the parental divorce. He said he felt very badly about leaving his mother and very concerned about her happiness. He said he talked to her twice a week by telephone and returned for the weekend at least twice a month. His mother was not doing well.

The New Couple. Presenting medical issues are male and female problems, obstetrics, and prenatal and postnatal care. The related psychologic issues may have to do with courtship, early marriage, and gender empathy. Clinical examples follow:

1. A couple in their twenties came to the office together, the wife presenting with "painful intercourse." They both indicated that they were anxious to have a pregnancy and a first child. The physical evaluation proved negative. In conversation about their relationship it became clear that the woman felt very emotionally inhibited, controlled, and regulated by her husband, by the marriage, and by expectations from her parents. As they talked, both parties also seemed very fused to each other emotionally. Their shared dilemma was that she wanted to get pregnant but intercourse was too painful.

2. A 27-year-old woman presented for prenatal care. Her first pregnancy was aborted electively. The second pregnancy aborted spontaneously. The third pregnancy was ectopic. The patient did not want alpha fetoprotein screening. Her prenatal course was remarkable for multiple episodes of premature contractions, which were controlled with rest. The conversation revealed fear of having an abnormal baby, fear of being an inadequate parent, and fear of how the new baby would change the relationship between the patient and her husband and between herself and her mother.

The Family with Young Children. Presenting medical issues are childhood illnesses, infectious diseases, recurrent illnesses, and well baby check-up. The related psychologic issues pertain to early development and the emotionality of parenting. Clinical examples follow:

1. A 24-year-old mother, who had conceived a child out of wedlock, brought her 6-month-old infant for a well-baby check-up. The mother reported that the baby was having trouble sleeping. The conversation revealed that the mother herself had insomnia related to concerns about the current marital relationship and her abuse of drugs.

2. A 32-year-old mother of three children presented on an initial postpartum visit with a complaint of a problem with her "nerves." She added that her newborn was crying frequently, resulting in poor sleep for both the patient and her husband. Discussion of the problem revealed that she was having significant interpersonal problems with her mother, who although living in the same city had not yet seen the new baby, and the patient was unwilling to let her do so. Her husband was in disagreement with this.

The Family with Adolescents. Presenting medical issues are contraception, teenage pregnancy, acne, bodily fears, drugs and other addictive problems, eating disorders, and accidents. Related psychologic issues are identity questions, body-image, self-esteem, trauma, authority problems, scapegoating, impulse control, mid-life crises (of the parents), dependency and co-dependency. Clinical examples follow:

1. A 17-year-old male presented with headaches. The physical examination proved negative. Discussion of the problem revealed that he had moved from another state from his divorced father's home (where he was "very happy") back to his mother's home out of concern for his mother's well-being. His mother was currently in the process of a divorce from her second husband and had been calling the teenager daily on the phone, weeping and appealing for help. Since his stepfather was still in the home, the patient felt unable to leave either by day or night in order to provide continuous protection for his mother. He expressed great concern for his mother's happiness and also great regret that he had had to leave his father's house.

2. A 13-year-old female presented with intermittent abdominal pain consistent with gastritis, which had occurred during the past 2 months. Discussion of

the problem revealed that she was having intense conflict with her stepmother with whom she was living. This was temporally related to the onset of her symptoms. The girl's natural mother added that she had a personal history of a "nervous stomach" and identified with her daughter's symptoms, diagnosis, and treatment.

Launching Children. Presenting medical issues are hypertension, ulcers, colitis, anxiety, depression, obesity, hypochondriasis. Related psychologic issues are separation anxiety, empty nest syndrome, work success or failure, money problems, marital conflict, transmission of values, crises, and issues revolving around the family of origin. Clinical examples follow:

1. A 47-year-old widower presented with a new onset of hypertension. His younger daughter had recently married and his son had just moved out of state. Along with feeling these losses, he reported increased stress at work and increased financial worry.

2. A 23-year-old female presented with intermittent shortness of breath and epigastric pain. During the discussion of the problem, she spontaneously related her symptoms to stress at work and, more particularly, to intense ongoing conflict with a very domineering mother with whom she still lived.

The Family in Later Life. Presenting medical issues are cardiac problems, cancer, management of chronic illnesses (diabetes, arthritis, asthma), chronic problems of old age, and terminal illnesses. Related psychologic issues are control, rage, thought disorders, marital stagnation, life failure, and loss and grief. Clinical examples follow:

1. A 55-year-old male presented for continuing treatment of angina pectoris. He had previously declined heart catheterization, which was recommended after significant failure on the treadmill. During the discussion of the problem, he reported increasing dissatisfaction with his job as a stockbroker, which, although high-paying, was volatile and a "constant worry" to him. His wife had recently moved to another state, ostensibly as the beginning of relocation for the family. He missed her greatly and was not completely certain about the future of the marriage.

2. A 72-year-old woman presented with low back pain as a result of a recent fall. She was also taking medication for hypertension. Her husband had died a year earlier of myocardial infarction. During the discussion of the problem, she reported that she was continuing to grieve, was struggling with loneliness, and was having difficulty in readjusting to being by herself.

This schema does not allege linear causal relationships or necessary causal chronologic sequences. Rather, it does point to typical *contextual patterns* at different levels of human consciousness and at different life stages, which interact to create the human experiences of health and illness. Also, it centers on the fundamental and formidable issue of what to do. What data should be included and what excluded? What kind of therapy or treatment responses are necessary, useful, or possible? Which of these modes of therapy or treatment can or should the family physician offer? What are his or her options with regard to the others? These dilemmas underscore the value of a practice of collaborative health care between family physicians and family therapists as previously advocated by Glenn (1984). But the key word is "collaboration" and not "referral." Some understanding of *context, system,* and *pattern* facilitates more refined and comprehensive differential diagnoses. This, in turn, will generate more effective and far-reaching treatment interventions over time, whether the presenting situation is acute or chronic or preventive.

IV. The systemically oriented family physician *is an expert in crafting and using therapeutic language.* Language has been referred to earlier but is so crucial that it is worth returning to. Language is used to elicit the patient's story, the inner experience of the illness. Language is used to give feedback, i.e., the meaning and outcome, or the diagnosis and treatment recommendations. Language also creates the context of relationship that is the vehicle for both receiving and giving information. Consequently, the language used determines the nature of the relationship and, therefore, the character and impact of the intervention. This has considerable influence on patient satisfaction and compliance as well as outcome and prevention. As the vehicle for giving and receiving information and that connects all the parts, language is the medium whereby a treatment system is created and sustained or changed. The systemically oriented physician understands that the use of language itself is a *treatment intervention.* Consequently, it is a crucial aspect of the complex interactional system known as the medical interview. An effective language intervention is a treatment in and of itself. When spoken by a physician in a medical examination room, language has a special power and authority. When it occurs in the context of the examination room, it is not considered psychotherapy, although it may be psychotherapeutic. Rather, this is the practice of systemic family medicine.

V. The physician who practices with systemic understanding maintains *equal loyalty with all members of the family.* This is an important systemic principle practiced in family systems therapy (Boszormenyi-Nagy and Spark, 1973) but is still a novel idea in family practice. Although the family physician has an immediate medical responsibility to the individual family member who presents to the medical office, he or she nonetheless has a sense of continuing loyalty to all members of the entire family over time. He or she is aware that individual behaviors are simultaneously systemic family phenomena when viewed from another perspective. Therefore, when the physician responds biomedically (and attentively) to the physical presentation of the individual patient, at a psychologic level, he or she does not take sides with one spouse, or a parent, or a child in opposition to other members or other relationships within the family. When it is necessary to do so for the health of one family member, he or she will interview the individuals involved in the relationship in the office or the entire family. In doing so, the physician is not practicing family therapy but systemic family medicine.

VI. The systemic family physician *has an open mind and is capable of being flexible.* Rakel and Pisacano (1984) describe the personal attributes characterizing the family physician as including compassion, understanding, and patience "mixed with a high degree of intellectual honesty." Further, the physician must be thorough and have a keen sense of humor. He or she is driven by persistent curiosity.

The conception of the personal attributes of the systemic family physician builds upon this picture. Because the systemic family physician has a nonhierarchical and collaborative style, he or she is more emotionally available and intimate with patients. To have a systemic orientation, the physician needs an open mind and a flexible intellectual and psychologic makeup. He or she will need to be comfortable using methods and epistemologies that cross theoretical and interdisciplinary lines. He or she is able to practice comfortably in a profession in which there may not be an absolute answer to every problem. Consequently, the physician must be able to live with uncertainty, and to accept truth as simply a perspective and an ever-changing one at that. He or she will, therefore, need a strong sense of self, both personal and professional, and inner security and confidence in his or her clinical knowledge and competence as well as not being threatened by his or her limitations. The physician is skilled in using himself or herself as an evaluational tool as well as using the self as a vehicle of healing and treatment through the use of language as an intervention.

In light of this, the biggest pedagogic issue in the development of systemically oriented family physicians is not the amount of new information they must master or the amount of time needed for this kind of practice, although these are both relevant concerns. Rather, the biggest issue is the threat to identity, both personal and professional, posed by a systemic and consequently less well-defined epistemology that is likely to be experienced as discontinuous with prior medical education, mythology, and culture.

Systemic Family Medicine: The Choreography of the Dance

When a patient presents in the examination room, the family physician's first responsibility is to make a swift and accurate biomedical differential diagnosis. Second, the physician must become aware of the degree of the patient's distressed emotionality, knowing that both the physical and psychologic spheres will constantly be in interaction and that one may mask the other. Being alert diagnostically to a patient's immediate emotional state and level of stress as well as to signs of physical illness does not require the family physician to be a psychotherapist. Most patients presenting with psychologic problems are not seeking prolonged or formal psychotherapy. It has been noted that "skilled and insightful grandmothers have been doing a good job of this for centuries" (Sagan, 1987). On the other hand, eliminating psychologic considerations from the assessment and limiting the inquiry to biomedical information will encourage diagnostic error on the part of the physician, noncompliance with therapeutic regimens on the part of the patient, and outright treatment failures. Additionally, the diagnosis and treatment of a problem is more efficient when it makes sense to a patient, particularly if it can be linked to the patient's own beliefs about health and illness. By describing the illness and its treatment in terms the patient can understand, the family physician enhances the patient's sense of control over his or her own life and destiny and, thereby, discourages dependency. If no such description is made, then noncompliance or treatment failure is a more likely outcome.

Patients are often unreceptive to a more systemic approach because it means exploring issues other than those medical issues for which they presented initially. It is easier for patients as well as physicians to accept the "germ theory" of disease than it is to address more complex and challenging systemic parameters. The germ theory relieves patients of the need to become more aware and to review their life styles. It further relieves the physician of the same burden as well as having to move to a more complex level of intellectual perception and emotional connection in the relationship with the patient. Even when patients are initially unresponsive, it is possible for the physician to "plant a seed," that is to expand the patient's awareness of how body and mind are both involved in health problems, as is done in psychotherapy. Family physicians frequently are aware that the patient has not disclosed all relevant pieces of information. This occurs when signs and symptoms do not fit together or when there is no logical explanation for the symptom. Consequently, the family physician is a natural for this way of thinking and interviewing. Given the kind of person who voluntarily selects this discipline, he or she is likely to be gratified by making a personal connection with the patient at this deeper level of mind and spirit.

In the choreography for the dance and occurring over multiple visits, the physician moves through interviewing sequences using a series of leading questions in a particular chronology. Each builds on the one before and there are three different boundary lines or cut-off points at different stages (see Fig. 4–3). Consequently there are key decision moments in every interview in which the physician decides either to take the conversation across a boundary to another level of inquiry or else to limit the conversation at that point. There are three different boundary lines

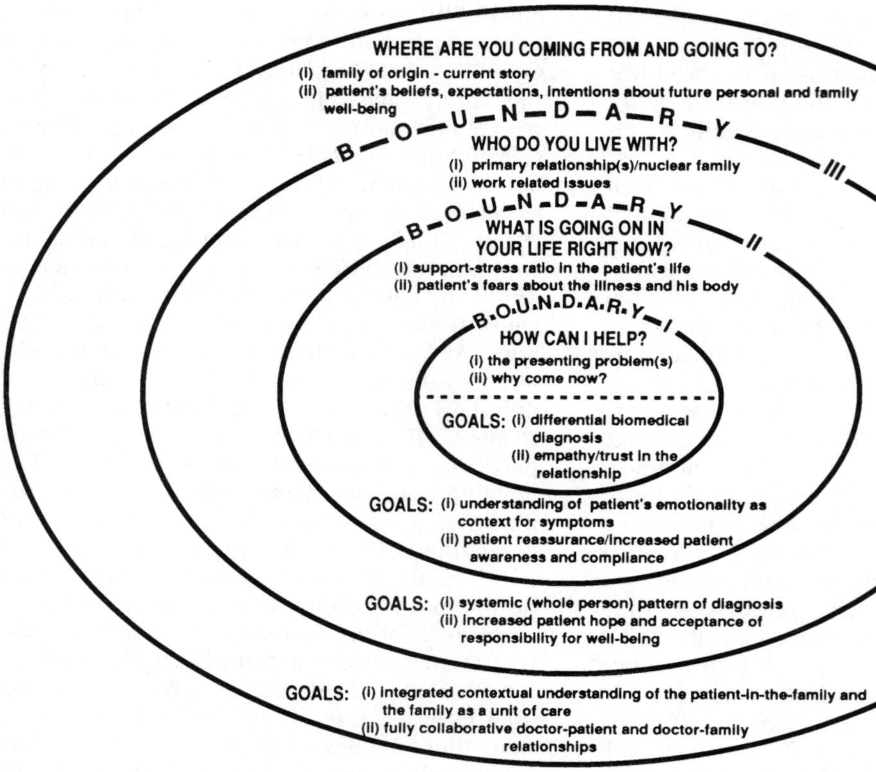

Figure 4–3. Context and boundary in systemic family practice.

and each of the four content areas is introduced by a particular question.

FIRST LEVEL OF INQUIRY

How can I help? This is the initial interview with the patient, which focuses on why he or she has come and what symptoms or distress he or she is experiencing. If it is a first visit, the conversation may include a medical history for both the patient and his or her family. Typically this is followed by the physical examination, during (or after) which the physician is usually already making a formulation or differential diagnosis. After this, he or she may decide to order further laboratory work or other tests and, depending upon outcome, he or she decides how to proceed next. First and foremost, the physician will inform and reassure the patient.

When the patient's condition is not an emergency and when other factors such as the time and energy and the emotional availability of both the patient and the physician will permit it, then the physician will cross the first boundary and proceed to the second level of inquiry.

SECOND LEVEL OF INQUIRY

What is going on in your life right now, including your thoughts and fears about your body and your presenting symptoms? At this point, the physician widens the context of the exploration. To begin with, the discussion now includes a discovery of the patient's emotional reactions toward his or her symptoms and health, both present and future. Second, the physician will explore the major sources of stress in the patient's life. This discussion proceeds in an unhurried and open-ended way, not suggesting responses and giving the patient time to relax and think about the answer and then respond. This is followed by an inquiry into the patient's major sources of social support. An evaluation of the current support-stress ratio in the patient's life is probably the single most revealing, productive, and relevant piece of contextual information about the patient, and is usually readily available to the physician. An empathic and reassuring acknowledgment of this emotionality is at the heart of a good physician-patient relationship.

THIRD LEVEL OF INQUIRY

Who do you live with? Next follows an exploration of the most significant relationship(s) in the patient's life, which for most adults is either the marriage or an ongoing love relationship if the patient is single. This inquiry frequently is a further development of the preceding discussion about major stress and major support systems. The discussion is continued by asking how the marriage (or relationship) is going. How happy, conflicted, joyful, playful, angry, worrisome, or disappointing is it? What is happening right now between the two members of the relationship? If the patient is not involved in an important ongoing relationship, then ask about the patient's dating practices. If the patient is not dating, then the obvious question should be raised about loneliness or fearfulness in relationships. On the other hand, if the patient is a parent, then the physician will inquire about parenting experiences and issues.

Second, the patient's ongoing work situation should be discussed, including work in the home. There is an awareness in the physician's mind that stress at work is often a re-creation of unresolved issues originating within the family sphere. However, this factor is a background assumption and is not a valid focus for discussion. Rather, the discussion focuses on the patient's enjoyment and satisfaction at work; feelings of stress; his or her sense of success or failure; feelings of being acknowledged and rewarded, both financially and through positive feedback; and his or her sense of social connection and friendship at work. Finally, the patient will be asked about his or her feelings of security or insecurity, or both, and whether the patient views his or her work situation as a long-term career or as a transitional point in the career path.

By now the physician has acquired a more systemic understanding of the individual patient as a total person and how this is a backdrop to his health problems. At the same time, the patient assumes more control and, therefore, more responsibility for his or her own physical health and general well-being. If the various circumstances again permit and encourage it, then the physician may continue across the third boundary to a new question and the final level of inquiry.

FOURTH LEVEL OF INQUIRY

Where are you coming from and going to? What is the current story of your family of origin? What are your beliefs, expectations, and intentions about future personal and family well-being? Now there is a brief discussion of the patient's family of origin, although the discussion is primarily focused *in the present.* When and how did the parents die if they are deceased? Did the patient resolve major life issues before the parents died as well as grieve appropriately after their death? Where are they living and what is the status of each one? Are the parents still together and, if so, what is the character of their ongoing relationship? What is the ongoing relationship of the patient to each parent? In general, how do things stand between the two generations today? All of this can be explored without moving into the emotionality of early family history, which may not be available, or simply may make the patient uncomfortable or occasionally trigger deeper upset.

The main reason for asking these questions is not to introduce an explicit therapeutic intervention, although empathic listening and acknowledgment are themselves therapeutic interventions. Rather, the reason is to enlarge and complete the contextual picture and, therefore, the physician's understanding of the patient's physical and social context. The goal over the long term is for the physician to master an integrated contextual understanding of the patient in his or her social world, including his or her social history. The physician gains this understanding by forming a mental picture and a record of the patient in relation to the family and the family as a unit of care. The physician will now be sensitized to the suprasystem or system of systems in which individual health problems occur (see Fig. 4–2). Over time, this allows the physician to repeatedly draw the patient's attention to the interactional patterns of health experiences at multiple levels of consciousness in his or her life. These interactional patterns occur most often between mind and body and between the self and others. The dynamics of both these spheres often result in unresolved conflicts that affect the patient's physical status in the form of symptoms, which then bring the patient to the examination room. As noted earlier, this style of practice gives a rich meaning to the phrase "continuity of care."

Finally, there is an open forum, however brief, in a patient-physician relationship, which is now ideally characterized by empathy, rapport, trust, and collaboration. This moment gives the patient an opportunity to identify any other areas of concern. Again, the purpose of the discussion is not so that the physician can take the responsibility for solutions but rather to increase the contextual understanding of the patient's life. The physician may now hear about the patient's thoughts and expectations with regard to his or her future, including the future of his or her health. This discussion frequently provides clues about the patient's intentions on both the conscious and unconscious levels. All of these factors facilitate the evolution of a collaborative relationship between the physician and the patient.

As a consequence of these intimate discussions, the physician develops a rich picture of the patient's belief systems and pattern of expectations, whereby the patient constructs a personal reality or epistemology. This personal reality includes the patient's view of the presenting symptoms as well as health and illness in general (for example whether this patient sees himself or herself at present as strong or weak, and as secure or vulnerable in the future). It includes personal issues such as how the patient fares in life in general, how the patient rates his or her performance or achievements, what his or her future possibilities are, and where the patient thinks the moral responsibility for all of this resides, including the illness. This sets up a context in which the physician can issue a *call to consciousness,* with an encouragement to both accountability and fulfillment of potential on the patient's part.

This kind of physician-patient relationship implies an intimate connection and creates a reservoir of relational goodwill. Considerable potential feedback is also now available that can be given to the patient over time, as it can be assimilated and used by him or her. On the physician's part, providing this feedback requires the ability to observe empathically and to integrate complex levels of information and experience. It is a challenge, it is the art of medicine, and it is of the essence of "family doctoring."

Systemic Family Medicine: a Co-Construction and a Co-Evolution

Despite the identity problems and political dilemmas still facing family medicine today, we are reminded by Stein (1987) that

> *few humans become ill, or can be made well, in isolation from those with whom they live . . . the formation, structure, health and pathology of the relationships between those who live together, and their influence on the individual's and the group's health will continue to constitute a domain of special knowledge.*

Perhaps the pivotal paradox facing the field at this time is the fact that family practice is the *specialty distinguished by its commitment to nonspecialization.* Consequently, there is the haunting identity issue facing the physician in family practice as well as the unending questions "who are you?" and "what do you do?" and even "what can you do?" and "what do you know?"

In response to these questions the expertise (if not the specialty) has been defined previously as

> *Patient management is the quintessential skill of clinical practice, and is the area of knowledge unique to family physicians. Family physicians know their patients, know their patients' families, know their practices, and know themselves . . . the true foundation of family medicine lies in the formalization and transmission of this knowledge (Stephens, 1982).*

Building on this concept, we suggest that family medicine as a specialty is defined not in terms of an organ system or even a set of skills, although the latter is clearly implicit, but rather in terms of its *epistemology*. This epistemology does not deny or contradict what has come before. Rather it builds upon it. It is the result of attempting a more radical application of systems thinking to the understanding of health and illness behaviors as patterns with exciting implications for practice.

Perhaps any physician not trained in the complexity of direct patient care and the subtleties of physician-patient interaction should have second thoughts about regular practice contact with patients. That is, he or she should be as careful about making direct psychologic contact with patients as the physician not trained in complicated surgery techniques is hesitant about taking a knife to major organs in the body. If the damage potential and the unhealed wounds in psychologic and social distress were as immediately visible as in many physical disorders, the "rules of engagement" would probably be just as rigorous.

Systemic family medicine is still a tentative and evolving idea. As a theoretical framework and as a resulting style of practice management, it is being co-constructed and is co-evolving through an intimate professional collaboration between family physicians and consulting family psychologists. The meeting point between the two disciplines centers around families and family well-being. The shared goal is to develop a systemic model of family-centered health care as a new mode of collaborative practice between these two disciplines. Systemic family medicine is the foundation of the practice, and systems theory is the intellectual foundation upon which it can be built.

References

Baird, M. A., Becker, L. A., and Doherty, W. J.: Family medicine and the biopsychosocial model: The road toward integration. *In* Doherty, W., Christianson, C. E., and Sussman, M. B. (Eds.) Family Medicine: The Maturing of a Discipline. New York, The Haworth Press, 1987, p. 65.

Bateson, G.: Steps to an Ecology of Mind. New York, Jason Aronson, 1972.

Bloch, D. A.: Family/disease/treatment systems: A coevolutionary model. Fam. Systems Med., *5*(3):277–292, 1987.

Boszormenyi-Nagy, I., and Spark, G.: Invisible Loyalties: Reciprocity in Intergenerational Family Therapy. New York, Harper and Row, 1973.

Bowen, M.: Family Therapy Clinical Practice. New York, Jason Aronson, 1978. *This is an excellent collection of most of the published papers of perhaps the most significant early theorist in the development of family systems theory. A good introduction to transgenerational family therapy theory.*

Callahan, D.: The WHO definition of "health." Hastings Cent Study *1*(3):77–88, 1973.

Christie-Seely, J. (Ed.): Working with the Family in Primary Care: A Systems Approach to Health and Illness. New York, Praeger Publishers, 1984. *An enlightening and exhaustive application of family systems thinking to an understanding of the processes of health and illness and family from the myriad medical perspectives of family practice.*

Crouch, M. A., and Roberts, L. (Eds): The Family in Medical Practice: A Family Systems Primer. New York, Springer-Verlag, 1987.

Doherty, W. J., and Baird, M. A.: Family-Centered Medical Care: A Clinical Casebook. New York, The Guilford Press, 1987. *This clinical casebook collects 71 colorful and compelling case histories and case descriptions contributed by family physicians collaborating with family therapists. There are useful commentaries on each case. This helps the reader apply the insights of family theory to family practice.*

Doherty, W. J., and Baird, M. A.: Family Therapy and Family Medicine. New York, The Guilford Press, 1983. *The first chapter title (In Search of the Family in Family Medicine) explains this book, which is a very good introduction to "family thinking" in general and to family practice in particular.*

Doherty, W. J., Christianson, C. E., and Sussman, M. B.: Family Medicine: The Maturing of a Discipline. New York, The Haworth Press, Inc., 1987. *This is a first rate philosophical overview and summary of the present standing of family medicine as a distinct discipline, acknowledging the paradoxes, dilemmas, and identity problems presently existing in the field as well as its exciting possibilities.*

Engel, G. L.: Need for a new medical model: A challenge for biomedicine. Science, *196:*129–134, 197, 1977. Copyright 1977 by the American Assn. for the Advancement of Science.

Erikson, M. H., and Rossi, E.: Hypnotherapy: An Exploratory Casebook. New York, Irvington, 1979.

Foss, L., and Rothenberg, K.: The Second Medical Revolution: From Biomedicine to Infomedicine. Boston, New Science Library: Shambhala, 1987, p. 205.

The Foundation for Inner Peace. The Course in Miracles. Tiburon, CA, The Foundation for Inner Peace, 1975, p. 144.

Glenn, M. L.: Collaborative Health Care: A Family-Oriented Model. New York, Praeger Publishers, 1987. *An excellent argument by one of the best and most cogent thinkers in the interdisciplinary area of family medicine and family therapy, who develops a concept for a program of intimate professional collaboration between family physicians and family therapists.*

Glenn, M. L.: On Diagnosis: A Systemic Approach. New York. Brunner/Mazel, Inc., 1984, pp. 41–42.

Haley, J.: Uncommon Therapy: The Psychiatric Techniques of Milton H. Erikson, M.D.: A Casebook of an Innovative Psychiatrist's Work in Short-Term Therapy. New York, W.W. Norton and Co., 1973.

Hawkins, S. W.: A Brief History of Time. New York, Bantam Books, 1988.

Huygen, F. J. A.: Family Medicine: The Medical Life History of Families. New York, Brunner/Mazel, Inc., 1982, pp. 147–148. *This was one of the very first genuinely family-oriented family medicine textbooks, written by a Dutch physician who kept detailed family case histories over several decades. Huygen takes the position that the family system is an important perspective that should be considered by family physicians.*

Justice, B.: Who Gets Sick: Thinking and Health. Houston, TX, Peaks Press, 1987, p. 13.

Kerr, M. E., and Bowen, M.: Family Evaluation: An Approach Based on Bowen Theory. New York, W.W. Norton and Co., 1988, pp. 14–24.

Rakel, R. E., and Pisacano, N. J.: The Family Physician. *In* Rakel, R. E. (Ed.): The Textbook of Family Practice. 3rd ed. Philadelphia, W.B. Saunders Co., 1984, pp. 3–11.

The Random House Dictionary of the English Language. 2nd ed., unabridged. New York, Random House, Inc., 1987, p. 1930.

Rasmussen, H.: Pharos *38:*53, 1975. Cited in Engel, G. L.: Need for a new medical model: A challenge for biomedicine. Science *196:*31, 1977.

Sagan, C.: Cosmos. New York, Random House, 1980. Cited in Kerr, M. E., and Bowen, M.: Family Evaluation: An Approach Based on Bowen Theory. New York, W.W. Norton and Co., 1988, p. 16.

Sagan, L. A.: The Health of Nations. New York, Basic Books, 1987.

Sawa, R. J.: Family Dynamics for Physicians: Guidelines to Assessment and Treatment. New York, The Edwin Mellen Press, 1985.

Selvini-Palazzoli, M., Boscolo, L., Cecchin, G., and Prata, G.: Hypothesizing-circularity-neutrality: Three guidelines for the conductor of the session. Fam. Process *19:*3–12, 1980.

Simon, F. B., Stierlin, H., and Wynne, L. C.: The Language of Family Therapy: A Systemic Vocabulary and Sourcebook. New York, Family Process Press, Inc., 1987, pp. 353–354. *An excellent—indeed the only existing—"dictionary" or lexicon of the new language of family therapy, consisting of helpful one to two page definitions of key terms and key concepts.*

Stein, H. F.: Polarities in the identity of family medicine: A psychocultural analysis. *In* Doherty, W. J., Christianson, C. E., and Sussman, M. B. (Eds.): Family Medicine: The Maturing of a Discipline. New York, The Haworth Press, Inc., 1987, pp. 213–215, 224.

Stephens, G. G.: The Intellectual Basis of Family Practice. Tucson, Arizona, Winter Publishing Co., Inc., 1982, p. 8.

Von Bertalanffy, L.: General Systems Theory. New York, George Braziller, 1968, p. 40.

Watzlawick, P., Weakland, J. H., and Fisch, R.: Change: Principles of Problem Formation and Problem Resolution. New York, W.W. Norton and Co., 1974. *This small book has been extremely influential in the field of systemic therapy and is a delightful introduction to both paradoxical and brief therapy.*

Williamson, D. S.: Personal authority via termination of the intergenerational hierarchical boundary; a "new" stage in the family life cycle. J. Marital Fam. Ther., *7:*441–452, 1981.

Williamson, D. S.: Personal authority via termination of the intergenerational hierarchical boundary: Part II. The consultation process and the therapeutic method. J. Marital Fam. Ther., *8:*25–37, 1982.

Williamson, D. S.: Personal authority via termination of the intergenerational hierarchical boundary: Part III. Personal authority defined and the power of play in the change process. J. Marital Fam. Ther., *8:*309–323, 1982.

5

The Impact of Illness on the Family

John S. Rolland

This chapter provides a family systems–oriented model for clinical practice with chronic and life-threatening illness. At the heart of all systems-oriented inquiry is the focus on *interaction*. In the arena of physical illness, particularly chronic disease, the focus is the systemic interaction of a disease with an individual, family, and other biopsychosocial systems (Engel, 1977, 1980). This chapter centers on the family level in recognition that the family is a system influenced heavily by a range of social, economic, institutional, and political forces in the larger environment. A scheme of the systemic interaction of family and illness might look like the diagram in Figure 5–1.

This diagram illustrates the three central constructs of the family systems–illness model that will be described: (1) psychosocial typology and time phases of illnesses and key time phases in their natural history, (2) interface of illness, individual, and family development, and (3) family health/illness belief system. (Rolland, 1984, 1987a, 1987b, 1987c, 1988, in press).

Psychosocial Typology of Illness

In order to think in an interactive or systemic manner about illness, individual and family, we need a way to characterize the illness in psychosocial terms over time. A schema, which conceptualizes chronic diseases, is required that remains simultaneously relevant to both the psychosocial and biological worlds and provides a common language that transforms or reclassifies our usual medical terminology. Better linkage of these two worlds will help to clarify the relationship between long-term illnesses and the family. There have been two major impediments to progress in this area. First, insufficient attention has been given to the areas of diversity and commonality inherent in different chronic illnesses. Second, there has been a glossing over of the qualitative and quantitative differences in how various diseases are manifest over the course of an illness. Chronic illnesses need to be conceptualized in a manner that organizes these similarities and differences over the disease course so that the type and degree of demands relevant to clinical practice are highlighted in a more useful way.

The great variability of chronic illnesses and how they evolve over time have presented a vexing problem to psychosocial investigators who have attempted to identify those psychosocial variables associated with disease course or treatment compliance. Recent reviews of the psychosocial modifiers of stress emphasize a variety of methodologic and conceptual problems (Elliot and Eisdorfer, 1982; Kasl, 1982; Weiss et al., 1981). One major difficulty may be the use of a disease classification based on purely biologic criteria that are clustered in ways to meet the needs of medicine. This nosology is most useful to establish

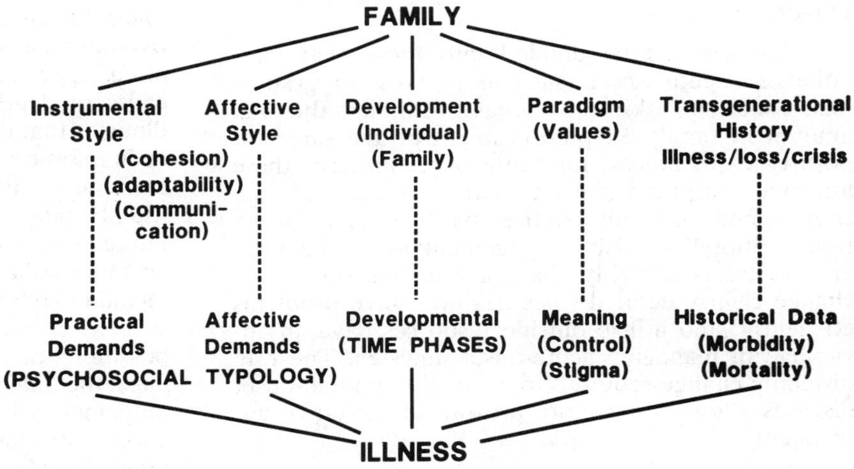

Figure 5–1. Interface of chronic illness and the family. (Modified from Rolland, J. S.: Family systems and chronic illness: A typological model. J. Psychother. Fam., 3(3):143–168, 1987.)

a medical diagnosis and formulate a medical, rather than a psychosocial, treatment plan.

Historically, this specific illness orientation has guided psychosocial research and clinical investigations toward opposite poles. Truths are sought either in each specific disease or in "illness" as a general, quasimetaphoric concept. Findings with one disease are then generalized to cover all illnesses indiscriminately. Or, findings are held to be not generalizable and researchers study each illness in a narrowly focused way. Both of these extremes hamper the clinician. Lacking guidelines to balance unifying principles and useful distinctions, clinicians can become bewildered by the wide variety of chronic illnesses. They may apply a monolithic treatment approach to all chronic illnesses. They may inappropriately transpose aspects of their clinical experience with psychiatric disorders. Extensive experience with a single kind of illness that requires intensive focus on issues of separation and loss, like terminal cancer, may get transferred to a chronic illness, like stroke, where other issues such as role reallocation predominate.

The psychosocial importance of different time phases of an illness is another poorly understood dimension. A major reason for this in research has been the relative predominance of cross-sectional, in contrast to longitudinal, studies. Likewise, clinicians often become involved in the care of an individual or family coping with a chronic illness at different points in the "illness life cycle." Understanding the evolution of a long-term illness is hindered because clinicians rarely follow the family through the complete life history of a disease.

A few studies have explored short-range psychosocial effects on disease course in rheumatoid arthritis (Modolfsky and Chester, 1970) and in diabetes and asthma (Minuchin et al., 1975; Baker et al., 1975; Bradley, 1979; Hamburg et al., 1980). Although these studies are important, they concern microfluctuations rather than broad-scale phases of an illness.

Only a few clinical studies have addressed the importance of broad-time phases of illness. One example has been studies that examine the adaptive versus the harmful role of denial—loosely defined as one's attempts to negate the existence of a problem—at different points of the disease course. For parents of a child with leukemia, denial may enable them adaptively to perform necessary duties during earlier phases of the illness but might lead to devastating consequences for the family if maintained during the terminal phase (Chodoff et al., 1964; Wolff et al., 1964). Likewise, denial may be functional for recovery on a coronary care unit after a myocardial infarction but harmful if this translates into ignoring medical advice vis-à-vis diet, exercise, and work stress over the long term (Croog et al., 1971; Hackett et al., 1968). Such studies highlight the importance of a longitudinal perspective.

The problems of illness variability and time phases are addressed on two separate dimensions: (1) chronic illnesses are grouped according to key biologic similarities and differences that dictate significantly distinct psychosocial demands for the ill individual and his/her family; (2) the prime developmental time phases in the natural evolution of chronic disease are identified.

PSYCHOSOCIAL TYPES OF ILLNESS

The goal of a psychosocial typology is to facilitate the creation of categories with similar psychosocial demands for a wide array of chronic illnesses. This typology is not intended for traditional medical purposes but to examine the relationship between family dynamics and chronic disease. It conceptualizes broad distinctions of (1) onset, (2) course, (3) outcome, and (4) degree of incapacitation of illness. For a broad range of diseases, these categories are hypothesized to be the most psychosocially significant. Although each variable is actually a continuum, it will be described here in a categorical manner by the selection of key anchor points along the continuum.

Onset

Illnesses can be divided into those that have either an acute onset, such as strokes, or gradual onset, such as Parkinson's disease. Although the total amount of family adaptation might be the same for both types of illness, for acute onset illnesses these affective and practical changes are compressed into a short time. This will require that the family more rapidly mobilize crisis management skills. Families able to tolerate highly charged affective states, exchange clearly defined roles flexibly, solve problems efficiently, and utilize outside resources have an advantage in managing acute-onset illnesses. The rate of family change required to cope with gradual-onset diseases allows for a more protracted period of adjustment.

Course

The course of chronic diseases can take three general forms: progressive, constant, or relapsing/episodic. A *progressive* disease (e.g., Alzheimer's disease, emphysema) is one that is continually or generally symptomatic and progresses in severity. The individual and family are faced with the effects of a perpetually symptomatic family member, where disability increases in a stepwise or progressive fashion. This means that a family must live with the prospect of continual role change and adaptation as the disease progresses. Periods of relief from the demands of the illness tend to be minimal. Increasing strain on family care-takers is caused by both exhaustion and the continual addition of new care-taking tasks over time.

A *constant* course illness is one where, typically, an initial event occurs after which the biologic course stabilizes. A single-episode myocardial infarction or spinal cord injury are two examples. Typically, after an initial period of recovery, the chronic phase is characterized by some clear-cut deficit or residual functional limitation. Recurrences can occur, but the individual or family is faced with a semipermanent change that is stable and predictable over a considerable time span. The potential for family exhaustion exists without the strain of new role demands over time.

A *relapsing* or *episodic* course in illnesses like ulcerative colitis and asthma is distinguished by the alternation of stable periods of varying length, characterized by a low level or absence of symptoms, with periods of flare-up or exacerbation. Strain on the family system is caused by both the frequency of transitions between crisis and noncrisis and the ongoing uncertainty of *when* a recurrence will occur. This requires a family flexibility for alternation between two forms of family organization. Also, the wide psychologic discrepancy between periods of normalcy versus illness is a particularly taxing feature unique to relapsing diseases.

Outcome

The extent to which a chronic illness is a likely cause of death and the degree to which it can shorten one's life span are critical features with profound psychosocial impact. The most crucial factor is the *initial expectation* of whether a disease is a likely cause of death. On one end of the continuum are illnesses that do not typically affect the life span, such as lumbosacral disc disease or arthritis. At the other extreme are illnesses that are clearly progressive and usually fatal such as metastatic cancer or acquired immune deficiency syndrome (AIDS). There is also an intermediate, and more unpredictable, category, including both illnesses that shorten the life span, such as cardiovascular disease, and those with the possibility of sudden death, such as hemophilia. Perhaps the major difference between these kinds of outcomes is the degree to which the family experiences anticipatory grief and its pervasive effects on family life (Davies et al., 1973; Derogatis et al., 1979; Schmale and Iker, 1971; Simonton et al., 1980).

When loss is less imminent or certain an outcome, illnesses that may shorten life or cause sudden death provide a fertile ground for idiosyncratic family interpretations. The "it could happen" nature of these illnesses creates a nidus for both overprotection by the family and powerful secondary gains for the ill member. This is particularly relevant to childhood illnesses, such as hemophilia, juvenile onset diabetes, and asthma (Baker et al., 1975; Herz, 1988; Minuchin et al., 1978; Minuchin et al., 1975).

Incapacitation

Incapacitation can result from impairment of cognition (e.g., Alzheimer's disease), sensation (e.g., blindness), movement (e.g., stroke with paralysis, multiple sclerosis), energy production (e.g., cardiovascular disease), and disfiguring (e.g., severe burns) diseases associated with social stigma (e.g., AIDS).

The extent, type, and timing of incapacitation imply sharp differences in the degree of stress facing a family. For instance, the combined cognitive and motor deficits of a person with a stroke necessitate greater family role reallocation than a spinal cord injured person who retains his or her cognitive abilities. For some illnesses, like stroke, incapacitation is often worst at the time of onset and would magnify family coping issues related to onset, expected course, and outcome. For progressive diseases, like Alzheimer's disease, disability looms as an increasing problem in later phases of the illness, allowing a family more time to prepare for anticipated changes. It provides an opportunity for the ill member to participate in disease-related family planning.

By combining the kinds of onset, course, outcome, and incapacitation into a grid format, we generate a typology with 32 potential psychosocial types of illness. This grid is shown in Table 5–1.

The predictability of an illness and the degree of uncertainty about the specific way or rate at which it unfolds overlay and color the other attributes: onset, course, outcome, and incapacitation. For illnesses with highly unpredictable courses, such as multiple

Table 5–1. CATEGORIZATION OF CHRONIC ILLNESSES BY PSYCHOSOCIAL TYPE.*

		Incapacitating		Nonincapacitating	
		Acute	*Gradual*	*Acute*	*Gradual*
PROGRESSIVE	FATAL		Lung cancer with CNS metastases AIDS Bone marrow failure Amyotrophic lateral sclerosis	Acute leukemia Pancreatic cancer Metastatic breast cancer Malignant melanoma Lung cancer Liver cancer, etc.	Cystic fibrosis†
RELAPSING	FATAL			Cancers in remission	
PROGRESSIVE	SHORTENED LIFE SPAN, POSSIBLY FATAL		Emphysema Alzheimer's disease Multi-infarct dementia Multiple sclerosis (late) Chronic alcoholism Huntington's chorea Scleroderma		Juvenile diabetes† Malignant hypertension Insulin-dependent adult onset diabetes
RELAPSING	SHORTENED LIFE SPAN, POSSIBLY FATAL	Angina	Early multiple sclerosis Episodic alcoholism	Sickle cell disease† Hemophilia†	Systemic lupus erythematosus†
CONSTANT	SHORTENED LIFE SPAN, POSSIBLY FATAL	Stroke Moderate severe myocardial infarction	P.K.U. and other inborn errors of metabolism	Mild myocardial infarction Cardiac arrhythmia	Hemodialysis treated renal failure Hodgkin's disease
PROGRESSIVE	NONFATAL		Parkinson's disease Rheumatoid arthritis Osteoarthritis		Noninsulin dependent adult onset diabetes
RELAPSING	NONFATAL	Lumbosacral disc disease		Kidney stones Gout Migraine Seasonal allergy Asthma Epilepsy	Peptic ulcer Ulcerative colitis Chronic bronchitis Other inflammatory bowel diseases Psoriasis
CONSTANT	NONFATAL	Congenital malformations Spinal cord injury Acute blindness Acute deafness Survived severe trauma and burns Posthypoxic syndrome	Nonprogressive mental retardation Cerebral palsy	Benign arrhythmia Congenital heart disease	Malabsorption syndromes Hyper-/Hypothyroidism Pernicious anemia Controlled hypertension Controlled glaucoma

*From Rolland, J. S., Fam. Systems Med. *2*(3):252–253, 1984.
†Early.

sclerosis, family coping and adaptation, especially future planning, is hindered by anticipatory anxiety and ambiguity about what they will actually have to deal with. Families unable to put long-term uncertainty into perspective are at high risk of exhaustion and dysfunction.

The complexity, frequency, and efficacy of a treatment regimen, the amount of home- versus hospital-based care required by the disease, and the frequency and intensity of symptoms vary widely across illnesses with important implications for individual and family adaptation. Some regimens require significant financial resources and care-giving time and energy (e.g., home kidney dialysis, cystic fibrosis). Treatments least likely to be adhered to are those that have a high impact on lifestyles, are difficult to accomplish, and have minimal effects on the level of symptoms or prognosis (Strauss, 1975). Although they reduce time-consuming dependence on medical centers, home-based treatments place heavier responsibility on patient and family. Therefore, the degree of family emotional support, role flexibility, effective problem solving, and communication in relation to these treatment factors will be crucial predictors of long-term treatment compliance.

It is important to consider the likelihood and severity of disease-related crises (Strauss, 1975) and associated family anxiety. A clinician should assess the family's understanding about the possibility, frequency, and lethality of a medical crisis. How congruent is the family's understanding with that of the medical team? Are their expectations catastrophic, or do they minimize real dangers? Are there clear warning signs that the patient or family can recognize? Can a medical crisis be prevented or mitigated by detection of early warning signs or institution of prompt treatment? When a patient or family heeds the early warning signs of a diabetes insulin reaction or asthma attack, a full blown crisis can usually be averted. How complex are the rescue operations? Do they require simple measures carried out at home (e.g., medication, bed rest), or do they necessitate outside assistance or hospitalization? How long can crises last before a family can resume "day-to-day" functioning? It is essential to ask a family about its planning for such crises and the extent and accuracy of their medical knowledge. How clearly has leadership, role reallocation, emotional support, and use of resources outside the family been formulated? If an illness began with an acute crisis (e.g., stroke), then assessment of that event provides useful information as to how that family handles *unexpected* crises. Evaluating the overall viability of the family's crisis planning is crucial.

TIME PHASES OF ILLNESS

In this psychosocial schema of chronic diseases, the developmental time phases of illness is a second dimension. The concept of time phases provides a way for the clinician to think longitudinally and to reach a fuller understanding of chronic illness as an ongoing process with landmarks, transitions, and changing demands. Each phase has its own unique psychosocial developmental tasks that require significantly different strengths, attitudes, or changes from a family. To capture the core psychosocial themes in the natural history of chronic disease, three major phases can be described: (1) crisis, (2) chronic, and (3) terminal. The relationship between a more detailed chronic disease time line and one grouped into broad time phases can be diagrammed as in Figure 5–2.

The *crisis* phase includes any symptomatic period before diagnosis and the initial period of readjustment and coping after the problem has been clarified through a diagnosis and initial treatment plan. This period holds a number of key tasks for the ill member and family. Moos (1984) describes certain universal practical illness-related tasks, including: (1) learning to deal with pain, incapacitation, or other illness-related symptoms; (2) learning to deal with the hospital environment and any disease-related treatment procedures; and (3) establishing and maintaining workable relationships with the health care team. In addition, there are critical tasks of a more general, sometimes existential, nature. The family needs to: (1) create a meaning for the illness event that maximizes a preservation of a sense of mastery and competency, (2) grieve for the loss of the preillness family identity, (3) gradually accept the illness as permanent while maintaining a sense of continuity between their past and future, (4) pull together to undergo short-term crisis reorganization, and (5) in the face of uncertainty, develop a system flexibility toward future goals.

During this initial crisis period, providers have enormous influence over a family's sense of competence and the methods devised to accomplish these developmental tasks. The initial meetings and advice given by providers at the time of diagnosis can be thought of as a "framing event." Because families are so vulnerable at this point, clinicians need to be extremely sensitive in their interactions with family members. Who is included or excluded (e.g., patient) from a discussion can be interpreted by the family as a message of how a family should plan their communication for the duration of the illness. Providers who—in some fashion—blame the patient, a family member, or the whole family for an illness (e.g., delay in seeking an appointment, negligence by parents, poor health habits) or distance themselves from a family may undercut a family's attempt to sustain a sense of competence.

The *chronic* phase, whether long or short, is the time span between the initial diagnosis and readjustment period and the third phase when issues of death and terminal illness predominate. This era can be marked by constancy, progression, or episodic change. Thus, its meaning cannot be grasped by simply knowing the biological behavior of an illness. Rather, it has been referred to as "the long haul," or "day-to-day living with chronic illness" phase. Often, the individual and family have come to grips psychologically and/or organizationally with the permanent changes presented by a chronic illness and have devised an ongoing modus operandi. The ability of the family to maintain the semblance of a normal life under the abnormal presence of a chronic illness and heightened uncertainty is a key task of this period. If the illness is potentially fatal, this is a time of "living in limbo." For certain highly debilitating but not clearly fatal illnesses, such as a massive stroke or dementia, the family can become saddled with an exhausting problem seemingly without end. Paradoxically, a family's hope to resume a normal life cycle might only be realized after the death of their ill member. This highlights another crucial task of this phase: the maintenance of maximal autonomy for *all* family members in the face of a pull toward mutual dependency and care-taking.

The last or *terminal* phase includes the preterminal stage of an illness where the inevitability of

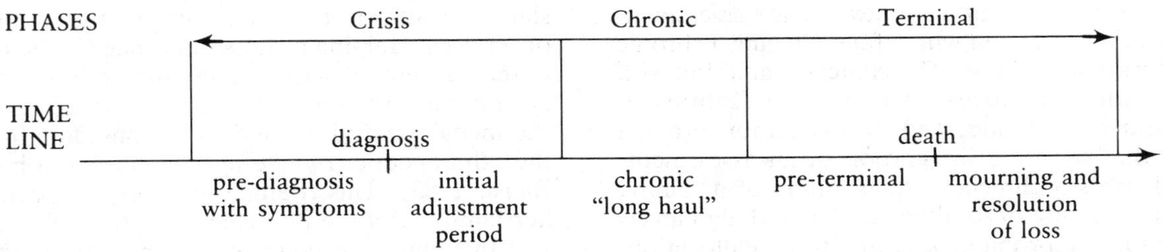

Figure 5–2. Psychosocial time phases of illness. (From Rolland, J. S.: Toward a psychosocial typology of chronic and life-threatening illness. Fam. Systems Med., 2(3):245–263, 1984.)

death becomes apparent and dominates family life. This phase is distinguished by issues surrounding separation, death, grief, resolution of mourning, and resumption of normal family life beyond the loss.

Critical transition periods link the three time phases. Carter and McGoldrick (1988) and Levinson (1978, 1986) have clarified the importance of transition periods in the family and adult life cycle literature. Transitions in the illness life cycle are times when families re-evaluate the appropriateness of their previous life structure in the face of new illness-related developmental demands. Unfinished business from the previous phase can complicate or block movement through the transitions. Families can become permanently frozen in an adaptive structure that has outlived its utility (Penn, 1983). For example, the usefulness of pulling together in the crisis period can become a maladaptive and stifling prison for all family members in the chronic phase. Enmeshed families would have difficulty negotiating this delicate transition.

The interaction of the time phases and typology of illness provide a framework for a chronic disease psychosocial developmental model that resembles models for human development. The time phases (crisis, chronic, and terminal) can be considered broad developmental periods in the natural history of chronic disease. Each period has certain basic tasks independent of the type of illness. Each "type" of illness has specific supplementary tasks. The basic tasks of the three illness phases and transitions recapitulate in many respects the unfolding of human development. For example, the crisis phase is similar in certain fundamental ways to the era of childhood and adolescence. Child development involves a prolonged period during which the child learns the fundamentals of life as parents temper other developmental plans (e.g., career) to accommodate raising children (Piaget, 1952). In an analogous way, the crisis phase is a period of socialization to the basics of living with chronic disease, when other life plans are frequently put on hold by the family to accommodate to the illness. Just as the transition from adolescence to adulthood is marked by the relinquishing of a moratorium in order to assume adult identity and responsibilities (Erikson, 1950), the transition to the chronic phase of illness emphasizes autonomy and the creation of a viable ongoing life given the realities of the illness. In the transition to the chronic phase, a "hold" or moratorium on other developmental tasks that served to protect the initial period of socialization/adaptation to life with chronic disease is re-evaluated. The separate developmental tasks of "living with chronic illness" and "living out the other parts of one's life" must be brought together.

The psychosocial types and phases of illness can be combined into a typology so that each "psychosocial type" of illness can be thought about in relation to each of the time phases. The addition of a family systems model creates a three-dimensional family systems–illness model (Fig. 5–3). Psychosocial illness types, illness time phases, and key family systems variables constitute the three dimensions. This model allows consideration of the importance of strengths and weaknesses in various components of family functioning in relation to different types of disease at different illness phases.

CLINICAL IMPLICATIONS

There are several important implications of this model for clinical practice. The components of the typology provide a means to grasp the character of a chronic illness in psychosocial terms. They provide a meaningful bridge for the clinician between the biologic

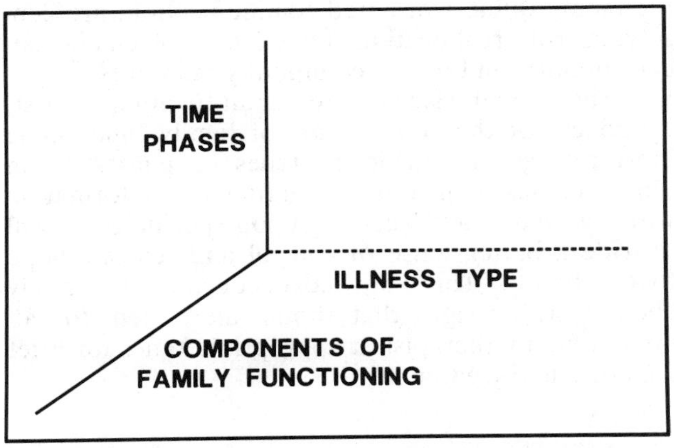

Figure 5–3. Three-dimensional model representing the relationship between illness type, time phases, and family functioning. (Modified from Rolland, J. S.: Chronic illness and the life cycle: A conceptual framework. Fam. Proc., 26(2):203–221, 1987.)

and psychosocial worlds. Perhaps the major contribution is the provision of a framework for assessment and clinical intervention with a family facing a chronic or life-threatening illness. The clinician can think with greater clarity and focus. Attention to features of onset, course, outcome, and incapacitation provide markers that facilitate integration of an assessment. This will focus a clinician's questioning of a family. For instance, acute onset illnesses demand high levels of adaptability, problem solving, role reallocation, and balanced cohesion. A high degree of family enmeshment might make a family less likely to be able to cope with these demands. Forethought on this issue would cue a clinician toward a more appropriate family evaluation.

The concept of time phases provides a way for the clinician to think longitudinally and to reach a fuller understanding of chronic illness as an ongoing process with landmarks, transition points, and changing demands. An illness time line delineates psychosocial developmental stages of an illness, each phase with its own unique developmental tasks. Kaplan (1968) has emphasized the importance of solving phase-related tasks within the time limits set by the duration of each successive developmental phase of an illness. The failure to resolve issues in this sequential manner can jeopardize the total coping process of the family. Therefore, attention to time allows the clinician to assess a family's strengths and vulnerabilities in relation to the present and future phases of the illness.

Taken together, the psychosocial types and time phases provide a context to integrate other aspects of a comprehensive assessment, involving a range of universal and illness-specific family dynamics. This could include assessment of a number of factors: the family's illness belief system; the meaning of the illness to the family; the interface of the illness with individual and family development; the family's transgenerational history of coping with illness, loss, and crisis; the family's medical crisis planning; the family's capacity to perform home-based medical care; and the family's illness-oriented communication, problem solving, role reallocation, affective involvement, social support, and use of community resources.

The model clarifies treatment planning. First, awareness of the components of family functioning most relevant to particular types or phases of an illness guides goal-setting. Sharing this information with the family and deciding upon specific goals will provide a better sense of control and realistic hope to the family. This knowledge educates the family about warning signs that should alert them to call upon a family therapist at appropriate times for brief goal-oriented treatment.

CLINICAL APPLICATIONS

Using the psychosocial typology of illness as a reference point has important implications for health services delivery both for the patient's/family's relationship to health professionals and for the organization of services. Helping professionals need to be included in the conceptualization of any therapeutic treatment system with a family. The application of this idea in the medical world has led to various descriptions of the "therapeutic triangle in medicine" (Doherty and Baird, 1983). This triangle includes the patient, his/her family, and the physician (health care team).

Including the concept of types of psychosocial illness into the scheme creates a four-member system composed of four interlocking triangles (Fig. 5–4). It is easier to conceptualize the illness as a fourth member if one pictures each illness type as having a personality (which includes the kind of onset, course, outcome, degree of incapacitation, and predictability) and particular developmental life course.

Using this four-sided diagram, one can see how the original therapeutic triangle is colored by different types of illness. For instance, consider the concept of locus of control in relation to disease (Wallston et al., 1976, 1978). This concept refers to how much an individual or family sees outcomes as being influenced by their own efforts. A family's beliefs about the potential to control biologic processes can vary along a continuum from an internal to external orientation. A certain minimal level of agreement concerning this kind of health belief is critical for the establishment of a viable therapeutic relationship between the patient, his or her family, and the health care team. The degree of consensus concerning locus of control can vary dramatically for this triad depending on the type of chronic disease. A particular family physician may have had a good working relationship with a family that had presented over the years with non–life-threatening and nonincapacitating illnesses. If the father suffers a serious heart attack and there are differences in beliefs about control that surface in relation to this more life-threatening and incapacitating illness, the stability of the long-standing therapeutic triangle might be threatened. If the physician checked his or her own beliefs and questioned the family about theirs in relation to a life-threatening incapacitating disease, a potential serious rift in this therapeutic system might be averted.

The illness time phases offer a framework for timing family psychosocial check-ups to coincide with key transition points in the illness life cycle. The typology facilitates the development of various preventively oriented psychoeducational or support groups for patients and their families. For example, groups could be designed to meet the needs of patients dealing with progressive, life-threatening diseases; relapsing disorders; acute onset, incapacitating illnesses; or the chronic phase of constant course diseases. Sometimes, there are not enough families involved with any particular disease to form such groups, particularly in more rural settings or for less common illnesses. Organizing group-oriented services in terms of illness types overcomes these obstacles while maintaining the groups' thematic coherence.

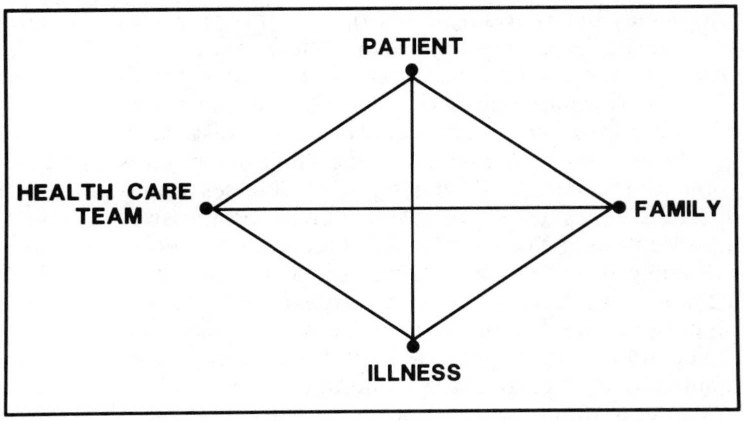

Figure 5–4. The therapeutic quadrangle. (Modified from Rolland, J. S.: A conceptual model of chronic and life-threatening illness and its impact on the family. *In* Chilman, C., Nunnally, E., and Cox, F. (Eds.): Chronic Illness and Disability: Families in Trouble. Beverly Hills, CA, Sage Publications, 1988.)

Also, packaging brief psychoeducational modules, timed for critical phases of particular "types" of diseases, enables families to digest manageable portions of a long-term coping process. Each module could be tailored to the particular phase of the illness life cycle and family coping skills necessary to confront disease-related demands. This would provide a cost-effective preventive service that could also aid in the detection of families at high risk for maladaptation to chronic illness.

Family Assessment

This section centers on illness-oriented family dynamics that concern belief systems and the dimension of time, and these dynamics are used to illustrate how one can apply the psychosocial typology of illness to family assessment more generally. There is a burgeoning literature that describes family coping and adaptation to a variety of normative and unexpected life stresses (Hill, 1949; Burr, 1973; McCubbin, 1979; McCubbin et al., 1980; Hansen and Johnson, 1979; Figley and McCubbin, 1983; McCubbin and Figley, 1983). Researchers and clinicians have documented key elements in successful family coping and adaptation to a specific type of stressor, such as chronic illness (Moos, 1984). Most endorse the notion that chronic illnesses become incorporated into the family system and its processes. Diseases interface with both general and illness-specific family dynamics, such as communication, problem solving, hierarchy, role reallocation, affective involvement, information gathering, social support, utilization of community resources, mastery of home-based medical care, medical crisis planning, and maintenance of self-esteem.

A developmental framework and family paradigms may provide the most useful view of family dynamics and long-term illness. Particular attention is given to (1) the family transgenerational history of coping with illness, loss, and crisis; (2) the interface of the illness with the individual and family life cycles and; (3) the family illness/health belief system. The interrelationship of the psychosocial types and illness phases with each of these components of family functioning is highlighted through clinical examples. These vignettes also suggest a broader application of the typology to other components of family functioning.

TRANSGENERATIONAL HISTORY OF ILLNESS, LOSS, AND CRISIS

Many systems-oriented practitioners have emphasized that a family's present behavior cannot be adequately comprehended apart from its history (Boszormenyi-Nagy, 1973; Bowen, 1978; Carter and McGoldrick, 1980; Framo, 1976; McGoldrick and Walsh, 1983). Historical questioning is a way to track key events and transitions to gain an understanding of a family's organizational shifts and coping strategies *as a system* in response to past stressors. This is not a cause and effect model but reflects a belief that such a historical search may help explain the family's current style of coping and adaptation. A historical systemic perspective involves more than simply deciphering how a family organized itself around past stressors; it also tracks the evolution of family adaptation over time. Patterns of adaptation, replications, discontinuities, shifts in relationships (i.e., alliances, triangles, cutoffs), and sense of competence are important considerations. These patterns are transmitted across generations as family myths, taboos, catastrophic expectations, and belief systems (McGoldrick and Walsh, 1983). By gathering this information, a clinician can create a family genogram (see McGoldrick and Gerson, 1985, and Chapter 74). A chronic illness–oriented genogram focuses on how a family organized itself as an evolving system specifically around previous illnesses and unexpected crises in the current and previous generations. A central goal is to bring to light the adults' "learned differences around illness" (Penn, 1983).

The psychosocial types and phases of illness are useful concepts in the family evaluation. Although a family may have certain standard ways of coping with any illness, there may be critical differences in their style and success in adaptation to different types of diseases. A family may show a disparity in their level of coping with one disease versus another, disregarding differences in demands. If the clinician inquires about the same and similar types of illnesses versus different types (e.g., relapsing versus progressive, life-threatening versus non-life-threatening), he/she will make better use of historical data. For instance, a family may have consistently organized itself successfully around non-life-threatening illnesses but reeled under the weight of metastatic cancer. This family might be particularly vulnerable if another life-threatening illness were to occur. A different family may only have had experience with non-life-threatening illnesses and be ignorant of how to cope with the uncertainties particular to life-threatening diseases. Cognizance of these facts will draw attention to areas of strength and vulnerability for a family facing cancer. A recent family consultation highlights the importance of tracking prior family illnesses.

Joe, his wife Ann, and their three teenage children presented for a family evaluation 10 months after Joe's diagnosis with moderate-severe asthma. Joe, age 44, had been successfully employed for many years as a spray painter. Apparently, exposure to a new chemical triggered the onset of asthmatic attacks that necessitated hospitalization and occupational disability. Although somewhat improved, he continued to have persistent and moderate respiratory symptoms. Initially, his physicians had predicted that improvement would occur but remained noncommittal as to the level of chronicity. Continued breathing difficulties contributed to increased symptoms of depression, uncharacteristic temperamental outbursts, alcohol abuse, and family discord.

In the initial assessment, I inquired as to their prior illness experience. This was the nuclear family's first encounter with chronic illness, and their families of origin had limited experience. Ann's father had died 7 years earlier of a sudden and unexpected heart attack. Joe's brother had died in an accidental drowning. Neither had experience with disease as an ongoing process. Joe had assumed that improvement meant "cure." Illness for both had meant either death or recovery. The physician/family system were not attuned to the hidden risks for this family coping with the transition from the crisis to chronic phase of his asthma—the juncture where the permanency of the disease needed to be addressed.

Tracking a family's coping capabilities in the crisis, chronic and terminal phases of previous chronic illnesses highlight complications in adaptation related to different points in the "illness life cycle." A family may have adapted well in the crisis phase of living with a spinal cord injury but failed to navigate the transition to a family organization consistent with long-haul adaptation. A rigidly enmeshed family may have become frozen in a crisis structure and may have been unable to deal appropriately with issues of maximizing individual and collective autonomy in the chronic phase. Another family with a member with chronic kidney failure may have functioned very well in handling the practicalities of home dialysis. However, in the terminal phase, their limitations around affective expression may have left a legacy of unresolved grief. A history of phase-specific difficulties can alert a clinician to potential vulnerable periods for a family over the course of the current chronic illness. The following case illustrates the interplay of problems coping with a current illness, fueled by unresolved issues related to a particular type and/or phase of disease in a family of origin.

Mary, her husband Bill, and their son Jim sought treatment 4 months after Mary had sustained a serious concussion in a life-threatening head-on auto collision caused by the driver of another vehicle. For several months, there was some concern by the medical team that she might have suffered a cerebral hemorrhage. Ultimately, it was clarified that this had not occurred. Over this time, Mary became increasingly depressed and, despite strong reassurance, continued to believe she had a life-threatening condition and would die from a brain hemorrhage.

In the initial evaluation, she revealed that she was experiencing vivid dreams of meeting her deceased father. Apparently, her father, with whom she had been extremely close, had died from a cerebral hemorrhage after a 4-year history of a progressive debilitating brain tumor, marked by progressive and uncontrolled epileptic seizures. Mary, 14 at the time, was the "baby" in the family; her two siblings were much older. The family had shielded her from his illness, culminating in her mother's decision that she not attend either the wake or the funeral. This event galvanized her position as the "child in need of protection"—a dynamic that carried over into her marriage. Despite her hurt, anger, and lack of acceptance of the death, she had avoided dealing with her feelings with her mother for over 20 years. Other family history revealed that her maternal grandfather had died when her mother was 7 years old. The mother had had to endure an open casket wake at home. This traumatic experience was a major factor in her mother's attempt to protect her daughter from the same kind of memory.

Mary's own life-threatening head injury had triggered a catastrophic reaction and dramatic resurfacing of previous losses involving similar types of illness and injury. Therapy focused on a series of tasks and rituals that involved her initiating conversations with her mother and visits to her father's gravesite.

The family's history of coping with crises in general, especially unanticipated ones, should be explored. Illnesses with acute onset (i.e., heart attack), moderate-severe sudden incapacitation (i.e., stroke), or rapid relapse (i.e., ulcerative colitis, diabetic insulin reaction, disc disease) demand in various ways rapid crisis mobilization skills. In these situations, the family needs to reorganize quickly and efficiently, shifting from its usual organization to a crisis structure. Other illnesses can create a crisis because of the continual demand for family stamina (i.e., spinal cord injury, rheumatoid arthritis, emphysema). The family history of coping with moderate-severe ongoing stressors is a good predictor of adjustment to these types of illness.

For any significant chronic illness in either adult's

family of origin, a clinician should try to get a picture of how those families organized to handle the range of disease-related affective and practical tasks. Also, it is important to find out what role each played in handling these emotional or practical tasks. Whether the parents (as children) were given too much responsibility (parentified) or shielded from involvement is of particular note. What did they learn from those experiences that influences how they think about the current illness? Whether they emerge with a strong sense of competence or failure is essential information. In one particular case involving a family with three generations of hemophilia transmitted through the mother's side, the father had been shielded from the knowledge that his older brother who died in adolescence had had a terminal form of kidney disease. Also, this man had not been allowed to attend his brother's funeral. From that trauma, he made a strong commitment to openness about disease-related issues with his two sons with hemophilia and his daughters who were genetic carriers.

By collecting such information about each adult's family of origin, one can anticipate areas of conflict and consensus. Unresolved issues related to illness and loss can remain dormant in a marriage and suddenly re-emerge triggered by a chronic illness in the current nuclear family (Penn, 1983; Walker, 1983). Penn describes how particular coalitions that emerge in the context of a chronic illness are isomorphs of those that existed in each adult's family of origin, as in the following vignette:

If a mother has been the long-time rescuer of her mother from a tyrannical husband, and then in her own family bears a son with hemophilia, she will become his rescuer, often against his father. In this manner she continues to rescue her mother but, oddly enough, now from her husband rather than from her own father. . . . In this family with a hemophiliac son, the father's father had been ill for a long period and had received all the mother's attention. In his present family, this father, though outwardly objecting to the coalition between his wife and son, honored that relationship, as if he hoped it would make up for the one he had once forfeited with his own mother. The coalition in the nuclear family looks open and adaptational (mother and son), but is fueled by coalitions in the past (mother with her mother, and father with his mother) (Penn, 1983).

The re-enactment of previous system configuration around illness can occur largely as an unconscious, automatic process. Further, the dysfunctional complementarity can emerge de novo specifically within the context of a chronic disease. On detailed inquiry, couples frequently reveal a tacit unspoken understanding that if an illness occurred they would reorganize to re-enact "unfinished business" from their families of origin. Typically, the role chosen represents a repetition or opposite role played by themselves or the same sex parent. A clinician needs to maintain some distinction between functional family process with and without chronic disease. For families that present in this manner, placing a primary therapeutic emphasis upon the resolution of family of origin issues might be the best approach to prevent or rectify an unhealthy triangle.

Families, like those just described, with encapsulated illness "time bombs" need to be distinguished from families with more pervasive, long-standing dysfunctional patterns where illnesses can become imbedded in a web of pre-existing fused family transactions. In the traditional sense of psychosomatic, a severely dysfunctional family often has a greater level of baseline reactivity such that when an illness enters their system, this reactivity is expressed somatically through a poor medical course and/or treatment noncompliance. These families lack the foundation of a functional nonillness system. The initial focus of therapeutic intervention may need to be targeted more on pragmatic immediate help rather than on family of origin work, with more limited therapeutic aims.

A third group of symptomatic families facing chronic disease are those without significant intra- or intergenerational family dysfunctional patterns. Any family may falter in the face of multiple superimposed disease and nondisease stressors that impact in a relatively short time. With progressive, incapacitating diseases or the concurrence of illnesses in several family members, a pragmatic approach that focuses on expanded or creative use of supports and resources outside the family is most productive.

INTERFACE OF THE ILLNESS, INDIVIDUAL, AND FAMILY LIFE CYCLES

To place the unfolding of chronic disease into a developmental context, it is crucial to understand the intertwining of three evolutionary threads: the illness, individual, and family life cycles (Rolland, 1987a, 1988). The psychosocial typology offers a language to characterize diseases in psychosocial and longitudinal terms—each illness having a particular pattern and expected developmental life course. Second, because an illness *is* part of an individual, it is essential to think simultaneously about the interaction of individual and family development.

The *life cycle* is a central concept for both family and individual development. Life cycle means there is a basic sequence and unfolding of the life course within which individual, family, or illness uniqueness occurs. A second key concept is the human *life structure.* Levinson (1978) described life structure to mean the design of a person's life at any given point in the life cycle. This design is made up of an individual's various commitments (e.g., work, family, religious affiliation, hobbies) and the relative importance of each commitment. The life structure mediates transactions between the individual/family and the environment. Although Levinson described the individual adult male life cycle, his concepts can be applied to the family as a unit.

Illness, individual, and family development have in common the notion of eras marked by the alternation of life structure–building/maintaining and life structure–changing (transitional) periods linking developmental eras. The primary goal of a structure–building/maintaining period is to form a life structure and enrich life within it based on the key choices an individual/family made during the preceding transition period. The delineation of separate eras derives from a set of developmental tasks associated with each. Transition periods are potentially the most vulnerable because previous individual, family, and illness life structures are reappraised in the face of new developmental tasks that may require major, discontinuous change rather than minor alterations (Hoffman, 1988). Levinson (1978) has described four major eras in individual life structure development: childhood and adolescence, early, middle, and late adulthood. Each era lasts approximately 20 years. Carter and McGoldrick (1988) have delineated the following six family life cycle stages: (1) the unattached young adult, (2) the newly married couple, (3) the family with young children, (4) the family with adolescents, (5) launching children and moving on, and (6) the family in later life.

A primary distinction between Levinson's and the family life cycle model described by Carter and McGoldrick is the focus on age-specific periods versus transitional marker events. In family models, marker events (e.g., marriage, birth of first child, last child leaving home) herald the transition from one stage to the next. Levinson's research elucidated a sequence of age-specific periods, 5 to 7 years in length, during which certain developmental tasks for adult males are addressed independent of marker events. In his model, marker events will both color the character of a developmental period and, in turn, be colored by their timing in the individual life cycle.

The concept of centripetal versus centrifugal family styles and phases in the family life cycle is particularly useful to the task of integrating illness, individual, and family development (Beavers, 1982; Beavers and Voeller, 1983). Applying this notion to the family life cycle, Combrinck-Graham (1985) describes a family life spiral model where she envisions a three-generational family system oscillating through time between periods of family closeness (centripetal) and periods of family disengagement (centrifugal). These periods coincide with oscillations between family developmental tasks that require intense bonding or high cohesion, like early child-rearing, and tasks that emphasize personal identity and autonomy, like adolescence. In a literal sense, centripetal and centrifugal describe a tendency to move respectively toward and away from a center. In life cycle terms, they connote a fit between family developmental tasks and the relative need for family members to direct their energies inside the family and work together to accomplish those tasks. During a centripetal period, both the individual member's and family unit's life structure emphasize internal family life. External boundaries around the family are tightened while personal boundaries between members are somewhat diffused to enhance family teamwork. In the transition to a centrifugal period, the family life structure shifts to accommodate goals that emphasize an individual family member's life outside the family. The external family boundary is loosened while separateness between some family members increases.

From this brief overview of life cycle models, we can cull out several key concepts that provide a foundation for discussion of chronic disease. The life cycle contains alternating transition and life structure–building/maintaining periods. Further, particular periods can be characterized as either centripetal or centrifugal in nature (Fig. 5–5).

The notion of centripetal and centrifugal modes is useful in linking the illness life cycle to the individual and family life cycles, from the vantage point of chronic illnesses in general or that of specific illness types or phases. In general, chronic disease exerts a centripetal pull on the family system. In family developmental models, centripetal periods begin with the addition of a new family member (infant) that propels the family into a prolonged period of socialization of children. In an analogous way, the occurrence of chronic illness in a family resembles the addition of a new member, which sets in motion for the family a centripetal process of socialization to illness. Symptoms, loss of function, the demands of shifting or new illness-related practical and affective roles, and the fear of loss through death all refocus a family inward.

If the onset of an illness coincides with a centrifugal period for the family, it can derail the family from its natural momentum. If a young adult becomes ill, he/she may need to return to the family of origin for disease-related care-taking. Each member's extrafamilial autonomy and individuation are at risk. The young adult's ability to establish a life away from home is threatened either temporarily or permanently. Both parents may have to relinquish interests outside the family. Family dynamics as well as disease severity will influence whether the family's reversion to a centripetal life structure is a temporary detour within their general movement outward or a permanent involutional shift. A highly cohesive or enmeshed family frequently faces the transition to a more autonomous period with trepidation. A chronic illness provides a sanctioned reason to return to the "safety" of the prior centripetal period. For some family members, the giving up of the building of a new life structure already in progress can be more devastating than when the family is still in a more centripetal period with more preliminary future plans. An analogy would be the difference between a couple discovering that they do not have enough money to build a house versus being forced to abandon their building project with the foundation already completed.

Disease onset that coincides with a centripetal period in the family life cycle (e.g., early child-rearing) can have several important consequences. At minimum, it can foster a prolongation of this

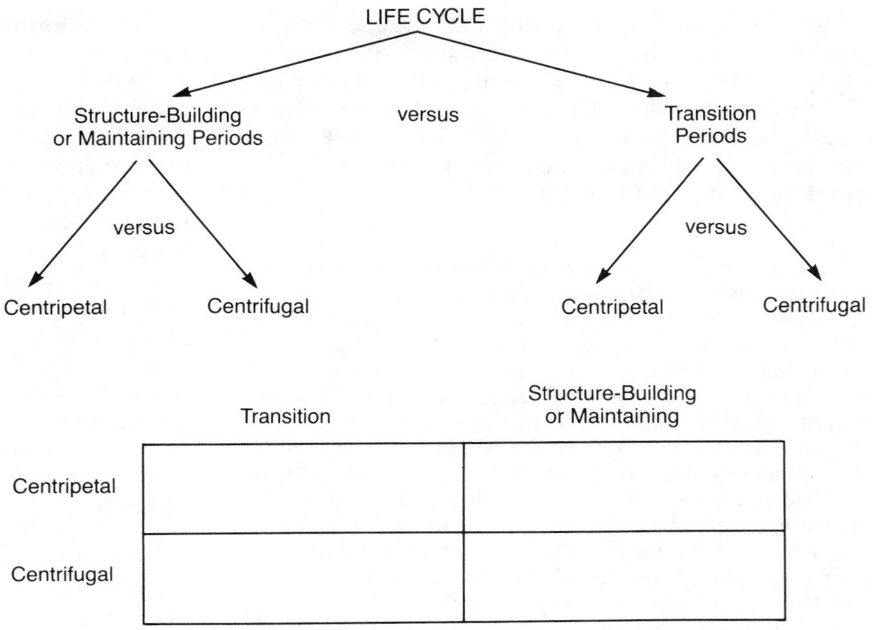

Figure 5–5. Periods in the family and individual life cycle. (Modified from Rolland, J. S.: Chronic illness and the life cycle: A conceptual framework. Fam. Proc., *26*(2):203–221, 1987.)

period. At worst, the family can become permanently stuck at this phase of development, when the inward pull of the illness and the phase of the life cycle coincide. The risk here is their tendency to amplify one another. For families that function marginally before an illness onset, this kind of mutual reinforcement can trigger a runaway process leading to overt family dysfunction. Minuchin's and colleagues' (1975, 1978) research of "psychosomatic" families has documented this process in several common childhood illnesses.

When a parent develops a chronic disease during this centripetal child-rearing phase of development, a family's ability to stay on course is severely taxed. The impact of the illness is like the addition of a new infant member with "special needs" competing for potentially scarce family resources. For psychosocially milder diseases, efficient role reallocation may suffice, as in the following case:

Tom and his wife Sally presented for treatment 6 months after Tom had sustained a severe burn injury to both hands that required skin grafting. A year of recuperation was necessary before Tom would be able to return to his job, which required physical labor and full use of his hands. Prior to this injury, his wife had been at home full time raising their two children, ages 3 and 5. Although Tom was temporarily handicapped in terms of his career, he was physically fit to assume the role of househusband. Initially, both Tom and Sally remained at home using his disability income to "get by." When Sally expressed an interest in finding a job to relieve financial pressures, Tom resisted and marital strain caused by his injury flared into dysfunctional conflict.

Sufficient resources were available in the system to accommodate the illness and ongoing child-bearing tasks. Their definition of marriage lacked the necessary role flexibility to master the problem. Treatment focused on rethinking his masculine and monolithic definition of "family provider," a definition that had, in fact, emerged in full force during this centripetal phase of the family life cycle.

If the disease affecting a parent is more debilitating (e.g., traumatic brain injury, cervical spinal cord injury), its impact on the child-rearing family is twofold. A "new" family member is added, a parent is "lost," and the semblance of a single-parent family with an added special needs child is created. For acute onset illnesses, when both events occur simultaneously, family resources may be inadequate to meet the combined child-rearing and care-taking demands. This situation is ripe for the emergence of a parentified child or the re-enlistment into active parenting of a grandparent. These forms of family adaptation are not inherently dysfunctional. A clinician needs to assess these structural realignments. Are certain individuals assigned rigid care-taking roles, or are they flexible and shared? Are care-taking roles viewed flexibly from a developmental vantage point? For an adolescent care-taker, this means the family being mindful of the approaching developmental transition to an independent life separate from the family. For grandparent care-takers, it means sensitivity to their increasing physical limitations or need to assist their own spouse.

The degree of centripetal/centrifugal pull varies enormously in different types and phases of illness. This variability has impact on the family life cycle independent of family dynamics. The tendency for a disease to pull a family inward increases with the level of incapacitation or risk of death. Progressive diseases over time are inherently more centripetal than constant course illnesses. The ongoing addition of new demands as an illness progresses keeps a family's energy focused inward. After a modus operandi has been forged, a constant course disease (excluding those with severe incapacitation) permits a family to enter or resume a more centrifugal phase of the life cycle. The added inward pull exerted by a progressive disease increases the risk of reversing normal family disengagement or freezing a family into a permanently fused state.

Mr. L., age 54, had become increasingly depressed as a result of severe and progressive complications of his adult-onset diabetes that had emerged over the past 5 years. These complications included a leg amputation and renal failure that recently required the instituting of home dialysis on a four times daily basis. For 20 years, Mr. L. had had an uncomplicated constant course, allowing him to lead a full active life. An excellent athlete, he engaged in a number of recreational group sports. Short- and long-term family planning had never focused around his illness. This optimistic attitude was reinforced by the fact that two people in Mrs. L.'s family of origin had had diabetes without complications. Their only child, a son age 26, had uneventfully left home after high school and had recently married. Mr. and Mrs. L. had a stable marriage, where both maintained many outside independent interests. In short, the family had moved smoothly through the transition to a more centrifugal phase of the family's life cycle.

His disease's transformation to a progressive course coupled with the incapacitating and life-shortening nature of his complications had reversed the normal process of family disengagement. His wife took a second job that necessitated her quitting her hobbies and civic involvements. Their son moved back home to help his mother take care of his father and the house. Mr. L., disabled from work and his athletic social network, felt a burden to everyone and blocked in his own mid-life development.

The essential goal of family treatment in developmental terms centered around reversing some of the system's centripetal over-reaction back to a more realistic balance. For Mr. L., this meant a reworking of his life structure to accommodate his real limitations while maximizing a return to his more independent style. For Mrs. L. and her son, this meant developing realistic expectations for Mr. L. and re-establishing key aspects of their autonomy within an illness/family system.

Relapsing illnesses alternate between periods of drawing a family inward and periods of release from the immediate demands of disease. However, the on-call state of preparedness dictated by many such illnesses keeps some part of the family in a centripetal mode despite medically asymptomatic periods, hindering the natural flow between phases of the family life cycle.

One way to think about the phases of illness is that they represent to the family a progression from a centripetal crisis phase to a more centrifugal chronic phase. The terminal phase, if it occurs, forces most families back into a more inward mode. The so-called illness life structure, developed by a family to accommodate each phase in the illness life cycle, is colored by each phase's inherent centripetal/centrifugal nature. For example, in a family where illness onset has coincided with a centrifugal phase of development, the transition to the chronic phase permits a family to resume more of its momentum.

One cannot overemphasize the need for clinicians to be mindful of the timing of the onset of a chronic illness, with individual/family transition and life structure building/maintaining periods of development. All *transitions* involve the basic processes of termination and initiation. Arrivals, departures, and losses are common life events, generating an undercurrent of preoccupation with death and finiteness (Levinson, 1978). Chronic and life-threatening illness precipitates the loss of the preillness identity of the family. It forces the family into a transition in which one of the family's main tasks is to accommodate the anticipation of further loss and possibly untimely death. When the onset of a chronic illness coincides with a transition in the individual or family life cycle, issues related to previous, current, and anticipated loss will be likely magnified. Transition periods are often characterized by upheaval, rethinking of prior commitments, and openness to change. As a result, those times hold a greater risk for the illness to become unnecessarily embedded or inappropriately ignored in planning for the next developmental period. During a transition period, the very process of loosening prior commitments creates a context for emergence of family rules regarding loyalty through sacrifice and care-taking. Indecision about one's future can be resolved by excessive focus on a family member's physical problems. This can be a major precursor of family dysfunction in the context of chronic disease. By adopting a longitudinal developmental perspective, a clinician will stay attuned to future transitions and their overlap.

An example can highlight the importance of the illness in relation to future developmental transitions. Imagine a family in which the father—a carpenter and primary financial provider—develops multiple sclerosis. At first, his level of impairment is mild and stabilized, allowing him to continue part-time work. Because their children are all teenagers, his wife is able to undertake part-time work to help maintain financial stability. The oldest son, age 15, seems relatively unaffected. Two years later, father experiences a rapid progression of his illness that leaves him totally disabled. His son, now 17, has dreams of going away to college to prepare for a science career. The specter of financial hardship and the perceived need for a "man in the family" creates a serious dilemma of choice for the son and the family. In this case, there is a fundamental clash between developmental issues of separation/individuation and the ongoing demands of progressive chronic disability upon the family. This vignette demonstrates the potential clash between simultaneous transition periods: the illness transition to a more incapacitating and progressive course, the adolescent son's transition to early adulthood, and the family's transition from the "living with teenagers" to "launching young adults" stage. Also, this example illustrates the significance of the type of illness. A less incapacitating or a relapsing illness (as opposed to a progressive or constant course disease) might interfere less with this young man's separation from his family. If his father had an intermittently incapacitating illness, like disc disease, the son might have moved out but tailored his choices to remain close by and thus available during acute flare-ups.

Illness onset may cause a different kind of disruption if it coincides with a *life structure building/maintaining period* in individual or family development. These periods are characterized by the living out of choices made during the preceding transition period. Relative to transition periods, family members try to protect their own and their family unit's current life structure. Diseases with only a mild level of psychosocial severity (e.g., nonfatal, none/mild incapacitation, nonprogressive) may require some revision of individual/family life structure but not a radical restructuring that would necessitate a return to a transitional phase of development. A chronic illness with a critical threshold of psychosocial severity will demand the re-establishment of a transitional form of life, at a time when individual/family inertia is to preserve the momentum of a stable period. An individual's or family's level of adaptability is a prime factor determining the successful navigation of this kind of crisis. In this context, family adaptability involves the ability to transform its entire life structure to a prolonged transitional state.

For instance, in the previous example, the father's multiple sclerosis rapidly progressed while the oldest son was in a transition period in his own development. The nature of the strain in developmental terms would be quite different if his father's disease progression had occurred when this young man was 26, had already left home, finished college and secured a first job, married and had a child. In the latter scenario, the oldest son's life structure is in a centripetal, structure-maintaining period within his newly formed nuclear family. To fully accommodate the needs of his family of origin could require a monumental shift of his developmental priorities. When this illness crisis coincided with a developmental transition period (age 17), although a dilemma of choice existed, the son was available and less fettered by commitments in progress. Later, at age 26, he has made commitments and is in the process of living them out with his newly formed family. To serve the demands of an illness transition, the son might need to shift his previously stable life structure back to a transitional state. And the shift would happen "out of phase" with the flow of his individual and nuclear family's development. One way to resolve this dilemma of divided loyalties might be the merging of the two households, thereby creating a single large centripetal family system.

This discussion raises several key clinical points. From a systems viewpoint, at the time of a chronic illness diagnosis it is important to know the phase of the family life cycle and the stage of individual development of all family members, not just the ill member. This is important information for several reasons. First, chronic disease in one family member can profoundly affect developmental goals of another member. For instance, a disabled infant can be a serious roadblock to a mother's mastery of child-rearing, or a life-threatening illness in a young adult can interfere with the spouse's task of beginning the phase of parenthood. Second, family members frequently do not adapt equally to chronic illness. Each member's ability to adapt and the rate at which they do so is related to the individual's own developmental stage and role in the family (Ireys and Burr, 1984). The oldest son in the previous example illustrates this point.

There exists a normative and non-normative timing of chronic illness in the life cycle. Coping with chronic illness and death are considered normally anticipated tasks in late adulthood. On the other hand, illnesses and losses that occur earlier are "out of phase" and tend to be developmentally more disruptive (Herz, 1988; Neugarten, 1976). As untimely events, chronic diseases can severely disrupt the usual sense of continuity and rhythm of the life cycle. The timing in the life cycle of an unexpected event, like a chronic illness, will shape the form of adaptation and the event's influence on subsequent development (Levinson, 1978).

The notion of "out of phase" illnesses can be conceptualized in a more refined way. First, since diseases have a centripetal influence on most families, they can be more disruptive to families in a centrifugal phase of development. Second, the onset of chronic disease tends to create a period of transition, the length or intensity of which depends upon the psychosocial type and phase of the illness. This forced transition is particularly "out of phase" if it coincides with a life structure building/maintaining period in the individual's or family's life cycle. Third, if the particular illness is progressive, relapsing, increasingly incapacitating and/or life threatening, then the phases in the unfolding of the disease will be punctuated by numerous transitions. Under these conditions, a family will need to more frequently alter their illness life structure to accommodate the shifting and often increasing demands of the disease. This level of demand and uncertainty keeps the illness in the forefront of a family's consciousness, constantly impinging upon their attempts to get back "in phase" developmentally. Finally, the transition from the crisis to the chronic phase of the illness life cycle is often the key juncture where the intensity of the family's socialization to living with chronic disease can be relaxed. In this sense, it offers a "window of opportunity" for the family to recover its developmental course.

Chronic diseases that occur for adults in the child-rearing period can be most devastating because of their potential impact on family financial and child-rearing responsibilities (Herz, 1988). Again, the actual impact will depend on the "type" of illness and preillness family roles. Families governed by rigid gender-defined roles, as to who should be the primary financial provider and care-taker of children, will potentially have the greatest problems with adjustment and need to be coached toward a more flexible view about role interchange.

In the face of chronic disease, an overarching goal is for a family to deal with the developmental demands presented by the illness without family members completely sacrificing their own or the family's development as a system. Therefore, it is vital to ask about what life plans had to be canceled, postponed, or altered as a result of the diagnosis. It is useful to know whose plans are most and least affected. By asking a family when and under what conditions they will resume plans, put on hold, or address future developmental tasks, a clinician can anticipate developmental crises related to "independence from" versus "subjugation to" the chronic illness. Family members can be helped to resume their life plans, at least to some extent, by helping them to resolve feelings of guilt, over-responsibility, and hopelessness and to find resources that are internal and external to the family for more freedom, both to pursue their own goals and provide needed care for the ill member.

Health/Illness Belief System

Each of us as an individual and as part of larger systems adopts a value orientation, belief system, or philosophy that shapes our patterns of behavior toward the common problems of daily life in society (Kluckhohn, 1960). Beliefs lend coherence to cognitive and affective dimensions of family life and temporal continuity to past, present, and future. Values provide a mode of approaching new and ambiguous situations. Depending on which system we are speaking of, this phenomenon can be labeled as values, culture, religion, belief system, world view, or family paradigm.

Reiss (1981) has argued that families as a unit develop paradigms for how the world operates. These models dictate how families interpret events and behaviors in their environment. One component of the family's overall construction of reality is their set of health/illness beliefs that will determine how they interpret illness events and guide their health-seeking behavior (Rolland, 1987b). Although individual family members can hold different beliefs, the values operative at the level of the whole family may be the most significant.

At the time of a medical diagnosis, a primary developmental task for the family is to create a meaning for the illness event that preserves a sense of competency and mastery in the context of partial loss, possible further physical compromise, and/or death. Chronic illness is both a betrayal of our fundamental trust in our bodies and belief in our invulnerability and immortality (Kleinman, 1988). At an existential level, family health beliefs are designed to grapple with dilemmas of our (1) universal fear of finiteness and mortality, (2) attempts to sustain our denial of death, and (3) attempts to reassert control over unjust suffering and untimely death. At a practical level, belief systems serve as a cognitive map guiding decisions and action.

It is essential for clinicians to inquire about a family's health beliefs as part of a routine evaluation, focusing on the following key components (Rolland, 1987b). First, one needs to ascertain the specific values to which a family adheres. These include assessment of (1) a family's basic belief about the relationship between mind and body, control and mastery, and change; (2) the meanings attached by a family, ethnic group, religion, or the wider culture to certain symptoms (e.g., chronic pain), types or time phases of illness (e.g., life-threatening disorders), or specific diseases; (3) the family's assumptions about what caused an illness and what will influence its course and outcome; (4) family of origin or nuclear family historical factors related to illness, loss, adversity, and crisis that have shaped a family's health beliefs, and (5) anticipated nodal points in the unfolding of the illness, individual, and family life cycle where health beliefs will be strained or need to shift. Second, a clinician needs to assess the fit of health beliefs (1) within the family and its various subsystems (e.g., spouse, parental, extended family); (2) between the family and provider system; and (3) between the family and wider culture.

THE FAMILY'S SENSE OF MASTERY OVER AN ILLNESS

A clinician needs to determine a family's beliefs about their competence to master health and illness from a biologic, psychologic, and social perspective. Mastery is similar to the concept of health locus of control (Lefcourt, 1982; Dohrenwend, 1981), which can be defined as the belief an individual or family has about their influence over the course/outcome of an illness. A family's place along the locus of control continuum is an important distinction with far-reaching clinical implications. Levenson (1973, 1974, 1975) described three basic loci of control orientations: internal, external by powerful others, and external by chance.

An internal locus of control orientation means that there is a belief that an individual/family can effect the outcome of a situation. Families with such a belief about their health will endorse such statements as, "I am directly responsible for my health," or "If I become sick, I have the power to make myself well again" (Wallston et al., 1976; Wallston and Wallston, 1978).

An external orientation entails a belief that outcomes are noncontingent upon the individual's or family's behavior. Families that view illness in terms of chance will agree with such statements as, "Luck plays a big part in determining how soon my family member will recover from an illness," or "When I become ill, it's a matter of fate." Individuals who see health control as in the hands of powerful others will see health professionals, God, or sometimes "powerful" family members, rather than themselves, as exerting control over their bodies. They will endorse statements such as, "Regarding my health, I can only do what my doctor tells me to do," or "My family has a lot to do with my becoming sick or staying healthy."

A family may adhere to a different set of values concerning control when dealing with a *biological* process as opposed to other day-to-day types of problem solving. Therefore, it is important to assess a family's basic value system first, then, with increasing specificity, assess notions about control for illnesses in general, chronic and life-threatening illness, and, finally, the specific disease facing the family. A family guided normally by an internal locus of control may switch to an external viewpoint when a member develops any chronic illness or perhaps only in the case of a life-threatening disease. Such a change might occur in a family with a strong need to remain in accord with society's values, a particular ethnic background, or a specific cross-generational experience with life-threatening diseases. One can inquire as to whether a family has any particular beliefs surrounding specific types of illnesses. Regardless of the actual severity in a particular instance, cancer may be equated with death or loss of control because of medical statistics, cultural myth, or prior family history. For many, certain types of heart disease with a similar life expectancy as certain forms of cancer could be seen as more manageable because of prevailing cultural beliefs. Imagine a family traditionally guided by a strong sense of personal control. If the paternal grandfather, the powerful patriarch of the family, died at midlife because of a rapidly progressive and painful form of cancer, the family may develop an encapsulated exception to their views about control that is specific for cancer or generalized to include all life-threatening illnesses.

It is critical to distinguish whether a family's belief system is based on the premise of internal control, external via chance, or external via powerful others. A family's value orientation about mastery strongly affects the nature of its relationship to an illness and to the health care system. A family's beliefs about control are a predictor of certain health behaviors, particularly treatment compliance, and suggest the family's preferences about participation in their family member's treatment and healing. In my experience, families that view disease course/outcome as a matter of chance tend to establish marginal relationships with health professionals largely because their belief system minimizes the importance of their own or a health professional's relationship to a disease process. Just as any psychotherapeutic relationship depends upon a shared belief system about what is therapeutic, a fit between the patient, his/her family, and the health care team in terms of these fundamental values is essential. Families that express feelings of being misunderstood by health professionals are often referring directly or indirectly to a lack of joining at this basic value level.

Variations in a family's beliefs about mastery can occur dependent on the time phase of the illness. For some illnesses, the crisis phase involves a lot of involvement outside the family. For instance, the crisis phase after a stroke may begin with an intensive care unit and months of extended care at a rehabilitation facility. This kind of protracted care outside the family's direct control may be stressful for a family that prefers to tackle its own problems with a minimum of outside leadership. For this family, the patient's return home may increase the workload but allow members to re-establish more fully their values concerning control. A family guided more by a preference for external control by experts will have greater difficulty when their family member returns home. For this family, leaving the rehabilitation hospital means the loss of their locus of competency—the professionals. Health providers' cognizance about this basic difference in belief about control can guide a psychosocial treatment plan tailored to each family's needs.

In the terminal phase of an illness, a family may feel least in control of the biologic course of the disease and the decision making regarding the overall care of their ill member. Families with a strong need to sustain their centrality may need to assert themselves more vigorously with health providers. Effective decision making regarding the extent of heroic medical efforts or whether a patient will die at home or in an institution or hospice requires an effective family/provider relationship that respects the family's basic beliefs.

THE FAMILY'S BELIEFS ABOUT THE ETIOLOGY OF AN ILLNESS

The context within which an illness event occurs is a very powerful organizer and mirror of a family's belief system. The limits of current medical knowledge mean that tremendous uncertainties persist about the relative importance of a myriad of biopsychosocial factors in disease onset. This fact allows individuals and families to make highly idiosyncratic attributions about what caused their family member's illness. Therefore, a family's beliefs about the etiology of an illness need to be assessed separately from its beliefs about control once an illness is present. One way to gather this information is to ask *each* family member for his or her explanation of the existence of the disease. Responses will reflect a combination of the current level of medical knowledge about the particular disease in concert with family mythology. This mythology might include punishment for prior misdeeds (e.g., an affair), blame of a particular family member ("Your drinking made me sick"), a sense of injustice ("Why am I being punished, I have been a good person"), genetics (e.g., cancer runs on one side of the family), negligence by the patient or parents (e.g., sudden infant death syndrome), or bad luck. Asking this question can function as an effective family Rorschach, bringing to light unresolved family conflicts.

Attributions about the cause of an illness that invoke blame, shame, or guilt are particularly important to uncover. Beliefs of this nature make it extremely difficult for a family to establish functional coping and adaptation to an illness. In the context of a life-threatening illness, the blamed family member is held accountable for potential murder if the patient dies. Decisions about treatment can become confounded and filled with tension. A mother who feels blamed by her husband for their son's leukemia may be less able to accept stopping a low-probability experimental treatment than the angry, blaming husband. A husband who believes his drinking caused his wife's coronary and subsequent death may have a pathologic grief reaction and may increase his drinking to mask his profound guilt.

In my clinical experience, families with the strongest, at times extreme, beliefs about personal responsibility, and those with the most severely dysfunctional patterns, will be those most likely to attribute the cause of an illness to a psychosocial factor. For high, internal locus-of-control families, an ethos of personal responsibility guides all facets of life, including the etiology of an illness. For these families, a relative lack of acknowledgment of "outrageous fortune" as a factor in illness events can create for these families a nidus for blame, shame, and guilt. For highly dysfunctional families, characterized by unresolved conflicts and intense blaming, attributions of what or who is responsible for an illness often becomes ammunition in long-term family power struggles.

It is difficult to characterize an "ideal" family health belief about mastery or control. On one hand, a major thesis of systems-oriented medicine is that there is always an interplay between disease and other levels of the system. On the other hand, illnesses and phases in the course of disease may vary considerably in their responsiveness to psychosocial factors versus their inherent nature. Distinctions need to be made between a family's beliefs about their overall participation in a long-term disease process, their beliefs about their ability to control the biologic unfolding of an illness, and the flexibility with which a family can apply these beliefs. An optimal expression of family competence or mastery would seem to depend on their grasp of these distinctions.

A family's belief in their participation in the total illness process can be thought of as independent from whether a disease is stable, improving, or in a terminal phase. Sometimes, mastery and the attempt to control biologic processes coincide. A family coping with a member who has cancer in remission may tailor its behavior to help maintain health. This might include changes in family roles, communication, diet, exercise, and balance between work and recreation. Suppose the ill family member loses remission and vigorous efforts to re-establish a remission fail. As the family enters the terminal phase of the illness, participation as an expression of mastery must now be transposed for a successful process of letting go.

The difference between a family experiencing a loss with a sense of competency versus profound failure is intimately connected to this kind of flexible use of their belief system. For instance, it can be helpful if clinicians recognize that the death of a patient, whose long debilitating illness has heavily burdened others, can be a matter of relief as well as sadness to some or all family members. Since a sense of relief over death goes against most conventions in our society, it can trigger massive guilt reactions that may be expressed tangentially through such symptoms as depression and negative family interactions. Clinicians will need to help family members accept, with a minimum of guilt and defensiveness, the naturalness of ambivalent feelings they may have for their deceased member.

Thus, flexibility within the family and the health-provider system may be the key variable in optimal family functioning. Families can view mastery in a rigid, circumscribed way that views biologic outcome as the sole determinant of success, or families can define control in a more "holistic" sense where involvement and participation in the overall process is the main criteria defining success. This is analogous to the distinction between healing the system and curing the disease. Healing the system may influence the course/outcome of an illness, but disease outcome is not necessary to a family's feeling successful. This flexible definition of mastery permits the quality of relations within the family or between the family and health providers to become more central to criteria of success. It permits the health provider's competence to be viewed from both a technical and caregiving perspective (Reiss, 1989) that is not linked only to the biological course of the disorder.

THE FAMILY'S ETHNIC, RELIGIOUS, AND CULTURAL BELIEFS

Ethnicity, race, and religion are major determinants of a family's belief concerning health and illness (McGoldrick et al., 1982; Zborowski, 1969). There are cultural differences in definitions of what constitutes a family in different ethnic, racial, and religious groups; what the responsibility of families is for the care of ill members; who in the family is chiefly responsible for this care (usually the wife/mother/daughter in traditional cultures); what the role of the extended family is in patient care, and so on. Health professionals need to familiarize themselves with belief systems of various ethnic, racial, and religious groups in their community, particularly as these translate into different behavioral patterns in regard to illness. For instance, it is customary for Italians and Jews to describe physical symptoms freely and in detail while individuals from Irish or white Anglo-

Saxon descent tend to deny or conceal ailments. One can surmise about the potential for misunderstanding and tension that could develop between Italian or Jewish health providers working with Irish or white Anglo-Saxon patients and their families. A mutually frustrating cycle of health providers pursuing a distancing family could develop. At minimum, dissatisfaction would ensue; at worst, a family might leave treatment, their negative experience reinforcing its alienation and isolation from adequate care. Clinicians need to be mindful of the cultural differences between themselves, the patient, and the family. Deference to these distinctions is a necessary step to forging a workable provider-patient-family alliance that can endure a long-term illness. Disregarding these issues can lead families to wall themselves off from health providers and available community resources—a major cause of noncompliance and treatment failure.

FAMILY AND FAMILY-PROVIDER HEALTH BELIEF CONGRUENCE

As family illness beliefs are articulated, a clinician should inquire about the degree of family consensus or congruence concerning a particular value, such as health locus of control. This is important because it is a common, but unfortunate, error to regard "the family" as a monolithic unit that feels, thinks, believes, and behaves as an undifferentiated whole.

In assessing the family's level of agreement, one should learn about the family's general tolerance for differences. What is the family rule? "We must agree on all/some values," or "diversity and different viewpoints are acceptable." Further, clinicians should determine whether the family policy about consensus is adhered to in relation to the prevailing cultural or societal beliefs. Can the family hold values that differ from the wider culture? The family's general rule has multiple determinants that include cultural norms, historical context (era of "family consensus" versus each member "doing his/her own thing"), and the beliefs of the adults' families of origin.

A family's rules about consensus can have profound implications for permissible options when a family faces chronic illness. If consensus is the rule, then individual differentiation implies deviance. If the guiding principle is, "we can hold different viewpoints," then diversity is allowed. When working with illness-related values in a family where consensus is the rule, attention to the entire family is mandatory. One treatment goal can be to help families negotiate their differences and support the separate identity, needs, and goals of each member. In a family where diversity is permitted, there may be greater latitude to work on certain disease-related psychosocial issues with the ill member alone or with particular members of the family without mobilizing family resistance.

Next, it is important to look into the *actual* level of agreement with regard to illness values both within the family and between the family and medical system. How congruent are the family's basic beliefs about control with their illness value system? A family that is uniformly external will generally adapt best if psychosocial interventions are tailored to that fact. On the other hand, a family that generally adheres to an internal locus of control but feels the opposite with a particular disease may, through exploration of underlying issues, be able to change its beliefs about illness. It is critical to keep in mind that beliefs about control refer to a family's beliefs about the importance of their *participation in the total illness process* rather than just their beliefs about a disease's curability.

It is important to analyze differences among family members in terms of illness values. Disparities in two- and three-person relationships involving the ill member are particularly significant. Consider a common situation in which there is a long-standing loyalty conflict for a man caught between his spouse and his mother. Both women vie for his devotion, while he is unable to define boundaries between his family of origin and nuclear family. This dysfunctional triangle may have smoldered for years in a precarious balance when the man develops a slowly progressive and debilitating illness, such as multiple sclerosis. If the man and his mother share a strong sense of internal control while his spouse grew up in a family that saw chronic illness as a matter of fate, an unbalancing of this triangle is likely to occur. The smoldering mother-son coalition now re-emerges in full force fueled by shared basic beliefs concerning mastery, while the marital couple is driven apart.

The different ethnic backgrounds of the adults in a family may be a primary reason for the kind of discrepancies about illness beliefs that emerge at the time of a major illness. Differences may occur in such areas as the definition of the appropriate sick role for the patient; the kind and degree of open communication about the disease; who should be included in the illness care-taking system (e.g., extended family, friends, professionals); and the kind of rituals viewed as normative at different stages of an illness (e.g., hospital bedside vigils, healing and funeral rituals). In families of mixed ethnic heritage, clinicians should assess these areas for consensus, disagreement, and negotiation.

It is common for differences in beliefs or attitudes between family members to erupt at major transition points in the treatment or disease course. For instance, in situations of severe disability or terminal illness, one member may want the patient to return home while another prefers extended hospitalization or transfer to an extended care facility. Since the chief task of patient care-taking is usually assigned to the wife/mother, she is the one most apt to bear the chief burdens in this regard. If this family also operates under the constraint of traditional role assignments where the wife/mother defers to her spouse as the family decision maker, she may not make her true feelings known and may become the family martyr, taking on the home nursing tasks without overt disagreement at the time critical decisions are made with health professionals. Clinicians can be misled by a family that presents this kind of united front. A careful and perceptive assessment can help avert the long-term consequences to such a family of role overload, resentment, and deteriorating family relationships.

It is essential to assess the fit between the belief systems of the family and the health care team. The same questions asked of the family are relevant to the medical team. What is the attitude of the health care team about their and the family's ability to influence the course/outcome of the disease? How does the health team see the balance between theirs versus the family's participation in the treatment and control of the disease? If basic differences in beliefs about health locus of control exist, it is critical to assess how to reconcile these differences. Because of the tendency of most health facilities to disempower individuals and thereby foster dependence, utmost sensitivity to family values is needed to create a therapeutic system. Many breakdowns in relationships between "noncompliant" or marginal patients and their health care providers are related to lack of agreement at this basic level.

The relative need for consensus will vary according to the illness phase. One point where a good fit of values is usually needed is during the initial crisis period when health providers engage in much high technology medicine and rapid decision-making and exchange of information, especially if life-threatening circumstances prevail. Teamwork is particularly important. Illnesses characterized by recurrent crises or key transitions have nodal points of stress where consensus will again become important.

One major transition is the often murky junction between the chronic and terminal phases of an illness. The attitudes and behaviors of the medical team can have a major influence in either facilitating or hindering this process for a family. A medical team that maintains heroic efforts to control the terminal phase of an illness can convey confusing messages. Families may not know how to interpret continued lifesaving efforts. Is there still real hope that should be taken by families as a message to redouble their faith in and support of medical improvement? Do the physicians feel bound to a technologic imperative that requires them to exhaust *all* possibilities at their disposal, regardless of the odds of success? Often, physicians feel committed to this course for ethical reasons, a "leave no stone unturned" philosophy, or because of fears concerning legal liability. Is the medical team having its own difficulties letting go? Strong relationships with certain patients can be fueled by identifications with losses, often unresolved, in the health providers' own lives. Health care professionals and institutions can collude in a pervasive societal wish to deny death as a natural process truly beyond technologic control (Becker, 1973). Endless treatment can represent the medical team's inability to separate a general value placed on controlling diseases from their beliefs about participation (separate from cure) in a patient's total care. Professionals need to closely examine their own motives for treatments geared towards cure rather than palliation, particularly when a patient may be entering a terminal phase. Professionals' self-examinations need to be done in concert with a careful understanding of the family's belief system.

Because information about and linkage to community resources and services is frequently valuable, the clinician must assess how family health beliefs influence their overall illness behavior within a community (Mechanic, 1978; Kleinman, 1975). Clinicians need to know the availability of and access to community resources relevant to the management of long-term illnesses. This includes a range of primary and tertiary medical, rehabilitation, respite, transportation, housing, institutional, and financial entitlement services. Also, it includes potential psychosocial support from friends, neighbors, self-help groups, and religious, ethnic/cultural, or other group affiliations. On the family side, one must inquire about a family's prior experience using such resources. Have these experiences been affirming or alienating? To what extent is the family adequately informed about potential outside sources of help? Ignorance may reflect family isolation from the community due to such things as geographical distance in a rural setting, lack of education (e.g., literacy), language barrier, poverty, race, and ethnic or religious distinctions from the wider culture. On the other side, a family's willingness to use outside resources may be limited by ethnic/cultural values, certain family dynamics, and their own illness paradigms.

For example, rigidly enmeshed families tend to view the world as dangerous and threatening to their fragile sense of autonomy. Individual autonomy is sacrificed to keep the family system intact. Their beliefs about control will need to be defined within a framework of family exclusiveness that minimizes the role of outsiders. The occurrence of a chronic illness presents a powerful dilemma for these families. The illness may necessitate frequent excursions beyond the family borders or require the inclusion of outside professionals in disease management. Any hope of establishing a viable family health care team relationship depends upon exquisite sensitivity to this interplay of dysfunctional family dynamics and their belief system.

Summary

This chapter has described a three-dimensional model for assessing the impact of illness on families. On the first dimension, psychosocial "types" of illnesses are based on four components: onset, course, outcome, and degree of incapacitation. The second dimension distinguishes three phases in the life history of chronic disease: crisis, chronic, and terminal. The third dimension includes various universal and illness specific components of family functioning. Particular attention is given to the family illness value system, transgenerational history of illness, loss, and crisis; and the interface of the individual and family life cycles with chronic disease. This model provides a framework for effective clinical intervention that takes into account the important interactions between illness, individual patients, and their families.

References

Baker, L., Minuchin, S., Milman, L., et al.: Psychosomatic aspects of juvenile diabetes mellitus: a progress report. In Modern Problems in Pediatrics. 12th ed. White Plains, NY, S. Karger, 1975.

Beavers, W. R.: Healthy, midrange, and severely dysfunctional families. In Walsh, F. (Ed.): Normal Family Processes. New York, Guilford Press, 1982.

Beavers, W. R., and Voeller, M. M.: Family models: comparing and contrasting the Olson Circumplex Model with the Beavers Systems Model. Family Process, *22:*85–98, 1983.

Becker, E.: The Denial of Death. New York, Free Press, 1973.

Boszormenyi-Nagy, I., and Spark, G.: Invisible Loyalties. New York, Harper and Row, 1973.

Bowen, M.: Theory in the practice of psychotherapy. In Bowen, M. (Ed.): Family Therapy in Clinical Practice. New York, Jason Aronson Inc., 1978.

Bradley, C.: Life events and the control of diabetes mellitus. J. Psychosom. Res., *23:*159–162, 1979.

Burr, W. R.: Theory Construction and the Sociology of the Family. New York, Wiley, 1973.

Carter, E. A., & McGoldrick, M. (Eds.): The Changing Family Life Cycle: A Framework for Family Therapy. 2nd ed. New York, Gardner Press, 1988. *The major text describing the family from a developmental and multigenerational perspective. The book includes chapters on the family life cycle in relation to chronic illness, death, and aging that are particularly important to the family practitioner.*

Chodoff, P., Friedman, S. B., and Hamburg, D. A.: Stress, defenses and coping behavior: observations in parents of children with malignant disease. Am. J. Psychiatry, 120:743–749, 1964.

Combrinck-Graham, L.: A developmental model for family systems. Family Process, *24:*2, 139–150, 1985.

Croog, S. H., Shapiro, D. S., and Levine, S.: Denial among male heart patients: an empirical study. Psychosom. Med., 33:385–397, 1971.

Davies, R. K., Quinlan, D. M., McKegney, P., and Kimball, C. P.: Organic factors and psychological adjustment in advanced cancer patients. Psychosom. Med., *35:*464–471, 1973.

Derogatis, L. R., Abeloff, M. D., and Melisartos, N.: Psychological coping mechanisms and survival time in metastatic breast cancer. J. A. M. A., *242:*1504–1508, 1979.

Doherty, W. J., and Baird, M. A.: Family Therapy and Family Medicine: Toward the Primary Care of Families. New York, Guilford Press, 1983. *An excellent text for practitioners that integrates a practical application of family systems theory into family medicine.*

Dohrenwend, B. S., and Dohrenwend, B. P. (Eds.): Stressful Life Events and Their Contexts. New York, Prodist, 1981.

Elliott, G. R., and Eisdorfer, C.: Stress and Human Health: Analysis and Implications of Research. New York, Springer, 1982.

Engel, G. H.: The need for a new medical model: a challenge for biomedicine. Science, *196:*129–136, 1977.

Engel, G. H.: The clinical application of the biopsychosocial model. Am. J. Psychiatry, *137:*535–544, 1980.

Erikson, E. H.: Childhood and Society. New York, Norton, 1950.

Figley, C. R., and McCubbin, H. I. (Eds.): Stress and the Family, Volume II: Coping with Catastrophe. New York, Brunner/Mazel, 1983.

Framo, J.: Family of origin as therapeutic resource for adults in marital and family therapy. Family Process, *15:*193–210, 1976. *This article describes the clinical importance of inquiry about adult family members' family of origin.*

Hackett, T. P., Cassem, N. H., and Wishnie, H. A.: The coronary-care unit: an appraisal of its psychologic hazards. N. Engl. J. Med. *279:*1365–1370, 1968.

Hamburg, B. A., Lipsett, L. F., Inoff, G. E., and Drash, A. L. (Eds.): Behavioral and Psychological Issues in Diabetes. U.S. Government Printing Office, NIH Publication No. 80–1993, 1980.

Hansen, D., and Johnson, V.: Rethinking family stress theory: definitional aspects. In Burr, W., Hill, R., Nye, I., and Reiss, I. (Eds.): Contemporary Theories of the Family. Vol. 1, New York, The Free Press, 1979.

Herz, F.: The impact of death and serious illness on the family life cycle. In Carter, E. A., and McGoldrick, M. (Eds.): The Changing Family Life Cycle: A Framework for Family Therapy. 2nd ed. New York, Gardner Press, 1988. *A well-written chapter that describes the effects of serious illness and loss on each spouse, on the couple's relationship, and on the family unit. These effects are discussed in terms of the timing of the illness event with the life cycle.*

Hill, R.: Families Under Stress. New York, Harper, 1949.

Hoffman, L.: The life cycle and discontinuous change. In Carter, E. A., and McGoldrick, M. (Eds.): The Changing Family Life Cycle: A Framework for Family Therapy. 2nd ed. New York, Gardner Press, 1988.

Ireys, H. T., and Burr, C. K.: Apart and a part: family issues for young adults with chronic illness and disability. In Eisenberg, M. G., Sutkin, L. C., and Jansen M. A. (Eds.): Chronic Illness and Disability through the Life Span: Effects on Self and Family. New York, Springer Publishing Inc., 1984. *This chapter gives a nice description of the impact of illness and disability on a young adult's development. In particular, it details how the normal developmental tasks of early adulthood need to be redefined in situations of illness and disability. Other chapters describe nicely the impact of illness timed at different points in the life cycle.*

Kaplan, D. M.: Observations on crisis theory and practice. Soc. Casework, *49:*151–155, 1968.

Kasl, S. V.: Social and psychological factors affecting the course of disease: an epidemiological perspective. In Mechanic, D. (Ed.): Handbook of Health, Health Care and the Health Profession. New York, Free Press, 1982.

Kleinman, A. M.: Explanatory models in health care relationships. In Health of the Family (National Council for International Health Symposium). Washington, D. C., National Council for International Health, 1975.

Kleinman, A. M.: The Illness Narratives: Suffering, Healing and the Human Condition. New York, Basic Books Inc., 1988. *Through the use of patient narratives, Kleinman describes the clinical importance of the personal and cultural meanings patients attach to symptoms and illnesses and the profound implications for patient-health provider relationships.*

Kluckhohn, F. R.: Variations in the basic values of family systems. In Bell N. W., and Vogel E. F. (Eds.): A Modern Introduction to the Family. Glencoe, IL, The Free Press, 1960. *Kluckhohn offers a useful, anthropologic framework for conceptualizing basic components of family belief systems. She describes basic human dilemmas for which all cultures and families need to develop a belief system. This cross-cultural orientation offers clinicians a practical way to think about paradigms.*

Lefcourt, H. M.: Locus of Control, 2nd ed. Hillsdale, N. J.: Lawrence Erlbaum Assoc., 1982.

Levenson, H.: Multidimensional locus of control in psychiatric patients. J. Consult. Clin. Psychol., *41:*397–404, 1973.

Levenson, H.: Activism and powerful others: distinctions within the concept of internal-external control. J. Pers. Assess., *38:*377–383, 1974.

Levenson, H.: Multidimensional locus of control in prison inmates. J. Appl. Soc. Psychol., *5:*342–347, 1975.

Levinson, D. J.: The Seasons of a Man's Life. New York, Knopf,

1978. *On the basis of his in-depth research of 40 men, Levinson describes his theory of adult (male) development. To date, this constitutes the most thorough and clinically useful model of adult development. I highly recommend practitioners to familiarize themselves with his concepts.*

Levinson, D. J.: A conception of adult development. Am. Psychol., 41, No. 1, 3–13, 1986.
A condensed version of Levinson's model of adult development. Well written.

McCubbin, H. I.: Integrating coping behavior in family stress theory. J. Marriage Fam., *41:*237–244, 1979.

McCubbin, H. I., and Figley, C. R.: Stress and the Family, Volume I: Coping with Normative Transitions. New York, Brunner/Mazel, 1983.

McCubbin, H. I., Joy, C. B., Cauble, A. E., et al.: Family stress and coping: a decade review. J. Marriage Fam., *42:*855–871, 1980.

McGoldrick, M., and Gerson, R.: Genograms in Family Assessment. New York, Norton Press, 1985. *This is a well-written, extremely practical book that describes the clinical utility of genograms and how to do them effectively. Clinical examples of famous people make it enjoyable. All family physicians should read this book.*

McGoldrick, M., Pearce, J. K., and Giordano, J.: Ethnicity and Family Therapy. New York, Guilford Press, 1982. *It is an excellent book. The only book of its kind. Separate chapters on a range of ethnic groups describe for each the key characteristics of family life.*

McGoldrick, M., and Walsh, F.: A systemic view of family history and loss. In Aronson, M., and Wolberg L. (Eds.): Group and Family Therapy, 1983. New York, Brunner/Mazel, 1983.

Mechanic, D.: Medical Sociology. 2nd ed. New York, Free Press, 1978.

Minuchin, S., Rosman, B. L., and Baker, L.: Psychosomatic Families. Cambridge, Harvard University Press, 1978. *A description of family research at the Philadelphia Child Guidance Clinic with children with asthma, diabetes, and anorexia nervosa. A structural model of intervention with these families is described using in-depth clinical examples.*

Minuchin, S., Baker, L., Rosman, B., et al.: A conceptual model of psychosomatic illness in children: family organization and family therapy. Arch. Gen. Psychiatry, *32:*1031–1038, 1975.

Moldofsky, H., and Chester, W. J.: Pain and mood patterns in patients with rheumatoid arthritis: a prospective study. Psychosom. Med. *32:*309–318, 1970.

Moos, R. H. (Ed.): Coping with Physical Ilness. Vol. 2: New Perspectives. New York, Plenum Publishing, 1984.

Neugarten, B.: Adaptation and the life cycle. The Counselling Psychologist, *6*(1):16–20, 1976.

Penn, P.: Coalitions and binding interactions in families with chronic illness. Fam. Systems Med., *1*(2):16–25, 1983. *Excellent article that describes dysfunctional patterns of family structure and interaction that can occur in situations of chronic illness. Includes discussion of intergenerational issues that indicate high-risk families.*

Piaget, J.: The Origins of Intelligence in Children. New York, International Press, 1952.

Reiss, D.: The Family's Construction of Reality. Cambridge, Harvard University Press, 1981.

Reiss, D.: The family and medical team in chronic illness: a transactional and developmental perspective. In Ramsey, Jr., C. N. (Ed.): Family Systems in Family Medicine. New York, Guilford Press. *Reiss uses a systems framework for describing in longitudinal terms the evolution of the family-provider system. Nodal points in the illness life cycle are discussed in relation to the relative need for providers to assume a technological versus a care-giver role.*

Rolland, J. S.: Toward a psychosocial typology of chronic and life-threatening illness. Fam. Systems Med., *2*(3):245–263. 1984. *This article describes in greater detail the psychosocial typology and time phases framework.*

Rolland, J. S.: Chronic illness and the life cycle: a conceptual framework. Family Process, *26*(2):203–221, 1987a. *This article describes in greater detail the integration of chronic illness (from a psychosocial typology/time phases perspective) with family and individual development. The clinical importance of transgenerational, present, and future life cycle issues are described.*

Rolland, J. S.: Chronic illness and the life cycle. In Carter, E. A., and McGoldrick, M. (Eds.): The Changing Family Life Cycle: A Framework for Family Therapy. 2nd ed. New York, Gardner Press, 1988.

Rolland, J. S.: Family illness paradigms: evolution and significance. Fam. Systems Med., *5*(4):467–486, 1987b. *This article describes in greater detail the clinical importance of family health and illness beliefs and a framework for assessment.*

Rolland, J. S.: Family systems and chronic illness: a typological model. J. Psychother. Fam., *3*(3):143–168, 1987c.

Rolland, J. S.: Helping Families with Chronic and Life-Threatening Disorders. New York, Basic Books, in press.

Schmale, A. H., and Iker, H.: Hopelessness as a predictor of cervical cancer. Soc. Sci. Med., *5:*95–100, 1971.

Simonton, C. O., Mathews-Simonton, S., and Sparks, T. F.: Psychological intervention in the treatment of cancer. Psychosom., *21*(3):226–233, 1980.

Strauss, A. L.: Chronic Illness and the Quality of Life. St. Louis, C. V. Mosby, 1975. *An excellent book that describes medical disorders in psychosocial terms. Some of the best chapters include: preventing and managing medical crises, managing the trajectory, a basic strategy—normalizing, the burden of rheumatoid arthritis, and management of regimens.*

Walker, G.: The pact: the caretaker-parent/ill-child coalition in families with chronic illness. Fam. Systems Med. *1*(4):6–30, 1983.

Wallston, B. S., Wallston, K. A., Kaplan, G. D., and Maides, S. A.: Development and validation of the health locus of control (HLC) scale. J. Consult. Clin. Psychol., *44:*580–585, 1976.

Wallston, K. A., and Wallston, B. S.: Development of the multidimensional health locus of control (MHLC) scales. Health Education Monographs, *6*(2):160–170, 1978.

Walsh, F., and McGoldrick, M.: Loss and the family life cycle. In Falicov, C. J. (Ed.): Family Transitions: Continuity and Change over the Life Cycle. New York, Guilford, 1985. *An excellent chapter that describes a systemic multigenerational view of loss and its impact on current family functioning. Issues related to unresolved loss, catastrophic expectations, family cutoffs, replications, and dysfunctional family patterns are addressed.*

Weiss, S. M., Herd, J. A., and Fox, B. H. (Eds.): Perspectives on Behavioral Medicine. New York, Academic Press, 1981.

Wolff, C. T., Friedman, S. B., Hofer, M. A., and Mason, J. W.: Relationship between psychological defenses and mean urinary 17-hydroxy corticosteroid excretion rate. I. A predictive study of parents of fatally ill children. Psychosom. Med., *26:*576–591, 1964.

Zborowski, M.: People in Pain. San Francisco, Jossey-Bass, 1969.

6

The Family's Influence on Health

Thomas L. Campbell
Donald F. Treat

Over the past decade, research on families and health has grown tremendously and improved in quality. Early research in this area came primarily from the fields of sociology and family therapy and often suffered from serious methodological problems (Campbell, 1986). More recently, high quality research on families and health is being conducted in all fields of social science and medicine including family medicine (Doherty and Campbell, 1988).

Based upon the rigorous studies on the influences of social support on compliance, the Working Group on Health Education and High Blood Pressure Control of the National Heart, Lung, and Blood Institute has recommended that all physicians use the following as one of three basic strategies for increasing adherence to prescribed antihypertensive regimes:

> *Enhance support from family members—identifying and involving one influential person, preferably someone living with the patient, who can provide encouragement, help support the behavior change, and, if necessary, remind the patient about the specifics of the regimen.*
>
> (WGHEHBPC, 1987)

This government guide, sent to all physicians in the United States, gives specific suggestions on how to enhance family support for each of the five most frequent behavior changes recommended for the hypertensive: taking medication daily, maintaining desirable weight, reducing dietary sodium, increasing vigorous exercise, and moderating alcohol consumption. Thus, well-designed research can lead to recognition of the importance of the family in health care and the implementation of family-oriented approaches (McDaniel et al., 1989).

Disease Prevention: The Family's Influence on Health Behaviors

A major challenge for medicine in the 1990's and beyond is the prevention of chronic illness. Most chronic illnesses result in part from unhealthy behaviors or risk factors that are difficult to change. This is particularly true for coronary heart disease—the leading cause of death in the United States. Most health behaviors, including diet, smoking, and exercise, develop within the family context and have been shown to be strongly influenced by the family (Sallis and Nader, 1988).

CARDIOVASCULAR RISK FACTORS

Numerous studies have shown that cardiovascular and other health risk factors tend to cluster within families (Baranowski et al., 1982). Family members are more likely to share the same risk factors than would be expected by chance: including smoking (Venters et al., 1984; National Institute of Education, 1979), obesity (Garn and Clark, 1976), hypercholesterolemia (Shear et al., 1978) lack of exercise (Sallis et al., 1988), and hypertension (Sackett et al., 1975). This sharing of risk factors occurs both between spouses and among parents and their children. For example, the Framingham Heart Study found a higher than expected concordance between spouses for blood pressure, cholesterol, triglyceride, blood sugar, smoking, and lung function (Sackett et al., 1975). Other studies have shown that parent-child blood pressure (Feinleib et al., 1980; Patterson et al., 1987), body fat (Garn et al., 1976), and cholesterol (Karlin et al., 1982) are significantly correlated.

Shared risk factors within families can be explained by several different mechanisms. Family members can influence each other's lifestyle and health habits. Adolescents are much more likely to smoke if either of their parents or an older sibling smokes (Bewley and Bland, 1977; National Institute of Education, 1979). A teenager who has a parent and older sibling who smoke is five times more likely to smoke than a teen from a nonsmoking family. Families usually eat a similar diet and, therefore, ingest similar amounts of salt (Venters et al., 1984), calories (Laskarzewski, 1980), cholesterol, and saturated fats (Eastwood et al., 1982). An emphasis on physical fitness and maintaining ideal body weight is often a shared family value. Parents' exercise habits and attitudes have a strong influence on their children's levels of physical activity (Gottlieb and Chen, 1985; Livingood et al., 1981).

Since genetics can influence some of these risk factors, similarities between parents and children may be inherited. While a recent study of adopted children concluded that obesity in children is largely determined by genetics (Stunkard et al., 1986), other studies have demonstrated a significant effect of the familial environment (Garn et al., 1976; Hartz et al., 1977). One study of twins demonstrated that most of the concordance of cholesterol levels is due to similar diets (Feinleib et al., 1977).

MATE SELECTION

Spouses may share cardiovascular risk factors because they married someone with similar habits. This tendency to marry someone with same traits or behaviors, called assortative mating, is quite common. Smokers tend to marry other smokers (Sutton, 1980), and couples tend to smoke the same number of cigarettes per day (Venters et al., 1984). Obese men tend to marry obese women. Marital partners may even choose each other (consciously or unconsciously) based upon their dietary or exercise habits. In the Framingham study, the concordance of risk factors between spouses did not increase over time, suggesting that these similarities existed at the time of marriage (Sackett et al., 1975).

FAMILY INFLUENCE

Whatever the cause of this phenomenon, it has major implications for health care providers. If one member of a family has a particular cardiovascular risk factor, other family members are likely to be more difficult to change if it is shared by other members of the family. Smokers are more likely to stop smoking if no one else in the family is a smoker (Price et al., 1981) and remain abstinent longer if their spouse or friends do not smoke (Lichtenstein, 1982; Ockene et al., 1981). Changing one member's risk factor may have a ripple effect and influence the entire family. For example, if one family member starts an exercise program, other family members may want to join in. Smoking couples tend to quit smoking at the same time (Venters et al., 1984). An intervention designed to change the risk factors within the family, rather than in only one individual, may be more successful, time efficient, and cost effective (Nader et al., 1983).

The ability of an individual to make life style changes and reduce the risk of cardiovascular disease is strongly influenced by the support of family members. In a study of an exercise program for men with multiple cardiac risk factors (Heinzelman and Bagley, 1970), men whose wives had positive attitudes about the program were twice as likely to complete the program than those whose wives were neutral or negative.

Support from the spouse is associated with successful smoking cessation (Graham and Gibson, 1971; Ockene et al., 1981). In two smoking cessation programs (Mermelstein et al., 1983; Coppotelli and Orleans, 1985), smokers who had the cooperation and reinforcement of their partner had lower relapse rates, while critical behaviors, such as nagging and policing by the partner, had the opposite effect. Unfortunately, intervention studies designed to enhance spousal support of smoking cessation have been unsuccessful (Lichtenstein et al., 1986).

CHOLESTEROL

The family's health beliefs about prevention will influence their support for changing risk factors. As part of a cholesterol reduction study, Doherty and colleagues (1983) examined the relationship of spouses' support and health beliefs to compliance with medication. The wife's belief regarding how susceptible she thought her husband was to elevated cholesterol was correlated with both her support and her husband's compliance with a cholesterol-lowering drug. In addition, the wife's "interest in the program" and "reminding him about medicine or diet" correlated with compliance, while "nagging about medicine" was negatively correlated with compliance.

EATING HABITS AND OBESITY

An unhealthy behavior sometimes plays a role within a family that can hinder attempts to change the behavior. For example, studies suggest that eating behavior and obesity play an important homeostatic function within many families (Barbarin and Tirado, 1984). In a survey of eating behavior within families, 25 per cent of mothers reported that they used food as a reward for their children, and 10 per cent used it as punishment (Bryan and Lowenberg, 1958). Parents' encouragement to eat has been shown to correlate with obesity in their children (Klesges et al., 1983). In one weight reduction program, 91 per cent of the spouses of obese women reported that they wished their wives would lose weight, but only 49 per cent were willing to help (Stuart and Davis, 1972). Fifty-three per cent of the men anticipated that weight loss would have an adverse effect on the marriage due to loss of eating as a shared activity, loss of power in marital conflicts, and concern over marital commitment and sexual fidelity. During recorded mealtime conversations, these husbands were seven times more likely to talk about food than their dieting wives and four times more likely to offer food to the other. The men criticized their dieting wives 12 times more often than they praised them. When health-related behaviors, such as eating, serve important functions in the family, these behaviors may be resistant to change unless attention is paid to how changing the behavior will affect the family.

The family can have a significant effect on the treatment of obesity. Several randomized controlled trials of weight reduction have demonstrated that spouse or partner involvement in weight reduction programs can significantly improve results (Brownell et al., 1978; Pearce et al., 1981; Saccone and Israel, 1978). These studies have used a behavioral paradigm in which family members provide immediate and long-term reinforcement for weight loss or dieting. When the partner participates in the weight reduction program, the obese individual is not only able to lose more weight but is able to maintain the weight loss.

HYPERTENSION

Despite the fact that hypertension is relatively easy to identify and treat and that adequate treatment significantly lowers the risk of heart attacks and strokes, only one fourth of all hypertensive individuals are under treatment and only one half of those under treatment have their blood pressure adequately controlled (McKenney et al., 1973). Compliance with medication is a major problem in the treatment of hypertension and reduction of cardiovascular disease. In a randomized, controlled study, Morisky and colleagues (1983) demonstrated a dramatic effect of family involvement on hypertension compliance and overall mortality. They studied the impact of three different educational interventions (brief individual counseling, instructing the spouse or significant other during a home visit, and small patient group sessions) on appointment keeping, weight control, and medication compliance. Involving the spouse not only improved overall compliance but resulted in a significant reduction in blood pressure and overall mortality. Overall, the experimental groups had a 57 per cent overall reduction in mortality compared to the controls and groups that received family education tended to do the best. The family intervention was included in this study after a survey indicated that 70 per cent of the clinic's hypertensive patients wished that family members knew more about hypertension (Levine et al., 1979). Based upon this and other studies of the role of social supports in improving compliance, the National Heart, Lung, and Blood Institute has stressed the importance of "the help that patients receive from their family and friends to carry on with their treatments" (Haynes et al., 1982).

There is strong evidence for both healthy and unhealthy influences by families on cardiovascular risk factors. Numerous randomized, controlled trials have demonstrated that family involvement improves the results of weight reduction, and one study shows a similar result for hypertension control. Similar studies are needed for exercise programs, smoking cessation, and dietary changes (low salt and cholesterol). Despite the proven efficacy of a family approach to prevention, health care providers remain focused on the individual. A major challenge to the health profession is to become more effective in health promotion and to incorporate a family approach to prevention.

Disease Onset: The Family's Influence on Susceptibility to Illness

FAMILY STRESS

While the idea that stress can cause illness is widely accepted by the lay public, it is difficult to demonstrate empirically. Stress is hard to define and study (Rabkin and Struening, 1976). Stress may refer to any of the three components of what has been called the stress process (Pearlin et al., 1981): (1) the stressors—environmental events experienced by an individual, (2) the physiologic response to the stressors, or (3) the health consequences of the stressors. The most successful method for studying stress and health has been to examine stressors, particularly the relationship of stressful life events to illness. Holmes and Rahe (1967) developed their life event scale by asking a random sample of the population to rank how stressful they perceived each of 43 common life events to be. Many retrospective and prospective studies using this scale have shown that an increase in stressful life events precedes the development of a wide range of diseases (Cohen, 1981). Life events that are perceived negatively or are not under the individual's control have the most adverse effect on health (Blake, 1988).

Most of the events on the Holmes and Rahe scale occur within the family, and 10 of the 15 most stressful events are family events. Since children are likely to be affected by this stress, a number of studies have looked at the relationship of family life events and child health. Meyer and Haggerty (1962) found that chronic stress was associated with higher rates of streptococcal pharyngitis, and that 30 per cent of the strep infections were preceded by a stressful family event. In a study of illness conducted in a day-care center, children who experience more stressful life events had longer but not more frequent respiratory illnesses (Boyce et al., 1977). A prospective study of over 1000 preschoolers found that family life events were strongly correlated with subsequent visits to the physician and hospital admissions for a wide range of conditions. Children from families with more than 12 life events during the 4-year study period were six times more likely to be hospitalized (Beautrais et al., 1982).

The *death of a spouse* is the most stressful common life event, and the health consequences of bereavement have been extensively studied (Jacobs and Ostfeld, 1977; Osterweis et al., 1984). From examining U.S. census data, Kraus and Lilienfeld (1959) found that young widowers had 10 times the normal death rate for many illnesses. In a classic prospective study, Parkes and coworkers (1969) followed London widowers for 9 years after the death of their spouses. The men had a 40 per cent higher mortality rate during the first 6 months of bereavement compared to the general population. A population study of 4032 widowed persons (Helsing and Szklo, 1981) found that when potential confounding variables (especially smoking and socioeconomic status) were controlled for, widowers, but not widows, had increased mortality rates, which persisted throughout the 10 years of the study. However, widowers who remarried had a lower death rate than the control, nonwidowed group, suggesting that marriage had a protective effect on health. In a study of 95,647 widowed persons in Finland, death rates were highest and twice the expected rate during the first week of bereavement (Kaprio et al., 1987). Studies suggest that the first 6 months is the period of highest risk of death for bereaved spouses. It is not known whether this increased mortality during bereavement is a result of the spouse's death or due to health risks shared with the spouse either from assortative mating or a shared physical environment (Campbell, 1986). However, studies of impaired immune functioning after bereavement (see below) suggest the former.

Divorce or marital separation is also an extremely stressful event and is ranked second on the Holmes and Rahe scale. Numerous studies have demonstrated that divorced or separated persons have poorer mental and physical health than comparable married, widowed, or single persons (Briscoe et al., 1973; Bachrach, 1975; Bloom et al., 1978). In several cross-sectional studies (Lynch, 1977; Verbrugge, 1977; Carter & Glick, 1970) divorcees have a higher death rate from all diseases. However, research has also shown that chronic physical illness has an adverse effect on marital satisfaction (Bruhn et al., 1977; Klein et al., 1968) and may eventually lead to divorce. Prospective studies of divorce and health are needed to determine which is cause or effect.

FAMILY SUPPORT

Research on social supports and health has burgeoned in the past decade and is the subject of several comprehensive reviews (Blake, 1988; Cohen and Syme, 1985; Ganster and Victor, 1988). Social support has been conceptualized in terms of its structure and function. Berkman (1984) defines structural social supports or social networks as "the web of social ties that surrounds an individual" and functional social supports as "the emotional, instrumental and financial aid that is obtained from one's social network." An extensive body of research has demonstrated that social support has a powerful influence on health (Broadhead et al., 1983; Cohen and Syme, 1985) and that the family has been found to be the most important source of social support. Furthermore, Cohen and Wills (1985) concluded from a review of this literature that structural components of social support (e.g., marital status, number of children) had a direct effect on health, while functional or perceived social support (e.g., quality of relationships) have an indirect effect by buffering stress.

Mortality

In a seminal study of over 6000 adults, Berkman and Syme (1979) showed that social networks were a major predictor of mortality over a 9-year period, independent of socioeconomic status, previous health status, or health practices. The most socially isolated adults had more than twice the death rate of the least isolated group. Marital status and contacts with relatives and friends were the most powerful predictors of health. A similar study (House et al., 1982) confirmed the strong association between social isolation and mortality but for men only. Again, the family components of social support were the most predictive. In a 6-year follow-up study of 17,433 Swedish men and women, those with the fewest available social contacts had over three times the death rate of those with the most social contacts (Orth-Gomer and Johnson, 1987).

Studies of social supports in the elderly have shown that the relative importance of different aspects of family support may change over the life span. Two studies found that older persons with impaired social supports have two to three times the death rate of those with good supports (Blazer, 1982; Zuckerman, et al., 1984). Unlike studies of younger populations, marital status was not associated with mortality. The presence and number of living children were the most powerful predictor of survival. This finding suggests that adult children become the most important source of social support in the elderly.

Pregnancy

Family supports play a particularly important role in the outcome of pregnancy. Highly stressed women with low family and social supports have higher rates of obstetrical complications (Nuckolls et al., 1972; Norbeck and Tolden, 1983). Women who live apart from their families deliver smaller babies than those who live with their partners or families of origin (Ramsey et al., 1986). However, women who are excessively close or enmeshed with their extended families also tend to deliver smaller babies, suggesting that the quality as well as the quantity of family support influences health. Ramsey and colleagues have hypothesized that the extended family's over-involvement during pregnancy may be detrimental by not allowing enough autonomy or psychological space for a new family member.

Clearly, family support and family stress, especially bereavement, can have a powerful influence on overall mortality. An understanding of the family and their potential sources of stress and support can provide the physician with ways to reduce family stress, bolster family supports, and improve health.

Disease Course: The Family's Influence on the Course of Illness

Research on families and chronic illness is gradually moving from looking at how families "cause" illness (a pathogenic model) to examining ways in which families influence, positively or negatively, the course of chronic illness (Walsh and Anderson, 1988). The success of this latter approach is best demonstrated in schizophrenia where the concept of the "schizophrenogenic" family has been largely abandoned, and numerous well-designed prospective studies have demonstrated how the emotional climate and patterns of communication powerfully affect relapse (Goldstein, 1987). Randomized, controlled trials of clinical interventions derived from these studies have shown that family psychoeducation dramatically improves the course of schizophrenia (Anderson et al., 1986; Walsh, 1988). As a result of this work, family interventions have become a standard part of the treatment of schizophrenia.

THE PSYCHOSOMATIC FAMILY

No such persuasive line of research exists in the work on families and chronic physical illness where the predominant clinical model remains a pathogenic one—that of the psychosomatic family. Minuchin and colleagues (1975) developed the concept of psychosomatic families from their experiences with the families of children with brittle diabetes, severe asthma, and anorexia nervosa at the Philadelphia Child Guidance Center. They observed a specific pattern of family interaction, characterized by enmeshment (high cohesion), overprotectiveness, rigidity, and conflict avoidance.

To determine how these family interactions can affect chronic illness, Minuchin and colleagues (1978) studied the physiologic responses of diabetic children to a stressful family interview. During the family interview, the children from psychosomatic families had a rapid rise in free fatty acids (a precursor to diabetic ketoacidosis), which persisted beyond the interview. The parents of these children exhibited an initial rise in FFA levels, which fell to normal when the diabetic child entered the room. Minuchin hypothesized that in psychosomatic families, parental conflict is detoured or defused through the chronically ill child, and the resulting stress leads to exacerbations of the illness. Minuchin (1975) also reported the successful treatment of brittle diabetes, severe asthma, and anorexia nervosa using structural family therapy to help establish more appropriate family boundaries. In all the treated cases, there was a dramatic improvement in the illnesses with fewer hospitalizations and less need for medication.

Minuchin's work on psychosomatic families has been criticized for conceptual (Kog et al., 1985) and methodologic reasons (Coyne and Anderson, 1988; Campbell, 1986). Problems include a lack of clear definitions of the central concepts, small number of subjects, lack of control groups, observer biases, and the absence of statistical analyses. Several studies of diabetics and their families do demonstrate that poor diabetic control is associated with family dysfunction (Grey et al., 1980; Koski and Kumento, 1977; Orr et al., 1983), but it is not known whether there is any cause or effect. Most of the families of 30 poorly controlled diabetic children studied by White and coworkers (1984) had numerous dysfunctional psychosocial factors, including absent fathers, poor living conditions, inadequate parental functioning, chronic family conflict, and lack of family involvement with the diabetes. On the other hand, clear organization in the family has been associated with good metabolic control (Shouval et al., 1982). High parental self-esteem is also associated with good control and is an important mediating factor between family functioning and diabetes (Grey et al., 1980).

DIABETES MELLITUS

How emotionally close or cohesive a family is seems to be particularly important for the care of diabetes. Both low cohesion or disengagement and high cohesion or enmeshment have been associated with poor blood sugar control. In a carefully controlled study, Anderson and colleagues (1981) found that low cohesion and high conflict were associated with poor diabetic control. Parental indifference can result in the worst diabetic control and lead to depression in the diabetic child (Khurana and White, 1970). Thus, in emotionally distant or disengaged families, inadequate supervision and parental support results in noncompliance with insulin and diet and poor diabetic control. In a large sample of diabetic families, Cederblad and colleagues (1982) demonstrated that high cohesion in the mother, rigidity in the father, and anxiety in the diabetic child were all associated with poor metabolic control.

These studies suggest that the mechanisms by which the family influences diabetic control may depend upon the style of family functioning, especially its cohesion. Both high and low cohesion are associated with poor diabetic control. In enmeshed families, diabetic control may be physiologically linked to emotional processes within the family. In disengaged families, inadequate family structure and support may result in noncompliance. Optimal management of diabetes requires the support and supervision of the family along with respect for individuality and age-appropriate autonomy. While these results suggest specific clinical interventions with each type of family, no controlled studies have been conducted.

ASTHMA

Studies of families with an asthmatic child have been too few to determine whether the illness is associated with family dysfunction or any family characteristic. Dubo and colleagues (1961) failed to find any relationship between the quality of family life and severity of asthma. In a study to specifically test the psychosomatic model in asthma, Burbeck (1979) found no relationship between any of the four family characteristics said to be characteristic of these families and the severity of asthma. Taking the concept of families as pathogenic to an extreme, Purcell and colleagues (1969) removed 25 severely asthmatic children from their families and observed that half of them improved. This uncontrolled and controversial study is fortunately not likely to be replicated.

Two randomized, controlled trials of family psychotherapy have demonstrated a beneficial effect on the course of asthma. Lask and Matthew (1979) randomly assigned 33 families with 37 asthmatic children to experimental and control groups. The experimental groups received a total of 6 hours of family therapy designed to improve the families' coping skills in dealing with acute attacks. At the end of 1 year, the children who received family therapy reported less wheezing and slightly improved pulmonary function tests. In a similar study, Gustafsson and colleagues (1986) found that children with severe asthma who received family therapy improved significantly on several measures while those who received conventional treatment did not improve. These two studies are the only randomized, controlled trials of family therapy for a physical illness in the literature.

Despite its popularity, the psychosomatic family model has yet to be validated. Similar to the concept of a schizophrenogenic family, this model tends to blame families for the chronic illness and alienate them from the health care system. There is currently no evidence that any particular type of family or style of family interaction is associated with a specific disease. This parallels the failure of psychosomatic researchers to find specific personality traits associated with specific diseases. Steinglass and Horan (1988) have raised the question of whether one should look for common themes across all chronic illnesses rather than looking just at specific illnesses.

More recent research on families and chronic illness has abandoned the concept that families can cause disease and has focused on how family processes can influence the course of an illness. In an elegant, but controversial, study, Reiss and his colleagues (1986), studied how family factors influence the survival of patients on chronic hemodialysis. Contrary to their initial hypotheses, they found that the patients from higher functioning families (better problem solving, higher accomplishments, and longer marriages) died sooner than those from less healthy families. In addition, they found that compliance with the medical treatments (assessed by multiple measures) was associated with early death and mediated the relationship between family factors and survival. From these results, the authors hypothesized that some healthy families extrude a terminally ill member to preserve the integrity of the family and that the patient may accept this extrusion by complying with the medical regimen. This study emphasizes the importance of measuring health outcomes in all family members and raises the ethical dilemma when the health of an individual is in conflict with the health of the rest of the family.

Mechanisms: How Families Influence Health

Excluding the transmission of infectious agents from one family member to another, there are two general pathways—psychophysiologic and behavioral—by which a family can influence the health of its members. In the psychophysiologic pathway, family factors, such as stress or life events, affect the emotional state of an individual family member resulting in direct physiologic changes that predispose the individual to becoming ill. With the behavioral pathway, the family influences the individual's health behaviors (such as diet, exercise, smoking, compliance with medical treatment, or visits to the physician), and these behaviors affect the individual's health. Understanding these processes will help in the development of clinical interventions to prevent adverse outcomes.

PSYCHOPHYSIOLOGIC PATHWAY

Early research on the psychophysiologic pathway emphasized the neuroendocrine connection. Stress researchers, such as Walter Cannon and Hans Selye, demonstrated that stressful stimuli lead to changes in the autonomic nervous system and the endocrine system. In the fight-flight response, large amounts of catecholamines are released into the bloodstream and result in a hyperalert state. Blood pressure and heart rate increase, pupils dilate, blood is shunted away from internal organs to skeletal muscles, and the individual feels fearful or anxious. While this is generally an adaptive response, it can be harmful. In persons with heart disease, the increased stress can lead to a heart attack, arrhythmias, or death (Lown et al., 1980). Engel (1971) studied 170 cases of sudden death and found that 39 per cent of the women and 11 per cent of the men died immediately following the death of someone close. He hypothesized that the deaths were due to cardiac arrests in individuals with pre-existing heart disease. In stressed diabetic patients, elevated epinephrine levels may increase glucose and free fatty acid production and worsen diabetic control. Minuchin and colleagues (1978) reported that in certain psychosomatic families of diabetics, conflict between family members can elevate fatty acids and precipitate ketoacidosis. Marital conflict and dissatisfaction has been shown to increase autonomic arousal and lead to poorer self-reported health (Levenson and Gottman, 1983, 1985).

Recent interest in biologic mechanisms has focused on the immune system and evolved into the development of the field of psychoimmunology. Studies in animals and humans reveal that stress can lead to immunosuppression and an increase in illness (Ader, 1981; Calabrese et al., 1987). Two well-controlled studies demonstrated a decrease in cellular immunity (T-lymphocyte stimulation) during bereavement (Bartrop et al., 1977; Schleifer et al., 1983). However, in a third study, T-cell function was reduced only in those bereaved subjects who were clinically depressed (Linn et al., 1984). Divorced or separated men and women have significantly poorer immune function than matched married controls (Kiecolt-Glaser et al., 1987; Kiecolt-Glaser et al., 1988). Among the married individuals in these studies, poor marital quality correlated with both depression and decreased immunity. Immune function is also impaired in major depression, and researchers have suggested that changes occurring in the central nervous system during depression may be a final common pathway (Calabrese et al., 1987).

BEHAVIORAL PATHWAY

The family may also influence health more indirectly by influencing health behaviors. For example, while the stress of bereavement may directly affect the immune system, it also results in profound behavioral changes, including an increase in smoking, alcohol consumption, and use of sedatives, all of which may result in poor health. Cirrhosis, accidents, and suicide account for a large proportion of the increased mortality after bereavement and are often the result of alcohol abuse. These changes in health behaviors may be more important clinically than the direct physiologic effects of bereavement.

Although more research has been done on the psychophysiologic pathway, it is likely that the behavioral pathway is a more important mechanism for the family's influence on health. Research suggests that health behaviors have a more powerful influence on health than emotional states. For example, behavioral cardiac risk factors, such as smoking, diet, and compliance with hypertension medication, are more important than emotional states, such as stress or Type A, in the development of heart disease. Similarly for diabetes, poor metabolic control appears to be primarily a result of poor compliance rather than emotional distress (Coyne, 1988). Knowing the mechanism by which families influence health will help guide the clinical interventions.

Clinical Implications

The research on the family's influence on health has important implications for the assessment of patients and their families and the choice of interventions. When interviewing one or more members of a family, the family physician should determine the amount of stress the family is experiencing, including any recent deaths, divorces, or separations, and any current illnesses, marital difficulties, or sexual dysfunctions. When the patient or family is experiencing a high level of stress, an assessment of coping mechanism should include how the family is coping with the current stressors and how they have dealt with crises in the past. Social and family supports are an important resource when a patient or family is in crisis and should be assessed. It is useful to know not only the availability and utilization of supports but how helpful the patient or family perceives the supports to be.

Because health risk factors tend to run in families, the entire family should be screened when an unhealthy behavior is detected in an individual. These risk factors include smoking, excess alcohol consumption, hypercholesterolemia, obesity, and hypertension. Education about these risk factors should include the entire family, not just the individual patient. Whenever possible, intervene at a family level. For example, the family physician can encourage both members of a couple to quit smoking or all members of a family to reduce their cholesterol intake. One should try to get the patient's spouse to actively support recommended life-style changes or compliance with medication. On the other hand, it is important to block any tendencies for a family member to nag or "police" the patient.

When working with patients who have a chronic illness, encourage the family to be involved in the management of illness, while supporting the patient's autonomy and ultimate responsibility for care. For distant or disengaged family members, this may involve asking them to accompany the patient for appointments and finding specific ways in which they can assist the patient. For enmeshed families, it is often necessary to help the patient and family negotiate which responsibilities will be the patient's and which will be the family's. Severely dysfunctional families with chronic illness should be referred to a family therapist and cared for jointly with the therapist's assistance. It is important not to blame family members for medical problems. Referrals should be presented as helping the family cope with the chronic illness.

Research on families and health demonstrate the powerful influence of the family on health and illness. Cardiovascular and other risk factors are often shared by family members, and a family approach is an effective way to change unhealthy life styles. Family stress and support have an effect on overall mortality. Bereavement is associated with an increased risk of death. Spousal support has a direct protective effect on health and buffers the impact of stress. Studies of chronic disease indicate that family dysfunction is associated with poor health outcomes.

We are just beginning to understand the relationship of families and health, and much more research is needed. This research should have a sound theoretical base and develop from clinical observations. It is well established that the family influences health and that a family approach is effective. We must now begin to test different types of family interventions in clinical practice to determine how best to work with families in family medicine (McDaniel et al., 1989).

References

Ader, R., (Ed.): Psychoneuroimmunology. New York, Academic Press, 1981.

Anderson, C. M., Reiss, D. J., and Hogarty, G.: Schizophrenia and the Family. New York, Guilford Press, 1986.

Anderson, B. J., Miller, J. P., Auslander, W. F., and Santiago, J. V.: Family characteristics of diabetic adolescents: Relationship to metabolic control. Diabetes Care *4*:586–594, 1970.

Bachrach, L. L.: Marital Status and Mental Disorder: An Analytical Review. Washington, D.C., US Government Printing Office, 1975.

Baranowski, T., Nader, P. R., Dunn, K., and Vanderpool, N. A.: Family self-help: Promoting changes in health behavior. J. Commun. *Summer*:161–172, 1982.

Barbarin, O. A., and Tirado, M.: Family involvement and successful treatment of obesity: A review. Fam. Systems Med. *2*:37–45, 1984.

Bartrop, R. W., Luckhurst, E., Lazarus, L., et al.: Depressed lymphocyte function after bereavement. Lancet *1*:834–836, 1977.

Beautrais, A. L., Fergusson, D. M., and Shannon, F. T.: Life events and childhood morbidity: A prospective study. Pediatrics *70*:935–940, 1982.

Berkman, L. F.: Assessing the physical health effects of social networks and social supports. Ann. Rev. Public Health *5*:413–432, 1984.

Berkman, L. F., and Syme, S. L.: Social networks, host resistance and mortality: A nine year follow-up study of Alameda County residents. Am. J. Epidemiol. *109*:186–204, 1979.

Bewley, B. R., and Bland, J. M.: Academic performance and social factors relating to cigarette smoking by school children. Br. J. Prev. Soc Med *31*:8–24, 1977.

Blake, R. L.: The effects of stress and social support on health: A research challenge for Family Medicine. Fam. Med. *20*:19–24, 1988.

Blazer, D. G.: Social support and mortality in an elderly community population. Am. J. Epidemiol. *115*:684–694, 1982.

Bloom, B. L., Asher, S. J., and White, S. W.: Marital disruption as a stressor: A review and analysis. Psychol. Bull. *85*:867–894, 1978.

Boyce, W. T., Jensen, E. W., Cassel, J. C., et al.: Influence of life events and family routines on childhood respiratory illness. Pediatrics *60*:609–615, 1977.

Briscoe, C. S., Smith, J. B., Robins, E., et al.: Divorce and psychiatric disease. Arch. Gen. Psychiatry *29*:119–125, 1973.

Broadhead, W. E., Kaplan, B. H., James, S. A., et al.: The epidemiologic evidence for a relationship between social support and health. Am. J. Epidemiol. *117*:521–537, 1983.

Brownell, K. D., Heckerman, C. L., Westlake, R. J., et al.: The effects of couples training and partner co-operativeness in the behavioral treatment of obesity. Behav. Res. Ther. *16*:323–333, 1978.

Bruhn, J. G.: Effects of chronic illness on the family. J. Fam. Prac. *4*:1057–1060, 1977.

Bryan, M. S., and Lowenberg, M. E.: The father's influence on young children's food preferences. J. Am. Diet. Assoc. *34*:30–35, 1958.

Burbeck, T. W.: An empirical investigation of the psychosomatogenic family model. J. Psychosom. Res. *23*:327–337, 1979.

Calabrese, J. R., Kling, M. A., and Gold, P. W.: Alterations in immunocompetence during stress, bereavement and depression: Focus on neuroendocrine regulation. Am. J. Psychiatry *144*(9):1123–1134, 1987.

Campbell, T. L.: Family's impact on health: A critical review and annotated bibliography, Fam. Systems Med. *4*(2&3):135–328, 1986.

Carter, H., and Glick, P. C.: Marriage and Divorce: A Social and Economic Study. Cambridge, Harvard University Press, 1970.

Cederblad, M., Helgesson, M., Larsson, Y., and Ludvigsson, J.: Family structure and diabetes in children. Pediatr. Adoles. Endocrin. *10*:94–98, 1982.

Cohen, S., and Wills, T. A.: Stress, social support, and the buffering hypothesis. Psychol. Bull. *98*:310–357, 1985.

Cohen, F.: Stress and bodily illness. Psychiatr. Clin. North Am. *4*:269–285, 1981.

Cohen, S., and Syme, S. L. (Eds.): Social Support and Health. Orlando, Academic Press, 1985.

Coppotelli, H. C., and Orleans, C. T.: Partner support and other determinants of smoking cessation among women. J. Consult. Clin. Psychol. *53*:455–460, 1985.

Coyne, J. C., and Anderson, B. J.: The "psychosomatic family" reconsidered: Diabetes in context. J. Mar. Fam. Ther. *14*:113–123, 1988.

Dishman, R. K., Sallis, J. F., and Orenstein, D. R.: The determinants of physical activity and exercise. Publ. Health Rep. *100*:158–171, 1985.

Doherty, W. J., and Campbell, T. L.: Families and Health. Families studies text series. Beverly Hills, Sage Publishing, 1988.

Doherty, W. J., Schrott, H. G., Metcalf, L., and Iassiello-Vailas, L.: Effect of spouse support and health beliefs on medication adherence. J. Fam. Pract. *17*:837–841, 1983.

Dubo, S., McLean, J. A., Ching, A. Y. T., et al.: A study of relationships between family situation, bronchial asthma, and personal adjustment in children. J. Pediatr. *59*:402–414, 1961.

Eastwood, M. A., Brydon, W. G., Smith, D. M., and Smith, J. H.: A study of diet, serum lipids and fecal constituents in spouses. Am. J. Clin. Nutr. *36*:290–293, 1982.

Engel, G. L.: Sudden and rapid death during psychological stress: Folk lore or folk wisdom. Ann. Int. Med. *74*:771–782, 1971.

Feinleib, M., Garrison, R. J., Fabsitz, R., et al.: The NHLBI twin study of cardiovascular disease risk factors: Methodology and summary of results. Am. J. Epidemiol. *106:*284–295, 1977.

Feinleib, M., Garrison, R. J., and Havlik, R. J.: Environmental and genetic factors affecting the distribution of blood pressure in children. In Lauer, R. M., Shekelle, R. B. (Eds.): Childhood Prevention of Atherosclerosis and Hypertension. New York, Raven Press, 1980.

Ganster, D. C., and Victor, B.: The impact of social support on mental and physical health. Br. J. Med. Psychol. *61:*17–36, 1988.

Garn, S. M., Cole, P. E., and Bailey, S. M.: Effect of parental fatness levels on fatness of biological and adoptive children. Ecol. Food Nutr. *6:*1–3, 1976.

Garn, S. M., and Clark, D. C.: Trends in fatness and the origins of obesity. Pediatrics *57:*443–456, 1976.

Goldstein, M.: Psychological issues. Schizophr. Bull. *13*(1):157–171, 1987.

Gottlieb, N. H., and Chen, M. S.: Sociocultural correlates of childhood sporting activities: Their implications for heart health. Soc. Sci. Med. *5:*533–539, 1985.

Graham, S., and Gibson, R. W.: Cessation of patterned behavior: Withdrawal from smoking. Soc. Sci. Med. *5:*319–337, 1971.

Grey, M. J., Genel, M., and Tamborlane, W. V.: Psychosocial adjustment of latency-age diabetics: Determinants and relationship to control. Pediatrics *65:*69–73, 1980.

Gustafsson, P. A., Kjellman, N. M., and Cederblad, M.: Family therapy in the treatment of severe childhood asthma. J. Psychosom. Res. *30:*369–374, 1986.

Hartz, A., Giefer, E., and Rimm, A. A.: Relative importance of the effect of family environment and heredity on obesity. Ann. Hum. Genet. *41:*185–193, 1977.

Haynes, R. B., Mattson, M. E., and Chobanian, A. V., et al.: Management of patient compliance in the treatment of hypertension: Report of the NHLBI working group. Hypertension *4:*415–423, 1982.

Heinzelman, F., and Bagley, R. W.: Response to physical activity programs and their effects on health behavior. Public Health Rep. *85:*905–911, 1970.

Helsing, K. J., and Szklo, M.: Mortality after bereavement. Am. J. Epidemiol. *114:*41–52, 1981.

Hepworth, J.: Families and chronic pain. In Rosenthal, D. (Ed.): Families in Stress, Family Therapy Collection, Rockville, MD, Aspen, 1987.

Holmes, T. H., and Rahe, R. H.: The social readjustment scale. J. Psychosom. Res. *39:*413–431, 1967.

House, J. S., Robbins, C., and Metzner, H. L.: The association of social relationships and activities with mortality: Prospective evidence from the Tecumseh Community Health Study. Am. J. Epidemiol. *116:*123–140, 1982.

Jacobs, S., and Ostfeld, A.: An epidemiological review of the mortality of bereavement. Psychosom. Med. *39:*344–357, 1977.

Kaprio, J., Koskenvou, M., and Rita, H.: Mortality after bereavement: A prospective study of 95,647 widowed persons. Am. J. Pub. Health *77:*283–287, 1987.

Karlin, S., Williams, P. T., Farquhar, J. W., et al.: Association arrays for the study of familial height, weight, lipid, and lipoprotein similarity in three west coast populations. Am. J. Epidemiol. *116:*1001–1021, 1982.

Keitner, G. I., Baldwin, L. M., Epstein, N. B., and Bishops, D. S.: Family functioning patients with affective disorders: A review. Inter. J. Fam. Psychiatry *6:*405–437, 1985.

Khurana, R., White, P.: Attitudes of the diabetic child and his parents towards his illness. Postgrad. Med. *48:*72–76, 1970.

Kiecolt-Glaser, J. K., Kennedy, S., Malkoff, S., et al.: Marital discord and immunity in males. Psychosom. Med. *50:*213–229, 1988.

Kiecolt-Glaser, J. K., Fisher, L. D., Ogrockl, P., et al.: Marital quality, marital disruption, and immune function. Psychosom. Med. *49*(1):13–32, 1987.

Klein, R., Dean, A., and Bogdanoff, M.: The impact of illness of the spouse. J. Chronic Dis. *20:*241–252, 1968.

Klesges, R. C., Coates, T. J., Brown, G., et al.: Parental influences on children's eating behavior and relative weight. J. Appl. Behav. Analy. *16:*371–378, 1983.

Kog, E., Vandereyecken, W., and Vertommen, H.: The psychosomatic family model: A critical analysis of family interaction concepts. J. Fam. Therapy. *7:*31–44, 1985.

Koski, M. L., and Kumento, A.: The interrelationship between diabetic control and family life. Pediatr. Adoles. Endocrin. *3:*41–45, 1977.

Kraus, A. S., and Lilienfeld A. M.: Some epidemiological aspects of the high mortality rate in the young widowed group. J. Chronic Dis. *10:*207–217, 1959.

Lask, B., and Matthew, D.: Childhood asthma: A controlled trial of family psychotherapy. Arch. Dis. Child *54:*116–119, 1979.

Laskarzewski, P., Morrison, J. A., Khoury, K., et al.: Parent-child nutrient intake relationship in school children ages 6 to 19: The Princeton School District Study. Am. J. Clin. Nutr. *33:*3250–3255, 1980.

Levenson, R. W., and Gottman, J. M.: Marital interaction: Physiological linkage and affective exchange. J. Person. Soc. Psychol. *3:*587–597, 1983.

Levenson, R. W., and Gottman, J. M.: Physiological and affective predictors of change in relationship satisfaction. J. Person Soc. Psychol. *49:*85–91, 1985.

Levine, D. M., Green, L. W., Deeds, S.G., et al.: Health education for hypertensive patients. J.A.M.A. *241:*1700–1703, 1979.

Lichtenstein, E., Glasgow, R. E., and Abrams, D. B.: Social support in smoking cessation: In search of effective interventions. Behav. Ther. *17:*606–619, 1986.

Lichtenstein, E.: The smoking problem: A behavioral perspective. J. Consult. Clin. Psychol. *50:*465–466, 1982.

Linn, M. W., Linn, B. S., and Jensen, J.: Stressful events, dysphoric mood, and immune responsiveness. Psychol. Rep. *54:*219–222, 1984.

Livingood, A. B., Goldwater, C., and Kurz, R. B.: Psychological aspects of sports participation in young children. Adv. Behav. Pediatr. *2:*141–169, 1981.

Lown, B., Desilva, R. A., Reich, P., and Murawski, B. J.: Psychophysiologic factors in sudden cardiac death. Am. J. Psychiatry *137:*1325–1335, 1980.

Lynch, J.: The Broken Heart: The Medical Consequences of Loneliness. New York, Basic Books, 1977.

Martin, J. E., Dubbert, P.: Exercise applications and promotion in behavioral medicine: Current status and future directions. J. Consult. Clin. Psychol. *50:*1004–1017, 1982.

McDaniel, S., Campbell, T., and Seaburn, D.: Family-oriented Primary Care: A Manual for Medical Providers. New York, Springer-Verlag, 1989.

McKenney, J. M., Slining, J. M., Henderson, H. R., et al.: The effect of clinical pharmacy services on patients with essential hypertension. Circulation *48:*1104–1111, 1973.

Mermelstein, R., Lichtenstein, and E., McIntyre, K.: Partner support and relapse in smoking cessation programs. J. Consult. Clin. Psychol. *51:*465–466, 1983.

Meyer, R. J., and Haggerty, R. J.: Streptococcal infections in families: factors altering individual susceptibility. Pediatrics *29:*539–549, 1962.

Minuchin, S., Baker, L., Rosman, B. L., et al.: A conceptual model of psychosomatic illness in children: family organization and family therapy. Arch. Gen. Psychiatry *32:*1031–1038, 1975.

Minuchin, S., Rosman, B. L., and Baker, L.: Psychosomatic Families. Cambridge, Harvard University Press, 1978.

Morisky, D. E., Levine, D. M., Green, L. W., et al.: Five year blood pressure control and mortality following health education for hypertensive patients. Am. J. Public Health *73:*153–162, 1983.

Nader, P. R., Baranowski, T., Vanderpool, N. A., et al.: The Family Health Project: Cardiovascular risk reduction education for children and parents. Develop. Behav. Pediatr. *4:*3–10, 1983.

National Institute of Education. Teenage Smoking: Immediate and Long-term Patterns. Washington, DC, US Government Printing Office, 1979.

Norbeck, J. S., and Tolden, V. P.: Life stress, social supports, and emotional disequilibrium in complications of pregnancy: A prospective, multivariate study. J. Health Soc. Behav. *24:*30–46, 1983.

Nuckolls, K. B., Cassel, J., and Kaplan, B. H.: Psychosocial assets, life crisis and the prognosis of pregnancy. Am. J. Epidemiol. *95:*431–441, 1972.

Ockene, J. K., Nuttall, R. L., Benfari, R. S., et al.: A psychosocial model of smoking cessation and maintenance of cessation. Prev. Med. *10:*623–638, 1981.

Orr, D. P., Golden, M. P., Myers, G., and Marrerro, D. G.: Characteristics of adolescents with poorly controlled diabetes referred to a tertiary care center. Diabetes Care *6:*170–175, 1983.

Orth-Gomer, K., and Johnson, J. V.: Social network interaction and mortality: A six year follow-up study of a random sample of the Swedish population. J. Chronic. Dis. *40:*949–957, 1987.

Osterweis, M., Solomon, F., Green, M. (Eds.). Bereavement: Reactions, Consequences, and Care. Washington DC, National Academy Press, 1984.

Parkes, C. M., Benjamin, B., and Fitzgerald, R. G.: Broken heart: A statistical study of increased mortality among widowers. Br. Med. J. *1:*740–743, 1969.

Patterson, T. L., Kaplan, R. M., Sallis, J. F., and Nader, P. R.: Aggregation of blood pressure in Anglo American and Mexican American families. Prev. Med. *16:*616–625, 1987.

Pearce, J. W., LeBow, M. D., and Orchard, J.: Role of spouse involvement in the behavioral treatment of overweight women. J. Consult. Clin. Psychol. *49:*236–244, 1981.

Pearlin, L. I., Menaghan, E. G., Lieberman, M. A., and Mullan, J. T.: The stress process. J. Health Soc. Behav. *22:*337–365, 1981.

Price, R. A., Chen, K. H., Cavallii, S. L., et al.: Models of spouse influence and their applications to smoking behavior. Soc. Biol. *28:*14–29, 1981.

Purcell, K., Brady, K., Chai, H., et al.: The effects of asthma in children of experimental separation from the family. Psychosom. Med. *31:*144–163, 1969.

Rabkin, J. G., and Struening, E. L.: Life events, stress and illness. Science *194:*1013–1020, 1976.

Ramsey, C. N., Abell, T. D., and Baker, L. C.: The relationship between family functioning, life events, family structure and the outcome of pregnancy. J. Fam. Prac. *22:*521–527, 1986.

Reiss, D., Gonzales, S., and Kramer, N.: Family process, chronic illness and death: On the weakness of strong bonds. Arch. Gen. Psychiatry *43:*795–804, 1986.

Saccone, A. J., and Israel, A. C.: Effects of experimental versus significant other-controlled reinforcement and choice of target behavior on weight loss. Beh. Ther. *9:*271–278, 1978.

Sackett, D. L., Anderson, G. D., Milner, R., et al.: Concordance for coronary risk factors among spouses. Circulation *52:*589–595, 1975.

Sallis, J. F., and Nader, P. R. Family determinants of health behaviors. In Gochman, D. S., (Ed.): Health Behavior. New York, Plenum Publishing Corp., 1988.

Sallis, J. F., Patterson, T. L., Buono, M. J., et al.: Aggregation of physical activity habits in Mexican-American and Anglo families. J. Behav. Med. *11:*31–41, 1988.

Schleifer, S. J., Keller, S. E., Camerino, M., et al.: Suppression of lymphocyte stimulation following bereavement. *250:*374–377, 1983.

Shear, C. L., Frerichs, R. R., Weinberg, R., and Berenson, G. S.: Childhood sibling aggregation of coronary artery disease risk factor variable in a biracial community. Am. J. Epidemiol. *107:*522–528, 1978.

Shouval, R., Ber, R., and Galatzer, A.: Family social climate and the health status and social adaptation of diabetic youth. Pediatr. Adoles. Endocrin. *10:*89–93, 1982.

Stanton, M. D.: Drugs and the family: A review of the recent literature. Marr. Fam. Rev. *2:*1–10, 1979.

Steinglass, P., and Robertson, A.: The alcoholic family. Biology of Alcoholism: Psychosocial Factors *VI:*243–307, 1983.

Steinglass, P., and Horan, M. E.: Families and chronic medical illness. In Walsh, F., and Anderson, C. M. (Eds.): Chronic Disorders and the Family. New York, Haworth Press, 1988.

Stuart, R. B., and Davis, B.: Slim Chance in a Fat World: Behavioral Control Obesity. Champaign, IL, Research Press, 1972.

Stunkard, A. J., Sorensen, T. I. A., Hanis, C., et al. An adoption study of human obesity. N. Engl. J. Med. *314:*193–201, 1986.

Sutton, G.: Assortive marriages for smoking habits. Ann. Hum. Biol. *7:*449–456, 1980.

Turk, D. C., and Kerns, R. D. (Eds.): Health, Illness, and Families: A Life-Span Perspective. New York, John Wiley & Sons, 1985.

Venters, M. H., Jacobs, D. R., Luepker, R. V., et al.: Spouse concordance of smoking patterns: The Minnesota heart survey. Am. J. Epidemiol. *120:*608–616, 1984.

Verbrugge, L. M.: Marital status and health. J. Marr. Fam. *7:*267–285, 1977.

Walsh, F.: New perspectives on schizophrenia and the family. In Walsh, F., Anderson, C. M. (Eds.): Chronic Disorders and the Family. New York, Haworth Press, 1988.

Walsh, F., Anderson, C. M. (Eds.): Chronic Disorders and the Family. New York, Haworth Press, 1988.

White, K., Kolman, M. L., Wexler, P., et al.: Unstable diabetes and unstable families: A psychosocial evaluation of diabetic children with recurrent ketoacidosis. Pediatrics *73:*749–755, 1984.

Working Group on Health Education and High Blood Pressure Control, National Institute of Heart, Lung, and Blood. The Physician's Guide: Improving Adherence Among Hypertensive Patients. Washington, DC, Government Printing Office, 1987.

Yager, J.: Family issues in the pathogenesis of anorexia nervosa. Psychosom. Med. *44:*43–59, 1982.

Zuckerman, D. M., Kasl, S. V., and Osterfeld, A. M.: Psychosocial predictors of mortality among the elderly poor: The role of religion, well-being, and social contact. Am. J. Epidemiol. *119:*410–423, 1984.

7

Impact of Divorce on the Family

James H. Bray

Separation and divorce have a major impact on the health and well-being of all family members. Divorce is best understood not as a single event but as a process of transition that continues for many years. Millions of children and adults are directly involved in the many stresses and changes caused by their family moving from a nuclear family to a postdivorce family to a stepfamily. Some will be involved in even more changes because of the multiple divorces and remarriages of one or more parents.

Demographic Changes

Although the divorce rate has decreased since 1979, it is better seen as leveling off rather than a major reduction. Despite this change, the divorce rate continues to be alarmingly high. It is estimated that up to 50 per cent of first marriages will end in divorce and approximately 60 per cent of all divorces involve children. Demographic estimates indicate that over 50 per cent of all children in the United States will be affected by their parents' separation and divorce during their childhood (Hetherington and Arasteh, 1988; Norton and Moorman, 1987).

Family changes do not stop after the divorce, because a large number of divorced men and women remarry. Estimates are that 80 per cent of divorced women and 83 per cent of divorced men will remarry, one half within 3 years postdivorce (Furstenberg and Spanier, 1984). Recent estimates indicate that remarriage rates are also changing; fewer adults may remarry, and they may wait longer periods after divorce to remarry.

Demographic projections suggest that in the 1990's, 50 per cent of all children will spend some time in a single parent home, and over 25 per cent of children will spend some time in a stepfamily (Glick, 1984). Divorce and remarriage involve a complex series of changes that often affect every aspect of family functioning. Divorce and remarriage affect parent-child relationships, parenting practices and effectiveness, family conflict, family income and residence, extended family relationships, and peer and social relationships. These changes may produce both short-term crises and long-term effects on individual family members. This chapter reviews the process of divorce and remarriage, how it affects family members, and the role a family physician can play in this process.

Families can be viewed as interdependent, interactional systems in which each family member affects and is affected by other members of the family system. It is assumed that change within one part of the family system produces change in other parts of the family through reciprocal feedback and interaction between family members. Families also go through a family life cycle with predictable and unpredictable developmental changes. Predictable changes include progression through the family life cycle transitions from single adulthood, marriage, family with children, families in later life, etc. Unpredictable changes include transitions caused by outside stressors, such as natural disasters, wars, unexpected deaths, etc., or breakup of the family through divorce. Divorce can be viewed as causing both kinds of changes because it is difficult to predict if and when a family will break up, but when families divorce and remarry they appear to go through a series of predictable transitions from family breakup and separation, binuclear, postdivorce family to remarried family.

However, individuals within a family may have very different *experiences* of a divorce, and these differences are important in understanding and helping them through this process. For example, a woman may be very unhappy in a marriage and psychologically divorcing her husband for years. Yet, the husband may be generally satisfied with the marriage and shocked and surprised when his wife tells him she wants a divorce. The children may each have different reactions and align with mother or father during the process. Thus, by the time of the actual legal divorce, the wife may have resolved much of her grief and negative feelings, but the husband and some of the children may be in the middle of emotional turmoil about the divorce process. The family physician needs to understand these differences to most effectively treat the individual family members and help the family through this process.

Divorce is not necessarily bad for family members. Staying together in an unhappy, conflictual marriage for the children's sake or any other reason may not be in their best interests. Children actually adjust better in a stable, divorced home than in an unhappy, highly conflictual intact home. Hetherington and colleagues (1978) stated, "Our study and previous research show that a conflict-ridden intact family is more deleterious to family members than a stable home situation in which parents are divorced. Divorce is often a positive solution to destructive family functioning" (p. 34). Hetherington and colleagues (1982, 1984) also found that some women benefit from a divorce and later develop better self-esteem, higher levels of competence, and career achievements. This is not to say that divorce is always good or that it is to be recommended in all cases. In fact, most research indicates that, in general, being married is associated with better outcomes and fewer health problems than being divorced or single.

Process of Separation and Divorce

The decision for adults to separate and ultimately divorce is a complex process that results in a high degree of emotional distress. During the deliberation period, prior to the separation, partners often quarrel, confront their partners with their unhappiness, seek outside assistance from friends, ministers, primary care physicians, and marital counselors (Kaslow, 1981). Many families turn to their family physician for support and assistance because the family physician is seen as someone who has unique knowledge of families. The physician's role is to decrease the psychologic risk of patients, to promote healthy methods of coping with stress, to teach parents ways of relating to their children that maximize their coping, and to make appropriate referrals for additional help.

Separation Reactions. During the early stages of marital distress, patients may present with anxiety, depression, impotence, ulcers, migraines, or other psychosomatic symptoms related to the stress of living with an unhappy relationship. Common feelings include disillusionment, alienation, anger, and general dissatisfaction. Conflict may escalate between the spouses, and children may become involved as a way of deflecting the marital conflict. Later, there is likely to be withdrawal, both emotional and physical, and a yo-yo effect in which partners may attempt to alternately deny problems and have intense emotional conversations to convince each other to stay in the marriage. Physicians should be prepared to recommend marriage counseling if patients present evidence of marital distress. In its early stages, deterioration of the relationship may be reversible. Early assessment, intervention, and, if necessary, referral to a marriage and family therapist can short-circuit the difficulty of a marital separation and help save the marriage. If reconciliation is not possible, counseling may allow the couple to negotiate the separation process with less distress to themselves and any children involved. It should be noted that not all couples who separate, or file for divorce, ultimately divorce. Many couples reconcile after a separation period, and the physician can help the family through this process with support and early intervention.

People decide to divorce for multiple reasons. Many couples divorce because of marital conflict, poor communication, child-related conflict, and problems with a spouse, such as abuse, violence, or emotional problems. However, several studies have found that 25 to 30 per cent of couples report no intense conflict prior to their divorce and decide to end their marriage "because there had been a gradual loss of love and mutual regard or a divergence in life-styles and values" (Kelly, 1988, p. 121). Thus, there is considerable heterogeneity in the reasons for and responses to divorce. Appreciating and understanding the variety of experiences is essential to help people through this process.

The stage of physical separation is particularly stressful. However, the degree and effects appear to differ for men and women. Women are more likely to terminate a marital relationship than men, and some research indicates that the person who seeks the divorce is able to cope better than the partner who does not seek the divorce. Bloom and Hodges (1981) found that women tend to develop more physical complaints and symptoms following a separation, while men are more likely to feel a loss of interpersonal gratifications. Gunn (1970) found that after the final separation, over half the respondents reported disturbances in work, sleep, and health status.

Children usually experience the separation as a crisis event. They often respond to this crisis with reactive depression and sadness, anxiety about their future and care, anger at one or both parents, loyalty conflicts, and decreased school performance. Preoccupation with their parents' separation and fantasies of reconciliation are often accompanied by the changes in academic performance and school behavior as the children withdraw into their fantasy world or act out their unhappiness with increased behavior problems.

Strong feelings of depression, anger, hopelessness, confusion, sadness, loneliness, and relief may be present during the litigation of the divorce. There are multiple aspects of the divorce process: the emotional divorce, legal divorce, economic divorce, and community divorce (Bohannon, 1973). Many of these aspects, such as the financial and emotional divorce, may continue long after the legal separation and divorce. Thus, a person or family may be coping with a divorce for many years after the legal termination of the marriage. The unresolved emotional attachment, usually in the form of anger and resentment, can have long-term effects on both adults and children.

POSTDIVORCE BINUCLEAR FAMILIES

Following the legal divorce, the family enters a phase in which they attempt to achieve a new equilibrium and stability. Most adults and children encounter many new problems and responsibilities following the breakup of the family. The term binuclear family (Ahrons, 1979) is used to describe these families rather than the traditional term, single-parent family, because the children continue to be linked to two families—the custodial and the noncustodial parent, and both families have an ongoing influence on family members. Although many fathers (up to 50 per cent) may stop visiting with their children following a divorce, their ghost and legacy and their extended family continue to exert an influence on the children.

Custodial Arrangements. There are two basic child custody arrangements following a divorce: sole custody and joint custody. By far the most common custodial pattern following a divorce is the sole managing conservatorship arrangement, commonly called sole custody. National estimates indicate that women retain custody of the children and men are noncustodial parents in 85 to 90 per cent of divorced families (U.S. Bureau of the Census, 1979). However, men are much more active in parenting and seek custody of their children more often now than in the past. States are changing their laws to support the continuing involvement of the noncustodial parent. Despite the increase in fathers' participation with their children after a divorce, there is still a bias toward having a single parent custody arrangement in the majority of contested and uncontested divorces.

Sole Custody. In the sole custody arrangement, the custodial parent retains custody of the children and the noncustodial parent has visitation with the children. The custodial parent retains all rights, privileges, duties, and powers to the exclusion of the other parent. The noncustodial parent retains a limited set of rights, privileges, duties, and powers. It should be noted that the noncustodial parent may be awarded additional rights and responsibilities either by agreement or by a judge. Usually, the custodial parent has the exclusive right to seek medical treatment for the children. This means that, without the permission of the custodial parent, the noncustodial parent can only seek medical treatment under emergency situations.

Joint Custody. There are many types of joint custody. In discussing this area, it is important to distinguish between joint legal custody and joint physical custody. The common element of the two types is that both parents retain the rights of a parent and have equal power and authority over their children's general welfare, education, and upbringing. This does not necessarily mean that the child will live with each parent the same amount of time or that there is an equal sharing of parental responsibilities. Practically speaking, one parent is usually given the sole right to determine the domicile of the children. In most cases of joint custody, the child has a primary residence or home base with one parent and lives with or has access to the other parent at specified time periods. In an ongoing study of custodial arrangements in California, the Stanford Child Custody Project (Maccoby et al., 1988) found that most joint custody arrangements functioned like sole custody arrangements despite the presumption and prescription of joint legal custody in the divorce decree.

With joint physical custody, both parents retain the rights, privileges, and duties of a parent, and the child lives with both parents on a shared basis. Joint physical custody usually requires more cooperation between the parents, particularly if the children move back and forth between each parent's home on a frequent basis. Kelly and colleagues (1988) found that many parents successfully negotiate and carry out a joint physical custody arrangement and report the arrangement to be satisfactory.

ADULTS' REACTIONS TO DIVORCE

The first year after divorce is highly stressful for adults. Both men and women report decreases in self-esteem, feelings of loss of control, loneliness, and isolation. Hetherington et al. (1982) found that adults frequently have "not me" experiences in which they engage in uncharacteristic behavior and may make major changes in life style and appearance. Adults come to physicians with complaints of fatigue, depression, and general somatic complaints. These are signs that the person is having difficulty coping with the family changes.

Marital disruption is the single most powerful sociodemographic predictor of stress-related physical illness (Somers, 1979). Separated individuals have 30 per cent more acute illness and physician visits than married adults. Separated and divorced adults have the highest rates of acute medical problems, chronic medical conditions that interfere with social activity, and disability. Divorced men have increased rates of suicide, admissions to mental hospitals, vulnerability to minor and major physical illness, and increased risk of being victims of violence (Bloom et al., 1978). Marital separation is associated with reduced qualitative and quantitative immune functioning in men and women compared with married controls. This may explain their increased risk of illness (Kiecolt-Glaser et al., 1987; Kiecolt-Glaser et al., 1988).

Within approximately 2 years after the divorce, most adults have adjusted to the marital breakup and developed a new stability in their lives. Many people expect to recover from the effects of divorce much faster than is realistic. The physician can advise the patient to set goals for recovery that are achievable rather than overwhelming. Hetherington and colleagues (1982, 1987) found that women tend to adjust faster and somewhat better than men. Women and men who have not remarried after 2 years of divorce, report a deep sense of loneliness. With time, feelings of well-being increase, and most adults experience more internal control and satisfaction in life.

EFFECTS OF DIVORCE ON CHILDREN

The process of divorce has wide-reaching influences on children. The effects vary depending on a number of factors that include sex of the child, age of the child, length of time since the divorce, postdivorce family relationships, and socioeconomic factors. Many studies have found that divorce is more difficult and traumatic for boys than for girls, and boys have more severe and enduring negative reactions to divorce than girls (Hetherington and Camara, 1984; Kelly, 1988). Boys tend to develop more behavior, sex-role adjustment, and academic problems than girls, and these problems often persist for 4 to 7 years postdivorce, particularly if the custodial mother remains single. There is some evidence that children tend to adjust best after a divorce when they live with the same sex parent. This pattern appears to reverse itself after the remarriage of the mother with girls having more behavior problems and adjustment difficulties than boys. Children's reactions to their parent's remarriage will be discussed later.

Age Differences. Children's ages at the time of the divorce influence the type and quality of reactions they have to their parents' divorce. Table 7–1 presents children's reactions based on age groups found by various studies (c.f., Hetherington and Camara, 1984; Kelly, 1988; Wallerstein et al., 1988; Wallerstein and Kelly, 1980 for reviews). It is important to point out that an individual child may have a wide range of reactions that include some or all of those problems listed in Table 7–1.

Children, 3 years old and below, are likely to regress in their behavior (e.g., bed wetting) and experience developmental delays, such as difficulty in toilet training. They are also likely to experience intensified separation anxiety when leaving the custodial parent or primary care-taker. Children at this age are highly influenced by their custodial parent and may respond to their parent's anxiety and fear of situations by becoming upset and anxious, particularly when children are left at day-care centers and when the noncustodial parent visits.

Preschool children, ages 4 to 6, are also likely to exhibit regressive behavior and have some developmental delays. They may be whiny and clinging. They will be more aware of and upset by the absence of a parent. Children's anxiety is influenced by their parent's feelings, and they will often respond to the parent's distress rather than other situational factors. Parents will often assume the child's distress is caused by visitation of the noncustodial parent, but if the child calms down rapidly (5 to 10 minutes) after the transition from one parent to the other, then the child is most likely responding to the parents' tension and anxiety around the transition.

School-aged children, ages 6 to 11, are likely to respond to the divorce with sadness and upset. Younger children, ages 6 to 8, are usually unable to completely understand the divorce process or separate themselves psychologically from their parents' influence and wishes. Thus, they may feel responsible for the divorce and blame themselves for the breakup of the family. Older children can understand more about the divorce process. Children at these ages often report frequent reconciliation fantasies. Boys are likely to have increased behavior problems and adjustment difficulties while girls are likely to internalize their feelings and be sad and withdrawn. However, girls may also have an increase in behavior problems as well.

Adolescents, ages 12 to 18, are usually able to separate themselves from their parents' divorce and not blame themselves for the breakup of the family. Anger, resentment, and hostility are common reactions to the divorce. Both boys and girls are likely to have more behavior problems and adjustment difficulties.

Long-Term Effects of Divorce. Several longitudinal studies of children's long-term responses to parental divorce indicate that boys from divorced homes continue to have more behavioral problems than boys in nuclear families or girls in divorced or nuclear families. These problems continue 6 to 10 years after their parents' divorce if their custodial mother does not remarry (Hetherington and Arasteh, 1988). There are generally few differences in behavior problems and adjustment found between girls in divorced and nuclear families. Children's behavioral adjustment changes after the remarriage of the custodial parent will be discussed in the next section.

Table 7–1. CHILDREN'S REACTIONS TO DIVORCE*

Age of Child	Reaction of Child	Expected Problems	Risk Factors	Advice to Parents
Infancy (0–3)	Perceives loss of parent	Regression and developmental delays Problems with feeding, sleeping and toileting Irritability, excessive crying Apathy, withdrawal	Loss of care-giver Diminished capacity of custodial parent Psychologic disturbance of custodial parent	Maintain predictable routines Expect normal separation anxiety to be exaggerated Support for parent caring for herself and baby Substitute care for infant if parent is seriously depressed
Preschool (3–5)	Fears of abandonment Fears loss of custodial parent Confusion	Whining, clinging, and fearful behavior Regression and developmental delays Nightmares, bewilderment, confusion, aggression Sadness, neediness, low self-esteem Denial, perfect behavior	Persistent or severe regression, nightmares, or separation anxiety Persistent encopresis with smearing Refusal of nonresident parent to visit or of resident parent to allow visits Inability of parent to enforce discipline	Both parents should tell children about divorce and what is occurring Establish daily routine Maintain consistent discipline Emphasize that children are not responsible for divorce Encourage involvement of both parents in children's lives
Early School Age (6–8)	Guilt, self-blame for divorce Sense of loss Feels betrayed, rejected Confusion	Sadness, crying, depression Longing for absent parent Anger, tantrums, acting out Asks for reconciliation Increased behavior problems	Developmental arrest, no new learning Loss of interest in peers and activities Other losses—friends, pet, relatives Changes in school or teacher	Regular frequent visits by noncustodial parent Shielding from parental hostility Involvement of both parents in child's care Consistent discipline Regular school attendance
Older School Age (9–11)	Can view divorce as parents' problem but needs to find blame or reason Feels shame, rejection, resentment, loneliness	Conflicting loyalties between parents Worry about custody Hostility towards one or both parents Dependency School problems Increased behavior problems	Ongoing hostility between parents Complete rejection of one parent Parents pressure child to take sides Decrease in school performance	Involvement of both parents Parents avoid blaming each other Parental honesty Defuse child's anger
Adolescence (12–18)	Concern about loss of family life Concern about own future Feels responsible for family members Anger, hostility	Immature behavior Early or late development of independence Overcloseness or competition with same sex parent Worry about own role as sexual or marital partner	Persistent academic failure Depression and suicide threats Delinquency or promiscuity Substance abuse	Maintain parent role with child Limit involvement in parent worries Child needs peer support Maintain consistent discipline Be aware of emotional ups and downs of adolescence—may be aggravated by stress of divorce

*Adapted from Rhyne, M. C.: Nurs. Practitioner, *11*(12):37–46, 1986; Rae-Grant, Q., and Robson, B. E.: Can. J. Psychiatr., *33(6)*:443–452, 1988; Ansett, R., and Lewis, B.: Postgrad. Med., *80*(2):137–140, 1986; Hetherington, E. M., and Camara, K.: In Parke, R. D. (Ed.): Review of Child Development Research. Vol. 7. The Family. Chicago, University of Chicago Press, 1984; and Wallerstein, J. S., and Kelly, J.: Surviving the Break-up: How Children and Parents Cope with Divorce. New York, Basic Books, 1980.

Wallerstein et al. (1988) reported that 10 years after their parents' divorce, children who were school-aged or adolescents at the time of the divorce still had vivid memories of the problems of their parents' divorce, were less likely to attend college, and reported significant concerns about having successful relationships and marriages. In contrast, children who were preschool aged at the time of their parents' divorce had few memories of the intact family and divorce process and reported few concerns about repeating their parents' mistakes in their own lives.

CHANGES IN FAMILY FUNCTIONING AFTER A DIVORCE

It takes about 2 years for the postdivorce family to stabilize and readjust to the disruption caused by divorce. This is a time of great change, upheaval, and opportunity for the family. The first year after the divorce is characterized as a crisis period in which the family undergoes major changes and restructuring. Parenting practices change, and children respond differently to their parents as the family struggles to find a new equilibrium. Parenting methods that worked prior to the divorce may not be effective after the divorce. Children, especially boys, are less compliant to their parent's discipline and parenting. Parents are less effective in their discipline, particularly custodial mothers with their sons. Parents are less effective for many reasons including changes in their parenting practices, guilt over the divorce, less structure and routine for the family, trouble coping with their own feelings over the divorce, and role overload. Between the first and second year after divorce, the family usually settles down and becomes stabilized in new patterns and roles. Parenting often improves and children respond more to their custodial parent's discipline. A number of potential problem areas remain for the binuclear family throughout this process.

Loss and Grief. All family members must deal with feelings of grief and loss in response to the divorce. Depression and sadness are common reactions and are most salient during the early adjustment period. Adults and older children may feel bad about feeling bad, which escalates and perpetuates the depression. Some family members may deal with the grief through denial and avoidance of the issues. One form of this denial in parent-child relationships is for each party to deny his or her own needs for the sake of the other person. This can build an unhealthy dependency that interferes with the resolution and adjustment of the family members. Others may deny their depression by becoming intensely involved in other relationships. Children may become attached to outside authority or parental figures, such as teachers or extended family members. Adults may become involved in one or a series of relationships but remain intensely involved with their former spouse, usually through anger and hostility.

Acknowledgment and open discussion by a family physician can short-circuit this vicious cycle and help the healing process. For example, empathically informing a patient that it is common to feel depressed after a divorce and that it is important to work through these feelings. Telling the patient, "I am not surprised that you are feeling blue or down in the dumps, and I am surprised that you are doing as well as you are given all of your stress," can help them work through this process and resolve the loss and grief by normalizing and validating their feelings.

Role Overload. Custodial parents, usually mothers, may feel particularly overloaded by all of the physical, emotional, and economic demands at a time when they are emotionally drained by the divorce process. The custodial mother is usually responsible for day-to-day demands of maintaining a household (earning a living, preparing meals, caring for the children) and is the sole focus for the children's emotional reactions. Parenting and disciplining the children must be carried out, often without the help and support of the noncustodial parent. In response to this stress, it is not uncommon for parents to ignore issues that need attention and for children to be in charge of areas that may be considered adult responsibilities in two-parent households.

Isolation. Social isolation can result from and contribute to problems in postdivorce adjustment. Many women reconnect with their parents for help after a divorce and may actually move in with them on a temporary basis. However, most adults and children experience a disruption in their peer and social relationships because of a move, lack of time, or lack of energy. This tends to put more pressure on family members to meet the social and emotional needs of each other, which may foster unhealthy dependencies. Helping family members reconnect with extended family members or joining social support groups can facilitate adjustment and decrease isolation (Hetherington and Camara, 1984).

Economic Hardships. Decreased economic resources for custodial mothers and children is a major short- and long-term stressor that is often overlooked. Many women and families fall below the poverty line following a divorce. In addition, children experience a dual loss if their mother begins outside employment immediately after a divorce (Hetherington et al., 1982). Poverty is usually not good for anyone and the lowered socioeconomic status of divorced families has been found to explain many, but not all, of the negative effects of living in a single-parent household.

Interparental Conflict. The relationships between biologic parents can strongly influence the adjustment of children after the divorce. Hostility and conflict between parents *that involves the child* make it much more difficult for the child to adjust. Children who are exposed to high levels of interparental conflict have significantly more behavior problems (Kelly, 1988). Boys are usually exposed to more interparental conflict than girls. Conflict also interferes with the parents working together and coparenting their children. Families with high levels of conflict may not be good candidates for custodial arrangements that require significant amounts of cooperative decision-making or access to each other (Johnston et al., 1988). It is clearly in children's best interests for their parents to be cooperative and work together for a better postdivorce adjustment. A family physician can facilitate this through educational guidance and a proactive stance for the children with the parents.

Relationship With the Noncustodial Parent. The relationships between parents and children usually change after the divorce. Most studies have found that there is no correlation between predivorce relationships between parent and child and postdivorce relationships between parent and child. Fathers who have been actively involved in their children's lives prior to the divorce may suddenly disappear and have little to do with their children. Likewise, fathers who had little contact with their children prior to the divorce may suddenly become very involved with the children after the separation.

Several studies indicate that continued contact and relationships between noncustodial parents and their children are related to better postdivorce adjustment for children (Guidubaldi et al., 1983; Hetherington et al., 1982; Wallerstein and Kelly, 1980).

The ongoing relationship with the noncustodial father is even more important for boys than girls. As noted above, the exception to this finding is when the parents have highly conflictual relationships that involve the children (Johnston et al., 1988). In these cases, less contact may actually be better for the children.

ROLE OF THE FAMILY PHYSICIAN

The concerned physician can offer a great deal to the divorcing family in the form of support and concern. To do this, the physician must not only have a general understanding of the situation but must also understand its particular significance to the individual. As noted before, people can have dramatically different *experiences* of a divorce process. Patients may not volunteer the information that they are contemplating or are involved in a divorce. They may wish to avoid embarrassment, protect their privacy, or assume that such information is irrelevant to their care. Inquiry by the physician opens the door and makes it clear that such changes are important to the ongoing care of the patient. Open-ended inquiries—"How have things been since our last appointment?" or "How are things going at home?"—are good ways to elicit information about such psychosocial changes. Once divorce has been identified, it should be noted in the chart either in the problem list or in the family genogram. If a patient presents who is already a single parent, it is important to ascertain if the patient is a single parent by choice and whether this came about by divorce, death, or other means. It is also important to know if the patient sees the transition to single parenthood as a positive or negative one. Questions, such as, "People have many reactions to a divorce; what has it been like for you and your children?" provide a way to elicit information without making biased assumptions about individual experiences.

Helping Adults. Adults may seek medical evaluation at the time of separation and want medication for their anxiety, depression, or sleep difficulties. Physicians can assist patients going through this process by considering the role of stress and grief in their problems and by making patients aware of their vulnerability during this time. Educating them about the effects of stress and negative life events can normalize their experiences and help them cope with some of the physical and emotional effects of divorce.

Anstett and Lewis (1986) found that single parents unanimously agreed that physicians gave advice *without* first learning about single parenthood and frequently *ignored* the problem altogether. The majority of single parents in their practice preferred that the physician just listen empathically rather than give advice concerning the problems of single parenthood. Most advice was seen as superficial and not really responsive to the particular needs of the individual. A more effective approach is to be an empathic listener and to reassure patients that their feelings are a normal part of a grief process and that this process is temporary and *will change* over time.

Helping Children. Children may be brought to the family physician for behavior and academic problems and stress-related somatic complaints. Parents may or may not recognize the possibility that divorce-related stress is involved. The family physician has the opportunity here to act as the child's advocate. As with other family members, it is important to determine the child's unique perception of events. How the child has been informed about the divorce and what it means is critical. Wallerstein and Kelly (1980) noted that less than 10 per cent of children had any adult talk to them about the divorce. Parents may even present unrealistic stories about why one parent has left the household. Physicians should ask parents how the divorce has been presented to the children. This will also give information about how the parents are handling it themselves.

Ideally, both parents should tell the child about the divorce and where the departing parent will be living in terms the children can understand. It should be emphasized that the parents are divorcing each other, not the children. All children should be reassured that they were not the cause of the divorce. Books about divorce are helpful for both older and younger children. Reassurances about continuity of the parent-child relationship and blamelessness of the children should be reiterated throughout the divorce process.

The physician needs to be alert to signs that a child is at risk for emotional and developmental damage. Suspicion should be aroused by depression, anxiety, vague somatic complaints, fatigue and boredom, a drop in school performance, irritability, and withdrawal from parents, friends, and usual social activities. More severe problems, such as running away, promiscuity, and alcohol and drug abuse, may also indicate problems adjusting to divorce that need professional intervention.

The physician can assist in prevention and management of problems by suggesting ways for parents to deal with their children during and after the divorce. Consistent parenting, maintaining discipline, and allowing children to express feelings should be encouraged. It should be acknowledged that effective parenting and emotionally supporting children may be difficult when the parent feels emotionally overwhelmed and drained since role overload is a major stress. Supportive encouragement should always include praise for the parent's concern and efforts. Patterns of behavior that suggest blurring of generational boundaries or inappropriate dependency between parent and child should be identified and discouraged. Both parents should be urged to stay involved with monitoring the children's well-being and planning for the future. The physician should discourage actions that force a child to take sides between parents or require the child to be a message bearer between parents.

The physician can assist the child directly during office visits. The child should be allowed to express his or her feelings and perceptions about the divorce. The physician can assist this process by asking how the child feels about his or her parent's divorce, and how life has been affected by it. If misperceptions and fears are revealed, the physician can act as the child's advocate and help the parents interpret the divorce more appropriately to the child (Musty, 1983).

If the child becomes seriously ill during the divorce, the physician should encourage both parents to provide support to the child. Divorced parents of hospitalized children have been shown to need more reassurance from the hospital staff because they often feel that they or the divorce contributed to the child's illness or accident (Ahrons and Arrn, 1981). Divorced couples may carry their interpersonal hostility into the hospital to the detriment of the child's interests. The physician may have to take responsibility for coordinating communication between the parents and encourage them to acknowledge their feelings so that they do not subvert efforts to care for the child.

Children can also develop physical and emotional problems as a way to keep their parents together. If the custodial parent calls the noncustodial parent because she cannot handle the child's problems, this reinforces the child to be sick or a problem. This indicates a lack of emotional divorce for the family. The family physician has a unique opportunity and authority to promote change in these situations through direct intervention. The following case exemplifies this.

A few years ago a six year old girl began visiting the pediatrician's office biweekly because of a variety of minor complaints that began soon after her parents' divorce. Everyone involved knew this was a highly stressful time for the family. During one visit the physician lifted her up on the examination table so she would be at eye level with him. He told her quietly and confidently that he had decided that, although her illnesses had been useful so far, she did not need to be sick anymore and indeed probably would not need to come back for another office visit for a long time. There was a remarkable improvement thereafter.

(Williamson and Bray, 1985, p. 105)

Remarried Families

THE DEVELOPING STEPFAMILY

Stepfamilies are quite diverse in their structure and membership. A stepfamily is formed when an adult with children from a previous relationship remarries. The adult with children may have been divorced, widowed, or never married. The new spouse or stepparent may or may not have been previously married and may or may not have children. The term *step* comes from an Anglo-Saxon term *steop* that means to make orphan or bereave. Prior to the turn of the century, most children entered a stepfamily due to the death of a parent (usually their mother), whereas most children now enter a stepfamily due to the breakup of their parents' marriage. Thus, stepfamilies are "born out of loss" (Visher and Visher, 1988) because of the death of a parent or parental marriage, and they are also "instantly formed families" because of the presence of children from the beginning of the marriage.

Since women retain custody of children in 85 to 90 per cent of divorce cases, the most common type of stepfamily is the stepfather family. Various terms have been used to describe these families, including stepfamily, remarried family, REM family, reconstituted family, or blended family. Despite the large increase in these types of families, the term "step" is still viewed as a pejorative term and is commonly used to denote something that is less than desired (Ganong and Coleman, 1984). In addition, common myths, fairy tales (such as Cinderella or Hansel and Gretel), and cartoons reinforce these negative perceptions, particularly for children. This issue is important to remember since many children have conscious and unconscious fears about joining a stepfamily because of these social myths and stories.

INTEGRATION TASKS

Stepfamilies also grow through a process with predictable and unpredictable changes and stresses. Three major tasks are required for stepfamilies during the first years of remarriage: (1) integrating the stepparent into the new family and negotiating parenting for the children, (2) developing a good marital bond and relationship, and (3) integrating the noncustodial parent and his or her kinship system into the stepfamily. Parenting stepchildren is a major task and stress for new stepfamilies. It is usually best if the stepparent plays a secondary parental role and supports the biologic parent in disciplining the children, rather than trying to move in and take over the parental and disciplinary functions early in the remarriage. It may take from 2 to 4 years for the stepparent to be accepted as a parental figure by the children in a stepfamily. This is likely to occur faster with younger children than with older children and adolescents. Boys seem to accept a stepfather faster and more easily than girls. Girls often have more conflict with their stepparent and have more negative relationships with their stepfathers.

Marital Relations. Forming a strong marital bond in an instantly formed stepfamily with children is no easy task. Because of the multiple demands and loyalty pulls between biologic parents and children and the stepparent, the new marriage can easily be neglected. However, the new marriage serves as a foundation for the new family, and it is critical to nurture this relationship (Visher and Visher, 1988). Early during remarriage, marital relations have little direct impact on children's adjustment. However, a good marital adjustment helps the parents work together on the other tasks of parenting children and integrating other family members into the stepfamily system. The Grant family is a good example of this process. Each parent had children from a previous marriage. They were too busy dealing with the kids to take a honeymoon and had not been out alone together since before their wedding 8 months previously. They were planning a 2-week vacation with all of the kids. It was suggested that they take one of those weeks for a honeymoon and invite the children for the second week. This allowed the couple to work out some issues and re-establish their marital bonds. They were also instructed to have a "date" with just the two of them at least every other week to solidify their marital relationship. Rapid improvement followed this intervention.

Noncustodial Parent. Integrating the noncustodial parent and his or her kinship system varies widely depending on their role prior to the remarriage. If the noncustodial parent was active in the children's lives prior to the remarriage, then he will need to be integrated into the current marriage. Noncustodial fathers are likely to decrease their involvement with their children after the remarriage. If the noncustodial parent had little or no contact with the children before the remarriage, then there is less integration required. However, it is quite common for the noncustodial parent to suddenly show up and want to visit with the children after a remarriage. This may be out of competition with the stepparent or because of legal action by the custodial parent to enforce child support payments. Old anger and resentments from the divorce often resurface at this point and need to be resolved in order to have a successful integration of both families (Visher and Visher, 1988).

It is important to understand that stepfamilies are much more complex, have more change, and are fundamentally different than nondivorced intact families. Accepting this continuing change, much of which is unpredictable, is one of the most difficult developmental tasks for stepfamilies. For example, it is common for remarried couples to have their weekend plans disrupted because the noncustodial parent does not pick up the children for a visitation. This constant change is a reminder that a stepfamily is not an intact nuclear family and trying to mold a stepfamily into one is like trying to force a square peg into a round hole; it just does not fit.

EFFECTS ON ADULTS AND CHILDREN

Early during the remarriage, there is considerable stress for parents and female children. The stresses are both positive and negative. The remarriage starts a series of changes for family members. For example, positive stresses often include moving to a new and better home, having more income, and having two adults to help with the children and household. However, moves are often negatively stressful—they require developing new friends and new schools and losing old friends and familiar surroundings for children. There is often conflict over parenting and deciding on household routines. The stress appears to decrease after 2 years as the family integrates and develops their own routines (Bray et al., 1988).

Children in stepfamilies have more behavior problems and adjustment difficulties than children in nuclear families. These problems vary with the age of the child. It appears that both boys and girls below the age of 9 have increased behavioral problems, and these problems decrease after about 2 years of remarriage (Bray, 1988; Bray et al., 1988). Children between 9 and 13 in stepfamilies also have more behavioral problems than children in nondivorced families, but girls have the most difficult time adjusting, and their problems persist for longer periods after remarriage (Hetherington, 1987; Hetherington et al., 1985). The problems are somewhat different after a remarriage than after a divorce. Children tend to act out, having more behavioral problems and conflicts with parents after a remarriage.

ROLE OF THE FAMILY PHYSICIAN

Family physicians can provide help to stepfamilies by anticipating problems and providing preventive guidance and counseling. A genogram is a good way for the physician to understand the new family relationships, and it will contribute to a thorough history (see chapter 71). The physician should inquire about behavioral changes and symptoms for each family member, including their temporal relationship to family transitions. Because remarriage entails more change for the family, including further alteration of social and life-style patterns, previous adjustment problems may re-emerge or intensify after the remarriage. Family members, especially children, may experience new grief because the new marriage underscores the permanence of the divorce (Visher and Visher, 1988).

As in the case of divorce, the physician can provide support and guidance to ease the impact of these stressors. An important aspect of this guidance is to debunk some of the myths about stepfamily formation that cause families to feel distress. These include the belief that formation of a stepfamily will bring an immediate increase in stability. Families may also believe that affection, respect, and love will occur instantly between new members, resulting in guilt, anger, and confusion when this does not occur (Visher and Visher, 1988; Wood and Poole, 1983).

The family physician can also recommend activities that will ease the transition into the new family and encourage the formation of appropriate bonds between its members. Validating and normalizing feelings of conflict will help families accept that they may feel grief, sadness, and anxiety in addition to positive feelings like hope, joy, and excitement at the new opportunities. Helping parents negotiate parenting and household responsibilities and helping the family develop their own rituals and rules can greatly facilitate adjustment within the stepfamily. The physician should encourage open communication about these feelings with patients during office visits and between family members.

New emotional bonds can be supported by having the family identify common interests and shared goals or values. New and old sources of social support should be fostered by adults and children. Younger children may need help from their parents to achieve this. The physician can also provide important assistance by attention to the often overlooked marriage bond. The new marriage is the basis of the new family, and its importance can become overshadowed by the stresses of family formation. Couples should be encouraged to take time for themselves without the children in order to renew their commitment to each other.

In the case of severe or long-standing adjustment problems, the family physician may choose to refer the family to a professional counselor. Wood and Poole (1983) recommend that physicians refer if there are multiple problems in the family, if there has been marital separation or family violence, if a child has repeatedly run away, or if any family members feel that the situation is hopeless. It is important to refer to a counselor who has specific experience with the problems encountered by stepfamilies.

Legal and Ethical Issues for the Family Physician

The complexity of the changes surrounding divorce and remarriage can present legal and ethical dilemmas for the family physician. During the litigation of a divorce, it is not uncommon for the family physician to be called upon as a witness in the trial. The physician may be called as a fact witness—someone who provides information to the court to verify parental involvement with children or information about medical treatment. The physician may also be called as an expert witness to render a professional opinion concerning topics such as parenting practices, proper medical care of the children, or physical and sexual abuse. Adults and their lawyers will attempt to force the physician to take sides and favor one parent over another, which may endanger the ongoing professional relationship with other family members. If a physician has no experience in courtroom testimony, it is highly recommended that he or she consult with a professional to help prepare for this work. The physician may also be called to testify in cases after a divorce as a witness concerning postdivorce problems, such as visitation issues or alleged abuse or neglect.

Sexual Abuse Allegations. Allegations of sexual abuse and neglect are frequently made during heated custody disputes both during and after the divorce. Allegations of sexual abuse during conflict over custody or visitation are substantiated less frequently than those without coexisting parental conflict; however, more than half are substantiated (Paradise et al., 1988). Fictitious accusations are uncommon, in general, but their exact frequency is unknown. Failure to substantiate does not necessarily mean that abuse did not occur or that falsehood was involved. Allegations involving younger children may be more difficult to substantiate because it is harder to elicit a sexual history from them.

A physician is often consulted to verify the abuse or neglect and may be unknowingly pulled into the conflict. To avoid these difficult situations it is recommended that the physician (1) ask about the reason for performing an evaluation of the child, (2) make sure the parent has the legal right to consent to evaluation and treatment of the child, and if the physician does not have the special training to diagnose abuse and neglect, (3) request that the case be referred to another physician or to the local child protective services agency for further assessment. If the parent states that they brought the child at the recommendation of their attorney, it is highly probable that the physician will be part of a lawsuit to substantiate any positive findings.

Child Snatching. Child snatching has been called "the ultimate in alienated action by divorcing parents" (Kappelman, 1985). It can have serious consequences for the well-being of the child involved. Even after resolution of the kidnapping incident, a high proportion of adverse effects, such as symptoms of post-traumatic stress syndrome and severe anxiety, may be common. Kappelman (1985) recommends communication with the parent's lawyer and clear advice to the parent at any suggestion of child snatching. Should kidnapping occur, the physician and lawyer should unite and advocate the immediate return of the child prior to negotiation of custody issues. After the return of the child, the physician should be alert to signs that the child may need treatment for emotional problems.

It is important to be familiar with the particular laws in a given state and jurisdiction as family law varies widely throughout the United States and the law continually changes. For example, in Texas, the custodial parent usually has the right to consent to medical treatment for their minor children. The noncustodial parent can usually consent to medical treatment for their children only under emergency situations. Physicians may need to document the emergency in order to protect themselves from a lawsuit from the custodial parent. Asking a parent if they have the right to consent to treatment or requesting a copy of the divorce decree are ways to verify this information. Physicians should also remember that, unless a legal adoption has taken place, a stepparent has no legal relationship to a child. This means that the stepparent does not have the legal authority to consent to medical procedures or to access the medical records of the child.

Conclusion

The process of separation, divorce, and remarriage is replete with potential pitfalls, stresses, problems, *and opportunities* to make positive changes in family members' lives. Understanding the unique experiences of each family member, providing an empathic listening ear, and acknowledging the stresses and problems they are experiencing can greatly contribute to helping family members cope with these life transitions. The family physician has an important role in this process by helping family members focus on the opportunities and options available to make a positive difference in their current lives and for their future health and well-being.

Acknowledgments

I would like to thank Alixandre Bennett for her contribution to the development and writing of this chapter. She was particularly helpful in preparation of Table 7–1 and suggestions for practice.

References

Ahrons, C. R.: The binuclear family: Two households, one family. Alternative Lifestyles, *2:*499–515, 1979.

Ahrons, C. R., and Arrn, S.: When children from divorced families are hospitalized: Issues for staff. Health Soc. Work, *6:*21–28, 1981. *Discusses common issues that may arise when a child from a divorced home is hospitalized.*

Anstett, R., and Lewis, B.: The single parent family: How an understanding physician can help. Postgrad. Med., *80*(2):137–140, 1986. *Gives some good advice and suggestions for physicians to help single-parent patients and their families.*

Bloom, B. L., and Hodges, W. F.: The predicament of the newly separated. Community Ment. Health J., *17:*277–293, 1981.

Bloom, B. L., Asher, S. J., and White, S. W.: Marital disruption as a stressor: A review and analysis. Psychol. Bull., *85:*867–894, 1978. *Excellent overview on marital separation. It may be a little dated now.*

Bohannan, P.: The six stations of divorce. In Lasswell, M. E., and Lasswell, T. E. (Eds.): Love, marriage and family: A developmental approach. Glenview, IL, Scott, Foresman and Co., 1973.

Bray, J. H.: Children's development during early remarriage. In Hetherington, E. M., and Arasteh, J. (Eds.): The impact of divorce, single-parenting and step-parenting on children. Hillsdale, NJ, LEA Publishers, 1988. *The articles by Bray and colleagues provide recent research on children in stepfamilies. They discuss family relationships and parenting practices about stepfamilies and intact families.*

Bray, J. H., and Anderson, H.: Strategic interventions with single-parent families. Psychother., 21:101–109, 1984.

Bray, J. H., Berger, S. H., Silverblatt, A. H., et al.: The developing stepfamily. Symposium papers presented at the American Psychological Association annual convention, Atlanta, Georgia, August, 1988.

Bray, J. H., Berger, S. H., Silverblatt, A., and Hollier, A.: Family process and organization during early remarriage: A preliminary analysis. In Vincent, J. P. (Ed.): Advances in family intervention, assessment and theory. Vol. 4. Greenwich, CT, JAI press, Inc., 1987.

Furstenberg, F. F. and Spanier, G. B.: Recycling the family: Remarriage after divorce. Beverly Hills, Sage Publications, 1984. *The book summarizes a longitudinal research project on divorce and remarriage.*

Ganong, L. H., and Coleman, M.: The effects of remarriage on children: A review of the empirical literature. Fam. Relations, *33:*389–406, 1984. *A good review of research on children in stepfamilies. The review is a little dated, since many new studies have been conducted and are in progress.*

Glick, P. C.: Prospective changes in marriage, divorce, and living arrangements. J. Fam. Issues *5:*7–26, 1984.

Guidubaldi, J., Cleminshaw, H. K., Perry, J. D., and McLoughlin, C. S.: The impact of parental divorce on children: Report of the nationwide NASP study. School Psychology Review *12:*300–323, 1983.

Hetherington, E. M.: Family relations six years after divorce. In Pasley, K., and Thinger-Tollman, M. (Eds.): Remarriage and stepparenting today: Research and theory. New York, Guilford Press, 1987. *Hetherington's and colleagues' research is some of the best on divorce and remarriage. She focuses on the longitudinal effects on children in divorced and remarried families. There are many practical implications of her work.*

Hetherington, E. M., and Arasteh, J. (Eds.): The impact of divorce, single-parenting and stepparenting on children. Hillsdale, NJ, LEA Publishers, 1988. *A new book that presents recent and state of the art research in this area.*

Hetherington, E. M., and Camara, K.: Families in transition: The processes of dissolution and reconstitution. In Parke, R. D. (Ed.): Review of Child Development Research. Vol. 7. The Family. Chicago, University of Chicago Press, 1984.

Hetherington, E. M., Cox, M., and Cox, R.: The aftermath of divorce. In Stevens, J. H., and Mathews, M. (Eds.): Mother-child, father-child relations. Washington, DC, NAEYC, 1978.

Hetherington, E. M., Cox, M., and Cox, R.: Effects of divorce on parents and children. In Lamb, M. E. (Ed.): Nontraditional families: Parenting and child development. Hillsdale, NJ, LEA, Publications, 1982.

Hetherington, E. M., Cox, M., and Cox, R.: Long-term effects of divorce and remarriage on the adjustment of children. J. Am. Acad. Child Psychiatry, *24:*518–530, 1985.

Kaslow, F. W.: Divorce and divorce therapy. In Gurman, A. S., and Kniskern, D. P. (Eds.): Handbook of family therapy. New York, Brunner/Mazel, 1981. *A good chapter on divorce and how to intervene. Author provides several models of the divorce process and practical implications.*

Kappelman, M. M.: Children of divorce: The pediatrician and the lawyer. Dev. Beh. Pediatr., *6*(2):104–106, 1985.

Kelly, J. B.: Longer-term adjustment in children of divorce. J. Fam. Psychology, *2:*119–140, 1988. *Excellent, up-to-date review of research. Kelly also reviews important factors that affect successful adjustment after divorce.*

Kiecolt-Glaser, J. K., Fisher, L. D., Ogrocki, P., et al.: Marital quality, marital disruption, and immune function. Psychosom. Med., *49*(1):13–34, 1987.

Kiecolt-Glaser, J. K., Fisher, L. D., Ogrocki, P., et al.: Marital discord and immunity in males. Psychosom. Med., *50*(3):213–229, 1988.

Maccoby, E., Depner, C., and Mnookin, M.: Longitudinal study of custodial arrangements following divorce. Presentation at the annual convention of the American Psychological Association, Atlanta, Georgia, August, 1988.

Musty, T. A.: Divorce in medical practice: Helping patients through the process. Ariz. Med., *6:*392–397, 1983.

Norton, A. J., and Moorman, J. E.: Marriage and divorce patterns of U.S. women. J. Marriage Fam., *49:*3–14, 1987.

Paradise, J. E., Rostain, A. L., and Nathanson, M.: Substantiation of sexual abuse charges when parents dispute custody or visitation. Pediatrics, *81*(6):836–839, 1988.

Rae-Grant, Q., and Robson, B. E.: Moderating the morbidity of divorce. Can. J. Psychiatr., *33*(6):443–452, 1988.

Rhyne, M. C.: Understanding and supporting families in the process of divorce. Nurs. Practitioner, *11*(12):37–46, 1986.

Somers, A. R.: Marital status, health, and the use of health services. J.A.M.A., *241:*1818–1822, 1979.

U.S. Bureau of the Census: Current population reports, divorce, child custody and child support (Series P-23, No. 84). Washington, DC, US Government Printing Office, 1979.

Visher, E. B., and Visher, J. S.: Old Loyalties, New Ties: Therapeutic Strategies with Stepfamilies. New York, Brunner/Mazel, 1988. *An excellent new book. Has a good review of the literature and good clinical material. Useful for professionals and patients.*

Wallerstein, J.S.: Children of divorce: Preliminary report of a ten-year follow-up of older children and adolescents. J. Am. Acad. Child Psychiatry, *24:*545–553, 1985.

Wallerstein, J. S., Corbin, S. B., and Lewis, J. M.: Children of divorce: A 10-year study. In Hetherington, E. M., and Arasteh, J. D. (Eds.): Impact of divorce, single parenting and stepparenting on children. Hillsdale, NJ, Lawrence Erlbaum Associates, 1988.

Wallerstein, J. S., and Kelly, J.: Surviving the Break-up: How Children and Parents Cope with Divorce. New York, Basic Books, 1980. *This book provides a summary of the longitudinal research conducted by the authors. Well written and practical. Because there was no intact family control group, some of their results need to be interpreted cautiously.*

Williamson, D. S., and Bray, J. H.: The intergenerational point of view. In Henao, S., and Grose, N. P. (Eds.): Principles of Family Systems in Family Medicine. New York, Brunner/Mazel, 1985.

Wood, L. E., and Poole, S. R.: Stepfamilies in family practice. J. Fam. Pract. *16*(4):739–744, 1983. *Good brief overview of stepfamilies and how physicians can help them in practice.*

8

Child Abuse and Sexual Assault

Child Abuse

Susan Schooley

The problem of child abuse has received dramatically increased attention, both medically and socially, in the last three decades. Changes in understanding, attitude, and response from year to year are difficult for practicing physicians to assimilate. Despite the dynamic nature of what is known about this problem, it is evident that child abuse exists in epidemic proportions. It is a major cause of morbidity and mortality in childhood and has devastating consequences for its victims, and even the generations that follow, throughout their lives. The prevalence of child abuse and the magnitude of its ill effects oblige family physicians to become adept at its recognition, treatment, and prevention.

Inadequate recognition and underreporting of child abuse are well-documented problems ascribed to medical professionals, family physicians among them (Chang et al., 1986). Reasons for this phenomenon include inexperience at eliciting or identifying clinical presentations, discomfort and denial on the part of the professional, mistaken assumptions about who may be at risk, discomfort at reporting incompletely substantiated suspicions, and lack of confidence in the child protective system. Family physicians may face some unique disincentives in that long-term relationships with families may mitigate their ability to recognize abuse or to function clearly as a child advocate when they also feel bound by an implicit contract to care for the abuser. In all states, physicians are mandated by law to report situations in which they *suspect* child abuse to the proper authorities. The physician may fear a disruption in his or her relationship with the family as a consequence of reporting, but families can often be convinced of the physician's professional and legal obligation and the nonadversarial nature of the subsequent investigation. The physician can offer continued support to the entire family through this difficult time while maintaining a primary posture of child advocacy. The horrible nature of child victimization, the grief and anger of families, and unfamiliarity with the forensic aspects of child abuse, such as testifying in court, make this particularly difficult clinical work. The consequences of failing to recognize or treat abuse, however, must persuade physicians to overcome these barriers through continuing education, frank discussions with other colleagues, and personal commitment.

Physical Abuse

Epidemiology of Physical Abuse. Estimates of the prevalence of nonaccidental injury to children are problematic. Data sets from which such estimates are derived contain significant inaccuracies. Problems with the definition of abuse, nongeneralizable cross-sectional studies, and reporting bias challenge attempts to define who is at risk (Jason, 1984). Reported cases may represent only a fraction of the total incidence of actual abuse, and the volume of reports increases annually. Regional variations are difficult to interpret and may reflect reporting bias rather than different demographic patterns. Earlier associations of child abuse with urban environments, single-mother and young-mother families, poverty, and race have not held up under methodological scrutiny. It would be prudent for family physicians to assume that all ages of victims and all families are potentially at risk, and that offenders can be family members, other acquaintances, or strangers.

Reports of child homicide show the United States to be second only to Northern Ireland in this extreme form of abuse. Nonaccidental injury is responsible for 3 per cent of all deaths in children aged 1 to 4 years and most often results from violence in the family (Christoffel, 1983). Infants are at particular risk for severe injury by virtue of their physical vulnerability (Jason, 1983).

The particular vulnerability of infants would imply that physicians who could identify risk factors prenatally or in the postpartum period might have access to preventive opportunities. Although demographic risk factors may not be helpful, personal and social factors identifiable during routine care may be predictive of risk. Abusive caretakers are more likely to exhibit poor self-esteem, a perception of parental deprivation or actual abuse in their own childhoods, and unrealistic expectations about early child development, for example, ascribing aggressive motives to crying infants. Physicians may witness evidence of poor impulse control, unmet dependency needs, or substance abuse that may put a parent at greater risk. Characteristics of child victims may also be risk factors: low birth weight and premature infants, those with congenital problems or chronic illness, and twins are at greater risk.

Family and social factors that the physician can use to predict risk include isolation, stress, and even cultural attitudes toward violence (Howze and Kotch, 1984). Identification of such risk factors during routine care offers the possibility of increased surveillance for abuse. Self-esteem, stress reduction, problem-solving skills, and social support can be enhanced by means of the relationship with the family physician and appropriate community referrals.

Identification of Physical Abuse. Lines between socially acceptable forms of child discipline and child abuse have changed over time but continue to be indistinct. Discrimination of nonaccidental trauma from normal childhood accidents also confounds the problem of diagnosis. When the history offered as to how an injury occurred is incompatible with the injury or when the stories of different witnesses are variable, suspicion should be aroused. Likewise, an injured child accompanied by a hostile, defensive, or unusually anxious parent may be suspect. The victim may also show evidence of abnormal behavior, such as overt fear of adults or caretakers or extreme passivity or inappropriate physical affection with strangers.

Physicians can enhance their ability to make the diagnosis by taking careful nonjudgmental histories of the injury from the parents or other pertinent adults and the child in separate interviews. Avoidance, delay, or discontinuity of medical attention or a previous history of other "accidents" can be important data.

The Physical Examination in Child Abuse (Table 8–1). Head trauma is common in child abuse, ranging from superficial injuries of the mouth and face from striking blows to severe intracerebral injury from blows or shaking. Infants are particularly vulnerable to severe head trauma and may not show obvious external signs. Their lack of independent mobility makes all such trauma suspect. Computed tomography of the head may be an appropriate screening tool

Table 8–1. PHYSICAL MANIFESTATIONS OF PHYSICAL CHILD ABUSE

Skin Findings
- ***Bruises and Welts***
  - Face, lips, mouth
  - Back, buttocks, thighs, torso
  - Clusters or regular patterns
  - Different stages of healing
- ***Burns***
  - Soles, palms, back, buttocks
  - Stocking and glove distribution
  - Donut-shaped areas
  - Unusual areas
  - Rope burns
- ***Alopecia***
  - Hair pulling
  - Occipital (infant neglect)
- ***Lacerations***
  - Back of arms, legs, torso
  - Genitalia
  - Mouth, lips, gums, eyes
  - Human bites

Fractures
- Epiphyseal-metaphyseal fractures, especially in infants
- Diaphyseal fractures, either spiral or oblique
- Skull fractures in infants
- Rib fractures
- Multiple fractures of different ages
- Skeletal trauma in combination with other injury

Head Trauma
- Skull fracture, linear
- Subdural hemorrhage
- Epidural hemorrhage (less common)
- Retinal hemorrhage, detachment
- Hyphema, dislocated lens
- Cerebral edema
- Cerebral contusion, hematoma

Blunt Abdominal Trauma
- Duodenal hematoma (x-ray study with contrast medium shows intramural mass, "coiled spring" mucosa)
- Pancreatitis, pancreatic pseudocyst
- Hepatic injury—lacerations

if another inflicted injury is documented (Merten, 1983).

Blunt abdominal trauma may be exhibited as internal bleeding, nonspecific pain, vomiting, or obstruction. Visceral injuries are associated with a high mortality rate and must be evaluated with appropriate thoroughness (Kirks, 1983).

Genital trauma in child sexual abuse requires special techniques and is covered in a subsequent portion of this chapter.

Musculoskeletal trauma is common in childhood from falls and other accidents, but some presentations are associated with inflicted injury. Fractures of the extremities are the most common form of bone injury in abuse, followed in order of occurrence by skull, rib, and clavicular fractures. Half of skeletal injuries in abuse occur in infants less than 1 year old (Leonidas, 1983).

Dermatologic abnormalities are among the most common findings in physical abuse, and a thorough careful examination with highly specific documentation is mandatory. Burns purposefully inflicted from lighted cigarettes as a form of punishment are common and leave round, bullous, scabbed, or scarred lesions. They must be distinguished from impetigo infections and accidental burns, the lesions of which are more often single, superficial, and irregular in shape. Immersion burns take on a stocking and glove shape, with symmetry, involving palms and soles, unlike most accidental burns. Dunking of the trunk causes burns to the buttocks and genitals, sparing protected areas of skin in folds or centrally (donut-shaped) where the skin contacts the cool tub. Forcible placing of the child against hot objects can leave symmetrical patterns in unusual places, such as the buttocks or the back. Restraint or gagging can leave marks at the wrists, ankles, and corners of the mouth.

The literature reflects increased numbers of cases of Munchausen's syndrome by proxy, in which an adult caretaker, often someone in a medical or paramedical profession, surreptitiously inflicts bizarre illness on a child to arouse medical concern and attention. Chronic poisoning, recurrent suffocation, or inflicted infections are examples of causes of illness that often initially escape the differential diagnosis of an unusual presentation (Richardson, 1987).

Acute Management of Physical Abuse. The family physician has three compelling objectives in the initial response to suspected child abuse. First, the specific injuries must be assessed and treated. Second, the child must be protected from further harm. The Child Protective System in most areas offers 24-hour availability for prompt notification and initiation of services. When the immediate protection of the child cannot be ensured in the care of his or her usual guardian or another family member, the child can be remanded into temporary custody of the state and emergency foster placement can be arranged through court order by the Department of Social Services. Sometimes admission to the hospital is warranted either because of the severity of the child's condition or until appropriate investigations or alternative placement arrangements can be made. This can be accomplished even against the parents' will through the hospital administrator and the judge by court order. Having to deal with extremely hostile parents may call for the assistance of the police or hospital security staff.

The third objective in the acute management of child abuse is careful documentation of the medical record. Ultimate protection of the child from further harm often depends on the legal system to intervene in defining the abuse as criminal. This can serve to limit access to the child by the abusing adult and can often help pay for treatment for the family. The thoroughness and specificity of the physician's account of the history and physical examination may be instrumental in helping agencies to document the nature and severity of abuse and succeed in the child's behalf. Verbatim accounts; precise descriptions, drawings, or photographs of injuries; and opinions as to the cause of injuries, to the extent that such opinions can be substantiated by the evidence, can be of importance to the subsequent process. Physicians with inadequate experience in assessing child abuse can harm the interests of the child by recording impressions with false certainty. Referral in such cases would be the appropriate response.

Long-term Role of the Physician in Child Abuse. The family physician who participates in the acute diagnosis and management of child abuse can also become a part of the therapeutic process for the child victim and family through the continuity of the physician-patient relationship. A child facing the turmoil of investigative procedures, court processes, or the temporary or permanent loss of an abusing parent can be soothed by ongoing contact with a familiar caring person. The focus of helping agencies on their roles as child advocates may mean that other family members, including the abuser, are neglected and must face the crisis on their own. The physician can lend support and legitimacy to the helping process. Some families are successfully rehabilitated, and the physician can be a member of the team that nurtures and monitors that process along with social workers, home health workers, counselors, and so on.

Primary Prevention of Child Abuse. Since child abuse is frequently a transgenerational phenomenon, one of the main preventive strategies is early recognition and intervention for the sake of the next generation. Besides being alert for the signs and symptoms of abuse, physicians can adjust their routine health maintenance visits for children to include inquiries about temper problems or violence in the household, assessments about developing self-esteem, and problem-solving flexibility. Prenatal care can include assessments of parental readiness, perceptions and experiences of nurturing in the parents' own past, and anticipatory guidance about child development and the stresses of child-rearing. Well-baby care should include education about the normalcy of occasional hostile feelings toward demanding infants and toddlers and contingency planning with the parents for periods of stress in which the parents feel anxiety about controlling such impulses. The physician can be available to the family for such times of crisis and can suspect and intervene in an impending crisis when there are frequent calls due to nonspecific complaints and other unusual behaviors. The physician can mobilize social and financial support from community agencies for families that lack adequate finances as well as serve as a part of that support network. Adults who were deprived in their own childhoods can experience a nurturing relationship with a family physician as a model of good parenting behavior, demonstrating acceptance and appropriate limits.

Sexual Abuse

Sexual Abuse of Children. The sexual abuse of children represents an entity distinct from physical abuse. In the last decade, it has evolved from a hidden problem to a subject of tremendous social, legal, scientific, and media concern. Reports of sexual abuse now exceed those of physical abuse in many departments of social service. Despite this increased attention, sexual abuse remains cloaked in secrecy, denial, and taboo and much of it goes undetected and unreported. Confusion as to what constitutes sexual abuse also compounds this problem. The range of exploitative sexual acts perpetrated on children is broad, including forcible violent rape; coercive, nonviolent anogenital penetration; orogenital contact; sexualized fondling and touching; and even noncontact exploitation. The use of children for prostitution or pornography is also a concern. Child abuse offenders may be strangers but more often are intimate acquaintances and family members, compounding the betrayal and confusion experienced by their victims. The consequences of sexual victimization in childhood are often devastating, with suicide, chronic mental illness, criminal behavior, substance abuse, sexual dysfunction, and incapacity for intimacy among its long-term sequelae. Sexually transmitted diseases and unwanted pregnancies are potential short-term outcomes. Although sexual abuse is rarely associated with life-threatening harm or violence, it may result in even more damage to the victim's self-concept and the ability to reach full adult potential.

Physicians' reluctance to diagnose and report sexual abuse is well described (James et al., 1978), but the importance of sexual abuse as a cause of significant functional and emotional harm dictates the need for familiarity with this problem and the effective responses to it.

Epidemiology of Sexual Abuse. Understanding about the prevalence of child sexual abuse suffers the same problems as other forms of child abuse, but social prohibitions, secrecy, and its subtle manifestations make sexual victimization even harder to identify. Children may be victims of chronic sexual abuse for years before they come to attention, if they ever do. Studies vary in their estimates of the prevalence of sexual abuse, but some reports of retrospective random cohorts of women declare that 43 to 63 per cent of the women in the sample have experienced some form of sexual abuse before the age of 18, depending on the type of abuse and age of the respondent (Wyatt and Peters, 1986; Russell, 1983). Only a small percentage of these events were reported.

Profiles of victims demonstrate a bimodal distribution of age, with a large proportion of victims being under 6 years of age. A second peak occurs for adolescent victims (Cupoli and Sewell, 1988). Currently, there are many more female victims diagnosed than male victims, but this may represent an artifact of silent suffering and nondetection rather than actual contrast in incidence (Vander Mey, 1988). Male victims tend to have younger abusers, and those victims who present for treatment have more frequently been sodomized and exposed to threats or violence (Reinhart, 1987; Pierce and Pierce, 1985). Child victims of both sexes often know their perpetrators, who are almost always men, with the majority being either biologic fathers or stepfathers and most of the others other close relatives or acquaintances (Kendall-Tackett and Simon, 1987). The distribution of the nature of abusive acts varies widely from study to study. Estimates of anal or vaginal penetration as part of the abuse are rising, but intercourse still accounts for only a portion of sexual abuse. The harmful consequences of sexual exploitation do not correlate well with the seriousness of the abusive act, and inappropriate touching, fondling, or even verbal exchange, although harder to prove, are as much a betrayal of trust as more invasive forms of abuse.

Identifying Sexual Abuse. Some victims of sexual abuse present for evaluation after a child has made specific disclosures about abusive events to a trusted adult. More commonly, however, such presentations may be masked, with disclosures from the child victim elicited with much difficulty. Shame, fear of reprisals, threats of family disruption, and promises of secrecy to the perpetrator may all contribute to reluctance to tell on the part of the child. This behooves the family physicians and others in the lives of children to be alert to more subtle clues to the occurrence of sexual abuse (Table 8–2).

Sexual abuse shares behavioral features with other forms of psychologic stress and should be considered as part of the differential diagnosis in nonspecific abnormal presentations. Sexual abuse victims, including very young ones, are more likely than other children to demonstrate age-inappropriate, abnormal sexualized activities, with a precocious understanding or role playing of sexual acts with playmates or other adults (Gale et al., 1988). Alertness to masked presentations makes it possible for physicians to explore more carefully for the presence of abuse in such cases (Hunter et al., 1985).

Table 8–2. POSSIBLE CLUES TO THE PRESENCE OF SEXUAL ABUSE

Infants and Toddlers
Intense fear of a person or place
Abrupt change in behavior
Sleep disturbances (bedwetting, insomnia, nightmares)
Withdrawal or depression
Developmental delays

Physical signs and symptoms
- Genital, rectal, or oral trauma or irritation
- Urinary tract infection
- Foreign bodies in the vagina, urethra, or rectum
- Other bruises, burns, or injuries
- Vaginitis, unusual vaginal odor or discharge
- Complaints of genital or rectal discomfort
- Excessive masturbation

Pre-School Children
All of the signs listed earlier plus:

A direct or coded statement indicating sexual hurt
Sexual acting out with peers or adults
Precocious knowledge of sexual activities
Excessive sexual curiosity

Physical signs and symptoms
- Enuresis, encopresis
- Regressive behavior
- Hyperactivity
- Somatic complaints—headache, abdominal pain, constipation

School-Aged Children
All of the signs listed earlier plus:

Disturbed peer interactions
Change in school performance
Mistrust of adults in general
Depression, withdrawal, sadness
Aggression, rage
Sleeping disorders—nightmares, insomnia
Avoidance of physical activity and undressing

Adolescents
All of the signs listed earlier plus:

Self-destructive activity or suicidal thoughts, gestures
Eating disorders (especially binging and purging)
Delinquent behavior or running away
Drug and alcohol use
Early pregnancy
Prostitution, promiscuous behavior, or other unusual sexual behavior

Genital complaints, an abnormal genital or rectal examination, or the presence of sexually transmitted diseases can also alert the physician to the existence of sexual abuse and are discussed later.

Interviewing Victims of Possible Sexual Abuse. Children are often reluctant to tell about sexual encounters, fearing punishment, retribution, disapproval, or abandonment. These obstacles pose a challenge to history-taking in suspected cases. Young children may not have an adequate understanding of what has happened to them to be able to provide coherent details, and some victims are too young to communicate verbally at all. As if these problems were not enough, the interviewing process is also subjected to strict requirements of technique, since such disclosures to the physician are often part of crucial legal testimony for use in protection of the child, and the physician's interview must be free of coercion or leading questions.

Sexually abused children have already had the boundaries of their privacy invaded by someone in authority. In such cases, the medical evaluation must balance the needs of the child for control with the need to gather information for the child's protection. The experience can be extremely anxiety producing for the victim and must be performed with extreme care and gentleness. Sometimes, the gender of the examiner can make a significant difference to the child.

If possible, the child should be interviewed alone. The physician can create an atmosphere of acceptance and calm. The child's verbal and cognitive maturity must guide the line of questioning, and when some kind of sexual contact is suspected, one of the first steps at eliciting information is discovery and use of the child's own vocabulary for body parts. Children can be given specific reassurance that the physician will not be angry with them no matter what they tell, that they have done nothing wrong, and that the physician wants to help the child. Children who have already disclosed details of sexual abuse to others may be ready to tell again with little prompting. In situations in which abuse is suspected but not corroborated by the child, disclosure to the physician may not occur during the first visit. In that case, if the child is capable of comprehending, the physician can describe a hypothetical situation of a child with a secret problem like sexual abuse. The physician can then ask what might happen if the child were to tell and who in the child's environment might he or she be able to tell such a secret. The specificity of the response to the hypothetical situation can give a clue about the child's reluctance and can also identify someone who may be more likely to be the recipient of a disclosure from the child. That individual can then be prepared to help the child tell.

Children can be encouraged to tell if they have had any problem with an adult in which the adult has touched them or hurt them or asked them to do something they did not want to do. The use of anatomically correct dolls has facilitated such interviews with young children who may be more comfortable showing what happened using the dolls. They can then be asked several questions. Did someone do that to you? Who was that? What else did he do? Where were you when that happened? Where was your mommy? What did he tell you? Did that happen any other time? This approach avoids complex questions, using the child's own words, and not leading the child with closed questions. Specialists in child sexual abuse are experienced and painstaking in this process and can be called on as consultants.

The Physical Examination. The physician must perform a detailed physical examination, with special attention to the genital and rectal areas for evidence of sexual trauma or infection. This examination can provoke anxiety in the child and in rare extreme cases needs to be performed under sedation. To lessen the possibility of discomfort, the physician should attend to reassuring and informing the child about the examination, attend to the child's modesty, and invite a trusted companion to accompany the child. Inspection of the child's vulvar area can be accomplished in either the lithotomy or the knee-chest position, with gentle lateral traction on the adjacent buttocks. The child can participate by performing this traction herself. Evidence of trauma or discharge should be sought and detailed (Emans et al., 1987) (Table 8–3). The transverse diameter of the vaginal orifice should be measured in millimeters, since an opening of greater than 4 mm in prepubertal girls is associated with sexual abuse at least 85 per cent of the time (Cantwell, 1983, 1987). Physicians must become familiar with the varied appearance of the normal prepubertal hymen in order to identify abnormalities and should make this inspection a routine part of all well child examinations. In most girls, the hymen is a very thin, pink crescent-shaped membrane, which is symmetric and regular. Some infantile hymens are circumferential and fimbriated, and careful traction must be applied for full inspection to rule out scarring or trauma.

Table 8–3. PHYSICAL FINDINGS IN SEXUAL ABUSE OF CHILDREN

Genital Fondling or Manipulation
Erythema
Perihymenal neovascularization
Hymenal rounding, microscarring
Clitoral hood hypertrophy
Introital synechiae
Hymenal or labial trauma above 3 o'clock and 9 o'clock positions
Vulvar Coitus
As listed earlier plus:
Perihymenal abrasions
Laceration or scarring of posterior fourchette
Vaginal Penetration—Acute
As listed earlier plus:
Labial contusion, ecchymosis
Introital abrasions
Vaginal abrasions
Fourchette or hymenal transection
Pubococcygeal spasm
Chronic Genital Sexual Abuse
Vulvar hypopigmentation, hyperpigmentation
Clitoral hood cutaneous hypertrophy
Introital scarring, neovascularization, synechiae
Fourchette scarring, deformity
Enlarged hymenal diameter
Vaginitis
Anal Penetration
Perianal edema, abrasions, petechiae
Acute anal fissures
Acute anal spasm
Chronic fissures with induration
Venous dilatation
Pigmentation changes
Perianal hyperkeratosis
Scarring, anal deformity
Skin tags
Funnel anus with laxity
Reflex dilatation of anal sphincter

The anus should be inspected for dilation, laxity, and trauma (Hobbs and Wynne, 1986). The use of the colposcope can greatly facilitate the discovery of subtle abnormalities of the physical examination and should be undertaken if possible (Woodling and Heger, 1986; Teixeira, 1981).

If acute sexual contact is suspected, forensic evidentiary protocols used in management of acute sexual assault should be performed (See page 132).

Laboratory Evaluation in Sexual Abuse. Adjunctive laboratory examination can assist in documenting the existence of sexual contact as well as determine potential harmful consequences of such contact, such as pregnancy or infection. A pubertal victim should have a sensitive urine pregnancy test. Three orifices, mouth, rectum, and vagina (or urethra in males), should be cultured for *Neisseria gonorrhoeae* and *Chlamydia trachomatis*. *Chlamydia* should be assayed by specific culture rather than direct specimen antigen methods. The presence of either of these infections in children can be considered presumptive evidence of sexual abuse (Ingram et al., 1984; Hammerschlag et al., 1984; Groothius et al., 1983). The small size of nasopharyngeal swabs on aluminum wires may be more tolerable to small children for specimen collection. They should see and touch the swabs beforehand to prepare them for the test.

Collections of vaginal secretions in saline to reveal *Trichomonas* or *Gardnerella* infections should be done, if indicated. Although these infections along with condyloma acuminatum have been documented to be transmitted to children in the absence of venereal contact, they are nevertheless suggestive of abuse and merit documentation and specific treatment (White et al., 1983; De Jong, 1985; Herskowitz, 1982).

As occurs in adults, cystitis and even upper urinary tract infection may represent ascending bacteriuria secondary to vaginitis or urethral trauma. The diagnosis of urinary tract infection in female children calls for careful inspection of the genitalia for evidence of sexual abuse or vaginitis.

Syphilis has increased in prevalence in adult venereal disease and can be expected to appear with increasing frequency in child victims. Serologic tests should be obtained. Human immunodeficiency virus (HIV) transmission to children by sexual contact is feasible and needs to be considered, although testing after acute contact would only document lack of preexisting viral exposure and needs to be delayed for several months.

Rare cases have come to attention because of symptoms of primary infection with herpesvirus II. Specific culture media are available.

Psychologic Treatment of Incestuous Families and Sexual Abuse Victims. Once sexual abuse is documented and the victim is protected from further exploitation, the healing process can begin. Single assaults in the context of a supportive family environment are rarely damaging to the developing child. Chronic sexual abuse by a family member is more insidious. Victims often have ambivalent feelings about the abuse itself, since there may be aspects of the close relationship with the abuser and the physical contact itself that may be associated with positive feelings for the child. Through treatment, it is hoped that victims gain insight into their lack of culpability despite their ambivalence; integrate ambivalent feelings for the abuser, including resolution of rage; and gradually gain confidence in their ability to control interpersonal boundaries in their lives while risking the loss of trust and intimacy with others.

Offenders have varying rates of rehabilitative success, depending on the etiology and nature of their disorders. Those who are compulsive child molesters, with multiple victims and who demonstrate a persistent sexual orientation toward children, are refractory to most treatment. Others who revert to child partners under times of stress, but who have the capacity to relate to adults normally, may be treatable.

Adult Victims of Previous Child Abuse. Among the adult patients of the family physician are likely to be many persons who have been victimized in their childhood, physically, sexually, or both, who have never been identified or treated. Some of the same behavioral indicators used as clues for the identification of child victims are pertinent for adults as well. Chronic somatic complaints with an unclear etiology, depression, substance abuse, and poor self-esteem can all be clues to prompt the physician to inquire about a history of abuse. Until victims acknowledge their childhood wounds, it is unlikely that they will be able to function in fully satisfied lives. Among populations of physicians themselves are former victims, whose histories may handicap them even further in their response to this important clinical situation. Once diagnosed, treatment can begin, with supportive listening, individual psychotherapy, and group work with other survivors of incest and other abuse.

Taking Care of the Caregivers. Professionals who deal with child victims are often profoundly emotionally affected by what they encounter. The innocence of the victims and the magnitude of their betrayal and harm are shocking and disturbing. Participation in the criminal justice system as accuser is also stressful and might not be a role physicians would otherwise choose. The importance of restoring such children to the possibility of normal lives warrants paying such a price and mandates physicians' involvement, but physicians need to attend to their own emotional needs in the process. They can benefit from contact with others with similar experiences to manage the emotional weight of their work.

References

Cantwell, H. B.: Vaginal inspection as it relates to child sexual abuse in girls under thirteen. Child Abuse Negl., 7:171–176, 1983.

Cantwell, H. B.: Update of vaginal inspection as it relates to child sexual abuse in girls under thirteen. Child Abuse Negl., *11*:545–546, 1987.

Chang, A., Oglesby, A. C., Wallace, H. M., et al.: Child abuse and neglect: Physicians' knowledge, attitudes, and experiences. Am. J. Pediatr. Hematol. Oncol., *66*:1199–1201, 1986.

Christoffel, K. K., and Liu, K.: Homicide death rates in childhood in 23 developed countries: U.S. rates atypically high. Child Abuse Negl., *7*:339, 1983.

Cupoli, J. M., and Sewell, P. M.: One thousand fifty-nine children with a chief complaint of sexual abuse. Child Abuse Negl., *12*:151–162, 1988. *Report of a large series of cases from a Tampa, Fla., Emergency Room.*

De Jong, A. R.: Vaginitis due to *Gardnerella vaginalis* and to *Candida albicans* in sexual abuse. Child Abuse Negl., *9*:27–29, 1985.

Emans, S. J., Woods, E. R., Flagg, N. T., et al.: Genital findings in sexually abused, symptomatic and asymptomatic, girls. Pediatrics, *79*:778–785, 1987. *Contains clear photographs depicting abnormalities in the inspection of genitalia of female children.*

Gale, J., Thompson, R. J. Moran, T., et al.: Sexual abuse in young children: its clinical presentation and characteristic patterns. Child Abuse Negl., *12*:163–170, 1988.

Groothius, J. R.: Pharyngeal gonorrhea in young children. Pediatr. Infect. Dis. J., *3*:99–101, 1983.

Hahn, Y. S., Raimondi, A. J., McLone, D. G., et al.: Traumatic mechanisms of head injury in child abuse. Child's Brain, *10*:229–241, 1983.

Hammerschlag, M. R.: Are rectovaginal chlamydial infections a marker of sexual abuse in children? Pediatr. Infect. Dis. J., *3*:100–104, 1984.

Herskowitz, L. J.: Condyloma acuminatum in the prepubescent child: report of a case. J. AOA, *82*:429–431, 1983.

Hobbs, C. J., and Wynne, J. M.: Buggery in childhood—a common syndrome of child abuse. Lancet, *ii*:792–796, 1986. *A controversial article describing the examination findings in children with alleged anal penetration, described in accompanying photographs. Debate about the prevalence of anal sexual abuse and the specificity of physical findings has been active in the subsequent literature.*

Howze, D. C., and Kotch, J. B.: Disentangling life events, stress, and social support: Implications for the primary prevention of child abuse and neglect. Child Abuse Negl., *8*:401–409, 1984.

Hunter, R. S., Kilstrom, N., Loda, F.: Sexually abused children: Identifying masked presentations in a medical setting. Child Abuse Negl., *8*:17–25, 1985.

Ingram, D. L., Runyan, D. K., Collins, A. D., et al.: Vaginal *Chlamydia trachomatis* infection in children with sexual contact. Pediatr. Infect. Dis. J., *3*:97–99, 1984.

James, J., Womack, W. M., and Strauss, F.: Physician reporting of sexual abuse of children. J.A.M.A., *240*:1145–1146, 1978.

Jason, J.: Fatal child abuse in Georgia: The epidemiology of severe physical child abuse. Child Abuse Negl., *7*:1–9, 1983.

Jason, J.: Centers for Disease Control and the epidemiology of violence. Child Abuse Negl., *8*:279–283, 1984. *Good summary of the inherent problems in epidemiologic investigations of child abuse.*

Kendall-Tackett, K. A., and Simon, A. F.: Perpetrators and their acts: Data from 365 adults molested as children. Child Abuse Negl., *11*:237–245, 1987.

Kirks, D. R.: Radiological evaluation of visceral injuries in the battered child syndrome. Pediatr. Ann., *12*:888–893, 1983. *Useful for information about which radiologic, ultrasonographic, or nuclear studies are useful in the assessment of various injuries.*

Leonidas, J. C.: Skeletal trauma in the child abuse syndrome. Pediatr. Ann., *12*:875–881, 1983.

Lynch, M. A.: Child abuse before Kempe: An historical literature review. Child Abuse Negl., *9*:7–14, 1985. *Establishes the contextual backdrop on which modern medical understanding has developed.*

Merten, D. F., and Osborne, D. R. S.: Craniocerebral trauma in the child abuse syndrome. Pediatr. Ann., *12*:882–887, 1983.

Pierce, R., and Pierce, L. H.: The sexually abused child: A comparison of male and female victims. Child Abuse Negl., *9*:191–199, 1985.

Reinhart, M. A.: Sexually abused boys. Child Abuse Negl., *11*:229–235, 1987.
Ricci, L. R.: Medical forensic photography of the sexually abused child. Child Abuse Negl., *12*:305–310, 1988. *Basic suggestions about forensic photography with examples.*
Richardson, G. F.: Munchausen syndrome by proxy. Am. Fam. Phys., *36*:119–123, 1987.
Russell, D. E. H.: The incidence and prevalence of intrafamilial and extrafamilial sexual abuse of female children. Child Abuse Negl., *7*:133, 1983.
Teixeira, W. R. G.: Hymenal colposcopic examination in sexual offenses. Am. J. Forensic Med. Path., *2*:209–215, 1981.
Vander Mey, B. J.: The sexual victimization of male children: a review of previous research. Child Abuse Negl., *12*:61, 1988.
White, S. T., Loda, F. A., Ingram, D. L., and Pearson, A.: Sexually transmitted diseases in sexually abused children. Pediatr., *72*:16, 1983.
Woodling, B. A., and Heger, A.: The use of the colposcope in the diagnosis of sexual abuse in the pediatric age group. Child Abuse Negl., *10*:111–114, 1986.
Wyatt, G. E., and Peters, S. D.: Methodological considerations in research on the prevalence of child sexual abuse. Child Abuse Negl., *10*:241–251, 1986. *This article reviews and critiques several important prevalence studies.*

Sexual Assault: Rape

Rebecca Jackson

Definition of Rape

Rape is a violent and traumatic act against a person intended to humiliate and disempower by shame, physical injury, emotional pain, transgression of sexual boundaries, and threat of death. Sex is used in the service of anger. The trauma of rape affects not only the victim but also the family, friends, those involved in providing care to the victim, and society as a whole (Pynoos and Nader, 1988).

The spectrum of sexual assault is broad, covering both sexes and all ages. Different types of rape apply to different circumstances: child sexual abuse, date rape, marital rape, and rape in prison. The effect of each type is devastating, however. Aspects that vary include the degree of relationship between the victim and the perpetrator, the type of coercion used, and the amount of physical and psychologic injury inflicted. Just as the circumstances of the assault may vary, so may the reactions of the survivors and their paths to recovery.

Social Context

Rape occurs in all cultures and all countries and has occurred for all time (Brownmiller, 1975). Incidence and reporting rates vary widely. In the United States one in three girls and one in seven boys will be sexually abused by the time they are 18. There is an association between cultural support for violence and the incidence of rape (Baron et al., 1988).

The Victims

Victims of sexual assault may be anyone—male or female, young or old—they only need to be vulnerable or at the wrong place at the right time. Those at risk include children; females; transients; the indigent; the mentally ill, including addicts and alcoholics; the mentally retarded; and prisoners. In a study of 6159 college students at 32 institutions of higher learning in the United States, one of every four women had experienced an episode of rape or attempted rape since the age of 14 (Koss et al., 1987). College males report an incidence of 7.3 per cent of childhood sexual abuse (Risin and Koss, 1987).

The Rapists

Sexual abusers tend to be male. In the study mentioned above, Koss and associates (1987) report a prevalence among college students of 1 in 15 men raping or attempting to rape since the age of 14. Females also sexually abuse.

A higher percentage of reported rapes are of the *blitz type*, i.e., a sudden attack by a rapist unknown to the victim. In the *confidence type* of rape, the rapist is known to the victim and the perception of danger is gradual, since nonviolent interaction precedes the rape (Silverman et al., 1988). Population-based studies suggest that confidence rapes (including marital and date rape) are much more common and are underreported (Kilpatrick et al., 1988). Sexual offenders are highly likely to have been sexually abused as children (Finkelhor and Lewis, 1988) at a rate that is nearly eight times that of a population of college males (Burgess et al., 1988).

Help-Seeking Behaviors of Survivors

Of those who report sexual assault immediately, the route to the medical facility may be via a relative, a friend, a Rape Crisis Center advocate, the police, or a school counselor. Some victims find themselves whisked into the medical setting by the police or an ambulance before they are ready to cope with another authoritarian figure. Others come alone, concerned about confidentiality.

Factors associated with not reporting include (1) close social relationship with the assailant, e.g., a family member, spouse, date, or ex-spouse; (2) fear of reprisal by the assailant, e.g., "If you tell anyone I will kill you," "I will kill your children," or, in the case of incest, "It will split up the family"; (3) feelings of shame; (4) feelings of powerlessness; (5) fear of being in another situation in which one might be powerless; (6) fear of blaming; (7) invalidating the response of the first person told; (8) not knowing whom to tell; and (9) shock, denial, dissociation, and amnesia (Kilpatrick et al., 1988; Rose, 1986; Kaszniak et al., 1988). Conversely, factors associated with reporting are similar to those associated with a higher likelihood of being believed (physical injury, social distance between the rapist and the survivor, or the presence of witnesses to the crime or a supportive person encouraging the victim to seek health care).

Male victims report at a lower rate than females. In one study, those who reported showed a higher incidence of physical trauma, suggesting that it is even more difficult for males to report sexual assault than females unless they have a legitimate reason to access the health care system (Kaufman et al., 1980).

The Physician's Response

PERSONAL RESPONSES

Issues of competence and *Primum non nocere* (First do no harm) raise questions such as "Can I care for this very hurt person without hurting him or her further?" Rape provokes an emotional response in which the physician may feel fear for personal safety and safety of loved ones, anger at the rapist for the hurt caused to the victim, and feelings of powerlessness. Dread of experiencing such feelings again may precede seeing a subsequent patient. Knowledge of the correct procedures for providing medical care and legal documentation and evidence collection will help in bolstering the physician's self-confidence. However, attending to one's own emotional needs is paramount in order not to act out one's feelings to the detriment of the patient. Physicians must have an opportunity to work through the trauma of caring for victims of sexual assault or they may burn out or revictimize the patient. In training programs in which a high volume of rape victims are seen by a relatively small number of providers, weekly or biweekly meetings for presenting cases, both to review procedures and share the emotional impact, are essential. Support from and good working relationships with rape victim advocates can be extremely helpful in sharing the burden of care and the trauma of the experience.

MEDICAL CARE OF THE RAPE SURVIVOR

Victims of sexual assault need help re-establishing a sense of safety, recovering self-esteem, revalidating the emotional self, regaining power and control, healing the physical body, and addressing the fear of sexually transmitted diseases and unwanted pregnancy.

Emergency departments are not the ideal place for rape victims to feel safe. They should be escorted to a private and quiet place, accompanied by a supportive relative until a victim advocate is available. Initial needs may include contacting a spouse or parent, or making sure that the children are safe. The rape victim may have spent an extended period of time in the custody of someone who has threatened to kill her or him. Regaining a sense of safety in human interactions is dependent on the successful communication of needs and emotions as well as minimizing further trauma during the vulnerable healing stages.

Caretakers often ask "What can I do?," "How can I help?" In these circumstances, the answer is listen, and to listen nonjudgmentally but critically. Rapists act irresponsibly, without regard for the victim. In the face of someone who refuses to accept responsibility for his or her actions, the victim, searching for an element of control, may begin to blame herself. Assignment of blame, while a common defense mechanism, may interfere with feeling the emotion of anger and prolong the grieving process. Anger in itself is a frightening feeling, particularly in the context of rape in which the rapist acts without acknowledgment of his own anger. The physician must be careful not to reinforce this inappropriate assignment of "behavioral self-blame."

It is important to be aware that family members or friends, in an effort to protect themselves, may listen eagerly for aspects of the story that prove that it could not happen to them. Parents who are grieving over their loss of ability to protect their teenagers may blame the victim, saying "How could you let this happen to you?" Family members may tell the victim not to think about it, thereby acting through denial. All of these aspects of grieving may be out of synchrony with the survivor's own healing process and may even be harmful.

The physician should be careful to offer knowledge, skill, and medicine in such a way that the patient can make healthful choices. Regaining choice and control is more important than whether or not evidence is collected exactly right. Who would choose to have a pelvic or rectal examination after being raped unless it were offered in the context of a clear benefit?

People who have been raped may be in the survival level of their recovery phase and may be totally unable to consider prosecution or to encounter in any way the rapist who has threatened to kill them. Therefore, they may not wish to allow evidence to be collected. Inform the survivor that although evidence is fragile and must be collected early to be of future use, the decision of whether or not to prosecute may be made at some time in the future when the victim is able to consider the possibility. Although serial rapists continue to rape until they are made to deal with their responsibility, usually only through incarceration or court-ordered treatment, do not put undue pressure on the victim. Good working relationships between rape crisis advocates, police, physicians, and district attorneys result in better care of survivors as well as more convictions.

Outline of Medical Care

OBTAINING THE HISTORY

Although it is difficult for the victim to recount exactly what happened, the process of telling the story to a nonjudgmental listener can be healing in itself. Details of the type of assault are important for both medical care and for legal documentation. *Where* the crime was initiated is necessary for jurisdiction assignment. *When* the assault occurred may be useful in interpreting evidence such as lack of sperm motility.

The experience of rape is often confusing. In confidence rapes, the victim may be in the assailant's custody for an extended period of time, and the rapist's behavior may change and include long apologies. The use of open-ended questions and the patient's own words are best for catharsis and for documentation for later use in court. Statements made for purposes of medical diagnosis or treatment are generally admissible in court as an exception to the hearsay rule (Federal Rules of Evidence, 1989). This also diminishes the need for the use of the word "alleged" throughout the history. If the patient cannot describe the rape or has difficulty talking about the issue, directed questions may be necessary, e.g., "Sometimes the rapist puts his penis in his victim's rectum, did this happen to you?," or "Sometimes the rapist does unusual things or things that don't make sense. Did anything like that happen to you?" The process of retelling, although painful, begins to allow the victim to make sense out of it. Be aware that victims in a state of shock may tell or withhold parts of the story that are most painful, thus distorting the sequence as it is finally revealed months later in the court. Allow the patient time to process feelings.

MEDICAL HISTORY

Inquire about any previous sexual assault or sexual abuse—sometimes a previous unreported event must be dealt with before the immediate event can be addressed. Obtain information about any other medical conditions, allergies, and gynecologic history, including the last intercourse to which the victim consented, contraceptive methods used, and contraindications to postcoital contraceptives. The victim's past sexual behavior is generally not admissible in court (Federal Rules of Evidence, 1989).

PHYSICAL EXAMINATION

Ask permission to examine the patient, recognizing that the victim's refusal to be examined may be an important part of re-establishing control over his or her body. Choosing to be examined may represent a healthful choice and may also enhance self-esteem. Treat the whole person not just an invaded orifice. Value the person as a whole. Recognize that touch can be healing. Begin with familiar, less-threatening parts of the examination such as taking pulses or examining the head. Look for injuries anywhere on the body for documentation as well as treatment. Explain the components of the genital examination, especially since it may differ from a routine exam, e.g., pubic hair combings, large numbers of swabs taken from the vagina, vaginal washings, and Wood's light examination for semen. If this is the patient's first genital examination, allow more time. Have appropriate assistance and chaperonage during the exam without having too many people in the room so as not to interfere with the patient's comfort.

LABORATORY AND EVIDENCE COLLECTION

Specimens that should be collected for evaluation are listed in Table 8–4. These include a Papanicolaou smear for cancer screening as well as evidence of sperm; a wet mount for evaluation for motile sperm; cultures for gonorrhea and *Chlamydia* from the cervix, urethra, rectum, and mouth (fluorescent antibody may be used for the cervix and urethra only); serologic tests for pre-existing syphilis and HIV; and a urine pregnancy test.

Know the requirements of the evidence kit being used, since many states and the Armed Services have their own. Kit components are listed in Table 8–5. Specimens should be preserved appropriately by drying or refrigeration. Be sure to maintain the chain of custody of the evidence to maintain its validity for

Table 8–4. HOSPITAL LAB SPECIMENS

Sensitive urine pregnancy test
Cultures for gonorrhea
Chlamydia slide for fluorescent antibody/viral cultures
Serology test for pre-existing syphilis
Baseline HIV serology test
Wet mount for sperm
Papanicolaou's smear

Table 8–5. COMPONENTS OF EVIDENCE KIT

Floor and table sheet for shed debris
Clothing, especially underpants
Fingernail scrapings
Debris, blood or semen on skin (use Wood's light)
Pubic hair combings
Slides for sperm, air dried
Swabs (air dried) and washings for semen, acid phosphatase and other prostatic fluid enzymes from mouth (gum line), vagina, and rectum as appropriate.
Controls
Plucked pubic and head hairs (15 to 20 each)
Saliva for blood type secretor status
Blood sample for blood type

the court. This means that evidence is never left unattended and can be accounted for from the time of collection to the time of evaluation in the forensic laboratory. It is appropriate to collect evidence up to 5 days after the assault; although some materials will not be intact, others will still be interpretable. Rectal swabs for sperm must be collected through an anoscope. The gumline plaque of the patient should be swabbed for evidence of ejaculation in the mouth. The forensic laboratory will analyze seminal fluid for subtypes of enzymes, including phosphoglyceromutase, esterase D, and peptidase A. Highly accurate but expensive DNA probes are available at three private laboratories and may become more available in the future.

PREGNANCY PREVENTION

The incidence of pregnancy after rape is approximately 5 per cent and is lower than that predicted for random intercourse, probably because of the sexual dysfunction of some rapists (Groth and Burgess, 1977). Fear of pregnancy as well as fear of not being able to become pregnant in the future may be a significant concern of the rape survivor. Postcoital contraceptives may be offered with the understanding that they are not ideal. Postcoital contraceptives cause nausea and are contraindicated in the presence of pre-existing pregnancy because of teratogenicity. They are thought to work by making the uterine lining inhospitable to implantation and must be started within 72 hours after the rape. As such, they must be considered to be abortifacients and may be unacceptable on religious or ethical grounds. One widely used but not FDA approved regimen includes Ovral, a combined estrogen and progesterone. The dose is four tablets given either as one tablet every 3 hours, or two tablets initially and then again 6 or 12 hours later.

Inquire about menstrual cycles, risk of pre-existing pregnancy, contraceptive methods currently in use, and the victim's desire for a postrape contraceptive. As a physician, it is helpful to be aware of one's own values and the choice one might make oneself. However, it is important for the patient to make her own choice.

SEXUALLY TRANSMITTED DISEASES

There are about 20 different kinds of sexually transmitted diseases. Some of these are not preventable once exposure has occurred and treatments are only palliative, e.g., herpes, hepatitis B, and HIV. Others may not become apparent until a follow-up examination, e.g., *Trichomonas vaginalis* infection and condyloma acuminatum. The incidence of sexually transmitted diseases after rape has been reported to be 5 to 30 per cent (Forster et al., 1986). At the present time, the Centers for Disease Control recommendations suggest prophylactic antibiotic regimens that treat gonorrhea, infection with *Chlamydia*, and incubating syphilis. A follow-up examination and serologic tests are also recommended.

Regimens for STD prevention are: ceftriaxone (Rocephin), 250 mg. intramuscularly; plus doxycycline (Vibramycin), 100 mg. orally twice a day for 7 days; or amoxicillin 3 gm., by mouth all at once; and probenecid, 1 gm.; plus tetracycline, 500 mg., by mouth four times a day for 7 days.

Legal Issues in the Rape Examination

The rules of the legal arena are different from those of the medical arena. The prospect of going to court at some time in the future may increase the reluctance of physicians to be involved in providing care for assaulted persons. Alternatively, this may be viewed as an opportunity to testify and to learn the process of the law. As a caretaker, it is difficult to change one's attitude and become a dispassionate technician and statistician. Meeting with the district attorney ahead of time is extremely important to clarify one's role.

One important role change is typified by the phrase "alleged sexual assault." Nowhere else in medicine do we modify our assessment in such a way—we do not prescribe treatments for alleged headaches or alleged back pain. Nor are we accustomed to write alleged gunshot wound or "alleged physical assault." In the case of sexual assault, we struggle to differentiate our diagnostic decision from a legal decision to be determined in the future by a jury. The issue at court is usually one of either identity or consent. If consent is the issue, the physician's testimony may be used to establish evidence of harm. If the identity of the suspect is the issue, providing the link in the chain of evidence will be important.

Clear, concise, detailed, preferably dictated notes of the initial and follow-up encounters are helpful because the trial occurs long after short-term memory has lapsed. Schematic drawings, such as those used for burned patients, or sketches to illustrate injuries are also useful. A complete evidence collection or clear explanation of any deletions is important. Medical records may be admissible as evidence and may be subpoenaed (Federal Rules of Evidence, 1989).

States that use uniform evidence collection kits have improved physician compliance in evidence collection and have increased the validity of evidence in court. New Mexico, for example, has developed its own kit that comes with instructions for the physician, which are updated as new techniques are developed.

Cross-Gender Issues

Some victims, particularly those who have not seen their assailant(s) because of blindfolds or darkness, have great difficulty encountering a physician who is the same sex as their assailant. As often as possible, a physician of the same sex as the victim should be sought. For other victims, a competent and caring interaction with a physician of the opposite sex may be a healing step. A useful first step is for the physician to ask the patient what he or she needs rather than to imply that the physician knows what is best.

Post-Trauma Syndromes

Since only a small percentage (one in three to one in thirty) of victims report sexual abuse, a large proportion of survivors have not revealed the event to anyone and may present to the physician with the sequelae of sexual abuse and sexual assault (Table 8–6). Dissociation and amnesia as well as minimization and denial may interfere with the patient's response to direct questioning. Perceptions of how the interviewer will respond as well as personal values also keep the patient from revealing previous traumatic histories. Nevertheless, resolution of the trauma itself may be necessary for recovery from post-trauma symptoms.

Table 8–6. SEQUELAE OF RAPE

Depression, eating disorders
Guilt
Feelings of inferiority and low self-esteem
Interpersonal problems
Delinquency
Substance abuse
High incidence of suicide and suicide attempts
Fear, anxiety, and chronic tension
Prostitution, rape, sexual dysfunction, pelvic pain syndromes
Repetition or revictimization
Anger
Ego constriction

Providing good care for the victim of sexual abuse at the time of the assault with referral for counseling is the ideal treatment. Patients who present at a later time do not have fewer symptoms merely through the passage of time (Frank et al., 1988). Types of therapy that have been helpful include cathartic grief work, desensitization, cognitive therapy, and psychodynamic psychotherapy.

References

Baron, L., Straus, M. A., and Jaffee, D.: Legitimate violence, violent attitudes, and rape: A test of the cultural spillover theory. Ann. N.Y. Acad. Sci., *528*:79–110, 1988. *This is a thought-provoking article that focuses on societal issues.*

Briere, J.: The long-term clinical correlates of childhood sexual victimization. Ann. N.Y. Acad. Sci., *528*:327–334, 1988.

Brownmiller, S.: Against Our Will: Men, Women and Rape. New York, Simon and Schuster, 1975. *A classic in the literature of rape.*

Burgess, A. W., Hazelwood, R. R., Rokous, F. E., et al.: Serial rapists and their victims: Reenactment and repetition. Ann. N.Y. Acad. Sci., *528*:277–295, 1988.

Burt, M. R., and Katz, B. L.: Coping strategies and recovery from rape. Ann. N.Y. Acad. Sci., *528*:345–358, 1988.

Conte, J. R.: The effects of sexual abuse on children: Results of a research project. Ann. N.Y. Acad. Sci., *528*:310–326, 1988.

D'Epiro, P.: Examining the rape victim. Patient Care, April 30, 1986.

Federal Rules of Evidence for United States Courts and Magistrates. Pub. L. 93–595, § 1, January 2, 1975, 88 stat, 1926. As amended to February 1, 1989 Rule 803(4), 803(3), 803(6), 803(7), Rule 412.

Finkelhor, D., and Lewis, I. A.: An epidemiologic approach to the study of child molestation. Ann. N.Y. Acad. Sci., *528*:64–78, 1988.

Forster, G. E., Pritchard, J., Munday, P. E., and Goldmeier, D.: Incidence of sexually transmitted diseases in rape victims during 1984. Genitourin. Med., *62*:4, 1986.

Frank, E., Anderson, B., Stewart, B. D., et al.: Immediate and delayed treatment of rape victims. Ann. N.Y. Acad. Sci., *528*:296–300, 1988.

Goodwin, J.: Trauma and post-trauma symptoms. Personal communication, 1985.

Groth, A. N., and Burgess, A. W.: Sexual dysfunction during rape. N. Engl. J. Med., *297*(14):764–766, 1977.

Heinrich, L. B.: Care of the female rape victim. Nurse Practitioner, November *12*(11):9, 10, 12, 16–18, 23, 26–27, 1987.

Jacobson, A., and Richardson, B.: Assault experiences of 100 psychiatric inpatients: evidence of the need for routine inquiry. Am. J. Psychiatry, *144*:7, 1987.

Kaszniak, A. W., Nussbaum, P. D., Berren, M. R., and Santiago, J.: Amnesia as a consequence of male rape: A case report. J. Abnorm. Psychol., *97*:1, 1988. *An interesting case study of an important defense.*

Kaufman, A., DiVasto, P. V., and Jackson, R.: Male rape victims: Non-institutionalized assault. Am. J. Psychiatry, *137*: 1980.

Keen-Payne, R.: Serving as an expert witness in rape cases. Nurse Practitioner, *13*:7, 1988. *This article is of value to anyone serving as an expert witness in a rape trial.*

Kilpatrick, D. G., Best, C. L., Saunders, B. E., and Veronen, L. J.: Rape in marriage and in dating relationships: How bad is it for mental health? Ann. N.Y. Acad. Sci., *528*:335–344, 1988. *A thoughtful and well written article.*

Koss, M. P., Gidycz, C. A., and Wisniewski, N.: The scope of rape incidence and prevalence of sexual aggression and victimization in a national sample of higher education students. J. Consult. Clin. Psychol., *55*:2, 1987. *A very large population study that is hard to deny.*

Meyer, C. B., and Taylor, S. E.: Adjustment to rape. J. Pers. Soc. Psychol., *50*:6, 1986.

Pynoos, R. S., and Nader, K.: Children who witness the sexual assaults of their mothers. J. Am. Acad. Child. Adolesc. Psychiatry, *27*:5, 1988. *A poignant and thought provoking study.*

Risin, L. I., and Koss, M. P.: Sexual abuse of boys: Prevalence and descriptive characteristics of childhood victimization. J. Interpers. Violence *2*:3, 1987. *Also a classic study in the field.*

Rose, D. S.: "Worse than death:" Psychodynamics of rape victims and the need for psychotherapy. Am. J. Psychiatry, *143*:7, 1986. *This is a valuable paper.*

Shearer, S. L., and Herbert, C. A.: Long-term effects of unresolved sexual trauma. Am. Fam. Phys., *36*:4, 1987.

Siegel, J. M., Sorenson, S. B., Golding, J. M., et al.: Resistance to sexual assault: Who resists and what happens? Am. J. Pediatr. Hematol. Oncol., *79*:1, 1989.

Silverman, D. C., Kalick, S. M., Bowie, S. I., and Edbril, S. D.: Blitz rape and confidence rape: A typology applied to 1,000 consecutive cases. Am. J. Psychiatry, *145*:11, 1988. *A large study from the Beth Israel Hospital, Boston.*

Vinogradov, S., Dishotsky, N. I., Doty, A. K., and Tinklenburg, J. R.: Patterns of behavior in adolescent rape. Am. J. Orthopsychiatry, *58*:2, 1988.

Weinstein, J. B., and Berger, M. A.: Weinstein's Evidence, Commentary on Rules of Evidence for the United States Courts and State Courts. Matthew Bender and Company, Inc., Albany, N.Y., 1988.

9

Spouse and Elder Abuse

Sandra K. Burge
David V. Espino

Spouse Abuse

Spouse abuse is a term that refers to intentional physical abuse by one's spouse or significant other that causes pain or injury (Pagelow, 1981). This gender-neutral term, however, implies a mutuality of violence that is unsubstantiated. Men inflict far more injuries than they receive (Straus et al., 1980); 91 to 95 per cent of all violent crimes between spouses are victimizations of wives by husbands (Browne, 1987). Therefore, the remainder of this discussion uses the terms battered women or wife abuse to more accurately represent the nature of this phenomenon.

PREVALENCE AND INCIDENCE

Straus and Gelles (1986) published a national probability survey that indicated a husband-to-wife violence rate of 11.3 per cent per year. The violent behavior included slapping, pushing, and throwing objects as well as more severe behavior such as punching, kicking, and using weapons. Three per cent of the wives in this study had been subjected to severe violence; this translates into 1.6 million severely abused wives per year. Assuming substantial underreporting by subjects, the investigators estimated that the actual incidence of wife abuse could be two times higher.

ETIOLOGY

Women who are chronically battered do not choose to be so. Most men do not hit women during courtship; instead, violence begins after both partners have developed a deep emotional investment in each other. The first violent incident comes as a complete surprise to the victim and is not recognized as a precursor to a violent pattern. However, the nature of aggression is such that it escalates over time. Thus, early injuries may be minor and the woman's commitment to her husband may outweigh the harm done to her. Later, as the violence increases in severity, the emotional investment may decrease but fear of further violence if she leaves, in combination with little help from social institutions, will keep a woman trapped in an abusive marriage (Browne, 1987).

Why does violent behavior occur? Violence has been attributed to the psychopathology of the abuser, examined as a behavior learned from one's family of origin, and explained as a phenomenon that serves a function in our society (Gelles and Straus, 1979). Certainly, several influences have an impact on the problem of wife abuse.

Gelles (1983) proposed a multifactorial theory that suggested that people use violence when the costs of being violent do not outweigh the rewards. He stated that men abuse their wives "because they can" (p. 157). For men, the rewards of wife abuse include stopping an emotional argument, providing an outlet for frustration, and getting one's wishes granted (Browne, 1987). In contrast, the costs of being violent are low. Wives are unable to retaliate, either physically or economically, and interference on the part of public agencies (e.g., legal authorities) is severely limited by our society's belief that what goes on inside a family is private business. Paradoxically, the most serious cost to an abuser of being violent, the loss of his spouse through divorce, is usually controlled with threats of further violence.

ABUSER AND VICTIM

Research has uncovered no "typical" battered woman (Browne, 1987; Walker, 1983). Expecting to find a "victim-prone" personality among battered women, Walker (1983) instead discovered that abused wives perceived themselves to be stronger, more independent, less traditional, and more sensitive than other women. Other researchers (Browne, 1987; Rosewater, 1988) have also discovered many strengths that allow a woman to function, nurture others, and survive in a violent environment.

Rather than using women's characteristics to predict their odds of being victimized by husbands, professionals are directed to look for specific qualities in the men (Pagelow, 1981; Browne, 1987). Batterers have certain identifiable characteristics: low self-esteem, traditional sex-role attitudes, other-directed blame, pathologic jealousy, Jekyll and Hyde personality, coping reactions to severe stress that involve wife assault and drinking, use of sex as an act of aggression, and unwillingness to take responsibility for violent behavior.

AFTERMATH OF VIOLENCE

The injuries of battered women look different from the injuries of accident victims. Battered women are more likely to have facial injuries and are 13 times more likely to have injuries on the chest, breasts, and abdomen (Stark et al., 1979). Additionally, they are more likely to present with multiple injuries than accident victims. Evidence of old and new injuries in the same location are common. Because of the repetitive, escalating pattern of violence that perpetrators tend to display, battered women's visits to physicians are repeated with increasingly severe injuries (Health Care Systems Committee of Tulsa, Oklahoma, 1984).

In addition to acute injuries, abused women have a higher prevalence of chronic health problems (Haber and Roos, 1985) and often turn to their family physicians for relief from vague but unremitting symptoms. Common complaints include somatic symptoms such as insomnia, fatigue, disturbing physical sensations, chronic pain, and anemia (Haber and Roos, 1985; Kerouac et al., 1986).

Battered women's psychologic reactions to violence are like other victims' reactions to catastrophe or threat (Browne, 1987). During the act of violence, the individual's focus is primarily on self-protection and survival. Reactions of shock, denial, disbelief, withdrawal, confusion, and fear are common. Long-term reactions include fear, confusion, and anger (Rosewater, 1988). Some victims remain withdrawn and passive and exhibit symptoms of depression and listlessness. Chronic fatigue and tension, intense startle reactions, sleeping and eating disturbances, and nightmares may be noted (Browne, 1987). Psychologic reactions can be severe and are sometimes misdiagnosed as schizophrenia or borderline personality. Rosewater (1988) advocates the avoidance of psychiatric labels and directs professionals to explore and treat the *source* of the problem (the battering) instead of the *symptoms*.

FAMILY PRACTICE INTERVENTIONS

The impact of continuing violence on a woman's health demands a response from physicians that addresses more than the treatment of acute injuries. Family physicians who offer continuing health care that focuses on the whole person are in an ideal position to assist battered women. Effective intervention requires an accepting, collaborative attitude in addition to the following actions:

The most important service a physician can perform for battered women is to *ask about the violence*: "Is anyone at home hitting you?" (Finkelhor and Yllo, 1985). Initiating the discussion communicates to the patient that: (1) this problem is not too shameful, deviant, insignificant, or irrelevant to talk about; (2) the patient's discomfort with and reactions to her husband's violence are understandable and rational; and (3) the situation is changeable, not hopeless. Furthermore, the information gathered helps the physician to find the appropriate diagnosis and to direct treatment.

The second step involves assessing the patient's current level of safety and collaboratively developing a concrete plan of safety that will allow her and her children to escape or avoid future violence. Discussion should address options relating to when to leave; where to stay; how to arrange transportation; how long to stay; getting legal protection; and so on. Many women have resources that allow some respite and protection (such as a relative who will temporarily shelter them), but others will need public assistance, such as that provided by battered women's shelters.

Third, a physician must guide battered women to appropriate referrals. In a study of women who "beat" wife-beating (Bowker, 1983), subjects recommended contacting social service agencies, women's self-help groups, and women's shelters; such agencies guide women to basic resources (food, shelter, jobs, legal assistance) and offer emotional support to the wives and interventions to violent husbands.

Finally, follow-up is necessary. Options discussed in the physician's office (such as legal intervention or psychotherapy for the husband) require contemplation, planning, and time on the part of the patient. One discussion generally does not cure violence in a family, but continuing communication, support, and exploration of options will empower women to make changes that eliminate violence from their lives.

Elder Abuse

Current awareness of the potential for violence within families, combined with the increasing numbers of frail elderly in our population (and the demands for care-giving that their presence signifies), has led researchers and clinicians to a recent focus on elder abuse and neglect.

Elder abuse lacks uniform classifications. The broadest area of agreement recognizes that elder abuse is characterized by fiscal, material, psychologic, and physical abuse and/or neglect (Trilling et al., 1987). Fiscal abuse entails misuse of the victim's financial resources, as in fraud and embezzlement. Material abuse involves the violation of the victim's material possessions, involving, for example, theft or misuse of property. Psychologic abuse includes environmental deprivation, verbal abuse, or a denial of rights. Physical abuse may include assault, rape, burns, starvation, or bondage. While our society's most common image of abuse results from such intentional physical violence, several scholars have noted that the most common form of elder abuse is neglect (Taler and Ansello, 1985). Neglect is characterized by inattention or isolation of the elderly individual; for those who are dependent upon others to provide daily necessities, this passive form of abuse can be very serious.

PREVALENCE

The difficulties with the definition and the reporting of elder abuse have led to a paucity of accurate data. Current estimates of the numbers of elderly who are maltreated vary from 0.5 to 2.5 million persons (Salond et al., 1984).

ETIOLOGY

The causes of elder abuse in the family, like other forms of violence, are multifactorial and, undoubtedly, interrelated. Risk factors that have been proposed include: (1) the development of a dependent relationship and consequent vulnerability on the part of the elder person; (2) lack of close family ties; (3) a history of family violence; (4) lack of financial resources; (5) psychopathology of the abuser and care-giver; and (6) a lack of community support (Hickey and Douglass, 1981; Kimsey et al., 1981).

VICTIM AND ABUSER

The typical abused elder is in poor health and is living with another person or persons (Wolf et al., 1984; Steinmetz and Amsden, 1983). Most have been subjected to a combination of the abuses described previously (Sengstock and Barnett, 1986). Approximately equal numbers of males and females in the population are abused; however, Pillemer and Finkelhor (1988) report that abused women suffer more physical and psychologic consequences from violence than victims who are men.

Most often, the abuser of the elder is a relative of the victim and has taken care of that person for a number of years. In many cases, the burden of care-giving overwhelms individuals to such an extent that they feel they are in an inextricable situation. Feeling trapped further increases the burden of care-giving, predisposing the individual to violent reactions.

A predominant image, reinforced by the media, is that abuse is committed by ungrateful children toward their unreasonable aging parents (Sengstock and Hwalek, 1987). This image has recently been challenged, however, with findings indicating that the more common perpetrator of elder abuse is the spouse (Wolf et al., 1984; Pillemer and Finkelhor, 1988). This suggests that elder abuse is often a form of wife abuse, indicating that clinical approaches to wife abuse are appropriate for many elderly victims.

AFTERMATH OF VIOLENCE

The abused elder may exhibit various indicators that, although not pathognomonic, should alert the family physician to the possibility of abuse or neglect. Common behavioral indicators of abuse, such as generalized fear, may be misinterpreted as paranoia related to dementia or a latent psychosis (Council on Scientific Affairs, 1987). Physical indicators of elder abuse are similar to those of wife abuse, with bruises, lacerations, multiple fractures to ribs or long bones, and rope burns being part of the initial presentation.

FAMILY PRACTICE INTERVENTIONS

The successful identification of abused elders and the development of effective prevention plans has been difficult to achieve. Unfavorable societal attitudes toward older persons, in combination with a culture-wide denial of the existence of abuse, means that many professionals will fail to identify elder abuse when it is present. The lack of uniform definitions of elder abuse further hinders efforts to identify it. Finally, inconsistent federal, state, and local approaches toward reporting elder abuse and enforcing legal protection of the abused have slowed preventive efforts.

To identify elder abuse, a high index of suspicion is recommended for the following findings: older persons with physical findings inconsistent with the medical history; care-givers with an absence of assisting behaviors; observation of angry, hostile, or abusive behavior on the part of the care-giver; observation of a care-giver obsessed with control, showing excessive concern, or harping on the burdens of care-giving (Taler and Ansello, 1985). Because research in this area is still rudimentary and inconclusive, physicians are directed to assume that the likelihood for abuse is equal for males and females, for dependent and independent individuals, and for those who live alone as well as for those who live with others. Whenever the diagnosis is in doubt, impartial third party cooperation is necessary.

Family physicians are in an ideal position to take the lead in developing a management plan for abused elders; however, it is important to utilize a multidisciplinary approach. Physicians should be familiar with the local services available to the aged (Salond et al., 1984). Social workers, mental health professionals, and other area agency professionals (such as representatives from legal aid, Meals-on-Wheels, or local adult protection agencies) can help ensure adequate continuity of care and the proper utilization of community resources.

References

Bowker, L. H.: Beating Wife-Beating. Lexington, MA, Lexington Books, 1983.

Browne, A.: When Battered Women Kill. New York, Free Press, 1987. *This book describes a study of 42 women charged with the death or serious injury of their husbands. Browne finds that these homicidal women are not very different from a control group of 205 self-identified battered women. Rather than presenting a collection of special cases of family violence, the author explores the progression from affection to violence that typifies battering relationships and describes relevant phenomena such as violence in childhood, the nature of aggression, fear and hopelessness, and survival and escape. This is compelling reading.*

Council on Scientific Affairs: Elder abuse and neglect. J.A.M.A., *257*:966–971, 1987. *This comprehensive article represents the latest findings on elder abuse and neglect.*

Finkelhor, D., and Yllo, K.: License to Rape: Sexual Abuse of Wives. New York, Free Press, 1985.

Gelles, R. J., and Straus, M. A.: Determinants of violence in the family: Toward a theoretical integration. *In* Burr, W. R., Hill, R., Nye, I., et al.: Contemporary Theories about the Family. Vol. I. New York, Free Press, 1979.

Gelles, R. J.: An exchange/social control theory. *In* Finkelhor, D., Gelles, R.J., Hotaling, G.T., et al. (Eds.): The Dark Side of Families: Current Family Violence Research. Beverly Hills, CA, Sage, 1983.

Haber, J. D., and Roos, C.: Effects of spouse abuse and/or sexual abuse in the development and maintenance of chronic pain in women. Adv. Pain Res. Therapy, *9*:889–895, 1985. *In a study of 151 women with chronic pain, the authors found that 53 per cent had been physically or sexually abused prior to the onset of pain. Further, abused women had significantly more medical problems than nonabused women. The authors suggested that abused subjects relied on somatization as a coping style, which explained why these women utilized the medical system more than those who were not abused.*

Health Care Systems Committee of Tulsa, Oklahoma: Adult Abuse and Neglect: Handbook for Medical Personnel. Health Care Systems Committee of Tulsa, Oklahoma, 1984.

Hickey, T., and Douglass, R. L.: Mistreatment of the elderly in the domestic setting: An exploratory study. Am. J. Public Health, *71*:500–507, 1981.

Kerouac, S., Taggart, M. E., Lescop, J., and Fortin, M. F.: Dimensions of health in violent families. Health Care Women Int., *7*:413–426, 1986.

Kimsey, L. R., Tarbon, A. R., and Bragg, D. F.: Abuse of the elder—the hidden agenda. I. The caretakers and the categories of abuse. J. Am. Geriatr. Soc., *29*:465–472, 1981. *This article reviews the care-giver role in the development of elder abuse.*

Pagelow, M. D.: Woman-battering: Victims and Their Experiences. Beverly Hills, CA, Sage, 1981.

Pillemer, K., and Finkelhor, D.: The prevalence of elder abuse: A random sample survey. Gerontologist, *28*:51–57, 1988. *This study represents the first large-scale effort to document the prevalence of elder abuse and neglect. From interviews conducted with 2020 elderly people, a prevalence rate of 32 per 1000 was determined. Spouses were found to be the most likely abusers, and roughly equal numbers of men and women were victims, although women suffered more serious abuse.*

Rosewater, L. B.: Battered or schizophrenic? Psychological tests can't tell. *In* Yllo, K., and Bograd, M. (Eds.): Feminist Perspectives on Wife Abuse. Newbury Park, CA, Sage, 1988. *This study sought to find if there was a "battered woman's MMPI profile." MMPI tests were administered to 118 battered women, and the results revealed a profile typically displayed by paranoid schizophrenics. Rosewater cautions against misdiagnosis and directs professionals to treat the source of the problem—the violence—not merely the symptoms.*

Salond, E., Kane, R. A., Satz, M., and Pynoos, J.: Elder abuse reporting; Limitations of statutes. Gerontologist, *24*(1):61–67, 1984.

Sengstock, M. C., and Barnett, S.: Elderly victims of family abuse, neglect, and maltreatment: Can legal assistance help? J. Gerontol. Social Work, *9*:43–61, 1986.

Sengstock, M. C., and Hwalek, M.: A review and analysis of measures for the identification of elder abuse. J. Gerontol. Social Work, *10*:21–36, 1987.

Stark, E., Flitcraft, A., and Frazier, W.: Medicine and patriarchal violence: The social construction of a "private" event. Int. J. Health Serv., *9*:461–493, 1979. *This study of 481 women using emergency services in a large metropolitan hospital discusses how ignoring evidence of wife-battering can perpetuate the violence.*

Steinmetz, S., and Amsden, D. J.: Dependent elders, family stress, and abuse. *In* Brubaker, T. H. (Ed.): Family Relationships in Later Life. Beverly Hills, CA, Sage Publications, 1983.

Straus, M. A., and Gelles, R. J.: Societal change and change in family violence from 1975 to 1985 as revealed by two national surveys. J. Marriage Family, *48*:465–479, 1986. *This article reports the results from two classic studies of family violence, investigating the incidence of parent-to-child, husband-to-wife, and wife-to-husband violence. Results indicate that, over the 10 years between 1975 and 1985, child abuse decreased by 47 per cent and wife abuse by 27 per cent.*

Straus, M. A., Gelles, R. J., and Steinmetz, S. K.: Behind Closed Doors: Violence in the American Family. Garden City, NY, Anchor Press, 1980.

Taler, G., and Ansello, E. F.: Elder abuse. Am. Fam. Phys., *32*(2):107–114, 1985. *This review of the literature on elder abuse includes information about prevalence and incidence, characteristics of victims and abusers, diagnosis and intervention strategies as well as legislative action.*

Trilling, J. S., Greenblatt, L., and Shepard, C.: Elder abuse and utilization of support services for elderly patients. J. Fam. Pract., *24*(6):581–587, 1987. *This article is valuable for its review of types of community resources that should be accessed in suspected elder abuse cases.*

Walker, L. E.: The battered woman syndrome study. *In* Finkelhor, D., Gelles, R.J., Hotaling, G.T., et al. (Eds.): The Dark Side of Families: Current Family Violence Research. Beverly Hills, CA, Sage, 1983. *In another classic study, Walker interviewed 403 self-identified battered women in order to study the natural history of wife abuse. Data confirmed the existence of a cyclical pattern of violent behavior, moving from tension-building to battering to loving contrition, back to tension-building again. Walker also confirmed that battered women display behaviors resembling learned helplessness, i.e., passivity learned in response to uncontrollable trauma.*

Wolf, R., Godkin, M., and Pillemer, K.: Elder abuse and neglect: Report from three model projects. Worcester, MA, University of Massachusetts Medical Center, 1984.

10

Caring for the Elderly

Mason P. Thompson
Joseph W. Tollison

"Do not cast me off in the time of old age; do not forsake me when my strength fails."

PSALMS 71:9 (ASV)

Life itself represents a progressive process of aging, heralded by the newborn's first breath. As Greenblatt noted (Feldman, 1983), the aging process begins with the first cry at birth, as if to be born is to start to die. Our role in caring for the elderly is to help ensure that aging is not synonymous with senescence and to assist people in living active, productive, and creative lives well into old age (Feldman, 1983). Remaining active, not merely alive, and experiencing the joy of their accomplishments has been a common denominator of those who have remained highly productive into their advanced years. In fact, a historical review of mankind's achievements reveals that some of society's most significant contributions have been from the aged. Michelangelo completed his work on St. Peter's Basilica at the age of 75. Grandma Moses, who began painting late in life, completed her most famous painting, "Christmas Eve," at the age of 100 (Libow and Sherman, 1981).

The elderly are not a homogenous group. Many believe that they represent the most diverse group within our population in the areas of biologic factors and pharmacokinetics, as well as in the psychosocial, pathophysiologic, and economic realms. It is therefore important to avoid stereotyping the elderly. Although their capacity to respond to the dynamics of our society varies, as many as 95 per cent of them are "up, out, and about" and not institutionalized.

The number of people in the United States over 65 is currently approaching 30 million and is increasing. This is greater than the total population of our largest state, California. During the past two decades, our elderly population grew at approximately twice the rate of the rest of the population. Of special importance is the increasing number of "older old" people (over 75 years old). The group over 75 comprised just 30 per cent of the U.S. population over 65 years of age in 1940 (Special Committee on Aging, 1979). By the year 2000, however, this group will constitute approximately 45 per cent of the elderly. The group 85 years old and above is expanding even more rapidly. By the year 2050, this group of "older old" is expected to have increased by approximately 700 per cent. This means that up to 50 per cent of our American population will be expected to live to their 85th birthday and beyond.

Women generally live longer, a fact which becomes increasingly apparent with each passing decade. For persons approaching age 70, there are approximately 80 men for every 100 women within the same age group. After age 85, the ratio of women to men is nearly double this number. Therefore, many women must face the prospect of living alone for the final years of their lives.

Another major consideration for the elderly population is the economic factor. For example, many older patients are on fixed incomes which may not have kept up with inflationary trends. The inability of the patient to afford necessary maintenance medication for chronic illnesses may present major problems. Life experience influences the lives of these older patients, as is depicted in Figure 10–1.

Another problem frequently encountered is one of attitude. Ageism is a pervasive prejudice which is not only manifested in younger people and among family members but also is often encountered among the elderly themselves. Ageism, as described by Butler, bears striking similarity to the prejudices of racism and sexism (Butler, 1985). This prejudice, based largely on the fear of growing old or dying, is very prominent in our Western culture. Respect for our elderly, providing them with appropriate roles, and quality of life, is important to their overall welfare and, in the long term, important in attempting to alter this prejudice.

Keeping them "up, out, and about" and involved is our goal. Involvement is crucial, for social isolation in the elderly is generally detrimental and often devastating. The training of a majority of today's health care providers did not emphasize care of the ambulatory elderly, but rather the 5 per cent who are institutionalized. Although the vast majority of elderly patients are ambulatory and alert and have varying degrees of self-sufficiency, 80 per cent nonetheless have some chronic medical condition (Brotman, 1979). The elderly may deny their illness and, therefore, delay seeking medical care. In contrast, there is a subgroup among elderly patients who have rather negative perceptions of their health and often make excessive physician visits (Levkoff et al., 1988).

The elderly, as a group, may be our most appreciative patients. They are, however, among those who require the greatest care in diagnosis and management for several reasons. Accumulation of medication is often an expectation, marginal nutrition is commonplace, and assistance with the activities of daily living may be necessary. Coping with these problems is particularly difficult in our society in which many families have become increasingly dependent on two incomes. Also, aging children must in more and more instances either provide or arrange care for "older old" parents.

Prejudices of Society

As more and more people live longer and longer, the elderly as a group are presenting new and far-reaching challenges for our health care system. This is influenced by factors reaching far beyond sheer numbers and complexity of problems. Prominent among these factors is the youth-oriented society in which we live. In spite of this youth orientation, the graying of America must be properly addressed. Maintaining health in an aging population benefits society as a whole and reduces the health care resource requirements.

Striving for improvement in life quality for those over 65 is a goal worthy of our best efforts. In caring for elderly patients, one of the greatest obstacles to effectiveness is the physician's difficulty in coming to grips with his or her own mortality. Overcoming this obstacle is required in order for him or her to be

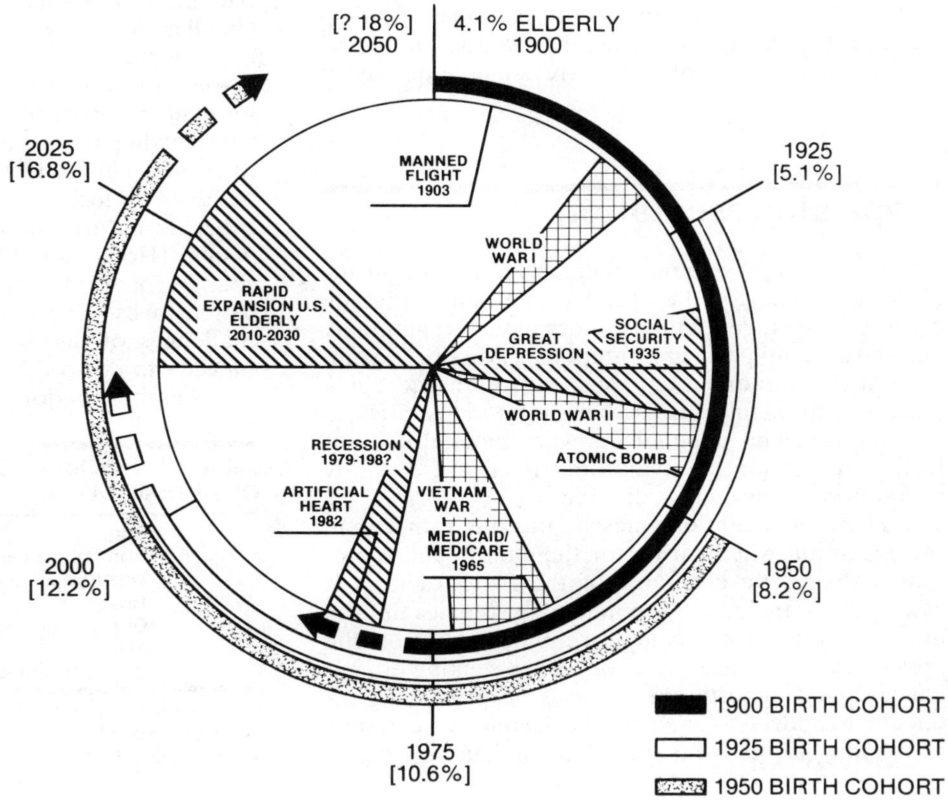

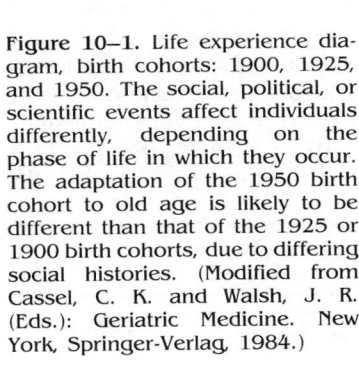

Figure 10–1. Life experience diagram, birth cohorts: 1900, 1925, and 1950. The social, political, or scientific events affect individuals differently, depending on the phase of life in which they occur. The adaptation of the 1950 birth cohort to old age is likely to be different than that of the 1925 or 1900 birth cohorts, due to differing social histories. (Modified from Cassel, C. K. and Walsh, J. R. (Eds.): Geriatric Medicine. New York, Springer-Verlag, 1984.)

maximally effective in caring for an aging patient population (Hazzard, 1983).

Another significant factor has been the orientation of physician training in the care of the elderly. Emphasis in training has long been on cure, which remains our ultimate goal in every possible instance. However, among the elderly, in whom chronic diseases and a decline in the proper functioning of organ systems are more prevalent, providing a cure may not be possible. Instead, control may be the ultimate goal. This requires adaptability of thought among health care providers. Quality of life issues come to the fore as do issues centering on functional status. Clinical emphasis on achieving the preillness functional status is a helpful and practical approach to care of older patients, rather than emphasizing only the traditional diagnosis-oriented approach.

Inevitability

Another product of many of our medical training backgrounds has been the concept of "inevitability." In the past, patients were sometimes seen with the prevailing thought that the disease process being viewed was a part of an inevitable aspect of aging. Therefore, therapy was not emphasized or was perhaps even deferred for certain problems (e.g., confusion, hypertension, heart disease). This view is now less commonly encountered. Most organ systems do undergo functional decline with aging, although none is compromised sufficiently, even at advanced ages, for death to result in the absence of disease (Schneier and Brody, 1983). In our care of patients, although we cannot ultimately deny death, our goal should be to delay it while maintaining a reasonable quality of life.

Atypical Presentation

There are two prominent challenges in the diagnostic phase of caring for the elderly. The first is that, in contrast to younger patients, older patients commonly demonstrate atypical presentations. "Missing" symptoms are commonplace. Thus, we often see aging patients with painless myocardial infarctions, afebrile pneumonias, and appendicitis with minimal discomfort. Attenuation of symptoms is also frequently encountered (Berman et al., 1987).

These presentations may be the rule rather than the exception when caring for the elderly and represent a diagnostic challenge of the first order. It is essential to include all potential etiologies in the differential diagnosis, being careful not to narrow the possibilities prematurely. For those seeking to enhance their diagnostic skills, this concept is an essential one to address. A nonspecific decline in a patient's status may result from infectious and noninfectious causes. Therefore, the challenge lies not only in dealing with the atypical presentation but also in trying to determine the etiology of a nonspecific decline in the health of an elderly patient (Table 10–1) (Berman et al., 1987).

Early Diagnosis

Another concept of equal importance is that of early diagnosis. Owing to expected changes in the immune system and in the decreased functioning reserve of the older patient, early diagnosis generally becomes more critical. Delay in diagnosis may result in an acute process often becoming overwhelming and thus increasing morbidity and mortality. The type of problems encountered in the elderly also differ in frequency from those found in younger patients, as noted in Table 10–2.

Another area of great importance is that of communication problems and disorders. As the elderly age, they are particularly prone to increasing sensory loss in vision, hearing, and touch, among others. This may create or contribute to a sense of isolation for the patient. It becomes increasingly important for the physician to ensure that problems with communication as stated by patients, or especially by family or friends, do not represent instead a modifiable communication disorder.

As noted earlier, emphasis on functional diagnosis is important to the overall health of the elderly patient. In assessing the functional status of the patient, rather than a simple diagnostic assessment (Fiedler et al., 1977 and Pfeiffer, 1976), it is necessary to know the degree of impairment caused by a specific disease or disorder (Tobias et al., 1988). There is normally a steady loss in organ reserve as the patient ages, leading to increased vulnerability and ultimately to death. This reduction in functional capacity may be due to loss of functioning cells, which is an expected occurrence throughout the life span of the patient (Hollander, 1970). Homeostasis, the ultimate goal, becomes increasingly difficult to maintain as the patient ages. The body attempts to respond to the challenges of disease but with an ever-diminishing capacity to do so (Table 10–3) (Zoller, 1987).

Another major consideration for care of the

Table 10–1. NONINFECTIVE CAUSES OF DETERIORATION*

Angina	3
Congestive cardiac failure	3
Fecal impaction	2
Drugs	2
Grand mal seizure	1
Stroke	1
Unknown cause	1

*From Berman, P., Hogan, D. B., and Fox, R. A.: The atypical presentation of infection in old age. Age Ageing, *16*:201–207, 1987.

Table 10–2. RATE OF FUNCTIONAL SYMPTOMS AND CONSEQUENT INTERVENTION IN YOUNG AND OLD HOSPITAL ADMISSIONS*

	Incidence (%)			Frequency (%)	
Functional Symptom	***Young***	***Old***	**Intervention**	***Young***	***Old***
Confusion	3.6	29.5	Psychotropic drugs	58.3	13.7
			Restraints	58.3	52.9
Not eating	1.8	15.6	Nasogastric tube	0	29.6
Incontinence	5.5	26.6	Foley catheter	11.1	15.2
Falling	0.9	5.2	None		—
At least one symptom	8.8	40.5	Any intervention	37.9	47.1

*From Kane, R. L., et al.: Essentials of Clinical Geriatrics. San Francisco, McGraw-Hill Book Company, 1984.

elderly centers on the various options to institutionalization. Although we have made significant progress in recent years in this area, nonetheless we have far to go. Home health care services have rapidly expanded in scope and availability. Supportive housing areas have become more available, as have congregate housing programs. Continued expansion of these and other support programs is severely needed. Alternatives to hospitalization should be considered wherever possible. And, when necessary, hospitalization should be for the shortest time possible.

The adverse potential of hospitalization was demonstrated in Reichel's study of 500 consecutive elderly inpatient admissions. In this study, 146 patients had a total of 193 reactions (Reichel, 1965). Adverse responses to medications and to procedures ranked as the first and third most commonly encountered problems, respectively. However, it is of importance to note that the second most common adverse effect was falls, possibly because of the unfamiliar environment or disorientation from the change of location. Acquired psychologic problems and acquired infections along with medical nursing errors were problems as well (Reichel, 1965). Of concern is the intercurrent diseases that develop during the patient's hospitalization. Table 10–4 lists various potential problems.

For the elderly, the familiar becomes all too unfamiliar after only modest changes in the environment. The potential for iatrogenic problems, in the areas of medication as well as in other areas of hospitalization for this age group, requires that careful thought be given to a situation prior to action. We must always consider what is done to our patients while making extreme efforts to do something for them. Not infrequently, invasive diagnostic studies as well as therapeutic interventions may be responsible for iatrogenic illness in the elderly (Libow and Sherman, 1981). Physicians have been encouraged to avoid the thought of a "complete workup" (Hardison, 1979) and to study each patient with the thought of "minimal interference" (Seegall, 1964). Table 10–5 details some of the most common iatrogenic problems.

Another approach that has been of benefit over the years is that of early discharge planning. When it is necessary to hospitalize an elderly patient, the fears that these patients often have concerning hospitalization may be ameliorated to some extent by discussing discharge planning prior to admission. Also, exercise, dietary arrangements, and other important aspects of the patient's daily life should be addressed, providing the patient with an expectation for life after hospitalization.

The team concept of health care can be extremely important in caring for the elderly. Its focus on the total patient challenges all members of the team to view the patient beyond his or her individual discipline. The physician's role is thus expanded or extended, and the patient as the primary beneficiary remains the focus.

Preventive health care for older citizens is another important concept, yet it has received insufficient emphasis in most circles in years past. Now, however, much more aggressive postures and approaches are often used in various chronic diseases, as well as in working actively toward preventing or delaying the onset of others. Thus, preventive gerontology has resulted in both improved quality and length of life for a number of our elderly. Also, exercise may be of significant help. Exercise for up to 45 minutes, three times per week, was associated with increased bone mineral content in one study of middle-aged women. This could have an important impact on the aging female (Barry, 1986). Overall, in dealing with problems common to the elderly, health professionals must "think elderly," thus heightening the index of suspicion for those problems prevalent in aging populations, and then work accordingly to prevent or delay their onset or progression.

Immune Systems in the Elderly

Alteration in the immune system is an expectation in the process of aging. This area has been the subject of intensive scientific study in recent years.

Involution of the thymus is a major factor in the aging immune system. It contributes to the reordered balance which occurs with aging. The per cent of peripheral blood T lymphocytes decreases with age, as does the absolute number (Nagel et al., 1983). The increased incidence in the elderly of both infectious and malignant diseases and disorders may well be a result of the progressive senescence of the immune system. Unquestionably, many diseases of the elderly are associated with alterations in immune

Table 10–3. STRUCTURAL/FUNCTIONAL AGE-RELATED CHANGES*

1. Cellular Level: Various morphologic changes in nucleus and cytoplasmic organelles; decreased cell number generally throughout tissues; deposition of lipofuscin pigment in both mitotic and postmitotic cells; decreased cell functions including oxidative phosphorylation. DNA and RNA synthesis and protein synthesis and decreased adrenergic responsiveness, changes in response to stress and functional effectiveness of enzyme systems.
2. Connective Tissue: Collagen-increased strength, stability, and increase in number of cross-links, resulting in greater stiffness; decreased tissue elasticity in skin, major blood vessels, heart, lungs, and ligaments.
3. Body Composition: Weight generally declines after age 50 in males while remaining relatively constant in females, decrease in lean body weight caused primarily by shrinkage of muscle mass reflected in decreased creatinine production (25% in males and 15% in females); organ size declines (muscles, liver, brain, kidneys) with some exceptions (prostate, lungs, heart, and (?) G.I. tract).
4. Cardiovascular: Cardiac output falls 1% per year after age 30, impaired heart rate increases to stress; stroke volume decreases 0.7% per year in resting state; heart rate declines; prolonged mechanical refractory period; ECG has small increases in PR, QRS, and QT intervals with decreased amplitude and left-shift of QRS; progressive elastocalcinosis of media of elastic arteries and elastic lamina of muscular arteries resulting in decreased distensibility and increased systolic blood pressure; decreased blood flow to various organs—less to kidney than heart or brain.
5. Excretory: Total nephron count decreases by 30 to 40% between ages 25 and 85; kidney weight decreases 30%; GFR decreases 46% and RPF 53% between ages 20 and 90; filtration fraction increases; a parallel reduction in renal tubular cell mass causes a 43% decrease in max. tubular resorption for glucose; decreased concentrating ability and a slower and prolonged response to acid and base loads; serum creatinine does not reflect creatinine clearance because of decreased production owing to smaller muscle mass; compensatory hypertrophy capabilities are decreased to a max. of 30% vs. 50% in a young kidney.
6. Respiratory: Increased A-P diameter, kyphosis, decreased strength of expiratory muscles = decreased compliance of chest wall; decreased number of alveoli owing to destruction of septa with dilatation of resp. bronchioles and alveolar ducts; increased rigidity of lungs and decreased compliance promotes airway collapse; increased RV, FRC with unchanged TLC; VC decreased 26 and 22 cc. per year in males and females, respectively; increased Aa_{O_2} difference (10 to 15%) due to V/Q abnormality with airway collapse in dependent but still perfused lung regions; no change in Pa_{CO_2}; all timed ventilatory functions decrease probably owing to decreased elastic recoil and early airway collapse with increased resistance to expiration; increased risk of pulmonary infection owing to decreased projective force of cough and mucociliary clearance rate, increased frequency of aspiration, and gram-colonization rate of oropharynx.
7. Gastrointestinal:
   - Dentition: Wearing of enamel and dentin on chewing surfaces; fibrosis and Ca^{++} of pulp space; root resorption and root dentin sclerosis; apical migration of supporting structures; all result in increased chance of loss of teeth—50% are without by age 65.
   - Esophagus: Decreased peristaltic response; increased nonperistaltic generalized contractions (corkscrew esophagus on barium swallow); delayed transit time; decreased LES relaxation following swallowing-achalasia; increased incidence of H.H; increase in columnar epithelium in lower esophagus.
   - Stomach: Decreased secretion of acid to 20% of volumes in youth; increased intestinal metaplasia and polyposis; increased incidence of atrophic gastritis (Scandinavian study—40% after age 65), but this is probably a genetically determined age-related pathologic process.
   - Sm. Intestine: Decreased Peyer's patches and lymphoid tissue; with exception of decreased absorption of Ca^{++} (active transport), which may be affected by endocrine function, and possibly Fe^{++}, which is related to gastric acidity, no significant changes in absorptive function have been noted.
   - Colon: Thickened muscularis mucosa; increased incidence of diverticulosis over 50% by age 80; decreased intestinal motility (increased hypotonia and decreased peristalsis), resulting in increased storage and dehydration of stool, leading to constipation; increased incidence of fecal incontinence owing to decreased external sphincter tone—assoc. (+/−) with neurologic disease and responds to feedback training.
   - Liver: Weight decreased by 20% by age 50; albumin is decreased and globulin is increased with no change in total protein; remainder of common LFT's are normal (bil, SGPT, SGOT, and alk. phos.); there is slow metabolism of several drugs owing to decreased efficiency of enzyme systems.
   - Gallbladder: Increased incidence of stones to 40% by age 80 possibly owing to decreasing cholesterol stabilization mechanisms.
   - Pancreas: No change in organ weight but possibly decreased functional tissue: trypsin decreased but bicarbonate, lipase, and amylase (with stimulation) are all normal; insulin—see Endocrine.
8. Endocrine:
   - Pituitary: ACTH response to stress is possibly decreased; ADH response to hyperosmolarity is increased, resulting in an increased incidence of SIADH.
   - Thyroid: T4 and TSH are normal while T3 is decreased 25 to 40% after age 60, ^{131}I uptake rate is decreased as is T4 metabolism by the liver, response to stress is normal, therefore reduced turnover rates reflect decreased BMR and peripheral need owing to decreased lean body weight.
   - Parathyroid: Reports are equivocal as to PTH levels.
   - Pancreas: Decreased number and function of insulin-secreting cells; a greater proportion of insulin secreted is in inactive precursor proinsulin form; progressive peripheral insulin resistance owing to relative increase in body fat in relation to decrease in LBW—as stable number of fat cells increase in size there is a decrease in insulin receptor effectiveness; all this results in an increased glucose response to an oral GTT but a normal fasting glucose.
   - Adrenals: Glucocorticoid levels retain normal diurnal rhythms with decreased secretion and excretion rates—i.e., a slower turnover; response to stress is normal to decreased; there are decreased levels of adrenal androgens (50%); estrogens are all adrenal in origin after menopause and are 5 to 10% of normal in females and unchanged in males; testosterone metabolism and production rates both decrease while binding globulin increases—these changes result in decreased free testosterone.

Table 10–3. STRUCTURAL/FUNCTIONAL AGE-RELATED CHANGES* *Continued*

9. Hematopoietic and Immune: Red cell line is normal, including a normal hematocrit; Fe^{++} absorption is reduced as are serum Fe^{++} and TIBC slightly; platelets are normal; fibrinogen levels are increased, and consequently, the ESR can be increased up to 40 mm. per hour; phagocytic function is normal; IgA and IgG are normal while IgM may be decreased; number of B cells is normal but response to antigen challenge of vaccination is reduced possibly owing to decreased T cell function; there is a reduced ability of T cells to proliferate in response to challenge possibly owing to changes in cell subpopulations, i.e., an increase in suppressor cells; there is decreased delayed hypersensitivity in elderly; complement levels are normal.
10. Neurologic: Variable degree of neuronal dropout, depending on location and individual differences; decreased interconnections between dendrites with presumed decrease in number of transmitted impulses; lipofuscin pigment accumulation and degeneration of Nissl substance; geometric increase in number of senile plaques, neurofibrillary tangles and granulovacuolar degeneration; cerebral blood flow declines with age; 15% decrease in nerve conduction velocities with a decrease in motor and sensory latency; increased MAO's and serotonin with possible decreased catechol levels; progressive loss of stage 4 sleep with numerous brief arousals with slight decrease in total sleep giving the impression of sleeplessness; sedatives decrease the latency to sleep and periods of arousal but only temporarily, with return of usual pattern after a few days; a 7% decline in brain weight by age 80; 20% decrease in blood flow to CNS by age 70.
11. Special Senses:
    - Sight: Decreased visual acuity, visual fields, and speed of dark adaptation; increased minimal light threshold reception, and greater loss of VA with dim illumination; increased discoloration and rigidity of lens nucleus, resulting in decreased accommodative ability; pupillary response to light and accommodation decrease so that by age 85 only ⅓ respond to light and none to accommodation; increased frequency of chronic glaucoma owing to decreased reabsorption of intraocular fluid; increased lens size and abnormalities of shape lead to astigmatism and myopia; increased incidence of cataracts (? pathologic condition).
    - Hearing: Tympanic membrane flexibility declines; increased mean pure tone threshold with age for all frequencies, especially for 4000 cps in males after 60; more important is the loss in speech reception and discrimination thresholds.
    - Taste: Decrease in number and functional status of taste buds; saliva flow is decreased by ⅔, leading to dry mouth and decreased taste sense; taste also affected by state of oral hygiene and use of dental prostheses.
    - Smell: Decreased to same extent as taste (one study with only 22% normal).
    - Touch: Decreased touch acuity; pain sensors appear to be intact.
12. Musculoskeletal:
    - Stature: Height progressively decreases primarily owing to shortening of the vertebral column from narrowing of the intervertebral disks and a decrease in vertebral height; there is kyphosis as well; long bones are relatively preserved in length; total height loss is 2 inches between ages 20 and 70.
    - Bones: Bone loss is universal beginning after age 40, accelerated in females after menopause and totaling 25% in females and 12% in males; those with the smallest bone mass at maturity are affected most; etiology is still unclear; there is continued appositional bone growth on outside surfaces, resulting in wider hollowed out bones; there is loss of trabeculae along with apatite and protein matrix; increased risk of fracture is present and incidence of vertebral collapse and femur fractures is significantly increased; edentulous state leads to progressive mandibular resorption.
    - Joints: Dehydration of intervertebral disks and joint cartilage with wear and tear atrophy (fibrillar degeneration); exposure of subchondral bone leads to ebumation and spur formation at sites of trauma; changes affect weight-bearing joints most but also the glenoid and others; pain is a concomitant symptom.
    - Muscles: Decreased number of cells; increased fat content in muscle bundles; decreased numbers of capillaries and neurons per motor unit; increased lipofuscin pigment deposition; decreased myosis-ATPase activity; progressive loss of muscular strength and mechanical efficiency.

*Adapted from Kallenberg, G. A., and Beck, J. C.: Care of the geriatric patient. *In* Rakel, R. E. (Ed.): Textbook of Family Practice. Philadelphia, W. B. Saunders Co., 1984, pp. 248–249.

function (Powers et al., 1987). Autoantibodies and circulating immune complexes which have the potential to damage tissues and organs may contribute to the pathologic changes of aging (Stiles et al., 1984). However, it is not yet confirmed whether senescence of the immune system in the elderly patient is a primary or secondary factor. In general, however, the patients who are among the "older old" are those in whom the least decrease in immune response has occurred (Murasko et al., 1986).

The role of emotion in disease is as important a factor in the elderly as it is among younger patients (Plotnikoff et al., 1986). This has been recognized for many years. Osler, the father of modern medicine, noted that it is equally important to understand the emotions within a man as it is to predict the outcome of his disease.

Psychoneuroimmunology, a rapidly expanding field, focuses on the study of the effects of emotions and stress on immune function and the role of the central nervous system in alteration of immune function (Plotkinoff et al., 1986). Studies in the mediation

Table 10–4. 44 INTERCURRENT DISEASE PROCESSES DEVELOPING DURING HOSPITALIZATION (500 PATIENTS)*

Disease Process	No. of Cases
Pulmonary embolization and infarction	16
Aspiration pneumonia	15
Fecal impaction	2
Decubitus ulcer	2
Parotitis	2
Urinary retention	7
TOTAL	44

*Reichel, W.: Complications in the care of five hundred elderly hospitalized patients. J. Am. Geriatr. Soc., *13*:973–981, 1965.

of and resistance to disease through the immune system are among the most dynamic in medicine today and will provide vital information for the future care of our patients. Increasing knowledge in this area and the ability to alter defined defects may provide practical application for aging patients in the future (Stiles et al., 1984).

Premorbid personality traits may have some predictive value in certain patients with diseases such as arthritis and autoimmune disorders. Factors that may influence this include life change stress (Locke, 1984) and maintenance of a viable social support network which may be protective for patients encountering overwhelming stress (Cobb, 1976).

Drug Action in the Aging Patient

The elderly, currently comprising more than 11 per cent of the population, account for 29 per cent of the total personal health care expenditures. They also receive over 25 per cent of all prescriptions and take an even larger percentage of nonprescribed medication, particularly in the expanding over-the-counter market (Special Committee on Aging, 1979 and Rabin, 1972). Taking medications on their own that have "worked" for family or friends is also relatively common. The high incidence of chronic disease in the elderly accounts for much of this drug use (O'Brien and Kursch, 1987). The expected physiologic changes in the aging patient in relation to drug kinetics involve the key alterations of function outlined in Table 10–6Another significant age-related alteration is in response to medications. This is complicated by the fact that up to 60 per cent of medications taken by the elderly are purchased over-the-counter and often are not reported to the physician, sometimes even with a careful drug history. Some of these over-the-counter medications, such as antihistamines, have cumulative anticholinergic effects, producing acute confusion, worsening of dementia or a hypertensive event, or possible sequelae (Everitt and Avorn, 1986).

Those agents that are lipophilic or hydrophilic are normally affected by the predictable changes in body status. For example, an increase in total body fat increases the distribution of lipophilic medications. Psychotherapeutic agents, most of which are lipophilic, are stored in increasing amounts. Also, with less protein binding capacity, the unbound, or pharmacologically active, fraction may cause increased toxicity.

Most antidepressants have anticholinergic properties and thus may produce postural hypertension. Desipramine and nortriptyline are less likely to cause postural hypotension, whereas amitriptyline is more likely to do so (O'Brien and Kursch, 1987).

With less protein binding, as well as reduced glomerular filtration rate, the result is a reduction in excretion. The major resulting pharmacokinetic alteration noted in the aging patient is the decrease in excretory ability (Lamy, 1986). Medications often take longer to reach peak effect, remain active longer, and have a greater effect, milligram for milligram, than occurs in younger patients. Therefore, drug accumulation is the expectation in the elderly. Recent studies support the hypothesis that both the autonomic effects and sedative effects of psychotherapeutic medications increase the likelihood of falling and subsequent fractures in older patients (Ray et al., 1987). Dosing intervals are therefore of critical importance in elderly patients, as is appropriate selection of pharmaceutical agent and proper dosage. A "start low, go slow" approach is generally optimal, with periodic reassessment of all medications being a critical factor in the patient's overall care. In the elderly, with most chronic medications tending to accumulate, a beginning dose of one third to one half

Table 10–5. COMMON IATROGENIC PROBLEMS OF THE ELDERLY*

Overzealous labeling
Dementia
Incontinence
Bed rest
Polypharmacy
Enforced dependency
Transfer trauma

*From Kane, R. L., et al.: Essentials of Clinical Geriatrics. San Francisco, McGraw-Hill Book Company, 1984.

Table 10–6. AGE-RELATED PHYSIOLOGIC CHANGES*

Decrease	Increase
Total body water	Body fat
Lean body mass	
Serum albumin	
Splanchnic blood flow	
Liver mass	
Renal plasma flow	
Glomerular filtration rate	
Renal tubular function	

*From Roe, D. A. (Ed.): Drugs and Nutrition in the Geriatric Patient. New York, Churchill Livingstone, Inc., 1984.

that of younger patients should be strongly considered. In prescribing medications, as in other diagnostic or therapeutic decisions, the physician must always consider the worst possible result related to his choices and actions (Reichel, 1965).

The critical nature of physiologic changes and the expected impact on the aging human organism are shown in Figure 10–2.

Age-Associated Mental Change

As in physical parameters, there are expected changes in mental status in aging patients. A nonprogressive, mild memory impairment, largely associated with recent memory, is commonly seen among the elderly (Libow, 1981). A second change in the elderly involves the intellectual changes of aging, which normally includes a decline in the speed of response. The third expectation is alterations in creativity and originality (Libow and Sherman, 1981).

Lehman's work demonstrated that originality and creativity tended to reach their zenith between the ages of 30 and 40. On the other hand, activities and one's knowledge of politics, literature, metaphysics, history, and philosophy continue to improve slightly with aging. Psychologic testing among the elderly confirms that their thinking in general is more stereotyped, routine, and "concrete" (Libow and Sherman, 1981). Nonetheless, creativity is frequently preserved.

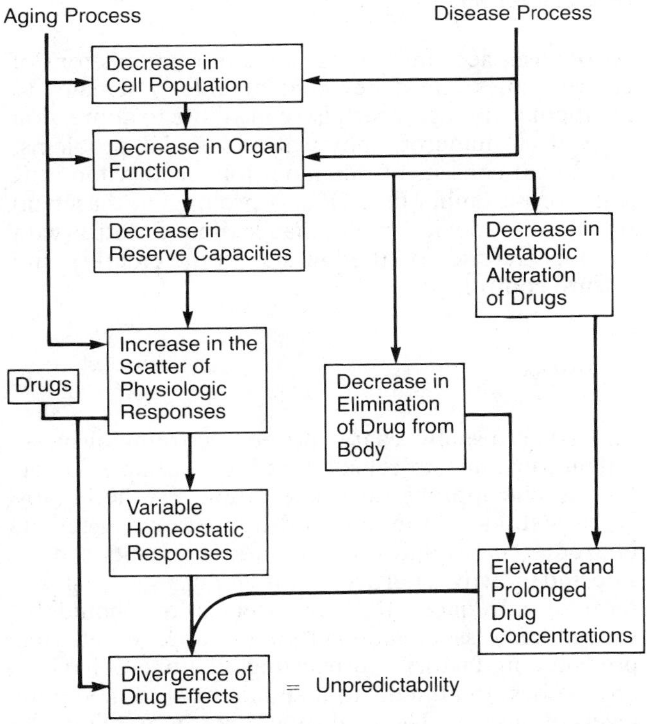

Figure 10–2. Flow diagram indicating factors that lead to unpredictability of drug effects in the aged. (From Riley, G. A.: The influence of aging on drug therapy. U.S. Pharmacist, 2(10):28, 1977.)

The fourth expected change involves learning time. Learning in the elderly is slower than in the young (Libow and Sherman, 1981). The fifth major change is that of a decline in psychomotor skills, which suggests that older patients should not be placed in situations requiring continuous rapid motion (Libow and Sherman, 1981). However, the elderly tend to compensate for this with greater attention to detail. Therefore, older workers are no less productive than younger workers (U.S. Department of Labor).

Among the emotional changes of aging, a change in motivation (generally decreasing with age) is commonly noted. Therefore, many elderly people may need strong incentives, emotional support, and ongoing encouragement to venture into new areas. The second major emotional change is the trend toward avoidance and substitution or even withdrawal (Libow and Sherman, 1981). This is termed disengagement (Busse and Pfeiffer, 1977) and may be largely influenced by factors such as socioeconomic forces or the previous life style of the patient (Libow and Sherman, 1981). As a part of this, the elderly become more preoccupied with their bodily functions. Thus, excessive body awareness seems to occur in some patients.

Also, a reduction in sexual activity is noted with age. For example, about half of patients up to age 70 have regular intercourse, whereas only approximately 20 per cent remain active over 75 (Pfeiffer et al., 1968 and Kinsey et al., 1948). Change in tempo is also an expected occurrence. The elderly oftentimes find alternate ways (e.g., hugging, holding, caressing, words of endearment) of expressing intimacy with their mates.

Mental and Nervous Disorders

Although the elderly normally undergo some expected changes in mental status, the emotional condition among the elderly is often quite diverse. The elderly are stereotyped as being inflexible, fragile, and susceptible, but commonly they can be extremely strong in adversity. Most are able to cope with social, financial, and health problems as effectively as when they were younger. The person's emotional status during these earlier years may provide much information in this consideration. However, if the emotional reserve of an individual is minimal, this balance can give way to anxiety and depression when one is stressed. For example, a minor change in a chronic disease of an elderly patient may provoke significant emotional complications. Dehydration, fever, or infection can further aggravate the problem (Bianchine et al., 1981).

Such elderly patients may require disproportionately large amounts of time and energy from health care providers (McKegney, 1975). They may be labeled as "crocks" and then become a considerable health risk because they alienate personnel and may receive little attention for their psychologic or biologic needs. They show muted anger, often focused on previous medical care. Unfortunately, a large percentage of persons over the age of 60 are often placed on psychotropic medications in order "to treat" such disorders (Eisdorfer and Fann, 1973).

It is helpful to give these patients emotional reinforcement by commending them for their rising above hardship, for their dedication and self-sacrifice, and for their strengths. Many respond to this approach. It is also important to encourage them to fight their illness, to be a "soldier," to try to get along without medicine, and so forth (McKegney, 1975). They even can be encouraged to "be your own doctor," provided visits continue and they are not discharged.

DEPRESSION

Mood disorders are more common among older individuals than in other age groups (Ruegg et al., 1988). Elderly patients, however, are also likely to mask depression by complaining of physical problems. Pseudodementia is a term used to refer to a reversible global impairment owing to a mental illness, most commonly depression. Pseudodementia is characterized by reasonably good orientation and intact memory. "I don't know" and "I can't remember" are common answers to questions. By contrast, patients with dementia often give wrong or confabulatory answers (Wells, 1979). On the other hand, the elderly can conceal physical ailments owing to fear of being old and useless. They may conceal true medical problems such as weight loss, bleeding, or breast lumps.

The severity of depression in the elderly can vary greatly. The potential of suicide is four times greater among elderly patients than in younger adults, especially among white males (Butler, 1985; Pfeiffer and Busse, 1973). The difference in incidence between males and females increases with age, with the male rate climbing sharply at middle age and continuing to rise. Reasons for suicide include depression associated with physical illness or disability, change of role, isolation, and rigidity (Breed and Huffine, 1979).

Always do a thorough physical evaluation of the elderly depressed patient. Medical problems that can be associated with depression are cancers (especially of the pancreas), occult infection, arthritis, and endocrine problems such as hypothyroidism or even apathetic hyperthyroidism, especially if associated with excessive weight loss. Patients with neurologic diseases associated with dementia such as Alzheimer's, multi-infarct dementia, Parkinson's, and Huntington's chorea often have some manifestation of associated depression (Alexopoulos et al., 1988). Also, determine if medications are being taken or alcohol consumed, as these may be other possible causes of depression.

Depression is frequently associated with stroke. Right hemispheric injury has been commonly associated with impaired ability to accurately communicate or to understand. The cognitive syndromes associated with strokes involving the left hemisphere are well known. Although studies have not been totally consistent, some associated impairment in the ability to express affect and mood has also been associated with left-sided injuries (Dupont et al., 1988).

Treatment of Depression

Treatment of depression has been clearly described, but there are some special features of therapy in the elderly. Mild depression should always be treated initially with psychotherapy. The use of antidepressants in the elderly is complicated by coexisting medical illnesses, other concurrent medications, and the high incidence of side effects. Antidepressants can, however, be well tolerated in the elderly if titrated slowly and monitored closely. They frequently are quite effective.

The agent selected does require some special consideration. Sedation, anticholinergic effects, and postural hypotension are three major concerns. Minimizing these effects in the selection of agents for elderly patients can avoid possible serious side effects. Trazodone, desipramine hydrochloride, and nortriptyline are commonly used agents in the elderly (Blazer, 1989).

ALCOHOLISM

Alcoholism accounts for 12 per cent of admissions of elderly males and 4 per cent of elderly females to inpatient facilities. It can also contribute to depression as well as numerous physical and social problems. Treatment consists of thiamine, folic acid, vitamin K if the prothrombin time (PT) is prolonged, diazepam or chlordiazepoxide, maintenance of fluid status (with caution exercised on the low side in the elderly), and seizure control.

ANXIETY

Anxiety is usually characterized by tremulousness, fatigue, inability to relax, sweating, dizziness, palpitations, and apprehensive expectation. Psychotherapy is the first line of therapy. If drug therapy is needed, benzodiazepines and tricyclic antidepressants can be safe and effective, particularly if emphasis is on short-term or infrequent therapy. Medication should be viewed only as an adjunct to therapy. Identifying precipitating factors and learning adaptive behaviors are the best treatments to maintain mild to moderate levels of anxiety. The goal should not be to eliminate all anxiety, as an acceptable level of anxiety appears to be necessary to cope with the problems of daily living.

SLEEP DISORDERS

Decreased sleep time is associated with normal aging: increased number of awakenings, decreased deep sleep, and a decrease in REM sleep. Treatment consists of avoidance of sleeping during the day or early evening. Activity levels should be increased for persons having difficulty sleeping. Reading before bed and drinking a warm, nonstimulant beverage can also be helpful. Sedatives should be used only for short-term therapy since they are potentially addicting both physically and psychologically.

CENTRAL NERVOUS SYSTEM

It has been stated that "no pharmacologic agent has been proven to be of definitive value in reversing, or even slowing, the progressive cognitive deficit that sometimes occurs with aging" (Medical Letter, 1976). This statement remains true.

MEMORY LOSS

The key aspects of memory loss are difficulties with registration of information, retention, and recall. Medication toxicity, hypothyroidism and other metabolic disorders, depression, and CNS lesions are the most common causes of reversible memory loss in the elderly (Larson et al., 1987). Stress, occult disease, and alcoholism may also cause memory loss.

DEMENTIA

Alzheimer's disease accounts for approximately 50 per cent of dementia, and vascular problems cause about 17 per cent (Tomlinson et al., 1968 and 1970). A combination of the two make up an additional 18 per cent. Senile dementia of the Binswanger type is one example of vascular dementia. Pseudodementia and normal pressure hydrocephalus are also potential causes of syndromes suggesting dementia.

Accurate diagnosis of dementia is difficult. Possible reversible causes should be actively sought. The diagnostic procedures used to evaluate dementia are shown in Table 10–7. There are possibly three major diagnostic errors: failure to recognize depression, especially in the presence of mild organic brain disease; equating brain atrophy on the CT scan with clinical dementia; and failure to distinguish focal from global intellectual impairment (Garcia et al., 1981).

Senile dementia of the Binswanger type is a vascular ischemia affecting the periventricular white matter. It may cause disconnection of a relatively intact cerebral cortex, resulting in true subcortical dementia. A clinical feature is that it occurs only in patients 50 years or older.

Hypertension, diabetes, cardiovascular disease, and often recurrent hypotension are frequent risk factors. A history of repeated small strokes (commonly lacunae) with discrete neurologic deficits is common. The clinical spectrum can extend from asymptomatic or minimally symptomatic disease with only radiologic signs, to patients with a slow, progressive dementia associated with memory loss, emotional instability, gait problems, and urinary incontinence (Roman, 1987).

DELIRIUM

While delirium can occur at any age, its incidence is highest among elderly persons. It is a transient disorder of cognition and attention. Delirium is commonly accompanied by disturbances of the sleep-wake cycle and psychomotor behavior (American Psychiatric Association, 1980).

Delirium usually begins acutely and is first noticed mostly at night. The confusional state is short, lasting from several days up to a month. Most patients recover fully; however, approximately 20 to 30 per cent die most commonly from the disease process that precipitated the delirium. Hallucinations and delusions are common. Illnesses or toxicities that are known to occur with or that precipitate delirium are common. The most common cause of delirium in the geriatric patient is medications. Usually, those medications involved have anticholinergic properties that are cumulative (Table 10–8) (Lipowski, 1983).

PSYCHOSIS

Psychosis can be produced by a wide range of neurologic, metabolic, and toxic disorders including physical and mental stresses. The elderly are especially susceptible. The most common variety of delusion manifested by patients involves ideas of reference, false beliefs of persecution, and fears of injury or death (Cummings, 1986).

Diagnosis requires careful study of potential disorders associated with psychosis. CNS disorders, systemic illnesses, vitamin deficiency states, electrolyte disorders, medications (Wood et al., 1988), and toxins are suspected categories. Appropriate testing is required for ones that are suspected. Treatment is aimed at alleviating any identifiable primary cause that may be reversible.

Diagnosis

There is no available specific test to diagnose mental disorders in the elderly patient. A detailed history including medication and family history followed by a mental status exam are the most important components of evaluation. Dementia and delirium often occur together. A mini mental state test (Folstein et al., 1975) may help elicit cognitive and attention deficits but cannot distinguish delirium from dementia. The differential diagnosis among dementia,

TABLE 10–7. DIAGNOSTIC PROCEDURES FOR THE EVALUATION OF DEMENTIA*

Procedures	Rationale
Initial studies	
Urine drug screen for sedatives	Unknown drug use or cumulated metabolites
CBC	Anemia, infection, leukemia
Psychometrics	Confirmation of cognitive dysfunction and the degree of dysfunction
Automated chemistry	
Electrolytes (Na, K, CO_2, Cl, Ca, PO_4, Mg)	Pulmonary, renal, or endocrine dysfunction, occult malignancy, alcoholism, dehydration
BUN/creatinine	Renal dysfunction, dehydration
Liver function tests	Hepatic dysfunction, metastatic lesions, nutritional status
Thyroid function tests	Hyperthyroidism/hypothyroidism
Erythrocyte sedimentation rate	Collagen vascular disease, occult malignancy, inflammation
B_{12}, folate	Deficiency, pernicious anemia
Serologic test for syphillis	Neurosyphillis
Electroencephalogram	Focal or diffuse cerebral dysfunction
Computed tomographic scan	Intracranial masses, epidural or subdural hematoma, old infarcts, hydrocephalus, focal or diffuse cerebral atrophy
Additional studies (as indicated)	
Urinalysis	Renal, hepatic, or endocrine disease
Chest x-ray	Infection, chronic lung disease, primary or metastatic tumor
Electrocardiogram	Arrhythmias, heart block
Drug levels (barbiturates, bromides)	Drug intoxication
Heavy metal screens (blood, urine)	Heavy metal poisoning
Lumbar puncture	Infection, neoplasm, inflammation
Arteriography	Intracranial bleed, neoplasm
Serum cortisol	Cushing's disease, Addison's disease
Blood cultures	Infection, sepsis
Arterial blood gas	Pulmonary disease, hypoxia

*Modified from Black, K. S., and Hughes, P. L.: Alzheimer's disease: Making the diagnosis. Am. Fam. Physician, *36*:199, 1987.

delirium, and psychosis may therefore be difficult, but certain characteristics, if present, are helpful (Table 10–9).

A history of progressive intellectual decline is suggestive of dementia (Lipowski, 1987). A demented patient is usually normally alert and aware of his or her surroundings, has a fairly constant level of awareness during daytime, and shows defective knowledge of commonly known facts. However, acute deterioration in a known demented patient suggests delirium. Such a situation warrants an investigation to determine its cause. A patient with psychosis is likely to have a past history of psychiatric illness, tends to have markedly depressive or manic behavior and systematized rather than fleeting delusions, and does not have the characteristic worsening of symptoms at night (Lipowski, 1989).

Treatment

Symptomatic and supportive therapy for mental disorders is important. In cases of delirium, specific treatment of any underlying organic cause or the withholding of any potential medication causing intoxication is necessary for recovery. A controlled environment in a quiet, well-lighted room, appropriate sedation, and good nursing care are essential requirements for patients with any mental disturbance. Reassurance and orientation from one or two attentive family members are helpful.

Sedation may be necessary to relieve severe agitation, insomnia, or both. Haloperidol is usually the safest and most effective drug for this purpose; however, therapy must be monitored. Fluid and electrolyte balance, nutrition, and adequate vitamin supply are important. In alcohol withdrawal, benzodiazepines are the drugs of choice. In severe anticholinergic intoxication, physostigmine salicylate should be used parenterally.

Movement Disorders Associated with Aging

Several movement disorders are believed to be related to aging. Senile tremor is probably the most common, and usually involves the mouth, lips, head, and voice. Senile chorea occurs in the mouth, lips, tongue, and face and is similar to tardive dyskinesia. It occurs in patients who have never been exposed to neuroleptic drugs. Senile tremor and senile chorea are often associated with other chronic medical illnesses.

Neuroleptic medications used in the elderly mainly for psychosis cause a number of extrapyramidal side effects that include dystonic reactions, parkinsonism, and akathisia, as well as potentially irreversible disorders such as tardive dyskinesia (Lohr and Bracha, 1988). These reactions may occur in 50 per cent of patients treated with neuroleptics.

Other movement disorders can occur in Parkin-

Table 10–8. ORGANIC CAUSES OF DELIRIUM*

Primary Intracranial Disease
Structural brain disease
Stroke
Epilepsy
Systemic Disease That Affects the Brain
Infections involving any organ system
Cancer
Congestive heart failure
Hypoxia
Myocardial infarction
Hypertensive encephalopathy
Orthostatic hypotension
Uremia
Hepatic failure
Diabetes
Hypoglycemia
Malnutrition—especially B vitamins
Dehydration
Sodium depletion
Hypokalemia
Exogenous Toxic Agents
Anticholinergic drugs
Diuretics
Digoxin
Cimetidine
Antihypertensive drugs
Antiarrhythmic drugs
Benzodiazepines
Nonsteroidal anti-inflammatory agents
Neuroleptics
Analgesics
Substance Withdrawal
Alcohol
Sedatives
Hypnotics
Stress
General surgery
Burns
Fever
Pain
Femoral neck fractures
Impairment of vision and hearing
Sleep loss
Sensory deprivation
Sensory overload
Bereavement
Relocation
Hypothermia
Heat stroke

*Adapted from Lipowski, Z. J.: Delirium in the elderly patient. N. Engl. J. Med., *320*:578–582, 1989.

son's disease, Huntington's disease, and Wilson's disease. They can also be seen in Alzheimer's disease, catatonic schizophrenia, and psychotic depression. Movement disorders can also be associated with the use of other medications such as L-dopa, benzodiazepines, lithium, and carbamazepine.

PARKINSON'S DISEASE

Parkinson's disease usually appears in the latter decades of life. It produces a slowly progressive movement disorder that causes increasing disability. The disease usually has four primary clinical features: tremor, bradykinesia, rigidity, and disturbance of posture (Bianchine, 1976). Depression commonly accompanies Parkinson's disease and may require treatment also.

The basal ganglia in the brain show a loss of dopamine neurons and neuromelanin pigment. Parkinson's disease is considered to be a dopamine-deficiency state in which neural cell bodies and their dopamine receptors are damaged in a fashion similar to the aging process elsewhere in the brain. The clinical efficacy of dopamine analogues such as bromocryptine in the treatment of parkinsonism further validates this hypothesis (Bianchine, 1976).

The introduction of levodopa, or 3,4 dihydroxyphenylalanine, the metabolic precursor to dopamine, has shown significant promise in the treatment of Parkinson's disease. Approximately 75 per cent of patients with parkinsonism respond reasonably well to levodopa. Improvement in the movement disorder associated with parkinsonism accompanies overall improvement in functional ability. Secondary motor manifestations such as disturbances in posture, gait, associated movements, facial expression, speech, handwriting, swallowing, and respiration are also improved.

A combination of levodopa and carbidopa, a peripheral decarboxilase inhibitor, is the most effective drug available in the United States for treatment of Parkinson's disease (Medical Letter, 1988b). Carbidopa prevents many of the adverse effects caused by dopamine after peripheral decarboxylation of levodopa. The usual dosage range is 300 to 1000 mg. of levodopa. Muenter (1982) described in detail a treatment regimen of levodopa and carbidopa combination. Relatively complete inhibition of peripheral decarboxylase requires at least 75 mg. per day of carbidopa; some patients may require much larger doses.

After 2 to 5 years of treatment, the benefit from each dose becomes shorter. Some believe that levodopa may have a time limit on its effectiveness; therefore, it should be reserved for severe forms of the disease (Duvoisin, 1987). The most disturbing long-term effects of levodopa are frequent, abnormal, involuntary movements which usually are dose-related. The drug may also cause unpleasant dreams, hallucinations, and other mental changes. Temporary withdrawal of the drug (a "drug holiday") for 4 to 14 days may cause a dangerous return of parkinsonian symptoms and should be avoided if possible.

Bromocriptine is a dopamine agonist that can also be used in Parkinson's disease. It has less effect than levodopa when used alone, but it may cause fewer involuntary movements and has a longer duration of action. The best results with bromocriptine have occurred early in treatment when the drug was given concurrently with Sinemet. Low doses of bromocriptine (less than 30 mg. per day) combined with Sinemet can ameliorate the "wearing off" and "on-off" effects after prolonged use of levodopa (Rinne, 1987). Also, lower dosages of levodopa may also achieve the therapeutic goal.

Table 10–9. CLINICAL FEATURES OF DELIRIUM, DEMENTIA, AND ACUTE FUNCTIONAL PSYCHOSIS*

Characteristic	Delirium	Dementia	Acute Functional Psychosis
Onset	Sudden	Insidious	Sudden
Course over 24 hr.	Fluctuating, with nocturnal exacerbation	Stable	Stable
Consciousness	Reduced	Clear	Clear
Attention	Globally disordered	Normal, except in severe cases	May be disordered
Cognition	Globally disordered	Globally impaired	May be selectively impaired
Hallucinations	Usually visual or visual and auditory	Usually none	Predominantly auditory
Delusions	Fleeting, poorly systematized	Often absent	Sustained, systematized
Orientation	Usually impaired, at least for a time	Often impaired	May be impaired
Psychomotor activity	Increased, reduced, or shifting unpredictably	Often normal	Varies from psychomotor retardation to severe hyperactivity, depends on type of psychosis
Speech	Often incoherent, slow, or rapid	Patient has difficulty finding words	Normal, slow, or rapid
Involuntary movements	Often asterixis or coarse tremor	Often absent	Usually absent
Physical illness or drug toxicity	One or both are present	Often absent, especially in senile dementia of Alzheimer's type	Usually absent

*From Lipowski, Z. J.: Delirium in the elderly patient. N. Engl. J. Med., *320*:580, 1989.

Nausea and orthostatic hypotension may occur early in treatment. These side effects possibly can be avoided by increasing the dosage slowly. The main disadvantage of bromocriptine is the frequent occurrence of mental disturbances, including nightmares, agitation, hallucinations, and paranoid delusions, especially in elderly patients.

Anticholinergic agents were used alone to treat Parkinson's disease before levodopa. They are still useful, especially for tremor. Although they are not as effective, they may be used with levodopa to offer an effect. Side effects include dry mouth, constipation, urinary retention, aggravation of glaucoma, impaired memory, confusion, and hallucinations.

Amantadine may be effective by increasing dopamine in the brain. It is also used as an antiviral drug in Type A influenza. Amantadine is generally used alone, in a dosage of 100 mg. two or three times a day early in the disease or as an adjunct in later stages. A 2-week trial is usually needed to determine its effectiveness. Confusion and hallucinations, ankle edema, and livedo reticularis can occur. Adverse effects of amantadine and anticholinergics may be additive.

Sensory Changes

VISUAL

Normal, expected changes in an aging sensory system include reduction in pain sensitivity and sense of touch. There are also potential reductions in taste and odor perception. Reflexes and reaction times are reduced.

Thus, as a person approaches advanced age and loses much of the ability to perform physically as in earlier years, he or she becomes more of an observer of others' participation. It is one of the ironies of human existence that at this critical time, the likelihood of disturbances in visual acuity increases significantly. Reading and traveling, watching television, and other activities often have a reduced level of enjoyment for the elderly who are not able to see well. Preservation of vision becomes a goal to be actively sought (Reichel, 1983). Eye problems common to elderly patients and their associated signs and symptoms are outlined in Table 10–10.

Although the majority of older patients preserve functional vision throughout life, fear of blindness is understandable among elderly patients. Causes of visual impairment are outlined in Table 10–11.

Both entropion and ectropion often occur during the aging process. Either disorder may expose the globe to trauma through direct damage or to alteration of the integrity of the tissue with subsequent secondary viral or bacterial infection. Although often requiring surgical correction in the final analysis, the entropion may be temporarily treated with taping of the lid to the cheek to evert the lid edges.

Glaucoma is also increasingly prevalent among aging patients. In any situation involving a red, painful eye, elevated intraocular pressure, and a fixed, somewhat dilated pupil, acute angle glaucoma is the diagnosis until proven otherwise. Ophthalmologic referral is strongly recommended. However, if consultation is not immediately available, instillation of 2 per cent pilocarpine should be initiated (Libow and Sherman, 1981). Fortunately, acute angle glaucoma is uncommon, whereas chronic, open angle glaucoma is relatively common, affecting approximately 5 per

Table 10–10. SIGNS AND SYMPTOMS ASSOCIATED WITH COMMON VISUAL PROBLEMS IN THE ELDERLY*

Signs and Symptoms	Cataracts	Open-angle Glaucoma	Angle-closure Glaucoma	Macular Degeneration	Temporal Arteritis	Diabetic Retinopathy
Pain			X		X	
Red eye			X			
Fixed pupil			X			
Retinal vessel changes					X	X
Retinal exudates				X		X
Optic disc changes		X			X	
Sudden visual loss			X		X	
Loss of peripheral vision		X				
Glare intolerance	X					
Elevated intraocular pressure		X	X			
Loss of visual acuity	X			X		X

*From Kane, R. L., et al.: Essentials of Clinical Geriatrics. San Francisco, McGraw-Hill Book Company, 1984.

cent of those over 70. It is an insidious process which may often be symptom free in the early stages. Periodic assessment of intraocular pressure is important. Family history is also often positive in these patients. A major differential diagnosis is benign ocular hypertension in which the peripheral fields and optic disks remain unchanged (Libow and Sherman, 1981). Ocular hypertension may not require intervention, whereas chronic glaucoma requires ongoing therapy.

Opacities of the lens are another problem frequently associated with aging. Modern techniques of microsurgery have made cataract surgery available to essentially all patients. The decision to operate, however, is generally based on limitation of vision more than the state of the cataract. Components of the basic ophthalmologic examination are shown in Table 10–12.

HEARING

Hearing impairment is common among elderly patients. Approximately 90 per cent of the elderly living in nursing homes have hearing deficiencies (Chafee, 1967). Of importance is that hearing loss also involves emotional problems related to isolation which may arise including withdrawal, depression, and paranoia.

Table 10–11. VISUAL IMPAIRMENT: COMMON CAUSES OF VISUAL FAILURE IN THE ELDERLY*

Rapid Onset	Gradual Onset
Retinal detachment	Cataract
Vascular occlusion	Macular degeneration
Ischemic optic neuropathy	Chronic glaucoma
Acute glaucoma	Diabetic retinopathy

*From Pathy, M. S. J. (Ed.): Principles and Practice of Geriatric Medicine. London, John Wiley & Sons, Ltd., 1985.

Also, because of hearing loss, physical risk for the patient is increased outside the home. Many pedestrian accidents occur secondary to this problem (Libow and Sherman, 1981).

There are three types of hearing loss: conductive, sensorineural, and mixed. Conductive losses are precipitated by abnormalities in the outer or middle ear. Sensorineural losses occur as a result of changes within the cochlea and cranial nerve VIII neural connections. Combinations of these two are defined as mixed. Air conduction is used to measure the overall auditory system (Libow and Sherman, 1981). The cochlea and cranial nerve VIII or its connections are measured by testing bone conduction. Ranges of hearing loss are shown in Figure 10–3.

Conductive hearing loss is characterized by the patient's speaking in a relatively quiet voice (Libow and Sherman, 1981). The patient generally understands very well what he hears and often can hear better in the presence of noise than a person with normal hearing. Tinnitus is commonly associated. In contrast, the patient with a sensorineural hearing loss often speaks in a very loud voice because he is unable to hear his own voice normally (Libow and Sherman, 1981). This patient, as contrasted with one with conductive loss, often has difficulty in understanding what others are saying and is sensitive to loud noises. Tinnitus is again often present but may be of a higher pitch than in conductive type loss.

Leading causes of conductive hearing loss include excess cerumen in the ear, acute otitis media, serious

Table 10–12. OPHTHALMOLOGIC SCREENING*

Visual acuity	Ability to read newspaper-sized print
Lens, fundus	Ophthalmoscopic examination
Intraocular pressure	Tonometry
	Visual fields

*From Kane, R. L., et al.: Essentials of Clinical Geriatrics. 2nd ed. New York, McGraw-Hill Book Company, 1989.

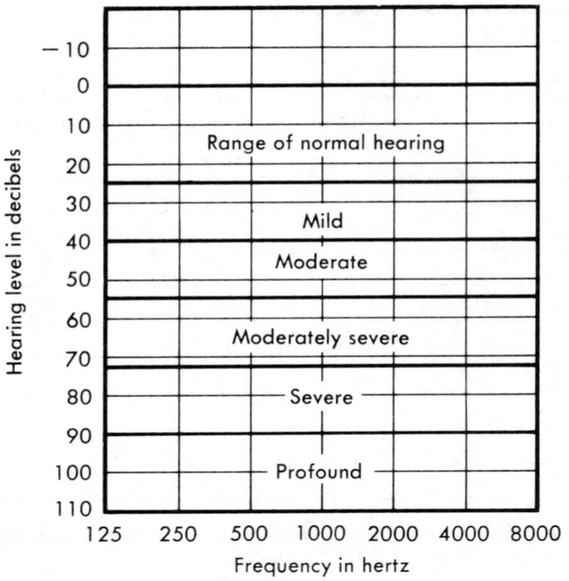

Figure 10–3. Audiogram showing ranges of hearing loss. (From Libow, L. S., and Sherman, F. T.: The Core of Geriatric Medicine—A Guide for Students and Practitioners. St. Louis, C. V. Mosby Company, 1981.)

otitis media, and cholesteatomas (Libow and Sherman, 1981). Other causes of conductive loss include Paget's disease and otosclerosis. Otosclerosis, a hereditary phenomenon, results in fixation of the stapes. It represents a frequent cause of progressive conductive deafness in older adults.

Sensorineural hearing loss may result from age-related normal changes or pathologic processes which may affect the inner ear (Libow and Sherman, 1981). Presbycusis is the leading cause in the elderly. Other causes include noise trauma, ototoxicity from various drugs, and involvement of the acoustic nerve by both benign and malignant neoplasms. Another possibility is otosclerosis (Libow and Sherman, 1981). Patients with this type loss generally ask for repetition of statements. "What?" or "I beg your pardon" is often heard (Libow and Sherman, 1981). Ototoxic drugs include gentamycin (Libow and Sherman, 1981), bolus doses of furosemide, and aspirin ingestion. Tumors capable of producing a sensorineural loss include acoustic neuromas and metastatic tumors. Clues to this may be conduction differences between ears as well as audiogram variances. See Figures 10–4 to 10–6 for examples of types of hearing loss patterns.

Unilateral hearing loss is seldom due to presbycusis. Nor is it a factor in elderly hearing loss isolated to one ear unless significant trauma can be determined. Acoustic neuroma should be the diagnosis in this circumstance until proven otherwise. Neuroradiologic techniques have greatly enhanced diagnosis of this disorder. Sudden hearing loss, on the other hand, is infrequently due to congestion. Perilymphatic fistula must be considered. Bed rest may be attempted in this disorder; however, if correction does not occur rapidly, surgical intervention must be considered. A consultation with an otolaryngologist is necessary for definitive therapeutic intervention in this disorder. Another possible etiology is vascular occlusion of the labyrinthine artery which often responds to vasodilator therapy (Fitzgerald, 1985).

Modern hearing aids can be an immense benefit to many of these patients and should be encouraged wherever applicable. Hearing aids have improved significantly in recent years. They amplify better, can filter out background noises better, and are cosmetically more acceptable. Sensory deprivation is a concern for elderly patients who have had long-standing hearing losses. Early diagnosis again becomes critical to help the patients at a time when the hearing impairment is still mild to moderate and the overall surrounding problems less complicated (Miller, 1986). Some hearing loss is expected as a result of aging,

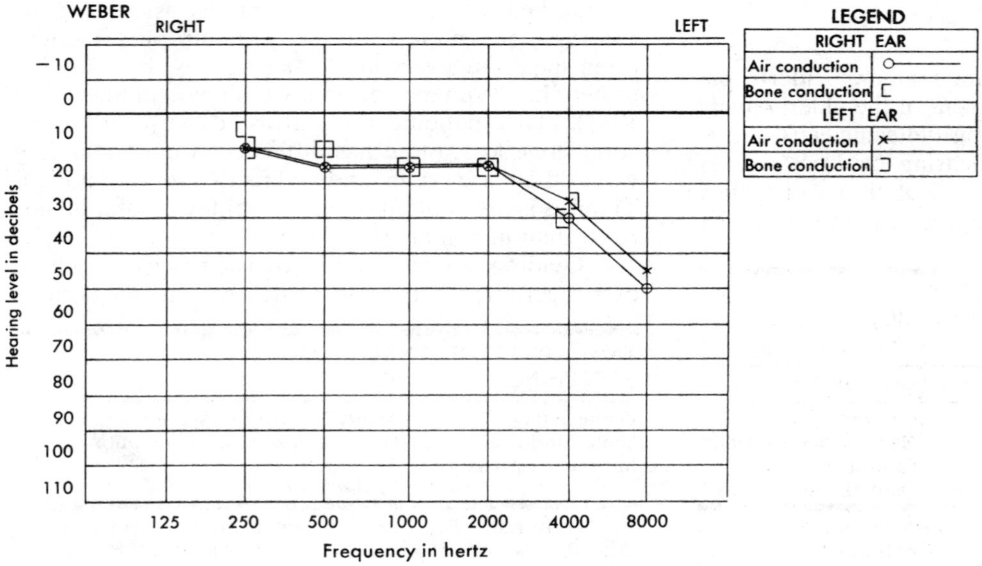

Figure 10–4. Audiogram showing early presbycusis with hearing loss in the higher frequencies bilaterally and normal hearing in the low and middle frequencies. This loss is typical of early presbycusis. Note that air and bone conduction tests are the same, showing that the loss is purely sensorineural. (From Libow, L. S., and Sherman, F. T.: The Core of Geriatric Medicine—A Guide for Students and Practitioners. St. Louis, C. V. Mosby Company, 1981.)

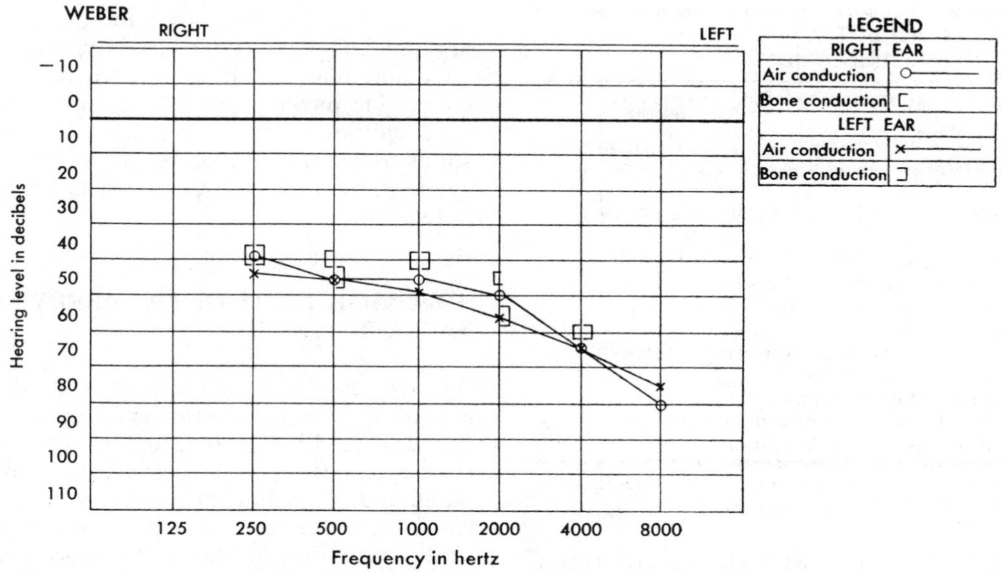

Figure 10–5. Moderately advanced presbycusis. This pure-tone audiogram shows bilaterally symmetrical moderate sensorineural hearing loss dropping to moderately severe in high frequencies. (From Libow, L. S., and Sherman, F. T.: The Core of Geriatric Medicine—A Guide for Students and Practitioners. St. Louis, C. V. Mosby Company, 1981.)

but even sensorineural hearing loss does not preclude the use of amplification (Table 10–13) (Reichel, 1983).

Cardiovascular Disease

Cardiovascular disease has received a great deal of attention in medicine for the past several decades. Tremendous progress has been made in prevention, diagnosis, and treatment of cardiovascular disease; however, the elderly do remain a population at risk for heart and vascular disease.

SYSTOLIC MURMURS

Auscultation of the heart is very important in the regular evaluation of the elderly patient. However, heart sounds are sometimes misinterpreted. The diagnosis of aortic stenosis is one of the more common errors made when the systolic murmur heard is actually caused by degenerative calcific valvular disease. A serious error in prognosis can be made in these persons, who actually have mild or no heart disease (Luisada, 1970).

The systolic murmur of degenerative calcific valvular disease is best heard at the third left and second right interspaces. The murmur is usually Grade 1 or 2, the second sound is single or normally split, and

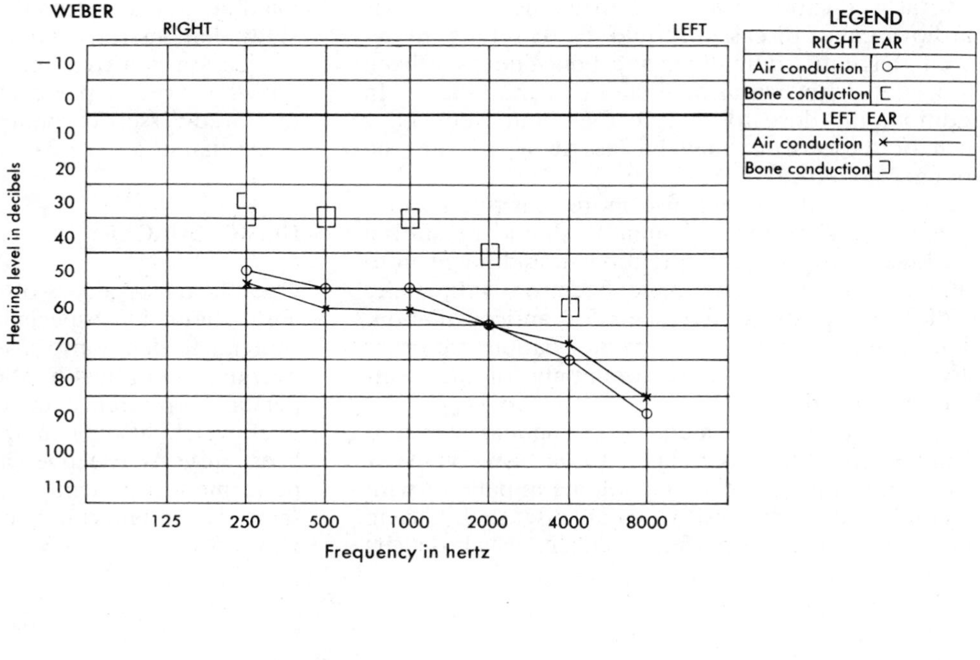

Figure 10–6. Mixed hearing loss. This audiogram shows a bilateral mixed hearing loss such as would be seen in an elderly individual with presbycusis (the sensorineural component) and impacted cerumen (the conductive component). The brackets are the results of bone conduction hearing testing, and the circle and *x* are the results of air conduction tests. The difference between them is the conductive loss. (From Libow, L. S., and Sherman, F. T.: The Core of Geriatric Medicine—A Guide for Students and Practitioners. St. Louis, C. V. Mosby Company, 1981.)

Table 10–13. FACTORS IN THE EVALUATION FOR A HEARING AID*

Exclude contraindicating medical or other correctable problem.
Greatest satisfaction is achieved with aid if loss is between 55 and 80 dB. There is only partial help if loss is greater than 80 dB.
Less satisfaction is achieved when poor discrimination is present.
Aid is specifically designed for face-to-face conversation; patient's expectations should be realistic.
Loudness perception abnormalities may make aid unacceptable.
More severe hearing loss requires aid worn on the body rather than behind-the-ear device.
Assess for monaural or binaural aids.
Assess for patient's ability to handle aid independently.
Assess patient's motivation for using an aid.

*From Kane, R. L., et al.: Essentials of Clinical Geriatrics. San Francisco, McGraw-Hill Book Company, 1984.

there is no palpable thrill. The electrocardiogram shows no evidence of left ventricular hypertrophy.

The best method used in physical examination to differentiate aortic stenosis from degenerative disease is palpation of the carotid artery. In aortic sclerosis, there is a normal rise, while in aortic stenosis there is a slow rise in the palpated pulse (Constant, 1976).

Phonocardiography can also help in the differentiation. The best information to be obtained short of catheterization is an echocardiogram (Wong et al., 1983). Correlations done at autopsy show that the problem is common but rarely causes significant dysfunction. Therefore, systolic murmurs in the elderly do not fully define the pathology and should be investigated further before management decisions or prognoses are decided.

ADVERSE REACTIONS OF CARDIOTROPIC MEDICATIONS

Several medications used in the treatment of various cardiovascular diseases should be carefully monitored. Digitalis, quinidine, and lidocaine have been associated with confusional states in the elderly. In addition, the dose to achieve therapeutic effect for each of these drugs may be less than that for the younger patient.

Elderly patients are also more sensitive to anticoagulants. Therefore, Coumadin should be started at a lower dose. Careful attention should be given to patients who may also have been on antiplatelet medications prior to the need for anticoagulation. Many elderly patients use such medications for other vascular problems or more commonly for the treatment of arthritis.

Antihypertensive medications should be used cautiously in elderly patients with occlusive vascular disease. Dropping circulating volume in patients with cerebral and peripheral vascular disease by using diuretics can lead to perfusion deficits. Such deficits can produce ischemic extremities, confusion, lethargy, and even coma. Postural hypotension can cause falls that may result in hip fractures. Angiotensin converting enzyme (ACE) inhibitors should also be used cautiously in the elderly. Improving volume status by withholding diuretics prior to starting these agents may avoid the acute onset of significant hypotension.

ADVERSE EFFECTS OF ANTIARRHYTHMIC THERAPY

An age-associated increase in both the prevalence and complexity of ventricular ectopic beats has been found (Fleg, 1988). Care must be taken in considering therapy for the elderly because they have a greater likelihood of significant adverse effects from antiarrhythmic drugs than younger patients. Reasons include reductions in lean body mass, renal function, and hepatic blood flow associated with older age. The elderly also tend to be on other medications which can potentially interact adversely with antiarrhythmic drugs.

Antiarrhythmic therapy should be limited to elderly patients with known organic heart disease and frequent ventricular ectopy consisting of couplets, runs of ventricular tachycardia, or a history of syncope or prior cardiac arrest. A 75 per cent reduction in premature ventricular beats and elimination of ventricular couplets or runs of ventricular tachycardia should be documented on a 24-hour ambulatory ECG for justification of continued therapy with a specific antiarrhythmic.

DIAGNOSING ANGINA

Noninvasive approaches to diagnosing angina such as exercise testing alone or combined with radionuclide angiography may offer more information for decision-making short of coronary catheterization. The Duke study demonstrated good correlations between catheterization and treadmill and radionuclide angiography; however, 5 per cent of patients with left main or three-vessel coronary disease may be missed (Christian et al., 1983).

HEART SURGERY

Open heart surgery is obviously a major decision for any patient, but especially so for an elderly patient. Individual decisions based on a patient's present overall state of health, ability to tolerate surgery, and personal preference in available treatment alternatives weigh heavily in the choice to undergo open heart surgery. Elective cardiac operations have been performed in patients over 80 years of age with the same risk and mortality as in patients between 70 and 79 years of age (Silvay et al., 1988).

Elderly patients, in general, do require experienced anesthetic management, intensive monitoring, and careful postoperative care. Association between mortality and prolonged endotracheal intubation is usually due to complications encountered such as pneumonia, heart failure, arrhythmias, and septicemia. Emergency operation, cachexia, NYHA Class IV disease, and previous myocardial infarction are independent risk factors for early death (Edmunds et al., 1988).

An aggressive surgical approach in elderly patients may offer significant symptomatic benefit, and age alone should not be a contraindication for cardiac operations. Furthermore, in patients age 65 and over, the Coronary Artery Surgery Study documented a favorable outcome at 6 years with coronary artery bypass surgery (Gersh et al., 1985). If coronary artery lesions are not amenable to angioplasty, carefully selected older patients with this disorder can be surgical candidates (Table 10–14).

TREATMENT OF HYPERCHOLESTEROLEMIA

Elevated cholesterol has been associated with elevated morbidity and mortality, and its treatment has demonstrated reductions in vascular events. Studies, however, have concentrated on middle-aged men. A low-cholesterol diet is important to all individuals, as is appropriate weight loss and discontinuance of smoking.

Treatment with cholesterol-lowering medications which may produce intolerable or detrimental side effects remain to be extensively studied in the older patient. Oster and Epstein (1987) found that for patients over 65 years of age, the cost-effectiveness of therapy with cholestyramine was below the standard of other accepted medical practices. Therefore, treatment decisions based on level of cholesterol, existing vascular disease, and cost should be made on an individual basis for elderly patients.

Table 10–14. INDICATORS FOR SURGICAL THERAPY IN CORONARY ARTERY DISEASE*

Criteria that may be used in selecting continued medical therapy in preference to surgical therapy for coronary artery disease include:

1. The absence of impaired ventricular function.
2. The presence of remediable, precipitating factors for angina.
3. Performance on treadmill exercise testing, including duration, rate/pressure product achieved, and absence of inducible ventricular arrhythmia.
4. Ease of instituting a medical program that would be readily adhered to without compromise of quality of life.
5. The absence of critical (>70%) left main coronary artery stenosis.

*Adapted from Graboys, T. B., Headley, A., Lown, B., et al.: Results of a second-opinion program for coronary artery bypass graft surgery. J.A.M.A., *258*:1612, 1987.

HYPERTENSION

Therapy for hypertension in the elderly has many potential pitfalls. Adverse reactions occur more frequently, having a detrimental effect on the daily functioning of older patients. For the physician, the therapeutic decision of whether or not to treat presents the classical question of risk versus therapeutic reward. The reward of both diagnosis and therapy must be weighed against the incumbent risks. In doing so, the physician must always consider the worst possible resulting events related to his or her choices and actions (Reichel, 1965).

Reduction of significantly elevated blood pressure is of unquestionable benefit to aging patients. However, the mildly hypertensive older patient remains a source of study. Therefore, in "borderline" hypertension, even greater care must be taken in selecting therapy. Nonpharmacologic therapy is often recommended for initial hypertension among the elderly. However, attempts at weight loss have varying long-term success. Most clinicians believe in only moderate sodium restriction, and the goal of reducing excessive salt ingestion by one half is encouraged. In addition, exercise should also be of a moderate nature (Moser, 1987). Nonetheless, one cannot afford the possibility of waiting years for development of an end-organ effect. Therapy must be initiated to include carefully selected medications and dosages as appropriate.

Among the potential adverse effects, postural hypotension ranks as a major hazard associated with antihypertensive therapy. Many medications may exacerbate these problems. Postural hypotension also occurs with many anticholinergic or hypotension-inducing therapies. An important concept is that the effect of these agents is cumulative.

Antihypertensive agents with proven efficacy overall may have heightened downside effects in the elderly (e.g., CNS effects of central agents or hypokalemia with diuretics). Depression is a common side effect of a number of antihypertensive medications, including beta blockers, and some of the central agents (Butler, 1985). These agents may have the advantage of cost and long experience, but the newer agents (e.g., calcium channel blockers and ACE inhibitors) may demonstrate a reduction in adverse effects as well as produce favorable or desired cardiovascular effects.

The use of diuretics among elderly hypertensives has been frequently discussed in recent years. Advocates of diuretics still contend that low dose diuretics are acceptable first line therapy among selected elderly hypertensives. Potential hypokalemia is a major concern. Recent clinical trials with these medications appear to confirm that elderly patients complied well with therapy, their adverse reactions were mild, their metabolic alterations were relatively easily manageable, and postural hypertension was not overly significant.

Some strongly advocate angiotensin converting

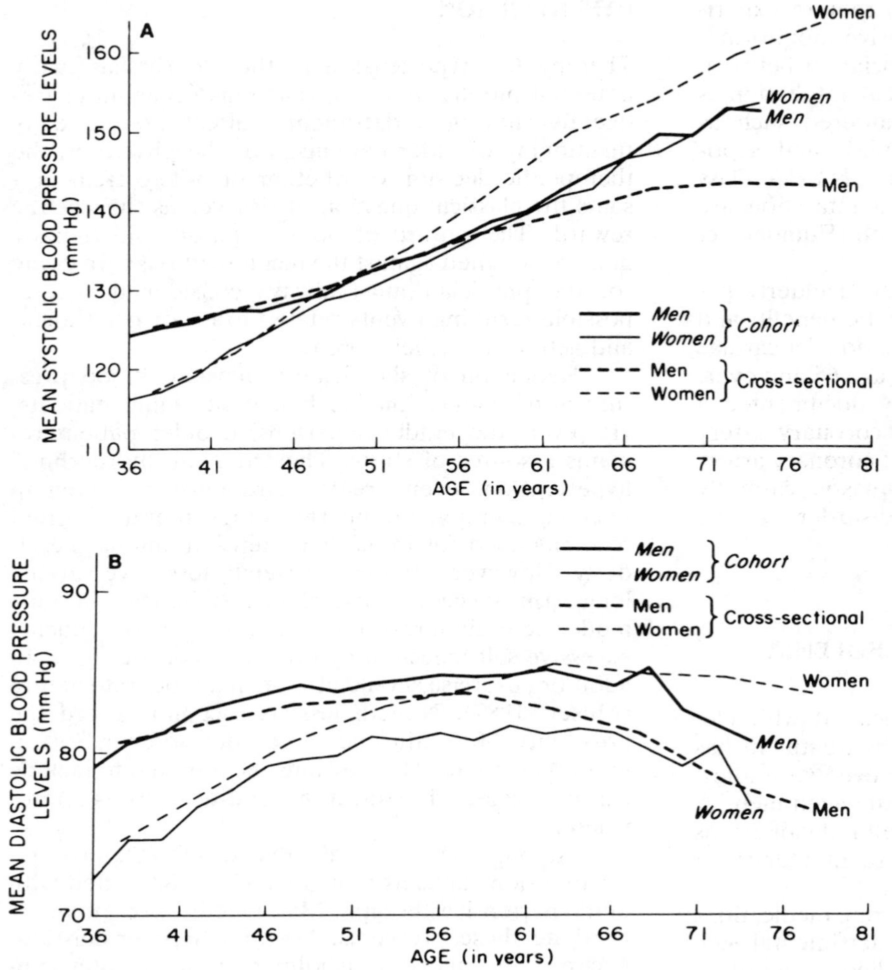

Figure 10–7. *A,* Average age trends in systolic blood pressure for cross-sectional and cohort data (Framingham Study, Examinations 3 to 10). *B,* Average age trends in diastolic blood pressure levels for cross-sectional and cohort data (Framingham Study, Examinations 3 to 10). (From Caird, F. I., Dall, J. L. C., and Kennedy, R. D.: Cardiology in Old Age. New York, Plenum Press, 1976.)

enzyme inhibitors or calcium channel blocking agents for antihypertensive therapy in older patients, while others advocate cardioselective beta blockers. The cardiac and peripheral effects which may be more pronounced in the elderly for each type of medication must be given careful thought in the individual patient. The rationale for the choice of cardioselective beta blockers is that in elderly hypertensive patients, symptoms of pump failure might be induced through inadequate filling in the rather stiff heart. In using a cardioselective beta blocker, diastole can be prolonged, improving filling and stroke volume (Moser, 1987). Another major aspect of this type agent is its ability to reduce left ventricular wall stress and left ventricular hypertrophy. Certainly in the patient with angina pectoris, ischemic heart disease, or myocardial infarction, cardioselective beta blockers may well be selected as a first line agent (Moser, 1987). Expense of these various drugs is a factor for many patients since they are usually more costly.

Systolic blood pressure generally increases with age as is outlined in Figure 10–7*A* and *B*.

Oral Care

TEETH

The digestive process begins with the act of chewing. Assessment of the teeth and the mechanics of chewing is an important part of ensuring proper digestion in elderly patients who tend to seek dental care much less often than medical care (Chauncey and House, 1977). In addition, it was estimated in the early 1970's that approximately 50 per cent of all persons 65 and over had lost all of their teeth. This figure has been declining as more attention has been given to overall health care including oral care in the younger years.

Because physicians often have more frequent patient contact, they have greater opportunity to identify the dental needs of the geriatric patient. The dietary preferences of the elderly change with their progressively declining ability to chew. These changes may result in a nutritionally depleted patient, often also at risk for bacteremia from associated dental infections.

Loss of the teeth is the most common dental problem encountered among the elderly. Dental caries and periodontal disease are the major diseases that result in wastage of teeth. Cavities are the result of acid made by bacteria such as *Streptococcus mutans* within dental plaque. The low pH produced causes demineralization of the tooth enamel. Cavities have been shown by the National Center for Health Statistics Survey (1971–1973) and the National Institute of Dental Research (1979–1980) to be significantly altered by ingesting appropriate amounts of fluoride while the teeth are developing (MMWR, 1985). The optimal amount of fluoride necessary to reduce the most dental decay with the least risk of dental fluorosis is 0.7 to 1.2 parts fluoride per 1 million parts water.

Chronic periodontal disease (periodontitis) is responsible for the loss of more teeth than dental caries in the older patient. It begins as gingivitis usually during childhood and adolescence manifested by slight bleeding after eating or brushing. This process slowly spreads to involve the underlying periodontal ligament, alveolar bone, and cementum (Megran and Chow, 1986). The alveolar bone is slowly resorbed and results in loss of the periodontal ligament attachment from the tooth to the bone. The separation of soft tissue from the tooth results in a "pocket" where further food debris and bacteria can collect. Pus may form, causing further destruction, and the teeth may become mobile resulting in ultimate loss of teeth.

The type, extent, and improper function of dental prostheses can produce marked changes in food choices of the older patient toward softer, more liquid types of food. Not only may a problem exist with the mechanics of chewing, but there may also be a significant change in the taste of food associated with the wearing of dental prostheses. These may all contribute to a nutritionally inadequate diet.

ORAL CAVITY

Halitosis can be a challenging complaint from family members of older patients, as well as from the patients themselves. It can lead to social withdrawal if not properly treated. Halitosis can occur in patients who experience chronic dental infections or chronic infections of the upper respiratory tract or who have coatings on the tongue. Treatment is directed toward the particular infection if one is detected or to the light brushing of the tongue with a toothbrush if a tongue coating is suspected. In some patients, no cause can be detected.

Certain vitamin deficiencies can present as irritation of the oral mucosa and tongue. The most notable are deficiencies of the B vitamins and folate which are manifested by soreness of the mouth, with a red, swollen, and painful tongue and mucous membranes. Angular stomatitis can occur but is not specific. Severe vitamin C deficiency (scurvy) is manifested by bleeding gums, gingivitis, and loosening of teeth as well as other systemic symptoms including perifollicular hemorrhages.

Angular cheilitis is usually due to deepened facial folds secondary to loss of connective tissue support with pooling of saliva, poorly fitting dentures, pernicious anemia and other vitamin B deficiencies, and monilial infection (Koopmann and Coulthard, 1982). Nicotinic stomatitis can occur as a result of smoking or chewing tobacco (Bhaskar, 1968).

All chronic ulcerative lesions of the oral cavity should be biopsied if they do not heal in approximately 2 weeks. Cancers of the oral cavity are common and should be carefully searched for in the elderly patient including under dental prostheses during an exam. Malignant tumors are frequently found on the tongue or under it in the floor of the mouth. Squamous cell carcinoma is the most commonly found intraoral malignancy, accounting for over 90 per cent of malignant tumors (Koopmann and Coulthard, 1982), and is found 95 per cent of the time on the lower lip. An increased incidence of oral cancer is found in patients with long histories of alcohol and tobacco abuse. Other implicated causes are poor oral hygiene, poorly fitted dentures causing chronic irritation of tissues, and chronic exposure to actinic radiation. Basal cell carcinoma occurs more commonly on the upper lip.

DISEASES OF THE SALIVARY GLANDS

Xerostomia, or dryness of the mouth, is due to salivary gland dysfunction as may be seen in elderly persons, duct blockage from sialolithiasis or tumor, excessive mouth breathing, or emotional stress. It may be caused by primary gland failure as seen in Sjögren's syndrome (Condemi, 1987) or in infection of the glands. Xerostomia can also be secondary to drugs that are drying such as diuretics, antihypertensive agents, nicotine, antihistamines, tricyclic antidepressants, antipsychotics, hypnotics, or antiparkinsonism drugs. It also can result from irradiation of the head and neck for treatment of malignancy. Saliva protects the teeth through several mechanisms including neutralizing dental plaque acids (Council on Dental Therapeutics, 1988). The lack of it can result in large numbers of dental caries.

The diagnosis of xerostomia is primarily based on evidence derived from the patient's history, an examination of the oral cavity, and sialometry (a simple office procedure that measures the flow rate of saliva). The technique of sialometry is described by Sreebny and Valdini (1987). The symptoms and signs of xerostomia are caused by low salivary flow. They include stomatitis, glossitis, chelitis, mucosal ulcers, dental caries, candidiasis, speech and mastication difficulties, problems with taste and swallowing, and pain.

For treatment, patients can take frequent sips of water, suck ice chips, or coat mucous membranes with petrolatum. Chewing stimulates the flow of saliva. Because affected patients are highly susceptible to dental caries, they should not use sugar-containing foods or acidic foods to stimulate salivary flow. Patients can eat bulky foods which are low in sugar. They can also chew sugarless gum. They should have regular dental checks and possibly topical application of fluoride, which may help them avoid caries. Commercial nonprescription solutions used to lubricate the oral tissues may be the only effective treatment for patients whose glands cannot respond to stimulation (Medical Letter, 1988c).

Gastrointestinal System

ESOPHAGEAL DISORDERS

Reflux

Esophageal reflux is the regurgitation of gastric contents into the esophagus. The most important determinant of reflux into the esophagus seems to be an inadequate lower esophageal sphincter. The common symptoms of reflux are "heartburn," chest pain, or a sour taste coming into the mouth after a large meal or while bending over. It may also occur while lying down or wearing tight fitting garments. Well-publicized treatments are directed at preventing reflux, abolishing symptoms, and preventing stricture formation. Aspiration may become a significant problem in the older patient with a decreased level of consciousness or in the presence of an esophageal stricture. The reoccurrence of pneumonia should lead one to suspect these esophageal problems in the elderly and to prompt investigation.

Presbyesophagus

Presbyesophagus is the clinical syndrome of abnormal esophageal motility attributable to the aging process (Chopra and Curtis, 1985). Manometric studies have demonstrated individuals older than 70 years who have a diminished amplitude of propulsive contractions but in whom the remainder of the peristaltic complex of the esophagus is intact. This suggests that changes in motility may be due to diverse illnesses associated with aging such as diabetes mellitus, Parkinson's disease, peripheral neuropathy, and senile dementia.

Dysphagia

Dysphagia is the subjective awareness of solid or liquid food being lodged in the esophagus. A patient's complaint of dysphagia should never be considered psychogenic without adequate investigation. Its presence warrants a systematic search for the etiology. It may be the result of disordered motility or of mechanical obstruction.

Difficulty in swallowing only solid foods suggests a mechanical obstruction. As the degree of obstruction advances, the patient begins to have trouble with liquids as well as solids. The clinical course of dysphagia is helpful. Dysphagia that lasts just a short time may be due to a transient, inflammatory process in the esophagus. Progressive dysphagia that worsens over several weeks or months suggests carcinoma of the esophagus. Recurrences of dysphagia with solid foods over several years without clinical deterioration of the patient implies more benign mechanical problems.

Carcinoma is the most common cause of progressive dysphagia in the elderly. Treatment of esophageal cancer in general is palliative since about only 20 per cent of patients are candidates for surgical cure (Chopra and Curtis, 1985). Other possible mechanical causes of dysphagia include webs, rings, Zenker's diverticulum, and benign esophageal strictures. Extrinsic compression by tumors or aberrant large vessels is rare. Elderly patients may present only with a history of subsisting on a diet of baby food or liquids and with significant weight loss.

Several neuromuscular disorders can interfere with esophageal function. Evaluations should carefully search for signs of polymyositis, myasthenia gravis, stroke, Parkinson's disease, and poliomyelitis (Pope, 1977). The skin over the hands and the fingers should be carefully examined for signs of scleroderma or dermatomyositis.

Achalasia

The presenting symptoms of achalasia are often dysphagia, occasionally pain on swallowing, and possibly weight loss. The lower esophageal sphincter during manometry shows a persisting high resting pressure. Achalasia is a disorder of the esophageal smooth muscle. Cricopharyngeal achalasia, in contrast, is almost exclusively a disorder affecting elderly patients. A prominent indentation of the barium column during barium swallow is seen at the level of the cricopharyngeal muscle. If the condition causes recurrent pulmonary aspiration, cricopharyngeal myotomy is the treatment of choice.

EVALUATION

Barium swallow is usually the first step in identifying potential structural problems. This is followed by endoscopy with biopsy and brush cytology if indicated. Cineradiography providing a visual image and esophageal manometry which measures pressures simultaneously at different levels of the esophagus may offer assistance in motor disorders.

GASTRITIS AND PEPTIC ULCER

Indigestion is a common complaint, manifested by lower chest and upper abdominal discomfort associated with the ingestion of food. The sensation may be the result of esophageal reflux, direct mucosal injury secondary to foods or medications (especially arthritis medications that may be taken near meals), food intolerance, or gas. Spicy foods are blamed for the majority of occurrences of indigestion.

The clinical presentation of peptic ulcer disease can vary greatly in the elderly, making recognition more difficult (Jacknowitz, 1984). The patients may not recall any previous classic symptoms. If symptoms are present, they tend to be vague and often atypical. A pattern of pain may be difficult to define and localize. Instead, loss of appetite, nausea, vomiting, and weight loss may be the dominant symptoms. The vagueness of the symptoms may not prompt appropriate investigation.

The elderly patient is more likely to present with a major complication as the first indication of an ulcer. Hospitalization for gastrointestinal hemorrhage, perforation, persistent nausea and vomiting from pyloric obstruction, or large loss of weight accompanied by weakness, or anorexia not controlled by diet or drug therapy are likely presentations. Bleeding is the most common complication of peptic ulcer in the elderly and accounts for one half to two thirds of all fatal cases (Sterup and Mosbeck, 1973).

Treatment

Patient compliance and cost are major problems with antacid use in elderly patients. Patients take only an average of 30 to 45 per cent of the amount of antacid recommended when they are not subjected to rigorously controlled clinical trials (McCarthy, 1979). In addition, aluminum hydroxide may be neurotoxic in patients with chronic renal failure and can produce a syndrome compatible with Alzheimer's disease. Sucralfate causes few adverse effects because it is not absorbed. It can be combined with antacids if pain relief is needed, but antacids should not be given within 30 minutes of sucralfate administration because of possible interference in the binding action with proteinacious material and the formation of a protective barrier at the site of the ulcer. Sucralfate does not neutralize gastric acid. No significant interactions with other drugs have been reported.

Cimetidine, an H_2-receptor antagonist, inhibits the secretion of gastric acid. Its use is occasionally associated with mental confusion which usually begins within 24 to 48 hours after the first dose with symptoms of flushing, sweating, confusion, disorientation, and agitation. Hallucinations, focal twitching, seizures, and unresponsiveness may also occur.

Ranitidine has a long duration of action with a twice daily dosage regimen, relatively low interaction potential, and an apparently low level of adverse effects, all of which make it also an excellent therapy. Famotidine and nizatidine are other H_2-receptor antagonists and are used for treatment and maintenance therapy for active duodenal ulcer. They do not apparently interfere with the hepatic metabolism of various other drugs such as anticoagulants and theophylline (Medical Letter, 1988a).

GALLBLADDER DISEASE

Cholelithiasis and cholecystitis are the problems most often seen in the elderly involving the biliary tract. The present opinion is that elective cholecystectomy for asymptomatic gallstones should usually be reserved for patients under the age of 60. The only exceptions are those older patients with diabetes mellitus. If the patient is an appropriate candidate, the treatment of symptomatic cholelithiasis is surgery.

In patients who have a functioning gallbladder, treatment with medications to dissolve gallstones along with lithotripsy will become more available. Choledocholithiasis is also common in the geriatric population and may present more commonly with obstructive jaundice but without the typical biliary colic. Fiberoptic endoscopic papillotomy to remove gallstones at the lower end of the common bile duct is particularly valuable in older patients who may be poor risks for surgery (Cohen, 1980). It should be remembered also that painless jaundice may be the result of malignant obstruction of the biliary tract. Hepatocellular disease is the cause of jaundice in only about 16 per cent of elderly patients. Other potential causes of jaundice are hemolytic disease and drugs causing hepatotoxicity. Primary carcinoma of the liver is rare. The liver, however, is a very common site for metastases from many primary malignancies.

VASCULAR DISEASE OF THE BOWEL

Abdominal angina is manifested by intermittent dull or cramping abdominal pain (Chopra and Curtis, 1985). It usually occurs 10 to 15 minutes after a meal and may last for several hours. Most patients are elderly and have evidence of arteriosclerotic disease in other places in the vascular system. A fear of eating develops with resulting significant weight loss. Barium studies are of little help early. Angiography is the most helpful test but is invasive. Involvement of the three major splanchnic vessels (celiac, superior mesenteric, and inferior mesenteric arteries) may show significant levels of obstruction. Angiography, however, only supports a clinical diagnosis. The decision to operate is a difficult one and should be based on a combination of careful clinical evaluation and angiographic findings. Other pathologic conditions have to be excluded.

Mesenteric embolization is most commonly seen in patients with rheumatic or postmyocardial infarction or in patients with mural thrombi. Occasionally emboli come from vegetations of bacterial endocarditis, valvular prostheses, arteriosclerotic plaques, or, rarely, atrial myxomas. The onset of symptoms is usually acute and consists of severe abdominal pain, nausea, vomiting, and diarrhea which becomes Hemoccult positive with bowel infarction. Gastrointestinal bleeding and evidence of intestinal obstruction may not be present initially. Physical findings may be minimal, with few abdominal signs at early presentation.

Preoperative angiography should be carried out early. Laparotomy and embolectomy should be performed on an emergency basis if vascular obstruction is found. A "second look" operation may be necessary for persistent abdominal symptoms to recheck intestinal viability.

Because pre-existing collateral blood flow is often present, mesenteric thrombosis has a less sudden onset than mesenteric arterial embolism. Approximately 50 per cent of patients with acute thrombotic infarction of the intestine will give a history of previous abdominal angina. In nonocclusive intestinal infarction, there is no occlusion of major arteries. There is, however, involvement of the smaller arterioles, capillaries, and venules. Most patients are elderly and have severe congestive heart failure, significant hypotension, or hypoxemia. Digitalis, known to cause mesenteric vasoconstriction, may be a potential etiology. The clinical presentation is similar to that of occlusion. Angiography may be beneficial in excluding large thrombotic or embolic occlusions and give an angiographic pattern relatively specific for this syndrome. Mortality is very high owing to the presence of complicating illnesses and lack of effective therapy.

The acute onset of lower abdominal pain and diarrhea in an elderly patient is more likely to represent an episode of ischemic colitis than one of inflammatory bowel disease. It may be confused with diverticulitis. Sigmoidoscopy, however, reveals the presence of proctitis, mucosal ulceration, or bluish-black nodular lesions. Rectal biopsy may show ischemic necrosis but is often nonspecific. "Thumbprinting" is seen on plain films or barium enema. The acute onset and rapid resolution help separate this diagnosis from inflammatory bowel disease. Patients usually recover from ischemic colitis, but they may occasionally develop strictures.

Polyarteritis nodosa, a systemic vasculitis, can present in the older or younger adult. The presenting syndrome depends on the distribution, the vessels involved, and the collateral blood supply that may have developed. Frequently the patient presents with symptoms of intermittent small bowel obstruction.

DIVERTICULAR DISEASE

Diverticula of the colon are uncommon in the adult below the age of 40. They occur in 20 to 30 per cent of people over age 60 and are found in more than 40 per cent of persons over age 80. Diverticula are usually asymptomatic but can present with classic pain. They represent a confusing and complicated intra-abdominal process in the elderly. The presence of diverticula is usually established by a barium enema. This should not be performed during a suspected attack because of the potential of complications. Diverticula can also be identified during sigmoidoscopy or colonoscopy (Cohen, 1980).

CONSTIPATION

Constipation is defined as a decrease in the frequency of bowel movements accompanied by difficult passage of hard stool or bowel movements followed by a sensation of incomplete evacuation (Derezin, 1974). The most common cause of true constipation is failure to pass the stool when the urge to pass stool is precipitated by rectal distention. This sensation may not be recognized in the immobile or otherwise compromised older patient.

Many elderly have strong beliefs that a daily bowel movement is necessary to good health. In one study over 98 per cent of 1455 patients, which included elderly patients, had bowel movements in the range of three per day to three per week. (Connel, 1965). A bowel movement that occurs at least once a week is still considered to be within the normal range. A major factor leading to constipation in the elderly is lack of mobility owing to stroke, depression, senility, or other chronic debilitating diseases. Poor nutrition and a decreased fluid intake may also produce constipation.

Numerous medications taken for chronic illnesses may also contribute significantly to constipation. Verapamil, anticholinergics, phenothiazines, tricyclic antidepressants, sedatives, opiates (especially codeine), iron salts, and calcium-containing antacids are a few. Continuous abuse of laxatives by patients or continued use by a health care facility is another cause of constipation. Other causes include hypothyroidism, hypercalcemia, or intestinal obstruction.

Complications of chronic constipation include fecal impaction and megacolon (Elliot et al., 1983). Severe fecal impaction can rarely lead to intestinal obstruction or intestinal perforation. However, more complications result from chronic laxative use than from constipation. Chronic use of stimulant laxatives may result in the "cathartic colon." Electrolyte disorders can also be caused by frequent laxative use. Melanosis coli is dark pigmentation of the mucosa of the colon from use of anthracene derivatives such as cascara, senna, or aloe. The pigmentation will resolve from 4 months to 20 months following discontinuation of the laxative.

Treatment

A moderate increase in the amount of bran or other dietary fiber in the daily diet can be an effective treatment for constipation. One to 2 tablespoonfuls daily in orange juice can be helpful. Patients with an atonic colon are not always responsive to treatment with bran, since such therapy may actually add to the problem by increasing the bulk in an already distended colon. Atonic colon is usually treated by enemas or manual disimpaction. One regimen may be to give an enema (such as a hypertonic phosphate enema) daily for a period of approximately 7 to 10 days. Once this form of constipation has been relieved, the weekly use of an enema or a bisacodyl or glycerin suppository may be all that is necessary.

Bulk-forming laxatives include methylcellulose, sodium carboxymethylcellulose, polycarbophil, and psyllium. They cause retention of large amounts of water, thus preventing constipation, and paradoxically may also be effective in the management of diarrhea. Hyperosmotic laxatives are glycerin and lactulose. Glycerin is used only in the suppository form since it is rapidly absorbed when taken orally. Lactulose, previously used only in hepatic encephalopathy, has few side effects and is useful in treating constipation in the elderly. Surfactant laxatives such as dioctyl sulfosuccinates allow the fecal material to be penetrated by water and fat. Use of emollient laxatives such as mineral oil can result in deficiencies of the fat soluble vitamins A, D, E, and K. Aspiration of the mineral oil may produce pneumonitis and pulmonary fibrosis (Jacknowitz, 1984).

FECAL INCONTINENCE

Fecal incontinence is frequently seen in elderly patients, particularly in association with dementia (Smith, 1983). It can result from diseases affecting the colon, fecal stasis, or neurologic disorders.

FECAL STASIS

Fecal stasis is by far the most common single cause of fecal incontinence in the elderly. It is associated with immobility and is commonly seen in hospitalized and nursing home patients. Ninety-eight per cent of fecal impaction is rectal and is easily diagnosed by digital examination.

NEUROLOGIC DISORDERS OF THE GI SYSTEM

Local

Change can occur in the normal anorectal function when prolonged straining at stool causes the syndrome of the descending perineum (Parkes et al., 1966). Also, prolonged use of laxatives or other drugs such as anticholinergics and phenothiazines can result in toxic damage to the nerve plexus. The resulting laxity in the sphincter muscles and the loss of the anal reflex leads to a reduction in loss of angulation of the anal canal (Smith, 1983).

Central

Loss of central inhibition to the defecation reflex from severe mental impairment is much more common than local change. The patient is unable to inhibit intrinsic rectal contractions that result from rectal distention (Brocklehurst, 1972). The resulting symptoms are passage of formed stool once or twice daily in the bed or clothing, usually followed by the gastrocolic reflex.

Management

Immediate. It is essential to exclude reversible disease as a possible cause of fecal incontinence. A careful evaluation, including history of the current use of prescribed and nonprescribed medications, should be done. A thorough physical, including neurologic exam, sigmoidoscopy, and possibly a barium enema, is recommended. A mental status exam is necessary and assists greatly in choosing the treatment plan and determining ultimate prognosis.

Treatment of associated disease states that may be found, such as carcinoma, ischemic colitis, or diverticular disease may be helpful. Drugs felt to be contributing to the problem should be stopped if possible. Fecal stasis can be resolved using small bulk enemas. Regular bowel movements should be encouraged using a standard bowel elimination program.

Long Term. Establish a regular toilet pattern. It is possible to use the physiologic gastrocolic reflex to establish a regular pattern of bowel emptying. Retraining is done by attempting to pass stool regularly after meals. Increase dietary fiber and ensure food and fluid intake of at least 2 liters per day. Mobility should be maintained as much as possible.

In patients in whom there is a local neurologic cause of fecal incontinence, surgical repair of rectal prolapse is successful in 70 per cent of cases (Keighley et al., 1980). If the uninhibited neurogenic rectum exists, the proper treatment is to use a constipating agent in the morning and a purgative at night (Jarratt and Exton-Smith, 1960) or a constipating agent daily with twice weekly enemas or manual removal after use of a stool softener (Brocklehurst, 1972). These measures have been found to be helpful in controlling the number of incontinent episodes. Toileting after meals reinforced with a suppository or small bulk enema may also be effective in mild cases.

VOLVULUS

Volvulus of the colon occurs mostly in elderly patients, usually over 70. Abdominal distention, pain, and constipation may be deceptively mild in the older patient. Abdominal x-rays usually suggest volvulus. Sigmoidoscopy or a barium enema can often reduce the volvulus. Surgery may not be necessary if the volvulus is not recurrent (Cohen, 1980).

CARCINOMA OF THE COLON

Carcinoma of the colon is predominantly a disease of the aged and seems to be increasing in incidence

(Cohen, 1980). Regular evaluation according to guidelines for screening should be followed. Family history of colon cancer is also a factor. Aggressive screening and evaluation of change in bowel habits or bleeding are indicated in the elderly.

Genitourinary Tract Problems

Genitourinary tract disorders constitute a major health problem. They are the most common problems among nursing home residents, exceeding even heart disease (Resnick et al, 1989). Most urinary tract infections in the elderly, however, are asymptomatic. Also, women may complain of dysuria, frequency, and incontinence, but not have an infection when a urine culture is obtained. However, patients who do have symptomatic infections should be treated.

URINARY TRACT INFECTIONS IN WOMEN

The diagnosis of urinary tract infection in all age groups is usually determined by quantitative cultures of clean catch midstream urine specimens. One culture with greater than 10^5 bacteria per ml. has an 80 per cent probability of indicating infection. Two cultures with titers reading greater than 10^5 of the same bacteria have a 95 per cent probability of indicating urinary tract infection. However, these statistics have been challenged and may not apply in elderly women.

Comparison (Moore-Smith, 1972) of midstream and suprapubic urine cultures from elderly hospitalized women (mean age 79) found 30 per cent positive by midstream culture, but only 13 per cent positive by suprapubic aspirate. This yields a 57 per cent false-positive rate or only a 43 per cent probability of indicating infection. Other studies (Klarsov, 1976) report much lower false-positive midstream quantitative cultures (e.g., 10 per cent in elderly women).

The accuracy of midstream urine cultures from elderly women is undoubtedly related to the degree of effort given in obtaining a true midstream urine specimen after proper cleansing. This can be better facilitated with the help of assistants to collect the specimen (Lye, 1978). If it is impossible to obtain a satisfactory midstream specimen, catheterization may be done or suprapubic aspiration. The latter, however, is technically demanding and causes some discomfort in the elderly.

The prevalence of asymptomatic urinary tract infection in predominantly ambulatory and self-sufficient elderly women is approximately 13 per cent (Bertakis and Ross, 1987). However, almost all women who have symptomatic urinary tract infections have recurrent infections instead of persistent infections. One study concluded that radiologic and endoscopic examination of the urinary tract will rarely uncover abnormalities that alter the management of recurrent urinary tract infections in women. In 104 excretory urograms, renal cell carcinoma was a finding in only one patient. Among 75 cystograms and 74 cystoscopic examinations, there were three urethral diverticuli found and one case of transitional cell carcinoma of the bladder (Fowler and Pulaski, 1981).

ACUTE SYMPTOMATIC URINARY TRACT INFECTIONS

As in younger people, dysuria and increased urinary frequency are the most common symptoms of cystitis. However signs and symptoms of an upper urinary tract infection may be vague or absent. The patient may not experience fever, chills, flank pain, costovertebral angle tenderness, and dysuria. They may present only with a history of decreased oral intake and lethargy. Tachypnea, tachycardia, vague abdominal pain, and abrupt mental status changes may be the only symptoms. Urinalysis and culture are essential to proper diagnosis. Elevated white blood cell counts with a left shift associated with systemic symptoms indicate pyelonephritis. Blood cultures are also helpful in the care of these patients.

E. coli remains the most common cause of infection in the elderly. The gram-positive coccus *Enterococcus* is also more common in elderly patients than in younger patients. Other potential organisms are *Klebsiella, Enterobacter, Proteus mirabilis,* and *Pseudomonas aeruginosa*. When the urine pH is above 7, the infecting organism is usually proteus. The high pH is due to the production of urease, which degrades urea to ammonia. High urine pH is also associated with the formation of renal stones.

Treatment

Cystitis in the elderly patient is usually resolved with an oral antibiotic. Treatment regimens include single-dose therapy, a 3-day regimen, and 7 to 14 day regimens. Trimethoprim/sulfamethoxazole, trimethoprim alone, and amoxicillin or ampicillin are useful. Other useful options are amoxicillin/potassium clavulanate, a first-generation cephalosporin, a sulfonamide, or a tetracycline.

Pyelonephritis always warrants hospital admission in elderly patients and aggressive therapy with intravenous antibiotics. The choice of trimethoprim/sulfamethoxazole, an aminoglycoside, or a cephalosporin is usually adequate as initial therapy. Ampicillin should never be used alone initially but may be used in combination or later when sensitivities prove efficacy.

The quinolone antibiotics norfloxacin and ciprofloxacin HCl are newly marketed. They are more effective with gram-negative organisms then other oral antibiotics. Norfloxacin is not indicated for patients with suspected bacteremia. The dosage of norfloxacin is 400 mg. two times a day and for ciprofloxacin, 250 to 500 mg. two times a day.

Investigation of the urinary tract is generally unnecessary unless fever persists. If the patient does not improve or sepsis worsens, obtain a renal ultrasound to look for possible obstruction or perinephric abscesses. Close following of pyelonephritis is essential to a positive outcome in the elderly.

Asymptomatic bacteriuria occurs frequently in noncatheterized elderly men and women. Almost all patients with catheters become colonized. Although the management of asymptomatic bacteriuria has been controversial, it is unusual that such infections become symptomatic, and there does not seem to be any association with the subsequent development of renal failure. Mortality also does not seem to be affected. If treatment is tried, more resistant organisms become dominant. Physicians should consider treating asymptomatic patients who have diabetes mellitus and those with urinary tract obstructions.

CHRONIC URINARY TRACT INFECTIONS

The prevalence of bacteriuria increases with age, and in the elderly, the prevalence also increases with advancing functional disability (Kaye, 1980; Lye, 1978). Of possible factors precipitating the initial development of bacteriuria in a population, concurrent illness is the most frequent. The mechanism by which illness precipitates bacteriuria is not known, but decreased mobility with impaired bladder emptying is a possible explanation (Nicolle et al., 1983). Institution of condom drainage in male patients for the management of incontinence also tends to precipitate bacteriuria (Hirsh et al., 1979).

Although evidence regarding increased morbidity and mortality associated with bacteriuria (Dontas et al., 1981) is conflicting, most authors (Kaye, 1981) do not recommend treating the asymptomatic patient. In the absence of underlying structural abnormalities, bacteriuria does not contribute to renal failure. Therapy is often ineffective in eliminating bacteriuria and does not change morbidity or total mortality from infection. Attempts at therapy may result in superinfection, emergence of resistant organisms, or drug-related side effects. Thus, asymptomatic bacteriuria in the majority of elderly men appears to be a benign condition (Freedman, 1975).

RECURRENT URINARY TRACT INFECTIONS

Persons who have infrequent infections are easily treated. If reinfections are frequent and symptomatic, prophylactic therapy should be used following treatment of the last acute infection. Long-term prophylaxis should be followed with urine cultures obtained monthly. Therapy should be adjusted if bacteriuria recurs.

URINARY INCONTINENCE

It appears that 10 to 20 per cent of the elderly living in the community and close to 50 per cent of elderly patients in nursing homes have some degree of urinary incontinence (Mohide, 1986; Yarnell and St Leger, 1979). Functional disabilities (other than incontinence) and impaired cognitive function common among hospitalized elderly patients are strongly associated with incontinence (Sier et al., 1987). Urinary incontinence is a pathologic condition that, when rationally approached, can usually be ameliorated or cured, often without invasive tests or surgery and almost invariable without an indwelling catheter (Marron et al., 1983).

Urge Incontinence

Urge incontinence, the most common type in the elderly (Resnick et al., 1989), occurs when involuntary voiding is preceded by a warning of a few seconds to a few minutes. Leakage is periodic but frequent. The usual cause is detrusor overactivity, a condition in which the bladder escapes central inhibition and contracts reflexively. Other causes include a local bladder disorder such as acute or interstitial cystitis, carcinoma-in-situ, or radiation-induced irritation of the bladder. In addition, central nervous system damage owing to stroke, Alzheimer's disease, brain tumor, or Parkinson's disease, and interference with spinal inhibitory pathways owing to spondylolysis or metastasis can cause urge incontinence.

Initial management involves identification and treatment of reversible causes. Many causes, however, are not responsive to specific therapy. Simple measures such as providing a bedside commode or a urinal, as well as asking the patient to void more frequently, are often successful. Toileting regimens may be useful in patients with advanced cognitive impairment.

Pharmacologic intervention can be added, although little data are available regarding efficacy and toxicity. Smooth-muscle relaxants such as flavoxate (300 to 800 mg. per day in divided doses) and calcium channel blockers have been used, as have anticholinergic agents such as propantheline (15 to 120 mg. per day). Oxybutynin (5 to 20 mg. per day), combining both smooth-muscle-relaxant and anticholinergic properties, and imipramine (50 to 150 mg. per day) are frequently successful. All drugs are given in divided doses. Potential adverse effects must be weighed against desired results. Postvoiding residual volume and common indices of renal function (BUN, serum creatinine, and urine output) should be monitored, since urinary retention may develop with these medications.

Reflex Incontinence

Reflex incontinence is present when no stress or warning precedes involuntary voiding. Voiding is frequent all during the day and the volume is moderate (Resnick and Yalla, 1985). Classically, reflex incontinence is due to a suprasacral spinal-cord lesion above the voiding reflex arc. The most common cause is trauma, but it can also be caused by tumor or multiple sclerosis. The potential of infection, hydronephrosis, stone formation, and ultimate renal damage is high (Tanagho, 1978). However, severe cortical damage in the elderly may also simulate this condition.

The goal of treatment is to maintain the best possible functional capacity while controlling infection and incontinence and preserving renal function. Attempts at control of incontinence should not be detrimental to the preservation of renal function. Attempts at management are largely dependent on the capacity of the bladder. It is sometimes possible for patients with large capacities to train bladder emptying by developing a trigger maneuver such as applying lower abdominal pressure with the hand or squeezing the genitalia. Those with very low capacities cannot successfully do bladder training. A permanent catheter or surgical drainage system can be used. Parasympatholytic drugs such as propantheline bromide may be tried, but they are effective only in selected patients.

Stress Incontinence

Involuntary leakage that occurs only during stress such as coughing, laughing, or rising from a chair is common in elderly women but unusual in men unless the sphincter has been damaged during prior urinary tract surgery. Stress incontinence is characterized by daytime loss of small amounts of urine and infrequent incontinence while lying down. There is usually a low postvoiding residual volume. The most common cause is urethral hypermobility owing to pelvic floor weakness.

Stress incontinence is improved through weight loss if the patient is obese or by treatment of conditions that precipitate incontinence such as cough or atrophic vaginitis. Pelvic-floor exercises have been used and are frequently effective, especially if combined with estrogen applied locally or given orally.

If urethral hypermobility is diagnosed, surgery can correct the problem and is successful in the majority of elderly patients. An alpha-adrenergic agonist such as phenylpropanolamine (50 to 100 mg. per day in divided doses) can be useful. If all other interventions fail or are contraindicated, intravaginal devices, such as a pessary, may be useful. These devices require periodic inspection of the vaginal wall to monitor for irritation and ulceration. Condom catheters or penile clamps may be useful for men. Pads and diapers are helpful measures, but their use can depress or limit patients who desire to remain socially active.

Overflow Incontinence

Overflow incontinence occurs when the weight of urine in a distended bladder equals outlet resistance. This condition causes constant leakage of small amounts of urine throughout the day and night. The patient may also have a need to strain, a diminished urine flow, and a sense of incomplete emptying. The residual urine volume is large, and the bladder may be palpable or seen on an abdominal x-ray.

In males, outlet obstruction is caused by prostatic hypertrophy or urethral stricture. Outlet obstruction is uncommon in females but can be caused by an underactive detrusor secondary to muscle or neurogenic factors such as a disc or peripheral neuropathy associated with diabetes mellitus, vitamin B_{12} deficiency, or tabes dorsalis. Since obstruction can cause renal damage and clinical diagnosis is difficult, urologic investigation is indicated.

If obstruction is excluded, the first step is to use indwelling or intermittent catheterization to decompress the bladder for at least 10 to 14 days. A check should be made for potential infection. If decompressing the bladder does not cause bladder function to return, augmented voiding techniques such as double voiding and the use of the Credé or Valsalva maneuver may be helpful.

If the cause of obstruction can be surgically corrected, surgery is the treatment of choice. If surgery is contraindicated, several medications can be helpful. Prazosin is an alpha blocker and can reduce outlet resistance in order to further facilitate emptying. It is given at a dosage of 3 to 12 mg. per day in divided doses. Bethanechol (40 to 200 mg. per day in divided doses) is occasionally useful in the patient whose bladder contracts poorly. Again, potential adverse effects must be carefully considered prior to using these medications in elderly patients.

If the postvoiding residual volume remains high, intermittent catheterization is indicated. The goal is to keep urine volume below 300 ml. Prophylaxis against urinary infection is warranted. If an indwelling catheter is used, neither antibiotic nor antiseptic prophylaxis for urinary infection appears to be helpful (Warren et al., 1981).

LONG-TERM URETHRAL CATHETERS IN OLDER PATIENTS

When such measures as behavioral training, drugs, special clothing, and nursing care fail to keep a patient dry, some type of urine-collecting device may be needed. For men, the condom catheter has been used for decades. An indwelling catheter may be considered.

However, long-term catheterization for both men and women entails the possibility of several complications (Table 10–15). Bacteriuria invariably develops with a closed system catheter which has been in place for 30 days or more (Munchie and Warren, 1988; Warren et al., 1982b). At present, the most effective method of preventing bacterial entry is careful maintenance of the closed catheter system. The administration of a systemic antibiotic intermittently or over

Table 10–15. COMPLICATIONS OF LONG-TERM URETHRAL CATHETERIZATION*

Acute
Bacteremia
Fever
Pyelonephritis
Chronic
Local infections
Urinary tract stones
Vesicoureteral reflux
Tubulointerstitial nephritis
Renal failure

*From Munchie, H. L., and Warren, J. W.: Long-term urethral catheters in older women. Am. Fam. Physician, 37:107, 1988.

a prolonged period is not useful clinically and may lead to infection with antibiotic-resistant organisms (Warren et al., 1982a; Warren et al., 1981).

SEXUALITY

Drug-induced sexual dysfunction in males is a secondary cause of sexual dysfunction and is becoming increasingly apparent. Drug-related sexual dysfunction also applies to women and is usually related to vaginitis causing dyspareunia or to a decrease in libido. This fact is usually not mentioned in articles on the subject (Medical Letter, 1987a). Drugs that cause sexual dysfunction are listed in Table 10–16.

Antihypertensive agents probably interfere with sexual function more than any other type of drug, but dysfunction that occurs with one antihypertensive drug may not recur with another (Medical Letter, 1987b). Antihypertensive drugs generally thought not to cause sexual dysfunction include the angiotensin-converting enzyme inhibitors (captopril and enalapril), calcium-channel blockers (verapamil), and the arteriolar dilating agent (hydralazine).

The four most common causes of sexual dysfunction in men, other than drugs, are vascular, endocrine, neurologic, and psychogenic. Other nondrug causes are end-organ problems such as Peyronie's disease and chordee (Nelson, 1987). There is frequently an overlap, as in diabetic patients who have both vascular and neurologic components. Complete history and physical examination is always appropriate for the initial evaluation of sexual dysfunction.

Laboratory Tests

The following laboratory tests can be used to determine underlying causes of sexual dysfunction:

- CBC
- SMA-12 (liver function, cholesterol, and creatinine)
- urinalysis
- serum testosterone (if low or low normal, measure serum prolactin, FSH, and LH) (Nelson, 1987)

Special Tests

1. Penile blood pressures measured with Doppler of the cavernosal arteries on the right and left dorsum of the coronal sulcus and compared with the brachial systolic pressure, giving a penile brachial index (PBI, normal >0.8)
2. Nocturnal penile tumescence
3. Video monitoring with a bend test
4. Evoked response nerve conduction delay
5. Arteriography
6. Cavernosography (Nelson, 1987)

Advances in surgical oncology, which reduce the incidence of impotence after prostatectomy and cystectomy, and increasing knowledge in the neurophysiology of erection may reduce the incidence of impotency and the need for penile prosthesis (Walsh and Mostwin, 1984; Walsh and Donker, 1982).

Goals for Use of Penile Implants

1. Determine the primary complaint and the cause of the patient's sexual dysfunction (includes factors that initially caused the problem and then maintained the dysfunction, in addition to the spouse's reaction to the problem and the patient's overall relationship with his spouse or his sexual partner).
2. Identify which patients will benefit from nonsurgical treatment such as psychologic therapy, marital counseling, sexual counseling, medical treatment, penile pumps, or pharmacologic corporeal injections.
3. Assuming that organic causes have been documented, the next step is to evaluate the patient's motivation for surgery and to outline the patient's and his partner's expectations, particularly those of penile size and concealability.
4. Identify patients who, although motivated for surgery, will not respond well, as when surgery might precipitate emotional problems, especially if complications arise.
5. After complete evaluation for surgical implantation, the patient must be prepared for postoperative adjustments, such as routine postoperative care and dealing with his partner's fears about other sexual partners or whether the patient will sufficiently involve himself in his partner's arousal before penetration (Nelson, 1987).

Physicians must assess carefully their patient's candidacy for a penile prosthesis and, just as important, noncandidacy, as malpractice claims involving sexual dysfunction are now the third highest in the field of urology (Malloy, 1984).

RENAL FAILURE

The family physician should periodically monitor renal function in elderly patients and work to avoid potential preventable causes of acute and chronic renal failure. First, older patients have a reduced

Table 10–16. DRUG-INDUCED SEXUAL DYSFUNCTION*

acetozolamide	loss of libido; decreased potency
alcohol	decreases libido; causes gynecomastia; and interferes with sperm production
alprazolam	inhibition of orgasm; delayed or no ejaculation
amitriptyline	loss of libido; impotence; no ejaculation
anticholinergic tricyclic antidepressants	block dilation of the arterial supply to the corpus cavernosum and corpus spongiosum
amiloride	impotence; decreased libido
amoxapine	raises prolactin level
barbiturates	decreased libido; impotence
beta blockers	penetrate CNS because they are lipophilic, causing central sympatholytic effects
carbamazepine	impotence
central sympatholytic agents (e.g., clonidine, guanethidine, methyldopa, reserpine)	through peripheral or central adrenergic blockage interferes with dilation of the arteries supplying the corpora and possibly blocks autonomic transmission needed for emission and antegrade ejaculation
chlorpromazine	decreased libido; impotence; no ejaculation; priapism
chorthalidone	decreased libido; impotence
cimetidine	antiandrogen
clofibrate	antiandrogen
clonidine	impotence; delayed or retrograde ejaculation
CNS depressants	impotence; decreased libido
cocaine	causes ejaculatory disturbances; decreased libido with chronic use
diazepam	decreased libido; delayed ejaculation; retarded or no orgasm in women
digoxin	interferes with libido
hydralazine	impotence; priapism
indomethacin	interferes with libido
ketoconazole	impotence
levodopa	increased libido
lithium	decreased libido; impotence
marijuana	decreases libido; causes gynecomastia; and interferes with sperm production
methyldopa	elevates serum prolactin levels; decreased libido; impotence; impaired ejaculation
metoclopramide HCl	increases prolactin secretion; impotence; decreased libido
metronidazole	interferes with libido
opiates	increases prolactin levels
phenothiazide antipsychotics	block dilation of the arterial supply to the corpus cavernosum and corpus spongiosum
phenytoin	interferes with libido
prazosin	impotence; priapism
propranolol	loss of libido; impotence
ranitidine	loss of libido; impotence
reserpine	elevates serum prolactin levels
spironolactone	causes gynecomastia; decreases libido
thiazide diuretics	impotence
thioridazine	impotence; priapism; delayed, decreased, painful, retrograde, or no ejaculation
tobacco smoking	affects small peripheral vasculature, documented by statistically significant abnormal penile brachial index values
trazodone	priapism
verapamil	impotence

*Adapted from Med. Lett. Drugs Ther.: Drugs that cause sexual dysfunction. *29*:66–70, 1987; and Nelson, R. P.: Male sexual dysfunction: Evaluation and treatment. South. Med. J., *80*:70, 1987.

nephron mass and function compared with younger patients (Tinetti, 1983). In addition, older patients are more susceptible to dehydration, congestive heart failure, infection, hypertension, stress of surgery, and urinary obstruction.

Medications such as nonsteroidal anti-inflammatory drugs (NSAIDs) cause prerenal azotemia by a decrease in renal perfusion. The reduced perfusion is secondary to reduced synthesis of vasodilatory prostaglandins (Humes and Weinberg, 1986). Chronic tubulointerstitial nephritis can be caused by analgesic abuse.

Antibiotics are also commonly implicated. Aminoglycosides can cause a direct toxic effect on renal tubular epithelium (Cooper and Bennett, 1987). Immunologic hypersensitivity reactions causing allergic interstitial nephritis can be observed with numerous drugs including often used penicillin derivatives, sulfonamides, and diuretics. A primary glomerulopathy can result from gold therapy and captopril. Numerous drugs used in congestive heart failure and hypertension can interfere with fluid and electrolyte balance.

In general, radiocontrast agents are safe, but the elderly are especially susceptible to acute renal injury owing to dehydration, diabetes mellitus, or the presence of pre-existing chronic renal failure. The current agents contain iodine and are water soluble and hypertonic. They are used in intravenous urography, computed tomography, angiography, and venography and are primarily excreted by the kidney. The serum creatinine usually rises slightly and returns to normal; however, some patients may experience the oliguric phase of acute tubular necrosis, requiring careful fluid management and possibly dialysis.

The major treatment is prevention. Avoidance of known toxic drugs is important if possible. Should their use be necessary, close monitoring is important and changes should be made as indicated. Adequate treatment of infections and hypertension along with avoidance of serious dehydration will protect the elderly from the development of renal failure. Adequate fluid intake in elderly patients, who have a reduced sense of thirst, is important.

STONES

Although most renal stones are associated with a younger age group, stone formation with possible urinary obstruction may go unnoticed in the elderly. They may be discovered on abdominal x-rays done for other complaints, in evaluation of chronic or recurrent renal infections or renal failure, and during the emergency investigation of sepsis. General sepsis in the face of complete urinary obstruction is a urologic emergency. Dehydration, immobility, and infection with bacteria that produce urease, usually *Proteus* species, may all contribute to the development of stones in the elderly.

CANCER

Malignancy has been described in almost every part of the genitourinary tract. More common sites are the prostate, bladder, and kidney. The cancers are often diagnosed late. Gross or continued microscopic hematuria requires urologic investigation. Pain, dysuria, masses, increased hematocrit in the absence of lung disease, anemia, and undiagnosed fever can also be potential presenting symptoms. Treatment decisions are based on type of tumor, location, stage of disease, and functional capacity of the patient.

Osteoporosis

Osteoporosis is a generic term for an abnormally low total bone mass (i.e., bone matrix and mineral) (Bellantoni and Blackman, 1988). Accelerated bone loss during menopause appears to be related to estrogen deficiency. Not all women develop significant osteoporosis. Those who are thin, are Caucasian, have less bone mass, are smokers, and drink more than two alcoholic drinks per day appear to have a higher risk of osteoporosis and fractures.

Fractures that are commonly associated with osteoporosis in the elderly are hip, Colles', and spinal fractures. The differential diagnosis includes osteomalacia, primary hyperparathyroidism, hyperthyroidism, Cushing's syndrome, and multiple myeloma. Numerous techniques to evaluate bone mass have been devised. These include x-rays of the hand and spine, CT scan, x-ray photon densitometry, and single-beam and dual-beam photon absorptiometry.

Serum levels of calcium, phosphorus, alkaline phosphatase, and parathormone and urine excretion of calcium are also helpful. Iliac crest biopsies are also used in difficult cases. Serum electrophoresis, urine immunoelectrophoresis, and bone marrow examination should be done if multiple myeloma is suspected.

Exercise and good nutrition with adequate intake of calcium may be the best measures to prevent postmenopausal osteoporosis (Figure 10–8). Attention to prevention of falls is also an important preventive therapy. Medications, both prescribed and over-the-counter, can be a factor here. The proper use of assistance devices for persons with an unstable gait and the assessment of the home for hazards such as throw rugs, poorly lighted stairways, and low objects in walkways can protect the osteopenic elderly person from fall-related fractures (Bellantoni and Blackman, 1988).

At menopause, estrogen is the most effective drug for preventing the accelerated progression of osteoporosis. Estrogen replacement therapy that is begun at menopause slows bone loss and decreases the incidence of fractures (Ettinger et al., 1985). Many clinicians now add a progestin to cyclic estrogen to ensure more complete shedding of the endometrium to prevent endometrial hyperplasia and possibly carcinoma. The disadvantages of taking a progestin are light to moderate menstrual periods and possibly elevations in lipid profiles, which have been associated with an increased risk of cardiovascular disease (Gambrell, 1987; Whitehead and Fraser, 1987).

Once osteoporosis is present, sodium fluoride may prove helpful in increasing bone mass (Riggs et al., 1982). Recent studies have not provided strong support for the growing use of calcium supplements to retard postmenopausal bone loss (Stevenson et al., 1988). However, combined use with 0.3 mg. per day of conjugated estrogens (about half the usual dosage) with calcium was effective (Ettinger et al., 1987). Nevertheless, many Medical Letter consultants (1987b) believe a high calcium intake may prove helpful in preventing postmenopausal osteoporosis, especially if begun years before menopause. The required daily amount for adults is 800 mg. Higher amounts may be required in older patients, who do not absorb calcium as well from the gastrointestinal tract.

At the present time, it seems prudent to use these relatively inexpensive preventive therapies in

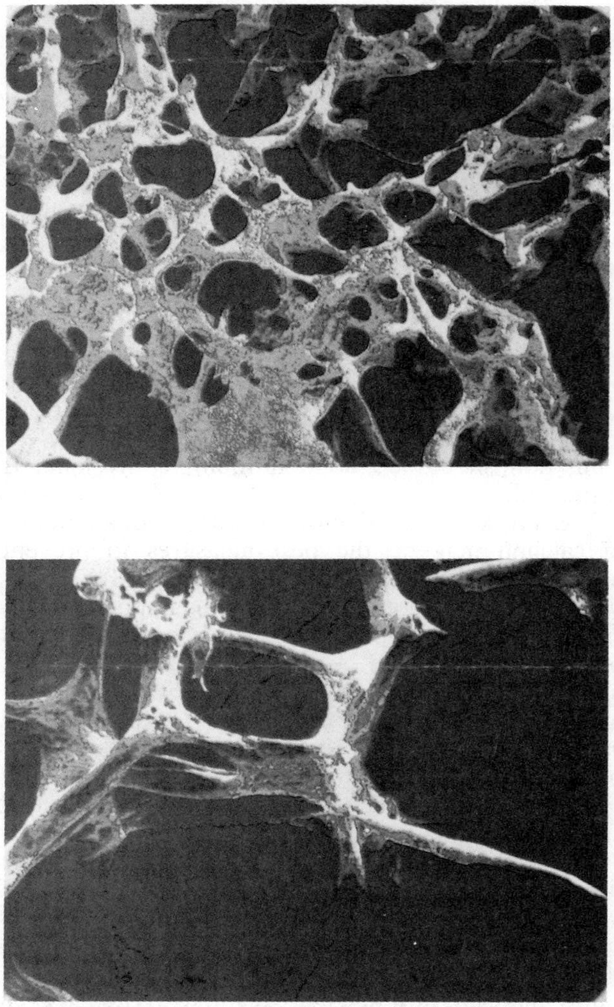

Figure 10–8. A scanning electron micrograph of trabecular bone from a healthy 40-year-old woman *(top)* shows the honeycomb array characteristic of the axial skeleton. Another color-enhanced electron micrograph at the same magnification shows trabecular bone from a 67-year-old woman with osteoporosis *(bottom)*. Although there is a major depletion of bone substance, the remaining trabeculae appear to be qualitatively normal. (From Marcus, R.: Osteoporosis alert: Clues to thinning bone. Diagnosis, August 1985, pp. 60–74.)

all elderly patients, rather than to do serial, expensive, sophisticated testing which has proven valuable as research documentation of osteoporosis (Bellantoni and Blackman, 1988). Advising aging patients on exercise, nutrition, and evaluation for estrogen replacement is the main component of management. Prevention of falls is imperative in the patient with an unstable gait.

Age-Related Pathologic Change: Skin Problems

Dermatitis in the elderly manifests two differences from that in younger patients. It is generally more

Table 10–17. PHYSIOLOGIC PARAMETERS IN HUMAN SKIN THAT DECLINE WITH AGE*

Growth rate	Immunosurveillance
Injury response	Vascular responsiveness
Barrier function	Thermoregulation
Chemical clearance rates	Sweat production
Sensory perception	Sebum production

*From Gilchrest, B. A.: Age-associated changes in the skin. J. Am. Geriatr. Soc., *30*:139, 1982.

resistant to treatment, and it often produces more significant distress for the patient. Expected alterations in elderly skin that accompany aging are noted on Table 10–17.

The "barnacles of life" also arise with age. However, most of these lesions are benign. Other disorders commonly listed are actinic keratoses, tinea pedis, contact dermatitis, seborrheic dermatitis, stasis dermatitis, and skin cancer (Beauregard and Gilchrest, 1987). The types of skin growths that commonly occur or increase with age are listed in Table 10–18.

Many benign skin lesions are associated with age, ranging from skin tags to keratoses and others. Senile keratosis, epithelioma, seborrheic keratosis, eczema, and contact dermatitis are common conditions which bring elderly patients to the physician. On the other hand, conditions such as alopecia and impetigo and other bacterial dermatitides are less frequently noted (Lane and Rockwood, 1949). Of major concern are malignant neoplasms which often are age- and sun-related. These include basal cell carcinoma, squamous cell carcinoma, and malignant melanoma. A high index of suspicion is the most able defense we have in regard to these disorders. Early biopsy of suspicious lesions or lesions responding poorly to topical therapy is strongly recommended. Some have the potential to be life-threatening. The majority of malignant skin lesions are basal cell epitheliomas which appear early as firm opalescent or "pearly" papules with fine telangiectases readily visible (Calkins et al., 1986). Most basal cell lesions occur in exposed areas and often in fair-skinned individuals with a history of excessive sun exposure.

Squamous cell skin cancers also occur largely in fair-skinned patients and also generally in heavily

Table 10–18. PROLIFERATIVE GROWTH ASSOCIATED WITH AGING IN HUMAN SKIN*

Lesion	Participating Cells or Tissue
Acrochrodon (skin tag)	Dermis, keratinocytes, melanocytes
Cherry angioma	Capillaries
Seborrheic keratosis	Dermis, keratinocytes, melanocytes
Lentigo	Melanocytes
Sebaceous hyperplasia	Sebaceous glands

*From Gilchrest, B. A.: Age-associated changes in the skin. J. Am. Geriatr. Soc., *30*:139, 1982.

sun-exposed areas. They appear early as asymptomatic firm red papules or plaques generally with a scaly surface. A more advanced lesion may appear as an ulcerated area that does not respond readily to conservative therapy or which on initial evaluation appears to deserve further definition (Calkins et al., 1986). In many of the lesions of the elderly, biopsy should be an early consideration.

The third major malignant neoplasm of grave concern is melanoma, which has been increasing by epidemic proportions in recent years. The previously defined malignancies, basal cell and squamous cell carcinoma, grow quite slowly and can be resolved definitively early to midcourse. However, early recognition is the absolute key to survival in malignant melanoma. Advancing age is commonly associated with poor prognosis in malignant melanoma. In the elderly, melanoma is characterized by an increasing proportion of deeper penetrating lesions (Cohen et al., 1987).

Diagnostic clues for melanoma include size (greater than 7 mm.), variation in color such as red, blue, or white in association with a black-brown lesion, brown irregular borders, and irregular surface. Seborrheic lesions, by contrast, can often be differentiated by their "stuck on" quality, their even brown pigmentation, and their regularly "irregular" surface (Sober et al., 1979, and Mihm et al., 1973). The key to therapy for basal cell and squamous cell lesions may include excision, liquid nitrogen, Moh's surgery, or electrodesiccation and currettage (Albright, 1979). However, for melanoma the only advisable therapy is excision, and this as early as possible.

Pruritus is another common complaint among elderly patients, both localized and generalized (Table 10–19). It is the most frequent complaint concerning the skin among elderly patients (Beauregard, 1987). The incidence of underlying systemic disease ranges up to 50 per cent (Rajka, 1966; Lyell, 1972).

If topical therapy for pruritus is not helpful, a relatively basic diagnostic evaluation is recommended, including serum creatinine, blood urea nitrogen, bilirubin, and liver enzymes and a CBC. A chest x-ray may also be justified in screening for malignancies (Calkins et al., 1986). The application of moisturizers promptly after bathing, while the skin is hydrated, is highly recommended for those with xerosis.

Table 10–19. SYSTEMIC DISORDERS SOMETIMES ASSOCIATED WITH PRURITUS IN THE ELDERLY*

Renal	Chronic renal failure
Hepatic	Extrahepatic bilary obstruction
	Hepatitis
	Drug ingestion
Hematopoietic	Polycythemia vera
	Hodgkin's disease
	Other lymphomas and leukemias
	Multiple myeloma
	Iron deficiency anemia
Endocrine	Hyperthyroidism
	Diabetes mellitus
Miscellaneous	Visceral malignancies
	Opiate ingestion
	Drug ingestion
	Psychosis

*From Gilchrest, B. A.: Pruritus pathogenesis therapy and significance in systemic disease states. Arch. Intern. Med., *142*:101, 1982.

Infections

There are several factors distinctive to elderly patients that make diagnosis of infections important to their care. As has been mentioned, there is a decline in immune status associated with age as well as in association with chronic disease. In addition, elderly patients are more likely to delay seeking treatment. Initially, the symptoms of infection may be significantly blunted, and the patient and family members may not recognize the severity of illness. The fever may not be high, the cough may not be significant, or the pain may not be intense.

Delay in seeking treatment also can be attributed to reluctance to leave home, a fear or dislike of hospitalization, or inability to pay for medical care. Elderly patients may feel that going to a hospital might be a prelude to death. In addition, the physicians might find a disabling or catastrophic disease not already diagnosed (Albano et al., 1975).

Elderly people who reside in nursing homes are more likely to contract an infection than those who live in the community (Abrutyn et al., 1988). The close environment is convenient for person-to-person spread of contagious disease. Respiratory syncytial virus, influenza, gastrointestinal viruses, and other infections can be rapidly spread in a nursing home population. Nursing homes are an ideal setting for the spread of communicable illnesses, but other factors include chronic debility and immobility, poor nutrition, and a declining immune system.

Consideration of several other infectious diseases is particularly important to the elderly person in terms of morbidity and mortality (Yoshikawa, 1981). Other than respiratory illnesses, geriatric patients are susceptible to urinary tract infection, skin and soft tissue infection, herpes zoster, intra-abdominal sepsis, and gram-negative bacteremia. Less common infections are bacterial arthritis, bacterial meningitis, infective endocarditis, and tuberculosis.

INFLUENZA

Influenza in the elderly may present with classic symptoms but may also present with an acute decompensation of a chronic illness such as lung or heart disease. Patients should be immunized against influenza during autumn, preceding the influenza season. Amantadine may be used for prophylaxis during influenza A epidemics, but this does not supersede recommendations for vaccination. Elderly patients should be cautioned against exposure to influenza if possible. If they do develop influenza, they should be monitored closely for the development of complications by family members, friends, and health care providers.

PNEUMONIA

Physical examination may give more information than a chest x-ray early in the course of pneumonia (Louria, 1986). Fever, cough, pleuritic chest pain, focal rales, and dullness to percussion should prompt one to begin therapy since x-ray findings may lag behind. Chest x-rays can also be falsely negative if the patient is significantly dehydrated. Delay in therapy by several hours in a bacteremic patient may have serious effects on patient outcome.

As in the community (Garb et al., 1978), *Streptococcus pneumoniae* is the most common cause of bacterial pneumonia (Berk et al., 1981) in nursing home patients. Splenectomy, chronic obstructive pulmonary disease (COPD), and multiple myeloma predispose patients to pneumococcal disease. Other gram-positive etiologic bacteria may be *Staphylococcus aureus* and, occasionally, Groups A and B streptococci.

Hospitalized patients and nursing home residents are more subject to aerobic gram-negative bacilli, particularly *Escherichia coli, Klebsiella pneumoniae*, and *Enterobacter* (Ebright and Rytel, 1980). *Legionella pneumophilia* and bacterial pneumonias complicating influenza are also common in these patients. *Branhamella catarrhalis* has also been recognized in nursing home residents. Reactivation of or primary tuberculosis should always be a suspect in the clinical setting of a respiratory infection that does not follow a normal course of resolution.

Mixed pneumonia caused by anaerobes and gram-negative bacilli is also common in older individuals because of their tendency to aspirate, especially those who have dysphagia, those who have a decreased level of consciousness, or those who are undergoing nasogastric feedings (Horton and Pankey, 1982). The most common anaerobes are *Peptococcus* and *Bacteroides* species. Achlorhydria in the elderly and those who are on antacids and H_2 inhibitors may play a role as well.

A chest x-ray should always be done at the initial visit if a patient is suspected of having pnuemonia. It not only assists with the diagnosis of pneumonia but also defines the extent of the disease and may give a suggestion of the possible organisms involved based on the location and appearance of the infiltrate.

A Gram's stain of an adequate sputum sample is imperative in the initial antibiotic selection of any patient with pneumonia. An adequate sputum sample is defined as more than 25 to 50 polymorphonuclear leukocytes and less than 5 to 10 squamous epithelial cells per low power field (10×). These characteristics suggest that the sample did originate from the lower respiratory tract and not the oropharynx. This definition is an especially important consideration in the evaluation of the elderly since they may commonly produce an inadequate sample without several attempts and much encouragement.

If the patient cannot readily produce a sputum sample, it may be necessary to rehydrate the patient. A mist tent will also provide moisture to the airways and promote sputum mobilization. If these measures fail, consider either endotracheal suction or transtracheal aspiration. Bronchoscopy is not usually indicated unless the clinical situation warrants invasive action.

Blood cultures should be done in all elderly patients with pneumonia. If an adequate sputum cannot be obtained, the blood culture may be the best source of information about the infecting organism. Pleural effusions should be tapped for diagnostic tests.

Suspected bacteremia is an indication for hospitalization. Other indications include increased respiratory rate, cyanosis, and serious chronic disease. A lobar pattern on x-ray should also signify need for admission. Any patient who is at risk of respiratory failure or the adult respiratory syndrome should be admitted directly to intensive care.

TREATMENT

Penicillin is the drug of choice for pneumococcal pneumonia. Erythromycin may be used if mycoplasma pneumonia or Legionnaire's disease is suspected. *Haemophilus influenzae* should be tested for sensitivity to ampicillin. If B-lactamase positive, a second-generation or third-generation cephalosporin is indicated. Trimethoprim/sulfamethoxazole can also be used.

Anaerobic organisms, *Branhamella catarrhalis, E. coli, Klebsiella pneumoniae, Pseudomonas,* and *Staphylococcus* are other potential infecting agents requiring specific therapies for adequate coverage. Ciprofloxacin HCl, a new quinolone antibiotic, demonstrates promise in treating more patients with gram-negative organisms.

In general, chest x-rays and other tests should be repeated only if the patient fails to improve or if the clinical status of the patient deteriorates. A chest x-ray should be done in follow-up if tumor involvement is suspected. If the subsequent film shows complete resolution, tumor is unlikely.

IMMUNIZATION

Pneumococcal vaccine should be recommended to all elderly immunocompetent persons who are at an increased risk of infection (Health and Public Policy Committee, American College of Physicians, 1986). It should be offered to other elderly patients who are without underlying disease, and it may be offered to immunodeficient patients, although response here is unpredictable.

The current vaccine is a 23-valent vaccine that has replaced the previous 14-valent vaccine. This new vaccine contains antigens to pneumococcal types that cause approximately 85 per cent of bacteremic pneumococcal pneumonias. The vaccine is safe and is approximately 70 per cent effective in immunocompetent adults. Revaccination with the new vaccine later in life is not routinely recommended.

INTRA-ABDOMINAL INFECTIONS

Many changes related to aging make the elderly susceptible to intra-abdominal sepsis. Disorders commonly associated with sepsis are gastric ulcer, GI tract cancers, cholelithiasis, diverticulosis, and ischemic bowel disease. Biliary sepsis, acute diverticulitis, intestinal infarction with peritonitis, acute appendicitis, and abscess formations can present as major life-threatening illnesses in the elderly.

The incidence of gallstones increases as people get older. Approximately 30 per cent of persons over the age of 70 years have gallstones (Amberg and Zboralske, 1965). Gallbladders have already been removed in 5.7 per cent of persons. Amberg and Zboralske (1965) found that gallbladder disease was apparently the prime cause of death in 8.1 per cent of autopsied patients. From this date, elective cholecystectomy is suggested only for those patients after age 70 with severe symptoms.

Facultative anaerobic or aerobic bacteria are the most frequent organisms isolated from patients who have biliary sepsis. In descending order of frequency, the major organisms isolated are *Escherichia coli, Staphylococci,* Klebsiella-Enterobacter group, diphtheroids, *Enterococcus,* and *Clostridium perfringens,* followed by alpha streptococci (Fukunaga, 1973).

The role of anaerobic bacteria in biliary sepsis has become more apparent. Current studies show that *Bacteroides fragilis* is the dominant anaerobe in patients who have biliary infections (England and Rosenblatt, 1977). *Clostridium* species have also been described. Complicating factors such as prior surgery on the biliary tract, carcinoma of the gallbladder, or biliary obstruction are other determinants of anaerobic infections. Antibiotic choices in these situations should cover the possibility of anaerobic involvement (Table 10–20).

Empyema, gangrene, and perforation are frequent complications in acute cholecystitis in the elderly (Fry et al., 1981). Elderly patients with suspected acute cholecystitis should have the following: (1) ultrasonography and radionuclide scanning of the gallbladder to assist with the diagnosis; (2) prompt stabilization of cardiopulmonary status; (3) blood cultures; (4) appropriate intravenous antibiotics; and (5) cholecystectomy with intraoperative Gram's stain and culture of bile as early as possible. In these patients, medical management alone is almost always unsuccessful (Morrow et al., 1978). Delays in diagnosis and definitive surgery are common. They are the result of deceptively benign clinical presentations and often require emergency resuscitation in many patients before a definitive surgical procedure can be performed.

Approximately 7 per cent of the general population will develop acute appendicitis some time during their lifetime. Appendicitis more commonly affects young persons than elderly patients. The elderly account for only approximately 5 per cent of all cases (Peltokallio and Jauhiainen, 1970); however, elderly patients with appendicitis constitute the majority of all deaths from this disease. In select reports, the mortality rates for appendicitis in the elderly (60 years or older) has varied from 2 to 14 per cent since the 1950's.

The symptoms of appendicitis in aged persons do not seem to differ from the usual symptoms of the disease, but the number of perforations is much higher (Thorbjarnarson and Loehr, 1967). Rupture of the appendix may be as high as 70 per cent of patients overall. This is related chiefly to delays in elderly patients seeking medical care and to a lesser extent delays in surgery after hospitalization (Owens and Hamit, 1978). Reasons for delays center on problems in communication, obtaining excessive laboratory tests and x-rays, excessive consultation, attempting to obtain "optimum" condition, and reluctance to operate because of age (Albano et al., 1975).

The majority of elderly persons who have appendicitis will complain of some abdominal pain, usually in the right lower quadrant in two thirds to three fourths of patients. Nausea, vomiting, diarrhea, constipation, fever, and leukocytosis vary greatly. Elderly patients who become confused owing to sepsis or who are demented present special diagnostic problems.

As a general recommendation, appendicitis should be considered in every elderly patient who has unexplained abdominal pain of recent onset or who demonstrates an acute confusional state associated with an apparent infection and who has not had appendectomy (Norman, 1983). Management should include early diagnosis, avoidance of relying on diagnostic studies, and prompt surgery.

DIVERTICULITIS

The incidence of diverticulosis ranges from 5 per cent of the population in the 5th decade to 50 per cent in the 9th decade of life. Diverticulitis, the most common complication of diverticulosis, will occur at some period in 10 to 25 per cent of all patients who have diverticulosis. Disordered motility is one of the major theories of pathogenesis. When manometry and cineradiography were combined, waves of high pressure coincided with bandlike contractions that occluded short segments of the bowel (Painter et al., 1965). Herniation of the mucosa seemed to result from the especially high pressures in these confined spaces. The second possible factor in diverticular formation is a relative weakness of the colonic wall (Almy and Howell, 1980).

Clinical findings for elderly patients may be nonspecific, atypical, or even absent in the early presentation. Most patients do experience some gastrointestinal symptoms, usually left lower quadrant pain. A change in bowel habits such as constipation or even diarrhea may occur. Physical findings include left lower quadrant tenderness associated with guarding and rebound and diminished bowel sounds. There may be a tender mass present.

Diffuse guarding, ileus, free air, and clinical findings of sepsis are hallmarks of more complicated disease. Such findings suggest perforation of the diverticulum. Diverticulitis may be confused with gynecologic disorders in elderly women, Crohn's disease, and ulcerative colitis (Almy and Howell, 1980).

Most patients are treated medically and will not experience another episode. Patients with mild cases of diverticulitis may be treated as outpatients. Such patients may benefit from high-fiber diets. Carrots, apples, and oranges are considered especially valuable on the basis of water-adsorptive capacity. Hydrophilic colloids such as psyllium and methylcellulose are also used.

Antibiotics such as ampicillin are used. More severely ill patients should be hospitalized and treated by nasogastric suction, intravenous fluids, and parenteral antibiotics. A combination of ampicillin, aminoglycoside, and clindamycin is often used to increase coverage (Almy and Howell, 1980). Mefoxitin may also be used alone or in combination with other agents. Surgical intervention is necessary in those who fail to respond or for those who develop an abscess, generalized peritonitis, fistula formation, or bowel obstruction. Patients who are suspected of having co-existing carcinoma also require surgery.

TUBERCULOSIS

Tuberculosis is an important infectious disease of the elderly. The Centers for Disease Control has reported that the attack rate of tuberculosis in the United States between 1953 and 1979 was highest in persons 65 years old and older (Powell and Farer, 1980). Less than one third of the increase in newly reported cases is attributable to the larger number of elderly people.

Preventive therapy with isoniazid is not recommended for most tuberculin-positive persons older than 35 years because of the risk of adverse reactions, especially hepatitis. Older persons who do have identifiable risk factors such as recent tuberculous infection should receive preventive therapy with isoniazid. However, most older persons are at low risk of infection and are not candidates for preventive therapy.

HERPES ZOSTER

Herpes zoster is a commonly encountered skin disorder which has greater incidence in older patients. Over two thirds of cases occur in patients older than 50 years (Calkins et al., 1986). It is the result of reactivation of latent herpes virus in the dorsal root ganglia. The diagnosis is not difficult when the typical vesicular lesions break out in a dermatome distribution. It becomes more difficult when pain syndromes develop prior to the development of the rash. The more common complication of the disease in the elderly is the occurrence of postherpetic neuralgia. Another significant complication is trigeminal involvement.

Treatment is centered on good local care of the vesicles and pain control with analgesics. Corticosteroids have been used in an attempt to resolve skin lesions and to reduce the incidence of postherpetic neuralgia (Sultzberger et al., 1951; Eaglstein et al., 1970; Keczkes and Basheer, 1980), but their efficacy is questioned. The administration of acyclovir in the immunocompromised host can accelerate resolution of the rash and possibly prevent complications from the virus (Peterslund et al., 1981).

SEPTIC ARTHRITIS IN THE ELDERLY

About 25 per cent of patients who develop septic arthritis are over age 60 (Rosenthal et al., 1980). Chronic joint disease has been shown to be a definite risk factor for the development of septic joints in the elderly (McGuire and Kauffman, 1985). The knee and the hip are the most common joints to become infected. *S. aureus* is usually the most common organism and not *Neisseria gonorrhoeae* as seen in younger populations. Another difference from younger populations is the large incidence of gram-negative infections, often associated with bacteremias originating in the urinary tract (Kreger, 1980). *Escherichia coli* is the most frequent gram-negative organism, followed in frequency by *Klebsiella, Enterobacter,* and *Serratia* species, *Pseudomonas aeruginosa, Proteus* and *Providencia* species, and species of *Bacteroides*.

The signs and symptoms of septic arthritis appear similar to those in other age groups. Swelling and redness are common, except when joints such as the hip are involved. Fever was noted in only 56 per cent of patients in this series at the time of presentation (Rosenthal et al., 1980). The average duration of symptoms before diagnosis was 14 days (range 1 to 180 days). In most cases, the synovial fluid reveals leukocytosis with a predominance of segmented neutrophils. A Gram's stain should be done on all synovial fluid samples but may not always be positive, especially when gram-negative bacilli are the pathogens (McGuire and Kauffman, 1985).

Early diagnosis of septic arthritis is important to the ultimate outcome of the joint. Making the diagnosis early is aided by maintaining a sufficient index of suspicion whenever there are signs of an inflamed joint in an elderly patient. Initial antibiotic coverage should include nafcillin or a first-generation cephalosporin combined with an aminoglycoside. Antibiotic coverage may be altered when the culture and sensitivity results are obtained.

VACCINATION AGAINST AND PREVENTION OF INFECTIOUS DISEASE

In addition to the diagnosis and treatment of infectious diseases in the elderly, it is equally if not more important to prevent infectious illnesses if possible. A number of approaches can be pursued in an effort to decrease the frequency, morbidity, and mortality of infections in the aged (Yoshikawa, 1983). Currently, immunization has been the major approach to preventing infections.

Vaccines against influenza and *S. pneumoniae* infections are available. In the future, rejuvenation of the immune system may be potentially another approach. Finally, prevention of microbial attachment to mucosal surfaces appears to be a rational approach to prevention of infection (Beachey, 1981).

Nutrition

Many aspects of nutrition among the elderly are of concern (Feldman, 1983). Those living alone often relate how difficult it is to cook for only one and the lack of social activities that eating frequently involves. Also of importance are the cultural aspects that are carried over into the aging process. A review of factors often involved or associated with poor nutrition is listed in Figure 10–9.

As noted earlier, poor dentition is an important potential cause of commonly found nutritional problems of the elderly. The inability to chew properly may result in inadequate nutrients. The reduction in appetite that commonly occurs in the aging process may also play a role, as may the availability of perishable and other foods or the resources with which to purchase them. One would expect that in this country food would be reasonably available. However, reduced mobility, economic problems, reduced purchasing power, and CNS problems including reduction in short-term memory may all adversely influence the elderly patient (Stiles et al., 1984). It has been estimated that up to 50 per cent of the elderly do not get essential nutrients on a daily basis and that up to 40 per cent of the elderly are iron deficient with resulting anemia. In addition, up to 30 per cent of the noninstitutionalized elderly suffer from Vitamin B_{12} and folic acid deficiencies, while other vitamin and mineral deficiencies may account for symptoms such as loss of appetite and confusion

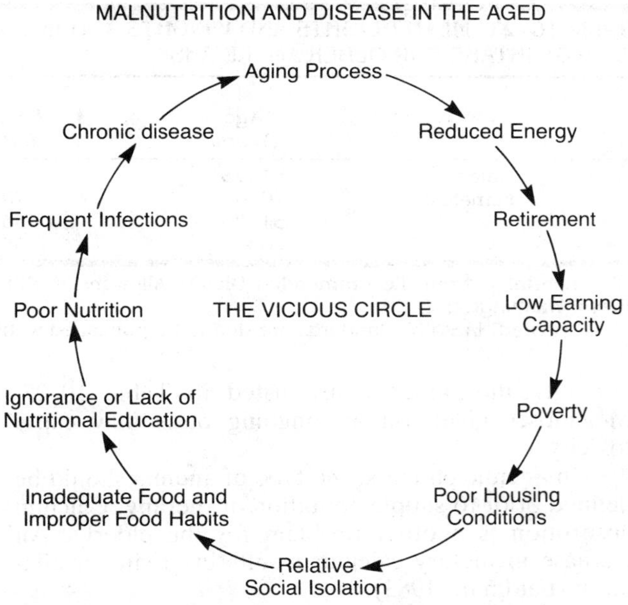

Figure 10–9. Interrelation of health, economics, social conditions, and disease in the aged. (From Rao, D. B.: Problems of nutrition in the aged. J. Am. Geriatr. Soc., *21*:362, 1973.)

(Stiles et al., 1984). The basic caloric needs of the elderly are shown in Table 10–21.

Twelve per cent of the calories for the elderly patient should consist of protein. This will meet basic protein needs of the aging patient without being excessive (Feldman, 1983). Other requirements are listed in Table 10–22.

Adequate, though not excessive, amounts of

Table 10–20. ANTIMICROBIAL CHEMOTHERAPY FOR BILIARY SEPSIS OF ELDERLY PATIENTS*

	Recommended Drug(s)†
Acute cholecystitis	
No sepsis or hypotension	1. Cefoxitin
	2. Cefamandole and clindamycin (or metronidazole)
	3. Cefoperazone
	4. Piperacillin (or mezlocillin)
	5. Ampicillin and any first- or second-generation cephalosporin
Sepsis or hypotension	1. Ampicillin, clindamycin (or metronidazole), and aminoglycoside‡
	2. Ampicillin, cefamandole, and clindamycin (or metronidazole)
	3. Ampicillin and cefoxitin
	4. Piperacillin (or mezlocillin) and aminoglycoside‡
Acute suppurative cholangitis	1. Same as regimens for acute cholecystitis with sepsis or hypotension

*From Norman, D. C., and Yoshikawa, T. T.: Intraabdominal infections in the elderly. J. Am. Geriatr. Soc., *31*:679, 1983.

†Recommendations are not necessarily in order of preference.

‡Gentamicin, tobramycin, amikacin, or netilmicin.

Table 10–21. MEAN HEIGHTS AND WEIGHTS AND RECOMMENDED ENERGY INTAKE FOR OLDER AMERICANS*

	Age *(Years)*	Weight *(kg.)*	Height *(cm.)*	Energy Needs (with range) *(kcal.)*
Males:	51–75	70	178	2400 (2000–2800)
	76+	70	178	2050 (1650–2450)
Females:	51–75	55	163	1800 (1400–2200)
	76+	55	163	1600 (1200–2000)

*Reprinted from: Recommended Dietary Allowances. 9th ed. (revised). 1980, with permission from the National Academy Press, Washington, D.C.

(Updated NAS/NRC standards are due to be published within this year.)

vitamins and minerals are listed in Table 10–23. Megadoses given on an ongoing basis may cause toxicity.

In anemic patients, the type of anemia should be defined prior to supplementation or therapy. Calcium absorption is another problem for the elderly. An increase in dietary calcium results in greater availability (Feldman, 1983).

Alcoholism remains a major cause of nutritional deficiencies in the population at large and certainly among elderly. It is much more common than is often recognized, believed to involve between 1 and 10 per cent of the elderly population (Feldman, 1983). This would mean that there are between 1 and 2 million elderly alcoholics in this country (Feldman, 1983).

Nutritional deficiencies among alcoholics represent a critical impediment to their rehabilitation. Vitamin deficiencies are also present. A critical area to assess is that of fat and protein supplementation (Feldman, 1983). These nutrients often must be increased very gradually in order not to precipitate hepatic encephalopathy or steatorrhea (Feldman, 1983). In the presence of hepatic involvement, 0.8 grams per kg. of protein is adequate, with greater amounts increasing the risk of encephalopathy (Feldman, 1983).

Table 10–22. RECOMMENDED DIETARY ALLOWANCES FOR ADULTS 51 YEARS OF AGE OR OLDER

	Men (70 kg.)	Women (55 kg.)
Energy (kcal)	2400	1800
Protein (g)	56	44
Vitamin A (μg. RE)[a]	1000	800
Vitamin D (μg.)[b]	5	5
Vitamin E (mg. T.E.)[c]	10	8
Vitamin C (mg.)	60	60
Thiamin (mg.)	1.2	1.0
Riboflavin (mg.)	1.4	1.2
Niacin (mg. N.E.)[d]	16	13
Pyridoxine (mg.)	2.2	2.0
Folacin (μg.)	400	400
Vitamin B_{12} (μg.)	3.0	3.0
Calcium (mg.)	800	800
Phosphorus (mg.)	800	800
Magnesium (mg.)	350	300
Iron (mg.)	10	10
Zinc (mg.)	15	15
Iodine (μg.)	150	150

[a]retinol equivalent: 1 μg. retinol or 6 μg. betacarotene
[b]as cholecaliferol: 1 μg. = 400 I.U. vitamin D
[c]a-tocopherol equivalents
[d]niacin equivalent: 1 mg. niacin or 60 mg. tryptophan

Reprinted from: Recommended Dietary Allowances. 9th ed. (revised). 1980, with permission from the National Academy Press, Washington, D.C.

(Updated NAS/NRC standards are due to be published within this year.)

Table 10–23. ESTIMATED SAFE AND ADEQUATE DAILY INTAKES FOR ADULTS OF ADDITIONAL SELECTED VITAMINS AND MINERALS[a]

Vitamins	Intake
Vitamin K (μg.)	70–140
Biotin (μg.)	100–200
Pantothenic acid (mg.)	4–7
Trace Minerals[b]	
Copper (mg.)	2.0–3.0
Manganese (mg.)	2.5–5.0
Fluoride (mg.)	1.5–4.0
Chromium (mg.)	0.05–0.2
Selenium (mg.)	0.05–0.2
Molybdenum (mg.)	0.15–0.5
Electrolytes	
Sodium (mg.)	1100–3300
Potassium (mg.)	1875–5625
Chloride (mg.)	1700–5100

[a]Because there is less information on which to base these allowances, these figures are not given in the main table of the RDA and are provided as ranges of recommended intakes.
[b]Since toxic levels for many trace elements may be only several times the usual intakes, the upper levels of intake for the trace minerals should not be exceeded habitually.

Reprinted from: Recommended Dietary Allowances. 9th ed. (revised). 1980, with permission from the National Academy Press, Washington, D.C.

(Updated NAS/NRC standards are due to be published within this year.)

References

Abrutyn, E., Berk, S., and Raff, M. J.: High-risk infections in the elderly. (Desmond, M., Ed.). Patient Care, *22*:32–50, March 30, 1988.

Albano, W. A., Zielinski, C. M., and Organ, C. H.: Is appendicitis in the aged really different? Geriatrics, *30*:81, 1975.

Albright, S. D., III: Treatment of skin cancer using multiple modalities. J. Am. Acad. Dermatol., *73*:39, 1979.

Alexopoulos, G. S., Young, R. C., Meyers, B. S., et al.: Late-onset depression. Psychiatr. Clin. North Am., *11*:101–115, 1988.

Almy, T. P., and Howell, D. A.: Diverticular disease of the colon. N. Engl. J. Med., *302*:324–330, 1980. *An excellent review of diverticular disease including pathogenesis, differential diagnosis, treatment, and complications including hemorrhage.*

Amberg, J. R., and Zboralske, F. F.: Gallstones after 70. Requiescat in pace. Geriatrics, *20*:539–542, 1965.

American Psychiatric Association: Diagnostic and Statistical Manual of Mental Disorders. 3rd ed. Washington, D.C., 1980.

Barry, H. C.: Exercise prescriptions for the elderly. Am. Fam. Physician, *34*(3):155–162, 1986.

Beachey, E. H.: Bacterial adherence: Adhesin-receptor interactions mediating the attachment of bacteria to mucosal surfaces. J. Infect. Dis., *143*:325–345, 1981.

Beauregard, S., and Gilchrest, B. A.: A survey of skin problems and skin care regimens in the elderly. Arch. Dermatol., *123*:1638–1643, 1987.

Bellantoni, M. F., and Blackman, M. R.: Osteoporosis: Diagnostic screening and its place in current care. Geriatrics, *43*:63–70, 1988.

Berk, S. L., Gallemore, G. M., and Smith, J. K.: Nosocomial pneumococcal pneumonia in the elderly. J. Am. Geriatr. Soc., *29*:319–321, 1981.

Berman, P., Hogan, D. B., and Fox, R. A.: The atypical presentation of infection in old age. Age Ageing, *16*:201–207, 1987.

Bertakis, K. D., and Ross, J. L.: Office evaluation of urinary tract infections in elderly women. J. Fam. Pract., *24*:72–75, 1987.

Bhaskar, S. N.: Oral lesions in the aged population: Survey of 785 cases. Geriatrics, *23*:137–149, October 1968.

Bianchine, J. R.: Drug therapy of Parkinsonism. N. Engl. J. Med., *295*:814–818, 1976.

Bianchine, J. R., Gerber, N., and Andresen, B. D.: Geriatric Medicine—Current Concepts. Kalamazoo, Upjohn, 1981, p. 9.

Blazer, D.: Depression in the elderly. N. Engl. J. Med., *320*:164–166, 1989.

Breed, W., and Huffine, C. L.: Psychopathology of Aging. New York, Academic Press, 1979, pp. 289–309.

Brocklehurst, J. C.: Bowel management in the neurologically disabled. The problems in old age. Proc. R. Soc. Med., *65*:65, 1972.

Brotman, H.: Every ninth American. Developments in aging: 1978. A Report of the Special Committee on Aging, United States Senate, Washington, D.C., U.S. Government Printing Office, 1979.

Bureau of the Census: Population characteristics of the United States. Age, sex, race and Spanish origin of the population by regions, divisions, and states. Supplementary reports, 1980 census of population, 1981.

Busse, E. W., and Pfeiffer, E.: Behavior and Adaptation in Late Life. 2nd ed. Boston, Little, Brown, & Co., Inc., 1977.

Butler, R. N.: Why Survive? Being Old in America. New York, Harper & Row Publishers, Inc., 1975.

Butler, R. N.: Geriatric psychiatry. *In* Kaplan, H. T., and Sadock, B. J. (Eds.): Comprehensive Textbook of Psychiatry. 4th ed. Baltimore, Williams & Wilkins, 1985, pp. 1953–1959.

Calkins, E., et al.: The Practice of Geriatrics. Philadelphia, W. B. Saunders Company, 1986.

Cape, R. D. T. (Ed.), et al.: Fundamentals of Geriatric Medicine. New York, Raven Press, 1983.

Cassel, C. K., and Walsh, J. R. (Eds.): Geriatric Medicine. Volume II. New York, Springer-Verlag, 1984.

Chafee, C. E.: Rehabilitation needs of nursing home patients. Rehabilitation Lit., *18*:377, 1967.

Chauncey, H. H. and House, J. E.: Dental problems in the elderly. Hosp. Pract., *12*:81–86, December 1977. *An important statement regarding the dental needs of elderly patients.*

Chopra, S., and Curtis, R.: Manual of Clinical Problems in Geriatric Medicine. Boston/Toronto, T. M. Walshe, 1985, pp. 183–206.

Christian, T., et al.: Comparison of rest and exercise radionuclide angiocardiography and exercise treadmill testing for diagnosis of anatomically extensive coronary artery disease. Circulation, *67*:1204–1210, 1983.

Cobb, S.: Social support as a moderator of life stress. Psychosom. Med., *38*:300–314, 1976.

Cohen, N.: Gastroenterology in the aged. Mt. Sinai J. Med. (NY), *47*:142–149, 1980.

Cohen, H. J., Cox, E., Manton, K., et al.: Malignant melanoma in the elderly. J. Clin. Oncol., *5*:100–106, 1987.

Condemi, J. J.: The autoimmune diseases. J.A.M.A., *258*:2920–2929, 1987.

Connel, A. M. C.: Variations of bowel habit in two population samples. Br. Med. J., *2*:1095–1099, 1965.

Constant, J.: Bedside Cardiology. Boston, Little, Brown, & Co., Inc., 1976, p. 274.

Cooper, K., and Bennett, W. M.: Nephrotoxicity of commonly used drugs in clinical practice. Arch. Intern. Med., *147*:1213–1218, 1987. *An excellent overview of nephrotoxic drugs with emphasis on NSAIDs, antibiotics, and radiocontrast agents.*

Council on Dental Therapeutics: Consensus: Oral health effects of products that increase salivary flow rate. J. Am. Dent. Assoc., *116*:757, 1988.

Cummings, J. L.: Organic psychoses: Delusional disorders and secondary mania. Psychiatr. Clin. North Am., *9*:293–310, 1986.

Derezin, M.: Laxatives and fecal modifiers. Am. Fam. Physician, *10*:126–128, 1974.

Dontas, A. S., Kasviki-Charvati, P., Papanayiotou, P. C., et al.: Bacteriuria and survival in old age. N. Engl. J. Med., *304*:939–943, 1981.

Dupont, R. M., Cullum, C. M., and Jeste, D. V.: Poststroke depressions and psychosis. Psychiatr. Clin. North Am., *11*:101–115, 1988.

Duvoisin, R. C.: To treat early or to treat late? Ann. Neurol., *22*:2–3, 1987.

Eaglstein, W. H., Katz, R., and Brown, J. A.: The effects of corticosteroid therapy on the skin eruption and pain of herpes zoster. J.A.M.A., *211*:1681, 1970.

Ebright, J. R., and Rytel, M. W.: Bacterial pneumonia in the elderly. J. Am. Geriatr. Soc., *28*:220–223, 1980.

Edmunds, L. H., Stephenson, L. W., Edie, R. N., et al.: Open-heart surgery in octogenarians. N. Engl. J. Med., *319*:131–136, 1988. *A summary of outcome in 100 patients 80 years or older who underwent open heart surgery.*

Eisdorfer, C. and Fann, W. E. (Eds.): Psychopharmacology and Aging. New York, Plenum Press, 1973.

Elliot, D. L., Watts, W. J., and Girard, D. E.: Constipation: Mechanisms and management of a common clinical problem. Postgrad. Med., *74*:143–149, 1983.

England, D. M., and Rosenblatt, J. E.: Anaerobes in human biliary tracts. J. Clin. Microbiol., *6*:494–498, 1977.

Ettinger, B., Genant, H. K., and Cann, C. E.: Long-term estrogen replacement therapy prevents bone loss and fractures. Ann. Intern. Med., *102*:319–324, 1985.

Ettinger, B., Genant, H. K., and Cann, C. E.: Postmenopausal bone loss is prevented by treatment with low-dosage estrogen with calcium. Ann. Intern. Med., *106*:40–45, 1987.

Everitt, D. E. and Avorn, J.: Drug prescribing for the elderly. Arch. Intern. Med., *146*:2393–2396, 1986.

Feldman, E. B. (Ed.). Nutrition in the Middle and Later Years. Boston, John Wright, 1983.

Fiedler, K., Kaufman, A., Johnston, T., et al.: Undergraduate medical education in geriatrics: Nursing home experience. J. Fam. Pract., *4*:869, 1977.

Fitzgerald, D. C.: The aging ear. Am. Fam. Physician, *31*:225–232, 1985.

Fleg, J. L.: Ventricular arrhythmias in the elderly: Prevalence, mechanisms, and therapeutic implications. Geriatrics, *43*:23–29, 1988.

Folstein, M. F., Folstein, S. E., and McHugh, P. R.: "Mini-mental state": A practical method of grading the cognitive state of patients for the clinician. J. Psychiatr. Res., *12*:189–198, 1975.

Fowler, J. E. and Pulaski, E. T.: Excretory urography, cystography, and cystoscopy in the evaluation of women with urinary-tract infection. N. Engl. J. Med., *304*:462–465, 1981.

Freedman, L. R.: Natural history of urinary infection in adults. Kidney Int. [Suppl], *8*S:96–100, 1975.

Fries, J. F.: Aging, natural death, and the compression of morbidity. N. Engl. J. Med., *303*:130–135, 1980.

Fry, D. E., Cox, R. A., and Harbrecht, P. J.: Gangrene of the gallbladder: A complication of acute cholecystitis. South. Med. J., *74*:666–668, 1981.

Fukunaga, F. H.: Gallbladder bacteriology, histology, and gallstones. Study of unselected cholecystectomy specimens in Honolulu. Arch. Surg., *106*:169–171, 1973.

Gambrell, R. D., Jr.: Use of progestogen therapy. Am. J. Obstet. Gynecol., *156*:1304–1313, 1987.

Garb, J. L., Brown, R. B., Garb, J. R., et al.: Differences in etiology of pneumonias in nursing home and community patients. J.A.M.A., *240*:2169–2172, 1978.

Garcia, C. A., Reding, M. J., and Blass, J. P.: Overdiagnosis of dementia. J. Am. Geriatr. Soc., *29*:407–410, 1981.

Gersh, B. J., Kronmal, R. A., Schaff, H. V., et al.: Comparison of coronary artery bypass surgery and medical therapy in patients 65 years of age or older: A nonrandomized study from the coronary artery surgery study (CASS) registry. N. Engl. J. Med., *313*:217–224, 1985.

Graboys, T. B., Headley, A., Lown, B., et al.: Results of a second-opinion program for coronary artery bypass graft surgery. J.A.M.A., *258*:1611–1614, 1987.

Hardison, J. E.: To be complete. N. Engl. J. Med., *300*:193–194, 1979.

Hazzard, W. R.: Preventive gerontology: Strategies for healthy aging. Postgrad. Med., *74*:279–287, 1983.

Health and Public Policy Committee, American College of Physicians: Pneumococcal vaccine. Ann. Intern. Med., *104*:118–120, 1986. *A position paper on pneumoccal vaccine.*

Hirsh, D. D., Fainstein, V., and Musher, D. M.: Do condom catheter collecting systems cause urinary tract infection? J.A.M.A., *242*:340–341, 1979.

Hollander, C. F.: Functional and cellular aspects of organ aging. Exp. Gerontol., *5*:313–321, 1970.

Horton, J. M., and Pankey, G. A.: Pneumonia in the elderly. Postgrad. Med., *71*:114–123, 1982.

Humes, H. D. and Weinberg, J. M.: The Kidney. Philadelphia, B. M. Brenner and F. C. Rector, 1986.

Jacknowitz, A. I.: Current Geriatric Therapy. Philadelphia, W. B. Saunders, 1984, pp. 182–183.

Jarratt, A. S., and Exton-Smith, A. N.: Treatment of fecal incontinence. Lancet, *1*:925, 1960.

Kane, R. L., et al.: Essentials of Clinical Geriatrics. San Francisco, McGraw-Hill Book Company, 1984.

Kaye, D.: Urinary tract infections in the elderly. Bull. N.Y. Acad. Med., *56*:209–220, 1980.

Keczkes, K. and Basheer, A. M.: Do corticosteroids prevent postherpetic neuralgia? Br. J. Dermatol., *102*:551, 1980.

Keighley, M. R. B., Makuria, T., Alexander-Williams, J., et al.: Clinical and manometric evaluation of rectal prolapse and incontinence. Br. J. Surg., *67*:54–56, 1980.

Kennie, D. C.: Good health care for the aged. J.A.M.A., *249*:770–773, 1983.

Kinsey, A. C., Pameroy, W. B., and Martin, C. R.: Sexual Behavior in the Human Male. Philadelphia, W. B. Saunders Co., 1948.

Klarskov, P.: Bacteriuria in elderly women. Dan. Med. Bull., *23*:200–204, 1976.

Koopman, C. F. and Coulthard, S. W.: The oral cavity and aging. Otolaryngol. Clin. North Am., *15*:293–312, 1982. *A good overview of problems that are commonly seen in the elderly with accompanying photographs of lesions.*

Kreger, B. E., Craven, D. E., Carling, P. C., et al.: Gram-negative bacteremia. III. Reassessment of etiology, epidemiology, and ecology in 612 patients. Am. J. Med., *68*:332–343, 1980.

Lamy, Peter P.: Prescribing for the Elderly. Littleton, Mass., PSG Publishing Company, Inc., 1980.

Lamy, P. P.: Geriatric drug therapy. Am. Fam. Physician, *34*:118–124, 1986.

Lane, C. G., and Rockwood, E. M.: Geriatric dermatoses. N. Engl. J. Med., *241*:772–777, 1949.

Larson, E. B., LaRue, A., and Wyma, D.: Memory loss: Is it reversible? (Desmond, M., Ed.) Patient Care, *21*:54–66, April 30, 1987.

Levkoff, S. E., Cleary, P. D., Wetle, T., et al.: Illness behavior in the aged: Implications for clinicians. J. Am. Geriatr. Soc., *36*:662–629, 1988.

Libow, L. S., and Sherman, F. T.: The Core of Geriatric Medicine. St. Louis, C. V. Mosby Co., 1981.

Lipowski, Z. J.: Transient cognitive disorders (delirium, acute confusional states) in the elderly. Am. J. Psychiatry, *140*:1426–1436, 1983.

Lipowski, Z. J.: Delirium (acute confusional states). J.A.M.A., *258*:1789–1792, 1987.

Lipowski, Z. J.: Delirium in the elderly patient. N. Engl. J. Med., *320*:578–582, 1989.

Lipschitz, D. A., Goldstein, S., Reis, R., et al.: Cancer in the elderly: Basic science and clinical aspects. Ann. Intern. Med., *102*:218–228, 1985.

Locke, S. E., Kraus, L., and Leserman, J.: Life change stress, psychiatric symptoms and natural killer cell activity. Psychosom. Med., *46*:441–453, 1984.

Lohr, J. B. and Bracha, S.: Association of psychosis and movement disorders in the elderly. Psychiatr. Clin. North Am., *11*:61–80, 1988.

Louria, D. B.: Pneumonia in the severely ill patient. Infect. Med., 234–244, July/August 1986.

Luisada, A. A.: Auscultation of the senile heart. Postgrad. Med., *48*:255–259, September 1970.

Lye, M.: Defining and treating urinary infections. Geriatrics, *33*(3):71–77, 1978.

Lyell, A.: The itching patient: A review of the cause of pruritus. Scott. Med. J., *17*:324, 1972.

Malloy, T.: Treatment of Peyronie's disease. Presented at Mayo Clinic Sexual Dysfunction Symposium, September 1984.

Marcus, R.: Osteoporosis alert: Clues to thinning bone. Diagnosis, August, 1985, pp. 60–74.

Marron, K. R., Fillit, H., Peskowitz, M., et al.: The nonuse of urethral catheterization in the management of urinary incontinence in the teaching nursing home. J. Am. Geriatr. Soc., *31*:278–281, 1983.

McCarthy, D. M.: Peptic ulcer: Antacids or cimetidine? Hosp. Pract., *14*:52–64, December 1979.

McGuire, N. M., and Kauffman, C. A.: Septic arthritis in the elderly. J. Am. Geriatr. Soc., *33*:170–174, 1985. *A summary of 23 elderly patients with septic joints specifying the frequency of joints involved, the organisms, and patient outcome.*

McKegney, F. P.: Psychosomatic aspects of gastrointestinal disease. Postgrad. Med., *57*:43–47, 1975.

Med. Lett. Drugs Ther.: Drugs for improvement of cerebral function in the elderly. *18*:38–39, 1976.

Med. Lett. Drugs Ther.: Drugs that cause sexual dysfunction. *29*:65–70, 1987a. *An excellent listing of the drugs that may cause sexual dysfunction.*

Med. Lett. Drugs Ther.: Prevention and treatment of postmenopausal osteoporosis. *29*:75–78. 1987b.

Med. Lett. Drugs Ther.: Nizatdine (Axid). *30*:77–78, 1988a.

Med. Lett. Drugs Ther.: Drugs for Parkinsonism. *30*:113–116, 1988b.

Med. Lett. Drugs Ther.: Treatment for xerostomia. *30*:74–76, 1988c. *Summarizes treatment for a common geriatric problem for which helpful information is often difficult to find.*

Megran, D. W. and Chow, A. W.: Averting complications of tooth and gum infections. Diagnosis, 100–111, March 1986.

Mihm, M. C., Jr., Fitzpatrick, T. B., and Lane-Brown, M. M.: Early detection of primary cutaneous malignant melanoma: A color atlas. N. Engl. J. Med., *289*:989, 1973.

Miller, M. H.: Restoring hearing to the older patient: The physician's role. Geriatrics, *41*:75–88, 1986.

Morbidity and Mortality Weekly Report: Dental caries and community water fluoridation trends—United States. *34*:77–80, 1985.

Mohide, E. A.: The prevalence and scope of urinary incontinence. Clin. Geriatr. Med., *2*:639–656, 1986.

Moore, J. T.: Functional disability of geriatric patients in a family medicine program: Implications for patient care, education, and research. J. Fam. Pract., *7*:1159–1166, 1978.

Moore-Smith, B.: Bacteriuria in elderly women. (Letter) Lancet, *2*:827, 1972.

Morrow, D. J., Thompson, J., and Wilson, S. E.: Acute cholecystitis in the elderly: A surgical emergency. Arch. Surg., *113*:1149–1152, 1978.

Moser, M.: Diuretics and alternative drugs in geriatric hypertension. Geriatrics, *42*:39–49, 1987.

Muenter, M. D.: Current Therapy 1982. Philadelphia, W. B. Saunders, 1982, pp. 766–772. *A well-organized approach to the treatment of Parkinson's disease.*

Munchie, H. L., and Warren, J. W.: Long-term urethral catheters in older women. Am. Fam. Physician, *37*:103–109, 1988.

Murasko, D. M., Nelson, B. J., Silver, R., et al.: Immunologic response in an elderly population with a mean age of 85. Am. J. Med., *81*:612–618, 1986.

Nagel, J. E., Chrest, F. J., Pyle, R. S., et al.: Monoclonal antibody analysis of T-lymphocyte subsets in young and aged adults. Immunol. Commun., *12*:223–237, 1983.

Nelson, R. P.: Male sexual dysfunction: Evaluation and treatment. South. Med. J., *80*:69–74, 1987. *An excellent discussion of the evaluation and treatment of sexual dysfunction in the male.*

Nicolle, L. E., Bjornson, J., Harding, G. K. M., et al.: Bacteriuria in elderly institutionalized men. N. Engl. J. Med., *309*:1420–1425, 1983.

Norman, D. C., and Yoshikawa, T. T.: Intraabdominal infections in the elderly. J. Am. Geriatr. Soc., *31*:679, 1983.

O'Brien, J. G., and Kursch, J. E.: Healthy prescribing for the elderly. Postgrad. Med., *82*:147–157, 1987.

Oster, G., and Epstein, A. M.: Cost-effectiveness of antihyperlipemic therapy in the prevention of coronary heart disease: The case of cholestyramine. J.A.M.A., *258*:2381–2387, 1987.

Owens, B. J., and Hamit, H. F.: Appendicitis in the elderly. Ann. Surg., *187*:392–396, 1978. *A study of 68 patients between the ages of 65 and 99 years of age.*

Painter, N. S., Truelove, S. C., Ardran, G. M., et al.: Segmentation and the localization of intraluminal pressures in the human colon, with special reference to the pathogenesis of colonic diverticula. Gastroenterology, *49*:169–177, 1965.

Parkes, A. G., Porter, N. H., and Hardcastle, J.: The syndrome of the descending perineum. Proc. R. Soc. Med., *59*:477–482, 1966.

Pathy, M. S. J. (Ed.). Principles and Practice of Geriatric Medicine. London, John Wiley & Sons Ltd, 1985.

Peltokallio, P., and Jauhianen, K.: Acute appendicitis in the aged patient. Arch. Surg., *100*:140, 1970.

Peterslund, N. A., Ipsen, J., Schonheyder, H., et al.: Acyclovir in herpes zoster. Lancet, *2*:827, 1981.

Pfeiffer, E.: Multidimensional functional assessment: Why and how. *In* Pfeiffer, E. (Ed.): Multidimensional Functional Assessment: The OARS Methodology. Durham, N.C., Center for the Study of Aging and Human Development, Duke University, 1976.

Pfeiffer, E., and Busse, E. W.: Affective Disorder, Mental Illness in Later Life. Washington D.C., American Psychiatric Association, 1973, pp. 109–644.

Pfeiffer, E., Verwoerdt, A., and Wang, H. S.: The natural history of sexual behavior in aged men and women. Arch. Gen. Psychiatry, *19*:753, 1968.

Plotnikoff, N. P. (Ed.) et al.: Enkephalins and Endorphins: Stress and the Immune System. New York, Plenum Press, 1986.

Pope, C. E.: Symposium: Motor disorders of the esophagus. Postgrad. Med., *61*:118–126, 1977. *The first article in a series of articles on disorder of the esophagus in this symposium issue.*

Powell, K. E., and Farer, L. S.: The rising age of the tuberculosis patient: A sign of success and failure. J. Infect. Dis., *142*:946–948, 1980.

Powers, D. C., Nagel, J. E., Hoh, J., et al.: Immune function in the elderly. Postgrad. Med., *81*:355–377, 1987.

Rabin, D. W.: Use of medicine: A review of prescribed and nonprescription medicine use. 1972 Reprint Series, DHEW Pub. No. HSM 73-3012, U.S. Department of Health, Education, and Welfare.

Rajka, G.: Investigation of patients suffering from generalized pruritus with special reference to systemic disease. Acta Derm. Venereol., *49*:190, 1966.

Ray, W. A., Griffin, M. R., Schaffner, W., et al.: Psychotropic drug use and the risk of hip fracture. N. Engl. J. Med., *316*:363–369, 1987.

Reichel, W.: Complications in the care of five hundred elderly hospitalized patients. J. Am. Geriatr. Soc., *13*:973–981, 1965.

Reichel, W. (Ed.) Clinical Aspects of Aging. Baltimore, Williams & Wilkins, 1983.

Resnick, N. M., and Yalla, S. V.: Management of urinary incontinence in the elderly. N. Engl. J. Med., *313*:800–805, 1985. *A well-organized summary of the different types of urinary incontinence in the elderly with discussions of therapy for each type.*

Resnick, N. M., Yalla, S. V., and Laurino, E.: The pathophysiology of urinary incontinence among institutionalized elderly persons. N. Engl. J. Med., *320*:1–7, 1989.

Riggs, B. L., Seeman, E., Hodgson, S. F., et al.: Effect of the fluoride/calcium regimen on vertebral fracture occurrence in postmenopausal osteoporosis—Comparison with conventional therapy. N. Engl. J. Med., *306*:446–450, 1982.

Rinne, U. K.: Early combination of bromocriptine and levodopa in the treatment of Parkinson's disease: A 5-year follow-up. Neurology, *37*:826–828, 1987.

Roe, D. A. (Ed.): Drugs and Nutrition in the Geriatric Patient. New York, Churchill Livingston, Inc., 1984.

Roman, G. C.: Senile dementia of the Binswanger type: A vascular form of dementia in the elderly. J.A.M.A., *258*:1782–1788, 1987.

Rosenthal, J., Bole, G. G., and Robinson, W. D.: Acute nongonococcal infectious arthritis: Evaluation of risk factors, therapy, and outcome. Arthritis Rheum., *23*:889–897, 1980.

Rousseau, P.: Hearing loss in the elderly. Am. Fam. Physician, *36*:107–113, 1987.

Ruegg, R. G., Zisook, S., and Swerdlow, N.: Depression in the aged: An overview. Psychiatr. Clin. North Am., *11*:83–98, 1988.

Schneier, E. L., and Brody, J. A.: Aging, natural death, and compression of morbidity: Another view. N. Engl. J. Med., *309*:854–855, 1983.

Seegall, D.: The principle of minimal interference in the management of the elderly. J. Chronic Dis., *17*:299–300, 1964.

Shock, N. W.: Systems integration. *In* Finch, C. E., and Hayflick, L. (Eds.): Handbook of the Biology of Aging. New York, Van Nostrand Reinhold, 1977, pp. 639–665.

Sier, H., Ouslander, J., and Orzeck, S.: Urinary incontinence among geriatric patients in an acute-care hospital. J.A.M.A., *257*:1767–1771, 1987.

Silvay, G. S., Bodner, N., Koffsky, R. N., et al.: Open heart surgery in patients in the eight and ninth decades of life. J. Am. Geriatr. Soc., *36*:1123–1124, 1988.

Smith, E. L., Smith, P. E., Ensign, C. J., et al.: Bone involution decrease in exercising middle-aged women. Calcif. Tissue Int., *36*:S129–138, 1984.

Smith, R. G.: Fecal incontinence. J. Am. Geriatr. Soc., *31*:694–697, 1983.

Sober, A. J., Mihm, M. C., Jr., Fitzpatrick, T. B., et al.: Malignant melanoma of the skin, and benign neoplasms and hyperplasias of melanocytes in the skin. *In* Fitzpatrick, T. B., Eisen, A. Z., Wolff, Y., et al. (Eds.): Dermatology in General Medicine. New York, McGraw-Hill, 1979, p. 630.

Special Committee on Aging: Developments in aging: 1978. United States Senate, Washington, D.C., U.S. Government Printing Office, 1979.

Sreenby, L. M., and Valdini, A.: Xerostomia: A neglected symptom. Arch. Intern. Med., *147*:1333–1337, 1987. *A complete description of xerostomia.*

Sterup, K., and Mosbeck, J.: Trends in the mortality from peptic ulcer in Denmark. Scand. J. Gastroenterol., *8*:49–53, 1973.

Stevenson, J. C., Whitehead, M. I., Padwick, M., et al.: Dietary intake of calcium and postmenopausal bone loss. Br. Med. J., *297*:15–17, 1988. *A 12-month study examining the influence of dietary intake of calcium on bone by taking skeletal measurements and independently assessing cortical and trabecular bone.*

Stiles, D. P., et al.: Basic and Clinical Immunology. Los Altos, Calif., Lange Medical Publications, 1984.

Sultzberger, M. B., Sauter, G. C., Herrmann, F., et al.: Effects of ACTH and cortisone on certain diseases and physiological functions of the skin. I. Effects of ACTH. J. Invest. Dermatol., *16*:323, 1951.

Tanagho, E. A.: General Urology. Los Altos, Calif., D. R. Smith, 1978, pp. 333–353.

Thorbjarnarson, B., and Loehr, W. J.: Acute appendicitis in patients over the age of sixty. Surg. Gynecol. Obstet., *125*:1277–1280, 1967.

Tinetti, M. E.: Clinical conference: Effects of stress on renal function in the elderly. Bentley, D. E., Williams, M. E., and Williams, T. F. (Eds.). J. Am. Geriatr. Soc., *31*:174–180, 1983.

Tobias, C. R., Turns, D. M., Lippman, S., et al.: Psychiatric disorders in the elderly. Postgrad. Med., *83*:313–319, 1988.

Tomlinson, B. E., Blessed, G., and Roth, M.: Observations on the brains of demented old people. J. Neurol. Sci., *7*:331–356, 1968.

Tomlinson, B. E., Blessed, G., and Roth, M.: Observations on the brains of demented old people. J. Neurol. Sci., *11*:205–242, 1970.

United States Department of Health, Education, and Welfare: Prevalence of chronic conditions and impairments. National Health Survey, PHS Pub. No. 10000, Series 12, No. 8, 1967.

United States Department of Labor, Bureau of Statistics: The employment problems of older workers, Bulletin 1721.

United States National Center for Health Statistics: Changes in mortality among the elderly: United States, 1940, 1978. Hyattsville, Md.: National Center for Health Statistics, 1982 (Vital and health statistics. Analytical Studies. Series 3. No. 22). (DHHS publication no. (PHS)82–146).

Walford, R. L., Gottesman, S. R., Windruch, R. H., et al.: Immunopathology of aging. *In* Eisdorfer, C. (Ed.): Annual Review of Gerontology and Geriatrics. Vol 2. New York, Springer-Verlag, 1981, pp. 3–48.

Walsh, P. C., and Donker, P. J.: Impotency following radical prostatectomy: Insight into etiology and prevention. J. Urol., *128*:492–497, 1982.

Walsh, P. C., and Mostwin, J. L.: Radical prostatectomy and cystoprostatectomy with preservation of potency. Results using a new nerve sparing technique. Br. J. Urol., *56*:694–697, 1984.

Warren, J. W., Muncie, H. L., Jr., Bergquist, E. J., et al.: Sequelae and management of urinary infection in the patient requiring chronic catheterization. J. Urol., *125*:1–8, 1981.

Warren, J. W., Anthony, W. C., and Hoopes, J. M., et al.: Cephalexin for susceptible bacteriuria in afebrile, long-term catheterized patients. J.A.M.A., *248*:454–458, 1982a.

Warren, J. W., Tenney, J. H., Hoopes, J. M., et al.: A prospective microbiologic study of bacteriuria in patients with chronic indwelling urethral catheters. J. Infect. Dis., *146*:719–723, 1982b.

Wells, C. E.: Pseudodementia. Am. J. Psychiatry, *136*:398–900, 1979.

Whitehead, M. I., and Fraser, D.: Controversies concerning the safety of estrogen replacement therapy. Am. J. Obstet. Gynecol., *156*:1313, 1987.

Wong, M., Chuwa, T., and Shah, P. M.: Degenerative calcific valvular disease and systolic murmurs in the elderly. J. Am. Geriatr. Soc., *31*:156–163, 1983.

Wood, K. A., Harris, M. J., Morreale, A., et al.: Drug-induced psychosis and depression in the elderly. Psychiatr. Clin. North Am., *11*:167–193, 1988.

Yarnell, J. W. G., and St. Leger, A. J.: The prevalence, severity and factors associated with urinary incontinence in a random sample of the elderly. Age Ageing, *8*:81–85, 1979.

Yoshikawa, T. T.: Important infections in elderly persons. West. J. Med., *135*:441–445, 1981.

Yoshikawa, T. T.: Geriatric infectious diseases: An emerging problem. J. Am. Geriatr. Soc., *31*:34–39, 1983.

Zoller, D. P.: The physiology of aging. Am. Fam. Physician, *36*:112–116, 1987.

11

Care of the Dying Patient

Robert E. Rakel
Porter Storey

In previous centuries, it was assumed that one's whole life should be so lived that one would be able to "die well," but contemporary American culture has refused to accept death as a normal occurrence. Children and young adults have been conditioned to consider death from the viewpoint of the observer or disinterested third party. An individual's attitude toward his or her own death depends to a large extent on the experiences of dealing with the death of relatives or friends. However, too often what would naturally be a very personal encounter has been depersonalized by the removal of the dying patient to an institutional setting.

Rather than being a time of despair, sickness may be used as an opportunity for reflection. For some patients, it may be the first time they have faced their own mortality.

Informed physicians, family, and friends can do much to help the terminal patient die with integrity and with dignity. However, if dying is really to be accepted as a normal component of the life cycle, then reintegration of the dying patient into the routine course of living is necessary.

The concept of quality care does not always demand that death be regarded as an enemy to be fought with every weapon at a physician's disposal. An obsession with quantity of life can adversely affect its quality . . . there are times when graceful death with dignity is preferable to lingering torment.

LORAN COMMISSION REPORT, 1989

The Physician's Attitude

Too often, care of a terminally ill patient centers primarily on the disease, and the patient as a whole person is neglected. The value of treatment must be interpreted on the basis of its net value to the individual. When additional treatments no longer provide benefits, the patient then needs concerned care from someone who provides personalized care with attention to the patient's emotional as well as physical comfort. The dying person is often physically and emotionally isolated from familiar surroundings and placed in a social setting that gives very low priority to individual personality, fears, and past experiences. In some ways, terminal illness is more taxing on the physician than sudden and unexpected death.

It is not surprising for an empathic family physician who has enjoyed a long and close relationship with a patient to be uncomfortable in dealing with the patient's impending death. While expressing concern and compassion for a terminal patient, the family physician must still maintain composure and objectivity to remain effective. Osler (1904) refers to this as "calm equanimity" and adds, "Our equanimity is chiefly exercised in enabling us to bear with composure the misfortunes of our neighbors." Medicine has long emphasized the need for physicians to remain objective and deal with problems factually; but if a physician is unable to do so effectively, attempts to hide emotion may lead the physician to adopt a facade that appears unsympathetic and insensitive to the patient's needs. Such a physician fears rejection and alienation. During the terminal stages of a fatal illness, it is vital to the dying patient that the family physician maintain a warm and caring relationship and through the strength of the doctor-patient bond provide support for the patient.

Physicians are most uncomfortable when they feel helpless. Unfortunately, this leads to withdrawal from the patient who is terminally ill because the physician inappropriately feels helpless and impotent when in fact a great deal of comfort and help can be provided. A son reported that "With the worsening of my father's condition, the physician stopped being friendly and warm; his visits became rare and brief; his manner became quite detached, almost angry" (Servalli, 1988).

Physicians sometimes lose enthusiasm for care once an illness has been recognized as incurable and inevitably fatal. If this occurs, interaction with the patient diminishes at the very time emotional support is needed most and the patient's fear of abandonment is greatest. Time-and-motion studies indicate that nurses and other ward personnel also spend less time with the terminally ill patient when giving baths and providing routine care.

The physician who is uncomfortable discussing impending death can discourage conversation in many subtle ways. Hospital rounds are made rapidly, perhaps in a superficial, lighthearted manner, never pausing long enough to give the patient an opportunity to express fears and concerns. Comments such as "Everything will be all right" effectively close lines of communication with an intelligent patient who is fully aware of the seriousness of the situation. When the physician tells a patient, "Don't worry," the patient interprets this as, "Don't bother me." Patients are unlikely to initiate discussions regarding their fears of death or feelings of helplessness under such circumstances and will remain silent or avoid these issues unless they feel the physician is willing to listen and is interested in them. The physician can easily squelch such conversation; but a slight indication of willingness to discuss the problems disturbing the patient often results in frank conversations, which relieve much of the patient's anxiety and bring into the open concerns that can be shared with no one other than the physician.

THE "RIGHT TIME" TO DIE

Simpson (1976) describes the "how dare you die on me" syndrome, in which the patient has the effrontery to die before medical and nursing staff have used all the treatments in their repertoire. The patient is supposed to die "at the right time;" neither before all potential effective therapies have been tried nor too long after all palliative procedures have been utilized. Health professionals often have a need to feel that everything possible was done for the patient prior to death. These attitudes have developed because the health care process too often focuses more on the health professionals' expectations than on the patients' needs.

> *We might consider what we have done to the patient who dies in the isolation of a laminar flow room, without having been able to touch another person's hand during his last few weeks of life. Such treatment is a false-positive, a treatment inappropriate to the real needs of the patient.*
>
> SAUNDERS, 1976

It is, however, impossible for physicians to provide adequate support during this difficult time unless they have come to terms with their own mortality.

> *Studies by the Group for the Advancement of Psychiatry have revealed that physicians are afraid of death in greater proportion than controls of patients.*
>
> ARING, 1971

What better defense against death than to spend one's full-time vocation fighting it? Confronting and accepting one's mortality is good mental health practice for anyone, but it is professionally necessary for all who deal regularly with death: physicians, clergy, counselors, police, nurses, firefighters, funeral directors, ambulance drivers, and so on.

Prognosticating

One of the most difficult tasks in medicine is predicting how long someone with a terminal illness will live. People enjoy repeating stories of patients who survived long after the date their doctor predicted. In most cases, however, physicians tend to be overly optimistic, and short estimates are more accurate than longer ones (Evans and McCarthy, 1985). Attempts have been made to develop indexes (e.g., the Karnofsky index) that assist the physician in making objective estimates that correlate with actual survival. However, no accurate method is currently available, largely because of the multiple variables that influence when a patient dies. A good policy is to provide a conservative estimate. It is better to have the patient and family proud that they "beat the odds" or exceeded the physician's prediction than to have the patient die earlier than everyone anticipated.

Communication: When to Tell the Patient

The issue today is not so much whether or not to tell patients they have a terminal illness but how to share this information with them—since most patients know the nature of their disease process to some degree. Because family physicians know their patients well, they should be able to gauge patients' desire to be told and their capacity to withstand the shock of disclosure.

A frank discussion of death or of how long the patient is expected to live may not be necessary or even indicated. A good understanding between doctor and patient may make open disclosure unnecessary. The physician's role may be primarily one of supporting patients during the progressive terminal course of their illness. Such a situation should not be used by the physician who is uncomfortable with the subject as an excuse to avoid discussing the issue, however. The family physician's primary responsibility is to take the time to evaluate the situation, make sure the patient's true desires have been assessed correctly, and provide whatever support is needed, based on the patient's concepts and needs rather than those of the physician.

The physician who can deal with death honestly is able to focus more attention on the patient and can determine the patient's level of awareness by listening and observing nonverbal cues. Clues to the patient's wish to discuss his or her condition may be nothing more than an deep sigh, a tear, or a shaky voice. The physician must be alert during busy hospital rounds for these or similar signs. If time permits, the physician can pause to sit and encourage conversation or return later when more time is available. Whenever possible, however, the response should be at that moment, since the patient is more likely to communicate freely in a spontaneous situation. A physician who is uncomfortable in this situation may be found insulating himself from the issue during hospital rounds by checking every inch of the IV tubing for air bubbles or otherwise directing his attention away from the patient, effectively ignoring overt as well as subtle clues to the patient's needs.

When the patient is ready to discuss his or her impending death, physician and patient are probably past the most difficult stage and the physician needs merely to listen, accept the patient's feelings, and respond to questions honestly.

Most patients will raise questions that indicate how much they wish to know, provided the physician gives them the opportunity. These openings or invitations may take the form of the physician asking "How do you feel you are progressing" or "Do you have any questions or worries?" (Spilling, 1986).

Patients will also usually indicate when they would like to discuss their prognosis, and will also let the physician know when they would like to avoid the subject altogether and focus on more pleasant topics. Even patients who have reached a full level of acceptance of their terminal illness cannot remain constantly focused on that subject and must divert their attention to more satisfying issues from time to time. Physicians should honor and respond to this need, just as they would respond to a desire to discuss pain or other problems.

What physicians say to dying patients is not nearly as important as physicians' willingness to listen. One of the most comforting steps physicians can take in caring for the dying is to allow them to talk about their fears, frustrations, hopes, needs and desires. *Talking about problems can be very therapeutic.* Patients who are permitted to examine and discuss their feelings about death and dying are grateful for the opportunity and usually become less anxious, experience less pain, and accept their situation more easily. If they are denied this opportunity, especially when the terminal process is obvious, they may be convinced that the time remaining is too terrible to be discussed and their anxiety will be significantly increased.

Often, the terminally ill are more fearful of the manner in which their death will occur (e.g., painful, alone and abandoned, weak and helpless) than they are of death itself.

Do all patients wish to be told of their fatal illness, however? Surveys indicate that 80 to 90 per cent of patients say they wish to be told, whereas many physicians prefer not to tell a patient that he or she is dying. A study by Ward (1974) revealed that family physicians are more likely to discuss a fatal diagnosis with women than with men (22 per cent versus 7.5 per cent) and more often with patients in the upper social class than the lower social class (24 per cent versus 5 per cent for men and 30 per cent versus 26 per cent for women). Many physicians who state they theoretically believe in telling the patient of the terminal nature of his or her illness employ evasion in their actual practice as often as most other physicians. Because of this reluctance, which may be based on discomfort with the issue emanating from intensive conditioning to preserve health and maintain life, future medical students must be trained more adequately in assisting patients with the process of living just prior to death.

Most physicians will tell a patient that he or she has terminal cancer if the patient asks a direct question but otherwise will evade the issue and discuss it openly only with the family. There are many occasions when this is the most appropriate course of action; patients are not infrequently encountered who clearly indicate they cannot and do not wish to face the fact that they have an incurable disease. It is essential, however, that the physician evaluate the true nature of the patient's desire in the matter and neither avoid the issue when the patient wishes to discuss it or force a discussion upon an unwilling individual.

> *When the task of telling a patient about an onerous diagnosis is too easy, the doctor has become callous. When it is too difficult, he needs to examine his own guilt or anxiety.*
>
> WEISMAN AND BRETTELL, 1978

Patients should be given adequate time to absorb the knowledge of the terminal nature of their illness and the opportunity to react appropriately before death intervenes. This is not possible if the physician procrastinates or rationalizes that it is better not to inform the patient. The process should not be allowed to advance to so final a stage that there is inadequate time remaining for the individual to react appropriately and put his or her affairs in order.

There is no need to answer questions the patient has not yet asked. One way to approach the subject is to ask the patient what he thinks the problem is, or how sick he thinks he really is. The response may be straightforward "I think I have cancer"; or the patient may indicate a wish to avoid the issue by saying, "I hope it's nothing serious." The patient's condition can be revealed gradually or in stages, such as telling him or her following surgery that there is a suspicion of cancer but that further information will have to wait for the pathology report. Observe the patient's response to this initial hint and, based upon that reaction, choose a method for presenting subsequent information. Tumulty (1973) supports the concept of gradualism in informing a patient and the family of the terminal nature of the illness:

> *The total truth is revealed in small doses as the illness unfolds, affording the family the opportunity to get its feet under itself before another blow falls . . . The patient and the family need to be eased into the truth . . . not slugged with it.*

Such a gradual disclosure is likely to lead to acceptance, whereas a harsh, sudden, or abrupt disclosure is likely to result in denial or severe depression. If the patient appears reluctant to accept the information, do not push the issue; merely make sure that openings for discussion are periodically made available and further information provided when the patient is ready.

When sharing information regarding a fatal diagnosis with a patient, eye contact, touch, and personal closeness are important. If possible, sit with the patient and hold his hand or touch his forearm. Such gestures convey a sense of support, closeness, and compassion, reinforcing verbal assurance that he or she will not be abandoned during the difficult time remaining. Sitting with the patient on the bed or at the bedside rather than standing puts the physician on the same level and conveys in a clear, nonverbal manner a willingness to talk and listen. A study was done in which physicians visited with hospitalized patients for exactly 3 minutes. Half of the time they sat down and the other half they remained standing, a little removed from the bed.

> *Every one of the patients where the physician had sat down thought the physician had stayed at least 10 minutes. None of the ones where the physician remained standing estimated that it was as long.*
>
> KÜBLER-ROSS, 1975

Conspiracy of Silence

Honesty with the terminal patient will provide the greatest benefits. However, the physician is frequently torn between patient and family, with the patient saying, "Don't tell my wife because she can't handle it," while simultaneously the wife is saying, "Don't tell my husband because he can't handle it." Although the wishes and desires of the family must be considered when deciding how to care for a dying patient, the physician's primary obligation is to the patient. The method of management must be based upon the physician's knowledge of the patient and insight into his or her desires, feelings and approach to life. Despite all efforts at deception, the patient knows or will soon learn about the condition anyway.

By cooperating with the family in a conspiracy of silence, information that really belongs to the patient is withheld. Only if the physician believes the patient is not yet ready to cope with the information or sincerely wishes not to be told should the information be withheld. This is more often the exception than the rule, however. One patient said, "I knew it was cancer from the moment they started lying to me" (Lamerton, 1976). Simpson (1976) describes a 63-year-old woman whose family insisted she knew nothing of her inoperable gastric carcinoma. When visited by the physician, "She gave a dry chuckle: 'Only a little ulcer . . . and my relatives down from Wales to see me for the first time in 15 years, and the priest here at 6 in the morning?' " Obviously the patient knew the seriousness of her condition, and the mutual deception was nothing more than a charade. When such a game continues, a terminally ill patient becomes more and more isolated because he is unable to communicate honestly and openly with those closest to him about his concerns and fears. The elaborate schemes some families and physicians develop to "protect" the patient lead to a great deal of tension within the family, as everyone attempts to perpetuate the lie while continuing to interact with the patient.

Similarly, failure to provide the information to the patient's family can lead to a decrease in the quality of their relationship in the time remaining, since tensions and fears felt by the patient are not understood by those close to him or her. Dunphy (1976) describes an incident in which a patient with terminal cancer asked that his wife not be told. He then quickly planned a world cruise, which they had wanted to take for some time. The wife, unaware of the reason for the hasty departure, was unhappy and complaining throughout the trip, while the husband saw himself as a silent martyr, trying to provide a final measure of happiness for his wife. Only after returning home and reminiscing on this miserable cruise was his wife told the truth and the reason for the precipitous departure. Had she been told earlier, each one of their final days together could have been a pleasant and memorable experience.

Denial

Most patients tend to deny the reality of their situation after being made aware of the terminal nature of their illness. Denial is one way of coping with or protecting oneself against overwhelming anxiety, which could otherwise be incapacitating. This reaction is more marked in the patient who is told abruptly without being adequately prepared beforehand. Although denial is noted primarily when the patient first learns of his or her impending death, it can appear in different degrees at different times. Even patients who have reached the level of acceptance of the terminal nature of their illness will need to employ denial periodically to avoid feelings of hopelessness. The mental burden of impending death is too heavy to carry all the time, and periodic relief is necessary in order to carry on customary activities and enjoy the limited time left. As Aring (1971) notes, La Rochefoucauld said: "Neither the sun nor death can be looked at steadily."

A patient who avoids asking about his or her illness or prognosis when the physician offers every opportunity to do so is normally experiencing denial. Excessive denial usually means that the patient subconsciously knows the truth but wishes to avoid facing it consciously. Even when repeatedly given the accurate diagnosis, some patients deny ever having been told. This denial provides constant emotional protection until the patient is ready to face the truth.

Watch With Me

The greatest fear of the dying patient is that of suffering alone and being deserted. There is less fear of a painful death than of the loneliness and alienation that may accompany it. A patient particularly dreads being abandoned by the physician in the face of death, and may need increasing levels of professional support as the illness progresses. This is particularly true if family and friends are not able to cope with the deteriorating condition and begin to avoid contact, thus contributing further to the patient's feelings of loneliness and abandonment. If the patient feels he has no one with whom to discuss his condition or to relate in an open and honest fashion, despair is likely to ensue. The patient's fear of the unknown is easier to cope with if his or her apprehension can be shared with a caring physician who provides comfort, support, encouragement, and even a modicum of hope.

Each new problem of the dying patient should be viewed as a nuisance requiring relief or removal and approached with the vigor that one would devote to an acute, short-term illness. Whenever a fresh complaint arises, the patient should be reexamined and attempts made to relieve the symptom so the patient will not feel unworthy of further attention. If everyday nuisances can be controlled or lessened, the patient will feel there is sincere concern for making his or her remaining life pleasant. The physician should give attention to details such as improving the taste of food by fixing or replacing dentures, stimulating the patient's appetite, eliminating foul odors, or suggesting occupational therapy in an attempt to avoid boredom. The physician should take advantage of every opportunity to touch and examine the patient rather than standing apart. Gentle palpation of areas of pain or merely taking a pulse can convey a sense of concern and warmth and provide comfort for an apprehensive and lonely patient. The physician and other health professionals can provide a great deal of support merely through conversation. The tendency to withdraw and reduce conversation contributes to the patient's sense of loneliness. Silence is an enemy of the dying and serves to widen their separation from society. Conversation is a social bond that affirms life and reduces anxiety by providing a means of catharsis. Saunders (1976) sums up the need of a dying patient with the words of one patient, "Watch with me," asking that he not be abandoned in his final days. The readiness to listen and the personal caring contact is a comfort that cannot be matched by our modern wonder drugs and procedures.

When a dying patient notices that people are avoiding him, he may interpret it as rejection because he has failed to get better or see it as the loss of love from family and friends. The last-mentioned situation is particularly traumatic, since it tends to negate relationships the patient has cherished throughout life. The pleasures and joys of a rewarding life can suddenly appear to lose their value as the dying patient reflects over past events if he or she is ignored or avoided during these final days. The dying patient's contentment is dependent on maintaining warm relationships with loved ones as well as continuing other satisfying interpersonal relationships—such as with the physician. If physicians and others withdraw from interaction with the terminally ill patient, much of the motivation for living disappears and is replaced by despair or terminal depression. The following plea to fellow health professionals is from a young student nurse who is terminally ill (Kübler-Ross, 1975):

> *I know you feel insecure, don't know what to say, don't know what to do. But please believe me, if you care, you can't go wrong. Just admit that you care . . . All I want to know is that there will be someone to hold my hand when I need it. I am afraid. Death may get to be a routine to you, but it is new to me. You may not see me as unique! . . . If only we could be honest, both admit of our fears, touch one another. If you really care, would you lose so much of your valuable professionalism if you even cried with me? Just person to person? Then, it might not be so hard to die—in a hospital—with friends close by.*

Patient Control

Terminally ill patients have a need to believe that they are still in control of their affairs as far as possible, even though they have lost control of their bodies. They should be given the freedom to make choices and assume responsibility over as many aspects of their existence as possible. For many individuals, this is an essential part of living and its loss may destroy their motivation to live. A terminally ill patient should be helped to focus on and cope with the realities of daily living, since these problems remain very real and can serve as a diversion from constant preoccupation with the prospect of death. When a patient has understanding and insight into the treatment and feels he still has some control over the decision-making process regarding his life, he is more likely to cooperate with prescribed treatment regimens. It is often fear of the unknown that makes a patient suspicious and resistant to therapy. The patient should also be given the opportunity to settle his or her affairs. Concentration on preparing his or her financial business and putting the house in order is a pragmatic approach to active participation in the decision-making process. Some patients may have a burning desire to complete a cherished project, reconcile an estranged relationship, or visit particular places before they die. Positive motivation can be maintained by assisting them to focus on and deal with these issues.

A sense of control is more possible for the patient if pain is controlled and he or she is made comfortable. Sleep should not be forced with medication, because some patients resist going to sleep fearing they may never awaken, whereas others frequently have terrifying dreams.

Hope

Hope is one of the essential ingredients of human existence, without which life is dark and cold and frustrating. It maintains strength and gives substance to courage. In the presence of hope, suffering of all sorts still has some positive qualities. In its absence, suffering is a completely negative experience.

TUMULTY, 1973

Twycross (1986) defines hope as having "an expectation greater than zero of achieving a desired goal." The physician should not raise false hopes or be overly aggressive in treating a terminal illness to help the patient maintain hope. Advanced cancer patients can, however, maintain a positive outlook on life. The physician can help direct a patient toward an achievable goal such as pain relief, support for the family from a hospice service, or making a trip to visit relatives.

Hope increases when honest information is provided, and it is reduced when information is withheld.

Even when death is near, the patient can hope for a measure of happiness during the amount of time remaining. The physician can support the patient's hope for a good quality of life in the remaining time, for spiritual healing, and for a final phase of life that has integrity and dignity.

Prolonging Living or Prolonging Dying?

It has been a long time since pneumonia was accepted as "the old man's friend." As one organic system after another slowed to a halt, the aged person was released from nausea, pain, delirium, and the degradation of lingering deterioration by finally developing pneumonia and dying. The family doctor merely showed concern and support; before antibiotics there was not much to do but stand by and "let nature take its course." With improved medical care, it is possible that a person whose dying process might have taken only a few days in previous years can now have the unrewarding dying experience dragged out for months (Veatch, 1972). Modern technology makes it possible to carry the benefits of improved medical care to unrealistic extremes; one person was kept alive in a vegetative state for over 37 years (LORAN Commission Report, 1989).

Protraction of the dying process is a modern epidemic. Some physicians seem to forget that their primary responsibility is to relieve suffering, not to prolong it. Greater clinical skill is often required to provide daily supportive care than to cure acute illness. Tenderness and caring must be included in the protocols of the terminally ill so that the ravaged patient is allowed to die peacefully, without tubing and respirators. Patients should

be allowed to experience those waning moments unencumbered by high-tech devices that serve only to impede their capacity for human interaction. Here it is the patient's comfort, not the caregiver's need "to do something" that should prevail.

LORAN COMMISSION REPORT, 1989

Sometimes therapeutic restraint is necessary to permit a patient to die with dignity. When a cure is no longer possible, care should focus on the comfort of patient and family. At St. Christopher's Hospice in London, medical equipment is shunned and feeding is provided by human hands instead of nasogastric or intravenous tubes—"even if the patient does not get enough physical nourishment, he or she gets what is more important—the personal nourishment of someone who cares enough to sit by the bed several hours each day" (Nelson and Rohricht, 1973).

Management of Symptoms

A great deal can be done to help a patient whose disease is incurable. The family physician can help alleviate the fear, symptoms, and family stress that so often make this a distressing time. Care of the dying patient can be one of the most rewarding aspects of the family physician's practice. Yet, too often, the physician's discomfort with this stage of life contributes to the isolation and discouragement of the terminally ill patient. Unwarranted fears of respiratory depression, addiction, or tolerance prevent the prescribing of adequate amounts of analgesics. The resulting uncontrolled pain makes those final weeks a nightmare for all. Families may disintegrate as a result of the sleepless nights, fears, and guilt that come from trying to cope with the uncontrolled symptoms. Who needs a physician more than this family?

Good control of pain, nausea, and dyspnea can enable patients to die in the place of their choosing with comfort and dignity. Families can cope with their responsibilities and carry good memories of their loved one's final weeks. Physicians can feel gratified at the excellent relief from distress they can provide in this trying time.

The keys to symptom control, as in all areas of medicine, are a careful history and physical examination to determine the various causes of discomfort, and a broad knowledge of the therapeutic agents available.

PAIN CONTROL

Chronic pain is influenced by memories of past pain and by the anticipation of pain yet to come. The fear of worsening pain may color the present perception of discomfort. Frustration and anxiety may accentuate the pain. All of these factors can lower the patient's pain threshold so that even minor disturbances take on immense proportions (Twycross, 1978).

Failure to treat the whole person often results in inadequate pain control for patients with terminal cancer. Fatigue, insomnia, anxiety, boredom, and anger all contribute to a lower threshold of pain. Rest, sleep, diversion, and companionship all help to increase the patient's tolerance for pain.

Analgesics should be given in adequate amounts to provide comfort (Angell, 1982). The approach to analgesic medication in which doses are given as needed should be abandoned in the treatment of dying patients, since it contributes to a lower pain threshold and a need for increasing doses of medication to relieve the pain. When medication is given regularly in adequate doses, the anxiety and fear that accentuate pain are avoided and lower doses of the drug are effective, since the patient no longer fears recurrence or "break through" of the pain.

High doses of narcotics may be necessary to obtain initial pain control in a patient with severe pain. Dependence is rarely a problem in patients who receive appropriate narcotic doses for chronic severe cancer pain. When medication is given *prior* to the recurrence of pain, craving for medication does not occur. After several weeks of freedom from chronic pain, the dose of medication can be reduced in a stepwise fashion without the appearance of withdrawal phenomena. There should be no more than a 20 per cent reduction in dosage in any 2-day period, otherwise withdrawal symptoms may occur.

Narcotics. A symptom-oriented history and careful examination may reveal a number of different sources of pain. Oral candidiasis, decubitus ulcers, constipation, and infected wounds all have specific remedies. Most patients with pain from cancer (and many patients with pain from non-neoplastic illnesses) will require a narcotic analgesic. Narcotics are often the safest analgesics available, usually causing only temporary sedation and increased need for laxatives.

Concerns about addiction, respiratory depression, and tolerance are usually unwarranted in these patients (Twycross and Lack, 1983; Walsh et al., 1981). If the dose is carefully titrated, the patient's pain (or dyspnea) can usually be completely controlled and the patient can still be alert and mentally clear on even hundreds of milligrams of oral morphine given every 4 hours. Underprescribing, however, remains extremely common.

A number of effective oral narcotic preparations are available (Table 11–1). If codeine, 30 to 60 mg. every 4 hours is not adequate, oxycodone, 5 to 10 mg. every 4 hours should be used. Oral morphine, beginning with 10 to 15 mg. every 4 hours, is usually the next step. The morphine dose should be titrated upward until analgesia lasts the full 4 hours, even if a dose of 200 mg. every 4 hours is required.

The particular drug used is less important than the method of administration. In order to *prevent* pain and end the cycle of uncontrolled pain followed by oversedation, an oral narcotic should be administered on a regular schedule around the clock. "Booster" doses equal to about half of the regular 4-

Table 11–1. SELECTED ORAL NARCOTICS

	Oral Morphine Equivalent (mg.)
Codeine 30 mg. and acetaminophen 300 mg (Tylenol #3)	1 to 2
Hydrocodone 5 mg. + homatropine (Hycodan)	1 to 2
Hydrocodone 5 mg. + acetaminophen 500 mg (Vicodin)	1 to 2
Oxycodone 5 mg. + aspirin 325 mg (Percodan)	5
Oxycodone 5 mg. + acetaminophen 325 mg (Percocet)	5
Oxycodone 5 mg. per 5 ml. (Roxicodone)	5 mg. per 5 ml.
Hydromorphone 2 mg. (Dilaudid)	10
Morphine slow release 30 mg. (M S Contin 30 mg., Roxanol SR)	10 mg. q 4 hr. × 3
Morphine	
Tablets (Lilly, Roxane, Purdue-Frederick)	10, 15, or 30 mg.
Syrup (Roxane, Purdue-Frederick)	10 or 20 mg. per 5 ml.
Solution (Roxane, Purdue-Frederick)	20 mg. per ml.

hour dose can be used as needed for breakthrough pain. Long-acting drugs like methadone (half-life, 48 to 72 hours) can be prescribed every 6 to 8 hours, but are unsuitable for "booster" doses. They will accumulate over several days and are difficult to titrate, especially in patients who have fluctuating levels of pain or deteriorating renal or hepatic function. Slow-release morphine preparations such as MS Contin and Roxanol SR can provide excellent analgesia for 8 to 12 hours but are expensive and unsuitable for "booster" doses. These tablets are also useless when the patient cannot swallow because they must not be crushed. Small, soluble tablets or concentrated solutions of morphine or hydromorphone can be given sublingually when the patient is too weak to swallow, and can be used for both 4-hour and booster doses. There is no need to use injections when an adequate dose by mouth will work as well. Table 11–2 provides a checklist of items to remember when prescribing a narcotic.

Two narcotic agents that are also available orally are not recommended for cancer pain. Meperidine (Demerol) has a very low oral potency, a short duration of action, and a toxic metabolite that can cause tremors or even seizures (Kaiko et al., 1983). Pentazocine (Talwin, Talacen) is an agonist-antagonist agent that is no more potent than aspirin with codeine and has a high incidence of psychotomimetic effects (hallucinations, confusion) in cancer patients.

Co-Analgesics. Co-analgesics are drugs that potentiate the analgesic effects of narcotics for particular types of pain (Table 11–3). Nonsteroidal anti-inflammatory drugs are quite helpful in the alleviation of pain from lesions in bones or skeletal muscles. The nonacetylated salicylates (e.g., salsalate [Disalcid], choline magnesium trisalicylate [Trilisate]) are less toxic to the gastric mucosa and do not inhibit platelet function (Zucker and Rothwell, 1978) but are less potent analgesics. The newer nonsalicylate nonsteroidal anti-inflammatory drugs are more potent, more convenient, more expensive, and less toxic than aspirin. Although no single agent has been shown to be consistently more efficacious, particular patients do seem to favor one drug over another. If swallowing large tablets becomes a problem, piroxicam (Feldene) capsules, naproxen (Naprosyn) suspension, or indomethacin (Indocin) rectal suppositories may be used.

For the burning, stabbing, or shooting pain caused by nerve damage, a tricyclic antidepressant or an anticonvulsant may be a useful addition. Amitriptyline, in doses smaller than those used to treat depression (10 to 50 mg. at bedtime), is often effective. If swallowing problems arise, doxepin (Sinequan) solution should be used. The addition of carbamazepine (200 mg. three times daily) should be considered if the tricyclic agent alone is not adequate. A short course of steroids has also been helpful in treating difficult, narcotic-resistant pain.

Table 11–2. PHYSICIAN'S CHECKLIST WHEN PRESCRIBING NARCOTICS*

1. Has an appropriate starting dose been determined?
2. Is a co-analgesic needed?
3. Is an antiemetic needed?
4. Has a laxative been prescribed?
5. Is the drug regimen written out in sufficient detail?
6. Has the patient been warned about possible side effects that might occur initially?
7. Do the patient and family know what to do if the pain remains uncontrolled?
8. Have arrangements been made for follow-up after 1, 3, and 7 days—either by the physician or a trained hospice nurse?
9. Does the patient know what to do if he or she needs help or advice before the next follow-up visit?
10. Is the patient confident that the pain will improve considerably, probably within a few days, certainly within 1 or 2 weeks?

*Modified from Twycross, R. G., and Lack, S. A.: Symptoms Control in Far Advanced Cancer: Pain Relief. London, Pitman, 1983.

VISCERAL OR BLADDER SPASMS

These spasms are best treated with an anticholinergic agent like dicyclomine (Bentyl) or oxybutynin (Ditropan). If only small doses are needed, Transderm Scop patches may be useful. For more severe cases, the addition of 0.8 to 2.0 mg. of scopolamine to a 24-hour subcutaneous infusion of a narcotic should be used.

ANXIETY

If anxiety is severe enough to require drug therapy, consider hydroxyzine (Atarax or Vistaril), 10 to 50 mg. orally every 4 to 8 hours. This drug has also been shown to potentiate morphine in large doses. If a parenteral agent is needed, use methotrimeprazine (Levoprome). This is the only phenothiazine with analgesic activity, and it is a potent sedative and antiemetic as well. An intramuscular injection of 20 to 30 mg. will usually calm a crisis, and 50 to 300 mg. per day can be given by subcutaneous infusion. Orthostatic hypotension and irritation at the injection site are possible side effects.

DYSPNEA

Like pain, dyspnea can have a multitude of causes. When anemia, bronchospasm, and heart failure have been excluded or treated, the focus should be on symptom control. Oxygen can be helpful but is much less effective than narcotics for controlling this distressing symptom. When the dose of narcotic is carefully titrated to control the pain and the narcotic is administered on a regular schedule with "booster doses" available, the patient can experience excellent relief without significant respiratory depression (Twycross and Lack, 1983; Walsh et al., 1981). Careful

Table 11–3. CO-ANALGESICS

Pain Source	Pain Character	Drug Class	Examples	
Bone or soft tissue	Tenderness over bone or joint Pain on movement	NSAID	Ibuprofen 400 mg. q 4 hrs	inexpensive, *big* pills
			Sulindac (Clinoril) 200 mg. q 12 hrs	well tolerated, preferred in renal impairment
			Naproxen (Naprosyn susp) 125 mg. per 5 ml, 15 ml. q 8 hrs	liquid preparation
			Indomethacin (Indocin 50 mg.) caps *or* supp. q 8 hrs	suppository, more gastritis?
			Piroxicam (Feldene 20 mg.) capsules, 1 q d	easiest to swallow, more gastritis?
			Choline Mg. Trisalicylate (Trilisate susp) 500 mg. per 5 ml., 15 ml. q 12 hrs	no platelet dysfunction, less problem with gastritis, less effective
Nerve damage or dysaesthesia	Burning or shooting pain radiating from plexis or spinal root	Tricyclic antidepressant	Amitriptyline (Elavil 10 to 50 mg. q hs) or	best studied, sedating, start with low dose
		alone or with	Doxepin (Sinequan 10–50 mg. q hs) or	10 mg. per ml. susp. available
			Trazodone (Desyrel 25–150 mg. q hs)	less anticholinergic effect, ⅓ as potent as amitriptyline
		Anticonvulsant	Carbamazepine (Tegretol 200 mg. q 6 to 12 hrs)	absorbed from rectum, unlike phenytoin
Smooth muscle spasms	Colic—cramping abdominal pain bladder spasms	Anticholinergic	Scopolamine (Transderm-Scōp 1 to 2 patches q 3 d)	may also be mixed with narcotic in SQ infusion, 0.8–2.0 mg. per d
			Dicyclomine (Bentyl 10 mg. q 4–8 hrs)	Capsules
			Oxybutynin (Ditropan 5–10 mg. q 8 hrs)	Tablets
Anxiety	Generalized restlessness and discomfort	Antihistamine	Hydroxyzine (Atarax or Vistaril 10 to 50 mg. q 4 hrs)	PO or by SQ infusion
		Phenothiazine	Methotrimeprazine (Levoprome 50–300 mg. per d)	IM or SQ infusion only

consideration should be given to the use of antibiotics for pneumonia in the terminally ill patient. Since dyspnea can be well controlled without antibiotics, the physician must decide whether the antibiotics will improve the quality of life or just prolong dying.

CONSTIPATION

When mobility and oral intake decrease and narcotic analgesics are required, virtually every patient will require regular doses of laxatives to avoid distressing constipation. The laxative should be given once or twice *every* day and the amount increased until an effective dose is found. Bulk laxatives are poorly tolerated and are rarely adequate for those patients. If docusate (Colace), 100 to 200 mg. twice daily, is not effective, add senna (Senokot) or bisacodyl (Dulcolax), 1 to 4 tablets twice daily. Lactulose (Chronulac) should be added in doses of 15 to 45 ml. two or three times per day if the tablets are inadequate or cause excessive cramping. If a patient has gone several days without a bowel movement or is having small, frequent, liquid stools, an impaction may require manual removal. Bisacodyl suppositories or enemas may be needed occasionally until an effective oral regimen is found.

NAUSEA AND VOMITING

In patients with nausea and vomiting, first look for a reversible cause such as constipation or gastritis from nonsteroidal anti-inflammatory drugs. If increased intracranial pressure is the cause, then the patient may require steroids. Overfeeding may be the problem if a nasogastric or gastrostomy tube is in place. Metoclopramide (Reglan) is the agent of choice when an enormous liver limits gastric emptying. Many patients whose nausea and vomiting have not responded to prochlorperazine (Compazine) or promethazine (Phenergan) will be relieved by haloperidol (Haldol), 0.5 to 2 mg. every 8 hours.

Like persistent pain, persistent nausea should be treated with regularly scheduled doses. Combinations of antiemetics that have different modes of action may be needed. A combination of haloperidol with metoclopramide or cyclizine (Marezine) is effective. When oral antiemetics cannot be tolerated, rectal suppositories can be tried but rarely provide adequate control for persistent nausea and vomiting. Continuous subcutaneous infusions of metoclopramide, haloperidol, or methotrimeprazine (Levoprome) are more effective (Baines, 1988). Even vomiting associated with complete bowel obstruction can be controlled *without* a nasogastric tube or gastrostomy with a continuous subcutaneous infusion of narcotics, antiemetics, and anticholinergic agents (Baines et al., 1985).

HICCUP

Persistent hiccuping can be caused by any lesion affecting the phrenic nerve and by gastric distention or systemic problems such as uremia. Treatment can consist of chlorpromazine (Thorazine), 25 to 50 mg. orally every 4 to 6 hours; metoclopromide (Reglan), 10 to 20 mg. orally every 6 to 8 hours; or haloperidol (Haldol), 1 to 2 mg. orally every 4 to 6 hours.

Subcutaneous Infusions

When oral narcotics or antiemetics cannot be tolerated because of nausea, vomiting, stupor, or extreme weakness, parenteral medications may be needed. Frequent intramuscular injections or frequently restarting intravenous infusions can be painful and difficult to manage at home. Up to 50 ml. of medication per day can be infused through a small gauge butterfly needle under the skin of the upper chest, arms, abdomen, or thighs, using a miniature pump (Figure 11–1). Morphine and hydromorphone (Dilaudid) have been shown to be safe and effective when administered by this route (Bruera et al., 1988). Metoclopramide (Reglan), 60 to 90 mg. per day; methotrimeprazine (Levoprome), 50 to 300 mg. per day; and scopolamine, 0.4 to 2.0 mg. per day, can be combined with a narcotic for control of nausea, colic, and secretions. Haloperidol can also be combined with the narcotic and infused by this route, but a white crystalline precipitate of pure haloperidol sometimes forms in the syringe at higher (> 1.5 mg. per ml.) concentrations. This infusion is usually started in the hospital or hospice inpatient unit to ensure proper dose selection. The family can be taught to maintain the infusion and give "booster" doses as needed, either with the pump or sublingually.

Nutrition

Although uncontrolled pain is the principal complaint of many patients, their family's principal concern is often how little they are eating. The causes of cancer cachexia are still unknown. Since patients seem to stop eating, lose weight, and eventually die, the natural assumption has been made that even if we cannot effectively treat the cancer, we can at least treat malnutrition and thereby delay death.

The problem is that more harm than good can come from aggressive dietary therapy. Families are sometimes referred to aggressive dieticians who emphasize the need for multiple cans of supplement each day so strongly that the family feels responsible if the patient loses weight and dies. Unfortunately, the patient's final weeks become a struggle with the family over how much they have eaten. One patient said, "Tell her to stop pushing that spoon into my face, I don't want any more!" This can be carried to extremes such as inserting nasogastric tubes in patients who "do not cooperate." Their hands are even tied to bed rails if the tube is tugged on. A study of tube feedings in elderly patients revealed that within 2 weeks, 67 per cent of patients with nasogastric tubes had attempted self-extubation and 43 per cent had aspiration pneumonia! Gastric or jejunal tubes had a lower self-extubation rate (44 per cent), but 56 per cent of the patients had aspiration pneumonia, 31 per cent had a leak or infection at the insertion site, and 50 per cent had a clogged or kinked tube (Ciocion et al., 1988). Large volumes of supplemental feeding can cause painful gastric distention, nausea, diarrhea, and copious pulmonary secretions.

There is no evidence that forced feeding really prolongs life. Careful metabolic studies on force-fed cancer patients at the National Institutes of Health showed irreversibly increased metabolic rates from force feeding. It was speculated that tumor growth was accelerated (Terepka and Waterhouse, 1956). Animal experiments have shown that growth rates of a variety of different cancers are nutrient dependent—the growth rate slows down with fasting or protein-free diets and speeds up with total parenteral nutrition (Buzby et al., 1980; Stragand et al., 1979). Several trials have been conducted in which patients receiving total parenteral nutrition plus chemotherapy were compared with those receiving chemotherapy alone. The group receiving total parenteral nutrition died faster. This was especially true for patients with adenocarcinoma of the lung (Jordan et al., 1981), colorectal cancer (Nixon et al., 1981), and small cell lung cancer (Shike et al., 1984). When Klein and associates (1986) pooled the data from papers written on total parenteral nutrition and cancer through 1985, they found that infections were more common in patients receiving total parenteral nutrition, and that these patients were less responsive to chemotherapy and had shortened survival times.

After reviewing all of the clinical trials of parenteral nutrition in patients receiving cancer chemotherapy, the American College of Physicians (1989) concluded:

> *The evidence suggests that parenteral nutritional support was associated with net harm, and no conditions could be defined in which such treatment appeared to be of benefit. Thus, the routine use of parenteral nutrition for patients undergoing chemotherapy should be strongly discouraged.*

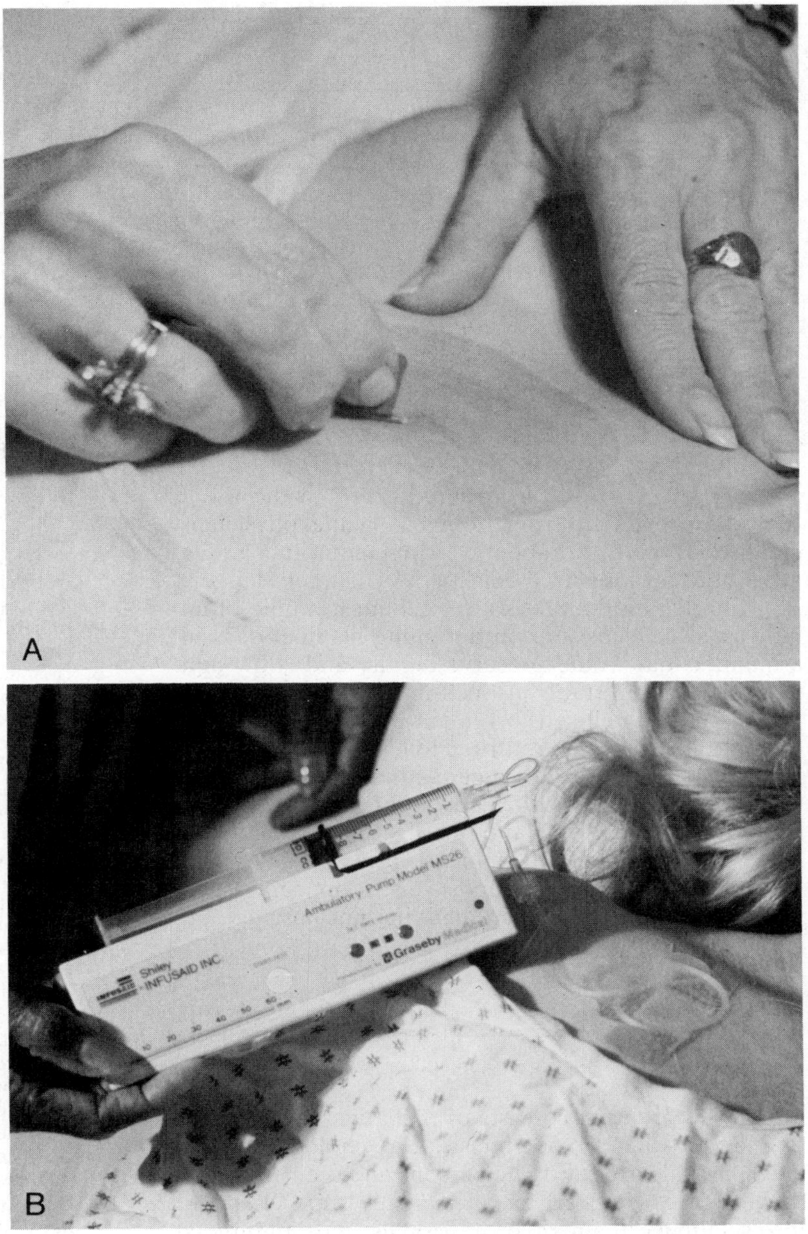

Figure 11–1. *A,* Application of subcutaneous infusion. *B,* Syringe driver in place for subcutaneous infusion. (Photos by Mildred Duelberg.)

What should be done to relieve the anorexia of advanced cancer? Table 11–4 lists a number of treatable causes of anorexia. Uncontrolled pain blunts anyone's appetite and can be alleviated. Low level nausea, oral candidiasis, and constipation can certainly interfere with eating and all are easily treated. Families can be taught how to relieve xerostomia (dry mouth) with a small syringe filled with water or juice and how to prepare soft foods. Corticosteroids have been beneficial to some. The most important service the family physician can provide is to allay guilt. An appropriate statement would be: "I do *not* feel that how much time your husband has or how comfortable he is depends on how much he eats."

Where to Die

Death with dignity is easiest to accomplish when the patient dies amidst the surroundings that gave meaning to his or her life and in the company of those whose companionship provided most of the rewards of living. Physicians too often deny this, however, in the medically conditioned struggle to prolong life. Medical technology has advanced to the point that few patients are permitted to die at home, even though improved diagnostic techniques identify the irreversible nature of a terminal process at an earlier stage. A sorry commentary, reflecting the abuse of technology, is the case of a man who had built his

Table 11–4. MANAGEMENT OF ANOREXIA

Treat "Anorexia"
- Aches and pains
- Nausea
- Oral candidiasis
- Reactive depression
- Evacuation problems (constipation)
- Xerostomia (dry mouth)
- Iatrogenic problems (from chemotherapy or radiation therapy)
- Acid problems (gastric, ulcers)

Teach the family to prepare soft, easy-to-swallow foods
Consider steroids
Avoid nasogastric or gastrostomy tubes or hyperalimentation
Allay guilt

house with his own hands and wanted to die there but was prevented from doing so while physicians exhausted their therapeutic armamentarium in an attempt to prolong his life a few days or weeks longer.

Charles Lindbergh is an excellent example of an individual who insisted on designing his final days in a manner that would preserve dignity and allow him to die as comfortably as possible. When dying of lymphoma, he refused to remain in a medical center on the East Coast and returned to his home in Hawaii, where he made final arrangements regarding his estate and discussed with friends and family the details of his memorial service and burial site. His death was as he preferred—quiet, dignified, private, and in the company of family and friends—a striking contrast to what it would have been had he not insisted on leaving the medical center.

Hospice Care

A hospice program consists of palliative and supportive services that provide physical, psychologic, social, and spiritual care for dying persons and their families. Services are provided by a medically supervised interdisciplinary team of professionals and volunteers and are available both in the home and in an inpatient setting. Home care is provided as necessary—on a part-time, intermittent, regularly scheduled, or around-the-clock on-call basis. The hospice concept is directed toward providing

> *. . . support and care for persons in the last phases of incurable diseases so that they might live as fully and as comfortably as possible . . . (and) that, through appropriate care the promotion of a caring community sensitive to their needs, patients and families may be free to attain a degree of mental and spiritual preparation for death that is satisfactory to them.*
>
> NATIONAL HOSPICE ORGANIZATION, 1979

Hospice care is not focused only on the patient; the unit of care is the patient and family. The physical, psychologic, and interpersonal needs of both the patient and the family are addressed.

Admission to a hospice program requires that a person have an inevitable fatal illness with a prognosis of weeks or months, that a request be made for the services, and that the attending physician consent to and cooperate with the hospice care. Table 11–5 lists the standards of a hospice program as developed by the National Hospice Organization.

The interdisciplinary hospice team consists of a patient care coordinator, a nurse, a physician, a counselor, a volunteer coordinator, and spiritual sup-

Table 11–5. NHO STANDARDS OF HOSPICE PROGRAM OF CARE*

1. Appropriate therapy is the goal of hospice care.
2. Palliative care is the most appropriate form of care when cure is no longer possible.
3. The goal of palliative care is the prevention of distress from chronic signs and symptoms.
4. Admission to a hospice program of care is dependent on patient and family needs and their expressed request for care.
5. Hospice care consists of a blending of professional and nonprofessional services.
6. Hospice care considers all aspects of the lives of patients and their families as valid areas of therapeutic concern.
7. Hospice care is respectful of all patient and family belief systems, and will employ resources to meet the personal philosophic, moral, and religious needs of patients and their families.
8. Hospice care provides continuity of care.
9. The hospice care program considers the patient and the family together as the unit of care.
10. The patient's family is considered to be a central part of the hospice care team.
11. Hospice care programs seek to identify, coordinate, and supervise persons who can give care to patients who do not have a family member available to take on the responsibility of giving care.
12. Hospice care for the family continues into the bereavement period.
13. Hospice care is available 24 hours a day, 7 days a week.
14. Hospice care is provided by an interdisciplinary team.
15. Hospice programs will have structured and informal means of providing support to staff.
16. Hospice programs will be in compliance with the Standards of the National Hospice Organization and the applicable laws and regulations governing the organization and delivery of care to patients and families.
17. The services of the hospice program are coordinated under a central administration.
18. The optimal control of distressful symptoms is an essential part of the hospice care program requiring medical, nursing, and other services of the interdisciplinary team.
19. The hospice care team will have:
    a. a medical director on staff
    b. physicians on staff
    c. a working relationship with the patient's physician
20. Based on the patient's needs and preferences as determining factors in the setting and location for care, a hospice program provides inpatient care and care in the home setting.
21. Education, training, and evaluation of hospice services in an ongoing activity of a hospice care program.
22. Accurate and current records are kept on all patients.

*From the NHO Standards Document, National Hospice Organization.

port. Medical services are on call 24 hours a day, 7 days a week. Continuity of care by the same group of team members provides a familiarity that is comforting to the patient. Volunteers are an integral part of the program and provide many helpful services.

SUPPORT FOR THE FAMILY

Following a patient's death, family members experience increased morbidity and mortality, emphasizing the need for greater family support from the physician. Unfortunately, most physicians do not routinely contact the family following a patient's death, so this need often goes unrecognized (Tolle et al., 1984).

The hospice team provides follow-up bereavement care to the family for up to 1 year after the patient's death. Family members who experience grief following the death of a loved one are more vulnerable to physical and other emotional disturbances than at any other time in their lives. They need help dealing with the grief, guilt, and the symptoms associated with this emotional turmoil. The bereavement services of a hospice team can minimize these problems and can help family members cope with the pain of memories that arise from time to time, especially at holidays, birthdays, and other stressful occasions.

One man who was dying of cancer kept it a secret from family and friends in order to spare them having to suffer with him. After his death some admired his ability to suffer in silence but many were angry and hurt, interpreting his actions to mean that he did not feel they were strong enough to suffer with him. The survivors were not only angry because he did not appear to need them, but also hurt because he did not even say good-bye (New Age Hospice Horizons, 1989).

The most remarkable contribution of the hospice movement is not that it provides a special and compassionate setting in which terminally ill persons can die without heroic measures being applied to them, but that the family becomes involved and comfortable in caring for the ill member.

With the rapid increase of scientific and technologic competence in the field of medicine, families feel increasingly incompetent and impotent to deal with dying. The hospice movement has reversed that trend and helps family members to work with community support services to provide home care for many of these patients. When symptoms cannot be controlled at home, the hospice inpatient unit can provide medical and nursing expertise in a "homelike" setting.

The hospice concept can benefit patients and families wherever death takes place. What is important is a network of support for all concerned. However, there should not be an arbitrary judgment as to what is best for all people. Some patients do not want to be a burden to their family and pride themselves on being able to afford hospitalization or nursing home care. For some of these patients, the gradual withdrawal from family may be an emotional "letting go" that is necessary for all concerned in their particular family and circumstances. On the other hand, there may be a spouse of a perfectly good marriage who is simply not equipped either physically or psychologically to deal with the loved one dying right there in the house over a 2-month period. The family physician will be sensitive to the style of living and the style of dying that seems most appropriate in a given case once the options have been explained to the family.

SELECTING A HOSPICE

Most cities now have more than one hospice. Some organizations consist of good-hearted volunteers with little or no medical expertise. Others have free-standing inpatient units and their own medical staffs. The following questions will help in the selection of a hospice:

1. Is the hospice certified by Medicare and the Joint Commission on Accreditation of Health Care Organizations?
2. Does the hospice employ its own staff to provide home and inpatient care? (A hospice is more than a billing agreement.)
3. Does the hospice employ a physician who will be able to help with particularly difficult problems?

Social Support and Resources in the Community

In addition to the extended family, there are many other resources that the family physician can use in the care of the dying patient. Reference has already been made to the visiting or public health nurse. Most county social service departments have some form of homemaker service. Social workers from both public and private agencies can assist the patient and family in dealing with negative feelings, hostile relationships, economic planning, and financial assistance programs. The social worker is often the key to obtaining tangible assistance such as wheelchairs, walkers, and hospital beds and adapting the home for the handicapped.

For the sensorily deprived there are talking books, tape cassettes, and other aides from the local public library and the library of the State Commission for the Blind. The chronically and terminally ill child of school age can have a teacher for the homebound to keep up with his peers, making every day count in as positive a manner as possible. The patient avoids the burden of feeling rejected because of the stigma of dying. In-home assistance also increases the number of natural interpersonal relationships, avoiding further isolation of a person who already is limited in locomotion and outreach.

Some persons have built close relationships through membership in churches or synagogues, service clubs, choirs, prayer groups, athletic teams, professional associations, hobby clubs, and so on. If these friends and associates do not show up, it may be, as Orville Kelly found before he organized Make Today Count, that they are embarrassed and insecure in the face of the impending death of a friend, or that they hesitate to intrude. This malady need not go untreated. The family physician does not have time to be a social coordinator, but a brief call to a minister, social worker, or family member can usually start the wheels of social interaction moving again. The physician is simply the catalyst.

Every religion pays special attention to the dying person. Support comes from the priest, minister, or rabbi who can help the patient work through basic issues of the meaning of life. The question of "why?" and the confusion of guilt that plagues some patients may benefit most from a religious counselor. Even if a particular unresolved issue that now surfaces is in no way related scientifically or medically to the illness, it is still a great relief to get it resolved, whether through confession, sacramental absolution, restitution, or reconciliation with a significant other. This can be fully as important as medication in the care of the whole person. Bereavement on the part of family members or friends is also eased when things are "made right."

The priest, minister, or rabbi not only serves as a symbol of a community of faith that cares about the sick and dying but also represents a belief system that nurtures hope and trust.

The task of the minister (or priest or rabbi) is both to sustain and nurture hope through the dying process, and to help the person who is dying surrender the unrealistic forms of hope in favor of more appropriate forms as death draws near.

PATERSON, 1981

Euthanasia or Assisted Suicide

Virtually every dying patient thinks about suicide and many ask their physician to help them. The greatest difficulties in dying are sometimes seen in patients who linger much longer than expected—so-called "post-mature" deaths. How should the caring physician respond?

In any areas in which medicine intersects moral codes, there are bound to be diverse opinions and heated debate. The distinction between "active" and "passive" euthanasia should be kept in mind. "Active" euthanasia involves the purposeful administration of drugs to end life. It is common practice in Holland but unlawful in the United States. "Passive" euthanasia involves the withholding of drugs and permitting the disease to run its course. "Assisted suicide" involves the prescribing of large quantities of sedatives for the purpose of empowering a patient to take his or her own life.

The principal reason for most patients wanting to end their lives is the high degree of suffering—usually because of uncontrolled pain or intolerable debilitation. However, much can be done to relieve pain, and support systems can be devised to provide the necessary care for an incapacitated patient. One experience of being thanked for *not* agreeing to assist in suicide by a patient whose pain was previously intolerable but is now well controlled makes any physician hesitate before agreeing to participate in assisted suicide. Permanent solutions to temporary problems should be avoided.

The notion that any treatable complication of a terminal illness *must* be treated because it *can* be treated is also wrong. Most patients don't want to die but they are just as concerned about the *quality* of their time remaining as they are about the *quantity*. The physician may rescue an advanced cancer patient from one potentially lethal complication, only to find that another, which may cause much worse suffering, will end the person's life. Hippocrates' admonition "primum non nocere" (first do no harm) may apply to treatments that are often helpful, such as antibiotics and percutaneous ureterostomies.

LIVING WILL

The version of the Living Will shown in Figure 11–2 has several advantages over others. While it makes very clear the person's wishes, it is also fair to the physician and hospital administration. Instead of locking things arbitrarily in place, it leaves two witnesses as guardians of the individual's wishes and intentions with discretion to use their judgment in the specific circumstances. A statement that simply says "no reasonable expectation of my recovery from physical or mental disability" seems too vague and broad. It is also difficult to define so general a term as "artificial means" that is included in other Living Wills. This statement presumes good will on all sides and should be helpful to all concerned.

Although over 75 per cent of states have laws permitting living wills, only 9 per cent of Americans have one.

LEGISLATION: "NATURAL DEATH" LAWS

Beginning in 1976 with the California Natural Death Act, legislation has been enacted or proposed in many states to provide a more structured and legally binding provision for what the Living Will accomplishes on an individual basis. The California law not only mandates that the wishes of the signer of such a document must be granted but also holds the physician immune from prosecution for malpractice for fulfilling the stipulation of the document. The law varies somewhat from state to state and each physi-

I wish to live a full and long life, but not at all costs. If my death is near and cannot be avoided, and if I have lost the ability to interact with others and have no reasonable chance of regaining this ability, or if my suffering is intense and irreversible, I do not want to have my life prolonged. I would then ask not to be subjected to surgery or resuscitation. Nor would I then wish to have life support from mechanical ventilators, intensive care services, or other life prolonging procedures. I would wish, rather, to have care which gives comfort and support, which facilitates my interaction with others to the extent that this is possible, and which brings peace.

In order to carry out these instructions and to interpret them, I authorize ____________________ to accept, plan, and refuse treatment on my behalf in cooperation with attending physicians and health personnel. This person knows how I value the experience of living, and how I would weigh incompetence, suffering, and dying. Should it be impossible to reach this person, I authorize ____________________ to make such choices for me. I have discussed my desires concerning terminal care with them, and I trust their judgment on my behalf.

In addition, I have discussed with them the following specific instructions regarding my care:

Date ____________ Signed ______________________________

Witnessed by ______________________________ and by ______________

Figure 11–2

cian should become acquainted with the local legislation.

Because family physicians know the patient within the familial context and the community ethos, and provide greater continuity of care than large tertiary care centers, there should be less of a need to rely upon legislation to protect the patient's rights or to guarantee voluntary informed consent. Over a period of time, the family physician can build the kind of relationship of trust wherein a consensus is naturally understood. When such a covenant exists, an adversarial relationship usually does not arise. Although public policy statements and guidelines have their place, they are no substitute for the trust and mutual respect that should characterize the doctor-patient relationship.

"DO NOT RESUSCITATE" ORDERS

Obviously, one will die if the heart stops working; yet cardiac arrest happens in persons who need not die, because the incident is a temporary crisis and is reversible, sometimes even by the intervention of a lay person trained in cardiopulmonary resuscitation. At the other end of the spectrum, it is technically possible with heart-lung machinery and a pacemaker to keep a heart stimulated or keep the blood circulating in a body to which, according to consensus, consciousness will never return. Neither of these extremes presents a major problem in medical ethics. Decision-making is more difficult in the gray area between these two extremes. There are complex moral and legal issues involved in decisions not to treat or not to resuscitate, or in so-called "no code" orders (Wong and Swazey, 1981).

The physician should be acquainted with any policy statement or guidelines that have been developed by the hospital. In or out of the hospital, persons with unexpected cardiac arrest should be resuscitated because it is an emergency and there is no time to assess the cause or attendant circumstances. It is not wise to allow age, mental retardation, or other "quality of life" issues to enter at this time. In the case of a patient with no response on an electroencephalogram, the physician should be alert to the possibility that drug overdose, hypothermia, or barbiturate therapy may be responsible. It is entirely within the physician's prerogative to determine the care that is medically appropriate for a patient. An attending physician may determine that a patient is irreversibly terminally ill and that no course of therapy offers any reasonable expectation of remission or cure of the terminal condition. Once this determination has been made, then the decision not to resuscitate may be appropriate. The essence of terminal illness is the expectation that death is imminent "within a short time." Since it is not possible to predict the time of death precisely, the decision is based on medical judgment. Consultation with a medical colleague should be sought if there is any doubt about the status of the patient. This consultation may also provide reassurance for the family in certain instances.

The patient may request that no cardiopulmonary resuscitation be initiated in case of an arrest, raising the issue of "voluntary informed consent" and the patient's rights. The physician needs to assess the mental status of the patient to ascertain that there are no extenuating circumstances such as disorientation due to chemotherapy, metabolic abnormalities, or psychosocial factors. (One patient developed a sudden loss of interest in living when served with divorce papers while receiving treatment in the hospital.)

One way to avoid confusion or misinterpretation is to talk frankly with the terminally ill patient some time prior to the end stage of an illness. The following is an example of a frank but sympathetic approach.

As you know, we have used medicine A, which gave you some relief for a time; then we changed to treatment B, which has not helped you as much as we had hoped it would. We have no cure for this illness but will continue to do what we can to keep you going and comfortable as possible for as long as you have yet to live. Do you have any questions about what I have said so far? . . . Now I want to explain what else we could do for you. Your heart is very weak and may fail to work. I recall you said you hoped that your son could come to visit you and that he is seeking an emergency furlough from his Army duty overseas. You also mentioned that you are so tired of this illness and pain that you are ready to die. If your heart should stop working, we could try to start it again and keep it going with a special treatment. What do you think of this? . . .

The above conversation takes into account the illness, past treatment, future prospects, and interpersonal relationships. It acknowledges individual values and gives the patient a chance to participate in the decision-making process. Meanwhile, the physician does not lose professional standing or authority or the opportunity to provide scientific and medical expertise as the patient's valued consultant and guide.

It is not pleasant to talk about dying. If one perseveres and overrides the initial reticence, however, the rewards of this kind of interaction are great. Many physicians report that their most meaningful relationships with patients have been precisely those that involved deep and personal sharing about the meaning of life that was allowed to surface by facing death together. There are issues to be considered other than pleasure and the avoidance of pain. Being truly human means being open to all the meanings of existence.

References

American College of Physicians Position Paper: Parenteral nutrition in patients receiving cancer chemotherapy. Ann. Intern. Med., *110*(9):734–736, 1989.

Angell, M.: The quality of mercy. N. Engl. J. Med., *306*:98, 1982. *In this brief but strongly stated case for a more compassionate approach to pain relief, a specific suggestion is made involving a change in the regimen of administering medications as needed.*

Aring, C. D.: The Understanding Physician. Detroit, Wayne State University Press, 1971.

Baines, M.: Nausea and vomiting in the patient with advanced cancer. J. Pain Symptoms Manage. *3*:81–85, 1988. *Thorough review of the etiology and treatment of these distressing symptoms by a dedicated physician who has worked with Cicely Saunders at the St. Christopher's Hospice for over 20 years.*

Baines, M., Oliver, D. J., and Carter, R. L.: Medical management of intestinal obstruction in patients with advanced malignant disease. Lancet, *2*(8462):990–993, 1985. *A series of 38 laparotomy-documented cases of bowel obstruction are successfully treated medically without an I.V. and without an N.G. tube. Several patients lived more than 7 months.*

Bruera, E., Brenneis, C., Michaud, M., et al.: Use of subcutaneous route for administration of narcotics in patients with cancer pain. Cancer *62*(2):407–411, 1988. *A series of 108 patients treated with continuous subcutaneous infusions of morphine or hydromorphone is reviewed.*

Buzby, G. P., Mullen, J. L., Stein, T. P., et al.: Host-tumor interaction and nutrient supply. Cancer *45*:2940–2948, 1980.

Ciocon, J. O., Silverstone, F. A., Grouer, M., et al.: Tube feedings in elderly patients. Arch. Intern. Med., *148*:429–433, 1988.

Coping with Cancer; a Resource for the Health Professional. Prepared by the Office of Cancer Communication. Bethesda, Md., National Cancer Institute, September 1980 (NIH Pub. No. 80–2080). *Examines how patients and family members respond to cancer and, where feasible, suggests ways of identifying and meeting their needs. Includes extensive references from behavioral sciences literature about living with cancer.*

Davidson, G. W.: Living With Dying. Minneapolis, Augsburg Publishing House, 1975. *A useful paperback for family and friends of the dying, which helps them deal with issues such as loss, change, conflict, and suffering. It also provides positive practical suggestions for support of the patient and the family.*

Driscoll, C. E.: Pain management. Prim. Care, *14*(2):337–352, 1987.

Driscoll, C. E.: Symptom control in terminal illness. Prim. Care, *14*(2):353–363, 1987.

Dunphy, J. E.: On caring for the patient with cancer. N. Engl. J. Med., *295*:313, 1976.

Evans, C., and McCarthy, M.: Prognostic uncertainty in terminal care: Can the Karnofsky index help? Lancet, *1*(8439):1204–1206, 1985.

Graham, J.: In the Company of Others. New York, Harcourt Brace Jovanovich, 1982. *Written by a victim of terminal cancer for other patients, their families, and friends. A common sense approach to living with cancer.*

Hively, J. (Ed.): Hospice of Marin Information Handbook. 2d ed. San Rafael, CA, Hospice of Marin, November 1981. *An excellent source of information on hospice philosophy, standards, and practicalities of management.*

Jordan, W. M., Valdivreso, M., Frankmann, C., et al.: Treatment of advanced adenocarcinoma of the lungs with ftoratur, doxorubicin, cyclophosphamide and cisplatin (FACP) and intensive I.V. hyperalimentation. Cancer Treat. Rep., *65*:197–205, 1981.

Kaiko, R. F., Foley, K. M., Gravinsky, P. L. J., et al.: Central nervous system excitatory effects of meperidine in cancer patients. Ann. Neurol., *13*:180–185, 1983.

Kelly, O. E., and Murray, W. C.: Make Today Count. New York, Delacorte Press, 1975. *The author, a patient with lymphoma, started the organization Make Today Count for patients, their families, and interested individuals to serve as a forum for discussion of problems besetting terminally ill patients. It focuses on ways of helping them and others to face their problems and make the most of the days remaining. The book describes Mr. Kelly's personal background and the origins of the organization. Recommended reading for all health professionals, especially students of medicine.*

Klein, S., Simes, J., and Blackburn, G. L.: Total parenteral nutrition and cancer clinical trials. Cancer *58*:1378–1386, 1986. *Meta-analysis of all studies on total parenteral nutrition and cancer provides a helpful and important summary of data.*

Kübler-Ross, E.: Death: The Final Stage of Growth. Englewood Cliffs, NJ, Prentice-Hall, 1975. *A compilation of writings by a variety of authors, focusing on cultural attitudes influencing death and on the positive aspects of dying. If one has lived life to its fullest, he or she leaves love and respect for life behind. Includes editorial comments and occasional papers by Kübler-Ross. Easy reading.*

Kübler-Ross, E.: On Death and Dying. New York, Macmillan, 1969. *This is the classic that stimulated renewed interest in care of the dying patient. It is primarily a compilation of case reports obtained when dying patients were interviewed as part of a research project and class for theology students. From this study arose a description of the five stages in the dying process. Valuable reading for all students and available in paperback.*

Kushner H. S.: When Bad Things Happen to Good People. New York, Schocken Books, 1981. *A moving and thoughtful account of a personal encounter with the issue expressed in the title by a rabbi whose son was a victim of progeria.*

Lamerton, R.: Care of the Dying. Westport, Conn., Technomic Publishing Co., 1976.

Lindemann, E.: Symptomatology and management of acute grief. Am. J. Psych., *101*:141, 1944. *This is the pioneer article on grief reactions and the need to work through the agony of loss as well as the hazards of repression and avoidance.*

Lipman, A. G.: Drug therapy in cancer pain. Cancer Nurs., *3*:39, 1980. *Expert, practical, and specific advice from a pharmacologist with extensive hospice experience.*

LORAN Commission: A Report to the Community. Brookline, Mass, Harvard Community Health Plan, 1989.

National Hospice Organization. Hospice Principles and Standards. 6th ed. Vienna, VA, National Hospice Organization, 1979.

Nelson, J. B.: Human Medicine: Ethical Perspectives on New Medical Issues. Minneapolis, Augsburg Publishing House, 1973. *Chapter 6, Humanizing the Dying Process, is especially recommended. A good book for staff discussion in a clinic or hospital continuing education program. Easy to read and available in paperback.*

Nelson, J. B., and Rohricht, J. S.: Human Medicine: Ethical Perspectives on Today's Medical Issues. Minneapolis, Augsburg Publishing House, 1984.

New Age Hospice Horizons. Houston, Texas, New Age Hospice, 1989.

Nixon, D. W., Moffit, S., Lawson, D. H., et al.: Total parenteral nutrition as an adjunct to chemotherapy of metastatic colorectal cancer. Cancer Treat. Rep., *65*(suppl 5):121–128, 1981.

Osler, W.: Aequanimitas. Philadelphia, P. Blakiston's Son and Co., 1904.

Paterson, G.: Death, dying, and the elderly. *In* Clements, W. M. (Ed.): Ministry with the Aging. New York, Harper and Row, 1981, pp. 227–228.

Pearson, L. (ed.): Death and Dying. Cleveland, The Press of Case Western Reserve University, 1969. *An edited text. The chapter by Cicely Saunders entitled "Care of the Dying Person" is especially worthwhile, as is the chapter by Richard Kalish entitled "The Effects of Death Upon the Family." There is a large annotated bibliography on death and dying by Pearson.*

Saunders, C.: Living with dying. Man Med., *1*:227, 1976.

Seravalli, E. P.: The dying patient, the physician and the fear of death. N. Engl. J. Med., *319*:1728–1730, 1988.

Shike, M., Russell, D.McR., Detsky, A. S., et al.: Changes in body composition in patients with small-cell lung cancer—the effects of TPN as an adjunct to chemotherapy. Ann. Intern. Med., *101*:303–309, 1984.

Shimm, D. S., Logue, G. L., Maltie A. A., et al.: Medical management of chronic cancer pain. J.A.M.A., *241*:2408, 1979. *A useful discussion of narcotic analgesics and psychoactive drugs, with some suggestions for patient evaluation.*

Simpson, M. A.: The Facts of Death. Englewood Cliffs, NJ, Prentice-Hall, 1979. *Subtitled "A Complete Guide for Being Prepared," this book offers a practical approach to coping with the psychosocial aspects of dying and caring for the dying and their families. For example, the chapter on "Euthanasia and the 'Living Will' " succinctly summarizes relevant ethical and legal questions and reproduces pertinent documents limiting treatment.*

Simpson, M. A.: Planning for terminal care. Lancet, *2*:192, 1976.

Spilling, R.: Terminal Care at Home. Oxford, Oxford University Press, 1986.

Snow, L. W.: A Death with Dignity: When the Chinese Came. New York, Random House, 1974. *A personal memoir by Edgar Snow's wife Lois of how a medical team from China helped him and his family face his final illness.*

Stedeford, A.: Couples facing death. II. Unsatisfactory communication. Br. Med. J., *238*:1098, 1981. *Considerable suffering, much of which is unavoidable, is caused by poor communication—whether between physician and patient, physician and family, staff and patient, or patient and family.*

Stragand, J. J., Braunschweiger, P. G., Pollice A. A., et al.: Cell kinetic alterations in marine mammary tumors following fasting and refeeding. Eur. J. Cancer, *15*:218–286, 1979.

Switzer, D. K.: The Dynamics of Death. New York, Abingdon Press, 1970. *Views grief as the anxiety resulting from damage to one's own identity through the loss of someone with whom there was a close emotional relationship.*

Terepka, A. R., and Waterhouse, C.: Metabolic observations during forced feedings of patients with cancer. Am. J. Med., *20*:225, 1956.

Tolle, S. W., Elliot, D. L., and Hickam, D. H.: Physician attitudes and practices at the time of patient death. Arch. Intern. Med., *144*:2389–2391, 1984.

Tumulty, P. A.: The Effective Clinician. Philadelphia, W. B. Saunders Co., 1973.

Twycross, R. G.: Hospice care. *In* Spilling, R. (Ed.): Terminal Care at Home. Oxford. Oxford University Press, 1986, p. 105.

Twycross, R. C.: Principles and practice of pain relief in terminal cancer. *In* Corr, C. A. (Ed.): Hospice Care—Principles and Practice. New York, Springer Publishing, 1983.

Twycross, R. G.: The assessment of pain in advanced cancer. J. Med. Ethics, *4*:112, 1978. *The author, a recognized expert in the relief of cancer pain and currently director of Sir Michael Sobell House in Oxford, argues that complete assessment includes both diagnosis and initiation of appropriate treatment. A recommended procedure is outlined.*

Twycross, R. G., and Lack, S. A.: Symptoms Control in Far Advanced Cancer: Pain Relief. London, Pitman, 1983. *Highly recommended reference text with chapters on "Myths about Morphine" and other important aspects of pain control.*

Veatch, R. M.: Choosing not to prolong dying. Med. Dimensions, December: 1972.

Volkan, V.: Typical findings in pathological grief. Psychiatr. Q., *44*:231, 1970. *An older but still useful review of pathologic grief from a psychoanalytical perspective.*

Walsh, T. D., Baxter, R., Bowman, K., et al.: High-dose morphine and respiratory function in chronic cancer pain. Pain, *1*(Suppl):39, 1981.

Ward, A.: Telling the patient. J. R. Coll. Gen. Pract., *24*:465, 1974.

Weisman, A., and Brettell, H. R.: The pre-terminal and terminal patient. *In* Rakel, R. E., and Conn, H. (Eds.): Family Practice. 2nd ed. Philadelphia, W. B. Saunders Co., 1978.

White, R. B., and Gathman, L. T.: The syndrome of ordinary grief. Am. Fam. Physician, *8*:96, 1973. *A practical approach to managing patients in grief and a review of the grieving process.*

Wong, C. B., and Swazey, J. P. (Eds.): Dilemmas of Dying: Policies and Procedures for Decisions Not to Treat. Boston, G. K. Hall & Co., 1981. *Proceedings of a 1979 conference sponsored by Medicine in the Public Interest, Inc. Physicians, medical ethicists, and legal experts discuss the competent patient and the right to refuse treatment, rights and responsibilities in connection with incompetent patients, and the implications of significant judicial events such as the Saikiewicz and Dinnerstein decisions.*

Zucker, M. B., and Rothwell, K. G.: Differential influences of salicylate compounds on platelet aggregation and serotonin release. Curr. Ther. Res., *23*:194–199, 1978.

12

Ethics in Primary Care Medicine

Warren L. Holleman
Baruch A. Brody

Economic, social, legal, and political factors have combined, in recent years, to effect major changes in medical practice and health care policy. Concern for patient rights and patient autonomy, as well as the demands of third party payers, have transformed the practice of medicine. The ethical issues discussed in this chapter have taken on new dimensions as a result of this transformation.

Medicine as a Relationship and as a Profession

At its most fundamental level, the practice of medicine should not be regarded as a science, an art, or a business, even though each of these elements is essential. The practice of medicine—particularly primary care medicine—is rooted, instead, in a relationship between the patient as person and the physician as professional (Jonsen, Siegler, and Winslade, 1986; Smith and Churchill, 1986; Siegler, 1985). Two problems currently threaten the quality of that relationship: a misunderstanding of patient autonomy and inappropriate third party intervention.

When physicians respect the autonomy of their patients so that patients take control of their health care, the physician is in danger of becoming a hired hand of the patient and the physician-patient relationship is in danger of degenerating into a purely commercial relationship. Patients "own" their bodies but they should not "own" their physicians. Physicians have an obligation to practice within professional standards of care as well as a right to refrain from doing anything that would violate their own moral and religious conventions (Christie and Hoffmaster, 1986). Physicians must respect the autonomy of their patients, but they must also avoid the temptation to shirk their own professional and moral responsibilities and must nurture a cooperative relationship with the patient. This is no easy task, but it is through cooperation that the physician and the patient can best work together toward a common goal—to maintain the health of the patient.

The physician-patient relationship also suffers when outside parties interfere inappropriately. When third party payers set the standard of care, the physician is in danger of becoming a hired hand of the third party. The physician must balance competing loyalties between patients and third parties as well as between professional standards and personal beliefs. In this era of third party payers, the physician-patient relationship can no longer be exclusive, but it must remain primary. In the remainder of this section, we examine two areas in which these problems are particularly prominent: work-related visits and benefits-related visits.

WORK- AND SCHOOL-RELATED EVALUATIONS

Pre-employment examinations, work release evaluations, school absence excuses, and athletic physicals comprise a major component of many primary care practices. Inappropriate third party interventions in this area challenge the primacy of the physician-patient relationship and the integrity of the medical profession. The following guidelines have been suggested (Holleman and Holleman, 1988; Rosenstock and Hagopian, 1987; Kelman, 1985) and should help alleviate some of the problems most commonly associated with these evaluations.

The purpose of the pre-employment examination is to determine a person's fitness for work, to protect workers from illnesses and injuries, to protect employers from the costs of preventable job-related illnesses and injuries, and to collect baseline data for the future treatment of such illnesses and injuries. To enable the physician to make such an evaluation, the employer must provide the physician with a detailed job description, including physical requirements, psychologic strains, and exposures to toxins. The physician should then tell the employer whether the prospective employee can perform the job without posing a risk to the self or others. As discussed below, the physician should not release any medical records to the employer but should keep them on file as baseline data. At the beginning of the evaluation, the physician should advise the patient of the investigative nature of the visit. The physician must warn the prospective employee regarding health risks of the particular occupation (e.g., toxins affecting pregnancies, stresses affecting hypertensive patients) and must tell him or her of any problems detected in the course of the evaluation, regardless of their effect on job performance.

Work release evaluations, school release evaluations, and athletic physicals should be performed in accordance with the same guidelines as pre-employment physicals, but they do present some additional problems of their own. Most work and school release evaluations involve short-term absences for minor problems for which there are few, if any, objective findings. Often, workers and students present after their illness or injury has resolved. These absences often reflect personal, family, or job-related problems that are not strictly medical in nature. Investigating such problems for employers and school administrators damages the physician-patient relationship and discredits medicine as a healing profession. Patients will have difficulty trusting a physician who investigates on one occasion but offers therapy on another. We recommend that physicians encourage employers and school administrators to develop nonmedical strategies for policing casual absenteeism. Physicians who do perform these evaluations should minimize the harm to the physician-patient relationship and to the integrity of the profession by evaluating only in the context of treatment and by refusing to release confidential medical information to employers and school administrators.

Many patients present to primary care physicians seeking to be certified as eligible for worker's compensation, long-term disability, group or individual medical insurance, Medicare, Medicaid, and veteran's benefits. Many others have already been certified and are seeking proper care under the terms of these programs. Physicians must be familiar with the details of the various programs so as to enable their patients to benefit appropriately from them. Physicians must also be aware of the potential abuses of such programs so as to help protect those who legitimately qualify from being harmed by those who do not. For example, if a patient presents with an on-the-job injury but also requests treatment for some other problem, the physician should file separate bills so that the worker's compensation fund only pays for job-related illnesses and injuries. Physicians who detect intentional abuse should attempt to identify the reasons for the abuse, particularly in the case of habitual, long-term abusers (Alexander, 1980; Whiting, 1977). Long-term abuse of benefits programs can be prevented only if primary care physicians insist that patients receive continuing comprehensive care from one physician or from a small team of physicians who know the patient well.

Special Problems in Primary Care Settings

Having introduced the concept of medicine as a relationship and as a profession and having seen what this concept means in many primary care contexts, we turn in the next sections to problem areas that challenge our understanding of the physician-patient relation and of the professional character of medicine.

CONFIDENTIALITY

The principle of confidentiality is one of the most widely accepted and historically influential principles governing the patient-physician relationship in western cultures. The Hippocratic oath mandates that the physician not divulge "whatsoever I shall see or hear in the course of my profession as well as outside my profession in my intercourse with men, if it be what should not be published abroad." The 1980 Principles of Medical Ethics of the American Medical Association mandate that the physician "shall safeguard patient confidences within the constraints of the law."

Confidentiality is important as a way of encouraging patients to be frank in their communications with physicians, as a way of physicians keeping an implicit promise to patients that their confidence will be respected, and as a way of emphasizing the patient's right to privacy. In all of these ways, preserving confidentiality strengthens the relationship between an autonomous patient and a professional physician.

As the delivery of health care has changed from the model of a single physician caring for individual patients to the model of a team of health care workers in an institutional setting providing care to a wide variety of patients, the mandate of confidentiality has changed. The emphasis has switched from physicians keeping secrets to information about patients being divulged only to those members of the health care team and those institutional employees who have a need for the information, either to provide appropriate care or to meet appropriate institutional needs (e.g., monitoring of quality of care or organizing reimbursement). The underlying theme remains that information should not be provided to anyone else without the patient's consent.

This last point deserves special emphasis because it structures the decision as to when it is appropriate to provide information about the patient to insurance companies and to employers. Providing such information is perfectly appropriate if the patient consents; otherwise, it is not. For this reason, patients are commonly asked to authorize the release of information to particular individuals; the principle of confidentiality is not breached if information is provided pursuant to such a release (Bruce, 1984). However, the scope of information supplied and the persons to whom it is supplied are determined by the patient's instructions. Thus, if a patient requests a statement certifying that he or she is fit to return to work, it is not appropriate for the physician to provide to the employer a full account of the patient's illness and treatment; all that should be provided is the requested statement about the patient's fitness to return to work.

There are circumstances in which our society has judged that the need for information outweighs the principle of confidentiality; these are the circumstances in which the physician is required by law to disclose otherwise confidential information regardless of the wishes of the patient. The exact circumstances vary from jurisdiction to jurisdiction and are determined by state statutes and court decisions. Common circumstances include certain types of judicial proceedings, suspected abuse of dependent individuals such as children and the frail elderly, venereal and communicable diseases, and gunshot wounds (Bruce, 1984). In recent years, following the Tarasoff decision in California (Tarasoff, 1974), the concept has emerged that physicians are obligated to warn and/or to take measures to protect third parties threatened by the behavior of their patients, even if doing so involves a breach of confidentiality. The scope of that principle is far from clear (Mills et al., 1987); one obvious controversial example is whether physicians should warn the spouses or regular sexual partners of patients who test positively for the AIDS virus about the threat this illness poses to them (Dickens, 1988).

The principle of confidentiality extends to not providing information to family members of competent adult patients unless the patients want the information to be shared. Often, it will be clear that the patient has no concern about the sharing of information with his or her family. In cases of doubt, the patient should be consulted, especially if the information is of a sensitive nature or if there is evidence of family discord. An appropriate practice upon admitting a patient to a hospital is to ask the patient to identify a particular family member, if any, to whom information should be provided for distribution to the family if the patient is not capable of fulfilling that role (e.g., in the immediate postsurgical period).

Certain cases are particularly troublesome. Among the most troublesome are those involving teenage patients. Information about pediatric patients is, of course, provided directly to the parents of the patients and not to the patients themselves; information about adult patients is, of course, provided directly to the patient and not the patient's parents. What about teenage patients seeking abortions, contraceptive advice, or treatment for venereal diseases, substance abuse, or psychiatric problems? Unless confidentiality can be guaranteed, such patients may not seek out the care they need. If confidentiality is protected, such patients may not get the parental counseling and support from which they could also benefit. Considerable confusion exists about the morally appropriate and legally mandated approach to confidentiality of information involving adolescent patients (Holder, 1985; Morrissey et al., 1986). Equally troubling are cases involving elderly patients who are less than fully competent but far from totally demented. Families of such patients often ask physicians to provide them with information about the patient's condition, information that they may not want to share with the patient. Such a request may be perfectly appropriate for the clearly incompetent demented patient, whereas it is obviously inappropriate for normal geriatric patients. How to handle cases that fall between these two extremes is unclear.

INFORMED CONSENT

The principle of informed consent is a much more recently articulated principle than the principle of confidentiality; the actual phrase "informed consent" first appeared in 1957 in the court case Salgo v. Leland Stanford Jr. University Board of Trustees. It has come, however, to be accepted as a fundamental principle governing the relation between patients and physicians.

The principle's basic mandate is that a physician must obtain the free and informed consent of a patient, if the patient is competent to give that consent, or of the patient's surrogate, if the patient is not competent, before medical treatment is provided. Two exceptions are normally recognized. The first (the emergency exception) is invoked when emergency treatment is necessary to protect the patient's life or health and consent cannot be obtained in a timely fashion. The second (the therapeutic privilege) is invoked when there is strong reason to believe that the very attempt to obtain consent will be harmful to the patient because of the psychologic impact of the information conveyed (Rozovsky, 1984).

Several complementary accounts of the significance of the principle of informed consent are available. One stresses the clinical benefits (in terms of building trust and obtaining compliance) from a therapeutic regimen begun as a result of a joint patient-physician decision rather than as a result of a unilateral physician decision. The other stresses the patient's right to control what happens to his or her body; the resulting obligation of the physician to obtain informed consent is the way in which the physician respects that right.

The standard practice in many institutions is to obtain written documentation of informed consent primarily (if not exclusively) in cases of invasive procedures. This practice should not be understood to mean that the principle of informed consent does not apply to other medical interventions; it applies to all of them. Signed consent forms are merely written evidence of the informed consent already obtained, and the practice reflects the prudent desire to obtain written documentation in cases in which potential liability is highest. Informed consent, as opposed to the written documentation of that consent, should be obtained in all cases, both as a way of obtaining clinical benefits and as a way of respecting patient's rights.

There has been considerable disagreement about the amount and type of information that must be supplied to the patient. Obviously, only a portion of the relevant information known by the physician can be conveyed to the patient. Moreover, any attempt to provide too much information may result in the physician overwhelming and confusing the patient. Some selection of information is required, and the disagreement centers around which principle of selection to adopt.

Two different proposals have been adopted by America's courts (Rozovsky, 1984). The first is the *professional practice standard*, which maintains that a consent is informed if the patient has been provided the information that reasonable medical practitioners would normally provide under similar circumstances. The second is the *reasonable person standard*, which maintains that a consent is informed if the patient has been provided the information that a reasonable person would need to have in order to make a decision about whether to undergo the therapy in question. The information to be provided would presumably fall under the categories shown in Table 12–1.

Most commentators have argued for the second standard, since it best corresponds to the goals of informed consent, but a majority of courts have adopted the usually less demanding professional practice standard (Rozovsky, 1984). Clinicians are, we believe, best advised to adopt the usually more stringent reasonable person standard, since it provides all the clinical and moral benefits of obtaining informed consent while firmly ensuring that the legal requirement of informed consent is satisfied. Clinicians must also be careful to provide that information using terminology that patients are likely to understand.

Table 12–1. ELEMENTS OF INFORMED CONSENT UNDER REASONABLE PERSON STANDARD

Nature of the patient's condition (e.g., hypertension)
Description of the treatment proposed (e.g., particular medication)
Benefits of proposed treatment (e.g., control of hypertension and resulting lowering of risk of disease)
Risks of proposed treatment (e.g., side effects for that medication)
Alternatives (e.g., other medications, diet and exercise, no intervention)
Costs of proposed treatment

A very difficult problem arises when one is dealing with patients whose competency is impaired. Informed consent is obtained from the patient when the patient is clearly competent and from the patient's surrogate (a legally appointed guardian, if available, or the closest family member) if the patient is clearly incompetent. What, however, should one do when the patient's mental capacities are clearly impaired but present to some degree? This problem is partially alleviated when one remembers that the assessment of the patient's competency is not an assessment of the patient's total ability to manage all of his or her affairs; it is just the assessment of whether at this moment the patient can: (1) receive the information relevant to giving or refusing informed consent for this particular treatment; (2) remember that information; (3) appropriately assess and use that information to make a decision; and (4) make a decision (Brody, 1988). Although no formal test exists to ensure that the patient has the capacity to perform items 1 to 4 in the list, a careful discussion with the patient will usually enable the physician to ascertain whether these criteria are satisfied. If doubt remains, one should obtain consent from both the patient and the surrogate.

A second difficulty involves teenage patients. Informed consent is obtained from parents before one treats children, but from patients once they become adults. How should physicians treat teenage patients? Most states have passed special laws allowing physicians to treat them after obtaining only their consent when: (1) the treatment is for venereal disease, pregnancy or contraception, or drug-related problems; (2) they are living away from their parents and are responsible for their own affairs; or (3) they are married. Other cases (particularly abortion) are more problematic (Holder, 1985; Morrissey et al., 1986).

THE NONCOMPLIANT PATIENT

Implicit in the principle of informed consent, the principle that medical treatment can only be provided after the patient has freely and knowingly consented to it, is the concept that a patient may choose not to comply with the physician's recommendations and that the choice not to comply must be respected. This concept can easily be misunderstood, however, leading to a quick and facile acceptance of a patient's noncompliance before its meaning is properly understood.

Several studies of noncompliance (Applebaum and Roth, 1983; Connelly and Campbell, 1987) have indicated that the majority of cases of noncompliance involve failures of communication, lack of trust due to previous bad experiences with the physician in question or others, and psychologic and psychopathologic factors. Only a minority of cases involve a true value difference between the physician and the patient. This finding has profound implications for the clinical management of noncompliance. Physicians confronting noncompliant patients need to assess the noncompliance, evaluate its cause, and react appropriately. Table 12–2 indicates how such a noncompliance assessment would proceed. In short, morality does not call upon the physician to accept at face value every episode of noncompliance on the part of the patient. Doing so may in fact constitute a form of disrespect for the patient. What morality does call for is a full evaluation of the cause of the noncompliance, appropriate responses where possible to eliminate the cause, and respect for the patient's noncompliance only when it is an informed and competent refusal that is based upon a difference between the patient's and the physician's values.

Even in those cases in which noncompliance represents an informed and competent refusal of the physician's recommendations because the patient's values differ, there may well exist alternative second-best forms of treatment that could be mutually acceptable. Consider a patient who refuses to stay in a hospital for a full evaluation because the patient is concerned about the need to be home to handle personal problems. Such a patient should be scheduled for an outpatient evaluation, even if it is not as satisfactory as a full evaluation in the hospital. (More examples of such compromises are provided later.) Respecting patient values in cases of noncompliance is not a matter of letting the patient win a power struggle; it is, more often, finding a mutually acceptable (even though not necessarily optimal) course of action. A failure to seek out such alternatives may often represent a lack of respect for the patient.

A form of noncompliance that deserves special attention is the patient who doesn't fill the prescription the doctor writes. This is sometimes due to the patient's financial condition. The optimal medication, from the physician's perspective, may cost too much from the patient's perspective. Particularly when dealing with patients who have high medication bills because they need so many drugs or with patients who have very limited means, physicians should raise the question of cost frankly and explore less expensive but satisfactory (even if not optimal) medications.

A similar problem often arises when one considers the question of side effects of various drugs. Different patients with different values and different tolerances may find certain side effects unacceptable. The physician should certainly not assume that a pattern of side effects that are acceptable to the physician will be acceptable to the patient. An important recent study (Croog et al., 1988) has stressed the significance of these matters in connection with the choice of antihypertensive agents, considering the implications of different agents for sexual dysfunction. Taking the patient's values into account in deciding which antihypertensive medication to order is a far clearer example of respecting the patient's values than simply accepting a patient's noncompliance with a prescription for a particular antihypertensive medication. This point can, of course, be generalized to other cases.

Table 12–2. EVALUATION OF NONCOMPLIANCE

Cause	Clinical Response
Problem in communication	Patient should be reinformed about the need for treatment
Failure of trust	Address question of mistrust Involve other physicians who may be trusted
Psychologic factors	Treat anxiety, depression, and so on
Value conflict	Respect patient wishes

Special Problems in Tertiary Care Settings

Quality of care can be improved by careful attention to the components examined thus far: the physician-patient relation, medicine as a profession, confidentiality, informed consent, and the promotion of patient compliance. When the focus shifts from primary care provided by the family physician to care provided by subspecialists in tertiary care settings, new problems arise and old problems become even more complicated. The next two sections examine ways of resolving some of these problems.

REFERRALS

Decisions regarding referrals are often accompanied by great confusion. Referrals to subspecialists practicing in tertiary care institutions can provoke anxiety on the part of patients. The referring physician risks losing a patient and a substantial amount of money and is subject to embarrassment if a mistake is discovered. Referrals sometimes degenerate into power struggles between subspecialists and generalists. Because primary care is a community-based discipline, there is much debate and little consensus as to the primary care physician's role in the tertiary care setting (Christie and Hoffmaster, 1986). The following guidelines about appropriate referrals and about continuity through referrals are intended to help clarify these responsibilities and thus ease the tension and improve the quality of care.

Decisions to refer should be based upon a realistic assessment of the potentialities and limitations of family medicine as a discipline, of oneself as a physician, and of the facilities available in one's geographic region. Unfortunately, a number of other factors (financial and institutional as well as medical) often cloud the decision-making process and disrupt relations between primary and tertiary care physicians (Weiss, 1986; Weiss, 1985).

Many subspecialists in oversubscribed areas have taken it upon themselves to practice primary care as a means of bolstering their incomes, despite their inadequate training in this area (Sigel and Sigel, 1980; Aiken et al., 1979; Gillette, 1979). Conversely, primary care physicians sometimes feel pressured to go beyond their areas of expertise for financial and professional reasons: they fear losing the patient and the income and fear that their seeking consultation might reinforce the misconception that primary care physicians are inferior (Perkoff, 1986; Weary, 1984; Sussman et al., 1982).

Knowing when to refer requires courage and humility. Courage is the ability to act competently and wisely without being swayed by irrational fears. Some primary care physicians, motivated by unrealistic fears of mistakes and exposure, refer too early. Humility, on the other hand, is the willingness to recognize one's *actual* limitations and to act accordingly. Some primary care physicians, unaware of their limitations, refer too late. A proper combination of courage and humility, along with good working relationships with subspecialists, can prevent most of the problems involved in referring too early or too late.

Even if the primary care physician does decide to refer the patient, he or she remains the patient's primary physician (Christie and Hoffmaster, 1986). Equipped with a strong knowledge of general medicine, of the patient's medical history, and of the patient's personal traits and committed to treating the disease in the context of the person and the person in the context of the family, the primary care physician is ideally suited to manage the patient throughout the referral.

When initiating a referral, the primary care physician's responsibilities are to educate the patient as to the reasons for referral, to recommend a subspecialist or treatment center best suited to the patient's medical and personal needs, to prepare the patient for what lies ahead, and to provide the specialist with data relevant to the patient's illness. Even after the referral, the primary care physician remains responsible for the quality of the patient's care. This may require translating medical jargon to patients or patient preferences to subspecialists and hospital staff, coordinating the activities of the various consultants, mediating disputes between consultants, ensuring that confidentiality is maintained by the health care team, and counseling patients and their families. The referral process is not complete until the subspecialist and the primary physician have discussed all findings, treatments, results, and recommendations and the patient has discussed these with the primary care physician (Christie and Hoffmaster, 1986; McPhee et al., 1984; Rakel and Williamson, 1984).

Sometimes, subspecialists disagree as to how to manage a particular disorder. Consider the different way that surgeons and cardiologists may treat carotid artery disease. Or consider the range of approaches, within particular subspecialties, in treating certain disorders: differences among gynecologists regarding indications for a hysterectomy, and differences among neonatologists in managing severely handicapped infants. This makes the referring physician's task a difficult and delicate one. The referring physician must be aware of the differences between subspecialties and between particular physicians within a subspecialty. The referring physician must know the patient and the patient's family well enough to recommend the appropriate subspecialist. In many cases, the principle of informed consent will mandate that the referring physician educate the patient and the family to the strengths and weaknesses of the available options. Primary care physicians should help their patients find a subspecialist who will be appropriate to both their medical needs and their personal preferences (Froom et al., 1984).

FINANCIAL GATEKEEPING

The soaring costs of health care have led corporations and government agencies to develop prospective payment systems and capitation plans, with primary care physicians often serving as gatekeepers of the health care network. It is hoped that this will save money and streamline the referral process. On the other hand, this might drive a bureaucratic wedge into the physician-patient relationship, allow money to compete with quality in determining the standard of care, and inhibit the physician's freedom to practice an individualized style of medicine.

Prospective reimbursement systems (such as the Medicare Diagnosis-Related Group system) save money by limiting the reimbursement available to physicians, thereby encouraging them to do less. Designers of such systems have the legitimate right to require physicians to avoid wasteful procedures and referrals; this prevents unnecessary expenditures and ensures a more just distribution of health care expenditures. Such limitations do not, however, preclude the physician's responsibility to offer the patient the best possible care within the limitations set by those policies. When particular patients require care in excess of the normal level of reimbursement, the primary care physician confronts a major ethical dilemma.

Considerable controversy exists as to whether physicians should do everything that they believe may benefit each patient without regard to costs or other societal considerations (Levinsky, 1984) or whether physicians must not be allowed to ignore the bottom line (Aaron and Schwartz, 1984). Traditionalists tend to ignore the fact that financial considerations have always limited the quality of care available to the poor. The question we are now confronting is whether these considerations may legitimately limit the quality of care available to everyone.

In caring for individual patients, physicians should distinguish between providing what the patient wants and what the patient needs. The controversy concerns whether all procedures and services likely to benefit the patient—as evidenced by outcome data—should be made available to the patient. When patients request unnecessary or marginally beneficial procedures and services, however, physicians must refuse.

It is often recommended (Fried, 1975) that if societal costs necessitate that care be withdrawn from or limited for certain patients, these decisions must be made not at the bedside but at the policy level, prior to and apart from particular situations and applications. Such difficult policy decisions should not be made by physicians alone but should be negotiated at the policy level by the three major competing parties in the health care delivery system: institutional representatives, whose concern it is that the bills be paid; physicians, whose interest is professional integrity and personal income; and patients, who want the best care and the maximum choice at the lowest price (Pellegrino and Thomasma, 1981). It is an open question whether these recommendations are reasonable, realistic, and appropriate (Brody, 1988).

The Physician as Human Being

The medical profession has, in the past few decades, achieved truly impressive gains in the battle against sickness, suffering, and death. Diseases that killed their victims just a generation ago are now manageable, curable, or even preventable. Yet physicians seem remarkably inept at maintaining their own health and well-being; they suffer high rates of alcoholism, substance abuse, divorce, burnout, and suicide (Hilfiker, 1985; Jonsen, 1983). Why can't the healers heal themselves, and what can they do to get on the road to recovery? To deal with these problems, we recommend that physicians learn to distinguish between competence and perfectionism, dedication and workaholism, and compassion and sentimentalism.

In medical school and residency, young doctors often learn to put their careers ahead of self and family (Gerber, 1983). This dedication is, in some ways, good. Young physicians want to do everything they can to help their patients. But this is often coupled with an unrealistic perception of their capabilities and those of their profession. They allow their egos to become too closely identified with their successes and failures. They become obsessed with insecurity (they are not good enough) and guilt (they do not work hard enough). They worry that they might have missed a diagnosis and fear that their patients will die or suffer unnecessarily. Physicians are not supposed to make mistakes, but they do. Their profession requires staying on top of an ever-expanding field of knowledge, adeptness at a wide range of techniques and skills, making the right decision when fatigued or hassled or angry, picking up on subtle clues or poorly articulated symptoms, and juggling a plethora of human needs at once. Mistakes are inevitable, but talking about them is taboo. The only place mistakes are openly discussed, it seems, is the courtroom (Hilfiker, 1985). To be more effective clinicians, physicians must learn to acknowledge their capacity to err and must learn to discuss errors in a constructive manner. Physicians who do not admit their mistakes are doomed to repeat them. Physicians who discuss their mistakes can learn from them and experience healing in the process.

The physician who takes the time to care for personal and family needs is a more effective clinician because he or she is better able to cope with the stresses and strains of a demanding profession. And, in the case of primary care physicians whose patients know them well, the physician will become a role model for personal health and fitness.

Another area in which physicians must learn to accept their humanity, and the humanity of their patients, is in the area of emotions. Clinicians must help patients recognize, express, and interpret their emotions. Clinicians must become aware of their own emotions, recognize their clinical value, and learn how to express and interpret them. The physician who ignores the emotions dehumanizes the physician-patient relationship. The primary care physician who improperly expresses, utilizes, or interprets emotional factors deprofessionalizes that relationship (Zinn, 1988; Frankel, 1986; Katz, 1963). Traditionally, physicians have been trained to maintain objectivity, affective neutrality, and clinical detachment. To be scientific, however, does not preclude recognizing the legitimacy of emotions or the necessity of empathy as a legitimate clinical and moral response to suffering. Sometimes a patient's feelings offer a clue to his or her symptoms. Sometimes a physician's feelings in response to a patient offer a clue to the patient's problem (Zinn, 1988). Suffering patients need a physician who will suffer alongside them and who will help them to express and interpret their feelings (Reich, 1989). When their patients suffer, physicians suffer too. The physician who suffers alongside a suffering patient or family allows the opportunity for healing of self as well as of the patient or family. Many of the physician's feelings, however, cannot be appropriately expressed in the clinical encounter. To maintain personal well-being, therefore, the physician must find appropriate outlets for expression and interpretation.

Conclusion

The ethical questions faced by physicians have been transformed, in ways we have indicated, by changing economic, social, legal, and political factors. In the end, however, the ethics of medicine remains committed to a view of the patient-physician relationship as a relationship between two autonomous human beings—a patient who is suffering and seeks help, and a physician who maintains his or her humanity as well as his or her professionalism.

References

Aaron, H., and Schwartz, W.: The Painful Prescription: Rationing Hospital Care. Washington, D.C., Brookings Institute, 1984.

Aiken, L. H., Lewis, C. E., Craig, J., et al.: The contributions of specialists to the delivery of primary care: A new perspective. N. Engl. J. Med., *300*:1363–1370, 1979.

Alexander, E., Jr.: A "truth in mending" act (commentary). J.A.M.A., *243*:1239–1240, 1980.

Applebaum, P., and Roth, L.: Patients who refuse treatment in medical hospitals. J.A.M.A., *250*:1296–1301, 1983. *A careful study of the incidence of noncompliance in hospitals. The authors identify a variety of causes for this noncompliance, and they develop clinical strategies for dealing with the different cases.*

Brody, B. A.: Life and Death Decision Making. New York, Oxford University Press, 1988. *An overview of the many different cases in which physicians have to decide between prolonging life and allowing patients to die. The author presents a new framework for resolving the disputes that arise in such cases.*

Bruce, J. A.: Privacy and Confidentiality of Health Care Information. Chicago, American Hospital Association, 1984. *A comprehensive treatment of confidentiality and privacy, with special emphasis on appropriate policies for protecting patient records. Of special value is the discussion of the disclosure of information to third parties.*

Christie, R. J., and Hoffmaster, C. B.: Ethical Issues in Family Medicine. New York, Oxford University Press, 1986. *An examination of ethical issues arising in the everyday practice of family medicine. Of special value are the many case studies and the thorough overview of the literature in the field.*

Connelly, J., and Campbell, C.: Patients who refuse treatment in medical offices. Arch. Intern. Med., *147*:1829–1833, 1987. *A careful study of the incidence of noncompliance in the ambulatory setting. The authors identify a variety of causes for this noncompliance, and they develop clinical strategies for dealing with the different cases.*

Croog, S., et al.: Sexual symptoms in hypertensive patients. Arch. Intern. Med., *148*:788–794, 1988.

Dickens, B. M.: Legal limits of AIDS confidentiality. J.A.M.A., *259*:3449–3451, 1988.

Eastaugh, S. R.: Financing Health Care: Economic Efficiency and Equity. Dover, MA, Auburn House Publishing Company, 1987.

Frankel, B. L.: Affective neutrality (A Piece of My Mind). J.A.M.A., *256*:515, 1986.

Fried, C.: Rights and health care—Beyond equity and efficiency. N. Engl. J. Med., *293*:241–245, 1975.

Froom, J., Feinbloom, R. I., and Rosen, M. G.: Risks of referral. J. Fam. Pract., *18*:623–626, 1984.

Gerber, L. A.: Married to Their Careers: Career and Family Dilemmas in Doctors' Lives. New York, Tavistock Publications, 1983.

Gillette, R. D.: The delivery of "primary care" by specialists. N. Engl. J. Med., *301*:893–894, 1979.

Hilfiker, D.: A Physician Looks at His Work. New York, Pantheon Books, 1985.

Holder, A.: Legal Issues in Pediatrics and Adolescent Medicine. New Haven, CT, Yale University Press, 1985. *A comprehensive discussion of the legal treatment of the many ethical issues raised in the management of pediatric patients.*

Holleman, W. L., and Holleman, M. C.: School and work release evaluations. J.A.M.A., 1988; *260*:3629-3634. *This study identifies ethical issues arising in the performance of school and work release evaluations. It proposes ways of resolving these difficult issues.*

Jonsen, A. R., Siegler, M., and Winslade, W. J.: Clinical Ethics: A Practical Approach to Ethical Decisions in Clinical Medicine. 2nd ed. New York, Macmillan Publishing Company, 1986. *A manual of ethical and legal principles and of their application to many clinical situations. It has both the merits and shortcomings of brief manuals.*

Jonsen, A. R.: Watching the doctor. N. Engl. J. Med., *308*:1531–1535, 1983.

Katz, R. L.: Empathy: Its Nature and Uses. London, The Free Press of Glencoe, Collier-Macmillan Limited, 1963.

Kelman, G. R.: The pre-employment medical examination. Lancet, *2*:1231–1233, 1985.

Levinsky, N. G.: The doctor's master. N. Engl. J. Med., *311*:1573–1575, 1984. *This article presents the problems posed by the physician as a gatekeeper and argues that physicians must be concerned solely with the welfare of their patients; social cost considerations should not be considered by physicians.*

McPhee, S. J., Lo, B., Saika, G. Y., and Meltzer, R.: How good is communication between primary care physicians and subspecialty consultants? (Special report.) Arch. Intern. Med., *144*:1265–1268, 1984. *This articles examines the often-neglected question of the relation between primary care physicians and subspecialist consultants. Of special importance is its discussion of communication between these physicians.*

Mills, M., Sullivan, G., and Eth, S.: Protecting third parties: A decade after Tarasoff. Am. J. Psychiatry, *144*:68–74, 1987.

Morrissey, J., Hofmann, A., and Thrope, J.: Consent and Confidentiality in the Health Care of Children and Adolescents. New York, The Free Press, 1986. *A comprehensive discussion of the legal treatment of the ethical issues surrounding informed consent and confidentiality when dealing with nonadult patients. Of special importance is its discussion of adolescents.*

Pellegrino, E. G., and Thomasma, D. C.: A Philosophical Basis of Medical Practice: Toward a Philosophy and Ethic of the Healing Professions. New York, Oxford University Press, 1981.

Perkoff, G. T.: Ethical aspects of the physician surplus: Implications for family practice. J. Fam. Pract., *22*:455–460, 1986.

Rakel, R. E., and Williamson, P. S.: Use of consultants. *In* Rakel, R. E.: Textbook of Family Practice. 3rd ed. Philadelphia, W. B. Saunders Company, 1984, pp. 190–197.

Reich, W. T.: Speaking of suffering: A moral account of compassion. Soundings, 72:83-108. *A phenomenological analysis of the phases of suffering undergone by patients and of the corresponding need for phases of compassion by physicians.*

Rosenstock, L., and Hagopian, A.: Ethical dilemmas in providing health care to workers. Ann. Intern. Med., *107*:575–580, 1987.

Rozovsky, F.: Consent to Treatment: A Practical Guide. Boston, Little Brown, 1984. *An extremely comprehensive treatment of all aspects of the doctrine of informed consent. Of special value is its discussion of the implications of that doctrine for different areas of medicine.*

Siegler, M.: The progression of medicine: From physician paternalism to patient autonomy to bureaucratic parsimony. Arch. Intern. Med., *145*:713, 1985.

Sigel, L., and Sigel, B.: The role of subspecialists in primary medical care. Perspect. Biol. Med., *24*:122–128, 1980.

Smith, H. L., and Churchill, L. R.: Professional Ethics and Primary Care Medicine: Beyond Dilemmas and Decorum. Durham, NC, Duke University Press, 1986. *An exploration of philosophical and moral issues raised by the interface of persons and values in primary care medicine. More philosophical but less clinically oriented than Christie and Hoffmaster's Ethical Issues in Family Medicine.*

Sussman, E. J., Tsiaras, W. G., and Soper, K. A.: Diagnosis of diabetic eye disease. J.A.M.A., *247*:3231–3234, 1982.

Tarasoff v. Regents of California 118 Cal. Rptr. 129 (1974).

Weary, P. E.: Behold, the gatekeeper cometh. (Commentary). Int. J. Dermatol., *23*:33–35, 1984.

Weiss, B. D.: Family practice in hospitals. (Commentary.) J.A.M.A., *253*:549–550, 1985.

Weiss, B. D.: The effect of malpractice insurance costs on family physicians' hospital practices. J. Fam. Pract., *23*:55–58, 1986.

Whiting, R. K.: The anxious manipulator and disability. (Letter.) J. Occup. Med., *19*:655, 1977.

Zinn, W. M.: Doctors have feelings too. J.A.M.A., *259*:3296–3298, 1988.

Part II

Community Medicine

13

The Periodic Health Examination

Renaldo N. Battista
Walter O. Spitzer
Jean Haggerty

The family physician must be an able practitioner of preventive medicine; competence as a prognostician is essential in order to apply the principles of preventive medicine to a person or a family. Thus, the family physician must perform complete work-ups and also be highly sophisticated in performing preventive check-ups.

The approach proposed for the periodic health examination is based on a set of age- and sex-related health protection packages and aims at creating a lifetime health care plan. This strategy results from shortcomings discovered in the conventional annual check-up. The scope and the frequency of examinations included in the conventional check-up are challenged on grounds that they bear little relation to the needs of different age and sex groups. Moreover, most of the tests and procedures included in routine examinations have not been demonstrated to be efficacious or effective and the optimal frequency of their administration has not been ascertained. The health protection package approach addresses these two main criticisms by being specifically targeted to age and sex groups and by being restricted to procedures about which we have some evidence of efficacy and effectiveness.

Theoretical Foundation of the Periodic Health Examination

DEFINITION OF TERMS

Periodic Health Examination. The periodic health examination is composed of a group of tasks designed either to determine the risk of subsequent disease or to identify disease in its early, symptomless state. Other interventions, such as injections for immunization and counseling for the prevention of disease or the maintenance of health, are also covered by the definition.

Health Protection Package. Health protection packages are sets of procedures that are particularly applicable to the periodic health examination at certain ages and in certain "at-risk" groups.

Preventive Intervention. There are basically two types of preventive intervention—primary and secondary. The aim of *primary prevention* is to prevent the occurrence of disease by modifying exposure to ill health behaviors or risk factors; the aim of *secondary prevention* is to identify a disease at such an early stage that application of a subsequent intervention could affect the ultimate outcome positively. Although secondary prevention and early detection are often used interchangeably, a secondary preventive intervention subsumes the application of an early detection procedure followed by the appropriate primary preventive or curative intervention. Detection of disease or even risk factors for a disease by health workers in patients who consult physicians for unrelated symptoms is also referred to as **case finding.** **Screening** is the application of procedures to populations or subpopulations in order to classify them into two groups: one with a high probability of being affected by fatal or disabling conditions, the other with a low probability of incurring the same conditions. Those with a high probability are then referred to a physician for further diagnosis or consultation. Poor compliance with the second step will compromise the effectiveness of screening; case finding is favored because the subsequent referral process is unnecessary.

Efficacy. The attribute of an intervention or maneuver that results in more good than harm to those who accept and comply with the intervention and subsequent treatment.

Effectiveness. The attribute of an intervention or maneuver that results in more good than harm to those to whom it is offered.

Efficiency. The attribute of an effective intervention that optimizes the use of limited resources.

SCIENTIFIC PRINCIPLES OF EVALUATION OF PREVENTIVE SERVICES

The efficacy and effectiveness of preventive interventions are best ascertained through the same approaches used to evaluate any therapeutic intervention. The randomized controlled trial remains the preferred strategy of evaluation whenever feasible. Other approaches are the cohort study, the case-control study, quasi-experimental designs such as time series, and descriptive studies or case reports (see Chapter 82). Measuring health outcomes is a difficult and common problem whatever design is chosen. Ideally, an intervention should be evaluated in terms of such outcomes as mortality, morbidity, or the resulting quality of life.

An early detection procedure can be a history item, a physical examination, or a laboratory test; ideally it should be accurate, safe, simple, inexpensive, acceptable to both patients and clinicians, and positive (or neutral) in its psychologic labeling effects. The performance characteristics of early detection procedures can be determined. *Sensitivity* is defined as the proportion of diseased individuals correctly identified by the procedure; *specificity* is the proportion of healthy individuals correctly classified as disease free by the technique. The positive and negative predictive values of each test should also be ascertained, if at all possible, since they are of utmost importance to the clinician. The *positive predictive value* is that proportion of individuals having a positive test who are actually affected by the disease in question, whereas the *negative predictive value* of a test is the proportion of subjects with a negative test who are free of the disease. When the prevalence of a particular disease is low, the positive predictive value of relevant detection tests will be low, even when they have high sensitivity and high specificity, whereas the negative predictive values will be high. When asymptomatic subjects are being examined, high performance on all of these test properties is crucial to early detection. The principles involved are discussed at length in the epidemiologic literature (Vecchio, 1966; McNeil et al., 1975; Sackett et al., 1985; Fletcher et al., 1982).

Several methodological snares can jeopardize the evaluation of secondary preventive interventions, particularly in the domain of chronic diseases. The advantage sought by early detection is improvement of life expectancy and quality of life, but commonly used indices, such as the 5-year survival from time of diagnosis, can be very deceptive in this context. Early detection does not, in itself, ensure any deferral of the time of death: It may only lengthen the illness by making people aware of their disease sooner. Proper evaluation of secondary preventive strategies should always correct for this potential *"lead-time" bias*. Detection procedures probably identify slowly evolving conditions more easily than rapidly progressing ones. The more likely identification of conditions with longer natural histories and better prognoses may make a preventive procedure appear to have a better performance than it actually has *(length bias)* (Cole and Morrison, 1980; Sackett et al., 1985).

When the efficacy and effectiveness of preventive interventions have been ascertained, their cost-benefit and/or cost-effectiveness ratios should be assessed since the increasing scarcity of resources for health care make societal choices necessary. Decision-makers can then recommend choices from among those with comparable effectiveness but different degrees of efficiency (Weinstein and Stason, 1977; Russell, 1986). Sound practice recommendations should also take into account issues of safety, availability, and acceptability of effective or efficacious interventions.

FORMULATION PROCESS OF PRACTICE RECOMMENDATIONS

The Canadian Task Force on the Periodic Health Examination developed a clinical-epidemiologic approach in making recommendations for the periodic health examination. This process was subsequently adopted and amended by the United States Preventive Services Task Force at its initiation in 1984. The task forces identified potentially preventable target conditions that might be assessed during a periodic health examination. Each of the candidate conditions was assessed according to the following criteria:

- the *current burden of illness* attributable to it, taking account of years of life lost, amount of disability, pain and discomfort, out-of-pocket and indirect cost of treatment, and the effect on families
- when applicable, the performance characteristics of early detection procedures (sensitivity, specificity, and predictive values)
- the effectiveness of primary and/or secondary preventive interventions as well as safety, acceptability, labeling, and cost issues

The most important consideration when deciding whether or not to include a preventive intervention in a periodic health examination is its effectiveness in preventing the target medical condition weighted against the potential risks of the intervention itself. Table 13–1 lists clinical procedures that have been shown to be ineffective in preventing or improving the outcome of the target condition.

The evidence as to the effectiveness of each preventive intervention is graded by the two task forces according to the quality of evidence found in the world medical literature. Quality of study design is an important consideration, with randomized clinical trials at the top of the hierarchy and descriptive studies at the bottom. Within each study, the quality of information is assessed by considering potential for bias, adequacy of statistical power, and data analysis. Other important considerations are the general applicability of results and the potential for the use of labeling.

For each condition, the information on the burden of illness, the accuracy of the early detection procedure, the effectiveness of the primary or sec-

Table 13–1. PREVENTIVE INTERVENTIONS THAT SHOULD *NOT* BE PERFORMED IN THE PERIODIC HEALTH EXAMINATION OF ASYMPTOMATIC PERSONS

Clinical Procedure	Target Condition	Comments	Grade*	Reference
Chest x-ray studies, sputum cytology	Lung cancer (bronchogenic carcinoma)	No clinical maneuver has been validated for early detection	D	CTF,† 1979
Photofluorography, saline wash, and cytologic examination of gastric contents	Cancer of the stomach	Early treatment does not alter the natural history of the disease High-risk region: Newfoundland Some evidence of value of early detection	C	CTF, 1979
Endometrial biopsy; cytologic examination of endometrium	Endometrial cancer	Unreliable early detection maneuvers for benign hyperplasia. Effectiveness of screening unknown. No controlled studies on the effectiveness of early treatment	D	CTF, 1987
Urinalysis	Urinary tract infection	Screening detects some cases, but yield is low. Reinfection often follows treatment	D	CTF, 1979
Thyroid function tests, T4 elevation	Hyperthyroidism	Effectiveness of detection and treatment of presymptomatic disease unknown; symptoms manifest rapidly	D	CTF, 1988
Funduscopy, measurement of intraocular pressure, visual field testing	Primary open-angle glaucoma	Disc-cup ratio measured by funduscopy is the most accurate detection maneuver but only when done by ophthalmologists	C	CTF, 1986
Psychiatric assessment	Psychiatric disorders (affective disorders and suicide)	For psychotic affective disorders, treatment is efficacious. For neurotic or reactive affective disorders, treatment is of uncertain efficacy. For suicide, the value of prevention has not been demonstrated	D	CTF, 1979
Preschool developmental screening with Denver Development Test	Developmental delay	Improved school performance through early intervention has not been demonstrated; however, parental anxiety is decreased	D	CTF, (in press)
Bone densitometry	Osteoporosis	Clinical maneuver is expensive and not widely available. Bone mass is not a sufficiently accurate predictor or fracture incidence	D	CTF, 1988
Cytologic examination of the urine	Bladder cancer	There is no evidence that early detection improves the prognosis	D	CTF, 1979

*See Table 14–5, page 227, for explanation of grades assigned by the Canadian and United States Task Forces.
†Canadian Task Force on the Periodic Health Examination.

ondary preventive intervention, and the quality of the evidence is synthesized. A graded recommendation for inclusion or exclusion of the procedure in the search for that condition in the periodic health examination is made as follows:

A. There is *good* evidence to support the recommendation that the condition be *included* in a periodic health examination.

B. There is *fair* evidence to support the recommendation that the condition be *included* in a periodic health examination.

C. There is *poor* evidence regarding either the inclusion or exclusion of the condition in a periodic health examination, and recommendations may be made on other grounds.

D. There is *fair* evidence to support the recommendation that the condition be *excluded* from consideration in a periodic health examination.

E. There is *good* evidence to support the recommendation that the condition be *excluded* from consideration in a periodic health examination.

Graded recommendations explicitly acknowledge the different degrees of current scientific certainty about different preventive services. Grades help clinicians attach priorities to preventive activities in their practices. Graded recommendations may also help point the way for reimbursement agencies when considering which procedures to reimburse. Finally, by making explicit the areas where evidence is weak, problems are highlighted for future research agendas.

The Practice of the Periodic Health Examination

RECOMMENDATIONS AND HEALTH PROTECTION PACKAGES

One should reiterate that primary and secondary preventive measures are performed when a patient comes in to see the physician for intercurrent illness or problems. These are patient-initiated encounters. The patient is given an explanation of the purpose of the procedures and counseling. Over time, it is hoped that a family physician's practice would become "educated" to this lifetime strategy of prevention.

Tables 13–2 through 13–8 are guidelines for preventive interventions that should be included in the periodic health examination of different patient groups; they summarize the findings of the Canadian Task Force on the Periodic Health Examination and the United States Preventive Services Task Force. For each age group, the tables indicate whether the procedure is primary or secondary prevention, whether or not it should be directed at high risk persons, and when possible, its frequency. The references given are for the respective task force publications, which, in turn, contain all the key references used in making the final recommendations and assigning the grades.

In the following section, we offer three sample cases of case finding and the practice of the periodic health examination. There are several common themes of preventive practice that pervade all three examples:

1. Prevention was done in the course of management of intercurrent health problems frequently handled by the family physician.
2. Guidelines such as those shown in the tables in this chapter or adaptations of such guidelines created by physicians for their own patient population should be subjected to clinical judgment, based on knowledge of the patient.
3. The presence of a high-risk situation (for instance, the man occupationally exposed to loud noise or the woman with heavy ultraviolet light exposure) should influence the preventive schedule adopted.
4. Although most of these activities can be done in the context of patient-triggered encounters, exceptions need to be recognized. For instance, a recall system for patients who would benefit from mammography on an annual basis would be essential to ensure adequate patient adherence to the preventive schedule.
5. Much of what can and should be done in preventive medicine is appropriately undertaken by allied health professionals working with the family physician, especially if the physician works in settings with a team approach.

Physicians involved in lifetime health maintenance should adopt or design flowsheets compatible with their own practices and charting systems. Such flowsheets make it very easy to check the "health protection status" of patients when they come in for any problem (see Fig. 11 A & B chapter 73).

Clinical Examples

Consider these examples of health protection tactics:

CASE 1

A 42-year-old male, who has been known to the physician for 12 years but has not been seen for 3 years, comes in to have pain at the bottom of his spine checked. He has had it for 5 days following a fall on the ice. A physical examination by the physician reveals a possible fracture of the tip of the coccyx with very localized tenderness. Appropriate advice is given for this problem as well as reassurance. While the patient is in the physician's office, his blood pressure is measured (it is within normal limits) and clinical assessment of hearing is done, since this man is a foreman in a lumber processing mill of northern Quebec; the physician stresses the value of wearing ear protection to prevent hearing loss. Alcohol does not appear to be a problem, and the physician reinforces with satisfaction the patient's continuing 6-year abstinence from smoking. The physician notes that 5 years ago, the patient's plasma cholesterol was within normal limits; another nonfasting total plasma cholesterol measure is ordered. The patient has been a strong advocate of mandatory seatbelts for a long time and has been to the dentist within 12 months. His family situation seems to be healthy.

Table 13–2. PREVENTIVE INTERVENTIONS THAT ARE TO BE INCLUDED IN THE *PRENATAL* PERIODIC HEALTH EXAMINATION

Clinical Procedure	Target Condition	Recommendation and Comments	Grade*	Reference
Blood pressure measurement	Hypertension	At every visit	A	CTF,† 1984
Microbiologic examination of the urine	Bacteriuria	Secondary prevention. Screen once in each trimester, and 6 weeks postpartum	B	CTF, 1979
Blood typing, Rh antibody test	Blood group incompatibility	Secondary prevention. Screen at first prenatal visit	A	CTF, 1979
Fasting and oral glucose tolerance test	Gestational diabetes	Primary prevention of macrosomia. Perform OGTT at 24–28 weeks' gestation. Most patients achieve glucose control by dietary management	B‡	CTF, 1979
Cultures of cervical and urethral smears	Gonorrhea	Primary prevention of ophthalmia neonatorum	A A	CTF, 1979 USTF§ Horsburgh, 1987
Cultures of cervical and urethral smears	Chlamydial genital infection	Primary prevention of chlamydial conjunctivitis. Efficacy of treatment during pregnancy not yet proved	B B	CTF, 1984 USTF Horsburgh, 1987
VDRL blood test	Syphilis	Primary prevention of congenital syphilis. Target at high risk women. Recommendation based on severe effects of untreated syphilis	A B	CTF, 1979 USTF Horsburgh, 1987
Counseling	Breast-feeding	Primary prevention. Provide appropriate information about all infant feeding methods. Breast-feeding is recommended for baby's health	B	CTF, 1984
Counseling, nutritional history, weighing	Low birth weight	Primary prevention. Ensure adequate protein and caloric intake by mother. Possibly determine serum protein. Advise to stop smoking	B	CTF, 1979
Counseling and advice	Alcohol consumption	Primary prevention. Inform women of consequences of alcohol consumption. Advise to reduce consumption	B	CTF, 1979
Family assessment	Parenting problems	Primary prevention. Identify families in need of more than usual amount of services; promote early parent-infant interaction through early contact, rooming-in, and breast-feeding	B	CTF, 1979
Counseling, referral for serum α-fetoprotein test	Neural tube defect	Secondary prevention. A positive test may imply the need for therapeutic abortion. Women should be informed of all the alternatives before they are screened, and follow-up arrangements should be made	B	CTF, 1979
Genetic counseling, amniocentesis	Down's syndrome	**High-risk women *only:*** a) one parent known carrier of faulty chromosome, b) previous child with Down's syndrome, c) familial history of Down's, d) maternal age >35 years Secondary prevention. Positive result may imply the need for therapeutic abortion	B	CTF, 1979
Counseling, serologic testing for *Toxoplasma gondii*	Toxoplasmosis	**High-risk women *only:*** women with cat at home or who eat raw meat. Primary and secondary prevention. Nonimmune (seronegative) women should be tested each trimester, counseled to avoid cat litter and raw meat. Treat with spiramycin in case of seroconversion	A	CTF, 1979
Cerclage of cervix	Preterm labour	**High-risk women *only*:** history of incompetence of the cervix Primary prevention	B	CTF, 1979
History and counseling	Postnatal asphyxia	Primary prevention. Counseling to promote intrauterine growth through smoking cessation, adequate rest, and good nutrition. Physician can diagnose diseases early and prevent complications	B	CTF, 1979
History and counseling	Electronic fetal monitoring during labor	**High-risk women *only*:** women with toxemia, hypertension, renal disease, heart disease, diabetes mellitus, endocrine ablation, previous blood group incompatibility, previous pregnancy problems, or anatomic disorders of pregnancy. Secondary prevention	C	CTF (in press)

*See Table 14–5, page 227, for explanation of grades assigned by the Canadian and United States Task Forces.
†Canadian Task Force on the Periodic Health Examination.
‡Recommendation currently under review; recommendation may change.
§United States Preventive Services Task Force position paper, 1989.

Table 13–3. CONDITIONS THAT ARE TARGETS FOR SEARCH IN THE PERIODIC HEALTH EXAMINATION OF *NEONATES AND INFANTS* (0–18 months)

Clinical Procedure	Target Condition	Recommendation and Comments	Grade*	Reference
I. Preventive Interventions at Birth				
Silver nitrate eye drops	Ophthalmia neonatorum	Potential secondary prevention of gonococcal infection	A	CTF,† 1979
VDRL of cord blood	Congenital syphilis	Secondary prevention	B	CTF, 1979
T4 testing from heel prick	Neonatal hypothyroidism	Secondary prevention. Part of mass screening programs at hospitals	A	CTF (in press)
Intramuscular vitamin K	Hemorrhagic disease of the newborn	Primary prevention. 1 mg. at birth	B	CTF, 1979
II. Preventive Interventions for Neonates				
Ortonlani's maneuver, hip flexion abduction	Congenital hip dislocation	Secondary prevention. Perform in first week of life	B	CTF, 1979
Clinical examination, history-taking	Intraventricular septal defect	Secondary prevention. Perform at discharge from nursery and at 6 weeks. Accurate diagnosis important in view of documented labeling effects	B	CTF, 1979
Guthrie test, fluorometric test	Phenylketonuria	Secondary prevention. Accuracy of screening test depends on baby's age; repeat and supplemental tests may be necessary	B	CTF, 1979
III. Preventive Interventions for Infants				
History and physical examination	Hearing impairment	Secondary prevention. Elicit history of failure to "babble" or to demonstrate a startle or turning response to noise outside their field of vision.	B	CTF, 1979
Serial height and weight measures	Physical growth disorders	Secondary prevention. At each well baby visit. Investigate infants under the 3rd or above the 97th percentile	B	CTF, 1979
Eye inspection, cover-uncover test	Strabismus	Secondary prevention. Age at which early detection should occur is unclear. Treatment is effective	B	CTF, 1979
DPT, polio, and MMR vaccination	Vaccine for preventable infectious diseases	Primary prevention. DPT and polio performed in first 6 months of life; MMR between 12 to 15 months. Caution is advised in infants allergic to egg protein	A A	CTF, 1979 USTF‡ LaForce, 1987
Sweat test on at least two occasions	Cystic fibrosis	**High-risk infants *only:*** siblings of cystic fibrosis patients Secondary prevention. Treatment in first year of life enhances survival and prognosis	B	CTF, 1979
Family function assessment	Child abuse	Primary prevention. Ask about parents' coping ability, stresses, and supports. Identify families in need of more than usual services	A	CTF, 1979
Counseling, anticipatory guidance	Night-time crying	Secondary prevention. At 6-month visit, if parents distressed by infant not sleeping through the night, recommend systematic ignoring		CTF§
Counseling and advice	Motor vehicle accidents	Primary prevention. Counsel parents to use proper car seats when transporting child	B	USTF Pollen, 1988
Counseling	Accidental injury in the home	Primary prevention. Advise to reduce exposure to accident risk factors by reducing hot water to <54.4° C. (130° F.), safety-proofing cupboards, electrical outlets, and drawers with poisonous substances or sharp objects, putting gates over stairs		CTF[4]

*See Table 14–5, page 227, for explanation of grades of recommendation assigned by the Canadian and United States Task Forces.

†Canadian Task Force on the Periodic Health Examination.

‡United States Preventive Services Task Force position paper, 1989.

§Recommendation currently under review; final grade has not been assigned.

Table 13–4. PREVENTIVE INTERVENTIONS RECOMMENDED FOR THE PERIODIC HEALTH EXAMINATION OF *CHILDREN AND ADOLESCENTS* (age 1½ to 19 years)

Clinical Procedure	Target Condition	Recommendation and Comments	Grade*	Reference
Serial height and weight measurement	Physical growth disorders	Secondary prevention. Further investigation in children under the 3rd or above the 97th percentile	B	CTF,† 1979
	Obesity	Primary and secondary prevention. Encourage daily physical activity and appropriate caloric intake	C	CTF, 1979
	Malnutrition	Primary and secondary prevention. Adolescent girls are at high risk for malnutrition. Enquire into eating habits, possibly determine serum protein concentration	B	CTF (in press)
Visual acuity testing. Cover-uncover test	Refractive defects, strabismus, amblyopia	Secondary prevention. Routine screening in preschool years decreases the prevalence of uncorrected disorders	B	CTF, 1989b
Vaccination history	Rubella, diphtheria, and tetanus	Primary prevention. Ensure that prepubertal girls are vaccinated for rubella. Ensure that diphtheria and tetanus booster are given 10 years after full immunization	A A	CTF, 1979; USTF‡ Laforce, 1987
Most recent influenza vaccine	Influenza	**High-risk Persons *only*:** Children with metabolic disease, immunosuppression, or renal dysfunction. Primary prevention	A	USTF LaForce, 1987
Rifampin chemoprophylaxis	Meningococcal meningitis	Primary prevention in **high-risk groups:** infants who have had close contact with patients with meningococcal infection	A	USTF LaForce, 1987
Counseling	Motor vehicle accidents	Primary and secondary prevention. Advise parents to use car seat and seat belts for children. Education of parents in medical setting shown to increase use	B	USTF Pollen, 1988
Contraceptive counseling	Unwanted teenage pregnancy	Primary prevention. Identify sexually active adolescents, inform of contraceptive methods, prescribe if necessary	B	CTF, 1988
Dental history and counseling	Dental caries, malocclusion	Primary prevention. Enquire about last dental visit, encourage regular visits and consultation with dentists	B	CTF, 1979

*See Table 14–5, page 227, for explanation of grade of recommendation assigned by the Canadian and United States Task Forces.

†Canadian Task Force on the Periodic Health Examination.

‡United States Preventive Services Task Force position paper.

CASE 2

A 65-year-old woman consults her physician about headaches she has had for 4 months. This results in three visits in which a careful investigation of the problem is carried out. On the third visit the physician undertakes health protection activities. The decision to defer prevention to the third visit was taken because the patient was known to adhere strongly to recommendations of physicians. Otherwise, the package would have been administered earlier in the process. The patient's blood pressure is checked. The skin is examined carefully because this patient spends 7 or 8 months of the year in the hot sun of Alabama; she is encouraged to routinely use sun screens. A physical examination of the breasts is done and arrangements are made for a mammography study. She is strongly urged to return for a further physical examination and mammography in approximately 1 year. The practice nurse has a recall card system for that purpose. The patient gives a history of being under dental care every 8 weeks because of bridge work. A tetanus booster is given in accordance with her mid-decade examination. A Papanicolaou smear is performed because the last one had been performed when she was age 60. The importance of wearing seatbelts is reinforced by the physician, since she is resistant to this practice.

CASE 3

A 16-year-old girl comes to the physician on referral by a friend to receive a certificate of health as a requirement for attending a basketball camp. Her history reveals that she has not been immunized against rubella, and since she has not seen a physician for several years, she did not receive her mid-decade tetanus-diphtheria booster when she was

Table 13–5. PREVENTIVE INTERVENTIONS TO BE INCLUDED IN THE PERIODIC HEALTH EXAMINATION OF *ALL ADULTS* (age 20 to 64 years)

Clinical Procedure	Target Condition	Recommendation and Comments	Grade*	Reference
Blood pressure measurement	Hypertension	Primary prevention of stroke. Measure at every visit	A	CTF,† 1984
Clinical breast examination, mammography	Breast cancer	Secondary prevention. Perform annually for women aged >50 years; consider for women aged 35+ with positive family history	A	CTF, 1986 USTF‡ O'Malley, 1987
Papanicolaou smear	Cervical cancer	Secondary prevention. Perform annually following initiation of sexual activity until the age of 35 years; every 2 to 3 years until age 60, then decrease frequency to every 5 years	B	USTF, 1982 Miller, 1988
Nonfasting total plasma cholesterol measurement, counseling	Hypercholesterolemia	Primary prevention of coronary heart disease. Perform in all men age 30 to 59 (see intervention for high-risk adults for all others). If elevated (>240 mg./dl.), advocate low-fat diet and monitor progress. Drug therapy effective for nonresponders to diet	B	CTF (in press)
Estrogen replacement therapy, calcium supplementation	Osteoporotic fractures	Primary prevention. Weigh against possible risk of endometrial cancer; consider for postmenopausal women with the following **risk factors:** white race, low body weight for height, smoking. Measurement of bone mass is *not* recommended	C	CTF, 1988
Tetanus booster	Tetanus	Primary prevention. Mid-decade birthday is the suggested marker for boost	A	USTF Laforce, 1987
Counseling and follow-up	Smoking cessation	Primary prevention. Inform about the risks of smoking and the available smoking cessation strategies available; schedule follow-up visits to reinforce advice. Prescribe nicotine gum only as an adjunct	A	CTF, 1986 USTF Kottke et al., 1988
	Problem drinking	Primary prevention. Advise heavy drinkers to reduce alcohol consumption, and monitor their progress. Recommend that men drink no more than 3 to 5 drinks per day and women, 2 to 3 drinks per day	B	CTF, 1989

*See Table 14–5, page 227, for explanation of grades of recommendation assigned by the Canadian and United States Task Forces.

†Canadian Task Force on the Periodic Health Examination.

‡United States Preventive Services Task Force position paper.

15 years old; appropriate vaccinations are given. She is slightly underweight for her height but on inquiry into her eating habits and dieting practices, the physician is assured that her diet is adequate. She wears orthodontic braces and has received regular dental care; the physician suggests that she consult her dentist regarding dental sealants, and that she wear teeth guards while playing basketball. She is commended for not smoking and given advice about seat-belt use. She denies being sexually active; the physician urges her to seek contraceptive advice when she is ready to be sexually involved.

Facilitating the Implementation of Preventive Services in Primary Care

COGNITIVE FACTORS

Information that is acceptable to all recommending bodies on preventive services is certainly a necessary but not a sufficient condition for implementation. The process followed by the Canadian Task Force on the Periodic Health Examination and the United States Preventive Services Task Force is structured and uses explicit rules of evidence and criteria to formulate recommendations. From the clinician's perspective, a problem arises when alternative recommendations on the same issues are offered by other recommending bodies, such as specialty organizations and the National Institutes of Health Consensus Development Conferences (Jacoby, 1985). These bodies often use other approaches for which the process is less structured and may be more heuristic. Potential conflicts and controversies centering around recommendations have a major impact on beliefs of clinicians.

In addition, the common diffusion pathways used to convey such recommendations, namely continuing medical education activities, journals, and seminars, might not be sufficient to shape the beliefs and attitudes of clinicians and affect their behaviors (Lomas and Haynes, 1988). Indeed, other factors are

Table 13–6. PREVENTIVE INTERVENTIONS TO BE INCLUDED IN THE PERIODIC HEALTH EXAMINATION OF *HIGH-RISK ADULTS ONLY*

Clinical Procedure	Target Condition	Recommendation and Comments	Grade*	Reference
Inspection of the skin	Skin cancer	Secondary prevention **High-risk persons:** those with heavy exposure to ultraviolet light or in contact with polycyclic aromatic hydrocarbons; first-degree relatives of patients with dysplastic nevi	B	CTF,† 1984
Counseling	Skin cancer	Primary prevention. Counsel to reduce exposure to ultraviolet light		
History and counseling	Noise-induced hearing impairment	Primary prevention by promoting use of ear protection in those with occupational or leisure-time exposure to loud noise	A	CTF, 1984
History, otoscopy, referral for audiometry		Secondary prevention **High-risk persons:** those with a positive family history and a history of ear problems. Early detection and correction of impairment is possible	B	CTF, 1984
Nonfasting plasma cholesterol, counseling	Hypercholesterolemia	Primary prevention of coronary heart disease **High-risk:** women of all ages and men under age 30 or over age 60 with coronary heart disease risk factors: positive family history or early coronary heart disease, severe obesity; and presence of xanthomas, hypertension, smoking. Advise to lower dietary fat, and monitor progress. Drug therapy not evaluated for this population	C	CTF (in press)
Flexible sigmoidoscopy, Hemoccult	Colorectal cancer	Secondary prevention **High risk:** first-degree relatives of colorectal cancer patients, patients with history of breast or cervical cancer **Highest risk:** Patients with ulcerative colitis, patients with familial polyposis syndrome	C	CTF, 1989a; USTF‡ Knight, 1989; Selby, 1989;
Fasting and oral glucose tolerance test	Diabetes mellitus	Secondary prevention **High risk:** positive family history, circulatory dysfunction and frank vascular impairments, obstetrical history of birth weight over 4 kg., stillbirth, recurrent abortion, or fetal abnormalities	B	CTF, 1979
Culture of cervical or urethral swab, or micromethod	Chlamydial genital infection	Secondary prevention **High risk:** sexual partners of patients with nongonococcal urethritis, those with multiple sexual partners. Treatment is effective	B	CTF, 1984
Culture of cervical or urethral swab	Gonorrhea	Secondary prevention **High risk:** persons with multiple sexual partners, in active military service, at work camps, or in prisons; homosexuals	A	CTF, 1979; USTF Horsburgh, 1987
Syphilis	VDRL and ART blood tests	Secondary prevention **High risk:** homosexuals; those with multiple sexual partners, in active military service, at work camps, or in prisons	A	CTF, 1979; USTF Horsburgh, 1987
Hepatitis B vaccination	Hepatitis B	Primary prevention **High risk:** dialysis patients; patients receiving multiple blood products; health care personnel exposed to blood or blood products; patients entering institutions for mentally retarded; drug addicts; homosexuals; those in contact with patients or carriers Three doses recommended: 2 one month apart, third after 6 months	A	CTF, 1984
BCG vaccine	Tuberculosis	Primary prevention **High risk:** those in contact with tuberculosis patient; communities or groups with high infection rate	A	CTF, 1979 USTF LaForce, 1987
Isoniazid chemoprophylaxis	Tuberculosis	Secondary prevention **High risk:** positive tuberculin reactors who: recently converted; have inactive disease; are being treated with corticosteroids; have reticuloendothelial system disease; have severe, unstable diabetes	A	CTF, 1979 USTF LaForce, 1987

*See Table 14–5, page 227, for explanation of grades of recommendation assigned by the Canadian and United States Task Forces.
†Canadian Task Force on the Periodic Health Examination.
‡United States Preventive Services Task Force position paper.

Table 13–7. PREVENTIVE INTERVENTIONS TO BE APPLIED TO THE *OLDER ADULT* (>65 years of age)*

Clinical Procedure	Target Condition	Recommendation and Comments	Grade†	Reference
History, referral for auditory testing	Hearing impairment	Secondary prevention. Identify those with a history of occupational or leisure-time exposure to loud noise, or who present with loud speech, tinnitus, or need to have words repeated	B	CTF,‡ 1984
Visual acuity testing	Refractive defects	Secondary prevention. Correction of refractive disorders may facilitate activities of daily living	C	CTF, 1979
Physical appraisal, detailed clinical inquiry	Functional incapacity with aging	Secondary prevention. Detect impairment in sensory function, psychologic function, locomotion, and activities of daily living (including personal cleanliness and continence). Preferably done in the home setting, otherwise gain familiarity with home conditions. Include general symptom inquiry by focusing on each body system	B	CTF, 1979
Anti-influenza vaccination	Influenza	Primary prevention. Use most recent influenza vaccine annually in the fall. **Contraindication:** allergy to egg or egg products	A	CTF, 1979 USTF§ LaForce, 1987
Diphtheria/tetanus vaccination	Diphtheria, tetanus	Primary prevention. Td booster every 10 years. In recent years, attack rates have shifted toward the elderly population	A	USTF LaForce, 1987
Pneumococcal vaccination	Pneumococcal infections	Primary prevention. Persons over 65 should be vaccinated once	B	USTF LaForce, 1987
Nutritional history, height and weight measurement	Malnutrition	Secondary prevention for those at **high risk:** elderly persons living alone. Home visits may be useful	B	CTF, 1979

*To be performed in addition to procedures recommended in the adult health examination.

†See Table 14–5, page 227, for explanation of grades of recommendation assigned by the Canadian and United States Task Forces.

‡Canadian Task Force on the Periodic Health Examination.

§United States Preventive Services Task Force position paper.

Table 13–8. PREVENTIVE INTERVENTIONS THAT REMAIN CONTROVERSIAL AS TO INCLUSION IN OR EXCLUSION FROM THE PERIODIC HEALTH EXAMINATION

Clinical Procedure	Nature of the Controversy
Fecal occult blood screening in all adults over 45 years of age	Effectiveness in early detection of colorectal cancer is not established; awaiting results from ongoing trials. Problems exist with accuracy of the test and the rate of patient compliance
Digital rectal examination for early detection of prostate cancer in the older men	The sensitivity and specificity of the maneuver have not been established. The prevalence of prostatic cancer increases with age but may not always be life-threatening. The evidence supporting radical surgery is inconclusive
Teaching breast self-examination for early detection of breast cancer	There is insufficient evidence that breast self-examination reduces mortality; awaiting results from ongoing trial. Breast self-examination may produce anxiety, or cause the performance of unnecessary diagnostic procedures in young women, in whom the incidence of breast cancer is very low. There is insufficient evidence to recommend exclusion of this practice where it already exists
Stress ECG for detection of asymptomatic coronary artery disease	There is no evidence regarding the effectiveness of treatment of coronary artery disease in asymptomatic patients. The test requires considerable expenditure of time and resources. There is a heavy risk of burdening the patient with the possibility of sudden cardiac death in the absence of efficacious prevention
Neck auscultation for detection of cervical carotid bruits	The efficacy of early detection and treatment for preventing stroke in asymptomatic patients is not established
Scoliosis screening	There is lack of sound evidence about the efficacy of treatment, even when scoliosis is detected at an earlier and less severe stage
HIV screening in pregnant women	Objective is primary prevention of AIDS in the unborn baby; no efficacious treatment of the mother is available. May be applied to high-risk women; positive result may imply the need for therapeutic abortion

perceived to be essential in bringing recommendations into practice. Activities with which clinicians would personally comply or that they would offer to their family members also are priorities in their practice. Perception of their efficacy in administering such services would also seem to be an important determinant of their patterns of preventive practice (Green et al., 1988).

SOCIODEMOGRAPHIC CHARACTERISTICS OF PROVIDERS

Despite major differences between the Canadian and the American health care systems, the level of integration of preventive services into primary care seems to be comparable in these two countries (Lewis, 1988; Bass and Elford, 1988).

The importance of the periodic health examination was reaffirmed in the 1970's, and it is therefore not surprising to observe that younger physicians are more likely to comply with such practice recommendations. In one study, women physicians have been found to be more likely to include preventive activities in their clinical practice (Battista et al., 1986). Greater awareness of the consequences of specific conditions such as cervical and breast cancers could explain this different pattern of practice. However, other investigators assessing the beliefs and attitudes of medical students toward prevention did not find this gender difference (Maheux et al., 1987). The issue is, therefore, controversial.

Other factors that have been suggested to have an impact on practice behaviors include past medical training, residency training, and licensures (Peterson et al., 1956; Clute, 1963). Although very little evidence would support that differences in practice patterns result from differences in past medical training, recent evidence from a study conducted in Canada would seem to support the hypothesis that practitioners who went through family medicine residency training are more likely to include preventive services into their clinical practice (Borgiel et al., 1989).

ORGANIZATIONAL FACTORS

Most of the available empirical evidence concurs that the most important determinant of practice behavior is the practice environment in which clinicians work. Cognitive and sociodemographic factors are certainly important elements in successful implementation of preventive services, but these factors are not sufficient without a supportive environment that will ultimately shape the practice of clinicians (Inui et al., 1981; Carter et al., 1981). Several types of organizational factors are considered, including operational tools, practice settings, and reimbursement modalities.

Operational Tools

The translation of practice recommendations into practical instruments that will make them more accessible to the practicing clinician is an idea that has definite merit and that has already been successfully tested (Cohen et al., 1982; Knight et al., 1987). Instruments such as flow sheets or health charts can be introduced in medical records so as to alert the clinicians to the activities that should be offered for specific age or sex categories of patients (see Tables 13–20 and 13–21, and Chapter 73, Fig. 73-11*A* and *B*). Specific reminders could also be used to convey such information, such as with the use of computer software on the periodic health examination. The use of these provider-oriented instruments could be further enhanced by an appropriate recall system.

An important avenue to explore is the development and distribution of patient-oriented instruments, such as health passports or magnetic health cards, that would convey the same information to patients and thus create a common base of knowledge for interactions between providers and consumers (Skilsa, 1984). The creation of a unified system in preventive medicine, including instruments developed for providers and patients, would seem a natural extension of the concept of the periodic health examination.

Practice Settings

The structural features of practice settings would certainly have an impact on patterns of practice. Peer pressure in a group practice is usually an element that shapes practice behavior. Settings such as the community health centers (CLSC) in Canada or the health maintenance organizations (HMO) in the United States are examples of organizations that would carry a more specific preventive orientation. Although the level of integration of preventive services into primary care has been demonstrated to be higher in CLSCs as compared with fee-for-service practices (Battista and Spitzer, 1983), similar evidence pertaining to HMOs is controversial (Wilner, 1986).

Time is certainly an important limiting factor in the integration of preventive services into primary care. Preventive services compete with curative services, and time pressures are much greater in fee-for-service practices. This might explain the greater difficulty of integration in such practices. In addition, a limited number of preventive activities can be offered during an encounter. In effect, with respect to counseling activities, there is certainly a limit to the number of topics that can be discussed in one visit.

Reimbursement Modalities

Discussion of the impact of the practice setting on practice behaviors cannot be disassociated from consideration of the reimbursement modalities under which clinicians practice. Although some evidence exists that fee-for-service practices are less conducive to the offering of preventive services as compared with those practices in which physicians are paid either on a salary or a sessional basis (Pineault, 1976; Manning et al., 1984), the absence of specific incentives for preventive services in the fee-for-service schedule impedes us from concluding that a given mode of reimbursement carries an inherent advantage in this respect. Some evidence from an ongoing study supports the hypothesis that fee-for-service physicians provided with the appropriate monetary incentives for prevention would actually devote more time to offering preventive services (Logsdon and Rosen, 1984).

Implementing preventive services into primary care is a complex exercise. Successful implementation of preventive services should result from a balanced and artful orchestration of the several factors discussed. In effect, it has been shown that the importance of all of these determinants would vary according to the specific condition being considered (Battista et al., 1986).

Future Trends

Current recommendations must evolve continually, since new evidence on the effectiveness of primary and secondary preventive measures emerges constantly. Moreover, changing social and economic circumstances in Canada and in the United States may require reconsideration of the recommendations and of the strategy that has been advocated in this chapter.

Our current state of knowledge makes it impossible to make absolute recommendations about most disorders. For certain important preventive interventions, the evidence is either controversial or incomplete (Table 13–8), and bodies such as the Canadian and United States Task Forces cannot make recommendations on the basis that a particular preventive measure *might* be beneficial. For stronger recommendations, more definitive evidence is required to strengthen the scientific basis of preventive practice in family medicine.

In the *The Logic of Medicine*, Murphy (1979) offers a pertinent admonishment:

If we can never know the answer, let us be honest and admit that we cannot. If we cannot produce proof, let us withhold the final stamp of intellectual approval until we do. It is better to be an agnostic forever than to worship false gods.

The authors of this chapter adopted a similar stand, and have attempted to justify it in an earlier section. But what of the harried clinician who must act now and cannot wait for the conclusive evidence to be gathered and disseminated.

Thoughtful clinicians act daily on the basis of incomplete evidence, executing those clinical maneuvers that they think are in their patients' best interest. So, too, with the preventive interventions discussed in this chapter. Those that have been found, on rigorous validation, to do more good than harm are unequivocally recommended. The rest are presented with open and candid uncertainty as to their value. The worst disservice to the harried clinician would be to fail to distinguish between unquestionably beneficial detection maneuvers and those of dubious value, and to withhold the evidence associated with each preventive act that a family physician contemplates as she or he cares for patients and seeks to protect their health.

Although the clinically based approach to prevention is a worthwhile preventive strategy, clinicians must remember that their efforts should be construed as part of a whole that includes community-based preventive interventions and, even more broadly, provincial or state and national policies in prevention. The contribution of primary care physicians to the good health of their patients can be tremendous, especially if it is harmoniously and adequately articulated with preventive efforts emanating from Community Health or Public Health Programs.

References

Bass, M. J., and Elford, R. W.: Preventive practice patterns of Canadian primary care physicians. Am. J. Prev. Med., *4*(Suppl):17, 1988.

Battista, R. N., and Spitzer, W. O.: Adult cancer prevention in primary care: Contrasts among primary care practice settings in Québec. Am. J. Public Health, *73*:1040, 1983.

Battista, R. N., Williams, J. I., and MacFarlane, L. A.: Determinants of primary medical practice in adult cancer prevention. Med. Care, *24*:216–224, 1986.

Borgiel, A. E. M., Williams, J. I., Bass, M. J., et al.: Quality of care in family practice: Does residency training make a difference? Can. Med. Assoc. J., *140*:1035, 1989.

Canadian Task Force on Cervical Cancer Screening Programs. Summary of the 1982 Canadian Task Force Report. Can. Med. Assoc. J., *127*:581, 1982. *The Canadian Task Force on Cervical Cancer Screening Programs examined measures to improve the quality and sensitivity of screening programs in Canada. Their recommendation was to concentrate on reaching high-risk women rather than increasing the frequency of screening in previously screened women.*

Canadian Task Force on the Periodic Health Examination: The periodic health examination. Can. Med. Assoc. J., *121*:1196, 1979. *This article is the brief summary of the Task Force recommendations on the 78 conditions. The findings are in tabular format with key references; the recommendations are synthesized into health protection plans according to age and sex. Though not as complete as the PHE Monograph, it is an excellent overview of the recommendations.*

Canadian Task Force on the Periodic Health Examination: The periodic health examination 2. 1984 update. Can. Med. Assoc. J., *130*:1278, 1984. *This report re-examines the evidence on conditions covered in the 1979 report: chlamydial genital infection, hearing impairment in adults, hypertension, skin cancer, and scoliosis. It also gives recommendations on new conditions: asymptomatic coronary artery disease, asymptomatic cervical corotid bruit, testicular cancer, hepatitis B, and breast-feeding.*

Canadian Task Force on the Periodic Health Examination: The periodic health examination 2. 1985 update. Can. Med. Assoc. J., *135*:724, 1986. *This report outlines practice recommendations for early detection of breast cancer, smoking cessation counseling, and detection of primary open-angle glaucoma. The evidence on detection of breast cancer is examined in detail.*

Canadian Task Force on the Periodic Health Examination: The periodic health examination 2. 1987 update. Can. Med. Assoc. J., *138*:618, 1988. *This report updates and amplifies the 1979 recommendation on prevention of unwanted teenage pregnancy. It also addresses early detection of endometrial cancer and prevention of osteoporotic fractures. The evidence on the latter condition is complex, but this article gives an excellent overview of the issues that must be considered in making individual practice decisions.*

Canadian Task Force on the Periodic Health Examination: The periodic health examination 2. 1988 update. Can. Med. Assoc. J., (in press). *This report updates the 1979 recommendation on early detection of colorectal cancer, the detection and early treatment of problem drinking, and the early detection of hyperthyroidism and hypothyroidism.*

Canadian Task Force on the Periodic Health Examination: The periodic health examination 2. 1989 update. Can. Med. Assoc. J., *141*:209, 1989. *This report focuses on prenatal and pediatric prevention strategies. Recommendations are made on preschool screening for developmental delay, visual deficits, and hearing problems. The evidence is examined regarding the effectiveness of serial ultrasound studies for detecting intrauterine growth retardation, of intrapartum electronic fetal monitoring, and of screening for congenital hypothyroidism.*

Carter, W. B., Belcher, D. W., and Inui, T. S.: Implementing preventive care in clinical practice. II. Problems for managers clinicians and patients. Med. Care Rev., *38*:195, 1981.

Clute, K. F.: The general practitioner. A study of medical education and practice in Ontario and Nova Scotia. Toronto, University of Toronto Press, 1963.

Cohen, D. I., Littenberg, B., Wetzel, C., and Neuhauser, D.: Improving physician compliance with preventive medicine guidelines. Med. Care, *20*:1040, 1982.

Cole, P., and Morrison, A. S.: Basic issues in population screening for cancer. J. Natl. Cancer Inst., *64*:1263, 1980.

Fletcher, R. H., Fletcher, S. W., and Wagner, E.: Clinical Epidemiology—The Essentials. Baltimore, Williams & Wilkins, 1988, pp. 41–58.

Green, L. W., Eriksen, M. P., and Schor, E. L.: Preventive practices by physicians: Behavioral determinants and potential interventions. Am. J. Prev. Med., *4*(Suppl):101, 1988. *Using the framework of predisposing, enabling, and reinforcing factors for behavioral change, Green reviews the literature and proposes strategies to enhance the implementation of preventive activities among physicians.*

Horsburgh, C. R., Douglas, J. M., and LaForce, F. M.: Preventive stategies in sexually transmitted diseases for the primary care physician. J.A.M.A., *258*:814, 1987. *This article outlines the practice recommendations of the United States Preventive Services Task Force for the prevention of sexually transmitted diseases in neonates and adults. The sexually transmitted diseases covered are gonorrhea, syphilis, enteric infections, and infections with human immunodeficiency virus, human papilloma virus, herpes simplex virus, and* Chlamydia trachomatis.

Inui, T. S., Belcher, D. W., and Carter, W. B.: Implementing preventive care in clinical practice. I. Organizational issues and strategies. Med. Care Rev., *38*:129, 1981.

Jacoby, I.: The consensus development program of the National Institutes of Health—current practices and historical perspectives? Int. J. of Technology Assessment in Health Care, *1*:420, 1985.

Knight, B. P., O'Malley, M. S., and Fletcher, S. W.: Physician acceptance of a computerized health maintenance promoting program. Am. J. Prev. Med., *3*:19, 1987.

Knight, K. K., Fielding, J. E., and Battista, R. N.: Occult blood screening for colorectal cancer. J.A.M.A., *261*:587, 1989. *This is the paper stating the position of the United States Preventive Services Task Force on the early detection of colorectal cancer.*

Kottke, T. E., Battista, R. N., DeFriese, G. H., and Brekke, M. L.: Attributes of successful smoking cessation interventions in medical practice. J.A.M.A., *259*:2882, 1988. *This position paper for the United States Preventive Services Task Force was based on a meta-analysis of 39 controlled smoking cessation trials. It outlines the common factors that predict success in physicians' advising their patients to quit smoking.*

LaForce, M. F.: Immunizations, immunoprophylaxis and chemoprophylaxis to prevent selected infections. J.A.M.A., *257*:2464, 1987. *This is the paper stating the position of the United States Preventive Services Task Force on indications, contraindications, efficacy, and strategies for childhood and adult immunizations.*

Lawrence, R. S., and Mickalide, A. D.: Preventive services in clinical practice: Designing the periodic health examination. J.A.M.A., *257*:2205, 1987.

Lewis, C. E.: Disease prevention and health promotion practices of primary care physicians in the United States. Am. J. Prev. Med., *4*(Suppl):9, 1988.

Logsdon, D. N., and Rosen, M. A.: The cost of preventive health services in primary medical care and implications for health insurance coverage. J. Ambulatory Care Management, *7*:46, 1984.

Lomas, J., and Haynes, R. B.: A taxonomy and critical review of tested strategies for the application of clinical practice recommendations: From "official" to "individual" clinical policy. Am. J. Prev. Med., *4*(Suppl):77, 1988.

Maheux, B., Pineault, R., and Béland, F.: Factors influencing physicians' orientation toward prevention. Am. J. Prev. Med., *3*:12, 1987.

Manning, W. G., Leibowitz, A., Goldberg, G. A., et al.: A controlled trial of the effect of a prepaid group practice on use of services. N. Engl. J. Med., *310*:1505, 1984.

McNeil, B. J., Keeler, E., and Adelstein, S. J.: Primer on certain elements of medical decision-making. N. Engl. J. Med., *193*:212, 1975. *This article discusses diagnostic tests that have a continuous scale of values. The concept of a receiver-operating-curve is introduced to illustrate the effect of altering cut-off points on the sensitivity, specificity, and impact on larger issues such as cost-effectiveness.*

Miller, A. B.: Cervical cancer screening: A time for reappraisal in Canada. Can. J. Pub. Health, *79*:90, 1988. *Current cervical cancer screening approaches are critically examined, and new recommendations of frequency are made. This is the position represented in this chapter.*

Mullan, F., and Jacoby, I.: The town meeting for technology—The maturation of consensus conferences. J.A.M.A., *254*:1068, 1985.

Murphy, E.: The Logic of Medicine. Baltimore, The Johns Hopkins University Press, 1979.

O'Malley, M. S., and Fletcher, S. W.: Screening for breast cancer with breast self-examination: A critical review. J.A.M.A., *257*:2197, 1987. *The United States Preventive Services Task Force mandated this critical review of the literature on breast self-examination. It found no evidence of its benefit in reducing breast cancer mortality. In making individual practice policy decisions, physicians must weigh its potential as a screening method against factors such as potentially negative psychologic effects.*

Periodic Health Examination Monograph—Report of a Task Force to The Conference of Deputy Ministers of Health. Ottawa, Ontario, Canada. Health services and promotion branch, Department of Health and Welfare Canada, 1980. Catalogue No. H39-3/1980E. pp. 18–78. *This monograph outlines the preventive practice recommendation of the Canadian Periodic Health Examination Task Force regarding 78 conditions. A statement on each condition summarizes the major findings of the task force and their reasons for assigning the graded recommendations. Key references are annotated, and the recommendations are compiled into health protection plans for age and sex groups.*

The monograph is available from Publications Unit, Health and Welfare Canada, Tunney's Pasture, Ottawa, Ontario, K1A 1B4, Canada.

Peterson, O. L., Andrews, L. P., Spain, R. S., et al.: An analytic study of North Carolina general practice. J. Med. Educ., *31*:1, 1956.

Pineault, R.: The effect of prepaid group practice on physicians' utilization behavior. Med. Care, *14*:121, 1976.

Polen, M. R., and Friedman, G. D.: Automobile injury—selected risk factors and prevention in health care setting. J.A.M.A., *259*:76, 1988. *This review for the United States Preventive Services Task Force found evidence supporting the effectiveness of physicians' advice to parents to use occupant restraints for their children. Other programs have been poorly evaluated, but recommendations are made on the basis of prudence.*

Russell, L. B.: Is Prevention Better than Cure? Washington, D.C., The Brookings Institution, 1986. *This 130-page paperback uses the principles of economic analysis to counter the myth that preventive medicine is a means of cutting health care costs. Prevention offers better health but at an additional cost.*

Sackett, D. L., Haynes, R. B., and Tugwell, P.: Clinical Epidemiology: A Basic Science for Clinical Medicine. Boston, MA, Little, Brown and Co., 1985, pp. 59–155. *An excellent primer, designed for self-teaching, for those wishing to learn the basic principles of clinical epidemiology.*

Selby, J. V., and Friedman, G. D.: Sigmoidoscopy in the periodic health examination of asymptomatic adults. J.A.M.A., *261*:599, 1989. *This is the paper stating the position of the United States Preventive Services Task Force on early detection of colorectal cancer by sigmoidoscopy.*

Skilsa, L. W.: Patient-retained records—the health identity card. J. Royal College of General Practitioners, *34*:104, 1984.

U.S. Preventive Services Task Force: Recommendations for breast cancer screening. J.A.M.A., *257*:2196, 1987.

Vecchio, T. J.: Predictive value of a diagnositic test in unselected populations. N. Engl. J. Med., *174*:1171, 1966.

Weinstein, M. C., and Stason, W. B.: Foundations of cost-effectiveness analysis for health and medical practice. N. Engl. J. Med., *296*:716, 1977. *The authors offer a concise overview of the basic approaches to economic analysis and its application to health policy.*

Wilner, S.: Health promotion and disease prevention in HMOs. Health Aff., *5*(1):122, 1986.

14

Preventive Health Care in Family Practice

R. Michael Morse
Warren A. Heffron

Role of the Family Physician

Of all specialists, the family physician has a unique opportunity to be an effective force in disease prevention and health promotion. As the primary care provider for all ages in family units, the family physician can most effectively screen for a broad range of risk factors associated with preventable diseases and encourage appropriate preventive measures such as proper diet and exercise. To be most effective, many preventive activities will need to be applied to an entire family unit. These broader, family-wide, disease prevention and health promotion activities can then serve as the foundation for more age-specific recommendations and interventions for individual members.

Although other medical and surgical problems may occasionally require subspecialty consultation, the family physician is the specialist to whom patients and other specialists look for provision of this broad range of health promotion and disease prevention activities.

Preventive activities are traditionally classified to the phase of the disease process in which intervention occurs: tertiary (disease diagnosed and symptoms present), secondary (disease present and diagnosable, but no symptoms present), and primary (no diagnosable disease and no symptoms present).

The bulk of medical education relates to the patient who is already ill (tertiary prevention); progressively less time is spent on secondary and primary prevention. This leads physicians to provide evaluation and treatment in "reaction" to patient symptoms rather than in a "proactive" mode of care—that is, in attempting to anticipate problems and prevent them.

Physicians may encounter a variety of obstacles to providing comprehensive preventive health services, including severe demands on the physician's time by patients already ill, lack of financial resources in the patient population, and negative patient and third party attitudes toward preventive care. The information provided in this chapter needs to be tailored to each physician's practice.

Evaluating Preventive Activities

Not all diseases lend themselves well to the shift from medical intervention at the tertiary level to the secondary or primary level. Several parameters are used to determine the validity of such a shift for each disease and to determine the population group to whom the intervention should be applied. The general criteria are:

1. Is the disease worth screening for? Does it have a significant impact on the quality or quantity

of life, and is it of sufficient prevalence in the population to justify screening?

2. Is sufficient information available to accurately identify, using risk factors and screening tests, the individual or groups likely to develop the disease? Or by using diagnostic tests, is it possible to identify those likely to already have the disease at a presymptomatic stage?

3. Are the tests that are used to accomplish the screening or early detection acceptable to the patient and physician in terms of accuracy, morbidity, and cost?

4. If it is possible to predict the disease or diagnose it prior to the onset of symptoms, is there a known intervention that will significantly alter the course of the disease?

5. Is the intervention or treatment acceptable in terms of proven effectiveness, risk, morbidity, cost, and patient acceptability?

To help answer these questions, a number of measures are used.

Incidence. This is the rate of onset of a disease in a population; it is usually expressed as the number of persons developing the disease per a given number of persons (typically, cases per 100,000 per year). Incidence expresses the risk of developing the disease in the general population. If the incidence is very low, the benefits of mass screening may also be very low. However, the incidence may be high enough in a subgroup (specific age groups, certain nationalities, a specific sex, and so on) to qualify for prevention in that specific group.

Mortality. The death rate of a disease is expressed as the number of persons dying from the disease per population at risk (usually 100,000) per year. Since a disease may not be fatal but may still be preventable, mortality statistics are not as useful by themselves but are generally more available and accurate. Incidence statistically represents the onset of a disease; mortality represents the end-point of fatal illnesses.

Table 14–1 shows a typical mortality table.

Table 14–1. MAJOR CAUSES OF MORTALITY IN THE UNITED STATES—1985*

Rank	Cause of Death	Number of Deaths	Death Rate per 100,000 Population	Percent of Total Deaths
	All Causes	2,086,440	739.0	100.0
1.	Heart diseases	771,113	261.4	37.0
2.	Cancer	461,563	170.5	22.1
3.	Cerebrovascular diseases	153,050	51.0	7.3
4.	Accidents	93,457	36.0	4.5
5.	Chronic obstructive lung diseases	71,047	25.0	3.4
6.	Pneumonia and influenza	67,615	22.0	3.2
7.	Diabetes mellitus	36,969	13.1	1.8
8.	Suicide	29,453	11.2	1.4
9.	Cirrhosis of liver	26,767	10.6	1.3
10.	Arteriosclerosis	23,926	7.6	1.1
11.	Nephritis	21,349	7.3	1.0
12.	Homicide	19,893	7.5	1.0
13.	Diseases of infancy	19,246	8.8	0.9
14.	Septicemia and pyemia	17,182	6.0	0.8
15.	Aortic aneurysm	15,112	5.3	0.7
	Other and ill-defined	258,698	96.1	12.5

*As published by the American Cancer Society from Vital Statistics of the United States, 1985.

Prevalence. Prevalence is the proportion of individuals with a trait or disease in the population at a given time. Prevalence statistically represents the interval between onset and end of a given disease process and increases proportionally with the length of the disease. When evaluating screening procedures, this is a critical value for predicting the efficacy of screening.

Sensitivity. Sensitivity is the value derived by applying a test to a group of individuals *known to have a trait or disease* and is expressed as a percentage of positive tests in that tested group. Thus, sensitivity tells one about a test but is not helpful by itself in interpreting that test for an individual in whom the presence of disease is unknown. The value tells nothing about the results when applied to an undifferentiated population.

Specificity. Specificity is the complement of the sensitivity and is derived by applying a test to a population *known not to have a trait or disease.* It is expressed as a percentage of the disease-free group with a negative test.

Positive Predictive Value. This value is more useful when interpreting a positive test performed on a particular individual. Positive predictive value tells one about the test when applied to a mixed population of individuals both with and without the disease. It is expressed as a percentage of all the positive tests that will be true positives. Thus, it expresses the likelihood of a disease truly being present in an individual when a test is positive.

Negative Predictive Value. This is the converse of the positive predictive value and is expressed as the percentage of negative tests in a mixed population that will be true negatives. Thus, it expresses the likelihood of a negative test representing the absence of a disease.

The sensitivity and specificity are constants that are always true of a certain test when it is properly performed, regardless of the population tested. However, the positive predictive value and the negative predictive value *are dependent on the prevalence of disease* in the population tested. The relationship between sensitivity, specificity, positive predictive value, and negative predictive value can be shown in a four-square table (Table 14–2).

Table 14–3 demonstrates the interdependence of positive predictive value, negative predictive value, and prevalence. By following each value in the table, the sequence of completing a four-square table can be understood. (Each item number below refers to the same number in the table.)

Table 14–2. THE FOUR-SQUARE TABLE*

	Positive tests	Negative tests	
Prevalence =			
Population with disease =	TP	FN	Sensitivity = $\frac{TP}{TP+FN} \times 100$
Population without disease =	FP	TN	Specificity = $\frac{TN}{FP+TN} \times 100$
	PPV = $\frac{TP}{TP+FP}$	NPV = $\frac{TN}{TN+FN}$	

*TP, true positive; FN, false negative; FP, false positive; TN, true negative; PPV, positive predictive value; NPV, negative predictive value.

1. Assume we know the screening test we are interested in is known to be 95 per cent sensitive (95 per cent of patients known to have the disease will have a positive test) and . . .

2. Ninety per cent specific (90 per cent of patients known not to have the disease will have a negative test).

3. Assume that we wish to screen a population with a 1 per cent prevalence of the screened disease.

4. In screening 10,000 individuals, 100 persons would in fact have the disease (prevalence of 1 per cent × 10,000 individuals to be screened).

5. With a sensitivity of 95 per cent, performing this test on this group of 100 with the disease should yield 95 positive tests and . . .

6. Five false negatives.

7. Similarly, there will be 9900 patients without the disease . . .

8. of which 8910 (specificity of 90 per cent × 9900 patients) will be true negatives . . .

9. and the rest (990) will be false positives. Unfortunately, we usually do not have the luxury of knowing who has or does not have the disease prior to testing. Therefore, we will only know whether a given individual is positive or negative for the test. To interpret this positive or negative test for a likelihood that the patient does or does not have the disease, we need to derive the positive predictive value and the negative predictive value using the four-square table.

10. Using the values now entered in the table, it can be seen that there will be 1085 (95+990) positive tests of which only 95 (9 per cent of the total) are true positives.

It can be seen that this test has a positive predictive value of only 9 per cent and will be very poor at best under most circumstances. This test could conceivably be useful if there were an *additional test* that could be easily applied to the original test-positive population and that would have a much higher positive predictive value.

11. In a similar manner, the negative predictive value can be calculated to be 99 per cent. But, one must remember that with a prevalence of 1 per cent, any random patient will have a 99 per cent likelihood of not having the disease *with no testing at all.*

However, assume it is possible to select out a high-risk group (individuals with a risk factor) for testing that has a significantly higher prevalence of perhaps 25 per cent. The four-square table would be as shown in Table 14–4.

Thus, as shown on the table, by screening a high-risk population (i.e., with a higher prevalence of disease), the positive predictive value increases dramatically despite no change in sensitivity or specificity. This is essentially "Bayes' theorem." Bayes' theorem also takes into account the other ways of increasing the positive predictive value of a test: to increase the sensitivity or increase the specificity, or both. In general, for diseases of low prevalence, the sensitivity and especially the specificity must be very good for a screening test to be valuable. A screening test with very high specificity will accurately define a population that needs no further screening, i.e., a very low likelihood of anyone in that negative-test population having the disease. The positive-test group may or may not need to be screened further, depending on the test's sensitivity (i.e., to be positive only for those with the disease).

Cut Points. These issues become important con-

Table 14–3. EXAMPLE OF CALCULATIONS IN A FOUR-SQUARE TABLE*

	Positive tests	Negative tests	
Prevalence = 1 per cent[3]			
Population with disease = 100[4]	TP[5] 95	FN[6] 5	Sensitivity = 95 per cent[1]
Population without disease = 9900[7]	FP[9] 990	TN[8] 8910	Specificity = 90 per cent[2]
	PPV = 9 per cent[10]	NPV = 99 per cent[11]	

*TP, true positive; FN, false negative; FP, false positive; TN, true negative; PPV, positive predictive value; NPV, negative predictive value.

Table 14–4.* CHANGE IN PREDICTIVE VALUES AS A RESULT OF CHANGE IN PREVALENCE

Prevalence = 25 per cent	Positive tests	Negative tests	
Population with disease = 2500	TP 2375	FN 125	Sensitivity = 95 per cent
Population without disease = 7500	FP 750	TN 6750	Specificity = 90 per cent
	PPV = 76 per cent	NPV = 98 per cent	

*TR, true positive; FN, false negative; FP, false positive; TN, true negative; PPV, positive predictive value; NPV, negative predictive value.

siderations when defining the "cut points" for a test—the value at which the test becomes positive. Almost all tests have a range of possible values. Even tests that are reported as positive or negative (e.g., stool guaiac cards, urine pregnancy tests, strep antigen) must have a cut point defined during the basic development and refinement of the test. The decision of what value will be called positive must take into account the test's sensitivity and specificity at that value and, moreover, the positive predictive value when applied to the prevalence in the population to be screened.

Risk Factors. A risk factor is a value or condition that, if present, significantly alters the likelihood of a disease occurring when compared with the likelihood for the population.

A risk factor does not necessarily imply a cause-and-effect relationship between the factor and the disease. It may be simply a statistical association. To substantiate such a cause-and-effect relationship, a study must modify a single risk factor and show, as a result, a statistically significant change in the incidence, morbidity, or mortality of the disease being studied. The proportion of risk for a particular disease that can thus be "attributed" to a specific factor is known as the *attributable risk.*

When mulitiple risk factors are present, their cumulative effect is most often additive but in some cases may be multiplicative. Likewise, modification of risk factors usually reduces risk in a subtractive manner.

Interventions. When testing the effectiveness of an intervention, the type of study and how well it is designed will determine the believability of the results. Both the Canadian Task Force and the United States Preventive Services Task Force have embraced a common method of rating the effectiveness of interventions (Table 14–5). These ratings are assigned after a thorough review of all the evidence available. They provide specialty groups and individual physicians with critical information to help make judgments concerning the value of various preventive care activities.

Recommendations. Both the Canadian Task Force and the United States Preventive Services Task Force have likewise endorsed and used a rating system to classify recommendations for inclusion of the *disease or condition* in a screening program (Table 14–5).

Prevention Applied to Specific Diseases

ATHEROSCLEROTIC DISEASES

Coronary Heart Disease

Incidence. An adult male in the United States has a one in five chance of having a myocardial infarction by 60 years of age, which is twice that of females. The yearly incidence of myocardial infarction is 1.5 million.

The yearly incidence of newly diagnosed coronary heart disease is shown in Table 14–6. Males, between the ages of 35 and 84, have myocardial infarction or sudden death as their *initial* onset of symptoms 67 per cent of time. This is the presenting event for a lesser percentage (43 per cent) of females.

Prevalence. By 20 to 24 years of age, about 44 per cent of white males, 34 per cent of black males, 11 per cent of white females, and 43 per cent of black females will have raised lesions in their coronary arteries. By self-report in a 1982 survey, 2.7 per cent or over six million Americans have symptomatic coronary heart disease.

Although difficult, predicting the prevalence in *asymptomatic* adults is of importance if early aggressive intervention is to be targeted to the appropriate patients. In addition, 20 per cent of myocardial infarctions are either asymptomatic or so atypical as to be unrecognized by the patient (Kannel et al., 1986). A number of studies of angiographic and autopsy data estimate a prevalence of significant coronary heart disease (50 per cent stenosis of at least one major vessel) in 4 to 4.5 per cent of all asymptomatic adults. Since the positive predictive value of screening procedures rises significantly when a group with a high prevalence is screened, it is of importance to know the prevalence in population subgroups. These autopsy studies show a range of 1.9 per cent in 30- to 39-year-old men to 12.3 per cent for men 60 to 69. Women in the same age groups ranged from 0.3 per cent to 7.5 per cent, respectively.

Cost and Impact on Society. It is estimated that the cost of all cardiovascular disease to our society in 1983 was $102 billion, $48 billion in direct costs and $54 billion in indirect costs.

Morbidity and Mortality. Framingham data place

Table 14–5. UNITED STATES PREVENTIVE SERVICES TASK FORCE CLASSIFICATION CODES

Effectiveness of Intervention	Classification of Recommendations
I: Evidence obtained from at least one properly randomized trial	A: There is good evidence to support the recommendation that the condition be specifically considered in a periodic health examination
II-1: Evidence from well-designed controlled trials without randomization	B: There is fair evidence for inclusion
II-2: Evidence obtained from well-designed cohort or case-control analytic studies, preferably from more than one center or research group	C: There is poor evidence for inclusion
II-3: Evidence obtained from multiple time series studies with or without the intervention	D: There is fair evidence to support the recommendation that the condition be excluded from consideration in a periodic health examination
III: Opinions of respected authorities based on clinical experience, descriptive studies, or reports of expert committees	E: There is good evidence to exclude the condition from consideration in a periodic health examination

the mortality due to coronary heart disease at 434 per 100,000 persons aged 35 to 74 per year, and 28 per cent of *all* deaths. Even more striking is the fact that 40 per cent of all deaths in the 35- to 64-year-old age group are secondary to coronary heart disease. The overall case fatality rate is 30 per cent for the first myocardial infarction and 50 per cent for subsequent infarctions. Of those surviving, 13 per cent of males and 40 per cent of females will have a second infarct within 5 years. The 10-year survival rate for males is 50 per cent and for females, 30 per cent. Two thirds of patients with myocardial infarction do not make a complete recovery, although 88 per cent of those under age 65 are able to return to work (Kannel et al., 1986).

Important Facts Relevant to Prevention

1. Risk factor reduction will lessen the incidence of coronary heart disease, especially when concentrated on blood cholesterol levels, hypertension, and cigarette smoking.

2. Changing the American diet to a low-saturated fat, low-cholesterol diet will reduce the levels of serum cholesterol.

3. No population in the world has been found with a combination of high total serum cholesterol levels and low rates of coronary heart disease.

4. Recently, a 4.8-year study has shown that aspirin, in dosages of 325 mg. every other day, can reduce the incidence of myocardial infarction by nearly half. Total vascular-related deaths were reduced by 23 per cent. Although this study included only male physicians who were 40 to 84 years of age and in otherwise fairly good health, it may have significant relevance to much broader groups. (Steering Committee of the Physicians' Health Study Research Group, 1988)

Table 14–6. INCIDENCE RATES PER 100,000 OF NEW ONSET CORONARY HEART DISEASE BY PRESENTING SIGNS AND SYMPTOMS IN THE UNITED STATES, PERSONS AGED 35–84*

	Male	Female
Angina	420	370
Myocardial infarction	710	220
Sudden death	160	60
Total	1290	650

*Framingham Study data, Kannel, W.B., Thom, T.J., and Hurst, J.W.: Incidence, prevalence, and mortality of cardiovascular diseases. *In* Hurst, J.W.: The Heart. New York, McGraw-Hill, 1986.

Risk factors for coronary heart disease as they apply to determining LDL cholesterol cutpoints are listed in Table 14–7.

Screening Test Recommendations. For the general population:

1. Measure low-density lipoprotein and high-density lipoprotein cholesterol between 20 and 30 years of age and at least every 5 years thereafter.

2. Measure blood pressure each office visit.

3. Update family and smoking history in previous nonsmokers every 5 years.

4. Measure fasting blood sugar every 5 years. The presence of diabetes is a major independent risk factor.

5. Monitor activity levels at least every 5 years for every patient for the recommended 30 minutes of aerobic activity three times weekly.

6. Evaluate for obesity (greater than 20 to 30 per cent over ideal body weight) yearly.

7. Monitor stress levels (family and occupational) yearly.

Preventive Activities Recommendations. All risk factors noted in Table 14–7 should be modified whenever possible.

Cholesterol Control

1. Physicians should prescribe a healthy diet to decrease the risk of heart disease for all patients. It is particularly important that children learn healthy eating habits early in life. For patients less likely or able to follow the more extensive dietary instructions of the Step 1 Diet, Table 14–8 gives very general guidelines that most patients can easily progressively implement.

2. All patients should be screened for risk status.

Table 14–7. LDL CHOLESTEROL CUTPOINTS BASED ON PRESENCE OF RISK FACTORS FOR CORONARY HEART DISEASE

LDL cholesterol >160 in any patient
Low-density lipoprotein cholesterol >130 in any patient with two or more of the following:
Prior history of coronary heart disease
Male sex
Family history of premature coronary heart disease (less than 55 years of age)
Cigarette smoker (greater than 10 per day)
Hypertension
High-density lipoprotein cholesterol level less than 35
History of any occlusive vascular disease
Severe obesity (more than 30 per cent overweight)
Other risk factors:
High stress personality profile (probable)
Inactivity (probable)
Oral contraceptive use in smokers over 35 years of age

The presence of other risk factors is used to determine the low-density lipoprotein intervention levels. Table 14–9 shows these recommendations for intervention with diet and medications.

Epidemiologic data show a significant protective effect against coronary heart disease in populations consuming three or more servings of fish weekly. Also, a diet high in soluble fiber (oat bran products, legumes, and fruits) has been shown to reduce serum cholesterol, whereas nonsoluble fiber (present primarily in wheat, vegetables, and fruits) has no effect on cholesterol.

Other methods of altering risk secondary to hypercholesterolemia include weight control, exercise (to increase high-density lipoproteins), and drug therapy.

Control of Hypertension. Aggressive treatment of all patients with a systolic pressure greater than 140 or a diastolic pressure greater than 90 is essential. Risk is proportional to blood pressure even at diastolic levels between 80 and 90.

Prior to institution of drug therapy for hypertension, nonpharmacologic methods should be considered. These include salt restriction, weight reduction, reduction or elimination of alcohol intake, biofeedback, and regular aerobic exercise.

Smoking Cessation. Control of smoking may be the most correctable risk factor for coronary heart disease. Each physician should have a plan for assisting patients in smoking cessation that includes the following elements:

1. Patient recognition of smoking as a health problem.
2. A firm stance by the physician against smoking.
3. Encouraging the patient to make the decision to stop.
4. Setting a target date for starting the program.
5. Multiple methodologies available depending on patient needs and preferences: tapering, "cold turkey," substitution (e.g., nicotine gum), counseling, hypnosis, support groups, buddy systems, and acupuncture.
6. Structured long-term follow-up with maximal support and encouragement from physician and office staff.

Other Preventive Activities. It is recommended that physicians assist all patients to avoid risk factor development through encouragement of healthy life styles. Education to prevent smoking, promotion of physical activity, promotion of stress reduction, maintenance of ideal body weight, and provision of periodic preventive health care should be made available to patients.

RELATED ISSUES. The incidence of coronary heart disease in this country has decreased 40 per cent between 1964 and 1984. It is estimated that 60 per cent of this reduction is due to life style changes, especially diet modification and smoking cessation. This encouraging information alone provides physicians sufficient reason to pursue further aggressive risk factor prevention and modification on a population-wide basis.

Although total cholesterol measurement is appropriate for mass public screening, use of low-density lipoprotein and high-density lipoprotein levels is more appropriate when determining risk for individual patients. These two values have a predictive power approximately 10 times that of total cholesterol alone (Castelli, 1984).

Most authorities believe that the monounsaturated fats (olive oil, canola oil) should be increasingly recommended to patients in their proportion of the total dietary fat allowance. This is based on epidemiologic studies and on the observation that these oils reduce low-density lipoprotein cholesterol at least as much as the polyunsaturated fatty acids when substituted in the diet for saturated fats. Further, they do not lower high-density lipoprotein levels as do the polyunsaturated fats.

The issue of the effect of personality characteristics on the risk of coronary heart disease is poorly understood. Although traditionally the Type A personality (highly stressed, constantly pushed for time, highly competitive, often intolerant of others) has been implicated as a risk factor, recent studies raise serious doubts about this concept.

Treadmill exercise stress testing has been advocated as both a screening test and a diagnostic test. Because of a generally low sensitivity and a prohibitively high false-positive rate, this test has not found a clear indication as a screening test. The only current recommended use for exercise stress testing is for previously inactive males over 40 years of age wishing to embark on a new vigorous exercise program.

IMPACT ON THE FAMILY UNIT. The life styles that are important for prevention of coronary heart disease cannot be easily implemented by an individual without due consideration of the person's family and environment. The chances of the patient quitting

Table 14–8. SIMPLIFIED GUIDELINES TO HELP PATIENTS BEGIN LOWERING CHOLESTEROL AND FAT IN THEIR DIET

Foods to Reduce or Eliminate	Recommended Substitutions
Whole eggs	Egg whites (2 whites/whole egg) Egg substitute
Cheese	Whey cheeses Low-fat cottage cheese Low-fat (part skim) cheeses Nondairy cheese
Whole milk	Low-fat or skim milk
Butter	Soft margarines Powdered butter flavoring
Ice cream	Sherbets, sorbets Ice milks Vegetable oil–based frozen dessert Tofu-based "ice cream"
Fatty meats, hot dogs, luncheon sausage, bacon, poultry skin, internal organ meats	Lean varieties of red meats, meats less often and in smaller (3 oz.) portions Skinned chicken and turkey Fish Avoid frying Nonmeat meals Textured vegetable-based meat substitutes
Shellfish	Reduced portions, if used Use lower cholesterol varieties (crab, clams, scallops) Fish-based mock crab legs
Chocolate	Cocoa
Highly refined prepared foods	Whole grain varieties, fresh fruits and vegetables
High-fat prepared foods (bakery items, foods prepared with coconut, palm, palm kernel, or hydrogenated vegetable oils or animal fat or lard)	Homemade or prepared low-fat varieties, using the unsaturated vegetable oils (soybean, canola or rapeseed, olive, corn, safflower, sesame, sunflower)

smoking are dimmed considerably when there are other smokers in the home. Dietary changes, especially, cannot be effectively implemented for only one individual in a family unit. Major changes in knowledge, attitudes, and habits of the entire family are often required so that the desirable foods can be purchased, properly prepared, and consumed with an agreed-upon common goal of improved health. Anything less can lead to resentment, confusion, and outright rebellion.

When a family member needs dietary therapy, a family meeting at the beginning will enhance the chances of long-term success. This meeting can be used to educate the family about risk and diet, enlist all family members' cooperation and support, and make plans for flexibility to meet everyone's needs. Fortunately, the diets recommended by the American Heart Association are nutritionally well balanced and can be recommended to all individuals, regardless of risk status.

Very helpful guidelines and educational materials are available from the American Heart Association through local and state chapters. Several excellent cookbooks are also widely available (Conner and Conner, 1986; Brody, 1985; Eshleman, 1984).

Cerebrovascular Disease

Incidence. Incidence of stroke is 140 in 100,000 persons per year, resulting in a total of 500,000 strokes per year. The yearly incidence increases with age from 100 in 100,000 persons between the ages of

Table 14–9. GUIDELINES FOR TREATMENT OF CORONARY HEART DISEASE RISK BASED ON LOW-DENSITY LIPOPROTEIN* LEVELS

Risk Group	Initiate Diet	Initiate Medication†	Goal
No coronary heart disease and less than two risk factors	160 mg./dl.	190 mg./dl.	<160 mg./dl.
Known coronary heart disease or two or more risk factors	130 mg./dl.	160 mg./dl.	130 mg./dl.

*Medication started only if step 1 and 2 diets fail to achieve goal.
†National Cholesterol Education Program, 1988.

45 and 54 to 900 in 100,000 persons between the ages of 65 and 74 and, ultimately, to 1800 in 100,000 persons at age 85. This translates into a 1 in 20 chance of having a stroke prior to age 70 for both males and females (Kannel et al., 1986).

Prevalence. There are nearly 2 million stroke victims still alive for a population prevalence for completed stroke of 800 in 100,000 persons. This, of course, does not include the millions of individuals with significant atherosclerotic cerebrovascular disease who are at an extremely high risk for stroke.

Cost and Impact on Society. The cost of stroke is estimated at $7.3 billion (Preziosi, 1986).

Morbidity and Mortality. Stroke is the third leading cause of death in the United States after coronary heart disease and cancer. The mortality rate is 69 in 100,000 persons per year, resulting in a total of 155,000 deaths in 1984. Thirty per cent of stroke victims die within 30 days and 43 per cent by 6 months of the original event.

In addition to the high mortality rate, stroke carries a very high morbidity. Forty per cent of stroke victims currently alive require special services and 10 per cent require total care (Kannel et al., 1986). The morbidity rate also rises dramatically with age.

Important Facts Relevant to Prevention. The major risk factor for stroke is hypertension. The other risk factors for coronary heart disease are less predictive for stroke risk. However, the known presence of heart disease carries a high risk, with an estimated 20 to 34 per cent of cerebral infarcts resulting from cardiac embolism. Diabetes mellitus, even when mild, carries a significant increased risk. This risk rises dramatically if both hypertension and diabetes are present.

Transient ischemic attacks confer a high risk of subsequent stroke. One out of five stroke victims has had one of four major symptoms suggestive of a transient ischemic attack in the previous year: (1) temporary loss of vision (especially in one eye), (2) unilateral numbness, (3) aphasia, and (4) focal weakness.

Patients with carotid bruits have a 2 per cent incidence of stroke per year, but infarcted areas are often not supplied by the affected artery (Wolf et al., 1981). These patients are also at significantly increased risk for myocardial infarction. Although most experts recommend prophylactic aspirin therapy, the current data are not sufficient to show that treatment with aspirin, anticoagulants, or surgery will effectively reduce the risk of stroke in patients with asymptomatic carotid bruits. Such studies are in progress and will provide further guidance in the future.

Other risk factors for stroke include family history of stroke, cigarette smoking, oral contraceptive use, hyperlipidemia, and elevated hematocrit.

Screening Test Recommendations. Elevated blood pressure, systolic *or* diastolic, is the single greatest risk factor for stroke and should be evaluated at each office visit.

Other risk factors for atherosclerosis should be sought as previously recommended under coronary heart disease.

The patient should be checked for the presence of carotid bruits every 5 years after age 40.

Preventive Activities Recommendations. Prevention of stroke is aimed primarily at prevention of sustained, even mild hypertension. Promotion of the healthy life-style habits discussed for coronary heart disease is likely, although unproven, to be of benefit. Smokers, in particular, should be strongly advised to stop. Secondary prevention of completed stroke in patients with transient ischemic attacks may include aspirin prophylaxis, anticoagulation, or carotid endarterectomy, depending on the clinical circumstances.

Discussion. The most important reason to listen for carotid bruits is to document the existence of significant atherosclerosis and, therefore, to alert the physician of the need to more aggressively modify risk factors. There is a risk, however, of initiating a process leading to unnecessary angiography and endarterectomy, which carry substantial risk.

Impact on Family Unit. The common results of stroke—physical disability, intellectual disability, and depression—often cause a loss of independence. The family or friends are suddenly forced to help make parental-type decisions. Active participation in the rehabilitation and care of a stroke victim can create enormous stress, both financially and emotionally, on the family unit. Placement of the patient in a nursing home, however rational, will require a resolution of guilt within the family. The family physician plays a critical central role in the coordination of rehabilitation with the family and in helping the family to resolve conflicting feelings.

SUBSTANCE ABUSE: ALCOHOLISM AND OTHER DRUG DEPENDENCY

Incidence. Difficulties in clearly identifying the point in time when an individual becomes an alcoholic make incidence rates very difficult to reliably determine. A rough estimate of incidence is 310 in 100,000 persons per year, which is derived by using prevalence rates and the average of 12 to 15 years of untreated alcoholism from onset to death.

Prevalence. Alcoholism affects at least 18 million Americans for a prevalence of 7500 in 100,000 persons or 7.5 per cent of the entire population. In an ambulatory medical setting, the prevalence of alcoholism is at least 10 per cent (Whitfield et al., 1986). The rates for dependency on other drugs is about 2 per cent (2000 in 100,000 persons). The rates of drug use and abuse in adolescents and young adults is particularly striking, as shown in Table 14–10.

Cost and Impact on Society. Estimated cost of alcohol abuse in the United States in 1983 was $117 billion: $71 billion from lost employment and reduced productivity and $15 billion in health care costs (Petrakis et al., 1987). Estimated 1983 total costs for illicit drug abuse were $60 billion.

Table 14–10. PERCENTAGE OF ILLICIT USE OF DRUGS BY YOUTHS AND YOUNG ADULTS, 1982*

	12–17 Years		18–25 Years	
	Ever Used	*Current Use*	*Ever Used*	*Current Use*
Alcohol	65	27	95	68
Cigarettes	50	15	77	40
Marijuana/hashish	27	12	64	27
Hallucinogens	5	1	21	2
Cocaine	7	2	28	7
Stimulants	7	3	18	5
Sedatives	6	1	19	3
Tranquilizers	5	1	15	2

*Adapted from Miller, J. D., Cisin, I. H., Gardner-Keating, H., et al: National Survey of Drug Abuse: Main Findings, 1982. Washington, D.C., US Government Printing Office, 1983.

Morbidity and Mortality. Patients with alcoholism have an overall risk of mortality of 2.5 times that of the normal population. An estimate for alcohol-related deaths in 1982 was 138,027 or 7.6 per cent of all deaths that year.

The morbidity for chemical dependency (alcohol and drug abuse) is substantial, ranging from the extremely high association with crime to the incidence of cirrhosis, psychosis, depression, cardiomyopathy, peptic ulcer disease, overdose, cancer of directly exposed organs (lips, mouth, larynx, pharynx, esophagus, stomach, and liver), pancreatitis, suicide, various infections (hepatitis, AIDS, endocarditis, and pneumonia), fetal alcohol syndrome, and accidents of all types.

Important Facts Relevant to Prevention. The most useful definition of chemical dependency is: The continued habitual use of a substance by a person despite resultant serious adverse effects on that person's life.

Measures to increase enforcement of drinking and driving laws, to increase prices for alcoholic beverages, and to increase the minimum drinking age have been shown either to reduce consumption or to reduce frequency of the legal consequences of drinking. Whether education will, in fact, reduce the rate of alcoholism is not known. Strong cultural biases (e.g., Orthodox Jews) against drunkenness have a strong effect on the reduction of the prevalence of dependency.

Children of alcoholics are at a three times greater risk of becoming alcoholics, whether or not they are raised by their biologic parents (Petrakis et al., 1987).

While spontaneous recovery of alcoholism is reported in 4 to 26 per cent of patients, treatment can result in a 70 per cent recovery rate (Whitfield, 1986). It is unrealistic, dangerous, and delusional for an alcoholic to ever attempt controlled drinking.

Screening Test Recommendations. All patients over 12 years of age should be screened regularly for alcohol and substance abuse. A yearly frequency of Annual screenings will deliver a strong educational message to the patient.

Probably the single best screening questions are: "Have you ever had a health, legal, or personal problem as a result of drinking alcohol?" This should be followed by: "When was your last drink?" (The answer is positive if the last drink occurred within 24 hours.) In a high-risk population with a prevalence of 20 per cent (e.g., the average inpatient population), affirmative answers to *either* of these two questions has a diagnostic accuracy as follows: sensitivity of 91.5 per cent, specificity of 89.7 per cent, positive predictive value of 69.4 per cent, and negative predictive value of 97.6 per cent (Cyr and Wartman, 1988). Two positive answers on the CAGE questions (Table 14–11) are also highly suggestive, with a 66 per cent positive predictive value (Bush et al., 1987). The MAST (Michigan Alcohol Screening Test), as shown in Table 14–12, can also be helpful in the diagnostic evaluation (Selzer, 1971).

The presence or absence of alcoholism in first-degree relatives should be a part of the family history. All patients, including children, should be asked yearly if there are any problems within the family that involve alcohol.

Preventive Activities Recommendations. Literature concerning the warning signs of alcoholism and sources of help should be freely available in every medical office. If the subject of chemical dependency is dealt with openly, there is an increased likelihood that the affected individual will seek help through the family physician.

Patients with a family history of alcoholism should be counseled concerning their high-risk status and encouraged to become a member of Alanon or the Children of Alcoholics Foundation.

Related Issues. The same questions used for alcohol may be equally applicable to drug abuse.

Certain cues found in alcoholics and other drug-

Table 14–11. CAGE SCREENING TEST FOR ALCOHOLISM*

CAGE Questions:	
C	utting down?
A	nnoyed by criticism of your drinking?
G	uilty about your drinking?
E	ye opener ever?

*Positive answers to any two questions point to a diagnosis of alcoholism.

Table 14–12. THE MICHIGAN ALCOHOLISM SCREENING TEST (MAST)*†

Question	Yes	No
Do you enjoy having a drink now and then?	0	____
Do you feel you are a normal drinker? (By normal we mean you drink less than or as much as most other people and you have not gotten into any recurring trouble while drinking)	____	2
Have you ever awakened the morning after some drinking the night before and found that you could not remember part of the evening?	2	____
Do either of your parents or any near relative, or your spouse or any girlfriend or boyfriend every worry or complain about your drinking?	1	____
Can you stop drinking without a struggle after one or two drinks?	____	2
Do you feel guilty about your drinking?	1	____
Do friends or relatives think you are a normal drinker?	____	2
Are you able to stop drinking when you want to?	____	2
Have you ever attended a meeting of Alcoholics Anonymous (AA)?	5	____
Have you gotten into physical fights when you have been drinking?	1	____
Has your drinking ever created problems between you and either of your parents, or another relative, your spouse, or any girlfriend or boyfriend?	2	____
Has any member of your family ever gone to anyone for help about your drinking?	2	____
Have you ever lost friends because of your drinking?	2	____
Have you ever been in trouble at work or school because of your drinking?	2	____
Have you ever lost a job because of drinking?	2	____
Have you ever neglected your obligations, your school work, your family, or your job for two or more days in a row because you were drinking?	2	____
Do you drink before noon fairly often?	1	____
Have you ever been told you had liver trouble or cirrhosis?	2	____
After heavy drinking have you ever had severe shaking or heard voices or seen things that really were't there? 2 (5 Delirium tremens)	____	
Have you ever gone to anyone for help about your drinking?	5	____
Have you ever been in a hospital because of drinking?	5	____
Have you ever been a patient in a psychiatric hospital or a psychiatric ward of a general hospital where drinking was part of the problem that resulted in hospitalization?	2	____
Have you ever been seen at a psychiatric or mental health clinic or gone to any doctor, social worker, or clergy for help with any emotional problem where drinking was a part of the problem?	2	____
Have you ever been arrested for drunk driving, driving while intoxicated, or driving under the influence of alcoholic beverages or any other drug? If yes, how many times?	2 each	____
Have you ever been arrested or taken into custody even for a few hours because of other drunk behavior, whether due to alcohol or another drug? If yes, how many times?	2 each	____

*Each response scores the number of points listed. A total of 0 to 3 = probable normal drinker; 4 = borderline; 5 to 9 = 80 per cent likelihood of dependence; and 10 or more = 100 per cent likelihood.

†From Selzer, M. L.: The Michigan alcoholism screening test: The quest for a new diagnostic instrument. Am. J. Psychiatry, *127*:1653, 1971.

dependent patients will help lead to the correct diagnosis: problems with children, separation, divorce, job changes, depression, anxiety, hypertension, macrocytosis of red blood cells, low resistance to infections, recurrent accidents, any trouble with legal authorities (including driving while intoxicated), upper gastrointestinal complaints, and abnormal liver enzymes.

Impact on the Family Unit. The family is at the epicenter of the alcoholic earthquake. As the rumblings of the disease progress, so does pathology within the family. Most prominent is the role of the "co-alcoholic" or "enabler" who assumes the abnegated responsibilities of the alcoholic, covers for the alcoholic, and makes possible the alcoholic's continued drinking. This person is often the major focus of the alcoholic's hostility. Treatment should include healing of the entire family.

CANCER

General Cancer Information

Incidence. Estimated new cancer cases for 1988 (excluding carcinoma-in-situ and nonmelanotic skin cancers) is 985,000 or 402 per 100,000 persons. The six cancers with the highest incidence (excluding skin cancers) are cancers of the lung, the colon-rectum, the breast, the prostate, the urinary tract, and the uterus. Thirty per cent of all Americans will eventually develop cancer.

Prevalence. There are over 5 million people alive today with a history of cancer. No data are available to indicate how many Americans have undiagnosed cancer at this time.

Cost and Impact on Society. Estimated total cost of medical care for cancer is over $10 billion per year. An additional $25 billion is lost in income.

Morbidity and Mortality. Cancer mortality is second only to cardiovascular diseases in the United States, and cancer is responsible for over 22 per cent of all deaths. Estimated mortality for 1988 is 494,000 or 202 per 100,000 persons. The six leading causes of cancer death are cancers of the lung, the colon-rectum, the breast, the prostate, the pancreas, and the urinary system.

From 1930 to 1985, the mortality rate for cancer in the United States rose from 130 to 171 per 100,000 persons. This rise has been primarily due to the continuing rise of mortality from cancer of the lung.

Important Facts Relevant to Prevention. Seventy-five million Americans (30 per cent of the population) now living will eventually have cancer. Thirty-five per cent of all cancer deaths are thought to be related to diet (including obesity) (Doll and Peto, 1981). Obese individuals have increased risk of colon, breast, and uterine cancers. High-fat diets are a risk factor for prostate, breast, and colon cancer. Foods rich in vitamins A (dark green and deep yellow vegetables and fruits) and C (citrus fruits, strawberries, and sweet peppers) and cruciferous vegetables (cabbage, broccoli, brussel sprouts, and cauliflower) are all believed to have protective effects for various cancers. Salt-cured, smoked, and nitrite-cured foods increase the risk of upper gastrointestinal cancers.

Smoking accounts for 30 per cent of cancer deaths, primarily cancer of the lung, the urinary bladder, the mouth, the throat, and the larynx, whereas alcohol is responsible for approximately 3 per cent and occupational exposures are responsible for 5 per cent of cancer mortality.

Therefore, diet, smoking, alcohol, and occupational exposures appear to account for over 73 per cent of all cancer mortality. These are potentially preventable causes and are amenable to intervention by the family physician.

Early diagnosis and treatment (secondary prevention) is also of great benefit. Currently, 40 per cent of newly diagnosed cancer victims have a 5-year survival. Of the 494,000 individuals who have died from cancer, 174,000 might have been saved by earlier diagnosis and treatment.

Related Issues. The prevention of cancer takes on a new urgency when one considers the likely doubling of the incidence and morbidity of cancer by the year 2000 due to the increasing number of elderly and success with decreasing mortality due to other causes.

Life-style modification plus early diagnosis through screening could potentially reduce cancer mortality by 80 to 90 per cent (Doll, 1981).

Impact on the Family Unit. For many of the cancers, a positive family history is a significant risk factor that requires the physician to emphasize prevention and early detection for these families. Also, it may create a variety of behavioral problems within the family. Members of families caring for cancer patients may experience hypochondriasis, depression, phobic disorders, generalized anxiety, and anger and hostility. These may be precipitated when issues of illness and death are being dealt with in the family.

Because of the great importance of life style in the prevention of cancer, family health habits are the major source of potential successful cancer prevention. When one considers the fact that cancer will strike three out of four families, the value of generally applied preventive health measures within every family practice becomes evident.

Colorectal Cancer

Incidence. Colorectal cancer has the second highest incidence of all cancers. The American Cancer Society estimated 147,000 new cases in 1988 for an incidence of 60 in 100,000 persons. The incidence of colorectal cancer begins to rise after age 40, roughly doubling each decade. Ninety per cent occur in the population over 50.

Prevalence. The exact prevalence in the population is not known. Most screening trials find one to two cancers and 80 polyps per 1000 screened patients.

Morbidity and Mortality. Mortality has been steady for almost 30 years at approximately 50 per cent (62,000 deaths in 1988), despite the increasing vigilance of screening by physicians. This may be explained in part by the shift of lesions from the rectum and sigmoid colon to the right colon, where early detection with sigmoidoscopy is not possible.

The survival rate varies dramatically with the stage of the cancer, as shown in Table 14–13.

Important Facts Relevant to Prevention. Colorectal cancer appears to arise almost exclusively from benign adenomatous polyps over a period of 5 to 10 years. However, only 20 to 30 per cent of polyps are adenomas, and only 5 to 10 per cent of adenomatous polyps become malignant (Riegelman et al., 1988). The initial appearance of adenomas occurs primarily between 40 and 45 years of age, with a significant increase in colorectal cancer every 5 to 10 years after that.

Polyps less than 1.0 cm. are malignant 1 to 2 per cent of the time, those 1.0 to 2.0 cm. in size are malignant 5 to 10 per cent of the time, those 2.0 to 4.0 cm. are malignant 40 per cent of the time, and those greater than 4.0 cm. are malignant 60 per cent of the time (Bader, 1986).

When compared with pathology found on colonoscopy, stool guaiac specimens (Hemoccult II, not rehydrated, two stool samples daily for three consecutive days) were 91 per cent specific for no pathology of any type, and they were 52 per cent sensitive for carcinoma, 23 per cent sensitive for polyps greater than 1.0 cm., and 4.4 per cent sensitive for polyps less than 1.0 cm. (Crowly et al., 1983). A major prospective study (uncontrolled) of over 20,000 patients, followed for up to 25 years and screened periodically with only a 25-cm. scope, showed a 50 per cent reduction of incidence of bowel cancers over that predicted (Gilbertson and Nelms, 1978).

Although there has been a progressive change toward polyps occurring higher in the large bowel, over 60 per cent are still within reach of the 60-cm. flexible sigmoidoscope.

Compared with the current 5-year survival rate of 55 per cent, it is estimated that potentially 80 to 90 per cent of all colon cancers could be prevented by screening and removal of adenomatous polyps.

Twenty per cent of colorectal cancers can be attributed to a dietary cause, especially to lack of fiber in the diet. High-fat diets have also been implicated.

Risk factors for colorectal cancer are found in

Table 14–13. FIVE-YEAR SURVIVAL RATE FOR COLORECTAL CANCER

		Per Cent Survival		
Surgical Pathology	**Dukes Stage**	*1**	*2†*	*3‡*
In situ, mucosal invasion only	A	100	88	80
Muscular invasion	B	60	61	61
Local nodes	C	22 to 43	26	40
Distant spread	D	4	1	2

*Astler and Coller, 1961
†Jarvinen and Turunen, 1984
‡Turunen and Peltokallio, 1983

Table 14–14. RISK FACTORS FOR COLORECTAL CANCER

Age >50
History of adenomas
Personal or family history of colorectal cancer or polyps
Ulcerative colitis
Crohn's disease affecting the colon
Personal or family history of genital or breast cancer in females

Table 14–14. Other risk factors that are less well established are cutaneous papillomas, a history of cholecystectomy, extensive work-related handling of synthetic fibers, and a history of ureterosigmoidostomy.

Screening Test Recommendations

1. Rectal examination and a 6-slide fecal occult blood test on all patients yearly over 40 years of age.

2. Flexible sigmoidoscopy every 3 to 5 years on all adults starting after age 40 and no later than age 50. (American Cancer Society recommends two yearly examinations starting at age 50 and every 3 to 5 years thereafter.)

Preventive Activities Recommendations. Risk factor analysis should be performed when the patient is at least 40 years of age. Preventive activities include the surveillance, noted earlier, which includes searching for presymptomatic carcinomas and lesions with malignant potential (adenomas). All patients, regardless of age, should be encouraged to eat a high-fiber, low-fat diet.

Related Issues. The ideal screening method would be to perform periodic colonoscopy on all high-risk persons. This method is not practical, cost-effective, or acceptable to patients.

Knowing the 5- to 10-year natural history of progression from adenoma to cancer, one could reasonably begin primary prevention at least this long prior to the age of 50 when the most dramatic increase in actual cancer incidence occurs.

The frequency of testing patients every 5 years is favored for the general population. More frequent testing of those believed to have significant risk factors is justified. It may be possible to define a very low-risk population in which flexible sigmoidoscopy is no longer beneficial by using the risk criteria and perhaps a given number of negative examinations.

Impact on the Family Unit. Since family history is a major risk factor, information obtained by the family physician should be used for family education concerning prevention.

Breast Cancer

Incidence. The age-adjusted breast cancer incidence rate was 92.1 per 100,000 white females and 81.8 for black females in 1983, and has increased only slightly since that time. In 1988, there were an estimated 135,000 new cases of invasive breast cancer and an additional 5000 cases of carcinoma-in-situ. The lifetime incidence of breast cancer for females is 1 in 10 and appears to be slowly increasing. Twenty-eight per cent of all new female cancers are breast cancers, compared with 16 per cent for colorectal cancer, the next most common cancer in females.

Prevalence. Based on incidence and mortality statistics, the estimated number of patients with previously diagnosed breast cancer who are currently living is 432,000.

Morbidity and Mortality. The mortality rates for breast cancer from 1974 to 1985 has been stable at approximately 27 per 100,000 women or 39,000 deaths. This accounts for 18 per cent of all female cancer deaths, which is now second to the 20 per cent of female cancer deaths caused by lung cancer. The 5-year survival rate for localized breast cancer is 90 per cent compared with 78 per cent in the 1940's. In situ breast cancer has a cure rate approaching 100 per cent. The survival rates at 5, 8, and 10 years were 88 per cent, 83 per cent, and 79 per cent, respectively, for breast cancers diagnosed through screening in the Breast Cancer Detection Demonstration Project (Seidman, 1987).

Important Facts Relevant to Prevention. The major accepted risk factors are listed in Table 14–15. In addition, there have been suggested associations between breast cancer and certain diets: high fat, low fiber, and moderate alcohol. Despite evaluation of risk factors, 75 per cent of women with breast cancer

Table 14–15. RISK FACTORS FOR BREAST CANCER*

Factor	Relative Risk
†Atypical hyperplasia and family history	11
†Family history of premenopausal bilateral breast cancer	9
†Family history of premenopausal breast cancer	1.5
Family history of postmenopausal breast cancer	1.5
Family history of bilateral breast cancer	5
†History of previous personal breast cancer	5
Fibrocystic disease, proliferative type on biopsy	1.5 to 4
†Lobular carcinoma-in-situ	7.2
†Intraductal carcinoma-in-situ (risk > lobular carcinoma-in-situ)	N/A
†Atypical lobular or ductal hyperplasia on biopsy	N/A
First pregnancy after age 35	2 to 3
Nulliparous	3
Early menarche or late menopause	1.3 to 2.0
Increasing age	
Factors with Unclear Status	
Alcohol intake	
High-fat, low-fiber diet	
Obesity	
History of ovarian, endometrial, salivary cancers	

*Modified from Love, S. M., Gelman, R. S., and Silen, W.: Fibrocystic disease of the breast—a non-disease? Reprinted with permission from N. Engl. J. Med., *312*(3):146, 1985.

†Factors for which there is a consensus to place a patient in a high-risk group needing special attention.

will have no risk factor other than their age. The risk rises progressively with age. A female of 65 to 69 years old has over 200 times the risk of a female 20 to 24 years old and over four times the risk of a female 35 to 39 years old.

Breast self-examination alone has a sensitivity of 26 per cent compared with 45 per cent for clinical breast examination, 71 per cent for mammography, and 75 per cent for a combination of mammography and clinical breast examination (O'Malley and Fletcher, 1987). Of significance, however, is the fact that in the Breast Cancer Detection Demonstration Project, 690 of the total 2675 breast cancers diagnosed were found by breast self-examination between screening visits. Nevertheless, a definitive study showing a lowered mortality rate for those performing breast self-examination has not been done.

Clinical breast examination is believed to be useful. Up to 16 per cent of cancers may be missed if no breast examination is included in screening. Half of these are minimal cancers and, therefore, highly curable (Potchen, 1987).

The Breast Cancer Detection Demonstration Project was conducted over 5 years with 280,000 women, aged 35 to 74, participating to evaluate a mass screening program for breast cancer. It demonstrated that screening 40- to 50-year-old women was as effective in long-term survival rates as screening those over 50 (Seidman, 1987). However, the Health Insurance Plan of New York study failed to show a statistically significant decrease in mortality for the age group under 50 years of age, although there was a trend in that direction. The most important conclusion from the Health Insurance Plan of New York study is that early detection of breast cancer does significantly decrease mortality (Potchen, 1987).

A number of factors have been shown not to alter the risk of breast cancer. These include breast trauma, fibroadenomas, fibrocystic breast disease of the nonproliferative type, caffeine consumption, mastodynia with negative mammographic and clinical examination, breast-feeding, and use of birth control pills or postmenopausal estrogen therapy.

Screening Test Recommendations. Table 14–16 outlines the official guidelines of the United States Preventive Health Services Task Force, the American Academy of Family Physicians, and the American Cancer Society. These recommendations range from conservative to aggressive. Table 14–5, discussed earlier, explains the classifications used by the United States Preventive Services Task Force. Each physician must decide the appropriate level of preventive care to implement in his or her practice. The United States Preventive Health Service Task Force guidelines represent the minimum level of preventive health care expected of primary care physicians.

Preventive Activities Recommendations. Very little has been proved concerning the primary prevention of breast cancer. Diet may have a significant role. Patients should be advised of the concern raised as a result of the association of moderate alcohol ingestion, high-fat diets, and low-fiber diets with breast cancer. These dietary recommendations can be made on other grounds and are considered to be of general benefit. Therefore, physicians may wish to make these recommendations before a direct cause and effect relationship is firmly established.

Although of unproven benefit, breast self-examination is a logical, low-risk, no-cost activity. It should be taught to each female at the time of her first gynecologic examination and reviewed at each subsequent examination.

Every female should have an initial documented evaluation of risk factors for breast cancer at or before age 30. A long-term program for screening should be determined at that time.

Secondary prevention is the goal of current major screening recommendations and is focused on the early detection of disease prior to symptoms. All lesions of the breast should be promptly investigated. Any mass found on physician examination or on mammography should be evaluated by needle aspiration, needle biopsy, or open excisional biopsy, depending on the clinical circumstances. A negative mammogram or a negative clinical examination alone is never fully adequate to rule out cancer.

Related Issues. Environmental factors deserve more attention. The Japanese have very low incidence of breast cancer. However, subsequent generations of Japanese immigrants to the United States have increasing incidence rates, eventually equaling the high levels in the United States. Several recent studies have suggested a strong association between alcohol ingestion and breast cancer (O'Connell, 1987).

Who should be placed in a high-risk group and receive special attention is controversial. Certain factors as noted in Table 14–15 are considered adequate to place a female in the high-risk group. For instance, a mother and sister with premenopausal bilateral breast cancer imparts a lifetime risk of 30 per cent (McLellan, 1988).

Screening mammography in the 40- to 50-year-old group remains controversial. There is good reason to do this in the high-risk group, with many experts recommending yearly mammography starting at age 35. Many physicians will offer screening mammography every 1 to 2 years to all women in this age group.

The positive predictive value of abnormal results (positive clinical breast examination or positive mammography interpretation) of the Breast Cancer Detection Demonstration Project screening program is very low (approximately 15.5 per cent) due primarily to a low sensitivity of 87 per cent (Reigelman, 1988). However, the specificity is very high. Therefore, by using this screening program, very few women with carcinoma of the breast will be missed, but a large number of women will be falsely positive and need to be evaluated with further diagnostic work-up, such as needle aspiration, needle biopsy, or open biopsy.

The costs of mammographic screening remain a major concern. The 10-year cost of annual screening

Table 14–16. OFFICIAL RECOMMENDATIONS FOR BREAST CANCER SCREENING

		American Academy of Family Physicians and the American Cancer Society	United States Preventive Services Task Force		
Age	*Test*	*Frequency*	*Frequency*	*Category of Evidence*	*Recommendations*
20 to 34	BSE	Monthly			
	CBE	q3 Years			
35 to 39	BSE	Monthly			
	CBE	q3 Years			
	Mamm	Once			
40 to 49	BSE	Monthly		III	C
	CBE	Yearly	Yearly	III	C
	Mamm	q1–2 Years			
50 to 59	BSE	Monthly		III	C
	CBE	Yearly	Yearly	I	A
	Mamm	Yearly	Yearly	I	A
60+	BSE	Monthly		III	C
	CBE	Yearly	Yearly	II-2	B
	Mamm	Yearly	Yearly	II-2	B

BSE, breast self-examination; CBE, clinical breast examination; Mamm, mammography.

of only 25 per cent of all women in the 40- to 49-year age range would be $402 million, with a total 373 lives saved by the year 2000 (Eddy, 1988). Even limiting mammography to those over 50 years of age would result in a cost of $3.3 billion at the current average cost of $100 per examination. This is by far the most expensive preventive health care activity recommended.

The smaller the tumor when discovered, the better the prognosis. A review of several studies shows that nonpalpable mammographically detected cancers have a 13 to 20 per cent incidence of metastatic spread, whereas those found by palpation have positive nodes 40 to 55 per cent of the time (McLellan, 1988). It has been calculated that the average time between the ability of mammography to first detect the cancer and the ability of the physician to palpate the mass is 2 years, which may be of some value in estimating the optimal interval for mammography.

Impact on the Family Unit. The fear of breast cancer can produce a great deal of anxiety. This fear is substantially heightened by a strong family history. As with other diseases with a strong familial predisposition, the elements of guilt and resentment can have a profound effect on family functioning.

A major fear is associated with the patient's and the husband's perceived loss of feminine identity. This can be allayed in part by a knowledgeable physician willing to openly discuss these issues and inform the patient and husband of the variety of improved treatment alternatives now available. These include consideration of limited surgical procedures, radiation, and prosthesis implantation.

Once cancer has been diagnosed and a treatment plan decided upon, the family physician can play a critical role in preventing subsequent family dysfunction (Gates, 1988). The patient will need help in dealing with anger, helplessness, fear of recurrence, and the ill effects of treatment. Once cancer has been diagnosed, the emotional life of the family is changed forever. The family as a unit will require guidance and understanding.

Lung Cancer

Incidence. Lung cancer now has the highest cancer incidence for both males and females in the United States. In 1988, the estimated number of new cases was 152,000.

Morbidity and Mortality. Lung cancer is the leading cause of cancer mortality for both males and females. The estimated number of deaths in 1988 was 139,000. Comparing the similarity of the incidence and mortality statistics, the grim nature of the prognosis is apparent, reflected in a 13 per cent 5-year survival.

Important Facts Relevant to Prevention. Except for the small minority of cases secondary to industrial exposure, the only known way to prevent lung cancer is to not smoke. Eighty-three per cent of all lung cancers are directly attributable to smoking.

Screening Test Recommendations. Although chest x-ray studies or sputum cytology may detect lung cancer at a presymptomatic stage, there is no study that shows a resultant improvement in the prognosis.

Preventive Activities Recommendations. Patients at all ages should receive a strong health message from their physician concerning smoking: "It's addicting. Don't start. If you have started, stop." All preventive health checks should include an inquiry concerning smoking.

Related Issues. It is ironic that lung cancer has the highest incidence and mortality rate of all cancers and yet is one of the most preventable. Physicians can continue to have a major impact on the risk of this disease through community and patient intervention and education. Excellent support materials are available from the American Academy of Family Physicians, the American Cancer Society, and the American Heart Association. Physician recommendation has a great potential impact on patients' decisions to stop smoking.

Impact on the Family Unit. A single smoker in a family can be a source of secondary smoke exposure for the rest of the family. Angina and respiratory symptoms may worsen. Children from households with smokers have a higher school absentee rate. Couples who smoke create a special problem for the physician who wishes to help. It is difficult to persuade one smoker to quit while the other continues, and it is equally problematic to bring two smokers to the point of wishing to stop at the same time. The withdrawal period is one of great stress and requires family education and support.

Carcinoma of the Cervix

Incidence. The incidence of invasive cervical carcinoma is declining. There are now approximately 12,900 new cases of invasive cancer yearly. The incidence rises steadily through age 50 and then remains steady. Worldwide, cervical carcinoma is the most common malignancy in women, whereas in the United States it ranks seventh among all cancers.

Morbidity and Mortality. The mortality for invasive carcinoma of the cervix is 7000 persons per year. The preinvasive cancer lesion of cervical intraepithelial neoplasia (CIN III or carcinoma-in-situ) has a 100 per cent cure rate with proper treatment, whereas stage 1 disease has an 80 per cent 5-year survival and stage 3, a 30 per cent 5-year survival. Overall, the 5-year survival rate is 66 per cent. The death rate has dropped 70 per cent in the last 40 years. This is primarily a result of Papanicolaou's smear screening programs detecting this disease at earlier stages when cure rates are higher.

Important Facts Relevant to Prevention. Squamous cell carcinoma of the cervix occurs almost exclusively in women who have had coitus.

Although the mean time for progression from mild dysplasia (CIN I) to severe dysplasia or carcinoma-in-situ (CIN III) is 5.8 years and the mean time for further progression to invasive carcinoma is an additional 10 years (Richart, 1981), the rate of progression for any one individual is unpredictable. Carcinoma-in-situ may regress spontaneously in 30 to 50 per cent of cases. At least 30 per cent of patients with CIN III will have progression to invasive carcinoma (Hudson, 1988).

Major risk factors are early age for first intercourse, multiple sexual partners, herpes simplex virus infection, and history of condylomata (human papillomavirus) infection. Early sexual intercourse has an especially dramatic effect on risk. Females who have had coitus less than one year after menarche are 26 times as likely to eventually develop cervical carcinoma as the general population.

Fifteen to twenty per cent of American women do not undergo regular Papanicolaou's tests and they account for the majority of cases of carcinoma of the cervix. The Papanicolaou's test is demonstrated to be 70 per cent sensitive (30 per cent of cases are missed) (Richart, 1981).

Screening Test Recommendations. All women should begin having Papanicolaou's smears when sexual activity begins but no later than age 18. The American Cancer Society recommends that each woman should have at least three negative annual Papanicolaou's smears, at which time frequency may be reduced at the discretion of the physician. Many physicians continue to advocate yearly screening. As yet, there appears to be no justification for screening high-risk groups more frequently. However, the 33 per cent incidence of CIN in patients with human papillomavirus infections may represent a high-risk subgroup requiring more frequent monitoring. The authors would support those who wish to continue yearly screening in their practice.

Preventive Activities Recommendations. Risk status should be re-evaluated at each preventive health visit, especially in groups who may have an increased likelihood of multiple sexual partners. Women should be advised of their risk status with emphasis on the importance of regular re-evaluation. Although barrier contraception has only theoretical benefit, it can also be strongly recommended to help prevent sexually transmitted diseases.

Related Issues. There are other good reasons to see many women more often than every 3 years, such as monitoring use of birth control pills, breast cancer screening, dietary advice, contraceptive counseling, and prepregnancy counseling. It may be only a minority of women who will need to visit their physician less often than once yearly. Women have been educated for many years that the yearly Papanicolaou's test is essential but *not* that there are other important issues to be dealt with during these visits.

Impact on the Family Unit. The occurrence of invasive cervical cancer during the childbearing years will usually be treated surgically, ending chances of future pregnancy. This will have a profound effect on a single female's approach to possible marriage and on a married couple's plans and relationship. The family physician's role only begins with referral for appropriate treatment. Preventive counseling is necessary in these situations. Women past the childbearing years may still suffer a loss of identity, similar to but not as intense as the breast cancer victim.

Skin Cancer

Incidence. There are 500,000 cases of skin cancer each year, of which 27,000 are malignant melanoma. This is over twice the incidence of cancer in any other organ system. The incidence continues to rise dramatically.

Morbidity and Mortality. Of the 7800 deaths each year, 5800 are from malignant melanoma.

Important Facts Relevant to Prevention. The major risk factor for all skin cancer is exposure to ultraviolet light. Those who have had severe exposures as children and those with fair complexion are at particular risk. Occupational exposures to coal tar, pitch, arsenic, radium, and creosote all increase risk. A prior history of local treatment with ionizing radiation increases chances of localized skin cancers 25 to 30 years later.

Screening Test Recommendations. During regular preventive health examinations, the skin should be thoroughly examined for suspicious lesions. All lesions suspicious for malignancy should be prophylactically excised and submitted for pathologic interpretation.

Preventive Activities Recommendations. For primary prevention, all patients at risk should be counseled in measures for avoidance of ultraviolet light (sun or artificial tanning), protection with higher number sunscreens (level 15 or greater), and use of protective clothing. Secondary prevention includes regular self-examination. This is a logical activity, especially for patients with already existing melanotic nevi.

The physician should also be alert to actinic keratoses and treat these as appropriate with 5-fluorouracil topical application when generalized or with cryocautery when localized.

Endometrial Cancer

Incidence. Nineteen per 100,000 persons (47,000 cases per year).

Morbidity and Mortality. Four per 100,000 persons (10,000 cases per year).

Important Facts Relevant to Prevention. Endometrial cancer is primarily a postmenopausal disease. The major etiologic factor appears to be the presence of unopposed estrogen, whether physiologic or iatrogenic. The most important early warning sign is abnormal vaginal bleeding. Risk factors are obesity, prolonged treatment with estrogen alone, age, chronic anovulation. Hypertension and diabetes are less strongly associated with risk, probably because of the prevalence of obesity in these patients.

Screening Test Recommendations. Abnormal endometrial cells are occasionally found on Papanicolaou's smear, but this is not an adequate screen. Any endometrial cells found on a postmenopausal Papanicolaou's smear should be considered abnormal.

All postmenopausal females with bleeding of any amount must have endometrial sampling performed.

Preventive Activities Recommendations. Risk factors should be established at menopause and modified when possible.

All females treated with estrogen replacement therapy also should be cycled with a progestational agent.

Cancer of the Prostate

There is no known prevention for cancer of the prostate. Early detection has not been shown to alter the prognosis.

Rectal examination has already been recommended as part of the screening for colorectal cancer. The prostate should be examined at that time with the hope that there is a subset of patients that may benefit from early detection.

OTHER PREVENTABLE DISEASES

Osteoporosis

Incidence. The incidence of fractures secondary to osteoporosis is 1 million per year. By extreme old age, one in every three women and one in every six men will have had a hip fracture, and one in three women over 65 will have vertebral fractures (Riggs, 1986).

Prevalence. It is estimated that 15 to 20 million Americans have osteoporosis and are, therefore, at markedly increased risk for fractures.

Cost and Impact on Society. The direct and indirect costs of caring for patients suffering fractures secondary to osteoporosis is $6 billion each year (National Institutes of Health, 1984).

Morbidity and Mortality. Between 12 and 20 per cent of hip fractures lead to death and 50 per cent lead to significant disability.

Important Facts Relevant to Prevention. Bone mass peaks in human beings at approximately 30 years of age. Caucasian females have significantly lower peaks than males or darker skinned females. In females, after age 30, there is a 0.3 to 0.5 per cent loss of bone mass yearly that abruptly increases to 2 to 3 per cent per year at menopause and then, over the next 10 years, gradually returns to premenopausal rates. The rates of loss of trabecular bone and cortical bone (the hip contains both) are somewhat different. Trabecular bone loss (vertebra, distal radius) occurs earlier and in greater proportion during the menopausal years than cortical bone (long bones) (Riggs, 1986). Men follow a similar sequence but without the accelerated phase. Total loss of bone mass in males is about two thirds that of females.

Prior to 30 years of age, adequacy of calcium intake will affect the peak bone mass and after 30 will affect the rate of loss of bone mass. All women and men need 1.0 gm. of elemental calcium to maintain a zero calcium balance. In postmenopausal women not receiving estrogen replacement therapy, increasing this amount to 1.5 gm will still not maintain zero calcium balance, will have no effect on trabecular bone, and will have only a minimal effect on cortical bone (Riis et al., 1987). There is an 80 per cent prevalence of inadequate calcium intake among females.

Estrogen replacement therapy is the most effective method of preventing the accelerated phase of bone mass loss after menopause. Case control studies have shown significant decreases in postmenopausal fracture rates with estrogen replacement therapy (Riggs, 1986). Discontinuation of estrogen therapy results in a prompt return of accelerated bone loss. Other methods of maximizing peak mass and slowing bone mass loss include regular weight-bearing exercise. Actual gains in lumbar bone mass have been demonstrated in postmenopausal women placed on a weight-bearing exercise regimen, as long as exercise was continued (Dalsky et al., 1988).

There are many primary risk factors for osteoporosis and multiple additional medical conditions that may place an individual at higher risk (Table 14–17). Contributing factors may be easily overlooked when an illness that may increase risk of osteoporosis consumes the focus of attention. A good example might be the elderly white female in otherwise good health who develops polymyalgia rheumatica. The diagnosis and treatment with corticosteroids becomes the major focus. It is easy to forget that such a person, 2 years later, may be free of symptoms of polymyalgia rheumatica but be debilitated by vertebral fractures.

Screening Test Recommendations. No screening test can be recommended. Specifically, densitometry has no place in routine preventive health care at this time.

Preventive Activities Recommendations. All patients, especially females, should be educated regarding the recommended intake of 1000 mg. of dietary calcium. Postmenopausal females not receiving postmenopausal estrogens should increase that amount to 1500 mg. Major nutritional sources of calcium are listed in Table 14–18. Recommendations for use of dairy products include the advice to use low-fat alternatives wherever possible as part of the overall prudent diet. Females of any age unable to meet minimal calcium needs through diet should be advised to use supplemental calcium.

Risk status should be determined for all females, preferably at menarche, and should be re-evaluated at the time of routine preventive health visits. Additional counseling concerning osteoporosis prevention should be given to those at higher risk.

Every female should be thoroughly evaluated at menopause for risk factors and possible estrogen replacement therapy. In general, most white females with any other risk factors are candidates unless there are specific contraindications. Therapy should be life long.

All patients should be counseled to maintain regular aerobic weight-bearing activity as part of the overall program for general preventive health care. Although 50 to 60 minutes of exercise performed three times weekly has been shown to increase bone mass, the minimum levels necessary have not been determined (Dalsky, 1988).

Related Issues. When prescribing estrogen replacement therapy, a daily dosage equivalent to 0.625 mg. of conjugated estrogen has been documented to be effective; 0.3 mg. may be equally effective. It is desirable to add progesterone for at least the last 10 days of each estrogen cycle, followed by 5 to 7 days without either hormone. Progesterone reduces or eliminates the increased risk of endometrial cancer associated with unopposed estrogen therapy. Although estrogen replacement therapy appears to favorably affect the lipid profile, the effects of progesterone may partially negate this, and therefore should be used in the lowest effective dose—the equivalent of 5 mg. of medroxyprogesterone acetate.

Impact on the Family Unit. Family eating patterns will primarily determine the peak bone mass achieved. Therefore, counseling of women in the childbearing years should include recommendations for the entire family.

Elderly patients who are already at high risk create a dilemma for the family physician. There is little that is of proven value in replacing bone mass that is already lost. The process may be slowed with calcium, estrogens, and exercise. Exercise, in particular, places the osteoporotic patient at some increased risk for fractures. The resulting sudden loss of independence in an elderly family member suffering from a serious fracture has a great impact on the family in emotional, organizational, and financial terms. The major decisions that must be made as a result of the condition often reverse the parent-child roles.

Intimate knowledge of the elderly patient, his or her functional capacities, and the living situation place the family physician in a pivotal role in the prevention of fractures.

Table 14–17. RISK FACTORS FOR OSTEOPOROSIS

Positive family history
Advancing age
Female
Caucasian or Asian
Early menopause (including surgically induced)
Underweight
Cigarette smoking
History of dietary calcium deficiency
Hypogonadism (males)
Sedentary life style
Alcohol consumption
Subtotal gastrectomy
Hyperthyroidism
Hemiplegia
Chronic obstructive pulmonary disease
Glucocorticoid therapy
Anticonvulsant therapy

Table 14–18. NUTRITIONAL SOURCES OF CALCIUM

Food	Serving Size	Calcium (mg.)
Milk	1 cup	300
Cheese (low fat)	1 oz.	185
Yogurt (nonfat)	1 cup	450
Yogurt (whole milk)	1 cup	275
Cottage cheese (1 per cent)	½ cup	70
Dark leafy greens	½ cup	150 to 180
Other vegetables	½ cup	30 to 100
Fruits	average serving	<25

Sexually Transmitted Diseases

Incidence. The peak incidence of sexually transmitted diseases is in teenagers and young adults; teenagers alone account for 2.5 million cases. The reported incidence of gonorrhea has dropped from a peak in 1974 to current levels of 375 per 100,000 persons (total cases, 879,000), with marked clustering in metropolitan areas. True incidence may be twice the actual reported incidence. Estimated yearly incidence figures for chlamydial infection is an astounding 4.65 million cases. Each year, 120,000 infants are infected with *Chlamydia* at birth. There are an estimated 724,000 new cases of herpes genitalis each year.

Prevalence. Because of the long duration of infection, the two most prevalent sexually transmitted diseases are herpes simplex virus and human papillomavirus. The cumulative prevalence of herpes simplex virus genitalis alone is 20 million cases at this time. Because of the asymptomatic nature of many chlamydial infections, it is estimated that the prevalence in the general population is 5 per cent.

Cost and Impact on Society. For pelvic inflammatory disease alone, the costs per year are $2.6 billion.

Morbidity and Mortality. Over 200,000 women per year, one fifth of those with pelvic inflammatory disease, become infertile, and 50 per cent of all ectopic pregnancies are a result of pelvic inflammatory disease (Washington et al., 1986). Twenty per cent of females with one episode of pelvic inflammatory disease will develop chronic pain.

Important Facts Relevant to Prevention. All of the sexually transmitted diseases have a high asymptomatic carrier rate, making prevention of transmission very difficult. Therefore, the single major risk factor is multiple sexual partners. Only abstinence, monogamy, or condoms will dramatically affect the risk.

Screening Test Recommendations. No screening tests are recommended for the general population. A screening gonorrhea culture test and a direct fluorescent antibody test or enzyme-linked immunoassay for *Chlamydia* should be performed in patients from high-risk groups at the time of routine pelvic examination. Persons with multiple sexual partners should be examined yearly.

Preventive Activities Recommendations. Education should begin before or at the beginning of sexual activity. All sexually active patients should be encouraged to seek medical evaluation for even apparently minor genital tract symptoms.

Related Issues. Physicians must maintain a high index of suspicion for all sexually transmitted diseases since there is a very high percentage of asymptomatic and minimally symptomatic patients. In high-risk populations, presumptive treatment for chlamydial infection, even with minimal signs or symptoms, is recommended by many experts. Treatment recommendations for gonorrhea now include coverage for *Chlamydia* as well for all patients.

Impact on the Family Unit. The incrimination that can result when a husband or wife is diagnosed with a sexually transmitted disease may lead to major family disruption. The physician will play the key role in interpreting the meaning of such an episode and bringing the couple to a mutual understanding. It is, therefore, critical that the physician know the natural course of the disease. For instance, 30 per cent of women with gonorrhea may be asymptomatic carriers (in some populations, men may also be almost this high), 70 per cent of patients with genital herpes have no symptoms, and 70 per cent of female lower genital tract infections with *Chlamydia* are asymptomatic (Office of Disease Prevention/Health Promotion, 1988).

Human Immunodeficiency Virus Infection

Incidence. The incidence of AIDS secondary to human immunodeficiency virus infection was estimated at 1.43 per 100,000 persons in 1984. The reported 3-year incidence of AIDS in subjects who were seropositive for human immunodeficiency virus has ranged from 8.0 to 34.2 per cent.

Prevalence. The Centers for Disease Control estimates that human immunodeficiency virus had infected 1.5 million Americans by 1987. The prevalence of AIDS was estimated at 9.5 per 100,000 persons in 1986, with 200,000 cases projected by 1991.

Cost and Impact on Society. The Centers for Disease Control estimates total direct and indirect costs in 1984 were $1.9 billion, representing a total health care cost to the country of $692 billion.

Morbidity and Mortality. The case fatality rate

is over 75 per cent for persons diagnosed with AIDS after 2 years.

Important Facts Relevant to Prevention. The groups with the highest prevalence are hemophiliacs, homosexual males, intravenous drug users, individuals with multiple sexual partners, patients with multiple blood transfusions after 1977 and prior to blood screening in 1985, and babies born to infected mothers.

Screening Test Recommendations. All patients should be screened for risk status. The frequency of screening will vary depending on the particular patient population. Patients in high-risk groups should be strongly encouraged to be screened for antibodies to human immunodeficiency virus. One major reason for screening is to identify those individuals who are already infected so that intervention may be instituted to halt the further spread of the virus.

Preventive Activities Recommendations. Education of patients is the first priority for the individual family physician. At this time, the only real chance for meaningful intervention is to prevent exposure to individuals infected with human immunodeficiency virus. Children and teenagers, in particular, must be helped to understand the reality of the risks of sexual contact (especially when condoms are not used) and intravenous drug use (especially using shared needles or syringes).

Women at high risk in the childbearing years should be considered for yearly human immunodeficiency virus antibody screening. Any of these women found to be positive for human immunodeficiency virus should be strongly counseled against conception.

Within the office, the physician has a responsibility to employees and other patients to implement recommended measures to ensure protection from inadvertent transmission.

Related Issues. In addition to individual action, there is a need for immediate, aggressive public health measures. These have been well outlined on the "Report of the Presidential Commission on the Human Immunodeficiency Virus Epidemic," June 24, 1988. Major preventive recommendations in this report include (1) institution of a confidential system whereby an exposed partner would be notified; (2) notification of all persons having received blood transfusions between 1977 and 1985 that they should be tested; (3) prevention and treatment of intravenous drug abuse as a top national priority; (4) prevention of drug and alcohol abuse (considered a factor for potential exposure to human immunodeficiency virus) should be aggressively pursued, especially through education of the nation's young people; (5) continual monitoring of blood supplies for safety; and (6) prevention of spread within health care facilities.

Secondary prevention will become increasingly important if methods to stop or retard disease progression in its presymptomatic stages become accessible and affordable.

Impact on the Family Unit. A special tragedy is the 65 per cent possibility that human immunodeficiency virus will be transmitted from the mother to an unborn baby. Many of these infected babies are now left abandoned in the hospital.

Accidents

Incidence. The estimated number of accidents in 1982 was almost 60 million, reflecting a rate of nonfatal injury of 26,400 per 100,000 persons. The highest rate was found in the 18- to 24-year-old group.

Cost and Impact on Society. Estimated direct and indirect costs of injury in 1984 were nearly $97 million.

Morbidity and Mortality. Accidents are the fourth leading cause of death in the United States. The rate was 61 per 100,000 persons in 1983. Almost half were secondary to automobile accidents. A distant second cause is falls, but these accidents are remarkable in that over 70 per cent of them occur in individuals over age 65. The third most frequent cause of accidental death is drowning.

Important Facts Relevant to Prevention. Homes are the most common site of overall injuries, whereas the automobile is the most common site for fatal injury. It is estimated that over half of all fatal automobile accidents involve a driver that has been drinking.

Screening Test Recommendations. Screening for alcohol abuse is of top priority. Not only is it the major cause of traffic fatalities, it is also a major factor in all other types of traumatic accidents. Patients should be asked at the time of routine preventive health checks whether or not they regularly use seat belts.

Preventive Activities Recommendations. The guidelines for prevention listed under the sections for alcohol abuse and osteoporosis should be followed. Parents should be encouraged to ensure that all children are taught to swim. Homes should be safety-proofed, especially when small children and the elderly live within the home. Use of seat belts and child restraint devices should be strongly encouraged.

Impact on the Family Unit. In addition to the immediate trauma suffered, nonfatal accidents have a direct impact on the individual and the family. An issue that must be confronted is the injured person's and the other family members' own mortality. Although some families will come closer at these times, others may distance themselves from the patient as a defense mechanism.

Fatal accidents present a special problem. The loss is unexpected, and often occurs in those who are otherwise young and healthy. For the family, the process of grieving may become particularly difficult or pathologic.

Glaucoma

Prevalence. The prevalence of increased intraocular pressure rises with age, from 5 per cent at 40 years of age to 15 per cent at 70 to 75 years of age.

About 10 per cent of those with increased pressure will have glaucoma.

Important Facts Relevant to Prevention. The ultimate result of untreated glaucoma is blindness. The most common type of glaucoma, primary open angle, is asymptomatic until severe, when irreversible damage has often occurred.

The three major criteria for diagnosis are elevated intraocular pressure, visual field defects, and optic disc pallor and cupping. In glaucoma, the cup's diameter is 30 per cent greater than that of the disc. The funduscopic changes on direct ophthalmoscopy are best seen with a red filter.

Patients with upper normal intraocular pressure can have glaucoma and suffer from secondary blindness, whereas other patients can have elevated pressures without glaucoma. Both of these groups represent exceptions to the usual course of the condition.

The risk factors for glaucoma are family history, black race, diabetes mellitus, and age.

Screening Test Recommendations. The value of screening for elevated intraocular pressure with the Schiøtz tonometer is controversial. If the family physician elects to use this method, patients should be screened starting at 40 and every 5 years thereafter until age 60, at which time the screening interval should be reduced to every 2 to 3 years. Funduscopic evaluation by a well-trained physician at the time of tonometry will increase the sensitivity of screening.

Preventive Activities Recommendations. No primary preventive measures are available. Secondary prevention consists of educating patients of the need for regular evaluation for early detection and the warning signs of progressive glaucoma (e.g., blurring of vision and halos around lights).

Discussion. Schiøtz tonometry, although an accurate measure of intraocular presure, has only a sensitivity of only 66 per cent and a specificity of 91 per cent. Therefore, one third of the patients with glaucoma will have normal tonometry readings and will be missed. Also, 9 per cent of those with elevated measurements will not have glaucoma. These facts make it imperative that high-risk patients receive more extensive screening by an ophthalmologist and that patients who are screened are advised that they are still at risk. The major value in screening is to detect those individuals with presymptomatic disease who would not ordinarily see an ophthalmologist. These individuals can then be referred for additional testing.

Diabetes Mellitus

Diabetes mellitus does not meet the criteria for mass screening, despite its high prevalence, high morbidity and mortality, long presymptomatic stage, and ease of diagnosis. Early diagnosis and treatment has not been shown to alter the prognosis. Nevertheless, screening has been advocated in the recommendations for coronary heart disease because the presence of diabetes is a major risk factor in that evaluation.

The only exception in which screening for diabetes provides clear direct benefit is during pregnancy.

Life Styles for Health

When one reviews the diseases discussed in this chapter, there is a strikingly common theme in their etiology and prevention: An individual's life style is the major modifiable determinant of health.

Proper diet is of paramount importance to prevent the nation's number one killer, coronary heart disease; and it is estimated that 35 per cent of cancers, the nation's number two killer, is secondary to diet (Doll, 1981). Fortunately, the specific dietary components that are recommended for prevention of one disease are also beneficial in general. Therefore, it is possible to make broad prudent dietary recommendations as a base on which all physicians and patients can build, including (1) total calories to achieve and maintain ideal body weight; (2) fat intake of less than 30 per cent of total calories; (3) saturated fat intake of less than 10 per cent of total calories; (4) cholesterol intake of less than 300 mg. per day; (5) carbohydrate intake of 50 to 60 per cent of total calories, emphasizing the need for complex carbohydrates; (6) maximal fiber intake in the diet, with emphasis on the need for soluble fiber sources; (7) minimum calcium intake of 1000 mg. daily; and (8) sodium chloride intake of less than 3 gm. of sodium (7.5 gm. of salt).

The importance of stress reduction and exercise in preventing disease is a subject of great interest. There is general agreement that they are of real importance. Their benefits are difficult to quantitate in disease prevention.

Another common theme is the critical importance of avoiding toxins, especially the addictive substances, nicotine and alcohol. Smoking accounts for 30 per cent of all cancer deaths and is a major factor in coronary heart disease. It is related to 320,000 deaths each year. It is estimated that each pack of cigarettes sold results in a cost of $2.17 in medical care and lost productivity. The pervasive social and health effects of alcohol on individuals and society have been outlined.

Table 14–19 shows the major diseases discussed and the most common risk factors.

Developing a Preventive Health Care Flow Sheet

A simple and flexible flow sheet is essential for the continuity and comprehensiveness of preventive

Table 14–19. RELATIONSHIP BETWEEN COMMON PREVENTABLE DISEASES AND THE MOST COMMON RISK FACTORS

Risk Factor	Diet	Hyper-lipidemia	Obesity	Hyper-tension	Smoking	Alcohol	Sedentary Life Style	Heredity	Stress and Depression
Coronary heart disease	■	■	■	■	■		■	■	■
Stroke	■	■	■	■	■		■	■	■
Chemical dependence						■		■	■
Osteoporosis	■							■	
Accident/suicide						■		■	■
Sexually transmitted diseases and human immunodeficiency virus infection						■			
Lung cancer					■				
Breast cancer	■					■?		■	
Colon cancer	■								
Cervical cancer									
Endometrial cancer			■						

Table 14–20. PREVENTIVE HEALTH CARE FLOW SHEET, DEPARTMENT OF FAMILY MEDICINE, UNIVERSITY OF VIRGINIA

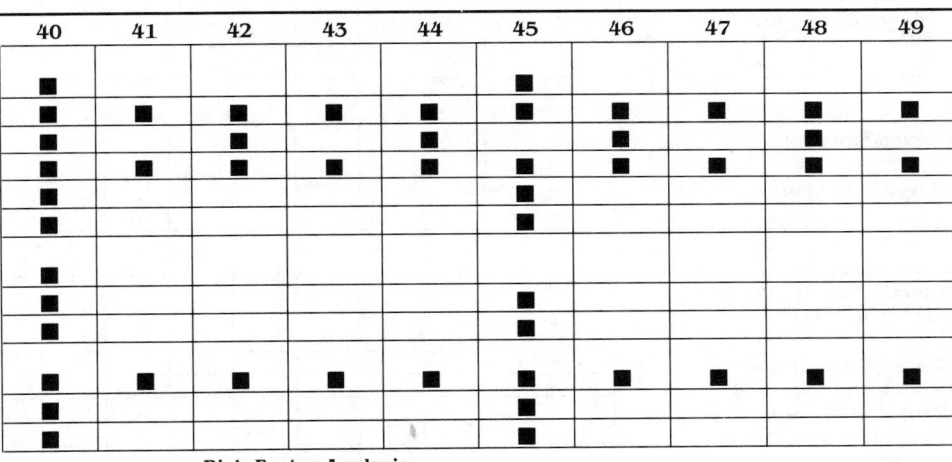

	40	41	42	43	44	45	46	47	48	49
Cholesterol and high-density lipoprotein	■					■				
Breast examination	■	■	■	■	■	■	■	■	■	■
Mammogram	■		■		■		■		■	
Papanicolaou's smear	■	■	■	■	■	■	■	■	■	■
Urinalysis	■					■				
Hematocrit	■					■				
Tetanus, diphtheria (adult) toxoid	■									
Fasting blood sugar	■					■				
Tonometry and fundus	■					■				
Stool guaiac and rectal examination	■	■	■	■	■	■	■	■	■	■
Flexible sigmoidoscopy	■					■				
Life style and risk	■					■				

Risk Factor Analysis

Coronary heart disease and stroke
Positive family history
Hyperlipidemia
Tobacco use
HTN
Diabetes mellitus
Obesity
Stress
Male
Sedentary
Birth control pill use > 35 years old

Osteoporosis
< 1 gm. calcium per day
Sedentary life style
Positive family history
Thin physical stature
White/Oriental
Tobacco use

Alcohol abuse
Felt like cutting down
Annoyed by criticism
Guilty about drinking
Eye opener
Positive family history
Drink in past 24 hr.
History of legal, personal, or health problems due to alcohol use

Cervical cancer
Condyloma history
Herpes history
Multiple partners
Early intercourse

Sexually transmitted diseases and human immunodeficiency virus
Blood transfusions
Multiple sexual partners
Bisexual/homosexual
Nonbarrier contraceptive use

Suicide
Previous attempt
Positive family history
Depression

Accidents
Drink and drive
Seat belt use

Breast cancer
Positive family history
Nulliparous
Primigravida, > 35 years old
Previous high risk biopsy results

Glaucoma
Positive family history
Diabetes mellitus
Black

Lung cancer
Tobacco use

Table 14–21. EXAMPLE OF HEALTH SCREENING FLOW SHEET USED IN THE DEPARTMENT OF FAMILY MEDICINE, UNIVERSITY OF NEW MEXICO

Categories	Age Date	36	37	38	39	40	41	42	43	44	45	46	47	48	49	50
History and Physical Examination																
Blood pressure measured every year																
Dental examination every year																
Teach breast self-examination																
Menopause symptoms (present?)																
Contraceptive needs reviewed every year																
Laboratory Tests																
Baseline mammogram (under age 50)																
Cholesterol and high-density lipoprotein (baseline)																
Papanicolaou's smear (every 2 years—American Cancer Society; every 5 years Canada)																
Immunization																
Td (every 10 years)																
Counsel/Patient Education (Annually)																
Cigarette smoking																
Alcohol use																
Occupational hazards																
Skin cancer protection																
Seat belt use																
Exercise																
Life stages: career/achievement, family social stability																
Calcium supplementation																

health care. This form can be effectively used as a tool for educating patients concerning their preventive health care needs. Patients at high risk for certain illnesses may need to have increased frequency of screening tests or special tests added. Also, recommendations for preventive activities will change as new information becomes available. An inflexible form will be of little use after 5 to 10 years.

An *informative* flow sheet will alert the physician to risk factors that have not been identified and procedures that have not been accomplished. Missing pieces of information should be obvious on even a cursory review of the form.

A deterrent to the use of any form or flow sheet is a need to duplicate information that is available elsewhere in the record. Therefore, the more data entry that is *unique* to the form, the more likely it is to be used.

Tables 14–20 and 14–21 show examples of flow sheets that the family physician may wish to modify for a particular practice.

Getting Started

A comprehensive preventive health program is difficult to implement all at once in a busy physician's office. It often requires adopting a new perspective for the physician and the staff, a supporting set of educational materials and referral sources, and equipment. Adding new elements, one at a time, will obviate much of the potential threat posed by such a major undertaking. The office may decide to emphasize lipid screening or colorectal cancer screening at the beginning. Necessary staff and physician education, selection of appropriate educational materials, purchase of equipment, and implementation of the program can then take place in a longitudinal fashion at a comfortable pace. Once this is done to everyone's satisfaction, additional screening and preventive modules can be added, once again, one at a time.

The important thing is to begin.

References

American Heart Association: An Eating Plan for Healthy Americans. Dallas, TX, American Heart Association, 1985. *This is roughly the equivalent of the Phase One therapeutic diet but is presented in terms that are understandable and useable by the general population. It is highly recommended for general availability in each office.*

American Heart Association: Dietary Treatment of Hypercholesterolemia—A Manual for Patients. Dallas, TX, American Heart Association, 1988. *This guide was developed in cooperation with the National Heart, Lung, and Blood Institute. It is the latest and best in a long series of patient dietary guides by these organizations. It clearly defines the specifics for a step 1 (mildly restrictive) and step 2 (moderately restrictive) diet. This publication is strongly recommended as the basic dietary manual for physicians to make available to patients with dyslipidemia.*

Astler, V. B., and Coller, F. A.: The prognostic significance of direct extension of carcinoma of the colon and rectum. Ann. Surg., *139*:846–851, 1951.

Bader, J.P.: Screening of colorectal cancer. Dig. Dis. Sci., *31*:9, Suppl., 1986. *This is a thorough and thoughtful review of all the important data to date on screening for colorectal cancer. It clearly identifies what is known and what is only assumed.*

Brody, J.: Good Food Book. New York, W.W. Norton and Co., 1985. *This is an excellent cookbook with emphasis on high complex carbohydrates and low saturated fat and salt. Occasional recipes require some modification to meet Phase One goals in the American Heart Association Diet. In general, patients will be pleased that this cookbook allows them to cook many of their favorite dishes in a more healthy way.*

Bush, B., Shaw, S., Cleary, P., et al.; Screening for alcohol abuse using the CAGE questionaire; Am. J. Med., *82*:231, 1987.

Castelli, W.P.: Epidemiology of coronary heart disease: The Framingham Study. Am. J. Med., *76*:4–12, 1984.

Centers for Disease Control: Recommendations for prevention of HIV infection in the health care setting. M.M.W.R., *36*(2S)1–18, 1987. *All physicians should read this report and implement the recommended changes within their offices and hospitals.*

Conner, W.E., and Conner, S.L.: The New American Diet. New York, Simon and Schuster, 1986. *An excellent cookbook with many truly innovative recipes. The first half is well presented educational material. It does not take into account the newest information concerning monounsaturated fats.*

Cyr, M. G. and Wartman, S. A.: The effectiveness of routine screening questions in the detection of alcoholism. J.A.M.A., *259*(1):51, 1988.

Dalsky, G.P., Stocke, K.S., Ehsani, A.A., et al.: Weight-bearing exercise training and lumbar bone mineral content in postmenopausal women. Ann. Intern. Med., *108*(6):824–828, 1988.

Doll, R., and Peto R.: The Causes of Cancer: Quantitative Estimates of Avoidable Risks of Cancer in the United States Today. New York, Oxford Medical Publications; Oxford University Press, 1981.

Eddy, D.M.: The value of mammography screening in women under age 50 years. J.A.M.A., *259*(10):1512–1519, 1988.

Eshleman, R.: The American Heart Association Cookbook. New York, David McKay Co., 1984.

Frame, P.S.: A critical review of adult health maintenance. J. Fam. Pract., (4):341–346, (5):417–422, (6):511–520, 23, (1):29–39, 1986. *A succinct review of the evidence for various preventive health care activities with recommendations from the author. The opinions are conservative and represent only those recommendations that can be made based on solid scientific data.*

Gates, C.C.: The "most-significant other" in the care of the breast cancer patient. Cancer, *38*(3): 146–153, 1988. *A valuable review of the important role the physician can play in the care of not only the breast cancer patient but in the care of all terminally ill patients.*

Gilbertson, V.A., and Nelms, J.M.: The prevention of invasive cancer. Cancer, *41*:1137–1139, 1978.

Gullino, P.M.: Natural history of breast cancer: Progression from hyperplasia to neoplasia as predicted by angiogenesis. Cancer Res., *35*:512–516, 1975.

Harvey, E.B., Schairer, C., Brinton, L. A., et al: Alcohol consumption and breast cancer. J. Natl. Cancer Inst. *78*(4):657–661, 1987.

Hudson, T.W., et al.: Clinical Preventive Medicine: Health Promotion and Disease Prevention. Boston, Little, Brown & Co., Inc., 1988.

Jarvinen, H. J., and Turunen, M. J.: Colorectal carcinoma before 40 years of age: Prognosis and predisposing conditions. Scand. J. Gastroenterol., *19*:634–638, 1984.

Kannel, W.B., Thom, T.J., and Hurst, J.W.: Incidence, prevalence, and mortality of cardiovascular diseases. *In* Hurst, J.W. (Ed.): The Heart. New York, McGraw-Hill, 1986.

Love, S.M., Gelman, R.S., and Silen, W.: Fibrocystic disease of the breast—a non-disease? N. Engl. J. Med., *312*(3):146, 1985.

McLellan, G.L.: Screening and early diagnosis of breast cancer. J. Fam. Prac., *26*(5):561–568, 1988. *An excellent, brief state of the art review with an extensive bibliography.*

Miller, J. D., and Cisin, I. H., Gardner-Keating, H., et al.: National Survey of Drug Abuse: Main Findings 1982. Washington, D.C., U.S. Gov. Printing Office, 1983.

National Heart, Blood and Lung Institute: National Cholesterol Education Program. Bethesda, MD, National Institutes of Health, 1987.

National Institutes of Health: Osteoporosis—consensus development conference statement. Washington, D.C., United States Government Printing Office, 1984. *A comprehensive review of all the data concerning osteoporosis with clinical recommendations.*

O'Connell, D.L., Hulka, B.S., Chambless, L.E., et al.: Cigarette smoking, alcohol consumption, and breast cancer risk. J. Natl. Cancer Inst., *78*(2):229–234, 1987.

O'Malley, M.S., and Fletcher, S.W.: Screening for breast cancer with breast self-examination: A critical review. J.A.M.A., *257*:16, 1987.

Office of Disease Prevention and Health Promotion, United States Public Health Service: Disease Prevention/Health Promotion: The Facts. Palo Alto, CA, Bull Publishing Co., 1988. *A single source for the most recent data relating to the major preventable diseases. Emphasis is on epidemiology.*

Petrakis, P.L., et al.: Sixth Special Report to the U.S. Congress on Alcohol and Health. Washington, D.C., United States Government Printing Office, 1987. *Petrakis was the lead writer and editor of this monograph. There are many other contributors listed as writers of various chapters.*

Preziozi, T. J., and Barker, L. R.: Cerebrovascular Disease in Principles of Ambulatory Care. Baltimore, Williams & Wilkins, 1986.

Potchen, E.J., and Sierra, A.E.: The detection and cure of breast cancer. Obstet. Gynecol. Clin. North Am., *14*(3):667–684, 1987. *This article reviews all the major international studies of secondary prevention of breast cancer. It is recommended reading for the physician who wishes a succinct review of the major preventive studies.*

Richart, R. M., Barron, B. A., et al.: Screening strategies for cervical cancer and cervical intraepithelial neoplasia. Cancer, *47:*1176–1181, 1981.

Riegelman, R. K., and Povar, G. J.: Putting Prevention into Practice. Boston, Little, Brown & Co., Inc., 1988. *An excellent introduction to the methodology of evaluating preventive activities presented in an instructional format. Continuing education hours available for completion. Contains highly instructive analyses of the prevention of colorectal cancer, breast cancer, and coronary heart disease.*

Riggs, B.L., and Melton, L.J.: Involutional osteoporosis. N. Engl. J. Med., *314*(26):1676–1686, 1986. *Reviews the pathophysiology of osteoporosis and defines two major categories of disease: Postmenopausal and senile.*

Riis, B., Thomsen, K., and Christiansen, C.: Does calcium supplementation prevent postmenopausal bone loss? A double-blind, controlled clinical study. N. Engl. J. Med., *36*(4):173–177, 1987.

Seidman, H., Gelb, S. K., Silverberg, E., et al.: Survival experience in the Breast Cancer Detection Demonstration Project. Cancer, *37:*259, 1987.

Selzer, M.L.: The Michigan alcoholism screening test: The quest for a new diagnostic instrument. Am. J. Psychiatry, *127:*1653, 1971.

Steering Committee of the Physicians' Health Study Research Group, Preliminary Report: Findings from the aspirin component of the ongoing Physicians' Health Study. N. Engl. J. Med., *318:*4, 1988.

Turunen, M. J., and Peltokallio, P.: Surgical results in 657 patients with colorectal cancer. Dis. Colon Rectum *26:*606–612, 1983.

U.S. Preventive Services Task Force: Guide to Clinical Preventive Services. Baltimore, Williams and Wilkins, 1989.

Whitfield, C.L., Davis, J.E., and Barker, L.R.: Alcoholism: Principles of Ambulatory Medicine. Baltimore, Williams and Wilkins, 1986.

Wolf, P.A., Kannel, W.B., Sorlie, P., et al.: Asymptomatic carotid bruit and risk of stroke. J.A.M.A., *245:*1442–1445, 1981.

15

Use of Consultants

Robert E. Rakel

All physicians, regardless of their specialty, turn to another physician at some time for advice. This process necessarily became formalized as physicians focused their training and limited their practice to a particular segment of medicine. The first specialty board, the American Board of Ophthalmology, was formed in 1917, and by 1989, there were 23 specialty boards and 51 subspecialty boards. The American Board of Family Practice was established in 1969 as the 20th primary specialty.

It is a common misconception of medical students that subspecialists know more than generalists. The fact is that the amount of information required to practice each of the 74 specialties and subspecialties is clearly defined and is equivalent. What varies is the degree of breadth and depth in each. In addition to being trained in a wide variety of clinical areas, family physicians are also trained to coordinate the care of seriously ill individuals who require a variety of consultants, orchestrating the skills of each to achieve optimum patient care and satisfaction (see Chapter 1). "Every patient should have a primary care physician who not only sees him for first-contact care, but who actively participates in his secondary and tertiary care by arranging and coordinating his consultant needs, by providing continuity, and by taking the patient back" (Stephens, 1982).

The appropriate use of the consultation process is an art that contributes to improved patient care when utilized properly by family physicians. Although there is a definite distinction between consultation and referral, the terms are often used interchangeably. Consultation is by definition the practice of one physician asking another for an opinion or assistance, whereas referral is the transfer of responsibility to another physician for the care of a specific problem. Referral usually involves one physician requesting the services of another for a particular purpose and for a limited time, such as referral to a surgeon for a cholecystectomy or to a cardiologist for coronary angiography. On the other hand, consultation is the process whereby one physician requests the opinion of a colleague regarding the diagnosis or management of a patient's problem. Regardless of this distinction, the physician initiating either process is spoken of as the referring physician, and the physician who is consulted or to whom the patient is referred is called the consultant.

In a study of patterns of consultation and referral, Geyman and associates (1976) found that 97 per cent of the exchanges between family physicians and other specialists were referrals and only 3 per cent were consultations. Fry (1971) notes with regret that consultation is no longer a deliberation between colleagues about diagnosis or proper treatment. He says, "We have come to view our specialist colleagues more as expert 'technicians' than as consultants." Although the system in the United Kingdom has been described as the specialist controlling the hospital and the general practitioner controlling the patient, this separation avoids much of the rivalry over patient care that occurs in the United States. Horder (1977) believes that, " . . . patients look to all of us for the same two things, technical competence and personal care. I believe that, at present, we have more cause to be concerned about the supply of personal care than technical competence."

When to Refer

Dixon (1976) lists five reasons for referral: (1) diagnosis, (2) management, (3) diagnosis and management, (4) patient request, and (5) reinforcement or confirmation of a diagnosis or plan of management.

It is wise to ask for a consultation whenever the patient or family expresses doubt or shows lack of confidence in the diagnosis or management. It is sometimes wise to obtain a second opinion for patients who have a life-threatening illness or a disease with a poor prognosis. Brock (1977) found that 62 per cent of referrals in a Canadian community occurred because the community lacked required facilities or skills, 72 per cent were for a second opinion regarding management, and 45 per cent were for a second opinion regarding diagnosis (more than one category could be selected in the survey).

Consultation should also be considered when the family physician is dissatisfied with the patient's progress or is unsure of the diagnosis. Sometimes an agency or special unit has a capability of providing better service, such as in drug detoxification. One rarely gets in trouble asking for help with a difficult problem, but every experienced physician can remember at least one case in which a consultation should have been obtained. A consultation should be promptly initiated any time the patient or family requests or hints that they would like to have one. The physician must be alert to subtle clues of doubt indicating the desire for another opinion. If these clues are recognized and acted upon, confidence in the family physician increases. If not recognized, patient dissatisfaction leading to malpractice litigation may result. When doubt is recognized, the patient or family member should be encouraged to discuss this openly; consultation is then often unnecessary.

An early consultation is much less likely to damage patient confidence than a delayed one. The confident and secure physician who considers patient welfare to be of the utmost importance is not threatened and freely utilizes consultants at the appropriate, sometimes early, stage of a problem, before it has progressed to serious proportions that are more difficult to manage.

The patient's family is more apt to display doubt regarding the management of a case than is the patient. The physician who communicates easily with members of the family and is aware of their feelings will detect this insecurity earlier than the physician who is familiar only with the patient. The patient is less likely than other family members to express doubt regarding a diagnosis or method of management for fear of offending the physician. Whenever doubt is noted among the family members, the physician should suggest that the opinion of another physician be obtained.

Responsibilities of the Referring Physician

The consultation process involves approximately 12 decision points, beginning with the family physician's decision to refer and concluding with the family physician's providing feedback to the consultant regarding the eventual outcome (Table 15–1).

Selection of the Consultant. The referring physician is responsible for the selection of the proper consultant for a particular patient. The family physician whose comprehensive training involves a broad range of disciplines has the insight needed to select the appropriate consultant for a specific problem. Care must be taken to select a consultant who has knowledge and skills appropriate to the patient's need, a personality compatible with that of the patient, availability, competency maintained by frequent use of the required skills, and the ability to work well with the referring physician. Compatibility of personalities is an especially important factor to be considered, if at all possible, when selecting a consultant. A surgeon who alienates the patient, no matter how skilled, will be less effective than one who establishes good rapport and has the patient's confidence and cooperation.

Referrals to a psychiatrist sometimes pose special problems. Some patients resist such a referral and the family physician may also feel uncomfortable making the suggestion. However, the patient frequently welcomes psychiatric help and may be relieved by the recommendation. In a review of psy-

Table 15–1. THE CONSULTATION PROCESS*

1. The decision is made to refer.
2. Consideration is given to the patient's medical, emotional, cultural, and socioeconomic background.
3. Selection of the appropriate discipline (specialty field).
4. Selection of the appropriate physician in that field.
5. Preparation of both the patient and family for the consultation.
6. Preparation of the consultant.
7. The consultant provides feedback to the patient and family.
8. The consultant provides feedback to the family physician.
9. The family physician evaluates the appropriateness of the consultant's recommendations.
10. The family physician facilitates the patient and the family's acceptance of recommendations.
11. The family physician acts on the recommendations or selects another consultant in the same or a different field.
12. The family physician provides feedback to the consultant regarding eventual outcome.

*Modified from Barnett, B. L., Jr., and Collins, J. J., Jr.: A new look at the consultation continuum. J. Fam. Pract., 5:665, 1977.

chiatric problems encountered in hospitalized patients (Steinberg et al, 1980), 50 per cent of the patients for whom psychiatric consultation would have been helpful did not receive it because of physician resistance or failure to recognize the psychiatric problem. In those patients who later received psychiatric care, most of them accepted it well.

Patients are likely to benefit more from a psychiatric referral if they enter into the consultation with a positive frame of mind. Once the need for a psychiatric referral has been determined, the patient should be told the reason in an honest, straightforward manner. Questions about psychosocial problems should be incorporated into the history from the beginning of an illness, since they are a part of every problem, rather than being avoided until organic possibilities have been exhausted, resulting in the interpretation by the patient that "the problem is all in my head."

A perceptive family physician—through knowledge of the patient's personality, life style, and previous reaction to similar situations—can best select the consultant and clinical setting to which the patient will respond positively. Occasionally, it is necessary for the family physician to emphasize the consultant's excellent technical skills and forewarn the patient of possible personality differences or other idiosyncrasies. Patient and family confidence can play a major role in the effectiveness of that consultant. This confidence will be enhanced if the referring physician shows respect for the consultant's skills and makes the recommendation with enthusiasm.

Adequate Transfer of Information. The referring physician must be sure that the referral contract is clearly understood by the consultant. If the referring physician wants help with a diagnosis but does not say so, the consultant may assume that the request is for help with management, leading to dissatisfaction and unwarranted charges of "patient stealing." The referring physician should state the reason for the request and the action desired so that the consultant knows clearly whether the request is for an opinion only or also involves management.

The most common breakdowns of communication between referring and consulting physicians are the consultation request and the consultant's report. The referring physician must evaluate the problem adequately and transmit all necessary information to the consultant. Complete and accurate background information should avoid unnecessary duplication of diagnostic tests. Adequate transfer of information does not consist of a few notes scribbled on a prescription blank, nor is it proper to provide the consultant only with sketchy details by telephone.

The process of information transfer varies with the nature of the problem. Some are straightforward, as for example a 67-year-old patient with an intertrochanteric fracture. If there are no medical problems and the patient is a good surgical risk, the transfer report can be brief. Other problems may require a complete summary of the office record, as in the referral of a 9-year-old patient for recurring fever that lasts approximately 1 week every month despite negative laboratory studies.

An outpatient referral is facilitated by using a standard form such as that shown in Figure 15–1*A*. It should be in the mail within 24 hours or, better still, carried by the patient to the consultant, accompanied by a copy of the problem list and other pertinent items from the data base, including recent progress notes, laboratory reports, and x-ray films. The problem-oriented medical record is ideally suited to this, since it summarizes all major disorders affecting the individual and alerts the consultant to other past and potentially significant complications that should be considered in the management of the patient's current situation. An extensive referral note is not needed when adequate information is provided by the medical record.

Patient Preparation and Compliance. Ten per cent of all patients never keep the appointment with the consultant (Cummins et al., 1980). Patient compliance may be improved if the patient feels more involved in the referral process. First, the referring physician should adequately inform the patient regarding the need for referral and ensure his or her understanding and cooperation. (The consent is particularly important if the patient is hospitalized, since almost half of the complaints to medical society grievance committees stem from patients receiving bills for hospital consultations that they had not authorized.) The informed patient understands what will occur and that the family physician will remain in charge or will resume responsibility at the conclusion of the referral. The understanding is important if the patient is to avoid feeling rejected or "sent away."

It is also likely that compliance will be increased if the patient is given some choice of consultants and control over the time of appointment. When the family physician recommends a consultation, the patient should be asked if a specific consultant is preferred. If not, then three qualified individuals should be suggested, with the positive features of each being identified. If the patient does not indicate a preference, then the family physician should make the final decision. Hines and Curry (1978) encourage the patient to review the referral form and accompanying materials when carrying them to the consultant. They feel this increases patient insight and cooperation, reducing "no shows" in the consultant's office.

Details about the appointment with the consultant may be difficult for the patient to remember, so providing a written note containing the consultant's name, address, and telephone number is helpful. It may also help to include directions to the consultant's office and discuss with the patient what to expect during the visit, especially the amount of time it will take.

Evaluation of Information. It is the family physician's responsibility to continue to interact with the physician to whom the patient is referred and to lend

BAYLOR FAMILY PRACTICE CENTER
5510 Greenbriar
Houston, Texas 77005
(713) 798-7700

DATE: ____________________

TO: ____________________

FROM: ____________________

PLEASE SEE: ____________________

REGARDING: ____________________

____

____

____

____
BAYLOR FAMILY PRACTICE DOCTOR'S SIGNATURE

INITIAL RESULTS OF CONSULTATION: ____________________

____

____

____

____

____
CONSULTANT'S SIGNATURE

A PLEASE SEND A NARRATIVE WITH FINAL REPORT.

Figure 15–1. *A*, Standard Physician Referral Form. (Used with permission from Baylor College of Medicine, Department of Family Medicine, Houston, TX.)

SANUS NEW YORK LIFE
A New York Life Company

SANUS/NEW YORK LIFE HEALTH PLAN, INC.
3800 Buffalo Speedway, Suite 230
Houston, TX 77098-9998
(713) 993-9520; Toll-free: 1-800-833-5318

PRIMARY PHYSICIAN REFERRAL

This referral form is authorized for use for ambulatory office visits or diagnostic tests only. All outpatient surgical or invasive diagnostic procedures in hospitals or surgery centers or elective inpatient admissions must first be precertified by SANUS/NEW YORK LIFE.
This referral is valid for services authorized for either the number of visits indicated below or 60 days, whichever occurs first. The first visit must occur within thirty (30) days from the date of this referral otherwise this referral is void.

REFERRAL TO:

Name: ______________________

Address: ______________________

Telephone No.: ______________________

REFERRAL FROM: (PRIMARY PHYSICIAN ONLY)

Name: ______________________

Address: ______________________

Telephone No.: ______________________

PLAN TYPE:

☐ Sanus/New York Life
☐ Sanus/NY Life 65 (Medicare)

MEMBER NAME:

MEMBER NUMBER:

REASON FOR REFERRAL: ENCLOSE PERTINENT LAB, X-RAY AND OTHER DIAGNOSTIC RESULTS

____

____

____

____

____

____

SERVICE(S) REQUESTED

☐ Evaluation only; all services must be directly provided by Physician in the Physician's Office

☐ Diagnostic Test(s), Specify: ______________________

____

☐ Treatment for indicated condition ☐ Other

VISITS

This referral is for one (1) visit unless otherwise indicated below.

☐ 2 visits ☐ 4 visits
☐ 3 visits ☐ 5 visits

Primary Physician Signature ______________________ Date ______________________

IMPORTANT NOTICE

PRIMARY CARE PHYSICIAN: Please make sure the "referred to" consultant/specialist physician is a participating provider of the SANUS/NEW YORK LIFE HEALTH PLAN. Referral to a physician who is not a member of the SANUS/NEW YORK LIFE HEALTH PLAN requires the approval of the SANUS/NEW YORK LIFE HEALTH PLAN Medical Director prior to the referral being made.

CONSULTANT PHYSICIAN: Make certain you are currently contracted with the SANUS/NEW YORK LIFE HEALTH PLAN. A copy of this referral form must accompany your bill to the SANUS/NEW YORK LIFE HEALTH PLAN in order to obtain payment for services. Only those services and/or visits authorized by the primary care physician or the Medical Director of the SANUS/NEW YORK LIFE HEALTH PLAN are payable.

NON-PARTICIPATING PHYSICIAN: This form is not valid for services provided by non-participating physicians. Non-participating provider referrals require the prior approval of the SANUS/NEW YORK LIFE HEALTH PLAN Medical Director.

SECONDARY REFERRAL: Specialist/Consultant providers may not issue a secondary referral to any provider unless he/she has written authorization or telephone approval from the primary care physician.

PPR-06/89

B WHITE COPY: Consultant/Specialist send with bill or claim YELLOW COPY: Consultant/Specialist keep PINK COPY: Primary Physician keep

Figure 15–1 *Continued B,* Physician Referral Form used by a Health Maintenance Organization. (Used with permission from SANUS/New York Life Health Plan, Inc.)

assistance in the management of the case to the degree that is necessary for the best care of the patient. Even referrals that are for specific surgical procedures require that the family physician remain involved to manage concomitant medical problems, especially if they require cooperation from other family members. Carson (1982) found that only 7.8 per cent of referrals were for the purpose of establishing a diagnosis. As in other studies, most referrals were for specific procedures, in this case to orthopedists, obstetricians, general surgeons, and dermatologists. Even when the consultation involves surgical or other technical skills, the family physician is responsible for ensuring that other aspects of the patient's medical background are not ignored and that the family is kept adequately informed.

Newly discovered information needs to be coordinated with that already recorded. When information is received from the consultant, the family physician must evaluate it within the context of the individual patient and the patient's family situation, work environment, expectations, and ability to comply. The family physician should also guide the consultant in the amount of information that should be given to the patient and family, being aware of how much information the family can tolerate and how it should be provided in order to enlist maximum support. Continued involvement of the family physician improves compliance with the treatment program and facilitates long-term rehabilitation.

Feedback to Consultants. It may be of value to keep a log of all referrals. Such a log, containing the patient's name, name of consultant, and date of referral, could then be checked when the report is returned to ensure that the patient actually sees the consultant and that a report is obtained. It would also help identify consultants who do not return information about patients. The log could be reviewed weekly and the consultant or patient contacted if no information is received after a specified time.

Family physicians should give feedback to the consultant regarding the outcome of an unusual case and not leave the consultant wondering whether the diagnosis was correct or the treatment successful. This is an especially appropriate courtesy if the consultant was prompt in reporting and in returning the patient. If the consultant has not provided information of value in managing the patient, then a second consultation should be seriously considered. Clarfield (1980) found that referring physicians felt that one third of the time (31 per cent of consultations) they had learned nothing of value from the referral. It is also important to let the consultant know if the consultation was inadequate. Experienced family physicians can help young consultants improve their "art of consultation" and should accept this as a responsibility, since consultants are rarely taught this skill during residency training. Bates (1979) believes that "nothing better expresses the ideal fraternity of medicine than an older family doctor helping a young specialist with professional relationships."

Suspecting that faulty consultation practices may be learned during residency training, McPhee and colleagues (1984) studied the communication between 27 general internists at a university medical center and their subspecialty colleagues who practiced in the same building in San Francisco. Even in this close academic setting where the referral rate was 9.4 per cent, the referring physician did not receive a report 45 per cent of the time. The poorest responding consultants were in ophthalmology (no response 69 per cent of the time), obstetrics and gynecology (61 per cent), orthopedics (57 per cent), and dermatology (52 per cent). A response was most likely to be received if the referring physician personally contacted the consultant and if the patient had a return appointment.

Responsibilities of the Consultant

The consultant is expected to provide a prompt and concise report to the referring physician. The specific questions posed on the consultation request should be addressed and action limited to the amount of involvement requested. When the consultation involves a hospitalized patient, the consultant should see the patient promptly; provide an opinion and give therapeutic suggestions in a concise note on the consultation sheet; and, in general, should not write orders unless requested to do so by the referring physician.

The consultant has a responsibility to the patient and the referring physician to avoid unnecessary expense through duplication of studies recently obtained by the primary physician, unless there is good reason to doubt the results or there is sufficient need to repeat the test. Of course, the referring physician must have included the actual x-rays and adequate laboratory data as part of the referral document if such duplication is to be avoided. Adequate communication via the consultation request is essential, so that the consultant is made aware of the tests that already have been performed, the methods used, and the results obtained. The consultant's obligation is to build on this information, repeating procedures only when necessary to verify an abnormality or evaluate a change.

When a patient is referred for care, the consultant should remain in contact with the referring physician throughout the period of care and return the patient with a full written report when the problem is resolved or when no further involvement by the consultant is warranted.

A consultant should not refer patients to other consultants without the knowledge and consent of the primary physician, who should be coordinating or at least closely involved with this process. When the consultant is trying to decide whether the referring physician is capable of resuming care of the patient, the wisest course may be simply to ask rather than run the risk of underestimating or overestimating the family physician's level of competency or desire to resume care at that point.

The most common reason for discontinuing referrals to a particular consultant is failure to receive adequate reports or failure of the consultant to return the patient for continuing care. The latter occurs most frequently when physicians who also function as primary physicians are used as consultants. The patient may "stay on" for continuing care if the consultant does not encourage his or her return to the referring physician. Even though a specific request was made for follow-up information, Cummins and associates (1980) received a report from the consultant only 62 per cent of the time. Seventy-eight per cent of consultants who were in private practice responded, but only 59 per cent of those in university clinics did so. It was disappointing to note that the follow-up information was not better for patients who required continuing care by the family physician than for those with self-limiting problems. Even though one university stressed to its staff the importance of providing such follow-up information, the faculty did so only 75 per cent of the time. It is distressing for the family physician who is responsible for continuing care of the patient to have the patient return after being hospitalized at a university center with no information having been sent regarding the treatment given or plans for follow-up. It is even more embarrassing to learn from a family member that a patient who was recently referred to a nearby medical center has died.

Curry and associates (1980) found that enclosing a return mailer with the consultation request (including a stamped, self-addressed envelope and a form specifically requesting feedback from the consultant) increased the percentage of consultant feedback from 39 per cent to 60 per cent and also increased the speed of the reply. These rates were significantly higher if the lack of reply from Veterans Administration Hospitals was excluded. Even with the higher response rate, it is unfortunate that 40 per cent of the referrals resulted in no report to the referring physician. Another method that may improve the response rate is to use a two-part pressure-sensitive form, the top half of which includes the referring physician's information. The bottom half is then available for the consultant's report (Fig. 15–1*A*).

Providing appropriate feedback to both patient and referring physician is a talent possessed by too few referral centers. The Mayo Clinic has an excellent reputation for providing good feedback to the referring physician. The Clinic also has a talent for maintaining or bolstering patients' respect for their family physician. Bates (1979) says, "The top notch consultant will render a report that informs without patronizing, educates without lecturing, directs without ordering and—sometimes most difficult of all—solves the problem without making the referring physician appear to be stupid. The real stars in this play are the consultants who discuss the differential diagnosis in such a way that they make a good case for the referring physician's previous diagnosis even when it was wrong."

Although most consultation requests instruct the consultant to proceed with diagnosis and treatment of a problem, this should not be assumed unless specifically indicated. Tumulty (1973) outlines the basic code of ethics for a consultant as follows:

> *After completing his examination, the consultant should simply state to the patient and to his family that he will thoroughly discuss the problem with the responsible physician . . . Under no circumstances at this time should a consultant give to a patient or his family any information of a specific nature relating to diagnosis, treatment, or prognosis unless he is directly requested to do so by the primary physician.*

The consultant's opinion should be weighed by the referring physician and the appropriate action taken, depending on the conclusions reached. The family physician may have already considered many of the recommendations the consultant makes but discarded them based on factors that may be unknown to the consultant.

Shortell and Anderson (1971) describe the rewards for both referring physician and consultant when their exchange is effective. For the referring physician, it is a positive and rewarding experience, knowing that the patient has received proper treatment. It will be a negative experience if the patient does not return or is disappointed with the consultant. The consultant will be flattered at being chosen as an expert and will enjoy receiving a well-prepared, cooperative patient. This could change to a negative feeling if the consultant receives an unpleasant, problem patient because the family physician does not want to be "bothered" any longer (i.e., the "dumping syndrome"), or if the consultant is called upon to treat patients without having been provided with adequate background information.

Referral Rates

Rates of referral by family physicians in the United States and Canada average 2.7 per cent, with a range of 1.0 to 5.4 per cent, as shown in Table 15–2 and 15–3. Referral rates are greater for women than men and are highest in 15- to 44-year-old individuals (Mayer, 1982). The National Ambulatory Medical Care Survey (1985) noted a 4.2 per cent consultation rate in general and family practice.

Lawler found a referral rate of only 1.31 per cent among 2nd- and 3rd-year family practice residents. Second-year residents had lower referral rates than third-year residents, supposedly because of differences in case mix and a lack of referral experience by second-year residents (Lawler, 1987).

The largest study of outpatient consultation rates by family physicians has been conducted by Crump

Table 15–2. TYPES AND RATES OF REFERRAL FOR THE UNITED STATES

	Crump and Massengill	Dolezal et al.	Geyman et al.	Glenn et al.	Mayer	Metcalfe and Sischy	Moscovice et al.	Ruane	Schmidt	White
Location	Alabama	South Dakota	California	Missouri	Minnesota	New York	Washington	Vermont	Massachusetts	Illinois
Year conducted	1977 to 1985	1977 to 1978	1974	1977 to 1979	1978	1973	1978	1978	1972 to 1973	1984
Length of study	9 years	1 year	2 months	3 years	1 year	1.5 months	3 months	7 months	1 year	2 months
Number of family physicians	161*	27*	8	> 20†	3	4	6 and 1 surgeon	* + +	1	17
Total number of patient visits during study period	177,838	15,609	6409 (office and hospital)	30,131	12,228	4604	6586	7220	5814 (office and hospital)	3975
Referral rate (per cent)	1.4	1	1.6	1.65	3.85	2.2	2.4	1.5	3	2.97

Ranking of Top Five Specialties Consulted

Crump	*Per Cent*	*Dolezal*	*Per Cent*	*Geyman*	*Per Cent*	*Metcalfe*	*Per Cent*	*Moscovice*	*Per Cent*
ENT	13.4	Ortho.	17.9	Gen. Surg.	20.6	Gen. Surg.	25.5	Ortho.	21.2
Ortho.	13.3	OB-Gyn	17.3	Ortho.	15.8	OB-Gyn	10.8	Surg.	19.3
OB-Gyn	12.2	Gen. Surg.	15.4	OB-Gyn	11.9	Ortho.	9.8	ENT	10.6
Gen. Surg.	12.1	ENT	13.0	Ophthal.	11.1	ENT	9.8	Neurol.	7.5
Neurol.	8.0	Ophthal.	8.0	Urology	7.9	Urology	7.8	Gynecol.	5.0

				Mayer					
Ruane	*Per Cent*	*Glenn*	*Per Cent*	Fee-for-Service	Per Cent	HMO	Per Cent	*White*	*Per Cent*
Gen. Surg.	22.0	Gen. Surg.	13.7	Gen. Surg.	17.3	Gen. Surg.	14.8	ENT	+ +
Ortho.	13.7	OB-Gyn	12.9	ENT	13.1	ENT	13.4	Surgery	+ +
ENT	12.7	ENT	11.9	Ortho.	12.5	Derm.	10.6	Neurol.	+ +
Univ. Hosp. Emerg. Dept.	10.8	Ortho.	10.5	OB-Gyn	10.7	OB-Gyn	9.5	OB-Gyn	+ +
Ophthal.	8.8	Ophthal.	7.9	Derm.	8.9	Ortho.	8.1	Ortho.	+ +
Derm.	6.9							Ophthal.	+ +

+ + Number not specified
*Residents and faculty.
†Residents, faculty, and nurse practitioners.

Table 15–3. TYPES AND RATES OF REFERRAL FOR CANADA

	Brock		Dixon		Hines and Curry	
Location	Ontario (London)		Ontario (Rainy River)		Ontario (Toronto)	
Year conducted	1975		1975		1975 to 1976	
Length of study	1 month		1 year		1 year	
Number of family physicians	39 (8 private practice; 31 residents and faculty)		1.7 (1 full time; 1 for 8 months)		3 Family Practice teaching units 9 full time faculty 17 part time faculty, residents and students	
Total number of patient visits during study period	8616		6584 (estimated)		35,351	
Referral rate (per cent)	5.4		3.3		5.3	
	Ranking of Top Five Specialties Consulted					
		Per Cent		*Per Cent*		*Per Cent*
	OB-Gyn	18.0	Gen. Surg.	35.9	Ophthal.	12.1
	Gen. Surg.	13.0	Ortho.	16.6	OB-Gyn	10.9
	Ophthal.	13.0	OB-Gyn	13.8	Gen. Surg.	10.2
	Int. Med.	11.0	Int. Med.	12.4	ENT	9.2
	ENT	8.0	ENT	6.0	Ortho.	8.3

and Massengill (1988) at the University of Alabama in Huntsville. This was a nine-year study involving 177,838 patient visits to 143 residents and 18 faculty members. The overall consultation rate was 1.4 per cent; little year-to-year variation was noted (range 1.1 to 1.6 per cent). Most of the referrals were to specialists in otolaryngology and orthopedics, followed by obstetrics and gynecology, general surgery, neurology, and urology.

In pediatrics and internal medicine, the two other primary care specialties, referral rates are somewhat higher. Internal medicine has a referral rate of 2.2 to 18.2 per cent, and pediatrics has a range of 1.0 to 9.5 per cent (Penchansky and Fox, 1970); however, the referral process in these specialties has not been studied in as much detail. It appears that this difference in rates can be explained by the less comprehensive nature of internists' and pediatricians' practices and their need for assistance in fields peripheral to areas of major emphasis in training. As noted in Table 15–2, most referrals are to a surgical specialty for a diagnostic procedure or specific therapy.

Ruane (1979) reviewed 108 consecutive referrals in a family practice and found a 1.5 per cent referral rate. He noted that, "The well trained family physician provides definitive care for the vast majority (in this study 98.4 per cent) of patient encounters, contrary to the cherished beliefs of many medical school faculty." Twenty per cent of the referrals were for the specific treatment of clear-cut problems (usually surgery). Sixty-four per cent were for diagnostic tests not available to the primary care physician, such as allergy testing or arthrography. One family physician in his third year of practice found that less than one half of 1 per cent of patients were referred to a tertiary care center and these were usually for the management of uncommon problems such as leukemia, sepsis, bone tumor, or cardiac bypass rather than for diagnosis (Schmidt, 1977). Dixon (1976) studied a small rural community in Ontario (referral rate of 3.3 per cent) and found that referrals were primarily to specialists in general surgery, orthopedics, and obstetrics for specific surgical procedures such as appendectomy, cholecystectomy, and cesarean section.

Consultations in a rural practice have been documented according to the International Classification of Health Problems in Primary Care (Glenn et al., 1983). By far, the most frequent problems requiring consultation involved the nervous system and sense organs. More than 86 per cent of these problems were referred to specialists in neurology, ophthalmology, or otolaryngology. The second most common problems that needed referral were those associated with the genitourinary system, requiring consultation from a urologist or gynecologist. Data of this type may assist residency directors in emphasizing those areas during graduate training, although most referrals will continue to be for specific subspecialty procedures.

When referral rates for fee-for-service patients were compared with those for members of a health maintenance organization (HMO) in Minnesota (Mayer, 1982), the fee-for-service patients had a lower referral rate (3.19 per cent) than the HMO patients (4.46 per cent). Although the percentages of referral differed, the rank order of specialties that problems were referred to was remarkably similar and matched the specialties referred to most commonly in other studies (see Table 15–2).

What is not clear is whether a low rate of referral indicates that the physician is competent and requires assistance infrequently or whether that physician is incompetent and does not recognize problems that require referral. Other factors may play a role as well; the practice may consist mostly of healthy young adults, or consultants may not be available and referral may be difficult.

Self-Referral by Patients

Patient self-referral plays a large role in the number of patients seen by physicians in consulting specialties in the United States. Thirty-two per cent to seventy per cent of patients seen by subspecialists in fields such as cardiology, gastroenterology, surgery, urology, and proctology are self-referred rather than being referred by a primary care physician (Shortell and Anderson, 1971).

Self-Referral by Physicians

Physicians have come under considerable criticism when suspected of referring patients to colleagues or laboratories in which they have an interest or from which they derive some financial benefit as a result of the referral. Professional "kickbacks" in which the physician is paid for referring a patient have long been unethical. Receiving or paying a kickback for referring a Medicare patient is now a felony in the United States. Although few physicians would refer a patient to a poor quality physician or laboratory purely because of a financial kickback, it is also clear that "anyone's judgment can be subtly influenced by financial interests" (Stark, 1989). Any time a physician referral is thought to be in the physician's best interest rather than the patient's, the profession of medicine is at risk of losing its valued place in society. Physicians must avoid any referral that involves personal gain since this practice runs the risk of influencing decisions and affecting patient care. The most common types of self-referral are those to laboratories or medical equipment suppliers in which the physician has a significant investment.

The Teacher-Pupil Relationship

The consultation process works best when two physicians work together as colleagues to solve a difficult patient problem. Since the process is usually a learning opportunity for the referring physician, it is easy for the consultant to assume the role of teacher and the referring physician the role of pupil. However, the process is not a superior-inferior or teacher-pupil relationship but rather two skilled physicians working together. The consultant has the responsibility to confirm the findings of the referring physician if no new information is detected. The consultant should not enter into a series of exotic tests merely because it is thought to be "expected" or because of fear that his or her prestige as a consultant will be jeopardized. The family physician may have requested another opinion primarily to confirm the diagnosis, perhaps wishing to obtain reassurance before telling the patient he or she has a permanent and incurable disease. Merely informing the patient of a relatively benign diagnosis of chronic disease such as hypertension results in an increased amount of time lost from work due to the patient's assuming the "sick" role.

If the referring physician places the consultant in the role of "teacher," the consultant may feel obliged to make comments or recommendations that may not be necessary. The "pupil" likewise feels obliged to follow these recommendations. If the consultant's report is superficial, the referring physician is obliged to take only those actions that he or she feels are in the best interest of the patient. The family physician should accept full responsibility for interpreting and using the opinions of the consultant, in a manner similar to the evaluation of laboratory test results. The referring physician is as free to ignore the consultant's advice as to solicit it in the first place.

Balint (1964) feels that this teacher-pupil relationship interferes with patient care if the family physician is dissatisfied with the consultant's report but follows the advice solely out of respect for the consultant as the "expert." The consultant may have formed an opinion based on insufficient information or without total knowledge of the patient's emotional and medical background; or the opinion may have been generated, or even manufactured, as a result of having little additional information to offer. A good consultant will admit when he has nothing further that needs to be done and will not pursue unnecessary additional testing.

The consultation process is more successful when there is a personal interchange between two physicians rather than when communication is solely by letter. When the referring physician responds only to recommendations made in a report without the opportunity to discuss them with the consultant, inappropriate assumptions may be made. The more personal the interchange that occurs between the two physicians, the more effective will be the consultation.

Collusion of Anonymity

A "collusion of anonymity" exists when neither the referring physician nor the consultant accepts responsibility for the patient (Balint, 1964). Inappropriate decisions regarding patient care can be made when neither physician accepts full responsibility. The problem is amplified when the family physician turns to a variety of consultants for advice, yielding to each, with no one person accepting ongoing responsibility for the patient. The consultation process is not a ritual of "passing the buck" but an integral part of the family physician's continuing responsibility for patient care. If the consultant does not provide meaningful or useful information, then additional consultations must be obtained until the problem is satisfactorily resolved. The term primary physician implies primary responsibility for the patient, not just physician of first contact.

The Family Physician as a Consultant

It is unfortunate that too much responsibility for primary care is burdening many subspecialists. Cardiologists who treat acne and general surgeons who remove ingrown toenails are wasting years of specialized training. Referrals to family physicians are frequently made by physicians in the surgical disciplines for the care of families when psychosocial problems are prominent, for geriatric care, for the long-term management of a chronic illness, and for medical emergencies. Pediatricians frequently refer teenagers or young adults who have outgrown their practice.

In a survey of family physicians from five midwestern states, Amundson and Vogt (1989) found that 35 per cent of the respondents received consultations and referrals from other generalist specialists and 28 per cent received them from subspecialists. The most common reason for the referral was that the patient did not have a family physician, but the second most common reason, when the referring physician was another generalist, was for a procedure such as flexible sigmoidoscopy or vasectomy. One of the most common reasons for referral overall was for the family physician to serve as a coordinator of care (i.e., "captain of the ship").

The family physician can be a valuable consultant when comprehensive and continuing health care is in the patient's best interest or when there is a need for a physician skilled in coordinating the care of multiple specialists.

References

Amundson, L. H., and Vogt, H. B.: The consultant family physician. J. Am. Board Fam. Pract., *2*(1):34–36, 1989.

Balint, M.: The Doctor, His Patient, and the Illness. London, Sir Isaac Pitman and Sons, 1964. *This classic text on psychotherapy in family practice is the basis for "Balint groups" in many residency programs. Although the text focuses on psychotherapy, three chapters discuss the relationship between referring physician and consultant, namely the collusion of anonymity, the general practitioner and his consultants, and the perpetuation of the teacher-pupil relationship.*

Barnett, B. L., Jr., and Collins, J. J., Jr.: A new look at the consultation continuum. J. Fam. Pract., *5*:665, 1977. *A clear and concise overview of the consultation process.*

Bates, R. C.: The two sides of very successful consultation. Med. Econ., *56*:172, 1979.

Brock, C.: Consultation and referral patterns of family physicians. J. Fam. Pract., *4*:1129, 1977. *This study of referral patterns involved 39 family physicians, most of whom were residents and staff at the University of Western Ontario. Reasons for the referral and for choosing a specific consultant or agency were analyzed. Specialties referred to were compared with Geyman's and Metcalfe's studies.*

Carson, M. E.: The referral process. Med. J. Aust., *1*:180, 1982. *This Australian study illustrates the problem of comparing referrals between countries. Because the health care system required physicians' referrals for refraction, 21.6 per cent of referrals were for refraction only. Also, 6.5 per cent of the referrals had already taken place and the referring physician was asked to back-date the referral certificate.*

Clarfield, A. M.: A study of all referrals from a family practice unit. Can. Fam. Physician, *26*:527, 1980.

Crump, W. J., and Massengill, P.: Outpatient consultations from a family practice residency program: Nine years' experience. J. Am. Board Fam. Pract., *1*(3):164–166, 1988.

Cummins, R. O., Smith, R. W., and Inui, T. S.: Communication failure in primary care: Failure of consultants to provide follow-up information. J.A.M.A., *243*:1650, 1980.

Curry, R. W., Jr., Crandall, L. A., and Coggins, W. The referral process: A study of one method for improving communication between rural practitioners and consultants. J. Fam. Pract., *10*:287, 1980.

Dixon, A. S.: Survey of a rural practice: Rainy River 1975. Can. Fam. Phys., *22*:693, 1976. *This is a thorough 1-year study of family practice in a small, rural community in northwestern Ontario. Analysis includes problems seen in the office and hospital plus patterns of referral. A comparison is made among the illnesses encountered in this practice with those seen in an urban Canadian practice and a rural practice in New Zealand.*

Dolezal, J. M., Amundson, L. H., Sinning, N. J., et al.: Pricare and ambulatory referrals. Cont. Educ. Fam. Physician, 12:84–94, 1980. *A study of outpatient referrals by residents and faculty at the Sioux Falls Family Practice Center. The one per cent referral rate excluded referrals made on hospitalized patients. No report was received from 30 per cent of the consultants, most of whom were in orthopedics, gynecology, and general surgery.*

Everett, G. E., Parsons, T. J., and Christensen, A. L.: Educational influences on consultation rates of house staff physicians in a primary care clinic. J. Med. Educ., *59*:479–486, 1984.

Fry, J.: Hospital referrals: Must they go up? Changing patterns over 20 years. Lancet, *2*:148, 1971.

Geyman, J. P., Brown, R. C., and Rivers, K.: Referrals in family practice: A comparative study by geographic region and practice setting. J. Fam. Pract., *3*:163, 1976. *This study compared referrals from eight family physicians in solo and group practices in urban, suburban, and rural northern and central California. Results were compared with the Metcalfe and Sischy study in New York, and suggest that family physicians provide definitive care for as many as 98 per cent of patient visits in daily practice. The majority of referrals involved sharing patient care responsibility. Most were to surgical fields and obstetrics and gynecology. There were significant but unexplained seasonal differences in referral rates.*

Glenn, J. K., Hofmeister, R. W., Neikirk, H., and Wright, H.: Continuity of care in the referral process: An analysis of family physicians' expectations of consultants. J. Fam. Pract., *16*:329–334, 1983.

Hines, R. M., and Curry, O. J.: The consultation process and physician satisfaction: Review of referral patterns in three urban family practice units. Can. Med. Assoc. J., *118*:1065, 1978. *This review showed that involving the patient in the referral process can improve compliance and the response rate from consultants (92 per cent in this study).*

Horder, J. P.: Physicians and family doctors: A new relationship. J. R. Coll. Gen. Pract., *27*:391, 1977.

Lawler, F. H.: Referral rates of senior family practice residents in an ambulatory care clinic. J. Med. Educ., *62*:177–182, 1987.

Mayer, T. R.: Family practice referral patterns in a health maintenance organization. J. Fam. Pract., *14*:315, 1982. *A comparison of the referral patterns of fee-for-service patients and members of a health maintenance organization (HMO). The HMO patients constituted 52.3 per cent of patient visits and 60.5 per cent of referrals. Most referrals in each group were to specialists in general surgery, otolaryngology, and orthopedics.*

McPhee, S. J., Lo, B., Saika, G. Y., and Meltzer, R.: How good is communication between primary care physicians and subspecialty consultants? Arch. Intern. Med., *144*:1265–1268, 1984.

Metcalfe, D. H., and Sischy, D.: Patterns of referral from family practice. NY State J. Med., *73*:1690, 1973. *One of the first studies of referral rates from private physicians in the United States, involving four practices in Rochester, New York. The main reasons for referral were for technical assistance rather than diagnosis. No reports were received from consultants in 18.5 per cent of the cases.*

Moscovice, I., Schwartz, C. W., and Shortell, S. M.: Referral patterns of family physicians in an underserved rural area. J. Fam. Pract., *9*:677, 1979.

National Center for Health Statistics: Unpublished data from 1985. National Ambulatory Medical Care Survey.

Nyma, K. C.: Referral patterns in general practice. Aust. Fam. Physician, *2*:173, 1973.

Penchansky, R., and Fox, D.: Frequency of referral and patient characteristics in group practice. Med. Care, *8*:368, 1970. *Compares the referral rates of family physicians, internists, and pediatricians. Also, looks at variations according to urban, suburban, and rural settings; sex; race; age; and method of payment.*

Phelps, L. A., and Renner, J. H.: The development of a "Statement of policy regarding consultations." J. Fam. Pract., *5*:979, 1977. *Describes the policy on the use of consultants developed by the Department of Family Medicine and Practice at the University of Wisconsin. Includes an illustration of their patient referral form.*

Price, P. B., Loughmiller, G. C., and Murray, S. L.: Attributes of a good practicing physician. J. Med. Educ., *46*:229, 1971.

Ruane, T. J.: Consultation and referral in a Vermont family practice: A study of utilization, specialty distribution, and outcome. J. Fam. Pract., *8*:1037, 1979. *A referral rate of 1.5 per cent was noted in a rural family practice office located 17 miles from the University of Vermont Medical Center. There was a 24-per cent nonresponse rate from consultants.*

Saunders, R. C.: Consultation-referral among physicians: Practice and process. J. Fam. Pract., *6*:123, 1978.

Schmidt, D. D.: Referral patterns in an individual family practice. J. Fam. Pract. *5*:401, 1977.

Shortell, S. M., and Anderson, O. W.: The physician referral process: A theoretical perspective. Health Serv. Res., *6*:39, 1971.

Stark, E. H.: Ethics in patient referrals. Acad. Med., 64:146–147, 1989.

Steinberg, H., Torem, M., and Saravey, S. M.: An analysis of physician resistance to psychiatric consultations. Arch Gen. Psych. *37*:1007, 1980.

Stephens, G. G.: The Intellectual Basis of Family Practice. Tucson, AZ, Winter Publishing Company, 1982.

Tenney, J. B., White, K. L., and Williamson, J. W.: NAMC: Background and methodology. Vital and Health Statistics, Series 2, No. 61, DHEW Publication (HRA) 74-1335, 1974.

Tumulty, P. A.: The Effective Clinician. Philadelphia, W. B. Saunders Co., 1973.

White, F. Z.: Referral patterns among family practitioners. I. M. J. *166*(1):31–33, 1984.

16

Family Practice Around the World

United States

David N. Sundwall

Overview of the Current U.S. Health Care System*

The health care system in the United States is not a single system but, in fact, many. It has been described as a pluralistic system, having multiple organizations and entities that deliver health services.

However, it is fair to say that a distinguishing characteristic of the U.S. system has been the patient's freedom of choice of providers. Although certain elements of the system have become much more highly organized and integrated in the past decade (for instance, the development of health maintenance organizations and hospital-based group practices), it is still the patient's decision regarding the choice of providers that is the most common element of the system.

Over the past half century, a pattern of physician practice has developed, with physicians, either singly or in groups, seeking to provide a defined set of services to a population that is geographically congruent. Although the patient-physician relationship has remained of primary importance, other entities in the health care system have also developed an increasingly important role in determining the types and quality of care delivered. Of particular note are the roles of group purchasers of health insurance (primarily business concerns and governmental units) and the insurance industry, which provides interface between beneficiary and provider. The growth of coverage of health insurance—in terms of both indi-

*These sections present material written for a previous edition by Robert Graham, M.D., and updated by David N. Sundwall, M.D.

viduals participating and scope of services—has been explosive in the last 20 years; it is now estimated that over 80 per cent of U.S. citizens are covered by some type of health insurance, paid for out of public or private funds. There still remains, however, a group of over 30 million who are uninsured. Current policy debate focuses on how to provide coverage for both the poor, nonworking population and the working uninsured (Wilensky, 1988).

FEDERAL ROLE

Although the great majority of industrialized nations have developed some type of federal or governmental role for coordination and payment of health care services, the federal role in the United States has remained relatively constant over the last 20 years. Historically, the federal government has undertaken the responsibility of providing direct services for a relatively small number of individuals—most significantly American Indians and Alaskan Natives, merchant seamen, active military personnel and their dependents, and veterans. In the mid-1960's, there was an expansion of federal responsibility for the payment of services provided by the private sector to the elderly (Medicare) and the medically indigent (Medicaid). There was also limited provision of direct care services in geographic regions considered to have a significant deficiency of medical services through federally funded community and migrant health centers and by providing needed health professionals (National Health Service Corps). Since the early 1970's, the most significant expansion of the federal role in health care was the passage of the Medicare Catastrophic Coverage Act of 1988, which provided additional hospital, physician, and drug benefits to some 33 million elderly and disabled Medicare beneficiaries.

Major Organizational Elements

PRIMARY CARE

The basic organizational element for the delivery of care is the primary care physician. This individual is typically office based, serves a geographically defined community, provides a wide range of services (including some in-hospital treatment), and sees his or her patients at a frequency that is largely determined by the patient's own perception of need for medical care. The vast majority of such primary care physicians are engaged in private practice, whether solo or in association with a group. The growth of organized primary practice (for instance, health maintenance organizations) began modestly but has increased in recent years and has been concentrated in the more densely populated urban areas. Federal financing through special project support has been particularly important in the initiation of a large number of the health maintenance organizations (HMOs) and community health centers, and the provision of Medicare and Medicaid reimbursement to previously medically indigent individuals has markedly expanded the number of individuals now able to receive primary care services from a provider of their choice.

SECONDARY CARE

The next level of care, that of secondary care, consists of a heterogeneous mix of hospital-oriented specialty and subspecialty services. The mixture of community-based secondary care hospitals in the United States includes voluntary (not for profit), proprietary (for profit), and public institutions. Most of these institutions have, over the past decade, provided the nidus around which numerous specialty and subspecialty group practices have been organized to provide consultative and referral services to the primary care community of practitioners. There is now a geographic distribution of such secondary hospitals throughout the country, and the increasing scientific knowledge of recent medical school graduates has assured a generally high level of advanced medical care available for patients at the community level.

TERTIARY CARE

The site of the most complex medical care, tertiary care, is generally in one of the relatively few large hospitals that are associated with academic medical centers, voluntary hospitals, or local units of the government (public facilities). These hospitals, of which there are fewer than 200 in the United States, are the location for the training of the vast majority of medical residents and advanced specialists. Most of the centers are located in or around large metropolitan areas. These centers, like the secondary care centers, also serve as a nidus for the organization of specialty and subspecialty group practices. With the exception of primary care training programs, however, practicing primary care physicians with staff privileges are less likely to be found in such tertiary care hospitals. Patients in these hospitals tend to be the most critically and acutely ill, and the hospitals put a heavy emphasis on provision of the newer technologically complex procedures and on research. These hospitals, as a result of their mission and their geographic locations, frequently provide a large percentage of care to Medicare and Medicaid beneficiaries or to individuals who are medically indigent.

SYSTEM INTEGRATION

With this abbreviated description of the three-tiered system in the United States, it is still clear that the glue holding the disparate institutional elements of the system together is composed of the patients, the physicians, and the payers. The decision about the site of care is most commonly a joint decision on the part of the physician and the patient. It depends on factors such as severity of the illness, patient preference, physician hospital staff privileges, and availability of needed services. Payment for such services is most commonly determined by the health insurance coverage of the individual patient. There are a wide variety of private insurance plans and insurers, and as noted above, over 80 per cent of the U.S. population is covered by some kind of medical care insurance. Most commonly, insurance plans are negotiated on a group basis by the employer and tend to give fullest coverage to nonprimary care costs of ailments. Many insurance plans either provide limited or no coverage for preventive services. Some insurance plans do provide for substantial latitude in patient contribution for costs (for instance, coinsurance or deductible), and patients who are totally without insurance still must bear the costs of physician and hospital services themselves or seek care provided in public facilities.

Historical Overview of the Role of the Federal Government in Health

Although the federal government has had some involvement in health care almost since its inception, it is useful to divide this involvement into five phases: before 1900, 1900 to 1940, post World War II to 1960, 1960's to the mid-1970's, and the mid-1970's forward.

BEFORE 1900: LIMITED GOVERNMENT INVOLVEMENT

By today's standards, medicine can be considered primitive before the 1900's. Although there were a few highly regarded centers of medical science in the United States, they were independent of federal funding and overview.

Nonetheless, concern for public well-being has always been a part of our collective conscience, as evidenced by discussions recorded in the Annals of Congress during their first session. On July 20, 1789, it was "ordered that a Committee be appointed to bring in a bill or bills providing for the establishment of hospitals for sick and disabled seamen." President John Adams, who was a member of the Boston Marine Society, signed the act in 1798, which directed the master of every U.S. ship entering a U.S. port to pay to the collector of customs a sum equal to 20 cents a month for each of the members of the crew, to be deducted from the seaman's wages. Hospitals were built with these funds, and directors were appointed in the principal ports by the President of the United States (Thurm, 1970).

This act initiated the beginning of our present Public Health Service (PHS). However, in its first century, the PHS's activities were limited to the establishment of marine hospitals. It was not until 1870 that the Marine Hospital Service was formally organized as a national agency with central headquarters in Washington, D.C. Many of the hospitals had grown obsolete and many of the personnel who staffed them were found to have inadequate training and abilities. Therefore, new regulations were established governing the appointment and promotion of physicians within the marine hospital service. This paved the way for the establishment in 1889 of the Commissioned Corps of the Public Health Service (Raffel, 1980).

1900 TO 1940: EMERGING MEDICAL SCIENCE—INCREASED FEDERAL INVOLVEMENT

The latter part of the 19th century was a period of major advances in medical science. The most dramatic strides were in surgery, with the development of antiseptic techniques and anesthesia and the elaboration of the germ theory that spurred the development of the science of microbiology and techniques for vaccination. One of the first scientific laboratories to be established in this country was at the Marine Hospital on Staten Island.

In 1891, the laboratory was moved to service headquarters in Washington, D.C. and expanded to include departments of pathology, chemistry, pharmacology, and zoology. In 1930, the Hygienic Laboratory became known as the National Institute of Health (NIH) with a broad mandate of ascertaining the cause, prevention, and cure of disease (DHEW Publication No. [HRA]76-616).

The trend of increasing federal involvement during this period can be seen in some of the major health-related legislation passed during this period, including the Biologics Control Act of 1902, the Federal Food and Drug Act of 1906, the involvement in the study of water pollution and other sanitation problems, the National Cancer Act of 1937, and the Venereal Disease Control Act.

WORLD WAR II TO 1960: BIOMEDICAL SCIENCE AND THE FEDERAL GOVERNMENT—A NEW HEALTH PARTNERSHIP

Research conducted during World War II had a major impact on the health sciences, and the interest in biomedical research proved to be the most logical focus for new interests in health issues by the federal government. During this period, the NIH grew rapidly. Federal dollars multiplied from a few million in the early war years to more than $3.5 billion in 1981. By 1965, the government contributed 65 per cent of the total U.S. funding for medical research and development. Thus, in response to congressional mandate, the federal government became the major supporter of biomedical research (Mider, 1976). Although this era in our nation's history was dominated by the development of high-quality and effective biomedical research, the federal government was busy on many other fronts as well. In 1946, two major new programs were initiated through legislation: (1) the National Surveying Construction Program (Hill-Burton), which provided federal support to states to assist in building hospitals, and (2) the National Mental Health Act, a broad program providing grants for research, training, and community health services. PHS activities were further expanded into areas of environmental health (Water Pollution Act, 1948), care of American Indians and Alaskan Natives (Indian Health Service, 1955), ambulatory care services (Community, Health Services and Facilities Act, 1961), and nationwide immunization programs (Vaccination Assistance Act, 1962) (Raffel, 1980).

1960's TO THE MID-1970's: THE FEDERAL GOVERNMENT TAKES THE LEAD

In the 1960's, the federal government added a wide range of health programs to its previous efforts. It became involved with training health professionals, assessing the health manpower needs of the nation, providing guidelines for occupational safety, and, most importantly, becoming a major purchaser of health care services with the enactment of Medicare and Medicaid legislation. These efforts resulted in a dramatic increase in the federal expenditures for health (Russell and Burke, 1978). In 1965, the federal government accounted for more than 13.2 per cent of health expenditures; by 1986, it accounted for 29.4 per cent of the expenditures (Health Care Financing Administration, 1987).

The extraordinary costs incurred are related to multiple legislative initiatives. Although the major increases were related to Medicare and Medicaid, legislative initiatives in the training area were also taking place. Most important to the discipline of family medicine were the passage of the Health Professions Education Assistance Act of 1963 and the Nurse Training Act of 1964. These acts, and subsequent amendments, provided money for the construction of health professional schools, money for operating expenses, and loans for scholarship programs to encourage students to enter these professions. These initiatives were created in response to data suggesting that the United States was suffering from significant shortages in health manpower. Specific activity relevant to family practice is discussed further in the section on Federal Role in Promoting Family Practice.

Coincident with the federal interest in training health professionals to meet our nation's needs was an escalation in providing services to underserved populations, either directly or indirectly, through multiple community-based programs. These programs included rural health programs, community and migrant health centers, and maternal and child health programs.

All of these efforts in education and service are overshadowed in terms of costs, however, by the Medicare and Medicaid legislation, which became law in 1966. Medicare provides a comprehensive two-part health insurance plan for the elderly (those over 65 years of age). Part A covers the cost of institutional care, primarily in the hospital, and Part B pays for physician care and for certain outpatient services. In 1973, Medicare benefits were extended to include the disabled and persons suffering from chronic kidney disease.

Medicaid began as an expansion of the already existing welfare program to pay for the health care of the poor. This program was designed to be a partnership effort with states: the federal government provides financial assistance to the states to meet the medical costs of people receiving assistance under the federal-state welfare system, for instance, the aged, the poor, the blind, the disabled, and families with dependent children (Russell and Burke, 1978).

Although the cost of Medicare and Medicaid has greatly exceeded in total costs all other health programs, they are not the only federal health care assistance programs. Others include maternal and child health programs, expansion of the Department of Defense's supplementary programs to pay for care provided in the private sector (CHAMPUS Program), and expanded care for veterans' families by the Department of Veterans' Affairs.

THE MID-1970's FORWARD: ADVANCED TECHNOLOGY OUTSTRIPS RESOURCES AND STATE INVOLVEMENT INCREASES

In the past decade or so, health experts have occasionally issued warnings that health rationing might occur. This issue gets raised particularly in terms of the intensity of care provided to the chronically ill elderly. We have, in fact, reached the age wherein we have outstripped our ability to pay for the myriad of medical wonders that we are theoretically capable of providing.

While most of the rise in health care expenditures has been attributed to general inflation, as much as 40 per cent of the increase has been attributed to factors having to do with increased intensity of services, increased utilization, and medical care sector-specific inflation, most of which are influenced by technology (Garrison and Wilensky, 1986).

The accomplishments of research scientists continue at a dazzling rate. Recent improvements have been made in the treatment of cancer and cardiovascular diseases, as well as depression and other forms of severe mental illness. Activity in genetic engineering research and development suggests that we are entering a new era of more effective and safer biologic products.

An example of how technology may have outstripped our resources is the area of human organ transplantation. The end-stage renal disease program enacted into law in 1972 was projected at that time to cost $200 million per year. Actual costs are now approximately fifteen times that. In the past decade, improved immunosuppressive drugs have made it possible to transplant several vital organs in addition to kidneys. However, with the cost of a liver transplant exceeding $100,000 per patient, payers are reluctant to provide complete coverage for these costly, albeit lifesaving, procedures.

Those who fear that new knowledge might only be translated into more costly applied technology, however, fail to understand the potential for cost savings as we learn how to prevent debilitating diseases and premature death. But regardless of the promises held out by scientific advances, the current phase of federal health policy will of necessity be characterized by painful competition for limited resources.

The recent changes in the Medicare reimbursement system reflect this new imperative. The previous cost-based, third-party reimbursement policy tended to provide incentives to adopt cost-increasing technologies. The switch to a prospective payment system in 1983 for inpatient hospital services has tended to change the incentives. The incentives have become those of minimizing treatment costs per admission, consistent with high-quality care, and focusing particularly on technology that is cost saving.

The new era of limited resources is also giving impetus to renewed interest in preventive medicine and health promotion. Sound research in disease prevention and better education of our citizens to assume responsibility for their health are likely to be areas with high payoff.

The most significant change in the Medicare program in two decades is the Medicare Catastrophic Coverage Act of 1988. Provisions of the Act will protect 31 million elderly and disabled Americans from excessive hospital, physician, and outpatient prescription drug bills. Medicare coverage of hospitalization will be expanded to 365 days, with cost sharing kept to one first-day deductible.

Supply of Primary Care vs. Specialty Physicians

DEVELOPMENTS IN PHYSICIAN SUPPLY

Since 1970, the number of physicians has grown faster than the overall population. Data from the American Medical Association (AMA) show that as of December 31, 1985, there were 552,716 total allopathic physicians in the United States, over half of whom were board certified. The physician/population ratio has increased from 202 to 228 per 100,000 between 1980 and 1985. In 1986, there were an additional 25,479 osteopathic (D.O.) physicians in the United States (U.S. DHHS, 1988).

SPECIALIZATION

The ranking of the specialties shows a relatively larger growth for internal medicine among the primary care specialties. In 1985, internal medicine had the largest number of practitioners, followed by general/family practice, general surgery, pediatrics, psychiatry, obstetrics/gynecology, anesthesiology, orthopedic surgery, and pathology. Table 16–1 summarizes the number of physicians by major specialty.

Although the actual number of general/family practitioners has increased with overall growth, there has been a decline in the percentage of general/family practitioners among all medical doctors (MDs), most recently falling from 12.5 per cent in 1981 to 12.1 per cent in 1985. Among osteopathic physicians with board certification, more than half are in primary care.

ACTIVITY STATUS

Patient care MDs have accounted for approximately 80 per cent of the total physician population during the 1970's and 1980's, while nonpatient care MDs have ranged from 7 to 10 per cent, with the rest unclassified. Particularly large gains have been shown between 1975 and 1985 in the office-based category, which grew by 53.2 per cent, and in research, which grew by 192.9 per cent (U.S. DHHS, 1988).

Physicians are increasingly becoming employed rather than self-employed, reflecting the growth of alternative delivery systems such as HMOs and prepaid care. Employed, nonfederal physicians in patient care grew from 23.4 per cent in 1983 to 25.7 per cent in 1985. This is particularly true for younger physicians and for female physicians.

EDUCATIONAL DEVELOPMENTS

As of 1988 there were 127 allopathic medical schools in the United States. Enrollment appears to have peaked, reaching a total of 67,327 in 1983 and 1984, with a slight decline since then. The size of first-year classes has also shown a slight drop, from a peak of 17,268 in 1981 and 1982 to a level of 16,819 in 1986 and 1987. Table 16–2 shows total U.S. medical school enrollment, by gender.

There are an additional 15 U.S. schools of osteopathic medicine. In academic year 1984 and 1985, first-year enrollment was 1,750 and total enrollment was 6,547.

With regard to graduate medical education, the total number of allopathic residents on duty was at

Table 16–1. LARGEST 1985 SPECIALTIES: NUMBER OF MDs AND RANK, 1970 AND 1985*

	1970		1985		1980–1985
Specialty	*Number*	*Rank*	*Number*	*Rank*	*Annual Rate (Per Cent) of Change*
Internal Medicine	41,872	2	90,417	1	4.8
General/family practice	57,948	1	67,051	2	2.2
General surgery	29,761	3	38,169	3	2.3
Pediatrics	17,941	6	35,617	4	4.7
Psychiatry	21,146	4	32,255	5	3.3
Obstetrics/gynecology	18,876	5	30,867	6	3.3
Anesthesiology	10,860	7	22,021	7	6.7
Orthopedic surgery	9,620	9	17,166	8	6.7
Pathology	10,283	8	15,456	9	2.9

*From American Medical Association: *Physician Characteristics and Distribution, 1986 Edition* and previous editions, as reported in U.S. Department of Health and Human Services: Chronology-Health Professions Legislation 1956–1979 (Publication No. [HRA] 80–69). Rockville, MD, 1980.

76,815, as of September 1, 1986. This included some 6,332 accredited programs. In 1986 and 1987, nearly 45 per cent of all residents were in training in internal medicine, general/family practice, and pediatrics. This compares to only 26 per cent being trained in these specialties in 1970. Between 1976 and 1986, the number of general/family practice programs increased from 346 to 383. Residents in general/family practice programs declined from 7,600 in 1984 to 7,200 in 1986. Table 16–3 shows the number of residents for the top eight specialties in 1986.

In addition, the American Osteopathic Association (AOA) reports that there were 1,250 residents in AOA-approved osteopathic programs in the academic year 1986 and 1987.

Development of Family Medicine as a Specialty

In order for a primary medical certifying board to be established, petitioners must gain approval of the Advisory Board for Medical Specialties and the American Medical Association Council on Medical Education. Necessary steps are discussed in the document, "Essentials for Approval of Examining Boards in Medical Specialties" (American Academy of Family Physicians, 1980).

Petitioners for the American Board of Family Practice proceeded through these prescribed steps and obtained official recognition for the board on February 8, 1969. There was a fairly long and involved process to reach that stage, which is discussed in a publication entitled "Family Practice: Creation of a Specialty" (American Academy of Family Physicians, 1980).

The effort to obtain a certifying board in family practice began in the 1940's and required the participation of the American Academy of General Practice (now the American Academy of Family Physicians) and the Section on General Practice of the American Medical Association (later the AMA Section on Family and General Practice).

Although serious efforts to establish a certifying board did not begin until the mid-1950's, the first apparent call for a certifying board occurred in the AMA House of Delegates in 1941. In that year, the AMA was presented a resolution requesting that they study the matter of developing standards and means "by which certification may be given in recognition of special training, experience and fitness, and special qualifications for general practice" (American Academy of Family Physicians, 1980).

Table 16–2. TOTAL U.S. MEDICAL SCHOOL ENROLLMENT, BY GENDER, SELECTED YEARS 1978–1979 THROUGH 1984–1985*

	1979–1980 (126 Schools)		1983–1984 (127 Schools)		1986–1987 (127 Schools)	
Gender	*Number*	*Per Cent*	*Number*	*Per Cent*	*Number*	*Per Cent*
Men	47,651	74.7	46,692	69.4	44,025	66.6
Women	16,149	25.3	20,635	30.6	22,100	33.4
Total	63,800	100.0	67,327	100.0	66,125	100.0

*From Fall Enrollment Survey, Association of American Medical Colleges, as reported in U.S. Department of Health and Human Services: Chronology-Health Professions Legislation 1956–1979 (Publication No. [HRA] 80–69). Rockville, MD, 1980.

Table 16–3. NUMBER OF RESIDENTS, RANK-ORDERED FOR TOP EIGHT SPECIALTIES, 1986*

Specialty	Total† Number of Residents	Per Cent of Total Residents	Cumulative Per Cent
1. Internal medicine	20,633	26.9	26.9
IM subspecialties	2,517		
2. Surgery	7,982	10.4	37.3
Surgical subspecialties	102		
3. Family practice	7,238	9.4	46.7
4. Pediatrics	6,503	8.5	55.2
Pediatric subspecialties	686		
5. Ob/Gyn	4,525	5.9	61.1
5. Psychiatry	5,494	7.2	68.3
Child psychiatry	602		
7. Anesthesiology	3,864	5.0	73.3
8. Radiology, diagnostic	3,095	4.0	77.3
All others	17,763	22.7	100.0
Total	76,815		

*From American Medical Association: 1987–1988 Directory of Graduate Medical Education Programs. Chicago, 1987, as reported in U.S. Department of Health and Human Services: Chronology-Health Professions Legislation 1956–1979 (Publication No. [HRA] 80–69). Rockville, MD, 1980.

†Totals for each specialty also include subspecialties.

Federal Role in Promoting Family Medicine

The development of family medicine as a discipline and family practice as a medical specialty in the United States has been assisted to a great extent by federal legislation.

With the Health Professions Educational Assistance Act of 1963, funding was authorized for assistance to increase the opportunities for training of physicians, dentists, and selected other health professions personnel. Funds were provided for construction of teaching facilities and for grants to school loan funds. That involvement was expanded in 1965 to include improvements in the quality of educational programs and to provide incentives to expand enrollment.

The Comprehensive Health Manpower Training Act of 1971 provided for capitation grants to a variety of health professions schools, again with incentives to increase enrollment. Specific authority was provided for start-up awards to new schools of medicine, as well as conversion of 2-year schools. This Act also authorized a new program of grants to public and nonprofit private hospitals for professional training programs in the field of family medicine for medical students, interns, residents, or practicing physicians; for traineeships and fellowships for participants in such programs who plan to enter the practice of family medicine; and for other approved training programs in the field of family medicine.

Under the Health Professions Educational Assistance Act of 1976, an expanded set of family medicine training programs was put into place. Eligibility (previously limited to hospitals) was broadened to include schools of medicine or osteopathy, or other public or private nonprofit entities. Contract authority was added. Authority was added for training of physicians to teach family medicine and for traineeships and fellowships to such physicians. Osteopathic internship training specifically was made eligible for assistance. New categorical authority was also added for project grants to schools of medicine and osteopathy to establish and maintain academic administrative units or family medicine departments to provide clinical instruction in family medicine. The goal was to create units that would be comparable to those for other major clinical specialties in status, faculty, and curriculum.

With passage of the Omnibus Budget Reconciliation Act of 1981, support was ended for the major programs to expand medical school enrollment. Authorization for programs of capitation and construction grants were deleted from the law. Grants for family medicine residency programs and family medicine departments were extended. The focus of legislation shifted to solving targeted problems of specialty and geographic distribution. The Health Professions Training Assistance Act of 1985 continued this focus on targeted project grants.

The expansion of the federal programs and activities related to this legislation is documented in Chronology-Health Professions Legislation 1956–1979 (DHHS Publication No. [HRA] 80–69, 8/1980).

In terms of overall support of family medicine initiatives, the major program components have accomplished the following:

- *Predoctoral training*. Since 1978, predoctoral training grants have been awarded to allopathic and osteopathic medical educational institutions. From 1978 through 1986, awards totaling $61.2 million were made to 95 different institutions. An estimated 95,041 trainees have been involved in clerkship activities, preceptorship experience, and student assistantships.
- *Faculty development*. The faculty development grant program was designed to increase the number of physician faculty available to teach in allopathic

and osteopathic family medicine training programs. Faculty from every level of the medical education pathway were recruited to participate in short- and long-term (3 to 12 months) traineeships, master's degree programs, workshops, and seminars. Since the program's inception through fiscal year (FY) 1986, approximately $32.3 million has been spent to train 15,196 physician and nonphysician family medicine faculty.

- *Family medicine academic units*. In an effort to strengthen the family medicine academic unit, Grants for Establishment of Departments of Family Medicine were initiated in FY 1980. The goal of these grants is to help family medicine academic units become comparable to the other major clinical disciplines in allopathic and osteopathic institutions. The grants are somewhat flexible in order to respond to a particular applicant's needs. Projects may be geared toward undergraduate program development, residency programs, faculty enrichment needs (research, teaching, administration), or overall departmental reorganization. During the first 6 years of the program's operation, 85 medical education institutions received funding that totaled $53.9 million.
- *Graduate medical education*. Efforts in graduate family medicine education have been directed toward increasing the numbers and affecting the geographic distribution of family medicine practitioners and in the planning, development, and operation of the programs themselves.

From 1972 through 1986, the federal government awarded nearly $299.6 million for graduate family medicine training activities. During this period, the number of accredited family practice residency programs increased from 117 to 383, and each year an average of 54 per cent of all residents were in supported programs. In 1986, 142 allopathic and 16 osteopathic programs with a total of 3,422 residents in training received $17.7 million (U.S. DHHS, 1988).

Current Issues Regarding Family Practice

FINANCING GRADUATE MEDICAL EDUCATION

In recent years, there has been increased pressure to limit increases in educational expenditures as part of the overall effort to moderate increases in health care costs. At the same time, there is a growing recognition of the importance of training in ambulatory settings as part of graduate medical education (GME). Patients are increasingly receiving their health care in ambulatory settings. Specialties, such as family practice and pediatrics, have historically been oriented to ambulatory practice and training.

A recent report of the Council on Graduate Medical Education concluded that a concerted emphasis on training in ambulatory settings is warranted: "There are difficulties in financing GME in ambulatory settings, related to lower levels of payment by third parties and to increased logistical problems in teaching. The current financing of GME results in disincentives for ambulatory training" (Council on Graduate Medical Education, 1988).

The overall pattern of reimbursement tends to discourage GME in ambulatory settings. There is usually less third-party coverage of the population for ambulatory care. Payment levels are often lower for similar services when provided in ambulatory settings as opposed to inpatient settings. In addition, patients using ambulatory settings generally have to pay a greater share of payments or, in many cases, have no insurance. The Council found that it is difficult for ambulatory facilities and entities other than those owned or operated by hospitals to secure financing for the additional cost of operating in the presence of a teaching program.

QUALITY ASSURANCE/MALPRACTICE ISSUES

Physician credentialing ensures physician competency and protects the public through a complex arena of processes and decisions that include (1) accrediting over 6000 programs through which allopathic and osteopathic physicians are educated, (2) evaluating their competency to receive and continue to hold licenses, (3) determining their qualifications for and awarding specialty certification, and (4) specifying their hospital privileges.

With regard to the licensure and discipline of physicians, each state legislature has enacted a medical practice act to provide statutory authority to carry out these functions. The practice acts generally charge the state board with the primary responsibility and obligation of protecting the public through its licensure and discipline of physicians. Most other aspects of physician credentialing are the domain of the private sector. The federal government also maintains policies relative to the credentialing and discipline of federally employed physicians.

In the last few years, there has been widespread public and professional concern about the issues of medical liability and malpractice. Insurance premiums have been rising substantially. In some states and for selected specialties, they have risen to a level that appears to be interfering with the availability of care for certain portions of the population. One of the damaging effects of rising insurance costs is the practice of defensive medicine.

As early as 1974, physicians in several states began to experience problems in obtaining malpractice insurance. The average premium cost for all physicians increased by 81 per cent between 1982 and 1985, and for some specialties, such as obstetrics, average premium costs rose by 113 per cent.

The American Academy of Family Physicians reported in a 1984 survey that 21 per cent of respondents had restricted their obstetrics practice. This was apparently a result of certain insurers' reclassification of family physicians who provide obstetric care from a low-premium category to a higher category assigned to obstetricians/gynecologists, as well as family physicians often lacking a sufficient number of deliveries per year to compensate for the increased insurance costs (U.S. DHHS, Report of the Task Force on Medical Liability and Malpractice, 1987).

One of the steps being taken in this area is the establishment of a National Practitioner Data Bank, authorized by the Health Care Quality Improvement Act of 1916. This data bank will contain information on substandard professional performance and is intended to lessen the possibility that incompetent physicians and dentists may move their practices from state to state without detection.

PROVIDING SERVICE TO UNDERSERVED AREAS

Although there has been an increase in the supply of physicians generally, and primary care physicians specifically, there are still areas in the United States that are medically underserved. It is difficult for market forces to meet the needs of this residual core of shortage areas because of their remote location, extreme poverty, lack of cultural amenities, and other socioeconomic factors. Programs, such as the National Health Service Corps, Community and Migrant Health Centers, and the Area Health Education Centers, have been designed to help alleviate this problem.

In addition, the federal commitment to promote predoctoral, residency, and faculty development programs in the specialty of family practice has helped lead to a rapid expansion in the number of physicians in family medicine and, concomitantly, an increase in physicians in rural areas. One study concluded that:

Family physicians appear to locate in the more rural areas in much greater numbers than any other medical specialty, including general practitioners, heretofore the major provider of medical care in rural areas. They are also locating in nonmetropolitan urban areas to a much greater degree. Since the bias of more recent graduates would be for family physicians to be found in the location of their residency programs—most of which are in metropolitan areas—those differences are notable (U.S. DHHS, 1980).

A 1986 survey of graduates of family practice residency programs indicates that these graduates expect to establish practice outside urban areas or in rural communities at an annual rate of about one and one half times that at which they expect to locate in urban settings. Family physicians also appear to be locating more than other specialties in both physician-short, nonmetropolitan and whole-county shortage areas, although the total number of graduates establishing practice in rural areas still remains comparatively small.

PRIMARY CARE CURRICULA

A major issue for the future is whether the current family medicine/primary care curricula are being adapted to changing circumstances and emerging problems. The Health Resources and Services Administration, which administers the grant programs fostering family medicine training, held a conference in early 1988 on Future Directions in Primary Care. The question was raised about the extent to which primary care curricula meet current needs. Among relevant questions:

- Is there sufficient focus on disease prevention and health promotion?
- How adaptable has the curriculum been to such issues and problems as substance abuse, acquired immune deficiency syndrome (AIDS), geriatrics, and related issues such as Alzheimer's disease?
- How are competencies in mental health, geriatrics, nutrition, and patient education being developed?
- Does the curriculum prepare physicians to use and apply techniques important to the practice of community-oriented primary care?
- Are physicians being taught the concepts necessary for managed and coordinated care practice?

The conference participants recognized that the world in which the primary care physician practices is changing rapidly. Technologies that recently were available only in leading academic medical centers are often now available in community hospitals and physicians' offices. An aging population will change the patient mix and the clinical problems that a primary care practitioner will see. Changes in reimbursement patterns are likely to put more constraints on physician income, while increasing the complexity of the reimbursement process (Ginsburg and Falkson, 1988). It is clear that as the environment for primary care changes, primary care educational programs will face new and increasing challenges, and inevitably the federal role to support the training of primary care physicians will continue only if society values the results.

References

American Academy of Family Physicians: Family Practice—Creation of a Specialty. Kansas City, MO, 1980.

Council on Graduate Medical Education: First Report of the Council. Vol. 1. Rockville, MD, 1988.

Garrison, L. Jr., and Wilensky, G.: Cost containment and incentives for technology. Health Affairs, 5:2, 1986.

Ginsburg, S., and Falkson, J.: Future Directions in Primary Care—An Overview of the Issues. Prepared for a conference sponsored by the Health Resources and Services Administration, DHHS, 1988.

Health Care Financing Administration: National health expenditures, 1986–2000. Health Care Financ. Rev. *8*:4, 1987.
Mider, G. B.: The federal impact on biomedical research. Adv. Am. Med.: Essays at the Bicentennial, *2*:806, 1976.
Raffel, M. W.: The U.S. Health System: Origins and Functions. New York, John Wiley and Sons Inc., 1980.
Russell, L. B., and Burke, C. S.: The political economy of federal health programs in the United States: An historical review. Int. J. Health Serv., *8*:55, 1978.
Thurm, R. H.: Early history of the U.S. Public Health Service (marine) hospitals: The first federal prepaid medical care plan. Mt. Sinai J. Med. *37*:568, 1970.
U.S. Department of Health and Human Services: Chronology-Health Professions Legislation 1956–1979 (Publication No. [HRA] 80–69). Rockville, MD, 1980.
U.S. Department of Health and Human Services: Report of the Task Force on Medical Liability and Malpractice. Washington, D.C., U.S. Government Printing Office, 1987. *The report reviews the problems related to medical liability and malpractice, including relevant aspects of health care, professional liability law, and the insurance industry.*
U.S. Department of Health and Human Services: Sixth Report to the President and Congress on the Status of Health Personnel in the United States. Rockville, MD, 1988. *This provides a substantial amount of data and analysis on trends relating to the education, supply, and distribution of physicians and other health personnel.*
U.S. Department of Health and Human Services, Bureau of Health Professions: The Location of Family Practitioners and Other Medical Specialists in Shortage and Rural Areas. Report No. DHPA 81–6, Hyattsville, MD, December, 1980.
Wilensky, G. R.: Filling the gaps in health insurance: Impact on competition. Health Affairs, *7*:3, 1988. *This provides an overview of recent trends in the uninsured population and potential strategies for reducing gaps in coverage for the uninsured.*

Canada

Reg L. Perkin

Canada As A Country

Canada is the largest country in the western hemisphere and second largest in the world. Its territory is diverse, ranging from wide fertile prairies and farm lands, large areas of mountains, rocks and lakes, to northern wilderness and arctic tundra. The greatest north-south distance is 4,634 km., and the greatest east-west distance is 5,514 km. The total area of land and fresh water is 9.97 million square km (Statistics Canada).

The climate is extremely variable. Most areas experience four seasons, with warm dry summers and cold snowy winters. The winters are milder in the southern half of British Columbia. Arctic conditions prevail across the northern parts of Canada.

There is no permanent settlement in approximately 89 per cent of Canada. Only the smallest province, Prince Edward Island, is completely occupied. Canada has a population of 26 million. Most of these people live in a narrow band to the north of the U.S. border. Toronto, Montréal, and Vancouver—the three largest metropolitan areas—have a combined population of 8 million people that represents 30 per cent of Canada's population.

As in other parts of the western world, birth rates dropped in Canada in the late 1960's and during the 1970's and have now stabilized. The net result is that the number of young children is stabilizing, but the population in the age group 14 to 24 is lower. The adult population continues to increase, particularly in the older age groups. The number of citizens over the age of 65 has doubled in the past 25 years, and the rate of increase in this age group is twice that of the population as a whole.

More than four of five (84 per cent) of Canadians live in families. Although the proportion of Canadians in families has been gradually declining, the number of families is increasing at a rate slightly greater than 1 per cent per year and currently stands at approximately 7 million. The typical Canadian family is now smaller, having decreased from an average size of 3.9 people 25 years ago to 3.1 at the present time.

Historically, Canada is a bilingual country—15.3 million people (61 per cent of the population) report English as their only mother tongue, and 6.2 million (24 per cent of the population) speak French. The francophone population is concentrated in the Province of Québec. Some of the native population of North American Indians and Inuit continue to live in the north and on reservations, while others have integrated into urban areas and other communities across the country. Canada has attracted a large number of immigrants from all parts of the world and 2.9 million people (11 per cent of the population) report a language other than English or French as their mother tongue. In recent years, immigrants from Asia have outnumbered those from Europe by a ratio of 2:1.

Medical Manpower

In the decade from 1975 to 1985, there was an increase of 33 per cent in the number of physicians while the population grew only 11.4 per cent. During this period, the 16 Canadian medical schools were graduating a total of 1,750 students per year, and the number of immigrant physicians averaged approximately 350 per year. Excluding interns and residents, the 1985 population per physician ratio ranged between 511:1 in British Columbia and 820:1 in New Brunswick.

Maneuvers to prevent an oversupply of physicians have already taken place. Medical school enrollment has been reduced so that the graduating class is now less than 1600 per year. Physician immigration has also been curtailed. In some provinces, there have been cutbacks in the number of funded postgraduate training positions in the residency programs.

Canada maintains a 50:50 ratio between family physicians and consultant specialists. In the decade from 1955 to 1965, when the population of Canada increased by 18 per cent, the number of specialists increased by 94 per cent and the number of family physicians by only 4 per cent (Perkin, 1967). One of the important factors in this trend away from family practice was the lack of family physician teachers in the Canadian medical schools. With the introduction of family medicine departments into the medical schools in the late 1960's and early 1970's, this trend was reversed, and an equal ratio between family physicians and consultant specialists was maintained.

Distribution of physician manpower continues to be a problem in Canada. Incentive schemes in some provinces have been successful in encouraging physicians to practice in more remote areas. British Columbia introduced a system of restrictive billing numbers in order to control the number of physicians in the heavily populated lower mainland of that province, but this legislation has now been reversed by the courts. Innovative methods of communication and support, such as telemedicine and ambulance services, have been instituted to assist physicians practicing in remote areas.

Generally speaking, the physician population in Canada is appropriate to the needs of the Canadian people. The increasing number of female physicians, who for personal and family reasons work less than their male counterparts, will require that the supply of physicians be maintained at least at the present level. Forty per cent of the graduating medical class in Canada is female, and it is anticipated that this will increase to at least 50 per cent by the year 2000. Recent studies have indicated that the female physician on the average provides 70 per cent of the patient care services of the average male physician (Moore, 1982; Woodward and Adams, 1985).

Medical Education and Academic Family Medicine

GENERAL INFORMATION

There are 16 medical schools in Canada, graduating a total of 1600 students per year. Three schools in the Province of Québec are francophone. All undergraduate programs are of 4 years in duration, except for one school which has a 5-year program and two schools that have 3-year programs with an extended academic year.

The undergraduate programs are accredited in a manner comparable to medical schools in the United States. The postgraduate programs in family medicine are accredited by the College of Family Physicians of Canada (CFPC) and those in the other specialty disciplines by the Royal College of Physicians and Surgeons of Canada (RCPSC). Beginning in 1986, joint accreditation of postgraduate programs has been undertaken by the CFPC and RCPSC in conjunction with the licensing bodies in each province, thereby streamlining the accreditation process for the medical schools.

Medical education in Canada is funded by the provinces through the ministries of education and health. The educational costs for medical students are heavily subsidized, and postgraduate trainees are paid a salary by the provincial government. The majority of faculty members receive only partial income from the university for their teaching and administrative responsibilities, supplementing their income with fee-for-service patient care dollars and research funds.

FAMILY PRACTICE RESIDENCY PROGRAMS

The declining interest in family practice as a career, demonstrated by medical students during the 1950's and 1960's, led to the development of family medicine departments in the 16 medical schools in the late 1960's and early 1970's. The initial activities of these new academic departments focused on providing postgraduate training. The first three family practice residency programs began in 1966 at the University of Calgary, McMaster University, and the University of Western Ontario. They were initially of 3 years' duration but were reduced to 2 years beginning in 1970.

By the mid-1970's, there were family practice residency programs in all 16 medical schools. The programs are based on educational objectives, developed by each medical school in cooperation with the CFPC. The basic format of the 2-year program consists of 8 months of family medicine, 12 months of appropriate hospital rotations, and 4 months of elective time. Additional experience in a third-year program is available for a small percentage of trainees who require extra training to practice in rural or remote areas or who wish to pursue an academic career or an area of special interest, such as emergency medicine or geriatrics.

Family practice teaching takes place in family practice units, established in conjunction with the teaching hospitals, and also in community health centers and the medical practices of community-based family physician teachers. Community hospitals are also used to supplement the experience available in the teaching hospitals.

Continuing involvement with a group of patients is a prominent feature of family practice residency training in Canada. This allows the resident to experience continuing comprehensive care under supervision, including learning experiences, such as following an obstetrical patient through the prenatal period, doing the delivery, and then looking after the mother and newborn. Teaching in the family practice units includes intensive supervision using videotape and one-way glass. There is a strong didactic program of seminars and other learning experiences. In-training evaluation is carried out at regular intervals and residents who achieve the educational objectives are recommended by the university program director following the 2 years of training to take the certification examination of the CFPC.

Family practice residency programs in Canada are graduating approximately 450 family physicians per year. This represents slightly more than half of the 50 per cent of medical school graduates who choose family practice as a career. Some Canadian graduates still enter family practice following a 1-year internship or a portion of an RCPSC specialty program. It is anticipated that within the next 3 years there will be sufficient family practice residency training positions available in Canada to accommodate all trainees proceeding to a career in family practice.

UNDERGRADUATE MEDICAL EDUCATION

Increasing involvement in the undergraduate curriculum has been a major focus of academic family medicine in Canada in recent years. A family medicine clerkship is now part of the core curriculum in the final year in all but four Canadian medical schools, where it is still an elective. The family medicine clerkship is usually of 4 to 6 weeks' duration and takes place in family practice units or community teaching practices. The CFPC currently has a Task Force on Undergraduate Education, which is assisting medical schools to strengthen their undergraduate programs.

In those medical schools where the family medicine clerkship is well established, family physician teachers have become more extensively involved with the curriculum in the earlier undergraduate years. This includes teaching interviewing skills, physical examination, ethical issues, and the clinical relevance of the body systems' approach in the other disciplines. Family medicine electives have been developed that allow students to gain ambulatory clinical experience, participate in family medicine research, and explore family practice as a career in different community settings.

FAMILY PRACTICE RESEARCH

The bedrock and lifeblood of any academic discipline is research. Now that family medicine departments are more firmly established in the Canadian medical schools, and some of the early priorities and pressures are past, a great deal more attention is being focused on research and other scholarly activities. Academic family physicians, working through the university departments of family medicine with the collaboration of the CFPC and other international groups such as the North American Primary Care Research Group (NAPCRG), have started to contribute very significantly to medical research in Canada.

The CFPC has developed a national sentinel network of community family physicians, the National Research System (NaReS). Freestanding papers by family physician researchers now constitute one of the most popular sessions on the program of national and chapter annual scientific assemblies of the CFPC. Specific research projects, such as the CFPC Quality of Care Study that established a very sophisticated protocol for peer review assessment of a family physician's office practice, have excited international interest.

FACULTY DEVELOPMENT

Special graduate programs leading to a Master's degree have been developed at the University of Western Ontario and McGill University.

The CFPC has developed a Section of Teachers as a semiautonomous branch within the College that provides a focus for full-time and part-time academic family physicians, as well as non-MD teachers in our university programs. The Section conducts faculty development workshops on a regular basis.

CONTINUING MEDICAL EDUCATION

Since its inception in 1954, the CFPC has required a minimum of 50 hours of approved CME annually to maintain membership. The CFPC still provides direct CME through its annual scientific assemblies at both the national and provincial level, as well as other educational programs. However, there are now a large number of CME providers in Canada, primarily at the 16 medical schools, and the CFPC accredits the CME programs produced by these bodies.

Certificants in family medicine are required to do a Maintenance of Certification Program every 5 years, under the supervision of the CFPC. This is a CME program in which participation is required to maintain certification in family medicine, but there is no pass/fail decision made on each physician.

The CFPC also offers a Self-evaluation Program in both a print and computer format. Computerized patient management problems are also being developed and will soon be generally available.

The Health Care Delivery System

Responsibility for health care is shared between the federal and provincial governments, with the major responsibility resting with each province. The federal government through Health and Welfare Canada is responsible for providing health care to Indians and Inuit, public servants, certain immigrant and refugee groups, and residents of the Yukon and Northwest Territories.

Health insurance is universal in Canada through a series of interlocking provincial plans all of which share the common elements of comprehensiveness of services, universal population coverage, reasonable accessibility to services, portability of benefits, and nonprofit administration by a public agency. The plans are designed to give all Canadians access, on a prepaid basis, to needed medical and hospital care. A formal structure of committees at each level provides the mechanism for federal/provincial cooperation.

Financing is through federal/provincial cost-sharing formulae and direct provincial funding through general revenue, supplemented by premiums in four jurisdictions (Ontario, Alberta, British Columbia, and the Yukon).

Payments for physician services are negotiated in each province between government and the medical association. The majority of Canadian physicians are paid on a fee-for-service basis, accounting for 95 per cent of the payments nationally. There is increasing interest in alternate payment mechanisms, which exist only to a minor degree at the present time.

The overall cost of health care in Canada, including expenditures by all levels of government and the private sector, reached $39.2 billion in 1985. This calculates to $1554 per person.

Many battles have been fought in Canada between physicians and the government over the extra billing issue, and the government has won every time. Since 1987, physicians must accept the fee provided by the provincial medical care plan as full payment for insured professional services, and extra billing is not allowed.

The major concern of physicians and other health care workers in Canada is that the amount of funding available from the public purse will not be sufficient to provide the quality of medical care that will be demanded by Canadian patients. At the same time, there is consensus that Canada has a good health care system at the present time. What is required in the future is a willingness on the part of government to look at innovative ways of supplementing the public funding with money from the private sector in a way that will maintain quality and still preserve the principles inherent in the Canadian health care delivery system.

Scope of Family Practice in Canada

The 50:50 ratio between family physicians and consultant specialists in Canada results in a situation where most of the primary care is delivered by family physicians. They offer a broad range of clinical services in the community, the hospital, and other health care facilities. Canadian family physicians continue to have good access to the country's hospitals.

The majority of babies are still delivered by family physicians, 56 per cent of whom continue to offer obstetrical care and do an average of 32 deliveries per year. The majority of family physicians work part time in the emergency department, and most admit their own patients to the hospital and participate appropriately in their in-hospital care. Very little major surgery is now done in Canada by family physicians, but they continue to be important providers of anesthesia services. In 1986, 26 per cent of the anesthesia services in Canada were provided by family physician anesthetists (Canadian Medical Association).

The scope of family practice varies from one geographic region to another. In the large cities, family physicians are mostly office and community based, less likely to look after their own patients in the hospital, and involved to a lesser degree in obstetrics and emergency care. The smaller centers, including the community hospitals, are often staffed entirely by family physicians, and in those settings, family physicians provide a broad range of services including obstetrics, emergency surgery, and anesthesia. Suburban areas and larger towns would include a mixture of these practice patterns.

Current Trends and Future Prospects

There is a major move at the present time in Canadian medical education to enlarge the resources for family practice residency training to provide sufficient positions for the 50 per cent of graduates choosing family medicine to take the 2-year family practice residency program. More attention is also being directed towards additional training in such areas as obstetrics and anesthesia, necessary for trainees planning to practice in remote areas.

There is more research activity in family medicine. Quality assurance and peer review are attracting much more attention. Hospital care is being deemphasized, and more effort directed to providing care in the community. This results in the role of the family physician being more important to the health care system, particularly in directing the extension into the community of services previously provided in hospital. Health maintenance, care of the elderly, and palliative care are finally gaining the recognition that they deserve.

The major challenge for family medicine in Canada is to predict the type of family physician that will be required to serve the needs of Canadian patients in the 21st century and to determine that the training being provided for students now is appropriate to their anticipated role in the future.

References

Canadian Medical Association: Report on the Training of General/Family Practitioners to Provide Anaesthesia Services. Ottawa, CMA, May 1988.

College of Family Physicians of Canada: Canadian Family Medicine. Educational Objectives for Certification in Family Medicine, 2nd ed. Toronto, CFPC, 1981.

Moore, C. A.: Family physician manpower: Poor planning with inaccurate data. Can. Med. Assoc. J., *127*:1180, 1982.

Perkin, R. L.: Medical manpower in general practice. Can. Med. Assoc. J., *97*:1569–1572, 1967.

Statistics Canada: Canada Year Book 1988. Ottawa, Statistics Canada, 1987.

Woodward, C., and Adams, O.: Physician resource databank: Numbers, distribution and activities of Canada's physicians. Can. Med. Assoc. J., 132(10):1175–1178, 1182–1188, 1985.

Britain

John Fry

Three fundamental facts must be borne in mind when looking at any national health care delivery system.

1. There are four inevitable and essential levels of care, each with its own roles, skills, techniques, and educational needs; these include self-care, primary professional health care (including family practice), general specialist care, and subspecialist care.
2. There is no single best-buy system that can be applied and accepted universally.
3. Each system evolves historically and is influenced by social customs and culture, economic wealth, geography, and even religion and politics.

The United Kingdom

The United Kingdom is an old country with new roles and problems. It has lost its great empire and the wealth from it and has become a densely populated offshore island of Western Europe. A democratic parliamentary monarchy, the United Kingdom's recorded history goes back more than 2000 years. The United Kingdom now includes England, Wales, Scotland, and Northern Ireland. Its population is 57 million, including 5 per cent recent immigrants from the West Indies, Asia, and Africa. A strong liberal and social philosophy has permeated each of the three main political parties (the Conservative, Labour, and Liberal parties), and a national social welfare and health system is accepted by all of them.

SOCIAL CHANGES

Major social changes have taken place and are taking place. Birth rate has fallen to 13 per 1000 from 17 per 1000 in the 1960's. Life expectancy (at birth) now is 72 years for males and 78 years for females; 15 per cent of the population is over 65 and 3 per cent over 85 (numbers over 85 are predicted to double over the next 40 years).

Families are becoming smaller, with less than 2 children per married couple, and more dispersed, so care for the elderly is less by the family, particularly as more than one half of married women are working.

One child in 10 lives with a single parent, and the divorce rate has increased so that one out of three marriages are likely to end in a divorce. Cohabitation is rife, and one out of five births is illegitimate; in two thirds of these, there is a stable relationship.

Although 10 per cent of the working force is unemployed, more wealth, personal amenities, and comforts exist than ever before, but crime has increased, with more violence and vandalism.

Health is improving, smoking has been cut by one half over the past 20 years, only one third of adults smoke (with higher rates in young women).

THE NATIONAL HEALTH SERVICE (NHS)

When it was introduced on July 5, 1948, the NHS was not a new system. I have been in my practice in Beckenham since 1947; on July 6, the only dramatic change was that no longer did I have to bill my patients. Since 1948, I have received regular remuneration based on capitation fees—a set annual fee for each person registered with me and for whom I undertake to provide continuing care—plus other fees for special services, such as obstetrics, immunization, cervical cytology, family planning, and night visits. In addition, I am reimbursed for the rental and rates (local taxes) of my premises, and for 70 per cent of the wages of the staff that I employ. If I am appointed as a *trainer* of family medicine residents (trainees) or if I work in a group practice of three or more family physicians, I am paid extra. I am also paid expenses for continuing medical education courses. This many-faceted system of payments has evolved from negotiations between the profession (British Medical Association) and the government (Department of Health).

The British general practitioner is well paid compared with other professionals. His or her job is secure, and he or she receives a generous pension from the NHS upon retirement, based on total career income.

It must be emphasised that the British citizen is free to choose freely any general practitioner of her or his choice; vice versa, the general practitioner is free to accept or reject patients. There is no compulsion or restriction from any bureaucracy. In fact, there is relatively little bureaucracy in the NHS as far as general practice is concerned.

The NHS organization and administration are in the hands of Parliament. NHS is paid for out of direct and indirect taxation. The national administration includes 15 regional health authorities and some 140 district health authorities. Each region and district administers and organizes hospitals—specialist, general practice, and public health community services.

The whole population is covered by the NHS, which is now 41 years old. Although free at the time of delivery, the NHS costs 6 per cent of the Gross Domestic Product (GDP) annually or $750 per person. In the United States, health care costs almost 12 per cent of the gross national product and over $1600 per person per year. However, 10 per cent of the British population is covered by private health insurance in addition. Most are a part of extra work benefits with premiums paid by employers. The services used are mainly for elective surgery and the benefits are shorter waiting times for admission to hospital and more luxurious facilities.

General medical care (family practice) makes up almost 20 per cent of the NHS costs—8 per cent to physicians and 12 per cent for their prescribing costs.

GENERAL PRACTICE AND HOSPITALS

Except in some rural areas, there is generally a clear distinction between the hospital specialist service and general practice. The hospital service is staffed medically by trained, appointed specialists and junior residents. General practitioners do not have hospital privileges to care for their own patients.

Referral

When a patient requires specialist advice and attention or hospitalization, I refer that patient with a referral letter to one of my hospital specialist colleagues. These colleagues carry out their tasks and then refer the patient back to my care with a full report. This report is filed in the patient's lifelong records, but they are the property of the NHS. When a patient moves and registers with a new family practitioner, the records are sent on to the new doctor. There is no patient self-referral to a hospital, except for accidents or emergencies. General practitioners can refer their patients directly to local hospital departments for full pathologic and radiologic studies with no cost to themselves or to their patients.

Although in only 1 out of 10 of consultations does the general practitioner refer the patient to hospital, the proportions of the population who use the hospital service are high. Thus, 13 per cent of the population were hospitalized in 1988, 18 per cent were referred for an ambulatory specialist consultation, and 22 per cent were treated in hospital emergency rooms.

Trends in General Practice in NHS: Facts and Figures

There is one general practitioner to 2000 persons. The maximum number of patients allowed per general practitioner is 3500. As in the United States, Canada, Western Europe, and Australia, we are approaching a situation in which there may be a surplus of physicians. The numbers of general practitioners are increasing annually.

THE PRACTICE

Most of the 30,000 general practitioners in the United Kingdom work in small groups. Only 10 per cent are in solo practice. The mean number of general practitioners per group is between four and five. This trend toward group practice has been dramatic because, in 1950, well over half of the general practitioners were working solo.

Most (75 per cent) general practitioners work from premises that they own and for whose buildings and arrangements they are responsible. But there are over 1000 health centers. These are specially constructed buildings in the community designed to accommodate not only general practitioners but other social and nursing health workers as well. Over 6000 general practitioners now work from such health centers. Recently, the building of such new health centers has slowed because of current national political decisions. Health centers are built and owned by local government authorities; the practitioners are tenants.

THE TEAM

A significant trend over the past 15 years has been the evolution of the primary health team. The concept is to provide shared medical and health care in the community through general practitioners' working with nurses, public health nurses (health visitors), midwives, social workers, and practice medical secretaries—all based on the practice unit and premises.

Most practices now utilize such paramedical colleagues. The nurses, health workers, midwives, and social workers are employed by the NHS and not by the practice. Such associations have worked well and have brought an extension of joint care into the community and better collaboration with local hospitals.

Recently, there has been a change and practices are employing their own practice nurses (for whom they receive a reimbursement of 70 per cent of their salaries). These nurses work in the practice treatment room and have taken on a considerable amount of follow-up care, screening, and health promotion. There are now over 6000 practice nurses.

PRACTICE VOLUME

The volume of work in a typical practice is as follows:

1. Some 70 per cent of the practice population will consult one or more times each year.
2. The mean consultation rate is three to four consultations per person.
3. The weekly total of consultations is approximately 155 (this includes 15 to 20 home visits and a few hospital visits).

TEACHING AND TRAINING

There has been a preceptor type of training for general practice for many centuries. General practice is now recognized as a special field of medical work requiring special skills and training. It is the largest field of medical work—almost half of all practicing physicians in the NHS are general practitioners.

Education and training in general practice in the United Kingdom now encompasses one's entire professional lifetime. All undergraduate programs in medical schools include a set period of teaching on general practice during the 5-year curriculum, and most have their own faculty departments. For those who decide on a career in general practice, there is a 3-year mandatory period of vocational training (residency). One year is spent in an approved training practice, during which time the trainee is attached to a trainer. The 2-year hospital period is spent in selected specialties, such as obstetrics and gynecology, psychiatry, or pediatrics. Continuing medical education is well organized in the NHS. Each district general hospital has its own postgraduate medical center with library, lecture hall, seminar rooms, and catering facilities at which regular meetings, courses, and so forth are arranged almost daily.

THE FUTURE

In 1989, the Conservative government, following its policy of getting better value for money, put forward discussion proposals for changing general practice. These included better services for the public, which included more information for patients about the practice, more public participation, and better access to and availability of care. There were proposals to make general practice more efficient and cost effective with more supervision and controls to promote better quality and standards of care through changes in remuneration acting as suitable incentives.

Thus, more health checks, screening, computerization, better surveillance of child development, and care of the elderly were proposed. To achieve these, more teamwork and role sharing (with nurses and others) was suggested. Premises were to be visited regularly to comply with suitable standards, and general practitioners were to be made to retire at 70 years. (It is said that a number aged 90 and over are still practicing!)

In spite of these changes, general practitioners will remain as independent contractors running their practices as they wish in keeping with agreed standards.

THE NHS: ADVANTAGES AND DISADVANTAGES

In summary, it is useful to note the pros and cons of the NHS in an honest and constructive manner. On the positive side, the NHS provides a well-organized national health service that is available to all at no cost at the time of care, a strong general (family) practice component with its own education and training programs, referral system to hospital specialist services, family medicine as a general rather than a specialized discipline, primary care teamwork, and full access to hospital pathology and radiology facilities. The negative aspects of the NHS include poor incentives and rewards for good quality care by the general practitioner, exclusion of general practitioners from hospital bed privileges, insufficient control and coordination of primary care with possibly too much clinical independence and freedom, waste of resources, lack of operational data on which to base policy decisions, and hospital waiting lists for admission (for elective surgery) that may be 3 to 12 months.

Australia

Wesley E. Fabb

The Country

Australia, the world's largest island, is 3 million square miles in area but populated by only 16 million people. Contrary to the popular image of Australia as a land of rural dwellers, all but 14 per cent live in urban areas stretched mainly in a coastal belt from the far north of Queensland to the southwest of Western Australia. Over the last 30 years, there has been a large urban shift of population parallel with the growth of industry and commerce. Australia is now one of the most highly industrialized nations in the world, with the attendant problems of environmental pollution and heavy population density.

The People

Australia has a mixed ethnic population; over 50 ethnic groups are represented in considerable numbers. Of the 21 per cent of Australians who are born overseas, 7 per cent come from the United Kingdom; 7 per cent from Greece, Italy, Yugoslavia, and other European countries; and, more recently, increasing numbers have come from Southeast Asian countries (Australian Bureau of Statistics, 1987a). Australia's original inhabitants, the aborigines, number only 206,000, with less than half of these people living in their tribal areas.

The population is aging. Thirty years ago, only 8 per cent of the population were over 65, but by the end of this century, the figure will be at least 12 per cent (Cameron, 1980). Most Australians live in separate or semidetached housing. Only 2 per cent live in high-rise apartments. Fifty-seven per cent of families own or are buying their own home (Australian Bureau of Statistics, 1987b).

In providing health care, the significant social factors to be considered are the increasing age of the population, the high level of urbanization, the geographic remoteness of a small part of the population, the presence of significant unemployment, and the existence of areas of poverty that affect the health of a small proportion of the population.

Australia's Health Care System

When the colony was founded 200 years ago, hospitals became a central element in the provision of health care. Alongside these, private practice and public health services gradually emerged. After World War II, the Commonwealth Government introduced a pharmaceutical benefits scheme, which made some prescription drugs available at little or no cost; a medical benefits scheme, which provided refunds of part of the doctor's fee; hospital benefits, which subsidized hospital care; and a pensioner medical service, which provided free medical services for retired persons. A number of voluntary health insurance agencies arose to provide private health insurance.

In 1974, a universal health insurance program, Medibank, funded by the Commonwealth Government, was introduced. It covered a wide range of pharmaceutical, medical, and hospital benefits. Since 1976, this has been progressively dismantled, and now health insurance is provided only by private funds. About 50 per cent of Australians are covered by this private insurance (Commonwealth Department of Health, 1986). In 1984, the government introduced Medicare, which provides a rebate of 85 per cent of family physicians' consultation fees and a higher proportion of specialist fees, and free hospital accommodation for people using public hospital facilities. It is funded by a taxation levy. About 20 per cent of the population—pensioners, single parents, and the socially disadvantaged—have been issued a Health Benefits Card by which they receive free health care.

There is a strong public hospital system in each of the six states and two territories, which is administered by state health departments. Although previously providing free services to all, some charges are now being levied for persons who are not Health Card holders. Services are provided by salaried or sessionally paid medical and nursing staff.

Municipal health services provide infant welfare, public health, and supportive services, such as home help and meals on wheels.

The Doctors

A strong private sector exists in Australia. Seventy per cent of all consultations take place in private consulting rooms, and a further 11 per cent in the home (Australian Bureau of Statistics, 1980). The family physician conducts about 78 per cent of the consultations in the community, specialists 12 per cent, and hospital doctors 10 per cent. With the growth of specialization, the proportion of family physicians dropped to a low of 33 per cent in 1978 but is now over 40 per cent and rising steadily. In 1986, there were over 34,000 doctors in Australia, of which over 14,000 were family physicians, 10,000 specialists in private practice, and the rest were hospital doctors, administrators, or researchers. Twenty-two per cent of all doctors, and 25 per cent of family physicians, were female (Commonwealth of Australia, 1988a). The family physician-to-population ratio was about 1:1100.

The Costs

The cost of providing health care has risen from $2 billion (Australian dollars) in financial year 1970 and 1971 to $11 billion (Australian dollars) in 1981 and 1982 (Australian Institute of Health, 1985a). In 1981 to 1982, expenditure on health care was 7.6 per cent of the gross domestic product, of which 47 per cent was spent on hospitals, 9 per cent on nursing homes, 17 per cent on medical services, and 9 per cent on pharmaceuticals. Only 0.6 per cent was spent on health promotion and illness prevention (Australian Institute of Health, 1985b).

Medical Education in Australia

Australia has 10 medical schools. The annual output of Australian resident graduates is declining from over 1300 graduates in 1985 to a projected 1160 in 1994 (Commonwealth of Australia, 1988b). Of new enrollments in medical schools in the 1980s, about 40 per cent were women (Commonwealth of Australia, 1988c). Medical schools have, in general, developed along traditional lines, and it was not until the mid-1970's that undergraduate departments—variously called community practice, community health, community medicine, or general practice—were established in all medical schools. Unfortunately, these departments emerged at a time when funding was becoming restricted and their development has been constrained (Saint, 1981). Nonetheless, they have engendered a heightened awareness of the opportunities available in family practice, and increasing numbers of students have chosen this vocation on graduation from medical school. Nine medical schools have 6-year courses; one has a 5-year course.

Almost all postgraduate vocational (residency) education and continuing education in the specialties, including family practice, are the responsibility of the academic colleges, which are independent of the universities. The first of these to be established was the Royal Australasian College of Surgeons in 1928; since then, the number of specialist colleges has risen to 11. The Royal Australian College of General Practitioners was founded in 1958 and is a leader in the field of medical education in Australia. It has a widely read monthly journal, innovative national and local educational programs, a well-regarded fellowship examination, and, since 1973, a vocational training program for family practice—the Family Medicine Program. College membership has grown to about 6000, including almost 2000 fellows by examination.

The Australian Medical Association, although not an academic body, has had a vast influence on the practice of medicine in Australia. About 50 per cent of Australia's doctors are members.

Inquiry into Medical Education

In April 1988, a Committee of Inquiry into Medical Education and Medical Workforce submitted its report to the Commonwealth Government (Commonwealth of Australia, 1988d). It made a number of recommendations about medical education: the fostering of self-directed learning in medical schools; early exposure of undergraduates to family practice and the provision of funding to achieve this; assessment of attitudes, skills, and problem solving as well as knowledge in medical schools; the better training of undergraduate teachers; more opportunities for medical and public health research; and the greater use of computer-aided instruction.

It also recommended the compulsory completion of two postgraduate years before registration for unsupervised practice, the introduction during these years of an educational program and a 3-month community placement for all graduates to give experience in community practice, and the provision of adequate funding to support these developments.

The Committee's recommendations concerning graduate or vocational training included: the continuance of Commonwealth Government funding for vocational training for family physicians, stronger links between universities and vocational training programs, and the development of educational programs in community services, health promotion, disease prevention, efficient health care delivery, Aboriginal health, and social and mental health. The Committee felt unable to recommend mandatory training for all entering family practice but recommended a review of the need for mandatory training in 5 years.

The Committee endorsed the need for continuing education based upon physicians' needs and recommended the greater use of computer and satellite networks. The Committee embraced the concept of self-directed learning and the need for quality assurance and research.

On the issue of the medical workforce, the Committee recommended the establishment of a Medical Workforce Review Committee to analyze workforce data and to maintain an output of Australian resident graduates appropriate to the health care needs of the community. The Committee recommended that medical schools investigate alternative means of selecting medical students, broaden the socioeconomic mix of students, and analyze the effect of the admission of mature students.

How many of these recommendations will be implemented remains to be seen.

Family Practice in Australia

The pattern of morbidity, as established by the Australian General Practice Morbidity and Prescribing Survey 1969 to 1974, shows morbidity similar to other developed countries (Bridges-Webb, 1976). The survey showed that for every episode of illness, just over 2.5 doctor contacts were made. Eighty per cent of these were in physicians' offices, 12 per cent in the home, and the rest were indirect contacts. Visits to the middle-aged and elderly constituted 70 per cent of the home visits.

The over-65 age group had the most doctor contacts, with the middle-aged and young adult groups not far behind. The most common presenting conditions in children were respiratory diseases, accounting for 50 per cent of morbidity in the pediatric group; whereas, in the geriatric group, 26 per cent presented with cardiovascular conditions, 12 per cent with respiratory conditions, and 11 per cent with musculoskeletal conditions.

A survey by the Australian Bureau of Statistics on doctors' consultations in 1983 showed that in the 2 weeks before the survey 18 per cent of the sample surveyed had consulted a doctor, of which 89.5 per cent presented for illness or injury, 5.5 per cent for a check-up, 3.5 per cent for pre- or postnatal care, and 1.5 per cent for immunizations (Australian Bureau of Statistics, 1986). The relatively small proportion presenting for preventive care is noteworthy, as it points to a deficiency that still exists in Australia's health care system. However, there are increasing signs of public interest in prevention and health promotion, and doctors are responding by providing information and by installing surveillance programs in their practices.

The use of medical services varies with age and sex: infants average 10 consultations per year, preschool children seven, school children and adult males three, adult females six, and the elderly seven (Australian Bureau of Statistics, 1980; Bridges-Webb, 1973 and 1974). The average number of visits to the family physician per capita of population per year is 4.5 (Bridges-Webb, 1981). In the Australian Bureau of Statistics study mentioned previously, 65 per cent of the population surveyed had seen a doctor within the last 6 months, and almost 80 per cent in the last 12 months. These figures indicate the opportunities available for preventive care and health promotion.

THE FAMILY PHYSICIAN

In the late 1960's and early 1970's (when there was a shortage of family physicians), the average number of patient contacts per week was 160 (Bridges-Webb, 1981). By 1980, the number of contacts had dropped to 130 per week, and it continues to fall as the number of family physicians increases. The average urban physician works 50 hours per week, of which 40 hours are devoted to clinical work (Bridges-Webb, 1981).

Although group practice has grown over the last 30 years, there are still many solo practitioners; perhaps as many as 40 per cent of family physicians are in solo practice. Locum or deputizing services became established in the late 1960's during the family physician shortage, and, although now operating at a lower level of activity, these services continue to provide some out-of-hours care in the large cities. Home visits, always a feature of Australian family practice, are coming back into vogue after almost disappearing during the family physician shortage. Recently, a number of 24-hour clinics have appeared in the larger cities, usually funded by entrepreneurs and staffed by family physicians and specialists. Pathology and radiology services are usually provided on site. These convenience clinics provide prompt service for urgent and episodic illness, but cater less for chronic problems. They have made substantial inroads into the practices of nearby doctors.

VOCATIONAL TRAINING FOR FAMILY PRACTICE IN AUSTRALIA

Training for family practice in Australia is the responsibility of The Royal Australian College of General Practitioners, which is supported financially by a Commonwealth Government grant to conduct its family medicine program. The course is of 4 years' duration, of which 1 year is spent in hospital posts following the intern year, 2 years in family practice posts, including 6 months in accredited teaching family practices, and 1 year in an elective post (The Royal Australian College of General Practitioners, 1988). Educational resources are available for use in the educational program accompanying in-service training and for personal study.

The family medicine program adopts a self-directed learning philosophy. Trainees are encouraged to take responsibility for their own learning. Program staff assist trainees in determining their personal program of learning, which is documented in the form of a learning plan negotiated between the trainee and the trainee's advisor. Formative assessment is carried out throughout training to assist trainees to identify strengths and weaknesses. A Certificate of Satisfactory Completion of Training is awarded to those who satisfy the program's requirements. In 1989, a program of progressive summative assessment was introduced, and after 1992, the Fellowship of The Royal Australian College of General Practitioners will be awarded to those who meet the standards set by the College.

There are 1850 trainees in the family medicine program, of which over 1400 are full-time trainees.

There are over 700 accredited family practices and over 150 hospital programs. The family medicine program is decentralized into almost 90 training areas. Each area has a coordinator—usually a practicing family physician—who oversees the training process in his or her area and conducts an educational program. In the larger states, areas are grouped into regions supervised by a regional coordinator. The regional and area activities are coordinated by seven state offices. In turn, the state offices are coordinated by a national office that provides educational and administrative support and a large resource center that houses over 90 per cent of the family medicine program's educational resources. These are available on loan anywhere in Australia. A television studio produces audiovisual materials specific to the needs of Australian trainees. The family medicine program operates with the equivalent of only 24 full-time academic staff members. It relies heavily on its large contingent of part-time area and regional coordinators, training advisors, and family physician supervisors, who oversee the training in accredited family practices.

Although there is no compulsion to take training for family practice, about 80 per cent of those who enter it do so through the family medicine program.

CERTIFICATION IN FAMILY PRACTICE

The Royal Australian College of General Practitioners conducts a fellowship examination, which is the certifying examination in family practice. The examination consists of eight tests: case commentaries, multiple choice, clinical interpretation, patient management problems, diagnostic interviews, management interviews, physical examination, and practice assessment. Most trainees in the family medicine program see the fellowship as the end point of their training, and from 1992 many will obtain their fellowship through progressive summative assessment rather than the examination.

The Future of Health Care in Australia

In planning health care for the future in Australia, attention needs to be paid to a number of contemporary issues: the escalating cost of health care and the concern of governments with cost effectiveness; the overemphasis on hospital care and high technology and the low priority given to community-based health care; the changing needs and expectations of the community; the increasing public interest in self-care, prevention, and health promotion; the increasing number of aged and disabled; the increasing number of doctors—especially women; the rise in the number of allied health professionals; the demand for a quality assurance mechanism linked to continuing medical education; the low priority given to research, especially community-oriented research; and the inadequate funding of training for family practice.

It seems clear that what is needed in the decades ahead is a reorientation of medicine toward the promotion of health, health education, and the prevention of illness and disability and a greater involvement of the patient in taking responsibility for his or her own health care. There will need to be a move away from hospital-based high technology to the care that can be provided by family physicians and other community-based health care workers. This trend is already apparent.

The training of family physicians should equip them to provide preventive and promotive services as well as the traditional curative and rehabilitative services. However, the full potential of family physicians in providing preventive care and in promoting health will not be realized until there is proper funding of these activities.

Now that an adequacy of family physicians seems assured for the next decade or two, they need to be trained and deployed in a way that enables them to meet the current and emerging needs of the community. It is up to training programs in family medicine to ensure that this challenge is met.

References

Australian Bureau of Statistics: 1986 Census of Population and Housing Australia, Canberra, ABS, 1987a, p. 173.

Australian Bureau of Statistics: 1986 Census of Population and Housing Australia, Canberra, ABS, 1987b, p. 188.

Australian Bureau of Statistics: Australian Health Survey 1983 Canberra, ABS, Cat. No. 4311.0, 1986, p. 24.

Australian Bureau of Statistics: Australian Health Survey 1977–78 Doctor Consultations, Canberra, ABS, Cat. No. 4319.0, 1980.

Australian Institute of Health: Australian Health Expenditure, Canberra, AIH, 1985a, p. 6.

Australian Institute of Health: Australian Health Expenditure, Canberra, AIH, 1985b, p. 23.

Bridges-Webb, C. (Ed.): The Australian general practice morbidity and prescribing survey, 1969–1974. Med. J. Aust., Special Supplement, October 2, 1976, p. 9. *This was the first thorough survey of morbidity patterns and prescribing in Australia. It enabled researchers to compare and contrast morbidity in Australia with that in other countries.*

Bridges-Webb, C.: The Traralgon Health and Illness Survey. Int. J. Epidemiol., *2*:67, 1973.

Bridges-Webb, C.: The Traralgon Health and Illness Survey. Int. J. Epidemiol., *3*:37, 1974.

Bridges-Webb, C.: How many GP's is enough? Aust. Fam. Physician, *10*:678, 1981.

Cameron, R. J.: Social Indicators Australia, No. 3. Canberra, AGPS, Australian Bureau of Statistics, 1980, p. 8.

Commonwealth Department of Health: Annual Report 1985–86, Canberra, AGPS, 1986, p. 118.

Commonwealth of Australia: Australian Medical Education and Workforce into the 21st Century, Committee of Inquiry into Medical Education and Medical Workforce, Canberra, AGPS, 1988a, p. 371, 382. *This is the largest survey of undergraduate, vocational, and continuing medical education in Australia. In a volume of over 600 pages, it describes the views of the hundreds of groups and individuals that made submissions to the Committee of Inquiry and the conclusions and recommen-*

dations drawn by the Committee from them. It focuses too on medical manpower needs in Australia into the 21st Century. It has become a standard reference work for health planners and medical educators.

Commonwealth of Australia: Australian Medical Education and Workforce into the 21st Century, Committee of Inquiry into Medical Education and Medical Workforce, Canberra, AGPS, 1988b, p. XXVIII.

Commonwealth of Australia: Australian Medical Education and Workforce into the 21st Century, Committee of Inquiry into Medical Education and Medical Workforce, Canberra, AGPS, 1988c, p. 522.

Commonwealth of Australia: Australian Medical Education and Workforce into the 21st Century, Committee of Inquiry into Medical Education and Medical Workforce, Canberra, AGPS, 1988d.

Royal Australian College of General Practitioners: Training for General Family Practice with the Family Medicine Programme. Melbourne, RACGP, 1988, pp. 5–37. *This booklet describes the features of the Family Medicine Programme of The Royal Australian College of General Practitioners, which is responsible for training Australia's family physicians. Recently updated, it describes all aspects of the programme for intending applicants, trainees entering the programme, and those interested in vocational training for family practice.*

Saint, E. G.: Community Practice in Australian Medical Schools. Tertiary Education Commission Evaluative Studies Program, Canberra, AGPS, 1981. *This report describes the development of departments of community practice in Australian medical schools since their inception in the mid-1970's.*

New Zealand

John Richards

New Zealand general practice owes much to the British tradition. It remains the most widely practiced medical discipline with approximately 40 per cent of all medical graduates selecting general practice as a career.

The major difference from North American family practice is the absence of hospital privileges. With a few exceptions, once a general practitioner admits a patient to the hospital, that patient is totally under the care of the hospital specialists. The notable exceptions to this rule are certain geriatric hospitals and some obstetric units.

This means that the New Zealand general practitioner is denied the stimulus to keep up to date that is fostered by a close association with hospital peers. Other sources of postgraduate education have to be sought. Fortunately, there is no shortage of these.

Nature of the Practice

As a further compensation, the New Zealand general practitioner tends to be more heavily involved in domiciliary care, although even this has tended to diminish because of the demands it makes on time and the high cost of gasoline. Nevertheless, most general practitioners would make at least three house calls each day, which on average represents about 10 per cent of the total daily consultations. There is even some domiciliary obstetrics.

Training

Today, most general practitioners complete the obligatory 6 years of medical school training and follow that with 2 years of hospital residencies and 1 year of specific vocational training before embarking on independent practice.

In fact, New Zealand legislation permits a physician to enter general practice after only 1 year of hospital-based postgraduate experience, but this is frowned upon and is uncommon.

THE ROYAL NEW ZEALAND COLLEGE OF GENERAL PRACTITIONERS (RNZCGP)

This college is the local equivalent of the American Academy of Family Physicians. Now completely independent, it arose originally as an offshoot of the United Kingdom's College of General Practitioners.

This organization has as its principal objective the furtherance of general practice and, in particular, is dedicated to ensuring the best possible patient care. It also strives to facilitate good working conditions for physicians as a means to that end. The RNZCGP has been responsible for the development of what is known as the Family Medicine Training Programme (FMTP), which has been successful in securing state funding.

FAMILY MEDICINE TRAINING PROGRAMME (FMTP)

Trainees are eligible to enter this 1-year program of vocational training, provided they have completed 2 years of hospital-based rotating residencies.

The FMTP training varies slightly from year to year and from place to place. In general, it affords 6 to 9 months of supervised general practice experience in an approved practice in the community and 3 to 6 months of further hospital residency. During this latter residency, it is hoped to fill any training gaps that remain after the previous 2 years of hospital experience.

It is hoped that one or two of the trainees, who are known as registrars, will spend this time in an academic department of general practice, rather than the hospital. Such trainees will assist in the teaching programme for undergraduates and undertake some research. This, it is hoped, will provide a first step towards developing a cadre of appropriately trained academics as the future teachers of family practice.

Throughout the whole of the year, FMTP registrars are released from their other work for a half day, during which, usually accompanied by their general practice supervisors, they attend a series of seminars designed to further their knowledge and understanding of the discipline.

The registrars are also encouraged to take a half day each week to attend some other service that is likely to benefit their overall education (e.g., visits to family planning clinics or to dermatology outpatient clinics etc.).

Membership of the RNZCGP is not obligatory for general practitioners, but well over 50 per cent of all general practitioners are either fellows, members, or associates.

Today, entrance to the College is primarily by examination, and candidates who complete the FMTP find they have fulfilled all the prerequisites to enable them to take this examination. However, physicians who have completed at least 2 years of relevant hospital experience and at least 6 months of general practice experience are also eligible to take this examination without formal postgraduate training.

The examination is looked upon as a benchmark of competence in general practice and the pass rate is high.

Candidates who pass the examination are invited to become associates of the College but are not admitted to full membership of the College until they have completed a further 2 years of general practice experience and have submitted themselves to further evaluation procedures that do not include a formal examination. In fact, the most significant part of this final evaluation is a practice visit by a senior College member who reviews the candidate's practice facilities and equipment; ensures that the practice organizes appropriate out-of-hours cover for emergency calls and additionally sits in with the candidate during a half day of consultations.

General practitioners who have had more than 10 years of practice experience can apply for this second part of the evaluation without having to submit to the more formidable first part. This is not an uncommon method of entry to membership of the College.

Members of the College at the time of their entry undertake to maintain continuing education, but there is as yet no formal requirement and no ongoing assessment of competence.

ACADEMIC DEPARTMENTS OF GENERAL PRACTICE

Undergraduate training for general practice has been provided since the early 1970's. The strength of the teaching departments has recently been enhanced by the endowment by one individual—a retired elderly woman general practitioner, Dr Elaine Gurr—of two chairs of General Practice: the first at the Otago School and the second at Auckland.

It should be noted that there are also departments of general practice at the clinical schools in Wellington and Christchurch but these, as yet, lack a professor.

Practice Arrangements

A majority of general practitioners in New Zealand work in groups. Many of these are two-person practices. Very few practices would have more than five physicians. It is usual to employ a receptionist and a practice nurse although in a few small practices this role is filled by one person. Occasional, larger practices employ a practice manager and, even more rarely, a trained counselor. Such staff are usually paid a salary by the doctor, and the doctor is paid a fee for service by the patient.

Methods of Payment

Many years ago, the government undertook to subsidize general practice services, and a subsidy was introduced (at the time, this equated about three quarters of the usual fee). Despite government promises, this subsidy has been allowed to fall far behind inflation and now, for a working adult, represents about 5 per cent of the physician's fee. The situation for the elderly and for children is slightly better but not good.

Obstetric services by general practitioners have always been fully subsidized, and no fee can be charged. The payment here has been upgraded from time to time but is still not an adequate compensation for the care given and responsibility taken. Laboratory investigations and most pharmaceuticals are also free to the patient except for a one dollar charge per prescription.

ACCIDENT COMPENSATION

In 1974, legislation was introduced that sought to do away with all litigation in accident cases. The aim was to provide complete medical care for all accident victims without cost to the patient. Eighty per cent of the victim's usual income was to be paid throughout the time of incapacity.

For some years, a 100 per cent subsidy of doctors' fees was paid by the Accident Compensation Corporation—the body set up by the government to organize this. The 100 per cent subsidy was conditional on the physician's charging a fee that was considered reasonable by New Zealand standards. After some years and with dwindling reserves, the corporation began to dispute the quantum of fee considered to be reasonable, and this soon fell to an obviously unrealistic figure. So, physicians began to charge their patients again—albeit, only the difference between the subsidy the corporation was willing to pay and their usual fee. The situation remains unresolved but it seems likely that the corporation will be required to increase the subsidy.

From the foregoing, it is clear that the whole question of how the physician is paid needs careful review. With this in mind, a Health Benefits Review Committee was set up in 1986, and it brought down an analysis of possible future options in a report entitled "Choices for Health Care." So far no action has been taken on this report.

PRIVATE INSURANCE

Because of the failure of the subsidies for medical care to keep pace with inflation, many members of the public have sought to bridge the gap with private insurance. Almost one third of the population now has some form of private medical insurance.

Practice Location

Despite considerable subsidization, the New Zealand general practitioner maintains a substantial measure of independence. General practitioners are free to practice where they like and patients are free to choose any general practitioner at any time. The Department of Health provides a loose surveillance of practitioners but has virtually no powers to implement any measures designed to ensure adequate practice standards although some control over extravagant prescribing is possible, and, occasionally, the subsidy has been removed temporarily if a physician is considered to be seeing excessive numbers of patients.

In the future, many of the health department functions are likely to devolve onto local area health boards, and it is possible that physicians will contract with these Boards to provide primary health care services. If and when this occurs, a variety of payment systems may be introduced.

Referral

The general practitioner is perceived as the gatekeeper to medical care, and specialist services are almost always dependent upon general practitioner referral. Specialists who see patients without referral are viewed with strong disapproval. Seen in this light, general practice may, in the future, be the key to maintaining the costs of health care within acceptable limits.

References

Choices for Health Care. Report of the Health Benefits Review Committee, 1986.

Geyman, J. P., and Fry, J.: Family Practice: An International Perspective in Developed Countries. East Norwalk, CT, Appleton-Century-Crofts, 1983. *The section on family practice in New Zealand, written by the present author, covers in more detail the present situation of general practice in that country.*

Israel

Max R. Polliack

The same social, cultural, and economic changes that characterized the development of modern, industrialized societies have been reflected and compressed into the 40 years that have elapsed since the State of Israel was re-established in 1948. During this brief period, the Jewish population has increased sevenfold, due mainly to successive waves of immigrants and refugees from the holocaust of war-time Europe and the Middle East. During the first 3 years, over 650,000 refugees were admitted, exceeding in number the total Jewish population at the time. Concomitantly, and despite the recurrent wars and economic crises, the country has raced through an accelerated process of modernization, industrialization, and urbanization based on extensive educational, social, and technological programs that have transformed the parched deserts, eroded hills, and malarious swamps into a flourishing modern Welfare State.

These changes and the rapid development of comprehensive hospital and community health services have eradicated the major infectious and tropical diseases endemic in this region. Maternal mortality is almost zero, and infant mortality has dropped to 11.4 per 1,000 live births. Life expectancy at birth for Jewish men and women (73.9 and 77.3 years respectively), and for non-Jews (72.0 and 75.8 years respectively), compares favorably with most developed countries. Today's population numbers 4.3 million of whom 83 per cent are Jews, 14 per cent Moslems, 2 per cent Christians, and 1 per cent Druses and other religions. Of these, 55 per cent were born in Israel, 25 per cent in Europe or America, and 20 per cent in Asia or Africa. Eleven per cent are over the age of 65 years (Statistical Abstract, 1987).

Primary Health Care Services

Almost 96 per cent of the population are covered by prepaid health insurance. Premiums based on income, with fixed maximums, entitle all members to extensive social and medical benefits and to the full range of primary and hospitalization services. The Kupat Holim Health Insurance Institution provides comprehensive health insurance and medical services to 80 per cent of the population in its own network of clinics and hospitals throughout the country. Four small Sick Funds provide health insurance and primary care services to 16 per cent of the population, mainly in urban areas. The Health Ministry, Hadassah Organization, Malben Joint Distribution Committee, local health authorities, and other agencies also maintain extensive hospital facilities and additional services, especially for the aged and the handicapped.

Primary health care (Polliack, 1986) is provided in rural areas by doctor-nurse teams in local clinics or in large centers serving 2000 to 3000 residents of nearby settlements. In urban areas, services are based on clinics serving 5000 to 20,000 people, with laboratory and radiologic facilities, and specialist consultants accessible in the clinic or in larger regional clinics or hospital outpatient departments. Most family physicians work in multidisciplinary teams with nurses and allied health personnel, with an average practice panel of 1500 to 2000 patients. The Sick Funds also contract with independent doctors who usually practice from modest premises or their own homes. Overt private practice is increasing but mainly limited to patients seeking additional opinions or endeavoring to bypass the queues and prolonged waiting times that typify the freely available health services.

Israel is well endowed with medical manpower (doctor:population ratio = 1:450), maintained by immigration and by four medical schools that graduate 300 doctors annually. Nevertheless, our health services have long faced serious organizational problems especially at the community level. These have been aggravated by the structural split between preventive and curative services, fragmentation and lack of coordination, overutilization in the absence of cost containment measures, and an irrational bias in the distribution of medical resources toward the hospital services. These and other factors have contributed to producing a major crisis in the health services (Professional Public Commission, 1988).

Development of Family Medicine

The concept of community-oriented health care was envisaged in 1953, when the pioneer Health Centre, staffed by doctors and allied health personnel, was established in Kiryat Hayovel in Jerusalem as a model teaching unit for the University Department of Social Medicine (Kark, 1974; Abramson et al., 1981). General practice was already recognized as an independent medical specialty in 1963, thus preceding most, if not all, other countries in this respect (Scientific Council, 1963). Its status was, however, clearly inferior to that of other specialties, and it failed to attract local graduates.

The need for family physicians led to the establishment of the first Department of Family Medicine, in the Tel-Aviv University Sackler Medical School, with an obligatory clinical clerkship for all students (Medalie et al., 1969) and an innovative 4-year residency training program (Polliack and Medalie, 1969). Since then, and for many years as the sole academic department in Israel, it provided the major impetus to the renaissance of family medicine as an independent medical specialty. Further impetus was provided in later years by the establishment of academic departments in the medical schools in Jerusalem, Haifa and Beer Sheba, the latter with an integrative community-oriented undergraduate curriculum (Segall et al., 1978). These departments are now increasingly involved in student teaching and residency training in five regions (see table at bottom of page).

National Examination Boards were established in 1975, followed by the founding of the Israel Association of Family Physicians in 1977. In 1980, the Tel-Aviv Department introduced the first academic study program leading to a postgraduate diploma and a Master's degree in family medicine. During this period, the Kupat Holim Sick Fund has played a

	Tel-Aviv	Haifa	Jerusalem	Afula	Beer Sheba	Total
Accredited trainers	43	8	6	5	4	66
Residents	110	39	34	30	24	237

crucial role by investing considerable budgets and expanding training and practice facilities for residents in its clinics.

Residency Training Programs

Residency training is provided within the service framework of Kupat Holim by whom the residents are employed and under the auspices of the University Departments of Family Medicine in each region. The Scientific Council of the Israel Medical Association (IMA) has statutory responsibility for accrediting and monitoring all programs. The curriculum extends over a 4-year period after completion of the mandatory internship year and consists of (IAFP, 1984):

1. 27 months of full-time hospital rotations: internal medicine (12 months); pediatrics (6 months); mental health (3 months); two electives (3 months each) in either dermatology, ophthalmology, gynecology, otorhinolaryngology, geriatrics, orthopedics, rehabilitation, or emergency care.
2. 21 months full-time clinical practice: assistantship in the tutor's practice (9 months); independent practice with tutelage (12 months).
3. Postgraduate diploma studies provided by an academic department of family medicine comprising: comprehensive clinical management, interpersonal concepts and skills, family and community-oriented health care, and practice organization.
4. Board examinations: primary—written, and final—oral clinical assessments.

Successful completion of the program entitles residents to specialist certification by the Health Ministry.

Licensure and Certification

Recent government legislation requires mandatory examination as a precondition for medical licensure or residency training, except for physicians who have completed recognized preinternship examination or who have practiced continuously for 20 years. Specialists whose primary and final Board examinations are recognized by the Scientific Council of the IMA, or who have practiced as specialists for 5 years and been exempted from the primary Board examinations of the Scientific Council, may also apply for exemption from licensure examination. Practice eligibility is not recognizable for specialist certification in family medicine. The Scientific Council is, however, prepared to recognize and accredit equivalent components of overseas residency programs but requires completion of those components not accredited, prior to recognizing Board eligibility or specialist certification.

Future Trends

Several commissions have recommended the reassessment of the traditional roles of the Health Authorities and Sick Funds and a radical reorganization of the health care system with increased priority and resources for family and primary medicine (Scientific Council, 1977; Professional Public Commission, 1988; Workshop, 1988). If these are to be implemented, several major issues must be addressed.

The Continuum of Medical Education. Because future health needs are not easily predictable, it is undesirable to orient medical students toward one branch of medicine, albeit hospital- or community-based. The universal trend towards specialization has effectively lengthened formal medical education to 11 years or more, of which the undergraduate period is common to all physicians and residency training specific to each specialty. There is also an inevitable trend to link continuing medical education (CME) with continuing medical practice. These trends will increasingly obligate academic departments to accept teaching responsibility throughout the full continuum of medical education, and to provide appropriate educational programs at all levels. They also obligate academic departments to develop a cadre of family physician-tutors with clinical, teaching, and research skills commensurate with accepted academic criteria. Medical school priorities and resources for Family Medicine must increasingly reflect these trends.

Improved Residency Training. Traditional hospital rotations are more oriented toward service commitments than toward the objectives of residency training. Their relevance should be reviewed in relation to the clinic setting in which the residents will ultimately practice. All residents should be affiliated with University Departments of Family Medicine that should assume responsibility for the quality of training programs in their region. Department facilities must be decentralized and supplemented by greatly expanded outreach and teaching activities in the accredited practices and in regional clinics accessible to tutors and residents in the area. Without negating the complementary role of full-time hospital and university faculty and model clinics, it seems essential that academic family physicians must also be perceived as clinical role models in the normal service setting, if they are to maintain their credibility in the eyes of their residents and colleagues. Health Service authorities must, therefore, recognize the principle that academic activities are an integral part of the work of the family physician-tutor, and his service commitments should reflect and facilitate these objectives. There is, thus, an urgent need to establish a formal framework within which academic departments and Health Service authorities could coordinate their activities as legitimate partners in improving facilities for effective residency training in the clinics.

Maintaining Professional Competence. All physicians employed in Kupat Holim Clinics are entitled to regular paid study leave and organized CME is readily available. Weekly academic studies, lectures, seminars, and clinical sessions are provided by the Department of Family Medicine in Tel Aviv and are attended by over 200 family physicians and general physicians. Weekly academic courses and regular study days are also provided by the Departments of Family Medicine in Jerusalem, Haifa, and Beer Sheba. The Israel Association of Family Physicians and the Postgraduate Institute for Medical Studies of Kupat Holim and the Hebrew University provide regular study days and meetings for family physicians and general physicians. Although recertification is not mandatory for maintaining professional licensure or specialist certification, the Scientific Council of the IMA has acknowledged the importance of regular CME in maintaining professional competence. Its Education Committee has already established the criteria and framework for accrediting and monitoring CME and for certifying physicians who complete these requirements. The linkage of such certification with professional and academic advancement could facilitate and encourage all physicians to demonstrate and verify their commitment to ongoing education.

Improved Practice Facilities. Progress in the development of family medicine as an independent academic and clinical specialty has been most impressive during the past decade. Future progress, however, ultimately depends on the formulation of national policies and priorities by the Health Service Authorities and Sick Funds to ensure an organizational framework in which residency-trained family physicians could work effectively and provide comprehensive family-oriented health care to their practice populations.

If these challenges are effectively addressed, family medicine could continue to provide an efficient and cost-effective foundation for the health care system in Israel.

References

Abramson, J. H., Gofin, R., Hopp, C., et al.: Evaluation of a community program for the control of cardiovascular risk factors: The CHAD program in Jerusalem. Israel J. Med. Sci., *17*:201–212, 1981.

I.A.F.P. (Israel Association of Family Physicians): The content of residency training for family medicine. Fam. Phys. (Israel), (Suppl), *12*:(2): 1–47, 1984.

Kark, S. L.: The development of community medicine and primary health care in a neighbourhood. *In* Epidemiology and Community Medicine. New-York, Appleton-Century-Crofts, 1974, pp. 334–348. *A classic book presenting innovative concepts of the community determinants of health and disease, community health and diagnosis, based on the author's extensive experience in integrating public health practice with comprehensive personal care, and the practical application of these concepts in a pioneer health center established in an immigrant community setting in Jerusalem in 1953.*

Medalie, J. H., de Vries, A., and Shachor, S.: The department of family medicine in the Tel-Aviv University Medical School. Lancet *2*:979–981, 1969.

Polliack, M. R., and Medalie, J. H.: Programme for specialization in family medicine. Br. Med. J., *4*:487–489, 1969.

Polliack, M. R.: National perspectives in Israel. *In* Fry, J., and Hasler, J. C. (Eds.): Primary Health Care 2000. London, Churchill Livingstone, 1986, pp. 295–308. *An international team of 31 contributors, each with a special interest in primary health care, review progress and common issues, problems and needs for action in achieving the aim of the World Health Organization (WHO) program of health for all by the year 2000, launched at the Alma-Ata conference in 1978.*

Professional Public Commission for Establishing Policy, Organizational and Functional Reform of the Health Care System: Recommendations of the Trainin Commission. Jerusalem, Health Ministry, 1988. *This report of a governmental enquiry commission presents a comprehensive analysis of the crisis in the health care system. It proposes that the Health Ministry dispose of its hospitals to an independent nongovernment Hospital Authority, and restrict its responsibility to legislative and supervisory aspects. It also recommends increased resources and priorities for community health services based on residency-trained family physicians.*

Scientific Council of the Israel Medical Association: Manual for Specialty Training and Residents. Jerusalem, Israel Medical Association, 1963.

Scientific Council of the Israel Medical Association: Report of the commission on the organization of medical services in the community. Fam. Phys. (Israel), *7*:342–354, 1977. *This report, also published in English, establishes guidelines and proposals for the reorganization of medical services based on residency-trained family physicians working in multidisciplinary health care teams and coordinated with community and hospital services.*

Segall, A., Prywes, M., Benor, D. E., and Susskind, O.: University Centre for Health Sciences, Ben Gurion University of the Negev. An Interim Perspective. *In* Katz, F. M., and Fulop, T. (Eds.): Personnel for Health Care: Case Studies of Educational Programs. Geneva, WHO, 1978, p. 111.

Statistical Abstract of Israel, No. 38. Jerusalem, Central Bureau of Statistics, 1987.

Workshop for Problems of the Economy: Report on the Economic Aspect of the Public Health Services. Van Leer Jerusalem Institute, January 1988, pp. 1–98.

17

Sociocultural Influences on Medicine and Health

Kent D. Bergh
Donald S. Asp
Kathleen A. Culhane-Pera

Understanding Sickness and Healing

In this chapter, we will examine how cultural beliefs influence the meaning of sickness episodes for patients and physicians, how the social environment shapes the incidence and consequences of sickness and the process of medical care, and how both patients and physicians seek to prevent and relieve suffering due to sickness. We will address how physicians can use an awareness of these aspects of sickness to best advantage when caring for patients (including those who speak another language), perceive their illness from an unfamiliar cultural viewpoint, or are subject to social circumstances remote from those in the physicians' own experiences. We will also examine how physicians can apply this awareness to understand how their own cultural and social viewpoint influences their effectiveness and their experiences as physicians.

Sociocultural processes influence sickness at the level at which the whole person interacts with the beliefs of others and institutions. The phenomena described by biochemical, histologic, physiologic, psychologic, cultural, and sociologic levels of analysis can be thought of as interacting with each other in a hierarchy of progressively greater complexity. Such a concept of sickness as a complex, multilevel system has been termed a *biopsychosocial* model (Engel, 1977).

We will refer to the pathophysiologic abnormality perceived by clinical medicine as the *disease*, the unpleasant, culturally defined state of being experienced by sick people as the *illness*, and the resulting disturbances of social roles and interactions as *sickness*, which will also serve as an inclusive term (Twaddle, 1979; Eisenberg, 1980).

Pathophysiologically based approaches to medicine treat diseases as real entities. A disease is not an observed fact, however; it is a description of observed processes accepted by some observer, often for complex social or cultural reasons. For example, some consider starvation or a hangover to be diseases while others do not (Campbell et al., 1979). Medicine's clinical approach arose from values and beliefs about the nature of reality promoted by social changes during the industrial revolution. Our medical perceptions continue to be influenced by experiences as members of stratified, intricately subspecialized, and bureaucratically organized societies (Foucault, 1973).

The values and perceptions of clinical medicine are not always shared by patients from other cultural or social backgrounds. Their sickness experience is correspondingly different. It can be translated, but we interpret it as outsiders, using analogies (Geertz, 1973). When immigrant people like the Hmong describe "soul loss" as a cause of sickness, American physicians can only approximately translate this concept into our medical model of disease or our conventional sense of reality.

Physicians may be unable to help patients even from their own society if they attend only to their physical or psychologic diseases. Apparently normal people present symptoms that cannot be explained physiologically (although we may say they are somaticizing); they complain of conditions that physicians do not accept as real diseases (i.e., folk illnesses); they unexpectedly fail to follow our advice (noncompliance); or they react to our diagnoses or advice in ways we find inexplicable (persisting, for instance, in taking medications that we believe cannot possibly be of value). Events such as these are due to the pervasive influence of sociocultural processes in sickness and in medical encounters. For many common problems in ambulatory care settings—from headache to abdominal symptoms—technical proficiency and adherence to protocol bear less relationship to good outcome than does the ability of the physician and patient to agree on the nature of the problem presented and to attend to its psychosocial aspects (Bass et al., 1986).

Most patients have their own ideas about what is wrong with them, fears about what may be wrong, interpretations about what this means and what may occur because of it, and hopes and expectations about what should be done about their illness. Difficulties arise when physicians make inaccurate assumptions about these matters (Beckman and Frankel, 1984). Patients in such instances are generally dissatisfied with their care, and physicians may feel they have wasted much time and effort. The sociocultural factors in medical care are so important that it is reasonable for the physician to consistently seek to learn from the patient about the illness, and consider its social consequences, before attempting to settle on a management plan, even in everyday illness encounters.

Illness as a Cultural Phenomenon

Cultural gaps affect the physician's and patient's ability to communicate, to agree upon the nature of the problem and settle upon a mutually acceptable treatment plan. When refugees or foreign students arrive at a clinic, or when a physician practices in a foreign country, the cultural differences between patients and physicians are often easily recognized. Cultural differences also influence the clinical interactions between patient and physician who superficially share the same cultural background.

Helman (1984) defines culture as "a set of guidelines (both explicit and implicit) which an individual inherits as a member of a particular society, and which tell him how to view the world, and how to behave in it in relation to other people, to supernatural forces or gods, and to the natural environment." Cultural knowledge is learned and constantly changes. Every subgroup in society is identifiable because it develops some cultural uniqueness. Groups and individuals within groups have multiple, varying, and often conflicting views. Cultural views are like lenses or veils through which people perceive, understand, and interpret the world. We are so accustomed and have so adjusted to our own cultures that often we cannot notice their influence. We each assume our interpretations about the world are accurate, although they are necessarily shaped by the lenses or veils through which we see.

CULTURAL MODELS OF ILLNESS

All societies have medical models that instruct their members how to interpret bodily functions and malfunctions, often with analogies from everyday life. As western society developed machinery, people utilized the current models to explain the body (Scheper-Hughes and Lock, 1987). In the past, the brain has been explained in mechanistic terms of gears, levers, and steam, later in electrical terms of circuits, wires, and currents, and more recently in the popular idiom of computers. Cultural metaphors are resources for action. Scientists, physicians, and patients with a culturally mechanistic model of the body perceived the possibility of replaceable parts, which led to the technology of prosthetics and organ transplants.

Cultures' models of the body and of illness are related to their descriptions of the physical, social, and spiritual aspects of reality. The anthropologic literature provides many descriptions of these models. The Quollahuaya-Andean Indians understand a mountain's structure in terms of human anatomy and explain human malfunctions in terms of landslides and earthquakes. Classical Chinese theory blended Taoist cosmology and Confucian social ideals into a system of harmony, balance, and mutual interdependence, which explained social interactions as well as organ interactions (Scheper-Hughes and Lock, 1987). Concepts of optimal balance are common in many cultural models of illness; balance between humors, illnesses, foods, and medicines with hot and cold properties have been described throughout the world.

Patients' cultural models of the body's structure and function influence their interpretations of bodily symptoms as well as their interpretations of physicians' actions, descriptions, and recommendations.

For example, Asian patients influenced by the Chinese humoral model react negatively to venipunctures since they believe they weaken the body and that loss of an irreplaceable vital substance unbalances the humors within. The Hispanic model of balance between hot and cold may require that a hot condition receive a cold treatment. A hot antibiotic may be perceived as increasing the imbalance, worsening rather than improving the illness (Harwood, 1981).

Most cultures believe that impaired relationships between the sick person and family members, society, or spirits can lead to illness, while harmonious relations contribute to health. Often in traditional societies, "(t)he body . . . is dependent upon, and vulnerable to, the feelings, wishes, and actions of others, including spirits and dead ancestors" (Scheper-Hughes and Lock, 1987). For Southeast Asians with animist beliefs, good relations with ancestral spirits need to be maintained so the ancestors can protect their descendents from attacks by evil spirits (Muecke, 1983). Disagreements with neighbors and family members in some black American social networks may result in hexes or curses (Mathews, 1987). Stress and contagion are often perceived as social causes of illness in both British and American cultures (Helman, 1978; Gillick, 1985).

INDIVIDUAL EXPLANATORY MODELS OF ILLNESS

Learning a society's predominant popular medical models does not ensure success at interpreting any given person's illness model because there is much variation in any culture (Good and delVecchio-Good, 1980). Families have their own health cultures, which produce variations in belief within ethnic groups (Guarnaccia, et al., 1985). Individuals have varied understandings and perspectives, depending on their special social roles (such as occupation, caste, education) and on their age, sex, or individual history (Fabrega and Hunter, 1978; Garro, 1988).

A set of ideas about an illness can be considered an explanatory model of the illness. Kleinman has suggested that explanatory models of illness deal with five main issues: (1) etiology, (2) timing and mode of onset of symptoms, (3) pathophysiology or other mode of action, (4) expected course and consequences, and (5) preferred treatment (Kleinman, 1980). The explanation gives the illness a culturally appropriate personal meaning and guides the health care seeking process. Patients, like physicians, often consider several models to be possible explanations of an illness—some of which they deem particularly likely and some more threatening or uncertain (Tuckett et al., 1985).

Patients' explanatory models can be quite different from the physicians' medical models. Blumhagen (1980) found that patients in a Seattle Veterans Administration hypertension clinic interpreted their disorder as due to anxiety, resulting in too much tension, for instance, while lay models of fevers and colds in Great Britain appear to indicate that the medical concept of bacterial infection has been transformed in popular belief to be consistent with older folk ideas contrasting cold and wet with hot and dry illnesses (Helman, 1978).

Sickness as a Social Phenomenon

The social circumstance of illness has been called the *illness predicament*. The illness predicament influences the role the sick person plays as events unfold. Following abdominal surgery, an elderly member in one family is placed in a nursing home; in another, he or she receives home visits by nurses and physicians; and in another, the family manages with the help of each other and folk healers. This variation is not all due to cultural factors. The resources available and beliefs of other people in the patient's social environment can be as important to the illness outcome as the diagnosis or the patient's own explanatory model. The illness predicament and the sick role reflect both large- and small-scale social processes.

HEALTH CONSEQUENCES OF SOCIOECONOMIC STRATIFICATION

The level of economic prosperity and the public health measures of a society have historically had more impact upon the health status of populations than individual medical care. Within populations, health often varies most strongly with socioeconomic status (DHEW, 1986). Since socioeconomic status (or social class) reflects a person's command of society's resources, those with greater resources can use them to avoid health risks as well as to obtain needed medical care. Those with fewer resources may be devastated by the demands of an illness. The links between socioeconomic status, the incidence of disease, the consequences of disease, and the usage of health care are complex, but a basic understanding of these relationships is important for understanding the differing meanings of sickness for individual patients in a medical practice.

The 1980 Black Report found that the premature death rate for the lowest social class in Britain was 2½ times that of the highest classes. Even conditions often considered characteristic of high social status (such as coronary artery disease, cancer, and stroke) produce higher premature mortality rates among the lower socioeconomic classes (Gray, 1982). Perinatal and neonatal mortality rates are most strongly associated with low income, family disorganization, and lack of education (Lieberman et al., 1987; Honigfield and Kaplan, 1987). In addition, infections, malnutrition, homicide, and accidents are associated with lower socioeconomic status worldwide (WHO, 1986).

The association between lower socioeconomic status and poor health is due to several factors. The occupations open to the less educated are more dangerous. Lower status social environments are also more hazardous. Falls, fires and pedestrian-vehicle accidents appear to be factors in the higher death rates of children from urban lower socioeconomic status families (Egbuonu and Starfield, 1982) and suicide, homicide, chemical dependency, and accidents are major socially influenced problems for lower socioeconomic status young adults (Amler and Dull, 1984). In many parts of the world, the social environment fails to consistently provide adequate or affordable food, water, housing, or sanitation. Interethnic, interracial, and interclass discrimination often accentuates the economic disadvantage and vulnerability of less powerful social groups (Wise et al., 1985). Warfare, armed robbery, refugees, and victims of torture are grave reminders of the health consequences of failures of social control over injustice and intergroup conflict around the world.

Peoples' access to health care varies with social status. In many areas of the world, access to primary health care is restricted by inadequate numbers of practitioners, inadequate facilities, long distances, and transportation difficulties. The choice of physicians or traditional folk healers in one rural Mexican region depended partly on how easy it was to get to a clinic (Young, 1981). In the United States, about 20 per cent of the population (primarily the working poor) cannot afford health insurance and are not included in public health plans, such as Medicare and Medicaid (DHEW, 1986). Members of this group are often forced to make direct choices between medical care and other basic needs. Lower socioeconomic status persons also may have fewer opportunities to master the jargon and language styles necessary to communicate their needs to bureaucrats or professionals who might help.

Limitation of access to medical care leads to increased morbidity and mortality (Aiken and Mechanic, 1986). Patients dropped from Medicaid in California developed poorer health within a year (Lurie et al., 1984). Both the individual and society may be poorly served by policies restricting access to care. For example, insurance company and government policies may require medical evidence of permanent disability for patients to qualify for income maintenance after work-related injuries but require evidence of potential for recovery to qualify for rehabilitation programs. Such limitations may increase the prevalence of chronic disability (Institute of Medicine, 1987).

Public decisions on industrial, social, and environmental policy can powerfully influence the health of individuals and populations. Such decisions often involve potential conflict between what is good for the majority and what would be best for particular subgroups or for individuals (Milio, 1983). Physicians can use the information they gain about the personal consequences of policies on individuals of different social circumstance and culture to help conflicting social and cultural groups embrace health-protective public policies in ways that balance group and individual interests.

SOCIAL NETWORKS AND SOCIAL SUPPORT DURING SICKNESS

When people are sick, the reactions of their personal social network are among the most important consequences of their illness. We identify with family, friends, or fellow employees, and with larger social groups, based on similarities of gender, age, race, or profession. We value approval from those with whom we identify; indeed, we value the disapproval of members of groups who compete, conflict, or otherwise are in contrast with our own group. We receive support for beliefs and habits characteristic of our group; they are among the prime criteria for group identity and membership (Totman, 1985; Brown and Levinson, 1987).

People with strong social networks have more opportunity to learn and identify with their own social group's cultural beliefs about illness, which may support or conflict with medical advice (Geertsen et al., 1975). Social support and peer pressure influence many behavioral risk factors for illness for better or for worse (Sorenson et al., 1986; Brown and Gary, 1987). Social support from families and religious groups generally inhibits smoking, drinking, and drug use (Jarvis and Northcott, 1987), but spouses, coworkers, or friends can make it harder to quit cigarettes or give up other habits associated with health risks (Sorenson et al., 1986; Brown and Gary, 1987).

Social networks help define the meanings of stressful life events, including illnesses, as well as provide social support for members during stressful events. Adequate social network support appears to decrease the risk of disease and death and improve disease outcomes and mortality—at least for diseases in which the individuals' behavior can influence the outcome (Berkman and Syme, 1979; Orth-Gomer and Johnson, 1987). Social support or the lack of it appears to be associated with ischemic heart disease, premature labor, alcoholism, depression, cancer, hypertensive stroke, accidents, and ulcers (Brown and Harris, 1978). Feeling valued and receiving help from social networks seem to buffer people against social stress. For instance, it appears to increase resistance to coronary artery disease (Seeman and Berkman, 1988).

In the face of increased threats to their health, the poor also have diminished resources. Medical care is costly, and illness further depletes financial resources (Eisenberg and Kleinman, 1980). The tangible assistance that social networks provide can be critical for persons with limited means. Networks are "the most adaptable and responsive" source of support for older people (Wentowski, 1981). People trade services such as nursing help, rides, temporary shelter, and short-term loans that otherwise may be prohibitively expensive.

Personal networks do require reciprocity, both to obligate others and to maintain participants' self-respect and sense of shared identity (Stoller, 1984). For those most dependent upon them, social network maintenance can consume a large proportion of available time and resources. When people become ill, their ability to maintain their networks by reciprocity may be threatened unless they have invested enough emotional and social capital in their networks to see them through. The physician can reduce the social costs of illness for the patient by inquiring about and considering the effects of his or her choices of diagnostic wording, explanations, and treatment plans on the patients' obligations to their personal network.

It is also useful to ask patients how their sickness might influence their ability to work, keep employment, and comply with work rules about illness absences. Powerlessness and poverty have destructive effects on social networks and social supports. Job insecurity can threaten self-esteem, and job stress has been found to deplete reserves of social support from coworkers and spouses. These processes increase the fragility of poor families (Marcellisen, 1988; Atkinson et al., 1986).

The Cultural Meanings and Social Environment of Medical Care

THE DECISION TO SEEK HELP

Patients' explanatory models of their illnesses include expectations about appropriate treatment for their conditions. Patients' social environments influence the therapeutic resources they have to choose from. The processes of health seeking and healing are complex. In this section, we will first explore the sociocultural factors that influence health-seeking behaviors and then we will turn our attention to those that influence healing and the medical care system itself.

Identifying an illness and seeking help can be thought of as a culturally defined sequence of stages for dealing with sickness. These include prevention, identifying symptoms and illnesses, anticipating prognoses, seeking the help, and managing the consequences, including recovery, disability, and death (Chrisman, 1977; Twaddle, 1979).

Almost every day, people experience possible symptoms that they first note, then monitor, interpret, and evaluate for familiarity, seriousness, and social acceptability. We think, perhaps, "What is this pain? Is it just a normal headache? Because it is bothersome, should I take the medicine I have at home? Since it hasn't gone away and is disturbing my work, is it serious enough to ask someone else for help?" This interpretation and evaluation of symptoms is influenced by the person's ethnic background, medical models, personal experiences, and social networks (Mechanic, 1972).

Once a symptom arouses concern, people may treat themselves or turn for help to their lay referral network—a social network of family members and friends thought best informed about illnesses, who may help with home remedies or over-the-counter medications (Chrisman, 1977). Most symptoms either respond or resolve spontaneously (Verbrugge and Ascione, 1987). If an illness seems persistent, serious, or embarrassing enough, people usually seek help from someone with specialized knowledge of healing—a folk or professional therapist (Kleinman et al. 1978, Kleinman, 1980).

Folk healers include herbalists, masseuses, spiritual healers, and practitioners of many other traditions. A healer's explanatory models of the patient's illness often derive from traditional cultural knowledge and from personal experience. Healers often have specialized folk knowledge or relative expertise in the general medical culture of a group, although not necessarily of the one to which their patient belongs (Staiano, 1981; Helman, 1984).

Patients' and families' lay referral networks continue to advise them while they seek help. They can promote, assist, delay, or discourage the referral of their members to folk healers or professional services. Social networks can establish expectations about the patient-provider encounter and about the outcome of the visit, influencing patient satisfaction. Members of a person's social network also evaluate the professionals' actions and plans after an interaction (Freidson, 1970; Chrisman, 1977).

If the physician's diagnosis and plan do not produce overall improvement within the total context of the person's life, including effects on self-image and standing with others, the advice will be rejected. People may find that following a treatment recommendation is incompatible with important social roles, contradicts beliefs shared with others who are important to them, or requires face-threatening actions. To wear a motorcycle helmet or to take regular medication may be to risk ostracism from certain social groups (Eisenberg, 1980). It may often be easier for a physician and patient to agree on how to proceed with an illness if the physician has first elicited a sense of the makeup and values of the patient's group of lay advisers.

People consider the benefits and costs of any culturally defined sick roles available to them when deciding where, when, and with whom to seek care. When people are sick, their behavior becomes deviant, in that they cannot meet normal cultural expectations. The acutely ill are often exempted from obligations and not held responsible for their deviance, but they are expected to want to and try to get well. Western society, for instance, distinguishes nonconformity labeled as sickness from the deviant behaviors labeled as crime, sin, and disloyalty. Those who make such distinctions are the status definers of the sick role. When the sick person and the status definers disagree, the person may be labeled as malingering or denying the illness. A person's different social identities are often associated with conflicting cultural definitions of sickness and expectations about how to conduct oneself while sick. People who assume some sick roles can be deprived of status and power, feelings of self-efficacy, and even their sense of identity. In the patient sick role, people may be expected to relinquish control over their own situation and give physicians autonomous power to help them (Freidson, 1970; Twaddle, 1979).

Physical barriers (such as location, availability, ease and cost of transportation), financial considerations (the costs of missing work or of baby-sitting, as well as direct costs for medical services), and social barriers (language, racial, ethnic, and social class differences between the providers and the patients) also contribute to people's decisions about adopting a sick role or becoming a patient (Berkanovic et al., 1981). Social barriers may have considerable impact on access to care, as patients from different social and cultural groups often feel alienated, unwelcome, and discriminated against in mainstream institutional settings. Physicians can lobby their affiliated institutions for action to decrease this alienation (for instance, through community involvement, bilingual and ethnic staff, culture brokers and patient advocates (Anderson et al., 1982). Physicians can help individual patients by asking about the interaction of the patient role with other roles the patient must fulfill and by attending to the often emotional responses of patients whose other social roles have unintentionally been compromised by the patient role.

HEALING AS A CULTURAL PHENOMENON

The social and cultural act of healing is not well understood, despite its familiarity. Healing is not an absolute event; rather, it is a subjective assessment that a treatment directed at an illness has been adequate. A physiologic disease process may be cured while the patient remains ill, while an illness may be healed, subjectively, without a physiologic cure. Healing is a cultural process involving the values and the explanatory illness models of the participants. It is influenced by the expectations of the social network, by socioeconomic class, and by the social relationships between healers, patients, and their family members (Eisenberg, 1980).

Healers of many cultural backgrounds use "psychosocial support therapies" that deal not only with illness "within the patients' body but also with his relationship with his society, and perhaps, dysfunctions as well within the society itself" (Foster and Anderson, 1978). Hence, one function of the healer may be to repair any perceived disorder in social and spiritual life. Healers may manipulate the symbolic nature of the illness as a psychotherapeutic strategy (Laderman, 1987; Turner, 1967). Both the "manipulation of important cultural symbols and the restoration of social harmony are critical elements in the healing process" (Johannes, 1980).

What healers actually do varies widely. Family physicians heal patients by doing a complete examination and providing a medical explanation and a prescription. An American faith healer might pray with a sinner before his congregation; a traditional Chinese physician might examine the pulse and prescribe herbal medicines; a rural Mexican healer might ritually sweep evil from a victim; and a shaman might suck an angry spirit from a person's body or transfer it to an animal sacrifice.

All healers seem to be more successful in dealing with patients' experiences of their illness and in promoting well-being when they share the patients' cultural world view, elicit the patients' explanatory models, and deal directly with their patients' experience of the sickness event. Physicians' successes at curing disease require close attention to pathophysiologic processes. Successful healing of illness requires similar attention to experiences or meanings of sicknesses. A poorly treated illness can unexpectedly and adversely affect even the best treatment of the patient's disease (Kleinman, 1980).

THE PHYSICIAN AND THE CULTURES OF MEDICINE

Physicians perceive patients' illness beliefs and predicaments through the lenses of their own particular personal and professional cultures (Hooper et al., 1982) (also see Chapter 4). Physicians use explanatory models of illness drawn from their formal academic training, the informal culture of clinical medicine, and their interpretations of the lay beliefs of their families and communities. The concerns, treatments, and criteria for success implicit in these models are not always congruent with each other.

Despite medicine's professional emphasis on independence from the patient, physicians' practices are often strongly, if naively, influenced by patients' lay expectations, particularly when competition is strong and peer support weak (Starr, 1982). Specialties and local practice communities also develop their own clinical practice styles, which are, in part, local, cultural responses to physicians' needs for social peer support, often for decisions they must make in the face of medical uncertainty (Wennberg et al., 1982; Eddy, 1984).

Academic medical education, by contrast, emphasizes the pathophysiologic management of acute disease by technical means. Sociocultural reasons for prevailing practices (and limitations on their value) are infrequently discussed (Freidson, 1970; Foucault, 1973; Starr, 1982). As a result, conflicts over values, power, and resources within medicine are usually presented as disputes over technical competence (delVecchio-Good, 1980; Bosk, 1986). In the socioeconomic hierarchy of specialties that has evolved in this cultural environment, family practice has a relatively low status and is poorly reimbursed. This sometimes inhibits even family physicians from giving adequate attention to the sociocultural aspects of patient care.

Fear of lawsuits may further deter physicians from attending to sociocultural factors if they believe peer recognition of their competence depends on displaying a disease focus. Paradoxically, this may discourage genuinely informed consent. Fear of malpractice encourages risk sharing through the overuse of consultants, leading at times to a "collusion of anonymity" in which no one is fully responsible for a patient's care (Balint, 1964).

The social position of the medical profession influences physicians' abilities to attend to the sociocultural dimension of illness. All social groups have culturally shared, generally self-justifying beliefs about how to interpret social reality (de Kadt, 1982). Since physicians often affiliate with socially dominant groups, their peers may encourage them to attribute the uneven distribution of sickness in society to biologic or psychologic causes rather than to social or cultural inequities (Cafferata, 1981).

Academic and clinical interest in the application of sociocultural approaches to health services and medical practice is potentially a source of substantial, relatively unpredictable change in the culture of medicine itself. Primary care physicians trained to investigate the social, economic, and cultural causes and consequences of the illness episodes of their patients share the interests of both traditional healers and clinical epidemiologists, while occupying a key place as the gatekeepers between lay medicine and the largely disease-oriented, bureaucratically organized specialty referral system.

Social and Cultural Interactions in Family Practice

Family Medicine ". . . emphasizes the importance of understanding the complex interaction between physical, psychological, and social elements of illness. It examines how illness is organized and presented by patients and interpreted and managed by doctors; and the importance of culture, community, and family in determining attitudes and values to health and illness (Howie, 1984)."

As Howie has so articulately stated, the integration of sociocultural knowledge of illness into practice is a major goal of family medicine. Family physicians have a responsibility to incorporate and apply even more knowledge about the impact of sociocultural factors on sickness and healing into our training programs, our clinical practices, and our lobbying efforts. We can and must improve our ability to meet patients' needs by providing culturally sensitive and socially conscious health care as individual clinicians and members of a professional group.

Physicians in all countries are increasingly likely to deal with patients from substantially different backgrounds from their own. A White House Commission on Immigration and Refugee Policy report indicated that by the end of the century 39 per cent of the U.S. population will again be members of immigrant families. A century from now, half of all Americans may be Afro-American, Hispanic, or Asian (Like and Steiner, 1986). Cross-cultural and cross-social class practices present particularly complex challenges for comprehensive care.

THE PHYSICIAN-PATIENT VISIT

When patients and physicians have substantially different cultural and social backgrounds that influence their different perspectives and explanations about illness, these differences contribute to misunderstandings and suboptimal patient care. Complications may arise between the patient's folk medical knowledge and the doctor's biomedical knowledge and between the patient's and the doctor's folk ways. Regardless of background, patients rarely are experts in medicine, which like all specialized occupations has its own culture, language, values, beliefs, and behavioral norms not shared by lay people. Physicians are sometimes well versed in their own lay culture's medical knowledge, acquired from their own families and from previous patients, which they rely upon in addition to their formal medical knowledge. Treating colds with cough syrup, for instance, is accorded greater validity in the British physician's folk culture than in formal medical culture (Helman, 1978). Applying this folk cultural knowledge to a member of another cultural group may, however, produce conflict.

Most clinical encounters also occur across social classes. The imbalance of social status adds to the physicians' potential for control of the professional-client relationship. This authority can benefit patients whose culture expects this of physicians. Family physicians should attempt to avoid giving a message that only their own knowledge and viewpoints are valid and valuable or that the patient's illness experience is unimportant (Harwood, 1981).

Primary care physicians must recognize that their patients are cultural experts on their own language of symptoms, on the social and economic risks of their environment, and on the influence of illness on their own social networks. If physicians actively seek the patients' expertise, agreement on the problem and reduction of disability from the illness are more attainable; patients also feel more valued, and the detrimental effects of cultural and social gaps can be diminished. It is also important to explain diagnoses and treatments in the patients' own concepts and to check that this has been understood (Tuckett et al., 1985). Physicians try to influence patients who are their social peers by establishing trust and displaying expertise. Patients of high social status receive more information and attention than lower status patients. There is no difference in people's desire for information or attention by social class, however, or in the physician's responsibility to provide it (Waitzkin, 1984).

Physicians collaborate with patients in defining the moral dimension of illness as well as the limits of sick roles. One of a healer's primary tasks is to mend the social conflicts that sickness exposes (Turner, 1967). Physicians diagnose diseases on cultural and social as well as technical grounds. "The doctor and the patient are curing the threat posed to convention and to society" (Taussig, 1980). When physicians' professional actions involve legal authority, such as police holds, reporting of venereal diseases, workers' compensation, or driver's license certifications, the physician must recognize a parallel responsibility to help patients protect their self-esteem within their own moral system.

Family physicians' ability to perform useful work within the ambulatory care setting depends, then, not exclusively upon their knowledge of medical technology. It also depends on their knowledge of the experience of illness in the numerous social circumstances of everyday life, as it is interpreted within the diverse cultural belief systems of patients. This expertise requires that the family physician devote a substantial effort to listening, both intellectually and emotionally, to patients, and to talking with patients within the context of their experience and not just as a technician (Cassell, 1985).

There are several specific ways to improve physician-patient communication as well as patient satisfaction in most encounter situations. Four areas in which physicians can improve their clinical interactions with patients of different ethnic groups and social classes are using medical interpreters, eliciting patients' explanatory models and patients' requests, negotiating treatment plans, and cultural self-awareness.

USING INTERPRETERS

Language barriers are a major detriment to communication. Learning even a few words in a patient's native language enhances the potential for understanding because a message of respect, interest, and desire to learn from the patients is conveyed. When a clinical practice includes a substantial number of patients who are not fluent in the physician's language, it is essential to employ a medically trained interpreter in order to optimize communication. Family members are often a poor choice to act as interpreter.

The physician must teach pertinent medical and cultural information to the interpreter, since many concepts do not have equivalents in other cultures. The interpreter needs to teach the physician about specific cultural views of the body, disease, and treatment. The physician should speak to the patient, not to the interpreter. The physician must keep in mind the different types of roles that interpreters play, including that of patient advocate and cultural broker. Interpreters may be in a position of considerable power because they are the only ones who can communicate verbally and nonverbally with both the provider and the patient. It is helpful to treat each other as coworkers and colleagues with the joint goal of understanding patients (Putsch, 1985).

TALKING WITH PATIENTS ABOUT ILLNESS AND DISEASE

The patient is expert about his or her own illness and life-world, just as the physician is expert about clinical medicine (Tuckett et al., 1985). Patients usually have expectations about what will occur in the clinical encounter. They have hopes they consider unrealistic or fears about their illness. Often there are strong and specific feelings about the doctor-patient interface itself. Patients make both explicit and implicit requests of their physicians based upon these expectations.

Good and delVecchio-Good (1980) found that patients request explanations twice as often as tests and "half again as frequently as medication" in a primary care outpatient clinic. At other times, patients' explicit requests (chief complaints) are only a "ticket of admission" to see a physician about a hidden agenda that is too embarrassing or threatening to bring up directly (Jarsky, 1981). In cross-cultural encounters, special efforts are necessary to understand patients' requests, needs, fears, and expectations, but the ability to recognize these is important in the care of all patients, even those of cultural backgrounds similar to the physicians' own.

Physicians need to acquire three basic skills in order to deal with illnesses in the wider context we have discussed in this chapter. First is the ability to elicit from patients their knowledge of and response to the illness and its social, cultural, and economic context. Second is the ability to explain the physician's diagnosis and advice to the patient, and to check to see that they have understood it within their cultural context. Third is the ability to negotiate a resolution when there is conflict between the physicians' and the patients' judgments of the situation.

Eliciting patients' explanatory models can be an important first step in understanding patients' views of their problem. Physicians should ask the patient about his or her explanatory model of the illness before presenting their own, since patients may fear the consequences of appearing to contradict the doctor (Tuckett et al., 1985). Questions should be flexibly directed towards learning what the patient thinks about the etiology, timing, and mode of onset, mode of action, expected course, and possible treatments of the illness. Kleinman (1980; Kleinman et al., 1978) has proposed a set of questions that may help to elicit the individual's explanatory model:

1. What do you call your problem?
2. What do you think has caused your problem?
3. Why do you think it started when it did?
4. What does your sickness do to you?
5. How severe is it?
6. Will it have a short or long course?
7. What do you fear most about your sickness?
8. What are the chief problems your sickness has caused for you?
9. What kind of treatment do you think you should receive?

Good and delVecchio-Good (1980) proposed that clinicians view the clinical encounter as fundamentally interpretive. In this meaning-centered approach, clinicians are encouraged to elicit the patient's personal meaning of the symptoms in addition to eliciting the patient's explanatory model of the sickness. This information would increase the clinician's understanding of the patient's illness experience, which strongly influences the sickness behaviors, including choosing treatment plans. With this increased understanding of the patient's illness experience, reaching agreements about diagnoses and treatments through negotiation would be greatly facilitated.

Active listening to the patient's description of the illness may be more effective if the physician adopts a patient-centered style of communication. The physician needs to be facilitative, encouraging the patient with open-ended questions or reflections. It is helpful to give verbal acknowledgment that the patient is being heard and to avoid cutting off a patient's offers of information by, for instance, changing the subject. When misunderstanding appears possible, the physician needs to reopen or return to the relevant parts of the previous discussion for clarification.

Once a physician is comfortable with the patient-centered approach, it improves patient satisfaction and both physician and patient compliance with each other's requests. Patients perceive that the physician has understood their concerns, and visits are only slightly longer. Training is required to master the skill, however, just as it is to become comfortable with eliciting patients' explanatory models. Physicians just beginning to apply these concepts will seem clumsy, awkward, and slow, just as do beginning students in physical diagnosis (Stewart, 1987).

Other important components of active listening include directing attention to patient's tone of voice, vocal rhythm, word choices, logic, and story line (Cassell, 1985) and to the nonverbal, physical communications of both doctor and patient (Friedman and diMatteo, 1982) (see Chapter 26). Patients and physicians culturally differ from one another in all these areas, and our ability to work together during an illness episode depends on learning from one another in all of them.

NEGOTIATING WITH PATIENTS

Once patients' perspectives have been elicited, including their concerns and their treatment desires, the patient's and the physician's explanatory models can be clearly compared and contrasted. Different views of the problem to be addressed and of the treatments to be initiated can be dealt with directly. Negotiating these points may be the crux of optimal cross-cultural interactions. Negotiating and reconciling differences in explanatory models are the most important physician-controllable predictor of a good outcome in ambulatory care of common problems (Bass et al., 1986). Indeed, if conflicting perceptions of illnesses are inherent in the clinical interaction, then "conflict resolution by negotiation is a critical part of successful helping relationships" (Lazare, 1979).

Usually, patients and physicians have different explanatory models about an individual sickness. Unless differences are recognized, they contribute to different expectations, misunderstandings, and conflicts between them, making negotiation extremely difficult. If, for example, a Hmong patient views the etiology of his or her sickness as soul loss, while the physician believes it is an infection, disagreement may contribute to disputes over the optimal therapeutic approaches; should resources be spent on a shaman's ceremony, or on a lumbar puncture and antibiotics? Recognition of the differences may allow compromises to be reached so that the pathophysiologically diagnosed disease and the experienced illness can both be treated.

Negotiations require that at least one party be willing to learn about the others' needs and views in order to overcome differences. This is why elicitation from patients of their cultural expectations and the social context of their illness is so important. Negotiation also requires that the initiating party be willing to be explicitly aware of his or her own needs in the interaction and of their best options if an agreement cannot be reached (Fisher and Ury, 1981).

Physicians have their own explanatory models of the patient's sickness that have been influenced by their cultural background, medical cultural beliefs, and their idiosyncratic experiences (Helman, 1984). Delivery of socioculturally appropriate medical care requires that we become aware of our own cultural veil and our own social prejudices and that we realize how we are defined by socially shared cultural beliefs and behaviors (Stein, 1985). Caring for seriously ill people who lack critical resources, or who have different perceptions of reality and different values, can unsettle our sense of self and produce powerful emotional defenses. The most critical response we can make is to use these occasions to further our own self-awareness. These painful times are opportunities to understand the role of culture, social identity, and social support in our own lives and in our responses to sickness and the difficulties of cross-cultural translation.

Physicians are expected to negotiate for their patients' best interest. When conflict with the patient arises because of the patient's cultural beliefs, and particularly when the illness has evoked strong, emotionally laden responses in the patient (such as denial, anger, fear, or indecision), physicians may discover that their own response includes protection of their own emotional equilibrium, self-esteem, or reputation. Negotiation will be more likely to succeed where such implicit needs are acknowledged, at least to oneself.

THE PREVENTION OF ILLNESS

The prevention of illness is an important concern of family physicians. Sociocultural factors are important in prevention as well. Patients must make sense of their physicians' preventive advice on smoking cessation, infant car seats, condom use, exercise, and prudent diets within the context of what they already know about illness prevention. Folk and popular medical practices are also often intended to prevent illness. Sweat baths, vitamins, antibiotics, and hats are all used to prevent lung trouble in different cultures, based on people's explanatory models of the causes of respiratory illness. Physician-recommended preventive practices are perhaps only adopted when patients succeed in justifying them within some acceptable explanatory model. Since common practices are used for different purposes with different justifications in many cultures, it is best to elicit the explanatory model rather than rely on stereotyped assumptions about what a given piece of advice will mean to someone.

Many preventable illnesses are at least partially due to social and cultural causes, and prevention on an individual basis requires sociocultural change. Family food traditions that create coronary disease risks may also be important elements of ethnic group identity. The physician's advice may require patients to make difficult, even painful choices. Preventive programs based on life style interventions are always potentially invasive of the identities and personal lives of patients and other people in their social network. Physicians need to ask about the potential cultural and social consequences of their preventive advice in order to know what medical information will most help the patient to make sound decisions.

Patients can only follow preventive advice within the constraints of their cultural, social, and economic circumstances. Family physicians need to be aware of the potential risk of victim blaming in preventive health care. If an illness is preventable by individual initiative, sickness often seems to imply moral failure. It is often important, then, even at the level of individual patient care, for the physician to be aware of, and committed to, public health approaches to disease prevention that address sociocultural factors in disease incidence beyond the patient's control. Family physicians who regularly inquire into the cultural values and illness predicaments of their patients can collectively provide important support, and socioculturally sensitive direction, to public policies that can promote health.

Medical anthropology, medical sociology, epidemiology, and many related social science disciplines have studied the influence of cultural patterning and social processes upon people's health, disease rates, illness experiences, and preferred treatments. In addition, they have studied the effects of patients' and doctors' different cultural orientations and social status upon their relationship. We feel that much of this literature can be helpful to family physicians and expect that family physician researchers and practitioners will further explore these avenues.

References

Aiken, L. H., and Mechanic, D. (Eds.): Applications of Social Science to Clinical Medicine and Health Policy. New Brunswick, NJ, Rutgers University Press, 1986. *Aiken and Mechanic provide a useful set of review essays by noted sociologists that could be a useful initial reference point for the family physician attempting to gain a social perspective on medical practice.*

Amler, R. W., and Dull, H. B. (Eds.): Closing the Gap: The Burden of Unnecessary Illness. New York, Oxford University Press, 1984. *A review of the major preventable causes of morbidity and mortality in the United States demonstrates the importance of sociocultural factors and the role of community medicine and other social interventions in diminishing their impact.*

Anderson, B. G., Toledo, J. R., and Hazam, N.: An approach to the resolution of Mexican-American resistance to diagnostic and remedial pediatric heart care. *In* Chrisman, N. J., and Maretzki, T. W. (Eds.): Clinically Applied Anthropology: Anthropologists in Health Science Settings. Dordrecht, Holland, D. Reidel Publishing Co., 1982.

Atkinson, T., Liem, R., and Liem, J. H.: The social costs of unemployment: Implications for social support. J. Health Soc. Behav., *27*:317–331, 1986.

Balint, M.: The Doctor, the Patient, and his Illness. London, Tavistock, 1964. *A classic examination of needs and possibilities for a psychosocial approach to illness in primary care written by a British psychiatrist who developed a training program to help general practitioners make better use of themselves as a "doctor drug" with their difficult patients.*

Bass, M. J., Buck, C., Turner, L., et al.: The physician's actions and the outcome of illness in family practice. J. Fam. Practice, *23*:43–47, 1986. *A Canadian study of symptom resolution in several common ambulatory conditions found that psychosocial problems and psychosocial management were respectively the most important patient and physician variables. More traditional medical quality-of-care measures failed to predict outcome.*

Beckman, H., and Frankel, R.: The effect of physician behavior on the collection of data. Ann. Intern. Med., *101*:692–696, 1984. *Describes the effects of physician overcontrol during medical visits.*

Berkanovic, E. C., Telesky, C., and Reeder, S.: Structural and social psychological factors in the decision to seek medical care for symptoms. Med. Care, *19*:693–709, 1981.

Berkman, L. F., and Syme, L. S.: Social networks, host resistance, and mortality: A nine-year follow-up study of Alameda County residents. Am. J. Epidemiol., *109*:186–204, 1979. *This examination of social support networks is a classic of epidemiological study design and has been part of the foundation of most work since.*

Blumhagen, D.: Hyper-tension: A folk illness with a medical name. Cult. Med. Psychiatry, *4*:1979–2027, 1980.

Brown, D. R., and Gary, L. E.: Stressful life events, social support networks, and the physical and mental health of urban black adults. J. Human Stress, *13*:165–174, 1987.

Brown, G. W., and Harris, T.: Social Origins of Depression. New York, Free Press, 1978. *This British study linking depression with socioeconomic deprivation is accepted on both sides of the debate about the usefulness of the concept of social stress.*

Brown, P., and Levinson, S. C.: Politeness. Cambridge, Cambridge University Press, 1987. *An important work of sociolinguistic theory that proposes that universal rules govern the ways people threaten, defend, and protect each other's identity or face and underlie the culturally diverse forms of politeness. The essential ideas are of great potential usefulness in primary care.*

Cafferata, G.: The ideology of the American medical profession: An attribution perspective. Soc. Sci. Med., *15A*:689–699, 1981.

Campbell, E. M. J., Scadding, J. G., and Roberts, R. S.: The concept of disease. Br. Med. J., *2*:757–762, 1979.

Cassell, E.: Talking with Patients. Cambridge, MIT Press, 1985. *Very useful two-volume work explores the theory and practice of how effective clinicians use language in medical care. It is an excellent, very readable introduction to clinical listening and talking, particularly valuable for its discussions of clinical acumen, patients' narratives, and paralanguage.*

Chrisman, N. J.: The health seeking process: An approach to the natural history of illness. Cult. Med. Psychiatry, *1*:351–377, 1977. *Describes a lay medical decision-making model that attempts to link the social psychology of symptom definition, the social process of role change in sickness, and anthropological concepts of lay consultation and referral.*

Chrisman, N. J., and Maretzki, T. W. (Eds.): Clinically Applied Anthropology: Anthropologists in Health Science Settings. Dordrecht, Holland, D. Reidel Publishing Co., 1982.

de Kadt, E.: Ideology, social policy, health, and health services: A field of complex interactions. Soc. Sci. Med., *16*:741–752, 1982.

Department of Health, Education and Welfare—Public Health Service: Health Status of Minorities and Low-Income Groups. Washington DC, U.S. Government Printing Office, 1986.

Eddy, D. M.: Variations in physician practice: the role of uncertainty. Health Care, *3*:74–89, 1984.

Egbuonu, L., and Starfield, B.: Child health and social status. Pediatrics, *69*:550–557, 1982.

Eisenberg, L.: What makes persons 'patients' and patients 'well'? Am. J. Med., *69*:277–286, 1980. *A classic exposition of the difference between disease and illness.*

Eisenberg, L., and Kleinman, A. (Eds.): The Relevance of Social Science for Medicine. Dordrecht, Holland, Reidel Publishing Co., 1980. *This volume contains a number of excellent survey essays on various sociocultural aspects of medical practice.*

Engel, G. L.: The need for a new medical model: A challenge for biomedicine. Science, *196*:129–136, 1977. *A widely cited attempt to integrate biologic and social science approaches to medicine by seeing them each as appropriate to different levels of phenomena, using the concepts and language of general systems theory.*

Fabrega, H., Jr., and Hunter, J. E.: Judgments about disease: A case study involving Ladinos of Chiapas. Soc. Sci. Med., *12*:1–10, 1978.

Fisher, R., and Ury, W.: Getting to Yes: Negotiating Agreement Without Giving In. Boston, Houghton Mifflin, 1981. *A popular paperback manual that guides the reader through the basic concepts of negotiating agreement in conflict situations.*

Foster, G. M., and Anderson, B. G.: Medical Anthropology. New York, John Wiley and Sons, 1978. *A general textbook of the field of medical anthropology.*

Foucault, M.: The Birth of the Clinic: An Archaeology of Medical Perception. New York, Pantheon, 1973.

Freidson, E.: Profession of Medicine: A Study of the Sociology of Applied Knowledge. New York, Harper and Row, 1970. *An influential work that examines medical professional autonomy and dominance, the sick role, lay referral networks, and patient-physician relations.*

Friedman, H. S., and diMatteo, M. R. (Eds.): Interpersonal Issues in Health Care. New York, Academic Press, 1982. *Includes an excellent discussion of both verbal and nonverbal communication in clinical medicine.*

Garro, L. C.: Explaining high blood pressure: variation in knowledge about illness. Am. Ethnol., *15*(1):98–119, 1988.

Geertsen, R., Klauber, M. R., Kindflesh, M., et al.: A reexamination of Suchman's views on social factors in health care utilization. J. Health Soc. Behav., *16*:226–237, 1975.

Geertz, C.: The Interpretation of Cultures. New York, Basic Books, 1973.

Gillick, M.: Common sense models of health and disease. N. Engl. J. Med., *313*:700, 1985.

Good, B. J., and delVecchio-Good, M.: The meaning of symptoms: A cultural hermeneutic model for clinical practice. *In* Eisenberg, L., and Kleinman, A. (Eds.): The Relevance of Social Science for Medicine. Dordrecht, Holland, Reidel Publishing Co., 1980.

Gray, A. M.: Inequalities in health—the Black Report: A summary and comment. Intl. J. Health Serv., *12*:349–381, 1982. *A useful summary of the contents of a major British government study of the persistence and possible increase of social inequalities in sickness and health care under the National Health Service.*

Guarnaccia, P. J., Pelto, P. J., and Schensul, S. L.: Family health culture, ethnicity, and asthma: Coping with illness. Med. Anthro., *9*:203–224, 1985.

Hahn, R. A., and Gaines, A. (Eds.): Physicians of Western Medicine: Anthropological Approaches to Theory and Practice. Dordrecht, Holland, Reidel Publishing Co., 1985.

Harwood, A. (Ed.): Ethnicity and Medical Care. Cambridge, Harvard University Press, 1981. *Both a summary of the popular medical cultural beliefs of seven major ethnic minorities of the United States, and a helpful general discussion of ethnicity and medicine.*

Helman, C. G.: 'Feed a cold, starve a fever'-folk models of infection in an English suburban community, and their relation to medical treatment. Cult. Med. Psychiatry, *2*:107–137, 1978.

Helman, C. G.: Culture, Health, and Illness: An Introduction for Health Professionals. Bristol, UK, Wright PSG, 1984. *An excellent overview of different cultures' perceptions of anatomy and physiology, diet and nutrition, pain, doctor-patient interactions, and importance of rituals.*

Honigfield, L. S., and Kaplan, D. W.: Native American postneonatal mortality. Pediatrics, *80*:575–578, 1987.

Hooper, E. M., et al.: Patient characteristics that influence physician behavior. Med. Care, *20*:630–638, 1982.

Howie, J.: Research in general practice: Pursuit of knowledge or defence of wisdom? Br. Med. J., *289*:1770–1773, 1984.

Institute of Medicine: Pain and Disability: Clinical, Behavioral, and Public Policy Perspectives. Washington, National Academy Press, 1987. *The problems of chronic illness demonstrate the complexity of the interactions of psychology and biology with sociocultural, political, and economic factors.*

Jarsky, A.: Hidden reasons some patients visit doctors. Ann. Int. Med., *94*:492, 1981.

Jarvis, G. K., and Northcott, H. C.: Religion and differences in morbidity and mortality. Soc. Sci. Med., *25*:813–824, 1987.

Johannes, A.: Many medicines in one: Curing in the eastern highlands of Papua New Guinea. Cult. Med. Psychiatry, *4*:43–70, 1980.

Kleinman, A., Eisenberg, L., and Good, B.: Culture, illness and care: Clinical lessons from anthropological and cross-cultural research. Ann. Int. Med., *88*:251–258, 1978. *A compact exposition of explanatory models and the clinical importance of sociocultural factors.*

Kleinman, A.: Patients and Healers in the Context of Culture. Berkeley, University of California Press, 1980. *A study of Taiwanese healers in which the concept of explanatory models is fully elaborated.*

Laderman, C.: The ambiguity of symbols in the structure of healing. Soc. Sci. Med., *24*(4):293–301, 1987.

Lazare, A. (Ed.): Outpatient Psychiatry: Diagnosis and Treatment. Baltimore, Williams and Wilkins, 1979.

Lieberman, E., Ryan, K. J., Monson, R. R., et al.: Risk factors accounting for racial differences in the rate of premature birth. N. Engl. J. Med., *317*:743–748, 1987.

Like, R., and Steiner, R.: Medical anthropology and the family physician. Fam. Med., *18*:87–92, 1986.

Lurie, N., Ward, N. B., and Shapiro, M. F.: Termination from Medi-Cal: Does it affect health? N. Engl. J. Med., *311*:480–484, 1984.

Marcellisen, F. M. G.: Social support and occupational stress: A causal analysis. Soc. Sci. Med., *26*:365–373, 1988.

Mathews, H. F.: Rootwork: Description of an ethnomedical system in the American south. South. Med. J., *80*(7):885–891, 1987.

Mechanic, D.: Social psychologic factors affecting the presentation of bodily complaints. N. Engl. J. Med., *286*:1132–1139, 1972. *A classic article that discusses a large number of social psychologic processes involved in the perception, definition, and public acknowledgment of symptoms and illnesses.*

Milio, N.: Primary Care and the Public's Health. Lexington, MA, Lexington Books, 1983.

Muecke, M.: In search of healers: Southeast Asians in the American health care system. West. J. Med., *139*(6):835–840, 1983.

Orth-Gomer, K., and Johnson, J. V.: Social network interaction and mortality: A six-year follow-up study of a random sample of the Swedish population. J. Chron. Dis., *40*:949–957, 1987.

Putsch, R.: Cross-cultural communication: The special case of interpreters in health care. J.A.M.A., *254*:3344–3348, 1985.

Scheper-Hughes, N., and Lock, M.: The mindful body: a prologomenon to future work in medical anthropology. Med. Anthrop. Quart., *17*(5):128–129, 1987. *A review of the relationship of emotions and cultural concepts of the body and of society.*

Seeman, T. E., and Berkman, L. F.: Structural characteristics of social networks and their relationship with social support in the elderly: Who provides support? Soc. Sci. Med., *26*:737–749, 1988.

Sorensen, G., Pechacek, T., and Pallonen, U.: Occupational and worksite norms and attitudes about smoking cessation. Am. J. Publ. Health, *76*:544–549, 1986.

Staiano, K. V.: Alternative therapeutic systems in Belize: A semiotic framework. Soc. Sci. Med., *15B*:317–332, 1981.

Starr, P.: The Social Transformation of American Medicine. New York, Basic Books, 1982. *An institutional history of medicine as a profession and as an industry in the United States over the past century that argues that a transition is underway from professional dominance in medicine to bureaucratic medical care systems.*

Stein, H. F.: The Psychodynamics of Medical Practice: Unconscious Factors in Patient Care. Berkeley, University of California, 1985.

Stewart, M.: Studies in the patient-centered approach. Paper presented at the conference Communicating with Patients, Tampa, 1987.

Stoller, E. P.: Self-assessments of health by the elderly: The impact of informal assistance. J. Health Soc. Behav., *25*:260–270, 1984.

Taussig, M.: Reification and the consciousness of the patient. Soc. Sci. Med., *14B*:3–13, 1980.

Totman, R.: Social and Biological Roles of Language: The Psychology of Justification. London, Academic Press, 1985. *A theoretical explanation of social support in terms of the social psychological concepts of cognitive dissonance and social influence.*

Tuckett, D., Boultan, M., Olson, C., et al.: Meetings Between Experts: An Approach to Sharing Ideas in Medical Consultations. London, Tavistock Publications, 1985. *A well-conducted, large-scale quantitative study done for the British Health Education Council that confirms the importance of many of the approaches discussed in the present chapter. The notes include a useful summary of their approach to assisting physicians to improve their consulting skills.*

Turner, V.: Forest of Symbols. Ithaca, NY, Cornell University Press, 1967. *A classic anthropological examination of the role of symbols and the importance of the community in healing in the traditional culture of a tribal African society.*

Twaddle, A. C.: Sickness Behavior and the Sick Role. Boston, G. K. Hall, 1979. *A clear exposition of key concepts of medical sociology derived from the work of Parsons and Freidson.*

Verbrugge, L. M., and Ascione, F. J.: Exploring the iceberg: Common symptoms and how people care for them. Med. Care, *25*:539–569, 1987. *One of a series of social epidemiologic survey studies that examine the relationship of symptoms to illness episodes, self-care, and the use of medical services.*

Waitzkin, M.: Doctor-patient communication: Clinical implications of social scientific research. J.A.M.A., *252*:2441–2446, 1984. *A review of how, and to whom, physicians give information during office visits, including a number of surprising findings about the relationship of the physician's own social background and information-giving behavior.*

Wennberg, J. E., Barnes, B. A., and Zubkoff, M.: Professional uncertainty and the problem of supplier-induced demand. Soc. Sci. Med., *16*:811–824, 1982. *Wennberg and colleagues use "small-areas variations analysis" to examine how physician practice styles differ between medical communities, raising important questions about the relationship of local medical cultures to treatment outcomes.*

Wentowski, G. J.: Reciprocity and the coping strategies of older people: Cultural dimensions of network building. Gerontologist, *21*:600–609, 1981.

Wise, P. H., Kotelchuck, M., Wilson, M. L., et al.: Racial and socioeconomic disparities in childhood mortality in Boston. N. Engl. J. Med., *313*:360–366, 1985.

World Health Organization: World Health Statistics Annual. Geneva, World Health Organization, 1986.

Young, J. C.: Medical Choice in a Mexican Village. New Brunswick, NJ, Rutgers University Press, 1981.

18

Psychosocial Influences on Health

Gabriel Smilkstein

The biopsychosocial model elaborated by Engel (1977, 1980) details the biomedical and psychosocial influences that have an impact on a patient's health. Although family medicine has accepted this integrated approach to health care as a central tenet of the discipline, a pragmatic scheme for the employment of the model still needs to be developed.

Much has been done to advance knowledge of the model's psychosocial risk component. For example, there is considerable literature that relates family function to health outcome (Pratt, 1976; Smilkstein, 1984). Application of this knowledge to clinical practice, however, requires that knowledge of a patient's family function be integrated into a dynamic view of the patient's psychosocial risk. That is, family function should be viewed as only one of the many psychosocial variables that influence the patient's health. The conceptual framework for this approach to patient care is outlined by Engel (1980).

". . . the investigator . . . is obliged to select one system level on which to concentrate. . . . For the physician that system is always the patient. . . . [The physician should] elicit simultaneously information needed to characterize [the patient] as a person and to evaluate the status of [the medical problem]. For the biomedically trained physician, judgments . . . bearing on . . . social aspects of patients' lives commonly are made with minimum information about people, relationships, and circumstances involved. . . . The biopsychosocially oriented physician . . . identifies and evaluates the stabilizing and destabilizing potential of events and relationships in the patient's environment."

Thus, according to Engel, a physician's understanding of the stabilizing and destabilizing events and relationships in the life of a patient is central to the successful application of the biopsychosocial model in health care. In this paper, stabilizing and destabilizing forces are equated with social support resources and emotional stressors, respectively. Although psychosocial risk will be highlighted, Engel's admonition to "simultaneously" explore a patient's health problem and personal status should always be respected. Restated, optimum health care requires that physicians address both emotional and physical determinants (Levi, 1979; Girard et al., 1985). Although biomedical risk assessment techniques are well known to all students and practitioners of medicine, less well known are the strategies needed to assess psychosocial risk (Smilkstein, 1983).

A Cycle of Psychosocial Risk: An Assessment Model

A model is needed that forms into a cohesive unit the components that contribute to psychosocial risk. A cyclic model of psychosocial risk will be presented that displays emotional responses reported to occur when an individual perceives a life experience as a stressor (Fig. 18–1). The purpose of the model is to facilitate an understanding of the forces that influence the relationship between psychosocial risk and health.

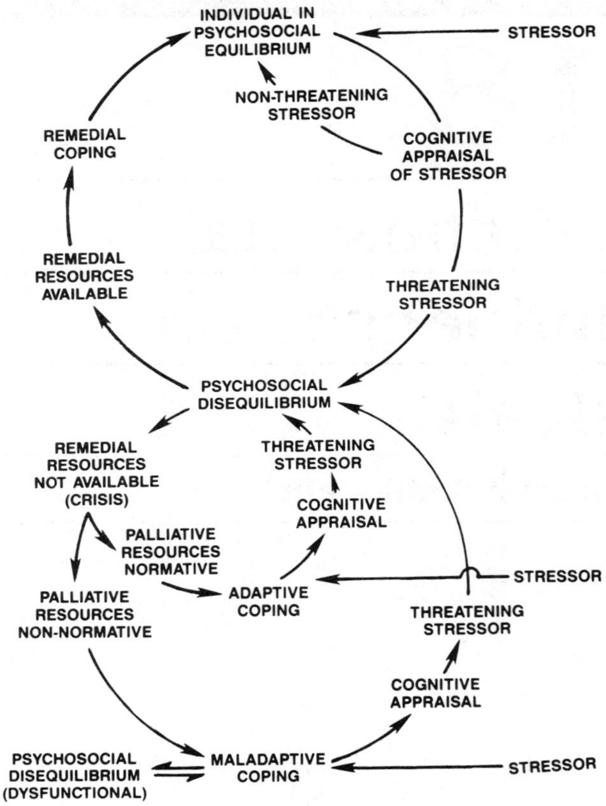

Figure 18–1. Cycle of Psychosocial Risk.

The fundamental structure of this model is drawn from the Cycle of Family Function, which offers a conceptual framework for viewing the responses of a family when it experiences a stressful life event (Smilkstein, 1980). Although the Cycle of Family Function was built on the contributions of many social scientists, Hill's (1965) studies of families under stress were seminal for this paper. Hill's ABCX formula offered the following conceptual framework: "A (the event); interacting with B (the family's crisis-meeting resources); interacting with C (the definition the family makes of the event); produces X (the crisis)." In this paper, Hill's formula is interpreted as a stressor/resources interaction (modified by idiosyncratic coping mechanism), producing a qualitatively predictable alteration in an individual's emotional homeostasis.

This model focuses on an individual's response to life stressors and demonstrates how an individual's psychosocial equilibrium may be influenced by an interaction of stressors, social support, and coping strategies. A definition of terms used in the cycle is given in Table 18–1.

THE UPPER CYCLE: STRESSOR RESOLUTION

Multiple stressors impact upon an individual's psyche each day (Hinkle, 1973; Dohrenwend and Dohrenwend, 1984). These stressors are received and processed, and a response is generated that reflects the individual's cognitive appraisal of the stressor (Lazarus and Folkman, 1984). Cognitive appraisal is influenced by many factors. Among these factors are the individual's psychosocial equilibrium at the time the stressor is received, the individual's past experience with similar stressors, the number and intensity of other stressors being processed by the individual, and the perceived threat to relationships and self-esteem (Lazarus et al., 1974).

Not all stressors stimulate an alarm reaction. Cognitive appraisal may result in a view of the stressor as nonthreatening. This response usually occurs when past experience with the stressor has been favorable, and when resources are deemed to be available. Nonstressful experiences will not significantly alter psychosocial equilibrium (Holmes and Rahe, 1967; Masuda and Holmes, 1978).

If, however, the stressors are perceived as threatening (based on past experience or knowledge that needed resources may not be available), the individual moves into a state of psychosocial disequilibrium (Cassel, 1974; Pearlin et al., 1981). Because of the "dis-ease" associated with psychosocial disequilibrium, resources are sought to neutralize or buffer the stressor (Cobb, 1976). A number of psychosocial resource categories have been identified—social, cultural, religious, educational, economic, environmental, and medical (Smilkstein, 1983). Of these, social support from family members, friends, and work supervisors appears to be the most influential in altering psychosocial risk (Cassel, 1976; Cohen et al., 1986). If resources are available and remedial coping strategies are employed, the individual will usually experience stressor resolution and a return to psychosocial equilibrium.

THE LOWER CYCLE: UNRESOLVED STRESSORS

The downward spiral in the cycle occurs when individuals experience threatening psychosocial stressors and find their resources or coping mechanisms inadequate for stressor resolution (Thoits, 1986; Shonkoff, 1985). An inability to identify or utilize the resources needed to solve a problem results in a crisis state (Baldwin, 1978). Crisis is usually associated with anxiety (Spielberger, 1972). This concept of anxiety as an outcome of crisis or emotional disequilibrium is of central importance, since studies have shown that anxiety is the primary emotional mediator of neuroendocrinologic and neuroimmunologic system changes that alter health outcome (Ader and Cohen, 1975; Stein et al., 1976; Borysenko and Borysenko, 1982).

In the absence of problem-solving resources, individuals choose some form of palliative coping to obtain relief from anxiety and to maintain ongoing function. Some individuals temporize and gain release

Table 18–1. DEFINITION OF TERMS FROM THE CYCLE OF PSYCHOSOCIAL RISK

Stressors	A stressor is a life experience that may disrupt or endanger an individual's personal and social values and relationships. (This definition is in accordance with Selye's language of stress, in which the noxious stimulating condition or stressor has the potential for producing emotional disequilibrium or stress.) Stressors are divided into two categories: (1) life change events and (2) role strains or chronic life situations
Psychosocial Equilibrium	A state of psychologic homeostasis in which resources are available to meet the routine challenges of life's stressors
Cognitive Appraisal	The process by which an individual evaluates a life event or role strain in terms of the impact of the experience on his or her emotional and social integrity
Threatening Stressor	A life event or role strain that represents a danger or challenge to a relationship or self-esteem
Psychosocial Disequilibrium	A state of impaired emotional and social functioning that occurs when an individual's resources are inadequate or unavailable to meet an intense stressor or an accumulation of stressors
Resources, Social Support	Those assets that serve to nurture an individual and that supply the means for solving stressor-induced problems. Resources fall into the general categories of social, cultural, religious, economic, educational, environmental, and medical support systems
Remedial Coping	The process by which an individual uses resources and adaptive strategies to maintain some degree of psychosocial function when resources are inadequate or not available to solve a stressor-induced problem
Crisis	A state of emotional disequilibrium, usually becoming manifest by anxiety that results from the failure of an individual to identify or use resources to resolve a stressor-induced problem
Maladaptive Coping	The use of pathologic defense mechanisms to escape from an unresolved crisis, resulting in a state of impaired emotional and social functioning. In a medical setting, the most commonly seen pathologic defenses are projection and somatization
Chronic Psychosocial Disequilibrium	A state of emotional and social dysfunction, usually becoming manifest by an individual's inability to cope with life's responsibilities such as work, home, or school. The dysfunctional state is characterized by responses such as depression, panic attacks, and disabling somatization

from the emotional tensions induced by an unresolved stressor through activities such as taking time-out, physical exercise, and relaxation through behavior modification (Kobosa et al., 1982; Martin and Coates, 1987). These palliative coping techniques permit transient equilibrium and modified function in the face of an unresolved stressor. A host of psychologic defense mechanisms may be used on a short-term basis to bide time while seeking resources to manage the stressor. Avoidance, denial, projection, and somatization are examples of psychologic defense mechanisms that may be employed to gain relief from the pressure of an unresolved, anxiety-producing stressor.

Not all stressors are resolvable. For example, after the death of a spouse, there is a period of bereavement with its concomitant psychologic disequilibrium and dysfunction. Yet individuals find it necessary to get on with life. In general, those who return to psychologic equilibrium the soonest are those who have social support and use "mature" coping strategies (Walker et al., 1977). Some of the "mature" strategies used for both remedial and palliative coping are altruism, anticipation, humor, resource sharing, role adjustment, sublimation, and time-out (Smilkstein, 1985).

Knowledge of a patient's social support, coping strategies, and stressors will enhance the physician's ability to understand an individual's psychosocial risk. But the idiosyncratic effect of personal resources must also be considered when assessing the quality of a patient's ability to manage stressors. Kobosa and colleagues (1982) applied the term "hardiness" to the subjects in their studies who demonstrated a low incidence of illness in the face of high stress. The developmental history of hardiness has not been elaborated; however, individuals so labeled have been characterized as having (1) a greater sense of control over what occurs in their lives, (2) a feeling of commitment to the various activities in which they are engaged, (3) a view of change as a challenge rather than a threat, and (4) a sense of a meaningfulness to their lives. It is likely that hardiness reflects past successes in employing resources to overcome life stressors. A postulate that needs examination is that hardiness will erode if an individual experiences a series of coping failures due to unresolvable stressors and the loss of social support.

THE LOWER CYCLE: LONG-TERM MALADAPTIVE PSYCHOSOCIAL EQUILIBRIUM

When stressors present an overwhelming threat or become chronic, individuals seek long-term defense strategies to modify anxiety. That is, individuals use strategies that permit them to retain self-esteem and maintain relationships, even though their function in assigned roles may be impaired (Bowden, 1983).

The strategies chosen to address anxiety-provoking stressors may be consciously planned, initiated with only partial awareness, or generated from an unconscious level. Although many psychologic defense mechanisms may be seen in a health care setting, the ones with somatic manifestations attract the most interest. Two of the more frequently encountered are projection and somatization (Ford, 1983).

Projection is most commonly seen in families. A child with a health problem may become the identified patient upon whom the unresolved family problems are transferred. The greater the number and intensity of the family stressors, the more likely the child is to appear in the clinic and hospital (Beautrais et al., 1982).

Somatization occurs when an individual consciously or unconsciously employs physical symptoms to address the anxiety of an unresolved stressor. The physical symptoms are usually associated with an existing health problem, but they may also be related to a past personal or family experience with illness or physical disability (Mechanic, 1972; Rosen et al., 1982). Somatization in one of its many forms (such as chronic low back pain) is among the most common problems seen by physicians (Nachemson, 1984). Somatization is an expedient defense mechanism because it places individuals in the sick role. And individuals who are granted the sick role are usually released from responsibilities associated with work, school, and home. Furthermore, they are also permitted to be cared for by others (Parsons, 1958).

A Dynamic Model

The Cycle of Psychosocial Risk represents pathways that may be followed as an individual strives for emotional homeostasis. The dynamic nature of the cycle reflects the ever-changing pressures of unresolved stressors, the impact of new stressors, and changes in the quality, quantity, and availability of resources.

If and when new resources for coping are discovered, the individual can be expected to cycle upward to a higher level of functional equilibrium. At other times, when the number and intensity of stressors increase, a resource-poor person may move from long-term maladaptive coping into the dysfunctional state of chronic disequilibrium. Those who move into this category are usually unable to carry on tasks of daily living. Major therapeutic intervention is usually required to bring individuals out of chronic disequilibrium and into the emotional homeostasis that is required for positive functioning both as an individual as well as with family, friends, and community.

Clinical Applications

The physician who is receptive to psychosocial cues and willing to intervene should establish dual therapeutic goals. The first should be to offer short-term symptomatic relief from the disabling anxiety that is usually associated with psychosocial disequilibrium. Such relief from anxiety may be obtained with the use of palliative coping techniques. These include supportive interventions such as the ancient art of listening to the patient as well as instructing the patient in health-promoting activities (exercise, regular sleep, and balanced diet) (Fordyce, 1976). And since the impact of stressors on the patient may be buffered by social support, the patient should be counseled to seek aid from family and friends. But assessment of the quality of the patient's social support is also needed. Although family and friends are usually recognized as the first line of social support, the quality of these resources must be investigated, for family and friends may also be the source of stress for the patient. In addition, psychotropic medication should be prescribed when needed to augment the above program.

A companion therapeutic goal should be long-term problem resolution or remedial coping. This activity requires the identification and assessment of stressors such as life change events and role strains (chronic life situations) (Pearlin and Johnson, 1977).

To help the patient achieve an adequate level of remedial coping ability, the physician's challenge is to determine the resources that will help the patient manage stressors. Figure 18–2 is a biopsychosocial computational model that can be used to make an empirical determination of health outcome. The psychosocial risk portion of the equation demonstrates an interactive relationship between stressors and resources (Sarason et al., 1985). For example, psychosocial risk is heightened when there is an increase in stressors (numerator) and a decrease in resources (denominator). This simple arithmetic model can be applied in routine practice situations. Support for application of this model can be found in health outcome studies that have examined such health problems as complications of pregnancy (Smilkstein, 1984; Reeb et al., 1987) and cardiovascular disease (Medalie and Goldbourt, 1976; Haynes et al., 1980).

How does a physician identify the patient whose health problem indicates that assessment of psychosocial risk is appropriate? Since, in this cyclic model,

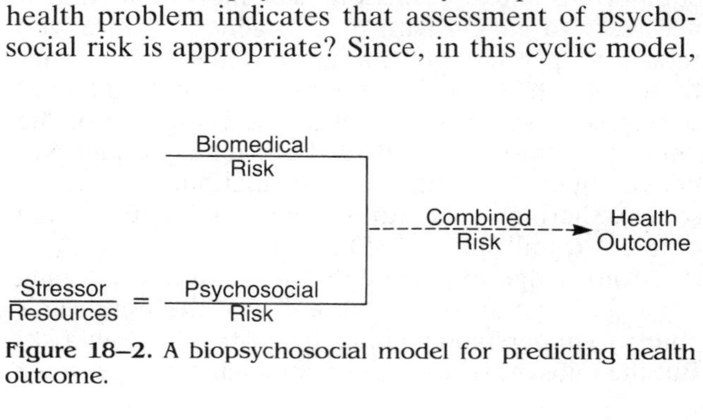

Figure 18–2. A biopsychosocial model for predicting health outcome.

Table 18–2. EXAMPLES OF OVERT CUES OF PSYCHOSOCIAL DISEQUILIBRIUM OR MALADAPTATION

Depression	Family member abuse (child, spouse, elder)
Panic attacks	Delinquency
History of alcohol or substance abuse	Run-away
Sexual dysfunction	School behavior problem
Divorce/separation	School failure
Incest	

psychosocial risk relates primarily to emotional disequilibrium caused by a rise in stressor intensity or a loss of social support, or both, a physician must be attitudinally prepared to recognize emotional disequilibrium. To do this, the physician must be able to receive cues from patients that reflect psychosocial risk. Tables 18–2 and 18–3 list examples of overt and covert cues that suggest significant disturbances in the patient's psychosocial equilibrium.

APPLICATION OF THE BIOPSYCHOSOCIAL MODEL

When the patient presents with both biomedical and psychosocial risks, rational responses are necessary. The medical, economic, and temporal resources of the patient, physician, and health system must be used appropriately and frugally if the biopsychosocial approach to health care is to be accepted. Present medical training and practice highlight biomedical factors so strongly that iatrogenic reinforcement of a patient's somatization frequently occurs. This problem, which has been labeled as "somatic fixation" (Van Eijk et al., 1983), is the process by which a patient becomes locked into a physical problem with the support of a physician who pursues a patient's persistent or exaggerated physical symptoms through an escalation of laboratory tests, office visits, and consultations. It is true that good medical practice requires a relevant pursuit of persistent or exaggerated physical symptoms with follow-up visits, objective studies, and second opinions. A study of physicians involved in "somatic fixation," however, suggests that their patients would have experienced emotional and economic benefits if psychosocial risks had been examined along with biomedical risk.

Table 18–3. EXAMPLES OF COVERT CUES OF PSYCHOSOCIAL DISEQUILIBRIUM OR MALADAPTATION

- Somatization
- Excessive utilization of health care facilities
- Noncompliance with use of medications or instructions for self-care
- History of multiple surgeries
- Chronic pain
- Failure to thrive
- Recurrent childhood poisonings
- Shopping for different physicians

CASE DISCUSSION

Figure 18–3 illustrates psychosocial risk assessment applied to a case study using the Cycle of Psychosocial Risk. The psychosocial risk assessment was carried out in harmony with biomedical studies. The dynamically interrelated components revealed by this assessment can be observed by following the Cycle of Psychosocial Risk pathways.

The patient initially reported anxiety due to chest pain. He admitted to a fear that chest pain was associated with heart problems and death. The physician also learned that within the last year the patient had experienced a series of stressful life events that challenged his emotional homeostasis—a major move, a painful divorce, and a new job. The job was a daily hassle due to conflicts with the boss and the patient's concern regarding the adequacy of his job performance.

Life change events, such as those experienced by the patient in this case study, have been studied extensively over the past 30 years. This research has established that life change events are significantly associated with adverse health outcomes such as cardiovascular disease (Ostfeld et al., 1985). Such findings emphasize the value of a biopsychosocial approach, especially when anxiety is expressed along with the presenting complaint.

Although all life events have an impact on a patient's psychosocial equilibrium, negative life experiences seem to cause the most intense responses (Sarason et al., 1978). These include loss of relationships (especially of family members and friends), loss of self-esteem, loss or decrease in body function, major economic reversals, and change of home site (Masuda and Holmes, 1978). Identification of high-impact stressors is important, but the physician should also seek to identify other life change events that may be troubling the patient, for in some patients it will be a "pile-up" of life change events that causes emotional disequilibrium (Patterson, 1988).

The second category of stressors that contributes to psychosocial risk includes role strains or chronic life situations associated with an individual's position as a parent, friend, patient, employee, student, or member of a family or group (Pearlin and Johnson, 1977). Conflicts in role relationships, such as with one's boss, may severely challenge an individual's psychosocial equilibrium and have a negative impact on health (Hamburg and Killilea, 1979).

The physician who is able to identify role strains and stressful life events that contribute to a patient's maladaptive behavior is in a position to combine biomedical and psychosocial interventions to the patient's advantage. In all psychosocial risk studies, however, it is not enough to identify stressors. The physician must also assess the significance of stressors

CASE HISTORY: A 35-year-old, white, divorced, male computer scientist, who recently moved to a new city, reported to his physician the recent onset of chest pain and anxiety. Psychosocial assessment is shown below following the pathways of the Cycle of Psychosocial Risk. Biomedical assessment, which was also completed by his physician, did not reveal any organic pathology.

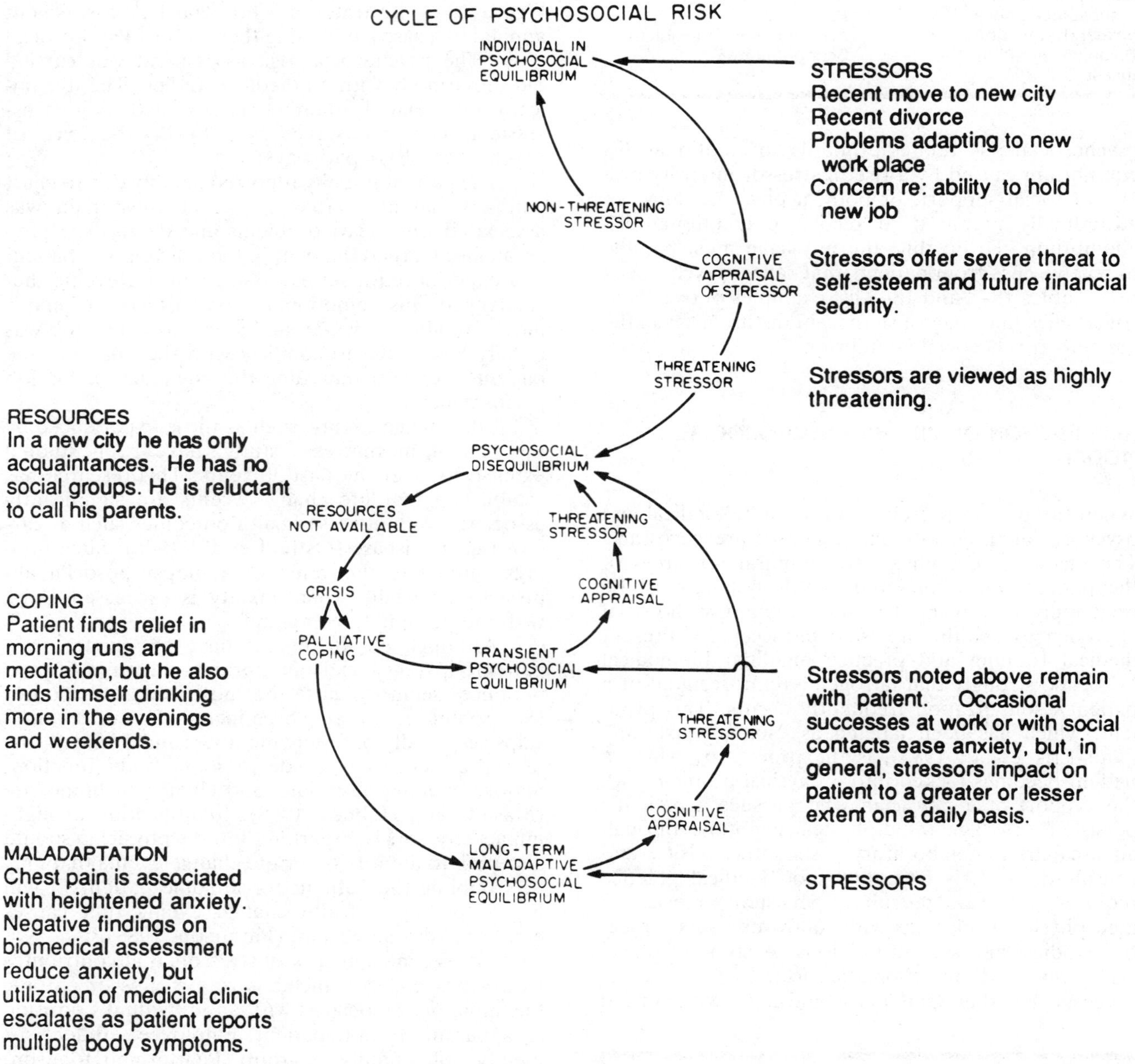
CYCLE OF PSYCHOSOCIAL RISK
INDIVIDUAL IN PSYCHOSOCIAL EQUILIBRIUM
STRESSORS
Recent move to new city
Recent divorce
Problems adapting to new work place
Concern re: ability to hold new job
NON-THREATENING STRESSOR
COGNITIVE APPRAISAL OF STRESSOR
Stressors offer severe threat to self-esteem and future financial security.
THREATENING STRESSOR
Stressors are viewed as highly threatening.
RESOURCES
In a new city he has only acquaintances. He has no social groups. He is reluctant to call his parents.
PSYCHOSOCIAL DISEQUILIBRIUM
RESOURCES NOT AVAILABLE
THREATENING STRESSOR
COGNITIVE APPRAISAL
CRISIS
COPING
Patient finds relief in morning runs and meditation, but he also finds himself drinking more in the evenings and weekends.
PALLIATIVE COPING
TRANSIENT PSYCHOSOCIAL EQUILIBRIUM
Stressors noted above remain with patient. Occasional successes at work or with social contacts ease anxiety, but, in general, stressors impact on patient to a greater or lesser extent on a daily basis.
THREATENING STRESSOR
COGNITIVE APPRAISAL
MALADAPTATION
Chest pain is associated with heightened anxiety. Negative findings on biomedical assessment reduce anxiety, but utilization of medical clinic escalates as patient reports multiple body symptoms.
LONG-TERM MALADAPTIVE PSYCHOSOCIAL EQUILIBRIUM
STRESSORS

Figure 18–3. Psychosocial stressors and resources are given empiric values so that psychosocial risk may be calculated. The interactive effect of biomedical and psychosocial risk yields a combined risk. Knowledge of a combined risk enhances the physician's ability to predict health outcome.

to the patient (Kleinman and Smilkstein, 1980). This is, perhaps, the most problematic aspect of psychosocial assessment because physicians often assume they understand the intensity of a patient's stressors based on their own experiences. Such an attitude fails to recognize that differences in cultural and social backgrounds of physicians and patients result in physicians and patients making different cognitive appraisals of stressors. In order for the physician's response to be effective, the physician need not agree with the patient regarding the significance of the stressor; however, when the physician accurately understands the patient's idiosyncratic cognitive appraisal of the stressor, therapeutic intervention will be facilitated.

Figure 18–3 traces the patient's movement into the lower cycle of unresolved stressors. He traveled this route primarily because his resources were inadequate and his coping strategies did permit use of available social support, such as his parents. Although palliative coping techniques (exercise and meditation) gave some relief, the strain of the unresolved stressors remained.

The appearance of the chest pain significantly altered the patient's homeostasis. As a somatic representation of the patient's heightened anxiety, the chest pain denied the patient the option of exercise for palliative coping. The perceived physical problem did, however, lead the patient to the physician.

The physician thoroughly investigated the biomedical aspects of the case. But when the physical and laboratory findings were reported to the patient as normal, the reassurance did not relieve the patient's anxiety. Psychotropic drugs were prescribed to relieve this anxiety; however, the physician's records showed an increase in office visits, with the patient reporting early morning wakening and loss of appetite.

Management of individuals at high psychosocial risk is challenging. Physicians frequently find that the care of these patients is characterized, as in this case, by high utilization and poor compliance (Becker and Maiman, 1975). As stress takes its toll, depression becomes more evident and often requires intense biopsychosocial intervention by the physician to maintain function and, at times, to prevent suicide.

When it became evident from the psychosocial risk assessment that this patient's anxiety and depression were a major problem, interventions based on the cyclic model were designed. These included interventions that specifically addressed components of the cyclic model, e.g., regular scheduled office visits to the physician, listening time by the physician to identify work and home problems, reassurance regarding the patient's heart status, and counseling to encourage use of support from family and friends.

After the biopsychosocial therapeutic interventions were initiated by the physician, changes were observed in the patient that suggested improvement. He identified a few individuals in the community with whom he shared common interests. He realistically examined his stressors to determine whether they were resolvable, and he voluntarily discontinued his psychotropic drugs and decreased the number of his office visits.

In general, as clarified by the cyclic model, movement toward psychosocial equilibrium can be measured by a patient's ability to recognize the stressors that are jeopardizing emotional stability, to identify resources and employ them appropriately, to move away from drug and physician assistance, and to employ coping strategies that advance physical and emotional health.

Principles of Psychosocial Intervention

The physician who wishes to identify the psychosocial risks that may influence health care or health outcome must assess the patient's stressors and resources (Hinkle, 1987). The process is initiated when a cue suggests overt or covert evidence for psychosocial dysfunction. A willingness to listen to the patient will usually facilitate the identification of major stressors. Once the stressor or stressors have been identified, the physician should ask the patient to estimate the importance of the stressor(s) in his or her life.

The second part of the psychosocial risk equation requires the assessment of resources. It is not enough to establish that the patient has family and friends. The resource person(s) must be available and valued by the patient.

For those patients who are identified as having anxiety due to high psychosocial risk, short-term intervention requires consideration of appropriate medications and techniques for palliative coping (e.g., time-out, aerobic exercises, and behavior modification).

In the office or clinic, behavior modification has special merit. If continuity of care can be effected, wellness activities can be substituted for dysfunctional behavior such as high utilization and somatization.

An outline of behavior modification includes the following agenda: physical activity is chosen that is acceptable to the patient (e.g., walking); time or distance goals, or both, are set; reinforcement of the activity is carried out by family, friends, and physician; the activity is rehearsed, monitored, and shaped to advance the patient's performance and improve the patient's self-esteem. Central to the success of behavior modification is the identification of appropriate goals and the encouragement given by the patient's social support system (Martin and Coates, 1987).

Whenever possible, remedial coping should be the long-range goal of the physician and patient partnership. This long-term intervention requires identification of resources that may be directed toward the management of anxiety-producing stressors (e.g., use of counseling, educational programs, social agencies, and psychotherapy).

Physicians should recognize that they are major resources in the treatment of patients at psychosocial risk. But even with optimal physician assistance, high-risk patients with poor social support, whose lives are characterized by an accumulation of high-intensity stressors, frequently experience an accentuation of physical and emotional health problems. The most effective treatment for such patients may be long-term, supportive therapy. This therapy involves three strategies: (1) offering regular appointments at which time positive feedback is given to bolster self-esteem (usually focusing on behavior modification); (2) addressing stressors as contributors to illness problems;

and (3) searching for new resources at each patient encounter.

References

Ader, R., and Cohen, N.: Behaviorally conditioned immunosuppression. Psychosom. Med., *37:*333–340, 1975.

Baldwin, B.A.: A paradigm for the classification of emotional crisis: Implications for crisis intervention. Am. J. Orthopsychiatry, *48:*438–551, 1978.

Beautrais, A.L., Fergusson, B.A., and Shannon, F.T.: Life events and childhood morbidity: A prospective study. Pediatrics, *70:*935–940, 1982. *This study relates stressful life events to childhood illnesses and hospitalizations. Significant relationships are demonstrated between stressors and childhood illnesses.*

Becker, M.H., and Maiman, L.A.: Sociobehavioral determinants of compliance with health care recommendations. Med. Care, *13:*10–14, 1975.

Borysenko, M., and Borysenko, J.: Stress, behavior and immunity: Animal models and mediating mechanics. Gen. Hosp. Psychiatry, *4:*59–67, 1982.

Bowden, C.L.: Anxiety defenses and adaptation. *In* Bowden, C.L., and Burstein, A.G. (Eds.): Psychosocial Basis of Health Care. 3rd ed. Baltimore, Williams & Wilkins, 1983.

Cassel, J.C.: Psychosocial processes and stress: A theoretical formulation. Int. Health Serv., *3:*471–482, 1974.

Cassel, J: The contributions of social environments to host resistance. Am. J. Epidemiol., *104:*107–123, 1976.

Cobb, S: Social support as a moderator of life stress. Psychosom. Med. *38:*300–314, 1976.

Cohen, S., Sherrod, D.R., and Clark, M.S.: Social skills and the stress-protection role of social support. J. Pers. Soc. Psychol., *50:*963–973, 1986.

Dohrenwend, B.S., and Dohrenwend, B.P.: Stressful Life Events and Their Contexts. New Brunswick, Rutgers University Press, 1984. *These authors have been responsible for a number of critical reports on stressful life events. They have carefully reviewed the impact of stressful life events on health. The reader of this book will be able to put stressful life event research in perspective.*

Eisenberg, L., and Kleinman, A. (Eds.): The Relevance of Social Science for Medicine. Boston, D. Reidel, 1981, p. 12.

Engel, G.L.: The need for a new medical model: A challenge for biomedicine. Science, *196:*129–136, 1977.

Engel, G.L.: The clinical application of the bio-psychosocial model. Am. J. Psychol., *137:*535–544, 1980. *This paper, along with Dr. Engel's 1977 article in* Science, *"The Need for a new Medical Model: A Challenge for Biomedicine," offers a scientific rationale for physicians assessing both biomedical and psychosocial risk. A case study is used to identify the biopsychosocial forces that influence a patient's health outcome.*

Ford, C.V.: The Somatizing Disorders: Illness as a Way of Life. New York, Elsevier Biomedical, 1983.

Fordyce, W.E.: Behavioral Methods for Chronic Pain and Illness. St. Louis, C.V. Mosby, 1976.

Girard, D.E., Arthur, R.J., and Reler, J.B.: Psychosocial events and subsequent illness: A review. West. J. Med., *142:*358–363, 1985.

Hamburg, B.A., and Killilea, M.: Relation of social support, stress, illness and use of health services. *In* The Surgeon General's Report/Institute of Medicine. Washington, D.C., U.S. Government Printing Office, 1979, pp. 253–276.

Haynes, S.G., Feinleib, M., and Kannel, W.B.: The relationship of psychosocial factors to coronary heart disease in the Framingham study: III. Eight-year incidence of coronary heart disease. Am. J. Epidemiol., *111:*37–58, 1980.

Hill, R.: Generic features of families under stress. In Parad, H.J. (ed). Crisis Intervention: Selected Readings. New York. Family Service Association of America, 1965, pp. 32–52. *This article describes the family crisis ("X") that results from an interaction among "A" (Stressor), with "B" (Interpretation of Stressor) and, "C" (Social Support Resources). This ABCX formula has served as the template for a number of family studies since 1965.*

Hinkle, L.E., Jr.: The concepts of stress in the biologic and social sciences. Sci. Med. Man, *1:*31–48, 1973.

Hinkle, L.E., Jr.: Stress and disease: The concept after 50 years. Soc. Sci. Med., *25:*561–566, 1987. *An excellent review article for those studying the relationship of stress and disease by an author with 30 years of experience in psychosocial risk research. Present evidence suggests that stress does contribute to health impairment; however, a number of other variables may buffer or accentuate the stress effect. The dynamic nature of psychosocial risk represents a major challenge for biopsychosocial research.*

Holmes, T.H., and Rahe, R.H.: The social readjustment rating scale. J. Psychosom. Res., *11:*213–218, 1967.

Kleinman, A., and Smilkstein, G.: Psychosocial issues. *In* Rosen, G.M., Geyman, J.P., and Layton, R.H. (Eds.): Behavioral Science in Family Practice. New York, Appleton-Century-Crofts, 1980. *The value of this chapter lies in the review of illness as an expression of psychosocial risk. Illness problems are frequently associated with the "difficult" patient; therefore, understanding psychosocial risk can facilitate the management of illness problems.*

Kobosa, S.C., Maddi, S.R., and Kahn, S.: Hardiness and health: A prospective study. J. Pers. Soc. Psychol., *42:*168–177, 1982. *Emotional hardiness may be a factor in maintaining health. The authors identify the characteristics of hardiness, but they do not report how it is achieved. Hardiness is a function of commitment, internal locus of control and challenging difficult life situations. In the study, hardy people had fewer health problems than controls.*

Lazarus, R.S., Averill, J.R., and Opton, E.M., Jr.: The psychology of coping: Issues of research and assessment. *In* Coelho, G.V., Hamburg, D.A., and Adams, J.E. (Eds.): Coping and Adaptation. New York, Basic Books, 1974, p. 264.

Lazarus, R.S., and Folkman, S.: Stress, Appraisal and Coping. New York, Springer, 1984, pp. 266–270.

Levi, L.: Psychosocial factors in preventive medicine. *In* The Surgeon General's Report/Institute of Medicine: Healthy People. Washington, D.C., U.S. Government Printing Office, 1979, pp. 207–252.

Martin, A.R., and Coates, T.J.: A clinician's guide to helping patients change behavior. West. J. Med., *146:*751–753, 1987.

Masuda, M., and Holmes, T.H.: Life events: Perceptions and frequencies. Psychosom. Med., *40:*236–261, 1978.

Mechanic, D.: Social psychologic factors affecting the presentation of bodily complaints. N. Engl. J. Med., *286:*1132–1139, 1972.

Medalie, J.A., and Goldbourt, U.: Angina pectoris among 10,000 men: II. Psychosocial and other risk factors as evidenced by a multivariate analysis of a five-year incidence study. Am. J. Med., *60:*910–921, 1976. *This paper reports one of the earliest studies that related social support to health outcome. Angina pectoris was found to be significantly related to dysfunctional social support.*

Nachemson, A.: Prevention of chronic back pain: The orthopedic challenge for the '80's. Bull. Hosp. Jt. Dis. Orthop. Inst., *44:*1–15, 1984. *This paper reflects the studies of an internationally prominent investigator of diseases of the spine. Diagnostic difficulties are identified and related to problems in the assessment of low back pain in the somatizing patient.*

Ostfeld, A.M., Berkman, L.F., Kahn, R.L., et al.: Social support and social networks. *In* Ostfeld, A.M., and Eaker, E.D. (Eds.): Measuring Psychosocial Variables in Epidemiologic Studies of Cardiovascular Disease. Washington, D.C., NIH Publication No. 85-2270, U.S. Government Printing Office, 1985, pp. 49–101.

Parsons, T.: Definitions of health and illness in the light of American values and social structure. *In* Jaco, E.G. (Ed.): Patients, Physicians, and Illness. Glencoe, Illinois, The Free Press, 1958.

Patterson, J.M.: Families experiencing stress. Fam. Systems Med., *6:*202–237, 1988.

Pearlin, L.I., and Johnson, J.S.: Marital status, life-strains and depression. Am. Soc. Rev., *42:*704–715, 1977.

Pearlin, L., Menaghan, E., Lieberman, M., and Mullan, J.T.: The stress process. J. Health Soc. Behav., *22:*237–356, 1981. *This paper enlarges one's view of life's stressors. In addition to* *stressful life events, the authors discuss the contributions of chronic life events that are persistent and stressful.*

Pratt, L.: Family structure and effective health behavior: The energized family. Boston, Houghton Mifflin, 1976. *This book features an epidemiologic study of families. A relationship is demonstrated between cohesive-functional families and decreased use of the health care system. The study described in this book was one of the earliest to correlate family function with health of family members.*

Reeb, K., Graham, A., Zyzanski, S., and Kitson, G.: Predicting low birthweight and complicated labor in urban black women: A biopsychosocial perspective. Soc. Sci. Med., *25*(12):1321–1327, 1987. *Biopsychosocial studies in pregnancy offer increased understanding of pregnancy outcome. This paper reports pregnancy outcome in a selected population; however, the research design identifies the critical variables central to biopsychosocial research in pregnancy.*

Rosen, G., Kleinman, A., and Katon, W.: Somatization in family practice: A biopsychosocial approach. J. Fam. Pract., *14:*493–502, 1982. *This paper offers a basic review of somatization in primary care. The authors, a family physician and two psychiatrists (one with international credentials in medical authropology) offer a balanced view of the biomedical and psychosocial assessment of the somatizing patient.*

Sarason, I.G., Johnson, J., and Siegel, J: Assessing the impact of life changes: Development of the life experiences survey. J. Consult. Clin. Psychol., *46:*932–946, 1978.

Sarason, I.G., Sarason, B.R., Potter, E.H., and Antoni, M.H.: Life events, social support and illness. Psychosom. Med. *47:*156–163, 1985. *These authors review the relationship of stressful life events and social support to illness. The strength of the paper is the authors' knowledge of the studies related to social support and health.*

Shonkoff, J.P.: Social support and vulnerability to stress: A pediatric perspective. Pediatr. Ann., *14:*550–554, 1985.

Smilkstein, G.: The cycle of family function. A conceptual model for family medicine. J. Fam. Pract., *11:*223–232, 1980.

Smilkstein, G.: The unity of biomedical and psychosocial issues in individual and family health care. *In* Carr, J.E. and Dengerink, H.A. (Eds.): Behavioral Science in the Practice of Medicine. Elsevier Biomedical, New York, 1983, pp. 168–183. *This is a survey paper that reviews the literature that relates biopsychosocial risk factors of stress and social support to health outcome.*

Smilkstein, G.: The physician and family function assessment. Fam. Systems Med., *2:*263–278, 1984.

Smilkstein, G., Helsper-Lucas, A., Ashworth, C., et al.: Prediction of pregnancy complications: An application of the biopsychosocial model. Soc. Sci. Med., *18:*315–321, 1984.

Smilkstein, G.: Family assessment tools. *In* Henao, S. and Grose, N.P. (Eds.): Principles of Family Systems in Family Medicine, New York, Brunner/Mazel, Inc., 1985, pp. 372–389. *Hundreds of instruments have been devised to test family function, yet few are applicable to clinical situations. This paper reviews some of the more pragmatic family function tools.*

Spielberger, C.D.: Anxiety: Current Trends in Theory and Research. Vols. 1 and 2. New York, Academic Press, 1972, pp. 23–49. *Spielberger's State-Trait Anxiety Scale (STA) is one of the most commonly used questionnaires to evaluate anxiety. The text reviews the basic studies that relate to anxiety research.*

Stein, M., Schiavi, R.C., and Camerino, M.: Influence of brain and behavior on the immune system. Science, *191:*435–439, 1976.

Thoits, P.S.: Social support as coping assistance. J. Consult. Clin. Psychol., *54:*416–423, 1986. *Thoits reviews data that gives credence to the role of social support as a stressor buffer. The author also gives appropriate reference to the limitations of these studies.*

Van Eijk, J.Th.M., Grol, R.P.T.M., Hugen, F.J.A., et al.: The family doctor and the prevention of somatic fixation. Fam. Systems Med., *2:*5–15, 1983. *Somatic fixation is a theory that relates somatization to the overenthusiastic application of the biomedical model by physicians. Although further studies are needed to clarify the role of the physician in somatization, the implication of excessive use of biomedical interventions makes the physician highly suspect.*

Walker, K.N., MacBride, A., and Vachon, M.S.S.: Social support networks and the crisis of bereavement. Soc. Sci. Med., *11:*35–41, 1977.

19

Community-Oriented Primary Care

Paul A. Nutting
Larry A. Green

An unprecedented growth in knowledge and technology since the mid-1940's has engulfed the medical profession, producing many miracles of modern medicine but also leading to an unfortunate overemphasis on the biotechnology of health care. By the mid-1960's this technological revolution had nearly eliminated the practice of primary care, but fortunately the pendulum has begun to reverse its swing, aided by the timely development and growth of family medicine. Over its nearly 20 years, family medicine has been uniquely committed to providing primary care to individuals and family units. Compared with other disciplines, family medicine makes no claim to subspecialty care but rather devotes its energies to practicing, teaching, and developing the knowledge base of primary care, an all-encompassing field that focuses on the patient and his or her problems. With the growing strength of family medicine, primary care is slowly becoming once again the foundation of the health care system in the United States.

As primary care has begun to gain prominence, renewed interest is also being given to community-oriented primary care (COPC). Once considered to be the domain of publicly funded health programs treating underprivileged populations, the principles of COPC are now being embraced by private practices and for-profit health programs as well. *Community-oriented primary care is a modification of the traditional model of primary care in which a primary care practice or program systematically identifies and addresses the health problems of a defined population.* This is accomplished by combining primary care skills and the principles of epidemiology. Although not the prevailing form of primary care in this country, the challenges of COPC are increasingly attracting the interest and attention of primary care physicians, educators, and researchers.

COPC has only recently become part of the vocabulary of primary care, but the underlying concepts have been expressed by primary care advocates in the United States for some time (White, et al., 1961; Sheps, 1978; Geiger, 1967; Haggerty et al., 1975). These and other proponents of primary care have stressed the need to harness and direct the technical capability of our health care system toward addressing the health care needs of defined populations. Each has argued for a central strategy that combines epidemiology and primary medical care. Sidney Kark first introduced the term COPC to primary care literature in describing his work first in South Africa and more recently in Israel (Kark, 1981). He defines COPC as "a strategy whereby elements of primary health care and of community medicine are systematically developed and brought together in a coordinated practice." Writing on the topic in the context of the United States, Donald Madison characterizes a community-responsive practice as "one which assumes a larger than ordinary share of responsibility for safeguarding the health of a community, and which follows through on this responsibility by taking action beyond the traditional mode of treating the complaints and problems of patients as they approach the practice one-by-one" (Madison and Shenkin, 1978). In describing the future of COPC in the United States, Fitzhugh Mullan characterizes COPC as "the reunion of the traditions of public health and personal clinical health services" (Mullan, 1982).

The principles of COPC have a long-standing tradition, having provided the philosophical foundation for publicly funded health programs for many years. As one example, community health centers strive to address the health problems of the local communities in underprivileged areas and target primary care services toward medically needy populations. On another front, the Indian Health Service has delivered health care services to American Indians and Alaskan natives since 1955. Over a 30-year period, a comprehensive, integrated primary care program has been developed that operates within and is tailored to the health needs of particular Indian communities. Community involvement has been an integral philosophical underpinning of both the community health centers and the Indian Health Service.

More recently, the mainstream of primary care has begun to adopt elements of COPC as well. A recent study from the Institute of Medicine described the implementation of COPC principles in different primary care settings in the United States. The study concluded that although it is not a prevalent form of primary care practice, the approach of COPC offers great promise as a form of primary care that is responsive to the health care needs of defined populations, ranging from geopolitical communities to the enrolled populations of prepaid health plans (Institute of Medicine, 1984a). Seven case studies demonstrated the feasibility, if not always the practicality, of COPC in vastly different health care environments, illustrating the spectrum of COPC utilization in settings typical of today's health care system (Institute of Medicine, 1984b). This is particularly the case with prepaid group practices, an increasingly common form of service delivery over the last decade. With a contractual obligation to a fixed enrollment, Health Maintenance Organizations (HMOs) have an economic incentive to respond to the perceived health needs of their enrolled communities.

In recent years, family physicians have begun to shift their focus from care of unusual problems to the care of common maladies, from the care of specific organ systems to the care of the entire individual, and from care limited by artificial boundaries dividing specialties to problems as they occur in the community. This broadened focus offers a rich substrate for the principles of COPC to take root and grow. Although family medicine has no monopoly on COPC, it represents the most promising opportunities for growth because its broad mandate permits a physician to be attentive to problems such as unplanned pregnancy, child abuse, hypercholesterolemia, somatization, inadequate immunization, and substance abuse. In summary, family medicine offers the best hope for incorporating the central principles of COPC into the mainstream of primary care.

Why Community-Oriented Primary Care?

COPC is a process by which physicians examine their practice for the purpose of improving the health of their communities. Inevitably, after adopting this perspective, the physician discovers unmet needs that differ from service demands and finds that the existing knowledge base is insufficient to define or address important problems within the community. Herein lies the untapped intellectual challenge that combines the fulfillment of community practice with the adventure of exploring one's world.

COPC provides a strategy for defining and addressing a target population and an opportunity to market primary care services that are responsive not only to the demands but also to the health care needs of that population. Although most family physicians are hesitant to join the competitive marketplace with overt marketing practices, COPC provides a patient-oriented strategy for defining persons in need of care and for offering an appropriate mix of medical care services. Ironically, primary care and COPC may become financially more attractive to subspecialty physicians as third party payers consider remodeling the relative value scale for physicians' fees. The attractiveness of COPC to patients may also attract new devotees in light of the projected excess of physicians in some specialties and the resulting competition for patients. Practices with the competitive edge are likely to be those that have captured and served a target population well, and in this regard COPC offers a distinct advantage.

In an educational setting, COPC can provide the structure for defining and exploring the health problems of a population, an intellectual perspective that acknowledges the full range of the common problems that patients bring to a primary care practice. Students and residents should be trained to treat the community as a living laboratory, one that requires a probing, active physician and that needs to be understood and managed. The myopic view of the community as the sum of active patients needs to be strongly discouraged. Instead, physicians-in-training need to be offered the skills that will permit them to accept the community as the appropriate focus of their primary care efforts.

In summary COPC offers a context for the physician to expand beyond the focus of the examining room and to systematically consider the larger population from which active patients emerge for care. COPC offers a set of strategies and techniques that can assist any family physician to define and respond to the priority health problems of the community.

Moreover, the fundamental principles of COPC serve as a catalyst for a physician to become involved in a community and to confront the myriad health care issues that are relevant to that community. Perhaps most importantly, engaging in a COPC practice can lead the family physician to a deeper sense of satisfaction with the practice of primary care. In a health care arena that undervalues primary care, COPC offers an opportunity to act fully on the important principles that have guided the practice of medicine for centuries.

COPC as a Form of Practice-Based Research

There is a pressing need to develop the knowledge base of primary care—that system of theory and fact upon which primary care as a scientific discipline will eventually rest. A portion of this foundation will derive from research in the actual practice settings of primary care. The rich tradition of practice-based research that exists in the United Kingdom is only now beginning in the United States. For example, the seminal work of practice networks, such as the Ambulatory Sentinel Practice Network, has started to contribute to an understanding of primary care (Iverson et al., 1988). The great value of such practice networks lies in their potential to function as a laboratory with access to the relevant phenomena of community life and family practice. They have also demonstrated that primary care research networks are feasible and offer opportunities for uniting clinicians, academicians, and others concerned about public welfare. Moreover, the knowledge emerging from this work that addresses questions relevant to practice should be useful in other community practice settings. Issues that remain to be explored through practice networks include analyses of the distribution of care and the patterns of care-seeking behavior in a primary care population, the natural history or concerns that people bring to primary care physicians, studies of referral patterns and methods for achieving coordinated care, specific interventions that show promise of relieving suffering at the level of primary care, and investigations of the distribution of functionality versus dysfunctionality within a primary care population. Those family practices that identify and collect data on their denominator populations are in an ideal occupation to engage in and contribute to the kind of population-based research so necessary to building the knowledge base for primary care.

The simultaneous re-emergence of interest in COPC and practice-based research in the 1980's is probably not accidental. Both represent corrective actions to the extraordinary success of the modern health science center, with its unforeseen adverse consequences. These centers have emphasized the unusual phenomena in medicine; that which Last refers to as the "tip of the iceberg" (Last, 1963), and which White characterizes as "the smallest box in the ecology of medical care" (White et al., 1961), leaving in relative neglect the common concerns of patients. In response, family practice leaders are recognizing the urgent need to apply with greater vigor the methods of science to phenomena occurring at the level of the community. Of course, all practice-based research is not part of COPC and the major thrust of COPC is not research; but they are syntonic in their intent and process, and they both seek to overcome similar selection and observer biases by concentrating attention on a defined population. Because of this common interest, progress in practice-based research is likely to fuel COPC, and the COPC process will, in turn, stimulate critical inquiry into the clinical problems people most commonly have.

The Components of COPC

The basic elements of COPC are simple and consist of (1) a primary care practice or program, (2) a defined population that the practice wishes to serve, and (3) a process by which the major health problems of the target population are addressed. Given the dramatic variations in the organization and financing of primary care, it is not surprising that the basic elements have been widely adapted to the practice environments of different communities, as demonstrated by the case studies in the Institute of Medicine report on COPC (Institute of Medicine, 1984b). A model of COPC has been proposed that accommodates different utilizations of COPC while providing enough structure to support research, education, and practice (Nutting, 1986).

PRIMARY CARE PRACTICE OR PROGRAM

The face of primary care in the United States continues to evolve with new practice plans constantly being developed. Practices that differ in their organizational structure and methods of financing will nonetheless find that the COPC model is flexible enough to accommodate a vast range of organizational characteristics. The only requirement is that the practice meet the basic characteristics of primary care; namely, that it *offer an array of personal health services that are accessible and acceptable to the patient, comprehensive in scope, coordinated and continuous over time, and for which the physician is accountable for the quality and potential effects of services offered*. The primary care component of the model addresses the services a practice provides but not the composition or organization of the physicians or the manner by which the costs are reimbursed (directly or indirectly by the patient, patient groups, or third parties).

THE COMMUNITY OR TARGET POPULATION

There is a myth that there is an ideal definition of a community. In reality, the target population changes continually and usually requires an explicit definition before a particular program can be mounted or a study question can be answered. For example, a practice might define its population as all patients seen in the past 2 years. Even this simple population will change each day as some patients leave and others join. In accepting ongoing changes in this population, such a definition might be relevant to an immunization campaign. In comparison, however, a program used to detect early developmental delays would need to focus on a subset of the population. The critical concept is not to define the particular population but to define a relevant population and accept responsibility at some level for offering a mix of health services that are relevant to its needs and demands.

In some settings, the COPC practice will address true communities, those sharing common social, cultural, economic, and political systems. In other cases, the community may consist of less clearly defined and perhaps less organized groups such as individuals enrolled in a health plan, occupational or workplace populations, or school populations. Where the community is difficult to define, the practice may choose to limit its focus to its active patient population or more broadly to its practice population, the latter consisting of all members of households of active patients.

Involving the community or members of the target population in the process is an important feature of COPC and one to be encouraged where possible. However, the manner and extent to which it is feasible for the community participants to collaborate in the process of COPC will vary widely across different settings, whether they are small fee-for-service practices in rural areas, large urban HMOs, or publicly funded community health centers. Although a fee-for-service suburban practice would appear to be the least conducive to community participation, at least one excellent example has been described (Seifert, 1987).

The range of variation for community participation can be thought of in terms of (1) the organization and mechanisms of input, (2) the level of involvement, and (3) the focus of attention. Of these factors, the focus of attention is perhaps the most critical. Just as physicians have a tendency to focus their attention on their most active patients (the numerator of the practice), the community participants also often develop a "numerator bias." For example, the consumer boards of federally funded community health centers frequently focus on administrative issues surrounding the daily operation of the health facility. When attention is broadened to the "denominator" population, community involvement can add a distinctly new and vitally important dimension to the identification of community health problems. For example, group consensus techniques can enhance the involvement of consumers and physicians in setting priorities among competing health needs and in allocating constrained resources among competing health programs (Horowitz and Gallagher, 1987). *The critical role for the patient and community participants is to develop a "denominator bias" and to represent the interests of the entire target population while participating in the functions of the COPC process.*

THE COPC PROCESS

The third component of the model is the process by which the major health problems of the community are identified and systematically addressed. This process can be described as a set of activities that fall into four functional categories, and each can be accomplished through a variety of strategies (Nutting, 1987).

Defining and Characterizing the Community. The tradition of primary care has stressed the importance of understanding the community from which individual patients present for care. The COPC model extends this notion to the denominator group, recommending that the health status of the population be analyzed with the same rigor that the physician uses when approaching the individual patient. The physician needs to know who the individuals are who compose the denominator population, where they live, how their behavior influences their health, where and when they seek care for ailments, and how they perceive and finance their care.

Through years of practice and observation, many family physicians will have developed a basic knowledge of their community based on subjective analysis of information gained from patients and the fact of living and often raising a family in the community. In the absence of a systematic approach to collecting and analyzing the data on the community, however, family physicians may erroneously generalize patterns of health and health behavior from their most familiar patients (the numerator) to the target community (the denominator). Most physicians can recall from their training examples of this error made by specialists who assume the importance of some obscure disease that appears commonly in their specialty practice.

In many instances valuable information on the community can be derived from secondary data obtained from the local health department. Census and vital statistics can also be useful in the early development of an information base on the community, and these statistics are clearly most relevant when drawn from a population that corresponds closely to the target population of the practice.

Identifying the Community Health Problems. The second step follows logically from the first and includes the activities necessary to identify the major health problems of the community, characterize their determinants and correlates, and set priorities among them. Initially, it may be appropriate to identify important problems based on the physician's practice impressions and the perceptions of community members. The use of group process techniques can improve the rigor of these activities (Horowitz and Gallagher, 1987). In addition, information can often be obtained at reasonable expense through secondary data sources (vital statistics and epidemiologic studies).

Community surveys can be helpful and potentially yield important information, but they are expensive and time consuming, and too often the momentum for COPC dissipates during the long process of designing, conducting, and analyzing survey information. It is important to realize that in the nearly 60 examples of community problems addressed by 26 programs and practices surveyed during the Institute of Medicine study (Institute of Medicine, 1984a), not a single health problem was discovered from primary data collection that was not previously suspected by either the physicians or the community (Nutting et al., 1985). This is not to suggest that primary data collection may not be important in the COPC process. New data are often needed to clarify the extent and severity of the problem and to develop an intervention that will be successful within that particular population. At the same time, however, when primary data collection is not feasible, impressions derived from experience in the practice and secondary data can help delineate health problems that warrant the practice's attention.

Most practices that undertake this process will find a number of important health problems, and some attention will be required to set priorities among them. For the family physician this may require deciding between such disparate problems as teen pregnancy, breast cancer screening, or *Haemophilus influenzae* immunization in children.

Modifying Practice Patterns. Once a priority health problem has been identified, the COPC practice should develop an intervention strategy to better address the problem. In practice, these strategies generally fall into two categories. First, the physician can initiate an emphasis program entirely within the practice by modifying practice patterns. In this case, the emphasis program will consist largely of varying the mix and array of services provided, targeting services toward high-risk individuals, or changing patterns of accessibility to services. Second, the physician can develop or collaborate in an emphasis program beyond the scope of the practice. In this case, the physician may retain the traditional role of the physician or may assume the role of an active citizen. The active COPC physician will be involved simultaneously in emphasis programs that mix both categories.

Most interventions are not intended to blanket all members of the community, nor are they intended to be limited to those individuals who present for or request certain services. Often those individuals who might benefit most from the emphasis program are not active users of the health care system at all. In this case, efforts to target high-risk individuals and mount aggressive outreach activities may be necessary to achieve the desired effect. Even simple interventions may have a dramatic impact when successfully targeted toward specific individuals at increased risk (Nutting et al., 1975).

Monitoring Impact of Program Modifications. Of the four COPC functions, this is the one that is most often neglected. Although it is tempting to move to the next health problem, some level of effort should be devoted to assessing the impact of practice modifications. In addition to identifying refinements that may increase the impact of emphasis programs, monitoring practice activities permits elimination of those activities that may already have served their purpose with little or no continuing benefit, thus freeing up energies and resources for program activities with potentially higher impact.

In reality, all programs are evaluated on a subjective level. Practitioners and patients alike form opinions of new programs and both are often vocal in their views. Where more formal evaluation and primary data collection are needed, the evaluation plan should be simple enough to be realistically implemented but rigorous enough to provide information that is useful in determining the future of the local intervention effort under study. The first and most important step in accomplishing this is to state as precisely as possible the evaluation question to be addressed and to frame it in the context of the entire denominator population. Too often emphasis programs are designed to address an important problem within the target population, but evaluation efforts focus only on those individuals who emerge from the community as active users of the practice. Evaluations that are "numerator based" can lead to erroneous judgments of program benefit (Nutting, 1987b).

Problems and Obstacles

The development of a COPC practice or program will entail several difficult problems (Madison, 1983; Rogers, 1982) that will vary with the practice setting. First, for many practices the community may be extremely complex and difficult to define, particularly in urban areas in which the community can be subdivided into neighborhoods, each with a unique ethnic and social structure. Many communities, especially suburban communities, are served by a multitude of practices and health programs, making it difficult for physicians to distinguish their own community from those of other practices. Indeed, many families and individuals do not look to a single practice or program for all of their health care services, using several physicians instead.

Most physicians have a limited set of resources at their disposal that can be directed to COPC activities. It is uncommon to find a primary care practice that has an abundance of financial reserves, staff commitment, or time and energy to be devoted to activities beyond direct patient care.

Most practices have only a basic data system, in many cases limited to the hard copy of the medical record. Although many practices are converting to data automation, most computer systems in primary care are devoted to billing and other practice management tasks. Even those practices with well-developed patient care information systems often find that data are limited to their active patients and do not serve well in identifying and characterizing the health problems of the larger target population.

Primary care physicians generally lack specific skills, knowledge, and experience in the principles, strategies, and methods of COPC. This lack is reminiscent of the predicament of the medical graduates of two decades ago. Upon entering a primary care practice, physicians found that they lacked many of the skills necessary to provide care for those common problems that were prevalent in their patient population but that were rare in the teaching curriculum of the tertiary care centers where they trained. The current dilemma is an extension of the old problem: although training programs in primary care are now providing improved training in the treatment of primary care problems, they are deficient in training physicians how to define and respond to health problems within their target populations or communities. Much has been accomplished through academic departments of community medicine, but regrettable gaps remain between the training for primary care, community medicine, and public health.

Quantitative tools and techniques that are feasible for COPC activities are lacking in most primary care settings. Although methods have been well developed in the parent disciplines of demography, epidemiology, anthropology, health services and evaluation research, and biostatistics, they have not been distilled and fitted to the unique needs of the busy primary care setting. To be useful and to support the practice of COPC, tools and techniques must strike a careful balance between the ease and simplicity with which they can be used and the rigor required to confidently alter the health care program. To use a clinical analogy, working diagnoses are made with an information base that could be challenged if submitted for publication in a leading medical journal. Nonetheless, they are quite adequate in the primary care setting in which care is continuous and vigilant enough to detect early changes in a patient's health status.

Finally, the most vexing problem facing COPC, and indeed facing all of primary care, is that the current mechanisms of reimbursement do not support, much less encourage, the additional activities of COPC. Many new forms of practice are developing in an attempt to gain an edge in the increasingly competitive medical care marketplace; unfortunately, none provide clear incentives for the additional activities of COPC. Even HMOs do not provide a clear incentive to act prospectively to improve the health of a population that is free to disenroll before the impact of an emphasis program may be realized.

Taking an Incremental Approach to COPC

Clearly, there are significant impediments to implementing a COPC practice, yet it is quite possible to integrate the COPC principles into the practice of primary care in an incremental fashion. To many physicians, the decision to develop a COPC practice is seen as one requiring momentous and largely irreversible changes in the practice or program. Since the COPC literature in the last several years has described relatively well-developed forms of COPC, many physicians perceive a gulf between their current practices and the COPC practice model, which has, in turn, discouraged many potential COPC physicians from taking the first steps. In reality, the transition to a COPC practice involves the addition of only two elements to a primary care practice—a definition of the target population and the development of activities that systematically address the health problems of that population. Both of these additional elements can be approached incrementally and at a pace appropriate to the individual setting.

START WITH A DEFINABLE TARGET POPULATION

Many physicians may find it difficult to address the health problems of their total community. The characteristics of the community may appear overwhelmingly complex, with a bewildering mix of ethnic groups and political factions. In addition, the presence of other primary care programs may complicate efforts to distinguish one practice population from another and call into question the appropriateness of the physician's assuming responsibility for patients presumably cared for through another practice or program. In such cases, the COPC process might be started by targeting a community consisting of the active patients of the practice or a "practice community," consisting of the active patients and all members of their households. Similarly, other target populations may be addressed, such as populations defined by location (e.g., school or workplace), by health problem (e.g., hypertension, homeless), age group (e.g., elderly, infants), or risk group (e.g., teenage pregnancy). COPC is an iterative process, and the practice starting with a small subset of the community can expand its scope later.

START WITH SIMPLE TOOLS

Similarly, the process adopted for addressing the community's health problems can vary widely. Each of the four functions can be approached using different degrees of rigor at different costs and with different requirements for physician time and energy. At the most basic level, the physician can rely on subjective information gleaned from the practice impressions of professional colleagues and the wealth of information that can be mined from the opinions and experience of individuals from the community. Subjective information of this sort can be obtained with little expense, and the combined wisdom of the health professional and the consumer offers a richness of information not often possible with quantitative data alone. Moreover, through collaboration, professional and consumers can cooperatively approach the difficult task of setting priorities among competing health problems.

The use of secondary (or existing) data offers another inexpensive alternative for initiating the COPC program. Most communities have a wealth of data available, ranging from census data to vital statistics. The appropriateness of secondary data will, of course, vary across settings and will largely be a function of the "fit" between the target population of the practice and the population for which the data were collected. Increasingly, basic socioeconomic data are becoming available by zip code, enabling many practices with a billing system to estimate some population parameters for their active patients.

These two strategies offer the practice ways of moving toward a more mature COPC model, as shown in Table 19–1. On one level, the increasing rigor of the processes of COPC can be described in terms of the scope of input information used. At Stage 1, the practice may be characterizing the community and identifying health problems using the subjective impressions of the physicians, patients, or both. At Stage 2, secondary data may be used; whereas at Stage 3, new data are collected and analyzed to describe the community and its health problems.

On another level, a COPC practice can define its denominator population at three levels. The first is the population of active patients, defined as all individuals who have contacted the practice within the previous 2 years. The next level is the practice community, which includes all members of the household to which active patients belong. Finally, there is the larger population encompassing, for example, school populations, the enrolled members of a health plan, participants in a health program in the workplace, or a geographic community.

Viewed in this context, physicians may locate their current pattern of practice and identify feasible steps toward a more rigorous practice of COPC. Many practices may be operating simultaneously in more than one section of the matrix. For example, a practice that has a strong quality assurance activity may be engaged in activities at Stage 3 in examining the quality of care provided for dysuria among the working women in the practice. At the same time, the physicians may be concerned about members of the practice community with undiagnosed or untreated hypertension, based on prevalence figures extrapolated from secondary data (Stage 2). Finally, the practice may be collaborating with other community programs to address the problem of unwanted teenage pregnancy based on subjective information within the larger community (Stage 1). If the practice is involved in an HMO or has a contract with a major employer in the community for occupational health services, other denominator populations may be addressed at differing stages of implementation of the COPC process.

Although the matrix scheme of Table 19–1 implies a value associated with higher degrees of rigor, the appropriateness of COPC activities on either level will vary with the issues and will be specific to local resources and requirements. In some settings, the philosophy of the physicians or the needs of the area may argue for defining the denominator population as a social, cultural, or geographic community, whereas other practices or programs may find it more appropriate to address a practice community. On the other level, Stage 3 may represent a high level of development for a given function, but attaining the ideal in a practical world may not always be worth the marginal cost. For example, some programs may be able to extract more information about their community from the diligent use of secondary data than from the use of a sophisticated but undoubtedly more expensive data system.

Getting Started

For physicians interested in incorporating some of the principles of COPC into their practice, a preparatory inventory may be made by seriously reflecting on five questions.

Table 19–1. AN ITERATIVE APPROACH TO COPC*

	Levels of the Target Population		
	Active Patients	*Practice Community*	*Total Community*
Stage 1: use of subjective information			teenage pregnancy
Stage 2: use of secondary data		hypertension	
Stage 3: use of newly collected and analyzed data	dysuria in working women		

*A practice may address different target populations, with methods requiring different levels of quantitative rigor.

How Committed Am I to Trying COPC?

One's own personal commitment is critical and should be judged objectively and without bias. Initiating a COPC practice requires a great deal of time and personal commitment and requires individual leadership from at least one physician in the practice.

Do I Have Professional Colleagues Who Are Equally Committed?

The commitment of other professionals on the staff is important. At least one other fellow traveler committed to the principles of COPC can make the journey through largely uncharted terrain less hazardous and more stimulating. Also, the division of labor that colleagues within the practice or in other community programs permit may allow more time for alternative pursuits.

Is the Practice or Program on Reasonably Stable Ground, Both in Terms of Financial and Professional Growth?

The costs of initiating COPC activities have not been calculated, and the practice may not generate additional income. The practice that is struggling financially or that is in a period of rapid transition in terms of personnel, physical facilities, or definition of goals may have a full agenda without taking on the challenges of COPC. On the other hand, physicians who have established their practice and are looking for further challenge in their professional life may find that moving toward a COPC model is less expensive and professionally more rewarding than embarking, for example, on an expensive hobby.

Is There Sufficient Interest and Commitment Among the Community or Target Population That the Physician Would Address?

Important allies in the COPC process, often not relied upon heavily enough in the early phases of COPC, are the patients and community participants. What constitutes the community and who the key participants are must be defined early in the process, and will vary greatly among practices. The commitment of the target population and its major participants can be an extremely important resource to recognize and incorporate at the time of the initial decision to implement COPC.

Do I Have Access to a Reasonable Amount of Data on the Target Population?

Depending on how the target community is defined, there may or may not be a great deal of data available, a difference that can be critical in the early stages of defining and characterizing the community and identifying its major health problems. For practices that plan to start with the active patient population, it is helpful (but certainly not necessary) to have an operational data system within the practice. For those planning to address a geographic community, a few hours spent with an epidemiologist at the local health department can provide an important reconnaissance of the available data and a reasonable assessment of the additional effort that will be required in early COPC activities.

If this initial inventory of resources affirms moving toward the COPC model, the following suggestions may be useful.

1. *Define your community in a manageable way.* Initially, starting with the active patients of your practice or with the households of your active patients may be a more than adequate challenge. Later, an expansion of the definition of the community will be relatively easy.

2. *Develop allies for the COPC effort within your practice or program, within the community you plan to address, and wherever possible among other practices and community programs.* Developing allies means gaining partners, an important asset even at the price of possible modification in initial goals or timetables. Remember, however, that the practice of COPC is a continuing journey. Fellow travelers are important and usually well worth the inconvenience of altering the initial travel plan.

3. *Take your time and don't rush—maintain modest and achievable expectations.* Although difficult to appreciate at the beginning, many of the early successes will appear small but will be viewed later as the most critical in the history of your efforts. Plan them carefully and enjoy accomplishing them well. Subsequent progress and success will build on these initial efforts.

4. *Plan for initial success.* Nothing reinforces commitment and generates new allies like an initial success. Taking on the most critical and often the most vexing health problem of the community at the outset is risky. A good strategy is to direct initial efforts at a visible problem for which there is considerable concern but particularly one for which a positive impact is achievable in a relatively short period of time and will be apparent when achieved. Attempting to reduce cardiac mortality, for example, through a community-based blood pressure control program is a frequently selected COPC emphasis program. However, it may be an unsatisfactory problem *for the initial* effort, since success, even if achieved, will occur so far in the future and may be modest relative to the community's total cardiac mortality. Long before the data show that the initial efforts had an important impact, you and your allies may have moved on to other areas of personal interest.

5. *Maintain a healthy perspective.* You are among the first to discover and explore the territory of COPC. Those few that have gone before you are the pioneers—and you are one of the early settlers. There is not a great deal known on how to accomplish COPC in your setting. You will rapidly become an

expert. Document your experiences and share them with others, for you are helping to develop the field.

The Outlook for COPC

There remains a general malaise among physicians and a remarkable lack of recognition concerning the great potential in COPC and practice-based research. There are few organizational supports for a practice inclined to pursue a better understanding of a community and its problems, and appropriate quantitative tools applicable to practice settings are lacking. More importantly, other than the fees for services that may be incidentally billable as part of customary care, there are virtually no financial incentives for physicians to adopt COPC. This same malaise and organizational inertia discourage the enthusiastic pursuit of knowledge about such common problems as headaches, fatigue, and sleeplessness; problems that do not now fit neatly into the specific organ systems that are the focus of medical specialties.

Now that the principles of COPC and the promise of practice-based research have been conceived and realized in some settings, further progress is critical and indicated. Advancements depend in part on physicians being able to recognize the inadequacy of the biomedical model alone and to accept the challenge to enrich it with the methods and fruits of practice-based research and COPC. If these opportunities are ignored, the interface between people and their personal physicians will indeed remain ill-defined and poorly understood. If the opportunities are realized, patients in their communities should get the care they need rather than what we simply have to offer, and the care they get should be more demonstrably effective and ultimately more personally satisfying.

References

Geiger, H. J.: The neighborhood health center. Arch. Envir. Health, *14*:912, 1967.

Haggerty, R. J., Roghmann, K. J., and Pless, I. B.: Child Health and the Community. New York, John Wiley and Sons, 1975. *Describes work carried out in the late 1960's and early 1970's in Monroe County, New York, by a team of physicians and researchers. Although focusing on health of children, the principles of COPC are clearly demonstrated. This work is an excellent example of COPC and is well worth carefully reading.*

Horowitz, C., and Gallagher, K. M.: Group process techniques for COPC practice. *In* Nutting, P. A. (Ed.): Community-Oriented Primary Care: From Principle to Practice. Pub No HRS-A-PE 86–1. Washington, D.C., U.S. Government Printing Office, 1987.

Institute of Medicine: Community-Oriented Primary Care: A Practical Assessment, Vol. I, The Committee Report. Washington, D.C., National Academy Press, 1984a.

Institute of Medicine: Community-oriented Primary Care: A Practical Assessment, Vol. II, The Case Studies. Washington, D.C., National Academy Press, 1984b. *Describes the seven case studies that formed the basis of the Institute of Medicine report on COPC. The case studies are notable in their representation of the varied settings in which primary care is practiced in the U.S., and includes a private family practice.*

Iverson, D. C., Calonge, B. N., Miller, R. S., et al.: The development and management of a primary care research network, 1978–87. Family Med., *20*:177, 1988. *This paper describes the development and progress of the largest of the primary care research networks in the United States and provides a rich reference list for tracing the progress of practice-based research in the United States, Canada, Australia, and Europe.*

Kark, S. L.: Community-Oriented Primary Health Care. New York, Appleton-Century-Crofts, 1981. *The author describes the principles of COPC through the use of examples from his work in a neighborhood in Jerusalem. This is a classic book by the physician who first coined the term COPC.*

Last, J. M.: The iceberg: Completing the clinical picture in general practice. Lancet, *2*:28, 1963.

Madison, D. L.: The case for community-oriented primary care. J. A. M. A., *249*:1279, 1983. *An analysis of the problems and opportunities for integrating COPC into the practice of primary care.*

Madison, D. L., and Shenkin, B. N.: Leadership for Community-Responsive Practice. Chapel Hill, N.C., The Rural Practice Project, 1978.

Mullan, F.: Community-oriented primary care: An agenda for the '80s. N. Engl. J. Med., *307*:1076, 1982.

Nutting, P. A., Strotz, C., and Shorr, G. I.: Reduction of gastroenteritis morbidity in high risk infants. Pediatrics, *55*:354, 1975.

Nutting, P. A., Wood, M., and Conner, E. M.: Community-oriented primary care in the United States. J. A. M. A., *253*:1763, 1985.

Nutting, P. A.: Community-oriented primary care: An integrated model for practice, research, and education. Am. J. Prev. Med., *2*:140, 1986. *Provides a complete description of the COPC model, including the levels of development and criteria for each of the steps in the COPC process.*

Nutting, P. A. (Ed): Community-Oriented Primary Care: From Principle to Practice. Pub No HRS-A-PE 86–1. Washington, D.C., U.S. Government Printing Office. 1987. *A rich source of descriptive material on the tools and techniques of COPC. The text includes contributions from over 70 authors with experience in applying the principles of COPC in different practice settings.*

Nutting, P. A.: The evaluation function in COPC: Quality assurance for the community. *In* Nutting, P. A. (Ed.): Community-Oriented Primary Care: From Principle to Practice. Publication No. HRS-A-PE 86–1. Washington, D.C., U.S. Government Printing Office, 1987.

Rogers, D. E.: Community-oriented primary care. J. A. M. A., *248*:1622–1625, 1982. *Describes the barriers to applying COPC in the current policy climate in the United States. Much of the discussion applies equally to the environment of primary care in general.*

Seifert, M. H.: An incremental patient participation model. *In* Nutting, P. A. (Ed.): Community-Oriented Primary Care: From Principle to Practice. Publication No. HRS-A-PE 86–1. Washington, D.C., U.S. Government Printing Office, 1987. *A fascinating description of one family physician's development of a patient advisory council within his practice population. The author provides a stepwise approach to developing an advisory council and many of the activities that may be undertaken to the benefit of the practice and its patients.*

Sheps, C. G.: Primary care—The problem and the prospect. Ann. N.Y. Acad. Sci., *310*:265, 1978.

White, K. L., Williams, T. F., and Greenburg, B. G.: The ecology of medical care. N. Engl. J. Med., *265*:885, 1961. *This frequently referenced paper has become a classic in primary care. Using data from several sources, the authors describe the illness rates in the community and the disproportionately small number of patients that come to a university medical center. Although the authors point out that this provides an inappropriate case load for teaching primary care, it is equally clear that research involving such a highly selected population cannot be generalized as a reflection of most primary care physicians' practice experience.*

20

Patient Advisory Councils

Peter Pritchard

"I spend all day listening to my patients. They would tell me if anything was wrong with the organization of the practice. So why should I waste time and energy listening to them in a group?" These are understandable, if negative, remarks of a busy family physician faced with the idea of starting a patient advisory council.

What Are Patient Advisory Councils and Why Have They Come About?

Such groups, known in Britain as patient participation groups, have been forming—and failing (Mann, 1985)—in the past 15 years in a number of countries.

Participation of various kinds has developed in parallel in the United States and Britain starting in the early 1970's when the consumer movement was strong. Since one of the earliest British groups was formed in 1972 (Pritchard, 1975), the number has increased gradually so that there are about 125 such groups in Britain today, representing less than 1.5 per cent of general practices. This is slow progress, but many physicians find it a threatening notion to join with their patients in evaluating and improving the service they provide. Consumer involvement in any professional field does not happen spontaneously. So why have these groups arisen at all?

Family physicians are now being trained to listen, and to have a more patient-centered style (Byrne and Long, 1976). This was difficult to apply when the organizational setting was not equally patient-centered, so the extension of the counseling style to the organization was a logical if not a generally accepted step. A second influence was the spread of management knowledge into medical organizations. Physicians who tried to adopt a participative style of practice management and to build a "learning organization" (Argyris and Schon, 1978) soon discovered a missing dimension, namely feedback from patients. Patient feedback fits with an "open systems" model of family practice, and two of the first three groups to begin in Britain between 1972 and 1974 were of this type.

A further influence had to do with a change from the traditional way of meeting expressed demand to a more population-oriented approach. For the doctor to take the initiative in health promotion and to screen people who felt perfectly well required a renegotiation of the doctor's role. These three influences were at work in different degrees in different settings, and so it is no surprise that established patient advisory councils follow many different models.

Gradations of consumer participation are clearly set out in Arnstein's (1969) "ladder of citizen participation." The top rung represents citizen control. Next is delegated power, the second from the top is partnership, and this seems the appropriate level for doctors and patients to communicate, with neither side losing their autonomy. Arnstein has five levels below partnership that she characterizes as tokenism, or nonparticipation—in other words, a facade to disguise "placation" or "manipulation," which are the lowest levels in Arnstein's model.

What Do Patient Advisory Councils Do?

Patient advisory councils vary in their focus of attention from the narrower focus of producing a good service to attending patients, to the broader focus of looking into the health problems of a local population, or to the extreme of a holistic approach to health promotion of an entire local population. Which is chosen may well depend on the structure of local health care. But councils may prefer to start with modest aims that are likely to succeed and use the incremental approach described by Seifert (1987). He outlines three steps. First, to collect data on the standing of the practice and of local health needs; second, to enhance the doctor/staff/patient relationship; and third, to organize the staff/patient group partnership in the light of the data collected.

Each council exists to reflect local needs and aspirations as they affect the practice, so the wide range of activities such as those found in British patient participation groups is set out below.

The key activity of a patient group is to hold a dialogue with service providers. This will work only if each side is prepared to listen. For some patients, to be asked for advice about the way the practice is organized is such a surprise that they are speechless. But the surprise is pleasurable and releases much energy and goodwill. This dialogue must be open and equal and in terms that all can understand. It opens up pathways for action by the group that are compatible with perceived priorities and needs.

Physicians, too, may get some surprises. For example, at one of the first meetings of the group in the author's practice, a request was made for a booklet to be available in the waiting room so that people could find out ways of avoiding visits to the doctor. A booklet, "Hints on Keeping Well," was duly written, which not only gave guidelines on life style but also set out the practice philosophy on such things as smoking, dieting, and sleeping pills. This area of health promotion, about which we had considerable anxieties, was handed to us on a plate. In the process of writing the booklet, physicians and nursing staff had to share ideas in order to produce a consensus about policies, which were then discussed with patients.

The introduction of teaching in the practice produced problems with which we needed guidance. The responses were very clear. There was no objection raised by the patients to medical students or trainees joining a doctor-patient consultation, provided there was advance warning, including the gender of the visitor, and the patient had an opportunity to refuse. Social work or nursing students were not acceptable except in special clinics. There were strong reservations about the use of a video camera during consultations. Agreement was reluctantly given, provided that there was due warning, the circumstances in which recordings were played back or destroyed were specified, and there were safeguards about confidentiality. Patients' reluctance was not based on any opposition to change but on the very high value they placed on the one-to-one consultation that they did not want to be compromised.

Who should set the goals of the practice—the physicians alone or the staff and patients? This issue was explored in a questionnaire to patients and staff in which they were asked to rank eight possible goals in order of importance (Pritchard, 1981). All agreed that the primary goal was to "make the right diagnosis and provide the right treatment," but thereafter views diverged widely. For example, physicians thought that their referral to specialists was adequate (ranked 8), whereas patients ranked "more frequent referral to specialists" third in importance. Not only did the results give the doctors and staff much food for thought, but the resulting dialogue with patients produced a serious reappraisal of physicians' roles and goals.

A patient group can report on underprivileged people in the locality such as the elderly people who are housebound or ethnic minorities. They would then take practical steps, with professional support, to implement remedies. Groups could help to design acceptable screening programs; for example, their rewording of the invitation to patients doubled the use of Papanicolaou's smears in the author's practice. Members of patient advisory councils are often members of other organizations, and these connections between very complex community networks can be very helpful in arranging appropriate care.

Physicians tend to follow a biomedical model of thinking that guides their actions. Patients often think differently. So any opportunity for gaining an understanding of patients' health beliefs (King, 1983) can benefit the planning of health education and promotion programs. Patient advisory councils often play a very active part in these programs, which makes them more relevant and more likely to achieve behavioral change. Physicians need to decide if they wish to be involved in helping people to take responsibility for their own health or leaving it entirely to the patient to take the "flight into health" (Suchman, 1967).

Doctors in Britain acting alone have often failed to prevent the closure of community hospitals and the withdrawal of ambulances or to achieve the setting up of new services. However, joint action with a patient group has been successful in achieving these goals. Such joint action is helpful for community-based public services that, in contrast to the powerful voice of hospital medicine, are rarely heard.

Other activities (Paine, 1982) have included support for volunteer services in the community, support for the practice (e.g., voluntary car services or purchase of equipment), special interest and self-help groups, fact-finding, providing information for patients about services and diseases, handling complaints, and fund raising.

Participation as a Principle of Effective Health Care

The widespread growth of consumerism in the past two decades has attempted to alleviate patients' lack of power to influence the kind of services that were provided, ostensibly for their benefit. The World Health Organization in the Declaration of Alma-Ata (WHO/UNICEF 1978) went further by stating that "people have the right and duty to participate individually and collectively in the planning and implementation of their health care."

This principle of participation as a central strategy for health care has been restated in the literature relating to community-oriented primary care in the United States (Nutting, 1987) (see Chapter 19) and by the Rockefeller Foundation (Halstead et al., 1985) in relation to cost-effective health services in the developing world. Carlson and Rosenqvist (1988) showed convincingly that local worker and consumer participation improved diabetic care. Staff members were given feedback for planning and were made more aware of psychologic and social problems encountered by the diabetic patient, and patients were able to contribute their own skills to improve the work design process. This study emphasized the importance of participative organization design rather than conforming to centrally generated protocols.

The opportunity for participation should not be open only to the poor but is a basic ingredient of human autonomy and dignity. Physicians cannot assume ownership of the patient's illness and health care any more than they can of the patient's body. Participation implies a negotiated agreement on the professional boundaries within which doctors are accountable.

The extent and effectiveness of participation has been hard to measure owing to lack of indicators of process and outcome. However, recent studies based mainly on Third World settings (Rifkin et al., 1988) have considerable relevance for family practice in industrialized countries. These authors used five indicators of participation, namely needs assessment, leadership, organization, resource mobilization, and management. Each of these indicators was rated on a five point scale in light of a series of questions that present a challenge to those involved in patient advisory councils in family practice.

Do Patient Advisory Councils Help or Hinder Family Practice?

Wood and Metcalfe (1980) asked a group of British general practitioner teachers who had no experience with a patient advisory council what effect it might have on their practice. They replied that it would "increase friction, decrease effectiveness, limit the doctor's role, and was an unnecessary fad." But the same questions to general practitioners who had experience with such a group in their practice produced the replies that the group "reduced friction, increased understanding, improved effectiveness, extended their role, and was an essential tool."

The most thorough research study in Britain was that performed by Richardson and Bray (1987) in which the activities of 63 patient participation groups were studied. Their characteristics were very similar to patient advisory councils in the United States (Early and Seifert, 1981). They stated that "there can be little question that, taken as a whole, patient participation groups had many visible achievements to their credit." Two thirds of the groups considered that "they had achieved greater awareness of health issues among patients, that doctors had become more aware of patients' needs, and that doctor-patient relationships had improved."

On the negative side, nearly two thirds of groups recorded poor attendance at meetings. A few felt that the doctors were not involved enough or, on the other hand, tended to dominate the group. Several groups felt they did not attract the right people. Some respondents felt that doctors were reluctant to make changes, but doctors did not see these groups as impinging on their professional freedom and most viewed them positively.

Richardson and Bray concluded that "they were a worthwhile exercise and overall seemed worth a try, and were an impetus for quality assessment." These groups are, in the final analysis, "one means of mobilizing ordinary people in the interests of the health of their community and some input to their practice. That they do so with difficulty, and varying success, can come as no surprise. That they do so at all is a matter for congratulation."

In giving information to patients, sharing ideas, and making themselves open to criticism, physicians may feel a loss of power. This argument has some force. But a profession that is isolated intellectually and socially from the public may end up with no power and eventually no role. So the contrary hypothesis would be that physicians working in a partnership with patients increases power and effectiveness of both parties.

Future Prospects for Patient Involvement in Health Care

The trend toward patients assuming personal responsibility for health seems to be growing. This does not mean that physicians can relax and leave all the decisions to the patient, but rather that they must work in a closer and more equal partnership. This partnership is already becoming the norm in the one-to-one consultation format but is developing more slowly at the level of management in organization and decision-making. At the same time, the scope of family practice is expanding to include fields such as health promotion and the prevention of ill health, which need new skills in communication and management and can succeed best with public involvement.

The combined demands for professional accountability and quality assurance are on the rise and can only be met by asking for input from patients. Patient advisory councils can be particularly useful in providing such feedback. Research into their nature and effectiveness is particularly difficult, but this represents an important task for the future.

Family physicians have a developing role of almost limitless scope. The patient advisory council is a party used to negotiate role boundaries and to help patients take more responsibility for their own health. This is all part of the learning process that is part of the pursuit of health. But it is a mutual process. Doctors can learn from patients who themselves learn from other patients as well as from health professionals. Patient advisory councils are nothing for physicians to fear—quite the reverse—they become a helpful resource. But they are not easy to set up or maintain, and different communication skills are needed for the success of all parties involved in the "partnership for health."

References

Argyris, C. and Schon, D. S.: Organizational Learning: A Theory of Action Perspective. Reading, MA, Addison-Wesley, 1978.

Arnstein, S.: A ladder of citizen participation. Am. Inst. Planners J., *53*:216–224, 1969.

Byrne, P. S., and Long, B. E.: Doctors talking to patients. A study of the verbal behaviour of general practitioners consulting in their surgeries. London, Her Majesty's Stationery Office, 1976.

Carlson, A., and Rosenqvist, U.: Locally developed plans for quality diabetes care: on worker and consumer participation in the public health care system. *In* Luft, R., Bajaj, J., and Rosenqvist, U.(Eds.): Diabetes care as a model for primary health care. Elsevier, Amsterdam, 1988. *One of a series of important research papers from Sweden, in which objective outcome measures were related to processes of care such as communication and participation and the presence of community support networks.*

Curtis, P., Berolzheimer, N., Evens, S., et al.: Patient participation in a medical education environment. J. Fam. Pract., *13*:247–253, 1981.

Early, F., and Seifert, M. H.: Starting Your Own Patient Advisory Council. Spring Park, MN, M.D. Publishing Co., 1981.

Halstead, S. B., Walsh, J. A., and Warren, K. S.: Good Health at Low Cost. New York, The Rockefeller Foundation, 1985. *This report considered the health systems of four relatively poor countries that had achieved considerable success in improving the health care of their populations. Common factors were equitable distribution of health care or education; political will and public participation; and investment in primary health care.*

King, J.: Health beliefs in the consultation. *In* Pendleton, D., and Hasler, J. (Eds.): Doctor-Patient Communication. London, Academic Press, 1983.

Mann, R. G.: Why patient participation groups stop functioning: General practitioners' viewpoint. Br. Med. J., *290*:209–211, 1985.

Nutting, P. A.: Community-Oriented Primary Care: From Principle to Practice. Washington, D.C., U.S. Department of Health and Human Services, 1987. *A valuable source book of articles about population-based primary care, including seven papers on patient and community involvement.*

Paine, T.: Survey of patient participation groups in the United Kingdom. Br. Med. J., *286*:768–772, 847–849, 1982.

Pritchard, P. M. M.: Community participation in primary health care. Br. Med. J., *3*:585–587, 1975.

Pritchard, P. M. M.: Manual of Primary Health Care: Its Nature and Organization. 2nd ed. Oxford, Oxford University Press, 1981.

Richardson, A., and Bray, C.: Promoting Health Through Participation: Experience of Groups for Patient Participation in General Practice. Research report No 659. London, Policy Studies Institute (100 Park Village East, London NW1 3SR, UK), 1987. *One of few research studies of patient participation in Britain by a leading researcher into participation in many fields of activity, including health, resulting in a very balanced view of the issues and problems raised.*

Rifkin, S. B., Muller, F., and Bichmann, W.: Primary health care: On measuring participation. Soc. Sci. Med., *26*:931–940, 1988.

Seifert, M. H., Jr.: An incremental patient participation model. *In* Nutting, P. A. (Ed.): Community-Oriented Primary Care: From Principle to Practice. Washington, D.C., U.S. Department of Health and Human Services, 1987, pp. 379–383.

Suchman, E. A.: Health attitudes and behavior. J. Health Soc. Behav., *8*:197–209. 1967.

WHO/UNICEF: Primary health care. Report of the International Conference on primary health care, Alma-Ata USSR. 6–12 September 1978. Geneva, World Health Organization, 1978. *The report of a conference that surprised everyone by its success. Representatives of 134 governments signed the Declaration, which is still having a profound effect on health policies worldwide.*

Wood, J., and Metcalfe, D.: Professional attitudes to patient participation groups: An exploratory study. J. R. Coll. Gen. Pract., *30*:538–541, 1980.

21

Utilization of Community Resources

John E. Arradondo

Increasingly, the family physician is the first health professional to whom individuals and families turn for help in solving complex medical and health problems. Frequently, these problems involve not only disease or infirmity but also the physical, social, or mental well-being of the individual and family. Accordingly, the family physician is challenged to recognize and mobilize a broad and continuing array of community resources to address the problems presented. Additionally, the family physician should integrate the use of community resources into his or her regular problem-solving process. Finally, the physician must follow up the patient's or family's use of community resources to monitor their accessibility, cost, and usefulness.

As the specialty geared to providing both the broad array of disease treatment and management services as well as a comprehensive set of behaviorally oriented health promotion and disease prevention services, family practice attracts patients whose problems require both kinds of services. Several examples illustrate the point. A person who abuses drugs (prescription, illicit, or alcohol) inevitably presents with psychologic, social, or physical problems that demand the use of secondary and sometimes tertiary (institution-based) care services (see Figure 21–1.) The obese person with diabetes mellitus usually requires the use of multiple health service providers outside of the physician's office: the opthalmologist may assist to prevent or delay blindness; the physiatrist may aid in weight reduction or in preventing early deterioration from neuromuscular complications; and the health educator, social worker, or psychologist may utilize support groups to aid in the patient's attempts to reduce weight, eat properly, or achieve and maintain cardiovascular fitness and musculoskeletal flexibility. The person with human immunodeficiency virus (HIV) infection, or AIDS, very likely will require use of many of the medical, surgical, dental, and psychologic health services. Beyond those services, this person will often need the services of social workers, nutritionists, special laboratories, housing and legal experts, and others. Frequently, people in the terminal stages of HIV infection require assistance in all these areas and more. The final example is the child with a chronic disease, e.g., asthma, sickle cell disease, or mild mental retardation. The child and the family require the caring, compassion, and problem-solving capabilities of a family physician who is willing and able to use the full range of community resources.

Utilizing the Health Care Team

In recognizing the broad array of available community resources, family physicians can attempt to solve more than just the patient's immediate physical complaint. They can offer a formidable array of services aimed at solving any patient problem. One way to view medical health services is to divide them into three categories: primary, secondary, and tertiary health care services. Primary health care services are those that provide (1) early access to the system, (2) continuing care by the same provider or part of the system, (3) comprehensive care within the system, and (4) personalized, humane care. For most people, primary care can be delivered by a physician specializing in family practice. For selected groups of people (women, children, adults), primary care may be provided by a gynecologist, general pediatrician, or general internist. Secondary health care services are those that provide a second opinion, a consultation, or a more intensive attention to a problem. Such services are more apt to use hospital-based activities. The tertiary health care services are those that provide a consultation to both the primary care and secondary care providers. They pay significant attention to relatively narrowly based problems, often focusing on a single bodily organ or organ system. These services are usually hospital based and often require hospital-based equipment and technology.

Just as health care can be categorized as primary, secondary or tertiary, providers and agencies delivering the services can be grouped into primary care teams, secondary care teams, or tertiary care teams. Figure 21–1 depicts the members of the medical and health care teams. Some function on one or more teams because of the variation in the breadth and depth of services they can provide. In Figure 21–1, the generalists are included in the primary circle with the patient, the family, and the family physician. The medical subspecialists, surgeons, psychiatrists, and Human Services Agencies are all shown as being able to provide two levels of care: some office-based secondary care and some institution-based tertiary care. Providers of other disciplines (legal, religious, and housing) are included to the extent they become involved in promoting the physical, social, and mental well-being of patients and assist them in preventing disease or infirmity. It should be recalled that other providers (social workers, clergy, psychologists, and various counselors) may provide first access to the patient and, as a part of the system, manage the person's entire receipt of health services. In Figure 21–1, the family physician provides and manages the full range of services to the patient. In promoting health and preventing or managing chronic disease, the patient is often the most important member of the primary care team.

In mobilizing community resources (as in managing many complex patient problems), a physician is influenced by several personal and procedural characteristics.

First, the physician should be willing to accept the members of the secondary and tertiary care teams as colleagues or peers in the care of his or her patients. When chosen properly, their expertise is comparable to the physician's.

Second, physicians themselves must be aware of their biases, habits under stress, and feelings and reactions to certain problems and people. Reaching logical conclusions and providing nonjudgmental advice and therapy is a prudent place to begin. A physician's (or other team member's) inappropriate response to the problems of a person presenting with

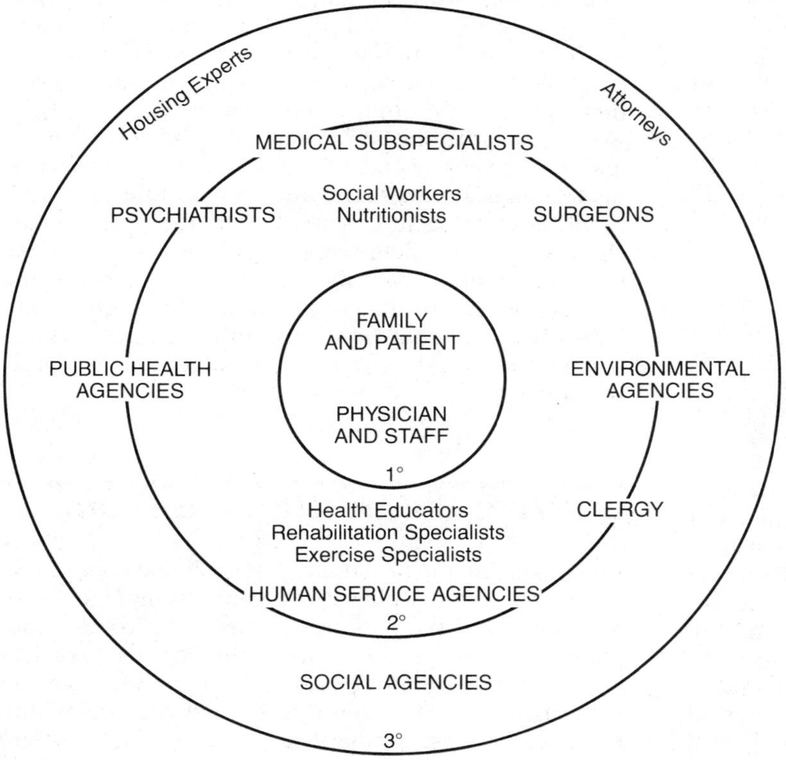

Figure 21–1. Recognizing members of the medical/health team: The three circles encompass primary, secondary, and tertiary care team members, starting in the center and moving outward. Some members function in two areas.

alcoholism, sexually transmitted disease, obesity, or emotional imbalance can neutralize or misdirect the result of a consultation from or referral to another member of the health care team.

Third, the physician who appreciates the capabilities and limitations of the different resources or members of the health team is more likely to satisfy the patient, regardless of the objective outcome of the referral. This knowledge of the limitations of the various resources ranges from weighing the merits of surgical versus medical therapy of coronary artery disease to the benefits of a health educator, nutritionist, or an exercise physiologist for an obese diabetic to the overall effectiveness of an emergency room versus a public health clinic in the therapy and secondary prevention of sexually transmitted diseases.

The **fourth** characteristic is an understanding of the process of general communications and risk communications in managing care for a complex problem. For simple communication, the rate of error in transmitting the message increases astronomically as the number of involved people increases. Since the frequent use of community resources requires interacting with many people, the likelihood of communication error is relatively high. Therefore, concise, precise messages are most useful.

Finally, the ability to communicate to patients the kind and magnitude of the health risk they face is an art requiring constant vigilance for the opportunity to communicate effectively. The family practice of the future is likely to emphasize risk communication as much as it stresses interpersonal skills. Assessing and communicating risk necessitates a physician having an epidemiologic-based knowledge of the "universe" of patients from which each patient comes or the universe of problems similar to the one presented. The less a physician knows about the patient or problem the more he must rely on sound problem-solving techniques.

Solving a Problem

Problem solving is a generic and ancient matter. During the last 20 years, the problem-solving technique has increasingly been applied to individual and family problems. In the current health delivery system, patients come to primary care physicians in many ways; yet most have a problem or complaint that serves as their reason for admission to a particular set of services. The problem-solving process has several attributes and several steps. The process needs to be as factual as possible. The patient should be made aware of the steps. The physician needs to recognize that the process succeeds at varying rates.

The problem-solving process has several steps. **First,** agree on the complaint, preferably in the patient's language, and its meaning. For example, the complaint, "Doctor, I've lost my nature," quickly leads to an understanding of male sexual impotence and a query about medications and diseases causing this. Similarly, a complaint of "feeling tired" could lead to an understanding of weakness, sleeplessness, or intolerance.

Second, clarify the problem. How does it relate to other problems, activities, beliefs, health practices? What has been done about it? Who has helped? What have been the outcomes of these interventions? This should lead to a clearer definition of the problem. The man who lost his nature could have had a prior prescription of pills for "sugar in the urine" and make the physician focus on diabetes. Alternatively, he could notice his symptom only when he takes his antihypertension medication, which involves a different probable outcome.

A **third** step examines the possible courses of action: from further history through the physical examination and other data-collecting activities to a specific formulation of the course of action for the most likely cause of the patient's original complaint. Some activities are so routine that the physician and patient proceed tacitly (such as the physical examination and laboratory studies). Others are so unusual that the patient may require a family member's presence (referral to special agencies or tertiary care surgical specialists). Self-awareness is an important attribute of the physician, which is needed to render nonjudgmental advice to a patient.

The **fourth** step lets the physician and patient jointly select a course of action. This degree of patient involvement increases patient compliance yet does not diminish the physician's value as the primary care provider. Showing respect for the expertise of the other team members and anticipating a satisfactory interaction between the patient and the new team member increases patient compliance and the likelihood of a successful outcome.

The **fifth** step implements the agreed-upon plan and begins the monitoring and follow-up processes.

The Consultation/Referral Process

In using community resources, the referral or consultation process becomes an integral part of the problem-solving process. It ranges from (1) merely getting and following advice from a consultant to (2) having the consultant check the patient and initiate therapy before returning the patient to (3) the consultant providing an entire episode of therapy or service before the patient returns to the primary physician. In item 2, the health care team members often share in the care of the patient, a process demanding precise, concise, and continuing communication.

A pregnant teenager offers an instructive situation for describing a referral. **First,** the physician or the staff can check the availability of teen care services in the phone book, the Community Services or Social Services directory, or by calling a clinical social worker who specializes in care for teenagers. Usually this step reveals the appropriate resource. **Second,** the physician's staff can call any of several information and referral agencies. Often such information and referral resources are available through a "crisis call" hot-line, the local United Way or Community Council, or the local Public Health or Human Services department. **Third,** the staff can call an institution that works with a particular kind of problem (high-risk pregnancy) or with a particular demographic group (teenage girls). These include the school system (principal, counselor, or nurse), various religious organizations or associations, hospital social workers, welfare case workers, mental health centers, and others. While seeking information from which to make a referral decision, the physician should begin building a data base of people, agencies, and facilities that provide various services that the patient might require. This eases the process the next time the problem arises. This data base should include:

- Name of agency or provider
- Qualifications of provider(s)
- Accessibility: costs, hours, and locations
- Procedure for setting appointments
- Kind of feedback to primary providers

This kind of data collection procedure should become a skill of more than one staff member of each practice. The information can be kept in a "Consultation and Referral Index—Problems" file (Table 21–1).

Similarly, the family physician should keep a list of agencies with (1) the problems they address, (2) the areas they serve, (3) the locations and hours of service, (4) the programs and activities, (5) the eligibility criteria, (6) fees, and (7) referring procedures. For each agency, list the name, address, phone number, and contact person. See Table 21–2 for a list of resources by agency type.

Table 21–1. CONSULTATION AND REFERRAL INDEX—PROBLEMS

Abortion	Family planning
Adoption	Family services
Alcoholism	Financial aid
Cancer	Food, clothing, shelter
Children	Health education
Abuse and neglect	Housing
Behavior	Information and referral library
Growth and development	Legal
Handicapped	Mental health and retardation
Communicable disease follow-up	Nursing
Day care	Public health
Disability	Rehabilitation
Drug abuse	Reportable disease follow-up
Education	Shelter
Emergency services	Speech and hearing
Medical	Transportation
Mental	Unwed Parents
Social	Volunteering
Employment	Welfare
Environmental health	Others

The consultation and referral process is dynamic. It should be pro-active. The primary physician and the patients get the most from the process when consultations are for precise reasons and prompt feedback is provided. This precision of thought and expectation simplifies an otherwise complex system of available community resources.

Community Resources

Utilization of community resources proceeds most efficiently and effectively when the primary care provider knows the community, is aware of its many needs, and recognizes its resources. The parallel concepts of community-oriented primary care (see Chapter 19) and community-oriented family care em-

Table 21–2. CONSULTATION AND REFERRAL INDEX—AGENCIES

I. Public agencies
  A. Educational resources
    1. Schools
      a. Testing, counseling, special classes
      b. Libraries
      c. Agriculture extension services
        (1) Homemaking
        (2) Nutrition
    2. School nurses
  B. Health services
    1. Department of Public Health
      a. Epidemiology
      b. Disease surveillance
      c. Public health nursing
      d. Mental health and guidance
      e. Screening
      f. Disease prevention
      g. Communicable disease follow-up
      h. Laboratory
      i. Infants and children's program
      j. Housing inspection
    2. Hospitals
  C. Financial—social services
    1. Welfare department
    2. State employment office
    3. Office of Social Security
    4. Child protective services
    5. Human services department
    6. Area agency on aging
  D. Employment services
  E. Public safety services
  F. Legal services
II. Private (not for profit) agencies
  A. Volunteer organizations
    1. Self-help
    2. Neighborhood or community organizations
  B. Sectarian
    1. Nursing homes
    2. Churches, temples, synagogues
    3. Charitable agencies
  C. Nonsectarian
    1. Nursing homes for aged
    2. Specific disease associations
    3. Financial counselors
    4. Hospitals and clinics
    5. Education agencies

phasize the use of epidemiologic-based knowledge of the community to chart its needs and the knowledge of community resources to aid families and individuals in addressing their medical and health problems.

A physician can increase his or her knowledge of and contacts within community resource agencies on an "as-needed" basis when patients demonstrate a need. Keeping a problem-oriented index of resources (as in Table 21–1) is very helpful. *In addition, physicians should develop a list of services and agencies in order to become acquainted with the services available in a community.* Table 21–2 lists community resources worthy of a family physician's attention. Some residency programs train physicians in a technique called "community diagnosis" or assessment. This process assesses most aspects of the health services in a community. It examines the hospital, pharmacy, dental, nursing home, insurance, medical society, health department, pharmaceutical companies, equipment and furniture distributors, financial institutions, mental health institutions, and voluntary health organizations within a community and determines whether opening a practice in the community is wise. Such an assessment would reveal, among other things, resources and agencies shown in Table 21–2.

Many of the agencies will be listed in a directory of social service agencies or of community resource agencies. Using these agencies expands the problem-solving ability of the primary care provider.

Evaluating the Outcome

Patients and families can get lost in the maze of social services agencies and health services agencies and providers. The skilled family physician records these consultations and referrals in the medical record. Good outcomes are noted in the resource file. Poor outcomes are cited as a caution in the resource file. This completes the circle of problem solving, therapy, referral, and follow-up. It aids patient compliance and provides a sense of satisfaction to the busy practitioner.

References

Mullin, F.: Community-Oriented Primary Care. Institute of Medicine, National Science Foundation. Washington, D.C., U.S. Government Printing Office, 1983. *Proceedings of a symposium retreat containing papers on community assessment, matching resources to family and community needs and alternative styles of practice.*

Treat, D. F., and Hank, M. L.: Utilization of community resources. *In* Rakel, R. E., and Conn, H. F. (Eds.): Family Practice, 2nd ed. Philadelphia, W. B. Saunders Co., 1978.

22

Occupational Medicine

Carolyn C. Lopez
Kevin M. Sherin

History of Occupational Medicine

The origins of occupational medicine can be traced to Hippocrates, but it is Bernardo Ramazzini (1633–1714) who has been called the father of occupational medicine. Ramazzini described diseases of tradesmen and promoted the concept of being able to work without acquiring a disabling illness (Rom, 1983).

The industrial revolution, with its impact on workers' health, served as the impetus for modern efforts in the area of occupational medicine. In England, the interrelationship of industry, health, and governmental regulation was recognized and reforms were advanced in this context (Smith, 1988).

In the United States, Alice Hamilton (1869–1970) was inspired by the work done in Europe by Sir Thomas Oliver and others. From the early 1900's until her death in 1970, Dr. Hamilton dedicated herself to the advancement of occupational medicine in the United States.

Incidence of Occupational Disease in the United States

Conflicting data exist in the examination of the morbidity and mortality of occupational disease. Estimates of the number of workers killed on the job vary widely and are based on a variety of incomplete data sources (National Safety Council, 1985).

In 1984, the number of traumatic occupational fatalities in the United States was estimated at 3740 (Cotter, 1987); 4960 (National Safety Council, 1985) and 11,500 (MMWR, 1988) respectively. Improved surveillance systems at the National Institute of Safety and Health (NIOSH) and the Bureau of Labor Statistics may help close this information gap (Wiegand, 1988). These improved reporting capabilities record a greater burden of occupationally related deaths than previously recorded. Death rates per 100,000 workers were highest in mining, construction and agriculture, and forestry and fishing in rank order based on the NIOSH system (Wiegand, 1988).

The Bureau of Labor Statistics produces national estimates of occupational fatalities based on an annual survey of 280,000 private sector establishments with 11 or more employees. Concern exists about underreporting and overreporting of employers (Pollack and Keimig, 1987; Seligman et al., 1988). Of greater concern is that an underreporting of occupational disease exists related to (1) lack of knowledge, (2) poor surveillance, and (3) fear of job loss. Estimates of the annual cost of this health burden have been placed at 30 billion dollars for deaths and injuries (Hines, 1982). In 1982, NIOSH developed a list of the 10 leading work-related diseases and injuries in the United States (Table 22–1). Among occupational injuries, back, hand, and eye injuries are the most frequently reported.

The Role of the Family Physician in Occupational Medicine

Patients may preferentially seek diagnosis and management for their known job-related illness or injury

Table 22–1. TEN LEADING OCCUPATIONAL DISORDERS IN THE UNITED STATES (1982)

Occupational lung diseases
Musculoskeletal injuries
Occupational cancers
Amputations, fractures, eye loss, lacerations, and traumatic death
Cardiovascular diseases
Disorders of reproduction
Neurotoxic disorders
Noise-induced loss of hearing
Dermatologic conditions
Psychologic disorders

from their family physicians. In the course of routine care, the family physician may be the first to identify a job-related problem. Even when the medical problems are not job-related, when physicians certify their patients for return to work after an illness they are practicing occupational medicine. Thus, it is imperative that family physicians have an understanding of this important aspect of practice.

Family physicians may also elect to take on a more formal role as occupational physician. Being a "company physician" may be a part-time role (intended to augment income) or a full-time involvement. These roles have different stresses and pressures than the more traditional roles listed above. These physicians may find themselves under pressure from the company to minimize injuries or illness or to return employees to work sooner (or later) than is medically indicated.

Approach to the Patient

The approach to the patient in occupational medicine varies with the type of encounter. Pre-employment screening is matter of fact. Hidden issues, however, may include substance abuse or occult injuries that require more careful reading of nonverbal cues or physical signs. Routine nonoccupational medical evaluations of adults should include an occupational history, which is one of the most neglected areas of the clinical history (Felton, 1980). Employees with job-related injuries or illness on duty require careful scrutiny for hidden agendas, including (1) job dissatisfaction, (2) conscious disability, and (3) unconscious disability.

Objective evaluations of occupational medical encounters require the physician to assume a different role than one limited to patient advocacy. The approach to the occupational health problem requires the consideration of the entire work environment, including safety as well as the individual's motivations vis-à-vis possible secondary gains through the system of compensation or disability benefits. Here, the family physician may be called upon to be more of a "company doctor," and be required to be an advocate for the employer as well as the employee.

The Occupational History

The fundamental question that all too frequently goes unasked is "What do you do?" Physicians also make the mistake of failing to get specific details of the work actually being done. As a consequence, we may not obtain information valuable in arriving at a correct diagnosis or prescribing the appropriate treatment.

A thorough history includes the length of time spent at this particular type of work, any known exposures to hazardous conditions (e.g., noise) or materials (e.g., chemicals), a general description of the work environment (indoor or outdoor, sitting, standing, and so on), the timing of symptoms in relation to work, and the existence of symptoms in coworkers (if known). Similar questioning may be necessary regarding past employment.

Pre-Employment Screening

The pre-employment physical examination is often viewed by the physician as boring and by the prospective employee as a potential impediment to employment. This can result in a process that serves no one well. In the ideal situation, the prospective employee will honestly reveal all health information and the physician will have all details related to the physical demands of the job. In this way the health and safety of the worker can best be protected.

Unfortunately, specific job information is frequently unavailable to the examining physician. In addition, prospective employees may fail to disclose pertinent health information, believing it may cost them a job.

Nevertheless, industry often demands that such examinations be done. A careful occupational history is just as important, perhaps more so, in this setting as in any other. The physical examination should pay special attention to those organ systems likely to be stressed by the type of work that will be done.

Laboratory and x-ray studies may or may not be necessary. If done, they should not be based on blanket screening but should rather be based on selective studies.

SCREENING ISSUES

Screening for asymptomatic occupational disease has significant cost-benefit potential for progressively oriented industries. Screening, the secondary level of prevention, attempts to identify early disease in more treatable stages before significant clinical damage has occurred. The ideal screening test (1) is sensitive with a high predictive value, (2) detects early disease with a high potential for morbidity and mortality, (3) has a high acceptability for patients, (4) has a low cost, and (5) detects disease for which an efficacious intervention exists (Last, 1986). The ideal occupational disease screening test should, therefore, possess all of the above characteristics.

An example of the type of occupational screening that can be applied in the family practice setting is office spirometry screening for occupational pulmonary disease. Whether spirometry is predictive of possible occupational disease is a matter of some debate (Eisen, 1987). Industries at risk for these disorders should include spirometry or pulmonary function tests as a baseline against which to measure possible future work-related lung injury evaluation. Office spirometry remains an inexpensive, fairly reliable technique capable of demonstrating restrictive and obstructive deficits. Baseline audiometry is another reasonable occupational screening test in jobs in which noise trauma may be significant.

Occupational Injury

Thousands of work-related deaths and millions of disabling injuries occur in the United States each year. For the purpose of discussion here, occupational injury and trauma are considered to be equivalent.

Occupational trauma may be acute or chronic. Examples of acute trauma may include but are not limited to muscle strain (or even ruptures), fractures, eye injuries, and lacerations. Examples of chronic trauma include injuries from repetitive activities (such as carpal tunnel syndrome), hearing loss from chronic noise exposure, and degenerative joint disease.

Industry losses from worker injuries run in the tens of billions of dollars annually. The loss in terms of human suffering is more difficult to measure but no less profound.

OCCUPATIONAL LUNG DISEASE

All too often occupational pulmonary disease is a retrospective diagnosis. Greater attention to prevention is required by all concerned. The family physician must always be attuned to industrial exposure to dusts, gases, vapors, and fumes. Occupational asthma is precipitated by exposure to such diverse substances as Freon, cobalt, coffee beans, hops, flour, ethylenediamine, penicillin, and adhesives (Lam, 1987). Employees of industries such as bakeries, breweries, cosmetics factories, metal plants, agricultural occupations, textile mills, forestry occupations, and factories that manufacture plastics and detergents should be screened for these disorders. Many patients present with recurring attacks of bronchitis. To qualify as having occupational asthma, individuals must not have had a bronchospastic disorder prior to exposure to noxious chemicals in the workplace. Most often, immunologic mechanisms appear to mediate occupational asthma.

Other major varieties of occupational lung disease include silicosis, hard metal dust exposure, occupational lung cancer, acute inhalation injury, pleural asbestosis, and agricultural or organic chemical lung disease (Rosenstock, 1987). Carcinogens of pulmonary tissues include acrilonitrile, arsenic, beryllium, bischloromethyl ether, cadmium, chromium, nickel, radon, and vinyl chloride (Cone, 1987). The synergy between tobacco and asbestos exposure that results in cancer is well known. The incidence of silicosis appears to have declined in recent years, although new cases continue to be reported in foundry workers, sand blasters, and packers of silica flour (Landrigan, 1987). Interstitial pulmonary fibrosis has been associated with hard metal dust such as tungsten, carbide, and cobalt (Balmes 1987). Chlorine gas exposure is also a familiar form of acute inhalational injury.

OTHER OCCUPATIONAL DISORDERS

Occupational disorders cover the spectrum of problems from dermatoses to problems related to the physical and chemical environment. Two of the more troubling are low back pain and work-related stress.

The cost of occupational low back pain is staggering. Of note is that the cost is not distributed uniformly; that is, much of the expense can be traced to a small number of high-cost cases (Snook and Jensen, 1984). Also significant is the fact that direct medical costs (such as physician fees, diagnostic tests, drugs, and so on) account for only one third of the cost related to low back pain (Leavitt et al., 1971). Disability payments account for the remainder. Indirect costs such as wages for replacement workers and accident investigations are more difficult to quantify but are omnipresent. It is critical, therefore, that the evaluation and treatment of patients with low back pain be optimal.

Optimal management of low back pain includes early identification, differentiation between discogenic and musculoligamentous pain, appropriate analgesics, and physical therapy. Prolonged bed rest is generally not helpful. Surgery may be beneficial when appropriate indications exist.

Job-related stress has been recognized as having a potentially deleterious effect on workers' health. Although this is intuitively accepted, the cost is less well defined than the cost of low back pain.

There are many factors in the work site that can cause stress. Stressors have been defined as factors triggering physiologic, psychologic, or behavioral responses (Berggren et al., 1988). Stressors include job and task requirements as well as role conflict. Individual coping strategies and personality characteristics must also be considered part of the picture. All of these factors must be taken into account when evaluating a patient for job-related stress so that potential areas of intervention can be identified. Just as work stress may be detrimental to worker health, modification of the work environment may be beneficial (Berggren et al., 1988).

Other occupational disorders include hearing impairment, a variety of skin disorders, and neuropathies. Problems such as hearing impairment and dermatoses can be helped by utilizing appropriate protective equipment and clothing, such as personal hearing protection devices and gloves. In some cases, federal and state regulations mandate that employers provide their workers with this equipment (Olishifski, 1988). In all cases, however, early identification of these problems can prevent or decrease the severity of any disability.

Workers' Compensation

Workers' compensation provides for the cost of medical care and rehabilitation as well as lost wages for workers who suffer a work-related illness or injury. In the United States, the first workers' compensation laws were passed in 1911 (Rom, 1983). The concept of employer responsibility for worker injuries, however, dates back to the middle ages in English law (King, 1986). Laws governing worker compensation are all state laws, and as a result, there is some variability from state to state. However, they all share a "no-fault" philosophy (King, 1986).

In addition to compensating injured employees, workers' compensation programs also provide an incentive to employers to optimize job safety and health conditions (Ashford and Andrews, 1983). Companies may provide benefits through a commercial insurance policy or by setting aside money for self-insurance.

Although the philosophy of workers' compensation laws is based on a "no fault" policy, in order to receive benefits the worker must establish a causal connection between the work performed and the injury or illness. This is not always easy, particularly in the case of occupational diseases. The medical report may be helpful in clarifying this point.

It is essential for the medical records and reports to be clear and for them to be handled with the same regard for confidentiality as other medical documents.

Management of the Acute Injury

The medical management of acute occupational injuries differs little from the approach to nonwork-related trauma. The differences are related to the work setting and the systems that have an impact on the injured employee, especially workers' compensation. One key determination in the initial evaluation is whether a work-related injury actually occurred and not that it was an injury occurring elsewhere that was then blamed on the workplace. Secondary gains include (1) time away from work or boss and (2) pay benefits.

After the determination of a true work-related injury and circumstances is made, a thorough examination is undertaken. Signs of swelling, point tenderness, loss of range of motion, and functional limitations (including visual acuity if applicable) are accurately recorded using diagrams where appropriate.

Bed rest for several days is a reasonable initial intervention for acute back injury. Prompt follow-up in 48 hours is important to monitor progress or further investigation or referral. Subacutely injured employees often can participate in light duty programs that greatly reduce costs (see the section on Light Duty Programs). Subacute injuries with disproportionate residual complaints that are persistent should receive further evaluation for conscious or unconscious disability (Florence and Miller, 1985). Soft tissue injections are sometimes helpful in relieving pain and reducing morbidity in back injuries (Medical World News, 1987).

Patterns of Response to Treatment

Patterns of response to treatment of work-related injuries are as follows:

Stoic. This individual desires to return to work before he or she is fully recovered. Possible motivations may include fear of job loss, either real or imagined; compulsiveness for work achievement; or high pain thresholds, either culturally or physiologically based. In any event the clinician needs to decipher these messages to avoid further injury in the face of partial recovery. Short-term utilization of light duty programs may be a satisfactory half-step measure.

Subconscious Disability. Here, the employee has a disproportionate degree of residual pain for which he or she seeks relief, with an absence of or minimal objective signs. Often, the history is vague and frankly inaccurate. This individual may assume that the clinician "always knows" the history (Florence, 1985). The physical examination is often inconsistent, although the individual readily submits to a thorough examination. Frequently, hysteria, depression, or anxiety may be present and readily uncovered by simple history-taking. These individuals are passive and often respond well to physical therapy. Antidepressants may also be helpful. A lack of concern for documentation or legal involvement is present.

Conscious Disability. This patient presents with a complete history, a positive chart sign, and a demanding attitude. Often, he or she demands surgery while reciting a litany against the previous treating physician. Legal material may also be presented. This patient doesn't want the clinician to miss any of the critical information. The appearance of being "coached" may be evident. Sometimes there may be a reluctance to submit to a complete examination. The patient states, "I've been through all this before and you can't help me anyway" (Florence and Miller, 1985). Marked defensiveness and anger may be another sign. Conscious disability patients resist family involvement. The term "malingerer" should be avoided in their care. Interventions and diagnostic work-ups often lead to complications and should be avoided. These patients resist new interventions.

Approach to Disability

Work-related disability has a myriad of implications for the health care provider. Most significant of all to the patient is the loss of function that they have suffered. People overcoming disability prefer the term "physically challenged" as opposed to disabled or handicapped. Work-related disability has additional implications often including prolonged settlement through the worker's compensation process. During this period, the challenge to the family doctor is to help patients maximize their potential by availing themselves of all diagnostic treatment and rehabilitation approaches while the system slowly comes to terms with settlement.

Since the family physician may play a significant role in disability determination, knowledge of correct terminology and definitions is required. A *disability* is a "deficit in performance that represents a restriction in the manner or range of activities considered normal within the context of the physical and social environment" (Calkins, 1986). A *handicap* is a "social disadvantage an individual experiences in fulfilling roles that are considered normal." An *impairment* is "an anatomic, physiologic, mental, or psychologic deficit that represents an organic dysfunction coded in ICD-9-CM. Standardized disability determination guides are available from the American Medical Association. When objective signs are lacking, healthy skepticism is not unreasonable. Vocational testing and rehabilitation are necessary for follow-up care.

Chronic Pain Syndromes

The family physician's approach to work-related chronic pain should temper concern with thoroughness. Chronic pain should be suspected when pain persists longer than 30 days. The physician should attempt to maintain an attitude of concern regardless of etiology. Approaches to unconscious disability have already been outlined. Chronic pain may also include a developing true disability, which can be missed by concentrating on the subacute injury.

REFLEX SYMPATHETIC DYSTROPHY

One form of pain syndrome which has the potential to become permanent is reflex sympathetic dystrophy (Borenstein, 1986). Reflex sympathetic dystrophy is a syndrome characterized by severe burning pain (causalgia), vasomotor instability, trophic skin changes, and changes on x-ray studies indicative of osteopenia. Pain related to reflex sympathetic dystrophy persists long after a wound is healed. Sensory C fibers and sympathetic efferent stimulation are believed to be causative factors. Fractures and hand injuries are among the occupational traumas prone to this complication. Reflex sympathetic dystrophy is characterized by burning pain, dysesthesia, temperature and color changes, and edema. Treatment must be initiated immediately and includes nonsteroidal anti-inflammatory drugs, temperature modalities, exercises during the early period, and local steroid injection. Sympathetic blockades, surgical or medical, may be tried for relief in the later phases.

MANAGEMENT OF CHRONIC PAIN SYNDROMES

The vast majority of chronic pain syndromes can be managed by the family physician with consultation from a physical medicine and rehabilitation specialist. Thorough functional and physical examination, including a neurologic and motor examination, is a cardinal rule for every office visit. Particular attention must be paid to actual functional limitations. Activities of daily living should be reviewed. The effect of the chronic pain on the patient's psyche and family and social spheres must be considered. Aggressive and early physical therapy should be pursued to maximize outcome. Chronic pain often responds to nonsteroidal anti-inflammatory drugs or amitriptyline (Elavil) or other antidepressants.

If motor or sensory deficits are identified, these should be pursued with electromyelography and nerve conduction studies. If deficits are in turn identified, they should be pursued as to etiology with computed tomography or magnetic resonance imaging. Fibromyalgia can complicate unconscious or true disability and further complicate chronic pain management. A full range of physical medicine modalities may be of benefit for fibrositis and may include (1) spray and stretch techniques, (2) local lidocaine (Xylocaine) injection, (3) ultrasound, (4) whirlpool, (5) massage, and (6) range of motion and strengthening exercises. All may be of benefit and help the patient to reduce his or her level of deficit despite the persistence of pain. A holistic approach would include stress reduction and psychologic evaluation and treatment, which may help to reduce the perception of chronic pain.

Environmental Diseases in the Workplace

THE IMPACT OF CHEMICALS ON WORKERS' HEALTH

Many of the chemicals used in the workplace have been associated with health disorders. Lead, manganese, and other metals found in industry can also cause health problems in workers. The nature of the problem may be dependent on a variety of factors, including the route of exposure, the intensity and duration of the exposure, the frequency of exposure, and, of course, the material itself.

Examples of environmental diseases in the workplace include lead poisoning, arsenical poisoning, and other heavy metal poisoning. These poisonings can occur in acute or chronic forms. Neurologic disorders may result as a consequence of exposure to carbon monoxide and organophosphate insecticides. Blood disorders, including anemia and polycythemia, may result from exposure to benzene. Some of these materials have been found to be carcinogenic as well.

Ethical Issues

There is the risk of succumbing to pressures that put the interests of the company above the health of the worker. The challenges in this area are so great that, in 1976, the American Occupational Medicine Association drafted a "Code of Ethical Conduct for Physicians Providing Occupational Medical Services." This document was subsequently approved by the Board of the American Academy of Occupational Medicine.

Hospital Employee Health

It has been said that health care is one of the last industries to establish standards for occupational health. The subject of hospital employee health has recently been extensively reviewed (Patterson, 1985). Most accidents occur while personnel are manipulating people or equipment. The greatest percentage of injuries involve back trauma among nursing staff. Laundry personnel are also at higher risk for injury. Among infection control issues to consider are the employees' immunity status, especially to rubella and varicella. Considerable morbidity occurs with lost work time related to varicella exposure. Recombivax R is recommended for all high-risk personnel, including surgery, emergency room, obstetrics, dialysis, and intensive care staff. The risk of transmission of the AIDS virus by puncture appears minimal, but universal precautions and confidential testing programs are now in place in many institutions in the United States (McCray, 1986). Surveillance of employees for other infectious diseases such as tuberculosis is ongoing in pre-employment screening. Scabies remains a pernicious problem for health care workers. Significant chemical hazards exist in hospitals and are underrecognized by employees. Important considerations here include ethylene oxide (gas sterilizers), formaldehyde (used in laboratory and pathology testing), anesthetic gases, and chemotherapeutic agents (used in oncology and pharmacology). The full impact of these toxic agents is not known. Eighty per cent of all health care workers are female, many of whom are of child-bearing age. Monitoring systems exist, but enforcement varies depending on location. Many smaller hospitals have nurse-only employee health units.

Ergonomics

Ergonomics, the study of work, deals with the impact of work activities on the worker's health (Armstrong and Langolf, 1983). It crosses over several disciplines, including engineering and biologic and behavioral sciences (Dickerson and Baker, 1988).

There is an interrelationship between the worker, the task, the work station design and the tools being used as well as the physicial environment (Dickerson and Baker, 1988). Because of this interrelatedness, problems in any one of these areas may result in problems throughout the system. Productivity and worker health may be hurt.

Conversely, when all these parts are functioning optimally, worker health, satisfaction, and productivity should also be optimal. Thus, the application of ergonomic principles represents a significant contribution to occupational health (Dickerson and Baker, 1988).

One can work toward optimal functioning of the workplace from the direction of workplace design (or redesign) or from worker selection (Nordin and Frankel, 1987). The family physician may have limited input into workplace design unless employed by industry. Nevertheless, if the family physician becomes aware of a workplace condition that jeopardizes health, attempts should be made to advise appropriate company officials.

In the context of the pre-employment physical, the family physician is more routinely in a position to have an impact on the system. As an adjunct to the physical examination, a physician may order specific strength testing. Various devices exist that measure strength. Guides such as the Ergonomics Guide for the Assessment of Human Static Strength (Chaffin, 1975) may be used by physicians to better understand and utilize strength testing. It is essential for the family physician to have as much information as possible regarding the physical requirements of the job.

Community and Regulatory Issues

In 1970, the United States Congress enacted the Occupational Safety and Health Act, which formed the Occupational Safety and Health Administration (abbreviated as OSHA) (MMWR 1988). This agency is the regulatory agent for occupational safety and health in the United States. Other agencies act in a collaborative fashion and include the National Safety Council. The Bureau of Labor Statistics compiles data and also acts collaboratively in surveillance activities. The Occupational Safety and Health Administration has made significant strides in improving workplace safety by regulation and enforcement. Recently, however, the Occupational Safety and Health Administration has scaled back its work force and has begun to contract for inspection services with state regulatory agencies. Yet another division, the Mine Safety and Health Administration (abbreviated as MSHA), regulates mines through the United States Department of Labor. The National Safety Council, in turn, works closely with the Centers for Disease Control and compiles recommendations and occupational safety and health standards. The Morbidity and Mortality Weekly Report (MMWR), published by the Centers For Disease Control, provides a source of data for the family physician on special hazards, alerts, and guidelines regarding particular occupational health issues. Definitions of all the standards and terms are listed in the MMWR's National Safety Council supplement issue (MMWR, 1988).

Perhaps in no other area is there such an opportunity to maximize our impact on overall community health than in the workplace. There are over 110 million members of the work force in the United States who spend a third or more of their day in the workplace. Community health attempts to benefit the larger group that shares a particular location. Occupational safety and health improvements, therefore, benefit large numbers of individuals. Workplace health concerns can extend beyond safety and environmental issues to chronic disease screening and health promotion activities. Since there is a shortage of physicians to provide occupational health care, this burden is largely addressed by family physicians. The family doctor interested in occupational health can have a great impact when he or she becomes involved with local companies to provide pre-employment screening and handle work-related injuries. Family physicians have been instrumental in improving overall plant safety and in providing industry with cost savings in work-related–injury care and workers' compensation, while helping to improve the overall community's health.

Work Site Fitness Programs

In a continued effort to curb rising health care costs, a number of major corporations in the United States have implemented worksite wellness programs. Companies such as AT&T, General Motors, and Johnson & Johnson offer such programs as smoking cessation, early disease detection, weight reduction, and exercise (Goldsmith, 1986).

The actual impact of such programs remains unclear. Although one study found lower rates of absenteeism and health care costs in workers who exercised, the change was not significant, leading to the conclusion that the differences were related to personality traits rather than the exercise program itself (Braun et al., 1986).

One analysis of Johnson & Johnson's Live for Life program suggests lower hospital costs for participants versus nonparticipants (Bly et al., 1986). Concerns regarding methodology, however, raise some questions as to the validity of these results (Sciacca et al., 1987).

Although their actual benefit remains to be determined, interest in these programs continues to be strong. As programs proliferate, it will be important to monitor their outcome to make a valid cost-benefit determination.

Work Capacity Testing and Work Hardening Programs

Work capacity testing and work hardening programs are an integral part of the disability rehabilitation process. Work capacity testing is the determination of an individual's ability to perform work tasks. Work hardening programs are programs of intensive rehabilitation keyed to job-specific physical requirements and designed to return the individual to his or her own job. Work capacity testing should be considered for all personnel who have been disabled or who have been away from work for prolonged periods. The latter group may be tested with a work tolerance screen that takes less than a day to complete. Full work capacity testing must be completed for individuals with significant loss of function either from work-related disability, non-work–related disability, or chronic diseases impairing work capacity. Work hardening programs may be contracted with rehabilitation programs for larger employers. A 6-week program may allow the disabled person to gradually increase his or her work capacity while independent medical evaluations confirm progress.

Fitness for Duty—Drug and Alcohol Use in the Workplace

When an employee's work performance is at issue, drug and alcohol use in the workplace may need to be addressed. The issue of drug testing remains controversial. Some would argue that random workplace screening probably should be avoided because of low predictive value (Last, 1986). Others defend random screening as the best available mechanism for dealing with a known problem (Goldsmith, 1988). Still others acknowledge that people often change their behavior when they know they are being observed (Lundberg, 1986). When transportation workers are involved, the courts take a more activist position. If an employee is intoxicated, the chances of injury are greatly increased. The employee can also irreversibly harm others or products produced. Employees who have the odor of alcohol on their breath at work before lunch are virtually certain to be alcoholics. Signs of impairment at work may include (1) absenteeism, (2) late arrival, (3) frequent injuries, and (4) declining performance. Medical evaluation should attempt to corroborate the etiology of impairment by focusing the history and physical on substance abuse and its targets. Laboratory work-up can be pursued depending on company policies and the individual's consent. A referral to an employee assistance program can facilitate rehabilitation of the employee if chemical dependency or impairment related to other issues is determined.

The pressures for drug screening are increasing as the business community's concern with the drug problem increases. There are essential elements that any screening program should contain whether it is a pre-employment, for cause, or random screening program. These elements include interpretation of the test results by a physician (Goldsmith, 1988) and use of the best available technology to ensure reliability and accuracy and to ensure due process for those being tested (Lundberg, 1986). A fair policy should exist, of which drug testing is only one component. Supervisor training and employee education assistance, counseling and treatment, and disciplinary procedures should also be part of the policy (Goldsmith, 1988).

Light Duty Programs

Light duty programs have been shown to be effective in reducing workers' compensation costs. Employees with unconscious or true disability or those who are stoics may be candidates for light duty programs. Light duty pools allow the employee to work in a low-risk setting, have limitations on endurance or work times that are flexible, get the employee away from the drudgery of home to therapy and home again, and allow them to perform a useful service while being paid through workers' compensation.

Health Objectives for the Nation

"Healthy People: The Surgeon General's Report on Health Promotion and Disease Prevention" (1979) listed occupational safety and health as an "action" of major importance in protecting the lives of all Americans (Miller, 1983). The United States Public Health Service established 20 objectives specifically in occupational safety and health for achievement by 1990 (United States Government Printing Office, 1980). These are summarized as follows:

A. Improved health status
- By 1990, workplace deaths in firms with 11 or more employees should be reduced to less than 3750 per year.
- By 1990, the rate of work-related injuries should be reduced to 3.3 cases per 100 full-time workers.
- By 1990, among workers newly exposed after 1985, there should be virtually no new cases of four preventable occupational diseases—asbestosis, byssinosis, silicosis, and coal-related pneumoconiosis.
- By 1990, occupational heavy metal poisoning (lead, arsenic, zinc) should be virtually eliminated.

B. Reduced risk factors
- By 1990, all firms with more than 500 employees should have an improved plan of hazard control for all new processes, equipment, and new installations.
- By 1990, at least 25 per cent of workers should be able to state the nature of their occupational health and safety risks and their potential consequences prior to employment as well as be informed of changes in these risks while employed.

C. Improved services and protection

D. Improved surveillance and evaluation

RIGHT-TO-KNOW LAWS

Consistent with objective B above, some states have enacted "right-to-know laws" that have implications for physicians to inform patients about toxic work-related exposures (Himmelstein and Franklin, 1985). OSHA, state, and local regulations are now promulgating these rules. Employers post material safety data sheets to make employees more aware of hazards resulting from 600 basic chemicals. Some state requirements increase this list to 30,000 chemicals.

The physician may be called upon to help provide specific answers about the neoplastic potential or other long-term effects of particular substances, conditions, or equipment. Physicians may be required to include routine screening histories as to occupational exposures listed within the medical record. The physician can obtain material safety data sheets from the patient who copies it from the employer or directly from the employer by written request. Referencing work and data base acquisition will be required of the family physician to perform this interpretive function when the material safety data sheets are received.

References

American Occupational Medical Association: Ethical Guidelines. Chicago, 1976.

Armstrong, T. J., and Langolf, G. D.: Ergonomics and occupational safety and health. *In* Rom, W. N. (Ed.): Environmental and Occupational Medicine. Boston, MA, Little, Brown and Company, 1983.

Ashford, N. A., and Andrews, R. A.: Workers' compensation. *In* Rom, W. N. (Ed.): Environmental and Occupational Medicine. Boston, MA, Little, Brown and Company, 1983.
Balmes, J.: Respiratory effects of hard metal dust exposure. State of the Art Reviews: Occupational Medicine, 2:2, 1987. *A comprehensive review series which is an important reference for occupational medicine.*
Berggren, T., Hane, M., Ekberg, K., et al.: Stress at work: An interactive model for work environment analysis. *In* Occupational Medicine—Principles and Practical Applications. Chicago, IL, Year Book Medical Publishers, 1988.
Bly, J. L., Jones, R. C., and Richardson, J. E.: Impact of worksite health promotion on health care costs and utilization. Evaluation of Johnson & Johnson's Live for Life program. J.A.M.A., *256*(23):3235–3240, 1986.
Borenstein, D.: Reflex sympathetic dystrophy. Drug Ther, *16*:64–67, 1986.
Braun, W. B., Bernacki, E. J., and Tssi, S. P.: A preliminary investigation: effect of a corporate fitness program on absenteeism and health care cost. J. Occup. Med., *28*(1):1986.
Calkins, E., Davis, P., and Ford, A. (Eds.): The Practice of Geriatrics. Philadelphia, W.B. Saunders, 1986.
Campbell, V., and Nicolle, F.: Occupational and Environmental Diseases in Family Practice. J. Fam. Pract., *13*(1):118–119, 1981.
Centers for Disease Control: MMWR 1983, Leading Work-Related Diseases in Industries in the United States. M.M.W.R., *32*:24–26, 1983.
Chaffin, D.: Ergonomics guide for the assessment of human static strength. Am. Ind. Hyg. Assoc. J., *36*(7):505–511, 1975.
Committee on Ethical Practice in Occupational Medicine of the American Medical Association: Drug screening in the workplace: ethical guidelines. J. Occup. Med., *28*(12):1240, 1986. *A useful guide in helping physicians find their way through the maze presented by the troublesome and challenging problems of chemical dependency in the workplace.*
Cone, J.: Occupational Lung Cancer. State of the Art Reviews: Occupational Medicine, 2:2, 1987.
Cotter, D. M., and Macon, J. A.: Death in industry, 1985: BLS survey findings, MO Labor Rev., *77*:45–47, 1987.
Cowart, V.: Drug use, no matter why, raises ethical issues. J.A.M.A., *256*:2649, 2653–2654, 1986. *A brief but excellent summary of some of the ethical issues in drug use and the physician's role in diagnosis and treatment.*
Dickerson, O. B., and Baker, W. E.: Practical ergonomics and work with video display terminals. *In* Zenz, C. (Ed.): Occupational Medicine—Principles and Practical Applications. Chicago, IL, Year Book Medical Publishers, 1988.
Eisen, E.: Standardizing spirometry: problems and prospects. State of the Art Reviews: Occupational Medicine, *2*:213, 1987.
Felton, J. S.: The occupational history, a neglected area in the clinical history. J. Fam. Pract., *11*:33, 1980.
Florence, D. W., and Miller, T. C.: Functional overlay in work-related injury. Postgrad. Med., *77*(8):87–106, 1985.
Frank, A.: The occupational history and examination. *In* Rom, W. N. (Ed.): Environmental and Occupational Medicine. Boston, MA, Little, Brown and Company, 1983.
Goldsmith, M. F.: Worksite wellness programs: latest wrinkle to smooth health care costs. J.A.M.A., *256*(9):1089–1091, 1095, 1986.
Goldsmith, M. F.: Drug testing upheld, decried; physicians asked to help decide. J.A.M.A., *259*:2341–2342, 1988.
Healthy People: The Surgeon General's Report on Health Promotion and Disease Prevention (1979) vs. Department of Health Publication No., Washington, D.C., U.S. Government Printing Office. *A comprehensive report of hospital employee health.*
Himmelstein, J., and Franklin, H.: Special article—The right to know about toxic exposures—Implications for physicians N. Engl. J. Med., *312*(11):687–690, 1985.
Hines, T.: When accidents happen. Fortune, *106*(5):62–68, 1982.
King, N.: Practical consideration for the physician concerning worker's compensation law. Hand Clin. *2*(3):603–610, 1986. *An excellent review of an important topic physicians deal with often, but understand little.*
Kvale G.: Occupational exposure and lung cancer risk. Int. J. Cancer, *37*:185–193, 1986.
Lam, Chan-Yeung: Occupational asthma: Natural history, evaluation and management. State of the Art Reviews: Occupational Medicine, *2*:2, pp. 373–380, 1987.
Landrigan, P.: Silicosis. State of the Art Reviews: Occupational Medicine, *2*:2, 1987.
Last, J. (Ed.): Preventive Medicine and Public Health. Maxcy and Rousseau: Public Health and Preventive Medicine. 12th ed. Appleton-Century-Crofts, 1986, p. 40.
Leavitt, S. S., Johnston, T. L., and Beyer, R. D.: The process of recovery: Patterns in industrial back injury. Part I: Cost and other quantitative measures of effort. Ind. Med. Surg., *40*(8):7–14, 1971.
Lundberg, G. D.: Mandatory unindicated urine drug screening: Still chemical McCarthyism. J.A.M.A., *256*:3003–3005, 1986.
McCray, E.: Special report: Occupational risk of acquired immunodeficiency syndrome for health care workers. N. Engl. J. Med., *314*(17):1127–1132, 1986.
Medical World News: Soft tissue injections studied for back pain. September 28, 1987, p. 15.
Miller, J., and Myers, M.: Occupational safety and health: Progress toward the 1990 objectives for the nation. Public Health Rep., *98*(4):324–335, 1983.
NIOSH Recommendations for occupational safety and health standards. M.M.W.R., *37*(5–7), 1988.
Olishifski, J. B.: Occupational hearing loss, noise, and hearing conservation. In Zenz, C. (Ed.): Occupational Medicine—Principles and Practical Applications. Chicago, IL, Year Book Medical Publishers, 1988.
Patterson, W. B.: Occupational hazards to hospital personnel. Ann. Intern. Med., *102*:658–80, 1985. *A comprehensive report of hospital employee health.*
Pollack, E. S., and Keimig, D. G. (Ed.): Counting Injuries and Illnesses in the Workplace: Proposals for a Better System. Washington, D.C., National Academy Press, 1987.
Pope, M. H., Frymoyer, J., and Andersson, G. (Eds.): Occupational Low Back Pain. New York, Praeger Publishers, 1984. *This short book is an outstanding reference clearly and concisely covering all aspects of this important problem.*
Rom, W. N. (Ed.): Environmental and Occupational Medicine. Boston, MA, Little, Brown and Company, 1983.
Rosenstock, L., (Ed.): Occupational Pulmonary Disease. State of the Art Reviews: Occupational Medicine, *2*:2, 1987.
Sciacca, J. P., Black, D. R., and Seehafer, R. W.: Worksite health promotion and health care costs and utilization (letter). J.A.M.A., *258*(17):2379, 1987.
Seligman, P. J., Sieber, W. K., Pedersen, D. H., et al.: Compliance with OSHA record-keeping requirements, Am. J. Public Health, *78*:1218–1219, 1988.
Smith, F. R.: A paradigm for perspective. Occupational medicine in a deregulatory era: the beginnings 1835–1970. Edwin Chadwick John Farr through Alice Hamilton. J. Occup. Med., *30*(5):425-E, 1988. *A concise work which provides the reader a historical background from which to view occupational medicine.*
Snook, S. H., and Jensen, R. C.: Cost. *In* Pope, M. H., Frymoyer, J., and Andersson, G. (Eds.): Occupational Low Back Pain. New York, Praeger Publishers, 1984.
United States Government Printing Office: Department of Health and Human Services: Promoting health/preventing disease—Objectives for the Nation. Washington, D.C., U.S. Government Printing Office, 1980, pp. 39–43.
Wiegand, N.: Fatal occupational injuries in U.S. industries: Comparison of two national surveillance systems. Am. J. Public Health, *78*(9):1215–1217, 1984.
Zenz, C. (Ed.): Occupational Medicine—Principles and Practical Applications. Chicago, IL, Year Book Medical Publishers, 1988. *This is a classic textbook on occupational medicine.*

23

Assessment of Functional Health Status

Patrick J. O'Connor
Sydney H. Croog

The maintenance and improvement of patients' functional status is often one of the fundamental goals of the family physician (Katz, 1987). In order to do this effectively, the physician must have a practical and accurate method of screening and assessing function. At present, many methods of screening and assessing patients' functional status are available, including the physician's traditional approach of questions and observations as well as standardized scales and measures that have recently been developed.

In primary care office practice, however, the presence of functional impairment in many patients as well as marked time constraints create a persisting clinical dilemma. How can the busy physician accurately detect significant functional impairment in a routine office visit that may necessarily be very brief?

The need for functional assessment has stimulated the recent development of a number of innovative methods of screening and assessing functional status in the office. The explosion of information on functional status presents clinicians with many new options (McDowell, 1987). However, given this array of options, how effective are the various methods? Can they be used on large numbers of patients daily in office practice without disrupting patient flow? Should they be applied to all patients or only to those at greatest risk of functional impairment? Finally, what advantages, if any, do these newer techniques have over traditional clinical methods of screening and assessing functional impairment?

Definition and Clinical Significance of Functional Status

The definition of functional status is a matter of some controversy. This derives in part from semantic confusion in the use of certain terms (WHO, 1980) and in part from differences in the theoretical concepts of functional status (Ware, 1987).

Functional status, as considered in this chapter, includes those dimensions of health that extend beyond but are related to the purely biologic dimension. Considering functional status as a multidimensional construct, there is general agreement that physical, emotional, cognitive, and social function are critical components. Physical function is a measure of the ability to perform certain activities, such as bathing, toileting, cooking, eating, walking, climbing stairs, dressing, and peeling an apple. Emotional status may include measures of depression, anxiety, self-esteem, and coping. Cognitive function includes measures of orientation, memory, language, reasoning, judgment, attention span, and alertness. Social function includes measures of the intactness and extent of a person's interpersonal contacts, social resources, and performance of usual role activities (Levine and Croog, 1984; Ware, 1987) and sexual function (Croog et al., 1988).

Other dimensions sometimes included in functional status are feelings of well-being and satisfaction and inventories of symptoms or assessment of pain (Stewart et al., 1988; Nelson et al., 1987).

Functional status is related to but not necessarily dependent upon physiologic homeostasis. For example, two persons with diabetes of similar type and duration and with similar treatment, control, and complications may have quite different configurations of functional status. One person may have made appropriate family and life-style adjustments and maintained work and social involvements. The other may have greater difficulty adjusting to the disease and may have stopped working and may have reduced social involvements. A thorough grasp of the patient's physiologic state does not necessarily provide accurate knowledge of functional status.

Historically, clinical assessment of those dimensions of health referred to as functional status has always been an important part of primary care (Novak, 1987), and many clinicians use questions to probe these dimensions. Yet in office practice, time pressures often limit the depth of exploration of physical, emotional, cognitive, and social functions. Organic problems (such as elevated blood pressure or serum glucose) demand time and attention, and the average time spent by family physicians in an office visit with most patients is less than 15 minutes, even for patients with complex medical problems (Radecki et al., 1988).

Much acute illness can indeed be dealt with purely in terms of the biomedical model; i.e., no extended inquiry into functional status is required. However, for the chronically ill, the elderly, the caretakers of these patients, and some other special groups of patients, *screening* for functional deficits or change in functional status may be critical in providing good care. When functional impairments are identified by screening, *comprehensive functional assessment* followed by specific treatment or *intervention strategies* are warranted.

A Systematic Approach to Screening and Assessment of Functional Status

In office practice, traditional clinical techniques of questioning and observation are usually effective in evaluating the nature and severity of functional impairment. However, under some circumstances, a substantial proportion of functional impairment may elude detection. For example, Nelson and associates (1983, 1987), using a sophisticated method of assessing functional status in a network of primary care practices, found that 32 per cent of patients reported moderate or major limitations of physical function, 45 per cent of patients reported moderate or major limitation of emotional function, and 34 per cent of patients reported moderate or major limitations of social function. However, only about half of these functional limitations were recognized by the patients' regular physicians. The implications of these discrepancies for functional outcomes, patient satisfaction, and doctor-patient relationships clearly merit consideration.

In a sense, functional impairment is a problem or "disease" in its own right. Hence, standard criteria for screening, diagnosis, and treatment have been developed for functional impairment just as they have for other diseases (Feinstein, 1987). However, because data suggest that existing informal methods of screening and diagnosis of functional impairment are not always sufficiently effective in office practice, we advocate use of a three-step formal approach, leading from screening to assessment to treatment.

1. *Office-based screening* of selected high-risk groups of patients can be incorporated using brief, standardized, self-administered instruments. (These data can be viewed, perhaps, as analogous to an additional vital sign.)

2. *Comprehensive functional assessment* (CFA) can be used for those individuals who are identified by screening to have a significant functional impairment. The physician can construct a "functional problem list" based on the CFA and include it along with the usual medical problem list of the problem-oriented medical record.

3. An *effective treatment or intervention strategy,* guided by the functional problem list, can be used to stabilize or improve the functional status of the patient.

Systematic screening methods can provide an effective, brief way of identifying functional impairment in office practice. At present, many useful CFA methods are available for physical, emotional, cognitive, and social functional assessment (Duke University, 1978; Kane and Kane, 1981; Granger et al., 1987). Such problems, once identified, may also merit more in-depth assessment. Detailed evaluation of the patient and the construction of a functional problem list can thus provide a rational basis for treatment or intervention strategies. When employing these or other methods, the physician carrying out CFA of a particular patient should first focus on those functional dimensions that are most important to the patient.

CFA can often be done by the physician alone, but it may sometimes require a multidisciplinary team. Moreover, while many intervention strategies cannot be carried out solely by the physician, the physician is often in the best position to screen for functional problems, initiate CFA, and coordinate referral to other services.

Given the current state of the art, it is often difficult to demonstrate specifically that detection of more subtle functional impairments leads to better health outcomes. However, a considerable body of data suggests that certain interventions, when applied appropriately and early, may lead to better functional outcomes. Such interventions include changing pharmacotherapy to reduce functional impairment (Croog et al., 1986; Jachuck et al., 1982), emotional support by physicians and other health professionals (Novak,

1987), disease-specific patient and caretaker support groups (Poulshock, 1984), and caretaker education groups. They may also include physical therapy or job retraining (Granger et al., 1987), family therapy or individual counseling (Cartwright, 1982), respite care, hospice care, visiting nurse support, special transportation services, or systematic intervention based on CFA (Rubenstein et al., 1985; Rubenstein, 1987; Teasdale et al., 1983; Narain et al., 1988).

Thus, efficient screening, comprehensive assessment, and effective treatment and intervention strategies can improve functional status. In particular, screening for functional status seems justified in certain high-risk groups, according to Frame's screening criteria (1986):

1. The condition must have a significant impact on a person's health or well-being.
2. The incidence of the condition must be sufficient to justify the cost of screening.
3. Screening tests that are acceptable to patients must be available at a reasonable cost to detect the condition accurately in the subclinical period.
4. Intervention or treatment strategies of proven effectiveness must be available for use.
5. The condition must have a subclinical period during which early detection and treatment can be effective.
6. Initiation of treatment in the subclinical period should yield a better outcome than that obtained by delaying treatment.

Working with Groups at Highest Risk of Functional Impairment

Several groups of patients are at high risk for impaired physical, emotional, cognitive, or social function. These include the elderly, the chronically ill, the caretakers of the elderly and the chronically ill, and patients being treated with pharmacologic agents that may impair function.

THE CHRONICALLY ILL

Cluff (1981) estimates that 30 to 50 million people in the United States suffer some dysfunction related to chronic disease or the sequelae of injuries. About 15 million people have dysfunction that is severe enough to cause limitation in their work or school performance or their ability to run a household. The rates of functional impairment are highest in the elderly: 12 per cent of the population over age 65 accounts for about 33 per cent of disabilities. However, about two thirds of those with limitations are found in younger age groups, particularly among the chronically ill and survivors of serious injuries.

In addition to the studies of Nelson and associates (1983, 1987), data from other sources confirm high rates of functional impairment in the primary care setting. A survey of 11,186 patients of 526 physicians in three regions of the United States found that 45 per cent reported limited physical function, 28 per cent had limited role function, 9 per cent had limited social function, 31 per cent had limited mental function, 52 per cent had low health perceptions, and 29 per cent reported moderate or greater pain (Stewart et al., 1988). Each of these levels of impairment was much greater than those reported in a general population survey of 2008 patients using the same questions. Parkerson and coworkers (1981), using the Duke University of North Carolina Health Profile (in which 1 represents optimal function), observed that the mean function score for all adult patients attending a family medicine center in North Carolina was 0.72 for physical abilities, 0.77 for emotional status, and 0.74 for social function. Although using different approaches, these four studies indicate very high levels of functional impairment in many dimensions among patients seeking primary medical care.

Screening of chronically ill patients, particularly patients who have more than one disease, is important because of the functional impact of the diseases (which may act synergistically) and the sometimes veiled functional impacts of therapy (Jachuck et al., 1982; Croog et al., 1986 and 1988). CFA can then be brought to bear on these multiple identified problems.

The impact of chronic diseases on physical function has been well described, and evaluation of physical function in patients with rheumatic disease and cardiac disease (Feinstein, 1987) has proved to be of great clinical utility. However, functional measures that tap emotional, cognitive, and social dimensions in patients with chronic diseases are less developed.

THE ELDERLY

Among the elderly, in particular, functional status is commonly impaired. As many as 50 per cent of elderly living at home may have some physical disability that interferes with performing activities of daily living, and nearly 80 per cent of those over 65 years old suffer at least one chronic illness (Rowe and Besdine, 1988).

Systematic screening of functional status in the elderly can be usefully applied in the office as (1) an aid in diagnosis, (2) a way to anticipate needed social interventions, and (3) a guide in developing plans for treatment and approaching possible institutionalization of an elderly person.

Functional status provides an empirical yardstick against which to measure risks and benefits of alternative therapeutic strategies. But an additional advantage of systematic and periodic functional assessment of the elderly is that the process may facilitate communication among various specialists or disciplines involved in care of the elderly.

An axiom of geriatric medicine is that reliable and objective screening of functional status should be done at regular intervals, and that this screening should be supplemented by CFA whenever problems are detected. Dimensions of function that may require particular attention include vision, hearing, physical, emotional, cognitive, and social function as well as general well-being. Such screening and assessment are needed not only because they help to determine the best supportive strategies to compensate for loss of function over time but also because subtle deterioration in function (e.g., mobility, mental status, continence, or intake) may herald the onset of serious new disease or worsening of chronic disease (Besdine, 1983).

However, realistic and accurate screening for functional impairment in the elderly may be difficult. Visual and auditory deficits or impaired cognitive status may make data from examinations, interviews, or questionnaires unattainable or inaccurate. Hence, it may be necessary to question caretakers and family members in order to obtain a clinically useful picture of a patient's functional status.

CARETAKERS OF THE CHRONICALLY ILL AND ELDERLY

Another group at high risk of functional impairment is the caretaker, spouse, or family of an elderly or chronically ill patient. Although the phenomenon was not systematically examined until recently, there is now an expanding literature on the stress and health risks to people in caretaker roles (Andolsek et al., 1988). The expression "hidden patient" has been used to describe their situation. These persons are *themselves* often at high risk for impairment of emotional status (depression, anxiety, and exhaustion) and of social function (sleep deprivation, missed work, inability to leave the home, and so on). Although some physicians question whether searching for such problem situations is their proper role or prerogative (Brody, 1980), others strongly argue that this is a vitally important role for which the family physician in particular is ideally suited (Cartwright, 1982).

Making a home visit or getting the "hidden patient" to accompany the identified patient on office visits can provide valuable information about caretaker function and coping as well as give additional information about the identified patient. Information provided by relatives, neighbors, or clergy may also be useful. Such data can lead to more informed management of both the patient and the caretaker in the context of the family system; they can help avoid disasters such as undetected depression or suicide of a caretaker (Cohen et al., 1988) and premature or delayed institutionalization of the identified patient.

OTHER GROUPS AT HIGH RISK OF FUNCTIONAL IMPAIRMENT

Patients with acute conditions who are being treated with drugs that might impair walking, memory, sleep, vision, sexual function, continence, or appetite form another group at high risk of functional impairment. Even a short course of medication for an acute problem can cause significant emotional or social dysfunction, occasional physical injury, or serious adverse drug effects. For example, among patients being treated with psychotropic medications, there is an increased risk of functional impairment ranging from drowsiness to falls with associated hip fractures (Ray et al., 1987). Thus, continuing evaluation of changes in functional status of patients being treated for acute illness may provide data that help the clinician choose treatments that are both biologically and functionally optimal.

Overview of Available Instruments to Screen for Functional Status in the Office Setting

Pioneer multidisciplinary research teams have developed a number of comprehensive instruments to assess functional health status for research purposes. Three of the most comprehensive are the Sickness Impact Profile (Bergner et al., 1981), the Rand Adult Health Status Measures (Brook et al., 1979), and the Older American Resource Survey (OARS) (Duke University, 1978). Because of their length, none of these instruments is appropriate for routine screening in the office setting, but some have been used in CFA protocols. Many of the short, practical office methods of assessing functional status discussed in the following sections were derived from these longer instruments or standardized against them.

A number of *disease-specific* multidimensional measures of functional status are available. These include instruments designed for musculoskeletal conditions, cardiac disease, and cancer. Instruments are being developed for use with diabetes and other diseases but are not yet ready for widespread clinical application. Although some of these measures are useful, they will not be discussed here, since we will focus on global measures of functional status rather than disease-specific ones.

Several relatively short, global, multidimensional functional scales are useful to the busy office-based practitioner who wants to assess functional status in a quantitative and objective fashion (Table 23–1). Most of the instruments discussed here can be self-administered or administered by office personnel. Most were developed and tested for use in primary care settings. All have been shown to be useful in assessing functional status at one point in time; more data are needed to determine which are useful in assessing changes over time.

The Duke University of North Carolina Health Profile

The Duke University of North Carolina Health Profile was developed by a team of family physicians,

Table 23–1. SUMMARY OF GLOBAL MULTIDIMENSIONAL FUNCTIONAL STATUS MEASURES*†

Reference	Number of Items	Can Be Self-Administered by the Patient	Easy to Understand	Reliability	
				Internal Consistency Cronbach Alpha‡	*Test-Retest Reliability*
Duke University of North Carolina Health Profile (Parkerson et al., 1981)	63	Yes	Yes	0.85	0.53–0.82
Rand Short Form General Health Survey (Stewart et al., 1988)	20	Yes	Yes	0.81–0.88	Not reported
Dartmouth Cooperative Charts (Nelson et al., 1987)	9 charts	Yes	Yes	Insufficient scale size	Not reported
Nottingham Health Index (Hunt et al., 1985)	38	Yes	Variable	0.90–0.94	0.75–0.88
Functional Status Questionnaire (Jette et al., 1986)	34	Yes	Variable	0.64–0.82	Not reported
Functional Status Index (MacKenzie et al., 1986)	3 areas	No	Variable	0.85	0.76

*These measures may be useful in office-based screening for functional impairment.
†Measures of validity vary and appear in detail in the original references.
‡The closer this coefficient is to 1.0, the more likely the measure can be used repeatedly to assess changes over time.

internists, and health service researchers for use in primary care (Parkerson et al., 1981). It is a 63-item scale that takes 10 to 15 minutes to complete and measures four dimensions of function: physical, emotional, social, and symptom status.

The Health Profile was tested on 395 ambulatory adult patients in a family medicine center. Reliability measures were good and there was good convergent, discriminant, and construct validity. The Health Profile has not been extensively tested for its ability to detect change in functional status in individual patients over time. It does identify areas of concern, allowing the clinician to delve further into problems as he or she sees fit.

The Rand Short Form General Health Survey

This 20-item instrument measures functional status in six dimensions: physical functioning, role functioning, social functioning, mental health, health perceptions, and pain. This screening instrument was derived from the much longer Adult Health Status Measures fielded by the Rand Institute in the late 1970's as part of the Health Insurance Study (Brook et al., 1979).

The Short Form has been tested by phone interviews with a national sample of 2008 adults and also with 11,186 patients of 526 health care providers in three communities (Stewart et al., 1988). Correlation among health measures, comparison of patient and general population samples, and correlations between health measures and sociodemographic traits all suggested adequate to good scale validity. This instrument covers a broad range of functional dimensions in reasonable depth, can be self-administered in an average of 3 to 4 minutes, and appears to be useful for screening functional status. However, the number of items may be too small for it to be useful as a measure of change in functional status over time. Data to decide the last point are available but have not yet been published. Selected questions from this instrument are shown in Table 23–2.

The Dartmouth Cooperative Chart Method

Nelson and coworkers (1987) have developed a system of assessing functional status using nine pictorial charts. Patients view each chart and then select one of five choices reflecting varying levels of function. The charts cover physical condition, emotional condition, daily work, social activities, pain, change in conditions, overall condition, social support, and quality of life. A sample chart is shown in Figure 23–1.

The charts have been tested on 117 patients in two practices. They can be self-administered or staff-administered in only 2 minutes at the time usual vital signs are taken. The authors claim they are acceptable to patients, office staff, and physicians, based on pilot testing with 112 patients. No data are presented on the test-retest reliability of the method. The sensitivity of the charts to change over time was not assessed, but is likely to be suboptimal; internal consistency reliability measures are not applicable because each dimension is scored by only one response (one chart). Validity was assessed by comparing patients' Dartmouth Cooperative Chart responses with scores on the Functional Status Questionnaire (Jette et al., 1987). Convergent validity ranged from 0.40 to 0.74 and averaged 0.64. Discriminant validity was good except for some collinearity between physical and role function scores (r = 0.50). The authors believe that the charts have good face validity, improve

Table 23–2. RAND SHORT-FORM HEALTH SURVEY: MEDICAL OUTCOMES STUDY

In general, would you say your health is:

1 ☐ Excellent
2 ☐ Very good
3 ☐ Good
4 ☐ Fair
5 ☐ Poor

How much bodily pain have you had during the past 4 weeks?

1 ☐ None
2 ☐ Very mild
3 ☐ Mild
4 ☐ Moderate
5 ☐ Severe

For how long (if at all) has your health limited you in each of the following activities? (Check One Box on Each Line)

	Limited for more than 3 months 1	Limited for 3 months or less 2	Not limited at all 3
a. The kinds or amounts of vigorous activities you can do, like lifting heavy objects, running, or participating in strenuous sports	☐	☐	☐
b. The kinds or amounts of moderate activities you can do, like moving a table, carrying groceries, or bowling	☐	☐	☐
c. Walking uphill or climbing a few flights of stairs	☐	☐	☐
d. Bending, lifting, or stooping	☐	☐	☐
e. Walking one block	☐	☐	☐
f. Eating, dressing, bathing, or using the toilet	☐	☐	☐

Does your health keep you from working at a job, doing work around the house, or going to school?

1 ☐ Yes, for more than 3 months
2 ☐ Yes, for 3 months or less
3 ☐ No

Have you been unable to do certain kinds or amounts of work, housework, or schoolwork because of your health?

1 ☐ Yes, for more than 3 months
2 ☐ Yes, for 3 months or less
3 ☐ No

For each of the following questions, please check the box for the one answer that comes closest to the way you have been feeling during the past month. (Check One Box on Each Line)

	All of the Time 1	Most of the Time 2	A Good Bit of the Time 3	Some of the Time 4	A Little of the Time 5	None of the Time 6
How much of the time, during the past month, has your health limited your social activities (like visiting with friends or close relatives)?	☐	☐	☐	☐	☐	☐
How much of the time, during the past month, have you been a very nervous person?	☐	☐	☐	☐	☐	☐
During the past month, how much of the time have you felt calm and peaceful?	☐	☐	☐	☐	☐	☐
How much of the time, during the past month, have you felt downhearted and blue?	☐	☐	☐	☐	☐	☐
During the past month, how much of the time have you been a happy person?	☐	☐	☐	☐	☐	☐
How often, during the past month, have you felt so down in the dumps that nothing could cheer you up?	☐	☐	☐	☐	☐	☐

Please check the box that best describes whether each of the following statements is true or false for you. (Check One Box on Each Line)

	Definitely True 1	Mostly True 2	Not Sure 3	Mostly False 4	Definitely False 5
a. I am somewhat ill	☐	☐	☐	☐	☐
b. I am as healthy as anybody I know	☐	☐	☐	☐	☐
c. My health is excellent	☐	☐	☐	☐	☐
d. I have been feeling bad lately	☐	☐	☐	☐	☐

From Stewart et al., 1988. Copyright Rand Corporation.

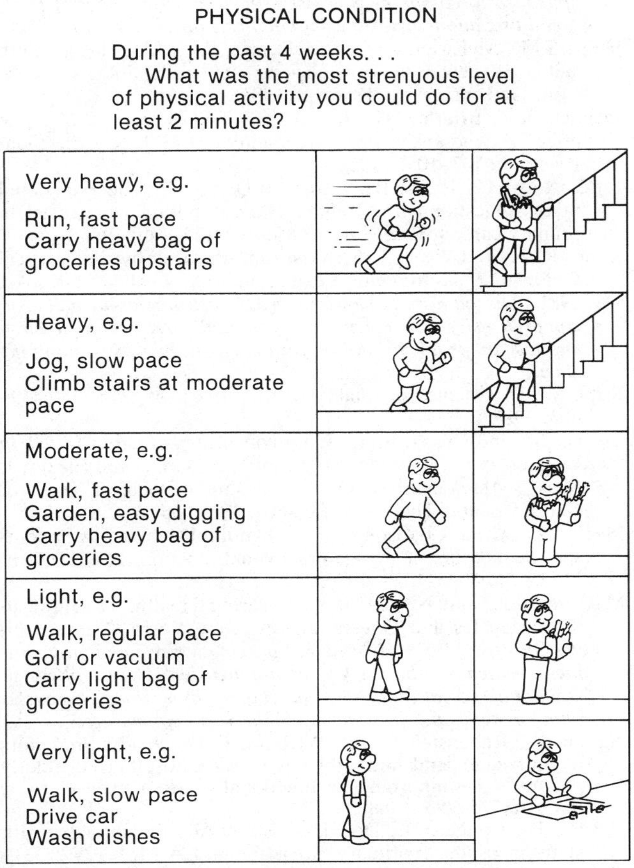

Figure 23–1. Sample Dartmouth Cooperative Chart to measure physical function. Copyright Trustees of Dartmouth College.

physician-patient communication, and lead to discovery of treatable problems that, in turn, lead to changes in management and possibly better patient outcomes. The authors included two patients' stories to support these assertions; more work is needed to refine the Dartmouth Cooperative Charts and to further assess their utility in office practice.

Nottingham Health Profile

Hunt and associates (1985) have developed and tested in several practice settings a 38-item instrument that evaluates six functional dimensions: energy level, pain, emotional reactions, sleep, social isolation, and physical abilities. The instrument can be self-administered in less than 10 minutes; each item presents a statement (e.g., "I soon run out of energy.") to which the patient answers yes or no.

The Nottingham Health Profile is well-suited for screening, since around 60 per cent of patients show no functional impairment on the scale. On the other hand, the Nottingham Health Profile may be insensitive to subtle impairment in status and is unlikely to be sensitive to subtle change over time. Scoring is complicated, and summary scores over the six dimensions are not advised, since their meaning would be unclear.

Functional Status Questionnaire

Jette and coworkers (1986) have developed the Functional Status Questionnaire collaborating with researchers at Rand. This 34-item instrument is designed to screen for disability and to monitor change in functional status. Dimensions measured include physical function, psychologic function, social function, and role function. The Functional Status Questionnaire was tested on 1153 patients in hospital clinics in Boston and private practices in California.

The Functional Status Questionnaire scale scores had relatively low correlation with such health-related measures as bed disability days (0.15 to 0.28) and restricted activity days (0.15 to 0.28). Higher correlation was noted between Functional Status Questionnaire scale scores and work role limitations (0.25 to 0.61). Correlation of Functional Status Questionnaire scale scores with that of other functional status measures has not been reported. Thus, the validity of the Functional Status Questionnaire has not been well established, and for some scales, the internal consistency is so low that the ability of the Functional Status Questionnaire to accurately detect change over time is questioned by its authors.

Functional Status Index

The Functional Status Index has been recently developed by MacKenzie and associates (1986) at Cornell University Medical Center. This simple index is designed to be sensitive to change in maximal function over time in individual patients. It starts with a "baseline component;" changes from baseline are detected using a "transition component." The index has three dimensions: physical, mental, and emotional.

Maximal functional status is scored as better, the same as, or worse than baseline. Validity was measured against Sickness Impact Profile scores, and the Functional Status Index scores were well-correlated with Sickness Impact Profile scores over time for the physical dimension. The validity of the emotional and mental dimensions has not been reported.

The Functional Status Index is limited by the fact that only *directionality* of change in maximal function is indicated; the magnitude of the change cannot be measured. There are only three dimensions in the Functional Status Index; thus it lacks the breadth of other scales such as the Rand Short Form General Health Survey and Duke University Health Profile. Nevertheless, the method is innovative and appears promising, since the office-based practitioner is often interested in changes in functional status over time.

Summary

Of the six global multidimensional instruments reviewed here, the Duke University Health Profile and the Rand Short Form General Health Survey

(Table 23–2) appear most promising for office-based screening of adult patients at highest risk for functional impairment. The Dartmouth Cooperative Charts and the Functional Status Index suggest creative and promising new directions that deserve further development.

As these instruments and others are used more in the future, specific recommendations may change. A major issue awaiting further evaluation is how sensitive the different instruments are in detecting changes in an individual patient's functional status over time. Further experience with a formal and systematized method of screening, assessing, and treating functional impairment will provide the ultimate test of their effectiveness as a means of improving the health status of patients.

References

Andolesek, K.M., Clapp-Channing, N.E., Gehlbach, S.H., et al.: Caregivers and elderly relatives: The prevalence of caregiving in a family practice. Arch. Int. Med., *148:*2177–2180, 1988. *Random survey of adults over 40 years of age attending a family practice, which showed that over 20 per cent were caregivers for noninstitutionalized relatives. Sixty per cent of these relatives were functionally impaired, and 40 per cent were substantially impaired. The clinical implications are discussed.*

Bergner, M., Bobbitt, R.A., Carter, W.B., and Gilson, B.S.: The Sickness Impact Profile: Development and final revision of a health status measure. Med. Care, *19:*787–805, 1981.

Besdine, R.W.: Educational utility of comprehensive functional assessment in the elderly. J. Am. Geriatr. Soc., *31:*651–656, 1983.

Brody, D.S.: Physician recognition of behavioral, psychological, and social aspects of medical care. Arch. Int. Med., *140:*1286–1289, 1980.

Brook, R.H., and Kamberg, C.J.: General health status measures and outcome measurement: A commentary on measuring functional health status. J. Chronic Dis., *40*(Suppl. 1):131S–136S, 1987.

Brook, R.H., Ware, J.E., Davies-Avery, A., et al.: Overview of adult health status measures fielded in Rand's Health Insurance Study. Med. Care, *17*(Suppl):1–131, 1979.

Cartwright, A.: The role of the general practitioner in helping the elderly widowed. J. Roy. Col. Gen. Pract., *32:*215–227, 1982.

Cluff, L.E.: Chronic disease, function, and quality of care. J. Chronic Dis., *34:*299–304, 1981.

Cohen, D., and Eisdorfer, C.: Depression in family members caring for a relative with Alzheimer's Disease. J. Am. Geriatr. Soc., *36:*885–889, 1988.

Croog, S.H., Levine, S., Testa, M.A., et al.: The effects of antihypertensive therapy on the quality of life. N. Engl. J. Med., *314:*1657–1664, 1986.

Croog, S.H., Levine, S., Sudliovsky, A., et al.: Sexual symptoms in hypertensive patients: A clinical trial of antihypertensive agents. Arch. Intern. Med., *148:*788–794, 1988.

Duke University Center for the Study of Aging and Human Development: Multidimensional Functional Assessment: the OARS Methodology. 2nd ed. Durham, NC, Duke University Press, 1978.

Feinstein, A.R.: Clinimetrics. New Haven, Yale University Press, 1987. *A fascinating book in which a distinguished author argues for an improved understanding and unified approach to clinical measures and provides a theoretical framework to achieve this goal.*

Frame, P.S.: A critical review of adult health maintenance. Parts 1–4. J. Fam. Pract., *22:*341–346, 417–422, 511–520; and *23:*29–39, 1986.

Granger, C.U., Seltzer, G.B., and Fishbein, C.F.: Primary care of the functionally disabled: Assessment and management. Philadelphia, J.B. Lippincott Company, 1987. *A systematic approach to comprehensive assessment and treatment of functional limitations, with special emphasis on physical function.*

Hunt, S.M., McEwan, J., and McKenna, S.P.: Measuring health status: A new tool for clinicians and epidemiologists. J.R. Coll. Gen. Pract., *35:*185–188, 1985.

Jachuck, S.J., Brierley, H., Jachuck, S., and Willcox, P.M.: The effect of hypotensive drugs on quality of life. J. R. Coll. Gen. Pract., *32:*103–105, 1982.

Jette, A.M., Davies, A.R., Cleary, P.D., et al.: The Functional Status Questionnaire: Reliability and validity when used in primary care. J. Gen. Intern. Med., 1:143–149, 1986.

Kane, R.A., and Kane, R.L.: Assessing the Elderly: A Practical Guide to Measurement. Lexington, MA, Lexington Books, 1981. *The authors review numerous instruments available to comprehensively assess physical, mental, and social function and discuss problems and opportunities in their use among the elderly.*

Katz, S.: The science of quality of life. J. Chron. Dis., *40:*459–463, 1987.

Levine, S., and Croog, S.H.: What constitutes quality of life? *In* Wegner, N.K., Mattson, M.E., Furberg, C.D., and Elison, J. (Eds.): Assessment of Quality of Life in Clinical Trials of Cardiovascular Therapies. Le Jacq, 1984, pp. 46–58.

MacKenzie, C.R., Charlson, M.E., DiGiola, D., et al.: A patient-specific measure of change in maximal function. Arch. Intern. Med., *146:*1325–1329, 1986.

McDowell, I., and Newell, C.: Measuring Health: A Guide to Rating Scales and Questionnaires. New York, Oxford University Press, 1987. *Helpful and pragmatic review of 50 instruments which can be used to comprehensively assess physical, emotional, social, and other functional dimensions. Discusses both strengths and weaknesses of the various measures.*

Narain, P., Rubenstein, L.Z., Wieland, G.D., et al.: Predictors of immediate and 6-month outcomes in hospitalized elderly patients. The importance of functional status. J. Am. Geriatr. Soc., *36:*775–783, 1988.

Nelson, E., Conger, B., Douglass, R., et al.: Functional health status measures of primary care patients. J.A.M.A., *249:*3331–3338, 1983.

Nelson, E., Wasson, J., Kirk, J., et al.: Assessment of function in routine clinical practice: Description of the COOP chart method and preliminary findings. J. Chronic Dis., *40:*51; 55S–63S, 1987.

Novak, D.H.: Therapeutic aspects of the clinical encounter. J. Gen. Intern. Med., *2:*346–355, 1987.

Parkerson, G.R., Gehlbach, S.H., Wagner, E.H., et al.: The Duke-UNC Health Profile: An adult health status instrument for primary care. Med. Care, *19:*806–828, 1981.

Poulshock, S.W., and Deimling, G.T.: Families caring for elders in residence: Issues in the measurement of burden. J. Gerontol., *39:*230–239, 1984.

Radecki, S.E., Kane, R.L., Solomon, D.H., et al.: Do physicians spend less time with older patients? J. Am. Geriatr. Soc., *36:*713, 1988.

Ray, W.A., Griffin, M.R., Schaffner, W., et al.: Psychotropic drug use and the risk of hip fracture. N. Engl. J. Med., *316:*363, 1987.

Rowe, J.W., Besdine, R.W. (Eds.): Geriatric Medicine. 2nd ed. Boston, Little, Brown and Company, 1988.

Rubenstein, L.V., Calkins, D.R., Fink, A., et al.: Topics in primary care medicine: How to help your patients function better. West. J. Med., *143:*114–117, 1985.

Rubenstein, L.Z.: Geriatric assessment: An overview of its impacts. Clin. Geriatr. Med., *3:*1, 1987.

Stewart, A.L., Hays, R.D., and Ware, J.E., Jr.: The Medical Outcome Study (MOS) Short-Form General Health Survey: Reliability and validity in a patient population. Med. Care, *26:*724, 1988.

Teasdale, T.A., Schuman, L., Snow, E., et al.: A comparison of placement outcomes of geriatric cohorts receiving care in a geriatric assessment unit and on general medicine floors. J. Am. Geriatr. Soc., *31:*529, 1983.

Ware, J.E., Jr.: Standards for validating health measures: Definition and content. J. Chron. Dis., *40:*473, 1987.

World Health Organization: International classification of impairments, disabilities and handicaps. Geneva, World Health Organization, 1980.

24

Home Care

Lawrence H. Bernstein

Today, home care is being discussed as if it were an entirely new concept invented by this generation of health care providers. Thirty-five years ago, when I was 8 years old, I would sometimes wait in the car while my father, a general practitioner carrying a black bag, made house calls. Much of what needed to be done diagnostically and therapeutically was available in that bag. An examination, a simple test, and a shot were often the order of business.

Today, as a family physician, I do home care, rarely carry a black bag, and frequently rely on technologic advances like cardiac telemetry to assist me. Tests are sent off to the hospital or brought back to the office, and it would be unusual for me to visit the home specifically to give an injection.

Even though our generation, like generations in the past, prefers to think we evented the concept of home care, we didn't. Home care is a new term for an old idea that is an important part of the style and art of medical practice. Yes, physicians are beginning to make house calls again. And, when it is feasible and when given a choice, most patients would prefer being treated at home.

Yet, with the pressures of increasingly complex technologies and with our dependence on acute care hospitals, we have gotten away from thinking about caring for patients in their homes as an expected part of patient care. We tend to view home care as an exception.

The Lost Art

A number of factors explain why home care has been removed from the mainstream of medical practice.

TRAINING

With few exceptions, physicians practicing today have had little hands-on experience with caring for patients in the home. The experience they have is often focused more on *observing*, from a distance, the functioning of a home care team. The physician is not taught to perceive himself or herself as an active participant in the process or to explore the unique skills the physician can bring to the encounter. And the lessons learned from home care are not commonly extrapolated to the office setting.

ROLE MODELS

In the tertiary care teaching setting, students and house staff are unlikely to encounter the primary care physician who makes house calls. This type of physician is often viewed as the antithesis of the more highly regarded specialists who publish, obtain grants, and teach. Fortunately, there is a teaching role for both kinds of practitioners. Physicians at all levels of practice can learn a great deal about caring for people from academicians and black bag toting doctors alike.

LITERATURE

The nursing literature is filled with excellent articles on caring for patients at home, but the medical literature (defined as articles a doctor will read) has almost none. The same applies to continuing medical education courses. As a result, we have not provided the opportunity for physicians to learn about home care or even to make an informed choice about whether this is a style of medicine they would like to adapt.

HOUSE CALLS

There's no doubt that physicians make far fewer house calls than they did 20 to 30 years ago, although this is beginning to change. Obviously, this trend means that we are far less comfortable and less experienced dealing with patients in their homes.

Home care is measured more by a physician's practice style and approach to patients than the number of house calls made. In fact, most of the in-home work is done by nurses and therapists. Implicit in caring for patients at home is demonstrating a concerned, caring, competent response to a broad spectrum of patients' needs. By managing patients with other members of the home care team, the amount of time the physician devotes to house calls can be minimized.

REIMBURSEMENT

A major reason for lack of physician interest in home care is financial since payment is considerably less than for an equal amount of time in the office or hospital. However, the burden on the physician's time can be minimized by working with home care personnel and learning how to maximize their capabilities.

RESPONDING TO PATIENTS' NEEDS

Home care helps the family physician respond to some of the fundamental human needs of patients, whether they are independent functional patients seen in the office or severely dysfunctional homebound patients. Most patients want to maximize independence, remain at home if they can, and live with a sense of safety and security. For this, and other reasons, home care is often just plain good medicine.

FINANCIAL CONSTRAINTS

Managed care systems—health maintenance organizations (HMOs), preferred provider organizations (PPOs), etc.—are a dominant theme in medicine, and their influence is growing. One of the major goals of these insurance entities is the search for alternatives to institutionalization. In addition, PPO schemes, such as diagnosis-related groups (DRGs), have pressured us into discharging patients from the hospital sooner than ever before—the quicker and sicker discharge. Because lengths of stay are decreasing, many patients go home with problems requiring further resolution. Home care can be part of the process of continuing medical care after discharge. Not only is this good medical practice, it is also a specific response to a major source of patient anxiety.

DEMOGRAPHICS

America is graying. Not only is the 85-plus age group the fastest growing segment of the population, but the ratio of elderly persons to persons of working age has tripled in this century and is continuing to rise. Society is slowly coming to grips with the problems of caring for an increasingly older population with chronic care needs. Home care has a special place in this effort, along with nursing homes, hospices, and other approaches to the long-term care issues of caring for the elderly.

TECHNOLOGIC CHANGES

Hospital technology has moved into the home. Patients who require respirators or central venous catheters for a prolonged period can be effectively, safely, and economically managed at home. Similarly, an increasingly broad spectrum of infectious disease, such as endocarditis, orthopedic prostheses infections, and osteomyelitis, are being treated in the home with parenteral antibiotics. Space age technology will increasingly be applied to the care of patients in the home and at remote sites using sophisticated equipment that permits improved patient monitoring and greater patient independence.

Definition

Home care is usually defined in terms of the *resources* provided to the patients in the home. These include:

- Personnel services, such as those offered by visiting nurses, physical or occupational therapy, homemakers, aides, and intravenous therapists.
- Consumable supplies, such as protection or collection devices for incontinence (adult diapers or pads), dressings, and ostomy equipment.
- Durable medical equipment (DME) includes commodes, transfer benches, and hospital beds.

For some people, home care is defined by *ambulatory* status—if a patient is bedbound but not eligible for nursing home or hospital care, he or she is a home care patient. However, both the resource based and ambulatory status definitions place artificial constraints on the patient population we can serve with home care.

Thus, I propose the following broad definition of home care:

Home care is caring for patients in the home, and home-care patients are patients with home-care needs.

The inherent simplicity of this definition is explained by concentrating on the patient's needs *in functional terms relevant to the patient*. For example, when using this definition, the most important questions to answer in deciding whether the patient is a candidate for home care are:

- How does the problem affect the patient's life?
- How has this problem affected the patient's ability to perform the basic activities of daily living (ADLs)?
- If the patient were to wish for but one change in his or her situation, what would it be?
- Is there a home-care treatment modality, equipment, or personnel that can help with these problems?

If the answer to this last question is "yes," the patient is a home-care patient regardless of most other constraints on the definition.

Whether the patient is ambulatory or bedbound is largely irrelevant for the family physician's involvement in home care. If we concentrate on a patient's *functional requirements* instead of *ambulatory status*, it makes sense that we shouldn't deny patients access to home care *because* they are ambulatory and functional. For example, even though a patient can drive to the office does that mean we shouldn't provide home-care modalitites (like a homemaker or bathroom safety devices) for the patient's arthritis. But before one can identify functional requirements there should be a structure and format to carry out the history taking process.

Assessment of the ADLs and instrumental activities of daily living (IADLs) is the first step in understanding patients' functional needs (Table 24–1). ADLs span a spectrum from very basic functions, such as eating, bathing, and toileting, to more complex IADLs like shopping, managing medications, or using the telephone.

These specific functions, taken together, determine a person's ability to perform more general functions, such as living at home with minimal assistance and a sense of security; feeling competent about personal abilities; appropriately utilizing available community and family resources; and anticipating future needs.

Table 24–1. FUNCTIONAL ASSESSMENT

Activities of Daily Living
- Ambulation
- Toileting
- Grooming
- Dressing
- Feeding
- Bathing and hygiene
- Continence

Instrumental Activities of Daily Living
- Writing
- Finances
- Shopping
- Housekeeping
- Telephoning
- Travel outside the home
- Reading

While the ADLs provide a construct for assessing specific functions, the PULSES profile can help further delineate specific deficits responsible for a functional problem (Table 24–2).

The ADLs, IADLs, and PULSES profile, together, provide a structured format that determines more than just the ability of the patient to perform a series of tasks. It gives a picture of how the patient lives at home: What is it like for this person? How does it feel? What are the patient's anxieties? What are the disappointments? What should be changed?

While a comprehensive functional evaluation is clearly important, the more important goal is learning what a specific disease, disability, or functional deficit means to the patient, what is the impact on his or her life, and what facets of the disability are of greatest concern.

In the office setting, this is especially important because, in the typical brief office visit, the physician's evaluation is usually going to be tightly focused. The patient is in the office with a very specific problem and expects the physician to provide some preliminary answers—answers that respond to what the patient thinks is the salient problem.

I keep returning to the *patient's perspective* because this is often forgotten when using the traditional history and review of systems taught in medical school. For example, a gentleman presenting in the office with minimal nighttime urinary incontinence will require a history, physical examination, and appropriate laboratory testing. The review of systems includes queries about dysuria, urgency, pyuria, hesitancy, strength of stream, and so on. An intravenous pyelogram and urology consult may be required to arrive at a precise diagnosis and appropriate therapy.

However, what is the most important dimension of the problem to the patient? Are there other concerns, often left unanswered, because we didn't ask the right questions? Consider, in addition to the textbook pursuit of the diagnosis, asking the patient "What is it like when you get up to urinate at 2 o'clock in the morning?" (This is a patient seen in the office and would not be conventionally thought of as a home-care patient.) "Well, to tell you the truth, doc, I get kind of dizzy when I try to stand up at night and I'm afraid I might fall. Besides, I hate waking my wife because she has such trouble getting back to sleep because of her arthritis, and she really can't keep going up and down the stairs doing the

Table 24–2. PULSES PROFILE

P	physical condition: general health status
U	upper limb functions: self-care activities (eating, drinking, dressing, etc.)
L	lower limb functions: the ability to walk, transfer from bed to chair, from chair to toilet, etc.
S	sensory functions: sight, hearing, ability to communicate, etc.
E	excretory functions
S	support factors: psychologic supports, family structure, social and financial supports, etc.

wash all the time. It's a long walk to the bathroom and the hallway is dark because I can't change the light bulb in the ceiling fixture. And, to top it off, last Sunday my daughter stopped by and told us that if she smelled urine in the house one more time she would probably put me in a nursing home."

Now we know what *really* concerns this gentleman. At the moment, his major concern is not whether or not he needs a prostatectomy. He simply wants to stay dry! Our obligation, then, in addition to providing standard medical care, is to provide a bedside commode, or urinal, or adequate adult diapers, or protective pads. If we don't acknowledge and provide for these needs, we have missed a very important part of caring for this patient.

These are home-care needs, and this is a home-care patient, even though he may be functional in all other regards. It is important to note that obtaining this sort of information and providing this kind of care is neither inconsistent nor incompatible with a compulsive medical evaluation and a definitive therapeutic approach.

Another example is the patient with arthritis who lives alone and functions well. Because physicians are often uncomfortable with functional assessment, there is a tendency to concentrate on relieving pain and prescribing the correct anti-inflammatory drug. However, there are other aspects to caring for this person. On initial observation in the office, it may be noted that the patient is having difficulty climbing onto the examination table. Based on this observation, the physician may then discover that the patient has a fear of bathing because he might fall, problems cooking because of weak hands, or poor nutrition because of an inability to go shopping.

The solutions to these problems are often in the domain of home care, despite the fact that this is not a conventionally defined home-care patient. Furthermore, the concept of delving into functional capacity is as applicable to the severely disabled patient as it is to the average ambulatory patient.

In addition to patients with well-defined problems, many have a pervasive, gradually diminishing global loss of function. For lack of a more apt phrase, this group is often referred to as having the dwindles.

Because these people may be confused at times, feel unsafe in the kitchen, have inadequate nutrition and poor hygiene, and rarely leave the house, they frequently find themselves living precariously. Even though they may not be safe, comfortable, and competent living alone they usually don't want or need to be in an institution. They would openly admit that they would rather die than go to a nursing home. This is not an indictment of long-term care facilities. But, for patients in the dwindling category, nursing homes are usually inappropriate.

The physician should assess daily functioning using the ADLs as a structure for the interview and then consider making a referral to the local visiting nurse agency or for-profit home care company.

What are some specific things that will affect these people's ability to continue living independently?

- If the patient is arthritic and fears falling in the shower or tub, provide a shower transfer bench or grab bars. Poor hygiene may merely be a result of fear of falling.
- Urinary incontinence may be functional, meaning that if adequate toilet facilities were within the patient's reach (based on both cognitive and physical abilities), the patient would be able to remain dry. To maintain both urinary and fecal continence, the patient must be able to get to the toilet or commode.
- If cooking and shopping are difficult, arrange for Meals-on-Wheels or a homemaker or aide. Often, poor nutrition is a result of simply not being able to go shopping.
- An occupational therapist can come into the home and show the patient how to efficiently and effectively accommodate many of the deficiencies resulting from arthritis. For example, there is an impressive array of cleverly designed, inexpensive equipment designed to accommodate the needs of arthritics who have trouble dressing, opening tight jars, or handling small utensils. Using this equipment, a talented therapist can significantly enhance the patient's ability to eat, dress, and bathe.
- If mobility is impaired, an individual with a two-story house can safely live on the first floor and sleep, bathe, and use the toilet upstairs by using an electric stair.

The Home as a Clinical Setting

The home has an enormous positive emotional significance to patients. Butler (1986) describes this feeling succinctly: "The place where one lives is connected with *who* one is, and how one expresses this sense of *self*. Many older people associate home with autonomy and control." In contrast, the office or hospital usually engenders a neutral or even negative response.

When physicians make house calls, we enter a world that is entirely the patient's. This is the place where that patient likely spends all or almost all of his or her time. It is the place where the patient rightly assumes control. Physicians are accustomed to being in control of encounters with patients. In the office, the patient is the physician's guest and in the hospital feels more like a captive. But in the home, the physician becomes the patient's guest. This turning of the tables carries with it certain expectations regarding behavior.

Because the patient is in a comfortable environment and is at ease, the patient feels a greater sense of being able to influence what happens. It is worthwhile acknowledging this and emphasizing to patients the areas in which they *do* have some control. For example, in the hospital, meals are served at specified times—whether one is hungry or not. It is unreasonable to assume that a patient will suddenly change a 70-year habit of getting out of bed at 6 A.M., having a cup of coffee, reading the paper, and then eating breakfast at 9 A.M. In the home, this is easily accommodated: in the hospital, it is impossible to imagine.

Following hospitalization, patients and family easily reassume their accustomed roles in the home. Sometimes the family needs help successfully accomplishing this transition back to previous roles. It is important for the physician to support these changes because patients sometimes sustain the role of patient long after it is appropriate to do so. Being a part of this process provides enormous insight into the family's dynamics and the impact the illness has had on the family unit.

The house call provides the opportunity to glimpse the family as they really are, not as they appear in the office or in the hospital or as the physician wants them to be. In the first few minutes in the home, the physician can glean more about family structure and function than in multiple visits in other settings.

Cultural Influences on Home Care

The influences of a patient's culture on the doctor-patient relationship are important in all areas of medicine but have a special poignancy for home care. Cultural influences are pervasive, affecting virtually every aspect of the patient's daily life. Since home care requires the physician to understand and become a part of the patient's world more than in the office or hospital setting, it is necessary to be sensitive to the patient's culture. Culture can be loosely defined as what can be done, what should be done, what cannot be done, and what must be done.

Cultural perceptions can affect things like receptivity to professional advice, compliance with dietary instructions, the degree to which patient and family actively or passively partake in the treatment process, and the ability of the patient or family to perform specific tasks.

For example, gender role expectations vary from culture to culture. In a strongly patriarchal society or culture, it may be difficult for the male to assume the dependent role of patient and allow a female to, of necessity, manage household finances. Anger directed at the wife may be a manifestation of the frustration and inability to be the passive recipient of care.

Cultural food preferences require a different kind of sensitivity on the part of the physician. Consider the elderly Jewish grandmother with congestive heart failure who insists on eating heavily salted chicken soup because of its alleged therapeutic effects. Could the patient be better off eating the soup? Especially if we increase the diuretic dosage to compensate? If we forbid this dietary indiscretion, two things will happen: First, we will lose credibility because *everyone knows* chicken soup has a certain therapeutic efficacy. Second, she probably won't listen to us anyway!

In some cultures, disease is viewed as a matter of fate. This will affect the patient's receptivity to interventions that are intended to alter the disease course. For example, a patient recovering from a stroke may adapt a passive noninvolved attitude toward rehabilitation. Physicians, largely middle-class, goal-oriented, type-A personalities, may interpret this as laziness or depression. However, if we understand the patient's belief system, his or her response makes sense. If the patient feels disease is inevitable and the process inexorable, then there really is no reason to believe that the physician can change the course of events. The patient sees the logical extension as: Why bother with rehabilitation if I'm going to end up with the same result anyway? This is not to deny the possibility of clinical depression.

Dealing with these issues requires a degree of introspection on the part of the physician. If the patient is only minimally involving himself in a rehabilitation program, is it unfair for the physician to call it laziness? By imposing a personal value system on the patient, the physician has done an injustice. If, for example, because of my compulsiveness, I inappropriately push the patient harder than is reasonable for his culture, then I have behaved unfairly and insensitively.

The more we are able to look at ourselves and our attitudes before we evaluate and treat the patient the more compassionate will be our care. We need to understand ourselves while we are trying to understand the patient. As we become more human to the patient, we will both become more humane to each other. Although this is particularly important for home care, it is broadly applicable to all areas of medicine.

Caring for patients in the home imposes a new and different set of issues.

The Past as Prologue

Part of caring for a family is knowing about their past. Although we may have cared for a family for a few weeks, months, or even years, we sometimes forget that these people have lived together for perhaps 20 or 30 years. A great deal of history has likely preceded the acute illness. Before we assume certain expectations for the family's behavior or pass judgment on their actions, it is important that we know more about their relationships *before* we became the family's physician. Because illness and disability are very disruptive of past patterns, the window we are permitted to glimpse through may well provide a view atypical of how they have lived in the past. The new equilibrium, even though it may appear normal, may have been attained at a great cost.

For example, the quadriplegic seen in bed at home may appear mild mannered, compliant, and quite the perfect gentleman. And, because of this perception, the physician may have trouble understanding the wife's reluctance (or even refusal) to fully participate in the care plan—a plan requiring intermittent bladder catheterization and changing soiled bed linen. The reason may be obvious if we know what the marriage was like *before* the accident that left her husband with a C3–4 quadriplegia. In the past, this patient may have been abusive, a heavy drinker, and a somewhat less-than-faithful spouse. As a result, the treatment plan may need to be adjusted and the family will probably need more help than originally anticipated.

The Care-Partner as Patient

In most home-care situations, there is both an identified and an unidentified patient. The identified home-care patient is obvious. But the unidentified patient—the primary care-partner—deserves to be a patient in his or her own right as well. Being treated as a patient implies being treated as an individual—not just an extension of the identified patient. The phrase *care-partner*, coined by Anthony Grieco (Bernstein, 1987), is used instead of *care-giver* because of the *partnership* relationship between patient, spouse, family, doctor, etc. Partnership also implies an active interaction instead of a passive relationship between people.

In the example of a woman caring for a quadriplegic husband, both she and her husband have an agenda of problems that are both congruent and separate. Because of our intense focus on the identified patient's problems, we tend to view the wife only as the woman caring for her husband. But Mrs. Smith is still Mrs. Smith, a woman with her own concerns—anger, hostility, ambivalence, etc. If we ignore these, and only treat her as an extension of her husband, we have not treated her *or* her husband adequately. Thus, treating her as a patient is an integral part of the care plan for her husband.

To accomplish this it is sometimes necessary to set aside a separate appointment time to sit down with Mrs. Smith to talk about her problems without reference to her husband. Although at times this may seem somewhat artificial, it can be very productive. She can be encouraged to talk about her anger and ambivalence. The conversation should focus on her own identity and not on the identity of a person caring for a quadriplegic. In all likelihood, she spends too much time thinking about the latter and too little time thinking about the former.

In the process of talking with Mrs. Smith, the message should be that it is understandable that she feels angry. An attempt should be made to establish, or re-establish, her identity as a person. Even though caring for her husband seems like an overwhelming chore, she should realize the importance of recognizing her own personal needs.

Immobility

The ability to maneuver in the home or in the community is a function of physical and cognitive abilities. The family physician is likely to care for a large number of patients with modest mobility problems who do not necessarily need physical therapy (PT) or occupational therapy (OT). What can the family physician offer these patients with modest deficits? The patients whose needs are *least* likely to be met are moderately independent office patients who have no medical contact other than their family physician. If they were more restricted, they would probably have already been involved with PT or OT.

Physicians must first be sensitive to the problems: What does it mean to you when you can't walk as well as you used to? What things can't you do that you really enjoy? In general, how does this affect your life? By asking these questions, the physician is telling the patient that the physician considers these problems at least as important as ordering computerized tomography scans, using the latest generation of cephalosporins, or ordering exotic blood tests. That is an important message, especially when so many patients start the conversation with, "I don't want to bother you with this. I know how busy you are, but I just can't get around like I used to and, for me, a messy house is intolerable."

Practical help can be provided by recommending a homemaker a few days a week. In addition, *in-home* PT or OT evaluation can help devise simple solutions to vexing problems, such as reaching top shelves, making beds, cooking, and dressing. Home-care agencies welcome referrals and handle all of the logistical and insurance problems, draw up a care plan, and stay in contact with the referring physician.

In addition, there are local services provided by national associations, such as the Arthritis Foundation, American Cancer Society, and the American Society for the Blind. Sometimes we think of the services provided by these organizations as suitable only for the more severely impaired patients. It is true that the severely impaired certainly need this help, but the more modestly affected will also benefit. This highlights a dominant theme in the family physician's role in home care: Because the more minimally impaired patient is likely to have fewer medical encounters, the doctor's responsibility to this patient is arguably greater.

Skin Care

Decubitus ulcers are a major cause of morbidity and mortality in homebound, immobile patients. The incidence of decubiti in patients with spinal cord injuries ranges from 25 per cent to 85 per cent. Decubitus ulcers are caused by four basic processes:

- Pressure
- Shearing forces
- Friction
- Moisture

Although all four factors are important, pressure, especially over bony prominences, is the most critical issue. Pressure is a function of both the absolute pressure and the duration of *unrelieved* pressure. If pressure is relieved, the body can tolerate even large pressures for brief periods of time. For example, when we walk, our feet are subjected to a load several times body weight, but the pressure is relieved at regular intervals.

The reason unrelieved pressure is so important is that it requires only 17 mm Hg of pressure to obstruct local capillary flow. Compare this with an average skin pressure of 164 mm Hg on a mattress and 260 mm Hg on a hard surface. On these surfaces, irreversible skin damage can occur after only 2 hours of unrelieved pressure. In addition, poor nutrition, anemia, edema, and other conditions common in the debilitated elderly contribute to the likelihood of decubitus development.

Since the major factor in preventing pressure sores is *pressure relief*, pressure-relieving methods should be used if a patient is bedridden or immobile for long periods. Examples of such methods include alternating pressure mattresses, gel pads, and rotating the patient from side to side. Keep in mind that these principles apply to prolonged sitting as well. In particular, wheelchair sling seats—a common cause of trochanteric decubiti—should be used for only very brief periods of sitting. For prolonged sitting, an adequate chair should be used or, alternatively, an appropriate wheelchair pad.

The physician has a major role educating the family about the importance of inspecting the skin daily for the telltale sign of redness. A decubitus is pyramid shaped with the apex at the skin surface. Because the redness seen on the surface represents only a fraction of what is occurring underneath, a little redness over a bony prominence may indicate a major problem and should be approached aggressively. The family should be instructed to call at the first sign of skin reddening.

When the skin begins to break down, debridement may be indicated. If debridement is necessary, this can be accomplished painlessly with forceps and scissors at home. Even though enzymatic debriding agents are useful, a greater amount of necrotic tissue can be snipped away in a few minutes than can be dissolved away in a week. Bedside debridement is easy and has few, if any, major pitfalls.

If a dressing is necessary, two types of new dressings are worth considering. As alternatives to gauze and tape, one can use hydrocolloid-occlusive dressings or a vapor-permeable dressing. These dressings aid debridement, prevent infection, and promote tissue growth and faster healing. The total amount of patient care and cost is diminished, because the dressings are waterproof and can be left on for up to 1 week without changing (Fellin, 1984; Sebern, 1986). They are also cosmetically appealing and do not interfere with bathing.

Preventive and Anticipatory Care

While preventive and anticipatory care is such an integral part of family medicine in the office, it is usually inaccessible to home care patients. However, access to immunizations, dental care, mammography, etc. should not be based solely on ambulatory or functional status.

Patients who are unable to leave the home because of modest or major disabilities have the same incidence as other patients of most of the diseases for which screening is available and appropriate. For example, a middle-aged woman with multiple sclerosis does not have a decreased need for routine screening mammography in accordance with American Cancer Society guidelines. Being homebound does not confer protection against breast cancer. The problem is partly logistic. But it is more a matter of thinking about it. Similar principles apply to Pap smears. The nurse can easily do a Pap smear in the home with a flashlight and disposable plastic speculum.

The same is true for dental care. Although there can be logistical problems in maneuvering some home-care patients into a dental chair, these can often be solved with some planning. Many elderly patients, in fact, have nutritional difficulties because of dental problems. To some extent, these may be avoided with regular dental care and hygiene.

Anticipatory guidance is as important for the elderly as it is for the mother with a new baby. The elderly's greatest fear is the nursing home. And one of the greatest burdens for middle-aged couples is caring for their aging parents at the same time that they care for school-aged children—a problem known as the sandwich phenomenom.

Anticipating the functional needs of elderly patients is good medical care. But it also addresses their real fears and anxieties. Sometimes a simple gesture or suggestion can provide needed care, be a stimulus for additional services, and, at the same time, give the message that these aspects of their life are as important to you as their blood pressure, diabetes, or angina.

References

Bernstein, L., Griew, A., and Dete, M.: Primary Care in the Home. Philadelphia, J.B. Lippincott, 1987.

Butler, R.: The aging process. *In* Rossman, I. (Ed.): Clinical Geriatrics. 3rd ed. Philadelphia, J.B. Lippincott, 1986.

Fellin, R.: Managing decubitus ulcers. Nurs. Management, *15*:29, 1984.

Friedman, J.: Home Health Care. New York, Norton, 1986.

Granger, C.V., Albrecht, G.L., and Hamilton, B.B.: Outcomes of comprehensive medical rehabilitation; measurement by PULSES profile and the Bartel index. Arch. Phys. Med. Rehabil., *60*:145, 1979.

Kramer, A. M., Shaughnessy, P. W., and Peltigrew, M.: Cost effectiveness implications based on a comparison of nursing home and home case mix. Health Serv. Res., *20*:387, 1985.

Physician's Guide to Home Care. Chicago, American Medical Association, 1989. *Published by the AMA, this is a concise guide with clinical and economic discussions of home care.*

Portnow, J., and Houtman, M.: Home Care for the Elderly. New York, McGraw-Hill, 1987. *This book, written for patients, has a great deal of practical nuts-and-bolts clinical material for practicing physicians.*

Rossman, I.: The geriatrician and the homebound patient. J. Am. Geriatr. Soc., *36*:348, 1988. *Dr. Rossman is the physician with the greatest breadth of experience with home care in the United States.*

Sebern, M.: Pressure ulcer management in home health care: efficacy and cost effectiveness of moisture vapor permeable dressing. Arch. Phys. Med. Rehabil., *67*:726, 1986.

Steel, K.: Physician-directed long-term home health care for the elderly: a century-long experience. J. Geriatr. Soc. *35*:264, 1987.

Part III

Communication in Family Medicine

25

Establishing Rapport

Robert E. Rakel

Compassion, interest, and thoroughness are essential components of successful patient care. These features have been traditionally embodied in the term bedside manner, which also connotes qualities of concern, kindness, friendliness, wit, and cheerfulness, all of which result in an atmosphere of trust and confidence between physician and patient. The physician with the best bedside manner may actually be the one who makes no special effort to communicate these feelings but simply acts in a concerned, natural, and comfortable manner.

Since the health care relationship involves trust and a certain degree of control over another person, the provider must be skilled and effective in the requisite technical services. Charm, a warm bedside manner, or a pleasant personality, in the absence of skill, sound judgment, and knowledge, is hollow. On the other hand, competence of the highest level, in the absence of rapport, results in less than optimal clinical outcome. Patients and staff may tolerate a boorish, tactless, and insensitive physician of exceptional ability, but such relationships are usually characterized by friction, anxiety, anger, and, sooner or later, disloyalty.

Oliver Wendell Holmes said that the physician, in order to be effective, should "speak softly, be well-dressed, have quiet ways and have eyes that do not wander." A good first impression is certainly a great help in establishing rapport. The physician should approach the patient in an assured, confident (but not cocky or arrogant) manner, and present a personal appearance that is acceptable to the patient. Empathetic frankness and honesty are also important factors in instilling confidence and trust.

Personal appearance is a significant part of nonverbal communication. Patients consider house staff who wear white coats with conventional street clothes as more competent than those who wear scrub suits. Negative attitudes toward physicians are associated with casual clothing (such as blue jeans, athletic shoes, and clogs), with overly feminine items such as prominent ruffles and dangling earrings, and with temporarily fashionable items (such as long hair on men, male earrings, and patterned hose on women) (Gjerdingen et al., 1987).

A genuine smile can be helpful in quickly establishing a friendly atmosphere and developing a warm interpersonal relationship. A grin can be the physician's most effective weapon for breaking down resistance or apprehension in patients, especially children or young adults. Posture is also important in conveying an image of confidence and competence. Standing erect, moving briskly with head up and stomach in, is better than slouching. Energetic people seldom slump; they sit upright and appear alert. A listless or lethargic appearance can be interpreted as lack of concern.

Before entering the examining room or hospital room to see a patient, review the chart briefly and become familiar with the patient's name and its proper pronunciation. If the pronunciation is either unusual or difficult, place phonetic markings on the chart as a reminder for future use. Review the chart also for particular aspects of the previous visit that should be remembered and commented upon, such as the illness treated at that time, family conditions, or other personal problems. Patients will feel that the well-informed physician is truly interested in them. Additional courtesy, such as opening the door and assisting patients with their coats, especially an elderly patient, shows a consideration that aids in establishing and maintaining rapport.

Respect

The greatest deterrent to establishing patient rapport is an attitude of indifference or lack of interest by the physician. Patients should feel that their comments are being listened to, carefully considered, and taken seriously. They must feel that the physician values their comments and opinions before trusting him or her with information of a more personal nature. As long as the physician's attitude toward the patient embodies respect, concern, and kindness and a sincere effort is made to understand the patient's difficulties, the patient will overlook or forgive a myriad of other problems.

Oliver Wendell Holmes advised patients to

choose a man who is personally agreeable, for a daily visit from a intelligent, amiable, pleasant, sympathetic person will cost you no more than one from a sloven or a boor, and his presence will do more for you than any prescription the other will order.

Ideally, there will be a bond of mutual respect between physician and patient. A physician can show his respect for patients, and accept their respect for him, only insofar as respect is an integral part of his personality. There must be a concept of self-respect before one can respect others. When one is secure and satisified with one's self, one is then able to relate comfortably with warmth and feeling to another person.

It may be that it is the lack of this security rather than an excess of it that leads physicians to appear aloof and unconcerned. Too often physicians feel that a godlike image of omnipotence is necessary for the maintenance of patient respect and confidence. It is usually a lack of self-confidence that causes physicians to retreat behind this protective image, which in turn limits their ability to help. Secure physicians are more free to establish close personal relationships with patients without fearing their position will be threatened. A physician with a positive self-image is also willing to recognize and admit the limits of personal competence and feels comfortable seeking help from a colleague when such consultation is of value to the patient's care.

The bond of mutual respect is enhanced if the physician makes positive statements about other people. Patients find it difficult to respect a physician who is regularly detractive, making negative statements about other people or other physicians. Any comments that can be interpreted as "building yourself up by tearing someone else down" merely accomplish the reverse.

The effectiveness of physicians depends upon the degree of their insight into the limitations of their personalities and the psychologic defenses that distort their perceptions of patients. Physicians must recognize those situations or patients that make them unreasonably angry or provoked (for example, a whining, complaining individual who shows no interest in being rehabilitated, preferring a role of social dependency). Obviously, the physician's emotions, if they go unrecognized, can serve as a barrier to the development of mutual respect. If the physician is aware of negative feelings toward a patient, an effort can be made to avoid showing signs of irritation or anger. It has been said that clenching of the physician's fist is a clinical sign of the hysterical patient. The physician should attempt to remain objective and analyze the situation for its diagnostic value.

Patients with trivial complaints or somatic manifestations of emotional disease are sometimes given less attention than those with clear-cut organic abnormalities. The frequency with which a physician complains about the triviality and inappropriateness of patients' problems has been found to be related to the volume of patients seen and the degree to which the physician feels overburdened. The more patients that physicians see and the more overloaded their practices, the more likely they are to describe patient complaints as trivial, inappropriate, or bothersome. Physicians who either have more time or take more time per patient and investigate the patient's complaints more thoroughly frequently uncover significant factors and have less tendency to view the complaints as trivial. Respect for patients involves taking their fears and apprehensions seriously and withholding value judgments. Patients who frequently seek help for nonspecific somatic and functional complaints may be depressed (Widmer, 1980).

Communication and Rapport

Even the most knowledgeable and skilled physician will have limited effectiveness if unable to develop rapport with patients. Unfortunately, rapport is one of those intangibles that is more than the sum of its parts. Rapport is not easily analyzed within any one body of knowledge. Yet it is fair to say that the basis of rapport is the development of communication skills that instill in patients a sense of confidence and trust by conveying sincerity and an interest in their care and well-being. The patient's satisfaction and compliance with the physician's instructions (both measures of rapport, so to speak) depend upon the ability of the physician to communicate understanding, compassion, and genuine interest in the patient and to display a thorough approach to solving the patient's problems. Patient satisfaction is also related to the physician's talent for educating patients regarding the disease process and for motivating them to participate in their treatment.

The majority of complaints against physicians—and those that all too frequently lead to legal action—are simply the result of a lack of communication between doctor and patient. The potential for a serious problem always exists when a patient is inadequately informed regarding a diagnostic procedure, treatment, prognosis, or anticipated cost. The misunderstandings that result cause a great deal of unnecessary expense and grief for both parties.

Similarly, the worries that result from distorted information can severely jeopardize the doctor-patient relationship. When a patient is discussed on hospital rounds or with a colleague in the office, take care that the discussion is not within the patient's hearing distance or within that of other patients. Another patient, overhearing the conversation, may believe that the comments apply to him, or he may know the patient involved and relay the information in a distorted manner. Fragments of such conversations, overheard by the patient or others, are too easily taken out of context and can become the focus of fearful fantasies that only serve to increase uneasiness and apprehension.

Failure of communication between physician and patient can also affect the outcome of treatment, often as seriously as can an error in treatment. More complaints against physicians result from a breakdown of the caring aspect of the doctor-patient relationship than from the technical quality of treatment.

Unfortunately, there are no criteria for the establishment of rapport, as there are criteria for the diagnosis of this or that disease. Each physician must develop his or her own unique style. However, communications theory identifies most of the major elements of rapport and a brief acquaintance with relevant portions of that theory may be helpful.

First, communication suggests an exchange of information between persons over some type of channel. Establishing an open channel is the first element of the communication process and influences all that follows. In the clinical setting, the channel is the face-to-face conversation of patient and clinician in the interview or examination; the telephone is an important secondary channel.

Establishing communication means that the patient can gain access to the clinician—on the phone or by an early appointment—without having to run an obstacle course created by an overly protective staff. Delay in returning a phone call may result in a patient remaining home all day waiting; if the call is not returned at all, the negative effect on rapport is great.

Unwillingness to make communication convenient for the patient usually results in a spiral of increasingly frequent attempts to reach the physician and mounting frustration for everyone. On the other hand, physicians who give a high priority to communicating discover that most patients are considerate and even protective of the physician's time. At the beginning of a practice, a certain amount of testing is done by patients to determine how accessible a physician is; those who pass the test find that they are rarely inconvenienced by unnecessary calls or visits.

In any face-to-face encounter, communication is both intended and unintended, and the distinction is important. *Intended* messages are verbal statements that transmit fact and nonverbal messages that the sender hopes will elicit predictable responses from the receiver. One patient, for example, may enact by a sophisticated blend of verbal and nonverbal communications the role of "strong, brave, unafraid, and willing to face reality." Another patient (or, indeed, the same patient in another setting) may communicate verbally and nonverbally a message of "weak, helpless, needing support and sympathy." Such a performance is not the result of a well thought out, conscious decision; it results mostly from learned processes that are unconscious but accessible to scientific analysis.

Unintended communication refers to messages that are given off by individuals beyond their awareness. Subtle clues are, however, perceptible to the astute observer. The patient who wishes to create an impression of bravery, for example, may contradict the intended message by a slight hand tremor, a barely noticeable weakness of the voice, or beads of perspiration on the forehead. In clinical practice, the recognition of the patient's true thoughts and feelings is a central skill in establishing and maintaining rapport.

VERBAL COMMUNICATION

Much of the communication process in the clinical interview centers on verbal interchange. Symptoms, past medical history, family medical history, and psychosocial data are transmitted primarily by verbal means (see Chapter 28, Interviewing Techniques). Some aspects of verbal communication play an important role in establishing and maintaining rapport. Slips of the tongue or major areas of omission (for example, a married person who never mentions a spouse) may signify problem areas that, when explored, help establish the interviewer as a perceptive person who understands what lies beneath the surface. The interviewer must constantly consider: Why is the patient telling me that? Even simple, casual remarks may be the patient's way of sending up a trial balloon about issues of great concern—for example, the patient who says, "Oh, by the way, a friend of mine has been having some chest pain when he walks a lot—do you think that sounds serious?" may be actually talking about a concern of his own that he is unable to face directly. Or, a child may be brought to the office with a trivial problem in order that the mother might have a chance to discuss with the physician something that is troubling her; the child is a calling card, signaling the need to open the communication channel. The physician who is sensitive to these subtle clues and encourages the patient to discuss what is actually troublesome will find that the rapport thus established allows future interviews to be much more open and direct.

Physicians in practice who have established rapport during an ongoing relationship with patients communicate more easily than do physicians seeing a patient for the first time in an emergency department. Studies by Korsch and Negrete (1972) showed that doctors in an emergency room did more talking than the patients although their perception was just the opposite. This was attributed to interaction with unfamiliar patients by house staff in a setting in which the stress level is high and the orientation therapeutic. Yet Arntson and Philipsborn (1982) found that physicians in private practice for 26 years, who knew the patients and saw them in a low stress situation for diagnosis or health maintenance, also talked more than the patients (twice as long). One difference in the two settings, however, was that in the private office there was a strong reciprocal affective relationship between doctor and patient. If either made an affective statement, the other would respond similarly; whereas in the emergency room, mothers expressed twice as many affective statements as did the physicians.

Vocabulary

The use of appropriate vocabulary assists in establishing rapport by ensuring easy and accurate communication. Phrasing questions in simple language appropriate to the patient's level of understanding and avoidance of medical jargon help establish a sense of working together. The patient's cultural background and educational level should be considered, and the physician should avoid using slang (or a contrived accent), since the patient will detect the artificiality and consider this patronizing. However, a language style can easily be assumed that is different from the physician's normal speech yet natural and comfortable for both physician and patient.

Medical terminology should be avoided unless it is familiar to the patient. More than once a lumbar puncture has been interpreted by the patient to mean an operation to drain the lungs. No longer does the physician gain a therapeutic advantage by writing prescriptions in Latin or impressing the patient with medical words. Today's patients prefer to be enlightened and demand maximum insight into their care. It is best to start all explanations at a basic level and proceed only as rapidly as patient understanding permits.

Physicians should also be sure of what patients mean to convey by their word selection and make certain that they are operating at a common level of understanding. When the patient says he "drinks a little," inquire further to find out what is meant by a little; or if he "spits up blood," determine whether he is truly spitting or vomiting. A major barrier to accurate interpersonal communication is the tendency of people to react to a statement from their own points of view, rather than attempting to interpret it from the speaker's vantage point. If a question exists regarding the clarity of the interpretation, it is best to repeat it to the speaker's satisfaction. Contract negotiators have found that when parties in a dispute realize that they are being understood and each party sees how the situation appears to the other, there is less need to exaggerate and act defensively.

Korsch and Negrete (1972) found that some of the longest interviews between physician and patient were due to failures in communication; the doctor and patient had to spend considerable time trying to get on the same wavelength. An analysis of the conversations revealed that less than 5 per cent of the physician's conversation was personal or friendly in nature and that although most of the physicians believed that they had been friendly, fewer than half of the patients had this impression. The following partial transcript of an interview from Korsch and Negrete (1972) is a vivid illustration of failure to communicate because of inappropriate vocabulary and lack of attention to patient understanding.

Father: How does his heart sound?

Doctor: Sounds pretty good. He's got a little murmur there. I'm not sure what it is. It's . . . it uh . . . could just be a little hole in his heart.

Mother: Is that very dangerous when you have a hole in your heart?

Doctor: No, because I think it's the upper chamber, and if it's the upper chamber then it means nothing.

Mother: Oh.

Doctor: Otherwise they just grow up and they repair them.

Mother: What would cause the hole in his heart?

Doctor: H'm?

Mother: What was it that caused the hole in his heart?

Doctor: It's 'cause . . . uh . . . just developmental, when their uh . . .

Mother: M-h'm.

Doctor: There's a little membrane that comes down, and if it's the upper chamber, there's a membrane that comes down, one from each direction. And sometimes they don't quite meet, and so there's either a hole at the top or a hole at the bottom and then . . . it's really . . . uh . . . almost never causes any trouble.

Mother: Oh.

Doctor: It's uh . . . one thing that they never get SBE from . . . it's the only heart lesion in which they don't.

Mother: Uh-huh.

Doctor: And uh . . . they grow up to be normal.

Mother: Oh, good.

Doctor: And uh . . . if anything happens they can always catheterize them and make sure that's what it is, or do heart surgery.

Mother: Yeah.

Doctor: Really no problem with it. They almost never get into trouble so . . .

Mother: Do you think he might have developed the murmur being that my husband and I both have a murmur?

Doctor: No.

Mother: No. Oh, it's not hereditary, then?

Doctor: No.

Mother: Oh, I see. (Someone whistling in the room)

Doctor: It is true that certain people . . . tendency to rheumatic fever, for instance.

Mother: H'mm.

Doctor: There is a tendency for the abnormal antigen-antibody reaction to be inherited, and therefore they can sometimes be more susceptible.

Mother: Oh, I see. That wouldn't mean anything if uh . . . I would . . . I'm Rh negative and he's positive. It wouldn't mean anything in that line, would it?

Doctor: Uh-huh.

Mother: No? Okay.

Doctor: No. The only thing you have to worry about is other babies.

Mother: M'h'm.

Doctor: Watch your Coombs' and things.

Mother: Watch my what?

Doctor: Watch your Coombs' and things.

Mother: Oh, yeah.

Doctor: Your titres, Coombs' titres.

NONVERBAL COMMUNICATION

Verbal communication occupies so much of daily social interaction that nonverbal communication is often ignored. However, much that is said is unspoken. Communication specialists have convincingly demonstrated the major importance nonverbal messages have in validating or contradicting verbal messages, and their enormous influence as communication symbols in their own right.

Communication between two people is usually one-third nonverbal. What is said verbally is often emphasized nonverbally, and personal attitudes and emotions are usually communicated at the nonverbal level. Since nonverbal communicative signals are under less censorship from conscious control than are verbal messages, they are likely to be more genuine.

Charles Darwin held that there is a unique pattern of nonverbal actions for each emotion. In *Expressions of the Emotions in Man and Animals* (1872), Darwin suggested that emotional expressions are evolutionary remnants of previous adaptive behavior that persist even though currently useless. Snarling as a sign of aggression is one example. While more recent knowledge indicates that emotional expression is learned as well as genetically mediated, Darwin's idea of a unique pattern of actions has been shown for depression and anxiety and is likely in the future to be demonstrated for other emotional states as well.

The elements of nonverbal communication have been classified in the following categories (Knapp, 1978): *Body language* or *kinesics* (including gestures and facial expressions), *physical characteristics* (such as age, skin coloration, evidence of health), *touching, paralanguage* (tone of voice, rate of speech, and so on), *proxemics* (spatial factors), *artifacts* (clothing and accessories), and *environmental factors* (furniture, decor, and so on). All of these aspects of nonverbal communication have relevance for the physician-patient encounter.

Paralanguage

Paralanguage is the voice effect that accompanies or modifies talking and often communicates meaning. It includes velocity of speech (fast, slow, hesitant), tone and volume of voice, sighs and grunts, pauses, and inflections. Urgency, sincerity, confidence, hesitation, thoughtfulness, gaity, sadness, and apprehension are all conveyed by qualities of voice. McCaskey (1979) feels that the literal interpretation (definition) of words accounts for only 10 per cent of communication between two people, while facial expression and tone of voice account for up to 90 per cent of the communication.

Certainly there is a real difference between verbal and vocal information. The verbal message refers to the words literally transmitted. The vocal message includes the emotional quality, the tone of voice, and the frequency and length of pauses—information that is lost when the words are written. Tone of voice, for example, can actually reverse the meaning of words. Comparative studies have shown that when the vocal and verbal messages transmit contradictory information, the vocal is more accurate. Sarcasm is a common example of a contradiction between vocal and verbal messages.

Physicians should be alert to subtle changes of tone, such as when patients ask whether everything will be all right. Are they asking for reassurance, showing fear, or doubting the diagnosis? Rather than concentrate exclusively on *what* patients are saying, the astute physician will concentrate on *how* they are saying it.

Touch

A close personal interest in the patient can be communicated by the appropriate use of touch. The most socially acceptable method in this country is a handshake, enabling the physician to establish early contact with the patient. The handshake, properly used, can convey to the patient sincerity and interest as well as security and poise. It is an inoffensive intrusion into the other person's area of privacy and can be extended under certain circumstances to include the application of the left hand to the upper or lower arm. This technique is often used by politicians to emphasize sincerity and concern.

The handshake as a traditional greeting of friendship began by the raising of exposed hands by two approaching individuals to give evidence that they held no weapons. This proceeded to the grasping of hands, or in the Roman society, the forearms. In the United States, a firm handshake is most acceptable. Usually, the limp or "wet dishrag" handshake indicates lack of interest or insincerity, especially if it is rapidly withdrawn. A moist palm is a sign of nervousness or apprehension, and the "halfwaythere," fingers-only handshake indicates reluctance or indecision. But the handshake continues to be culturally modified, and one should be extremely wary of misinterpreting another person's handshake without understanding his or her cultural background.

In China, the Confucian code of etiquette dictated that there should never be a touching of persons, and even today Chinese officials may appear reluctant to grasp an extended hand (a Chinese formerly shook his own hand) (Butterfield, 1982). Some young people in the United States have modified the traditional palm-to-palm handshake to a grasping of the thumb and thenar eminence and continue to develop new variations reminiscent of the secret handshakes of fraternal groups.

Touching can be an effective method for communicating concern or compassion and can break down some of the defensive barriers to communication. Caution should be exercised, however, not to use it excessively or earlier than is socially permissible. If used without adequate preparation, touch can be interpreted as an invasion of privacy and a forward and inconsiderate act. Touch by a physician can be viewed as aggressive behavior if it is used before rapport is established. During the physical examination, it is best to talk before touching by explaining to the patient what will be done next. Studies of primates have shown that touching gestures are usually considered nonaggressive and calming in nature. When used properly by the physician, touch can be facilitative and welcome.

The tremendous symbolic value of touch as a healing power was demonstrated during the Middle Ages when people sought relief from scrofula (tuberculous lymphadenitis) through the King's touch, or royal touch, in spite of the notoriously low cure rates. This power has been transferred to physicians, and patients often feel better after a routine physical examination. Friedman (1979) states that 85 per cent of patients leaving a physician's office feel better even if they have not received medication or treatment, and 50 per cent of patients in the waiting room feel better in anticipation of the help they will receive.

Touch, or laying on of the hands, may indeed promote healing, especially if it is imbued by the patient with a special symbolic value. Franz Mesmer (1734–1815) was among the first to emphasize the medical importance of "laying on of the hands." Mesmer, however, believed that there was a magnetic power in his hands, which he called animal magnetism and which he applied to ailing individuals. His theory was unscientific, and although he became famous for successfully treating a number of hysterical patients, he was finally discredited by a committee that included Benjamin Franklin and Antoine Lavoisier. They found his treatments to be without magnetism and essentially useless. They did agree, however, that he had helped many people and had brought about many cures. They attributed these cures to as yet unknown factors rather than to the animal magnetism he claimed. Incidentally, mesmerism was the forerunner of hypnosis (initially called artificial somnambulism), which was developed by Puysegur, a disciple of Mesmer.

The magic of touch can be good medicine, especially when combined with concern, support, and reassurance. Stroking, a special kind of touching, describes a physical or symbolic recognition of a person's finer attributes. A stroke may be a kind word, a warm gesture, or a simple touch of the hand. Infants deprived of touch and stroking suffer mental and physical deterioration. Adults also require stroking to maintain a healthy emotional state. Stroking occurs whenever an interchange between two people leaves one or both with a good, or fulfilled, feeling.

Kinesics (Body Language)

The astute physician will cultivate observational skills that enable the detection of hidden or subtle clues to diagnosis contained in the patient's nonverbal behavior. Kinesics is the study of nonverbal gestures, or body movements, and their meaning as a form of communication. It is essential to remember, however, that specific gestures and their interpretation are of importance only when judged in the context of the circumstances surrounding them. Body language alone does not reveal the entire behavioral image any more than does verbal language alone. Just as one word does not make a sentence or even have much meaning without the sentence, a single gesture has clinical relevance only as part of a sequence of actions. Although individual signs have significance, they are not reliable when they stand alone; they are meaningful only when considered in the context of a person's total behavioral pattern.

When there is congruence between the verbal and nonverbal message—that is, when the gesture conveys the same message as the spoken word—communication and its meaning are almost sure to be in agreement. When one indicates something different from the other, however, the nonverbal message will usually be the more accurate.

Attempts by the patient to mask feelings can be readily detected by observing body behavior. True feelings are more likely to leak through conscious efforts to conceal one's feelings. Likewise, a physician's attempt at deception will be detected by patients and can destroy confidence and damage rapport. Positive verbal communication such as "You're looking better today" when accompanied by negative nonverbal cues will be interpreted by the patient as insincere. For example, a patient who is not told the true nature of a terminal illness usually knows it anyway and may distrust family, friends, and physician if they persist in the charade.

Reassuring a patient that "nothing is wrong," rather than putting the patient at ease because the physician found nothing abnormal, may instead be interpreted as "the doctor is unable to make me better." Premature reassurance may be interpreted as rejection. If reassurance is used, it must be genuine and realistic and given only after a thorough evaluation of the problem (Lau, 1989).

Alan Alda (1979) in a medical school commencement address, challenged new physicians to be able to read a patient's involuntary muscles as well as their x-ray studies. He said, "Can you see the fear and uncertainty in my face? If I tell you where it hurts, can you hear in my voice where I ache? I show you my body, but I bring you my person. Will you tell me what you are doing and in words I can understand? Will you tell me when you don't know what to do?" The physician will see the fear and uncertainty in the patient's face only if he is looking at the patient rather than the medical record. Alda's statement reflects the concern and compassion that patients desire. By using appropriate body language, the physician can convey this attention and concern in the most effective manner possible.

Body Position. The body position when sitting can show varying degrees of tension or relaxation. The tense person sits erect with a fairly rigid posture. One who is moderately relaxed has a forward lean of approximately 20 degrees and a side lean of up to 10 degrees. A very relaxed position (usually too relaxed for physicians interacting with patients) is a backward lean (recline) of 20 degrees and a sideways lean of over 10 degrees.

Higher patient satisfaction is associated with forward body lean and rotation of the torso toward the patient. Larsen and Smith (1981) found that "the patient also responds more favorably to the physician who relaxes his chin in his hands and gazes directly at the patient, rather than a physician who elevates his chin (unsupported) as if to imply a more superior status." Physicians whose communication styles have been considered patient oriented have been noted to change body position more frequently than physicians whose conversations were physician centered.

An attempt should be made, whenever possible, to sit rather than stand when interviewing a patient. Rapport is improved if the physician does not intimidate patients by placing them in a submissive position. Patients feel more comfortable, and less helpless, speaking in a sitting position rather than prone. Sitting on the patient's bed has been frowned upon, but for some patients it is an effective means of establishing closeness and conveying warmth in a relaxed yet attentive manner.

Mirroring. When good rapport exists between two people, each will mirror the other's movements. Some people consciously try to establish rapport with another by mirroring that person's body posture (Fig. 25–1). Disruptions in this mirroring may signal that one member disagrees with what the other has said or feels betrayed or insulted but cannot express this verbally. If the physician notices this sudden disruption of mirroring activity by the patient, more attention should be focused on the comment that led to the change of position. Renegotiation or further explanation may be indicated.

Head Position. Typically, the head is held forward in anger and back in defiance, anxiety, or fear. It is down or bowed in sadness, submissiveness, shame, or guilt. The head tilted to one side indicates interest and attention (Fig. 25–2); and when circumstances are appropriate, it can be a flirtation. The head erect indicates self-confidence and maturity.

When listening to a patient, the physician should show interest and concern by an attentive position—best illustrated by sitting forward in the chair with an interested, attentive facial expression and the head slightly tilted. Darwin was one of the first to note that animals assume a head tilt when listening intently.

Face. Darwin (1872) proposed that cultures throughout the world express similar emotions or states of mind with remarkably uniform body movements. His information was gathered from missionary friends working with aborigines, persons under hypnosis, infants, and the insane. He also studied the

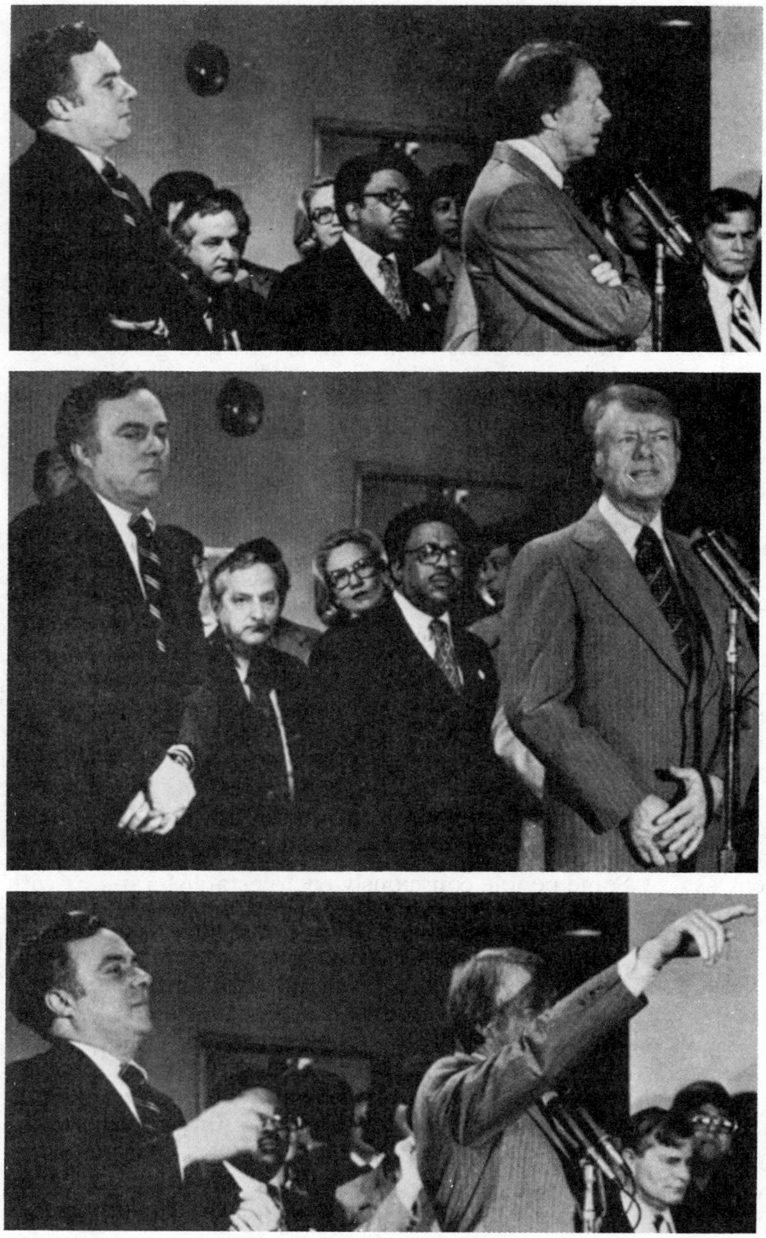

Figure 25–1. Joseph Califano *(left)*, Secretary of Health, Education and Welfare, mirrors his boss, President Jimmy Carter, through his posture and gestures. (From Key, M. R. (Ed.): The Relationship of Verbal and Nonverbal Communication. New York, Mouton Publishers, 1980.)

blind and deaf, who, without benefit of learning from others, were noted to raise eyebrows when surprised and shrug their shoulders to indicate helplessness.

Darwin held that the facial expression of emotion when undisguised is independent of culture and is identical throughout the world. Thus, the facial expressions of joy, sadness, and anger are the same in the Australian aborigine, the American farmer, and the Norwegian fisherman. Various cultures, however, do disguise the facial expression in different ways. In the American culture, the mouth is most commonly used to disguise feelings. A person in a social gathering may be smiling, although inwardly sad or angry. The eyebrows, eyes, and forehead are least affected by these cultural disguises and are the most consistently dependable indicators of emotion. As Shakespeare wrote, "I saw his heart in his face" (The Winter's Tale, Act I, Scene II).

Ekman and Friesen (1975) found that the facial expressions of fear, disgust, happiness, and anger were the same in countries with widely disparate language and culture. They also found that these expressions involve both sides of the face, but contempt involves only one side, such as tightening one corner of the mouth. Videotapes of college students in the United States and Japan, taken without their knowledge while they were watching a stress-inducing film, showed identical facial expressions of disgust. When they discussed the film with other people, however, the Japanese masked their facial expres-

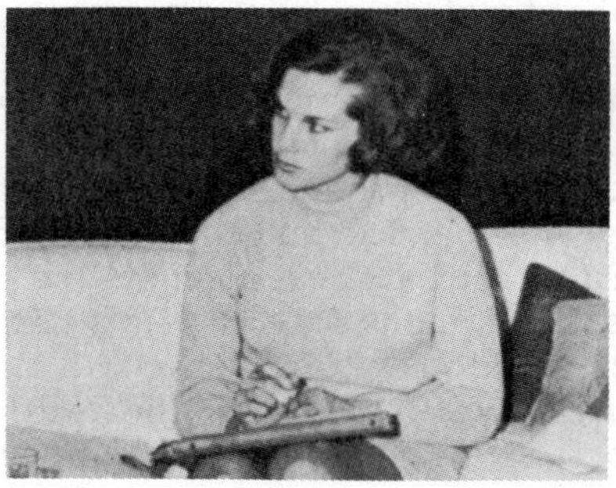

Figure 25–2. This woman signals attentiveness and seriousness by holding very still, cocking her head, and looking intently at the speaker. (From Scheflen, A. E.: Body Language and the Social Order—Communication as Behavioral Control. Englewood Cliffs, NJ, Prentice-Hall, Inc., 1972.)

sions of unpleasant feelings much more than did the Americans.

Ekman and Friesen used composite facial photographs to show how each part of the face contributes to the expressions of emotion, especially surprise, fear, disgust, anger, happiness, and sadness (see Fig. 25–3).

In our culture when someone wishes to disguise their true feelings and convey an impression that is more socially acceptable, they do so by smiling. This may be especially true in patients who are sad or depressed. Figure 25–4 is a composite showing sadness in the eyes, brow, and forehead being masked by a smile.

Formerly, infants were thought to be unable to imitate facial gestures until 8 months of age. Meltzoff (1977) showed that infants 2 to 3 weeks old were able to do this (Fig. 25–5).

Micro-expressions. Ekman and Friesen also described micro-expressions, a valuable indication of masking or deception. "Micro-expressions are caused by the face's all too rapid efficiency in registering inner feelings" (Morris, 1977). Most facial expressions last more than 1 second, but micro-expressions last only one fifth to one twenty-fifth of a second. This is approximately the time it takes to blink an eye and can easily be missed if the physician is not carefully observing the patient. Micro-expressions occur when the patient begins to show a true facial expression, senses this, and immediately neutralizes or masks the expression. Some micro-expressions are complete enough to show the true emotion felt, but many times they are squelched to such extent that the physician has only a clue that patients are managing their facial expressions.

Eyes. The eyes are probably the principal organs of expression. They are so important to a person's appearance that when anonymity is desired, only the eyes need to be covered. The eyebrows have been shown to have 40 different positions of expression and the eyelids 23. Consider the magnitude of possible combinations when all facial elements are involved as indicators of expression. The message conveyed by each position can be further modified by the length of a glance and its intensity.

The eyes can give more information for some emotions than others. Knapp (1978) found that the eyes were better than the brow, forehead, or lower face for the accurate portrayal of fear but were less accurate for anger and disgust. Even the lower eyelid alone can convey considerable information. In Figure 25–6, it is apparent that B depicts more sadness than A, but the pictures differ only in one respect—the lower eyelid.

It has long been known that *pupils* dilate when the person sees something pleasant and contract when he sees something unpleasant. This involuntary signal

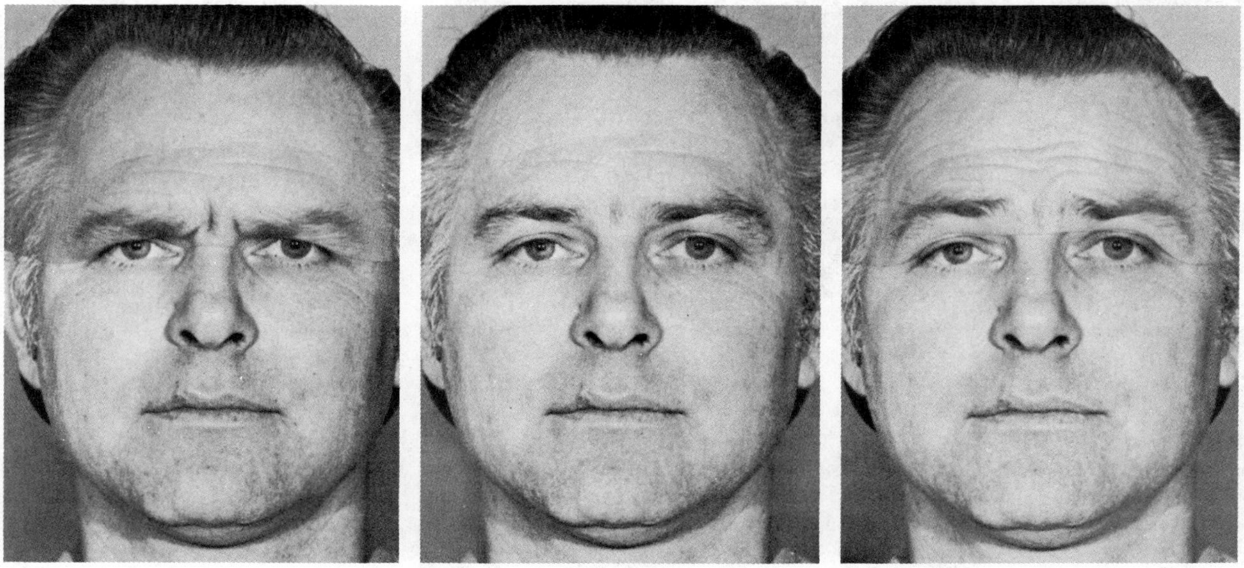

A B C

Figure 25–3. This man shows the anger brow with the rest of the face uninvolved *(A)*; a neutral face *(B)*; and, for comparison, the fear brow with the rest of the face uninvolved *(C)*. (From Ekman, P., and Friesen, W. V.: Unmasking the Face: A Guide to Recognizing Emotions from Facial Clues. Englewood Cliffs, NJ, Prentice-Hall, Inc., 1975.)

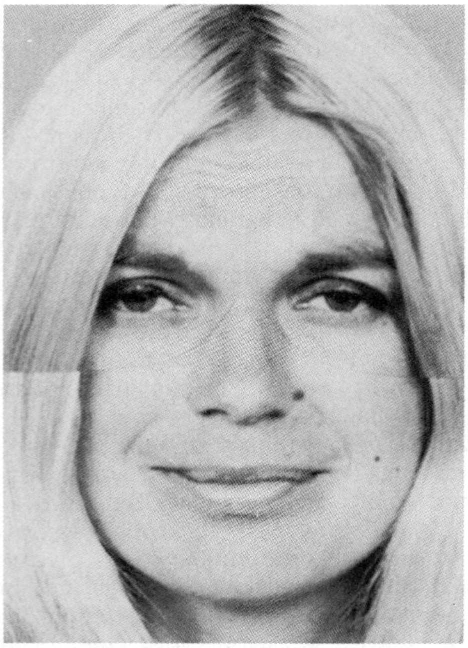

Figure 25–4. Masking of sadness by smiling (see eyes and forehead). (From Ekman, P., and Friesen, W. V.: Unmasking the Face: A Guide to Recognizing Emotions from Facial Clues. Englewood Cliffs, NJ, Prentice-Hall, Inc., 1975.)

can be a valuable indication of what is really going on. Oriental jade dealers wore dark glasses so that no one could see their pupils dilate when they discovered an especially valuable piece of jade. Likewise, a magician doing card tricks can tell when a preselected card is seen by a subject because of the sudden pupil enlargement. In one experiment (Hess, 1975), the pupils of males dilated when the men were shown photographs of nude females and constricted for nude males. Homosexuals demonstrated the opposite. Baby pictures produced pupil dilation in both single and married women and in married men with children. The pictures produced pupil constriction in single men and married but childless men. Dilated pupils can also indicate that listeners are interested, while constricted pupils suggest that they do not like what is being said (as well as viewed).

Sincerity is expressed with the eyes. The best method for conveying sincerity is frequent eye contact, a technique most appropriately used when listening to the other person. One trait of good listeners is that they constantly look at the speaker. A listener who does not maintain eye contact, but continues to look down or away from the speaker, may be shy, depressed, or indicating rejection of either the speaker or the comments being made. One patient recently said, "I had one student doctor who looked at his toes instead of me. If he ever opens a practice, I don't believe I would trust him." On the other hand, speakers may frequently break eye contact when talking and are permitted a distant stare when formulating ideas and selecting phrases. But they should still try to make frequent, though less prolonged and intense, eye contact.

A special kind of human-to-human awareness is conveyed by eye contact. Prolonged eye contact, or staring, can be offensive. Monkeys can be provoked to combat by a person staring at them because of the threat of aggression that this represents. Under other circumstances, however, staring can be flirtatious, emphasizing that the meaning of eye behavior depends upon other factors in the situation.

The acceptability of eye contact varies significantly among different cultures. In the United States,

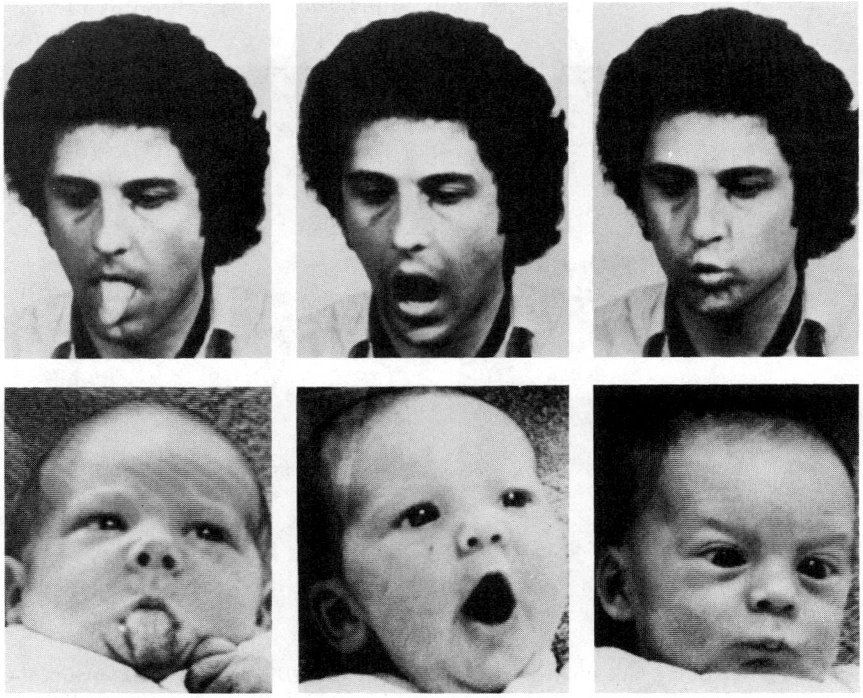

Figure 25–5. Psychologist Andrew Meltzoff *(top row)* makes a series of faces at infants, whose responses are shown in the bottom row. (From Meltzoff A. N., and Moore, M. K.: Imitation of facial and manual gestures by human neonates. Science, *198*:75–78, 1977).

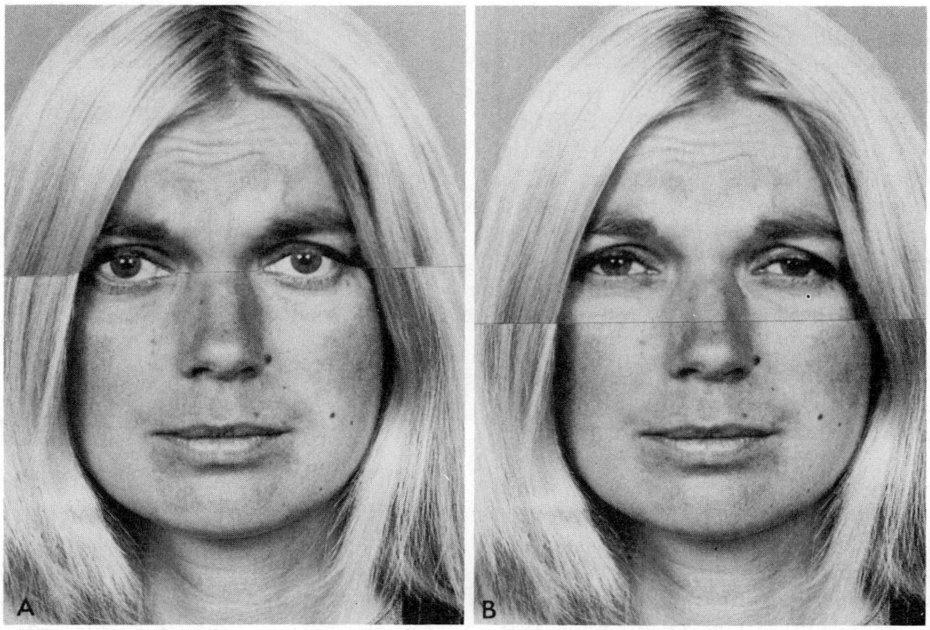

Figure 25–6. Sadness shown in the eyes and forehead (the mouth is neutral). The importance of the eyelids can be seen since *B* is obviously sadder than *A* but differs only in that a sad lower eyelid has been substituted for a neutral lower eyelid. (From Ekman, P., and Friesen, W. V.: Unmasking the Face: A Guide to Recognizing Emotions from Facial Clues. Englewood Cliffs, NJ, Prentice-Hall, Inc., 1975.)

focusing one's eyes on the speaker indicates respect and attention regardless of the age of the individuals involved. However, Mexican-Americans and blacks tend not to maintain as much eye contact while listening as do other Americans and may look away from the speaker more often. This is not a sign of disrespect or inattention. In Latin American countries, a younger person may be thought disrespectful if his eyes meet those of the adult who is speaking. A physician could be considered seductive in that culture if he maintained steady eye contact while talking to a patient. In the United States, it is impolite to maintain eye contact with a stranger for more than 3 seconds, but Europeans feel that longer periods of eye contact are perfectly normal. Obviously, then, the physician needs to consider the patient's cultural background when interpreting the meaning of eye contact behavior. Looking away from the speaker from time to time may be a sign of respect and sensitivity rather than the opposite. At the same time, the physician's failure to look a patient in the eye can be dehumanizing and cause the patient to feel more like an object than a person. Patients are most comfortable when the physician looks at them approximately 50 per cent of the time and are uncomfortable when eye contact is avoided. The physician may want to sit at the same level as the patient but just to the side, so the patient can comfortably look away while talking.

The frequency of eye contact can also provide clues to whether the patient is anxious or depressed. Waxer (1977) demonstrated that both the presence of anxiety and its intensity could be determined on the basis of nonverbal cues alone. Prominent cues involved the hands, mouth, and torso. Anxious patients generated more stroking of themselves, such as hand on hand or hand on face, and had more twitches and tremors. They smiled less, and their torsos were stiff and rigid as though they were afraid to move. They also had a more rapid respiratory rate. The eyes of anxious patients blinked frequently or darted back and forth. They looked at the interviewer as frequently as low-anxiety patients but maintained eye contact for less time on each gaze. (Similarly, the patient may interpret the physician's lack of eye contact as indicative of anxiety or discomfort, even rejection.)

Depressed patients also maintain eye contact only one fourth of the time of nondepressed patients. Downward contraction of the mouth and a downward angling of the head are also cues to depression. As with the anxious patient, there is no difference in frequency of eye contact in the depressed patient; the difference is only in the duration of contact.

Patients with abdominal pain that is due to organic disease are more likely to keep their eyes open during palpation of the abdomen than those with nonspecific pain (Gray et al., 1988). This may be because the patient with genuine abdominal tenderness apprehensively watches the doctor's hand as it approaches the tender area.

Hands. The hands will be droopy and flaccid with sadness, fidgety or grasping in anxiety, and—when responding to anger—will form clenched fists, often moving in a pounding fashion with the index finger extended. When a speaker joins his hands, with fingers extended and fingertips touching, it is called steepling and indicates confidence and assurance in the comments being made (Fig. 25–7).

Palms are usually held in the palm-in position. Turning the palms outward can be a subtle courting behavior (usually used by women) but more likely indicates a warm and friendly greeting (Davis, 1975).

The hands of an anxious patient can be noted to shake when holding a pen or cigarette, to twitch, or to be braced unnaturally. The white knuckle pose of tightly locked fingers can be an effort to mask the jitters. Patients with clenched fists, tight masseters, and frowns may be depressed, especially if they show evidence of turning anger upon themselves by scratching the back of their hands.

Hands can also be a subtle indicator of the urge to interrupt. Be alert for this sign in a patient so that important information will not be suppressed, and the patient can be given every opportunity to supply valuable information. Indications of this urge to interrupt are a slight raising of the hand or perhaps the index finger only, pulling at the ear lobe, or raising the index finger to the lips. The latter may also indicate an attempt to suppress a comment and should alert the physician to inquire further and elicit the hidden information. A patient listening in "The Thinker" position, with the index finger across the lips or extended along the cheek, or one sitting with elbows on the table and hands clenched in front of the mouth, although listening intently, may not be buying what the physician is saying (Fig. 25–8). Take additional time to amplify the issue or explain the diagnosis or treatment regimen further.

Arms. Although folded arms are found in all cultures, this is considered a discovered action rather than an inborn trait, since it is a natural position of comfort that is as easily discovered by the African tribesman as the New York banker. It is the subtle ways in which the arms are held that can give clues to underlying emotions. Crossed arms can be a defensive posture, indicating disagreement with another's view, or it can be a sign of insecurity. It can also be nothing more than a position of comfort and

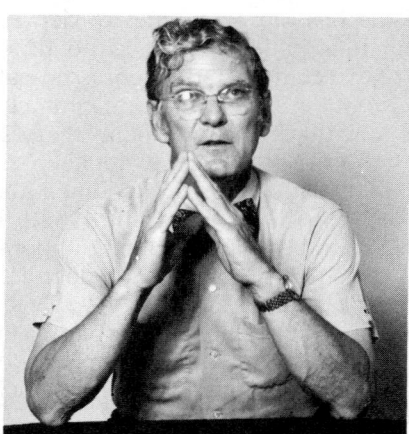

Figure 25–7. Steepling.

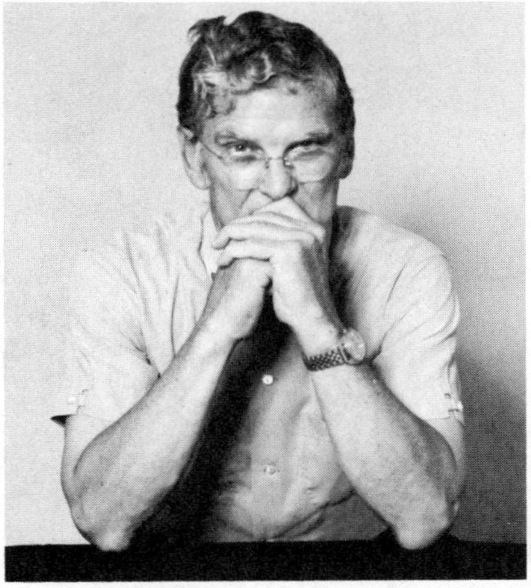

Figure 25–8. The defensive or "doubting Thomas" position.

should, as with all other signs, be considered in the context of the individual's total behavior.

Note the manner in which the arms are crossed. Are they relaxed in the normal position of comfort, or are they in a hugging posture, reflecting insecurity or sadness and indicating a need for reassurance? Anger can be seen in clenched fists that are held tightly against the body in a holding back manner, preventing them from hitting (Fig. 25–9). If the patient has assumed a position of resistance or defensiveness, sitting with arms and legs crossed and perhaps with body turned away, search for the reason for this defensiveness and try to eliminate it. Perhaps a recommendation that the patient stop smoking is threatening and difficult to accept. In that case, it is important to make an additional effort to explain the

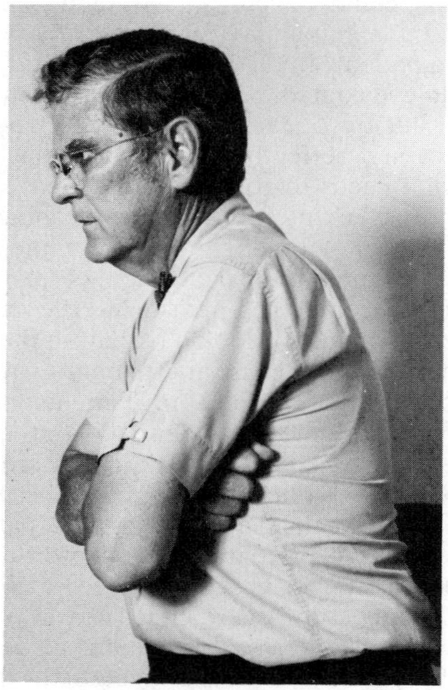

Figure 25–9. The resistant position, suggesting suppressed anger.

rationale for the recommendation; do not hurry over it with a brief comment or admonition.

Legs. Although crossing the legs is a common position of comfort, it can also indicate a shutting out of, or protection against, the outside world. If crossed legs in a patient confirm the total kinesic picture of resistance, including crossed arms and other signals discussed earlier, make every effort to identify the reason for the resistance and correct it before proceeding further (Fig. 25–10). Diagnostic information obtained from a resistant patient is likely to be incomplete, and instructions are unlikely to be followed.

Note also the position of the feet and their movement. Just as anxiety is associated with fidgety hand movements, so it is with the fidgety, constantly moving foot. An anxious or scared person may sit forward in the chair with feet placed in the ready-to-run position, one foot in front of the other. The angry person is more likely to place the feet widely apart in a position of stability, while the feet of a sad person tend to move in a slow, circular pattern.

Preening Gestures. Preening gestures, such as the male pulling up socks, adjusting tie, or combing hair, and female adjusting clothing or using a mirror to review makeup may not necessarily be seductive in nature but can be an attempt to establish rapport and good interpersonal relations. If the preening is intended to be flirtatious, however, the woman may cross her legs, place a hand on the hip, caress her leg, or stroke the arm or thigh in some fashion. The flirtatious male will usually utilize gaze holding and head tilt to accentuate normal preening gestures. The physician should remain alert to the accentuation of normal preening gestures into courtship actions in order to identify the seductive patient and deal with the issue early, before unknowingly encouraging the patient to proceed further along this course.

Respiratory Avoidance Response. The respiratory avoidance response involves a frequent clearing of the throat when no phlegm or mucus is present. All animals exhibit a respiratory avoidance response as a means of clearing something unpleasant or undesirable from the respiratory tract. This action can also be a nonverbal indication of disgust or rejection. When physicians find themselves doing this, they should observe the accompanying circumstances and note whether posterior pharyngeal mucus is truly present.

Another component of the respiratory avoidance syndrome is the nose rub (Fig. 25–11). This involves a light or subtle rub of the nose with the index finger and signals rejection of a statement being made either by the subject or by another individual. The nose rub to relieve an itch is usually vigorous and involves a repeated series of rubs, whereas that of the respiratory avoidance response is soft and consists of one or two light strokes, often involving nothing more than a light flick of the nose.

Morris (1977) describes the nose flick as "a reflection of the fact that a split is being forced between inner thoughts and outward action." It can

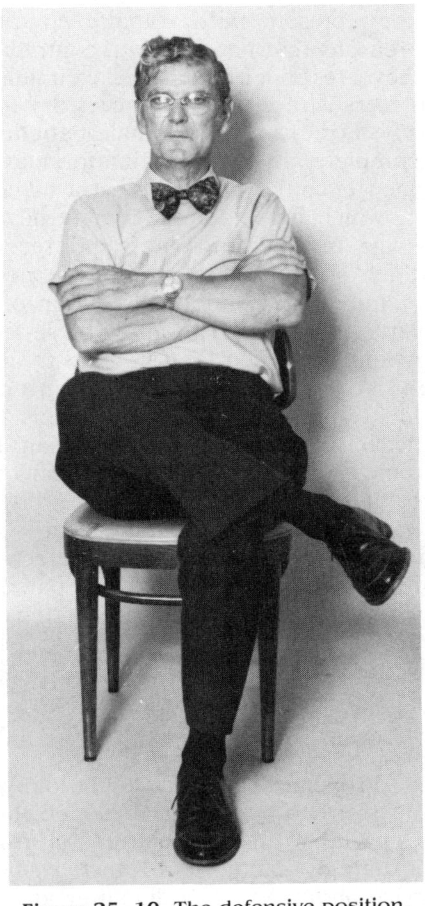

Figure 25–10. The defensive position.

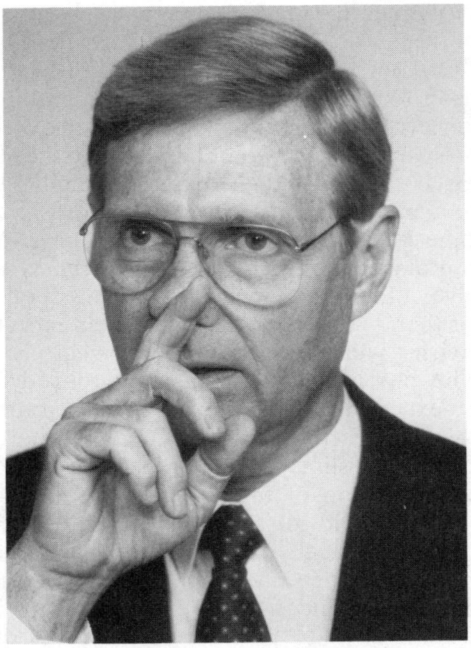

Figure 25–11. The nose rub, a variation of the respiratory avoidance response.

be associated with lying or with the struggle to appear calm while suppressing anger or discomfort.

This sign can be quite useful in patient interviewing. For example, the physician may ask a patient, "How are things at home?" He may answer, "Fine," then clear his throat and lightly rub his nose with the index finger. He is actually saying, "I don't like what you are asking me," or "I feel uncomfortable with my answer; things really aren't going very well at home." If there is a cause to pursue the issue further, a simple comment such as "Really?" or "You mean not even an occasional argument?" may lead to a flood of information masked by the previous response.

Another example that what a patient is saying may be in conflict with what is being felt is a "verbal-nonverbal mismatch," for example, when the patient answers "fine" to "how are things between you and your husband" while looking sad and avoiding eye contact (Quill, 1989).

Other clues that the patient may not be telling the truth or that there are repressed feelings are asymmetrical facial expressions and a prolonged smile or expression of amazement. Almost all authentic facial expressions fade after 4 or 5 seconds (Ekman, 1985).

Hidden (or Masked) Communication

Although the average person has a symptom about every 6 days, he visits a physician only once every 4 months. Some people will visit a physician much more frequently than others, for the same symptom. The group that visits more frequently tends to have a higher level of anxiety, fear, grief, or frustration. It is the physician's responsibility to search for, identify, and treat organic disease if it is present, yet in about half of the cases none will be found. Of course, it is equally important to identify the reason for these visits—the basis for the heightened concern or increased anxiety. A person may see a minor symptom as a potential catastrophe if he or she feels it may be a sign of cancer similar to that causing a parent's death. In other words, patients may come because of what they imagine is causing the symptoms rather than because of the symptoms themselves. Identifying what patients hope can be done for them—that is, focusing on their expectations for the visit—will often reveal hidden reasons for the visit. The physician should be sure to address the patient's expectations and make certain that the interpretation is correct. Is the patient really there "just for a blood pressure check" or because of concern over the condition of his coronary arteries since a friend recently had an acute myocardial infarction? If the physician deals only with the symptoms, the real concerns may go undetected, and the result will be a dissatisfied and noncompliant patient. Barsky (1981) cautions that "patients who express dissatisfaction with their medical care should be questioned about this, as they may be dissatisfied because their real motivation in seeking care has not been illuminated." He also advises the physician to investigate the patient's current life stresses when visits are made when there is no change in clinical status.

Hand on the Doorknob Syndrome. The patient's parting phrase is sometimes a clue to the primary reason for the visit, or it may reflect another issue of great concern that is emotionally threatening and could not be voiced until adequate courage was summoned at the moment of departure. It sometimes finally surfaces as a last, desperate attempt to communicate—since, with hand on door, escape is readily accessible if the physician's reaction is unfavorable. Reasons for this hidden communication by the patient are important and must be recognized and dealt with. Because of fear of rejection or humilation, the patient may test the physician with minor complaints before mentioning the real reason for the visit (Quill, 1989). Be alert to any unusual behavior during an interview, such as slips of the tongue, unexpected responses, and overly enthusiastic denials. Search further for the underlying reason for the visit when a patient presents with a trivial complaint that appears inappropriate at that time. It is a good practice to routinely ask the patient at the end of a visit "Is there anything we have not covered or anything else you would like to ask me?"

Patients with a fear of cancer, for instance, are often unable to voice their concern to the physician. Instead, they present with somatic complaints or contrived reasons that necessitate a complete examination. They are hopeful that the examination will allay their fears without it being necessary to express them openly. For example, a female patient presenting for a complete physical examination may actually be concerned over the possibility of a carcinoma of the breast, which her elder sister may have had at the same age or for which a friend recently had surgery. Such situations emphasize the need for a complete family history and a discussion of any patient concerns, in an effort to allow these feelings to surface. Attention should then be paid to alleviating the anxiety. Apprehension regarding cancer is widespread, and often the only cure for this fear is a therapeutic conversation with the physician. It is very likely that most patients harbor some fear of cancer, and, therefore, following a complete history and physical examination, specific mention should be made that no signs of cancer can be detected at this time. If this precaution is not taken, a patient with a hidden anxiety or fear of cancer may remain suspicious that a cancer could be present, since there was no apparent attempt to look specifically for it.

Proxemics (Spatial Factors)

Space. Proxemics is the study of how people unconsciously structure the space around them. This structuring varies with every culture. North Americans, for example, maintain a protective "body bubble" of space about 2 feet in diameter around them when they interact with strangers or casual acquaintances. Violators of that space are considered intruders and cause the person to become defensive (Fig. 25–12). In the Middle East, no such bubble exists, and it is proper to invade this area. In fact, not to do so may be interpreted as unfriendly and standoffish. Arabs prefer to stand close enough to touch and smell the other person. Americans, however, if forced to stand close together, as on a crowded subway, will use their eyes (distant gaze) to maintain a more proper distance. An arm's length is a good measure of the appropriate personal distance for most people. A wife can stand inside her husband's bubble, but she will be unhappy if another woman invades this sphere of privacy (and vice versa).

Robert Frost said that "good fences make good neighbors." In suburbs and small towns, people are more likely to talk to each other while in their backyards if a fence indicates the boundary than if there is a communal yard (McCaskey, 1979). Marking the boundary helps maintain territoriality and actually brings the neighbors closer together than when there is no fence.

Intimate space has been classified as that ranging from close physical contact to 18 inches, *personal* space from 18 inches to 4 feet, *social* space from 4 feet to 12 feet, and *public* space 12 feet and beyond. Placing a desk between two people shifts personal space to social space. The office desk can also be a barrier to communication when it is placed between the physician and patient, thereby emphasizing the illusion of the physician's importance and power. There may be occasions when this is desired, but it usually is not necessary in a family physician's office. Office furniture should be arranged so that a minimum number of obstacles lie between physician and patient. The patient should also be made to feel as comfortable as possible, with a minimum of bright lights, smoke, and other irritating stimuli present in the room.

Listening Well

A good family physician must be a good listener. Of all the communication skills essential to rapport, the ability to listen well is probably the most impo tant. All the information in the world about body language, vocal messages, and nonverbal cues is of limited value unless it helps the family physician be a better listener.

Physicians should listen to patients in an alert and uncritical manner. They should appear relaxed yet attentive. They should be nonjudgmental, so as not to inhibit the patient's expression and willingness to relate problems of a sensitive nature.

Analyses of doctor-patient interviews reveal that on the average the doctor rather than the patient does most of the talking, although the physicians, when questioned, usually imagine the reverse. In general, the less the physician says during an interview, the more the patient will say. Silence can be as effective a means of eliciting further information as direct questions. The timing is important, however, and silence should be used as a technique only when the physician is relatively certain that there is more information to follow the last statement. A shift of position, or a nod and a smile, properly timed and coupled with silence can be more effective than an encouraging comment. Nonverbal encouragement to continue is less distracting and may be more facilitative than the verbal. The patient may be following a line of thought and may be about to open up more but must stop and refocus on the physician if he "captures" the patient's attention with a verbal state-

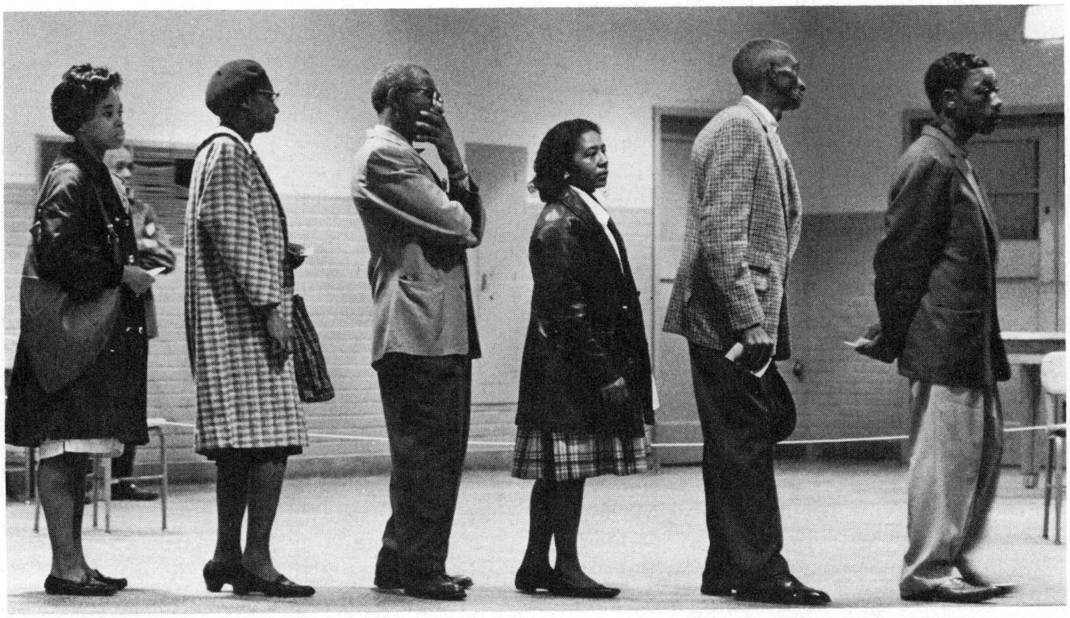

Figure 25–12. The "body bubble" surrounding strangers in a queue. (By permission of Magnum Photos, Inc., New York.)

ment. The physician should interrupt a patient's statement only if it is necessary to change the conversation to a new topic, clarify an issue, elicit information not produced spontaneously, offer reassurance, or reduce patient anxiety.

The appearance of readiness to listen is aided by bending forward and maintaining eye contact. The physician can discourage a patient from talking simply by looking away or writing in the medical record. Well-chosen questions can be rendered useless by inappropriate nonverbal behavior.

Interviewing Effectively

The skilled family physician can spend 10 minutes with a patient, and the patient feels it was 20. This is far better than the physician who spends 20 minutes but leaves patients feeling that the physician was in a hurry and they were encroaching on the physician's precious time every minute of the visit.

Overly brief or abrupt conversations in the office or at the bedside can severely damage rapport. Physicians signal how much time they plan to spend by a variety of nonverbal cues, and patients rarely have the courage to counter this by asking for more time. The physician who hurriedly asks "How are you?" while flipping through a chart with only a quick glance at the patient destroys communication. Even the busiest physicians can accomplish wonders in a very few minutes by indicating that their full attention is on the patient: Everyone remembers an outstanding physician who, for whatever time was available, would, by a relaxed posture and attentive manner, truly communicate with the patient.

The interesting and revealing study by Korsh and Negrete (1972), involving analysis of taped doctor-patient encounters in a pediatric clinic, revealed that many of the mothers were dissatisfied because the physician paid too little attention to their concern and apprehension about their child. Their attitude had little relationship to the amount of attention that the physician actually paid to the infant, which was usually very adequate.

Even in an established family practice where essentially none of the patients was dissatisfied with the physician, 54 per cent of the patients either forgot to mention something of concern or misunderstood facts about diagnosis or treatment (Snyder et al., 1976). Twenty-nine of the 84 patients forgot to tell the physician something that was bothering them. This illustrates the wisdom of concluding every interview with the statement "Is there anything else bothering you that we haven't discussed?" Snyder suggests that "the physician will be well advised to consciously underestimate his ability to communicate." Rather than assume that patients have understood the instructions, ask them to repeat the instructions as they understood them. Patients with chronic illnesses, and those visiting the physician for the first time, are most likely to misunderstand treatment instructions. When seeing a patient with a chronic illness, assess the patient's understanding of instructions given at a previous visit by asking, "What medications are you taking?" or "How are you taking your medication?" A patient seen for the first time can be asked, "How have you been treating this problem?"

When meeting a new patient, the method used to address the patient during the introduction can help establish rapport by conveying an atmosphere of mutual respect. Use the patient's name during the introduction, during the interview, and upon leaving. An appropriate introduction would be, "Good morning, Mrs. Brown, I'm Dr. ____ ." or "Good morning, Mrs. Brown. I'm ____ ____ , a second year medical student, and I'll be taking your medical history and examining you today."

Rapport can be influenced positively or negatively by how the physician addresses the patient. Although the majority of patients prefer to be addressed by their first name, some may be irritated by this if sufficient familiarity has not been established. A good policy is to ask the patient what they prefer to be called (e.g., by a nickname) and note this in the chart, or wait until adequate familiarity has been established. Bergman et al. (1988) found that 96 per cent of patients preferred to be addressed by their first name, and 40 per cent preferred to address the physician by first name although only 14 per cent actually did so.

Facilitating Techniques. In addition to the nonverbal facilitating techniques of silence and body positioning mentioned previously, patients can be encouraged to talk further with simple comments such as, "And then?" or by repeating a portion of the statement just made. For example:

Patient: I have been very nervous lately.

Doctor: Nervous?

Confrontation. Confrontation, wisely used, can help establish communication and rapport. Statements such as "you look unhappy" or "you appear very anxious" are based on the physician's observation of the patient. If the physician has been unable to establish rapport, it may help to approach the issue openly and frankly, "We don't seem to be communicating very well. Can you tell me what is wrong?" This is also a useful maneuver when a previously good relationship suddenly turns sour.

Summarization (or Paraphrasing). Summarization is a brief restatement of what the patient has said and gives both the interviewer and patient a chance to correct errors or misunderstanding. It demonstrates the physician's interest in the patient's history and his or her effort to collect the facts accurately. The physician can restate what the patient has said and emphasize the important points to assure clear understanding. Summarization assures that both parties are using the same definitions and minimizes inappropriate assumptions. "Let me see if I have understood you correctly" or "Am I understanding this correctly?" are good ways to introduce a paraphrase.

Concluding a History. In an effort to avoid leaving gaps in the history or allowing patient concerns to go unattended, it is wise to conclude every complete history with the statement, "Is there anything else you would like to mention?" or "Is there anything that we have not discussed?"

Open-Ended Questions. Probably the single most valuable rapport-promoting element of verbal communication is the use of open-ended questions at the onset of an interview. "Tell me more about it" is both an interview technique and a state of mind. The physician who understands that no check list of "yes-no" questions can possibly portray the patient as a unique human being will create an atmosphere of sensitivity and interest that contributes greatly to the early establishment of rapport. Once the broad outlines of the patient's unique situation are indicated, detailed questioning moves along quickly.

Specific questions beget specific answers and rarely anything more. However, the physician may wish to use this technique on occasion, as when dealing with the verbose, rambling patient who refuses to stick to the point or when specific information is needed. When more general or hidden data are sought, however, the physician must choose questions and gestures that offer the maximal potential for obtaining information. In order to be effective, open-ended questioning requires that the physician appear relaxed and ready to listen regardless of the amount of pressure from waiting patients. Once it becomes apparent that more time is necessary than is available, a new appointment should be made so that adequate time is assured.

Signals That Discourage Communication. While appearing to respond affirmatively and facilitate the conversation, people can in fact turn off the speaker if they frequently comment "yes" in a manner that conveys disinterest or impatience. Everyone has experienced the person who says "yes" before the sentence is finished or the point made. Patients can be subdued and reduced to silence in a similar manner—intentionally or unintentionally.

The physician should also avoid putting his hands to the mouth or face when speaking, since this may indicate indecision, nervousness, or defensiveness. Such signs, when recognized, even unconsciously, by the patient serve as a barrier to establishing rapport.

Confidentiality. Confidentiality is a cardinal principle of professionalism. Effective communication requires that the patient feel secure in the knowledge that all information will be kept strictly confidential. It is the ethical responsibility of each physician to maintain this bond of confidentiality. The family physician must appreciate this intimate and confidential bond and avoid any threat to its dissolution. Hippocrates said, "And whatever I shall see or hear in the course of my profession, as well as outside my profession in my intercourse with men, if it be what should not be published abroad, I will never divulge, holding such things to be holy secrets."

Assurance that all information and actions will be kept confidential is especially important when dealing with adolescents. They may not be aware of this basic ethical principle in the medical profession or realize that it applies to them. They may be reluctant to share information and trust completely for fear that parents or peers may find out. A 16-year-old girl may not communicate her desire for information about birth control methods if she anticipates that the request will be made known to her parents.

Complex problems of confidentiality can arise for the physician who cares for several members of the same family. Family members can often provide important information that supplements what the clinician learns directly from the patient. Unfortunately, information may sometimes be offered only on the promise that it will not be disclosed to the patient. Remembering who said what and about whom and what information is privileged and what is not can quickly result in an impossible situation for the family physician. Secrets rarely can be kept for long; the patient sooner or later learns what has been confided, thus straining the bonds of trust. In general, it is best not to be a party to secrets but rather to find a way to discuss sensitive material. Not infrequently, the very issues about which secrecy is requested are central to the patient's problem. If rapport is to be maintained, the physician must diplomatically explore the possibility of dealing with such problems in a constructive fashion as soon as the patient's situation permits.

Rapport with Families

No patient exists in a social vacuum. Visible or invisible, family and friends provide a social environment that exerts an important influence on the clinical course of disease. Since the family usually has a stronger emotional influence on the patient than does the physician, effective communication with the patient's family is an important element in successful patient care. Their positive support is necessary if the physician's plan of management is to be carried out. Family support of the physician's treatment regimen can help ensure that a patient remains on a prescribed diet, takes medication as instructed, rests appropriately, or maintains a proper exercise program. An unsupportive family attitude could negate or severely jeopardize previous gains in treatment.

A supportive social environment may permit some patients who ordinarily require hospitalization to be cared for at home. The family physician is in a good position to assess the contribution the family can make to the care of the patient. Family strengths must be carefully evaluated. The healthy family can buffer the impact of disability and contribute in a substantial way to the patient's recovery. The unhealthy family, on the other hand, may create major problems for the patient and the health care team. It is an all too common occurrence for family members or friends to bring food, alcohol, or cigarettes surreptitiously to patients who should not have them. Sometimes troubling news is tactlessly communicated without realizing the impact on the patient. At times, the conclusion seems inescapable that some members of the social environment are unconsciously countering the patient's efforts to get well.

Family, friends, and colleagues can be valuable sources of important information regarding the patient's illness beyond that given by the patient, including facts that were forgotten, repressed, or even unknown to the patient. Communication should be established through the most responsible family member (other than the patient). However, it is important that such discussion be known to patients and a summary of the discussion shared with them by the physician to avoid a misunderstanding or conflict of ideas when patients and family members interact. If the patient and the family have different sets of information, they may become suspicious of future communications with the physician. Any frustration on the patient's part resulting from inadequate communication will be considerably magnified by family members. Any defect in family communication can create difficulties directly related to the number of interested individuals within the family, often causing a small problem to reach enormous proportions.

Communication with concerned family and friends need not be time consuming. If a serious or prolonged illness is involved, a family conference can outline what can be expected and what will be done. It is usually possible to identify one family member as the communication channel to whom future reports will be given, thus avoiding frequent and repetitious calls. Many clinicians find that optimal control and satisfaction is achieved by initiating the calls themselves on a regular schedule.

Rapport with Children

Working with children is one of the delights of practice. Children have a quality of freshness and directness that adults often lack. There are no secret formulae for interacting with the young, although there are cautions to be observed. Most procedures are not uncomfortable if one exercises patience, but forced gaiety and false promises that "it won't hurt" are immediately perceived as dishonest, and once trust is destroyed, it may never be regained by any physician. It is usually possible to find ways to elicit the cooperation of the apprehensive child. A separate pediatric examination room, with appropriate decor, is reassuring. White coats need not be worn if the child has unpleasant associations with such uniforms. Examining the ear of the mother or an older sibling, for example, before examining the child often allays anxiety. Let the child handle the stethoscope or otoscope. Simple rewards can also make the physician's office a place of interest for the child. Accompanying other members of the family on visits to the physician helps the child gain familiarity with the office and staff. The physician who spends a few extra minutes with children and family early in the professional relationship will reap enormous dividends in years to come.

Rapport with the Elderly

The older patient is becoming an increasingly large part of the typical family practice. Treating the senior citizen can be rewarding if viewed with a positive attitude. The basis of such a perspective is a sound knowledge of geriatric medicine that offers creative approaches for dealing with problems once viewed as frustrating or hopeless.

Elderly patients may feel that their lives are empty or meaningless and may seek satisfaction in memories of past accomplishments; usually, they are appreciative of any attention paid to these meaningful segments of their lives. Whenever possible, preserve their sense of dignity and foster their feeling of continuing usefulness. Loneliness, depression, and increased dependency, where they exist, must be addressed in any treatment plan. The effort to see beyond the patient's immediate problem to the strengths and accomplishments of the older individual can lay the foundation for a positive relationship based on mutual respect. A house call can establish rapport as nothing else can; the physician gains an important perspective on the patient as a person. Any danger of creating an unhealthy state of dependency can be avoided by tactful conversation with the patient and family about what should be expected as part of the physician's routine services.

A few geriatric patients can be difficult to deal with on a creative basis; the vast majority, however, will enrich a practice by bringing to it all the wisdom, insight, and maturity that comes with having successfully lived through the difficulties and gratifications that are an inevitable part of our era.

Care with Caring

One of the essential qualities of the clinician is interest in humanity, for the secret of the care of the patient is in caring for the patient.

This statement by Francis Peabody in 1923 could well serve as the maxim for establishing patient rapport. While continuing to emphasize the curing aspects of medicine, family medicine places increased emphasis upon its caring aspects. Caring is the opposite of apathy and implies the application of human tenderness and compassion to the curing of individuals. It involves respect for the individual as a human being and enables the physician to motivate patients to participate in their care. Physicians must convince the patient that they care and are sincerely interested in providing help.

Allen Gregg has said that more mistakes in medicine are made by those who do not care than by those who do not know. The caring implies an empathetic relationship between physician and patient. Empathy is the capacity of physicians to participate in the feelings of the patient and is best accomplished if physicians place themselves in the role of patients in an effort to understand their feelings. This does not imply a sharing of feelings with the patient (sympathy), since the physician would then become emotionally affected. Empathy involves only insight into the patient's feelings. It is best that the physician avoid becoming emotionally involved in order to maintain professional equanimity and objectivity when caring for the patient.

Chekov, a physician himself, felt that medical students should spend half of their time learning what it feels like to be ill. Although this may be an extreme method for developing empathy, it is important that the student, before becoming immersed in the technical and cognitive aspects of medicine, be able to identify with the patient's feelings, fears, apprehensions, and expectations so that the knowledge acquired during medical school can be applied meaningfully in the context of these needs. Exposing students to patients in the first year of medical school, before they have been preoccupied with the diagnosis and treatment of disease, offers them an opportunity, under the watchful gaze of an instructor, to focus on the process of communication. Barriers to effective communication can then be identified. For example, a student may have difficulty permitting a patient with terminal cancer to talk about the disease or his impending death. More than one student has been known to convey his discomfort nonverbally by conducting the interview standing at the foot of the hospital bed, adjacent to the door, ready to escape.

Although the physician may be able to cure a disease only occasionally, he can always console the patient. An unknown French author has admonished the medical profession "to cure sometimes, to relieve often, to comfort always." The family physician provides personalized patient care and attempts to minimize the often frightening and dehumanizing experience to which patients are subjected in our highly structured modern medical system. The physician must constantly strive to preserve personal dignity for patients, especially when their identities are threatened by a strange and somewhat frightening hospital environment. Care *for* a patient is more personal than the care *of* a patient.

References

Alda, A. Time, May 28, 1979, p. 68.

Arnston, P. H., and Philipsborn, H. G.: Pediatrician-parent communication in a continuity-of-care setting. Clin. Pediatr., *21*:302, 1982.

Barsky, A. J.: Hidden reasons some patients visit doctors. Ann. Intern. Med. *94*:492, 1981.

Bergman, J. J., Eggertsen, S. C., Phillips, W. R., et al.: How patients and physicians address each other in the office. J. Fam. Pract., *27*:399–402, 1988.

Brotschi, E.: Taking care of the hateful patient (Letter). N. Engl. J. Med., *299*:367, 1978.

Browne, K., and Freeling, P.: The doctor-patient relationship. Edinburgh and London, E & S Livingston Ltd., 1967. *This small text (73 pp.) contains much material of value to the student. Of greatest interest are the introduction and the chapters The Sixth Sense, Communication and Language, and Skills and Tricks.*

Butterfield, F.: China: Alive in the Bitter Sea. New York, Times Books, 1982.

Coble, R. J., Sinnott, S. K., and Walz, T. H.: The family physician's office: proposed design criteria for family centered medical care. J. Fam. Pract., *14*:77, 1982.

Davis, F.: Inside Intuition. New York, New American Library, 1975.

Derek, W. R., Gray, J., Dixon, M., and Collin, J.: The closed eyes sign: an aid to diagnosing non-specific abdominal pain. Br. Med. J. *297*:837, 1988.

Ekman, P.: Telling Lies. New York, W. W. Norton, 1985.

Ekman, P., and Friesen, W. V.: Unmasking the Face: A Guide to Recognizing Emotions From Facial Clues. Englewood Cliffs, New Jersey, Prentice-Hall, 1975. *A classic text in facial expression and emotion. Uses composite photographs to show the importance of one area such as the brow, eyes, or mouth. A chapter on facial deceit helps recognize clues to facial deception when someone is trying to mask emotions. The chapter on sadness shows how to recognize depression masked by a smile.*

Friedman, H. S.: Nonverbal communication between patients and medical practitioners. J. Soc. Issues, *35*:82, 1979.

Gjerdingen, D. K., Simpson, D. E., and Titus, S. L.: Patients' and physicians' attitudes regarding the physicians' professional appearance. Arch. Intern. Med. *147*:1209–1212, 1987.

Goffman, E.: The Presentation of Self in Everyday Life. New York, Doubleday, 1959. *Deals with human behavior in social situations from the perspectives of role and communication theory. A brilliant study written in a highly entertaining style.*

Groves, J. E.: Taking care of the hateful patient. N. Engl. J. Med. *298*:883, 1978.

Hess, E. T.: The Telltale Eye. New York, Van Nostrand Reinhold, 1975.

Holmes, O. W.: Medical Essays: 1842–1882. Boston and New York, Houghton Mifflin Company (The Riverside Press, Cambridge), 1911.

Kent, G. G., Clark, P., and Dalrymple-Smith, D.: The patient is the expert: a technique for teaching interviewing skills. Med. Educ., *15*:38, 1981.

Key, M. R.: The Relationship of Verbal and Nonverbal Communication. New York, Mouton Publishers, 1980.

Knapp, M. L.: Nonverbal Communication in Human Interaction. 2nd ed. New York, Holt, Reinhart and Winston, 1978. *A comprehensive review of nonverbal communication. Extensive bibliography.*

Korsch, B. M., and Negrete, V.: Doctor-patient communication. Sci. Am., *227*:66, 1972. *Describes patient dissatisfaction resulting from the use of medical jargon by physicians and inadequate attention to patient concerns and expectations. The studies involved the parents of children brought to the emergency clinic of the Children's Hospital of Los Angeles.*

Larson, K. M., and Smith, C. K.: Assessment of nonverbal communication in patient-physician interview. J. Fam. Pract., *12*:481, 1981.

Lau, B. W. K.: Reassurance does not always help. Can. Fam. Physic., *35*:1161–1163, 1989.

Levinson, D.: A Guide to the Clinical Interview. Philadelphia, W. B. Saunders Company, 1987. *An excellent soft-back publication on basic interviewing and problem-solving techniques.*

McCaskey, M. B.: The hidden messages managers send. Harv. Bus. Rev., Nov.-Dec., 1979, p. 135.

Meltzoff, A. N., and Moore, M. K.: Imitation of facial and manual gestures by human neonates. Science, *198*:75–78, 1977.

Morris, D.: Manwatching: A Field Guide to Human Behavior. New York, Harry N. Abrams, 1977. *A cross-cultural look at behavior, with excellent illustrations, especially regarding gestures, signals, and other nonverbal means of communication.*

Nierenberg, G. I., and Calero, H. H.: How to Read a Person Like a Book. New York, Hawthorn Books, Inc., 1917. *One of the more useful books on body language. Contains many specifics of value to the physician in reading the nonverbal messages from patients.*

Peabody, F. W.: Doctor and Patient. New York, The Macmillan Co., 1930.

Peck, S. R.: Atlas of Facial Expression. New York, Oxford University Press, 1987.

Pendleton, D., and Hasler, J.: Doctor-Patient Communication. London, Academic Press, 1983.

Polhemus, T. (Ed.): The Body Reader: Social Aspects of the Human Body. New York, Pantheon Books, 1978. *Discusses in detail the universality of body language and similarities that indicate a common ancestry for all cultures. The importance of environment and other factors is presented in the form of selected papers by leading investigators including Birdwhistell, Efron, Mead, and Darwin.*

Quill, T. E.: Recognizing and adjusting to barriers in doctor-patient communication. Ann. Intern. Med., *111*:51–57, 1989.

Reiser, D. E., and Schroder, A. K.: Patient Interviewing: The Human Dimension. Baltimore, Williams and Wilkins, 1980. *Much more than a discussion of interviewing technique. Numerous extended case studies lead the reader to consider some of the basic emotions of both physician and patient in a variety of life situations. Rewarding reading.*

Scheflen, A. E.: Body Language and the Social Order—Communication as Behavioral Control. Englewood Cliffs, New Jersey, Prentice-Hall, Inc., 1972.

Snyder, D., Lynch, J. J., and Gruss, L.: Doctor-patient communication in a private family practice. J. Fam. Pract., *3*:271, 1976.

Stein, H. F.: Toward a life of dialogue: Therapeutic communication and the meaning of medicine. Cont. Ed. Fam. Phys., *16*:29, 1982.

Teller, J.: Taking care of the hateful patient (Letter). N. Engl. J. Med., *299*:367, 1978.

Waxer, P. H.: Nonverbal cues for anxiety: An examination of emotional leakage. J. Abnorm. Psychol., *86*:306, 1977. *Silent video segments of patients with varying levels of anxiety were viewed by 46 raters. They were able to discriminate varying intensities of anxiety on the basis of nonverbal cues alone.*

Widmer, R. B., and Cadoret, R. J.: Depression in primary care: Changes in pattern of patients visits and complaints during a developing depression. J. Fam. Pract., *7*:293, 1978. *Changes in patient behavior associated with a developing depression were recorded. Visits to the clinic, somatic complaints, and anxiety were significantly increased during the 6 months before the diagnosis of depression was made.*

Widmer, R. B., Cadoret, R. J., and North, C. S.: Depression in family practice: Some effects on spouses and children. J. Fam. Pract., *10*:45, 1980. *Medical complaints and office visits of spouses and children of depressed patients were examined and compared with a matched comparison group of spouses and children of nondepressed patients. Several significant changes were found.*

26

Patient Compliance

C. Edward Evans
R. Brian Haynes

Introduction

[The physician] should keep aware of the fact that patients often lie when they state that they have taken certain medicines.

HIPPOCRATES

The recognition of poor compliance in ancient times belies the fact that over 90 per cent of the literature on compliance has been published since the early 1970's. Thus, although physicians have dispensed medicines and potions through the centuries in vast quantities, it is only in recent years that there has been systematic examination of whether patients actually take the treatment.

This interest in patient compliance seems to parallel the introduction of more and more efficacious medications. Whether this is fortuitous or not, it was perhaps to the patient's benefit in the past that little attention was paid to compliance, as poor compliance probably saved the patient's life on many occasions. Some treatments, especially the massive purges and bleeding of the 18th century and arsenic and hydrochloric acid of this century, certainly had lethal rather than therapeutic potential. Such lessons of the past should not be forgotten in considering compliance today, as we still prescribe many treatments of dubious value. Nevertheless, our armamentarium of useful treatments is now sizeable and expanding rapidly; low patient compliance stands squarely in the way of achieving the full benefit of modern therapy.

The extent of poor compliance is distressing. Fifty per cent is a representative compliance figure for many classes of long-term therapy. Only about two thirds of those who continue under care take enough of their prescribed medication to achieve adequate blood pressure control (Haynes et al., 1979). If we look at compliance with diets and lifestyle changes, such as smoking cessation, the figures are even more dismal (Best and Block, 1979).

Added to this, physicians—even family physicians—are not good at estimating compliance levels in patients (Gilbert et al., 1980). Physicians have a strong tendency to overestimate the compliance of their own patients and are usually unable to predict which patients will comply with treatment.

Fortunately, the story does not end here. There are practical methods of detecting poor compliance and strategies for improving it, as we shall see as this chapter unfolds.

Definitions

The trend in medicine, and particularly in family medicine, is away from the authoritarian care-giver towards a more democratic role that involves the patient in decisions. Thus, the use of the word *compliance* has raised objections from many physicians because it implies obedience to a superior will or intellect and anything but an adult-to-adult relationship between physician and patient. Unfortunately, no better term has surfaced. Adherence and defaulting are probably the most common alternatives, but they still carry many negative connotations. While we recognize the problems and sympathize with the views of those who oppose the term, we will use *compliance* throughout this chapter because it is widely used and generally accepted.

Compliance has been defined as the extent to which a person's behavior (in terms of keeping appointments, taking medications, and executing lifestyle changes) coincides with medical advice (Sackett, 1976). Poor compliance is more difficult to define. What percentage of prescribed medication can a patient forget or omit before being classed as a poor complier? How are patients who take too much medication classified? These are questions without simple, straightforward answers. One way of looking at the problem is to use patient outcomes as a guide. For instance, in hypertension studies, patients taking 80 per cent or more of prescribed medication were considered compliant because this amount of medication is required to produce systematic blood pressure reduction (Sackett et al., 1975). It makes sense that efforts directed at poor compliers should be concentrated on those not achieving therapeutic goals. This obviously makes for more efficient use of resources. However, this pragmatic approach is not entirely satisfactory in that some patients who respond to treatment may be doing so because of overprescribing rather than good compliance. In the event that these patients are hospitalized or placed in some other situation in which compliance may be near to 100 per cent, they may well run into serious effects of overdose.

Factors Influencing Compliance

Many approaches, ranging from complex psychologic theories to simplistic or intuitive ideas, have been taken to explain compliance behavior. None is entirely satisfactory, and many are lamentably wrong (Leventhal and Cameron, 1987).

In looking at the many factors involved, there is a natural tendency for the physician to feel that poor compliance is the patient's fault. In the final analysis, this may be true. After all, it is the patient who must swallow the pill, but there are many other factors leading up to the final act of pill taking that need to be considered. For instance, what about the disease or condition being treated: Is it symptomatic or asymptomatic, life threatening, or purely a nuisance? What about the treatment itself: Is it unpleasant to take, inconvenient, or expensive? Does it work? Is the environment in which the treatment is prescribed conducive to regular follow-up? Does the physician inspire confidence in the treatment? Do his attitudes interfere with compliance? All of these factors could have important effects on compliance behavior, but, as we shall see, only some of them do.

THE PATIENT

The sociodemographic characteristics or attitudes of the patient have received a great deal of attention, and such attributes as age, sex, marital status, education, intelligence, and economic status bear no consistent relationship to compliance. Two exceptions are the very young and the very old, whose compliance characteristics tend to conform to those of their care-takers.

Perhaps the most widely held theory of compliance behavior, probably because of its intuitive appeal, is that of the communications approach (Leventhal et al., 1984). In this model, it is proposed that patients generally do not know enough about their illness or treatment and that it is this ignorance that leads to poor compliance. It follows that adequate instruction or message generation and reception, comprehension, and retention of the message should result in improved compliance. While it appears that this is true for short-term treatments (less than 2 weeks in duration), knowledge bears little relationship to compliance with chronic disease regimens (Haynes, 1979).

Another popular theory looks at patient motivation and beliefs. The Health Belief Model (Becker, 1976) argues that the likelihood of an individual undertaking a recommended health action is dependent on his perception of the level of personal susceptibility to the particular illness or condition; the degree of severity of the consequences of contracting the condition; the potential benefits or efficacy of the treatment in preventing or reducing susceptibility and/or severity; and the physical, psychologic, financial, and other barriers or costs involved in initiating or continuing the treatment. The model also requires a stimulus or cue to action to trigger the appropriate behavior (compliance); this cue can be either internal (e.g., a symptom) or external (e.g., screening campaign or physician's advice). This model has been shown to have predictive value for some preventive and short-term, therapeutic health actions, such as immunizations and medical regimens for acute disease, but the extent of its predictive value is modest at best (Janz and Becker, 1984).

Other models have been studied, including the behavioral learning model, which is based on cognitive and social learning theory, and the self-regulating model. As yet, no model has been developed that adequately explains a person's compliance behavior or gives a clear rationale for modifying it (Haynes et al., 1982).

THE DISEASE

In general, disease factors are relatively unimportant as determinants of compliance. There are, however, a few exceptions to this generalization. Psychiatric patients with schizophrenia, paranoid features, and personality disorders are less compliant than other psychiatric patients—a fact that probably reduces the compliance of psychiatric patients as a whole below that of patients with nonpsychiatric disorders.

Surprisingly, no relationship has been demonstrated between the severity of symptoms and compliance, but the *more* symptoms a patient reports, the *lower* his compliance is likely to be. On the other hand, increasing disability produced by a disease appears to be associated with better compliance. Whether this is a result of increased severity of disease or simply the result of the *increased supervision* that often accompanies increased disability has not been examined directly.

Chronic diseases requiring long-term treatment have been clearly shown to result in increasingly poor compliance. This fact is of great clinical importance in such potentially serious diseases as tuberculosis and hypertension and is more likely to be a function of the duration of the *treatment* regimen than the duration of the *disease* itself.

THE REGIMEN

On the whole, the greater the behavioral demands of a treatment, the poorer the compliance. This means that regimens requiring changes in life style, such as dieting, exercising, and stopping bad habits, result in much poorer compliance than simply taking pills, because of the substantially greater behavioral changes demanded.

Nevertheless, it is quite clear that the greater the number of drugs or treatments prescribed for a patient, the greater the probability of poor compliance. This includes both errors of omission and commission. While the frequency of pill taking is not so important, it also has an effect in that patients are less likely to comply with a regimen requiring four or more doses a day than with one requiring one or two daily doses.

Although alternative oral medications for the same condition do not appear to result in substantial differences in compliance, there does appear to be a difference between different treatments for different problems. This ranges from 17 per cent compliance with antacids to 89 per cent with cardiac drugs (Closson and Kikugawa, 1975).

One form of alternative treatment that has been shown to have a beneficial effect is the injection of long-acting parenteral preparations. Examples of this are the use of benzathine penicillin for acute streptococcal pharyngitis and rheumatic fever prophylaxis and long-acting phenothiazines for schizophrenia, both of which have been shown to be acceptable to patients and more successful than oral preparations. This has also been demonstrated with twice weekly injections of streptomycin for tuberculosis. The fact that diabetics comply so poorly with self-injected insulin suggests that the success of long-acting preparations is less likely to be due to their parenteral nature than to result from the medical supervision necessary to administer them.

Another disappointment for intuitive reasoning is the fact that there is very little evidence that side effects of treatment are a major cause of poor compliance. Studies have shown that there is no difference in the reported frequency of side effects between compliers and noncompliers (Latiolais and Berry, 1969; Willcox et al., 1965). In studies in which patients were asked for reasons for their noncompliance, only 5 to 10 per cent implicated side effects (Glick, 1965; Rickels et al., 1964).

The cost of treatment is an important barrier to compliance for many people, although the total effect of cost is not obvious as might first appear. For instance, one study showed that hospital admissions *increased* among psychiatric outpatients given drugs at nominal cost compared to a group paying regular prices (Cody and Robinson, 1977).

THE PHYSICIAN

The physician is obviously in a key position to influence compliance. After all, it is the physician who initiates the treatment in the majority of cases. For example, if the frequency of dose affects compliance, then by the very act of prescribing a four times a day regimen the physician is potentially reducing compliance below the level achievable with a prescription requiring a single daily dose.

More complex than the mechanics of prescribing, however, is the interaction between physician and patient. Patients are more likely to comply with treatment if their expectations are met by the visit and if they are well satisfied with their care (Francis et al., 1969; Kincey, 1975). The concept of a personal physician or the feeling of knowing a physician well has also been associated with increased compliance (Ettlinger and Freeman, 1981). The problem is that dissecting the physician-patient relationship and measuring factors resulting in increased satisfaction are not easy. This is demonstrated in one study in which some patients felt they knew their physician *well* after only one visit, while others felt they still did not know their physicians after as many as *14* visits (Ettlinger and Freeman, 1981).

It is conceivable that a long-term relationship between physician and patient might even result in decreased knowledge by the physician of the patient's level of compliance. A long-time patient may not want to hurt his or her physician by admitting to poor compliance. Certainly, there is evidence that physicians are no better at estimating compliance in patients they have known for more than 5 years compared to those they have known for shorter periods; they do abysmally with both groups (Gilbert et al., 1980).

Detection of Poor Compliance

CLINICAL JUDGMENT

Most of us would like to believe that a good physician can detect poor compliance in his patients; surely, this goes along with increasing clinical experience. Unfortunately, studies have shown that this is not the case: Using clinical judgment has been shown to be no better than flipping a coin as a detection method. The first studies demonstrating this were carried out in specialty settings and with physicians who did not have an ongoing relationship with patients. Unfortunately, the hope that family physicians with their ongoing relationships with their patients might be in a better position to make predictions has also been dispelled. Family physicians were not only unable to detect poor compliers among their patients, but the length of time they had known their patients had no effect on their ability to predict.

The emphasis of the unreliability of clinical judgment is important in that it serves to direct us to a more systematic approach towards detection of poor compliance.

MONITORING ATTENDANCE

As referred to previously, over 50 per cent of hypertensives stop visiting their physicians within a year of starting treatment, and patients who do not show up for follow-up appointments are unlikely to be in a position to be good compliers with treatment. What is not so obvious, however, is that many physicians are unable to detect this type of noncompliance because their appointment systems are inadequate or because the patients do not take the step of making an appointment in the first place.

It follows, then, that an important method of detecting poor compliance is to watch the appointment book and day sheet. While there is no guarantee that patients who keep appointments will comply with treatment, there is no doubt that those who do not appear for follow-up will not be in a position to comply with treatment. The importance of monitoring attendance cannot be overstressed: Dropping out of care is one of the most frequent and most severe forms of noncompliance.

RESPONSE TO TREATMENT

Provided that the treatment prescribed is known to be efficacious, failure of a patient to respond to treatment can be used as a readily available indicator of compliance levels. However, this method of assessing compliance is not infallible. For example, patients who appear to respond to treatment may do so because they were misdiagnosed and do not have the condition of interest or because their physicians' overprescribing is compensating for their poor compliance. Nevertheless, from the compliance perspective at least, there is little need to be concerned about patients who have reached the therapeutic goal. On the other hand, patients not showing a response to treatment will include patients who genuinely do not respond to therapy or who have been prescribed inadequate amounts and will also include a high proportion of poor compliers or noncompliers. Further detection methods are desirable to positively identify the latter.

ASKING THE PATIENT

Although it is not always reliable, asking the patient directly about compliance can be a very valuable and practical way of determining the pattern of medication consumption (Table 26–1). When asked directly, about half of noncompliant patients will admit to missing at least some medication (Haynes et al., 1980). One can be assured that it is highly improbable that a *compliant* patient will admit to poor compliance, so patients admitting to missing medication have a very high likelihood of being poor compliers. The converse is not true, however, as even under optimal interview conditions about half of noncompliant patients will deny the fact. Patients who admit to missing medication generally overestimate the amount of medication they do take. In one study, the average overestimate was in the region of 20 per cent.

It must be emphasized that the method of questioning is of paramount importance. Asking in a threatening or belligerent manner will result in reflex denial. Approaching the patient with a face-saving, nonthreatening, nonjudgmental question will yield a higher proportion of accurate responses. One way of doing this is to use an approach such as the following, "Many people find it difficult to remember to take medicines: About how often do you forget yours?" Taking into account the tendency to overestimate compliance, admission of any noncompliance thus implies a compliance rate of less than 80 per cent or as low as 40 per cent on average.

The methods of detecting low compliance described so far can be easily applied in any treatment setting and, if applied with care, will detect the majority of poor compliers. The following methods may be of help in detecting some of the remainder.

Table 26–1. A SIMPLE METHOD TO DETECT NONCOMPLIANCE

Asking the Patient
The easiest way to detect medication noncompliance is to ask the patient.
About 50 per cent of noncompliant patients will admit to missing at least some medication.
If patients admit to noncompliance, you can believe them.
Patients admitting to poor compliance are most responsive to attempts to improve compliance.
How to Ask
Use a matter-of-fact, nonjudgmental, nonthreatening manner.
Use an introduction that allows a patient to save face: "Many people find it difficult to remember to take medicines: About how often do you forget yours?"

COUNTING PILLS

As a method of proving a quantitative estimate of compliance over a period of time, pill counts can be relatively reliable so long as they are carried out in the patient's home with strict attention to bookkeeping (Haynes et al., 1980). Unless the count can be carried out in such a manner that the patient is unaware of what is going on, it becomes a one-time-only procedure. It follows that while pill counts are very important research tools, they are not very practical for most clinical situations. It can be reasoned that using pill counts in the office or clinic will result in a bias in the direction of overestimating compliance in that patients will consciously or unconsciously only bring *some* of their unused pills with them, giving the appearance that they have taken more of the medication than is actually the case. It is virtually impossible for the bias to go in the opposite direction unless the patient is receiving the same prescriptions from two or more physicians at the same time.

In general, pill counts give higher estimates of compliance than quantitative drug assays and lower (but more accurate) estimates than patient self-reports.

DRUG LEVELS

A laboratory test to detect the presence or absence of good compliance is an unrealistic dream. But for some drugs, especially those with long serum half-lives resulting in relatively steady serum levels, the measurement of serum levels can be an extremely useful indication of compliance. The best examples of this are digoxin and phenytoin, for which plasma levels have been used successfully to both monitor compliance and improve it through feedback to the patient. Other drugs commonly measured in this way are phenobarbitone and other anticonvulsants, theophylline, tricyclic antidepressants, lithium, and a variety of cardiac drugs. The caution is, however, that there is a great deal of individual variation in drug absorption, metabolism, and excretion. In addition, serum levels of drugs with short half-lives only indicate how recently a dose was taken and give no information on long-term compliance.

Drug levels in urine have also been used as compliance indicators. For instance, the presence or absence of penicillin can be easily detected using inhibition of growth of a microorganism, *Sarcina lutea*. While these methods and others involving inactive markers such as riboflavin and carbon 14 have been used in research, they are not practical methods for the clinician. What is more, single qualitative assessments of urine samples have been shown to be inferior measures of compliance to simply asking the patient (Haynes et al., 1980).

Prevention and Treatment of Poor Compliance

MISCONCEPTIONS

Before discussing prevention and treatment, it is worthwhile to re-examine some popular misconceptions about compliance.

The first misconception is that a good clinician can identify poor compliers. In fact, clinical judgment has a poor record of detecting compliance levels. *There is no stereotypical poor complier.* This is very important, because restricting prevention and treatment strategies to patients thought to be potentially poor compliers must result in neglect of a large number of patients who need attention as well as unnecessary attention to some patients who do not require it.

Another popular and important misconception is that all that stops patients from being near-perfect compliers is their ignorance of either the condition being treated or the treatment being used. While there is some evidence that written instructions help improve compliance for short-term regimens, even mastery learning, in which patients were given detailed step-by-step instruction on hypertension, had no beneficial effect on long-term compliance (Sackett et al., 1975). The belief that it is possible to scare a patient into complying with treatment has also been dispelled (Leventhal et al., 1967).

Although these popular beliefs have been discredited, Logan (1978), in a survey of primary care physicians, has shown that the methods they employed to improve compliance were predominantly those that have been found lacking. What is more, methods that *have* been shown to be effective were not generally applied. Furthermore, changing the long-term behavior of physicians to manage compliance successfully cannot be done by simply informing or instructing them about efficacious interventions (Evans et al., 1984; Haynes et al., 1984).

PREVENTION

The main thrust in the prevention of poor compliance is to remove barriers to compliance. Preventing patients from dropping out from care is of primary importance. Longer waiting times are associated with higher no-show rates (Rockart and Hoffman, 1969) so that one aim is to keep patient waiting time to a minimum. Individual appointments at mutually convenient times help to achieve this goal. A system for follow-up, ensuring that patients leave the office with a *specific time* for a future appointment rather than with instructions to call for an appointment in, for example, 3 months, makes detection of those who do drop out much easier.

Simplifying the treatment regimen will remove another barrier to compliance. An essential element of this approach is to *eliminate unnecessary medications*. In addition, medications should be prescribed that need to be taken as few times daily as possible. The frequency of dosing with many drugs can be reduced below usually prescribed levels with no reduction in efficacy. For example, tricyclic antidepressants can be given as a single bedtime dose, thus reducing dosing frequency and timing side effects so that they occur mainly during sleep. A final strategy is to prescribe the least amount of medication necessary to achieve the therapeutic goal.

It has been shown that patients who feel that they are actively involved in their own care are better compliers than those who do not (Schulman, 1979). Studies have also shown that negotiating care with the patient rather than simply dictating or prescribing it results in better compliance (Eisenthal et al., 1979; Tracy, 1977). Encouraging patients to take greater responsibility for their care by asking more questions of their physicians results in improved attendance (Roter, 1977). It follows that encouraging patients to participate in and take more responsibility for their own care is another strategy for preventing poor compliance, and it not only makes scientific sense but follows contemporary trends in physician-patient relationships.

TREATMENT (Table 26–2)

Dropping out of care constitutes a *compliance crisis*. Mail and telephone reminders to increase attendance, at least in the short term, can help prevent dropout. If the patient does fail to attend, it calls for prompt action by the receptionist or office nurse to reschedule nonattenders (Takala et al., 1979). A simple method of identifying those patients for whom compliance is important, e.g., the use of chart stickers or special symbols on the day sheet, may make the receptionists's task simpler. Personal contact of persistent nonattenders by the physician himself and the use of outreach services such as public health nurses are other ways of "treating" nonattendance.

Table 26–2. KEYS TO SUCCESSFUL COMPLIANCE MANAGEMENT

Detection
Monitor attendance and achievement of the therapeutic goal.
Ask the patient.
Prevention
Make appointments convenient.
Simplify the regimen.
Give clear instructions, preferably written.
Make the patient an active participant.
Treatment
Follow up nonattenders.
increase attention and supervision.
Use cueing, feedback, and positive reinforcement.
Titrate frequency of visits to compliance need.
Involve spouse or other partner.
Maintain compliance interventions as long as compliance is desirable.

Low compliance is a chronic condition without a "one-shot" cure, so treatment of poor compliance must continue as long as the regimen of prescribed treatment. To make matters worse, none of the following has improved compliance when tested alone: special learning packages (Sackett et al., 1975) and pamphlets (Swain and Steckel, 1981); special unit dose reminder pill packaging (Becker et al., 1986); counseling about medication and compliance by a health educator (Levine et al., 1979) or by nurses (Shepard et al., 1979); visits to patients' homes (Johnson et al., 1978); provision of care at the worksite (Sackett et al., 1975); self-monitoring of blood pressure (Johnson et al., 1978; Shepard et al., 1979); tangible rewards (Shepard et al., 1979); and group discussions (Shepard et al., 1979). Although these tactics have not worked alone, many have been part of more complex interventions that have been successful; whether they are essential parts of these complex interventions or just along for the ride is difficult to say.

Most successful compliance interventions have two features in common: increased supervision of, or attention to, the patient; and intentional reinforcement, reward, or encouragement of compliance (Haynes, 1987).

A variety of inducements to comply have been used, including feedback of blood pressure response to hypertensive patients either by the provider (McKenney et al., 1973; Takala et al., 1979) or patients taking their own blood pressure (Haynes et al., 1976; Nessman et al., 1980); small tangible rewards for improved compliance and/or therapeutic response (Haynes et al., 1976; Shepard et al., 1979; Swain and Steckel, 1981); medication tailored to daily schedules to decrease forgetting and inconvenience (Haynes et al., 1976; Logan et al., 1979); encouragement of family support (Levine et al., 1979); stimulation of self-help through group support and discussion (Levine et al., 1979; Nessman et al., 1980); negotiation of a brief written contract with the patient to improve health behavior (Swain and Steckel, 1981); and calling back patients who miss appointments (Bass et al., 1986; Peterson et al., 1984; Takala et al., 1979).

It is important to note here that there are many individuals other than physicians who have taken an effective part in this process. In addition to physicians, nurses, pharmacists, health educators, a psychologist, and even an individual with no formal health training have played a key role in successful interventions.

In summary, the treatment of poor compliance involves many approaches. For short-term treatments, simple clear instructions are sufficient. For longer-term treatments, there must be follow-up of nonattenders by telephone or mailed reminders. In addition, the practitioner must increase attention to and supervision of poor compliers and provide rewards or positive reinforcement for good compliance that could include, among other simple maneuvers, simple praise and extending the time between appointments for those responding to treatment. Inui and colleagues (1976) have shown that most of these maneuvers can be incorporated with success into regular practice by simple focusing on compliance for a few moments during each encounter with the patient, emphasizing the importance of following the regimen and tailoring medication to daily routines. This can be accomplished without necessarily prolonging the visit. And, most important, it is clear that all compliance interventions applied to noncompliers must be maintained as long as treatment is prescribed.

ETHICAL ISSUES

"Am I my brother's keeper?" (Genesis 4:9). This question highlights the dilemma in which most physicians find themselves when they are pressed to extend their compliance-improving strategies beyond a simple office visit. As with most questions of ethics, there is no easy answer.

The decision to apply tactics deliberately designed to change the compliance behavior of patients should meet several ethical standards that apply to all therapeutic interventions (Levine, 1980). First, the diagnosis must be correct. Second, the therapy to be complied with must be of established efficacy. Third, neither the illness nor the proposed treatment should be trivial. Fourth, the patient must be an informed and willing partner in any attempt to alter his or her compliance. Finally, the method employed to improve compliance must also be of demonstrated effectiveness.

Having applied these standards and embarked upon a course of treatment, it makes no sense, ethically or otherwise, for the physician to abandon a patient at the first sign of poor compliance. Most physicians consider it *unethical* to withhold efficacious treatment from a patient with a serious physical disease. Why then should it be *ethical* to consider withholding treatment when the condition is *noncompliance*?

FUTURE TRENDS

The advent of the personal computer has resulted in increasing use of microcomputers and microcomputer networks in physicians' offices. While initial applications have been for business and office management purposes, the computerization of health records affords a potential for monitoring patient compliance and assisting in the management of poor compliers (Haynes and Walker, 1987).

Computerized appointment systems make it possible to provide patients with appointment times for long periods ahead and can easily be modified to flag nonattenders and produce automatic reminders. The ability to record age, sex, and diagnoses makes it possible to design a system that can improve *provider* compliance with screening and preventive maneuvers (Bypass et al., 1988). Medication systems that store prescribing information can form the basis of a system that monitors whether patients are at least requesting prescription refills on time (Steiner et al., 1988). The potential is great, but it will require both effort and expense by physicians to make it work.

What of other advancements? The technology that brought us the efficacious treatments is also helping with compliance—drugs with long half-lives, long-acting parenteral preparations, conjunctival inserts, continuous transcutaneous absorption. The next, but perhaps more disturbing, stage could be the use of high technology. An artificial pancreas is under development and will not only dispense insulin but adjust the dose according to blood levels. What is to stop the development of implanted arterial pressure sensors with automatic dispensing of parenteral antihypertensives? These thoughts make concerns about telephoning nonattenders seem trifling.

Conclusion

In dealing with compliance, we have consciously concentrated on compliance with medication, emphasizing long-term medications. This is not because we feel that compliance with short-term medications is inconsequential or that there is no problem of compliance with life-style or other behavioral changes. On the contrary, both of these areas are very important and, in fact, noncompliance with life-style changes is a monster yet to be tamed.

It is our hope that we have raised the level of compliance consciousness in the reader. Being aware of the problem and the difficulties in detecting it are essential before any treatment can be carried out.

The approaches to treatment we suggest are practical and well within the reach of practicing physicians. At last, after centuries of ineffectual ministrations, we have treatments that actually work; it behooves us as providers of those treatments to give them every opportunity to be effective.

The past decade, more than any other, has brought the therapist together with the patient, the family, and other members of the health care team in jointly working towards the full effectiveness of potent treatments. The rewards of this alliance are great—reduction of morbidity, disability, and preventable deaths. The family physician is in an ideal position to share in these rewards.

References

Bass, M. J., McWhinney, I. R., and Donner, A.: Do family physicians need medical assistants to detect and manage hypertension? Can. Med. Assoc. J., *134*:1247–1255, 1986. *A randomized trial of medical assistants in community-based family practice.*

Becker, L. A., Glanz, K., Sobel, E., et al.: A randomized trial of special packaging of antihypertensive medications. J. Fam.

Pract. 22:357–361, 1986. *A study of foil-backed blister packaging compared to regular medication vials. No significant difference in blood pressure control or compliance.*

Becker, M. H.: Sociobehavioral determinants of compliance. *In* Sackett, D. L., and Haynes, R. B. (Eds.): Compliance with Therapeutic Regimens. Baltimore, Johns Hopkins University Press, 1976, pp. 40–49.

Best, J. A., and Block, M.: Compliance in the control of cigarette smoking. *In* Haynes, R. B., Taylor, D. W., and Sackett, D. L. (Eds.): Compliance in Health Care. Baltimore, John Hopkins University Press, 1979, pp. 202–222. *An extensive review of strategies employed in attempting to modify smoking behavior.*

Bypass, P., Hanlon, P. W., Hanlon, L. C. S., et al.: Microcomputer management of a vaccine trial. Comput. Biol. Med. *18*:179–193, 1988. *A study involving a microcomputer for call and recall of infants due for vaccination in a trial of rotavirus vaccine in Africa.*

Closson, R., and Kikugawa, C.: Non-compliance varies with drug class. Hospitals, *49*:89, 1975. *A study in a Veterans Administration population.*

Cody, J., and Robinson, A.: The effect of low-cost maintenance medication on the rehospitalization of schizophrenic outpatients. Am. J. Psych., *134*:73, 1977.

Eisenthal, S., Emery, R., Lazare, A., et al.: "Adherence" and the negotiated approach to patienthood. Arch. Gen Psych., *36*:393, 1979.

Ettlinger, P. R. A., and Freeman, G. K.: General practice compliance study: Is it worth being a personal doctor? Br. Med. J., *282*:1192, 1981. *A general practice study involving two group practices. Compliance with antimicrobial prescription was assessed at an unannounced home visit and was found to be strongly associated with whether the patient thought that he knew the prescribing doctor well.*

Evans, C. E., Haynes, R. B., Birkett, N. J., et al.: Does a mailed continuing education program improve physician performance? Results of a randomized trial in antihypertensive care. J.A.M.A. *255*:501–504, 1984. *A population-based study of the effect of mailed continuing medical education material on hypertension treatment and control.*

Francis, V., Korsch, B. M., and Morris, M. J.: Gaps in doctor-patient communication. N. Engl. J. Med., *280*:535, 1969. *Pediatric patient population. The effects of doctor-patient communication on patient/parent satisfaction, reassurance, and compliance were assessed.*

Gilbert, J. R., Evans, C. E., Haynes, R. B., et al.: Predicting compliance with a regimen of digoxin therapy in a family practice. Can. Med. Assoc. J., *123*:119, 1980. *This study involved 10 family physicians who were asked to predict the compliance of randomly selected patients on digoxin. Compliance was assessed by pill counts, serum levels, and patient report.*

Glick, B. S.: Dropout in an outpatient, double-blind drug study. Psychosomatics, *6*:44, 1965.

Haynes, R. B.: Determinants of compliance: The disease and the mechanics of treatment. *In* Haynes, R. B., Taylor, D. W., and Sackett, D. L. (Eds.): Compliance in Health Care. Baltimore, Johns Hopkins University Press, 1979, pp. 49–62. *A review of factors that have been studied in relation to their influence on compliance.*

Haynes, R. B., Davis, D. A., McKibbon, A., et al.: A critical appraisal of the efficacy of continuing medical education. J.A.M.A., *251*:61–64, 1984.

Haynes, R. B., Sackett, D. L., and Taylor, D. W.: Practical management of low compliance with antihypertensive therapy: A guide for the busy practitioner. Clin. Invest. Med., *1*:175, 1979. *A "how to do it" review.*

Haynes, R. B., Mattson, M. E., Chobanian, A. V., et al.: Management of patient compliance in the treatment of hypertension. Hypertension, *4*:415, 1982.

Haynes, R. B., Sackett, D. L., Gibson, E. S., et al.: Improvement of medication compliance in uncontrolled hypertension. Lancet, *1*:1265, 1976. *Report of a randomized control trial of a behaviorally oriented strategy for improving compliance, including blood pressure, self-monitoring, and tailoring treatment to daily habits.*

Haynes, R. B., Taylor, D. W., Sackett, D. L., et al.: Can simple clinical measurements detect patient non-compliance? Hypertension, *2*:757, 1980. *A comparison of several methods of measuring compliance with antihypertensive medication including pill counts, urine drug levels, patient self-reports, changes in uric acid and potassium, and blood pressure response.*

Haynes, R. B., and Walker, C. J.: Computer-aided quality assurance: A critical appraisal. Arch. Intern. Med., *147*:1297–1301, 1987.

Haynes, R. B., Wang, E., Gomes, M. D.: A critical review of interventions to improve compliance with prescribed medications. Patient Educ. Counseling, *10*:155–166, 1987. *A review of scientifically sound investigations testing strategies intended to improve compliance.*

Inui, T., Yourtee, E., and Williamson, J.: Improved outcomes in hypertension after physician tutorials. Ann. Intern. Med., *84*:646, 1976. *Report of the effect of tutorials for physicians on the compliance of their hypertensive patients in a general medical outpatient clinic.*

Janz, N., and Becker, M.: The health belief model: A decade later. Health Educ. Q., *11*:1–47, 1984.

Johnson, A. L., Taylor, D. W., Sackett, D. L., et al.: Self-recording of blood pressure in the management of hypertension. Can. Med. Assoc. J., *119*:1034, 1978.

Kincey, J., Bradshaw, P., and Ley, P.: Patients' satisfaction and reported acceptance of advice in general practice. J. R. Coll. Gen. Pract., *25*:558, 1975. *A general practice study evaluating patients' satisfaction with medical advice and the relationship between satisfaction and compliance.*

Latiolais, C. J., Berry, C. C.: Misuse of prescription medication by outpatients. Drug Intell Clin Pharmacy 1969; *3*:270–277.

Leventhal, H., Watts, J., and Pagano, F.: Effects of fear and instructions on how to cope with danger. J Pers Soc Psychol 1967; *6*:313–321.

Leventhal, H., Zimmerman, R., Gutman, M.: Compliance: A self-regulation perspective. *In*: Gentry, D. (Ed.): Handbook of Behavioral Medicine. New York, Pergamon Press, 1984, pp. 369–434.

Leventhal, H., and Cameron, L.: Behavioral theories and the problem of compliance. Patient Educ. Counseling, *10*:117–138, 1987. *An excellent review of behavioral theories related to compliance, outlining the strengths and deficiencies of each.*

Levine, D. M., Green, L. W., Deeds, S. G., et al.: Health education for hypertensive patients. J.A.M.A., *241*:1700, 1979.

Levine, R. J.: Ethical considerations in the development and application of compliance strategies for the treatment of hypertension. *In*: Haynes, R. B., Matteson, M. E., and Engebretson, T. O., Jr. (Eds.): Patient Compliance to Prescribed Antihypertensive Regimens. Washington, D.C., U.S. Department of Health and Human Services, N.I.H. Publication No. 81–2102, 1980, pp. 229–246.

Logan, A. S.: Investigation of Toronto general practitioners' treatment of patients with hypertension. Canadian Facts, Toronto, 1978.

Logan, A. S., Milne, B. J., Achber, C., et al.: Worksite treatment of hypertension by specially trained nurses: A controlled trial. Lancet, *2*:1175, 1979.

McKenney, J. M., Slining, J. M., Henderson, H. R., et al.: The effect of clinical pharmacy services on patients with essential hypertension. Circulation, *48*:1104, 1973. *A controlled study of the use of clinical pharmacists who educated patients, monitored blood pressure control, and assisted in the management of questions and problems that arose.*

Nessman, D. G., Carnahan, J. E., and Nugent, C. A.: Improving compliance: Patient-operated hypertension groups. Arch. Intern. Med., *140*:1427, 1980.

Peterson, G. M., McLean, S., and Millingen, K. S.: A randomized trial of strategies to improve patient compliance with anticonvulsant therapy. Epilepsia, *25*(4):412–417, 1984. *A randomized study of a combination of patient counseling, special medication containers, self-recording of medication intake and seizures, and mailed reminders to collect prescription refills and attend clinic appointments.*

Rickels, K., Boren, R., and Stuart, H. M.: Controlled psycho-

pharmacological research in general practice. J. New Drugs, *4*:138, 1964.
Rockart, J. F., and Hoffman, P. B.: Physician and patient behavior under different scheduling systems in a hospital outpatient department. Med. Care, *7*:463, 1969. *A descriptive study of patient mean arrival time, waiting time, and no-show rate and of physician mean arrival time at several outpatient departments using different scheduling methods.*
Roter, D.: Patient participation in the patient-provider interaction: The effects of patient question asking on the quality of interaction, satisfaction and compliance. Health Educ. Monogr., *5*:281, 1977.
Sackett, D. L., Haynes, R. B., Gibson, E. S., et al.: Randomized clinical trial of strategies for improving medication compliance in primary hypertension. Lancet, *1*:1205, 1975. *An evaluation of the effect on compliance of treatment at the worksite and of a special education program about new hypertensives.*
Sackett, D. L.: Introduction. *In* Sackett, D. L., Haynes, R. B. (Eds.): Compliance with Therapeutic Regimens. Baltimore, Johns Hopkins University Press, 1976, p. 1.
Schulman, B.: Active patient orientation and outcomes in hypertensive treatment. Med. Care, *17*:267, 1979.
Shepard, D. S., Foster, S. B., Stason, W. B., et al.: Cost-effectiveness of interventions to improve compliance with antihypertensive therapy. Prev. Med., *8*:229, 1979.
Steiner, J. F., Koepsall, T. D., Fihn, S. D., et al.: A general method of compliance assessment using centralized pharmacy records: Description and validation. Med. Care, *26*(8):814–823, 1988. *A comparison of central pharmacy records with serum drug levels and patient outcomes.*
Swain, M. A., and Steckel, S. B.: Influencing adherence among hypertensives. Res Nurs Health 1981; *4*:213–218.
Takala, J., Niemela, N., Rosti, J., and Sivers, K.: Improving compliance with therapeutic regimens in hypertensive patients in a community health center. Circulation, *59*:540, 1979. *A controlled trial of a very practical approach to improving compliance in primary care, including written directions, called back nonattenders, and feeding back blood pressure levels at visits.*
Tracy, J.: Impact of intake procedures upon client attrition in a community mental health centre. J. Consult. Clin. Psychol., *45*:192, 1977.
Willcox, D. R., Gillan, R., and Hare, E. H.: Do psychiatric outpatients take their drugs? Br. Med. J., *2*:790, 1965.

27

Patient Education

Donna R. Falvo
Donald A. Bosshart

Patient Education

Patient education, as a distinct component of quality medical care, has received increased recognition from practicing physicians over the last decade. Giving patients information about their health and treatment of course isn't a new concept. Physicians have been giving instructions to patients since medical practice began. As medical practice has changed in complexity and sophistication, however, so has the focus and need for effective patient education.

In earlier days, when much of medical care took place in patients' homes, information was based on the physician's experience with and exposure to patients in their home environment. Information given was intuitively derived from observation of patients and their families in the home and from an intimate knowledge of the social context of patients within the community. Most patients were unsophisticated in matters of health and disease and looked to the physician as the major authority in health care matters. Little could be done to prevent or to combat the progression of many diseases. Consequently, neither patient nor physician had much control over health outcomes. Patient teaching was often as much a matter of providing hope and support as it was directing patients toward cure or control of disease. Scientific and technologic advances have changed medical practice considerably. Infectious diseases about which little was empirically known are largely now nonexistent in western cultures or can be prevented and cured. Morbidity and mortality have changed significantly. Major health concerns now focus largely on chronic, degenerative health problems that carry with them a tremendous physical, emotional, and financial cost. Consequently, today, information given to patients by physicians takes on even greater importance.

RATIONALE FOR PATIENT EDUCATION

As a result of the increasing complexity of medical care, medical practice has shifted from patients' homes to the physician's office. Information and insight about patients, their family, and their environment, which previously helped physicians determine patient education needs, are not as readily available. The amount, scope, and breadth of information patients need to understand and to manage their condition is also more complex.

Patient Factors

Patients have become more sophisticated about health care. As a result of the consumer movement and the self-help movement, patients no longer look to physicians as the ultimate authority in health care matters. Rather than being passive recipients of medical care, patients often expect or demand information about and involvement in medical care they receive. Patient satisfaction has been linked to the patients' perceptions that their informational needs have been met by physicians (Falvo, et al., 1980; Francis, et al., 1969; Korsch, et al., 1968). The Patient's Bill of Rights, adopted by the American Hospital Association in 1973, states:

> *The patient has the right to obtain from his physician complete current information concerning his diagnosis, treatment, and prognosis in terms the patient can reasonably understand*
>
> AMERICAN HOSPITAL ASSOCIATION, 1975

The Patient's Bill of Rights has since been accepted by a number of professional associations, including the American Medical Association (American Medical Association, 1975).

Legal Factors

The doctrine of informed consent, although often only thought of as a formal agreement between physicians and patients before a procedure is performed, has a broader meaning that is increasingly being enforced. Patient education is now more consistently thought of as a necessary part of quality patient care. The doctrine imposes a legal obligation on physicians to assure that patients understand their condition and treatment as well as risks and benefits of following or not following treatment recommendations. This includes information about conditions, prescriptions, or tests that once may have been considered too routine to discuss. But now such discussion is considered the physician's responsibility. Physicians can now be held legally responsible for acts of omission or commission with regard to education of patients and their families. Physicians' legal responsibilities to adequately educate patients was substantiated in a ruling in an Iowa Court in 1974 when the court ruled that a physician who had failed to advise a patient adequately could be tried for negligence (Krosnick, 1974).

Economic Factors

The containment of medical costs has become a national imperative. Patient education is one way physicians can limit the cost of care. Many harmful effects of disease and other potentially disabling conditions are preventable or treatable, yet patients continue to be incapacitated or disabled by conditions for which effective treatments are available. Although a variety of factors can explain this phenomenon, one simple explanation is that a large number of patients simply do not follow physicians' recommendations. Noncompliance can produce substantial adverse effects on quality and cost of care. Some noncompliance is a result of poor patient education that does not clearly outline what patients are to do or outline the potential benefits of therapies or preventive measures. Although knowledge alone does not guarantee compliance, patients cannot follow instructions that they do not understand or that they are unable to carry out. Spending sufficient time educating patients about their condition and treatment, identifying barriers that prevent patients from following treatment recommendations, and making appropriate alterations in treatment recommendations might help to obviate many factors that contribute to patient noncompliance.

SHARED RESPONSIBILITY FOR PATIENT EDUCATION

The foundation of patient education includes philosophic, legal, economic, and practical components. Although patient education can be a means of patient support, it also provides patients with information they need and, often expect, to prevent or control disease. Patient education can create an atmosphere of shared responsibility between patients and physicians, providing patients with a basis on which to make choices about their health and health care.

Physicians have the responsibility of giving patients accurate, appropriate information about care and treatment. Patients also have the major responsibility for carrying out that plan of care. Actively involving patients in decisions about their care and treatment communicates this attitude of shared responsibility. (See section on Patient Advisory Councils at the end of this chapter.) Given this situation, skills in patient education are fundamental to effective office practice. In order for patient teaching to be most effective, it must be more than simply transferring information or facts. It must also facilitate learning and problem solving, helping patients to clarify issues and reach decisions that are compatible with their own priorities and life styles. Initiatives in patient education should be directed toward maintaining and maximizing the well state, preventing the likelihood of illness, and helping patients make the required changes in life styles or activities.

PATIENT EDUCATION IN CLINICAL ENCOUNTERS

The most important strategy for teaching effectiveness is creating an atmosphere that encourages active patient involvement. By far the most frequent patient teaching occurs during one-to-one interaction with a physician. Without an effective start in this patient teaching arena, all other strategies and supporting instructional materials become superfluous. The physicians' role and influence in conducting effective one-to-one patient teaching is absolutely critical.

Patient education is most frequently an exchange between patients and physicians during a regular clinical encounter. The goal of patient teaching in this setting, as well as in any other, is to communicate knowledge, skills, and attitudes to patients with the hope that they will be incorporated and put to use. Merely giving information to patients is insufficient. To be effective, information must be presented in a way that makes it relevant and comprehensive. This means physicians must not only identify the information needs of individual patients but also consider patients' feelings, perceptions, and motivation. Goals for patient education should be realistic and appropriate for individual patients. If expectations are unrealistic and goals not feasible, the result can be disillusionment and disappointment for both parties.

Viewed in this context, patient education requires the same problem-solving skills as any other clinical intervention. Just as diagnosis is not made without first gathering sufficient data on which to base the diagnosis, patient education cannot be conducted effectively without first gathering information about the individual patient to whom the teaching is to be directed. Just as the same treatment may not be prescribed for all patients with the same condition, neither can all patients with the same condition receive the same type of information. A simple way to assess patients' views is by asking questions such as:

1. What do you think the problem might be?
2. What do you think may be causing the problem?
3. Do you know anyone else with a similar problem? If so, what happened?

Patients' responses to these questions can give physicians insight into patients' reasoning and approaches to their illness.

The type and amount of information given depends on the needs, interest, and circumstances of the patient. Conducting patient education in this manner need not be a time-consuming process. Studies indicate that physicians devote about one fourth of their time with patients in the office, giving information and counseling about a variety of health matters (Flynn, 1980) yet often these efforts are ineffective (Cassileth, 1980). In most instances, this doesn't mean that more time should be spent conducting patient teaching. It may, however, mean that there are ways to conduct patient education in a more efficient and effective manner.

TIPS FOR EFFECTIVE PATIENT EDUCATION

Creating an Atmosphere of Acceptance

Patient education is most dependent upon the effective exchange of information. This is most readily accomplished if the physician has the ability to make patients feel cared for and respected as individuals. The degree to which patients feel comfortable sharing information about themselves, as well as their receptivity to information given them by physicians, is determined to a great extent by an atmosphere of acceptance and understanding. The quality of the relationship can have a significant impact on the outcome of treatment and on the patients' abilities and willingness to carry out recommendations.

Establishing such an atmosphere implies that physicians are able to accept patients' views, although different from their own, and that they are able to communicate a nonjudgmental attitude. Acceptance is not synonymous with approval. An attitude of acceptance does, however, establish an atmosphere in which patients can openly share feelings and concerns. Physicians must also be able to communicate an understanding of patients' concerns. Understanding is demonstrated by the physician's ability to grasp patients' perspectives and to interpret the meaning of their words and behavior accurately. In order to demonstrate acceptance and understanding, physicians must be attentive to what patients say, not only in terms of words, and ideas but also in terms of what patients may be expressing through their behavior.

Initiating Patient Education

In general, patient education should be conducted any time the need arises. There are instances when a time should be set aside specifically for patient education, such as at the time of initial diagnosis or any time patients are given treatment recommendations. There are, however, opportunities for patient education in every clinical encounter. Seizing these opportunities can help set the stage for additional information and help physicians assess a patient's general level of understanding and concern. For example, patients may be given explanations of findings while a physical examination is being performed. Although additional or more detailed information may be given after the examination is completed, giving information during the examination requires little additional time and establishes a basis for patient understanding of any treatment recommendations that may later be warranted.

Patient education may also be initiated when a patient's need for information is unexpectedly identified. For example, although a middle-aged woman may be seen for evaluation of a sore throat, if during the visit she asks in passing about screening mammography, the physician has an additional opportunity to conduct patient teaching. Being sensitive to a patient's information needs takes little additional time. Such sensitivity also helps to establish additional trust and rapport with patients that, in turn, increases the probability that they will feel more at ease asking for information in the future.

In other instances, physicians may identify the need for additional information. For example, although a child may present at the clinic for evaluation of otitis media, if at the same time the physician notes from the chart that the child's immunizations are not up to date, an additional need for patient education has been identified. In other instances, the physician may identify age-related learning needs of patients. For example, performing a routine school physical on a preadolescent patient may also provide the physician an opportunity to discuss changes to be anticipated during puberty. Performing a routine work physical also provides physicians with the opportunity to evaluate patients' life-style practices and to conduct teaching about the value of routine exercise.

Patient education need not take place in a formal teaching setting in order to be effective. Every interaction with patients is an opportunity for patient teaching. When teaching is a routine part of an office visit, or medical procedure, there is no reason to delimit the teaching portion of the interaction. Under these circumstances, patient education becomes a normal part of communication between physicians and patients. Even under these circumstances, however, the need for presentation of information in a clear, organized manner based on a patient's level of need and receptivity should not be minimized.

Determining when to conduct patient education

is dependent on the physician's ability to accurately assess the patient's physical and emotional state. Patients who are physically uncomfortable or in pain will be distracted, and even the most organized presentation of information will be ineffective. Patients who are upset or anxious because of their diagnosis, or because of other circumstances, will not hear, much less incorporate, the information that the physician has given. In these instances, a more effective approach to patient education would be to reschedule patient teaching at a later date or to return to patient teaching at a time when the patient is more receptive. In instances when patient education cannot wait, physicians should prioritize the information, giving crucial information first and arranging for additional information to be given at a later time. When the patient is not receptive to receiving information that is necessary for their well-being, the physician should include family members who can assist in carrying out the care.

Quantifying Information Given

Not all patients need or want the same amount of information. There is no need to present information that patients already know. Presenting information that patients do not feel is needed is unproductive. In order to conduct patient education most efficiently and effectively, physicians must be able to assess the patient's information needs and tailor the presentation appropriately.

In general, all patients should be given sufficient information to have a working understanding of their condition and treatment as well as an understanding of possible consequences of following or not following medical advice. Overly detailed information may confuse some patients, while information that is too sparse may not provide them with sufficient information to carry out medical advice. Patients who are more medically knowledgable may want more detailed information while other patients may only want rudimentary details. Coercing patients into receiving information they are not ready to receive or in which they are disinterested serves no purpose other than to frustrate physicians and alienate patients.

When determining the amount of information the patient should be given, physicians should ask themselves:

1. What information does the patient need in order to be able to follow the treatment recommendations?
2. What information does the patient currently possess?
3. What is the patient's level of interest/receptivity?
4. How much information is the patient able to retain at one time?

Assessing Patient Needs

Much objective and subjective information about patients can be gained during the routine clinic visit. Observation of a patient's appearance, posture, facial expression, and reactions to information can tell physicians much about their emotional and physical state and, consequently, about their readiness to receive information.

Through simple verbal interchange, physicians can gain insight into a patient's potential learning capabilities by noting language structure and level of communication. Through this same interchange, physicians can determine anger, anxiety, or sadness from a patient's tone of voice as well as from words spoken. Through casual conversation, physicians may begin to note clues about life styles, support systems, attitude, feelings about their condition, and treatment as well as about their receptivity to patient education. Identifying patients' particular fears or concerns about their condition or treatment can be extremely important.

Although some assessment of patient needs may involve formal interviews, skilled observation can be a valuable tool when combined with other sources of data such as the medical record. Information can be obtained from patients any time there is contact, such as while preparing patients for an exam, during procedures, or during the physical examination. Assessing the patient's information needs in the normal context of patient care requires no extra time.

Gaining Patient Cooperation

Physicians may not perceive medical recommendations as being difficult or unreasonable to carry out; however, patients may view them in quite a different light. To conduct education without considering the impact of the recommendations on patients' lives is to discount the patient's point of view. Values held by the physician may not be the same as those held by the patient. Recommendations that seem simple to the physician may be overwhelming to patients initially or when patients are trying to implement them. Patient education outcomes held as ideal by physicians may not be outcomes that patients value.

The degree to which patients are willing to follow recommended regimens is related somewhat to their perception of the cost associated with following instructions. Cost, to patients, takes the form of financial cost as well as the cost of pain, discomfort, loss of function, and loss of self-esteem. This evaluation of cost by patients is subjective. A patient's assessment of their physician's recommendations are made in terms of their own lives and the impact that following or not following recommendations might have.

Physicians should be aware of the problems or perceptions patients may have with regard to the recommendations given. Lecturing patients, attempting to coerce cooperation by use of fear, or threatening patients with abandonment does little to gain cooperation and can alienate them. A physician's best tact, when patient views differ, may be to investigate other medically accepted alternatives to the recommended treatment. In so doing, physicians communicate understanding and concern for patients' positions that may, in turn, facilitate patient cooperation. Without such flexibility additional time and effort conducting patient education is both inefficient and ineffective. Even though patients may be able to regurgitate information given, such regurgitation doesn't guarantee that recommendations will be followed.

Maintaining the flexibility that considers patients' needs, perceptions, and feelings does not mean that patients determine all of their own treatment recommendations. Instead, maintaining flexibility emphasizes shared responsibility in which patient and physician discuss potential compromises in order to reach mutually acceptable goals, with each maintaining their own particular standards. Some medical conditions or some circumstances will preclude compromise. The most productive means for handling these situations may be for the physician to accept the fact that the patient will not follow the regimen recommended. Efforts can then be devoted toward working with the patient in areas of the treatment regimen in which there is cooperation. In so doing, the physician is able to continue to monitor the patient's progress, remaining available to answer questions and offering alternatives when and if the patient is ready to accept them. This approach does not necessarily demonstrate the physician's approval of the patient's behavior. Physicians may still be honest with patients about why they feel the recommendations should be followed. Respecting patients' points of view, however, keeps channels of communication open, enhancing the possibility of further education and influence.

Physicians should be realistic in relaying consequences of following or not following instructions. Reasons for following instructions should be based on facts rather than making promises based on personal bias or conjecture. For example, a statement such as "If you don't stop smoking, you'll die of lung cancer" is ineffective in persuading patients to quit smoking. The patient has only to know one other person who has smoked heavily and didn't develop lung cancer in order to dispute the statement. A more effective way to approach the problem may be a statement, such as, "Given the information we have at this time, the chances of developing lung cancer are increased considerably by smoking." The information is conveyed to the patient in a factual and unbiased way that cannot be easily dismissed or challenged.

Using the Family as a Resource

Patients' families are also of central importance in patient education. It is important to assess how patients define their own family unit rather than making assumptions about traditional family organization. How the family functions has an influence on the health of its members as well as on how individuals react to illness and treatment recommendations. A physician's ability to effectively teach patients to maintain or restore health also depends upon understanding patients' relationships with their families.

In many instances, involving families in patient education can enhance communication between patients and physicians. Family members can help to clarify information patients may have difficulty understanding. Facilitating discussion between family members may be beneficial throughout the course of patient management.

Physicians should capitalize on assistance from family members who can be a source of support. However, physicians should also remember that not all families can or do provide the needed support and encouragement. Families may undermine recommendations. In the case of chronic illness, some families may not have the emotional stability to cope with changes the illness has brought about, much less with the recommendations prescribed.

When teaching patients and families, it is important to identify patterns of relationships and attitudes of family members. One way physicians can assess these attitudes and relationships is by asking questions, such as:

1. Who have you talked with about your symptoms (problem)?
2. What did they say?
3. Who do you generally turn to for help?

Physicians may also ask family members questions such as:

1. What do you believe is causing the symptoms (problem)?
2. What are your major concerns?
3. What can be done to help?

Identifying resources and helping family members to mobilize their resources so treatment recommendations may be followed is a crucial part of patient education. It is also important to remember, however, that the purpose of including families in patient education is to gain their support, not to remove responsibility from patients.

Physicians should be alert to family receptivity to patient education. Apprehension or resistance to learning about patients' conditions or treatments may have implications for the degree of support patients will receive from family members when attempting to follow the treatment recommendations. In these instances, physicians must either help families deal with their anxiety or consider other resources to be used in helping patients follow the treatment recommendations.

Family members who are anxious and under stress may have a tendency to misunderstand or misinterpret what they are told. Family members may distort information, turning it into what they want to hear. Such occurrences can cause conflict between patients and their families and can interfere with follow through of treatment recommendations. Physicians should give information in a positive way and should help family members develop realistic expectations.

PITFALLS IN PATIENT EDUCATION

Using Fear to Motivate

Although fear and anxiety at certain levels can be motivating, at certain levels they can also be immobilizing. Severe anxiety can lead to denial. When the following or not following of instructions seems critical to a patient's well-being, physicians may be tempted to use threat and fear arousal in an attempt to motivate patients to follow recommendations. Studies indicate, however, that as the degree of fear is increased, adherence to recommendations decreases (Leventhal, 1970; Leventhal, et al., 1965). Fear arousal can raise patients' anxiety levels to a degree that they deny that the threat exists in order to protect themselves from increased anxiety. As a result, patients may totally ignore health advice rather than admitting the seriousness of their condition. Use of fear as a strategy in patient education to gain cooperation is usually ineffective.

Using Jargon

Giving patients information in language they cannot understand is an inefficient use of time and is also unlikely to achieve the desired results. The patients' educational levels are frequently not an indication of their grasp of medical terminology. Often, physicians assume patients understand medical terminology when they do not. Whenever possible, physicians should use lay terms and analogies when giving explanations. In some situations, using lay terms in conjunction with medical terms is a way of teaching medical terminology as well as avoiding the appearance of talking down to patients. For example, explanation of an arteriogram may include a statement, such as, "This test will help us to determine the degree of *stenosis* or *narrowing* of the vessels." This technique serves to acquaint patients with the medical terminology while still conveying the content of the message.

Making Assumptions

Assumptions about a patient's understanding of his or her condition or treatment should not be based solely on that individual's previous experience. Although some patients may have had a similar condition in the past or had similar treatment prescribed, physicians cannot assume that patients were given correct information in the past or that they correctly interpreted information they were given. A patient's level of understanding and interpretation of his or her condition and treatment should always be assessed before determining whether or not additional patient education is necessary.

Giving Vague Instructions

The more specific instructions are, the greater the probability that patients will follow them accurately. Although physicians may believe they are being clear in their explanation, the information may still not be sufficient to convey understanding. Instructions, such as, "Cut down on the cholesterol in your diet," are of little help if patients are unaware of specific foods that are high in cholesterol. Likewise, vague instructions—for example, "avoid heavy lifting,"—may be interpreted in different ways. In order to enhance the possibility that patients will follow instructions accurately, instructions should be as specific as possible. For example, instead of instructing patients to "take the medication four times a day," specific times the medication is to be taken should be given. Specific instructions prevent another interpretation of the treatment recommendations: "The medication is to be taken four times a day—at 6 in the morning, 12 noon, 6 in the evening, and 12 midnight." As another example, before instructing patients to take medication before meals, there should be clarification of how often meals are consumed. Patients eating only one meal a day may perceive that they are following recommendations accurately when, in fact, they are not following them within the actual context of the physician's recommendation.

The more specific physicians can be in giving patients information, the more likely patients are to have a clear understanding of what they are to do and the more likely they are to carry out instructions accurately.

Failing to Check Understanding

Throughout the teaching interaction, a patient's understanding and interpretation of the information presented should be evaluated. Patients should be encouraged to ask questions. A simple question—"Are there points I have made that are not clear, or that you would like to talk about some more?"—give patients the opportunity to clarify any information of which they are uncertain.

Checking for a patient's understanding of information before he or she leaves the office is crucial if recommendations are to be followed accurately. It is insufficient to merely ask patients, "Do you understand what you are to do?" Not only is such a question likely to result in an affirmative response regardless of the level of understanding, but patients may believe they understood the recommendations when, in actuality, they did not. Asking patients to repeat or to paraphrase the information they have been given takes little time and can reveal significant information gaps or misconceptions. This provides the opportunity for immediate correction or reinforcement of the information. Physicians can assess a patient's level of understanding in a short amount of time without being condescending with a simple statement: "Just so I can be sure that I've been clear about the information I've given you, would you repeat back in your own words what you are to do?"

USING INSTRUCTIONAL AIDS

There are numerous instructional materials in the form of pamphlets, audiovisual aids, and fact sheets that physicians can use to supplement information given to patients in the one-to-one interaction. The effectiveness of these instructional materials as teaching aids, however, is dependent upon their appropriate use.

Teaching aids should be used only to reinforce information given by physicians, not as a replacement for personal interaction. Instructional materials are most effective if patients view them as an extension of information given to them by physicians rather than as a substitute. Information presented in instructional materials should be consistent and complementary to the information given by physicians. Physicians should also remember that just as they are responsible for the accuracy of information given to patients verbally so are they responsible for content contained within instructional aids used. Consequently, physicians should take time to choose instructional aids carefully, reviewing and updating them periodically.

Using Material Effectively

In order to be an effective teaching aid in patient education, instructional materials need not be elaborate or costly. Often, simple written instructions or simple drawings may be sufficient depending on the needs of the patient.

The same type of instructional material may not be appropriate for all patients with the same disease or problem. Instructional materials should be geared to the reading and comprehension level of the patient and perhaps family members. The type of instructional materials chosen for office practice should be based on the patient population served and by the conditions that occur most frequently. Because of the number of materials available, there are significant advantages of creating a system for determining what materials will be used on a regular basis in the practice. If the number of materials is not limited, there is high probability that materials will be distributed sporadically, creating a less than optimal effect. The number of instructional materials possessed is not nearly as important as the quality and applicability of the material to the specific situation.

The manner in which instructional materials are used is often as important, if not more important, as the instructional material itself. Patients will take the instructional material more seriously if physicians take time to point out major areas in the material that are of particular importance. An example of appropriate presentation of instructional material might be the following statement: "This pamphlet outlines some of the things we've talked about today. In particular, it lists the foods we talked about that you should avoid. I'd like you to take this home with you as a reminder of our discussion. If there are things you're still not clear about after reviewing the pamphlet, please feel free to give me or my nurse a call."

The statement clarifies how the patient is to use the instructional material and also serves as reassurance that the information contained in it is consistent with the information received from the physician. The statement also communicates openness to further questions if the material contained within the pamphlet is unclear. It is often helpful to place the physician's name and phone number on the material in the event of questions.

Choosing Professionally Developed Instructional Aids

A variety of professionally developed instructional materials are available at variable cost. Commercially prepared written materials are frequently less expensive if purchased in large quantities. Many excellent written materials may be obtained free of charge from local or national voluntary organizations or from governmental or private sources. The most expensive instructional aids are not necessarily the best. More important are the materials' accuracy, consistency, and the likelihood that patients can understand the information contained within.

Written material should be structured in a logical way that patients are able to follow. In general, written material should be presented in sequence, starting with simple concepts and moving to more complex issues. Subheadings that separate major content areas may be useful in helping patients understand one concept before moving on to another. When assessing written instructional aids, physicians should also consider readability for the majority of patients in their practice. In general, written materials will be more useful if sentences are short and simple, using common words rather than medical jargon. Usually, the longer and more complicated the written aid, the less likely patients are to read or understand it. Physicians can obtain professional guidance about the readability of materials by consulting junior high or high school teachers or librarians.

Visual aids can be helpful in illustrating points, especially for patients who are unfamiliar with various anatomic structures and the terms that describe them. Often, simple line drawings by physicians will suffice. In other instances, models or pictures may be used to help patients understand their condition or treatment. Audiovisual aids, such as videotapes, audiotapes, or movies, can also serve as supplements to the information given by physicians. As with written materials, the effectiveness of audiovisual aids is dependent on their accuracy and completeness as well as on how they are used. The use of audiovisual aids can be costly. Films and tapes are usually available either for purchase or rent but at considerable expense. Use of audiovisual aids also requires special equipment, such as projector or video monitor. Before choosing an audiovisual aid, the physician should check whether the number of patients for whom the aid will be used is sufficient to warrant the total purchase cost.

No matter what type of teaching aid is used in patient education physicians should take time to select the materials themselves, making sure information contained within the material is consistent with information given the patient. Instructional materials should reinforce the teaching done by the physician, not confuse it. In choosing instructional materials, the physician should also make sure that material is presented objectively without bias or distortion.

EVALUATING PATIENT EDUCATION EFFECTIVENESS

Unless patient teaching is evaluated, there is no way of knowing whether or not it was effective. Evaluation of patient education on a short-term basis may measure the effectiveness of the immediate interaction in terms of patient understanding or effectiveness of the development of a mutually acceptable plan by which patients will be most able to follow the recommendations given. The ultimate, long-term goal of patient education is usually that patients incorporate information into their life style in their home environment away from supervision of physicians. Long-term effectiveness of patient education may be evaluated by measuring the extent to which patients actually follow the recommendations given.

Surprisingly, many physicians fail to check on how patients follow through with medical recommendations. In some instances, follow-up may not be possible or practical; however, in other instances, follow-up is merely neglected. It takes little time, for example, at subsequent visits to ask patients how they are managing the recommendations made at a previous visit. This not only communicates to patients that the recommendation was important, but it also enables physicians to identify problems that patients may have encountered in carrying out the recommendations. In other instances, such follow-up may help physicians identify the need for additional patient education.

Evaluating patient education effectiveness—by assessing the degree to which the patient followed recommendations—is productive only if accurate information is gained. Merely asking patients whether or not they followed the treatment plan is insufficient. Such a question will probably result in an affirmative response regardless of the patient's actual level of compliance. The question may also preclude obtaining further information that may have identified the need for an alteration of the recommendations or the need for additional patient education. Less direct questions, such as "Tell me how you've been taking your medication," or "How many pills do you have left," are less threatening to patients and also have a higher probability of providing physicians with more accurate information.

Evaluating patient education is a way to identify problems that may have prevented the patient from following recommendations. It is important for physicians to remember that the purpose of patient education is to teach patients the knowledge, skills, or attitudes that will enable them to carry out recommendations. If the original patient education was not effective, then additional means may be needed to accomplish the desired goals.

DOCUMENTATION OF PATIENT EDUCATION

It is routinely accepted that the medical record is important as a means to help physicians to monitor care, convey patient management to other health professionals, and as a source of protection against litigation. Just as documentation of physical findings and treatment prescribed is necessary in the provision of quality patient care so is the documentation of patient education activities.

Concise documentation is important for several reasons. First, communication with others on the health care team is essential if there is to be a coordinated, consistent approach to patient teaching. Documentation is a way of communicating what has been taught, the patient's level of understanding, and what further teaching or reinforcement of information may need to be performed. Such information prevents redundancy and can assist in the evaluative process. Documentation of patient teaching helps other health professionals reinforce information given and provides an opportunity to gather further information or to identify additional problems.

In instances when patient teaching may continue through several clinic visits, documentation helps to remind physicians what has been covered at previous visits and what needs to be covered in the future. In addition, documentation serves as a reminder to follow up, evaluate, and reinforce a patient's success with the previous recommendations given.

To be useful, documentation need not be elaborate nor need it take an inordinate amount of time. In some instances, when information is complex or is given often to many patients with similar conditions, documentation may consist of a simple check sheet that can be placed on the chart with space for comments about individual patients. In other instances, documentation may consist of a simple note in the progress notes recording information that patients were given, patients' reactions or responses to the information, any specific problems or barriers that were identified, as well as strategies devised to solve the problem.

INTEGRATING PATIENT EDUCATION INTO OFFICE PRACTICE

Incorporating patient education into the general atmosphere of office practice can enhance the overall patient education effort. From the moment patients enter physicians' offices, they should be exposed to an environment that facilitates learning and interest in good health care. The reception area itself may set the tone. A number of journals and periodicals that address health issues are available from governmental, voluntary health organizations, and private publishers. Pamphlet racks in the waiting area, as well as in other locations throughout the office, offer patients the opportunity to choose from a variety of materials in order to enhance their knowledge of specific conditions or health practices.

Physicians and their office staff may consider designing displays on a bulletin board in the main reception area that provide up-to-date information on recent health-related topics of concern. Providing lists of health-related programs available within the community or on radio or television are ways of informing patients about specific patient education programs.

Materials that may be used in the clinical encounter with patients for specific conditions should be kept in individual examining rooms or in a central area that is easily accessible to physicians. All printed patient education materials should be cataloged for easy selection and retrieval.

Coordination of general patient education efforts within the office practice should be delegated to one person who is responsible for organizing, restocking, and reordering patient education materials. New materials may be reviewed and evaluated by a patient education committee composed of office staff members. However, all materials should be reviewed and evaluated by physicians before distribution to ensure that information is accurate and is congruent with their clinical approach. The overall patient education effort in office practice can be enhanced by actively involving all members of the office staff. Nurses can enhance the effectiveness of patient education efforts by reinforcing information given to patients by physicians or, in many instances, supplementing it. In these instances, it is important that good communication between the physician and nurse exist so the information the patient has been told, or should be told, can be delineated. Monitoring the effects of patient education conducted by members of the physician's team remains a critical element of the physician's responsibility.

It is not sufficient to only delegate components of patient education to other members of the health care team. Patient education must be managed just as other components of practice are managed. This means monitoring performance and providing appropriate reinforcement to staff members to whom the responsibility has been delegated. When outcomes do not meet expectations, corrective activity is needed.

In addition to patient education resources in practice, resources within the community can be used to enhance overall patient education effectiveness. Many hospitals have educational programs targeted at specific diseases. Various local volunteer organizations may also offer educational programs or groups that can lend patients additional support. As with other adjunctive patient education activities, use of such groups should not be made indiscriminately. To use these resources effectively, it is helpful for physicians to actually attend some sessions to meet the individuals responsible for conducting the program as well as to assess the content presented.

Patient Education Resources

1. National Health Information Clearing House Office of Disease Prevention and Health Promotion
   U.S. Department of Health and Human Services
   P.O. Box 1133
   Washington, DC 20013-1133
   Phone: 800-336-4797
   A health information referral service that provides health information resource guides on numerous topics: women's health, exercise for older Americans, on-line data bases, toll-free numbers for health-related information.
2. Huffington Library of the Family Health Foundation
   American Academy of Family Practice
   8880 Ward Parkway
   Kansas City, MO 64414-2797
   Phone: 816-333-9700
   Provides information on patient education materials. Offers a data base that describes and directs the user to favorably evaluated patient education materials in 24 subject areas (e.g., arthritis, diabetes mellitus).
3. Sources: A catalog of information materials on medicine and health.
   Pharmaceutical Manufacturing Association
   1100 15th Street, N.W.
   Washington, DC 20005
   Phone: 202-835-3463
   A guide booklet to 438 materials that provides useful health and drug information (updated periodically). Arranged by categories of diseases or conditions. Includes a brief description of each material and the name of the distributor. Ordering information can be found at the end of the catalog. No charge for most materials.
4. Medical Information Sources: A Referral Directory
   (1988 American Medical Association)
   Division of Library and Information Management
   P.O. Box 10623
   Chicago, IL 60610
   Quick and convenient directory of medical and health-related topics, and medically related agencies, associations, and hotlines. Arranged by subject from AIDS to women's health. Based on most

frequently asked health-related questions by physicians, businesses, and the public. National in scope. Over 1000 referrals sources listed.

5. Voluntary Health Organizations: A Guide to Patient Services (1987)
   Scheinberg, L., and Schneider, D.
   Demos Publishing Publications, Inc.
   156 5th Avenue, Suite 108
   New York, NY 10010
   Lists national addresses and phone numbers, descriptions of organizations, and what they do. Breaks down services provided at national and local level.
6. Encyclopedia of Associations
   Koek, K. E., Martin, S. B., Novallo, A. (Eds.)
   Gale Research Inc.
   Booktower
   Detroit, MI 48226
   A series of reference books found in most public libraries that provides information about over 2500 national and international organizations including many in the health field (also includes many non-health-related organizations). Listed by name and key words.

References

American Hospital Association. A Patient's Bill of Rights. Chicago, American Hospital Association, 1975.

American Medical Association. Statement on Patient Education. Chicago, American Medical Association, 1975.

Cassileth, B. R., Zupkis, R. V., Sutton-Smith, K., et al. Informed consent: why are its goals imperfectly realized? N. Engl. J. Med., *302*:896–902, 1980.

Falvo, D. R., Woehlke, P., and Deichmann, J.: Physician behavior and its relationship to patient compliance. Patient Counseling Health Ed., *2*:185–187, 1980.

Flynn, B.: Completion of referrals for hypertension screening. Phys. Patient Ed. News Lett., December, 1980.

Francis, V., Korsch, B. M., Morris, M. J.: Gaps in doctor-patient communication: Patients' response to medical advice. N. Engl. J. Med., *280*:535–540, 1969.

Korsch, B. M., Gozzi, E. K., Francis, V.: Gaps in doctor-patient communication. I. Doctor-patient interaction and patient satisfaction. Pediatrics, *42*:855–871, 1968.

Krosnick, A.: Failure to educate patients may lead to charge of physician negligence. Diab. Out. *9*(4):27, 1974.

Leventhal, H.: Findings and theory in the study of fear communication. Adv. Exp. Soc. Psych. *5*:119–186, 1970.

Leventhal, H., Singer, R. P., and Jones, S.: Effects of fear and specificity of recommendations upon attitudes and behavior. J. Personal. Soc. Psych., *2*:20–29, 1965.

28

Interviewing Techniques

F. Marian Bishop
Robert E. Froelich

The Purpose of the Interview

The interview has several purposes. The one most often identified is that of gathering data from the patient that will lead to an understanding of the disease process and the underlying physiologic status. Equally important is the purpose of establishing a relationship and a treatment contract between the patient and the physician and the physician's staff. This relationship and the associated treatment contract is an essential common element of all successful patient care.

Prior to establishing a successful contract with a patient, another purpose of the interview takes place. The assessment of the patient's attitudes, beliefs, understandings, and biases as they relate to his or her illness, the role of medications, and the patient role is necessary for successful treatment. In the extreme situation, a patient may understand the role of patient as a passive recipient of care, while the physician may expect the patient to take active care of himself. If this difference in expectations is not understood, the chance of successful treatment is endangered.

The final purpose of the interview is to meet the needs of the patient and the needs of the physician. In most patient visits, when the physician and patient are from the same cultural background, their expectations are harmonious and synchronized to the point that their individual needs never enter conscious awareness. Only when the expectations are not harmonious, when there are friction, discomfort, and noncompliance, do the needs and expectations of the patient and physician come into awareness and become an issue for discussion, working through, and resolution.

The Communication Process

Given the barrage of mass communication on the lives of most individuals in today's environment, it is useful to consider some points about mass communications before considering the medical interview.

The commercialization of mass communication has led to a depersonalization of human relations and to a glorification of cliches and slogans. The standardized response begins more and more to substitute for deeply felt, personalized expression, . . . the human ear has adapted itself to sort ***and disregard*** *a considerable number of verbal messages that emerge from radio loudspeakers and the television sets, just as it formerly accommodated itself to the task of absorbing what was being said by patients.*

RUESCH AND KEES, 1970

These observations suggest that interviewers have been unconsciously trained by mass communication media to not hear and have the task of retraining themselves to hear what is being said by patients.

In daily life human beings are rarely able to do more than hint at what they desire to express, inasmuch as the very nature of their needs often forces them to exchange messages without delay in time. Thus it is left to the receiver to fill in unexpressed details.

RUESCH AND KEES, 1970

The interviewer has the problem of being sure that when he "fills in the unexpressed" from the patient, it is filled in accurately.

The nonverbal accompaniment to the words (the context, the voice quality, and emphasis; the facial expression, the body posture, the setting, the attire, the patient's age and culture) help the interviewer fill in the unexpressed. However, the only way to be sure that this understanding is accurate is for the interviewer to check it with the patient. The use of summary statements and asking, "What I hear you saying is . . . am I correct?" is an effective technique to be sure that the patient is being heard correctly.

The communication process is further understood when we realize that "if words are to be used significantly, they must still evoke pictorial images in the mind of a reader or listener . . . " and "that only through the use of words that evoke exact and striking images can an emotional response be produced in the reader" (Ruesch and Kees, 1970). The reverse of this statement is that no communication occurs when the listener has no experience or image to connect to the words being spoken. "We do not first experience or understand some reality and then find words to name that understanding. We understand in and through the languages available to us. . . . " (Tracy, 1987.)

If we understand that we see out of our eyes and hear out of our ears (i.e., we do not see or hear that which we are not trained or set to see or hear), we begin to focus our attention in interviewing on seeing and listening, rather than asking. To be open to hearing whatever is said and to see whatever happens is a most difficult task. Once we begin to seeing and hear what is not familiar, then the next task begins—that of giving meaning to these observations. It is only through time spent with patients that we finally understand their communication and what meaning to apply to it.

Semantics As a Foundation for Communication

Semantics is a basic study of all verbal communication (Hayakawa, 1964). Time after time, students listen to a word a patient says and jump to the conclusion that they understand what the patient meant by the word. A common misconception of all interviewers is the belief that the patient is using a word to mean what the interviewer believes it to mean. To illustrate this point, let us consider the professor who writes, rewrites, and reviews a test question on a topic that he and his students have been discussing for several weeks. They have been using a set of words common to the field of study. What happens when the professor puts the question on a test? Without a doubt, some of the students will misinterpret the question and answer with a meaning that the professor had no intention of asking.

Greater opportunity for confusion is present if the question was not previously written, was not reviewed for possible misinterpretations, and is only presented in the oral form. This is the precise situation of an interview. Taken one step further, let us say that the question can be answered with a "yes" or "no." How much misinformation can be developed by such a question and answer?

A basic semantic concept is that a word is to what it represents as a map is to a territory. No map *is* the territory. No two maps of the same territory are the same. Each map is a unique abstraction of that territory. As an illustration, consider a sensation that a patient notes and refers to as pain. The sensation the patient experiences is the territory. The patient's description of the pain is a map of the territory. The words paint the verbal picture of the sensation. It is only through clarification of the patient's use of the words that an interviewer can get a relatively accurate idea of what the territory is.

Most diagnoses can be made if one is able to get an accurate description of the patient's internal sensation or territory. Consider the situation where 10 neurons from deep pain fibers are firing into the spinal cord dorsal root. One person may refer to this sensation as very painful while a second person may refer to it as an ache. The territory is the same, and each uses a different map to represent the territory.

Every communication has two components. One component is the cognitive, dictionary definition of the words that make up the communication—the description of the territory. The second component is the affective or emotional tone of the communication. It is important to hear both components and to have the ability to respond to either component. For example, when people are angry, the dictionary definitions of their words may convey very little of the intended message. To react only to the words may completely miss the message.

The Questionnaire Compared with the Interview

Though a written questionnaire given to a patient may result in information, there is no relationship established between a patient and a questionnaire. Since the relationship is important to the treatment of the patient and the patient's cooperation, the human interview is an essential element of the patient's visit.

The questionnaire completed by a patient (either on paper or from the interviewer's memory) is quite different from an interview. They differ in two major ways. First, the questionnaire (either in the interviewer's memory or on paper) lacks the human qualities of a human interaction—a constantly renegotiated give and take. It lacks all of the nonverbal aspects of meaningful communication. Second, the questionnaire lacks the ability to make meaning out of the patient's responses. Without meaning, the physician has limited or no use of the information. To illustrate, the datum that a patient was married at age 15 is of little use in and of itself. However, knowing the circumstances surrounding the decision to get married at age 15 may have profound meaning in understanding the patient's reactions to a present illness. The raw datum, "married age 15," is made meaningful and useful in the present context by elaboration in the interview.

The Computerized History Compared with the Personal Interview

The major activity of the interviewer is to make meaning out of the words chosen by the patient. Only after the meaning is confirmed by the interviewer can the physiologic processes be understood.

It is crucial not to put man-machine interaction and human dialogue on the same footing. A computer is quite unable to understand anything, but it can help health professionals in gathering medical history data.

HOUZIAUX, 1986

By not being able to make meaning out of the patient's words, the computerized histories have the semantic problems of not being able to further explain to the patient just what is meant by the question being asked and the reverse of not being able to ask the patient just what was meant by what was said. A study of computerized histories found that only "68% (of patients) could express all or most of their complaints, but some of their physical complaints could not be entered (at all)." Only "52% of the women" and "74% of the male patients found the range of answers from which to choose sufficient" (Quaak et al., 1986). As the authors of this chapter found as early as 1968, the computer is unable to understand a patient's communication since communicating includes verbal and nonverbal messages. The meaning of the words is shaded by the nonverbal as well as the linguistic aspects of the message, and the computer is unable to pick up this meaning.

Pitfalls in Interviewing

A good interview should result in an accurate and comprehensive story of the patient's situation. This story is sometimes referred to as the medical history. A commonplace phrase is "taking a medical history."

But medical histories, like written histories of nations or institutions, are not taken but made . . . made from oral accounts of the patient's present and past illnesses by the patient, family, and friends, as well as the oral and written statements of colleagues, records of previous hospitalizations, and so on. Selection, interpretation, and ordering of information pervade the process of writing the case history. The point of all of this is that medical histories are created, not found.

DONNELLY, 1988

The effectiveness of an interviewer to conduct a good medical interview and to create and make a medical history is dependent in part upon the ability to avoid some of the following common pitfalls. These pitfalls can, at times, become an unconscious detriment of both the experienced and the novice interviewer. With attention and vigilance, they can be appropriately utilized rather than routinely utilized.

DIRECT QUESTIONS

The temptation to resort to direct questions is probably the major pitfall for the inexperienced interviewer and the interviewer who lets skills languish. An interview made up of direct questions gathers little information per unit time, since most of the time is spent by the interviewer framing and asking questions, each of which gives a specific bit of information.

The direct question approach does not permit patients to give information as they have experienced it, and interviewers may never obtain the piece of information the patients wanted to give. That is, unless interviewers just happen to ask the one specific question that tapped the information. Remember the problem of the computer interview noted earlier in the chapter. Computer-generated questions, by necessity, must be direct questions since the computer is unable to accept dialogue as a response.

"WHY" QUESTIONS

A second pitfall is asking "why" questions. "Why did you take that medicine?" "Why did you leave work?" "Why did you get a divorce?"

What is wrong with these questions? They call on patients to account for their behavior and encourage defensive attitudes. "Why" questions to a patient imply that the patient did something wrong. Since much of patient behavior may be derived from the unconscious or be related to reasons that are not socially acceptable, patients may be antagonized by the implication in the question that they did something wrong. Patients may feel that such a question finds fault with them and may thus become irritated or annoyed. It is difficult to ask a "why" question and avoid the overtones of accusation. In addition, questions come from a whining transactional position on the part of the interviewer. The whining position may be described as a position of helplessness, pleading, or angry frustration.

The above questions could be rephrased as: "Tell me about taking that medicine." "You needed to leave work?" "Are you willing to tell me about the divorce?"

SUGGESTIVE QUESTIONS

A third pitfall is a question which has the answer within it. This is called a suggestive question. An example is, "When you discussed your problem, your breathing was a little rapid. Were you a little nervous at the time?" What choice does the patient have in responding to such a question? Obviously, much misinformation can be obtained by using suggestive questions. This is especially true when the patient feels put down or inferior to the physician and feels a need to be compliant.

YES AND NO QUESTIONS

With many patients there is a danger in using questions requiring yes and no answers. The patient's answer may be more dependent on the immediate milieu than on the facts. When a question is answered with a "Yes," it is not clear what the "Yes" means. Is it given to please, to give the interviewer what the patient thinks the interviewer wants to hear, to avoid discussing an area that the patient wants to avoid, or is it a factual response?

Similarly, when the question can be answered with a "No," the patient may just wish to disagree, wish to please, wish to avoid discussing a topic, or wish to give a factual response. Much inaccurate information can be obtained by using this type of question. Even an experienced interviewer can get misinformation from any patient by a question that can be most appropriately be answered by a "Yes" or "No."

UNSIGNALED TOPIC CHANGES

When the physician asks the patient for information and there is a longer than usual pause before answering, the topic has probably been changed without signaling this intention to the patient. This interviewing pitfall slows the interviewing process and, because the topic change is unsignaled, gives the patient the impression that the interviewer has no clear plan of action. When it is time to change a topic, it is best to use a bridging phrase, such as "Let's shift to talking about . . . ," to guide the patient in the direction the interview is to go.

LACK OF EYE CONTACT

A pitfall that is sometimes forgotten is that lack of eye contact through concentration on a note pad, a chart, or a referral note will greatly affect the information obtained from a patient. In addition to giving the message that the paper is more important than the patient, the interviewer misses out on all of the gestures, facial expressions, and shifts in position that add so much to the meaning of what is said. At times when listening to only the words, the interviewer even misses the intonation of the voice, the guttural emphasis, the slight laugh, or the held back cry.

LACK OF FEEDBACK TO PATIENTS

Giving no feedback to the patient is an interviewing pitfall that will interfere with the doctor-patient relationship. Giving no feedback is impossible if both the doctor and the patient are in the same room in view of each other and able to hear each other. As one patient said to her physician, "I knew how you felt about that by your raised eyebrows." The physician, however, had been unaware of any eyebrow movement. Whatever we do is interpreted by the patient as either encouraging or discouraging his or her current responses. With practice and videotape review of interviews, an interviewer can gain increasing conscious control of the nonverbal feedback given to the patient.

While there are other potential interviewing problems that could be reviewed, direct questions, "Why" questions, suggestive questions, unsignaled topic changes, lack of eye contact, and lack of feedback to the patient are some of the more common pitfalls that, with practice and conscious effort, can be avoided.

Organizing the Medical Interview

A broad point of view suggests that the interchange between physician and patient is a problem-solving process made up of seven or eight steps, depending upon the definition of each step. From this perspective, the medical interview can be organized as follows.

STEP 1: PURPOSE AND WILLINGNESS TO CONSIDER PROBLEMS

By seeing the physician, the patient expresses a willingness to talk about an acute or chronic problem, illness, or discomfort with the physician. Occasionally, the patient comes for other reasons, such as to get out of work or obtain disability. The session can be frustrating if its purpose is not clear to both the patient and the physician.

By seeing the patient, the physician expresses a willingness to consider and deal with the patient's problems. Some physicians have other reasons like earning a living or fulfilling an educational requirement. If one of these other reasons prevails, the session may be very frustrating to the patient.

STEP 2: GREETING AND SIZING UP

In the first 20 seconds, visual input dominates the awareness of the two participants. For the patient, the warmth or coldness of the room's decor, the light level, and the privacy or lack of it are important first impressions. Next, the posture, dress, attitude, physical distance, sex, age, and body build of the physician are noted. The physician's voice pitch, volume, and expression are judged by the patient and fitted into prejudices built up by past experiences. What the physician actually says is then judged in this context. Thus, who says it, how it is said, and when it is said play as big a role as what is said.

Similarly, the physician judges the patient's body build, posture, sex, age, dress, and gestures. Quickly, the physician imagines the patient is sick, a complainer, an alcoholic, and so on and guesses the patient's economic resources and type of work the patient does. Based upon past experiences, the physician also stereotypes the patient before a word is spoken. With a new patient, it is probably best for the physician to be quiet for 5 seconds to allow this sizing up process to take place.

STEP 3: THE PROBLEM OR CHIEF COMPLAINT

Opening the medical interview varies with the setting and style of the physician. Generally, a nurse, clerk, or secretary obtains descriptive data about a patient, such as name, address, age, other family members, medical insurance, and telephone number, before the interview. Some physicians prefer to acquire this information themselves as a way to open an interview on a nonthreatening topic. By gathering this information firsthand, the physician can also observe and obtain information concerning the patient's memory, orientation, and problem relationships.

Once the descriptive data are obtained, the next step is to ask what led the patient to make an appointment. Usually, the record will indicate a reason for the visit. It is best to remember that a patient needs an admission ticket to see a physician. An admission ticket is a socially and medically acceptable excuse for the visit. But it may be just that, an excuse. To find the real reason, it is helpful to ask for the chief complaint, using a facilitation or an open-ended question, not a specific question. For example, "What is the situation that brings you here today?" rather than "The nurse says you have an earache. What seems to be the trouble?"

Once the chief complaint is identified and clarified, the patient and physician need to agree that both are willing to share information, to explore the complaint, and to do what is necessary to understand, diagnose, or treat it. Ideally, the contract also defines the type of relationship they will have, i.e., they are going to relate as a superior and an inferior, as two equals, as a teacher and a student, or as two advocates with veto power over the other's decision.

Most often, the contract is understood by behavior and willingness to respond to each other. However, when there is hesitancy to respond, when the patient asks questions of the physician, or when either person is uncomfortable, it is important to verbally define a contract and see if the other will agree. For example, "You seem a bit hesitant to answer my questions. Are you willing to share information with me about this problem?" Such a question will bring out what each expects and is willing to do. If the answer is "No," the next question might be "What are you willing to do?"

The type of relationship is usually established by the style and personality of the physician. But the physician can learn to adapt and modify the approach to best meet the needs of each patient. Sometimes the type of relationship contract is established and agreed to nonverbally through posture, tone of voice, relative physical positions, and the medical problem.

STEP 4: DATA GATHERING

Once the chief complaint is understood and clarified, data concerning the present illness are encouraged and elicited from the patient. The interview process for a simple acute problem is generally limited to several specific questions, such as "Where did the fall occur?" or "How did the cut happen?" The interview process for a complex or chronic condition usually follows an overall guideline of obtaining specific details of the present symptoms, related diet, exercise, medications, work and home environments, social stresses, financial stresses, the emotional and behavioral reactions to the symptoms, and what the patient does to alleviate them.

The successful, efficient process for a medical interview has been described as: open the topic with open-ended questions followed by facilitations, reflections, emphatic replies, and silences to learn as much as the patient is able to tell without physician suggestion and interference (Enelow et al., 1986). Once patients have said as much as they can, patients are facilitated further by laundry list questions, direct questions, yes-no questions, and summary statements of clarification. The topic is closed and a bridging comment is made to move to the next topic. This process is repeated many times during a medical interview in dealing with each topic.

Once the present condition is defined, the onset of the problem should be dealt with. The physician needs a detailed description of the symptoms, how they were precipitated, how they progressed, and any data associated with each period of symptoms up to the present time. Table 28–1 sets out the types of

Table 28–1. PHYSICIAN INTERVENTIONS FOR PHASES OF THE MEDICAL INTERVIEW

I.	**Opening a Topic**
	Facilitation
	Open-ended question
	Bridging phrase
II.	**Assisting the Patient's Narrative**
	Support and reassurance
	Empathy
	Confrontation
	Reflection
	Interpretation
	Silence
	Modified laundry list
III.	**Focusing upon a Topic**
	Confrontation
	Reflection
	Probing
	Interpretation
	Summation
IV.	**Obtaining Specific Information**
	Direct question
	Yes-no question
	Probing
	Problem question
	Laundry list
V.	**Closing Topic or Interview**
	Summation
	Prescription for action

From Froelich, R. E., and Bishop, F. M.: Clinical Interviewing Skills. 3rd ed. St. Louis, C. V. Mosby Co., 1977.

physician interventions most suited for each phase of medical interview topic exploration.

The most common mistake in medical interviewing is for the physician to deal with the onset of the illness before knowing enough about the patient's present state to have a good idea of which organ is involved. Without this understanding, the physician does not know where to focus attention in obtaining details of the progression of the present illness. If it is not known whether the pain described in the chest is cardiac, esophageal, or chest wall, it is not known on which organ to focus the review of the present illness.

Relevant data from the past medical, social, work, and family histories are obtained using the same techniques and process of opening the topic, assisting the narrative, closing the topic, and bridging a new topic (Table 28–1).

STEP 5: ANALYSIS AND DEFINITION OF THE PROBLEM

Once the data are obtained, they must be analyzed to give meaning to the symptoms, history, and associated data. This analysis defines the patient's discomforts as a physiologic or disease process. Thus, a tentative diagnosis is formed. Though dependent upon the interview, the diagnostic process is related to training, information, and abilities to synthesize numerous types of data.

STEP 6: TREATMENT ALTERNATIVES AND DECISIONS

After the physiologic process is defined, diagnostic or treatment alternatives are considered. In the ideal problem-solving process, the patient has enough understanding to suggest some of the diagnostic or treatment alternatives. The physician presents suggestions and alternatives along with their probable outcomes, cost, and side effects. Ideally, this decision is a joint decision between the physician and the patient.

STEP 7: ACTION AND EVALUATION

The diagnostic or treatment alternative is instituted and the results are evaluated by both the physician and the patient. If the decision involves a treatment and it solves the problem, this episode of health care for this patient is concluded with questions and suggestions of how to avoid similar illnesses in the future. If the decision is a diagnostic activity or an unsuccessful treatment, the physician and patient return to **Step 3** or **Step 4** with the new data.

Problem Patients

The effectiveness of an interviewer, in large part, is dependent upon the number and variety of interviewing techniques the physician can utilize to meet the variety of situations that arise in an interview. For example, the same techniques will not work with the overtalkative and the reticent, the sad and the angry, or the frightened and the stoic patient.

Some of the interviewing literature focuses upon problem patients. While this focus has led to some meaningful understandings, the broader view of the problem patient being a part of an interview system has led to additional insights with a focus on the physician as well as the patient. A problem patient to one physician may be an ideal patient to the next physician. This section will focus on both the patient and the physician, using a personalized approach to attitudes and feelings of the physician in the discussion.

DEFENSIVE PATIENT

Patients are usually defensive because of an expected negative outcome if they were to talk freely about the topic at hand. For instance, the patient may expect anger, rejection, blame, or ridicule, and there is fear or anxiety about the expected outcome. Several techniques may be used to deal with defensiveness and the obstacle it poses to evaluation and diagnosis.

One technique is to ask, "What might happen if you were to talk about . . . ?" The patient's answer is pursued until the physician understands the fear. In rare instances, the physician may agree that the expected outcome is a probable outcome, e.g., information used in a pending lawsuit, and that the patient should not discuss the topic. More likely, once the outcome is discussed, it becomes evident to the patient that nothing bad will happen if the topic is discussed. As the topic is dealt with, the defensiveness begins to melt away.

A second technique is to ask, "What is the worst possible thing or catastrophic fear that could happen if you talked about . . . ?" Again, the physician may agree that the catastrophe might occur or, as is more usually the case, the patient will realize the unlikeliness of the catastrophic action actually taking place.

A third technique, especially if the patient is teasing or appears to be suggesting there is important information and then withholds the information, is to agree not to discuss the topic and go on to another one. If this is a tease, the topic will be brought up later in the session or in the next session if it is of great importance to the patient. By not responding, the physician reinforces a straightforward open discussion rather than a continuation of teasing innuendos.

A fourth technique is to comment on the defensiveness, such as: "You seem very reluctant to discuss this topic," followed initially by silence on the physician's part. If the patient does not respond, the physician may proceed with, "Is there anything that will make it easier for you to discuss this topic?" or "Are there any questions you want to ask before proceeding?" or "Can you identify your concerns in talking about this topic?" And, finally, the physician might ask, "Is there something about your trusting me with the information about this topic?" or "Is there something that concerns you about my reaction to or feelings toward you if we discuss this topic?"

Should any of the latter questions be asked, the physician needs to be prepared to discuss the patient's replies honestly, directly, objectively, and without personal distance in the sense that the patient is reacting to the person in the physician role. The first time the relationship between the physician and the patient is focused on it may be helpful to record the session on tape and review the session with a peer or supervisor who can provide some objective observations on the doctor-patient relationship. When dealing with defensiveness, it is a transference problem rather than a reality problem most of the time.

FEARFUL PATIENT

One can produce anxiety in one's self with a scary thought and restricted breathing. By doing the opposite, relaxing the breathing and avoiding the fear-producing thoughts, anxiety can be controlled.

A decision needs to be made as to whether the patient's fear is related to a real threat, sometimes referred to as reality fear, or to an imagined threat, referred to as neurotic fear. Fear associated with a real threat is considered healthy. Relaxation techniques, focusing the person's attention away from the threat, and caring support are useful ways to comfort these patients. It is important to let patients experience their real fear and help them through it.

The neurotic fear of an imagined threat should be handled through exploration of the threat and the probability that it would actually occur along with the consequences if it did occur. Again, what is the catastrophic fear, and how realistic or likely is it to happen? The question "So what if it does happen?" may help. This process confronts the unreality of the fear and imagined threat.

The next step is to encourage the patient to agree to breathe slowly and deeply and to stop the scary thoughts. The patient should focus on some pleasant thoughts instead. This uses a positive approach rather than a negative approach.

ANGRY PATIENT

Several issues are raised when dealing with an angry patient: (1) What is the direction and quality of the anger? (2) Can the physician accept or allow the patient to be angry? (3) Is the patient's anger affecting the medical problem? (4) How is the patient justifying the anger? (5) Is the anger due to frustration, or is it a cover-up for sadness?

In the normal, healthy person, anger is the natural result of frustration. To overcome the frustration in a socially acceptable manner, the anger takes the form of aggression. Once the anger changes to hostility, it becomes destructive rather than constructive and is considered maladaptive.

Physicians vary widely in their ability to recognize anger and tolerate it in a patient. One physician may enjoy the spunk of the angry patient while another fears, withdraws from, or denies a patient's anger. The issue is, how can the physician be comfortable with an angry patient? Is the physician willing to learn how to be comfortable with an angry patient? Some physicians answer this question with, "Yes, if I am sure the patient is in control of himself and will not hurt me." This is a diagnostic decision that needs to be addressed.

Whether or not a person is angry at a given moment is under his own control. A person who chooses not to be angry cannot be made angry. Invitations to be angry may be ignored or viewed as just idiosyncrasies. Also, attention can be focused on what might motivate others to send out such behavioral signals or invitations. Any of these techniques will effectively help a person avoid becoming angry.

Understanding anger as a feeling under the control of the individual suggests a way to manage it. An additional factor to consider is how the person uses anger in the interpersonal process. Anger is frequently used as blackmail; e.g., "If you do . . . I will be angry and when I get angry you better watch out."

Anger is also frequently used as an attempt to control the behavior of others. Thus, the treatment of anger is to acknowledge it and then ignore it with such a statement as "You sure are angry. If you want to be angry it's OK with me." And if it fits, "I really think it is kind of stupid to stay angry in this situation."

These statements acknowledge the anger, accept the patient being angry, and avoid being a part of the game with subsequent payoff. The physician might follow these statements with "If you want to look at how you make yourself so angry, I am willing to look at it with you," or "I will be happy to refer you to someone who will help you find a way to be more comfortable rather than angry."

MANIPULATIVE OR DEMANDING PATIENT

A manipulative patient is skilled in getting something wanted from other people by using a variety of artful maneuvers, such as threats to produce a fit of temper, attempts at suicide that are aimed at influencing others, and behavior that otherwise plays on the guilt of others, such as seduction.

The issue is "Can I accept the patient's being manipulative?" or "Can I outmanipulate the patient for his own good?" The issue of manipulation becomes potentially pathologic when the patient becomes dishonest or deceives the physician as a way to obtain more drugs, hospital admission, unwarranted surgery, or some special treatment. At this level of manipulation, consultation with a psychiatrist or someone who knows how to manage such patients may be needed. Most manipulative patients can be managed by the family physician by the use of a very specific contract regarding the issues of discomfort, such as demands to be seen after hours or unnecessary night calls.

CHANGING REACTIONS TO PROBLEM PATIENTS

The key to changing behavior is answered by the question "How?" When the process, mechanism, or procedure for the behavior, in this case interview style, is understood, it is possible to change some part or all of the process, mechanism, or procedure in order to initiate a new behavior.

For example, if a physician becomes angry with a patient and wishes to change this feeling, the question should be asked, "How did I make myself angry?" or "How did I interpret the patient's statements or behavior to make myself angry?" or "What meaning did I assign to the patient's behavior?" Once these "how" and "what" questions are answered, the physician can ask, "Is there another way to interpret the patient's behavior?" or "Would I still be angry if I interpreted the behavior another way and gave it a different meaning?"

The conclusive step to institute change is to decide to interpret the behavior in another way and decide to feel something other than anger the next time the physician is faced with the patient's behavior. This process involves asking: (1) How do the physician's behavior or feelings come about? (2) What meaning is assigned to the patient's behavior? (3) How can the perception of the behavior be interpreted differently? The process also involves deciding on an alternate way to interpret the behavior to initiate change. In learning medical interviewing, this process of change is key to improving medical interviewing skills.

References

American Medical Association: Physician/Patient Communication (Video Clinic Series). Chicago, IL, American Medical Association, 1987. *For those who are visually oriented this 50-minute, color, 3/4" VHS/BETA videotape provides a review of basic communication concepts, factors that have both a negative and positive effect on the effective communication, and samples of techniques that can promote patient cooperation. While subjects are not covered in depth, there is a breadth of review that the videotape learner will find useful.*

Bernstein, L., and Bernstein, R. S.: Interviewing: A Guide for Health Professionals, 4th ed. East Norwalk, CT, Appleton-Century-Crofts, 1985. *This volume is intended primarily for students in schools of medicine and nursing and provides some interesting and useful interpretations of specific interviewers' interventions, such as the hostile response, the reassuring response, and the understanding response. For those interested, there is a chapter on family interviewing, along with a sample family interview.*

Coulehan, J. L., and Block, M. R.: Medical Interview: A Primer for Students of the Art. Philadelphia, F. A. Davis Co., 1987. *Though primarily written as a textbook for medical students, this 195-page book can be reviewed by the practitioner in sections that are relevant for specific patient encounters. There is an interesting attempt to bridge the system's review information with medical interview skills. The book is easy to read with numerous examples of doctor-patient interactions.*

Deckert, G.: Videotaping Presentations on Interpreting Body Language in Everyday Practice. Los Angeles, CA, Professional Research, Inc., 1974. *A 25-minute color videotape cassette designed to teach observational skills that assist in interpreting the meaning of a patient's body language, emphasizing the emotions of anxiety, anger, and sadness.*

Donnelly, W. J.: Righting the medical record: Transforming the chronicle into story. J.A.M.A., *260*:6, 1988.

Eckman, P., and Frierson, W.: Unmasking the Face. Englewood Cliffs, NJ, Prentice-Hall, Inc., 1975. *The implications of body language are discussed along with a pictorial guide to understanding the emotions depicted in facial expressions. This is a classic presentation on nonverbal behavior.*

Enelow, A. J., and Swisher, S. N.: Interviewing and Patient Care. New York, Oxford University Press, 1986. *This continues to be a useful review of basic interviewing skills including the variety of interviewing responses that are available to the experienced interviewer.*

Froelich, R. E., and Bishop, F. M.: Clinical Interviewing Skills: A Programmed Manual. 3rd ed. St. Louis, C. V. Mosby Co., 1977. *A programmed manual with definitions and illustrations of interviewing interventions and a guide for organizing a medical interview. Practice interviews of a general nature and of so-called problem patients are provided so that the reader can self-pace. The appendix includes forms and exercises for the teacher to use with students.*

Hardt, E. J.: The Bilingual Medical Interview. Boston, Area Health Education Center, 1987. *For the family physician with a bilingual patient population, this is one of the few learning packages that address the issues of interviewing and providing health care to people of different languages and cultures. This 30-minute, 1/2", 3/4" VHS comes with a 67-page Discussion Leader's Guide for four vignettes involving patients who speak Spanish, Vietnamese, and French-Creole. The use of a translator system is also presented.*

Hayakawa, S. I.: Language in Thought and Action. New York, Harcourt, Brace & World, 1964.

Henderson, G. (Ed.): Physician-Patient Communications, Readings and Recommendations. Springfield, IL, Charles C Thomas, 1981. *Chapters on special communication exchanges with persons with hearing disabilities, arthritis, alcoholism, and spinal cord injuries are unique contributions. The chapter on techniques for communicating with elderly patients is useful to the practice of family medicine.*

Houziaux, M. O.: Historical and methodological aspects of computer-assisted medical history-taking. Med. Inf. (London), *11*(2):129–143, 1986.

Kagen, N.: Influencing human interaction: eleven years with IPR. Canadian Counselor, *9*:74, 1975. *A discussion of the Interpersonal Process Recall as an evaluation technique along with an analysis of the principles of human interaction and motivation that form the basis of why IPR works.*

National Medical Audiovisual Center: The Teaching of Interpersonal Skills to Health Professionals: A Series of Five Manuals. Amherst, MA, Carkhuff Associates, Inc., 1978. *The National Library of Medicine; National Institutes of Health; and Department of Health, Education, and Welfare funded this series of five instructional manuals. Family physicians interested in improving interviewing skills will be interested in No. 1, How to Set Instructional Goals; No. 2, How to Involve Students in the Learning Process; and No. 5, How to Use Videotechnology.*

Quaak, M. J., Westerman, R. F., Schouten, J. A., et al.: Appraisal of computerized medical histories: Comparisons between computerized and conventional records. Comput-Biomed-Research, *19*(6):551–564, 1986.

Ruesch, J., and Kees, W.: Nonverbal Communication. Berkeley, University of California Press, 1970, pp. 3–7.

Satir, V.: Peoplemaking. Palo Alto, CA, Science and Behavior Books, Inc., 1972. *Although written in the early seventies, this book remains a valuable basic text for understanding families. Of particular value are chapters on Patterns of Communication and Special Families: One-Parent and Blended. This excellent primer is easy to read and understand.*

Tracy, D.: Plurality and Ambiguity: Hermeneutics, Religion, Hope. New York, Harper and Row Publishers, Inc., 1987, p. 48.

Part IV

Practice of Family Medicine

29

Clinical Problem-Solving in Family Practice

I. R. McWhinney

Although the general principles of problem-solving are the same in all branches of medicine, each discipline has its own way of applying them. The differences between disciplines result from differences in the problems they encounter and from differences in their roles within the health care system. The problem-solving strategies of family physicians have evolved in response to a number of special features of family practice:

1. The pattern of illness in family practice approximates the pattern of illness in the community. This means that there is a high incidence of acute, short-term illness, much of it transient and self-limiting; a high prevalence of chronic illness; and a high prevalence of behavioral problems. Contrary to the conventional view, patients do not present with either physical or behavioral problems. They come with problems that are often a complex mixture of physical, psychologic, and social elements.

The incidence and prevalence of disease in family practice have, as we will see, an important effect on the predictive value of symptoms and tests. To deal successfully with this pattern of problems, the family physician's problem-solving strategies must be especially adapted for two purposes. First, they must be capable of distinguishing, in the early stages of illness, the serious and life-threatening diseases from the transient and minor ones. Since patients with serious diseases are examined in the midst of patients with more common minor and transient illnesses and since the symptoms are often very similar, this is no easy task. Second, they must be capable of determining the specific physical, social, and psychologic elements of the patient's problem.

2. When the patient first sees the family physician for a new episode of illness, the illness is likely to be both undifferentiated and unorganized. The meaning of these concepts is discussed later.

3. Since the family physician is available for all types of problems, no prior assumptions can be made about the type of problems likely to be encountered. Problem-solving methods must, therefore, be adaptable enough to deal with any health-related problem. Since the family physician's commitment to patients is unconditional, he or she cannot exclude the analysis of a problem because it does not fall within one's field as can organ and system specialists.

4. In family practice, disease is often seen in the early stages, before the full clinical picture has developed. Information on which to base a precise diagnosis—the kind of information discussed in textbooks—is often not available to the family physician when the patient is first seen. Decisions have to be made with fewer cues than are available in the later stages of disease. They also have to be made with different cues. Symptoms change as an illness advances. The symptoms and tests that have diagnostic value in the early stages may be quite different from those that have diagnostic value in later stages.

5. The family physician's relationship with patients is continuous and transcends individual episodes of illness. This has two important consequences. Since the relationship is open-ended, the physician does not need to be in a hurry to solve all the patient's

problems in one or two visits. Observation over time can be used as a method for testing hypotheses, assessing probabilities, and attempting to understand the context of problems.

6. Since family physicians are directly available to their patients, their workload can be predicted and planned only to a limited extent. This means that decisions often have to be made under pressure of time. To be effective decision-makers under these conditions, family physicians must be particularly skilled in ascertaining at an early stage what the patient's main problem is. They must develop the skills of formulating a strategy for dealing with the problem in the time available, focusing on the decisions that have to be made immediately, selecting the most efficient strategy for arriving at these decisions and devising a plan for long-term assessment and management of the problem. Finally, the physician must set priorities for other problems and devise a similar plan for their long-term assessment and management.

Undifferentiated Illness

By undifferentiated illness we mean an illness that has not previously been assessed, categorized, and named by a physician. First, in the process of diagnosis, the physician takes the raw data presented by the patient, adds the data acquired by his own search, and tries to fit the illness into a disease category within his or her own frame of reference. In this way, many of the patients presenting to family physicians have the raw data of their illnesses differentiated into well-known disease categories.

On the other hand, many patients have illnesses that defy this kind of differentiation. There are at least four reasons why this may be so. First, an illness may be transient and self-limiting, creating a functional disturbance that clears completely, leaving no evidence on which a diagnosis can be based. These illnesses are usually short lived, but not invariably so. Sometimes, a patient may suffer for months from an illness that eventually clears without ever having been diagnosed.

Second, there are, at the edge of every disease category, borderline and intermediate conditions that are difficult or impossible to classify. Our disease categories are not as sharply outlined as we sometimes think. In his book, *Anatomy of an Illness,* Norman Cousins (1979) describes his personal experience with a serious illness that was never precisely diagnosed. Since family physicians see all variants of disease, they are especially liable to encounter patients with milder variants and borderline conditions that may never be referred to the system specialist.

Third, an illness may remain undifferentiated for many years before its true nature unfolds in time. For example, it may be years before an attack of transient blurring of vision is followed by other evidence of multiple sclerosis.

Fourth, an illness may be so closely interwoven with the personality and personal life of the patient—so individual—that it defies classification. Chronic pain is often an example of this type of illness.

The family physician's assessment of an illness may, therefore, have a number of outcomes. Some illnesses will be diagnosed in the conventional manner in a comparatively short period of time; some will eventually be diagnosed after a longer period of observation; some will come and go without ever being diagnosed; some will never be diagnosed because they defy classification. Whatever type of illness is being dealt with, the family physician must have a strategy that is appropriate for the problem. Harm may be done if the wrong strategy is used. For example, the use of the conventional diagnostic strategy in a patient with an ill-defined pain syndrome may result in a spurious "diagnosis," overinvestigation, overmedication, and iatrogenic disease. Using data from the National Ambulatory Care Survey, Carmichael (1967) has calculated that only in half the ambulatory encounters with the family physician does the patient have an illness with objective evidence of physical pathology. Of the other half, the majority are in the affective domain, and many of the remainder are visits for preventive or administrative purposes. Carmichael argues that for self-limiting and behavioral problems and for preventive services (between them accounting for 80 per cent of all encounters), the crucial factor is the relationship between the patient and the physician rather than the action of the physician.

Unorganized Illness

The concept of the organization of illness is an important one for family medicine. When patients first tell a physician about their problems and symptoms, they usually do so with little insight into their nature or cause. A patient who has had malaise, anorexia, and discolored urine for 5 days and a 3-month history of fatigue, depression, and headaches does not know that in the physician's mind these add up to two clusters of symptoms—one suggesting hepatitis, the other depression. When these problems are presented for the first time, they will not usually come out in an orderly sequence that reflects a clear concept of their nature and cause. The patient may, of course, have his or her own ideas about the significance of the symptoms, but these will often be very different from the assessment made by the physician. The way the symptoms are presented is also strongly influenced by the patient's fears and anxieties and by his or her ability to describe these sensations.

Once the patient has been through the process of assessment by a physician, the situation changes.

The patient learns that the malaise, anorexia, and discolored urine are not isolated phenomena but a cluster of symptoms associated with hepatitis. He or she learns that the tiredness is related to depression, that the headaches are tension headaches, and that these are quite separate problems from hepatitis. If we now imagine that the hepatitis becomes worse and the patient is referred to a specialist, it is not difficult to see that the history given to the specialist will be quite different from the one given to the family physician. It will be "organized" around the concepts of infectious hepatitis and depression.

Five facts contribute to the lack of organization in the data presented to the family physician:

1. Patients often present more than one problem at the same visit.
2. The problems are often not presented in order of priority. The most serious problem may be left until last or not even mentioned at all.
3. The most sensitive problems may be expressed in indirect or metaphoric language.
4. The problem is not necessarily the same as the disease.
5. Much of the information presented by the patient is "noise," i.e., it is not useful in solving the patient's presenting problems. At this stage, the patient usually has little insight into the significance of the data he or she is presenting. Even "noise," however, may be useful to the physician as background information.

Diagnosis

Although there is no agreed-upon definition of the terms "diagnosis" and "making a diagnosis," in modern usage they usually refer to the process of classifying a patient's illness into one of the recognized disease categories. This has not always been so. In other periods of history, diagnosis meant diagnosis of a patient rather than diagnosis of a disease. Nevertheless, I think it is better to adhere to modern usage and define diagnosis (the process) as "the assignment of a patient's illness to a category that links the symptoms with a pathologic process, a known outcome, and—whenever possible—a cause."

Successful classification of the illness has four very important results. First, by knowing the natural history of the disease category, the clinician can predict the outcome of the illness if it remains untreated. Second, he or she can make inferences about the cause or causes of the illness. Third, he or she can make inferences about the patient that go beyond the evidence determined by the senses. And fourth, the physician can, by using the common taxonomic language of medicine, communicate the findings to other clinicians. If for example, a patient with fatigue, pallor, and loss of weight is classified as having "pernicious anemia," the clinician can infer that the patient is deficient in intrinsic factor, will die if untreated, and will respond rapidly to injection of vitamin B_{12}.

It will be clear that classification is a very powerful tool. The successful application of technology to medicine depends on it, for unless physicians can predict the outcome of untreated illness, they cannot know whether or not their interventions are effective. It helps physicians organize their thoughts about the phenomena of illness. As we shall see, it also helps physicians organize their thoughts about human behavior. While recognizing the central role of classification, however, physicians must not lose sight of its limitations. Classification is a generalizing process that tacitly ignores individual differences. It works by reducing the complex phenomena of illness or behavior to relatively simple categories. Neither illness nor behavior, however, is as simple as this. No two patients are the same, and no two illnesses are the same. In making clinical decisions, therefore, the clinician has to go through two processes at the same time: one is a generalizing process, the other an individualizing process. As we shall see when we discuss management decisions, this can lead to different management decisions for patients with the same "diagnosis" or disease label. The distinction between illness and disease, which is discussed later, provides physicians with a useful conceptual framework for thinking about these complex phenomena.

Diagnosing (classifying and naming) the patient's illness is a crucial part of the problem-solving process, but it by no means represents the whole process. At the same time, the clinician has to assess the personal and environmental context of the illness. This will involve the individual description of a unique person as well as other types of classification. The clinician also has to make complex management decisions in which risk and benefit, prognostic, and ethical calculations play a part.

The family physician learns, to an extent few other physician do, the limitations of the conventional classification system. It is estimated that in only about 50 per cent of patients seen by family physicians is it possible to make a diagnosis in the sense I have defined it. The reasons for this have already been given. Of course, conditions that cannot be diagnosed can always be given labels like "low back syndrome" or "pleurodynia," but this is not diagnosis as defined above and labels of this type have little predictive value. Even when a diagnosis is made, the family physician also knows that the problem may not have been solved, for the problem may be different from the diagnosis.

Howie (1973) has provided evidence that with some types of illness, family physicians base their management decisions on the presence or absence of certain clinical features rather than on the diagnostic label applied. In a large study done in 62 general practices, 1000 patients with respiratory illness were reported. Cough and chest signs were present in 163, and of these, 152 (93 per cent) received an antibiotic. The presence of cough and chest signs, therefore, had a predictive value for antibiotic treatment of 0.93. Twelve different diagnostic labels were applied to the conditions of 163 patients. Five of the labels had a predictive value of only 0.45. It appears, therefore, that family physicians, when dealing with certain kinds of illness, make management decisions based on their clinical findings and then apply a diagnostic label after the decision is made.

Illness and Disease

The conceptual distinction between illness and disease is a useful one for the family physician (Kleinman et al., 1978). An illness may be described as all the sensations of a patient and all the ramifications of the disorder. It includes symptoms, feelings, discomforts, disabilities, defenses and supports, attitudes toward the condition and the physician, and the effect of the disorder on personal relationships and work. A disease is a theoretical construct that a physician uses to explain something about a patient's illness. Given a certain constellation of findings we say, for example, that a patient has a disease called pernicious anemia. The category "pernicious anemia" is a useful conceptual tool that enables us to make certain inferences and predictions about the patient.

As I have defined them, disease and illness belong to two different universes of discourse: one to the world of theory, the other to the world of experience. The patient experiences the illness: the physician diagnoses the disease, i.e., puts the illness into his or her own explanatory frame of reference. It is important to note that the patient may have his or her own explanatory frame of reference, which may be derived from the patient's culture, religion, social class, or personal experience (Kleinman et al., 1978).

Understanding Patients' Behavior

From all that has been said so far, it is clear that an understanding of patients' behavior is crucial to the accurate identification of undifferentiated clinical problems. For any patient visit, the physician should be able to answer the following questions:

1. Why did the patient come?
2. Why did the patient come at this particular time?
3. What does the patient mean by these complaints? What type of language is the patient using?
4. What is the patient's own perception of the problem(s)?
5. What is the chief problem?
6. What is the context of the problem(s)? How does it relate to the patient's life situation and stage of development?

The process of finding answers to the questions often goes on in parallel with the process of clinical diagnosis. The steps in the first process are essentially the same as those in the second: the physician responds to certain cues, formulates a hypothesis about the patient's behavior, and then conducts a search to verify the hypothesis. The difference between the two processes is that in clinical diagnosis the physician has as a guide a precise and universally recognized classification of disease. For patient behavior, we have no such universally agreed-upon schema.

It is helpful, however, to formulate simple classification systems that can help us identify patient behavior just as classifications of disease help us identify pathology. One schema of this kind describes five categories of patient behavior at the point of contact with the physician (McWhinney, 1972):

Limit of Tolerance. The patient comes because pain, discomfort, or disability has become intolerable.

Limit of Anxiety. The patient comes not because the symptoms are causing distress but because he or she is anxious about their implications, for example, slight hemoptysis.

Problems of Living that Present as Symptoms. The patient's symptoms are a form of communication by which he tries to convey some personal distress that he is unable to convey in words.

Administrative Needs. This category covers doctor-patient contacts with mainly an administrative purpose, even though the patient is ill, e.g., the provision of a certificate for a transient illness that would not otherwise lead to a demand of service.

No Illness. This category includes all attendances for preventive purposes when no symptoms are present.

Figure 29–1 provides an example of how a physician reaches an understanding of the patient's behavior by formulating and testing behavioral hypotheses.

In the course of problem-solving, the family physician makes use of categories that are different from the recognized taxa of disease. In the early part of the process, for example, he or she may have to place the illness into one of two broad categories: A/B and A/Not A. Examples are given in Figure 29–2.

Several points should be borne in mind about this binary categorization:

1. Although many patients can be usefully categorized in this way, the physician must always remember that patients' problems may fall into both categories, such as psychogenic and organic or upper and lower respiratory infection.
2. This broad categorization is used early in the problem-solving process. Obviously if a patient falls into some of the categories, the process will continue toward a much more precise clinical diagnosis.
3. On the other hand, if the illness is categorized as "not an acute abdomen" or "virus infection (not serious)," the clinician may discontinue the search and observe the patient, since the illness is expected to be minor and self-limiting. In these cases, the clinician can achieve his or her objective by defining

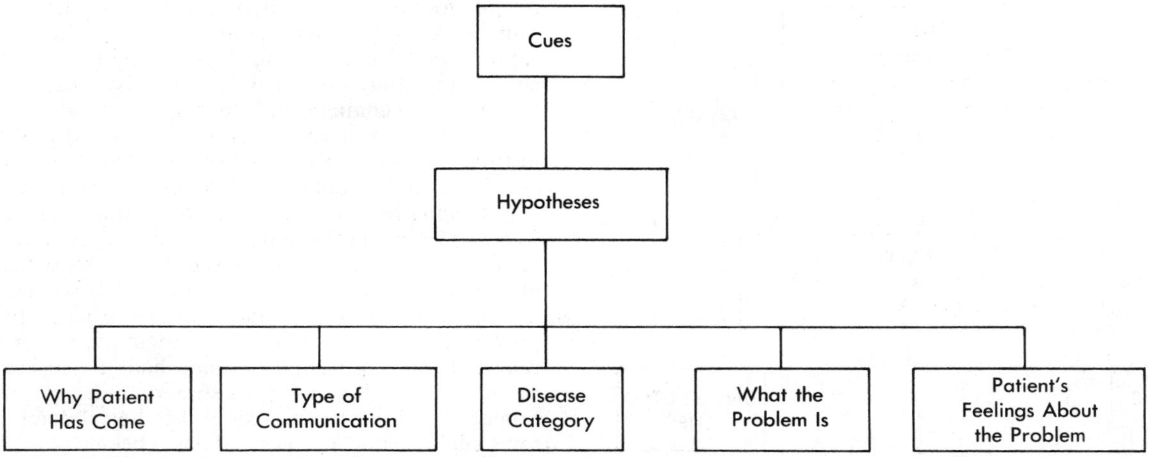

Figure 29–1. Variety of hypotheses formed by the family physician. (From McWhinney, I. R.: An Introduction to Family Medicine. New York, Oxford University Press, 1981. By permission.)

what the patient does not have—the so-called eliminative diagnosis of Crombie (1963).

4. If the illness is categorized as "psychogenic," this may be the end of the classification process. The physician may then proceed to explore the individual aspects of the illness.

5. The tests that are useful for differentiating illnesses into these broad categories are different from those that are useful for attaining a precise clinical diagnosis. The erythrocyte sedimentation rate (ESR), for example, is a very useful test for discriminating between categories like psychogenic or organic and active rheumatism or no active rheumatism; it is much less useful for distinguishing between the categories of rheumatic disease.

One of the reasons that family practice is so confusing to new students and residents is that the descriptions of disease they study in standard medical textbooks are based on observations made in the advanced stages of disease. The family physician works at the other end of the time scale, where the pattern is very different and much less complete. The first stage of the problem-solving process, in this situation, is to identify cues to the patient's illness.

The Problem-Solving Process

Figure 29–3 shows a model of the process of clinical problem-solving that applies to all fields of medicine. The model is based on the work of Elstein and associates (1978). When presented with a problem, the clinician responds to cues by forming one or more hypotheses about what is wrong with the patient. He or she then embarks on a search (the history, examination, and investigation) to test the hypothesis. In the course of the search, the physician looks for positive (confirming) and negative (nonconfirming) evidence. If the evidence does not confirm the hypothesis, the hypothesis is revised and the search begins again. As indicated by the feedback loop in Figure 29–3, the process is a cyclical one, the clinician constantly revising, testing, and further revising the

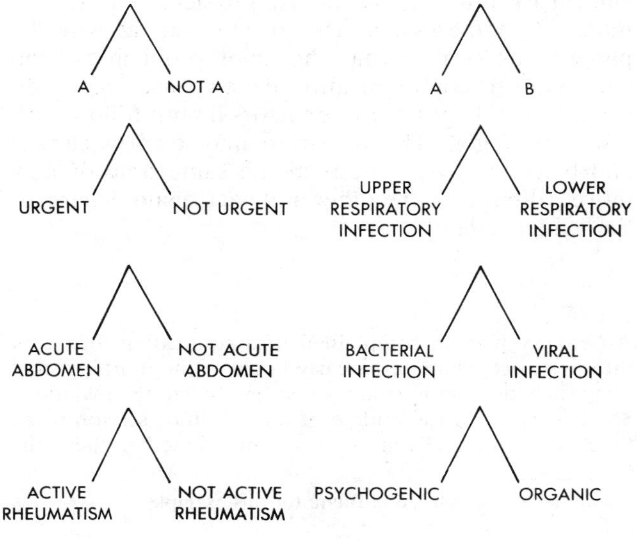

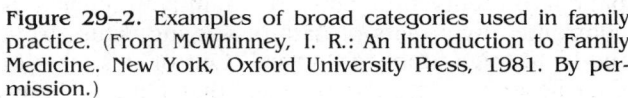

Figure 29–2. Examples of broad categories used in family practice. (From McWhinney, I. R.: An Introduction to Family Medicine. New York, Oxford University Press, 1981. By permission.)

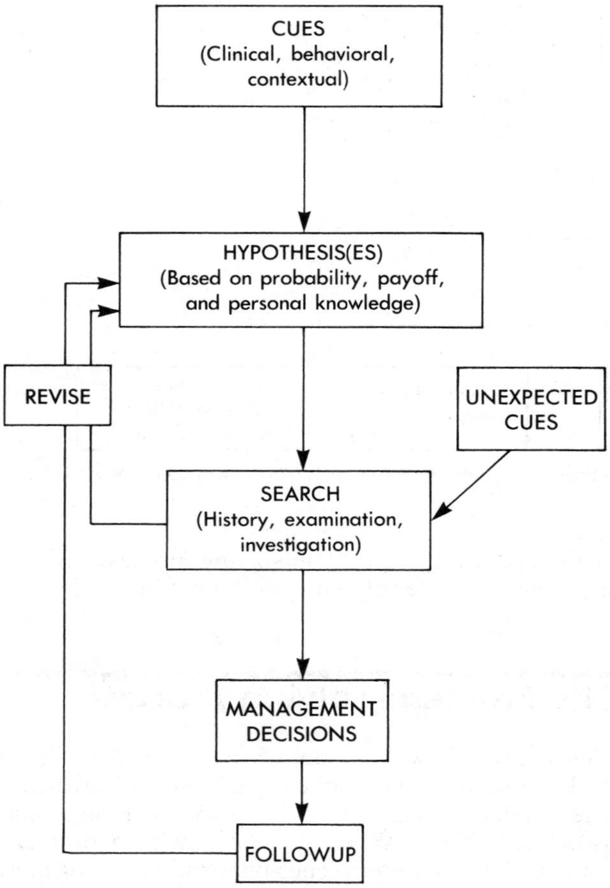

Figure 29–3. Model of the diagnostic process. (From McWhinney, I. R.: An Introduction to Family Medicine. New York, Oxford University Press, 1981. By permission.)

hypothesis until it has been refined to the point at which he or she feels justified in making management decisions. Even after this point, the clinician must still be prepared to revise the hypothesis if the progress of the patient is not proceeding as predicted.

Figure 29–1 illustrates the variety of hypotheses formed by family physicians. Besides the conventional clinical hypotheses, the family physician has to formulate hypotheses about such questions as why the patient has come, what the chief problem is, and what kind of communication is being used. As indicated in the diagram, these factors do not follow each other in stages. The physician may form a clinical and behavioral hypothesis at the same time or may move from one to the other and back again, wherever the evidence leads.

*CASE 1**

An elderly woman complained of a suffocating feeling in the chest, occurring in the early hours of the morning, that was relieved to some extent by sitting by an open window. She first came in the middle of a busy office session when time was short. Given the cues mentioned earlier, the doctor formed a first hypothesis of nocturnal cardiac asthma. After a physical examination revealed no signs to support the diagnosis, the doctor sent the patient for a chest x-ray study. When this, too, was normal, he asked the patient to come in for a longer interview.

At the second visit the doctor obtained the following history. The patient's main complaint was of very active peristalsis and abdominal discomfort, occurring at night and keeping her awake. After lying awake for hours, she would become more and more tense, get a suffocating feeling, and have to get up and go to the window. The abdominal symptoms had been present for twenty years, but the insomnia was of more recent origin. Many years previously she had had a cholecystectomy, which failed to relieve her symptoms, and later had a mastectomy for carcinoma. She had a fear of surgery and, on direct questioning, admitted to an anxiety that her abdominal symptoms might be due to cancer. She had been widowed several years and lived in an apartment by herself. Recently her landlord had raised her rent without giving her any notice. Her two children were both married and were living far away. Recently her daughter had moved near to her after living further away for some years. During the interview, she expressed hostility toward her landlord, who, she believed, had been very unfair to her.

The physician's hypotheses as he went through this process can be represented in a flow diagram (Figure 29–4).

*I am indebted to Dr. John Biehn for this example.

This example illustrates a number of important points:

1. Under pressure of time, the physician focused on the hypothesis with the highest payoff: cardiac asthma.

2. Because of his knowledge of the patient, he was able to move easily between physical and behavioral hypotheses as cues were received.

3. Some other cues were symptoms—others were contextual (why did the patient come in after 20 years?).

4. Correct formulation of the problem was the key to successful management, even with this relatively minor problem. If the physician had focused on the abdominal symptoms and not picked up the behavioral cues, the patient might have been subjected to a series of uncomfortable, expensive, and redundant investigations. As it was, explanation and reassurance, together with a short period on an anxiolytic drug, led to a resolution of the problem.

5. There is no diagnosis in the conventional sense of the term.

Cues. A cue is an item of information. When a patient presents problems, the family physician is confronted by a mass of data of varying value, from the highly significant to "noise." Out of this mass of data he or she responds to cues that have meaning because they give him or her an idea about what is wrong with the patient.

Cues can be classified in a number of ways:

1. Single or multiple. Sometimes there is only a single cue. More often they form a cluster, so that the physician responds to a pattern.

2. Symptom cues, sign cues, behavioral cues,

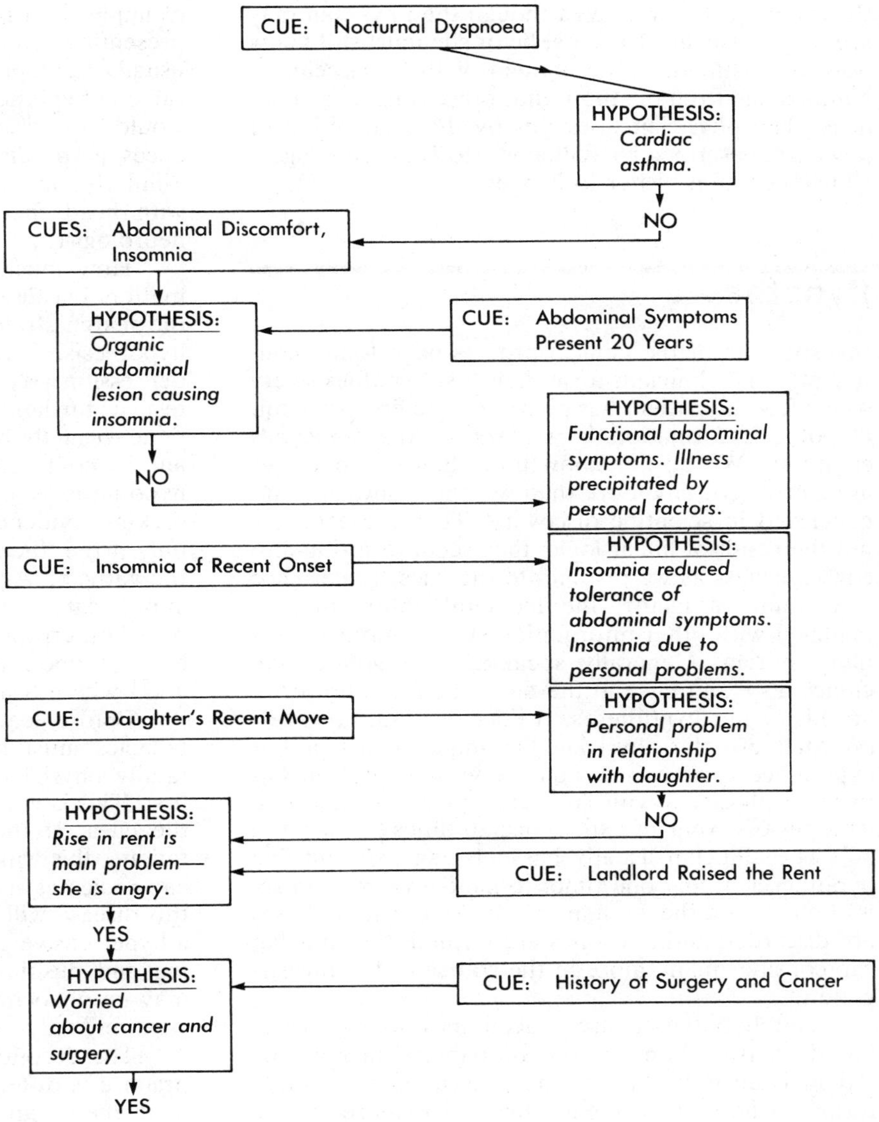

Figure 29–4. Flow diagram to illustrate hypothesis testing in a case. (From McWhinney, I. R.: An Introduction to Family Medicine. New York, Oxford University Press, 1981. By permission.)

contextual cues. Symptom and sign cues need no explanation. Behavioral cues are those the physician receives from the patient's behavior or from his or her subjective sensations. "I feel I could cry" is a cue to the patient's emotional state. "This patient makes me feel depressed" may be a cue to the patient's mood. Contextual cues are those that come from some incongruity the physician senses in the whole pattern of the consultation. For example: "Why did the patient not mention her husband?"

3. Certain and probabilistic cues. A certain cue enables the physician to say with certainty what is wrong with the patient. This is what we usually mean by a spot diagnosis. Unfortunately, certain cues are rare in family practice, as they are in most fields of medicine. Most cues are probabilistic, i.e., they may indicate a number of different diseases with varying probabilities, and the physician can only formulate hypotheses about what is wrong with the patient. The hypotheses then have to be tested by a search for further information.

Of all the cues presented to family physicians, symptoms are the most important. In the early stage of illness, and in the varieties of illness seen by the family physician, signs are less frequently available. The family physician is especially concerned with two aspects of a symptom. One is its capacity to bring the patient to the office (i.e., its significance for the patient). This has been called by Feinstein (1967) the "iatrotrophic stimulus." For example, hemoptysis has a greater value as an iatrotrophic stimulus than cough. The other is the sensitivity, specificity, and predictive value of the symptom in the early stages of illness. These terms will be defined later when the search is discussed. All of them are measures of how effective a symptom or test is in identifying a disease and in discriminating between it and other diseases or a state of health.

To learn family medicine, one must learn the value of symptoms in the early stages of illness. Naturally, cues to the early detection of serious and life-threatening illness are of special importance for the family physician. Even though the physician may see only one every 10 years, he or she must still know how to distinguish the patient with subarachnoid hemorrhage from the thousands presenting with headache. The physician does this by the recognition of key cues, described by Williams (1977) as "red flags," which alert him or her to danger.

Hypotheses

Investigators of the clinical process have found consistently that clinicians form their first hypothesis very soon after the patient has presented the first problem. Hypothesis formation is a mark of the clinician's creativity. We do not know how clinical hypotheses are generated, any more than we know how they are generated in scientific discovery. They are certainly not the result of linear logic: they seem to spring into consciousness as we respond to the cues. Experience is certainly a factor: the incoming information is matched with other information stored in our mind's filing system. Generally speaking, the greater the clinician's experience in the field, the more powerful are his or her hypotheses. It does depend, however, on what use the physician has made of his or her experience. There is a well known comparison between a physician with 20 years' experience and one who has one year of experience 20 times.

The clinician usually has between two and five hypotheses at any one time: to handle more than six is difficult for the human mind. As old hypotheses are discarded and new ones are formed, the clinician can consider many more in the course of the investigation.

The hypotheses are placed in ranking order, based on two main criteria: probability and payoff. Payoff is an indication of the consequences of diagnosing or not diagnosing a disease. The more serious a disease and the more it is amenable to treatment, the greater the positive payoff of making the diagnosis and the greater the negative payoff of missing it. If a disease has a high payoff, it may be ranked high on the clinician's list, even though it has a low probability. In a child with abdominal pain, for example, acute appendicitis may be ranked high—even though of low probability—because of the high positive value of an early diagnosis.

If considerations of pay-off do not arise, the hypotheses are ranked in order of probability. Note that this is not the prior probability (the prevalence of the disease in the practice population) but *the conditional probability* (the probability of the presence of the disease, given the patient's symptoms). A synonym for conditional probability is predictive value: the predictive value of symptom x for disease A.

Predictive value varies with prevalence. Because of differences in disease prevalence, there may be a big difference between the predictive values of the *same symptom* in family and specialty practices. For example, in a patient with fatigue but with no other presenting data, my first-ranking hypothesis would usually be depression. For a hematologist, the first-ranking hypothesis might be anemia. Each hypothesis would be correct in its own context, given the differences in predictive value of the symptom fatigue. Similarly, my first-ranking hypothesis in a patient with headache might be different from that of a neurologist.

How much does the ranking order matter? It matters because the order of hypotheses determines the search strategy. If depression is my first-ranking hypothesis, I would begin by seeking evidence of depression. If my hypothesis is supported I would test it further by ruling out other causes of fatigue—usually by a few simple and economical tests and by continuing observation over time. If my first hypothesis is a blood disorder, I would begin by seeking evidence for this and consider depression only if the findings were negative or did not explain the fatigue. Again, each search strategy would be appropriate in its context. However, a search strategy based on erroneous ranking (assuming payoff factors are not operative) can lead to waste of resources and—where tests carry a risk—harm to the patient.

Before leaving the subject of hypotheses, two fallacies must be mentioned. The first is that the family physician always thinks of common diseases first. This is not necessarily so: it depends entirely on the cues. If the cues are highly probabilistic, like fatigue, this will hold true. If, on the other hand, the cue indicates a rare disease with relative certainty, this disease will be the physician's first hypothesis. If a hypertensive patient complains of attacks of sweating and flushing, for example, the first hypothesis may be pheochromocytoma, even though the physician may only see one case in a whole lifetime.

The second fallacy is that diagnosis in family practice is different from diagnosis in other fields of medicine because it is probabilistic. All clinical diagnosis is probabilistic. Where family practice differs is that it deals in the relatively low levels of probability at which many decisions have to be made.

The Search. The purpose of the search is twofold: to test and validate the physician's hypothesis(es) and to bring to light new and unexpected cues. These purposes are fulfilled respectively by the directed and the routine search.

The Directed Search. Since the purpose of the directed search is to test the physician's initial hypothesis, it follows that the search strategy will vary with the hypothesis. In selecting a search strategy, the family physician has to make two kinds of choices: which tests to use and what the extent of the search should be.

The word "tests" embraces history questions, items included in the physical examination, and laboratory and imaging investigations. Tests are selected according to two kinds of criteria. First, the capacity of the test to change the prior or pre-test probability that the patient has or does not have the disease in question. Second, the risks and benefits of doing the test. The measures used to determine the usefulness of a test are its sensitivity, specificity, and predictive value.

One way of understanding these indices is by means of a 2 × 2 grid, illustrated in Table 29–1. Patients with the disease (e.g., infectious mononucleosis) are in the two left-hand boxes, those without the disease in the two right-hand boxes. Patients with positive test results (with the Monospot test) are in the upper two boxes, those with negative test results are in the lower two boxes. The boxes are identified from the upper left as a, b, c, and d. Box a contains those patients who have the disease and who have positive test results (true positives). Box b contains those patients without the disease with positive test results (false positives). Box c contains those patients with the disease who have negative test results (false negatives). Box d contains those patients without the disease who have negative test results (true negatives).

With the help of the table, we can now look at the meaning of the three indices.

SENSITIVITY

Sensitivity is the proportion of patients with the disease who have a positive test result, which has been called "positivity in disease" (Galen and Gambino, 1975). In the table, boxes a + c give us those patients with the disease and box a gives us those with the disease who have positive test results. Therefore, sensitivity expressed as a percentage is

$$\frac{a}{a + c} \times 100$$

Another way of putting this would be

$$\text{Sensitivity} = \frac{\text{True positives (TP)}}{\text{True positives (TP)} + \text{False negatives (FN)}} \times 100$$

In Table 29–1, the boxes have been completed for the Monospot test used in infectious mononucleosis. The sensitivity of the test is

$$\frac{17}{17 + 3} \times 100 = 85 \text{ per cent}$$

Some factors about sensitivity are especially important for family physicians. A highly sensitive test is very good for ruling out hypotheses. If we have a test that is 100 per cent sensitive, and the patient has negative test results, we can say with confidence that the patient does not have the disease. Since the test is 100 per cent sensitive, we know that there are no false negatives. A positive test, however, is not so helpful, because we do not know whether it is a true or false positive. If a test is 100 per cent sensitive, it will certainly not be 100 per cent specific and there will be some false positives. Let us consider some examples.

In a study of headache in family practice, we found that tenderness on pressure over the sinuses was 100 per cent sensitive for sinusitis. Absence of tenderness ruled out sinusitis. Presence of tenderness, however, was of little value because so many patients without sinusitis had positive test results. In patients over the age of 50 with headache, an erythrocyte sedimentation rate of >50 mm. in 1 hour was 100 per cent sensitive for cranial arteritis. This is very tentative since the disease is rare and there was only one case among the 272 patients in the study. There was also only one false positive, a patient who turned out to have pernicious anemia. Our study supported a clinical impression that the test is very useful for ruling out cranial arteritis.

Table 29–1. SENSITIVITY, SPECIFICITY, AND PREDICTIVE VALUE OF THE MONOSPOT TEST FOR INFECTIOUS MONONUCLEOSIS IN PATIENTS WITH SORE THROAT*

		Infectious mononucleosis	
		Present	Absent
Monospot test	Positive	17 (a)	69 (b)
	Negative	3 (c)	911 (d)
		20	980

$$\text{Sensitivity} = \frac{a}{a + c} \times 100 = \frac{17}{20} \times 100 = 85 \text{ per cent}$$

$$\text{Specificity} = \frac{d}{b + d} \times 100 = \frac{911}{69 + 911} \times 100 = 93 \text{ per cent}$$

$$\text{Positive Predictive Value} = \frac{a}{a + b} \times 100 = \frac{17}{17 + 69} \times 100 = 19 \text{ per cent}$$

*Prevalence of IM in patients with sore throat = 20/1000.

Sensitivity Varies with the Stage of the Disease. Failure to understand this factor can lead to difficulties for the newcomer to family medicine.

CASE 2

A second year resident saw a 12-year-old boy in the office during his morning session. The boy had complained of continuous central abdominal pain for several hours. On examination, there was no abdominal tenderness and the temperature was normal. Since there was some frequency of micturition, the resident diagnosed a urinary infection. That same evening, the mother called the doctor on duty because the pain was worse and the boy was vomiting. Examination of the abdomen showed tenderness and muscular rigidity in all areas. A perforated appendix was diagnosed and the boy made a full recovery after emergency surgery.

The pitfall here was that abdominal tenderness and pyrexia, although sensitive signs in the later stages of appendicitis, are not 100 per cent sensitive in the early stages. The family physician cannot, therefore, rely on these for ruling out appendicitis. In this case, the history of continuous abdominal pain should have been sufficient to require re-examination of the patient within 4 hours. An additional error was to make urinary infection a top-ranking hypothesis, since it is uncommon in males of this age and not usually associated with continuous abdominal pain.

This variation of sensitivity with evolution of a disease is apparent in many diagnostic tests: the chest x-ray film in pneumonia, lung cancer, and pulmonary embolus; the electrocardiogram in myocardial infarction; and splenic enlargement in infectious mononucleosis. Few are well documented; textbooks are not written about the early stages of illness.

SPECIFICITY

Specificity is the proportion of patients without the disease who have a negative test result. This is sometimes referred to as "negativity in health" (Galen and Gambino, 1975), but note that absence of the disease in question is not synonymous with health. The patient may have some other disease. In Table 29–1, boxes b and d represent those patients without the disease and box d represents those without the disease who have negative test results. Specificity, therefore, expressed as a percentage is

$$\frac{d}{b + d} \times 100$$

Another way of putting this would be

$$\frac{\text{True negatives (TN)}}{\text{True negatives (TN)} + \text{False positives (FP)}}$$

In Table 29–1, the specificity of the Monospot test is

$$\frac{911}{69 + 911} \times 100 = 93 \text{ per cent}$$

A highly specific test is very good for selecting possible hypotheses. If a test is 100 per cent specific and the patient has a positive test result, we can say with certainty that the patient has the disease. Since the test is 100 per cent specific, we know that there are no false positives. The test is diagnostic. A negative test, however, is less helpful, because we do not know whether or not it is a true or false negative. If a test is 100 per cent specific, it will almost certainly not be 100 per cent sensitive.

PREDICTIVE VALUE

As we have seen, sensitivity tells us nothing about the false positives and specificity tells us nothing about the false negatives. Yet it is important for us to know about them. The trouble about false positives and false negatives is that both carry penalties for the patient. A false positive can be hazardous in two ways: by imposing a disease label on a healthy person and by exposing him or her to risky investigations and therapies. A false negative carries a penalty since it misses the diagnosis in a sick patient. Thus, we need a measure that tells us about the false positives and negatives. The predictive value provides us with this information.

The positive predictive value is the proportion of positive test results that are true positives (note that + ve = positive and − ve = negative):

$$\text{PV} + \text{ve} = \frac{\text{TP}}{\text{TP} + \text{FP}} \times 100$$

The negative predictive value is the proportion of negative test results that are true negatives:

$$\text{PV} - \text{ve} = \frac{\text{TN}}{\text{TN} + \text{FN}} \times 100$$

The denominator in each case is the number of positive or negative test results rather than the number of patients with or without the disease. In Table 29–1, the positive predictive value is

$$\frac{a}{a + b}$$

The negative predictive value is

$$\frac{d}{c + d}$$

Synonyms for positive predictive value are the conditional probability of a positive test result and the post-test probability of disease following a positive result. Synonyms for negative predictive value are the conditional probability of a negative test result and the post-test probability of no disease following a negative result.

In Table 29–1, the predictive value positive of the Monospot test is:

$$\frac{17}{17 + 69} \times 100 = 19.7 \text{ per cent}$$

The predictive value negative of the Monospot test is:

$$\frac{911}{3 + 911} \times 100 = 99 \text{ per cent}$$

The predictive value is a key index because it tells us the power of a test to change the probability that the patient has the disease in question. There is, however, something very important to bear in mind. We have already mentioned it: The predictive value varies with the prevalence of the disease. Let us see how this works in the case of the Monospot test. In Table 29–1, the prevalence of mononucleosis in patients with sore throat is 2 per cent.

In Table 29–2, the prevalence is 10 per cent. The difference in prevalence could be the difference between a family practice and a student health service practice. The effect of this is to increase the positive predictive value to 58 per cent, whereas the sensitivity and specificity remain virtually the same. The reason is that, as the prevalence increases, the proportion of people with the disease increases and the number of false positives decreases.

The variation of predictive value with prevalence can mean that a test that is indicated in a specialty clinic may be contraindicated in family practice.

Having said that predictive value varies with prevalence, we must go on to say that there is one exception. If the sensitivity of a test is 100 per cent, the predictive value of a negative test does not vary with prevalence. There are no false negatives and the negative predictive value is also 100 per cent. Conversely, if the specificity of a test is 100 per cent, the predictive value of a positive test does not vary with prevalence. There are no false positives and the predictive value of a positive test is also 100 per cent. Unfortunately, there are not many tests that reach 100 per cent either for sensitivity or specificity. Those tests that we have that reach 100 per cent we treasure for their capacity to rule out or to rule in a diagnosis.

For the more common tests with sensitivity and specificity of between 80 and 95 per cent, the variation with prevalence is important. Table 29–3 shows how predictive value changes with prevalence for a test that has 95 per cent sensitivity and specificity. Note that a test has greater power to change the pre-test or prior probability in the middle ranges of prevalence (40 to 80 per cent). When we get to prevalence rates of 90 per cent and 10 per cent, the change in pre-test probability is less than 10 per cent. Whether or not this makes the test justifiable depends on the payoff of the diagnosis and the risk of the test. A disease may be so devastating if undiagnosed and so amenable to treatment that we do the test even though the disease has a very low prevalence. The test for phenylketonuria is an example of this.

A reminder is in order here. Remember that our definition of a test includes elements of the history, examination, and investigation. The experienced clinician selects questions and items of physical examination for their capacity to change the prior probability. Even before the physician begins, the patient's presenting symptoms have changed the prior probability in some way.

Despite the panoply of investigations available to us, the history and physical examination—espe-

Table 29–2. SENSITIVITY, SPECIFICITY, AND PREDICTIVE VALUE OF THE MONOSPOT TEST FOR INFECTIOUS MONONUCLEOSIS IN PATIENTS WITH SORE THROAT*

		Infectious mononucleosis: Present	Infectious mononucleosis: Absent
Monospot test	Positive	86 (a)	63 (b)
	Negative	14 (c)	837 (d)
		100	900

$$\text{Sensitivity} = \frac{a}{a + c} \times 100 = \frac{86}{86 + 14} \times 100 = 86 \text{ per cent}$$

$$\text{Specificity} = \frac{d}{b + d} \times 100 = \frac{837}{63 + 837} \times 100 = 93 \text{ per cent}$$

$$\text{Positive Predictive Value} = \frac{a}{a + b} \times 100 = \frac{86}{86 + 63} \times 100 = 58 \text{ per cent}$$

*Prevalence of IM in patients with sore throat = 100/1000.

Table 29–3. THE EFFECT OF PREVALENCE ON THE PREDICTIVE VALUE OF AN EXCELLENT SIGN, SYMPTOM, OR LABORATORY TEST*†

Prevalence (Pre-test likelihood or prior probability of disease)	99 per cent	95 per cent	90 per cent	80 per cent	70 per cent	60 per cent	50 per cent	40 per cent	30 per cent	20 per cent	10 per cent	5 per cent	1 per cent	0.5 per cent	0.1 per cent
Predictive value of a positive test (Posterior probability of disease following a positive test result)	99.9 per cent	99.7 per cent	99.4 per cent	99 per cent	98 per cent	97 per cent	95 per cent	93 per cent	89 per cent	83 per cent	68 per cent	50 per cent	16 per cent	9 per cent	2 per cent
Predictive value of a negative test (Posterior probability of *no* disease following a negative test result)	16 per cent	50 per cent	68 per cent	83 per cent	89 per cent	93 per cent	95 per cent	97 per cent	98 per cent	99 per cent	99.4 per cent	99.7 per cent	99.9 per cent	99.97 per cent	99.99 per cent
(Posterior probability *of* disease following a negative test result)	84 per cent	50 per cent	32 per cent	17 per cent	11 per cent	7 per cent	5 per cent	3 per cent	2 per cent	1 per cent	0.6 per cent	0.3 per cent	0.1 per cent	0.03 per cent	0.01 per cent

*From Sackett D. L., Hayes R. B., and Tugwell, P.: Clinical Epidemiology: A Basic Science for Clinical Medicine. Little, Brown & Co., Inc., Boston: 1985. Reproduced with permission.

†Both sensitivity and specificity equal 95 per cent in every case.

cially the history in family practice—are still the most effective ways of increasing the probability. Let us see how this works in the case of a patient with chest pain.*

Suppose we have a middle-aged man who presents with a typical history of angina of effort: tight substernal pain that comes on after a fixed amount of exertion and is relieved within 5 minutes of rest. The probability of coronary disease, given these symptoms (conditional probability) is about 90 per cent (Diamond and Forrester, 1979). By taking the history alone, we have raised the probability from the prevalence of coronary disease in males of his age group in our practice (about 5 per cent) to 90 per cent. Now, will an exercise electrocardiogram help define the condition further? The positive predictive value at this prevalence rate is 98 per cent, a small increase in the previous figure; the negative predictive value is 20 per cent; that is, even if the test is negative there is still an 80 per cent probability of coronary disease. The sensitivity of the test is 60 per cent, and the specificity 91 per cent. Let us apply the acid test for an investigation: Will it change our management of the patient whatever the result? In this case, the answer is no. If the test is positive, we will still be certain of our diagnosis: but we were already certain. If the test is negative, it will not make any difference, since we will still go by our clinical assessment: with a 60 per cent sensitivity, the value of the test to rule out the disease is low.

Now suppose we have a 40-year-old man with vague left-sided chest pain, unrelated to exercise, but worse on some movements of the chest wall. The history is suggestive of intercostal muscle pain and has no features to indicate coronary disease, although the patient is worried about his heart. The probability of coronary disease in this patient is about the same as for any other male of his age in the practice population—about 5 per cent. The positive predictive value of an exercise electrocardiogram at this prevalence rate is only 26 per cent. The negative predictive value is 98 per cent, so only 2 per cent of the negatives will be false negatives. Will an exercise electrocardiogram define the condition further? A negative result will reinforce our opinion that the patient does not have coronary disease. A positive test will not help us, since 74 per cent of positives will be false positives. In fact, it will probably do harm since it will make it more difficult to reassure the patient that he does not have coronary disease—a big price to pay for a marginal benefit. The physician will do better to have confidence in his or her own clinical judgment.

Now suppose we have a middle-aged man with attacks of substernal pain for several months that occurs at rest and lasts from a few minutes to half an hour, sometimes related to exertion but not relieved by rest, and that has not worsened since the onset. The pre-test probability of coronary disease in a patient with this type of history is about 50 per cent. At this prevalence rate, the positive predictive value of the test is 87 per cent—a big increase in the probability of coronary disease. The negative predictive value is 69 per cent, so 31 per cent of negatives will be false negatives, a reduction of 19 per cent in the pre-test probability.

If positive, the test does help to clarify the management options. The physician will feel justified in treating the condition as ischemic heart disease with appropriate drugs and reduction of risk factors

*I have based this example on cases described by D. L. Sackett, R. B. Haynes, and P. Tugwell in their book *Clinical Epidemiology: A Basic Science for Clinical Medicine* (Little, Brown & Co., Inc., 1985).

and refer the patient for further investigation if there is a poor response or if the pain progresses. If negative, the test is less helpful.

In all these patients, the history alone has been enormously effective in assessing the probability of coronary disease. It has provided the family physician with most of what is needed for making good management decisions, and the exercise electrocardiogram does not have a great deal to add.

Before leaving the question of how to select tests, mention must be made of two other tools that help physicians make choices: likelihood ratios and decision analysis.

DECISION ANALYSIS

As a tool for helping physicians with decisions about individual patients, decision analysis has little application in family practice. It is useful mainly in developing optimal strategies for complex clinical conditions. Sackett and associates (1985) define decision analysis as "a method of describing complex clinical problems in an explicit fashion, identifying the available courses of action (both in terms of diagnosis and management), assessing the probability and value (or utility) of all possible outcomes, and then making a simple calculation to select the optimal course of action." For a description of how this tool works, see Sackett and associates (1985).

LIKELIHOOD RATIOS

Likelihood ratios are another way of expressing how good a test is for increasing the probability of a diagnosis. The calculation of the ratios uses indices with which we are already familiar: sensitivity and specificity. The likelihood ratio for a positive result is the odds that a test will be positive in a patient with the disease, in contrast to a patient without the disease. The likelihood ratio for a negative result is the odds that a test will be negative in a patient with the disease, contrasted with a patient without the disease.

The first figure in the likelihood ratio positive (positivity in disease, or true positive rate) is the sensitivity of the test. The second figure (positivity in non-disease, or false positive rate) is 100 minus the specificity (expressed as a percentage). For example, the likelihood ratio of a positive Monospot in infectious mononucleosis (from Table 29–1) is

$$\frac{a}{a + c} \times 100 \, / \, 100 - \left(\frac{d}{b + d} \times 100\right)$$

i.e.,

$$85 \, / \, 7 = 12{:}1$$

The odds of a patient with a positive test result having the disease are 12 to 1. By multiplying the ratio with the pre-test odds, we can arrive at the post-test odds for the diagnosis. The pre-test odds on a patient having infectious mononucleosis were 1:50, or 0.02:1. The post-test odds with a positive test are therefore 0.02 × 12 or 0.24:1. If we prefer to think in probabilities, odds can be converted to probability and vice versa. To convert odds to probability, we divide it by itself plus one. The post-test odds on infectious mononucleosis becomes a post-test probability of

$$\frac{0.24}{0.24 + 1} = 0.19 \text{ or } 19\%$$

To convert probabilities to odds, we divide the probability by its complement (one minus itself). The post-test probability of 94.7 per cent becomes a post-test odds of

$$\frac{0.19}{1 - 0.19} = \frac{0.19}{0.81} = 0.23$$

In this example, we have treated the test as if the result will be either positive or negative rather than as a continuous variable. It is also possible to express likelihood ratios for different levels of a test result that varies over a range. For the serum uric acid test, for example, we can express the likelihood ratio for gout at 7.0, 8.0, and 9.0 mg./100 ml.

Since likelihood ratios are calculated from sensitivity and specificity data, they do not vary with the prevalence of the disease. Like sensitivity and specificity, however, they do vary with the stage of the disease.

As time goes on, information about the likelihood ratios and predictive values of tests will probably become increasingly available. As family physicians, we should not only get to know these indices for the symptoms, signs, and tests we use ourselves but also become accustomed to asking our consultants for the likelihood ratios or predictive values of tests they recommend to us. As our patients become more informed, we may also find that they begin to ask these questions themselves.

In testing a hypothesis, the clinician seeks both positive and negative evidence: He or she seeks not only to support it but also to refute it; to rule it in and to rule it out. Suppose that the first two hypotheses in a patient with weight loss are thyrotoxicosis and diabetes. Suppose that the search has yielded evidence in support of thyrotoxicosis. The physician will then proceed with tests like urine and blood sugar, which should be negative if the first hypothesis is correct (unless both conditions are present). Studies of problem-solving have shown that clinicians, like problem-solvers in other fields, show a marked preference for positive over negative evidence. They would much rather try to support their hypothesis than to refute it. As Elstein and coworkers

(1978) have observed, this is an experimental confirmation of an observation made centuries ago by Francis Bacon: "It is the peculiar and perpetual error of the human intellect to be more moved and excited by affirmatives than by negatives." The testing of hypotheses raises the difficult question of when the directed search should be ended. When has the physician collected enough evidence? What is the appropriate level of probability?

The Last Part of the Search. This brings us face to face with the problem of uncertainty and with the potential conflict between precision on the one hand and the patient's well-being on the other. Uncertainty is inherent in medicine. The data we collect are of uncertain value; the observations we make and the tests we perform are subject to error; our diagnoses are probabilistic; and both the outcome of the patient's illness and the results of treatment are, to varying degrees, unknown. The main purpose of our search is to reduce uncertainty. The problem is introduced when we have to balance the pursuit of greater precision against the risk of further testing. In modern times, precision in medicine has been the overriding value. It is of course a great good and a worthy objective. But greater precision does not necessarily reduce uncertainty. The quest for precision can become mindless, as in the inexorable search for a diagnosis in a patient who is already recovering from an illness. The quest for precision can become a false trail when the true need is to gain a better understanding of the patient.

Until recently, an excessive pursuit of precision did not carry many risks. Now the technology of investigation has advanced so rapidly as to create many hazards, not to speak of enormous expense. Not the least of the hazards is that of finding a spurious abnormality, with all the attendant risks of inappropriate treatment.

The End-Point in Family Practice. Traditionally, the end-point of the search has been a diagnosis. In family practice, however, this is not always realistic. For reasons already discussed, many of the illnesses seen in family practice do not have a diagnosis in the strict sense of the term.

The illness may be at too early a stage for definitive diagnosis; it may clear spontaneously before diagnosis is possible; or it may be so interwoven with the personal life of the patient as to defy categorization.

In all patients, however, decisions have to be made, even if no diagnosis is possible. It is more helpful, therefore, to describe the end-point in terms of a management decision. The end-point of the search on any particular occasion is the point at which enough information is available for an informed decision to be made without avoidable risk to the patient.

It is important to understand that end-points are often different in family practice from those in referral specialties. A consultant seeing a referred patient will probably feel the need to make a definitive diagnosis before referring the patient back to his or her own physician. A family physician is not under the same constraint. The continuing relationship with patients means that not all problems have to be solved right away. Since the relationship itself has no formal end-point, the search can be discontinued and resumed according to need. In this sense, there is no final end-point, since the family physician should always be ready to revise the hypothesis if new evidence becomes available.

The family physician, because of his or her role, makes two types of decisions that do not arise as often in other branches of medicine:

1. The decision to wait. In making this decision, the physician is using the evolution of the illness over time as a test of the hypothesis. It is obviously inherent in this decision that no extra risk should be incurred by waiting. The use of time to validate hypotheses in this way can make many investigations redundant. One example of this decision is the eliminative diagnosis referred to earlier, in which the physician decides that the illness is transient and minor, then waits for the hypothesis to be verified.

2. The decision to refer. The end-point of a search may be the decision to consult with or refer the patient to another physician. This decision may have to be made before a definitive diagnosis is arrived at, for example, with a severely ill baby or a patient with an acute abdomen. It is clear that the objective of the family physician in these cases is different from that of the specialist. The family physician has fulfilled the obligation if he or she has decided to refer the patient in time to receive effective treatment. The physician has failed to fulfill his or her obligation if the outcome of the illness was worsened by delaying referral in an effort to provide a more definitive diagnosis.

The Routine Search. This comprises the routine systems inquiry and physical examination. The chief aims of the routine part of the search are to prompt alternative hypotheses by bringing to light cures that have not emerged in the directed part of the search, to collect baseline and background data on the patient, and to screen for symptomless conditions like hypertension.

The routine search is sometimes referred to as a complete history and physical. This is a misnomer, for even the routine search is a selection from a much larger number of possible tests. As in the directed search, the tests are selected for their usefulness in achieving the objective. Internists would probably include ophthalmoscopy in their routine, but not laryngoscopy—for the very good reason that ophthalmoscopy is more useful in generating new cues in patients seen by internists. For similar reasons, otolaryngologists would probably make the opposite choice.

For three reasons, the family physician tends to make different use of routine tests than some other clinicians. First, since the patient is usually well known to the physician, he or she may already have all the baseline data needed. Second, in minor and transient disorders, little in the way of a routine search is required. Third, since the physician deals with such a wide range of clinical problems, from minor to life threatening, no single routine is appropriate for every patient. Therefore, the physician develops different routine tests for different problems: one for sore throat, one for fatigue, one for dyspepsia, and so on.

Management Decisions. Diagnosis, as defined above, is a categorizing process. Its end-point is a probabilistic statement about what is wrong with the patient. A decision, on the other hand, cannot be probabalistic. A clinician cannot "probably" prescribe an antibiotic or "probably" refer a patient. Management decisions have to be either one way or the other. When the clinician arrives at such a decision, he or she takes the probabilistic statement and integrates it with a large number of other variables, many of them unique to the patient. Whereas diagnosis is a reductive, generalizing process, decision-making is a synthesizing, individualizing process.

Among the variables the clinician must take into account are the patient's wishes; the diagnosis of the patient's main problem; other problems the patient may have; the prognosis; the personality and life situation of the patient; the risks and benefits of the decision alternatives; the family's wishes; and ethical issues.

First on this list are the patient's wishes, because if we have a true regard for his or her autonomy, it is the patient who makes the decision on the advice of his physician after being as fully informed as possible about the alternatives.

The complexity of problems, the frequent difficulty in achieving diagnostic precision, and the close personal knowledge of patients combine to make management both the most challenging and the most rewarding part of family practice. Gayle Stephens (1975) has called it "the quintessential skill of clinical practice and the ground of what family physicians know that is unique." Management is probably more individualized in family practice than in any other field of medicine. Obviously, the more precisely defined the problem, the less scope for variation in management. If a patient has pernicious anemia, the treatment in all cases is vitamin B_{12}. Even in this case, however, there may be individual aspects of management that, if neglected, may lead to failure of treatment. For example, how likely is the patient to comply? What is to be done to ensure that he or she is followed up? Few problems in family practice are as easy to define as pernicious anemia.

Extraneous Factors in Clinical Decision-Making. In this chapter, emphasis has been placed on the logic of decision-making. The process has been presented as a rational one, with a logic arising out of the clinical situation itself. It is important to recognize, however, that factors outside the clinical situation may have a powerful influence on the process. Some of these factors are as follows:

1. Institutional factors. In deciding on a search strategy, a physician may be heavily influenced by the rules of the institution. Such rules, applied regardless of individual situations, lie behind some of the overinvestigation that is done in teaching hospitals. The rules are no less powerful for being unwritten.

2. Patients' expectations. As a result of reading medical articles in the press, or of hearsay, or of a belief that they are exercising their rights as consumers, patients may make demands for tests that the physician may find very difficult to resist, even though there is no logical justification for them.

3. Fear of litigation. The prevalence of malpractice suits has had a powerful influence on the search strategies of physicians, the effect being to encourage overinvestigation.

4. The physician's experience. Another influence on the diagnostic process is the physician's own personality, feelings, and experience. Physicians who feel insecure or who cannot tolerate uncertainty tend to carry out more tests than those who feel secure and tolerate uncertainty well. A physician's strategy may be influenced by feelings of anxiety about a particular patient or a type of problem. If a physician believes he or she has made past errors with a patient or with a particular problem, for example, he or she may tend to be overmeticulous in investigations or especially liable to refer the patient to a specialist.

Identification of Errors

It is important for both teacher and learner to be able to identify where in the process an error has occurred. Problem-solving errors in family practice can be classified according to the level at which they occur: cues, hypotheses, search, or management decisions. Some common examples are given below.

Cue Blindness. This describes the situation in which the clinician fails to respond to cues presented by the patient. The fault may be due to inexperience, as when the clinician does not recognize the information as a cue, or the cue may be "blocked out" for some reason. This is especially common with late cues. One example from my own experience was in a patient who for some time had had a fever of unknown origin, with a high erythrocyte sedimentation rate. Exhaustive investigation had failed to provide a diagnosis. After a time, the patient began to complain of headaches, a cue missed until a consultant recognized it as a predictor of cranial arteritis, a diagnosis that proved to be correct.

Another reason that cues are missed is the particular "mental set" of the clinician. The following story was told by a resident about a clinician he was working with. The patient suffered from anterior chest pain, and the clinician was taking a history with a diagnosis of ischemic heart disease in mind. Suddenly the patient interjected, "And I feel like crying all the time." The clinician failed to respond to this cue and continued to ask questions about the pain. The eventual diagnosis was depression. In this case the clinician had been "set" on a certain line of inquiry, which blinded him to the most valuable cue of all.

Premature Convergence on a Hypothesis. In the early stage of hypothesis formation, it is important for the clinician's thinking to be lateral and divergent, considering many possible explanations for the patient's symptoms. One common error at this level is premature convergence on a hypothesis of virus infection in a patient with a mild febrile illness. This leads to failure to test such alternative hypotheses as urinary tract infection.

Errors in the Search. Two opposite errors are common in the search strategy. The first is redundancy. In this case, investigations are continued far beyond the point necessary for making an informed decision. Overinvestigation is perhaps the most common error in medicine today, though it is more typically found in the teaching hospital than in family practice. Sometimes it is due to the inexorable search for a diagnosis in a patient who is already recovering from an illness. Another example of this error, often found early in the family medicine residency, is the use of investigations when clinical observation would provide a better search strategy. For many illnesses encountered in family practice, like herpes zoster and measles, clinical observation is the only way of making the diagnosis.

A second common error is inadequate testing. Sometimes very simple procedures will increase the validity of a diagnosis without additional risk or expense: a determination of the erythrocyte sedimentation rate in a patient with fatigue and depression; a rectal examination in a patient with abdominal pain; a urine analysis in a patient with fever. Yet these opportunities for validation are often not taken if the clinician feels that there is good positive evidence for the hypothesis. This is an example of the well-known preference of all problem solvers for positive rather than negative evidence.

Management Errors. A common fault in management is failure to consider some of the important variables that should enter into the decision, such as the risks of treatment or the ethical issues. The fault can often be identified by asking two questions: What were the decision alternatives? What is the evidence for and against each alternative? It is by reflecting on their decisions and the ensuing consequences that clinicians can continue to improve their skills.

Conclusion

The methods used by family physicians do not "come naturally"; they have to be learned. Nowadays students can be introduced to them as undergraduates and can learn them formally during vocational training. Formerly, young physicians were plunged into family practice after a hospital-based education and experienced the confusion described by Mackenzie (Mair, 1973):

> *I had not long been in the practice when I discovered how defective was my knowledge. I left college under the impression that every patient's condition could be diagnosed. For a long time I strove to make a diagnosis and assiduously studied my lectures and textbooks, without avail. . . . For some years I thought that this inability to diagnose my patients' complaints was due to personal defects, but gradually, through consultations and other ways, I came to recognize that the kind of information I wanted did not exist. . . .*

It has been erroneously assumed that clinical methods learned in a hospital, on selected patients with advanced disease, will be transferable to the problems encountered in family practice. All the evidence from experimental psychology is that such a transfer does not take place. The learning process must take place in an environment similar to the future environment of practice. Formerly, practitioners did learn eventually, but they did so by the slow and painful process of trial and error.

The description of the methods used by family physicians has been a liberating influence in family medicine. For years, it was assumed—even by family physicians themselves—that their methods were a debased form of the purer and more thorough methods used in other fields of medicine. Now we know that every field of medicine develops its own methods and that those of family medicine are admirably suited to the problems encountered in family practice.

The analysis of clinical decision-making has, therefore, been an important process for family medicine. We cannot teach or learn clinical family practice until we can anatomize the clinical process, give the reasons for our decisions, and identify and correct the errors. A physician who can examine his or her own decisions in this way will continue to grow in clinical wisdom throughout his or her career.

To achieve maximum benefit from this learning process, we must obviously review each case after we know its outcome. Since, in family practice, the interval between the onset of an illness and the outcome may be several years, a good record system is a necessity. Not only should individual patients' records be accurately kept but there should also be a diagnostic index by which the physician can review his or her experience of all patients within a single diagnostic rubric.

References

Bartlett, F.: Thinking. London, Allen and Unwin, 1958.

Bursztajn, H., Feinbloom, R.I., Hamm, A., et al.: Medical Choices, Medical Chances. How Patients, Families, and Physicians Can Cope with Uncertainty. New York, Delacorte Press, 1981. *An important book for family physicians. Bursztajn and his coauthors provide a critique of the conventional approach to clinical decision-making, based, they argue, on a mechanistic paradigm that is no longer valid.*

Carmichael, L.P.: The relational model: A paradigm of family medicine. J. Fla. Med. Assoc., *67*:860–862, 1980.

Cousins, N.: Anatomy of an illness as perceived by the patient. Reflections on Healing and Regeneration. New York, W.W. Norton and Co., 1979.

Crombie, D.L.: Diagnostic methods. Practitioner, *191*:539, 1963.

Diamond, G.A., and Forrester, J.S.: Analysis of probability as an aid in the clinical diagnosis of coronary artery disease. N. Engl. J. Med., *300*:1350–1358, 1979.

Elstein, A.S., Shulman, L.S., and Sprafha, S.A.: Medical Problem-Solving: An Analysis of Clinical Reasoning. Cambridge, Harvard University Press, 1978. *Elstein and his coworkers describe the results of their seminal work on the psychology of clinical reasoning. This work was influential in correcting the delusion that clinicians use an inductive rather than a hypothetic-deductive method for solving problems. It has far-reaching implications for clinical practice and medical education.*

Feinstein, A.: Clinical Judgement. Baltimore, Williams & Wilkins, 1967.

Galen, R.S. and Gambino, S.R.: Beyond Normality. The Predictive Value and Efficiency of Medical Diagnoses. New York, John Wiley, 1975. *A very readable introduction to the principles of clinical reasoning.*

Howie, J.G.R.: A new look at respiratory illness in general practice: A reclassification of respiratory illness based on antibiotic prescribing. J. R. Coll. Gen. Pract., *23*:895, 1973.

Kleinman, A., Eisenberg, L., and Good, B.: Culture, illness and care: Clinical lessons from anthropologic and cross-cultural research. Ann. Intern. Med., *88*:251, 1978. *This important paper proposes strategies for applying concepts from cultural anthropology to clinical medicine. The authors stress the importance of understanding the patient's own culturally determined interpretation of his illness.*

Mair, A.: Sir James Mackenzie, M.D., General Practioner, 1853–1925. Edinburgh, Churchill Livingstone, 1973.

McWhinney, I.R.: Beyond diagnosis. An approach to the integration of behavioral science and clinical medicine. N. Engl. J. Med., *287*:384, 1972.

McWhinney, I.R.: A Textbook of Family Medicine. New York, Oxford University Press, 1989. *Chapter 8 has a detailed discussion of clinical method in family practice.*

Sackett, D.L., Hayes, R.B., and Tugwell, P.: Clinical Epidemiology: A Basic Science for Clinical Medicine. Boston, Little, Brown, & Co., Inc., 1985. *An important source book, which is highly recommended.*

Stephens, G.G.: The intellectual basis of family practice. J. Fam. Pract., *2*:423, 1975.

Weinstein, M.C., Fineberg, H.V., Elstein, A.S., et al.: Clinical Decision Analysis. Philadelphia, W.B. Saunders Company, 1980. *An advanced and authoritative text on the application of decision analysis to clinical medicine. The authors describe how to construct a decision tree, using many clinical examples. Important chapters describe the application of probability theory to clinical medicine, including the use of diagnostic information to revise probabilities.*

Williams, T.: A strategy for defining the clinical content of family medicine. J. Fam. Pract., *4*:497, 1977.

30

Infectious Diseases

Michael F. Parry
Harold C. Neu

Antimicrobial Therapy

Successful treatment of an infectious disease requires early diagnosis and prompt administration of appropriate antimicrobial agents. Above and beyond this, however, the outcome of the illness depends to a considerable extent upon the nature of the infecting agent, its virulence, portal of entry, the natural history of the untreated infection, and the integrity of the host's defense mechanisms. Conditions present in the host, such as malnutrition, neutropenia, or undrained abscesses, are more important determinants of outcome than selection of a specific drug for treatment. Nevertheless, in patients with comparably severe underlying disease, the selection of an appropriate antibiotic clearly enhances outcome.

Antibiotic Susceptibility Testing. Tests of antimicrobial susceptibility provide useful information both to maximize the effectiveness of treatment and to minimize toxicity by enabling the physician to select the most appropriate drug, dose, and route of administration. Susceptibility testing is indicated for all organisms that contribute to an infectious process when the susceptibilities cannot be uniformly predicted on the basis of species identification. Such organisms include members of the *Enterobacteriaceae* (gram-negative enteric bacilli), staphylococci, and nonfermentative gram-negative bacilli, such as *Pseudomonas.*

Techniques for determining antibiotic susceptibility fall into two broad categories: dilution tests and diffusion tests. *Diffusion susceptibility testing* (the Kirby-Bauer method) has been a widely available procedure since the mid 1960's. The principle of the method is that drug, contained in filter paper discs and applied to an agar surface, will diffuse into the surrounding medium and generate a gradient of concentrations from the disc's edge. Zones of inhibition occur where antibiotic concentrations are just sufficient to inhibit bacterial growth on the agar surface. The diameter of the zone produced varies inversely with the concentration of the drug needed to inhibit growth. Results are thus reported as sensitive, moderately sensitive, or resistant in relationship to antimicrobial drug concentrations that are easily achievable in blood or urine with standard doses of a given agent.

In contrast to the disc diffusion method, which is qualitative and reflects bacterial inhibition rather than killing, *broth dilution methods* are quantitative and can be used to determine killing as well as inhibition. Tubes or wells of broth containing an antibiotic are inoculated with a suspension of bacteria and examined for growth, or turbidity, after overnight incubation. Failure of growth to occur indicates effective inhibition, and the lowest concentration of drug inhibiting bacterial growth is called the *minimum inhibitory concentration* or MIC. Bacterial killing can be assessed by subculturing samples from the tubes or wells without apparent growth to see if viable organisms remain. The lowest concentration of drug at which killing is achieved is called the *minimum bactericidal concentration* or MBC. Results reported as MIC values can be directly related to achievable blood, urine, or tissue concentrations of antimicrobial agent. Blood, urine, and cerebrospinal fluid (CSF) concentrations that can be achieved with standard doses of most antimicrobial agents are listed in Table 30–1. Wherever possible, concentrations of the drug at the site of infection should be greater than or equal to eight times the MIC value of the offending organism(s).

It is important for the microbiology laboratory to test bacterial susceptibility to antimicrobial agents known to be representative of other compounds in their class. For example, routine susceptibility testing of *Staphylococcus aureus* includes only one penicillinase-resistant penicillin derivative, such as oxacillin. The class representative, oxacillin, indicates susceptibility to nafcillin and methicillin and the oral agents cloxacillin and dicloxacillin as well.

Cephalosporin antibiotics have been fashionably classified into first-, second-, and third-generation derivatives. All first-generation cephalosporins (e.g., cephalothin, cefazolin, cephradine, cephapirin, cephalexin, and cefaclor) have a similar spectrum of activity and are represented by the class agent, cefazolin. Second-generation cephalosporin derivatives (cefuroxime, cefamandole, cefotetan, and cefoxitin) have expanded but different spectra and need separate susceptibility testing when the organism in question is resistant to a first-generation derivative. Third-generation cephalosporins (e.g., cefotaxime, ceftriaxone, cefoperazone, ceftazidime) offer a further expanded spectrum and need specific susceptibility testing when resistance is encountered to earlier-generation cephalosporin derivatives.

Aminoglycoside antibiotics, although chemically related, differ in their antimicrobial spectrum. Members of this class, such as gentamicin and amikacin, must be tested separately. Tobramycin susceptibilities are quite similar to those of gentamicin, and, except for some nonfermentative bacilli (such as *Pseudomonas* and *Acinetobacter*), susceptibility to tobramycin is indicated by susceptibility to gentamicin and vice versa.

Antibiotic Selection. Organism-specific therapy is the ultimate goal of antimicrobial selection. The use of several, or broader spectrum, agents will be less cost effective, may increase the risk of toxicity, and may actually increase the incidence of superinfection.

The choice between bactericidal and bacteriostatic antibiotics has plagued clinicians for years. Despite theoretical advantages (with certain exceptions, such as infective endocarditis, meningitis, and infections in the neutropenic patient), bactericidal drugs have not proved clinically superior to bacteriostatic compounds. In the aforementioned exceptions, bactericidal drugs (such as penicillins or cephalosporins) are necessary because of impaired host defenses or sites of infection that are inaccessible to normal host defenses. A two-drug regimen is sometimes necessary in order to assure bactericidal activity. Enterococci are not killed by penicillin alone, and enterococcal endocarditis requires treatment with a combination of a penicillin plus an aminoglycoside antibiotic. Two-drug therapy may also be indicated in situations where either drug is only marginally effective against the offending pathogen but where the two drugs together may be many fold more active than either drug alone (i.e., they may be synergistic).

Ultimately, the choice of antimicrobial agent is based on past clinical experience as well as upon the results of antimicrobial susceptibility testing. Some drugs, such as penicillin or cephalosporin derivatives, can be given in extremely high doses with little toxicity; this is not true of others such as aminoglycoside antibiotics. Additional concerns may include degree of protein binding, lipid solubility, routes of excretion and metabolism, and available modes of administration. Failure to cure typhoidal *Salmonella* infections with aminoglycoside antibiotics despite in vitro susceptibilities emphasizes the difficulties encountered in interpreting laboratory data without a clinical correlation. The preferred drugs for treatment of specific microorganisms are listed in Table 30–2.

Antimicrobial Prophylaxis. Controlled clinical trials have clearly demonstrated the value of prophylactic antibiotics in reducing the incidence of postoperative infection in certain situations. Unfortunately, much prophylaxis is inappropriately administered, resulting in excessive costs and the risks of superinfection and drug toxicity.

Perioperative infections usually arise from contamination of the wound or operative site by microorganisms from contiguous skin or mucosal surfaces transected during surgery. Less commonly, exogenous sources, such as unsterile equipment or airborne bacteria, are to blame. Factors influencing the development of wound infection include local conditions, such as the number of bacteria inoculated into the wound, the adequacy of local defense mechanisms, and the condition of the tissue with respect to necrosis, debris, or ischemia; and systemic factors, such as obesity, old age, malnutrition, prolonged preoperative hospitalization, or lengthy operative procedures.

The principle of antimicrobial prophylaxis is that antibiotics administered at the time of, or immediately before, inoculation of bacteria into the wound will prevent infection. Administration of antimicrobial prophylaxis after inoculation is ineffective. Accordingly, administration of prophylactic antibiotics is best achieved by a single preoperative dose. Maintenance of intraoperative antibiotic levels may require redosing during prolonged surgical procedures, but the value of continuing antibiotics after surgery has not been convincingly demonstrated. If antibiotics are continued, their administration should be limited to 48 hours postoperatively.

The indications for perioperative prophylaxis are listed in Table 30–3. Prophylaxis is indicated in certain situations only for high-risk patients. For example, prophylaxis is not indicated for most gastroduodenal surgery unless bleeding, obstruction, or achlorhydria (e.g., chronic antacid or H_2-receptor–blocking therapy) is a factor. High-risk patients for infection after biliary surgery include those individu-

Text continued on page 428

Table 30–1. ANTIMICROBIAL DRUG THERAPY

	Dosage*					
	Newborn (age)		*Children*		*Adults*	
DRUG	7 DAYS	7–30 DAYS	ORAL	PARENTERAL	ORAL	PARENTERAL
Acyclovir (Zovirax)	30 mg./kg./day q. 8 h.	30 mg./kg./day q. 8 h.	ND	30 mg./kg./day q. 8 h.	1000 mg./day q. 4 h.	15–30 mg./kg./day q. 8 h.
Amdinocillin (Coactin)	ND	ND	—	ND	—	40–60 mg./kg./day q. 6 h.
Amikacin (Amikin)	15 mg./kg./day q. 12 h.	15 mg./kg./day q. 12 h.	—	15 mg./kg./day q. 8–12 h.	—	15 mg./kg./day q. 8–12 h.
Amoxicillin plus clavulanic acid (Augmentin)	ND	ND	20–40 mg./kg./day q. 8 h.	—	750–1500 mg./day q. 8 h.	—
Amoxicillin (Amoxil, others)	ND	ND	20–40 mg./kg./day q. 8 h.	—	750–1500 mg./day q. 8 h.	—
Amphotericin B (Fungizone)	0.25–1.0 mg./kg./day	0.25–1.0 mg./kg./day	—	0.25–1.0 mg./kg./day	—	0.25–1.0 mg./kg./day
Ampicillin	50–100 mg./kg./day q. 12 h.	100–200 mg./kg./day q. 8 h.	50–100 mg./kg./day q. 6 h.	100–200 mg./kg./day q. 4–6 h.	1–4 gm./day q. 4–6 h.	2–12 gm./day q. 4–6 h.
Ampicillin plus sulbactam (Unasyn)	ND	ND	—	100–200 mg./kg./day q. 6 h.	—	3–12 gm./day q. 6 h.
Azlocillin (Azlin)	ND	ND	—	100–300 mg./kg./day q. 4–6 h.	—	100–300 mg./kg./day q. 4–6 h.
Aztreonam (Azactam)	ND	ND	—	50–150 mg./kg./day q. 6 h.	—	2–8 gm./day q. 6 h.
Bacampicillin (Spectrobid)	—	—	800 mg./day q. 12 h	—	800–1600 mg./day q. 12 h.	—
Carbenicillin (Geocillin, Pyopen, others)	200–300 mg./kg./day q. 8–12 h.	300–400 mg./kg./day q. 6–8 h.	50–65 mg./kg./day q. 6 h.	200–600 mg./kg./day q. 4–6 h.	1.5–3.0 gm. (4–8 tabs/day) q. 6 h.	30–40 gm./day q. 4–6 h.
Cefaclor (Ceclor)	—	—	20–60 mg./kg./day q. 6 h.	—	1.0–2.0 gm./day q. 6 h.	—
Cefadroxil (Duricef)	—	—	20–60 mg./kg./day q. 12 h.	—	1.0–2.0 gm./day q. 12 h.	—
Cefamandole (Mandol)	ND	ND	—	50–150 mg./kg./day q. 4–6 h.	—	2–12 gm./day q. 4–6 h.
Cefazolin (Ancef, Kefzol)	30 mg./kg./day q. 12 h.	30–60 mg./kg./day q. 8 h.	—	25–100 mg./kg./day q. 8 h.	—	1–6 gm./day q. 8 h.
Cefoperazone (Cefobid)	50–100 mg./kg./day q. 12 h.	50–100 mg./kg./day q. 12 h.	—	50–150 mg./kg./day q. 6–12 h.	—	2–12 gm./day q. 6–12 h.
Ceforanide (Precef)	ND	ND	—	20–40 mg./kg./day q. 12 h.	—	1–2 gm./day q. 12 h.
Cefotaxime (Claforan)	100 mg./kg./day q. 12 h.	100–200 mg./kg./day q. 8 h.	—	50–150 mg./kg./day q. 8 h.	—	2–12 gm./day q. 4–6 h.
Cefotetan (Cefotan)	ND	ND	—	ND	—	2–6 gm./day q. 12 h.
Cefoxitin (Mefoxin)	40 mg./kg./day q. 12 h.	50–150 mg./kg./day q. 6 h.	—	50–150 mg./kg./day q. 4–6 h.	—	2–12 gm./day q. 4–6 h.
Ceftazidime (Fortaz, others)	60 mg./kg./day q. 12 h.	60 mg./kg./day q. 12 h.	—	50–150 mg./kg./day q. 6–12 h.	—	2–12 gm./day q. 6–8 h.
Cefuroxime (Zinacef, Ceftin)	ND	ND	250–500 mg./day q. 12 h.	50–100 mg./kg./day q. 8 h.	250–1000 mg./day q. 12 h.	2.25–4.5 gm./day q. 8 h.
Cephalexin (Keflex)	—	—	25–50 mg./kg./day q. 6 h.	—	1–4 gm./day q. 6 h.	—

*Doses are expressed as total daily dose and normal dosing intervals
ND = no data or insufficient data for comment
†NC, no change
‡Peak adult body fluid levels for dose and route given
||Cerebrospinal fluid levels are those achievable in the presence of inflammation
§mg./kg. dosing data are expressed as mg. of trimethoprim component

Modifications in Renal Failure† Creatinine Clearance (ml./min.)				Peak Adult Body Fluid Levels‡ (mcg./ml.)		
30–60	10–30	< 10	Dose	Blood	Urine	CSF
5 mg./kg. q. 12 h.	5 mg./kg. q. 24 h.	2.5 mg./kg. q. 24 h.	5 mg./kg. I.V.	10	—	5
NC	NC	q. 8 h.	10 mg./kg. I.V.	50	1000	—
5 mg./kg. q. 12–16 h.	2.5 mg./kg. q. 12–16 h.	2.5 mg./kg. q. 24–36 h.	7.5 mg./kg. I.M. or I.V.	25	400	2
NC	q. 12 h.	q. 24 h.	500 mg. P.O.	10	500	—
NC	q. 12 h.	q. 24 h.	500 mg. P.O.	10	500	—
NC	NC	NC	0.5 mg./kg. I.V.	1–2	2	0.1
NC	q. 8 h.	q. 12 h.	500 mg. P.O. 1.0 gm. I.V.	5 25	400 500	— 4
NC	q. 8–12 h.	q. 12–24 h.	1.5 gm. I.V.	25	500	4
NC	q. 6–8 h.	q. 8–12 h.	3.0 gm. I.V.	200	3000	10
q. 8 h.	q. 12 h.	q. 24 h.	1.0 gm. I.V.	90	1000	3
NC	NC	400–800 mg./day	400 mg. P.O.	6–8	100	—
q. 6 h.	2–4 gm. q. 8 h.	2 gm. q. 12 h.	500 mg. P.O. 4.0 gm. I.V.	10 250	400 5000	— 20
NC	NC	NC	500 mg. P.O.	12	400	—
NC	q. 12–24 h.	q. 24–36 h.	500 mg.	15	400	—
q. 6 h.	q. 8 h.	q. 12 h.	1.0 gm. I.V.	65	1000	—
q. 8 h.	5–10 mg./kg. q. 12 h.	5–10 mg./kg. q. 24 h.	1.0 gm. I.V.	100	1500	—
NC	NC	NC	2.0 gm. I.V.	250	1000	1–20
NC	q. 24 h.	q. 48 h.	1.0 mg. I.V.	125	2000	—
NC	NC	q. 6–8 h.	1.0 gm. I.V.	70	2000	1–20
NC	q. 24 h.	q. 48 h.	1.0 gm. I.V.	125	2000	—
q. 8 h.	q. 12 h.	q. 24 h.	1.0 gm. I.V.	50	2000	2
q. 8 h.	q. 12 h.	q. 24 h.	1.0 gm.	80	2000	2–15
NC	q. 12 h.	q. 24 h.	1.5 gm. I.V.	100	2000	10
NC	q. 12 h.	q. 24 h.	500 mg. P.O.	16	400	—

Table continued on following page

Table 30–1. ANTIMICROBIAL DRUG THERAPY *Continued*

	Dosage*					
	Newborn (age)		*Children*		*Adults*	
DRUG	7 DAYS	7–30 DAYS	ORAL	PARENTERAL	ORAL	PARENTERAL
Cephalothin (Keflin, others)	40 mg./kg./day q. 12 h.	60 mg./kg./day q. 8 h.	—	60–100 mg./kg./day q. 4–6 h.	—	2–12 gm./day q. 4–6 h.
Cephapirin (Cefadyl)	ND	ND	—	40–80 mg./kg./day q. 4–6 h.	—	2–12 gm./day q. 4–6 h.
Cephradine (Anspor, Velosef)	ND	ND	25–50 mg./kg./day q. 6 h.	50–100 mg./kg./day q. 4–6 h.	1–4 gm./day q. 6 h.	2–12 gm./day q. 4–6 h.
Chloramphenicol (Chloromycetin)	25 mg./kg./day q. 12 h.	50 mg./kg./day q. 12 h.	50 mg./kg./day q. 6 h.	50–100 mg./kg./day q. 6 h.	1–2 gm./day q. 6 h.	1–4 gm./day q. 6 h.
Ciprofloxacin (Cipro)	—	—	—	—	500–1500 mg./day q. 12 h.	—
Clindamycin (Cleocin)	ND	ND	10–20 mg./kg./day q. 8 h.	15–40 mg./kg./day q. 8 h.	450–1200 mg./day q. 8 h.	900–2700 mg./day q. 8 h.
Cloxacillin (Tegopen, others)	—	—	50–100 mg./kg./day q. 6 h.	—	2–4 gm./day q. 6 h.	—
Cyclacillin (Cyclapen)	—	—	50–100 mg./kg./day q. 6 h.	—	1–2 gm./day q. 6 h.	—
Dicloxacillin (Dynapen, others)	—	—	25–50 mg./kg./day q. 6 h.	—	1–2 gm./day q. 6 h.	—
Doxycycline (Vibramycin)	—	—	—	—	100–200 mg./day q. 12–24 h.	100–200 mg./day q. 12–24 h.
Erythromycin (Erythrocin, E-mycin, others)	20–40 mg./kg./day q. 6–8 h.	20–40 mg./kg./day q. 6–8 h.	30–50 mg./kg./day q. 6–8 h.	15–50 mg./kg./day q. 6–8 h.	1–2 gm./day q. 6–8 h.	1–4 gm./day q. 6–8 h.
Ethambutol (Myambutol)	—	—	15 mg./kg./day q. day	—	15 mg./kg./day q. day	—
Flucytosine (Ancobon)	—	—	50–200 mg./kg./day q. 6 h.	—	50–200 mg./kg./day q. 6 h.	—
Gentamicin (Garamycin, others)	5 mg./kg./day q. 12 h.	7.5 mg./kg./day q. 12 h.	—	3.0–7.5 mg./kg./day q. 8 h.	—	3.0–5.0 mg./kg./day q. 8 h.
Imipenem plus Cilastatin (Primaxin)	ND	ND	—	10–40 mg./kg./day q. 6 h.	—	1–4 gm./day q. 6 h.
Isoniazid	5–10 mg./kg./day q. day	5–10 mg./kg./day q. day	10 mg./kg./day q. day	10 mg./kg./day q. day	300 mg./day q. day	300 mg./day q. day
Kanamycin (Kantrex)	15–20 mg./kg./day q. 12 h.	15–20 mg./kg./day q. 8 h.	—	15–20 mg./kg./day q. 8–12 h.	—	15 mg./kg./day q. 8–12 h.
Ketoconazole (Nizoral)	—	—	200–400 mg./day q. day	—	200–400 mg./day q. day	—
Methicillin (Staphcillin, others)	50–100 mg./kg./day q. 12 h.	100–200 mg./kg./day q. 6 h.	—	100–200 mg./kg./day q. 4–6 h.	—	4–12 gm./day q. 4–6 h.
Metronidazole (Flagyl, others)	ND	ND	30—50 mg./kg./day q. 6–12 h.	30–50 mg./kg./day q. 6–12 h.	1–3 gm./day q. 6–12 h.	1–3 gm./day q. 6–12 h.
Mezlocillin (Mezlin)	150 mg./kg./day q. 12 h.	300 mg./kg./day q. 6 h.	—	100–300 mg./kg./day q. 4–6 h.	—	6–24 gm./day q. 4–6 h.
Miconazole (Monistat)	ND	ND	—	20–40 mg./kg./day q. 8 h.	—	200–3600 mg./day q. 8 h.
Minocycline (Minocin)	—	—	—	—	100–200 mg./day q. 12–24 h.	100–200 mg./day q. 12–24 h.
Moxalactam (Moxam)	100–150 mg./kg./day q. 8–12 h.	100–150 mg./kg./day q. 6–8 h.	—	50—150 mg./kg./day q. 6–8 h.	—	2–8 gm./day q. 6–8 h.

*Doses are expressed as total daily dose and normal dosing intervals
ND = no data or insufficient data for comment
†NC, no change
‡Peak adult body fluid levels for dose and route given
‖Cerebrospinal fluid levels are those achievable in the presence of inflammation
§mg./kg. dosing data are expressed as mg. of trimethoprim component

Color Plates

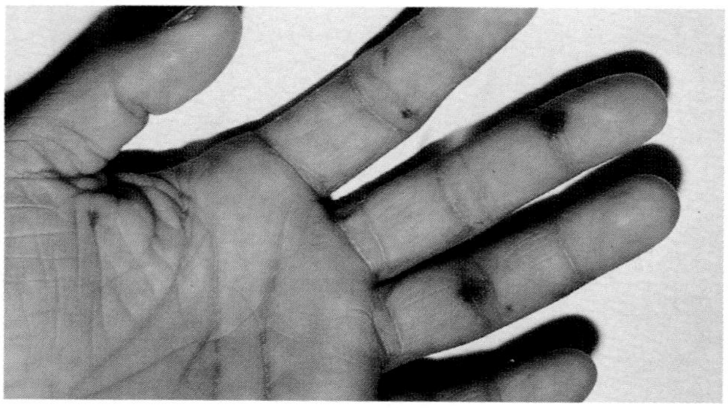

Plate IA

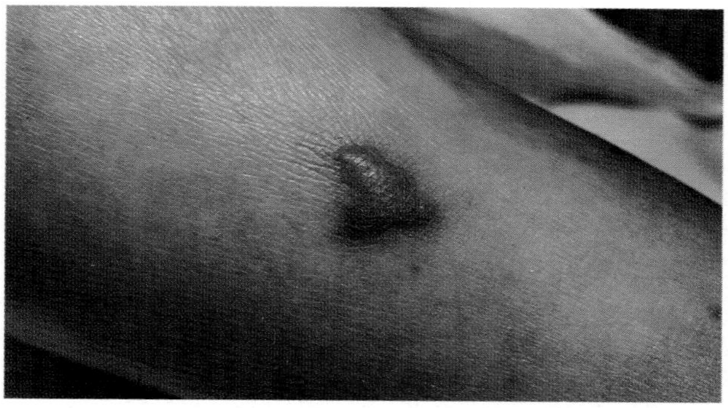

Plate IB

Plate I. Hemorrhagic vesicopustules on the hand *(A)* and hemorrhagic bullae on the ankle *(B)* in a case of gonococcal bacteremia.

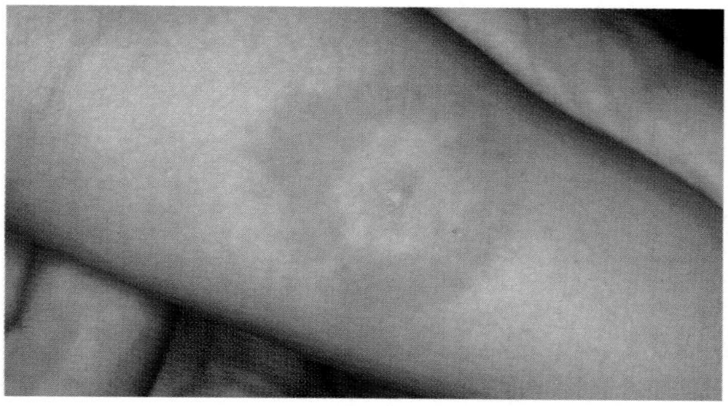

Plate IIA

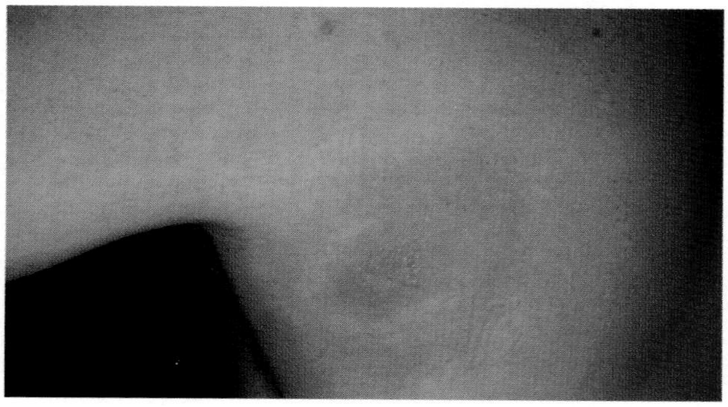

Plate IIB

Plate II. Erythema chronicum migrans on the forearm of a four-year-old child *(A)* and the shoulder of a 25-year-old man *(B)*. Note the central vesiculation.

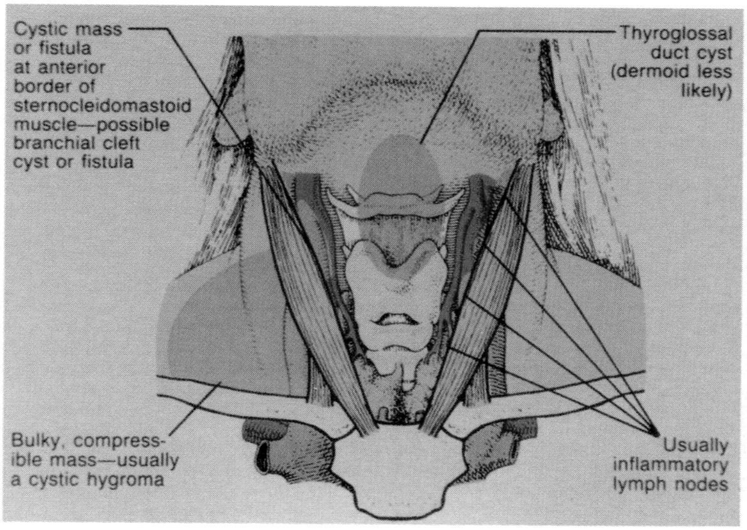

Plate III. Common neck masses in children.

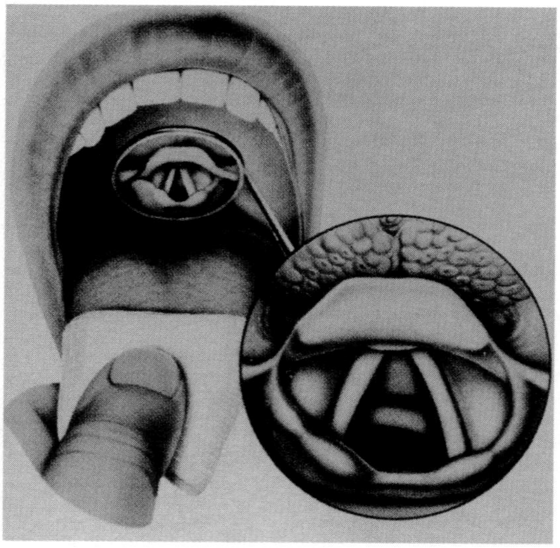

Plate IV. The hypopharynx should be examined, at least by indirect and preferably also by direct laryngoscopy, because of the high frequency of involvement of these sites by primary squamous cell carcinoma. (From Clark, W. D., and Bailey, B. J.: Diagnosis: Evaluation of neck masses. Hosp. Med., August 1983, p. 64.)

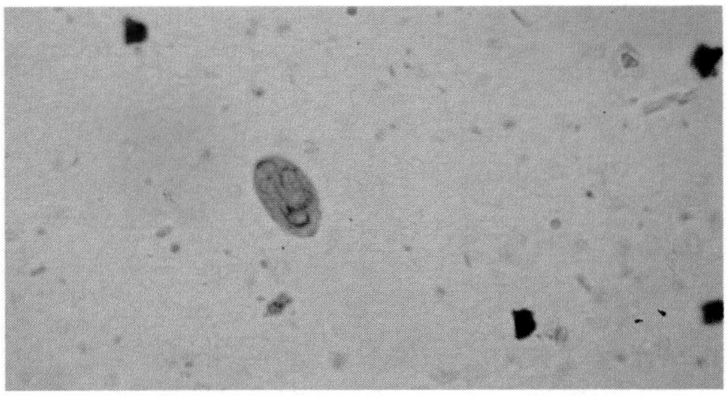

Plate V. *Giardia lamblia* cyst. Iodine stain. Showing ovoid shape and small nuclei. This form is the most likely to be seen in fecal material.

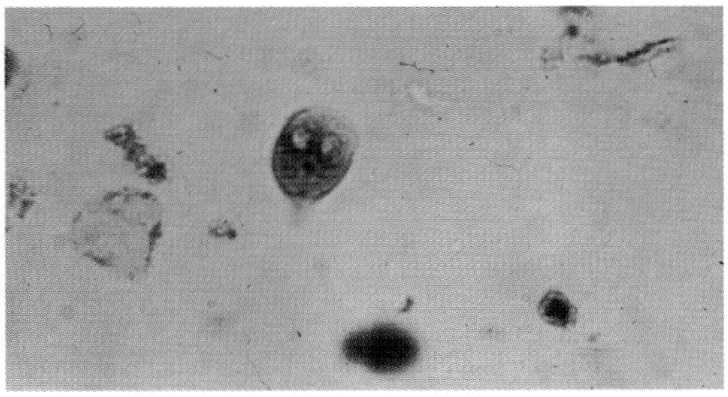

Plate VI. *Giardia lamblia* trophozoite. Showing pear-shape and characteristic "monkey face" appearance.

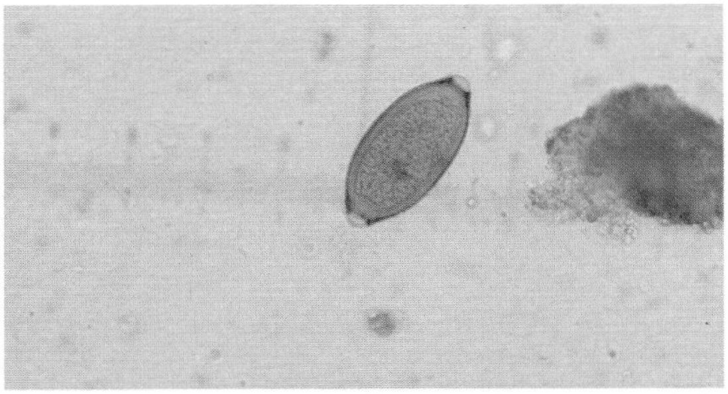

Plate VII. *Trichuris trichiura* ovum. Characteristic shape and bipolar plugs demonstrated.

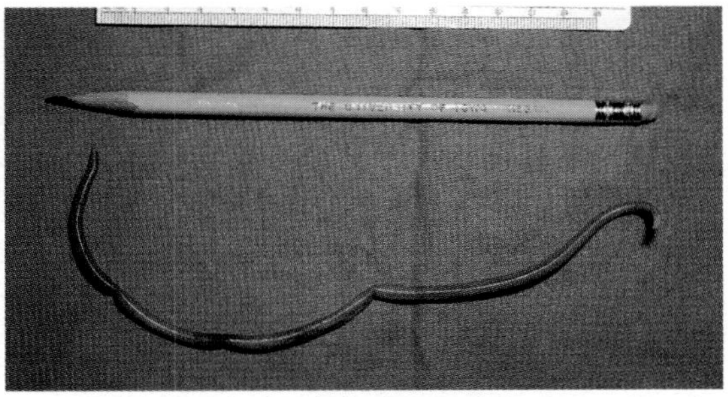

Plate VIII. *Ascaris lumbricoides* adult. Large "earthworm" appearance. (Reprinted from Jones, J. E.: Office parasitology. Am. Fam. Physician, Summer, 1981 issue, published by the American Academy of Family Physicians.)

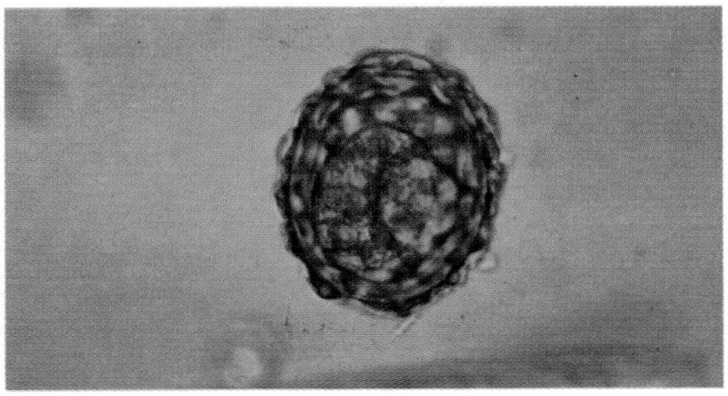

Plate IX. *Ascaris lumbricoides* fertilized ovum demonstrates distinct corticated shell. This shell protects the egg for up to 2 years in the environment. (Reprinted from Jones, J. E.: Office parasitology. Am. Fam. Physician *22*:86, 1980, published by the American Academy of Family Physicians.)

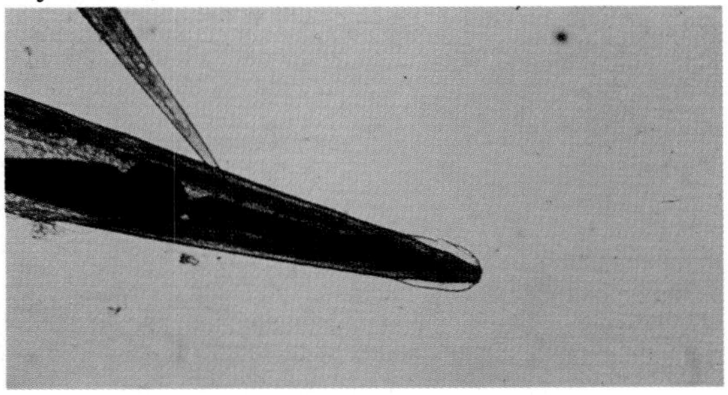

Plate X. *Enterobius vermicularis* adult. Notice mouth parts called alae or wings. This finding may be useful in differentiating this species from the larval stages of other parasites. (Reprinted from Jones, J. E.: Office parasitology. Am. Fam. Physician, *22*:86, 1980, published by the American Academy of Family Physicians.)

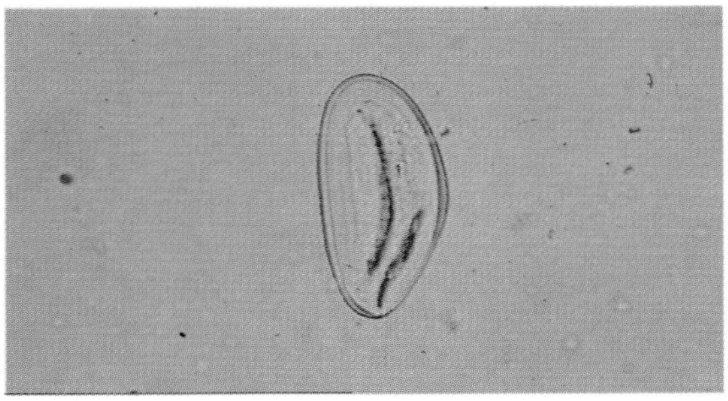

Plate XI. *Enterobius vermicularis* ovum. Illustration shows characteristic shape with developing larva inside. Note irregularly shaped edge on one side of the shell.

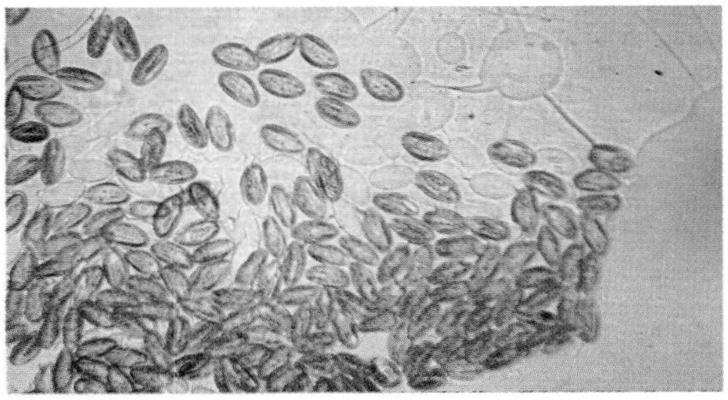

Plate XII. *Enterobius vermicularis* ova. Adhesive tape test demonstrating appearance of many eggs on low power. For details of technique, see text.

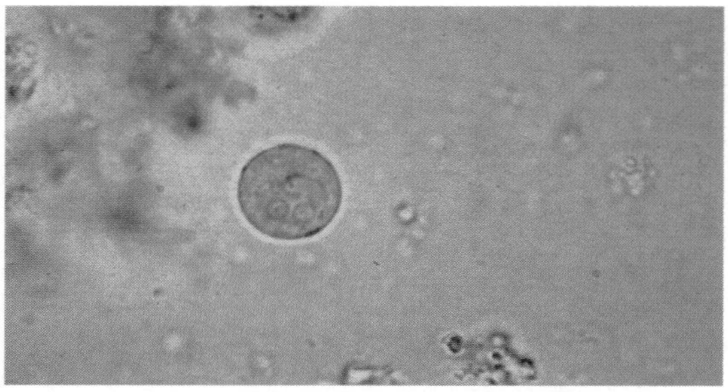

Plate XIII. *Entamoeba histolytica* cyst. Iodine stain. Illustration demonstrates four nuclei. The number of nuclei aids in species identification.

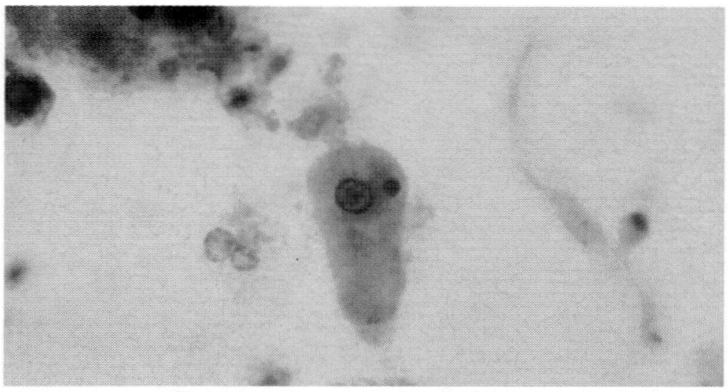

Plate XIV. *Entamoeba histolytica* trophozoite. Illustration shows the ameboid shape, single nucleus, and ingested red blood cell.

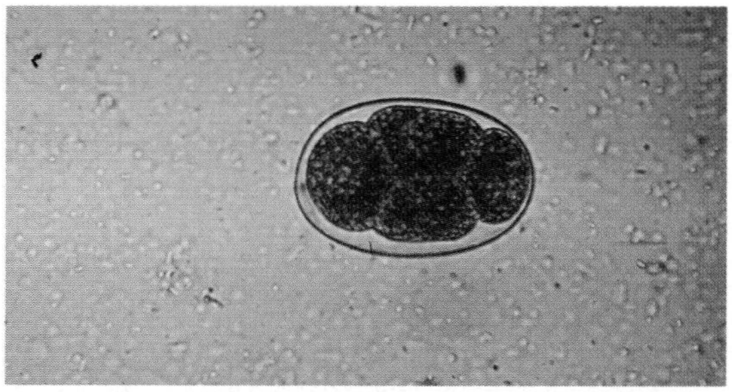

Plate XV. Hookworm species ovum. Demonstrates four-stage morula. This is the usual level of development when passed in feces. (Reprinted from Jones, J. E.: Office parasitology. Am. Fam. Physician, *22*:86, 1980, published by the American Academy of Family Physicians.)

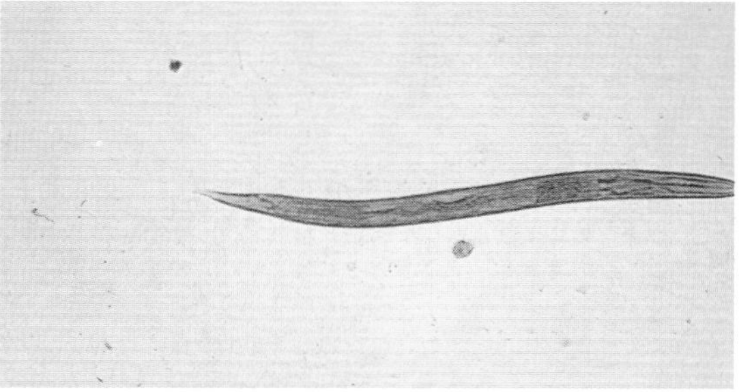

Plate XVI. *Strongyloides stercoralis* larva. Low-power view showing rhabditiform larva. This is the stage that is usually seen on stool examinations. (Reprinted from Jones, J. E.: Office parasitology. Am. Fam. Physician, *22*:86, 1980, published by the American Academy of Family Physicians.)

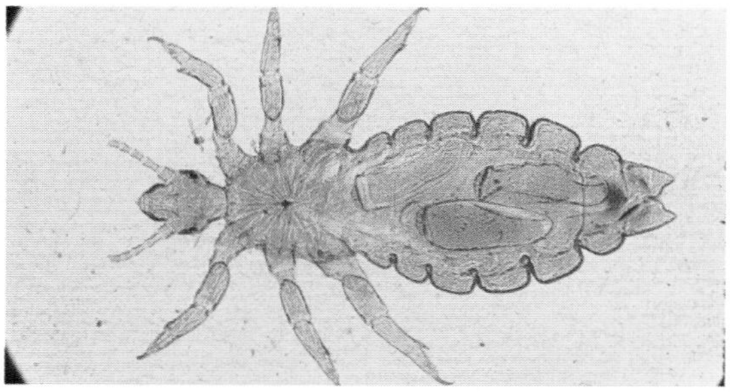

Plate XVII. *Pediculus humanus capitis.* Female adult. Note diamond-shaped head with abdomen wider than thorax.

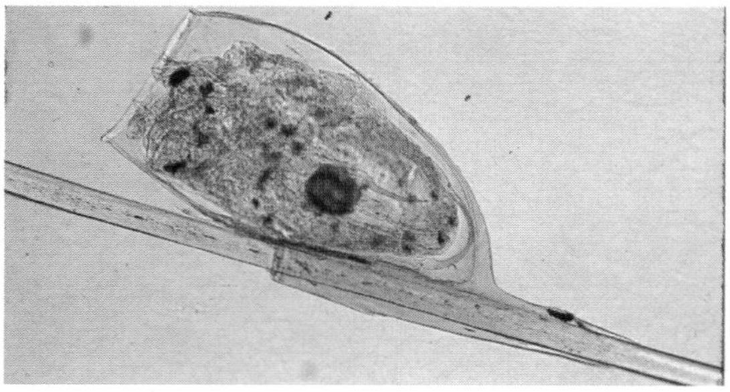

Plate XVIII. *Pediculus humanus capitis* nit. Egg sac attached to hair shaft. Notice extent of attachment to hair fiber. May first be thought to be flecks of dandruff.

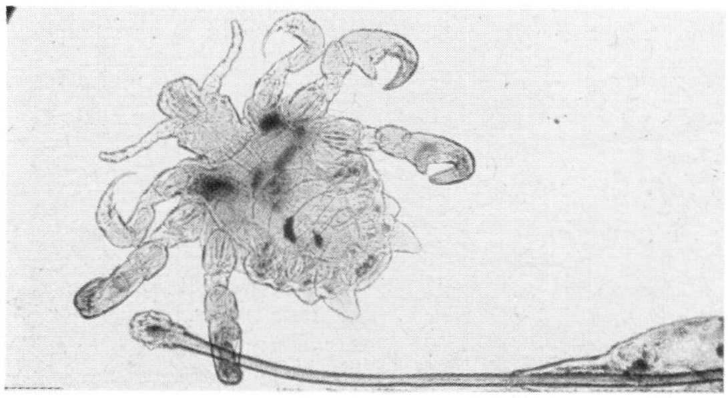

Plate XIX. *Phthirus pubis.* Adult attached by claw to hair shaft. Note turtle shape, rectangular neck, and short abdomen.

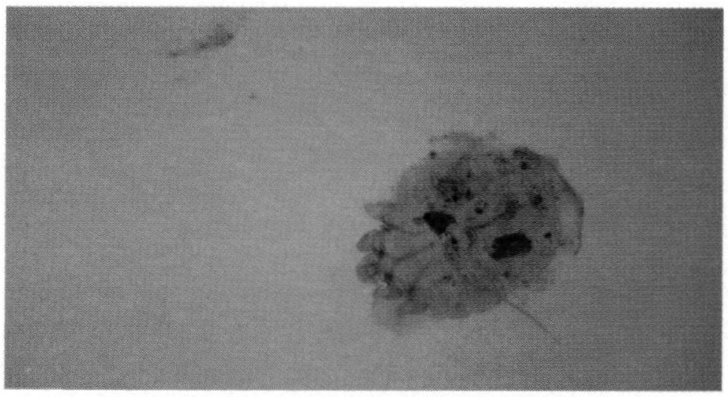

Plate XX. The *Sarcoptes scabiei* mite is small and rounded and has four pair of legs, two pair anterior and two pair posterior.

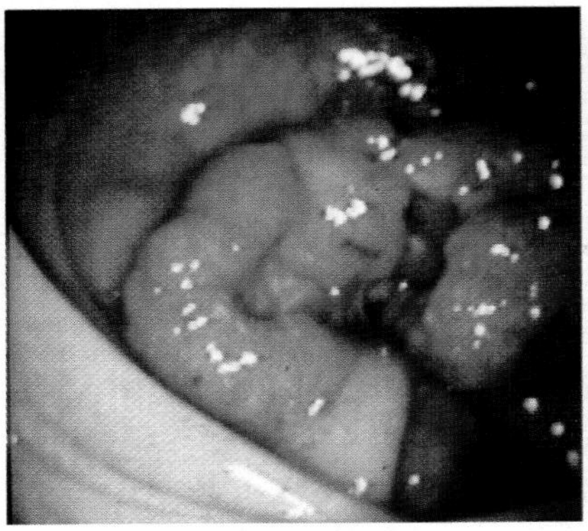

Plate XXI

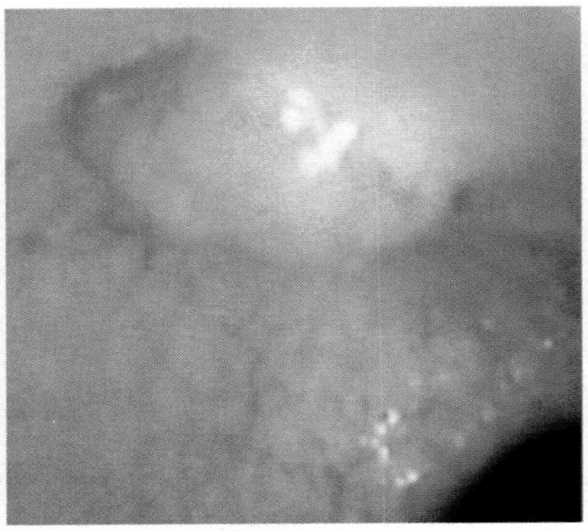

Plate XXII

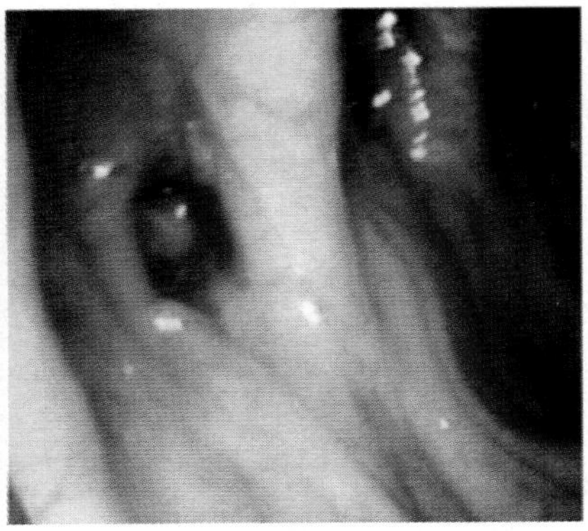

Plate XXIII

Plate XXI. This constricting annular lesion was detected by flexible sigmoidoscopy. Analysis of the colectomy specimen determined the staging and diagnosis to be Dukes B adenocarcinoma.
Plate XXII. Note the broad base of a smooth, nonfriable 6 mm. lesion, which was located at 18 cm. of insertion depth. The lesion was later removed by an electrocautery snare, and the pathologist described it as being a benign adenoma.
Plate XXIII. Diverticulosis has many appearances, but all suggest an outpouching of colonic mucosa.

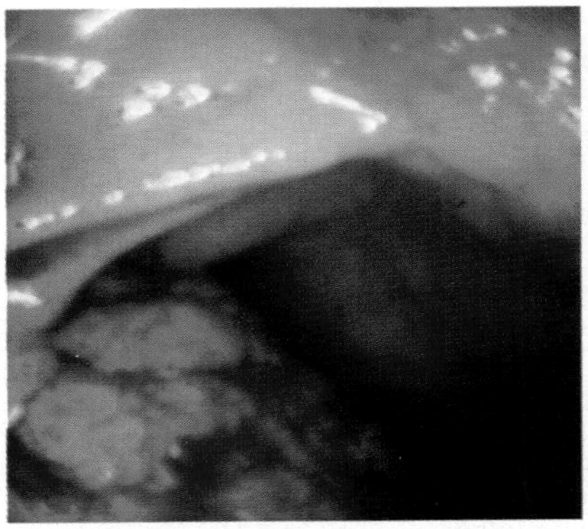

Plate XXIV

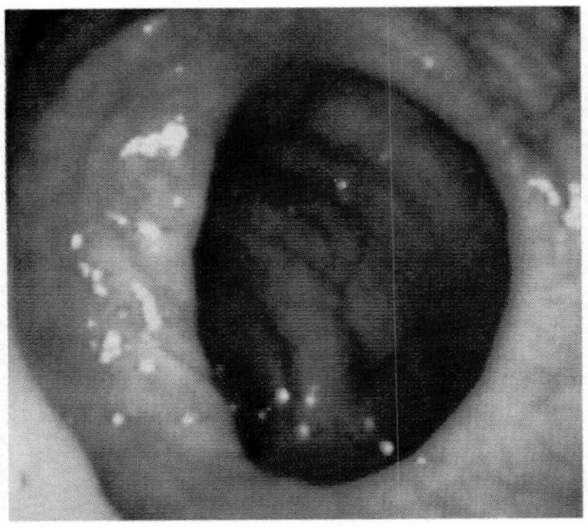

Plate XXV

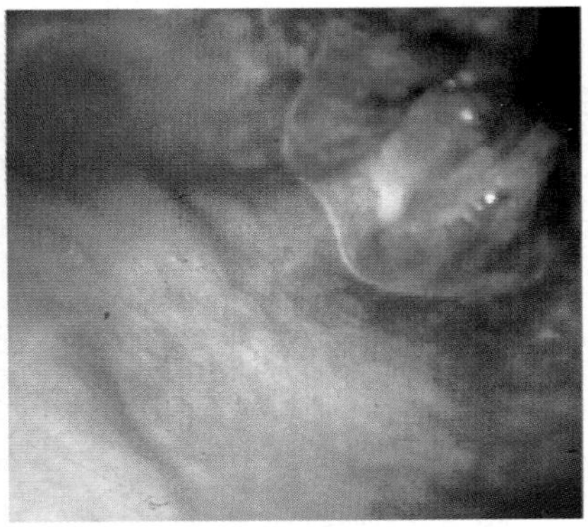

Plate XXVI

Plate XXIV. An exophytic friable lesion found in the transverse colon was removed at laparotomy. This adenocarcinoma was placed at Stage B.
Plate XXV. A prominent vascular pattern was located at the rectosigmoid junction, but a biopsy was not taken.
Plate XXVI. This is a turnaround view, and the scope shaft can be seen in the upper right-hand corner of the picture. These are internal hemorrhoids that appear to be covered by a tightly adherent white epithelium that is sharply demarcated at its proximal extent. This epithelium probably represents a transitional epithelium, which is much like a squamous metaplasia. In this case, there is a pseudodentate line, which appears to have migrated cephalad above these internal hemorrhoids. This demonstrates some of the anatomic variability of this region. The terms basaloid epithelium or cuboidal epithelium may apply.

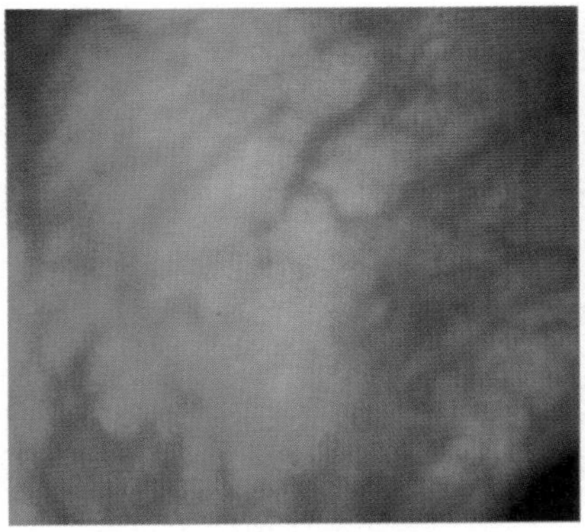

Plate XXVII

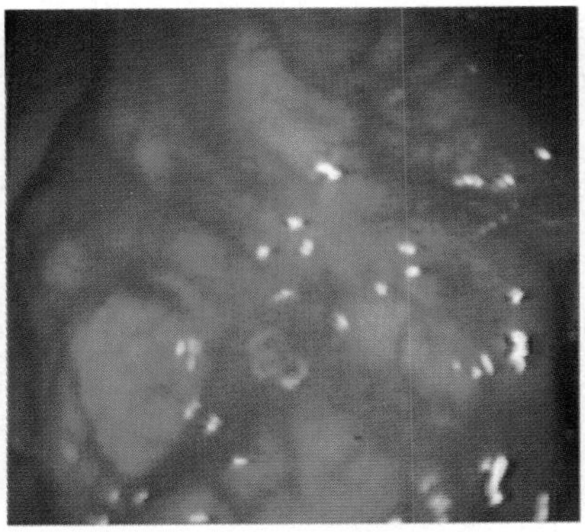

Plate XXVIII

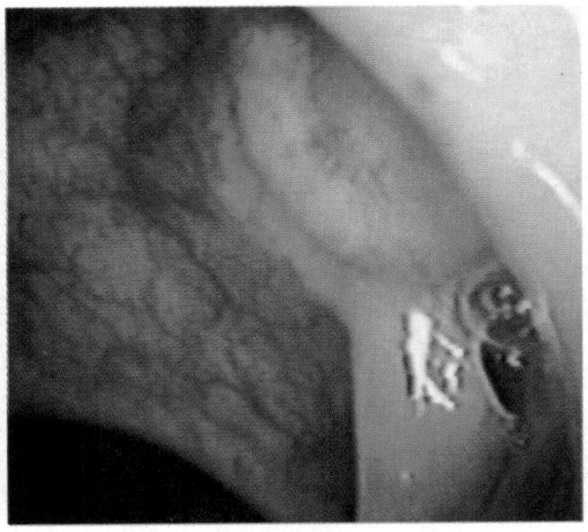

Plate XXIX

Plate XXVII. A solitary aphthous ulcer at an insertion depth of 18 cm. The biopsy sample from the edge was consistent with Crohn's disease.
Plate XXVIII. These vessels in the rectal canal are sufficiently large to be called varices. A biopsy would be contraindicated.
Plate XXIX. An adenomatous polyp on a stalk is partially hidden by one of the rectal valves. Since polypectomy is indicated, a biopsy of this lesion will not be helpful.

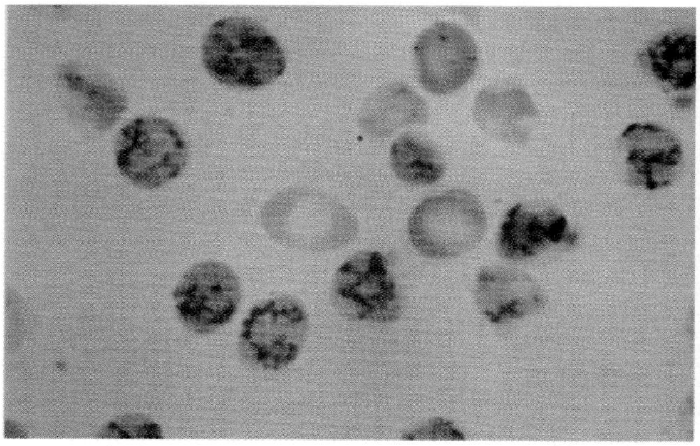

Plate XXX. Reticulocytes with methylene blue staining in a patient with a immunohemolytic anemia. (From Hobbs J. The hemolytic anemias. Am. Fam. Physician, *20*(1):85, July 1979. Permission pending.)

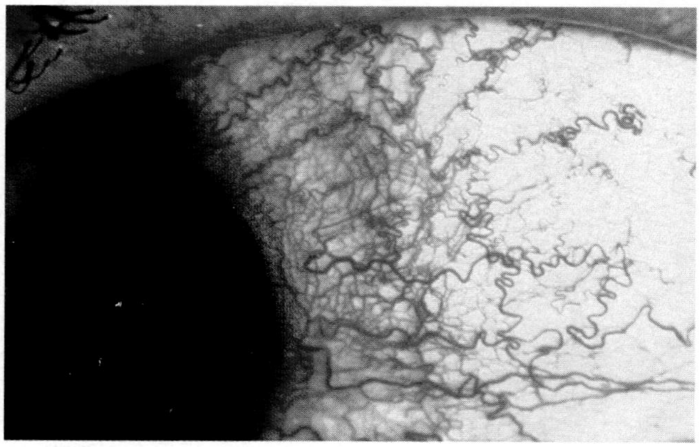

Plate XXXI. Circumcorneal (ciliary) injection is a danger sign indicating corneal involvement, iritis, or angle-closure glaucoma. (From *The Red Eye,* American Academy of Ophthalmology, Professional Information Committee, San Francisco, California, 1982.)

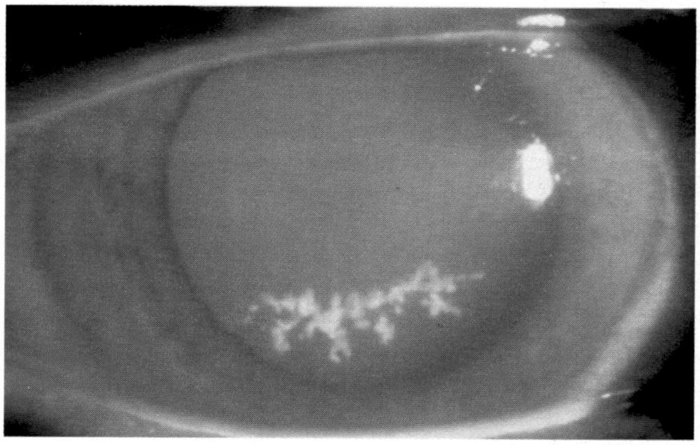

Plate XXXII. Corneal staining can indicate a corneal abrasion or a herpetic dendritic ulcer.

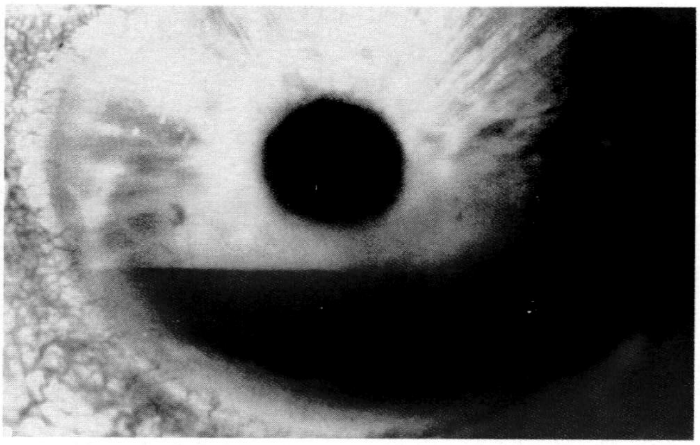

Plate XXXIII. Traumatic hyphema can threaten vision and cause corneal blood staining, glaucoma, and optic atrophy. (From *The Red Eye,* American Academy of Ophthalmology, Professional Information Committee, San Francisco, California, 1982.)

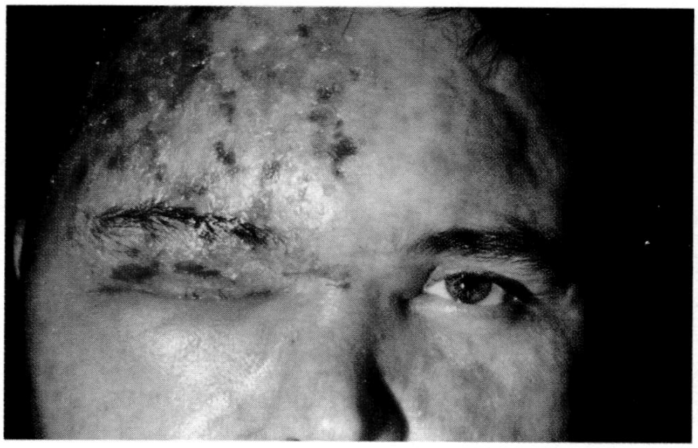

Plate XXXIV. This is a 28-year-old patient with herpes zoster of the trigeminal nerve.

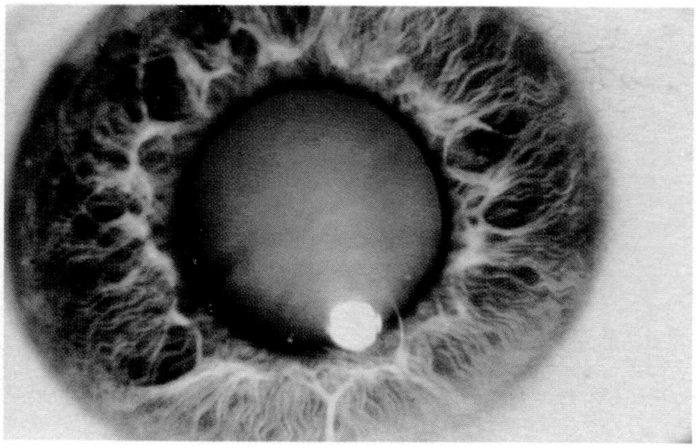

Plate XXXV. This 60-year-old patient had reduced vision to 20/400 because of a mature cataract.

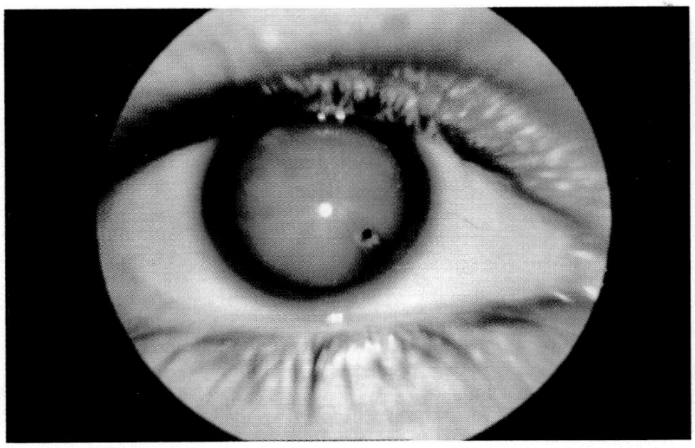

Plate XXXVI. This is a 22-year-old roofer who presented with a history of reduced vision in his right eye. Note the lens opacity and intralenticular metal from his roofing accident, which resulted in traumatic cataract.

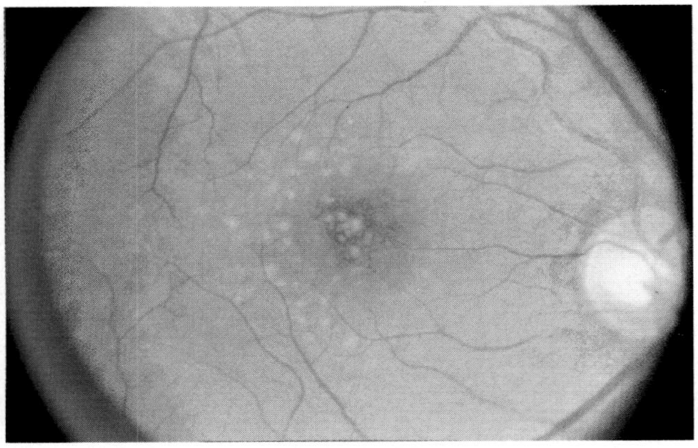

Plate XXXVII. Age-related maculopathy (macular degeneration) can often be associated with drusen. (From *The Aging Eye,* American Academy of Ophthalmology, Professional Information Committee, San Francisco, California, 1982.)

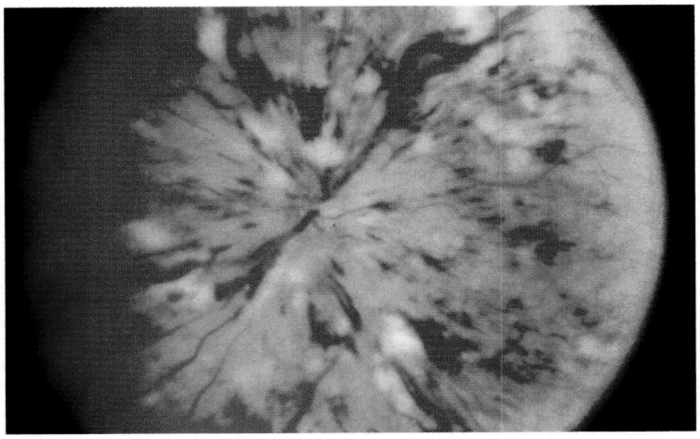

Plate XXXVIII. Retinopathy with hemorrhages and exudates secondary to hypertension. (From *The Aging Eye,* American Academy of Ophthalmology, Professional Information Committee, San Francisco, California, 1982.)

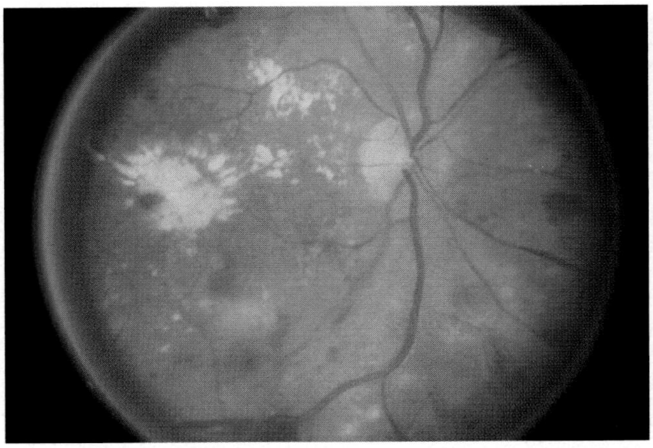

Plate XXXIX. Hypertensive retinopathy. Note the increased light reflex on the retinal arteries as well as the flamed-shaped hemorrhages in the nerve fiber layer. In addition, there is a moderate amount of exudate concentrated in the macular area. (Courtesy of William T. Humphrey, M.D., Director of Retinal Service, Eastern Virginia Medical School.)

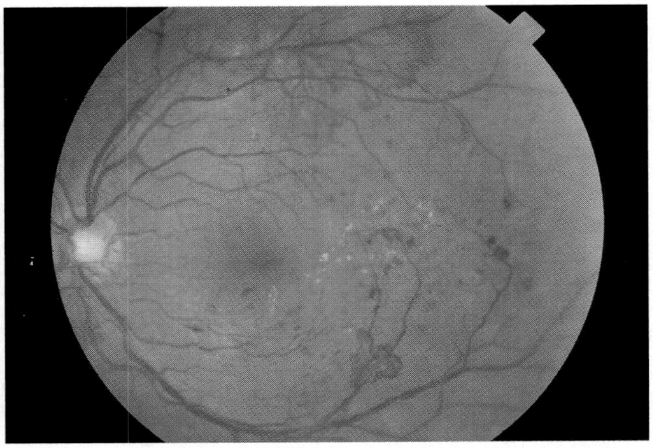

Plate XL. Proliferative diabetic retinopathy. Note the scattered retinal hemorrhages and exudates. In addition, there is new vessel formation, or neovascularization, of the retina as well as the optic disc. In addition, notice that there is some degree of vitreous beading. (Courtesy of William T. Humphrey, M.D., Director of Retinal Service, Eastern Virginia Medical School.)

Modifications in Renal Failure† *Creatinine Clearance (ml./min.)*				Peak Adult Body Fluid Levels‡ *(mcg./ml.)*		
30–60	10–30	< 10	Dose	Blood	Urine	CSF
q. 6 h.	q. 8 h.	q. 12 h.	1.0 gm. I.V.	50	1000	—
q. 6 h.	q. 8 h.	q. 12 h.	1.0 gm. I.V.	50	1000	—
q. 6 h.	q. 12–24 h.	q. 36 h.	1.0 gm. I.V.	50	1000	—
NC	NC	NC	1.0 gm.	10	100	5
NC	NC	q. 24 h.	500 mg. P.O.	3	600	0.3
NC	NC	NC	150 mg. P.O. 600 mg. I.V.	2.5 10	60 200	— —
NC	NC	NC	500 mg. P.O.	8	300	—
NC	q. 8–12 h.	q. 24 h.	500 mg.	12	200	—
NC	NC	NC	250 mg. P.O.	8	500	—
NC	NC	NC	100 mg. P.O. 100 mg. I.V.	2–4 6–8	— —	— —
NC	NC	NC	500 mg. P.O. 500 mg. I.V.	1–4 10–20	15 40	— —
NC	10 mg./kg./day	5 mg./kg./day	15 mg./kg. P.O.	3	—	—
q. 12 h.	q. 24 h.	q. 48 h.	2.0 gm. P.O.	45	1000	40
1.5 mg./kg. q. 12–16 h.	0.75 mg./kg. q. 12–16 h.	0.75 mg./kg. q. 24–36 h.	1.5 mg./kg. I.M. or I.V.	6	60	0.3
NC	q. 8–12 h.	q. 12–24 h.	500 mg. I.V.	40	200	6
NC	NC	200–300 mg./day	300 mg. P.O.	1–2	—	1
5 mg./kg. q. 16 h.	2.5 mg./kg. q. 16–24 h.	2.5 mg./kg. q. 24–48 h.	500 mg. I.M.	20	200	2
NC	NC	NC	200 mg. P.O.	3	—	0.2
NC	q. 6 h.	q. 8 h.	1.0 gm. I.V.	25	400	4
NC	NC	q. 8–12 h.	500 mg. P.O. 500 mg. I.V.	12 25	50 50	4 15
NC	q. 6 h.	q. 8 h.	3.0 gm. I.V.	200	3000	20
NC	NC	NC	200 mg. I.V.	1–2	—	—
NC	NC	NC	100 mg. P.O.	2–3	—	—
q. 8 h.	q. 12–16 h.	q. 24 h.	2.0 gm. I.V.	120	2000	1–20

Table continued on following page

Table 30–1. ANTIMICROBIAL DRUG THERAPY *Continued*

	Dosage*					
	Newborn (age)		*Children*		*Adults*	
Drug	7 Days	7–30 Days	Oral	Parenteral	Oral	Parenteral
Nafcillin (Nafcil, Unipen)	40 mg./kg./day q. 12 h.	60 mg./kg./day q. 8 h.	25–50 mg./kg./day q. 6 h.	50–200 mg./kg./day q. 4–6 h.	2–4 gm./day q. 6 h.	2–12 gm./day q. 4–6 h.
Nalidixic acid (NegGram)	—	—	—	—	4 gm./day q. 6 h.	—
Netilmicin (Netromycin)	4–6.5 mg./kg./day q. 12 h.	4–6.5 mg./kg./day q. 12 h.	—	3–6 mg./kg./day q. 8–12 h.	—	3–6 mg./kg./day q. 8–12 h.
Nitrofurantoin (Furadantin, others)	—	—	5–7 mg./kg./day q. 6 h.	—	200–400 mg./day q. 6 h.	—
Norfloxacin (Noroxin)	—	—	—	—	800 mg./day q. 12 h.	—
Oxacillin (Prostaphlin, others)	50–75 mg./kg./day q. 12 h.	75–100 mg./kg./day q. 8 h.	25–75 mg./kg./day q. 6 h.	100–200 mg./kg./day q. 4–6 h.	2–4 gm./day q. 6 h.	2–12 gm./day q. 4–6 h.
Penicillin G	50,000–100,000 U/kg./day q. 12 h.	100,000–200,000 U/kg./day q. 6 h.	—	50,000–250,000 U/kg./day q. 4 h.	—	2–24 million U/day q. 4 h.
Penicillin V	—	—	25,000—100,000 U/kg./day q. 6 h.	—	2–4 gm./day q. 6 h.	—
Piperacillin (Pipracil)	ND	ND	—	100–300 mg./kg./day q. 4–6 h.	—	6–24 gm./day q. 4–6 h.
Rifampin (Rifadin, Rimactane)	—	—	10–20 mg./kg./day q. day	—	600 mg./day q. day	—
Spectinomycin (Trobicin)	—	—	40 mg./kg. once	—	2.0 gm. once	—
Streptomycin	ND	ND	—	20–30 mg./kg./day q. 12–24 h.	—	1–2 gm./day q. 12–24 h.
Sulfonamides (Gantanol, Gantrisin)	—	—	150 mg./kg./day q. 6 h.	100 mg./kg./day q. 6 h.	2–4 gm./day q. 6 h.	100 mg./kg./day q. 6 h.
Tetracycline (Achromycin, others)	—	—	—	—	1–2 gm./day q. 6 h.	Use doxycycline or minocycline
Ticarcillin (Ticar)	225 mg./kg./day q. 8–12 h.	200–300 mg./kg./day q. 8 h.	—	200–300 mg./kg./day q. 4–6 h.	—	200–300 mg./kg./day q. 4–6 h.
Ticarcillin plus clavulanic acid (Timentin)	ND	ND	—	200–300 mg./kg./day q. 6 h.	—	12.4 gm./day q. 6 h.
Tobramycin (Nebcin)	5 mg./kg./day q. 12 h.	7.5 mg./kg./day q. 8 h.	—	5 mg./kg./day q. 8 h.	—	3–5 mg./kg./day q. 8 h.
Trimethoprim (Proloprim, Trimpex)	—	—	8–10 mg./kg./day q. 12 h.	—	200 mg./day q. 12 h.	—
Trimethoprim-Sulfamethoxazole§ (Bactrim, Septra)	—	—	5–10 mg./kg./day q. 12 h.	5–20 mg./kg./day q. 6–12 h.	320/1600 mg./day (2 DS tabs) q. 12 h.	5–20 mg./kg./day q. 6–12 h.
Vancomycin (Vancocin, Vancoled)	30 mg./kg./day q. 12 h.	40 mg./kg./day q. 8 h.	0.5–1.0 gm./day q. 6 h.	40 mg./kg./day q. 6–12 h.	1.0 gm./day q. 6 h.	2.0 gm./day q. 6–12 h.
Zidovudine (Azidothymidine, Retrovir)	ND	ND	ND	ND	400–1200 mg./day q. 4–6 h.	ND

*Doses are expressed as total daily dose and normal dosing intervals
ND = no data or insufficient data for comment
†NC, no change
‡Peak adult body fluid levels for dose and route given
||Cerebrospinal fluid levels are those achievable in the presence of inflammation
§mg./kg. dosing data are expressed as mg. of trimethoprim component

Modifications in Renal Failure† *Creatinine Clearance (ml./min.)*				Peak Adult Body Fluid Levels‡ *(mcg./ml.)*		
30–60	10–30	< 10	Dose	Blood	Urine	CSF
NC	NC	NC	1.0 gm. I.V.	25	500	1
NC	Avoid	Avoid	1.0 gm. P.O.	—	15	—
1.7 mg./kg. q. 12–16 h.	0.8 mg./kg. q. 12–16 h.	0.8 mg./kg. q. 24–36 h.	1.7 mg./kg. I.V.	7	60	—
NC	Avoid	Avoid	100 mg. P.O.	—	150	—
NC	q. 12–24 h.	q. 24 h.	400 mg. P.O.	2	400	—
NC	NC	NC	1.0 gm. I.V.	30	500	1
NC	2–10 M.U./day	1–4 M.U./day	1.0 M.U. aqueous I.V.	20	1000	3
			1.2 M.U. procaine I.M.	5	500	—
NC	q. 8 h.	q. 12 h.	250 mg. P.O.	3	300	—
NC	q. 8 h.	q. 12 h.	4.0 gm. I.V.	180	5000	1–20
NC	NC	NC	600 mg. P.O.	7	70	3
NC	Avoid	Avoid	2.0 gm. I.M.	100	—	—
q. 24 h.	q. 48 h.	q. 72–96 h.	1.0 gm. I.M.	40	800	—
q. 8 h.	q. 12 h.	q. 24 h.	1.0 gm. P.O.	20	500	10
NC	Avoid	Avoid	500 mg. P.O.	5	200	2
q. 6 h.	q. 8 h.	q. 12 h.	3.0 gm. I.V.	200	3000	20
NC	q. 8 h.	q. 12 h.	3.1 gm. I.V.	200	3000	20
1.5 mg./kg. q. 12–16 h.	0.75 mg./kg. q. 12–16 h.	0.75 mg./kg. q. 24–36 h.	1.5 mg./kg. I.M. or I.V.	6	60	0.3
NC	100 mg./day	Avoid	100 mg. P.O.	1	150	—
NC	4–10 mg./kg. (1 DS tab) per day	Avoid	160/800 mg. P.O.	2/40	100/1000	2/20
1.0 gm. q. 24–36 h.	1.0 gm. q. 48–72 h.	1.0 gm. q. 5–7 days	500 mg. I.V.	10	200	2
NC	NC	NC	200 mg. P.O.	0.6	—	0.1

Table 30–2. ANTIMICROBIAL AGENTS OF CHOICE FOR THE TREATMENT OF SPECIFIC MICROORGANISMS

Infecting Organism	Morphology*	Drug of First Choice†	Alternate Choices†
Acinetobacter‡	GNB	APP	Aminoglycoside, amp/sulb, imipenem, quinolone, ceftazidime
Actinomyces	GPB	Penicillin G	Clindamycin, tetracycline
Aeromonas‡	GNB	Quinolone	Aminoglycoside, TGC, TMP/SMX
Bacteroides fragilis‡	GNB	Metronidazole	Clindamycin, BLI + P, cefoxitin, cefotetan, imipenem, APP
Bacteroides other than *B. fragilis*‡	GNB	Clindamycin	Penicillin, APP, BLI + P, cefoxitin, cefotetan, metronidazole
Bordetella	GNCB	Erythromycin	Ampicillin, tetracycline
Borrelia burgdorferi	GNS	Penicillin or tetracycline	Ceftriaxone
Borrelia recurrentis	GNS	Tetracycline	Chloramphenicol
Brucella	GNB	TMP/SMX	Tetracycline + streptomycin, quinolone
Campylobacter jejuni	GNB	Quinolone	Erythromcyin, gentamicin, TGC
Chlamydia	NA	Tetracycline	Erythromycin, sulfonamide, quinolone
Citrobacter diversus‡	GNB	TGC	Aminoglycoside, aztreonam, quinolone, BLI + P, TMP/SMX, imipenem
Citrobacter freundii‡	GNB	Imipenem or APP or aminoglycoside	TGC, TMP/SMX, aztreonam, quinolone
Clostridium botulinum	GPB	Antitoxin	
Clostridium difficile	GPB	Vancomycin (PO) or metronidazole	Bacitracin (PO)
Clostridium perfringens	GPB	Penicillin G	Cephalosporin, clindamycin, metronidazole
Clostridium tetani	GPB	Antitoxin plus immunization	
Corynebacterium diphtheriae (illness)	GPB	Antitoxin plus erythromycin	Penicillin G
Corynebacterium diphtheriae (carrier)	GPB	Erythromycin	Clindamycin
Corynebacterium species JK	GPB	Vancomycin	
Eikenella corrodens	GNB	BLI + P	Penicillin G, cefoxitin, TGC, imipenem
Enterobacter‡	GNB	Aminoglycoside or APP or imipenem	TGC, aztreonam, quinolone, TMP/SMX
Enterococcus	GPC	Ampicillin ± gentamicin	Vancomycin ± gentamicin, quinolone (urine)
Escherichia coli‡ (community acquired)	GNB	Cephalosporin	Ampicillin, TMP/SMX, quinolone
Escherichia coli‡ (hospital acquired)	GNB	TGC	Ampicillin, aminoglycoside, aztreonam, BLI + P, imipenem, quinolone, TMP/SMX
Eubacterium	GPB	Penicillin G	Clindamycin, tetracycline
Flavobacterium‡	GNB	Aminoglycoside	APP, TGC, TMP/SMX
Francisella tularensis	GNCB	Streptomycin ± tetracycline	Tetracycline, chloramphenicol
Fusobacterium	GNB	Penicillin G	Clindamycin, metronidazole, BLI + P, APP, imipenem
Gardnerella vaginalis	GVB	Metronidazole	
Haemophilus influenzae‡ (systemic infection)	GNCB	TGC	Ampicillin, chloramphenicol, TMP/SMX, cefuroxime, BLI + P, quinolone
Haemophilus influenzae‡ (other)	GNCB	Amoxicillin	Quinolone, TMP/SMX, BLI + P
Haemophilus ducreyi	GNCB	Ceftriaxone	TMP/SMX, quinolone, erythromycin
Herpes simplex (ocular)	Virus	Trifluridine	Vidarabine, IUDR
Herpes simplex (other)	Virus	Acyclovir	Vidarabine
Influenza A	Virus	Amantidine	
Klebsiella‡	GNB	Cephalosporin	Aminoglycoside, TMP/SMX, BLI + P, aztreonam, imipenem, quinolone
Legionella	GNB	Erythromycin	Rifampin, quinolone, TMP/SMX, tetracycline
Leptospira	GNS	TGC	Penicillin, tetracycline
Listeria monocytogenes	GPB	Ampicillin ± aminoglycoside	TMP/SMX, erythromycin
Morganella morganii‡	GNB	TGC	Aminoglycoside, APP, aztreonam, imipenem, quinolone, TMP/SMX
Mycoplasma pneumoniae	NA	Erythromycin	Tetracycline, quinolone
Mycobacterium leprae	AFB	Dapsone + rifampin	Clofazimine
Mycobacterium marinum‡	AFB	Rifampin + ethambutol	Minocycline
Mycobacterium tuberculosis‡	AFB	Isoniazid + rifampin ± pyrazinamide	Ethambutol, streptomycin, PAS
Neisseria gonorrhoeae‡	GNC	Ceftriaxone	Ampicillin, penicillin, spectinomycin, BLI + P, quinolone
Neisseria meningitidis (illness)	GNC	Penicillin G	TGC

Table 30–2. ANTIMICROBIAL AGENTS OF CHOICE FOR THE TREATMENT OF SPECIFIC MICROORGANISMS *Continued*

Infecting Organism	Morphology*	Drug of First Choice†	Alternate Choices†
Neisseria meningitidis (carrier)	GNC	Rifampin	Quinolone, minocycline, sulfonamide
Nocardia	GPB	Sulfonamide	TMP/SMX, minocycline, imipenem
Pasteurella multocida	GNCB	Penicillin G	Tetracycline, TMP/SMX, quinolone, TGC
Peptococcus	GBC	Penicillin G	Clindamycin, erythromycin, vancomycin, cephalosporin
Peptostreptococcus	GPC	Penicillin G	Clindamycin, erythromycin, vancomycin, cephalosporin
Proprionibacterium acnes	GPB	Tetracycline	Clindamycin (topical), erythromycin
Proteus mirabilis‡	GNB	Ampicillin	TGC, aminoglycoside, BLI+P, aztreonam, TMP/SMX, imipenem, quinolone
Proteus vulgaris‡	GNB	TGC or aztreonam	Aminoglycoside, APP, imipenem, quinolone, TMP/SMX
Providencia‡	GNB	TGC or aztreonam	Aminoglycoside, imipenem, APP, quinolone, TMP/SMX
Pseudomonas aeruginosa‡ (in neutropenia)	GNB	Aminoglycoside + APP or ceftazidime	Aminoglycoside + cefoperazone, imipenem, or aztreonam; quinolone
Pseudomonas aeruginosa‡ (other systemic)	GNB	APP or imipenem or ceftazidime or cefoperazone or aztreonam or quinolone ± aminoglycoside	Aminoglycoside
Pseudomonas aeruginosa‡ (urinary tract)	GNB	Quinolone	Aminoglycoside, APP, ceftazidime, aztreonam, cefoperazone, imipenem
Pseudomonas cepacia‡	GNB	TMP/SMX	
Pseudomonas maltophilia‡	GNB	TMP/SMX	Ticarcillin + clavulanic acid, quinolone
Rickettsia	GNCB	Tetracycline	Chloramphenicol
Salmonella typhi‡	GNB	Amoxicillin or quinolone	Chloramphenicol, TMP/SMX
Salmonella, nontyphi‡	GNB	Quinolone	TMP/SMX, ampicillin, amoxicillin
Serratia‡	GNB	TGC	Aminoglycoside, aztreonam, APP, imipenem, quinolone, TMP/SMX
Shigella‡	GNB	Quinolone	Ampicillin, TMP/SMX
Spirillum	GNS	Penicillin G	Tetracycline
Staphylococcus aureus‡ Methicillin sensitive	GPC	PRP	Cephalosporin, vancomycin, clindamycin, erythromycin, TMP/SMX, imipenem, quinolone
Staphylococcus aureus‡ Methicillin resistant	GPC	Vancomycin	Quinolone, TMP/SMX
Staphylococcus epidermidis‡	GPC	Vancomycin	PRP, cephalosporin, imipenem, quinolone, TMP/SMX
Streptobacillus	GPB	Penicillin G	Tetracycline
Streptococcus agalactiae (Group B)	GPC	Penicillin G	Erythromycin, cephalosporin, vancomycin
Streptococcus bovis (Group D)	GPC	Penicillin G	Cephalosporin, vancomycin
Streptococcus pneumoniae	GPC	Penicillin G	Cephalosporin, erythromycin, clindamycin, vancomycin
Streptococcus pyogenes (Group A)	GPC	Penicillin G	Erythromycin, cephalosporin, clindamycin, vancomycin
Streptococcus viridans group	GPC	Penicillin G	Cephalosporin, vancomycin
Treponema pallidum	GNS	Penicillin G	Erythromycin, tetracycline
Ureaplasma	NA	Tetracycline	Erythromycin, quinolone
Vibrio vulnificus	GNB	Tetracycline	Ampicillin, quinolone
Vibrio cholerae	GNB	Tetracycline	Quinolone
Vibrio parahaemolyticus	GNB	Quinolone	Tetracycline, ampicillin
Yersinia enterocolitica‡	GNB	TGC	Cefoxitin, TMP/SMX, quinolone
Yersinia pestis	GNB	Streptomycin	Tetracycline, chloramphenicol
		FUNGI	
Aspergillus		Amphotericin B	
Blastomyces		Amphotericin B	Ketoconazole
Candida species			
Systemic		Amphotericin B ± 5-FC	Miconazole, ketoconazole
Urinary		Amphotericin B (single dose) 5-FC	
Chronic mucocutaneous		Ketoconazole	
Cutaneous		Clotrimazole (topical)	Miconazole (topical), ketoconazole

Table continued on following page

Table 30–2. ANTIMICROBIAL AGENTS OF CHOICE FOR THE TREATMENT OF SPECIFIC MICROORGANISMS *Continued*

Infecting Organism	Morphology*	Drug of First Choice†	Alternate Choices†
Coccidioides		Amphotericin B	Ketoconazole, miconazole
Cryptococcus		Amphotericin B ± 5-FC	Fluconazole
Chromoblastomycosis		5-FC	Amphotericin B
Dermatophytes		Ketoconazole (systemic)	
		Clotrimazole (topical)	Miconazole, tolnaftate, econazole, tioconazole
Histoplasma capsulatum		Amphotericin B	Ketoconazole
Paracoccidioides		Ketoconazole	Amphotericin
Sporothrix schenckii		Iodides	Amphotericin B
Zygomycoses (Mucor)		Amphotericin B	

*Morphology: GNB = gram-negative bacillus; GNCB = gram-negative coccobacillus; GNS = gram-negative spirillary organism or spirochete; GVB = gram-variable bacillus; GNC = gram-negative coccus; GPC = gram-positive coccus; GPB = gram-positive bacillus; NA = not applicable.

†Antimicrobial agents: APP = antipseudomonal penicillin (carbenicillin, ticarcillin, mezlocillin, azlocillin, piperacillin); PRP = penicillinase-resistant penicillin (oxacillin, nafcillin, methicillin, cloxacillin, dicloxacillin); BLI + P = beta-lactamase inhibitor plus a penicillin combination (ampicillin + sulbactam, amoxicillin + clavulanic acid, ticarcillin + clavulanic acid); TGC = third-generation cephalosporin (cefotaxime, ceftizoxime, ceftazidime, cefoperazone, ceftiaxone); TMP/SMX = trimethoprim + sulfamethoxazole; 5-FC = 5-flucytosine.

‡Susceptibilities vary; alter therapy according to antimicrobial susceptibility test results.

als over 70 years of age, patients with obstructive jaundice or previous biliary tract surgery, patients with common duct stones, and patients operated upon for or during acute cholecystitis. The indications for prophylactic antibiotics in ceasarean section include patients in labor, patients with ruptured membranes, and those who have had internal fetal monitoring during labor prior to cesarean section. Patients receiving antibiotics while undergoing surgery for traumatic wounds or a ruptured viscus are considered to be receiving treatment rather than prophylaxis. Accordingly, therapy is usually continued for some time after surgery.

Patients with valvular heart disease, who may be predisposed to bacterial endocarditis after bacteremia associated with manipulation of infected or potentially infected tissues, should receive prophylaxis directed against organisms that produce endocarditis. This may require a regimen different from the standard surgical prophylactic program listed in Table 34–3 and is discussed in the section on cardiovascular infections.

Aminoglycoside Antibiotics. Aminoglycoside antibiotics are complex amino-sugars produced by a variety of fungi. They are active against most aerobic gram-negative bacilli and staphylococci. Gentamicin, the most commonly used derivative, is active against nearly all strains of *Escherichia coli, Klebsiella,* and *Proteus* as well as *Pseudomonas* and other nonfermentative gram-negative bacilli. Streptococci and anaerobes, however, are intrinsically resistant to aminoglycoside antibiotics.

Aminoglycosides work by binding to ribosomes. Such binding is usually irreversible, and, therefore, these drugs are bactericidal. Resistance to aminoglycoside antibiotics is mediated either by a decrease in permeability to the compound (streptococci and anaerobes) or by enzymatic inactivation (which may be plasmid mediated and, therefore, transferable from one organism to another) in gram-negative bacilli. Amikacin is less susceptible to such inactivation and, therefore, is of value when gentamicin- and tobramycin-resistant strains are frequent.

Aminoglycoside antibiotics are not absorbed after oral administration. After parenteral administration, they are not metabolized and are excreted by glomerular filtration. Impairment of renal function profoundly affects the excretion of these compounds, and dosage modification is necessary (see Table 30–1). In order to assure adequate blood and tissue levels and to avoid toxicity, measurement of blood concentrations is recommended in all patients receiving aminoglycoside antibiotics for systemic infections. Gentamicin or tobramycin peak blood concentrations should be maintained between 4 and 8 μg./ml., and trough levels between 1 and 2 μg./ml. for patients with normal renal function. The tissue penetration of aminoglycoside antibiotics is poor, and CSF concentrations are generally subtherapeutic even in the presence of inflammation.

Toxicity is the major drawback to the use of aminoglycoside antibiotics. Ototoxicity, both auditory and vestibular, neuromuscular blockade, and nephrotoxicity are the major problems. Ototoxicity is most frequently seen in patients with underlying renal disease and pre-existing auditory disease, and its occurrence is related to the total dose received, duration of therapy, and treatment with other ototoxic drugs, particularly prior aminoglycoside antibiotics or loop diuretics. Neuromuscular blockade is occasionally seen after surgical procedures, where prolonged muscular weakness after anesthesia is the presentation. Occasionally, acute neurologic deterioration is seen in patients with other neuromuscular disorders, such as myasthenia gravis.

Nephrotoxicity is the most frequently encountered adverse effect of aminoglycoside antibiotics. It is usually seen after prolonged administration (over 2 weeks) to elderly patients with pre-existing renal disease. Typically, it is nonoliguric renal failure, with

Table 30–3. PREVENTION OF WOUND INFECTIONS AND SEPSIS IN SURGICAL PATIENTS

Nature of Surgery	Most Common Pathogens	Recommended Drugs	Preoperative Adult Dose*
Cardiovascular			
Prosthetic valve insertion	*S. aureus, S. epidermidis, diphtheroids*	Cephalosporin,† or penicillinase-resistant penicillin, or vancomycin	1 gm. I.M./I.V. 1 gm. I.M./I.V. 1 gm. I.V.
Arterial Reconstructive			
Involving an aortic prosthesis or a groin incision	*S. aureus, S. epidermidis,* enteric gram-negative, enterococci	Cephalosporin, or vancomycin	1 gm. I.M./I.V. 1 gm. I.V.
Noncardiac Thoracic			
With bronchial transection	*Staphylococcus, Streptococcus, Haemophilus*	Cephalosporin	1 gm. I.M./I.V.
Orthopedic			
Total hip replacement Internal fixation	*S. aureus, S. epidermidis*	Cephalosporin, or penicillinase-resistant penicillin, or vancomycin	1 gm I.M./I.V. 1 gm. I.M./I.V. 1 gm. I.V.
Head and Neck			
With mucosal incision	*S. aureus, Streptococcus,* oral anaerobes, *Klebsiella*	Cephalosporin	1 gm. I.M./I.V.
Gastroduodenal			
(high-risk patients)	*Streptococcus,* enteric gram-negative, oral anaerobes	Cephalosporin	1 gm. I.M./I.V.
Biliary Tract			
(high-risk patients)	Enteric gram-negative, *Streptococcus*	Cephalosporin	1 gm. I.M./I.V.
Colorectal	Enteric gram-negative, *Streptococcus,* anaerobes, especially *B. fragilis*	Oral neomycin plus erythromycin WITH OR WITHOUT Cefoxitin, or cefotetan, or clindamycin plus gentamicin or metronidazole plus gentamicin	1 gm. of each at 1 P.M., 2 P.M. and 11 P.M. the day before surgery 1 gm. I.V. 600 mg. I.V. 1.5 mg./kg. I.M./I.V. 500 mg. I.V. 1.5 mg./kg. I.M./I.V.
Hysterectomy			
Vaginal or abdominal	Enteric gram-negative, anaerobes, *Streptococcus*	Cephalosporin	1 gm. I.M./I.V.
Cesarean Section			
(high risk, primary)	Enteric gram-negative anaerobes, *Streptococcus*	Cephalosporin	1 gm. I.M./I.V. after cord clamping

*If surgery is prolonged, additional doses of antimicrobial agent should be given q. 4–6 h. during surgery. For a discussion of the value of continuing antibiotics postoperatively, see text.

†A first-generation cephalosporin, such as cefazolin, is preferred in most instances.

variable urinary microscopic findings, and a gradually rising blood urea nitrogen (BUN) and creatinine. Azotemia is usually reversible if the drug is stopped early and if other complicating factors, such as septic shock, are absent.

Aminoglycoside antibiotics are of value because of their very broad aerobic gram-negative spectrum. Their clinical use is primarily for the empiric treatment of gram-negative bacillary infections, for the treatment of difficult infections due to gram-negative bacilli in combination with a beta-lactam antibiotic, and with ampicillin or penicillin for the treatment of serious enterococcal infections. Although rarely drugs of first choice because of their toxicity, they are frequently necessary in the hospital setting because of multiresistant organism infection.

Cephalosporins. Cephalosporins are beta-lactam antibiotics, active by virtue of their interference with the synthesis of bacterial cell wall components and are bactericidal for most susceptible microorganisms. The multitude of cephalosporin derivatives has been popularly divided into first-, second-, and third-generation derivatives based on the timing of their development and their spectrum of activity.

Cefazolin is the workhorse first-generation derivative and has a spectrum of activity similar to cephapirin, cephradine, and cephalothin. It is active against most gram-positive cocci, with the exception of enterococci; most gram-positive anaerobes; many strains of *E. coli, Klebsiella,* and *Proteus mirabilis;* and some gram-negative anaerobes but not *Bacteroides fragilis.* Cefuroxime and cefamandole are second-generation cephalosporin derivatives, possessing the same basic spectrum as cefazolin but are also active against *Branhamella, Haemophilus,* and some other gram-negative bacilli. Cefoxitin and cefotetan, because of resistance to gram-negative beta-lactamases, are active against *Bacteroides fragilis* and many strains of enteric gram-negative bacilli that are resistant to first-generation cephalosporins. However, they possess weaker activity than other second-generation derivatives against gram-positive bacteria and *Haemophilus*.

Ongoing development of cephalosporins has created third-generation derivatives, such as cefotaxime, ceftizoxime, ceftriaxone, cefoperazone, and ceftazidime. These drugs are significantly more active against members of the Enterobacteriaceae and hemolytic streptococci. Cefoperazone and ceftazidime also have activity against many strains of *Pseudomonas*. In addition, they are all very active against *Neisseria, Branhamella,* and *Haemophilus* species, including ampicillin-resistant strains, but have weaker activity against staphylococci than the earlier cephalosporins. None of these derivatives have activity against enterococcus, and their anaerobic coverage is variable.

Cephalosporin pharmacokinetics vary from one derivative to another (see Table 30–1). Most are renally excreted; some have considerable biliary excretion; others are metabolized (particularly cephalothin and cefotaxime). The third-generation derivatives penetrate the blood-CSF barrier and achieve CSF concentrations effective for the treatment of gram-negative bacillary meningitis. Except for cefuroxime, first- and second-generation derivatives do not enter the CSF and should not be used for the treatment of meningitis.

Cephalosporins retain, along with penicillins, relative freedom from major toxicity. Hypersensitivity reactions, local reactions to infusion or injection, and rare instances of leukopenia, thrombocytopenia, or hemolytic anemia are occasionally seen. Cefamandole, moxalactam, cefotetan, and cefoperazone possess a unique side chain that has weak antivitamin K activity. Patients on a vitamin K-deficient diet (such as postoperative patients or patients on hyperalimentation) may experience unexpected rises in prothrombin time and bleeding correctible by administration of vitamin K. These agents can also produce an Antabuse-like reaction if a patient drinks alcohol.

The cephalosporins are of clinical value for a wide variety of infections because they lack major toxicity, are bactericidal, and have a broad spectrum of activity. They are useful for prophylaxis, are of value in complicated and mixed infections, and are effectively used as substitutes for penicillin in some patients allergic to penicillin. Third-generation cephalosporins are the drugs of choice for resistant *Haemophilus* and gram-negative bacillary meningitis.

Chloramphenicol. Chloramphenicol is an antibiotic isolated from *Streptomyces*. It inhibits protein synthesis at a ribosomal level and is either bactericidal or bacteriostatic depending upon the particular isolate involved. Chloramphenicol has a broad spectrum of activity. It is active against most gram-positive cocci including *S. pneumoniae*. Its activity against aerobic gram-negative bacteria is also broad and includes *Haemophilus* species, most *E. coli, Enterobacter, Klebsiella, Proteus, Serratia,* and *Salmonella*. It is not active against *Pseudomonas*. Chloramphenicol is active against the majority of anaerobes, including *B. fragilis*.

Chloramphenicol yields better plasma levels after oral compared to parenteral administration. Its lipid solubility accounts for its ability to cross the blood-brain barrier, thereby achieving CSF concentrations adequate to treat some forms of meningitis.

Although an extremely active compound, chloramphenicol is potentially toxic. Bone marrow depression is the major adverse reaction. This may be a dose-related, reversible phenomenon, seen with administration of large doses for a prolonged time period, usually in excess of 14 days of parenteral therapy. Pancytopenia or selective cytopenias are seen but are reversible on withdrawing the drug. A more severe, aplastic anemia is seen as an idiosyncratic reaction, independent of dose, and occurs with a frequency of approximately 1 in 50,000. Although it is said to occur primarily after oral administration, this may be a statistical artifact based on the relative preponderance of patients who received oral chloramphenicol in the past. It seems impossible to predict who will develop marrow aplasia due to chloramphenicol. At least triweekly blood counts are indicated in all patients receiving chloramphenicol, with termination of therapy if white blood cell counts fall to $<4000/mm.^3$ or platelet counts to $<120{,}000/mm.^3$ Because of its toxicity, it should not be used for trivial infections.

Other side effects of chloramphenicol include the gray baby syndrome (circulatory collapse in premature and newborn infants related to high levels of unconjugated chloramphenicol), optic neuritis after prolonged oral administration, and, rarely, hypersensitivity reactions. Chloramphenicol inhibits the activity of microsomal liver enzymes, thereby interfering with the metabolism of other drugs, particularly phenytoin and warfarin. It may thereby induce toxicity to either of these drugs.

With the development of safer and more potent antimicrobial agents, chloramphenicol has been relegated to a role of largely historical interest. However, it remains useful for the treatment of systemic *Salmonella* infections and rickettsial infections. Because of its central nervous system penetration, it is a useful alternative to penicillin G or cephalosporins for the treatment of gram-positive meningitis, brain abscesses, and *H. influenzae* infections of the central nervous system.

The Lincinoids. Lincomycin and clindamycin are antibiotics similar in activity to erythromycin. They act by competitively binding to ribosomes, thereby inhibiting protein synthesis. They appear to occupy the same binding sites as erythromycin so that concomitant administration of both drugs results in antagonism. The spectrum of activity of clindamycin and lincomycin includes most gram-positive bacteria, with the exception of enterococci, and most anaerobes, including *B. fragilis.* Clindamycin is much more potent in the latter regard and lincomycin is no longer used. Neither drug is active against aerobic gram-negative bacilli.

Clindamycin is well absorbed orally and parenterally. It is distributed throughout the body but does not reach adequate levels in CSF. Clindamycin is excreted primarily through the liver and the normal half-life is not appreciably altered in patients with renal impairment (see Table 30–1). Only small amounts are excreted in the urine.

The major toxicity of clindamycin is gastrointestinal. Diarrhea occurs in 10 per cent and pseudomembranous colitis, due to overgrowth of *Clostridium difficile,* occurs in perhaps 1 per cent of patients. It occurs as frequently with parenteral therapy as with oral, is not related to duration of therapy, and may be exacerbated or precipitated by coadministration of antiperistaltic drugs, such as diphenoxylate (Lomotil). Hypersensitivity reactions and hepatotoxicity are seen on rare occasions.

Clindamycin is valuable for the treatment of staphylococcal and streptococcal infections, particularly in bone and soft tissue. Clindamycin is also useful for the treatment of anaerobic infections, particularly those due to *B. fragilis.* Since it is ineffective against aerobic gram-negative bacilli, it must usually be used in combination with other drugs for the treatment of infradiaphragmatic infections. As an alternate to penicillin G, it is excellent for the treatment of anaerobic and mixed aerobic and anaerobic pleuropulmonary infections.

Macrolide Antibiotics. Erythromycin is a broad-spectrum macrocyclic antibiotic. It is active against many staphylococci and most streptococci, excluding enterococci. In addition, it is active against many gram-positive bacilli, including anaerobes, *Listeria,* and *Corynebacterium.* Gram-negative organisms are infrequently sensitive, although some strains of *Haemophilus* and *Bacteroides* may be effectively inhibited. *Treponema pallidum, Mycoplasma, Chlamydia,* and *Rickettsia* are susceptible to erythromycin. It is the agent of choice for the treatment of *Legionella* infections. Erythromycin acts by inhibiting protein synthesis in susceptible microorganisms by binding competitively to ribosomal proteins, thereby inhibiting protein synthesis.

Erythromycin is well absorbed after oral or parenteral administration. A variety of oral forms are available, and it has not been established that any of the various erythromycin salts, esters, or base preparations has a clinical advantage over any other in the treatment of infections due to susceptible microorganisms. Erythromycin distributes well to most body tissues except the CSF. It is excreted primarily in the bile and penetrates prostatic fluid, but urinary levels are marginal (see Table 30–1).

Erythromycin has minimal serious toxicity. Nausea, vomiting, and abdominal cramps are fairly frequent. Cholestatic hepatitis may follow use of the estolate. Hypersensitivity reactions are unusual. Phlebitis after intravenous administration is common. Transient sensorineural hearing loss has appeared as a very rare complication of high-dose intravenous therapy.

Clinical uses of erythromycin include treatment of gram-positive infections, particularly in penicillin-allergic patients; treatment of *Legionella* and mycoplasma infections; an alternate to penicillin for the treatment of *Chlamydia* and uncomplicated syphilis in penicillin-allergic patients; and as a valuable agent for the treatment of *Corynebacterium diphtheriae* infections.

Metronidazole. Metronidazole is an imidazole derivative with unique activity against certain protozoa *(Trichomonas, Entamoeba,* and *Giardia)* and anaerobic bacteria, including *B. fragilis.* It has no activity against aerobic microorganisms and in the treatment of mixed infections must be used with an antibiotic effective against aerobes. Metronidazole interferes with DNA synthesis and is bactericidal against susceptible microorganisms.

Metronidazole is well absorbed after oral or intravenous administration. It penetrates all body tissues well and reaches a particularly high concentration in the brain and CSF. Metronidazole is excreted primarily unchanged in the urine, although a considerable proportion is metabolized in the liver and excreted in the urine as inactive metabolites.

Metronidazole is well tolerated but can cause gastrointestinal upset and rarely leukopenia, peripheral neuropathy, and seizures. Although extensive studies have not shown an increase in bacterial mutation or carcinogenicity in humans, it should not be used in pregnant women. Metronidazole interferes with ethanol metabolism producing an Antabuse-like reaction and may also inhibit the metabolism of warfarin and phenytoin.

Metronidazole is of great clinical use for the treatment of protozoal infections, particularly trichomoniasis, amebiasis, and giardiasis. It is not a very effective intraluminal amebacide and, therefore, must be followed by an effective intraluminal drug, such as diiodohydroxyquin (Diodoquin). Metronidazole is very valuable for the treatment of anaerobic infections, but when a mixed infection is present, it must be combined with an antibiotic effective against aerobic bacteria. Metronidazole is the agent of choice for the treatment of anaerobic infections of the central nervous system (such as brain abscesses).

Penicillin Derivatives. Penicillin and its many derivatives remain safe, effective, and potent despite the appearance of beta-lactam destroying enzymes in many genera of gram-positive and gram-negative bacteria. Derived from the *Penicillium* group of fungi, penicillins are bactericidal inhibitors of cell wall synthesis.

Penicillin G is becoming less active against gram-positive bacteria. Ninety per cent of staphylococci are resistant. Penicillins are not bactericidal for enterococci, and certain strains of *Streptococcus pneumoniae* have become resistant to penicillin G. Although the majority of these pneumococcal strains can be killed by high doses of penicillin G, some isolates are totally resistant to penicillin. Ampicillin and amoxicillin are more active against gram-negative bacilli and are effective for the treatment of many infections due to non-beta-lactamase producing *Haemophilus, E. coli, P. mirabilis,* and *Salmonella* species.

Methicillin, nafcillin, and oxacillin are resistant to the hydrolytic action of gram-positive beta-lactamases. Accordingly, these derivatives have become the drugs of choice for treating infections due to staphylococci. They are less active than penicillin G against other gram-positive organisms and have inadequate activity against anaerobes and gram-negative microorganisms.

Carbenicillin, ticarcillin, mezlocillin, azlocillin, and piperacillin are antipseudomonal penicillins active against a wide variety of gram-negative microorganisms. They have a spectrum of activity similar to ampicillin and, in addition, are effective against many strains of *Enterobacter, Serratia, Acinetobacter, Morganella,* and *Pseudomonas*. Piperacillin and mezlocillin are also active against 60 to 80 per cent of community-acquired *Klebsiella* species and have better enterococcal activity than other members of this group. In the order listed, they have increasing in vitro potency against *Pseudomonas aeruginosa,* although none has convincingly been shown to be superior to another for the treatment of clinical infections due to *Pseudomonas*.

In order to expand the spectrum and retain the usefulness of some penicillin derivatives threatened by the increased prevalence of beta-lactamase production in both gram-positive and gram-negative bacteria, the beta-lactamase inhibitors clavulanic acid and sulbactam were developed. These compounds effectively block the activity of staphylococcal beta-lactamases and many gram-negative beta-lactamases, allowing the parent—penicillinase-susceptible derivative ampicillin, amoxicillin, or ticarcillin—to regain activity against previously resistant bacteria. Thus, Augmentin (amoxicillin-clavulate), Unasyn (ampicillin-sulbactam), and Timentin (ticarcillin-clavulanate) (see Table 30–1) are active against beta-lactamase producing *Staphylococci, Haemophilus, Branhamella, Neisseria gonorrhoeae, Bacteroides, E. coli,* and *Klebsiella.* Microorganisms producing primarily cephalosporinases of the type 1 variety are not susceptible to this inhibitory function, and these combinations offer no advantage over amoxicillin, ampicillin, or ticarcillin alone. Such microorganisms include *Enterobacter, Serratia, Morganella,* and *Pseudomonas*. Owing to the clinical distribution of beta-lactamases, the beta-lactamase blocking compounds provide broad-spectrum, polymicrobial coverage in skin and soft tissue infections, intra-abdominal and pelvic infections, and upper and lower respiratory infections.

Penicillin derivatives are excreted primarily in urine, although the antistaphylococcal penicillins, mezlocillin, and piperacillin are metabolized in the liver and excreted in the bile (see Table 30–1). Penicillin G is not acid stable and, therefore, penicillin V is the form of choice for oral administration. Amoxicillin is better absorbed orally and reaches twice the blood level of ampicillin at equivalent doses. The tissue penetration of these compounds is good, but CSF levels are low in the absence of inflammation. The concentrations of amoxicillin in sinus and middle ear fluids are greater than those achieved by ampicillin, making it preferable for the treatment in otitis media and sinusitis.

Penicillin derivatives are free from major toxicity. Anaphylaxis is the most serious adverse reaction, occurring in approximately 0.05 per cent of penicillin-treated patients. Other hypersensitivity reactions include eosinophilia, interstitial nephritis, maculopapular skin eruptions, and serum sickness. High doses of penicillin derivatives, particularly in the presence of renal failure, can produce myoclonus and seizures. Inadvertent intravenous injection of procaine penicillin produces acute procaine toxicity with fever, tachycardia, anxiety, and hallucinations.

When ticarcillin and carbenicillin are administered in large doses, inhibition of platelet aggregation may occur, and clinical bleeding is observed in from 1 to 10 per cent of patients treated with these compounds. Hypokalemia is also seen due to the effect of nonreabsorbable anion and resultant hyperkaluria. The amount of sodium in ticarcillin and carbenicillin is approximately 5 mEq/gram and may occasionally be sufficient to exacerbate congestive heart failure. Rarely, leukopenia, hemolytic anemia, and thrombocytopenia are seen due to the administration of penicillins.

Patients reporting allergy to penicillin often lack true hypersensitivity. Some reactions to ampicillin and methicillin are not immunologically mediated and do not recur on re-exposure. Late hypersensitivity reactions (i.e., occurring several days or weeks after starting penicillin) are IgG mediated and are not usually dangerous. Penicillin may be continued if necessary with symptomatic treatment of the rash and pruritus. In this setting, however, the occurrence of clinically significant serum sickness, interstitial nephritis, or exfoliation should prompt withdrawal of the drug. Immediate hypersensitivity reactions, mediated by IgE, are rare and represent true hypersensitivity. Such reactions can usually be detected by skin testing with penicilloyl-polylysine (commercially available as Prepen) and a dilute mixture of penicillin G, known as minor determinant mixture. A positive reaction to these tests has a high predictive value for immediate hypersensitivity and contraindicates the use of penicillin. If absolutely necessary, desensitization may be undertaken by a trained allergist or infectious disease specialist.

The incidence of cross-allergenicity with cephalosporin derivatives is frequently debated but is probably less than 5 per cent. In general, patients with true anaphylaxis to penicillin G should not be given cephalosporin antibiotics without extreme caution. Patients with late reactions to penicillin derivatives can usually be given cephalosporin derivatives without incident, and the cephalosporins play a valuable role in this situation.

Aztreonam. Aztreonam is the first of a group of monocyclic beta-lactam antibiotics, also known as the monobactams. These antibiotics are potent, bactericidal drugs active against most aerobic gram-negative bacilli, including aminoglycoside-resistant strains, and *P. aeruginosa.* Aztreonam is also active against *Neisseria* species and *Haemophilus,* including beta-lactamase producing strains. It has no activity against gram-positive bacteria or anaerobes.

Aztreonam is not orally bioavailable. Intravenous or intramuscular administration produces effective blood and tissue concentrations for 4 to 6 hours in patients with normal renal function. There is insignificant metabolism, and the drug is excreted almost entirely in the urine, requiring dosage adjustment in renal failure (see Table 30–1).

Due to its unique spectrum, aztreonam has proved a useful, albeit more costly, replacement for aminoglycoside antibiotics in many clinical situations. It has proven effective for the treatment of urinary tract infections, lower respiratory tract infections, skin and soft tissue, and bone and joint infections as a single agent. In polymicrobial infections or where gram-positive or anaerobic bacteria are suspected, a second agent to cover these additional pathogens must be used in addition.

The adverse effects associated with the use of aztreonam are similar to those seen with other beta-lactams. Aztreonam is not nephrotoxic or ototoxic, and, due to its lack of anaerobic activity, diarrhea is uncommon. A major advantage of aztreonam is its lack of immunologic cross-reactivity with penicillin and cephalosporin derivatives. It has been used without incident to treat infections in patients with positive penicillin skin tests and a documented history of anaphylactic reaction to these agents.

Imipenem. Imipenem is a carbapenem, a semisynthetic beta-lactam with an unusually broad spectrum of activity. It is active against all gram-negative bacilli including *Pseudomonas aeruginosa,* most gram-positive bacteria, except for methicillin-resistant staphylococci and some enterococci, and all anaerobic bacteria, including *Bacteroides fragilis.* Cross-resistance with other penicillins occurs rarely, so it is useful for the treatment of infections due to multidrug-resistant flora.

No oral formulation of imipenem is available. When administered intravenously, it undergoes rapid inactivation by renal peptidases. This inactivation is effectively inhibited by combining imipenem with cilastatin, an enzyme inhibitor, to provide a clinically useful combination, known commercially as Primaxin. The pharmocokinetics of this combination are similar to those of other beta-lactams, achieving good concentrations in most body fluids except the central nervous system. Renal dysfunction requires dosage adjustment (see Table 30–1).

Imipenem is useful for a wide variety of bacterial infections, particularly polymicrobial infections where aerobes and anaerobes are present. Intra-abdominal and soft tissue infections are examples. Due to its broad spectrum, imipenem has an important role in treating drug-resistant nosocomial infections. For this reason, together with concerns about its cost and toxicity, many specialists reserve Primaxin for use in exceptional clinical situations.

Primaxin, like other beta-lactams, is usually well tolerated. Cross-allergenicity with penicillins does occur. Administration of large doses in renal failure may produce seizures, so close monitoring of renal function and appropriate dose adjustment is necessary (see Table 30–1). The maximum daily dose of Primaxin should not exceed 4 grams, and it cannot be used to treat meningitis.

Quinolones. The newly introduced fluorinated quinolones are synthetic antimicrobial agents. They are bactericidal compounds, inhibiting DNA gyrase, an enzyme crucial to bacterial cell function and replication. They are highly active in vitro against enteric gram-negative bacilli such as *E. coli* and *Klebsiella* and also against nonfermenters such as *Pseudomonas* and *Aeromonas.* They possess relatively good activity against staphylococci, including methicillin-resistant strains. Activity against enterococci and other streptococci is somewhat less, and their therapeutic value in infections caused by these microorganisms is less well established. The anaerobic activity of most quinolones is weak and probably not clinically valuable. Quinolones are also active against *Legionella, Mycoplasma, Haemophilus,* and *Neisseria* species. They possess variable activity against *Chlamydia, Ureaplasma,* and *Mycobacteria.*

Resistance to the fluoroquinolones is rare. A community hospital study of over 2400 aerobic bacterial isolates revealed that less than 1 per cent were resistant to ciprofloxacin; most of these were enterococci and *Pseudomonas* species other than *P. aeruginosa.* Cross-resistance to other classes of antimicrobial agents, such as beta-lactam or aminoglycoside antibiotics, is not observed so that these compounds are useful for the treatment of infections due to multidrug-resistant pathogens.

The quinolones are readily absorbed after oral administration. Their relatively small molecular weight and low degree of protein-binding results in excellent tissue penetration. Particularly high concentrations are achieved within phagocytic cells and in prostatic tissue, bronchial epithelium, bile, urine, and stool. The serum half-lives of these antimicrobial agents are long, permitting dosing intervals of 8 to 12 hours or more. Although metabolized to varying degrees in the liver, urinary concentrations of active drug are high at all levels of renal function, far in excess of those needed to inhibit most urinary pathogens.

Ciprofloxacin and norfloxacin are the quinolone

derivatives currently in use. Both compounds are effective orally for the treatment of uncomplicated and complicated urinary tract infections, including prostatitis and infections due to *Pseudomonas*. These drugs are also agents of choice for the treatment of infectious diarrhea since they inhibit essentially all enteric pathogens except *Clostridium difficile*. Ciprofloxacin has also been shown to be effective in skin, soft tissue, bone and joint, and lower respiratory infections due to susceptible pathogens, particularly gram-negative bacilli. In these roles as oral agents, quinolones may shorten the course of, or replace entirely, intravenous antimicrobial therapy of certain infections.

Quinolones are well tolerated. The most frequent adverse reactions are gastrointestinal, chiefly nausea, occurring in 8 to 10 per cent of patients. Vomiting and diarrhea occur less frequently. Some patients experience central nervous system effects, such as headache, dizziness, restlessness, or tremor. These reactions are seen most frequently in patients taking theophylline or caffeinated beverages. Other adverse reactions, such as drug fever, rash, and pruritus, occur in 1 to 2 per cent of patients. Due to fetal and juvenile cartilage toxicity in some animal models, administration of these agents to pregnant or lactating women is contraindicated, and no pediatric indication currently exists.

A significant drug interaction between fluoroquinolones and xanthine derivatives results in increased serum concentrations of theophylline and caffeine during therapy. All antacids have been shown to decrease the absorption of the quinolones due to their chelation by magnesium, aluminum, and calcium. Concomitant administration of H_2 antagonists, however, does not significantly alter antimicrobial serum concentrations.

Sulfonamides and Trimethoprim. The sulfonamides, first synthesized for clinical use in 1935, initiated a new era in the chemotherapy of infectious diseases. They are bacteriostatic compounds and act by inhibiting dihydrofolate synthetase activity, since they are structural analogues for its substrate, para-aminobenzoic acid. In combination with trimethoprim, which inhibits the next step in purine synthesis, dihydrofolate reductase, they are frequently synergistic.

Sulfonamides are active against a wide variety of gram-positive bacteria, except enterococci and gram-negative organisms. Most members of the Enterobacteriaceae are susceptible. In addition, *Chlamydia, Nocardia,* and *Toxoplasma* are inhibited. Trimethoprim has a similar range of activity against aerobic gram-positive and gram-negative bacteria. Because of their sequential activity in blocking bacterial purine synthesis, sulfamethoxazole and trimethoprim (Bactrim, Septra) are synergistically active against the vast majority of susceptible microorganisms, particularly *H. influenzae,* staphylococci, and members of Enterobacteriaceae species. *Pseudomonas aeruginosa* and enterococci are not effectively inhibited.

Both sulfonamides and trimethoprim are well absorbed after oral administration and penetrate well to all body tissues, including the central nervous system. Trimethoprim penetrates prostatic tissue particularly well and, either alone or in combination with sulfamethoxazole, is a drug of choice for the treatment of bacterial prostatitis. Both drugs are excreted predominantly in the urine, reaching levels higher than those found in serum (see Table 30–1).

Adverse reactions due to sulfonamides and trimethoprim are primarily those of hypersensitivity: a variety of cutaneous eruptions and serum sickness. Erythema multiforme, or the Stevens-Johnson syndrome, is the most severe form of hypersensitivity, and can be seen with either drug. It is particularly severe with long-acting sulfonamides. Therefore, short-acting sulfonamides (sulfisoxazole or sulfamethoxazole) are the derivatives of choice for the treatment of most infections. Drug fever, nausea, vomiting, diarrhea, pulmonary reactions, and hypersensitivity meningitis are seen on rare occasions. Agranulocytosis due to sulfonamide derivatives has been described, and megaloblastic anemia due to inhibition of human dihydrofolate reductase is occasionally seen in patients receiving trimethoprim chronically or in large doses. These patients are usually malnourished or receiving other antifolates for the treatment of malignancy. Administration of folinic acid (Leukovorin) will readily reverse the folic acid deficiency induced by these agents.

The clinical utility of sulfonamides and/or trimethoprim is primarily in the treatment of urinary tract infections. However, in combination, these drugs are particularly effective for the treatment of upper and lower respiratory tract infections due to pneumococcus, *Branhamella,* or *Haemophilus* species, including sinusitis, otitis media, and exacerbations of chronic bronchitis. The combination is also effective for the treatment of *Nocardia* infections, infections due to *Pneumocystis carinii,* certain drug-resistant malaria infections, chlamydial infections, and perhaps also toxoplasmosis. Because of bacterial resistance, the sulfonamides are no longer drugs of choice for the treatment or prophylaxis of meningococcal infections. Trimethoprim plus sulfamethoxazole is a popular choice for the treatment of enteric infections, particularly those due to *Salmonella* or *Shigella.*

Tetracyclines. The tetracyclines are complex compounds with a broad range of activity. They are primarily bacteriostatic and act by inhibiting protein synthesis at a ribosomal level. Tetracyclines are active against many gram-positive bacteria, including *S. aureus,* and gram-negative bacteria, including most members of the Enterobacteriaceae, except *Proteus* species. Many other gram-negative bacteria are also susceptible, including *Haemophilus* species, *Neisseria* species, and some nonfermentative bacteria (but not *P. aeruginosa*) at achievable serum levels. The tetracyclines are also active against a wide variety of other microorganisms, including *Rickettsia, Chlamydia,* and *Mycoplasma.*

Tetracyclines are well absorbed orally, except in the presence of food or divalent cations, such as antacids or ferrous compounds. Minocycline and doxycycline, however, are less affected by such agents and are essentially completely absorbed, even in the presence of food. Doxycycline and minocycline are excreted primarily by the liver and not in the urine (see Table 30–1). All other tetracyclines are excreted to a large extent in urine and are effective for the treatment of some urinary tract infections. Tetracyclines penetrate fairly well into all body fluids. Doxycycline and minocycline are more lipid soluble, an important property in determining their tissue penetration.

The side effects of tetracycline are primarily gastrointestinal, with nausea, vomiting, and diarrhea common. Hypersensitivity reactions are uncommon. Photosensitivity, however, is particularly troublesome, although it is attributed more commonly to demethylchlortetracycline than any other derivative. Tooth discoloration contraindicates the use of tetracyclines in pregnancy and under the age of 10 years. Hepatotoxicity may be seen with intravenous tetracycline, particularly during pregnancy or in renal failure. Doxycycline and minocycline are the parenteral tetracyclines of choice, since they are excreted by extrarenal means and have not been associated with hepatotoxicity. Minocycline is unique in the production of reversible vestibular toxicity, seen in up to 80 per cent of patients, particularly females.

Tetracyclines have a broad clinical role. They are useful for the treatment of a variety of respiratory tract infections, particularly exacerbations of chronic bronchitis associated with *Haemophilus* infection. They are effective for the treatment of mycoplasma and staphylococcal infections, uncomplicated urinary tract infections, prostatitis, and infections due to *Rickettsia*. Tetracyclines are effective drugs for the treatment of chlamydial infections, particularly nongonococcal urethritis. In enteric infections, tetracyclines are effective against some *Shigella* species, and doxycycline has been shown to be somewhat effective for the prophylaxis of traveler's diarrhea. In the latter instance, however, it increases the risk of infection with tetracycline-resistant organisms, owing to elimination of protective normal flora.

Vancomycin. Vancomycin use has had a resurgence due to the increased prevalence of methicillin-resistant staphylococci. Its mode of action is the bactericidal inhibition of cell wall synthesis. It is active against most gram-positive bacteria, including staphylococcal species, *Corynebacteria,* enterococci, and *Clostridia*. It is not active against gram-negative bacteria.

Vancomycin is not absorbed after oral administration, and parenteral administration is not effective for the treatment of *C. difficile* colitis. The drug is not metabolized but is excreted by the kidneys in unchanged form. Vancomycin diffuses into most body compartments except the cerebrospinal fluid. Because of its total dependence on the kidney for excretion, major adjustments in dose are necessary in the presence of renal insufficiency (see Table 30–1).

Deafness is the most serious adverse effect of vancomycin administration. It is most common in the elderly and in those with renal insufficiency. Ototoxicity is related to excessively high serum levels. Blood levels of vancomycin must be monitored during therapy. Occasional hypersensitivity reactions are seen, and thrombophlebitis is frequently troublesome. Too rapid infusion produces facial and upper body flushing and pruritus (red neck syndrome) due to histamine release.

Vancomycin is a valuable drug for the treatment of staphylococcal infections, particularly those due to methicillin-resistant staphylococci or serious staphylococcal infections in penicillin-allergic patients. It is also very useful for the treatment of enterococcal endocarditis infections as an alternative to penicillin. Vancomycin is a drug of choice for the treatment of pseudomembranous colitis (due to *C. difficile*), for which it must be administered orally in a dose of 125 to 250 mg. every 6 hours, since parenteral administration does not result in measurable fecal concentrations of vancomycin.

The following sections discuss important clinical entities which may be encountered by the family practitioner with emphasis on common pathogens, methods of diagnosis and treatment.

Bone and Joint Infections

INFECTIOUS ARTHRITIS

Infectious arthritis may be of hematogenous origin, due to direct percutaneous inoculation of a joint, or secondary to a contiguous focus of infection in adjacent soft tissues or bone. In children below 1 year of age, septic arthritis is usually spread from adjacent osteomyelitis, since capillaries perforate the epiphyseal growth plate, allowing infection to spread from bone to joint. Over the age of 1 year, infection is likely to be localized to the joint without concomitant osteomyelitis. Distant infection, trauma, and preexisting osteoarthritis or rheumatoid arthritis are common predisposing risks for the development of septic arthritis. Arthritis may be seen in certain systemic infections, such as meningococcemia, due to immune complex disease rather than joint infection. The arthritis that follows *Salmonella, Shigella,* or *Yersinia* intestinal infection is immunologically similar, and occurs most often in persons with histocompatibility antigen (HLA) type W27.

The frequency with which certain microorganisms cause arthritis is dependent upon the patient's age (Table 30–4). In the newborn, group B streptococci and staphylococci are most common, although some gram-negative bacilli such as *E. coli* may cause septic arthritis as a consequence of bacteremia. The most common organisms in children between the age of 2 months and 2 years are *H. influenzae* and streptococcal species. After 2 years of age, *S. aureus* causes most bacterial arthritis. In adults from ages 15 to 50, *Neisseria gonorrhoeae* is the most common agent. Lyme disease is a common cause of large joint monarticular arthritis at all ages, particularly in southern Connecticut, southeastern New York, and the north central states. Gram-negative bacilli are uncommonly implicated as a cause of infectious arthritis in all age groups. Most afflicted patients have underlying disease or long-standing arthritis in the affected joint. Intravenous drug users are likely to develop *Pseudomonas* septic arthritis, particularly in sternoclavicular and sacroiliac joints. *Salmonella* arthritis occurs in individuals with hemolytic disorders, such as sickle cell disease. Anaerobes, although uncommonly reported, appear to be important causes of septic arthritis in the elderly. Mycobacteria characteristically produce an indolent monoarticular arthritis of the knees. Such infections may also involve tendon sheaths. *Sporothrix schenkii* is the most common fungus isolated from infected joints, particularly the knee and wrist. Monarticular arthritis also occurs with other fungi such as *Coccidioides immitis.*

Individuals with septic arthritis present with fever, pain, limitation of motion, swelling, and redness of the joint. Small children may only have limited movement of the joint and appear to have paralysis. In the majority of cases, an effusion will be demonstrable, although the hip may be difficult to evaluate. The knee is the most common joint affected in both children and adults (Table 30–5).

Laboratory findings in septic arthritis are nonspecific. The sedimentation rate and white blood cell count are usually elevated. Anemia may be present but is more likely related to the underlying disease. Examination of the joint aspirate reveals purulent fluid with a leukocyte count usually over $50{,}000/mm^3$. Joint fluid protein is elevated and the glucose will usually be less than 40 mg. per dl., although in children it may be normal. Gram-stained smears of joint fluid will show the organism in most cases of staphylococcal arthritis but in less than 30 per cent of cases of arthritis due to other organisms. Cultures should be performed using special media for fastidious organisms, such as *Haemophilus* and *Neisseria,* and blood cultures are indicated since they will be positive in many patients. Counterimmunoelectrophoresis or latex agglutination is a useful supplementary tool to identify bacterial antigen in joint fluid. X-ray studies are not helpful unless concomitant osteomyelitis exists.

Table 30–4. MICROBIOLOGIC ETIOLOGY OF INFECTIOUS ARTHRITIS BY AGE

	Age (years)			
Organism	*< 2*	*2–14*	*15–40*	*> 40*
Staphylococcus aureus	45%	60%	20%	70%
Haemophilus influenzae	30	10	< 1	< 1
Streptococcus	20	20	15	15
Neisseria gonorrhoeae	< 1	5	60	< 1
Gram-negative bacilli	5	5	5	10
Anaerobes	< 1	< 1	< 1	5

Table 30–5. FREQUENCY OF JOINT INVOLVEMENT IN INFECTIOUS ARTHRITIS

Joint	Children	Adults
Knee	40%	50%
Hip	20	25
Ankle	15	7
Elbow	15	10
Wrist	5	7
Shoulder	5	15
Interphalangeal, metacarpal	1	1
Sternoclavicular	1	8
Sacroiliac	< 1	2

Although all individuals who present with acute monoarticular arthritis should be evaluated for a bacterial etiology, other diseases may mimic septic arthritis. Rheumatoid arthritis, osteoarthritis, gout, pseudogout, acute flares of systemic lupus erythematosus, and hemarthroses all produce similar findings. A high polymorphonuclear leukocyte count in synovial fluid is seen in many of these diseases, particularly gout and pseudogout. Joint fluid must be examined for crystals, glucose, protein, and cell count as well as culture and Gram's stain.

After proper joint fluid examination and culture, therapy is initiated based on the results of the Gram's stain and the anticipated pathogens. Empiric therapy should be begun immediately without waiting for culture confirmation to avoid joint destruction and should be tailored to the isolated microorganism. Infectious arthritis is generally treated for 3 to 4 weeks, usually with parenteral antibiotics, although recent studies indicate that oral therapy in children is effective after 1 week of parenteral therapy. Antibiotics penetrate joint fluid well, and intra-articular administration is of no additional value. Infected joint fluid should be removed as it accumulates to prevent leukocyte enzyme destruction of articular cartilage. Closed-needle aspiration is the preferred mode of drainage and appears to result in greater recovery of joint function than open drainage. The exception to this is in septic hip infection in which the mechanical difficulties of closed needle aspiration make open drainage preferred.

LYME DISEASE

Lyme disease is a multisystem disorder with prominent rheumatologic and cutaneous manifestations.

Originally recognized in 1975 as a cluster of pediatric arthritis in Lyme, Connecticut, it has become clear in the last decade that Lyme disease is a common illness with protean manifestations affecting adults as well as children throughout the world. It is a spirochetal infection, caused by a newly recognized pathogen, *Borrelia burgdorferi,* and is transmitted primarily by ticks of the *Ixodes dammini* species (the deer tick). Subsequent to inoculation, the illness of Lyme disease appears in three stages, occurring in roughly chronologic order.

Stage one of the illness is manifest by rash—erythema chronicum migrans (Plate I), a flu-like syndrome with malaise and fatigue, and low-grade fever. Many patients do not recall the tick bite since the deer tick is so small. With a median incubation period of 7 days (range 5 to 21 days), a small, red macule or papule appears, expanding with a flat or raised red border to a diameter of up to 20 or more centimeters. The center may become pale, vesicular, or hemorrhagic. Subsequent to the initial lesion, approximately 50 per cent of patients develop smaller, secondary annular lesions, but, in total, less than 50 per cent of infected patients develop any rash. The appearance of erythema chronicum migrans is almost pathognomonic for Lyme disease, but atypical forms occur and may be mistaken for cellulitis, traumatic lesions, or allergic rashes.

Subsequent to the initial infection, and a variable latent period of well-being, neurologic manifestations may appear. These may take the form of aseptic meningitis, neuritis with cranial nerve palsies such as Bell's palsy, motor or sensory peripheral neuropathies, or demyelinating-like syndromes. Up to two thirds of patients exhibit subtle signs of encephalitis, such as memory loss, emotional lability, irritability, fatigue, depression, and headache. Cardiac abnormalities manifest by rhythm disturbances, atrial ventricular block, myocarditis, or pericarditis.

Late Lyme disease, or stage three disease, is usually manifested by arthritis. This occurs weeks, months, or even years after the initial infection and presents as a monarticular or oligoarticular arthritis affecting primarily large joints. Arthritis may migrate, fluctuate in intensity, and, in children, may be accompanied by significant fever. In untreated patients, the arthritis becomes chronic, resulting in erosive joint damage and disability. Late neurologic manifestations include multiple sclerosis-like illness, seizures, dementia, or psychiatric illness.

The diagnosis of Lyme disease depends upon a high index of clinical suspicion, particularly for the multisystem manifestations of the disease. Serologic testing is readily available, but tests are frequently negative in early disease; false positive tests may occur in patients with hypergammaglobulinemia, other spirochetal diseases, and perhaps autoimmune disease and infectious mononucleosis. Isolation of the spirochete from blood or body fluids is difficult and impractical.

The treatment of Lyme disease depends upon its stage. In early disease associated with erythema chronicum migrans, tetracycline or penicillin V administered for 14 days is generally curative. Lower cure rates are observed with erythromycin. Patients with more advanced disease may require intravenous antibiotics or longer courses (e.g., 30 days) of oral agents. If neurologic involvement, carditis, or established arthritis is present, or if the patient has failed to respond to an adequate course of oral agents, then parenteral therapy is preferred. High-dose intravenous penicillin or ceftriaxone has proven effective. With early and aggressive treatment, the prognosis in early Lyme disease (stage one) is excellent. The response rates in later stages are lower, in part due to lingering fatigue and arthralgia that commonly occur after an adequate course of antibiotic therapy. Adjunctive therapy with nonsteroidal anti-inflammatory agents, antidepressants, and psychologic support may be helpful. Adrenocortical steroid therapy is not advised.

OSTEOMYELITIS

Osteomyelitis can be divided into categories by pathogenesis. Hematogenous osteomyelitis is blood borne from a distant source, contiguous osteomyelitis develops from an adjacent soft tissue infection, and traumatic osteomyelitis develops from surgical or nonsurgical trauma.

Hematogenous Osteomyelitis

Acute hematogenous osteomyelitis occurs primarily in children. Seventy per cent of such cases occur before the age of 10 years. The favorite anatomic site for hematogenous osteomyelitis in children is rapidly growing long bones, most frequently the distal epiphyses of the lower extremities. Bacteria are seeded into the dilated capillary loops of the metaphysis where sluggish and turbulent blood flow allows bacterial growth. The infective process may cross the epiphyseal plate in infants, resulting in joint space infection. Many studies report notable, but physically minor, trauma immediately prior to the onset of symptoms.

Infecting microorganisms, as in septic arthritis, depend upon the age of the patient (Table 30–6). In infantile osteomyelitis, *H. influenzae,* group B streptococci, and staphylococci are important pathogens. In childhood hematogenous osteomyelitis, *S. aureus* is overwhelmingly predominant. In adults, hematogenous osteomyelitis is infrequent, and its occurrence is associated with severe debility or parenteral narcotic abuse. *S. aureus* remains the most common isolate, but gram-negative organisms, particularly *Pseudomonas,* are found with increased frequency, especially in vertebral osteomyelitis associated with drug abuse.

The presenting signs and symptoms of hematogenous osteomyelitis vary from minimal to pronounced

Table 30–6. ETIOLOGIC AGENTS OF ACUTE HEMATOGENOUS OSTEOMYELITIS BY PATIENT AGE

	Age (years)					
Organisms	< 2	2–5	6–10	11–15	Adult	Average
S. aureus	33%	60%	76%	73%	62%	61%
S. epidermidis	14	0	0	8	2	5
Streptococcus	16	11	5	8	5	9
S. pneumoniae	5	0	0	0	2	1.5
H. influenzae	11	2	0	0	0	2.5
P. aeruginosa	0	2	2	4	3	2
Enterobacteriaceae	3	0	2	0	2	1.5
Salmonella	0	3	0	0	2	1
E. coli, Proteus	0	3	0	0	7	2
Mixed						
Staphylococci and others	9	2	0	0	1	2.8
Pseudomonas and others	0	2	0	0	1	0.6
Unknown	18	19	15	7	15	15

depending upon site of involvement, age of the patient, and severity of illness. In the newborn and infant, physical findings are few. Clinical illness ranges from a benign form with minimal symptoms to a fulminant disease with symptoms due to bacteremia rather than to osteomyelitis itself. Physical examination may show edema and tenderness over the entire extremity, making localization difficult. Less severely involved infants will guard the affected limb, especially if septic arthritis is present as well. A high index of suspicion must be maintained in the infant who refuses to use a limb or who has tenderness and swelling of a limb.

Despite difficulties in interpretation due to new bone formation in infants, x-ray studies frequently show soft tissue swelling, foci of necrosis, and rarefaction in the metaphysis adjoining the epiphyseal plates. X-ray study changes occur earlier in infants than in older children and may appear within 7 to 10 days of onset.

Most hematogenous osteomyelitis in older children occurs in males between the ages of 1 and 14. Forty per cent have a history of preceding minor trauma. The distal femur, proximal and distal tibia and fibula, foot, and proximal humerus are involved in 80 per cent. History and physical findings in this age group lend themselves to earlier diagnosis, although many cases remain unsuspected and result in avoidable disability. Most patients have fever and chills. Limping, regional bone pain, localized swelling, warmth, erythema, and guarding of the affected limb are found in most patients. Pain may be severe enough to cause pseudoparalysis of the affected member. Specific physical localization can be difficult before the process involves a subperiosteal area, allowing discrete pain.

The diagnosis in all ages is facilitated by the use of bone scanning. Technetium-labeled polyphosphate compounds accumulate in areas of rapid bone turnover and may define an area of involvement within 48 hours of the onset of symptoms. However, a negative bone scan does not rule out osteomyelitis, and a positive bone scan is not pathognomonic for infection. Bone lysis on the x-ray study appears at 14 to 21 days, although x-ray study changes may never develop if antibiotics are administered early.

Hematogenous osteomyelitis in adults frequently involves the spine. The vertebral body is the prime focus, with the lumbar area most frequently involved. Patients usually present with nondescript complaints of fever, chills, and backache. Paravertebral spasm may be present. Paraspinal abscesses frequently occur and result in serious neurologic deficits that require emergent myelography and decompression. Laboratory findings are limited, but the white blood cell count and sedimentation rate are usually elevated. X-ray studies, bone scan, and computerized tomography are usually needed to confirm the diagnosis.

The prognosis of hematogenous osteomyelitis is good if the diagnosis is made early. With proper therapy, cure rates of over 90 per cent can be expected. Disability is usually related to delayed diagnosis. This is particularly true in infants whose epiphyseal growth plate may be disturbed due to the infection. In adults, the frequent presence of underlying debilitating disease makes overall outcome worse.

Contiguous and Traumatic Osteomyelitis

Contiguous osteomyelitis usually affects patients over 50 years of age who have an adjacent soft tissue infection or an infected surgical wound extending directly to bone. Surgical procedures most often implicated are open reduction of fractures, insertion of prosthetic devices, or spinal surgery. Soft tissue infections causing contiguous osteomyelitis include lung abscesses spreading to ribs or spine, infected teeth resulting in mandibular infections, sinus or ear infections leading to involvement of the skull and mastoid, and diabetic foot infections.

Staphylococcus is the primary pathogen in 65 per cent of cases, but gram-negative enteric bacteria and anaerobes are also isolated with regularity (Table 30–7). The bacteriology is reflective of the particular contiguous focus: e.g., osteomyelitis of the mandible is caused by mouth flora such as streptococci and anaerobes, and gram-negative microorganisms and staphylococci are implicated in infections involving the feet.

Physical examination is the key to diagnosing contiguous osteomyelitis. Pain, swelling, and erythema developing in the postoperative period or after initial control of a soft tissue infection should arouse the suspicion of osteomyelitis. An x-ray study is the cornerstone of diagnosis, with rarefaction, periosteal reaction, and necrosis of bone. Radionuclide scans are difficult to interpret, since postoperative changes or contiguous soft tissue inflammation may give mis-

Table 30–7. MICROORGANISMS RECOVERED FROM OSTEOMYELITIS DUE TO A CONTIGUOUS FOCUS OF INFECTION

Microorganism	Average Per Cent
Staphylococcus aureus	49
Staphylococcus epidermidis	2
Streptococcus	9
Anaerobes	15
Pseudomonas	7
Other aerobic gram-negative bacilli	16
Other	8
Mixed	8
Unknown	12

leading results. If the diagnosis is delayed, continued pain and swelling with development of sinus tracts and persistent drainage are the usual complaints. Fever is not usually present. At this stage, the diagnosis is obvious.

Traumatic osteomyelitis most commonly follows compound fractures, surgical procedures, and puncture wounds where the underlying bone is traumatized. Males, ages 15 to 30, constitute the majority of patients. Bacteria involved are primarily skin flora, such as staphylococci and occasionally gram-negative environmental organisms. Osteomyelitis of the foot following puncture wounds, particularly in children, requires special consideration since *P. aeruginosa* is a common isolate due to its propensity for growing in the soles of tennis shoes.

Chronic Osteomyelitis

Irrespective of the primary cause, once osteomyelitis becomes established it is self-sustaining. Chronic osteomyelitis occurs most frequently in situations in which blood supply is compromised, as in diabetes mellitus or atherosclerotic peripheral vascular disease.

Clinically, the picture is one of long-standing induration with draining sinuses and open wounds. Systemic symptoms are usually absent. X-ray studies reveal devitalized bone, new bone formation, sequestra, and soft tissue swelling. If an underlying foreign body, such as a plate or pin, is present, loosening of the pin or screw may be evident on x-ray. Sinus tract and wound cultures in patients with underlying chronic osteomyelitis are not helpful, since the wound or sinus tract is frequently colonized by irrelevant microorganisms. Cultures must be obtained directly from the involved bone.

Treatment

Surgical therapy is frequently required to establish a diagnosis, to drain collections of pus, and to remove dead bone and other foreign material. Failure of response to appropriate antibiotic therapy, continued pain, swelling, fever, and a persistently elevated sedimentation rate may also be clues to the need for surgery. In vertebral osteomyelitis, neurologic compromise requires immediate surgical intervention to relieve cord compression. Surgery should be used to drain an infected hip joint when it complicates osteomyelitis, but closed-needle aspiration is usually adequate to drain septic arthritis in other joints when it accompanies osteomyelitis.

Antibiotic therapy is a cornerstone of therapy. In acute hematogenous osteomyelitis, antibiotics are frequently effective alone if given before extensive bone damage has occurred. In contrast, in chronic osteomyelitis or osteomyelitis associated with a foreign body, antibiotics alone are of little value unless all dead bone and foreign bodies are removed. Antibiotic therapy is selected based on the pathogens isolated from bone culture and is generally continued in high doses for 4 to 6 weeks parenterally. Oral antibiotic therapy for acute hematogenous osteomyelitis in children has been of value, although it requires careful attention to clinical follow-up, good compliance, and the measurement of serum antibiotic levels and bactericidal activity. Empiric therapy is frequently needed, however, since cultures are commonly not available or are negative, perhaps owing to prior administration of outpatient antibiotics.

Cardiovascular Infections

INFECTIVE ENDOCARDITIS

Endocarditis is an infection of the heart valves or endocardium. It may present as an acute, fulminant illness with rapid valve destruction and severe systemic toxicity. More frequently, however, it presents as an indolent illness, with weeks or months of predominantly constitutional symptoms, and, in this form, is known as subacute endocarditis. Although an appreciation of the tempo of illness is helpful in understanding its pathogenesis and the organisms involved, there is great variation from case to case.

Infective endocarditis is not uncommon, accounting for 1 to 2 per 1000 hospital admissions. In recent years, rheumatic heart disease has become a less important predisposition to endocarditis than drug addiction, prosthetic heart valves, or atherosclerotic valvular disease. With increasing longevity and cardiovascular surgery, the relative shift in predisposing conditions will probably continue. There has also been an increase in aortic valve involvement although mitral valve infections remain the most common.

Pathogenesis

The pathogenesis of endocarditis as it occurs on a previously damaged valve is well understood. The pre-existing valve lesion creates turbulent flow, which produces endothelial damage and the formation of sterile platelet-fibrin thrombi. Bacteremia with an organism that has the ability to adhere to endothelium or platelet-fibrin thrombi may result in infection. Since phagocytosis does not occur on valve leaflets, bacteria multiply within the thrombus to form a vegetation.

Understanding the pathogenesis of endocarditis explains a number of clinical observations. Patients with chronic congestive heart failure, atrial septal defects, chronic atrial fibrillation, or purely stenotic valvular lesions generally have low pressure gradients and, therefore, less turbulent flow. These lesions are all low risk for infective endocarditis. In contrast, insufficient valvular lesions associated with a high-pressure gradient and markedly turbulent flow are at greater risk. Patients with mitral valve prolapse are at greater risk if a regurgitant murmur is audible than if only a click is present. The predominant right heart involvement in intravenous drug abusers suggests that tricuspid valve damage may occur due to injected particulate material.

As the infection progresses, it may extend into supporting valve structures, leading to further damage and compromised valve function. Vegetations may embolize, resulting in vascular occlusion. Suppurative metastatic lesions may follow these embolic phenomena, particularly if gram-negative bacilli or staphylococci are the etiologic agents. Infections with more indolent organisms, such as *Streptococcus viridans* group (*Streptococcus mutans, Streptococcus sanguis,* etc.) are associated not with suppuration but with immunologic events (vide infra).

The sources of the infecting bacteria in endocarditis are usually mucosal surfaces with transient bacteremia precipitated by local trauma. Bacterial seeding from the gums, sinuses, genitourinary tract, or gastrointestinal tract may precipitate endocarditis. Intravenous drug abuse or indwelling intravenous catheters may also produce bacteremia and endocarditis.

Clinical Presentation

The clinical presentations of endocarditis vary widely. Indolent onset, with low-grade fever, constitutional and musculoskeletal symptoms, weight loss, malaise, easy fatigability, and anorexia are common in patients with subacute infection. In contrast, patients with acute endocarditis present with high fever, systemic toxicity, and shaking chills of short duration. Many patients will have suppurative or embolic extracardiac manifestations, such as a focal central nervous system deficit, pleuritis, meningitis, flank pain and pyuria, cough and hemoptysis, abdominal pain, or acute cardiac decompensation.

Up to 10 per cent of patients have no audible murmur. This is particularly true for individuals with endocarditis involving only the tricuspid valve. Petechiae may be visible in the nail beds, conjunctivae, and other mucous membranes. They are due to small vessel infarction or emboli and when seen in the retina are particularly striking. Retinal infarcts, referred to as Roth spots, appear as oval hemorrhages with pale centers. They are not pathognomonic for endocarditis but can be seen in other vascular diseases, such as systemic lupus erythematosus. Janeway lesions are large nontender macules occurring on the palms or soles and probably represent embolic phenomena. Osler's nodes are tender subcutaneous erythematous nodules in the pulp of the fingers or toes. They may represent either antigen-antibody complex vasculitis with infarct or embolic phenomena. Similar to Roth spots, they are not pathognomonic for endocarditis. Clubbing and splenomegaly are rarely seen nowadays except in neglected, untreated cases of subacute endocarditis and indicate a disease process of over 6 weeks duration.

Laboratory Findings

Anemia is the most common hematologic abnormality in endocarditis. It is normochromic and normocytic and is usually due to marrow suppression associated with infection. Hemolysis is unusual in endocarditis involving natural heart valves but is frequently seen in prosthetic valvular endocarditis. The white blood cell count is elevated in acute infections but may be normal in subacute infections. The erythrocyte sedimentation rate is elevated in almost all patients. The rheumatoid factor may be positive, particularly in patients with long-standing disease. This is a nonspecific finding and is due to elevated IgM anti-IgG. Serum complement levels are usually elevated as acute phase reactants but may be depressed if antigen-antibody complex disease is present. Cryoglobulins are positive in many patients and represent circulating immune complexes. Other nonspecific immunologic events may be seen, including a false positive Veneral Disease Research Laboratories (VDRL) test, and antinuclear antibody. The urinalysis frequently shows proteinuria and microscopic hematuria. Microscopic hematuria may be due to immune-complex glomerulonephritis and may be associated with red blood cell casts.

Blood cultures are positive in greater than 90 per cent of patients with endocarditis. Numerous studies have shown that three blood cultures will yield the causative organism in over 95 per cent of culture-positive cases. The bacteremia of endocarditis is continual; therefore, random cultures are most appropriate, the diagnosis being dependent on the volume of blood drawn rather than the number of cultures performed. In suspected endocarditis, therefore, three samples should be obtained prior to initiation of therapy. Each sample should be taken by separate venipuncture.

Despite improved techniques and special media, 15 per cent of cases of bacterial endocarditis will be culture negative. High levels of antibacterial antibody, poor viability of the microorganism, cell wall deficient or particularly fastidious microorganisms, and prior antibiotic therapy all cause culture-negative endocarditis. If clinical evidence is particularly strong, empiric therapy may be indicated.

It should be stressed that a single positive blood culture is inadequate to make the diagnosis of endocarditis. Endocarditis represents a sustained bacteremia and should be so documented. A single blood culture positive for the group *S. viridans* or coagulase-negative staphylococci could represent transient bacteremia from the mouth, intestine, or skin, rather than endocarditis.

Microbiology

Streptococci and staphylococci account for 80 per cent of cases of endocarditis on natural heart valves (Table 30–8). Although the *S. viridans* group of presumably oral origin still account for the majority of cases, recent dental work can be implicated in only 10 per cent. Group D streptococci have become increasingly important in recent years, owing to the increased frequency of elderly patients with underlying genitourinary or gastrointestinal disease. *S. bovis,* a nonenterococcal group D streptococcus, is associated with occult colonic neoplasia in over 50 per cent of cases. Staphylococci are also found with increased frequency due to the prevalence of intravenous drug users and patients with prosthetic heart valves. Gram-negative endocarditis remains uncommon but is a particular problem for patients with prosthetic heart valves and intravenous drug users. The reason for the preponderance of streptococci in infective endocarditis is due to their ability to adhere to valve tissue. Gram-negative bacilli adhere poorly and explain the paucity of cases of gram-negative endocarditis despite the fact that these organisms commonly cause bacteremia.

Fungal endocarditis occurs only in specific settings. Open heart surgery patients, patients receiving prolonged intravenous therapy, particularly total parenteral nutrition, and intravenous drug abusers are prone to fungal endocarditis. *Candida* species are most commonly isolated, although *Aspergillus* may cause infection as well. Most fungal infection on prosthetic valves is acquired in the operating room. Fungal endocarditis in drug addicts is usually related to prolonged intravenous therapy for a preceding bacterial infection. The diagnosis of fungal endocarditis is very difficult because blood cultures may be negative. However, bulky vegetations frequently produce major organ emboli, the pathology of which may make a diagnosis.

Prosthetic valve endocarditis may be temporally divided into two groups: early infection, occurring less than 60 days, and late infections, occurring more than 60 days postoperatively (see Table 30–8). Early prosthetic valve infections are due to organisms acquired perioperatively including fungi, staphylococcal species, and gram-negative bacilli. These microorganisms may be acquired intraoperatively or in the perioperative period, owing to intubation and prolonged use of indwelling intravenous and bladder catheters. Late infections occur after the valve has become epithelialized and resemble natural valve infections in their microbiology (see Table 30–8).

Table 30–8. MICROBIOLOGY OF HEART VALVE INFECTIONS

	Per Cent of Isolates			
Microorganism	*Natural Valve*	*Intravenous Drug User*	*Early Prosthetic Valve*	*Late Prosthetic Valve*
S. viridans group	35	5	5	30
Group D streptococci	25	10	10	20
Enterococci	10	8	8	10
Nonenterococci	15	2	2	10
S. aureus	15	60	10	10
S. epidermidis	2		30	20
Gram-negative bacilli	5	10	20	5
Fungi	3	10	20	5
Others*	15	5	5	10

*Includes diphtheroids, other streptococci, and *Haemophilus.*

Treatment

The treatment of infective endocarditis is with microbicidal antibiotics. Since neutrophils are not involved in the resolution of endocarditis, antibiotics alone are the mainstay of therapy. Treatment must be prolonged to kill those microorganisms resting deep within the vegetation. Acute endocarditis should be treated as soon as blood cultures are obtained without waiting for culture results in order to minimize valve destruction and spread of infection to the supporting valve structures. In subacute endocarditis, treatment can usually be delayed for 1 or 2 days until blood cultures are known to be positive. Effective programs for the treatment of endocarditis are outlined in Table 30–9.

Most *S. viridans* and *S. bovis* are exquisitely sensitive to penicillin G. Recent experience with the combination of penicillin plus an aminoglycoside has not shown convincing superiority to penicillin G alone. It may, however, allow a shorter course of parenteral therapy with completion using an oral regimen. In contrast, enterococci are not killed by penicillin or ampicillin alone and require, in addition, a synergistic aminoglycoside antibiotic, such as gentamicin. For enterococcal endocarditis in the penicillin-allergic patient, vancomycin plus an aminoglycoside antibiotic is the preferred treatment. Duration of symptoms, valvular calcification, the recent emergence of multiply-resistant strains and other factors impact on the selection and duration of therapy, and infectious disease consultation should be sought.

The role of testing for serum bactericidal activity is controversial. Tests are difficult to perform and poorly predictive. They are probably only of value in selected cases due to unusual microorganisms.

Staphylococci should be considered penicillin-

Table 30–9. TREATMENT OF ENDOCARDITIS

Microorganism	Preferred Regimen	Penicillin Allergic
Streptococcus viridans group for 3–4 weeks	Penicillin G 12–18 million units/day for 3–4 weeks OR Penicillin G 12–18 million units/day plus streptomycin 1 gm. (or 15 mg./kg.)/day for 2 weeks	Cefazolin 6 gm./day or vancomycin 2 gm./day
Group D streptococci		
(a) *S. bovis*	Same as *S. viridans*	Same as *S. viridans* group
(b) Enterococcus	Penicillin G 18–24 million units/day plus gentamicin 4–5 mg./kg.day for 4–6 weeks	Vancomycin 2 gm./day plus gentamicin 4–5 mg./kg./day for 4–6 weeks
Staphylococci		
(a) Nonpenicillinase producing	Penicillin G 18–24 million units/day for 4–6 weeks	Cefazolin 6 gm./day or vancomycin 2 gm./day for 4–6 weeks
(b) Penicillinase producing	Oxacillin 12 gm./day or nafcillin 12 gm./day for 4–6 weeks	Cefazolin 6 gm./day or vancomycin 2 gm./day for 4–6 weeks
Pneumococci or beta-hemolytic streptococci	Penicillin G 18–24 million units/day for 4–6 weeks	Cefazolin 6 gm./day or vancomycin 2 gm./day for 4–6 weeks
Haemophilus species, *Actinobacillus* or *Cardiobacterium*	A third-generation cephalosporin for 4–6 weeks	Ampicillin 12 gm./day plus gentamicin 5 gm./kg./day for 4–6 weeks
Gram-negative bacillus	A beta-lactam antibiotic plus an aminoglycoside antibiotic according to susceptibility tests for 4–6 weeks. Surgery probably also required.	
Fungus	Amphotericin B plus early surgery. 5-Flucytosine, fluconazole or ketoconazole may be useful adjuncts.	

resistant until susceptibility tests prove otherwise. Staphylococcal endocarditis must be treated for 6 weeks for optimal results. The addition of an aminoglycoside antibiotic for synergy has not been shown to enhance cure rates in the treatment of staphylococcal endocarditis. Gram-negative and fungal endocarditis present extremely difficult problems. Surgery is almost always necessary for cure and should be performed early to avoid irreversible damage to the valve and supporting structures.

The management of prosthetic valve infections is difficult. Early prosthetic valve infection occurring within 60 days of surgery almost always requires valve replacement in addition to antibiotic therapy. However, late prosthetic valve infections, particularly when these infections are due to penicillin-sensitive streptococci, frequently respond to medical therapy alone. The need for surgery is dictated by the response to medical therapy.

Ancillary therapy should include cardiovascular support as necessary. Corticosteroid therapy is of no value. Anticoagulants should be used as needed for thromboembolic events and are not specifically contraindicated.

Surgical removal of infected valves plays an increasingly important role in the treatment of endocarditis. Indications for surgery include persistent infection despite appropriate antibiotic therapy (e.g., for fungal or gram-negative endocarditis), intractable or progressive congestive heart failure unresponsive to standard cardiotonic regimens, and major organ emboli. Patients with bulky vegetations seen on echocardiogram, particularly if they involve the aortic valve, may be candidates for early surgery in the absence of these indications. Early valve replacement is not associated with an increased risk of infection as long as effective antimicrobial agents are being administered at the time of surgery.

Even after effective therapy is instituted, the patient may remain febrile for some time. Prolonged or recurrent fever should prompt re-evaluation for a febrile drug reaction, thrombophlebitis, embolization, or superinfection. However, prolonged fever in endocarditis is not unusual and may be related to the endocarditis itself or the therapy thereof. Embolic phenomena may occur late, despite adequate therapy, and are not an indication of failure to achieve adequate killing with the antimicrobial regimen.

Differential Diagnosis

A variety of conditions mimic infective endocarditis. The prolonged fever and constitutional symptoms typical of subacute endocarditis may be due to such conditions as neoplasia, tuberculosis, viral infection, or collagen vascular disease. Prolonged fever in the patient with rheumatic heart disease may be rheumatic fever itself. Fever after open heart surgery may have many causes other than an infected prosthesis, including pneumonia, postpericardiotomy syndrome, urinary tract infection, or thrombophlebitis. Acute endocarditis, which frequently presents with extracardiac manifestations, may be mistaken for a primary pulmonary infection, meningitis, cerebrovascular accident, or pyelonephritis. Attention to the cardiovascular examination and clinical situation together with appropriate cultures of blood and other body fluids should help in the diagnosis, as long as the possibility of endocarditis is at least considered.

Prevention

Bacteremia is the prerequisite for endocarditis. When bacteremia is anticipated, prophylactic antibiotics should be administered to prevent endocarditis in patients with pre-existing valvular lesions. Prophylaxis must be administered so that *peak blood levels* are achieved at the time of anticipated bacteremia. This concept differs from that of surgical wound prophylaxis, in which *tissue levels* are required at the time of surgery. Antibiotics are selected to kill the microorganisms most likely to produce bacteremia and endocarditis from a given source. In the mouth, this is the *S. viridans* group and in the gastrointestinal and genitourinary tract, enterococci. Prophylactic antibiotics should be administered immediately prior to the procedure and may be repeated once 6 to 8 hours later (Table 30–10). Cephalosporins should not be used. Administration of antibiotics for several days prior to the procedure promotes the emergence of resistant microorganisms and decreases the effectiveness of prophylaxis.

PERICARDITIS AND MYOCARDITIS

Pericarditis is an inflammation of the visceral and parietal pericardium. A variety of agents are associated with infectious pericarditis; most are viral (Table 30–11). Fever, chest pain, and fatigue may be the presenting problem. The chest pain is usually retrosternal, with radiation to the neck and arms. It may be increased by inspiration or motion and is frequently lessened by sitting or leaning forward. In chronic pericarditis, however, pain may not be present, and the manifestations may be only those of increasing congestive heart failure due to constriction.

The diagnosis of pericarditis is based on clinical suspicion, electrocardiographic abnormalities suggesting pericarditis, echocardiography, and a chest x-ray showing cardiac enlargement. It should be noted that in constrictive pericarditis cardiac enlargement may not be marked.

Coxsackie B virus infections are the best documented causes of viral pericarditis. Coxsackieviruses are ubiquitous, and infections due to these agents are prevalent in the summer and early fall. Children and young adults are most commonly affected and frequently have a history of cough and coryza 10 to 14 days prior to the onset of pericarditis. Diagnosis is made by virus isolation, but because of the late onset of pericarditis, the virus may not be recovered. Serodiagnosis is usually not practical because of multiple antigenically different serotypes of coxsackievirus.

Purulent pericarditis is a medical and surgical emergency. It may be due to bacteremic seeding of the pericardium or contiguous spread from a pulmonary or mediastinal focus. *S. aureus, H. influenzae,* and pneumococci account for the majority of cases.

The differential diagnosis of infectious pericarditis should include noninfectious etiologies such as systemic lupus erythematosus, congestive heart failure, uremia, radiation pericarditis, trauma, myocardial infarction, pulmonary emboli, nephrosis, neoplasia, or acute rheumatic fever. Myxedema, rheumatoid arthritis, serum sickness, and other connective tissue diseases should also be considered.

Agents responsible for myocarditis are usually those responsible for pericarditis (Table 30–12). Both myocarditis and pericarditis may occur in the same patient, and the differential diagnosis is similar. Most cardiomyopathies in adults are idiopathic, but some may originate from a primary infectious process.

Management of pericarditis or myocarditis should be directed at treatment for the causative agent (if applicable) and maintenance of a stable cardiovascular status by bed rest and cardiotonic drugs. The role of steroids remains controversial, particularly in individuals for whom infection can be documented. Pericardiotomy may be indicated if effusions prove persistent. No specific drug therapy is available for most viral causes of pericarditis or myocarditis, but specific antimicrobial therapy is clearly indicated in bacterial and tuberculous pericarditis and may be of value in Chagas' disease, toxoplasmosis, and fungal infections.

Central Nervous System Infections

BACTERIAL MENINGITIS

Pathophysiology

Despite advances in the prevention and treatment of many infectious diseases, meningitis remains a profoundly serious infection, and its impact on the afflicted individual has been tempered little by recent developments. Death and serious disability from bacterial meningitis are decreased only by early recognition and the immediate institution of appropriate antimicrobial therapy.

Microorganisms reach the central nervous system by one of two routes: direct extension from an extra-

Table 30–10. PROPHYLAXIS OF ENDOCARDITIS IN PATIENTS WITH VALVULAR HEART DISEASE

For Dental and Upper Respiratory Tract Procedures		
Parenteral		
Ampicillin	2 gm. I.M. or I.V.	30 minutes before procedure
plus gentamicin	1.5 mg./kg. I.M. or I.V.	
OR		
Vancomycin	1 gm. I.V.	Infused over 1 hour before procedure
Oral		
Penicillin V	2 gm. P.O.	60–90 minutes before procedure
then Penicillin V	1 gm. P.O.	6 hours later
OR		
Erythromycin	1 gm. P.O.	90–120 minutes before procedure
then erythromycin	500 mg. P.O.	6 hours later
Gastrointestinal and Genitourinary Procedures		
Parenteral		
Ampicillin	2 gm. I.M. or I.V.	30 minutes before procedure
plus gentamicin	1.5 mg./kg. I.M. or I.V.	
OR		
Vancomycin	1 gm. I.V.	Infused over 1 hour
plus gentamicin	1.5 mg./kg. I.M. or I.V.	1 hour before procedure
Oral		
Amoxicillin	3 gm. P.O.	1 hour before procedure
then amoxicillin	1.5 gm. P.O.	6 hours later

Parenteral regimens are more likely to be effective and are recommended especially for patients with prosthetic heart valves, prior endocarditis, or those taking penicillin for rheumatic fever prophylaxis.

cerebral source or hematogenous spread from a remote focus of infection. Remote foci are often the lung, bowel, skin, and heart. Local foci of infection include the paranasal sinuses, ears, and other facial areas. Most meningitis nowadays is hematogenous in origin. Organisms reaching the spinal fluid spread rapidly throughout the subarachnoid space. The brain itself is remarkably resistant to bacterial infection, although cortical vasculitis with small vessel thromboses may produce focal signs.

The cellular response to infection in the subarachnoid space is polymorphonuclear, if bacterial, and mononuclear, if fungal, tuberculous, or viral. The cellular response, particularly if polymorphonuclear, may produce disturbances in cerebrospinal fluid production and flow, resulting in hydrocephalus. In small children, inflammation in the subdural space may produce subdural effusions. Cerebral edema secondary to cortical vasculitis may produce herniation and brainstem compression.

Normal spinal fluid glucose is greater than 40 per cent of simultaneous blood glucose, although at values over 250 mg./dl. this relationship may no longer hold true. The decrease in CSF glucose concentration

Table 30–11. CAUSES OF INFECTIOUS PERICARDITIS

Viral	**Bacterial**
Adenovirus	*Borrelia burgdorferi*
Coxsackievirus A, B	*Francisella*
Cytomegalovirus	Gonococcus
Echovirus	*Haemophilus*
Epstein-Barr virus	*Legionella*
Influenza virus	Meningococcus
Mumps virus	*M. tuberculosis*
Varicella virus	Pneumococcus
	Staphylococcus
	Streptococcus
Fungal	**Protozoal**
Aspergillus	*Entamoeba*
Blastomyces	*Toxoplasma*
Coccidioides	*Trypanosoma*
Cryptococcus	
Histoplasma	

Table 30–12. INFECTIOUS CAUSES OF MYOCARDITIS

Viral	**Bacterial**
Adenovirus	*Borrelia burgdorferi*
Arbovirus	*Chlamydia psittaci*
Coxsackievirus A, B	*C. diphtheriae*
Cytomegalovirus	*Leptospira*
Echovirus	Meningococcus
Epstein-Barr virus	*M. tuberculosis*
Hepatitis B virus	*Treponema pallidum*
Herpesvirus	
Human immunodeficiency virus	**Parasitic**
Influenza virus	*Toxoplasma*
Lymphocytic choriomeningitis virus	Trichinae
Measles virus	*Trypanosoma*
Mumps virus	**Fungal**
Poliovirus	*Aspergillus*
Rabies virus	*Coccidioides*
Rubella virus	*Histoplasma*
Varicella virus	

seen in meningitis is a result of both a decrease in the active transport of glucose into the CSF and the interaction of bacteria and leukocytes, resulting in glucose consumption because of phagocytosis. In viral meningitis, the mononuclear cell response does not usually result in a fall in CSF glucose concentrations. CSF protein levels in meningitis are increased due to the entry of plasma proteins by alteration in the permeability of the blood-brain-CSF barrier. Cellular response is dictated by the infecting organism (Table 30–13).

Neonates

Neonatal meningitis occurs in one to two per thousand births. Risk factors include maternal infection, prematurity, small size, complicated delivery, and prolonged (over 24 hours) rupture of membranes. The organisms responsible for neonatal meningitis are usually those acquired from the maternal vaginal flora. Occasionally, they may be acquired from the nursery environment during prolonged hospital stay.

Group B streptococci account for 30 to 40 per cent of cases of neonatal meningitis. Fifty per cent of babies born to mothers colonized with group B streptococci will be themselves colonized, and one per hundred colonized babies will become ill. *E. coli* are the next most common cause and 80 per cent of the responsible *E. coli* strains have K1 capsular polysaccharide, compared to less than 15 per cent of *E. coli* strains isolated from septicemic adults. Organisms such as *Klebsiella, Proteus, Enterobacter,* and *Citrobacter* may be acquired at birth as are most *E. coli,* but they are more likely due to colonization within the nursery or neonatal intensive care unit. Such organisms may be multi-drug-resistant and present major treatment problems.

The clinical presentation of neonatal meningitis is subtle. Irritability, lethargy, changes in feeding habits, respiratory distress, or periodic apnea may be the only manifestations. Neck stiffness is rarely seen. Bulging fontanelles and seizures are late phenomena and, if present, associated with high mortality.

The laboratory features of neonatal sepsis and meningitis are few. The peripheral white blood cell count is rarely helpful. Lumbar puncture is usually diagnostic. Results, however, must be interpreted in light of the fact that normal neonatal cerebrospinal fluid contains up to 30 white blood cells and has a protein content of up to 120 mg./dl. Gram's stain and cultures should be promptly performed and ancillary tests, such as bacterial antigen detection in spinal fluid, may be useful. Blood cultures are frequently positive.

The empiric treatment of neonatal meningitis traditionally consisted of a combination of ampicillin plus an aminoglycoside antibiotic to cover the likely gram-positive and gram-negative microorganisms. A combination of ampicillin plus a third-generation cephalosporin, such as cefotaxime, is now preferred. Treatment should be continued for a minimum of 3 weeks. Despite effective therapy, however, the mortality in both group B streptococcal and *E. coli* meningitis occurring in the first week of life is close to 50 per cent. Fifty per cent of the survivors will have major neurologic residual, such as mental retardation, seizure disorders, and learning disability.

Children

Bacterial meningitis in children aged 2 months to 10 years is due to *H. influenzae, N. meningitidis,* or *S. pneumoniae.* All these organisms possess a polysaccharide capsule that contributes to their pathogenicity. Asymptomatic nasopharyngeal carrier rates range from 5 to 50 per cent depending upon the time of year and age of the patient. Bacterial meningitis peaks in incidence from December to April and parallels the frequency of pharyngeal colonization with each organism. The factors that cause a colonized individual to develop meningitis are unknown, although antecedent viral infection is probably important.

Haemophilus influenzae, type b, is the main cause of meningitis from 3 months to 3 years in the United States. Protective maternal antibody falls between 3 and 6 months of age and corresponds to the increasing incidence of meningitis. *N. meningitidis* peaks in incidence at age 1 to 4 years and again at age 15 to 30 years. Capsular types B, C, and Y have been the most common causes of meningitis in recent years. As with immunity to *Haemophilus,* immunity to *Neisseria* species is stimulated by exposure to other, cross-reacting, microorganisms. Although development of antibody protects against bacteremia and meningitis, it does not prevent nasopharyngeal colonization with either *Haemophilus* species or *N. meningitidis.* Such colonized, but immune, individuals

Table 30–13. CEREBROSPINAL FLUID PROFILES IN MENINGITIS

	Bacterial Meningitis	Viral Meningitis	Fungal/TB Meningitis
Pressure	Increased	Normal or slightly increased	Increased
Protein	> 300 mg./dl.	50–150 mg./dl.	> 300 mg./dl.
Glucose	< 40 mg./dl.	Normal	< 40 mg./dl.
Cells	> 500/mm.^{3} > 90% neutrophils	< 500/mm.^{3} > 50% mononuclear	20–400/mm.^{3} > 50% mononuclear

remain a reservoir for these organisms within the family and population at large.

Pneumococcal meningitis may develop as a primary bacteremic illness or as a complication of pneumonia, otitis, mastoiditis, or sinusitis. Hypogammaglobulinemia, the absence of the spleen, or concomitant sickle cell disease predisposes to pneumococcal bacteremia and meningitis. The large number of pneumococcal serotypes, 82, means that infection with one type does not confer protection against future infections with another type. The incidence of pneumococcal meningitis peaks later in life than that for *Haemophilus* or *Neisseria* infection and is the most common cause of meningitis over age 10.

The clinical manifestations of meningitis in the older infant and child are more dramatic than those of the neonate. Fever, headache, confusion, lethargy, vomiting, or convulsions may be the presenting signs. Physical examination may reveal altered consciousness and a stiff neck. The presence of a petechial or purpuric rash should suggest *Neisseria,* although *Haemophilus,* pneumococcus and *Staphylococcus aureus* can occasionally produce this rash. Coexistent pneumonitis, sinusitis, or otitis should suggest pneumococcal or *Haemophilus meningitis.*

Table 30–14. CEREBROSPINAL FLUID PROFILES

Purulent Profile (polymorphonuclear leukocytes)
Bacterial meningitis
Early viral meningitis
Embolic cerebral infarction in endocarditis
Parameningeal infections (brain abscess, subdural empyema, venous sinus thrombophlebitis)
Chemical meningitis
Lymphocytic Low-glucose Profile
Tuberculous meningitis
Fungal meningitis
Partially treated bacterial meningitis
Certain bacterial meningitis (spirochetal, *Listeria,* Lyme disease)
Certain viral meningitides (mumps, lymphocytic choriomeningitis, herpes simplex, varicella-zoster)
Sarcoidosis
Carcinomatous meningitis
Lymphocytic Normal-glucose Profile
Viral meningitis or encephalitis
Postinfectious or postvaccinal encephalomyelitis
Parameningeal infection (brain abscess, subdural empyema, epidural abscess, venous sinus thrombophlebitis)
Early fungal meningitis
Early tuberculous meningitis
Parasitic infection (e.g., toxoplasmosis)

Adults

Bacterial meningitis in the adult is overwhelmingly likely to be due to *Streptococcus pneumoniae.* In certain settings, however, staphylococci (after trauma or associated with intravenous drug use) or gram-negative bacilli (after neurosurgery or in immunosuppressed individuals) may produce meningitis. *Cryptococcus* and *Listeria* must be considered in the differential diagnosis of patients with depressed cell-mediated immunity as seen in lymphoma and HIV infection. The presentation of meningitis in the older, particularly immunosuppressed, adult may be atypical. Mental confusion, absence of fever, or lack of a stiff neck may make the diagnosis difficult.

The laboratory diagnosis of meningitis is made by examining the cerebrospinal fluid (see Table 30–13). Normal cerebrospinal fluid should contain less than four cells, all lymphocytes. Gram's stain should be performed on the centrifuged sediment and must be interpreted with caution. Detection of bacterial antigen by latex agglutination may provide some help in assisting with rapid diagnosis.

Purulent spinal fluid, associated with hypoglycorrhachia, is characteristic of untreated bacterial meningitis but may also be seen with parameningeal infections or meningeal carcinomatosis. Conversely, partially treated bacterial meningitis may have a lymphocytic predominance (Table 30–14).

Treatment

The prognosis in meningitis is dependent upon the speed with which appropriate therapy is initiated. If the clinical setting and examination of the spinal fluid give a clue to the specific organism, treatment based on past experience and known susceptibility patterns can be initiated promptly. If the diagnosis is unknown, empiric therapy must be begun.

In neonates, treatment must cover *E. coli* and group B streptococcus. Recent experience suggests that a third-generation cephalosporin with concomitant ampicillin is appropriate. In young children, the organisms to be considered are *Haemophilus,* meningococcus, and pneumococcus, and since many (perhaps 20 per cent) strains of *Haemophilus* are ampicillin-resistant, initial therapy should be with cefuroxime, cefotaxime, or ceftriaxone. In the adolescent and adult, pneumococcus or meningococcus is the most likely microorganism and empiric treatment with penicillin G is usually adequate. The presence of immunosuppression, intravenous drug abuse, or recent neurosurgery should raise consideration of more unusual microorganisms, and therapy should be selected on the basis of likely pathogens. Most meningitis should be treated parenterally for a minimum of 10 days. Gram-negative meningitis requires a minimum of 3 weeks. Intrathecal or intraventricular antibiotics are not indicated except for fungal or multidrug-resistant gram-negative meningitis.

Prophylaxis

The occurrence of meningococcal disease requires contact prophylaxis. Both group A and group C meningococcal vaccines are available and very effective in epidemic settings. Family members, nursery school, and intimate contacts of cases of meningococcal disease should be treated prophylactically with rifampin or minocycline. Rifampin, 10 mg./kg.

(maximum 600 mg.) every 12 hours for 4 doses, is preferred, owing to the vestibular side effects associated with minocycline administration. Casual contact and contacts in the hospital setting (unless mouth-to-mouth resuscitation or pipetting accidents have occurred) do not require prophylaxis. Family contacts, and perhaps close and nursery school contacts of patients with invasive *Haemophilus* infections (such as meningitis), also warrant rifampin prophylaxis: 20 mg./kg./day for 4 days.

ASEPTIC MENINGITIS

Viral infections of the central nervous system occur at all ages and are most commonly seen in the summer and early fall. Aseptic meningitis is usually an illness of abrupt onset and short duration. Fever, headache, nausea and vomiting, and neck stiffness are the cardinal manifestations. Children show irritability with drowsiness or lethargy. Multiple attacks of aseptic meningitis, although uncommon, do occur. A variety of agents are implicated (Table 30–15). It is important to remember that Lyme disease and syphilis are causes of aseptic meningitis.

Laboratory abnormalities include a relatively normal peripheral white blood cell count and a CSF pleocytosis that is predominantly mononuclear (see Table 30–13). However, polymorphonuclear leukocytes may predominate in the first several hours of a viral infection and repeat lumbar puncture in 12 hours may be necessary to clarify the etiology. In some cases of mumps, lymphocytic choriomeningitis, and herpes infection, hypoglycorrhachia may occur (see Table 30–14).

The differental diagnosis of aseptic meningitis includes tuberculous meningitis, cryptococcal meningitis, brain abscess or other parameningeal infection, endocarditis, and hypersensitivity meningoencephalitis (see Table 30–14). Occasionally, neoplastic involvement of the meninges can mimic aseptic meningitis.

Agents causing aseptic meningitis may also produce encephalitis (see Table 30–15). The distinction among aseptic meningitis, meningoencephalitis, and encephalitis is primarily clinical. Coxsackievirus and echovirus usually produce aseptic meningitis rather than encephalitis. Arboviruses produce primarily encephalitis. Herpes simplex virus 1, the cause of most oral infections, produces characteristic frontotemporal encephalitis. The prognosis is poor, and treatment with parenteral acyclovir is only partially effective. In contrast, herpes simplex virus 2, the cause of most genital infections, produces primarily aseptic meningitis.

The management of aseptic meningitis and encephalitis, with the exception of herpes virus or bacterial etiologies (see Table 30–15) is purely supportive. The outcome of viral meningitis and encephalitis is extremely variable. Mortality in herpes simplex encephalitis is high, but the morbidity in mumps meningitis is extremely low. In general, the very young and the very old have a greater morbidity.

Table 30–15. CAUSATIVE AGENTS OF ASEPTIC MENINGITIS AND ENCEPHALITIS

- Adenovirus
- Arthropod-borne (arbovirus) viruses
  - California encephalitis
  - Eastern equine encephalitis
  - Western equine encephalitis
  - St. Louis encephalitis
- *Borrelia* (Lyme disease)
- *Brucella*
- Cytomegalovirus
- Epstein-Barr virus
- Enterovirus
  - Echovirus, types 1–33
  - Coxsackieviruses A and B
  - Polioviruses
- Herpes simplex viruses 1 and 2
- Human immunodeficiency virus
- *Leptospira*
- Lymphocytic choriomeningitis virus
- Mumps virus
- *Mycoplasma pneumoniae*
- *Rickettsia rickettsii* (Rocky Mountain spotted fever)
- *Treponema pallidum* (syphilis)
- Varicella-zoster virus

PARAMENINGEAL INFECTIONS

Subdural empyema and brain abscess are parameningeal collections that manifest themselves primarily as central nervous system mass lesions. Infection may occur by direct extension from a contiguous focus, such as sinusitis or otitis; septic thrombosis of a penetrating venous system from an underlying focus of infection; or hematogenous seeding from a distant focus, such as a pulmonary infection, endocarditis, or skin infection.

The organisms implicated in infection depend upon the source. If the source is sinusitis or otitis, streptococci (including *S. pneumoniae*), anaerobes, and *S. aureus* predominate. After intracranial surgery or head trauma, staphylococcal species and gram-negative bacilli are the likely organisms. Hematogenous seeding implicates *S. aureus,* streptococci, anaerobes, and the *Enterobacteriaceae*. Most cryptogenic brain abscesses of unknown primary origin are due to streptococcal species and anaerobes. Mixed infections are common, and gram-stained smears of abscess material should always be made, since 20 per cent of cultures fail to grow any organism.

Subdural empyema presents with abrupt onset of fever and headache. Altered consciousness and seizures may be present. Signs of meningeal irritation are frequently found. In contrast, parenchymal brain abscesses present insidiously, with drowsiness, confusion, vomiting, seizures, and focal neurologic signs. Fever is uncommonly prominent in brain abscesses, with 50 per cent of patients having fever less than 100.5° F. Because of the absence of fever, the diagnosis of brain abscess is frequently overlooked, with early diagnoses primarily those of a neoplastic lesion or psychiatric disturbance.

Laboratory data are not particularly helpful in the diagnosis of parameningeal infections. The peripheral white blood cell count and sedimentation rate may be normal or elevated. Cerebrospinal fluid reveals moderately elevated protein and a mild pleocytosis of mixed cell type. Caution must be exercised in performing a lumbar puncture, since pressure may precipitate herniation. Computerized tomography (CT) scan, magnetic resonance imaging (MRI), and arteriography are helpful in localizing the infectious process.

The management of subdural empyema and brain abscess is twofold. Antibiotic therapy should be directed against the likely microorganisms, with surgical intervention timed appropriately. Early surgical drainage is the keystone of therapy for subdural empyema, and antibiotics should be continued a minimum of 3 weeks after surgery. The timing of surgical intervention for brain abscesses is more controversial. Experts favor either complete excision of the abscess cavity and abscess wall or stereotactic needle aspiration. A small abscess, particularly when due to *S. aureus,* may resolve with medical therapy alone. Signs of increased intracranial pressure are an indication for early surgical intervention, but it may be desirable to delay surgery until there is evidence of abscess encapsulation. Antibiotics should be initiated as soon as a diagnosis is considered and should be continued for at least 2 weeks postoperatively. The role of steroids is also controversial, but their use should be minimized, since they may interfere with adequate encapsulation and resolution of the infection.

The empiric selection of antibiotics is difficult. Since anaerobes are so commonly involved in brain abscesses, metronidazole is favored as part of the initial regimen. Ampicillin, oxacillin, and third-generation cephalosporins are also valuable and should be used in addition to metronidazole, pending the results of microbiologic studies. It should be remembered that metronidazole has purely anaerobic activity and that most intracranial paramenigeal infections are mixed aerobic and anaerobic infections.

Fever

Fever is the most celebrated manifestation of infectious disease and the foremost patient complaint. Studies performed in the 1800's showed that fever could be produced by the injection of microbial-free extracts of human cells and Beeson demonstrated in 1948 that fever associated with infection was due primarily to a substance isolated from human phagocytic cells. This mediator, initially named endogenous pyrogen, later known as the lymphocyte-activating factor or leukocytic pyrogen, is now known as interleukin-1.

PATHOGENESIS OF FEVER

A variety of experimental and clinical data clearly define the role of interleukin-1 in the production of fever. It is a heat-labile protein, synthesized and released by monocytes and tissue macrophages. Interleukin-1 production can be evoked by a variety of both microbial and nonmicrobial stimuli. The systemic effects of this mediator include fever due to the action of interleukin-1 on the thermal regulatory center in the brain, an increase in the number of neutrophils due to a direct action on the bone marrow, and modulation of a variety of subcellular acute phase responses. The fact that fever is a regular occurrence in patients with agranulocytosis, certain blood dyscrasias, viral infections, and granulomatous infections, supports the role of monocytes and tissue macrophages as the most prominent inflammatory cells responsible for releasing pyrogen. Lymphocytes do not produce pyrogenic substances. However, they have a role in the production of fever associated with pure delayed hypersensitivity phenomena or viral infections by releasing substances (lymphokines) that stimulate macrophages to release interleukin-1.

Interleukin-1 stimulates thermosensitive neurons in the preoptic region of the anterior hypothalamus to initiate changes in body temperature. This interaction is reflected by an abrupt increase in the synthesis of prostaglandins in the anterior hypothalamus. The antipyretic action of salicylates and nonsteroidal anti-inflammatory agents seems directly related to their antiprostaglandin effect.

The regulation of body temperature is performed mostly by the autonomic nervous system that adjusts blood flow to body surfaces, thereby regulating the amount of heat lost or gained by vasodilatation or vasoconstriction. Normally, humans generate body heat from the metabolism of dietary fats, proteins, and carbohydrates. At rest, the viscera supplies 60 per cent of body heat; during exercise, up to 90 per cent of body heat may be generated by muscular activity. Shivering produces a four-fold increase in heat production. Heat loss from the body occurs primarily through radiation or evaporation, as in sweating.

The hypothalamus normally maintains body temperature at 98.6° F or 37° C. The equilibrium between heat production and heat loss in healthy people is tightly regulated with a normal diurnal variation producing peak temperatures in late afternoon and early evening. Fever, resulting from the effect of interleukin-1 upon the hypothalamus, raises the body's temperature to a new set point around which the new temperature is regulated. When interleukin-1 is withdrawn, the set point is lowered, the body sweats, the skin vasodilates, and the temperature falls.

Although fever physiologically follows the effect

of pyrogen upon the hypothalamus, there are situations in which normal mechanisms do not function. In thyrotoxicosis, metabolic activity and heat production exceed the body's ability to dissipate heat by vasodilatation and sweating, resulting in fever. In heat stroke, environmental temperature overwhelms the body's ability to dissipate heat, and the regulatory function of the hypothalamus is impaired resulting in high fever without effective vasodilatation or sweating. Finally, central nervous system lesions due to tumors or vascular disease may produce fever due to direct malfunction of the hypothalamic regulatory centers. Patients with central fever usually manifest wide swings of temperature without a diurnal pattern.

Fever is not usually harmful to the host, with some exceptions. Sustained core temperatures over 105° F (40.5° C) may produce cerebral damage. Intracranial pressure rises with increases in body temperature; in patients with central nervous system mass lesions, such as a brain abscess, fever may exacerbate the increased intracranial pressure. The metabolic demands of fever may be detrimental to patients with acute myocardial infarction, and febrile seizures are seen in young children. In these situations, fever may need to be specifically treated. In other circumstances, administration of antipyretic drugs frequently does more to confuse than to help the clinical situation.

PATTERNS OF FEVER

In health, body temperature has a diurnal variation. That is, temperatures are higher in late afternoon and lowest in early morning, consistent with the daily variation in corticosteroid production. Most patients with a febrile illness will maintain this diurnal variation. Night sweats represent defervescence through sweating at a time when the temperature ordinarily drops to a diurnal low point. Absence of diurnal variation suggests hypothalamic derangement or factitious fever.

Physiologic fever may occur in response to normal physical stresses, after a meal, after exercise, or with dehydration, and rarely exceeds 100° F. Infants may develop higher temperatures with dehydration, occasionally exceeding 103° F. Physiologic variation in temperature occurs with the menstrual cycle, and there is a slight elevation in body temperature during the early stages of pregnancy.

FEVER OF UNKNOWN ORIGIN

Fever of unknown origin (FUO) has been defined as an illness of at least 3 weeks' duration with a temperature exceeding 101° F or 38.3° C on several occasions and with no established diagnosis after 1 week of evaluation in the hospital. This definition, proposed in 1960, may not be applicable today, since patients are more extensively and promptly evaluated by better laboratory screening and more sophisticated radiologic procedures. Nevertheless, it serves as a useful categorization for febrile illnesses of long duration. It should be noted that febrile illnesses of short duration are most often due to infection, whereas prolonged fevers are frequently noninfectious.

Diagnostic categories of fever of unknown origin vary in frequency according to the age and population group. Approximately 40 per cent of fevers of unknown origin are due to infectious diseases; 20 per cent are due to neoplasia; 15 per cent are due to collagen vascular diseases; and 15 per cent are due to miscellaneous causes. Approximately 10 per cent of FUOs remain undiagnosed. In pediatric populations, infection represents a greater percentage and neoplasia a smaller percentage of the total cases when compared with adults.

Infection is the most common single cause of prolonged fever (Table 30–16). *Tuberculosis* remains a major cause of FUO. Many such patients are elderly and have a negative chest x-ray and a negative purified protein derivative (PPD). A single organ, such as the endometrium or kidney, may be involved. Biopsy and culture of lymph node, bone marrow, and liver are helpful diagnostically, as are a history of foreign birth, family history of tuberculosis, and prior episode of prolonged pulmonary infection.

Infective endocarditis is a frequent cause of FUO. In recent studies, patients are more likely to be elderly, may or may not have a heart murmur, and usually do not have the classic manifestations of embolic phenomena, splinter hemorrhages, or splenomegaly. Multiple blood cultures, echocardiograms, and repeated careful physical examinations are most helpful in diagnosis.

Table 30–16. DIAGNOSTIC CATEGORIES OF FEVER OF UNDETERMINED ORIGIN

I. Infection
- A. Systemic infection
  - 1. Tuberculosis
  - 2. Infective endocarditis
  - 3. Miscellaneous infections: cytomegalovirus, Epstein-Barr virus, toxoplasmosis, HIV, disseminated mycoses, malaria, babesiosis, brucellosis
- B. Localized infection
  - 1. Hepatic infection (liver abscess, cholangitis)
  - 2. Other visceral infections (pancreatic abscess, tubo-ovarian abscess, psoas abscess)
  - 3. Urinary tract infections (pyelonephritis, renal carbuncle, perinephric abscess, prostatic abscess)

II. Neoplasms

III. Collagen-vascular Disorders

IV. Miscellaneous Causes
- A. Inflammatory bowel disease
- B. Pulmonary emboli
- C. Granulomatous disorders
- D. Drug fever
- E. Factitious fever
- F. Hepatic cirrhosis with active hepatocellular necrosis
- G. Miscellaneous rare causes (familial Mediterranean fever, Whipple's disease)

V. Undiagnosed

Viral infections, especially human immunodeficiency virus, cytomegalovirus, or Epstein-Barr virus, are common causes of prolonged fever. In the pediatric age group, viral infections are the single most common cause of FUO.

Visceral abscesses may present as a fever of unknown origin. Perirectal abscesses are commonly a focus of infection in the neutropenic patient, and subphrenic or pelvic abscesses are common causes in the postoperative patient. Liver abscesses should be considered, especially in travelers (amoebic) or in individuals with biliary disease. Perinephric abscesses occur in patients with a history of urinary tract infection, especially in young women, or in patients with obstructive uropathy or calculous disease. Prostatic abscesses should be considered in older men with underlying prostatic disease. Abscesses presenting as an FUO may be manifest not by localized pain, tenderness, or mass but as fever alone in the appropriate historical setting.

Fever may be due to *neoplasia* without infection. Such is commonly the case with reticuloendothelial neoplasms. In lymphoma, fever is often remittent, irregular, or spiking and accompanied by night sweats. Fever responds to appropriate chemotherapy, and its reappearance may suggest recurrent disease. When fever in acute leukemia is present on admission or at discovery of disease, it is usually associated with a readily diagnosable localized infection or is due to the leukemia itself. Fever occurring upon induction of chemotherapy may be self-limited and due to lysis of malignant cells. Fever occurring after the onset of marrow aplasia and granulocytopenia is likely to be associated with bacteremia and a high mortality. Fever may also be associated with nonreticuloendothelial tumors. Renal cell tumors and hepatoma are particularly noteworthy. Atrial myxoma may present as fever, anemia, and a heart murmur and must be differentiated from infective endocarditis. Fever frequently accompanies the liver metastases of any primary neoplasm.

Collagen-vascular diseases may present with prolonged fever. Juvenile rheumatoid arthritis is one of the two most common causes of FUO in children, the other being viral infection. In adults, rheumatoid arthritis frequently presents with fever, and temporal arteritis or polymyalgia rheumatica may present with prolonged fever in the older adult. Systemic lupus erythematosus may be manifest by fever and should be suspected when rash, leukopenia, and serositis are also present. Most of these collagen vascular diseases have prominent constitutional and musculoskeletal symptoms and markedly elevated sedimentation rates, suggesting their diagnosis.

Drug fever is particularly common, not only as a cause of FUO but also as a cause of short-term fever. Other manifestations of hypersensitivity, such as rash and eosinophilia, may or may not be present. Fever may be due to an allergic or direct effect of the drug. Phenothiazines, for example, impair temperature regulation through their effects on the autonomic nervous system. Drugs most commonly associated with fever are antiarrhythmic drugs, such as procainamide and quinidine; anticonvulsants, particularly phenytoin; antimicrobial agents, especially penicillins, cephalosporins, isoniazid, and sulfonamides; the antihypertensives, hydralazine, and alpha-methyldopa; bleomycin, iodides, and cimetidine. Fever is usually low grade, but may be spiking, and is usually associated with a normal white blood cell count.

Fevers are frequently associated with a variety of *granulomatous disorders,* such as sarcoidosis, Wegener's granulomatosis, granulomatous hepatitis, and infectious diseases, such as fungal disease or tuberculosis. The diagnosis may be difficult, and tissue diagnosis is frequently necessary.

Inflammatory bowel disease should always be considered in the differential diagnosis of an FUO. There may be few bowel symptoms, and, thus, the diagnosis may be elusive. Joint symptoms may predominate, particularly in Crohn's disease or Whipple's disease.

Pulmonary emboli, especially small and multiple, are frequently overlooked as the cause of prolonged fever. Such patients may have a normal chest x-ray and no evidence of thrombophlebitis. Predisposing factors include recent surgery, venous disease, prolonged inactivity, and prostatic or pelvic inflammatory disease.

Factitious fever (Table 30–17) should always be considered, particularly in young, usually female, often paramedical personnel, who have prolonged fever without evidence of weight loss and a relatively good appearance. It should be remembered, however, that factitious fever may appear on a background of organic disease so that such patients may already have a distracting, alternative diagnosis. Factitious fever may be falsified, through manipulating the thermometer, or may be created through self-injection of foreign material. Clues to the diagnosis of falsified fever are listed in Table 30–17. Factitious fever has traditionally been the diagnosis of 1 to 2 per cent of all patients with fever of unknown origin.

In the evaluation of a patient with fever of unknown origin, a thorough history and physical examination are of utmost importance. Detailed

Table 30–17. EVALUATION OF FACTITIOUS (FALSIFIED) FEVER

Clinical Clues
- Pulse-temperature dissociation
- High temperature (> 106° F)
- Lack of diurnal variation
- Absence of sweating or shivering
- Well looking, no weight loss
- Normal laboratory data

Diagnostic Clues
- Oral/rectal temperature discrepancy
- No fever when under direct observation, as when taken electronically
- Temperature of freshly voided urine

travel, drug use, animal and sexual exposure, and occupational histories are mandatory. Important symptoms to elicit are the presence of weight loss, subtle gastrointestinal or genitourinary symptoms, myalgias, arthralgias, or rash. Repeated physical exams must be performed to detect the presence of adenopathy, splenomegaly, abdominal tenderness, abnormalities of joints or skin, heart murmurs, and fleeting findings on funduscopic exam. The lack of an adequate history and physical examination is responsible for the fact that 50 per cent of prolonged fevers are undiagnosed. Other omissions, such as failure to perform an indicated laboratory test or ignoring an abnormal test, account for another 20 per cent of misdiagnosis. Two thirds of patients with prolonged fever can be diagnosed with reasonable certainty by paying meticulous attention to the patient's history and physical examination.

If the diagnosis of prolonged fever is not established after a thorough history and physical examination, standard laboratory and x-ray studies, including abdominal CT scan, and tissue biopsy will frequently secure a diagnosis. Blind biopsies are not usually helpful, but they should be guided by abnormal laboratory tests, symptoms, or physical findings. Liver biopsy and bone marrow biopsy are useful in certain settings. Therapeutic trials of antibiotics are indicated when the index of suspicion is high but cultures are negative.

Finally, it is important to realize that patients presenting with prolonged fever usually have common illnesses with atypical presentations rather than exotic diseases. In all cases, it behooves the clinician to pursue the diagnosis, since most patients with prolonged fever recover only after a specific diagnosis is made and therapy tailored to that diagnosis is administered.

Gastrointestinal Infections

Diarrheal disease is a topic of passing interest to many physicians. Indeed, in industrial nations, it is considered more a nuisance than a serious illness. However, in the United States, diarrheal diseases are among the five leading causes of death in small children, and in underdeveloped countries, diarrheal disease results in more infant deaths than any other cause.

DIARRHEAL DISEASE

Pathogenesis

Although systemic conditions, such as age and nutritional status, are important protective factors, the gastrointestinal tract itself plays the most important role in protection from exogenous infection (Table 30–18). The first line defense is *gastric acid,* which destroys most ingested bacteria. Gastric surgery or prolonged administration of antacids or histamine antagonists will increase susceptibility to infection with ingested microorganisms. The *indigenous intestinal flora,* from stomach to colon, maintains ecologic stability of the gastrointestinal tract and interferes with the establishment of residence by invading microorganisms. This seems to be accomplished by competition for essential nutrients, by the production of toxic metabolites, such as short-chain fatty acids, and by competition for epithelial cell-binding sites by which disease is mediated. Bile acids, deconjugated by enteric bacteria, are inhibitory to other microorganisms and probably play a significant role in the maintenance of normal intestinal flora. *Bowel motility* is an important element of protection, since it moves bacteria along the intestinal tract, inhibiting attachment to and penetration of the gastrointestinal epithelium. Interference with bowel motility by administration of antiperistaltic drugs can significantly worsen the course of an established enteritis. *Local immunity* with production of secretory IgA is important for protection against invading microorganisms. Secretory IgA prevents attachment of the organisms to the epithelial cell surface and aids in their immobilization within the intestinal mucus. The secretion of *digestive proteases* or enzymes into the lumen of the intestine destroys toxins elaborated by pathogenic organisms.

Table 30–18. HOST DEFENSES AGAINST GASTROINTESTINAL INFECTION

Gastric acid	Secretory immunoglobulin
Indigenous flora	Digestive proteases
Bowel motility	

Acute diarrheal disease may be caused by a variety of different bacteria, fungi, parasites, and viruses. Each agent has distinct epidemiologic and clinical features that aid in diagnosis. Diarrhea may occur in epidemics, as in food-borne outbreaks, or as a sporadic illness without a clear-cut vehicle. Almost all diarrheal disease is due to fecal-oral transmission, directly or indirectly.

Common etiologic agents of diarrheal disease are listed in Table 30–19. However, it is important to note that in up to 50 per cent of diarrheal outbreaks, no pathogen is isolated. Whether these are chemical, viral, or due to other unidentifiable or unrecognizable pathogens is not clear. The type and severity of diarrheal illness will be determined by the age and underlying disease of the patient, the geographic location and time of year, the patient's dietary and personal hygiene habits, and the economic development and industrialization of the country of origin.

There are a number of properties of microorganisms that enable them to cause diarrheal illness. Many microorganisms elaborate toxins that produce disease. Preformed toxins (Table 30–20) are frequently neurotoxins and produce their effects through activity

Table 30–19. COMMON ETIOLOGIC AGENTS OF DIARRHEAL DISEASE

Bacillus cereus	Foods (cereal products, fried rice)
Campylobacter	Foods (poultry), animals
Clostridium difficile	Environmental, person to person
Clostridium perfringens	Foods (prepared meat dishes)
Entamoeba histolytica	Water, person to person, institutions
Escherichia coli, toxigenic	Foods, water
Escherichia coli, verotoxin	Foods (hamburger)
Giardia	Water, foods, person to person
Parvovirus	Person to person
Rotavirus	Person to person, institutions
Salmonella	Foods (eggs, poultry), animals
Shigella	Person to person, foods, institutions
Staphylococcus aureus	Foods (prepared dishes)
Vibrio cholerae	Water, shellfish
Vibrio parahaemolyticus	Shellfish
Yersinia	Foods, water, person to person

on the central nervous system. Enterotoxins stimulate secretion of electrolytes and/or fluids by the intestinal mucosa. There is no inflammation associated with enterotoxin production. In contrast, some enteric pathogens produce cytopathic toxins that cause mucosal destruction and inflammatory colitis. Some organisms invade the epithelium and cause tissue destruction locally (e.g., *Shigella*) while others invade without much inflammatory response (e.g., *Salmonella*). An important virulence factor is the ability of the microorganism to adhere to the intestinal mucosa, even for those agents that produce disease by toxin elaboration (e.g., *Vibrio cholerae*).

Approach to Diarrheal Disease

An adequate history is the best approach to the differential diagnosis of diarrheal illness. The patient's age and the severity, type, and duration of illness are all important. The presence or absence of fever, severe abdominal pain, and hematochezia suggest different pathogens than those for profuse, watery diarrhea without pain, blood, or fever (see Table 30–20). A detailed history of prior antibiotic use, travel, contact with illness, and diet (see Table 30–19) is necessary. Physical examination should be done promptly to determine the degree of fluid loss, particularly in children.

Stool must be examined to provide objective evidence of illness. Whether it is watery, mucoid, or bloody provides specific information as to etiology. Microscopic examination will show fecal leukocytes in invasive disease (see Table 30–20). Cultures should be obtained promptly. This is particularly true if *Shigella* is suspected, since this organism will not survive even short periods of storage. It is essential to notify the laboratory if certain organisms are suspected, since *Vibrio, Clostridium difficile,* and *Yersinia* require specific and selective culture techniques.

Diarrhea in the Infant

Diarrhea in newborn infants usually occurs in epidemic situations and is frequently due to rotaviruses or toxin-producing strains of *E. coli.* Occasionally, *Shigella, Salmonella, Campylobacter,* and other viral enteritides occur in infants, particularly during institutional outbreaks. In the index cases in such outbreaks, the child may have acquired the infection at birth through contact with maternal fecal or perineal flora. Since the majority of diarrheal disease in infants is not invasive, septic complications are unusual and dehydration is the major clinical problem. The use of antimicrobial agents or antimotility and antisecretory drugs is rarely necessary or successful.

Treatment of diarrhea in infants and young children is primarily with fluids and electrolyte replacement. Oral rehydration therapy is satisfactory unless dehydration is severe. Recommended solutions are highly effective, inexpensive, and readily available. The oral rehydration solution recommended by the World Health Organization contains 3.5 grams NaCl, 1.5 grams KCl, 2.5 grams $NaHCO_3$, and 20 grams glucose per liter. The active intestinal transport of

Table 30–20. TYPES OF ENTERIC DISEASE

Mechanism	Preformed toxin Noninflammatory	Enterotoxin Noninflammatory	Invasion/cytotoxin Inflammatory	Invasion Penetrating
Location of effect	Central nervous system	Small bowel, proximal	Colon	Small bowel, distal
Microorganisms	*S. aureus* *Bacillus cereus*	*Vibrio cholerae* *E. coli* *Salmonella* spp. *Vibrio parahaemolyticus* *Clostridium perfringens* *Bacillus cereus* *Shigella dysenteriae* *Campylobacter*	*Shigella* *E. coli* *Campylobacter* *Clostridium difficile* *Salmonella* spp. *Entamoeba histolytica*	*Salmonella typhi* *Salmonella paratyphi* *Yersinia*
Illness	Vomiting, watery diarrhea	Watery diarrhea	Fever, dysentery, diarrhea	Fever, diarrhea
Stools	No leukocytes	No leukocytes	Fecal polymorphonuclear leukocytes	Fecal monocytes and PMNs

glucose promotes coupled absorption of sodium and water, thereby accelerating the replenishment of fluid and electrolytes. Oral rehydration should begin at 15 to 25 ml./kg./hour for 4 hours for mild to moderate dehydration, and be followed by maintenance fluids equivalent to measured stool, urine, and insensible losses. Oral intake of food, including breast milk, should continue if clinically possible.

Diarrhea in Children

Children aged 6 months to 5 years represent the bulk of patients with infectious diarrhea. Organisms of particular importance in this age group include rotavirus, *Salmonella,* and *Shigella.*

Rotaviruses are the main cause of winter gastroenteritis in children in temperate climates. After an incubation period of 48 hours, vomiting and diarrhea begin suddenly and may last from 2 to 14 days. Fever is unusual. Stools are watery with mucus but do not contain blood or leukocytes. Treatment is supportive using the oral rehydration therapy described for infant diarrhea. The role of milk products in therapy is controversial owing to the appearance of a temporary lactase deficiency in viral gastroenteritis.

Shigellosis occurs in this same age group, particularly in a family milieu or institutional setting. The incubation period is 2 to 4 days, followed by fever, diarrhea, and dysentery (bloody stools of small volume). Vomiting may occur in younger children, and respiratory symptoms are also frequent at this age. Meningismus may be present. The abdominal findings in shigellosis are typical of invasive disease. Tenderness, hyperactive bowel sounds, and even rebound tenderness are occasionally seen. Sigmoidoscopy shows intense hyperemia with mucus, pus, and multiple ulcerations. Microscopic examination of the stool reveals large numbers of polymorphonuclear leukocytes.

Individuals with shigellosis should be treated according to the severity of their illness. The drug of choice at present is trimethoprim-sulfamethoxazole for children or ciprofloxacin or norfloxacin for adults. Ampicillin or tetracycline may be of value if the isolate is shown to be susceptible. In recent years, antibiotic-resistant *Shigella* species have become common. Treatment of shigellosis substantially shortens the period of diarrhea and fever compared with placebo treatment. Antiperistaltic drugs, such as diphenoxylate, lopexamide, or opiates are contraindicated in invasive diarrheal diseases.

The highest incidence of *Salmonella* gastroenteritis is in children between the ages of 6 months and 2 years. House pets, from dogs to turtles, and food products, particularly poultry and egg products, are the major reservoirs. Person-to-person transmission is also implicated occasionally.

Seventy per cent of *Salmonella* infections manifest themselves as diarrheal disease. The incubation period is 8 to 48 hours, and symptoms include abdominal cramps, vomiting, and fever. Stools are foul smelling and bile colored. Bacteremia is more common in children less than 1 year of age, and respiratory symptoms and meningismus also occur in this age group. Physical examination shows mild abdominal tenderness and hyperactive bowel sounds. Examination of the stool may reveal a few white cells, and, occasionally, blood will be found.

Salmonella enteritis is self-limited except when bacteremia occurs. In children below 3 years of age, blood cultures should always be obtained. Treatment is indicated if bacteremia is present or the illness is prolonged. Oral antibiotics may prolong the carrier state and increase the risk of person-to-person transmission because of prolonged fecal carriage. The drugs of choice for treatment of *Salmonella* infections in children include trimethoprim-sulfamethoxazole, ampicillin, and amoxicillin. Cephalosporins and aminoglycoside antibiotics, although active in vitro, are not effective.

When bacteremia occurs with *Salmonella* in this age group, a typhoidal illness is not usually seen. Salmonella may, however, seed discrete organs, such as bone, spleen, or liver particularly in children with hematologic disorders. This may result in focal *Salmonella* infections requiring specific medical and/or surgical therapy or may result in a chronic fecal carrier state.

Diarrheal Disease in Older Children and Adults

Viral diarrhea occurs regularly in adolescents and young adults. Epidemics occur in late fall and early winter. The clinical features include various combinations of diarrhea, nausea, vomiting, low-grade fever, abdominal cramps, headache, and malaise lasting 24 to 48 hours. The agents most frequently implicated are calciviruses such as the Norwalk agent, and the treatment is symptomatic. Stool examination shows no leukocytes, thereby ruling out invasive bacterial infection.

Shigellosis and salmonellosis also occur in adults, particularly those having traveled to foreign countries. The clinical manifestations are similar to those in children and most cases are self-limited but protracted or severe illness should be treated with a quinolone antimicrobial (norfloxacin or ciprofloxacin). Salmonella bacteremia in older adults has an unfortunate predilection for vascular endothelium with the development of mycotic aneurysms.

S. typhi infections in adults may present a clinical syndrome called typhoid fever. The incubation period varies from 8 to 14 days. Onset of illness is gradual with headache, anorexia, lethargy, and malaise. Nonproductive cough is common but only 20 per cent have diarrhea. Constipation is a more frequent complaint. Fever fluctuates between 102 and 105° F for 2 to 3 weeks in untreated patients. Physical findings are variable, but the pulse may be slow, there may be scattered rhonchi, and splenomegaly is frequently present. Laboratory data show leukopenia and sometimes thrombocytopenia. *S. typhi* can be isolated from the stool at any time in the illness and from the blood in 90 per cent of the patients during the first week. *Salmonella* agglutinins are helpful but not definitive, and a diagnosis must be based on culture. While a number of antimicrobial agents are effective in vitro against *S. typhi* infections, only chloramphenicol, ampicillin (and amoxicillin), trimethoprim-sulfamethoxazole, and the quinolones are clinically useful. An individual who continues to excrete *S. typhi* in the stool may respond to prolonged ciprofloxacin therapy or require cholecystectomy.

Campylobacter jejuni is a short, curve-shaped, gram-negative bacillus and a major cause of bacterial diarrhea in humans. Commonly acquired from sick pets, unpasteurized milk, or ill-prepared poultry products, it produces an acute illness with frequently bloody diarrhea, fever, and tenesmus. Abdominal pain may be severe. Symptoms last from 2 to 7 days but may be more protracted. Sigmoidoscopy is not specific and appearance on biopsy may be indistinguishable from that of ulcerative colitis. The treatment of choice is a quinolone antibiotic or erythromycin by mouth. Occasionally, septicemia is present and requires parenteral therapy with a third-generation cephalosporin, imipenem, or a quinolone.

Yersinia enterocolitica is an organism responsible for a variety of clinical syndromes. In children less than 5 years old, fever and gastroenteritis may occur. In older children and adolescents, abdominal pain is the most prominent feature and is due to suppurative mesenteric lymphadenitis. This may mimic appendicitis and has prompted appendectomy on many an occasion. A self-limited diarrheal illness may also be seen.

Vibrio species are halophilic, gram-negative rods found in marine water and shellfish throughout the world. *V. parahaemolyticus* is the most common species seen in the United States, where it produces outbreaks of illness in the summer. *V. parahaemolyticus* may produce a toxigenic illness similar to that produced by *E. coli* or an invasive illness similar to shigellosis. In contrast, *V. cholerae* produces only a toxigenic diarrhea. Cholera is rare in the United States, although the organism is endemic in the Gulf Coast and may be found in crustaceans and shellfish harvested from this area.

Traveler's diarrhea is an illness acquired by travelers to tropical or semitropical countries. Toxigenic *E. coli* is the most frequent pathogen, although viruses, *Shigella, Salmonella, Entamoeba,* and *Giardia* are all seen in this setting (Table 30–21). Toxigenic *E. coli* produces watery diarrhea of sudden onset, with abdominal cramps but no fever and no tenesmus. Stools are watery and free of blood and fecal leukocytes. Treatment is symptomatic. Prophylactic Pepto-Bismol has been found to be useful, but prophylactic antibiotics may predispose to infection with drug-resistant organisms and are not routinely recommended. Empiric treatment with trimethoprim-sulfamethoxazole or a quinolone will shorten the course of severe illness.

Table 30–21. ENTERIC PATHOGENS AND TRAVELER'S DIARRHEA

Etiologic Agents	Frequency of Association With Traveler's Diarrhea
Enterotoxigenic *E. coli*	30–60
Shigella	5–10
Campylobacter jejuni	5–15
Salmonella strains	3–5
Aeromonas hydrophila	1–5
Rotavirus	1–5
Norwalk agent	1–5
Cryptosporidia	1–5
Giardia	1–3
Multiple agents	5–15
Unknown	15–25

Antibiotic-associated diarrhea is common. Most cases are self-limited and not associated with significant colitis. True pseudomembranous colitis is rare. It has been most commonly associated with clindamycin administration (perhaps 1 per cent of those receiving clindamycin develop this condition), although it is now seen with a variety of beta-lactam antibiotics, tetracyclines, and sulfonamides. Pseudomembranous colitis is due to overgrowth of antibiotic-resistant *C. difficile,* which produces a cytopathic toxin. The clinical findings are those of diarrhea, fever, abdominal pain, distention, and systemic toxicity. Stools are usually watery and mucoid and may contain blood and fecal leukocytes. The treatment of choice is oral vancomycin 125 to 250 mg. 4 times a day or metronidazole 500 mg. 3 times a day. Parenteral vancomycin does not enter the intestinal lumen and is not effective.

INTRA-ABDOMINAL INFECTIONS

Intraperitoneal infections may be generalized or localized depending upon the host response and pathogenesis. Since intraperitoneal recesses all interconnect, infection in one area may spread to another during the course of any intra-abdominal infection.

Primary peritonitis occurs without a definite cause. It is seen at all ages, particularly in children with nephrotic syndrome and in adults with alcoholic cirrhosis. About 10 per cent of patients with alcoholic cirrhosis and ascites will develop primary peritonitis although the diagnosis may be difficult due to subtle physical signs.

The most common agents in children are *S. pneumoniae* and group A streptococci. In adults, *E. coli* is most common followed by *S. pneumoniae, Bacteroides,* and other bowel flora. Streptococcal infection is usually considered to be hematogenous while infection due to bowel flora suggests an intestinal transmural route as well. Clinical manifestations include fever, distention, and abdominal tenderness. Rigidity and/or paralytic ileus may be present. Children show more signs of inflammation than the adult cirrhotic is apt to. Ascitic fluid protein content is of little help in the diagnosis, but the peritoneal white blood cell count is usually over 300 per cubic millimeter.

Secondary peritonitis usually occurs as a result of injury to the gastrointestinal tract, such as perforated ulcer, ischemic bowel, or diverticulitis, or as a result of the spread from infection originating in an intra-abdominal or juxtaperitoneal organ, such as the uterus, fallopian tube, or appendix. Most cases of secondary peritonitis are caused by microorganisms from a ruptured viscus. The stomach, duodendum, and upper small bowel contain mouth flora, such as *S. viridans,* staphylococci, and oral anaerobes (Table 30–22). Some individuals, particularly those with gastric outlet obstruction, achlorhydria, bleeding, or prolonged administration of antacids or H_2 blockers may also be colonized with colonic flora such as *E. coli, Klebsiella,* enterococci, and *B. fragilis*. The flora of the colon is primarily anaerobic (see Table 30–22).

Intraperitoneal abscesses frequently follow peritonitis, particularly in cases of appendicitis or diverticulitis, or after bowel surgery. Characteristically, as with peritonitis, infections are polymicrobial with anaerobes predominating, particularly *B. fragilis* and anaerobic streptococci.

The clinical manifestations of secondary peritonitis are usually dramatic and of sudden onset. Abdominal pain is severe and aggravated by motion and palpation. The patient is febrile and toxic. Tachycardia, tachypnea, and shock may be present. The abdomen shows marked distention with direct and rebound tenderness to palpation. Rigidity of the abdominal wall may be present, and the bowel sounds will usually be absent. The presence of bloody stools suggests ischemic or inflammatory bowel disease as the primary problem, while findings such as cervical tenderness, cul-de-sac fullness, or vaginal discharge may provide a clue to the etiology. It should be noted that patients receiving steroids and elderly patients may have a paucity of clinical findings.

The clinical manifestations of intra-abdominal abscess are less dramatic. Pain may or may not be present, and tenderness is less impressive than in peritonitis. The appearance of fever and chills 5 to 7 days after bowel surgery should suggest a localized area of peritonitis or abscess due to an anastomotic leak.

Table 30–22. FLORA OF THE INTESTINAL TRACT

Aerobes	Anaerobes
Mouth, Esophagus, and Proximal Small Bowel	
Streptococcus	*Bacteroides oralis*
Staphylococcus	*Bacteroides melaninogenicus*
Neisseria	*Fusobacterium* species
Haemophilus	*Peptococcus*
Lactobacillus	*Peptostreptococcus*
Colon and Distal Small Bowel	
E. coli	*Bacteroides fragilis*
Klebsiella	*Clostridium* species
Proteus	*Peptostreptococcus*
Enterobacter species	*Peptococcus*
Enterococci	*Eubacterium*
	Bifidobacterium

The clinical diagnosis of secondary peritonitis is usually not difficult except in the compromised host where physical findings may be blunted. There is usually leukocytosis, and there may be evidence of hemoconcentration due to pooling of fluid in the intestine or abdomen. X-rays reveal distention of the bowel, and if a viscus has ruptured, free air may be seen below the diaphragms. Needle aspiration of the abdomen may yield cloudy fluid with leukocytes and bacteria on smear.

The diagnosis of intra-abdominal abscess may be more difficult. This is particularly true in the postsurgical patient, in whom physical findings are obscured by recent surgery. Gallium scan is of limited value due to postsurgical inflammation. The use of ultrasound, radionuclide, and CT or MRI scanning may be necessary in combination to determine the presence or absence of an abscess.

The treatment of intraperitoneal infection secondary to bowel flora requires aggressive surgical correction of the primary lesion, drainage of sequestered collections of pus, and administration of appropriate antimicrobial agents. Since most such infections are polymicrobial, broad-spectrum therapy is indicated to cover aerobic and anaerobic gram-positive and gram-negative microorganisms if and until definite cultures are available. Many fastidious anaerobes may not be recovered, and empiric therapy for anaerobes often must be continued even in the face of negative cultures. Gram-stained smears of peritoneal exudate will assist in determining the likely pathogens. Equally effective antimicrobial regimens include clindamycin or metronidazole plus an aminoglycoside, cefoxitin, or cefotetan ticarcillin plus clavulanic acid or ampicillin plus sulbactam, or imipenem. The selection is made by personal preference, severity of illness, relative risks of drug toxicity, the results of gram-stained smears and cultures, and cost. Duration of therapy varies with clinical circumstances but is generally continued until the white blood cell count is normal and the patient has been afebrile for 3 to 5 days.

Infection in the Compromised Host

Individuals with altered host defenses comprise a significant proportion of the hospital population and are increasingly being cared for by family practitioners. Patients may be compromised in a variety of ways and be susceptible to different pathogens according to the type of immunosuppression (Tables 30–23 and 30–24). Bacteria, fungi, viruses, or para-

Table 30–23. HOST DEFENSE SYSTEMS

1. Anatomic barriers and secretions (integument, mucosal surfaces)
2. Normal bacterial flora
3. Phagocytes (granulocytes, monocytes, macrophages)
4. Reticuloendothelial system (spleen, liver, tissue macrophages)
5. Complement system
6. Cell-mediated immunity (T-lymphocyte, macrophage)
7. Humoral immunity (immunoglobulin, B-lymphocyte)

sites may be responsible for disease, depending upon the particular defect in host defense (Table 30–24). For example, the use of indwelling percutaneous catheters provides a means by which bacteria or fungi may circumvent normal skin barriers and enter the vascular system. The patient infected with the human immunodeficiency virus (HIV) has depressed cellular immunity resulting in an increased risk of infection with fungi, protozoa, and intracellular bacteria such as *Salmonella* and mycobacteria. Many diseases, such as hematologic malignancies treated with steroids and chemotherapy, compromise multiple defense systems and, therefore, render the patient susceptible to a wide variety of bacteria, fungi, viruses, and parasites.

MECHANISMS OF IMMUNE DEFENSE

Phagocytes and immunoglobulin are important for protection against bacterial infection. In neutropenic patients, the majority of infections are caused by bacteria, particularly *S. aureus* and gram-negative bacilli. Humoral immunity is important for protection against encapsulated microorganisms, such as *S. pneumoniae* and *H. influenzae*. In the absence of preexisting antibody, the spleen has a special role in clearing the blood stream of such organisms. Overwhelming sepsis due to these organisms may occur in asplenic individuals, particularly children. T-lymphocytes are important in a permissive role for the development of humoral immunity by facilitating B-cell differentiation to antibody-producing plasma cells. Defects in cell-mediated immunity, therefore, may also predispose to bacterial infection, such as pneumococcal sepsis, as seen, for example, in HIV infection. The intimate relationship between B-cells, T-cells, and macrophages makes isolated deficiencies uncommon.

Protection of the host from invasive fungal infections involves multiple systems. Fungi such as *Candida, Aspergillus,* and *Mucor* generally produce systemic infection only in those individuals with absent normal flora, damaged cutaneous defenses, defective humoral and cell-mediated immunity, and abnormal leukocyte function. Serious infections due to *Candida,* for example, are seen in patients receiving antibiotics, thereby suppressing normal flora; individuals with surgical or ulcerative disruption of the gastrointestinal mucosa, allowing *Candida* to enter the blood stream; and in patients receiving corticosteroid therapy whose cell-mediated immunity and neutrophil function are compromised. In individuals with depressed immunity due to HIV infection, neoplasia, and/or cancer chemotherapy, *Aspergillus, Cryptococcus, Histoplasma,* and *Coccidioides* may produce disease. The diagnosis of such infections requires a high index of suspicion, appropriate cultures (which frequently require tissue biopsy), and attempts at serologic diagnosis.

Viral infections occur primarily in individuals with depressed cell-mediated immunity. Infections in this category include herpes viruses (both varicella zoster and herpes simplex), cytomegalovirus, and hepatitis virus. The defenses against protozoal and parasitic infections are combined humoral, phagocytic, and cell mediated. Cell-mediated immunity appears to play the most important role in the control of infection by most of these pathogens, particularly *Pneumocystis carinii, Toxoplasma gondii,* and *Strongyloides stercoralis*. However, since most disease is associated with multiple immune defects, the differential diagnosis is wide and should not be limited by such categorization.

Table 30–24. COMMON PATHOGENS IN IMMUNOSUPPRESSED PATIENTS WITH SPECIFIC IMMUNOLOGIC DEFECTS

Depression of	Pathogens
Humoral immune response (globulins, B-cell)	*Pneumococcus, Haemophilus, Pseudomonas,* gram-negative bacilli
Cellular immune response (macrophage, T-cell)	Mycobacteria, *Candida, Cryptococcus, Salmonella, Legionella, Listeria* Toxoplasma, herpes, cytomegalovirus *Pneumocystis*
Polymorphonuclear leukocyte function	Staphylococci, gram-negative bacilli, *Candida, Aspergillus, Mucor*
Reticuloendothelial system (splenectomy)	*Pneumococcus, Haemophilus,* gram-negative bacilli

TREATMENT

It is clear that in patients with neoplastic disease, infection is still the leading cause of death, and the risk of bacterial infection is proportional to the degree of neutropenia in such patients (Table 30–25). The treatment of infection in the compromised host requires a precise diagnosis because of the wide variety of microorganisms that may be implicated. An understanding of the type of immune defect in the individual will help to suggest particular pathogens.

In severe neutropenia, systemic bacterial infection must be suspected and empiric therapy begun at the onset of fever. Failure to do so may result in death from overwhelming infection. The initial regimen should consist of two antibiotics, an aminoglycoside (either gentamicin, tobramycin, or amikacin)

Table 30–25. RISK OF INFECTION IN NEUTROPENIA ASSOCIATED WITH MALIGNANCY

Neutrophil Count	Number of Episodes of Infection Per 1000 Days
< 100/mm.^{3}	45
100–500/mm.^{3}	20
500–1000/mm.^{3}	10
> 1000/mm.^{3}	5

plus a beta-lactam (such as ticarcillin, mezlocillin, ceftazidime, or a cefoperazone). A double-beta-lactam regimen (e.g., piperacillin plus cefotaxime) may also be used. Monotherapy with a single broad-spectrum antibiotic, such as ceftazidime or imipenem has recently become popular but is not to be used without caution. Vancomycin may be a useful adjunct when methicillin-resistant diphtheroids or staphylococci are suspected, as in patients with indwelling central venous catheters.

Blood and other accessible body fluids (or tissues) should be obtained for culture prior to initiation of therapy; serologic studies should be performed when indicated for fungi; and a history of exposure to tuberculosis, parasites, or animals should be documented. Intravenous and bladder catheters should be cultured and changed or removed since they may be the source of infection. If the infection is associated with a pulmonary focus, fiberoptic bronchoscopy and lavage, shielded brushing, or biopsy may be necessary to identify the pathogen. Failure to identify an offending pathogen may result in lack of response to therapy and worsening of the patient's condition. If an etiology is not established by routine work-up, physical examination, and repeated x-ray studies and cultures, additional empiric therapy in the face of continued immunosuppression may be indicated. For example, failure to respond to a combination of antibiotics in neutropenia may warrant the addition of empiric antifungal therapy. Neutropenic patients who become afebrile on empiric antibiotic therapy, even if a microorganism is not isolated, should be treated for a minimum of 14 days. While neutropenic, they will continue to be at risk of additional serious systemic bacterial or fungal infections. Clinical recovery is ultimately dependent upon bone marrow recovery.

Prophylactic oral antibiotics are beneficial but other ancillary measures, such as granulocyte transfusions and protected environments (reverse isolation), are of questionable value. Supplemental immunoglobulin therapy is valuable for patients whose IgG level is less than 300 mg./dl., and careful attention to maintenance of normal skin and mucous membrane integrity is vital. Further prevention of infection may be achieved by good nutrition; avoidance of invasive procedures and the indiscriminate use of antibiotics; avoidance of unnecessary hospitalization, when increased colonization with gram-negative, frequently multi-drug-resistant, bacilli may occur; and decreasing or eliminating immunosuppressive therapy as soon as possible.

Respiratory Tract Infection

Respiratory tract infection is one of the most common illnesses seen by the family physician. Ten per cent of hospital admissions are for the treatment of serious respiratory tract infections and such infections are a major cause of mortality, particularly in those with underlying cardiopulmonary disease or alcoholism. Despite the introduction of antimicrobial agents, a large number of patients still die of pneumonia. These patients are usually elderly, with a variety of associated diseases, and present complex diagnostic and therapeutic problems.

HOST DEFENSES AGAINST RESPIRATORY INFECTION

Pneumonia develops when there is a breakdown of normal host defense mechanisms. A variety of protective factors exist that prevent respiratory infections and maintain normal functioning of the bronchopulmonary tree (Table 30–26).

The mouth, nasopharynx, and oropharynx are colonized by a variety of normal flora. Large numbers of aerobic gram-positive cocci (particularly group *S. viridans*) and gram-negative cocci (*Neisseria* species) as well as anaerobic bacteria (*Fusobacterium*, anaerobic streptococci, and oral *Bacteroides* species) maintain the integrity of a mucosal defense system. Interference with this normal flora, such as by administering antibiotics, can increase susceptibility to colonization with more pathogenic organisms. Seasonal changes in normal flora do occur, with *S. pneumoniae* colonizing 25 to 40 per cent of normal individuals during the winter months. Expectorated sputum samples from such individuals may grow *S. pneumoniae*, reflecting only pharyngeal colonization.

Bronchial mucous secretion and ciliated respiratory epithelium immobilize and remove most bacteria and fungi. In addition, secretory immunoglobulin (IgA) immobilizes bacteria and prevents their invasion. Absence of IgA, and disrupted bronchial mu-

Table 30–26. HOST DEFENSES AGAINST RESPIRATORY TRACT INFECTION

Nasal filter
Normal flora
Cough reflex
Epiglottic reflex
Mucociliary clearance
Secretory immunoglobulin (IgA)
Alveolar macrophages, neutrophils, lymphocytes, circulating immunoglobulin (IgG, IgM)

cosa and ciliated epithelium, as is found in chronic obstructive pulmonary disease, cystic fibrosis, or bronchiectasis, increases the risk of pulmonary infection.

The cough and epiglottic reflexes prevent particulate matter from entering the lower respiratory tract. Impairment of these reflexes occurs in individuals with neurologic disease, alcoholism, or drug overdose and may lead to aspiration pneumonia.

The final line of defense is alveolar macrophages, lymphocytes, neutrophils, and circulating immunoglobulin. Pneumonia can also develop when there is a breakdown of any of these elements, such as in systemic immunodeficiency, neutropenia, or congestive heart failure with accumulation of alveolar fluid.

Viral infections probably predispose to bacterial pulmonary infections by damaging the bronchial epithelium, with a resultant decrease in mucociliary clearance and precipitation of infection by small amounts of aspirated oral flora. Small-volume aspiration is a common phenomenon in most individuals, but normal clearance mechanisms usually prevent disease.

RESPIRATORY INFECTIONS IN THE NEWBORN

Bronchopulmonary infections are an important cause of death in infants. Risk factors include prematurity and prolonged rupture of membranes prior to delivery. Congenital pneumonia, seen within the first few days of life, is either transplacentally acquired or from aspiration of infected amniotic or vaginal fluid. The latter is more common and is usually due to gram-negative bacilli (particularly *E. coli*) or group B streptococci. Occasionally, staphylococci, other gram-negative bacilli, or *Chlamydia* may be the cause (Table 30–27).

Hospital-acquired neonatal pneumonia usually occurs between 2 and 14 days after birth. In these instances, pneumonia is usually the result of resuscitation efforts or contamination of infants by bacteria present on the hands of personnel in the nursery. Occasionally, it is due to hematogenous spread of organisms from infected sites, such as the umbilicus or an intravenous catheter. Staphylococci and gram-negative bacilli are the predominant pathogens.

Table 30–27. TYPES OF PNEUMONITIS ACCORDING TO AGE

Newborn	*Escherichia coli,* group B streptococci, *Staphylococcus aureus, Chlamydia*
Children Aged 1 to 8 Years	Viruses, *Streptococcus pneumoniae, Haemophilus influenzae*
Older Children, Young Adults	*Mycoplasma pneumoniae,* adenovirus, *Streptococcus pneumoniae*
Adults	*Streptococcus pneumoniae, Haemophilus influenzae,* oral anaerobes, *Staphylococcus aureus, Klebsiella, Legionella pneumophila, Mycoplasma pneumoniae*
Immunocompromised Patient	All the above microorganisms, *Pneumocystis carinii, Nocardia asteroides, Aspergillus, Candida, Cryptococcus,* cytomegalovirus

The presentation of pneumonia in the newborn is one of respiratory distress. The neonate may be cyanotic, may or may not be febrile, and usually has minimal sputum production. Grunting, intercostal retraction, and nasal flaring may be present. X-ray studies show patchy infiltrates and are crucial for diagnosis because of the paucity of physical findings.

Chlamydial pneumonitis usually occurs between 3 and 6 weeks after birth. The onset is gradual with a dry cough. The child is usually afebrile but has tachypnea and rales, and x-ray studies show hyperinflated lungs with patchy infiltrates. Conjunctivitis may be present, and eosinophilia is frequent. The diagnosis may be established by culture or by demonstrating intracytoplasmic inclusions in cells from the conjunctivae or nasopharynx.

Bacteriologic diagnosis of pneumonitis in the newborn is necessary for specific therapy. Blood cultures, Gram's stain, and cultures of tracheal or gastric aspirates are frequently helpful in diagnosis. Initial therapy should be directed at likely pathogens, including group B streptococci and gram-negative bacilli. Ampicillin and gentamicin is the most commonly used regimen but should be altered according to the results of culture and susceptibility tests. Chlamydial pneumonitis is treated with erythromycin.

RESPIRATORY INFECTIONS IN CHILDREN AGED 2 MONTHS TO 12 YEARS

Upper and lower respiratory tract infections account for 80 per cent of illnesses experienced by children. Normal children aged 3 to 5 years have six to eight infections per year, ranging from pharyngitis and otitis to pneumonia. Most lower respiratory tract infections in this age group are due to viruses, particularly respiratory syncytial virus (RSV), parainfluenza viruses, and adenovirus. Of these, RSV and parainfluenza viruses are responsible for most lower respiratory tract illnesses below the age of 2 years. *Mycoplasma pneumoniae* produces most disease in the preadolescent and adolescent age group. HIV-infected children will usually develop respiratory infections after 6 months of age. Recurrent infections due to *H. influenzae* or pneumococcus or diffuse lung infiltrates compatible with lymphoid interstitial pneumonia or *Pneumocystis,* should prompt a search for HIV infection (see Chapter 32).

Croup occurs primarily in children 3 months to 3 years of age. It usually begins with a mild but distinctive cough that progressively worsens. There is little sputum production, but low-grade fever and associated coryza are present. The disease is primarily subepiglottic and the epiglottis is not markedly inflamed or edematous. Croup is most often due to parainfluenza virus infection. Treatment is symptomatic, with a stress on humidification. Antibiotics are not indicated, since this is a viral infection.

Epiglottitis occurs primarily in children 2 to 7 years of age. The illness is of sudden onset, with sore throat, high fever, hoarseness, dysphagia, drooling, and respiratory distress. Stridor may develop. Cough is not prominent, in contrast to croup. The epiglottis is edematous and cherry red. It should not be repeatedly examined, since this may precipitate acute airway obstruction. Lateral soft tissue x-ray studies of the neck demonstrate an enlarged epiglottis. The etiology is usually *H. influenzae,* type b, and cultures of pharynx and blood are frequently positive. The treatment of choice is cefuroxime, cefotaxime, or ceftriaxone initially, modified when culture and susceptibility results are available.

Bronchiolitis occurs in children 6 months to 2 years of age and is most commonly due to respiratory syncytial virus. It begins with a mild cough, coryza, and rhinorrhea, progressing to tachypnea, wheezing, and respiratory distress. Rales and rhonchi may be evident. X-ray studies show hyperinflation, peribronchial cuffing, and perihilar infiltrates. The disease may be particularly severe in infants less than 1 year of age and may lead to respiratory failure. Treatment is primarily humidification and bronchodilation, with antibiotics reserved for bacterial superinfection.

Pneumonia in children is usually viral. When bacterial, *S. pneumoniae* and *H. influenzae* are the main causes. Mycoplasma in the child produces a tracheobronchitis rather than the pneumonia typical of young adulthood. Children with sickle cell disease are predisposed to particularly severe pneumococcal or mycoplasma pneumonia. Treatment of viral pneumonia is symptomatic. Treatment of bacterial pneumonia depends upon the etiologic diagnosis, with appropriate antibiotics based on that diagnosis.

RESPIRATORY INFECTIONS IN THE ADULT

Acute bronchitis is an inflammation of the tracheobronchial tree. In patients without underlying lung disease, it is predominantly due to viruses, such as influenza, adenovirus, and parainfluenza virus, occasionally mycoplasma and, less frequently, bacterial pathogens. The illness usually begins with rhinorrhea, sore throat, and coryza. Cough follows quickly and may persist after many of the upper respiratory symptoms have abated. Sputum production increases with duration of the illness, particularly in those who are smokers.

Physical examination reveals rhonchi and occasional wheezes. Rales and signs of consolidation are not present unless concomitant pneumonia exists. Fever is usually less than 101° F. Chest x-ray studies reveal no pulmonary infiltrates but may show peribronchial cuffing or hyperinflation. Laboratory studies are usually unremarkable.

Treatment should consist of hydration and possibly expectorants. Bronchodilators may be necessary if wheezing occurs. The role of antibiotics is not clear, but they are not indicated if the illness is of viral etiology. If examination of the sputum reveals bacterial pathogens on Gram's stain or culture, antibiotics will then be useful.

Acute bacterial exacerbations of chronic bronchitis in patients with structural disease of the tracheobronchial tree represent a different problem. Most of these patients have a history of smoking, have chronic cough and sputum production, and may have attendant pulmonary or cardiac insufficiency. These exacerbations are frequently manifest by an increase in sputum production with or without upper respiratory tract symptoms, change in viscosity and color of sputum, and increasing dyspnea and wheezing. Most patients do not have chills, fever, or leukocytosis.

Evaluation of such patients is difficult. The sputum is usually full of leukocytes in the absence of acute exacerbation. Organisms may also be present in such secretions. Although the exacerbations may be precipitated by viral infection, a concomitant increase in leukocytosis and bacterial counts in the sputum of such patients suggests a bacterial component. Since *Haemophilus* species and pneumococci are the most commonly isolated organisms, antibiotic administration should be directed at these pathogens and is of value. Perhaps more important is attention to pulmonary toilet, discontinuance of smoking, bronchodilators, and humidification. Cough suppressants, antihistamines, and other drying agents should be avoided. Occasionally, pathogens other than *Haemophilus* species and *S. pneumoniae* may be present and may need alternative therapy, including parenteral antibiotics. Useful empiric agents include amoxicillin, tetracycline, and trimethoprim-sulfamethoxazole. If resistant flora are isolated, more potent oral agents, such as cefuroxime, amoxicillin plus clavulanic acid, or ciprofloxacin, may be effective.

Prophylactic administration of antibiotics to patients with a history of chronic bronchitis is of value in those individuals with severe underlying lung disease who have a history of repeated decompensation during the winter months. Cyclic antibiotic regimens include any of the previously mentioned three agents.

PNEUMONIA IN THE ADULT

Identification of the etiologic agent of pneumonia is frequently difficult and requires a thorough history, physical examination, and thoughtful interpretation of Gram's stains, cultures, and x-ray studies. Important clues to the diagnosis are patient age (see Table 30–27), season, duration of illness, and concomitant clinical features, such as alcoholism, loss of consciousness, underlying cardiac disease, travel history, exposure to birds or animals, recent surgical procedure or hospitalization, and concomitant extrapulmonary disease. Physical examination and x-ray findings are rarely specific, although certain suggestive features may emerge (Tables 30–28 and 30–29).

Influenza is an illness of short incubation and rapid onset. Cough, malaise, chills, severe headache and retro-orbital pain, coryza, rhinorrhea, and watery eyes are common. Myalgias are marked, particularly in the low back and legs. Fever is prominent and may be as high as 104° F. Cough is usually nonproductive. Influenza occurs in epidemics—an important clue to its diagnosis.

The early phase of the illness is due to a bronchitis, and there is decreased mucociliary clearance due to the direct effects of viral infection on the respiratory epithelium. These abnormalities predispose to bacterial superinfection. Typically, this occurs after 5 to 7 days of illness, at which time the patient has begun to improve, when purulent sputum and return of fever suddenly develop. Physical examination now reveals signs of pneumonia. Organisms most commonly implicated include *S. pneumoniae, H. influenzae,* and *S. aureus.* Occasionally, *Klebsiella* or *Branhamella* is a secondary infecting organism. Bacterial superinfection occurs particularly in smokers and in individuals with chronic bronchitis.

Influenza may require 2 to 4 weeks to resolve in the absence of superinfection, and postviral fatigue may be prominent, particularly in the elderly. Although no specific therapy of established infection is available, amantidine hydrochloride (Symmetrel) may be of value in speeding defervesence and decreasing the degree of peripheral airway resistance.

Consideration should be given to prophylaxis of influenza by *annual* vaccination (in October or November) of susceptible individuals (Table 30–30). Current vaccines are safe and effective. After vaccination, 2 to 3 weeks are required for immunity to develop. Amantidine is a less satisfactory but also effective method of prevention of influenza A infection. It must be taken daily (200 mg. per day) to be effective. Pneumococcal vaccine should also be ad-

Table 30–28. DIFFERENTIAL CHARACTERISTICS OF BACTERIAL AND VIRAL OR *MYCOPLASMA* PNEUMONIA*

Feature	Bacterial	*Mycoplasma*/Viral
Onset	Sudden	Gradual
Shaking chills	Common	Uncommon
Cough	Variable	Prominent
Fever	High	Low-grade, < 102° F
Tachycardia > 120	Common	Uncommon
Tachypnea > 30	Common	Uncommon
Chest pain	Common	Uncommon
Sputum	Purulent	Scant, mucoid
X-ray consolidation	Frequent	Unusual
Pleural effusion	Occasional-large	Infrequent-small
Leukocytosis	Frequent	Rarely > 12,000/mm.^{3}

*None of these characteristics are absolute; they are most useful in the nondebilitated or nonimmunosuppressed host without significant underlying pulmonary disease.

Table 30–29. X-RAY FINDINGS IN PNEUMONIA

Bacterial Pneumonia	
Pneumococcus	Usually RLL or LLL infiltrate or consolidation in healthy adult; bronchopneumonia in alcoholics or debilitated patients
Staphylococcus	Multiple infiltrates, early abscess formation, pneumatoceles
Klebsiella	Upper or RML consolidation, loss of volume, bulging fissure, early abscess formation
Haemophilus	Bronchopneumonia
Pseudomonas	Usually lower lobes, multiple small abscesses, perihilar infiltrates, wedge shaped
Anaerobes	Dependent areas, lower lobes, right greater than left, empyema, abscess
Legionella	Patchy alveolar infiltrates, lobar or segmental
Nonbacterial Pneumonia	
Adenovirus	Diffuse interstitial infiltrates
Cytomegalovirus	Diffuse interstitial infiltrates
Influenza virus	Diffuse interstitial infiltrates
Varicella-zoster virus	Fine, widespread nodular infiltrates, especially lower lobes
Chlamydia psittaci	Perihilar infiltrates, often bilateral
Mycoplasma	Scattered patchy infiltrates, small effusions, rare consolidation
Mycobacterium tuberculosis	Child: lower or middle lobe infiltrate, hilar adenopathy; adult: upper lobe, cavitary
Fungal Pneumonia	
Aspergillus	Perihilar, necrotizing, wedge-shaped (infarct)
Histoplasma	Perihilar and diffuse with adenopathy; calcifications; upper lobe, cavitary
Cryptococcus	Basilar streaky to dense infiltrate
Coccidioides	Multiple infiltrates, pleural effusions, thin-walled cavities
Other	
Pneumocystis	Perihilar and interstitial infiltrates, ground glass, bilateral, extensive

Table 30–30. TARGET GROUPS FOR INFLUENZA VACCINE

Groups at Greatest Risk of Influenza-related Complications
1) Adults and children with chronic cardiovascular or pulmonary diseases
2) Residents of nursing homes or other chronic care facilities

Groups at Modest Risk of Influenza-related Complications
1) Otherwise healthy individuals over 65 years of age
2) Adults and children with diabetes mellitus, renal dysfunction, anemia, immunosuppression or immunodeficiency (including HIV infection)
3) Children (6 months through 18 years of age) receiving long-term aspirin therapy

Groups Capable of Nosocomial Transmission
1) Physicians, nurses, and other medical care personnel having extensive contact with high-risk patients
2) Providers to high-risk patients in the home care setting, including family members

Any Individual Who Wishes to Receive Vaccine to Reduce the Chance of Acquiring Influenza Infection

ministered to those who require influenza vaccine, as well as to asplenic patients. One dose of pneumococcal vaccine provides effective immunity for at least 5 years after administration. It does not need to be repeated annually.

Mycoplasma pneumonia occurs most frequently in young adults, although recent reports suggest that it occurs occasionally in middle-aged and older adults as well. The onset is gradual, with a hacking nonproductive cough. Later, scant, white, then purulent, sputum appears as bronchial epithelial cells slough and initiate a polymorphonuclear leukocyte response. At this time, differentiation from bacterial disease may be difficult. Systemic symptoms are prominent and include malaise, headache, and fever between 100° and 103° F. Rash, serous otitis, and joint symptoms may occasionally accompany the pulmonary complaints. Additionally, helpful diagnostic features include occurrence in the late summer and early fall, associated family cluster of respiratory complaints, or an outbreak in a summer camp or similar institution.

Physical findings may be unremarkable. Auscultation of the chest reveals only scattered rhonchi or fine localized rales in most cases. The x-ray study, in contradistinction to the benign physical exam, is often impressive, with fine or patchy lower lobe or perihilar infiltrates. Consolidation may occur, particularly in older patients, and small pleural effusions are not uncommon. Laboratory data reveal a white blood cell count of 10,000 to 15,000/mm.[3] with a polymorphonuclear leukocyte predominance. Cold agglutinin titers may be helpful early in the disease but are not specific and are negative in approximately one third of cases. The diagnosis is confirmed by acute and convalescent *Mycoplasma* complement fixation titers. Although cultures can be performed, they are uncommonly available.

The treatment of choice is erythromycin or, alternatively, tetracycline. Symptomatic improvement occurs with administration of either of these agents, but cough and malaise may persist. Therapy should continue for 3 weeks. The organism is not eradicated from the sputum, and, therefore, secondary cases in the family may still occur. Even in the absence of treatment, resolution is spontaneous in the vast majority of patients.

Other, nonbacterial pneumonias may be seen in both children and adults. *Adenoviral* pneumonia cannot be differentiated clinically or radiographically from *Mycoplasma* pneumonia. *Psittacosis* occurs in individuals exposed to infected birds. Sporadic cases are most frequently associated with parrots or parakeets, although outbreaks occasionally occur in poultry processing plants or from contacts with infected turkeys. The onset is usually abrupt, with prominent dry cough and severe headache. Temperature-pulse dissociation is frequent, and infiltrates may be perihilar or peripheral. The infection responds promptly to administration of tetracycline.

Q-fever is a similar illness presenting in individuals exposed to infected animals, particularly cattle or the meat or excreta thereof. It is a rickettsial illness but, unlike other rickettsial diseases, is not associated with rash. Liver function test abnormalities are prominent. Tetracycline is again the drug of choice.

Tularemia, associated with inhalation of aerosols from infected rabbit or other rodent tissue, may produce a fulminant pneumonia with severe systemic symptoms. Treatment of choice is streptomycin.

Fungal pneumonia should be considered in the differential diagnosis of nonbacterial pneumonia. Travel to the southwest should suggest coccidioidomycosis. Exposure to bird droppings, chickens, or starlings should suggest histoplasmosis. Cryptococcal pulmonary disease should also be suggested in this setting. All of these illnesses present with moderate fever, flu-like symptoms, and a nonproductive cough. Their presence or absence should be considered by appropriate history. The diagnosis is made serologically and by examination of lung tissue. Cultures are rarely positive in the early stages of such illnesses.

Pneumocystis pneumonia must be considered in the young adult with fever and nonproductive cough, especially when a history of sexual promiscuity or intravenous drug abuse is elicited. Findings from chest x-ray studies may be subtle but dyspnea, hypoxemia, thrush, and other signs of HIV infection may be present.

Legionella infection is relatively common, accounting for approximately 1 to 2 per cent of community-acquired pneumonias. *Legionella* may also cause a hospital-acquired pneumonia, particularly in immunosuppressed or transplant patients. *Legionella pneumophila* is a weakly gram-negative staining bacillus whose source is usually water (e.g., cooling towers or shower heads) and soil (particularly in areas of excavation). Person-to-person transmission is not important. Disease is most common in the spring, summer, and fall when air conditioning systems and cooling towers are in use.

Fever, myalgias, chills, and a nonproductive cough occur 2 to 10 days after exposure. Abdominal pain, nausea, vomiting, and confusion may be prominent. Most patients are male, elderly, and smokers. Physical examination reveals an acutely ill patient with a temperature of 103 to 105° F. Rales and rhonchi may be present, but signs of consolidation are not found early. Findings from x-ray studies vary from patchy infiltrates to lobar consolidation. Solitary lung abscesses have been reported, and pleural effusions may occur.

Laboratory data reveal a leukocytosis, sometimes exceeding 20,000/ml.[3] Other findings are proteinuria, hyponatremia, and hypophosphatemia. Sputum Gram's stains are negative, but fluorescent antibody stains and DNA probes are available to identify the organisms in respiratory secretions. Special media (charcoal yeast extract agar) is necessary to isolate the organism, with greatest yields obtained from lung biopsy, lung aspirate, or transtracheal aspirates. The diagnosis can be confirmed serologically, allowing 3 weeks between acute and convalescent serology and demonstrating a four-fold antibody rise.

Legionella infections carry a high mortality, in part because of delayed diagnosis and because the infection is frequent in elderly and immunosuppressed patients. The diagnosis should be considered in an individual with rapidly progressive pneumonia and no organisms isolated by standard culture techniques and who does not respond to usual antibiotic therapy. Mortality in the absence of specific therapy is over 50 per cent. With appropriate antibiotics, this mortality can be reduced to 10 per cent. Erythromycin is the drug of choice, administered at a dose of 3 to 4 gm./day, intravenous initially, for 3 weeks. Rifampin, trimethoprim-sulfamethoxazole, tetracycline, or a quinolone may be useful alternative agents.

S. pneumoniae (pneumococcus) is the most common cause of pneumonia in the adult, with an incidence of one to two cases per thousand individuals per year. Pneumococcal pneumonia is also common in small children, especially those with sickle cell disease or immunoglobulin dysfunction. Underlying diseases in the adult, such as chronic lung or cardiac disorders, alcoholism with cirrhosis, and diabetes mellitus, predispose to illness. Pneumococcal pneumonia is most frequent during the winter months.

The classic presentation of pneumococcal pneumonia is a sudden onset of fever, pleuritic chest pain, and cough with purulent or rusty sputum. Antecedent viral upper or lower respiratory tract infection is present in many cases. However, atypical presentations are common, particularly in the elderly and alcoholic population. In such patients, fever may be low grade, behavior disturbances may seem more significant than respiratory symptoms, and cough may not be prominent. Patients appear acutely ill, frequently with dyspnea and chest splinting. Signs of consolidation are frequently present, a pleural friction rub or signs of pleural fluid may be present, and there may be abdominal pain and ileus.

Laboratory findings include an elevated white blood cell count with a left shift. In the elderly or alcoholic, however, the white count may be normal or depressed. Chest x-ray studies usually show disease confined to one lobe, frequently a lower lobe, but several lobes may be involved with either consolidation or bronchopneumonia. Chronic changes in the lung architecture in chronic lung disease make both auscultation and radiographic analysis difficult, so the presence of pneumonia may be unclear. Gram's stain of the sputum will show polymorphonuclear leukocytes and lancet-shaped gram-positive diplococci. However, up to 40 per cent of patients with bacteremic pneumococcal pneumonia will have negative sputum cultures so that blood cultures should be obtained in all patients. Since bacteremia is so common and since meningitis or other metastatic foci of infection may also occur, alteration in mental status should be viewed with suspicion and lumbar punctures performed in such cases.

The treatment of uncomplicated pneumococcal pneumonia is with parenteral penicillin G, 3 to 6 million units/day until afebrile. When bacteremia or metastatic foci of infection are suspected, or until the limited nature of the pneumonia is confirmed, parenteral aqueous penicillin G, 12 to 18 million units per day, is indicated. In the penicillin-allergic patient, erythromycin, or a first-generation cephalosporin (e.g., cefazolin) may be used. Attention should be paid to adequate hydration, oxygenation and ventilatory support, postural drainage, and adequate humidification. Pleural effusions, if present, should be diagnostically aspirated and empyemas drained.

Staphylococcal pneumonia accounts for less than 5 per cent of adult pneumonia but carries a high mortality. It is seen particularly in the wake of influenza and as a hospital-acquired infection. In addition, staphylococcal pneumonia is seen as a consequence of bacteremic spread from another focus of infection, particularly tricuspid valve endocarditis in the intravenous drug user.

The clinical features of staphylococcal pneumonia are frequently more striking than the x-ray examination. Recurrent chills, high spiking fever, dyspnea, cyanosis, and pleuritic chest pain are common. Sputum is frequently purulent with blood streaking. Physical findings are variable, but a pleural effusion and pleural friction rub are frequently detected. Leukocytosis is usually marked. Chest x-ray findings include multiple infiltrates with abscess formation, empyema, pyopneumothorax, and pneumatoceles (thin-walled cavities). Sputum examination usually shows many polymorphonuclear leukocytes and gram-positive cocci in clusters. However, in bacteremic staphylococcal pneumonia, the sputum may be normal.

The treatment of staphylococcal pneumonia is with parenteral administration of an antistaphylococcal penicillin, such as oxacillin, in a dose of 8 to 12 grams per day in the adult and 100 to 200 mg./kg./day in the child. Cephalosporins or vancomycin are alternative therapy. Blood cultures should always be performed prior to therapy. Tricuspid valve endocarditis should always be considered in the intravenous drug user. The presence of pleural fluid should prompt evaluation for empyema, with surgical drainage as necessary. Despite effective therapy, the severity of illness and the rapidity of its progression contribute to the still high mortality of 20 to 30 per cent.

Aerobic gram-negative bacillary pneumonia accounts for less than 20 per cent of community-acquired pneumonia but for 50 per cent or more of hospital-associated cases. Most pneumonia deaths in the hospital setting are due to these organisms. Gram-negative pneumonia is usually acquired by aspiration of endogenous oropharyngeal flora in those individuals colonized with gram-negative bacilli. It is less commonly seen as a complication of contaminated aerosols, particularly in patients on ventilatory support for other pulmonary conditions, or as a complication of bacteremia from an extrapulmonary source. Pharyngeal colonization with gram-negative bacilli varies from less than 10 per cent in the normal host to over 50 per cent in the debilitated, hospitalized, elderly, particularly bedridden, individual. Twenty-five per cent of colonized and intubated patients will develop gram-negative pneumonia.

A precise bacteriologic diagnosis may be difficult. The diagnosis is obviously secure in patients with bacteremia, but a positive sputum culture may reflect only pharyngeal colonization. Appropriate x-ray findings (see Table 30–29), a Gram's stain showing many polymorphonuclear leukocytes and gram-negative bacilli, and an absence of oropharyngeal epithelial cells help to confirm the diagnosis in the absence of bacteremia.

H. influenzae produces pneumonia in infants and children and in the elderly. As a cause of childhood pneumonia, it is frequently associated with bacteremia. In elderly patients, chronic bronchitis and alcoholism are usual concomitant illnesses. X-rays show patchy, bilateral infiltrates, and the sputum Gram's stain is usually diagnostic.

Klebsiella pneumonia is typically seen in elderly males with a history of alcoholism or other underlying lung disease. It is also an important cause of pneumonia in nursing homes and in hospitalized patients. The onset is sudden with severe toxicity. Pleuritic chest pain and hemoptysis are features. Sputum is thick, often with blood, but in only 25 per cent is it the characteristic currant-jelly sputum. Pneumonia due to *E. coli* is most often a bacteremic pneumonia, with an extrapulmonary source, such as the genitourinary or gastrointestinal tract.

Pseudomonas pulmonary infections occur due to aspiration of pharyngeal flora, seeding of the lung due to bacteremia from distant foci, and from aerosols of contaminated solutions. *Pseudomonas* pneumonia associated with bacteremia occurs in individuals with severely compromised host defenses, such as neoplasia with neutropenia, severe burns, or prolonged confinement in an intensive care unit. The mortality in bacteremic *Pseudomonas* pneumonia is over 75 per cent. This is primarily a reflection of severity of underlying disease in the host rather than an attribute of the microorganism per se.

The successful treatment of gram-negative pneumonia has traditionally required a two-drug regimen, such as a beta-lactam antibiotic plus an aminoglycoside. In *Pseudomonas* pneumonia, the combination of ticarcillin plus tobramycin has been efficacious as has the combination of a cephalosporin plus an aminoglycoside for *Klebsiella* pneumonia. Therapy of all gram-negative bacillary pneumonia, however, depends upon the antimicrobial susceptibility of the involved microorganisms, and single drug therapy particularly with newer and more potent agents will be adequate in many cases. In addition to specific antibiotic therapy, adequate humidification, oxygenation, and ventilation is necessary. Intubation may be appropriate for such patients but provides an added risk of superinfection.

ANAEROBIC LUNG DISEASE

Anaerobic lung infection is usually due to aspiration or oral microorganisms, although occasionally metastatic foci from an anaerobic infection distant to the lung may be the cause. Predisposing factors to anaerobic pleuropulmonary infections include those conditions that result in altered consciousness or dysphagia and are primarily structural or functional rather than immunologic. Alcoholism, seizure disorders, narcotic addiction, sedative overdose, esophageal dysfunction due to tumor or motility disorder, cerebrovascular accidents, gastrointestinal disease with prolonged vomiting, or neurologic defects are frequently present. Local pulmonary conditions, such as infarction, obstruction due to carcinoma, bronchiectasis, or foreign bodies, are also important risk factors. Anaerobic pulmonary infections are located in dependent segments, particularly the posterior segments of the upper lobes and the superior segments of the lower lobes.

Pleuropulmonary disease due to anaerobes may take several forms. Simple pneumonitis, necrotizing pneumonia, lung abscess, or empyema may occur. Necrotizing pneumonia may be rapidly progressive, whereas lung abscesses are usually indolent. The majority of patients with lung abscesses have symptoms for over 7 days; fever, weight loss, and other constitutional symptoms are common. Foul-smelling sputum is a helpful sign, but its absence does not rule out an anaerobic pulmonary infection. Furthermore, although aspiration pneumonia is usually due to anaerobes, the edentulous patient, lacking gingivae that are the source of anaerobes, may have an aerobic pneumonia due to aspiration. In hospitalized patients, although anaerobes may be present, colonizing gram-negative aerobes may be important copathogens.

Penicillin G or clindamycin is the antibiotic of choice for anaerobic pleuropulmonary infections. Tetracycline, erythromycin, and cephalosporin derivatives may also be effective in some patients. Patients with lung abscesses usually have adequate drainage via the bronchial tree by expectoration of sputum. If there is obstruction, however, drainage may need to be surgically established. Anaerobic empyema demands surgical drainage.

THE LABORATORY DIAGNOSIS OF PNEUMONIA

Sputum examination and culture are essential for appropriate diagnosis of pneumonia. Saliva or nasopharyngeal secretions are of little value in determining the etiology, since colonization with gram-negative bacilli and other organisms is frequent. Whether secretions are obtained by expectoration, endotracheal suction, or transtracheal aspiration, such material must be confirmed adequate by smear. If there are more than 25 squamous epithelial cells per low-power field of specimen, such material should be considered inadequate for culture because it represents oral flora. Expectorated sputum is adequate for culture if fewer than 10 epithelial cells are present per low-power field and polymorphonuclear leukocytes are seen. The neutropenic patient may have no neutrophils seen on smear but should have no epithelial cells in the specimen. The morphology of a microorganism may enable a presumptive diagnosis from Gram's stain alone, but it is not distinctive in most instances. Cultures should be performed on blood agar, chocolate agar, and a selective gram-negative agar. Transtracheal cultures or bronchoscopic specimens obtained by shielded brush techniques may be cultured anaerobically or for fastidious organisms such as *Legionella*. Anaerobic cultures of expectorated sputum or unshielded bronchoscopic samples are of no value, since they contain oral anaerobic flora.

DIFFERENTIAL DIAGNOSIS OF PNEUMONIA

Other conditions may mimic the signs and symptoms of pneumonia. *Pulmonary emboli* should be considered, particularly in individuals with prolonged bed rest, recent immobilization, or intra-abdominal or pelvic surgery. *Atelectasis* in the postoperative patient may present with fever and linear infiltrates. *Mucous plugging* may cause segmental or lobar atelectasis with or without infection. *Pulmonary contusion* secondary to trauma may present as pleuritic chest pain, fever, and tachypnea with infiltrates on a chest x-ray study. *Congestive heart failure* may be manifest by nonproductive cough and dyspnea. However, fever is unusual, sputum production is minimal, and cardiomegaly is usually present on x-ray study.

Sepsis and Bacteremia

EPIDEMIOLOGY

In the 1930's and 1940's, 90 per cent of all bacteremia was due to gram-positive microorganisms; most of these were due to streptococci and staphylococci. After the introduction of penicillin and streptomycin in the 1940's, the rate of gram-positive sepsis fell markedly relative to gram-negative sepsis. Approximately three fourths of all bacteremia is now due to gram-negative bacilli, and between one half and three fourths of all gram-negative bacteremia occurs in the hospital rather than in the community. Between 10 and 12 cases occur for every thousand hospital admissions. This is double the rate for 1970 and ten times the rate for 1950. Although the percentage of fatalities due to gram-negative sepsis is slightly less than in previous years, the number of fatalities has increased due to an overall rise in the incidence of gram-negative sepsis. *E. coli* is the single most common isolate, accounting for 30 to 40 per cent of cases followed by *Klebsiella, Pseudomonas,* and *Bacteroides* (Table 30–31). Approximately 10 per cent of patients have polymicrobial bacteremia.

Table 30–31. GRAM-NEGATIVE BACTEREMIA IN THE UNITED STATES

Microorganism	Per Cent of Cases	Per Cent Mortality
E. coli	35	30
Klebsiella	25	38
Pseudomonas	15	54
Bacteroides	10	30
Proteus	10	33
Enterobacter	5	25
Serratia	4	37

Reasons for the increased incidence of gram-negative infections are multiple and include a larger percentage of patients with severe underlying disease, an increased age of patient population, a greater use of invasive surgical procedures, more frequent antibiotic treatment, and an increased use of adrenocortical steroids and cytotoxic drugs in the population at risk.

Knowing the source of bacteremia allows one to predict the pathogen (Table 30–32). Genitourinary tract infections cause 40 per cent of all septic episodes, usually due to *E. coli, Proteus,* or *Pseudomonas*. The gastrointestinal tract, respiratory tract, skin, and soft tissues are additional sources in decreasing order of frequency. Soft tissue infections include such sources as decubitus or venous stasis ulcers, subcutaneous abscesses, and cellulitis from I.V. sites (Plate I, *A* and *B*).

SEPTIC SHOCK

Not all gram-negative sepsis is accompanied by clinical shock. The factors that determine whether shock will occur are not clearly understood, although it is the cell wall lipopolysaccharide, or endotoxin, that provokes most of the biochemical, functional, and clinical changes that characterize septic shock. Endotoxin directly injures endothelial cells resulting in

Table 30–32. SOURCE OF GRAM-NEGATIVE SEPSIS AND ISOLATED PATHOGENS

Source	Per Cent of Cases	Most Common Pathogens
Genitourinary tract	40	*E. coli, Proteus mirabilis, Pseudomonas*
Gastrointestinal tract	25	*E. coli, Klebsiella, Bacteroides*
Respiratory tract	20	*Pseudomonas, Enterobacter, Klebsiella*
Skin and soft tissue	15	*E. coli, Enterobacter, Pseudomonas, Bacteroides*

prostaglandin synthesis, exposure of vascular collagen, and activation of Hageman factor with subsequent complement, kinin, and clotting factor consumption. Endotoxin also interacts with macrophages to release interleukin 1, which causes fever and leukocytosis, and tumor necrosis factor or cachectin, which further activates prostaglandin and leukotriene systems. The resultant endothelial damage, vascular dilatation, vascular permeability, and capillary occlusion diminishes microcirculation to vital organs with resultant tissue hypoxia. Peripheral oxygen utilization is decreased, lactic acidosis develops, and if the process continues, cell death and patient demise will follow.

The clinical manifestations of septicemia may be subtle (Table 30–33). In early septic shock, the patient is warm, vasodilated, hypotensive, tachycardic, and tachypneic. The patient may or may not be febrile. As a consequence of tissue hypoxia, the patient may be agitated or confused. The urine output in early septic shock may be good, but the central venous pressure will be low, reflecting a decreased intravascular volume due to venous pooling and loss of fluid through damaged vessel walls. As septic shock progresses, vasoconstriction supervenes. The patient becomes cold, mottled, and dusky. Blood pressure remains low, the pulse is weak, and myocardial contractility is now impaired. The patient becomes more acidotic, tachypneic, and confused. Urine output decreases, and a paralytic ileus may be prominent. Diffuse rales are audible throughout the lungs and reflect a combination of cardiac and noncardiac pulmonary edema due to vascular damage.

The laboratory findings in septic shock are numerous. The most reproducible hematologic abnormality is thrombocytopenia due to disseminated intravascular coagulation. Elevated prothrombin time and thrombin time and increased fibrin-split products are observed. Although the biochemical parameters of disseminated intravascular coagulation are reversed with heparin, the use of heparin does not decrease the mortality or morbidity of septic shock. Other hematologic abnormalities in sepsis include an early rise in hematocrit due to hemoconcentration and a later fall due to hemolysis in conjunction with disseminated intravascular coagulation. The white blood cell count initially falls due to margination of cells and perhaps as a direct effect of endotoxin on the release of neutrophils from the bone marrow. Subsequently, the white count should rise in a response appropriate to the severity of infection.

Table 30–33. THE VARIED CLINICAL MANIFESTATIONS OF SEPSIS

Chills, fever, hypotension
Hyperpnea, tachypnea, respiratory alkalosis
Unexplained confusion, agitation
Oliguria or anuria
Thrombocytopenia
Tachycardia
Paralytic ileus
Metabolic acidosis

The hemodynamics of septic shock change with time. Early on, the total peripheral resistance is low and the cardiac output is normal or high. Central venous and pulmonary artery pressures are low due to venous pooling and vasodilation. As septic shock progresses, total peripheral resistance rises and cardiac output falls. The central venous and pulmonary artery pressures may remain low if fluid losses are not replaced.

The pulmonary findings in septic shock are those of noncardiac pulmonary edema, or adult respiratory distress syndrome, due to vascular damage with leakage of intravascular fluid into interstitial spaces. Intravascular aggregates of platelets, neutrophils, and fibrin are observed microscopically. Arterial blood gases initially show a respiratory alkalosis with decreased P_{CO_2} and decreased P_{O_2} due to ventilation-perfusion abnormalities and interstitial edema. Subsequently, metabolic acidosis appears, due to accumulation of lactic acid.

Renal function in septic shock remains normal early. Renal blood flow and urine flow decrease later. Oliguric renal failure in septic shock has an extremely poor prognosis, with a mortality greater than 65 per cent in most series.

The Treatment of Septic Shock

The treatment of septic shock is logical if one understands its pathophysiology. Treatment is twofold: (1) restoration of the microcirculation and (2) elimination of the microorganism. Attempts to modulate the effects of endotoxin and other biochemical mediators of septic shock are subjects of active study but have not yet proven clinically valuable.

Intravenous fluids are important early in treatment. They are administered aggressively while monitoring central venous or pulmonary artery pressure and urine output. Intravascular volume measurements are particularly important in late septic shock, when myocardial depression and/or renal failure may have developed. The fluid deficit may be several liters prior to adequate repletion of intravascular volume. Isotonic saline is the preferred solution. Supplemental colloid in the form of albumin, fresh frozen plasma, or whole blood may also be of value.

Partial correction of metabolic acidosis should be attempted. Overcorrection may lead to cerebral vasoconstriction, hypokalemia, and a leftward shift in the oxyhemoglobin dissociation curve, with decreased oxygen delivery to vital tissues. The role of corticosteroids in septic shock is controversial. Recent evidence suggests they may worsen outcome if administered to septic patients with impaired renal function.

Vasopressors are secondary to fluid replacement in importance. Administration in the face of inadequate intravascular volume will exacerbate vasoconstriction and worsen tissue hypoxia. Dopamine is the preferred agent, since it produces less renal vasoconstriction than other compounds when used in the correct dosage.

Antibiotics are selected based on the spectrum of activity necessary to cover most anticipated pathogens (see Table 30–32). They are always given intravenously to assure total and adequate absorption. A two-drug or even three-drug regimen may be necessary to assure adequate coverage of potential gram-negative and gram-positive (particularly *S. aureus* and *Streptococcus* species) pathogens based on their anticipated susceptibility patterns (see Table 30–2). One must also look for a correctable lesion, such as an abscess, an obstructing ureteral stone, or an infected intravenous site, that can be eliminated.

The prognosis in gram-negative sepsis is primarily dependent upon the severity of the host's underlying disease. Patients with rapidly fatal underlying disease (such as acute leukemia or acute renal failure) have a mortality of up to 80 per cent, compared with patients with nonfatal underlying disease (such as trauma or surgery), where the mortality is 20 per cent. Mortality increases with age, a gastrointestinal or respiratory tract source versus a genitourinary tract source, and acquisition of infection within rather than outside the hospital. Finally, prognosis is also dependent on early recognition of infection, vigorous treatment of shock, and prompt administration of an appropriate antimicrobial agent.

TOXIC SHOCK SYNDROME

Several toxin-mediated syndromes appear clinically similar to septic shock. Staphylococcal toxic shock syndrome is the most well recognized of these. Originally described in 1978, toxic shock syndrome received more widespread publicity in 1980 when its association with tampon use became evident. Despite changes in tampon use and structure, several hundred cases of toxic shock syndrome occur annually, now equally divided between menstrual and nonmenstrual cases. Nonmenstrual cases are equally divided between men and women.

Essentially, all patients with staphylococcal toxic shock syndrome have focal infection or colonization with toxin-producing strains of *S. aureus.* Such localized infections may include pharyngitis, vaginitis, proctitis, community-acquired skin and soft tissue infections, nosocomial staphylococcal wound infections, staphylococcal pneumonia complicating intravenous drug use or postinfluenza, and primary bacteremia.

The clinical manifestations of toxic shock syndrome vary from fulminant shock with multiple organ failure to milder cases manifest primarily by fever and cutaneous abnormalities. A temperature of over 102° F., diffuse erythroderma with subsequent palmar desquamation, and symptomatic hypotension occur in most patients. Diarrhea, nausea, and vomiting are common. Conjunctivitis and oral hyperemia are seen in over three quarters of patients. Myalgia is also common and frequently complicated by elevated creatinine phosphokinase (CPK) values. Central nervous system manifestations include disorientation and lethargy, but generally no focal findings or signs of meningitis. Abnormal renal and hepatic function occur in over 50 per cent of patients, and thrombocytopenia is common. Additional clinical findings of importance include headache, edema of the hands and feet, abdominal pain, and patchy hair or nail loss subsequent to recovery.

The treatment of toxic shock syndrome is primarily hemodynamic support, removal of any sequestered focus of staphylococci (such as tampon removal or abscess drainage), and the administration of an effective antistaphylococcal antibiotic. Aggressive treatment usually leads to full recovery. The risk of recurrence in menstrually associated toxic shock syndrome varies from 20 to 40 per cent and should interdict future tampon use. The role of adrenocortical steroids in the treatment of this disease has not been well studied.

The differential diagnosis of toxic shock syndrome should include other hypotensive illnesses, such as septicemic or hemorrhagic shock, and illnesses associated with similar cutaneous manifestations, such as measles, leptospirosis, scarlet fever, Kawasaki's disease, and drug eruptions. Appropriate cultures, serologic testing, history and physical exam, and appreciation of the spectrum of illness of toxic shock syndrome should allow differentiation between these various illnesses.

Sexually Transmitted Diseases

Although syphilis and gonorrhea are considered the prototypic venereal diseases, it is clear that a host of viral, bacterial, and protozoal pathogens may be transmitted by sexual activity. This is particularly true for anal sex. Furthermore, the incidence of most sexually transmitted diseases (STDs) is increasing annually despite educational programs stemming from the AIDS epidemic (see Chapter 31). Pathogens with documented sexual transmission are listed in Table 30–34. It is useful to approach the differential diagnosis of STDs by the manifestations of infection (Table 30–35), whether they be exudative or ulcerative.

GONORRHEA

Although second in frequency to nongonococcal urethritis in the male, gonorrhea remains a major public health problem with serious systemic consequences, particularly in the female. Seventy per cent of infected females are asymptomatic and represent the reservoir for the heterosexual population. About 10 per cent of heterosexual males are also asymptomatic, as are homosexual males who engage in anal intercourse. The disease transmits almost entirely by sexual means, since the gonococcus is unable to survive even

Table 30–34. SEXUALLY TRANSMITTED DISEASES

Agent	Disease
Bacteria	
Neisseria gonorrhoeae	Gonorrhea
Treponema pallidum	Syphilis
Haemophilus ducreyi	Chancroid
Calymmatobacterium granulomatis	Granuloma inguinale
Gardnerella (prev. *Corynebacterium* or *Haemophilus*) *vaginalis*	Nonspecific vaginitis
Shigella, Salmonella	Gastroenteritis
Campylobacter species (prev. *Vibrio*)	Gastroenteritis, proctitis
Mycobacterium tuberculosis	Genital tuberculosis
Chlamydia/Ureaplasma	
C. trachomatis (serotypes L_1-L_3)	Lymphogranuloma venereum
C. trachomatis (serotypes D-K)	Nongonococcal urethritis, cervicitis
U. (prev. *Mycoplasma*) *urealyticum*	Nongonococcal urethritis
Viruses	
Herpes simplex virus	Herpes genitalis
Papillomavirus	Genital warts
Poxvirus (?)	Molluscum contagiosum
Cytomegalovirus (CMV)	CMV mononucleosis
Hepatitis B virus	Hepatitis B (serum hepatitis)
Human immunodeficiency virus	AIDS
Fungi	
Candida species	Vaginitis; balanitis
Parasites	
Trichomonas vaginalis	Trichomonas vaginitis
Giardia lamblia	Giardiasis
Entamoeba histolytica	Amebiasis
Enterobius vermicularis	Vaginitis (pinworm)
Phthirus pubis	Pediculosis pubis
Sarcoptes scabei	Scabies

short periods outside the human body. Uninfected women exposed to infected men during sexual intercourse will become infected 50 to 70 per cent of the time. In contrast, only 20 to 30 per cent of men exposed to infected women will become infected. Gonorrhea is an illness that fails to confer immunity; therefore, reinfection is the rule.

Local symptoms in the male occur after an incubation period of 3 to 7 days. Typically, urethritis is manifest by burning on urination and a spontaneous, purulent penile discharge. Urethritis uncommonly occurs in the female. Individuals engaging in anal intercourse may develop proctitis, although the majority of rectally infected individuals are asymptomatic. Proctitis is manifested by tenesmus and pain or burning on defecation. Anoscopy reveals punctate ulcerations and intraluminal pus. Most anal symptoms in individuals engaging in rectal intercourse are due to local trauma or fissures rather than proctitis. Pharyngitis may occur in individuals engaging in oral/genital sex, although many of these individuals will also be asymptomatic. There are no characteristic clinical manifestations of gonococcal pharyngitis, and the appearance of the throat is variable. Conjunctivitis may occur due to direct inoculation of gonococcus into the conjunctivae. Rapid progression and corneal ulceration ensue if treatment is not prompt.

Table 30–35. MANIFESTATIONS OF SEXUALLY TRANSMISSIBLE DISEASE

Diseases Manifest by Discharges
- Gonorrhea
- Nongonococcal urethritis

Diseases Manifest by Ulcers
- Syphilis
- Herpes simplex
- Chancroid
- Granuloma inguinale

Diseases Manifest by Nodules
- Molluscum contagiosum
- Genital warts
- Secondary syphilis (condylomata lata)

Failure of treatment in the male may result in spread of infection to the posterior urethra, prostate, seminal vesicles, and epididymis. Untreated urethritis may result in urethral stricture and the later sequelae of obstructive uropathy.

Localized cervical and vaginal colonization is the rule in infected females. Neither vaginitis nor urethritis occurs. Spread to the uterine cavity and fallopian tubes may follow, particularly at the time of menstruation, and result in acute salpingitis and pelvic peritonitis. The exact role of the gonococcus in the production of pelvic inflammatory disease, however, is unclear. Anaerobes and enteric gram-negative bacilli may be more important and lead to superinfection, abscess formation, tubal stricture, and sterility. Gonococci are rarely recovered from such infections.

Gonococci may disseminate in both males and females. Systemic gonococcal infection, however, is rarely seen in males, owing to the local symptoms that prompt early treatment in contrast to the asymptomatic nature of infection in females. Gonococcemia may be manifest as the gonococcal arthritis-dermatitis syndrome. Bacteremia with fever, chills, and characteristic hemorrhagic, vesicopustular skin lesions occurs (Plate II). Tenosynovitis, particularly of the small joints of the hands and feet, is seen frequently. Skin lesions are painful and may evolve into a necrotic eschar. Blood cultures are usually positive and joint fluid aspirates are negative in this syndrome but organisms may be recovered from the skin lesions. Occasionally, monarticular arthritis is the presenting manifestation of disseminated gonococcal infection, and the skin lesions, bacteremia, and tenosynovitis are not present. In these cases, gonococci can usually be recovered from the joint fluid but not the blood.

Disseminated gonococcal infection may produce endocarditis, although this is very uncommon. Perihepatic involvement may occur by direct spread from infected fallopian tubes. Right upper quadrant pain and tenderness are the manifestations, making the disorder difficult to distinguish from acute cholecystitis. Blood cultures are usually negative, but fine, filmy, banjo-string adhesions may be seen on peritoneoscopy. This presentation is frequently referred to as the Fitzhugh-Curtis syndrome and should be considered in the differential diagnosis of right upper quadrant pain and fever in sexually active women.

Gonococcal ophthalmia, as it may occur in the adult, may also occur in the newborn who acquires the microorganism from contact with infected vaginal secretions. The disease is prevented by prophylactic administration of erythromycin or silver nitrate eye drops. Genital gonococcal infections in children are usually due to sexual abuse by an infected adult, usually a relative.

Gram's stain of urethral exudate is an accepted technique for diagnosis of gonorrhea in the male. In the female, however, only a minority of cases can be diagnosed correctly because of confusing normal flora. Cultures should be taken from the cervix, rectum (not contaminated with feces), and pharynx of women suspected of having gonorrhea. Culture of urethral exudate in males is adequate to confirm the diagnosis, except in homosexual males from whom oral and anal cultures should also be obtained. In disseminated infection, cultures of cul-de-sac fluid, joint fluid, and aspirates of skin lesions should be performed and inoculated onto chocolate agar. Cultures taken from the areas with normal flora (pharynx, rectum, or female genital tract) should be inoculated onto Thayer-Martin, Transgrow, or other selective media to inhibit growth of competing normal bacterial flora. Cultures should be inoculated promptly and placed in a high carbon dioxide atmosphere. Refrigeration of specimens will kill the gonococcus.

In recent years, *N. gonorrhoeae* has become more resistant to penicillin. Even relatively sensitive strains require high doses of penicillin for cure. However, strains of gonococci that disseminate tend to remain more penicillin-sensitive than those causing purely local disease. In the last 10 years, many strains of *N. gonorrhoeae* have become totally resistant to penicillin by production of a beta-lactamase (penicillinase). These PPNG strains comprise up to 5 per cent of isolates in some regions and account for 1 to 2 per cent of isolates nationwide. For this reason, penicillin G can no longer be considered the drug of choice for the treatment of infections due to *N. gonorrhoeae.*

Treatment regimens are outlined in Table 30–36. Men and women *exposed* to gonorrhea should be examined, cultured, and treated at once with any of the primary treatment regimens. Ceftriaxone is preferred, particularly in individuals with anorectal or pharyngeal infection. Pharyngeal infections are difficult to treat, and high failure rates are reported with both oral amoxicillin and intramuscular spectinomycin. Gonococcal regimens should be followed by tetracycline or doxycycline for 1 week to eliminate potentially coexistent *Chlamydia* or *Ureaplasma* infection. Follow-up cultures should be obtained 3 to 7 days after completion of treatment for all cases of uncomplicated gonorrhea. Long-acting forms of penicillin G (i.e., benzathine penicillin) are effective for the treatment of syphilis but have no role in the treatment of gonorrhea. Oral penicillin V is similarly ineffective. Patients with incubating syphilis are likely to be cured by all treatment regimens for uncomplicated gonorrhea except for spectinomycin, and serologic tests for syphilis should be done for all patients with suspected STD.

In treating pelvic inflammatory disease, early hospitalization and intravenous therapy should be considered to prevent tubal scarring and infertility or when an abscess is suspected, when the patient is toxic or unable to take oral medication, or when the diagnosis is uncertain. An intrauterine device, if present, should be removed. For disseminated gonococcal infection, hospitalization is indicated for those who may be unreliable or who have uncertain diagnoses. Open drainage of infected joints other than the hip is not indicated. Follow-up examination and cultures should be performed in all instances.

CHLAMYDIA INFECTIONS

With the advent of reliable culture techniques, enzyme immunoassay, and monoclonal antibody methods, the spectrum of disease produced by *Chlamydia* has broadened. These organisms are obligate intracellular bacteria divisible into two species: *Chlamydia psittaci,* the cause of psittacosis, and *Chlamydia trachomatis.* Several serovars of *C. trachomatis,* designated A through L, have been described and are responsible for a multitude of clinical conditions including trachoma, nongonococcal urethritis, mucopurulent cervicitis, inclusion conjunctivitis, proctitis, epididymitis, prostatitis, salpingitis, endometritis, perihepatitis, neonatal conjunctivitis and pneumonitis, and lymphogranuloma venereum.

Nongonococcal urethritis (NGU) is probably more prevalent than gonorrhea. However, it is not a reportable disease so the exact incidence is unknown; estimates range from 3 to 5 million new cases annually. *C. trachomatis* is isolated from 50 per cent of NGU cases, although many men with *Chlamydia* urethritis are asymptomatic. Symptoms, when present, are those of dysuria and discharge. The urethral exudate is usually scant and mucoid in contrast to the spontaneous and purulent discharge of gonorrhea. Epididymitis and prostatitis may follow untreated infection. Concurrent conjunctivitis due to self-inoculation is not uncommon.

Chlamydial infections in women produce a mucopurulent cervicitis and acute dysuria (the urethral syndrome). Dysuria due to *Chlamydia* causes pyuria without bacteriuria. Mucopurulent cervicitis is diagnosed by the presence of mucopurulent endocervical secretions seen on swab and confirmed on Gram's stain, together with cervical erythema and friability. As a consequence of ascending infection, *Chlamydia* are thought to cause up to 50 per cent of the 1 million

Table 30–36. RECOMMENDED TREATMENT SCHEDULES FOR THE TREATMENT OF GONORRHEA AND PELVIC INFLAMMATORY DISEASE*

Condition	Drug of Choice	Dosage	Alternatives
Gonorrhea			
Urethritis or cervicitis	Ceftriaxone	125–250 mg. I.M. once	Amoxicillin 3 gm. P.O. once plus probenecid 1 gm. P.O. once Spectinomycin 2 gm. I.M. once
Rectal	Ceftriaxone	125–250 mg. I.M. once	Procaine penicillin G 4.8 M.U. I.M. once plus probenecid 1 gm. P.O. once Spectinomycin 2 gm. I.M. once
Pharyngeal	Ceftriaxone	125–250 mg. I.M. once	Procaine penicillin G 4.8 M.U. I.M. once plus probenecid 1 gm. P.O. once Trimethoprim-sulfamethoxazole 9 tabs daily in one dose for 5 days
Ophthalmia (adults)	Ceftriaxone plus saline irrigation	1 gm. I.M. daily for 5 days	Penicillin G 10 M.U. I.V. daily for 5 days plus saline irrigation
Bacteremia and arthritis	Ceftriaxone	1 gm. I.V. daily for 7 days	Penicillin G 10 M.U. I.V. daily for 3 days then amoxicillin 500 mg. P.O. q.i.d. for 4 days Doxycycline 100 mg. P.O. b.i.d. for 7 days
Neonatal			
Ophthalmia	Cefotaxime plus saline irrigation OR ceftriaxone plus saline irrigation	25 mg./kg. q. 8–12 h. for 7 days 125 mg. I.M. once	Penicillin G 100,000 U/kg./day I.V. in 4 doses for 7 days plus saline irrigation
Arthritis and septicemia	Cefotaxime	25–50 mg./kg. q. 8–12 h. I.V. for 10–14 days	Penicillin G 100,000 U/kg./day I.V. in 4 doses for 7 days
Children			
Urogenital, rectal, and pharyngeal	Ceftriaxone	125 mg. I.M. once	Amoxicillin 50 mg./kg. P.O. once plus probenecid 25 mg./kg. (max. 1 gm.) Procaine penicillin G 100,000 U/kg. I.M. once plus probenecid 25 mg./kg. (max. 1 gm.) once Spectinomycin 40 mg./kg. I.M. once
Arthritis and septicemia	Ceftriaxone OR Cefotaxime	50 mg./kg./day (max. 2 gm.) I.V. for 7 days 50 mg./kg./day I.V. for 7 days	Penicillin G 150,000 U/kg./day I.V. for 7 days Tetracycline (over 8 y.o.) 10 mg./kg. P.O. q.i.d. for 7 days
Chlamydia trachomatis Infection			
Urethritis or cervicitis	Doxycycline OR Erythromycin	100 mg. b.i.d. for 7 days 500 mg. P.O. q.i.d. for 7 days	Sulfisoxazole 500 mg. P.O. q.i.d. for 10 days
Neonatal			
Ophthalmia	Erythromycin	12.5 mg./kg. P.O. or I.V. q.i.d. for 14 days	
Pneumonia	Erythromycin	12.5 mg./kg. P.O. or I.V. q.i.d. for 14 days	Sulfisoxazole 100 mg./kg./day P.O. or I.V. in divided doses (after 4 weeks of age)
Epididymitis	Ceftriaxone followed by doxycycline	250 mg. I.M. once 100 mg. P.O. b.i.d. for 10 days	Amoxicillin 3 gm. P.O. once plus probenecid 1 gm. P.O. once followed by doxycycline 100 mg. P.O. b.i.d. for 10 days
Pelvic Inflammatory Disease			
Outpatients	Cefoxitin plus probenecid OR ceftriaxone, either one followed by doxycycline	2 gm. I.M. once 1 gm. P.O. once 250 mg. I.M. once 100 mg. P.O. b.i.d. for 10 days	
Hospitalized patients	Cefoxitin plus doxycycline followed by doxycycline	2 gm. I.V. q.i.d. 100 mg. I.V. b.i.d. until improvement 100 mg. P.O. b.i.d. to complete 10 days	Clindamycin 600 mg. I.V. q.i.d. plus gentamicin 2 mg./kg. once followed by gentamicin 1.5 mg./kg. I.V. q. 8 h. until improvement, followed by clindamycin 450 mg. P.O. q.i.d. to complete 10–14 days

*Modified from: Centers for Disease Control: Sexually transmitted disease treatment guidelines, 1988. Morbidity and Mortality Weekly Report 30:5, 1988.

annual cases of pelvic inflammatory disease in the United States. In this role, it is implicated as a cause of infertility, premature delivery, postpartum and neonatal infections.

The diagnosis of chlamydial infection must be made primarily on clinical grounds since laboratory methods are imperfect. Cell culture, although most sensitive, is not widely available. Direct fluorescent antibody testing is useful but of low sensitivity, particularly in screening low-risk populations. Enzyme immunoassay is more sensitive but less specific; false positive tests occur in women with heavy bacterial growth. Serologic testing is rarely useful.

Drugs of choice for the treatment of *Chlamydia* infections are tetracycline or erythromycin, the former being preferred. Sulfonamides are also useful. Tetracycline hydrochloride 500 mg. four times a day or doxycycline 100 mg. twice a day for a minimum of 7 days is required for uncomplicated infections or documented exposure. Longer courses of therapy should be given for complicated infections, such as epididymitis or salpingitis.

SYPHILIS

Syphilis remains a widespread disease. Reported cases of both primary and secondary syphilis have shown no decrease in recent years. In 1986, 28,000 cases were reported to public health authorities, an increase of over 17 per cent since 1976. Most cases are reported from large urban areas.

Primary syphilis occurs 10 to 90 days after sexual contact. The typical chancre is single, indurated, and nonpainful. Regional lymphadenopathy is usually present. Although most occur in the genital area, lesions may occur on the lip, tongue, breast, and elsewhere. Dark-field examination is positive, but serologic tests do not become reactive until the chancre begins to heal. The FTA-absorption test becomes positive earliest, but by the fourth week, both the VDRL (ART and RPR tests) and FTA absorption tests are usually reactive.

Secondary syphilis develops 2 to 6 weeks after the primary infection. It is manifest by a flu-like illness with headache, malaise, generalized lymphadenopathy, arthralgia, and rash. Cutaneous lesions are bilateral, involve the palms and soles, and are nonpruritic; they may be pustular, anular, or follicular. Mucous membranes are involved, with a thin gray exudate (mucous patches) or broad-based, wart-like lesion (condyloma lata). Such lesions are teeming with spirochetes and highly contagious. Nephritis, meningitis, uveitis, and hepatitis may also occur at this stage. Lesions resolve spontaneously in 2 to 5 weeks, although relapses may occur within the first 2 years. Serology is always positive in secondary syphilis, the VDRL frequently in high titer.

Late syphilis may be symptomatic or asymptomatic. In asymptomatic late syphilis, there are no signs or symptoms of infection. Diagnosis is made by routine serology. Symptomatic late syphilis may present with skin lesions, usually gummas, which are painless, ulcerating lesions particularly of the face and palate. Skeletal lesions, either Charcot joints or osteomyelitis, may occur. Cardiovascular syphilis, involving the aortic ring with the development of aortic regurgitation, is well appreciated.

Central nervous system involvement in late syphilis may be meningeal (most commonly seen in early late or secondary syphilis), parenchymatous (as tabes dorsalis or general paresis), or asymptomatic. Meningeal involvement is associated with a positive serology in both the blood and spinal fluid and is reversible with treatment. Late asymptomatic parenchymatous syphilis is frequently associated with a negative serum VDRL, and a high index of suspicion must, therefore, be maintained to make the diagnosis. The spinal fluid VDRL will frequently be positive. Response to treatment is variable in late parenchymatous central nervous system infections.

The diagnosis of syphilis in the primary stage is made by dark-field examination. In subsequent stages, the diagnosis is made on clinical grounds and by serology. Two basic tests are available: (1) nonspecific antibody tests directed against cross-reacting lipid antigens of the treponema and (2) specific antitreponemal antibody tests. The VDRL (or its simplified counterparts the ART and RPR) is the standard flocculation test for nontreponemal antibody. It is used as a screening test in most laboratories. The FTA-ABS test (fluorescent treponemal antibody absorption) test is the specific antitreponemal antibody test most frequently used (Table 30–37).

The FTA-ABS test is positive in 85 per cent of late primary syphilis and in 99 per cent of other forms. The FTA-ABS may be positive in early syphilis when VDRL is still negative, and in late syphilis, VDRL may become negative while the FTA-ABS will remain positive. The VDRL titer is most useful in following response to treatment, but patients with long-standing positive serologies may remain positive even in the face of adequate treatment (i.e., they are serofast). As with all serologic reactions, the VDRL is subject to false positive tests (Table 30–38). Although false positive reactions of the FTA-ABS do occur, they are rare, are associated with abnormal globulins, and can frequently be distinguished technically from true positives. A positive VDRL, ART, or RPR in the face of a negative FTA-ABS test is due to disease other than syphilis and is referred to as a biologic false positive.

Table 30–37. RESULTS OF COMMONLY USED SEROLOGIC TESTS FOR SYPHILIS

Test	Frequency of Positivity by Stage (%) Primary	Secondary	Late
VDRL	70	99	70
ART or RPR	80	99	70
FTA-ABS	85	100	98

Table 30–38. CONDITIONS REPORTED TO CAUSE FALSE-POSITIVE VDRL

Addison's disease	Lymphosarcoma
Atopic dermatitis	Malaria
Brucellosis	Measles
Chancroid	Mumps
Cirrhosis	Multiple myeloma
Coccidioidomycosis	Myocardial infarction
Cryoglobulinemia	Narcotic addiction
Dermatomyositis	Pellagra
Diabetes mellitus	Pemphigus
Diphtheria	Pernicious anemia
Epstein-Barr virus infection	Pneumonia
Acute glomerulonephritis	Pregnancy
Hashimoto's thyroiditis	Polyarteritis nodosa
Hemolytic anemia	Rat-bite fever
Hepatitis	Relapsing fever
Histoplasmosis	Rheumatic fever
Human immunodeficiency virus infection	Sarcoidosis
Idiopathic thrombocytopenic purpura	Scleroderma
Infectious mononucleosis	Subacute bacterial endocarditis
Influenza	Systemic lupus erythematosus
Leprosy	Trypanosomiasis
Leptospirosis	Tuberculosis
Lymphocytic leukemia	Typhus
Lymphogranuloma venereum	Vaccinia
	Varicella
	Vincent's angina

Penicillin is the preferential agent for the treatment of all forms of syphilis (Table 30–39). The VDRL will usually become negative 6 to 12 months after effective treatment of primary syphilis and 1 to 2 years after treatment of secondary syphilis but may remain positive for life after treatment of late syphilis. Since penetration of the central nervous system by benzathine penicillin is essentially nil, intravenous aqueous penicillin G is preferred for the treatment of active neurosyphilis.

Approximately 50 per cent of patients with early forms of syphilis will develop fever, malaise, myalgia, and a flare of cutaneous lesions after penicillin treatment. This is referred to as a Jarisch-Herxheimer reaction and is due to systemic release of treponemal antigens. Very early treatment of primary or incubating syphilis, before the development of a significant antibody response, may create a negative serology and an individual who has no protective antibody.

HERPES SIMPLEX INFECTIONS

It is estimated that genital herpes occurs with an annual incidence of 700,000 primary cases and 20 million recurrences. Most infections are caused by herpes simplex virus 2, although herpes simplex virus 1 has become increasingly common, accounting for 10 to 15 per cent of all cases.

The manifestations of illness are multiple vesicular lesions that develop on the external or internal genitalia with an incubation period of approximately 1 week. Vesicles in moist areas ulcerate and become exquisitely painful. First infections are usually more severe and may be accompanied by considerable fever and autonomic neuropathy with urinary retention. Dysuria, pain, and paresthesias are the local manifestations in women, whereas in men the lesions are less prone to ulcerate and are less painful. Active genital herpes in the parturient female is an indication for cesarean section, since the morbidity and mortality of disseminated herpes infection in the neonate is extremely high.

The diagnosis of herpes simplex is made by observing the characteristically multiple vesicles or ulcers and by examining Giemsa-stained scrapings or Pap smears made from the base of the lesions. Intranuclear inclusions or multinucleated giant cells can be seen. Viral cultures are useful to confirm the diagnosis.

Acyclovir is the only effective therapy for HSV infections currently available. It is most efficacious by the parenteral route, for primary infections, and

Table 30–39. RECOMMENDED TREATMENT SCHEDULES FOR SYPHILIS

Stage	Preferred Treatment	Alternative Treatment
Early syphilis (primary, secondary, latent less than 1 year duration)	Benzathine penicillin G, 2.4 million units intramuscularly once	Tetracycline hydrochloride 0.5 gm. orally 4 times a day for 15 days OR Erythromycin, 0.5 gm. orally 4 times a day for 15 days
Late syphilis (more than 1 year's duration, cardiovascular)	Benzathine penicillin G, 2.4 million units intramuscularly weekly for 3 doses	Tetracycline hydrochloride, 0.5 gm. 4 times a day orally for 30 days OR Erythromycin, 0.5 gm. 4 times a day orally for 30 days
Neurosyphilis	Aqueous penicillin G, 12–24 million units/day intravenously divided every 4 hours for 10 days	Tetracycline hydrochloride, 0.5 gm. 4 times a day orally for 30 days OR Erythromycin, 0.5 gm. 4 times a day orally for 30 days
Congenital syphilis	Aqueous penicillin G, 25,000 units/kg. intramuscularly or intravenously twice a day for 10 days OR Procaine penicillin G, 50,000 units/kg. intramuscularly daily for 10 days	

for prevention of frequent recurrences. It is of questionable value for treatment of symptomatic recurrences but does decrease viral shedding, perhaps important for minimizing transmission. Current treatment recommendations are listed in Table 30–40.

PAPILLOMAVIRUS INFECTIONS

Genital human papillomavirus (HPV) infections are increasing in frequency and are now the most common viral STD, twice as common as genital herpes virus infections. With recognition that most genital HPV infections are subclinical, their epidemiologic and clinical significance has been redefined.

Long considered a nuisance STD, it is now clear that certain DNA types of HPV possess tissue specificity and potential oncogenicity. HPV types 6 and 11 are most prevalent in exophytic genital warts and HPV types 16 and 18 are most commonly associated with cervical neoplasia. Indeed, the prevalence of HPV type 16 or 18 in cervical dysplasia (CIN I) is 70 per cent, and in carcinoma-in-situ (CIN III), it is 85 per cent. The prevalence of HPV DNA in sexually active females is high even without clinical disease: 5 to 15 per cent of cytologically (Pap smear) normal women possess HPV DNA in cervical cells.

The spectrum of clinical illness produced by HPV ranges from asymptomatic infection to exuberantly hypertrophic warts. Condylomata acuminata are usually flesh colored but may be hyperpigmented, with plaques, papules, and pointed (acuminate) projections. Flatter, sessile lesions may also occur and are easily overlooked. Warts occur predominantly on the vulva and cervix in females and on the penile shaft in males. Anal and oral warts are seen in relationship to specific sexual practices. HPV infections of the cervix and vagina are usually subclinical. Their presence is suspected by colposcopic application of 3 to 5 per cent acetic acid, resulting in the appearance of white lesions, or by cytology. Serologic studies and direct antibody staining of infected tissues are insensitive and of limited availability.

All modes of treatment suffer from a high relapse rate after apparently successful therapy. Podophyllin, a resin extract of the May apple, has been most widely used but is followed by a relapse rate of 60 to 70 per cent. Cryotherapy is more successful but usually requires several treatments for cure. Surgery or laser ablation are useful adjuncts but recurrence rates are also high, particularly for laser therapy. The roles of 5-fluorouracil and interferon compared to or combined with standard therapy are not clear.

CHANCROID

Chancroid is a localized, ulcerative lesion of the genitalia of increasing frequency. The ulcers are usually multiple, painful, and soft with associated adenopathy. Mucous membranes are not affected, and the disease is caused by a fastidious gram-negative rod, *Haemophilus ducreyi*. The organism is rarely grown or cultured but can be suspected on Gram's stain. The treatment of choice is ceftriaxone or trimethoprim-sulfamethoxazole. The major differential diagnosis is syphilis, which, in contrast, to chancroid, is usually painless and associated with a positive darkfield examination.

LYMPHOGRANULOMA VENEREUM

Lymphogranuloma venereum is a chronic lymphadenitis caused by *Chlamydia trachomatis*. Lymphadenopathy, fever, chills, arthralgias, and headache are

Table 30–40. TREATMENT RECOMMENDATIONS FOR GENITAL HERPES SIMPLEX INFECTIONS*

1. Immunocompetent host	
(a) First episodes	• Acyclovir, 200 mg. P.O. 5 times/day for 10 days, or • Acyclovir, 5 mg./kg. body weight IV q. 8 h. for 5–7 days (for severe local or systemic symptoms, neurologic complications, or dissemination)
(b) Symptomatic recurrences of genital HSV infection	• Acyclovir, 200 mg. P.O. 5 times/day for 5 days, if associated with significant symptoms (of uncertain benefit)
(c) Suppression of recurrent genital HSV infection	• Acyclovir, 200 mg. P.O. 3–5 times daily for up to 12 months, intended for patients with frequent (> 6 times per year) symptomatic recurrences
2. Immunosuppressed host	
(a) First episodes or symptomatic recurrences	• Acyclovir, 200–400 mg. P.O. 5 times/day for 7–10 days, or • Acyclovir, 5 mg./kg. body weight IV q. 8 h. for 7 days
(b) Suppression of reactivation of HSV infection during periods of immunosuppression	• Acyclovir, 2.5–5 mg./kg. body weight IV q. 8 h. for high-risk periods
3. Genital HSV infection during pregnancy	• Acyclovir not indicated

*Modified from Webb, D. H., and Fife, K. H.: Genital herpes simplex virus infections. Inf. Dis. Clin. N.A., *1*:97, 1987.

prominent. Obliterative lymphadenitis of the penis or vulva, and rectal strictures develop. The diagnosis is made serologically and clinically, and treatment of choice is with tetracycline 2 grams/day for 2 weeks.

GRANULOMA INGUINALE

Granuloma inguinale is a chronic granulomatous disease of the skin and lymphatics of the groin and perineum. Lesions have a foul odor with a beefy-red, ulcerated appearance. Adenitis is less impressive than with lymphogranuloma venereum. The diagnosis is made clinically and histologically by the appearance of Donovan bodies in large mononuclear cells obtained from biopsied lesions. The disease is rare but responds to prolonged administration of tetracycline.

MOLLUSCUM CONTAGIOSUM

Molluscum contagiosum is a viral illness presenting with grouped, umbilicated papules on genital skin. Occasionally, these lesions may appear on the limbs or trunk and are spread by contact, with an incubation period of 6 to 8 weeks. The lesions are painless and asymptomatic. The diagnosis is made clinically and established by crushing a lesion and examining the contents for intracytoplasmic inclusions. Treatment is by desiccation or cryosurgery, although lesions usually regress spontaneously over several weeks to months.

VAGINITIS

Vulvovaginitis in females may be due to a variety of organisms. *C. albicans, Trichomonas vaginalis,* and *Gardnerella vaginalis* are most common. Clinical distinction between these various etiologies may be difficult, and smears and cultures are helpful in making a definitive diagnosis. Mixed infections are frequent. Although the type of discharge varies from one individual to another, *Trichomonas* generally causes a profuse, frothy, malodorous discharge, and *Candida* causes a scant, thick, and cheesy-white exudate.

Smears of vaginal exudate will show yeast and pseudohyphae in vaginal candidiasis and clue cells, vaginal epithelial cells coated with masses of gram-variable coccobacilli, in *Gardnerella* infection (also known as nonspecific vaginitis or bacterial vaginosis). Cultures are necessary to rule out *N. gonorrhoeae.* The treatment of *Trichomonas* and *Gardnerella* vaginitis is with metronidazole. Treatment of *Candida* is best accomplished with intravaginal nystatin, miconazole, or ketoconazole. Oral treatment with ketoconazole is reserved for refractory cases due to its potential hepatotoxicity.

Skin and Soft Tissue Infections

Skin and soft tissue infections are an important cause of visits to the family physician. They can best be classified by their clinical appearance and can be grouped together as pyodermas, a term signifying bacterial infections of the skin and sometimes underlying subcutaneous tissues.

Impetigo is a disease of the superficial layers of skin. It begins as a vesicular eruption, which becomes pustular, then crusted. Many are mixed infections, although *S. pyogenes* (group A) is implicated in most cases. *S. aureus* is involved in 10 to 20 per cent. The presence of bulli should suggest infection primarily due to *S. aureus.* Impetiginous lesions may occasionally be confused with herpes simplex, particularly when they occur around the lips and chin. Most impetigo occurs in children and is probably precipitated by a skin abrasion or insect bite. A nonsuppurative complication of concern is acute poststreptococcal glomerulonephritis. Strains of group A streptococci causing skin infections are different serologic types from those causing pharyngeal infection, and they do not, in general, cause acute rheumatic fever.

Furunculosis is usually due to *S. aureus.* Infections may vary from a small pimple to a deep, multipocketed carbuncle extending into the subcutaneous fat. Furuncles and carbuncles occur at areas of perspiration and friction, such as the neck, axillae, thighs, and buttocks. The lesions are more common in individuals with diabetes or obesity, in those receiving corticosteroids, and in individuals with defects of phagocytic cell function. Whereas furuncles are well localized and may drain spontaneously, carbuncles are more indurated and may spread in deep tissue planes. Bacteremia may accompany the latter.

Erysipelas is a superficial infection of the skin with extensive lymphatic involvement, usually due to group A streptococci. It occurs more often in infants, children, and the elderly. There is frequently an antecedent upper respiratory tract infection, and the lesion tends to reoccur in the same site. Erysipelas is an expanding, red, edematous lesion with a sharply raised border. Leukocytosis is common, and bacteremia may be present. Streptococci may be cultured from the advancing edge of the lesion.

Cellulitis is a spreading infection of deep skin layers usually caused by *S. aureus* or group A streptococcus. There is frequently a history of trauma with a puncture wound or laceration. The patient complains of local tenderness, erythema, and pain. Fever, chills, and malaise are frequent. Ascending lymphangitis or regional adenopathy may also be present. Occasionally, septic thrombophlebitis may occur.

Under certain circumstances organisms other than staphylococci and streptococci may cause cellulitis. *Erysipelothrix* causes cellulitis after handling contaminated fish or pork products. Gram-negative bacteria such as *E. coli* or *Proteus* may be involved after abdominal or perineal surgery or, together with anaerobes, in cellulitis associated with foot ulcers. *Aeromonas hydrophila* is an important cause of cellulitis after injuries in fresh water. Injuries associated with salt water activity may result in cellulitis due to *Vibrio* species. Cellulitis associated with cat or dog bites, particularly if ascending lymphangitis is present, is likely to be due to *Pasteurella multocida.* Cellulitis from human bites involves anaerobic bacteria such as *Fusobacterium* as well as staphylococci or streptococci. Culture and Gram's stain of the lesions, particularly if there is a history of trauma, will help to elucidate the pathogen(s) and allow appropriate and specific therapy.

Certain skin lesions are accompanied by extensive necrosis, marked systemic toxicity, and rapid progression. The classification of these necrotizing infections is sometimes difficult because of the multiple organisms involved and their varied clinical presentation. An attempt at classification is shown in Table 30–41. Necrotizing infections frequently follow contaminated wounds or abdominal or perineal surgery. Predisposing factors in addition to surgery include diabetes, devitalized tissue, and blunt trauma with hematoma infection. Multiple organisms are frequently involved and utmost attempts should be made to define the infecting pathogens by biopsy or tissue aspiration, Gram's stain, and blood cultures. The presence of gas within the wound does not necessarily imply *Clostridia* (Table 30–41). The majority of gas-forming infections are nonclostridial, owing to a mixed flora of anaerobes, microaerophilic streptococci, and enteric gram-negative bacilli.

The treatment of skin and subcutaneous infections is dictated by their depth and severity. Superficial infections, such as impetigo and erysipelas, usually respond to conservative therapy with penicillin. In the penicillin-allergic patient, erythromycin or clindamycin is usually effective.

Surgical drainage alone is frequently adequate for the treatment of furuncles and carbuncles. If antibiotics are necessary, an oral penicillinase-resistant penicillin, such as cloxacillin, is the drug of choice, since staphylococci are the most common pathogens. In the penicillin-allergic patient, erythromycin, tetracycline, clindamycin, or a cephalosporin may be used.

The treatment of cellulitis depends upon the pathogen. Since a variety of microorganisms may be present, a thorough history and Gram's stain of wound exudate will be valuable in selecting appropriate initial therapy. All such lesions should be cultured aerobically and anaerobically. Empiric antimicrobial therapy should be directed at staphylococci and streptococci if no other pathogens are suspect. In bite wounds, infection with mouth anaerobes must be considered and all human bite victims should receive prophylactic antibiotics.

The treatment of necrotizing skin and subcutaneous infections is also dependent upon definition of the pathogens. Urgent surgical debridement is an absolute essential. All necrotic tissue must be excised and fasciotomies are crucial to decompress and drain swollen fascial compartments if infection extends beneath the subcutaneous tissue. Antibiotic therapy should be directed at multiple pathogens (see Table 30–41) with initial therapy assisted by Gram's stain of wound exudate. Blood cultures should be obtained, since bacteremia is present in many patients with necrotizing infections. It is essential to remember that all necrotic tissue must be removed. Attempts to save nonviable tissue invariably end in disaster.

Tuberculosis

The incidence of tuberculosis has declined in recent decades owing to improvements in socioeconomic conditions and nutrition. Mortality has also declined due to the introduction of effective chemotherapy. However, it remains a prevalent disease, particularly in HIV-infected persons, immigrants, and older, nonwhite males. New cases are seen with regularity in urban populations. Although extrapulmonary tuberculosis is becoming more prevalent in HIV-infected patients, 80 to 90% of clinical tuberculosis is pulmonary disease.

PATHOPHYSIOLOGY OF TUBERCULOSIS

Most human tuberculosis is due to *Mycobacterium tuberculosis.* Infection is acquired through inhalation of aerosolized droplets of sputum known as droplet nuclei, which, when inhaled, pass through terminal airways and are deposited in the alveolae. Fomites (inanimate objects) generally do not transmit tuberculosis. Following deposition in alveolae, the bacteria multiply without extensive tissue reaction, spreading through regional lymphatics to the hilar lymph nodes and then the bloodstream. During this asymptomatic blood stream dissemination, mycobacteria are seeded to all parts of the body. Tuberculin-delayed hypersensitivity, representing the establishment of cell-mediated immunity, develops between 2 to 10 weeks after acquisition of infection.

As the primary focus resolves, infected lymph nodes may calcify, yielding a Ghon complex. Subsequent, postprimary disease is the form of tuberculosis most commonly recognized. It represents reactivation of dormant foci inoculated at the time of primary bacteremia. Reactivation usually occurs months to years after the primary infection and is usually precipitated by depression in cell-mediated immunity due to intercurrent disease or administration of immunosuppressive drugs.

CLINICAL MANIFESTATIONS OF PULMONARY TUBERCULOSIS

Primary pulmonary tuberculosis is usually a disease of children and young adults when it is manifest as a

Table 30–41. DIFFERENTIAL DIAGNOSIS OF NECROTIZING INFECTIONS OF SKIN AND SOFT TISSUE

Type of Infection	Predisposing Factors	Progression	Systemic Toxicity	Pain	Skin Changes	Odor of Exudate	Tissue Gas	Muscle Involvement	Anticipated Pathogens
Necrotizing Fasciitis (Streptococcal)	Local trauma	Rapid	Marked	Moderate to severe	Variable erythema, anesthesia, and gangrene with extensive undermining	Little	Absent	None	Group A streptococci
Necrotizing Fasciitis (Mixed)	Diabetes mellitus; abdominal surgery perirectal infection	Rapid	Marked	Moderate to severe	Variable erythema, anesthesia, and gangrene with extensive undermining, patchy necrosis of skin	Foul	Variable	None	*S. aureus*, Enterobacteriaceae, Anaerobes, *Streptococcus* species
Infected Vascular Gangrene	Diabetes mellitus; peripheral arterial insufficiency	Slow	Minimal	Variable	Discolored, often black	Foul	Frequent	Variable	Anaerobes, Enterobacteriaceae, Pseudomonas, *Staphylococcus*, enterococci
Progressive Bacterial Synergistic Gangrene	Surgery; draining sinus	Slow	Minimal	Moderate	Shaggy ulcer with gangrenous margin and erythematous periphery	Variable	Variable	None	Anaerobes, *Staphylococcus*, Enterobacteriaceae
Clostridial Cellulitis	Local trauma; surgery	May be rapid	Minimal	Mild	Minimal discoloration	Variable	Extensive	None	*Clostridium*
Nonclostridial Anaerobic Cellulitis	Diabetes mellitus; pre-existing local infection	May be rapid	Moderate	Mild	Minimal discoloration	Foul	Extensive	None	Anaerobes, Enterobacteriaceae, *Streptococcus* species, *Staphylococcus*
Clostridial Myonecrosis (Gas Gangrene)	Trauma surgery; bowel pathology	Very rapid	Prominent	Severe	Bronze discoloration, edema, bullae	Little	Slight	Yes	*Clostridium*
Nonclostridial Myositis	Trauma	Moderate	Late	Moderate	Erythema	Variable	Rare	Yes	Anaerobic streptococci, Group A streptococci, Enterobacteriaceae

flu-like illness. A brassy cough with scant sputum production, myalgias, low-grade fever, and malaise may last only a few days. Auscultation is usually unremarkable and chest x-ray studies may show a small, lower lung field infiltrate with hilar adenopathy. Acid-fast bacilli are usually not demonstrable on smears at this time, although the tuberculin skin test will be positive at the time of clinical illness.

Postprimary pulmonary disease is usually upper lobe and represents reactivation of dormant foci. However, atypical radiographic findings may include lower lobe infection, multiple lobe involvement, or primarily pleural disease. The onset is usually insidious, with constitutional symptoms predominating. Anorexia, weight loss, fatigue, fever, chills, and night sweats are common. Occasionally, patients do not realize they are ill, and the disease is incidentally discovered on a chest x-ray study. When cough and sputum production develop, they are frequently not severe at onset. Hemoptysis may occur if ulceration of a bronchial wall or blood vessel occurs. Pleuritic pain may be present if the pleura is involved in the inflammatory response.

Physical examination in postprimary disease is often of little value unless there is a large cavity or extensive pneumonitis. Laboratory data are also of little assistance, although there may be anemia, elevated sedimentation rate, and mild leukocytosis. Sputum Gram's stains are unrevealing, but acid-fast smears will be positive. Invasive techniques may be necessary to demonstrate the organism if expectorated sputum is scant or if smears are negative.

THE TUBERCULIN SKIN TEST

The tuberculin skin test contains an extract prepared from culture filtrates of tubercle bacilli. It is called purified protein derivative (PPD) and is administered intradermally to evaluate delayed hypersensitivity. Intermediate PPD (the usual skin test preparation, representing 5 tine units) is injected as 0.1 ml. of solution, and the injection site is evaluated at 48 to 72 hours for induration. Induration greater than 10 mm. is interpreted as a positive test; induration 5 to 9 mm. as a doubtful or borderline test; and less than 5 mm. as negative.

Approximately 10 per cent of normal individuals with culture- and biopsy-proven tuberculosis are skin test negative. A negative skin test, therefore, does not conclusively eliminate the diagnosis. Patients with a borderline reaction may represent prior tuberculosis exposure with no recent antigenic stimulus or atypical mycobacterial infection. A second intermediate PPD, performed 1 week after the initial test, will be positive in those individuals with true *M. tuberculosis* exposure. A significantly higher incidence of active tuberculous disease is seen in those individuals with PPD reactions in excess of 15 mm. First test strength (1 tine unit) or second test strength (250 tine units) PPDs have little role to play in the diagnosis of most forms of tuberculosis.

Interpretation of tuberculin reactions in individuals who have received bacille Calmette-Guérin (BCG) vaccine is often difficult. These patients usually have positive tests for 6 to 7 years after immunization. However, strongly positive tests more than 10 years after immunization, provided the individual has not been regularly skin tested, should suggest new infection with *M. tuberculosis*. Falsely negative tuberculin tests may be seen with old PPD preparations; intercurrent viral illness, vaccination, or other intracellular infection; inadequate application of the test material; overwhelming illness; concomitant administration of adrenal corticosteroids or immunosuppressive drugs; or diseases such as malnutrition, HIV infection, or neoplasia.

EXTRAPULMONARY TUBERCULOSIS

Although pulmonary tuberculosis accounts for most mycobacterial infection, extrapulmonary forms of the disease present both diagnostic and therapeutic problems (Table 30–42). Extrapulmonary tuberculosis represents reactivation of dormant foci seeded at the time of primary bacteremia.

Genital tuberculosis in the male is usually secondary to renal involvement with foci in the kidney, seminal vesicles, prostate, or epididymis. Genital lesions presenting with swelling and tenderness may suggest neoplasm or bacterial infection. In the female, genital tuberculosis also results from reactivation and involves the fallopian tubes most commonly. Symptoms are nonspecific, and the diagnosis is frequently made during evaluation for sterility. The majority of patients with genitourinary tuberculosis are of foreign birth and nonwhite. Fifty per cent have normal chest x-ray studies, and the diagnosis is made by biopsy of involved tissue or by urine cultures for evaluation of culture-negative pyuria. Urine cultures must be processed immediately, since storage of urine will result in death of the mycobacteria.

Table 30–42. DISTRIBUTION OF EXTRAPULMONARY TUBERCULOSIS

Location	Frequency
Lymph node	26
Pleural	18
Genitourinary	16
Miliary	14
Bone and joint	10
Meningeal	9
Peritoneal	5
Pericardial	2
Skin	1
Other	1

Lymph node tuberculosis is the most common form of extrapulmonary disease, due to reactivation of organisms hematogenously disseminated at the time of the primary pulmonary infection. The usual presentation is a painless swelling of the anterior cervical lymph nodes. Posterior cervical, mediastinal, and supraclavicular lymph nodes are less frequently involved. Fever, weight loss, and pain are usually not present. Laboratory evaluation is normal and biopsy is needed for diagnosis.

Tuberculous peritonitis is a disease of insidious onset, uncommon in the United States, with a predilection for females of foreign birth. The hallmarks are abdominal pain, fever, and exudative ascites. Organisms seed the peritoneal cavity from hematogenous spread during primary tuberculosis or from contiguous spread from infected peritoneal lymph nodes, fallopian tubes, or intestinal foci. Ascites is prominent on physical examination and an abdominal mass may be palpated due to adhesions of bowel, omentum, and mesentery. Laboratory values reveal anemia, a normal white blood cell count, and elevated sedimentation rate. As in genitourinary tuberculosis, the chest x-ray is normal in 50 per cent of patients. The diagnosis is dependent upon culture and histologic examination of the peritoneum. Ascitic fluid smears and cultures are usually negative.

Tuberculous pericarditis may develop from reactivation of dormant foci or from contiguous spread from infected mediastinal lymph nodes. The peak incidence is in the fourth to fifth decades of life and the presenting symptoms are cough, dyspnea, fever, and chest pain. Cardiomegaly is present in 95 per cent, but pulmonary infiltrates or evidence of active pulmonary tuberculosis is present in less than one half. A positive tuberculin test is present in 85 per cent, and the diagnosis is made by culture of pericardial tissue obtained at surgery.

Skeletal and joint tuberculosis is uncommon. In the United States, it is primarily a disease of older adults, intravenous drug users, or HIV-infected patients. Organisms reach the bones during the hematogenous phase of primary tuberculosis. The spine is most frequently involved, followed by the hip and knee. Immunosuppressed patients may have numerous sites of involvement, with rib involvement predominating. Tuberculous arthritis is monoarticular, characteristically involving the weight-bearing joints. Diagnosis can be established only by biopsy.

Tuberculous meningitis is a disease of older adults and young children. Headache, weight loss, night sweats, and other vague symptoms are the presenting complaints. Classic signs of meningitis may or may not be present. The cerebrospinal fluid profile is mononuclear and low glucose.

Miliary tuberculosis results from massive hematogenous dissemination of tubercle bacilli from an established, reactivated focus. Numerous lesions of the same age and size occur in many organs of the body. Characteristically, the large numbers of granulomata seen in the lungs on chest x-ray are likened to millet seeds. It is a disease of middle-aged or elderly, frequently malnourished, individuals. The presenting manifestations are vague, and the diagnosis is difficult. Weakness, anorexia, weight loss, and fever are present in over 50 per cent of patients. Nonproductive cough, fever, and weight loss are present in only 50 per cent, and the tuberculin skin test is positive in only half the patients. X-ray studies may not show miliary lesions at the outset, and sputum analysis is not helpful, since cavitary disease with endobronchial microorganisms is not present. Diagnosis must be made by lung biopsy, bone marrow biopsy, or liver biopsy obtained for histology and culture.

DISEASES DUE TO OTHER MYCOBACTERIA

It has long been known that acid-fast microorganisms other than *M. tuberculosis* can cause clinical disease. The current classification of mycobacteria and the diseases they may cause are listed in Table 30–43. *M. kansasii* may cause pulmonary disease identical to that of *M. tuberculosis,* and frequently responds to chemotherapy. *M. avium* and *M. intracellulare* are frequent contaminants in the processing of cultures for mycobacteria but can occasionally cause pulmonary infections in patients with structural lung disease, particularly pneumoconiosis and in patients infected with human immunodeficiency virus. In the latter group, infection may be manifest as bacteremia, intestinal, pulmonary, lymph node, or multiple organ involvement. *M. avium-intracellulare* is multidrug resistant and responds poorly to any chemotherapeutic regimen. *M. scrofulaceum* produces cervical adenitis, primarily in children under 2 years of age, and is treated by excision of the involved lymph nodes. Lymphadenitis in adults is usually due to *M. tuberculosis. M. marinum* is a cause of granulomatous skin lesions, nodular lymphangitis, and soft tissue infection after trauma sustained in fresh or salt water, particularly while handling fish, and usually responds well to antimicrobial therapy.

Table 30–43 CLASSIFICATION OF ATYPICAL MYCOBACTERIA AND THE DISEASES THEY MAY CAUSE

Organisms	Disease
I. Slow-growing Potential Pathogens	
A. *M. avium-intracellulare*	Lymphadenitis, pulmonary, disseminated
B. *M. scrofulaceum*	Lymphadenitis
C. *M. kansasii*	Pulmonary and disseminated
D. *M. ulcerans*	Cutaneous and soft tissue
E. *M. marinum*	Cutaneous and soft tissue
F. *M. xenopi*	Pulmonary
G. *M. szulgai*	Very rare
H. *M. simiae*	Very rare
II. Rapid-growing Potential Pathogens	
A. *M. fortuitum*	Soft tissue, bone, pulmonary
B. *M. chelonei*	Soft tissue

CHEMOTHERAPY OF TUBERCULOSIS

The goal of chemotherapy in tuberculosis is to administer enough agents to prevent the emergence of resistant microorganisms and to administer them for an adequate period of time to prevent relapse. A two-drug regimen is adequate for the treatment of most minimal to moderate active pulmonary disease due to *M. tuberculosis.* Isoniazid and rifampin are the drugs of choice and are administered for 9 months. Recent data suggest that a three-drug regimen using isoniazid, rifampin, and pyrazinamide for 2 months and isoniazid and rifampin for the remainder of a 6-month course yields equivalent cure rates. In extensive pulmonary tuberculosis, a three-drug or four-drug regimen should be used, adding either ethambutol or pyrazinamide, to continue for 9 to 12 months. Susceptibility tests should be performed on all isolates of *M. tuberculosis,* since drug resistance occurs in up to 15 per cent. Surgery is rarely necessary except in the face of multiple-drug resistance or far advanced, cavitary disease. Attention must also be given to nutrition, psychologic, and sociologic problems that coexist. Every attempt must be made to assure that the medications are taken for the prescribed amount of time, and intermittent, supervised therapy may be useful. Extrapulmonary tuberculosis is treated in the same fashion as pulmonary tuberculosis except meningitis or miliary disease that may require more aggressive therapy.

The family and contacts of active cases must be evaluated, skin tested, and/or x-rayed. Certain contacts will benefit from prophylactic treatment with isoniazid. The conversion of a negative to positive skin test carries a high risk of developing active tuberculosis within 2 years. The benefits of prophylaxis must be weighed against the risks of INH toxicity (i.e., hepatitis), which is seen in approximately 1 per cent of all patients but is lowest in individuals under 35 years of age. Administration of isoniazid seems to decrease the risk of reactivation, although its actual effect on dormant bacilli is not known. Based on these principles, isoniazid prophylaxis is recommended for those individuals listed in Table 30–44. In these patients, the risk of developing active disease is high, and INH is administered to eradicate the small numbers of actively growing bacilli living in sequestered foci. Isoniazid is administered in a dose of 300 mg./day for 1 year in these situations.

Urinary Tract Infections

Urinary tract infections are second in frequency only to respiratory tract infections as a clinical problem encountered by the practicing physician. Our understanding of the etiology, pathogenesis, and natural history of urinary tract infections has improved in recent years and a more rational approach to therapy has been developed both for the management of acute infections and for the prevention of recurrent infections.

TERMINOLOGY

Traditionally, urinary tract infections are designated as pyelonephritis or cystitis based on purely clinical criteria without objective evidence to indicate whether the infection is confined to the kidney or urinary bladder. However, in order to utilize the best therapeutic regimen, it is essential to understand where the infection is localized.

Cystitis describes a *clinical* symptom complex of dysuria, frequency, urgency, and suprapubic tenderness. This symptom complex may be caused by urethritis, bacterial infection of the bladder, local infection due to herpes simplex, or other inflammatory conditions. *Acute pyelonephritis* describes a syndrome of flank pain, costovertebral angle tenderness, and fever, with or without the symptoms of cystitis or urethritis. The clinical manifestations of pyelonephritis, however, can be mimicked by renal infarction, renal calculi, or ureteral obstruction without infection and are sometimes seen with purely bladder bacteriuria.

Table 30–44. CRITERIA FOR ISONIAZID (INH) PROPHYLAXIS

1. Recent (< 2 years) converters of any age
2. Tuberculin (intermediate PPD) reactors below age 35
3. Household contacts of infectious cases, particularly if children less than 4 years of age
4. Immunosuppressed patients with a positive intermediate PPD if never previously treated
5. Any age patient with a positive intermediate PPD and old granulomatous disease on chest x-ray (not a Ghon complex) who has never been treated

Repeated episodes of urinary tract infection may be *relapses* or *reinfections.* Relapse indicates reoccurrence of infection with the same microorganism. Reinfection means that bacteriuria is due to a microorganism different from the preceding one. Relapse suggests either inadequate therapy due to an inappropriate drug or duration of therapy, or a focus of infection not adequately treated by antimicrobial therapy alone, such as a calculus, stricture, diverticulum, or other obstructive uropathy. Reinfection implies predisposition to infection from an exogenous source without structural disease. Patients with *asymptomatic bacteriuria* have significant numbers of organisms in the urine without symptoms. *Symptomatic bacteriuria* or the *urethral syndrome,* refers to lower tract symptoms without organisms being cultured from the urine. *Chronic pyelonephritis* does not necessarily mean infection but is a pathologic diagnosis. It is most often due to vascular disease, analgesic abuse, or uric acid nephropathy. It may or may not be complicated by infection.

PATHOGENESIS OF URINARY TRACT INFECTION

Ascending infection is the major route of entry for microorganisms into the urinary tract. Hematogenous seeding of the urinary tract is a rare event, except with bacteremia due to *Staphylococcus aureus.*

The bladder itself is normally sterile. It is removed from contact with bacteria by the urethra. The distal urethra has a normal bacterial flora composed of diphtheroids, lactobacilli, streptococci, and coagulase-negative staphylococci. In females, gram-negative bacteria from the colon colonize the anterior vagina, vulva, and subsequently the distal urethra. Microorganisms then migrate into the bladder, sometimes with the help of mechanical massage as occurs in sexual intercourse. Failure to remove all of the bacteria with urination, particularly if there is residual urine in the bladder, allows multiplication of microorganisms within the bladder and subsequent infection. The short urethra of the female, its closeness to the perirectal area, and the nature of sexual intercourse make colonization of the female lower urinary tract easy.

Both bacterial and host factors are important in the pathogenesis of urinary tract infection. Although there are many different strains of *E. coli,* only a small proportion of these strains cause infection. The presence of surface proteins or adhesions on the surface of such bacteria allows them to attach to vaginal, vulvar, and uroepithelial cells. Adherence occurs by attachment of these bacterial surface proteins to epithelial cell surface glycolipid receptors (also known as the glycocalyx). Adhesive capacity is associated with the severity of infection and the propensity of a given strain of *E. coli* to cause pyelonephritis rather than cystitis or asymptomatic bacteriuria.

Host factors also contribute to the pathogenesis of, or protection from, urinary tract infection. It has been shown that *E. coli* organisms adhere more avidly to the uroepithelial cells of women who develop recurrent infection than to the cells of women who do not. Thus, a combination of bacteria with surface proteins of high affinity for certain types of epithelial cell surface receptors and the presence of such receptive cells in a specific individual will predispose to urinary tract infection.

Protective elements that inhibit growth of bacteria in the urine include a high urea concentration, high osmolality, and low pH. The bladder mucosa itself has antibacterial activity, which, combined with the removal of bacteria by urination, acts as a major protective factor. The low pH of vaginal secretions and the presence of cervicovaginal antibody in some women also protects against perineal colonization by fecal bacteria and decreases the risk of infection.

Structural abnormalities in the urinary tract interfere with these protective functions. Most important is obstruction to flow due to such conditions as urethral valves, urethral strictures, calculi, retroperitoneal fibrosis, uterine enlargement, tumors, prostatic hypertrophy, and neurologic disease. Furthermore, intraluminal lesions, such as calculi or diverticuli, may provide a residual focus in which bacteria may survive, sequestered from the effects of antimicrobial therapy.

Vesicoureteral reflux due to congenital abnormalities or bladder distention provides an easy route for bacteria to reach the kidney. Incomplete emptying of the bladder, whether due to obstruction or neurologic disease, promotes urinary stasis, allowing growth of microorganisms. Patients with obstruction or stasis often have bacteria introduced by cystoscopy or bladder catheterization—therapy producing an infection that is difficult to eradicate.

BACTERIA INVOLVED

E. coli is by far the most common pathogen. In female outpatients, more than 85 per cent of infections are due to *E. coli,* whether first-time infections or recurrences. The remaining 15 per cent of infections are due to *P. mirabilis, Klebsiella* species, and *Staphylococcus* species. It is exceedingly rare for an outpatient to develop infection due to *Pseudomonas, Serratia,* or *Enterobacter.* These organisms cause infection primarily in hospitalized patients after instrumentation of the urinary tract. Occasionally, however, these organisms may occur without instrumentation in the bedridden patient who is ill and incontinent and has received antibiotics that alter the bowel and perineal flora. Nonetheless, even as a cause of nosocomial (hospital-acquired) infection, *E. coli* is more frequent than *Klebsiella, Proteus,* or *Pseudomonas.*

It has become apparent in recent years that coagulase-negative staphylococci may produce symptomatic urinary tract infections. *S. saprophyticus* is the chief culprit and can be differentiated from *S. epidermidis* by its resistance to novobiocin. It causes bladder infections, primarily in young women, with a seasonal preponderance in the summer months. *S. aureus* present in a urine culture should prompt a search for distant foci of infection with secondary bacteremic seeding of the urinary tract. *Chlamydia* are also an important cause of lower urinary tract symptoms in young women whose urine is culture negative and who have primarily urethritis. *P. mirabilis* is most frequently seen in patients with urinary tract calculi, and its presence should be suspected in this setting. The production of a urease by *P. mirabilis* results in an abnormally high urine pH, which is a clue to its presence.

EPIDEMIOLOGY OF URINARY TRACT INFECTION

Although the prevalence of bacteriuria increases with age, urinary tract infections occur at all ages (Table 30–45). In the neonate, the frequency of bacteriuria is approximately 1 per cent. The majority of such children are male, and the bacteriuria is usually associated with congenital abnormalities of the urinary tract. During the preschool and school years, urinary tract infection is more common in girls than boys. Large surveys have found from 1 to 5 per cent prevalence of bacteriuria in female school children (see Table 30–45). Infection in either boys or girls in the preschool age is frequently associated with structural lesions or vesicoureteral reflux and may be responsible for significant renal damage in this situation.

From age 5 to 15, between 5 and 6 per cent of girls will have at least one episode of bacteriuria. Each year approximately 25 per cent of those bacteriuric will spontaneously cure, or be treated and cured, but a similar proportion will become bacteriuric. It is clear from long-term studies that bacteriuria in young girls defines a person who is at greater risk of developing symptomatic urinary tract infections later in life, but it is not clear that, in the absence of obstruc-

Table 30–45. PREVALENCE OF BACTERIURIA

Age Group	Females (%)	Males (%)
Newborn	< 0.5	0.5–1
Preschool	3–5	< 0.5
School	1–5	< 0.5
Adults 15–50 years old		< 0.5
Sexually active	4–8	
Nuns	0.5–2	
Adults over 60 years old	10–20	2–10

tion or major degrees of vesicoureteral reflux, there is any risk of permanent, clinically significant renal damage.

In adults, the frequency of bacteriuria increases with sexual activity. Between 4 and 8 per cent of sexually active young women have bacteriuria, a percentage that increases with increasing age, debility, and bed rest. At least 20 per cent of women will have a urinary tract infection at some time in their life, whether symptomatic or asymptomatic.

During pregnancy, there is a much higher frequency of symptomatic upper tract infection due to a number of physiologic changes that occur during the last trimester. Ureteral compression and hydronephrosis due to uterine enlargement and decreased ureteral peristalsis occur. In addition to the risk of renal infection, there is an increased risk of prematurity, perinatal death, stillbirth, and intrauterine growth retardation in pregnant bacteriuric women. Routine screening of all pregnant women for bacteriuria is justified, since treatment can reduce the risk of pyelonephritis and perinatal complications.

Bacteriuria is rarely seen in males between the ages of 1 and 50 in the absence of instrumentation. However, about 3 to 4 per cent of men over 70 years of age have bacteriuria, and 10 per cent of hospitalized elderly males are bacteriuric. This increase is due to the presence of prostatic disease.

CLINICAL PRESENTATIONS

The manifestations of urinary tract infection vary with age. Neonates and children younger than 2 years of age do not complain of dysuria but present with fever, failure to thrive, and vomiting. Dysuria and abdominal or back pain are complaints of children over 3 years of age. In adults, the symptoms of lower tract infection are frequent urination of small amounts, urgency, dysuria, and suprapubic pain. Upper tract infection (acute pyelonephritis) usually presents with fever and chills, flank pain, and nausea. Frequency, urgency, and dysuria of lower tract origin may or may not be present.

Acute dysuria in young women does not always signify bacterial cystitis (Table 30–46). Indeed, 10 per cent of such women have symptoms due to local disease, such as vaginitis or herpes simplex infection. An additional 40 per cent have either bladder bacteriuria with numbers smaller than the benchmark 10^5 organisms per ml., or they have isolated urethritis, usually due to *Chlamydia*. Appropriate clinical and microbiologic evaluation must be made to distinguish between these etiologies.

Not every patient with a urinary tract infection will have classic symptoms. Many will be asymptomatic, and many symptomatic patients present in atypical fashion. An individual may feel tired. A child who is toilet trained may wet her bed. A man may have low back pain. The illness may present as a fever of unknown origin. Pain may be referred to the right lower quadrant or anterior abdomen rather than the flank. Paralytic ileus may be the most prominent finding. A diagnosis of urinary tract infection should obviously be considered in all these situations.

DIAGNOSIS

A diagnosis of urinary tract infection is made by examining the urine. A clean, voided, midstream urine specimen is the method of choice, since it has no morbidity. Attention should be paid to the technique of collection, since poor technique may lead to misdiagnosis.

Microscopic examination of the urine is performed after centrifugation at 3000 rpm for 5 minutes. The sediment is resuspended after decanting the supernatant and is examined under high dry-power. The presence of 5 to 10 leukocytes per high-power field represents 50 to 100 cells per cubic millimeter, and white blood cell casts indicate renal parenchymal injury. Pyuria (over 10 leukocytes per high-power field), however, is an unreliable prediction of infection (i.e., bacteriuria) since both false positive (30 per cent) and false negative (30 per cent) results are frequent.

Hematuria and proteinuria may occur in urinary tract infections. Most patients, however, excrete only small amounts of protein (less than 1 gram per 24 hours) unless concomitant glomerular disease is present.

The most useful rapid test for presumptive diagnosis of a urinary tract infection is the presence of bacteria on a smear of unspun urine. Place a drop of fresh urine on a glass slide, allow to dry, and then proceed with Gram's stain. More than one organism visible per oil field indicates over 10^5 organisms per ml. of urine. It is absolutely essential that the urine be processed immediately, since the number of bac-

Table 30–46. DISTRIBUTION OF DIAGNOSIS IN 200 OTHERWISE HEALTHY ADULT WOMEN PRESENTING WITH FREQUENCY AND DYSURIA*

Local Disease	Cystitis	Pyelonephritis	Urethral Syndrome
Herpes simplex infection	$> 10^5$ bacteria per ml. of urine	$> 10^5$ bacteria per ml. of urine	$< 10^5$ per ml. of urine (bladder infection)
Vaginitis of various causes	Lower tract infection	Upper tract infection	*Chlamydia* urethritis
10%	40%	10%	40%

*Modified after Stamm, W. E., Wagner, K. F., Amsel, R., et al.: N. Engl. J. Med., 303:409, 1980.

teria changes with time. The visibility of bacteria on *spun* urine specimens is inappropriate for quantitation.

Urine culture is ultimately necessary to definitively diagnose a urinary tract infection. A midstream specimen of urine is collected in order to wash urethral bacteria and obtain normally sterile bladder urine. Numerous studies have established that greater than 10^5 bacteria per milliliter of urine is indicative of infection. However, 10^3 to 10^5 bacteria may occasionally be significant, since other factors, such as degree of hydration, prior antibiotic administration, and methods of collection, also influence the number of bacteria present.

Urine samples should be obtained in a sterile container and promptly processed. A dip-slide method has become popular in which an agar slant is inoculated with a thin film of freshly voided urine at the bedside. This latter method avoids changes in bacterial counts associated with transportation or storage. Urine that cannot be inoculated immediately should be refrigerated until processing. For male patients in whom prostatitis is suspected, a divided urine specimen is necessary. The first voided 10 ml. represents urethral flora. A midstream collection is then obtained, representing bladder flora. Prostatic massage is performed, and the following 10 ml. of urine collected represents prostatic flora. Infection can be easily localized by comparing quantitative cultures of the aforementioned specimens.

In children with urinary tract infections, particularly neonates, suprapubic aspiration of the bladder is a simple and useful method. Even small numbers of bacteria, e.g., 10^2 to 10^4, are indicative of infection if obtained by subrapubic aspiration.

Urethral catheterization may be necessary if an adequately voided specimen cannot be obtained. However, one should realize that this carries a risk of introducing infection. Catheterization must be done with close attention to sterile technique. The risk of infection following single catheterization depends upon the patient population, with a low of 1 per cent in a healthy, young, female outpatient to a high of 10 per cent in an elderly bedridden female.

LOCALIZATION OF INFECTION

The most reliable method of demonstrating whether bacteria come from the bladder or kidney is to perform ureteral catheterization (Table 30–47). Alternatively, bladder catheterization, washout with an antibiotic solution followed by rinsing with sterile water, and serial collection of subsequent urine samples can localize the infection. If bacterial concentrations increase promptly in serial samples, bacteriuria is of renal origin. Neither ureteral catheterization nor bladder washout methods are practical or necessary.

Other methods of localization are available. Clinical parameters, as mentioned previously, are unreliable. The presence of white blood cell casts or tissue fragments may indicate renal damage, but they are frequently not present. Serologic methods, functional tests, radionuclide scans, and enzymatic testing have been utilized but are not reproducible enough to differentiate renal from bladder bacteriuria.

Table 30–47. METHODS OF LOCALIZATION OF URINARY TRACT INFECTION

Direct
Ureteral catheterization
Bladder washout method
Clinical
Fever, flank pain
Dysuria, frequency, urgency, suprapubic pain
Microscopic: white blood cell casts, tissue fragments
Serologic: antibody to bacterial antigens
Functional: loss of concentrating ability
Detection of urinary enzyme excretion
Radionuclide scanning
Antibody coating of urinary bacteria
Response to single-dose antimicrobial therapy

Examination of the urine for antibody-coated bacteria has proved useful in some settings. Fluorescein-conjugated antihuman globulin is added to urine containing bacteria. Bacterial fluorescence indicates antibody coating that suggests their renal origin. False positives do occur, however, particularly in patients with hemorrhagic cystitis, neurogenic bladder, long-term indwelling catheters, or postrenal transplant infections and in men with prostatitis. Conversely, infants and 10 per cent of unselected patients may have renal bacteriuria without antibody coating.

Finally, one can utilize the principle that a single large dose of an antimicrobial agent will reliably eradicate bladder bacteriuria but not renal bacteriuria. Examination of the urine 3 to 5 days after single-dose therapy will indicate bladder bacteriuria if sterility has been achieved.

TREATMENT

The goals for treatment of urinary tract infection are (1) resolution of the acute infection and (2) prevention of irreversible renal damage.

Patients with asymptomatic bacteriuria in the absence of pregnancy, obstruction, or gross vesicoureteral reflux, although at increased risk of symptomatic urinary tract infections, do not appear to suffer any adverse long-term consequences of their bacteriuria. Patients with asymptomatic bacteriuria who clearly need treatment include (1) pregnant women, (2) males, (3) children with vesicoureteral reflux, and (4) individuals with obstructive uropathy. There is also some evidence to suggest that diabetics and elderly nursing home patients with asymptomatic bacteriuria may benefit from treatment to reduce both morbidity and mortality.

Acute symptomatic infections in outpatients without underlying urologic pathology are usually caused by *E. coli* sensitive to all antibiotics. This is particularly true for young women. Each episode should, therefore, be treated with the least expensive, most readily available agent, such as trimethoprim-sulfamethoxazole or ampicillin. For difficult infections, including failure of primary therapy, relapse, or infection due to resistant microorganisms, a quinolone may be indicated. In those individuals with recurrent symptomatic episodes, long-term prophylaxis may be indicated. Such prophylaxis will decrease the risk of recurrent symptomatic episodes as long as it is continued. However, after terminating prophylaxis, bacteriuria will return. A variety of prophylactic regimens have been found to be effective and are listed in Table 30–48.

The doses of antimicrobial agent necessary to treat a lower urinary tract infection may be lower than those normally used for systemic infection. The response of a lower tract infection is dependent upon urine concentration rather than on serum concentration of drug. Therefore, organisms that may appear resistant at serum concentrations may be susceptible to urinary levels of the drug as illustrated in Table 30–1.

The duration of treatment needed to cure a urinary tract infection depends upon the site of infection. Acute dysuria in young women is usually of bladder or urethral origin and will likely respond to single-dose therapy as suggested previously. Proven regimens include oral amoxicillin, 3 grams; sulfisoxazole, 2 grams; trimethoprim-sulfamethoxazole, 2 DS tablets; or trimethoprim 400 mg. Single-dose therapy should not be used even in uncomplicated infections without careful attention to follow-up. Due to the controversy surrounding single-dose therapy and the possibility of unforeseen complicating clinical features (Table 30–49), many specialists recommend a 3-day short course program to minimize the risk of treatment failure. These regimens have a low rate of adverse reactions and a cure rate equal to that achieved with longer courses of treatment. Such programs include ampicillin 500 mg. every 6 hours, trimethoprim-sulfamethoxazole 1 DS every 12 hours, sulfisoxazole 500 mg. every 6 hours, norfloxacin 400 mg. every 12 hours, and ciprofloxacin 250 mg. every 12 hours.

Complicated urinary tract infections (see Table 30–49) require longer courses of treatment and the presumption of upper tract infection (pyelonephritis). Antimicrobial therapy for acute pyelonephritis is best selected from drug susceptibility testing results and continued for 14 days. Parenteral therapy is needed for septicemia, extreme illness, dehydration, or concomitant paralytic ileus. Courses of treatment longer than 14 days may be required for relapse of pyelonephritis or persistent prostatic foci of infection.

The role of ancillary measures is unclear. Although adequate hydration is important, the role of forced diuresis is unknown. Indeed, increasing urine output decreases the urinary concentration of antimicrobial agent and so may actually be counterproductive. Attention should be paid to good voiding habits, with avoidance of prolonged voluntary deferral of micturition, voiding after intercourse if sexual habits seem to promote recurrent infections, and maintenance of adequate hydration. Perineal cleansing after defecation should be established as a front-to-back maneuver to minimize fecal contamination of the periurethral area. Attention to such detail has been shown to be of some value in preventing recurrent infections.

Finally, the management of patients with infected urine and an indwelling bladder catheter must be discussed. Treatment of asymptomatic bacteriuria in such patients is not indicated because it will select out resistant microorganisms as long as the catheter remains in place. Removal of the catheter will usually result in spontaneous elimination of bacteriuria. If such is not the case, specific therapy can then be administered. Treatment of bacteriuria in patients with indwelling catheters should be reserved for symptomatic episodes. Avoidance of catheterization is the best method of preventing catheter-associated infections.

Table 30–48. EFFECTS OF LOW-DOSE, PROPHYLACTIC ANTIBIOTIC REGIMENS ON RECURRENT BACTERIURIA

Regimen	Episodes/Patient/Year
None	2.8–4.2
Sulfamethoxazole 500 mg. q.i.d.	2.0–2.5
Methenamine plus ascorbic acid q.i.d.	1.6–2.0
Sulfamethoxazole + trimethoprim ½ tab. q.i.d.	< 0.2
Nitrofurantoin 100 mg. q.d.	< 0.2
Trimethoprim 100 mg. q.d.	< 0.2

Table 30–49. RISK FACTORS FOR COMPLICATED URINARY TRACT INFECTIONS

Male
Age < 12, > 65 years
Hospital-acquired infection
Known urologic abnormality or stone
Indwelling catheter
Recent instrumentation
Diabetes mellitus
Prior relapse after treatment
History of recent pyelonephritis
Symptoms for < 7 days pretreatment
Persistent symptoms (> 4 days) during therapy
Pregnancy

Virus Infection

Viruses are obligate intracellular parasites and are, therefore, transmitted by close contact between an immunologically naive and an infected host (human or otherwise). Failure to respond to antimicrobial agents and difficulties in cultivation make the diag-

Table 30–50. DISEASES CAUSED BY VIRUSES—THEIR MODES OF TRANSMISSION, THEIR PREVENTION, AND THEIR TREATMENT

Disease State	Virus	Transmission	Prevention*	Treatment†
Bronchitis	Parainfluenza virus	Respiratory	None	None
	Adenovirus	Respiratory	Vaccination (military use only)	None
	Influenza virus	Respiratory	Vaccination, amantidine (type A only)	Amantidine
	Respiratory syncytial virus	Respiratory, hands	Hand washing	None
Bronchiolitis	Respiratory syncytial virus	Respiratory, hands	Hand washing	Ribavirin
Common cold	Rhinovirus	Hands, respiratory	Hand washing	None
	Coronavirus	Hands, respiratory	Hand washing	None
Conjunctivitis/keratitis	Coxsackievirus A	Hands, direct contact, ophthalmologic instruments	Hand washing	None
	Enterovirus 70		Hand washing	None
	Adenovirus		Hand washing	None
	Herpes simplex virus		Hand washing	Topical adenine arabinoside or trifluridine
Croup	Parainfluenza virus	Respiratory	None	None
Diarrhea	Rotavirus	Fecal-oral	Hand washing, sanitation	None
	Parvovirus	Fecal-oral	Hand washing, sanitation	None
Febrile exanthem	Coxsackievirus	Fecal-oral, respiratory	Hand washing	None
	Echovirus	Fecal-oral, respiratory	Hand washing	None
	Measles virus	Respiratory	Vaccination	None
	Rubella virus	Respiratory	Vaccination	None
	Roseola virus	Respiratory	None	None
	Fifth disease virus	Respiratory	None	None
Hemorrhagic fevers	Marburg virus	Person to person	None	None
	Ebola virus	Person to person	None	None
	Dengue virus	Mosquito	Repellants	None
	Yellow fever virus	Mosquito	Repellants, vaccine	None
	Miscellaneous geographically localized hemorrhagic fevers virus	Uncertain, rodent	None	None
Hepatitis	Hepatitis A virus	Fecal-oral	Passive antibody (ISG)	None
	Hepatitis B virus	Blood, secretions	Passive antibody (HIBG) vaccination	None
	Epstein-Barr virus	Respiratory, blood	None	None
	Cytomegalovirus	Respiratory, blood	None	Ganciclovir, ISG
	Yellow fever virus	Mosquito	Repellants, vaccination	None
	Non-A, non-B hepatitis virus	Blood	? Passive antibody (ISG)	None
Influenza	Influenza A virus	Respiratory	Vaccination, amantidine	? Amantidine
	Influenza B virus	Respiratory	Vaccination	None
Lymphadenopathy	Epstein-Barr virus	Respiratory, blood	None	None
	Cytomegalovirus	Respiratory, blood	None	None
	Human immunodeficiency virus	Blood, sexual	Condoms, blood precautions	Zidovudine
Meningitis/encephalitis	Coxsackieviruses A, B	Fecal-oral, respiratory	Hand washing	None
	Echovirus	Fecal-oral, respiratory	Hand washing	None
	Mumps virus	Respiratory	Vaccination	None
	Rabies virus	Bite or saliva of infected animal	Vaccination, passive antibody	None
	Herpes simplex virus	Respiratory, contact	None	Acyclovir
	Human immunodeficiency virus	Blood, sexual	Condoms, blood precautions	Zidovudine
	Lymphocytic chloriomeningitis virus	None	None	Respiratory (rodent)
	Arbovirus(es)	Mosquito	Repellants	None
Paralytic illness	Poliovirus	Fecal-oral	Vaccination	Bed rest
	Coxsackievirus	Fecal-oral, respiratory	Hand washing	None
	Echovirus	Fecal-oral, respiratory	Hand washing	None
Parotitis	Mumps vorus	Respiratory	Vaccination	None
	Coxsackievirus	Fecal-oral, respiratory	Hand washing	None

Table continued on following page

Table 30–50. DISEASES CAUSED BY VIRUSES—THEIR MODES OF TRANSMISSION, THEIR PREVENTION, AND THEIR TREATMENT *Continued*

Disease State	Virus	Transmission	Prevention*	Treatment†
Pharyngitis	Coxsackievirus A	Fecal-oral, respiratory	Hand washing	None
	Coxsackievirus B	Fecal-oral, respiratory	Hand washing	None
	Echovirus	Fecal-oral, respiratory	Hand washing	None
	Cytomegalovirus	Respiratory, blood	None	None
	Epstein-Barr virus	Respiratory, blood	None	None
	Adenovirus	Respiratory	Vaccination (military only)	None
Pharyngitis, vesicular	Coxsackievirus A (herpangina)	Fecal-oral, respiratory	Hand washing	None
	Herpes simplex virus	Contact	None	Acyclovir
Pleuritis	Coxsackievirus B	Fecal-oral, respiratory	Hand washing	None
Pneumonia	Influenza virus	Respiratory	Vaccination Amantidine (A only)	? Amantidine (A only)
	Adenovirus	Respiratory	Vaccination (military only)	None
	Cytomegalovirus	Respiratory, blood	None	Ganciclovir, ISG
Vesicular exanthem	Herpes simplex virus	Contact	None	Acyclovir
	Varicella-zoster virus	Respiratory, contact	None	Acyclovir
	Echovirus 9	Fecal-oral, respiratory	Hand washing	None
	Smallpox virus	Respiratory, contact	Vaccination	Methisazone

*Diseases spread by respiratory routes or direct contact may be prevented in some cases by isolation of infected patients.
†Supportive treatment (e.g., intravenous fluids, oxygen, and so on) may be indicated but is not listed as specific antiviral therapy.

nosis of most viral infections a presumptive one based on the presenting clinical syndrome. Although many of these viruses, particularly enteroviruses and HIV, produce an illness of protean manifestations, certain characteristic clinical and epidemiologic features help us to determine the likely etiology and more appropriately manage infection due to these agents. Table 30–50 summarizes the spectrum of illness produced by most human viruses according to their clinical presentation and outlines their modes of transmission, prevention, and treatment.

References

General

Benenson, A.S., (Ed.): Control of Communicable Diseases in Man. 14th ed. Washington, D.C., American Public Health Association, 1985.

Bennett, J.V., and Brachman, P.S. (Eds.): Hospital Infections. 2nd ed. Boston, Little, Brown and Co., 1986. *This is an important text for all physicians who treat hospitalized patients. It is a complete discussion of the epidemiology and management of hospital-acquired infections.*

Grieco, M.H. (Ed.): Infections in the Abnormal Host. New York, Yorke Medical Books, 1980.

Hoeprich, P.D. (Ed.): Infectious Diseases. 3rd ed. Philadelphia, Harper and Row, Inc., 1983.

Krugman, S., and Katz, S.L. (Eds.): Infectious Diseases of Children. 8th ed. St. Louis, C.V. Mosby Co., 1985.

Mandell, G.L., Douglas, R.G., Jr., and Bennett, J.E. (Eds.): Principles and Practice of Infectious Diseases. 2nd ed. New York, John Wiley and Sons, 1985. *This is the most complete textbook of infectious diseases available. Organized by both disease and microorganism, it is written by the foremost authorities in the field.*

Remington, J.S., and Klein, J.O. (Eds.): Infectious Diseases of the Fetus and Newborn Infant. 2nd ed. Philadelphia, W.B. Saunders Co., 1983. *An exhaustive review of the topic and a valuable reference work. Dr. Remington's discussion of toxoplasmosis is most complete.*

Warren, K.S., and Mahmoud, A.A.F. (Eds.): Geographic Medicine for the Practitioner. 2nd ed. New York, Springer-Verlag, 1985. *An algorithmic approach to the diagnosis and treatment of a variety of common infectious diseases that may be acquired by both foreign and domestic travel.*

Antibiotics

Garrod, L.P., Lambert, H.P., and O'Grady, F.: Antibiotic and Chemotherapy. 5th ed. New York, Churchill Livingstone, Inc., 1981.

Hirschmann, J.V., and Inui, T.S. Antimicrobial prophylaxis: A critique of recent trials. Rev. Infect. Dis., *2*:1, 1980. *This review puts prophylaxis into perspective and gives the best information on the role and value of prophylactic antibiotics.*

Kucers, A., and Bennett, N.M.: The Use of Antibiotics. 4th ed. Philadelphia, J.B. Lippincott, 1987. *This is a complete textbook of antimicrobial therapy, thoroughly referenced from the world's literature. Each chapter is logically organized and contains particularly practical information regarding toxicity and clinical use of the drugs.*

McCracken, G.H. Jr., and Nelson, J.D.: Antimicrobial Therapy for Newborns. 2nd ed. New York, Grune and Stratton, 1983.

Medical Letter: The Medical Letter Handbook of Antimicrobial Therapy. New Rochelle, New York, The Medical Letter, 1988. *Very useful reference guide for dosages, preferred drugs for treatment, and adverse reactions.*

Neu, H.C. (Ed.): Update on antibiotics I and II. Med. Clin. North Am., *71*:1051, 1987; *72*:555, 1988.

Bone and Joint Infection

Chandrasekar, P.H., and Narula, A.R.: Bone and joint infections in intravenous drug abusers. Rev. Infect. Dis. *8*:904, 1986.

Emslie, K.R., and Nade, S.: Pathogenesis and treatment of acute hematogenous osteomyelitis. Rev. Infect. Dis. *8*:841, 1986.

Goldenberg, D.L., Brandt, K.D., Cohen, A. S., et al.: Treatment of septic arthritis: Comparison of needle aspiration and surgery as initial modes of joint drainage. Arth. Rheum., *18*:83, 1975.

Mackowiak, P.A., Jones, S.R., and Smith, J.W.: Diagnostic value of sinus-tract cultures in chronic osteomyelitis. J.A.M.A., *239*:2772, 1978. *This study is important because it documents the futility of sinus tract cultures as a means of isolating the microorganism responsible for chronic osteomyelitis. Less than 50 per cent of sinus tract cultures contained the isolate recovered operatively from bone, and many irrelevant microorganisms were recovered.*

Stechenberg, B.W.: Lyme disease: The latest great imitator. Pediat. Infect. Dis. J. 7:402, 1988. *The diversity of presentation and clinical features of Lyme disease are reviewed. This is an excellent and well-referenced review for the family practitioner.*

Steere, A.C., Schoen, R.T., and Taylor E.: The clinical evolution of Lyme arthritis. Ann. Intern. Med. *107:*725, 1987.

Waldvogel, F.A., and Vasey, H.: Osteomyelitis: The past decade. N. Engl. J. Med., *303:*360, 1980. *A sequel to Dr. Waldvogel's review 10 years earlier, this recent perspective stresses newer insights into the pathogenesis, diagnosis, and treatment of osteomyelitis.*

Cardiovascular Infections

Churchill, M.A., Geraci, J.E., and Hunder, G.G.: Musculoskeletal manifestations of bacterial endocarditis. Ann. Intern. Med., *87:*754, 1977.

Garvey, G.J., and Neu, H.C.: Infective endocarditis—an evolving disease. Medicine, *57:*105, 1978. *This review stresses the changes that have occurred in the spectrum and distribution of patients with infective endocarditis. In particular, the factors associated with an increased risk of mortality are discussed in detail.*

Karchmer, A.W., Dismukes, W.E., Buckley, M.J., et al.: Late prosthetic valvular endocarditis. Am. J. Med., *64:*199, 1978. *Late prosthetic valvular endocarditis due to streptococci frequently responds to medical therapy alone. Nonstreptococcal etiology, a new regurgitant murmur, or moderate to severe congestive heart failure suggests an unlikely response to medical therapy and a need for early surgical intervention.*

Pesanti, E.L., and Smith, I.M.: Infective endocarditis with negative blood cultures: An analysis of 52 cases. Am. J. Med., *66:*43, 1979.

Venezio, F.R., Westenfelder, G.O., Cook, F.V., et al.: Infective endocarditis in a community hospital. Arch. Int. Med., *142:*789, 1982.

Wilson, W.R., and Geraci, J.E.: Treatment of streptococcal infective endocarditis. Am. J. Med. *78*(suppl 6B):128, 1985. *A 2-week regimen of penicillin plus streptomycin appears effective for penicillin-susceptible streptococcal endocarditis. However, enterococcal endocarditis with symptoms for >3 months or mitral valve involvement requires 6 weeks of penicillin plus an aminoglycoside.*

Central Nervous System Infections

deLouvois, J.: The bacteriology and chemotherapy of brain abscesses. J. Antimicrob. Chemother., *4:*395, 1978.

Geiseler, P.J., Nelson, K.E., Levin, S., et al.: Community-acquired purulent meningitis: A review of 1316 cases during the antibiotic era, 1954–1976. Rev. Infect. Dis., *2:*725, 1980. *A comprehensive survey of the epidemiology, clinical and laboratory features, and outcome of bacterial meningitis seen over a 20-year period in Chicago.*

Overturf, G.D.: Treatment of the child with bacterial meningitis. *In* Remington, J.S., and Swartz, M.N. (Eds.): Current Clinical Topics in Infectious Diseases. Vol. 3. New York, McGraw-Hill, 1982.

Sande, M.A.: Antibiotic therapy of bacterial meningitis: Lessons we've learned. Am. J. Med., *71:*507, 1981. *Dr. Sande reviews our experience in the chemotherapy of bacterial meningitis with particular reference to the treatment of gram-negative meningitis. The role of third-generation cephalosporins in the treatment of gram-negative meningitis is emphasized.*

Fever

Bernheim, H.A., Block, L.H., and Atkins, E.: Fever: Pathogenesis, pathophysiology and purpose. Ann. Intern. Med., *91:*261, 1979.

Dinarello, C.A., Cannon, J.G., and Wolff, S.M.: New Concepts on the Pathogenesis of Fever. Rev. Infect. Dis. *10:*168, 1988. *It is now clear that interleukin 1 is primarily responsible for fever production. This exhaustive review summarizes our current knowledge of temperature regulation in humans.*

Esposito, A.L., and Gleckman, R.A.: A diagnostic approach to the adult with fever of unknown origin. Arch. Intern. Med., *139:*575, 1979.

Mackowiak, P.A. and LeMaistre, C.F.: Drug fever: A critical appraisal of conventional concepts. Ann. Intern. Med., *106:*728, 1987.

McNeil, B.J., Sanders, R., Anderson, P.O., et al.: A prospective study of computed tomography, ultrasound and gallium imaging in patients with fever. Radiology, *139:*647, 1981.

Petersdorf, R.G., and Beeson, P.B.: Fever of unexplained origin: Report of 100 cases. Medicine, *40:*1, 1961. *This review defines F.U.O. and remains the classic thesis on its causes.*

Pizzo, P.A., Lovejoy, F.H., and Smith, D.H.: Prolonged fever in children: Review of 100 cases. Pediatrics, *55:*468, 1975.

Gastrointestinal Infection

Bartlett, J.G., Chang, T.W., Gurwith, M., et al.: Antibiotic-associated pseudomembranous colitis due to toxin-producing *Clostridia.* N. Engl. J. Med., *298:*531, 1978. *Cytopathic toxin produced by* Clostridium difficile *is discovered to be the cause of pseudomembranous colitis associated with antibiotic administration.*

Blacklow, N.R., and Cukor, G.: Viral gastroenteritis. N. Engl. J. Med., *304:*397, 1981.

Cantey, J.R.: Infectious diarrhea: Pathogenesis and risk factors. Am. J. Med., *78:*65, 1985.

Ericsson, C.D., and DuPont, H.L.: Traveler's diarrhea: Recent developments. Infect. Dis. Clin. N.A., *2:*66, 1985.

Guerrant, R.L., Shields, D.S., Thorsan, S.M., et al.: Evaluation and diagnosis of acute infectious diarrhea. Am. J. Med., *78*(suppl 6B):91, 1985. *A practical and algorithmic approach to the clinical and laboratory evaluation of infectious diarrhea, this review is of special interest to the family practitioner since acute enteric illnesses are second only in frequency to the common cold.*

Ryser, R.J., and Hornick, R.B.: A review of "new" bacterial strains causing diarrhea. *In* Remington, J.S., and Swartz, M.N. (Eds.): Current Clinical Topics in Infectious Diseases. Vol. 2. New York, McGraw-Hill, Inc., 1980. *A comprehensive review of diarrheal disease due to* Campylobacter, Yersinia, *and* Vibrio parahaemolyticus.

Infection in the Compromised Host

Bodey, G.P.: Antimicrobial prophylaxis for infection in neutropenic patients. Curr. Clin. Top. Infect. Dis. *9:*1, 1988.

Glenn, J., Cotton, D., Wesley, R., et al.: Anorectal infections in patients with malignant diseases. Rev. Infect. Dis., *10:*42, 1988. *Anorectal infections are a frequent source of sepsis in neutropenia and, if not quickly diagnosed and aggressively managed, can possess a mortality of >50 per cent in this population.*

Kurrle, E., Bhaduri, S., Krieger, D., et al.: Risk factors for infections or the oropharynx and the respiratory tract in patients with acute leukemia. J. Infect. Dis., *144:*128, 1981. *This is a detailed study of risks of respiratory tract infection in leukemic patients. Pharyngeal colonization with gram-negative bacilli and the degree of neutropenia are the most significant risk factors.*

Meunier-Carpentier, F., Kiehn, T.E., Armstrong, D.: Fungemia in the immunocompromised host. Am. J. Med., *71:*363, 1981.

Pizzo, P.A.: Infectious complications in the child with cancer. I. Pathophysiology of the compromised host and the initial evaluation and management of the febrile cancer patient. J. Pediatr., *98:*341, 1981.

Sickles, E.A., Greene, W.H., and Wiernik, P.H.: Clinical presentations of infection in granulocytopenic patients. Arch. Intern. Med., *135:*715, 1975. *Physical findings in the absence of neutrophils are blunted although fever and bacteremia occur more frequently than in nongranulocytopenic patients. The presentations of specific infections are discussed in detail.*

Young, L.S.: Nosocomial infections in the immunocompromised adult. Am. J. Med., *70:*398, 1981.

Respiratory Infections

Ching, W.T., and Meyer, R.D.: *Legionella* Infections. Infect. Dis. Clin. N.A., *1:*595, 1987. *A variety of* Legionella *species can cause both pneumonia and extrapulmonary infections in both epidemic and sporadic forms. Their propensity to cause nosocomial infection should be remembered.*

England, A.C., et al.: Sporadic legionellosis in the United States: The first thousand cases. Ann. Intern. Med., *94:*164, 1981. *Accounting for perhaps 2 to 5 per cent of community-acquired pneumonia, the characteristics of* Legionella *pneumonia are well described. Mortality averages 20 per cent, even in patients treated with effective antimicrobial agents.*

Finland, M.: Pneumonia and pneumococcal infections with special reference to pneumococcal pneumonia. Am. Rev. Resp. Dis., *120:*481, 1979.

McGowan, J.E.: Respiratory tract infections due to *Branhamella catarrhalis* and *Neisseria* species. Curr. Clin. Top. Infect. Dis., *8:*181, 1987.

Murphy, T.F., Henderson, F.W., Clyde, W.A., Jr., et al.: Pneumonia: An eleven-year study in a pediatric practice. Am. J. Epidemiol., *113:*12, 1981. *A decade-long study of lower respiratory tract infections in children reveals the vast majority are due to nonbacterial agents. Respiratory syncytial and parainfluenza viruses are the major causes in children less than 5 years of age, while mycoplasma are most important over 5 years of age.*

Reyes, M.P.: The aerobic gram-negative bacillary pneumonias. Med. Clin. North Am., *64:*363, 1980.

Sepsis

Freedman, R.M., Ingram, D.L., Gross, I., et al.: A half-century of neonatal sepsis at Yale. Am. J. Dis. Child., *135:*140, 1981.

Klein, J.O.: Bacteremia in febrile children managed out of hospital. Curr. Clin. Top. Infect. Dis., *6:*184, 1985.

Kreger, B.E., Craven, D.E., Carling, P.C., et al.: Gram-negative bacteremia. III. Reassessment of etiology, epidemiology and ecology in 612 patients. Am. J. Med., *68:*332, 1980. *An increased incidence of gram-negative sepsis is noted over the 10-year period of 1965–1974. Fatality rates most closely parallelled the severity of the host's underlying disease rather than the selection of specific antimicrobial agents.*

Kreger, B.E., Craven, D.E., and McCabe, W.R.: Gram-negative bacteremia. IV. Reevaluation of clinical features and treatment in 612 patients. Am. J. Med., *68:*344, 1980.

Setia, U., and Gross, P.A.: Bacteremia in a community hospital. Arch. Intern. Med., *137:*1698, 1977.

Todd, J.K.: Staphylococcal toxin syndromes. Ann. Rev. Med., *36:*337, 1985. *Staphyloccal toxins cause such diverse illnesses as food poisoning, scalded skin syndrome, bullous impetigo, and toxic shock syndrome.*

Sexually Transmitted Diseases

Brogadir, S.P., Schimmer, B.M., and Myers, A.R.: Spectrum of the gonococcal arthritis-dermatitis syndrome. Semin. Arth. Rheum., *8:*177, 1979.

Handsfield, H.H.: Gonorrhea and non-gonococcal urethritis: Recent advances. Med. Clin. North Am., *62:*925, 1978. *Excellent review of the clinical features and differential diagnosis of urethritis. Emphasizes the importance of asymptomatic gonococcal urethritis in males.*

Handsfield, H.H. (Ed.): Sexually transmitted diseases. Infect. Dis. Clin. North Am., *1:*1, 1987. *This clinics issue is devoted entirely to an update on all aspects of sexually transmitted diseases (STDs).*

Mertz, G.J., Jones, C.C., Mills, J., et al.: Long-term acyclovir suppression of frequently recurring genital herpes simplex virus infection. J.A.M.A., *260:*201, 1988.

Quinn, T.C., Corey, L., Chaffee, R.G., et al.: The etiology of anorectal infections in homosexual men. Am. J. Med., *71:*395, 1981.

Skin and Soft Tissue Infections

Cruse, P.J.E., and Foord, R.: The epidemiology of wound infection: A 10-year prospective study of 62,939 wounds. Surg. Clin. North Am., *60:*27, 1980. *This is a monumental analysis of the risk factors associated with development of surgical wound infections. It is worth careful reading by all physicians who care for surgical patients.*

Feingold, D.S.: The diagnosis and treatment of gangrenous and crepitant cellulitis. *In* Remington, J.S., and Swartz, M.N. (Eds.): Current Clinical Topics in Infectious Diseases. Vol. 2. New York, McGraw-Hill, 1981. *A thorough clinical review and classification of all types of necrotizing infections involving the skin and subcutaneous tissues.*

Fleisher, G., Ludwig, S., and Campos, J.: Cellulitis: Bacterial etiology, clinical features and laboratory findings. J. Pediatr., *97:*591, 1980.

McDonough, J.J., Stern, P.J., and Alexander, J.W.: Management of animal and human bites and resulting human infections. Curr. Clin. Top. Infect. Dis., *8:*11, 1987.

Meislin, H.W., Lerner, S.A., Graves, M.H., et al.: Cutaneous abscesses: Anaerobic and aerobic bacteriology and outpatient management. Ann. Intern. Med., *87:*145, 1977. *This article evaluates 135 cutaneous abscesses in outpatients. Primary management included incision and drainage, and antibiotics were not considered of value for such localized infections in patients with presumably normal host defenses.*

Musher, D.M.: Cutaneous and soft-tissue manifestations of sepsis due to gram-negative enteric bacilli. Rev. Infect. Dis., *2:*854, 1980.

Tuberculosis

American Thoracic Society/Centers for Disease Control: Treatment of tuberculosis and tuberculous infection in adults and children. Am. Rev. Resp. Dis., *134:*355, 1986. *The state of art in all aspects of tuberculous chemotherapy.*

Glassroth, J., Robins, A.G., and Snider, D.E., Jr.: Tuberculosis in the 1980's. N. Engl. J. Med., *302:*1441, 1980. *A thoroughly referenced update on the diagnosis, treatment, and prevention of tuberculosis.*

Slavin, R.E., Walsh, T.J., and Pollack, A.D.: Late generalized tuberculosis. Medicine, *59:*352, 1980.

Snider, D.E., Rieder, H.L., Combs, D., et al.: Tuberculosis in children. Pediatr. Infect. Dis., *7:*271, 1988.

Woods, G.L., and Washington, J.A.: Mycobacteria other than *Mycobacterium tuberculosis:* Review of Microbiologic and Clinical Aspects. Rev. Infect. Dis., *9:*275, 1987.

Urinary Tract Infection

Andriole, V.T.: Urinary tract infections. Infect. Dis. Clin. North Am., *1:*713, 1987. *A current review of all aspects of urinary tract infection with particularly useful sections on therapy and prophylaxis.*

Gillenwater, J.Y., Harrison, R.B., and Kunin, C.M.: Natural history of bacteriuria in schoolgirls. N. Engl. J. Med., *301:*396, 1979. *This is an important study that clarifies that girls with asymptomatic bacteriuria are at high risk of recurrent symptomatic infections but, in the absence of obstruction or major degrees of reflux, are at very low risk of reduced renal function.*

Kunin, C.M.: Detection, Prevention and Management of Urinary Tract Infections. 4th ed. Philadelphia, Lea and Febiger, 1987.

Souney, P., and Polk, B.F.: Single-dose antimicrobial therapy for urinary tract infections in women. Rev. Infect. Dis., *4:*29, 1982.

Stamm, W.E.: Guidelines for prevention of catheter-associated urinary tract infections. Ann. Intern. Med., *82:*386, 1975.

Stamm, W.E., Wagner, K.F., Amsel, R., et al.: Causes of the acute urethral syndrome in women. N. Engl. J. Med., *303:*409, 1980. *A prospective evaluation of over 200 women presenting with dysuria and frequency. Clarifies the etiology of culture-negative symptoms in such patients.*

Stamm, W.E.: Diagnosis of *Chlamydia trachomatis* genitourinary infections. Ann. Intern. Med., *108:*710, 1988.

31

Ambulatory Management of AIDS

Susan M. Miller

Acquired immunodeficiency syndrome (AIDS) has become the most frightening, controversial, and lethal pandemic of modern medicine. The Centers for Disease Control estimate that 270,000 cumulative cases of AIDS will occur in the United States by the year 1991 (Coolfont, 1986). Epidemiologic, clinical, and virologic evidence has identified the RNA retrovirus, human immunodeficiency virus (HIV), as the etiologic agent of AIDS. Although the strict taxonomic classification is controversial, HIV is considered by most investigators to be a member of the lentivirus subfamily. Retroviruses have an unusual replicative enzyme known as reverse transcriptase (RNA-directed DNA polymerase) that is not found in normal eukaryotic cells. This enzyme allows the virus to copy its own RNA into DNA precursors. The proviral DNA thus formed has the ability to permanently incorporate itself into host cell chromosomes, thereby protecting the HIV's DNA from host cell defenses and guaranteeing its survival by transmission through germ lines.

Etiology and Pathogenesis

The first step in the immunopathogenesis of AIDS is infection by HIV. This infection is characterized by a chronic, progressive, and potentially fatal clinical course. The biologic features of HIV that trigger immune suppression and disease progression remain an enigma and are the subject of intensive research.

Studies have shown that HIV preferentially infects monocytes, macrophages, and helper T lymphocytes. In addition, HIV may affect other host cells, including B cells, bone marrow precursors, Langerhans' cells, and glial cells.

There are two overlapping arms of the immune response: humoral and cellular. The humoral (antibody) response consists of B lymphocytes. The cellular arm, on the other hand, is composed of all subsets of T lymphocytes and monocytes and macrophages.

The subpopulation of T lymphocytes known as helper T cells are the primary regulators of the immune response and proliferate in response to antigenic stimulation. Furthermore, HIV-infected helper T cells are susceptible to cytopathic effects and resultant cellular depletion. Recent evidence suggests that T lymphocyte progenitor cells in the bone marrow are also infected by HIV (Folkes et al., 1988).

Monocytes and macrophages are essential in activating the immune response and may be necessary for the development of antibody responses in addition to their traditional role of scavengers. Infected macrophages also have the ability to cross the blood-brain barrier and may be a mechanism for central nervous system penetration by HIV.

In order to conceptualize the clinical picture of this disease, an understanding of the replicative process of HIV is essential. First, HIV preferentially infects cells with a specific protein receptor known as the OKT4 antigen. Once HIV has entered the cell cytoplasm, it either actively replicates or becomes integrated into host cell DNA. HIV progeny released from cells then elicit either an antibody response or infect other susceptible cells.

After HIV infection is established, it persists throughout the lifetime of the infected person, avoiding clearance by the host immune response. With repetitive and sequential replication of HIV, however, a subsequent depletion of T4 lymphocytes occurs that results in disarray of cell-mediated immune responses. This depletion of T4 lymphocytes is a slow process without spontaneous reversal and parallels the prolonged clinical course between the appearance of antibodies to HIV (acute seroconversion) and the appearance of an AIDS-defining illness. The longer an individual is infected with HIV, the greater the risk of disease progression. Studies by Lui and associates estimate a mean incubation period for progression in homosexual men of 7.8 years. Their statistical analysis further predicts that 99 per cent of HIV-infected individuals will develop AIDS (90 per cent confidence interval, ranging from 0.38 to 1). An asymptomatic carrier state has not been identified.

The Centers for Disease Control have established a classification system for HIV infection based on the natural history of this illness. The categories in this definition have been standardized to gather epidemiologic data and to simplify the clinical description in local and national reporting (Centers for Disease Control, 1985, 1987).

Fortunately, HIV is not an easily transmissible disease. Its communicability is related to an individual's behavior that may ultimately place that person in high-risk categories. These behaviors include sexual intercourse (i.e., homosexual, bisexual, or heterosexual), parenteral exposure (i.e., intravenous drug use, blood, blood products, or organ transplantation), and vertical transmission (i.e., perinatal and transplacental). Human breast milk and oral sex have been implicated as a mechanism of infection in rare instances. The occupational risk of a transmission to health care providers is less than 0.1 per cent per year of exposure (four cases per approximately 4000 subjects per 3 years) (Sande and Volberding, 1989). Reasonable precautions include avoidance of needle sticks and use of disposable gloves if there is a chance of exposure to infected substances. If a surface has been contaminated with HIV, ordinary household bleach will rapidly destroy the virus. In addition, HIV is not transmitted by hepatitis B vaccine, RhoGAM, heat-treated Factor VIII, or immunoglobulin preparations. Furthermore, insect vectors, casual contact (e.g., environmental surface, skin, sweat, tears, changing diapers), and social contact (e.g., hugging, sneezing, coughing, shaking hands) have not been implicated as routes of transmission in empirical investigations (Sande and Volberding, 1988).

Ambulatory Management

The first step in the management of HIV-infected individuals involves primary care physicians educating themselves and their staff about recommendations of the Centers for Disease Control governing universal precautions (Centers for Disease Control, 1987, 1988). Adherence to these guidelines will minimize occupational risk for the health care provider.

Diagnosis. Identification of individuals with past (e.g., blood transfusion), current (e.g., intravenous drug use), and potential (e.g., adolescent) high-risk status is imperative. Physicians need to assess whether individual situations warrant testing or contact tracing. Numerous immunodiagnostic tests to ascertain HIV have been developed for laboratory and clinical use. For example, viral presence can be detected by viral co-cultures or polymerase chain reaction (amplification of nucleic acid sequences) techniques. These methods are not commercially available and are impractical in the ambulatory environment.

Antigen Testing. P24 antigen testing, a test for direct viral presence, is widely available. Although its sensitivity and specificity are presently unknown, an elevated level indicates (1) early infection (prior to an antibody response) or (2) reactivation of disease. A decrease in p24 antigen level may have potential predictive ability in measuring clinical response to antiviral therapy.

Antibody Testing. To date, the most commonly utilized HIV-specific detection techniques are the enzyme-linked immunosorbent assay (ELISA) and Western immunoblotting antibody tests. Enzyme-linked immunosorbent assay is used in blood screening because it is inexpensive and simple to perform. Although the Western blot test is technically more difficult to interpret, under optimal laboratory conditions its sensitivity is comparable to or greater than that of reactive enzyme immunoassays. If used correctly, Western blot analysis will increase the predictive value of a positive test and can be used to aid in the confirmation of a positive enzyme-linked immunosorbent assay screening test. Indeterminate results of a Western blot test need to be repeated with subsequent patient sampling. Antibody and antigen tests identify individuals with prior HIV infection, but do not measure host immunity. Furthermore, they cannot predict the moment of initial infection or the patient's remaining life expectancy.

Antibody tests are not 100 per cent sensitive or specific; false positive and false negative results occur. A list of possible associative causes for false positive and false negative results and recommendations for testing are provided in Tables 31–1 and 31–2.

Baseline Evaluation of the HIV-Infected Person. After detection of HIV infection by ELISA screening, with confirmation by an independent testing method (e.g., Western immunoblot technique), a baseline evaluation incorporating the following procedures is suggested.

Medical History. Obtain the following information for clinical classification or delineation of potential cofactors of disease progression: recent herpes zoster infection, Bell's palsy, sexually transmitted disease history, health of significant others, arthral-

Table 31–1. POTENTIAL SOURCES OF FALSE POSITIVE OR FALSE NEGATIVE ANTIBODY TESTS

False Positive	False Negative
Populations with low seroprevalence Passive transfer of antibody in immunoglobulin preparations Cross-reactive antibodies secondary to multiple blood transfusions, serum proteins (cryoglobulins, rheumatoid factor), other retroviruses, or human leukocyte antigens Transplacental transfer of maternal antibody Laboratory error	Prior to host antibody response (i.e., "window period") Late infection, resulting from deterioration of host antibody response Laboratory error

gias, myalgias, possession of household pets, prior hepatitis B or vaccination, foreign travel, drug allergies, contraceptive use, previous research treatment, risk factor(s) for HIV, advanced HIV symptoms (e.g., weight loss, chronic diarrhea, night sweats, fever), change in personality, and a medical review of symptoms.

Physical Findings. Accurate staging of disease will alert the clinician to potential complications of HIV infection and guide the choice of therapeutic options. The following physical abnormalities may be clinical features associated with HIV infection and should suggest the need for HIV serologic testing: oral candidiasis, recurrent tinea infections, seborrheic dermatitis, molluscum contagiosum, psoriasis, Reiter's syndrome, periodontal disease, oral hairy leukoplakia, staphylococcal folliculitis, extrainguinal lymphadenopathy, retinal abnormalities, hepatosplenomegaly, Kaposi's sarcoma, perioral or perianal herpes, peripheral neuropathy, cognitive changes, myopathy, parotid gland enlargement, and chronic sinusitis. A subset of these symptoms is highly predictive of the development of AIDS (e.g., oral candidiasis, hairy leukoplakia, generalized wasting, and dermatomal zoster). Sande and Volberding provide an excellent review of clinical symptoms and physical findings. Staging of HIV infection may be simplified by the use of the Centers for Disease Control classification schema for HIV infection (Table 31–3).

Baseline Laboratory Analysis. Obtain the following laboratory studies: complete blood count (to rule out HIV-associated anemia, thrombocytopenia, and granulocytopenia); absolute T4 lymphocyte count (to assess degree of relative immune suppression); chemistry profile (e.g., an elevated lactate dehydrogenase level may be associated with *Pneumocystis carinii* pneumonia); and a rapid plasma reagin test (latent syphilis may be difficult to diagnose with concurrent HIV infection). A baseline application of five tuberculin units of purified protein derivative and a screening chest roentgenogram are suggested to rule out occult tuberculosis.

Prognostic Markers. In patients with advanced immune dysfunction, studies that may indicate a

Table 31–2. ADULT HIV SEROLOGIC TESTING—UNITED STATES RECOMMENDATIONS

Pre-Test and Post-Test Counseling

Pre-test and post-test counseling must address the following issues: determination of individual potential risk status (past, current, future); implications of positive, negative, and indeterminate test results; pregnancy and contraception issues; behavior modification to reduce risk; low-risk sexual activities; and referral to appropriate agencies for follow-up.

Note: Pre-test and post-test counseling provides an opportunity to tailor risk reduction education. Health care providers may wish to consider the use of an informed consent form. Finally, a sample that is repetitively positive needs to be confirmed by an independent antibody assay.

Anonymous or Confidential Testing

A system must be implemented that has the ability to protect the anonymity and confidentiality of test specimens and results. Preferably, results of testing are given in a face-to-face encounter.

Note: If testing is performed in a private office, the physician may wish to use numerically coded samples. If this is not feasible, use of alternative testing sites may be advisable.

Voluntary versus Mandatory Testing

Although voluntary testing is preferable, in certain situations mandatory testing is performed.

Mandatory testing: Testing of blood, plasma, sperm, and organ donation. Mandatory testing also occurs within the military, and in specific legal interactions.

Voluntary testing: Previous or current high-risk behavior, prior blood transfusion, occupational exposure, new-onset tuberculosis, syphilis, and public health surveillance. Voluntary testing is also used to confirm a clinical diagnosis.

Interpretation of Results

A negative enzyme-linked immunosorbent assay screen and absence of antibody bands on the Western immunoblot test at 3, 6, 9, and 12 weeks provide evidence that no immune response to HIV has occurred. Indeterminate test results need to be followed closely. Polymerase chain reaction testing may have a role in confirmation.

Table 31–3. CENTERS FOR DISEASE CONTROL CLASSIFICATION SCHEMA FOR ADULT HIV INFECTION

Group I*	Acute HIV infection: Transient illness resembling infectious mononucleosis with development of positive antibody test
Group II	Asymptomatic HIV infection: May or may not have had a history of Group I symptoms; positive antibody test; possible abnormal lymphocyte testing
Group III	Persistent generalized lymphadenopathy: Lymphadenopathy (>1 cm diameter) at 2 or more extrainguinal locations for greater than 3 months' duration
Group IV	Other types of HIV infection:
	Subgroup A: Constitutional disease. Fever for >1 month, involuntary weight loss >10 per cent, persistent diarrhea for >1 month, absence of other illnesses that could explain symptoms
	Subgroup B: Neurologic disease. Dementia, myopathy, or peripheral neuropathy, absence of other illnesses that could explain symptoms
	Subgroup C: Secondary infectious diseases
	C-1: Any one of the following indicator diseases for AIDS: *Pneumocystis carinii* pneumonia, toxoplasmosis, crytococcosis, histoplasmosis, candidiasis (esophagus, trachea, bronchi, lungs), cytomegalovirus infection, chronic cryptosporidiosis, isosporiasis, chronic mucocutaneous herpes simplex, *Mycobacterium avium* complex or *M. kansasii* disease, extrapulmonic *Mycobacterium* tuberculosis, extraintestinal strongyloidiasis, or progressive multifocal leukoencephalopathy
	C-2: Symptomatic or invasive disease or one of the following: oral hairy leukoplakia, oral candidiasis, multidermatomal herpes zoster, recurrent *Salmonella* bacteremia, nocardiosis
	Subgroup D: Secondary cancers. Kaposi's sarcoma, non-Hodgkin's lymphoma, or primary lymphoma of the brain
	Subgroup E: Miscellaneous. May include the following: HIV-wasting syndrome, lymphoid interstitial pneumonitis

*These definitions are intended to provide consistent statistical data for public health purposes. Criteria exist for presumptive diagnoses of illnesses indicative of AIDS (e.g., cytomegalovirus retinitis, CNS toxoplasmosis without biopsy).

short-term risk of developing AIDS are elevated p24 antigen, neopterin, or β_2 microglobulin levels (Moss, 1988) or a decrease in antibody levels to p24 antigen.

Laboratory Abnormalities. It is often difficult to interpret nonspecific symptoms or physical findings in HIV infection. After completion of an HIV-oriented review of the patient's symptoms, the following laboratory studies may have diagnostic utility based on individual symptomatology. Patients with central nervous system complaints may require a cryptococcal antigen test, toxoplasmosis titer, lumbar puncture, computerized axial tomography scan, or magnetic resonance imaging studies. Patients with prior serologic evidence of toxoplasmosis are at increased risk for reactivation of disease. If a patient complains of shortness of breath or a chronic, nonproductive cough, measurement of arterial blood gases, gallium scanning, or a bronchoscopy may clarify the clinical diagnosis. Female patients need relatively frequent Papanicolaou's smears to screen for cervical carcinoma and require serum pregnancy tests before the initiation of many therapies.

Acute or chronic gastrointestinal symptoms commonly have a treatable etiology. Hence, stool studies for amoeba, *Mycobacteria, Shigella, Salmonella, Isospora, Cryptosporidium,* or *Clostridium difficile* toxin may be warranted. Finally, suspicious skin lesions or lymph nodes need to be biopsied.

Tests that are not routinely helpful include cytomegalovirus titers, Epstein-Barr virus titers, and *Pneumocystis carinii* antigen and antibody tests.

Immunization. Determine the patient's vaccination status. Adult recommendations for symptomatic and asymptomatic individuals are listed in Table 31–4. After a baseline medical evaluation, patients should be seen at regular intervals to assess any changes in their clinical status.

Psychosocial Issues

In addition to treating intercurrent medical sequelae, the primary physician is in an excellent position to prospectively anticipate the myriad psychosocial is-

Table 31–4. IMMUNIZATION OF ADULTS INFECTED WITH HIV— UNITED STATES RECOMMENDATIONS

Vaccine	Asymptomatic or Symptomatic**
Pneumovax*	Yes
Influenza	Yes
Hepatitis B†	Yes
Tetanus toxoid	Yes
Yellow fever	No
Oral poliovirus‡	No
Smallpox	N/A
Cholera	N/E
Typhoid	N/E
Rabies§	Yes
TB (bacille Calmette-Guérin)	No
HbCV	‖
HIV	N/A
Rubeola	¶

*Especially in splenectomized patients; may not induce an immune response in symptomatic persons.

†In high risk individuals, it may be prudent to check serology first; this is especially important for individuals who continue to practice high risk behavior, and for health care workers.

‡Oral, attenuated poliovirus vaccine; should not be administered to an immunosuppressed individual if not vaccinated as a child; consider IPV, inactivated polio vaccine.

§Use of this vaccine must be given in a context of administration; pre-exposure in an asymptomatic individual where job exposure is likely, may be warranted; post-exposure vaccination is recommended.

‖*Haemophilus* b conjugate vaccine; although current recommendations are only for pediatric patients, future recommendations may include use for adult and elderly patient populations.

¶Administration of single antigen vaccine to HIV-infected adults is controversial. The safest course is to update immune status of non-infected family members. Pre-exposure: individuals born before 1957 are considered "immune" regardless of their clinical history; Post exposure: gamma globulin 0.5 cc/kg (maximum dose 15 cc) within 6 days of exposure.

**Yes, safe to administer; No, do not administer; N/A, not available; N/E, not efficacious. Note: Vaccination of an HIV-infected individual may not provoke protective or measurable antibody titers.

sues that confront patients with HIV infection. Although referral for counseling may be necessary in some situations, the clinician may alleviate a majority of these concerns by addressing these issues within the framework of longitudinal care. The following organization of psychosocial issues may assist physicians and their support staff in providing concrete assistance to patients and families.

Issues Directly Related to the Patient. Numerous psychologic issues interface with the medical complications of HIV infection. Upon initial discovery of seropositivity, the patient may experience a spectrum of psychologic responses ranging from fear, denial, and anxiety to guilt, depression, and suicidal ideation. Unless these emotional responses are acknowledged, they have the potential to undermine patient care by confounding the presentation of clinical illness.

Family Issues. As in other chronic diseases, the family may not have the capacity to offer unconditional support. Oftentimes, these families have been unaware of the individual's risk behavior and may, once informed, exhibit anger, blame, hostility, or abandonment. Frequently, they need reassurance concerning their own safety and perceived risk of infection. In addition, peer or societal alienation may further stigmatize and isolate the family. The physician can serve a valuable role in addressing these concerns.

Legal Issues. The debate concerning legal issues is exacerbated by rapidly changing public policy. Legal guidelines governing informed consent in serologic testing and disability definitions remain in transition. Controversies surrounding mandatory testing, quarantine, confidentiality, and duties to warn close contacts and family members further compromise the public health response to this epidemic. The judicial system is in the process of clarifying these dilemmas. Frequently in the preterminal stages of HIV infection, neurologic impairment or dementia occurs. Prior to this complication, the patient needs to obtain a will and durable power of attorney. Documentation of advance directives for resuscitation can assist the physician in abiding with the patient's wishes.

Adjuvants to Care. Patient education that focuses on holistic care may diminish the desperation and hopelessness observed in many patients. For this educational process to be credible, it should address alcohol and drug abuse, the existence of alternative treatment regimens, and special needs of minority populations. However, patients need to understand that quack regimens (e.g., ozone enemas) are ubiquitous and potentially harmful. In addition, individual and family therapy, assessment of spiritual needs, and nutritional counseling will facilitate management of this disease.

Palliation. The role of palliation for primary care providers is determined by the clinical stage of HIV infection. A patient with a relatively intact immune system will require treatment interventions that stabilize and maintain health. Those patients with acute infectious emergencies require aggressive medical management. Eventually, however, some patients in the terminal stage of their illness will decline further treatment. In this scenario, pain control management and palliation supersede other concerns.

Treatment

No curative antiviral therapy or vaccine for HIV is anticipated in the near future. The scientific obstacles to vaccine development include transmission of HIV as a free or cell-bound virus, genetic diversity of isolates, lack of neutralizing antibody response, potential enhancing antibody response, and establishment of latent infections (Fauci, 1988; Dalgleish and Malkovsky, 1988).

The inherent difficulties in treating HIV-infected

Table 31–5. PRIMARY AND PROPHYLACTIC TREATMENT OF OPPORTUNISTIC INFECTIONS IN AIDS

Standard Adult Therapy (Daily Dose)	Alternative Therapy	Prophylactic or Maintenance Therapy
Pneumocystis carinii pneumonia		
Pentamidine isethionate (3 to 4 mg. per kg.)	Pentamidine isethionate (aerosolized)	Pentamidine isethionate (aerosolized)
Trimethoprim-sulfamethoxazole (15 to 20/75 to 100 mg. per kg.)	Trimethoprim and dapsone	Trimethoprim-sulfamethoxazole
	Trimetrexate and leucovorin (investigational)	Dapsone
	Difluoromethyl ornithine (investigational)	Sulfadoxine and pyrimethamine (Fansidar)
Toxoplasma gondii encephalitis		
Pyrimethamine (75 mg. once, then 25 mg.) *plus* leucovorin (folinic acid) (5 to 10 mg.) *plus* sulfadiazine (4 to 6 gm.)	Clindamycin	Suppressive therapy required: pyrimethamine (25 mg.) *plus* leucovorin (folinic acid) *plus* sulfadiazine (2 to 4 gm.)
Cryptosporidium colitis		
None	None (Supportive care: fluids, analgesics, antispasmodics, opiate-derived antidiarrheals)	None
Isospora belli enteritis		
Trimethoprim-sulfamethoxazole (640 mg. per 3.2 gm.)	Pyrimethamine (75-mg. loading dose, then 25 mg.) *plus* leucovorin (5 to 10 mg.)	Suppressive therapy with trimethoprim-sulfamethoxazole or sulfadoxine and pyrimethamine (Fansidar) may be necessary
Mycobacterium tuberculosis		
Isoniazid (300 mg.) *plus* pyridoxine (50 mg.) *plus* rifampin (600 mg.) *plus* ethambutol (15 mg. per kg.)	Pyrazinamide Streptomycin	Minimum duration of therapy is 1 year after culture results are negative; therapy based on clinical sensitivities
Mycobacterium avium-intracellulare infection		
None	Clofazimine Rifabutin Amikacin Ciprofloxacin Ethambutol Ethionamide Cycloserine	Maintenance therapy required; duration unknown
Candida stomatitis		
Clotrimazole (30 to 50 mg.) Nystatin (3 × 10^6 units) Ketoconazole (200 to 400 mg.)	Fluconazole	Maintenance therapy required
Candida esophagitis		
Ketoconazole (400 to 600 mg.) Amphotericin B (5 to 15 mg.)	Fluconazole	Maintenance therapy required
Cryptococcosis		
Amphotericin B (0.5 to 0.7 mg. per kg.)	Fluconazole	Maintenance therapy after 1- to 2-gm. dosing with amphotericin B
Histoplasmosis		
Amphotericin B (0.3 to 0.6 mg. per kg.)	None	Maintenance therapy with ketoconazole (400 mg.) or amphotericin B (1 mg. per kg. per wk.)
Coccidioidomycosis		
Amphotericin B (0.3 to 0.6 mg. per kg.)	None	Same as for histoplasmosis

Table 31–5. PRIMARY AND PROPHYLACTIC TREATMENT OF OPPORTUNISTIC INFECTIONS IN AIDS *Continued*

Standard Adult Therapy (Daily Dose)	Alternative Therapy	Prophylactic or Maintenance Therapy
Herpes simplex		
Acyclovir ointment 5 per cent (5 ×)		Suppressive therapy may be necessary
Acyclovir (15 mg. per kg.)	Vidarabine	
Herpes zoster		
None	High-dose (30 mg. per kg.) acyclovir	None
Epstein-Barr virus infection		
None	Desciclovir (investigational)	None
Epstein-Barr virus infection: oral hairy leukoplakia		
None	Acyclovir	None
Cytomegalovirus		
Ganciclovir (DHPG) (induction: 5 mg. per kg. per b.i.d.)	Foscarnet (investigational)	Suppressive therapy needed to treat recurrent disease (5 mg. per kg., 5 to 7 days per week)
Salmonella infection		
Ampicillin (2 to 12 gm.)	Ciprofloxacin (investigational)	Relapse common; maintenance therapy required
Trimethoprim-sulfamethoxazole (10 mg. to 50 mg.)	Cefotaxime	
Chloramphenicol (2 to 8 mg.)		

Pneumocystis carinii pneumonia: Empiric therapy is a temporary measure until a diagnostic procedure can be performed. Simultaneous use of two treatment regimens does not increase survival. Alternatives for failed initial therapy may involve changing from one conventional regimen to another and repeating the bronchoscopy to rule out a second opportunistic infection. Prophylaxis may be initiated in patients with T4 counts $<200/mm^3$. The clinician may wish to monitor serum sulfamethoxazole levels. A brief course of high-dose steroids may be helpful.

Toxoplasma gondii encephalitis: Folic acid prevents action of pyrimethamine. Folinic acid decreases toxicity of pyrimethamine.

Mycobacterium tuberculosis: HIV-seropositive patients with positive skin tests need 6 months of INH/pyridoxine prophylaxis. An absence of skin test reactivity, however, is not exclusionary. Pyrazinamide and ethambutol treatment is continued for 2 months. Report cases to health department. Therapeutic failures occur when isoniazid and rifampin are coadministered with ketoconazole because of drug interactions. Rifampin may increase methadone maintenance requirements.

Mycobacterium avium-intracellulare infection: Tailor therapy based on in vitro sensitivities. Rifabutin is available from Adrian Labs (Columbus, OH). Amikacin may require 6 weeks of intravenous therapy.

Herpes simplex: Vidarabine is used to treat acyclovir-resistant herpes simplex.

Salmonella infection: Therapy is indicated in immunosuppressed HIV patients. An increased incidence of bacteremia is seen.

Candida infection: Ketoconazole requires a low gastric pH for absorption. Premedications for amphotericin B may include diphenhydramine, meperidine, or low-dose corticosteroids. Heparin may decrease incidence of thrombophlebitis.

patients are related to the increased severity of opportunistic infections, increased frequency of adverse reactions to standard doses of medications (e.g., sulfa compounds), multiplicity of infections, and the likelihood of recurrent infections. Because of the high relapse rate after successful treatment, prophylactic therapy is becoming a standard therapeutic option. However, the use of prophylaxis creates a problem of polypharmacy, with its attendant risk of drug toxicities and interactions.

Research interventions, antiviral therapy, and opportunistic infection prophlylaxis are usually guided by the patient's T4 lymphocyte or clinical classification status.

Opportunistic Infections. In addition, because there is a lack of successful treatment for certain viral (e.g., HIV, CMV), protozoal (e.g., *Cryptosporidium*), and bacterial (e.g., atypical *Mycobacteria*) infections, there is a continued need for either research medications or research applications of previously approved medications (e.g., aerosolized pentamidine). A summary of treatment guidelines for the most common opportunistic infections is listed in Table 31–5 (Sande and Volberding, 1988; DeVita et al., 1988; Glatt et al., 1988; Kaplan et al., 1987).

Zidovudine. Zidovudine (Retrovir, AZT), a reverse transcriptase inhibitor, is the only licensed antiretroviral therapy. Zidovudine is virustatic, not virucidal. Administration is also associated with significant toxicity. The standard dosage regimen is 100 mg. orally every 4 hours for individuals with a prior opportunistic infection, AIDS-related Kaposi's sarcoma, or an absolute T4 lymphocyte count of less than 200. Future indications for zidovudine therapy may include AIDS dementia complex, HIV-associated psoriasis, HIV-associated thrombocytopenia, and pediatric patients (Bartlett, 1988). Clinicians are beginning to administer zidovudine to patients with T4 counts between 200 and 250. Clinical trials are in progress to determine whether or not zidovudine stabilizes the immune system at these and higher T4 levels. Preliminary evidence suggests that although it may also improve cognitive and immune function, significant toxicity continues to occur. Until these

Table 31–6. MAJOR TOXICITIES ASSOCIATED WITH TREATMENT MODALITIES

Therapeutic Agent	Toxicity
Acyclovir	High doses may be associated with thrombocytopenia, renal insufficiency, central nervous system depression, seizures, encephalopathy, phlebitis, hives
Amikacin	Ototoxicity, nephrotoxicity
Amphotericin B	Renal failure, hypokalemia (check magnesium level), thrombophlebitis, marrow suppression
Ampicillin	Anaphylaxis, rash, marrow suppression, epigastric distress, pseudomembranous colitis
Cefotaxime	Hypersensitivity, pseudomembranous colitis, marrow suppression, elevated liver enzymes, positive direct Coombs' test
Ciprofloxacin	Nausea, vomiting, abdominal pain, pruritus, central nervous system effects, arthralgias
Clindamycin	Pseudomembranous colitis, rash, increased hepatic enzymes
Clofazimine	Abdominal pain, blue discoloration of skin, gastrointestinal obstruction, splenic infarction
Chloramphenicol	Pseudomembranous colitis, anaphylaxis, rash, polyarthritis
Clotrimazole	Elevated liver enzymes; dextrose component may contribute to dental caries
Cycloserine	Hypersensitivity, central nervous system effects (seizures, mental status changes, vertigo), hepatic enzyme elevation
Dapsone	Anemia, rash, renal, increased methemoglobin
Ethambutol	Optic neuritis, anaphylaxis, epigastric distress, peripheral neuritis, skin rash
Ethionamide	Epigastric distress, peripheral neuritis, optic neuritis, jaundice
Fluconazole	Elevated hepatic enzymes, seizures
Foscarnet	Anemia, liver enzyme elevation, increased Ca^{++} levels, renal failure. Dosage based on creatinine clearance, not serum creatinine
Ganciclovir	Dose adjustment necessary for renal insufficiency. Neutropenia, thrombocytopenia, confusion, epigastric distress
Isoniazid	Hepatitis (risk increased with alcohol), peripheral neuropathy, nausea, epigastric distress, diarrhea
Ketoconazole	Adrenal suppression, hepatotoxicity, anaphylaxis
Nystatin	Diarrhea, nausea, vomiting
Pentamidine isethionate (intravenous)	Renal, pancreatic, and hepatic toxicities; bone marrow insufficiency; nephritis; hypotension; hypoglycemia; diabetes
Pentamidine isethionate (aerosolized)	Bronchospasm, cough, metal taste in mouth, increased triglycerides
Pyrazinamide	Hepatotoxicity, epigastric distress, rash, arthalgias, hyperuricemia
Pyrimethamine	Thrombocytopenia, neutropenia
Rifampin	Hepatic dysfunction, epigastric distress, headache, thrombocytopenia (especially when combined with ethambutol), hypersensitivity, reddish or orange discoloration of urine and body secretions
Streptomycin	Ototoxicity, nephrotoxicity
Sulfadiazine	Thrombocytopenia, neutropenia, rash, acute renal failure
Sulfadoxine and pyrimethamine (Fansidar)	Stevens-Johnson syndrome, bone marrow suppression
Trimethoprim-sulfamethoxazole	Drug fever, nausea, rash, neutropenia, thrombocytopenia
Vidarabine	Epigastric distress, central nervous system disturbances, marrow suppression

research protocols are completed, routine administration of full-dose zidovudine to patients with T4 lymphocyte counts >200 is not recommended.

Although human DNA polymerases are less sensitive to chain termination by zidovudine as compared with the HIV reverse transcriptase, drug administration is associated with significant toxicity (Table 31–6). Forty per cent of patients develop anemia that requires either a reduction in dose or a transfusion. Leukopenia, especially with granulocytopenia, occurs in 40 per cent of patients. Within 2 weeks of initiation of therapy, patients develop a megaloblastic anemia. If folate or serum B_{12} levels are normal, no reduction in dosing is necessary (Bartlett, 1988; Richman et al., 1987).

If hemoglobin levels are less than 7.5 grams per dl. or neutropenia (<750 neutrophils per mm.^{3}) occurs, an interruption in dosing until evidence of bone marrow recovery is required. After recovery, a titration in dose to 100 mg. every 4 hours may be attempted. In less severe marrow suppression, the physician may wish to either reduce dosing without interruption of therapy or to give a transfusion with CMV-screened packed red blood cells. The efficacy of reduced-dose zidovudine is not known. During initiation of therapy, it is recommended to obtain a complete blood count every 2 weeks to determine bone marrow stability. Anemia usually occurs within the first 6 weeks of therapy, and neutropenia occurs within the first 8 weeks. If after 8 weeks of therapy the marrow is stable, hematology studies can usually be conducted on a monthly schedule. The clinical response to zidovudine therapy usually lasts 6 months to a year.

Drug Interactions. When using zidovudine, the patient must avoid the concomitant use of medications that affect hepatic glucuronidation such as acetaminophen, morphine, probenecid, and nonsteroidal anti-inflammatory agents. These medications may increase the toxicity of zidovudine. Other indications of toxicity seen with zidovudine include hepatic insufficiency, anxiety, headache, nausea, fatigue, weakness, polymyositis, allergic reactions, seizures, and cardiomyopathy. These adverse drug reactions may be greater than the antiviral effect and may preclude the long-term administration of zidovudine to the majority of patients. However, in spite of this toxicity, zidovudine appears to prolong the lives of patients and is a viable alternative until more effective therapies are developed.

Future Studies. Studies examining other reverse transcriptase inhibitors, immunomodulators, zidovudine dosing, vaccines, HIV-blocking agents (CD4), and the use of combination therapy are in progress. Many of the secondary infections require treatment with experimental or nonapproved protocols. Eligible patients can be referred to respective research centers for consultation with subspecialists in the treatment of these opportunistic infections and malignancies.

References

Barre-Sinoussi, F., Chermann, J.C., Rey, F., et al.: Isolation of a T-lymphotropic retrovirus from a patient at risk for acquired immunodeficiency syndrome (AIDS). Science, *220:*868–871, 1983.

Bartlett, J.A.: HIV therapeutics: An emerging science. J.A.M.A., *260:*3051–3052, 1988. *An overview describing the potential uses of zidovudine.*

Centers for Disease Control: Revision of the CDC surveillance case definition of acquired immunodeficiency syndrome for national reporting—United States. M.M.W.R., *34:*373–375, 1985.

Centers for Disease Control: Revision of the CDC surveillance case definition of acquired immune deficiency syndrome. M.M.W.R., *36:*Suppl:1S–15S, 1987.

Centers for Disease Control: Recommendations for prevention of HIV transmission in health-care settings. M.M.W.R., *36:*1S–18S, 1987. *Essential reading.*

Centers for Disease Control: Update: Universal precautions for prevention of transmission of human immunodeficiency virus, hepatitis B virus, and other bloodborne pathogens in health-care settings. M.M.W.R., *37:*377–387, 1988. *Essential reading.*

Centers for Disease Control: Public Health Service guidelines for counseling and antibody testing to prevent HIV infection and AIDS. M.M.W.R., *36:*509–515, 1987. *Essential reading.*

Coolfont report: A PHS plan for prevention and control of AIDS and the AIDS virus. Public Health Rep., 101:341–348, 1986.

Dalgleish, A., and Malkovsky, M.: Advances in human retroviruses. Adv. Cancer Res., *51:*307–360, 1988.

DeVita, V.T., Hellman, S., and Rosenberg, S.A.: AIDS: Etiology, Diagnosis, Treatment, and Prevention. Philadelphia, J.B. Lippincott Co., 1988. *An excellent, comprehensive reference that covers etiology, epidemiology, clinical management, and public health issues in the human immunodeficiency virus epidemic.*

Dournon, E., Rozenbaum, W., Michon, C., et al.: Effects of zidovudine in 365 consecutive patients with AIDS or AIDS-related complex. Lancet, *i:*1297–1302, 1988. *An additional study examining the effects of zidovudine.*

Fauci, A.S.: The human immunodeficiency virus: Infectivity and mechanisms of pathogenesis. Science, *239:*617–622, 1988.

Federle, M.P., Megibow, A.J., Naidich, D.P. (Eds.): The Radiology of AIDS. New York, Raven Press, 1988. *A superlative reference book that provides a comprehensive overview of the radiologic findings and imaging strategies relevant to HIV infection.*

Fischl, M.A., Richman, D.D., Grieco, M.H., et al.: The efficacy of azidothymidine (AZT) in the treatment of patients with AIDS and AIDS-related complex: A double-blind, placebo-controlled trial. N. Engl. J. Med., *317:*192–197, 1987. *The original article describing efficacy of zidovudine (AZT).*

Folkes, T.M., Kessler, S.W., Orenstein, J.M., et al.: Infection and replication of HIV-1 in purified progenitor cells of normal human bone marrow. Science, *242:*919–922, 1988.

Gallo, R.C., Salahuddin, S.Z., Popovic, M., et al.: Frequent detection and isolation of cytopathic retroviruses (HTLV-III) from patients with AIDS and at risk for AIDS. Science, *224:*500–503, 1984.

Gartner, S., Markovits, P., Markovitz, D.M., et al.: The role of mononuclear phagocytes in HTLV-III/LAV infection. Science, *233:*215–219, 1986.

Glatt, A.E., Chirgwin, K., and Landesman, S.H.: Treatment of infections associated with human immunodeficiency virus. N. Engl. J. Med., *318:*1439–1448, 1988.

Kaplan, L.D., Wofsy, C.B., and Volberding, P.A.: Treatment of patients with acquired immunodeficiency syndrome and associated manifestations. J.A.M.A., *257:*1367–1374, 1987.

Klatzmann, D., Barre-Sinoussi, F., Nugeyre, M.T., et al.: Selective tropism of lymphadenopathy-associated virus (LAV) for helper-inducer T-lymphocytes. Science, *225:*59–64, 1984.

Lui, K.J., Darrow, W.W., and Rutherford, G.W.: A model-based estimate of the mean incubation period for AIDS in homosexual men. Science, *240:*1333–1335, 1988.

Moss, A.R.: Predicting who will progress to AIDS—at least four laboratory predictors available. Br. Med. J., *297:*1067–1068, 1988.

Richman, D.D., Fischl, M.A., Grieco, M.H., et al.: The toxicity of azidothymidine (AZT) in the treatment of patients with AIDS and AIDS-related complex: A double-blind, placebo-controlled trial. N. Engl. J. Med. *317:*192–197. *The original article describing the toxicity associated with zidovudine (AZT).*

Sande, M.A., and Volberding, P.A.: The Medical Management of AIDS. Philadelphia, W.B. Saunders Co., 1988. *An excellent review of the clinical spectrum and management of HIV infection. Clear diagnosis and treatment guidelines are included. Recommended as a basic reference for the primary care provider.*

Spickett, G.P., and Dalgleish, A.G.: Cellular immunology of HIV-infection. Clin. Exp. Immunol., *71:*1–7, 1988.

What science knows about AIDS. Sci. Am. *259:*4, 1988. *A comprehensive issue on the current status of research and understanding of acquired immunodeficiency syndrome. The contributing authors are recognized experts in the field.*

32

Pulmonary Medicine

John G. Prichard
Lawrence M. Tierney, Jr.

Most respiratory illnesses encountered in family medicine practice are benign and self-limited. It is the great challenge of a generalist's practice to distinguish those milder afflictions from serious diseases that often present in an undifferentiated form. As in all areas of practice, it is the ability to note unique susceptibilities of one's patients and to find in the multitude of historical points, physical findings, and laboratory data those often small pieces of information that set apart one disease process from another.

The diagnosis and management of respiratory illnesses require knowledge of the epidemiology of diseases of the chest, an understanding of the natural history of individual disorders, and an ability to enable patients to note deviations from expected clinical courses of self-limiting diseases. For example, the knowledge that influenza activity is beginning within the community often allows one to make a presumptive diagnosis given the proper clinical setting. As complications of this disease are few, patients or their family must, under the direction and guidance of the physician, observe the course of the illness and report findings or symptoms that may forewarn of complications. It is frequently the passage of time, and the persistence of a particular symptom, that becomes the only reasonable way to distinguish it as having a possibly serious underlying cause.

The prevention of respiratory disease is an especially important responsibility of the family physician. The prevention of pertussis and diphtheria, now taken to be routine, may presently be extended to include the prevention of influenza, tuberculosis, pneumococcal pneumonia, and infections caused by *Haemophilus influenzae*. Nearly all cases of lung cancer and the majority of cases of chronic obstructive lung disease could be eliminated by smoking prevention. Efforts in this regard, as in environmental air pollution, are a form of preventive medicine that must be pursued on an individual basis with our patients and in the community as both a social and political problem.

To review in detail even the most common of respiratory illnesses seen in the family physician's office would be a formidable undertaking. We therefore have limited the text to areas of pulmonary medicine where diagnosis or management has recently changed or is controversial. We have also elected to include entities that, though perhaps uncommon, represent diagnostic dilemmas or are not discussed in other readily available sources.

Radiology

As most of the chest is hidden, even to those most accomplished in auscultation, x-ray studies are a crucial part of our diagnostic armamentarium. The radiologist's ability to provide a reasonable differential diagnosis based on the pattern of x-ray abnormalities is greatly hampered by the absence of historical information. Under ideal circumstances, an x-ray study is ordered to solve a clinical difficulty. The radiologist then reviews the film and notes a particular pattern from which a differential diagnosis may be generated. That list is further refined, ideally in consultation with the family physician, by distinguishing features in the history and physical examination. Supplemental radiographic studies may then be chosen and, depending on the results of those studies, further diagnostic interventions or treatment undertaken.

Chest radiographs ordered in asymptomatic people are not helpful as part of routine screening for the early diagnosis of lung cancer in smokers or as a means of screening for tuberculosis. Additionally, routine chest x-ray films do not influence the overall management of patients with chronic lung diseases such as asthma, or chronic bronchitis-emphysema, unless there is clinical evidence indicating worsening.

On the other hand, the chest x-ray can be of immense value in attempting to sort out the cause of persistent cough, the origin of fever in a young child or elderly person, or distinguishing between acute bronchitis and pneumonia. If chest x-rays are ordered, the aim should be toward resolving a particular clinical problem, or in a complex patient for whom the chest x-ray allows us to investigate clinically unapproachable or silent areas.

Tests of Respiratory Function

Spirometric units that measure the forced expiratory volume in one second (FEV_1) and the forced vital capacity (FVC) are satisfactory for office testing of respiratory function. Reliable and inexpensive spirometers are now readily available. For children or young adults, hand-held peak flow meters can be easily used and give reproducible results. Standard reference tables for normal values (as functions of age, height, and sex) are often available from instrument manufacturers or may be found in standard texts of respiratory disease.

Oximetry is becoming widely used in hospital emergency rooms and outpatient respiratory therapy departments. Pulse oximetry is a useful and noninvasive method of determining the percent oxygen saturation. Its greatest use is in evaluating patients with acute respiratory illness, such as pneumonia, where the need for supplemental oxygen must be assessed. It is also useful for patients with chronic respiratory disease in whom there has been a worsening of symptoms. Oximetry results may, at times, be helpful in deciding upon admission to the hospital or the need for supplemental home oxygen therapy for patients with obstructive lung disease or to document desaturation for insurance or disability purposes.

Arterial blood gases are invaluable for the evaluation of patients with pulmonary disease. Blood gases allow a determination as to the presence or absence of hypoxemia, the adequacy of ventilation and the degree of metabolic compensation for respiratory dysfunction. Though expensive and uncomfortable for patients, compared with oximetry, arterial blood gases provide more information and are very precise. Determination of the partial pressures of oxygen and carbon dioxide is especially useful in the initial evaluation of patients with chronic obstructive or restrictive lung disease, both to assess the severity of disease and as a baseline to which one can later refer during periods of clinical deterioration or improvement.

Persistent Cough Without Apparent Cause

Persistent cough is a common complaint in ambulatory practice. Nonproductive but persistent cough in children is most frequently due to allergy or recurrent viral infections. In both children and adults, a persistent cough may follow a lower respiratory tract viral infection. In this circumstance, the cough is most often due to otherwise clinically silent reactive airways. The symptoms can frequently be managed with a combination of bronchodilator and a cough suppressant, such as dextromethorphan or codeine.

Environmental changes may bring about a persistent cough; chemical pollutants, such as smoke from a wood-burning stove or fireplace, tobacco smoke, or industrial exposures may produce cough that remits only with a change in climate or location of work. An atmosphere of very low humidity, whether occurring naturally at higher altitudes or as a consequence of home heating, may produce tracheobronchial irritation and subsequent cough. In younger children, a bronchial foreign body, or foreign body lodged deep within the ear canal, may produce a persistent cough.

An evening cough is particularly associated with reactive airways, especially in children. Similarly, an evening cough may be associated with postnasal discharge due to respiratory allergy. In these instances, an empiric trial of a bronchodilator or antihistamine may bring relief.

Disease of the pulmonary interstitium, congestive heart failure, and pulmonary neoplasms may produce chronic cough. The chest x-ray is crucial diagnostically and should be employed early in evaluating persistent cough, particularly if initial empiric therapy fails.

Endobronchial disease (tuberculosis, tumors) may cause persistent nonproductive cough without abnormalities on chest x-ray. Hence, occasional patients with persistent cough will eventually require bronchoscopy for diagnosis. Bronchoscopy should be advised early if there are worrisome symptoms, such as hemoptysis, fever, or weight loss, associated with the persistent cough.

Angiotensin-converting enzyme inhibitors (enalapril, captopril) may produce cough in certain susceptible individuals; however, the underlying mechanism is not presently understood. Lastly, a persistent cough may represent a tic or habit cough. Psychogenic coughs are related to anxiety and questioning may reveal, particularly in the adolescent, signs of adjustment difficulty in several areas. Clues to the nature of the cough may include its disappearance during sleep or its resolution during weekends or school holidays.

In most instances, a chronic cough will respond to empiric therapy with antihistamines and/or bronchodilators or resolve spontaneously without treatment. Otherwise, a chest x-ray, and occasionally bronchoscopy, will provide answers to its cause. In rare circumstances, despite one's best efforts at history taking and various diagnostic maneuvers, the cause of cough remains obscure. In this instance, it is best to start the diagnostic process over again with particular attention to recognizable exacerbating factors, recent environmental changes, and a survey of all medications consumed. A thorough ear-nose-throat examination and repeat x-ray examination of the chest may prove helpful. Pulmonary function tests may demonstrate abnormalities of diffusing capacity (interstitial lung disease), or spirometry may reveal reversible bronchospasm that may then justify an intensive course of brochodilator therapy.

Pleural Effusion

Diagnostic approaches to pleural effusion have not changed substantially over the last several years. The history, physical examination, chest radiograph, and laboratory analysis of pleural fluid yield a definitive or presumptive diagnosis in over 90 per cent of the cases. Pleural effusions are expected in many clinical settings and often may be followed until the underlying condition is controlled and resolution occurs.

Pathophysiologic mechanisms in pleural fluid accumulation are generally well understood. In the individual patient, however, they are often multiple. These mechanisms, with a single example, are presented in Table 32–1.

Table 32–1. MECHANISMS UNDERLYING PLEURAL FLUID COLLECTIONS

Mechanism	Example	Type of Effusion
Increase in hydrostatic pressure	Congestive heart failure	Transudate
Decrease in oncotic pressure	Nephrotic syndrome (hypoalbuminemia)	Transudate
Increased negative intrapleural pressure	Atelectasis	Transudate
Increased capillary permeability	Infection	Exudate
Decreased lymphatic drainage	Obstruction of lymphatics due to malignancy	Exudate
Increased transport of fluid across diaphragm	Pancreatitis	Exudate

Physical findings in cases of pleural effusion are well known and are not recounted here. Signs are not likely to be elicited unless the effusion is greater than 300 ml. Patients with pleural effusion are most commonly seen in consultation because of the underlying disorder associated with, or directly producing, the effusion. Symptoms and signs associated with the present illness guide the immediacy with which the effusion must be evaluated and determine approaches to diagnosis. Depending upon its cause, pleuritic pain may be present and moderate effusions (800 to 1000 ml.) may be associated with breathlessness.

In defining the cause of an effusion, attention should be directed to associated complaints of the patient. Pleuritic pain, fever, and the production of purulent sputum would make a diagnosis of parapneumonic effusion likely. Worsening dyspnea on exertion, paroxysmal nocturnal dyspnea, and clinical signs of right-sided heart failure will implicate increased hydrostatic pressure. Weight loss and a recent or remote history of breast malignancy would suggest a malignant effusion.

Pleural fluid first accumulates in the most dependent regions of the thorax, recesses that lie posteriorly. With increasing amounts, the lateral recesses, and eventually the anterior recess, will be occupied as well. Occasionally, pleural fluid accumulates between the lung and the hemidiaphragm rather than the posterior or lateral sulcus. Subpulmonary collections may be quite large. Once suspected, lateral decubitus views confirm the suspicion of fluid.

Occasionally, pleural collections may become encapsulated between fissures and form a tumor-like, rounded density. In the majority of cases, such pseudotumors occur at the horizontal fissure and vanish with control of the underlying cause, congestive heart failure in most cases. In addition to defining the amount of pleural fluid and its precise location, associated parenchymal infiltrates, or congestive heart failure, x-ray studies may also provide clues to the presence of subdiaphragmatic pathology. Bilateral decubitus views will sometimes allow imaging of the entire ipsilateral lung.

In most instances, analysis of pleural fluid obtained by thoracentesis will define the cause of the collection. Because there are many biochemical, cytologic, and microbiologic tests obtainable on pleural fluid, test selection must evolve from the clinical setting. Table 32–2 briefly lists various tests and their significance. In some instances, the clinical circumstances point so strongly toward a particular etiology that ordering specific tests with the initial thoracentesis is justified.

When the clinical picture is less obvious, the most useful tests are those that allow one to distinguish between exudative and transudative effusions. This is best done by obtaining total protein and lactate dehydrogenase simultaneously on the pleural fluid and serum. Table 32–3 shows the values for these

Table 32–2. LABORATORY FINDINGS ON PLEURAL FLUID AND THEIR SIGNIFICANCE

Test	Significance and Special Instruction
Total protein	Obtain serum protein determination. An exudative effusion is defined by a pleural fluid protein divided by serum protein equaling 0.5 or more.
Lactate dehydrogenase	Obtain serum LDH level. An exudate is indicated if pleural fluid LDH divided by serum LDH = 0.6 or greater, or LDH more than two thirds above upper limit of normal for serum.
Differential count	Collect in tube with anticoagulant.
Red cells	Frankly bloody effusions suggest malignancy, lung infarct, or trauma.
White cells	Total count of 10,000 is common in many causes of exudative effusions. Very large numbers seen with empyema.
Lymphocytes	If lymphocytes predominate (≧ 50 per cent), malignancy or tuberculosis is most likely. Pleural biopsy and/or cytologic studies should follow.
Mesothelial cells	Presence of mesothelial cells common; absence is of more importance. Tuberculosis very unlikely if large numbers are present and *is* likely in lymphocyte predominant exudates with few or no mesothelial cells.
Plasma cells	Seen in association with many causes of exudative effusions, including trauma. Very large numbers may suggest myeloma.
Eosinophils	Associated with pulmonary embolus, malignancy, hemothorax, resolving parapneumonic effusion, viral pleuritis, tuberculosis, and coccidioidomycosis.
Glucose	Useful if effusion is thought to be associated with rheumatoid disease, in which case the value is usually 30 mg. per dl. or less.
Amylase	Elevated in pancreatic disease, esophageal rupture and, occasionally, in nonpancreatic malignancies.
pH	Draw into heparinized blood gas syringe. Obtain only when pneumonia present. A value of 7.20 or less is indication for chest tube but only if effusion is due to bacterial infection.
Gram's stain	If positive, very useful in parapneumonic effusion. Will help guide antimicrobial therapy.
Acid-fast stain	Almost *never* positive even in proven cases. Histology and culture of pleural biopsy preferred. If pleural fluid cultured for AFB—send *large* volume (300 ml.).
Cytology	Add heparin to collection tube or place directly in fixative such as 60 per cent ethanol. Volume needed will depend upon method cytologist uses.
Cell block	Often very helpful addition to cytology. Larger volumes required—discuss with pathologist before thoracentesis performed.
Cultures	Preferable to collect in syringe, exclude remaining air. Take to laboratory with covered new needle. Be selective in ordering fungal and AFB cultures.

Table 32–3. ANALYSIS OF PLEURAL FLUID: EXUDATIVE VS. TRANSUDATIVE EFFUSION

Laboratory	Transudate	Exudate
Pleural fluid protein divided by serum protein	< 0.5	> 0.5
Pleural fluid LDH divided by serum LDH	< 0.6	> 0.6

findings that will allow a confident separation into the two types of effusions.

Transudative effusions occur in conditions in which intravascular oncotic pressures are diminished (nephrotic syndrome, advanced liver disease) or in circumstances of elevated venous pressures (congestive heart failure, constrictive pericarditis). Transudative effusions are more frequently bilateral and can, in the majority of cases, be confidently observed while managing the underlying cause. In contradistinction, exudative effusions are almost invariably caused by one of the following serious illnesses:

- Malignancy
- Infections
    - Bacterial parapneumonic effusion
    - Viral
    - Tuberculosis
    - Fungal (rare)
    - Parasitic (rare)
- Serositis
    - Rheumatic pleuritis
    - Lupus erythematosus
    - Drug hypersensitivity
- Pulmonary infarction
- Trauma
- Subdiaphragmatic disorders
    - Pancreatitis
    - Peritoneal carcinomatosis
    - Peritonitis
    - Subphrenic abscess
    - Subphrenic trauma (e.g., spleen hematoma)
    - Hepatic abscesses
- Miscellaneous disorders
    - Uremia
    - Sarcoidosis (rare)
    - Meigs' syndrome
    - Postradiation therapy
    - Chronic atelectasis
    - Abnormalities of lymphatic drainage
    - Benign effusion with asbestos

The pH of pleural fluid should be obtained in cases where an effusion complicating bacterial pneumonia is the principal diagnostic consideration. There is general agreement that a pleural fluid pH of 7.20 or less indicates need for tube thoracostomy. Draining the pleural space obviates the development of empyema thoracis or loculation of parapneumonic fluid. The pH of pleural fluid in circumstances other than underlying bacterial pneumonia has no prognostic or diagnostic significance.

Cytologic analysis of pleural fluid has become the cornerstone of diagnosis in malignant effusions. Combining the examination of Papanicolaou stained smears and sections prepared from paraffin-imbedded cell buttons yields a diagnosis in more than 90 per cent of cases. False positive results are occasionally reported, usually due to misinterpretation of reactive mesothelial cells as malignant. If initial studies are negative or inconclusive, and malignant effusion remains the principal clinical diagnosis, repeated cytologic studies are warranted.

Needle biopsy of the pleura finds its greatest use in circumstances where a pleural effusion is exudative, lymphocyte-predominant, and relatively lacking in mesothelial cells. These findings are characteristic, but not diagnostic, of pleural tuberculosis. If pleural biopsy specimens are examined histologically and cultured, this more than doubles the diagnostic yield over culturing pleural fluid only. By combining all three methods, a definitive diagnosis of tuberculosis can be achieved in roughly 80 per cent of cases. Pleural biopsy also improves diagnostic accuracy in cases of malignant effusion. As pleural biopsy is not without risk and is frequently uncomfortable, it is probably best reserved for cases of suspected tuberculosis or suspected malignant effusions when initial cytologic studies are inconclusive.

Pleural effusion due to malignancy is most often a consequence of primary tumors having their origin in the lung. Breast malignancy and tumors arising from the lymphoreticular system are the second and third most common cause, respectively. Adenocarcinoma of unknown primary site produces malignant effusions at a rate comparable to that for tumors arising in the lymphatic system (12 per cent). Primary tumors of the genitourinary or gastrointestinal tract involve the pleura less often.

Pleural effusions associated with malignancies other than breast or lymphoma signify advanced disease and a poor prognosis. If the tumor is responsive to chemotherapy, the collection may resolve and not recur. Frequently, management will require removal of the collection by tube thoracostomy followed by pleurodesis. Tube drainage can be accomplished with relative comfort if a small bore chest tube is placed under adequate systemic and local analgesia. When drainage is minimal (less than 50 ml. in 24 hours), pleurodesis may be undertaken. This is most often accomplished by instillation of 500 to 1500 mg. of intrapleural tetracycline. Some patients tolerate this procedure well while others find it very painful. Thus, every effort should be made to ensure adequate intrapleural analgesia. Recent studies have shown that a dose of 250 mg. of lidocaine in a 1 or ½ per cent solution will achieve good pleural anesthesia without toxic serum levels. Insuring contact of the lidocaine solution with all pleural surfaces is essential before instilling the tetracycline solution. Local pleural anesthesia should be augmented by systemic analgesia with opiates. Effective pleurolysis can be expected in the majority of patients. On the occasions when this method fails, repeated application of tetracycline is often effective.

Tuberculous effusions may be seen in the absence of underlying parenchymal disease. These effusions occur as a consequence of rupture of a caseous focus subjacent to the pleura. A low-grade fever is frequently present and, unless the collection represents an empyema, the skin test is almost invariably positive. The collection is exudative and usually, though not exclusively, lymphocytes predominate. Treatment is identical to that used for pulmonary tuberculosis.

Effusion commonly occurs coincident with pneumonia. Initially, the fluid is thin with a relatively low number of inflammatory cells. With prompt antibiotic therapy, such effusions are arrested and resorb without further difficulty. Effusions associated with more virulent organisms, or in cases in which treatment is delayed, become more heavily laden with inflammatory cells and fibrin. These effusions may form loculated collections in dependent, posterior regions of the chest. If loculations are small, unassociated with persistent fever, and painless, they will likely cause no great difficulty and resorb with time. Conversely, large collections and persistent fever are indications for drainage. Localization of loculated collections is easily defined by ultrasound. Percutaneous drainage often brings dramatic resolution of fever and x-ray abnormalities.

Empyema, or the appearance of grossly purulent material and viable organisms in the pleural space, may occur following a parapneumonic effusion or rupture of a tuberculous or bacterial abscess into the pleural space. Aerobic organisms are the cause in 40 per cent of cases and streptococcal species are most frequently isolated. Mixed anaerobes are exclusively found in 30 per cent of cases with *Bacteroides* species being the predominant organism.

When a parapneumonic effusion is noted, early thoracentesis may have valuable diagnostic as well as therapeutic implications. A Gram's stain may detect organisms and direct specific antibiotic therapy. In a nonloculated effusion, pleural pH will help guide the immediacy with which tube thoracostomy may be necessary.

A minority of patients with pleural effusion will remain undiagnosed following initial endeavors at defining its etiology. Recent studies have suggested certain criteria that, if present, strongly predict an underlying malignant or other treatable cause. Those patients with small exudative effusions (800 ml. or less), and who are not associated with the criteria set forth in Table 32–4, may be followed expectantly. Should the clinical circumstance change, then further diagnostic efforts are warranted. The use of fiberoptic bronchoscopy in the evaluation of pleural effusion of unknown cause provides a very low diagnostic yield.

Interstitial Lung Diseases

The interstitium of the lung may be defined as that part of the alveolar wall that separates the capillary endothelial cells from alveolar epithelial cells. In excess of 125 different diseases have been considered to be interstitial when they involve the lung, though it is to be recognized that many involve other tissues and organ systems. As regards chronic diffuse diseases of the lung, then, they may be principally interstitial; mainly alveolar filling; or, more often, a combination of both. Thus, the term interstitial lung diseases can be confusing to the clinician but perhaps less so if it is remembered that these processes are uncommonly restricted specifically to that part of the pulmonary anatomy.

The so-called interstitial diseases, irrespective of their cause, tend to show either inflammation or fibrosis pathologically and often both; when inflammation dominates, the process is frequently termed alveolitis. Any number of different cells of inflammation may be observed, including mononuclear cells, lymphocytes, polymorphonuclear neutrophils, and eosinophils, with the prevalence of one or another determined by the cause of the disease. In addition, an important feature of some interstitial lung diseases is the presence of granulomas; sarcoidosis (see later) is an example. However, most interstitial lung diseases may be separated from each other with difficulty based solely on histopathologic examination. Thus, only in certain circumstances is it necessary to obtain biopsy material in the assessment of interstitial lung disease. The pathogenesis of all these conditions may be summed up by considering that an abnormal inflammatory response exists in the pulmonary interstitium, that it may be initiated by numerous processes—some known but others idiopathic, that varying types of histology may be observed in the acute phase (but with the two broad groups being lymphocytic/granulomatous and neutrophilic), and that all ultimately may result in pulmonary fibrosis.

As might be anticipated by this localization of the pathology within the lung, interstitial lung diseases share many functional abnormalities. Lungs affected with these conditions show consistently decreased compliance; the lungs are stiff, and require greater pressures to achieve any volume of expansion, resulting in an increased work of breathing. At the same time, the higher pressures required for expansion secondarily result in a lower lung volume and lower total lung capacity. Damage to the exchange surface between the circulation and the inspired air results in impairment of diffusion capacity, because of a reduced total area for effective gas exchange. Together, these result in a typical pattern seen in interstitial lung diseases of hypoxia with slight reduction in PCO_2. Though diffusion is impaired as noted above, the hypoxia more likely results from impairment of the matching of ventilation and perfusion than it does from abnormal diffusion as had been believed previously. The hypoxia and hypocarbia tend to be progressive, and when oxygen saturation of hemoglobin is consistently below 90 per cent, which occurs at a PO_2 of approximately 50 to 55 mm. Hg then consequent pulmonary hypertension may be expected. This in turn exacerbates the process by inflicting additional trauma upon the pulmonary microvasculature.

Many observers prefer to differentiate interstitial lung diseases into those of known and unknown causes (Table 32–5), and it is clearly in the patient's best interest for a meticulous search to be carried out for any potentially reversible cause. The general

Table 32–4. FACTORS INDICATING UNDERLYING MALIGNANT OR TREATABLE INFECTIOUS CAUSES OF EXUDATIVE PLEURAL EFFUSION (SEE TEXT)

Weight loss of 4.5 kg. or more
Fever
Large effusion
Reactive tuberculin test
>95 per cent lymphocytes in pleural fluid

Table 32–5. CAUSES OF INTERSTITIAL PULMONARY DISEASE

Known Cause	Unknown Cause
Inorganic dusts	Idiopathic pulmonary fibrosis
Silica	Sarcoidosis
Silicates (including asbestos)	Eosinophilic granuloma
Beryllium	Rheumatic disease associated
Hard metal dusts	Goodpasture's syndrome
Organic dusts (hypersensitivity pneumonitis)	Idiopathic pulmonary hemosiderosis
Gases, fumes, vapors	Wegener's granulomatosis
Chlorine	Angioimmunoblastic lymphadenopathy
Sulfur dioxide	Ankylosing spondylitis
Mercury	Amyloidosis
Drugs	Pulmonary lymphangiomyomatosis
Antineoplastic agents	Whipple's disease
Antibiotics	Alveolar proteinosis
• Sulfonamides	Inflammatory bowel disease associated
• Nitrofurantoin	
Drugs inducing lupus erythematosus	
Sulfonylureas	
Gold	
Phenytoin	
Amiodarone	
Poisons	
Paraquat	
Radiation	
Infections	
Disseminated mycobacterial or fungal infections	
Viral pneumonia	
Pneumocystis carinii pneumonia	
Residue of active infection of any type	
Pulmonary edema	
Lymphangitic carcinoma	

history obtained from the patient with suspected interstitial lung disease, therefore, is directed in a fashion aimed at identifying such causes. The specific pulmonary symptoms, however, are remarkably similar irrespective of cause; the typical patient notes the insidious onset of dyspnea, usually exertional; the breathlessness is not episodic, and orthopnea is not a feature. Depending upon the rate of progression, the patient may be dyspneic at rest when first observed, but the considerable majority of patients have a more indolent onset of this complaint. The other common symptom is cough. This is typically dry and nonproductive. Hemoptysis is seldom present unless extensive fibrosis has occurred. On physical examination, the patient usually appears comfortable, although very slight tachypnea may be observed if the respiratory rate is counted over a minute. The only finding on auscultation is inspiratory crackles, most often appreciated at both bases. Some clinicians believe the dry rales to be characteristic of an interstitial process.

In clinical practice, the combination of a complaint of dyspnea and/or cough, with or without the presence of crackles on physical examination, is sufficient reason to obtain a roentgenogram of the chest. It is at this point that the interstitial nature of the process is appreciated, and further historical inquiries are typically made. Likewise, additional abnormalities on the chest film, when present, allow the clinician to narrow the differential considerably.

As concerns additional history, there are several fruitful areas of inquiry. For example, the presence of symptoms suggesting a systemic autoimmune disease, such as dermatomyositis or lupus erythematosus, would lead the clinician to recognize that this would be interstitial lung disease complicating those disorders. Many drugs have been reported to cause interstitial pneumonitis; the most typical encountered in family practice would likely be nitrofurantoin, though numerous antineoplastic agents, gold, and even radiation itself can produce the same process. An occupational history is quite important in the patient with an interstitial abnormality on chest x-ray. Exposure to metals (such as beryllium, silica, coal, and asbestos) or organic matter (such as sugar cane, hay, or sawdust, and many others) may cause this. Similarly, the presence of additional systemic symptoms, such as fever, may lead the clinician to consider more seriously an infectious etiology. Tuberculosis, fungal diseases (such as histoplasmosis and coccidioidomycosis), many viral infections, and atypical pneumonitides (such as Q fever) may result in an interstitial process.

Given implications for therapy, it is of special importance to consider infection (Table 32–6) in all such cases. Of particular interest in the patient's history is the presence or absence of risk factors for AIDS; additional inquiries could concern the presence or absence of pets, especially birds; a previous history of malignancy might alert the physician to the presence of lymphangitic carcinoma presenting as an interstitial radiologic pattern. Other aspects of the physical examination, once the clinician is aware of the presence of interstitial radiographic diseases, become important. Lymphadenopathy, synovitis, hepatomegaly, a palpable spleen, and evidence of cardiomegaly all can help the clinician assign priorities to various etiologies in order to tailor the subsequent investigation.

Table 32–6. INFECTIOUS CAUSES OF INTERSTITIAL LUNG DISEASES

Bacterial chlamydial:	tuberculosis, atypical mycobacteriosis, actinomycosis, *Nocardia* infection, psittacosis, leptospirosis, Whipple's disease, Lyme disease, Legionnaires' disease (occasionally), mycoplasma (occasionally) infections
Viral:	acute HIV, Epstein-Barr virus, cytomegalovirus, herpes simplex virus infections
Parasitic:	*Pneumocystis carinii, Echinococcus* infections
Fungal:	sporotrichosis, histoplasmosis, coccidioidomycosis
Rickettsial:	Q fever

Additional evaluation of the chest film itself also provides additional clues. Of prime importance is the initial distinction between a mostly interstitial abnormality and one that is primarily caused by an alveolar filling process. Though most of the latter are associated with more acute illnesses, such as bacterial pneumonia or pulmonary edema, there are several chronic abnormalities of alveolar filling that clinically resemble the interstitial lung diseases. These include alveolar proteinosis, Goodpasture's syndrome, and eosinophilic pneumonia; all are quite rare. Roentgenographically, an alveolar abnormality results in the loss of the distinction of adjacent parenchymal vessels and of the boundaries of neighboring structures such as the heart border or diaphragm. The infiltrate of interstitial diseases, by contrast, appears in the early phase as linear, or sometimes nodular, with many patients showing elements of both. With chronicity of disease, scarring and retraction may result in an appearance referred to as honey-combing, which is the development of small cystic spaces throughout the lungs. Prominent pulmonary arteries are also noted in this late stage of interstitial lung disease.

Associated abnormalities may be quite helpful in diagnosis. If there is concomitant pleural thickening or effusion, then considerations such as the interstitial diseases associated with autoimmune processes, asbestosis, lymphangitic carcinomatosis, and nitrofurantoin lung are more likely. Associated hilar and/or mediastinal lymphadenopathy favor sarcoidosis, lymphoma with lymphangitic involvement, primary or metastatic lung carcinoma, or pneumoconiosis, particularly berylliosis. If pneumothorax is present, then eosinophilic granuloma is worthy of consideration; the latter is also associated with lytic bone lesions that can be appreciated in ribs. Interstitial disease that is most prominent in the upper lung fields suggests end-stage sarcoidosis; infections such as tuberculosis; and pneumoconiosis, particularly silicosis. When cardiomegaly is present with an interstitial lower lobe infiltrate, the clinician should keep congestive heart failure in mind; in this case, the infiltrates are linear and subpleural, the so-called Kerly B lines. Finally, approximately 10 per cent of patients who ultimately develop roentgenographically abnormal interstitial lung disease may be symptomatic with a normal chest film at the time of first presentation; this can be observed in small recurrent pulmonary embolization and *Pneumocystis* pneumonia.

In short, the combination of numerous details of history, physical examination, and thorough inspection of the chest x-ray allow the physician a reasonable opportunity to establish the diagnosis and, more importantly, to select subsequent studies of higher predictive value. Any subsequent investigation of interstitial lung diseases is tempered by the fact that in more than two thirds of cases, no identifiable cause will be found. Similarly, though many conditions have been reported to be associated with an interstitial abnormality by x-ray, in many of these conditions, this pattern is an atypical or unusual manifestation. Thus, a panel of studies obtained on a routine basis is to be avoided. For example, culture of the expectorated sputum for typical bacterial pathogens, as well as for fungus and tuberculosis, is seldom likely to be helpful. Hematologic studies are usually within normal limits; the occasional patient with long-standing hypoxia may show erythrocytosis, but the white cell count is usually within normal limits. Chemistries are only revealing when certain conditions are under active consideration; for instance, the elevated alkaline phosphatase and hypercalcemia of sarcoidosis may be illuminating, as is the elevated lactate dehydrogenase of *Pneumocystis* pneumonia, but these studies are only supportive of an hypothesis and not diagnostic. As implied above, examination of expectorated sputum is in general not helpful. In many centers, however, the diagnosis of *Pneumocystis* pneumonia may be made after sputum induction by ultrasonic nebulization; in this instance, the patient may be spared more invasive studies.

The principal conundrum in the approach to interstitial lung diseases relates to the appropriateness of bronchoscopy, bronchoalveolar lavage, and open lung biopsy in patients with this problem. Thus, a preprocedure assessment of the likelihood of finding a treatable lesion, and consideration of whether the patient is a candidate for such treatment, is prudent. Occasionally, invasive diagnostic studies are employed to establish a diagnosis related to occupational exposure for purposes of compensation; asbestosis is an example.

Of these studies, an open lung biopsy is the most sensitive and specific. It is excellent in identifying infectious or neoplastic causes of interstitial lung disease, demonstrates granulomas when they are present, and is also accurate for many other parenchymal processes. A biopsy also allows the clinician the opportunity to determine how much a roentgenographic process is contributed to by active inflammation, and how much by fibrosis, even if the specific etiology of the process cannot be determined. Open lung biopsy, on the other hand, requires general anesthesia and, thus, carries a small but finite risk of significant morbidity or even mortality; similarly, recuperation requires a chest thoracostomy tube. Further, the majority of open lung biopsies will not yield a specific cause of the problem. This has led clinicians to attempt to employ less invasive studies, which invariably are less sensitive diagnostically. A transbronchial lung biopsy, though highly sensitive for sarcoidosis and *Pneumocystis* pneumonia, is less likely to reveal definitive information about other parenchymal processes. Complications of transbronchial biopsy include hemoptysis, pneumothorax (in about 5 per cent of cases), and the worsening of hypoxia. Pulmonary hypertension and coagulation disorders constitute contraindications. Another study performed in increasing numbers of centers is bronchoalveolar lavage. In this procedure, irrigation of the distal airways is carried out by bronchoscopy, and an analysis of the fluid for the type of cells present is carried out. Predominance of lymphocytes suggests a granulomatous process such as sarcoidosis; increased numbers of neutrophils are observed in idiopathic pulmonary fibrosis. It is safe to say, however, that this procedure is not in widespread use and remains more of a research tool than a clinically useful investigation. In short, an open lung biopsy is more sensitive and specific but more invasive; transbronchial biopsy is diagnostic in certain conditions but is less useful in many diffuse pulmonary processes in which involvement of the lung is patchy.

As certain causes of interstitial pulmonary diseases are of particular interest, they will be discussed individually, starting with several conditions of identified cause. Silicosis results from the inhalation of silicon dioxide and occurs in sand blasters and quarry workers. The development of pulmonary disease requires many years of exposure, and the highest doses occur with occupations such as sand blasting. Early in the disease, there are small nodular densities distributed interstitially in the lungs; these nodules become larger over time. Silicosis is more prominent in the upper lobes, and it is often associated with dense calcification of regional hilar nodes. Patients with silicosis also have a very much higher risk for the development of tuberculosis. The diagnosis can generally be made from the history along with a plain chest film; more invasive investigation is seldom necessary.

Although its major effects are pulmonary, *sarcoidosis* is a systemic disease of unknown cause. It most commonly affects blacks and is more frequent among women than men; it is a young person's disease. Because of its systemic nature, the clinical manifestations are protean. Pulmonary sarcoidosis may present with bilateral hilar adenopathy alone (stage I), hilar adenopathy plus parenchymal interstitial disease (II), or parenchymal disease by itself (III). It is likely that the disorder progresses through all three stages, but the occasional patient may not come to medical attention until it is rather advanced, at which time it is also more difficult to diagnose.

Unusual pulmonary manifestations include nodules, with or without cavitation, and, rarely, pleural effusions. Extrapulmonary manifestations and indications for steroid therapy include hypercalcemia, due to granulomatous elaboration of a vitamin-D–like substance, granulomatous hepatitis, arthritis, iritis, carditis (characterized typically by conduction disturbance abnormalities), and nodular skin lesions. All or none of these may be present in the patients with pulmonary involvement. Most observers would favor establishing a histologic diagnosis, even with quite high pretest probability, and sarcoidosis is a condition in which transbronchial biopsy demonstrative of noncaseating granulomas has high sensitivity. This is not as specific given the many causes of granulomas, such as tuberculosis. Generally, the combination of this pathology in the proper clinical situation allows the clinician to establish the diagnosis. Approximately three quarters of patients with sarcoidosis have skin test anergy, a sometimes useful feature helping to separate this process from similar conditions.

Asbestosis is another common interstitial lung disease. Asbestos also is capable of causing mesotheliomas of pleura and peritoneum and is synergistic with cigarette smoke in inducing bronchogenic neoplasm. Patients who have exposure to asbestos include shipyard and construction workers, and those who have worked extensively with brake linings. Inadvertent exposure may still occur in the remodeling of buildings where asbestos had been used during construction. The chest x-ray in asbestosis shows prominent bibasilar nodular streaking. Typically, associated pleural disease is present, including calcification of the diaphragmatic pleura, and irregular thickening of the pleura elsewhere in the lung. Asbestosis may also be associated with a benign exudative pleural effusion, with or without interstitial lung disease. In general, the diagnosis of asbestosis may be made by the clinical history in concert with the chest film, though the occasional patient may require histologic confirmation; asbestos fibers may be readily identified in histologic specimens, but this requires electron microscopic analysis.

Hypersensitivity pneumonitis is perhaps an unfortunate term, but this condition is one in which immunologic attack on inhaled particles occurs in the interstitium of the lung. The inhaled antigens in hypersensitivity pneumonitis are invariably organic, being derived from nonpathogenic micro-organisms or plant or animal proteins. The list of such antigens is now a long one, although the prototype disease of this category is *farmer's lung,* in which the presence of micro-organisms in damp hay are inhaled and produce immunologic pulmonary injury. Clinically, the dyspnea in hypersensitivity pneumonitis is typically episodic, occurring shortly after exposure. In some cases, however, inhalation and symptoms may not be temporally related. In this case, it may be difficult to appreciate the relationship between the exposure and the illness and thus requires a higher index of suspicion on the part of the physician. Hypersensitivity pneumonitis is thus an example of the importance of a detailed occupational history in all patients presenting with interstitial abnormality by chest x-ray. Histopathologically, one observes prominent lymphocytic infiltration in the interstitium as well as occasional poorly formed granulomas, which may thus be distinguished from those seen in sarcoidosis. This correlates with the belief that the pathogenesis of this condition is related to a cell-mediated immune response to the antigen. Though it might be anticipated that corticosteroids would be of some value in this condition, the most obvious therapeutic intervention is the alteration or discontinuation of the patients' exposure to the responsible antigen.

Interstitial lung disease induced by radiation is seen in up to 10 per cent of patients who receive therapeutic radiation for lymphomas and carcinomas involving thoracic structures. Symptoms may begin as early as 1 month after the completion of treatment, in which case symptoms are more acute, although the indolent onset of dyspnea may reflect a more fibrotic process and may not present until a year after the radiation. In the early phase, patients may be febrile in addition to experiencing pulmonary symptoms. Radiation pneumonitis is characteristically not confined to an anatomical segment of lung but rather involves the part that receives the radiation. Perhaps the biggest dilemma facing the clinician in this situation is whether the pulmonary infiltrate is due to radiation, to concomitantly administered chemotherapy, to recurrence of the tumor itself, or to superimposed infection. Steroids may be effective for early occurring disease but are less valuable if fibrosis is present.

As has been noted previously, though there are many identifiable causative agents of interstitial lung diseases, and many other diseases with which interstitial lung disease is associated, the majority of interstitial lung disease encountered by the clinician is of unknown cause and is generally termed idiopathic pulmonary fibrosis. The diagnosis of this process, by definition, is one of exclusion. If this criterion is adhered to, then patients who present with idiopathic pulmonary fibrosis are usually in the fifth to seventh decades of life, with an equal incidence in both sexes. In addition to the symptoms of dyspnea and cough, the occasional patient will have fever and arthralgias; on exam, clubbing of the fingers may be present in addition to basilar crackles. It is believed by many that idiopathic pulmonary fibrosis is a process that undergoes an evolution from desquamative interstitial pneumonitis, in which inflammatory cells in the interstitium and in the alveolar spaces are observed, through a picture of usual interstitial pneumonitis, where the most notable pathologic abnormality is fibrosis. Other investigators believe these are two separate processes. In any event, theories advanced to account for either possibility invariably conclude that some unknown antigen initiates the disease, and that antigen-antibody complexes are important in its pathogenesis. This view would also hold that these complexes stimulate the activation of macrophages, which in turn release chemotactic factors for neutrophils and perhaps other mediators of inflammation. Though neutrophils are not prominent histopathologically, they are more numerous on bronchoalveolar lavage than in other forms of interstitial lung disease. Many patients with idiopathic pulmonary fibrosis have nonspecifically positive studies for antinuclear antibodies and rheumatoid factors. It is to be underscored that these test abnormalities occur in the absence of other more specific clinical evidence for autoimmune diseases; at the same time, several primary immunologic diseases may in fact be associated with interstitial pulmonary disease. It can be appreciated that a biopsy of the lung in idiopathic pulmonary fibrosis will review the nonspecific findings that have been referred to, and such a study is more important for excluding other etiologies. If granulomas are present, idiopathic pulmonary fibrosis is excluded. The prognosis for this problem is better for patients whose initial biopsy specimens reveal more active inflammation than fibrosis, and many clinicians believe that this group responds more favorably to treatment with immunosuppressive agents, particularly corticosteroids.

The treatment of interstitial lung diseases, then, depends entirely upon the cause. In those instances in which a specific infectious cause can be demonstrated, the outlook is excellent. Similarly, in those cases in which an inhalant or drug is responsible, therapy consists of withdrawing the offending agent. In the majority of cases, however, the clinician is left without an identifiable etiology and must decide whether to institute steroids empirically or to proceed to an open lung biopsy first. Given the fact that response to this type of treatment is inconsistent, and in view of the long-term toxicity of steroids, empiric treatment is unwise for most patients. Similarly, there is little correlation between the roentgenographic appearance and the histologic presence or absence of fibrosis. For all these reasons, there are few instances in which histologic confirmation is not obtained. Occasionally, very rapid progressive interstitial pulmonary fibrosis, or other immunologically mediated lung disease, may progress rapidly enough to render the patient a poor candidate for either open lung biopsy or bronchoscopy. In these few patients, a course of steroids may be attempted, but it is often necessary to treat simultaneously for infectious diseases. Otherwise, the treatment is entirely supportive, with supplemental oxygen of value if patients are symptomatic at rest or whose ambient Po_2 concentrations are consistently less than 55 mm. Hg.

Disorders of the Proximal Airways

Most of the disorders of the proximal airways encountered in ambulatory practice affect children. The proximal airways and larynx of the child have a small surface area with an extensive submucosal vasculature. Infection or inflammation of these structures results in edema with consequent narrowing of the lumina. The most common disorders affecting the proximal airways in childhood and adolescence include *epiglottitis* (see chapter on Otolaryngology), *laryngotracheitis, bacterial tracheitis*, and *laryngotracheobronchitis*. While the above-mentioned diseases have factors in common and may overlap in terms of severity, a diagnosis can usually be made on the basis of history, physical findings, and the results of therapeutic interventions.

Laryngotracheitis (spasmotic croup) is most commonly encountered in the fall and winter months and usually affects children between 1 and 4 years of age. The onset of the illness is usually sudden, predominantly nocturnal, and characterized by a barking cough. There is a paucity of prodromal or concurrent symptoms of upper respiratory tract infection, and fever is usually absent. The disorder is considered to be caused by a viral infection or allergy causing subglottic edema. Exposure to humidified air, cold or warm, often brings relief of cough and stridor promptly. Hence, children brought to the hospital for evaluation may be rendered nearly free of symptoms simply by exposure to the evening or night air.

Viral laryngotracheitis must be distinguished from a bronchial foreign body, angioneurotic edema, extrinsic or intrinsic laryngeal or tracheal masses. The onset of the illness and surrounding circumstances can usually lead to the exclusion of these disorders. Laryngotracheitis is distinguished from epiglottitis by the latter's association with a somewhat less precipitous onset, fever, and a toxic appearance. Treatment includes the provision of humidified air, whether at home or in the hospital. Corticosteroids have shown benefit in decreasing the duration of symptoms.

In laryngotracheobronchitis, cough becomes associated with symptoms and signs of a viral upper respiratory tract infection. Cough progresses in severity and becomes associated with stridor, bronchospasm, and fever. Signs and symptoms frequently worsen in the evening hours. Although the illness is more frequently encountered in winter, it may be seen during any season, and most commonly between the age of 3 months and 3 years. The syndrome may accompany outbreaks of influenza virus, respiratory syncytial virus, and other viral respiratory pathogens.

Physical examination reveals a febrile child with a croup-like cough. Respiratory distress may be manifested by retractions, and stridor may be present to a minor or marked degree. There are usually signs indicating upper respiratory tract inflammation including rhinorrhea. Audible wheezing is usually present and a chest x-ray may show narrowing of the tracheal shadow. Differential diagnosis includes epiglottitis, inhaled foreign body, and spasmodic croup.

Therapy consists of humidified air and oxygen therapy. Racemic epinephrine, given by aerosol, is indicated in other than mild cases and may bring rapid, albeit transient, relief. Repeated aerosol treatments may be warranted but refractiveness to this modality may occur. Although benefit is not proven, some clinicians occasionally employ corticosteroids as some children seem to respond. In the minority of cases, airway narrowing progresses and respiratory distress worsens. Nasotracheal intubation may be required, and the tube may need to be left in place for several days.

Occasionally, children thought to have laryngotracheobronchitis are found, at the time of intubation, to have purulent secretions in the airway. Bacterial cultures may grow *Staphylococcus aureus*. Bacterial tracheitis may occur as a primary event but is generally thought to occur following viral injury to the proximal airway. Treatment usually involves placing a nasotracheal tube, providing supplemental oxygen, humidification of inspired air, and a beta-lactamase–resistant penicillin or a cephalosporin.

Acute Bronchitis

Acute bronchitis is the fifth most commonly diagnosed illness by family physicians. This condition accounts for an enormous amount of time missed from work and school. During particular seasonal outbreaks, especially influenza, acute bronchitis can account for more than half of telephone consultations and one third of office visits.

Viruses cause the vast majority of episodes of acute bronchitis with influenza A and B, and respiratory syncytial virus being associated with distinct seasonal outbreaks. Adenoviruses, rhinoviruses, coxsackievirus, and parainfluenza viruses also cause episodes of acute tracheobronchitis. In young adults, *Mycoplasma pneumoniae* and a particular strain of *Chlamydia psittaci* have been documented to cause a small proportion of cases of acute bronchitis in young adults.

With the exception of *Bordetella pertussis*, the etiologic agent of whooping cough, bacterial agents are more difficult to incriminate as definite causes of bronchitis. Most of the organisms thus far incriminated (*H. influenzae, Streptococcus pneumoniae*, and *B. catarrhalis*) are part of normal flora of the upper respiratory tract. The isolation of these organisms in cases of acute bronchitis is therefore expected. However, their presence in increased numbers in persons with chronic disease of smaller airways and their common association with pneumonia lend credence to their presumed role as causative agents of acute bronchitis.

The diagnosis of acute bronchitis usually rests upon clinical grounds. Patients complain of acute, usually productive cough and, occasionally, minimal hemoptysis, frequently in association with mild to moderate fever, chills (without true rigors), myalgias, and fatigue. In many cases, pharyngitis and/or rhinitis either precedes or accompanies the lower respiratory tract symptoms. Persons who smoke develop acute bronchitis more frequently, with more severe and persistent symptoms.

On examination of the chest, signs of consolidation are absent. Fine crackles, representing secretions in the airways, may be demonstrated and wheezing may be evident or discovered only upon auscultation during forced expiration. In the elderly febrile patient, and occasionally in febrile infants and children with signs and symptoms of bronchitis, a chest x-ray is warranted to differentiate acute bronchitis from pneumonia. In most patients, neither x-ray studies nor additional laboratory tests, such as leukocyte counts, are of value.

Treatment of acute bronchitis remains largely symptomatic. For those in whom cough is severe, and wheezing can be demonstrated, temporary use of inhaled bronchodilators may be of benefit. If the cough is associated with substernal pain and lack of sleep, a cough suppressant, such as dextromethorphan or codeine, may bring improvement. For patients with rhinitis, the addition of an antihistamine may be helpful. Acetaminophen or other nonsteroidal anti-inflammatory agents may help control fever and myalgias.

Antibiotics are frequently prescribed for acute bronchitis though their benefit remains unproven. Although bronchitis may be a harbinger of pneumonia, this is an infrequent complication and antibiotic therapy has not been shown to decrease the frequency with which it evolves.

The use of antibiotic therapy in acute bronchitis, though often demanded by patients, is both elective and empiric. The choice of antibiotic in acute bronchitis is also problematic. Clinical syndromes overlap sufficiently that one cannot easily distinguish between potential causative agents, and no laboratory tests can reliably differentiate among the various pathogens. Although serologic tests and viral cultures are available, these are not practical in the ambulatory setting.

Erythromycin is frequently prescribed; however, there is an increasing rate of resistance to this agent among strains of *H. influenzae* and a high rate of discontinuance owing to gastric intolerance, even with enteric-coated formulations. Erythromycin and tetracycline have been shown to decrease the duration of illnesses caused by *Mycoplasma*; however, there is no reliable constellation of symptoms or signs that favor *Mycoplasma* over other agents as the cause of bronchitis.

If antibiotic therapy is elected, a Gram's stain of sputum may be helpful in guiding selection of an antimicrobial. If *S. pneumoniae* or *Haemophilus* is recognized, then trimethoprim-sulfa or amoxicillin-clavulinate represent rational choices. If the patient is between 5 and 40 years of age, has purulent sputum without a predominant organism on Gram's stain, or lives in a relatively closed environment in which *Mycoplasma* illness has been documented in others, erythromycin may then be prescribed.

During outbreaks of influenza A activity, patients

with compatible symptoms may reasonably be treated with amantadine. To be effective it must be instituted within the first 72 hours of illness.

Bronchiolitis

Acute bronchiolitis is a febrile disease of infancy and early childhood due to infection of the respiratory epithelium of smaller airways. Peribronchial edema and inflammatory cell infiltration occur, becoming associated with obstruction of small airways from cellular debris and mucous plugs.

The disease is most commonly encountered in children from 2 to 12 months. During epidemics of bronchiolitis, which occur predominantly between January and May, more than 80 per cent of cases are due to respiratory syncytial virus. During nonepidemic outbreaks, respiratory syncytial virus is found in slightly over 50 per cent of cases, with parainfluenza viruses, adenoviruses, influenza viruses, rhinoviruses, and *Mycoplasma* being associated with the remainder of cases. Concomitant infection with either another virus or bacteria occurs in roughly 5 per cent of cases.

Following an incubation period of 5 to 7 days, the child develops fever, often associated with signs of upper respiratory tract infection, and copious production of tenacious nasal secretions. Progressive cough and dyspnea then ensue during the first 5 days of illness. Irritability and respiratory distress usually bring the child to medical attention.

On examination, the most striking findings are rhinorrhea, respiratory distress, and wheezing. The chest x-ray may show marked hyperinflation with depression of both diaphragms, thereby explaining the frequent ability to palpate both spleen and liver on physical examination. Peribronchial and interstitial infiltrates may be noted in multiple lobes in addition to atelectasis.

The differential diagnosis includes gastric aspiration, inhaled foreign body, and asthma associated with viral infection. Pneumonia is often considered because of the high frequency of abnormal chest x-rays associated with respiratory syncytial virus infection. The white blood cell count may be elevated, and in some children a left shift is seen. An initial episode of asthma precipitated by a viral infection may not be distinguishable from bronchiolitis on clinical grounds. Definitive etiologic diagnosis is possible using viral cultures or immunofluorescence assays on nasopharyngeal secretions; however, these studies are rarely ordered outside of research or teaching institutions.

The treatment of bronchiolitis is aimed at the management of respiratory distress. Supplemental oxygen is provided and antibiotics are sometimes prescribed owing to the uncertainty concerning bacterial pneumonia. Though children less than 2 years old are relatively unresponsive to inhaled beta-agonist therapy, this is often provided along with intravenous theophylline to seriously ill children. The mortality rate in large series varies from 0.5 to 5 per cent with death more likely in children with pre-existing lung disease (i.e., bronchopulmonary dysplasia) or heart disease.

It has long been recognized that children with severe bronchiolitis, once recovered, may have persistent chest symptoms several years hence. Recurrent lower respiratory tract infections with evidence of airway obstruction may occur and mandate readmission. Because of these findings, an etiologic role of respiratory syncytial virus in the pathogenesis of asthma has been postulated. Current evidence does not support an association of recurrent chest symptoms following bronchiolitis with a family history of asthma or evidence of atopy. The extent to which antiviral therapy is effective in treating bronchiolitis or in preventing its sequelae is presently unknown. For children who experience wheezing following bronchiolitis, most episodes can be shown to be precipitated by a recurrent viral illness. Additionally, most of these children have come from homes where parents smoke.

Pneumonia

The term pneumonia encompasses an extraordinary range of severity of illness and of causative agents. Though here we are concerned mainly with infectious causes of pneumonia, the same symptoms and signs can be caused by a host of noninfectious illnesses including inhaled chemicals, hypersensitivity disorders, and other noninfectious inflammatory disorders such as sarcoidosis. Certainly, most cases of pneumonia are transient, self-resolving infections that go unrecognized or respond to empiric therapy on an outpatient basis. In the majority of instances, even among hospitalized patients, no etiologic agent is identified.

Given the variety of organisms capable of causing pneumonia, and the overlapping clinical and radiographic findings caused by them, a clinical diagnosis based solely on possible etiologic agents will be unrewarding. For example, *S. pneumoniae*, the most common cause of community-acquired pneumonia in hospitalized patients, may produce a relatively mild illness with inflammation limited to a single lobe. This same organism may also cause an overwhelming illness with panlobar involvement, bacteremia, and multiple distant sites of infection.

Radiographic patterns are extremely helpful in the diagnosis of pneumonia (Figs. 32–1 to 32–4). Although certain patterns may be characteristic of a particular pathogen, none are pathognomonic. Similarly, laboratory studies, such as the white blood cell count or degree of left shift, offer only general guidance. Most laboratory tests are nonspecific and a good deal of variation is to be expected.

Hence, whereas knowledge of the usual pattern

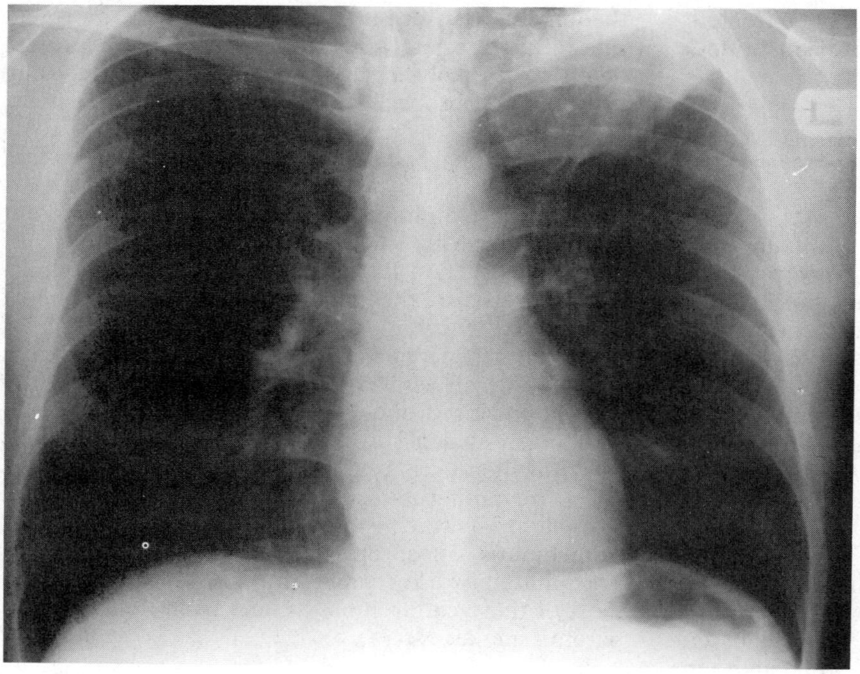

Figure 32–1. Segmental density, left upper lobe: The alveolar infiltrate is uniform and is compatible with pneumonia. The radiographic appearance is, however, nonspecific. The clinical history suggested an indolent rather than an acute infection, which proved to be due to *Cryptococcus neoformans.*

of illness caused by distinct pathogens is essential in the evaluation of an individual patient with pneumonia, an epidemiologic approach is more useful. Factors that bear upon unique susceptibilities and influence the presentation or likely course are found in the patient's history; age, race, occupation, local endemicity, associated illnesses such as diabetes, HIV infection, or a recent episode of influenza each may help to incriminate a particular pathogen.

Subjective data will lead one to suspect an *acute* or *chronic* pneumonia—a distinction that carries great etiologic significance. Whether the disease was *acquired in the hospital* or in the *community* raises suspicion for certain pathogens and the likelihood that the organism will be resistant to antibiotics.

Combining epidemiologic, historical, and clinical information with specific patterns found on the chest x-ray is enormously helpful. Whether the lung involvement is localized or diffuse, is associated with effusion, predominantly cavitary, or demonstrates involvement far out of proportion to the degree of illness influences one's further diagnostic attempts. A recent history of altered consciousness (e.g., seizure) and the finding of pulmonary infiltrates in dependent

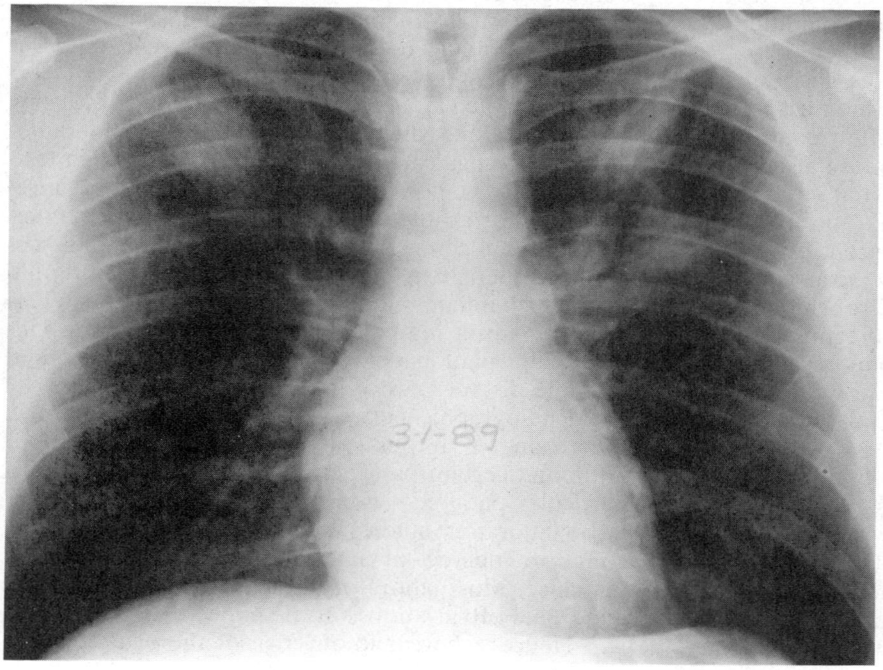

Figure 32–2. Multifocal, ill-defined densities in both upper lobes: The radiographic findings are consistent with an atypical pneumonia with a broad differential diagnosis. The x-ray film is that of a young man with cough and dyspnea for several weeks. He was moderately ill and known to have an infection with human immunodeficiency virus. The clinical setting and severity of the illness prompted a diagnostic bronchoscopy, which provided a diagnosis of *Pneumocystis carinii* pneumonia.

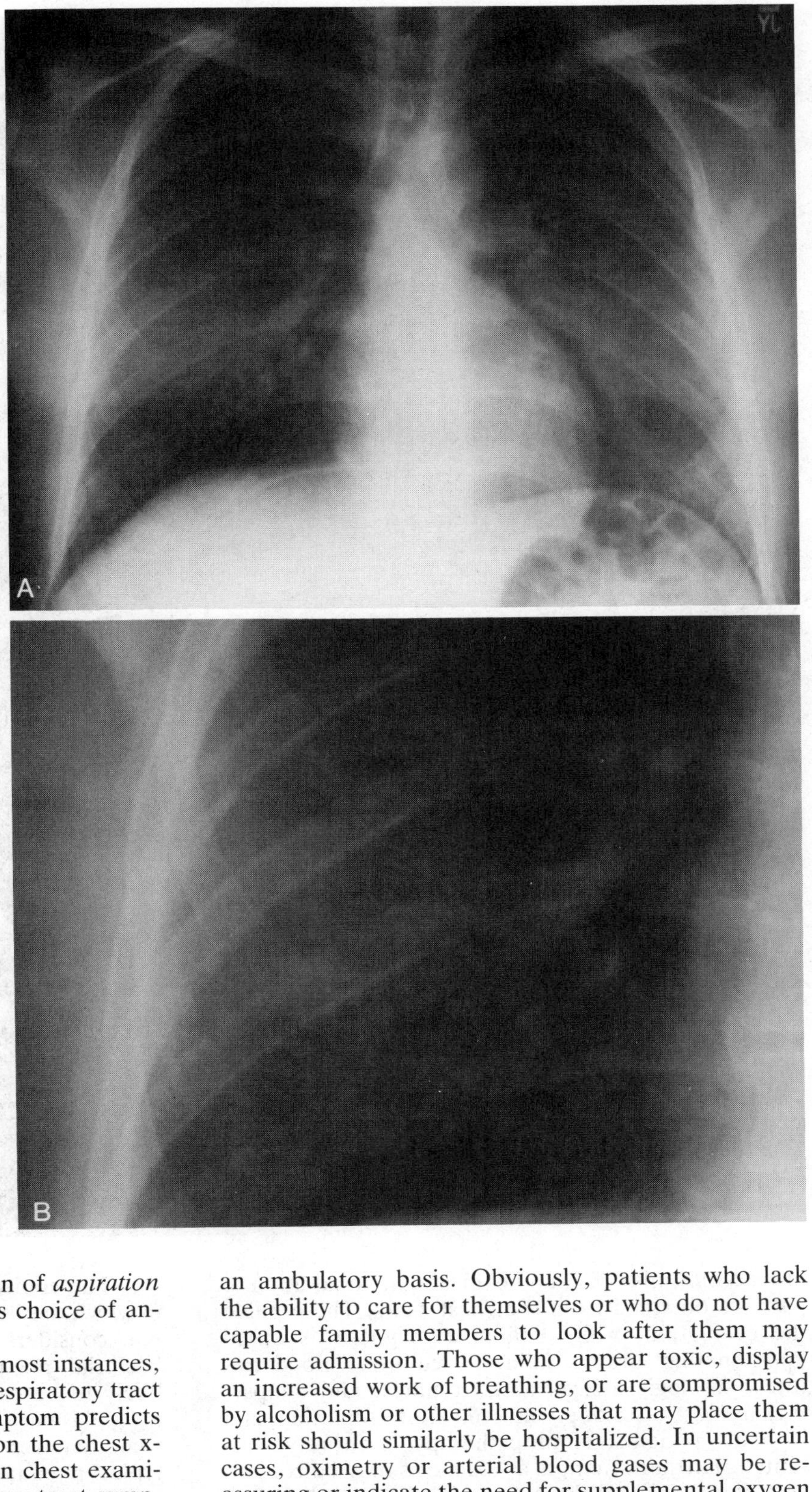

Figure 32–3. *A* and *B*, Diffuse, fine nodular densities: The densities are sometimes better seen on a lateral film in the retrosternal or retrocardiac region. This pattern may be seen, in febrile patients, with hypersensitivity pneumonia, tuberculosis, fungal or viral infections. The patient came from an endemic region for tuberculosis, and the Mantoux test was reactive. Sputum examination yielded rare acid-fast bacilli.

segments leads one to the consideration of *aspiration* pneumonia and immediately influences choice of antibiotic therapy.

The diagnosis of pneumonia is, in most instances, made clinically on the basis of lower respiratory tract signs. No single clinical sign or symptom predicts accurately the presence of infiltrates on the chest x-ray. Abnormal auscultatory findings on chest examination, in patients with acute respiratory tract symptoms, are, however, most predictive of an abnormal chest x-ray.

The most immediate difficulty in managing patients with pneumonia is the decision whether to admit the patient to the hospital or begin therapy on an ambulatory basis. Obviously, patients who lack the ability to care for themselves or who do not have capable family members to look after them may require admission. Those who appear toxic, display an increased work of breathing, or are compromised by alcoholism or other illnesses that may place them at risk should similarly be hospitalized. In uncertain cases, oximetry or arterial blood gases may be reassuring or indicate the need for supplemental oxygen therapy in the hospital. Reasonable and insightful patients who have concerned family members to supervise their course can be managed satisfactorily as outpatients.

The etiologic diagnosis of pneumonia must take

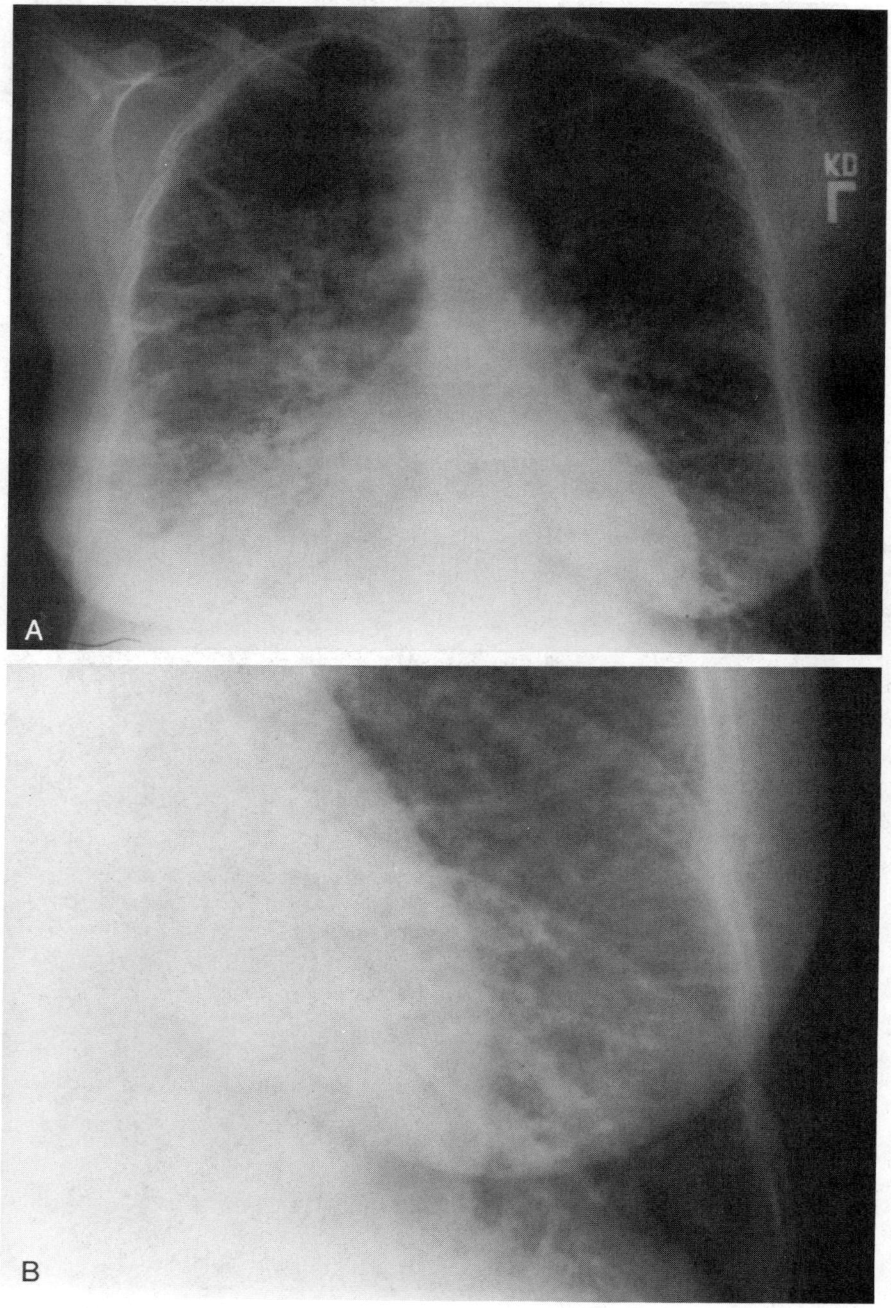

Figure 32–4. *A* and *B,* Reticular densities: The interstitial pattern is commonly seen in pulmonary edema. Thickened interlobular septa are best seen in the costophrenic angles *(B)*. This pattern is also seen with atypical, acute pneumonias caused by viruses and *Mycoplasma*. The x-ray film is that of a young woman with influenza pneumonia.

into account historical and clinical data in addition to patterns obtained from the chest x-ray. These guide the evaluation, while definitive diagnosis is based upon sputum Gram's stain and cultures, blood cultures, serologic assays, and, at times, lung biopsy. Again, most cases of pneumonia are self-limiting, and in many patients, empiric therapy is entirely warranted. Further attempts at diagnosis may be reasonable only if empiric therapy is failing or the diagnosis can be obtained by relatively simple and inexpensive diagnostic tests. Urgent and invasive diagnostic methods may, however, be necessary, either because of the severity of illness or the setting in which it is evolving.

The choice of laboratory tests and the sequence in which they are employed will depend upon whether one considers the pneumonia to represent typical bacterial pneumonia or an atypical process more likely to be caused by mycobacteria, viruses, fungi, mycoplasma, or parasitic disease. Table 32–7 lists some features helpful in distinguishing atypical from typical pneumonia in older children or adult patients.

Despite efforts to identify clinical and laboratory factors that might aid in differentiating bacterial pneumonia from viral pneumonia in children, the positive predictive value of any single finding or group of combined laboratory and clinical findings is poor. Judgment as to the severity of illness within the

Table 32–7. FEATURES DIFFERENTIATING TYPICAL AND ATYPICAL PNEUMONIA

Feature	Typical	Atypical
Prodromal illness	+ +	+ + +
Sudden onset (or sudden worsening of prodrome)	+ + +	+
Rigors	+ + + +	+ − + +
Chest pain	+ + + +	+ − + +
Fever (> 102° F)	+ + + +	+ +
Purulent sputum	+ + + +	+ +
White cell count with left shift	+ + + +	+ +
Dyspnea	+ + +	+ − + +
Degree of illness	+ + +	+ − + +
X-ray study worse than anticipated	+ − + +	+ + + − + + + +
Lobar distribution of infiltrate	+ + + +	+
Pleural effusion	+ + + +	+

context of the patient and his or her community has been consistently found to be of greater importance than any single laboratory determination, or group of laboratory findings, in deciding proper disposition of the patient. Factors that favor the bacterial cause of pneumonia rather than the viral include the following: age greater than 6 months, fever greater or equal to 103° F, and total band count greater than 500. Certain roentgenographic features may also be helpful: if a single lobe is involved with a definite infiltrate or if multiple lobes are involved by well-defined infiltrates, this favors a bacterial etiology. The presence of pleural effusion, pneumatoceles, or abscesses each favors a bacterial cause as well. On the other hand, interstitial or peribronchial infiltrates that involve multiple sites associated with segmental atelectasis favor a viral etiology.

Whether one evaluates a child with a lower respiratory tract infection by a formal scoring system, or a more global clinical evaluation based on clinical experience and judgment, is less important than recognizing that viral or bacterial causes of lower respiratory tract infections are not mutually exclusive. Indeed, most bacterial infections of the lower respiratory tract probably arise as a consequence of disordered local defense mechanisms induced by a viral infection. Hence, whether one elects to admit a child with a respiratory tract infection or manage its care on an outpatient basis, *re-evaluation* of the child's clinical course in response to therapy is most crucial.

As most cases of community-acquired pneumonia are likely to be due to either *S. pneumoniae* or *H. influenzae*, oral agents chosen for treatment should cover these bacteria. Beta-lactamase–producing strains of *H. influenzae* are increasingly isolated; thus amoxicillin-clavulinic acid represents a reasonable first choice for oral therapy. Trimethoprim-sulfamethoxazole and erythromycin-sulfisoxazole represent satisfactory alternatives.

The course of *Mycoplasma* pneumonia can be shortened by treatment with erythromycin. Tetracycline is an alternative agent, except in children. Unfortunately, the diagnosis is difficult; there are no reliable clinical or radiologic findings, either in children or adults, that can distinguish *Mycoplasma* from other causes of atypical pneumonia, especially early in its course (Table 32–8). A cold-agglutinin titer of 1:32 or greater is supportive of the diagnosis but is nonspecific. Complement fixation titers may not increase to a diagnostic level until the second or third week of illness. Culture of sputum for *Mycoplasma* is difficult and is not helpful in deciding upon initial antibiotic therapy. Hence, erythromycin may be reasonable empiric therapy in young patients with an atypical pneumonia syndrome, a compatible chest x-ray, and whose sputum shows leukocytes but no evident pathogens on Gram's stain.

In the management of adults with community-acquired pneumonia, there may be instances when oral antibiotic therapy is not deemed adequate. Yet, for a variety of reasons, hospitalization may not be desirable, or the patient may refuse admission. In these circumstances, parenteral therapy may be initiated using a long half-life cephalosporin (e.g., cefonicid) administered once every 24 hours by the intramuscular route or via an indwelling heparin lock. Parenteral therapy may be discontinued and replaced with oral therapy as soon as the patient's clinical course indicates that the pneumonic process is resolving.

The extent to which efforts should be directed toward etiologic diagnosis before beginning therapy will be influenced both by the severity of illness and the relative likelihood of complications. Tests, such as the total leucocyte count, are nonspecific and provide little insight as to potential pathogens. A Gram's stain and culture of adequate sputum specimens are most useful; if adequate specimens cannot be produced spontaneously, they can often be obtained by saline aerosol induction. If positive, blood cultures provide highly specific information and should be considered, particularly for patients who are to receive parenteral therapy for pneumonia on an outpatient basis.

Table 32–8. SIGNS AND SYMPTOMS ASSOCIATED WITH *MYCOPLASMA PNEUMONIAE* PNEUMONIA*

Symptom or Finding	Expected Occurrence (Per Cent)
Cough	90
Fever	80
Sore throat	50
Injected pharynx	45
Nausea, vomiting	40
Headache	30
Chills	30
Otitis, myringitis	30
Chest pain	25
Muscle aches	25
Lung consolidation	25
Dyspnea	25
Adenopathy (cervical)	25

*Adapted from Mansel, J. U., Rosenow, E. C., Smith, T. F., and Martin, J. W.: Chest, *95*:639, 1989.

Tuberculosis

Tuberculosis is a chronic, relapsing, systemic illness that is transmitted almost exclusively via the respiratory route. Similar to other chronic granulomatous diseases of the lung, such as histoplasmosis or coccidioidomycosis, a primary infection is followed by healing in the majority of cases: only 15 per cent of infected individuals develop an illness that will be, at some time, diagnosed as tuberculosis.

In most of the world, infection is acquired during childhood, though a new infection may occur at any age. Symptoms following initial infection are usually mild and, unless suspicion is aroused because of additional epidemiologic or skin test data, often do not lead to further investigation. Cough may or may not be present and constitutional symptoms are highly variable, being less frequently seen in the very young or elderly.

Concomitant with the development of pneumonia, there is subclinical dissemination of *Mycobacterium tuberculosis* to virtually all organs. Within 6 weeks following infection, delayed hypersensitivity develops with arrest of bacterial replication. From time to time, however, factors that enforce local control at such infected sites may falter. Mycobacterial replication may resume and a variety of syndromes may then occur, depending upon the location of bacterial regrowth. Reactivation of tuberculosis usually occurs in the lung, resulting in so-called reactivation-type tuberculosis. Infiltrates are most commonly seen in the upper lobes, often with cavities. Formation of the latter requires some degree of hypersensitivity. In some patients, cavitation does not occur, and the infiltrates may take on the appearance of pneumonia of any cause or may appear as nodules simulating neoplasm.

As evidenced by the foregoing, the diagnosis of tuberculosis is often made by inference; taking the history, epidemiologic clues, clinical, and radiographic information into account. In children, the finding of a reactive tuberculin skin test in association with an abnormal chest x-ray is usually grounds for a full course of antituberculosis chemotherapy. If warranted (uncertain diagnosis, suspicion of resistant organisms), three successive early morning gastric aspirates may be obtained. In those able to cooperate, the induction of sputum samples using hypertonic saline is superior to spontaneously produced sputum in terms of recovery of organisms.

Biopsy of affected organs (pleura, lymph nodes, or bone) may be required to obtain a histologic diagnosis and for cultures. At times, despite one's best efforts, treatment must proceed on an empiric basis. This is nearly always the case in smear-negative pulmonary tuberculosis, as cultures often take as long as 6 weeks before definitive identification is possible. Recent advances using fluorescent microscopy and newer methods of culture have, however, greatly improved the rapidity with which definitive diagnosis can be made.

The treatment of pulmonary and extrapulmonary tuberculosis affecting children or adults is outlined in Table 32–9. Complications and drug interactions of the most commonly used chemotherapeutic agents are outlined in Table 32–10. In circumstances where the patient's illness is complicated by renal insufficiency, adjustment of drug doses need be made only in the case of ethambutol or aminoglycosides. The dose of ethambutol should be 10 to 15 mg./kg. per day with a 50 per cent decrement in renal function. Renal insufficiency greatly prolongs the half-life of aminoglycosides, and, therefore, the dosage interval must be increased.

During pregnancy, isoniazid and rifampin may be used without concern for teratogenicity and if resistance is suspected, ethambutol should be added. Duration of therapy using isoniazid and rifampin combinations, in the setting of susceptible organisms, is 9 months. Therapy is necessarily longer if drug resistance is encountered or a concomitant infection with the human immunodeficiency virus is present. In the latter instance, the precise duration of therapy is not known though might reasonably be continued for at least 9 to 12 months following conversion of sputum samples to negative.

The prevention of tuberculosis is acomplished not only by the treatment of contagious patients but by the identification of infected, asymptomatic individuals as well. The tuberculin skin test may identify individuals who have been infected with tuberculosis, but it cannot distinguish between those with active or inactive disease. Current recommendations, for otherwise well individuals, suggest screening with intradermal or multipuncture skin tests at 1 year of age, again at the time of entry to preschool or kindergarten, and at some point during adolescence. Tuberculin skin testing should also be considered for all new immigrants and young people planning to study or travel extensively in areas where tuberculosis is endemic.

As a result of screening either in the office or by school health services, the physician may be confronted with the patient who is well but has a reactive tuberculin skin test. Figures 32–5 and 32–6 suggest a management scheme for asymptomatic children and adults. Though 10 mm. of induration at 48 to 72 hours is usually taken to represent a prior tuberculosis infection, this threshold may properly be lowered to 5 mm. For example, a 5 mm. area of induration in a 6-month-old child known to have been exposed to a family member with active pulmonary tuberculosis might well be considered to indicate infection. It is especially the case in a young adult or child that a reactive tuberculin skin test indicates the presence of an infectious individual in the young person's environment. Hence, the reactive tuberculin test represents a sentinel event that should prompt investigation of the child's siblings, parents, or other persons with whom significant contact has been made.

The decision to use preventative therapy, usually isoniazid, presumes that active disease has been rea-

Table 32–9. EQUIVALENT STANDARD THERAPEUTIC REGIMENS FOR *MYCOBACTERIUM TUBERCULOSIS* INFECTIONS

Type and Duration	Drug and Dosage: Adult		Drug and Dosage: Pediatric	Comment
I. Continuous (9 months)	INH 300 mg. Rif 600 mg.	Daily	INH 10–15 mg./kg. (max. 300 mg.) Rif 10–15 mg./kg. (max. 600 mg.)	Recommended for cooperative patients with little chance of resistant organisms. Add PZA 30 mg./kg./day (3.0 gm. max.) for children or adults if resistance anticipated. In pregnant patients with possible resistant organisms add EMB 15–20 mg./kg./day. May discontinue PZA or EMB abruptly if organisms found to be sensitive.
II. Intermittent (9 months) 4 weeks:	INH 300 mg. Rif 600 mg.	Daily	As above	Consider for patients who are forgetful or require medicines to be dispensed, children or adults whose compliance may be incomplete. Add PZA 30 mg./kg./day or EMB 15–20 mg./kg/day if resistant organisms suspected.
then 8 months	INH 15 mg./kg. (max. 900 mg.) Rif 600 mg.	Twice weekly	INH 15 mg./kg. (max. 900 mg.) Rif 10–15 mg./kg. (max. 600 mg.)	
III. Continuous (6 months) 8 weeks:	INH 300 mg. Rif 600 mg. PZA 30 mg./kg.	Daily	INH 10–15 mg./kg. (max. 300 mg.) Rif 10–15 mg./kg. (max. 600 mg.) PZA 30 mg./kg. (max. 3.0 gm.)	Consider for compliant patients when shorter course desirable. Add EMB 15–20 mg./kg./day if resistance suspected.
then 4 months	INH 300 mg. Rif 600 mg.	Daily	INH 10–15 mg./kg. (max. 300 mg.) Rif 10–15 mg./kg. (max. 600 mg.)	
IV. Intermittent (6 months) 8 weeks:	INH 300 mg. Rif 600 mg. PZA 30 mg./kg.	Daily	As in III above	Good regimen for unaccommodating patients. Add EMB 15–20 mg./kg./day initially if drug resistance suspected.
then 4 months	INH 15 mg./kg. (max. 900 mg.) Rif 600 mg.	Twice weekly	INH 10–15 mg./kg. (max. 900 mg.) Rif 10–15 mg./kg. (max. 600 mg.)	

Key: INH = Isoniazid; Rif = rifampin; PZA = pyrazinamide; EMB = ethambutol.

These agents may be given once daily as single dose. For children: INH elixir available (10 mg./5 ml.) and rifampin suspension (10 mg./5 ml.) can be formulated by pharmacist.

From Prichard, J. G. and Raleigh, J. W.: Tuberculosis and other mycobacterial diseases. *In* Rakel, R. E. (Ed.): Conn's Current Therapy. Philadelphia, W. B. Saunders Company, 1988, pp. 167–174.

sonably eliminated and compliance with either a year-long or 6-month regime can be anticipated. Isoniazid is usually very well tolerated, though parents occasionally complain that a child may seem somewhat hyperactive. This can usually be satisfactorily resolved by providing the drug in the evening hours. Though drug-induced hepatitis represents a rare complication of isoniazid therapy, it is an age-related phenomenon usually occurring in older individuals. Periodic determinations of hepatic transaminase in an otherwise well individual is generally not warranted.

Chronic Disorders of the Airways

Three disorders are commonly recognized under the term chronic obstructive pulmonary disease (COPD): chronic bronchitis, asthma, and emphysema. Though often thought of as mutually exclusive and distinct clinical entities, they share either common precipitants, pathophysiology, or response to therapeutic intervention. Obstruction to airflow can be demonstrated in each as can anatomic abnormalities, such as bronchial muscle hypertrophy, glandular hypertro-

Table 32–10. SIDE EFFECTS AND DRUG INTERACTIONS OF THE MAJOR ANTITUBERCULOSIS AGENTS

Drug	Associated Side Effects	Other Drugs With Which Clinically Significant Interactions May Occur	Consequence
Isoniazid	Rash, lightheadedness, hepatotoxicity, peripheral neuropathy, hypersensitivity reactions (e.g., fever, urticaria, red cell aplasia), optic neuritis, seizures	Disulfiram	Psychotic episodes
		Dilantin	↑ Blood levels of phenytoin
		Aluminum-containing antacids	↓ Absorption of INH
		Ketoconazole	↓ Blood levels of ketoconazole
Rifampin	Orange color in urine, tears, hepatotoxicity, thrombocytopenia, anemia, renal failure Flu-like illness (myalgias, chills, fever, arthralgias, vomiting, diarrhea)	Trimethoprim Warfarin Oral hypoglycemic agents Methadone Oral contraceptives Digitalis Theophylline Dilantin Glucocorticoids Verapamil	↓ Blood levels or effectiveness
		Ketoconazole	↓ Blood levels of rifampin and/or ketoconazole
Ethambutol	Optic neuritis Hyperuricemia Hypersensitivity reactions Peripheral neuropathy	Aluminum-containing antacids	↓ Absorption
Pyrazinamide	Hepatotoxicity Arthralgia Hyperuricemia Nausea Acute gouty arthritis Fever Flushing		
Streptomycin	Vestibular toxicity, auditory dysfunction Renal toxicity Rash	Loop diuretics Other nephrotoxic drugs Curare-like agents	May augment auditory toxicity May augment renal toxicity Prolong neuromuscular blockage

From Prichard, J. G. and Raleigh, J. W.: Tuberculosis and other mycobacterial diseases. *In* Rakel, R. E. (Ed.): Conn's Current Therapy. Philadelphia, W. B. Saunders Company, 1988, pp. 167–174.

phy, and varying degrees of airway narrowing. Therapeutic interventions, specifically cessation of smoking, and the use of various bronchodilating drugs may have a salutary effect.

Though asthma is typically regarded as paroxysmal episodes of reversible bronchospasm, in some the obstruction to airflow eventually becomes less reversible, resembling patients with chronic bronchitis.

In some individuals who smoke, an increase in elastase and various mediators of the inflammatory response can be demonstrated within alveoli. The result is the destruction of very small distal airways and a concomitant increase in the size of alveolar spaces. Though rare patients may be demonstrated to have relatively pure emphysema (e.g., alpha 1-antitrypsin deficiency), most can be demonstrated to have bronchorrhea and reversible limitations of airflow.

The terms blue bloater and pink puffer are occasionally used to distinguish between, respectively, individuals with chronic bronchitis and emphysema. Anatomic studies have, however, shown more similarities than differences between these two clini-

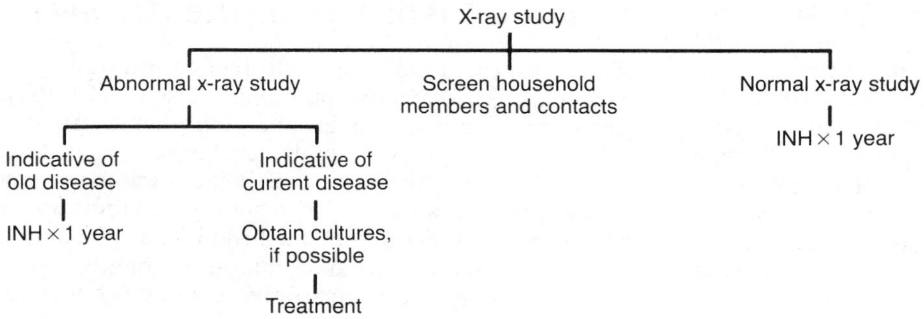

Figure 32–5. Management of tuberculin-positive asymptomatic children or young adults.

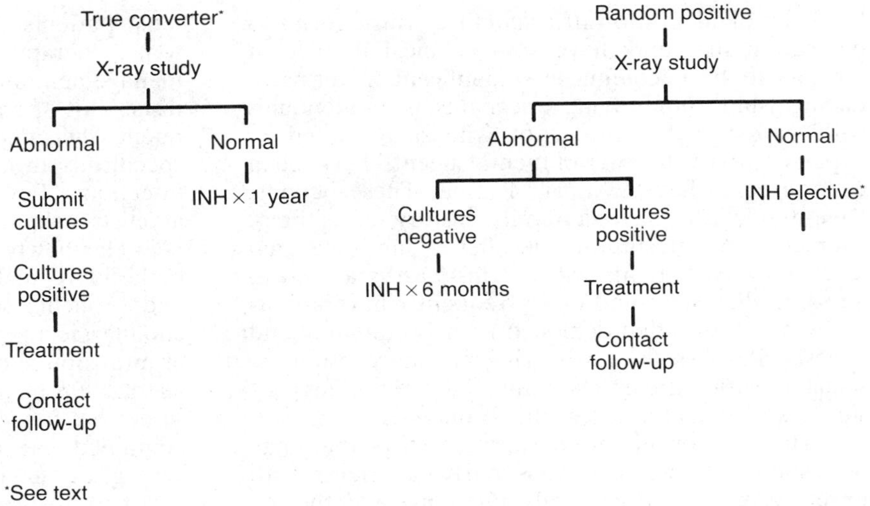

Figure 32–6. Management of tuberculin-positive asymptomatic adults.

cally identifiable groups. It appears that the clinical abnormalities in these groups can be attributed to differing central responses to hypoxemia, rather than fundamental differences in type or severity of pulmonary disease.

Asthma

Asthma is defined by several criteria and must be differentiated from other causes of paroxysmal dyspnea. In childhood, asthma must be distinguished from acute bronchiolitis, lower respiratory tract infections, cystic fibrosis, congestive heart failure, recurrent pulmonary aspiration, and retained bronchial foreign body. Asthma attacks are characteristically paroxysmal and may bear temporal relationships to environmental or emotional stimuli or become manifest only with upper or lower respiratory tract infections. There may be a seasonal incidence with return of normal respiratory function during interval periods. A family history of asthma or a personal history of eczema or other atopic phenonema may support a diagnosis of asthma.

Physical examination may show wheezing during all phases or only part of the respiratory cycle that usually clears promptly with institution of treatment and remains clear during asymptomatic intervals. The chest x-ray is characteristically normal during asymptomatic periods. Eosinophils may or may not be found in sputum and are sometimes increased on the differential white cell count.

Since 1979, there has been a consistent increase in the reported number of deaths due to asthma, only in part explained by a change in disease classification and reporting. Increases in asthma mortality have been reported from other countries as well and have been most striking within the age group 5 to 34 years. The rising mortality in metropolitan areas may be in part related to increasing air pollution, however, as indicated by asthma death rates in Montana (third highest rate in United States); other factors are also important. A lack of definite seasonal variation in mortality argues against viral infections or environmental allergens playing a significant role.

Studies from New Zealand, where the highest increase in death rate has thus far been reported, showed that more than 50 per cent of those who died were *in extremis* at the time of presentation to the hospital. As testimony to their circumstances, no deaths occurred in those surviving more than 30 minutes after reaching the emergency room.

In childhood cases that have been intensively reviewed, certain high risk factors have emerged; discontinuity of medical supervision, nearly exclusive reliance on emergency rooms for asthma care, and frequent admissions for status asthmaticus. Recent hospitalization, tapering of relatively high steroid doses, and minority racial status are also associated with the higher likelihood of sudden death due to asthma. A dysfunctional family circumstance or an expressed wish to die has been documented in a number of adolescent asthma deaths. Overreliance upon the use of inhaled beta-mimetic agents and a tendency to delay seeking emergency care appear to contribute to a large proportion of deaths due to asthma.

Long clinical experience clearly supports the notion that asthma is a paroxysmal illness that, with each episode, represents a potential threat to life. Most asthma attacks are readily terminated. This usual experience may lull patients, their families—and even their care-givers—into a false sense of security. On the other hand, unpredictable attacks of breathlessness, especially in children, may cause great anxiety. Thus, in the care of asthmatic patients and their families, the physician must walk the narrow path of providing confidence and competency to the patient and family, while at the same time acknowledging concern and the importance of seeking care urgently.

Asthma is a heterogeneous disorder, both in severity and natural history, that is multifactorial in its causation and persistence. Traditionally, asthma has been divided into intrinsic and extrinsic forms, a distinction that may have some clinical merit, but appears to be becoming less significant in terms of distinguishing underlying mechanisms. Individuals with paroxysmal episodes of wheezing related to hypersensitivity to environmental agents have been considered to have extrinsic asthma. These patients have tended to have a family history of asthma, cutaneous manifestations of allergy, and elevated levels of IgE. Patients with intrinsic asthma tend to be somewhat older and more frequently have abnormal x-ray studies that demonstrate hyperinflation and fibrosis. Paroxysms of wheezing are more often associated with purulent sputum and their illness assumes a course akin to chronic bronchitis.

The relationship to heritable factors that may predispose to reactive airways, early experience with lower respiratory tract viral infections, and the acquisition of hypersensitivity in the development of asthmatic syndromes remain unknown. Recent data indicate a very strong association between asthma prevalence and increasing age-specific IgE levels. However, among unselected individuals with very high IgE levels only a minority suffer from asthma. Clearly then, there are other factors that predispose to the onset of asthma and perpetuate its occurrence. As many as one third of asthma attacks in childhood and adulthood can be shown to be associated with lower respiratory tract viral infections, especially those caused by respiratory syncytial virus (RSV). The majority of children recovering from RSV infections will experience lower respiratory tract symptoms over the succeeding several years.

The therapy of asthma involves use of pharmacologic and nonpharmacologic therapy that is based upon an understanding of precipitating factors and the severity and constancy of symptoms. There is considerable individual variation in the degree to which pharmacologic therapy is tolerated and effective. Therefore, therapy proceeds in a stepped manner, using objective methods (e.g., FEV_1, peak flow rates) to monitor benefits while noting drug-associated toxicity.

For patients with asthma who smoke, persistent efforts toward achieving complete cessation should be undertaken. Specific precipitating events, drugs, or environmental circumstances are alleviated when possible. Intensive efforts toward home dust control by the use of air purifiers are expensive and disruptive and are of unproven benefit. The value of dietary restrictions, allergy testing, and immunotherapy remains controversial. The latter are time consuming and expensive. Their use might be considered in circumstances in which there is evidence of other immune-mediated disorders, such as atopy or allergic rhinitis, and pharmacotherapy has not satisfactorily controlled wheezing. Indeed, referral to a pediatrician or pulmonary physician experienced in the treatment of asthma should precede referral for immunotherapy.

With respect to pharmacotherapy, inasmuch as most patients with asthma have intermittent symptoms, therapy need not be continuous. First-line management involves the use of inhaled beta-agonists. This often suffices alone for patients with infrequent wheezing or those who develop bronchospasm specifically in association with viral respiratory tract infections. For younger children, the use of beta-agonists, taken orally, are effective as well.

The newly recognized significance of parasympathetic regulation of both bronchodilatation and endobronchial secretion has increased interest in anticholinergic agents. New derivatives of atropine, such as ipratropium bromide, are effective bronchodilating agents. Onset is rapid following inhalation and lasts somewhat longer than sympathomimetic agents. The combined use of these drugs may be additive or synergistic, having both an increased bronchodilating effect and duration. Additive effects of anticholinergics with oral theophylline have been documented as well. The use of spacers or reservoirs with metered dose inhalers improves drug delivery and ease of use.

Various theophylline preparations have been used for years in the management of asthma and have their most useful place in circumstances in which asthma attacks are prolonged or occur with great frequency. When long-term and continuous use is anticipated, long half-life preparations should be used that allow once or, most commonly, twice daily dosing schedules. When theophylline is used intermittently, shorter half-life preparations should be used so that effective blood levels may be reached more quickly. Theophylline may be used in addition to inhaled sympathomimetic and/or anticholinergic agents.

The use of long-term theophylline treatment is not without its difficulties. Blood levels should be determined to ensure a therapeutic range of 10 to 20 μg. per ml. Various dosing schemes have been devised to ensure adequate, nontoxic blood theophylline levels. Table 32–11 lists some of the factors known to influence theophylline pharmacokinetics.

Children or adults who are free of bronchospasm during daytime hours, but develop it at night, may be better served by discontinuous administration of theophylline. In this circumstance, short half-life agents given in the late afternoon or evening may effectively relieve bronchospasm, with less need for

Table 32–11. DRUGS AFFECTING SERUM THEOPHYLLINE LEVELS

Drug	Effect on Blood Level
Allopurinol	Increased
Cimetidine	Increased
Ciprofloxacin	Increased
Erythromycin	Increased
Influenza vaccine	Increased
Propranolol	Increased
Rifampin	Decreased

Hydrocarbons in tobacco smoke increase clearance of theophylline (decreased blood levels). Hepatic disease and congestive heart failure may be associated with decreased clearance and elevated blood levels.

monitoring of blood levels. In circumstances in which exercise or exposure to cold air appears to be a precipitant of bronchospasm, the effect of such stimuli may be modified by the prophylactic use of inhaled cromolyn sodium. Even in the absence of clear asthma precipitants, a trial of cromolyn is warranted if wheezing is not controlled by beta-agonists and/or theophylline. Such a trial should continue for several weeks before assessing its effectiveness.

Corticosteroids are also effective, both in the acute management of asthma and as part of long-term therapy. Single oral doses of corticosteroids have been shown to have prompt beneficial effects both in children and adults. Early use of oral or intravenous steroids in severe bouts of asthma decreases both the duration of illness and need for hospitalization. The short-term use of oral corticosteroids has also been noted to be effective in children who predictably have bouts of wheezing associated with viral respiratory tract infections. Long-term use of oral corticosteroids should be avoided, particularly in childhood. On the other hand, prolonged use of inhaled corticosteroids has been shown to be efficacious and safe and may completely replace the need for an oral drug in the majority of patients.

In cases of severe or persistent bronchospasm, all of the agents mentioned above may come to be utilized sequentially or continuously. With an increasing number of drugs utilized, the potential for toxicity also increases. An indicator of the successful management of asthma is not simply the absence of bronchospasm but also the minimizing of disruption of school performance and other aspects of daily living brought about by therapy. Asthma represents a variety of syndromes, the course of which will change from time to time owing to a host of factors; the therapy one employs must change accordingly.

Chronic Bronchitis-Emphysema

Patients with persistent airway obstruction, chronic production of sputum, and usually a long history of cigarette use are commonly considered to have chronic bronchitis-emphysema. Postmortem studies have shown both airspace destruction and airways disease, thereby justifying inclusion of both disorders under the term COPD. Studies concerning the natural history of chronic airway obstruction have demonstrated a dismal prognosis. Ten-year survival data varied little between those nonatopic smokers with chronic sputum production and those with a more pure form of emphysema who also were smokers. These findings were in sharp distinction to nonsmoking asthmatics whose 10-year survival was excellent.

Despite the fact that COPD is not a reversible disease process, both the duration and quality of life can be improved upon with careful management. The single, most important factor slowing the inevitable decline in FEV_1 is complete cessation of smoking. Though numerous clinical trials using varied modalities for smoking cessation have been conducted, it appears that consistent advice from a concerned physician to both the patient and his or her family is as effective as any other type of intervention. However, some patients appear to respond to adjunctive measures, such as smoking cessation classes or pharmacologic interventions.

Bronchodilators have been the mainstay of pharmacotherapy for COPD. It has long been stated that theophylline should be prescribed only to those patients who have at least a 15 per cent improvement in FEV_1 following administration of an inhaled sympathomimetic agent. Recent studies have shown that the acute response to bronchodilator therapy is an imperfect predictor of the long-term effects of therapy either in terms of lessening airflow obstruction or improving functional abilities. The lack of concordance between the acute response to bronchodilator and long-term benefits derived from therapy may be in part related to effects of these drugs on organs other than small airways, such as the heart and respiratory muscles.

As some airway obstruction in COPD is always present, though with periods of exacerbation and improvement, continuous bronchodilator therapy is rational. This can be accomplished by prescribing long half-life theophylline preparations, administered once or twice daily, with serum levels maintained between 10 and 20 μg./ml. Theophylline is, however, a drug with potential for serious toxicity, particularly in the elderly. Additionally, there is an ever-increasing number of interacting drugs that may enhance its accumulation and result in fatal complications (see Table 32–11). Hence, many clinicians favor the use of inhaled, selective beta-agonists as initial therapy in COPD. Extrapolating from data obtained from asthmatic subjects, it is reasonable to presume that the additive effects of selective beta-agonists (e.g., albuterol) and theophylline would be efficacious in patients with COPD as well. Beta-2-agonists are best delivered topically by inhalation, as higher drug concentrations can be delivered while avoiding side effects often encountered with oral administration. Reservoir devices may be used in conjunction with metered dose inhalers to enhance deposition of drug into the smaller airways.

Therapy should be continued for several weeks to months, even in patients showing no acute response to the bronchodilator in the pulmonary function laboratory. Functional improvement, such as ability to carry out activities of daily living and exercise tolerance, should be noted in addition to objective measurements of airflow, such as repeated office spirometry (FEV_1). Overreliance on objective measurements should not, however, extend to ignoring subjectively reported benefits.

Long-term use of oral corticosteroids in doses of 10 to 15 mg. per day may decrease the rate at which FEV_1 declines in patients with COPD. Use of steroids in higher doses is beneficial during exacerbation of chronic bronchitis. Inhaled corticosteroids may completely, and safely, replace the use of systemic corticosteroids even over the long term. Inhaled corticosteroids also obviate the deleterious effects of systemic corticosteroids on target organs such as osteoporosis, acne, capillary fragility, glucose intolerance, and adrenal suppression. Maximum pharmacotherapy thus includes the use of an inhaled beta-2-agonist, and long half-life theophylline preparations. Some patients will receive added benefit by the addition of topical anticholinergics or inhaled corticosteroids.

Exacerbations of chronic bronchitis-emphysema are perhaps the most common reason for hospitalization among patients with COPD. Environmental irritants (such as air pollution), viral infections, or inappropriate discontinuance of medications may precipitate worsening of bronchospasm. Many patients report an increase in both quantity and purulence of secretions during these episodes. The role of antimicrobial therapy during exacerbations of COPD remains controversial. Studies of prophylactic antimicrobial therapy in COPD have yielded variable results though clinicians have noted that occasional patients respond to orally administered antibiotics.

Two major organisms are found in the airways of patients with COPD: *Streptococcus pneumoniae* and *Haemophilus influenzae*. Thus, antimicrobial agents selected for either prophylaxis or treatment of exacerbations should cover these organisms. Trimethoprim-sulfamethoxazole and a beta-lactamase–resistant penicillin derivative (amoxicillin-clavulinic acid) represent logical choices. Those patients who find that exacerbations become associated with increasingly purulent sputum may benefit from a trial of self-administered oral antimicrobial therapy. Should this maneuver appear effective, patients may be provided prescriptions, or supplies of drug, such that the antimicrobial can be taken when increasing airway resistance and change in sputum is first noted.

The development of acute lower respiratory tract infection in the setting of moderate to severe COPD carries a very serious prognosis. Providing yearly influenza vaccine and immunizing with polyvalent pneumococcal vaccine should be carried out in patients with chronic lung disease and may reduce the incidence or severity of this complication.

Rehabilitation of the patient with severe chronic obstructive lung disease is an important aspect of overall management; benefit may be noted by both objective and subjective determinants such as improved ability to carry out activities of daily living, improved self-esteem, and lessening of depression. Pulmonary rehabilitation programs may be prescribed through nonprofit community organizations or through hospitals that sponsor such programs.

Patients with chronic bronchitis-emphysema have a sustained increased work of breathing. It is particularly the pink-puffer who is frequently noted to be thin and undernourished. It has long been considered that this may contribute to poor respiratory muscle function; indeed, recent weight loss is a poor prognostic sign. In undernourished patients with severe airflow obstruction, supplementing the diet improves respiratory muscle power, breathlessness scores, and a sense of well-being. Individuals who are 90 per cent or less of their ideal weight should receive oral nutritional supplements to increase their daily total protein intake to 25 to 50 per cent greater than average for moderately active men and women.

The natural history of chronic bronchitis-emphysema is one of an inexorable decline in FEV_1. In some individuals, the work of breathing is not maintained, resulting in hypercarbia and sustained hypoxemia. These patients are often overweight, edematous, cyanotic, and have elevated hematocrits (blue-bloaters). Right heart failure, which produces edema, hepatomegaly, and jugular venous distention, is a direct consequence of pulmonary hypertension induced by chronic hypoxemia.

Long-term oxygen therapy, when used at least 15 to 18 hours a day, has clearly been shown to improve both the quality of life and its duration. In addition to long-term bronchodilator therapy, cessation of smoking and control of purulent secretions, long-term home oxygen therapy should be prescribed for those patients with sustained arterial Po_2 below 55 mm. Hg. If cor pulmonale is evident, and can be attributed to sustained hypoxemia, home oxygen therapy should be prescribed, even if daytime arterial blood gas determinations show a Po_2 greater than 55 mm. Hg. The reason for the latter is that some patients desaturate during sleep for sufficiently long periods to produce pulmonary hypertension. Despite the long-term benefits of oxygen therapy, it is expensive and cumbersome. Newer methods of home oxygen delivery can, however, improve patient mobility and efficiency of oxygen use at reasonable cost.

Bronchopulmonary Dysplasia

Family physicians are increasingly responsible for the care of preterm infants following their discharge from the neonatal intensive care setting. Bronchopulmonary dysplasia is a disorder occurring chiefly because preterm infants have received technologically advanced treatment that has allowed their survival. It is a disorder wherein airway obstruction due to retained bronchial secretions, bronchospasm, smooth muscle hypertrophy, underdevelopment of alveolar spaces, atelectasis, and pulmonary hypertension related to chronic hypoxemia are found. Key risk factors in its development are the degree of prematurity, mechanical ventilation, and degree of birth asphyxia. It is likely that mechanical ventilation is more important than the actual concentration of inspired oxygen. The chest x-ray frequently shows hyperexpansion, cystic changes, pulmonary infiltrates, and areas of atelectasis.

These infants and young children may be readmitted to the hospital because of recurrent bacterial pneumonia and/or deterioration of pulmonary function during lower respiratory tract viral infections. Because of the increased work of breathing, growth and development are slowed. Reactive airway disease and recurrent lung injury lead to hypoxemia, pulmonary hypertension, and heart failure. Treatment will depend upon the severity of disease. Theophylline decreases bronchospasm and may have additional benefits with respect to diaphragmatic and cardiac function. Diuretic therapy increases pulmonary compliance by decreasing interstitial pulmonary edema, and supplemental oxygen therapy will decrease the work of breathing and nutritional expenditures and prevent pulmonary hypertension.

The prognosis is quite variable; in some children with severe disease and cor pulmonale, the prognosis is poor. However, for those with milder disease, though persistently reactive airways may be found, lung development may gradually improve, with growth and developmental milestones eventually returning to normal.

Bronchiectasis

Bronchiectasis occurs as a consequence of weakness of the bronchial wall brought about by inflammation. Persistent inflammation and obstruction contribute to atelectasis, retained secretions, and repeated episodes of focal pneumonia. Subsequent healing and fibrosis places traction on bronchial walls resulting in further dilation. External compression of the bronchi, usually as a consequence of adjacent nodal inflammation, may also cause obstruction. The disorder is decreasing in prevalence owing to more effective treatment of pneumonias and the less frequent occurrence of tuberculosis.

Bronchiectasis may be diffuse or focal: Diffuse bronchiectasis may occur consequent to massive gastric aspiration, chemical injury, severe episodes of tuberculosis, staphylococcal pneumonia, fungal pneumonias, or allergic bronchopulmonary aspergillosis. Focal disease may be due to retention of an aspirated foreign body, obstruction by endobronchial tumors, localized pneumonia, or recurrent pulmonary aspiration of gastric contents.

Chronic productive cough associated with intermittent, minor hemoptysis is now the most frequent presentation. Recurrent bouts of fever with purulent secretions may occur and, with progressive disease, dyspnea, weight loss, and fatigue may supervene.

Physical findings will vary depending upon the stage of disease; however, wheezing, coarse rales, and clubbing may be noted. Laboratory studies may reveal leukocytosis if an intercurrent pneumonia is present. A mild anemia, hyperglobulinemia, or an elevated erythrocyte sedementation rate may be present. A chest x-ray may show evidence of localized or diffuse disease. The diagnosis may be confirmed by CT scan of the chest, which can nicely demonstrate segments of lung involvement.

Bronchoscopy is usually of limited value unless there is focal bronchiectasis, and a tumor or retained foreign body is to be excluded. Bronchography is now rarely performed but occasionally is used to define bronchial anatomy in preparation for surgical management. Pulmonary function tests will vary with the extent of disease but usually show a combined obstructive and restrictive defect.

In younger patients, bronchiectasis is commonly seen as a manifestation of an underlying systemic disorder rather than a consequence of prolonged or recurrent bouts of pneumonia. Impaired immune function (hypogammaglobulinemia), dysfunction of mucociliary transport (cystic fibrosis, Kartagener's syndrome), or reactive airways disease (asthma-bronchopulmonary aspergillosis) may be associated with diffuse bronchiectasis.

An approach to the patient with bronchiectasis should include securing anatomical proof of diagnosis by the least invasive method and ceasing cigarette use. A historical review, searching for precipitating events (recurrent pneumonias, tuberculosis) or conditions known to predispose to bronchiectasis should be undertaken.

Long-term treatment is aimed both at management of the underlying disorder, antibiotics to control infections, and effecting drainage of secretions. One should immunize patients against influenza and pneumococcal pneumonia and promptly treat bacterial infections when they occur. Reversing bronchospasm will be important in certain patients as well as maintaining an adequate level of nutrition. In patients with localized disease who experience repeated hemoptysis or pneumonia, surgical treatment should be considered.

Cystic Fibrosis

During the past two decades, the median survival of patients with cystic fibrosis (CF) has increased dramatically. Most affected children will now live to age 24—roughly twice the life expectancy of 20 years ago. Such progress is owed chiefly to the establishment of subspecialty centers. Improved management of nutrition and pulmonary infections largely accounts for the enhanced quality and duration of life. Despite centralization of their care, most patients with CF will identify two physicians as their caregivers—a family physician or pediatrician and their cystic fibrosis center doctor.

The family physician has an important role in the diagnosis of CF, treatment of non-CF illnesses, and a shared responsibility in the management of its complications. CF is an autosomal recessive disorder, occurring once in 2000 live births and may be suspected by a variety of signs or symptoms (Table 32–12). Though most cases are diagnosed before age 3,

Table 32–12. PRESENTING SIGNS AND SYMPTOMS OF CYSTIC FIBROSIS

Infancy	Meconium ileus
	Rectal prolapse
	Failure to thrive
	Recurrent pneumonia
	Diarrhea
	Persistent cough
	Hyponatremia
	Heat prostration
Childhood	Intussusception
	Constipation
	Abnormal stools
	Bowel obstruction
Adolescence	Sputum cultures positive for *Pseudomonas*
	Short stature
	Delayed sexual development
Adulthood	Infertility
	Steatorrhea-malnutrition
	Bronchiectasis

depending upon severity of disease, it may not be considered until adolescence or, in rare circumstances, adulthood.

Once the diagnosis is considered, the patient should be referred to a CF center for determination of sweat electrolyte concentration. Though these tests are time honored and standardized, they are not without problems; indeterminant results are found in a small percentage of subsequently proven cases, and false positive tests, though rare, do occur. Thus, if follow-up indicates a course other than expected for CF, the diagnosis should be reconsidered.

Patients with CF, and their families, face enormous burdens; daily management of the disorder itself, an almost constant fear of loss of life, delayed maturation, hampered development of physical and social skills, isolation, poor self-esteem, and unpredictable crises brought about by pulmonary infections are issues that the family physician must be prepared to help manage.

Particularly early on in the course of the illness, parents will be especially perceptive of any area of disagreement, no matter how trivial, between their personal physician and the CF center's staff. Opinions regarding the care of patients with CF differ even among those well experienced in its management. Hence, issues such as timing of immunizations, use of antibiotics during minor respiratory tract infections, nutrition, participation in school exercise programs, and genetic counseling of siblings or parents should be mutually agreed upon by the primary care physician and the subspecialist. Indeed, the successful long-term management of these children, and even their eventual loss, is eased tremendously by the experience and compassion of their team of physicians.

Pneumothorax

In ambulatory practice, pneumothorax is most often seen as a spontaneous and idiopathic event. Occasionally, patients with emphysema will develop pneumothorax, often associated with acute bronchitis. Deceleration injuries, thought to be minor at the time of their occurrence, may shortly be followed by dyspnea and/or chest pain and a pneumothorax subsequently recognized on a chest x-ray film, even in the absence of rib fractures.

Patients with expanding pneumothoraces, or those with limited respiratory reserve, may require immediate tube thoracostomy. On the other hand, there are instances when a pneumothorax may be managed expectantly. Individuals who have excellent respiratory reserve, are minimally symptomatic, and generally responsible may be observed by frequent radiographs until it is quite clear that the pneumothorax is stable. Depending on its size, a pneumothorax may resolve over days to weeks.

In acute cases of spontaneous pneumothorax in which tube thoracostomy is not immediately indicated, a series of x-ray studies, following hours upon the initial one, would seem prudent to ensure its stability before discharging the patient for expectant management. Occasionally, one may wish to attempt aspirating free air from within the pleural space using a small-bore catheter and syringe with stopcock. When successful, this technique is far less costly than tube thoracostomy and hospitalization. Whether one elects catheter aspiration or expectant management will depend entirely upon the degree to which the patient is symptomatic and can gain immediate care should the need occur.

Lung Cancer

Carcinoma of the lung remains the leading cause of death due to malignancy in the United States in both sexes. As of the late 1980s, there were approximately 150,000 new cases diagnosed yearly, of which about two thirds were in men. The incidence in both sexes has been rising dramatically, more so than in any other malignant neoplasm. Despite advances in diagnostic technology and in therapy for many diseases, there had been little change in the outlook for patients with lung cancer, 90 per cent of whom will die of their disease. Thus, this constitutes a major health risk, especially in light of the fact that as many as 80 or 90 per cent of these tumors can be prevented.

Causes for bronchogenic carcinoma are several, with cigarette smoking topping the list; nine cases in ten are directly linked to their use. Other exposures producing malignant deterioration of bronchial epithelium include asbestos, radiation (uranium), and chemicals such as nickel and chromic acid. Further, the occasional tumor arises in an area of the lung scarred from previous injury. As regards the association with smoking, the risk relates to total exposure as measured by the number of years a person has smoked, the total number of cigarettes smoked, the age at initiation of the habit, whether or not the person inhales, and the concentration of carcinogen in the smoke. After discontinuation, the risk decreases slowly, and after 10 to 15 years, reaches the level observed in individuals who have never smoked. The role of passive smoking is controversial. Though passive smoke may contain even higher levels of carcinogen, there has not been a consistent positive association between passive smoking and new cases of lung cancer, though many epidemiologists believe it exists. Special mention of the risk of asbestos is merited. Those nonsmokers exposed to it have a several-fold increase in the incidence of bronchogenic carcinoma, which rises to nearly 100 times control in individuals exposed to the substance who also smoke.

There are four commonly encountered histologic types of carcinoma of the lung: adenocarcinoma, squamous cell carcinoma, large cell carcinoma, and small cell carcinoma. Adenocarcinoma and squamous cell each represent approximately one third of the total, with small cell accounting for another one fifth or so. The remainder are large cell, with an additional 1 per cent (approximately) caused by other types, such as bronchoalveolar carcinoma. The individual cell types are associated with characteristic clinical behavior, though none is sufficiently distinctive to allow separation on any basis other than histopathologic analysis.

There are a number of clinical manifestations encountered in these patients. Tumors arising within the lung parenchyma produce symptoms through involvement of a bronchus, distant metastasis, or extension into mediastinal or chest wall structures. Less than 10 per cent of patients are totally asymptomatic at the time of diagnosis; in these, a chest x-ray has been obtained for other purposes, and the abnormality is an incidental finding. A subset of this group includes patients with asymptomatic coin lesions (see below). Common symptoms caused by the primary tumor include a persistent cough, with or without hemoptysis. Many patients have dull and poorly characterized chest pain. Nonspecific complaints include weight loss, fatigue, and malaise. The occasional patient will come to attention because of the symptoms of pneumonia caused by the tumor obstruction of a bronchus. If the primary tumor is located in the apex of the lung, symptoms caused by invasion of the brachial plexus, such as pain in the arm, may be reported. In fewer patients, medical attention is sought because of symptoms produced by metastasis. Many lung cancers spread to the central nervous system, and a seizure or stroke may be the first sign of this problem; similarly, bone pain or abdominal discomfort caused by hepatomegaly may bring the patient to a physician. Other manifestations caused by intrathoracic invasiveness of the tumor include hoarseness, caused by the compromise of the left recurrent laryngeal nerve, or facial or conjunctival suffusion on the basis of superior vena cava syndrome. Less commonly, a paraneoplastic syndrome is the presenting problem; the polyuria and constipation of hypercalcemia or the abnormal mental status or seizure caused by the hyponatremia of the syndrome of inappropriate antidiuretic hormone are examples.

The physical examination may be entirely within normal limits in patients with lung cancer, but most have one or another abnormality helpful in diagnosis. There may be temporal wasting due to weight loss, and evidence for COPD, with hyperexpanded lung fields and reduced breath sounds. Rales in the chest are almost never heard in patients with obstructed bronchi; their presence favors an infectious cause of a pulmonary process. Helpful when present are localized wheezes on auscultation and/or evidence for atelectasis or pleural effusion (reduced breath sounds, diminished percussion note). Finger clubbing is a common skeletal sign of bronchogenic carcinoma; interestingly, this seldom is observed in small cell cancer and tends to be confined to the other three histologic types. Physical examination may also reveal the neck vein prominence indicative of superior vena cava compromise or the Horner's syndrome associated with apical tumor. Finally, there may be evidence on exam of metastasis in the form of focal neurologic signs, bony tenderness, or hepatomegaly.

The study leading to the diagnosis of lung cancer is in nearly all instances the plain chest x-ray. Though it has had some advocates in the past, doing routine chest x-rays, even in patients at higher risk (e.g., cigarette smoker over the age of 40) does not result in a survival advantage related to early diagnosis. An asymptomatic patient with a small peripheral nodule that turns out to be malignant is in a better prognostic group, but the incidence of this type of presentation is not sufficiently great to justify the chest x-ray as a screening procedure. The radiographic changes of primary lung cancer are diverse. A hilar prominence or mass is characteristic of squamous cell and small cell carcinoma; a peripheral nodule is more likely to be adenocarcinoma. Any type may result in atelectasis of a lobe by occlusion of the bronchus; cavitation is most often observed in squamous cell. Large cell carcinoma often begins as a peripheral nodule but grows rapidly and is often a large mass by the time of presentation; like small cell, it spreads early to hilar and mediastinal lymph nodes. Any of the cell types may compromise a bronchus sufficiently to result in pneumonia, which may obscure the primary lesion. A large pleural effusion may be the only visible abnormality on plain chest film in patients presenting with lung cancer. Blood studies are frequently performed in these patients, but few are genuinely helpful. Many patients have a mild anemia, some have pseudonormal abnormalities due to preexisting erythrocytosis from chronic hypoxia associated with COPD. Occasionally, the first clue to a lung primary may be the hyponatremia or hypercalcemia caused by ectopic hormone production by the tumor.

Once suspected, the histologic diagnosis of lung cancer may be made in a number of ways. The least invasive test available is expectorated sputum cytology. Maximum yield is reached by obtaining three first morning specimens. Though this should be an ideal study to perform on an outpatient, most institutions report a higher yield from inpatients. This is likely due to more prompt processing of specimens once obtained. Sputum cytology has an excellent yield in proximal tumors but is rarely if ever positive in peripheral coin lesions. Like the routine chest x-ray, obtaining random sputum cytologies in an asymptomatic patient at high risk confers no survival advantage due to early diagnosis. In theory, because small cell carcinoma of the lung is almost invariably metastatic by the time of diagnosis, a positive expectorated sputum cytology for this cell type could save more invasive diagnostic procedures, such as bronchoscopy, in such patients. In practice, however, many patients with an unexplained pulmonary process in which lung carcinoma is in the differential diagnosis will undergo bronchoscopy. Thus, in practice, the role of sputum cytology is chiefly in stable, ambulatory patients. Definitive histologic diagnosis is frequently made by the bronchoscopic approach. Squamous carcinoma may often be visualized in this fashion as an exophytic mass, and brush biopsy for cytologic study is obtained directly. In small cell carcinoma, subepithelial invasion is common, and the bronchus may appear to be extrinsically compressed. For more peripheral lesions, a fine needle aspiration of the lung may be performed, which in experienced hands has a high yield. The complications of bronchoscopy are few, the main one being bleeding from a tumor or postprocedural bronchospasm; needle aspirations, however, frequently result in pneumothorax. Further, with fine needle aspiration, a negative result does not in all cases assure the clinician that the lesion is benign and, thus, may not ultimately change the clinical approach. In patients who are not surgical candidates, a diagnosis obtained in this way may guide subsequent nonsurgical therapies; likewise, the occasional patient who is resistant to undergoing surgery may find histologic proof of malignancy persuasive.

Once a histologic diagnosis is secure, it becomes essential to stage the extent of tumor in order to plan therapy. Because of the aforementioned propensity of small cell carcinoma to be metastatic at the time of diagnosis, a staging system is most pertinent for nonsmall cell tumors. In widespread usage is the TNM method, in which the primary neoplasm (T), nodal involvement (N), and metastasis (M) are separately assessed, with resultant grouping into three stages. *Stage I tumors*, in general, are confined to the pulmonary parenchyma without mediastinal node involvement. *Stage II* describes larger tumors with positive hilar nodes, but without mediastinal spread; *stage III* includes tumors extending locally beyond the lung, and those with mediastinal spread; *stage IV* indicates distant metastasis. Some controversy exists regarding patients with stage III disease and their suitability for surgical therapy. Occasionally, stage III disease is operable, but it is not characterized by metastasis to the contralateral thoracic nodes or to supraclavicular nodes, as well as invasive within the chest. In general, the TNM system reflects increasingly more extensive disease as the number rises. For instance, T1 disease is a tumor of less than 3 cm. in size not extending proximal to a lobar bronchus; N1 disease is metastatic to hilar nodes only.

It can be seen from the above that the principal areas of concern in this staging process, for the most part, are intrathoracic structures in the hilum and mediastinum. Thoracic computerized tomographic (CT) scans are now nearly invariably obtained, even if the plain chest film does not indicate hilar or mediastinal involvement. CT scan with contrast allows distinction of tumor masses and involved lymph nodes from vasculature and gives the clinician more information on which to base decisions concerning further invasive procedures. When hilar or mediastinal nodes are abnormal, but still of the size at which infectious or inflammatory etiologies could be present (1.5 cm. or less), then mediastinoscopy or limited surgical exploration through a small parasternal incision may be performed. Occasionally, this may be scheduled as a preliminary to more definitive surgery, and if the results indicate operability, an immediate thoracotomy may be performed, with the intent for curative resection.

Obviously, the presence of any distant metastases in nonsmall cell, or any small cell, lung cancer renders the patient inoperable. As a result, many patients are subjected to extensive diagnostic investigations of distant sites searching for a metastasis. The most common sites for metastasis of lung cancer are brain and bone. For obscure reasons, up to 30 per cent of all lung cancers also metastasize to the adrenal glands. There is no general agreement about the applicability of diagnostic studies in these patients. In general, any test, such as a CT scan of the brain, is more apt to be positive if symptoms or signs suggest a focal lesion to begin with. Similarly, a bone scan is more likely to show involvement if the patient has symptoms referable to the skeleton. Thus, many clinicians would obtain a brain CT scan, bone scan, or abdominal CT scan only if symptoms, signs, or initial blood studies indicate a higher likelihood of metastasis; others believe these studies should be performed on all patients, because of the occasional asymptomatic individual with subsequently proven metastasis. The disadvantage of imaging studies in patients with lower pretest probabilities of metastasis is that the incidence of a false positive test increases. For example, CT scanning of the normal population demonstrates adrenal abnormalities in approximately 5 per cent of normals; this is particularly troublesome in that the adrenals are (in most centers) now routinely visualized as part of the thoracic CT scan performed in nearly all patients with lung cancer. Thus, the issue of assessment for distant metastasis is not settled, but suffice to say that it is of crucial importance to establish its presence in the staging process, in view of the considerable effect it has on subsequent management.

With respect to small cell carcinoma, the TNM staging does not correlate as well with prognosis. Most observers prefer to view small cell carcinoma, once diagnosed, in one of two ways: clinically limited disease, in which there is no gross tumor in the contralateral lung or in distant sites, or extensive disease, when there is considerable tumor obvious even on the initial chest x-ray or in which distant metastasis is clinically obvious.

In sum, the diagnostic assessment of carcinoma of the lung is of considerable importance in planning therapy. In certain clinical situations, the assessment may consist simply of history and physical examination, chest film, and positive expectorated sputum cytologies; and in others, more extensive and invasive diagnostic studies are indicated.

The differential diagnosis of lung cancer includes several considerations. Most important to exclude are infectious processes mimicking a tumor. Cavitary lung abscess or tuberculosis may look quite similar to bronchogenic carcinoma; it should be noted that in the *edentulous* person, bacterial lung abscess is a rare event, and a cavity almost always indicates tumor. Pulmonary embolism may sometimes resemble lung cancer, especially when chest pain and hemoptysis are prominent. The occasional patient with autoimmune diseases, such as rheumatoid arthritis with pleural effusion, may be felt to have a bronchogenic neoplasm. In patients with trauma, a bloody pleural effusion may resemble one which is malignant. Perhaps of most concern is the assumption that any persistent cough reflects either a smoker's cough or bronchitis, delaying the proper assessment for a potential malignancy. Other conditions similar to primary bronchogenic carcinoma include other tumors metastatic to lung or lymphoma originating in the hilar or mediastinal nodes; in these patients, diagnostic assessment and treatment are altered considerably. Sarcoidosis, particularly when hilar adenopathy is prominent, may also be confused with malignancy. Any pulmonary process in smoking patients over 40 should always be regarded as potentially reflecting lung cancer.

The ideal treatment of bronchogenic carcinoma is surgical, and though only a small percentage of patients are cured of this disease, the appreciable majority of those that are owe this cure to surgical resection of the tumor. Given the patient population at risk, many patients with lung cancer have coincident coronary artery disease and obstructive lung disease; in addition, some are quite elderly. Thus, it can reasonably be argued that an assessment of suitability for operative approach should precede any extensive diagnostic and staging work-up. In patients with COPD, a forced expiratory volume of 2 liters or more in 1 second indicates that a pneumonectomy would be tolerated; if this figure is less than 1 liter, surgical treatment is relatively contraindicated. In those patients whose FEV_1 is between 1 and 2 liters, a ventilation perfusion scan may be helpful in predicting how much function will remain after resection of a lung. An FEV_1 of 750 ml. or more is ordinarily compatible with tolerable function so that a calculation using the percentage of contribution to the total FEV_1 of the segment in question may be made and subtracted from the overall FEV_1 to determine acceptability. This method of estimating postoperative pulmonary status is more reliable for pneumonectomy than for resection of smaller amounts of lung. Some clinicians merely prefer to walk with patients up two or more flights of stairs and observe whether or not the individual is still able to carry on a normal conversation; if so, these clinicians believe that the risk for pneumonectomy is acceptable. In addition to limited pulmonary reserve, patients with obstructive lung disease are more likely to experience postoperative complications, such as infection, atelectasis, or bronchopleural fistula, further compounding the difficulty of making this decision. As concerns the coexistence of coronary artery disease, though this increases the risk for surgery and for additional postoperative complications, it does not pose an absolute contraindication to operation.

The surgical outcome in nonsmall cell cancer, not surprisingly, is closely related to the TNM stage, and thus to the extent of disease. In addition to the contraindications noted above, a malignant pleural effusion, primary tumor within 2 cm. of the hilum, or tumor directly invading the chest wall, diaphragm, medastinum, or pericardium constitutes a contraindication to surgery. Exceptions to this rule are peripheral tumors involving the chest wall without pleural effusion and those that arise in the apex. Controversy remains about the surgical management of cases with ipsilateral mediastinal node positivity, in whom many clinicians favor surgical removal of the primary, with mediastinal lymph node dissection, followed by postoperative radiotherapy. Others consider these patients to be inoperable. For patients with stage I and II diseases, who undergo thoracotomy and in whom no additional positive lymph nodes are found, the 5-year survival is between 40 and 80 per cent. In the occasional stage III patient who is offered operative therapy, this figure slips to 20 to 40 per cent.

The nonoperative treatment of patients with nonsmall cell cancer is not gratifying. A number of regimens of combination chemotherapy have been tried, though benefits have been modest. Radiotherapy is applied more often in a palliative fashion and may be effective in selected patients in whom hemoptysis or bronchial obstruction poses clinical difficulties. Similarly, it may be valuable in providing a temporary remission in patients with superior vena cava syndrome, and it is the modality of choice for epidural metastases with threatened compromise of spinal cord function. Radiation therapy may also be valuable in relieving the pain associated with osseous metastasis. Radiation therapy is also used as an initial therapy in cancer rising in the superior sulcus, which is followed by surgical removal; despite the local invasivity, the prognosis with this treatment is quite good.

The management of small cell cancer differs appreciably from the above, with the exception of the radiation therapy applied to symptomatic bony, nervous system, or mediastinal lesions. In small cell carcinoma, systemic combination chemotherapy is the principal treatment. With modern regimes, many including drugs such as cisplatin and doxorubicin, 15 to 20 per cent of patients who have disease clinically localized to one hemithorax will enjoy a survival in excess of 2 years. A higher percentage than this obtains symptomatic relief, because of the relative sensitivity of this tumor; however, recurrence tends to be the rule. The role of radiation therapy in patients with clinically localized disease is under active investigation. Empiric radiation therapy of the brain reduces the incidence of clinically evident cerebral metastasis in patients who have obtained remission of disease elsewhere through chemotherapy. Very occasionally, subsequent surgical removal of a primary tumor is carried out if a mass has shrunk appreciably, but has not entirely disappeared, by chemotherapy. Similarly, in the very unusual patient with small cell cancer presenting as an asymptomatic coin lesion, primary surgical resection may be attempted. Those patients with small cell carcinoma who have extensive disease at the time of presentation have a very bleak outlook. Here, nearly all treatment is palliative, and less than 5 per cent survive for more than 2 years.

In sum, carcinoma of the lung remains a daunting clinical problem. Its natural history and prognosis are quite dependent upon cell type, but the overall survival still is in the range of 10 to 15 per cent for 5 years. Patients with squamous cell carcinoma do well if hilar nodes are histologically negative; many dying of the disease do so with tumors still confined to the chest, where it tends to be locally invasive. Individuals with small cell carcinoma, though having a poor overall prognosis because of the propensity for the disease to metastasize widely early in the course, may do well if they are free of disease 2 years after the institution of therapies; in them, treatment is, with few exceptions, nonsurgical. Adenocarcinoma of the lung remains unpredictable; though numerous surgical cures have been reported, absence of disease in the lymph nodes is not as good a predictor of subsequent recurrence elsewhere in the body as it is in squamous cell carcinoma. For large cell carcinoma, it too is a rapid growing neoplasm, and though surgical therapy remains the treatment of first choice, the outcome is seldom a good one.

Solitary Pulmonary Nodule

A commonly encountered problem in primary care practice is the asymptomatic pulmonary nodule. The clinician typically encounters this problem on a chest x-ray obtained as a matter of routine, or for some other indication, such as on a pre-employment examination. The approach to the asymptomatic pulmonary coin lesion is aimed at stratifying the risk of cancer and removing it in those patients in whom carcinoma cannot be safely excluded by clinical evaluation. Factors favoring malignancy in an asymptomatic person include age over 35, absence of calcification, size greater than 4 cm., history of smoking, and chest film showing recent growth. Such lesions are likely benign if they have shown no growth in the previous 2 years, if the lesion has sharp margins, if it occurs in a young patient, and if it has a high density on CT scan. Solid calcification and stability in size over 5 years indicate near certain benignity. Other factors important in stratifying risk include residence of the patient, since some areas of the country are endemic for histoplasmosis and coccidioidomycosis; this is particularly helpful in the young patient who is not a smoker. Other aspects of the history and the physical examination are seldom valuable. In young men, particular attention should be paid to examination of the testicles, however, because of the major implications for treatment in the presence of a gonadal tumor. Coexistence of rheumatoid arthritis is important, especially in the presence of peripheral rheumatoid nodules, as they may also occur within the lung parenchyma.

Diagnostic investigation of the solitary pulmonary nodule need not be extensive. Unless the history and physical examination, and inexpensive tests such as blood count, urine analysis, and basic study of serum chemistries are abnormal, the coin lesion is very unlikely to represent metastasis from an extrapulmonary primary tumor. For this reason, extensive imaging studies of the gastrointestinal tract and genitourinary systems are rarely indicated. Indeed, many would argue that the most direct approach in a patient in whom lung cancer is a serious consideration is immediate resection of the nodule. Fine needle aspiration, positive or negative, does not change the necessity for resection when the clinical indications are present, unless the patient requires histologic confirmation before consenting to operation.

In poor risk surgical candidates, it may be justified to observe the nodule with serial x-ray studies for growth, before taking the risk of surgery; since many years are necessary for the roentgenographic appearance of tumor, it appears that an additional 2 or 3 months does not affect the long-term prognosis. Studies commonly performed in the evaluation of pulmonary coin lesions include skin tests, sputum cultures, and cytologic examination of the sputum; these are seldom of diagnostic value. Likewise, bronchoscopic investigation is unlikely to result in diagnosis. Probably the most important, and most commonly overlooked, aspect of the investigation of the asymptomatic pulmonary nodule is a vigorous attempt to recover previous chest x-rays. Often the entire question can be rendered moot by finding the presence of a similar abnormality on studies performed years earlier (Fig. 32–7).

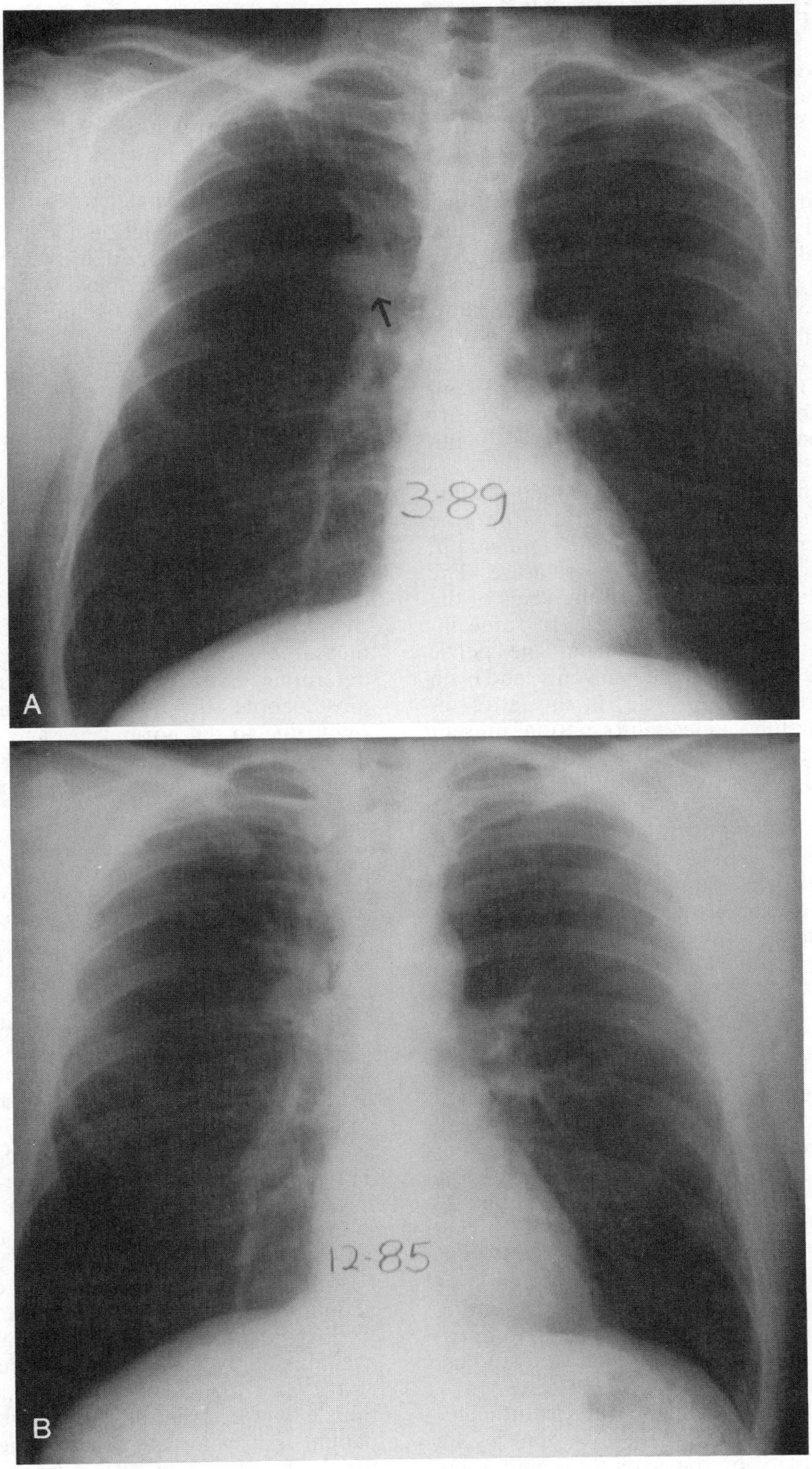

Figure 32–7. *A*, A right hilar nodule was noted on a pre-employment chest x-ray film taken in 1989. The issue of possible malignancy was raised and a search for old films ensued. A previous study was located *(B)* that revealed an essentially unchanged hilar nodule. The patient had worked in an endemic area for coccidioidomycosis. The nodule (and upper lobe fibrous strands) likely represent residual effects of a fungal pneumonia.

Pulmonary Embolism

Pulmonary embolism remains a daunting illness of high morbidity and mortality for all physicians. Autopsy studies have revealed that as many as 20 per cent of all deaths are at least associated with this finding; estimates of incidence indicate that over 600,000 occur yearly in the United States, with perhaps a third of these resulting in the death of the patient. What makes pulmonary embolization challenging for the physician is the difficulty in establishing the diagnosis, as well as the risks of therapy. Many episodes take place in already terminally ill patients in whom this problem is agonal; however, a majority are observed in patients who have a temporary predisposing factor and in whom recovery from the embolism is associated with good health subsequent to it.

Pulmonary embolism may be defined as the transfer of thrombus or other material from the systemic venous circulation, through the right side of the heart, and into the pulmonary vasculature. The majority of such thrombi originate in the veins of the lower extremities, above the popliteal. In some instances, embolization may occur from the pelvic veins, periprostatic plexus, subclavian veins, and even from the right atrium or ventricle; in the latter instances, there is often clinical information present leading the clinician to suspect these sources. There are several types of patients in whom pulmonary embolization from veins of the pelvis and the legs is more likely to occur. Deep venous thrombophlebitis is a common example, and, likewise, patients with any kind of major pelvic trauma, either spontaneous or surgical, fall into this group. Chronic venous insufficiency (postphlebitic syndrome) may also give rise to pulmonary embolization, and prolonged immobility for any reason is associated with both venous thrombosis and pulmonary embolization.

Patients with congestive heart failure, and its associated stagnation of the venous circulation, are more apt to suffer pulmonary embolization, and symptoms may be very difficult to separate from those of the primary cardiac condition. Systemic hypercoagulability—as observed in patients with malignancy, various congenital defects (such as antithrombin III deficiency), and, in particular, in women receiving oral contraceptive pills is also associated with both deep venous thrombosis and pulmonary embolization. Indeed, the past history of the patient presenting with suspected pulmonary embolization is an important determinant of the utility of diagnostic studies, as will be described below.

It has long been noted that the major difficulty in the diagnosis of pulmonary embolization results from the nonspecificity of the symptoms and signs associated with it. Indeed, the most common symptom is dyspnea, which itself has countless other causes. Chest pain, often pleuritic in quality, is frequent but not constant; the same is true of cough, and less commonly, hemoptysis, the latter when pulmonary infarction has taken place. The onset of the above symptoms is typically crisp, but recurrent episodes may result in the patient's perception that the onset of these complaints was gradual. There is little correlation between the severity of symptoms and the size of the embolus; in the rare patient in whom syncope is caused by pulmonary embolization, it is more likely to be massive.

Physical examination may be no more rewarding. Most commonly found are tachycardia and tachypnea, both of which have numerous other causes. Fever, most often low grade but occasionally more than 39°C., is observed in less than half of patients. Occasionally, adventitious sounds or pleural friction rub may be appreciated; more often, they are absent. Evidence of right ventricular overload, such as a palpable systolic parasternal lift and an increased intensity of the second heart sound, is seldom present but highly suggestive of the diagnosis when it is. Also helpful on physical examination is a search for a potential source, such as thrombophlebitis; however, physical signs for that condition are themselves undependable, with numerous false positives and negatives being encountered. The clinician occasionally measures the diameter of the lower extremities to determine if venous obstruction might be present; in most people, the left leg is slightly larger than the right, due to the normal passage of the left common iliac vein under the aorta. In short, the symptoms and signs of pulmonary embolization are seldom discriminant diagnostically.

As might be anticipated, the differential diagnosis of suspected pulmonary embolization is broad. Pneumonia, especially with pleural involvement, is a typical mimic; the pneumococcus is particularly apt to do this. Other infections causing pleuritic chest pain and dyspnea include epidemic pleurodynia. Episodic shortness of breath may also be caused by left ventricular dysfunction due to primary heart disease; when chest pain is not pleuritic, then myocardial infarction may be suspected. It has been stated that pulmonary embolization may also result in bronchospasm, thus producing confusion between it and asthma and/or COPD; this probably occurs rarely. The differential diagnosis may be summed by saying that nearly any cardiac or pulmonary disease, of any etiology, may be confused with pulmonary embolization; perhaps more importantly, pulmonary embolization may coexist with these conditions, further adding to the diagnostician's dilemma.

A wide variety of diagnostic imaging studies are available to investigate potential pulmonary embolism and its sources. Prior to undertaking any investigation, however, the physician should decide if the patient is a candidate for treatment, which consists for the most part of systemic anticoagulation. Commonly performed blood studies are usually not helpful; there may be mild leukocytosis and, very rarely, a slight elevation in serum bilirubin and lactic dehydrogenase (LDH) if pulmonary infarction has taken place. Arterial blood gases typically show slight hypoxemia and, with it, some hypocarbia, resulting in an increased A-a gradient. The electrocardiogram most often shows sinus tachycardia; evidence of right ventricular conduction disturbance, though helpful diagnostically, is usually absent. The plain chest x-ray may be completely normal; the most common abnormality is simple plate-like atelectasis and an elevation of one hemidiaphragm. Less frequent are reduced blood flow into the embolized lung and a prominent pulmonary artery on the affected side. Pleural effusions are occasionally observed. A wedge-shaped peripheral infiltrate in the lung parenchyma that is pleural based and pointing toward the ipsilateral hilum (Hompton's hump), though helpful when present, is most often absent.

The radionuclide ventilation-perfusion lung scan is the most useful imaging study. This is an extremely sensitive test, and a perfectly normal perfusion scan excludes any consideration of pulmonary embolism. However, abnormalities may be caused by numerous cardiopulmonary processes, including COPD and congestive heart failure. For this reason, a ventilation scan of the lung is compared with perfusion abnormalities. This study has its highest predictive value when there is a large (lobar) perfusion defect associated with normal ventilation; 90 per cent of such patients have pulmonary embolism at arteriography. Many variations, however, of this pattern are seen. Segmental or subsegmental unmatched perfusion defects make pulmonary embolism less likely; if the defects are matched by reduced ventilation, it is less likely still, with subsegmental matched defects representing a likelihood in the range of 10 per cent for pulmonary embolization. It is in this instance that consideration of the clinical likelihood of embolization guides the clinician. For example, the complete absence of any predisposing factors toward embolism may lead the physician to discontinue investigation after a low probability scan; other studies may be considered if one or more risk factors have been documented.

The gold standard for the diagnosis of pulmonary embolism is a pulmonary arteriogram. This is appreciably more invasive and expensive than the ventilation-perfusion scan, exposes the patient to radiation and intravenous contrasts, and carries with it the risk of potential cardiovascular abnormalities associated with the passage of the catheter through the right ventricle. A pulmonary angiogram never needs to be performed if a perfusion lung scan has been normal, and when abnormal, the scan may direct the radiologist to the affected parts of the lung, thus minimizing the exposure to contrast. The presence of pulmonary hypertension constitutes a relative contraindication to this study. Precise guidelines on when to perform pulmonary angiogram are difficult to enumerate, and it is often left to the clinician to weigh the risk of empiric anticoagulation for 3 to 6 months against the risk of the procedure. In most instances, it is performed in patients who constitute moderate anticoagulation risks. When anticoagulation is absolutely contraindicated, this study may be performed if the physician considers the patient a candidate for vena caval interruption (vide infra). Though there is considerable interest in such techniques as magnetic resonance imaging to visualize major proximal pulmonary emboli, these investigations are not applied widely for the diagnosis of pulmonary embolism at this time.

An alternative, and sometime supplemental, approach to the diagnosis of pulmonary embolism involves identifying a potential source. Since over 90 per cent of these emboli originate from the deep venous system of the pelvis and lower extremities, diagnostic techniques aimed at studying these vessels can be used with much efficacy to stratify the risk for embolism in a given patient. For example, the combination of a low or moderate probability ventilation-perfusion scan in a patient possessing one or more risk factors for pulmonary embolism and a positive study indicating deep venous thrombosis may be sufficient reason to anticoagulate the patient, obviating the need for pulmonary angiography.

The procedure that is most sensitive and specific for evaluating deep venous thrombosis in the legs is contrast venography. At the same time, this study is expensive. It is at times difficult to perform, requires an experienced radiologist to interpret, and exposes the patient to both contrast and radiation. Two types of less invasive studies are in widespread use: Doppler ultrasonography and impedance plethysmography. Both studies are painless and may be performed repetitively and on an outpatient basis. The sensitivity of both of these studies approaches 90 per cent for the presence of impaired flow of blood in the deep femoral systems. Of the two, Doppler is more sensitive in the calf veins, though these are rarely the source of a pulmonary embolism. Some clinicians prefer the use of both studies, believing that the sensitivity and specificity is increased. Doppler ultrasonography has the added advantage of being able to diagnose valvular incompetence in the venous system, but at the same time the interpretation of any Doppler study is operator dependent, thus requiring experience. Increasingly, advances are being made in noninvasive visualization of vascular structures, and it can be expected that duplex ultrasonography, which combines imaging plus the use of ultrasonography, will provide additional diagnostic information.

In short, many patients with pulmonary embolism may be diagnosed exclusively on noninvasive grounds. The most important aspect of the process is the pretest assessment by the clinician of the probability of the clinical event, plus a risk benefit analysis of treatment in a given patient. Thus, in some patients, the clinician may choose not to perform even a simple lung scan, if the patient is not a candidate for any therapy; in others, any combination of the above-described studies may be employed. Above all, it is important to consider each patient individually, rather than obtaining all possible studies on any patient with suspected pulmonary embolism.

The treatment of pulmonary embolism is systemic anticoagulation, though it still remains an area of some debate. Indeed, there exist very few studies, likely for ethical reasons, comparing the natural history of untreated pulmonary embolism with that of anticoagulated patients. Nevertheless, anticoagulation is widely accepted as a standard of care in the community. In nearly all patients, the initial therapy of pulmonary embolism is intravenous heparin, administered in a dose aimed at maintaining the patient's partial thromboplastin time (PTT) between 1.5 and 2 times the patient's baseline level; for patients with baselines higher than a laboratory's control values, it should be assumed to be in the middle of the laboratory range; when a patient's PTT is below the control range, then the clinician should aim for a therapeutic value of at least twice that baseline. Doses necessary to achieve this level of anticoagulation vary from patient to patient and may vary within the same patient during an episode of treatment. Clinically, patients appear more resistant to the anticoagulant effects of heparin in the early days after pulmonary embolization so that the clinician should be wary of an increasing PTT on a stable dose of heparin. A standard maintenance dose of heparin is generally in the range of 1000 units per hour, after a loading dose of 10,000 units; most prefer to administer it by constant infusion. Although the proper duration of intravenous heparin remains uncertain, most physicians settle on a 7- to 10-day course, followed by 3 to 6 months of additional anticoagulation. This may be accomplished by intermittent subcutaneous heparin in doses adequate to prolong the PTT to 1.5 times control halfway between doses or warfarin in doses capable of prolonging the patient's prothrombin time to 1.5 times control. It appears that little additional value, but a considerably increased bleeding tendency, is observed if the prothrombin time is between 1.5 and 2 times control so that a range between 1.3 and 1.5 is ideal. When warfarin is used for subsequent anticoagulation, it is generally instituted a few days before the intended discontinuation of heparin; this drug is contraindicated in pregnancy because of its toxicity to the fetus and because of teratogenicity so that subcutaneous heparin is administered in this instance. Though 3 to 6 months of anticoagulation is frequently the rule in these patients, assuming there are no contraindications, this is by no means proved. A shorter duration may be chosen for a person with risk factors that may be transient; in some instances, prolonged or even permanent anticoagulation might be chosen for other patients. This latter group might include those with permanent immobilization, previous episodes of pulmonary thromboembolic disease, or rare inherited clotting tendencies, such as antithrombin III deficiency.

The occasional patient with pulmonary embolization may be a candidate for thrombolytic therapy, either streptokinase or urokinase. Though no survival advantage has been shown for these therapies, it is agreed that there is more rapid resolution of symptoms and signs, especially of large and potentially life-threatening emboli. Thus, this type of treatment is best reserved for patients who are judged to have massive embolization by imaging studies or those who showed unstable cardiovascular systems (i.e., hypotension requiring pressors). It can be anticipated that there may be a role for tissue plasminogen activator in the future in this condition, but at the moment, it is largely an experimental agent for this indication.

Finally, vena caval interruption may be performed in certain circumstances. In patients with proved pulmonary embolization with absolute contraindications to anticoagulation, this is a valuable therapy; additionally, in those in whom documented recurrence of embolization occurs despite at least 24 to 48 hours of adequate anticoagulation, this may be offered. The mode of interruption in most widespread application is the Greenfield filter, which may be inserted through a neck vein, advancing through the superior vena cava to the inferior vena cava and positioned just below the renal veins. The filter remains in place permanently and, in experienced hands, is relatively easy to insert. However, complications reported have included tearing of the vena cava, or embolization of the filter itself, so it is important that it be reserved for the precise indications noted.

Considerable attention has been paid in recent years to the prevention of pulmonary embolization, and there is general agreement on the classes of patients to whom this should be offered. Prevention may be carried out by several therapies: low-dose subcutaneous heparin, full heparin anticoagulation, and external pneumatic compression of the lower extremities. Elastic stockings and early ambulation after a surgical procedure are less useful. The highest risk for pulmonary embolization exists in patients with femoral fractures or those having orthopedic operations on the pelvis or legs. The risk is lower, but still increased, for gynecologic, abdominal, or urologic surgery. Less well studied, but assumed to be a higher risk, are medical patients who will be at prolonged bed rest. There are a variety of other conditions, including neoplasms and acquired anticoagulation (which paradoxically produces an *increased* clotting tendency, such as the lupus anticoagulant), that usually do not receive prophylaxis therapy. The following constitute prophylactic recommendations.

For patients undergoing orthopedic procedures on the hip or femur, heparin should be given in doses sufficient to anticoagulate in the same way as described for acute pulmonary embolization above. Pneumatic compression is also helpful; low-dose subcutaneous heparin is ineffective in this group. For a patient undergoing gynecologic, abdominal, or urologic surgery, low-dose heparin (5000 units every 12 hours) affords protection. It has been suggested that pneumatic compression may be substituted for low-dose heparin in these patients, and it may prove to be equally as efficacious. Though there is less information to justify it, the same low-dose heparin therapy is often administered to patients with medical conditions at bed rest, particularly those with acute myocardial infarction, but also in those with chronic congestive heart failure or septicemia. Concerning neurosurgical procedures, any anticoagulation, including low-dose heparin, is contraindicated; here, external pneumatic compression is the therapy of choice.

The contraindications to full-dose anticoagulation, which would interdict either heparin or warfarin, include recent trauma, bacterial endocarditis, advanced diabetic retinopathy, recent or contemplated neurosurgery, and recent gastrointestinal bleeding (10 to 14 days).

References

Radiology

Oboler, S. Y., and LaForce, F. M.: The periodic physical examination in asymptomatic adults. Ann. Intern. Med., *110*:214, 1989.

Owens, M. W., Kinasewitz, G. T., Lambert, R. S., et al.: Influence of spirometry and chest radiograph on the management of pulmonary outpatients. Arch. Intern. Med., *147*:1966, 1987.

Persistent Cough

Boulet, L. P., Milot, J., Lampron, N., and Lacourciere, Y.: Pulmonary function and airway responsiveness during long term therapy with captopril. J.A.M.A., *261*:413–416, 1989.

Morgan, W. J., and Taussig, L. M.: The child with persistent cough. Pediatr. Rev., *8*:249–253, 1987.

Stulbarg, M.: Evaluating and treating intractable cough. West. J. Med., *143*:223–228, 1985.

Pleural Effusion

Feinsilver, S. H., Barrows, A. A., and Buaman, S. S.: Fiberoptic bronchoscopy and pleural effusion of unknown origin. Chest, *90*:516, 1986.

Himelman, R. B., and Callen, P. W.: The prognostic value of loculations in parapneumonic pleural effusions. Chest, *90*:852, 1986.

Irani, R., Underwood, R. D., and Johnson, E. H.: Malignant pleural effusion: clinical pathophysiologic study. Arch. Intern. Med., *147*:1133, 1987.

Leslie, W. K., and Kinasewitz, G. T.: Clinical characteristics of the patient with nonspecific pleuritis. Chest, *94*:603, 1988.

Light, R. W., Girard, W. M., and Jenkinson, S. G.: Parapneumonic effusions. Am. J. Med., *69*:507, 1980.

Prakash, U. B. S., and Reiman, H. M.: Comparison of needle biopsy with cytologic analysis for the evaluation of pleural effusion: analysis of 414 cases. Mayo Clin. Proc., *60*:158–164, 1985.

Sherman, S., Ravikrishnan, K. P., and Patel, A. S.: Optimum anesthesia with intrapleural lidocaine during chemical pleurodesis with tetracycline. Chest, *93*:153, 1988.

Sieskin, A., and Hirasuna, J.: Evaluation of pleural effusion. Med. Rounds, *1*:54, 1988.

Varkey, B., Rose, H. D., and Kutty, C. P.: Empyema thoracis during a ten-year period. Arch. Intern. Med., *141*:1771, 1981.

Interstitial Lung Disease

Hunninghake, G. W., Garrett, U. C., Richerson, H. B., et al.: Pathogenesis of the granulatomous lung diseases. Am. Rev. Respir. Dis., *130*:476, 1984.

Schwarz, M. I.: Idiopathic pulmonary fibrosis [Medical Staff Conference]. West. J. Med., *149*:199, 1988.

Weinberger, S. E.: Principles of Pulmonary Medicine. Philadelphia, W. B. Saunders Co., 1986, pp. 122–155.

Disorders of the Proximal Airways

Denny, F. W., Murphy, T. F., Clyde, W. A., et al.: Croup: an 11-year-study in a pediatric practice. Pediatr., *71*:871–876, 1983.

Koren, G., Frand, M., Barzilay, Z., and MacLeod, M.: Corticosteroid treatment of laryngotracheitis v. spasmodic croup. Am. J. Dis. Child., *137*:941–944, 1983.

McLaine, L. G.: Croup syndrome. A.F.P., *36*:207–214, 1987.

Nelson, W. E.: Bacterial croup: a historical perspective. J. Pediatr., *105*:52–55, 1984.

Acute Bronchitis

Dunlay, J., Reinhardt, R., and Roi, L. D.: A placebo-controlled, double-blind trial of erythromycin in adults with acute bronchitis. J. Fam. Pract., *25*:137–141, 1987.

Rodnick, J. E., and Gude, J. K.: The use of antibiotics in acute bronchitis and acute exacerbations of chronic bronchitis. West. J. Med., *149*:347–351, 1988.

Bronchiolitis

Khamapirad, T., and Glezen, W. P.: Clinical and radiographic assessment of acute lower respiratory tract disease in infants and children. Sem. Resp. Infect., *2*:130–144, 1987.

Tristram, D. A., Miller, R. W., McMillan, J. A., and Weiner, L. B.: Simultaneous infection with respiratory syncytial virus and other respiratory pathogens. Am. J. Dis. Child., *142*:834–836, 1988.

Webb, M. S. C., Henry, R. L., Milner, A. D., et al.: Continuing respiratory problems three and a half years after acute viral bronchiolitis. Arch. Dis. Child., *60*:1064–1067, 1985.

Pneumonia

Fraser, R. G., et al.: Infectious diseases of the lungs. *In* Fraser, R. G., Pare, J. A. P., Pare, P. D., et al. (Eds.): Diagnosis of Diseases of the Chest. Vol. II. Philadelphia, W. B. Saunders Co., 1989, pp. 807–827.

Grossman, L. K., and Caplan, S. E.: Clinical, laboratory and radiological information in the diagnosis of pneumonia in children. Ann. Emerg. Med., *17*:43–46, 1988.

Heckerling, P. S.: The need for chest roentgenograms in adults with acute respiratory illness: clinical predictors. Arch. Intern. Med., *146*:1321–1324, 1986.

Khamapirad, T., and Glezen, W. P.: Clinical and radiographic assessment of acute lower respiratory tract disease in infants and children. Semin. Resp. Infect., *2*:130, 1987.

Mansel, J. U., Rosenow, E. C., Smith, T. F., and Martin, J. W.: *Mycoplasma pneumoniae* pneumonia. Chest, *95*:639, 1989.

Prichard, J. G.: Role of long-acting cephalosporins in ambulatory therapy. Clin. Therapeut., *10*:688–693, 1988.

Shapiro, M. F., and Greenfield, S.: The complete blood count and leukocyte differential count: an approach to their rational application. Ann. Intern. Med., *106*:65, 1987.

Tristram, D. A., Miller, R. W., McMillan, J. A., and Weiner, L. B.: Simultaneous infection with respiratory syncytial virus and other respiratory pathogens. Am. J. Dis. Child., *142*:834–836, 1988.

Tuberculosis

Prichard, J. G.: Pulmonary tuberculosis. Med. Rounds, *1*:107–120, 1988.

Stead, W. W., To, T., Harrison, R. W., and Abraham, J. H.: Benefit-risk considerations in preventive treatment for tuberculosis in elderly persons. Ann. Intern. Med., *107*:843–845, 1987.

Asthma

Bavuer, A. F.: Strategies in managing asthma. West. J. Med., *150*:303–308, 1989.

Broder, I., Tarlo, S. M., Davies, G. M., et al.: Safety and efficacy of long-term treatment with inhaled beclomethasone dipropionate in steroid-dependent asthma. Can. Med. Assoc. J., *136*:129–135, 1987.

Burrows, B., Martinez, F. D., Halonen, M., et al.: Association of asthma with serum IgE levels and skin-test reactivity to allergens. N. Engl. J. Med., *324*:271–277, 1989.

Li, J. T. C., and Reed, C. E.: Proper use of aerosol corticosteroids to control asthma. Mayo Clin. Proc., *64*:205, 1989.
Milavetz, G., Vaughan, L. M., Weinberger, M. M., and Hendeles, L.: Evaluation of a scheme for establishing and maintaining dosage of theophylline in ambulatory patients with chronic asthma. J. Pediatr., *109*:351–354, 1986.
Sly, R. M.: Mortality from asthma 1979–1984. J. Allergy Clin. Immun., *82*:705–716, 1988.
Storr, J., Barry, W., Barrel, E., et al.: Effect of a single oral dose of prednisolone in acute childhood asthma. Lancet, *1*:879–882, 1987.
Strunk, R. C., Mrzaek, D. A., Wolfson-Furhann, G. S., and LaBrecque, J. F.: Physiologic and psychological characteristics associated with deaths due to asthma. J.A.M.A., *154*:1193–1198, 1985.
Webb, M. S. C., Henry, R. L., Milner, A. D., et al.: Continuing respiratory problems three and one-half years after acute viral broncholitis. Arch. Dis. Child., *60*:1064–1067, 1985.

Chronic Bronchitis-Emphysema

Efthimiou, J., Fleming, J., Gomes, C., and Spiro, S. G.: The effect of supplementary oral nutrition in poorly nourished patients with chronic obstructive pulmonary disease. Am. Rev. Respir. Dis., *137*:1075, 1988.
Guyatt, G. H., Townsend, M., Nogradi, S., et al.: Acute response to bronchodilator: an imperfect guide for bronchodilator therapy in chronic airflow limitation. Arch. Intern. Med., *148*:1949, 1988.
Heimloch, J. H.: Oxygen delivery for ambulatory patients. Postgrad. Med., *84*:68, 1988.
Petty, T. L.: Home oxygen therapy. Mayo Clin. Proc., *62*:841, 1987.
Rodnick, J. E., and Gude, J. K.: The use of antibiotics in acute bronchitis and acute exacerbations of chronic bronchitis. West. J. Med., *149*:347, 1988.

Bronchopulmonary Dysplasia

Swanson, J. A., and Berseth, C. L.: Continuing care for the preterm infant after dismissal from the neonatal intensive care unit. Mayo Clin. Proc., *62*:613, 1987.

Bronchiectasis

Barker, A. F., and Bardana, E. J.: Bronchiectasis: update of an orphan disease. Am. Rev. Respir. Dis., *137*:969–978, 1988.

Cystic Fibrosis

Landon, C., and Rosenfeld, R. G.: Short stature and pubertal delay in cystic fibrosis. Pediatr., *14*:253, 1987.
Rosenstein, B. J., and Langbaum, T. S.: Misdiagnosis of cystic fibrosis: need for continued follow-up and reevaluation. Clin. Pediatr., *26*:78, 1987.
Stern, R. C.: The primary care physician and the patient with cystic fibrosis. J. Pediatr., *114*:31, 1989.

Pneumothorax

Obeid, F. N., Shapiro, M. J., Richardson, H. H., et al.: Catheter aspiration for simple pneumothorax (CASP) in the outpatient management of simple traumatic pneumothorax. J. Trauma, *25*:882–886, 1985.

Lung Cancer

Filderman, A. E., Shaw, C., and Matthay, R. A.: Lung cancer. II. Staging and therapy. Invest. Radiol., *21*:80, 173, 1986.
Iannuzzi, M. C., and Scoggin, C. H.: Small cell lung cancer. Am. Rev. Respir. Dis., *34*:595, 1986.
Weinberger, S. E.: Principles of Pulmonary Medicine. Philadelphia, W. B. Saunders Co., 1986, pp. 226–248.

Solitary Pulmonary Nodule

Chaffey, M. H.: The role of the percutaneous lung biopsy in the workup of a solitary pulmonary nodule. West. J. Med., *148*:176–181, 1988.

Pulmonary Embolism

Coon, W. W.: Venous thromboembolism: prevalence, risk factors and prevention. Clin. Chest. Med., *5*:391, 1984.
Hirsh, J.: Venous thromboembolism: prevention, diagnosis and treatment. Chest, *89*:369s, 1986.
Weinberger, S. E.: Principles of Pulmonary Medicine. Philadelphia, W. B. Saunders Co., 1986, pp. 160–168.

33

Otolaryngology

Byron J. Bailey
Chester L. Strunk
Charles W. Smith, Jr.

Emergencies

CROUP

Croup is a syndrome characterized by inspiratory stridor, most often caused by parainfluenza virus. It is most likely to occur in children under the age of 2 years, in late fall or early winter epidemics (Strome et al., 1985). The trachea is inflamed below the glottis, usually sparing the lungs, distal bronchi, and the supraglottic regions.

Children with *croup* usually develop fever, a barking cough, *inspiratory stridor*, and hoarseness over a 24-hour period. Physical findings include *inspiratory* (and occasionally expiratory) *stridor* and *tachypnea*. The diagnosis is made clinically, but a lateral neck radiograph may help to differentiate *croup* from *supraglottitis* or *foreign body aspiration*. Blood gases should always be obtained if signs of respiratory distress are present.

The most important treatment decision is whether or not to hospitalize the child. Generally, children with a respiratory rate under 40 per minute can be managed on an outpatient basis if the parents are reliable and if the child is able to maintain hydration. Relief may be obtained by using a hot shower to generate humidification. A cool mist ultrasonic humidifier should be also run constantly for several days until symptoms abate.

Patients who are hospitalized should receive intravenous fluid replacement and humidified air. *Racemic epinephrine* (0.25–0.5 ml., mixed with 2 ml. normal saline by nebulization) may be repeated every 30 to 60 minutes as needed to relieve respiratory distress. The use of *steroids* is controversial because the data are conflicting as to their effectiveness. If steroids are used, the recommended dosage is dexamethasone 0.5 to 1 mg. per kg. I.V. or I.M. as a single treatment. If the above-mentioned treatment fails to result in improvement, intubation or tracheotomy is required.

The decision whether to intubate or to perform a tracheotomy is always difficult. Intubation is less invasive but may be complicated because of the age of the child and the degree of subglottic edema. *Nasotracheal intubation* is preferred, with emergency tracheotomy capability immediately available if the attempt is unsuccessful.

SUPRAGLOTTITIS

Supraglottitis (epiglottitis) is an acute infection of the larynx above the vocal cords, usually caused by bacteria. The majority of cases occur in children under the age of 6 years, and are almost always the result of *Haemophilus influenzae* infections. In adults, however, *β-hemolytic streptococci, pneumococcus*, or *Staphylococcus aureus* may also be causative (Dayal, 1981).

The illness is characterized by the abrupt onset of high fever (38.9° C [> 102° F]) and a severe, often progressive course. Severe throat pain is present, which makes it difficult for the patient to swallow secretions. Respiratory difficulty is an ominous sign and may begin to occur a short time after the onset of symptoms. The rapidity of the progression of symptoms is dependent on the age of the child and the virulence of the organism involved. The diagnosis should be strongly suspected whenever fever, dysphagia, and respiratory difficulty are seen simultaneously.

On physical examination, the patient appears acutely ill, and may have difficulty swallowing secretions. Nuchal rigidity may occasionally be seen, raising the possibility of meningitis. Tachypnea and use of accessory muscles of respiration may be seen. Severe cases may also be accompanied by cyanosis.

The presumptive diagnosis should be made from the history and general appearance of the patient and should be confirmed at the time the airway is secured. Once an airway is in place, laryngeal secretions should be obtained for culture. Blood cultures and serologic antigen studies should also be performed.

Antibiotics should be given to ensure coverage against the relatively common occurrence of ampicillin-resistant *H. influenzae*. Acceptable initial choices include *ampicillin* and *chloramphenicol* or a *third-generation cephalosporin* such as *cephtriaxone*. Therapy should be continued for at least 7 days. In addition to antibiotics, humidified air—usually with low-flow oxygen—should also be administered. The prognosis for recovery is excellent. Virtually all deaths occur because of respiratory embarrassment from inadequate airway management.

PERITONSILLAR ABSCESS

Abscesses in the *peritonsillar space* are most commonly a complication of *acute tonsillopharyngitis* and, thus, are almost always due to infection with *group A beta-hemolytic streptococci*. Symptoms of acute pharyngitis progress to severe unilateral throat pain and difficulty swallowing. Severe pain may limit oral intake and may cause drooling from pooled saliva and muffled speech, sometimes referred to as a "hot potato" voice.

Examination usually reveals a patient with fever, mild dehydration, increased oral secretions, and difficulty opening the mouth (trismus). The involved tonsil is swollen and displaced toward the midline and downward. It may be difficult to determine whether swelling is due to an abscess or cellulitis. Palpation of a fluctuant area with a gloved finger is useful to confirm an abscess. Other diagnostic possibilities include infectious mononucleosis, other parapharyngeal space infections, and tonsillar or pharyngeal tumors. Diagnostic tests should include a throat culture or a latex slide test for streptococcus, a culture of any aspirated material, a complete blood count, and a mono spot test.

All children should be admitted to the hospital. Adults who have significant dehydration or who cannot cooperate with outpatient drainage procedures must also be admitted. Others may be managed as outpatients with either needle *aspiration* or outpatient *incision* and *drainage*. After topical anesthesia with benzocaine or lidocaine, an 18-gauge spinal needle is inserted into the area of fluctuance. The patient should then be placed on oral penicillin, 500 mg. Q.I.D., for 10 to 14 days or until the episode resolves. If symptoms recur, the patient should be hospitalized for incision and drainage and treated with *intravenous antibiotics*. *Tonsillectomy* is recommended following resolution because of the tendency for recurrence.

FOREIGN BODY ASPIRATION

Foreign body aspiration is most commonly seen in small children, but may occur at any age. Objects may become lodged in the *pharynx, larynx, trachea*, or *bronchi*. Symptoms depend on the site of the foreign body. *Pharyngeal* locations primarily produce discomfort, whereas *laryngeal* foreign bodies cause total or near total occlusion. *Tracheobronchial* occlusions cause coughing and intermittent or constant stridor, wheezing, and cyanosis. More distal foreign bodies may initially go unnoticed but subsequently result in wheezing, respiratory distress, and pneumonia.

Physical findings are variable and also depend on the location and the severity of respiratory obstruction. Any combination of *tachypnea, cyanosis, stridor,* and *wheezing* may be found. Obstruction of the *right mainstem bronchus* causes decreased breath sounds and reduced chest expansion. A one-way ball valve effect may occur, resulting in hyperexpansion and hyperresonance to percussion.

The chest x-ray film may show signs of local, lobar, or whole lung atelectasis, and if the object is radiopaque, it may also be seen. If sufficient time has elapsed (usually 24 hours or more), pneumonic infiltrates may be present. *Anteroposterior* and *lateral views* of the neck should also be obtained. If the diagnosis is still in doubt, *fluoroscopy* often allows the site of obstruction to be localized.

Management involves maintenance of the airway and removal of the foreign body. Pharyngeal objects can usually be removed with a mirror and forceps. *Laryngoscopy* or *endoscopy*, used under anesthesia, is required for removal at the level of the larynx and beyond. Removal is usually followed by immediate relief of symptoms, unless infection is present.

HEAD AND NECK TRAUMA AND RESPIRATORY EMBARRASSMENT

Trauma to the head and neck region may cause respiratory difficulty in a number of ways, including *dislodged dentures, aspiration of blood and mucus, tongue trauma,* or *laceration of the airway*. Patients presenting with facial trauma and respiratory distress must be immediately assessed, suctioned, and given an oral or nasopharyngeal airway. If the patient is still in distress, an *emergency tracheotomy* or *cricothyrotomy* should be performed. Once the airway is stabilized, attention can be directed to other traumatized areas.

Laryngeal trauma will result in local pain and

dysphonia. *Laryngoscopy* should be performed to confirm the diagnosis and assess the damage. A *tracheostomy* should be performed if the airway is unstable. *Tracheal trauma* or *separation* may result in similar signs and symptoms, including *subcutaneous emphysema*. In addition to respiratory endoscopy, the *esophagus* should also be assessed for concomitant injury. A tracheotomy should be placed as far from the site of the injury as possible, and the tracheal separation repaired surgically.

EPISTAXIS

Epistaxis, or nosebleed, most commonly originates from the rich capillary network in the anterior septum known as *Kiesselbach's plexus*. In hypertensive and elderly patients, it may occur posteriorly in areas of the nose that are very difficult to visualize. The most common causes of nosebleed are drying of the nasal mucosa and trauma from picking the nose (Kirchner, 1982).

If *manual pressure*, applied to the nasal septum with the head upright for 10 full minutes, does not stop the bleeding, careful examination and identification of the point of bleeding is required. Proper equipment and lighting is an absolute must and should include a *nasal speculum, bayonet forceps,* and *suction capability* (Johnson, 1981). The physician must first determine whether the bleeding is anterior or posterior. If the bleeding site is not readily apparent, nasal vasoconstriction is accomplished with cotton balls impregnated with 5 per cent cocaine solution or a mixture of 4 per cent lidocaine and 1/100,000 epinephrine. After several minutes, the bleeding should be slowed so that identification of the bleeding point is possible. *Cautery* with 25 per cent *trichloroacetic acid* or *silver nitrate* is usually effective in controlling bleeding. Care should be taken to dry the nasal mucosa prior to cauterization. A silver nitrate stick should be applied to the bleeding site for about 20 seconds (Johnson, 1981). Following cauterization, patients should be advised not to blow the nose, to open the mouth when sneezing, to avoid aspirin, to use a cool-mist humidifier, and to apply antibiotic ointment or petroleum jelly to the nose several times per day.

If cautery is unsuccessful, half-inch iodoform gauze should be impregnated with petroleum jelly or antibiotic ointment and inserted into the nose in layers with bayonet forceps. As much packing as possible should be used without deforming the septum, and should be left in place for 2 to 5 days. Patients who have nasal packing in place should generally be treated with antibiotics because of the high likelihood of sinusitis. Pain medication is often necessary. Patients should be cautioned that nasal obstruction often persists for several days after the packing has been removed. An alternative to the use of gauze packing is the use of an *epistaxis balloon*, which is inserted into the nose and filled with air or saline.

If the bleeding originates from a posterior location, packing must be performed differently. A *posterior pack* is fashioned using two or three 4-inch gauze pads with three silk sutures tied around the middle. A soft, rubber catheter is introduced into the nose, grasped by a hemostat, and pulled from the nasopharynx through the mouth. Two of the sutures are tied to the end of the catheter, which is then pulled back through the nose, bringing the posterior pack into the nasopharynx. It is usually necessary to guide the pack into the nasopharynx with a finger. The third suture is left trailing from the mouth. A firm anterior pack is then placed, followed by a rolled gauze pad across the nose, secured by the two sutures hanging from the nose, which also secures the posterior pack firmly in place. Epistaxis catheters or Foley catheters may also be used to control bleeding from a posterior site; however, excessive pressure on the nasal ala or columella will cause tissue necrosis.

If bleeding cannot be controlled by any of the above-mentioned methods, or if it is recurrent, a referral for *arterial ligation* must be considered.

The Ear

SIGNS AND SYMPTOMS

Otalgia

Otalgia (ear pain, earache) is a symptom and not a diagnosis. Otalgia can be either primary or secondary. Primary otalgia arises from pathologic conditions of the ear itself. Secondary otalgia originates at periauricular sites or is referred from a distant origin. More than 50 per cent of cases of otalgia originates from a source other than the ear. The intensity of the otalgia is not necessarily proportional in seriousness to the disease causing it; mild otalgia or vague pain may result from laryngeal or esophageal carcinoma, whereas dental caries may cause severe pain.

The cause of pain originating from the external ear and canal will be obvious from inspection in most instances, e.g., a furuncle of the external canal or otitis externa. Exceptions include an early neoplasm of the external canal or the neuralgia of herpes zoster oticus. Otalgia of middle ear origin should be readily apparent. Tic-like pain may originate from the geniculate complex of the seventh nerve or the tympanic branch of the ninth nerve. The most common periauricular causes of otalgia include parotitis, lymphadenitis, and temporomandibular joint dysfunction. Periauricular lymphadenitis may arise from lesions in the scalp.

Temporomandibular joint dysfunction is a common cause of otalgia and is often a result of faulty dental occlusion or excessive jaw movement.

Lesions in the area of the palatine, pharyngeal,

and lingual tonsils, as well as those adjacent to the tongue, may cause ear pain via the glossopharyngeal nerve. Squamous cell carcinoma of the base of the tongue may be associated with referred otalgia and require palpation and biopsy for diagnosis. Laryngeal, hypopharyngeal, esophageal, and lung lesions may cause secondary otalgia from branches of the vagus nerve.

If the cause of otalgia is not readily apparent from a routine otorhinolaryngologic examination, then office laryngoscopy followed by a chest x-ray study and barium swallow may be required (Paparella, 1980).

Otorrhea

Drainage from the ear is a common otologic complaint. It is important to document the nature of the otorrhea, related symptoms, and possible causative events such as trauma. The most common cause of otorrhea is *cerumen*, which may range from pale yellow to dark brown and from liquid to solid. Profuse bleeding from the ear is rare except in cases of severe trauma or in patients with clotting disorders. Middle ear and mastoid infections, acute perforations, tumors, and external otitis may be associated with mild bleeding. Serous drainage may occur with bleb rupture from bullous myringitis, otitis externa, or external canal dermatitis. Purulent otorrhea indicates infection. The color may range from yellow to green. A malodorous discharge is associated with tissue necrosis and is usually found in an infected cholesteatoma. A mucoid discharge without odor is an indication of middle ear mucosal disease or eustachian tube dysfunction, or both, which is often of a temporary nature.

Spontaneous cerebrospinal fluid otorrhea is rare. It may accompany a temporal bone fracture or may be secondary to a tumor or surgery. The fluid is clear and the diagnosis may be confirmed by analysis of sugar, protein, sodium, and cells. Cerebrospinal fluid also produces a halo sign when a drop is placed on filter paper. The halo sign is a ring of clear fluid surrounding a circle of blood-stained moisture, produced by the greater diffusion of spinal fluid than blood.

EXAMINATION OF THE EAR

Otoscopy

The most convenient method to illuminate the external canal and tympanic membrane is the diagnostic otoscope (Fig. 33–1). It includes a halogen light source, an air-sealed head, and rubber tubing for pneumatic otoscopy. An open operating head should be available for removal of cerumen. When performing otoscopy, the physician should remember that the bony canal is very tender when manipulated. Prior to any instrumentation of the ear canal, the patient should be warned to prevent a sudden head movement. Infants should be examined while in the parent's arms. A bottle or pacifier may help to distract the infant. Young children will often respond positively to games such as watching the "Tinkerbell" otoscope light, blowing out the light, and looking for "bunnies in the ears." Every effort should be made to avoid a red eardrum produced by the child's crying. To visualize the tympanic membrane, the pinna must be pulled posteriorly and superiorly. The entire annulus should be seen, including the pars flaccida. The largest speculum possible should be used in order to obtain a tight seal for pneumatic otoscopy. A hand-held bulb or tubing in the mouth is used for changing pressure in the external canal. The flexibility of the normal tympanic membrane and middle ear allows the eardrum to move crisply in both directions. A weak tympanic membrane or one affected by negative middle ear pressure moves out with negative pressure, then passively returns without the need of positive pressure. The malleus should be examined for fixation or diminished mobility. With a retracted tympanic membrane, the short process of the malleus is very prominent, while the manubrium becomes more horizontal and foreshortened. The tympanic membrane in serous otitis changes from a shiny gray to amber, sometimes with air bubbles. Pus produces a white color in the tympanic membrane and causes it to bulge and lose landmarks. Blood causes the tympanic membrane to appear blue. Dense white plaques represent tympanosclerosis and indicate healed otitis media. In many normal ears, the incus can be seen shining through the posterosuperior quadrant of the drumhead (Strome, 1985).

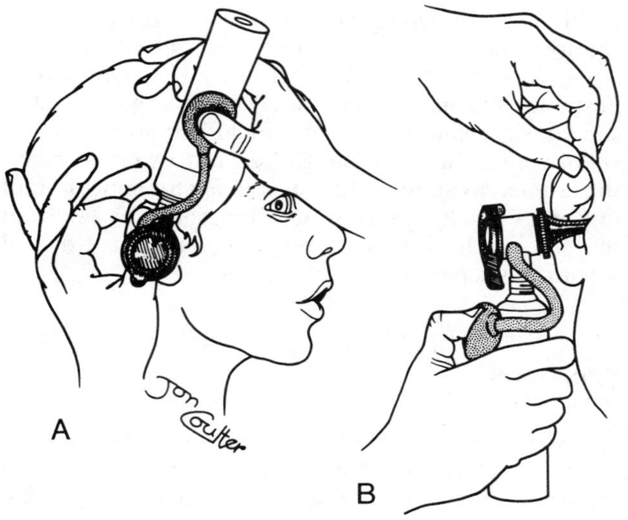

Figure 33–1. Methods of positioning the otoscope to enhance visualization and to minimize the chance that head movement will result in trauma to the ear canal. Both of the otoscopist's hands can be used *(A)*, or when the child is cooperative, a finger touching the child's cheek is sufficient *(B)*. (From Bluestone, C. D., and Stool, S. E. [Eds.]: Pediatric Otolaryngology. Philadelphia, W. B. Saunders Company, 1983, p. 142.)

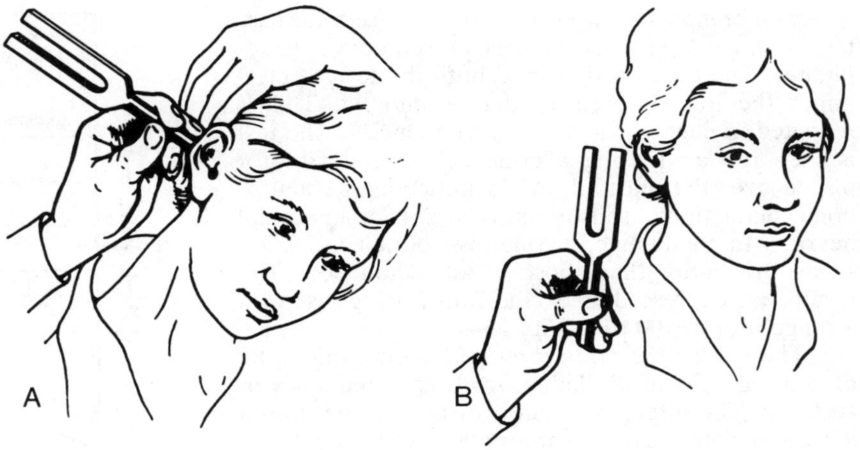

Figure 33–2. The Rinne test. (From Paparella, M. M., and Shumrick, D. A. [Eds.]: Otolaryngology. Vol. II. Philadelphia, W. B. Saunders Company, 1980, p. 1175.)

Hearing Evaluation

An office hearing evaluation consists of tuning fork tests and clinical speech testing. *Tuning fork tests* help detect abnormal hearing and differentiate conductive loss from sensorineural loss. These tests provide a gross estimate of hearing but are not as accurate as an audiogram. Tuning fork tests are not usually successful in children less than 4 years of age.

Clinical speech testing may be performed in patients over 5 years of age. The whispered voice test is performed by using bisyllabic words of equal stress, such as baseball, airplane, cowboy, railroad, eardrum, ice cream, and hot dog. The opposite ear is masked by using a Bárány's box or a partially occluded suction tubing. The hand should be held in such a way as to prevent the patient from lip reading. The results of the test should be expressed as normal hearing or as mild to moderate or severe hearing loss.

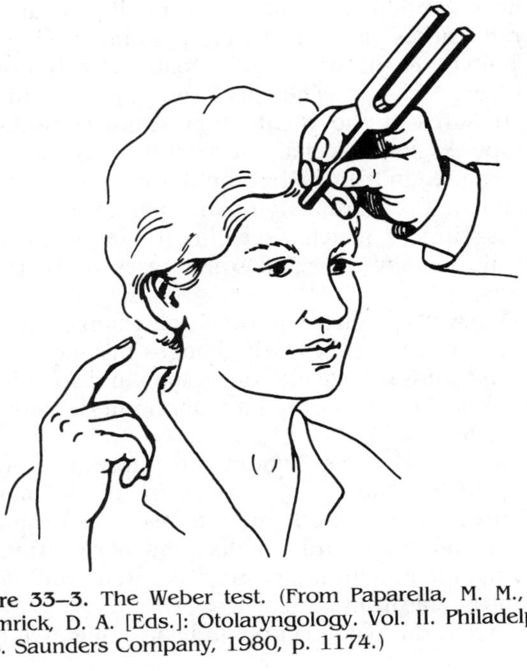

Figure 33–3. The Weber test. (From Paparella, M. M., and Shumrick, D. A. [Eds.]: Otolaryngology. Vol. II. Philadelphia, W. B. Saunders Company, 1980, p. 1174.)

This type of testing is much more accurate than the use of a watch tick. For children, calibrated noise makers are available that give some frequency information. Again, one must be careful to shield the noise maker from the visual field of the child to eliminate visual cues.

Another indirect measure of hearing in a young child is an assessment of their speech. If a child by 18 months of age has not said at least one word that is intelligible to an outsider, then hearing impairment should be considered as a possible cause. By age 2 years, a child should be able to put two words together and be understood. By age 3 years, the child should be able to put three-word sentences together.

Audiometric Diagnosis. A hearing evaluation should be an extension of a physical examination and can range in complexity from a simple office evaluation to sophisticated audiometry.

Tuning fork tests using a *512-Hz.* tuning fork should always be performed and can define normal from abnormal hearing, conductive loss versus sensorineural loss, and the frequency range of the loss. These tests provide a gross estimate and are not a substitute for an audiogram.

The *Rinne test* (Fig. 33–2) is performed by first placing the tuning fork on the mastoid tip (Fig. 33–2*A*), then aligning the prongs next to the meatus and parallel to the ear canal (Fig. 33–2*B*). The patient is asked which position sounds louder. If the air-conducted sound is louder than the bone-conducted sound, then the hearing is either normal or there is a sensorineural loss. If the bone-conducted sound is louder than the air-conducted sound, then there is a conductive loss in that ear.

The *Weber test* (Fig. 33–3) evaluates symmetry of hearing by placing the 512-Hz. fork on the forehead or central incisors. The patient reports whether the sound is heard loudest in the middle or whether it lateralizes to one ear or the other. If the tone is loudest in the middle, then either the hearing is normal or the hearing loss is symmetrical. Lateralization indicates a conductive hearing loss in that ear or a significant sensorineural loss in the opposite ear.

Basic audiometry involves *pure-tone testing* and

speech reception threshold testing. In pure-tone testing, a single frequency tone is presented via headphones. The intensity is varied until the tester determines the lowest intensity that is audible. This is repeated in each ear at various frequencies. The test is then repeated using a bone conduction vibrator placed over the mastoid. Air conduction is equal to bone conduction in sensorineural losses and in normal hearing. In conductive hearing loss, bone conduction scores are better than those of air conduction. The results are expressed as decibels of hearing loss with a range of 0 to 100 dB. (Fig. 33–4).

The *speech reception threshold* is determined by presenting a list of bisyllabic words at a frequency of 1000 Hz. The intensity of the words is varied until a level is reached at which the patient can repeat half of the test items.

The speech reception threshold for each ear should approximate the average of the pure tones at 500, 1000, and 2000 Hz. (± dB.) in each ear.

Speech discrimination tests are used to test the clarity of articulated speech. A list of monosyllabic words is given at 40 dB. above the speech reception threshold. The results are reported as a percentage of the words of the list that are repeated correctly. Normal discrimination scores are 90 per cent or above.

There are special audiometric tests to determine whether a hearing loss is caused by a cochlear or retrocochlear lesion (eighth nerve to auditory cortex). Other than auditory brainstem response, tone decay and reflex decay tests are the most commonly used basic audiometric tests for a retrocochlear lesion.

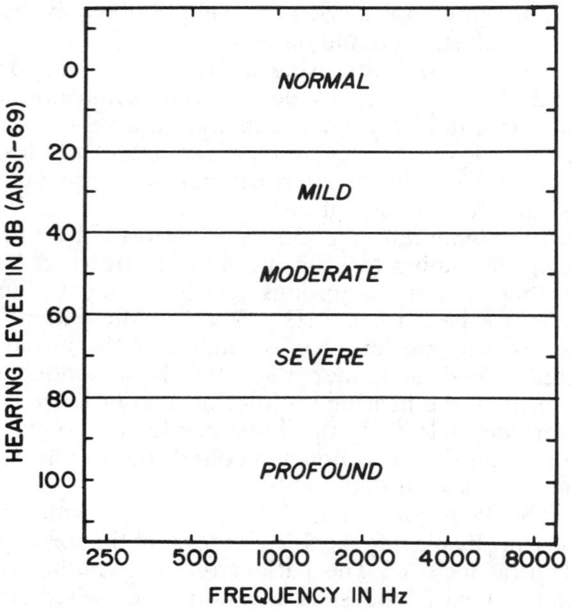

Figure 33–4. An audiogram form. The frequency scale ranges from 250 to 8000 Hz. The intensity scale ranges from − 10 to 110 dB. The five general categories used to classify a patient's hearing loss according to degree of impairment are illustrated. (From Paparella, M. M., and Shumrick, D. A. [Eds.]: Otolaryngology. Vol. II. Philadelphia, W. B. Saunders Company, 1980, p. 1226.)

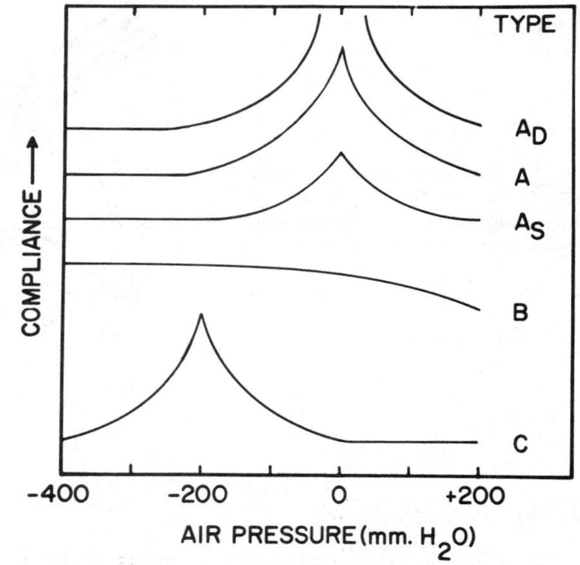

Figure 33–5. The three basic tympanometric shapes. (From Paparella, M. M., and Shumrick, D. A. [Eds.]: Otolaryngology. Vol. II. Philadelphia, W. B. Saunders Company, 1980, p. 1232.)

Impedance Audiometry. There are three important components of impedance audiometry. These three components include tympanometry, physical volume test, and acoustic reflex threshold.

Tympanometry is an objective measure of the compliance of the tympanic membrane as a function of mechanically varied air pressures in the external auditory canal. Tympanic membrane mobility reflects pathology of the middle ear space. With eustachian tube obstruction, there is absorption of the static air in the middle ear space by blood vessels. This creates negative air pressure in the middle ear space, followed by a transudation of fluid and retraction of the tympanic membrane. This negative middle ear pressure can be identified by tympanometry. There are five different curves produced by tympanometry (Fig. 33–5). The type A curve is found in patients with normal middle ear function. The curve shows normal middle ear pressures at the point of maximal compliance. The type As curve is characterized by normal middle ear pressure and limited compliance relative to the mobility of the normal tympanic membrane. The s denotes stiffness, which is seen in otosclerosis, scarred tympanic membranes, and some cases of tympanosclerosis.

The Ad type curve shows large changes in compliance with relatively small changes in air pressure. The d indicates disarticulation as seen in discontinuity of the ossicular chain or in large monomeric tympanic membranes.

The type B curve demonstrates little or no compliance with changes in air pressure in the middle ear. This type of curve is seen in instances of middle ear fluid, adhesive otitis media, and perforations of the tympanic membrane or with a patent ventilating tube in the eardrum.

Finally, the type C curve indicates negative middle ear pressure of −200 mm. H_2O. This may or may not indicate the presence of middle ear fluid.

The *physical volume test* will help clarify the etiology responsible for B type tympanograms. A type B tympanogram with volumes larger than 2.0 ml. in children is usually indicative of a perforation or patent ventilation tube. Type B tympanograms with a normal volume measurement is indicative of a nonmobile intact tympanic membrane.

The *acoustic reflex threshold* is a measurement of the level at which the stapedial muscle contracts. The individual with normal hearing produces an acoustic reflex with pure tone signals between 70 and 100 dB. hearing threshold level (HTL). Because the acoustic reflex is mediated by loudness, it is a sensitive indicator of cochlear pathology. The acoustic reflex test can also be used to confirm the presence of a conductive hearing loss. Another application of the acoustic reflex test is for the detection of retrocochlear pathology.

Auditory Brainstem Response Audiometry. *Auditory brainstem response audiometry* is an objective auditory test that does not require a subjective response from the patient. The aim of the auditory brainstem response audiometry is to record the potentials that arise in the auditory system as a result of sound stimulation. This test can be used to assess or approximate the threshold of hearing in the higher frequencies. *Auditory brainstem response audiometry* is also useful in detecting retrocochlear lesions such as an acoustic neuroma. The patient with multiple sclerosis and hearing loss may also demonstrate an abnormal auditory brainstem response.

SENSORINEURAL HEARING LOSS IN CHILDREN

Sensorineural hearing loss in childhood may go undetected for years, particularly if it is restricted to the high frequencies. This can result in speech and language difficulties that can have a profound effect on intellectual development. It is important to detect these losses at an early age so that corrective measures can be undertaken.

Hearing actually begins in utero. It has been shown clinically that a 3-month-old infant responds preferentially to a tape recording of his mother's voice. The first word is spoken at about 1 year, with two-word sentences being spoken by age 2 years. By age 4 years, the basic steps to normal language acquisition have been completed.

It is important to determine the cause of a hearing loss in children. This begins with a detailed interview with the parents covering the gestational, perinatal, postnatal, and family histories. The gestational history should seek to uncover maternal infection, trauma, immunologic disorders, nutritional disturbances, or endocrine imbalance. Maternal infections that can affect the fetus include rubella, cytomegalovirus, toxoplasmosis, influenza, syphilis, and herpes types 1 and 2. Maternal trauma may take the form of a disturbance in the placenta or umbilical cord, irradiation, drug ingestion, maternal alcoholism, and associated nutritional disturbances.

Endocrine disturbances of the mother such as thyrotoxicosis, diabetes, and pseudohypoparathyroidism may also predispose the fetus to aural damage.

Perinatal events that lead to hypoxia and hearing loss include placenta previa, abruptio placentae, prolonged difficult labor, nuchal or prolapsed cord, and prematurity. Neonatal jaundice and an unconjugated bilirubin of greater than 25 mg. per 100 ml. may lead to hearing loss. The use of aminoglycosides to treat septicemia or meningitis in an infant with an immature renal system may also cause a hearing loss.

The postnatal history must include a careful questioning of the response of the infant to sound and the onset of vocalization. Postnatal viral infections that cause hearing loss include adenovirus, chickenpox, Epstein-Barr virus, herpes zoster oticus, influenza, measles, mumps, encephalitis, and viral hepatitis. Of these, *mumps* is the leading cause of acquired unilateral sensorineural hearing loss in children. Bacterial meningitis may cause either a unilateral or bilateral sensorineural hearing loss.

The *family history* is very important since congenital deafness is inherited in 50 per cent of cases. Up to 80 per cent are inherited as an autosomal recessive trait, and 20 per cent as an autosomal dominant trait. The majority of these cases represent single-gene mendelian inheritance and not part of a recognizable syndrome associated with malformations of other organs or body systems. Autosomal dominant hearing loss is usually mild, flat, and progressive when compared with autosomal recessive losses. Only 1 to 3 per cent of genetic deafness is caused by x-linked inheritance.

The *physical examination* should include a thorough inspection of the pinna. The tympanic membranes should be examined with the pneumatic otoscope or the microscope. An effort should be made to uncover a recognized syndrome by using an organ system approach. A search for craniofacial, dental, cardiac, and renal abnormalities should be undertaken. In addition, endocrine dysfunction, neurologic disease, dermal abnormalities, and skeletal dysplasia may be found. Finally, a consideration of metabolic storage disease and chromosome abnormalities completes the evaluation.

A hearing evaluation using auditory brainstem response should be obtained in all high-risk newborn infants.

Medication Ototoxicity

Ototoxic drugs used in clinical practice include aminoglycosides, furosemide, ethacrynic acid, salicylates, *cis*-platinum, and erythromycin.

The aminoglycoside antibiotics destroy the hair cells and stria vascularis of the inner ear, resulting in irreversible hearing loss. The degree of ototoxicity is increased by noise exposure and use with other ototoxic drugs.

Streptomycin, gentamicin, and tobramycin are primarily vestibulotoxic. Netilmicin is a new synthetic aminoglycoside that is apparently less ototoxic than any of the presently available aminoglycosides. The effect of most aminoglycosides is insidious. Hearing loss may not become apparent until weeks or months after therapy has been discontinued. Early effects can be detected by high-frequency audiometry and electronystagmography. Since aminoglycosides are excreted by the kidney, renal impairment renders a patient much more susceptible to these ototoxic drugs. Aminoglycosides can cross the placental barrier, resulting in hearing loss in unborn children. Monitoring peak and trough blood levels when administering these medications is helpful in preventing toxicity.

Quinine can be the cause of temporary or permanent sensorineural hearing loss. Elderly patients taking quinine for leg cramps may develop tinnitus and hearing loss from this medication. The ingestion of therapeutic doses of quinine by the pregnant woman may cause severe bilateral sensorineural hearing loss in the fetus.

Salicylates cause reversible hearing loss and tinnitus. The salicylates block an enzyme system within the inner ear, resulting in the uncoupling of oxidative phosphorylation within the cochlea. Normal hearing returns 24 to 72 hours after discontinuation of the drug. Ingestion of 6 to 8 grams per day is required to produce toxicity. Hearing loss occurs whenever salicylate serum levels reach 20 mg. per cent or above.

Cis-platinum has both auditory and vestibular toxicity. The hearing loss is usually bilateral and appears first at high frequencies (6000 and 8000 Hz.). The hearing loss may be asymmetric and may not appear until several days after treatment.

Patients at high risk for ototoxicity from erythromycin include individuals with hepatic or renal failure or those with Legionnaires' disease. The daily dose of erythromycin should not exceed 1.5 grams if the serum creatinine concentration is above 1.8 mg. per cent. The otoneurologic changes observed with erythromycin administration are reversible following cessation of therapy (Meyerhoff, 1984).

CHRONIC OTITIS MEDIA WITH EFFUSION

Chronic otitis media with effusion develops secondary to eustachian tube obstruction, barotrauma, or radiotherapy. The fluid may be either serous or mucoid. Clinical experience and experimental evidence suggest that a continuum of serous to mucoid fluid is seen. The pathogenesis of serous effusions involves negative pressure within the middle ear, which occurs as the result of mucosal absorption of middle ear gas, which causes transudation of fluid from the blood vessels of the mucoperiosteum. *Serous otitis media* is the most common cause of hearing loss in children. More than 30 per cent of all children have had three or more episodes of otitis by their second birthday. If the effusion persists, secondary infection can develop and results in proliferation and activation of secretory cells in the middle ear.

As the fluid thickens, it is then known as a mucoid effusion. The patient with chronic otitis media with effusion presents with hearing loss and a fullness or pressure in the involved ear. Infants and toddlers with the disorder may present with pulling at the ears, *nocturnal awakening*, and general fussiness.

Physical examination reveals retracted eardrums and fluid, with or without bubbles. With serous fluid, the tympanic membrane is amber, whereas mucoid effusion is associated with a dull-appearing drum but with distinct margins. Pneumatic otoscopy reveals little or no movement. Tuning fork tests and audiometry show a conductive hearing loss that rarely exceeds 40 dB. Management involves the removal or elimination of any precipitating factors, including sinusitis, allergic rhinitis, and obstructing or chronically infected adenoid tissue. Eighty per cent of patients with otitis media with effusion are free of effusion within 2 months of an episode of acute otitis media or upper respiratory infection. If the effusion is still present at 2 months, then a 2-week trial of an antimicrobial agent effective against beta-lactamase–producing bacteria might be of benefit prior to consideration for surgery. Decongestants and antihistamines have not proved to be effective management for effusions; however, they may be helpful in patients with documented nasal allergy. The insertion of pressure-equalizing tubes is indicated if an effusion persists for 3 months or longer (Fig. 33–6). Approx-

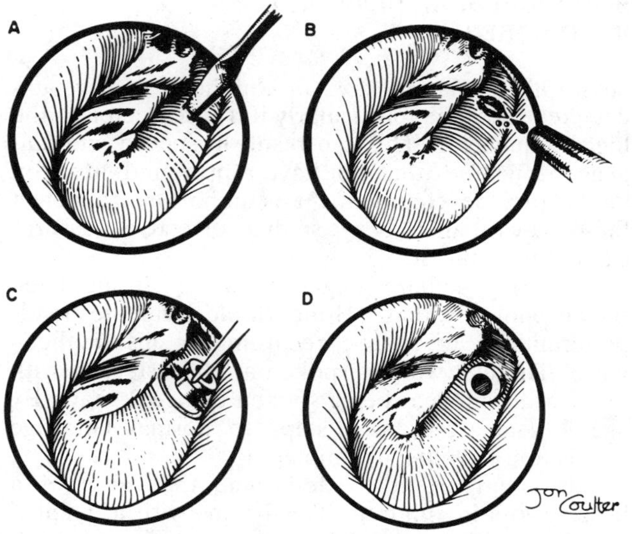

Figure 33–6. Method of insertion of a tympanostomy tube. *A*, Radial incision in the tympanic membrane. *B*, Middle ear effusion is aspirated. *C*, Short biflanged tympanostomy tube (Armstrong type) is inserted using alligator forceps. *D*, Tube is positioned in the anterosuperior portion of tympanic membrane. (From Bluestone, C. D., and Klein, J. O. [Eds.]: Otitis Media in Infants and Children. Philadelphia, W. B. Saunders Company, 1988, p. 179.)

imately 80 per cent of patients with pressure equalizing tubes respond after one insertion and require no further therapy. The child with a persistent conductive hearing loss secondary to otitis media with effusion is at risk for cognitive and language delay. The nasopharynx of adults with a unilateral effusion should be carefully examined for a nasopharyngeal carcinoma (Bluestone, 1988).

EVALUATION OF DIZZINESS

The office evaluation of the patient who has a chief complaint of dizziness begins with a detailed history. The history can be conveniently divided into five parts. First is the differentiation of true vertigo from lightheadedness or disequilibrium. True vertigo has a rotational component that can be in the form of objects spinning or turning around the individual, or severe spinning or turning feeling from inside. This is to be differentiated from the lightheadedness, giddiness, or "swimming-type" of sensation in the head. True vertigo is most often associated with a disorder of the vestibular system. Rarely is loss of consciousness associated with a vestibular disorder. Inquiries regarding the association of the vertigo with nausea or vomiting are important to ascertain the severity of the vertigo.

The second part involves gathering information about associated phenomena, participating factors, the periodicity of the attacks, and their frequency. Allergies, head injuries, position change, hyperventilation, fatigue, neck injury, and history of seizures are also important events that may be associated with dizziness.

The next part is specific for symptoms of ear disease. Questions about hearing, tinnitus, fullness or stuffiness in the ears, otalgia or discharge from the ears should be asked.

The fourth part attempts to rule out associated brainstem phenomena such as double vision, numbness of the arms, face, legs, or weakness of the arms or legs, difficulty with speech, confusion, or loss of consciousness.

The final part involves questions about high blood pressure, diabetes, or previous ear surgery.

After a thorough history, the physical examination should begin with the recording of vital signs, including blood pressure in the supine, sitting, and standing positions. The pulse should be taken carefully to evaluate arrhythmias. A thorough ear, nose, and throat evaluation is next. Tuning fork evaluation, including the Weber and Rinne tests, should also be performed. The eyes should be carefully examined for nystagmus, and the fundi should be examined carefully for papilledema. A neuro-otologic evaluation should include a careful examination of the cranial nerves, followed by cerebellar testing. Rhomberg testing should be performed as well as tandem walk, heel walk, and toe walk. If there is a positional component to the dizziness, then a test involving rapid position changes should be performed to aid in the search for nystagmus and evidence of benign paroxysmal positional vertigo. Further tests should usually include an audiogram. If there is a vertiginous component to the dizziness, then an electronystagmogram should also be considered. Additional tests will be directed by the findings of the history and physical examinations but may include magnetic resonance imaging, computerized tomography, and various blood tests such as FTA-Abs and erythocyte sedimentation rate.

Electronystagmography

Electronystagmography is an objective study of the vestibular system, based on the principle that the eye is a dipole with a positive charge at the cornea and a negative charge at the retina. Electrodes are placed about the eye to detect any movement of the eye such as might occur with nystagmus. Nystagmus may be either spontaneous or induced by a position change or a caloric stimulus. By comparing one ear with the other, a relative hypofunction can be identified. Other tests within the electronystagmography battery include positional testing, optokinetic testing, pendulum tracing, and spontaneous nystagmus.

Electronystagmography will not provide a diagnosis for vertigo but will help localize the lesion if it is in the vestibular system.

DISORDERS ASSOCIATED WITH DIZZINESS

Meniere's Disease

Meniere's disease is a term for the coexistence of recurrent vertigo, tinnitus, and hearing loss. Although the cause is uncertain, symptoms are produced by distention and pressure buildup in the vestibular and cochlear apparatus of the inner ear. The disease most commonly occurs in women around the age of 50, and often progresses from isolated vertigo to include tinnitus and hearing loss. Although the vertigo tends to lessen over time, the hearing loss tends to worsen because of gradual destruction of the vestibular and cochlear receptor sites.

The episodes of vertigo occur suddenly and without warning and are often accompanied by nausea and vomiting. Dizziness may last from a few minutes up to several hours, but patients often report feeling unsteady for several days. Although most patients have disease on one side only, about one third will eventually have a bilateral condition. The results of examination between attacks are normal, except for hearing loss, if present. During attacks, nystagmus that is directed away from the involved ear may be seen.

No effective cure for Meniere's disease exists. Management of an acute attack of vertigo includes bed rest and antivertiginous medication. Severe attacks may require hospitalization for parenteral fluids and medication. Long-term management strategies to reduce frequency of attacks include cessation of smoking, decreased caffeine consumption, and a low salt diet. Several surgical approaches have been used to treat intractable cases. About 10 per cent of patients eventually require surgery, primarily because of frequent uncontrolled attacks of vertigo. A decompressive shunt procedure performed on the endolymphatic sac resolves the vertigo in two thirds of patients, while allowing the patient to retain reasonable hearing ability. A vestibular nerve section resolves the vertigo in 95 per cent of patients but does not improve the hearing loss. No current operation consistently improves the hearing loss. Confirmation of the effectiveness of these procedures is still in progress.

Vestibular Neuronitis

Vestibular neuronitis primarily affects adults, causing the abrupt onset of severe vertigo, nausea, and vomiting without hearing loss. Although proof is lacking, it is thought to be a viral infection of the labyrinth and is self-limited, usually lasting a few days. Like most patients with acute vertigo, a change of head position markedly exacerbates symptoms. Patients may experience residual vertigo for several weeks.

Examination usually reveals only horizontal nystagmus. Caloric testing shows depression of the vestibular response. Treatment should include antihistamines, bed rest, and hydration. Progressive positional exercises should be performed once the acute vertigo is gone. The Cawthorne-Cooksey exercises are designed to retrain the eye and body musculature to use vision and proprioceptive signals to compensate for the lost vestibular signals (Table 33–1).

Table 33–1. CAWTHORNE-COOKSEY EXERCISES FOR PATIENT WITH VERTIGO

May Be Done in Bed, During Acute Phase
Eye movements, first slow, then fast
Up and down
Side to side
Focus on a finger from 10 to 30 cm from face
Head movements, first slow, then fast, then with eyes closed
Forward and backward
Side to side
Should Be Done While Sitting
Head movements as above
Shoulder shrugging and circling
Bending forward to pick up objects from the ground
Should Be Done While Standing
Eye and head movements, shoulder shrugging and circling as above
Go from sitting to standing position with eyes open, then closed
Throw small balls from hand to hand above eye level
Throw ball from hand to hand under knee
Change from sitting to standing position, turning around in between
Moving About
Circling around center person who throws large ball to and fro
Walking across room with eyes open, then closed
Walk up and down slope with eyes open, then closed
Walk up and down steps with eyes open, then closed
Perform a game involving stooping and stretching and aiming, such as skittles, bowling, or basketball.

Adapted from Baloh, R. W.: The dizzy patient. Symptomatic treatment of vertigo. Postgrad. Med., 73(5):317–324, 1983.

Benign Paroxysmal Positional Vertigo

Benign paroxysmal positional vertigo is the most common cause of vertigo in the elderly and is thought to be the result of stimulation of the labyrinthine mechanism from displacement of some of the otoconia, which rest atop hair cells in that organ (Slater, 1988). Initially, vertigo may be severe but gradually improves over several weeks to months. Examination reveals nystagmus in the affected head position characterized by a 2 to 20 second latent period and fatigue after 20 to 30 seconds. Since the nystagmus may be subtle and brief, it may not be detectable with the naked eye. The use of Frenzel glasses can help the physician make the diagnosis of this form of nystagmus. Many believe that the condition will resolve more quickly if the patient continually stimulates the vertigo by putting the head into the precipitating position. Patients should be instructed not to avoid the offending head position. Positional exercises are also helpful, presumably by helping the patient adapt to the asymmetrical input from the two labyrinths.

Labyrinthitis

Labyrinthitis is the *most frequent complication of otitis media*, owing to extension of infection within the temporal bone. There are three types of labyrinthitis that include, in order of descending severity, perilabyrinthitis, serous labyrinthitis, and suppurative labyrinthitis. Perilabyrinthitis, or labyrinthine fistula, which may be produced surgically, occurs secondary to bone erosion by a cholesteatoma or develops after a Valsalva maneuver or an explosion. The patient complains of dizziness or hearing loss, or both, particularly if he or she presses against the tragus, manipulates the auricle, or quickly turns the head. A Valsalva-type maneuver may reproduce the dizziness, and a loud noise may also cause vertigo momentarily. A positive fistula test is present in two thirds of the patients with a labyrinthine fistula. The positive fistula test consists of nystagmus and vertigo and is produced when positive and negative pressure is applied to the soft tissue covering the fistula. A strong positive fistula test is always an indication for surgical examination of the labyrinth. When erosion is associated with chronic otitis media, then a radical or modified-radical mastoidectomy is performed.

Serous labyrinthitis is due to diffuse intralabyrinthine inflammation without pus formation and is not followed by permanent loss of auditory and vestibular function. Serous labyrinthitis may be secondary to acute or chronic otitis media, with or without cholesteatoma formation. Serous labyrinthitis in acute otitis media is treated with intravenous injection of antibiotics and a myringotomy for drainage. Serous labyrinthitis secondary to chronic otitis media usually requires surgical intervention for drainage of the suppurative process or removal of the cholesteatoma matrix.

Suppurative labyrinthitis is a diffuse intralabyrinthine infection with pus formation and is associated with permanent loss of auditory and vestibular function. Suppurative labyrinthitis may be secondary to direct extension of the purulent process in the middle ear or from the spread of meningeal inflammation into the labyrinth through the internal auditory canal or, less frequently, the cochlear aqueduct. Clinical symptoms include nausea and vomiting, intense vertigo, tinnitus, hearing loss, and nystagmus. Treatment consists of intense antibiotic treatment and surgical drainage of the labyrinth.

Herpes Zoster Oticus

Herpes zoster oticus *(Ramsay Hunt syndrome)* is characterized by cutaneous eruptions about the auricle and external ear canal, facial nerve paralysis or palsy, vertigo, and hearing loss. There may be a prodromal period of general malaise and neuralgia prior to the onset of cutaneous eruption. The facial paralysis, hearing loss, and vertigo may occur alone or in various combinations after the onset of pain. The management consists of topical or systemic antibiotic therapy for control of any secondary bacterial infection. Systemic analgesics may also be necessary for pain control. The role of corticosteroids in the management of herpes zoster oticus has not been well established. Acyclovir may be helpful in decreasing the healing time and lessening the pain associated with these lesions. The facial paralysis of herpes zoster oticus is generally more severe than that seen in Bell's palsy and may be persistent. Sensorineural hearing loss may also persist following the resolution of the infection.

OTITIS EXTERNA

Otitis externa (swimmer's ear) commonly occurs during the summer months. Moisture from frequent swimming in combination with high temperatures creates optimum conditions for growth of bacteria in the external canal. Another common cause of recurrent otitis externa is due to excessive cleaning of the protective cerumen in the canal (Bell, 1985). The bacteria most commonly responsible for otitis are *Pseudomonas, Proteus*, and, occasionally, *Staphylococcus* and *Streptococcus*. The patient first experiences itching that usually progresses to ear pain, occasionally becoming quite severe. In addition, the patient often complains of a plugged sensation that also may be quite bothersome.

The most common physical finding is pain on traction of the external ear. The canal is erythematous and edematous, and may contain whitish exudate and desquamated debris.

Treatment should begin with gentle cleansing and suction of the ear canal. In cooperative patients, this can often be accomplished with the use of a small tuft of cotton on a wire applicator. Instillation of antibiotic-steroid drops (e.g., polymyxin B–neomycin–hydrocortisone), four to five times a day, usually results in healing within a few days. Marcy (1985) notes that 2 to 5 per cent acetic acid ear drops are also effective in eliminating the infectious agent. If severe swelling is present, a cotton wick should be inserted so that the drops can penetrate the canal. The wick may then be removed by the patient in 1 or 2 days. If cellulitis is present in the periauricular area, an oral antibiotic such as cephalexin should be prescribed.

An unusual form of external otitis is referred to as necrotizing (or malignant) external otitis. This entity is most often seen in diabetic patients and is due to *Pseudomonas* or *Proteus* infection. It usually involves not only the canal but the surrounding subcutaneous tissues and, often, the bone. Pain is usually more severe and examination may reveal granulation tissue on the floor of the ear canal at the bony cartilaginous junction. A diabetic or immunosuppressed individual with swimmer's ear deserves careful consideration to exclude this entity. Management requires long-term parenteral antibiotics and judicious debridement in an inpatient setting.

OTOMYCOSIS

Individuals especially susceptible to otomycotic external infections include hearing aid users, immunocompromised persons, or those who have undergone open cavity mastoidectomies. The organisms are usually saprophytes rather than pathogens and occur superimposed on an underlying bacterial infection of the external or middle ear. Fungal infections occur more frequently in tropical or subtropical climates and are associated with intense heat and humidity. Among the more commonly seen fungi are the *Aspergillus, Mucor,* yeast-like fungi, dermatophytes, and actinomyces. Itching is the initial and most prominent symptom, followed by fullness, hearing loss, and pain. The ear canals of such patients are mildly erythematous and may have a moist accumulation of debris. The primary management of saprophytic fungal infections is complete cleansing and debridement of the ear canal. This is usually performed under microscopic control with suction or irrigation and instruments, or both. The canal is then wiped with m-cresyl-acetate or 1 per cent thymol and 70% alcohol. After cleansing, the insufflation of 5 per cent iodochlorhydroxyquin in boric acid powder is effective in preventing a recurrence. This treatment may have to be repeated at weekly intervals for 1 or 2 weeks.

FURUNCLES OF THE EXTERNAL AUDITORY CANAL

Furuncles are staphylococcal infections of the pilosebaceous units of the outer third of the external auditory canal. They present as localized swellings that may become fluctuant and extremely tender. Early lesions are treated with local heat and antistaphylococcal antibiotics. Fluctuant lesions should be drained. Narcotics may be necessary for the first 24 to 48 hours for pain control.

EXTERNAL AUDITORY CANAL FOREIGN BODY

Impacted cerumen is one of the most common ear complaints in family practice. Prevention should always be stressed by discouraging the use of cotton tipped applicators. Even for patients who produce large amounts of cerumen, avoiding insertion of objects smaller than the little finger will usually result in flaking and natural extrusion. Once impaction has occurred, cerumen may be removed by an ear curette or by irrigation. Irrigation should not be used if there is a history of a draining ear or a perforation of the tympanic membrane. Use of body temperature water (37° C [98.6° F]) will help prevent the occurrence of vertigo (Black, 1986). A large amount of dry cerumen may need to be softened with triethanolamine polypeptide oleate-condensate (Cerumenex) or a similar preparation. Patients with very hard, dry wax may require the use of drops for several days prior to irrigation. A combination of curetting and irrigation may also be employed in difficult cases. If minor trauma results, antibiotic-steroid ear drops should be used for 24 to 48 hours.

BULLOUS MYRINGITIS

Bullous myringitis is most commonly associated with a viral or mycoplasmal upper respiratory infection. Symptoms are usually limited to mild to moderate ear pain or a sensation of ear fullness. Examination reveals blebs on the surface of the tympanic membrane, which have thin walls and contain fluid. The pain usually subsides in 1 or 2 days. If it is difficult to determine whether an associated otitis media is present, antibiotics should be prescribed followed by re-examination in 48 to 72 hours.

ACUTE OTITIS MEDIA

Acute otitis media is second only to viral upper respiratory infections in prevalence during childhood. Over two thirds of all children experience at least one episode of otitis media during the first 3 years of life. At least 10 per cent of these children have persistent effusions lasting 3 months or more. Most cases occur during the winter and early spring months and are associated with respiratory syncytial virus, influenza virus, and adenovirus infections (Henderson, 1982). The most common causative organism, accounting for about one third of cases, is pneumococcus, followed by *H. influenzae* and *Branhamella catarrhalis* (about 20 per cent each). Streptococci, staphylococci, and viruses are responsible for the remainder. Bodor (1982) reported that when otitis media was accompanied by purulent conjunctivitis, 73 per cent of patients had *H. influenzae* infections.

Symptoms of acute otitis media consist of ear pain, mild to moderate fever, and unilateral hearing loss. Diagnosis depends on careful examination of the tympanic membrane. Erythema, bulging of the tympanic membrane with distortion of landmarks, and discoloration from middle ear fluid are diagnostic of acute otitis. Patients who are acutely ill, newborns, and those who have not responded satisfactorily to antibiotic treatment should be considered for tympanocentesis.

Since the organism is not usually known, the choice of antibiotic is empiric. The initial drug of choice is amoxicillin (20 to 50 mg. per kg. per day). If the patient does not respond to this antibiotic, alternatives include erythromycin (30 to 50 mg. per kg. per day) combined with sulfamethoxazole (50 to 100 mg. per kg. per day) in four divided doses; trimethoprim-sulfisoxazole (8 and 40 mg. per kg. per day) in two divided doses; cefaclor (40 mg. per kg. per day); or amoxicillin-K clavulanate (40 mg. per kg. per day) in three divided doses. Follow-up examination should be performed 2 to 3 weeks later. In patients who have early recurrences on otitis, Carlin and colleagues (1987) noted that patients were more likely to be harboring a different organism than the one that caused the initial infection. Persistence of middle ear fluid is common, but gradual progress toward resolution should be expected. In patients with middle ear effusion, decongestants or another course of antibiotic therapy may be tried. Cantekin and associates (1983) showed in a double-blind, randomized trial that use of decongestants resulted in no better results than giving a placebo. Most clinicians prefer a conservative, noninterventional approach unless the patient continues to have significant symptoms. The decision to place ventilation tubes or to perform tonsillectomy or adenoidectomy, or both, is very subjective and difficult to make. If significant hearing loss or speech delay is present following recurrent otitis media, or if resolution of effusion is delayed longer than 12 weeks, consideration should be given to performing ventilating procedure (Ghory, 1982).

CHRONIC OTITIS MEDIA

Chronic otitis media describes a process whereby irreversible changes have occurred in the tympanic membrane, middle ear, or mastoid. This is a disease that requires surgery, which may vary from the correction of a small central perforation to the removal of an extensive cholesteatoma and drainage of a posterior fossa abscess. (Chronic otitis media can be active, with continuous suppuration, or inactive, representing the sequelae of previous infections.)

The cause of *chronic otitis media* is usually eustachian tube dysfunction or trauma and involves a defect in the structure of the tympanic membrane. The eustachian tube dysfunction may be a result of a cleft palate, obstructing adenoids, tumor, chronic sinusitis, allergic rhinitis, hypothyroidism, smoking, or collagen diseases.

Chronic otitis media can be further divided into tubotympanic disease and attic-antrum disease. Tubotympanic disease may be either a permanent perforation or a persistent tubotympanic mucosal infection. In a persistent perforation, there is a hole in the pars tensa, in which the margin is completely covered with healed epithelium. The ear is usually dry, although it may produce discharge intermittently secondary to water passing through the external meatus or from the spread of mucus through the eustachian tube from nose-blowing or sneezing. When the middle ear is infected, the mucosa is red and edematous and the discharge is mucopurulent and odorless. Hearing loss depends on the size and location of the perforation. Hearing may be normal in a small anterior perforation. Large posterior perforations cause a greater degree of hearing loss. A hearing loss of greater than 30 dB. usually indicates ossicular involvement.

The patient should be instructed to avoid getting water in the ear by plugging it with a molded wax plug or with a tightly fitted petrolatum cotton plug. Any pathology of the nose, paranasal sinuses, or nasopharynx should be treated. The ear that produces discharge should be cultured and cleaned, preferably with a microscope and suction or alternatively with the operating head of an otoscope and a cotton-tipped applicator. Appropriate antibiotic drops or powder, or both, may then be used in the ear.

Small, predominantly dry, central perforations that do not interfere with hearing may never need to be closed surgically. However, if the patient wishes to be active in water sports, then repair is preferable. The small-to-medium–sized perforation sometimes closes with a paperpatch procedure (the application of a thin piece of sterile paper to cover the perforation while closure occurs from epithelial migration) performed in the office. The ear should be free of infection for a few months prior to any procedure. Closure of a perforation prevents recurrent infections that cause mucosal changes of the windows and ossicles that may "stiffen" them or lead to disruption of the ossicular chain.

The chronically draining ear without a cholesteatoma exhibits an odorless mucopurulent discharge through a near-total defect in the tympanic membrane. The exposed ossicles are buried in a thick, exuberant, red mucosa. Polyps may be present and should not be removed except under microscopic control. Any pathology of the nose, paranasal sinuses, or nasopharynx must be corrected. Patients with this condition typically do not have otalgia, fever, or vertigo.

Cultures of the discharge should be obtained and appropriate antimicrobial drops and daily middle ear suctioning begun. Alternatively, the patient can be hospitalized and administered a parenteral beta-lactam antipseudomonal drug. The patient who does not respond to this regimen or develops an intratemporal suppurative complication requires surgery of the middle ear and mastoid.

Complications of Otitis Media

Suppurative intracranial complications of otitis media have decreased with the advent of antimicrobial agents. The complications that do occur are more often associated with chronic suppurative otitis media and mastoiditis, with or without a cholesteatoma. The middle ear and mastoid air cell system is adjacent to many important structures, including the sigmoid sinus, the posterior fossa dura, and the middle fossa dura. Suppuration in the middle ear and mastoid may spread to these structures, resulting in the following intracranial complications: meningitis, extradural abscess, subdural empyema, focal encephalitis, brain abscess, lateral sinus thrombosis, and otitic hydrocephalus (Fig. 33–7). The patient who has acute or chronic otitis media and develops one or more of the following signs or symptoms—especially while receiving medical therapy—should be suspected of having a suppurative intracranial complication: *persistent headache, lethargy, malaise, irritability, severe otalgia, onset of fever, nausea,* and *vomiting*. The following would be signs and symptoms demanding an intensive search for an intracranial complication: stiff neck, focal seizures, ataxia, blurred vision, papilledema, diplopia, hemiplegia, aphasia, dysdiadochokinesia, intention tremor, dysmetria, and hemianopsia. Fever is common with acute otitis media, but persistent or recurrent fever, particularly after the administration of appropriate antimicrobial therapy, may be a sign of the spread of the infection.

Meningitis is the *most common* intracranial suppurative complication of acute and chronic otitis media. The most common cause of meningitis is an upper respiratory infection with a simultaneous middle ear infection. When meningitis is suspected, tympanocentesis and myringotomy should be performed for identification of the causative organism and establishment of drainage.

Extradural abscess develops from either a cholesteatoma or infection, causing destruction of bone adjacent to the dura. This results in granulation tissue and purulent material collecting between the lateral aspect of the dura and the adjacent temporal bone. Symptoms can include severe earache, low-grade fever, and headache in the temporal region, with deep,

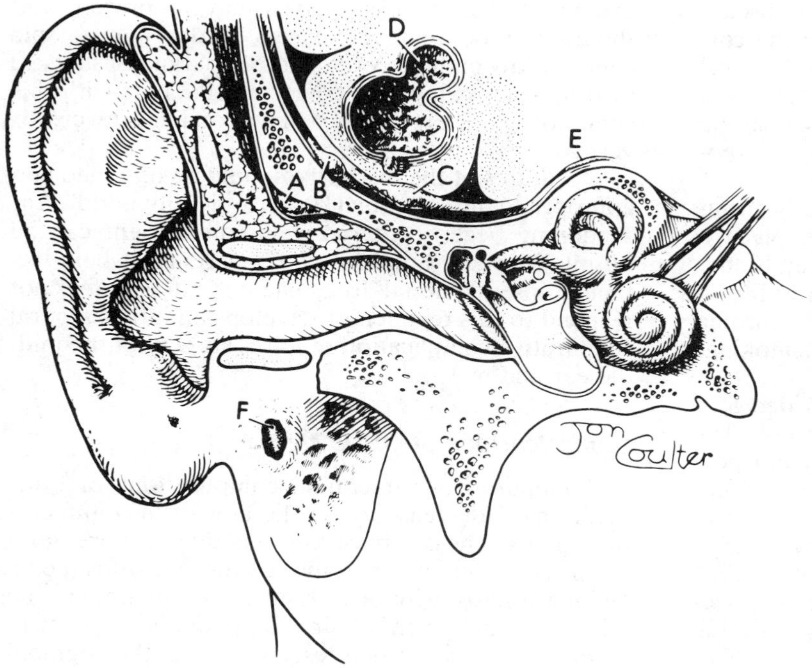

Figure 33–7. Suppurative complications of otitis media and mastoiditis. *A*, Subperiosteal abscess; *B*, extradural abscess; *C*, subdural empyema; *D*, brain abscesses; *E*, meningitis; and *F*, lateral sinus thrombosis. (From Bluestone, C. D., and Stool, S. E. [Eds.]: Pediatric Otolaryngology. Philadelphia, W. B. Saunders Company, 1983, p. 566.)

local, throbbing pain. Otorrhea may accompany the extradural abscess and is characteristically profuse, creamy, and pulsatile. Computerized tomography may reveal a sizeable extradural abscess. Treatment consists of appropriate antimicrobial therapy and surgical drainage, including a mastoidectomy.

Subdural empyema is a collection of purulent material between the dura externally and the subarachnoid membrane internally. This can occur by direct extension or, more rarely, by thrombophlebitis through venous channels. Patients with empyema are very toxic, are febrile, and have severe headache in the temporoparietal region. Central nervous system findings may include seizures, hemiplegia, dysmetria, belligerent behavior, somnolence, stupor, deviation of the eye, dysphagia, sensory deficits, stiff neck, and a positive Kernig's sign. Hemiplegia and recurrent seizures in a patient with suppurative middle ear and mastoid disease are indicative of a subdural empyema. A subdural empyema may be confirmed with computerized tomography. Treatment includes intensive intravenous antimicrobial therapy and neurosurgical drainage.

Otogenic abscess of the brain may follow from acute or chronic middle ear and mastoid infections, or follow the development of an adjacent infection such as lateral sinus thrombophlebitis, petrositis, or meningitis. Temporal lobe abscesses are more common than cerebellar abscesses. Signs of invasion of the central nervous system occur about a month after an episode of acute otitis media or an acute exacerbation of chronic otitis media. Systemic signs include fever and chills. Signs of generalized central nervous system infection may occur and include severe headache, vomiting, drowsiness, seizures, irritability, personality changes, altered levels of consciousness, anorexia, weight loss, and meningismus. In addition, there may be specific signs of temporal or cerebellar involvement, such as vertigo, focal seizures, visual field defects, and nystagmus. Temporal lobe abscesses may be completely silent. Terminal signs include coma, papilledema, or cardiovascular changes. Treatment consists of antimicrobial agents and drainage or resection of the brain abscess, or both, as well as surgical debridement of the primary focus, either the mastoid or adjacent infected tissues.

Lateral sinus thrombophlebitis results from inflammation of the adjacent mastoid. The mastoid infection in contact with the sinus walls produces inflammation of the adventitia, followed by penetration of the vein. The mural thrombus may become infected and may propagate to occlude the lumen. Clinical signs include high, spiking fevers and chills and signs of increased intracranial pressure, including altered states of consciousness, headache, papilledema, and seizures. Bacteremia is frequent and may result in spread of infected thrombi causing pneumonia and empyema, bone and joint infection, and, less commonly, thyroiditis, endocarditis, and abscess of the kidney. Computerized tomography is an invaluable aid in making the diagnosis and should precede a lumbar puncture. Management includes appropriate use of antimicrobial agents. The sinus should be uncovered and any perisinus abscess drained. The lateral sinus should be opened and the thrombus removed. On rare occasions, the internal jugular vein may have to be ligated.

TYMPANIC MEMBRANE PERFORATIONS

Tympanic membrane perforations may be secondary to infection or trauma or may be iatrogenically produced by a ventilating tube. A perforation due to acute otitis media is pinpoint in size and occurs in the pars tensa region. These perforations heal within 24 hours and are of no clinical significance. They are often so small that tympanometry is required to detect their presence. Rarely, acute otitis media may produce a larger perforation. Traumatic perforations produce a perforation of the pars tensa. These perforations are often large and are accompanied by pain, bleeding, a hollow feeling in the ear, and hearing loss. Patients with these perforations require careful examination and audiometric evaluation to rule out an ossicular chain discontinuity or sensorineural hearing loss. Associated vertigo must be investigated to rule out a problem at the oval or round windows. Uncomplicated pars tensa perforations are treated expectantly. If the perforation does not heal spontaneously in 3 months, then it may require surgical closure. Antibiotic drops are indicated only if there has been contamination by water or debris. Systemic antibiotics are not necessary, but pain medication may be required for the first few days. The patient should be cautioned to avoid water contamination of the middle ear by using cotton impregnated with petroleum jelly for plugging of the ear. An audiogram should be obtained at the end of treatment to document the return of hearing.

Perforations may also occur secondary to placement of ventilating tubes for middle ear effusions or infections, or both. These perforations occur when large-diameter or "long-term" tubes are used. They occur more commonly in patients who have had a tube in place for 2 years or longer. These perforations can be repaired when the underlying eustachian tube dysfunction has resolved.

ACUTE MASTOIDITIS

Acute mastoiditis consists of three stages. The *first stage* involves signs and symptoms consistent with acute otitis media. There are pain, fever, and hearing loss. X-ray studies of the mastoid air cell system shows clouding. If resolution does not occur at this stage, then it may progress to the *second stage, acute mastoiditis* with *periostitis*. At this stage, the infection has spread to the periosteum covering the mastoid process. Patients with acute mastoiditis with periostitis have fever, otalgia and postauricular erythema, tenderness, and slight swelling. The pinna may be displaced inferiorly and anteriorly, with loss of the postauricular crease. X-ray studies again show clouding of the mastoid air cell system. Patients with their condition should be hospitalized and have a tympanocentesis, followed by a myringotomy for drainage and perhaps insertion of a tympanostomy tube. They are placed on appropriate antimicrobial therapy and observed for the first 24 to 48 hours. Most patients improve, but if they do not, a complete simple mastoidectomy is performed.

The most advanced stage of acute mastoiditis is *acute mastoid osteitis*. Patients with this condition present with swelling, redness, and tenderness to touch over the mastoid bone. The pinna is displaced outward and downward, and swelling or sagging of the posterosuperior canal wall is present. Purulent discharge may issue through a tympanic membrane perforation. An occasional patient with acute mastoid osteitis may present with a normal-appearing middle ear and tympanic membrane. In these patients, the middle ear involvement drains through the eustachian tube. Computed tomography shows the haziness and distortion of the mastoid air cell system. There is loss of the sharpness of the shadows of the cellular walls owing to demineralization, atrophy, and ischemia of the bony septa. When this occurs, the process is known as coalescent mastoiditis. Management of acute coalescent mastoiditis involves a complete simple cortical mastoidectomy with an accompanying myringotomy and drainage of the middle ear air cell system. Intravenous antibiotic therapy is also administered.

CONGENITAL AND ACQUIRED CHOLESTEATOMA

Keratinizing stratified squamous epithelium within the middle ear or other pneumatized portions of the temporal bone is called a *keratoma* or a *cholesteatoma*. Cholesteatomas may be either congenital or acquired. A *congenital cholesteatoma* represents a congenital cyst of epithelial tissue and appears as a white, cyst-like structure within the middle ear or temporal bone. The most common cholesteatoma is the acquired type, which is secondary to middle ear disease. Seventy-five per cent of the acquired cholesteatomas are located in the attic or posterior superior quadrant. The pathogenesis involves a functional obstruction of the eustachian tube due to constriction rather than dilatation of the tube during swallowing. This results in impaired ventilation of the middle ear–mastoid air cell system, which in turns causes fluctuating or sustained high-negative middle ear pressure. The tympanic membrane becomes flaccid and eventually collapses onto the ossicles and medial wall of the middle ear. The most flaccid parts are the posterosuperior and pars flaccida areas. A retraction pocket develops that may become adherent to the ossicles or surrounding structures, or both. Cholesteatoma formation can then occur as demonstrated in Figure 33–8.

The signs and symptoms of cholesteatoma may be completely absent for many years. Recurrent or continuous foul-smelling discharge and progressive hearing loss are the usual presenting signs. Children do not usually complain of hearing loss, tinnitus, or fullness in the ear, particularly if the lesion is unilateral. Otalgia and fever may signify the development of a suppurative intratemporal or intracranial complication. Similarly, facial paralysis, severe vertigo,

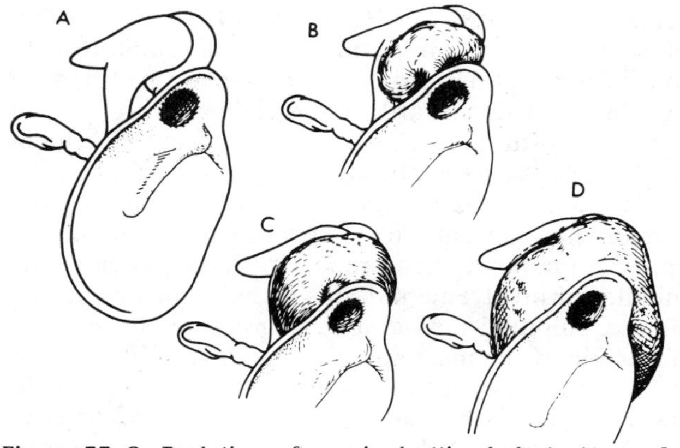

Figure 33–8. Evolution of acquired attic cholesteatoma. *A*, Attic retraction pocket that appears on otoscopic examination to be a "perforation." *B*, A narrow neck sac is developing. *C*, Enlargement of the sac with erosion of the ossicles. *D*, A large cholesteatoma sac, a portion of which can be seen through the eardrum. (From Bluestone, C. D., and Stool, S. E. [Eds.]: Pediatric Otolaryngology. Philadelphia, W. B. Saunders Company, 1983, p. 534.)

headache, and vomiting signify a suppurative complication.

Cholesteatomas appear as white, shiny, greasy flakes of debris in the attic or posterosuperior quadrant of the tympanic membrane. They may also be accompanied by polyps and a foul-smelling discharge.

The audiogram usually reveals a conductive hearing loss, although hearing may be normal. A mixed conductive and sensorineural hearing loss may also be present. The sensorineural component may be due to a serous labyrinthitis or a fistula.

Cholesteatomas are managed *surgically*. It is beyond the scope of this writing to describe the various surgical approaches used in the management of cholesteatoma. The goals of surgery are listed from most important to least important as follows: (1) to give a dry, safe ear, (2) preservation of hearing, and (3) improvement of hearing. One or more operations may be required to achieve these results (Bluestone, 1988).

OTOSCLEROSIS

Otosclerosis is an inherited autosomal dominant trait with poor penetrance that is much more common in Caucasians, less common in blacks, and rare in orientals. A positive family history is elicited in 50 to 70 per cent of the cases. About 10 per cent of Caucasians develop otosclerosis and 1 per cent become symptomatic. Women present clinically with otosclerosis twice as often as men, and most of the patients present between the ages of 11 and 30 years. Eighty per cent of cases eventually become bilateral. Pregnancy seems to accelerate the process. Patients with otosclerosis present with hearing loss. The otoscopic examination is usually unremarkable, but tuning fork tests usually confirm the diagnosis. A conductive or mixed hearing loss is detected. The conductive component will vary between 10 and 50 dB., depending on the degree of fixation. If there is cochlear involvement, the hearing loss will either be flat or sloping down across all frequencies, or have a "cookie-bite" configuration. There are generally four management options to consider in otosclerosis: (1) Observation, particularly if the hearing loss is mild. (2) The option of the use of a hearing aid to improve the hearing should always be discussed with the patient. (3) Sodium fluoride has been recommended as a medication that might halt or retard the progression of otosclerosis. (4) Surgery is the final option. The aim of surgical management is to restore a mobile mechanism for transmitting sound vibrations to the inner ear. Stapedectomy or stapedotomy is highly successful in the properly prepared and selected patient.

BENIGN TUMORS OF THE EAR

Benign tumors of the ear include *osteoma, exostosis, Winkler's disease, keratosis obturans,* and *glomus jugulare* tumors.

Osteomas consist of cancellous bone that arises as a pedunculated tumor from either the tympanosquamous suture or the tyampanomastoid suture. Symptoms include hearing loss and discomfort. Surgical treatment is only necessary when the lesion is symptomatic.

Exostoses are dense compact bone and are the most common tumors of the external auditory canal. They become symptomatic when they cause an accumulation of debris in the canal, resulting in infection or obstruction. The one causative factor is believed to be prolonged swimming in cold salt water.

Winkler's disease consists of a benign nodular painful growth on the helical rim, most often occurring in men. The nodule is tender, preventing some patients from sleeping on the affected side. Treatment consists of cortisone injections. Surgical excision may be required if cortisone does not relieve the pain.

Keratosis obturans is a rare collection or accumulation of large plugs of desquamating squamous epithelium deep within the external auditory canal. This process may cause an erosion of the bony portion of the external auditory canal. It is associated with chronic pulmonary disease, sinusitis, and bronchiectasis. Pain is the presenting complaint. The cause is unknown but is believed to result from faulty migration of squamous epithelium. Treatment consists of periodic debridement of the desquamated squamous epithelium.

Glomus jugulare tumors, also called nonchromaffin perigangliomas, arise from glomus bodies located in the adventitia of the dome of the jugular bulb or along branches of the tympanic plexus. These tumors grow slowly but are destructive by invasion of surrounding structures. They are sometimes multicentric in origin; up to 10 per cent have a definite association with carotid body tumors. The tumor typically is associated with a pulsating tinnitus, followed by hearing loss, and finally, invasion of the tympanic membrane. An isolated facial paralysis may develop, followed by multiple cranial nerve involvement, including nerves IX, X, XI, and XII. Examination in the early stages may reveal a reddish swelling behind the tympanic membrane, which pulsates. Radiologic techniques employed for diagnosis include high-resolution computerized tomography scanning, arteriography, and jugular venography. Unless there are contraindications, glomus tumors should be surgically removed. If there are contraindications to surgery, then radiotherapy may arrest tumor growth.

ACOUSTIC NEUROMA

Acoustic neuroma (schwannoma) accounts for approximately *8 per cent* of all brain tumors and *80 per cent* of all posterior fossa tumors. Patients with acoustic neuromas typically present with a gradual, progressive, unilateral sensorineural hearing loss with poor speech discrimination. At first, patients may only notice the accompanying unilateral tinnitus and not the hearing loss. Therefore, any unexplained unilateral, progressive hearing loss, and tinnitus should raise suspicion of an acoustic neuroma. Approximately 10 per cent of patients with an acoustic neuroma present with a sudden unilateral sensorineural hearing loss. Any patient who presents with an unexplained unilateral sensorineural hearing loss with a duration of 1 month or longer should undergo contrast-enhanced computerized tomography or a magnetic resonance imaging study. Approximately *10 per cent* of patients with acoustic neuroma present with episodic vertigo. More commonly, the vestibular presentation is one of unsteadiness rather than true vertigo. The majority of acoustic neuromas arise from the vestibular division of the eighth cranial nerve. The tumors damage vestibular function slowly enough for compensation of the resulting asymmetry to occur. Acoustic neuromas are usually removed surgically, although poor surgical candidates with small tumors may undergo *gamma knife* radiation therapy. Schwannomas may also arise from other sites, as indicated in the magnetic resonance imaging scan in Figure 33–9.

MALIGNANT NEOPLASMS OF THE EAR

Eighty-five per cent of ear malignancies involve the auricle, 10 per cent involve the external auditory canal, and only 5 per cent involve the middle ear and mastoid. *Otorrhea* and pain are the earliest symptoms. The pain is often intense and out of proportion to the pathologic and clinical findings. Bleeding, fullness in the ear, and conductive hearing loss may also be present. Late findings include perceptive deafness (15 per cent), vertigo (13 per cent), and facial nerve paralysis (13 to 35 per cent). Squamous cell carcinoma constitutes two thirds of the malignancies of the external ear, whereas basal cell carcinoma constitutes the remaining one third. In general, surgical resection provides a better prognosis than radiotherapy. The most common tumor of the middle ear is squamous cell carcinoma. Computerized tomography is useful in delineating the extent of bone destruction in carcinoma of the ear. Early attempts at treatment of cancer of the temporal bone consisted of radical mastoidectomy, followed by radiotherapy, and resulted in a 5-year cure rate of less than 25 per cent. Recent development of temporal bone resection techniques has increased the 5-year cure rate to 44 per cent.

AURICLE TRAUMA

Auricle trauma can be categorized as lacerations, hematoma, burns, and frostbite. Lacerations can range from simple lacerations to complete avulsions and are often associated with multiple trauma. The ear should be carefully cleaned of all foreign debris. Cartilage should not be sutured except to re-form the contour of the ear. Perichondrium should be closed using fine absorbable suture. The skin should be approximated using interrupted 6–0 monofilament nylon, and a sterile mastoid dressing should be applied. An avulsed auricle should be repaired in the operating room. The auricle can be preserved in sterile iced saline.

Hematomas are usually secondary to blunt trauma that produces a collection of blood between the perichondrium and the cartilage and presents as a smooth blue mass. Prompt drainage is required to prevent aseptic necrosis of the underlying cartilage. If hematomas or seromas are seen early before clot formation, they may be aspirated with an 18-gauge needle and a pressure dressing applied. If they recur or cannot be aspirated, they should be opened, drained, and compressed. The dressing rolls should be left undisturbed for 1 week and the patient placed on an antistaphylococcal antibiotic.

Emergency management of the burned auricle involves gentle local cleansing, topical antibiotic application, and the avoidance of any pressure on the ear. Late complications include perichondritis and chondritis, which require intravenous antibiotics and drainage if fluctuance develops.

Frostbite of the auricle occurs particularly when the temperature falls below 10° C (34° F), which blocks the sensory nerve input, depriving the patient of the warning of impending danger. The ear becomes white and shiny with bulla formation. Rapid rewarming is necessary with compresses at a temperature of 38° to 42° C (100.4° to 107.6° F). The ear is then treated like a burn by applying antibiotic cream to any breaks in the skin and avoiding any pressure. No debridement should be performed until lack of viability is determined with certainty.

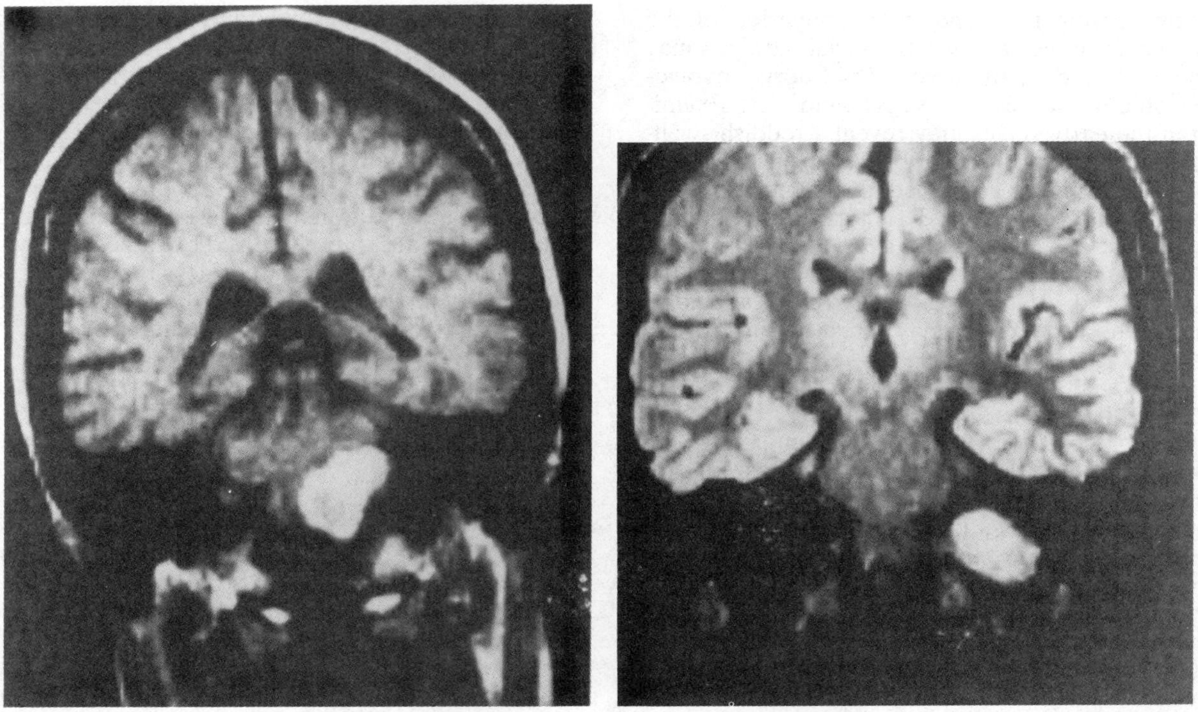

Figure 33–9. Schwannomas of the jugular foramen demonstrated by magnetic resonance imaging. *A,* Hemorrhagic schwannoma of left CN XI is seen as a high intensity mass in the region of the jugular foramen. *B,* High intensity mass within jugular foramen represents a schwannoma of CN XII. Both views are in coronal projection, with imaging performed on 0.35 Tesla Diasonics unit. (From Cummings, C. W., Fredrickson, J. M., Harker, L. A., et al. [Eds.]: Otolaryngology—Head and Neck Surgery. Vol. 4. St. Louis, MO, C. V. Mosby Company, 1986, p. 2858.)

BAROTRAUMA

Barotrauma results from a change in atmospheric pressure while the eustachian tube is occluded. Barotrauma is increasing in frequency because of increased air travel and scuba diving.

The eustachian tube functions as a one-way valve. Air can leave the middle ear passively, but an active process is required for air to enter the middle ear. Airplane ascent produces a decrease in pressure, leading to an increased volume of air. Descent leads to an increase in ambient pressure, which collapses the cartilaginous portion of the eustachian tube.

Factors that favor the development of barotitis include swelling of the nasopharyngeal end of the eustachian tube secondary to an upper respiratory infection or allergy, ignorance of the need to equalize pressure, rapid rate of descent, and sleeping during descent.

With moderate barotrauma, there is vascular engorgement and mild hemorrhage in the tympanic membrane. With more severe barotrauma, hemotympanum or perforation of the tympanic membrane may result. Symptoms vary with the severity of the barotrauma, and may include severe pain, decreased hearing, fullness, low-pitched tinnitus and, occasionally, vertigo.

The condition may be treated by performing a Valsalva maneuver when a sensation of fullness is first noted. Topical and systemic decongestants may be helpful. For hemotympanum, a myringotomy is performed only if the individual is a pilot and must immediately return to flying. Perforations are repaired only if they have not healed within 3 months.

Recurrent barotitis should be treated by eliminating any underlying pathology in the nose or sinuses, such as severe septal deviation, hypertrophic lymphoid tissue, allergic rhinitis, and chronic sinusitis. Insertion of ventilation tubes may be necessary for barotitis secondary to flying.

HEARING LOSS FROM ACOUSTIC ENERGY

Hearing loss from acoustic energy is the most commonly acquired and preventable cause of sensorineural hearing loss. The hearing loss may be secondary to extremely high levels of acoustic energy, e.g., an explosion or chronic noise exposure in excess of 80 dB. At least 10 million people in industry suffer from noise-induced hearing loss. Noise may be recreational, military, environmental, or social in origin and may produce either temporary or permanent hearing loss. Temporary threshold shifts last less than 16 hours and have their greatest effect at 4000 Hz. With continued exposure, the audiogram at 4000 Hz becomes deeper and wider until high-frequency perception is completely lost, then low frequencies are increasingly affected. A 16-hour interval is required between the last noise exposure and the measurement of hearing. For compensation purposes, at least 1 month should lapse between last exposure and final assessment. There is no age or sex difference in susceptibility to noise-induced hearing loss. When noise is combined with ototoxic drugs, there is more organic damage than either would produce alone. There is no evidence that a person with pre-existing sensorineural hearing loss is more susceptible to noise-induced hearing loss. There is a large amount of individual variation in susceptibility to noise-induced hearing loss.

Other factors that must be considered before attributing a sensorineural hearing loss to noise include presbycusis, ototoxic chemicals and drugs, familial hearing loss, trauma, and chronic otitis media.

There is no treatment that reverses a *permanent* threshold shift. Hearing aid amplification and lipreading are of benefit. Prevention is the key to reducing the incidence of noise-induced hearing loss. Reduction of the source of the noise would be best but is also the most difficult to achieve. The best ear protection is a combination of earplugs and fluid-sealed muffs. Cotton is not effective as an earplug. A hearing conservation program should be instituted if difficulty in hearing occurs while in a noisy environment, if tinnitus develops after working in noise, or if there is a temporary loss of hearing perceived by the worker.

TEMPORAL BONE FRACTURES AND LABYRINTHINE CONCUSSION

Temporal bone fractures are described as being either *longitudinal, transverse,* or *mixed.* Longitudinal fractures constitute 80 per cent of temporal bone fractures and result from direct lateral blunt trauma to the skull in the parietal region of the head. The fracture extends from the squamous portion of the temporal bone, along the roof of the external auditory canal. These fractures often disrupt the tympanic membrane, resulting in bleeding from the ear. There may be conductive hearing loss secondary to disruption of the ossicles of the middle ear. Spinal fluid leaks are rare in longitudinal fractures. Vestibular and cochlear function are usually preserved, although mild high-frequency sensorineural hearing loss is sometimes seen secondary to the concussive effect. Facial paralysis is rare and, if present, is often delayed in onset, since it is secondary to trauma and edema instead of interruption of the nerve.

Transverse fractures account for approximately 20 per cent of temporal bone fractures and are usually caused by a severe blow to the occipital portion of the skull. They occur in severely injured patients and result in profound sensorineural hearing loss and total loss of vestibular function. Facial paralysis may be present in up to 50 per cent of the cases and is usually caused by interruption of the facial nerve. Transverse fractures result in a hemotympanum rather than exterior bleeding. Cerebral spinal fluid leaks are frequently seen in transverse fractures and are detected when clear fluid drains from the eustachian tube into the nasopharynx. Labyrinthine concussion is secondary to head injury. The patient complains of mild unsteadiness or lightheadedness, particularly with change of head position. Audiometric testing reveals a high-frequency hearing loss. The electronystagmogram may show spontaneous or positional nystagmus. Occasionally, the caloric response is hypoactive.

SUDDEN SENSORINEURAL HEARING LOSS

One definition of sudden sensorineural hearing loss is a loss that is greater than 30 dB. in three contiguous frequencies that occurs in less than 3 days. In the majority of patients, the hearing loss occurs suddenly and the cause is not clinically apparent. Approximately half of the patients have some associated imbalance or vertigo. The reported incidence of 1:10,000 persons per year is probably lower than the true incidence, since many people recover before seeking medical attention. The prognosis for recovery is poor in those patients with vertigo or profound hearing loss, or in those who are older than 40 years of age.

The most common cause of idiopathic sensorineural hearing loss is viral cochleitis. Multiple viruses including mumps, influenza B, rubeola, and cytomegalo virus have been found to be responsible for idiopathic sensorineural hearing loss. Partial or complete occlusion of the cochlear vasculature that may occur in Waldenström's macroglobulinemia, polycythemia vera, or sickle cell anemia, or following cardiopulmonary bypass surgery can result in sudden hearing loss. Cochlear membrane breaks are also potential causes of sudden hearing loss. Round or oval window fistulas may occur following abrupt compression or decompression of the ears, head injuries, heavy lifting, and straining. Physical findings include fluctuating hearing and/or tinnitus, which may improve overnight and worsen during the day.

The initial work-up should include a history, otologic and neurologic examinations, audiologic testing, and laboratory studies. See Table 33–2 for a list of suggested tests. If hearing loss does not return in 1 month or is progressive, then computerized tomography with contrast or magnetic resonance imaging is obtained.

Patients with moderate hearing loss of presumed viral etiology who have no vestibular symptoms may respond to steroid therapy. Carbogen (5 per cent CO_2 and 95 per cent O_2) has been found to improve perilymphatic oxygen levels. There is evidence to suggest that this treatment may help improve hearing in the speech frequencies.

Finally, patients who have a definite history of antecedent barotrauma should have an immediate exploration of the middle ear to repair a fistula. Patients with an uncertain diagnosis of a fistula should be placed on bed rest with the head elevated.

Table 33–2. ASSESSMENT OF PATIENTS WITH SUDDEN HEARING LOSS

Initial Assessment (Within 2 Weeks of Hearing Loss)
History and otoneurologic examination
Laboratory data
Complete blood count (CBC)
Complete erythrocyte sedimentation rate (CESR)
Glucose
Glucose tolerance test (TT) or Hb A_{1c} (optional)
Fluorescent treponemal antibody-absorption test
Cholesterol level
Triglyceride level
Acute and convalescent sera for viral antibody titers (optional)
Audiologic evaluation
Air and bone conduction
Speech audiometry
Alternate binaural loudness balance
Auditory brainstem response
Upright and recumbent audiograms (for suspected fistulas only)
Hallpike's caloric test with electronystagmography; positional tests, fistula test, or ENG with impedance testing (for suspected fistulas only)
Further Evaluation if Hearing Loss Does Not Return in 1 Month, or if Hearing Loss Progresses
Radiographic views of internal auditory meatus
Computerized tomography scan, with contrast

PRESBYCUSIS

Presbycusis is defined as the effect of aging on the auditory system, characteristically resulting in a bilateral symmetrical neurosensory hearing loss in the frequencies above 2000 Hz., although other patterns occur. At first, conversation is not impaired because the frequencies involved are typically above those of speech, which is 500 to 2000 Hz. As the upper frequencies become involved, the patient typically complains of the inability to understand speech. This lack of understanding is the result of a decreased ability to discriminate consonants, particularly those spoken by women and children. When speech discrimination begins to fail, then conversation becomes more and more difficult, particularly in a group setting. The ability to ignore competing speech also becomes impaired and maintaining communication becomes increasingly more and more difficult, which often results in isolation of the individual. Approximately *one third* of the population over age 65 has a significant hearing impairment. It is difficult to ascertain what portion of hearing impairment is caused by aging of the auditory system and what portion is caused by other traumatic or metabolic factors. Efforts have been made to identify histologic and audiologic correlates. Schuknecht has divided presbycusis into four types: sensory presbycusis, neural presbycusis, strial presbycusis, and cochlear presbycusis. Whatever type of presbycusis is present, the individual can be helped with a properly fitted hearing aid. There are also many less expensive *assistive listening devices* available on the market that may be helpful in certain listening situations. There is current research involving an implantable hearing device which would drive the ossicular chain by electromagnetic means. This may become available in the near future to improve sensorineural hearing loss from many causes.

FACIAL NERVE PARALYSIS

Though trauma or surgery can result in facial nerve paralysis, the cause is usually never determined and the condition is referred to as Bell's palsy. Current theories favor a viral etiology (Olsen, 1984). It is relatively common, affecting about one in 60 or 70 persons. Paralysis occurs abruptly and is complete within 48 hours of onset. About 80 per cent of patients recover complete function within a few weeks or months, but recurrences are seen in about 10 per cent.

Examination reveals partial or complete paralysis in all branches of the seventh nerve. A complete neurologic examination should be performed. Electroneurography performed within the first 2 weeks may help determine the prognosis. Evidence of denervation on electroneurography indicates that a much longer recovery period is expected. Treatment should include protecting and splinting of the eye, massaging facial muscles, and administering corticosteroids.

Corticosteroids (e.g., prednisone, 60 to 80 mg. daily), given during the first 5 days and tapered over the next 5 days, may help to shorten and lessen the paralysis. If the patient does not seek treatment before 48 hours, the use of prednisone is probably not worthwhile. If complete facial paralysis lasts longer than 2 weeks, electroneurography provides some degree of prognostic information. Surgical decompression of the facial nerve has been performed in patients with severe denervation, but results are inconsistent and controversial.

The Nose and Sinuses

CHOANAL ATRESIA

Choanal atresia is a unilateral or bilateral obstruction of the posterior choanae (opening from the posterior of the nose to nasopharynx). The condition occurs in 1 per 5000 to 8000 births, and the obstructing tissue may be membranous only (10 per cent) but is usually osseous (90 per cent). It usually occurs in females and is usually unilateral. During prenatal development, the nasal cavities form as the nasal placodes invaginate posteriorly until they encounter the nasobuccal membrane, which usually attenuates and ruptures around the 6th week of gestation. Theories as to the cause of choanal atresia include persistence of the buccopharyngeal membrane, persistence of the nasobuccal membrane, and misdirection of mesodermal elements in the choanal region.

Neonates are obligate nasal breathers, and acute respiratory distress, which may be life threatening, usually occurs with bilateral atresia. Adaptation to oral breathing may take several weeks. Unilateral atresia can be overlooked until it is diagnosed later in life on the basis of persistent unilateral nasal discharge. There are often associated anomalies, including the CHARGE syndrome (coloboma, cardiac [heart], choanal atresia, retarded growth, genital, and ear).

Diagnosis requires a high index of suspicion. A wisp of cotton or a cold mirror will demonstrate lack of air flow through the nose. A No. 6 French catheter does not pass 3 to 4 cm. from the nostril, and radiopaque dye reveals the nature of the obstruction. Treatment usually requires emergency airway management, and a small oral airway is effective for a short time. As soon as the infant can safely tolerate general anesthesia, a transnasal, transseptal, or transpalatal approach is employed by the surgeon to open the choanal region.

ALLERGIC RHINITIS

Allergic rhinitis is commonly encountered in family practice and usually begins in patients younger than 20 years of age (Busse, 1983). It may occur seasonally from pollen allergies, or perennially from allergy to house dust, animal dander, or food. Patients usually present with itching of the nose and eyes, sneezing, nasal obstruction, watery nasal discharge, and increased lacrimation.

Examination reveals narrowing of the nasal airway with a pale, purplish hue to the mucosa and a clear, watery discharge. Nasal polyps may also be noted. Diagnosis is usually evident from a careful history of the relationship of symptoms to allergen exposure. A nasal smear for eosinophils may help in differentiating this condition from nonallergic nasal problems. Other helpful diagnostic procedures may include skin tests and radioallergosorbent tests.

Treatment requires a multifactorial approach, including elimination of exposure, desensitization therapy, antihistamines, and nasal instillation of corticosteroids. Recently a nasal preparation of cromolyn has become available that may help to prevent symptoms when used prior to exposure. In severe cases and for episodes that are limited to short periods during the year, a short course of systemic corticosteroids may be very helpful. Topical steroid sprays such as beclomethasone and flunisolide are also helpful for patients whose symptoms have not responded to antihistamines. Concomitant bacterial infection, especially sinusitis, is common.

NASAL POLYPOSIS

Nasal obstruction, partial or complete, may be caused by *nasal polyps*. These polyps are soft, smooth, translucent, lobulated tissue masses that arise from nasal or sinus mucosa. They consist of edematous mucosa and submucosa and may be unilateral or bilateral, single or multiple. They are the most commonly seen intranasal masses, occurring with equal frequency in both sexes and at any age.

Nasal polyps usually occur in association with other specific clinical entities such as allergic disorders, cystic fibrosis, aspirin-induced asthma, chronic sinus infection, and the recently described syndrome of recurrent respiratory disease, azoospermia, and nasal polyposis. There is a particularly high correlation between polyps and allergic rhinitis, with about half of these patients developing significant nasal polyposis. Also, over half of the patients with aspirin intolerance and asthma are noted to have nasal polyposis.

Diagnosis is made on the basis of the history and physical examination. Polyps differ from most other nasal masses because of their pale, wet appearance and because they are mobile, insensitive to pain, and do not bleed. Sinus roentgenograms are indicated to assess the degree of associated sinus disease so that an effective management plan can be undertaken. A sweat test should be performed in any child with polyposis in order to rule out cystic fibrosis. The differential diagnosis includes encephalocele, inverting papilloma, carcinoma, olfactory neuroblastoma, and angiofibroma.

The first approach in therapy should be medical, using antibiotics, antihistamines, steroids, and allergic hyposensitization, as appropriate. Surgical management is used secondarily and may include polypectomy, ethmoidectomy, and possibly other surgical techniques for the sinuses.

VASOMOTOR RHINITIS

Vasomotor rhinitis is a misnomer since it is not a type of inflammation. It is due to dilation of the nasal vessels and consequent nasal discharge. The condition appears to be more common in patients who are suffering from chronic anxiety states. Many of these patients may simply be intolerant of the normal production of nasal mucus (500 to 700 ml. per day). The condition occurs more commonly in adolescents and young adults and is more common in women. Patients primarily complain of nasal obstruction and clear nasal discharge. Examination often reveals mild swelling of the nasal mucosa. Systemic decongestants and antihistamines are the primary treatment for this condition. Patients must be educated about the deleterious effects of long-term use of topical decongestants. Patients who present with chronic, intractable symptoms may be considered candidates for submucous resection or cryosurgery of the nasal turbinates.

RHINITIS MEDICAMENTOSA

Rhinitis medicamentosa is not an inflammatory condition but a chronic, reactive vasodilation due to excessive use of topical nasal vasoconstrictors. After several days' use of topical vasoconstrictors, a rebound phenomenon occurs that consists of rhinorrhea, edema, and loss of ciliary function. A vicious circle develops that leads to increasingly frequent use of the offending medication. Patients soon come to feel addicted to the use of the nasal drops or sprays and typically have a great deal of trouble discontinuing their use. The patient's only recourse is to suffer nasal obstruction for about 2 to 3 weeks, after which time the normal tone returns to the nasal vasculature. Systemic decongestants, nasal instillation of normal saline, and aerosolized nasal corticosteroids may help to relieve symptoms during this period of withdrawal from the medication.

VIRAL RHINITIS

Colds are the most common type of infection in humans, occurring at least once or twice a year in adults and five to eight times per year in children. Although they are little more than a nuisance in the adult, they are often accompanied by sinusitis and middle ear infections in children. The main causative factor is one of many strains of rhinovirus. Other agents may cause a similar condition and include *Mycoplasma, Neisseria, Haemophilus influenzae*, and *Staphylococcus aureus*. Peak occurrences of viral rhinitis occur in September, January, and April.

A low-grade fever is rapidly followed by irritability, sneezing, and nasal discharge. Nasal secretions become progressively thicker, often purulent. Myalgias, headache, and a nonproductive cough are also common.

Treatment recommendations include acetaminophen, fluids, rest, and decongestants. Aspirin should not be given to children because of the increased risk of Reye's syndrome in cases of influenza or varicella infections. Instillation of nasal decongestants is useful for infants who have trouble breathing and eating from nasal obstruction. Saline or 0.125 to 0.25 per cent phenylephrine may be used. Symptoms rarely last for more than a week.

ACUTE SINUSITIS

Acute sinusitis may involve any or all of the paranasal sinuses, which include the frontal, maxillary, sphenoid, and ethmoids. Acute sinusitis, in contrast to subacute and chronic infections, is defined as lasting from 1 day to 3 weeks. It most commonly follows nasal obstruction from viral rhinitis. Mucosal swelling causes blockage of the ostia, resulting in obstruction and subsequent progression of the infection. Other predisposing causes include allergic rhinitis, deviated nasal septum, foreign body, and frequent swimming. Systemic predisposing factors include diabetes, malnutrition, and blood dyscrasias (Kern, 1988). The most common organisms found are streptococci, pneumococci, *H. influenzae*, and staphylococci. Sinusitis may occasionally be caused by gram-negative and anaerobic organisms, fungi, and mycobacteria.

The early symptoms of sinusitis are those of viral rhinitis, followed by a feeling of fullness over one side of the face or a dull, localized headache. Frontal involvement is often associated with a generalized headache and may progress rapidly. Maxillary sinusitis often causes radiation of pain to the teeth. Ethmoid sinusitis results in pain over the bridge of the nose and behind the eye. Sphenoid involvement also causes retro-orbital pain and may cause an occipital headache. On examination, patients may also have evidence of periostitis, leading to swelling and erythema over the involved sinus. The nasal mucosa is often erythematous and edematous, and purulent nasal drainage is often present. Tenderness to palpation may be present over the frontal or maxillary sinus.

Sinus x-ray studies are helpful in confirming questionable cases and may show mucosal thickening or air-fluid levels. If symptoms are limited to the maxillary sinus, a simple Waters view will usually suffice. Cultures may be taken from the posterior nasopharynx, but their usefulness is debated.

Treatment is directed at the infection itself and toward relieving congestion of the nasal mucosa to allow drainage of the involved sinus. Either ampicillin or erythromycin is effective against the majority of organisms causing sinusitis (Table 33–3). Treatment should be continued for a minimum of 10 days and, for recalcitrant cases, may need to be continued for as long as 21 days. A topical nasal decongestant spray should be used three times a day for a maximum of 5 days. Systemic decongestants may also be used.

Ethmoid Sinusitis

The ethmoid sinus complex is the primary key to the health of the nose and the other pairs of sinuses. Ethmoid sinus development begins with the

Table 33–3. CAUSATIVE ORGANISMS IN ACUTE SINUSITIS

Agent	Incidence (Per Cent of Cases)
Bacteria	30
Streptococcus pneumoniae	30
Haemophilus influenzae	20
Anaerobic bacteria	10
Staphylococcus aureus	4
Streptococcus pyogenes	2
Branhamella catarrhalis	2
Aerobic gram-negative bacteria	9
Viruses	
Rhinovirus	15
Influenza	5
Parainfluenza	3
Adenovirus	< 1

Adapted from Kern, E. B.: Suppurative (bacterial) sinusitis. Postgrad. Med., *81*(4):194–210, 1988.

appearance of small slits along the lateral wall of the nose during the 5th month of fetal development. At birth, the maxillary and ethmoid sinuses are the only sinus cavities, and during childhood these two groups are responsible for most of the complications of sinusitis occurring in children. Each ethmoid sinus complex consists of 4 to 17 cells, with the anterior group draining into the recess just beneath the middle turbinate and the posterior group beneath the superior turbinate.

Clinical manifestations of *ethmoid sinusitis* include upper facial pain, discharge, visual dysfunction, headaches, fever, and chronic cough. Because only a thin bony wall separates the ethmoid complex from the eye and the brain, complications of ethmoiditis may threaten both of these regions.

In addition to the history and physical examination, radiographic studies are essential for adequate assessment of the ethmoid sinuses. The computerized tomography scan has become the gold standard for precise evaluation.

Medical management includes antibiotics, antihistamines, decongestants, topical steroids, and allergic hyposensitization as appropriate for each individual patient. The goal is to relieve sinus obstruction and re-establish drainage and aeration of these cells. Usually, this can be accomplished with medical management, but when this fails, surgical intervention is indicated to avoid complications.

Chronic Nasal and Sinus Infection

Chronic or recurrent infection involving the nose and paranasal sinuses (Fig. 33–10) is a common and often frustrating challenge for primary physicians and otolaryngologists. Most instances of *chronic rhinosinusitis* are the result of pathologic conditions in the nasal airway, and many patients with these conditions cannot be controlled by medical management alone. With time, chronic infection results in disruption of normal airflow patterns (obstructed nasal breathing) and nasal ciliary clearance of mucus (anterior and posterior nasal discharge). When this occurs, more serious and even life-threatening complications become likely.

In some patients, the predisposing causes of the chronic condition are correctable. These include such factors as environmental smoke, dust, fumes, and pollen—all of which must be assessed and limited or controlled. Trauma to the nose or abnormal growth/development may result in internal deformity of the nasal septum, a problem that is reviewed later.

Endoscopic nasal and sinus diagnosis and surgery provide an important advance in this field. The ability to precisely identify the source and nature of the pathology is now linked with new techniques that permit removal of abnormal tissue and preservation of areas that can regain their normal function. Procedures are now performed on an outpatient basis that are safer and more effective than prior operations that required several days of hospitalization.

Acute and Chronic Frontal Sinusitis

The frontal sinus begins to develop between the 1st and 2nd years after birth and reaches its full size by about age 20. This sinus drains into the middle meatus under the middle turbinate.

Acute frontal sinusitis may develop secondary to various conditions that interfere with adequate sinus aeration and drainage. Typical predisposing problems are allergic rhinitis, polyps, septal deviation, tumors, or nasal infection. Common symptoms are headaches that are worse in the morning, mucopurulent discharge, and fever. Examination often reveals edema and tenderness over the sinus. Radiographic studies may show an air-fluid level or complete opacification of the sinuses. Complications include osteomyelitis, Pott's puffy tumor of the forehead, orbital cellulitis, and intracranial infection.

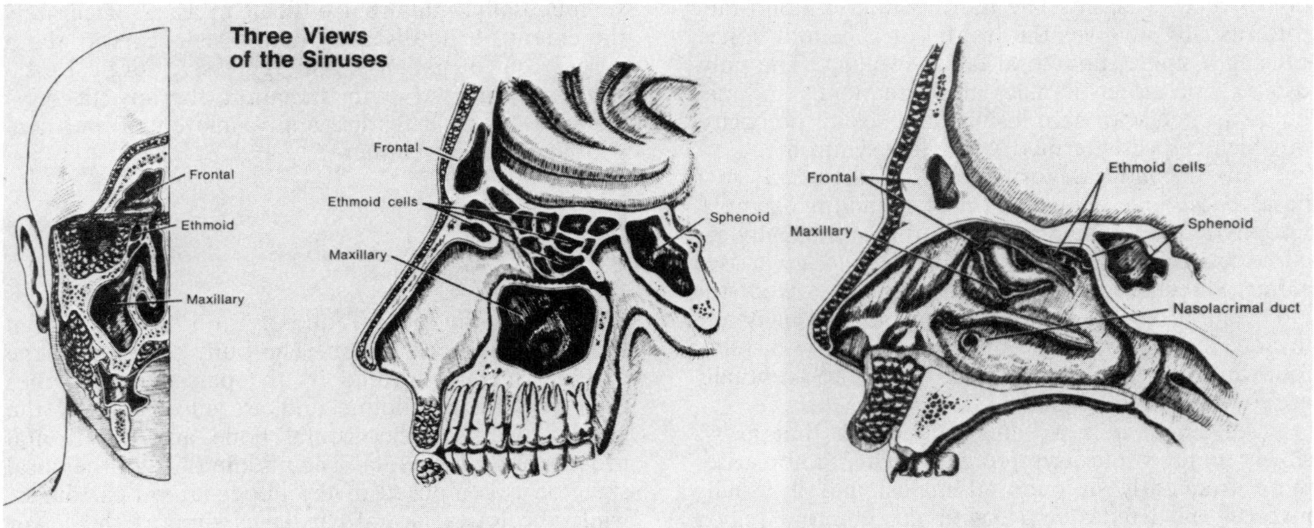

Figure 33–10. Three views of the paranasal sinuses.

Treatment of acute frontal sinusitis is directed at re-establishing sinus drainage using topical and systemic decongestants along with antibiotic therapy. Heat, humidified air, and rest are often helpful adjunctive measures. When medical management fails, the frontal sinus may require a drainage procedure (trephination).

Chronic frontal sinusitis may result from inadequately treated acute frontal sinusitis and is a surgical problem. The common symptoms are nasal discharge and frontal headaches. Roentgenograms show thickened mucosa or bony sclerosis, or both. The surgical procedure used is osteoplastic fat obliteration.

NASAL TUMORS

Tumors of the nasal passage and sinuses, other than polyps, are uncommon but of considerable importance because of their location and their tendency to impair nasal function. They usually become symptomatic by causing obstruction, pressure, or bleeding. Radiographic studies are useful in determining tumor extension to adjacent sites, and a biopsy is required to define the precise nature of the growth.

The first category of nasal masses is *tumor-like lesions* of the nose and paranasal sinuses. *Giant cell reparative granuloma* is felt to be an aberrant form of the local reparative reaction in response to an inflammatory process. This lesion may occur in any of the sinuses, but it is most commonly found in the maxillary or ethmoid region and is seen more frequently in young patients.

Ossifying fibroma is a cellular fibroma that produces calcified intercellular material. Seen most often in children as a painless cheek mass, it can expand and obliterate the maxillary sinus. Excision usually results in cure. A similar disorder, *fibrous dysplasia*, differs in that it arises from the proliferation of fibro-osseous tissue inside the affected facial bones and is not a true neoplasm. The more common monostatic form usually involves the frontal or sphenoid bones, causing a single, unilateral facial swelling. The polyostatic form affects females more frequently and may be associated with skin lesions and sexual precocity, in which case it is termed Albright's syndrome.

The second category is *benign neoplasm*, with nasal *papilloma* being the most common example. Exophytic papillomata are very firm and usually are cured by simple excision. *Inverting papilloma* is a softer, verrucous lesion that usually arises from the lateral nasal wall. These neoplasms grow slowly and invade the underlying bone. They tend to recur following excision, and 4 to 15 per cent eventually are found to be malignant.

An *osteoma* is a benign neoplasm that grows slowly and is often asymptomatic. This tumor arises more frequently in pubertal males, and it usually involves the frontal sinus, with the ethmoid region being the next most common site. Surgical excision is necessary if the osteoma grows sufficiently large to obstruct the sinus ostium.

Malignant neoplasms are the third category, and these are relatively rare, accounting for about 3 per cent of all upper aerodigestive tract cancers. Known etiologic factors are nickel, wood dust, and Thorotrast. Most patients are over the age of 50, most of these tumors arise in the maxillary sinus, and over half of the tumors are advanced (T_3 or T_4) when the diagnosis is made. *Squamous cell carcinoma* is the most common histologic type, and combined surgery and radiation therapy are employed in managing patients with these lesions. Cure rates of about 30 per cent are reported.

Adenocarcinoma is found predominately in the ethmoid sinuses. The patients are slightly younger, the tumors are somewhat more slow growing, and the prognosis is slightly better than for squamous cell carcinoma.

Lymphoma may arise in extranodal form in the nose or paranasal sinuses. Subclasses of nasal lymphoma include reticulosarcoma, lymphosarcoma, and plasmacytoma. Most of these tumors arise in the maxillary antrum, and they occur in patients at a younger age than most carcinomas. Unlike lymphoma elsewhere in the body, dissemination of sinus tumors is not common, and the prognosis is better than for other lymphomas and carcinomas.

Melanoma is rare and is found in older patients, with a mean age of about 75. These tumors tend to arise high in the nasal cavity and tend to invade the ethmoid sinuses. In contrast to skin melanoma, these malignancies do not appear to arise in pre-existing lesions and many of them may remain localized for a prolonged period. However, they carry a very poor prognosis, with a 5-year survival rate of about 5 per cent.

Esthesioneuroblastoma is a rare tumor arising in the roof of the nose. It usually occurs in young adults, and the common symptoms are nasal obstruction and loss of sense of smell. These tumors tend to spread submucosally, making it difficult to assess accurately the extent of the disease. Metastasis occurs in about 20 per cent of patients, and aggressive surgical excision is combined with radiation therapy in most instances. Cure rates are approximately 50 per cent with aggressive treatment.

NASAL TRAUMA

The nose is the most frequently injured structure in the head and neck region. The bony skeleton of the external nose is formed by the paired nasal bones that join in the midline and are supported by the nasal process of the frontal bone and the frontal process of each maxilla. The middle third of the nasal skeleton is composed of the upper lateral cartilages, while the lower lateral cartilages support the lower third. Internal nasal structures of importance are the

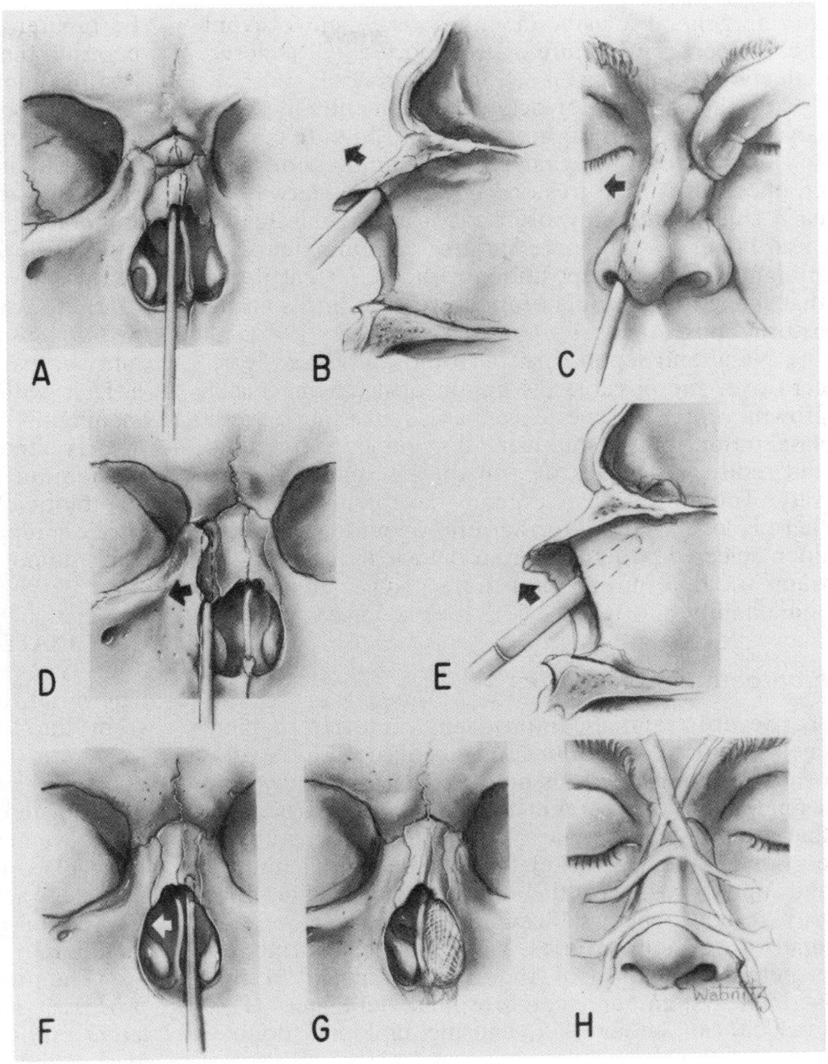

Figure 33–11. *A*, Elevator inserted into right nares. *B*, Narrow edge is placed high in nasal pyramid. *C*, With counterpressure on the laterally displaced left nasal bone, the elevator is moved outward, forward, and laterally. *D*, The elevator is inserted into the right nares. *E*, The elevator is thrust outward and laterally. *F*, Reduction of the nasal septum with medial pressure. *G*, Nasal packing with 1/2-inch gauze strip. *H*, Aluminum, foam rubber–covered splint or dental molding compound is used for severe comminution. (From Lore, J. M., Jr. [Ed.]: An Atlas of Head and Neck Surgery. Vol. I. Philadelphia, W. B. Saunders Company, 1973, p. 415.)

quadrangular cartilage and the bony vomer upon which it rests.

In adults, the nasal bones remain attached to each other when fractured, whereas they frequently separate in children. Therefore, unilateral depressed *nasal bone fractures* are much less common in adults than in children. Inside the nose, displacement of the quadrangular cartilage from the vomer or angulation of the quadrangular cartilage is a common occurrence in response to a strong anterior blow. Hematoma formation is common at these various fracture sites, making these areas susceptible to infection after a few days. In most cases, fibroblasts are activated but are quickly replaced by osteoblasts, which begin to lay down callus, leading to overall thickening of the bone and rapid healing that is quite advanced within 10 days.

Diagnosis of fracture is made on the basis of a visually apparent deformity or the palpation of loose or displaced fragments. Prior studies have shown that less than half of these patients have had an intranasal examination, an essential component of a thorough work-up and an important step in planning the proper treatment. Radiographic studies usually are not helpful and may be confusing.

In the absence of a significant septal fracture, reduction of displaced nasal bones can be accomplished using regional anesthesia (Bailey, 1982). Reduction is best performed between 3 and 7 days after injury. Intranasal packing is required for 7 to 10 days and an external splint is useful to maintain the reduction (Fig. 33–11).

If there is a concomitant *fracture of the nasal septum* with the external pyramid, alignment of the septum must be accomplished and maintained to prevent a later shift of the external nose by the internal structures. In the case of an isolated fracture-dislocation of the quadrangular cartilage, reduction is necessary to prevent the late complication of nasal airway obstruction. Open reduction, sometimes requiring general anesthesia, may be needed to avoid the 40 per cent failure rate reported with closed reduction techniques.

In the instance of delayed treatment for septal deviation, the goals of surgery are two-fold: to correct any dorsal deviation that gives the impression of a crooked nose and to restore a patent nasal airway on each side. Osteotomy or refracturing of misaligned nasal bones may be necessary, often combined with straightening and repositioning the nasal cartilages that shape the contours of the lower two thirds of the external nose.

Nasal and septal surgery in the child raises concern over the possible disruption of nasal and facial growth centers. Experience has shown that severe nasal trauma may displace and disrupt nasal structures and redirect the lines of growth, resulting in deformity. Therefore, most surgeons have concluded that there is less potential for harm in operating carefully upon selected patients than in delaying correction of traumatic deformities until these young patients become adults.

Frontoethmoid Fractures

Severe traumatic injury may result from high energy impact at the junction of the nose and forehead. Anatomically, this nasal complex region is not a single unit but a combination of adjacent structures that are relatively fragile. When fractured, the upper portion of the nasal skeleton can be driven inward and superiorly toward the anterior cranial fossa. This may result in heavy bleeding from tearing of the anterior ethmoid arteries, disruption of the medial palpebral ligaments of the eyelids, injury to the lacrimal system, and cerebrospinal fluid leak. The trochlea can be avulsed, causing diplopia (double vision).

On clinical examination, the cardinal sign of this injury is a broad, flat, depressed, and unstable nasal dorsum. There is usually a laceration over the nasal bridge and considerable edema of the adjacent soft tissue. There may be epistaxis and nasal obstruction as well.

Ophthalmologic assessment is a mandatory step for any patient with an injury in this area, to detect any associated eye injuries. Radiographic studies are necessary to define the exact status of the facial bones and skull base.

Definitive repair of *ethmoid complex fractures* is accomplished quickly, before fragments become fixed and healed in a poor position. Open reduction techniques with wiring of fractures and repair of the palpebral ligaments and reconstruction of the other soft tissue elements is required to prevent serious late complications.

Traumatic CSF Leak

Cerebrospinal fluid otorrhea occurs in about 6 per cent of cases involving basilar skull surgery. Fortunately, 90 per cent of these leaks close spontaneously, but persistent cerebrospinal fluid otorrhea is not uncommon following longitudinal fractures of the temporal bone. The diagnosis is made on the basis of chemical testing of the fluid, which reveals a glucose content that is two thirds of the blood glucose level. The most accurate test involves identifying two electrophoretic bands of transferrin.

Cerebrospinal fluid rhinorrhea may follow closed head injury or midfacial fractures. About 80 per cent of these cerebrospinal fluid leaks will be evident within 48 hours. A high index of suspicion is important because 20 per cent of the patients found to have a leak within 1 week of the injury will develop meningitis.

Treatment of cerebrospinal fluid leak is usually carried out by otolaryngologists and neurosurgeons. Antibiotic coverage is usually employed initially, and surgical repair is indicated for those patients whose leaks do not cease spontaneously in a timely manner.

TURBINATE DYSFUNCTION

The nasal turbinates are three shelf-like projections from the lateral wall of the nose. Their mucous membrane covering is lined with pseudostratified, columnar ciliated epithelium. The turbinates warm and moisten the inspired air, and they participate in the movement of the blanket of mucus that acts as a filter by catching and holding 95 per cent of the particles in the inspired air. By this function, they play a vital role in the body's overall defense against infection.

The turbinates become involved in many disease processes such as *acute rhinitis* (common cold), *allergic rhinitis, vasomotor rhinitis* (autonomic imbalance), and *rhinitis medicamentosa* (abuse of nose drops).

Chronic hypertrophic rhinitis is the end stage of the above types of rhinitis, and it is characterized by enlarged, meaty, obstructive turbinates. The diagnosis is confirmed by spraying the nose with a topical sympathomimetic solution (ephedrine) and observing the lack of a decongesting effect. Surgical management is the only effective treatment for this problem.

Oral Cavity and Pharynx

ACUTE PHARYNGITIS AND TONSILLITIS

Acute pharyngitis is one of the most common reasons patients visit the family physician. The two most common causes are viral and streptococcal. Recently the role of other agents such as *Chlamydia* and *Mycoplasma* has been debated. McMillan and colleagues (1986) reported that 40 per cent of 320 patients with sore throat had positive strep cultures compared with 11.9 per cent of controls. Sixteen per cent had positive viral cultures compared with 2.9 per cent of controls. While 15.8 per cent were positive for *Mycoplasma*, 17.6 per cent of controls also had positive cultures. This study supports the common belief that beta-hemolytic streptococci represent the major cause of significant bacterial pharyngitis (Mandel, 1985).

Patients with streptococcal pharyngitis present with sore throat, fever, and odynophagia. Myalgias, arthralgias, abdominal pain, headache, and vomiting may also occur. When cough and rhinorrhea are present, a viral etiology is much more likely. Physical examination reveals pharyngeal erythema, often with a patchy, purulent tonsillar exudate. Petechiae in the soft palate and tender anterior cervical lymph nodes are often present.

Diagnosis is made by either a throat culture or a latex fixation test for streptococcal antigen (rapid strep test). Recent evidence suggests that this technique is as sensitive and specific as the throat culture and, thus, is likely to replace that procedure in the near future (Fischer, 1986). Rapid identification allows early treatment of streptococcal pharyngitis, which can reduce the duration of symptoms to less than 24 hours (Bass, 1986). DeNeef (1986) notes that use of the rapid test minimizes costs and time away from work. When the rapid test is negative, a culture should generally be performed to clarify the diagnosis, since false-negative rates have been reported to range between 5 and 10 per cent.

Treatment consists of increased fluids, acetaminophen, warm saline gargles, and antibiotics. Penicillin is the drug of choice. If oral medication is preferred, penicillin V 250 Q.I.D. for 10 days should be given to adults and about 50,000 units (15 to 50 mg.) per kg. per day should be given in four divided doses to children. Alternatively, intramuscular benzathine penicillin may be given according to the following guidelines: 600,000 units for children under 6 years of age; 900,000 units for children between 6 and 9 years of age; and 1.2 million units for anyone over 9 years of age. Erythromycin is the drug of choice for patients who are allergic to penicillin.

STOMATITIS AND ORAL MANIFESTATIONS OF SYSTEMIC DISEASE

Many oral problems are localized and are not associated with systemic diseases (e.g., gingivitis, glossitis). In other instances, disease processes involving the rest of the body affect the mouth. It may be difficult to differentiate between these two categories and to decide which consultant to involve.

Infection of the oral cavity may be of bacterial etiology. *Streptococcal gingivostomatitis* is an example and is caused by *Streptococcus viridans* or β-hemolytic streptococcus. It differs from other forms of gingivitis in that it does not result in loss of gingival tissue. *Tuberculosis* may be associated with the oral cavity on rare occasions, with a predilection for the dorsum of the tongue. In other instances, the palate or the gingiva will be primary sites.

Viral stomatitis may take several forms, including *herpes zoster, herpes labialis* (herpes simplex virus), *herpangina* (Coxsackie virus), or a *viral wart.*

Acute necrotizing gingivitis (trench mouth) is a fusospirochetal infection that causes a grayish-yellow pseudomembrane that bleeds easily, fetid breath, fever, and cervical lymphadenopathy. It causes necrosis of the interdental papillae and recession of the gingival margin. *Oral syphilis* is rare, but may be associated with tertiary syphilis as a palatal perforation or a tongue mass.

Mycotic stomatitis is a category that includes acute and chronic conditions. *Acute pseudomembranous candidiasis* (thrush) is caused by *Candida albicans* and is seen most often in infants and debilitated, diabetic, or immunocompromised patients. It may occur as a side effect of the administration of antibiotics, corticosteroids, or cytotoxic drugs. *Chronic hyperplastic candidiasis* is signaled by an isolated white patch resembling oral leukoplakia. Both of these infections respond to antifungal agents such as nystatin or miconazole.

Actinomycosis (lumpy jaw) is a chronic infectious–granulomatous disease usually caused by *Actinomyces israelii* and characterized by tissue invasion and spread, with the formation of multiple sinus tracts. It presents as a bluish swelling of the tongue or gum or as a palpable neck mass. It is quite responsive to treatment with penicillin or ampicillin.

Several categories of systemic diseases may cause lesions in the oral cavity. These categories include endocrine, nutritional, and metabolic system diseases as well as hematopoietic system disorders and nervous system disorders. *Diabetes mellitus* may cause tongue dryness in addition to gingival bleeding hypertrophy and purple discoloration. *Addison's disease* often results in changes of oral mucosal pigmentation (white or very dark-appearing areas). *Acromegaly* is associated with mandibular hyperplasia and marked enlargement of the tongue (macroglossia). *Ascorbic acid deficiency* (scurvy) causes the gingival tissue to become quite swollen and to bleed easily. *Severe protein depletion* (kwashiorkor) results in an acute necrotizing gingivitis, candidiasis, atrophy of the tongue papillae, and cracking of the skin at the angles of the mouth. *Waldenström's macroglobulinemia* may be associated with the mucosal purpura and bleeding gums. *Amyloidosis* is associated with tongue enlargement.

Other systemic diseases causing oral cavity abnormalities are summarized in Table 33–4.

DEEP NECK INFECTIONS

The deep cervical fascia completely envelopes the neck, extending from the nuchal line of the skull and the cervical spine and wrapping around to attach to the hyoid bone and the clavicle (Figs. 33–12 and 33–13). In the preantibiotic era, nearly all of the deep

Table 33–4. DISEASES THAT CAUSE ABNORMALITIES OF THE ORAL CAVITY

Hematopoietic System	
Iron deficiency anemia	Loss of lingual papillae Pale or fiery red tongue
Sideropenic dysphagia (Plummer-Vinson syndrome)	Angular cheilosis Thin vermilia Atrophy of lingual papillae Esophageal webs
Pernicious anemia	Oral cavity paresthesias Taste disturbances Xerostomia (dry mouth) Lobulated tongue, loss of papillae
Thrombocytopenia	Bleeding, ecchymoses, purpura, and petechiae
Malignant neutropenia (may be drug induced)	Infective ulcerations Fever, sore throat, sweating, headache, and prostration
Chronic idiopathic neutropenia	Subacute gingivitis Loosening of teeth Recurrent aphthous ulcers
Nervous System	
Melkersson-Rosenthal syndrome	Unilateral facial paralysis Facial swelling Fissured tongue
Musculoskeletal System	
Dermatomyositis	Gingival edema
Scleroderma	Fibrotic, rigid lips Pale oral mucosa Immobility of tongue
Sjögren's syndrome (sicca syndrome)	Xerostomia Enlarged salivary glands Keratoconjunctivitis
Mikulicz's disease	Enlarged salivary glands
Skin	
Pemphigus vulgaris	Large bullae oral cavity
Erythema multiforme (Stevens-Johnson syndrome)	Stomatitis Skin bullae
Discoid lupus erythematosus	Erythematous lesions, followed by scaling, then atrophic lesions
Psoriasis vulgaris	Geographic tongue
Reticular lichen planus	Delicate white-gray buccal lesions

neck infections originated in the pharynx and tonsils, but now dental, otologic, nasal, and salivary gland origins are quite common. Most deep neck infections are caused by Streptococcus spp., but *Staphylococcus aureus* and anaerobes are also significant pathogens. There are five major distinct types of deep neck infections; pharyngomaxillary, retropharyngeal, submandibular, parotid, and masticator space infections.

Pharyngomaxillary space infections arise in the space bounded by the hyoid bone, the temporal bone, the lateral pharyngeal wall, and the mandible. The most common sources are infections of the pharynx and tonsils. Initial manifestations include fever, sore throat, and pain on swallowing (odynophagia). Trismus and medial displacement of the tonsil soon follow. Treatment for this abscess is intravenous antibiotics and drainage through an incision made below the angle of the mandible.

Retropharyngeal space infection occurs in the region deep to the posterior pharyngeal wall. Sites of origin include the nose, sinuses, and adenoids and nasopharynx. These abscesses are usually seen in children younger than 4 years of age, and when seen in adults, the physician should consider tuberculosis. Early signs and symptoms include refusal of food, followed by fever and respiratory obstruction. Later signs are neck extension and tilting of the head toward the side of less involvement. The infection may spread into the mediastinum. Intravenous antibiotics, incision and drainage, and, occasionally, a tracheotomy are the main therapeutic steps.

Submandibular space infections involve the anatomic space bounded by the floor of the mouth and the deep cervical fascia between the mandible and the hyoid bone. Most follow dental infections or a tooth extraction. There may be skin redness and fluctuance or mouth and tongue swelling. The tongue may be sufficiently displaced posteriorly to require a tracheotomy for airway obstruction. Intravenous antibiotics and incision and drainage are mainstays of therapy.

Parotid space infections usually follow acute parotitis, often in postoperative, dehydrated, or debilitated patients. There is pain, swelling, and warmth over the parotid gland. *Staphylococcus aureus* is a common pathogen, and successful treatment may require intravenous antibiotics, hydration, sialagogues, low dose radiotherapy, and incision and drainage.

Masticator space infections involve the region just anterior to the pharyngomaxillary space and often result from infection around an impacted third molar. There is trismus and swelling over the angle of the mandible. Intravenous antibiotics and incision and drainage are the therapeutic choices.

JUVENILE NASOPHARYNGEAL ANGIOFIBROMA

Juvenile nasopharyngeal angiofibroma is a highly vascular, locally aggressive tumor that is found almost exclusively in adolescent males. Grossly, the tumor is a reddish purple, lobulated, sessile mass arising in the roof of the nasopharynx. As it enlarges, it causes progressive nasal obstruction and spontaneous epistaxis. Hearing loss, sinusitis, cranial nerve deficits, and even facial swelling may be noted as the tumor expansion continues. Roentgenograms reveal anterior bowing of the posterior wall of the maxillary sinus, posterior bowing of the anterior wall of the pterygopalatine fissure, and a characteristic tumor blush on angiography. Biopsy is quite hazardous because of the potential for very heavy bleeding. The differential diagnosis includes a nasopharyngeal polyp, lymphoepithelioma, craniopharyngioma, chordoma, and dermoid cyst. Treatment is surgical excision, sometimes preceded by hormonal therapy or embolization as steps used to reduce the operative blood loss. Radio-

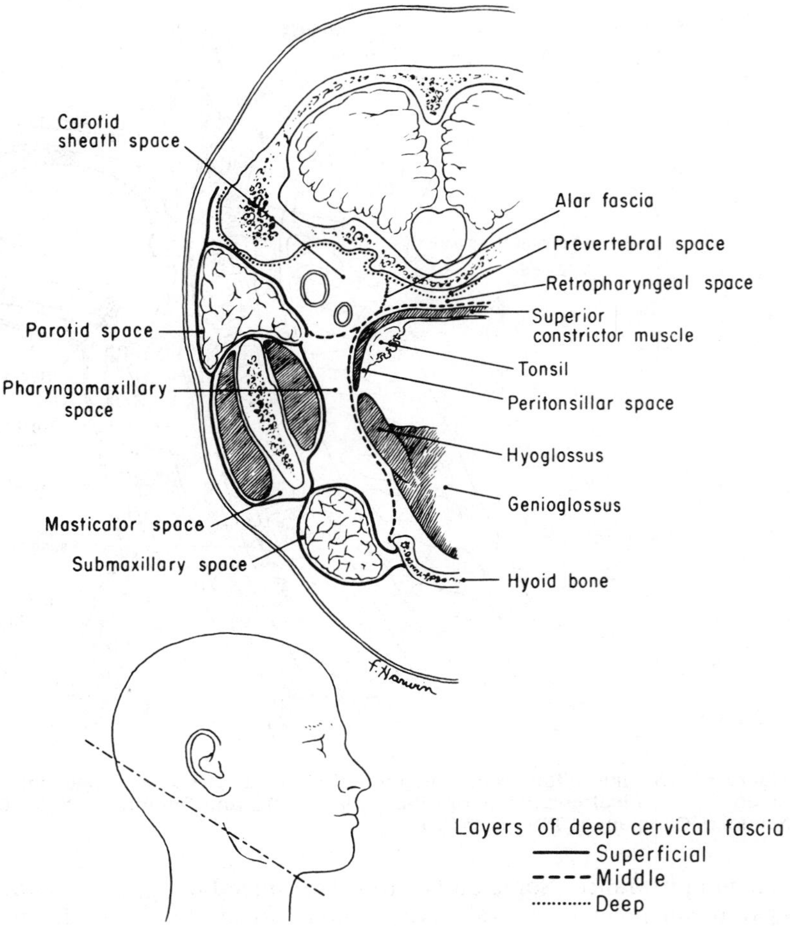

Figure 33–12. Cross section of the neck at the level of the oropharynx. Potential spaces bounded by deep cervical fascia are depicted. (From Paparella, M. M., and Shumrick, D. A. [Eds.]: Otolaryngology. Vol. III. Philadelphia, W. B. Saunders Company, 1980, p. 2313.)

therapy is reserved for those tumors that are unresectable because of intracranial expansion.

ORAL CAVITY MALIGNANCY

Squamous cell carcinoma of the *tongue* and *floor of the mouth* are the most common malignancies of the oral cavity. These tumors comprise 7 per cent of all cancers in the United States and 45 per cent of all cancers in Bombay, India. Alcohol and tobacco are the most important etiologic factors and act synergistically to induce the development of oral squamous cell carcinoma. These growths are usually preceded by an area of superficial leukoplakia (white patch) that is easily detected during a thorough examination. Bimanual palpation of the tongue and floor of the mouth should be routine during the examination of all patients older than 40 years of age. Diagnosis is confirmed by biopsy, and treatment planning must include assessment of the adjacent mandible and the cervical lymph nodes. Small, superficial cancers in this area can be managed by wide local excision. Larger tumors usually require combined surgery and radiation therapy.

Carcinoma of the palate is usually of the squamous cell type and usually arises near the posterior, free edge of the soft palate. The lesions are ulcerative and cause pain, odynophagia, and a sensation of a mass in the palate. Trismus is a late sign and indicates a poor prognosis. Surgery is utilized for early lesions and is combined with radiotherapy for advanced tumors. After resection, the anatomic and functional palatal defect is rehabilitated by a prosthesis. Prognosis depends upon the stage of the malignancy and ranges from 65–95 per cent for T_1 lesions to 30 per cent for T_3 lesions.

Minor salivary gland cancer commonly occurs on the palate and is exhibited as an asymptomatic, mucosa-covered mass. These tumors grow slowly and are not considered to be curable by radiotherapy. Surgical resection is the therapeutic mainstay.

Buccal (cheek) carcinoma usually occurs in older patients (60 or 70 years of age) with a history of smoking or chewing tobacco. These tumors may be either the superficial verrucous form or deeply invasive. About a third of the patients present with disease limited to the cheek, but unfortunately, patients frequently ignore early symptoms until the lesion passes beyond the point of curability. Small tumors may be cured by using either surgery or radiotherapy.

Malignant melanoma of the oral cavity arises most often on the palate. Grossly, the lesions appear brownish gray with a smooth, lacy pattern, giving a

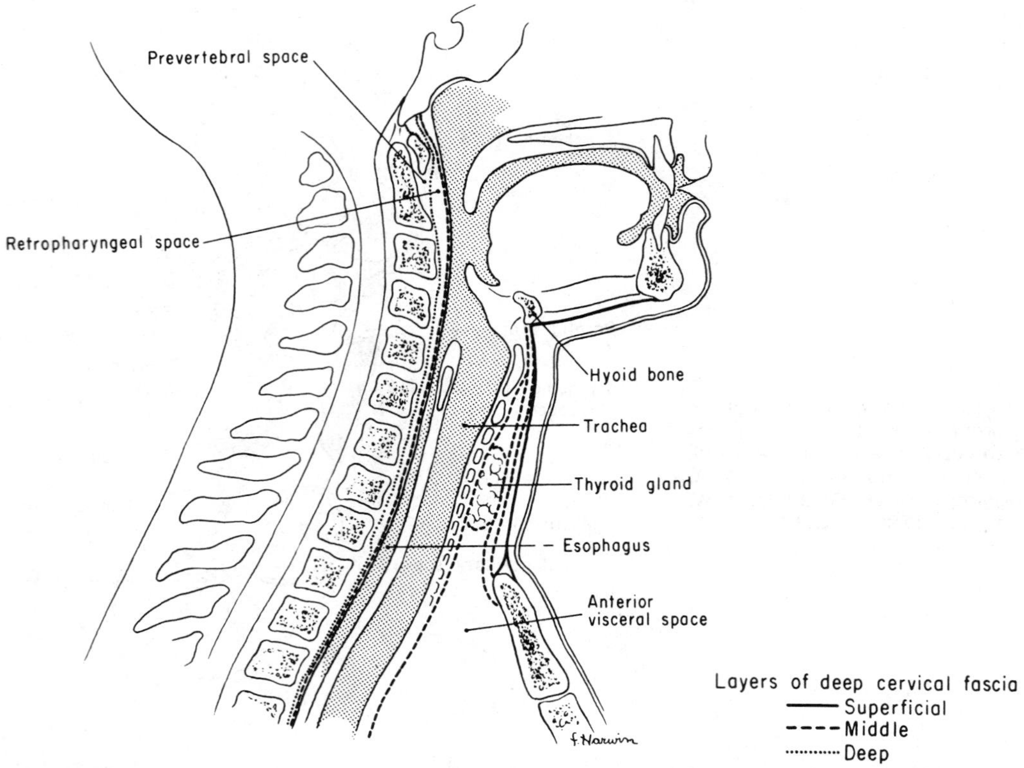

Figure 33–13. Midsagittal section diagram of the neck. Deep-neck space infections can progress inferiorly into the mediastinum or down the spinal column (From Paparella, M. M., and Shumrick, D. A. [Eds.]: Otolaryngology. Vol. III. Philadelphia, W. B. Saunders Company, 1980, p. 2312.)

benign appearance. Some authorities recommend biopsy of all pigmented oral cavity lesions arising in Caucasian patients. Treatment is surgical, and the 5-year survival rates are very low at 10 to 15 per cent.

SWALLOWING DISORDERS (DYSPHAGIA)

Dysphagia is a very common complaint, especially among the older patient population. Advances in the field of endoscopy and radiology have increased our understanding of the act of swallowing and our ability to assess individual patients. The most common disorders that cause disturbances of swallowing include achalasia, diffuse spasm, esophagitis, diverticulae, and tumors.

Achalasia is a disorder of esophageal motility involving the body of the esophagus and the lower esophageal sphincter. It is characterized by a decreased number of ganglion cells in Auerbach's myenteric plexus. This defect causes diminished or absent peristalsis and failure of the lower esophageal sphincter to relax. As the disease progresses, the esophagus becomes increasingly dilated until an entire meal may be lodged in its lumen. The onset of achalasia is usually insidious and the most common is a sensation of food "sticking" in the lower esophagus. Pain is infrequent, and regurgitation is common. Treatment consists of dilation in milder cases and an esophagomyotomy in more intractable cases.

Diffuse spasm of the esophagus is characterized by failure of the muscular contractions to follow the usual progressive peristaltic pattern in the distal half. The normal pattern is replaced by a series of repetitive contractions. The cause is unclear but is believed to be a disturbance of vagal tone. Histologically, there is an extreme degree of muscular hypertrophy. Diagnosis is based largely upon radiologic studies that document the functional disturbance. Patients complain of dysphagia and substernal pain that may radiate to the jaw or arms, in some cases mimicking angina. Treatment is similar to that for achalasia.

Esophagitis may be caused by chemical agents (alcohol, spices, tobacco), physical trauma (thermal injury, foreign body), infection (bacterial, viral, *Candida*, parasites), or radiation. Systemic disease may be a factor in some patients (blood dyscrasias, scleroderma, pemphigus, or immunosuppression). Therapy depends on the predisposing factors.

Diverticulae are pouches that form as the result of increased luminal pressure (pulsion diverticulum) or external pulling forces on the esophageal wall (traction diverticulum). *Zenker's diverticulum* is a pharyngoesophageal pouch that is usually seen in elderly males. These pouches cause regurgitation of food, foul odor, dysphagia, and aspiration. The treatment is surgical excision.

Benign esophageal tumors are uncommon and usually present after the 4th decade. They usually give no symptoms when they are small, so consequently they are usually quite large when diagnosed. *Leiomyoma* is the most common of the benign tumors, with cysts, papillomas, polyps, and hemangiomas being rare. Endoscopic excision is a possible treatment for these benign tumors.

Malignant esophageal tumors usually occur in male patients in the 50- to 70-year-old age group. Squamous cell carcinoma is the most common malignancy, and symptoms include dysphagia (with solids initially, then liquids), weight loss, hoarseness (recurrent laryngeal nerve involvement), cough, and pneumonia. Radiographic studies and esophagoscopy are employed for diagnosis. Radiation therapy or surgery may be utilized for treatment, but cure rates are only 10 to 15 per cent.

The Larynx

EXAMINATION OF THE LARYNX

Fiberoptic and Mirror Laryngoscopy

Mirror laryngoscopy can be accomplished in most patients unless they have a very sensitive gag reflex. Better visibility is gained by using the largest mirror that can be tolerated by the patient (Johnson, 1984). Spraying the throat with pontocaine or lidocaine prior to examination may help, but if the examination is still difficult, 2 to 5 mg. of intravenous *diazepam* will facilitate the process. The patient should be seated upright, leaning forward slightly. The mirror should be warmed slightly to prevent fogging. The tongue should be grasped with a gauze pad and the mirror introduced until it just touches the soft palate. The patient may be asked to "pant like a dog" to suppress the gag reflex, and to say "eee" to approximate the cords and facilitate visualization of the anterior larynx. If only the base of the tongue is visible, it is probably because the patient is not leaning far enough forward.

Both rigid and fiberoptic laryngoscopes are also available for office use. The flexible instrument is inserted through the nose, whereas the rigid scope is inserted through the mouth. The flexible scope is a small version of the flexible fiberoptic sigmoidoscope and is being used increasingly by primary care physicians as a diagnostic instrument. An additional benefit of the fiberoptic scope is the ability to photograph lesions for documentation or future consultation purposes (Dewitt, 1988).

DISORDERS OF THE LARYNX

Acute Laryngitis

Acute laryngitis in children usually becomes manifest as croup and was discussed earlier. Acute laryngitis in the adult is usually viral in etiology and is a mild, self-limited illness. Patients develop hoarseness, cough, and often become gradually unable to talk above a whisper. Fluids, humidification, and allowing the voice to rest should be advised until symptoms have resolved.

Chronic Laryngitis

Chronic laryngitis is primarily a problem of adults who use their voice for speaking or singing. An acute inflammation is often aggravated by an inadequate period of rest. Chronic bronchitis, excessive alcohol ingestion, and cigarette smoking are also frequent contributing factors. Examination usually reveals edema and, occasionally, thickening or nodularity of the cords. Therapy must focus on removal of all irritating factors and resting the voice, to which the patient is often resistant. A beclomethasone inhaler may help to decrease the inflammation.

Airway Obstruction in the Neonate

Airway obstruction in neonates is characterized by stridor, a rasping, rattling, or musical sound that coincides with the respiratory effort. *Inspiratory stridor* suggests a high obstruction (tongue, pharynx, supraglottis), whereas *expiratory stridor* indicates obstruction of the intrathoracic trachea or bronchi. The most likely causes for neonatal stridor are laryngomalacia, subglottic stenosis, vocal cord paralysis, and vascular ring anomalies.

The nature of the stridor differs with each of the above-mentioned disorders, and careful analysis of the stridor may be pathognomonic.

Laryngomalacia is characterized by a soft, floppy laryngeal skeleton and immaturity of neuromuscular function. Airway intervention is not usually necessary, and the problem resolves by 12 to 18 months of age. *Laryngomalacia* causes a coarse inspiratory stridor, but the vocalizing sounds of the infant are normal. Because of the redundant nature of the arytenoid and aryepiglottic mucosa, the neonate's cry may have a harsh component that is relieved in a prone position.

A neonate with *subglottic stenosis* will have normal-sounding but weak vocalizations obscured by stridor. The cry may be weakened by poor air exchange. The subglottic stenosis usually appears to be concentric, and the point of greatest obstruction is about 2 to 3 mm. below the true cords.

Vocal cord paralysis represents about 10 per cent of all congenital laryngeal abnormalities, with unilateral paralysis being more common than bilateral paralysis. Tracheotomy is often required in the case of bilateral paralysis. *Unilateral vocal cord paralysis* usually results in a breathy cry only, but if stridor is present it is usually louder when awake and may be positional. The infant may sleep quietly when lying on the side of the paralysis and become stridulous when placed on the other side.

Laryngeal webs may cause changes ranging from mild hoarseness to aphonia and from mild stridor and cough to gross obstruction with severe distress. The severity of the stridor and the obstruction are proportional to the degree of webbing anteriorly. About three fourths of the webs are glottic, with the remainder divided equally between supraglottic and subglottic webs. Gradual onset and progression of stridor suggests the possibility of an enlarging mass, such as a *subglottic hemangioma*. Feeding difficulties that cause aspiration or cyanosis suggest that the sphincteric mechanism of the laryngeal muscles is deficient (neurologic sensory or motor deficit). *Subglottic hemangiomas* usually become symptomatic within the first 6 months of life. They occur more commonly in females and more often on the left side. About half of neonates with this condition will have skin hemangiomas. Laser excision is currently recommended as the treatment of choice.

Unsuspected foreign bodies may be another possibility for these problems in neonates and infants. Radiographic studies and endoscopy are often essential steps in pinpointing the exact cause for stridor in this age group.

Among slightly older infants and children, acquired processes become more important as causes for airway obstruction. Prominent among these airway disorders are *viral laryngotracheobronchitis, bacterial tracheitis* (usually *Staphylococcus aureus*), *spasmodic croup*, and *epiglottitis*.

Laryngeal Trauma

Laryngeal trauma can be categorized according to the mechanism of tissue injury as *blunt trauma, penetrating injuries, thermal burns*, and *radiation* injuries. Each of these groups poses special problems in diagnosis and management.

The cartilaginous skeleton of the larynx is suspended from the hyoid bone and generally serves to support and protect the airway. The thyroid cartilage is composed of two halves that join in the midline in a keel-like configuration to form the prominence, or Adam's apple. The cricoid cartilage is shaped like a signet ring and completely encircles the subglottic lumen, the smallest area of the upper airway.

Blunt external trauma is the most common form of laryngeal trauma, and it may result in cartilage fractures. Often, in a motor vehicle accident, the neck is extended and the laryngeal region impacts the dashboard or steering wheel, driving it posteriorly and compressing it against the cervical spine. Patients who sustain this type of accident may fracture the thyroid or cricoid cartilages and lacerate the soft tissue inside the cartilages. Common symptoms are voice changes (hoarseness, aphonia), dysphagia, stridor, pain, local tenderness, subcutaneous emphysema (air in the neck tissues), and hemoptysis. Radiographic studies are essential to rule out cervical spine fracture, and a computerized tomography scan is best for assessing the degree of laryngeal injury.

After the airway is secured, laryngoscopy may be required to clarify the need for surgical repair. In general, surgical exploration is necessary if there is evidence of airway obstruction, subcutaneous emphysema, vocal cord paralysis, mucosal laceration, arytenoid displacement, or cartilage fracture.

Penetrating trauma usually results from a stab or gunshot wound. The signs and symptoms are similar to those of blunt external trauma, the difference being the presence of an obvious neck wound on physical examination. All penetrating laryngeal injuries require operative exploration and repair, along with antibiotic coverage and tetanus prophylaxis.

Thermal laryngeal injuries are usually caused by the aspiration of hot or caustic liquids or by inhalation. These injuries produce an intense inflammatory response with the larynx, often compromising the airway. Intubation is generally required for airway maintenance for the initial postinjury period. Thermal injuries may produce severe pulmonary damage as well. Baseline arterial blood gases, antibiotics, fluid replacement, aminophylline, steroids, and ventilatory support are components of the complex therapeutic regimen that is required in these circumstances.

Radiation injury is an uncommon complication of radiation therapy, but when it is encountered, it requires immediate recognition and treatment. Chondritis and cartilage necrosis have the potential to cripple the larynx or even require its removal. Antibiotics, steroids, and tracheotomy are used to manage this problem.

Laryngeal Papillomatosis

Juvenile laryngeal papillomatosis is the most common benign neoplasm of the larynx in children. It is caused by the human papillomaviruses, a group of related DNA viruses that also cause cutaneous and genital warts. The lesions are red, sessile lesions of the glottis primarily, but often involve the palate, tonsil, pharynx, and nose. The two clinical forms are juvenile onset and adult onset. The juvenile-onset type almost always presents by age 4 and usually is associated with a history of maternal genital warts. The lesions are almost always multiple, aggressive, and recurrent.

The adult-onset type presents in two patterns: as multiple lesions in young adults or as single warts in older adults.

Laryngeal papillomas almost always cause major voice changes and hoarseness. They may become obstructive and at times will also cause problems with aspiration. Laryngoscopy and laser excision is the customary treatment. Interferon has been shown to produce remission and regression of the process, but the effect is temporary and progression resumes when the interferon is discontinued.

Laryngeal Malignancy

Laryngeal carcinoma (almost exclusively squamous cell carcinoma) affects over 10,000 persons in the United States each year. Cigarette smoking and alcohol consumption are the major causative factors. Most laryngeal tumors originate on the true vocal cords (glottic), with nearly all of the remainder involving the false cords and epiglottis (supraglottic) or the pyriform sinuses and vallecula (marginal). The symptoms, signs, treatment, and prognosis differ for each of these sites.

Glottic carcinoma causes hoarseness as an early sign due to the interference with vocal fold movement and glottic closure. Indirect laryngoscopy reveals an irregular, red or white growth (Plate III). Direct laryngoscopy provides an opportunity for biopsy confirmation of the diagnosis and for planning the most appropriate therapy. Early lesions of the true cords can be managed by endoscopic excision, intermediate lesions by partial laryngectomy (Fig. 33–14), and advanced lesions by total laryngectomy or radiotherapy, or both. Cure rates range from over 90 per cent for T_1 glottic carcinoma to about 50 per cent for T_4 lesions.

Supraglottic and marginal zone laryngeal cancer usually is associated with a sensation of a lump in the throat, dysphagia, or an asymptomatic neck node mass. The supraglottic lymphatics are much more plentiful, and early spread to cervical lymph nodes is much more common than with glottic carcinoma. Early tumors can be treated by supraglottic partial laryngectomy, whereas more advanced lesions require total laryngectomy or radiotherapy, or both. Cure rates for supraglottic cancer range from 85 per cent for T_1 lesions to about 40 per cent for T_4 tumors.

The bottom line for primary physicians is the maintenance of a high index of suspicion for laryngeal cancer in patients past 40 years of age. The history of smoking should represent a red flag in the case of older patients with any voice change, dysphagia, sore throat, or neck mass. Persistence of symptoms beyond 2 weeks shifts the burden of proof to the primary physician to rule out the diagnosis of malignancy.

Subglottic (Laryngotracheal) Stenosis

The cross-sectional area of the airway is proportional to the fourth power of the radius of the lumen, so that small changes produced by edema or scarring (particularly in the infant larynx) are greatly magnified. For example, 1 mm. of edema in the normal neonatal subglottic larynx reduces the airway by 32 per cent. The subglottic region is particularly prone to damage from an endotracheal tube because the cricoid cartilage is the only rigid structure completely encircling the airway and the submucosa is particularly susceptible to an edematous inflammatory reaction.

Acquired laryngotracheal stenosis has increased in incidence over the past two decades following the

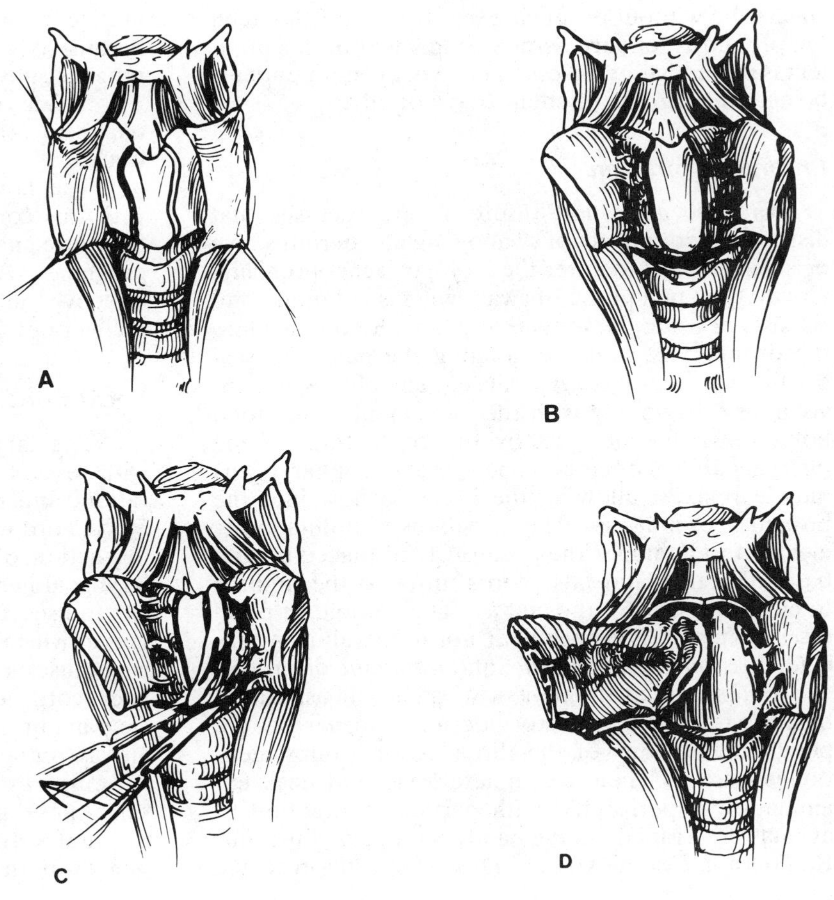

Figure 33–14. *A*, Creation of a central cartilage segment in patients with anterior commissure carcinoma. *B*, Elevation of the internal thyroid perichondrium on both sides. *C*, Laryngeal entry away from the tumor is shown as the first step in resection. *D*, Primary tumor is resected with adequate margins as exposure is gained. (From Bailey, B. J., and Stiernberg, C. M.: Extended partial laryngeal surgery. *In* Jacobs, C. [Ed.], Cancers of the Head and Neck. Boston, Martinus Nijhoff Publishers, 1987, p. 36.)

widespread use of prolonged intubation of neonates, especially those with prematurity and even smaller larynges. Use of a ventilator adds a piston-like action to the injury caused by an endotracheal tube. Birth weight, tube size, duration of intubation, multiple intubations, and infection are key factors in producing subglottic stenosis. Congenital stenosis has also been a major factor in some reported series.

The usual clinical picture involves an infant who cannot be extubated after prolonged intubation. Other causative factors predominate in older age groups, with external trauma, burns, and granulomatous disease leading the list of causes. Stridor is a common sign, often being biphasic and somewhat subtle at rest, but obvious with crying or exertion. Radiographic studies are helpful in localizing and evaluating the extent of the stenosis. The final step in assessment is endoscopic inspection of the subglottic region to establish the exact nature and configuration of the stenosis.

Treatment methods include dilation and the injection of steroids to decrease obstructive scar formation. Serial laser excision of cicatrix is useful in some instances. Severe stenosis requires open surgical resection of scar and reconstruction of the subglottic region. For neonates, the anterior cricoid splitting procedure has proved to be useful as an early measure for the infant who fails extubation. By releasing the constraint of the cricoid ring, the subglottic dimensions can be increased to accommodate the endotracheal tube without producing scar tissue. Fortunately, the prognosis for successful management of this problem is quite high, with less than 10 per cent of patients being left with a permanent tracheotomy.

Chronic Aspiration

Chronic aspiration results from processes that disrupt the normal act of swallowing and permit saliva or ingested food to enter the laryngotracheobronchial airway. The first phase of swallowing is voluntary and consists of using the tongue to push a food bolus into the oropharynx while contracting the palate to seal off the nasopharynx. All subsequent phases are involuntary, beginning with the movement of the food bolus down the pharynx by the contraction of the pharyngeal constrictors. Then the cricopharyngeus muscle relaxes, allowing the bolus to flow into the proximal esophagus. The larynx is simultaneously elevated to lie under the posteriorly displaced tongue base. The true and false cords move to the midline to close and protect the airway. The pathologic processes that may interfere with normal swallowing include *neurologic, neoplastic*, and *traumatic* disorders.

Evaluation of the patient with chronic aspiration begins with a careful history designed to narrow the possibilities to one of the three major groups mentioned earlier. Then a complete head and neck examination is performed with particular attention to evaluating cranial nerve and laryngeal function. Radiographic studies (especially a cine fluoroscopic examination) and endoscopic examination may be necessary to define precisely the nature of the problem.

Many patients with this condition are elderly and weak, and the major risk to their survival is *aspiration pneumonia*. In this group, the use of small feeding tubes, raising the head of the bed at a 45-degree angle, and changing their habits to reduce bolus size can be effective therapy.

Surgical therapy must be considered if the patient cannot be managed successfully by medical means. The need for this consideration could be shown by signs of pneumonia or could develop as a requirement for improved alimentation. The type of procedure chosen must be appropriate for the cause of the aspiration, the therapeutic objective, and the prognosis for recovery.

Surgical options include the following:

1. Tracheotomy and an inflated balloon cuff around the tracheostomy tube are used to prevent aspiration. This is a short-term solution for patients who can be expected to regain normal swallowing ability.
2. Hypopharyngostomy or esophagostomy is a surgical opening made for temporary or permanent feeding purposes.
3. Teflon injection into a paralyzed vocal cord expands the cord medially to close any opening that permits aspiration.
4. Cricopharyngeal myotomy is a cutting of the muscle fibers in those patients who are aspirating because of a holdup of the bolus caused by cricopharyngeus spasm or paralysis.
5. Laryngeal closure procedures plus tracheotomy seal off the larynx surgically to prevent aspiration.

The key to successful management of patients with this condition lies in the precise assessment of the cause and thoughtful consideration of the patient's prognosis. A plan must be chosen that is safe and effective but potentially reversible in the event of recovery of function.

Vocal Cord Paralysis

The larynx is a complex neuromuscular organ with several key functions, such as phonation, respiration, and protection of the lungs, to name a few. Vocal cord movement is controlled by the coordinating action of the vagus nerve through the superior laryngeal nerve, which supplies the cricothyroid muscle (tenses the cords), and the recurrent laryngeal nerve, which innervates the remaining intrinsic laryngeal muscles. Only one pair of muscles act to pull the vocal cords apart for breathing, whereas several muscle pairs bring them to the midline for phonation and airway protection.

Superior laryngeal nerve paralysis may be subtle, since there are remaining muscles to compensate for the motor function loss. It produces a paralysis of one or both cricothyroid muscles, which results in bowing of the true vocal cord on phonation. Inability to tense the cord causes a loss of ability to sing or speak in the higher pitch range. There may be mild problems with aspiration, but these are usually transient.

Unilateral recurrent laryngeal nerve paralysis usually produces an immobile vocal cord situated in a position just off the midline. Patients may have a hoarse and breathy voice and may have a weakened cough and may aspirate. In many cases, there is a gradual compensation process, with the opposite cord taking up much of the slack. If compensation is incomplete, teflon injection of the paralyzed cord is indicated.

Bilateral recurrent laryngeal nerve paralysis usually is associated with airway obstruction with stridor. The voice is usually strong because the cords are paralyzed near the midline of the airway. Tracheotomy is necessary if the airway obstruction is severe.

In general, vocal cord paralysis is classified as being either central or peripheral in origin. *Central paralysis* is caused by diabetic neuropathy, aortic aneurysm, inflammatory disease (from a virus, influenza, tuberculosis), bronchogenic carcinoma, esophageal cancer, thyroid tumors, mediastinal or neck metastatic cancer, surgical trauma (thyroidectomy), basal skull fracture, chest surgery, or penetrating neck trauma. Therefore, the work-up must include a comprehensive history and physical examination with particular attention to neurologic problems. Chest, skull base, esophageal and neck roentgenograms may be necessary. Lab studies include complete blood count, venereal disease testing, fasting blood sugar, viral antibody titers, rheumatoid factor, and a heavy metal screen.

Management options include watchful waiting, tracheotomy, neck exploration for trauma, teflon injection, and arytenoidectomy. Neuromuscular pedicle reinnervation techniques show promise for restoring laryngeal function in many patients, but these procedures are still in the process of clinical refinement and are not universally accepted.

The Neck

CONGENITAL NECK CYSTS AND SINUSES

The branchial apparatus is a system of segmental arches separated by external grooves and internal pouches that develop during the 4th week of intrauterine life. Grossly, this apparatus resembles a system of gill slits, and in some children, disorders of development result in the appearance of cysts, draining sinuses, or lymphatic vascular tumors. The most common of these lesions are *branchial cleft cysts, thyroglossal duct cysts*, and *lymphangiomas* (Plate IV).

Branchial cleft cyst usually appears as a smooth, round, nontender mass along the anterior border of the sternocleidomastoid muscle and deep to that muscle. These cysts usually do not become apparent until the second decade of life, when the slow accumulation of fluid or the onset of infection involving the cyst calls attention to its presence. These cysts are generally lined by stratified squamous epithelium with hair follicles and sweat and sebaceous glands. Cysts are more common than fistulas or sinus tracts. The exact location of the cyst and its associated tract varies depending on which branchial cleft is the origin. Diagnosis is based on the history of a progressively enlarging neck mass that is not consistent with cervical lymphadenopathy and is located in an appropriate site. Treatment is by surgical excision of the cyst and its tract, and postoperative recurrence is uncommon.

Thyroglossal duct cyst is a remnant of the descent of the mesodermal tissues in the region of the ventral (thyroid) diverticulum to its final developmental status as the thyroid gland. Along the way, this tissue passes through the hyoid bone region, and occasionally, duct tissue remnants are left along the route and form midline cysts. These cysts are usually located immediately inferior to the hyoid bone, but they may be located anywhere from the submental region to the suprasternal notch. The cysts are lined by squamous, ciliated, or transitional epithelium and are surrounded by a fibrous tissue capsule. The cyst fluid is mucinous and often contains cholesterol crystals. About half of these cysts become apparent prior to the age of 10 years as a painless, midline neck mass. Protrusion of the tongue usually causes the mass to move superiorly. Treatment consists of complete excision of the cyst and its tract in patients with infection or cosmetically unacceptable appearance. The procedure includes removal of the central portion of the hyoid bone and deep cone of midline tongue tissue. These steps have greatly reduced the incidence of cyst recurrence (from nearly 50 per cent in earlier years to less than 5 per cent).

The third most common congenital neck mass is *cystic hygroma* (often used synonymously with *lymphangioma*). This tumor is composed of lymphatic elements that are arranged like a cluster of grapes to form a soft, usually compressible mass that can be located at any level between the maxilla and the axilla. Typically, the mass is situated in the lower half of the neck and is noted during the neonatal period. Another pattern of presentation is that of a smaller mass located in the upper neck or lower portion of the face that becomes apparent after the age of 3 to 4 years.

Diagnosis is made on the basis of the painless, progressive enlargement in size and the typical physical findings. Treatment is through surgical excision, with great care taken to avoid injury to important head and neck structures.

SALIVARY GLAND DISEASE IN CHILDREN

With the exception of mumps, salivary gland disorders are more common in adults than in children.

Most pediatric salivary gland problems are characterized by a painful swelling or a gradually enlarging mass. The parotid gland and the submandibular gland are both surrounded by capsules that tend to constrain any swelling or infection that arises within the gland. Each gland is composed of a set of lobulated glandular units that drain through a branching series of ducts into one main excretory duct. This arrangement predisposes the gland to recurrent infection if there is blockage of a major duct by inflammation or a stone. The sole function of the salivary glands is the production of saliva for hydration, lubrication, and digestion. Glandular secretion results from both sympathetic and parasympathetic stimulation.

The most common cause of parotid gland swelling in children is *acute viral parotitis*, or mumps, which is a febrile illness that causes painful parotid enlargement. The physical examination reveals a red punctum (opening of a duct inside the cheek) with clear saliva. The disease is usually caused by mumps virus, but it may be caused by echovirus or Coxsackie virus A. There is an 18- to 21-day incubation period after exposure. Often, all four salivary glands are involved, and important complications include encephalitis, orchitis, pancreatitis, and deafness (usually unilateral).

Lymphoma, sarcoidosis, and *granulomatous diseases* (tuberculosis, infection with atypical *Mycobacteria*, actinomycosis, or cat-scratch disease) are related pathologic changes involving adjacent lymph nodes, and any of these conditions may mimic salivary gland disease. Also, several endocrine and metabolic diseases (such as *Sjögren's syndrome, cystic fibrosis*, and *allergic disorders*) may be difficult to differentiate from salivary gland disease.

Several noninfectious, primary, non-neoplastic diseases may cause swelling of the salivary gland in children. *Sialectasia* is a condition in which congenital, saccular degeneration of the smallest set of ducts causes stasis of the saliva and recurrent parotitis. The exacerbations are usually unilateral, last about a week, recur in 3 or 4 months, and are generally considered to be self-limiting. Diagnosis is by sialography, a radiographic dye study. *Sialolithiasis*, an inflammatory disease caused by an obstructing stone in the main duct, is more common in the submandibular salivary glands than in the parotid glands. Search for and removal of the offending stone is the management strategy.

Hemangioma and *lymphangioma* are the most common neoplasms of the salivary glands in children. *Benign mixed tumor* (pleomorphic adenoma) is essentially the only benign, solid, neoplastic mass in children.

SALIVARY GLAND DISEASE IN ADULTS

Sjögren's syndrome is characterized by a triad of xerostomia, keratoconjunctivitis, and a connective tissue disorder (usually rheumatoid arthritis). The presumptive diagnosis is made when two of these three features are present. On the physical examination there is a dry mouth (xerostomia) secondary to a decrease in salivary flow. The parotid glands are enlarged bilaterally, with a diffuse, firm, irregular contour. Fever and glandular tenderness are common. Patients complain of dryness of the eyes with a burning sensation and photosensitivity. On inspection there is often a superficial ocular keratitis. Dryness and scaling of the skin is common. Diagnosis is confirmed by increased gamma globulins, rheumatoid factor, and antinuclear antibodies. Biopsy of the lip shows histopathologic changes similar to those of the salivary glands (acinar atrophy, lymphocytic sialoadenitis, and ductal hyperplasia). Early treatment with corticosteroids is recommended.

Salivary gland neoplasms are characterized by the appearance of a slowly enlarging, painless mass in most instances. A *mixed tumor (pleomorphic adenoma)* is the most common. Salivary gland tumors represent about 65 per cent of all parotid tumors and 50 per cent of all submandibular gland neoplasms. Mixed tumors are more common in female patients and usually are present during the fifth decade of life. They are almost always limited to the superficial lobe in the parotid and superficial parotid lobectomy is nearly always curative.

Warthin's tumor represents about 5 per cent of all parotid tumors and is the second most common parotid neoplasm. It most frequently arises in older males and is felt as a rubbery, smooth mass in the tail of the gland (posteriorly and inferiorly). Surgical excision is curative in almost all instances.

Other important benign tumors are *oncocytoma, monomorphic adenoma,* and *sebaceous lymphadenoma.*

The most common malignancy of the parotid gland is *mucoepidermoid carcinoma*, a tumor that most often is exhibited in middle-aged women. Surgical excision carries a 90 per cent 5-year survival for low-grade tumors and a 40 to 50 per cent 5-year survival for high-grade malignancy.

Adenoid cystic carcinoma is the most common malignant tumor of the submandibular and minor salivary glands. Sexual distribution is about equal, and the patients are usually in their 40's. Treatment is through surgical excision, but postoperative radiation therapy is frequently employed because of the high percentage of late tumor recurrence. About 40 per cent of patients with this condition develop distant metastases (usually to the lungs); the 5-year survival is 65 per cent, but the 20-year survival is only about 15 per cent.

Other significant malignant neoplasms include *acinous cell carcinoma, malignant mixed tumor* (or carcinoma ex pleomorphic adenoma), *squamous cell carcinoma, adenocarcinoma, undifferentiated carcinoma,* and *lymphoma.*

SALIVARY GLAND TRAUMA

Salivary gland injuries are serious and frequently associated with long-term morbidity. Unfortunately, they are often overlooked or underestimated in patients who have suffered multiple traumas. These injuries are classified as *acute trauma* (blunt, lacerating, penetrating, avulsion, or blast) or as *chronic trauma* (irritation from dentures, foreign bodies, stones, or irradiation). The origin of the injury may be primarily external, intraoral, or both. A careful history and a thorough physical examination are necessary to clarify the exact injury to adjacent soft tissue, muscle, nerve, vascular tissues, and facial skeleton. A laceration of the salivary gland or main duct usually results in the presence of saliva in the wound. Ductal injuries should be repaired, if at all possible, prior to any efforts to repair concomitant facial lacerations.

Facial nerve injuries are also of great importance, and careful assessment of facial muscle function is a high priority—with attention to the forehead, eyes, nose, and mouth. The patient should be asked to smile, show the teeth, pucker the lips, close the eyes tightly, and wrinkle the forehead. All details should be recorded as soon as possible to avoid confusion concerning neurologic deficits that might occur at a later date after the injury (and, therefore, carry a different significance).

Penetrating wounds of the lower face carry a high potential for injury to the parotid or submandibular glands. Knife or shotgun wounds and human or animal bites place the site of the wound at risk for serious infection. In addition to the management of the initial injury, the job is not complete until tetanus prophylaxis (and rabies investigation in appropriate circumstances) has been considered.

The major point to be emphasized in assessing and treating lacerations around the parotid is that early recognition and repair of major salivary ducts or primary branches of the facial nerve is the key to a successful outcome (Fig. 33–15). These surgical methods require the use of microsurgical techniques, and referral to an otolaryngologist and head and neck surgeon is appropriate.

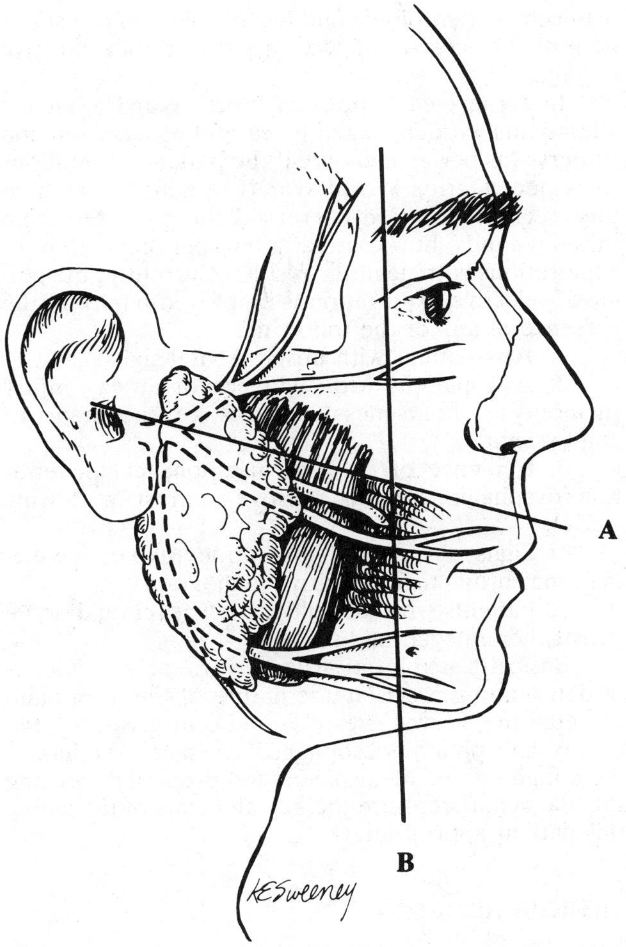

Figure 33–15. Line A, marking position of the parotid duct, extends from the tragus to the middle of the upper lip. The duct occupies the central third of this line. The buccal branch of the facial nerve runs parallel to line A near the duct. Line B runs from the lateral canthus vertically to the mental foramen. Fibers of the facial nerve anterior to line B need not be repaired and recover function if soft tissues are accurately approximated in layers. (Reproduced by permission from Cummings, C. W., Frederickson, J. M., et al. [Eds.]: Otolaryngology—Head and Neck Surgery. Vol. 2. St. Louis, 1986, The C. V. Mosby Company.)

PENETRATING NECK INJURIES

Stab and gunshot wounds are the main causes of *penetrating neck injuries*. Emergency management of patients with these injuries focuses upon protecting or restoring the airway, control of bleeding, and prevention or treatment of hypovolemic shock during the initial minutes of stabilization and evaluation.

Attention is then focused on assessment of the exact nature of the deeper injuries, with particular attention directed to systems that may be disrupted. Airway injury is indicated by hemoptysis, hoarseness, crepitus, or sucking wounds. Pharyngeal and esophageal injury is suggested by dysphagia, crepitus, tachycardia, and fever. The findings with vascular injury are an expanding hematoma, central nervous system deficit, pulse deficit, thrills, bruits, shock, or persistent bleeding. Particular importance should be attached to hoarseness, cranial nerve deficit, or hemiplegia.

In addition to the careful history and physical examination, direct laryngoscopy may be necessary to rule out lacerations of the larynx or pharynx and injury of the recurrent laryngeal nerves.

Radiographic assessment of the pharynx or esophagus is accomplished by having the patient swallow contrast material (thin barium still used most commonly). Angiography is valuable for diagnosis and may be useful in treatment when embolizing techniques are needed. Even though nearly all (92 per cent) of the carotid arteriograms will be negative in these patients, this study is indicated in all patients with central neurologic findings (if their clinical status permits it) because of the importance of a positive finding.

In earlier years (prior to World War II), almost all patients were managed by careful observation and surgery was performed only if the patients' conditions worsened. During World War II, a policy of mandatory neck exploration decreased the mortality from these wounds but carried a 60 per cent rate of explorations with negative results. Currently, the policy of selective exploration is employed based on the presence of any of the following:

1. Any patient with unstable vital signs.
2. Any patient with evidence of airway injury (hemoptysis, hoarseness, crepitus, or subcutaneous emphysema).
3. Evidence of pharyngeal-esophageal penetration (dysphagia, crepitus, positive contrast swallowing study).
4. Signs of vascular disruption (expanding hematoma, bruit, thrill, positive angiogram).
5. Patients with neurologic deficit (cranial nerve deficit, hemiplegia, and so on).

Basically, exploration is performed as a means of determining precisely the nature of the injury and of repairing nerves, vessels, and soft tissue of the airway and pharyngoesophageal passages. Maintaining a high degree of suspicion and promptly pursuing the diagnostic steps are the key elements of managing this patient appropriately.

THYROID NODULES

Thyroid nodules are most often due to single or multiple colloid goiters. Other causes include thyroglossal duct cysts, toxic nodular goiters, adenomas, and thyroid carcinoma. Benign tumors must be differentiated from thyroid malignancies. Palpation of a thyroid nodule should be followed by performance of a radioiodine scan to determine whether the lesion is "hot" or "cold." Cold nodules absolutely require either fine needle aspiration or open biopsy to determine the histology of the lesion.

THYROID CARCINOMA

Thyroid carcinoma arises from either epithelial or medullary tissue. Epithelial carcinomas are of three types: (1) papillary, (2) follicular, and (3) anaplastic. The great majority of lesions are papillary; both follicular and anaplastic lesions are unusual. Anaplastic lesions are most commonly seen in elderly patients and have very poor prognosis. Most other thyroid malignancies are treated surgically and have a relatively favorable prognosis.

References

Bailey, B. J.: Management of maxillofacial trauma. Res. Staff Physician, *29*:57–68, 1982.

Bailey, B. J.: Management of sinus infections. Am. Fam. Physician, *7*(6):100–107, 1973.

Bailey, B. J.: Trauma. *In* Cummings, C. W., et al. (Eds.): Otolaryngology—Head and Neck Surgery. Vol. 2. St. Louis, C. V. Mosby Company, 1986, pp. 1015–1026.

Bailey, B. J., and Stiernberg, C. M.: Extended partial laryngeal surgery. *In* Jacobs, C.: Cancers of the Head and Neck. Boston, Martinus Nijhoff Publishers, 1987.

Baloh, R. W.: The dizzy patient. Symptomatic treatment of vertigo. Postgrad. Med., *73*(5):317–324, 1983.

Bass, J. W.: Treatment of streptococcal pharyngitis revisited. J.A.M.A., *256*(6):740–743, 1986. *Traces the history of penicillin use for streptococcal pharyngitis, and discusses evidence for the importance of early treatment.*

Bell, D. N.: Otitis externa. A common, often self-inflicted condition. Postgrad. Med., *78*(3):101–106, 1985.

Black, B.: Cleaning the ear. Aust. Fam. Phys. *15*(10):1354–1357, 1986. *A well-written practical guide that contains some nice diagrams for preparation of swabs.*

Bluestone, C., and Klein, J.: Otitis Media in Infants and Children. Philadelphia, W. B. Saunders Company, 1988, pp. 217–229. *Covers otitis media from basic anatomy and pathogenesis through treatment and complications.*

Bodor, F. F.: Conjunctivitis-otitis syndrome. Pediatrics, *69*:695–698, 1982. *The author discusses the still somewhat speculative, but attractive hypothesis of the association of conjunctivitis with* H. influenzae *infections.*

Busse, W. W.: Chronic rhinitis. A systematic approach to diagnosis and treatment. Postgrad. Med., *73*(2):325–335, 1983.

Cantekin, E. I., Mandel, E. M., Bluestone, C. D., et al.: Lack of efficacy of a decongestant-antihistamine combination for otitis media with effusion in children. N. Engl. J. Med., *308*:298–301, 1983. *A "classic" article that effectively killed an age-old bias of the family physician—that decongestants were one of the cornerstones of treatment of otitis media.*

Carlin, S. A., Marchant, C. D., Shurin, P. A., et al.: Early recurrences of otitis media: Reinfection or relapse? J. Pediatr., *110*(1):20–25, 1987. *An important concept in the decision of whether an abnormal ear on follow-up is a reinfection or a relapse. The authors say it is more likely a reinfection. Therefore, it should be treated the same way it was the first time.*

Clark, W. D., and Bailey, B. J.: Diagnosis: Evaluation of neck masses. Hosp. Med., August: *19*(8):57–70, 1983.

Clark, W. W., and Bohne, B. A.: The effects of noise on hearing and the ear. Med. Times, December: *112*:17fm–22fm, 1984.

Dayal, V. S.: Clinical Otolaryngology. Philadelphia: J. B. Lippincott Company, 1981, p. 213.

DeNeef, P.: Comparison of tests for streptococcal pharyngitis. J. Fam. Pract., *23*(6):551–555, 1986.

DeWitt, D. E.: Fiberoptic rhinolaryngoscopy in primary care. Postgrad. Med., *84*(5):125–144, 1988. *Discusses the history of the use of this instrument and describes the technique for the use of the procedure as a diagnostic adjunct in the examination of the nose, throat, pharynx, and larynx.*

Fischer, P. M., and Mentrup, P. L.: Comparison of throat culture and latex agglutination test for streptococcal pharyngitis. J. Fam. Pract., *22*(3):245–248, 1986.

Ghory, J. E.: OME: Leading cause of preventable hearing loss. J. Resp. Dis., *3*(10):127–142, 1982.

Guralnick, W., Kaban, L. B., and Merrill, R. G.: Temporomandibular joint afflications. N. Engl. J. Med., *299*:123–129, 1978.

Henderson, F. W., Collier, A. M., Sanyal, M. A., et al: A longitudinal study of respiratory viruses and bacteria in the etiology of acute otitis media with effusion. N. Engl. J. Med., *306*:1277–1383, 1982.

Johnson, J. T.: Indirect laryngoscopy. Fam. Pract. Recert., *6*(9):23–26, 1984.

Johnson, J. T., and Rood, S. R.: Epistaxis management. Postgrad. Med., *70*(5):231–235, 1981.

Kern, E. B.: Suppurative (bacterial) sinusitis. Postgrad. Med., *81*(4):194–210, 1988.

Kirchner, J. A.: Current concepts in otolaryngology. Epistaxis. N. Engl. J. Med., *307*(18):1126–1128, 1982.

Mandel, J. H.: Pharyngeal infections. Postgrad. Med., *77*(3):187–199, 1985.

Marcy, S. M.: Infections of the external ear. Pediatr. Infect. Dis. J., *4*(2):192–201, 1985. *An excellent, comprehensive review of this common family practice problem.*

McMillan, J. A., Sandstrom, C., Weiner, L. B., et al.: Viral and bacterial organisms associated with acute pharyngitis in a school-aged population. J. Pediatr., *109*(5):747–752, 1986.

Meyerhoff, W. L.: Diagnosis and Management of Hearing Loss. Philadelphia, W. B. Saunders Company, 1984, pp. 74–75. *A handy reference, particularly for management of sudden hearing loss, vertigo, and tinnitus.*

Olsen, K. D.: Facial nerve paralysis. General evaluation, Bell's palsy. Postgrad. Med., *75*(8):219–225, 1984.

Paparella, M. M., and Shumrick, D. A.: Otolaryngology (The Ear). Volume II. Philadelphia: W. B. Saunders Company, 1980, pp. 1354–1357.

Rose, D. E.: Noise and hearing loss. Postgrad. Med., *70*:119–129, 1981.

Slater, R.: Vertigo. How serious are recurrent and single attacks? Postgrad. Med., *84*(5):58–67, 1988.

Strome, M., Kelly, J., and Fried, M.: Manual of Otolaryngology. Diagnosis and Therapy. Boston, Little, Brown and Company, 1985, pp. 4–7. *This is an outstanding addition to the Little, Brown spiral handbook series. The information is easy to find and contains practical advice for the treatment of most problems of the ear, nose, and throat. Would be an excellent edition for any practicing family physician's office library.*

Talaat, A. M., El-Dibany, M. M., and El-Garf, A.: Physical therapy in the management of myofacial pain dysfunction syndrome. Ann. Otol. Rhinol. Laryngol., *95*:225–227, 1986.

34

Allergy

Paul P. VanArsdel, Jr.
Greg L. Ledgerwood

Definition and Classification

Originally, immunology meant the study of immunity: the resistance to microbial infection acquired as a result of natural or deliberate exposure. Such immunity can be mediated either by circulating antibody, by cells (T lymphocytes), or by both. In any event, the reaction is with the organism or antigenic substance involved. This is called specific immunity. The scope of immunology expanded in the last century when scientists began to inject foreign proteins into animals and man in order to produce active or passive immunity. Unanticipated adverse reactions occurred. Portier and Richet described anaphylaxis in 1902 in dogs. With Schick, von Pirquet described serum sickness in 1905 and coined the word allergy in 1906. Today, the word *anaphylaxis* is generally used as it was originally, to designate an acquired adverse reactivity to a foreign substance, manifested by the rapid onset of generalized symptoms that may be fatal. It may also be applied to any reaction due to antigen-induced mediator release, even a positive immediate-type skin test (see below). *Allergy* on the other hand has acquired a broader connotation. Any injurious reaction due to acquired sensitivity (appearance of specific blood antibody or T cell) is an allergic reaction. Some prefer the word *hypersensitivity*, feeling that the meaning of the term *allergy* has degenerated through inappropriate usage. *Atopy* was coined in the early 1920's to designate a subset of allergic patients who had acquired sensitivity to environmental substances (pollens, mold spores, house dust, animal danders, foods, and so on) that were innocuous for most people. This type of sensitivity is familial and is manifested most often by asthma, allergic rhinitis, and infantile eczema affecting from 15 to 20 per cent of the population. The mode of genetic transmission is complex (Marsh and Bias, 1988).

What has happened to the word *immunology* since the 19th century? It is now used for all conditions (termed immunologic diseases) in which antibodies or T cells are helpful, harmful, or deficient. The first category, representing the original basis for immunology, is a component of preventive medicine and is covered in that chapter.

Coombs and Gell (1975) enhanced our understanding of harmful allergic reactions by developing a well-known classification that has come into general medical use (Table 34–1). The most frequent problems faced by the clinical allergist are in Type 1 (immediate hypersensitivity). When exposed to antigens (allergens) by inhalation, ingestion, or injection, allergic patients develop vascular dilatation, edema, glandular hypersecretion, and smooth muscle spasm; symptoms may be local (asthma, hay fever) or systemic (urticaria, anaphylactic shock). These symptoms are produced by the reaction of allergens with specific antibodies of the immunoglobulin E (IgE) class that are bound to receptors on tissue mast cells and blood basophils, resulting in a release of chemical mediators. Some mediators are pre formed (histamine, chemotactic factors), whereas others (leukotrienes, platelet-activating factor) are newly generated from membrane lipids and are extremely potent. Platelet-activating factor (PAF) may be 1000 times as potent as histamine and is produced by human mast cells as well as neutrophils, monocytes, and platelets (Serafin and Austen, 1987).

Type II reactions are primarily hematologic and are usually complement dependent. Allergic drug reactions may or may not be complement dependent. Penicillin can induce hemolytic anemia in patients who develop antibodies to red cell–bound penicillin

Table 34–1. THE COOMBS AND GELL CLASSIFICATION

Type	Antigen	Antibody	Mechanism	Clinical Problems
I	Free, soluble	IgE bound to mast cells, basophils	Release or synthesis of several potent chemical mediators	Anaphylaxis, allergic rhinitis
II	Cellular, or bound to cells	Circulating IgG, IgM, complement-activation	Complement-induced tissue injury	Transfusion reactions, autoimmune anemia
III	Bound to antibody in blood as complex lattice	Circulating IgG, IgM complement-activation	Complement-induced tissue injury	Serum sickness, systemic lupus erythematosus
IV	Any, except polysaccharides	None	Sensitive T-lymphocytes release mediators ("lymphokines")	Contact dermatitis, tissue graft reactions

determinants without complement activation. In another type, though, methyldopa can result in a complement-dependent autoimmune reaction through the production of antibodies with Rh specificity (VanArsdel, 1988).

Type III reactions produce various antigen-antibody complex diseases. Systemic lupus erythematosus is the prime example. Although most are autoimmune, some, such as bacterial endocarditis, involve microbial antigens. With most of the nonhuman (xenogeneic) therapeutic antitoxic sera having been supplanted by those of human origin, most serum sickness now occurs in transplant patients receiving antithymocyte globulin.

Finally, Type IV reactions are dependent on the acquisition of specific sensitivity by the T (i.e., thymus-derived) lymphocytes. Such cell-mediated sensitivity is an exaggeration of the normal host protective response to foreign substances. It can result in contact dermatitis when low molecular weight chemicals in contact with the skin conjugate with skin proteins to become active sensitizers. Cell-mediated sensitivity is also responsible in part for tissue graft rejection.

General Evaluation of the Patient

The *history* is usually the most important component in the evaluation of a patient suspected of having an allergic problem. In interviewing a new patient, the physician takes care to identify any previous allergic problems in the patient and also the presence of allergy in close family members. This is particularly helpful in providing support for the diagnosis of an atopic disease. A careful search of environmental factors should be undertaken. Variation in symptoms with the seasons and with changes in location should be carefully recorded. The patient should be questioned in detail regarding the home environment: location, type of heating, type and quality of construction, insulation, humidity, nature of furnishings, draperies and bedding, pets and their habits, method of house cleaning, cigarette smoking, and so on. The work environment needs to be examined for air pollution, other exposure to chemical irritants or sensitizers, physical demands, and job stresses. Sometimes the patient's clothing habits need to be recorded, and a dietary history should not be overlooked—especially in children. Finally, previous and present use of drugs should be noted, including laxatives, antacids, and other over-the-counter remedies that the patient may not recognize as drugs.

Most allergic problems involve the skin or respiratory tract, and these should receive the most attention on the physical examination. The location of skin lesions as well as their description should be recorded, and urticarial lesions, if present, should be outlined in ink to aid in determining whether they are evanescent or persistent. The nose is often overlooked or is given only a cursory examination. The color and degree of swelling of its mucous membrane, the amount and consistency of secretions, and the presence or absence of polyps (not to be confused with turbinates!) should be noted. The lungs, if free of rales, should be examined during forced expiration, which may bring out asthmatic wheezing.

The atopic child may have dark circles under the eyes (allergic shiners) and a transverse crease above the tip of the nose from frequent nose rubbing. Of particular importance in children is the observation of the tympanic membrane and its motility using a tympanometer or the pneumatic otoscope (see later), or both.

A few general *laboratory* procedures may be helpful, such as the nasal or sputum smear, which should be examined for eosinophils. Eosinophils are best visualized with an eosin-methylene blue stain (Hansel's). Blood eosinophilia is helpful if present, but its absence does not exclude allergic disease. The measurement of total serum IgE is of limited value and is rarely worth the expense.

For further evaluation of obstructive airways disease, several recording spirometers are simple, durable, and accurate. We use the Vitalograph spirometer extensively for the purposes of (1) confirming or ruling out airway disease, (2) establishing the degree of response to an inhaled bronchodilator, and (3) monitoring the progress of the patient. Several inexpensive peak-flow meters are also available for monitoring patients' progress.

Provocation testing involves the measurement of ventilatory function before or after some stimulus. It can be used by most physicians as an aid in diagnosing exercise bronchospasm. However, the methacholine provocation test, which is useful in doubtful situations to confirm or exclude the diagnosis of asthma in general, is time consuming and rather risky, so it is best left to experienced laboratories.

Skin testing should be selective and based on clues provided by the history whenever possible. In adults, testing is limited to pollens, house dust (dust mite), feathers, animal danders, and mold spores. If the history is suggestive, skin tests to some foods may also be done. Food testing is more useful in young children. The *prick test* is performed by placing a drop of 1:10 or 1:20 allergen extract on the skin and then "tenting" up the skin under the drop with the tip of a lancet or small needle until the tip pops free. The excess allergen is blotted off and the site is inspected for the development of a wheal-and-erythema reaction 15 minutes later. The prick test is sufficiently sensitive to identify practically all pollen or food allergies. However, if the prick test is negative or equivocal, the intradermal test may be needed to identify dust mite, dander, or mold allergies. This is performed by injecting just enough of a dilute, sterile solution (prepared by the manufacturer specifically for intradermal testing) to produce a 1- to 2-mm. bleb. The positive result again is a whealing reaction that should have a diameter at least 5 mm. but preferably 10 mm. greater than that of the control.

Specific IgE antibodies to a variety of antigens can be measured using the radioallergosorbent test, but this test is expensive and provides no more information than skin testing. The physician who is not equipped to do skin testing may get helpful information by sending a patient's serum to a laboratory that does the radioallergosorbent test, but results are not always reliable.

Some other procedures purported to identify allergy, particularly food allergy, have received considerable attention recently in the lay press. These are cytotoxic testing, subcutaneous or sublingual provocation testing, and neutralization testing. None of these has been established as reliable in properly controlled trials (VanArsdel and Larson, 1989).

The Role of the Family Physician in Allergy Diagnosis and Management

Never in the recent history of medicine has a field such as allergy, with its basis in immunology, expanded so much in scientific development and in treatment options as in the last 2 decades. Unfortunately the field of allergy has also been subject to a comparable expansion in questionable practices, including the inappropriate or controversial use of new technology. The family physician is deluged with new information on a daily basis. With this new information, the family physician's role in diagnosing and treating allergic conditions has expanded greatly. Reference laboratories have provided "kits" for allergy testing and "in-house" evaluation studies utilizing radioallergosorbent methods, which are all too commonplace. Therefore, it becomes important for the family physician to understand the limitations of the testing when applied to the allergic patient. Foremost in importance should be the careful history and physical examination and the use of appropriate medications prior to even considering diagnostic testing such as radioallergosorbent testing or skin testing. Even in qualified hands, these tests alone are not diagnostic, since they are subject to the interpretation by the person performing the test, and can lead the most well-meaning physician astray. The family physician can manage a great deal of the allergic problems presented to him or her but when conservative methods fail to control symptoms, one must consider referral.

Allergic Rhinitis

Allergic rhinitis is a symptom complex due to airborne allergens. It occurs as *seasonal rhinitis* (hay fever) when pollens are in high concentration in the air. It may be intermittent or continuous without seasonal variation, and it is then termed *perennial allergic rhinitis*. Occurring often in families with an allergic history and estimated to occur in eight to ten per cent of the population under 20 years of age, seasonal allergic rhinitis was found to occur twice as commonly as perennial allergic rhinitis (Broder, 1974).

Manifestations. In *seasonal allergic rhinitis*, exposure is followed by complaints of paroxysmal sneezing, a watery nasal discharge with congestion, and nasal itching. Conjunctival and pharyngeal itching is often present. Less specific symptoms are postnasal drainage with a sense of fullness or aching in the frontal areas.

In children, nasal irritation may result in nose picking and recurrent epistaxis. Parents may complain of restless sleeping, snoring, or night-time coughing associated with postnasal mucous drainage and mild hoarseness. As a result of a lack of smell, appetite may be decreased. An allergic "salute" may be present as seen by the upward thrust of the palm against the nares to relieve itching and to open the nasal airways. A gaping expression from mouth breathing is common, as are allergic shiners (described above). Denne's line (a wrinkle beneath the lower lid) is described as being associated with allergic rhinitis and atopic dermatitis. Speech may have a nasal quality. The nasal mucosa is typically moist, with enlarged pale turbinates and a serous discharge.

In *perennial allergic rhinitis*, nasal congestion, itching, obstruction, and the need to constantly sniff may be associated with a loss of sense of taste or smell and a feeling of being "stuffed up," with decreased hearing and a popping sensation in the ears. A lower sneezing threshold often occurs with altered autonomic reflexes in perennial allergic rhinitis so that paroxysms of sneezing and rhinorrhea may result from changes in ambient temperature, head movement, odors, perfume, tobacco smoke, irritants, alcohol, and exposure to small quantities of antigen. Exercise reverses nasal congestion temporarily, from minutes to hours.

The turbinates are usually swollen and edematous and may be mistaken for nasal polyps, which are pearl-gray gelatinous masses and are unusual in uncomplicated allergic rhinitis. Below the turbinates, the floor of the nostril is often prominent as a result of mucosal edema. In one third to one half of children with allergic rhinitis, eustachian tube obstruction may be present, with resultant serous otitis. Otoscopy may reveal a retracted or bulging tympanic membrane, impaired mobility, or a fluid level. In patients with intact tympanic membranes, tympanometry to measure middle ear pressures provides an indirect measurement of eustachian tube function (Bluestone and Cantekin, 1981). The edematous nasal mucosa may obstruct sinus ostia, resulting in congestion or sinusitis with pressure symptoms or headache, which is particularly notable when bending down.

Diagnosis. A seasonal history or an association with an inhaled allergen is helpful. It is often difficult to associate specific allergens with perennial rhinitis. Occasionally, a change in environment, such as a vacation, may point to the existence of environmental allergens. For confirmation of an allergic state, a nasal smear of secretions is easily made by having the patient blow the nose directly onto a sheet of plastic with transfer of secretions to a glass slide, which is than stained with Hansel's stain. An eosinophil count greater than 10 per cent of the total white cells indicates a probable allergic cause, whereas 80 to 90 per cent eosinophils are diagnostic of an allergic state. A peripheral eosinophil count when elevated is helpful; however, this is of limited use, since marked allergic symptoms can occur in the absence of blood eosinophilia.

Treatment of Allergic Rhinitis

Nonspecific. Removal of exposure to known allergens is of prime importance, since this will eliminate symptoms. When exposure is unavoidable, *environmental control* should reduce symptoms and prevent exacerbations. General measures such as the use of an air conditioner or electronic filters can reduce the number of particulate allergens. The use of a mask over the nose and mouth with replaceable microfoam filters significantly reduces the effects of a temporary exposure to inhaled allergens.

It is the patient or the family who must assume responsibility for environmental control, so that it is helpful to provide an understanding of allergens. Commonly inhaled allergens include pollens, which are widely recognized as producing symptoms of seasonal allergic rhinitis; conjunctivitis; and asthma. Allergenic pollens are produced by trees, grass, and weeds. Pollens from flowering plants are insect-borne and are not generally important allergens. In general, there is a direct relationship between pollen exposure and allergic symptoms. However, the intensity of reaction to pollen exposure is increased by recent exposure to other allergens, which appear to "prime" the nasal mucosa. Hence, the best indication of intensity is the symptom not the pollen count. Pollen prevalence is commonly determined by the use of "gravity" slides, which sample pollen fallout without regard to environmental wind direction, speed, and turbulence, so that reports of pollen prevalence in daily news media often do not reflect the true concentration in the air or individual exposure. Inhaled fungal allergens in fungus-sensitive subjects may produce seasonal symptoms during situations that promote fungal growth, such as humid and rainy weather and exposure to hay, mulches, commercial peat moss, compost piles, and leaf litter. Indoors, areas of spore formation can be identified at sites of water condensation such as shower curtains, window moldings, and damp basements. In addition, it may be important to recognize that cool mist vaporizers can be contaminated and serve as sources of fungal contamination.

A prime role for the patient and family is in the environmental control of house dust, which, though a heterogeneous mixture of bacteria, fibrous matter of plant and animal origin, human epidermis, food remnants, fungi, insect debris, and animal danders, contains one major source of antigen, the dust mite. Mites are ubiquitously in households and are most prevalent in bedding, mattresses, carpeting and upholstered furniture, particularly where warmth and humidity are high (Platts-Mills and Chapman, 1987). Animal allergens are derived from dried saliva on the shed fur of cats, rodent urine, and epidermal material from farm animals. The allergic respiratory reactions produced by animal allergens are species specific. Finished furs and wool are not allergenic. Feathers are often nonallergic when fresh and produce allergic symptoms only after degradation. A careful history used to identify environmental allergens is an important element in advising avoidance and treatment. When explanations for allergic exacerbations are provided by the physician to the patient, frustration can be decreased.

Control of Symptoms. Antihistamines are effective for symptomatic control of allergic rhinitis, whether seasonal or perennial. For optimal results, they should be used before exposure to the known allergen. Complete control may not be achieved with many patients who use antihistamines only sporadically. During the implicated season, an around-the-clock administration provides maximal symptomatic relief. To improve compliance to encourage continued use, one should explain that mild drowsiness and other side effects may subside after a few days of continual antihistamine therapy. If more significant side effects occur, such as somnolence, excitation, nervousness, palpitations, and dryness of the mouth, the dose might be reduced or the patient switched to one of the new nonsedating antihistamines. If allergic rhinitis is associated with asthma, the use of antihistamines during acute attacks of asthma should be used with care, since they occasionally worsen the inspissation of bronchial secretions.

In general, antihistamines are less effective alone than when used in combination with alpha-adrenergic decongestant drugs in controlling nasal obstruction, which may be the main problem in chronic perennial allergic rhinitis. Alpha-adrenergic drugs are effective not only in combination with antihistamines but also topically. Topical vasoconstrictors (sprays and drops) are best restricted to temporary use, e.g., when taking an airplane trip or during a severe temporary flare-up of symptoms. For more sustained control of chronic nasal obstruction unresponsive to oral anti-histamine-decongestants, the topical glucocorticoids beclomethasone and flunisolide are effective, and they produce no adrenal suppression when properly used. Their therapeutic effects are not immediate. This should be explained to the patient in order to ensure cooperation and continuation of treatment. One to three weeks may be required for some patients to achieve maximum benefit. If no improvement is evident by 3 to 4 weeks, the glucocorticoid should be discontinued. When symptoms are severe and non-responsive to trials of therapy as outlined above, oral glucocorticoid therapy can be used as a last resort and only for a limited duration, as for the remainder of a pollen season. The rationale for glucocorticoid therapy for allergic rhinitis is that the condition, though IgE-antibody mediated, has a dual component: the immediate phase of edema and hypersecretion and a late inflammatory phase (Bascom et al., 1988). This dual reation occurs in asthma as well (see later).

Specific Therapy. Upon identification by skin tests of sensitivity to an unavoidable inhalant allergen, immunotherapy may be indicated in the treatment of allergic rhinitis. Its efficacy has been shown to be 80 per cent for pollen symptom control and 60 per cent for molds and house dust symptom control. It is, therefore, more effective in seasonal allergic rhinitis than in perennial allergic rhinitis. In the consideration of the use of immunotherapy, the ease of control using other therapy should be weighed in respect to the frequency and severity of symptoms.

Nasal Polyps

Perennial allergic rhinitis may be associated with nasal polyps, but usually only when complicated by sinus infection. In the adult, the presence of polyps may be associated with a sensitivity to aspirin that becomes manifest by aggravation of rhinitis, asthma, and even shock. Nasal polyps often develop in the absence of or only coincidentally with allergy. They arise from infected ethmoid or maxillary sinuses and are easily visible in the nasal cavity. They can cause obstruction and aggravate the pre-existing sinus disease. The size of nasal polyps may be reduced by treating the patient briefly with systemic glucocorticoids or by using topical glucocorticoids two or three times daily for 3 or 4 weeks and then once daily for a longer period. If sinus infection or the underlying allergic factors are not appropriately controlled, polypectomy may be necessary. Unfortunately, this procedure, without sinus surgery, often is not curative, and polyps tend to recur.

Sinusitis

Chronic allergic rhinitis predisposes the patient to sinus disease, although as implied earlier, sinus disease can develop in the absence of allergy. Acute sinusitis is characterized by persistent rhinorrhea, postnasal drip, purulent discharge after an upper respiratory tract infection, and a dull throbbing pain over the affected sinus with fever. In younger children, the ethmoid sinuses are commonly involved; whereas in older children and adults, the maxillary and frontal sinuses are most frequently infected. Such acute sinusitis is usually caused by bacterial infection and is associated with pain and pressure over sinuses, headaches, and fever. When complicating allergic rhinitis, sinus disease may be associated with a sore throat, middle ear disease, and characteristically a persistent cough, especially at night. Periorbital edema, facial pallor, and circles under the eyes may be striking. The nasal mucosa is covered with purulent discharge, and a coexisting serous otitis media may be present. With persistent postnasal discharge, bacterial seeding from infected sinuses may result in recurrent bronchitis. Examination of the chest may reveal some wheezing due to a reflex bronchospasm. In the presence of acute bacterial sinusitis, the nasal smear will show a large number of neutrophils rather than the eosinophils of pre-existing allergic disease. Transillumination of the sinuses, though helpful, is not always reliable. Sinus x-rays may reveal opacification, air-fluid level, or marked membrane thickening. However, even in the presence of severe allergic mucosal edema with or without secretions, radiologic changes may be minimal. Chronic antihistamine therapy and topical glucocorticoids may be helpful in preventing recurrent episodes of sinusitis in patients with chronic allergic rhinitis.

Eosinophilic Nonallergic Rhinitis

Some patients with perennial rhinitis are not atopic by history or skin testing. Chronic nasal obstruction is the predominating symptom, and the condition may be associated with sinus disease and nasal polyps. Although there is no evidence of allergy by skin testing, numerous eosinophils are present, and the diagnosis is readily made by examining the nasal secretions for eosinophils (Mullarkey, 1988). The condition is also called nonallergic rhinitis with eosinophilia. Topical glucocorticoid therapy is much more effective than antihistamines or decongestants. As with asthmatics, the patients with associated sinus disease and nasal polyps are at risk for adverse reactions to aspirin and nonsteroidal anti-inflammatory agents.

Vasomotor Rhinitis

A substantial number of patients have chronic rhinitis with rhinorrhea, postnasal drainage, and chronic or intermittent nasal obstruction. Symptoms are aggravated by many factors of a physical or irritating character, such as cold air, odors, and smoke. Skin tests are negative, and there are no eosinophils in the tissues or secretions. No drug therapy is particularly satisfactory, although some patients benefit from antihistamine-decongestant combinations. The regular use of buffered saline lavages may be the most satisfactory treatment.

Allergy in the Eye

Conjunctivitis is the usual ocular reaction to airborne allergens. Itching is the first symptom and may be associated with lacrimation. Dilation of the conjunctival blood vessels produces a red eye. Transudation of fluid through vessel walls results in edema of the conjunctiva, while exuded cells with increased glandular mucous secretion result in ocular "discharge." In most atopic patients, conjunctivitis and allergic rhinitis occur together but some may be bothered only by the eye symptoms. In contrast to other forms of conjunctivitis, the secretions contain eosinophils.

Vernal conjunctivitis is so called because of its occurrence in spring and summer months. It is characterized by a bilateral recurrent inflammation of the conjunctiva. Vernal conjunctivitis commonly occurs between the ages of 5 and 20 years. It often spontaneously resolves in 5 to 10 years. More than 50 per cent of children with vernal conjunctivitis also have an atopic disorder such as allergic rhinitis, eczema, or asthma. Acute itching, tearing, and photophobia occur with excess mucus production. Frequently, a sense of a foreign body in the eye is present. The typical conjunctival appearance as described establishes the diagnosis, which is confirmed by cytologic smears showing numerous eosinophils. In the tarsal (palpebral) form, there are flat-top cobblestone papillae; in the limbal form, gelatinous hypertrophy may be present, with limbal papillary hypertrophy frequently associated with white dots (Trantas' spots). Despite the seasonal nature and the predilection for atopic patients, no allergens have been identified as causal or aggravating factors.

The usual therapy of atopic conjunctivitis is an oral antihistamine and a topical decongestant. Cromolyn (4 per cent ophthalmic solution) is also effective, particularly in preventing the development of anticipated symptoms. Contact lenses should not be worn. In severe cases and in vernal conjunctivitis, a soluble steroid such as a fluorometholone ophthalmic solution is effective. The dose should be titrated to the minimum required to control symptoms. Use should be intermittent, since glucocorticoids can lead to the development of cataracts, can potentiate secondary bacterial infection or a herpes simplex keratitis, and can increase intraocular pressure.

The eyelids rather than the conjunctiva are likely to be involved in angioedema or urticaria. Contact (Type IV) allergy may be caused by various chemicals that may be conveyed by the fingers to the eyelids. Obviously, though, contact allergy to ophthalmic solutions will involve the conjunctiva as well as the eyelids.

Asthma

Asthma is a reversible obstructive disorder of the tracheobronchial tree, characterized by paroxysmal episodes of respiratory distress, often interspersed with periods of apparent well-being. It can begin at any age but most often appears in childhood. It commonly has a familial predisposition; the majority of childhood-onset cases begin between 3 and 6 years of age, and the onset is often associated with a respiratory infection. When the onset is early, prognosis is excellent and most patients improve at puberty. Until puberty, asthma is twice as common among males as females. This distribution reverses between puberty and early adulthood, so that among adults with asthma, females are affected more frequently than males. In many children who have outgrown asthma in puberty there may be a recurrence of asthmatic symptoms later in life. When asthma appears in the adult, remission is less common than in children. Asthma can be conveniently differentiated by etiologic factors into two main groups, as seen in Table 34–2. In *intrinsic asthma* (most commonly seen in adults), symptoms are provoked and worsened by infection, exertion, emotion, and nonspecific environmental factors and are not related to allergen exposure. The majority of *extrinsic* asthma patients are atopic, with symptoms related to environmental allergens. The remaining nonatopic patients have extrinsic asthma related to occupational factors.

Pathophysiology. The characteristic physiologic change in asthma is airway obstruction due to bronchial smooth muscle spasm, mucous plugging, edema, and inflammation of the bronchial wall. As a result of such airway narrowing, inspiration and expiration are impeded. Obstruction of air flow results in air trapping and hyperinflation of lungs. Smooth muscle spasm can occur in the large, medium, or small airways. This airway hyperreactivity is associated with

Table 34–2. CLINICAL FEATURES OF EXTRINSIC AND INTRINSIC ASTHMA

	Extrinsic Asthma		Intrinsic Asthma (idiopathic)
	Atopic	*Nonatopic*	
Age of Onset	Usually childhood	Adult	Usually after age 25
Symptoms	Variable with environment and season	Usually occupation related	Unpredictable fluctuations, often chronic
Associated conditions	Allergic rhinitis, atopic dermatitis	None	Bronchitis, sinusitis, nasal polyps
Family history of atopic disease	Strong	Minor	Asthma only (?)
Skin tests (wheal-erythema)	Several positive, related to history	Negative, or one reaction only	Usually negative
Total IgE	High	Usually normal	Normal
Eosinophilia	High during allergen exposure	Sometimes high during allergen exposure	High
Prognosis	Good, especially with allergen avoidance	Good, especially with allergen avoidance	Fair, remissions uncommon

and probably aggravated by injury to and loss of the epithelial cell lining. When large airways are involved (50 per cent of asthmatic patients), wheezing predominates. When small airways are involved, the predominant symptoms are dyspnea and cough rather than wheezing. With air flow obstruction during an asthmatic attack, there is an increase in residual volume and a decrease in vital capacity proportionate to the degree of severity. With uneven airway obstruction in various parts of the lung, air flow is not uniform, while blood perfusion of the lungs continues through the poorly ventilated segments. The result is arterial hypoxemia, as seen in a reduced PaO_2. In subclinical asthma, the reduced PaO_2 may be the only abnormality. In mild to moderate asthma, the ventilation rate is increased and $PaCO_2$ is reduced while the pH remains normal, expressing compensated respiratory alkalosis. In more severe attacks, with impending respiratory failure, there is alveolar hypoventilation with a rise in $PaCO_2$ and a fall in pH, resulting in a respiratory acidosis. Pulmonary artery pressure increases as a result of air trapping and hyperinflation. In acute and rapidly reversible attacks, bronchospasm is the most significant abnormality; in chronic asthma and more prolonged irreversible acute attacks, dysfunction is due to mucus plugging, edema, and inflammation of the bronchial wall.

It is becoming clear that asthma has both immediate (bronchospastic) and late-phase (inflammatory) components in the response to inhaled allergens and certain other provoking agents (Cockcroft, 1988). The occurrence of this dual asthmatic response has important therapeutic implications.

Approach to the Patient. The history often provides a diagnosis. Asthma should be suspected in any person with unexplained episodes of dyspnea, cough, repeated chest colds, or bronchitis, particularly in children. Even cough by itself may be a symptom of asthma. In evaluation of the acute attack, severity is related to frequency, duration, intensity, response to previous medication with side effects, as well as symptom-free intervals. When symptoms are chronic or continuous, the condition may be confused with irreversible chronic obstructive pulmonary disease. A family history may be positive for asthma or atopy and a search for provocative environmental factors, including occupational exposure, smoking, stress, infection, exercise, and medication (aspirin, propranolol), may yield important information.

Signs. In the symptom-free uncomplicated asthmatic individual, there are no specific findings. However, examination of the upper respiratory tract may reveal signs of allergic rhinitis or the presence of nasal polyps. In children, a comparison of the growth grid is important, since growth retardation may be caused by chronic hypoxemia or previous medication with glucocorticoids, or both. Recording the blood pressure is important, since steroids, adrenergic agents, and theophylline may elevate blood pressure. During an asthmatic episode, the patient presents with difficulty in respiration with an increased respiratory rate, using accessory muscles with suprasternal retraction, pursed lip expiration, and flaring of the nostrils. Cyanosis may be present. Expiration is prolonged with intercostal retraction. There may be evidence of hyperinflation with an increased anteroposterior diameter, hyperresonance, and reduced diaphragmatic excursion. On auscultation, an unevenness of ventilation may be present with high-pitched inspiratory and expiratory dry rales. Rhonchi are accentuated during forced expiration. In children, compression of the chest during expiration may produce latent wheezing. It may be difficult to persuade older children and adolescents to exhale forcefully to induce latent wheezing, since the patient has learned that this might induce coughing and increase bronchial constriction. In patients with marked hyperinflation in whom there is little air exchange, wheezing may be absent. Cardiac dullness may be decreased and the liver edge may be palpable owing to a lowered diaphragm from pulmonary hyperexpansion.

Assessment. To supplement the *history and physical examination*, the response to a bronchial dilator may be used to establish the presence of reversible obstructive lung disease. To do this, the ventilatory function, using a forced expiration volume in one second (FEV_1), is measured before and after the patient inhales an aerosol of a bronchodilator drug. If there is no change, the patient may be retested after a subcutaneous injection of 1:1000 epinephrine. Examination of sputum is simple and can be done quickly. A predominance of lymphocytes suggest viral respiratory infection, whereas a predominance of neutrophils and ingested bacteria is indicative of secondary infection. Sputum analysis in an acute attack in the absence of infection usually shows some ciliated columnar epithelial cells, eosinophilia greater than 20 per cent, and varying amounts of neutrophils. With bronchial or bronchopulmonary infection, neutrophils predominate with lower ranges of eosinophils (5 to 20 per cent). Worsening of asthma symptoms is usually accompanied by an increase in total blood eosinophil count. Depression of the blood eosinophil count and sputum eosinophilia is seen with glucocorticoid therapy, and this response is occasionally used to assess the adequacy of the dosage.

The complete blood count is often normal. Moderate leukocytosis does not necessarily indicate infection. Inflammation and stress of the disease, fear or crying in a young individual, and epinephrine administration all can elevate the white count. Although blood eosinophilia is common in asthma, it may be suppressed by stress, epinephrine, or steroid therapy at the time the patient is being assessed.

A chest x-ray study is not often helpful in the evaluation of noncomplicated asthma, since it is usually normal. However, it provides a baseline for future comparison. In adults, chest x-ray studies may not be necessary with each episode in patients with predictable recurrent attacks. However, in young children first presenting with asthma, it is important to differentiate asthma from bronchiolitis in infancy. A chest x-ray study is also useful in ruling out a congenital anomaly or the presence of a foreign body. If the asthmatic attack is sufficiently severe to require hospitalization, an admitting chest x-ray study is advisable to rule out infiltrates, atelectasis, and free air in the chest, mediastinum, or soft tissues. A majority of asthmatics will show hyperinflation with increased bronchial markings and flattening of the diaphragm during an acute episode.

The total serum IgE is not particularly useful information for the management of asthma. It is normal in intrinsic asthma but not always elevated in extrinsic asthma. Its main significance is as an aid in diagnosing bronchopulmonary aspergillosis, which commonly has markedly elevated serum IgE levels.

Skin tests are selected according to the information obtained from the history. Obvious limitations are present, since some ubiquitous allergens may not be identified by history alone. The value of skin testing is greatest in the extrinsic asthmatic patient when respirable allergens are suspected from the history to be clinically significant causative agents. When all tests are negative, skin testing helps to establish the diagnosis of intrinsic asthma.

Pulmonary Function Tests. Pulmonary function tests provide information important in assessing airway function in the long-term evaluation of bronchial asthma. In the use of office spirometry, it is important to determine the "normal" pulmonary function value for each individual, since predicted limits are derived from a normal reference population and the individual's asymptomatic normal value may not conform with that population. In general, determination of pulmonary function in children less than 5 to 6 years of age is not practical, since cooperation may not be optimal.

The clinical picture of obstructive airways disease is characterized by a slow loss of ability to expel air from the lung. The decreased maximum expiratory flow rate can be measured by spirometry in the office setting. In the use of spirometry, the patient is first instructed thoroughly in the performance of the test. Conditions during testing should be consistent. Test results are valid only if the patient developed a maximal expiratory effort following full inspiration. The technician operating the pulmonary function equipment should first demonstrate how to perform the test. Reliable spirometric tests depend on individual motivation in addition to proper technique. When the patient has pain or a coughing spasm, maximal expiratory effort is not achieved. Premature termination of expiration or a Valsalva maneuver during the expiration produces errors. In general, no more than three consecutive spirometry tests are advisable for measuring pulmonary functions at any given time, since additional effort by an asthmatic patient can induce bronchospasm with progressive decrease in the flow rate.

Since an important use of pulmonary function tests is to determine the degree of reversibility of airways obstruction, bronchodilating medication should be discontinued at least 6 hours before this test. A baseline pulmonary function is first obtained and then repeated 15 minutes after inhaling a bronchodilating drug. In normal subjects, no change is observed in pulmonary function after the inhalation of a bronchodilator. In patients with reversible obstructive airways disease and a low baseline flow rate, significant improvement should occur (more than 15 to 20 per cent in the FEV_1, or peak flow rate). If no change occurs after inhalation of the bronchodilator, the patient may have irreversible airway disease (chronic bronchitis and emphysema) or the airway obstruction may be primarily due to inflammation and respond only to glucocorticoid therapy.

In patients who do not have abnormal pulmonary function when examined but complain of symptoms occurring at other times that suggest asthma, a bronchial challenge with histamine or methacholine (Provocholine) may be useful. Although bronchial challenge can be used to demonstrate that the bronchi are or are not hyperactive, which can rule out the diagnosis of asthma, such testing when positive is potentially dangerous and should be done only by experienced, properly equipped personnel. It can be particularly useful in consideration of occupational asthma. The bronchoprovocation test using inhaled allergen is rarely necessary. It may produce an immediate fall in lung function but may also produce a 6- to 8-hour delayed response. Again it should be undertaken only by experts in a controlled setting.

Differential Diagnosis. In children, it is important to differentiate asthma from bronchiolitis in infancy, bronchitis, croup, epiglottitis, and aspiration of a foreign body. An inspiratory stridor differentiates hypertrophic tonsils, laryngeal disease, subglottic stenosis, or a foreign body from asthma. Among the chronic conditions, childhood cystic fibrosis is distinguished by malabsorption and failure to thrive and a sweat chloride concentration greater than 60 mEq./l. In young adults, hyperventilation is generally associated with anxiety and nonpulmonary symptoms, and its relief through relaxation with reassurance often differentiates it from asthma. Rebreathing from a bag is helpful, though this is not advisable during an acute attack or when hypoxemia is suspected. In the older patients, pulmonary embolism may be differentiated by a history of predisposing factors (thrombophlebitis, cardiac failure, oral contraceptives, prolonged bedrest, or malignancy). Cardiac asthma may be associated with a history of cardiac disease, moist rales in the chest, and a third heart sound, which distinguish it from asthma. Cardiac asthma is usually exhibited as such in a patient with underlying obstructive lung disease who develops heart failure.

Management. The aim of management is to keep the patient as symptom-free as possible with minimal medication. It is essential that the patient understand the disease and its precipitating and aggravating factors and recognize its early manifestations so that an acute episode can be treated early in order to forestall hospitalization. Recognition of the emotional impact of asthma from a personal, family, and work standpoint can facilitate an acceptance of the limitations of the disease without overreaction and frustration. In school children, problems can be reduced by providing guidelines to parents and teachers in relation to appropriate activity. Asthmatic patients can be taught to practice relaxed breathing in association with meditation or autohypnosis to decrease the anxiety and to prevent the panic that is often associated with the onset of acute symptoms. Breathing instructions include conscious slow exhalation through pursed lips while allowing the abdominal muscles to relax and, at the same time, monitoring diaphragmatic movement with a hand placed on the upper abdomen. In children, if major allergens identified cannot be eliminated or avoided, immunotherapy can be useful. Compliance in drug therapy is particularly important.

For a patient with mild paroxysmal asthma, a beta_2-adrenergic bronchodilator, such as metaproterenol or albuterol, administered by a metered dose inhaler (1 to 3 inhalations, spaced 5 minutes apart) usually provides relief for at least 6 hours. More sustained relief, especially at night, can be provided with a long-acting (8- to 12-hour) theophylline preparation given around the clock. An oral beta_2-adrenergic drug may provide some additional benefit, but usually has no advantage over and more side effects than the same drug given by inhalation. Patient response determines the duration of treatment, which is best continued for 2 to 3 days during which the patient is symptom free.

When the patient with an acute attack of asthma does not respond to the measures outlined above, management should proceed in a controlled setting such as an emergency room of a hospital. Measurements of blood gases are obtained to assess the severity of the attack. The patient is treated first with a nebulized beta-adrenergic bronchodilator. In younger adults and in the absence of cardiac disease, this treatment can be supplemented with subcutaneous epinephrine or terbutaline if necessary. The nebulizer treatment can be repeated hourly and the subcutaneous drug once in 20 to 30 minutes. Improvement in bronchospasm is usually rapid. If response is sustained, the patient can be discharged on oral and inhaled bronchodilator therapy with appropriate follow-up. If the PaO_2 is below 60 mm. of mercury, supplemental humidified oxygen is administered at 2 to 4 l. per minute and blood gases should be re-evaluated to maintain the PaO_2 level above 65 torr. Intravenous fluids should then be given. Aminophylline may be added, I.V., although there is now mounting evidence that it offers no additional benefit over adequate adrenergic therapy in emergency room management. The usual loading dose of aminophylline is 6 mg. per kg. over 20 to 30 minutes, with a lower dosage used if oral theophylline has been taken recently. Infusion of aminophylline in a maintenance dose of 0.5 mg. per kg. per hour is continued with monitoring of serum theophylline levels. In patients who have needed glucocorticoid therapy in the past or are on a maintenance regimen of glucocorticoid, an intravenous infusion of methylprednisolone of 125 mg. is advisable. When sufficiently improved, the patient can be sent home with instructions to take oral steroid and bronchodilator drugs regularly for several days with appropriate follow-up. If the patient is not responsive to therapy as outlined, hospitalization for status asthmaticus is required for more intense management. A typical asthma therapy flow chart for emergency room use is depicted in Figure 34–1.

Status Asthmaticus. A patient is considered to have status asthmaticus when severe asthma is unresponsive to the usual emergency methods of treatment and ventilatory failure is imminent. Status asthmaticus has a 1 to 3 per cent mortality risk and is a medical emergency requiring prompt hospital management. While there may be no obvious precipitating factors, status asthmaticus may be triggered by inhaled allergens or irritants, a viral respiratory infection, an emotional crisis, or medication (especially steroid) withdrawal. Some patients may have a premonitory pattern, with increasing disability and wheezing associated with scantier, more tenacious

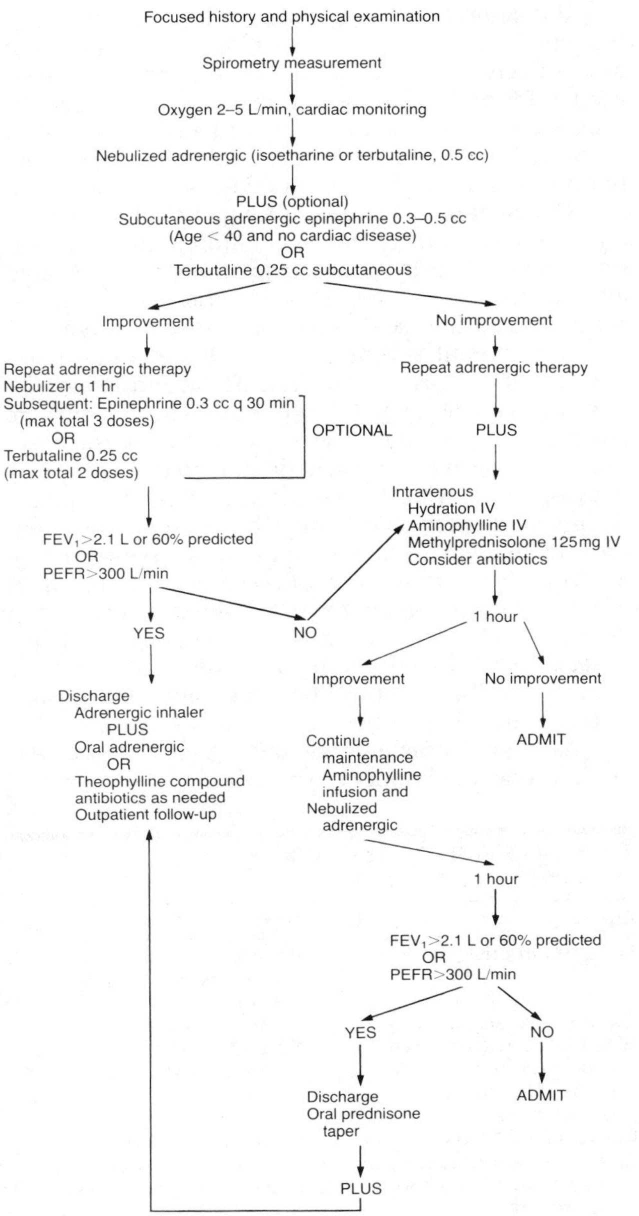

Figure 34–1. Flow chart for management of acute asthma. (From Eisenberg, M. S., and Copass, M. K. [Eds.]: Emergency Medical Therapy. 3rd ed. Philadelphia, W. B. Saunders Co., 1988, p. 454.)

sputum and a decreased efficacy of maintenance therapy. The patient is usually anxious, irritable, and tachypneic, with tachycardia and impaired speech due to labored breathing.

Status asthmaticus must be aggressively treated. The following changes provide an indication of severity. A paradoxical pulse correlates with an FEV_1 of less than 20 per cent of the predicted level. An arterial blood PCO_2 of 45 mm. Hg or more and a PO_2 of 60 mm. Hg or less indicates the patient has developed alveolar hypoventilation due to either fatigue of the respiratory muscle or a depression of respiratory-centered drive. This is an ominous sign. If the patient is able to cooperate, pulmonary function tests before and after treatment with a bronchodilator also provide information on severity, since an FEV_1 of less than 10 per cent of the predicted level, nonresponsive to bronchodilator therapy in the presence of hypoxemia and metabolic acidosis, indicates ventilatory failure requiring intubation and intensive care therapy. Other obvious parameters for hospitalization and intensive care are disturbance of consciousness; a "silent chest," in which air movement is too inadequate to generate a wheeze; and obvious pneumothorax or pneumomediastinum.

In general, sedation should be avoided, especially if the $PaCO_2$ is normal or elevated, to prevent depression of a central ventilatory drive, which can augment hypoventilation and cause respiratory acidosis. If necessary, hydroxyzine or benzodiazepine may be used cautiously for severe anxiety or to counteract the central effects of drug therapy. Barbiturates and phenothiazines are contraindicated, since they can depress the respiratory center and bronchial reflexes and often add to a confusional state secondary to decreased cerebral blood flow.

Management of Chronic Asthma. Asthma is chronic if the patient has daily symptoms and requires regular medication to remain symptom free. Management includes oral theophylline on a regular schedule, sufficient to achieve a therapeutic serum level of 10 to 20 μg./ml., which may need close monitoring for compliance. Acute symptoms can be treated as needed with a $beta_2$-adrenergic agonist delivered from a metered-dose inhaler. Cromolyn sodium can be used in the patient with extrinsic asthma either to prevent allergen-induced attacks or after steroids have produced maximal improvement and are being tapered. If effective, treatment can be continued, with regular attempts to lower the dosage by dropping one dose every 1 to 2 weeks. Cromolyn sodium should be discontinued in an acute asthmatic attack. In the chronic patient who is resistant to bronchodilator therapy and threatened with steroid dependence, a trial of beclomethasone inhalation for 4 weeks (2 to 4 inhalations, i.e., 100 to 200 μg., four times daily) can be effective if given when ventilatory function is still fairly good. Such inhalations can be given in conjunction with oral glucocorticoids to reduce the systemic dosage. If these inhalations themselves cause bronchospasm, pretreatment with a metaproterenol or albuterol inhalation (15 to 20 minutes before the beclomethasone inhalation) can facilitate peripheral penetration. Rinsing of the throat and mouth after inhalations of beclomethasone can decrease risks of oropharyngeal candidiasis. If continuous oral glucocorticoid therapy is necessary, giving the drug on alternate days will minimize side effects; however, asthma often appears on the day when the drug is not given. In the patient with chronic asthma who has thick tenacious sputum, maintenance of a high fluid intake is important.

In the long-term management of chronic asthma with frequent flare-ups related to hyperreactive airways, the value of long-term use of cromolyn and glucocorticoid therapy is just now being appreciated. Both drugs inhibit the late, or inflammatory, phase of asthma, whereas beta-adrenergic bronchodilators and theophylline do not. Cromolyn may have some advantage over glucocorticoids because of its complete lack of systemic side effects, but glucocorticoids are effective in a higher proportion of patients. Whether treatment with both drugs together has any advantage over either one alone has yet to be determined (König, 1988).

Some other drugs are used under special or investigative circumstances for treatment of patients with severe, chronic steroid-dependent asthma. These include troleandomycin (with methylprednisolone), methotrexate, and gold salts. Their use is beyond the scope of this chapter.

One other drug should be mentioned in part because it has recently been approved by the FDA for use. Ipratropium bromide is an anticholinergic bronchodilator available in this country in a metered-dose inhaler. Its main usefulness is in treatment of patients with bronchospasm associated with chronic bronchitis and emphysema (Gross, 1988). Its effect in asthmatic patients is variable; generally it is less effective than an adrenergic agent, and it has no effect on the late-phase asthmatic reaction. Being available only in a metered-dose inhaler, it is not very useful for emergency treatment.

Exercise-Induced Asthma. Asthma following exercise is common in children and young adults. It is usually brief and indistinguishable from asthma due to other causes. Some patients have asthma only after exercise. Patients may complain of mild chest tightness, irritation, and cough, or they may wheeze overtly and become severely short of breath and disabled when severe hypoxia may be present.

The most reliable method for evaluation of exercise-induced asthma is an exercise challenge, which can be easily performed in an office setting. Pulmonary functions using a peak flow meter or spirometer are usually measured before exercise. The pulmonary response is assessed after 5 to 8 minutes of a slow run. A decrease of 10 per cent in the peak expiratory flow rate or 12 to 15 per cent in the FEV_1 is considered abnormal. A change of 30 to 45 per cent is considered a moderately severe response and a change greater than 45 per cent, a severe response. Epinephrine and oxygen should be on hand for rare emergencies during exercise testing.

Treatment of Exercise-Induced Asthma. In general, exercise-induced asthma is not a contraindication to activity. Particularly in children in whom physical activity is a major part of normal development, counseling can provide a choice for an appropriate activity that is least likely to induce asthma. Swimming, baseball, gymnastics, and golf are usually well-tolerated. In general, some individuals may need to have restrictions from time to time, particularly on cold days or when environmental pollution or the pollen load is heavy. Such restrictions when adequately understood are usually accepted.

Premedication can prevent asthmatic attacks by the inhalation of cromolyn or an adrenergic drug immediately before exercise. When theophylline is used 1 1/2 to 2 hours before exercise, a therapeutic drug level is achieved for full effectiveness at the time of exercise. For international athletic competition, the use of adrenergic bronchodilators is not allowed.

Occupational Asthma. Occupational asthma is due to an agent or agents encountered at work. It is often aggravated by nonspecific stimuli such as cold air, exercise, smoking, and respiratory infections. Symptoms such as acute bronchospasm or cough may not appear until several hours after the worker has left the place of work, so that the diagnosis may be difficult. Cough may be superimposed on chronic obstructive pulmonary disease, with airways obstruction unresponsive to bronchodilators in the workplace but responsive when tested outside of the workplace. Recurrent "chest colds" may be present, with improvement away from work and recrudescence 1 to 2 weeks after returning to work. The deleterious effect of the work environment is determined by measuring the peak expiratory flow rate at regular intervals for 2 weeks at work and 1 week at home, differentiating between work exposure values and nonwork exposure values. Table 34–3 lists common causal agents.

Allergic Bronchopulmonary Aspergillosis. Allergic bronchopulmonary aspergillosis is an immedi-

Table 34–3. AGENTS THAT CAUSE OCCUPATIONAL ASTHMA

Agents	Workers at Risk
Flour, grain dust, mites	Bakers, millers, dock workers, farmers, silo workers
Cotton, flax, sisal, hemp	Textile workers
Wood dusts (western red cedar, redwood, mahogany, other hardwoods)	Sawmill workers, carpenters, builders
Cork dust (suberosis)	Cork makers, lumbermen
Epoxy resins (phthalic anhydride, triethylene tetramine)	Plastics, adhesives, synthetic rubber makers
Metals (nickel, cobalt, platinum, chromates)	Metal and chromium platers, metal refiners, grinders, jewelers
Enzymes (*Bacillus subtilis*)	Detergent industry workers
Coffee bean dust	Coffee workers
Polyvinyl chloride	Meat wrappers
Ammonia, chlorine, sulfur dioxide, hydrochloric acid	Chemical, petroleum, and papermill workers
Henna extracts, persulfates	Hairdressers
Organic phosphorus	Farmers
Soldering fluxes, rosin (colophony)	Electrical solderers, hot-melt glue workers, chemists, feather pluckers
Formaldehyde, formalin, toluene diisocyanate	Plastic molders, medical technicians
Penicillin, sulfonamides, piperazine, cimetidine, propranolol	Pharmaceutical workers
Animal dander, rat urine protein	Laboratory technicians, veterinarians, farmers

ate hypersensitivity and immune complex disease caused by *Aspergillus fumigatus*. It is associated with a history of asthma in atopic adult patients. It presents with episodes of wheezing, fever, cough productive of brownish plugs, and dyspnea. Leukocytosis and eosinophilia occur in both blood and sputum. Microscopy of the sputum often yields the fungus. Culture when repeatedly positive suggests the diagnosis. Transient or fixed pulmonary infiltrates are seen radiologically. Bronchoscopy or tomograms often reveal proximal bronchiectasis. The prick skin test with *Aspergillus* antigen is positive in 15 minutes.An intradermal test, if done, may produce a dual reaction at 15 minutes and in 6 to 8 hours. Precipitating antibodies to *Aspergillus* and elevated serum IgE confirm the diagnosis.

During acute episodes, bronchodilators (and antibiotics, if bacterial infection is present) are helpful in controlling symptoms, but oral prednisone, 25 to 50 mg. per day, is the treatment of choice. After 2 weeks, this can be tapered to an alternate-day regimen and stopped after 3 months. Repeat courses of steroids may be necessary. When untreated, destruction of lung tissue progresses to recurrent irreversible bronchiectasis and pulmonary fibrosis with eventual respiratory failure (Patterson et al., 1986).

Drug Treatment and Pregnancy

During pregnancy, the increase in chorionic gonadotropin and plasma cortisol and a slight increase in cyclic AMP combine to reduce the effects of histamine release. In addition, serum IgE levels tend to decrease in pregnancy. Asthma improves in approximately one third of pregnant asthmatic patients, slightly more than one third remain the same, and less than one third worsen. In women with mild asthma prior to pregnancy, there is likely to be little change or some improvement during pregnancy. In women with severe asthma, there is a tendency for the condition to worsen during pregnancy. If asthma worsened during the initial pregnancy, it is likely to worsen during subsequent pregnancies, and this may reflect a general worsening of asthma with time.

Treatment in the first trimester should be limited to essential medications to prevent maternal hypoxemia. Uncontrolled asthma leading to hypoxemia is a greater risk to the fetus than any of the usual drugs. Conventional therapy with theophylline is not associated with teratogenic effects, and cromolyn sodium can be used for prevention of attacks. Glucocorticoids should be used only when absolutely necessary to control asthma adequately. If steroids have been used during pregnancy, supplemental steroids may be necessary at delivery. An acceptable schedule is hydrocortisone acetate 100 mg. intramuscularly every 8 hours through labor and delivery. Newborns of mothers treated with high-dose glucocorticoid therapy should be observed for adrenal insufficiency.

Decongestants have not been established as safe during pregnancy. If used, they should be used sparingly and given topically if possible. Pseudoephedrine may be the safest oral decongestant. Judicious use of some antihistamines such as diphenhydramine (Benadryl), tripelennamine (Pyribenzamine), and chlorpheniramine (Chlor-Trimeton) is considered acceptable during pregnancy, but all should be used sparingly, especially during the first trimester (Weber and Nelson, 1986).

Severe antigen-induced systemic reactions during immunotherapy have produced lower abdominal cramping and uterine bleeding. Although no adverse fetal effects have been reported, immunotherapy should not be started during pregnancy, and the dose of each ongoing immunotherapy injection should be kept constant or decreased during the pregnancy (Weber and Nelson, 1986).

Breastfeeding. Less than 1 per cent of oral theophylline appears in the breast milk. At therapeutic blood levels in the mother, the infant would receive only about 2 mg. per kg. per 24 hours. Occasionally, infant hyperirritability has been attributed to maternal theophylline therapy. No known adverse effects have been related to beta-adrenergic bronchodilators in the breast milk. Although secreted in trace amounts in breast milk, antihistamines do not have adverse effects on the infant other than sleepiness. Secretion of glucocorticoids in breast milk is less than 1 per cent of the administered dose and never approaches the normal amount produced by the fetus. There is no contraindication to immunotherapy of the nursing mother. Antigens used may be secreted in trace amounts; however, absorption by the infant is considered to be clinically unimportant.

Hypersensitivity Pneumonitis

Hypersensitivity pneumonitis is an infiltrative lung disease caused by inhaled antigen and may become manifest as a combination of Type 3 (immune complex) and Type 4 (delayed or cellular hypersensitivity) immunologic reactions. Individual susceptibility varies. Clinical manifestations include fever, chills, malaise, and cough rather than bronchospasm and wheezing, developing 4 to 6 hours after exposure to the antigen. Pulmonary function tests reveal restrictive rather than obstructive lung disease, and the chest x-ray film will show signs of alveolitis. Examples of commonly seen conditions produced by the antigens are mushroom worker's disease, farmer's lung, maple bark stripper's disease, cheese workers's lung, and pigeon breeder's disease. A high index of suspicion often leads to the diagnosis. Environmental caution and the use of glucocorticoids are the mainstays of management.

Atopic Dermatitis

Atopic dermatitis is a chronic or relapsing, highly pruritic skin eruption that usually develops in patients with a personal or family history of respiratory atopic problems. The problem usually develops in infancy or early childhood. Onset occurs after the age of 5 in only about 10 per cent of cases. In contrast with other forms of infantile eczema, atopic dermatitis rarely appears before the infant is 2 months old.

The pathogenesis of atopic dermatitis is complex and only partially understood. The physiologic response of the skin is abnormal. There is an increased tendency for diaphoresis, yet sebum production is low and generalized dryness is often a problem. The response of the cutaneous vasculature is diagnostic. Stroking the skin produces vasoconstriction rather than vasodilation (white dermographism) and injection of methacholine produces the gradual appearance of vasoconstriction (the "delayed blanch" phenomenon) rather than erythema and wheal formation. Usually, there is no flare response to histamine either. In addition, there is some experimental evidence, mostly indirect, that the skin responds abnormally to adrenergic stimuli (Hanifin, 1982).

The central problem is itch. The above-described abnormalities are contributory to, or at least associated with, a low itch threshold. Any stimuli, including allergens, irritants, emotional stress, and the irritation produced by scratching, can aggravate itching. Once the skin is inflamed, it is entirely possible that the itch-scratch cycle can lead to a chronic problem in the absence of any other aggravating factors. Allergens are not of primary importance in the pathogenesis of atopic dermatitis, since as many as 20 per cent of patients have low serum levels of IgE and few, if any, positive allergen skin test reactions. However, allergens, especially foods, can induce or aggravate symptoms such as pruritus, erythema and edema, as determined by double-blind oral challenge studies (Sampson, 1986).

The clinical features vary with age. In infants, the lesions often appear on the face first and may extend to the scalp, trunk, and extensor aspects of the extremities. Vesiculation, oozing, and crusting are prominent, and secondary infection is common. In older children, the lesions tend to localize in flexural sites: the antecubital and popliteal fossae and the neck in particular. Vesiculation is less prominent; the lesions are papular and with time become lichenified. Generalized dryness of the skin is a common problem. If remission does not occur and the inflammation is not adequately controlled, the lesions become progressively lichenified—especially in the flexural area—and scattered excoriated, crusted papules commonly occur on the face, forearms, and hands, and even the wrists. The lesions of about 80 per cent of children under 2 years of age with atopic dermatitis will gradually clear up as they get older, but the remainder will have a chronic relapsing problem indefinitely, often into adult life. The clinical appearance is similar in adults.

Resistance to infection is impaired in some patients in proportion to the severity of the disease. The more severe cases of atopic dermatitis may be associated with host-defense deficiencies, but how these relate to the pathogenesis is uncertain. There is no doubt that many patients with atopic dermatitis have impaired T-cell function and relative cutaneous anergy and, thus, are at considerable risk for development of disseminated viral or fungal infection. An impaired T-cell suppressor function may be one of the reasons for elevated IgE production. During severe atopic dermatitis, neutrophil and monocyte chemotaxis is also impaired. Generalized vaccinia, sometimes fatal, was a serious risk when smallpox vaccination was in common use. Generalized herpetic infection is still a threat; and the susceptibility to other viruses—for example, warts and molluscum contagiosum—is substantial. Excoriations, vesiculation, and probably the chemotactic defects mentioned earlier render patients vulnerable to superficial staphylococcal or streptoccal infections.

Acute lesions, especially in infants, contain vesicles, and in chronic lesions, hyperkeratosis is prominent and there is an increased number of mast cells in the tissue. The histopathologic appearance of atopic dermatitis is inflammatory with mononuclear cells and occasional plasma cells. Only a small proportion of infiltrating cells are eosinophils or basophils.

The laboratory is of limited value in making the diagnosis of atopic dermatitis. An increased blood eosinophil count or serum IgE level, or both, may be helpful, for example, in excluding the diagnosis of seborrheic dermatitis in an infant; but the diagnosis can usually be made on clinical grounds. One would expect skin tests for IgE-mediated sensitivity to be positive to several inhaled and ingested allergens in these patients, and such information may be helpful in confirming the atopic state but not in establishing the cause.

Treatment is directed at relieving pruritus, controlling infection, and promoting healing. The patient or parent must understand that topical therapy is of primary importance in management. Acute, vesicular, exudative, crusting dermatitis is treated with cool dressings of Burow's solution several times daily. An oral antihistaminic such as diphenhydramine (Benadryl) or hydroxyzine (Atarax) aids in relieving pruritus. Scratching may be minimized by trimming fingernails or having the patient wear cotton gloves at night. A short course of systemic glucocorticoid therapy may be necessary. Appropriate antibacterial therapy may hasten recovery.

Except during the acute exudative phase, the foundation of topical therapy consists of an emollient for dry skin and a glucocorticoid for inflammation. There are many emollient creams, lotions, and ointments available, and the patient should be advised to obtain small supplies of several types of emollients to find out which is most effective. Preparations containing 10 per cent urea may be particularly effective in treatment of dry skin. A fluorinated steroid cream or ointment (whichever one of the many on the market is chosen) should be used in the lowest effective concentration available to minimize both side effects and cost. Because of the risk of skin atrophy and telangiectasis as local side effects of the fluorinated steroids, they should not be used on the face; hydrocortisone or a similar nonfluorinated steroid cream should be used instead. Conventional bathing, which promotes dry skin, should be avoided. Instead, the patient should use a nonlipid cleansing solution such as Cetaphil. Regular use of hydroxyzine as an oral antipruritic drug is often helpful; antihistamines should never be applied topically.

Most patients with atopic dermatitis will be sensitive to some allergens as determined by skin tests. As an adjunct to topical therapy, an empirical trial of environmental control (minimizing contact with dust, feathers, animals, and irritant substances such as wool garments) may be worthwhile. Also, a trial elimination of foods, such as wheat, eggs, nuts, and legumes, may be helpful—especially in youngsters below age 2. Skin testing for food and inhalant allergens might add some information if the empiric trials are inconclusive, but positive tests should be interpreted conservatively and in a way consistent with the history and, perhaps, food-challenge testing (Sampson, 1986).

Urticaria and Angioedema

The pruritic evanescent, edematous, erythematous, and circumscribed lesions (or hives) are familiar to physician and layman alike. They can vary widely in size, from pinhead-sized papules to the size of a rather large pancake. Angioedema may occur alone, but often occurs with urticaria. It is deeper, more diffuse, and likely to develop in thin, distensible, subcutaneous tissue such as lips, eyelids, genitalia, and mucous membranes.

The appearance of the lesions suggests that the pathogenesis of urticaria involves a Type I hypersensitivity mechanism: the IgE antibody-antigen triggering of the release of histamine and other vasoactive mediators from mast cells. This is often the case in acute urticaria, but in many cases of acute, and most of chronic, urticaria the trigger responsible for mediator release is unknown. The histologic appearance of urticaria is usually simple. Edema fluid separates collagen fibers and bundles, particularly in the reticular dermis. There are few inflammatory cells, and those that exist are perivascular. In a few cases, the biopsy shows vasculitis in addition to edema.

About 20 per cent of the population has experienced acute urticaria at least once. However, at any given time, the prevalence is little more than 1 in 1000. Of these, about two thirds have chronic urticaria. Whether the problem is acute or chronic, each urticarial wheal develops and then fades away over a space of a few hours. Persisting lesions should raise the question of vasculitis.

Urticaria is a disease of diversity, and its complex classification is outlined in Table 34–4. Allergic urticaria is usually acute and mediated by IgE antibody. By far the most common cases are reactions to drugs, stinging insect venoms, and allergenic extracts used in immunotherapy. In older children and adults, the skin and gastrointestinal tract are fairly effective barriers to allergens. Only the atopic person who is extremely sensitive is likely to react to an ingested food or to contact of an allergen with the unbroken skin. Urticaria due to an inhaled allergen is extremely rare.

Certain drugs can cause release of histamine directly; allergy is not involved. Radiographic contrast media, polymyxins, tubocurarine, and opiates can produce such toxic-idiosyncratic reactions. Contact urticaria can be a toxic effect of dimethyl sulfoxide and formaldehyde. Shellfish and certain fruits, when eaten in large amounts, can produce "urticaria

Table 34–4. CLASSIFICATION OF URTICARIA AND ANGIOEDEMA

I. Allergic
- a. Drugs
- b. Foods, food additives
- c. Contact allergens
- d. Inhaled allergens
- e. Venoms and other injectables

II. Toxic
- a. Histamine-releasing drugs and chemicals
- b. Foods

III. Intrinsic Host Abnormalities
- a. Increased stores of mediator
  - Urticaria pigmentosa
  - Systemic mastocytosis
- b. Physical sensitivity, nonfamilial
  - Cholinergic
  - Cold: Sporadic—IgE; Secondary
  - Light: 6 types—IgE
  - Dermographism—IgE
  - Pressure
  - Aquagenic
  - Decompression
- c. Genetic (all autosomal dominant traits)
  - Familial cold
  - Localized heat
  - Vibratory
  - Urticaria with deafness, limb pain, and amyloidosis
  - Erythropoietic protoporphyria
  - Hereditary angioedema

IV. Underlying Disease
- a. Infection
  - Viral: Hepatitis B, infectious mononucleosis, rubella, Coxsackie virus
  - Fungal: *Candida albicans*
  - Parasitic
- b. Other
  - Malignancy, especially lymphomas
  - Systemic lupus erythematosus
  - Vasculitis
  - Polycythemia vera
  - Porphyria
  - Sjögren's syndrome

V. Contributing Factors
- Alcohol ingestion
- Coffee and other stimulants
- Exercise
- Fever
- Emotional stress, depression
- Hyperthyroidism
- Pregnancy

VI. Unknown
- Idiopathic mast cell lability (?)

of gluttony." Coffee, alcoholic beverages, and aspirin may aggravate urticaria on a nonallergic basis.

The physical urticarias include three fairly common ones that can be mediated by IgE antibodies. It is thought that the antibodies are directed at some dermal proteins that are altered by the physical trauma and thus appear to be "foreign." Cholinergic urticaria is also fairly common. It is a unique generalized eruption consisting of highly pruritic small wheals that are often surrounded by a large flare. The eruption can be provoked by emotional stress, heat, or exercise. Indeed, an exercise test is the most reliable way to confirm the diagnosis.

All the familial conditions are rare. Hereditary angioedema is discussed here because it may be life threatening and can be very effectively treated. It is characterized by an indurated, edematous, subcutaneous swelling that develops spontaneously or following trauma or infection. The reaction is not pruritic. It may be preceded by evanescent reticulate erythema but is never associated with urticaria. It may occur in any cutaneous or mucous membrane location, including the bowel. Crampy gastrointestinal symptoms, sometimes mimicking bowel obstruction, occur at one time or another in almost everyone with the disease. Although it is hereditary, the family history may be negative; and the first symptoms do not necessarily appear during childhood.

The inherited defect in hereditary angioedema is a lack or dysfunction of a serum inhibitor of the activated first component of complement (C1 esterase). When complement is activated, the reaction accelerates without restraint in the absence of this inhibitor and leads to generation of potent vasoactive kinins. The diagnosis can be made by assay for inhibitor function or by measuring C4 (the fourth component of complement), which is almost always low, even between attacks. Treatment is specific and highly effective. The impeded androgens stanozolol and danazol prevent attacks by improving synthesis of the functional inhibitor (Sheffer et al., 1987).

Acute urticaria is a fairly common event during viral infections. It may be the first sign of hepatitis B infection; the surface antigen has been identified in the dermis of some patients. However, infection is an unusual cause of chronic urticaria. Although some have claimed that many cases are caused by sensitivity to a low-grade *Candida* infection, that occurrence has not been our experience. Also, a search for a parasitic disease is rarely productive.

Urticaria may be the first sign of some other underlying disease, such as lymphoma and systemic lupus erythematosus. Invariably, other manifestations of these diseases will soon appear. Cutaneous vasculitis, diagnosed by the presence of persistent lesions and a positive biopsy, should produce other lesions such as palpable purpura in due time, but sometimes urticaria remains the only visible manifestation. It is not known whether or not the prognosis for this type of urticaria differs from that for chronic urticaria.

Among the contributing factors, emotional stress is often discussed. In fact, it is not often a recognizable problem except in patients with cholinergic urticaria.

No cause can be identified in about 75 per cent of patients with chronic urticaria (Monroe, 1981). Once established, it may continue as an annoying but benign disease for several years.

In evaluating the patient with acute urticaria and angioedema, one should expect the cause to be fairly obvious from the history alone in many patients. If a viral infection is responsible, time alone will provide the answer. (Incidentally, the first signs of infection may precede the appearance of urticaria by several days. If an antibiotic is given before urticaria appears, the eruption may be falsely attributed to drug allergy.) Occasionally skin testing is helpful to differentiate food allergy from overindulgence. Perhaps half the cases of acute urticaria will not have an identifiable cause.

The patient with chronic urticaria should be questioned carefully about the chronic use of drugs and remedies and foods containing dyes, preservatives, and other additives. Skin testing for Type I allergy is rarely helpful. Underlying disease should be excluded by means of a thorough physical examination and routine screening laboratory tests. However, such screening tests and the more specialized serum complement tests so rarely detect an underlying disease that their cost effectiveness is questionable (Jacobson et al., 1980).

Treatment of acute urticaria, whether the cause is identified or not, consists of hydroxyzine or diphenhydramine to relieve itching. Since it is nonsedating, terfenadine may be more acceptable for some patients but is likely to be less effective than the others. If the reaction is severe, especially if angioedema threatens the airway, then subcutaneous and topical epinephrine should also be given (which is discussed in the systemic allergy section). Hydroxyzine is an effective drug for treatment of most patients with chronic or recurrent urticaria. Cyproheptadine may be more effective in some patients, particularly those with cold urticaria. Doxepin may be effective in others. Patients who are not well controlled by one of these drugs sometimes have been helped by the addition of an H_2-antihistamine or the beta-adrenergic drug terbutaline; in our experience, though, the results have been disappointing. Patients should be counseled to try to avoid aggravating factors such as coffee, aspirin, and stress and should be reassured about the benign nature of chronic urticaria, which often remits spontaneously.

Allergic Contact Dermatitis

This is a pruritic eruption that progresses from erythema and induration to a vesiculobullous state if contact with the offending substance continues. It is produced by substances that are not primary skin irritants or are irritating to the skin only in unusually high concentrations. As with any allergic state, contact dermatitis develops only after prior exposure of from a few days to several years. This acquired sensitivity is of the delayed or T lymphocyte–mediated type. Most sensitizers are low molecular weight chemicals and are not capable of eliciting reactions directly. Instead, it is thought that they conjugate to some dermal protein and function as allergenic *haptens* rendered active by the carrier protein. Certain dendritic cells in the epidermis, called Langerhans' cells, have been recognized as probably being responsible for the hapten processing that leads to sensitization (Thiers, 1982). The microscopic appearance consists of intracellular edema, round cell infiltration, and epidermal vesiculation.

Clinically, the erythematous, vesicular lesion proceeds to a weeping and crusting stage and may become secondarily infected. Occasionally the reaction develops slowly with induration, fissuring, lichenification, and pigmentation rather than vesiculation (Fisher, 1986). The location of the lesion, as much as its appearance, may suggest the diagnosis. Forearms, ears, eyelids, lips, groin, and dorsa of the feet are frequently involved. The eyelids are particularly sensitive and may react to a substance rubbed on them by the fingers, which do not react.

A few substances will sensitize almost everyone. These include the *Rhus* oleoresins (poison ivy, oak, and sumac) and a few chemicals, one of which, dinitrochlorobenzene, is used to induce sensitivity as a test for cell-mediated immune competence. Other common sensitizers affecting 1 to 10 per cent of the population are dyes, especially paraphenylenediamine; chromates used as tanning agents; rubber compounds; nickel found in costume jewelry and in garmet fastenings; and mercury. Among drugs, the more common are ethylenediamine, a stabilizer in some creams that cross reacts with aminophylline, the preservatives thimerosal and parabens, bacitracin, benzocaine, formaldehyde (also a primary irritant), idoxuridine, neomycin, sunscreen lotions, and therapeutic dyes.

Other substances produce photoreactivity. Some have this property as an inherent toxicity and thus will affect susceptible people on the first application. These include psoralens, eosin, and other dyes used in cosmetics and coal tar derivatives and residues. Others need to be applied for a while before an allergic, cell-mediated reaction develops on exposure to sunlight. The more common substances are the halogenated salicylanilides (found in some deodorant soaps) and stilbenes (textile whitening). No topical medicine now available in the United States is known to induce photoallergy.

The treatment of contact dermatitis is similar to that for atopic dermatitis, except that one can use systemic glucocorticoids with less concern about side effects, since it should be a self-limited condition. If the reaction is detected early enough, recognizing and removing the offending contactant may be all that is necessary. If doubt exists about the cause, then patch tests can be done with the suspected substances.

The patch test is carried out by placing each substance in question in contact with a small 5- to 6-mm. area of the skin and keeping it in place with hypoallergenic tape. It may be practical to use a small amount of the actual substance, but in some situations one must obtain specially prepared solutions made up in subirritating concentrations. A detailed listing of chemicals and other substances suitable for patch testing and the appropriate dilutions and diluents can be found in a book entitled *Contact Dermatitis* by Fisher (1986). The patches are left on for 48 hours or longer, and the patient warned to remove and wash off any site that begins to itch or burn before that time. A positive test at 48 hours is a reproduction in miniature of the original lesion: erythema, induration, and vesiculation. Occasionally a borderline reaction evolves into a definite positive result over the next day or two. The risks of patch testing consist of ulceration at the site of an intense reaction and a flaring of the original skin lesions.

Systemic Allergy

Anaphylaxis is any clinical reaction caused by the potent vasoactive mediators that are released explosively after triggering of IgE antibody–sensitized mast cells by an allergen (Type I reaction). *Systemic* or generalized anaphylaxis is a potentially life-threatening reaction to injected or ingested allergens. It can be caused by insect venoms, allergenic extracts used for immunotherapy, drugs (especially injected enzymes or horse antisera and oral or injected penicillin), and certain foods (shellfish, nuts, legumes, egg, and, rarely, others). Some other agents can produce a similar clinical reaction in the absence of allergic sensitivity because they cause the direct release of histamine from mast cells. The most important are the radiographic contrast media, which also generate vasoactive kinins. Such reactions are referred to as *anaphylactoid* rather than *anaphylactic*, because of the lack of evidence for allergy. In recent years, an increasing number of anaphylactoid reactions have been reported that are exercise-induced (Sheffer et al., 1985), and there are even more that have no identifiable cause (Boxer et al., 1987).

Any substance that can produce urticaria can produce systemic reactions if the dose, rate of administration, or reactivity of the recipient is great enough. Fortunately, most are not sufficiently potent to do this when given or taken in the customary way. Massive and explosive mediator release affects not only the skin but also the respiratory tract, the gastrointestinal tract, and the circulation. Angioedema may obstruct the upper airway to such an extreme that the patient is asphyxiated. This is the major recognizable cause of death found at autopsy (James and Austen, 1964). Anaphylactic *shock* primarily is the result of a drop in plasma volume due to a loss of vascular integrity. If the reaction is sufficiently severe and not treated, cardiogenic shock may develop.

The symptoms of systemic anaphylaxis are, in the usual order of progression, a feeling of apprehension, tingling of the extremities, a flushing sensation, itching, palpitations, urticaria, angioedema, nausea, abdominal or uterine cramps, cough, difficulty in breathing, vomiting, diarrhea, incontinence, convulsions, coma, and death. On examination, the typical patient has a generalized flush, with some urticarial wheals beginning to develop. The pulse is rapid, and the blood pressure is initially normal. Later, with sustained hypotension and compensatory peripheral vasoconstriction, the patient may appear pale.

The risk of anaphylaxis can be reduced by taking certain precautions. Gathering a careful history of the patient's previous adverse drug reactions is important. As many as 25 per cent of anaphylactic deaths from penicillin occurred in patients who were not asked about previous reactions, according to a World Health Association report. Skin testing to detect IgE-mediated sensitivity is advisable before giving anyone xenogenic serum, parenteral enzymes, or polypeptide hormones and should be performed also before administering penicillin to a person with a history suggestive of a previous reaction or before administering a chick embryo vaccine to a person with a history of egg sensitivity. The patient with a history of reaction to radiographic contrast media can be premedicated if another procedure is needed. The person who has had a systemic reaction to an insect sting should obtain an emergency kit that contains a prefilled syringe of epinephrine and should be trained in its use. Immunotherapy against the appropriate venom, starting with the injection of a fraction of a microgram and gradually increasing the dose to 100 μg., is highly effective in preventing reactions to subsequent stings (Valentine and Lichtenstein, 1987). Patients at risk for adverse drug reactions should wear a warning identification bracelet such as those provided by Medic-Alert.

The treatment of anaphylaxis is summarized in Table 34–5. Note that epinephrine is central to all aspects. If a reaction is developing from an injection or sting in an extremity, it can often be aborted by the prompt application of a tourniquet above the site of the injection and administration of 0.3 ml of 1:1000 epinephrine (0.01 ml. per kg. in children) in a different extremity. The site of injection can also be infiltrated with about 0.2 ml. of epinephrine in the same dilution to retard absorption. An intravenous line should be inserted and a glucose-saline solution administered. If the blood pressure begins to fall, the fluid should be run in rapidly. Several liters sometimes must be given to maintain or restore the blood pressure. The patient should be monitored to detect saline overload. Use of a colloid solution or a vasopressor drug is rarely necessary. Epinephrine injection can be repeated as early as 15 minutes after the initial dose. If the patient is in shock, it should be given slowly intravenously, 0.25 mg. to 0.5 mg in a 1:100,000 solution at 5 to 10 μg. per minute. If there is any hint of respiratory embarrassment, the patient should be given oxygen. Oropharyngeal angioedema can be treated topically with an aerosol application of epinephrine. Diphenhydramine, 50 to 100 mg. (adult dose), intravenously, may also be helpful. If upper airway obstruction is imminent, insertion of an airway (difficult!) or a tracheostomy may be necessary. If there is any sign of bronchospasm, intravenous aminophylline, 6 mg. per kg., should be given. Very rarely, one may need to give a direct beta-adrenergic stimulant, such as isoproterenol, which has an advantage over dopamine or dobutamine, since it is also a bronchodilator. Glucocorticoid therapy provides no benefit over the critical first few minutes. When all other appropriate therapy has been given, it would be prudent to give a glucocorticoid over the next 24 hours to suppress any late phase reaction (usually localized urticaria, but may become generalized) that may develop.

Table 34–5. TREATMENT OF ANAPHYLAXIS

Isolate antigen
Tourniquet
Epinephrine
Maintain or restore plasma volume
Epinephrine: (I.V. if B.P. ↓)
I.V. fluids
Maintain airway, give oxygen
Upper: Add topical epinephrine
I.V. antihistamine
Lower: Add theophylline
Restore cardiac output
Epinephrine
Theophylline
Isoproterenol

Drug Allergy

Most adverse drug reactions result from excessive intake (toxicity) or unusual susceptibility to the toxic effects of a substance. Some patients are unusually susceptible because of underlying disease, and some are unusually susceptible for unknown reasons. Their reactions are called *intolerance* if the adverse event is an expected pharmacologic effect of the drug and *idiosyncrasy* if it is substantially different.

Allergic drug reactions usually can be differentiated from the others by means of the features listed in Table 34–6. One of special importance is that the risk of allergic reaction exists far below the therapeutic range. If one can establish that the reaction to a drug is toxic-idiosyncratic, then treatment with a modest reduction in dose may be successful. This stratagem is unlikely to be successful, and may be dangerous, if the reaction is allergic.

Testing for drug allergy is reliable only in special circumstances. These have been alluded to earlier.

Table 34–6. FEATURES OF ALLERGIC DRUG REACTIONS

A. Prior exposure (usually for treatment) occurs without adverse effects
B. The reactions usually appear only after several days of treatment after first exposure to the drug
C. The risk of reaction still exists at doses far below the therapeutic range
D. Clinical manifestations do not resemble the general pharmacologic effects of the drug and cannot be predicted from animal testing
E. The reactions occur in a small proportion of the population
F. The reactions usually are restricted to a limited number of syndromes generally accepted as allergic in nature
G. In a few instances, antibodies of T lymphocytes have been identified that react specifically with the drug or a metabolite
H. The same reactions can be reproduced on administering a small amount of the suspected drug or drugs of similar chemical structure

Skin testing for immediate sensitivity does identify allergy to high molecular weight protein or polypeptide substances. However, most drugs have a low molecular weight, usually less than 1000 daltons, and thus can only sensitize by forming a firm covalent bond with a large carrier protein. This cannot happen directly; it occurs only after the drug has been modified in the body to a chemically reactive intermediate. The intermediates of penicillin are the only ones to have been definitely identified so far. One has been conjugated with polylysine to form penicilloyl-polylysine. It is available commercially for skin testing as Pre-pen. Unfortunately, penicilloyl-polylysine skin testing usually fails to identify those few patients at risk for systemic anaphylaxis. They have positive skin reactions to what are called the minor determinants, but the minor determinant mixture for skin testing is not yet on the market. Until it is, penicillin allergy can be excluded most of the time, when the need for treatment with one of the penicillins is especially pressing, by testing with penicilloyl-polylysine and a solution of 1000 units per ml. penicillin G (prick test first, followed by intradermal testing, if necessary). If the skin tests are negative, treatment can be cautiously started, using a small test dose first.

Except for some technically difficult tests that can be used to confirm hematologic drug reactions, in vitro tests that have been proposed for the diagnosis of drug allergy are unreliable. These include the radioallergosorbent test (with the single exception of penicilloyl-polylysine), lymphocyte stimulation, basophil or mast cell histamine release, and leukocyte cytotoxicity. This is not surprising, since the appropriate conjugates capable of producing specific immunologic reactions have not been identified, except for penicillin (VanArsdel, 1982).

The most reliable test is to readminister the drug to see if the clinical reaction can be reproduced. As mentioned earlier, this is the purpose of the patch test. Otherwise, the risk of doing so is usually unacceptable unless treatment is essential and no alternative drug is available.

Other types of clinical reactions than those discussed above are reviewed in detail elsewhere (VanArsdel, 1988), so they will be mentioned only briefly here. *Serum sickness* probably depends on both Type I and Type III (immune complex) mechanisms. Fever, adenopathy, and arthralgias occur with an urticarial rash when the reaction is due to foreign serum. A reaction similar to serum sickness may occur during or after treatment with a penicillin (or homologue), sulfonamide, or hydralazine, but it is distinctly uncommon.

"Rashes" are the erythematous maculopapular or morbilliform eruptions that are sometimes only minimally pruritic. Close to half of the drug reactions presumed to be allergic fall into this category. The most common substances involved are the semisynthetic penicillins, sulfonamides (especially trimethoprim-sulfamethoxazole), blood products, dipyrone, cephalosporins, allopurinol, and acetylcysteine (Bigby et al., 1986).

Fixed eruptions are pigmented macules that sometimes are eczematous. They can be produced by metronidazole, penicillins, sulfonamides, some analgesics and sedatives, gold salts, and even phenolphthalein. Reproducing the reaction by giving the drug again confirms the diagnosis.

Vasculitis most characteristically appears as an erythematous eruption that may become tender, purpuric, and palpable. Sometimes other organ systems besides the skin are affected. Allopurinol, cimetidine, furosemide, hydantoins, penicillins, and sulfonamides are commonly used drugs that can produce vasculitis. However, only about ten per cent of reported cases of vasculitis seem to be drug-induced, so any association may be coincidental.

Fever alone may be produced by allopurinol, cephalosporins, penicillins, barbiturates, methyldopa, phenytoin, procainamide, and quinidine. It is sometimes not associated with constitutional symptoms, so the patient may not be aware of it. The diagnosis is supported if treatment with the suspected drug is stopped and the temperature drops to normal within 48 hours (except for phenytoin, for which this drop may take several days). The diagnosis is confirmed, if necessary, by readministering a small dose of the drug; this is reasonably safe.

Pulmonary reactions are bronchospastic or infiltrative. *Asthma* is very rare except in association with systemic anaphylaxis. *Interstitial pneumonitis* develops with cough, dyspnea, fever, and malaise and is produced most often by gold salts, nitrofurantoin and thiazide diuretics. *Eosinophilic pneumonitis* is less symptomatic but is associated with blood eosinophilia. It can be produced by gold salts, penicillin, and sulfonamides.

Hepatic reactions can be primarily cholestatic and relatively benign or primarily hepatocellular and potentially fatal. The former can be caused by erythromycins (particularly the estolate), phenothiazines, imipramine, nalidixic acid, and nitrofurantoin. The latter can be produced by allopurinol, hydantoins, isoniazid, methyldopa, monoamine oxidase inhibitors, rifampin, sulfonamides, and valproic acid.

Interstitial nephritis is the usual allergic renal reaction, and the best-known responsible drug is methicillin. But other penicillins, cephalosporins, and sulfonamides have been implicated as well as cimetidine, diuretics, nonsteroidal antirheumatic drugs, and allopurinol.

Systemic lupus erythematosus is a self-limited reaction similar to the natural disease (but lacking the cerebral, cutaneous, and renal changes) and is associated with the appearance of circulating antinuclear antibodies. It often develops during treatment with hydralazine or procainamide and less frequently with chlorpromazine, isoniazid, penicillamine, and phenytoin treatment.

Hematologic reactions include blood *eosinophilia* alone (antimicrobials, digitalis glycosides, allopurinol, penicillamine, and phenothiazines), *hemolytic anemia* (high-dose penicillin, chlorpromazine, isoniazid, quinidine, rifampin, and sulfonamides), *thrombocytopenia* due to immune destruction (quinine, quinidine, cephalosporins, gold salts, hydantoins, antituberculous drugs, analgesics, sulfonamides, and thiazide diuretics), and *granulocytopenia* due to immune destruction (chlorpromazine, gold salts, phenylbutazone, procainamide, quinidine, and sulfonamides).

Toxic epidermal necrolysis is a rare but potentially fatal reaction that may be related to drugs such as allopurinol, penicillins, phenytoin, sulfonamides, and sulindac. Reactions that are occasionally drug induced but are more commonly related to infection or unknown causes include *exfoliative dermatitis* and *erythema multiforme*. There is no good evidence that *erythema nodosum* or *Henoch-Schoñlein purpura* are drug induced.

Pseudoallergic drug reactions are reactions due to the pharmacologic or toxic action of certain drugs. Reactions due to histamine-releasing drugs were mentioned earlier. Rhinitis is a well-recognized side effect of reserpine but can also be found during treatment with other antihypertensive drugs. Asthma is a recognized side effect of treatment with beta-blocking drugs, even timolol eye drops.

The prevention and treatment of allergic drug reactions is reviewed elsewhere (VanArsdel, 1988). Briefly, if a reaction occurs, the suspected drug or drugs should be stopped immediately. Symptoms should be treated with antipruritic and analgesic drugs as needed. If these are inadequate, a glucocorticoid drug should be given in ample doses.

Food Allergy

There are few topics so subject to confusion, misinterpretation, argument and outright exploitation as that of food allergy. The word *allergy* itself is used so indiscriminantly by laymen and professionals alike when food is involved that substitute words such as *sensitivity* and *hypersensitivity* have been proposed as being more precise. However, allergy, as it was originally intended and as it has been used in this chapter, refers only to conditions due to antibody-mediated or lymphocyte-mediated tissue injury following contact with a specific allergen.

Allergy mediated by IgE antifood antibodies usually develops in infancy as the diet is liberalized. There is some evidence also that some foods eaten by the mother appear in her milk and can sensitize the nursing infant. As expected, the individual with a strong family history of atopy is likely to acquire sensitivity to some foods, but which ones are determined largely by chance and by the age at which the food is introduced. The infant's incomplete digestion, high mucosal permeability, and perhaps weak immunologic defense (by secretory IgA) favor both sensitization and the production of symptoms after sensitization has been established. As the young child grows older, food-induced symptoms become less significant, probably because of maturation of the digestive action of the gastrointestinal tract. However, the IgE antibodies may persist for many years. Skin tests to the originally allergenic foods may remain positive long after those foods have ceased to cause symptoms.

The evidence that immunologic mechanisms other than IgE play a role is not impressive. Several gastrointestinal diseases have been associated with IgG antibodies in the serum, especially to milk, but these antibodies are probably secondary to the diseases rather than causative. Celiac sprue, caused by sensitivity to wheat gluten, is one example of food sensitivity that is probably due to an IgG antigluten antibody. Delayed or cell-mediated sensitivity may be involved in some adverse food reactions, but these reactions are not associated with positive delayed skin tests; supporting evidence is entirely circumstantial.

Some of the atopic diseases associated with food allergy were discussed earlier. Atopic dermatitis can be aggravated by food allergens, and asthma and allergic rhinitis can be provoked by them as well. Gastrointestinal symptoms—nausea, vomiting, abdominal cramps, and diarrhea—may occur alone, but more often they accompany respiratory and cutaneous symptoms in the atopic patient with or without atopic dermatitis.

The manifestations of food allergy noted earlier are most common in early childhood, but the highly allergic person may continue to have trouble into adult life. Indeed, such a person, if highly sensitive to some food, runs a risk of systemic anaphylaxis from that food that does not seem to diminish with time.

The importance of gastrointestinal digestion in preventing symptoms from ingested food allergens is best brought out by the many examples of patients who react on contact or inhalation of a particular food that gives a positive skin test but have no trouble in eating it. "Baker's asthma," due to inhaled wheat flour, is the best-known example.

Another interesting though rare disease that can occur in adults as well as children is eosinophilic gastroenteritis, a chronic disease associated with anemia and protein-losing enteropathy. It is made worse by ingestion of food allergens but, unfortunately, usually persists to a certain degree even if no recognizable allergens are eaten.

Other symptoms that are occasionally provoked by food allergens are headache, irritability, malaise, myalgias, or arthralgias. Usually, each accompanies one or more of the major symptoms rather than being the only symptom of food allergy.

The most common food allergens are milk, eggs, nuts and legumes, shellfish and other fish, wheat, chocolate, and pork, but any food is potentially allergenic.

Food *intolerance* is a condition in which the adverse reaction is based on a nonallergic mechanism or in which the mechanism is unknown. Thus, cow's milk intolerance, responsible for gastrointestinal symptoms, may be due to an intestinal deficiency in disaccharidase, but milk can also produce gastrointestinal and even respiratory symptoms in a few patients for no identifiable reason (Lessof et al., 1980). It has even been found to be responsible for intestinal blood loss in infants sufficient to cause significant anemia. The mechanism responsible for intolerance to some food additives or coloring agents is also unknown, but it is probably pharmacologic rather than immunologic. Asthma related to food ingestion may actually be produced by the yellow food dye tartrazine.

Food allergy or intolerance has been blamed for certain other conditions. The so-called allergic tension-fatigue syndrome is an example. Enuresis is another, and the "total allergy syndrome" (multiple symptoms attributed to allergy to practically everything) is a third that has received a good deal of attention by the press. Much publicity has also been given to the claim that abnormal hyperactivity in children is often due to food additives. All these alleged associations are controversial, since they have not yet been supported by any well-controlled clinical trials.

The diagnosis of food allergy depends to a great extent on the history. Symptoms should be recorded in terms of both time and severity in relationship with the types and amount of food ingested. This may best be done by asking the patient to keep a food-symptom diary over a 2-week period, being careful to note all ingredients of any given item. Any suspicious foods are then eliminated from the diet for 2 weeks. If improvement occurs, they are added back to the diet one at a time until symptoms reappear or get worse. If several items are suspected, one should look for a common allergenic ingredient, such as soybean. If no improvement occurs or the history is not helpful, an empiric elimination diet can be used to restrict the patient to one food in each category (grain, vegetable, fruit, meat) switching to a different food after 1 week. If the elimination diet is successful, then the one-by-one reintroduction of additional food proceeds as before until symptoms are provoked (Dong, 1984).

If the empiric diet adjustment is not successful, then testing for IgE food antibodies should be done. The prick test, using a 1:10 or 1:20 glycerinated extract, correlates well with true clinical food allergy, as proved by double-blind placebo-controlled oral challenge experiments (Bock, 1980). Intradermal testing can result in positive skin tests at levels of sensitivity insufficient to be responsible for the symptoms of most patients. The radioallergosorbent test offers no advantage over skin testing unless dermatitis is so extensive that the skin cannot be used. No other tests are advisable. Serum precipitating antibodies to milk or wheat, for example, do not indicate allergy. Other tests, such as cutaneous or sublingual provocation, the pulse and leukopenic test, and the leukocytotoxic serum test, have not been validated by acceptable scientific means.

The obvious treatment for food allergy or intolerance is to avoid the offending food. However, when allergy to many foods is suspected, one may need to establish which are clinically important by placebo-controlled blind challenges. These may become necessary if the alternative is a nutritionally deficient diet. Drug treatment of the cutaneous or respiratory symptoms of food allergy has been covered in earlier sections. The original hope that oral cromolyn sodium would not only control gastrointestinal symptoms but block food allergen absorption has not been realized, and immunotherapy to food allergens is risky and probably ineffective.

The greatest stumbling block that family physicians face in discussing food allergy is understanding what is and what is not food allergy. Unfortunately, the lay press along with popular talk shows have invited misunderstanding among patients. It becomes important for the family physician to become familiar with these misconceptions so that a sound and medically helpful evaluation can be done. The foregoing discussion is an attempt to clarify what, at this time, is medically known and understood.

References

Bascom, R., Pipkorn, U., Lichtenstein, L. M., and Naclerio, R. M.: The influx of inflammatory cells into nasal washings during the late response to antigen challenge: Effect of systemic steroid pretreatment. Am. Rev. Respir. Dis., *138*:406, 1988.

Bigby, M., Jick, S., Jick, H., and Arndt, K.: Drug-induced cutaneous reactions: A report from the Boston collaborative drug surveillance program on 15,438 consecutive inpatients, 1975 to 1982. J.A.M.A., *256*:3358, 1986.

Bluestone, R. D., and Cantekin, E. I.: Panel of experience with testing eustachian tube function. Ann. Otol. Rhinol. Laryngol., *90*:552, 1981.

Bock, S. A.: Food sensitivity: A critical review and practical approach. Am. J. Dis. Child., *134*:973, 1980.

Boxer, M., Greenberger, P. A., and Patterson, R.: Clinical summary and course of idiopathic anaphylaxis in 73 patients. Arch. Intern. Med., *147*:269, 1987. *This article summarizes the clinical experience with 73 patients seen and followed at Northwestern University Medical School in whom no identifyable precipitating cause could be identified. The report is optimistic. No fatal reactions have occurred, many have improved with time, and about 15 per cent have become asymptomatic.*

Broder, I., Higgins, M. W., Mathews, H. P., and Keller, J. B.: Epidemiology of asthma and allergic rhinitis in a total community, Tecumseh, Michigan. J. Allergy Clin. Immunol., *54*:100, 1974.

Cockcroft, D. W.: Airway hyperresponsiveness and late asthmatic responses. Chest, *94*:178, 1988.

Coombs, R. R. A., and Gell, P. G. H.: Classification of allergic reactions responsible for clinical hypersensitivity and disease. *In* Gell, P. G. H., and Coombs, R. R. A. (Eds.): Clinical Aspects of Immunology. 3rd ed. Oxford, England, Blackwell Scientific Publications, 1975.

Dong, F. M.: All About Food Allergy. Philadelphia, George F. Stickley Company, 1984. *This is an informative and sensible book written by a nutritionist for the layperson. She discusses the role of the dietician in helping the physician in diagnosis and diet management and also provides a critical section on controversial diagnosis and management programs.*

Fisher, A. A.: Contact Dermatitis. 3rd ed. Philadelphia, Lea & Febiger, 1986. *This is the definitive reference book on contact dermatitis. It has a 66-page appendix that is a quick-reference list of over 800 contact allergens, their source, and the appropriate concentrations and vehicles for patch testing.*

Gross, N. J.: Ipratropium bromide. N. Engl. J. Med., *319*:486, 1988.

Hanifin, J. M.: Atopic dermatitis. J. Am. Acad. Dermatol., *6*:1, 1982. *This article covers the clinical features, natural history, and, in particular detail, the investigational studies that are beginning to enlighten us regarding the pathogenesis of this puzzling condition.*

Hendeles, L.: Asthma therapy: State of the art, 1988. J. Respir. Dis., *9*:82, 1988. *A comprehensive review of drug therapy for asthma, written by a clinical pharmacist with extensive research experience. He provided over 100 references.*

Jacobson, K. W., Branch, L. B., and Nelson, H. S.: Laboratory tests in chronic urticaria. J.A.M.A., *243*:1644, 1980.

James, L. P., Jr., and Austen, K. F.: Fatal systemic anaphylaxis in man. N. Engl. J. Med., *270*:597, 1964.

König, P.: Inhaled corticosteroids—their present and future role in the management of asthma. J. Allergy Clin. Immunol., *82*:297, 1988.

Lessof, M. H., Wraith, D. G., Merrett, T. G., et al.: Food allergy and intolerance in 100 patients—local and systemic effects. Q. J. Med., *49*:259, 1980. *This is one of the best examples of how the diagnosis of food allergy is made or ruled out in a critical, unbiased manner.*

Marsh, D. G., and Bias, W. B.: The genetics of atopic allergy. *In* Samter, M., Talmage, D. W., Frank, M. M., et al. (Eds.): Immunological Diseases. 4th ed. Boston, Little, Brown & Co. Inc., 1988, p. 1027.

Monroe, E. W.: Urticaria. Int. J. Dermatol., *20*:32, 1981.

Mullarkey, M. F.: Eosinophilic nonallergic rhinitis. J. Allergy Clin. Immunol., *82*:941, 1988.

Patterson, R., Greenberger, P. A., Halwig, J. M., et al.: Allergic bronchopulmonary aspergillosis. Natural history and classification of early disease by serologic and roentgenographic studies. Arch. Intern. Med., *146*:916, 1986.

Platts-Mills, T. A. E., and Chapman, M. D.: Dust mites: Immunology, allergic disease, and environmental control. J. Allergy Clin. Immunol., *80*:755, 1987.

Sampson, H. A.: Food hypersensitivity as a pathogenic factor in atopic dermatitis. New Engl. Reg. Allergy Proc., *7*:511, 1986. *The author and colleagues have studied carefully the role of food hypersensitivity in children with atopic dermatitis by performing 458 double-blind, placebo-controlled oral food challenges in 132 children. At least one positive clinical reaction occurred in 59 per cent of the subjects. The symptoms consisted of a pruritic erythematous, macular, or morbilliform rash associated in over half the cases with gastrointestinal symptoms and in 36 per cent with respiratory symptoms. Elimination of the positive-challenge foods resulted in significant clinical improvement. (See also Sampson and McCaskill, J. Pediatr. 107*:669, 1985.)

Serafin, W. E., and Austen, K. F.: Mediators of immediate hypersensitivity reactions. N. Engl. J. Med., *317*:30, 1987.

Sheffer, A. L., Tong, A. K. F., Murphy, G. F., et al.: Exercise-induced anaphylaxis: A serious form of physical allergy associated with mast cell degranulation. J. Allergy Clin. Immunol., *75*:479, 1985.

Sheffer, A. L., Fearon, D. T., and Austen, K. F.: Hereditary angioedema. A decade of management with stanozolol. J. Allergy Clin. Immunol., *80*:855, 1987.

Thiers, B. H.: The Langerhans cell. J. Am. Acad. Dermatol., *6*:519, 1982.

Valentine, M. D., and Lichtenstein, L. M.: Anaphylaxis and stinging insect hypersensitivity. J.A.M.A., *258*:2881, 1987.

VanArsdel, P. P., Jr.: Diagnosing drug allergy. J.A.M.A., *247*:2576, 1982.

VanArsdel, P. P., Jr.: Drug hypersensitivity. *In* Bierman, C. W., Pearlman, D. S. (Eds.): Allergic Diseases from Infancy to Adulthood. 2nd ed. Philadelphia, W. B. Saunders Company, 1988, p. 684.

VanArsdel, P. P., Jr., and Larson, E. B.: Diagnostic tests for patients with suspected allergic disease: Utility and limitations. Ann. Intern. Med., *110*:304, 1989. *A critical review of allergy testing based on the existing medical literature. It is part of the Clinical Efficacy Assessment Project (CEAP); Health and Public Policy Committee, American College of Physicians.*

Weber, R. W., and Nelson, H. S.: Immunologic and atopic aspects of pregnancy and lactation. Ann. Allergy, *57*:159, 1986. *An informative and well-referenced review article that covers not only the appropriate medical management of allergic diseases during pregnancy, but also discusses the endocrinologic and immunologic changes during pregnancy, the immunity of lactation, and the excretion of drugs in breast milk.*

35

Parasitology

Jerry E. Jones

"To decide the uncertainty where worms are suspected, and effectually to expel them where they are known to exist in the human body, is not the least embarrassment of the physician's occupation."

THE AMERICAN TRANSLATER, 1817

Parasitic diseases are caused by organisms that live in or on another organism. In man, they can be grouped as protozoans, helminths, or anthropods and vary in size from several microns to more than 25 meters. They may occupy a variety of body tissues or organs and, as a direct result, generate a host of different signs and symptoms. The specific clustering of signs and symptoms for each parasitic disease reflects the parasite's size, location in the body of the host, life cycle, and numbers present within the host. The mode of attack may vary as well, producing the potential for a multitude of seemingly unrelated complaints and physical findings.

Terms that are frequently misunderstood are ova and cyst, larvae and trophozoite, and definitive host and intermediate host. Ovum (plural, ova) describes the egg or female sexual cell from which a new parasite develops following union with the male element. This life stage is often found in the stool, but in some species is found in certain tissues. A cyst refers to the nonmotile, asexual form of the protozoa, which forms from the adults and provides a survival mechanism for the parasite away from the host. Both ovum and cyst are the most common means by which parasites are transmitted to a new individual. The cyst does not need a male element for a new parasite to develop. Larva (plural, larvae) describes the developing young of the helminths and arthropods that differ in form from the parent. Protozoa do not have larvae. Larvae may be found in the stool and tissue and are generally responsible for the migrating phrase of most parasites. Trophozoite refers to the motile stage of a protozoan, which feeds, multiplies, and maintains the colony within humans. In most cases, it is the trophozoite stage of the protozoa that produces the symptoms. The definitive host refers to the host that harbors the sexual stage of the parasite. An intermediate host harbors the larval or asexual stages of the parasite. Humans may be both definitive and intermediate hosts.

Clinical Approach to Common Parasitic Diseases

Realizing that the probability of making a specific diagnosis varies directly with one's index of suspicion for the disease in question, one must think of parasites in order to recognize and treat infections that may present in typical, atypical, or even bizarre ways. The clinical history is the first step. A history of the patient's travel, as an integral part of the patient's history, may yield valuable data leading to a diagnosis. It is not enough to inquire as to where the patient has been lately, since some parasites have remarkably long life spans in their human hosts—as long as from 6 months to 4 years or more, depending on the species. It is important to ascertain whether the patient has been exposed to certain parasites. For example, has the patient been drinking untreated or potentially contaminated water (resulting in giardiasis or amebiasis) or walking in his or her bare feet (resulting in infection with hookworm or strongyloides)?

Knowledge of the endemic parasites in your practice area is necessary. Endemicity depends upon suitable environmental conditions as well as the presence of intermediate hosts, vectors when required, and definitive hosts. Annual information is available nationally for intestinal parasites from the Intestinal Parasite Surveillance Program at the Centers for Disease Control.

SIGNS AND SYMPTOMS

The presence of certain signs and symptoms should alert the physician to the diagnostic possibilities of parasitic diseases. However, very few of the signs and symptoms evoked by infection with parasitic organisms can be said to be pathognomonic. Only those conditions most likely to be encountered in the office setting are presented in this chapter.

Diarrhea. Diarrhea is frequently the earliest symptom of intestinal parasitic infection. Although transient diarrhea is common among persons who have traveled outside the country, it resolves within a few days without the need to identify the cause. Continuing diarrhea in mild, moderate, or explosive forms should alert clinicians to possible parasitic infections—whether or not the patient has been traveling. The most common parasitic cause of diarrheal disease in the United States is *Giardia lamblia.* Most intestinal helminths, however, do not cause diarrhea. Exceptions to this general rule are heavy infections with *Trichuris trichiura,* and *Strongyloides stercoralis.* Large numbers of diarrheal stools associated with blood or mucus suggest *Entamoeba histolytica.*

Eosinophilia. Eosinophilia has been thought to be an unfailing marker of parasitic infection. However, not all parasites cause eosinophilia, and the degree of eosinophilia usually depends on the degree of tissue invasion by the parasite. With one exception (toxoplasmosis), protozoan infections generally do not produce a peripheral eosinophilia. Likewise, purely lumen-dwelling parasites that do not invade tissue are rarely associated with eosinophilia. In contrast, parasites that have a larval migration phase through tissue are associated with eosinophilia. Marked eosinophilia (20 to 70 per cent) occurring in persons without a history of foreign travel suggests trichinosis, strongyloidosis, visceral larva migrans, or, in some areas of the United States, hookworm. Mild to moderate eosinophilia (6 to 20 per cent) suggests migrating larvae of helminths.

Abdominal Pain. Abdominal pain is seldom seen in light intestinal worm infections. However, *Ascaris* can cause intestinal biliary obstruction, producing signs and symptoms that mimic obstruction from other causes. *Strongyloides stercoralis* may cause severe duodenitis or jejunitis if heavy numbers invade the muscle wall. Visceral larva migrans may cause severe abdominal pain, often indistinguishable from acute appendicitis. Moderate to heavy eosinophilia generally accompanies either of these worm infections. Crampy, midepigastric pain may appear with giardiasis. It is usually mild but may occasionally be severe. Lower abdominal pain may characterize amebic colitis with tenesmus if the ulcerations of amebiasis involve the rectal area. Right upper quadrant pain may be seen if an amebic abscess of the liver develops.

Fever. Fever may be seen with the larval migration phase of roundworms. More classically, fever in an individual returning from a malarious area must be considered an indication of malaria unless proved otherwise. All four species of malaria act in a similar manner, producing chills, headache, and myalgia associated with fever. In the early stages of this disease, it may take several days before a classic fever pattern appears.

Cough. Cough secondary to pneumonitis may be seen as a presenting symptom. Often this is attributed to bronchitis or viral pneumonia. The migrating phase of certain roundworms, especially hookworms; *Ascaris;* and *S. stercoralis* will cause cough. *Ascaris* tends to stimulate more coughing than either hookworm or *Strongyloides* because of the larger size of its migratory larvae.

Anemia. Microcytic, hypochromic anemia has been classically associated with hookworm disease. Today, most cases seen in the United States are usually too light to produce significant blood loss. Heavy whipworm (*T. trichiura*) infections in children have also been reported to produce anemia. A moderate to severe hemolytic anemia may be found with falciparum malaria. The anemia occurring with the other three species of malaria is usually mild.

Splenomegaly. Splenomegaly accompanies many acute and chronic infectious processes. Parasites endemic within the United States do not produce splenomegaly, except for rare infections with *Echinococcus.* However, splenomegaly may occur with malaria, leishmaniasis, or trypanosomiasis.

Hepatomegaly. Enlargement of the liver may be caused by any parasite involving that organ. Endemic parasites that may involve the liver are *Entamoeba histolytica* (amebic hepatitis, liver abscess) and visceral larva migrans (*Toxocara*). Liver fluke infections and early schistosomiasis, although imported, are also characterized by an enlarged and tender liver.

Dermatitis. Dermatitis caused by parasites is most frequently the result of *Sarcoptes scabiei,* the itch mite. These mites invade the upper layer of the epidermis and cause intense itching. Secondary infection often occurs following scratching. Body and head lice may also cause dermatitis. In some areas of the country, bird schistosomes may cause dermatitis in persons bathing in fresh or marine water. The larval stage enters the skin, causing an allergic reaction characterized by intense itching and a reddish macular or maculopapular rash, or hives. The lesions appear within minutes to hours after exposure and may persist for several days. Another parasite limited to the skin is cutaneous larva migrans (creeping eruption). The larvae of the dog or cat hookworm are unable to complete their migratory cycle in humans but can penetrate the skin and produce visible crawl tracks under the surface.

OFFICE TECHNIQUES FOR DIAGNOSIS

The most important means of diagnosing most helminths is by direct inspection of the morphology of eggs and larval and adult forms. Similarly, most protozoa are identified by the morphology of their trophozoites and cysts. It is not unusual for the parasitized patient to bring his or her worm to your office, having passed it through the rectum. The physician should feel comfortable making an identification on gross specimens. At times, the evidence may be purely historical, with the person describing a worm-like object in an otherwise normal bowel movement. Size plays an important part in the identification of the parasite. If the worm is large (15 to 35 cm.), round, and looks like an earthworm, it must be *Ascaris lumbricoides.* This is generally the only worm that is known to be coughed up or vomited in the adult stage. The second most likely worm to be identified is the pinworm. It is small, 0.5 to 1 cm. in length, whitish in color, and often described as thin and thread-like and as wiggling in the stool. Mothers often see these parasites as they wipe or clean their children after a bowel movement. Other roundworms, such as the whipworm (*T. trichiura*), the hookworm, and *Strongyloides,* are rarely seen in the stool. However, they are similar in size to the pinworm and should not be confused with the giant *Ascaris.* Segments of tapeworms may also be passed in the stool. These adult helminths may be examined after being washed in a sodium chloride solution and after shaking the container vigorously to relax the organism.

If adult worm specimens are not available, it is frequently useful to obtain fecal material by digital rectal examination. By inserting the finger 3 to 5 cm. above the anal sphincter and rotating it 360 degrees, it is often possible to remove feces and debris containing the ova or cysts of the parasite. If the patient has diarrhea, only mucus and blood may be obtained, but this may be particularly helpful in identifying intestinal protozoa. The fecal material obtained by digital rectal examination is used to make a wet slide preparation by scraping the material from the tip of the glove with a wooden applicator stick or toothpick and placing it on a slide that has been prepared with two drops of normal saline. This is carefully mixed until the saline becomes cloudy. To avoid trapping air bubbles under the coverslip, place one edge of the coverslip at 45 degrees to the edge of the saline drop, allowing the mixture to run from end to end and then gently lowering it to the surface of the slide.

The fecal slide is examined under low-power magnification. Nematode ova can often be found by scanning the outer edges of the slide first. The entire slide should be examined under low-power magnification, changing to high-power to confirm the presence of or to identify the ova. Each species of roundworms has a distinctive ovum, which allows for specific diagnosis. When protozoa are suspected, high-power magnification will confirm the presence or absence of cysts. In some cases, it is possible to make species identification.

Pinworms can be identified using the "Scotch tape test." A plain microscopic slide is covered with a piece of transparent adhesive tape, adhesive-coated side out. About ¼ inch of the tape is pressed on one end of the slide and then folded backward over the end, with the sticky surface facing outward. The slide is gently directed into the anal verge so that the sticky surface of the tape touches the anus and the immediate perianal area. The tape is then placed sticky side down on the slide, smoothed out with tissue paper to remove air bubbles and wrinkles, and examined under the microscope for ova or fragments of the adult pinworm. Adult pinworms and eggs can also be removed from just above the anal verge using the digital rectal examination. After applying a small amount of lubricating jelly to the tip of a gloved little finger, the finger is inserted 1 to 2 cm. into the anus and rotated. A wet mount preparation is made as outlined above. This technique is often helpful when the "Scotch tape test" is negative as a result of the parent cleaning the perianal area before bringing the child to the office (Jones, 1988).

An anoscope or sigmoidoscope can be used for the collection of intestinal material and mucus, especially if intestinal protozoa are suspected. This material is prepared in the same manner as that derived from a digital rectal examination.

If fecal smears made from the procedures outlined are negative, multiple stool specimens should be collected and examined. Similarly, if a fecal smear made from digital examination is positive for one of the intestinal roundworms or protozoa, it may be necessary to rule out the presence of other intestinal parasites. Stool collection kits, usually containing a 10 per cent formalin solution and a polyvinyl-alcohol fixative as preservatives for cysts, ova, larvae, and trophozoites, are available commercially or from public health laboratories.

The patient is instructed to collect three separate stool specimens at home during a 3- or 5-day period. It is important to stress that the specimens should be taken from separate bowel movements. The stool specimens can be examined in the office or sent to a reference laboratory. If protozoan cysts are found, the specimen should be sent to a reference laboratory for staining.

Gastrointestinal x-ray studies should be delayed until after a stool examination for intestinal parasites, because barium will interfere with microscopic detection for up to 2 weeks. Antibiotics, antiparasitic drugs, laxatives, antidiarrheal agents, and enemas will also hamper the identification.

A final office procedure that may prove helpful if *G. lamblia* or *S. stercoralis* is suspected and cannot be found in repeated stool examinations is the "string test" or Entero-Test (Jones, 1986). After a 4- to 8-hour fast, the patient swallows a gelatin capsule containing a 90 cm. nylon string attached to a sterilized silicone-embedded lead weight. The capsule serves as an aid in swallowing the weight. The string extends through the capsule and the looped free end is held by the patient. The string unravels as the capsule is swallowed and the end is then taped to the cheek. The gelatin capsule dissolves in the stomach, allowing the weighted line to pass into the duodenum. Drinking water during the final 2 hours of the test helps the capsule pass through the patient's system. The line is withdrawn after 4 hours, and the distal end is checked for bile staining and pH. The intestinal secretion adhering to the nylon string can then be placed by glove onto a slide prepared with two drops of normal saline and examined under a microscope.

Certain serologic tests are also available to aid the diagnosis of parasites. In general, if they are positive, that patient has developed antibodies to a parasitic antigen. Care must be used in interpreting the results, since a positive titer does not indicate the numbers of parasites present or whether they are multiplying. The most useful serologic tests are those available for parasites that have tissue phases in man and would be difficult to diagnose by stool examination. Serologic tests are available for: (1) trichinosis, (2) echinococcosis, (3) amebiasis, (4) visceral larva migrans, and (5) schistosomiasis. Generally, specimens of serum should be sent to the State Health Department laboratory.

Nonpathogenic Protozoa

Nonpathogenic protozoa are frequently identified in stool examinations sent to the laboratory (Jones, 1983). Awareness of these species and their commensal role will aid the family physician in treatment decisions and with patient education.

Identification of this group of parasites is based on morphologic characteristics of the trophozoite stage or the cyst stage, or both. It is important that the laboratory use special staining techniques to make each species identification. Good communication with the reference laboratory personnel will help the physician ensure an accurate diagnosis.

Table 35–1 lists the eight intestinal protozoa that are widely accepted as nonpathogenic. The approximate sizes are listed for the trophozoites and cysts. This table should serve as a reference when the physician needs to identify a species as pathogenic or nonpathogenic.

Specific Parasites

Knowledge of the most frequent reported parasites within the United States is important when developing a differential diagnosis. Only the most commonly encountered parasite diseases are discussed in the following section.

GIARDIA LAMBLIA

Giardia lamblia is the most common pathogenic intestinal parasites in the United States and is usually caused by human or animal contamination of water supplies. It exists in two stages: an actively feeding trophozoite stage and a cyst stage. The hardy cysts live for months in the external environment, and routine chlorination procedures may not eliminate them. Although water filtration methods should be effective, several major outbreaks of giardiasis resulted from malfunctioning systems. Asymptomatic carriers may also be responsible for hand-to-food-to-mouth or hand-to-mouth transmission. Only recently has it become recognized that endemic giardiasis accounts for the vast majority of stools regularly found to be positive for cysts.

After a cyst is ingested, it divides into two trophozoites, which then multiply by binary fission. The trophozoites reproduce in the duodenum and proximal jejunum. The exact pathogenic mechanisms are unknown. The onset of acute symptoms usually occurs within 3 weeks after cyst ingestion. The hallmark symptom is explosive diarrhea, which may alternate with constipation. In children, the diarrhea may be steatorrheic. The stools are watery and characteristically foul. Many patients complain of a sulfur-like "rotten egg" taste in their mouths, a symptom that may help point to giardiasis. Flatulence, nausea, anorexia, headache, malaise, upper abdominal disten-

Table 35–1. NONPATHOGENIC INTESTINAL PROTOZOA OF HUMANS

	Organism	Stage of Organism: Trophozoite (Size in Microns)	Stage of Organism: Cyst (Size in Microns)
Amebae	*Entamoeba hartmanni*	3 to 12	4 to 10
	Entamoeba coli	15 to 50	10 to 35
	Iodamoeba butschlii	2 to 20	6 to 16
	Endolimax nana	5 to 12	5 to 12
Flagellates	*Chilomastix mesnili*	10 to 20	6 to 10
	Trichomonas hominis	7 to 15	no cyst
	Retortamonas intestinalis	4 to 10	4 to 7
	Enteromonas hominis	4 to 10	6 to 8

tion, pain, and tenderness are frequent complaints. The foul-smelling stools and flatus, a feeling of morbid distention, and the lack of blood and pus point to giardiasis rather than dysentery or inflammatory disease. Eosinophilia and an elevated white blood cell count are not present. At this stage, the infection may be confused with an ulcer, hiatal hernia, or gallbladder disease. Copious, light-colored, fatty stools, when severe, may lead to hypoproteinemia, hypoglobulinemia, and folic acid and fat-soluble vitamin deficiencies. Symptoms of the acute infection may persist for several days to 2 months.

A second type of presentation may be called the subacute or chronic form. This form may be the initial manifestation of giardiasis or may develop after an acute episode. Usually, a relentless or intermittent course of mushy stools, abdominal distention and flatulence, and a normal or slightly increased number of stools are noted. Associated anorexia and weight loss may be present. This phase of giardiasis may persist for months or years, with recurring exacerbations and remissions. Finally, an individual may become an asymptomatic cyst carrier. This form may be the most common and may be the major source of infection, especially in endemic areas.

Diagnosis usually depends upon identification of cysts from stools, since the trophozoites resist normal peristalsis. The office procedures outlined previously may be helpful in identifying the cysts, but detection varies with the skill of the examiner and the age of the specimen. The irregularity of cyst excretion is a major reason for variable detection. The cysts (Plate V) are ovoid in contour and slightly larger than white blood cells, 8 to 12 microns long and 6 to 10 microns wide. In the normal saline smear, the cysts appear as ovoid, colorless hyaline bodies with a thin cyst wall in which refractile structures, representing the axostyles and flagella, may be seen. With the addition of iodine, the cyst takes on a brownish color. Examination of multiple stools increases the detection rate. If giardiasis is suspected and multiple stools are negative, one may try to increase diagnostic yield by obtaining samples from the duodenum or proximal jejunum. The simplest and least invasive technique is the Entero-Test, outlined previously (Jones, 1986). Duodenal biopsy and aspiration are also useful, but they must be done by an endoscopist. The trophozoite (Plate VI) resembles a cut pear, 11 to 18 by 6 to 9 microns. In fresh untainted preparations, the trophozoite is actively motile, using a combination of irregular progression, rotation, and rocking movements. The cytoplasm is hyaline or finely granular in appearance, but the detailed structure is visible only in iron-hematoxylin preparations. The characteristic nuclei of the trophozoite cause it to take on a "monkey face" appearance. When repeated examinations do not reveal cysts and trophozoites and a high index of suspicion remains, a clinical trial of quinacrine or metronidazole (Flagyl) may be used.

Recommended treatment schedules are given in Table 35–2.

TRICHURIS TRICHIURA

T. trichiura (whipworm) represents the most frequently reported roundworm in the United States. Because of its smaller size, it is generally overshadowed by the largest roundworm, *A. lumbricoides*. The male whipworm measures 30 to 45 mm. in length and has a characteristic shape, resembling a "watch-spring" coil, at the posterior end. Females average 43 mm. in length. The more narrow anterior end gives the adult worm the appearance of a "whip." The head of the worm becomes embedded in the mucosa of the large bowel. It ingests minute amounts of blood, and anemia has been found in children with heavy infections. The adults may live for several years. The female worms will produce an average of 7500 eggs per day. These have a characteristic "barrel-shape," with transparent polar plugs (50 by 20 microns) (Plate VII). Once passed in the feces, 2 to 4 weeks are needed for embryonization. Once ingested in man, the embryonated eggs hatch in the small intestine and remain several days before slowly moving down the intestinal tract, where they develop into mature, egg-producing adults in 30 to 90 days.

The intensity of whipworm infection is greatest in children, with the highest rates found in 2- to 3-year-old children who most frequently come into contact with feces-contaminated soil. Light infections are usually asymptomatic. Heavy infections may present with lower abdominal pain and distention, tenesmus, nausea, vomiting, and weakness. The most dramatic sign of heavy infection is rectal prolapse secondary to rectal edema and straining at stool.

The diagnosis is made by identifying the characteristic eggs in feces. It is important to look for additional intestinal parasites when only light infections are found, since this parasite is generally associated with other roundworms and tends not to cause symptoms in light infections. Treatment is shown in Table 35-2.

ASCARIS LUMBRICOIDES

The largest of intestinal roundworms, *A. lumbricoides,* represents a significant parasite. Because of its size, it often creates a series of emotional reactions in the parents of children who pass this worm. The average adult male may be 15 to 30 cm. long and the adult female 20 to 30 cm. long (Plate VIII). The adult worms live in the lumen of the small intestine and resist peristalsis by their strong muscular design. The adults generally live for 1 year and, with light infections, produce no symptoms. Eggs are passed in feces and require 2 weeks' incubation before they become infective. One adult female may pass up to 200,000 eggs per day. Children are most often infected by hand-to-mouth transmission and are the chief source of soil contamination by defecating outdoors. Once the eggs are ingested, larvae hatch and penetrate the intestinal wall, entering the blood and lymphatics that

Table 35–2. DRUG TREATMENT OF COMMON HELMINTHIC AND PROTOZOAL INFECTION

	Adults	Children
Giardiasis *G. lamblia*	Quinacrine HCL, 100 mg. tid for 5 days or Metronidazole 250 mg. qid for 5 days or Furazolidone, 100 mg. qid for 7–10 days	2 mg per kg. tid for 5 days (max. 300 mg per day) or 5 mg. per kg. tid for 5 days or 1.25 mg. per kg. qid for 7 days
Enterobiasis *E. vermicularis*	Mebendazole, 100 mg. single dose or Pyrantel pamoate, 11 mg. per kg. single dose (max. 1 gram)	same > 2 yr or same
Ascariasis *A. lumbricoides*	Mebendazole 100 mg bid for 3 days or Pyrantel pamoate, 11 mg. per kg. single dose (max. 1 gram)	same > 2 yr or same
Strongyloidiasis *S. stercoralis*	Thiabendazole, 25 mg. per kg. bid for 2 days (max. 3 gram per day)	same
Trichuriasis *T. trichiura*	Mebendazole, 100 mg. bid for 3 days	same > 2 yr
Hookworm species	Mebendazole, 100 mg. bid for 3 days or Pyrantel pamoate, 11 mg. per kg. single dose (max. 1 gram)	same > 2 yr or same
Amebiasis *E. histolytica*	Asymptomatic patient Lodoquinol, 650 mg. tid for 20 days (max. 2 gram per day) Mild to moderate intestinal infection: Metronidazole, 750 mg. tid for 10 days, followed by lodoquinol per above dose Severe and extraintestinal infection: see medical letter reference	30 to 40 mg. per kg. per day in 3 doses for 20 days 30 to 50 mg. per kg. per day in 3 doses for 10 days

drain through the intestinal tract. These serve as portals for the transport of the larvae to the lungs via the portal circulation. The larvae are filtered out of the blood stream by the pulmonary capillary bed. The alveoli are then perforated, providing access to the respiratory passages. This stage produces a pneumonitis and stimulates a cough, fever, and eosinophilic response. Coughing brings the larvae to the epiglottis, and they are then swallowed, finally maturing in the intestine. This process takes approximately 60 days to complete. Once the worm is mature, characteristic eggs are passed, which may be fertilized or unfertilized. Each egg is surrounded by a thick outer shell and is highly resistant to environmental factors (Plate IX).

The symptoms of the initial phase of a moderate infection usually occur within 4 to 5 days of larval penetration of the intestinal tract. Fever from 39.6° to 41.2° C (103° to 105°F) may occur associated with frequent spasms of coughing, bronchial rales, and eosinophilia. There may be evidence of lobar consolidation on the chest roentgenogram. Occasionally, hemoptysis has been reported. This phase is easily misdiagnosed as bacterial or viral pneumonia.

The most common symptom in those infected with adult worms is abdominal pain, often without eosinophilia. The worms may migrate, and they show an affinity for small orifices. Major complications include invasion of the bile duct, liver, peritoneal cavity, and appendix. In heavy infections, volvulus, intussusception, and obstruction may occur. Intestinal obstruction seems more common in the United States, particularly among preschool children. It is important to look for *A. lumbricoides* before treatment is instituted for another intestinal parasite, because migration and obstruction of small orifices can result if ascariasis is partially treated with medication that is not specific for *A. lumbricoides.* The treatment of ascariasis is given in Table 35–2.

ENTEROBIUS VERMICULARIS

Perhaps the most common of all intestinal parasites is the pinworm. Exact figures on its prevalence and distribution are unknown. Often the parents have cleaned the anus and removed all traces of this parasite prior to bringing the child to the office. This tiny, white parasite (Plate X) has generated little medical concern because it produces minimal pathology, but it has generated a great deal of emotional and psychologic stress among the lay population.

The pinworm's life cycle is closely related to that of humans, its only known host. Gravid females (8 to 13 mm.) leave the intestinal tract by way of the anus, each depositing up to 17,000 eggs in the perianal area. The eggs (Plate XI) are transmitted to the mouth within a few hours by contaminated hands, food and drink, clothing, household items, or dust. Each egg contains a sticky surface, which aids in its transmission. Autoinfection is frequent, and pinworms quickly spread within families, schools, and institutions.

Eggs hatch in the duodenum, mature in 2 to 4 weeks, and reside primarily in the cecum and lower ileum before gravid females migrate out the anus. This migration causes the most common symptom, i.e., itching. The itching usually occurs at night when the female emerges to lay her eggs. The adults can be seen by the unaided eye and may be described as "thread size." The perianal deposition of ova permits use of the transparent adhesive tape test to obtain evidence of the parasite (Plate XII). The digital rectal examination is also helpful in making this diagnosis.

ENTAMOEBA HISTOLYTICA

One of the most diagnostically challenging protozoa, *E. histolytica,* although usually producing an asymptomatic condition, may cause diarrhea, bloody dysentery, liver abscesses, and metastatic complications throughout the body. The parasite is transmitted as small cysts, not much larger than a white cell, which are resistant to gastric juices as well as external treatment. They are passed mostly by asymptomatic carriers and persons with chronic infections (Plate XIII). Trophozoites may be seen in stools of persons with acute illness, but these are not infective.

After being ingested, the cyst ripens in the bowel lumen. Immature amebas then move to the cecal and sigmoidal regions, where they become active, vegetative (trophozoite) forms (see Plate XIV). This usually takes 4 to 6 weeks after the cysts are ingested. Once active, the trophozoite may invade the intestinal mucosa and undermine the mucous membrane. This trophozoite phase produces acute amebic colitis in some cases. The predominant symptom is diarrhea, usually accompanied by mucus and streaks of blood. The bowel movements are watery or mushy, can have an offensive odor, and may number 12 to 18 per day. Cramping lower abdominal pain frequently precedes the bowel movements. A few patients will have a low-grade fever, anorexia, nausea, vomiting, weakness, and abdominal tenderness. The acute symptomatic episode usually lasts 1 to 4 weeks. Once the acute phase passes, the individual may become asymptomatic but will begin to pass cysts in the stools.

Invasion of the blood stream and lymphatic system following erosion of the intestinal mucosa results in the transport of the trophozoites to the liver. The trophozoites become established in the lobules, resulting in necrosis of capillaries and parenchymal tissue. Symptoms of pain, fever, chills, and sweating develop. The liver usually becomes enlarged and tender, and a liver abscess may develop, often in the right lobe. Spread to the lungs and pleura is a possible complication in untreated patients.

Trophozoites may metastasize to other parts of the body, including the brain. Pericardial and dermatologica infections rarely occur.

The diagnosis depends on demonstrating cysts in formed stools (see Plate XIII), or trophozoites (see Plate XIV) in the mucoid and bloody diarrheal stools accompanying acute amebiasis. Either form is detectable in fresh specimens, but concentration methods will improve the chance of making a diagnosis. Particular attention to mucus or blood flakes in formed stools may also help in cyst identification.

White blood cells are commonly misidentified as *E. histolytica.* Differentiation from other species, particularly *Entamoeba coli,* a nonpathogenic, is necessary.

Visual examination of the colon by sigmoidoscopy may be helpful, since many patients with amebiasis have rectal lesions. Small, pinpoint ulcers may be seen, and material aspirated from these lesions may demonstrate trophozoites. Serologic tests are useful, particularly when extraintestinal amebiasis is suspected (92 to 98 per cent positive). They are slightly less positive for active intestinal infection (80 to 90 per cent positive).

HOOKWORM

Historically, hookworm is the most notorious of the roundworm species. Noted for years as a condition associated with poverty, lethargy, and anemia, it has received less and less attention owing to improved hygienic practices. *Necator americanus* is the prevailing species in the United States. It is still endemic in the Sunbelt and is found repeatedly in immigrant populations. *Ancylostoma duodenale,* the second species, may cause greater blood loss in the gastrointestinal tract.

The adult worms are grayish-white and are 5 to 13 microns long. They reside largely in the jejunum, where they attach to the mucosa by special mouth parts. Blood and mucosal substances are ingested. Studies have estimated that *N. Americanus* averages 0.03 ml. of intake of blood per worm per day, whereas *A. duodenale* averages 0.15 ml. of intake of blood per worm per day. The average life span of the adult is from 2 to 6 years.

The soil is contaminated by eggs passed in feces. Within 2 days, at optimal temperatures of 23° to 33° C (73.4 to 91.4° F) noninfective rhabditiform larvae are produced. They undergo a second molt into infective filariform larvae within 5 days, occupying the top half-inch of soil. Contact with contaminated soil for 5 to 10 minutes is required for skin penetration. Larvae penetrate man through hair follicles, pores, or unbroken skin, particularly on exposed hands and feet. Upon entering the blood stream, larvae migrate through the heart to the lungs, are coughed up, and are then swallowed. Within a week, they will have traveled to the upper small intestine.

Severe itching and erythema may occur at the site of penetration of the larvae. During larval migration, the host may be asymptomatic unless large numbers of worms are present, in which case pneumonitis may result from damage to the alveoli. Symptoms include fever, headache, nausea, dyspnea, and a nonproductive cough. In the intestinal tract, nonspecific gastrointestinal symptoms can occur, including nausea, vomiting, flatulence, diarrhea, and low-grade fever. If the worm burden is sufficient and there is no intervention, the microcytic hypochromic anemia of iron deficiency will result. Physical findings are usually present in hookworm disease only if there is significant anemia. These include pallor, tachycardia, increased precordial activity, systolic murmurs, slight hepatosplenomegaly, and dependent edema.

Eggs may be recovered daily from the feces and are recognizable by their symmetric shape, rounded ends, and thin, transparent, hyaline shells. The nuclear material is usually in its early-to-late morula stage of development (Plate XV). Hookworm larvae are rarely seen. For treatment see Table 35–2.

STRONGYLOIDES STERCORALIS

S. stercoralis is not as common as other roundworm infections, but it is significant because it is potentially lethal in susceptible hosts. Fatal disseminated *Strongyloides* infections have been reported in the compromised host, owing to the potential for autoinfection.

Adults are small (female 2.2 mm., male 0.7 mm.) and reside in the duodenum and upper jejunum. Thin-shelled eggs are laid in the epithelium and hatch within the intestine, producing the first-stage, rhabditiform larvae. It is this stage that is usually found in the stool (Plate XVI). Once passed, the rhabditiform larvae undergo metamorphosis to the infective (filariform) stage. This may occur within 24 hours. On contact with skin, the filariform larvae penetrate the epidermis, move to the small blood vessels, and are carried to the lungs. When they reach the pulmonary capillaries, they break out into the alveoli and proceed via the trachea to the intestine. Once in the intestine, they invade the epithelium of glands, molt twice, and reach maturity in about 2 weeks. In addition to this primary cycle, *S. stercoralis* may have an abbreviated cycle and a free-living cycle. In the abbreviated cycle, the metamorphosis to the filariform stage occurs within the intestinal canal or on the perianal skin. Here, reinfection takes place without the larvae leaving the body. The free-living cycle takes place in the soil. Here, the rhabditiform live in the soil and may then change into the filariform stage at a later date.

As with most of the intestinal parasites, individuals with light infections are asymptomatic. Penetration of the skin by the filariform larvae usually produces little reaction. However, repeated skin penetration may result in the development of a pruritic, papular, erythematous rash. Pulmonary signs reflect the severity of the infection. Cough, shortness of breath, wheezing, and fever may develop as the larvae migrate through the lungs. At this stage, transient pulmonary infiltrates have been observed on chest x-ray studies, and eosinophilia of 10 to 40 per cent may be found. Intestinal manifestations include burning abdominal pain, which is often epigastric. The pain may be exacerbated by food and is occasionally dull or crampy. Complaints of nausea and vomiting may be associated with the pain. The penetration of the intestinal mucosa by the adult worms may simulate ulcer disease, with symptoms being relatively acute in onset. Mucous diarrhea is common, sometimes alternating with constipation. A chronic pattern may develop, with periodic attacks occurring over many years. Generalized urticaria has been reported, although some patients may only show serpiginous wheals, beginning perianally and extending to the buttocks, abdomen, and thighs. The autoinfective cycle may lead to massive systemic strongyloidiasis. This is usually associated with severe, generalized abdominal pain, distention, shock, and a high fever. Massive larval migration to the lungs may result in cough, wheezing, and dyspnea. Polymorphonuclear leukocytosis is common, but eosinophilia frequently does not develop.

Identification of *S. stercoralis* rhabditiform larvae is diagnostic when found in fresh feces. Embryonated eggs may be seen in severe diarrheal stools and are differentiated from hookworm eggs by the well-developed larval phase within the egg shell. If the results of tests on stools remain negative when this roundworm infection is suggested, examination of duodenal fluid by the simple "string test" (Entero-Test) may yield diagnostic rhabditiform larvae.

HUMAN TOXOCARIASIS

The dog and cat roundworm may produce a disease process in man called visceral larva migrans. The parasite eggs are transferred with dog and cat feces to soil, sandboxes, and other points of human contact. When ingested by humans, usually young children, the larvae are unable to complete their development into adult roundworms in the human body. Instead, they migrate in the blood stream or intestine, producing the signs and symptoms of infection.

Toxocara canis (dog roundworm) has been found in more than 50 per cent of puppies and approximately 20 per cent of older dogs. *T. cati* has been reported in limited studies to be present in 10 to 75 per cent of cats examined. However, it is generally felt that the majority of infections in humans are due to *T. canis*.

The clinical picture reflects the mechanical damage caused by the migrating larvae and by the inflammatory response stimulated by them. The liver is most often involved, but any tissue can be invaded.

The invaded tissues will often show multiple eosinophilic abscesses and allergic-type eosinophilic granulomas. A peripheral eosinophilia of 50 to 90 per cent may be found with a leukocyte count of 30,000 to 100,000 per cubic millimeter.

Coughing, wheezing, pallor, malaise, irritability, and weight loss are common signs and symptoms. Pruritic eruptions have been reported to occur over the trunk and lower extremities accompanied by painful nodules. Joint pains, abdominal pain, nausea, and vomiting have also occurred. Neurologic disturbances, with convulsions and petit mal attacks, have occurred with nervous system migration. Ocular involvement, typically unilateral, has received increasing recognition. Common complaints at presentation include visual loss, strabismus, and, more rarely, eye pain. Some investigators believe that the eye involvement represents a different stage or phase of toxocariasis.

Overall, the infection with *Toxocara* usually runs a chronic-benign course but may last as long as 18 months. It is self-limited in the absence of reinfection. The severity of the infection depends on the number of larvae in the tissue and the immune state of the individual infected.

The diagnosis of this parasitic infection cannot be made by fecal examinations, since the parasite does not complete its life cycle in humans. A high and persistent eosinophilia in a child should arouse suspicion, particularly in patients with a history of eating dirt or playing on ground frequented by dogs or cats. Serologic tests are available but lack sensitivity. Newer serologic tests are becoming available and hold promise of greater sensitivity and specificity.

Treatment of light infections is generally felt to be unnecessary. However, concern over the possibility of eye involvement has led some to recommend treatment with thiabendazole (25 mg. per kg. twice a day for 5 days) or diethylcarbamazine (2 mg. per kg. three times a day for 30 days) (Markell and Voge, 1976).

ECTOPARASITES

Parasitic infections occurring on the surface of the body or articles in immediate contact with the body are defined as ectoparasites. Four ectoparasites are becoming increasingly more common in our office practice. Current epidemics of these parasites are confusing because they transcend the usual boundaries, affecting young and old, rich and poor, and clean and unclean. Their identification, however, allows for effective, straightforward treatment (Fisher et al., 1978).

Head Lice (*Pediculus capitus*). This ectoparasite has received increased attention from school officials and parents. School children are often brought to the office because someone noticed lice or their eggs—nits—in the hair. Only a few organisms (10 to 15 adults) are usually present, and the child is asymptomatic. Generally, the child has been infected a month or longer without realizing it. Small light-colored specks, which look like flakes of dandruff, can be seen. Transmission is through direct contact or by sharing close personal objects, such as combs and hats.

The adults are small (1.0 to 2.0 mm.), elongated, diamond-shaped insects with distinct body segments (Plate XVII). They favor the back of the neck and regularly feed on blood meals, thus generating focal irritation and itching.

When suspecting head lice, examine the occipital and postauricular regions of the scalp, using tongue blades to comb through the hair. Adults are rarely found but, if seen, confirm the diagnosis. Nits are apt to be more numerous and easily spotted. Confirm the diagnosis microscopically by examining a nit attached to a plucked hair under a low-power microscope (Plate XVIII).

Extensive scratching may lead to secondary scalp infections with lymph node involvement and fever. These complications generally occur in the late stages of the infection.

The use of gamma benzene hexachloride shampoo (Kwell), massaged into the premoistened scalp for 4 minutes before rinsing, is effective against head lice. Family members should be examined and treated if infestations are found. Personal items that may be shared should be disinfected and their use restricted.

Pubic Louse (*Phthirus pubis*). Generally considered to be sexually transmitted, this insect lives in the pubic area. Occasionally, it may be seen in the hairs of the axilla, thighs, trunk, eyelashes, and eyebrows. The beard and mustache of males can also be infected.

Itching is the major symptom and is likely to prompt the patient to seek help. Any sexually active patient with a pruritic eruption of the pubic region should be checked for *P. pubis*.

The patient will often report seeing the organism, and if so, the diagnosis is clear-cut. Otherwise, careful examination of the mons pubis may reveal nits or the crab-shaped adult lice. The adults (0.8 to 1.0 mm.) appear as black or rust-colored dots close to the skin surface. At first glance, they may be mistaken for freckles. The adults or nits may be removed with fine forceps and examined microscopically (Plate XIX).

Once a diagnosis of pubic crabs is made, other sexually transmitted diseases should be considered.

Excessive scratching may cause excoriations with secondary infection. This may confuse the picture and make diagnosis more difficult.

Treatment is the same as for head lice, except gamma benzene hexachloride lotion may be used instead of shampoo. It should be applied in a thin layer over the pubic mons and adjacent hairy areas. For eyelash infestations, however, nits and lice should be removed with forceps and petrolatum ophthalmic ointment applied daily for 8 to 10 days.

Body Lice (*Pediculus corporis*). The body louse is known as a vector of disease—typhus, trench fever, and relapsing fever. Unlike infections with the other forms of lice, it tends to correlate with the patient's attention to personal hygiene. The insect lives in the clothes—especially in the seams—and migrates to the body surface only to feed. The infestation is seen in individuals that wear only one set of clothes over a long period of time.

Hemorrhagic macules are formed at the site of a blood meal, usually in areas where the clothes fit tightly. In the late stages of infestations, eruptions are likely to be numerous and associated with excoriations due to intense itching.

Adults are generally not seen on body surfaces but may be found in the clothing along the seams or creases. Adults average 2 to 3 mm. in size and are the largest of the lice species.

Drug treatment is not required for management of body lice, since neither eggs, nymphs, nor adults survive personal cleanliness. The removal of infected clothing and bedclothes and the wearing of only freshly laundered clothes eliminate body lice. Strict personal hygiene should also pertain to family members. Clothing and immediate personal articles should be cleansed before reuse, since body lice may survive up to 1 week off the host. Clothing not easily washed or dry-cleaned may be deloused by sealing it tightly in a plastic bag for 10 days. After 10 days, lice and nits will be nonviable.

Scabies (*Sarcoptes scabiei*). *Sarcoptes scabiei* is the only itch or mange mite that commonly causes human disease. The small, rounded, four-legged mite (male, 200 to 250 mm.; female 300 to 450 mm.) burrows into the corneous layer of skin, particularly about the hands and wrists. The infection is characterized by pruritic papular lesions along burrows that house the female mite and her young. The female produces up to 50 eggs during her life span of about 1 month. The belt-line and thigh areas of men are especially susceptible, as are the nipples, abdomen, and lower buttocks of women. Since the eruptions are believed to be caused partly by hypersensitivity reactions, they may appear beyond sites of infestation. Lesions usually occur on the interdigital area of the hands, wrists, forearms, elbows, armpits and back, and in the inguinal and genital areas. Persons may be infested and capable of spreading the mites by close personal contact weeks before lesions appear.

The diagnosis of scabies is usually based upon the presence of intense itching at night and is confirmed by identification of mites using skin scrapings of papules or burrows. A No. 11 blade can be used to remove the parasite after identifying a papule or linear burrow (Plate XX). A strong light and magnifying lens may be helpful in detecting burrows, and the tunnel can be gently slit open. Material obtained on the tip of the blade is transferred to a glass slide for microscopic examination. The slide is prepared by adding two drops of 10 per cent potassium hydroxide to dissolve debris and then adding a coverslip.

This condition is extremely contagious, attacking infants and children as well as adults. In infants, the mite favors areas of the body that are easily exposed, particularly the face, scalp, palms, and soles. A high percentage of children develop persistent, reddish-brown infiltrate nodules, particularly on covered parts of the body. Intense scratching will lead to linear excoriations and secondary bacterial infections.

Treatment for adults requires applications of gamma benzene hexachloride lotion from the neck down following a warm bath. The lotion is left on the skin for 12 hours and then removed by showering or bathing. A second application may be needed in 6 days in heavy infections, since eggs may hatch in 4 to 5 days. In infested children or infants, 10 per cent crotamiton can be used or 6 to 10 per cent sulfur in petrolatum. These solutions also should be applied topically from the neck down after bathing. Although scabies is not transmitted 24 hours after therapy, pruritus and lesions may not disappear for several weeks because the patient remains hypersensitized. In severe reactions, antihistamines or salicylates may be required for relief, and systemic antibiotics may be required for secondary bacterial infections.

One should consider treating all members of the household and all sexual partners of an infected patient.

References

Benenson, A. S. (Ed.): Control of communicable diseases in man. 14th ed. Washington, D.C. American Public Health Association, 1985. *Paperback reference and pocket size. A good reference for office practice. Includes a brief discussion on major parasites of clinical importance.*

Blondell, R. D., and Dedman, E. B.: An extended family with giardiasis. J. Fam. Pract., *19*(3):388–392, 1984. *Discussion of impact that giardiasis can have on the family unit.*

Blumenthal, D. S.: Intestinal nematodes in the United States. N. Engl. J. Med., *297*:1437, 1977. *The five most common intestinal nematodes are briefly presented.*

Blumenthal, D. S., and Schultz, M. G.: Incidence of intestinal obstruction in children infected with *Ascaris lumbricoides*. Am. J. Trop. Med. Hyg., *24*:801, 1975. *A rare but potentially lethal complication of this intestinal roundworm.*

Bradley, S. L., Dines, D. E., and Brewer, N. S.: Disseminated *Strongyloides stercoralis* in an immunosuppressed host. Mayo Clinic. Proc., *53*:332, 1978. *Brief case report summarizing the major features of this often lethal manifestation of Strongyloides.*

Centers for Disease Control: Intestinal Parasite Surveillance. Annual Summary 1978. Issued August, 1979. *The last of a series of summaries published by the Centers for Disease Control. It contains a state-by-state report of intestinal parasites. Copies can be obtained by writing to Centers for Disease Control, Attention: Intestinal Parasite Surveillance, Parasitic Diseases Division, Bureau of Epidemiology, Atlanta, Georgia 30333.*

Craun, G. F.: Waterborne giardiasis in the United States: A review. Am. J. Public Health, *69*:817, 1979. *Increasing interest in this parasite has led to its general recognition as the major intestinal parasite of the 1970's. This article reviews the waterborne outbreaks of giardiasis. Most outbreaks occurred as the result of consuming untreated surface water or surface water with disinfection as the only treatment.*

Dupont, H. L., and Sullivan, P. S.: Giardiasis: The clinical spectrum, diagnosis and therapy. Pediatr. Infect. Dis., *5*(1):S131–S138, 1986. *A review of giardiasis from pediatric perspective.*

Fisher, A. A., Juranek, D., Maibach, H. I., et al.: Pediculosis:

Little lice can make mighty problems. Patient Care, *12*:240, 1978. *Practical discussion of this group of ectoparasites.*

Grove, D. I., Warren, K. S., Mahmoud, A. A. F: Algorithms in the diagnosis and management of exotic diseases. III. Strongyloidiasis. J. Infect. Dis., *131*:755, 1975.

Hurwitz, A. L., and Owen, R. L.: Venereal transmission of intestinal parasites. West. J. Med., *128*:89, 1978. *A review of parasites that can be transmitted by sexual contact.*

Jones, J. E.: Office parasitology. Am. Fam. Phys., *22*:86, 1980. *Photomicrographs of the most common intestinal parasites. Useful in the office laboratory for reference when looking for these parasites.*

Jones, J. E.: The royal roundworm: *Ascaris lumbricoides*. J. Fam. Pract., *13*:271, 1981. *A discussion of how this parasite can impact upon the family unit.*

Jones, J. E.: Identification of intestinal nematodes using the digital rectal examination. J. Fam. Pract., *12*:563, 1981. *A brief report on a small survey using the digital rectal examination as a method of obtaining samples for stool examinations.*

Jones, J. E.: The nonpathogenic intestinal protozoa. Am. Fam. Physician, *28*(3):215–218, 1983. *A good reference, with photographs of the nonpathogenic intestinal protozoa.*

Jones, J. E.: String test for diagnosing giardiasis. Am. Fam. Physician, *34*(2):123–126, 1986. *Step-by-step discussion of this single office procedure for the diagnosis of giardiasis.*

Jones, J. E.: Pinworms. Am. Fam. Physician, *38*(3):159–163, 1988. *Most common of all intestinal roundworms. Gives discussion of life-cycle and treatment.*

Kelly, M., and Keystone, J. S.: Travellers from the tropics—a practical approach to common problems. Can. Fam. Phys., *28*:387, 1980. *Straightforward approach to patients and their symptoms. Good reference to have.*

Krogstad, D. J., Spencer, H. C., Healy, G. R.: Amebiasis. N. Engl. J. Med., *298*:262–265, 1978.

Lozoff, B., Warren, K. S., Mahmoud, A. A. F.: Algorithms in the diagnosis and management of exotic diseases. VIII. Hookworm. J. Infect. Dis., *132*:606–610, 1975.

Markell, E. K.: Diagnosis of the more common parasitic diseases. Primary Care, *5*:57, 1978. *Excellent review of the signs and symptoms associated with parasitic diseases.*

Markell, E. K., and Voge, M.: Medical Parasitology. 4th ed. Philadelphia, W. B. Saunders Company, 1976.

Medical Letter: Drugs for Parasitic Infections. Vol. 30 (Issue 759), Feb. 12, 1988. *Complete listing of drug treatments and alternative drugs. A good reference to have for the office setting.*

Phillips, S. C., Milovan, D., William, D. C., et al.: Sexual transmission of enteric protozoa and helminths in a venereal disease–clinic population. N. Engl. J. Med., *305*:630, 1981.

Rosenthal, P., and Liebman, W. M.: Comparative study of stool examinations, duodenal aspiration and pediatric Entero-Test for giardiasis in children. J. Pediatr., *96*:278, 1980.

Schantz, P. M., and Glickman, L. T.: Toxocaral visceral larva migrans. N. Engl. J. Med., *298*:436, 1978.

Schantz, P. M. Weis, P. E., Pollard, Z. F., and White, M. C.: Risk factors for toxocaral ocular larva migrans: A case-control study. Am. J. Public Health, *70*:1269, 1980.

Stone, S. P.: Scabies. Am. Fam. Phys., *15*:152, 1977. *Brief but good discussion of this common ectoparasite.*

Strickland, G. T. (Ed.): Hunter's Tropical Medicine. Philadelphia, W. B. Saunders Co., 1976. *Perhaps the most readable of the larger tests on parasitic diseases. Highly recommended for those who wish to pursue deeper study of tropical medicine and parasitic diseases.*

Wolfe, M. S.: Giardiasis. N. Engl. J. Med., *298*:319, 1978.

36

Obstetrics

Kenneth L. Noller
Robert F. Avant

For years obstetric care has been an essential part of the practice of family medicine. The multiple changes of pregnancy have a significant effect on the pregnant patient and her family, and the addition of a new member has a multifactorial and long-lasting effect on the family unit. As stated by Candib (1976), "the longitudinal experience of knowing patients before they are pregnant, being the provider of the news that they are pregnant, dealing with the patient's fears and hopes about that process, following the changes in the patient's state of different stages of pregnancy, observing changing family dynamics with the expectation of the new baby, being present during the labor process, mediating that process to both mother and father and extended family, participating with the family in the delivery, assuring the family of normalcy or explaining the event of any abnormality in either mother of baby or the process itself, and, of course, following mother, baby, and family back into the home setting—this by nature longitudinal process is at the center of the experience of family practice."

Obstetric care is extremely important to the education of family physicians, as demonstrated by the requirements for training of the Residency Review Committee for Family Practice, which state that "the residents must be provided the instruction necessary to understand the biological and psychological impact of pregnancy, delivery, and care of the newborn upon a woman and her family. The residents should be taught technical skills and the provision of antepartum and postpartum care, and the normal delivery process as well as complications of pregnancy and their management" (Directory of Graduate Medical Education Programs, 1988–1989).

In addition, a joint effort by the American Academy of Family Physicians (AAFP) and the American College of Obstetricians and Gynecologists (ACOG) describes the basic minimal requirements for training in obstetrics and gynecology for family practice residents (ACOG-AAFP Recommended Core Curriculum and Hospital Practice Privileges in Obstetrics and Gynecology for Family Physicians).

Significant differences exist in the depth and breadth of obstetric care delivered by family physicians. In 1981, a study by the American Academy of Family Physicians indicated that residency-trained family physicians were more likely to include obstetrics in their practice, with 64.3 per cent of the respondents stating that they have hospital privileges for routine obstetric care. The range was from 93.1 per cent of physicians having routine obstetric privileges in the west and north-central regions, to 33.3 per cent in the middle atlantic region. The study also noted that only 1 per cent of those surveyed did not perform routine obstetrics because they were unable to obtain privileges. In that survey, 37.6 per cent of the respondents reported privileges in complicated obstetric care. Changes since the last edition of this textbook (primarily related to medical liability and malpractice premiums for physicians providing obstetric care) have had dramatic affects on the practice of obstetrics for both family physicians and obstetricians. A survey of 20,395 board-certified family physicians taking the American Board of Family Practice recertification examination and being in practice 6 years or longer demonstrate that 64.8 per cent of these family physicians do not perform obstetric care. In more recent years, family physicians who were recertified were asked about the numbers of deliveries that they perform. Of a total of 15,789 respondents, 10,012 (63.5%) do not perform obstetric care. Of the total respondents, 14.5 per cent perform 1 to 25 deliveries per year, 14.2 per cent perform 26 to 50 deliveries a year, and 7.8 per cent perform over 50 deliveries per year (Nicholas J. Pisacano, M.D., American Board of Family Practice, Lexington, KY).

This dramatic and rapid change in obstetric practice by family physicians will clearly have an effect on the future of family practice and obstetric care, and this chapter provides an outline of obstetrics for those family physicians continuing that important part of family practice. In view of the differences in obstetric practices among family physicians, the authors clearly recognize that some readers may find this chapter meets many of their needs, whereas others will need to refer to standard obstetric texts or current literature for more in-depth information.

Despite the changes in medical liability and malpractice insurance premiums, the recent movement toward more personalized family-oriented and less interventional obstetric care fits very well into the practice of family medicine, and one should expect a continued desire for patients to receive obstetrical care from their family physician. This factor, combined with the changes in obstetrical practice, including electronic fetal monitoring, ultrasonography, chemical determination of fetal maturity and neonatal intensive care, place significant demands on the physicians who provide obstetric care.

The early identification of high-risk obstetric patients, combined with the development of perinatal and neonatal centers, has had a significant effect on when and where high-risk patients should be delivered. It is extremely important for each family physician who provides obstetric care to identify sites with ready access to appropriate consultants in advance, so that prompt, efficient consultation or transfer of high-risk patients can be accomplished. Also, because of the dynamic nature of the birth process, it is extremely important that excellent communication between the family physician and obstetric consultant be maintained. Although pregnancy is a normal process and not a disease state, unexpected events can occur that may suddenly change the situation and jeopardize the health of the mother or infant.

Preparation for Pregnancy

Although pregnancy is a normal state for a woman, it makes a number of demands on the woman's organ systems. All organs or organ systems are affected by pregnancy. Although these stresses are easily accommodated by the normal adaptive mechanisms of pregnancy and result in no unusual morbidity, the additional stress of pregnancy can tax an unhealthy organ. Thus, preparation for pregnancy should become part of the routine health care of a woman.

In the past, very little consideration has been given to this aspect of health care. Although the decision to bear a child is one of the most important medical decisions a couple ever makes, it is rarely preceded by the medical screening and evaluation that many less important medical procedures would entail. For example, before a woman would be hospitalized for an elective surgical procedure such as tubal ligation, a thorough history and physical and basic laboratory tests would be obtained. Such evaluation is rarely accomplished before pregnancy. Yet the stress placed on the entire person is much greater in pregnancy than it is for the above-mentioned minor surgical procedure.

All women should be encouraged to have a general medical evaluation before becoming pregnant. The examination should include not only a routine pelvic examination but also an evaluation of the woman's general health status. Medical diseases of many organ systems may cause significant problems in pregnancy. For example, diseases of the cardiovascular system are among the most important to diagnose before conception. Despite this fact, nearly 50 per cent of all cardiac disease of adult women is diagnosed as a result of initial prenatal screening (Noller, 1981). With little expense in money and time, such a medical evaluation can be accomplished and appropriate evaluation and treatment initiated. This effort results in a better chance for a good outcome of pregnancy and a happier, healthier pregnant woman.

Certain general recommendations dealing with contraceptive practices, medications, habits, and social activities have special importance when preparing for pregnancy.

CONTRACEPTIVE PRACTICES

For many years, physicians and patients have suggested that the use of oral contraceptives should be discontinued for a few months before any attempts at conception. Although this is largely an empiric notion and the number of months was decided without any reliable basis, occasional studies have found that the occurrence of pregnancy immediately after discontinuing oral contraceptives is more frequently followed by an unfavorable pregnancy outcome (Janerich et al., 1980).

MEDICATIONS

When possible, the use of all medications should be eliminated during pregnancy. Therefore, any woman who is considering pregnancy should have a thorough evaluation of her need for medication before her pregnancy attempt. Women should be cautioned against the use of all prescription drugs, and many over-the-counter drugs should be restricted. For example, recent evidence shows that the use of aspirin-containing products may cause fetal problems in some circumstances.

HABITS

The use of tobacco during pregnancy should be avoided. There does not seem to be any "safe" level of tobacco use that can be documented to have no adverse fetal effects. Women should be encouraged to cease completely the use of tobacco-containing products before conception. Tobacco causes a decrease in the birth weight and an increase in abortion, premature birth, fetal death, placenta previa, and abruptio placenta. There is also documentation to suggest that toxemia, when it occurs in mothers who smoke, is a more serious disease than when it occurs in women who do not. Also, children born and raised in an environment of parents who smoke have a greater risk of pulmonary disease during their early months of life.

Alcohol consumption also should be discouraged during pregnancy. The fetal alcohol syndrome has now been described in women who consider themselves to be only "social" drinkers. Additionally, spontaneous abortion, mental retardation, low birth weight, and other birth defects have also been noted to be increased in the females who consume even "moderate" amounts of alcohol in pregnancy. Pregnant women should be counseled to avoid alcohol consumption.

Not all habits are necessarily bad. For example, a recent article has documented that coffee consumption in pregnancy does not lead to an increase in birth defects (Linn et al., 1982).

IMMUNIZATIONS

The preconception health evaluation also can serve to ensure that the woman who is considering pregnancy has been immunized. A rubella titer should be obtained, and if needed, immunization performed before conception.

DIET AND NUTRITION

Each woman's nutritional habits and present weight should be assessed at the prepregnancy health evaluation. Obesity should be corrected if possible by means of a reducing diet. In fact, morbid obesity may lead to infertility, since women who are grossly overweight frequently do not ovulate with regularity because of a "steady-state" estrogen level due to peripheral conversion and storage of estrogen.

Likewise, women who are extremely underweight may fail to ovulate because of a lack of the "critical body mass" (Frisch et al., 1980). Recently, a number of women who reduced their body fat to a minimal level have been shown to frequently experience amenorrhea and anovulation. Ballerinas and long-distance runners are examples of these types of women. This comment should not be interpreted to be "anti-exercise." However, the woman who exercises regularly (within reason) is able to tolerate the stresses of pregnancy much more readily than the woman who does not.

Some dietary instruction should be included in any discussion of preparation for pregnancy. In general, the common "middle class American diet" is satisfactory if it includes a representative sampling of all the major food groups. Although some may suggest that such a diet is too high in animal fats and carbohydrates, such a diet does include sufficient amounts of all of the essential nutrients for pregnancy, except iron and folic acid.

Diagnosis of Pregnancy

Anticipation and achievement of the first pregnancy is one of the most exciting and anxiety-producing events in a woman's life. It is no wonder then that the physician is often asked to diagnose a pregnancy very soon after conception. Although it is easy to do so once the presence of fetal movements or fetal heart sounds are evident to the examiner, most women request a positive diagnosis at a much earlier date.

A woman may perceive early signs of pregnancy within a few days of the first missed menstrual period. Usually, the earliest signs are (1) breast tenderness, (2) fatigue, and (3) some abnormal reaction to food. Although these three signs may not always be present or always be recognized by the woman even when they are present, they are common and are suggestive of intrauterine pregnancy. These symptoms are generally reliable indicators, even in women who have irregular menses and who frequently skip menstrual periods.

An examiner may have difficulty determining the presence of pregnancy in the first 6 to 8 weeks of gestation. Although the uterus is usually palpably enlarged and soft within 6 weeks from the last menstrual period, the exact size may not be easy to determine. This is particularly true in obese women and women who have had several children. The presence of Chadwick's sign—a purplish discoloration of the uterine cervix due to the increased blood supply—is often present by 6 weeks from the last menstrual period.

Rapid, inexpensive, and reliable urine pregnancy tests are now readily available from both medical laboratories and over-the-counter in most pharmacies. Each test has a slightly different sensitivity but most should be positive 14 days after the first missed menstrual period. Over-the-counter home pregnancy tests are reliable but are not infallible. Some women have difficulty interpreting the results of the test, and occasionally, false-positive results occur.

If a precise and accurate pregnancy test is needed, the amount of human chorionic gonadotropin present in the serum may be determined qualitatively or quantitatively. The qualitative blood pregnancy tests vary in sensitivity, depending on the source of the materials. The quantitative determination of human chorionic gonadotropin should not be used for routine pregnancy screening because it is time-consuming and expensive. However, when it is important to know the actual level (such as in the cases of hydatidiform mole or ectopic pregnancy), the level may be determined.

A reliable diagnosis of pregnancy also may be obtained by using pelvic ultrasonography. The test is too expensive to be used routinely for this purpose but may show intrauterine pregnancy when scanning because of symptoms suggestive of an ectopic pregnancy or an ovarian cyst. When signs and symptoms are suggestive of an ectopic pregnancy, confirmation of an intrauterine gestational sac by means of static or real-time B-scan ultrasonography can be useful. However, such a diagnosis may be difficult to make without the help of a skilled technician and should not be attempted casually or occasionally by an untrained examiner.The use of the vaginal probe ultrasound transducer has allowed even earlier diagnosis of pregnancy.

Accidents of Early Pregnancy

SPONTANEOUS ABORTION

Despite the best efforts of physicians and the hopes of parents, approximately one in six clinical pregnancies in the United States ends in spontaneous abortion (Barnes et al., 1980). When sensitive tests for pregnancy have been used for research purposes, it has been shown that up to one half of all human gestations end in abortion. These early losses result from many causes, but major chromosomal defects and poor implantation—causes not amenable to medical intervention—are believed to be the most frequent. Other causes, such as smoking, alcohol use, environmental toxins, drug exposure, and poor nutrition, can be reduced by medical intervention and counseling.

The term "spontaneous abortion" refers to the spontaneous passage of the products of conception. Such passage may be either complete or incomplete. If the products of conception are passed intact, if bleeding ceases promptly after such passage, and if the cervical canal and uterine size rapidly return to normal, the abortion is considered to be complete and manipulation of the uterus is not advised. To avoid continued bleeding, it has been general practice in the United States to use ergot derivatives such as methylergonovine, 0.2 mg four times a day for 2 to 3 days, unless a medical history of hypertension or asthma is present.

A woman often passes only part of the products of conception, and then the term "incomplete spontaneous abortion" is appropriate. Incomplete abortion is more likely if the pregnancy is of greater than 12 weeks' gestation or if infection has occurred. In these women, the endocervical canal usually remains dilated, fetal membranes or placental tissue may be seen in the canal, bleeding continues unabated, and the uterine size remains enlarged. Medications alone rarely cause complete uterine emptying. Therefore, it has been our practice to perform uterine evacuation when fragments of fetal tissue remain within the uterus. Evacuation of the uterus may be accomplished easily and safely by vacuum curettage if it is of less than 12 weeks' size. If the equipment for this procedure is not available, then curettage using sharp curettes may be accomplished. Dense uterine synechiae causing amenorrhea (Asherman's syndrome) and other complications of dilation and curettage occur more commonly after sharp curettage than after vacuum curettage. Oxytocin or ergot derivatives may be given to cause uterine contraction and to decrease the chances of perforation. Any uterus that is larger than 12 weeks' size presents a particular problem and is at high risk for perforation or rupture at evacuation.

THREATENED ABORTION

The term "threatened abortion" is defined as bleeding occurring during the first 4 months of pregnancy. Although nearly 50 per cent of all women who are pregnant will bleed some time during the pregnancy, bleeding is a sign that is suggestive of a high risk of fetal death. Although it is never easy to predict the outcome of threatened abortion, in general the amount of bleeding and the presence or absence of severe uterine cramping can be predictive signs. Thus, heavy bleeding and severe cramping are usually prodromal symptoms of impending spontaneous abortion.

In past years, women who have experienced a threatened abortion were often placed at bed rest or given medications to prevent spontaneous abortion. We now know that once bleeding has started, the use of medication and bed rest are of no benefit. Although a woman probably should be counseled against vigorous exercise or activities involving strenuous physical activity, data suggest that bed rest is not helpful. Similarly, avoidance of intercourse and the use of tampons do not increase the salvage rate. In fact, in most spontaneous abortions, fetal demise occurs days or weeks before the onset of vaginal bleeding.

Ectopic Pregnancy

Although the term "ectopic pregnancy" refers to a pregnancy that implants anywhere except the endometrial cavity, it is used almost synonymously with tubal pregnancy (Mattingly, 1977). Intra-abdominal and ovarian pregnancies do occur, but they are extremely rare.

An extrauterine pregnancy in the fallopian tube

occurs in approximately 1 of every 200 pregnancies, and its incidence is increasing at an alarming rate. Therefore, any physician who cares for pregnant women sees this complication with some frequency. The major contributing factor to this disease is the pre-existence of tubal scarring due to pelvic inflammatory disease. A second common factor is previous ectopic pregnancy, since women who have previously experienced this complication have approximately a 10-per cent chance of it occurring in subsequent pregnancies.

The presenting signs and symptoms in this disease usually are (1) pain, (2) vaginal bleeding, and (3) amenorrhea. This triad of symptoms is not always present, and other symptoms may be more important. These include those related to the presence or absence of frank rupture and the amount of intraperitoneal bleeding that is present. The woman with an ectopic pregnancy may experience several days of vaginal bleeding after a period of amenorrhea, accompanied by some mild abdominal discomfort. At some point, however, the pain usually becomes severe and tends to localize to the left or right side. Shoulder pain, indicating blood under the diaphragm, is frequent. Additionally, episodes of syncope are common.

On examination, the uterus usually will be slightly enlarged, an adnexal mass is often present, and cul-de-sac fullness may be evident. If the patient is not treated, profound shock may occur and death is possible if the treatment is not prompt.

A pregnancy test is helpful only if the result is positive. A rapid serum test that detects low levels of human chorionic gonadotropin often is more accurate than a urinary test. Many emergency rooms have such a test available on short notice. Ultrasonography can be helpful if it identifies an intrauterine gestational sac, since the presence of both an intrauterine and a tubal pregnancy is a very rare event. The use of the vaginal probe makes it possible to diagnose ectopic pregnancy with great reliability.

Laparoscopy is presently the diagnostic method of choice. An ectopic pregnancy can be easily and correctly differentiated from pelvic infectious disease and a ruptured corpus luteum cyst. Additionally, in the hands of an experienced operator, approximately 90 per cent of ectopic pregnancies can be managed by laparoscopy, thereby avoiding laparotomy. However, if this expertise is not available, following diagnostic laparoscopy, laparotomy should be performed immediately. Usually, if the operation is performed early, a salpingotomy with removal of the products of conception and repair of the tube is the procedure of choice. Indeed, removal of the tube should be done only rarely. Even if salpingectomy is necessary, the ovary should not be removed unless it is infarcted.

Prenatal Care

The importance of good prenatal care cannot be overemphasized. The practicing physician should not only be able to detect abnormalities of pregnancy as they occur but, based on a knowledge of risk factors of pregnancy, labor, and delivery, also *predict* these complications in most instances long before they occur. In order to do this, it is necessary to establish a method of "risk assessment." This has always been a part of routine prenatal care but has only recently been so named and formalized.

Pregnancy is a normal state for a woman, and pregnancy should not prevent a woman from leading a normal life, including working and exercising, unless complications occur.

RISK ASSESSMENT

Figure 36–1 shows the front page of a detailed prenatal risk assessment system that has been developed by C. Hobel and is used by many physicians and hospitals in the United States. The fact that such a detailed system is available underscores the importance of this aspect of prenatal care. Several other systems have been developed and are also in widespread use. Although some of these systems have been automated, at the present time they require large computer systems that are beyond the means of the usual private practitioner. However, it is likely that before this edition becomes obsolete, systems will be available that will run on office-based microcomputers.

Risk assessment has always been part of every initial obstetric visit. Physicians have always asked pertinent questions related to the patient's medical history, identified problems on the basis of physical examination and laboratory testing, and developed some decision about whether a patient should or should not be singled out for "special" care. The risk assessment form and techniques allow the physician to make an objective, relatively unbiased, assessment of the patient's risk. In addition, the risk assessment scores have been used on tens of thousands of pregnancies, and thus the correlation with pregnancy outcome is much more precise than that developed by any practitioner based on "experience."

The typical risk assessment forms are completed by making appropriate checkmarks, based on the history and physical findings, and the risk score is then tallied. Depending on the total score, the physician may decide that the patient is at low risk for complications of pregnancy and delivery, at medium risk and should be watched closely, or at high risk and consultation obtained from a physician who specializes in the treatment of high-risk obstetrical patients (Hobel et al., 1973; Sokol et al., 1979). Instruction manuals have been written that describe the scores that relate to low, medium, and high risk.

Of special concern to the family physician are those women who are in the category of "medium risk." These women require close observation throughout pregnancy and may require the use of specialized tests to ensure that the fetus and mother

PRESS HARD

YOU ARE MAKING EXTRA COPIES

INTAKE DATE & INITIALS:

OB INDEX

Age	Term	Premi	Ab-Ectop	Living

BIRTH CONTROL PILLS IN PAST YEAR ☐ Yes ☐ No

MENSES Onset / Int / Dur — CYCLES ☐ Regular ☐ Irregular

LMP: ☐ Normal ☐ Abnormal PMP: — EDC:

POSITIVE PREGNANCY TEST Date:

PAST PREGNANCIES

Pregnancy No.	Termination Date Mo.	Termination Date Yr.	EARLY LOSS <20 wks Spon	Ectop	Induced*	GA wks	≥20 wks LIVE OR STILLBORN Birth Wt	Sex	Living Y/N**	VAGINAL Spon Vtx	Br	Forceps	C-SECTION CPD	Fetal Distress	Abn Pres	Repeat	Other/Unk	ASSOCIATED PROBLEMS
1																		
2																		
3																		
4																		
5																		
6																		
7																		
8																		

*D&C S(Suction) Sa(Saline) P(Prostaglandin) H(Hysterotomy) O(Other) U(Unknown) **S(Stillbirth) N(Neonatal) I(Infant) C(Childhood)

HISTORICAL PROBLEMS

Prob. No.	±	Risk Value		
1		5		☐ AGE <17 ☐ AGE ≥35
2		5		MULTIPARITY (5 or more ≥20 weeks)
3		5		INDUCED ABORTION
4		10		HABITUAL ABORTION (3 or more)
5		10	PREVIOUS INFANTS	PREMATURE (<37 weeks) ☐ LGA
6		10		SGA (Small for Gestational Age)
7		5		BIRTH WEIGHT >4000 gms or 9 lbs
8		10		PERINATAL DEATH ☐ Stillborn ☐ Neonatal
9		5		POST NEONATAL PROBLEM ☐ Sudden Infant Death ☐ Neurologic Handicap ☐ Mental Retardation
10		10		NEONATAL JAUNDICE ☐ Rh ☐ ABO ☐ Physiologic ☐ Unknown ☐ Other:
11		5		GENETIC DISEASE ☐ Chromosomal ☐ CNS ☐ Inborn Errors of Metabolism ☐ Other: ☐ Structural Congenital Anomalies:
12		5	GYN	HISTORY OF INFERTILITY ☐ Primary ☐ Secondary ☐ Treated ☐ Untreated
13		10		UTERINE-CERVICAL ABNORMALITY ☐ Uterine Anomaly ☐ Corrected ☐ Incomp Cx ☐ Cerclage, Removed ☐ Yes ☐ No
14		5		PREVIOUS UTERINE SURGERY C-Section: ☐ Classical ☐ Low Trans ☐ Low Vert ☐ Unknown ☐ Hysterotomy ☐ Myomectomy
15		5	PREG. COMPLICATIONS	HEMORRHAGE ☐ Previa ☐ Abruptio ☐ Other 3rd Trimester ☐ Post Partum ☐ Transfusion
16		5		PREGNANCY-INDUCED HYPERTENSION ☐ Required Hosp ☐ Required Early Delivery ☐ Developed Eclampsia
17		10	MEDICAL-SURGICAL	CHRONIC HYPERTENSION (BP≥140/90 non-pregnant) ☐ On Drug Therapy:
18		10		HEART DISEASE ☐ Rheumatic ☐ Congenital ☐ Arteriosclerotic ☐ Other ☐ Surgical Correction ☐ Hx of CHF or Arrhythmia ☐ No limitation of physical activity ☐ Slight limitation ☐ Marked limitation ☐ Unable to carry on any physical activ. w/out discomfort
19		5		PULMONARY DISEASE ☐ Asthma ☐ Chronic Bronchitis ☐ Tuberculosis ☐ Other
20		5		GENITOURINARY INFECTIONS ☐ Asymptomatic Bacteruria ☐ Cystitis ☐ Pyelonephritis ☐ Gonorrhea ☐ Syphilis ☐ Genital Herpes
21		10		RENAL DISEASE ☐ Glomerulo ☐ Chronic Pyelo ☐ Diabetic ☐ Collagen-vas ☐ Calculi ☐ Other:
22		10		DIABETES ☐ A ☐ B ☐ C ☐ D ☐ F-R ☐ Insulin, Pre-preg Dosage:
23		10		THYROID DISEASE ☐ Hypo ☐ Thyroiditis ☐ Hyper: treated with ☐ Drugs ☐ Surgery ☐ I-131
24		10		OTHER MEDICAL ☐ Phlebitis ☐ Embolus ☐ Collagen-vas ☐ On Drug Therapy: ☐ Hematologic:
25		10		EPILEPSY ☐ On Therapy: ☐ Phenobarb ☐ Dilantin ☐ Mysoline ☐ Other:
26		5		PSYCHIATRIC ☐ Hospitalized ☐ On Drug Therapy:
27		5		PREVIOUS OPERATIONS ☐ Diag D&C ☐ Laparoscopy ☐ Appendectomy ☐ Cholecystectomy ☐ Other:
28		10	HABITS	EXCESSIVE USE ☐ Alcohol ☐ Tobacco ☐ Marijuana ☐ Narcotics:
29		5	FAMILY HISTORY	MATERNAL ONLY ☐ Hypertension ☐ Multiple Births ☐ Diabetes ☐ Hemoglobinopathy ☐ DES ☐ Other:
30		5		MAT. OR PATERNAL ☐ Mental Retardation ☐ Congen Anom ☐ Congen Hearing Loss ☐ Allergies ☐ Other:

HEALTH STATUS INDICATORS

YEARS OF EDUCATION Mother ______ Father ______

DIET (Ex, G, P, Undet) Calories ______ Protein ______ Iron ______

INSURANCE ☐ Public ☐ Private ☐ None

Carrier ______ # ______ # ______

Carrier ______ # ______ # ______

ALLERGIES

COMMENTS

SPECIAL COMMENTS FOR DATA ENTRY

Patient Address			City	State	Zip	Birth Date
Home Phone	Preferred Language	Marital Status M W D SEP S				
Contact Phone	Race-Ethnicity W B H I A O	Spouse's Name				
Referred By	Hospital of Delivery					

Last Name First Name Middle Initial

Pat Hosp # ______

Fam File Name ______ Pat Clinic # ______

Maiden Name Mother's Maiden Name

1 PRENATAL HISTORY

Figure 36–1. Prenatal History Form (POPRAS) includes risk-assessment scoring. (By permission of American International Perinatal Health, Inc., 2130 Professional Drive, Roseville, CA 95661.)

do well. These special tests often include nonstress and stress testing, amniocentesis, B-scan ultrasonography, and repetition of some of the common laboratory tests.

The risk assessment should be updated each time a new abnormality is found. Figure 36–2 shows the first page of the risk assessment form that should be completed at the onset of *labor*. The risk score should be tallied and the patient identified as being of low, medium, or high risk. By using forms such as those shown in Figures 36–1 and 36–2, almost all high-risk pregnancies can be identified before severe harm comes to the mother or fetus.

ROUTINE CARE (LOW-RISK PATIENT)

Elements included in the initial visit are the patient's history, the physical examination, and laboratory examinations. Pregnancy education and information on nutrition are scheduled for follow-up visits.

History. The first prenatal visit is extremely important not only in determining the health status of the pregnant patient but also in providing the opportunity for the family physician to initiate what will hopefully be a long relationship with this patient and her family. In a healthy primigravida patient, this office visit may be the first time that the woman has

PRESS HARD
YOU ARE MAKING EXTRA COPIES

OB INDEX	Weight	Height	Age	Term	Premi	Ab-Ectop	Living	LMP	EDC	GA wks	Fun Ht cms	Est Fetal Weight gms

ADMISSION NOTES

	DATE	TIME
ADMISSION TO LABOR	__/__/__	__:__
ONSET OF LABOR	__/__/__	__:__
MEMBRANES RUPTURED	__/__/__	__:__

PRENATAL CARE ☐Yes ☐No
PREPARED CHILDBIRTH ☐Yes ☐No
COACH IN DELIVERY ☐Yes ☐No
PRENATAL SCORE:________
CLINIC/PHYSICIAN:
ALLERGIES ________
PREFERRED LANGUAGE
RELIGION/CULTURE
Accompanied By: ☐Relative ☐Hosp Staff ☐Wheelchair ☐Other:
☐Dentures ☐Wig ☐Eyeglasses ☐Contacts
Communicable Disease:
Last Meal ☐Light ☐Heavy
Date: Time:
Dietary Restrictions:
Admitted by:

ROUTINE ADMISSION ORDERS
☐Prep
☐Enema
☐IV:
☐Serology/CBC/Hct/Hgb
☐Type & Rh
☐Crossmatch
☐Fetal Monitor ☐Int ☐Ext
☐NPO
☐Urine ☐Void ☐Catheter
☐Alternative Delivery
☐Repeat C-Section
☐BTL
☐Anesthesia:

Physician Signature
Nurse Signature

PHYSICAL and LAB

Normal	Yes	No		Yes	No		Yes	No	
HEENT			HEART			EXT GENITALS			DT REFLEXES ☐1+ ☐2+ ☐3+ ☐Clonus
LUNGS			ABDOMEN			VAGINA-CX			
BREASTS			EXTREMITIES			UTERUS			CONTRACTED PELVIS ☐Inlet ☐Mid ☐Outlet
NIPPLES			EDEMA			PELVIMETRY			

TYPE ☐A ☐B ☐O ☐AB
Rh ☐Neg ☐Pos
ANTIBODY SCREEN ☐Neg ☐Pos
HCT HGB

URINE: PROTEIN ☐Neg ☐Pos ☐1+ ☐2+ ☐3+
SUGAR ☐Neg ☐Light ☐Dark
MICRO ☐Neg ☐Pos:
CULTURE: ________

AMNIOTIC FLUID
NITRAZINE ☐Neg ☐Pos
FERN ☐Neg ☐Pos
MATURITY ☐Mature ☐Intermed ☐Immature

COMMENTS

ABNORMAL FINDINGS

EARLY LABOR PROBLEMS Include problems identified after last prenatal visit.

Prob. No.	±	Date Positive	Risk Val.	Problem
101				PRIOR HOSPITALIZATION ☐Prenatal ☐Intrapartum Transferred from:
102				ANTEPARTUM FETAL DEATH (Prior to labor)
103				ELECTIVE INDUCTION
104				FALSE LABOR
105			5	PREMATURE RUPTURE OF MEMBRANES ☐<12 hrs ☐>12 hrs prior to onset of labor
106			10	PREMATURE LABOR ≤37 Weeks Rx: ☐Alcohol ☐B-Mimetic ☐Other:
107			10	POLYHYDRAMNIOS
108			10	MULTIPLE PREGNANCY: Baby ☐A ☐B ☐C
109			10	ABNORMAL PRESENTATION ☐Breech ☐Face ☐Brow ☐Comp ☐Trans Lie
110			5	MEDICAL INDUCTION
111			10	DIABETES MELLITUS
112			10	ABNORMAL TEST for FETAL WELL-BEING ☐E-3 ☐HPL ☐Amnioscopy ☐Contraction Stress ☐Nonstress
113			10	POST TERM PREGNANCY ≥ 42 Wks
114			5	MECONIUM ☐LIGHT (light stained amniotic fluid, yellow or greenish)
115			10	MECONIUM ☐HEAVY (dark stained, usually dark green & tenacious)
116			10	HYPERTENSION CHRONIC
117			5	HYPERTENSION PREGNANCY-INDUCED ☐Mild
118			10	HYPERTENSION PREGNANCY-INDUCED ☐Severe ☐Superimposed
119			10	SUSPECTED IUGR
120			5	PROLONGED LATENT PHASE (>13 hrs multip, 20 hrs nullip)
121			10	UTERINE BLEEDING ☐Abruptio ☐Previa ☐Unknown

INTERIM LABOR PROBLEMS

Prob. No.	±	Risk Val.	Problem
122			MONITORING ☐External ☐Internal ☐Fetal Blood Sample
123		5	ABNORMAL PROGRESS OF LABOR: PRIMARY DYSFUNCTIONAL LABOR (Without oxytocin after 4 cm) ☐Nullipara, at least 1 cm p/hr ☐Multipara, 1.5 cm p/hr
124		10	ABNORMAL PROGRESS OF LABOR: SECONDARY ARREST OF DILATION (Failure to progress after 5 cm)
125		5	ABNORMAL PROGRESS OF LABOR: PROTRACTED DESCENT
126		5	ABNORMAL PROGRESS OF LABOR: PITOCIN AUGMENTATION OF LABOR
127		10	FETAL DISTRESS: BASELINE ☐Tachycardia ☐Bradycardia
128		10	FETAL DISTRESS: PERIODIC CHANGES ☐Early ☐Variable ☐Late
129		10	FETAL DISTRESS: DECREASED BASELINE VARIABILITY DUE TO: ☐Medication ☐Acidosis ☐Unknown
130		10	FETAL DISTRESS: ACIDOSIS ☐pH 7.20 – 7.25 ☐pH <7.20
131		10	CORD PROLAPSE
132		10	AMNIONITIS ☐Mat Temp ≥100.4°F ⁄ 38°C ☐Bacteria in Amniotic Fluid
133		10	SEIZURE ☐Eclampsia ☐Previous Seizure Disorder ☐Unknown

Last Name First Name Middle Initial
Pat Hosp #________
Pat Clinic #________
Family File Name ________ Birthdate ________

4 INTRAPARTUM PROBLEM LIST

Figure 36–2. Intrapartum Problem List (POPRAS) includes risk-assessment scoring. (By permission of American International Perinatal Health, Inc., 2130 Professional Drive, Roseville, CA 95661.)

sought medical advice since she was a child. In a multigravida patient, it is especially important to record any abnormalities that occurred during previous pregnancies. An accurate and thorough history is the most important aspect of the initial prenatal assessment.

The first items to be obtained in the patient's history pertain to the pregnancy. The date of the last menstrual period should be determined. If not known exactly, the date should be estimated. Very often, dates such as birthdays, national holidays, and school vacations will help pinpoint the date. Information about the length of the woman's normal menstrual cycle also should be obtained.

The usual method of determining an estimated date of confinement in the United States is to employ Nägele's rule. With this convention, the estimated date of confinement is determined by subtracting 3 months and adding 7 days to the date of the last menstrual period. However, extra days should be added for menstrual cycles that usually last longer than 28 days or subtracted for cycles that usually last less than 28 days. The patient should be questioned about methods of contraception that might have been employed during the time the pregnancy occurred. The estimated date of confinement that is determined in this manner should be considered to be tentative and may be changed at any time. The estimated date of confinement may be corrected if, on the basis of information learned later through observation of the uterus, the date of quickening, or ultrasonography, the original estimated date is obviously wrong. The estimated date of confinement is important because prolonged pregnancy is a high-risk situation. One of the most important milestones for confirmation of the estimated date of confinement is the perception of fetal activity by the pregnant woman. Generally, first movement will be noted by primigravida women at approximately 20 weeks of gestation; multigravida women usually will feel movement at approximately 16 weeks. Both of these dates are accurate within approximately 1 week. The commonly available gestational age wheels are perhaps the most useful equipment at a prenatal visit.

A thorough general medical history should be obtained. Of primary importance are any factors that may adversely affect the present pregnancy. The use of drugs by the patient ranks high on the list of important factors that must be determined. Many commonly used therapeutic agents may be teratogenic if administered in sufficient dosages during certain times of gestation. A few medications (for example, phenytoin, diethylstilbestrol, and methotrexate) have been shown, without question, to cause congenital malformations. Many more drugs have been associated with problems during pregnancy, but it is not certain that they can directly cause congenital abnormalities. A very few drugs (for example, penicillin and prednisone) do not seem to cause problems in the usual therapeutic doses. Most drugs, however, do not fit any of these categories; thus, all medication should be avoided during pregnancy unless indicated on the basis of significant clinical disease.

Illicit street drugs have become an increasingly important problem for all practicing physicians. Virtually all of the commonly available street drugs can have either teratogenic complications or lead to low birth weight, spontaneous abortion, or maternal complications. Although many women refuse to admit present usage of these drugs, they may state that they have used these drugs "in the past." This information should increase the physician's suspicion of present drug usage. Because drugs such as cocaine and the narcotics have such significant adverse effects on newborns, it is important for the physician to attempt to establish whether or not the pregnant woman is currently using these medications. When necessary and appropriate, urinary tests for drug residuals can be ordered. Even a history of past usage places these patients in the high-risk category.

The history should include notation of all previous operations and any serious medical illnesses. Respiratory disorders (such as asthma), heart disease, primary gastrointestinal disease (such as regional enteritis and chronic ulcerative colitis), metabolic diseases (such as diabetes), and neurologic diseases must be carefully noted. A family history should be obtained also because some medical disorders of close blood relatives are transmitted genetically. In case of serious or fatal illnesses in blood relatives, genetic counseling may be advisable.

The social history has been shown to be extremely important. In the past, this aspect of history-taking was often ignored. However, it is clear that patients are clearly at higher risk for complications of pregnancy if they are uneducated, of low socioeconomic class, under age 18 or over age 35, have a history of verbal or physical abuse, or are of certain ethnic backgrounds. There is very lengthy and detailed documentation that all of these factors can lead to unsuccessful outcomes of pregnancy. In fact, these items are of equal or greater importance than many common medical conditions.

Identification of these problems at the first visit is important because many studies have also shown that early intervention may reduce the perinatal morbidity associated with the presence of these factors. For example, the Special Supplemental Food Program for Women, Infants, and Children, Aid For Dependent Children, food stamps, and other local programs can help dramatically. Additionally, in the case of adolescent pregnancy, it is important for the physician to explore means for the pregnant teenager to continue her education during pregnancy. Lack of attention to educational needs often leads to another generation of socially deprived citizens.

Each patient must also be questioned about abuse. Although it is a hard question to ask at times, it has been our policy to ask every pregnant patient, regardless of her background, whether there has been physical or verbal abuse in her background or at the present time. All positive answers are treated as important information that places the patient at high risk.

Some physicians simply do not wish to become involved in the social aspects of prenatal care. If this is the case, the practicing physician must establish a close relationship with a social worker, public health nurse, or other health care provider who can appropriately respond to these nutritional, psychologic, environmental, and habit problems of the pregnant patient. This person should report to the physician at least monthly on the progress being made or new problems that have been identified. Prenatal care for a patient who is disadvantaged should include the "team" approach. The assistance of nurses and social workers is extremely helpful in the provision of prenatal care.

Physical Examination. A general examination should be performed. This should always include determining height, weight, and blood pressure as well as a complete and thorough physical examination.

A thorough pelvic examination is necessary. The external genitalia, vagina, and cervix should be carefully inspected for abnormalities that may lead to difficulties in pregnancy, labor, or delivery. A Papanicolaou smear should be obtained on every patient at her first prenatal visit unless a negative examination has been obtained during the last 6 months. Any evidence of vaginitis should be investigated thoroughly. However, some increase in vaginal discharge from the increased mucous production of the endocervical glands may be expected during pregnancy. It has become a common practice in many areas of the United States to routinely obtain an endocervical smear for *Neisseria gonorrhea* and *Chlamydia trachomatis* at the initial evaluation, but the absence of a positive culture at the first visit does not ensure that the disease will not be present later in pregnancy.

Uterine size should be carefully evaluated. During the first 14 weeks of pregnancy, the experienced examiner should be able to estimate the size of the uterus to within 2 weeks of gestational age (see Fig. 36–4). Any discrepancy between the size of the uterus and the last menstrual period should be noted, and the patient should be alerted to that fact. If, on a second visit the discrepancy is still noted, the patient should have ultrasonography for dating.

The most important prenatal technique that the examiner must learn is that of clinical pelvimetry. The diagonal conjugate is the most important pelvic measurement that must be taken by the examiner. In order to obtain this measurement correctly, the fingers of the examining hand must reach the promontory of the sacrum. At this point, the hand is elevated to the inferior aspect of the symphysis, and the distance between the tip of the middle finger and the symphysis is noted. All examiners who have an active obstetrical practice should be able to determine this measurement within a millimeter or two by noting where the symphysis touches the hand or knuckle.

Once the diagonal conjugate has been determined, the examining finger should trace the concavity of the sacrum. It is important to identify those women who have an unusual angulation of the sacrum. A flat or forward-pointing sacrum is a worrisome clinical sign, since it often represents a flattened posterior pelvic segment and a decreased likelihood of spontaneous vaginal delivery. The examining fingers should next trace the pelvic side walls on both sides. Any unusual shape should be noted. The side walls usually are gently curved inward. The fingers should then sweep between the ischial spines, and the distance between them should be estimated. The examining fingers may then be removed from the vagina, the ischial tuberosities identified, and the distance between them noted.

An inadequate pelvis for delivery should be suspected when the diagonal conjugate is less than 12 cm., the sacrum has an unusual shape, the pelvic side walls are straight, the distance between the ischial spines is less than 10 cm., or the medial aspects of the ischial tuberosities are less than 8 cm. apart (Pritchard and MacDonald, 1980).

Laboratory Examinations. A number of laboratory examinations should be done on a routine basis at the first prenatal visit (Table 36–1). There is no need for a routine chest roentgenogram unless the results of chest examination are abnormal or the patient is at high risk for tuberculosis (Bonebrake et al., 1978). Screening for AIDS is controversial. Some high-risk populations (e.g., intravenous drug abusers) in certain areas of the country are at such high risk that routine screening should be done. Other groups of patients (e.g., those in long-term monogamous relationship) are at such low risk that screening is not cost effective. Each physician must decide on the benefit of such testing based on the location and type of practice.

Pregnancy Education. The first prenatal visit is the physician's chance to discuss his or her attitude toward pregnancy, labor, and delivery with the patient and to inform her of the general restrictions that might apply to her. In a normal uncomplicated pregnancy in a healthy woman, these restrictions should be minimal. The patient should be informed of the importance of good nutrition, of maintaining adequate exercise and rest, of complete absence from smoking, abstinence from alcohol, and of reporting any symptoms of vaginitis or vulvitis (especially herpes).

Because of the recent increased interest in sports, many women are active in one or more individual or team sports. There appears to be no reason to limit any of these activities during pregnancy unless they are of a contact nature. For example, there is no reason to limit sports such as golf, tennis, or bowling, but sports in which there is a significant risk of serious injury, such as skiing, should be discouraged. Women who are not involved in a regular exercise program should be encouraged to do so, and jogging and swimming are among the best exercises for pregnant women.

The pregnant woman should be discouraged from believing the "old wives' tales" that she hears. Whenever she receives free *negative* advice from any relative or friend, she should first check the validity of the statement with her physician. Even in a relatively medically sophisticated society, some women may

Table 36–1. PRENATAL LABORATORY EXAMINATIONS

First Visit
Complete blood count (including platelets)
Urinalysis and culture
Blood group and Rh factor
Irregular antibody screen
Rubella immunity screen
Serology (syphilis screen)
Gonorrhea culture
Chlamydia culture
Hepatitis screen
AIDS screen
Ultrasonography prior to 18 weeks
Follow-Up Visits
Routine: urine for protein and white cells
28 weeks: complete blood count
1-hour glucose screen

believe that raising their hands above the top of their head will cause umbilical cord knots, that swimming in pregnancy is dangerous, and that coitus may damage the fetus.

At the first prenatal visit, many physicians find it helpful to distribute one of many excellent booklets that are available for the lay public. The American College of Obstetrics and Gynecology and the American Academy of Family Practice have many booklets available at a very low cost. The patient must be instructed to watch for the signs and symptoms of the complications of pregnancy (Table 36–2).

Nutrition. The growing fetus requires vitamins, minerals, amino acids, and sugar and can obtain these only from the maternal circulation. It is, therefore, important to stress to each pregnant woman that a well-balanced diet is essential during pregnancy. The physician should attempt to determine, in at least a general way, whether or not the patient practices general good nutritional habits. Many middle-class American women have an adequate diet, whereas others of all classes may rely on "junk food" or starches for their dietary intake. Many women do not require specific nutritional counseling or strict dietary control, whereas others may require early consultation with a dietician. If a good general diet is followed, there is no reason to encourage the avoidance of salt, ingestion of a large amount of calf's liver, or the necessity to drink a quart of cow's milk a day. The most important aspect of diet is that it be individualized, and the physician should discuss the importance with each patient frankly.

A pregnant woman in the United States should expect to gain approximately 25 lb. (11.4 kg.) during her pregnancy (Fig. 36–3). It has been shown clearly that gaining less than 20 lb. (9.1 kg.) often leads to a thin, malnourished fetus. *Physicians should be discouraged from limiting weight gain to less than 20 lb. (9.1 kg.).* This is true even if the woman is overweight at the beginning of her pregnancy. Although an overweight woman may mobilize many of her fat stores during pregnancy, her continuous acidotic state from such mobilization may be detrimental to the fetus. Likewise, the woman who gains more than 25 lb. (11.4 kg.) will retain the additional weight as fat and will have a unnecessarily heavy infant.

Table 36–2. SOME SIGNS AND SYMPTOMS OF PREGNANCY COMPLICATIONS

Severe headache
Blurring of vision
Fever > 38.3°C (101°F)
Swelling of the hands, feet, and face
Weight gain of more than 5 lb (2.3 kg.) in any week
Severe nausea and vomiting for more than 24 hours
Vaginal bleeding
Leakage of clear fluid from the vagina
Absence of fetal movements for more than 24 hours after the 5th month of pregnancy
Blood in the urine
Severe abdominal pain
Irregular heartbeat

Although it is common practice in the United States for physicians to routinely prescribe one of the many prenatal vitamin preparations, there is no reliable evidence that dietary supplementation is necessary, except for iron, folic acid, and perhaps calcium. Of interest is a recent study of mothers of patients with neural tube defects, indicating that the use of multivitamins during the periconceptual period may have a protective effect against the development of neural tube defects (Mulinare et al., 1988). Although the addition of other minerals included in such prenatal supplements does not seem to cause any adverse affects, they are probably not necessary in a well-nourished person.

The fetus and the other gestational tissues require approximately 800 mg. of iron during gestation (Levin and Algazy, 1975). The iron stores of most women are less than 2½ grams. If the needs of pregnancy were to be satisfied soley from the stores present at conception, the woman could become anemic during pregnancy. Also, it is almost impossible to obtain 800 mg. of iron from dietary sources alone. Therefore, virtually every pregnant woman should receive iron supplementation. Iron in various forms may be used for prophylaxis and is included in adequate amounts in all of the prenatal preparations. A simple ferrous sulfate tablet is still the least costly way of providing supplemental iron stores for the mother. However, it must be remembered that ferrous sulfate is toxic to small children who might ingest the tablets accidentally. If anemia is present at the start of pregnancy, larger amounts of supplemental iron will be needed, and one 325-mg. ferrous sulfate tablet taken three times a day usually rapidly corrects the anemia. Injected iron should not be used, since it may cause anaphylaxis, staining of the skin, and does not result in more rapid correction of anemia than oral supplements.

Folic acid is required by the fetus for growth and is usually present in large stores in most healthy women at the start of pregnancy. However, by the second half of pregnancy, these stores may be depleted and folic acid deficiency may occur. Therefore, folic acid should be taken throughout pregnancy in small amounts to prevent anemia. A daily amount of 500 μg. is sufficient to meet these needs but is not sufficient to treat folic acid anemia should it occur. Such anemia requires at least 1 mg. of folic acid daily.

The fetus requires large amounts of calcium for growth, but healthy adult women possess huge stores of calcium. Unless a woman has had many pregnancies in rapid succession or has a calcium-losing medical condition, she will not deplete her stores severely. Since virtually all prenatal preparations include some additional calcium and since calcium is readily available in many foodstuffs ingested by women in the United States (including milk), calcium deficiency is rarely, if ever, encountered in a healthy pregnant adult woman.

Follow-Up Visits. After an adequate evaluation at the initial prenatal visit, the follow-up examinations

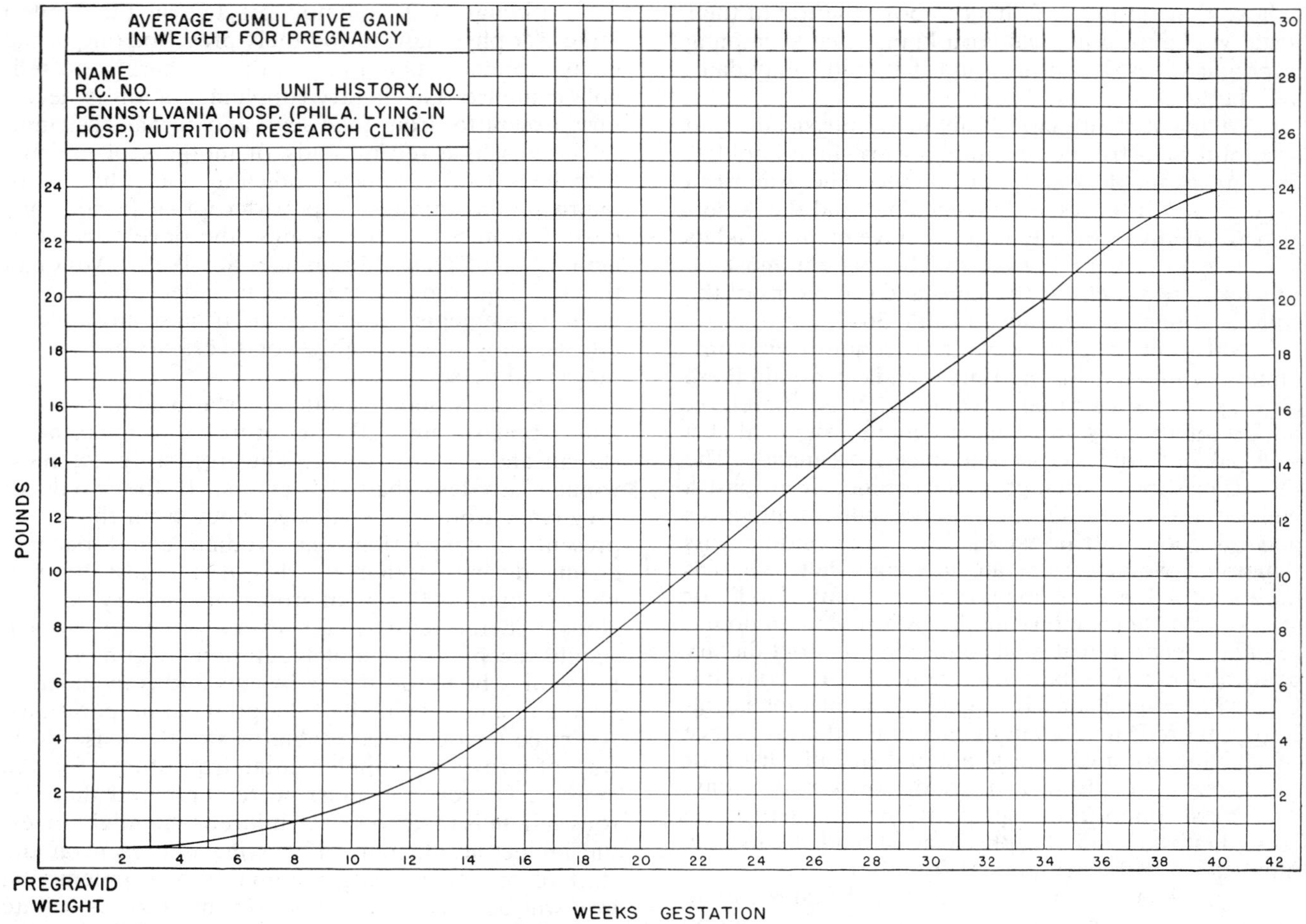

Figure 36–3. Prenatal weight gain grid. (From Lull, C. B., and Kimbrough, R. A.: Clinical Obstetrics. Philadelphia, J. B. Lippincott Company, 1953.)

may be short and limited to investigation of only a few items. Although the number of visits and their frequency should be individualized based on the patient's medical condition, it is common practice to schedule return visits approximately every month until the last 8 weeks of pregnancy, when the frequency should be increased. In uncomplicated pregnancies, our practice is to see all patients weekly, beginning at 36 weeks of gestation and continuing until spontaneous delivery or a decision has been made that the patient is postmature and requires induction of labor.

The history since the last visit is important. Generally, however, if the patient has been properly instructed, there is little to report, because any important events would have been telephoned to the physician. Specific information should be sought concerning any infections or medications used since the last visit.

The physical examination should be brief. The patient should be weighed and her blood pressure taken, preferably while in the left lateral recumbent position. The legs and hands should be checked for evidence of edema, and the extent of the edema should be noted. The uterus should be examined using Leopold's maneuvers at each visit (Fig. 36–4 and Table 36–3). Early in pregnancy, it will not be possible to determine the presenting fetal part, but at approximately 30 weeks, this should be easily determined. The height of the uterine fundus should be noted. Generally, the uterus should be half way between the symphysis pubis and the umbilicus at 16 weeks of gestation and at the umbilicus at 20 weeks of gestation (Fig. 36–5). McDonald's measurements

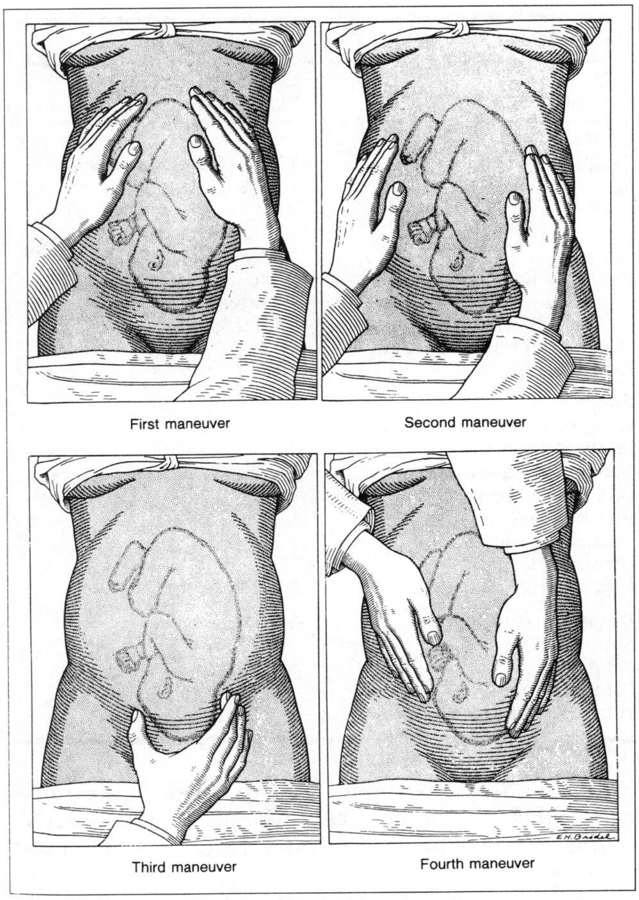

Figure 36–4. Palpation in left occiput anterior position. (From Cunningham, F. G., MacDonald, P. C., and Gant, N. F. [Eds.]: Williams Obstetrics. 18th ed. East Norwalk, CT, Appleton & Lange, 1989, p. 183. By permission.)

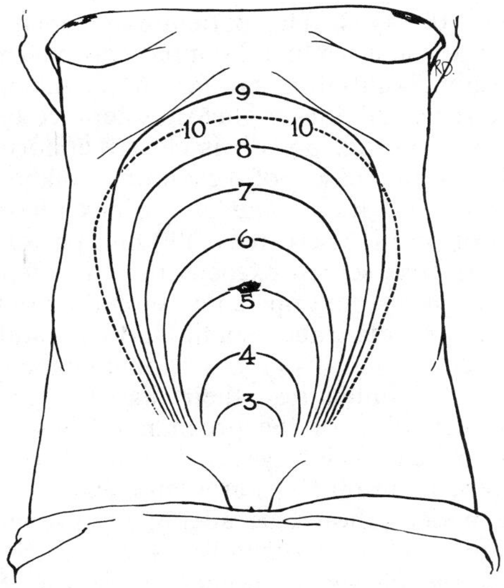

Figure 36–5. Relative height of the fundus at the various human months of pregnancy. (From Hellman, L. M., and Pritchard, J. A.: Williams Obstetrics. 14th ed. New York, Appleton-Century-Crofts, 1971, p. 280. By permission.)

of the uterine fundus are useful. This is done by measuring the distance from the top of the symphysis pubis to the top of the uterine fundus. Between 20 and 30 weeks of gestation, the height of the uterine fundus in centimeters should be approximately equal to the number of weeks' gestation. Any significant difference between the number of weeks and the uterine size should alert the physician to the possibility of multiple gestation if larger than expected or growth retardation if smaller than expected. Either

Table 36–3. LEOPOLD'S MANEUVERS

Maneuver	Action	Question
First	Examine the fundus	What fetal part is in the fundus?
Second	Palpate the lateral abdomen	Where is the fetal back?
Third	Palpate the suprapubic area	Is the presenting part engaged?
Fourth (vertex only)	Find the cephalic prominence	Is the head flexed?

condition may be more specifically defined by the use of B-scan ultrasonography.

Our practice is to perform vaginal examination for evaluation of the dilatation and effacement of the cervix and the position of the fetal presenting part weekly, beginning at 36 weeks of gestation. When previous premature labor or cervical dilatation has occurred, these vaginal examinations are begun earlier. It is important to use extreme gentleness and care in these examinations to avoid iatrogenic complications.

Laboratory evaluation at routine prenatal visits is minimal. Usually only an abbreviated urinalysis is necessary. The patient should be instructed to collect a first-voided urine sample the morning of the prenatal visit, and this should be checked for sugar, protein, leukocytes, and erythrocytes. A full microscopic evaluation need not be performed at each visit. The presence of blood, leukocytes, glucose, or protein suggests a need for further evaluation. Leukocytes in the urine may be the first sign of an asymptomatic urinary tract infection; glucosuria may represent the onset of gestational diabetes (though this is not reliable); and proteinuria may be the initial sign of toxemia.

If the initial determination of hemoglobin shows an adequate level with normal red cell indices, the determination need not be repeated at each visit if the patient has been taking iron and folic acid supplementation. We suggest a repeat hemoglobin determination at 28 weeks gestation. However, women who have evidence of anemia early in pregnancy should be monitored carefully to ensure that the anemia is corrected. Other laboratory tests are ordered only as indicated.

Also, at 28 weeks gestation it has become our practice to screen routinely for the development of gestational diabetes. The patient is given a 50-gm. glucose load and has a blood sample drawn 60 minutes later. Although authorities differ on the glucose level that requires a full 3-hour glucose tolerance test, any level above 150 mg. per dl. is clearly abnormal. At this level, some cases of gestational diabetes are overlooked, and thus some authorities recommend the level of positive screen be 140 mg. per dl. If the patient's glucose screen exceeds the cut-off point, a full 3-hour glucose tolerance test should be obtained. It is clear that fetal macrosomia and neonatal hypoglycemia can occur from gestational diabetes. Although most women lose their diabetic tendencies following cessation of the pregnancy, these women must be watched closely for the development of insulin-dependent diabetes at a later date.

The patient should be adequately prepared for parturition. At approximately 34 or 35 weeks of gestation, the physician should discuss the signs of the onset of labor and the appropriate actions to take, as well as the importance of rupture of membranes and the necessity for evaluation of the status of the fetus if rupture of the membranes should occur. Many physicians find it helpful for the father to be present at this session.

In many areas of the United States, classes are held for the purpose of preparing couples for childbirth. The physician should be familiar with the courses that are locally available, screen them carefully for appropriate content, and recommend them to patients who are in need of such detailed preparedness. Often, with proper preparation, a woman may be able to go through an entire labor and delivery experience without analgesia or anesthesia.

OBSTETRIC ULTRASOUND

B-scan ultrasonography has become one of the most useful techniques for the evaluation of the fetus and placenta in pregnancy. At the Mayo Clinic, we have performed B-scan ultrasonography on a routine basis on all pregnant women for the past 15 years. The information that we derive from this examination is of great benefit to us, to the fetus, and to the pregnant woman (Strassner et al., 1979). Since the initiation of ultrasonography, it has been possible to identify every case of multiple gestation in more than 20,000 live births prior to delivery. Additionally, all cases of total placenta previa have been identified, and in recent years patients with a low-lying placental margin also have been identified. At the present time, the technique has achieved sufficient quality to determine with great accuracy whether or not growth retardation is present and to detect many of the major fetal anomalies (Table 36–4).

Ultrasonography is also used for four of the five elements of the "Biophysical Profile." The fifth element is the nonstress test. This is a useful test of fetal well-being, which has largely supplanted the oxytocin challenge test. Whenever there is concern about fetal well-being (e.g., postmaturity, toxemia, medical disease), this test should be ordered. If the fetus is normal, it should be repeated twice a week until delivery.

Table 36–4. B-SCAN ULTRASONOGRAPHY

Indication	Optimal Time of Examination
General	
Pregnancy dating	14 to 16 weeks, repeat in 4 to 6 weeks (early scans are more accurate than later scans)
Placental localization	26 to 34 weeks (lower edge is seen best on later examinations)
Routine prenatal screening	16 to 20 weeks
Multiple gestation	After 12 weeks
Specific	
Cardiac anomalies	
Limb defects	
Spinal cord anomalies	
Umbilical cord problems	
Amniotic sac septum (multiple gestation)	
Growth retardation	
Macrosomia	After 28 weeks
Biophysical Profile	After 32 weeks
Amniotic fluid volume	
Fetal tone	
Fetal motion	
Fetal breathing	

Modern prenatal care cannot be satisfactorily accomplished without access to an adequate ultrasonographic examination. Unfortunately, there are many outdated, minimally clinically useful ultrasound machines being used by clinicians and radiologists throughout the United States. Ultrasonographic technology has advanced so rapidly that any equipment more than 3 years old is likely to be outdated and incapable of producing images of the desired quality. Additionally, it is important to note that not every radiologist, obstetrician, or family physician has the necessary training and skills to perform adequate ultrasound examinations. The technique requires many hours of training and practice. It cannot be emphasized enough that quality ultrasound examinations require both good equipment and excellent training.

COMPLICATIONS

Medical Complications. The list of all possible medical complications of pregnancy is too long to review in detail here. Texts are available for reference. However, some major problems are seen frequently enough to require special comment.

Cardiovascular System. Major cardiovascular complications are seen with sufficient frequency and are of sufficient severity to require special comment.

With the near disappearance of rheumatic heart disease in the United States, many fewer cases of organic heart disease are now seen than previously. In fact, mitral valve stenosis, the most frequent condition resulting from rheumatic heart disease, used to comprise nearly 90 per cent of all organic heart disease in pregnancy. This lesion now accounts for less than 50 per cent. Nonetheless, it is still the most frequently seen cardiac lesion in young pregnant women.

Mitral valve stenosis in young women presents a particular problem. In general, the cardiac muscle is still normal and the only lesion is the diseased mitral valve. Usually, there is good cardiac reserve. Although many sophisticated tests are available, the New York Heart Association Functional Classification of Cardiac Disease has remained a very useful, quick screen for the severity of cardiac disease (Table 36–5). However, patients still need appropriate cardiovascular testing to determine cardiac indices with some certainty.

Generally, patients with functional cardiac Class I disease should be managed with little interference except for adequate rest and monitoring of the hemoglobin. Class II cardiac patients also generally do well, although they should avoid strenuous exercise. Functional Class III and IV patients are at extremely high risk for fetal and maternal death. These patients are all in cardiac failure, and consultation with a high-risk perinatal center is strongly recommended.

The most important item to realize is that *cardiac disease should be diagnosed and treated before the onset of pregnancy*. The demands made on the heart by a normal pregnancy may cause heart failure in a person who has no particular difficulty except with extreme exercise (cardiac Class II). Patients with mitral valve stenosis may die if they suddenly have atrial fibrillation during pregnancy (Etheridge and Peperell, 1977). Because of the necessity of pumping large amounts of blood through a diseased valve, such an event may prevent adequate pumping or severe fatal pulmonary edema may occur.

The peripheral vascular system also presents particular problems in pregnancy, with the most frequent problem being varicose veins and their complications. Patients with varices or a family history of varices should be encouraged to wear good quality support panty hose throughout pregnancy. Patients should be instructed to wear these hose at all times when upright. Calf length and thigh high hose should be discouraged as the tight tops tend to cause distal edema. Frequent rest in the left lateral recumbent position may help drain the legs and prevent edema and venous stasis. All patients should be instructed in the signs of acute thrombophlebitis and should be advised to report any leg pain, red or warm areas, or obviously discolored areas over varices. Patients with varices also should be cautioned against riding in cars or airplanes for long periods without frequent breaks.

Table 36–5. NEW YORK HEART ASSOCIATION FUNCTIONAL CLASSIFICATION

Class	Criteria
I	No limitation of physical activity
II	No symptoms at rest Minor limitation of physical activity (fatigue, palpitations, minor dyspnea)
III	No symptoms at rest Marked limitation of physical activity due to symptoms of cardiac disease
IV	Symptoms at rest Discomfort increased with any physical activity

Mitral valve prolapse is a very common condition in young women. There continues to be controversy regarding the need for prophylaxis against bacterial endocarditis. If prophylaxis is to be used, great care must be taken to ensure that the antibiotic agents are safe for both the mother and the fetus.

Gastrointestinal System. Generally, only a few diseases of the gastrointestinal tract are common in pregnancy. Although some minor aversion to food is common during the early weeks of pregnancy, this is rarely of consequence. However, in a small percentage of pregnant patients, a severe form of pregnancy-related gastrointestinal disease occurs called hyperemesis gravidarum. It is characterized by loss of body weight, acidosis, and electrolyte imbalance. Prompt hospitalization and treatment with intravenous fluid is necessary for the safety of the patient and fetus. Although in the past, certain "aversion" techniques were used for the treatment of this disease, it is now recognized that most patients respond well to hospitalization, rest, intravenous fluids, and the passage of time. The patient should receive support from the physician and nursing staff and should be gradually restarted on a full diet. Most patients can be treated and, within a few days, leave the hospital and suffer no recurrence. No organic basis has been found for this disease. Support is probably the most important feature of treatment. Antiemetics are often utilized. However, none of these has been demonstrated to be safe for use in pregnancy.Psychiatric consultation is advised if there are recurrent episodes or if the initial event is serious and prolonged.

Pre-existing peptic ulcer disease generally becomes less symptomatic in pregnancy because there is a decrease in the hydrochloric acid secretion of the stomach. In fact, any time that ulcer disease is first diagnosed in pregnancy, the diagnosis is usually incorrect. In pre-existing disease, nonconstipating antacids may be used if symptoms do not abate with pregnancy.

Pancreatitis may occur in pregnancy and may be a life-threatening event if it is of the hemorrhagic type. Although this occurs predominantly in alcoholic women, the pregnancy-induced stasis of the biliary system may occasionally result in pancreatic enzyme reflux, causing a chemical pancreatitis that may be severe.

Regional enteritis may be severe in pregnancy. It is most important that good maternal nutrition be established and maintained throughout pregnancy when this disease is present (Homan and Thorbjarnarson, 1976). If the woman has severe disease and is in very poor nutritional balance, she probably will not become pregnant. However, if she does become pregnant, vigorous attempts to maintain adequate nutrition are essential.

Chronic ulcerative colitis also may present problems in pregnancy, but these are rarely as significant as regional enteritis. The patient should be followed with nutritional support and the fetus monitored carefully for evidence of growth retardation (Webb and Sedlack, 1974).

Hepatitis has become a common disease in the United States. In the past, most cases were considered to be hepatitis type A; it is now recognized that the most common form is hepatitis type B. Nutritional support is the most important element in the treatment of either disease in pregnancy (Hieber et al., 1977). Both the fetus and the mother will usually survive without sequelae if nutritional support is adequate (Noller, 1981). Acute fulminant hepatitis B is the only exception to this rule. This disease cannot be distinguished easily from the fatty necrosis of the liver that occurs infrequently in late pregnancy.

If a woman developes hepatitis B in pregnancy, the fetus is at risk for both active disease and carrier status (Table 36–6). At birth, the neonate should receive hyperimmune serum and the first dose of hepatitis vaccine. Although this may seem not to be indicated if the infant has active disease, there is some evidence that such treatment might shorten the disease course and prevent carrier status. In cases of hepatitis B, it is extremely important to take precautions against the spread of the virus to the medical and nursing personnel via the blood and amniotic fluid at delivery. This is especially important in dealing with certain high-risk patients such as intravenous drug users.

The second most common cause for jaundice in pregnancy is a disease that is identified by many names: the most accepted term at the present time is "cholestatic jaundice of pregnancy." This disease presents as pruritus in late pregnancy. Mild jaundice is often also present. This is an idiopathic disease usually occurring during the last 10 weeks of pregnancy. In the past, it was believed that the disease, while annoying, did not cause any significant fetal or maternal problems. However, it is now recognized that approximately 30 per cent of women with this disease have premature labor. The fetus is also at risk for asphyxia in late pregnancy and during labor and must be monitored closely. Therefore, all patients with cholestatic jaundice are, by definition, high risk and require close follow-up (Noller, 1981; Reid et al., 1976).

Table 36–6. HEPATITIS B STATUS OF NEONATE

Time of Maternal Infection	Neontal Status
Early pregnancy	Often no active disease; infant may be chronic carrier
Late pregnancy	Usually active disease; carrier status common
Positive "e" antigen	Usually active disease; carrier status common

Genitourinary System. The urinary system usually causes no significant problems during pregnancy. The most common important disease is acute infection of the bladder, ureters, or renal pelvis. Because of the dilated collecting system, even mild cystitis may develop into frank pyelonephritis in a few hours or days. The patient should be instructed at her initial visit to report any symptoms of dysuria to her physician who should immediately obtain a Gram stain and culture and determine sensitivities. Usually, these infections can be treated with antibiotics that are not contraindicated in pregnancy. Ampicillin and nitrofurantoin are commonly used and are effective for many infections. Sensitivity studies should be done to be sure that the correct antibiotic is chosen. The use of tetracycline or the sulfonamides should be avoided. Cephalosporin may be utilized, but the *Physicians' Desk Reference* should be consulted to avoid those few drugs with known or suspected fetal effects.

Asymptomatic bacteriuria is frequently present in pregnant women. Many studies have shown that women with this condition are at increased risk for developing pyelonephrits. It is generally recommended that a urine culture be obtained at the initial prenatal visit. If asymptomatic bacteriuria is present, it should be treated.

The genital tract rarely causes problems other than occasional acute vaginitis. When this occurs, infection with one of the yeast organisms is the most common cause. This condition usually responds well to a short course of treatment with miconazole, clotrimazole, or butaconazole. The male sexual partner(s) should also be treated to prevent reinfection.

Hematologic System. The most frequent problem with the hematologic system in pregnancy is anemia. Because the red blood cell mass expands approximately 30 per cent in pregnancy and the plasma volume expands about 50 per cent, some dilution and decrease in the hemoglobin and hematocrit values occurs. Therefore, it is important to differentiate dilutional effects from frank anemia. Mild anemia should not be diagnosed in pregnancy until the hemoglobin concentration decreases to less than 11 grams per dl., and the anemia is not severe until the level is less than 10 grams per dl. However, when the blood count falls below this lower limit, an attempt should be made to determine the cause. Acute loss of blood is uncommon in pregnancy and the cause should be evident. More commonly, a deficiency of iron or folic acid is present, and this can be determined by examination of the red blood cell indices. If appropriate therapy is instituted, the blood counts usually will return to normal. Therapy for iron deficiency anemia in pregnancy should be 325 mg. of ferrous sulfate taken two or three times a day; folic acid deficiency responds to 1 mg. of folic acid per day.

Rh Disease. Rh incompatibility between mother and fetus is largely a problem of the past. The pregnant woman's blood group and Rh factor should be determined at the first visit. All Rh-negative women should be counseled by their physicians about the process by which Rh sensitization occurs. Prophylaxis with Rh immune globulin is routinely performed at 28 weeks gestation, after any manipulation (amniocentesis, version), and after a significant bleeding episode. At birth, the Rh factor of the infant should be determined, and if it is positive, the mother should be treated with another dose of Rh immune globulin.

If a traumatic delivery has taken place, the Kleihauer test for fetal red cells in the maternal serum should be performed. This test is routinely available from most laboratories and can accurately determine the volume of fetal blood that has transferred into the mother's circulation. One vial of Rh immune globulin can neutralize 10 to 15 ml. of fetal blood. Traumatic deliveries include all operative deliveries—cesarean sections, mid-forceps deliveries, and manual removal of the placenta.

The D^u test is performed routinely in most laboratories but can only detect fetal-maternal bleeding in excess of 25 ml. Therefore, the test is not sensitive enough to identify bleeding of 15 to 25 ml. Two vials of Rh immune globulin are indicated for bleeding in this range.

There are some women who have been Rh sensitized in earlier pregnancies or who become sensitized through therapeutic abortion, spontaneous abortion, inadvertent transfusion with inappropriate blood, or spontaneously during an apparently normal gestation. When sensitization occurs, it is a very high-risk situation for the fetus, and consultation with a maternal-fetal medicine specialist is recommended. Frequent amniocenteses and fetal transfusion with red blood cells may be necessary.

Surgical Complications. Acute appendicitis remains the most common surgical complication in pregnant women. The disease is often misdiagnosed in early pregnancy as ectopic pregnancy, ruptured corpus luteum cyst, or hyperemesis gravidarum. The usual signs and symptoms are changed little from normal in early pregnancy, but the position of the pain may move away from McBurney's point, being displaced somewhat laterally and cephalad as the uterus grows. In acute appendicitis, the patient must undergo laparotomy with removal of the diseased appendix. This can be performed with ease early in pregnancy but becomes more difficult with advanced gestation.

Acute cholecystitis may occur in pregnancy but is rather rare. The biliary system dilates in pregnancy, and this process usually prevents cholecystitis. When the disease occurs, it is best managed medically if possible. However, if the signs and symptoms suggest a need for surgery to prevent a gangrenous gallbladder with ensuing peritonitis, it will be necessary to perform cholecystectomy. This procedure can be accomplished in pregnancy with no unusual difficulty (Hill et al., 1975).

Dental surgery is undoubtedly the most common operative manipulation in pregnancy. There is no contraindication to such therapy if (1) only local anesthesia is used (no inhalation agents), (2) prophylaxis against subacute bacterial endocarditis is provided when the woman has a cardiac disorder, and (3) the abdomen is shielded during all x-ray procedures.

Other causes for surgery in pregnancy include accidents requiring orthopedic or general surgery, primary gastrointestinal disease such as regional enteritis, and head and neck surgery. When general anesthesia is required, the anesthesiologist should be made aware of the patient's pregnant condition. A balanced general anesthesia using low-dose inhalation or narcotic agents should be used. When possible, the fetus should be electronically monitored throughout the duration of the administration of anesthesia.

Obstetrical Complications

Pregnancy-Induced Hypertension (also called toxemia of pregnancy). This disease of unknown origin is usually diagnosed on the basis of hypertension of greater than 140/90 mm. of mercury or an increase of 30/15 mm. of mercury from the previous baseline blood pressure determination on two occasions at least 6 hours apart. Edema, previously used as a marker for pregnancy-induced hypertension, has been shown to correlate poorly with the disease. Proteinuria with a loss of > 300 mg. in a 24-hour period is also usually present. Recently, it has been recognized that alternations in coagulation (especially a decrease in platelet concentration) and elevated liver enzymes are a consistent marker for severe disease. The basic underlying pathology is widespread vasospasm. The process, if severe, can be controlled only by removing the underlying cause, the placenta and fetus (Pritchard, 1980). It is primarily a disease of the first pregnancy, although it may occur in later pregnancies, especially in women who have previously experienced it.

Pregnancy-induced hypertension most commonly is exhibited by a slowly increasing blood pressure and increasing amounts of protein in the urine. A patient with these early manifestations should be educated concerning the symptoms of pregnancy-induced hypertension: severe headache, abdominal pain, nausea and vomiting, and rapidly worsening edema. The patient with pregnancy-induced hypertension should be placed at bed rest in the left lateral recumbent position. It has been our experience that, in reliable patients, bed rest at home often prevents progression of these symptoms and may effect some improvement.

It is important to recognize that patients with pregnancy-induced hypertension are actually hypovolemic despite their edema. There is no indication for the use of diuretics in the treatment of this disease; in fact, diuretics often accelerate the process.

Table 36–7. LABORATORY EXAMINATION REQUIRED TO ASSESS SEVERITY OF PREGNANCY-INDUCED HYPERTENSION

Urinary protein
Liver enzymes
Platelet concentration
Complete blood count
Uric acid
Electrolytes
Coagulation profile

Once pregnancy-induced hypertension has been diagnosed, the patient is at high risk for both maternal and fetal morbidity and mortality. The mother should be followed with very frequent examination or should be hospitalized. Frequent determination of the liver enzymes and platelets is important (Table 36–7).

A useful aid for monitoring the fetus is the nonstress test (see Figure 36–6). For nonstress testing, the patient is placed in a reclining position and the fetus is monitored for 20 minutes. The fetal heart rate pattern is observed after spontaneous fetal movement, and accelerations of the fetal heart rate of 15 beats or greater for more than 15 seconds should occur after movement on at least two occasions during the 20-minute test period. If the fetus does not react in this manner, the test is considered nonreactive and is suggestive of fetal sleep or fetal compromise. Nonreactive tests should be repeated in 8 hours, and if still nonreactive, they should be followed by a biophysical profile. The biophysical profile is a more sophisticated version of nonstress testing. Nonstress testing is performed in the usual fashion. Ultrasonography is then done to assess fetal breathing, tone, and motion, and the amniotic fluid volume is estimated. Scores of 0, 1, or 2 are given to each of these five variables (nonstress test, fluid volume, fetal tone, fetal breathing, and fetal motion) and a total of 10 indicates adequate placental perfusion. The biophysical profile has largely supplemented contraction stress testing in which low levels of oxytocin are used to cause at least three contractions in 10 minutes. Schemata for following patients by means of these tests are available (Jarrell and Sokol, 1979).

In addition to laboratory examination, the maternal condition should be followed by using measurements of weight and blood pressure and by determining the responsiveness of the reflexes. Increasing hyperreflexia, especially with clonus, is a worrisome finding.

If delivery must be effected because of the severity of the disease, vaginal delivery or cesarean section may be employed, depending of the severity of the condition. The major maternal risk is that of developing eclampsia (pregnancy-induced seizures). This is a life-threatening event and should be prevented. If the woman has hyperreflexia, magnesium

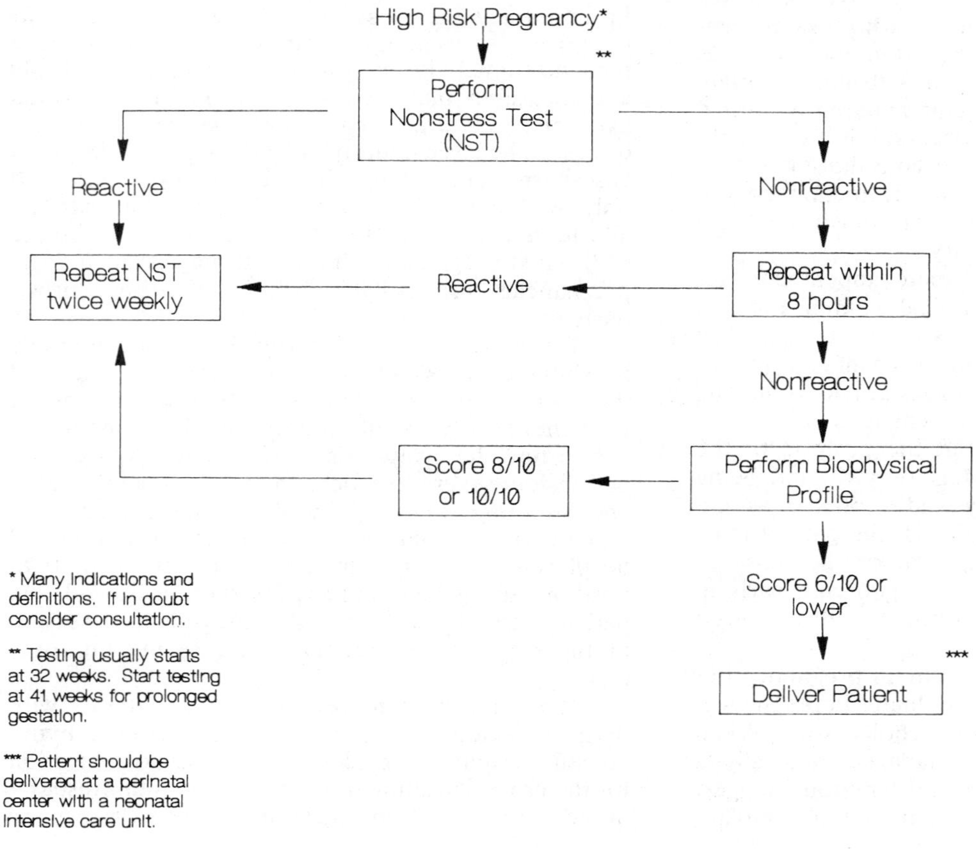

Figure 36–6. Nonstress test for fetal monitoring.

sulfate should be used to control reflexes and prevent seizures. Magnesium sulfate is a dangerous drug if used improperly. It should be given only (1) by the intravenous route, (2) with the aid of an infusion pump, and (3) where determination of maternal magnesium levels can be obtained rapidly. Dosages of magnesium sulfate must be individualized. Infusion rates may vary from 1 to 3 grams per hour. The exact rate needed depends on (1) the clinical condition of the patient, (2) the serum magnesium ion level, and (3) the urinary output. If the urinary output suddenly drops, the infusion rate should be immediately decreased or stopped while awaiting the serum level determination. Maternal asystole may occur with overdosage.

However, magnesium sulfate does little to control hypertension and, if the hypertension is severe, rapid-acting antihypertensives such as hydralazine should be used. Ten mg. of hydralazine may be given by slow intravenous push, if needed. The blood pressure must be watched very closely because of prolonged hypotension, which is occasionally observed after the use of this drug. The maximal effect will be seen within 20 minutes. Follow-up dosages must be given with care because of a potential additive effect.

In the past, when a pregnant woman with severe toxemia was admitted to the hospital, standard practice was to spend 24 hours "stabilizing" the patient before delivery was attempted. It is now clear that this only allows for progression of the disease process. In cases of severe disease, as soon as control of the reflexes and blood pressure has been established with magnesium sulfate and antihypertensive agents (usually in less than 2 hours), delivery should take place.

Many women with severe toxemia have disseminated intravascular coagulation. The platelet concentration and a coagulation profile should be obtained at admission for all women with this disease. If disseminated intravascular coagulation is profound, only delivery will correct the condition. Although there is no longer any indication for the use of fibrinogen, large amounts of platelet concentrate and fresh-frozen plasma should be available for use at the time of delivery, if necessary.

Third-Trimester Bleeding. This is a common complication of pregnancy and is usually the result of either placenta previa or abruptio placentae. Either condition may be a life-threatening situation for both mother and fetus. Electronic maternal and fetal monitoring should be instituted on admission. When ultrasound examination has been performed during prenatal care, the diagnosis of placenta previa can be excluded if a woman has vaginal bleeding when she enters the labor and delivery suite. If the placenta is not low-lying, vaginal examination may be undertaken. However, if ultrasonography has not been performed, vaginal examination should be deferred because a finger can be placed inadvertently through the placenta and can cause severe hemorrhage, with possible fetal and maternal death. Placenta previa requires cesarean section.

Abruptio placentae is similarly a life-threatening event for both mother and fetus. Depending on the portion of the placenta that has been torn from the uterine wall, the fetus may be little affected or may be dead. The area of placental separation often may be identified using real-time ultrasonography in the labor and delivery suite. Usually, the main symptom is pain and the signs are uterine tetany and vaginal bleeding. Large retroplacental hematomas may occur with sequestration of blood, depletion of the coagulation factors, and rapid onset of disseminated intravascular coagulation. Consideration should be given to immediate delivery, with blood products immediately available.

Vaginal delivery sometimes may be accomplished, but cesarean section is often needed. The fetus should be continuously monitored electronically with a scalp electrode because it may show signs of impending death during attempts at vaginal delivery. When treating a patient who has abruptio placentae, an efficient and fast hematologic laboratory should be available. Blood should be drawn for prothrombin time, fibrinogen levels, and a complete blood count. The treatment of choice is delivery. The patient need not be treated with blood products unless severe bleeding has occurred. Previously, it was believed that these patients should received heparin before delivery. However, it now has been shown that, if delivery can be effected quickly, the process can be rapidly reversed and heparin is rarely necessary. If loss of blood has been significant, whole blood, packed red blood cells, fresh-frozen plasma, and platelet concentrate can be used to restore the depleted blood and coagulation factors. Fibrinogen should not be administered because of the high risk of hepatitis.

Multiple Gestation. Twins occur spontaneously in approximately 1 in every 80 pregnancies in the United States. Triplets occur in approximately 1 in 6,500 to 8,000 pregnancies. Both of these are significant complications of pregnancy and require experience to deal with them properly. It used to be a commonly accepted fact that women with multiple gestation went into labor very early, with prematurity being the most common complication of twin birth. However, multiple gestation is usually identified early in pregnancy by means of ultrasonography, and if the patient is placed at bed rest, the woman will often carry to term. This will prevent prematurity and more likely ensure healthy neonates.

Cesarean section for twin deliveries is recommended unless both twins are in the vertex position, there are definitely two separate sacs, both twins are the same size (±300 grams), and electronic fetal monitoring is available. Electronic fetal monitoring of the second twin should be performed during and after delivery of the first twin.

Premature Labor. Prematurity is the most frequent cause of neonatal death in the United States. Certain women are at high risk for premature labor and deliveries (Table 36–8). Proper risk assessment

Table 36–8. FACTORS ASSOCIATED WITH INCREASED RISK OF PREMATURE DELIVERY

Medical	
	Primigravidity
	History of previous premature delivery
	In utero diethylstilbestrol exposure
	Maternal hypertension
	Multiple gestation
	Previous cervical manipulation (dilatation, conization)
	Sexually transmitted diseases
	Pyelonephritis
Social	
	Age < 18 or > 35
	Low level of education
	Nonmarried status
	Poor or absent prenatal care
	Low income
	Abusive relationship
Behavioral	
	Smoking
	Alcohol abuse
	Illicit drug use

at the time of the initial obstetric visit should identify most of these associated problems, if present.

If premature labor occurs, it should be documented carefully by means of external fetal monitoring. The diagnosis should not be made unless there is progressive cervical dilatation. If the gestation is of less than 36 weeks, consideration should be given to attempting to stop labor using beta-sympathomimetic agents or magnesium sulfate ($MgSO_4$). Currently, ritodrine is approved for this use. Table 36–9 shows the method of administration of this medication at the Mayo Clinic. We have found this method to be a very effective means of stopping labor, often for several weeks or months. Most women may be weaned from the intravenous solution to the oral medication and allowed to go home. Terbutaline is equally effective but requires a different regimen and is not marketed for this indication. $MgSO_4$ has become popular and, if used, must be given intravenously with all precautions as listed above in the section on pregnancy-induced hypertension.

When premature rupture of membranes without labor occurs before 34 weeks of gestation, the patient should be examined once with a sterile speculum on admission to the labor and delivery suite *and nothing further should be done.* In the past, it was frequently recommended that all of these women be delivered within 24 hours. At the present time, it is our practice to *not* induce labor if it does not occur spontaneously unless there are signs of infection. We have found that if vaginal examinations are excluded and coitus is prohibited, some of these women will carry to term, and many will not deliver for several days or weeks. Some women have carried for more than 10 weeks with no evidence of intrauterine infection. However, prolonged rupture of many weeks duration is associated with fetal pulmonary maldevelopment. Thus the patient should be informed about the possibility of the occurrence of this sometimes fatal event.

If an incompetent cervix is the cause of the premature labor and delivery, consideration should be given to the performance of a cerclage. The Shirodkar technique will often hold the cervix closed even if it had dilated 2 or 3 cm. before the procedure. This can be a difficult procedure and should be performed only by a physician very familiar with the technique. The McDonald technique is much less difficult but may not be as effective.

If signs of intrauterine infection are observed, broad-spectrum antibiotic treatment should be initiated and the patient delivered. Septic shock can occur rapidly in this situation.

The administration of corticosteroids in an attempt to induce fetal pulmonary maturation is common, although not all experts agree that it is effective. Corticosteroids should be used with caution if ritodrine or other beta-sympathomimetics are used because of the possibility of causing maternal pulmonary edema when the two medications are used together.

Intrauterine Growth Retardation. The astute physician can detect evidence of poor growth of the fetus in utero. In these situations, ultrasound should be obtained to document fetal size. A weight below the 10th percentile of expected weights for the population suggests intrauterine growth retardation. The estimate of weight requires measurement of the biparietal diameter, head and abdominal circumference, and femur length at a minimum. The measurements must be obtained in exactly the correct plane

Table 36–9. RITODRINE PROTOCOL

Patient placed in left lateral position
Obtain baseline K^+, glucose
Record: Maternal vital signs
  Blood pressure and pulse—baseline, then every 10 minutes until stabilized; then every 60 minutes
  Record input and output
Fetal heart rate
  Continuous electronic fetal monitoring
Start intravenous infusion with 5 per cent dextrose in lactated Ringer's solution
Administer ritodrine
- Infusion pump mandatory
- Piggyback to intravenous infusion
- Solution: 15 mg. ritodrine in 500 ml. 5 per cent dextrose (300 μg. per ml.)
- Infusion rate (μg. per minute): Increase until contractions cease
  - Initial: 0.3 ml (100 μg.)
  - 10 minutes: 0.5 (150 μg.)
  - 20 minutes: 0.7 (200 μg.)
  - 30 minutes: 0.9 (250 μg.)
  - 40 minutes: 1.0 (300 μg.)
  - 50 minutes: 1.2 (350 μg.)
- Do not exceed 350 μg. per minute

Maintain maternal: Pulse < 130 per minute
  Systolic blood pressure > 90 mm. Hg
Obtain K^+, glucose in 4 hours
Continue infusion for 12 hours after contractions cease
Maintenance schedule (after 12 hours without contractions)
- 10 mg. ritodrine orally
- Discontinue intravenous infusion 30 minutes later
- 10 mg. ritodrine orally every 2 hours for 24 hours
- 20 mg. ritodrine orally every 4 to 6 hours until delivery

to be meaningful. Only a trained ultrasonographer can accurately assess intrauterine fetal weight. However, with experience, the estimate is accurate to within a few grams.

If the fetus is not growing as expected, the cause may be intrinsic maternal or fetal disease or other extenuating circumstances such as smoking, alcoholism, malnutrition, or infection. In all cases, the fetus is considered at high risk and must be monitored closely for evidence of maladaptation to stress. Nonstress testing is indicated.

Postmaturity. Postmaturity is a life-threatening event for the fetus when the gestation is carried beyond 43 weeks. Nonstress testing should begin at 41 weeks gestation and should be performed at least twice weekly. Although some older texts suggest that a nonreactive nonstress test need be repeated only once a week, this is too optimistic. The biophysical profile has largely supplemented nonstress testing for following post-term pregnancies.

Induction of labor should be done before the 43rd week of gestation. If the cervix is not ripe, the use of prostaglandin gel on the cervix the night before the planned induction may greatly increase the success rate of induction.

Fetal Demise. Although fetal demise before viability (spontaneous abortion) is very common, losses in the late second and third trimesters are relatively rare. Appropriate management of coexistent medical diseases has greatly decreased fetal death due to these complications. Therefore, as part of the risk assessment at the first and subsequent prenatal visits, preexisting medical illnesses should be carefully reviewed to determine increased fetal risk.

A profound change has occurred in the frequency of intrapartum deaths during the past few years. Intrapartum deaths should rarely, if ever, occur. Electronic fetal monitoring has shown that deaths during labor and delivery do not occur suddenly. The fetus will exhibit evidence of its compromised state for many hours (even days) before death. In all cases of high-risk pregnancy, electronic fetal monitoring during labor is required.

Labor and Delivery

INITIAL ASSESSMENT OF THE PATIENT IN LABOR

Signs of Labor. Although many predictors of the onset of labor such as the estimated date of confinement, status of the cervix, and position of the presenting part are commonly used, the ability of the physician to predict the onset of labor is limited. Certain signs and symptoms may be helpful in determining whether labor is going to start soon or has actually started. Uterine contractions are most often used as the indicators of the onset of labor. Differentiation between the contractions of true and false labor is important in providing appropriate advice to patients during this time. The contractions of true labor are characterized by (1) regular occurrence, (2) gradually shortening intervals between them, and (3) an increasing intensity of pain located usually in the back and abdomen. The contractions of false labor differ in that (1) they occur at irregular intervals, (2) the intervals remain long, and (3) the intensity of the pain remains the same and is usually located in the lower abdomen. The character of the contractions plus other signs, such as passage of the mucus plug or leakage of amniotic fluid, may be indicators of the onset of labor that are helpful to the patient and her physician in deciding when the patient should report to the hospital.

In primigravid patients, the latent phase of labor may be long and may be best tolerated in the familiar atmosphere of the patient's home rather than the labor room. If a birthing room is available, the patient may wish to come to the hospital earlier in labor, since this atmosphere may combine the feeling of well-being afforded the patient by familiar surroundings with the security of being in the hospital environment. Signs and symptoms that should alert the patient to go immediately to the hospital are significant bleeding and unusual degrees of pain. Also, the patient with spontaneous rupture of the membranes should report to the hospital so that minimal time is lost if labor needs to be induced. We believe that the patient at term, 38 weeks or greater, should be delivered within 24 hours after the membranes have ruptured.

Progress of Labor. If the patient is in true labor or has had ruptured membranes, she should be given a thorough evaluation on arrival at the hospital. This is the time not only for the status of the fetus and the progress of labor to be assessed but also for a more thorough health evaluation. It may have been 6 or more months since a complete examination was done, and the ever-changing status of pregnancy requires that a thorough evaluation be done before delivery. It is assumed that the patient has been well educated regarding the management of her labor during the prenatal period, and this is a good time to review the status of the fetus and the expected progress of labor. A relaxed, confident patient with her personal physician at her side is more likely to have a smooth and shorter labor. This also is a time for the patient to be informed of the procedures that may be used during the labor. A very important way to prepare a patient is to have the patient involved with prenatal education classes. This is often done through prenatal classes given at the hospital or the physician's office.

Since the most accurate measurement of the progress of labor is the dilatation and effacement of the cervix plus descent of the presenting part, the cervix should be accurately evaluated at the outset of labor. Morbidity is no greater with vaginal checks than with rectal examination, except in the patient with ruptured membranes, who requires frequent vaginal examination and in whom the risk of infection may be increased slightly. If the patient's regular physician is not following the labor personally, the attending physician should understand what the other examiner's evaluations mean so that the progress of labor can be appropriately evaluated. The amount of dilatation of the cervix can be compared with values from charts, which should be in each labor area. Also, one should describe cervical effacement as uneffaced, partially effaced, or completely effaced rather than use percentages, which vary markedly from one examiner to another and are dependent on the thickness of the cervix before labor.

CONDUCT OF NORMAL LABOR

To be able to recognize quickly abnormalities in labor patterns, the physician should have a thorough knowledge of normal labor patterns and should record each patient's labor on a labor curve, which shows the patient's progress graphically. The frequency, duration, and intensity of contractions are not reliable measures of the progress of labor, and, therefore, labor curves are essential to monitor progress and to determine if labor is normal or abnormal (Fig. 36–7).

Classically, labor has been divided into three stages, with the first stage being the period from the onset of labor until the cervix has become completely dilated. The second stage of labor extends from the time of complete dilatation of the cervix until the delivery of the infant. The third stage is the time from the delivery of the infant to the delivery of the placenta.

The first stage of labor consists of latent and active phases, which also can be further subdivided into the acceleration phase, phase of maximal slope, and the deceleration phase. The latent phase of labor extends from the onset of regular contractions to the beginning of the active phase. During the latent phase, very little cervical dilatation occurs, but it is the time when uterine contractions are becoming more coordinated and prolonged and, therefore, more efficient. The cervix undergoes subtle changes that prepare it for the active phase. Normally, the latent phase of labor does not exceed 20 hours in nulliparous patients or 14 hours in multiparous patients. The length of the latent phase of labor does not correlate well with the length of the total labor, and latent phase is very sensitive to external factors. The most common problem seen in the latent phase concerns the premature use of analgesics. If analgesics are given during the latent phase, a series of events can occur. For example, if the latent phase becomes excessively prolonged, there may be confusion as to whether the patient is progressing or not, and augmentation of labor may be contemplated. Therefore, one should wait until the patient is in the active phase before using analgesics.

The active phase includes the acceleration phase, which is characterized by a rapid change in the rate of dilatation of the cervix. This is followed by the phase of maximal slope, which is characterized by the maximal rate of cervical dilatation and culminated in the deceleration phase, which is characterized by a slowing in the rate of dilatation until the cervix is completely dilated. The rate of cervical dilatation during the active phase is usually not less than 1.2 cm. per hour for nulliparous patients and not less than 2 cm. per hour in multiparous patients (Fig. 36–8).

The second stage of labor extends from the time of complete dilatation of the cervix to delivery of the infant. This is often the time when the patient wishes to bear down and experiences the urge to defecate. The average length of time for the second stage in primigravida patients is 1 hour and in multiparous patients, 1/2 hour. Usually, it should not last longer than 2 hours, but if the condition of the fetus is satisfactory, based on continuous electronic fetal monitoring, the second stage may be allowed to exceed 2 hours somewhat (Table 36–10).

In addition to risk assessment during the prenatal period, maternal and fetal risk should be assessed dynamically during labor. The system chosen by the Division of Family Medicine at the Mayo Clinic is a modification of the Hobel system of risk assessment.

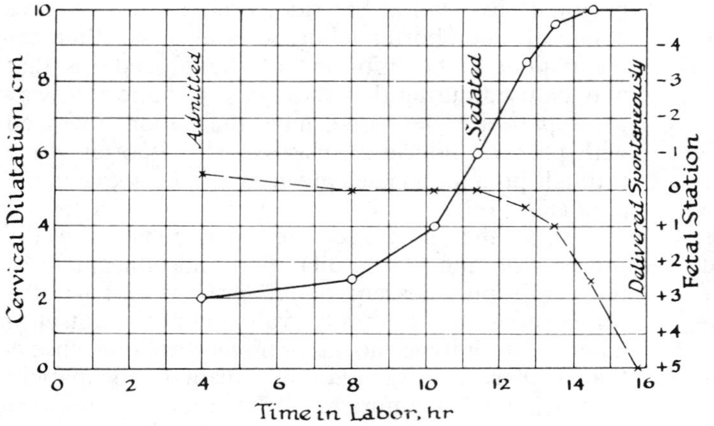

Figure 36–7. Evolution of normal patterns of cervical dilatation *(solid line)* and fetal descent *(broken line)*. Dilatation is plotted in centimeters (left scale) and entered according to the number of hours elapsed in the course of labor to trace the characteristic sigmoid curve shown, typical of all normal labors. Similarly, the hyperbolic curve of descent is traced in all normally progressive labors by plotting estimates of fetal station (right scale) against time in labor. (From Friedman, E. A.: Labor: Clinical Evaluation and Management. 2nd ed. New York, Appleton-Century-Crofts, 1978, p. 23. By permission.)

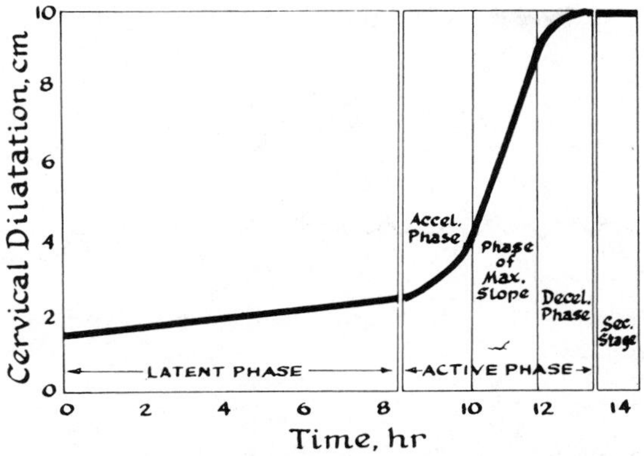

Figure 36–8. Composite of the average dilatation curve for nulliparous labor based on analysis of the data derived from the patterns traced by a large, nearly consecutive series of gravida patients. The first stage is divided into a relatively flat latent phase and a rapidly progressive active phase. The active phase has three identifiable component parts: an acceleration phase, a linear phase of maximal slope, and a deceleration phase. (From Friedman, E. A.: Labor: Clinical Evaluation and Management. 2nd ed. New York, Appleton-Century-Crofts, 1978, p. 33. By permission.)

For both the prenatal and the perinatal risk assessment, this system is a simple tool to determine whether or not patients should be placed in the high-risk category.

Upon admission of the patient to the labor room, the vital signs should be recorded and the prenatal record should be reviewed. Since the prenatal record is not generally available when the patient arrives at the labor room, the physician should send a copy of the prenatal record to the hospital at least 2 weeks before the estimated date of delivery. Special problems or requests of the patient when she arrives in labor should be mentioned on this copy. After the initial assessment, the mother and fetus should be evaluated thoroughly. Except when contraindicated, abdominal and pelvic examinations should be done to determine the relationship of the long axis of the fetus to the long axis of the mother (fetal lie). Also, the presentation of the fetus needs to be determined accurately, and the position of the presenting part within the pelvis should be described.

In preparing the patient for expected delivery, there has been a change from the routine full perineal shave and enema given all patients admitted to the labor room to a more individualized approach. During labor, the use of oral fluids should be limited because of delayed gastric emptying. It is our policy to start an intravenous line during labor not only to replace fluids lost during the labor but also to have immediate access for the rapid administration of medications, if this becomes necessary.

During this preparation, it is very important to review again with the patient the conduct of her labor and her expectations and desires regarding analgesia and anesthesia. A full explanation of all procedures contemplated and an explanation of the meanings and the results of the monitoring of the patient's blood pressure and the infant's fetal heart rate are important in producing the situation of a relaxed, confident, well-informed patient who thoroughly understands the process and procedures that she and her child are experiencing.

FETAL MONITORING

Monitoring of the fetus during labor and delivery has always been a part of the routine in labor and delivery suites. The current difference is that electronic methods often are now utilized instead of simple auscultation, and the precision and frequency of such monitoring have increased. A common misconception concerning fetal monitoring is very prevalent. It has been suggested that the recent rapid increase in the frequency of cesarean section has been due largely to the more liberal use of electronic fetal monitoring in the United States. There are now sufficient data to refute this statement. Where *correct interpretation* of the results of monitoring is performed, electronic

Table 36–10. THE PATTERNS OF ABNORMAL LABOR

Pattern	Diagnostic Criterion
Disorder of Preparatory Division of Labor	
Prolonged latent phase	
Nulliparas	Latent phase duration
Multiparas	Latent phase duration of 14 hr or more
Disorders of Dilatational Division of Labor	
Protracted active-phase dilatation	
Nulliparas	Maximum slope of dilatation of 1.2 cm. per hour or less
Multiparas	Maximum slope of descent of 2.0 cm. per hour or less
Disorders of Pelvic Division of Labor	
Prolonged deceleration phase	
Nulliparas	Deceleration phase duration of 3 hours or more
Multiparas	Deceleration phase duration of 1 hour or more
Secondary arrest of dilatation	Cessation of active-phase progression for 2 hours or more
Arrest of descent	Cessation of descent progression for 1 hour or more
Failure of descent	Lack of expected descent during deceleration phase and second stage
Precipitate Labor Disorders	
Precipitate dilatation	
Nulliparas	Maximum slope of dilatation of 5 cm. per hour or more
Multiparas	Maximum slope of dilatation of 10 cm. per hour or more
Precipitate Descent	
Nulliparas	Maximum slope of descent of 5 cm. per hour or more
Multiparas	Maximum slope of descent 10 cm. per hour or more

From Friedman, E. A.: Labor: Clinical Evaluation and Management. 2nd ed. New York, Appleton-Century-Crofts, 1978, p. 63. By permission.

fetal monitoring should only add approximately 1½ per cent to the primary cesarean section rate. In fact, even if utilized on a routine basis for all patients in labor, a rapid increase in the cesarean section rate should not occur. For more than 10 years, the Mayo Clinic staff has routinely used electronic fetal monitoring on all women in labor. The primary cesarean section rate on the obstetric service has remained low despite the large high-risk referral practice.

When the decision has been made to employ electronic fetal monitoring, the procedure should be discussed with the patient. If the patient is aware of the way in which the sensors pick up the fetal heart rate and contractions, she often can help in the maintenance of a quality signal. For those patients in whom it is sufficient to know the pattern of the fetal heart rate and only the occurrence of uterine contractions, external electronic fetal monitoring is sufficient. However, external monitoring gives no information concerning the strength of contractions. This can be obtained only by means of an intrauterine pressure monitor. It has been our experience that when electronic fetal monitoring is employed, external monitoring usually is sufficient. However, if worrisome patterns become evident, if it is essential to know the intrauterine pressure, or if there is great difficulty in establishing an adequate external signal, internal electronic fetal monitoring is employed.

A number of factors of the fetal heart beat are followed: the rate, the variability of the rate, and changes in the rate in relation to uterine contractions (Hill, 1979). In general, the fetal heart rate during active labor should be between 110 and 150 beats per minute. In a normal, uncompromised fetus, this rate will vary. In fact, lack of beat-to-beat variability of 10 to 15 per minute is suggestive of fetal compromise. However, many drugs—such as medications commonly used for analgesia—and fetal sleep may cause a temporary flattening of the normal variability. In the case of medication, this appears to be a direct effect of the maternal medication on the fetus through transplacental passage of the drug(s). Figure 36–9 demonstrates normal fetal heart rate variability, and Figure 36–10 shows an example of decreased variability.

The pattern of the fetal heart rate during and after uterine contractions gives the observer considerable information concerning the status of the fetus. Two patterns are considered normal. In many pregnancies, the fetal heart rate varies little, if any, during and just after uterine contractions. In others, a deceleration of the rate is noted that is coincident with the onset of the contraction and ceases at the time of relaxation of the uterus. These dips are a type of variable deceleration caused by contraction and are due to vagal stimulation caused by increased pressure on the fetal head during a uterine contraction (Fig. 36–11). These are considered a normal variant in most cases. However, if the decline is both profound and recurrent, it is worrisome, and the scalp pH should be measured.

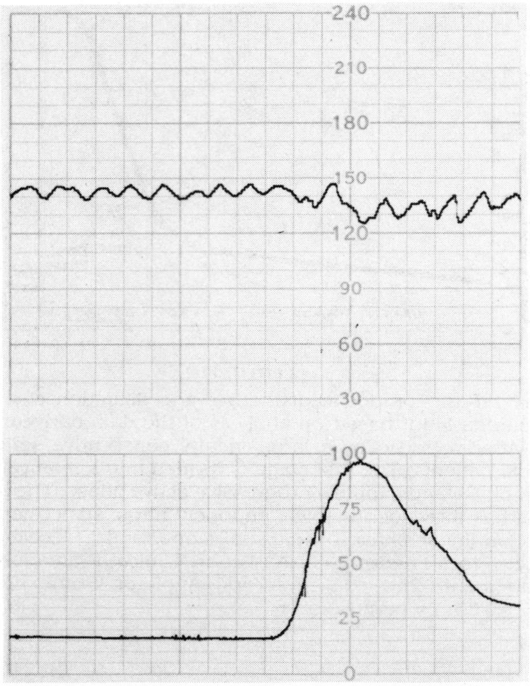

Figure 36–9. Normal fetal heart rate with normal beat-to-beat variability and a normal baseline (top line). The bottom line shows a normal uterine contraction. (From Hill, L. M.: Diagnosis and management of fetal distress. Mayo Clin. Proc., *54*:784, 1979. By permission.)

Two types of fetal decelerations are pathologic. Late decelerations are those that occur after uterine relaxation. These usually represent a central (neurologic) reaction to anoxic stress. The decelerations may be either dramatic or subtle (Fig. 36–12). The degree of deceleration is not directly indicative of the severity of the problem, and even small decelerations of the late type are worrisome.

The other pattern of possible pathologic fetal heart rate decelerations is the so-called variable deceleration (Fig. 36–13). In these cases, the fetal heart rate shows a mixed pattern of both decelerations and accelerations during and after the uterine contraction. The observed pattern varies from contraction to contraction. Cord compression and fetal anoxia are the cause of this heart rate pattern.

Variable decelerations present the greatest interpretive problem for the clinician. Although these decelerations may represent severe fetal compromise in some patients, in others long periods of variable decelerations do not result in the birth of a compromised fetus. When variable decelerations are present, fetal scalp pH can be a most useful adjunctive means of determining the true status of the fetus. The use of this test involves obtaining a small sample of blood from the fetal scalp in a heparinized capillary tube and determining the pH using a pH meter adapted for microvolumes. The technique of obtaining the sample is relatively simple. A scalp pH of between 7.25 and 7.45 is a reliable indication of fetal well-being. The clinician can be reassured that the variable

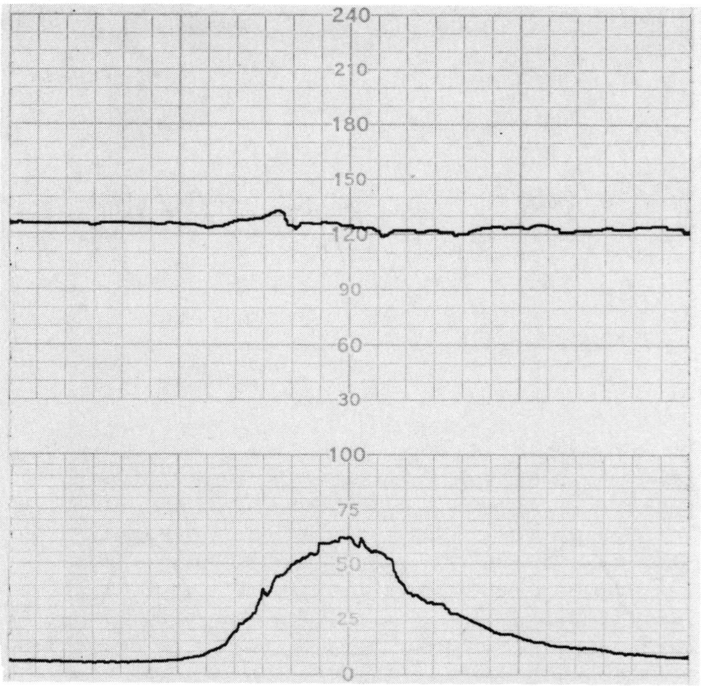

Figure 36–10. Decreased variability and normal baseline. This may be due to distress, medications, or fetal sleep. (From Hill, L. M.: Diagnosis and management of fetal distress. Mayo Clin. Proc., *54*:784, 1979. By permission.)

decelerations that are seen *at that time* have not caused fetal compromise. However, if the pattern continues, repeated scalp samples are advised.

If the scalp pH is 7.25 or less, another sample should be obtained to guard against laboratory error. If the second sample is also low or borderline, steps must be taken to either correct the acidosis or to deliver the fetus. At times, the use of oxygen by mask and changing the position of the woman resolves both the deceleration pattern and the acidosis. Once an abnormal pH sample is obtained, a repeat sample is indicated within a few minutes. In fact, it is always advisable to take a repeat sample if the pH is indicative of abnormality.

The status of the fetus cannot be determined on the basis of an isolated observation of a deceleration or of a single scalp sample alone. Interpretation of the findings must be individualized based on the risk status, the progress of labor, the use of analgesic drugs, and other known extrinsic factors. The decision to intervene should be made only after these factors have been carefully considered.

The end result of prolonged fetal compromise is predictable. If electronic fetal monitoring is employed, the fetus eventually experiences a terminal deceleration that will be profound and severe. The fetal heart rate may decrease to between 40 and 60 beats per minute and remain there for several minutes. Eventually, the heart rate will be lost completely. Once such a prolonged deceleration occurs, the only chance for fetal survival is immediate delivery either by emergency cesarean section or by forceps. Because many labor and delivery suites are not equipped to perform cesarean section within the 4 to 6 minutes that are required to increase the chances of fetal survival, steps should be taken to prevent this end point by early recognition of fetal distress.

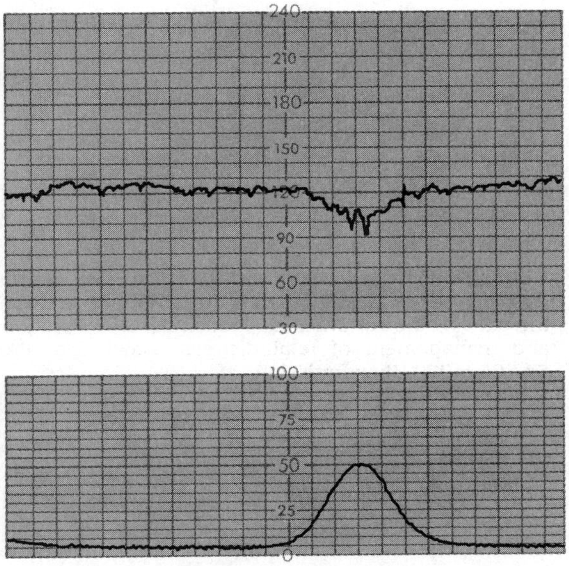

Figure 36–11. Normal baseline and variable deceleration with decreased variability. (From Hill, L. M.: Diagnosis and management of fetal distress. Mayo Clin. Proc., *54*:784, 1979. By permission.)

Electronic fetal monitoring should not be utilized unless the personnel observing the patterns are thoroughly familiar with its interpretation. Without these interpretive skills, a large number of inappropriate cesarean sections and difficult forceps deliveries will occur. Companies that market the technical equip-

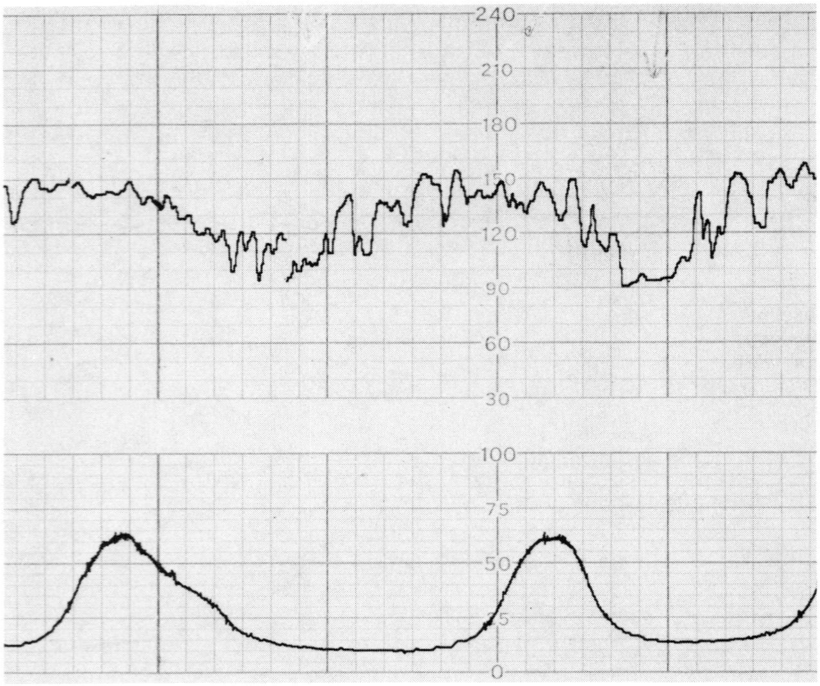

Figure 36–12. Internal monitor tracing showing persistent, severe late decelerations. (From Hill, L. M.: Diagnosis and management of fetal distress. Mayo Clin. Proc., *54*:784, 1979. By permission.)

ment for electronic fetal monitoring often provide detailed educational services for the paramedical and medical personnel who use the equipment.

NORMAL DELIVERY

Delivery of a normal healthy infant is a most rewarding experience for the patient, her family, and the physician. In recent years, the presence of the father at the time of delivery has become commonplace, adding an important dimension to this family event.

Delivery Room Set-Up. The delivery room not only must be organized in a manner that allows for easy delivery of the uncomplicated case but also must be adaptable so that management of sudden unexpected emergencies is possible. Physicians should

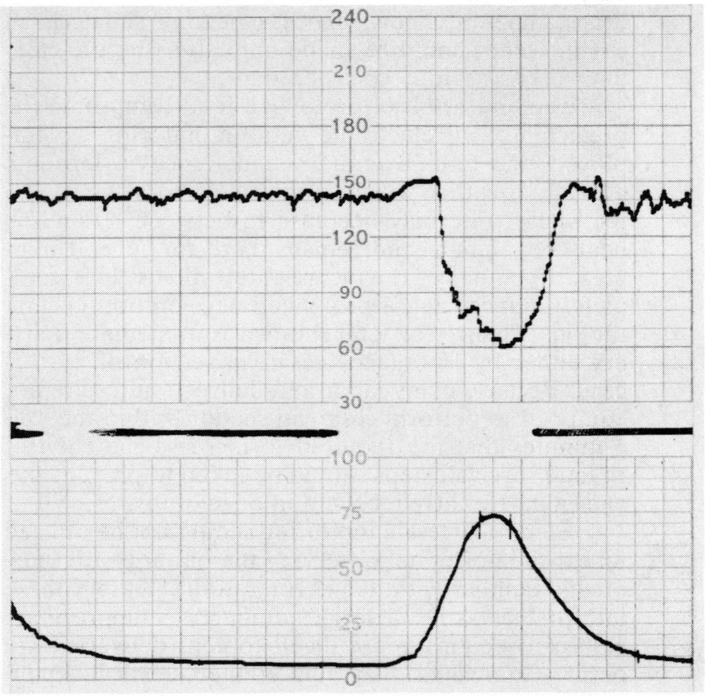

Figure 36–13. Decreased variability, normal baseline, and variable deceleration. Note the slight acceleration at the start of the contraction. (From Hill, L. M.: Diagnosis and management of fetal distress. Mayo Clin. Proc., *54*:784, 1979. By permission.)

urge their hospitals to equip all delivery rooms in a manner that makes it possible for cesarean sections to be performed. Unfortunately, too many hospital delivery rooms are not properly equipped and, even in an extremely emergent situation, the patient must be moved to a different room or even to a different floor for a cesarean section.

The type of delivery table, the patient drapes, and the instruments for a routine delivery are largely a matter of choice for the physician and hospital. The instruments should be set up using usual sterile techniques. Other instruments that may be needed for some deliveries should be either in the room or very near it. Forceps and instruments for repair of vaginal and perinatal lacerations should be readily available.

All delivery rooms must be properly equipped to manage the neonate during the first few minutes of life. An area must be provided where the neonate can be examined. All delivery rooms must have facilities immediately available for infant suction and intubation. Additionally, the infant should be placed in a warmer. Radiant warmers are superior to other types and should be the only type used. If a warm setting is not available for the infant, then the ambient temperature of the delivery room must be maintained at approximately 26.7° C (80° F). This temperature is generally uncomfortable for the patient, physician, and nursing staff, and infant warmers are a much better solution.

Birthing Room Alternatives. During the past few years, many women have requested that delivery be accomplished in a setting that is different from the traditional delivery room. Because of the different needs and desires of the patients, various facilities have been developed. The most popular alternative at the present time is that of a birthing room. At the Mayo Clinic approximately 2/3 of the normal vaginal deliveries now occur in a birthing room. Although many hospitals have rooms that have been so designated, it is important to remember that a birthing room is a concept, more than just a specific area in the hospital. A relaxed atmosphere can be provided in a traditional delivery room if the staff are aware of and participate in making this extremely important family event one that is personalized and comforting to the patient and her family.

The term birthing room usually refers to a room in which the patient can proceed through the total duration of labor and in which delivery can occur without the patient changing rooms or beds. These rooms are usually decorated to simulate a room at home and in many instances, with proper equipment, labor room delivery can be accomplished, providing many of the advantages of a birthing room. However, immediate access to a facility or room where cesarean section can be accomplished is essential.

Delivery of Infant. The decision to move the patient to the delivery room is one that is best made by an experienced nurse or physician. The woman who is about to deliver her first child generally can be taken to the delivery room between contractions after the infant's head is visible on the perineum. However, a multiparous woman should be taken much sooner. The woman should be placed in the dorsal lithotomy position and the legs placed in comfortable, padded stirrups or foot pads. Hand restraints should be avoided. It is our practice to begin oxygen by mask when the patient enters the delivery room and to continue oxygen administration at approximately 7 l. per minute until delivery of the infant and clamping of the cord have been accomplished.

Draping varies considerably among hospitals. There does not seem to be any drape that is clearly superior to another. The drapes should be used for the convenience of the patient, physician, and the nursing staff. They should provide the usual sterility. In general, cloth drapes are superior to paper drapes, though the latter are sometimes used because of fiscal considerations.

The woman should be asked to bear down with each contraction after the cervix is completely dilated. If the delivery room table is equipped with aids for bearing down, the woman may pull against these and push down into the perineal area with each contraction. Depending on the type of anesthesia, she may or may not have a considerable spontaneous urge to perform this maneuver. The fetal head should be allowed to distend the perineum. An episiotomy should not be performed unless it is obvious that perineal laceration will occur. A clean surgical incision with a scalpel or scissors is preferable to a jagged tear. There is no evidence to support the concept that episiotomy before distention will result in a more stable perineum in later years.

With very few exceptions, midline episiotomy is preferred. Compared with a mediolateral type, it is far easier to repair, blood loss is less, and the patient will be considerably more comfortable after delivery. However, a mediolateral episiotomy allows the operator much more room because it can be extended for a considerable distance. There is no indication for a midline episiotomy to include the rectal sphincter and mucosa. If bowel interruption is likely to occur when a midline episiotomy is performed, a mediolateral incision is preferable.

The infant's head should never be allowed to "pop" over the perinatal body. The fetal head should be delivered slowly and in a controlled fashion, and it often helps to ask the patient to push *between* (rather than with) contractions. Sudden delivery of the head can cause intercerebral bleeding and tentorial tears.

Immediately on delivery of the head, the physician's finger should be placed in the baby's mouth and the oral pharynx suctioned with either a bulb syringe or a DeLee suction. The nasal passages also should be cleared if there has been passage of meconium. After this maneuver, a hand is placed over the fetal head to the area of the neck and shoulders to determine whether or not the umbilical cord is around the neck. If it is, it can usually be easily slipped over the head. If this cannot be accomplished, the cord should be double clamped, cut between the clamps, and unwrapped from the fetal head.

If necessary, the shoulders should next be rotated gently to the anteroposterior position, and with *very gentle* traction on the head, the anterior shoulder should be delivered. On delivering the first shoulder, the infant is raised and the posterior shoulder usually delivers easily. The infant's body is then delivered.

Upon completion of the delivery, the infant's head should remain lower than the rest of the body and oral pharyngeal suction should be accomplished.

If the umbilical cord has not been cut previously, it should be clamped and cut. In the past, considerable debate has concerned the correct moment to clamp the umbilical cord. One group favored early clamping, another group favored late clamping, and a third group favored "stripping" of the cord. The "stripping" procedure should not be used, since overtransfusion often occurs. It has been our practice to clamp the cord after delivery of the infant and suctioning the oropharynx. There does not seem to be any advantage to slightly earlier or slightly later clamping.

If the amniotic fluid is contaminated with meconium, the delivery must be accomplished slightly differently. Immediately on delivery of the infant, the head should be kept down, the cord should be clamped, and the infant should be immediately placed in the warmer and intubated. Many instances of severe pneumonia in the newborn that have been seen in the past have been due to the aspiration of meconium. If meconium is at or below the vocal cords, intubation must be repeatedly performed until suctioning returns only clear fluid. In many infants, once the laryngoscope has been placed and no meconium can be seen in the pharynx, the procedure can be terminated. All physicians who deliver infants should be thoroughly familiar with this procedure.

Infant assessment should be accomplished at 1 and 5 minutes, and an Apgar score assigned. It has been repeatedly shown that the person performing the delivery should not assign the Apgar score, since the score could be falsely inflated. A nurse or other physician should assign the Apgar scores.

If the infant is in no acute distress, attention is then returned to the mother. The third stage of labor usually can be accomplished easily. If the mother is Rh negative, a sample of cord blood should be obtained and sent to the laboratory for determination of the Rh factor of the infant. After this sample has been obtained, the cord may be drained. *Gentle* traction on the cord is then used until the placenta separates, at which time it can be easily removed from the uterus and vagina. Strong traction should never be placed on the umbilical cord because inversion of the uterus may occur, and this is an extremely dangerous situation. The normal third stage of labor lasts less than 30 minutes. If the placenta does not spontaneously expel within this time, manual removal may be considered. This maneuver should be performed by someone who is familiar with the procedure since it is easy to leave cotyledons in place. After either spontaneous or manual removal of the placenta, it should be inspected carefully to ensure that removal is complete. Missing cotyledons suggest the necessity of intrauterine exploration.

Oxytocic agents should be used to help contract the uterus and minimize loss of blood after delivery of the placenta. It is our practice to use 20 or 30 units of oxytocin in a liter of the intravenous solution. Usually, we infuse 200 or 300 ml. of this solution rapidly and then decrease the rate to approximately 150 ml. per hour. This rate is continued for 4 or 5 hours after delivery.

Inspection of the cervix follows. The anterior lip should be grasped with a ring forceps and the cervix pulled into view. If any lacerations are present, they must be repaired immediately. Repair is done by placing absorbable sutures in a running-lock fashion. Generally, it is a difficult procedure to perform without assistance.

After inspection, the cervix should be pushed high into the vault, using sponges in a ring forceps, and the upper vault inspected for tears. Lateral forniceal tears are often difficult to detect. The lateral vagina should be inspected carefully for evidence of tears or extension of the episiotomy. The periurethral area should be carefully inspected.

Periurethral abrasions are common and need not be repaired unless heavy bleeding occurs. If there is heavy bleeding, suturing with a small gastrointestinal needle is useful. If the tear occurs near the urethral meatus, an indwelling Foley catheter should be placed in the urethra before the repair is accomplished.

Episiotomy repair has now been standardized throughout most of the United States (Fig. 36–14). Absorbable suture material should be used. Repair begins at the apex of the vaginal portion of the incision. The suture should be placed approximately 1 cm. above the apex and tied. The vagina is then closed using a running-lock suture. Tension should be maintained on the suture throughout this portion of the repair or bleeding from the epithelial edge may occur. If the epithelium has been undermined, interrupted sutures should be placed. The operator should always be careful to avoid placing a suture in the rectum. To avoid catching the rectum during the repair procedure, sewing should be from the midline to the lateral aspect of the incision.

The only landmark in the vagina is the hymenal ring. Once the vaginal repair has reached the hymenal ring, the suture should be either tied off or held out of the way while any necessary deep perineal sutures are placed. These may be either simple or figure-of-eight sutures and should accomplish hemostasis and provide good perineal support. Care must be taken so that the rectal mucosa is not perforated. It is very important to be certain that the rectal sphincter is intact. If it is not, it may be repaired by placing several figure-of-eight sutures in the fascial sheath surrounding the muscle.

After placement of the deep interrupted sutures,

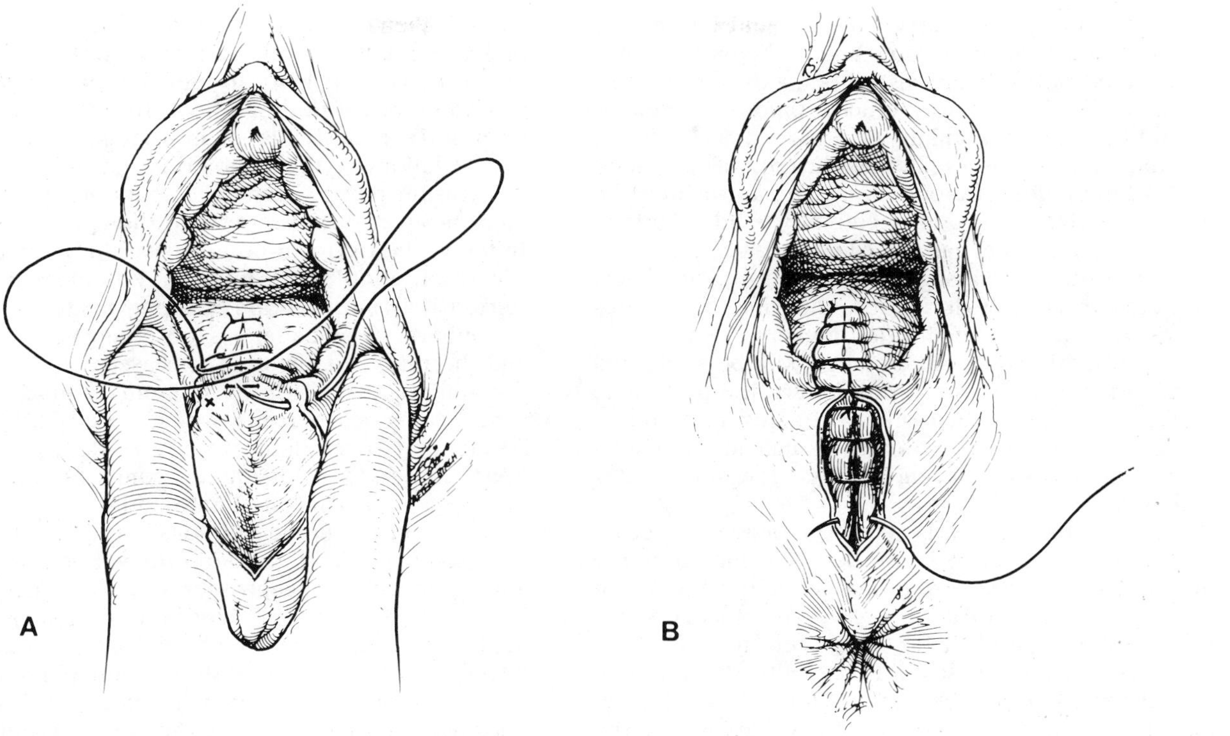

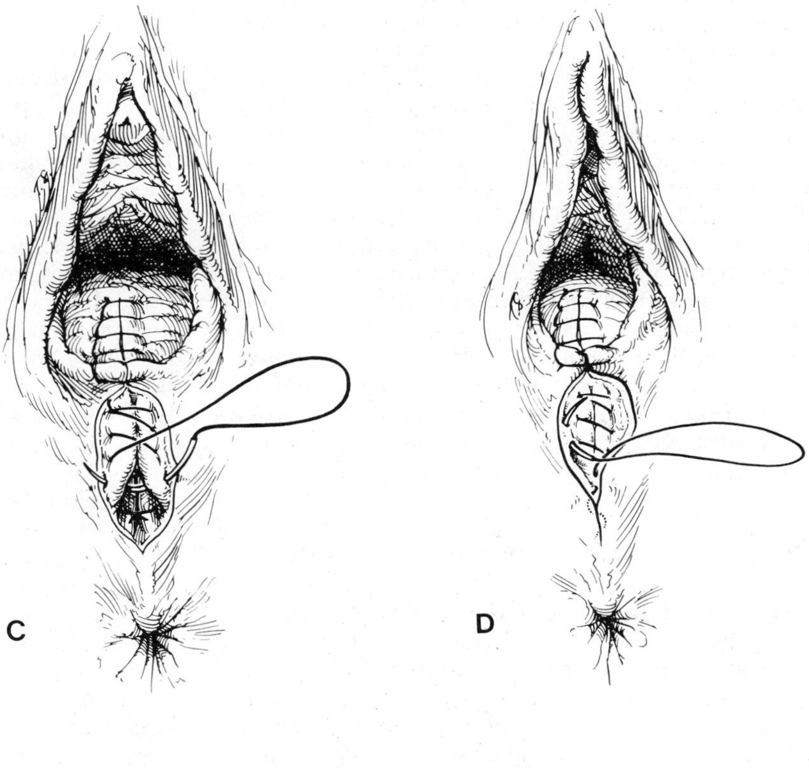

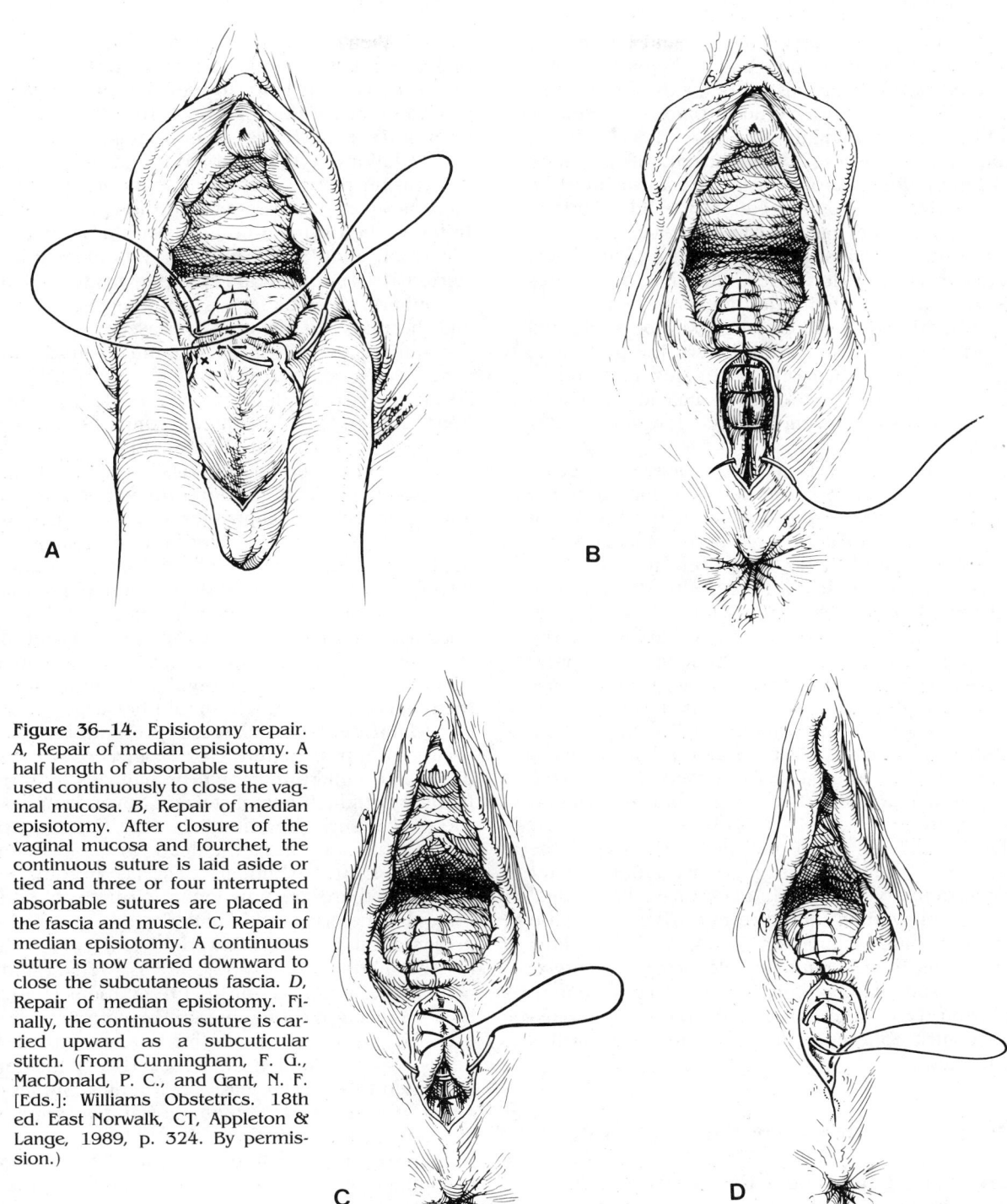

Figure 36–14. Episiotomy repair. *A*, Repair of median episiotomy. A half length of absorbable suture is used continuously to close the vaginal mucosa. *B*, Repair of median episiotomy. After closure of the vaginal mucosa and fourchet, the continuous suture is laid aside or tied and three or four interrupted absorbable sutures are placed in the fascia and muscle. *C*, Repair of median episiotomy. A continuous suture is now carried downward to close the subcutaneous fascia. *D*, Repair of median episiotomy. Finally, the continuous suture is carried upward as a subcuticular stitch. (From Cunningham, F. G., MacDonald, P. C., and Gant, N. F. [Eds.]: Williams Obstetrics. 18th ed. East Norwalk, CT, Appleton & Lange, 1989, p. 324. By permission.)

the same suture that was used for the vagina is usually extended down the perineal defect in the subcutaneous tissue until it reaches the bottom-most point of the incision. The suture is then turned around and brought up subcuticularly. The suture is tied at the hymenal ring.

After completion of the episiotomy repair, two final events should always occur: the uterus should be vigorously massaged to make certain that it is contracting well, and all blood clots should be removed from the vagina and cervix.

The patient's legs may now be placed back down on the table, and she should be transported to the recovery area.

All labor and delivery suites should be encouraged to have a recovery room where the patients may be watched carefully during the first 4 to 6 hours after delivery. This is a most crucial time. The fundus should be checked regularly. If the fundus is rising in the abdomen, this is a reliable indication of relaxation and accumulation of blood clots. The uterus must be massaged vigorously and frequently, and all blood clots expelled. The patient can be easily taught to help with uterine massage. The blood pressure must be watched carefully during recovery since some cases of severe toxemia appear *after* delivery.

The mother and infant need not be separated during the first few hours. And, in fact, it is preferable that they be near each other. Nursing may aid to contract the uterus somewhat, though many infants will not nurse well during the first few hours after delivery.

Before the woman is allowed to leave the recovery room for her postpartum bed, she should empty her bladder. After a very prolonged labor, the use of forceps, or periurethral or large perineal lacerations, it is frequently difficult for the patient to void spontaneously. In these cases, a Foley catheter should be placed for 24 hours. Once the patient is stable, she may be taken to her postpartum room, where she will stay for the remainder of her time in the hospital.

The length of the postpartum hospital stay has recently become a major issue. Some insurance carriers have set limits on the length of stay in the hospital. In most cases, 48 to 72 hours after delivery is sufficient time to allow for observation of the amount of lochia, lactation to begin, and stabilization of the infant.

During the last in-hospital postpartum visit, the woman should be given dismissal instructions. After a normal delivery, there is no reason to limit usual activities. The woman should refrain from coitus, use of tampons, or douching for 3 or 4 weeks to allow for healing of the perineum and closure of the cervix. It is also prudent to continue the prenatal vitamin preparation during the period of lactation. A discussion of contraception should be included during this last interview.

COMPLICATIONS OF LABOR AND DELIVERY

Premature Labor and Delivery. Prematurity is the most frequent cause of neonatal death in the United States. This unfortunate complication is often unpredictable. In the past, many agents have been used in the hope of stopping early premature labor. Presently, the beta-adrenergic drugs (beta-sympathomimetics) are effective for this purpose. These have been discussed previously in this chapter.

Prolonged or Arrested Labor. When labor is not progressing as expected, very frequently the cause is uterine inertia. Even an experienced examiner may have difficulty in being certain that contractions are of sufficient length and duration to effect a normal labor. Whenever labor is prolonged, an intrauterine pressure monitor should be placed. If the intrauterine pressure is not at least 50 mm. Hg, the contractions will not have the desired effect. In this case, oxytocin given intravenously may help to augment labor.

In labor, oxytocin should be given only through an infusion pump. Many accidents occur when oxytocin is given intravenously without such a device. Initially, the oxytocin infusion should be prepared at a concentration of 10 units in 1 l. of solution and started at an infusion rate of approximately 1 milliunit per minute. The patient is observed very carefully, and the rate of infusion is increased 1 to 2 milliunits per minute every 15 to 20 minutes until effective contractions occur. It is rarely necessary to go above 30 milliunits per minute to effect adequate contractions. In fact, if adequate contractions are not achieved at this infusion rate, other causes for the uterine inertia should be considered. If it appears that oxytocin at this infusion rate will be needed over a long time, the concentration should be increased to 20 or even 30 units per l. in order that smaller volumes of fluid will be given. Water intoxication can be a troublesome complication of long-augmented labors.

It is rare for a labor to not progress when documented strong contractions are present. If the fetal part does not descend despite contraction above 50 mm. Hg occurring at regular 3-minute intervals, then mechanical dystocia should be suspected.

Malpresentation. Breech presentation at term occurs in approximately 2 or 3 per cent of all deliveries. This condition should be handled by someone familiar with high-risk obstetrics. Several studies have shown that such presentation of the fetus in a primigravid woman suggests the need for cesarean section (Collea, 1980). Although this has become nearly doctrinal, there are now emerging data that suggest that, in some primigravid patients, an infant in breech presentation may be allowed to deliver vaginally if (1) the labor and delivery suite is prepared for immediate cesarean section, (2) the patient is attended by a physician thoroughly familiar with breech delivery, (3) x-ray pelvimetry has shown an adequate pelvis, (4) the fetal head is flexed, (5) the fetus is estimated to weigh at least 2,500 grams and less than 4,000 grams, and (6) neonatal care is immediately available (Collea, 1980; 1978).

However, breech presentation during labor is becoming a very rare event. External fetal version at 37 weeks gestation has become the norm when breech presentation is present in late pregnancy. Version can be accomplished safely in a delivery suite that is equipped with ultrasonography, electronic fetal monitoring, and facilities for the performance of immediate cesarean section if necessary. After a period of 15 to 20 minutes of external fetal monitoring to assess fetal stability, low doses of intravenous tocolytic agents are administered to completely relax the uterus. External version can then often be accomplished with ease. This usually requires two individuals to manipulate the fetus. Following version, the position of the fetus should be documented by ultrasonography, the tocolytic infusion stopped, and reassessment of fetal well-being using electronic fetal monitoring reinstituted. If the fetus shows signs of distress, the tocolytic agent should be started again and the fetus returned to breech presentation. This problem occurs rarely. If fetal heart rate deceleration persists, immediate cesarean section is indicated. Although this procedure is quite safe, it should be undertaken only by someone thoroughly familiar with the procedure and its risks.

Women who previously have had a vaginal delivery and who are in active labor at term with a breech fetus are at high risk for complications at delivery. However, the risk to the fetus in these women seems to be less than in primigravid women. If the labor is progressing well, if the pelvis is of adequate size, and if an operator experienced in delivery of infants from the breech position is present, labor can be allowed to proceed. However, if the labor becomes prolonged, cesarean section should be performed. With breech presentation, there is no need for induction of labor or aggressive stimulation of labor.

Breech delivery with a premature fetus is often followed by severe perinatal problems. A premature fetus in breech presentation should be delivered by cesarean section.

The most frequent malpresentation is transverse or posterior arrest of the fetal head in the mid pelvic region. A transverse position of the fetal head is normal as the infant is transversing the mid-pelvis, and should be considered abnormal only if it persists after complete dilatation and descent of the head below the spines. If this occurs, the patient should be taken to the delivery room and prepped and draped in a routine manner for vaginal delivery. In most patients, a transverse or posterior position may be corrected by manual rotation. If the woman is multiparous, she may then be allowed to push on the table and will usually deliver rapidly. If she is primiparous, it is often necessary to hold the head in the anterior position for some time while the patient continues to push the infant to the pelvic floor.

If the fetus is in good condition (as determined by electronic fetal monitoring), transverse positions may be watched without intervention. Continued pushing may effect rotation and delivery. Infants in the posterior position will usually persist but may occasionally deliver spontaneously.

Mid-forceps rotations were performed commonly in the past to correct transverse and posterior fetal positions. It is now clear that great harm can be done through the inappropriate use of these instruments (Friedman, 1973).

Cephalopelvic Disproportion. In this condition, the relationship between the size of the maternal pelvis and the infant's head size is the important factor. A large infant may easily pass through a very large pelvis, but a small pelvis can cause difficulties with the progression of labor of a large fetal head.

If cephalopelvic disproportion is present as demonstrated by lack of fetal descent despite documented adequate contractions, a cesarean section should be performed.

Toxemia. Although discussed in some detail earlier in this chapter, it is well to reconsider the possibility of toxemia occurring for the first time during and immediately after parturition. Severe pre-eclampsia is an indication for delivery. If the labor is progressing well, hyperreflexia should be controlled with the use of magnesium sulfate and severe hypertension should be controlled with the use of hydralazine or other appropriate antihypertensive drugs.

Fetal Distress. The use of the electronic fetal monitor and fetal scalp pH to evaluate fetal distress has been discussed. The delivering physician should consider the status of the fetus throughout labor and during delivery. It is unfortunate that many physicians who monitor women during labor remove the monitor when the patient is taken to the delivery room. Particularly in primigravid women, this period may exceed 1 hour, and severe fetal distress may occur without being detected.

Intrapartum and Postpartum Hemorrhage. Intrapartum hemorrhage is usually due to abruptio placentae. Should this occur, the status of the fetus must be monitored and the woman must be delivered as soon as possible.

Postpartum hemorrhage can be a life-threatening complication of delivery. When it occurs on the delivery table, it usually responds to vigorous uterine massage and the intravenous use of oxytocic agents. It is perhaps even more dangerous when it occurs after the woman has left the delivery room. In many hospitals, close observation of a normal patient does not occur. A woman may collect several units of blood in the uterus and vagina without feeling uncomfortable. Consequently, the fundus should be checked frequently.

If postpartum hemorrhage occurs during the first 4 to 6 hours, the most common cause is uterine relaxation. This condition should respond quickly to massage and oxytocic agents. If it does not, the possibility should be considered that a portion of the placenta has remained inside the uterus or that a previously unrecognized vaginal or cervical tear is present. The patient should be returned to the operating room and should be re-examined. Postpartum curettage should be avoided if possible because it can cause uterine perforation and scarring.

Uterine rupture is a rare cause of postpartum hemorrhage. Such rupture should be considered if a forceps delivery has been performed or if the woman has had a previous cesarean section.

Late postpartum hemorrhage also may occur. If it has been more than 24 hours since delivery, the most common cause is infection, and endometritis should be suspected. A retained placenta is second in frequency, and in this situation, curettage should be considered.

SURGICAL OBSTETRICS

Episiotomy and Repair. This procedure has been discussed earlier.

Cesarean Section. Cesarean section is a straightforward surgical procedure in the hands of an experienced, trained operator. It requires close cooperation with the anesthesiology and nursing staffs. The procedure should never be attempted in a setting where there is not adequate anesthesia coverage, a well-stocked blood bank, adequate neonatal care, and a physician experienced in performing the procedure. Anyone who performs this procedure should be prepared to perform a cesarean hysterectomy should the need arise. Although this step is rarely needed, occasionally it may be necessary. Usually, the patient cannot be moved.

Anesthesia must be individualized (Bonica, 1969). In the past, most cesarean sections have been performed with the patient under general anesthesia. This is safe for the fetus only if very low concentrations of inhalation and intravenous agents are used for a short time; all anesthetic agents rapidly cross the placenta and affect the fetus directly. Within minutes, the fetus can be anesthetized and will be at extreme risk for fetal distress and asphyxia. General anesthesia is now rarely used for cesarean section in the United States.

Spinal and epidural anesthesia techniques are the most common methods employed and are much safer for the fetus. However, hypotension must be carefully avoided, mostly by the use of intravenous fluids. Hypotension may be life threatening for the fetus.

Whenever possible, the cesarean section should be of the low cervical transverse type. In this procedure, the abdomen is opened either through a longitudinal low-midline incision or transversally through a Pfannenstiel incision. A bladder flap is then taken down from the lower uterine segment, and the uterus is opened transversally. Care must be taken that the incision does not extend into the area of the vessels of the broad ligament. In some cases, for example, when placenta previa has caused tremendous dilation of the vessels of the lower uterine segment, a low vertical incision is preferable.

Uterine Rupture. Spontaneous uterine rupture occurs very rarely. Most ruptures are the result of either overstimulation of the uterus from oxytocic agents or labor after classical cesarean section.

Time is essential in uterine rupture. The patient must undergo laparotomy as soon as possible. The fetus usually dies unless the rupture occurs in a hospital where cesarean section is available within a very few minutes. At the time of rupture, the patient will often relate a "tearing" feeling.

Uterine rupture may be repaired occasionally, but cesarean hysterectomy may need to be performed. This procedure requires the utmost care to prevent damage to the ureters or bladder, or both.

Vaginal Birth After Cesarean Section (VBAC). During the last several years it has been repeatedly demonstrated that vaginal birth may safely occur after cesarean section if the operation was performed transversely in the lower uterine segment. Both the American College of Obstetrics and Gynecology and the National Institutes of Health Consensus Conference Committee have stressed the need to employ VBAC in an attempt to lower the escalating rate of cesarean section in the United States. Whereas VBAC was performed in past years with great trepidation, it has been shown that VBAC is less likely to cause maternal complications than repeat cesarean section.

VBAC is indicated except in extremely unusual circumstances. Whenever the previous reason for cesarean section was a nonrepeated occurrence (for example, multiple gestation or breech presentation), VBAC is indicated. Other indications for cesarean section (for example, uterine inertia or cephalopelvic disproportion) are not contraindications since, in most cases, subsequent deliveries can occur vaginally. Only in the most unusal cases of pelvic deformity or gross fetal macrosomia would VBAC be contraindicated.

The labor and delivery suite attempting VBAC must, however, be prepared to perform emergency cesarean section on short notice. The anesthesia and operating teams must be present in the labor and delivery suite. Adequate supplies of replacement fluids and blood must be available.

Inverted Uterus. Spontaneous inversion of the uterus almost never occurs. In virtually all cases, inversion occurs as a complication of vigorous traction on the umbilical cord. Interestingly, severe maternal hypotension usually immediately follows uterine inversion.

The condition is corrected by immediately replacing the uterus, if possible. If the cervix has clamped down around the uterine fundus, inhalation agents can be used to relax the uterus, after which it may be replaced. In this case, uterine packing should be performed to maintain the uterus in place. Generally, these packs may be removed after 24 hours. Severe hemorrhage also may accompany this complication.

OBSTETRIC ANESTHESIA AND ANALGESIA

Analgesia. Narcotic medications have been used extensively for relief of pain in labor. Although these are effective for pain relief, they cross to the placenta rapidly and can depress the fetus or newborn. If needed for pain relief, these drugs should be given in only small doses (for example, 25 mg. of meperidine) and should be administered intravenously. Because these drugs and their metabolic products build up in the fetus, doses should not be repeated more than one or two times. These small dosages do not affect labor.

The timing of the peak action of the narcotic agent should be calculated so that is does not occur at the expected time of delivery. For example, meperidine has its peak action after an intravenous dose in about 30 minutes. If delivery occurs at this time, neonatal depression may be observed.

General Anesthesia. General anesthesia should be avoided. There is no place for the use of general anesthesia in routine deliveries. It should be reserved only for cesarean section when conduction anesthesia is not possible.

Regional Anesthesia

Pudendal. The most frequent form of anesthesia given to women in labor in the United States is the pudendal block. This block is accomplished by injection of approximately 10 ml. of a 1 per cent solution of an anesthetic agent such as lidocaine just medial and inferior to the ischial spine on each side of the pelvis. When properly performed, this will provide a good anesthetic effect in the posterior vulva, lower third of the vagina, and the area around the anus. This method allows for ease in delivery and episiotomy repair (Fig. 36–15).

Even in the hands of an experienced operator, the block is not always effective. It is common practice to repeat the injection at least once. However, anesthetic agents can reach maximal doses with repeated attempts at pudendal block. If the block cannot be accomplished on a single reinjection, the use of a local anesthesia should be considered.

Local. The use of local anesthesia for the repair of episiotomy has become more frequent during the past few years. Many women who wish a "natural" delivery prefer not to have a pudendal block. This is an adequate type of anesthesia for repair of episiotomy.

Paracervical Block. The use of paracervical block during labor has decreased throughout the United States. Paracervical block frequently causes prolonged fetal bradycardia. Although this generally does not result in serious fetal consequences, the bradycardia produced is of sufficient concern that this form of anesthesia should be avoided or used with great caution. Electronic fetal monitoring should always be used when paracervical block is administered.

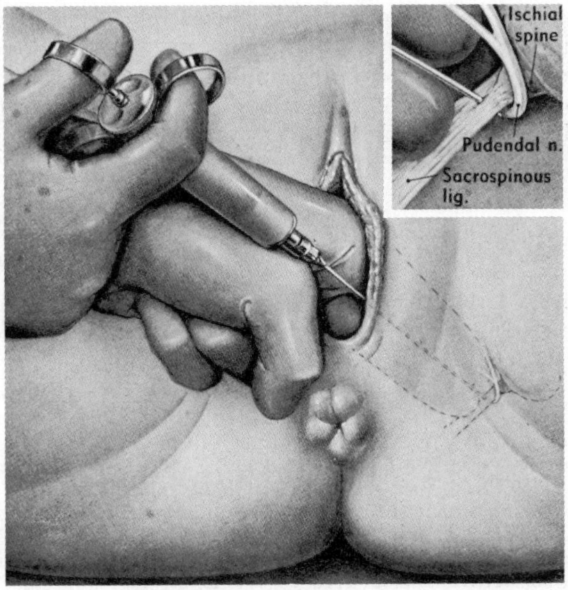

Figure 36–15. Technique of pudendal block. (From Bonica, J. J.: Principles and Practice of Obstetric Analgesia & Anesthesia. Vol. I. Philadelphia, F. A. Davis Company, 1967, p. 493. By permission.)

Epidural Block. Lumbar epidural block has become a very common anesthetic technique in the United States during the past 15 years. Correct utilization of this technique allows for adequate anesthesia during labor and delivery (Clark, 1981). A correctly placed epidural catheter can alleviate the pain from cervical dilatation in labor without affecting uterine contractions. When the patient is ready for the delivery room, she can be placed in an upright position, another injection given, and satisfactory perineal anesthesia accomplished.

This technique requires considerable experience for its safe use. One of the possible major complications is maternal hypotension with resultant fetal bradycardia and distress. This is almost never seen if the patient has been pretreated with an adequate fluid volume and is monitored closely. Maternal blood pressure should be measured every 5 minutes after institution of lumbar epidural block. If hypotension begins to develop, this can usually be corrected quickly by increasing the rate of intravenous fluid infusion. The lumbar epidural block also is ideal for cesarean section.

Spinal Anesthesia. In the past, spinal anesthesia was frequently employed for vaginal and cesarean births. The technique cannot be used during labor, because it is a single-injection technique that usually stops labor. Because of the frequent complication of severe spinal headache, spinal anesthesia has become less commonly used in the past few years. Additionally, the women must be monitored very closely and the blood pressure taken almost continuously once the agent has been placed in the subarachnoid space. This technique allows for good perineal relaxation but often completely blocks the patient's ability to push adequately.

The technique is sometimes used for cesarean section, but also in this situation, severe spinal headache may follow unless very small bore needles are used. For this reason, lumbar epidural anesthesia is superior.

Puerperium

HOSPITAL STAY

The hospital postpartum ward should be a place for both relaxation and education. The mother should be allowed to rest and relax but also should be introduced to the educational needs that are necessary for the care of her infant. Most primigravid women need to be shown the basic techniques of infant care. It is surprising that this is necessary even for those women who have previously aided in the care of younger siblings.

The woman has few medical needs postpartum. She may experience episiotomy pain, but this should be mild. Any severe perineal pain suggests the need for examination to rule out the possibility of a vaginal or vulvar hematoma. These are severe complications and must be managed by evacuation.

The routine hospital stay should vary according to the individual patient. In general, stays of less than 12 hours should be discouraged since a number of complications such as urinary retention and immediate postpartum hemorrhage can occur during this period. In most parts of the United States, the average stay is approximately 48 hours.

The nursing personnel should frequently check the patient for evidence of excessive blood loss or infection. Often, the first indication of endometritis is a slight increase in bleeding and a low-grade fever. These indications should be reported immediately to the physician, who can examine the patient and prescribe appropriate antibiotics if necessary.

In recent years, many more women have begun to breast-feed their infants. One cannot assume that the new mother has a thorough knowledge of how to nurse her infant. Therefore, it is important to provide patient education both prenatally and during the postpartum period. If the woman chooses not to nurse, various hormonal medications have been used to suppress lactation. However, these medications must be given in large dosages, are only partly effective, and have been associated with serious maternal complications.

Mastitis is a frequent complication experienced by women who are lactating. All women who choose to lactate should be instructed to immediately report to their physician any breast soreness accompanied by fever. These infections usually may be handled on an outpatient basis if treatment with the appropriate antibiotics is instituted immediately. Generally, a pie-shaped area of the breast extending from the nipple outward will be noticed to be tender, red, and thickened. Because most of these infections are due to *Staphylococcus aureus*, treatment should be instituted with a penicillinase-resistant antibiotic. This antibiotic should be given in high dosages and treatment continued for 7 days. If there is no pronounced improvement within 24 hours, the patient should be reexamined. A major complication that may occur from mastitis is a breast abscess. If present, an abscess must be opened and drained. In mild mastitis, lactation should be encouraged, since this process tends to help resolve the condition.

POSTPARTUM EXAMINATION

Traditionally in the United States, the postpartum examination is performed at 6 weeks. During this examination, the patient should be asked about any complications she experienced since leaving the hospital. If she is lactating, the breasts should be carefully examined for evidence of mastitis or problems with nipple care.

A complete pelvic examination is done, and a Papanicolaou smear obtained. The entire vaginal vault is carefully visualized, and the cervix inspected to ensure that it is well healed. It is important to thoroughly inspect the episiotomy site.

The postpartum examination is an excellent time to continue the discussion of contraceptive measures. Usually, the vaginal and perineal epithelial and deep structures have healed sufficiently within 3 or 4 weeks after delivery for patients to resume normal sexual activity. Therefore, it is important that the discussion of contraceptive measures be initiated while the patient is still in the hospital. Oral contraceptives may be started at any time, but there is more chance of difficulties with regulation and irregular bleeding if they are started before the first menstrual period. Although it has been recommended that women who breast-feed not use oral contraceptives, statements by the American Academy of Pediatrics indicate that the use of low dosage oral contraceptives in mothers who breast-feed does not create significant risk to the infant, although there is some evidence that lactation may be adversely affected (Committee on Drugs, 1981). The steroid hormones are excreted in small amounts in the breast milk and do reach the infant.

Diaphragms may be fitted with ease at the 6-week examination. The patient should be instructed thoroughly in the use of the diaphragm, with the help of visual aids in teaching the patient how to insert and use the diaphragm correctly.

Since the family physician generally cares for the infant, an opportunity is provided to check the status of the mother when the child is presented for well-baby examinations. Many family physicians have found it extremely advantageous to have the opportunity to care for both mother and infant and to observe the interactions of both whenever one or the other is the primary patient.

References

ACOG-AAFP Recommended Core Curriculum and Hospital Practice Privileges in Obstetrics-Gynecology for Family Physicians. AAFP reprint 261.

Barnes, A. B., Colton, T., Gundersen, J., et al.: Fertility and outcome of pregnancy in women exposed in utero to diethylstilbestrol. N. Engl. J. Med., *302*:609, 1980.

Bonebrake, C. R., Noller, K. L., Loehnen, C. P., et al.: Routine chest roentgenography in pregnancy. J.A.M.A., *240*:2747, 1978.

Bonica, J. J.: Principles and Practice of Obstetric Analgesia & Anesthesia. Vol. II. Philadelphia, F. A. Davis Company, 1969. *This is the reference text on the topic. Virtually every question about the safety (or lack of it) of anesthesia in obstetrics is covered in detail.*

Candib, L.: Obstetrics in family practice: A personal and political perspective. J. Fam. Pract., *3*:391, 1976.

Clark, R. B.: Conduction anesthesia. Clin. Obstet. Gynecol., *24*:601, 1981.

Collea, J. V.: Current management of breech presentation. Clin. Obstet. Gynecol., *23*:525, 1980.

Collea, J. V., Rabin, S. C., Weghorst, G. R., et al.: The randomized management of term frank breech presentation: Vaginal delivery vs. cesarean section. Am. J. Obstet. Gynecol., *131*:186, 1978.

Committee on Drugs: American Academy of Pediatrics: Breast feeding and contraception. Pediatrics, *68*:138, 1981.

'82–'83 Directory of Residency Training Programs (Accredited by the Accreditation Council for Graduate Medical Education). Chicago, American Medical Association, 1982, p. 18.

Etheridge, M. J., and Peperell, R. J.: Heart disease and pregnancy at the Royal Women's Hospital. Med. J. Aust., *2*:277, 1977.

Friedman, E. A.: Patterns of labor as indicators of risk. Clin. Obstet. Gynecol., *16*:172, 1973.

Frisch, R. E., Wyshak, G., and Vincent, L.: Delayed menarche and amenorrhea in ballet dancers. N. Engl. J. Med., *303*:17, 1980.

Hieber, J. P., Dalton, D., Shorey, J., et al.: Hepatitis and pregnancy. J. Pediatr., *91*:545, 1977.

Hill, L. M.: Diagnosis and management of fetal distress. Mayo Clin. Proc., *54*:784, 1979. *This is an excellent, brief review of the clinical role of EFM in the diagnosis of fetal distress. We are indebted to the author for his permission to use his figures in this chapter.*

Hill, L. M., Johnson, C. E., and Lee, R. A.: Cholecystectomy in pregnancy. Obstet. Gynecol., *46*:291, 1975.

Hobel, C. J., Hyvarine, M. A., Okada, D. M., et al.: Prenatal and intrapartum high-risk screening. I. Prediction of the high-risk neonate. Am. J. Obstet. Gynecol., *117*:1, 1973.

Homan, W. P., and Thorbjarnarson, B.: Crohn disease and pregnancy. Arch. Surg., *111*:545, 1976.

Iffy, L., and Kaminetzky, H. A. (Eds.): Principles and Practice of Obstetrics and Perinatology, Vol. I and II. New York, John Wiley & Sons, 1981. *This large reference includes chapters by many of the "giants" in the field of high-risk pregnancy. It is rather up-to-date for a field that is changing rapidly.*

Janerich, D. T., Piper, J. M., and Glebatis, D. M.: Oral contraceptives and birth defects. Am. J. Epidemiol., *112*:73, 1980.

Jarrell, S. E., and Sokol, R. J.: Clinical use of stressed and nonstressed monitoring techniques. Clin. Obstet. Gynecol., *22*:617, 1979. *This article is a good description of how and when to use nonstress testing and the oxytocin challenge test. However, it is now recognized that nonstress testing must be obtained more frequently than once weekly. At least twice-weekly tests are necessary.*

Levin, J., and Algazy, K. M.: Hematologic disorders. *In* Burrow, G. N., and Ferris, T. F. (Eds.): Medical Complications During Pregnancy. Philadelphia, W. B. Saunders Company, 1975, pp. 690–692.

Linn, S., Schoenbaum, S. C., Monson, R. R., et al.: No association between coffee consumption and adverse outcomes of pregnancy. N. Engl. J. Med., *306*:141, 1982.

Mattingly, R. F. (Ed.): Te Linde's Operative Gynecology. 5th ed. Philadelphia, J. B. Lippincott Company, 1977. *This text includes a very excellent section on ectopic pregnancy.*

Mulinare, J., Cordero, J. F., Erickson, J. D., and Berry, R.J.: Periconceptual use of multivitamins and the occurrence of neural tube defects. J.A.M.A., *260*(21):3141–3145, 1988.

Noller, K. L.: Heart disease and pregnancy. *In* Iffy, L., and Kaminetzky, H. A. (Ed.): Principles and Practice of Obstetrics and Perinatology. Vol. II. New York, John Wiley & Sons, 1981, p. 1314.

Noller, K. L.: Liver disease in pregnancy. *In* Iffy, L., and Kaminetzky, H. A. (Eds.): Principles and Practice of Obstetrics and Perinatology. Vol. II. New York, John Wiley & Sons, 1981, p. 1328; p. 1330.

Pisacano, N.J.: Personal communication.

Pritchard, J. A.: Management of preeclampsia and eclampsia. Kidney Int., *18*:259, 1980.

Pritchard, J. A., and MacDonald, P. C.: Williams Obstetrics. 16th ed. New York, Appleton-Century-Crofts, 1980. *This is the best known of the many texts on obstetrics. It has survived many editions and authors and still remains an excellent reference. Especially good are many of the illustrations demonstrating fetal positions, both normal and abnormal. The discussions of maternal hypertension and the proposed mechanisms for the onset of labor are also excellent. The section on clinical assessment of the pelvis deserves review.*

Reid, R., Ivey, K. J., Rencoret, R. H., et al.: Fetal complications of obstetric cholestasis. Br. Med. J., *1*:870, 1976.

Sokol, R. J., Stojkov, J., and Chik, L.: Maternal-fetal risk assessment: A clinical guide to monitoring. Clin. Obstet. Gynecol., *22*:547, 1979.

Stern, T. L., Schmittling, G., Clinton, C., et al.: Hospital privileges for graduates of family practice residency programs. J. Fam. Pract., *13*:1013, 1981.

Strassner, H. T., Platt, L. D., Whittle, M., et al.: Amniotic fluid phosphatidylglycerol and real-time ultrasonic cephalometry. Am. J. Obstet. Gynecol., *135*:804, 1979.

Webb, M. J., and Sedlack, R. E.: Ulcerative colitis in pregnancy. Med. Clin. North Am., *58*:823, 1974.

37

Care of the Newborn

R.H. Sprinkle

The well-trained family physician, among all potential caregivers, is best prepared to reduce perinatal risk by integrating the care of the sexually active adolescent, the expectant mother, and the newborn baby. When the same physician oversees pregnancy, labor, delivery, and newborn care, highly coherent perinatal management should result. When several physicians are involved, integrated management is less automatic but must still be sought, as it is the only acceptable standard of perinatal care.

Managing the Newborn Immediately after Delivery

DELIVERY ROOM ENVIRONMENT

To reduce cold stress to wet infants during transition from intrauterine to extrauterine life, ambient temperature should be adjusted to between 75° and 80° F (24° and 27° C) if possible. A radiant warmer, preferably self-regulating, should be brought to equilibrium. Warm sterile towels should be opened on the warmer. Oxygen masks, resuscitation bag and pressure manometer, oxygen flow, suction and suction catheter, laryngoscope blades and lights, bulb syringe, DeLee's catheter and trap, and several sizes of endotracheal tubes should be located, positively identified, and functionally confirmed.

INITIAL INSPECTION AND MANEUVERS

Blood and other fluids that staff may come in contact with in the delivery room may contain infectious agents; practices lessening, if not eliminating, skin and mucous-membrane contact with these substances should prevail.

The rough amount, color, gross contents, and odor of the amniotic fluid should be assessed during the delivery process. In selected cases, a sample of fluid should be dispatched for microscopic examination and culture or for lecithin/sphingomyelin determination.

First the oropharynx and then the nose should be suctioned on the perineum during or immediately after vaginal delivery or on the abdomen immediately after cesarean delivery. If thick meconium is present, routine oropharyngeal and nasal suctioning may be bypassed in favor of immediate laryngoscopic examination, ideally performed before the initial breath. If thick meconium is found, first the trachea and then the hypopharynx, oropharynx, and nose should be suctioned with a DeLee catheter or, preferably, through an endotracheal tube hooked up to a suction device. If standard suctioning is performed first in these high-risk babies, gagging, gasping, and deep inspiration of meconium may be stimulated. Aggressive suctioning of lightly stained infants is not advisable, however, and has been shown to cause more problems than it prevents (Linder et al., 1988) (Sepkowitz, 1987).

Neonatal blood volume is increased by stripping or "milking" the umbilical cord prior to clamping, holding the infant in a dependent position before clamping, or delaying clamping beyond the time needed to clear the infant's nasal and oropharyngeal secretions. These maneuvers are not ordinarily necessary and are not routinely advisable; they may increase iron stores at the price of hypervolemia or exaggerated neonatal jaundice. Cord-blood laboratory studies should be collected from the placental end of the cord.

The infant's umbilical cord stump should be clamped no closer than 2 cm. from the abdominal wall to facilitate umbilical vessel catheterization, should it become necessary.

The infant should be placed under a radiant warmer. A Trendelenburg position favors the suctioning of secretions and, if necessary, laryngoscopy and intubation.

The infant should be dried in a soft, prewarmed towel. This maneuver decreases evaporative heat loss and stimulates mildly depressed infants.

Sometimes, an otherwise normal infant will exhibit marked acrocyanosis immediately after delivery. Although central hypoxemia is seldom responsible, an oxygen stream is commonly directed at the baby's nose. This brief therapeutic maneuver may be harmless, but "wall oxygen" is typically pure oxygen, and even transient hyperoxemia may cause spasm of the retinal vasculature in the occasional infant. Blowing cold oxygen, air, or mist in the face may also stimulate a generalized vagal response.

At 1 minute and again at 5 minutes, the infant is given an Apgar score (Apgar, 1953). Criteria for Apgar scoring are presented in Table 37–1. A 1 minute Apgar score greater than 9 is rare, owing to physiologic acrocyanosis. Infants scoring 3 or less at 1 minute will probably need extended resuscitative efforts; those scoring from 4 to 6 may do well after vigorous stimulation or brief respiratory support; those scoring 7 and above will likely do well with no special treatment or with light or even incidental stimulation. Infants whose scores at 5 minutes have not risen to 7 or above and infants whose scores have actually fallen may be quite ill.

The placenta should be inspected for size and quality; infarcts, calcifications, and other defects; gross clotting; membrane cloudiness suggesting infection; umbilical cord length and number of vessels; and evidence of a pseudovascular umbilical structure suggesting a patent urachus or a freshly severed loop of bowel. The placenta should be preserved until the infant is discharged.

INITIAL PHYSICAL EXAMINATION

The initial examination includes birth weight and body measurements as well as the Apgar scores that predict clinical course. It provides a better opportunity to estimate gestational age than does an examination performed after an interval as short as 6 to 12 hours, because of rapid epidermal drying, although some neurologic aspects of the estimation may actually become clearer with time in the temporarily depressed infant. Patency of the nares may be demonstrated by passage of a no. 8 French catheter bilaterally, although this procedure need not be routine. Anal patency and the passage of meconium and urine should be noted, as should obvious birth trauma.

PARENTAL CONTACT AND PARTICIPATION

Unless the new mother is unconscious or unless, as a relinquishing mother, she has explicitly requested not to see her baby, the newborn should never leave the delivery room without being seen by and, if possible, touched by its mother. The same rule must apply to the father when present. No exception need be made even for severely ill infants. More happily, the vigorous newborn, dried and swaddled head to toe or dried and naked if ambient temperature permits, should be handed to a fully conscious mother and offered a first feeding while being cuddled against the breast.

PROPHYLACTIC MEASURES

Effective postexposure prophylaxis against *Neisseria gonorrhoeae* conjunctivitis can be achieved by the application of 1% silver nitrate, 0.5% erythromycin, or 1% tetracycline to the conjunctivae soon after delivery. Silver nitrate may be a superior prophylactic for penicillinase-producing *N. gonorrhoeae,* but tetracycline and erythromycin are superior for *Chlamydia trachomatis.* Silver nitrate works by stimulating an inflammatory response in the conjunctivae; a mild chemical conjunctivitis often results. Herpes simplex

Table 37–1. CRITERIA FOR APGAR SCORING

Sign	Score 0	1	2
Heart rate	Absent	Below 100 beats per minute	100 beats per minute or above
Respiratory effort	Absent	Hypoventilation or weak cry	Good effort or strong cry
Muscle tone	Absent	Some flexion or motion	Good flexion or active motion
Reflex irritability (to foot slap or nasal catheter)	Absent	Grimace only	Vigorous response, cry, sneeze, cough
Color	Blue all over or pale	Pink body and blue extremities	Pink all over

Adapted from Apgar, V.: A proposal for a new method of evaluation of the newborn infant. Curr. Res. Anesth. Analg., 32:260, 1953.

virus (HSV), another cause of ophthalmia neonatorum, is discussed in chapter 59.

Until the infant's gut is colonized by autochthonous flora, vitamin K cannot be produced and inactive forms of coagulation factors II, VII, IX, and X cannot be activated. Unless vitamin K is administered soon after birth, the infant will pass through several days unprotected from hemorrhagic disease of the newborn. Both intramuscular and oral forms of vitamin K are effective prophylactically, but the intramuscular form is better studied, and a needle mark in a standard site can serve as reassurance that vitamin K has in fact been given.

Ideally, all newborns should be actively immunized against hepatitis B virus (HBV) in regions where HBV is endemic (Moyes et al., 1987). Newborns known to be at risk for the vertical acquisition of HBV need both active and passive immunization in the delivery room.

Physiologic Adaptation from Intrauterine to Extrauterine Life

During fetal life, when circulation to the pulmonary bed is low, fluid produced in the lungs mostly flows out through the tracheobronchial tree to mix with fluid in the amniotic sac. During vaginal delivery but not during cesarean delivery, some residual pulmonary fluid is "squeezed out" through the nose and mouth. When the umbilical cord is clamped, cutting off the low-pressure placental circulatory bed, fetal cardiovascular systemic pressures rise abruptly, and complex events, many of them prostaglandin-mediated, take place. The lungs begin to fill with air when high negative pulmonary air pressure is generated by respiratory effort or, in the compromised infant, when high positive pulmonary air pressure is generated by resuscitative effort. Negative-pressure alveolar aeration contributes to a lowering of pulmonary vascular pressure. As the pulmonary vascular bed becomes more fully perfused, more residual lung fluid is resorbed into the circulation. Increasing pulmonary vascular return to the left atrium raises left atrial pressure, and this pressure rise effectively closes the foramen ovale. Progressive narrowing of the ductus arteriosus over the next several days then completes the functional separation of the higher-pressure systemic arterial circulation from the lower-pressure systemic venous and pulmonary circulations (Reller et al., 1988).

There are many potential impediments to normal physiologic adaptation. Cold stress is surely the commonest and the most easily prevented. Pulmonary surfactant deficiency or surfactant immaturity, corresponding roughly to a ratio of lecithin (phosphatidylcholine) to sphingomyelin less than 2.0, may not allow adequate alveolar inflation. Pulmonary hypoplasia, associated with diaphragmatic herniation or caused by low fetal urinary output or chronic amniotic fluid leakage through the mechanism of oligohydramnios, may make adequate gas exchange anatomically impossible. Cardiovascular malformations, the effects of cardiovascular-active drugs, and acquired problems, such as pulmonary infections or aspiration syndromes, may also prevent or impede successful adaptation.

Complete History and Physical Examination

The newborn's complete history is the full family history, the mother's preconception history, and the entire obstetrical history including any record of extrauterine or intrauterine fetal monitoring and the details of delivery and early neonatal life. These topics, excepting the last, have been covered in chapter 36. In practice, the newborn history can usually be written in a few short paragraphs and presented verbally in less than a minute.

The physician must record a full physical examination of the newborn within 24 hours of delivery. In babies not obviously the product of term gestations, a formal estimation of gestational age should be performed within 6 to 12 hours of delivery. The examiner must be attentive not only to significant pathology but also to trivial abnormalities and physiologic curiosities, since these lesser findings can needlessly cause parental anxiety if left undiscussed.

GENERAL INSPECTION

Size and Color

Even in the full-term baby, size may not be normal. A small or skinny baby may be the product of a poorly nourished, chronically diseased, or drug-abusing mother; or may have been maintained by an insufficient placenta; or may have been infected in utero; or may be expressing a chromosomal or metabolic abnormality. A postterm baby may appear long and thin, may have a "little old man" face, and may show dry, peeling skin and long fingernails and toenails, often stained green with meconium. Unusually large, fat babies may be the infants of diabetic mothers.

The normal newborn will almost always have a pink tongue. Unwrapped in a warm examination room and lying on a blanket, he may appear pink all over, or he may appear pink centrally while displaying bluish extremities. Acrocyanosis is common in the newborn period, especially under cold conditions, and is usually, though not always, physiologic. Acrocyanosis occurs when the concentration of reduced (unsaturated) hemoglobin reaches about 5 grams per dl. in capillary blood. Slow flow through the periphery will produce this condition, but slow flow through the periphery can be caused not only by cold stress but also by shock, heart failure, or vascular obstruction. Central cyanosis suggests the presence of about 3 grams per dl. of reduced hemoglobin in *arterial* blood. Central cyanosis persisting 20 minutes or so beyond delivery in a noncrying infant is not physiologic. Central cyanosis clearing only with crying—a paradoxical sign—suggests choanal atresia. Persistent central cyanosis implies an excess of reduced hemoglobin and can be caused by polycythemia, right-to-left shunting, heart failure with or without right-to-left shunting, pulmonary disease, central nervous system disease affecting respiratory drive, shock of any cause, or, rarely, methemoglobinemia. It should be noted that sick babies who happen to have relatively high concentrations of fetal hemoglobin may not display central cyanosis until their oxygen tensions reach dangerously low levels, so the absence of central cyanosis should not by itself deflect an investigation of oxygen delivery (Fanaroff and Martin, 1987).

Pale babies may be anemic. Plethoric babies, cyanotic or not, may be polycythemic. Icterus appearing on the first day of life suggests a hemolytic process, hepatitis, or hepatobiliary malformation.

Activity

The normal full-term newborn exhibits several patterns of activity, ranging from quiet sleep to crying. During the first day of extrauterine life, many babies are more alert than they will be later on in the first week, but some sleep almost constantly and show little interest in feeding. The term baby should exhibit flexor tone even during sleep and especially when agitated; babies born from abnormal presentations may not exhibit the usual flexor positions in all extremities; and babies of different races may vary markedly in tone. Jittery babies are usually perfectly normal, although their glucose, calcium, and magnesium levels are often checked, and they are sometimes held over for electroencephalography. Beyond the usual range of jitteriness is the baby withdrawing from a maternal drug of abuse. Inspection of the drug-withdrawing baby may also suggest other signs of autonomic dysfunction. Seizure activity in newborns is much different from seizure activity in older children and adults. Paroxysmal, repetitive activity of almost any sort can indicate abnormal discharge from the central nervous system.

Respirations and Phonations

Respirations should be quiet and unlabored, the chest and abdomen moving together. Normal respiratory rate varies from about 30 to 60 breaths per minute. Respiratory pattern also varies widely, with sporadic breath-to-breath intervals as long as 15 seconds, causing occasional false alarms. Nonstridorous, unlabored respirations and a lusty cry are strong evidence against airway obstruction, such as choanal atresia or laryngomalacia, and against significant pulmonary disease. Persistently weak or unusual cry suggests a broad range of pathologies. Tachypnea, retractions, nasal flaring, grunting, and, ultimately, cyanosis are the hallmarks of respiratory distress, although normal newborns in early transition to extrauterine life and hypothermic, hypoglycemic, anemic, or polycythemic newborns can show some or all of these signs as well.

Pulsations and Contours

Some congenital cardiovascular problems may be suggested by abnormally placed or abnormally timed superficial chest pulsations, pulsations sometimes better seen than felt. Unusually obvious peripheral arterial pulsations may be noticed in a baby whose ductus arteriosus remains patent; pulsations of the posterior tibial artery are often observable in this circumstance.

The abdomen may be rounded, flat, or scaphoid (meaning boatlike). Babies yet to pass their meconium may be a bit distended, as may be those who have swallowed large amounts of air during crying or during bag-and-mask ventilatory stimulation. The abdomen may be enlarged by an intra-abdominal solid mass; by a viscus distended with air, urine, or fluid; or by free intraperitoneal fluid. A scaphoid abdomen implies a deficiency of intra-abdominal contents, as in diaphragmatic herniation. If diaphragmatic herniation is suspected in a baby needing ventilatory resuscitation, intubation is required immediately since bag-and-mask ventilation may distend the intrathoracic gut with air, further compromising pulmonary function. Abdominal musculature may be incompletely approximated, as in diastasis recti or umbilical herniation.

Asymmetry of the head, neck, or extremities may suggest intrauterine molding, abnormal intrauterine lie, abnormal underlying structure, or birth trauma, such as brachial plexus injury or facial palsy. Symmetrical deformity of the feet or hips may also be due to molding or to abnormal intrauterine lie, respectively. Persistent tilting of the head to one side suggests fibrosed hemorrhage into the sternocleidomastoid muscle. The dorsa of the hands and feet or the skin over the pubis may be mildly edematous; marked edema of the dorsa of the feet in a phenotypic female should suggest Turner's syndrome.

VITAL SIGNS

Temperature

Normal newborn core temperature ranges from 36° to 37.5° C (96.8° to 99.6° F). In well babies, core temperature readings are often not taken. Axillary temperature readings are popular, although unreliable. Skin temperature readings are useful only in special care settings.

The newborn baby can compensate for evaporative, radiant, convective, and conductive heat loss over a narrower temperature range than adults. The newborn also makes relatively more use of nonshivering thermogenesis, accomplished predominantly by the catabolism of brown fat.

The thermal shock of delivery is a challenge to the baby's compensatory mechanisms. If left undried and unwrapped in a room made thermally comfortable for laboring adults, the newborn's core temperature can drop by 2° to 3° C. Cold stress can occur even if only the scalp is improperly dried and covered. Cold stress can present as an illness, such as respiratory distress or hypoglycemia, and it can make the course of any illness more difficult. Placing an infant in an incubator is not a guarantee that thermal neutrality will be achieved or maintained; improperly serviced or poorly designed incubators, many of obsolete, single-walled construction, are still in common use.

Hyperthermia is less frequently a problem and is more likely to be caused by high room temperature, equipment malfunction, or overwrapping than by infection, metabolic derangement, or brain injury. An environmentally overheated baby is vasodilated, and his extremities may not be much cooler than his trunk. A septic baby is likely to be vasoconstricted peripherally, at least at some stage in the course of his infection, and his extremities may be noticeably cooler than his trunk (Klaus and Fanaroff, 1986).

Pulse Rate

Pulse rate is rapid in the first few minutes after birth, normally topping 180 beats per minute. In the delivery room, the pulse is most conveniently felt at the umbilicus, but peripheral pulses should also be easy to feel since persistent flow through the ductus arteriosus produces a wide pulse pressure. By 20 minutes, heart rate is usually around 140 beats per minute. Mean peaks are lower for preterm infants. At no time in the delivery room should heart rate fall below 100 beats per minute. Heart rate is quite variable in the newborn period and can be expected to rise and fall quickly within broad limits with stimulation, irritation, or agitation and as a function of state of arousal. Most neonatal tachycardias and bradycardias are physiologic or procedure-related and are self-limited; others are caused by drugs or various pathologic conditions (Fanaroff and Martin, 1987).

Respiratory Rate

Respiratory rate and pattern have been described above.

Blood Pressure

Blood pressure should be measured in every newborn. The auscultatory or Doppler methods are usually employed; palpation readings are less reproducible and can approximate only the mean arterial pressure. Normal systolic pressure for term infants born by vaginal delivery is about 65 to 70 mm. Hg; for term infants delivered by cesarean section it is about 60 mm. Hg. Pressures for premature babies are somewhat lower. Aortic pressures obtained after catheterization of the umbilical artery (Fig. 37–1) have been used to establish reference values (Versmold, 1981). Since cuff pressures are commonly measured only in the arm in apparently normal babies and are not routinely measured in both arms and in one leg, it is unlikely that readings placed on the nursery day sheet will identify nonhypertensive babies with coarcted aortas.

MEASUREMENTS

Weight

Birth weight should be measured in metric units. Babies who weigh up to 1500 grams at delivery are very-low-birth-weight (VLBW) babies; those who weigh from 1501 to 2500 grams at delivery are low-birth-weight (LBW) babies; those who weigh from 2501 to 4000 grams are babies of normal birth weight. A baby of any birth weight up to 4000 grams may be described as "appropriate for gestational age" (AGA) or "small for gestational age" (SGA) or "large for gestational age" (LGA), according to reference values (Fig. 37–2). Babies who weigh 4001 grams or more are LGA and "macrosomic." AGA, SGA, and LGA determinations depend on sure knowledge of date of conception or on the result of an estimation of gestational age (EGA) by Dubowitz or Ballard criteria, as discussed below.

Most babies lose weight over the first three days of extrauterine life, an interval during which even vigorous babies may not feed avidly and mothers may find their milk has not yet "come in." In an otherwise well baby, this early weight loss, assuming it does not exceed about 7 per cent of birth weight, should be considered physiologic. Most of this weight loss is due to negative water balance, although brown fat is also expended. Head circumference, if carefully studied, can be shown to decrease during this period. Some small full-term AGA babies may fall below 2501 grams during the first few days; these babies do not become SGA.

Length

Length is usually measured incorrectly in the healthy, full-term baby because of hip and knee flexion, while usually being measured more accurately in the premature, sick, or floppy baby. Babies with good tone are best placed supine on a paper sheet; a vertically held pen can be used to mark the paper at the level of the baby's vertex; the hips and knees can then be straightened gently and another pen mark made at the level of the heel surfaces; the distance between the two marks can be measured in the baby's absence.

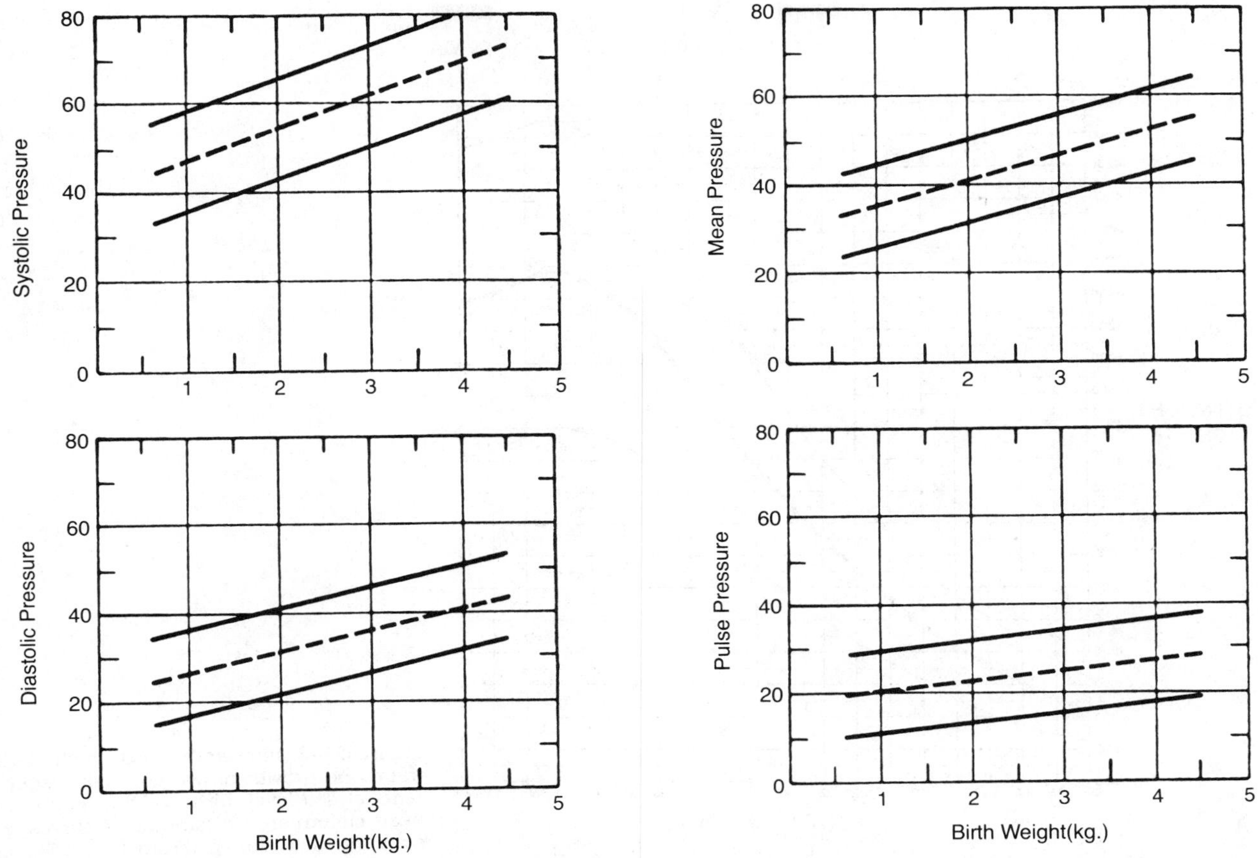

Figure 37–1. Arterial blood pressure values in newborns. Aortic pressures obtained by catheterization of the umbilical artery in stable infants of various weights within 12 hours of birth. (From Versmold, H.T., Kitterman, J.A., Phibbs, R.H., et al.: Aortic blood pressure during the first 12 hours of life in infants with birth weight 610 to 4,220 grams. Pediatrics, 67[5]:607–613, 1981.)

Head Circumference

The head is measured at its greatest circumference, the fronto-occipital circumference (FOC).

SKIN

Signs of Trauma and Stress

Babies normally suck on their fingers, hands, and forearms in utero, sometimes vigorously enough to cause sucking blisters. Many are monitored invasively during labor and show electrode screw marks on the skin of the presenting part, usually but not always the vertex. Forceps marks are often seen on the face, external ear, and scalp. Scalpel wounds are sometimes seen after cesarean deliveries. Ecchymoses are common on the scalp, face, neck, and extremities, especially in premature babies and after difficult or precipitous deliveries. Localized showers of petechiae suggest increased venous pressure, as may be found above a tight nuchal cord or in the presenting part. Inguinal petechiae are also common. Fixed petechial rashes must be distinguished from those that progress after delivery, as the latter suggest serious, evolving medical problems, such as sepsis, and not birth trauma. Nodular areas of subcutaneous fat necrosis are occasionally seen as early as the second day but are more often noticed after a week or so; they are most common at sites of trauma in large, difficult-to-deliver babies. A needle mark should be identified at the site of vitamin K administration. Meconium passed in utero may stain the skin and nails green.

Signs Correlated with Gestational Age

The skin of preterm babies is thin, smooth, and shiny; in particularly immature babies, the skin is translucent and almost gelatinous and is easily traumatized. The back, head, and even the face may be covered by a light growth of short, fine hairs called the lanugo.

The skin of freshly delivered full-term babies is pink, soft, well supported by subcutaneous fat but still easily wrinkled, and it is covered with a waxy, yellowish-whitish paste of dead cells and sebum called the vernix caseosa, or, literally from Latin, the "cheesy varnish."

Postterm babies lose subcutaneous fat and vernix caseosa and present as long, thin babies with loose, dry, already desquamating skin.

In full-term babies, desquamation typically begins after a physiologic reddening of the skin that begins within several hours of delivery and lasts

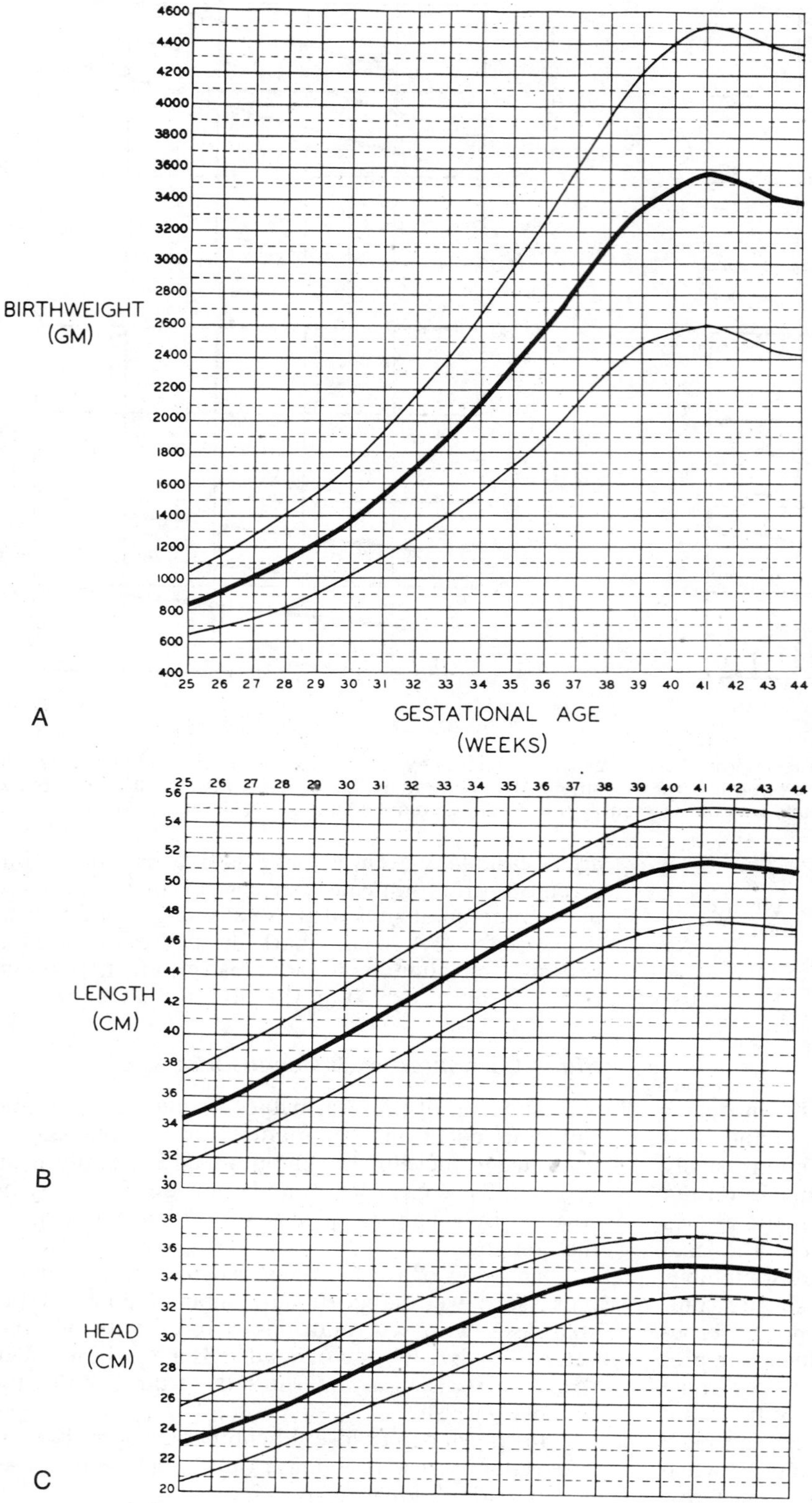

Figure 37–2. Intrauterine growth charts. Intrauterine growth of live-born caucasian infants at sea level: birth weight, length, and head circumference (smoothed curves ± 2 standard deviations). (From Usher, R., and McLean, F.: Intrauterine growth of live-born Caucasian infants at sea level: Standards obtained from measurements in 7 dimensions of infants born between 25 and 44 weeks of gestation. J. Pediatr., *74*[6]:901–910, 1969.)

several hours more. Livedo reticularis, a bluish mottling of the skin most prominent in a cool environment, may also follow this brief erythematous phase.

Appendages, Cysts, and Inclusions

Hair distribution and hair quality vary markedly in normal full-term newborns. Hypertrichosis, hypotrichosis, and abnormal appearance, texture, or morphology can be clues to the diagnosis of a range of congenital problems. Abnormalities in the other obvious skin appendages, the fingernails and the toenails, can similarly suggest specific diagnoses (Fanaroff and Martin, 1987).

Sweating is unusual during the first day, but facial sweating is commonly seen in warm or active babies by about the third day. Sebaceous glands are active in utero and continue to be active for the first few months or even the first few years; usually they then become dormant until puberty.

Tiny, firm, noninflammatory, yellowish-whitish keratogenous cysts are very often distributed over the forehead, nose, and cheeks. They are usually gone within the first month. Because they once brought to mind millet seeds scattered just below the surface of the skin, they were named "milia," plural form of milium, Latin for millet. Other, quite different lesions carry the name "miliaria" from febris miliarius, meaning "miliary fever," since some of these lesions were thought to be inflammatory forms of milia. They are not. Miliaria crystallina, miliaria pustularis, and miliaria rubra are all disorders of sweat retention, the first characterized by delicate clear vesicles, the second by delicate cloudy vesicles, and the third by crops of small reddish papules. This third version is often identified as a heat rash. Miliaria occurs in skin folds and over the face and scalp, particularly in warm, humid conditions. It is less common in the neonatal period than later on.

Squamous cell inclusions can be found in several areas, including the prepuce, where they can be confused with pustules.

Pigmentary Lesions

Babies are born with a full complement of melanocytes, regardless of race, but they are lighter-skinned than they will be in later childhood and adulthood. Bluish macular patches called Mongolian spots are common findings in most racial groups—Oriental, Black, American Indian, and Hispanic—and are also sometimes found in Caucasian babies. They are routinely seen in the lumbosacral area and usually disappear within a few years; Mongolian spots occurring elsewhere may more likely persist.

Café au lait spots, named for the color of coffee with cream, may be light to dark brown, depending on racial pigmentation. They are almost always inconsequential; small solitary spots are seen in as many as one fifth of normal newborns. Less dismissable are spots over 1.5 cm. in length, spots numbering more than six, or otherwise unremarkable spots noticed in the company of axillary freckles, which are actually tiny versions of the larger spots. Any of these three abnormal settings suggests neurofibromatosis. Some babies with tuberous sclerosis likewise present with abnormal café au lait spotting patterns, but they usually also display white macules shaped classically like slender, nondigitated leaves, often more easily seen under a Wood's lamp.

Nevi

Various nevi are seen in the newborn. Congenital pigmented nevi occur in 1 to 2 per cent of newborns. Small nevi can be distinguished from other brown spots by their texture or by their uneven color. Some of these lesions may undergo transformation to malignant melanomas in later life, so management options should be discussed sometime in childhood. Giant hairy nevi must be managed more aggressively. They are much more disfiguring, sometimes covering substantial areas of the trunk; they are often intensely pruritic; and they are much more prone to malignant transformation. They should be removed as soon as surgically feasible. Compound nevi and blue nevi also occur, are less ominous, but may still best be managed by surgical removal. Epidermal nevi are hamartomas made up of epidermis and epidermal appendages. They present as verrucous nevi of warty appearance or as sebaceous nevi of waxy appearance. Epidermal nevi may degenerate into basal cell carcinomas during puberty and so should be removed during early adolescence. Many if not most babies with large epidermal nevi will prove to have serious congenital defects on thorough examination.

Abnormal Vascular, Lymphatic, or Erythropoietic Structures

Vascular macules called "salmon patches"—irregular, flat, blanching spots on the forehead, glabella, eyelids, or the nape of the neck—are extremely common. They are transient capillary hemangiomas and usually disappear well within the first year, although marks on the neck, sometimes called "stork bites," may persist longer.

Unfortunately, the evocative term "nevus flammeus" or "flame nevus" has come to have two distinct uses. It is applied to transient capillary hemangiomas of the forehead, glabella, and eyelids, and it is also used as a synonym for "port-wine stain," a permanent lesion that may exist independently or may appear as part of an encephalofacial angiomatosis (Sturge-Weber syndrome) or as part of several other congenital syndromes (Fanaroff and Martin, 1987).

Cutaneous hemangiomas are capillary, cavernous, or mixed—the first kind constructed of dilated vessels superficially situated, the second containing blood-filled cavities deeper in the skin, the third showing both features histologically and grossly. Most of the cutaneous hemangiomas diagnosed are superficial, looking like single ripe strawberries stuck to the skin, often on the face and more often in girls than in boys. Many others are subcutaneous, looking mushy, lumpy, and bluish-red. Some are mixed, and some others are too deep to be detected except by palpation. Only about a quarter of the superficial lesions are apparent at birth (Tan and Gilchrest, 1988).

Cutaneous lymphangiomas, like cutaneous hemangiomas, can be superficial or cavernous. Most need not be treated in the newborn period but may eventually require surgery, often unsuccessful. Cystic hygromas are large lymphangiomas, usually in the neck. They often compress the airway acutely and, for many reasons, are extremely difficult to manage.

Purplish subcutaneous nodules may represent intradermal erythropoiesis associated with intrauterine infection, particularly congenital rubella, or may indicate congenital metastatic neuroblastoma. A baby so affected is often referred to as a "blueberry muffin baby."

Macules, Papules, Pustules, and Vesicles

Erythema toxicum neonatorum is, despite its name, a benign condition. It is observed almost exclusively in full-term babies, coming on in the first several days in one third to two thirds of a nursery's population and lasting from a few hours to a few weeks. Erythema toxicum is characterized by irregular erythematous macules and yellowish papules and pustules, the latter packed with eosinophils. Any part of the skin surface, usually excepting the palms and soles, can be involved, and the general appearance is well described as "flea-bitten." Flare reactions to touch are sometimes observed, and dermatographia can sometimes be elicited, suggesting an increased level of histamine in the skin of affected babies. Similar rashes in adults might be expected to stimulate complaints of pruritus, but there is no evidence that newborns are distressed by this eruption.

Transient neonatal pustular melanosis is an idiopathic vesiculopustular condition of intrauterine onset in which primary vesiculopustules form and resolve quickly, leaving behind postinflammatory hyperpigmented macules, briefly surrounded by the scaly remnants of the original lesions. The vesiculopustules may form on any skin surface, including palms, soles, and scalp, but often congregate on the forehead, under the chin, and on the lower back. They remain intact no more than a few days, but the macules they leave behind fade over several months; therefore, macules usually predominate, even at birth. The primary lesions can be distinguished from common bacterial pustules by noting that they contain no conventionally stainable organisms. They may be distinguished from the pustules of erythema toxicum by noting the neutrophilic staining of their polymorphonuclear leukocytes; unlike the pustules of erythema toxicum, they contain few if any eosinophils. If first noticed in its postvesiculopustular stage, this condition may cause some confusion, since its freckles may occasionally be misidentified as petechiae. Careful search for and characterization of a remaining vesiculopustule should help diagnose late-recognized cases.

Papules, pustules, and vesicles may be seen in miliaria, as discussed above. The skin lesions of HSV infection can be confused with benign conditions. See the section Infectious Problems below.

Dimples, Pits, and Sinuses

Lumbosacral dimples and pits are common and normal. However, lumbosacral sinuses, which may look like dimples or pits, suggest serious underlying abnormalities. Similarly, when found in the lumbosacral area or along the dorsal midline, skin tags, hairy patches other than hairy nevi, and discolorations other than Mongolian spots should prompt consideration of occult craniospinal defects.

Other Findings

Many other abnormalities of the skin occur as isolated minor abnormalities, as parts of recognizable patterns of malformation, or as distinct entities, sometimes tragically impressive. (See chapter 51.) Reference to specialized texts is also encouraged.

HEAD

Shape and Sutures

Babies delivered vaginally from a vertex presentation have characteristically long, pointed heads. Different molding patterns correspond to different presentations; molding is unlikely if cesarean delivery has been accomplished before pelvic head engagement.

The sagittal, coronal, lambdoid, and frontal sutures should be palpated. The anterior and posterior fontanelles should be located and measured. The posterior fontanelle is frequently not palpable in term babies. Wide sutures and large fontanelles may be associated with prematurity, increased intracranial pressure or other serious intracranial pathology, or congenital hypothyroidism; as isolated findings, though, they may be normal. Fused sutures are not normal.

Fractures

Skull fractures are infrequent because the cranial plates are relatively unmineralized in early life and because their joining by fibrous sutures allows overriding. All fractures are more common after difficult deliveries. Small, linear fractures predominate. Depressed fractures, which are easy to see and feel, are usually associated with forceps application. Basilar fractures are more difficult to diagnose. They often present as shock because of severe intracranial bleeding.

Craniotabes

Craniotabes is a physical sign elicited by indenting a resilient cranial plate. Craniotabes is most often physiologic and needs no work-up, especially when found only at a plate's periphery. But craniotabes can be a pathologic sign pointing to congenital syphilis (to which association it owes its name), osteogenesis imperfecta, or, in the older infant, rickets.

Caput Succedaneum

In vertex deliveries or cesarean deliveries achieved after engagement of the head, scalp edema may form a caput succedaneum, a boggy swelling often crossing suture lines and resolving spontaneously over a few days.

Cephalohematoma

Rupture of small, low-pressure subperiosteal vessels may produce a slowly enlarging cephalohematoma, a fluctuant outpouching of nondiscolored scalp confined within boundaries corresponding to suture lines. Cephalohematomas are most often found over the parietal bones but may appear over the occipital bone or even the frontal bones; they are typically single, but need not be. Boundaries may be surprisingly distinct and, later on, may even be ridgelike. Some physicians are made uneasy by their inability to palpate for a depressed skull fracture through a cephalohematoma, and about 1 in 20 cephalohematomas does indeed overlie a skull fracture, but these are almost always linear fractures needing no special treatment. More serious cranial and intracranial injuries may coexist with cephalohematomas, but in otherwise normal babies, routine radiographic examination is hard to justify. However, some authorities do advocate follow-up radiograms at four to six weeks to look for evidence of leptomeningeal cyst formation (Fanaroff and Martin, 1987). Resorption of old blood may accentuate or prolong neonatal jaundice, and slowly resolving cephalohematomas may become infected. Infection is especially correlated with attempts at aspiration or surgical drainage, so these procedures should be reserved for strong diagnostic and therapeutic indications, respectively. Cephalohematomas resolve over two weeks to three months, often leaving newly formed bone at the margins of the elevated periosteum.

FACE

In normal vertex deliveries, and especially when it has been the presenting part, the face can be bruised and abraded. It may display a petechial rash, reflecting functional obstruction to venous return from the skin and head during the second stage of labor, particularly if the umbilical cord has been wrapped tightly around the neck. Facial bones may occasionally have been fractured, and the cartilaginous nasal septum may have been dislocated, causing noisy respirations and even respiratory distress. Facial nerve palsies, best observed with crying, can follow either spontaneous or forceps-assisted deliveries but can also be atraumatic signs of Möbius's syndrome.

Many congenital disorders are first recognized by facial examination. The range and subtlety of facial signs defy summary, but a "normal facies" can be distinguished from an "abnormal facies" by any systematic observer.

EARS

External ears are apt to be traumatized during forceps application or traction. Hematomas must be evacuated to prevent "cauliflower" deformities of the cartilage.

The helix of the ear normally joins the scalp at a point on a horizontal line drawn from the lateral angle of the eye. Low position and posterior rotation of the ears may jointly result from premature arrest of tissue migration in embryonic life. Low-set, posteriorly rotated ears are often also small or malformed or "simplified."

Preauricular tags or pits can be associated with other specific abnormalities, but they are usually isolated findings in otherwise normal babies. Some preauricular pits can be the ostia of sinus tracks liable to become infected chronically in later life.

Abnormalities of the external ear should raise suspicions about ear canal patency and middle ear and inner ear function and, sometimes, renal function.

The tympanic membrane is often obscured by vernix and debris and is not usually worth examining in otherwise normal newborns. If examination is indicated, some peculiarities should be kept in mind. The pinna should be retracted inferiorly and posteriorly to straighten the ear canal, not superiorly and posteriorly as in older children. The tympanic membrane is whitish-gray, not pearly gray; it is normally opaque, not translucent; and it is normally highly vascular—which is to say that it looks edematous and injected by the standards of later childhood. Pneumo-otoscopy, which allows the examiner of older children to "palpate" the tympanic membrane visually, is less helpful in the newborn, since the more pliable canal walls expand and collapse with induced oscillations of air pressure, dampening the effect on the membrane and even obscuring it physically.

Hearing testing is possible in the newborn both by direct, nontechnical, behavioral means and by various technologically sophisticated means. Newborns who have been sick, especially those exposed to ototoxic or neurotoxic infectious agents or drugs, should be evaluated formally for hearing loss before or shortly after going home, as should babies with family histories of sensorineural hearing loss.

EYES

Comprehensive Versus Noncomprehensive Examination

In babies in whom nonocular congenital abnormalities have already been noticed or in whom intrauterine infection has been suspected or birth-related ocular trauma discovered, examination of the eyes should be comprehensive. Otherwise, noncomprehensive examination is reasonable and can be performed with just a few routines and maneuvers. Gross appearance, ocular size, position, symmetry, and extraocular details, such as palpebral fissure angle, should be noted. Behavioral reaction to light or visual stimulus and pupillary reaction to light should be elicited, and the gross functional integrity of the extraocular muscles confirmed by simple observation or by passive motion of the head. Congenital strabismus and nonphysiologic nystagmus are important findings. Conjunctival inflammation (common after prophylaxis for ophthalmia neonatorum) and conjunctival hemorrhage (common after vaginal delivery) should be recorded. Corneal size and clarity and defects of iris circularity or coloration should be noted. The pupil should be black on direct illumination and red when examined through an ophthalmoscope. The retina need not be examined in detail in the apparently normal baby.

Cornea, Lens, Vitreous, and Fundus

Normal corneas may be a bit cloudy for the first few days, more so in premature infants. Persistent cloudiness or marked cloudiness associated with an enlarged cornea should bring congenital glaucoma forcefully to mind. Suspect eyes must be examined by an ophthalmologist as soon as possible.

A cataract may be idiopathic; may be a sign of a genetic or inborn metabolic disease, intrauterine infection, or other congenital syndrome; or may be the result of trauma. Early evaluation is the key to preservation of sight. A cataract should always raise the possibility of congenital rubella or congenital cytomegalovirus infection.

Ectopia lentis, or dislocation of the lens, is often a sign of a recognizable syndrome or a sign of trauma.

Retinoblastoma, the most common malignant neonatal eye tumor, is well known as a cause of leukokoria and secondary glaucoma, but it often presents less strikingly. The opportunity to detect a premetastatic retinoblastoma should be a chief inducement to routine ophthalmoscopic examination.

Leukokoria, or white pupil, is easily noted in an alert newborn and always indicates an abnormality of the lens, vitreous, or fundus, fundus being the joint term for retina and choroid. However, the abnormalities to which diagnosis of leukokoria is such an obvious clue often do not in fact produce a grossly white pupil. A quick ophthalmoscopic examination must therefore be performed on every newborn. Primary description of an abnormal finding should note the level at which it comes into ophthalmoscopic focus: cornea, iris, lens, vitreous, or fundus. See chapter 59.

Sclera

The sclera is normally bluish-white to white in full-term newborns. The underdeveloped sclera of premature babies is more noticeably blue, as is the collagen-deficient sclera found in osteogenesis imperfecta, Marfan's syndrome, Ehlers-Danlos syndrome, and Crouzon's syndrome. Various scleral pigmentary abnormalities may occur as isolated defects.

Iris

Aniridia, or absence of the iris, unilateral or bilateral, may be associated with significant visual problems. It may also be associated with Wilm's tumor and, therefore, should prompt vigorous investigation.

Iris coloboma, an eccentric iris defect usually found in the inferonasal quadrant, is the most common congenital eye defect; it may or may not be associated with other eye defects or somatic syndromes.

Lid

Lid coloboma is a notchlike or larger defect of the eyelid. Some lid colobomas preclude full coverage of the cornea and must be repaired surgically.

Lid masses should easily be classifiable as hemangiomas, lymphangiomas, neurofibromas, or dermoid cysts, and they should be managed accordingly. Dermoid cysts are benign lesions found at the closure sites of embryonic clefts, typically in the lateral eyebrow or upper lid but sometimes occultly within the orbit itself. External dermoid cysts are firm, pealike masses attached to the underlying periosteum but unattached to the overlying skin. Since dermoid cysts may connect to the cranial, orbital, or sinus cavities, some authorities urge radiographic studies of the involved area. However, most experienced clinicians regard dermoid cysts of the brow or eyelid as incidental findings of little consequence.

Lid droop, or ptosis, if unilateral, suggests Horner's syndrome. In posttraumatic Horner's syndrome, iris pigmentation, to whatever extent it may be established at birth, should match bilaterally. If Horner's syndrome has developed in utero, as it might in the case of a congenital mediastinal neuroblastoma, for instance, ipsilateral iris pigmentation may not be occurring normally, and heterochromia may be apparent. Heterochromia may also be found in aganglionic megacolon (Hirschsprung's disease). Bilateral ptosis is more suggestive of a neonatal myasthenia gravis syndrome or abnormal innervation of both levator palpebrae superioris muscles.

NOSE

The newborn should be considered an obligate nose breather, although his nasal obligation is not absolute. Traumatic dislocations of the nasal septum can sometimes cause respiratory distress and can be reduced by lifting the nares with cotton swabs bilaterally or simply by grasping and lifting the nose with the fingers. Choanal atresia should be suspected in the otherwise normal but persistently stridorous or tachypneic infant and in the infant whose central cyanosis improves, rather than worsens, with crying. Nasal patency can be demonstrated indirectly in various ways—listening in a quiet room or fogging a cool mirror—and directly by passage of a no. 8 French catheter into the nasopharynx. Dogged pursuit of subtle findings may result in an iatrogenic obstruction caused by traumatic mucosal swelling.

Rhinorrhea is unusual early in the newborn period, and its differential diagnosis is not what it will be later on in life. Cerebrospinal fluid rhinorrhea can be a sign of basilar skull fracture. Syphilitic rhinitis, called "snuffles," can be present shortly after birth in transplacentally infected babies, although it more commonly presents after a few days to a few weeks or months; snuffling discharge should be considered potentially infective. Excoriating discharge from a saddle-shaped nose is a classic image that should always prompt consideration of congenital syphilis.

Bleeding from the newborn nose is almost always secondary to traumatic suctioning, sometimes performed reflexively by nursery staff in babies who sneeze, as babies do physiologically. Absent any sign of mucosal trauma, investigation should include confirmation of vitamin K administration and, perhaps, a platelet count.

The nose is deformed in many congenital syndromes.

JAW, LIP, PALATE, MOUTH, TONGUE, AND OROPHARYNX

Intrauterine molding of the jaw is common, a shoulder-shaped concavity being the usual sign. Affected babies may rest their heads toward the molded side preferentially.

Micrognathia, or very small jaw, is found in many syndromes. The Pierre Robin malformation complex is composed of micrognathia, glossoptosis, and a high-arched palate or U-shaped cleft palate. These babies may have serious difficulty breathing and nursing.

Cleft deformities range from isolated lip pitting and lip notching to isolated cleft of the upper lip or the palate to bilateral clefts of the upper lip extending through to the nose and combined with cleft palate. Bifid uvula suggests a submucous cleft of the hard palate. A gloved finger should be placed in the mouth in all babies to feel for a submucous cleft, whether or not the uvula is bifid.

Several intraoral lesions are fairly common. Natal teeth, usually lower central incisors, can interfere with nursing and can be aspirated when shed. They can also be signs of broader congenital problems (Leung, 1986). Ranulas are bluish sublingual salivary retention cysts that may need to be aspirated if they interfere with nursing. Lymphangiomas of the alveolar ridges, except for their location, look much the same; they usually regress. Bohn's nodules are nonmidline cysts of the hard palate or cysts of the alveolar ridges. Epstein's pearls, epithelial rests in the midline of the hard palate, are routine findings.

Macroglossia is seen in congenital hypothyroidism and various congenital syndromes, including mucopolysaccharidoses and Beckwith's syndrome.

The frenulum normally attaches nearly at the tip of the tongue; parents may need reassurance that the tongue does not have to be "untied" by frenulectomy.

Excessive oropharyngeal secretions may suggest a high gastrointestinal blockage, such as esophageal atresia.

NECK

Clavicular fractures are commonly of the greenstick variety, in which case they may be overlooked pending callus formation, but they may also be complete, in which case deformity and discoloration may be obvious and crepitus elicitable. Moro reflex may be asymmetrical in the presence of clavicular fracture. Another important sign of neck trauma is not seen in the neck but in the arm: brachial plexus injury. There are three patterns of brachial plexus injury. Only one, the Duchenne-Erb palsy of the upper arm, is common; it is caused by injury to cervical roots five and six. Babies with brachial plexus injuries sometimes have also sustained ipsilateral phrenic nerve injuries. Radiographic examination is recommended.

A firm, fusiform fibrous mass is sometimes found in the belly of one sternocleidomastoid muscle at birth or several weeks thereafter. Such masses have traditionally been assumed to be organizing or fibrosed traumatic hematomas, but this view no longer seems fully satisfactory. At any rate, this mass is associated with torticollis (Latin for "twisted neck"), whose common cosmetic result is wryneck and whose more extreme consequence is distortion of the face and skull. Early institution of physical therapy is advisable and can prove an adequate remedy, but parents should also be introduced to the idea that surgical resection may be needed within the first year.

Branchial cleft cysts also present in the area of the sternocleidomastoids. Cystic hygromas are large lymphangiomas arising in the anterior triangle of the neck. They can compress the airway acutely and often require complicated surgical and medical interventions during prolonged hospitalizations. Thyroglossal duct cysts present in the midline, as do congenital goiters.

The involution of ectatic lymphatic vessels results in webbing of the neck, a sign of several congenital syndromes, including Turner's, Noonan's, Klippel-Feil, and trisomies 18 and 21.

NIPPLES AND BREASTS

Supernumerary nipples occur in 2 to 3 per cent of newborns. They are found along the milk line from above the true breast toward the inguinal canal. They usually do not overlie breast tissue. Extra nipples are associated with renal anomalies; however, the association is a weak one in otherwise normal babies and in babies with recognizable malformations not independently associated with renal lesions (Kenney et al., 1987; Hersh et al., 1987).

Breast tissue may be present and may even excrete small amounts of milk ("witch's milk") if squeezed. Neonatal breast hypertrophy is a normal response to maternal hormone secretion; it may persist for weeks to months. If squeezed frequently, functioning neonatal breasts may more easily become infected and abscessed and, if abscessed, scarred. Parents should know that ignoring this oddity will hasten its resolution (Madlon-Kay, 1986).

CHEST

Inspection of the chest has been discussed above.

Palpation of the chest is performed as it would be in an adult patient except that the hand must be applied to several areas of interest at once. Abnormal cardiac pulsations, including thrills, should be noted.

Percussion is useful only for the assessment of gross pathology, such as pneumothorax or effusion or diaphragmatic hernia; newborn heart borders cannot easily be located by percussion.

Auscultation of the chest demonstrates shallow respirations punctuated by deep, noisy sighs and preponderantly tubular breath sounds transmitted through a thin chest wall. Localizing findings to a particular lobe is difficult. During transition from intrauterine to extrauterine life, retained lung fluid and still-unopened alveoli are associated with fine crepitant rales and some rhonchi, and flow through the ductus arteriosus may produce a characteristic murmur. The heart sounds should be identified and an attempt made to note splitting of the second sound; normal splitting is a good indicator of normal pulmonary circulation.

See also the section on Respiratory Problems below.

CARDIOVASCULAR SYSTEM

See chapter 46. See also the section on the chest above and the sections Femoral Arterial Pulses in Comparison with Other Arterial Pulses and Cardiovascular Problems later.

ABDOMEN

A warm-handed examiner can assess a sleeping or sucking newborn's abdomen quickly. Placing the nondominant hand behind the baby's flank allows bimanual examination. Alternatively, the hips can be flexed by lifting the ankles, and it is sometimes helpful to flex the spine by lifting the baby's neck and shoulders with the nonexamining hand. In an agitated baby, the examiner will have to divide his palpation between periods of inspiration when tension of the abdominal musculature relaxes momentarily; to take best advantage of these intervals, the hand should simply rest in the area of interest until a deep breath softens the belly.

Normal findings may include a smooth, soft liver edge several centimeters below the right costal margin; rarely, a spleen tip just within the left costal margin; vaguely palpable kidneys within the retroperitoneal wall; and a small bladder above the symphysis. Pathologic abdominal masses are mostly of renal and adrenal origin: horseshoe kidney, pelvic kidney, polycystic kidney, multicystic kidney, duplicated kidney, postobstructive hydronephrotic kidney, Wilm's tumor, neuroblastoma, and adrenal hemorrhage. Other lesions, such as choledochal cyst, are also found.

A stomach bubble may be felt, as may air-filled loops of bowel. Peristalsis may be observed, especially shortly after birth and in babies with thin abdominal walls. When air in a viscus causes concern, well-organized bowel sounds can be reassuring; reexamination in an hour or two will often demonstrate a change in pattern. The rectum must be inspected for patency and the day sheet checked to confirm passage of meconium; virtually all normal full-term babies will have passed a meconium stool by the end of their first 24 hours. A gloved, short-nailed fifth finger can safely examine a well-lubricated rectum up to several centimeters if necessary and may stimulate passage of a meconium plug. The stools of LBW babies and babies identified as ill will often be tested routinely for the presence of occult blood; occult hematochezia is surprisingly common in these babies and is usually not a sign of necrotizing enterocolitis (Abramo et al., 1988).

Emesis and excessive salivation may indicate gastrointestinal obstruction, especially in the setting of gestational polyhydramnios. To confirm esophageal patency, a feeding tube can be passed into the stomach and its presence confirmed by auscultation of injected air and by cross-table lateral radiography. (These maneuvers can confirm esophageal patency but cannot by themselves confirm tracheoesophageal integrity.) If an unexpectedly large amount of stomach fluid is found—over 30 ml. in a full-term baby—an upper gastrointestinal obstruction is likely, whether functional, as with an ileus, or mechanical. The source of bloody stomach fluid—swallowed maternal blood or gastrointestinal bleeding—can be differentiated by an Apt test.

UMBILICUS

The clamped cord should once again be inspected to confirm the presence of two arteries and one vein. Finding a single umbilical artery should prompt further investigation, particularly renal ultrasonography; in about one half of these babies, at least one additional congenital malformation can be identified (Leung and Robson, 1989). Rarely, a patent urachus or a severed loop of herniated bowel can be present in the umbilical stump; cord clamping makes discharge from these structures unlikely and careful inspection more critical. Mild erythema of the periumbilical skin is physiologic; frank erythema, classically in a triangular area above the umbilicus, purulent discharge, and putrid odor are signs of omphalitis. Umbilical herniation of various degree is common and is occasionally part of a recognizable syndrome. More striking errors in abdominal wall development require emergent fluid resuscitation, sterile regimen, and urgent surgical consultation: gastroschisis, a failure of closure on the right side of the umbilicus; omphalocele, a herniation of peritoneum-covered intra-abdominal contents, frequently malformed; and exstrophy of the bladder. Diastasis recti, manifested during crying by a midline abdominal outpouching, is normal and is not a mild form of failure of abdominal wall closure.

GENITALIA, PERINEUM, AND INGUINAL REGIONS

Almost all babies urinate within the first 24 hours. A dry diaper should prompt a look at the nursery day sheet; if urination has not been recorded, the examiner should repeat the abdominal examination to check bladder and kidney size.

On removing the baby's diaper, the examiner may notice a reddish stain at the point of urination. This is usually just a "red brick dust" stain caused by uric acid crystals; a hematest or guaiac test should be negative. Later on, vicarious menstruation may stain the diaper in girls. Like "red brick dust" staining, vicarious menstruation is physiologic.

The inguinal regions and the scrotum or labia majora should be checked for masses and indirect hernias. Inguinal hernias are more common in premature babies.

In males, inguinal herniation may be associated with cryptorchidism or with a hydrocele. Descended testicles may retract into the inguinal canal when cold or when examined. They can usually be coaxed back into the scrotum for examination. True bilateral cryptorchidism immediately raises doubts as to genotypic sex. Fluctuant, translucent scrotal masses are hydroceles, often bilateral. Most congenital hydroceles, as opposed to hydroceles of later onset, resolve spontaneously and do not indicate a coexistent inguinal hernia. Nontransilluminating scrotal masses may represent tumors or testicular torsion. Hypospadias comes in three degrees: first, urethral opening low on the ventral glans; second, urethral opening on the ventral penile shaft; third, urethral opening on the perineum at the base of the shaft. Epispadias exists when the urethra opens onto the dorsal surface of the shaft; epispadias is rare in otherwise normal babies. Circumcision should not be performed if the urethral meatus is not in the normal position since prepuce skin will be needed for surgical repair.

In females, the ovary may herniate into the labia majora, where there is some risk of its infarction. In the testicular feminization syndrome, an inguinal mass in a phenotypic female may in fact be a testicle. A vaginal tag may protrude from between the labia majora in normal females. A mucoid vaginal secretion is normal. Apparently, all otherwise normally formed females have hymens (Jenny, 1987; Mor and Merlob, 1988). Hydrometrocolpos presents as a white mass protuding from between the labia majora; spontaneous rupture or surgical incision releases the retained fluid.

Ambiguous genitalia must be described carefully and formal sex-determination procedures undertaken as soon as possible.

FEMORAL ARTERIAL PULSES IN COMPARISON WITH OTHER ARTERIAL PULSES

Patient palpation of the femoral triangles almost always locates femoral arterial pulses. Frustrated examiners sometimes find it reassuring to check arterial pulses in the lower legs before resuming their search. Once located, the femoral arteries must be palpated in simultaneous comparison to the brachial arteries, since "congenital" coarctation of the aorta may not yet be fully expressed. A baby's first complete physical examination should occur within 24 hours of birth; during this period, his ductus arteriosus may still be patent. A baby who will ultimately be recognized as having coarctation of the aorta may in fact have palpable femoral pulses on first examination either because blood still flows freely through the patent ductus or because the old distal opening of the now-closed ductus still distorts the aortic lumen just enough to allow blood temporarily to squirt around the impending coarctation (Thoele et al., 1987). Femoral arterial pulses may seem decreased only when compared with the brachial arterial pulse. Babies whose coarctations are proximal to the ductus may have full femoral arterial flow thanks to persistent ductal patency, but these babies should be recognizable on the basis of other findings.

SKELETON AND EXTREMITIES

The examiner should assure himself that the baby can move all extremities actively. He should note gross deformities and the effects of molding. Fixed joint deformities should be differentiated from passively reducible deformities.

Fracture of the clavicle, described above, is common. So is fracture of the humerus. Supernumerary digits, usually on the hands and more common in Blacks than in Whites, may or may not contain bone. If they do contain bone, their management requires orthopedic consultation; if not, they can be tied off with a ligature and left to necrose and shed. Constriction bands arising from a ruptured amnion may compromise an extremity; occasionally, an amniotic band may still be found at a constriction site.

Examination of skeleton and extremities could probably be carried out adequately by inspection alone were it not for the hips. Examination of the hip joints requires that the examiner perform Ortolani's reduction maneuver and Barlow's dislocation maneuver (Fig. 37–3). Very frequently, hip "clicks" stimulate requests for radiographic and orthopedic consultations. As in adults, clicks are caused by the movement of articular and periarticular parts. But the "clunks" attending subluxation and rearticulation are easily felt and often even grossly visible. Positive examinations should not be repeated excessively, as damage to the articular cartilage can result. See chapter 49.

NEUROLOGIC SYSTEM

As stressed above, sophisticated, systematic inspection satisfies most requirements of the neurologic examination.

Function and testing of the cranial nerves are summarized in Table 37–2.

Deep tendon reflexes should be elicited at the biceps, knee, and ankle. Ankle clonus should be unsustained, although it may sometimes be surprisingly prolonged in clearly normal babies.

Stroking the side of the mouth should stimulate a turning of the head toward the stimulus. Suck should be strong in alert babies.

The Moro and startle reflexes are elicited by physical shocks and sudden changes in support, such as first lifting slightly and then dropping one end of the examining table; the baby reaches out his arms and hands and then grasps in a manner recalling a lower primate offspring trying to regain a grip on its running mother's underbelly.

Placing a finger on the palm should elicit the palmar grasp reflex; the trunk and sometimes the head of a normal baby can be pulled off the examining table on the strength of his grasp. The plantar grasp reflex is more difficult to appreciate.

On picking up the baby, tone and head control should be noted. Holding him up under the chest and belly, the examiner should run a finger along either side of the back; the baby should squirm, his trunk becoming concave on the side of the stimulus.

The Babinski reflex, important in assessing upper motor neuron damage in older children and adults, is not reliable in newborns.

Seizure activity in newborns is more often tonic or clonic than tonic-clonic and is often subtle. Typical newborn seizures include abnormal movements or changes in tone in the trunk or extremities and rhythmic or tonic activity of the muscles innervated by the cranial nerves. The range of presentations includes—but is certainly not limited to—posturing, sucking or chewing, tonic deviation of the eyes or batting of the eyelids, bicycling movements of the legs, rhythmic twitching, and even apnea.

Depressed infants may have been neurologically devastated during the birth process, or they may be showing the effects of maternal anesthesia. Other seemingly depressed babies may actually be hypotonic, suffering from a myasthenic syndrome or a motor neuron disease. Highly agitated infants may be withdrawing from intrauterine habituation to a psychoactive drug.

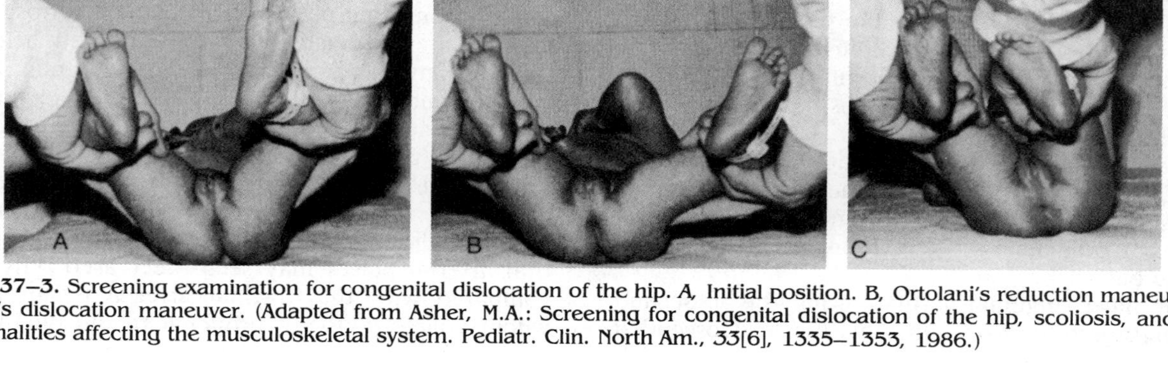

Figure 37–3. Screening examination for congenital dislocation of the hip. *A*, Initial position. *B*, Ortolani's reduction maneuver. *C*, Barlow's dislocation maneuver. (Adapted from Asher, M.A.: Screening for congenital dislocation of the hip, scoliosis, and other abnormalities affecting the musculoskeletal system. Pediatr. Clin. North Am., *33*[6], 1335–1353, 1986.)

Table 37–2. FUNCTION AND TESTING OF THE CRANIAL NERVES

Cranial Nerve	Name	Function and Testing
I	Olfactory	Smell—not tested. May use peppermint to stimulate sucking or an arousal-withdrawal response.
II	Optic	Vision—tested by blink response to light and by visual fixation with eyes following brightly colored object or examiner's face.
III IV VI	Oculomotor Trochlear Abducens	Control pupillary response to light (III) and extraocular muscle movements (III, IV, and VI). Latter may be tested by observing spontaneous eye movements or movements elicited by turning head from side to side (doll's eye maneuver).
V	Trigeminal	Sensory component displayed by rooting reflex and eye blink reflex. Strength of masseter and pterygoid muscles is best assessed by evaluation of suck and biting (motor V).
VII	Facial	Evaluated by carefully noting presence of nasolabial folds and position and movement of corners of mouth. Facial expressions are under control of VII.
VIII	Auditory	Vestibular component tested by rotating infant clockwise or counterclockwise and simultaneously noting that eyes turn in direction of rotation. Auditory component may be demonstrated by startle response to loud sound or simply speaking into one ear and noting infant's head turn toward voice.
IX	Glossopharyngeal	Tongue movement and taste—tested by gagging infant with tongue blade and noting normal midline positioning of uvula.
X	Vagus	Evaluated by noting normal cry and autonomic visceral functions.
XI	Accessory	Controls sternocleidomastoid muscle. Can be tested by observing the head move from side to side.
XII	Hypoglossal	Controls tongue movement. Tested by simply observing tongue thrusting and tongue movements when inspecting oropharynx.

From Coen, R. W., and Koffler, H.: Primary Care of the Newborn. Boston, Little, Brown & Co., Inc., 1987; adapted from Volpe, J. J.: Neurology of the Newborn, Philadelphia, W. B. Saunders Company, 1981.

Estimation of Gestational Age

Dubowitz's criteria for estimation of gestational age are presented in Table 37–3 and Figures 37–4 and 37–5. Ballard's simplified criteria are presented in Figure 37–6.

Routines for the First Few Days

OBSERVATION, STABILIZATION, AND SCREENING

The baby's physiologic transition period extends for many hours or even several days; it is made smoother by the maintenance of a neutral thermal environment. During the early transition period, vital signs should be checked hourly till stable. Ophthalmia neonatorum prophylaxis and vitamin K should be administered. Several routine laboratory studies should be performed on a lateral heel stick capillary blood sample: blood glucose, hematocrit, and thyroid stimulating hormone. Phenylalanine level, also performed on a heel stick sample, must follow the digestion of a milk feeding and therefore would be meaningless if collected immediately after delivery. Other studies run on cord blood should already have been dispatched from the delivery room: blood type and Coombs' test, a syphilis test, hemoglobin electrophoresis, and, at the physician's discretion, immunoglobulin M (IgM) level. Further discussion of these and additional tests routinely or frequently run on presumably normal newborns will appear below under Postnatal Screening. Routine body surface cultures yield no useful information (Evans et al., 1988).

BATHING

Preservation of the vernix caseosa makes good sense; it protects the skin from drying and is somewhat bacteriocidal. But its virtues are lost on most families, who usually think it unclean and unsightly, especially when mixed with maternal blood. So, after stabilization in a neutral thermal environment, the baby may be bathed with warm, freshly drawn, standing water. Bathing in running water is unwise, as it encourages observant mothers to adopt the practice at home, where careless attention to changing water temperature may result in burns, some severe. Soap (Morelli and Weston, 1987) is not necessary, except to suppress a documented nursery epidemic, such as bullous dermatitis or periumbilical cellulitis. Immersion above the umbilicus should be avoided until the umbilical stump has sloughed and the umbilicus has become covered in granulation tissue.

UMBILICAL CORD CARE

The umbilical cord stump may become colonized with pathogenic bacteria—typically streptococci, *Staphy-*

Table 37–3. DUBOWITZ CRITERIA FOR ESTIMATION OF GESTATIONAL AGE: EXTERNAL PHYSICAL FINDINGS

	Score*				
External Sign	*0*	*1*	*2*	*3*	*4*
Edema	Obvious edema of hands and feet; pitting over tibia	No obvious edema of hands and feet; pitting over tibia	No edema		
Skin texture	Very thin, gelatinous	Thin and smooth	Smooth; medium thickness; rash or superficial peeling	Slight thickening; superficial cracking and peeling, especially of hands and feet	Thick and parchment-like; superficial or deep cracking
Skin color	Dark red	Uniformly pink	Pale pink; variable over body	Pale; only pink over ears, lips, palms, or soles	
Skin opacity (trunk)	Numerous veins and venules clearly seen, especially over abdomen	Veins and tributaries seen	A few large vessels clearly seen over abdomen	A few large vessels seen indistinctly over abdomen	No blood vessels seen
Lanugo (over back)	No lanugo	Abundant; long and thick over whole back	Hair thinning, especially over lower back	Small amount of lanugo and bald areas	At least half of back devoid of lanugo
Plantar creases	No skin creases	Faint red marks over anterior half of sole	Definite red marks over > anterior half; indentations over < anterior third	Indentations over > anterior third	Definite deep indentations over > anterior third
Nipple formation	Nipple barely visible, no areola	Nipple well defined; areola smooth and flat, diameter < 0.75 cm.	Areola stippled, edge not raised, diameter < 0.75 cm.	Areola stippled, edge raised, diameter > 0.75 cm.	
Breast size	No breast tissue palpable	Breast tissue on one or both sides, < 0.5 cm. diameter	Breast tissue on both sides, one or both 0.5 to 1.0 cm.	Breast tissue on both sides, one or both > 1 cm.	
Ear form	Pinna flat and shapeless, little or no incurving of edge	Incurving of part of edge of pinna	Partial incurving of whole of upper pinna	Well-defined incurving of whole of upper pinna	
Ear firmness	Pinna soft, easily folded, no recoil	Pinna soft, easily folded, slow recoil	Cartilage to edge of pinna but soft in places, ready recoil	Pinna firm, cartilage to edge, instant recoil	
Genitals: Male	Neither testis in scrotum	At least one testis high in scrotum	At least one testis right down		
Genitals: Female (with hips half abducted)	Labia majora widely separated, labia minora protruding	Labia majora almost cover labia minora	Labia majora completely cover labia minora		

*For scoring see legend of Figure 37–5.

From Dubowitz, L. M., Dubowitz, V., and Goldberg, C.: Clinical assessment of gestational age in the newborn infant. J. Pediatr., 77:1–10, 1970; adapted from Farr, V., Kerridge, D. F., and Mitchell, R. G.: The definition of some external characteristics used in the assessment of gestational age of the newborn infant. Develop. Med. Child. Neurol., 8:507, 1966.

lococcus aureus, and coliforms—and may provide access for such organisms to the umbilicus itself, to the umbilical vein, to the anterior abdominal wall, and to the systemic circulation. It is advisable, then, to encourage drying and to apply to the stump an antiseptic agent, such as triple dye or alcohol, or an antibiotic ointment.

FIRST FEEDING

An "artificial" first feeding is a modern nursery tradition difficult to displace. Two justifications are commonly heard: some babies at risk for mild hypoglycemia may benefit from an "early" feeding of dextrose 5 per cent in water; some babies with upper

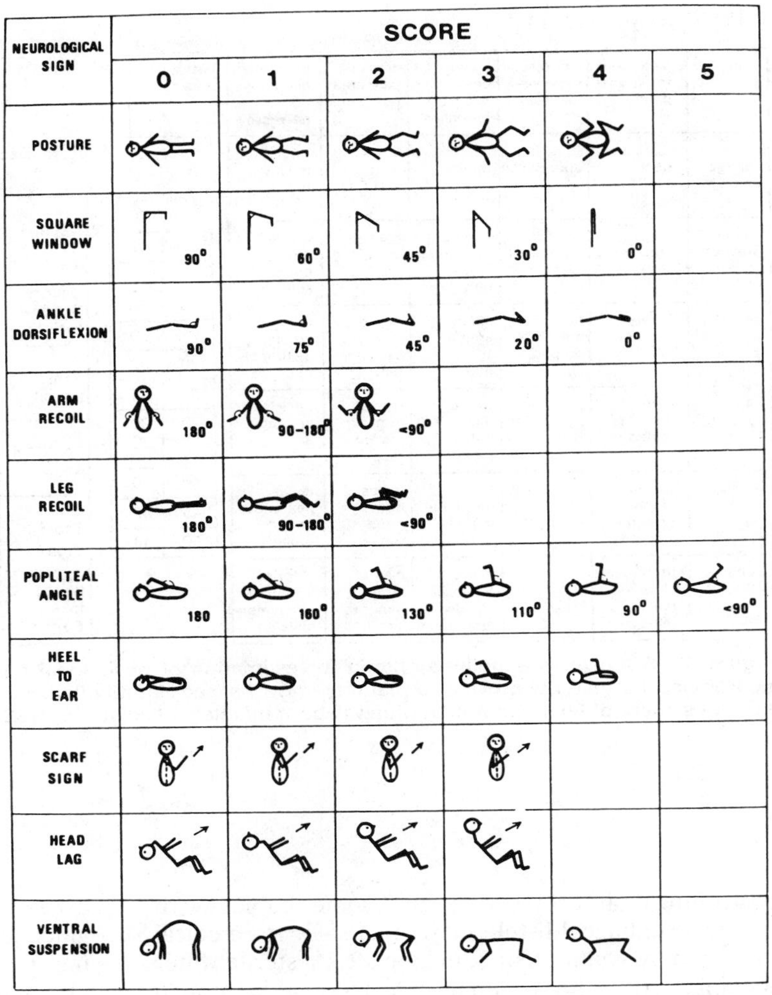
NEUROLOGICAL SIGN
SCORE
0
1
2
3
4
5
POSTURE
SQUARE WINDOW
90°
60°
45°
30°
0°
ANKLE DORSIFLEXION
90°
75°
45°
20°
0°
ARM RECOIL
180°
90-180°
<90°
LEG RECOIL
180°
90-180°
<90°
POPLITEAL ANGLE
180
160°
130°
110°
90°
<90°
HEEL TO EAR
SCARF SIGN
HEAD LAG
VENTRAL SUSPENSION

Figure 37–4. Dubowitz criteria for estimation of gestational age: neurological and neuromuscular findings. (From Dubowitz, L.M., Dubowitz, V., and Goldberg, C.: Clinical assessment of gestational age in the newborn infant. J. Pediatr., *77:*1–10, 1970; Amiel-Tison C.: Neurological evaluation of the maturity of newborn infants. Arch. Dis. Child., *43:*89, 1968.)

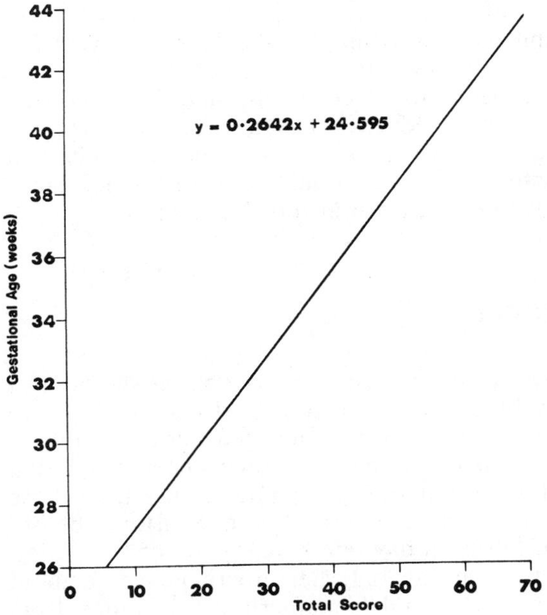

Figure 37–5. Dubowitz criteria for estimation of gestational age: gestational age scoring graph. Scoring: A maximum-score case would be arrived at by adding the Table 37–3 score (2+4+3+4+4+4+3+3+3+3+2=35) and the Figure 37–4 score (4+4+4+2+2+5+4+3+3+4=35). The total score of 70 (35+35), found in Figure 37–5, corresponds to a gestational age of 43 to 44 weeks. (From Dubowitz, M.L., Dubowitz, V., and Goldberg C.: Clinical assessment of gestational age in the newborn infant. J. Pediatr., *77:*1–10, 1970.)

PHYSICAL MATURITY

	0	1	2	3	4	5
Skin	gelatinous red, transparent	smooth pink, visible veins	superficial peeling &/or rash few veins	cracking pale area rare veins	parchment deep cracking no vessels	leathery cracked wrinkled
Lanugo	none	abundant	thinning	bald areas	mostly bald	
Plantar Creases	no crease	faint red marks	anterior transverse crease only	creases ant. 2/3	creases cover entire sole	
Breast	barely percept.	flat areola no bud	stippled areola 1–2 mm bud	raised areola 3–4 mm bud	full areola 5–10 mm bud	
Ear	pinna flat, stays folded	sl. curved pinna; soft with slow recoil	well-curv. pinna; soft but ready recoil	formed & firm with instant recoil	thick cartilage ear stiff	
Genitals ♂	scrotum empty no rugae		testes descending, few rugae	testes down good rugae	testes pendulous deep rugae	
Genitals ♀	prominent clitoris & labia minora		majora & minora equally prominent	majora large minora small	clitoris & minora completely covered	

MATURITY RATING

Score	Wks
5	26
10	28
15	30
20	32
25	34
30	36
35	38
40	40
45	42
50	44

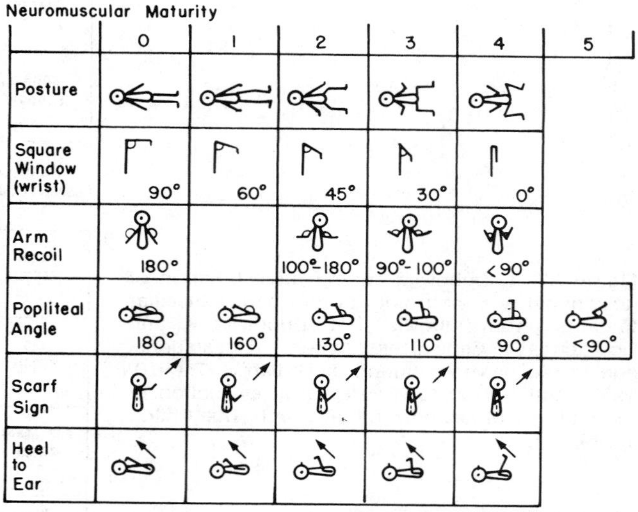

Neuromuscular Maturity
0
1
2
3
4
5
Posture
Square Window (wrist)
90°
60°
45°
30°
0°
Arm Recoil
180°
100°-180°
90°-100°
<90°
Popliteal Angle
180°
160°
130°
110°
90°
<90°
Scarf Sign
Heel to Ear

Figure 37–6. Ballard's simplified criteria for estimation of gestational age. The sum of scores on all items of physical and neuromuscular maturity provides a maturity in weeks (see Maturity Rating). (Modified from Ballard, J.L., et al.: A simplified score for assessment of fetal maturation of newly born infants. J. Pediatr., *95:*769–774, 1979.)

gastrointestinal obstruction and some babies with tracheoesophageal fistula may come safely to medical attention by vomiting or coughing after a sterile water feeding. Still, the optimal first feeding is human colostrum sucked immediately after delivery. The often negligible volume of this first feeding need not prompt supplementation. Normal, term babies are born fully hydrated; they come with a several days' supply of "excess" water already on board; it is this "excess" whose expenditure is primarily responsible for physiologic postnatal weight loss. If bottle feeding is the maternal choice, a standard formula can be offered.

Postnatal Screening

BLOOD GLUCOSE

At birth, blood glucose is about two thirds the mother's level. Within an hour or two, blood glucose falls to a level no lower than 35 to 40 mg. per dl. and then rises to a 6-hour value between 45 mg. per dl. and 60 mg. per dl. Levels in premature babies are a little lower, in part because glycogen stores are relatively deficient. Newborns normally consume glucose at about twice the adult rate; if they are physically stressed or if they are the hyperinsulinemic products of diabetic gestations, their glucose demand may exceed the supply deliverable by glycogenolysis and gluconeogenesis combined. Blood glucose below 40 mg. per dl. requires a diagnostic explanation. Hypoglycemic babies may be jittery and may even experience seizure, or they may be depressed. Most cases of transient neonatal hypoglycemia can be anticipated on the basis of prematurity or perinatal stress; early nutritive feeding or an intravenous dextrose infusion may prevent symptoms.

Capillary blood samples should be drawn from the side of the heel, to prevent scarring of the heel pad. The heel should be warm, since cold-induced vascular stasis produces a localized relative hypoglycemia. Samples should be analyzed immediately with fresh materials, or they should be placed on ice, since blood glucose levels fall at room temperature.

HEMATOCRIT

Peripheral vascular stasis increases the hematocrit of capillary blood obtained by lateral heel stick, more so if the leg and foot are squeezed during sampling. Hematocrits spun from freely flowing heel-stick blood are preferable but still give higher values than those spun from either peripheral venous or arterial blood. Average full-term day-one hematocrit is 53 per cent; by day two, the average hematocrit peaks at about 58 per cent. Normal hematocrit values range from about 45 to 60 per cent (hemoglobin from about 15 grams per dl. to 20 grams per dl.).

Hematocrit over 70 per cent defines polycythemia and implies hyperviscosity. Obviously, high capillary values must be checked with peripheral venous or arterial samples. Polycythemic babies are usually plethoric and may be lethargic. Immediate concerns are thrombosis and sludging, particularly in the brain. A partial exchange transfusion, not simple phlebotomy, may be indicated, although it has proved difficult to define babies whose ongoing risk from polycythemia exceeds their risk from therapy (Oh, 1986).

DIFFERENTIAL LEUKOCYTE COUNT

Neither total nor differential leukocyte counts should be considered routine postnatal screening tests. But babies coming to special attention because of perinatal history or physical examination should have these tests performed. An increased ratio of immature to total neutrophils may suggest acute systemic infection (Manroe et al., 1979).

BLOOD TYPE AND COOMBS' TEST

Maternal-infant ABO incompatibility or a positive direct Coombs' test should prompt serial hematocrits and indirect serum bilirubin levels. Severe ABO isoimmunization or Rh isoimmunization of any degree demands intermediate to intensive care.

SYPHILIS TEST

A positive serologic test for syphilis in an asymptomatic newborn may reflect antitreponemal IgG antibody acquired transplacentally from a treated or untreated mother. But this benign possibility cannot be confirmed on serologic grounds alone without observation of a fall in antitreponemal IgG titer over several months. Consequently, full syphilis work-up in the nursery is usually required. Physical examination must be repeated carefully (while wearing gloves). Darkfield examination of nasal discharge may be helpful; radiography of the long bones may show metaphyseal demineralization or periosteal bone formation. Cerebrospinal fluid (CSF) must be examined and a CSF fluorescent treponemal antibody absorption test (FTA-ABS) performed. A positive CSF FTA-ABS is not proof of congenital neurosyphilis, however; antitreponemal IgG antibody found in the CSF may have been transplacentally acquired. IgM antibody, in contrast to IgG antibody, does not cross the blood-brain barrier in newborns. Western blot analysis can now demonstrate specific antitreponemal IgM antibodies in CSF, confirming a diagnosis of congenital neurosyphilis (Sanchez, 1989). The Western blot technique should soon be widely available. Even when active congenital syphilis cannot be demonstrated definitively, antibiotic treatment of suspect cases is almost always advisable, and, in the context of parental unreliability, it is mandatory. See chapter 30.

HEMOGLOBIN ELECTROPHORESIS

Detection of sickle cell disease in the newborn period is very helpful (Vichinsky et al., 1988), since it allows early parental counselling and, most important, early initiation of daily oral penicillin prophylaxis against overwhelming sepsis. Several other hemoglobinopathies may also be detected by this test. See chapter 57.

THYROXINE (T_4) OR THYROID STIMULATING HORMONE (TSH)

In most North American jurisdictions, T_4 is the only thyroid screening test performed if it is normal; if it is low, a TSH is also run. Unfortunately, some babies with T_4 in the normal range will have an elevated TSH. In Japan and in most of Europe, the testing order is reversed. Neither policy is perfect; testing TSH first will not uncover babies with some of the more unusual congenital thyroid problems. Further problems result when early discharge or out-of-hospital delivery necessitates testing before three days of age, since TSH may be physiologically elevated during the first two days after delivery. Abnormal screening results should prompt immediate full maternal and infant evaluations and testing of both T_4 and TSH in a serum sample drawn from the baby's venous blood, not from another heel stick. Treatment for congenital hypothyroidism is with 1-thyroxine 10 to 15 micrograms per kg. per day, the goal being maintenance of T_4 levels in the upper half of the normal range throughout the first year of life (American Academy of Pediatrics and American Thyroid Association, 1987).

Nearly universal thyroid screening has been a great advance in developed countries, but it still misses from 6 to 12 per cent of congenitally hypothyroid babies and falsely implicates others. Congenital hypothyroidism must still be suspected on clinical grounds in babies who have large open fontanelles or umbilical hernias or who are hypothermic, hypotonic, macroglossic, excessively mottled, coarsely featured, somnolent, slow to feed, or persistently jaundiced, whether or not their thyroid glands are enlarged and whether or not their screening tests are normal.

PHENYLALANINE LEVEL

In classic phenylketonuria (PKU), phenylalanine hydroxylase activity is greatly decreased or absent, so dietary phenylalanine accumulates, and tyrosine, which is made from phenylalanine, is depressed. The affected baby is asymptomatic in the newborn period, but, if he has begun feeding, his blood phenylalanine level will be elevated, making him identifiable and making phenylalanine-related organ damage, particularly brain damage, largely preventable by dietary restriction.

GALACTOSEMIA

In babies with a deficiency of galactokinase, galactose accumulates in the lenses, causing cataracts. The urine of affected babies who are ingesting galactose or lactose (whose hydrolysis yields glucose and galactose) will contain a nonglucose reducing substance, specifically, galactose. Dietary restriction therapy is easy and effective if instituted early enough. Babies with a deficiency of galactokinase do not have classic galactosemia.

In babies with deficient activity of galactose-1-phosphate uridyl transferase, dietary galactose accumulates in and damages the liver and kidneys and eventually the brain and the lenses. The urine contains nonglucose reducing substances, specifically, galactose and galactose-1-phosphate. Affected babies appear normal at birth but become fulminantly ill within a few days and are usually assumed to be septic; occasionally, galactosemic babies are indeed septic as well as galactosemic. Others do not become critically ill but simply fail to thrive in the first year. Babies with a deficiency of galactose-1-phosphate uridyl transferase do have classic galactosemia.

Nonglucose reducing substances in the urine can be demonstrated by the combination of a negative Clinistix or Tes-Tape with a positive Clinitest.

IMMUNOGLOBULIN M (IgM) LEVEL

Cord blood IgM below 20 mg. per dl. is normal. Elevated values suggest fetal response to intrauterine infection.

OTHER POSTNATAL SCREENING TESTS

Other congenital problems for which screening tests were mandated in at least one United States jurisdiction in 1987 were these: maple syrup urine disease, homocystinuria, hyperleucinemia, histidinemia, adenosine deaminase deficiency, congenital hearing loss, intrauterine lead exposure, cystic fibrosis, and congenital adrenal hyperplasia (Caravella et al., 1987).

Circumcision

Circumcision should *never* be performed if there is any doubt whatsoever about the anatomic normality of the penis. Circumcision decreases the already small chance of urinary tract infection in the young male infant (Ginsburg and McCracken, 1982; Wiswell and Roscelli, 1986; Wiswell et al., 1988), but potential benefits must be weighed against known risks (Fergusson et al., 1988; Herzog and Alvarez, 1986; Brown and Brown 1987; Wallerstein, 1980). Free-hand circumcision is easily learned but is often abandoned in favor of Gomco or Plastibell techniques (Figs. 37–7 and 37–8).

Once the genital area is prepped and draped, a straight hemostat is inserted into the preputial orifice and the ring is gently dilated. A blunt flexible probe is inserted between the glans and the inner epithelium of the prepuce. To free the entire glans from the adherent prepuce, it usually is necessary to make a dorsal slit in the prepuce. This is accomplished by clamping a straight hemostat on the prepuce in the midline. The external urethral meatus should be identified clearly before placing the midline hemostat. After waiting approximately one minute, the hemostat is removed and the dorsal incision is made in the portion of the prepuce that was clamped. The incision is made to within 0.5 cm. of the coronal sulcus. The foreskin is pulled back and the blunt dissection continued until the entire glans is free of adhering tissue. Once this is accomplished the circumcision may be completed using either a Gomco clamp or a Plastibell.

If the Gomco clamp is used, it should be tightened for a minimum of five minutes before incising the foreskin. Once the clamp is removed, the penis should be wrapped with petroleum jelly gauze to protect it from adhering to a diaper.

Once a Plastibell is securely tightened in place, wait about five minutes and then incise the redundant foreskin. The Plastibell handle is separated from the cap, leaving the base of the foreskin fastened tightly to the cap. The opening in the cap permits urine to pass. Approximately 5 to 10 days later the cap and remaining foreskin fall off together.

Following the circumcision, it is necessary to instruct the parents to watch for signs of infection, problems in urination, and bleeding. Cleanliness is very important.

Circumcision is painful (Anand and Hickey, 1987); local anesthetic infiltration is a compassionate option.

Standard Care Through the First Month of Life

Many recommendations for standard newborn care are implicit or explicit in previous sections, especially Routines for the First Few Days.

SAFETY

In developed countries, the baby's trip home and all subsequent motorized trips should be taken in a well-designed and properly used infant car seat (Bull et al., 1988a; Bull et al., March, 1988b). Car-seat teaching can conveniently be managed postpartum by videotape, and car-seat office education can be accomplished cheaply and effectively (Hletko et al.,

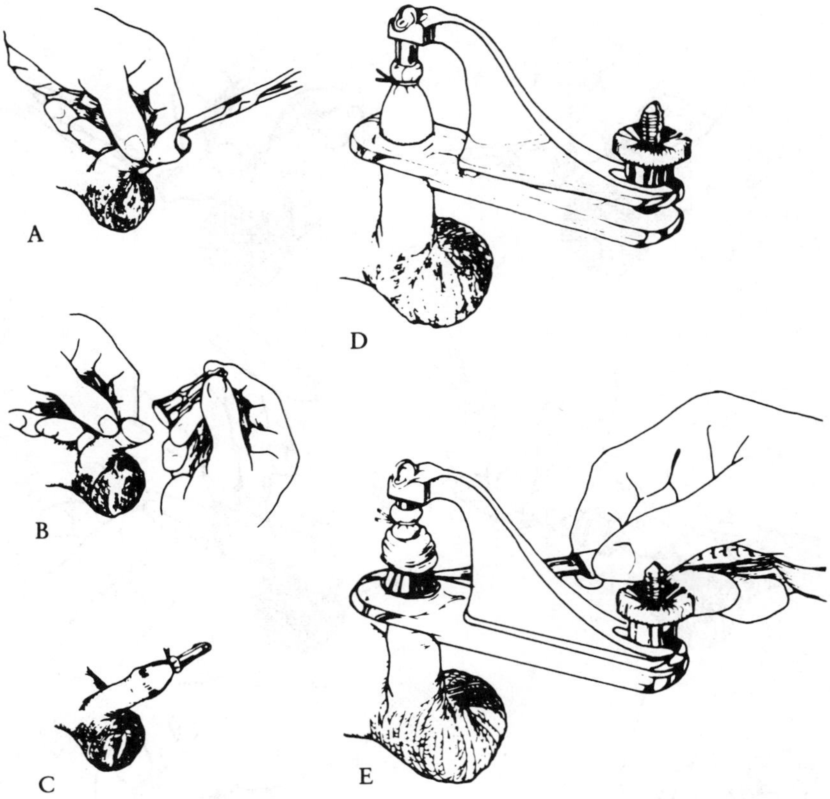

Figure 37–7. Gomco and circumcision technique (From Coen, R.W., and Koffler, H.: Primary Care of the Newborn. Boston, Little, Brown & Co., Inc., 1987; as adapted from Wallerstein, E.: Circumcision: An American Health Fallacy. New York, Springer, 1980.)

1987). Besides vehicular trauma, major safety risks during the first month of life include airway obstruction caused by defective multipiece pacifiers, airway compression caused by necklaces and pacifier strings, suffocation caused by improper bedding, thermal burns during bathing, pet and rat bites, hyperthermia from overwrapping in warm weather, and abusive reactions to crying.

DIAPERING AND CARE OF THE PERINEUM, UMBILICAL STUMP, AND PENIS

Diapering and its complications are discussed in chapter 51. Umbilical stump management is discussed above in Routines for the First Few Days. The uncircumcised penis should be cleaned carefully at each diaper change. The foreskin should not be fully retracted during the newborn period. Until healed, the circumcised penis should be wrapped in petroleum jelly gauze, changed with each diapering, or, at the very least, daily.

FEEDING ADVICE

Expectant mothers should strongly be encouraged to plan on nursing their babies. Exceptions to this rule are rare: mothers who may, in their breast milk, pass on the human immunodeficiency virus (HIV), the human T-cell leukemia-lymphoma virus (the human T-lymphotropic virus type I or HTLV-I), and, perhaps, the cytomegalovirus (CMV) (Oxtoby, 1988); mothers who have active pulmonary tuberculosis; mothers needing certain prescription drugs; mothers addicted to certain illicit substances; and mothers who, for whatever private reasons, clearly do not want to nurse. Even mothers from demographic groups with low breast-feeding rates can be influenced favorably by professional advice (Joffe and Radius, 1987; Kurinij et al., 1988; and Winikoff et al., 1987). Although they may not nurse for long, ambivalent breast feeders can still impart to their babies the immunologic advantages of colostrum and, apparently, the less well characterized advantages of transitional and mature milk.

Normal newborns, who are usually alert or easily arousable for an hour or so after birth, should be offered the breast as soon as possible. Suckling stimulates maternal secretion of oxytocin from the posterior pituitary and prolactin from the anterior pituitary. In the mother, oxytocin stimulates contraction of the myometrium, helping to prevent uterine hemorrhage, and stimulates contraction of the mammary myoepithelial cells, propelling milk toward and through the nipple. Prolactin stimulates milk production primarily.

The keys to successful lactation are the mother's confidence and the baby's sucking reflex. It is almost always the case that confident mothers have no serious problems nourishing alert, hungry, healthy babies. But maternal anxiety inhibits oxytocin-stimulated myoepithelial contraction, thus giving the impression that milk is not being produced in ade-

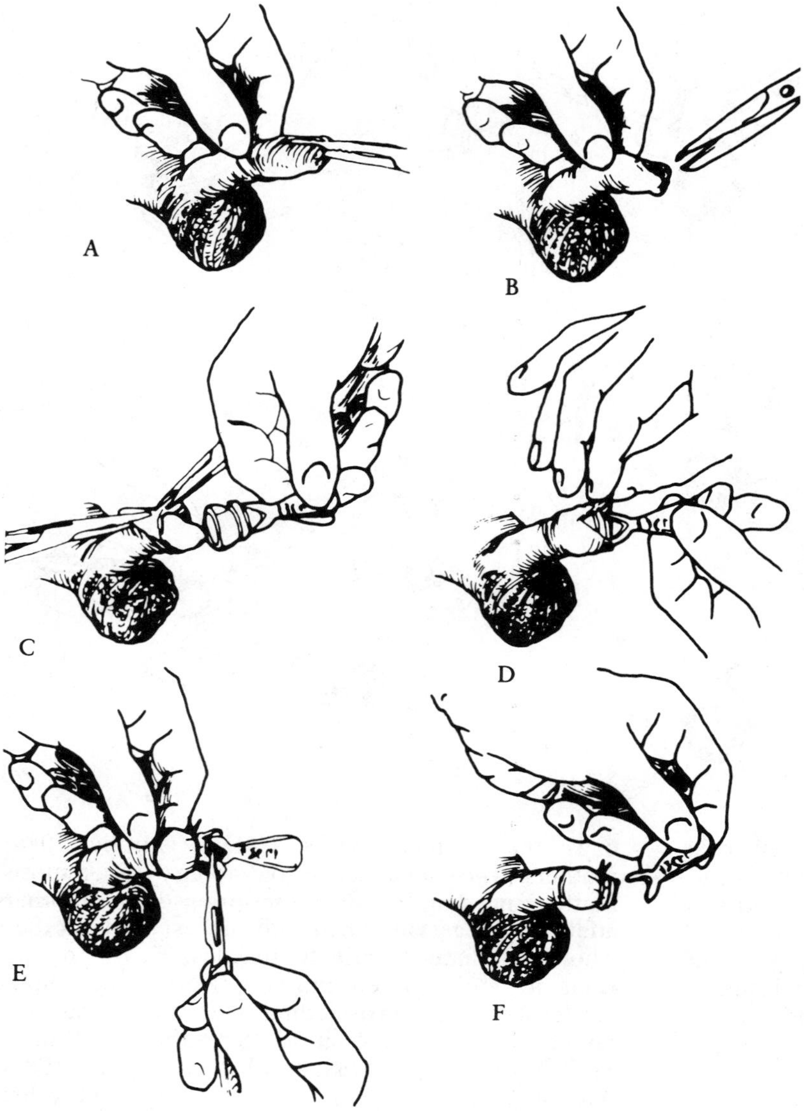

Figure 37–8. Plastibell circumcision technique. (From Coen, R.W., and Koffler, H.: Primary Care of the Newborn. Boston, Little, Brown & Co., Inc., 1987; as adapted from Wallerstein, E.: Circumcision: An American Health Fallacy. New York, Springer, 1980.)

quate quantity, further degrading self-assurance. Premature babies or babies with neurologic deficits or cardiovascular or pulmonary disease or sleepy babies not being fed "on demand" may not suck actively enough to maintain prolactin at levels sufficient to stimulate lactation. Breast pumping, breast milk storage or banking, and tube feedings may be indicated (Helsing and King, 1982).

"Demand" feeding matches milk supply to milk requirement physiologically, and it minimizes fussing by allowing the baby's circadian rhythm to mature smoothly. Trying to "normalize" a demand schedule too early is unwise, since it gives parents an opportunity to fail, an opportunity to think their baby is refusing to cooperate.

In the newborn period, energy requirement for growth is about 120 kcal. per kg. per day. Many competently composed and packaged nonhuman milk formulas are available, most providing about 0.6 to 0.7 kcal. per ml.; leading formulas are detailed in chapter 38. In developed countries, these formulas can be used safely as primary feedings or as convenient supplements to breast milk. In developing countries, they are usually transported dry and then mixed with local water, which is frequently not sterile (Habicht et al., 1988).

Iron supplementation of breast milk is not necessary in the newborn period, owing to enhanced iron absorption. Vitamin supplementation is sometimes provided. Iron supplementation of artificial formulas is desirable. The common suspicion that iron supplementation causes "colic" is unfounded (Nelson et al., 1988).

Neither human milk nor cow's milk contains a significant amount of fluoride, and an infant's intake of fluoridated tap water is hard to predict. Accordingly, fluoride intake must often be supplemented; two weeks of age is the recommended starting time and 0.25 mg. per day the recommended intake. But oversupplementation—even just twice the recommended daily intake—can discolor tooth enamel, so supplementation should be prescribed only for those babies unlikely to receive 0.25 mg. per day from diet and tap water (Herrmann and Roberts, 1987).

Colic connotes excessive, "unjustified" crying in otherwise healthy infants. The term is an antique and a misnomer; there is no colic in colic. Although a consensus on pathophysiology and behavioral dynamics is yet to form (Moore et al., 1988; Taubman et al., 1988; Woolridge and Fisher, 1988; and Schmitt, 1986), pharmacologic therapies for colic remain sharply inconsistent with most leading theories.

POSTPARTUM DEPRESSION

At some point before baby and parents go home, specific mention should be made of postpartum depression, a common phenomenon of largely somatic origin. The emerging neuroendocrine model of postpartum depression can be described in simple terms and should be stressed; older behavioral models are poorly supported scientifically, and their emphasis is ill-advised psychologically. Parents should know in advance that postpartum depression, in its myriad forms, may subtract from the happiness of early motherhood but does not imply maternal incapacity or unconscious rejection of infant or consort. Postpartum depression should not be feared, but it is unpleasant and even occasionally dangerous, and the physician should describe its symptoms and ask to be informed of their occurrence. See chapter 66.

THE FIRST RETURN VISIT

A short check-in at two weeks is advisable, especially for inexperienced parents. Nursery problems may need follow-up, and PKU and galactosemia screens may need repetition if hospital discharge preceded full feedings. In developing countries, bacille Calmette-Guérin (BCG) inoculation and rotavirus vaccination may be performed. This is the best time to discuss colic and the mother's plans, if any, to return to work outside the home.

FEVER IN THE FIRST MONTH OF LIFE

In-hospital parental teaching will often have included safe use of a thermometer, but temperature determination and interpretation in the baby's first month of life are so tricky that physicians should discourage parents from using thermometer readings when making care-seeking decisions. Most temperature elevations in the newborn period do not imply true emergencies, and rapidly progressive diseases, such as infection caused by the group B beta-hemolytic streptococcus, enteric bacteria, or *Streptococcus pneumoniae*, may present with elevated, depressed, or normal core temperature.

A well-wrapped baby normal on physical examination except for a mildly elevated core temperature should be re-examined after lying unwrapped on a blanket in a comfortably warm examining room. If, after an interval of 20 to 30 minutes, temperature normalizes, the parents may be reassured. They should be advised not to overwrap their baby and should be asked to report on their baby's condition after 6 to 12 hours. With this sole exception—environmental fever—prudent practice would dictate further diagnostic procedures, such as total and differential leukocyte counts, and, most important, re-examination in several hours—in other words, at the return of laboratory values—either in an outpatient or inpatient setting. Many physicians would also culture blood, examine and culture urine and cerebrospinal fluid, and perform a chest radiogram. Some physicians would, in addition, hospitalize all febrile babies under a month old and administer systemic antibiotics pending the maturation of cultures. All in all, meticulous physical examination and early repeat evaluation are the best guides to management.

No baby in the first month of life should have his fever evaluated over the telephone. No baby in the first month of life should have his fever treated with antipyretics. A baby in the first month of life whose fever needs symptomatic control is clearly sick enough to be hospitalized for definitive diagnosis and well-chosen therapy.

Making Sense of Shock, Distress, and Depression in the Newborn Period

TIMING

A baby depressed immediately after birth is likely to have been distressed in utero, injured in labor or delivery, or overwhelmed by the metabolic demands of the birth process. Explanations include placental insufficiency, placental hemorrhage or fetomaternal transfusion, hypoxic or traumatic encephalopathy, anesthetic or narcotic depression, acute ascending infection, lethal chromosomal defect, or secondary apnea from another cause. Many such babies, once removed from difficult intrauterine conditions, will improve, either spontaneously or with stimulation or, in the case of opioid depression, with naloxone. Others will respond only slowly or not at all to full ventilatory support and pharmacologic intervention.

A baby vigorous at birth but distressed shortly thereafter may be suffering the effects of prematurity generally, pulmonary immaturity specifically, a pulmonary malformation, a pulmonary aspiration syndrome, excess residual lung fluid, or a cardiovascular malformation or malfunction of little consequence under the conditions of fetal circulation but of much greater consequence in extrauterine life.

A baby apparently normal at birth but in trouble some hours or even a day or so later may be "running low" on a vital substance, such as glucose, calcium, magnesium, blood, or a dependency-producing drug; may be showing signs of infection; or may be evolving another type of pathology, such as cerebral edema from otherwise unsuspected head trauma or hypoxia.

A sick baby, particularly a premature baby, having unexpected problems after steady progress may be declaring a systemic infection, a gastrointestinal catastrophe (classically, necrotizing enterocolitis), a cerebral problem, such as a seizure, or a neurodevelopmental problem, such as an apneic spell.

A baby apparently normal at discharge from the nursery but now sick later in the first month of life may be demonstrating a problem previously overlooked, such as a congenital heart lesion, pulmonary malformation, or central nervous system defect, or may be presenting with a disease, usually infectious, that was acquired before, during, just after, or long after delivery. Late-onset group B beta-hemolytic streptococcal sepsis, listeriosis, chlamydial infection, and HSV infection, although acquired antepartum or intrapartum, may present after a considerable interval (as may other infections not so likely to cause shock, distress, or depression).

CLINICAL SETTING

Many problems predisposing to shock, distress, or depression can be anticipated antepartum: prematurity, postmaturity, intrauterine growth retardation from whatever cause (such as pregnancy-induced hypertension), multiple gestation, sonographically resolvable malformations, erythroblastosis fetalis, diabetic gestation, certain congenital and perinatally acquired infections, drug effect, and drug dependency. Other predispositions to shock, distress, or depression should come quickly to mind once delivery has been accomplished: hyaline membrane disease in the premature baby; meconium aspiration syndrome in the meconium-stained baby; intracranial hemorrhage in the traumatized baby; hypoglycemia in the premature, stressed, or macrosomic baby; addisonian crisis in the masculinized phenotypic female. Even after discharge, clinical setting can be a clue to diagnosis; pyloric stenosis (Breaux et al., 1988) in the thin but hungry first-born male is a classic example.

PREDOMINANT FINDING

Shock may be differentiated on clinical grounds into hypovolemic, cardiogenic, or septic varieties. Hypovolemic and cardiogenic shock are common final expressions of the full range of lethal pathologies; babies who are septic or who have sustained a critical cerebral insult may present in cardiovascular collapse.

Distress in the newborn is typically respiratory. The term respiratory distress connotes difficult air movement and suggests labored or stridorous breathing. The term respiratory distress syndrome (RDS) indicates hyaline membrane disease specifically and implies expiratory grunting, a classic RDS sign found also in pneumothorax, hypothermia, and polycythemia. Babies who are tachypneic are often in respiratory distress, although their distress may only be the transient tachypnea that marks the incomplete resorption of residual lung fluid. But tachypnea may also be seen in babies whose distress is not at all respiratory but, rather, metabolic, as in respiratory compensation of a metabolic acidosis, or neurologic, as in central hyperventilation.

Depression is a nonspecific sign and is best evaluated empirically. Babies who are easily stimulated physically or with a few positive-pressure breaths may be perfectly normal. Those responding to naloxone may need no special care beyond the first few hours. Those whose depression is not easily reversed or whose depression deepens are probably significantly damaged or seriously ill.

Other predominant signs, such as cyanosis, have been discussed in previous sections.

RESPONSE TO EARLY DIAGNOSTIC AND THERAPEUTIC INTERVENTIONS

Diagnostic procedures and therapeutic trials must be undertaken systematically. Their goals are the reliable narrowing of differential diagnoses. Their triple risks are the suggestion of unwarranted conclusions, the exacerbation of existing pathology, and the creation of iatrogenic damage.

Resuscitation of the Newborn

ATTITUDE

The amazing cost and the tragic outcome of many newborn hospitalizations have affected attitudes toward newborn resuscitation (Berseth et al., 1986). Intensive efforts applied to the newborn are sometimes misapplied, but resuscitation saves many babies who eventually will prove undamaged or only mildly damaged. An intraresuscitative re-evaluation may demonstrate the futility of full or continued efforts, particularly in very-low-birth-weight babies already receiving intensive support, but resuscitation should not be withheld entirely without compellingly humane cause. In the United States, the "Baby Doe" problem has complicated these decisions, although largely through misapprehension of the relevant rulings, regulations, and statutes (Todres et al., 1988, and Walters, 1988).

ADAPTING ADULT RESUSCITATIVE METHODS TO NEWBORNS

Physicians accustomed to the resuscitation of adults must thoughtfully adapt their critical-care practices to the resuscitation of newborns, in which population respiratory insufficiency predominates. Resuscitative habits acquired during the revival of asystolic, fibrillating, failing, or ischemic adult hearts will not save many babies. Primary cardiac arrest does occur in newborns, but it is rare. Acute cardiogenic pulmonary edema and acute pulmonary embolization are likewise much less common.

Response to volume expansion is not the same in newborns as in adults. Newborn stroke volume is practically fixed; therefore, cardiac output is rate-dependent and is not substantially increased by preload augmentation. Rapid volume expansion may cause the ductus arteriosus to dilate, producing a seemingly paradoxical hypotension. Rapid volume expansion, as might occur with sodium bicarbonate therapy for presumed metabolic acidosis, may cause periventricular or intraventricular hemorrhage, especially in premature babies. Nonmeticulous adult fluid practices are unacceptable in newborn resuscitation.

In adult resuscitations, hyperoxemia is a welcome sign that vigorous efforts, including the liberal use of supplemental oxygen, have been successful. In newborns, particularly prematures, supplemental oxygen must be administered more carefully, since even transient hyperoxemia increases the risk of blindness from retrolental fibroplasia, and hyperoxia of uncertain duration predisposes to bronchopulmonary dysplasia. That said, failure to administer sufficient supplemental oxygen in a resuscitation may result in brain damage or death.

Compared with adult resuscitation, acute vascular access is much more easily obtained in freshly delivered newborns with patent umbilical veins, but much more tediously secured if peripheral veins must be used or if central venous catheters must be placed at nonumbilical sites. Arterial blood gas sampling is harder, and acceptable sites are somewhat different: umbilical, radial, temporal, and posterior tibial arteries, but not brachial or femoral arteries. Smaller samples of both venous and arterial blood can be used for testing, and reported potassium values are much more likely to be spuriously high, reflecting erythrocyte lysis.

Carrying an age-appropriate "code card" can be reassuring (Rockney, 1988, and American Academy of Pediatrics, 1988).

STEP-BY-STEP RESUSCITATION IMMEDIATELY AFTER DELIVERY

Step 1. Consider Meconium Aspiration as a Risk in the Baby Needing Resuscitation

If thick meconium is evident, suction the trachea, hypopharynx, oropharynx, and mouth and then the nares and nasopharynx, preferably before stimulating a respiratory gasp and *always* before initiating positive-pressure ventilation. Asphyxia tolerance is greater in the newborn than in the older child or the adult, and extending asphyxia just long enough to prevent or lessen the severity of meconium aspiration is a good trade. If breathing has begun, suctioning should still be tried, since meconium may persist in accessible locations for 20 minutes or more. If a meconium-stained baby suddenly deteriorates, consider the possibility of a pulmonary air leak; percuss, ascultate, and transilluminate the chest for evidence of pneumothorax or pneumomediastinum.

Meconium is found in amniotic fluid in about 10 per cent of births; its "terminal" passage is usually not a respiratory risk; overly aggressive suctioning can itself cause trouble; and meconium-stained babies born apneic obviously have other serious problems as well. The risk of meconium aspiration should be assessed quickly, and retrieval maneuvers should either be skipped or performed efficiently.

Step 2. Check for Spontaneous Movement and Try to Elicit Spontaneous Respirations

The baby born totally limp, cyanotic, unresponsive, and bradycardic, although "stillborn" in the true sense of the word, can sometimes be resuscitated with reasonable results. If spontaneous respiratory movement can be elicited by sensory stimulation, the baby is exhibiting primary apnea and might begin gasping if left alone; if spontaneous respiratory movement cannot be elicited by sensory stimulation, the baby is exhibiting secondary apnea and would probably not gasp again without resuscitation. The majority of babies needing resuscitation are born in primary apnea. Although every depressed newborn deserves a resuscitative trial, those born in secondary apnea are less likely to respond and are less likely to recover without major sequelae. Quick, initial differentiation of primary from secondary apnea can help the resuscitating physician decide how long his efforts should persist.

Step 3. Dry the Skin and Hair

Cold stress is a frequently unremembered impediment to successful resuscitation. If the baby is lying on a blanket, drying can be incorporated into step 2 as the stimulatory maneuver used in the attempt to elicit spontaneous respirations. If not, a warm dry towel should be requested as step 4 is begun.

Step 4. Commence Bag-and-Mask Ventilation

The pharynx should be cleared of any obstruction and a birth-weight-appropriate mask fitted snuggly over the baby's nose and mouth, the baby held slightly head down and the head itself held in the "sniffing" position. Initial pressures of 20 to 30 cm. H_2O or higher may be needed. Compensatory hyperventilation—about 50 breaths per minute—is the best way to deal with metabolic acidosis during newborn resuscitation. However, rapid pH change, even rapid pH "improvement," is dangerous; steady, gradual raising of the pH should be the goal of compensatory hyperventilation.

Do not commence bag-and-mask ventilation if a scaphoid abdomen suggests diaphragmatic herniation, since air under pressure will enter the stomach and thence, perhaps, the intrathoracic gut, making the ventilation of presumably hypoplastic lungs even more difficult. If diaphragmatic herniation is suspected, proceed directly to tracheal intubation.

Depending on their configuration, self-inflating bags may not be able to deliver oxygen at high concentrations or any gas at high pressures. Anesthesia bags do not have the limitations of self-inflating bags, but their safe use requires prior familiarity and they *must* be used with pressure manometers. Pure oxygen is still the gas available in most delivery rooms; monitored retreat from 100 per cent supplemental oxygen is advisable to lessen the risks of retrolental fibroplasia and bronchopulmonary dysplasia.

Step 5. Commence External Cardiac Massage if the Heart Rate Does Not Rise Rapidly to Above 80 Beats per Minute Despite Adequate Ventilatory Support

A second operator is necessary if cardiac massage is required. Both thumbs should be placed over the midsternum and the other fingers placed under the spine; the two-handed, thumbs-on-the-sternum technique has been shown superior to the one-handed technique (David, 1988). Smooth compressions of 1 to 1.5 cm. should be made 100 to 120 times per minute. It is wise to coordinate ventilations and chest compressions to lessen the detrimental venous-return effect of positive-pressure ventilation and to lessen the risk of pneumothorax and pneumomediastinum; in practice, good coordination is hard to achieve. Heart rate is most easily monitored at the umbilicus, less easily at the femoral arteries.

Step 6. Intubate the Trachea if Bag-and-Mask Ventilation Seems Inadequate

A size 1 Miller laryngoscope blade—the term-infant-sized blade—can be used on babies of all sizes. Endotracheal tubes sized 2.5 mm., 3.0 mm., 3.5 mm., and 4.0 mm. should be available, as should a bendable metal obturator or stylette with which to stiffen the endotracheal tube for better control. An obturator can be dangerous; its tip must never extend beyond the end of the endotracheal tube; an obturated endotracheal tube must never be forced against tissue. Obturators are often used because endotracheal tubes, kept at the ready under radiant warmers, have become flaccid by the time they are needed. Keeping endotracheal tubes cool makes obturator use less of an issue. Sticking endotracheal tubes in a cup of sterile ice is very helpful, although a bit unorthodox.

As shown in Figure 37–9, take the laryngoscope in the left hand. Open the baby's mouth with the right hand. Slip the laryngoscope blade into the right side of the mouth and displace the tongue gently to the left. If it is comfortable to do so, place the fourth and fifth digits of the laryngoscope hand under the baby's chin or, in smaller babies, under the neck, and lift slightly. Visualize the epiglottis. Advance the blade tip into the vallecula (the "little valley" just anterior to the epiglottis itself); alternatively, "pick up" the epiglottis with the blade tip. Either way, lift straight up gently on the laryngoscope handle. Suctioning may be needed, and, sometimes, the light pressure of an assistant's finger on the trachea may be helpful.

The larynx must be visualized! Accept no substitutes! If the larynx cannot positively be identified, give up and return to bag-and-mask ventilation immediately. Try again after about 30 seconds. The endotracheal tube must be seen passing through the larynx and into the trachea. If the tube is not seen actually passing through the larynx, esophageal intubation must be assumed. Listening for ventilation sounds over the chest is a good habit but is not a definitive way to confirm endotracheal intubation in the newborn.

The endotracheal tube used should be the largest one that will allow an audible air leak at ventilatory pressures around 30 to 40 cm. of water. Some tubes are tapered at the optimal laryngeal level; nontapered tubes, which are generally preferred, are often marked with a black circle—the "vocal-cord line"—at this same level, the object being tube tip placement above the carina, not in the right main-stem bronchus. After securing the tube to the face with tape, compare breath sounds in the right lateral lung field to breath sounds in the left lateral lung field. If only the right lung is being ventilated, withdraw the tube a little, listen again, and retape. Eventually, safe tube position should be confirmed on a portable anteroposterior chest radiogram. Nasotracheal intubation, a procedure requiring the use of McGill forceps, may be preferred primarily in some babies with micrognathia or may be preferred generally to enhance tube stability.

Step 7. Insert an Orogastric Feeding Tube to Decompress the Stomach

Gastric distention can interfere with diaphragmatic excursion, and gastric contents can easily be aspirated, whether or not an endotracheal tube (always uncuffed in newborns) has been placed. Gastric content is relatively greater in babies born by cesarean section. Proper placement of an orogastric tube incidentally confirms esophageal patency.

Step 8. Assess Volume Status and Replete Absolute or Functional Deficiencies

Blood pressure is often difficult to measure during resuscitation. It is frequently very low, and even

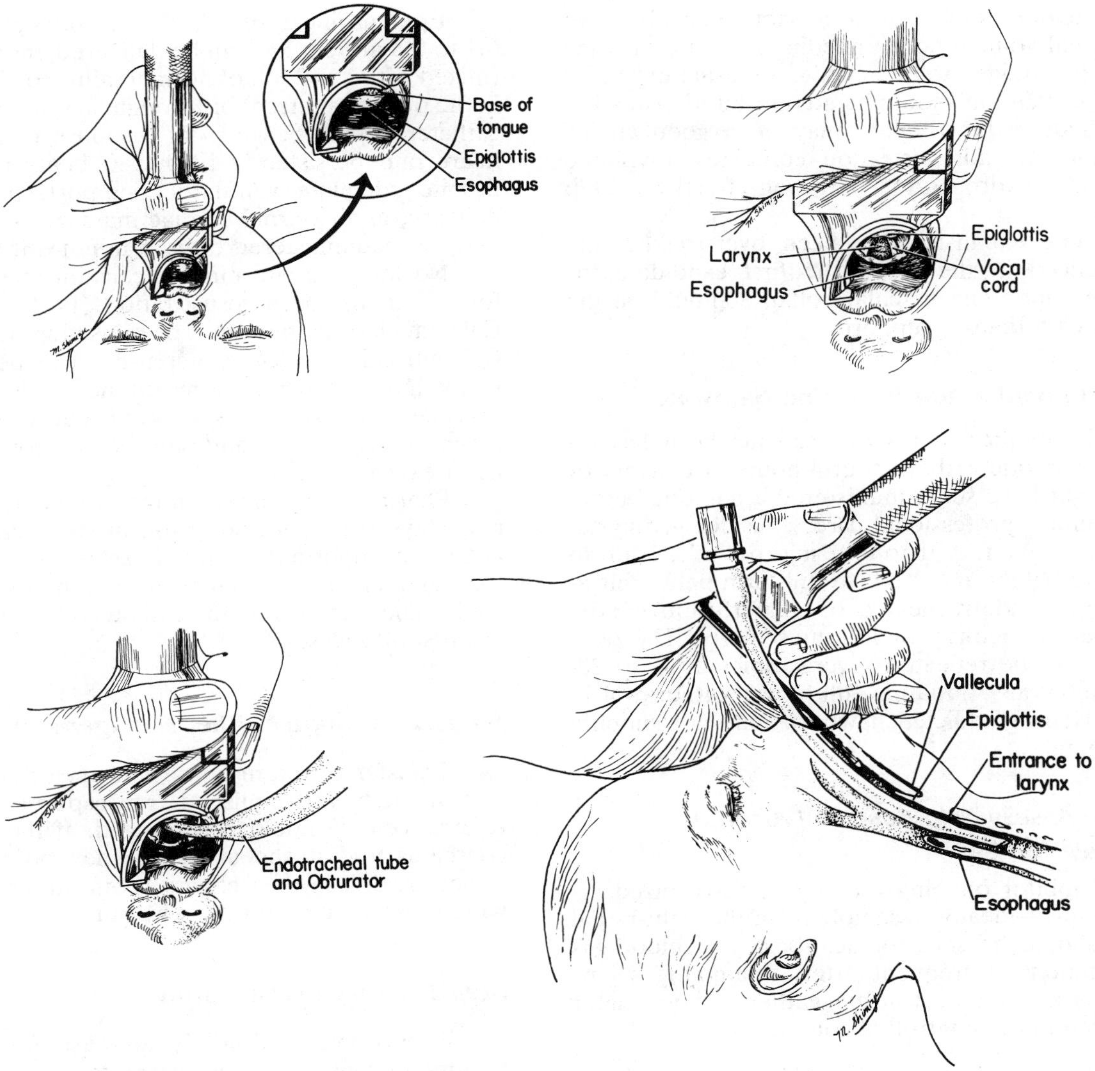

Figure 37–9. Direct laryngoscopy and intubation of the neonate. (From Klaus, M.H., and Fanaroff, A.A. [Eds.]: Care of the High-Risk Neonate. 3rd ed. Philadelphia, W.B. Saunders Company, 1986.)

when it is not low, auscultating Korotkoff sounds can be challenging, even when using a Doppler device. Hypotensive babies have weak peripheral pulses, but newborns with substantial right-to-left shunting have large pulse pressures and, so, may have pulses that are relatively easy to feel.

Respiratory support, with or without short-term external cardiac massage, should bring the heart rate to above 100 beats per minute in most newborns. When it does not, absolute or functional volume depletion should be considered. Using sterile technique, place a radio-opaque plastic catheter into the umbilical vein, no more than 5 cm. plus the umbilical stump length to avoid physical, osmotic, or pharmacologic trauma to the liver. Dispatch blood for a spun hematocrit, but remember that acute blood loss may not yet be reflected in the hematocrit. Consider inoculating a blood culture.

If acute blood loss is suspected (as it might be from inspection of the placenta) or if fetomaternal transfusion is suspected (as it might be after cesarean delivery because of cord clamping above the level of the placenta) or if massive hemolysis is suspected (as it should be in babies born to Rh-negative mothers), a transfusion of fresh whole blood, a plasma expander, Ringer's lactate, or normal saline should be considered. Low-antibody-titer, O-negative, fresh whole blood cross-matched against maternal blood is the volume expander of choice in this setting, but it is available only as a result of forethought. Blood can be drawn from the placental umbilical vein or from a vein on the placental surface. Placental blood is the baby's own blood and, barring ongoing immune-mediated hemolysis, is theoretically ideal. However, bacterial contamination and microembolization are risks; careful asepsis, use of a heparin-washed syringe, and interposition of a blood filter between syringe and catheter can reduce these risks. Whichever fluid is used, 10 ml. per kg. can be administered once or, as indicated, more than once.

Septic or otherwise-acidotic babies may also have a functional volume deficit needing repletion. If they are not also judged to be anemic, a plasma expander or a saline solution should be administered instead of blood. Sodium bicarbonate may be a good choice here, since its administration combines a volume effect and a hydrogen-ion buffering effect. See step 11 below.

Volume expansion has been overstressed and overpracticed in the past. The first candidate for blame in continuing vascular collapse should be the quality of ventilatory support.

Step 9. Consider Administering Naloxone

If the mother of a depressed newborn has received a narcotic within about 4 hours of delivery or if she might have self-administered a narcotic before coming under professional care, consider giving naloxone as Narcan, 0.01 to 0.02 mg. per ml., 1 ml. to premature babies and 2 ml. to full-term babies intravenously or endotracheally, or, if perfusion is adequate, subcutaneously or intramuscularly. The dose may have to be repeated several times at 5- to 20-minute intervals. Initiating full-blown withdrawal in a severely drug-addicted newborn may not simplify management.

Step 10. Assess Acid-Base and Arterial Blood Gas Status

To monitor ongoing therapy, a heparinized arterial sample—ideally, a sample from the right-radial artery—should be sent for acid-base and blood-gas determination. If frequent arterial sampling seems necessary, an umbilical artery catheter should later be inserted under controlled conditions.

Step 11. Consider Pharmacologic Intervention

Naloxone has been discussed in step 9.

Sodium bicarbonate can be used to treat primary metabolic acidosis or metabolic acidosis complicating prolonged resuscitation. However, in this second and more common case, its use is often inappropriate, since ventilatory insufficiency is a feature of most prolonged resuscitations, and ventilatory insufficiency precludes the hoped-for pH rise.

Sodium bicarbonate 1 mEq. per ml., 1 to 2 mEq. per kg. should be given slowly; some physicians prefer to dilute sodium bicarbonate 1:1 with sterile water; readministration every 5 minutes may be indicated. However, overadministration of sodium bicarbonate is dangerous; iatrogenic hyperosmolarity and alkalosis can damage or kill. Further treatment should be guided by arterial (or venous) pH determinations if available. Acidosis itself can sometimes elevate the blood pressure; alkali therapy in these cases may simultaneously correct the acidosis and drop the blood pressure.

Epinephrine 1:10,000, 0.01 to 0.03 mg. per kg., 0.1 to 0.3 ml. per kg. can be delivered endotracheally (mixed with 1 to 2 ml. of normal saline to aid dispersal in the pulmonary tree) or through an umbilical venous catheter. It can be given in response to asystole or heart rate persistently below 80 beats per minute despite adequate ventilatory support, pure-oxygen delivery, and external cardiac massage. Epinephrine may be readministered every 5 minutes if needed.

No longer is atropine or calcium recommended for use in newborn resuscitation (Peckham, 1986). Calcium chloride has often been used in desperation. Calcium chloride (or epinephrine) can be given directly into the heart in moribund babies, but this practice is almost never successful. Laceration of vital structures is routine and salvage of more than the heart extremely rare.

Pharmacologic interventions of many types are mainstays of modern newborn intensive care but are not often important in initial resuscitation. Ventilatory and circulatory support in a neutral thermal environment are surely the essential elements in most successful "saves."

Step 12. Arrange Further Management

Transfer to the in-house nursery or special-care unit should be accomplished or transport to a regional referral center should be arranged. If the mother is conscious and if she alone or she and the baby's father are still in the delivery room, move the infant within arm's length on the way out.

Step 13. Talk to the Family

Report events candidly and ask for whatever treatment consent seems warranted. If transfer to another institution seems necessary, assure the family that continuity of care will not suffer, either immediately or over the long term.

Step 14. Write Temporary Monitoring and Fluid Orders

Until disposition is fully determined, vital-sign and monitoring orders should be individualized to address anticipated risks.

Fully normal newborns can manage nicely with no fluid intake for well over a day; they do not need vascular access routes; they are not sick; and they have not just been resuscitated. But babies who have just been severely stressed or who are otherwise sick have particular needs, and fluid orders written for them must be individualized. Using "normal requirements" only as a guide, the physician must often compose fluids from scratch, ordering each constituent separately.

Newborn maintenance requirements are based on the following standards (Levin et al., 1984):

Water	100 ml. per kg. every 24 hours
Sodium (Na)	4 mEq. per kg. every 24 hours
Potassium (K)	2 mEq. per kg. every 24 hours
Chloride (Cl)	4 mEq. per kg. every 24 hours
Calcium (Ca)	50 to 200 mg. per kg. every 24 hours
Magnesium (Mg)	0.4 to 0.8 mEq. per kg. every 24 hours
Phosphate (PO_4)	15 to 50 mg. per kg. every 24 hours
Glucose	100 to 200 mg. per kg. every 24 hours

During the first day of life, water and glucose requirements would likely be met by a solution of dextrose 10 per cent and water pumped at 4 ml. per kg. per hour. But resuscitated babies should be fluid-restricted to no more than two thirds the water rate for at least the first postresuscitation day. Whether their base rate is full or restricted, babies under radiant warmers should be given 20 per cent more water and babies under bilirubin lights 10 per cent more water. Furthermore, babies whose rectal temperature varies above or below 37.8° C. should have their water rates compensated up or down 12 per cent per degree centigrade.

Blood glucose screening may prompt an adjustment in dextrose administration.

Calcium, as calcium gluconate, may or may not be required; until recently, calcium gluconate supplementation was provided compulsively to many babies who did not need it.

When urine is finally produced, isosthenuria suggests that "renal work" has been minimized by the administration of well-ordered fluids. Sodium, potassium, and chloride may be added on the second day of life if urination has begun. Regular serum sodium, potassium, and chloride measurements should guide further adjustments.

Respiratory Problems

THE RESPIRATORY DISTRESS SYNDROME (RDS) (HYALINE MEMBRANE DISEASE)

RDS is caused by surfactant deficiency or surfactant immaturity, perhaps exacerbated by pulmonary hypoperfusion (Klaus and Fanaroff, 1986). The classic histologic finding is a hyaline-staining pseudomembrane lining an uninflated alveolus. RDS affects about 10 per cent of all premature babies and some full-term babies as well. It is the greatest single cause of nursery mortality in developed countries.

RDS presents with difficulty initiating respirations, expiratory grunting or whining, sternal and intercostal retractions, nasal flaring, tachypnea or bradypnea, and, often, cyanosis. Chest radiography shows lung fields with a "ground-glass" appearance and air bronchograms (Fig. 37–10). Supplemental oxygen is sufficient for mildly affected babies, continuous positive airway pressure (CPAP) for some others, but many require mechanical ventilation (Carlo and Martin, 1986). Mild water and electrolyte restriction is helpful early in treatment. Frequent arterial blood gas determinations or some type of indirect continuous blood-gas monitoring is indispensable. Recovery occurs when endogenous surfactant production reaches adequate levels and is classically presaged by a spontaneous diuresis. Recovery is impeded by a host of common complicating problems, and slow pulmonary progress makes almost inevitable residual damage to lungs and, often, to other organs as well.

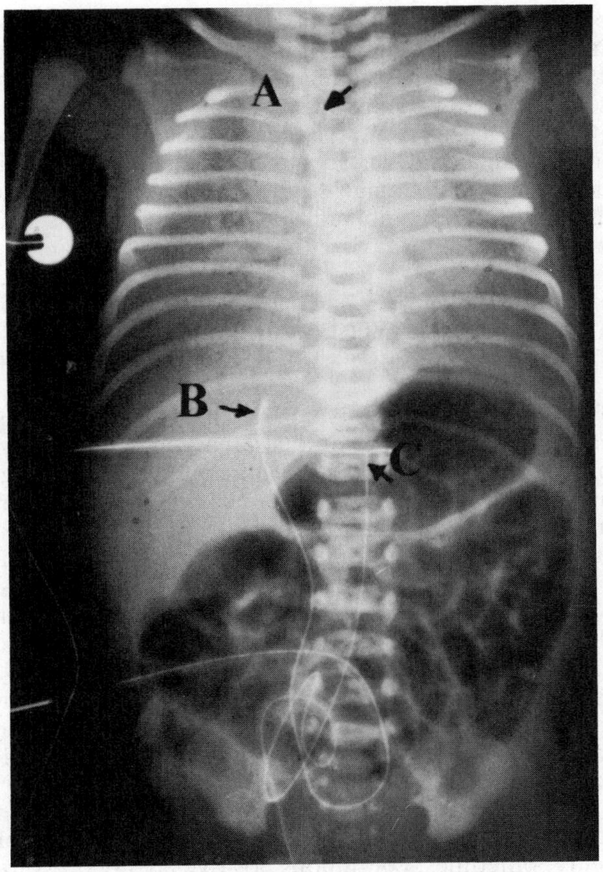

Figure 37–10. Anteroposterior roentgenogram of infant with hyaline membrane disease. Note granular lungs, air bronchogram, and air-filled esophagus. *A*, endotracheal tube; *B*, umbilical venous catheter at the junction of the umbilical vein ductus venosus, and portal vein. (From Behrman, R.E., and Vaughan, V.C., [Eds.]: Textbook of Pediatrics. 13th ed. Philadelphia, W.B. Saunders Company, 1987, p. 395.)

Many therapeutic innovations, intensive nutritional support chief among them, have improved salvage rates and quality. Novel ventilatory modes, such as high-frequency oscillatory ventilation, may or may not have a role (HIFI Study Group, 1989). Some severely affected babies can now be saved by the ventilatory rest achieved with extracorporeal membrane oxygenation (ECMO), but at significant risk to all organs other than the lungs, since thrombosis and thromboembolization are routine (Vogler et al., 1988), and at special risk to the brain, since ligation of the right internal carotid artery is currently necessary (Frattallone et al., 1988, and Schumacher et al., 1988). Despite these dangers, most ECMO survivors seem to be developing normally at 12 months of age (Glass et al., 1989). Therapeutic use of artificial and nonhuman animal surfactants has been disappointing; use of synthetic human surfactant, produced in large amounts by recombinant DNA techniques, seems more promising (Davis et al., 1988).

TRANSIENT TACHYPNEA OF THE NEWBORN (TTN)

The baby with TTN is typically otherwise normal and classically the product of a cesarean delivery. Tachypnea without distress, other than a little grunting, and usually without cyanosis, is observed; normal or mildly abnormal breath sounds are heard. Chest radiography shows central perihilar streaking and, often, a generous cardiac shadow.

Lack of a "vaginal squeeze" during cesarean delivery and incomplete resorption of fetal lung fluid are the reasons usually offered to explain TTN. Perihilar streaking may correspond to decreased pulmonary compliance. Tachypnea is presumably the most efficient way for these babies to minimize pulmonary work.

Special observation is needed, but either no treatment or just supplemental oxygen under 40 per cent. Sometimes, continuous positive airway pressure (CPAP) is indicated. Tachypnea persisting beyond 24 hours is not usually considered transient.

MECONIUM ASPIRATION

Meconium aspiration syndrome is caused by the presence of ball-valve collections of meconium in distal airways. Ventilation is made difficult primarily by airway obstruction and secondarily by air trapping and air leaking. Severely affected babies suffer multiple pneumothoraces and pneumomediastinum. Multiple complications make many of these babies unsalvageable. ECMO, despite its problems, has proved useful in otherwise hopeless cases.

PNEUMOTHORAX AND PNEUMOMEDIASTINUM

Pneumothorax or pneumomediastinum may be the first sign of the meconium aspiration syndrome. Spontaneous pneumothorax, if asymptomatic, requires no therapy. If associated with clinical signs of tension or other signs of respiratory distress, then evacuation is necessary. Chest radiography is needed, but, sometimes, action must be taken on clinical findings alone. A butterfly needle and catheter are used. The distal hub of the catheter is placed in a basin of sterile water, and the needle is introduced into the pneumothoracic region by "walking over" the appropriate rib, as if a pleural effusion were being tapped. Air under pressure will bubble into the basin. Alternatively, the hub can be connected to a two-way stopcock and the stopcock connected to a syringe containing a small amount of sterile water. The syringe can be used to evacuate several volumes of air. If air reaccumulates, chest tube placement becomes necessary. Breathing supplemental oxygen hastens absorption of pleural air (Klaus and Fanaroff, 1986).

PNEUMONIA

Perinatally acquired pneumonias, particularly group B beta-hemolytic streptococcal pneumonia, may closely resemble hyaline membrane disease. See Infectious Problems below and chapter 30.

Cardiovascular Problems

DISORDERS OF TRANSITION

Although fetal circulation may have been perfectly normal, the ductus arteriosus may close slowly, may close incompletely, may close and reopen during illness or during intravascular volume repletion or overexpansion, or may remain widely open for no apparent reason. Sick newborns with a patent ductus arteriosus (PDA) may develop congestive heart failure and may need pharmacologic PDA closure or surgical PDA ligation. Often, a mechanically ventilated baby failing to progress has an otherwise unsuspected PDA, at whose closure ventilatory support requirements start to decrease.

Persistent pulmonary hypertension of the newborn (PPHN) or "persistence of fetal circulation" may present idiopathically or in association with other serious illnesses. Affected babies are mostly full term. Pulmonary vascular resistance does not decline from, or it returns to, fetal levels, making adequate gas exchange impossible. Extremely intensive medical treatment is necessary in all cases; some babies sur(Levin et al., 1984).

CYANOTIC CONGENITAL HEART LESIONS

Central cyanosis should be evaluated as follows:

1. Physical examination should be performed with particular attention to breath sounds, arterial pulses, precordial configuration, precordial palpation and auscultation, and liver size.
2. A drop of blood should be smeared on a glass slide and exposed to 100 per cent oxygen. Color change to red excludes methemoglobinemia.
3. Hemoglobin and hematocrit should be measured, since polycythemia can cause both central cyanosis and congestive heart failure.

4. Arterial blood gas tensions and pH should be determined in room air (or at current supplemental oxygen settings) and then repeated in 100 per cent oxygen. In patients with cyanotic congenital heart disease, Pa_{O2} might rise by 10 to 15 mm. Hg but no higher. A rise of more than 25 mm. Hg suggests pulmonary disease.
5. A chest radiogram should be inspected for
   a. Primary pulmonary disease.
   b. Heart size.
   c. Heart shape.
   d. Pulmonary vascular markings, which should be classed as showing
      i. normal pulmonary blood flow.
      ii. increased pulmonary blood flow.
      iii. decreased pulmonary blood flow.
6. An electrocardiogram should be inspected for dysrhythmia and, with the help of a pediatric cardiologist, for other gross findings as well. Electrocardiograms performed or interpreted according to adult standards are useless except as rhythm strips.
7. An echocardiogram should be arranged at the earliest opportunity if it can be performed by an operator experienced with babies. Otherwise, echocardiography should be delayed pending transport to a regional center.
8. In babies with cyanotic congenital heart disease, cardiac catheterization (or, in special circumstances, a less invasive procedure) should be performed as soon as possible to define anatomy and guide therapy.

Cyanotic congenital heart lesions with diminished pulmonary blood flow include tetralogy of Fallot, pulmonary atresia with ventriculoseptal defect (pseudotruncus), pulmonary atresia without ventriculoseptal defect, critical pulmonary valvular stenosis, tricuspid atresia, Ebstein's anomaly of the tricuspid valve, and various other complex lesions.

Cyanotic congenital heart lesions with increased pulmonary blood flow include complete transposition of the great vessels, total anomalous pulmonary venous return, hypoplastic left heart syndrome, and persistent common truncus arteriosus (Levin et al., 1984).

NONCYANOTIC CONGENITAL HEART LESIONS

Noncyanotic congenital heart lesions include transposition of the great vessels with ventricular septal defect, isolated ventricular septal defect, aortic coarctation syndrome, and patent ductus arteriosus with pulmonary artery hypertension.

DYSRHYTHMIAS

Bradycardia can be seen in certain neurologic and metabolic disorders. Congenital heart block is usually seen in babies born to mothers with systemic lupus erythematosus; pacing is required. Paroxysmal atrial tachycardia (PAT), sometimes associated with Wolff-Parkinson-White syndrome, may convert to normal sinus rhythm with vagal stimulation, such as rectal examination or elicitation of the diving reflex (not recommended for the inexperienced). PAT requires digitalization and, often, cardioversion. Dysrhythmias should be treated in consultation with a pediatric cardiologist.

PERIPHERAL PULMONIC STENOSIS (PPS)

PPS is characterized by a soft systolic murmur heard best over the peripheral lung fields, usually in an otherwise normal newborn, often small. The PPS murmur is assumed to be due to turbulent flow in multiple branches of the pulmonary artery and is usually outgrown. Without other evidence of right-heart pressure elevation, PPS can be followed as a benign finding. PPS is much more commonly discussed in practice than in print.

Infectious Problems

Problems in newborns may be caused by maternal infection with or carriage of certain microorganisms:

1. Those known to be teratogenic—*Toxoplasma gondii,* rubella virus, CMV, HSV, *Treponema pallidum,* and HIV (known jointly as "TORCH-SH");

2. Those known to be acquired by otherwise normal babies either in utero or at delivery—*Chlamydia trachomatis,* pathogenic coliforms, CMV, HBV, HSV, HIV, *Listeria monocytogenes, Mycobacterium tuberculosis, Neisseria gonorrhoeae,* rubella virus, the group B beta-hemolytic streptococcus, *Toxoplasma gondii,* and *Treponema pallidum;* or

3. Those known to be or suspected of being passed in breast milk—CMV, HIV, HTLV-I.

Outside developed countries, additional infectious disease risks obtain.

Chorioamnionitis is a common cause of premature labor (Hillier, 1988) and neonatal infection. Babies born to mothers in whom chorioamnionitis has been suspected must be examined and observed carefully; total and differential leukocyte counts, blood cultures, and, often, lumbar punctures should be performed, and empirical administration of systemic antibiotics should be considered.

Babies born vaginally to mothers suffering a primary genital herpetic eruption are at high risk for serious herpetic infection. Babies born vaginally to mothers suffering a recurrent eruption are at lower risk (Brown et al., 1987a). However, neonatal herpetic infection also occurs in the offspring of unsuspected, asymptomatic HSV shedders (Prober et al., 1988). Babies delivered by cesarean section to avoid vaginal herpetic contact are not absolutely protected; rarely, ascending infection will prove already to have occurred. Any herpetiform skin lesion must be examined by Tzank preparation and viral culture, and every newborn with even one herpetic lesion must be treated expectantly for herpes encephalitis. The drug of choice is acyclovir.

Early-onset sepsis from perinatal acquisition of maternal organisms presents within 5 days of birth. Late-onset sepsis presents after 5 days and is likely to coexist with localized infection, such as meningitis. Organisms likely to cause early-onset sepsis include the group B beta-hemolytic streptococci (Payne et al., 1988), maternal gut bacteria, and *Listeria monocytogenes*. Organisms likely to cause late-onset sepsis include, in addition to the early-onset pathogens, *Haemophilus influenzae* and *Streptococcus pneumoniae*. Ampicillin and an aminoglycoside have long been first-choice antibiotics for both early-onset and late-onset sepsis, although newer agents, particularly cephalosporins, have come increasingly into use to cover strains less sensitive to older agents and to cover the wider variety of late-onset pathogens (Bradley, 1985).

The full range of intrauterine and newborn infections is extremely wide, both in terms of site and organism. See previous sections and chapter 30. Prophylactic and therapeutic protocols depend on local conditions and sensitivities; current recommendations should be followed in every case (Nelson, 1987).

Neurologic Problems

Hypoxic encephalopathy (Brann, 1986), periventricular and intraventricular hemorrhage (Allan and Volpe, 1986), and seizure disorders (Painter et al., 1986) require specialized evaluation and management.

Neonatal seizures always need to be explained as soon as possible but do not always need to be suppressed immediately. Traumatic, metabolic, toxic, infectious, and postasphyxial explanations should be considered quickly but as thoroughly as possible. When a correctable cause is discovered, such as hypoglycemia, seizure therapy can be definitive, not suppressive. But when neonatal seizures need to be suppressed, first therapy should be phenobarbital 10 to 20 mg. per kg. given intravenously over 5 to 10 minutes. If seizures persist or recur, an additional 10 mg. per kg. may be given an hour later and, if suppression is still inadequate, once more an hour after that. If phenobarbital maintenance seems necessary, 4 to 5 mg. per kg. per day may be given, intravenously or orally, divided into two doses. Phenytoin and other drugs must sometimes be added, but their use is more complicated. Prognosis for newborns with seizures is a function of ultimate diagnosis but is often optimistic. See chapter 60.

Drug withdrawal syndromes, characterized by jitteriness, irritability, hypertonicity, convulsions, hyperventilation, vomiting, diarrhea, and sweating, may occur in babies born to mothers taking various substances: narcotics (including methadone), benzodiazepines, phenobarbital, alcohol, pentazocine, cocaine, and others. Onset of symptoms is typically shortly after birth but in some cases of methadone withdrawal may be days or weeks later. Maternal history should be reviewed, and samples of blood and urine from mother and baby should be screened for narcotics and other toxic substances. Supportive care may have to be supplemented with phenobarbital or opiates and other depressants. Babies born to intravenous drug abusers should be evaluated for HBV and HIV exposure. Mothers being maintained on methadone should not breast feed their babies (Graef et al., 1988).

Cerebral palsy is a nonprogressive motor disorder with origins in pre- or perinatal life. It can often be anticipated. A low 5-minute Apgar score, seizure activity, and certain other neonatal signs are, taken together, significantly predictive (Ellenberg and Nelson, 1988). However, events occurring before labor and delivery are particularly important and relatively underappreciated (Ellis et al., 1988). Cerebral palsy can occur in infants and children with completely normal newborn histories (Nelson and Ellenberg, 1987).

Many embryopathies involving the central nervous system are recognized consequences of intrauterine infection or drug exposure. In developed countries, the fetal alcohol syndrome is the commonest preventable cause of mental retardation.

Metabolic Problems

Diabetic progeny require special evaluation and management. Residual hyperinsulinemia makes severe hypoglycemia a constant danger. Compulsive monitoring is required: blood glucose determinations at hours 0, 1, 2, 3, 6, 12, 24, and 48; serum calcium determinations at hours 6, 12, 24, and 48. Dextrose supplementation is required by the oral, the orogastric, or, usually, the intravenous route. Sometimes, while intravenous access is first being secured or after it has inadvertently been lost, glucagon 300 micrograms per kg. (maximum dose 1.0 mg.) can be given subcutaneously. Chronic hyperglycemia has many adverse effects, direct and indirect, and diabetic progeny have increased rates of specific congenital anomalies, perinatal asphyxia and trauma, RDS, polycythemia, hyperbilirubinemia, and other problems.

Congenital adrenal hyperplasia (CAH) is the outcome of various autosomally recessive defects in the enzymes needed to synthesize cortisol. Since pituitary feedback stimulation of the adrenal produces excess androgens, CAH often presents in the newborn period as virilization in the phenotypic female; in many phenotypic males the correct diagnosis is not made during life. In its common, salt-wasting form, CAH is caused by a deficiency of the enzyme 21-

hydroxylase. The affected baby is deficient in both hydrocortisone and aldosterone, and the renal distal tubular activity of whatever aldosterone is produced may be inhibited by 17-hydroxyprogesterone and progesterone. Presentation in addisonian crisis is therefore common. Emergent goals are the intravenous repletion of volume deficiency, initiation of glucocorticoid and mineralocorticoid maintenance therapy, and suppression of adrenocorticotropic hormone release. The most immediate needs are met by dextrose 5 per cent normal saline 20 ml. per kg. intravenously over 20 minutes, then hydrocortisone hemisuccinate (Solu-Cortef) 25 mg. by intravenous push, and then deoxycorticosterone acetate (DOCA) 1 mg. intramuscularly. Early consultation with a pediatric endocrinologist is essential.

Unexplained poor feeding, lethargy, irritability, convulsions, hypertonia, hypotonia, hyperventilation, or coma can be seen in babies whose blood ammonia is elevated. Many hyperammonemic babies lack specific urea cycle enzymes.

See also Postnatal Screening.

Gastrointestinal Problems

Many gastrointestinal problems have been described above. Management must often include pediatric subspecialists and pediatric surgeons. See chapter 55.

A meconium plug may obstruct the rectum or the distal colon (and even the entire colon and terminal ileum). A contrast enema may prove both diagnostic and therapeutic. Most babies with meconium plugs are otherwise normal, but a few will ultimately prove to have Hirschsprung's disease (congenital aganglionic megacolon). Some babies with meconium plugs really have the meconium ileus of cystic fibrosis.

Necrotizing enterocolitis (NEC) is classically seen in improving premature babies and often presents after the institution or advancement of enteral feedings. However, larger babies can also develop NEC, usually in combination with another illness. An insult to the bowel wall, perhaps an ischemic insult, may physically or immunologically compromise a section of mucosa, allowing bacterial entry. Vomiting or failure to digest an orogastric tube feeding is often the first sign, soon followed by abdominal distention, ileus, gastrointestinal bleeding, sepsis, gut perforation, peritonitis, abdominal wall inflammation, and death. Serial radiograms first may show a fixed loop of bowel, then air in the bowel wall (pneumatosis intestinalis), then air in the portal system and the liver. Initial stabilization involves gut rest, volume repletion, and antibiotics. Intensive medical support, including total parenteral nutrition, is always needed, and surgical intervention is often required on short notice. Consultation with a neonatologist is essential; transport to a Level III facility is usually necessary.

Neonatal hepatitis and biliary atresia usually present several weeks after birth as jaundice and hepatomegaly; their long-term management is complex.

Hematologic Problems

See also previous sections and chapter 57.

ERYTHROBLASTOSIS FETALIS

Erythroblastosis fetalis is caused by fetomaternal rhesus (Rh) incompatibility or ABO blood-group incompatibility. Obstetric management has been discussed in chapter 36.

Some Rh-positive babies born to Rh-negative mothers are only mildly affected, but severely affected babies are profoundly anemic, icteric, hydropic, and unstable. Rh-negative blood typed and cross-matched against maternal blood should be available in the delivery room and should be administered in a single-volume exchange transfusion as soon as an umbilical venous catheter can be placed. Subsequently, multiple double-volume exchange transfusions must be performed to prevent kernicterus, a clinical syndrome in which bilirubin crosses the blood-brain barrier.

Intrauterine death or hydrops at birth is rare in cases of ABO incompatibility, but hyperbilirubinemia is sometimes severe. Anti-A sensitization is more common and less dangerous than anti-B sensitization.

Rare blood-group incompatibilities can also sometimes cause severe hemolytic disease.

When rapidly deepening jaundice is caused by an ongoing hemolytic process, phototherapy cannot be considered an appropriate defense against kernicterus. Physical removal of sensitized erythrocytes, free hemoglobin, and hemoglobin's catabolites, including bilirubin, is necessary.

BLEEDING

Buchanan has suggested that the differential diagnosis of bleeding in the newborn can be simplified on clinical grounds. The most frequent causes of bleeding in "sick" newborns are disseminated intravascular coagulation, consumptive thrombocytopenia, and liver failure. The most frequent causes of bleeding in "well" newborns are immune thrombocytopenia, vitamin K deficiency, hemophilia (80 per cent A, 20 per cent B), and anatomic vascular disruption (such as in an ulcer or hemangioma). Work-up should include careful maternal and family histories, a careful physical examination of the baby, and, to begin with, a platelet count, prothrombin time, and partial thromboplastin time performed on the baby. Maternal laboratory work-up should be individualized (Buchanan, 1986).

Physiologic Jaundice

All bilirubin is derived from heme. In the newborn, bilirubin can be *overproduced* in cases of acute or chronic hemolysis, resorption of extravasated blood, and polycythemia. It can be *undersecreted* in metabolic or endocrine disorders or in biliary obstructive disorders. It can be *underexcreted* in cases of intestinal defect or obstruction, in which situations the enterohepatic circulation of bilirubin, in large part a hold-over from fetal life, may be accentuated, compounding the problem. And it can be overproduced, undersecreted, and underexcreted *simultaneously* in sick babies.

When, after the first day of extrauterine life, the hepatic conjugation of bilirubin is still too slow to prevent the accumulation of albumin-bound, lipid-soluble, unconjugated bilirubin in the serum, physiologic jaundice is described. When the serum level of unconjugated bilirubin threatens to exceed the bilirubin-binding capacity of albumin, exaggerated physiologic jaundice is described. When the serum level of unconjugated bilirubin does in fact exceed the bilirubin-binding capacity of albumin, kernicterus becomes a risk. In kernicterus, free lipid-soluble unconjugated bilirubin stains the basal ganglia and brainstem nuclei, and possible consequences range from a transient subclinical encephalopathy to neurologic devastation.

Jaundice occurs physiologically in half of all full-term babies and in more than half of all premature babies. It peaks and recedes within a week. Jaundice presenting during the first postpartum day is not physiologic. Unconjugated bilirubin levels exceeding 15 mg. per dl. in full-term babies and 10 mg. per dl. in premature babies are usually considered exaggerated and often prompt the institution of phototherapy. Kernicterus more often occurs occultly in premature than in full-term babies; autopsy evidence shows it to occur at lower serum levels in premature—or, at least, in sick premature—babies, even occurring at levels below 10 mg. per dl. Rules defining threshold levels for clinical response are arbitrary and often informal.

When exaggeration of physiologic jaundice occurs, history and physical examination must be reviewed. Samples must be collected for hematocrit, reticulocyte count, blood smear, and total and direct serum bilirubin concentration. Results of the direct Coombs' test and both the mother's and the baby's blood type and Rh factor must be retrieved and evaluated.

If exaggerated physiologic jaundice is diagnosed, several options may be considered:

1. The baby can be observed further. Intervention in the past has often been needlessly aggressive, particularly for full-term babies.
2. Feedings can be supplemented. Breast-fed babies may not yet be receiving enough milk to stimulate gut motility sufficiently to blunt the effectiveness of the enterohepatic circulation of bilirubin.
3. Breast feeding can be interrupted for a day or so. For a reason or reasons still obscure, breast feeding does contribute to physiologic jaundice in some babies.
4. Phototherapy can be initiated. Light in the 425 to 475 nm. range transforms unconjugated bilirubin into photoisomers that are more water soluble than the native species. These photoisomers must still pass through the liver, but they need not be conjugated by glucuronyl transferase to be secreted into the bile. Babies under "bililights" need a 10 per cent increment in their fluid maintenance; if they become temporarily lactose intolerant, as many do, they may need to be compensated for ongoing volume losses. Diarrhea under the lights is inconvenient, since diapers, which greatly decrease skin exposure to light, cannot be worn. Eyes must be covered, and the eye cover must not be allowed to work its way off the eyes or down over the nose. Some babies become "bronzed" during phototherapy, with unknown consequences.
5. Rarely, conservative steps cannot obviate the need for one or more double-volume exchange transfusions. Otherwise healthy term babies probably do not need exchange transfusions until their unconjugated bilirubin levels exceed 20 mg. per dl.; some physicians temporize until levels reach 25 mg. per dl. Exchange transfusions are not risk-free procedures.
6. In the near future, it may become common practice to slow bilirubin production by inhibiting heme oxygenase with tin-protoporphyrin, even in some cases of autoimmunization (Kappas et al., 1988).

Community Care of the Newborn Intensive Care Unit (NICU) Graduate

Family physicians are increasingly called on to care for NICU graduates, many of them former premature babies, many of them handicapped, most of them at increased risk of one sort or another (Trachtenberg and Miller, 1986). Failure to thrive is common, even when correction is made for gestational age. Bronchopulmonary dysplasia (BPD) often follows prolonged oxygen therapy or mechanical ventilation (Bancalari and Gerhardt, 1986). Babies with BPD often do poorly when infected with respiratory syncytial virus (RSV) (Groothuis et al., 1988) and other common pathogens; pertussis infection in these babies is extremely dangerous. Postintubation airway scarring and tracheomalacia increase many risks, especially respiratory infectious risks (Sotomayor et al., 1986). Weak suck, poorly coordinated swallowing, and gastroesophageal reflux (Giuffre et al., 1987) impede growth and increase the risk of pulmonary aspiration. Intestinal scarring can make common diarrheal illnesses difficult to manage. Sudden infant death syndrome (SIDS) is a well-known risk, as is child abuse. Nevertheless, most NICU graduates survive and most survivors ultimately thrive.

References

Abramo, T.J., et al.: Occult blood in stools and necrotizing enterocolitis: is there a relationship? Am. J. Dis. Child., *142:*451–452, 1988.

Allan, W.C., and Volpe, J.J.: Periventricular-intraventricular hemorrhage. Pediatr. Clin. North Am., *33:*1, 47–63, 1986.

American Academy of Pediatrics: Emergency drug doses for infants and children. Pediatrics, *81:*3, 462–465, 1988.

American Academy of Pediatrics and American College of Obstetricians and Gynecologists: Guidelines for Perinatal Care. 1988. *A helpful collection of current recommendations.*

American Academy of Pediatrics and American Thyroid Association: Newborn screening for congenital hypothyroidism: recommended guidelines. Pediatrics, *80:*5, 745–749, 1987.

Amiel-Tison, C.: Neurological evaluation of the maturity of newborn infants. Arch. Dis. Child. *43:*89, 1968.

Anand, K.J.S., and Hickey, P.R.: Pain and its effects in the human neonate and fetus. N. Engl. J. Med., *317:*21, 1321–1329, 1987.

Apgar, V.: A proposal for a new method of evaluation of the newborn infant. Curr. Res. Anesth. Analg., *32:*260, 1953. *Apgar is a surname, not an acronym, but is often used as a mnemonic.*

Athreya, B.H., and Silverman, B.K.: Pediatric Physical Diagnosis. Norwalk, Conn., Appleton-Century-Crofts, 1985. *A helpful guide.*

Ballard, J.L., et al.: A simplified score for assessment of fetal maturation of newly born infants. J. Pediatr., *95:*769–774, 1979.

Bancalari, E., and Gerhardt, T.: Bronchopulmonary dysplasia. Pediatr. Clin. North Am., *33:*1, 1–23, 1986.

Berseth, C.L., et al.: Longitudinal development in pediatric residents of attitudes toward neonatal resuscitation. Am. J. Dis. Child., *140:*766–769, 1986. *Among pediatric house officers, reluctance to initiate resuscitation of high-risk neonates increased with experience.*

Bradley, J.S.: Neonatal infections. Pediatr. Infect. Dis. J., *4:*3, 315–320, 1985.

Brann, A.W.: Hypoxic ischemic encephalopathy. Pediatr. Clin. North Am., *33:*3, 451–464, 1986.

Breaux, C.W., et al.: Changing patterns in the diagnosis of hypertrophic pyloric stenosis. Pediatrics, *81:*2, 213–217, 1988.

Brown, M.S., and Brown, C.A.: Circumcision decision: prominence of social concerns. Pediatrics *80:*2, 215–219, 1987.

Brown, Z.A., et al.: Effects on infants of a first episode of genital herpes during pregnancy. N. Engl. J. Med., *317:*20, 1246–1251, Nov. 12 1987.

Buchanan, G.R.: Coagulation disorders in the neonate. Pediatr. Clin. North Am., *33:*1, 203–220, 1986.

Bull, M.J., et al.: Misuse of car safety seats. Pediatrics, *81:*1, 98–101, 1988a.

Bull, M.J., et al.: Automotive restraint systems for premature infants. J. Pediatr., *112:*385–388, 1988b.

Caravella, S.J., et al.: Health codes for newborn care. Pediatrics, *80:*1, 1–5, 1987. *A survey of 52 United States jurisdictions.*

Carlo, W.A., and Martin, R.J.: Principles of neonatal assisted ventilation. Pediatr. Clin. North Am., *33:*1, 221–237, 1986.

Coen, R.W., and Koffler, H.: Primary Care of the Newborn. Boston, Little, Brown & Co., Inc., 1987. *A small but exceptionally valuable book concentrating on the management of normal newborns. Well designed, written, and illustrated, and supplemented with helpful appendices.*

David, R.: Closed chest cardiac massage in the newborn infant. Am. J. Dis. Child., *81:*4, 552–554, 1988.

Davis, J.M., et al.: Changes in pulmonary mechanics after the administration of surfactant to infants with respiratory distress syndrome. N. Engl. J. Med., *319:*8, 476–479, 1988.

Dubowitz, L.M., Dubowitz, V., and Goldberg, C.: Clinical assessment of gestational age in the newborn infant. J. Pediatr., *77:*1–10, 1970.

Ellenberg, J.H., and Nelson, K.B.: Cluster of perinatal events identifying infants at high risk for death or disability. J. Pediatr., *113:*3, 546–552, 1988.

Ellis, W.G., et al.: Neuropathologic documentation of prenatal brain damage. Am. J. Dis. Child., *142:*858–866, 1988.

Evans, M.E., et al.: Sensitivity, specificity, and predictive value of body surface cultures in a neonatal intensive care unit. J.A.M.A., *259:*249–253, 1988.

Fanaroff, A.A., and Martin, R.J., (Eds.): Neonatal-Perinatal Medicine: Diseases of the Fetus and Infant. 4th ed. St. Louis, C.V. Mosby, 1987. *A magnificent text: current, clear, and comprehensive.*

Farr, V., Kerridge, D.F., and Mitchell, R.G.: The definition of some external characteristics used in the assessment of gestational age of the newborn infant. Develop. Med. Child Neurol., *8:*507, 1966.

Fergusson, D.M., et al.: Neonatal circumcision and penile problems: an 8-year longitudinal study. Pediatrics, *81:*4, 537–541, 1988.

Frattallone, J.M., et al.: Management of pulmonary barotrauma by extracorporeal membrane oxygenation, apnea, and lung rest. J. Pediatr., *112:*5, 787–789, 1988.

Ginsburg, C.M., and McCracken, G.H.: Urinary tract infections in young infants. Pediatrics, *69:*409–412, 1982.

Giuffre, R.M., et al.: Antireflux surgery in infants with bronchopulmonary dysplasia. Am. J. Dis. Child., *141:*648–651, 1987.

Glass, P., et al.: Morbidity for survivors of extracorporeal membrane oxygenation: neurodevelopmental outcome at 1 year of age. Pediatrics, *83:*1, 72–78, 1989.

Graef, J.W., et al. (Eds.): Manual of Pediatric Therapeutics. 4th ed. Boston, Little, Brown & Co., Inc., 1988.

Groothuis, J.R., et al.: Respiratory syncytial virus infection in children with bronchopulmonary dysplasia. Pediatrics, *82:*2, 199–203, 1988.

Habicht, J-P., et al.: Mother's milk and sewage: their interactive effects on infant mortality. Pediatrics, *81:*3, 456–461, 1988. *In Malaysian households without piped water or a toilet, the death rate after one week of age among nonbreastfed infants was five times that among breastfed infants. In households with toilets, the death rate among nonbreastfed infants was two times that among breastfed infants. These data "confirm the pernicious synergistic effect of poor sanitation and nonbreastfeeding that was postulated previously on theoretical grounds."*

Helsing, E., and King, F.S.: Breast-feeding in Practice: A Manual for Health Workers. Oxford, Oxford University, 1982. *A complete guide to breast feeding in both developing and developed countries. Remarkably well done.*

Hensinger, R.N.: Congenital Dislocation of the Hip. Ciba Foundation Symposium *31:*5, 1979.

Herrmann, H.J., and Roberts, M.W.: Preventive dental care: the role of the pediatrician. Pediatrics, *80:*107–110, 1987.

Hersh, J.H., et al.: Does a supernumerary nipple/renal field defect exist? Am. J. Dis. Child., *141:*989–991, 1987.

Herzog, L.W., and Alvarez, S.R.: The frequency of foreskin problems in uncircumcised children. Am. J. Dis. Child., *140:*254–256, 1986.

HIFI Study Group: High-frequency oscillatory ventilation compared with conventional mechanical ventilation in the treatment of respiratory failure in preterm infants. N. Engl. J. Med., *320:*2, 88–93, 1989. *A large, prospective, randomized, multicenter trial showing significantly increased risk and no comparative benefit with high-frequency oscillatory ventilation.*

Hillier, S.L., et al.: A case-control study of chorioamnionic infection and histologic chorioamnionitis in prematurity. N. Engl. J. Med., *319:*15, 972–978, 1988.

Hletko, P.J., et al.: Infant safety seat use: reaching the hard to reach. Am. J. Dis. Child., *141:*1301–1304, 1987. *A successful interactive video infant-seat education program is described.*

Jenny, C., et al.: Hymens in newborn female infants. Pediatrics, *80:*3, 399–400, 1987.

Joffe, A., and Radius, S.M.: Breast versus bottle: correlates of adolescent mothers' infant-feeding practices. Pediatrics, *79:*5, 689–695, 1987. *Various breast-feeding encouragements are suggested by regression analysis of survey data.*

Kappas, A., et al.: Sn-protoporphyrin use in the management of hyperbilirubinemia in term newborns with direct Coombs-positive ABO incompatibility. Pediatrics, *81*:4, 485–497, 1988.

Kenny, R.D., et al.: Supernumerary nipples and renal anomalies in neonates. Am. J. Dis. Child., *141*:987–988, 1987.

Klaus, M.H., and Fanaroff, A.A. (Eds.): Care of the High-Risk Neonate. 3rd ed. Philadelphia, W.B. Saunders Company, 1986. *One of the most creative texts ever published in any clinical discipline. The book to buy and to read, cover-to-cover, for every physician responsible for the care of newborns. Indexing problems in the 2nd edition have been corrected.*

Kurinij, N., et al.: Breast-feeding incidence and duration in black and white women. Pediatrics, *81*:3, 365–371, 1988. *In-hospital formula supplementation of breast feedings is a major correlate of foreshortened breast feeding duration among black American urban women compared with caucasian American urban women.*

Leung, A.K.C.: Natal teeth. Am. J. Dis. Child., *140*:249–251, 1986.

Leung, A.K.C., and Robson, W.L.M.: Single umbilical artery: a report of 159 cases. Am. J. Dis. Child., *143*:108–111, 1989.

Levin, D.L., et al. (Ed.): A Practical Guide to Pediatric Intensive Care. 2nd ed. St. Louis, C.V. Mosby, 1984. *How and why to do nearly everything, one step at a time.*

Linder, N., et al.: Need for endotracheal intubation and suction in meconium-stained neonates. J. Pediatr., *112*:613–615, 1988. *In meconium-stained newborns with 1-minute Apgar score greater than 8, routine immediate tracheal suctioning caused more problems than it prevented.*

Madlon-Kay, D.J.: 'Witch's milk': galactorrhea in the newborn. Am. J. Dis. Child., *141*:252–253, 1986.

Manroe, B.L., et al.: The neonatal blood count in health and disease. I. Reference values for neutrophilic cells. J. Pediatr. *95*:89–98, 1979.

Moore, D.J., et al.: Breath hydrogen response to milk containing lactose in colicky and noncolicky infants. J. Pediatr. *113*:979–984, 1988. *Breath hydrogen was higher in colicky infants, both during fasting and postprandially, suggesting more colonic gas production.*

Mor, N., and Merlob, P.: Congenital absence of hymen only a rumor? Pediatrics, *82*:4, 679–680, 1988.

Morelli, J.G., and Weston, W.L.: Soaps and shampoos in pediatric practice. Pediatrics, *80*:5, 634–637, 1987.

Moyes, C.D., et al.: Very-low-dose hepatitis B vaccine in newborn infants: an economic option for control in endemic areas. Lancet, *1*:8523, 29–31, 1987.

Nelson, J.D.: 1987–1988 Pocketbook of Pediatric Antimicrobial Therapy. 7th ed. Baltimore, Williams & Wilkins. 1987. *The indispensible yellow book, updated every other year.*

Nelson, K.B., and Ellenberg, J.H.: The asymptomatic newborn and risk of cerebral palsy. Am. J. Dis. Child., *141*:1333–1335, 1987.

Nelson, S.E., et al.: Lack of adverse reactions to iron-fortified formula. Pediatrics, *81*:3, 360–364, 1988.

Oh, W.: Neonatal polycythemia and hyperviscosity. Pediatr. Clin. North Am., *33*:3, 523–532, 1986.

Oxtoby, M.J.: Human immunodeficiency virus and other viruses in human milk: placing the issues in broader perspective. Pediatr. Infect. Dis. J., *7*:825–835, 1988.

Painter, M.J., et al.: Neonatal seizures. Pediatr. Clin. North Am., *33*:1, 91–109, 1986.

Payne, N.R., et al: Correlation of clinical and pathologic findings in early onset neonatal Group B streptococcal infection with disease severity and prediction of outcome. Pediatr. Infect. Dis. J., *7*:12, 836–847, 1988.

Peckham, G.J., Chairman, Neonatal Resuscitation Committee, American Heart Association, et al.: Standards and guidelines for cardiopulmonary resuscitation (CPR) and emergency cardiac care (ECC): Part VI: Neonatal advanced life support. J.A.M.A., *255*:21, 2969–2973, 1986.

Prober, C.G., et al.: Use of routine viral cultures at delivery to identify neonates exposed to herpes simplex virus. N. Engl. J. Med., *318*:14, 887–891, 1988.

Reller, M.D., et al.: Duration of ductal shunting in healthy preterm infants: an echocardiographic color flow Doppler study. J. Pediatr., *112*:441–6, 1988. *Sixteen full-term newborns were studied as controls.*

Rockney, R.M.: Pediatric code cards. Am. J. Dis. Child., *142*:73–75, 1988. *A sample card is displayed ready for copying.*

Sanchez, P., cited in Nelson, J.D., and McCracken, G.H.: Pediatric Infectious Disease Journal Newsletter, *15*:1, 2, 1989, contained in Pediatr. Infect. Dis. J., *8*:1, Jan 1989. *"The yellow pages" in PIDJ are well worth regular reading, as is PIDJ itself.*

Schmitt, B.D.: The prevention of sleep problems and colic. Pediatr. Clin. North Am., *33*:4, 763–774, 1986.

Schumacher, R.E., et al.: Right-sided brain lesions in infants following extracorporeal membrane oxygenation. Pediatrics, *82*:2, 155–161, 1988.

Sepkowitz, S.: Influence of the legal imperative and medical guidelines on the incidence and management of the meconium-stained newborn. Am. J. Dis. Child., *141*:10, 1124–1127, 1987. *Meconium-related "diagnoses," "prophylactic" measures, and "therapies" in a community hospital increased sharply when litigation followed a meconium-aspiration death.*

Sotomayor, J.L., et al.: Large-airway collapse due to acquired tracheobronchomalacia in infancy. Am. J. Dis. Child., *140*:367–371, 1986.

Tan, O.T., and Gilchrest, B.A.: Laser therapy for selected cutaneous vascular lesions in the pediatric population: a review. Pediatrics, *82*:4, 652–662, 1988. *A well-illustrated discussion of the spider angioma, the strawberry hemangioma, and the port-wine stain; laser therapy is emphasized, but other therapeutic modalities are also discussed.*

Taubman, B.: Parental counselling compared with elimination of cow's milk or soy milk protein for the treatment of infant colic syndrome: a randomized trial. Pediatrics, *81*:6, 756–761, 1988. *Parental counselling seemed far more effective.*

Thoele, D.G., et al.: Recognition of coarctation of the aorta: a continuing challenge for the primary care physician. Am. J. Dis. Child., *141*:1201–1204, 1987.

Todres, I.D., et al.: Life-saving therapy for newborns: a questionnaire survey in the state of Massachusetts. Pediatrics, *81*:5, 643–649, 1988.

Trachtenberg, D.E., and Miller, T.C.: Office care of the premature infant. Am. Fam. Physician, *33*:5, 119–127, 1986.

Usher, R., and McLean, F.: Intrauterine growth of live-born Caucasian infants at sea level: standards obtained from measurements in 7 dimensions of infants born between 25 and 44 weeks of gestation. J. Pediatr., *74*(6):901–910, 1969.

Versmold, H.T., Kitterman, J.A., Phibbs, R.H., et al.: Aortic blood pressure during the first 12 hours of life in infants with birth weight 610 to 4,220 grams. Pediatrics, *67*(5): 607–613, 1981.

Vichinsky, E., et al.: Newborn screening for sickle cell disease: effect on mortality. Pediatrics, *81*:6, 749–755, 1988. *Newborn sickle-cell screening combined with proper case management—including penicillin prophylaxis—decreased mortality.*

Vogler, C., et al.: Aluminum-containing emboli in infants treated with extracorporeal membrane oxygenation. N. Engl. J. Med., *319*:2, 75–79, 1988. *Twenty-two of 23 autopsies showed fibrin thrombi or thromboemboli; 12 of the autopsies also showed emboli containing aluminum thought to be derived from the ECMO circuit.*

Volpe, J.J.: Neurology of the Newborn. Philadelphia, W.B. Saunders, 1981.

Wallerstein, E.: Circumcision: An American Health Fallacy. New York, Springer, 1980.

Walters, J.W.: Approaches to ethical decision making in the neonatal intensive care unit. Am. J. Dis. Child., *142*:825–830, 1988.

Winikoff, B., et al.: Overcoming obstacles to breast-feeding in a large municipal hospital: applications of lessons learned. Pediatrics, *80:*3, 423–433, 1987. *In-hospital formula supplementation of breast feedings most often followed a mother's perception that her milk volume was inadequate. Low milk volume and the impression that milk volume would not increase seemed related to inadequate encouragement from hospital staff.*

Wiswell, T.E. et al.: Effect of circumcision status on periurethral flora during the first year of life. J. Pediatr., *113:*3, 442–446, 1988.

Wiswell, T.E. and Roscelli, J.D.: Corroborative evidence for the decreased incidence of urinary tract infections in circumcised male infants. Pediatrics, *78:*96–99, 1986.

Woolridge, M.W., and Fisher, C.: Colic, "overfeeding," and symptoms of lactose malabsorption in the breast-fed baby: a possible artifact of feed management? Lancet, 8607, Aug. 13 1988. *Switching breasts before breast emptying, a common practice among mothers, means babies "overfeed" on low-calorie, low-fat foremilk, the possible result being a full stomach but inadequate calories and rapid gastric emptying and possibly also diarrhea.*

38

Growth and Development

Sanford R. Kimmel
Lorraine Fay

Growth is a dynamic process where increasing cell size and number in various tissues results in a physical increase in the size of the body as a whole. Simultaneously, development occurs as tissues differentiate in form and mature in function reflecting the individual's genetic heritage and environmental interaction. Nutritional, family, emotional, sociocultural, and community, as well as physical, factors play a role in shaping the child's psychologic and physiologic development (Vaughan, 1987). The child emotionally responds to a particular stimulus in an apparently innate and characteristic style that reflects his or her temperament (Sahler and McAnarney, 1981).

Knowledge of normal as well as abnormal patterns of growth and development enables the physician to assist the child in maximizing his or her fullest potential. Growth in height and weight are sensitive reflections of a child's general health (Green, 1986). Deviations from normal may reflect the presence of physical illness or a disturbance in the child's environment. Consequently, such deviations warrant an evaluation of those factors influencing growth and development (Table 38–1).

Measuring Physical Parameters of Growth

Weight, length, and head circumference are the most useful routine measurements in infants. The weight should be determined on a balance beam scale and recorded at each visit. Infants under 24 months should be weighed nude while older children may wear light clothing but not shoes.

Total body length in children under age 3 is most accurately obtained by placing them in the recumbent position and measuring from crown to heel. This procedure is facilitated in infants by the use of a measuring board or tray (Hoekelman, 1987). If this is not available, one may measure marks made on the examining table paper with a straight ruler placed between and perpendicular to the marks. Older children should have their shoeless standing height determined with heels, buttocks, scapulae, and occiput against a straight wall to which a fixed ruler has been attached. The child should look straight ahead while a right triangular board is placed firmly against the top of the head. The examiner then reads and records the height (Silverstein and Rosenbloom, 1988). The usual measuring rod attached to a weight scale is not precise (Green, 1986).

Head circumference reflects the growth of the cranium and its contents. It should be determined and recorded at all routine physical examinations during the first 2 years of life (AAP Committee on Psychosocial Aspects of Child and Family Health, 1985–1988, 1988). It may also be done as part of the initial exam at any age. A nonstretchable measuring tape (usually paper or soft plastic) is used to obtain the greatest circumference encompassing the occipital, parietal, and frontal prominences. A small head circumference or microcephaly may be familial or due to craniosynostosis, an underlying structural abnormality, or to congenital factors, such as infection. Large head circumference or macrocephaly may be

Table 38–1. FACTORS INFLUENCING PHYSICAL GROWTH

Genetic
1. Parental height
   a. Familial (tall or short) stature
   b. Constitutional growth delay
2. Chromosomal abnormalities
   a. Down's syndrome
   b. Turner's syndrome
   c. Other syndromes or disorders
3. Race

Environmental
1. Intrauterine
   a. Maternal size
   b. Maternal nutrition
   c. Maternal smoking and drug use
   d. Congenital infection
   e. Placental function
2. Postnatal
   a. Nutrition
   b. Socioeconomic status
   c. Cultural or home environment

Endocrinologic
1. Thyroid hormone
2. Cortisol
3. Androgens
4. Estrogens
5. Growth hormone-somatomedin axis
6. Diabetes mellitus (poorly controlled)

Chronic or recurrent systemic illness
1. Congenital heart disease
2. Central nervous system disease
3. Pulmonary disease
   a. Asthma
   b. Cystic fibrosis
4. Gastrointestinal disease
   a. Inflammatory bowel disease
   b. Malabsorption syndromes
5. Renal disease
   a. Chronic renal insufficiency
   b. Renal tubular acidosis
   c. Bartter's syndrome
   d. Nephrogenic diabetes insipidus

Metabolic disease or status
1. Chronic acidosis
2. Storage diseases

Chronic medications
1. Exogenous steroids

Adapted from Lipsky, M. S., and Horner, J. M.: Am. Fam. Phys., 37:230–233, 1988.

familial or due to hydrocephalus, intracranial bleeding, or masses or thickening of the skull (Green, 1986).

PROPER USE AND INTERPRETATION OF GROWTH CHARTS

The growth charts shown in Figure 38–1 are those constructed by the National Center for Health Statistics (NCHS) from a survey of generally well-nourished children representing a cross section of ethnic and economic groups in the United States (Vaughan, 1987). These graphs provide a normal range of weight and length or height for a given chronologic age. Recumbent length is recorded on the chart for children from birth to 36 months old, while standing height is recorded on the chart for children from 3 to 18 years old. Premature infants should have their chronologic age adjusted according to their degree of prematurity up to age 2 since most catch-up growth is complete by this time. Alternatively, an infant growth record beginning several months prior to term may be utilized for premature infants under 1 year of age (Fig. 38–2). Although a height or weight above the ninety-fifth percentile or below the fifth percentile should alert the physician to a possible problem, the child may represent the outer fringe of the normal range.

The growth curve constructed by a series of heights and weights taken over a period of time is more informative and allows the physician to compare the child's current growth with his previous pattern. A child whose growth curve parallels the normal curve regardless of his absolute percentile has a normal rate of growth for that particular child. In comparison, a child whose height or weight crosses multiple percentile lines or whose linear growth rate drops below 4 cm. per year after age 2 requires further evaluation for nutritional, psychosocial, or organic problems that could impede or accelerate growth (Lipsky and Horner, 1988). Children who are large at birth but destined to be small and children who are small but destined to be large will usually reach their genetic isobar on the growth chart by age 2 (Silverstein and Rosenbloom, 1988).

RULES OF THUMB

Although careful measuring and plotting of growth parameters is the most accurate method to follow a child's physical growth, rules of thumb are helpful to the physician in remembering and forming an overall impression of the child's progress (Table 38–2). The growth velocity or rate of gain in height or weight actually decreases from the time of birth until the onset of the pubertal growth spurt (Fig. 38–3).

FAMILIAL SHORT STATURE AND CONSTITUTIONAL GROWTH DELAY

Each child has a different rate of maturation or what Boas termed "tempo of growth" (Tanner, 1986). Consequently, if a child's growth falls outside the range of normal, it may be useful to obtain bone age films, usually of the hand and wrist. By comparing the development of ossification centers and epiphyseal-diaphyseal unions to known standards, it is possible to estimate skeletal maturity (Green, 1986). Some causes of retarded or accelerated bone age are listed in Table 38–3.

Calculation of midparental height also is useful in determining whether a child is or is not fulfilling his or her genetic potential. Midparental height is the average of the parents' heights, after adding 13 cm. to the mother's height for boys and subtracting

Text continued on page 680

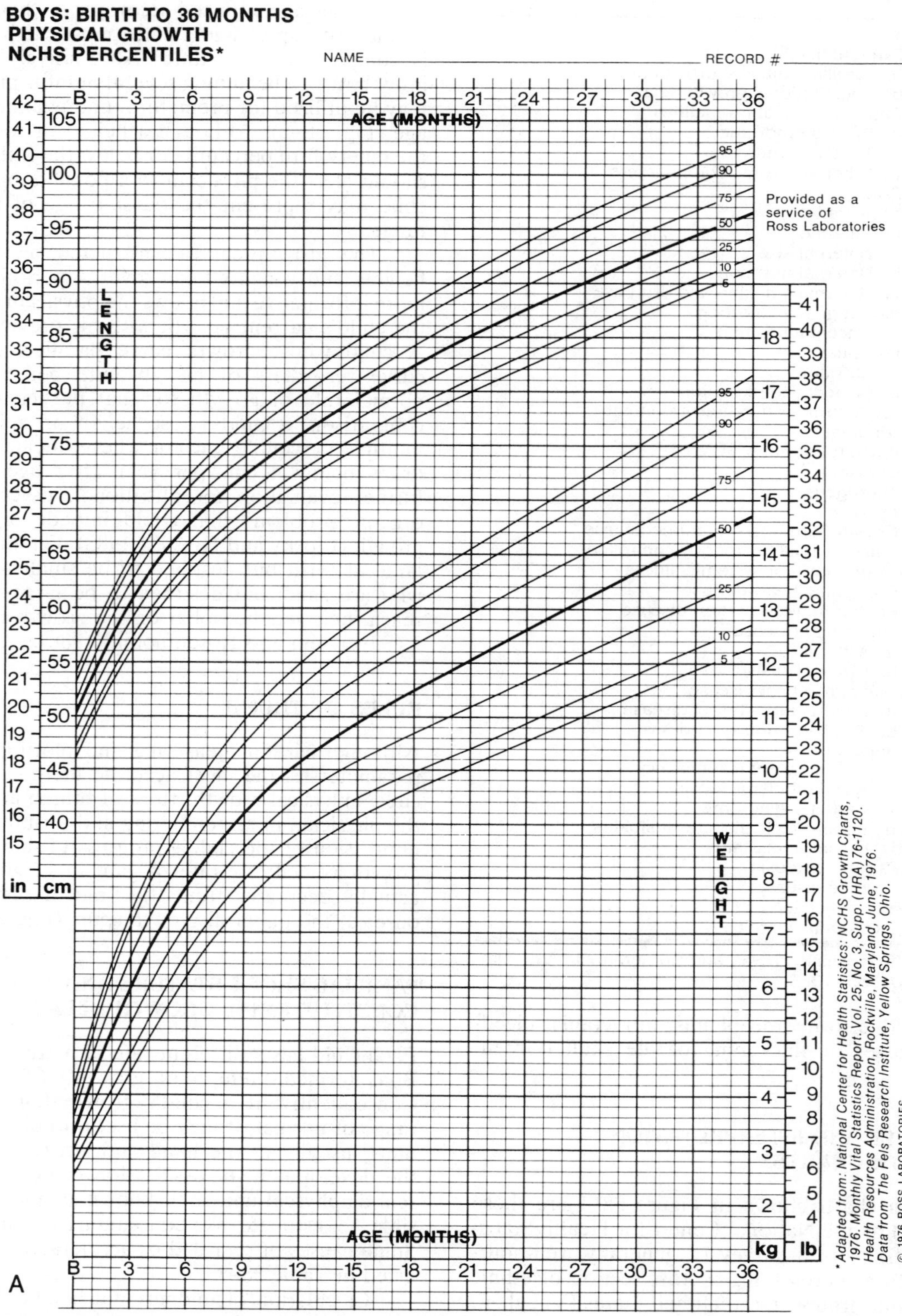

Figure 38–1. These growth charts for boys *(A, B)* and girls *(C, D)* plot length *(A, C)* or height *(B, D)* for age on their upper curves and weight for age on their lower curves. (Percentiles are constructed from NCHS data and reprinted with courteous permission from Ross Laboratories.)

BOYS: 2 TO 18 YEARS
PHYSICAL GROWTH
NCHS PERCENTILES*

NAME ______________________ RECORD # ____________

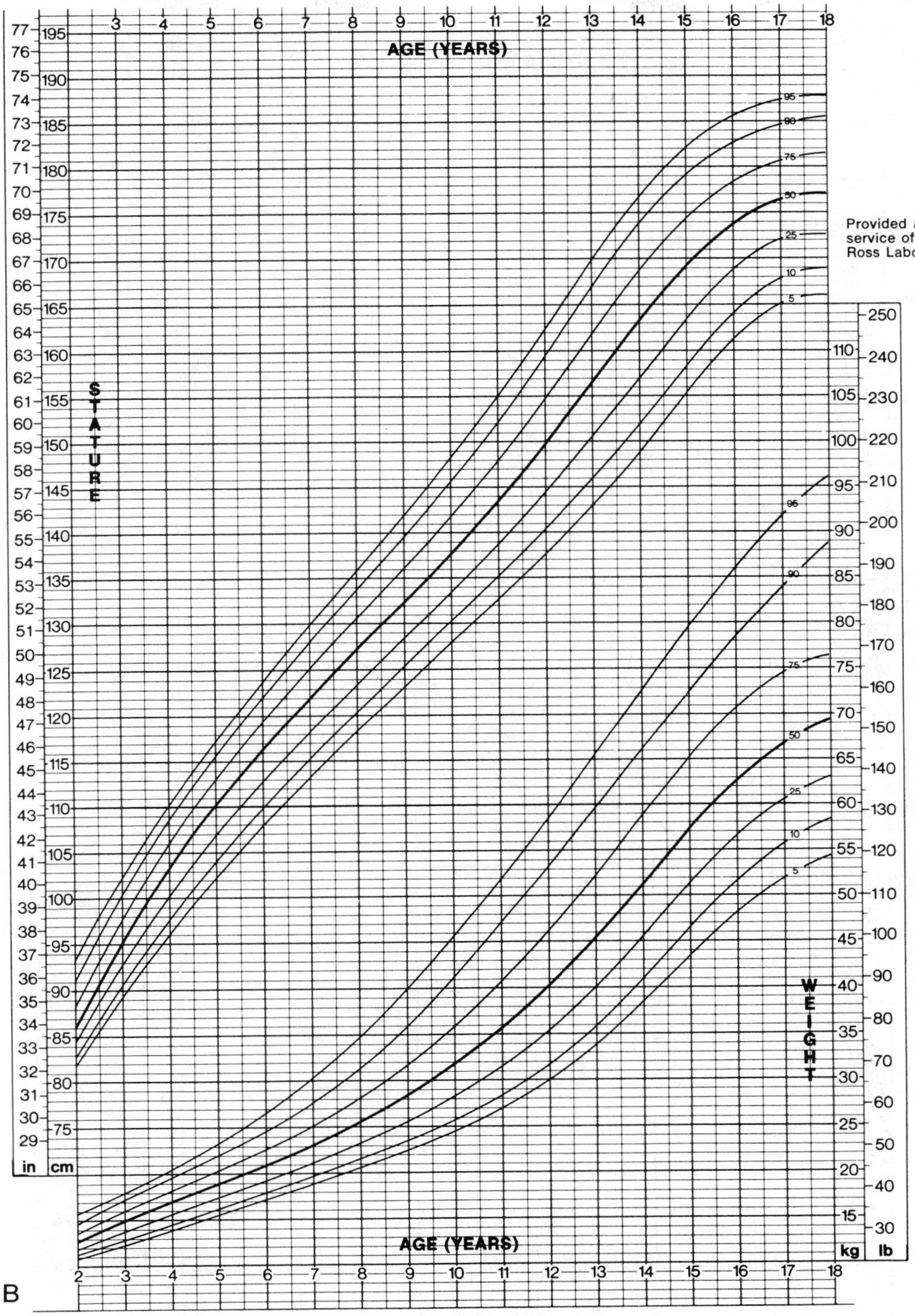

B

*Adapted from: National Center for Health Statistics: NCHS Growth Charts, 1976. Monthly Vital Statistics Report. Vol. 25, No. 3, Supp. (HRA) 76-1120. Health Resources Administration, Rockville, Maryland, June, 1976. Data from the National Center for Health Statistics.

Figure 38–1 *Continued*

Illustration continued on following page

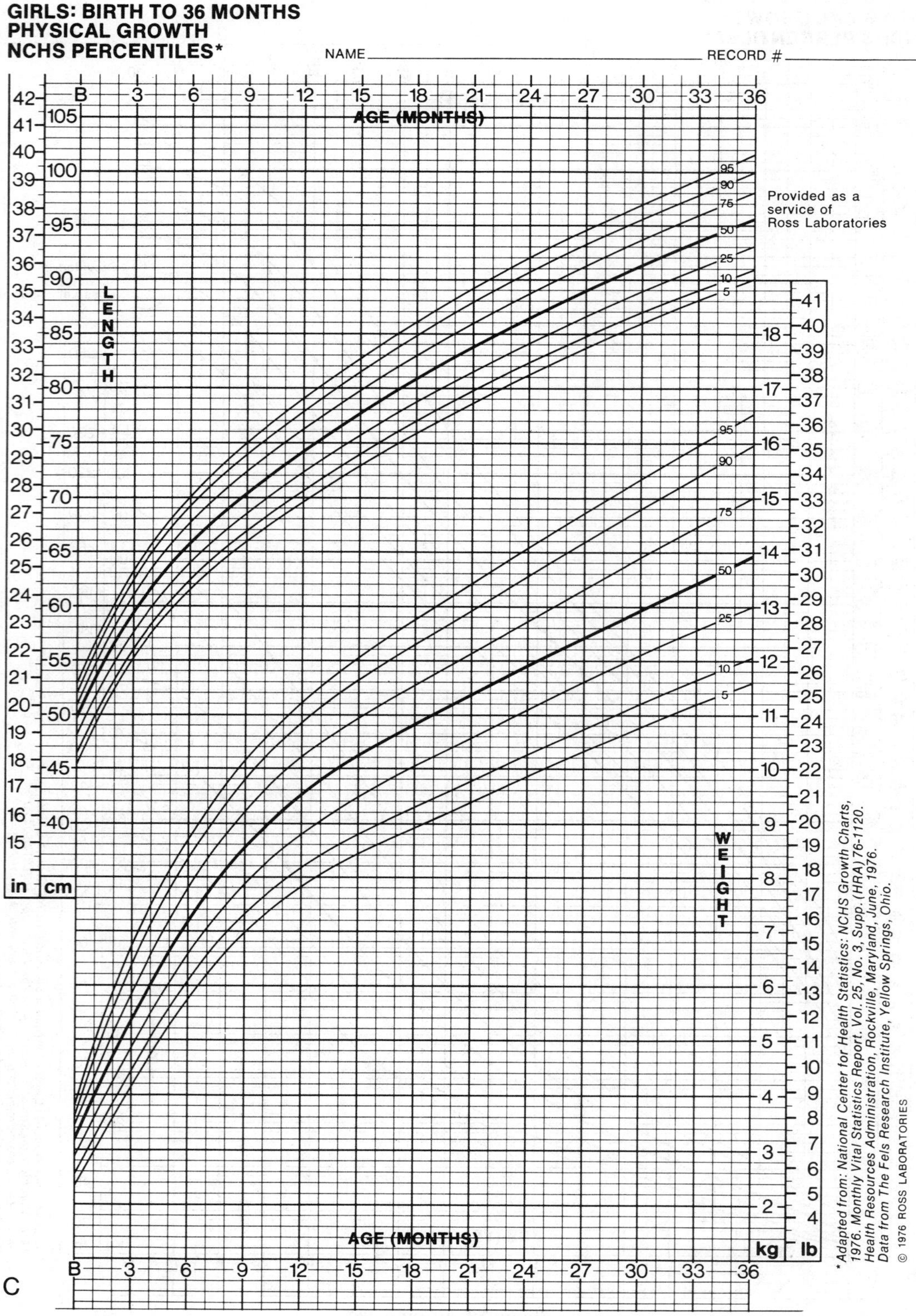
GIRLS: BIRTH TO 36 MONTHS
PHYSICAL GROWTH
NCHS PERCENTILES*
NAME
RECORD #
AGE (MONTHS)
LENGTH
WEIGHT
in
cm
kg
lb
Provided as a service of Ross Laboratories
*Adapted from: National Center for Health Statistics: NCHS Growth Charts, 1976. Monthly Vital Statistics Report. Vol. 25, No. 3, Supp. (HRA) 76-1120. Health Resources Administration, Rockville, Maryland, June, 1976. Data from The Fels Research Institute, Yellow Springs, Ohio.
© 1976 ROSS LABORATORIES
C

Figure 38–1 *Continued*

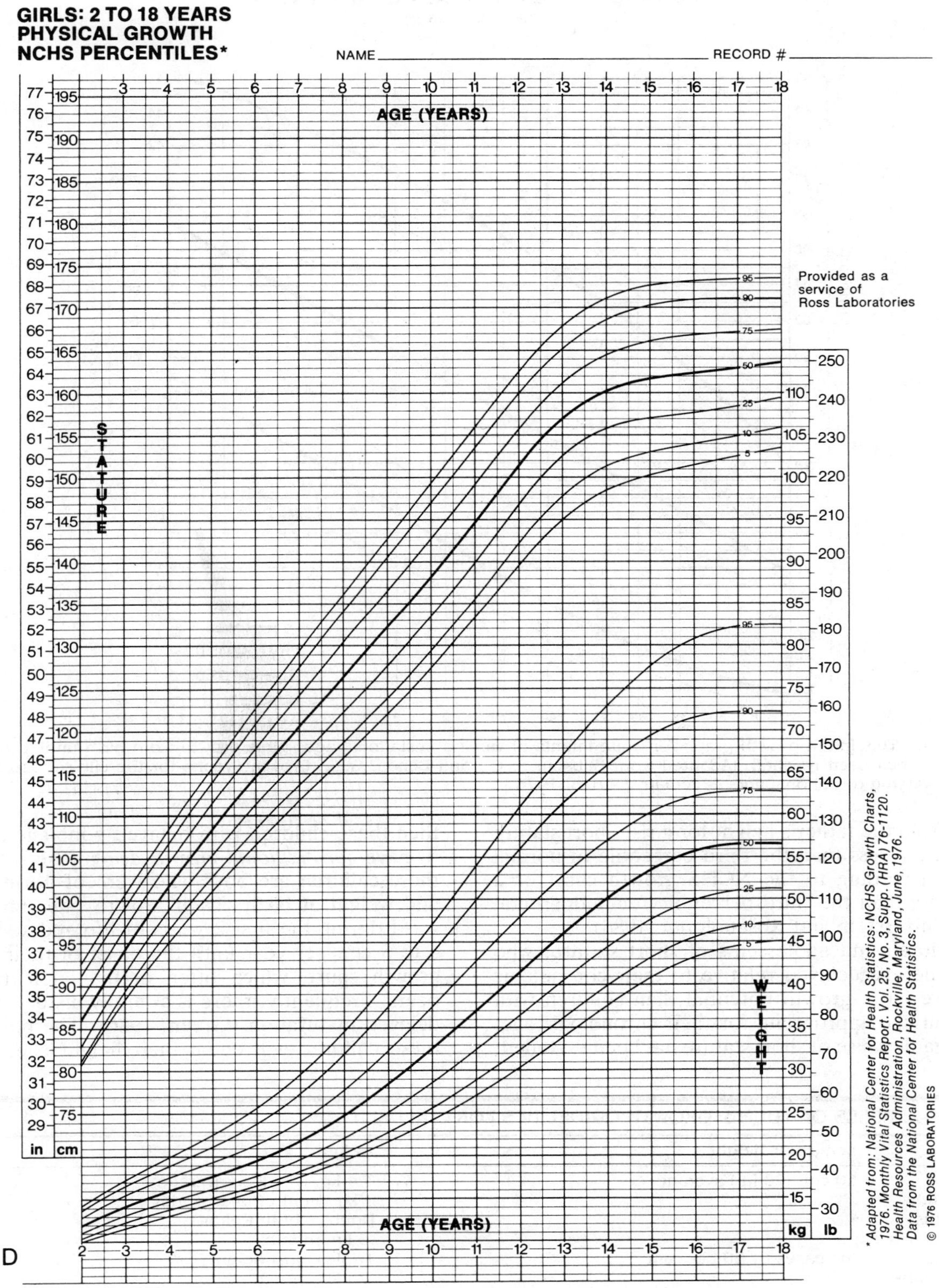

D

Figure 38–1 *Continued*

GROWTH RECORD FOR INFANTS
in relation to
GESTATIONAL AGE AND FETAL AND INFANT NORMS
(combined sexes)

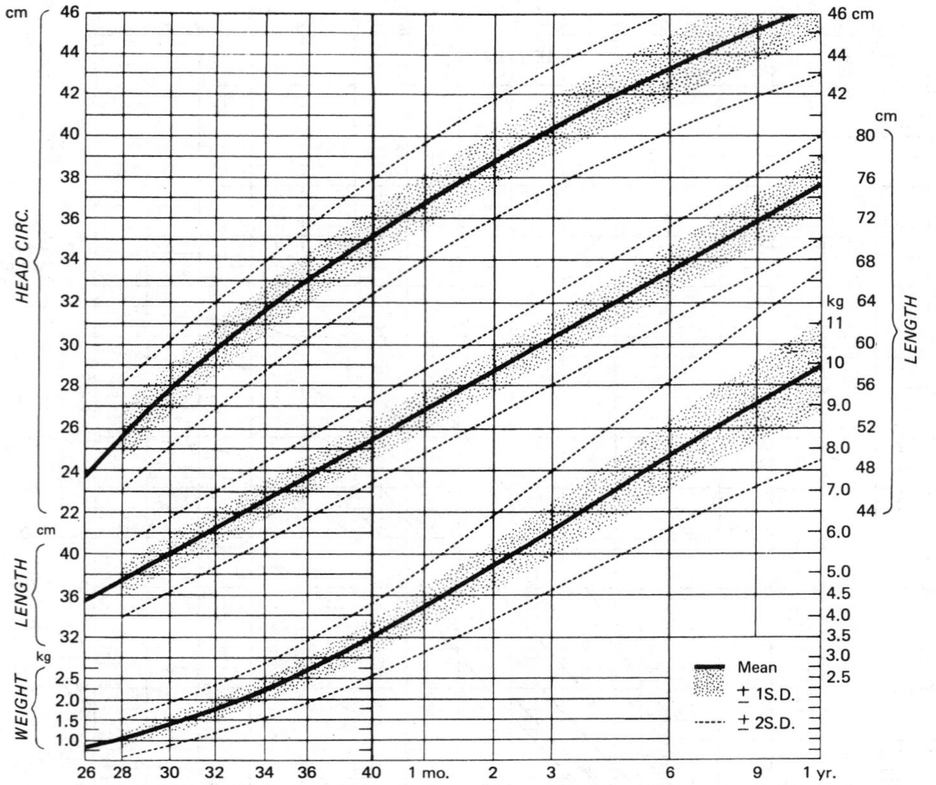

Figure 38–2. This infant growth graph for white infants of varying gestational ages plots growth from birth until 1 year of age after "term" has been reached. (Adapted from Babson, S. G., and Benda, G. I.: Growth graphs for the clinical assessment of infants of varying gestational age. J. Pediatr. *89*:815, 1976.)

13 cm. from the father's height for girls. Short stature is defined as less than the third percentile of normal for age according to the NCHS growth chart or a height less than the third percentile for midparental height (Silverstein and Rosenbloom, 1988).

Children and adolescents of short stature, who have bone age delayed relative to their chronologic age, have more growth potential than children with a skeletal age appropriate for their chronologic age. If an organic cause of short stature has been excluded, then these children with delayed bone age are likely to have *constitutional growth delay*. The majority of these children are boys who were of normal length and weight at birth. Their growth rate shifts downward during the first 2 years of life and stabilizes at 4 to 5 cm. per year until the onset of their pubertal growth spurt, which often occurs later than their peers. Frequently, there is a family history of similar delayed maturation (Green, 1986). The bone age of these children will equal their height age, which is

Table 38–2. RULES OF THUMB: GROWTH GUIDELINES FOR CHILDREN

Age	Length or Height	Weight
Newborn	50 cm. (20 in.) average	3.4 kg. (7½ lbs.) average
NB–3 months		1 kg./month (½–1 oz./day)
4–5 months		Doubles birth weight
6 months		.5 kg./month
12 months	Increases by 50 per cent	Triples birth weight
12–24 months		.25 kg./month
> 2 years	> 5 cm. (2 in.) per year until adolescent growth spurt	2.3 kg. (5 lb.) per year until adolescent growth spurt
4 years	Doubles (40 in. approximately)	40 lbs. approximately

Adapted from Keefer, C. H.: Normal growth and development: an overview. *In* Dershewitz, R. A. (Ed.): Ambulatory Pediatric Care. Philadelphia, J. B. Lippincott Co., 1988, p. 24.

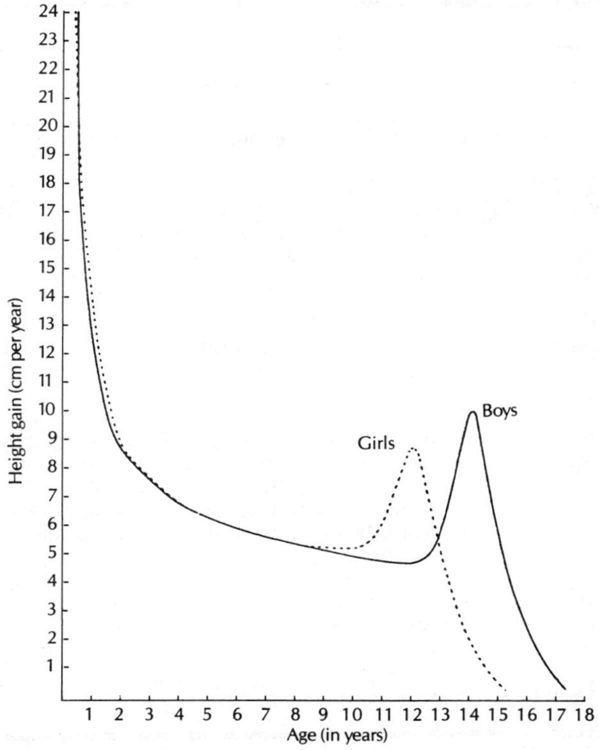

Figure 38–3. Average linear growth velocity curves for boys and girls from infancy through the pubertal growth spurt. Note the rapid deceleration of linear growth in infancy, its relative stability throughout childhood, and its rapid acceleration at puberty. Also note that the pubertal growth spurt in boys is later and greater than that in girls. As a result, the average adult stature of men is greater than that of women. (From Lipsky, M. S., and Horner, J. M.: The child with short stature. Am. Fam. Physician, 37:232, 1988.)

the age at which their height plots on the fiftieth percentile of the growth chart (Silverstein and Rosenbloom, 1988).

Children with *familial short stature* tend to be short at birth, follow the normal growth curve below the fifth percentile, have a bone age consistent with their chronologic age, and reach puberty at an appropriate time (Green, 1986). Usually, their parents or other close relatives are short, and when their height percentiles are corrected for midparental heights, they fall closer to the mean height percentile for age (Lipsky and Horner, 1988).

Table 38–3. CONDITIONS AFFECTING BONE AGE

A. Some Causes of Retarded Bone Age
1. Hypopituitarism
2. Hypothyroidism
3. Malnutrition
4. Constitutional dwarfism
5. Chronic disease
6. Severe illness
7. Male hypogonadism
8. Delayed adolescence

B. Some Causes of Accelerated Bone Age
1. Sexual precocity
2. Obesity

PUBERTAL GROWTH AND DEVELOPMENT

All children grow at a different tempo with some maturing earlier than others and some later. This difference is most apparent during puberty. As a result the usual NCHS growth charts are least able to account for variations in normality during this time. Tanner and Davies (1985) have taken the NCHS data and constructed height and height velocity curves for American boys and girls that account for the early and late maturers as shown in Figure 38–3. These charts also allow for notation of the various stages of puberty that have been described by Tanner (1986) (Table 38–4).

The onset of puberty generally occurs at age 9 in American girls with the peak height velocity occurring at age 11.5 years (range 9.7 to 13.5 years for early to late maturers), while American boys have onset of puberty at age 11 and peak height velocity at 13.5 years (range 11.7 to 15.3 years) (Tanner and Davies, 1985). Because boys have two additional years of prepubertal growth and a peak height velocity greater than girls, their ultimate height is usually taller. Head, hands, and feet are first to reach their adult size, followed by leg length, trunk length (which accounts for much of the spurt), and body breadth. Pubertal boys develop greater shoulder breadth than pubertal girls, who develop wider hips. Adolescents can be reassured that their body will eventually become more proportionate with their hands and feet. Boys ultimately gain greater muscle size and strength than girls while losing limb fat. This is due to their increased secretion of testosterone, which also increases red cell mass and hemoglobin (Tanner, 1986).

The adolescent growth spurt in skeletal and body dimensions is closely associated with the development of the reproductive system. Although the onset and rate of maturation varies according to the individual, the sequence is usually the same within sexes (Figs. 38–4 and 38–5).

The first sign of puberty in boys is an increase in growth of the testes and scrotum with reddening and wrinkling of the scrotal skin. Pubic hair appears within 6 months followed by phallic enlargement in 12 to 18 months and peak height velocity 2 to 2½ years after testicular enlargement (Copeland, 1986). Axillary hair usually appears two years after the beginning of pubic hair growth (stage four pubic hair), but there is considerable variability. Some boys may have enlargement of the breasts midway through adolescence. Following the attainment of peak height velocity, boys develop mature spermatozoa, full facial hair, and voice change. However, breaking of the voice is a late and often gradual process.

In girls, the breast bud is the first sign of puberty, and the pubertal growth spurt typically occurs concurrently, peaking at stage three breast and pubic

Table 38–4. SEXUAL MATURITY STAGES IN BOYS AND GIRLS

	Boys		Girls
Stage	*Male Genitalia*	*Pubic Hair*	*Breasts*
1.	Preadolescent—testes, scrotum, and penis are of childhood size	None; may be vellus hair, as over abdomen	Preadolescent, evaluation of papilla only
2.	Slight enlargement testes and scrotum; little or no enlargement of penis, reddening scrotal skin	Sparse growth long, slightly pigmented, downy hair, straight or slightly curled, primarily at base of penis or along labia	Breast bud stage; breast and papilla form a small mound; areolar diameter enlarges
3.	Further growth testes and scrotum; penis enlarges, mainly in length	Hair considerably darker, coarser, and more curled; spreads sparsely over junction of pubes	Further enlargement of breasts and areola with no separation of their contours
4.	Further growth testes and darkening of scrotum; penis enlarges, especially in breadth; glans develops	Adult type hair does not extend onto thighs, covering a smaller area than in adult	Areola and papilla project to form a secondary mound above the contour of the breast. Stage 4 development of the areolar mound does not occur in 10 per cent of girls and is slight in 20 per cent. When present, it may persist well into adulthood.
5.	Adult in size and shape	Adult in quantity and type with extension onto thighs but not up linea alba	Mature female; papilla projects and areola recesses to general contour of breast
6.		Spreads up linea alba (80 per cent men, 10 per cent women)	

Adapted from Tanner, J. M.: Clin. Endocrinol. Metab., *15*:436–440, 1986.

hair. The uterus and vagina develop simultaneously with the breast but menarche usually does not occur until stage four breast and pubic hair. Although the peak height velocity has been passed, girls may grow an average of 6 cm. more after menarche. Early cycles may be irregular and anovulatory, but early sterility should never be presupposed (Tanner, 1986).

Nutrition: From Infancy Through Adolescence

INTRODUCTION

Proper physical growth and appropriate cognitive development is clearly dependent upon adequate nutrition. In one study, treatment of a group of anemic children with iron and vitamin C resulted in an increased weight gain and slight improvement in achievement of new skills on the Denver Developmental Screening Exam (Aukett, et al., 1986). Meal time also represents a time for social interaction within the family unit, whether this be the bonding of mother and child during breast-feeding or discussion of the day's events during dinnertime.

Malnutrition is still a problem in the United States but inappropriate nutrition, especially calorie/nutrient imbalance, is even more commonplace. Frequent consumption of fast foods, although nutritionally adequate, often adds an excessive amount of calories to the diet in the form of fat. Information from population surveys, such as the National Health and Nutrition Examination Surveys (NHANES 1 and 2), documents a greatly increasing prevalence of obesity in the pediatric age group. This is associated with a greater risk of elevated systolic and diastolic blood pressure in obese children and adolescents (Gortmaker, et al., 1987).

Sociocultural factors, such as increased television viewing among young people, lead to decreased activity, excessive snacking on high-calorie junk foods, and subsequent obesity (Dietz and Gortmaker, 1985). In contrast, dieting in pursuit of the media's representation of the ideal woman may lead to eating disorders, such as bulimia and/or anorexia.

INFANTS AND TODDLERS

Infants require 80 to 120 kcal./kg./day to meet basal metabolic requirements and the energy demands of growth and activity during the first year of life. This decreases by about 10 kcal./kg./day for each subsequent *three*-year period. Increased physical activity or stress imposed by disease processes, such as fever, increase the body's basal energy requirements. For example, fever may increase basal caloric needs by 10 per cent for each degree centigrade while peak physical activity may double or triple the body's usual requirement of 15 to 25 kcal./kg./day. Human milk, most formulas, and a well-balanced diet usually have approximately 10 per cent of calories derived from protein, 50 per cent from carbohydrate, and 40 per

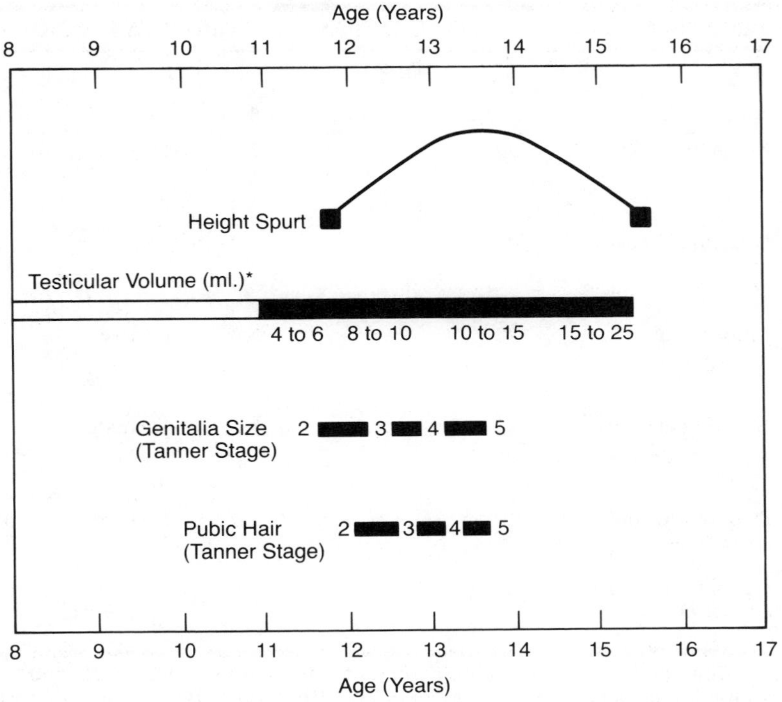

*Testicular volume less than ml. using orchidometer (Prader Beads) represents prepubertal stage.

Figure 38–4. Sequence of pubertal events in average American males. (Adapted from Brookman, R. R., Rauh, J. L., Morrison, J. A., et al.: The Princeton Maturation Study, 1976 unpublished data for adolescents in Cincinnati, Ohio. *In* Copeland, K. C., Brookman, R. R., and Rauh, J. L. [Eds.]: Assessment of Pubertal Development. Columbus, Ohio, Ross Laboratories, August, 1986.)

cent from fat (Barness, 1987). A comparison of some common milks and formulas is shown in Table 38–5.

The ideal food for full-term infants during the first 6 months of life is human milk. Oliver Wendell Holmes once noted, "A pair of substantial mammary glands has the advantage over the two hemispheres of the most learned professor's brain in the art of compounding a nutritious fluid for infants" (Cone,

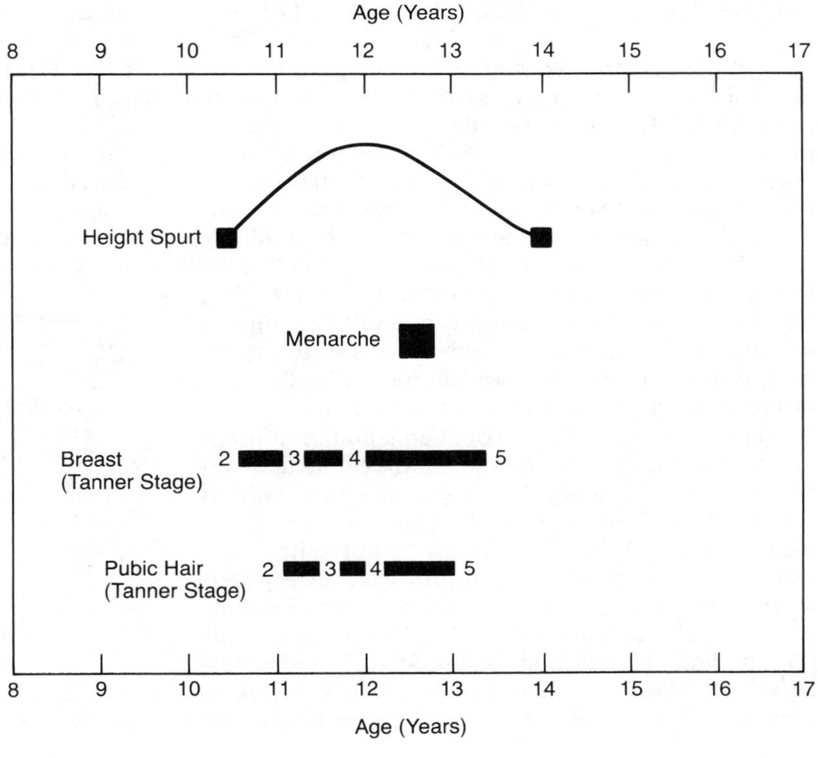

Figure 38–5. Sequence of pubertal events in average American females. (Adapted from Brookman, R. R., Rauh, J. L., Morrison, J. A., et al.: The Princeton Maturation Study, 1976 unpublished data for adolescents in Cincinnati, Ohio. *In* Copeland, K. C., Brookman, R. R., and Rauh, J. L. [Eds.]: Assessment of Pubertal Development. Columbus, Ohio, Ross Laboratories, August, 1986.)

Table 38–5. COMPARISON OF COMMON MILKS AND INFANT FORMULAS

Milk/Formula	Kcal./02	Protein gm./ 100 ml.	CHO gm./ 100 ml.	CHO Type	Fat (gm./ 100 ml.)	Fe Mg./L.	Comments
Human milk	22	1.1	7.0	Lactose	3.8	.3	Small flocculent curd: Iron easily absorbed. Low vitamin D (22 IU./L.) → Supplement or sunlight.
Pasteurized cow's milk	20	3.3	4.8	Lactose	3.7	.4	Tough curd. Do not use before age 6 months, then supplement with Fe and vitamin C.
Evaporated milk	22	3.8	5.4	Lactose	4.0	.4	Softer, smaller curd, less allergenic than whole cow's milk. Universal availability. Supplement with Fe.
Boiled goat's milk	21	3.7	4.6	Lactose	4.3	.5	Lower curd tension, more digestible fat. Must supplement with folic acid, vitamin D, and iron.
Prepared formula—cow's milk based	20	1.5	6.9–7.2	Lactose	3.6–3.8	1.1–1.5 12.0–12.7	Iron-fortified formula. Fluoride supplement if ready to feed formula.
Prepared formulas—soy based	20	1.8–2.1	6.6–6.9	Sucrose Corn syrup	3.6–3.9	12.0–12.7	25–40 per cent cross reactivity with cow's milk protein.

Compiled from Barness, L.: Formula feeding. *In* Berhman, R. E., and Vaughan, V. C. (Eds.): Nelson's Textbook of Pediatrics. 13th ed. Philadelphia, W. B. Saunders Co., 1987, pp. 131–132; and American Academy of Pediatrics Committee on Nutrition. *In* Forbes, G. B., and Woodruff, C. W. (Eds.): Pediatric Nutrition Handbook. Elk Grove Village, Illinois, American Academy of Pediatrics, 1985, p. 369.

1979). Human milk is fresh, readily available at the proper temperature, and generally free of contaminating bacteria. It contains macrophages, lactoferrin, a growth factor for *Lactobacillus bifidis*, and antibodies including secretory IgA (Barness, 1987). The protein in human milk is of higher quality than cow's milk and contains higher amounts of essential and sulfur-containing amino acids (Benkov and LeLeiko, 1987).

The lower protein content of human milk produces a lower renal solute load and a fluid requirement of 130 to 190 ml./kg./day for infants under 6 months of age (Barness, 1987). Commercial cow's milk and soy-based formulas must contain higher levels of protein to compensate for their lower quality (Table 38–5). However, they are quite acceptable for the mother who is unable to nurse her infant or for the parents who wish to bottle-feed their child. Since cow's milk and soy protein are potentially antigenic in some infants, it is advisable to use a protein hydrolysate formula in cases of true milk allergy or malabsorption (Benkov and LeLeiko, 1987).

Human breast milk or commercial infant formula is recommended for the first 6 months of life and may be continued throughout the first year if economically feasible or if there is a family history of allergic or atopic disease. Whole cow's milk is not suitable for infants under 6 months because of excessive protein intake, high renal solute load, poor mineral bioavailability, and increased risk for sensitization to milk protein and/or intestinal blood loss. Very low-fat milks are calorically inadequate and lack the polyunsaturated fats and cholesterol required for the developing nervous system. Whole cow's milk may be introduced after 6 months provided the child consumes one third of total calories as a variety of supplemental foods, including iron-fortified cereal, fruits, and vegetables (AAP Committee on Nutrition, 1986). The total intake of cow's milk or formula should be limited to 32 ounces per day so that other foods are not excluded from the diet.

Supplementation with 1 to 2 mg./kg./day of elemental iron should be considered for infants who are at high risk for iron deficiency (Table 38–6). Breast-fed infants and infants fed commercial ready-to-feed formula, who do not receive additional fluoridated water, may be given .25 mg./day of supplemental fluoride. The breast-fed infant, who receives little exposure to sunlight, may also benefit from an additional 400 units of vitamin D daily since this is present

Table 38–6. INFANTS AT HIGH RISK FOR IRON DEFICIENCY

Low birth weight
Perinatal bleeding
Low hemoglobin concentration at birth
High growth rate
Low socioeconomic status
Chronic hypoxia—high altitude
Frequent infections
Early cow's milk intake
Early solid food intake
Frequent tea intake
Low vitamin C intake
Low meat intake
Breast-feeding > 6 months without iron supplements

From Reeves, J. D.: Pediatr. Rev., *8*:179, 1986.

in small amounts in human milk (AAP Committee on Nutrition, 1980).

Solid foods are generally introduced between 4 to 6 months of age, when the extrusion reflex of early infancy has disappeared and the ability to swallow nonliquid foods has become established. Single-grain infant cereals, such as rice, are usually well tolerated and can provide a source of fortified iron. The order of introduction of other solid foods is generally not critical, but the child should be tried on each new single ingredient food for a week prior to introducing mixtures of foods. The high carbohydrate content of most infant foods balances the high protein content of a predominantly cow's milk diet while higher protein foods, such as meats, may be more appropriate to supplement the lower protein content of human milk. Homemade infant foods should not have salt or sugar added to suit adult tastes. Foods such as hot dogs, nuts, grapes, or rounded candies should not be offered to infants or toddlers because they pose the risks of choking, aspiration, and even death (AAP Committee on Nutrition, 1985).

The toddler's food intake may be quite variable from day to day or even meal to meal. An increasing variety in taste, color, consistency, and temperature will help to maintain an adequate nutritional intake (AAP Committee on Nutrition, 1985). Foods should include the basic four groups:

1. Meat, fish, poultry, eggs, legumes
2. Dairy products (i.e., milk, cheese, and other milk products)
3. Fruits and vegtables
4. Cereal grains, such as rice and potatoes

Parents should be counseled that children at this age are often picky eaters but generally grow well despite this. Parents need to guide children in their selection of food but should not turn mealtime into a battleground. Forcing the child to be a clean-plater does not benefit disadvantaged children and may serve to promote obesity in later life.

Children eating from the four basic food groups do not usually require a multivitamin supplement. Children who eat only vegetables but no dairy products, meat, or eggs require supplemental vitamin B_{12}. A dietitian should also be consulted since children following such a strict vegetarian diet may be lacking other nutrients. Children with malabsorption or hemolytic anemia may require additional folic acid (AAP Committee on Nutrition, 1985). Parents who insist on utilizing a vitamin supplement without any obvious deficiency on the part of the child should be counseled to use a preparation that does not exceed the recommended daily allowances (RDAs) of the National Research Council of the National Academy of Sciences. Vitamins A and D, in particular, can produce toxicity if given in excessive dosages.

ADOLESCENT NUTRITION

Although the common picture of a hungry teenage boy is one with his head immersed in a refrigerator or wolfing down a burger, adolescent boys have the same risk of developing iron-deficiency anemia as adolescent girls. This is due to their greater increase in lean body mass and blood volume. Teenage boys and girls often replace milk and juice with soft drinks, coffee, tea, and alcoholic beverages, thereby lowering their intake of calcium and vitamin C. Since girls are frequently dieting, their overall food intake is diminished in comparison to boys, who are attempting to gain weight and build muscle mass (AAP Committee on Nutrition, 1985).

Energy requirements vary greatly in adolescents, depending upon their activity and stage of adolescence. The athletic teenager at the peak of his or her growth spurt may require an additional 600 to 1200 kcal./day in comparison to the sedentary teenager who spends much of his or her time watching television and eating high-calorie snacks.

Special considerations include the pregnant teenage girl, the teenager following a vegetarian diet, or the teenager at risk for hyperlipidemia. In addition to the deficiencies in calcium, iron, and vitamin A common to adolescent diets, deficiencies of folate or zinc may occur, having a deleterious effect on the outcome of the pregnancy or maternal growth. The prenatal diet should be tailored to allow for a total weight gain of 11 to 13 kg. or an additional 300 kcal./day. The teenager following a strict vegetarian diet is also at risk for deficiencies of calcium, riboflavin, vitamin B_{12}, vitamin D, iron, zinc, and possibly other trace minerals (AAP Committee on Nutrition, 1985).

Routine screening for hyperlipidemias in children is controversial. Blood cholesterol determinations should be obtained in children who have a family history of premature coronary heart disease or hypercholesterolemia in parents, grandparents, and first-degree relatives. If the blood cholesterol exceeds the seventy-fifth percentile (approximately 170 mg./dl. for ages 2 to 19 years), total and high-density lipoprotein (HDL) cholesterol levels should be obtained. The older child or adolescent who is found to have a hyperlipidemia should be counseled to follow a diet lower in total and saturated fat as well as cholesterol, to lose weight if obese, to increase physical activity on a regular basis if sedentary, and to refrain from smoking (NIH Consensus Conference, 1985). Such advice is applicable to most teenagers.

Psychosocial Development

The physician caring for the growing child needs to be well versed in normal child development in order to provide anticipatory guidance to families and to ensure that a child is meeting his or her potential. Studies have indicated that early intervention programs are beneficial for children with developmental delays, regardless of whether the cause of their delays is organic, such as Down's syndrome, or cultural-familial in which the child's development is delayed in part because of unstimulating environment (Law and Frankenburg, 1983). Because the physician has frequent encounters with the young child, he or she is in a unique position to diagnose developmental delays and recommend that prompt intervention be provided.

THEORIES OF CHILD DEVELOPMENT

Individually, children develop at their own rate with a great deal of variability in the normal range.

Children do, however, follow a predictable sequence of acquisition of developmental tasks. For example, children do not learn to walk until they have mastered crawling and then standing. Although the majority of children are able to crawl by 9 months of age and walk by 14 1/2 months, even significantly delayed children will follow the sequence of crawl, stand, and walk (Milani-Comparetti and Gidoni, 1967). This information is important when providing guidance for parents about the development of their child or when prescribing intervention therapy for developmentally delayed youngsters. Regardless of the chronologic age of the child, intervention strategies must work with a child to attain the next step in sequence at his or her developmental age.

This predictable sequence is dictated not only by learning on the part of the child but by maturation of the central nervous system (CNS) as well (Springate, 1981). Prior to a critical stage in the maturation of the CNS, certain skills may not be learned regardless of the intellectual potential of the individual. For instance, nervous system control to the external anal sphincter is incomplete prior to 18 to 24 months of age. Therefore, before this, it is impossible to truly potty train a toddler, regardless of the emotional maturity of that child.

Developmental Screening

In the office setting, the most efficient way to ensure that children are developing to their fullest potential is by routine periodic administration of a standardized developmental screening test. One such screening test commonly in use is the Denver Developmental Screening Test (DDST). This test screens gross motor, fine motor, language, and personal social developmental skills (Fig. 38–6). A two-staged screening is recommended for cost/time effectiveness and to minimize false negatives and positives (Frankenburg, et al., 1983).

Stage I of the screening consists of either the abbreviated DDST or the Prescreening Developmental Questionnaire (PDQ) (Fig. 38–7). The abbreviated DDST is given by a staff member skilled in its administration. Twelve age-appropriate items, three in each section, are presented to each child. The PDQ is a parent questionnaire in which parents are asked 10 age-appropriate questions drawn from the standard DDST. The PDQ, as it requires less staff time, is the Stage I test of choice when parents have at least a high school education. Since results are less accurate with lesser educated parents, the abbreviated DDST is recommended in these cases.

Parents should be informed that this is a screening test, not an IQ test, and if the child does not do well, this does not automatically mean that handicap exists. Approximately 25 per cent of children will be suspect for developmental delay following administration of Stage I and will require Stage II screening. For parents with a high school education, this consists of repeating the PDQ in 2 to 3 weeks or immediate administration of the full DDST is recommended. The full DDST presents the child with additional items to clarify whether or not a delay exists and requires approximately 10 more minutes of the tester's time. Approximately 90 per cent of these testees will be nonsuspect following second stage screening. The other 10 per cent should repeat the full DDST in 2 months. Children who receive abnormal or questionable results on two consecutive DDSTs done 2 months apart should be referred to a child psychologist skilled in developmental assessment of preschoolers.

Other standardized tests exist to assist the practitioner in screening for developmental delays. The Clinical Linguistic and Auditory Milestones Scale (CLAMS) is a language screen based on parental report designed to screen cognitive delays in children with motor delays as well as screen language development in all children (Capute, et al., 1986).

The Milani-Comparetti is a scale of motor skills to identify motorically delayed children by assessing extinction of primitive reflexes, emergence of righting reflexes, and complex motor milestones (Milani-Comparetti and Gidoni, 1967). More recently, in 1978, Capute has published a scale of primitive reflexes and times of expected extinction.

Cognitive Development

Cognitive development, as well as motor development, appears to have certain stages prior to which certain concepts cannot be understood. Piaget has theorized about these stages, and they have become widely incorporated into the literature on child development and how they are relevant to the practitioner (Newman and Newman, 1979). Table 38–7 illustrates the salient features of Piaget's stages of cognitive development. Current researchers feel that these stages are not discrete and that they may overlap, with some children showing features of more than one cognitive stage at a given age. Based on Piaget's theory of cognitive development, children gradually become able to perceive their environment with less sensory input from the world. Familiarity with these stages provides the clinician with insight into not only what a child is learning but how he or she is processing incoming stimuli into knowledge.

The role of heredity and environment in predict-

DATE

NAME

DIRECTIONS BIRTHDATE

HOSP. NO.

1. Try to get child to smile by smiling, talking or waving to him. Do not touch him.
2. When child is playing with toy, pull it away from him. Pass if he resists.
3. Child does not have to be able to tie shoes or button in the back.
4. Move yarn slowly in an arc from one side to the other, about 6" above child's face. Pass if eyes follow 90° to midline. (Past midline; 180°)
5. Pass if child grasps rattle when it is touched to the backs or tips of fingers.
6. Pass if child continues to look where yarn disappeared or tries to see where it went. Yarn should be dropped quickly from sight from tester's hand without arm movement.
7. Pass if child picks up raisin with any part of thumb and a finger.
8. Pass if child picks up raisin with the ends of thumb and index finger using an over hand approach.

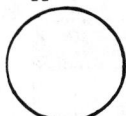

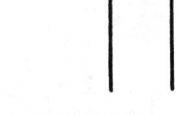

9. Pass any enclosed form. Fail continuous round motions.
10. Which line is longer? (Not bigger.) Turn paper upside down and repeat. (3/3 or 5/6)
11. Pass any crossing lines.
12. Have child copy first. If failed, demonstrate

When giving items 9, 11 and 12, do not name the forms. Do not demonstrate 9 and 11.

13. When scoring, each pair (2 arms, 2 legs, etc.) counts as one part.
14. Point to picture and have child name it. (No credit is given for sounds only.)

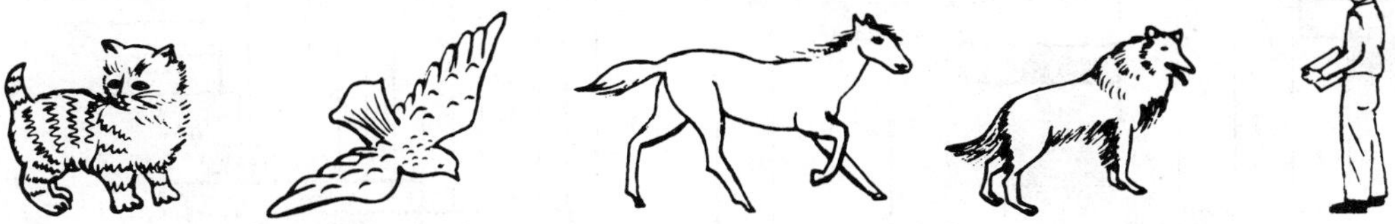

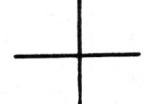

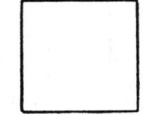

15. Tell child to: Give block to Mommie; put block on table; put block on floor. Pass 2 of 3. (Do not help child by pointing, moving head or eyes.)
16. Ask child: What do you do when you are cold? ..hungry? ..tired? Pass 2 of 3.
17. Tell child to: Put block <u>on</u> table; <u>under</u> table; <u>in front</u> of chair, <u>behind</u> chair. Pass 3 of 4. (Do not help child by pointing, moving head or eyes.)
18. Ask child: If fire is hot, ice is ?; Mother is a woman, Dad is a ?; a horse is big, a mouse is ?. Pass 2 of 3.
19. Ask child: What is a ball? ..lake? ..desk? ..house? ..banana? ..curtain? ..ceiling? ..hedge? ..pavement? Pass if defined in terms of use, shape, what it is made of or general category (such as banana is fruit, not just yellow). Pass 6 of 9.
20. Ask child: What is a spoon made of? ..a shoe made of? ..a door made of? (No other objects may be substituted.) Pass 3 of 3.
21. When placed on stomach, child lifts chest off table with support of forearms and/or hands.
22. When child is on back, grasp his hands and pull him to sitting. Pass if head does not hang back.
23. Child may use wall or rail only, not person. May not crawl.
24. Child must throw ball overhand 3 feet to within arm's reach of tester.
25. Child must perform standing broad jump over width of test sheet. (8-1/2 inches)
26. Tell child to walk forward, ⊂⊃⊂⊃⊂⊃⊂⊃→ heel within 1 inch of toe. Tester may demonstrate. Child must walk 4 consecutive steps, 2 out of 3 trials.
27. Bounce ball to child who should stand 3 feet away from tester. Child must catch ball with hands, not arms, 2 out of 3 trials.
28. Tell child to walk backward, ←⊂⊃⊂⊃⊂⊃⊂⊃ toe within 1 inch of heel. Tester may demonstrate. Child must walk 4 consecutive steps, 2 out of 3 trials.

<u>DATE AND BEHAVIORAL OBSERVATIONS</u> (how child feels at time of test, relation to tester, attention span, verbal behavior, self-confidence, etc,):

REVERSE OF DA FORM 5694, MAY 1988

Figure 38–6. The revised Denver Developmental Screening Test (DDST-R) screens developmental skills in children up to 6 years of age. Delays identified by the test require repeat or more definitive testing, since the test itself is not diagnostic. (From Frankenburg, W. K. Ladoca Publishing Foundation, Denver, Colorado, 1978.)

Illustration continued on following page

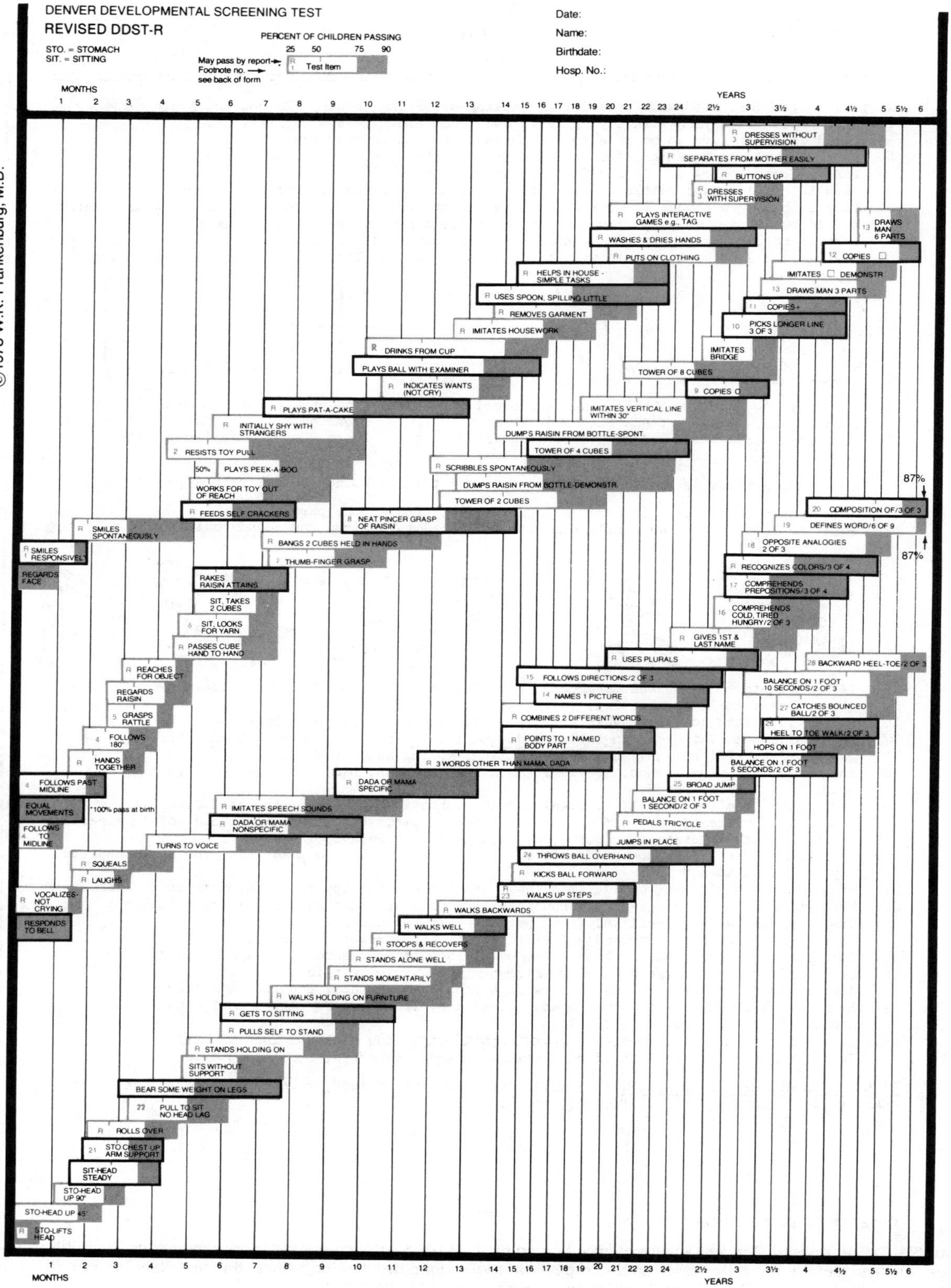

Figure 38–6 *Continued*

0-9 MONTHS (R-PDQ)

REVISED DENVER PRESCREENING DEVELOPMENTAL QUESTIONNAIRE

Child's Name ____________________

Person Completing R-PDQ: ____________________

Relation to Child: ____________________

For Office Use

Today's Date: ___ yr ___ mo ___ day

Child's Birthdate: ___ yr ___ mo ___ day

Subtract to get Child's Exact Age: ___ yr ___ mo ___ day

R-PDQ Age: (___ yr ___ mo ___ completed wks)

CONTINUE ANSWERING UNTIL 3 **"NOs"** ARE CIRCLED

Item			For Office Use
1. Equal Movements When your baby is lying on his/her back, can (s)he move each of his/her arms as easily as the other and each of the legs as easily as the other? Answer **No** if your child makes jerky or uncoordinated movements with one or both of his/her arms or legs.	**Yes**	**No**	(0) FMA
2. Stomach Lifts Head When your baby is on his/her stomach on a flat surface, can (s)he lift his/her head off the surface?	**Yes**	**No**	(0-3) GM

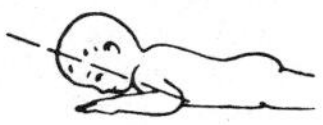

Item			For Office Use
3. Regards Face When your baby is lying on his/her back, can (s)he look at you and watch your face?	**Yes**	**No**	(1) PS
4. Follows To Midline When your child is on his/her back, can (s)he follow your movement by turning his/her head from one side to facing directly forward?	**Yes**	**No**	(1-1) FMA

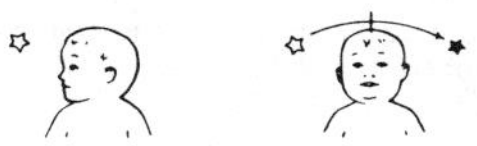

Item			For Office Use
5. Responds To Bell Does your child respond with eye movements, change in breathing or other change in activity to a bell or rattle sounded outside his/her line of vision?	**Yes**	**No**	(1-2) L
6. Vocalizes Not Crying Does your child make sounds other than crying, such as gurgling, cooing, or babbling?	**Yes**	**No**	(1-3) L
7. Smiles Responsively When you smile and talk to your baby, does (s)he smile back at you?	**Yes**	**No**	(1-3) PS
8. Follows Past Midline When your child is on his/her back, does (s)he follow your movement by turning his/her head from one side ***almost all the way to the other side?***	**Yes**	**No**	(2-2) FMA

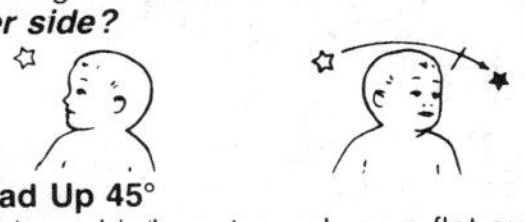

Item			For Office Use
9. Stomach, Head Up 45° When your baby is on his/her stomach on a flat surface, can (s)he lift his/her head 45°?	**Yes**	**No**	(2-2) GM

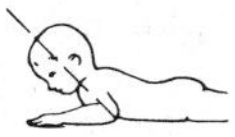

Item			For Office Use
10. Stomach, Head Up 90° When your baby is on his/her stomach on a flat surface, can (s)he lift his/her head 90°?	**Yes**	**No**	(3) GM

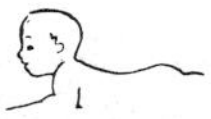

Item			For Office Use
11. Laughs Does your baby laugh out loud without being tickled or touched?	**Yes**	**No**	(3-1) L
12. Hands Together Does your baby play with his/her hands by touching them together?	**Yes**	**No**	(3-3) FMA
13. Follows 180° When your child is on his/her back, does (s)he follow your movement from one side ***all the way*** to the other side?	**Yes**	**No**	(4) FMA

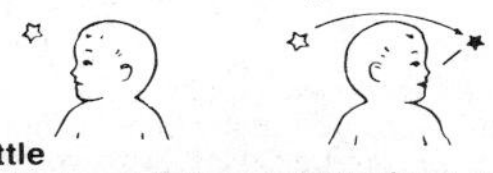

Item			For Office Use
14. Grasps Rattle ***It is important that you follow instructions carefully.*** Do ***not*** place the pencil in the palm of your child's hand. When you touch the pencil to the back or tips of your baby's fingers, does your baby grasp the pencil for a few seconds?	**Yes**	**No**	(4) FMA

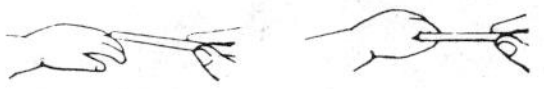

(Please turn page)

Figure 38–7. The Revised Denver Prescreening Developmental Questionnaire (R-PDQ) is administered in the physician's office to parents who have at least a high school education. (From Frankenburg, W. K. Ladoca Publishing Foundation, Denver, Colorado, 1986.)
Illustration continued on following page

ing potential has been widely argued. Most researchers in child development feel that developmental outcomes are a product of child factors, such as genetic predisposition and temperament; physical environmental factors, such as nutrition and playthings; cognitive levels; and values of the social milieu (Law and Frankenburg, 1982–1983).

Temperament. The concept of temperament is important in understanding a child's social and cognitive development.

Temperament is an inborn trait, influencing how infants interact with (and learn from) their environment. Simply expressed, temperament is the how of behavior as opposed to the why (motivation) or what (ability and content) (Thomas, et al., 1968). Temperament is composed of nine components (Table 38–8).

Three basic temperament profiles have been described, based on different combinations of these nine components.

Easy children are rhythmic, predictable, with a predominantly positive mood, and react to stimuli with moderate or low intensity. They readily approach new stimuli and adapt easily. These children are usually described by caregivers as good babies.

Difficult children are irregular with biologic functions, have predominantly negative moods with high intensity of expression, withdraw from new stimuli, and adapt slowly. This is a particularly high-risk group of children for which parental anticipatory guidance and behavioral counseling are extremely important to ensure good parent-child bonding and prevent behavior problems.

Slow-to-warm children typically withdraw from new stimuli and adapt slowly but are moderate to low in intensity. This child is often labeled anxious or fearful. By assuring parents that these children may take longer to adapt, but eventually gain pleasure from participation in new activities, undue parental anxiety and child behavior problems can be prevented.

These, of course, are broad generalizations. Each family's personal value system tempers that family's reaction to a child of a particular temperament. In a

0-9 MONTHS (R-PDQ)

Side #2

CONTINUE ANSWERING UNTIL **3 "NOs"** ARE CIRCLED

Item		For Office Use
15. Sits, Head Steady When sitting, can your child hold his/her head upright and steady? Answer **No** if his/her head falls to either side or upon his/her chest.	Yes No	(4) GM
16. Stomach Chest Up-Arm Support When your baby is on his/her stomach on a flat surface, can (s)he lift his/her chest using his/her arms for support?	Yes No	(4-1) GM

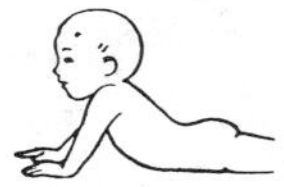

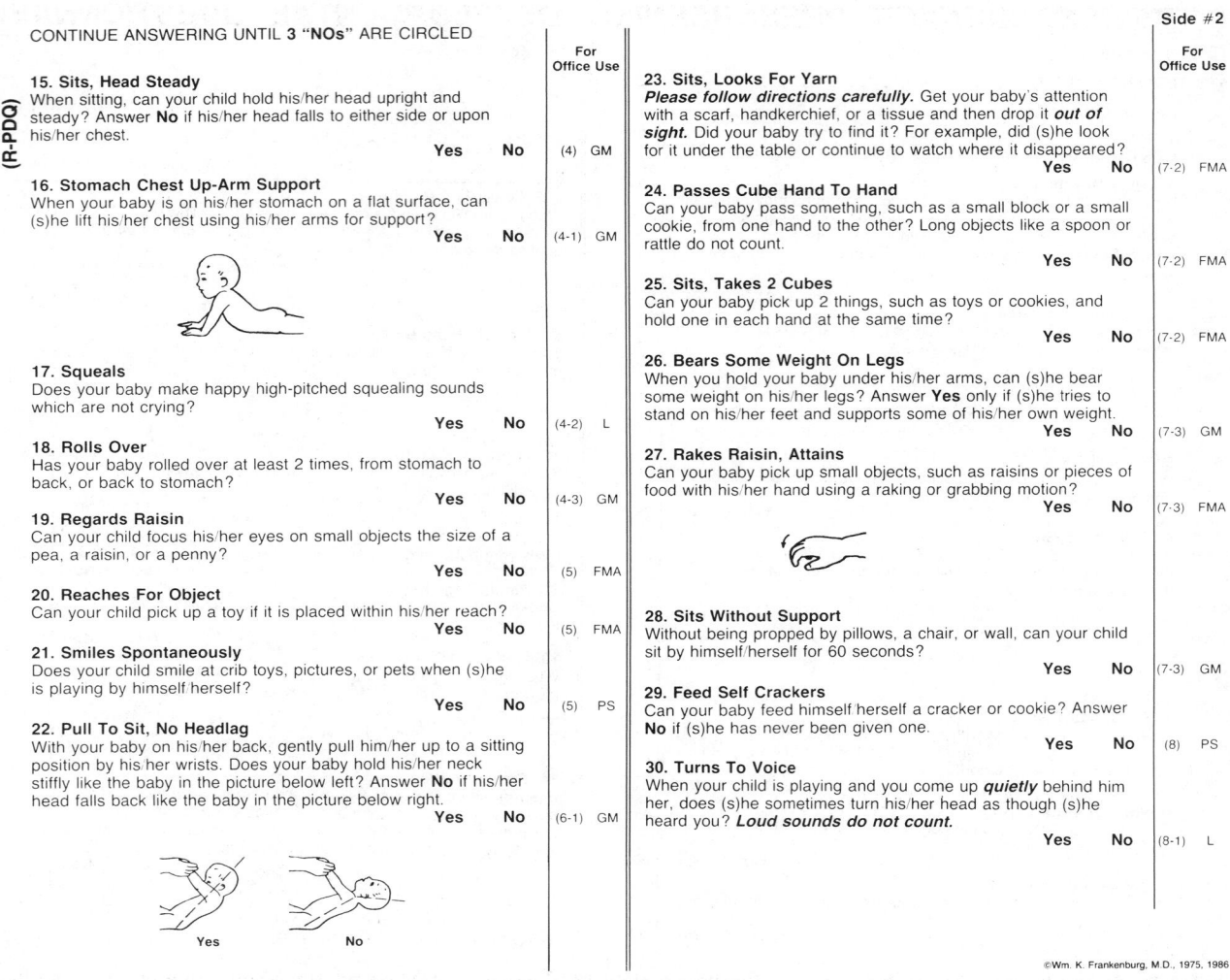

Item		For Office Use
17. Squeals Does your baby make happy high-pitched squealing sounds which are not crying?	Yes No	(4-2) L
18. Rolls Over Has your baby rolled over at least 2 times, from stomach to back, or back to stomach?	Yes No	(4-3) GM
19. Regards Raisin Can your child focus his/her eyes on small objects the size of a pea, a raisin, or a penny?	Yes No	(5) FMA
20. Reaches For Object Can your child pick up a toy if it is placed within his/her reach?	Yes No	(5) FMA
21. Smiles Spontaneously Does your child smile at crib toys, pictures, or pets when (s)he is playing by himself/herself?	Yes No	(5) PS
22. Pull To Sit, No Headlag With your baby on his/her back, gently pull him/her up to a sitting position by his/her wrists. Does your baby hold his/her neck stiffly like the baby in the picture below left? Answer **No** if his/her head falls back like the baby in the picture below right.	Yes No	(6-1) GM

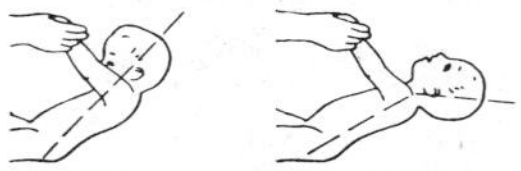

Item		For Office Use
23. Sits, Looks For Yarn ***Please follow directions carefully.*** Get your baby's attention with a scarf, handkerchief, or a tissue and then drop it ***out of sight.*** Did your baby try to find it? For example, did (s)he look for it under the table or continue to watch where it disappeared?	Yes No	(7-2) FMA
24. Passes Cube Hand To Hand Can your baby pass something, such as a small block or a small cookie, from one hand to the other? Long objects like a spoon or rattle do not count.	Yes No	(7-2) FMA
25. Sits, Takes 2 Cubes Can your baby pick up 2 things, such as toys or cookies, and hold one in each hand at the same time?	Yes No	(7-2) FMA
26. Bears Some Weight On Legs When you hold your baby under his/her arms, can (s)he bear some weight on his/her legs? Answer **Yes** only if (s)he tries to stand on his/her feet and supports some of his/her own weight.	Yes No	(7-3) GM
27. Rakes Raisin, Attains Can your baby pick up small objects, such as raisins or pieces of food with his/her hand using a raking or grabbing motion?	Yes No	(7-3) FMA

Item		For Office Use
28. Sits Without Support Without being propped by pillows, a chair, or wall, can your child sit by himself/herself for 60 seconds?	Yes No	(7-3) GM
29. Feed Self Crackers Can your baby feed himself/herself a cracker or cookie? Answer **No** if (s)he has never been given one.	Yes No	(8) PS
30. Turns To Voice When your child is playing and you come up ***quietly*** behind him/her, does (s)he sometimes turn his/her head as though (s)he heard you? ***Loud sounds do not count.***	Yes No	(8-1) L

Figure 38–7 *Continued*

highly competitive, athletically oriented family, for instance, high-energy, high-intensity characteristics in a child may be viewed more positively than in a family where academic achievement is valued. In families where conflict exists between parent and child temperament traits, it is helpful to counsel families about the inborn nature of temperament. This helps relieve unfounded guilt feelings that a parent somehow caused the child's temperament. The family can then work toward accepting the child's unique characteristics and helping him or her fit into the family.

Personality Development. It should be obvious by this point that a great deal of overlap exists in the development process of different facets of the human being. A child's motor, cognitive, and physical development all interrelate in complex ways, and temperament modifies how the development occurs.

Another aspect of the human being that grows and changes over time is personality. Personality is defined as the complex of characteristics that distinguishes an individual, especially the totality of an individual's behavior and emotional characteristics. Personality cannot be viewed totally independent of the other facets but as part of the whole.

One of the most comprehensive theories of personality development is Erikson's Psychosocial Theory. Erikson has broken down psychologic development into eight stages through life. At each stage, the individual is confronted with a crisis requiring integration of personal needs with sociocultural demands. Successful integration of needs and development indicates normal adaptation. Failure to integrate needs and demands represents maladaptive patterns that may persist through life. Knowledge of the stages allows the practitioner to counsel families about the psychosocial needs of a certain aged child and assist them in helping the child integrate societal demands (Table 38–9).

Certain vexing childhood behaviors, such as attachment to a blanket at age 1, negative behaviors and temper tantrums at age 2, and fear of the dark at age 3, are all normal expressions of a child's struggling to achieve age-appropriate developmental tasks. By understanding basic principles of a child's cognitive, emotional, and milestone development, the

Table 38–7. PIAGET'S STAGES OF DEVELOPMENT

Sensorimotor (Birth–18 months)—Patterns or schema of increasingly complex sensory and motor manipulations of the environment are seen. Language not involved.
- Examples:
  - *Cause and effect*—Drop a toy. It will make a sound.
  - *Object permanence*—When a toy is out of sight, it continues to exist.

Preoperational (2–7 years)—Child develops tools for making manipulations on objects symbolically rather than physically. Knowledge tied to our own experiences and requires use of language.
- Examples:
  - Use of imitation when model not present
  - *Symbolic play*—playing house; imaginary friend.

Concrete operational (7–12 years)—Child can perform actions on objects mentally rather than physically, thus can manipulate categories and hierarchies but needs very physical ties—no abstractions.
- Examples:
  - *Conservation*—Weight, mass, and volume of physical matter remain constant.
  - *Classification skills*—Group objects based on shared dimensions (i.e., all *red* objects).

Formal operations (12–late teens)—Thoughts governed more by logical principles than by own perceptions and experiences.
- Examples:
  - *Computational skills*—Ability to manipulate numbers (addition, subtraction, multiplication, division)
  - Manipulate more than two categories of variables simultaneously. Consider relationships between speed, distance, and time during travel.
  - Hypothesize possible changes in the future.
  - Anticipation of consequences of own actions.
  - Think of selves relative to cultural environment of which they are a part.

physician can, with confidence, reassure parents that their child is developing normally or, when deviations from normal do occur, be able to recognize and treat or refer for treatment.

Immunizations

INDICATIONS AND CONTRAINDICATIONS

Routine immunizations are essential for the control and prevention of previously common childhood infectious diseases. Experience has shown that when administration of vaccines, such as pertussis or measles, is allowed to decline or lapse, outbreaks of these diseases occur (Fulginiti, 1985). Most states also mandate routine childhood immunizations as a requirement for school admission. Since individuals vary in their immune and adverse responses to a vaccine, the potential risks to the child must be balanced against the potential benefit to the patient and community (Hess, 1988). Informed consent should be obtained from the patient, parent, or guardian. This should include the risks of the vaccine *and* the risks of the natural disease should the immunization not be given (Hess, 1988). Written information can be used to reinforce verbal communication and assist in documentation (Fulginiti, 1984).

Table 38–8. CHARACTERISTICS OF TEMPERAMENT

Activity	Frequency and speed of involvement
Rhythmicity	Regularity of physiologic functions such as hunger, sleep, elimination
Approach/Withdrawal	Immediate reaction of child to new stimuli
Adaptability	The degree of ease or difficulty with which child adjusts to new stimuli
Intensity	The energy level of responses, without regard to positive or negative quality of the response
Mood	Predominance of pleasant and friendly versus unfriendly behavior during waking
Attention Span/ Persistence	Length of time the child will engage in a single activity with or without interruption
Distractibility	Degree of ease with which extraneous stimuli interfere with child's task performance
Sensory Threshold	Amount of external stimulation required to evoke a response

Prior to vaccine administration, inquiry regarding the child's current state of health as well as that of other family members should be made. A pregnant, unimmunized or immunosuppressed member of the household may contraindicate the administration of certain live virus vaccines, such as polio. Inquiry should also be made regarding any adverse reactions to previously administered vaccines. Specifically, the following reactions contraindicate further administra-

Table 38–9. USING ERIKSON'S PSYCHOSOCIAL STAGES TO GUIDE DEVELOPMENT

Basic Trust vs. Mistrust (0–2 Years–infancy)—Parent can provide consistent nurturing to development of attitude of trust.

Autonomy vs. Shame and Doubt (2–4 Years)— Parent should allow safe exploration of environment and encourage decision making.

Initiative vs. Guilt (5–7 Years)—Limits on child should be for child's, family's, and society's protection and not random or condemning.

Industry vs. Inferiority (8–12 Years)—Caregiver must work with the school to assure that child is achieving to his or her abilities and feeling sense of competence vs. inferiority.

Identity vs. Role Confusion (13–17 Years)—Selection of career goal; establishment of relationship with opposite sex; independence from family should be encouraged by caregiver. Failures to adapt in previous stages make this stage more difficult.

Intimacy vs. Isolation (18–22 Years)—Need to make personal/occupational commitments.

tion of pertussis vaccine: (1) a severe neurological reaction, (2) persistent unconsolable screaming for 3 hours or more, (3) a hyporesponsive, shock-like state, (4) temperature of 40.5°C (105°F) or greater, unexplained by another cause within 48 hours following immunization, (5) a convulsion within 72 hours following immunizations, or (6) an allergic reaction to the vaccine (AAP Committee on Infectious Diseases, 1984). A history of anaphylactic reaction to egg ingestion may contraindicate the administration of measles, mumps, or influenza vaccine since embryonated chicken or duck eggs are used in their production. Skin testing and possible desensitization may be required before these vaccines can be given (Hess, 1988).

In general, vaccine administration should be postponed if the child has an underlying febrile illness, active infection, or has recently been exposed to an early childhood exanthem (Hess, 1988). Minor, nonfebrile illnesses should not contraindicate the use of vaccines, particularly in children who always seem to have an upper respiratory infection or allergic rhinitis (AAP Committee on Infectious Diseases, 1988).

VACCINE ADMINISTRATION

Most immunizations must be given by deep intramuscular injection or subcutaneous injection. Intramuscular injections should be given in the anterolateral thigh or the deltoid or triceps muscles of the upper arm. The sciatic nerve may be potentially injured by deep intragluteal injections. Live viral vaccines must be given simultaneously or at least 1 month apart. If gamma globulin is given, then further vaccine administration should be delayed for 3 months to allow optimal antibody production (Hess, 1988). Acetaminophen administered at the time of immunization in a dose of 10 to 15 mg./kg. and continued every 4 hours for up to 24 hours may moderate the fever, pain, and fussiness of diphtheria, tetanus, pertussis (DPT) vaccination (Lewis, 1988) but could obscure fever caused by concomitant, unrelated infection (AAP Committee on Infectious Diseases, 1988).

Schedule of Immunizations

The recommended schedule for active immunization of normal infants and children is given in Table 38–10. A lapse in the immunization schedule does not require starting over of the entire series. Doses of DTP or any vaccine should not be divided or reduced as this has not been shown to reduce side effects while preserving vaccine efficacy (AAP Committee on Infectious Diseases, 1988).

Every effort should be made to give the measles, mumps, and rubella (MMR) vaccine at 15 months of age. A second MMR is now recommended at entrance to elementary school or middle school, because outbreaks of measles still occur on college, high school, and junior high school campuses (AAP Committee on Infectious Diseases, 1989). MMR should be given at 12 months if there is a measles epidemic in the community. Children may be immunized with MMR even if there is a pregnant or immunosuppressed family member since the vaccine is not infectious to others (Phillips, 1988).

The *Haemophilus influenzae* b diphtheria toxoid conjugate vaccine (PRP-D) is given at 18 months because of its significantly greater ability to stimulate antibody production in younger children than the unconjugated vaccine and because the majority of disease due to *H. influenzae* type b occurs in children under the age of 2. Children with previous *H. influenzae* type b disease prior to age 2 usually do not develop protective antibodies and should also be immunized with PRP-D at 18 months (Phillips, 1988).

Booster Doses

Tetanus and diphtheria boosters (Td) are required every 10 years after the age of 5. If a wound appears particularly contaminated, the Td booster may be given if it has been 5 years since the previous immunization. Booster doses of inactivated polio vaccine must be given every 5 years while only one booster dose of oral polio vaccine (OPV) is required if traveling to an area where polio is endemic (Hess, 1988).

"Catching Up" with Immunizations

Unfortunately, physicians still encounter children who are lacking the appropriate immunizations for their age. At least 1 month is required between DTP doses and 6 to 8 weeks between OPV doses. For children who are at least 15 months old but less than 7 years of age, a tuberculosis skin test, DTP, OPV, and MMR can be given at the initial visit. A second DTP and OPV are given 2 months later and the PRP-D added for children from 18 to 60 months of age. A third DTP can be given 1 to 2 months later if needed to complete the primary series. Booster doses of DTP and OPV can be given 6 to 12 months after completion of the primary series and again between ages 4 to 6 prior to school entry. If compliance with future visits is uncertain, the PRP-D may be given in a separate site at the initial visit in the child who is at least 18 months of age. For the child 7 years old or older, the adult diphtheria-tetanus formulation (Td) is given in place of DTP.

Special Clinical Situations

Preterm infants should be immunized at the usual chronologic age (AAP Committee on Infectious Diseases, 1988).

Bacille Calmette-Guérin (BCG) and live viral

Table 38–10. RECOMMENDED SCHEDULE FOR ACTIVE IMMUNIZATION OF NORMAL INFANTS AND CHILDREN*

Recommended Age†	Vaccine(s)§	Comments
2 months	DTP#1¶, OPV#1**	OPV and DTP can be given earlier in areas of high endemicity
4 months	DTP#2, OPV#2	6-week to 2-month interval desired between OPV doses
6 months	DTP#3	An additional dose of OPV at this time is optional in areas with a high risk of poliovirus exposure
15 months††	MMR #1§§, DTP#4, OPV#3	Completion of primary series of DTP and OPV
18 months	HbCV¶¶	Conjugate preferred over polysaccharide vaccine***
4–6 years	DTP#5†††, OPV#4, MMR #2	At or before school entry
14–16 years	Td§§§	Repeat every 10 years throughout life

*Modified from the Centers for Disease Control: M.M.W.R., *38*:4, 1989.

†These recommended ages should not be construed as absolute, e.g., 2 months can be 6 to 10 weeks. However, MMR should not be given to children <12 months of age. If exposure to measles disease is considered likely, then children 6 through 11 months old may be immunized with single-antigen measles vaccine. These children should be reimmunized with MMR when they are approximately 15 months of age.

§For all products used, consult manufacturers' package enclosures for instructions regarding storage, handling, dosage, and administration. Immunobiologics prepared by different manufacturers can vary, and those of the same manufacturer can change from time to time. The package inserts are useful references for specific products, but they may not always be consistent with current ACIP and American Academy of Pediatrics immunization schedules.

¶DTP = Diphtheria and Tetanus Toxoids and Pertussis Vaccine Adsorbed. DTP may be used up to the seventh birthday. The first dose can be given at 6 weeks of age and the second and third doses given 4 to 8 weeks after the preceding dose.

**OPV = Poliovirus Vaccine Live Oral, Trivalent: contains poliovirus types 1, 2, and 3.

††Provided at least 6 months have elapsed since DTP#3 or, if fewer than 3 doses of DTP have been received, at least 6 weeks since the last previous dose of DTP or OPV. MMR vaccine should not be delayed to allow simultaneous administration with DTP and OPV. Administering MMR at 15 months and DTP#4 and OPV#3 at 18 months continues to be an acceptable alternative.

§§MMR = Measles, Mumps, and Rubella Virus Vaccine, Live. Counties that report ≥5 cases of measles among preschool children during each of the last 5 years should implement a routine 2-dose measles vaccination schedule for preschoolers. The first dose should be administered at 9 months or the first health-care contact thereafter. Infants vaccinated before their first birthday should receive a second dose at about 15 months of age. Single-antigen measles vaccine should be used for children aged <1 year and MMR for children vaccinated on or after their first birthday. If resources do not allow a routine 2-dose schedule, an acceptable alternative is to lower the routine age of MMR vaccination to 12 months.

¶¶HbCV = Vaccine composed of *Haemophilus influenzae* b polysaccharide antigen conjugated to a protein carrier. Children <5 years of age previously vaccinated with polysaccharide vaccine between the ages of 18 and 23 months should be revaccinated with a single dose of conjugate vaccine if at least 2 months have elapsed since the receipt of the polysaccharide vaccine.

***If HbCV is not available, an acceptable alternative is to give *Haemophilus influenzae* b polysaccharide vaccine (HbPV) at age ≥24 months. Children at high risk for *Haemophilus influenzae* type b disease where conjugate vaccine is not available may be vaccinated with HbPV at 18 months of age and revaccinated at 24 months.

†††Up to the seventh birthday.

§§§Td = Tetanus and Diphtheria Toxoids, Adsorbed (for use in persons aged ≥7 years): contains the same amount of tetanus toxoid as DTP or DT but a reduced dose of diphtheria toxoid.

vaccines such as oral polio vaccine are usually contraindicated in the patient who is immunocompromised or infected with human immunodeficiency virus (HIV) and in their household contacts. Enhanced-potency inactivated polio vaccine (IPV) should be given to these children (AAP Committee on Infectious Diseases, 1988). IPV should be given to previously unimmunized adult contacts, especially if pregnant. Because measles is a more serious disease in children with HIV infection than in normal children, MMR continues to be recommended for these children at 15 months or earlier if measles is present in the community (Phillips, 1988). If exposed to measles, these children should receive immune globulin at 0.5 ml./kg. to 15 ml maximum.

Inactivated influenzae vaccine and 23-valent pneumococcal vaccine are also recommended for children at increased risk of serious disease if they become infected. One dose of pneumococcal vaccine is given once to children 2 years and older who have sickle cell disease, functional or anatomic asplenia, nephrotic syndrome, HIV infection, or who are preparing to undergo chemo- or radiation therapy. Split virus influenzae vaccine may be given yearly to children over 6 months of age with chronic cardiac, pulmonary, renal, or metabolic conditions, and children with malignancy who are off chemotherapy or who have symptomatic HIV infection (AAP Committee on Infectious Diseases, 1988).

The infant born to a mother positive for hepatitis B_sAg should receive hepatitis B immune globulin (HBIG) 0.5 ml. intramuscularly within 12 to 24 hours after delivery. An initial dose of hepatitis B vaccine .5 ml intramuscularly (IM) should be given at a

Table 38–11. REPORTABLE EVENTS FOLLOWING VACCINATION*

Vaccine/Toxoid	Event	Interval from Vaccination
DTP, P, DTP/Polio Combined	A. Anaphylaxis or anaphylactic shock	24 hours
	B. Encephalopathy (or encephalitis)†	7 days
	C. Shock-collapse or hypotonic-hyporesponsive collapse†	7 days
	D. Residual seizure disorder†	(See Aids to Interpretation†)
	E. Any acute complication or sequela (including death) of above events	No limit
	F. Events in vaccinees described in manufacturer's package insert as contraindications to additional doses of vaccine‡ (such as convulsions)	(See package insert)
Measles, Mumps, and Rubella; DT, Td, Tetanus Toxoid	A. Anaphylaxis or anaphylactic shock	24 hours
	B. Encephalopathy (or encephalitis)†	15 days for measles, mumps, and rubella vaccines; 7 days for DT, Td, and T toxoids
	C. Residual seizure disorder†	(See Aids to Interpretation†)
	D. Any acute complication or sequela (including death) of above events	No limit
	E. Events in vaccinees described in manufacturer's package insert as contraindications to additional doses of vaccine‡	(See package insert)
Oral Polio Vaccine	A. Paralytic poliomyelitis	
	—in a non-immunodeficient recipient	30 days
	—in an immunodeficient recipient	6 months
	—in a vaccine-associated community case	No limit
	B. Any acute complication or sequela (including death) of above events	No limit
	C. Events in vaccinees described in manufacturer's package insert as contraindications to additional doses of vaccine‡	(See package insert)
Inactivated Polio Vaccine	A. Anaphylaxis or anaphylactic shock	24 hours
	B. Any acute complication or sequela (including death) of above event	No limit
	C. Events in vaccinees described in manufacturer's package insert as contraindications to additional doses of vaccine‡	(See package insert)

*From National Childhood Vaccine Injury Act: Requirements for permanent vaccination records and for reporting of selected events after vaccination. M.M.W.R., 37:198, 1988.

†Aids to Interpretation:

Shock-collapse or hypotonic-hyporesponsive collapse may be evidenced by signs or symptoms such as decrease in or loss of muscle tone, paralysis (partial or complete), hemiplegia, hemiparesis, loss of color or turning pale white or blue, unresponsiveness to environmental stimuli, depression of or loss of consciousness, prolonged sleeping with difficulty arousing, or cardiovascular or respiratory arrest.

Residual seizure disorder may be considered to have occurred if no other seizure or convulsion unaccompanied by fever or accompanied by a fever of less than 102°F occurred before the first seizure or convulsion after the administration of the vaccine involved,

AND, if in the case of measles-, mumps-, or rubella-containing vaccines, the first seizure or convulsion occurred within 15 days after vaccination OR in the case of any other vaccine, the first seizure or convulsion occurred within 3 days after vaccination,

AND, if two or more seizures or convulsions unaccompanied by fever or accompanied by a fever of less than 102°F occurred within 1 year after vaccination.

The terms seizure and convulsion include grand mal, petit mal, absence, myoclonic, tonic-clonic, and focal motor seizures and signs. Encephalopathy means any significant acquired abnormality of, injury to, or impairment of function of the brain. Among the frequent manifestations of encephalopathy are focal and diffuse neurologic signs, increased intracranial pressure, or changes lasting at least 6 hours in level of consciousness, with or without convulsions. The neurologic signs and symptoms of encephalopathy may be temporary with complete recovery, or they may result in various degrees of permanent impairment. Signs and symptoms such as high-pitched and unusual screaming, persistent unconsolable crying, and bulging fontanel are compatible with an encephalopathy, but in and of themselves are not conclusive evidence of encephalopathy. Encephalopathy usually can be documented by slow wave activity on an electroencephalogram.

‡The health-care provider must refer to the CONTRAINDICATION section of the manufacturer's package insert for each vaccine.

separate site within the first 7 days followed by repeat doses 1 and 6 months later (AAP Committee on Infectious Diseases, 1988).

FUTURE VACCINES

Varicella vaccine has been shown to be well tolerated in normal children and to provide long-lasting protection. Children with leukemia have more reactions to the vaccine and are less fully protected. However, their disease is milder if they develop chicken pox after having been immunized (Phillips, 1988). An acellular pertussis vaccine has demonstrated fewer local reactions, such as fever and fretfulness with good antibody response, in a neutralization test (Blennow, 1988). Protective efficacy accompanied by a significant decrease in serious adverse effects awaits further demonstration prior to general use in the United States.

THE NATIONAL CHILDHOOD VACCINE INJURY ACT

The National Childhood Vaccine Injury Act was passed to provide compensation for children inadvertently injured by any of the routinely recommended childhood vaccines and to provide liability protection for manufacturers and health care providers who administer the vaccines. The intent of the law is to ensure a stable supply of vaccine and allow routine immunizations to continue. The physician or other health care provider must maintain permanent documentation of the date, vaccine type, manufacturer, lot number, and name, address, and title of the person administering the vaccine. A list of reportable events is given in Table 38–11.

References

American Academy of Pediatrics Committee on Infectious Diseases: Pertussis vaccine. Pediatrics, *74*:303–305, 1984. *Discusses usage of pertussis vaccine and immunization deferred in children with neurologic problems.*

American Academy of Pediatrics Committee on Infectious Disease: Report of the Committee on Infectious Diseases (The Red Book). 21st ed. Elk Grove Village, American Academy of Pediatrics, 1988, pp. 14, 21, 41, 320. *Provides complete information on pediatric immunizations and infectious diseases of children. All physicians providing primary care for children should have a copy of this book.*

American Academy of Pediatrics Committee on Infectious Diseases: Measles: Reassessment of Current Immunization Policy. AAP News, *5*:6–7, 1989.

American Academy of Pediatrics Committee on Nutrition. *In* Forbes, G. B., and Woodruff, C. W. (Eds.): Pediatric Nutrition Handbook. 2nd ed. Elk Grove Village, American Academy of Pediatrics, 1985, pp. 2–65, 88–144, 213–220, 369. *Discusses pediatric nutrition from breast- and bottle-feeding to specific deficiencies or disease states.*

American Academy of Pediatrics Committee on Nutrition: Prudent life-style for children: dietary fat and cholesterol. Pediatrics, *78*:521–525, 1986. *The official recommendations of the AAP on this matter.*

American Academy of Pediatrics Committee on Nutrition: Vitamin and mineral supplement needs in normal children in the United States. Pediatrics, *66*:1015–1021, 1980.

American Academy of Pediatrics Committee on Psychosocial Aspects of Child and Family Health 1985–1988: Guidelines for Health Supervision II. Elk Grove Village, American Academy of Pediatrics, 1988, p. 59. *Covers historical information, physical exam items, screening tests, immunizations, and anticipatory guidance from prenatal visits to young adult exams.*

Aukett, M. A., Parks, Y. A., Scott, P. H., and Wharton, B. A.: Treatment with iron increases weight gain and psychomotor development. Arch. Dis. Child., *6*:849–857, 1986.

Barness, L. A.: Nutrition and nutritional disorders: *In* Behrman, R. E., and Vaughan, V. C. (Eds.): Nelson Textbook of Pediatrics. 13th ed. Philadelphia, W. B. Saunders Co., 1987, pp. 113–138.

Benkov, K. J., and LeLeiko, N. S.: A rational approach to infant formulas. Pediatr. Ann., *16*:225–230, 1987.

Blennow, M., Granstrom, M., Jaatmaa, E., and Olin, P.: Primary immunization of infants with an acellular pertussis vaccine in a double-blind randomized clinical trial. Pediatrics, *82*:293–299, 1988.

Capute, A., Accardo, P. J., Vinning, E., et al.: Primitive Reflex Profile. Baltimore, University Park Press, 1978.

Capute, A., Shapiro, B. K., Wachtel, R. C., Gunther, V. A., and Palmer, F. B.: The Clinical Linguistic and Auditory Milestone Scale (CLAMS). Am. J. Dis. Child., *140*:694, 1986.

Carey, W. B.: The Difficult Child. Pediatrics in Review, *81*(2):39, 1986.

Chess, S., and Hassibi, M.: Normal and abnormal psychological development. *In* Rudolph, A. M., Hoffman, J. I., and Axelrod, S. (Eds.): Pediatrics. 17th ed. Norwalk, CT, Appleton-Century-Crofts, 1982, pp. 43–81.

Cone, T. E.: History of American Pediatrics. Boston, Little, Brown, 1979, p. 138.

Copeland, K. C.: Variations in normal sexual development. Pediatrics in Review, *8*:47–55, 1986.

Dietz, W. H., and Gortmaker, S. L.: Do we fatten our children at the television set? Obesity and television viewing in children and adolescents. Pediatrics, *75*:807–812, 1985. *Correlates the prevalence of obesity with the hours of television watched per day. (Prevalence increased 2 per cent for each hourly increment of television.)*

Frankenburg, W. K., Sandal, A. W., and Kemper, M. B.: Developmental screening. *In* Frankenburg, W. K., Thornton, S. M., and Cohrs, M. (Eds.): Pediatric Developmental Diagnosis. Denver, Denver Developmental Materials Inc., 1987, pp. 15–27. *Basic overview of developmental screening in general practice, including chapters on developmental screening, neurologic evaluation, metabolic evaluation, and others.*

Fulginiti, V. A.: Patient education for immunizations. Pediatrics, *74*(Suppl):961–963, 1984.

Fulginiti, V. A.: Current topics in immunization. Pediatric Consult., *4*:1–6, 1985.

Gortmaker, S. L., Dietz, W. H., Sobol, A. M., and Wehler, C. A.: Increasing pediatric obesity in the United States. Am. J. Dis. Child., *141*:535–540, 1987.

Green, M. (Ed.): Pediatric Diagnosis. 4th ed. Philadelphia, W. B. Saunders Co., 1986, pp. 278–285. *Lists and discusses differential diagnoses for a variety of pediatric problems.*

Hamill, P. V. V., Drizd, T. A., Johnson, C. L., et al.: Physical growth: National Center for Health Statistics percentiles. Am. J. Clin. Nutr., *32*:607–629, 1979.

Hess, G. H.: Childhood immunizations. *In* Hess, G. H., and Van Buren, R. C. (Eds.): Immunization Guidelines. Kansas City, American Academy of Family Physicians, October, 1988, pp. 1–5. *Succinctly and practically summarizes immunization information.*

Hoekelman, R. A.: The physical examination of infants and children. *In* Bates, B.: A Guide to Physical Examination and History Taking. 4th ed. Philadelphia, J. B. Lippincott Co., 1987, pp. 544–546.

Keefer, C. H.: Normal growth and development: an overview. *In* Dershewitz, R. A., (Ed.): Ambulatory Pediatric Care. Philadelphia, J. B. Lippincott Co., 1988, pp. 23–27. *This textbook is an excellent reference for common office problems in pediatrics.*

Law, J., and Frankenburg, W. K.: Screening in pediatrics. *In* Kelley, V. C.: Practice of Pediatrics. Vol. 1. Philadelphia, Harper & Row, 1982–1983. *Excellent review of developmental screening.*

Levine, M. D., Carey, W. B., Crocker, A. C., and Gross, R. T.: Developmental-Behavioral Pediatrics. Philadelphia, W. B. Saunders Co., 1983.

Lewis, K., Cherry, J. D., Sachs, M. H., et al.: The effect of prophylactic acetaminophen administration on reactions to DTP vaccination. Am. J. Dis. Child., *142*:62–65, 1988.

Lipsky, M. S., and Horner, J. M.: The child with short stature. Am. Fam. Physician, *37*:230–241, 1988.

Milani-Comparetti, A., and Gidoni, E. A.: Routine developmental examination in normal and retarded children. Dev. Med. Child. Neurol., *9*:63, 1967. *A good objective screening test for motor development.*

Moore, W. M.: Physical growth. *In* Johnson, T. R., Moore, W. M., and Jeffries, J. E., (Eds.): Children Are Different:

Developmental Physiology. 2nd ed. Columbus, Ross Laboratories, 1978, pp. 2–23.

National Institutes of Health, Consensus Conference. Lowering blood cholesterol to prevent heart disease. J.A.M.A., *253*:2080–2086, 1985.

Newman, B. M., and Newman, P. R.: Development Through Life: A Psychosocial Approach. Homewood, IL, The Dorsey Press, 1979. *Psychology text that ties together the different psychosocial issues (temperament, cognitive development, emotional development, milestone development) for each age group throughout life and provides practical applications.*

Phillips, C. F.: Immunizations: let's keep kids on schedule. Contemporary Pediatrics, October, 1988, pp. 106–116.

Reeves, J. D.: Iron supplementation in infancy. Pediatr. Rev., *8*:177–184, 1986. *Discusses the evaluation of infants for iron deficiency and their management.*

Sahler, O. J., and McAnarney, E. R.: The Child from Three to Eighteen. St. Louis, The C. V. Mosby Co., 1981, pp. 3–20.

Silverstein, J. H., and Rosenbloom, A. L.: Evaluating growth failure: diagnostic tools. Fam. Pract. Recert., *10*:43–69, 1988. *Provides good clinical tips on assessing the child who fails to grow.*

Springate, J. E.: The neuroanatomic basis of early motor development: a review. Dev. Behav. Ped., *2*(4):146–149, 1981.

Tanner, J. M., and Davies, P. S. W.: Clinical longitudinal standards for height and height velocity for North American children. J. Pediatr., *107*:317–327, 1985. *Growth charts that account for early and late maturers during puberty may be obtained from Serono Laboratories, Inc., 280 Pond St., Randolph, MA 02368 or Castlemead Publications, Swains Mill, 4A Cranes Mead, Ware, Hertfordshire SG129PY, England.*

Tanner, J. M.: Normal growth and techniques of growth assessment. Clin. Endocrinol. Metab., *15*:411–450, 1986. *Focuses on appropriate methods of measuring physical growth, particularly pubertal growth.*

Thomas, A., Chess, S., and Birch, H. G.: Temperament and Behavior Disorder in Children. New York, New York University Press, 1968.

Vaughan, V. C.: Developmental pediatrics. *In* Behrman, R. E., and Vaughan, V. C. (Eds.): Nelson Textbook of Pediatrics. 13th ed. Philadelphia, W. B. Saunders Co., 1987, pp. 6–35.

39

Childhood and Adolescence

Christopher V. Chambers
Paul C. Brucker

One of the special joys of a family physician derives from providing care to children and adolescents in the context of their families. The family doctor functions not only as the health care provider and advocate for the child, but also as the physician for the entire family, thereby bringing a more global perspective to the issues of normal development and the disruptive effects of illness. Children and adolescents represent a significant portion of a family physician's practice. From 20 to 35 per cent of patient care activities of the average family physician are devoted to the care of children and young adults less than 21 years of age.

Pediatricians and other specialists also provide medical care for children and adolescents. According to one source, pediatricians provide most of the care given to infants and preschool children, but after age 4, the health care of children is nearly equally distributed between pediatricians and family physicians. After age 10, family physicians and general practitioners provide the great majority of care (Starfield et al., 1983).

The range of health care provided for children and adolescents by family physicians has been studied and is similar to that documented by primary care pediatricians. Table 39–1 presents data for the 25 most common diagnoses of children and adolescents (less than 18 years of age) seen in family practice, representing 77.5 per cent of all diagnoses made on these patients in one year (Poole et al., 1982). As evidenced from this table, family physicians provide a wide range of services, including health supervision, the diagnosis and management of acute and chronic medical problems, as well as the evaluation and management of emotional and social problems. The family physician must, therefore, possess broad-based clinical skills in order to be able to address the diversity of problems. The physician's practice must also make certain accommodations to appropriately meet the varied needs of these populations. The overall objective in providing medical care for children and adolescents should be to help them achieve their full potential in growth and development.

Routine Health Care of Children

UTILIZATION

The majority of health care for infants and toddlers is well-baby care, organized around recommended immunization schedules. Children under 2 make an average of 4 to 5 visits per year to physicians. For most children over the age of 2, the basic immunization schedules are nearly completed and most of the medical care provided to these children is for evaluation and management of acute or chronic medical problems. In general, this is a healthy group, and children between the ages of 2 and 14 make an average of less than two visits per year to physicians (National Ambulatory Medical Care Survey, 1978).

Nevertheless, there is much to be accomplished in the routine health supervision visit for children. In addition to obtaining an interval history, the child's growth and development are assessed by recording

Table 39–1. MOST COMMON DIAGNOSES IN CHILDREN (< 18 YEARS OLD) SEEN IN FAMILY PRACTICE

Diagnoses	Percent of All Pediatric Diagnoses	Percent of All Pediatric Patients
1. Well-child care	25.2	53.8
2. Upper respiratory tract infection	12.0	31.2
3. Acute otitis media	7.6	14.2
4. Prenatal care	4.3	3.5
5. Pharyngitis/tonsillitis	3.5	9.0
6. Laceration	2.7	6.5
7. Sprains/strains	2.0	4.8
8. Chronic or serous otitis media	1.9	4.8
9. Bronchitis/ bronchiolitis	1.8	4.8
10. Viral syndrome	1.4	4.6
11. Hay fever	1.3	2.5
12. Fracture	1.3	2.2
13. Bruise/contusion	1.2	4.0
14. Administrative*	1.2	3.6
15. Conjunctivitis	1.2	3.7
16. Infectious diarrhea	1.1	3.2
17. Abdominal pain (unknown etiology)	1.1	2.9
18. Warts	1.0	2.1
19. Cystitis	1.0	2.5
20. Asthma	0.9	1.7
21. Pneumonia	0.8	1.7
22. Eczema	0.7	2.0
23. Psychophysiologic gastrointestinal symptoms	0.7	1.8
24. Acne	0.6	1.6
25. Fever without an identified source	0.6	2.0
	77.5%	

From Poole, S. R., Morrison, J. D., Marshall, J., et al.: J. Fam. Pract., *15* (5):945, 1982.

*Administrative services for which the patient was billed, including filling out forms, writing letters, and making referrals.

the height and weight and systematically reviewing developmental and behavioral milestones. The child is examined and appropriate sensory screening is performed and recorded. Simple laboratory tests also have been recommended to screen for clinically unrecognized diseases, but the appropriate interval and frequency of screening remain elusive. At all visits, there is the opportunity to provide anticipatory guidance regarding future development and possible protection against illness.

There are no compelling guidelines regarding the frequency of routine visits for children over 2 years of age (Strain, 1984). Annual visits prior to each school year have been recommended, but visits may be most appropriate around the approach or arrival of other milestones. For older children in particular, the onset of puberty or menarche may be a good time for a visit to a trusted family physician. Although the best interval has not been determined, regular visits are recommended because they establish a trusted relationship for the discussion of future problems, and they allow the physician to assess a child's growth and development over time.

CONDUCT OF THE ROUTINE VISIT

Preschool and school-aged children are generally brought to the office by one or both of their parents. The parents should be given the opportunity to define the agenda. A simple question, such as "What had you hoped we would accomplish in today's visit?", may help to elicit any underlying concerns that the parent may have about the child's growth and development.

Although the parents provide the reason for the visit and most of the history, older children should be given the chance to tell the physician why they have come to the office. Even in the case of the young child, however, important nonverbal communication takes place during the first few minutes of the office visit. Preschool children keep a wary eye on the physician and make value judgments based on their perceptions of their parents' reactions to the physician. Because of this, it is a good idea to start off visits with small children by engaging in relaxed conversation with the parents and tentative playful interaction with the child in the parent's lap. Most of the physical examination of the 2- and 3-year-old child can be performed while the child is held by the parent. By alternating parts of the physical examination with playful conversation and gestures, a skillful clinician can examine even an ill 2- or 3-year-old without increasing the child's anxiety.

Older children are generally more comfortable in the physician's office, particularly if they have developed a sense of trust for the doctor. School-aged children usually enjoy telling the physician why they have come, and, conversely, it is a good idea for the physician to explain what is going to happen during each part of the visit. The physician's relationship with the adult members of the family, as well as the child's level of cooperation and maturity, helps to determine the best approach. Again, patience and flexibility are essential in evaluating children of various ages.

A brief mention should be made regarding physician availability for problems other than those addressed at regularly scheduled appointments. One of the most important factors in a parent's decision in choosing a physician for a child is the availability of the physician. As previously mentioned, the great majority of visits for the preschool-aged child, and to a lesser extent for the school-aged child, are for acute problems. The family physician taking care of children must have some available time in the practice schedule for seeing children on short notice. Availability by phone in off hours or during the day is also an issue. Although children over 2 are less likely to have urgent problems than infants and toddlers, there are still a great many questions that arise during the night. Many physicians have found it worthwhile to have a designated phone hour each morning before office hours begin to allow parents the chance to ask questions about less urgent problems or to discuss having their child seen that day for an unscheduled appointment.

GROWTH AND DEVELOPMENT MEASUREMENTS

During health supervision visits for children, growth and development are routinely assessed. Measurements are recorded and compared with published standards. The sequence of growth in children is usually uncomplicated and orderly. The challenge for the physician is to determine whether deviations from this orderly sequence are variations of normal or indications of an underlying problem. Any major variation from accepted standards becomes a red flag for the physician. The physician must then decide between watchful waiting—that is, a passive monitoring of indices of improvement or worsening—or diagnostic evaluation, looking for a specific diagnosis and a course of intervention. Often, the choice is a combination of the two.

Height and Weight

The height and weight of children should be recorded at least yearly after the age of 2. Routine head circumference measurements are no longer necessary unless there is specific clinical concern. The height and weight measurements should also be plotted on the standard growth curves and reviewed with parents. As an example, most parents find that visualizing the concept of tracking helps them understand how their child can be shorter than other children of the same age and still be growing normally.

Deviations from normal merit brief mention here. On one hand, growth curves can be used to identify the obese child in whom a more structured evaluation of diet should follow. Recent studies linking childhood obesity with risk factors for heart disease in adults suggest that there may be value in early identification and interventions for these children. Conversely, a very thin child may be found to have a calorie-poor diet and appropriate suggestions should be made for this child as well. Failure to grow or gain weight also can be a consequence of any of a number of physical and psychologic problems. There is no universally accepted definition for failure to thrive, but various authors have suggested that children with weight below the third percentile for age or children whose weights are significantly crossing percentiles should be considered to be failing to thrive (Berwick, 1980). When organic disease is not readily apparent by clinical examination, failure to thrive is an uncommon diagnosis in children over 2. In most instances, deviations from the accepted growth standards are the result of individual, familial, or ethnic variations from published charts. In general, clinical judgment dictates whether an aggressive medical evaluation or watchful waiting is appropriate.

Blood Pressure Monitoring

Although clinical hypertension is far less prevalent in children than in adults, there is increasing concern about the relationship between elevated blood pressure in youths and the development of essential hypertension and cardiovascular disease in adulthood. Consequently, recommendations for the regular monitoring of blood pressure have been established and standards for comparison are now available (Task Force on Blood Pressure Control, 1987).

It is generally accepted that routine monitoring of blood pressure as a part of continuing medical care should begin at age 3. For the normotensive child, annual measurements at the time of well-child visits are appropriate. Blood pressure measurements should also be made in the child over 3 at the time of presentation for acute illnesses such as poststreptococcal glomerulonephritis because increased blood pressure may complicate the primary illness.

Because of the rapid changes in growth during childhood, several different pediatric cuffs should be available. The appropriate size cuff should be long enough to completely encircle the circumference of the arm and wide enough to cover approximately three fourths of the upper arm between the shoulder and the olecranon. The bell of the stethoscope should fit comfortably in the antecubital fossa without being placed under the lower margin of the cuff.

The blood pressure in children is best measured when environmental stress and anxiety about the measurement have been reduced. Blood pressure in children is more labile than in adults and can be greatly affected by endogenous catecholamines. As a result, acute illness or even anxiety can lead to transient elevations of the blood pressure.

The blood pressure measurement should be recorded in the patient's chart and compared with standard nomograms (Fig. 39–1). These nomograms were compiled from cumulative data from several studies. Black, Mexican-American, and white children were represented in the studies sampled, and there were no differences in the blood pressure readings among these groups. The curves, therefore, appear applicable to all races.

In conjunction with the recommendations from the Task Force on Blood Pressure Control in Children published in 1987, normal blood pressure is defined as systolic and diastolic blood pressures less than the ninetieth percentile for age and sex. High normal blood pressure is defined as systolic and/or diastolic blood pressure between the ninetieth and ninety-fifth percentiles for age and sex. High blood pressure or hypertension is defined as average systolic and/or diastolic blood pressure equal to or greater than the ninety-fifth percentile for age and sex on at least three occasions. There are remarkable differences between children and adults with respect to the readings that

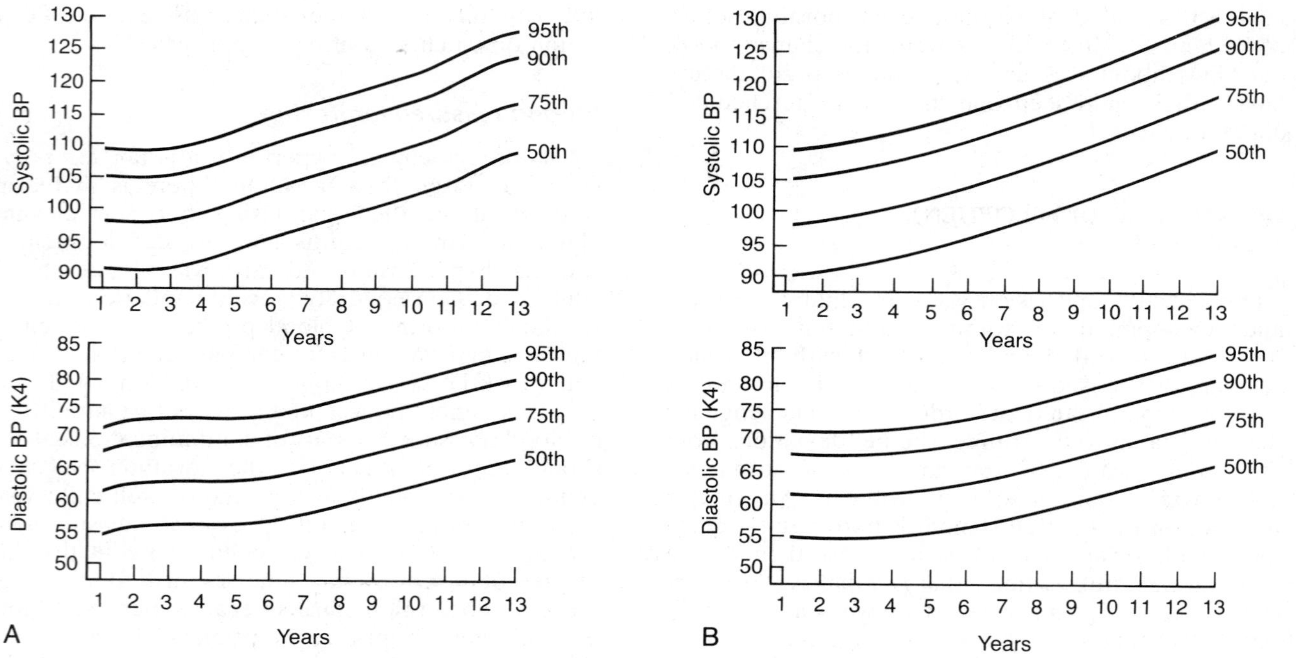

Figure 39–1. Age-specific percentiles of blood pressure measurements in *(A)* girls and *(B)* boys, 1 to 13 years of age; Korotkoff Phase IV (K4) used for diastolic blood pressure. (Redrawn from Task Force on Blood Pressure in Children.)

determine high blood pressure, and, consequently, comparisons to published standards must be done. For example, a systolic pressure of 111 mm. is in the ninetieth percentile for a 6-year-old boy.

Elevated Blood Pressure in Children

The significance of high blood pressure in children is often unclear. For young children, there is a poor correlation between high blood pressure measurements and the development of essential hypertension as an adult (Shear et al., 1986). It is not until the onset of puberty that elevated blood pressure predicts well the development of essential hypertension. There are no clear data regarding the number of children with high blood pressure in whom an underlying cause will be found. Previous studies that found secondary hypertension in 80 per cent or more of young children were studies of referral populations to specialty care. Good data regarding primary care populations are not available. However, it is still true that the younger the patient and the more severe the hypertension, the more likely one is to find an underlying cause of the elevated blood pressure.

In children under 6, the most common causes of chronic sustained hypertension are renal parenchymal disease, coarctation of the aorta, and renal artery stenosis. In the 6- to 10-year-old age group as a whole, renal artery stenosis is the most common cause of sustained hypertension followed by renal parenchymal disease and essential hypertension. However, this is skewed by the relatively large number of white females with renovascular or intrinsic renal disease. In 6- to 10-year-old white males and in black children of this age group of both sexes, essential hypertension is the most common diagnosis for sustained elevated blood pressures (Task Force on Blood Pressure, 1987).

It is readily apparent that the handling of a high blood pressure must be individualized for each patient and must take into account the age, race, sex, family history, and level of the blood pressure. Repeated blood pressure measurements are necessary to demonstrate that the elevation is sustained, but the extent of the medical evaluation will depend upon the severity of the elevation.

A detailed history and physical examination are necessary in the evaluation of children with sustained elevated blood pressure. The family history should elicit the presence of essential hypertension or other inherited diseases that may be underlying causes of secondary hypertension, as well as any family history of early complications of hypertension and the presence or absence of other coronary artery disease risk factors. Systemic symptoms suggestive of connective tissue disease or underlying endocrine problems should be reviewed when appropriate. In particular, the failure to grow or gain weight may be suggestive of renal parenchymal or renovascular disease.

On physical examination, attention should again be paid to detecting underlying causes of secondary hypertension, as well as documenting end organ disease from sustained elevated blood pressure. Aortic coarctation is suggested by absent or delayed femoral pulses and low leg blood pressure relative to arm blood pressure. An abdominal bruit may indicate the presence of renovascular disease. Young children should have a careful abdominal examination, looking for unilateral or bilateral masses found with Wilms' tumor, neuroblastoma, or polycystic kidneys. Physical findings related to less common problems of thyroid or adrenal function are generally apparent on examination. As in an older patient with high blood pressure, a funduscopic examination should be performed to look for changes consistent with chronic hypertension and a complete cardiac examination should be done, again looking for end organ disease.

The laboratory evaluation of the patient with hypertension should also be individualized. For many patients with mildly elevated blood pressure on a single measurement, the history and physical examination findings are noncontributory. However, given the common causes of hypertension in young children, it seems prudent to recommend a urinalysis to screen for underlying renal disease in every child with even one elevated reading. If the blood pressure remains elevated, the basic diagnostic studies recommended include a complete blood count (CBC), electrolytes, blood urea nitrogen (BUN) and creatinine, and a urine culture in all girls and selected boys with known urogenital pathology. The Task Force on Blood Pressure Control in Children also recommends an echocardiogram for children in whom drug therapy is being considered to establish baseline left ventricular mass, although data to support this recommendation are not available. Other diagnostic studies available for selected patients, including renal scans, renal ultrasounds, and the use of peripheral renins, should be considered in appropriate patients. Patients in whom a diagnosis of primary or essential hypertension is made should also have a fasting lipid panel done so that appropriate dietary interventions can be recommended.

The therapeutic interventions for children with persistent hypertension are dictated by the findings from the diagnostic evaluation. Patients with secondary hypertension generally require treatment of the underlying condition. For children in whom modest elevations of blood pressure are recorded without an underlying etiology, the appropriate course is often repeated visits with a greater emphasis on general counseling about cardiovascular risk factors, such as family history, obesity, lack of exercise, and use of tobacco. Oral contraceptives, if used, may need to be discontinued. Nonpharmacologic intervention strategies can often be introduced as the initial form of treatment and tailored to meet the needs of each patient. Antihypertensive drug therapy is generally reserved for patients with severe hypertension or when, after many months of nonpharmacologic therapy, the blood pressure remains significantly elevated.

SENSORY SCREENING

Evaluation of Hearing

Much of the early evaluation of hearing in infants and toddlers is based on subjective reports by the parents regarding the child's response to environmental sounds. However, the development of abnormal speech in the young child may make more formal evaluation appropriate. The human ear normally detects sounds in the range of 20 to 20,000 Hertz (Hz) but is most sensitive in the range of 1000 to 6000 Hz, the normal speech frequency. In this range, the normal ear has a threshold for sound levels near 0 decibels. The level of hearing loss that is measured is the threshold level measured in decibels relative to the normal hearing threshold. A typical hearing loss scale is given in Table 39–2.

Children under the age of 3 in whom a hearing loss is suspected should probably be referred to a hearing specialist for formal audiometry to quantify the hearing loss. Children over 3 years of age can generally be screened with the headphones used in routine office audiometry. An office audiometer is a relatively inexpensive item and minimal training is necessary for screening children. No clear guidelines regarding the frequency of testing are available, but two annual examinations prior to school seems reasonable. Testing is usually done at four different frequencies (500, 1000, 1500, 2000 Hz) for three different sound levels (25, 40, 60, dB) to quantify the extent of hearing loss, if any. The results of the audiometric evaluation can be recorded on a simple graph.

Children who have suspected middle ear disease may also be candidates for office tympanometry. This technique quantitates the change in tympanic membrane mobility or compliance as air pressure in the external ear canal is varied. The tympanic membrane is most compliant when the pressures on either side of it are equal. The test is performed by placing a three-channel probe into the ear canal to create a seal. A graph called a tympanogram is produced (Fig. 39–2).

In the normal or type A tympanogram, the point of peak tympanic membrane compliance is at the point where the air pressure in the ear canal varies from atmospheric pressure by less than 100 mm. water. Abnormal tympanograms that are flat (type B) or in which the peak compliance occurs when the air pressure within the ear canal is reduced (type C) may occur in the presence of a middle ear effusion or with other middle ear pathology.

Evaluation of Vision

Again, the evaluation of vision in children under 3 years of age is generally based on subjective reports

Table 39–2. HEARING LOSS SCALE

Hearing Impairment	Hearing Threshold (dB)
None	10–25
Mild	26–40
Moderate	41–55
Moderate to severe	56–70
Severe	71–90
Profound	>91

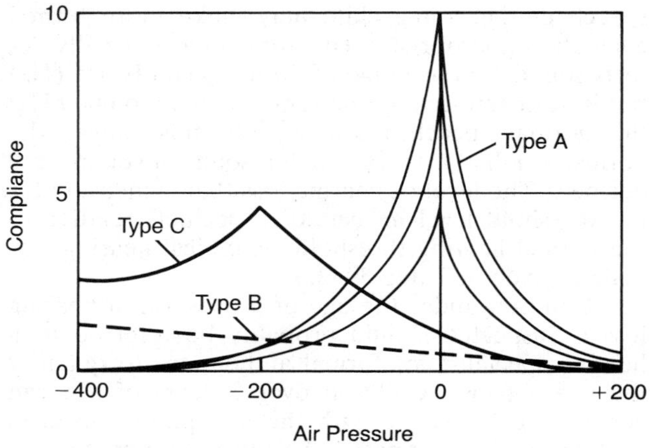

Figure 39–2. Common types of tympanograms. See text for explanation.

by the parent. More formal testing should begin routinely at age 3. Visual acuity may normally be in the 20/30 to 20/40 range at age 3 or 4 but improve to 20/20 by the age of 6 or 7. Squinting during testing, which creates a pinhole aperture effect, suggests the presence of an uncorrected refractive error. The family physician also may note strabismus, a misalignment of the eyes during testing. Strabismus may be intermittent and benign but, if it persists, can result in decreased visual acuity, i.e., amblyopia. Referral to an ophthalmologist is appropriate.

Allen Cards, which have pictures of easily recognized items, such as a telephone and a tree, can be used to test the visual acuity of children around 3 and 4 years of age. Once a child can read letters or numbers, acuity can be easily determined with the Snellen Chart. Interest and cooperation are obviously necessary to obtain optimal visual acuity. A difference between the right and left eye of more than one line on the chart is significant and should lead to further evaluation.

Routine screening should probably be performed annually for the preschool-aged child and for school-aged children through the second or third grade. Testing should again be recommended around the onset of puberty because of the increased likelihood of uncovering myopia around this stage of development.

Dental Screening

Primary dentition is usually complete by the age of 2 years. The permanent teeth generally begin erupting around the age of 6 or 7 years and are complete through the second molars by the age of 12 or 13. Children should be encouraged to brush their own teeth from 2 to 3 years of age, but parents should assist in the brushing. Most children lack the manual dexterity to brush satisfactorily until 6 years of age. Flossing is also difficult for children, and parents should take responsibility for flossing if there is tight contact between adjacent teeth. Routine dental appointments should begin at age 2 or 3 and are still recommended twice yearly by pediatric dentists.

SCREENING HEALTHY CHILDREN FOR DISEASE

Only a limited number of screening tests and procedures are recommended in the evaluation of the healthy child. The general purpose of a screening test is to identify normal individuals who have a disease or who are at high risk of getting that disease. This contrasts with a diagnostic test, which is used to confirm a clinical suspicion. A given test is, therefore, classified as screening or diagnostic depending on the purpose and clinical setting.

Iron Deficiency Anemia

The hemoglobin and hematocrit vary normally with age and, after the onset of puberty, are different for males and females. As seen in Table 39–3, the mean corpuscular volume (MCV) also increases with age. Although recent studies have documented a decline in the prevalence of anemia over the past decade (Yip et al., 1987), concerns regarding behavioral and developmental disturbances associated with iron deficiency and the availability of simple, inexpensive tests to identify this condition suggest that screening some populations is still appropriate (Stockman, 1987). Iron deficiency anemia is particularly prevalent in children with poor nutritional habits.

Several different tests can be used to screen for iron deficiency. The CBC or hematocrit, which can be performed in the office, detects iron deficiency at a late stage, well after iron stores are exhausted. The serum ferritin is a sensitive and specific test in children but is more expensive than these other tests. The free erythrocyte protoporphyrin (FEP) is more expensive than the office hematocrit but will detect iron deficiency at an earlier stage, before anemia occurs. It also has the advantage of screening for lead toxicity, another cause of microcytic anemias in children living

Table 39–3. VALUES (NORMAL MEAN AND LOWER LIMITS OF NORMAL) FOR HEMOGLOBIN, HEMATOCRIT, AND MCV DETERMINATIONS

	Hemoglobin (gm./dl.)		Hematocrit (%)		MCV (μ^3)	
Age (yr)	*Mean*	*Lower Limit*	*Mean*	*Lower Limit*	*Mean*	*Lower Limit*
0.5–1.9	12.5	11.0	37	33	77	70
2–4	12.5	11.0	38	34	79	73
5–7	13.0	11.5	39	35	81	75
8–11	13.5	12.0	40	36	83	76
12–14:						
Female	13.5	12.0	41	36	85	78
Male	14.0	12.5	43	37	84	77
15–17:						
Female	14.0	12.0	41	36	87	79
Male	15.0	13.0	46	38	86	78

Adapted from Oski, F. A., and Nathan, D. G. (Eds.): Hematology of Infancy and Childhood. Philadelphia, W.B. Saunders Co., 1987.

in urban areas. An FEP is recommended between 8 and 10 months as a routine screen of all children. Additional or annual testing should be performed on children at high risk as determined by environmental exposure or after nutritional assessment.

Children with an elevated FEP suggestive of an iron deficiency anemia can reasonably be given a trial of iron therapy. If the anemia is microcytic and not responsive to iron therapy, it probably represents a thalassemia syndrome, particularly if the family is of Mediterranean, Asian, or black heritage. In the healthy child, no further evaluation is generally necessary.

Routine Urinalysis

The most recent Guidelines for Health Supervision of Children and Youth (Strain, 1984) recommend a screening urinalysis at age 6 months and again during the preschool years. The rationale behind this recommendation is that abnormal findings may point to clinically undetected urinary tract infection or other renal disease, including nephropathy secondary to congenital anatomic anomalies. Although large trials have, in fact, detected cases of unrecognized infection (Kunin et al., 1962), the Canadian Task Force on the Periodic Health Examination (1979) concluded that the routine urinalysis should probably be eliminated from the periodic health maintenance visit in children.

Urinalysis testing is necessary when specific urinary symptoms are present or in the evaluation of a patient with nonspecific clinical indications, including fever or failure to thrive, for example. In these children with a higher probability of having urinary tract disease, the use of the urinalysis or other tests is more for diagnostic than for screening purposes.

Tuberculosis Screening

Routine screening for tuberculosis has been widely recommended in the past, due in part to the high effectiveness of antituberculous therapy in children. However, mass screening of children is not justified given the low prevalence of positive skin reactors in most communities and the high likelihood of false positive results due to previous exposure to atypical mycobacteria in the reactors. One study suggests that tuberculosis screening is not cost effective unless the prevalence of skin reactors is greater than 1 per cent (North, 1974). Therefore, a clinical history should be used to identify a population at risk. The most important criteria in defining a child who is at high risk is a clinical history of previous exposure to tuberculosis. There is also a higher prevalence of reactivity among children from Central America and Southeast Asia. In these children, screening for tuberculosis should be done using 5 tuberculin units (5 TU) of purified protein derivative (PPD) with interpretation at 48 to 72 hours. An area of induration of 5 to 9 mm. usually suggests exposure to atypical mycobacteria. Less than 5 mm. is a negative test. Tine (multipuncture) testing is not standardized and yields higher numbers of false-positive and false-negative results. Although it is an easier test to perform, it should be avoided. Repeat screening generally is not indicated unless there is evidence of new exposure to tuberculosis.

ANTICIPATORY GUIDANCE

In addition to monitoring growth and development, a portion of the routine visit for the preschool and school-aged child should be used to provide education about disease prevention.

Accident Prevention

One half of all deaths in childhood are attributable to accidents. There are more than 19 million medical visits by children for accidents and injury care each year, and 100,000 permanent disabilities result from accidents annually. The type of accidents that result in fatalities are most commonly motor vehicle accidents, followed by drownings, fires and burns, and aspirations and asphyxiations. Different aged children are more susceptible to each of these types of accidents, and the physician can take the opportunity at the routine screening visit to discuss measures that might help prevent future disability (Alpert and Guyer, 1985).

Automotive Safety

All states currently have laws requiring that infants and small children sit in appropriate safety seats while in a moving automobile. It is important for the physician to review with the parents the appropriate seat for their child. Children who are 17 to 20 pounds should sit in a toddler's seat. Once the child is 40 to 44 pounds, a booster seat or the seatbelt should be used. However, the shoulder harness is not appropriate until the child is at least 4 1/2 feet tall. Under no circumstances should a child be carried in a parent's lap while in a moving automobile.

One half of all traffic-related deaths in children are pedestrian deaths. Consequently, children above the age of 2 should be taught about street safety and the dangers of following thrown balls out into the street.

Drowning

Drowning is the second leading cause of death among children between 5 and 14. Most drownings take place in pools and in bathtubs. Therefore, younger children should be supervised at all times around the tub, and older children should be encouraged to develop their skills in swimming.

Fires and Burns

Parents should be instructed to equip their house with fire detectors and to regularly run through simulated fire drills. To prevent burns, hot water heaters should be set at 125°F. or less. Other burns occur near the stove, and parents should remember to turn pot handles away from the front of the stove so that toddlers and preschool children cannot overturn the pots and pans. Cigarette smoking is a common cause of house fires and yet another reason for physicians to recommend smoking cessation.

Aspiration

The foods that children most commonly aspirate are nuts, grapes, raisins, and other small, firm foodstuffs. Obviously, parents should be instructed to avoid giving these to young children. They should also be instructed in the basics of the Heimlich maneuver and the use of intrascapular blows to the back to dislodge aspirated food.

Poisonings

The parents of toddlers and young children should carefully examine their house and safety-proof their lower cabinets that contain poisonous cleansers and other substances. Houses with small children should have ipecac and activated charcoal available in the bathroom for use in emergencies, and the physician should review their use at the time of routine visits.

IMMUNIZATIONS

Preschool children who have received their previous immunizations require only the final diphtheria, pertussis, tetanus (DPT) and oral polio virus vaccine (OPV) boosters to complete the childhood schedules. These are given together between the ages of 3 and 5, prior to entering school or day care.

Immunization schedules for children who have not received their immunizations on time are listed in Tables 39–4 and 39–5.

Childhood Morbidity

Preschool and school-aged children make fewer visits than infants and toddlers to physicians for routine preventive health care. The great majority of office visits by children beyond the toddler stage are for the evaluation and treatment of minor, acute medical problems. As seen in Table 39–6, upper and lower respiratory problems account for a significant percentage of the visits to physicians by both preschool and school-aged children. A brief discussion of the evaluation and management of some of these common diagnoses follows.

OTITIS MEDIA

Acute otitis media, or purulent otitis media, is the most common medical diagnosis made in children (Paradise, 1980). By the age of 3, nearly three fourths of children have had at least one episode of otitis media and almost one third have had three or more episodes.

The pathophysiology of this disease seems to be related to eustachian tube dysfunction. The eustachian tube normally drains and ventilates the middle ear space. In children, the anatomy of the tube is different, and the function is often impaired. Viral infections may also affect the function of the eustachian tube apparatus. The role of allergies in predisposing children to middle ear infections is unclear.

Although viral infections are thought to predispose children to middle ear infections, viruses are rarely isolated from middle ear cultures. Bacterial infections are much more important as pathogens in otitis media. *Streptococcus pneumoniae* is the most important organism in children of all ages. *Haemophilus influenzae* and *Branhamella catarrhalis* are also important pathogens. Other bacteria, including group A *Streptococcus*, are less often isolated.

Clinically, children with otitis media usually have ear pain and often fever. Unlike smaller children, children over the age of 2 can generally localize the pain to the affected ear. Malaise, nausea and vomiting, or other less specific symptoms as presenting features are not as common as in younger children.

The diagnosis of otitis media is made by otoscopy. The classic findings include a bulging tympanic membrane with obscured bony landmarks. Diffuse or localized erythema is an inconsistent finding. Pneu-

Table 39–4. RECOMMENDED IMMUNIZATION SCHEDULE FOR INFANTS AND CHILDREN UP TO SEVENTH BIRTHDAY NOT IMMUNIZED AT THE RECOMMENDED TIME IN EARLY INFANCY

Timing	Vaccine(s)	Comments
First visit	DPT-1, OPV-1 (if child is ≥ 15 mo. of age, MMR)	DPT, OPV, and MMR can be administered simultaneously to children ≥ 15 mo. of age
2 mo. after first DPT, OPV	DPT, OPV-2	
2 mo. after second DPT	DPT-3	An additional dose of OPV at this time is optional for use in areas with a high risk of polio exposure
6–12 mo. after third DPT	DPT-4, OPV-3	
18 mo. (up to 60 mo.)	Hib	
Preschool (4–6 yr.)	DPT-5, OPV-4, MMR-2	Preferably at or before school entry
14–16 yr.	Td	Repeat every 10 years throughout life

Modified from the Centers for Disease Control: M.M.W.R., 38:4, 1989.

Table 39–5. RECOMMENDED IMMUNIZATION SCHEDULE FOR PERSONS 7 YEARS OF AGE OR OLDER

Timing	Vaccine(s)	Comments
First visit	Td-1, OPV-1 and MMR	OPV is not routinely administered to those ≥ 18 years of age
2 mo. after first Td, OPV	Td-2, OPV-2	
6–12 mo. after second Td, OPV	Td-3, OPV-3	OPV-3 may be given as soon as 6 weeks after OPV-2
10 years after Td-3	Td	Repeat every 10 years throughout life

Adapted from the Centers for Disease Control: M.M.W.R., 32:6, 1983.

matic otoscopy is less difficult than in the younger child and very helpful in the diagnosis. With a good seal, insufflation will reveal decreased or absent mobility of the tympanic membrane.

There are many options for treatment of acute otitis media. The choice of antibiotics is in part dependent on the importance of beta-lactamase producing *Haemophilus influenzae* and *Branhamella catarrhalis* in each geographic region. Nevertheless, amoxicillin has still proven to be a reasonable first-line antibiotic. Other first-line choices may include trimethoprim-sulfamethoxazole or erythromycin-sulfisoxazole. Cefaclor and the newer combination antibiotic—amoxicillin-clavulanate—also provide good coverage but are more expensive. In general, otitis media responds within 2 or 3 days. If there has been no adequate clinical response, then an empiric switch to a different antibiotic is appropriate.

Table 39–6. PERCENT AND CUMULATIVE PERCENT OF VISITS BY CHILDREN FOR MOST FREQUENT DIAGNOSES BY AGE

Age 2–5 Years	*Percent of Visits*	*Cumulative Percent of Visits*
General examination	19.7	19.7
Otitis media	16.9	36.6
URI	8.7	45.3
Pharyngitis	5.9	51.2
Tonsillitis	3.9	55.1
Bronchitis	3.9	59.0
Streptococcal pharyngitis	2.2	61.2
Asthma	2.2	63.4
Evaluation of suspected problem	2.0	65.4
Other viral illnesses	1.8	67.2

Age 6–10 Years	*Percent of Visits*	*Cumulative Percent of Visits*
General examination	15.2	15.2
Otitis media	9.2	24.4
Pharyngitis	8.0	32.4
URI	6.1	38.5
Asthma	4.6	43.1
Allergic rhinitis	4.3	47.4
Tonsillitis	4.1	51.5
Streptococcal pharyngitis	2.3	53.8
Bronchitis	2.2	56.0
Influenza	2.0	58.0

From National Center for Health Statistics. B. K. Cypress: Patterns of ambulatory care in pediatrics. The National Ambulatory Medical Care Survey, United States, January 1980–December 1981. Vital and Health Statistics. Series 13, No. 75, DHHS Pub. no. (PHS) 84-1736. Public Health Service, Washington, D.C., U.S. Government Printing Office, Oct., 1983.

Residual effusions after treatment of otitis media are common and up to 70 per cent of children will have an effusion still present at 2 weeks. Therefore, most experts recommend that follow-up examination in the patient with a satisfactory clinical response to antibiotic therapy be delayed until about 2 months after treatment. Any child who still has symptoms should, of course, be seen earlier. A follow-up tympanogram may be helpful to assess successful treatment.

Recurrences of otitis media within 1 month of the initial episode are frequently due to the same organism. Consequently, a change in the choice of antibiotics is probably indicated for early recurrences. Antibiotic prophylaxis should be considered for any child with multiple episodes of otitis media within a 6-month period. Effective antimicrobial choices include twice a day sulfisoxazole or once daily amoxicillin or trimethoprim-sulfamethoxazole. Antihistamines and decongestants have no proven benefit in the treatment of persistent middle ear effusions (Cantekin et al., 1983). The indications and relative benefits of surgical interventions for recurrent otitis media and persistent ear effusions have not been clearly defined.

VIRAL UPPER RESPIRATORY INFECTION (INCLUDING THE COMMON COLD)

Children of all ages get several colds per year with a slight increase in the number of infections during the winter time. Parents can anticipate that their child will get three to eight colds per year. There is some evidence that young children in day-care centers will experience more respiratory infections than children who remain at home, although this may be true only for the first year of day care. (Wald et al., 1988).

Many viruses cause colds in children. Rhinoviruses and coronaviruses are responsible for most of these infections. Other, less common causes of colds include parainfluenza, influenza, and respiratory syncytial viruses. Viruses appear to be transmitted by small droplets and by close contact. The viruses replicate in the upper respiratory epithelium and result in sloughing of the superficial layer of cells. Symptoms and viral shedding generally last for 3 days to a week or more.

The usual clinical symptoms of a cold include nasal congestion, cough, and fever of variable degree. The nasal discharge can be thin and clear or mucoid and purulent. Most viral upper respiratory infections (URIs) are uncomplicated but infrequent suppurative complications include otitis media, sinusitis, or lower respiratory bacterial infections, including bronchitis or pneumonia.

The nonspecific clinical presentation of a cold may mimic the prodrome of other childhood viral illnesses, including measles or chicken pox. In children with an allergic history, the nasal congestion of a URI should be distinguished from allergic rhinitis.

On physical examination, children with colds are not toxic appearing. The general appearance of a sick child should lead to a careful search for one of the suppurative complications listed above. The non–ill-appearing child should receive a careful head and neck examination as a minimum to rule out early otitis media. For the child with possible allergic rhinitis, a Wright's stain can be performed on the nasal discharge. The finding of many eosinophils suggests allergic rhinitis.

Colds resolve spontaneously without specific treatment, and either no treatment or only symptomatic relief should be recommended. Antibiotics have no benefit unless bacterial suprainfection has occurred. Acetaminophen is preferred over aspirin because of the association between the use of aspirin and certain viral illnesses and the subsequent development of Reye's syndrome. Decongestants and antihistamines often produce side effects worse than the symptoms for which they are prescribed. Antihistamines may provide some sedation for children in the evening. Older children may be able to use topical decongestants effectively without suffering systemic symptoms.

PHARYNGITIS AND TONSILLITIS

Sore throats are one of the most common problems among preschool and school-aged children. The peak incidence for sore throats occurs between the ages of 5 and 8 years old.

More than 80 per cent of all cases of pharyngitis are caused by viruses. A sore throat is often one of several symptoms associated with a viral URI. Occasionally, the sore throat is the predominant symptom. Adenoviruses may cause an exudative pharyngitis with or without other symptoms of nasal discharge and cough, particularly in younger children. *Herpangina*, which is due to Coxsackie virus or echovirus, is suggested by vesicles or small ulcers on the tonsillar pillars or soft palate. These may be accompanied by high fever and other symptoms, such as headache or malaise. One Coxsackie virus, type A16, is the agent responsible for *hand, foot, and mouth disease*. The pathognomonic findings include ulcerations of the buccal mucosa in conjunction with papulovesicular lesions on the palms of the hands and the soles of the feet. *Infectious mononucleosis* may also cause a sore throat and petechial lesions of the soft palate in addition to its characteristic posterior cervical adenopathy. Other viruses may cause pharyngitis but are less common.

Among the bacterial agents that cause pharyngitis, the most important is the *group A beta-hemolytic Streptococcus*, which may be responsible for as much as 15 per cent of this disease in children. Streptococcal pharyngitis remains important because untreated cases may infrequently be complicated by the development of acute rheumatic fever and acute glomerulonephritis. Strep throats are suggested by tonsillar erythema with exudates and an enanthem on the soft palate and, occasionally, clinically confirmed by the presence of the erythematous sandpaper-like rash of scarlet fever. Other bacterial infections causing pharyngitis are uncommon. Diphtheria causes a membranous exudate of the pharynx that is exceptionally rare in the immunized child. Gonorrhea and *Chlamydia* may be found in the sexually abused child and should always lead to a more comprehensive evaluation.

On physical examination, bacterial causes of pharyngitis are less likely if other symptoms of viral URI, such as cough and rhinorrhea, are present. The pharynx should be carefully examined to rule out uvular deviation seen with peritonsillar abscess or clinical signs consistent with epiglottitis.

Most children do not need a culture or quick antigen test for strep throat because of the low likelihood of infection. The strep culture should be used selectively based on clinical symptoms or signs in conjunction with a carefully obtained history of exposure and knowledge of regional epidemiology.

One of the difficult issues is the management of the child carrier of *Streptococcus*. About 50 per cent of children from whom *Streptococcus* is cultured have no serologic evidence of infection and, therefore, treatment is of no proven benefit. However, the problem is that at the time of evaluation, it is not known whether the patient is infected or merely a carrier who has symptoms of pharyngitis. In practice, the symptomatic carrier is routinely treated with antibiotics. The asymptomatic carrier, when discovered by culture, is also usually treated with antibiotics. Because the carrier state is difficult to eradicate and the risk of developing acute rheumatic fever for the carrier is unknown but appears low, experts are currently recommending that reculturing of children after completion of antibiotic therapy and culturing of asymptomatic contacts of children with streptococcal pharyngitis not be done routinely.

Recommended treatment for streptococcal pharyngitis is penicillin orally for 10 days. Erythromycin is an effective, inexpensive alternative for the child allergic to penicillin.

LOWER RESPIRATORY TRACT INFECTIONS

Lower respiratory tract infections are less common than upper respiratory tract infections in children.

Several clinical syndromes of lower respiratory tract infections in children are recognized (Table 39–7). Most children with lower respiratory tract infections are not ill enough to require hospitalization. Viruses and *Mycoplasma pneumoniae* are responsible for most of these infections, and antibiotics are, therefore, not required (Denny and Clyde, 1986).

Croup

Croup is a relatively common syndrome in children characterized by respiratory obstruction and a barking cough. Croup generally occurs in children aged 1 to 5 with a peak incidence during the second year of life. The cause of croup is generally viral, and the parainfluenza viruses have been implicated in up to 80 per cent of cases. Children with croup generally are afebrile or have low-grade fevers. The symptoms typically begin at night and recur nightly for several days. The symptoms can usually be improved by putting the child in the bathroom with the shower on or exposing him to the outside night air.

Tracheobronchitis

Tracheobronchitis is a syndrome involving the lower respiratory tract associated with a productive cough. On physical examination, there is no evidence of lung parenchymal involvement. Tracheobronchitis generally has a viral etiology, and secondary bacterial infection is rare. In a very ill child, a diagnosis of epiglottitis or bacterial tracheitis must be entertained, and urgent management including maintenance of the airway is essential.

Bronchiolitis

Bronchiolitis is a syndrome that occurs in small children and is unusual after the age of 2. It is generally viral in etiology. Respiratory syncytial viruses have been implicated in a large proportion of cases. Bronchiolitis can be difficult to differentiate from asthma. In borderline cases, it is useful to think of the pathophysiology as reactive airway disease associated with a lower respiratory infection. Recurrence of symptoms in a child with a family history of asthma suggests the possibility of asthma as the true diagnosis. An empiric trial of bronchodilator therapy is often useful.

Table 39–7. LOWER RESPIRATORY TRACT INFECTIONS IN CHILDREN

Croup	Hoarseness, cough, inspiratory stridor with laryngeal obstruction
Tracheobronchitis	Cough and rhonchi; no laryngeal obstruction or wheezing
Bronchiolitis	Expiratory wheezing with or without tachypnea, air trapping, and substernal retractions
Pneumonia	Rales or evidence of pulmonary consolidation on physical examination or radiograph

Pneumonia

The diagnosis of pneumonia is considered in the child with rales or clinical evidence of pulmonary consolidation. Most pneumonias in children are due to viruses and mycoplasma. Less than one third are bacterial in origin. In general, children with nonbacterial pneumonias have only mild respiratory distress, and chest x-ray, when obtained, shows hyperinflation, segmental atelectasis, and interstitial infiltrates. The child with bacterial pneumonia may appear more ill and have lobar consolidation. Small children generally cannot produce sputum and, therefore, sputum cultures and Gram's stains are not of benefit. For the older child with presumed bacterial pneumonia, erythromycin may be the appropriate antibiotic because of its effectiveness against pneumococcus and mycoplasma species.

ASTHMA

Asthma is one of the most common chronic medical conditions in childhood and is the most frequent cause for hospital admission among children. The prevalence of this disease in children is about 5 to 10 per cent. The incidence appears to be increasing among black children and in urban areas (Gergen et al., 1988). Most asthmatics have their first episode before the age of 3, although new cases are diagnosed at all ages, and the peak prevalence is among children age 10 to 12.

Asthma is defined as recurrent episodes of reactive airway disease. Common triggers of smooth muscle spasm in the distal airways include viral infections, environmental allergens, and exercise or cold weather. In some children, emotional factors may also precipitate bronchospasm.

The asthmatic child often presents 1 to 2 days following the onset of an upper respiratory infection. Less commonly, asthma is diagnosed in the child with recurrent cough, which typically is worse at night. Sometimes the diagnosis is suspected in the child with repeated viral infections associated with mild respiratory distress and confirmed by the empiric response to bronchodilator therapy.

On physical examination, there is a variable degree of respiratory distress and air hunger. Characteristic of the child with asthma is a prolonged expiratory phase. There may be use of accessory respiratory muscles.

The treatment of acute asthma has changed somewhat in the past few years. Because of a decrease in side effects, inhalation treatment with beta$_2$-adrenergic agents is preferred to subcutaneous epinephrine. Treatments may be repeated after 20 to 30 minutes for a total of 3 doses. If there is improvement, the child can be managed as an outpatient with oral beta-2 agents. Children over 8 can use metered-dose inhalers effectively. Children who have not improved after one or two inhalation treatments usually require intravenous theophylline and steroid therapy, as well as hospitalization.

Children with chronic asthma are usually maintained on an oral or inhaled $beta_2$ agonist. The long-acting theophylline preparations are often used for maintenance therapy, although their side effect profile and relatively narrow therapeutic window may make them a better second line medication. Children under 9 years of age are rapid metabolizers of theophylline and often need 20 to 24 mg./kg./day for maintenance therapy. Older children and adolescents are usually treated with doses of 300 to 400 mg. twice daily of a long-acting theophylline. For children on long-term theophylline therapy, a steady state level should be obtained and children should ideally be kept in the lower end of the therapeutic range of 10 to 20 mg. per ml. Several commonly prescribed drugs including erythromycin can interfere with the metabolism of theophylline and lead to toxic levels. Children on chronic theophylline therapy with steady state therapeutic levels should probably receive a reduced dose of their theophylline preparation when concomitant therapy with erythromycin is prescribed. Further adjustments in dosing can be determined by measured drug levels. Cromolyn has recently been suggested as a first-line medication. It can be given as a nebulized agent or with a metered-dose inhaler after bronchodilator therapy. Steroids are not recommended for routine use in asthmatics, except as indicated for hospitalized patients or for children with frequent exacerbations of asthma in spite of maximum treatment with other agents.

ATOPIC DERMATITIS

Atopic dermatitis is a chronic condition characterized by dry, eczematous skin in a typical distribution. This condition is often found in association with a personal or family history of other atopic disorders, including allergies and asthma. Atopic dermatitis affects between 1 and 3 per cent of children.

Atopic dermatitis generally begins during infancy but occasionally presents in the older child. By childhood, the rash most commonly involves the flexural surfaces of the antecubital and popliteal fossae, the wrist, and around the neck and face. Occasionally, small vesicles and pustules develop on the hands, particularly the interdigital areas. This dyshidrotic eczema is probably due to exposure to irritants in the child with atopy.

The most common complication of atopic dermatitis is secondary bacterial infection of affected areas. The infections are usually due to *Staphylococcus* or *Streptococcus* species.

The treatment of atopic dermatitis depends on the degree of inflammation present. Children should be instructed to avoid exacerbating irritants and to avoid frequent hand washing. Harsh, drying soaps should be replaced with mild, moisturizing soaps. Lubricants or moisturizing creams can be used following hand washing. Topical corticosteroid preparations are usually necessary to clear the inflammatory lesions. A general rule is to use the weakest preparation that will work. Fluorinated steroids should only be used for severe lesions and for short periods of time. One useful approach is to apply a small amount of a steroid cream and then cover the area with a lubricating agent. Systemic antibiotics may be necessary to clear up inflammatory lesions that have become secondarily infected.

GASTROENTERITIS

Gastroenteritis is a common problem in children with a decreasing incidence after the age of 2. In small children, most infections occur via the fecal/oral route. Not surprisingly, recent data have shown an increased likelihood of gastroenteritis in children attending day-care centers (Child Day Care Study Group, 1984). When looked for, a pathogen can be found in about one half of all cases. About 80 per cent of the pathogens identified are viral (Isaacs et al., 1986). In particular, the rotavirus has been implicated as a major cause of gastroenteritis in children.

Most cases of gastroenteritis in children over 2 are not severe and can be managed without medical intervention, often over the phone. In the otherwise healthy child, putting the bowel at rest with clear liquids for 24 to 48 hours is generally sufficient. Oral rehydration solutions have been used successfully in Third World nations and can be recommended for moderately dehydrated children. These solutions contain more sodium and less glucose than the oral electrolyte solutions that were previously available. Parents should be advised against feeding the child dairy products, since these often exacerbate the symptoms. The diet can slowly be advanced and dairy products added after 3 or 4 days.

Diarrhea and abdominal pain of nonviral etiology generally resolve without antibiotic therapy, as well. *Campylobacter* is now the most common bacterial cause of childhood diarrhea. Most episodes are of short duration, although the abdominal pain may be remarkable, and no therapy is indicated. Prolonged episodes with a positive culture should be treated with erythromycin. *Shigella* usually causes mild symptoms but may be associated with bloody diarrhea. Oral ampicillin or amoxicillin will shorten the duration of symptoms and lessen the period of infectivity to others. *Salmonella* usually causes relatively mild symptoms, and treatment is not indicated unless the child is at risk for invasive disease. *Giardia* is a protozoan that may cause diarrhea in children and has been found in up to 25 per cent of children in day-care centers, most of whom are asymptomatic. Treatment with quinacrine is probably indicated in most cases (Report of the Committee on Infectious Diseases, 1982). Metronidazole has not been approved for use in children under 12.

URINARY TRACT INFECTION

Urinary tract infections (UTIs) are relatively uncommon in children but require aggressive diagnostic and therapeutic management because of their potential to do renal damage. After infancy, girls are much more likely than boys to present with a UTI. Up to 90 per cent of first infections are caused by *Escherichia coli*. Other bacteria that may cause UTIs in children include *Klebsiella, Proteus*, Enterococci, and *Staphylococcus saprophyticus*. The clinical presentation of a UTI in children is dependent on the age of the child. Toddlers often present with nonspecific symptoms, including abdominal discomfort, fever, and a change in their voiding pattern. Preschool-aged children may have discomfort and secondary enuresis in addition to fever and abdominal pain. Older children are more likely to have the classic symptoms of a urinary tract infection including frequency, urgency, and dysuria.

Appropriate collection of a urine specimen in a child is difficult. Bagged urine is generally contaminated and can only be considered reliable if the specimen is sterile. Because of perineal contamination, a catheterized specimen may be necessary to confirm ambiguous results. After an appropriate collection, bacteria seen on an unspun specimen suggest infection. The number of white cells seen on a spun specimen is variable, but more than 5 to 10 per high power field implies inflammation.

A specimen for culture should be refrigerated until plated to prevent bacterial overgrowth. On a noncatheterized specimen, bacterial counts greater than 50,000 are consistent with an infection. On a catheterized specimen, any bacterial growth is significant.

Up to 50 per cent of children under age 4 or 5 will have some vesicoureteral reflux in conjunction with a urinary tract infection and fever. Therefore, treatment should be recommended for 10 to 14 days. Shorter courses in young children are not warranted. Older children and adolescents have had successful treatment with shorter courses of therapy.

The recommended further evaluation of children with UTIs is contingent on several factors. All males with a first UTI and females with repeat infection or clinical evidence of pyelonephritis or growth retardation should be further evaluated. The test of first choice would be a voiding cystourethrogram (VCUG) to look for reflux. The VCUG should be obtained 4 to 6 weeks after treatment of the acute infection because of the high incidence of reflux during a UTI in young children. Prophylactic antibiotics may be necessary to reduce the likelihood of recurrent infection until VCUG can be completed. The renal structure should also be evaluated with an intravenous pyelogram (IVP) or ultrasound. The finding of significant reflux or obstructive uropathy should result in referral to a urologist.

Adolescent Health Care

Family physicians are in a unique position to provide health care to adolescents during the transition from childhood to adulthood. Adolescence is often characterized as a period of chaotic development and risk-taking behaviors. Rapid changes in growth are accompanied by an increasing self-awareness and often self-doubt. In addition, influential forces, such as the media and peer pressure, conspire against a smooth assimilation of change. Finally, the family often has difficulty coping with these rapid, uneven changes. With the perspective that adolescence is one phase in the life cycle and not the culmination of development and with the understanding of the adolescent's family dynamics, the family physician has an opportunity to facilitate a teenager's evolution into adulthood that is not available to other specialists.

A common pitfall for physicians is to address adolescents' health needs based on their chronologic age. For the most part, our society groups adolescents by age or grade in school, assuming a progressive, linear increase in knowledge, maturity, and socialization skills. Development may be neither orderly nor even, and there may be disparities between physiologic and psychosocial growth in the same individual at a given time. The task of addressing adolescent health care needs requires sensitivity to the stage of development attained by the individual and the skills and emotional resources they have at their disposal. Tailoring health care delivery to find the most developmentally appropriate interventions may thus require assessments of the stage of maturity in several different areas.

By most criteria, adolescents are a healthy group with low morbidity and mortality. However, adolescents themselves report much greater concerns about their health than might be expected (Levenson et al., 1984). These concerns focus not only on medical problems per se but also on issues regarding interpersonal relationships, sexuality, substance abuse, and anxiety or nervousness. In other words, adolescents see themselves as needing more and broader professional care than they generally have access to.

There are many reasons for the apparent underutilization of health care by adolescents (Irwin, 1986). These barriers include the issue of confidentiality, given the physician's previous alignment with the patient's family, legal and ethical issues, and economics.

Confidentiality

Family physicians generally have ongoing relationships with the family members of an adolescent patient. Many studies have demonstrated that teenagers will not seek any or all of their health care from a physician if their parents have access to information about the visit (Herold and Goodwin, 1979). Adolescents are particularly reluctant to discuss issues of sexuality or contraception with a physician who has a previous alliance with the family. From the outset, the physician should establish that the doctor-patient relationship assures the patient's right to confidentiality. Occasionally, families prefer a two-physician arrangement to avoid conflict of allegiance. However, this represents an option of second choice and is generally unnecessary if the physician defines the ground rules from the start.

Legal and Ethical Issues

The adolescent's right to confidentiality must be balanced against the rights of the parents to supervise the health of their minor child and the physician's desire not to divide the family. Most states have laws that protect both adolescents and physicians regarding the provision of care without parental consent for specific health issues, including the diagnosis and management of pregnancy, the provision of contraception, the diagnosis and management of sexually transmitted diseases, substance use and abuse, and the initial evaluation and treatment of emotional illness. Without assurances of confidentiality, many of these problems would go unevaluated. These laws vary from state to state, and physicians should be familiar with the laws in their own state (Morrisey et al., 1986).

The mature minor doctrine states that minor individuals sufficiently mature to understand the benefits and risks of a medical evaluation and treatment are legally able to give valid informed consent (Hofmann, 1980). In most instances, the family physician should first gain the consent of the adolescent before sharing the information with the parents. This procedure empowers the adolescent but also keeps him or her a part of the larger family unit.

Economics

Although adolescents may desire confidentiality regarding their medical care, they often do not have financial resources to pay for their visits. If the physician has a good relationship with the parents, one possible arrangement is for the parents to agree to pay for medical visits that are deemed necessary by the physician. An alternative arrangement is for the teenager to assume part of the cost of each visit. In this era of third-party insurance, there are potential snags in the system to maintaining confidentiality. Bills listing procedures such as a dilatation and evacuation, Papanicolaou's smear, or the application of podophylline to venereal warts will be sent to the insured family member, usually a parent. If this arrangement is unsatisfactory, alternative plans must be made in advance.

CONDUCT OF THE VISIT WITH AN ADOLESCENT

Medical visits for adolescents are frequently more emotionally charged than visits for younger children. In some situations, the adolescent patient is distrustful of the physician, particularly of the potential for an alliance of the physician with the patient's parents. The doctor, on the other hand, must also be aware of certain emotions elicited by adolescent patients. Physicians often negatively stereotype adolescents as sexually promiscuous or as substance abusers. Alternatively, physicians may present themselves as more knowledgeable regarding salient adolescent issues than they really are. These judgmental attitudes increase the adolescent's distrust.

For these reasons, certain guidelines are helpful in the conduct of a medical visit for an adolescent. Most physicians who take care of adolescents see the patient with the parents for part of the visit and then the patient alone. This gives the mother and father an opportunity to discuss their concerns but still empowers the teenager as the patient. It is helpful to explain to the parents that issues discussed with the adolescent in privacy will be held confidential. Of course, the protection of information discussed does not hold in life-threatening situations, such as for the suicidal adolescent. Most parents are comfortable with this arrangement, particularly when it is laid out at the beginning of the visit. The purpose of this separation is not to divide the family. On the contrary, the family physician can often help the teenager figure out ways to discuss problems with the parents. Developmentally, however, it is often difficult for the teenager to openly discuss issues regarding sexuality and concerns about growth and development, for instance, in front of the parent.

This transition towards establishing increased responsibility regarding health care in the adolescent can be facilitated by establishing a similar pattern of visits for the older child and preadolescent patient. A few minutes of each routine visit can be set aside to allow the older child or preadolescent to discuss any concerns in private. This may foster a trusting relationship for the physician, patient, and family in years to come when developmental issues make confidentiality more important.

DEVELOPMENTAL ASSESSMENT

Assessment of Physical Development

Although the changes of puberty tend to follow a predictable sequence, they are highly variable on an individual basis. Chronologic age, therefore, correlates poorly with biologic maturity. A sexual maturity scale, such as the one developed by Tanner, can be used to assess the physical developmental stage of a patient. This scale assigns a Tanner stage of 1 (prepubertal) to 5 (adult) to girls based on breasts and pubic hair and to boys based on genitalia and pubic hair (Table 39–8).

Sexual development in the female is generally heralded by the finding of breast buds, a small amount of tissue beneath the nipple and areola, or thelarche

Table 39–8. CLASSIFICATION OF SEXUAL MATURITY STAGES IN GIRLS AND BOYS

Stage	Pubic Hair	Breasts
	Girls	
1	Preadolescent	Preadolescent
2	Sparse, lightly pigmented, straight, medial border of labia	Breast bud under areola
		Areolar diameter increased
3	Darker, beginning to curl, increased amount	Breast and areola enlarged, no contour separation
4	Coarse, curly, abundant but amount less than in adult	Areola and papillae form secondary mound
5	Adult feminine triangle, spread to medial surface of thighs	Mature, no contour separation, deepening color of areola
	Boys	
Stage	*Pubic Hair*	*Genitalia*
1	None	Preadolescent; testicles 1–2 cm.
2	Scanty, long, slightly pigmented	Testicles > 2 cm.; scrotum enlarged
3	Darker, starts to curl, small amount	Penis longer; testicles larger
4	Resembles adult type, but less in quantity; coarse, curly	Widening of glans; scrotum darker
5	Adult distribution, spread to medial surface of thighs	Adult

Adapted from Tanner, J. M.: Growth at Adolescence. 2nd ed. Oxford, England, Blackwell Scientific Publications, 1962.

(Fig. 39–3). The growth spurt generally occurs relatively early in puberty in females, around Tanner stage 3. Menarche typically occurs at the end of the growth spurt and signals closure of the epiphyseal growth plates. The mean age of menarche in the United States is 12.8 years, with only minor racial or regional variation.

In males, the first sign of puberty is testicular enlargement, which typically begins between 9½ and 13½ years of age. The growth spurt in males occurs late in puberty around Tanner stage 4. Therefore, males start puberty after females and have their growth spurt later in puberty.

There are many other somatic changes during puberty that are better correlated with sexual maturity than with age (Slap, 1986). Approximately 25 per cent of final adult height occurs during pubertal growth. Weight gain also increases appreciably during adolescence, and this change accounts for over 40 per cent of the ideal adult weight in both sexes. However, there are marked differences between males and females in terms of body composition. In girls, the lean body mass decreases from 80 per cent to 75 per cent, whereas in boys it increases from 80 to 90 per cent. Prior to the onset of puberty, males and females are similar in many physiologic measures. Due to the effects of testosterone, heart weight nearly doubles and vital capacity increases dramatically in boys. Blood volume, red blood cell mass, and hematocrit increase steadily throughout puberty in boys but remain fairly constant in girls, as shown in Figure 39–4.

Blood pressure measurements also change fairly dramatically with puberty. Systolic blood pressures rise rapidly in boys and reach a plateau in girls (Fig. 39–5). There is a much higher correlation between high blood pressure in adolescents of later maturity stages and adults than in young children. As a result, with each successive sexual maturity stage, a greater proportion of patients with high blood pressure will be found to have essential hypertension.

In addition to providing information regarding physiologic changes, the sexual maturity rating at the time of a visit can be used to help the adolescent with his or her concerns about normal development. For example, late developing males can be reassured that because of their early stage of development they still have several years of growth, including their growth spurt, ahead. As another example, males with gynecomastia can be told that nearly two thirds of boys have gynecomastia at Tanner stage 2 but that more than 95 per cent have resolution by the end of puberty. Adolescents who are most preoccupied with changes in their body and concerned about being examined generally benefit the greatest from information provided by physicians regarding normal developmental processes. Many physicians provide a running explanation of their findings during the physical examination of an adolescent.

Assessment of Psychosocial Development

Although biologic measures are the most obvious signs of puberty, the period of adolescence is, in fact, a complicated process where psychosocial growth is intertwined with physical development. Several tasks characterize this biopsychosocial process in adolescents. These tasks of adolescence include:

1. Emancipation from family and formation of self-identity
2. Sexual identification and achievement of intimacy
3. Future orientation and career choice

While adolescents are not a homogeneous group, Table 39–9 can be used to assess normal or abnormal development in adolescent patients.

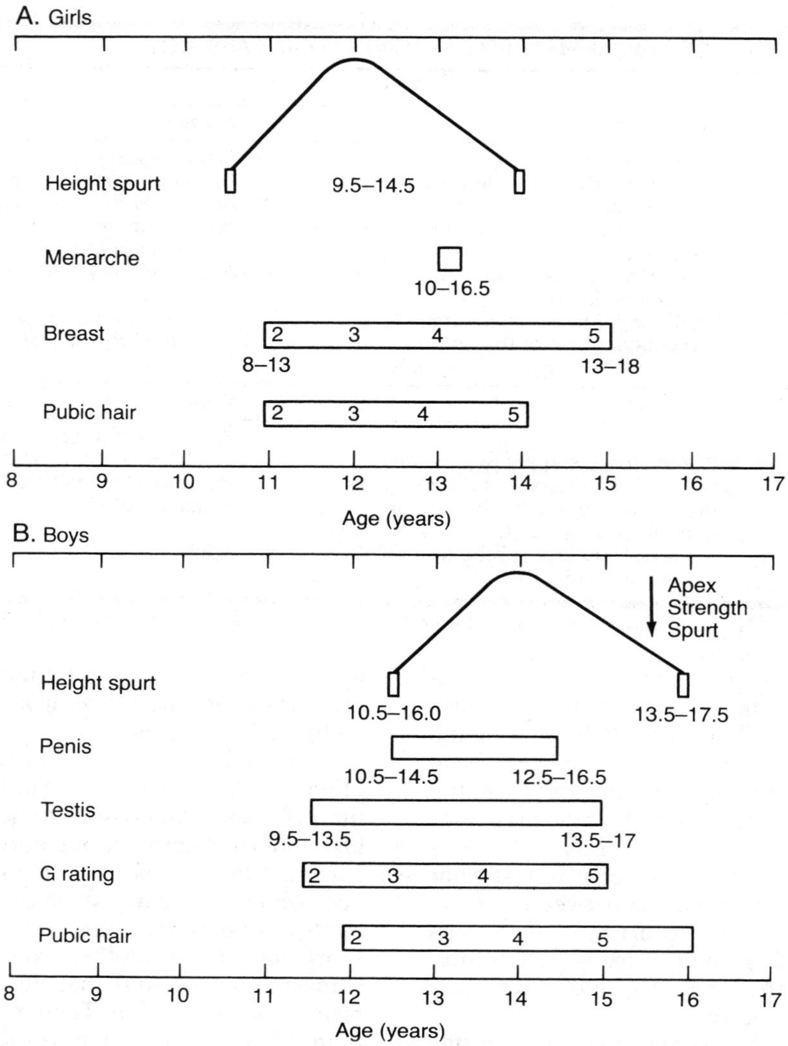

Figure 39–3. Sequence of events in puberty for (*A*) girls and (*B*) boys. (From Slap, G. B.: Normal physiological and psychosocial growth in the adolescent. J. Adolesc. Health Care, 7:135, 1986.)

Cognitive Development

The changes that occur in intellectual development during adolescence are harder to quantify than the sexual maturity ratings. In late childhood and early adolescence, concrete thought processes give way to more abstract thinking. This ability to think abstractly coincides with the introduction of courses in school, such as algebra and geometry. Consequently, teenagers who do not move beyond concrete thinking often manifest problems or frustrations with learning around the time of middle school or junior high school. This is an important time for knowledgeable physicians to intervene and help the slow learner find an appropriate educational pace.

The changes in cognition are also apparent in teenagers' future orientation and future events planning. With cognitive maturity comes the ability to set realistic life goals. The importance of future events planning often impacts on the medical system. Early adolescents have great difficulty in handling their own medications, not only because of issues of autonomy but also because they do not anticipate their own needs hours or days ahead.

Interpersonal/Social Development

One of the important tasks of adolescence is the establishment of autonomy, that is, the attainment of an identity separate from the family. The struggle usually begins early in adolescence with the adolescent showing less interest in family activities and perhaps substituting a close relationship with a same sex friend. Clinically, the early adolescent usually is brought in by the parent and sits there quietly while the physician and parent talk. By middle adolescence, the peer group has assumed greater importance, and the adolescent often conforms with peer group values. This often heightens any conflict with parental authority. These are the typical angry adolescents that are dragged into the office by a parent and, unless handled with care, refuse to talk or be examined. By late adolescence, the peer group is less important

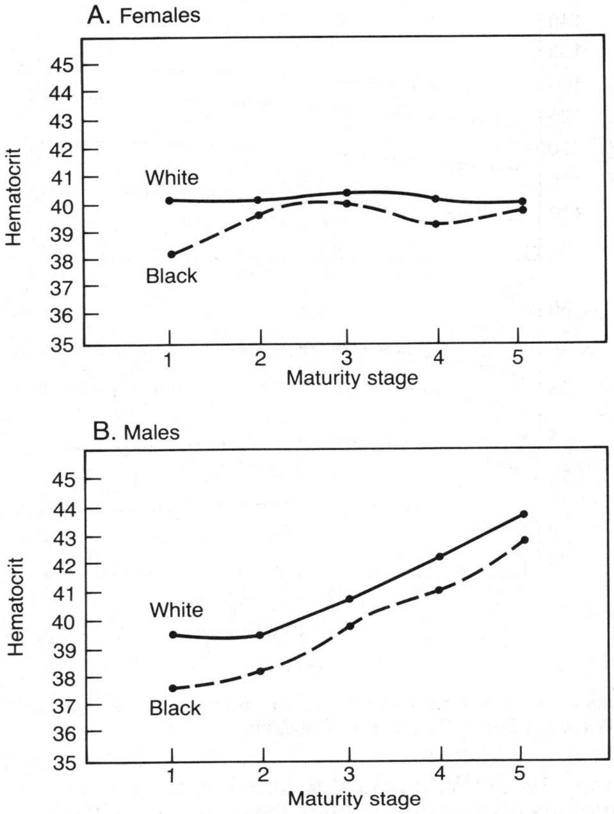

Figure 39–4. Hematocrit values for *(A)* females and *(B)* males, showing changes during puberty. (Reproduced by permission from Daniel, W. A., Jr.: Adolescents in health and disease. St. Louis, The C. V. Mosby Co., 1977.)

because the adolescent has established a more stable identity separate from the peer group or the family. With this increased maturity comes an ability to enter an intimate relationship. The relationship with the family is much less conflictual and the late adolescent can assimilate or let go of parental values. These patients often make their own appointments, or if the parent comes with them, they are comfortable letting the parent give his or her view of any problems.

Psychologic Development

Coincident with changes in cognitive function, the early adolescent frequently daydreams. The early adolescent often lives a personal fantasy and may feel that everyone is watching but that no one can understand his unique problems. This is the time when the adolescent is preoccupied with his body and the changes of puberty, the "Am I normal?" period. With midadolescence comes a greater acceptance of one's body and at times a feeling of being omnipotent. This is the time when many adolescents take great risks, either with experimentation of drugs or through sexual activity or, alternatively, with motor vehicles. By late adolescence, the body changes have been incorporated into a more stable identity and values from other parts of the adolescent's life help him to compromise and set limits in interpersonal settings.

SCREENING THE ADOLESCENT PATIENT

For developmental reasons, adolescents often have difficulty identifying a specific reason for their visit. Frequently, there is a hidden agenda that the physician must work to find. Furthermore, because many of the problems of adolescence relate to developmental issues, it is often helpful for the physician to review with the patient several important areas where adolescents frequently encounter problems. Most experts feel that the health care of adolescents should be comprehensive and not simply directed at the chief complaint. The essentials to be covered in the additional history taken from an adolescent are listed in Table 39–10. This list can be easily reviewed in a matter of minutes during each visit with an adolescent to see if there are any unrecognized problems.

Information about family interactions and peer relationships helps the physician understand how connected or isolated the adolescent feels. By reviewing school performance, the physician can see if the adolescent has the cognitive skills to handle abstract thinking required in many subjects beyond the sixth grade. If there are problems, the physician can work with the school to find a more appropriate learning plan. Intimate relationships and sexual activity, if any, should be discussed. Adolescents who are not sexually active should have the opportunity to discuss the pressures on them to become sexually active and supported in their decision not to be. Adolescents who are already sexually active should be offered contraception or referred elsewhere where they can receive appropriate counseling and contraception, if indicated. The last menstrual period should be noted for female adolescents who are sexually active. Concern about a possible pregnancy is a common reason for a visit among females. Drug and alcohol use should also be recorded and appropriate intervention planned for adolescents with identified problems. Other risk-taking behavior should be reviewed. This may include skate board and bicycle use in the younger adolescent and particularly risky behavior, such as drinking and driving, in the older adolescent.

ANTICIPATORY GUIDANCE

Adolescents worry about their health more than physicians realize. By self-report, fewer than 10 per cent of adolescents claim never to think about their health, but nearly 40 per cent think about it often, and 20 per cent worry about it all the time (Parcel et al., 1977). Through an understanding of normal developmental processes, family physicians may be able to allay some of this anxiety by reassuring the adolescent about normal physical findings at the time of examination and by discussing what changes the adolescent can expect in the months and years ahead. This is particularly true for the early to midadolescent who is so preoccupied with physical changes.

Following the developmental assessment and

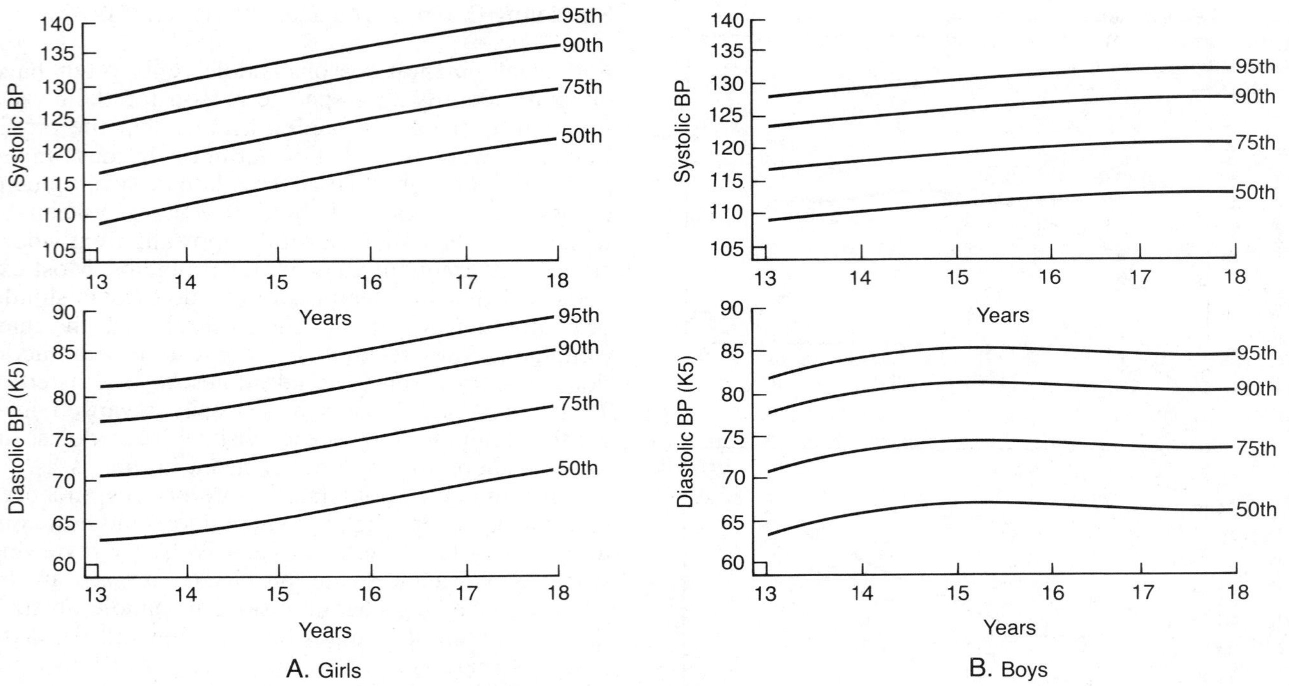

Figure 39–5. Age-specific percentiles of blood pressure measurements in *(A)* girls and *(B)* boys, 13 to 18 years of age; Korotkoff Phase V (K5) used for diastolic blood pressure. (Redrawn from Task Force on Blood Pressure in Children.)

physical examination, the physician can also provide appropriate information to help limit the teenager's future health risks. Adolescents who have a steady boyfriend or girlfriend and are in Tanner stage 4 or 5 are more likely to become sexually active in the near future. It is appropriate to review with the adolescent communication skills between partners regarding intimacy, the risks associated with sexual activity including pregnancy and sexually transmitted diseases, and the need for contraception. Similarly, adolescents who are engaged in one risk-taking behavior, such as smoking cigarettes, are at greater risk for experimenting with drugs and alcohol and the assumed risks should be discussed (Irwin and Millstein, 1986). With regard to anticipatory guidance for adolescents, several studies have shown that adolescents prefer a physician who offers information in a nonjudgmental way. Developmentally, it is difficult for an adolescent to ask the physician to discuss the risks of sexual activity or drug use, but most adolescents want to hear this information from an expert.

Morbidity and Mortality in Adolescence

Adolescence was the only age group in the United States that showed an increase in mortality from 1960

Table 39–9. PSYCHOSOCIAL DEVELOPMENT OF ADOLESCENTS

Area of Growth	Early Adolescence	Middle Adolescence	Late Adolescence
Family independence	Less interest in parental activities	Peak of parental conflicts	Reacceptance of parental advice and values
Body image	Preoccupation with self and pubertal changes	General acceptance of body	Acceptance of pubertal changes
	Uncertainty about appearance	Concern over making body more attractive	
Interpersonal relationships	Intense relationships with same sex	Peak of peer involvement	Peer group less important
		Conformity with peer values	More time spent in sharing intimate relationships
		Increased sexual activity and experimentation	
Self-perception (Identity)	Increased cognition—personal fantasy Idealistic vocational goals Increased need for privacy Lack of impulse control	Increased scope of feelings Increased intellectual ability Feelings of omnipotence Risk-taking behavior	Practical, realistic vocational goals; refinement of moral, religious and sexual values; ability to compromise and to set limits

Adapted from Neinstein, L.S.: Adolescent Health Care: A Practical Guide. Baltimore, Urban & Schwarzenberg, 1984.

Table 39–10. ESSENTIAL AREAS TO ADDRESS IN SCREENING THE ADOLESCENT PATIENT

1. Family interactions
2. Peer relationships
3. School performance
4. Intimacy/sexual activity
5. Drugs/other substance use
6. Other risk-taking behaviors

through 1981, a period of decreasing mortality for all other age groups. Approximately 75 per cent of the deaths in this group are due to accidents, homicide, and suicide. Accidents alone account for 60 per cent of the mortality during adolescence (Brown, 1979).

Data regarding morbidity during adolescence are harder to come by. The most common reason that adolescents seek medical care is for a comprehensive physical examination, generally for school or camp. Data from the National Ambulatory Health Statistics suggest that adolescents have many of the same problems as preadolescent patients. However, data from an office specifically directed to adolescent health care show that teenagers have several problems that are unique to their age group (Table 39–11). Some of the specific diagnoses are discussed in the following section.

ACCIDENTS

Accidents account for more than half of the mortality during adolescence. Motor vehicle accidents alone account for 37 per cent of teenage deaths (Brown, 1979). In addition, nonfatal injuries account for the largest number of hospital days among teenagers. National data show that accidents and poisonings account for about 15 per cent of ambulatory visits to physicians in adolescence.

There is evidence that the frequency of accidents in adolescents may be related to developmental issues (Brown, 1979). Mortality data regarding motor vehicle accidents cite excessive speed as a factor in more than half of accidents among adolescents compared to only 30 per cent of accidents among adults. Alcohol is also a more frequent contributing factor in motor vehicle fatalities among young drivers than it is in other age groups. Risk taking in adolescents serves to fulfill developmental needs related to autonomy and to mastery of new activities. Mastering a skill or activity requires experimentation and often involves testing limits and taking risks. Most teenagers do not have the cognitive ability and life experiences to understand the degree of risk associated with these behaviors. Experts have suggested that interventional strategies should include: (1) providing alternatives to the risk-taking behaviors that are safer and still fulfill the developmental needs and (2) insulating adolescents from the most negative consequences of risk-taking behaviors (Irwin and Millstein, 1986). An example of this would be to encourage the family of the young driver who is exposed to drinking at high school parties to sign a contract that will guarantee the young person a ride home from a party by an adult if the adolescent has been drinking.

SEXUAL ACTIVITY

Sexual activity among adolescents is common and is occurring at earlier ages than ever before. Nearly 60 per cent of females and 70 per cent of males report having had intercourse by the age of 18 (O'Reilly and Aral, 1985). Between 20 and 30 per cent of 15-year-olds are sexually active. Approximately one fifth of all sexually active females become pregnant each year, and half of these pregnancies occur within the first 6 months of sexual activity. Contraception is consistently used by only a small minority of teenagers. A combination of developmental factors, including misinformation, poor ability to plan for future events, inability to communicate with partner, and risk-taking behavior, as well as ambivalence in the female about the outcome of pregnancy, conspire against effective contraceptive use.

Provision of Contraception

A thorough developmental assessment is necessary before providing contraception to an adolescent. A discussion of the developmental advantages and disadvantages of some common contraceptive methods for adolescents follows (Gruber and Chambers, 1987).

Barrier methods pose no significant medical risk to adolescents and provide protection against acquisition of sexually transmitted diseases, as well as preventing pregnancy. Condoms are a nonprescription method of contraception that can be kept available relatively easily by the adolescent who typically has intercourse infrequently and sporadically. Additionally, it is the only method that allows the male to take primary responsibility for contraception, although females can also be encouraged to carry condoms. Unfortunately, this method requires con-

Table 39–11. SPECIFIC PROBLEMS IDENTIFIED DURING VISITS TO A TEEN HEALTH CENTER

Gynecologic	18%
Dermatologic	15%
Adolescent adjustment reaction	14%
Headache	10%
Obesity	8%
Endocrine	7%
Gastrointestinal	6%
Orthopedic	6%
Asthma	4%
Seizure disorder	4%

Adapted from Neinstein, L. S.: Adolescent Health Care: A Practical Guide. Baltimore, Urban & Schwarzenberg, 1984.

sistency of use and only a small percentage of males who use condoms at all report consistent use. Furthermore, use of the condom discourages use of more effective methods in some adolescents. The diaphragm has perhaps the lowest likelihood of continued use in adolescents for whom it is prescribed. Use of the diaphragm requires the female adolescent to have comfort with touching the genital area during insertion and generally requires that there is communication between partners regarding sexual activity. Clinical experience has shown that this method should only be recommended for relatively sophisticated, late adolescents in stable relationships with demonstrated communication skills.

When the intrauterine device (IUD) was first on the market, it seemed like an excellent contraceptive method for adolescents, since compliance was not an issue and no communication with the partner was necessary. However, there is an unacceptably high incidence of pelvic inflammatory disease and its sequelae of infertility and ectopic pregnancy related to use of this method, and the IUD cannot be recommended for teenagers.

Oral contraceptives containing 30 to 35 micrograms of estrogen are the contraceptive method of choice for the sexually active adolescent female. They can be safely recommended for most patients with only the usual absolute contraindications restricting their use.

Several practical issues are important for the physician who provides oral contraceptives to adolescents. Teenage females who by developmental assessment do not have good planning skills will need more frequent follow-up than adult patients for whom oral contraceptives are provided. All adolescents should be given more thorough counseling regarding the possibility of minor side effects, such as intramenstrual bleeding or nausea, that may cause the teenager to stop the pills. Similarly, the patient should be reassured that physiologic changes including small elevations in blood pressure or rashes are readily reversible. It is generally a good idea to allow the teenager to discuss any concerns that she has about taking the pill and to address each of the concerns carefully. Many offices benefit by having a nurse or other person designated to handle trouble shooting regarding oral contraceptive use by teenagers.

Sexually Transmitted Diseases

Sexually transmitted diseases (STDs) are a common problem among adolescents (McGregor, 1985). About one fifth of all cases of gonorrhea reported in the United States occur in teenagers. *Chlamydia*, which is not a reportable infection but which causes many of the same clinical syndromes as gonorrhea, is recognized as the most common STD in this age group. The importance of infections caused by the human papillomavirus (HPV) is unclear, but the number of teenagers infected with this agent appears to be increasing. Finally, although the acquired immune deficiency syndrome (AIDS) is uncommon among adolescents, the level of sexual activity in this group and the increasing incidence of other STDs suggest that individuals who develop AIDS in their third decade may have become infected during their teenage years.

There are many factors that may put teenagers at increased risk for acquiring STDs. Like other processes of adolescence, development of sexuality may be marked by experimentation and risk taking. Contraception (and relevant to STD transmission, barrier methods) is used infrequently. There may be multiple partners. There are biologic factors for this increased risk, as well. Both *Chlamydia* and gonorrhea have a predilection for the columnar epithelium on the immature cervix of an adolescent female. Moreover, adolescents have an unchallenged immune system that offers no local protection against STD agents.

Cervicitis in adolescent females is diagnosed by the finding of a mucopurulent cervical discharge and cervical friability. Cultures are positive for *Chlamydia* or gonorrhea in more than 50 per cent of cases. Herpes simplex is less commonly found. *Chlamydia trachomatis* has a reported prevalence of 8 to 33 per cent among sexually active adolescents and may be present without obvious clinical signs of cervicitis. Recent decision analysis studies recommend screening all sexually active females for *Chlamydia* if the prevalence of infection is greater than 7 per cent (Phillips et al., 1987).

The major concern regarding unrecognized and untreated cervical infections is related to the development of upper genital tract infection or pelvic inflammatory disease (PID). There is a 10 to 30 per cent chance of an ascending infection in females with cervical gonorrhea or *Chlamydia* (McGregor, 1985). One fifth of all cases of PID occur in adolescents (Washington et al., 1985). It is estimated that one out of eight sexually active 15-year-olds develops pelvic inflammatory disease yearly. Given the recognized sequelae of PID, including infertility, ectopic pregnancy, and chronic pelvic pain, sexually active adolescent females should be thoroughly evaluated for STDs and treated aggressively with careful follow-up.

HPV has been linked with cervical dysplasia. Until recently, HPV infection has been diagnosed by the finding of condylomata acuminata or indirectly on Papanicolaou's smear. Recent studies have isolated HPV from up to 33 per cent of sexually active adolescents (Rosenfeld et al., 1988). Only a small percentage of these patients had abnormal Papanicolaou's smears or genital warts. The current management of females with signs of HPV infection includes colposcopy. Papanicolaou's smears may be indicated more frequently in sexually active adolescents than in adult women.

Male adolescents may present for evaluation of symptoms of urethritis. Nongonococcal (generally chlamydial) urethritis is diagnosed when the Gram's stain of the urethral discharge, if present, shows no intracellular diplococci. Physicians may have some success in recommending the use of condoms for the egocentric male adolescent who has experienced an STD.

Although relatively few cases of AIDS have been diagnosed in adolescents, the number of people with AIDS between the ages of 20 and 29 comprise the second most common decade for this diagnosis. The current best estimate for the time between exposure to the human immunodeficiency virus (HIV) and the clinical diagnosis of AIDS is 5 to 7 years. Therefore, it is a safe assumption that many of the people who develop AIDS in their 20's contracted the virus during their teenage years. For these reasons, there is a greater urgency than ever before for physicians to counsel adolescents against behaviors that put them at risk. The means by which AIDS can and cannot be contracted should be discussed with all teenagers. Sexually active adolescents should be advised about responsible behavior, and barrier methods should be offered.

ACNE

Acne, which affects up to 85 per cent of all teenagers, is one of the most common medical problems for this age group. Although acne poses no serious medical risk, the psychologic effects of inflammatory lesions can be devastating. Lesions of acne may be as mild as an occasional papule or pustule or as severe as inflammatory, nodulocystic lesions. Areas commonly involved include the face, back, and upper chest.

The etiology of acne is well understood. Androgenic hormones stimulate a proliferation of sebaceous glands. These glands are colonized by skin bacteria including *Propionibacterium acnes*, which release lipases among other substances. These enzymes act on the sebum to release free fatty acids that cause inflammation in the dermis and act with other substances to produce abnormal keratinization of the glandular ducts.

Treatment of acne is directed by an understanding of the pathogenesis of this disease. Noninflammatory comedones can be treated with a topical keratolytic agent, such as benzoyl peroxide or retinoic acid. When inflammatory lesions are present, antibiotics are also indicated. Most physicians treat acne with a topical antibiotic, such as tetracycline, erythromycin, or clindamycin, and reserve systemic antibiotics for unresponsive cases. Severe cystic acne, which has the potential for long-term scarring, may require isotretinoin. Substantiated concerns regarding this drug's teratogenicity mitigate against its use in adolescent females. Regular monitoring of laboratory parameters, including liver and lipid profiles, is required when this drug is prescribed. This dangerous drug should only be considered in severe, refractory cases where careful follow-up is assured.

SPECIAL ORTHOPEDIC PROBLEMS

Scoliosis

Scoliosis, a side-to-side curvature of the spine, is found in 5 to 10 per cent of adolescents. It is usually noted on examination of the back by the finding of asymmetry of the hips, scapulae, or shoulders. Having the patient bend forward at the waist usually accentuates the asymmetry.

Scoliosis may be a result of an underlying problem; however, up to 70 per cent is idiopathic. This is particularly true in girls. Occasionally, the curvature in the spine is compensatory for a leg length discrepancy. This may be detected by differences in the height of the iliac crests. Congenital abnormalities of the spine, including occult spina bifida or hemivertebrae, are responsible for less than 10 per cent of cases. Neuromuscular abnormalities and other problems account for a very small percentage of cases.

The management of scoliosis depends on the degree of curve noted, as well as the sexual maturity rating of the adolescent. Teenagers in the early Tanner stages may require close follow-up because scoliosis tends to progress during the growth spurt. X-ray studies have been overused in the past and are generally not indicated when the physician is secure with the assessment. Similarly, exercises are of no proven benefit to halt the progression of scoliosis, although lower back exercises may strengthen muscles that easily fatique. X-ray studies are required when more aggressive interventions are being considered. The Cobb angle is determined by the intersecting lines extrapolated from the articular surfaces of the vertebral bodies that define the ends of the scoliotic curve. Adolescents with curvatures of more than 15 degrees who are entering a period of rapid growth probably warrant orthopedic evaluation. Braces are often prescribed for patients with scoliosis of greater than 20 degrees, but surgery is usually reserved for more severe cases.

Osgood-Schlatter Disease

Osgood-Schlatter disease is a painful swelling of the tibial tubercle at the insertion of the infrapatellar tendon. It is a common problem particularly in males in the early pubertal stages. Traction stress from the patellar tendon may lead to avulsion of small fragments of cartilage or of the ossification center.

This entity tends to occur in active adolescent males around Tanner stage 2 or 3. The pain is aggravated by activity and relieved by rest. On physical examination, there is soft tissue swelling and tenderness over the tibial tubercle. X-ray studies are not essential for the diagnosis and are only used to eliminate the possibility of other disease in atypical cases.

Treatment recommendations are easily made, but implementation is often difficult. Restriction of running and jumping activities is usually sufficient to allow improvement. However, most adolescent males are unwilling to completely stop their sports participation and a compromise must be met. Swimming and other sports that do not stress the area involved may be substituted. Ice applied to the area before and after activity and mild anti-inflammatories, such as aspirin, may provide some additional relief. If symptoms are severe or fail to respond to restriction of activity, rare cases may require immobilization.

SUBSTANCE USE AND ABUSE

Nationally obtained data substantiate high rates of substance use among both younger and older adolescents (Irwin and Millstein, 1986). In one study, cigarette smoking among 12- and 13-year-olds, 14- and 15-year-olds, and 16- and 17-year-olds was 3 per cent, 10 per cent, and 30 per cent, respectively. Alcohol use in these same three age groups was 10 per cent, 23 per cent, and 45 per cent. Marijuana use in these three groups was 2 per cent, 8 per cent, and 23 per cent. Other cross-sectional studies have confirmed these trends. In a survey of high school seniors in 1984, 93 per cent of the sample reported using alcohol (72 per cent within the past month), and 65 per cent reported using illicit drugs (Johnston et al., 1984).

Certain patterns regarding substance use occur in adolescence. Although many teenagers do not experiment with all of these substances, the use of alcohol or cigarettes is predictive of experimentation with marijuana or other drugs. Another interesting observation from these data is that the period around the seventh and eighth grade appears to be a critical time regarding an adolescent's experimentation or use of these potentially harmful substances. Physicians taking care of adolescents may be able to identify the teenager at risk for these behaviors and provide counseling and support.

PSYCHIATRIC DISEASE

Depression/Suicide

Suicide is the third leading cause of death in adolescents (Greydanus, 1986). The number of attempted suicides far exceeds the number of completed suicides with the ratio reported at between 50 and 120 to 1. Many deaths attributed to accidents may also be completed suicides. In general, female adolescents are more likely to make a suicidal gesture, and male adolescents are more likely to complete a suicide attempt. Suicide attempts in adolescents generally occur in the setting of chronic stresses, such as results from a broken family, a learning disability, or the diagnosis of a chronic disease. The acute precipitating event may be the break-up of a relationship or the concern about a pregnancy.

A depressed adolescent may present differently from the typical adult. While the older adolescent may have the classic vegetative signs of depression and report low self-esteem, depression in the younger adolescent may be marked by acting-out behavior, excessive anger, a fall-off in school performance, or new drug use. For developmental reasons, young adolescents are unable to articulate their troubles.

The physician should carefully evaluate a depressed teenager for the possibility of suicide. Direct questions about suicidal thoughts are appropriate. Similarly, any teenager who has made a suicide attempt or gesture should be handled seriously. Often, it is best to hospitalize such a teenager for 24 to 48 hours to cool off a volatile situation and to plan an appropriate evaluation and management.

EATING DISORDERS

Criteria for the diagnosis of anorexia nervosa include a weight loss of more than 25 per cent of original body weight, a disturbance of the body image, onset of the disease at less than 25 years of age, and no other illness that could account for the weight loss. Other commonly associated findings are amenorrhea, a ritualistic exercise history, and excessive preoccupation with food. This illness is far more common in females and occasionally coexists with bulimia. Bulimia is characterized by episodic binge eating followed by self-induced vomiting, use of laxatives, and often abdominal pain.

Patients with eating disorders first present to their family doctor. Although treatment of these illnesses is complicated, a thorough medical evaluation is the appropriate first step. Thereafter, the family physician may seek involvement of a psychiatrist or psychologist with expertise in treatment of eating disorders. Often, the treatment plan is three pronged and includes medical follow-up and individual as well as family counseling. Anorexia is a serious, potentially fatal diagnosis that requires long-term management.

References

Alpert, J. J., and Guyer, B. (Eds.): Injuries and injury prevention. Pediatr. Clin. North Am., *32*(1):5, 1985. *An excellent and practical presentation of the major areas in injury control.*

Berwick, D. M.: Non-organic failure to thrive. Pediatr. Rev., *1*:265, 1980. *A review article which stresses the need for a directed evaluation of children with FTT.*

Brown, S. S.: The health needs of adolescents in U.S. *In* Healthy people: The Surgeon General's report on health promotion and disease prevention, background papers. U.S. Dept. of Health, Education, and Welfare Publication No. (PHS) 79–55071A. Washington, D.C., Government Printing Office, 1979, pp. 333–364.

Canadian Task Force on the Periodic Health Examination: The periodic health examination. Can. Med. Assoc. J., *121*:1193, 1979. *This immense effort summarizes the data regarding the indications and recommended intervals for health screening interventions.*

Cantekin, E. I. Mandel, E. M., Bluestone, C. D., et al.: Lack of efficacy of a decongestant-antihistamine combination for otitis media with effusion ("secretory" otitis media) in children. N. Engl. J. Med., *308*:297, 1983.

Centers for Disease Control: General recommendations on immunization. M.M.W.R., *32*:5, 1983.

Daniel, W. A.: Adolescents in Health and Disease. St. Louis, C. V. Mosby Co., 1977. *A delightful text written in a practical style by a pediatrician who truly enjoys adolescent patients.*

Denny, F. W., and Clyde, W. A.: Acute lower respiratory tract infections in nonhospitalized children. J. Pediatr., *108*:635, 1986. *One of many excellent studies from a private pediatric practice in Chapel Hill, N.C.*

Dershewitz, R. A., (Ed.): Ambulatory Pediatric Care. Philadelphia, J. B. Lippincott, 1988. *An outstanding, encyclopedic reference text that lives up to its title and addresses issues from a primary care perspective.*

The Child Day Care Infectious Disease Study Group, Centers for Disease Control, Special Article: Public health considerations of infectious diseases in child day care centers. J. Pediatr., *105*:683, 1984.

Gergen, P. J., Mullally, D., and Evans, R.: National survey of prevalence of asthma among children in the United States, 1976 to 1980. Pediatrics, *81*:1, 1988.

Greydanus, D. E.: Depression in adolescence. J. Adolesc. Health Care, *7*:109S, 1986.

Gruber, E., and Chambers, C. V.: Cognitive development and adolescent contraception: integrating theory and practice. Adolescence, *XXII*:661, 1987. *Includes a useful table on the developmental advantages and disadvantages of various contraceptive methods.*

Herold, E. S., and Goodwin, M. S.: Why adolescents go to birth-control clinics rather than to their family physicians. Can. J. Pub. Health, *70*:317, 1979.

Hofmann, A. D.: A rational policy toward consent and confidentiality in adolescent health care. J. Adolesc. Health Care, *1*:9, 1980.

Irwin, C. E.: Why Adolescent Medicine? J. Adolesc. Health Care, *7*:2S, 1986. *This paper, by one of the leading advocates for adolescents nationally, reviews the history of this specialty. The entire volume is devoted to issues with implications for the practitioner.*

Irwin, C. E., and Millstein, S. G.: Biopsychosocial correlates of risk-taking behaviors during adolescence. J. Adolesc. Health Care, *7*:82S, 1986. *A developmental approach to understanding adolescent risk taking with recommended interventions for the practitioner.*

Isaacs, D., Day, D., and Crook, S.: Childhood gastroenteritis: a population study. Br. Med. J., *293*:545, 1986.

Johnston, L. D., Bachman, J. G., and O'Malley, P. M.: Use of licit and illicit drugs by America's high school students, 1975–84, U.S. Dept. of Health and Human Services Publication No. 85-1394. Rockville, MD, National Institute of Drug Abuse, 1984.

Kunin, C. M., Zacha, E., and Paquin, A. J.: Urinary tract infections in schoolchildren. N. Engl. J. Med., *266*:1287, 1962.

Levenson, P. M., Morrow, J. R., and Pfefferbaum, B. J.: Attitudes toward health and illness: a comparison of adolescent, physician, teacher, and school nurse views. J. Adolesc. Health Care, *5*:254, 1984.

McGregor, J. A.: Adolescent misadventures with urethritis and cervicitis. J. Adolesc. Health Care, *6*:286, 1985.

Morrissey, J. M., et al.: Consent and confidentiality in the health care of children and adolescents. New York, Free Press, 1986. *Includes a state-by-state review of laws regarding adolescents' rights to health care.*

National Center for Health Statistics. B. K. Cypress: Patterns of ambulatory care in pediatrics. The National Ambulatory Medical Care Survey, United States, January 1980–December 1981. Vital and Health Statistics. Series 13, No. 75, DHHS Pub. No. (PHS) 84-1736. Public Health Service, Washington, D.C., U.S. Government Printing Office, October, 1983.

National Center for Health Statistics. T. M. Ezzau: Ambulatory care utilization patterns of children and young adults. The National Ambulatory Medical Care Survey. United States. January–December 1975. Vital and Health Statistics. Series 13, No. 39. DHEW Pub. No. (PHS) 78-1790. Public Health Service. Washington, D.C., U.S. Government Printing Office, 1978.

Neinstein, L. S.: Adolescent Health Care: A Practical Guide. Baltimore, Urban & Schwarzenberg, 1984. *A handy text replete with tables and accessible outlines pertaining to adolescent health care issues.*

North, A. F.: Screening in child health care: where are we now and where are we going? Pediatrics, *5*:631, 1974.

O'Reilly, K. R., and Aral, S. O.: Adolescence and sexual behavior. J. Adolesc. Health Care, *6*:262, 1985.

Oski, F. A., and Nathan, D. G. (Eds.): Hematology of Infancy and Childhood. Philadelphia, W. B. Saunders Co., 1987.

Paradise, J. L.: Otitis media in infants and children. Pediatrics, *65*:917, 1980. *Outstanding review article covering all aspects of otitis media.*

Parcel, G. S., Nader, P. R., and Meyer, M. P.: Adolescent health concerns, problems and patterns of utilization in a triethnic urban population. Pediatrics, *60*:157, 1977.

Phillips, R. S., Aronson, M. D., Taylor, W. C., et al.: Should tests for *Chlamydia trachomatis* cervical infection be done during routine gynecologic visits? Ann. Int. Med., *107*:188, 1987.

Poole, S. R., Morrison, J. D., Marshall, J., et al.: Pediatric Health Care in Family Practice. J. Fam. Pract., *15*:945, 1982. *Data from 12 practice sites in Colorado are combined to evaluate the pediatric experience in family practice.*

Report of the Committee on Infectious Diseases: 1982 Red Book. Evanston, Ill., American Academy of Pediatrics, 1982.

Rosenfeld, W. D., Vermund, S. H., Wentz, S. J., et al.: Positive association of human papillomavirus with adolescent pregnancy. Society for Adolescent Medicine 15th Annual Research Meeting, New York City, March 24–27, 1988.

Shear, C. L., Burke, G. L., Freedman, D. S., et al.: Value of childhood blood pressure measurements and family history in predicting future blood pressure status: results from 8 years of follow-up in the Bogalusa Heart Study. Pediatrics, *77*:6, 1986.

Slap, G. B.: Normal physiological and psychosocial growth in the adolescent. J. Adolesc. Health Care, *7*:13S, 1986. *A succinct review of normal growth in adolescence with excellent tables and figures.*

Starfield, B., Hoekelman, R. A., McCormick, M., et al.: Who provides health care to children and adolescents in the U.S.? Pediatrics, *74*:991, 1983.

Stockman, J. A.: Iron deficiency anemia: have we come far enough? (Editorial) J.A.M.A., *258*:1645, 1987.

Strain, J. E.: AAP Periodicity Guidelines: a framework for educating patients. Pediatrics, *74*:924, 1984.

Tanner, J. M.: Growth at Adolescence. 2nd ed. Oxford, England, Blackwell Scientific Publications, 1962.

Task Force on Blood Pressure Control in Children, National Heart, Lung and Blood Institute: Report of the Second Task Force on blood pressure control in children—1987. Pediatrics, *79*:1, 1987. *An excellent position paper with useful nomograms and a reasonable review of the approach to the hypertensive child.*

Utilization of short-stay hospitals by adolescents. United States 1980, Advancedata Vital and Health Statistics, National Center for Health Statistics, Public Health Service Publication No. 93, 1983, pp. 1–5.

Wald, E. R., Dashefsky, B., Byers, C., et al.: Frequency and severity of infections in day care. J. Pediatr., *112*:540, 1988.

Washington, A. E., Sweet, R. L., and Shafer, M. B.: Pelvic inflammatory disease and its sequelae in adolescents. J. Adolesc. Health Care, *6*:298, 1985.

Yip, R., Binkin, N. J., Fleshood, L., et al.: Declining prevalence of anemia among low-income children in the United States. J.A.M.A., *258*:1619, 1987.

40

Behavioral Problems in Children and Adolescents

Robert W. Higgins
Alex R. Rodriguez

Among the most common problems that families will present to a family physician for attention and assistance are the range of child and adolescent behaviors that signal some concern about a possible emotional disturbance. Indeed, family emotional problems in general are among the most frequent in a family practice. To provide for an adequate evaluation and disposition of emotional disturbances in children and adolescents, it is essential that family physicians have a sound understanding of normal and pathologic mental functioning in children and adults, family interpersonal dynamics, and the effects of social and cultural factors in their psychosocial integration. The complex intertwining of biologic, psychologic, social, and spiritual aspects of an individual makes it necessary that each patient be viewed in an integrated and comprehensive fashion that takes into account all of these functional aspects of the individual.

Emotions are operant in all stages of health and illness. Clinical studies in what have been termed psychosomatic and somatopsychic conditions underlie the complex nature of emotions in conditions manifesting physical pathology. Neurobiologic and neuropsychologic research has advanced to the point that there is clear evidence that an individual's experiences have an evolving impact on neurologic development through organs of perception (Stark and Blum, 1986). Moreover, psychologic functioning—including the unique personality, emotional reactions, and mood disposition of each person—is itself an innate aspect of one's biologic make-up. In no individuals are these complex functions more in developmental flux than children. The role of a family physician in the monitoring of this development cannot be minimized. Knowledge of normal growth and development and ongoing psychologic evaluations of family members can be vital in preventing and minimizing emotional problems.

Epidemiology

Since behavioral problems of children and adolescents are not uncommon, the family physician can expect to see children presenting with manifestations of the various behavioral disorders on a regular basis (Rescorla, 1985). The overall prevalence rate of behavioral disorders is difficult to assess because of variance

The opinions and statements contained herein are those of the authors and are not to be construed as official or reflecting the views of the Department of Navy or the Department of Defense.

in definitions, sampling methods, and criteria for diagnosis. Another complicating factor is age, since the prevalence of most disorders changes with age. Nevertheless, many studies in preschool, elementary school, and junior high school age children show the overall rate of children with behavioral, educational, or social-family problems to be between 14 and 24 per cent (Noshpitz, 1979; American Psychiatric Association, 1987). Clinical studies further suggest that 60 per cent of children with behavioral problems have more than one problem. Some of the more common behavior problems that the family physician is likely to see are listed in Table 40–1.

Management of Common Behavioral Problems

The following section will discuss the more common behavioral problems occurring in childhood and adolescence that meet specific criteria for diagnosis in the *Diagnostic and Statistical Manual III, Revised (DSM-III-R)* (American Psychiatric Association, 1987). Specific diagnostic criteria from the *DSM-III-R* are not given. Some clues to therapy in the various disorders are given with an emphasis on the treatment of the family and not just the child or adolescent.

MENTAL RETARDATION

Mental retardation is a complex problem both diagnostically and in the management of those who fulfill the criteria for this diagnosis. Mental retardation implies an impairment of intelligence, usually from early life, with inadequate mental development and an impairment of adaptive behavior. There is presently no reliable or valid method of objectively measuring adaptive behavior, so it has traditionally been correlated with intelligence, as measured by one of the individually administered general intelligence tests, most commonly the Weschler Intelligence Scale for Children (WISC). The intelligence quotient (IQ), which is a ratio of mental age to chronologic age, is inaccurate but useful as a guide. It is generally thought to have an error of approximately five points, so any numerical value would represent an approximate intelligence range, i.e., an IQ of 70 would represent a range of 65 to 75. The subtypes of mental retardation are:

Mild (educable)	IQ 50–70
Moderate (trainable)	IQ 35–49
Severe	IQ 20–34
Profound	IQ below 20

The correlation of adaptive ability with IQ decreases as the IQ approaches 70. This is due in part to the fact that intelligence is not the result of a single mental process but is comprised of many facets, including memory, abstract thinking, causal reasoning, verbal expression, spatial comprehension, and other mental functions. It also is affected by experience and cultural background and may be modified by many factors, mostly environmental. There is a higher incidence of mental retardation in boys compared to girls, reported variously from 10 per cent greater incidence to twice the incidence. This may be due partly to biologic factors, i.e., sex-linked genetic disorders, and partly to different social expectations for boys and girls. The overall incidence is approximately 1 per cent of the general population.

The diagnosis is made regardless of coexisting mental or physical disorders. Since retarded children are more vulnerable to emotional problems and since children primarily with emotional problems may sometimes function at a retarded level, confusion in diagnosis may occur. The differential diagnosis includes those conditions that result in an interference in the capacity to learn or demonstrate intelligence on a structured test, resulting in a clinical picture of subaverage intellectual function.

Table 40–1. PREVALENCE RATES OF SOME COMMON CHILDHOOD BEHAVIORAL DISORDERS

Attention deficit disorder	1–5 per cent of prepubertal children
Anorexia Nervosa	0.5 per cent of girls age 12–18 years
Transient Tic Disorder	5–24 per cent of school children
Stuttering	8 per cent of all children
Functional Enuresis:	
Age 5 Years	7 per cent of boys, 3 per cent of girls
Age 10 Years	3 per cent of boys, 2 per cent of girls
Age 18 Years	1 per cent of boys, rare in girls
Sleepwalking Disorder	1–6 per cent of children at some time
Sleep Terror Disorder	1–4 per cent of children at some time
Articulation Disorder	10 per cent below 8 years, 5 per cent over the age of 8
Conduct Disorder	9 per cent of boys, 2 per cent of girls less than 18 years

MANAGEMENT

The physician who provides care for mentally retarded children will find this task complex but rewarding. It requires a multifaceted and continuing commitment involving not only health care for the retarded child but also providing education and support for the parents and coordination of community resources that promote education, socialization, and maximum autonomous functions.

Family physicians should be able to recognize developmental lags in infants and toddlers that may indicate mental retardation. When a presumptive diagnosis of mental retardation can be made, the family physician should provide an objective approach that is reassuring but not based upon unfounded opinions. The parents will be most comforted by positive information early on about what they can actively do to make the most of their child's potential, rather than adopting a wait-and-see attitude, which will only lead to frustration. It is imperative that both parents be included in discussions. Irregardless of when the diagnosis is made, the parents often experience some form of emotional reaction, which generally will include some levels and expressions of anger, anxiety, and depression. Further visits should be made available to help the parents deal with their anxieties. In cases where the diagnosis is not entirely clear, early multidisciplinary consultation (e.g., IQ testing, developmental evaluation by pediatric or child psychiatric specialist) is indicated.

In the child with mental retardation, a specific diagnosis will have important implications for prognosis and treatment of the child and genetic counseling of the parents. Helping parents obtain an adequate evaluation of their child while avoiding unnecessary expense is as much of an obligation of the physician as helping them accept the realities of their situation.

Retarded children require the same general health care that is desirable for all children. Many infants with varieties of brain damage are colicky, chronically irritable, difficult to feed, and have irregular sleep habits. The physician must assist the parents in coping with these problems to assure adequate nutrition and rest and to help minimize negative feelings by the parents toward the child. Providing reassurance about their need to have periodic child-care assistance and steering parents and siblings to local community support groups for families of retarded persons can often provide great relief.

Efforts to decrease disability and increase adaptive or functional ability are essential at all ages but are more effective at an early age when development is most rapid and learning capacity is most active. Close communication with the parents over realistic goals for their child is extremely important. These goals should be directed more towards development of effective work habits, development of some areas of ability (e.g., self-care, chores), and development of social interactions. These efforts will likely be multidisciplinary, involving various school and social service personnel.

The question of institutionalization versus care at home often arises and should be considered in assessment and treatment planning. The present trend is towards maintaining the child in a home environment with outside assistance. It seems clear that the continuing involvement of the parents results in the retarded child or adolescent having greater functional capacity, in contrast to those children who are institutionalized at an early age. It is ultimately the parents' decision, but they will need guidance and support from the physician. If there are few or no community services, if physical or emotional illness exists in a parent, or if there is some other family dysfunction, then institutionalization may be more indicated.

The family physician involved in the care of a retarded child must not only be aware of community resources but should be willing to help develop these resources if they do not exist. While the family physician would usually serve as coordinator and advocate in the care of the child, he or she should by no means be expected to provide for specialized services. In all instances, one should be willing to provide the ongoing support for the parents, as they deal with the often disappointing but often rewarding progress of their retarded child.

Disruptive Behavior Disorders

ATTENTION DEFICIT HYPERACTIVITY DISORDER

Attention deficit hyperactivity disorder (ADHD) is the current term referenced in the *DSM-III-R* to describe a cluster of clinically observable behavioral deviations among children. In the past, a series of terms have been used to describe this disorder, including: minimal brain damage, minimal brain dysfunction, hyperkinetic reaction of childhood, hyperkinetic syndrome, hyperkinetic impulse disorder, hyperactive child syndrome, minimal cerebral dysfunction, attention deficit disorder, and many others. This more recent focus in diagnostic nosology is the result of clinical observations that attentional difficulties are the most prominent characteristic among children with these diagnoses.

The essential features are signs of inappropriate expressions of inattention, impulsivity, and hyperactivity of at least 6 months duration where the onset occurs before age 7. Reference is made to the *DSM-III-R* for further delineation of diagnostic criteria and to other references for details related to clinical issues (Barkley, 1981; Bloomindale, 1985; Cantwell, 1984).

Typically, the signs and symptoms of this disorder in any one individual will vary with time and situation. Occasionally, their behavior will seemingly be well organized and appropriate in structured situations, such as in the physician's office, but may be distinctly abnormal in less structured or overstimulated situations. About 20 per cent of children will show behavior typical of the disorder in the physician's office. There are no generally recognized tests that are specific for the diagnosis of attention deficit disorder. Diagnosis can be made by direct observation, reports of significant observers (such as parents or teachers), and professional evaluations—correlated to the *DSM-III* diagnostic criteria. Certain rating scales (Gutterman et al., 1987; Beitchman et al., 1987) for the assessment of behavior can be helpful in the evaluation.

A developmental history can be of great value in arriving at a diagnosis. The parents typically relate a picture of an alert, active, demanding infant with feeding and sleeping difficulties, often in the first few months, who was slow to establish diurnal rhythms and commonly was colicky. The developmental milestones are usually normal or advanced. As toddlers, they frequently need a high level of supervision since they are physically active and constantly exploring, often to the point of causing damage to household objects or posing a danger to their security. Their behavior can often be very frustrating to parents and other care-takers, especially those with limited coping skills. Thus, the family physician should always be vigilant for potential child abuse in families with such children and be prepared to both assist and report where abuse exists (Council on Scientific Affairs [AMA], 1985).

Physical examination generally does not contribute to the diagnosis of attention deficit hyperactivity disorder (ADHD). However, the physician should be alert to certain signs, such as the reported increased frequency of minor congenital anomalies, including malformed ears, epicanthal folds, high arched palates, camptodactyly, and single palmar creases. There is also an increased frequency of what have been termed soft neurologic signs, such as mixed hand preference, and impairments of balance, stereognosis, graphesthesia, hand mobility, and finger localization.

Cognitive testing may contribute confirming data that may be useful in establishing the diagnosis. Children with ADHD may show circumscribed cognitive and perceptual deficiencies. Such testing should be provided by the local school district but, if not provided, *may* be reimbursed through health insurance. It is occasionally worthwhile to periodically repeat selected cognitive tests to correlate any functional gains that result from therapy and compare with the baseline evaluation.

The clinical course of this disorder is not clearly known, primarily because studies in the past have probably included children with other disorders, particularly conduct disorder, anxiety disorder, and oppositional disorder (Werry et al., 1987). In some instances, symptoms of ADHD persist into adolescence or adult life. In other situations, the disorder is self-limited, and most of the apparent symptoms disappear during puberty. It is important for the family physician to recognize that a significant proportion of boys with ADHD will be at risk for delinquency. This is likely related to the relatively high incidence of psychopathology in the parents of children with conduct disorder and ADHD (Lahey et al., 1988), particularly substance abuse, antisocial personality disorder, and somatization disorder. It is also important to recognize that depressive disorders may coexist with ADHD, either independently or dependently (Jensen et al., 1988; Costello, 1986). Whenever there is a dilemma over diagnosis or treatment in such situations, referral to or consultation from a child-adolescent psychiatrist is indicated.

In addition to difficulties in the diagnosis of this condition, questions have arisen over the specificity and efficacy of treatments. While the use of stimulant drugs has been controversial, this has largely been due to concerns about overprescription of stimulant medication. Recent studies would indicate a relatively clear, short-term, positive effect on hyperkinetic and inattentive behaviors, academic performance, and decreased family disruptions in both children and adolescents (Klorman et al., 1987). Stimulant drugs do exert some effect on interpersonal and affective functioning. Clinical impressions and studies have shown that children on stimulants may be less sociable and may seem less spontaneous or sad.

There has been a notable amount of clinical inquiry and professional and parental concern about the effects of stimulant drugs on physical growth. Recent studies confirm that there is a clear effect on weight increase (about 1.5 kg. less than expected over the first 2 years) with a small effect on increases in height (about 0.9 cm.). However, tolerance to this effect seems to develop about the third year, and longer term effects appear to be lessened, with no apparent effect on eventual adult stature or weight. Methylphenidate apparently has less effect than amphetamines on growth. Such side effects (e.g., gastrointestinal distress, as well as other factors, such as family disruptions) are among the reasons that compliance is commonly a problem, particularly when prescribed over long periods of time (Brown et al., 1987).

The authors recommend a treatment regimen that includes psychostimulant medication, psychosocial and academic interventions, and parental education and support. Stimulant drug therapy using methylphenidate (Ritalin) is recommended at an initial dose of 0.25 mg. per kg. daily, given in divided doses after breakfast and lunch. This may be increased up to 2 mg. per kg. daily (Campbell and Spencer, 1988; Rifkin et al., 1986). No doses should be given later than noon to avoid sleep problems. The drug should be given on school days but not on weekends, holidays, or during the summer school break in order to give the child a drug holiday. If a favorable change in behavior does occur, the drug should be continued preferably for the school year. At the beginning of the next school year, the drug should be withheld for several weeks to assess performance and behavior; if indicated, methylphenidate should be restarted for the school year. If a child does not respond to methylphenidate, a trial of dextroamphetamine at a dose of 0.2 mg. per kg. daily, may be indicated. If medication side effects should become severely distressing, then consideration should be given to reducing, changing, or discontinuing the medication. Close contact with parents and teachers must be established in order to adequately assess the effect of the drug. The use of a specific rating scale for the teacher will allow a more objective evaluation.

Approximately 75 per cent of attention-disordered children will respond to stimulant therapy. Overall, clinical research has not demonstrated the efficacy of other medications, such as imipramine (Pliszka, 1987) or clonidine. Additionally, research has shown no beneficial effect of additive-free diets (e.g., Feingold or K.P. diet) on the behavior of children with ADHD (Gross et al., 1987).

In addition to stimulant drug therapy, the child's educational problems must be addressed with the school system, and parents may need guidance regarding parenting strategies and other resources (e.g., parenting courses, handbooks). Psychotherapy may be indicated for the child and/or family, especially if the child displays serious antisocial or aggressive behavior or the parents and child experience interpersonal difficulties in adjusting to the behavioral problems. An important aspect of the successful treatment of these children is the need for the physician to view these children in a positive manner. Such an attitude should be conveyed to the parents, who in turn are encouraged to pass this attitude on to the child. If the child is taught to expect achievement of mastery over the environment, and has to invent unconventional strategies to achieve mastery, he or she may turn out to be a superior problem-solver.

CONDUCT DISORDER

The essential feature of a disorder of conduct is a repetitive and persistent pattern of behavior in which there is a basic violation of the rights of others or of societal norms or rules. There are basically three types of conduct disorders: those occurring as a part of a group (aggressive or nonaggressive), individually (generally aggressive), or as an undifferentiated mixture of behaviors.

It is important to keep in mind that this disorder characteristically is variable in severity of expression, is associated with major depression (16 to 23 per cent), is manifested over a period of at least 6 months, and is commonly associated with parental psychopathology. Moreover, such children have significantly greater tendencies to develop adult antisocial personality disorders and problems with delinquent behavior.

The term, juvenile delinquency, is frequently confused with or used synonymously with conduct disorder. A delinquent act by a child or adolescent is one that would be adjudged criminal if committed by an adult. Since children are not declared delinquent until a court has so adjudicated, juvenile delinquency, by definition, is a legal term. While some children and adolescents with a conduct disorder become juvenile delinquents, not all juvenile delinquents have a diagnosable conduct disorder. Some may commit an isolated antisocial act not related to a mental disorder, while others may act out psychologic conflicts through antisocial behavior. The coexistence of impulsivity and depression has been shown to result in greater suicidal risk than in children or adolescents with depression alone (Apter et al., 1987).

The family physician is in a unique position to have knowledge of the environment in which a child exists or will come into at birth. Parenting education support and monitoring are important aspects of prenatal and subsequent care for those parents identified as high risk for providing less than ideal parenting. In addition, psychiatric or social services referral of one or both parents in a high-risk family (e.g., significant psychiatric or substance abuse problems, family violence, antisocial behavior, single parent and illegitimate birth) may provide the opportunity for evaluation and treatment that can result in the potential for a more psychologically healthy environment and, subsequently, more psychologically promotive development of the child.

The family physician should always be aware that children and adolescents who fit the conduct disorder criteria can present with such underlying problems as venereal disease (especially at an early age and if two or more sexual partners are involved), unwanted early pregnancy, multiple episodes of injury from accident (including fighting, child abuse, and daredevil behavior), suicide behavior, and substance abuse. While none of these are pathognomonic of conduct disorder, they are nevertheless commonly associated behaviors.

If the family physician is asked to see a child or adolescent with a conduct disorder, it should be kept in mind that the patient needs and deserves a very careful work-up. This should include a detailed psychiatric history and mental status exam. Careful family, social, and medical history and complete physical exam are indicated, including a careful neurologic exam—with special attention for signs of intracranial mass lesions. Psychologic and educational evaluations should also be obtained. With data from this thorough work-up, some of the multiple factors correlated to the antisocial behavior may be clarified and potentially treatable disorders may be identified.

When the diagnosis of conduct disorder is made, it is important that the essential feature of a repetitive and persistent pattern of antisocial behavior be identified. Isolated acts of antisocial behavior should not be routinely diagnosed as conduct disorder but could be considered as childhood or adolescent antisocial behavior. Oppositional disorder may be confused with conduct disorder, in that the features of disobedience and opposition to authority figures are present, but basic rights of others and societal norms are not violated. ADHD and specific developmental disorder are commonly associated with conduct disorder and should also be noted in the diagnostic assessment when present.

Once the definitive or presumptive diagnosis of conduct disorder in children or adolescents is established, referral for specialized treatment should be made, since treatment is probably out of the realm of skills of most family physicians. Such a child might be treated effectively in outpatient psychotherapy but, in more dysfunctional children, might require residential treatment or inpatient care, where structure and therapeutic insight leading to behavior change and conflict resolution may occur. It should be emphasized that out of control behaviors that pose real harm to others (especially fire-setting and assaults) should be considered a psychiatric emergency

(Morrison, 1975; Bumpass et al., 1983). Such behaviors require immediate evaluation by a qualified child-adolescent psychiatrist and consideration of confinement in a psychiatric inpatient setting. If the origins of the antisocial behavior are in the family interactions, either concurrent treatment of the parent(s) or separation of the patient from the parent through group home placement might be indicated.

OPPOSITIONAL DEFIANT DISORDERS

Children with this disorder characteristically show a pattern of disobedient, negativistic, and provocative opposition to authority figures but do not violate the basic rights of others or of major age-appropriate norms or rules. The most striking feature is the persistence of the oppositional attitude even when it is clearly harmful to the apparent interests and well-being of the child. The oppositional attitude most frequently is directed toward family members. This child directs hostility indirectly—rather than directly—by procrastination, forgetting, dawdling, stubbornness, and resistance. When untreated, this disorder is usually chronic in nature and may be continuous with adult passive-aggressive personality disorder. Attention to manifested behaviors and affects is important in order to differentiate this disorder from others with similar characteristics, particularly attention deficit and conduct and anxiety disorders (Werry et al., 1987).

Treatment of children with oppositional disorder is usually difficult and usually requires professional psychiatric intervention. The family physician should encourage the parents to handle the oppositional behavior by setting firm, patient, and empathetic limits and expectations for the child. The parents and child should reach a decision on what his or her major tasks and responsibilities should be and a system set up for accomplishment and monitoring. A reward system for achievement—including praise, special time with parents, or privileges—is frequently helpful when the parents can be clear, consistent, and objective in working with the child. Resistances to minor tasks and responsibilities are best overlooked initially so that confrontations over less important issues are avoided and major goals can be focused upon. Age-appropriate assertiveness and independence should be clearly defined, encouraged, and rewarded. If these initial measures are unsuccessful, referral is indicated for the child and the parents.

Anxiety Disorders

Anxiety is a state of heightened tension accompanied by an inexpressible dread. There is an unpleasant sensation of apprehension, general irritability, often restlessness and fatigue, and occasionally associated visceral or somatic complaints. The symptoms of fear have much in common with anxiety. However, fear is an affective response to an actual, current, and external danger, whereas anxiety is a behavioral and psychophysiologic response to an internalized psychologic conflict triggered by certain situations.

Anxiety symptoms may be confused with those of certain medical conditions, such as hypoglycemia, pheochromocytoma, or hyperthyroidism. Similarly, children with a brain tumor or epilepsy may present with an unexplainable anxiety reaction. Therefore, a careful medical work-up, especially a history and physical exam, is important in the overall evaluation of the child presenting with anxiety symptoms.

The anxiety disorders of childhood or adolescence include three disorders in which anxiety is the predominant feature. In the separation anxiety disorder and avoidant disorder, the anxiety has a characteristic subjective and objective expression related to a specific conflictual focus, whereas in the overanxious disorder, the anxiety is generalized to a variety of situations.

SEPARATION ANXIETY DISORDER

The predominant disturbance in this disorder is excessive anxiety on separation from major attachment figures, from home, or from familiar surroundings. This is frequently associated with parents' own separation anxieties. The reaction to separation is beyond that expected for the child's level of development and can result in anxiety to the point of panic. It can become incapacitating to the point of the child's not being able to tolerate independent travel from home or from familiar locations—such as running errands, visiting at a friend's house, or attending camp or school. In more severe cases, they may not be able to tolerate staying in a room alone, preferring to cling to a parent even to the point of sleeping in or near the parent's bedroom (Van Winter and Strickler, 1984; Bernstein and Garfinkel, 1986).

School refusal is a prominent symptom of separation anxiety disorder. However, not all school refusal is due to separation anxiety. The problem with school attendance must be distinguished from school phobia. In school phobia, the child fears the school situation specifically, whether or not the parent is present—perhaps for realistic reasons such as a bully. When school refusal is due to separation anxiety, the child has difficulty in separating from home or parents. The treatment of school refusal is similar whether it is part of the symptom complex of separation anxiety disorder or is a school phobia, namely, *immediate* return to school unless the child is considered to be psychotic. While most cases of school phobia can successfully be treated by the family physician or pediatrician, children with separation anxiety disorder will most likely require referral for psychiatric evaluation and treatment. In such instances, coordination with the psychotherapist and school officials is essential.

There are many other manifestations of separation anxiety disorder. Children are often preoccupied with morbid fears that accidents or illness will occur—either to parents or themselves—resulting in separation. They may have unrealistic fears of such objects as monsters or animals or situations that they perceive as threatening the integrity of the family, such as burglars, kidnappers, car accidents, and plane travel. They may experience acute homesickness to the point of panic if they are away from home, and they may have specific fears, such as fear of the dark. On occasion, such symptoms can persist for many years and vary with evolving developmental demands, such as college attendance or employment. When no unusual demands for separation are made, children with this disorder usually display no particular interpersonal difficulties. The child may be brought to the family physician because of somatic complaints, such as nausea and vomiting, palpitations, headaches, or a variety of other somatic complaints. If a medical work-up fails to disclose a cause for the complaint, anxiety must be suspected and appropriate history obtained from the child, parent, and significant others, such as school teachers.

Treatment of this disorder can be difficult and involved in the more severe cases. Individual counseling for the child possibly may be helpful, especially if a good relationship can be established with the physician. Persistence of symptoms and resistance to a therapeutic alliance requires referral to a mental health professional. Family counseling is also essential and should be closely coordinated with the primary therapist of a child referred for individual psychotherapy. If there is a disparity between the parents over their ideas and methods of parenting, then parenting education or marital counseling may be indicated. Certainly, the school needs to be involved in cases of school refusal, both to obtain further history and to enlist parent cooperation in getting the child back in school. It is particularly important to insist that the child remain at school and for teachers to not overreact to somatic complaints by sending the child home or calling the parents.

AVOIDANT AND SCHIZOID DISORDERS OF CHILDHOOD OR ADOLESCENCE

This is an uncommon disorder characterized by an excessive and persistent shrinking in contact with strangers and occasionally with familiar persons. The essential elements are the avoidant behavior, severe enough to interfere with social functioning in peer and adult relationships, while maintaining a desire for affection and acceptance. They generally have warm and satisfying relations with family members and other familiar figures. Their social development within the family seems to be normal, though they are seen as timid and easily embarrassed. It is when they are confronted with someone outside of the family that they become extremely anxious and tearful and may even seem inarticulate or mute if social anxiety is severe, even though there is no impairment of communicative skills in nonstressful situations. These children are generally unassertive and lack self-confidence.

The course of this disorder is variable and not well known. Many improve spontaneously though some never form social bonds beyond the family, resulting in feelings of isolation and depression. Some children with this disorder may proceed to a chronic course into adult life, fulfilling the diagnostic criteria for Avoidant Personality Disorder.

The schizoid child, in contrast to the avoidant child, is characterized by having limited socialization skills and social-relational interests. Such a child is differentiated from the child with avoidant disorder of childhood, who desires socialization, but lacks self-assertion or support to achieve these skills. Schizoid children are not out of touch with reality, are not delusional, or do not experience hallucinations. Their interests do seem shallow and their energies are often constricted or limited. They have no close relationships other than (rarely) a relative or another socially isolated child. In adolescence, they are usually willfully oppositional or disobedient; insistent on doing what they want to do; moody; passively stubborn; resentful of advice or supervision; and easily offended. They often show a great interest in rites or cults.

This disorder always begins in childhood and can usually be diagnosed as early as 5 years of age, which differentiates it from normal social reticence. The course is not well known but usually results in continued or further withdrawal and detachment in adolescence, and eventual expression in adult symptoms indicating adult schizoid personality disorder or schizophrenia. In a few children, the disorder abates somewhat to allow self-limited but increased socialization during adolescence. This is usually the result of special efforts by caring persons, such as teachers.

The parents of such children should be referred for long-term guidance and assistance in providing experiences for the child that will facilitate socialization. Firm and caring insistence must be provided the child and parents for participation in activities that will enhance ego growth. Medication has proven of little or no value. It is important to recognize expressions of this disorder in a child as early as possible, since some studies suggest the outcome is more favorable if the child and parents receive professional assistance early in life. Early detection may be a problem in instances where the child might become obsessed with a limited activity and appear quite content to noninformed adults, resulting in their not being brought to the attention of the physician or other professional. Queries by the family physician about children's usual and unusual activities are always appropriate and may identify a child with this disorder.

OVERANXIOUS DISORDER

The essential features of this fairly common disorder are excessive worrying and fearful behaviors that are not focused on a specific situation or object. There is persistent anxiety, characterized by excessive fears, restless sleep, nightmares, and psychophysiologic symptoms. They often are seen by the parents as sensitive, shy, and aspiring. They usually feel inferior and submissive to others and worry about what others will think of their performance. These children may seem more mature than expected for their age because of their perfectionist tendencies and precocious concerns. There is sometimes an excess of nervous habits or restlessness, such as nail biting.

These children are frequently found in ambitious middle-class families who stress higher standards of achievement, even if the child is performing adequately. The children recognize that their acceptance within the family is contingent upon their continued superior performance. It is more commonly seen in eldest children and in small families and is apparently more common in boys.

Other Disorders of Infancy, Childhood, and Adolescence

REACTIVE ATTACHMENT DISORDER OF INFANCY

The essential features of this disorder are signs of poor emotional development and poor physical development, with onset before 8 months of age. The height and weight generally are below the third percentile for age, and bone age is retarded. It is considered to be due to lack of adequate care-taking and not primarily to physical disorder, mental retardation, or autistic disorder. The more severe cases of this disorder have also been called failure to thrive, though this term also refers collectively to failure of weight gain in an infant from any one of a variety of causes—either physical or psychosocial and with or without poor emotional development (Evans et al., 1972).

Infants with this disorder present with signs of poor social development. Normally, eye contact may be observed as early as 4 weeks of age and eye tracking and smile response by 2 months. As the baby grows older, the primary care-taker(s) become more influential stimuli for the social responses of smiling, looking, and anticipatory motor movements. By 6 months of age, hearing the voice of the care-taker elicits the same behavioral responses. In infants with Reactive Attachment Disorder, these social responses are minimal or absent, and the infant appears apathetic. Also commonly demonstrated are a weak cry, poor muscle tone, weak rooting and grasping reactions when feeding is attempted, a staring gaze, and low spontaneous mobility. Excessive sleep and a generalized lack of interest in the environment are frequently seen. The diagnosis can be made as early as the first month of life and onset of the disorder is always before 8 months, since early social attachments would usually be made by then if care-taking has been adequate.

Diagnosis is best made by hospitalization for evaluation and initial treatment. This provides an opportunity for quantitation of net caloric intake and for observation of interactions of the child during feeding and play with the mother or care-taker and with hospital personnel. Dramatic improvement in weight gain and social responsiveness often occurs in the hospital. A positive initial response like this usually makes it unnecessary to conduct an exhaustive and expensive search for an organic etiology of the presenting signs. Observation of the mother's interactions with the child, coupled with reports from friends, relatives, or neighbors, usually reveals the lack of adequate care provided for the infant. Clear evidence of this lack of a nurturing interaction is necessary to establish the diagnosis of Reactive Attachment Disorder of Infancy.

The course of this disorder is variable. If care remains grossly inadequate, malnutrition, intercurrent infection, and death can occur. Most children with this disorder eventually achieve physical development within normal range. If affectionate care is provided, the disorder is reversible, and the child may demonstrate minimal to no residual psychologic defect. However, about half will be identified as having neurotic traits or antisocial behavior, two thirds will manifest a delay in learning to read, and one third will have lower verbal than performance scores on IQ testing.

Prevention of this disorder is most effective when the physician recognizes characteristics and circumstances of parents that place infants at risk; this is increased with familiarity with the parents' circumstances. During the parents' prenatal visits, the family physician should assess the parenting attitudes, and cognitive and emotional adequacy of the mother-to-be to nurture. Education on parenting skills should be provided to those parents lacking knowledge. Close follow-up of the infants in whom prenatal conflicts are known to exist is imperative. Early counseling and adequate direct support in the care of the threatened child will help prevent development of this disorder.

When the diagnosis of reactive attachment disorder of infancy is made, prompt intervention is indicated for assuring the best outcome. This would be especially indicated in cases of extreme neglect, where severe physical complications can result in death quite rapidly. Most frequently, the diagnosis will be confirmed in the hospital setting, where a program of adequate care-taking can best be initiated. Sometimes, the period of hospitalization will be sufficient to relieve family tensions so that with advice, counseling, and support from a visiting nurse, social worker, or family service agency, sufficient adjustments in care-taking can be made to ensure adequate care of the child when returned home. If this is not feasible or successful, temporary or permanent placement in a foster home may be the best alternative.

ELECTIVE MUTISM

This rare disorder represents a condition in which the child limits verbal interactions to a few or all members of the family but steadfastly refuses to talk to other people. They may use gestures of various kinds to communicate or, in some cases, whisper. The situation occasionally comes to the physician's attention as the child enters school. In the school setting, they may attract attention to themselves by their lack of speech but soon become ostracized by their peers and a problem for the teacher. These children are usually shy, withdrawn, and socially isolated.

The disorder usually starts before age 5, though it will occur rarely in an older child who previously talked with others but suddenly stops. This acute onset is usually associated with some real or perceived traumatic event for the child. In most cases, this disorder lasts only a few weeks or months—with therapeutic intervention—although in rare cases it may persist for several years.

Many forms of therapy have been advocated, including long-term, outpatient therapy in a residential treatment center. For the family physician suspecting this condition, referral to a child psychiatrist or child psychologist is always indicated to minimize the potentially severely disabling consequences of this usually treatable disorder.

IDENTITY DISORDER

This disorder is characterized by excessive subjective distress arising from the inability of the individual to integrate and find fulfilling major aspects of his or her life, and develop an acceptable sense of self-identity. In the adolescent with identity disorder, the pathologic degree of uncertainty regarding long-term goals may be expressed as the dysfunctional inability to make a career choice or to decide the kinds of friends and the degree of intimacy to have. There may be inner conflicts over family and peer relationships, religious identification, patterns of sexual behavior, and moral issues.

Onset is most common in mid-to-late adolescence, when adolescents normally are establishing separate identities from their parents. It most frequently is first manifested by an acute or subacute onset of signs and symptoms (e.g., anxiety, moodiness, withdrawal, impulsive experimentation) that may resolve over time or may become chronic. Resolution of identity conflict is usually accomplished by the mid-twenties, with family support and counseling (psychologic, vocational, and/or religious). While occupational, academic and/or social dysfunction can be significant, it is not as severe as that seen with more severe disorders, such as Borderline Personality Disorder.

Eating Disorders

The eating disorders are a group of disorders characterized by a conspicuous disturbance in eating behavior. They are distinguished from peculiar eating behavior in patients with somatization disorders, affective disorders, and schizophrenic disorders. This is an important group of disorders with possible serious consequences, including death.

ANOREXIA NERVOSA

This disorder is seen primarily in teen-aged girls (rarely boys) with a prevalence that may be as high as 1 in 200 Caucasian girls but less frequent in other races. It is more common in middle- to upper-class families. It is characterized by an obsessive pursuit of thinness, disturbed attitude toward food and eating, disturbance of body image, strenuous physical activity until later stages, and amenorrhea in girls (Crisp, 1983; Herzog and Copeland, 1985). They often are hyperactive, awaken early with racing thoughts, have pressured speech, excel academically, and often seem euphoric to family and friends. They seemingly have a need for absolute control over their body. When the family insists on eating, they may hide the food, saying they have eaten it, or eat and then induce vomiting or use laxatives or enemas. There is a distortion of body image. Despite a frequent loss of at least 25 per cent of their body weight, they see themselves as overweight. Their preoccupation with body size leads to frequent gazing in a mirror. The weight loss is usually accomplished by reducing food intake—particularly carbohydrate and fat, strenuous exercise, use of laxatives and diuretics, and self-induced vomiting. Physical findings in anorexia nervosa are similar to those found in other starvation states. There is a decrease of both lean body mass and adipose tissue mass, dry skin, lanugo, cold intolerance, decreased skin and body core temperature, and acrocyanosis. Renal disturbances can be seen, as well as leukopenia, anemia, thrombocytopenia, and gastrointestinal malfunction, such as slow gastric emptying and duodenal-jejunal dilatation. Recently, it has been shown that patients with anorexia nervosa have hypercarotenemia, a finding that may be useful in supporting the diagnosis, since serum carotene levels tend to be decreased in other forms of malnutrition.

The course of this disorder is most commonly a single episode, with subsequent recovery, though it may be episodic or unremitting until death by starvation. The mortality has been variably reported to be between 3 and 21 per cent in different studies. The prodromal stage of anorexia nervosa is characterized by a loss of interest in peers; increasing isolation from the family; increased sensitivity to criticism, suggestion, or direction; diffuse stubbornness; and insensitivity to the consequences of eating behavior. An increased interest in physical exercise as well as amenorrhea may occur prior to actual dieting. Anxiety and depression often occur early also, mixed with signs of boredom, loneliness, and feeling of helplessness and uselessness. The actual dieting may start following an offhand remark about her weight by a family member or friend. Once started, the dieting course is usually relentless, until starvation and death, therapeutic intervention, or spontaneous reversal.

There has been recent interest in the delineation of two separate patterns seen in patients with this disorder, termed the restricting type and the bulimic type. The restricting type primarily lose weight through dietary restriction and exercise and, in general, seem to have a better prognosis. The bulimic type often overeat and then engage in vomiting and laxatives. They have frequently been obese, and approximately 50 per cent have a history of maternal obesity. They are generally more outgoing, less isolated, and more involved sexually than the restricting group. Their moods are frequently more labile, which may cause them to feel more out of control. Additionally, they may display harmful, impulsive behaviors, such as suicide attempts, self-mutilation, and stealing. They may abuse drugs and some may become alcoholic. The coincidence of such borderline personality behaviors usually complicates treatment and results in a poor long-term prognosis. These patterns should be kept in mind when counseling families with a child with disordered eating behavior. The families of such children can often be under great stress, and their defenses severely challenged. This frequently results in parental consternation and desperation, with increasing attempts to control the adolescent's behavior.

The treatment of patients with anorexia nervosa is aimed initially at restoring the nutritional state and may be lifesaving. Many treatment programs consider it unnecessary to use parenteral feeding or tube feeding, which may represent a perception of assault by the patient. Generally, treatment level and modalities are determined by severity of illness and capacity for compliance. Positive outcomes may be obtained with hospitalization using nursing care alone; or nursing care and psychotherapy; or nursing care and drug therapy, such as chlorpromazine; or behavior modification; or family therapy. Separation from the parents initially may be of benefit. Anorectic patients should be informed that they are expected to eat and that when an appropriate amount of weight is gained, discharge will occur. The patient should also be informed—firmly and without threat—that failure to eat and further weight loss will have to be treated by nasogastric tube feedings. Apart from this, the medical, nursing, and other staff should be instructed to adopt a matter-of-fact attitude toward the patient's eating behavior. Initial weight gain to more normal levels does not necessarily ensure long-term success, and relapses are fairly common. Long-term, outpatient, individual, and family therapies are usually indicated. This longer-term therapy should be directed at efforts to aid continued behavior integration, nutritional education, alleviation of associated psychosocial and medical disorders, and resumption of a viable family life.

BULIMIA NERVOSA

Patients with bulimia display an episodic pattern of planned or impulsive rapid consumption of a large amount of food (binge eating) in a discrete period of time—usually less than 2 hours. They are aware of the abnormal eating pattern and feel a loss of control over their ability to curb their binge eating. They have self-deprecation after episodes of binge eating, and repeatedly attempt to lose weight through strict dieting or fasting, vomiting, laxatives or diuretics, or vigorous exercise. However, fewer than 10 per cent of bulimic patients are overweight, and approximately 30 per cent are significantly underweight (10 to 20 per cent below normal). The termination of the binge is often accompanied by abdominal discomfort, excessive sleep, or self-induced vomiting. It was previously considered an uncommon disorder, though recent reports indicate that 4 to 4.5 per cent of university students may be bulimic.

The onset usually occurs in adolescence, predominantly in females. The course is chronic and intermittent over many years, with periods of normal eating, though in some severe cases there may be only binges and fasts with no normal eating periods. This behavior can lead to a number of medical complications, including fluid and electrolyte imbalances, gastric dilatation, and, rarely, gastric rupture that can be fatal.

Therapy of bulimia is not well established. Many claims that are positive but poorly documented are made by some inpatient eating disorder programs. There are reputable reports of successful intervention utilizing behavior therapy. There have been reports on the use of diphenhydramine (Benadryl) to control binge eating, but results are not conclusive. However, some improvement has been shown in patients whose binges are of short duration (1 hour or less). No improvement with diphenhydramine is likely in patients with an earlier history of anorexia nervosa. This condition is truly a disorder that has become more publicly prominent in the 1980's, emanating from Americans' peculiar fascination with diets and, in some instances, such underlying psychiatric conditions as major depression and borderline personality. Under any circumstances, it requires expert psychiatric intervention over time.

PICA

This is a disorder usually starting in infancy. It is characterized by the eating of such nonnutritive substances as plaster, charcoal, clay, paint, wool, ashes, and earth over a period of 1 month or more. The tasting or mouthing of objects by infants is a normal exploratory maneuver, but they usually do not eat these objects. It is between 12 and 18 months of age that some children begin to eat nonnutritious material; in some, this becomes a selective, purposeful, and habitual act. The eating of some materials, such as clay, can be associated with iron deficiency. One of the most serious and common consequences of pica is the eating of lead-based paint, which results in lead toxicity.

Pica is often associated with neglect or poor supervision, where the child may never have been taught that particular substances should not be eaten. It is associated also with family disorganization and emotional neglect. It is seen more commonly in lower socioeconomic families and may be associated with malnutrition. It is quite common in some areas of this country, affecting as many as 20 per cent of the children seen in mental health clinics in those areas.

Treatment must be directed to correction of underlying factors. In cases of neglect or retardation, training is necessary and should be constant and provided by someone able to establish warm contact with the child. Family evaluation, education, and psychotherapy, as indicated, are also required. In children with a history of pica, assessment of blood lead level is a necessary part of the evaluation.

RUMINATION DISORDER OF INFANCY (MERYCISM)

This is a rare and serious disorder in which an infant begins a pattern of chronic regurgitation after a period of normal feeding function. This behavior can lead to failure to thrive and to death in perhaps up to 25 per cent of cases. The onset usually occurs after 6 months of age but may be as early as 3 months or as late as 1 year. The infant displays chewing movements after feeding and typical arching of the back posture. Food may be brought up into the mouth without retching, though he or she may induce gagging with the tongue or fingers. The food is at least partially ejected from the mouth though some may be chewed or reswallowed. The infant seems to gain considerable satisfaction from this activity, which perhaps substitutes for lack of external stimuli.

The physician who sees an infant suspected of having this disorder must also rule out other causes of chronic regurgitation. A barium swallow and upper gastrointestinal radiographs will help rule out a hiatal hernia, esophageal stricture, chalasia, achalasia, or duodenal ulcer. The possibility of chronic renal disease must also be investigated.

Treatment of rumination disorder of infancy will almost always require the intervention of a child psychiatrist to coordinate the multiple interventions necessary in this condition. Treatment involves care of the infant by a care-taker who can provide a warm and appropriately intensive relationship. It has been noted that rumination ceases when eye and verbal contact are maintained until the stomach empties. This reduces regurgitation by the infant and allows weight gain. Therapy for the mother involves education, as well as support, in helping her overcome her feelings of inadequacy resulting from her infant's failure to thrive. If successful, she will begin to gain a sense of adequacy, establish a better maternal-infant relationship, and gradually take over care of her infant in the hospital, and eventually at home. This nurturing response usually results in a good prognosis for the infant. If the infant or mother cannot respond to intervention, placement in a foster home may be eventually required.

Other Disorders with Physical Manifestations

Many children are brought to the physician's office by parents because of social disturbances that have resulted from specific abnormalities of physical function. These common complaints center around speech difficulties, control of elimination functions, complex or simple tics, and sleep disturbances. This section will deal specifically with the more common disorders associated with these physically manifested problems, which represent a number of *DSM-III-R* categories. If these problems are left uncorrected, they can result in persistence of symptoms into adult life and possibly abnormal personality development.

STUTTERING (STAMMERING)

It is estimated that over 8 per cent of children in the United States have significant speech problems. The largest group have articulation difficulties, such as lisping, cluttering (abnormally rapid rate and erratic rhythm), and fluency disorders, mainly stuttering (5 per cent of children). The remainder have voice disorders, resonance disorders, or language comprehension disorders. Stuttering is usually considered to have a significant relationship to social difficulties and emotional disturbance.

Stuttering typically evolves between 2 to 3½ years, though ages 5 to 7 years comprise another onset period. It is characterized by blocks, repetitions, and prolongations of initial sounds and syllables. There are frequently secondary characteristics, such as grimacing and arm swinging, that accompany the stuttering. It is four times more common in boys, and, frequently, there is a familial history of stuttering. Many children may stutter for short periods of time between the ages of 2 and 4 years when their efforts at expression exceed their capacity to verbalize, but few go on to persistent stuttering. The course of this disorder may become chronic, extending throughout the individual's lifetime, but many studies show the spontaneous rate of remission without therapy to range from 50 to 80 per cent.

In those cases where stuttering persists, and particularly if the child is experiencing emotional disturbances, referral for speech therapy is indicated. It must be kept in mind that the child may also need psychotherapy to help him or her effectively deal with the anxiety, frustration, and lowered self-esteem that may result in impaired social functioning (Beitchman et al., 1986).

FUNCTIONAL ENURESIS

This very common problem is defined as the involuntary discharge of urine beyond the age when bladder control should be established. Approximately 80 per cent of children at age 2 years have ceased to wet themselves, and by age 3 years, the average child is usually able to keep his clothes and bed dry. For diagnostic purposes, involuntary wetting is classified as enuresis where the child is age 5 to 6 years and has two such episodes per month or one such episode per month after age 6. It may be nocturnal (nighttime), which is most common, diurnal (daytime), which is more common in girls, or may be both diurnal and nocturnal, which may indicate a more serious problem. Primary enuresis is diagnosed (before age 5 years) when the child has had no dry period greater than 1 year. Secondary enuresis is diagnosed (usually between ages 5 and 8) when bladder control has been achieved for a period of 1 year or more and then lost.

The diagnosis of functional enuresis is made by history, after the exclusion of an organic basis for the problem. There is a great deal of controversy in the medical literature over what constitutes an adequate and appropriate work-up to exclude an organic etiology. We believe the following approach is sensible and quite adequate (Redman and Seibert, 1979):

1. Enuretic children with symptoms of a possible urinary tract infection, such as dysuria, frequency, or urgency, should have a urinalysis and urine culture.

2. Those enuretic children with a previous history of a urinary tract infection or presently having a documented urinary tract infection should have an intravenous pyelogram and cystourethrogram.

3. Those enuretic children with symptoms of lower urinary tract obstruction, such as straining, intermittency, or small stream, should have a cystourethrogram. This implies that the physician should observe the child voiding.

4. The study of enuretic children with no associated symptoms seems unwarranted, except for a urinalysis following an overnight fast. Appropriate studies for other organic causes (e.g., diabetes, seizure disorder) should be done if symptoms or signs suggest this. The great majority of evaluated children will have functional enuresis.

There are many ways of treating the child with functional enuresis, but it seems reasonable to start with simple measures since the spontaneous cure rate approaches 15 per cent per year from age 5 to age 20 (Fournier et al., 1987). The exception to this advice is the enuretic child with a significant associated mental disorder who should have an early referral to a child psychiatrist. It is important to engage the parents to learn their perception of the problem and help them to establish an appropriate climate for the child's success in achieving bladder control. Punishment or humiliation by the parents or others should be strongly discouraged. It is important to enlist the child's cooperation and to help motivate the child to deal with the problem, such as by maintaining a daily chart, with rewards for one or two dry nights and larger rewards for greater success.

Withholding liquids after supper and having the child void at bedtime can be helpful. Repeated wakenings to void are usually not helpful and may be counterproductive. Older children should be expected to launder their own soiled bedclothes and pajamas. Undue praise for staying dry should be avoided since it may increase the child's feelings of shame and guilt. The important point is to get the parents and child working together on the problem in a matter-of-fact, nonemotional atmosphere.

The use of electric alarm pads has been popular but is usually not necessary except perhaps in refractory cases. Even then, such devices should be used only with the child's consent.

The use of tricyclic drugs, such as imipramine (Tofranil) or desipramine (Norpramin), is quite effective in helping the child have dry nights, but they do not cure the disorder. Most children relapse after cessation of therapy although delay in relapse may be seen. They should not be used in children under 6 years of age or over extended periods of time, i.e., over 8 weeks. The use of imipramine, 25 to 50 mg. at night, effectively reduces the incidence of bedwetting and may be appropriate for special nights, such as on a camping trip or staying at a friend's house. The prognosis for the child with functional enuresis is excellent for resolution, with only 1 per cent developing a chronic pattern into adult life. Thus, reassurance of the child and parents seems justified.

FUNCTIONAL ENCOPRESIS

The persistence of fecal soiling is far less common than enuresis but more disturbing to parents and those associated with the child. Functional encopresis denotes the absence of physiologic or anatomic defects as causes for the soiling. The child with functional encopresis is more likely to be emotionally disturbed than the enuretic child, and many will be found to have mental retardation or serious psychopathology. Approximately 90 per cent of children are continent of feces by age 3 years. Failure to achieve fecal continence after the age of 4 years is primary encopresis by definition and is present in approximately 1 per cent of children at age 5. Secondary encopresis usually begins between ages 4 and 8 years and is preceded by at least 1 year of fecal continence. Encopresis is further differentiated into two distinct groups, i.e., the retentive and nonretentive types. The child with retentive-type encopresis retains stool in the colon that becomes hard and impacted with continual leaking of fecal fluid around the hard stool. The child with nonretentive type encopresis passes normal, formed feces but deposits it in inappropriate places, such as in clothing or various parts of the house.

Measures similar to those used in treating enuresis may be helpful with encopretic children. It does tend to disappear with age, being very rarely seen after 16 years of age, but treatment is important as the symptom may seriously interfere with the normal socialization of the child. Early referral to a child psychiatrist is indicated, particularly in the nonretentive type of encopresis. Judicious use of laxatives or enemas may help in the retentive type, but the emotional struggle between the parents and child must be addressed with them. Behavior modification may be helpful early in the course before major parent-child conflicts are obvious.

SLEEPWALKING DISORDER (SOMNAMBULISM)

Sleepwalking is characterized by a sudden sitting up in bed that may or may not be followed by walking. Though the child's eyes are open, he does not appear to recognize people and is very hard to arouse. If the child walks, the movements appear to be purposeful in that he avoids obstacles, opens doors, but, contrary to public opinion, sleepwalkers are not careful and may be injured. Other actions may include dressing and eating. The episode may last from a few seconds to 30 minutes and usually ends with the child returning to bed or lying down elsewhere and continuing to sleep. There is usually total amnesia for the episode upon awakening, though some children may have a fragmentary recall. Sleepwalking may be associated with enuresis and sleep terror disorder, and some children talk while sleepwalking (Kales et al., 1987). It is estimated that 1 to 6 per cent of children have the disorder at some time; the incidence is higher if children with a single, isolated episode are included. The usual course results in onset between 6 and 12 years of age, with remission during adolescence. Frequency of episodes seems to have no relationship to age at which remission occurs. Recurrence during adult life may occur and results in a chronic course.

Sleepwalking appears to be a maturational defect in which action-oriented activity occurs during deep sleep, in contrast to the fantasy noted with dreaming sleep. It is unrelated to specific personality traits, may occur in children with any level of intelligence, and often occurs in children with little evidence of emotional disturbance.

There is no known treatment for sleepwalking disorder. Parents must be advised to make the environment as safe as possible to prevent serious injury during an episode. This would include sleeping on the ground floor, special bolts for doors and windows, and removal of sharp objects. If persistent into young adult life, it may preclude certain types of occupations, such as military service.

SLEEP TERROR DISORDER (NIGHT TERRORS, PAVOR NOCTURNUS)

Sleep terrors are nocturnal episodes of extreme terror and panic associated with intense motility and vocalization and high levels of autonomic discharge, lasting from 1 to several minutes. It appears to be an intense fight-flight response. The vocalization often starts with a piercing scream, and there is frequently cursing during the episode. The autonomic response results in a rapid increase in heart rate to 160 to 170 beats per minute within 15 to 30 seconds of onset of the episode, which is a greater response than with any other activity. The respiratory rate increases some, but the amplitude of respiration is markedly increased. In addition, pupil dilation, piloerection, and diaphoresis can be seen. Sleepwalking is also frequently associated. The child is confused and disoriented and has little or no recall of the episode either immediately after or the next morning.

It is important to differentiate between the relatively rare night terror and the far more common stage 2 or rapid eye movement (REM) nightmare. Table 40–2 compares these two sleep disturbances.

Management of the child with sleep terror disorder consists primarily of ensuring a safe environment as with sleepwalking because of the increased incidence of sleepwalking in children with sleep terror disorder. Benzodiazepam given at bedtime usually effectively controls night terrors. It is unclear whether the mechanism of action is through suppression of stage 4 sleep or by some more comprehensive biologic action. Suppression of stage 4 sleep for long periods of time in adults seems to cause no harmful effects, but the long-term effects in children are unknown. Thus, treatment of children with benzodiazepam is *not* recommended.

TIC DISORDERS

A tic is an "involuntary, sudden, rapid, recurrent, non-rhythmic, stereotyped motor movement or vocalization" (American Psychiatric Association, 1987). Tics may be expressed as:

Table 40–2. COMPARISONS OF SLEEP TERROR DISORDER WITH NIGHTMARE

Sleep Terror Disorder	Nightmare
1. Uncommon	1. Common
2. Occurs during arousal from stage 4 sleep	2. Occurs during stage 2 (REM) sleep
3. Occurs early in the night (within 15 minutes to 2 hours)	3. Occurs later in the night (after several hours)
4. Amnesic for the episode	4. Usually can recall some or all of dream
5. Intense autonomic discharge	5. Muted autonomic response
6. Severe anxiety	6. Mild anxiety
7. Intense vocalization with piercing scream	7. Absence of panicky scream
8. Sudden response to frightening terror	8. Gradual build-up of frightening content
9. High incidence of associated psychopathology (in adults)	9. Normal incidence of associated psychopathology
10. Very difficult to arouse during episode	10. Easily arousable

- Simple motor (e.g., eye blinking, neck jerking, shoulder shrugging, facial grimacing)
- Simple vocal (e.g., coughing, throat clearing, grunting, sniffing)
- Complex motor (e.g., facial gestures, hitting or biting self, jumping, touching)
- Complex vocal (e.g., repeating words or phrases out of context, using socially unacceptable words [coprolalia], repeating last-heard vocalizations of others [echolalia])

The tics generally are first manifested between 2 to 12 years of age, may be experienced as an irresistible but suppressible urge, are usually exacerbated by stress, and may be diminished during sleep and absorbing activities (e.g., reading, singing). They are characteristically differentiated from other movement disorders (e.g., choreiform, dystonic, atheoid, myoclonic, hemiballismic, dyskinetic, synkinetic, stereotyped, compulsive) and commonly associated with self-consciousness, depressed mood, social withdrawal, and related social, academic, and occupational dysfunctions. Categories include:

- Transient tic disorder: single or multiple motor and/or vocal, occurring several times daily for at least 2 weeks but not longer than 12 consecutive months, tending to disappear permanently or recur
- Chronic motor or vocal tic disorder: similar to Tourette's disorder except functionally less severe and characterized by motor or vocal expressions, but not both
- Tourette's disorder: Multiple motor and one or more vocal tics, usually several times daily, lifetime in duration, changing patterns (anatomic location, complexity, frequency, number), frequently associated with attention deficit hyperactivity disorder and obsessive-compulsive disorder

Evaluation of each disorder always requires a careful history and physical examination, especially a detailed neurologic evaluation. The common correlation of attentional, oppositional, and impulse control problems requires the family physician to be sensitive to both the presence of tics in children presenting with attentional and behavioral problems and the presence of such problems in children evaluated for tics (Sverd et al., 1988). Treatment is multifaceted, including behavioral modification, family supportive counseling, school consultation, and, for Tourette's disorder, pharmacologic treatment and family referral to a local Tourette Syndrome Association group or national office. Haloperidol (Haldol) (2 to 3 mg. per day) will be variably effective in reducing Tourette symptomatology. A cautious trial of stimulant medication can be utilized in children with Tourette's disorder and disruptive behavioral symptoms of inattentiveness, hyperactivity, and impulsivity. The family physician should be cognizant of the potential of stimulants to exacerbate tics in some children and of the potential for tardive dyskinesia with long-term use of haloperidol.

Pervasive Developmental Disorders

This is a group of disorders that are characterized by a distortion of development rather than a delay and by involvement of multiple functions rather than a specific function, thus differing from the specific developmental disorders. There are distortions in the development of the basic psychologic functions that are involved in the acquisition of social skills and language, such as attention, perception, reality testing, and motor movement. As such, these disorders represent a group of syndromes that are probably multivariate in etiology and are a source of considerable research and professional discussion, relative to nosology (Dahl et al., 1986) and relationship to such disorders as schizophrenia (Tanguay and Cantor, 1986).

AUTISTIC DISORDER

This severe and fortunately uncommon disorder of early development is characterized by: (1) onset before 30 months of age, (2) impaired interpersonal development seen as a failure to form normal social interactions, (3) impairment in verbal and nonverbal communication, (4) absence of imaginative activity, and (5) markedly restricted repertoire of activities and interests, such as stereotyped or repetitive behavior ranging from rocking and flicking to ritualistic play. Though many autistic children have mental retardation, some have average or above average intelligence, and some aspects of their psychologic development appear normal.

From their first weeks of life, autistic children may be noted by their parents to be inattentive to people and fixated on simple objects in their environment. By 7 or 8 months of age, disturbances are almost always apparent. The child seems inconsolable or unusually placid, inattentive, and socially distant. By the age of 1 year, the autistic child often becomes preoccupied with one object or toy and may spend hours looking at his fingers or banging his head against the crib. As he grows older, his failure to socially babble or use or be interested in speech may lead the family to suspect he is deaf. During the toddler years, increasing hyperactivity, aloofness, language difficulties, and odd mannerisms mark the child as distinctly abnormal. The preschool autistic child is unable to play imaginatively or share with others. The most devastating symptom is the child's inability to relate to other human beings in a normal, affectionate way. For the parents, the most painful aspect is the child's lack of concern for them or appreciation of their care-giving.

The family physician plays an important role in the early identification of this disorder and in helping to prevent the build-up of family stress. Early diagnosis can prevent false reassurances, keep parental guilt minimized, and help in early formulation of a therapeutic plan. Diagnosis is a two-step process with definitive diagnosis of autistic disorder as the first step. The second step is to evaluate the child's unique symptomatic characteristics and behaviors in order to plan individualized treatment. Referral to a child psychiatrist for this second step and definitive therapy or subsequent referral for specialized placement is always indicated (Wing, 1981).

The major roles of the family physician in the management of the autistic child and his family are to: (1) be an advocate for the family and assure that routine medical needs are met, (2) help monitor the use of psychopharmacologic agents, and (3) provide the family with some perspective regarding various controversial treatments of autism. This very serious condition requires significant family resources in time, emotions, and money. It is easy to refer the child to a psychiatric center, but the family needs the continuous and comprehensive care and support the family physician can often best provide. For physicians seeing this problem infrequently or for the first time, much information, such as appropriate services in his or her region, can be obtained from The National Society for Children and Adults with Autism (1234 Massachusetts Avenue, Washington, D.C., 20036).

The prognosis in autistic disorder is disheartening. About 15 per cent will be able to make an adequate social adjustment and be independent, another 15 per cent will make a fair adjustment, and the remainder continue to be severely handicapped and unable to lead an independent life (Cohen and Donnellan, 1986). The best predictors of outcome are the IQ score, language development, and the capacity for symbolic play. Short-term outcome is frequently much more favorable for, with appropriate management, most are able to show some improvement in adaptation, which can be very rewarding for the children and their families.

Specific Developmental Disorders

These are a group of disorders characterized by a delay in development of one area of function, such as language development or reading skills or math skills, but with normal function in other areas. These disorders are not recognized until the child reaches the age when the specific learning is expected to develop, such as language about age 3 years or reading at age 6 to 7 years. There is controversy over what degree of impaired development constitutes a learning disability and whether these dysfunctions constitute mental disorders as such. Children develop skills at different rates depending on genetic, biologic, psychologic, social, and environmental factors. Thus, at any one point in time it is difficult to judge if a child has a specific developmental disability or a delay in development. With the passage of Public Law 94-142, The Handicapped Children's Act of 1975, a much greater interest in learning disabilities was generated. Parallel to this legislation, changing criteria for inclusion in the group of individuals considered learning disabled resulted in larger numbers of children being so labeled. For many biologic and psychiatric parameters such as IQ, blood sugar, height, and weight, normal is usually defined as plus or minus two standard deviations from the mean. If this statistical approach was applied to parameters of learning, about 2 per cent of children would be included in the low standard deviation group, resulting in a large decrease in the number of children now labeled as learning disabled. This observation is made not to refute the validity of this group of disorders but, rather, to point out that there is a wide variation in the rates of development among children that may cause many more children than could be statistically identified in the general population to be considered developmentally delayed and requiring interventions. Thus, until specific etiologic factors for these disorders are identified that will allow further refinement of the diagnostic criteria, one should be careful in assigning the label of learning disabled to a child. The labeling of a child as anything but normal can result in his or her being treated as, and feeling like, a nonlearner. In time, this can become a self-fulfilling prophecy for the child. In a short space of time, even a few weeks, the child's life may be markedly changed from one of a satisfying existence to one of coerced involvement to perform in ways he or she finds difficult to do. Through some mechanism not fully appreciated by the child, he or she has become handicapped and disabled—in the eyes of others, in his or her own self-view, and finally in function. To the credit of many educators, special programs for children with specific developmental disorders are generally sensitive to this issue. The family physician can play a critical role in setting the tone of normal delay for the child, parents, and school in providing objective reassurances about placement and maturation of the child in such programs.

The three major areas of dysfunction subsumed under this broad category are disorders of academic skills, language and speech, and motor skills.

ACADEMIC SKILLS DISORDERS

Academic skills disorders include those associated with problems in reading, arithmetic skills and expressive writing. The condition of greatest relevance to a family physician is developmental reading disorder (Snyder, 1981).

This disorder has frequently been referred to as *dyslexia* and is characterized by significant impairment in the development of reading skills without concomitant impairment in other areas of function. Some children learn to read very early with little instruction while others do not develop these skills until they are nearly teenagers, even though they are expected to have this ability at age 7 or, regrettably, by some, as early as 5 years. In those children that have significant impairment (and not simply a delay) in the ability to develop reading skills, there is a tendency to show little improvement even into adulthood.

The physician has a role in the evaluation and management of children with this disorder. Treatable causes must be ascertained, such as hearing impairment or correctable visual defects. Counseling with the child and the family is essential to help place the problem in perspective. Close communication with the school is important to assure that appropriate help is being given. This would include encouraging educators to use audiovisual techniques and oral exams in school to help compensate for the effect of the reading disability and allow progress in other areas of the child's education. Psychologic evaluation and counseling should be considered if the child develops notable symptoms of an emotional disorder—not uncommon for learning disabled children.

LANGUAGE AND SPEECH DISORDERS

This group of disorders is characterized by a delay in language development in distinction to acquired language disorders, which are usually the result of trauma or neurologic disorders or of failure to acquire language, which is rare and usually associated with profound mental retardation. Language and speech disorders are relatively common disorders and involve dysfunctions in articulation (10 per cent of children below age 5), comprehension of language (receptive—3 to 10 per cent of school-aged children), or expressing language (expressive—3 to 10 per cent of school-aged children).

In the developmental receptive language disorder, there is a deficit in auditory or visual sensory perception, a deficit in integration of auditory and visual symbols and stored language recall. In developmental expressive language disorder, children can understand language seemingly but have difficulty finding words to express themselves. Commonly, articulation may be immature. These two types of language disorders must be differentiated from developmental articulation disorder, which is characterized by consistent failure to use developmentally expected speech sounds (e.g., p, b, and t in a 3-year old, and r, sh, th, f, z, and l in a 6-year old).

The language and speech disorders represent complex problems and need a multidisciplinary approach to management. There is a higher than normal prevalence of other mental disorders in children with these disorders. One study found 53 per cent of these children fit in another DSM-III diagnostic category, such as attention deficit disorder, oppositional disorder, conduct disorder, and various anxiety disorders (Beitchman et al., 1986). The family physician must stay involved with these children and families, as well as other treating specialist, to provide needed medical care and the continuing support of the child and his or her family.

MOTOR SKILLS DISORDER

The only disorder currently recognized in this category is developmental coordination disorder. This disorder is characterized by a pronounced impairment in motor coordination that interferes with activities of daily living or academic achievement. This diagnosis is only made after the family physician has ruled out mental retardation, attention deficit hyperactivity disorder, pervasive developmental disorder, and specific neurologic disorders (e.g., cerebral palsy, progressive cerebellar lesions). Prevalence is high (6 per cent of children between the ages of 5 and 11) and manifested by difficulties in fine motor and gross motor skills (e.g., buttoning, tying shoelaces, pivoting, writing-coloring). Early manifestations may be seen in delayed motor milestones (e.g., sitting, crawling, walking); awkwardness and clumsiness may persist into adolescence and adulthood in some instances. Treatment consists of practicing various fine or gross motor activities over time that will foster skills. The family physician's main contributions include reassuring the child and parents, cautioning the parents to not be negative or pressing in trying to force coordination, and providing assurance that appropriate special educational, recreational, and occupational therapies are provided to focus and support the child in skills development. It should be reassuring that many distinguished athletes, scholars, and family physicians had this condition as a child.

References

Adams, P. L.: Primer of Child Psychotherapy. 2nd ed. Boston, Little, Brown, 1982.

Adams, P. L., and Fras, I.: Beginning Child Psychiatry. New York, Brunner-Mazel, 1988.

American Psychiatric Association: Diagnostic and Statistical Manual of Mental Disorders. 3rd ed. revised. Washington, D.C., American Psychiatric Press, 1987. *An essential reference for all family physicians, this research diagnostic text is the standard nosology for psychiatric disorders. Family physicians should be thoroughly familiar with the contents.*

Apter, A., Bleich, A., Plutchik, R., et al.: Suicidal behavior, depression and conduct disorder in hospitalized adolescents. J. Am. Acad. Child Adolesc. Psychiatry, *27*(6):696–699, 1987.

Barkley, R. A.: Hyperactive Children: A Handbook for Diagnosis and Treatment. New York, Guilford Press, 1981.

Beitchman, J. H., Nair, R., Clegg, M., et al.: Prevalence of psychiatric disorders in children with speech and language disorders. J. Am. Acad. of Child Psychiatry, *25*(4):528–535, 1986.

Beitchman, J. H., Kruidenier, B., and Clegg, M.: The children's self-report rating scale: screening accuracy and predictive power reconsidered. J. Am. Acad. Child Adolesc. Psychiatry, *26*(1):49–52, 1987.

Bernstein, G. A., and Garfinkel, B. D.: School phobia: the overlap of affective and anxiety disorders. J. Am. Acad. of Child Psychiatry, *25*(2):235–241, 1986.

Bloomindale, L. M. (Ed.): Attention Deficit Disorder: Identification, Course and Rationale. New York, Spectrum, 1985.

Brown, R. T., Borden, K. A., Wynne, M. A., et al.: Compliance with pharmacological and cognitive treatments for attention deficit disorder. J. Am. Acad. Child Adolesc. Psychiatry, *26*(4):521–526, 1987.

Bumpass, E. R., Fagelman, F. D., and Brix, R. J.: Intervention with children who set fires. Am. J. Psychother., *37*:328–345, 1983.

Campbell, M., and Spencer, E. K.: Psychopharmacology in child and adolescent psychiatry: a review of the past five years. J. Am. Acad. Child Adolesc. Psychiatry, *27*(3):269–279, 1988. *An outstanding update of recent advances in and standard approaches to pharmacotherapy of child psychiatric disorders.*

Cantwell, D. P.: The attention deficit disorder syndrome: current knowledge, future needs. J. Am. Acad. Child Psychiatry, *23*:315–318, 1984.

Cohen, D. J., and Donnellan, A. (Eds.): Handbook of Autism. New York, John Wiley and Sons, 1986.

Costello, A. J.: Assessment and diagnosis of affective disorders in children. J. Child Psychol. Psychiatry, *27*:565–573, 1986.

Council on Scientific Affairs (American Medical Association): AMA diagnostic and treatment guidelines concerning child abuse and neglect. J.A.M.A., *254*:796–800, 1985.

Crisp, A. H.: Anorexia nervosa. Br. Med. J., *287*:855–858, 1983.

Dahl, E. K., Cohen, D. J., and Provence, S.: Clinical and multivariate approaches to nosology of pervasive developmental disorders. J. Am. Acad. Child Psychiatry, *25*:170–180, 1986.

Evans, S. L., Reinhart, J. B., and Succom, R. A.: Failure to thrive—a study of 45 children and their families. J. Am. Acad. Child Psychiatry, *11*:440, 1972. *Provides an excellent perspective of the family environment associated with this condition.*

Fournier, J. P., Garfinkel, B. D., Bond, A., et al.: Pharmacologic and behavioral management of enuresis. J. Am. Acad. Child Adolesc. Psychiatry, *26*(3):849–853, 1987.

Goodman, J. D., and Sours, J. A.: The Child Mental Status Examination. New York, Basic Books, 1967. *A basic reference for the physician examining the child's psychologic and cognitive functioning.*

Gross, M. D., Tofanelli, R. A., Butzirus, S. M., and Snodgrass, E. W.: The effects of diets rich in and free from additives on the behavior of children with hyperkinetic and learning disorders. J. Am. Acad. Child Adolesc. Psychiatry, *26*(1):53–55, 1987.

Gutterman, E. M., O'Brien, J. D., and Young, J. G.: Structured diagnostic interviews for children and adolescents: current status and future directions. J. Am. Acad. Child Adolesc. Psychiatry, *26*(5):621–630, 1987.

Herzog, D. B., and Copeland, P. M.: Eating disorders. N. Engl. J. Med., *313*:295–303, 1985. *An excellent overview of anorexia nervosa and bulimia.*

Jensen, J. B., Burke, N., and Garfinkel, B. D.: Depression and symptoms of attention deficit disorder with hyperactivity. J. Am. Acad. Child Adolesc. Psychiatry, *27*(6):742–747, 1988.

Kales, A., Soldatos, C. R., and Kales, J. D.: Sleep disorders: insomnia, sleepwalking, night terrors, nightmares and enuresis. Ann. Intern. Med., *106*:582–592, 1987.

Klorman, R., Coons, H. W. and Borgstedt, A. D.: Effects of methylphenidate on adolescents with a childhood history of attention deficit disorder. I. Clinical findings. J. Am. Acad. Child Adolesc. Psychiatry, *26*(3):363–367, 1987.

Lahey, B. B., Piacentini, J. C., McBurnett, K., et al.: Psychopathology in the parents of children with conduct disorder and hyperactivity. J. Am. Acad. Child Adolesc. Psychiatry, *27*(2):163–170, 1988.

Liebowitz, J. H., Rembar, J. C., Kernberg, P. F., et al.: Judging mental health sickness in children: development of a rating scale. J. Am. Acad. Child Adolesc. Psychiatry, *27*(2):193–199, 1988.

Lustick, M. J.: Bulimia in adolescents: a review. Pediatrics, *76*(suppl):685–690, 1985.

Morrison, G. D. (Ed.): Emergencies in Child Psychiatry. Springfield, IL, Charles C Thomas, 1975.

Nelson, W. M., Politano, P. M., Finch, A. J., et al.: Children's depression inventory: normative data and utility with emotionally disturbed children. J. Am. Acad. Child Adolesc. Psychiatry, *26*(1):43–48, 1987.

Noshpitz, J. D. (Ed.): Basic Handbook of Child Psychiatry, Vol. I and III. New York, Basic Books, 1979. *This book remains one of the major standard texts in child and adolescent psychiatry. It would serve as a comprehensive reference for most topics in the field except those related to more recent neurobiologic research and psychopharmacologic developments.*

Pliszka, S. R.: Tricyclic antidepressants in the treatment of children with attention deficit disorder. J. Am. Acad. Child Adolesc. Psychiatry, *26*(2):127–132, 1987.

Redman, J. F., and Seibert, J. J.: Uroradiographic evaluation of the enuretic child. J. Urol., *122*:799, 1979.

Rescorla, L. A.: Preschool psychiatric disorders: diagnostic classification and symptom patterns. J. Am. Acad. Child Psychiatry, *25*:162–169, 1985.

Rifkin, A., Wortman, R., Reardon, G., and Siris, S. G.: Psychotropic medication in adolescents: a review. J. Clin. Psychiatry, *47*:400–408, 1986. *An insightful and concise summary of clinical considerations in the use of medications for adolescent psychologic problems.*

Robson, K. S. (Ed.): Manual of Clinical Child Psychiatry. Washington, D.C., American Psychiatric Press, 1986.

Snyder, R. D.: A perspective on learning disabilities: the inefficient reader. J. Dev. Behav. Pediatr., *2*:49, 1981. *A very good review of learning disabilities.*

Stark, T., and Blum, R.: Psychosomatic illness in childhood and adolescence: clinical considerations. Clin. Pediatr. (Phila.), *25*:549–554, 1986. *This reference reports on a number of conditions (conversion, somatization, and factitious disorders, hypochondriasis, malingering) that represent 10 per cent of an outpatient pediatric population. Practical suggestions for management utilizing a number of interventions are discussed.*

Sverd, J., Curley, A. D., Jandorf, L., and Volkersz, L.: Behavior disorder and attention deficits in boys with Tourette Syndrome. J. Am. Acad. Child Adolesc. Psychiatry, *4*:413–417, 1988.

Tanguay, P. E., and Cantor, S. L.: Schizophrenia in children. J. Am. Acad. Child Psychiatry, *25*:591–594, 1986.

Van Winter, J. T., and Strickler, G. B.: Panic attack syndrome. J. Pediatr., *105*:661–665, 1984.

Werry, J. S., Reeves, J. C., and Elkind, G. S.: Attention deficit, conduct, oppositional and anxiety disorders in children. I. A review of research on differentiating characteristics. J. Am. Acad. Child Adolesc. Psychiatry, *26*(2):133–143, 1987.

Wing, L.: Management of early childhood autism. Br. J. Hosp. Med., *25*:353, 1981. *This reference contains practical information for the effective clinical management of the family with an autistic child.*

41

General Surgery

Christine C. Matson
Jon M. Burch
David V. Feliciano

The Family Physician as Diagnostician

Patients with surgical illnesses are a minority in a family physician's practice. On the other hand, the family physician is frequently the first to recognize a surgically correctable problem for which intervention can prevent catastrophic results. His knowledge of the family's threshold for sending a member to the doctor, stressful events or loss of supports that might alter this threshold, and the individual's relative stoicism are all helpful clues that aid in the assessment of the severity of pain or illness.

A request for surgical consultation may be warranted even when a surgically correctable condition is unlikely. The timing of a consultation request depends upon the potential for a life-threatening development, customary practice in the locality, and the family physician's relationship with the surgical consultant. The family physician may choose a consultant who takes a conservative approach to the management of fibrocystic disease of the breast when the goal is to reassure the patient with a second opinion.

Preoperative Assessment and Preparation

CLASSIFICATION OF RISK STATUS

Comprehensive preoperative evaluation of patients includes the following: (1) assessment of the patient's physical and emotional status, (2) identification of illness or other risk factors that would increase the risk of surgery for the patient, and (3) institution of prophylactic measures to decrease the risk of complications of surgery.

A thorough history and physical examination should enable the physician to distinguish between the healthy, low-risk patient and one at high risk because of health factors related or unrelated to the indication for surgery. An associated systemic disease significantly increases the patient's risk, especially if it is in the pulmonary, cardiac, renal, endocrine, or metabolic systems. The Physical Status Scale developed by the American Society of Anesthesiologists (ASA) is the most frequently utilized overall predictor of risk of surgery (Table 41–1) (Dripps et al., 1982; Feigal and Blaisdell, 1979).

Other factors increase surgical risk. Emergency surgery doubles the overall risk and increases the risk of myocardial infarction or cardiac death fourfold. If the operative site includes the thorax or upper abdomen, pulmonary complications are more likely. A poor preoperative psychologic adjustment, including marked depression, anxiety, or massive denial correlates with a poor outcome. The experience of the surgical team, quality of nursing care, and other hospital resources are also associated with outcome, whereas the type, route, and duration of anesthesia is inconsistently related to risk (Feigal et al., 1979; Cohen et al., 1988).

RISK FACTORS

Age

In general, surgical outcome relates more to the patient's ASA classification than to age, but age may

Table 41–1. CLASSIFICATION OF PREOPERATIVE PHYSICAL STATUS

I. **Good Risk:**
Surgical disorder without systemic effects (e.g., early acute appendicitis, hernia, or gallstones in otherwise healthy persons)

II. **Fair Risk:**
Surgical disorder with mild to moderate systemic disturbance or with a significant associated disease (e.g., simple small bowel obstruction, duodenal ulcer with hypertension or mild diabetes)

III. **Poor Risk:**
Severe systemic disturbance or disease with a related surgical disorder (e.g., perforated sigmoid diverticulitis with generalized peritonitis, groin hernia with severe chronic obstructive pulmonary disease

IV. **Extreme Risk:**
Life-threatening disturbance with a surgical disorder, the former not always being correctable by surgery (e.g., organic heart disease with intractable myocardial failure or angina, together with surgical disorder)

V. **Moribund Patient:**
(e.g., rupture of abdominal aortic aneurysm with profound shock.)

"E" is added to classification when the case is done as an emergency.

increase the dangers of other risk factors. Age greater than 75 years itself places the patient in class 2 of the ASA scale.

Physiologic assessment is especially important in the elderly, as decreases in functional reserve in several organ systems will increase susceptibility to the stress of surgery and surgical illness (Galazka, 1988). Age-related changes in the heart include a decreased cardiac output, a decreased response to sympathetic stimuli, and a greater incidence of ventricular hypertrophy and calcifications in the aortic and mitral valves. Decreased peripheral vascular resiliency increases susceptibility to fluid overload, along with decreased renal concentrating ability and tubular maximum for excretion. The decreased renal function resulting from age-related diminution in numbers of nephrons, renal blood flow, and glomerular filtration rate may not be reflected in serum creatinine levels, since muscle mass is also decreased in this population. Changes in the pulmonary system include a decrease in compliance of the lung parenchyma and thoracic cage. Functional residual capacity, residual volume, and dead space increase, while expiratory volume, peak expiratory flow rate, and arterial oxygen tension decrease. In the nervous system, decreased cerebral blood flow, decreased nerve conduction, and visual and hearing deficits increase the likelihood of difficulty in understanding and cooperating with instructions and treatments. Acute mental status changes frequently occur in the perioperative period, and pre-existing dementia is an independent risk factor for surgical complications.

Drug absorption may be either increased (cimetidine and propranolol) or decreased (quinidine) with age. Decreased total body water and lean body mass and a relative increase in body fat affect the volume of distribution and the half-life for both hydrophilic and lipophilic drugs. Decreased hepatic blood flow and metabolism may prolong the half-life of medications, while the decreased glomerular filtration rate slows excretion of drugs by the kidneys. Lastly, the decrease in plasma-binding proteins with age may result in an increase in the free fraction of highly bound drugs such as warfarin.

Careful preoperative assessment of the patient's functional and cognitive status includes recording the baseline ability to perform activities of daily living, both inside and outside the home, and quantification of cognitive function using a standardized instrument (Folstein et al., 1975; Pfeiffer, 1975). Assessment of the patient's emotional status, including expectations of the postoperative course and presence of personal and family support, is essential for planning postoperative rehabilitation.

Obesity

Because of the prevalence of obesity in the United States, surgical illness in an obese patient is a common occurrence. The most accurate determination of mild to moderate obesity is by measurement of triceps' skinfold thickness, since this method is less sensitive to increased muscle mass or edema. Morbid obesity is a condition defined by Krall (1983) as either 45 kg. (100 lb.) or 100 per cent above desirable weight, which increases perioperative risk of morbidity and mortality.

The prevalence of obesity varies by age group, ethnic origin, and geographic area, with estimates ranging from 10 to 50 per cent in some populations (DHEW Pub. No. HSM 72–8131, 1972; Holm et al., 1977). Moderate to severe obesity is associated with an increased risk of certain types of surgical disease, notably cholelithiasis and surgical intervention in obstetrics. Obese patients are more likely to have operative problems with the airway, ventilation, monitoring, and anesthetic requirement. Postoperative complications, such as hypoventilation, atelectasis, hypoxia, infections, and thromboembolic phenomena are also common. Because of the risks, careful consideration of the anticipated benefits of elective surgery versus the risks involved is mandatory.

If a morbidly obese patient requires an elective operation, weight loss prior to the procedure should be emphasized. When surgery is required and weight loss is unlikely, a thorough preoperative evaluation is required. The history should address risk factors and symptoms that might suggest the presence of pulmonary disease, sleep apnea syndromes, heart disease, hypertension, thromboembolic disease, and diabetes mellitus. The physical examination should focus particularly on the cardiovascular and pulmonary systems, as well as screening for any coexistent illness. Evaluation should include routine pulmonary function tests, an electrocardiogram, and a chest x-ray. Preoperative education in deep-breathing exercises and assisted coughing as well as a mandatory period without cigarettes can decrease the incidence of postoperative pulmonary complications. Unless contraindicated (e.g., ophthalmic or neurosurgical procedures), mini-dose heparin and early mobilization are recommended for prevention of thromboembolic complications. Heparin (5000 units) is begun subcutaneously 30 minutes before surgery and continued every 12 hours for 7 days. This regimen has been shown to decrease the incidence of deep venous thrombosis and pulmonary embolism in patients undergoing general thoracoabdominal surgery (Kakkar et al., 1975).

Nutritional Status

Surveys have shown that up to 50 per cent of patients presenting with a surgical illness may have one or more indicators of protein-calorie or vitamin malnutrition on admission, depending on the duration of symptoms, the concomitant illness, and the population studied. Those who present with malnutrition are more likely to have prolonged hospital stays and increased morbidity and mortality when compared with those without nutritional deficits.

Hospital stays may lead to or exacerbate malnutrition. The disease process itself may prevent oral nutrition or meals may be withheld for diagnostic testing. Nutritional support by other routes may be delayed or not considered. Acutely ill patients, especially those with burns, infection, or fever or those who undergo a major surgical procedure have greatly increased metabolic demands and, thus, may become rapidly depleted when nutrition is inadequate. This leads to more surgical infections, delayed wound healing, and prolonged convalescence (Cuthbertson, 1979).

Assessment of the patient's nutritional state on admission is critical in judging whether time should be allotted for correcting nutritional deficits prior to surgery, when possible, and allows for subsequent comparisons of the patient's status while in the hospital. A basic assessment consists of a dietary and weight history and measurement of height and weight, triceps' skinfold thickness, and midarm circumference. Additional tests, such as a 24-hour urine creatinine excretion, serum albumin level, and serum transferrin level, can provide more specific information. Serum albumin is affected by hepatic parenchymal dysfunction, transferrin by bone marrow iron stores, and both are affected by hemodilution. Cell-mediated immunity correlates with nutritional status and can be tested using common recall antigens, such as *Candida*, mumps, and tetanus. Total lymphocyte counts may also be helpful. Deficiencies of trace minerals or specific vitamins can be identified by determination of their blood or urine levels. If a vitamin deficiency is present, a multivitamin preparation, including vitamin C (which is required for wound healing), is given.

Vigilance regarding the patient's nutritional status includes daily charting of nutritional intake and weight, as well as recording anthropomorphic measurements and the aforementioned laboratory values at regular intervals. When malnutrition is identified, the cause should be sought and remedied when possible. Potential causes include the following: diminished intake (anorexia, mechanical difficulties in ingestion, or inadequacy of prescribed diet relative to requirements); increased losses (renal failure, diabetes, certain medications, gastrointestinal losses, or fluid loss through extensive burn); hypermetabolism; drug nutrient interactions (steroids, sedatives, antibiotics, anticonvulsants); and coexisting illnesses (Bolt, 1987).

When the need for perioperative nutritional support is identified, a variety of enteral and parenteral preparations are available. In the patient who is unable to ingest sufficient nutrients by mouth, liquid enteral mixtures delivered through narrow lumen nasoenteral tubes can help to restore positive nitrogen balance (Bolt, 1987). Use of the longer, weighted nasoenteral tubes helps to prevent aspiration of gastric contents. The position of the tube should always be confirmed by an abdominal x-ray prior to its use. Continuous delivery of the mixture with an infusion pump decreases abdominal cramping and occlusion of the tubing. Infusions of the enteral diet should begin at a low flow rate, and at one fourth to one half strength. Both flow rate and strength are increased to the desired levels over 3 to 4 days. Elevation of the head of the bed also decreases aspiration risk.

Three types of enteral mixtures are available.

1. Polymeric: low in osmolality, relatively inexpensive, and require normal proteolytic and lipolytic function
2. Monomeric (elemental): hypermolar, moderately expensive, do not require proteolytic or lipolytic function, and are useful in inflammatory bowel disease and enterocutaneous fistulas because of low residue
3. Modular: small volume, high caloric source

Diabetes

The preoperative preparation of the diabetic patient should focus on achieving stable control of serum glucose and optimal acid/base and electrolyte status. The patient's cardiovascular status and renal function should receive special attention including evaluation of the electrocardiogram for indicators of a recent silent myocardial infarction and precautions to avoid dye-induced nephropathy from diagnostic studies.

Maintaining adequate hydration is especially important in several groups:

1. Those with diabetic renovascular disease who are more susceptible to tubular necrosis
2. Those with low-renin hypoaldosteronism who may develop hyperkalemia when volume depleted
3. Those with autonomic neuropathy who may have abnormal vascular responses perioperatively

Postoperative management focuses on maintaining control in these areas as well as preventing infections or other complications that occur with a greater frequency in diabetic patients. Those with a history of stress-induced glucose intolerance, such as gestational diabetes, should be closely monitored for hyperglycemia. When an elective procedure is planned, a fasting blood sugar less than 250 mg. per dl. in the preoperative period is mandatory. Additional insulin may be required just because of the stress of the preoperative preparation and the patient's anxiety, resulting in the release of stress hormones with their anti-insulin effect. An anxiolytic agent as part of the preoperative medication decreases this effect. One other problem is that some anesthetic agents may increase glycogenolyis, inhibit glucose transport, and decrease insulin release.

When surgery is urgent or emergent because of the severity of the surgical illness, the risk of acid/base and electrolyte abnormalities is increased. Release of stress hormones, including catecholamines, adrenocorticotropic hormone, cortisol, glucagon, and growth hormone leads to inhibition of insulin release, increased insulin resistance, and increased gluconeogenesis and glycogenolysis. Should ketoacidosis result, an aggressive approach, including infusion of intravenous fluids and insulin with close monitoring and replacement of electrolytes (especially potassium), is required. Whenever possible, the patient's pH should be higher than 7.3 and bicarbonate higher than 20 mEq. per ml. before surgery is attempted. The possibility that ketoacidosis itself can mimic a surgical abdomen should be kept in mind. Hyperosmolar nonketotic states are more common in the diabetic patient and can be treated with fluids and smaller amounts of insulin.

The goal in the perioperative period is to maintain the blood glucose in the 150 to 250 mg. per dl. range to avoid the metabolic stresses of sustained hypo- or hyperglycemia. Diabetic patients should have their operations scheduled early in the day to prevent disruption of glucose control. For those with a fasting blood glucose less than 175 mg. per dl. who are undergoing minor procedures, monitoring the blood sugar before and after the procedure will suffice. Subcutaneous regular insulin (5 to 10 U.) can be used for glucose levels exceeding 250 mg. per dl.

For patients maintained on oral agents, the hypoglycemic agent can be held until after the procedure has been completed. Also, chlorpropamide should be discontinued 1 to 2 days prior to surgery because of its long half-life. Regular insulin should be substituted if major surgery is planned. An infusion of 5 per cent dextrose containing 10 U. regular insulin per liter at a rate of about 125 cc. per hour is begun the morning of surgery. The initial 50 cc. should be run through the tubing and discarded to minimize the effect of insulin binding to the plastic. This solution can be discontinued and the oral agent administered if the patient is able to eat following the procedure.

For patients previously maintained on insulin or for those undergoing major surgical procedures that preclude the early resumption of oral nutrition, several different approaches are available to deliver the insulin and provide the necessary calories for basic metabolic needs. Usually, one half of the regular dose of insulin is given subcutaneously as long-acting insulin on the morning of surgery. An infusion of 5 per cent dextrose containing 10 to 20 U. per L. of regular insulin, is begun as described above, depending on the patient's usual requirements. Serum glucose determinations are obtained at regular (2 to 6 hour) intervals, with insulin adjustments made either by subcutaneous administration or by altering the rate of the infusion. The accuracy of blood glucose levels, either by fingerstick or venipuncture, is far superior to urine determinations and should be exclusively used in this setting. The morning dose of long-acting insulin, along with the constant infusion of regular insulin, provides for the two thirds to three fourths of insulin needs that are basal and not related to meals.

Adequate carbohydrate must also be provided to give approximately 50 grams over 6 hours for each missed meal or 200 grams per day in the average sized adult. This can be given as 4 liters of D_5W, 2 liters of $D_{10}W$ or 400 cc. of $D_{50}W$. If the volume of D_5W required would be excessive, $D_{10}W$ can be substituted, or $D_{50}W$ piggybacked to provide adequate calories.

During the immediate postoperative course, the resolution of diabetogenic effects of anesthesia and the surgical illness, the decreased effect of anti-insulin hormones, and the patient's increasing activity usually decrease insulin demands. Premature discontinuation of intravenous calories prior to achieving adequate oral intake, however, can precipitate hypoglycemia. In contrast, cessation of intravenous insulin before subcutaneously administered insulin reaches appropriate levels can lead to hyperglycemia and the possibility of ketoacidosis. Close monitoring of glucose levels during this transition period can prevent either hypo- or hyperglycemia.

When subcutaneous insulin is begun following intravenous therapy as described above, approximately 0.15 U. per lb. of ideal body weight of long-acting insulin or 80 per cent of the previous day's total is given at breakfast. If two daily injections are planned, two thirds of the total is given before breakfast and one third before supper, with a mix of two thirds long-acting and one third regular. Additional regular insulin is then given based on plasma or serum glucose levels. The next day's dosage can be planned by incorporating 80 per cent of the additional insulin required the previous day. Because the effect of NPH and lente insulin extends beyond 24 hours, the frequency of changes in insulin doses should be judged accordingly.

Postoperative complications in diabetics should be anticipated and prevented whenever possible. Close control of blood glucose promotes wound healing and resistance to infection, as does early discontinuation of Foley catheters or other indwelling lines.

Autonomic neuropathies may present with complications, such as postural hypotension, gastric atony, and urinary retention. Attention to these problems as well as excellent skin care, early ambulation, and early diagnosis and treatment of infections will lead to an optimal outcome.

Cardiac

The assessment of cardiac risk factors prior to surgery is necessary in patients undergoing both cardiac and noncardiac surgery. Circulatory stress characterized by an increased myocardial oxygen demand and a decreased oxygen supply is present in the postoperative period. Increased sympathetic tone leading to tachycardia and hypertension, increased volume loading, postoperative shivering, and fever from atelectasis or infection all increase oxygen requirements. All anesthetic agents, most notably halothane and methoxyflurane, are myocardial depressants, and hypotension during anesthesia is not unusual. Bradyarrhythmias caused by increased vagal tone, hypoxemia from pre-existing pulmonary disease, upper abdominal or thoracic surgery, and uncorrected anemia all decrease oxygen supply to the myocardium, thereby increasing the risk of ischemia. All of these factors, which place increased stress on the heart, should be anticipated and avoided when possible.

Classification of cardiac risk in noncardiac surgery can be accomplished on the basis of readily available clinical evidence, including history and physical examination. The Cardiac Risk Index of Goldman et al. (1977) (Table 41–2), which was developed in a group of 1001 consecutive patients undergoing noncardiac surgery, has been shown to correlate with the likelihood of life-threatening cardiac complications, especially congestive failure, life-threatening arrhythmias, and myocardial infarction (Weitz and Goldman, 1987) (Table 41–3). As a corollary, the following independent risk factors were *not* found to be significantly correlated with an increased risk in noncardiac surgery: hyperlipidemia, smoking, diabetes, hypertension, stable angina, bundle branch blocks, peripheral vascular disorders, history of old myocardial infarction, ST-T changes, cardiomegaly, mitral valve disease, or congestive heart failure in the absence of an S_3 or jugular venous distention.

Table 41–2. COMPUTATION OF CARDIAC RISK INDEX

Criteria	Points
History	
Age > 70 year	5
Myocardial infarction in previous 6 months	10
Physical	
S_3 gallop or jugular venous distention	11
Important valvular aortic stenosis	3
Electrocardiogram	
Rhythm other than sinus or premature atrial contractions on preoperative electrocardiogram	7
> 5 premature ventricular contractions per minute at any time prior to surgery	7
General Status	3
$Po_2 < 60$ or $Pco_2 > 50$ mm. Hg	
$K > 3.0$ or $Hco_3 < 20$ mEq. per liter	
BUN > 50 or Cr > 3.0 mg. per dl.	
Abnormal SGOT	
Chronic liver disease	
Bedridden from noncardiac causes	
Operation	
Intraperitoneal, intrathoracic, or aortic surgery	3
Emergency surgery	4
Total points	53

Adapted from Goldman L., Caldera, D. L., Nussbaum, S. R. et al.: N. Engl. J. Med., *297*(16):845–850, 1977.

When initial evaluation reveals evidence of cardiovascular disease, further evaluation may be indicated prior to operation. Similarly, patients undergoing vascular surgery may be expected to have an increased risk of coronary artery disease. While diagnostic studies, such as exercise stress testing (McPhail et al., 1988) and thallium imaging (Morise et al., 1987), may help to assign patients to low- or high-risk groups, the strongest risk predictor is a history of myocardial infarction within the previous 6 months. Unless an operation is required for a life-threatening illness, patients with a history of infarction should not undergo surgery until 6 months post-infarction, when operative risk stabilizes. The value of coronary arteriography for preoperative risk assessment combined with prophylactic coronary revascularization has yet to be proven by controlled trial (Madlon-Kay, 1987). Patients with New York Heart Association class III and IV angina, however, should be considered for preoperative exercise testing and/or coronary arteriography. Additional preoperative measures that are indicated in the patient with heart disease include treatment of uncompensated congestive failure to obtain optimal function, evaluation of significant aortic valvular stenosis by cardiac catheterization, control of symptomatic ventricular arrhythmias, and control of unstable hypertension (diastolic pressure greater than 110 mm. Hg.). Patients in Goldman's classes III and IV (Table 41–3) should have intra-arterial and pulmonary artery hemodynamic monitoring intraoperatively.

Pulmonary Function

Factors associated with an increased risk of postoperative pulmonary complications include the site of incision, smoking history with productive cough, obstructive pulmonary disease, prolonged anesthesia time, and obesity (Jackson, 1988). A history of smoking, chronic cough, or other pulmonary disease is especially important and suggests that preoperative pulmonary function tests be performed. Other patients who should be considered for pulmonary function testing include patients who will have thoracic or upper abdominal surgery, obese patients, and those over 70 years of age. Any patient with a forced expiratory volume of less than 1 liter at 1 second (FEV_1) or a maximal breathing capacity less than 50

Table 41–3. CARDIAC RISK INDEX

Class	Point Total	No or Only Minor Complications	Life-Threatening Complications*	Cardiac Deaths
I	0–5	99%	0.7%	0.2%
II	6–12	93%	5%	2%
III	13–25	86%	11%	2%
IV	≥ 26	22%	22%	56%

*Myocardial infarction, pulmonary edema, or ventricular tachycardia
Adapted from Goldman L., Caldera, D. L., Nussbaum, S. R. et al.: N. Engl. J. Med., *297*:(16):845–850, 1977.

per cent of predicted is at high risk for perioperative complications. Arterial blood gases should be obtained in patients with moderate or severe spirometric deficits; the finding of hypercapnia also indicates significantly increased risk.

Physical examination can detect findings associated with chronic obstructive pulmonary disease including increased expiratory to inspiratory (E/I) ratio (normal 1:1), increased forced expiratory time (normal 3 to 4 seconds), and presence of wheezing, rales, or rhonchi.

When high-risk patients are identified by history, physical examination, or pulmonary function testing, measures should be initiated preoperatively to decrease the risk of complications in the postoperative period. Warner and colleagues (1984) observed that a statistically significant decrease in complications occurred in those who quit smoking a minimum of 8 weeks prior to surgery. Aggressive pulmonary toilet should be instituted in any patient with a chronic upper respiratory tract infection at least 3 to 4 days before surgery. Incentive spirometry, deep breathing exercises, or intermittent positive pressure breathing should be taught in the preoperative period as they may decrease atelectasis and promote clearance of secretions in the postoperative period. All of these modalities have been shown to decrease postoperative risk; however, intermittent positive pressure breathing is more expensive and has been associated with bloating and abdominal distention. Incentive spirometry appears to be the most effective of the three in decreasing length of hospital stay (Celli et al., 1984).

Postoperative hypoventilation is related to decreased tidal volume and increased splinting because of pain, suppression of coughing and normal intermittent sighing by narcotic analgesia, and probable diaphragmatic dysfunction after upper abdominal surgery. Physical therapy (including turning, coughing, deep breathing, and percussion or vibration) continues to be effective in limiting postoperative pulmonary complications.

Medications

Certain medications may pose a risk if continued up to or through the operative period. Antihypertensives, especially diuretics, may lead to problems of hypovolemia or hypokalemia; total body potassium may be depleted with only a slightly low serum value. With concomitant use of digitalis, the risk of intraoperative cardiac dysrhythmias is increased. Beta-blockers, such as propranolol, should be continued throughout the intra- and postoperative period to decrease the risk of arrhythmias precipitated by withdrawal. Calcium channel blockers should also be continued until the time of surgery in patients who require them; however, myocardial depression and hypotension secondary to decreased systemic vascular resistance from synergism with anesthetic agents is possible. Nitrates may also be continued through the operative period as nitropaste ointment or patch.

Antiplatelet agents and anticoagulants, on the other hand, should be discontinued prior to surgery. Aspirin, nonsteroidals, and other platelet inhibitors should be stopped at least 1 week before and warfarin 48 hours before surgery. Intravenous heparin may be substituted, when necessary. Patients taking oral contraceptive agents, who will be immobilized postoperatively, should stop their medication at least 1 month prior to elective surgery. Also, care is required when administering tricyclic antidepressants or monoamine oxidase inhibitors along with anesthetic agents.

Informed Consent/Patient Education

The process of obtaining informed consent for a surgical procedure provides an opportunity to discuss the patient's illness and to assess if expectations for surgery are realistic. This discussion should diminish the risk of postoperative psychologic or medicolegal complications (Celli et al., 1984). Informed consent can only be obtained from an individual who is legally competent, and competency is assumed unless substantial evidence to the contrary exists. The elements of informed consent, which have evolved from a series of judicial actions, include the following:

1. Nature and purpose of proposed procedure in lay language
2. Discussion of all risks, inconveniences, hazards, and problems in recuperation material to the decision of a reasonable person
3. Alternative treatments
4. Identity of surgeon
5. Opportunity for all questions to be answered.

It is appropriate for the surgeon who will be performing the procedure to obtain the consent, discuss the patient's understanding of the planned procedure, and address the patient's questions. The family physician's knowledge of the patient can facilitate this process, including consideration of the significance of the surgical illness and intervention for the patient and the family.

Preoperative Laboratory and Radiologic Evaluation

CHEST X-RAY

While the routine ordering of a preoperative chest x-ray is widespread, a large amount of data has been amassed that suggests that it is unnecessary. The percentage of abnormal findings that could not have been suspected from the history and physical is low (Loder, 1978; Sagel et al., 1974), and the findings that actually lead to changes in the management plan or cancellation of surgery are rare (Royal College of Radiologists, 1979; Tape and Mushlin, 1988). While the incidence of abnormal findings on a chest x-ray increases with age, these are just as likely to be clinically suspected in younger patients. An additional element in the argument against routine chest x-rays in a low-risk population is that the proportion of false positive interpretations is likely to be greater than true positives, leading to unnecessary diagnostic evaluations. One can, therefore, reasonably conclude that a preoperative chest x-ray should not be routine but should be obtained based on the following:

1. Indications determined from the history and physical examination
2. In those patients at greater risk of postoperative complications
3. In those from populations with a high prevalence of undiagnosed chest disease
4. Whenever the standard of care by the anesthesiology department in the hospital mandates a routine preoperative chest x-ray.

LABORATORY

The preoperative screening of all patients with a routine panel of laboratory evaluations has been demonstrated to lack cost effectiveness, to produce an unacceptable number of false positives in a low-risk population, and to result in only rare changes in management (Blery et al., 1986; Muskett and McGreevy, 1986; AMA, 1983). Certain tests can be recommended for all patients based on their low cost, prevalence of the conditions for which they screen, their implications for management of the surgical patient, and their specificity. These include a hemoglobin or hematocrit (anemia) and a urinalysis (diabetes, infection). Additionally, a urine pregnancy test should be obtained when indicated for females in the reproductive age group. Finally, an electrocardiogram should be obtained in patients over 50 years of age, who are at greater risk for myocardial infarction (Moorman et al., 1985).

Additional preoperative laboratory testing should be obtained based on indications determined from the history and physical. The family physician's knowledge of the patient may be valuable in directing additional investigations, such as obtaining electrolytes in a patient who uses diuretics or laxatives.

The Surgeon's Occupational Risk

HUMAN IMMUNODEFICIENCY VIRUS (HIV)

While the risk of acquiring HIV infection by occupational exposure is low for health care workers, the possibility raises significant anxiety. The issue especially concerns those involved in invasive procedures, since the risk of transmission of HIV infection by needlestick exposure is probably greater than by exposure of nonintact skin or mucous membranes. When a patient is known to be HIV positive, it is estimated that the rate of transmission of the virus by accidental needlestick exposure is less than 1 per cent. While this translates to a very low risk for health care workers, universal blood and body products precautions should be observed, including the use of gloves for all direct contact with a body substance. In addition, goggles should be added to the usual gowns and masks if excessive aerosolization or splattering of body substances is expected to occur during an operative procedure. Individuals handling needles or other sharp instruments should not recap these before dispensing of them in an appropriate container.

Because HIV positivity in a surgeon or other health care worker is not known to pose any significant risk to patients, individuals may continue their usual occupational activities, assuming their health status permits it. Double gloving should be practiced in operative procedures, and gloves should be worn if open or weeping lesions are present on the hands.

HEPATITIS B VIRUS

Exposure to the hepatitis B virus by needlestick is another occupational risk of those performing surgical procedures. The precautions described above will decrease this risk, as will immunization with hepatitis B vaccine prior to exposure.

Disorders of the Breast

GENERAL PRINCIPLES OF DIAGNOSIS

The very high prevalence of both benign and malignant breast disorders in women, combined with the individual and cultural meanings and significance associated with the female breast, assures that family physicians will regularly encounter patients concerned with an abnormal finding in the breast. Patients with a complaint related to the breast or in whom an abnormality is detected on physical examination should be approached with equal attentiveness to the emotional and physical aspects of the problem. Because of the importance of the patient's role in the early detection of breast cancer, the primary physician must regularly address educational and screening issues with patients and encourage self-breast examination.

PATIENT HISTORY

Patients should be asked about the onset, duration, and previous history of the problem. Breast symptoms, such as a lump, discharge, or pain, should also be related to the menstrual cycle, history of trauma, ingestion of drugs (including hormones or methylxanthines such as caffeine), and emotional state. The patient's parity, oral contraceptive use, history of breast-feeding, family history of breast or colon cancer, and her particular concerns regarding the symptom may also contribute.

Examination should be conducted in a warm, well-lighted examining room with attention to the patient's privacy and ongoing discussion of observations. The patient should be disrobed above the waist for the initial inspection portion of the exam. First the skin texture and color is observed, along with the symmetry and contours of the breasts. Next, the effect of isometric muscle contraction is observed while the patient presses down with hands on hips, then forward with hands behind the head. Dimpling, retraction, or asymmetry thus produced may indicate underlying tumor attachment or scarring. Palpation of the neck, supra- and infraclavicular areas, and axillae follow, with the patient in an upright and relaxed position. The robe is then replaced and used to cover the breast not currently being examined. With the patient in the supine position and her arm either at a right angle or placed above her head, each breast is carefully examined in turn, including the axillary tail of the breast and the infra-areolar area. If a discharge has been present by history, asking the patient to express fluid from the breast or gentle compression of the nipple by the physician may reveal the presence of discharge. If present, pressure by the examiner's thumb sequentially on each areolar quadrant toward the center may localize the source of discharge produced by an intraductal lesion. A mass associated with such a discharge should be specifically sought. The sensitivity of the examination to margins of a mass or thickening can be improved by using a surgical lubricant or lotion applied to the flat surfaces of the examiner's fingers. Recording findings in a sketch in the patient's record or on a written consultation request is useful for future reference.

The complete examination can be used as a method of instructing the patient in self-examination. Although relatively few patients perform their own examination regularly, even though informed in the technique (Scheuter, 1982), they are more likely to do so if they have been shown how and are confident in their skill (Bennett et al., 1983). Specifically asking the patient what hinders her from performing self-exam and addressing these areas may be helpful in facilitating self-screening.

Screening mammography has been shown to provide the best opportunity for decreasing mortality from breast cancer by detecting lesions with the best potential for cure (Shapiro et al., 1985; Baker, 1982). Recommendation for screening intervals are based on disease incidence and estimates of tumor doubling rates. Mammographic screening is less reliable in younger women in whom denser breasts afford less contrast, and many professional societies no longer recommend obtaining routine mammograms in low-risk women less than 40 years of age (King, 1989). The recommendation of the American Cancer Society given in Table 41–4 for asymptomatic, normal risk women remains as before. Screening intervals will vary in those with significant risk factors (see Risk Factors below).

While mammography alone is the single most sensitive means of identifying breast malignancies, some tumors would be missed if this technique were not combined with physical examination. Because of limitations in sensitivity, a biopsy must be performed when a suspicious mass is palpated even if the mammogram is negative. Although the technique has improved to allow detection of lesions approaching 2 mm. in size, significant limitations remain, including the variability in the radiologic interpretation of mammograms. The skill of the radiologist should be the major factor in deciding where to obtain mammograms for patients (Boyd et al., 1982). Noncompliance with screening guidelines, both by patients and physicians, also limits the attainment of the promise of early screening (Mann et al., 1987).

FIBROCYSTIC DISEASE

This entity is the most common benign breast disorder. A more appropriate designation may be fibrocystic changes, since a condition that is present in 53 per cent of clinically normal breasts and the majority

Table 41–4. GUIDELINES FOR SCREENING MAMMOGRAPHY IN ASYMPTOMATIC WOMEN*

Age	Interval
35–40	Baseline
41–49	1–2 years
≥ 50	Annually

*Recommendations of the American Cancer Society, 1989.

of women at some point in their reproductive period may not appropriately be called pathologic (Franz et al., 1951). Many other terms have been used, including fibroproliferative disease, cystic mastitis, and mammary dysplasia. These changes are produced by an exaggerated response to cyclic changes of estrogen and progesterone.

Three phases of the process that predominantly affect the upper outer quadrant of the breast are found at various stages of the life cycle (Droegemueller et al., 1987). The earliest stage is mastodynia, or breast pain, which usually first presents in young women in their 20's, and is characterized by stromal proliferation. Adenosis is more common in the decade of the 30's, resulting from proliferation of ducts, ductules, and alveolar cells. Multiple small nodules 2 to 10 mm. in size produce a lumpy-bumpy breast texture. As aging continues in the 40's, macrocysts and areas of gross nodularity may become prominent, primarily in the upper outer quadrant of the breast. The involved areas are frequently painful and tender, with premenstrual accentuation. A greenish or dark-colored nipple discharge may occasionally be noted in patients with fibrocystic changes.

Cyst Aspiration/Needle Biopsy

An isolated cyst may present as a dominant mass and is often detected by the patient. These cysts contain fluid that may be straw colored, dark brown, or green. Aspiration of the fluid in the office can provide immediate assurance as well as diagnosis. When a mass suggestive of a cyst is identified in an accessible location, aspiration of the cyst is discussed with the patient. Preparation consists of cleaning the overlying skin with povidone-iodine or alcohol. Injected anesthesia is not recommended since it would substitute one needlestick for another, and infiltration of an anesthetic may obscure the location of the mass. Ethyl chloride topical spray, however, may be helpful. The lesion is isolated with the thumb and forefinger of one hand and aspirated using a 20- or 22-gauge needle on an appropriate size syringe in the other. A vacuum is maintained as the cyst is approached, and a return of fluid signifies that the cyst has been entered. Aspiration of the fluid should result in complete collapse of the cyst. If a mass persists, has recurred at 1 month follow-up, or if the fluid is bloody, the patient should be immediately referred to a surgeon for consideration of biopsy. While cytologic examination of cyst fluid is rarely productive, it should be performed if the fluid has characteristics other than clear and straw colored.

If no fluid is obtained, a finer needle such as a 25-gauge may be passed several times into the mass through different tracts while aspirating, maintaining the vacuum while removing the needle. The contents are then expelled onto a slide for fixation with a cytologic spray. Such a fine needle aspiration may be helpful in planning the next step for diagnosis of a persistent mass (Lannin et al., 1986). While the false-negative rate of aspiration cytology is approximately 2 per cent in the hands of experienced operators (Goodson et al., 1987), the results depend on patient selection, the physician's experience, and the skill of the cytopathologist. A formal biopsy using a 14- or 16-gauge needle may also be used to determine whether to plan a definitive procedure as an outpatient or in the hospital.

Treatment

Initial management of the discomfort associated with fibrocystic changes includes physical measures, such as a well-fitted brassiere providing good support, local heat, and mild analgesics. Some women experience regression of symptoms when methylxanthines contained in coffee, tea, cola drinks, and some chocolates are limited, although the empiric validation of this recommendation is controversial. Minton and coworkers (1979) have proposed that eliminating cigarettes and methylxanthines and reducing stress quiets the cyclic adenosine monophosphate-guanosine monophosphate overactivity associated with fibrocystic breasts. Use of premenstrual diuretics or vitamin E (600 to 1800 I.U. daily) may be helpful. Most women experience decreased symptoms from suppression of ovarian function either by combination oral contraceptive agents or with a synthetic androgen, such as danazol (100 to 400 mg. daily for 4 to 6 months). Bromocriptine and tamoxifen have also been used for resistant cases.

While a history of fibrocystic changes in itself does not increase the risk of breast cancer, women in whom epithelial hyperplasia has been documented, including ductal or lobular hyperplasia with atypia, are considered to have up to five times the risk of breast cancer compared with women without these findings. Women with other histologic variants seen in the spectrum of fibrocystic changes are not at increased risk for cancer, but differentiating the recurrent nodules and cysts found in these women from breast malignancy can be frustrating and anxiety provoking, both for the patient and the physician. Cyst aspiration can be done repeatedly, using the same criteria to help decide on the need for biopsy. A noncystic dominant mass should always be viewed with suspicion, but observing the mass throughout the menstrual cycle may help decide whether biopsy is indicated. While regression of the lesion after the menses, history of rapid fluctuation of the mass, premenstrual tenderness, and presence of multiple masses in a woman are all supportive of a benign diagnosis, only an excisional biopsy is definitive in eliminating the possibility of malignancy.

FIBROADENOMA

A common benign tumor presenting in the breasts of young women in their teens or early 20's, this lesion is identified by its smooth, rubbery, sometimes lobulated characteristics, and is freely mobile within the surrounding breast tissue. It is usually painless and solitary but may be present with other similar tumors in 10 to 15 per cent of patients. Occasionally, a rapidly growing tumor called cystosarcoma phyllodes, which occasionally is malignant, may arise from a fibroadenoma; however, these tumors constitute only 1 per cent of breast malignancies. Because of the occasional tendency of fibroadenomas to enlarge rapidly, especially under the hormonal influence of pregnancy, as well as the small possibility of malignant disease, outpatient excisional biopsy is indicated under local anesthesia. Because the dense breasts of young women do not always allow for a clear-cut diagnosis on a xeromammogram and because malignancy is extremely rare in this age group, mammography is *not* recommended for the evaluation of fibroadenomas.

NIPPLE DISCHARGE

The patient's history combined with physical examination will usually distinguish between systemic or local causes of nipple discharge. The patient should be asked the duration of the discharge, events preceding its onset, whether unilateral or bilateral, whether spontaneous or not, its relationship to menses, and association with any medications. A bilateral serous or milky discharge that is positive for fat globules in a woman who has previously lactated is galactorrhea. A serum prolactin level can screen for increased pituitary secretion due to an adenoma or a variety of endocrine syndromes. The use of oral contraceptives or neuroleptics, as well as a variety of other medications, can be associated with galactorrhea. Chest trauma or surgery may also lead to bilateral nipple discharge. A discharge that is colored or bloody but may be serous, and which is unilateral but may be bilateral, suggests a local etiology. The most common cause of nipple discharge in the nonlactating breast is fibrocystic changes, followed by intraductal papilloma and carcinoma. As described under Patient History above, careful evaluation of the nipple, perhaps with a magnifying glass, will reveal whether a unilateral discharge emanates from a single duct or from multiple ducts. A spontaneous serous or serosanguinous discharge from a single duct is most often caused by an intraductal papilloma but may be an intraductal carcinoma. While a bloody discharge suggests cancer, even this finding is more commonly caused by an intraductal papilloma. The discharge should be submitted for cytologic examination and, if the color suggests the presence of heme, a test for occult blood should also be performed. Since the presence of a mass associated with a discharge is very significant, this finding should be carefully sought and is an indication for resection of the involved duct(s). When a persistent unilateral discharge is localized to a single duct or group of ducts, these ducts should be resected, even in the absence of a mass.

GYNECOMASTIA

Gynecomastia refers to an increase in glandular and stromal tissues in the male breast. It is distinguished from other causes of enlargement of the male breast, such as carcinoma or adiposity. Gynecomastia results in a palpable, firm mass centrally located in the subareolar region, which is usually bilateral but may be unilateral. Its incidence is bimodal, presenting in approximately 40 per cent of pubescent boys and in as many as 40 per cent of elderly men. Its cause is physiologic in these age groups, resulting from an altered estrogen/androgen ratio. Gynecomastia in the adolescent usually resolves within 2 years of onset, and observation and reassurance is all that is required. Occurrence of a breast mass in a male in other age ranges is more likely to result from a pathologic cause. The most common causes of nonphysiologic gynecomastia include drugs and alcoholic liver disease. Marijuana, psychotropic drugs, spironolactone, digitalis, cimetidine, and cytotoxic medications alter the estrogen/testosterone ratio by a variety of mechanisms. The administration of sex steroids, gonadotropins, or antiandrogen drugs have the same effect.

The pathologic causes of gynecomastia result from increased estrogen secretion (Klinefelter's syndrome, adrenal or testicular tumors), conversion of androgens to estrogens (liver disorders, thyrotoxicosis, or refeeding after starvation), decreased androgen secretion (hypogonadism), and decreased androgen activity due to receptor protein abnormalities (testicular feminization). Etiology of some cases of gynecomastia is unknown.

Diagnosis of gynecomastia can frequently be made from the history, such as in the case of an adolescent male or drug ingestion. Physical examination, in addition to defining local and axillary involvement, should focus on findings suggestive of systemic or neoplastic disease. Examples are eye findings consistent with pituitary tumor or thyroid disease; signs of liver failure; or testicular abnormality. Laboratory studies that may be useful (depending on the presentation) include liver function tests and hormonal assays (including estrone, estradiol, androstenedione, testosterone, luteinizing hormone, HCG, and urinary 17-ketosteroids). Free thyroxine index in the presence of signs of hyperthyroidism, or prolactin in the presence of galactorrea, may also be helpful.

Regression of gynecomastia occurs spontaneously in up to 90 per cent of adolescent males. If gynecomastia is of long standing, fibrotic changes may make the condition irreversible. Cosmetic mastectomy is occasionally indicated, depending on the patient's desires (Wyngaarden and Smith, 1985; Samiy et al., 1987).

BREAST CANCER

One of every 11 women in the United States will develop and be diagnosed with breast cancer during her lifetime (9 per cent lifetime risk). The risk to a woman with no identified risk factors is 6 per cent, and risk factors identify only 25 per cent of women who will develop breast cancer (Droegenmueller et al., 1987). Thus, every woman should be considered to be at significant risk for the development of breast cancer, with the accompanying responsibility of the family physician for patient education and emphasis on screening.

Risk Factors

The most significant risk factor for the development of breast cancer is a first-degree relative (mother or sister) with a history of breast cancer, especially if the cancer was premenopausal and/or bilateral. A family history of multiple individuals with cancers, especially adenocarcinomata, appears to increase risk. Interestingly, women who are diagnosed with a primary breast cancer are at twice the risk of developing a metachronous colorectal primary as controls and should, therefore, receive intensive screening in this area (Agarwal et al., 1986). The development of breast cancer is directly related to age, with only 2 per cent of diagnoses made before 30 years of age and the incidence continuing to increase with advancing age. Factors associated with increased risk of breast cancer are reproductive factors (early menarche, late menopause, nulligravid state, or first child after age 30), increased estrogen exposure (bilateral oophorectomy before 35 years of age with hormone replacement, persistent anovulation, obesity), personal history of breast cancer (annual risk of development of new cancer approximately 1 per cent), history of epithelial hyperplasia with atypia, exposure to ionizing radiation or other carcinogens, and certain dietary factors including fat and alcohol (see below). Long-term, regular exercise is associated with a reduced risk for breast cancer (Frisch et al., 1985) and may be related to a decreased percentage of body fat in athletes. The use of combination oral contraceptives has not been associated with increased risk in multiple large-scale studies, but the possibility of significantly increased risk for subgroups of women still exists. Postmenopausal estrogen use does not increase risk of breast cancer when administered cyclically and/or with medroxyprogesterone. As described above, a history of fibrocystic changes does not in itself increase risk, but documentation of epithelial hyperplasia with atypia does imply increased risk for the patient. The average doubling time of a breast tumor is 100 days, which means that a clinically detectable cancer has been present for at least 7 to 9 years when a malignancy is detected. This latent period makes study of the association of precipitating factors and disease difficult.

The only risk factor for breast cancer which is reasonably subject to modification is diet. A number of epidemiologic and animal studies have suggested that decreasing fat in the diet may decrease risk for breast cancer as well as other neoplasms. The American Cancer Society has recommended that the percentage of calories from fat in the diet be reduced to 30 per cent. The age threshold, if present, for such a reduction to be effective is unknown. Alcohol intake has been associated with increased risk in the large majority of studies in which it has been addressed, and a dose-response relationship has been demonstrated (Schatzkin, et al., 1987). The data appear sufficient to counsel patients with risk factors for breast cancer to limit the amount of fat and alcohol in their diets.

Detection

Carcinoma of the breast most frequently presents as a painless lump detected by the patient herself, although 20 per cent of patients complain of discomfort associated with their tumor. Additional findings may include a nipple discharge; retraction or dimpling; erythema, scaling, oozing, ulceration, or edema (peau d'orange) of the skin or nipple; axillary lymphadenopathy; or discovery of distant metastases. Excellent evidence supports the concept of self-breast exam in order to diagnose tumors at an earlier stage (Foster and Costanza, 1984). This method, if encouraged by physicians and widely practiced by women, is an extremely cost-effective way of decreasing the impact of breast cancer. The ideal frequency for self-breast examination is monthly, immediately following the menses in premenopausal women. Self-breast examination beginning at age 20, when combined with annual physician examination at least over the age of 30 for average risk women, significantly improves detection rates for breast cancer. More frequent physician examination may be indicated based on assessment of individual risk factors. Regular examination of the breasts should be included as part of the physical examination even in the patient with unrelated complaints if screening visits are not otherwise requested. The recording of risk factors for breast cancer on the patient's problem list serves to remind the physician of this need. Mammography complements self-breast examination and physician examination in the early detection of malignancy. Adherence to screening guidelines (Table 41–4) results in detection of smaller, presumably more curable lesions (Shapiro et al., 1985; Baker, 1982). With current mammographic techniques, the risk of radiation is negligible (0.1 to 0.8 rad for two views) relative to benefits and has been likened to the risk of smoking six cigarettes.

Diagnosis

Bilateral mammography is very useful in the work-up of a breast mass and is preferably done prior to any needle instrumentation, which may alter subtle diagnostic signs for the radiologist. Mammography should always be considered as complementary to and not a substitute for physical examination. Because of the significant incidence of false negative mammograms, biopsy of a clinically suspicious mass should never be deferred because of a negative mammogram. While ultrasonography may be useful when discordance exists between physical examination and mammographic findings, neither ultrasonography nor thermography has been proven as a screening modality.

Needle aspiration or biopsy, as described under the section on Fibrocystic Disease, can be readily performed in an outpatient setting to determine whether inpatient or outpatient open biopsy should be planned. An excisional biopsy is planned for the least objectionable scar in the event that no further surgery is required. It is helpful to mark the skin lines in the sitting position, since the lines of Langer may be distorted when the patient is supine. When the lesion to be biopsied is identified only by mammography, localizing needles may be inserted to assist the surgeon in locating the lesion, and the excised specimen should be submitted for radiologic examination to ensure that the lesion has been removed *in toto*. When a frozen section of the specimen is suspicious or confirmatory of malignancy, at least 500 mg. of tissue should be excised for submission for estrogen and progesterone receptor determination. Delay in definitive surgical therapy of up to 2 weeks does not adversely affect outcome and allows for complete discussion of options with the patient, her family, and perhaps other consultants. Exploration of the patient's psychologic state and support system (including marital relationship, which along with type of treatment have been shown to correlate with short-term psychiatric morbidity following mastectomy [Dean, 1987]) can be accomplished during this period. Discussion of the possibility of reconstructive surgery or use of a prosthesis can help the patient and family to prepare for the effect of surgery on body image. Careful study of permanent sections and hormone receptor status determination is also pertinent to making a decision regarding treatment options.

Histologic Type

The histologic type and clinical stage of breast cancer are highly correlated with prognosis. Host factors, including emotional arousal and immune competence, especially lymphocyte depletion or proliferation within axillary nodes, also contribute to outcome; but these factors are less well defined. The most common histologic types and percentages are given in Table 41–5. Based on a review of 1000 breast tumor specimens by the National Surgical Adjuvant Breast Project, 60 per cent were found to be of pure tumor types, whereas 40 per cent were of mixed types. Prognosis is that associated with the most aggressive cell type. Infiltrating ductal carcinoma is the most common and is characterized by a tendency to metastasize early. Other common types include medullary carcinoma, which has a better than average prognosis, and lobular carcinoma, which is frequently multicentric and bilateral.

Table 41–5. CLASSIFICATION OF MOST COMMON TYPES OF BREAST CARCINOMATA

Type	Per Cent of All Cases
Noninvasive	
Comedocarcinoma	1
Ductal papillary (in situ)	5
Lobular (in situ)	3
Invasive	
Infiltrating ductal carcinoma	70–80
Medullary	5–7
Lobular	5–10
Paget's, inflammatory, infiltrating papillary, tubular, mucinous	<5

Clinical Staging

It is now understood that the primary method of spread of most breast cancers is by microemboli through the circulatory system, rather than by local extension. While clinical staging classifies the disease presentation based on identifiable sites of spread, breast cancer can be best understood as a systemic disease, with the presence or absence of micrometastases at initial presentation based on the characteristics of the tumor type. Fifty per cent of women with carcinoma of the breast have metastatic disease, including positive axillary nodes, at presentation; two thirds will develop distant metastases in spite of therapy. The presence of positive axillary nodes is the most significant factor correlating with prognosis (Fig. 41–1). Gross and microscopic pathologic features that are associated with prognosis are listed in Table 41–6. The goal of clinical staging is to determine the local extent of disease, involvement of regional lymph nodes, the status of the opposite breast, and the likelihood of distant spread. Clinical staging allows appropriate therapy to be chosen based on the likelihood of disease spread and provides for an estimate of prognosis. The commonly used American Joint Committee for Cancer Staging and End Results Reporting Classification is shown in Table 41–7.

Staging begins with the history and physical examination, especially noting size of tumor, evidence of local spread, and presence of axillary nodes suspicious for tumor. Unfortunately, palpation for axillary nodes misses nodes that are histopathologically involved in about 40 per cent of patients (Baker, 1984); thus, microscopic examination of axillary nodes is required for accurate staging. Careful examination of the contralateral breast is essential. The investigation for systemic metastases is guided by the knowledge that breast cancer most commonly spreads to bone, especially the pelvis and spine, lungs, me-

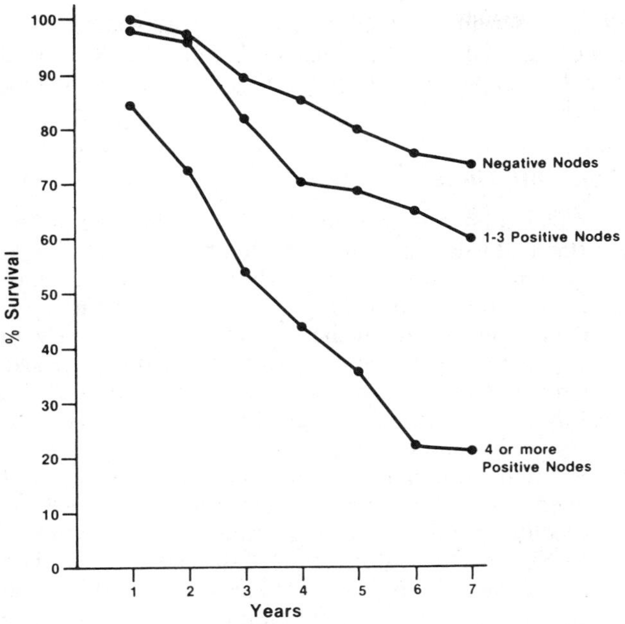

Figure 41–1. Per cent of survival according to nodal status. (By permission from Gambrell, R. D., Jr.: Proposal to decrease the risk and improve the prognosis of breast cancer. Am. J. Obstet. Gynecol. *150*:119–128, 1984.)

diastinal lymph nodes, and liver, although spread to almost any site is possible. A basic laboratory evaluation including a chest x-ray, complete blood count, alkaline phosphatase, and serum calcium is performed, with bone scan or biopsy indicated if bone pain is present or alkaline phosphatase is elevated. If

Table 41–6. TUMOR CHARACTERISTICS AND PROGNOSIS

1. **Histologic Grading**
   - Well-differentiated grade 1: undifferentiated grade 3
   - 70 per cent of cancers are grade 3
   - ER-negative associated with grade 3
2. **Nuclear Grade**
   - Well-differentiated grade 3: poorly differentiated grade 1
   - 10 per cent of cancers are grade 3: 30 per cent are grade 1
   - Relationship between grade 1 and poor prognosis
3. **Tumor size**
   - < 5 mm. is minimal cancer
   - Poorer survival is more related to node involvement than size
   - Larger tumors, more node positive, poorer survival
4. **Cell Reaction**
   - Lymphocytic infiltration usually means good prognosis
5. **Lymphatic and Blood Invasion**
   - Hard to determine and reproduce
   - Usually associated with poor prognosis
6. **Lymph Node Involvement**
   - 10-year prognosis related to number of nodes involved (in per cent)
   - 0 nodes 75
   - Positive nodes 25
   - ≥ 4 nodes 13

From Carbone, P. P.: Breast cancer. *In* Kahn, S. B. (Ed.): Concepts in Cancer Medicine. New York, Grune & Stratton, 1983, p. 404.

Table 41–7. BREAST CANCER STAGING

Tumor:	
T1	< 2 cm.
T2	2–5 cm.
T3	> 5 cm.
	T3b fixation to underlying fascia or muscle
T4	Tumor of any size with fixation and extension to chest wall, skin or inflammatory carcinoma
Nodes:	
N0	No palpable nodes
N1	Moveable nodes
	N1b felt to contain cancer
N2	Fixed, cancer-containing nodes
N3	Supraclavicular or infraclavicular nodes
Metastases:	
M0	No metastases
M1	Metastases

Stage I:
T1 N0 (N1a) M0
Stage II:
Any T1 or T2 with N1b or T2 with fixation to chest wall
Stage III:
T3, N1, or N2 M0
Stage IV:
T4, TN3, TM1

Adapted from Carbone, P. P.: *In* Kahn, S. B. (Ed.): Concepts in Cancer Medicine. New York, Grune & Stratton, 1983, p. 407.

the liver is enlarged or alkaline phosphatase elevated, a liver scan is indicated. The presence of neurologic symptoms mandates a brain scan. A carcinoembryonic antigen level may be done as a baseline or if the patient is likely to have advanced disease. The combination of an abnormal liver scan and elevated carcinoembryonic antigen is highly specific for the presence of hepatic metastases. Computed tomography of the liver is an alternative method of screening for hepatic metastases.

Blind, mirror-image biopsies of the opposite breast in the absence of clinical or radiographic evidence of malignancy should be considered only when the family history is strongly positive or when diffuse intraductal carcinoma or lobular carcinoma is present.

Surgical Options

The three major concerns in treating breast carcinoma include control of local disease, treatment of distant metastases, and improved quality of life for women treated for the disease. Presumably because of the high percentage of tumors that have metastasized at diagnosis, the most important prognostic factor is clinical stage at presentation. Thus, survival benefits do not appear to result from more aggressive efforts at local control. Local treatment for all but minimal breast cancer should primarily be aimed at removing or reducing tumor burden, allowing the host's defenses and adjuvant therapy to deal with residual tumor and any micrometastases, and at staging of the disease by the sampling of axillary nodes.

For more advanced cancers (stage III and IV),

the primary treatment is hormonal therapy if the receptor status is positive and chemotherapy and/or radiation if negative. Surgery is the primary treatment for stage I or II disease with or without radiation, hormonal therapy, or adjuvant chemotherapy.

Multiple surgical options are now available for both node-negative and node-positive breast carcinoma. While the modified radical mastectomy was the standard for many years, experience has shown that more limited procedures, when combined with radiation therapy and sometimes chemotherapy, is an acceptable alternative (Fisher et al., 1985).

Based on several recent reviews of clinical trials examining the outcome of conservative surgical therapy versus traditional, more radical techniques, a number of conclusions can be drawn (Tinker and Wise, 1987; Bosworth and Ghossein, 1984; Cuzick et al., 1987; Foster, 1984). First, survival is not improved by prophylactic treatment of regional nodes, either by surgical extirpation or by high-dose irradiation, versus subsequent nodal dissection for later involvement. Nevertheless, nodal dissection initially is important for clinical staging. Secondly, conservative techniques of dealing with local disease, such as lumpectomy, when combined with local prophylactic irradiation, do not adversely affect survival at 5- and 10-year intervals when compared to modified radical mastectomy. If local irradiation is omitted initially, the favorable outcome of subsequent ipsilateral recurrences treated by salvage mastectomy means that survival benefit is not compromised. However, because the long-term effects of irradiation of the breast are usually quite acceptable and because failure to use adjuvant radiation therapy results in a greater frequency of breast loss, local irradiation combined with conservative surgical therapy is recommended.

Several questions with regard to the technique of conservative therapy still remain, including the necessity of wide excision, the optimal combination of axillary dissection versus regional irradiation, and the long-term risk of ionizing radiation to the breast.

Given the options available for initial surgical therapy, when predicted outcomes are comparable, the patient should be the central participant in the decision regarding mode of therapy. Thorough discussion of options is even mandated by law in some states. Patients should be encouraged whenever possible to participate in treatment protocols that will ultimately define optimal therapy for each type of presentation. In some cases, however, medical factors limit available options. For instance, when the ratio of tumor to breast size or a central location of tumor would result in a cosmetically unacceptable result if breast conservation is attempted, an alternative procedure may be required. Examples would be a subcutaneous or modified radical mastectomy with delayed or immediate reconstruction or insertion of a subcutaneous prosthesis. If a multicentric tumor is present, breast-conservation therapy is not indicated. In summary, conservative management of stage I or II breast cancer with appropriate adjuvant therapy does not compromise survival, is associated with fewer surgical complications, and leads to a decreased negative impact on the patient's body image (Sanger and Reznekoff, 1981).

Adjuvant Therapy

The following are modified guidelines compiled by the National Institutes of Health Consensus Development Conference regarding adjuvant chemotherapy in hormonal therapy for breast cancer:

1. Combination chemotherapy reduces mortality in premenopausal women with positive nodes (Early Breast Cancer Trialists' Collaborative Group, 1988) and should be offered to this group regardless of hormone receptor status.
2. Women with negative nodes have generally not been offered adjuvant chemotherapy; however, recently published studies found the following:
   a. Significant prolongation of disease-free survival but no survival advantage was noted among both pre- and postmenopausal node-negative women given sequential combination chemotherapy. The effect was most notable in the older group (Fisher et al., 1989a).
   b. Significantly increased disease-free survival but no survival advantage was noted in pre- and postmenopausal node-negative, ER-positive women who received tamoxifen 10 mg. twice daily (Fisher et al., 1989b).
   c. Increased disease-free survival but no survival benefit was noted in node-negative women at high risk because of estrogen-receptor (ER)-negative tumor of any size or ER-positive tumor at least 3 cm. who received cyclic combination chemotherapy (Mansour et al., 1989).
   d. Both pre- and postmenopausal node-negative women had increased disease-free survival after receiving one course of perioperative adjuvant chemotherapy.

   These results suggest that node-negative women, who have approximately a 30 per cent risk of death due to breast cancer, can be offered adjuvant chemo- or hormonal therapy. The smallest number of women who do not require such adjuvant therapy will receive it if selection is made based on risk factors, including tumor size, hormone receptor status, cell type, proliferative rate, and nuclear ploidy.
3. Chemotherapy may be considered for postmenopausal women with positive nodes and negative hormone receptor levels—the group with poorest prognosis; however, chemotherapy has not been shown to be very effective in this group.
4. Tamoxifen is the treatment of choice for postmenopausal women with positive nodes and positive hormone receptor status.
5. The choice of drugs for adjuvant chemotherapy is best made with oncologic consultation. Combination chemotherapy appears much more effective than a single agent, but the most effective combi-

nation is still controversial. The most commonly used combination of drugs includes cyclophosphamide, methotrexate, and 5-fluorouracil (CMF), with prednisone and/or vincristine added as necessary. Adriamycin is helpful in combination with other medications, especially for induction therapy for inflammatory carcinoma.

Hormonal Therapy

Approximately 50 per cent of breast tumors are ER positive, with a lower incidence of 30 per cent in premenopausal versus 60 per cent in postmenopausal women. Eighty per cent of women whose tumors are ER positive respond to tamoxifen, while less than 10 per cent of ER-negative tumors respond. The presence of progesterone receptors also predicts a positive response to hormonal manipulation.

Rehabilitation and Follow-up

Psychologic adjustment after surgical treatment for breast cancer depends on the patient's premorbid psychologic adjustment, coping mechanisms and defenses used, social support including marital relationship, and the type of therapy offered. Recipients of conservative procedures are less likely to have an altered self-image and sexual dysfunction than patients who have undergone mastectomy. Breast reconstruction with a musculocutaneous flap, subcutaneous prosthesis, or external prosthesis can assist the patient in subsequent psychologic adjustment. The Reach for Recovery program sponsored by the American Cancer Society can provide a valuable resource for the patient adjusting to loss of a breast. Appropriate attention to physical rehabilitation and limitation of functional impairment should be provided.

Patients enrolled in specific protocols will have follow-up specified. Those who are not should be seen at 3-month intervals in the first 2 years following surgery, then at 6-month intervals indefinitely. Physical examination with attention to the most usual sites of recurrence (surgical scar, chest wall, axillary, infra- or supraclavicular areas, lungs, liver, and bone) is performed at each visit. Xeromammography is done biannually in a conserved breast or annually in the contralateral breast. Chest x-rays are done annually. Following laboratory parameters, such as alkaline phosphatase or carcinoembryonic antigen, may be useful.

Estrogen-containing medication should not be administered to a patient with a history of breast cancer, and pregnancy should be avoided for at least 2 years following completion of treatment.

Abdominal Pain

GENERAL APPROACH

The primary goal in evaluating a patient with acute abdominal pain is to make an earnest effort to determine the diagnosis (Table 41–8). When a diagnosis has been made and the condition of the patient assessed, a decision regarding the need for and timing of operative intervention is possible.

Most adult patients are aware that serious intra-abdominal conditions will require an exploratory laparotomy. This will expose them to the risks of general anesthesia, operative manipulation, and postoperative complications, as well as incapacitate them for 8 to 12 weeks. Recognizing the serious consequences, many patients presenting in the early stages of an acute abdominal illness may minimize their symptoms. Therefore, the physician should approach the patient presenting with abdominal pain in a concerned and compassionate way with attention to the patient's often unstated fears. He should also conduct the subsequent physical examination with the utmost care.

As with most disease processes, a diagnosis is most readily obtained through a comprehensive history, physical examination, appropriate laboratory tests, selected x-ray studies, and, finally, the use of a variety of adjunctive examinations.

The most critical items in the history include the mode of onset and the type, severity, and length of time that the abdominal pain has been present. For example, many of the more serious intra-abdominal conditions requiring emergency operation, such as perforation of a peptic ulcer, a superior mesenteric artery embolus, or rupture of an ectopic pregnancy, are all characterized by sudden onset and persistent severe pain. In contrast, some of the so-called urgent conditions requiring abdominal operation, such as obstruction of the small bowel, appendicitis, or cholecystitis, have a more gradual onset, the pain is moderately severe, and may actually resolve without surgical intervention. Severe abdominal pain of sudden onset that persists beyond 6 hours will most likely require surgical intervention, with the exception of pain in the upper abdomen caused by an intrathoracic process, such as a myocardial infarction, pneumonia, or pulmonary embolus.

In addition to the usual list of questions asked about an individual symptom, the physician should inquire about prior medical diseases that might mimic a surgical condition in the abdomen, the use of steroids that will severely mask intra-abdominal symptoms and often precipitate gastrointestinal perforation, and the self-administration of any antibiotics, which will also suppress the response to an infectious process in the abdomen.

The presence of associated symptoms in the gastrointestinal, genitourinary, and gynecologic systems should also be discussed with the patient. Vomiting, in particular, may reflect obstruction of an involuntary muscular tube (such as the gastrointestinal, biliary, or genitourinary tract) or may simply be a reflex response to irritation of the lining of the gastrointestinal tract.

Finally, the possibility of referred pain should be carefully investigated. Referred pain is that felt by

Table 41–8. SUMMARY OF CLASSIC SYMPTOMS AND SIGNS IN THE ACUTE SURGICAL ABDOMEN

Diagnosis	Symptoms	Signs
Acute appendicitis	Shifting of pain from epigastrium to right lower quadrant Loss of appetite Nausea and vomiting	Right lower quadrant abdominal tenderness
Perforated peptic ulcer	Sudden onset Severe generalized abdominal pain	Board-like rigidity on abdominal palpation Free air on upright x-ray
Intestinal obstruction	Crampy abdominal pain Nausea and vomiting Constipation	High-pitched peristaltic sounds Abdominal distention
Acute cholecystitis	History of biliary colic Right upper quadrant abdominal pain with radiation to right subscapular area	Right upper quadrant abdominal tenderness and guarding Murphy's sign
Acute pancreatitis	History of alcoholism or biliary colic Diffuse upper abdominal pain Persistent nausea and vomiting	Upper abdominal tenderness Elevation of serum or urinary amylase

the patient in one area of the body but which actually originates elsewhere. This migration of pain is based on the overlapping innervation of the two areas. The best known area of referred pain is that felt in the shoulder pad area after perforation of a peptic ulcer in the upper abdomen. Biliary colic from the passage of a gallstone through the cystic duct into the common bile duct is often referred to the right subscapular area, while the pain of acute pancreatitis or renal colic is frequently most severe in the back or flank. Lastly, pain may be referred to the testicle from pathology in the kidney or ureter or both.

In addition to the general observation of the patient, a comprehensive physical examination should emphasize the thorax, abdomen, genitalia, and rectal areas. The bases of the lungs are best auscultated with the patient seated if the patient's level of comfort permits it. Otherwise, the physical examination must be completed with the patient supine. Warming the examiner's hands and the bell of the stethoscope prior to the examination will prevent involuntary contraction of the abdominal muscles.

Examination of the pregnant patient is complicated as the patient nears term, and the physician must be aware that many intra-abdominal organs are displaced by the enlarging uterus. In particular, the location of the appendix is higher on the right side of the abdomen than in the nonpregnant patient.

Finally, it is best to examine an infant under light sedation, and it may be helpful to have the mother hold the child during the examination. Some intra-abdominal conditions, such as acute appendicitis, appear to progress more rapidly in infants and children. For this reason, it is mandatory to obtain a comprehensive examination of the abdomen by distraction, reassurance, and persistence.

The chest is carefully examined to rule out any signs of pneumonia, pleurisy, or a pulmonary embolus that might be suggested by the auscultation of rales or a pleural friction rub. The abdomen is carefully inspected and the presence of any scars, distention, or peristaltic movements of underlying bowel are noted. Auscultation is useful, particularly in patients with obstruction of the small intestine. In such patients, rushes and tinkles heard through the stethoscope at the same time the patient is having crampy abdominal pain is pathognomonic. On palpation, the physician should differentiate between superficial tenderness suggestive of severe peritoneal irritation, deep tenderness suggestive of the early phases of a surgical illness, and, finally, rebound tenderness also suggestive of peritoneal irritation. The patient's genitalia should be carefully examined since incarceration of any of the groin hernias can lead to small intestinal obstruction. Vaginal and rectal examinations are completed near the end of the examination as they are often uncomfortable for the patient. The vaginal examination may confirm the presence of pelvic inflammatory disease, while the rectal examination may suggest the presence of a pelvic abscess in a patient with a ruptured appendix or tenderness from the tip of a pelvic appendicitis.

Despite a comprehensive physical examination, the physician may still be confused about the source and location of the pain in some patients. Additional tests may then be used to help verify the presence of a common process, such as acute appendicitis. In the obturator test, rotation of the flexed thigh of the patient leading to hypogastric pain is suggestive of an inflammatory process adjacent to the fascia over the obturator internus muscle. A positive obturator sign can be caused by perforated appendicitis, local abscess, or an accumulation of fluid in the pelvis. The iliopsoas test is performed with the patient lying on the side opposite from his or her pain and extending the thigh on the affected side. Pain caused by this movement suggests retroperitoneal inflammation in the area of the psoas muscle.

Once the physical examination has been completed, appropriate laboratory tests are ordered, including a complete blood count with a differential, urinalysis, SMA-20, and a serum amylase. In the absence of known medical diseases, such as a coagulopathy, other laboratory tests are usually not indicated.

It is best to obtain both posterior-anterior and

lateral x-rays of the chest as well as flat and upright x-rays of the abdomen. This combination of films will reveal any intrathoracic pathology or the presence of a pneumoperitoneum. Some additional findings of surgical importance that may be revealed by abdominal films include ileus, dilatation of small or large bowel, an appendiceal fecalith, gallstones, thumbprinting on the colon, and elevation of a hemidiaphragm (Field, 1984). A barium or water-soluble iodinated contrast enema may be indicated to document the presence and location of a colonic obstruction. Radionuclide scanning with use of technetium 99m-labeled iminodiacetic acid derivatives is frequently utilized as acute cholecystitis is detected in approximately 98 per cent of cases with a specificity of 100 per cent (Suarez et al., 1980; Taylor et al., 1980). It is of most value when the ultrasound examination of the gallbladder is inconclusive. Computerized tomography scanning is rarely indicated in the diagnostic evaluation of acute abdominal pain but may be necessary should the pain become more chronic and the diagnosis remain unclear.

Finally, diagnostic adjuncts such as real-time ultrasound, diagnostic peritoneal lavage, and laparoscopy have been used with increasing frequency in recent years. The use of ultrasound is well recognized in patients with suspected symptomatic cholelithiasis, choledocholithiasis, pancreatitis, and, in recent years, acute appendicitis (Adams et al., 1988; Jeffrey et al., 1988). Diagnostic peritoneal lavage, a technique borrowed from trauma surgeons, appears to be useful in patients with abdominal pain and an altered sensorium, advanced age, or multiple medical problems (Richardson et al., 1983; Hoffman et al., 1988). The technique is performed by placing a nasogastric tube and urinary catheter in the patient to be evaluated and then making a short midline incision under local anesthesia approximately one third of the way down from the umbilicus. The peritoneal cavity is entered under direct vision and a peritoneal dialysis catheter is inserted. If blood-stained, purulent, or bile-stained, fluid is obtained, the diagnostic peritoneal tap is considered to be positive. Should the tap be nonrevealing, 1000 cc. of normal saline solution is infused into the peritoneal cavity. The patient is then rolled from side to side to ensure adequate mixing of the peritoneal fluid and the lavage fluid, and an effluent is removed through the siphon effect. A quantitative analysis of the effluent, which reveals cell counts > 100,000 RBC per mm.^{3} or > 500 WBC per mm.^{3} or organisms on a Gram's stain, is considered to be a positive lavage. Finally, diagnostic laparoscopy allows for an earlier diagnosis and institution of appropriate therapy for diseases of the female reproductive tract that simulate appendicitis (Whitworth et al., 1988).

Once a tentative diagnosis for the abdominal pain is established, the second major decision is whether or not surgery is indicated. Surgery will be indicated in the vast majority of conditions causing severe and persistent pain, with the exception of acute edematous pancreatitis that is treated conservatively.

Table 41–9. NEED FOR OPERATION IN PATIENTS WITH ABDOMINAL PAIN (NONTRAUMA)

Emergency Conditions (Immediate Operation)
- Gastrointestinal perforation
  - Appendicitis
  - Peptic ulcer
  - Colonic diverticulosis
- Intestinal infarction
  - Embolism or thrombosis of superior mesenteric artery
  - Strangulation (hernia; volvulus)
- Intra-abdominal hemorrhage
  - Ectopic pregnancy
  - Abdominal aortic aneurysm

Urgent Conditions (Surgery Within 6–10 Hours)
- Gastrointestinal obstruction
  - Adhesions
  - Incarcerated hernia
  - Tumor
- Acute inflammation
  - Appendicitis
  - Cholecystitis
- Gynecologic lesions
  - Twisted ovarian cyst
  - Twisted, pedunculated fibroid

The final decision for the physician is the timing of an operation should surgical intervention be necessary. Abdominal conditions requiring operation are generally described as either *emergent* (require immediate operation as soon as rapid resuscitation is performed) or *urgent* (operation delayed for 6 to 10 hours as patient is stabilized or prepared for surgery) (Table 41–9).

DIFFERENTIAL DIAGNOSIS—GENERAL

The most common acute abdominal conditions requiring laparotomy involve the gastrointestinal and biliary tracts (Table 41–10). There are, however, other medical and surgical conditions that will cause acute abdominal pain; hence, every attempt should be made to determine an accurate diagnosis in the individual patient.

A differential diagnosis is often suggested by the mode of onset or the severity of symptoms that the

Table 41–10. ABDOMINAL CONDITIONS (NONTRAUMA) REQUIRING EMERGENCY OPERATION IN 341 CONSECUTIVE PATIENTS, BEN TAUB GENERAL HOSPITAL, HOUSTON, TEXAS*

Condition	Number	Per Cent
Acute appendicitis	126	36.9
Intestinal obstruction	120	35.2
Perforated ulcer	28	8.2
Acute cholecystitis	21	6.2
Abscess	15	4.4
Pancreatitis	7	2.1
Diverticulitis	5	1.5
Others	19	5.5

*Modified from Jordan, G. L.: Adv. Surg., *14*:259–308, 1980.

patient describes. For example, patients who develop acute abdominal pain in the central abdomen are often found to have problems such as appendicitis or an obstruction of the small bowel; however, nonsurgical conditions (such as gastritis, enteritis, or edematous pancreatitis) may be present. *Severe* central abdominal pain associated with signs of shock is more likely to be caused by a mesenteric vascular catastrophe, intra-abdominal hemorrhage, or a more severe form of pancreatitis such as the necrotizing type.

Patients with severe central abdominal pain and a rigid abdominal wall are usually found to have a perforation of a peptic ulcer or some other lesion in the intestinal tract. Progressive abdominal pain associated with vomiting and distention, but without rigidity of the abdominal wall, is usually caused by obstruction of the small intestine or gastritis. Finally, patients who develop progressive abdominal pain associated with vomiting, increasing distention, and constipation frequently have an obstruction of the large bowel.

The differential diagnosis can also be based on the location of the abdominal pain. The most common location for abdominal pain is in the right lower quadrant. Acute appendicitis, regional ileitis, pyelonephritis, and pelvic inflammatory disease frequently present in this quadrant. The second most common location for abdominal pain is in the right upper quadrant where surgical problems (such as a penetrating or perforated duodenal ulcer, acute cholecystitis or choledocholithiasis, and a high appendicitis) may present. Medical conditions that may also cause pain in the right upper quadrant include right lower lobe bronchopneumonia, a pulmonary embolus, or pleurisy. The third most common location for abdominal pain is the left lower quadrant. In middle-aged or elderly male patients, sigmoid diverticulitis is the most likely diagnosis while ovarian pathology may present in this location in a female of reproductive age. Finally, left upper quadrant pain, relatively rare in the experience of most physicians, may be caused by a perforated gastric ulcer with soilage toward the left hemidiaphragm or spontaneous rupture of the spleen secondary to infectious mononucleosis.

DIFFERENTIAL DIAGNOSIS—SPECIFIC

Acute Appendicitis

This entity continues to be the most commonly encountered surgical condition of the abdomen in family practice. The majority of patients are in the second or third decade, and the disease is relatively uncommon in children under the age of 5. The disease tends to rapidly progress to perforation in children but may present more indolently with nonspecific symptoms in elderly patients, leading to significant morbidity and mortality associated with a delayed diagnosis.

To avoid the problems related to a missed diagnosis of acute appendicitis, especially one with perforation, it is generally accepted that surgery should be performed even when the diagnosis may not be completely clear; hence, approximately 15 to 20 per cent of appendectomies will result in the excision of a normal appendix. Conditions that may mimic the symptoms of appendicitis include mesenteric lymphadenitis, Meckel's diverticulitis, cecal diverticulitis, regional enteritis, passage of a right ureteral stone, acute pyelonephritis, *Campylobacter* ileocolitis, or *Yersinia* enteritis.

Diagnosis. The onset of acute appendicitis is often heralded by a day or two of malaise preceding the attack of abdominal pain. The patient may also notice some indigestion or gastritis as well as irregular bowel movements. Both constipation and diarrhea have been described, with the diarrhea presumably related to irritation of the rectosigmoid colon or rectum by the inflamed appendix. Most patients present with a reasonably classic progression of symptoms. Many awaken at night with the original symptom—a deep aching or ill-defined epigastric or periumbilical pain. Obstruction of the base of the appendix with either a fecalith or enlarged lymphatic tissue will then lead to nausea and vomiting, which is common in patients with distention of any hollow viscus. It is also at this point that the patient develops anorexia. The third symptom in progression is movement of the pain to the right lower quadrant as discrete peritonitis develops in the periappendiceal area. The location of pain will, of course, depend upon where the appendix is located. A retrocecal appendix may produce flank or loin pain and tenderness on physical examination associated with a positive psoas sign, while a pelvic appendix may present with continuing rectal symptoms and tenderness on the rectal examination. The patient's temperature will rise to 100 to 101°F. by the time he or she has developed right lower quadrant pain. Finally, leukocytosis in the range of 12,000 to 15,000/$mm.^3$ is usually noted when laboratory examinations are returned. Leukocytosis greater than 15,000/$mm.^3$ or a temperature significantly above 100 to 101° F. is atypical for uncomplicated appendicitis and suggests the possibility of rupture and peritonitis or abscess.

The diagnosis in young children or elderly patients can be extremely difficult. Classically, the young child is anorectic, lies quietly, and is quite irritable. Vomiting is usually prominent, and diarrhea is present in approximately 10 per cent of the patients. In the elderly patient, few symptoms other than indigestion and some abdominal distention may be present when the patient first visits his physician.

The presence of deep and rebound tenderness in the right lower quadrant, usually beneath the middle of a line between the umbilicus and the anterior superior iliac spine, is most characteristic of acute appendicitis. Significant tachycardia, shallow respirations, fever, and involuntary guarding suggest rupture with diffuse peritoneal contamination. Tenderness on rectal examination may suggest the presence of a retrocecal appendix or a pelvic abscess secondary to perforation.

As appendicitis is so common, but the diagnosis so often delayed in an outpatient setting, a number of diagnostic scoring systems have been developed in recent years (Teicher et al., 1983). Some authors have also attempted to define the reasons for delays in diagnosis (Buchman and Zuidema, 1984). The greatest recent advance in the diagnosis of acute appendicitis has been the use of high-resolution real-time ultrasonography (Adams et al., 1988; Jeffrey et al., 1988). A recent review of 250 patients with suspected appendicitis concluded that an adult patient without compelling clinical findings or a fecalith and with a maximal appendiceal diameter < 6 mm. should undergo a period of observation rather than immediate surgery (Jeffrey et al., 1988). Finally, diagnostic laparoscopy is used on many gynecologic and on some general surgery services to evaluate right lower quadrant pain in young women as previously noted (Whitworth et al., 1988).

Treatment. During the work-up of the patient with right lower quadrant pain suggestive of appendicitis, it is worthwhile to insert a nasogastric tube when vomiting is present and start an infusion of intravenous fluids for rehydration. When operation is indicated, broad-spectrum antibiotics with both aerobic and anaerobic coverage should be started in case perforation has occurred. The bacterial organisms that are most commonly found in patients with ruptured appendicitis include *E. coli*, enterococcus, and *B. fragilis*. While antibiotic combinations, such as gentamicin-clindamycin, have been used in the past, second- or third-generation cephalosporin antibiotics, such as cefoxitin or cefotaxime, have been used as single agents in recent years. It should be recognized, however, that cephalosporins do not adequately cover enterococci.

In the operating room, a short transverse incision is made lateral to the right rectus muscle, somewhat above the anterior superior iliac spine. The inflamed appendix is excised completely, the stump ligated or buried within the cecum, and the abdominal incision is treated depending upon the preference of the surgeon. Many surgeons choose to pack the subcutaneous tissue and skin of the incision open for a 5 to 6 day period when either acute gangrenous appendicitis with local or free perforation or an intra-abdominal abscess is found. Following the period of conversion of the bacterial flora in the open wound, a delayed primary closure can be performed prior to discharge from the hospital.

In the postoperative period, the nasogastric tube can often be removed on the day of operation, and oral feedings begun. Intravenous antibiotics are maintained only if the patient had an acute gangrenous appendicitis with or without perforation (Berne et al., 1982). In the former case, intravenous antibiotics are continued for 1 to 2 days in the postoperative period. Patients with diffuse peritonitis are generally treated for a 5 to 7 day period and then observed in the hospital for 24 to 48 hours following the cessation of the antibiotics. The physician's obligations in the postoperative period include carefully observing for the development of a wound infection, documenting that the patient's preoperative leukocytosis has resolved by the time antibiotic therapy is completed, and performing a rectal examination to verify that a pelvic abscess has not started to form should the patient still be in the hospital 4 or 5 days after surgery.

On occasion, a right lower quadrant or gutter abscess related to a previous perforation of an inflamed appendix will be so large that only drainage of the abscess can be performed at the first operation. If the appendix cannot be found at the original procedure, intra-abdominal drains are placed into the abscess cavity. If desired, an interval appendectomy is performed 6 weeks later.

Perforated Peptic Ulcer

In recent years, with the well-documented decline in the incidence of acid-peptic disease in men, fewer patients require operation. It is also true, however, that perforation of a peptic ulcer continues to account for about 15 per cent of all ulcer operations performed in general hospitals. Perforation occurs in approximately 5 to 10 per cent of patients with duodenal ulcers and is the first indication of an ulcer in about 2 per cent of patients.

Perforated Peptic Ulcer—Diagnosis. Patients with perforation of an acid-peptic ulcer note the sudden onset of severe, agonizing epigastric pain that may move to the right upper quadrant and subsequently involves the entire peritoneal cavity. In many patients, the acute perforation is preceded by at least several days of typical ulcer pain.

On physical examination, the abdominal wall is rigid and markedly tender in all quadrants, and hypoactive or absent bowel signs are noted. The diagnosis is generally confirmed by performing an upright abdominal x-ray study that shows free intraperitoneal air in approximately 70 to 75 per cent of patients. Should the patient have a history and symptoms compatible with perforation of a peptic ulcer, but free air is not present on the upright abdominal film, it may be worthwhile to insert a nasogastric tube. Then, either some air or water-soluble contrast material is gently injected to help document perforation rather than deep penetration.

Treatment. There continue to be isolated reports of nonsurgical treatment for patients with documented perforation of a peptic ulcer. This form of therapy should be reserved for patients who are truly too sick to undergo operation or for those whose presentation is so late that the perforation has sealed and the patient's symptoms are already resolving. In the remainder of patients, early operation is indicated as it confirms the diagnosis, allows for vigorous lavage of the peritoneal cavity, and eliminates a site of spillage from the gastrointestinal tract.

There is some controversy about the most appropriate operation for the patient with a perforated duodenal ulcer. Large review series in the past have documented that if patching with viable omentum alone is performed, two thirds of the patients will develop recurrent symptoms in the future and one half of these will eventually require a second operation (Jordan et al., 1974). For this reason, many centers have chosen to restrict the use of omental patching to patients with severe concomitant medical illnesses, intra-abdominal abscesses or severe peritonitis, or in those in whom the ulcer history is acute (less than 3 months) or medication induced. Other patients with more chronic histories, less contamination, and no other medical problems are probably best treated with a definitive operation. Truncal vagotomy and pyloroplasty have been used as definitive procedures in some centers (Kirkpatrick and Bouwman, 1980), while truncal vagotomy and antrectomy have been popular in others (Feliciano et al., 1984; Feliciano, 1987). In recent years, there have been a large number of reports about the usefulness of omental closure of the perforation followed by parietal cell vagotomy. In a recent series in which one half of the patients with perforation underwent closure and parietal cell vagotomy, the cumulative recurrence rate for a duodenal ulcer was 10.6 per cent at 3 years (Boey et al., 1988). Should the surgeon choose to use omental patch closure only for the perforation, then it is imperative to place the patient on vigorous antiulcer medical therapy in the postoperative period and schedule the patient for endoscopic follow-up within 4 to 8 weeks.

Patients with perforated gastric ulcers tend to be older, contamination is frequently greater, and the mortality for emergency operation is somewhat higher than in patients with perforated duodenal ulcers. While omental patching has been recommended by some, it is clear from recent data that definitive operation with resection of the area of perforation is well tolerated and curative in properly selected patients (Hodnett et al., 1988).

Intestinal Obstruction

Intestinal obstruction accounts for approximately 35 per cent of patients coming to operation for abdominal pain (see Table 41–10). In 75 per cent of patients with gastrointestinal obstruction, the small bowel is the primary site and, in one half of these, adhesions are the cause (Table 41–11). In contrast, approximately 70 per cent of obstructions of the large intestine are secondary to the presence of a colorectal carcinoma. The major source of morbidity and mortality in patients with intestinal obstruction is the added complication of strangulation of the area of obstruction, occurring in approximately 10 per cent of patients with a 30 per cent mortality.

Intestinal obstruction is an urgent surgical problem because of the tremendous loss of fluid into the bowel. This loss of fluid coupled with edema of the wall of the intestine, transudation of intraluminal fluid into the peritoneal cavity, vomiting, and nasogastric suction all contribute to profound dehydration and electrolyte imbalances in the patient who has been ill with an intestinal obstruction for several days. Should strangulation occur, more fluid is sequestered and lost in both the mesentery and the mesenteric veins.

Table 41–11. COMMON CAUSES OF MECHANICAL INTESTINAL OBSTRUCTION

	Small Bowel	Large Bowel
Adults	Adhesive bands* External hernia* Metastatic cancer Operative complications*	Colorectal cancer Diverticulitis Sigmoid and cecal volvulus*
Children	Incarcerated hernia* Intussusception* Meckel's diverticulum* Volvulus*	Hirschsprung's disease
Neonates	Intestinal atresia Midgut volvulus* Meconium ileus	Imperforate anus Hirschsprung's disease

*Risk of strangulation present.

Diagnosis. A patient with obstruction of the small bowel gradually develops epigastric or periumbilical pain that progresses to episodes of colicky pain lasting for 3 to 5 minutes at a time. This is associated with vomiting, constipation, and abdominal distention. Should the colicky pain change to steady pain, a closed loop obstruction (such as might be seen with an incarcerated hernia or volvulus) should be suspected.

On inspection of the abdomen, the presence of abdominal scars or hernias should be noted. Auscultation will reveal the presence of hyperactive and high-pitched bowel sounds (rushes and tinkles) associated with periods of colicky pain. On palpation, there may be localized tenderness over a dilated loop of small bowel or a palpable mass suggestive of a volvulus. In a child, the palpation of a sausage-shaped mass on the right lower quadrant strongly suggests the presence of ileocolic intussusception.

A routine blood count and urinalysis will often reveal an increased hematocrit as well as an increase in urine specific gravity, both reflective of dehydration. A leukocytosis and elevated amylase will also be present, particularly if the patient has a strangulation obstruction as well.

A flat plate of the abdomen in the patient with obstruction of the small bowel will show dilated loops of small intestine in the absence of colonic gas (Fig. 41–2), while the upright film will reveal multiple air-fluid levels. Depending on the number of dilated loops, the level of the obstruction may be estimated. In the patient with obstruction of the colon and an incompetent ileocecal valve, dilation of the colon and small intestine will be seen (Fig. 41–3). A barium or water-soluble iodinated contrast enema will document the level and extent of the obstruction.

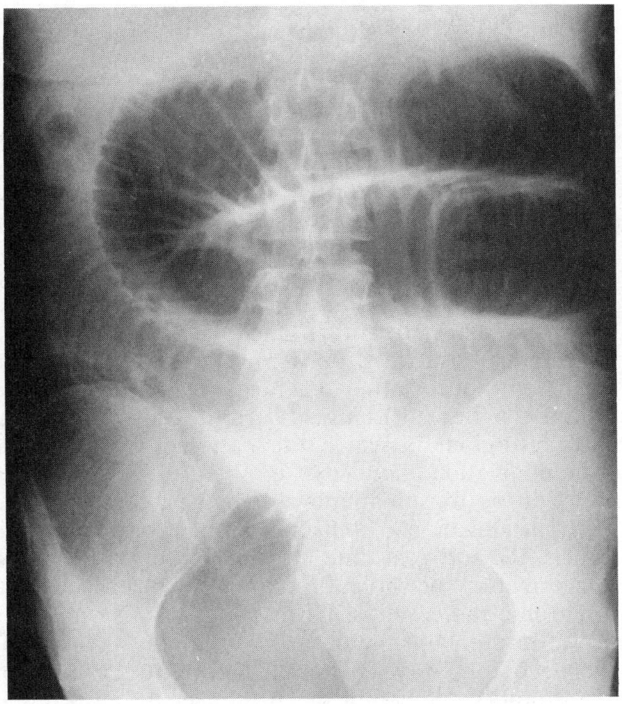

Figure 41–2. Flat plate showing small bowel obstruction.

Treatment. The priorities in treatment for the patient with a severe mechanical bowel obstruction are decompression of the proximal dilated bowel and restoration of fluid and electrolyte balance. A nasogastric tube is inserted, and intravenous fluids are infused until the patient is voiding 30 to 50 ml. of urine per hour. Potassium supplements are not placed in the intravenous resuscitation fluid until a good urine output is obtained.

If the patient has not passed flatus or has not had a bowel movement for a prolonged period of time, then a complete bowel obstruction is assumed to be present. In such a patient, an operation should be undertaken as soon as resuscitation has been completed. An early operation is also recommended for those patients who develop a closed loop obstruction, have a stepladder appearance of multiple dilated loops of small bowel on their abdominal x-ray, or who have any signs of strangulation obstruction. There is, however, a role for nasogastric or long tube (Miller-Abbott, Baker, Leonard, etc.) decompression in certain patients who have had multiple abdominal operations and previous episodes of partial small bowel obstruction (Bizer et al., 1981). Many of these patients will be able to describe how a previous episode of partial small bowel obstruction responded to conservative therapy with the passage of a short or long decompressing tube. There is no clear-cut evidence that the use of a long tube prevents any more operations than a nasogastric tube does, and this is particularly true in patients in whom the long tube never passes through the pylorus. If a long tube passes through the pylorus and the patient's symptoms do not resolve within 24 hours, then operation is indicated. Because of the possibility of strangulation obstruction in any patient with a small bowel obstruction, intravenous antibiotics covering both aerobic and anaerobic organisms are given in the preoperative period.

The most common cause of a small bowel obstruction is adhesions from a previous intra-abdominal operation, and these should be divided with a combination of sharp and blunt dissection (Hofstetter, 1981). Also, many surgeons will decompress the dilated loops of proximal bowel by squeezing intraluminal fluid back into the stomach where it can be aspirated with a large-bore tube. The second most common finding at operation for a small bowel obstruction is the presence of an inguinal or femoral hernia with an incarcerated loop of small bowel. The incarcerated bowel is reduced from the hernia ring, and its viability is determined. If the segment of small bowel is viable, a herniorrhaphy is then generally performed through the same incision. If the incarcerated bowel is necrotic, then the surgeon may perform a formal hernia repair but should pack the subcutaneous tissue and skin open.

An obstructing colorectal cancer is generally best treated with a proximal colostomy to allow for decompression and formal preparation of the colon (bowel prep) prior to an elective resection of the

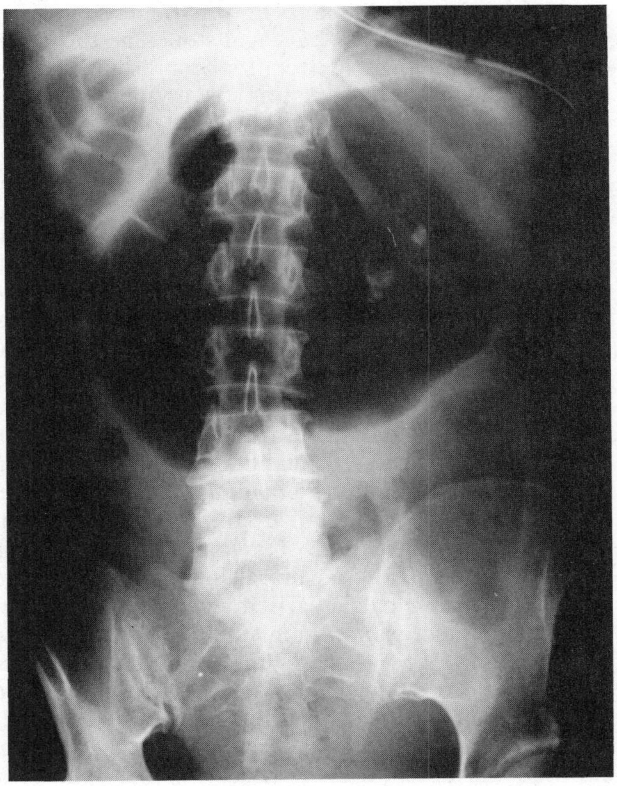

Figure 41–3. Flat plate of abdomen showing large bowel obstruction.

neoplasm within 10 to 14 days. If a sigmoid volvulus cannot be reduced in the preoperative period, it must be untwisted at laparotomy. A sigmoidopexy to the left lower quadrant peritoneum is then performed, or a rectal tube is placed through the anus to keep the sigmoid colon in place until an elective procedure can be performed after a colon prep within the next 10 days. A strangulated sigmoid volvulus is resected with creation of an end sigmoid colostomy and an oversewn distal rectal pouch. On the right side of the colon, incidental carcinoma is generally resected with a right hemicolectomy and an end-to-end ileotransversostomy, even without a bowel prep.

Cholelithiasis/Acute Cholecystitis

Approximately 20 million Americans have gallstones, and it is estimated that another million develop gallstones each year. At this time, there are approximately 700,000 cholecystectomies performed each year in the United States, thereby making it the most commonly performed intra-abdominal operation for the general surgeon.

Approximately 80 per cent of the gallstones seen in the United States are at least partially composed of cholesterol. The supersaturation of bile with cholesterol leads to precipitation of cholesterol crystals that subsequently act as a nidus for stone formation. Dietary modification alone does not appear to influence the incidence of cholesterol stones or mixed stones containing cholesterol.

Approximately 95 per cent of patients presenting with acute cholecystitis have gallstones as the etiology. The remaining 5 per cent who present with so-called acalculous cholecystitis have almost always suffered major trauma or undergone a major operation, associated with blood transfusion and the use of total parenteral nutrition in the postoperative period.

Diagnosis. There is a great deal of confusion with the terminology used to describe acute gallbladder problems. Biliary colic classically is paroxysmal pain associated with migration of gallstones into the cystic duct, resulting in temporary occlusion of the duct. The term has also been applied to attacks of dyspepsia, belching, nausea, or vomiting following a meal rich in fat. Should the stone remain in the cystic duct, the patient may have a more prolonged attack with steady epigastric or right upper quadrant pain radiating to the right subscapular area—a condition usually known as acute cholecystitis. The basic pathophysiology is obstruction of a hollow viscus that is trying to empty and transmural inflammation of the wall of the viscus, particularly if bacteria are present.

On physical examination, the patient with acute cholecystitis has voluntary guarding and tenderness in the right upper quadrant associated with a positive Murphy's sign and, on occasion, a palpable gallbladder. Laboratory tests will reveal leukocytosis, an elevated bilirubin (usually under 3.5 mg. per dl.), and perhaps an elevation of alkaline phosphatase and amylase.

It is important to make an accurate diagnosis in the patient with either biliary colic or acute cholecystitis as secondary complications (such as empyema, gangrene, or perforation of the gallbladder and formation of a pericholecystic abscess) can result from extension of the original attack.

The history, physical examination, and laboratory tests may all suggest the presence of some pathology in the biliary tree; however, documentation of the presence of gallstones will usually confirm the diagnosis of either biliary colic or acute cholecystitis. Only 15 to 20 per cent of gallstones are radiopaque and can be visualized on a routine flat plate of the abdomen; hence, other diagnostic tests are indicated in most patients (Laing, 1984). A traditional oral cholecystogram in which the patient ingests tablets containing radiopaque dye is not used in the acute situation as most patients are nauseated and some have an elevation of bilirubin as part of their acute attack. Rather, real-time ultrasonography is now the imaging study of choice in patients with either acute or chronic cholecystitis. Ultrasonography is especially useful in pregnant patients and children, as it avoids the need for x-ray exposure. The accuracy rate for ultrasound in detecting the presence of gallstones is approximately 90 to 95 per cent, with a 5 per cent false-negative rate. Ultrasound may also be useful in diagnosing a thickening of the wall of the gallbladder in patients with acute cholecystitis or the pericholecystic fluid collection in a patient with perforation. Finally, ultrasound can assess the diameter of the extrahepatic biliary ducts, as well as the presence of stones in these ducts.

In a patient with a suspected diagnosis of acute cholecystitis, but the absence of stones on an ultrasound, it may be worthwhile to order a radionuclide study such as a HIDA or PIPIDA scan (Hoffmann et al., 1988; Whitworth et al., 1988). These radioisotope scans will ordinarily show rapid filling of the gallbladder in a patient with a patent cystic duct. If the gallbladder does not fill with the radioisotope when the patient's gallbladder has been emptied by food in the gastrointestinal tract or the use of intravenous cholecystokinin, then acute cholecystitis is likely.

Treatment. The treatment of either biliary colic or acute cholecystitis includes the insertion of a nasogastric tube, administration of intravenous fluids, use of intravenous antibiotics with high biliary tract penetration, and early consultation with a surgeon. With rapid resolution of an attack of biliary colic, there is no urgency for cholecystectomy and operation can be performed at the patient's convenience. Using modern techniques of operation and postoperative care, discharge from the hospital within 24 hours of elective cholecystectomy can be expected in many patients (Moss, 1986). If the patient has acute cholecystitis and the attack persists for several days, then early surgical intervention on a semielective basis is worthwhile. This is particularly true if the patient is young and healthy or lives remote from medical care.

If an operation is chosen and if the patient is in reasonably stable condition, a cholecystectomy performed through an upper abdominal incision is the procedure of choice. Excision of an acutely inflamed gallbladder may be somewhat more difficult technically than excision of one that is not acutely inflamed. If the patient is thought to be too ill to tolerate a major abdominal operation under general anesthesia, then a small abdominal incision performed under local anesthesia can be made and a cholecystostomy performed. The stones in the gallbladder are extracted with stone forceps, and a drainage tube is inserted into the fundus of the gallbladder and fixed to the abdominal wall. Cholecystectomy can be performed when the patient's overall condition is improved. Finally, as common bile duct stones are present in approximately 15 to 18 per cent of those undergoing cholecystectomy, the surgeon must decide on whether to perform a cystic duct cholangiogram or proceed immediately to a common bile duct exploration. The only absolute indications for common bile duct exploration are a palpable stone in the common hepatic or bile duct or severe jaundice associated with a massively dilated bile duct. All other suggested indications (such as mild jaundice, recent history of gallstone pancreatitis, the presence of multiple small stones, and a large cystic duct) are considered to be relative indications for a common bile duct exploration. In patients with any of these, it is best to perform a cholangiogram first to verify the need for this procedure before proceeding with a common bile duct exploration for extraction of the stone. A rubber T-tube is inserted at completion, the common bile duct is sutured tightly around it, and a completion T-tube cholangiogram is performed before the patient leaves the operating room.

The family physician is frequently confronted with other patients who have had one episode of abdominal pain from biliary colic that resolved spontaneously. Patients with previous symptoms of biliary tract disease eventually have to undergo biliary tract operation 44 per cent of the time (McSherry et al., 1985). Hence, it is recommended that patients who develop any symptoms of abdominal pain from gallstones should have some type of therapy while they are still young and healthy. Alternative forms of therapy include oral agents (chenodiol or urssodiol) to dissolve cholesterol gallstones (Pitt et al., 1987), the use of percutaneous infusion of methyl tert-butyl ether into the gallbladder to dissolve cholesterol gallstones (Allen et al., 1985), and, finally, the use of biliary lithotripsy (Burhenne et al., 1988; Stahlgren, 1988).

Acute Pancreatitis

Acute pancreatitis as a cause of abdominal pain is a common indication for admission to general hospitals, but the need for operative intervention is rare. Acute alcoholism and gallstones cause most attacks of acute pancreatitis, with trauma, hyperlipemia, medications, etc. accounting for the remainder. Approximately 10 to 30 per cent of attacks have no obvious cause and are considered to be idiopathic.

There is a morphologic gradation of lesions in acute pancreatitis ranging from interstitial edema and mild peripancreatic fat necrosis (acute edematous) to parenchymal hemorrhage and necrosis with severe intrapancreatic and peripancreatic fat necrosis (acute hemorrhagic or necrotizing) (Singer and Gyr, 1985).

Diagnosis. Patients complain of steady, severe epigastric pain boring through to their backs and, usually, complains of nausea and persistent vomiting. They often have some hypertension and a low-grade fever. Examination of the abdomen reveals voluntary guarding, epigastric tenderness, and hypoactive bowel sounds. The diagnosis is strongly suggested by hyperamylasemia, hyperlipasemia, and an elevated 1-hour urinary amylase level; however, it is recognized that hyperamylasemia may be secondary to stimulation of salivary gland secretion by the ingestion of alcohol. When the diagnosis is in doubt, measurement of an amylase-to-creatinine clearance has been suggested, but this is nonspecific as well (Murray and Mackay, 1977). In rare instances, it may be necessary to separate serum isoamylases or measure a serum immunoreactive trypsin level.

Amylase levels in acute pancreatitis are usually higher than those found in patients with perforated peptic ulcers, strangulation obstruction, or acute cholecystitis. Also, amylase levels in patients with gallstone pancreatitis are initially higher and decrease more rapidly than those in patients with acute alcoholic pancreatitis (Hiatt et al., 1987).

The combination of certain physical and laboratory findings can be used as a prognostic indicator of the severity of an attack of acute pancreatitis. At the time of admission or diagnosis, these Ranson signs or criteria are age $>$ 55 years, WBC $>$ 16000 per mm^3, glucose $>$ 200 mg. per dl., LDH $>$ 350 mg. per dl., and SGOT $>$ 250 units. During the initial 48 hours, other Ranson signs are hematocrit falls $>$ 10 per cent, BUN rises $>$ 5 mg. per dl., calcium $<$ 8 mg. per dl., arterial $PO_2 < 60$ mm Hg, base deficit $>$ 4 mEq. per L., and estimated fluid sequestration $>$ 6000 ml. (Martin et al., 1984). The mortality rates for patients with 0 to 2 signs = 0.9 per cent, 3 to 4 = 16 per cent, 5 to 6 = 40 per cent, and 7 to 8 = 100 per cent in Ranson's 1974 report (Ranson et al., 1974).

The plain film of the abdomen may show a paralytic ileus or one dilated loop of small bowel (sentinel loop) in the upper abdomen. If calcifications are noted in the area of the pancreas, underlying chronic pancreatitis is likely. Either ultrasonography or computerized tomographic scanning can be used to document the type of pathology present in the pancreas and the progression of the disease process during a prolonged attack. A number of studies have documented that there is no correlation between the initial serum amylase level and the extent of the pancreatic process on computerized tomography (Clavien, 1988).

Treatment. The treatment of edematous pancreatitis is to make the patient NPO, insert a nasogastric tube, maintain normal hydration and electrolyte levels, and treat the epigastric pain with meperidine, which seems to cause less spasm of the sphincter of Oddi than morphine. Prospective randomized studies on the use of a nasogastric tube, cimetidine, anticholinergics, and aprotinin have shown no change in outcome with these adjuncts (Crist, 1987). The use of fresh frozen plasma, 5-fluorouracil, prostaglandins, somatostatin, glucagon, and heparin remains unclear at this time.

When Ranson's or other criteria suggest the presence of severe acute pancreatitis, the patient should be admitted to the intensive care unit because of possible pulmonary, cardiac, metabolic, renal, and hematologic problems. Intubation, ionotropic support, massive infusion of calcium, fluid resuscitation, and correction of coagulopathies may all be necessary. In the past, therapeutic peritoneal lavage has been suggested to improve the prognosis, but a recent randomized controlled clinical trial (Mayer et al., 1985) resulted in no decrease in complications or mortality.

Operative intervention is indicated in patients with progressive deterioration, sepsis originating in a pancreatic phlegmon or necrotizing pancreatitis, or a pancreatic abscess (Martin et al., 1984). The two most common approaches have been ostomy and drainage versus subtotal pancreatic resection. Ostomy and drainage refers to the insertion of gastrostomy, jejunostomy, and cholecystostomy tubes as well as peripancreatic drains. It allows for the removal of the nasogastric tube, feeding into the midgut, and decompression of the biliary tract (Lawson et al., 1970). Subtotal pancreatectomy has been used especially in England, France, Finland, and Germany (Beger et al., 1985) with an operative mortality of 25 to 40 per cent. Finally, the newest approach to patients with infected pancreatic necrosis or a pancreatic abscess is controlled open lesser sac drainage (open packing), which has resulted in a mortality of 11 to 18 per cent in recent studies (Pemberton et al., 1986; Bradley, 1987).

Gastrointestinal Bleeding

UPPER GASTROINTESTINAL BLEEDING

Upper gastrointestinal bleeding is suggested by the passage of melanotic stools or hematemesis. Also, it is generally accepted that massive bleeding from a duodenal ulcer in the foregut can also lead to the passage of bright red blood per the rectum, which is more commonly caused by lesions in the small bowel or colon.

In recent years, the most common causes of hemorrhage from the upper gastrointestinal tract have been peptic ulcer disease, which accounts for approximately 45 per cent of all patients seen, and acute erosive gastritis, which accounts for another 23 per cent (Table 41–12) (Silverstein et al., 1981; Greenburg, 1985). Bleeding from esophageal varices or Mallory-Weiss tears is much less common.

The major goals for the physician caring for the patient with upper gastrointestinal hemorrhage are to first treat the sequelae of the hemorrhage (such as hypovolemic shock), diagnose the source of the hemorrhage, and, finally, decide on whether surgical therapy is indicated.

Diagnosis

A careful history in the patient with upper gastrointestinal bleeding should include questions about a previous history of peptic ulcer disease, operations for the same problem, chronic alcoholism, previous episodes of hemorrhage, any history of a coagulation disorder, and whether or not vomiting or retching preceded an episode of hematemesis. The patient should also be carefully questioned about the recent ingestion of hemorrhage-inducing medications, such as aspirin or nonsteroidals, phenylbutazone, anticoagulants, or steroids.

On physical examination, the presence of epigastric tenderness would be suggestive of peptic ulcer disease, while the presence of a mass in the same location would more likely be a gastric carcinoma. The presence of hepatomegaly and splenomegaly is strongly suggestive of chronic alcoholic cirrhosis, while the presence of splenomegaly alone is more suggestive of a hematologic disorder or splenic vein thrombosis related to chronic pancreatitis.

It should be obvious that certain therapeutic maneuvers will have to be instituted as the history is taken from the patient. A nasogastric or large-bore tube is usually inserted shortly after admission. This tube will allow for the evacuation of clots from the upper gastrointestinal tract, aid in monitoring the rate of continuing hemorrhage, and allow for the infusion of agents that may help control mucosal hemorrhage. Once the stomach has been cleared by irrigation, fiberoptic endoscopy is indicated to define and localize the lesion (American Society for Gastrointestinal Endoscopy, 1988). It is true that numerous studies have shown no difference in outcome whether or not early endoscopy was performed; however, a decision on the need for and choice of surgical intervention

Table 41–12. CAUSES OF UPPER GASTROINTESTINAL HEMORRHAGE

Cause	Per Cent
Duodenal ulcer	24.3
Gastric erosion	23.4
Gastric ulcer	21.3
Esophageal varices	10.3
Mallory-Weiss tear	7.3

Modified from Silverstein, F. E., Gilbert, D. A., Tedesco, F. J., et al.: Gastrointest. Endosc. *27*:73–79, 1981.

following stabilization is easier to make if the site of hemorrhage has been identified. Fiberoptic endoscopy can be effective even if active hemorrhage is occurring. Important areas to be visualized are the distal esophagus for esophageal varices or a Mallory-Weiss tear, the lesser curvature of the stomach for a benign gastric ulcer at the incisura, the greater curvature of the stomach for an atypical gastric ulcer related to medication or malignancy, and the duodenal bulb for the presence of an actively bleeding duodenal ulcer.

Treatment

Once the stomach and upper duodenum have been emptied of the clot and a precise diagnosis made, medical therapy can be instituted in the patient who is hemodynamically stable or who has stopped bleeding. Should a duodenal or gastric ulcer be the source of hemorrhage, then a vigorous medical regimen of H_2 blockers and antacids can be used to lower the volume of acid secretion in the stomach and neutralize any residual acid that is present (Pingleton, 1983). An alternative approach for the treatment of a peptic ulcer is to use sucralfate, which will protect any injured mucosa from further damage by acid or bile. If acute erosive gastritis is present on endoscopy, then continued lavage of the stomach with iced saline through the nasogastric tube may be useful to cause some vasoconstriction of the gastric mucosa; however, some believe that this may make the gastric mucosa more susceptible to stress ulceration. When bleeding is controlled, a vigorous program of antacid administration coupled with H_2 blockers will once again allow for healing. It should also be remembered that acute erosive gastritis is frequently representative of other problems, such as atelectasis or pulmonary sepsis in the thorax or the presence of an occult intra-abdominal abscess in the abdomen. As acute erosive gastritis is somewhat difficult to manage at operation, continued hemorrhage can be treated by the interventional radiologist via insertion of a selective arterial catheter into the left gastric artery and a continuous infusion of vasopressin.

The medical treatment of varices generally involves a continuous infusion of pitressin (Conn et al., 1975), vigorous administration of coagulation factors (such as fresh frozen plasma, platelets, and vitamin K), and the insertion of a Sengstaken-Blakemore tube for persistent hemorrhage. The use of propranolol as an adjunct to decrease splanchnic venous pressure remains controversial.

In the patient who continues to hemorrhage, a decision must be reached on the need for and timing of operation. In general, the indications for early operative intervention in patients with upper gastrointestinal hemorrhage include:

- Patients over 50 who will not tolerate repeated episodes of hypotension
- Patients with recurrent bleeding during appropriate and vigorous medical therapy
- Patients with continued signs of hypovolemia
- Patients with $>$ 2000 ml. blood loss in the first 24 hours in the hospital
- Patients with a visible vessel in the base of an ulcer
- Patients who fail vigorous medical therapy for esophageal varices

The operation that is commonly chosen for the older patient with a bleeding duodenal ulcer is truncal vagotomy, opening of the duodenum and oversewing of the bleeding ulcer, and pyloroplasty. Truncal vagotomy, opening of the duodenum and oversewing of the bleeding ulcer, antrectomy, and gastrojejunostomy are more commonly performed in younger patients who are hemodynamically stable (Farnell and Larson, 1983). Vagotomy and pyloroplasty is a somewhat quicker operation and is ideal for the older patient; however, recurrence rates for stomal ulcers have been reported as high as 15 to 20 per cent. In the patient with a bleeding gastric ulcer, a gastrotomy should be performed, the bleeding gastric ulcer oversewn, and multiple biopsies from the quadrants of the ulcer taken for immediate frozen section. If the ulcer is benign, then a generous hemigastrectomy including the ulcer (as long as it is not part of the gastroesophageal junction) is curative in properly selected patients. If the ulcer is malignant, then the surgeon must make a decision on whether a more radical cancer-type operation should be performed in the face of acute hemorrhage.

An end-to-side portacaval shunt, which completely eliminates any portal venous flow to the liver, has long been the operation of choice in patients with exsanguinating hemorrhage from esophageal varices related to hepatic cirrhosis. While the mortality for an emergent procedure is much greater than that of an elective procedure, the successful end-to-side portacaval shunt permanently eliminates variceal hemorrhage. A major concern in patients who have such a fully diverting shunt is the life-long problem of hepatic encephalopathy in those who had some flow through the portal vein into the liver (hepatopetal flow) in the preoperative period. Under more elective circumstances, when variceal hemorrhage has ceased, many patients with normal or good hepatic function undergo selective celiac and superior mesenteric arteriography to determine whether venous flow in the portal vein proceeds in a hepatopetal or hepatofugal direction. Patients with hepatopetal flow who are not actively bleeding are perhaps best treated with a distal splenorenal shunt (Warren) or the insertion of an 8 mm. externally supported PTFE graft between the portal vein and the inferior vena cava. Both of these procedures will maintain hepatopetal flow to the liver for a certain number of years as long as a total coronary-azygous venous disconnection is added to the operation.

Mallory-Weiss tears spontaneously cease bleeding in 90 per cent of patients. On occasion, electrocoagulation or even insertion of a Sengstaken-Blakemore tube may be necessary. Persistent hemorrhage should prompt laparotomy, at which time a high gastrotomy with oversewing of the mucosal defect on the lesser curvature side of the gastroesophageal junction (83 per cent), is performed (Sugawa et al., 1983).

LOWER GASTROINTESTINAL BLEEDING

Patients with lower gastrointestinal hemorrhage present with hematochezia or bright red bleeding. In contrast to patients with upper gastrointestinal hemorrhage, the lesions responsible for lower gastrointestinal hemorrhage may be much more difficult to diagnose.

Diagnosis

The major questions to be asked in a patient with acute or chronic lower gastrointestinal hemorrhage are whether any previous episodes of bleeding have occurred, what the extent of the diagnostic work-up was at that time, and whether or not the patient has any known disease processes in the small bowel or colon (such as inflammatory bowel disease) that might precipitate the hemorrhage.

On physical examination, the presence of any stigmata of systemic syndromes (such as the lip freckling of Peutz-Jeghers) or inflammatory bowel disease (such as perianal sinuses) should be noted. Large hemorrhoids or other anorectal lesions are best detected on anoscopy.

The sequence and extent of the work-up in patients with lower gastrointestinal bleeding is age dependent (Table 41–13). In children, common causes of lower gastrointestinal bleeding include juvenile polyps (which will require colonoscopy for diagnosis), intussusception (which will usually present acutely), and an ileal lesion distal to a Meckel's diverticulum. In young adults, a Meckel's diverticulum and inflammatory bowel disease may both present with lower gastrointestinal hemorrhage. This is also the time period when many congenital arteriovenous malformations, such as hemangiomas or lymphangiomas of the small intestine, will first present with hemorrhage. Finally, lower gastrointestinal hemorrhage in the elderly patient is almost always due to diverticulosis, angiodysplasia, hemorrhoids, a colorectal neoplasm, or ischemic colitis. There is some dispute about whether visceral arteriography (with or without a preceding radionuclide scan with technetium-pertechnetate labeled red cells) or a colonoscopy should be performed. Arteriography is most helpful in patients who are actively bleeding. It allows for localization of the bleeding site as well as the option for the infusion of agents such as pitressin that will cause vasoconstriction or for embolization of the actual site of hemorrhage. In patients who are slowly bleeding, arteriography will never be positive, and colonoscopy may be more valuable in this group. Colonoscopy has the advantages of revealing a bleeding site in 50 to 70 per cent of patients examined, detecting lesions that are no longer bleeding and would not ordinarily be visualized on arteriography, and allowing for definitive treatment of mucosal lesions, such as bleeding polyps, or areas of angiodysplasia (American Society for Gastrointestinal Endoscopy, 1988).

Table 41–13. CAUSES OF LOWER GASTROINTESTINAL HEMORRHAGE

Elderly
Diverticulosis
Angiodysplasia (80 per cent in distal ileum, cecum, and ascending colon)
Hemorrhoids
Neoplasm
Ischemic colitis
Young Adult
Inflammatory bowel disease
Meckel's diverticulum
Congenital arteriovenous malformation
Children
Meckel's diverticulum
Juvenile polyps
Intussusception

Modified from Farnell, M. B., and Larson, D. E.: The investigation and management of gastrointestinal bleeding. *In* Irving, M., and Beart, R. W., Jr. (Eds.): Gastroenterological Surgery. London, Butterworths, 1983, pp. 118–157.

The more aggressive use of visceral arteriography in recent years has documented that many elderly patients previously thought to be bleeding from diverticulosis in the left colon are actually bleeding from a diverticular or angiodysplastic lesion in the right colon. Bleeding from a diverticulum is not associated with diverticulitis and recurs in approximately 25 per cent of patients without further therapy. Angiodysplasia of the right side of the colon is an acquired lesion related to the effects of colonic wall tension on the submucosal venous network. These interesting lesions, 80 per cent of which occur in the terminal ileum, cecum, or ascending colon, account for approximately one half the lesions found on arteriography in patients with chronic lower gastrointestinal bleeding. In addition, 25 per cent of the patients with angiodysplasia are also noted to have aortic stenosis.

In young adults, once inflammatory bowel disease has been ruled out arteriography may be necessary to document the presence of a congenital hemangioma or ileal lesion distal to a Meckel's diverticulum. A radionuclide scan may also be of value in localizing the presence of ectopic gastric mucosa in the Meckel's diverticulum. In children, the juvenile polyps previously mentioned are best diagnosed on colonoscopy.

Another lesion in the patient of any age is hereditary hemorrhagic telangiectasia (Osler-Weber-Rendu syndrome). Should this lesion be discovered, it is usually controlled by medication and repeated transfusion as the entire gastrointestinal tract is involved.

Treatment

The patient should be stabilized in the usual fashion and hypovolemia reversed, particularly in the elderly patient. If visceral arteriography is chosen as a diagnostic and therapeutic maneuver, a bleeding rate of 0.5 to 1.0 ml. per minute is required for the area of extravasation to be visualized. This is thought to approximate a transfusion requirement of 2 units of whole blood every 24 hours. Ongoing hemorrhage noted during arteriography will often respond to an infusion of vasopressin at 0.2 U. per minute into the superior mesenteric artery. Embolization through the same catheter may be a therapeutic alternative in patients with lesions in the small bowel; however, ischemia of the colon has resulted from this maneuver. If angiodysplasia is felt to be the source of bleeding on a visceral arteriogram and it can be accurately localized, then elective resection of the colon, usually a right hemicolectomy, is performed and is curative. The reason for aggressively approaching an operation in these lesions, in contrast to bleeding from what is thought to be colonic diverticulosis, is that rebleeding will occur in approximately 85 per cent of patients. In the patient whose lower gastrointestinal hemorrhage ceases before visceral arteriography can be performed, an elective work-up with sigmoidoscopy, colonoscopy, and gastroscopy should be performed. Barium studies are usually not performed early in the hospitalization because of the problem of making a diagnosis during a subsequent visceral arteriogram should bleeding recur during the work-up.

In elderly patients who have undergone a vigorous work-up for chronic lower gastrointestinal hemorrhage and no site has been found, iron supplementation and transfusions as needed are the only therapy. Should the patient develop an increased need for transfusion or have a sudden increase in the rate of hemorrhage, a repeat visceral arteriogram can be performed.

Hernias

A hernia is defined as a protrusion of a structure through the tissues that normally confine it. Hernias, therefore, can occur almost anywhere in the body; but, for the purposes of this chapter, the discussion will be limited to those involving the abdominal wall. Even in this region, the varieties of hernias are numerous.

Hernias of the groin include the indirect inguinal, the direct inguinal, and the femoral hernia (Fig. 41–4). Of these the indirect is the most common and is believed to occur in 1 to 2 per cent of males. By definition, an indirect inguinal hernia is one that

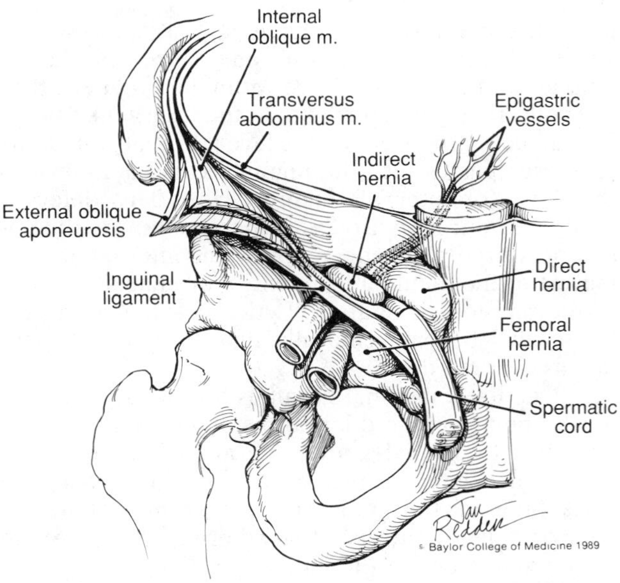

Figure 41–4. The relative locations of the three common groin hernias are shown. The importance of the transversus layer of the abdominal wall in the prevention and treatment of these hernias can be appreciated.

escapes the confinement of the abdominal wall just lateral to the inferior epigastric artery. The direct inguinal hernia, in contrast, occurs medial to the inferior epigastric artery through the region known as Hesselbach's triangle. These definitions, however, are misleading as they tend to stress the similarity of the lesions based on their relationship to a small artery; in fact, they have entirely different etiologies and treatments.

An indirect inguinal hernia begins as a congenital lesion: the patent processus vaginalis. This structure is a tube-shaped appendage of the peritoneum that accompanies the testicle during its descent into the scrotum. The processus normally becomes obliterated early in life, but, in about 20 per cent of males, it retains its lumen, which communicates with the peritoneal cavity (Morgan and Anson, 1942). Less often, women may also have a patent processus and develop indirect hernias.

Patients with a patent processus may remain asymptomatic as long as the musculoaponeurotic layers of the abdominal wall retain their integrity. The inner connective tissue layer of the abdominal wall is the first defense that must be breeched before a groin hernia develops. This tissue has, traditionally, been referred to as the transversalis fascia, based upon its relationship with the transversus abdominis muscle and aponeurosis. In reality, the transversalis fascia forms a sack that covers the entire abdominal cavity, just like the peritoneum, but is external to it. There are several thickenings of the transversalis fascia in the groin, such as the iliopubic tract, to which some surgeons attach considerable importance in the repair of hernias. More recently, the role of the transversus muscle and aponeurosis in the prevention and treatment of groin hernias has been emphasized (McVay, 1974). To avoid confusion, and since the fascia, muscle, and aponeurosis are intimately related, they will collectively be referred to as the transversus layer. The defect in the transversus layer through which the processus passes into the inguinal canal is known as the deep (or internal) inguinal ring. This defect is reinforced during episodes of increased intra-abdominal pressure by the apposition of the internal oblique muscle to the inguinal ligament, a mechanism known as the physiologic shutter (Lytle, 1945). An indirect hernia will become clinically manifest only if these defenses break down.

The direct inguinal hernia is felt by most authorities to be an acquired lesion resulting from wear and tear, usually in males after the age of 40 years and often much later. Direct hernias begin as a diffuse weakening of the transversus layer medial to the inferior epigastic artery. These hernias have a broad fascial defect unlike the indirect variety.

Most abdominal hernias tend to enlarge with time. In the case of the indirect hernia, the processus directs the contents of the hernia into the scrotum. The direct hernia usually enlarges anteriorly but may also progress into the scrotum. Very large, indirect hernias can dilate the internal ring and destroy the entire transversus layer in the inguinal region, thus resembling large direct hernias.

Femoral hernias are closely related to direct inguinal hernias since the basic defect is a weakening of the transversus layer just medial to the femoral vein. The difference between femoral and direct inguinal hernias is that the former occur below, rather than above, the inguinal ligament. Characteristically, a femoral hernia sac protrudes into the subcutaneous tissue of the upper thigh. Since the fascial defect between the inguinal ligament, femoral vein, and pubic ramus is small, femoral hernias are often small and may be hard to detect on a physical examination, especially in obese patients. Some are discovered incidentally at the time of laparotomy for a bowel obstruction. Although on a percentage basis femoral hernias occur more often in women than they do in men, the inguinal hernia is still the most common groin hernia in both sexes.

The diagnosis of a groin hernia is usually not difficult. Patients may give a history of a sharp, stabbing pain in the inguinal region that begins during exertion. With time, the pain may change in nature and be described as drawing or pulling and is often exacerbated by activity and relieved by rest. The history of an intermittent mass in the groin is also common.

On physical examination, the finding of a soft mass above the inguinal ligament, which disappears with manual pressure or recumbency, is virtually diagnostic. In obese patients, the detection of a small hernia may be challenging. Equally difficult is the diagnosis of a small, indirect inguinal hernia when the hernia sac is empty. In this situation, the examiner must attempt to demonstrate the patent processus of an indirect hernia or diffuse bulge of a direct hernia by having the patient strain or cough while palpating the inguinal region. This is accomplished in males by invaginating the skin of the scrotum over the index finger and carefully placing the tip of the finger into the external inguinal ring (a hole in the external oblique aponeurosis just lateral to the pubic tubercle through which the spermatic cord in men or round ligament in women passes). The patient is then instructed to cough or strain. This maneuver may produce an impulse on the tip of the examining finger representing a hernia. Considerable practice is required to diagnose inguinal hernias in this manner. Distinguishing whether the impulse is located on the tip or pad of the finger, although often mentioned as a method for differentiating direct from indirect hernias, is not as helpful as is knowing the patient's age. One word of caution in examining the external ring: this aponeurotic structure is extremely sensitive to stretch and careless examination will cause not only a sharp, lancinating pain but will also induce the patient to hop backward across the examining room.

Although inguinal hernias frequently descend into the scrotum, the presence of a scrotal mass is by no means pathognomonic of a hernia. These masses must be differentiated from hydroceles, varicoceles, testicular torsion, epididymo-orchitis, and even testicular carcinoma.

Hydroceles are related to indirect hernias in that they represent fluid accumulations within a processus that is obliterated proximally (a noncommunicating hydrocele) or one with a narrow, but patent, neck (a communicating hydrocele). In the majority of cases, a hydrocele is easily diagnosed by translumination.

A varicocele is a dilated plexus of veins that surrounds the testicle. For a number of anatomic reasons, it occurs almost exclusively on the left side. On physical examination, a varicocele resembles a bag of worms that disappears when the patient lies down. Varicoceles have no relationship to hernias but may be related to male infertility.

Testicular torsion causes a painful scrotal mass and jeopardizes the viability of the testicle. This is due to a twisting of the spermatic cord so that the testicle is elevated in the scrotum and lies transversely rather than in the normal anterior-posterior plane. Gentle elevation of the scrotum may help relieve the pain. Torsion is a surgical emergency.

Epididymo-orchitis is an inflammatory and probably infectious process of the testicle and/or epididymis that also causes a painful scrotal mass. Unlike torsion, the testicle is in the normal position, and the pain is not relieved by elevation. Both torsion and epididymo-orchitis must be differentiated from an incarcerated or strangulated hernia.

Testicular cancer presents as a rock hard scrotal mass intimately related to or obscuring the testicle. Its differentiation from a scrotal hernia should not be difficult.

Umbilical hernias are common hernias of the abdominal wall and occur through an open umbilical fascial ring. These lesions are particularly frequent in neonates and infants. It is estimated that 10 per cent of white babies and over 40 per cent of black babies have open umbilical rings at birth. As a rule, spontaneous closure of these defects occurs by 2 years of age. Because of the high rate of spontaneous closure, many authorities do not advocate surgical treatment of uncomplicated umbilical hernias during infancy or childhood. On the other hand, others believe that groups at high risk for complications can be identified, and prophylactic surgery can be recommended on a selective basis (Kiesewetter, 1961). The taping of umbilical hernias has been used to speed up spontaneous closure; it is unlikely to be of any benefit and may actually be harmful. In contrast to those in children, spontaneous closure of umbilical hernias does not occur in adults. Furthermore, they are prone to complications because of their small, rigid neck and thus should be repaired.

Incisional hernias, also known as ventral hernias, occur through surgical incisions and are iatrogenic complications. Although they are encountered somewhat more often in vertical as compared to horizontal incisions, the difference is not great enough to offset the advantages of vertical incisions. Risk factors for the development of these hernias include increased intra-abdominal pressure, infection, and poor surgical technique. The diagnosis is obvious in most cases since the fascial defect is often large. Small, satellite defects near the main hernia are common and are a potential source of complications.

All hernias of the abdominal wall have the potential for severe and life-threatening complications. Several well-known terms are used to describe these phenomena and are useful in communication with other physicians. A hernia that can be returned to the abdominal cavity by the patient or a physician is said to be *reducible*. When it cannot, it is *incarcerated*. When the contents of an incarcerated hernia become necrotic, it is *strangulated*. Incarcerated and strangulated hernias are surgical emergencies and must be operated upon promptly. If an incarcerated hernia can eventually be reduced, it should be operated upon soon since reincarceration is almost a certainty. Reducible hernias may be repaired electively but without undue delay. Optimal medical practice mandates the repair of abdominal wall hernias before incarceration (and, especially, strangulation) occur.

The complications of hernias occur when an intra-abdominal structure, usually a piece of intestine, becomes entrapped in the hernia sac. The unyielding borders of the musculoaponeurotic abdominal wall inhibit lymphatic and venous drainage of the bowel and cause swelling and entrapment outside the abdominal cavity. This results in a bowel obstruction with all its attendant metabolic consequences. If the hernia is treated at this point, morbidity and mortality should be minimal. Unfortunately, if repair is delayed and the arterial circulation of the intestine becomes compromised by the increasing venous pressure, necrosis of the bowel will occur. Because bacteria are present in high concentrations in obstructed bowel, and can migrate through the necrotic bowel wall, aggressive infections of the abdominal wall and feculent peritonitis rapidly ensue. These highly lethal complications can be prevented by elective repair of the hernia.

It is commonly taught that hernias with a small fascial ring (e.g., femoral, umbilical, and small indirect hernias) are more likely to cause incarceration than broad-based hernias, such as large direct or incisional hernias. Although these observations are generally true, it may be very difficult to differentiate direct from indirect hernias, and many incisional hernias contain strong fibrous bands or small fenestrations that can serve to cause strangulation. Therefore, as a general rule, all hernias of the abdominal wall should be considered indications for herniorrhaphy.

Clearly, this approach must be tempered by sound surgical judgment. There are patients whose operative risk is so great that the repair of any hernia may be contraindicated. In the same sense, not all incarcerated hernias require immediate surgery. Some incarcerated hernias may have been present for many years without causing symptoms. Although these too should be considered for repair, the urgency is less, and if the patient is feeble, repair may not be indicated. Decisions such as these should be made jointly with the patient and an experienced surgeon. Very large hernias may lose the right to domain with regard to the abdominal cavity (i.e., the volume of the abdominal cavity has decreased so there is no longer room for the hernia's contents). The repair of these hernias may require prolonged in-hospital preparation using techniques to stretch the abdominal wall prior to repair.

Hernias in the pediatric population require special consideration. Almost all groin hernias in children are of the indirect variety. Because of the increased patency of the processus in early infancy and the fact that the internal and external rings are located nearly on top of one another in infancy, the frequency of hernia in children is greater than in adults. Furthermore, the constantly improving survival of premature infants has increased the number of babies with a patent processus and, therefore, the number of potential hernias.

The diagnosis of an inguinal hernia in a child is usually suspected first by a parent who observes a swelling in the groin. As in adults, the mass may be intermittently present.

When examining the child, a warm environment, warm hands, the presence of a parent, and gaining the trust of the child are essential for success. It is wise to begin the examination with the parent holding the child in an upright position. If a reducible mass is present, the diagnosis is confirmed. If not, gentle manual pressure on the abdomen may produce a mass. The well-known silk sign—the palpation of two peritoneal surfaces gliding over one another—has not been shown to be of great value in the diagnosis of pediatric hernias (Gilbert and Chatworthy, 1979).

The scrotum must be examined carefully since the absence of a testicle raises the questions of an undescended testicle (cryptorchidism). Cryptorchidism is accompanied by a patent processus in about 90 per cent of cases. In addition to its association with hernias, the observation of cryptorchidism is an important finding since it is associated with a greatly increased risk of testicular cancer and male infertility.

Unless overwhelming reasons preclude surgery, the pediatric patient should undergo elective herniorrhaphy (with the exception of umbilical herniorrhaphy) as soon as possible. The reason for this approach is that the likelihood of both incarceration and strangulation are considerably greater than in adults, and the consequences may be more severe, especially in premature infants (Rowe and Chatworthy, 1970). If a child is found to have an incarcerated or strangulated hernia, a surgical emergency exists. In the care of surgeons and, particularly, anesthesiologists skilled in the care of pediatric patients, the success of repair should approach 100 per cent with a minimal risk.

An area of controversy remaining in pediatric surgery is the question of bilateral groin exploration when only one hernia is diagnosed. Approximately 50 per cent of infants, and slightly less in older children, will have a patent processus contralateral to the hernia at the time of initial exploration. If untreated, about half will become hernias; hence, this dilemma can be argued persuasively by surgeons who advocate or denounce simultaneous exploration. At this time, the majority of pediatric surgeons currently support bilateral exploration. An alternative approach is the use of herniography, the instillation of radiopaque dye into the peritoneal cavity to define the presence of a contralateral patent processus. Although intriguing, this method of diagnosis has not become widely accepted.

Today, most hernias can be successfully repaired with minimal associated morbidity or mortality. Many groin hernias are being electively repaired using local anesthesia in a day surgery setting. Large, complex hernias formerly required special techniques to close, and these were associated with a high recurrence rate. The introduction of Marlex and other meshes as well as Gore-Tex body patches to create an artificial musculoaponeurotic layer has simplified the repair of these hernias. At the present time, virtually all hernias of the abdominal wall can be repaired.

The use of a truss has no place in the care of patients with hernias. The truss, even when carefully designed and fitted, will not reliably prevent the life-threatening complications of incarceration or strangulation.

Cardiovascular Disorders

Cardiovascular disease includes both acute and chronic disorders of the arteries and veins. Although arteries and veins have similar functions, the clinical manifestations of arterial and venous disease are quite different. Occlusion of an artery causes ischemia of the tissue supplied by the artery. If the occlusion is acute, tissue necrosis is likely, whereas gradual occlusion may cause only minimal symptoms because of the collateral circulation that has developed. Arteries may also rupture due to aneurysms or undergo dissection of the wall of the vessel and create complex false lumens. In contrast, veins virtually never undergo chronic occlusion, rupture, or suffer dissection. Only rarely does acute occlusion of a vein result in tissue loss.

CHRONIC OCCLUSIVE ARTERIAL DISEASES

The etiologies of arterial diseases are numerous, but causes other than atherosclerosis are uncommon. When considering *all* disease processes, the consequences of atherosclerosis (i.e., myocardial infarction, stroke, and aortic aneurysm) are responsible for more deaths than any other disease process (National Center for Health Statistics, 1978)! Given the significance of atherosclerosis, most of this section will deal with the consequences of this disease.

The pathogenesis of atherosclerosis is incompletely understood. Most attention has been focused on complex biochemical interactions involving endothelial cells, blood-borne cells, lipid metabolism, and arterial smooth muscle (Ross, 1981). The common pathway leading to the eventual development of an atherosclerotic plaque is believed to be repeated endothelial injury—the injury hypothesis. Zarins (1986) has emphasized the development of plaques in regions of the arterial tree with either slow or turbulent blood flow. The biochemical and life-style risk factors associated with the development of atherosclerotic cardiovascular disease are addressed elsewhere.

CORONARY ARTERY DISEASE

The treatment of coronary artery disease (CAD) is constantly evolving. Data that were painstakingly accumulated in the recent past become irrelevant as new drugs, techniques, and operations are developed. The indications for the surgical treatment of CAD (i.e., coronary artery bypass [CAB]) are controversial. In order to test the efficacy of any treatment, whether medical or surgical, it is necessary to understand the natural history of the disease. Mortality due to CAD is related to ventricular function, as measured by ejection fraction, and the extent of atherosclerotic occlusions of the coronary arteries. The Coronary Artery Surgery Study (CASS), a multi-institutional investigation that began in the 1970's, demonstrated that medically treated patients with significant coronary occlusion ($>$ 70 per cent of the diameter) of a single coronary artery had a 92 per cent chance of surviving 4 years; with two-vessel occlusion, an 84 per cent chance; with three-vessel disease, a 68 per cent chance; and with isolated left main coronary stenosis, a 60 per cent chance (Mock et al., 1982). The quality of ventricular function was assessed separately. With an ejection fraction of > 50 per cent, approximately 90 per cent of patients survived 4 years, but with an ejection fraction of < 35 per cent the 4-year survival was only 58 per cent. When ventricular function and coronary artery status were considered together, patients with three coronary arteries involved but who had ejection fractions of >50 per cent faired well, with 79 per cent surviving for 4 years. In contrast, only 67 per cent of those with only single-vessel involvement, but impaired ventricular function (ejection fractions of < 50 per cent), survived for 4 years.

The treatment of patients with CAD has two goals: the relief of angina and increased longevity. That CAB is effective in the relief of angina is not disputed. At least 60 per cent of patients will have immediate and complete relief of angina and significant improvement will occur in another 35 per cent. In view of this fact, there is almost unanimous agreement that *angina refractory to medical management* is a clear indication for surgery. Although most patients with *unstable angina* will respond to intensive, in-hospital treatment, about 25 per cent will not and should be considered for prompt coronary arteriography and surgical treatment (Braumwald and Cohn, 1983). Based on data from the CASS study, there is general agreement that patients with left main coronary artery stenosis > 50 per cent should undergo CAB regardless of symptoms. Additional data from a randomized trial in the CASS study (Passamani et al., 1985) indicated that patients with triple-vessel disease and impaired ventricular function (ejection fraction of 35 to 49 per cent) survived longer with surgical than with medical treatment. Another group that appeared to benefit from surgical treatment were patients over the age of 64 who were at high risk for medical treatment failure: those with poor ventricular function, left main CAD, and moderate to severe angina. The appropriate treatment for patients with < 50 per cent occlusion of the left main coronary artery or involvement of fewer than three vessels with or without left ventricular dysfunction remains controversial and is continuing to evolve.

Two recent advances in surgical technique that may swing the pendulum to favor CAB in more patients are improvements in myocardial preservation during surgery (Fallette et al., 1978) and use of the internal mammary artery, which has a much better long-term patency rate than does the saphenous vein (Loop et al., 1986) (Fig. 41–5).

Contraindications to CAB are relatively few. Acute myocardial infarction is considered to be a contraindication to surgery. Even so, some centers with sophisticated resources and coordination have achieved reasonable results in this setting (Berg et al., 1982). Most surgeons prefer to wait 4 to 6 weeks

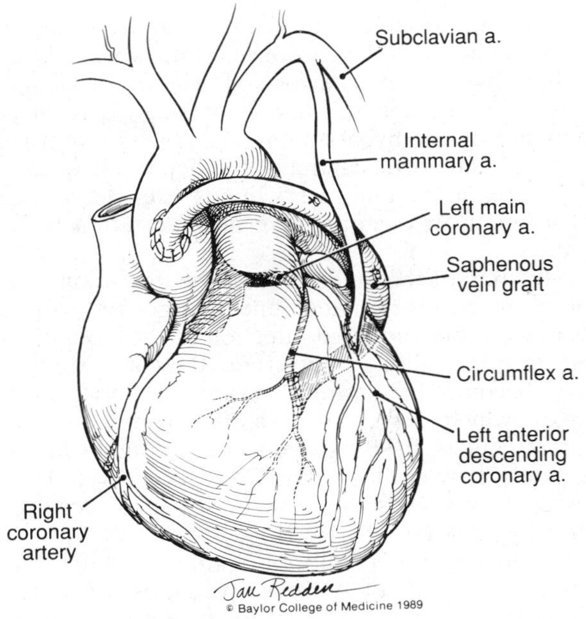

Figure 41–5. A completed coronary artery bypass. The left internal mammary artery has been anastomosed to the left anterior descending coronary artery, and a saphenous vein graft has been used to revascularize the circumflex artery.

after a myocardial infarction before considering surgery. Patients with chronic congestive heart failure manifested by pulmonary edema, hepatomegaly, and anasarca do not have an improvement in longevity, and have a significant operative mortality rate. They are not considered candidates for CAB (Spencer et al., 1971). A few patients with congestive heart failure may have ventricular aneurysms secondary to transmural myocardial infarcts. These patients may benefit from aneurysmectomy with or without CAB since the paradoxical motion of the aneurysm may contribute significantly to the congestive failure.

Coronary artery bypass is a complex operation that requires sophisticated equipment and personnel. The heart is exposed by an incision that longitudinally splits the sternum, and the patient is completely anticoagulated with heparin. Large cannulas are placed into the right atrium to remove venous blood returning to the heart, and a smaller cannula is placed into the descending aorta to return pressurized, oxygenated blood from the bypass pump to the arterial circulation. The pump is then turned on, and a clamp is placed between the aortic cannula and the heart so that no bleeding will occur when the coronary arteries are opened. To prevent ischemic injury to the heart during the bypass run, the patient's core body temperature is lowered to 25 to 30 °C, by a heat exchanger in the pump, and a cold cardioplegic solution is instilled into the coronary circulation to cool the myocardium and stop the heart from beating altogether—both of which further reduce the oxygen demand. Sites for bypass are then selected according to preoperative coronary arteriograms, and either the internal mammary arteries are sutured to the coronary arteries or saphenous veins are sutured from the ascending aorta to the coronary arteries. Usually two or three bypasses are performed. The aortic clamp is then removed, and the patient is weaned from dependence on the bypass pump. Following removal of the atrial and aortic cannulas, the heparin is reversed with protamine, and the wounds are closed. The usual length of postoperative hospitalization is 7 to 10 days.

In spite of the magnitude of the operation, complications are fortunately uncommon. As with all operations, bleeding and infection of the wounds can and do occur, though not often. Recently, surgeons have become increasingly aware of perioperative stroke, which can occur in a significant number of patients unless the surgeon is meticulous in its prevention (Shaw et al., 1986). Retrospective studies in this country suggest the rate of stroke is close to 1 per cent (Jones et al., 1984).

A low operative mortality rate is vital for the long-term results of CAB to surpass those of contemporary medical management. As demonstrated by the Veterans Administration Cooperative Study Group, the high operative mortality rate of 5.6 per cent easily offsets the 4-year surgical survival rate of 83 per cent compared to the 4-year survival rate of medically treated patients of 86 per cent (Read et al., 1978). In contrast, data from the CASS study demonstrated that a low operative mortality rate and excellent long-term survival could be achieved even in a multi-institutional study: 2.4 per cent and 90 per cent at 5 years, respectively (Myers et al., 1985).

Although long-term survival is the ultimate test of medical versus surgical treatment of CAD, graft patency, which correlates well with the relief of symptoms, is also an important factor. Loop et al. (1986) studied the long-term patency of 855 internal mammary artery grafts and 1445 saphenous vein grafts at intervals up to 13 years. The average patency rate at 10 years for internal mammary arteries was 96 per cent compared to 81 per cent for saphenous veins.

Antiplatelet therapy may also prolong bypass graft patency. A combination of aspirin and dipyridamole has been shown to reduce late graft occlusion to 16 per cent as compared to 27 per cent with a placebo (Chesebro et al., 1984).

While it is clear that CAB will significantly benefit selected patients with coronary artery disease, a new technique, balloon catheter angioplasty, has emerged that may alter the current role of CAB. This treatment, developed by Gruentzig (1978), involves mechanically dilating atherosclerotic plaques with a specially designed balloon catheter using a percutaneous approach. Ten years after he started this technique, Gruentzig (1987) published long-term follow-up of the initial 169 patients treated by angioplasty. The initial success rate was 79 per cent; however, restenosis occurred in 30 per cent of patients within 6 months; 27 per cent of the patients required repeat dilatation, and 19 per cent had a CAB. Early restenosis has been a common problem with angioplasty. The optimal candidate and timing for coronary angioplasty is still being studied (The TIMI Study Group, 1989).

CEREBROVASCULAR DISEASE

Cerebrovascular disease is second only to CAD in mortality and morbidity from cardiovascular disease. Atherosclerotic occlusive disease accounts for up to one third of all strokes (Mohr, 1978), about 60 per cent of which are preceded by premonitory symptoms. In that these lesions in the extracerebral carotid circulation are amenable to surgery, prevention is the main focus of the surgical approach.

Cerebral atherosclerotic occlusions tend to form at specific sites. The most common is in the carotid sinus, a bulbous dilatation at the origin of the internal carotid artery in the neck. Flow studies in glass models have revealed that the shape of the sinus changes the laminar nature of blood flow, thus predisposing to the development of an atherosclerotic plaque (Bharadvay et al., 1983).

The symptoms of atherosclerotic carotid artery disease range from fatal hemiplegic strokes to barely discernible focal deficits. It is generally agreed that a stroke occurs when thrombosis of the carotid artery or one of its intracranial branches reduces blood flow to a portion of the brain below that sufficient to meet its metabolic requirements. Clinical symptoms depend on the extent of collateral circulation; some patients with total occlusion of the internal carotid artery will be completely asymptomatic whereas others will suffer fatal hemiplegia.

The immediate mortality from an ischemic stroke is around 25 per cent and for those who survive, the risk of a recurrent stroke is about 10 per cent per year (Baker et al., 1968), with significant mortality.

In contrast to the devastating results of stroke are the *transient ischemic attacks* (TIAs). By definition, TIAs are ischemic neurologic deficits that may last minutes or hours but resolve completely within 24 hours of onset. They are often recurrent, almost always in the same anatomic distribution. The exact cause of TIAs is debatable. The two current theories are (1) they result from emboli arising from irregular atherosclerotic plaques in the carotid arteries that drift into the cerebral circulation and lodge in small cortical vessels or (2) stenosis of one of the vessels supplying blood to the brain results in regional transient ischemia. Currently, emboli from atherosclerotic plaques are believed to be responsible for the majority of TIAs (Moore and Hall, 1970).

The natural history of untreated TIAs has been well studied. Focal TIAs are associated with an increased risk of subsequent stroke between 30 to 40 per cent within 5 years (Whisnant et al., 1973; Loeb et al., 1978).

Amaurosis fugax is a unique variety of TIA caused by migration of emboli into the ophthalmic artery, which causes temporary monocular blindness. Classically, the patient describes a shade being pulled over the eye. As with other episodes of TIAs, this usually lasts only a few minutes, but in some instances, they may be prolonged. Patients that suffer from amaurosis have an increased risk of stroke, though not as great as patients with hemispheric TIAs. Although seemingly innocent compared to hemispheric TIAs, amaurosis can lead to permanent monocular blindness.

A stroke syndrome that lies somewhere between a TIA and a completed stroke is the *stroke-in-evolution*. This syndrome begins as a localized neurologic deficit, which over a matter of hours to days progresses with the development of additional neurologic deficits. The prognosis of stroke-in-evolution is quite poor: 60 per cent of patients suffer a severe neurologic deficit with an overall mortality of 15 per cent (Mentzer et al., 1981).

Another clinical presentation is the patient who has no discernible symptoms but is known to have an atherosclerotic plaque involving the carotid artery. Asymptomatic bruit has often been used to describe this lesion, but the term *asymptomatic stenosis* is more precise for an atherosclerotic plaque of the common or internal carotid artery. The use of noninvasive tests to follow the evolution of asymptomatic stenosis has revealed an approximate 4 per cent incidence of stroke per year with this lesion, provided the initial stenosis was greater than 50 per cent of the diameter of the involved vessel (Kartchner and McRae, 1977; Moore et al., 1985). In contrast, the annual rate of stroke with focal hemispheric TIA is in the range of 6 per cent per year. The carotid duplex scan is the best of several available noninvasive tests to evaluate asymptomatic stenosis, yielding both an image of the artery as well as physiologic data regarding the severity of the stenosis. The evaluation of TIAs or amaurosis should include an echocardiogram, searching for a source of emboli, and usually a computerized tomographic scan of the brain, which may detect hemorrhage from an intracerebral aneurysm or hypertensive stroke or even a brain tumor. Only if noninvasive tests are negative and the patient is being considered for surgery should a carotid arteriogram be performed, since this procedure carries with it a risk of stroke of somewhat less than 1 per cent.

The clearest indications for carotid surgery for the prevention of stroke are TIAs and amaurosis fugax. More controversial indications include (1) a patient with partial or complete recovery following a stroke, who has a carotid lesion in a patent artery corresponding to the side of the stroke; an increased risk of perioperative stroke limits operations for this indication; (2) an asymptomatic stenosis; surgery is considered when the stenosis is $\geq$ 50 per cent of the vessel diameter. Since the risk of stroke is not as great in these patients, the perioperative morbidity and mortality must be very low; (3) a stroke-in-evolution; this poses high risk for a further neurologic deficit. Although little surgical experience has been reported, some results have been excellent.

Acute stroke is considered a contraindication for carotid surgery, as is a completed hemiplegic stroke without return of function.

Some opponents of prophylactic carotid endarterectomy cite two series with notoriously poor results to support their opinion that the risk of surgery is worse than the natural history of the disease (Easton and Sherman, 1977; Brott and Thalinger, 1984).

These series stand in distinct contrast to numerous other series with outstanding long-term results and low operative morbidity and mortality (Thompson et al., 1978; Moore et al., 1979; Whitney et al., 1980; Ennix et al., 1979; Plecha et al., 1979). As in patients with coronary artery disease, careful patient selection is essential for good results.

Patients who recover from carotid artery surgery assume approximately the same stroke risk as age-matched patients without atherosclerotic lesions in the neck, slightly more than 1 per cent per year. Thus, a low operative stroke and mortality rate assures a favorable risk:benefit ratio for carotid artery surgery. Experienced vascular surgeons should be able to perform carotid endarterectomy with a combined stroke-mortality of 5 per cent or less. Many series with less than 3 per cent combined stroke-mortality have been published.

Carotid endarterectomy is carried out under general anesthesia with preparations to monitor the status of the patient's cerebral circulation during the operation (Fig. 41–6). An incision is made in the neck overlying the carotid artery, and the vessel is clamped. If monitoring indicates poor tolerance to clamping, a shunt is placed from the common to the internal carotid to insure adequate circulation during the remainder of the operation. The artery is then opened, and the atherosclerotic plaque is dissected from the outer layers of the vessel. The vessel is then closed. Although carotid endarterectomy is a simple procedure, absolutely meticulous technique is essential to avoid leaving any loose material or blood clots within the vessel lumen. Failure to do this almost always results in neurologic complications. Patients are hospitalized for 4 or 5 days, and if no complications occur, they may be discharged with few restrictions of their activity.

CHRONIC ATHEROSCLEROTIC OCCLUSION OF THE LOWER EXTREMITIES

Several patterns of occlusive disease are seen in the lower extremities. One involves the terminal abdominal aorta and the iliac arteries. In 1948, Rene Leriche (Leriche and Morel, 1948) described a syndrome associated with complete occlusion of the terminal aorta. Classically, patients develop the following signs and symptoms:

1. Profound weakness and fatigue of both lower extremities

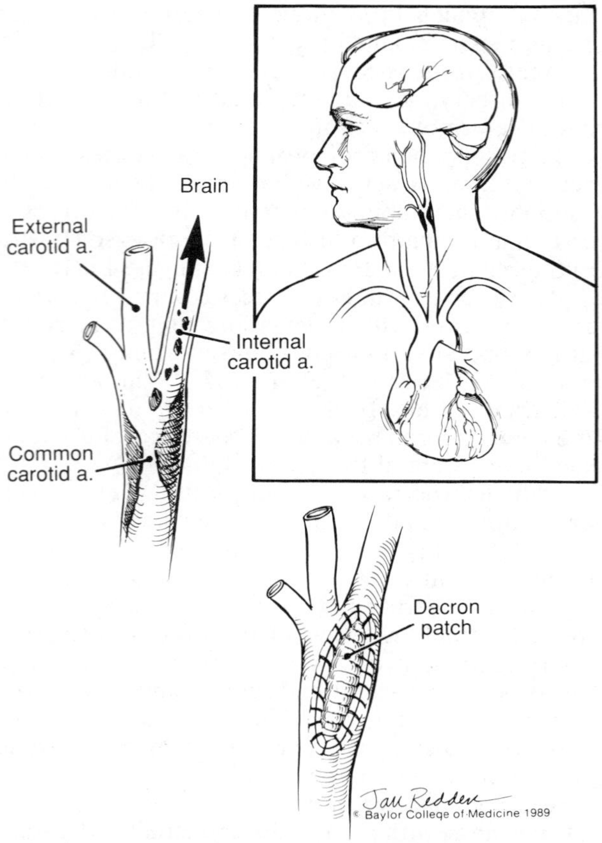

Figure 41–6. Many strokes are believed to result from small emboli that originate from the irregular surface of an atherosclerotic plaque in the carotid artery. The accessibilty of these lesions to surgical treatment is demonstated in the inset. Following the removal of the plaque, the arterial incision is often closed with a Dacron patch to prevent narrowing of the internal carotid artery.

2. Global atrophy of the leg
3. Absence of trophic changes in the skin of the lower extremities
4. Pallor of the legs even on standing
5. In males, inability to maintain a stable erection
6. Absence of femoral pulses

Of interest, Leriche stated specifically that these patients do not experience intermittent claudication, which is so characteristic of other occlusive lesions in the lower extremities.

More often, patients present with unilateral or bilateral iliac disease. These patients will suffer from intermittent claudication and usually describe cramping pain in the hips, thighs, and buttocks, when walking a particular distance, which is highly reproducible. Patients stop walking when the pain occurs; after a few minutes, they are able to resume walking again until the pain inevitably returns. Impotence may also be seen in this group of individuals if disease is present in any of the internal iliac arteries. The most common atherosclerotic lesion of the lower extremities is stenosis or occlusion of the superficial femoral artery. This produces intermittent claudication of the calf. The third site commonly involved is the tibial arteries. Lesions in this location are most prone to occur in elderly patients and those with diabetes.

Boyd (1960) studied the natural history of intermittent claudication, publishing the long-term follow-up of 1440 patients. After 5 years in his series, only 73 per cent of patients were alive; at 10 years, 38 per cent; and at 15 years, only 22 per cent. However, the chance of requiring a major amputation for necrosis was only 7 per cent at 5 years, and at 10 years, only 12 per cent. This study underscores the usually benign nature of intermittent claudication and emphasizes the fact that many of these patients have severe concomitant vascular disease. Although some patients improve without surgery (Imparato et al., 1975), approximately 20 per cent of patients with claudication will eventually require intervention.

A more severe symptom of lower extremity occlusive disease is rest pain. It is located either in the toes or the region of the metatarsal heads (Cranley, 1969) and, occasionally, is seen somewhat more proximally but *never* occurs above the ankle. Rest pain is burning in nature and often severe. So critical is the ischemia in these individuals that simply improving blood flow by making the feet dependent will often relieve the pain. Nocturnal calf cramps are never a sign of severe arterial insufficiency.

Patients with severe claudication and those with rest pain may exhibit the trophic changes including loss of hair, thinning of skin, and thickening of nails. In very advanced cases, painful ischemic ulcers may result. These are seen in the same distribution as rest pain. Necrosis of the toes or in areas subject to trauma, such as the medial and lateral aspects of the foot or the heel, can also occur. When examining an extremity for vascular disease, one should always examine the areas between the toes for ischemic lesions.

Dependent rubor is another sign of severe ischemia of the lower extremity. This finding is easily reproduced by simply having the patient sit with the legs dangling over the edge of the examining table. Within a few seconds or minutes, the affected extremity will become noticeably erythematous. Palpation of the pulses and auscultation for bruits provides important information. For instance, patients with only a single palpable pulse in the foot virtually never have rest pain. A few patients with isolated iliac or superficial femoral artery stenoses may have palpable pedal pulses and still claudicate. Most patients with claudication, however, will not have palpable pulses either in the popliteal fossa or the foot.

With the notable exception of aortic occlusion, the finding of an occluded artery is not itself an indication for surgery. In the case of aortic occlusion, the patient may have stable symptoms for several years, but in about one third of the patients, the thrombus will propagate proximally and cause thrombosis of the renal arteries (Starrett and Stoney, 1974). Therefore, patients with occlusion of the distal aorta, regardless of the symptoms, should be considered candidates for surgery.

Intermittent claudication is usually *not* considered an indication for surgery. Because of the increased risk of death due to other cardiovascular diseases, the physician should emphasize in these individuals the elimination of cardiovascular risk factors—in particular, the control of hypertension and the cessation of smoking. A regular exercise program of walking is also helpful. There are patients whose claudication is so severe that they are not able to work or to care for their daily needs or whose lives are made so miserable by limitation of their activities that they should also be considered for surgery. Ischemic rest pain, ischemic ulceration, and tissue necrosis are almost always indications for surgical intervention.

In most situations, a carefully performed history and physical will be all that is necessary to make a correct diagnosis and to determine whether a patient is in need of surgery. In some instances, however, the course may not be clear, and noninvasive tests are available that determine the severity of the occlusions and the adequacy of collateral circulation. The most popular of these is the ankle-brachial index. Using a blood pressure cuff and a Doppler flow detector, a blood pressure can be obtained in the lower extremity and divided by a blood pressure similarly obtained in the antecubital fossa. The fraction generated is known as the ankle-brachial index and correlates well with both the severity of the patient's symptoms and the extent of occlusion in the vessels above the blood pressure cuff.

In order to perform successful vascular surgery, high-quality arteriograms are essential. Although the risk of arteriography of the lower extremities is considerably less than in the coronary or cerebral circulation, complications can occur, notably acute renal failure and arterial trauma, in addition to the discomfort involved.

A commonly performed procedure for occlusive disease of the aorta and iliac arteries is an aortobilateral femoral bypass (Fig. 41–7). This operation is performed through an abdominal incision and a smaller incision in each groin. A Dacron tube, which has been knitted into the shape of the Y, is sutured from the aorta to both femoral arteries. For the treatment of occlusions in the superficial femoral artery, a femoral-popliteal bypass is performed. The choice of grafts includes the patient's own saphenous vein or a plastic conduit made of PTFE (Gore-tex).

For limb salvage bypasses below the knee, the saphenous vein is used almost exclusively. Postoperative recovery from reconstructions of the lower extremity may be lengthy. This is particularly true if patients have areas of necrosis and require simultaneous amputations. In uncomplicated cases, the postoperative stay is in the range of 1 to 2 weeks.

The most dreaded complication for reconstructive procedures of the lower extremities is infection

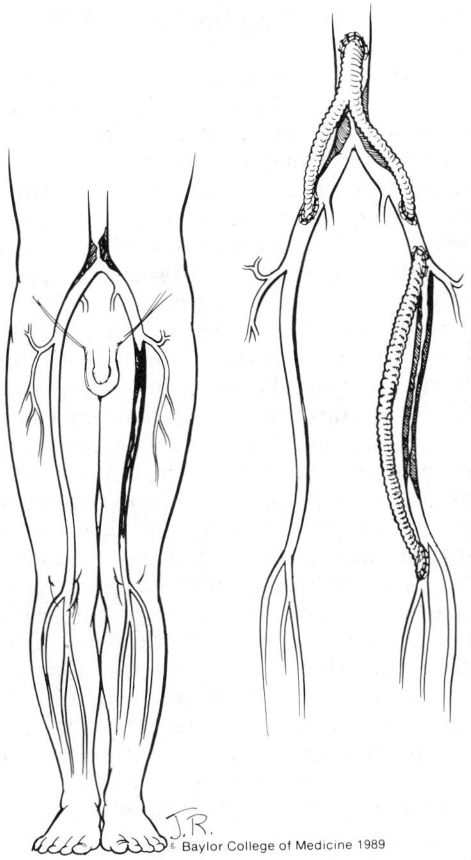

Figure 41–7. Two common sites of atherosclerosis affecting the lower extremities: the aortic-iliac segment and the superficial femoral artery. When sequential lesions occur, patients often experience pain at rest or tissue loss. Although an aortofemoral bypass and a femoropopliteal bypass are rarely performed simultaneously, these procedures may be indicated when pulsatile blood flow is necessary for healing, e.g., in cases of extensive necrosis of the foot.

in an artificial graft, which fortunately occurs in only 1 per cent of cases. When graft infection occurs in an aortoiliac graft, the overall mortality rate is at least 50 per cent and probably greater.

Furthermore, the risk of loss of an extremity is even higher. The mortality rate for aortic and iliac reconstruction is in the range of 2 to 3 per cent and the chances of a successful operation remaining functional for 5 years are in the range of 80 to 90 per cent (Kouchoukos et al., 1968; Moore et al., 1968).

Although the mortality rate for operations below the groin is similar to aortoiliac reconstructions, the long-term patency rates for these grafts is considerably lower, often in the range of 50 to 70 per cent at 5 years (Szilagyi et al., 1979; Veith et al., 1981; Bergan et al., 1982).

Because of the superior long-term results for operations on patients with aortoiliac disease, surgeons are more inclined to operate on those patients with less severe symptoms compared to those with femoral-popliteal disease.

ACUTE ARTERIAL OCCLUSION

There are three mechanisms by which acute arterial occlusion can occur. *Embolic occlusion* results from either a blood clot or valvular vegetation from the heart breaking off and drifting through the arterial circulation until it lodges at the site of a major arterial branching. The second mechanism of acute occlusion is *thrombosis*. Most cases of thrombosis occur when a previously narrowed atherosclerotic plaque becomes totally occluded. However, since the etiology of that presentation is atherosclerotic, it will not be considered in this section. Other causes for acute thrombosis are rare. These include hypercoagulable states, such as antithrombin III deficiency, protein S and C deficiency, and lupus anticoagulant. One other clinical setting responsible for thrombosis is the combination of estrogen-containing birth control pills and smoking in women. Hematologic diseases, such as polycythemia and disseminated intravascular coagulopathy, may predispose to thrombosis, and it can also occur in low-flow states, such as congestive heart failure or severe volume depletion. The third mechanism for acute occlusion is *trauma*. Traumatic thrombosis may be seen in blunt trauma where the stretching of arteries results in rupture of the arterial intima or in certain fractures, such as posterior dislocation of the elbow or knees and supracondylar fractures of the femur. Penetrating injuries (gunshot wounds and stab wounds) cause transections or damage to arteries that often result in thrombosis.

The rapidity of onset of acute occlusion leads to a far different clinical picture than chronic occlusion. In the cerebral circulation, an acute occlusion of the carotid artery almost always leads to an immediate severe stroke without prior warning. In the lower extremities, the symptoms are also dramatic. Classically, the patient presents with many of the well-known five (or six) P's:

- Pain
- Pallor
- Pulselessness
- Paresthesia
- Paralysis
- Poikilothermia

Most cases of acute occlusion are caused by embolism, and most emboli originate in the heart. The common sites of origin are in the left atrium, due to atrial fibrillation or rarely an atrial myxoma, and the left ventricle, due to a mural thrombus secondary to myocardial infarction. Less often, vegetations due to endocarditis can develop on the cardiac valves and embolize. Emboli can also originate from blood clots or debris caused by atherosclerotic plaques or aneurysms.

Once free in the arterial circulation, emboli frequently lodge in the large vessels leading to the lower extremities, the most common site being the femoral artery. Patients usually experience the acute onset of pain, which becomes severe within minutes to hours. The extremity also becomes anesthetic. When acute arterial occlusion initially occurs, pallor rather than cyanosis is seen. By the time that cyanotic mottling of the skin or paralysis develops, the ischemia is far advanced.

Since acute arterial occlusion immediately jeopardizes the viability of tissue, surgery is the only treatment available. It is generally believed that tissues of the extremities will tolerate acute ischemia for up to but not exceeding 6 hours. After that time, some tissue damage almost always results. In patients where the cause of acute occlusion is clearly embolic, such as those patients with atrial fibrillation or a recent myocardial infarction, extensive diagnostic work-ups are neither desirable or necessary. When the diagnosis is apparent in trauma patients, preoperative evaluation should also be kept to a minimum. In certain cases where the etiology may be obscure or the physician is not certain whether the acute event is a thrombosis of an existing stenotic lesion or an embolus, arteriography may be helpful in planning the surgery.

In patients suffering from emboli, the search for the origin of the embolus is important for three reasons:

1. The physician may uncover severe underlying disease, such as myocardial infarction.
2. The source may be eliminated, as with aneurysms or myxomas.
3. Life-long anticoagulation may be necessary.

An echocardiogram may be helpful in identifying intracardiac sources. If the cardiac evaluation is normal, peripheral arteriography should be considered to look for irregular vessels or aneurysms that may be the source of arterioarterial emboli. If no source can be identified, a work-up for hypercoagulable states is indicated.

Fogarty and colleagues (1963) developed an inflatable, balloon-tipped catheter that can slide by a thrombus or embolus while deflated. After inflation of the balloon, the catheter can be withdrawn removing the embolus with it. It is possible using this technique to remove emboli from most vessels in the body, with the notable exception of the intracranial vessels. This simple procedure can be performed under local anesthesia, which is a distinct benefit, since many patients have had a recent myocardial infarction.

The mortality rates for successful thrombectomy and embolectomy are high, near 20 per cent. This is due to serious concomitant diseases that either predispose to embolus or cause them. Limbs can be successfully salvaged in 85 per cent of survivors.

ANEURYSMS

An aneurysm is a pathologic dilatation of a blood vessel, usually an artery. Aneurysms occur most commonly in the abdominal aorta below the renal arteries and in other sites, including the popliteal, femoral, splenic, and renal arteries. Atherosclerosis is the most common cause of the aneurysmal disease that occurs in older patients. Diseases of collagen metabolism (e.g., Marfan's syndrome), infections, and trauma may also lead to aneurysms.

Aneurysms can be divided into several categories. A true aneurysm is one that contains all layers of the arterial wall. False aneurysms are those where most or all layers have been disrupted leaving only scar tissue to retain the blood stream. Another type of aneurysm is the dissecting aneurysm, resulting from dissection of the blood stream into the wall of the vessel and creation of a false passage (Fig. 41–8).

Aneurysms are prone to complications, including rupture, thrombosis, and embolism. Aneurysms of the thoracic, abdominal aorta, and visceral vessel are more likely to rupture, whereas femoral and popliteal aneurysms more often cause embolism and thrombosis.

The natural history of aortic aneurysms was accurately described by Estes (1950). In his series, only 19 per cent of patients with abdominal aortic aneurysm lived for 5 years or longer. Of the patients who died, 63 per cent died from rupture of the aneurysm. Although the incidence of complications from other aneurysms is not precisely known, their risk is sufficient to mandate repair of the aneurysm in most cases.

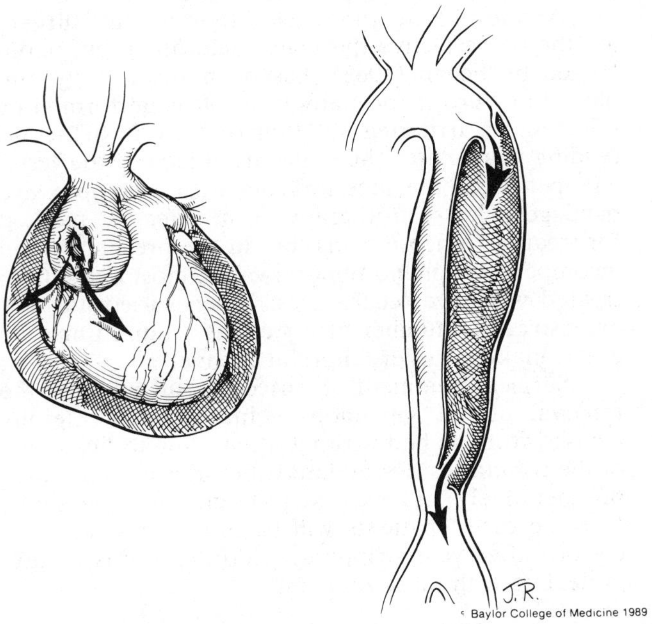

Figure 41–8. Two life-threatening complications of dissecting aortic aneurysms: On the left, an aneurysm has ruptured into the pericardium, causing acute cardiac tamponade; on the right, a dissecting aneurysm of the thoracic and abdominal aorta is shown with its false lumen. Dissections of the second type may cause visceral or extremity ischemia by compression of vessels that arise from the portion of the aorta involved by the dissection.

Patients with abdominal aortic aneurysms are usually asymptomatic but may present complaining of a lump in the abdomen that pulsates. The onset of abdominal or back pain is an ominous sign, which may signify the impending rupture of the lesion and should always be considered an emergency. On physical examination, the aneurysm should be palpated with one hand on each side of the lesion. The diagnosis is made if the hands are pushed apart with each pulse. In obese patients or those with small aneurysms, detection by physical examination may be difficult. Plain x-ray studies of the abdomen may reveal thin calcifications that define the size of the aneurysm. The best test available for diagnosing abdominal aortic aneurysms is ultrasound. Computerized tomographic scans have also been used but are of more value in planning an operation. Arteriograms should not be used for the diagnosis of an aneurysm but rather to evaluate concomitant vascular disease prior to surgery. The initial diagnosis of thoracic aneurysm is often made by a chest x-ray showing widening of the mediastinum. Aneurysms of the lower extremities are usually diagnosed by physical examination when the physician notices prominent pulses or a pulsatile mass. They may also be diagnosed by arteriography following acute thrombosis or embolism.

Considerable debate exists about the timing of surgery for small aortic aneurysms. The risk of rupture of an aortic aneurysm is related to its diameter (Rutherford, 1984). According to Rutherford, the risk of rupture of a 4 cm. aneurysm is less than 15 per cent compared to a 75 per cent risk for an 8 cm. aneurysm. Expectant management of small aneurysms (< 5 cm.) with serial ultrasound examinations may be considered, however, once rupture has occurred; the perioperative mortality rate is at least 50 per cent or more regardless of the size. When aneurysms are treated electively, the mortality rate is 2 to 3 per cent.

Because of the risk of sudden death, most aneurysms of the abdominal and thoracic aorta should be repaired unless serious concomitant illness contraindicates surgery (Fig. 41–9). For example, the operative risk for patients with myocardial infarction less than 6 months old or those with chronic congestive heart failure is usually prohibitive. Aneurysms that are *symptomatic* should be operated upon as emergencies.

Asymptomatic aneurysms of the popliteal and femoral arteries are operated upon electively except when thrombosis or embolus mandates immediate surgery to prevent limb loss. These procedures are quite simple with few contraindications.

The average length of hospitalization for abdominal aneurysm surgery is 7 to 10 days. For more complicated aneurysms involving both the thoracic and abdominal aorta, the usual hospitalization is much longer.

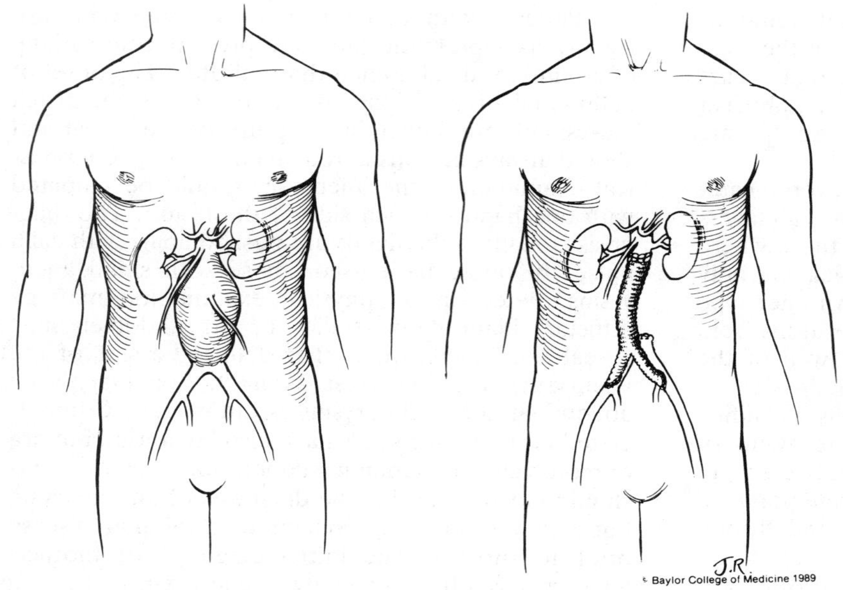

Figure 41–9. The figure on the left represents a typical infrarenal abdominal aortic aneurysm. On the right, the aneurysm has been resected and replaced with a Dacron bifurcation graft. Usually, the remaining aneurysm wall is sutured over the dacron graft to prevent the duodenum from being eroded by the aortic suture line. Such erosion can cause catastrophic hemorrhage or a graft infection.

VENOUS DISEASE

The physiology of the venous circulation is quite different from that of the arterial circulation. In veins, the pressure transmitted through the capillaries is too low to return blood to the heart of a standing adult. Therefore, veins are equipped with special dilatations and valves that, when compressed by the contraction of muscles, literally pump the blood back to the heart. Common presentations of venous disease include varicose veins, chronic venous insufficiency with postphlebitic syndrome, and deep venous thrombosis.

VARICOSE VEINS

The most familiar disease of the veins is varicose veins. These appear as serpentine dilatations most notably in the lower extremities below the knee. Not infrequently, varicosities are exacerbated or brought on by childbirth. Most patients with varicose veins are asymptomatic. However, some will suffer from cramping or burning pain, particularly after standing for long periods. Rarely, untreated varicose veins can lead to the formation of venous ulcers around the ankles.

The usual etiology is insufficiency of the valve located between the saphenous and femoral veins. Once the saphenous vein is exposed to higher pressure, successive failure of adjacent valves occurs. Because of its thick muscular wall, the saphenous vein is not likely to dilate. However, thin-walled venous tributaries leading to the saphenous vein are also exposed to higher pressure and do become dilated, resulting in the tortuous veins seen on physical examination. Some cases of varicose veins are caused by incompetence of tributaries connecting the deep venous system to the saphenous vein. Normally, blood flows from the superficial to the deep system, but if the valves of tributaries between the superficial and deep systems are damaged, blood flow is reversed.

Most cases of varicose veins do not require invasive treatment. Many patients are happy to wear support stockings. Nevertheless, some patients are concerned about the unsightly appearance of varicosities. These patients and those who are truly symptomatic should be considered for treatment.

At the present time, sclerotherapy and surgery are the two effective therapies. Sclerotherapy, popularized by Fegan (1963), has been successfully employed in Europe for many years. It is performed by injecting an irritating solution directly into the offending vein. After the veins are injected, the leg is wrapped from the toes to groin with a compressive bandage. The sclerotherapy is an effective method for treating varicose veins, but in the presence of an incompetent sapheno-femoral valve, most patients so treated will have recurrences. When varicosities are extensive, the number of injections required may be great, making surgery more attractive.

Surgical treatment of varicose veins involves the removal of the saphenous vein, which is literally avulsed from its bed without attempting to ligate any of the tributaries. Prominent tributaries are identified preoperatively and excised through small incisions. In some cases, patients will be left with small varicosities after vein stripping; sclerotherapy is helpful in dealing with these remnants.

CHRONIC VENOUS INSUFFICIENCY AND THE POSTPHLEBITIC SYNDROME

Two well-recognized etiologies for this disorder include (1) thrombosis of major proximal veins, such as the vena cava or iliac veins, and (2) the destruction of valves (in the deep venous system), including the iliac, femoral, and popliteal veins. The cause of both proximal venous thrombosis and valvular incompetence is thrombosis in the deep venous system. Following resolution of an acute attack, patients may be left with either permanent obstructions to flow caused by organizing thrombus or damaged valves as a result of inflammation and scarring. In the case of proximal thrombosis, collateral circulation quickly develops, and, in many cases, significant symptoms will not develop. Severe complications more often develop as a result of valvular insufficiency. When the valves are destroyed, the venous pump in the calves no longer works. Thus, as long as the legs are dependent, the veins and tissues of the lower legs are continuously exposed to high venous pressure that results in the postphlebitic syndrome. This syndrome is characterized by increasing pigmentation and thickening of the skin around the ankle, ulcerations, and chronic swelling of the extremity. Venous ulcerations are not nearly as painful as ischemic ulcers, though their appearance may be dramatic. Healing of a venous ulcer results in atrophic scarring, which is highly susceptible to recurrent injury. Consequently, patients have cycles of ulceration and healing. Most chronic venous ulcers are located around the ankle, usually on the medial side.

Although the diagnosis of chronic venous insufficiency is very clear, the etiology may not be. Since some cases of obstructive venous disease can be surgically treated, it is wise to document the cause of the venous insufficiency. For years, ascending and descending phlebography were the gold standards for diagnosing these disorders. However, phlebography is an invasive examination that carries with it a small but real risk of phlebitis and renal failure. For this reason, considerable effort has gone into the development of noninvasive tests. The best technique currently available for assessing chronic insufficiency due to obstructive disease is impedance plethysmography. This technique measures the changes of volume in the lower extremity following the application and release of proximal venous tourniquets. Photoplethysmography can be used to accurately diagnose valvular incompetence.

The treatment of chronic venous insufficiency due to outflow obstruction can be accomplished with custom fit graded compression hose or, in some cases, surgical bypass (Johnson et al., 1982; Palma and Esperon, 1960). The treatment of postphlebitic syndrome secondary to valvular incompetence is far more difficult and frustrating. Although it would seem logical to repair the damaged valves, the results have been poor. As a result, surgery plays a limited role, and both physician and patient must come to grips with the fact that the patient has a *chronic disease* that cannot be cured or treated with an operation. Patients must undergo a significant change in lifestyle: They must try to keep their legs elevated as often during the 24 hours of a day as possible, at least at the level of the heart. Patients who are obligated to work or to stand during the day should be custom fitted with compression stockings with an ankle pressure of at least 40 mm. Hg (Johnson et al., 1982). The stockings must be applied before getting out of bed in the morning and should be taken off before going to bed at night. In spite of the discomfort of these stockings, the consequences of not maintaining adequate compression during the day almost invariably results in severe ulceration.

Once ulceration occurs, the stockings are often inadequate for treatment. In this situation, the application of Unna's paste boot is necessary. This boot is actually a flexible walking cast that is applied after the patient has maintained the legs elevated to assure all edema is gone. Unna's paste is made from a combination of zinc oxide, glycerine, gelatin, and water. Using short strips of roller gauze, the custom fit boot can be rapidly applied. The boot should fit from the toes to just below the knee. A boot will last 1 or 2 weeks and should be reapplied as necessary until the ulcer is healed. With the use of Unna's paste boot, virtually all ulcerations will heal. Once the ulcers are healed, custom fitted high compression stockings must be worn as a routine. Parenthetically, it is remarkable how difficult it is to get patients with this syndrome to comply with the recommendations of their physician.

DEEP VENOUS THROMBOSIS

Deep venous thrombosis is caused by the acute formation of blood clots in the deep venous system of the lower extremities. Most cases occur in hospitalized patients. It is believed that deep venous thrombosis begins as blood clots in the tibial veins that progress proximally to involve the popliteal, femoral, and even iliac veins. The etiology of deep venous thrombosis is not known; however, the triad of stasis, endothelial injury, and hypercoagulability that Virchow (1856) described over a century ago is still considered central to the process. Hypercoagulable states clearly play a role in some patients and this diagnosis should be pursued in most patients with deep venous thrombosis. Risk factors in hospitalized patients include obesity, pelvic infection, advanced age, and malignancy.

Many patients with deep venous thrombosis do not have significant findings on physical examination. The typical signs and symptoms, when present, are aching or throbbing pain in the calf and tenderness to palpation in the calf and thigh. Homans' sign (pain on dorsal flexion of the foot) is of greater help when it coincides with other physical findings. Occasionally, a low-grade fever will be present. Rarely, venous occlusion will be so severe that pressure in the veins builds up to the point where it impedes arterial flow and jeopardizes the viability of the extremity. This condition is known as phlegmasia cerulia dolens. Because of the intense venous congestion in the tissues, the extremity takes on a purplish mottling. A somewhat less severe form of phlegmasia is known as phlegmasia alba dolens, where swelling of the entire lower extremity occurs, but the color of the leg remains normal and the limb is not jeopardized. All cases of phlegmasia involve thromboses in the femoral and iliac venous segments.

Physical examination has been notoriously unreliable to accurately diagnosis deep venous thrombosis. Since treatment carries a significant risk, accurate diagnosis is important. Two noninvasive tests have become popular for the diagnosis of deep venous thrombosis; these include the Doppler ultrasonic probe and impedance plethysmography. If noninvasive tests are equivocal or not available, a venogram should be considered. Evidence of DVT on noninvasive studies or venogram requires treatment. The goal of therapy is to avoid potentially lethal pulmonary embolism as well as crippling chronic venous insufficiency. Anticoagulation with heparin remains the treatment of choice in spite of recent advances in thrombolytic therapy. Heparin is usually given as a continuous infusion to maintain the partial thomboplastin time at least one and one half to two times the upper limit of normal. Heparin is continued for 7 to 10 days and during the last few days of heparinization, the patients are started on Coumadin. Recently there has been a trend toward initiating Coumadin simultaneously with heparin so as to reduce the overall length of hospital stay (Gallus et al., 1986). The prothrombin time is used to monitor Coumadin therapy, and it should be kept approximately one and one half to two times normal and be continued for 3 months. Chronic Coumadin therapy is potentially hazardous, and frequent office visits are necessary to avoid either inadequate or excessive anticoagulation.

Thrombolytic therapy with either streptokinase or urokinase is gaining more acceptance. Claims of a decreased incidence of postphlebitic syndrome are being made for this treatment. Unfortunately, streptokinase therapy is associated with a significant number of allergic reactions that may preclude treatment. Urokinase is at least as effective as streptokinase but is exceedingly expensive: the cost of treatment may exceed $1000 per day. Also, there is a risk of fatal hemorrhage with the use of either agent and precautions must be taken. The appropriate place for the use of these costly and sophisticated drugs remains to be defined.

Surgical treatment is rarely indicated for the treatment of deep venous thrombosis. The only indication with which most surgeons would agree is phlegmasia cerulia dolens, in which the patient's extremity is at risk.

References

Adams, D. H., Fine, C., Brooks, D. C. High-resolution real-time ultrasonography: a new tool in the diagnosis of acute appendicitis. Am. J. Surg., *155*:93–97, 1988.

Agarwal, N., Cayten, C. G., Ulahannan, M. J., et al.: Increased risk of colorectal cancer following breast cancer. Ann. Surg., *203*:307–310, 1986. *This retrospective analysis of 7605 cancer patients showed that patients with breast cancer have two times the usual risk of having a metachronous colon cancer, which is similar in magnitude to the risk following primary colon cancer (1.7).*

Albrechtsson, U., Anderson, J., Einarsson, E., et al.: Streptokinase treatment of deep venous thrombosis and its post-thrombotic syndrome: follow-up evaluation of venous function. Arch. Surg., *116*:33, 1981.

Allen, M. J., Borody, T. J., Bugliosi, T. F., et al.: Rapid dissolution of gallstones by methyl tert-butyl ether: preliminary observations. N. Engl. J. Med., *312*:217–220, 1985.

American Medical Association: Diagnostic and therapeutic technology assessment. J.A.M.A., *250*:540, 1983.

American Society for Gastrointestinal Endoscopy: The role of endoscopy in the management of upper gastrointestinal hemorrhage: guidelines for clinical application. Gastrointest. Endosc., *34*(Suppl.)45–55, 1988.

American Society for Gastrointestinal Endoscopy: The role of endoscopy in the patient with lower gastrointestinal bleeding: guidelines for clinical application. Gastrointest. Endosc., *34*(Suppl.):235–259, 1988. *Definitive statement on the role of colonoscopy in evaluating the patient with lower gastrointestinal bleeding.*

Baker, L. H.: Breast cancer demonstration project: 5 year summary report. Cancer, *32*:194–226, 1982. *This study detected 5.5 cancers per 100,000 women on first screen; the interval detection rate was 0.78 per 100,000.*

Baker, R. N., Schwartz, W. S., and Ramseyor, J. C.: Prognosis among survivors of ischemic stroke. Neurology *18*:933, 1968. *The grim prognosis for patients who survive ischemic strokes is little appreciated.*

Baker, R. R.: Preoperative assessment of the patient with breast cancer. Surg. Clin. North Am., *64*:1039–1059, 1984. *This review summarizes the literature on preoperative evaluation and staging of patients with breast cancer, including an assessment of the predictive value of commonly used laboratory tests and procedures.*

Beger, H. G., Krautzberger, W., Bittner, R., et al.: Results of surgical treatment of necrotizing pancreatitis. World J. Surg., *9*:972–979, 1985.

Bell, W. R., and Meek, A. G.: Guidelines for the use of thrombolytic agents. N. Engl. J. Med., *201*:1266, 1979.

Bennett, S. E., Lawrence, R. S., Fleischman, K. G., et al.: Profile of women practicing breast examination. J.A.M.A., *249*:488–491, 1983.

Berg, R. J., Selinger, S. C., Leonard, J. J., et al.: Surgical management of acute myocardial infarction. Cardiovasc. Clin. *12*:61, 1982.

Bergan, J. J., Veith, F. J., Berhard, V. M., et al.: Randomization of autogenous vein and polytetrafluoroethylene (PTFE) grafts in femoral-distal reconstruction. Surg., *92*:921, 1982.

Berne, T. V., Yellin, A. W., Appleman, M. D., and Heseltine, P. N. R.: Antibiotic management of surgically treated gangrenous or perforated appendicitis: comparison of gentamicin and clindamycin versus cefamandole versus cefoperazone. Am. J. Surg., *144*:8–13, 1982. *Gentamicin-clindamycin showed a clear advantage over cefamandole and cefoperazone in preventing infectious complications after surgical treatment of gangrenous or perforated appendicitis.*

Bharadvay, B. K., Zarins, C. K., and Giddens, D. P.: Carotid bifurcation atherosclerosis: quantitative correlation of plaque localization with flow velocity profiles and wall shear stress. Circ. Res. *53*:502, 1983.

Bizer, L. S., Liebling, R. W., Delany, H. M., and Gliedman, M. L.: Small bowel obstruction: the role of nonoperative treatment in simple intestinal obstruction and predictive criteria for strangulation obstruction. Surgery, *89*:407–413, 1981.

Blery, C., Charpak, Y., Szatan, M., et al.: Evaluation of a protocol for selective ordering of preoperative tests. Lancet, *1*:139–142, 1986.

Boey, J., Branicki, F. J., Alagaratnam, T. T., et al.: Proximal gastric vagotomy: the preferred operation for perforations in acute duodenal ulcer. Ann. Surg. *208*:169–174, 1988.

Bolt, R. J. (Ed.): Medical Evaluation of the Surgical Patient. Mt. Kisco, N.Y., Futura Publishing Co., 1987, pp. 12–14.

Bosworth, J. L., and Ghossein, N. A.: Limited surgery and radiotherapy in the treatment of localized breast cancer. Surg. Clin. North Am., *64*:1115–1123, 1984.

Boyd, A. M.: The natural course of arteriosclerosis of the lower extremities. Angiology, *11*:10–14, 1960. *Boyd's classic study of claudication serves as a perpetual reminder that the symptom is benign in most patients. Far more important is the risk these patients face from coronary and cerebral atherosclerosis.*

Boyd, N. F., Wolfson, C. K., Moskowitz, M., et al.: Observer variation in the interpretation of xeromammograms. J. Natl. Cancer Inst., *68*:357–363, 1982.

Bradley, E. L., III.: Management of infected pancreatic necrosis by open drainage. Ann. Surg., *206*:542–550, 1987.

Braumwald, E., and Cohn, P. F.: Ischemic heart disease. *In* Petersdorf, R. G. (Ed.): Harrison's Principles of Internal Medicine. 10th ed. New York, McGraw-Hill, 1983.

Brott, T., and Thalinger, K.: The practice of carotid endarterectomy in a large metropolitan area. Stroke *15*:950–955, 1984.

Buchman, T. G., and Zuidema, G. D.: Reasons for delay of the diagnosis of acute appendicitis. Surg. Gynecol. Obstet., *158*:260–266, 1984.

Burhenne, H. J., Fache, J. S., Gibney, R. G., et al.: Biliary lithotripsy by extracorporeal shock waves: integral part of nonsurgical intervention. A.J.R., *150*:1279–1283, 1988.

Celli, B. R., Rodriguez, K. S., and Shider, G. L.: A controlled trial of intermittent positive pressure breathing, incentive spirometry and deep breathing exercises in preventing pulmonary complications after abdominal surgery. Am. Rev. Resp. Dis., *130*:12–15, 1984. *In a prospective randomized study, comparing methods of preventing pulmonary complications, the frequency of complications was 48 per cent in the control group, 22 per cent in the IPPB group, 21 per cent in the incentive spirometry group, and 22 per cent in the deep breathing exercises group. Use of incentive spirometry decreased hospital stay in patients undergoing upper abdominal surgery by an average of 4.4 days versus controls.*

Chesebro, J., Fuster, V., Elveback, L., et al.: Effect of dipyridamole and aspirin on late vein graft patency after coronary bypass operations. N. Engl. J. Med., *310*:209–214, 1984.

Clavien, P. A., Hauser, H., Meyer, P., and Rohner, A.: Value of contrast-enhanced computerized tomography in the early diagnosis and prognosis of acute pancreatitis: a prospective study of 202 patients. Am. J. Surg., *155*:457–466, 1988.

Cohen, M. M., Duncan, P. G., and Tate, R. B.: Does anesthesia contribute to operative mortality? J.A.M.A., *260*(19):2859–2863, 1988. *A retrospective review found that advanced age, male gender, physical status, major surgery, emergency procedures, procedures performed in 1975 to 1979, intraoperative complications, narcotic techniques, and having one or two anesthetic drugs administered were associated with increased mortality.*

Conn, H. O., Ramsby, G. R., Storer, E. H., et al.: Intraarterial vasopressin in the treatment of upper gastrointestinal hemorrhage: a prospective, controlled clinical trial. Gastroenterology, *68*:211–221, 1975. *A prospective randomized trial comparing intraarterial vasopressin and conventional therapy in 60 episodes of upper gastrointestinal hemorrhage. Vasopressin was more effective in controlling hemorrhage from nonvariceal lesions ($p < 0.05$) and from varices ($p < 0.01$) than conventional therapy.*

Cranley, J. J.: Ischemic rest pain. Arch. Surg., *98*:187–188, 1969. *An excellent description of rest pain.*

Crist, D. W., and Cameron, J. L.: The current management of acute pancreatitis. Adv. Surg., *20*:69–123, 1987.

Cuthbertson, D. P.: Second annual Jonathan E. Rhoads lecture. The metabolic response to injury and its nutritional implications: retrospect and prospect. J. Parent. Enteral. Nutr., *3*(3):108–129, 1979.

Cuzick, J., Stewart, H., Peto, R., et al.: Overview of randomized trials comparing radical mastectomy without radiotherapy against simple mastectomy with radiotherapy in breast cancer. Cancer Treatment Reports *71*:7–14, 1987. *This summary of mature trials comparing radical mastectomy versus simple mastectomy plus irradiation (n=3236) shows no significant difference in survival.*

Dean, C.: Psychiatric morbidity following mastectomy: preoperative predictors and type of illness. J. Psychosom. Res. *31*:385–392, 1987. *Interviews with 122 women with primary operable breast cancer prior to 3- and 6-month postmastectomy showed 5 per cent with diagnosable psychiatric symptoms at 12 months postoperatively. Factors associated with risk of psychiatric illness postmastectomy were identified.*

DHEW Pub. No. HSM 72–8131: Ten-state Nutritional Survey, 1968–70. Washington, DC., U.S. Government Printing Office, 1972.

Dripps, R. D., Eckenhoff, J. E., and Vandam, L. D.: Introduction to Anesthesia: The Principles of Safe Practice. Philadelphia, W. B. Saunders, Co. 1982, pp. 16–17.

Droegemueller, W., Herbst, A. L., Mishell, D. R., and Stenchever, M. A.: Comprehensive Gynecology. St. Louis, The C. V. Mosby Co., 1987, p. 334.

Droegenmueller, W., Herbst, A. L., Mishell, D. R., and Stenchever, M. A.: Breast diseases. *In* Comprehensive Gynecology. St. Louis, The C. V. Mosby Co., 1987, p. 337.

Early Breast Cancer Trialists' Collaborative Group: Effects of adjuvant tamoxifen and of cytotoxic therapy on mortality in early breast cancer. N. Engl. J. Med., *319*:1681–1692, 1988. *In this summary of worldwide randomized trials begun before 1985 of adjuvant tamoxifen or cytotoxic therapy for early breast cancer (n=28,896), tamoxifen clearly reduced mortality in women > 50 years of age; chemotherapy clearly reduced mortality in women <50, and polychemotherapy was more effective than a single agent.*

Easton, J. D., and Sherman, D. G.: Stroke and mortality rate in carotid endarterectomy: 288 consecutive operations. Stroke *8*:565–568, 1977.

Ennix, C. L., Lawrie, G. M., Morris, G. C., et al.: Improved results of carotid endarterectomy in patients with symptomatic coronary disease: an analysis of 1,546 consecutive carotid operations. Stroke, *10*:122, 1979.

Estes, J. E.: Abdominal aortic aneurysm: a study of 102 cases. Circulation *2*:158–264, 1950.

Fallette, D. M., Fey, K., Mulder, D., et al.: Advantages of blood cardioplegia over intermittent ischemia during prolonged hypothermic aortic clamping. Circulation *58*(Suppl. 1):200, 1978.

Farnell, M. B., and Larson, D. E.: The investigation and management of gastrointestinal bleeding. *In* Irving M. H., and Beart, R. W., Jr.: Gastroenterological Surgery. London, Butterworths, 1983, pp. 118–153.

Fegan, W. G.: Continuous compression technique of injecting varicose veins. Lancet, *2*:109, 1963. *Fegan popularized sclerotherapy in Europe. The main benefit of this technique is that it leaves no surgical scars.*

Feigal, D. W., and Blaisdell, F. W. L.: The estimation of surgical risk. Med. Clin. North Am., *63*:1131–1143, 1979.

Feigal, D. W., Rose, S. D., Corman, L. C., et al.: Cardiac risk factors in patients undergoing noncardiac surgery. Med. Clin. North Am., *63*:1272–1287, 1979.

Feliciano, D. V.: Surgical options and results of treatment of perforated ulcers. Probl. Gen. Surg., *4*:301–307, 1987.

Feliciano, D. V., Bitondo, C. G., Burch, J. M., et al.: Emergency management of perforated peptic ulcers in the elderly patient. Am. J. Surg., *148*:764–767, 1984. *Elderly patients with previous symptoms of acid-peptic disease who do not have serious associated diseases that increase the risk of operation, generalized peritonitis, or localized abscesses can undergo definitive ulcer procedures for perforated peptic ulcers with satisfactory morbidity and low mortality rates.*

Field, S.: Plain films: the acute abdomen. Clin. Gastroenterol., *13*:3–40, 1984.

Fisher, B., Costantino, J., Redmond, C., et al.: A randomized clinical trial evaluating tamoxifen in the treatment of patients with node-negative breast cancer who have estrogen-receptor-positive tumors. N. Engl. J. Med., *320*:479–484, 1989.

Fisher, B., Redmond, C., Dimitrov, N. V., et al.: A randomized clinical trial evaluating sequential methotrexate and fluorouracil in the treatment of patients with node-negative breast cancer who have estrogen-receptor-negative tumors. N. Engl. J. Med., *320*:473–478, 1989.

Fisher, B., Redmond, C., Poisson, R., et al.: Eight-year results of a randomized clinical trial comparing total mastectomy and lumpectomy with or without irradiation in the treatment of breast cancer. N. Engl. J. Med., *312*:665–673, 1985. *Eight-year follow-up of 1843 women randomized to lumpectomy ± irradiation versus total mastectomy for stage I or II breast cancer showed no significant differences in rates of disease-free survival, distant disease-free survival, and overall survival. Irradiation reduced the probability of local recurrence following lumpectomy.*

Fogarty, T. J., Cranley, J. J., Krause, R. J., et al.: A method for extraction of arterial emboli and thrombi. Surg. Gynecol. Obstet., *116*:241, 1963. *The Fogarty catheter was a significant contribution to the treatment of thrombo-embolic disease. Prior to the introduction of this catheter there was no satisfactory method for extracting blood clots from vessels.*

Folstein, M. F., Folstein, S. E., and McHugh, P. R.: Mini-mental state: a practical method for grading the cognitive state of patients for the clinician. J. Psychiatr. Res. *12*:189–198, 1975.

Foster, R. S.: Surgery and radiotherapy for primary breast cancer. Surg. Clin. North Am., *64*:1125–1144, 1984.

Foster, R. S., and Costanza, M. C.: Breast self-examination practices and breast cancer survival. Cancer, *53*:999, 1984.

Franz, V. K., Pickren, J. W., Melcher, G. W., et al.: Incidence of chronic cystic disease in so-called "normal breasts." Cancer, *4*:762, 1951.

Frisch, R. E., Wyshak, G., Albright, N. L., et al.: Lower prevalence of breast cancer and cancers of the reproductive system among former college athletes compared to non-athletes. Br. J. Cancer *52*:885–891, 1985.

Galazka, S. S.: Preoperative evaluation of the elderly surgical patient. J. Fam. Pract., *27*(6):622–632, 1988. *This clinical review summarizes the contribution of age as an independent risk factor and describes a comprehensive preoperative assessment of the elderly individual.*

Gallus, A., Jackaman, J., Tillett, J., et al.: Safety and efficacy of Warfarin started early after submassive venous thrombosis or pulmonary embolism. Lancet, *2*:1293–1296, 1986.

Gambrell, R. D., Jr.: Proposal to decrease the risk and improve the prognosis of breast cancer. Am. J. Obstet. Gynecol., *150*:119–128, 1984.

Gilbert, M., and Clatworthy, H. W., Jr.: Bilateral operations for inguinal hernia and hydrocele in infancy and childhood. Am. J. Surg. *97*:255, 1979.

Goldman, L., Caldera, D. L., Nussbaum, S. R., et al.: Multifactorial index of cardiac risk in noncardiac surgical procedures. N. Engl. J. Med., *297*(16):845–850, 1977. *This prospective study of patients over 40 years of age using multivariate discriminant analysis is the classic study identifying independent correlates for fatal and life-threatening cardiac complications.*

Goodson, W. H., III, Mailman, R., and Miller, T. R.: Three year follow-up of benign fine-needle aspiration biopsies of the breast. Am. J. Surg., *154*:58–61, 1987. *Patients (285) whose fine-needle aspiration biopsy results were benign were followed for 3 years in order to determine a true false-negative rate for this procedure. Follow-up was obtained on 204 patients (71.5 per cent) of whom six were found to have invasive cancer and one lobular carcinoma in situ, in the hands of experienced operators.*

Greenburg, A. G., Saik, R. P., Bell, R. H., and Collins, G. M.: Changing patterns of gastrointestinal bleeding. Arch. Surg., *120*:341–344, 1985. *A retrospective analysis of 351 patients with gastrointestinal bleeding revealed that benign ulcer disease accounted for 86 per cent of emergency operations, stress bleeding as a surgical lesion has essentially disappeared, and lower gastrointestinal bleeding has a lower rate of operative intervention as compared to upper gastrointestinal lesions.*

Greuntzig, A.: Transluminal dilatation of coronary artery stenosis. Lancet, *1*:263, 1978. *Since Adreas Greuntzig first performed percutaneous transluminal coronary angioplasty, thousands of these procedures have been performed. Angioplasty is also performed for occlusive disease of the renal, iliac, femoral, and popliteal arteries. Early restenosis remains a significant problem.*

Gruentzig, A., King, S., Schlumpf, M., et al.: Long-term follow-up after percutaneous transluminal coronary angioplasty. N. Engl. J. Med., *316*:1127–1132, 1987.

Hiatt, J. R., Calabria, R. P., Passaro, E., Jr., and Wilson, S. E.: The amylase profile: a discriminant in biliary and pancreatic disease. Am. J. Surg., *154*:490–492, 1987. *A review of the different levels of amylase elevations in 35 patients with gallstone pancreatitis as compared to 50 patients with alcoholic pancreatitis.*

Hodnett, R. M., Gonzalez, F., Lee, W. C., et al.: The need for definitive therapy in the management of perforated gastric ulcers: review of 202 cases. Ann. Surg., *209*:36–39, 1988. *There was a definite difference in mortality among those patients treated with definitive operative procedures (11.3 per cent) versus those patients treated with nondefinitive surgery (22.9 per cent), even in the presence of purulent exudate in the abdominal cavity and among those patients presenting in shock.*

Hoffmann, J., Lanng, C., and Shokouh-Amiri, M. H.: Peritoneal lavage in the diagnosis of acute peritonitis. Am. J. Surg., *155*:359–360, 1988.

Hofstetter, S. R.: Acute adhesive obstruction of the small intestine. Surg. Gynecol. Obstet., *152*:141–144, 1981.

Holm, R., Rock, C., and Blumenstein, B.: A survey of 1000 outpatients seen at the Grady Memorial Hospital Medical Clinic, Emory University School of Medicine. Atlanta, Georgia. In-hospital data, 1977.

Imparato, A. M., Kim, G., Davidson, T., and Crowley, J.: Intermittent claudication: its natural course. Surgery, *78*:795–799, 1975.

Jackson, C. V.: Preoperative pulmonary evaluation. Arch. Int. Med., *148*:2120, 1988.

Jeffrey, R. B., Jr., Laing, F. C., and Townsend, R. R.: Acute appendicitis: sonographic criteria based on 250 cases. Radiology, *167*:327–329, 1988. *A review of high-resolution ultrasound in patients with suspected appendicitis. A diagnosis is confirmed in the patient with right lower quadrant pain and a visualized appendix greater than 6 mm. in diameter.*

Johnson, G., Jr., Kupper, C., Farrar, D. J., et al.: Graded compression stockings: custom vs. non-custom. Arch. Surg., *117*:69–72, 1982.

Jones, E., Craver, J., Michalik, R., et al.: Combined carotid and coronary operations: when are they necessary? J. Thorac. Cardiovasc. Surg. *87*:7–16, 1984.

Jordan, G. L., Jr., DeBakey, M. E., Duncan, J. M., Jr.: Surgical management of perforated peptic ulcer. Ann. Surg. *179*:628–633, 1974.

Kakkar, V. V., Carrigan, T. P., and Fossard, D. P.: Prevention of fatal postoperative pulmonary embolism by low doses of heparin: an international multicenter trial. Lancet, *2*:45–51, 1975.

Kartchner, M. M., and McRae, L. P.: Noninvasive evaluation and management of the "asymptomatic" of the carotid bruit. Surgery, *82*:840, 1977. *Noninvasive vascular studies have improved our understanding of the progression of carotid atherosclerosis and have provided an excellent screening tool for patients with cervical bruits. Kartchner and McRae are leaders in noninvasive testing.*

Kiesewetter, W. B.: Hernias–Inguinal and Umbilical. Am. J. Surg., *101*:656–663, 1961.

King, A. S.: Not everyone agrees with new mammographic screening guidelines designed to end confusion. J.A.M.A., *262*:1154–1155, 1989.

Kirkpatrick, J. R., and Bouwman, D. L.: A logical solution to the perforated ulcer controversy. Surg. Gynecol. Obstet., *150*:683–686, 1980.

Kouchoukos, N. T., Levy, J. F., Balfour, J. F., and Butcher, H. R.: Operative therapy for aortoiliac arterial occlusive disease: a comparison of therapeutic methods. Arch. Surg., *96*:628, 1968.

Krall, J. G. (Ed.): Surgical therapy in Greenwood MRC obesity. New York, Churchill Livingstone, 1983, pp. 25–38.

Laing, F. C.: Diagnostic evaluation of patients with suspected cholecystitis. Surg. Clin. North Am., *64*:3–22, 1984. *An excellent concise overview of radiologic options to confirm the diagnosis of cholecystitis.*

Lannin, D. R., Silverman, J. F., Walker, C., Povies, W. S.: Cost effectiveness of fine needle biopsy of the breast. Ann. Surg., *203*:474–480, 1986.

Lawson, D. W., Daggett, W. M., Civetta, J. M., et al.: Surgical treatment of acute necrotizing pancreatitis. Ann. Surg., *172*:602–615, 1970.

Leriche, R., and Morel, A.: The syndrome of thrombotic obliteration of the aortic bifurcation. Ann. Surg., *127*:193–206, 1948. *This is the first English language publication of Leriche's description of the syndrome that bears his name. At the time, Leriche believed that these patients suffered from a form of aortitis; we now know that these patients have early onset atherosclerosis.*

Loder, R. E.: Routine preoperative chest radiography: 1977 compared with 1955 at Peterborough District General Hospital. Anesthesia, *33*(10):972–974, 1978.

Loeb, C., Priano, A., and Albana, L.: Clinical features and long-term follow-up of patients with reversible ischemic attacks. Acta Neurol. Scand., *57*:471, 1978.

Loop, F., Lytle, B., Cosgrove, D., et al.: Influence of the internal mammary artery graft on 10-year survival and other cardiac events. N. Engl. J. Med., *314*:1–6, 1986. *The routine use of the internal mammary artery for coronary artery bypass may dramatically improve the long-term results of this operation. The average patency rate of 96 per cent over a 10-year follow-up is unparalleled in cardiovascular surgery.*

Lytle, W. J.: Internal inguinal ring. Br. J. Surg., *32*:441, 1945.

Madlon-Kay, R.: Evaluation of coronary artery disease in patients having non-cardiac surgery. South. Med. J., *80*(11):1366–1369, 1987. *This discussion of available methods for evaluation of patients with coronary artery disease describes the limitations of each method.*

Mann, L. C., Hawes, D. R., Ghods, M., et al.: Utilization of screening mammography: a comparison of different specialties. Radiology, *164*:121–122, 1987. *This study suggests that family physicians may be more vigilant in applying mammography screening guidelines than some other specialists.*

Mansour, E. G., Gray, R., Shatila, A. H., et al.: The efficacy of adjuvant chemotherapy in high-risk node-negative breast cancer. N. Engl. J. Med., *320*:485–490, 1989.

Martin, J. K., Jr., van Heerden, J. A., and Bess, M. A.: Surgical management of acute pancreatitis. Mayo Clin. Proc., *59*:259–267, 1984. *A review of 62 patients who underwent operation from a group of 222 patients who were treated for acute pancreatitis over a 2-year period at the Mayo Clinic. Biliary pancreatitis accounted for 63 per cent of operations, and the overall postoperative mortality was 24 per cent.*

Mayer, A. D., McMahon, M. J., Corfield, A. P., et al.: Controlled clinical trial of peritoneal lavage for the treatment of severe acute pancreatitis. N. Engl. J. Med., *312*:399–404, 1985.

McPhail, N., Calvin, J. E., Shariatmadar, A., et al.: The use of preoperative exercise testing to predict cardiac complications after arterial reconstruction. J. Vasc. Surg., *7*(1):60–66, 1988. *In this prospective study, 100 patients who achieved less than 85 per cent of their predicted maximum heart rate during exercise testing had a complication rate of 24 per cent, versus a 6 per cent complication rate in those who achieved more than 85 per cent of predicted maximum heart rate.*

McSherry, C. K., Ferstenberg, H., Calhoun, W. F., et al.: The natural history of diagnosed gallstone disease in symptomatic and asymptomatic patients. Ann. Surg., *202*:59–63, 1985.

McVay, C. B.: The anatomic basis for inguinal and femoral hernioplasty. Surg. Gynecol. Obstet., *139*:931, 1974. *Dr. McVay has made a life-long study of the anatomy of the abdominal wall and has spent almost as much time trying to teach surgeons to understand it. He also developed an elegant hernia repair for large or complex hernias of the groin. This repair bears his name.*

Mentzer, R. M., Finkelmeier, B. A., and Crosby, I. K.: Emergency carotid endarterectomy for fluctuating neurologic deficits. Surgery, *89*:60, 1981.

Minton, J. P., Foecking, M. K., Webster, D. J., et al.: Caffeine cyclic nucleotides and breast disease. Surgery, *86*:105, 1979.

Mock, M. B., Ringqvist, I., Fisher, L. D., et al.: Survival of medically treated patients in the Coronary Artery Surgery Study (CASS) Registry. Circulation, *66*:562, 1982.

Mohr, J. P., Caplan, L. R., Melski, J. W., et al.: The Harvard Cooperative Stroke Registry: a prospective registry. Neurology, *28*:754, 1978.

Moore, D. J., Miles, R. D., Gooley, N. A., and Sumner, D. S.: Non-invasive assessment of stroke risk in asymptomatic and nonhemispheric patients with suspected carotid disease: 5 year follow-up of 294 unoperated and 81 operated patients. Ann. Surg., *202*:491–504, 1985.

Moore, W. S., Boren, C., Malone, J. M., et al.: Asymptomatic carotid stenosis: immediate and long term results after prophylactic endarterectomy. Ann. Surg., *138*:228, 1979.

Moore, W. S., Cafferata, T., Hall, A. L., and Blaisdall, F. W.: In defense of grafts across the inguinal ligament: an evaluation of early and late results of aorto-femoral bypass grafts. Ann. Surg., *168*:207, 1968.

Moore, W. S., and Hall, A. D.: Importance of emboli from carotid bifurcation in pathogenesis of cerebral ischemic attacks. Arch. Surg., *101*:708, 1970.

Moorman, J. R., Hlatky, M. A., Eddy, D. M., et al.: The yield of the routine admission electrocardiogram. Ann. Int. Med., *103*:590–595, 1985.

Morgan, E. H., and Anson, B. J.: The anatomy of the region of inguinal hernia. IV. The internal surfaces of the parietal layers. Q. Bull. Northwest. Univ. Med. Sch., *16*:20, 1942.

Morise, A. P., McDowell, D. E., Savrin, R. A., et al.: The prediction of cardiac risk in patients undergoing vascular surgery. Am. J. Med. Sci., *293*(3):150–158, 1987.

Moss, G.: Discharge within 24 hours of elective cholecystectomy: the first 100 patients. Arch. Surg., *121*:1159–1161, 1986.

Murray, W. R., and Mackay, C.: The amylase creatinine clearance ratio in acute pancreatitis. Br. J. Surg., *64*:189–191, 1977.

Muskett, A. D., and McGreevy, J. M.: Rational preoperative evaluation. Postgrad. Med. J., *62*:925–928, 1986. *Clinical data from 200 consecutive patients on nine commonly ordered preoperative tests showed that 35.5 per cent of tests were abnormal, but only 5.9 per cent changed the patient's management before surgery; all but five of these were predictable, and all five were minor.*

Myers, W., Davis, K., and Foster, E.: Surgical survival in the Coronary Artery Surgery Study (CASS) Registry. Ann. Thorac. Surg., *40*:245–260, 1985.

National Center for Health Statistics: Vital statistics report: final mortality statistics. U.S. Dept. of Health and Human Services, Vol. II, Part A, 1978.

Nordestgaard, A. G., Wilson, S. E., and Williams, R. A.: Correlation of serum amylase levels with pancreatic pathology and pancreatitis etiology. Pancreas, *3*:159–162, 1988. *A prospective study in which 51 patients with acute pancreatitis underwent early computerized tomography. Within the etiologic subgroups—alcoholic = 28, gallstones = 14, cancer = 3, miscellaneous = 6—there was no correlation between the initial serum amylase level and the extent of pancreatic involvement visualized by computerized tomography.*

Palma, E. C., and Esperon, R.: Vein transplant and grafts in the surgical treatment in the post-phlebitic syndrome. J. Cardiovasc. Surg., *1*:94, 1960.

Passamani, E., Davis, K. B., Gillespie, M. J., et al.: A randomized trial of coronary artery bypass surgery: survival of patients with low ejection fractions. N. Engl. J. Med., *312*:1665–1671, 1985. *The Coronary Artery Surgery Study (CASS) has provided scientific documentation of the results of both the medical and surgical treatment of coronary artery disease. This particular randomized study showed a clear survival advantage for patients with impaired ventricular function and triple vessel disease when treated surgically.*

Pemberton, J. H., Nagorney, D. M., Becker, J. M., et al.: Controlled open lesser sac drainage for pancreatic abscess. Ann. Surg., *203*:600–604, 1986. *A retrospective review of 17 patients with pancreatic abscesses who were treated with controlled open lesser sac drainage as compared to another 64 patients treated with traditional closed drainage. In patients at increased risk of death (positive Ranson signs > 3), mortality after open drainage and closed drainage was 18 per cent and 70 per cent, respectively ($p < 0.05$).*

Pfeiffer, E.: A short portable mental status questionnaire for assessment of organic brain deficit in elderly patients. J. Am. Geriatr. Soc., *23*:433–441, 1975. *Use of either of these well-validated brief scales of mental status allows pre- and postoperative comparison of cognitive function.*

Pingleton, S. K.: Gastrointestinal hemorrhage. Med. Clin. North Am., *67*:1215–1228, 1983.

Pitt, H. A., McFadden, D. W., and Gadacz, T. R.: Agents for gallstone dissolution. Am. J. Surg., *153*:233–246, 1987. *A comprehensive review of currently available agents for dissolution of gallstones.*

Plecha, F. R., Abellone, J. C., and Beven, E. G.: A computerized vascular registry: experience of the Cleveland Vascular Society. Surgery, *86*:826, 1979.

Ranson, J. H. C., Rifkind, K. M., Roses, D. F., et al.: Prognostic signs and the role of operative management in acute pancreatitis. Surg. Gynecol. Obstet. *139*:69–81, 1974.

Read, R. C., Murphy, M. L., Hultgren, H. N., et al.: Survival of men treated for chronic stable angina-pectoris: a cooperative randomized study. J. Thorac. Cardiovasc. Surg., *75*:1, 1978. *The disappointing surgical results of this VA Cooperative Study were due in part to a high operative mortality rate. The technical expertise of those performing the procedures was questioned since, on the average, only one bypass was performed every 4 weeks.*

Richardson, J. D., Flint, L. M., and Polk, H. C., Jr.: Peritoneal lavage: a useful diagnostic adjunct for peritonitis. Surgery, *94*:826–829, 1983.

Ross, R.: Arteriosclerosis: a problem of the biology of arterial wall cells and their interactions with blood components. Arteriosclerosis, *1*:293–311, 1981. *A concise summary of the injury theory of atherogenesis.*

Rowe, M. I., and Clatworthy, J. W.: Incarcerated and strangulated hernias in children: a statistical study of high-risk factors. Arch. Surg., *101*:136, 1970.

Royal College of Radiologists: Preoperative chest radiology. Lancet, *2*:83–86, 1979.

Rutherford, R. B.: Infrarenal aortic aneurysms. *In* Rutherford, R. R., (Ed.): Vascular Surgery. Philadelphia, W. B. Saunders Co., 1984.

Sagel, S. S., Evens, R. G., Forrest, C. V., et al.: Efficacy of routine screening and lateral chest radiographs in a hospital-based population. N. Engl. J. Med., *291*(19):1001–1004, 1974.

Samiy, A. H., Douglas, R. G., and Barondess, J. A.: Textbook of diagnostic medicine. Philadelphia, Lea & Febiger, 1987, pp. 506–510.

Sanger, C. K., and Reznekoff, M.: A comparison of the psychologic effects of breast saving procedures with the modified radical mastectomy. Cancer, *48*:2341, 1981.

Schatzkin, A., Jones, D. Y., Hoover, R. N., et al.: Alcohol consumption and breast cancer in the epidemiologic follow up study of the first national health and nutrition examination survey. N. Engl. J. Med., *316*:1169–1173, 1987.

Scheuter, L. A.: Knowledge and beliefs about breast cancer and breast self-examinations among athletic and nonathletic women. Nurs. Res., *31*:348–353, 1982.

Shapiro, S., Venet, W., Strax, P., et al.: Selection, follow-up, and analysis in the Health Insurance Plan Study: a randomized trial with breast cancer screening. Natl. Cancer Inst. Monogr., *67*:65–74, 1985. *This is a follow-up study of the Health Insurance Plan Study, perhaps the single most important contribution to the control of breast cancer. A 40 per cent reduction in breast cancer mortality in women 50 years or older at entry was demonstrated at 9 years follow-up. Mortality was decreased by the early detection of preclinical disease.*

Shaw, P., Bates, D., Cartlidge, N., et al.: Neurological complications of coronary artery bypass graft surgery: six month follow-up study. Br. Med. J., *293*:165–167, 1986.

Silverstein, F. E., Gilbert, D. A., Tedesco, F. J., et al.: The national ASGE survey on upper gastrointestinal bleeding. I. Study design and baseline data. Gastrointest. Endosc., *27*:73–79, 1981.

Singer, M. V., and Gyr, K.: Revised classification of pancreatitis (Editorial). Gastroenterology, *89*:683–690, 1985.

Spencer, F., Green, G., Tice, D., et al.: Coronary artery bypass grafts for congestive heart failure: a report of experiences with 40 patients. J. Thorac. Cardiovasc. Surg., *62*:529, 1971.

Stahlgren, L. H.: Biliary lithotripsy. Am. J. Surg., *156*(Part 2):5B–8B, 1988. *A concise overview of the investigational status of biliary lithotripsy in the United States as of 1988.*

Starret, R. W., and Stoney, R. J.: Juxta-renal aortic occlusion. Surgery, *76*:890, 1974. *Many physicians have believed that chronic occlusion of the distal aorta was as benign as other causes of lower extremity ischemia we now recognize.*

Suarez, C., Block, F., Bernstein, D., et al.: The role of HIDA/PIPIDA scanning in diagnosing cystic duct obstruction. Ann. Surg., *191*:391–396, 1980. *One of the early reviews of radionuclide imaging in biliary tract disease that documents the excellent accuracy of the technique in confirming acute cholecystitis.*

Sugawa, C., Benishek, D., and Walt, A. J.: Mallory-Weiss syndrome: a study of 224 patients. Am. J. Surg., *145*:30–33, 1983.

Szilagyi, D. E., Haggman, J. H., Smith, R. F., et al.: Autogenous vein grafting in femoral-popliteal atherosclerosis: the limits of its effectiveness. Surgery, *86*:836, 1979.

Tape, T. G., and Mushlin, A. I.: How useful are routine chest x-rays of preoperative patients at risk for postoperative chest disease? J. Gen. Inter. Med., *3*:15–20, 1988. *A retrospective review of 341 admissions revealed a 40 per cent postoperative complication rate in patients with major chest x-ray abnormalities, versus 9 per cent with normal x-rays. Only nine patients had x-ray findings that led to clinical action, including three with potentially beneficial management changes, and six with potentially detrimental clinical action. No surgical cancellations occurred as a result of an abnormal x-ray.*

Taylor, T. V., Sumerling, M. D., Carter, D. C., et al.: An evaluation of 99 Tc^m-labelled HIDA in hepatobiliary scanning. Br. J. Surg., *67*:325–328, 1980.

Teicher, I., Landa, B., Cohen, M., et al.: Scoring system to aid in diagnoses of appendicitis. Ann. Surg., *198*:753–759, 1983.

Thompson, J. E., Patnam, R. D., and Talkington, C. M.: Asymptomatic carotid bruit: long term outcome of patients having endarterectomy compared with unoperated controls. Ann. Surg., *188*:308, 1978. *Jesse Thompson's superior results in carotid surgery have rarely been duplicated. In this article, he also calls attention to the risk of stroke in patients with asymptomatic bruits, about 17 per cent in 5 years.*

The TIMI Study Group: Comparison of invasive and conservative strategies after treatment with intravenous tissue plasminogen activator in acute myocardial infarction: Results in the Thrombolysis in Myocardial Infarction (TIMI) Phase II Trial. N. Engl. J. Med., *320*(10):618–627, 1989.

Tinker, M. A., and Wise, L.: The conservative management of breast cancer. Surg. Ann., *19*:279–315, 1987.

Veith, S. J., Gupta, S. K., Simpson, R. H., et al.: Progress in limb salvage by reconstructive arterial surgery combined with new and improved adjunctive procedures. Ann. Surg., *194*:386, 1981.

Virchow, R.: Neuer fall nontoedtlicher embolie der lungenarterien. Arch. Path. Anat. (Berlin), *10*:225, 1856.

Warner, M. H., Divertie, M. B., and Tinker, J. H.: Preoperative cessation of smoking and pulmonary complications in coronary artery bypass patients. Anesthesiology, *60*:380–383, 1984.

Weitz, H. H., and Goldman, L.: Noncardiac surgery in the patient with heart disease. Med. Clin. North Am., *71*(3):413–432, 1987.

Whisnant, J. P., Matsumoto, M., and Eleveback, L. R.: The effects of anticoagulant therapy on the prognosis of patients with transient cerebral ischemic attacks in a community—Rochester, Minnesota, 1965–1968. Mayo Clin. Proc. *48*:844, 1973. *This study provided important data on the natural history of transient ischemic attacks. Although the risk of stroke is significant, the annual rate of approximately 6 per cent mandates that prophylactic surgery be performed with a very low stroke/mortality rate.*

Whitney, D. G., Kahn, E. M., Estes, J. W., et al.: Carotid artery surgery without a temporary in-growing shunt: 1917 consecutive procedures. Arch. Surg., *115*:1393, 1980.

Whitworth, C. M., Whitworth, P. W., Sanfillipo, J., and Polk, H. C., Jr.: Value of diagnostic laparoscopy in young women with possible appendicitis. Surg. Gynecol. Obstet., *167*:187–190, 1988. *This prospective study documented the value of laparoscopy in permitting an earlier definitive diagnosis in patients with disease in the female reproductive tract. The negative appendectomy rate (33 per cent) in the institution did not change.*

Wyngaarden, J. B., and Smith, L. H. (Eds.): Cecil's Textbook of Medicine. Philadelphia, W. B. Saunders Co., 1985, pp. 1400–1401.

Zarins, C. K.: Hemodynamics in atherogenesis. *In* Moore, W. (Ed.): Vascular Surgery. Orlando, Florida, Grune & Stratton 1986. *Dr. Zarins' chapter on hemodynamics and atherosclerosis summarizes his intriguing alternative to the conventional theories of atherogenesis.*

42

Plastic and Reconstructive Surgery

Bonnie Baldwin
Samuel Stal
Christine C. Matson

The practice of plastic surgery offers to family physicians refined skills for their own use and surgical options for their patient's care. Four areas are of particular interest:

1. Concepts of tissue closure employed by plastic surgeons when applied by family physicians can minimize scar formation in repair of basic wounds.
2. Biopsy techniques, including punch biopsy and shave biopsy, can be useful to the family physician for the diagnosis of superficial skin lesions.
3. Large wounds, such as the decubitus ulcer, are frustrating but manageable with a clear strategy. Often these wounds will heal secondarily but may require well-planned surgical closure.
4. Patients have concerns about professional and personal stresses and success, and the possible role of aesthetic surgery. Guidance from the family physician plays an important role in patient care. Patients may consult their family physician when considering the possibility of aesthetic surgery. The family physician who is knowledgeable about the patient and the procedures can assess the patient's expectations and provide important guidance.

SURGICAL SCARS

Techniques of plastic surgery applied to the repair of lacerations produce a more aesthetic scar. Several factors contribute to the final appearance of the wound. Designing repairs to follow pre-existing skin lines, placing multiple sutures to relieve skin tension, and paying meticulous attention to skin edges are essential.

When the skin is cut, forces of tension separate the borders of the wound. In most regions of the body, the force of tension is greatest at right angles to the relaxed skin tension line (Borges, 1973). A wound inflicted perpendicular to the relaxed skin tension line will open widely, whereas a wound parallel to the tension line will remain narrow.

On the face, it is usually best to follow the visible wrinkle lines. In other areas of the body, these lines can be discerned by grasping the skin areas in a relaxed or flexed state, and observing which way the skin creases and folds. The folds are parallel to the tension lines. Designing the skin closure with its long axis parallel to these skin lines is desired for superior results (Figs. 42–1 and 42–2). There are areas of the body that form bad scars because of high tension in many directions. For example, patients should be warned that lacerations in the sternal and deltoid regions will develop wide scarring. Likewise, lacerations perpendicular to relaxed tension lines will heal with a more visible scar.

The term "atraumatic technique" in surgical repair is best visualized on a histologic level. Each cell layer, from the epidermis to the subcutaneous plane,

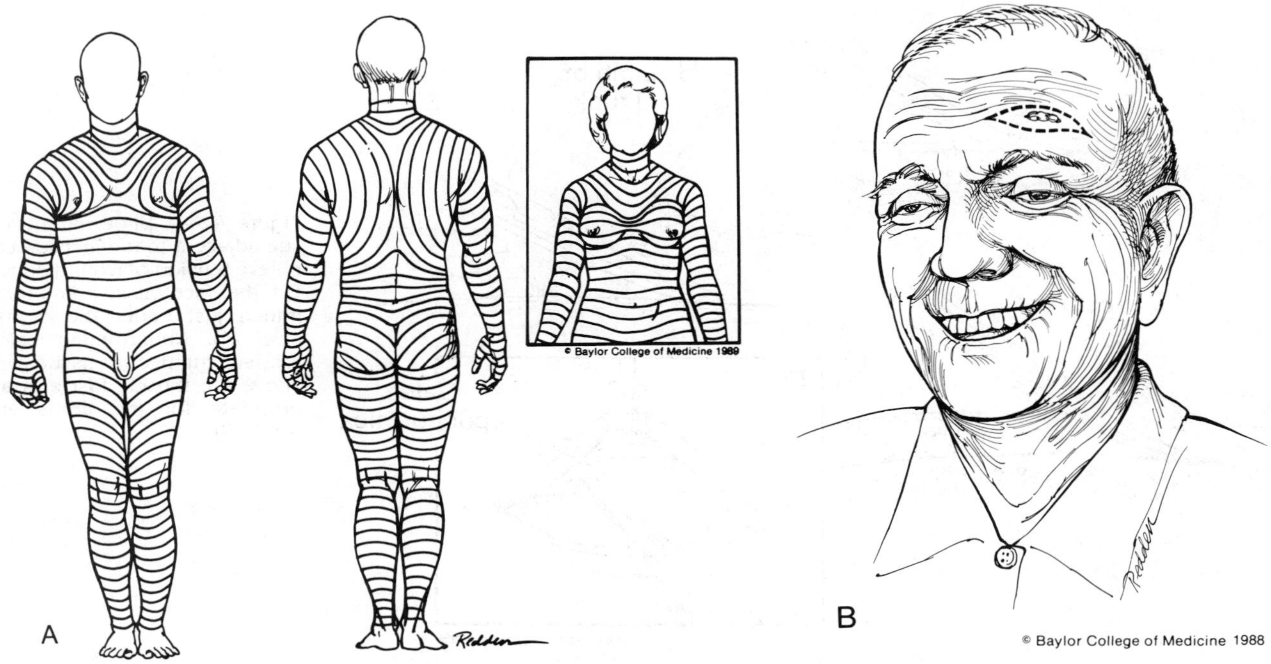

Figure 42–1. Relaxed skin tension lines on the face and body (*A*). Lesion on the forehead illustrates elliptical excision oriented with the tension lines (*B*).

depends on nutrients diffusing from capillaries into the surrounding tissue. The less pressure applied by pinching tissue with forceps or clamping dermal tissue with hemostats, the less cell damage is done. The more cleansing with a pulsatile flow of normal saline to remove foreign particles and nonviable tissue, the less diffusion barriers exist. If hemostasis is not achieved, a collection of blood between the upper skin layer and subcutaneous tissue will prevent capillary ingrowth into the epidermis and the skin will necrose at the wound edges. Close attention to these principles decreases the likelihood of a wound infection that results in a wider, thicker scar.

Several specific techniques aid in producing a fine, thin scar. As mentioned above, relief of tension

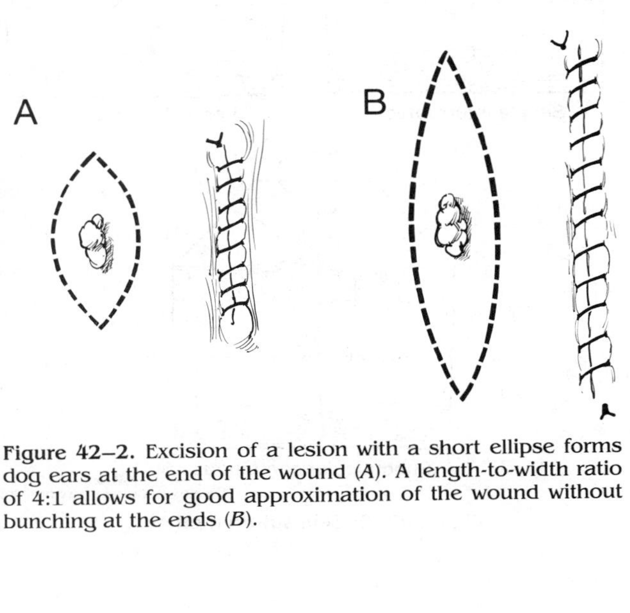

Figure 42–2. Excision of a lesion with a short ellipse forms dog ears at the end of the wound (*A*). A length-to-width ratio of 4:1 allows for good approximation of the wound without bunching at the ends (*B*).

on wound edges is of major importance. Careful approximation of the subdermal layers by suturing should allow the epidermal edges to lie closely together. If necessary, tension can be lessened by undermining the adjacent tissue (Fig. 42–3) (McGregor, 1975).

Slight eversion of the skin edges during repair allows healing of the epidermis as a flat scar, without a ridge. This can be accomplished both by the type of suture placed and the way each suture is placed. A simple interrupted suture will evert the epidermis when the needle enters the skin at an angle of 90 degrees or more. The needle passes into and across the dermis, exiting the skin the same distance from the wound edge as it entered. This suture is deeper than it is wide and includes a wider bite of the dermis than the epidermis (Fig. 42–4) (Spicer, 1982). Simple interrupted sutures placed 2 mm. from the wound edge are often used on the face.

A vertical mattress suture successfully everts the skin edge. It is technically the easiest method of wound edge eversion. This suture has more strength than a simple suture and is useful on the extremities. Commonly, a vertical mattress suture is alternated with a simple suture in wound closure. The subcuticular continuous suture provides good wound approximation and prolonged wound support (Fig. 42–5). The needle passes horizontally through the superficial dermis, with bites taken alternately on one side and then the other. Absorbable suture can be used, or one may choose to use a permanent monofilament, which is removed at 5 to 10 days. Epidermal approximation can be reinforced with microporous tapes (Steri Strips) (Fig. 42–6*D*).

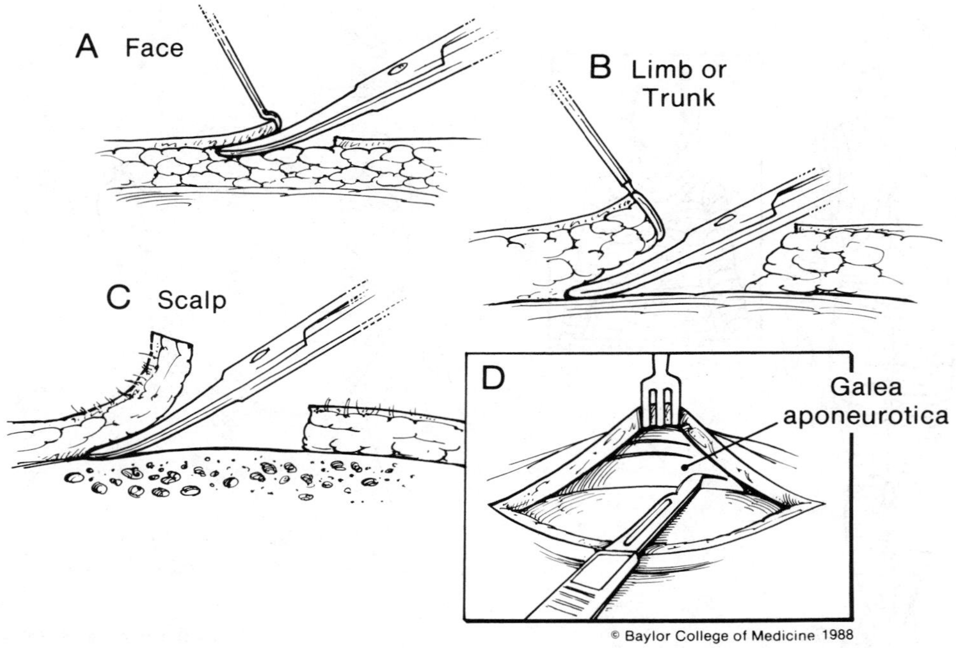

Figure 42–3. Undermining tissue adjacent to the incision can relieve tension of wound edges. On the face, tissue is undermined just under the dermal level (*A*). Undermining below the subcutaneous tissue and above the muscle fascia is appropriate for the limbs and trunk (*B*).

The technique of suture closure is more important to consider in relation to scar formation than the type of suture material. The deep layer of a wound is closed with absorbable suture (chromic catgut or polyglycolic acid), swedged on a ½ inch circle cutting needle, using a 4-0 or 5-0 suture on the face and a 2-0 or 3-0 suture on an extremity. A 4-0 or 5-0 polypropylene subcuticular suture can be passed through the skin every 5 to 8 cm. to facilitate removal in a long wound.

Prolonged placement of sutures results in scars at the suture tract sites. Facial sutures are removed at 3 to 5 days. Alternate sutures can be removed at 3 days, Steri Strips placed for reinforcement, and the remainder of the sutures removed at 5 days. Sutures on the extremities remain for 7 to 10 days. Again Steri Strips can be placed for support after suture removal. Skin suture marks are also more likely to occur if the suture is tied tightly or pulls laterally on

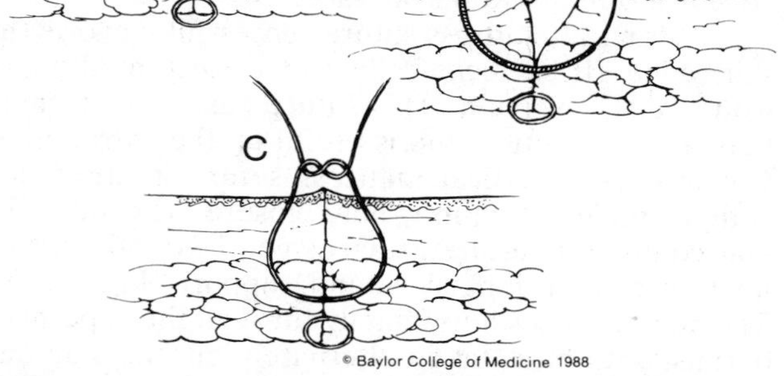

Figure 42–4. The simple interrupted suture is inserted with the needle entering the skin at an angle of 90 degrees or greater (*A*). This allows sufficient subcutaneous tissue to be included to encourage eversion of skin edges (*B*). The needle should exit with the same amount of tissue on each side of the suture (*C*).

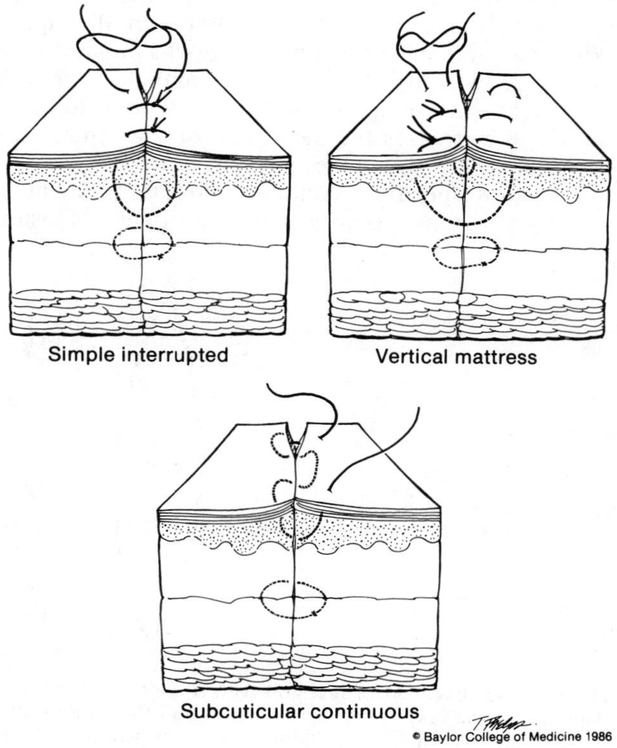

Figure 42–5. Skin suture methods.

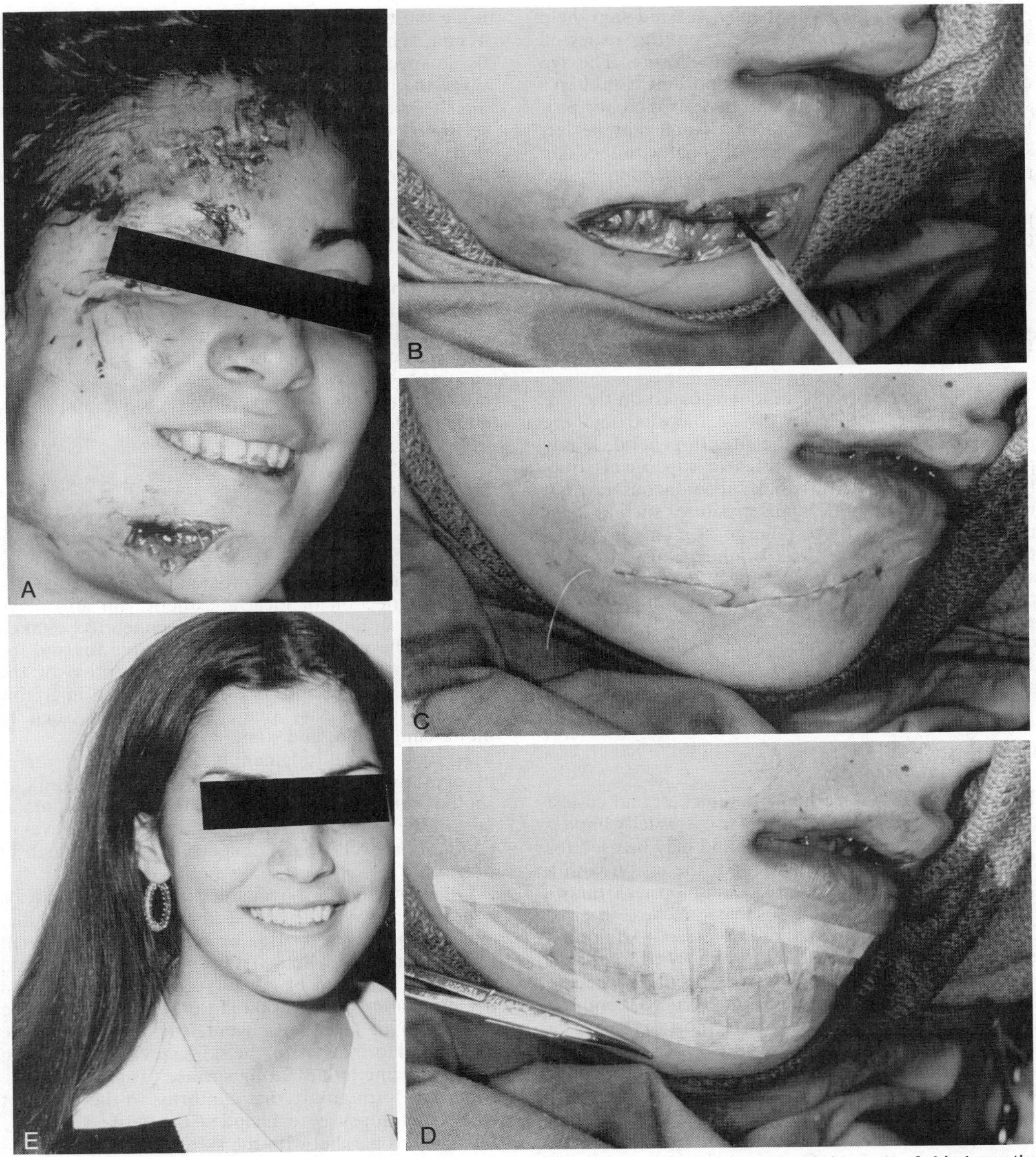

Figure 42–6. An 18-year-old patient involved in motor vehicle accident with facial lacerations (*A*). Debridement of chin laceration (*B*). Closure of wound with subcuticular closure (*C*). Bandage of Steri Strip tapes (*D*). Appearance of patient 1 year after wound closure.

the wound. Suture knots should be tied with only enough tension to approximate edges but not put pressure on the underlying tissue. Smaller tissue bites cause a smaller segment of tissue to be constricted (Grabb and Smith, 1979).

Skin type affects scar formation. Areas of thicker skin, such as that on the back, will form more noticeable scars. Very fine scars, however, form around the eyelids. Some individuals are predisposed to hypertrophic or keloid scars. Examination of the patient for other areas that have scarred may help the physician advise the patient on the expected outcome of the most recent wound closure. The age of the patient and the scar are important. Children's scars remain erythematous and hypertrophic for prolonged periods of time. The final result may be less satisfactory than in the older individual with less skin tension. All scars become less erythematous and hypertrophic as they mature, arriving at a final appearance only after 2 years. It is not until that time that scar revision should be considered (Figs. 42–6 and 42–7).

Biopsy Techniques

The choice of a biopsy technique is based on the size and location of the lesion to be biopsied and the thickness of the dermis at the site. In general, family physicians should limit biopsies to superficial structures (epidermis, dermis and subcutaneous layers), with care to avoid underlying structures such as large nerves, blood vessels, or tendons. Lesions involving the eyelids, nose, or fascia of the palms and soles should be referred to a specialist. Recognition that the dermis varies in thickness, from 1 mm. on the eyelid and 4 mm. on the back, to greatly thickened dermis on the palms and soles, will prevent the surgeon from obtaining only stratum corneum when performing a shave biopsy.

PUNCH BIOPSY

The punch biopsy is perhaps the quickest and easiest biopsy technique (Fig. 42–8). Its use is usually limited to lesions less than 5 millimeters and may be used for incisional (removing only a part of the lesion with a section of normal skin) or excisional biopsies (removing the entire lesion). Disposable punches, in sizes from 2 to 6 millimeters, are preferred. Additional equipment required includes a syringe with 1 per cent lidocaine, and a 27- or 30-gauge needle; a needle holder; suture material; and small curved pointed scissors such as iris scissors. Hemostasis may be obtained either with electrocautery or a chemical agent such as Monsel's solution (ferric subsulfate solution).

The biopsy site is prepared with an antimicrobial cleansing agent such as povidone-iodine. The area is then swabbed with 70 or 90 per cent isopropyl alcohol. An intradermal injection of 0.2 to 0.5 mm. of lidocaine is used to anesthetize the area and raise a skin wheal. Outward tension is applied to the skin with the thumb and forefinger of the physician's free hand, perpendicular to the natural skin tension lines. This produces an oval rather than a round defect. The punch is then applied firmly to the skin surface over the lesion, with the handle perpendicular to the skin. Firm downward pressure is applied in a rotary motion using the thumb and forefinger, to a depth of about 4 mm. The punch is removed and the cylindrical tissue specimen is elevated with a skin hook or the tip of the needle used for anesthesia, avoiding crushing the specimen. The base of the specimen is then sectioned with the scissors. Hemostasis may be obtained by direct pressure; usually one suture is adequate to oppose the edges and stop any bleeding. If the wound is larger or excessive bleeding occurs, Monsel's or other hemostatic agent can be applied.

In general, when an incisional biopsy is performed, including the expanding border of a lesion along with a section of normal tissue produces the most useful specimen for diagnosis. Attempts at excisional biopsies should be limited to those lesions whose lateral extent and depth can be completely encompassed by the punch biopsy. If this is not possible, an elliptical excisional biopsy should be done, as described above.

SHAVE BIOPSY

The shave biopsy technique may be useful when the exophytic nature of the lesion to be removed raises it above the plane of the surrounding tissue (Fig. 42–9). The injection of local anesthetic can also serve this purpose, allowing a biopsy specimen to be taken at a level between the deep papillary dermis and the midreticular dermis, parallel to the surface of the skin. The shave biopsy is especially useful in friable lesions with an easy plane of separation such as molluscum, milia, and some warts.

Good clinical judgment and a firm impression of preoperative diagnosis is required. This technique should not be utilized if a malignant melanoma is part of the differential diagnosis, because the level of penetration of the melanoma cells may be difficult to judge.

Two options are available for a shave biopsy: a hand-held razor blade or a scalpel blade on a handle. When using a razor blade, the blade is divided in half longitudinally and held between the forefinger and thumb. A thin film of anticorrosive oil containing a bacteriostatic agent is applied to the blade. After the infiltration of anesthetic agent, the physician's free thumb and forefinger roll the skin, elevating the lesion and producing a flat cutting surface. The razor blade is bent to form an arc that conforms to the depth of tissue the biopsy is to include. The curved blade is then moved parallel with the skin surface in a sweeping motion. Considerable skill is necessary to maintain control of the blade because of the tensile strength produced by the arc. The skillful use of the razor blade results in a good cosmetic result, with fine tapering of the edges of the biopsy.

For those who use this technique less frequently, a scalpel blade on a handle is a safe alternative. Elevation of the lesion with local anesthesia is used to contour the curved surfaces of the biopsy. A number 15 blade is applied parallel with the skin

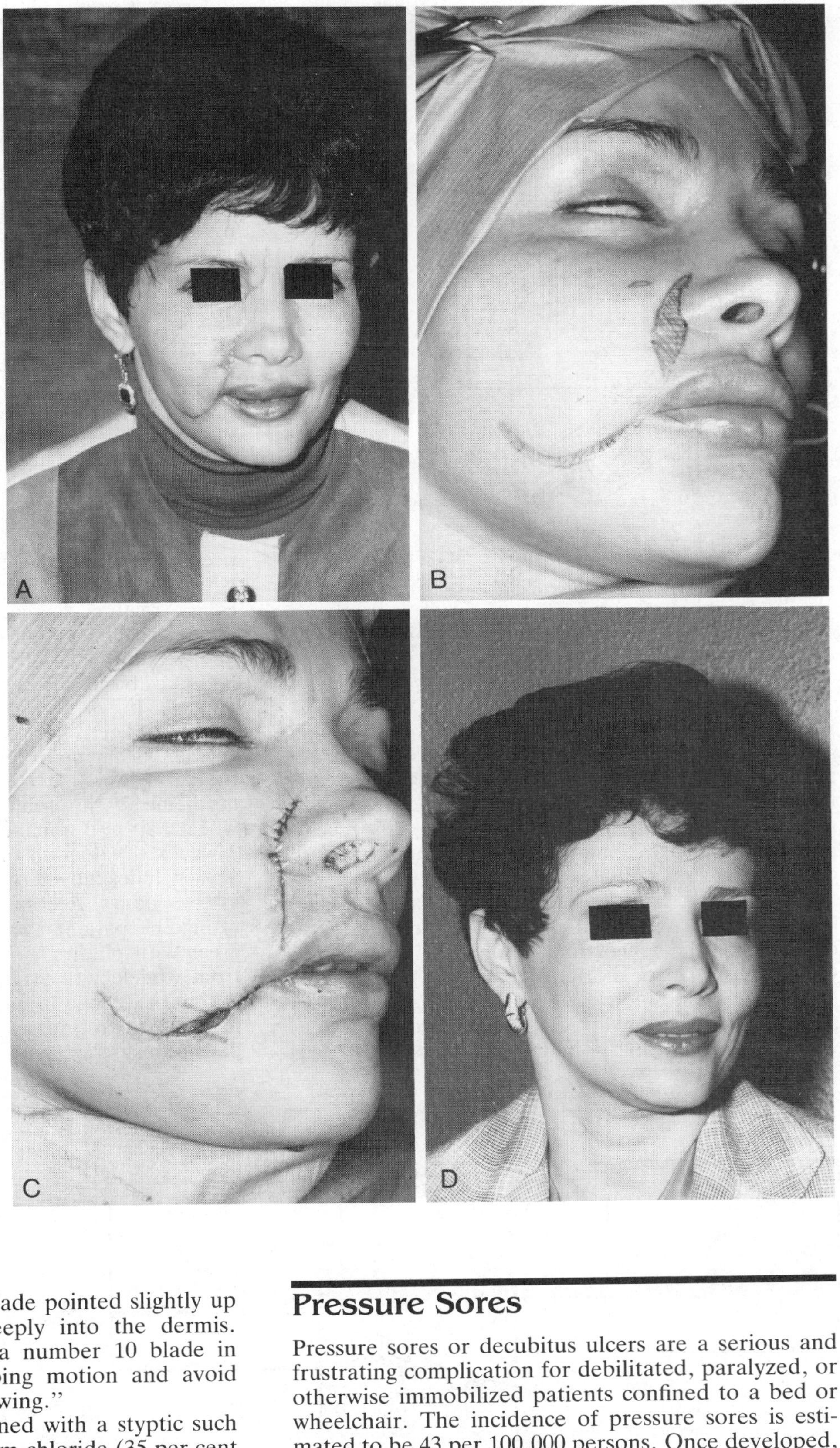

Figure 42–7. Secondary scar revision. Patient seen 1 year after facial laceration repair (*A*). Intraoperative markings and excision of the scar (*B* and *C*). Appearance one year after the operation (*D*).

surface, with the tip of the blade pointed slightly up to avoid penetrating too deeply into the dermis. Larger lesions may require a number 10 blade in order to use a single sweeping motion and avoid rough edges produced by "sawing."

Hemostasis can be obtained with a styptic such as Monsel's solution, aluminum chloride (35 per cent in 50 per cent isopropyl alcohol), or light electrodessication.

Pressure Sores

Pressure sores or decubitus ulcers are a serious and frustrating complication for debilitated, paralyzed, or otherwise immobilized patients confined to a bed or wheelchair. The incidence of pressure sores is estimated to be 43 per 100,000 persons. Once developed, a pressure ulcer substantially increases the need for nursing care and the cost of medical care (Linder and

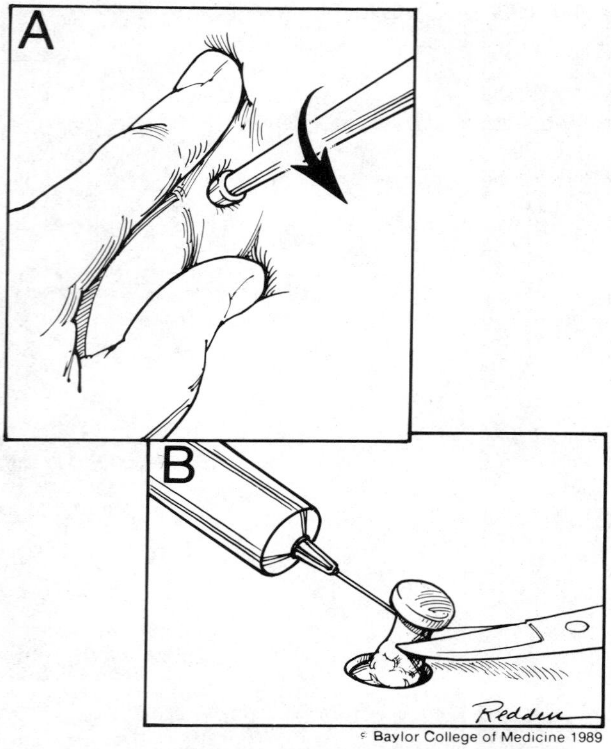

Figure 42–8. (*A* and *B*) Technique of punch biopsy.

Upton, 1984). In 1984, the median length of hospital stay for patients with pressure sores was 46 days and the median total cost of care was $27,000 (ranging from $3400 to $86,000) (Allman et al., 1986). Although prevention is the primary goal, early recognition of and a systematic therapeutic approach to decubitus ulcers facilitates early wound closure.

The basic cause of decubitus ulcers is tissue ischemia from physical forces of pressure. Pressure over bony prominences for a prolonged time (more than 2 hours), or for shorter repeated intervals results in breakdown at predictable sites (Fig. 42–10). In the presence of shearing forces, such as are generated when a person sitting in bed with the head elevated slides toward the foot of the bed, the amount of time or pressure required to produce ischemia is reduced (Bennett et al., 1969). In addition, frictional forces, especially when the skin surface is moist, contribute to superficial skin breakdown. Incontinence may increase the risk of pressure ulcer by 5.5 times (Lowthcan, 1976). The elderly are at particularly increased risk because of decreased spontaneous movements and age-related changes of the skin. Additional factors that increase the risk of pressure ulcers and the correction of which hasten healing include hypoalbuminemia and vitamin C deficiency (Allman et al., 1986; Husain, 1953; Taylor et al., 1974).

A standard classification for pressure sores was developed in 1975 (Shea, 1975). A Grade I lesion has erythema and induration of the skin, with the epidermis intact. If pressure is not relieved, this lesion progresses to Grade II ulceration, with epidermal and dermal breakdown to, but not including, subcutaneous tissues. A Grade III ulceration extends into the subcutaneous tissue but not through muscle. Extension down to the underlying bony prominence occurs in a Grade IV ulcer. A Grade V lesion occurs when an extensive ulcer spreads into a joint or body cavity (rectum, vagina, bladder) (Fig. 42–11).

The classification of pressure sores guides therapy. A superficial Grade I lesion requires re-examination of basic skin care. Those areas that are beginning to break down should respond to relief of pressure. The relief of pressure is continued until all erythema and induration has resolved, and is instituted 24 hours each day. A paraplegic patient with erythema of the ischial area should stay out of the wheelchair and remain prone for a minimum of 1 to 2 weeks. Evaluation of activity patterns is essential. This includes the understanding of rotation of position every 2 hours, release of pressure in a wheelchair by lifting the patient every 20 to 30 minutes, bridging areas with pillows, and avoiding traumatic transfers from wheelchairs (Staus and LaMantia, 1982). Additional therapeutic measures may include: (1) supplying an appropriate wheelchair cushion, air mattress bed, or egg-crate mattress; (2) supplying better nu-

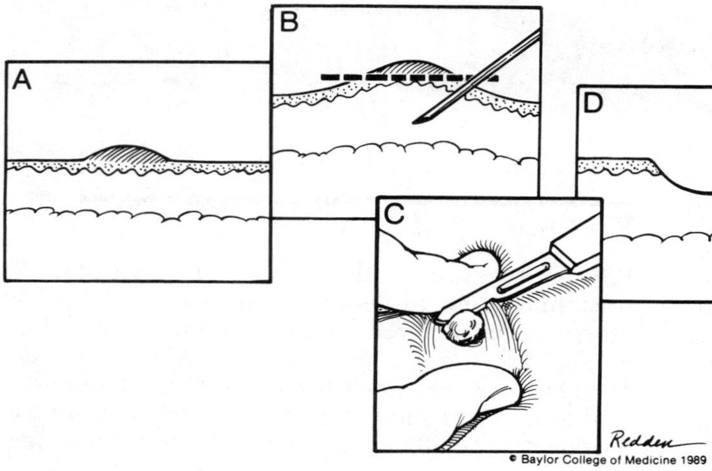

Figure 42–9. (*A* to *D*) Technique of shave biopsy.

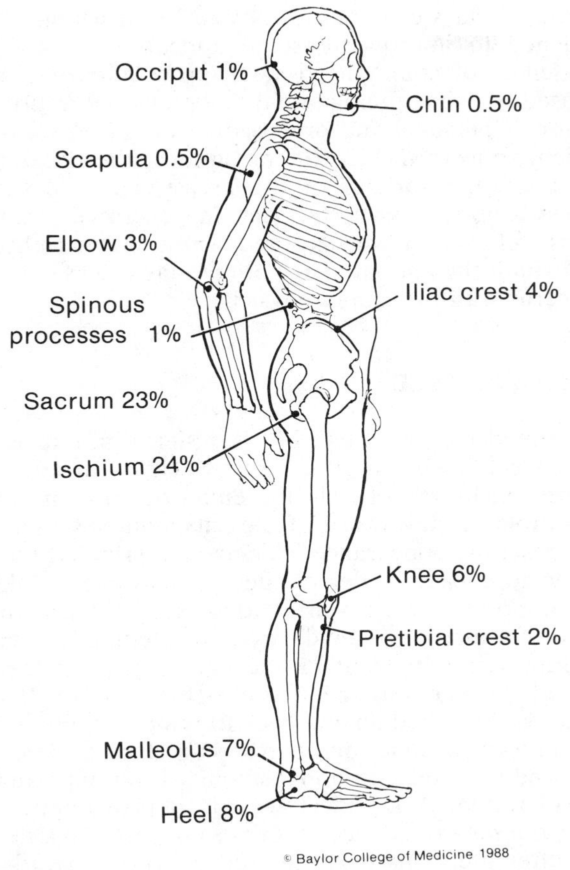

Figure 42–10. Areas of decubitus ulcer development and frequency of distribution.

trition for weight gain; (3) providing education concerning keeping the skin clean and dry and daily examination for skin breakdown; (4) wearing appropriate loose-fitting clothes; and (5) controlling spasms.

Grade II ulcers with erosion into the dermis require all the treatments listed earlier plus local wound care. Superficial lesions can be cleaned daily with a mild soap and left open to air. If trauma to the area is anticipated (i.e., ulceration under a halo jacket) the area may be covered with a dressing such as Duoderm or Opsite for short intervals. Deeper ulcers require regular local wound care. Although multiple topical agents are available for care of decubitis ulcers, the most basic and effective is wet to dry dressings with normal saline. A gauze material is dampened lightly and a layer of damp material is laid in the wound with dry gauze over this. This dressing is changed three to four times a day. The gauze dries between dressing changes. When removed, the dressing pulls off the fibrous tissue with it. This leaves a clean base for granulation tissue to form, allowing the wound to heal by secondary intention. If a superficial infection exists, the gauze can be dampened with dilute (½ strength) hypochlorite or Dakin's solution, or dilute povidone-iodine solution for a short time. Topical or systemic antibiotics have not proved to be effective and have specific toxicities (Longe, 1986).

Grade III to Grade V ulcers will usually require surgery. Necrotic tissue can be sharply debrided at the bedside. Because debridement may cause transient bacteremia, prophylaxis for bacterial endocarditis is advised in patients who have valvular lesions. Wet to dry dressings will mechanically debride the wound. Several chemical enzymatic preparations are available—collagenase, fibrinolysin, and trypsin. They have a questionable role in superficial debridement but have not been proved to promote wound healing. Whirlpool therapy is very effective in debridement and wound healing. After the debridement phase, a tissue growth environment is maintained with damp gauze dressings with normal saline, which are changed three to four times daily. However, if the wound is deeply necrotic and the patient is febrile and septic, hospitalization with intravenous antibiotics and sharp debridement is necessary.

In a Grade III ulcer, prolonged therapy with wet to dry dressings over several months with relief of all pressure may result in complete healing. The patient must remain off of the pressure points at all times. It is not adequate to continue normal daily activities. For example, in a paraplegic, the patient must stop work and recreational activities and remain out of the wheelchair until the wound is healed.

Surgical therapy provides procedures utilizing skin grafts, skin flaps, muscle flaps, musculocutaneous

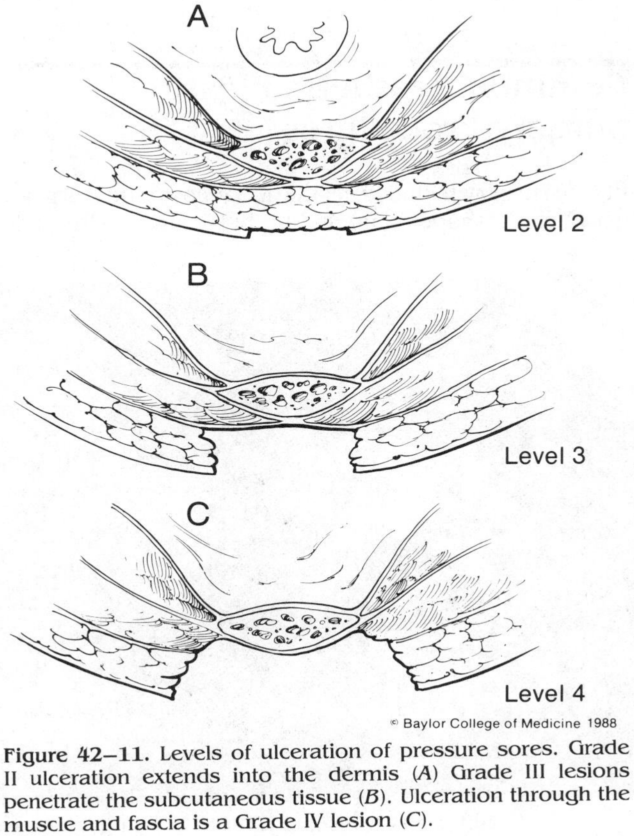

Figure 42–11. Levels of ulceration of pressure sores. Grade II ulceration extends into the dermis (*A*) Grade III lesions penetrate the subcutaneous tissue (*B*). Ulceration through the muscle and fascia is a Grade IV lesion (*C*).

flaps, neurovascular flaps, and free flaps for wound closure after excision of the ulcer (Fig. 42–12). There are several factors to be considered in preparing a patient for surgery. The patient must understand surgery is not a quick cure for the wound, and that four to six weeks of positioning to keep weight off the flap will be required postoperatively (Fig. 42–13). This often means being completely prone for that time. If a large amount of necrotic tissue is present, an initial extensive debridement in the operating room is most effective. This is followed by two to three weeks of local wound care to promote the beginning of healing through granulation tissue prior to wound coverage. Nutrition, pulmonary function, and spasm control should be optimal before surgery is performed. Plain x-ray studies of the involved area are used as a screening test for osteomyelitis. If deep or interconnecting Grade IV or V ulcers are present, a CT scan may be valuable to detect osteomyelitis; bone scans are less reliable (Sugarman et al., 1983). An open bone biopsy may be required for definitive diagnosis of osteomyelitis.

Basic skin care is the most important factor for long-term success of both operative wound closure and healing by secondary intention. The effectiveness of preventive management was shown by Krouskop et al. (1983) in an organized rehabilitation setting. Over a 4-year period, the recurrence rate of pressure sores was reduced from 32 per cent to 4 per cent. Their program provided and heavily reinforced patient education about skin care.

Common Aesthetic Plastic Surgery Procedures

Plastic surgery includes aesthetic, or cosmetic, surgery which can reshape facial and body features. Although it is not always essential for physical well-being, it is designed to improve personal appearance. Patient awareness of common cosmetic procedures has increased with continuing social acceptance of improving one's personal and professional image. Areas of patient concern include the aging face, the shape of the nose, the contour of the breast, and areas of excess adipose tissue. Surgery in several of these areas will also relieve signs and symptoms that physically limit the patient. The patient may discuss these concerns with the family physician.

THE AGING FACE

The rhytidectomy, or face lift, is designed to improve evidence of aging of the face. Much of the aging process includes not only loosening of the skin but also prolapse downward of the subcutaneous tissue. The resulting appearance is deepened wrinkled lines in the forehead, corner of the eye, nasolabial fold, and perioral area as well as loose skin folds in the neck. An incision is made from the temporal hair-bearing scalp, in front of the ear, and posteriorly behind the ear into the hairline (Fig. 42–14). The loose skin is pulled up and back to remove many, but not all, skin wrinkles and excess skin (Fig. 42–15).

The patient's emotional stability is an important consideration. A rhytidectomy can improve appearance and self-confidence, but does not result in a new or better life. This is considered a major operative procedure and is the equivalent of an abdominal operation. Good medical health is necessary. Many plastic surgeons will not perform a rhytidectomy on patients who smoke cigarettes. This problem as well as a history of bleeding disorders or a tendency to develop keloids or hypertrophic scars results in delayed healing or compromised surgical results.

The hospital stay averages 2 or 3 days. It may be performed under general or local anesthetic.

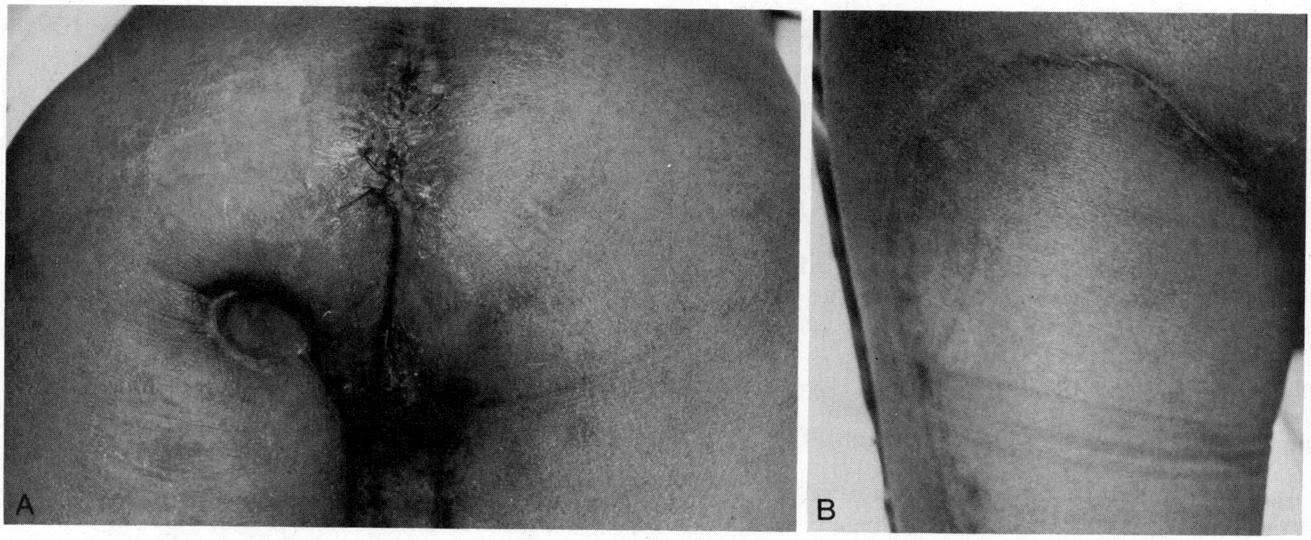

Figure 42–12. Ischial ulcer before surgery (*A*). Ischial ulcer after closure with posterior thigh flap (*B*).

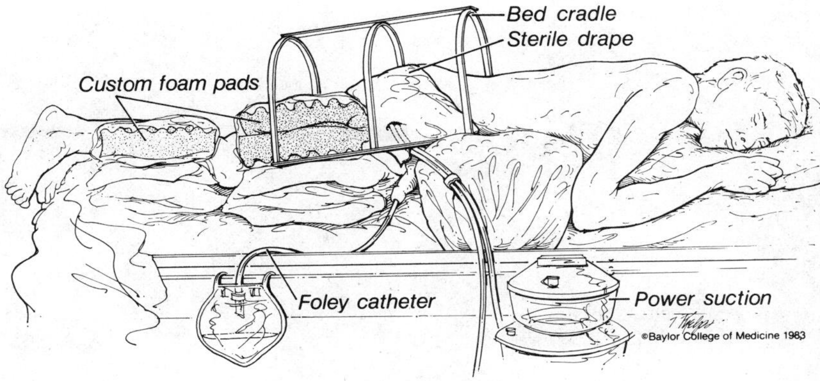

Figure 42–13. Postoperative positioning after surgical closure of decubitus ulcer. The patient is prone with wound drains, foley catheter, wound dressing, and bed cradle in place.

A blepharoplasty, or aesthetic eyelid surgery, may be performed alone or as a component of a rhytidectomy. The operation is designed to remove excess skin and fat on the upper and lower eyelids. It can help correct conditions of excess skin folds on the upper eyelid and bags under the eyes to help eliminate a tired look. Reconstructive blepharoplasty is performed when these conditions affect visual fields. This can be determined with visual field testing.

An incision is made in the crease of the upper eyelid and just below the lower lid lashes. Eyelid scarring is minimal. Swelling and discoloration last 5 to 8 days. The procedure may be performed on an inpatient or outpatient basis and under general or local anesthetic.

SURGERY OF THE NOSE

Aesthetic nasal surgery or rhinoplasty is reshaping the nose to improve its appearance. Reconstructive rhinoplasty is performed to recontour the external nose after injury or to alleviate congenital defects. Rhinoplasty is frequently combined with surgery to remove obstruction of the nasal airway if it exists. Possible improvements include reduction of the overall nose size, reshaping of the nasal tip, removal of the nasal hump, and improvement of the angle between the nose and upper lip. In most nasal surgery,

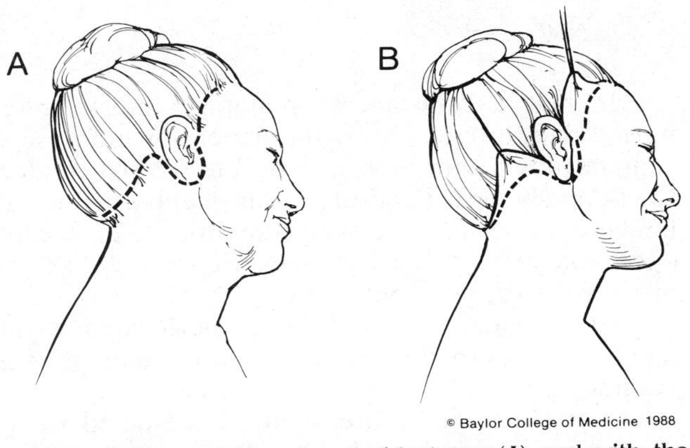

Figure 42–14. Incisions for rhytidectomy (*A*) and with the elevation of excess skin (*B*).

the incision is made inside the nostril. Additional cartilage from the ear or nasal septum or bone from the rib may be required for reconstructive nasal contouring.

As in a rhytidectomy, emotional stability is important. A recontoured nose will not reshape a life. The presence of airway obstruction can be determined on physical examination but will not always be relieved with surgery.

A rhinoplasty may be performed on an inpatient or outpatient basis, usually under local anesthetic. This cosmetic procedure is one of the most popular operations performed by plastic surgeons today.

CONTOUR OF THE BREAST

Cosmetic breast surgery addresses three patient concerns: the small breast, the overly large breast, and the ptotic breast.

Reduction mammoplasty, or reduction of large breasts, is performed to reduce weight-bearing pain in the breasts, pain in the upper portion of the neck and back, and to relieve discomfort caused by the pressure of brassiere straps across the shoulders. Breast reduction allows more comfort in physical activities and a wider range of clothes selection. Since these procedures are usually performed to relieve physical discomfort, costs may be partially or completely covered by insurance. A keyhole type of incision is made around the nipple and extends medially and laterally in the inframammary crease (Figs. 42–16 and 42–17). A vertical scar from the nipple to under the breast and a scar under the breast to the axilla remains.

Several important issues must be discussed with the surgeon. Ability to breast-feed after reduction is unpredictable. Usually, nipple sensation is decreased. A family history of breast cancer does not contraindicate cosmetic breast surgery; but a careful plan of preoperative and postoperative mammography and physical examination for breast disease is necessary.

The hospital stay is 2 to 3 days, with surgery performed under general anesthesia.

Augmentation mammoplasty, or breast augmentation with a Silastic breast prosthesis, is performed

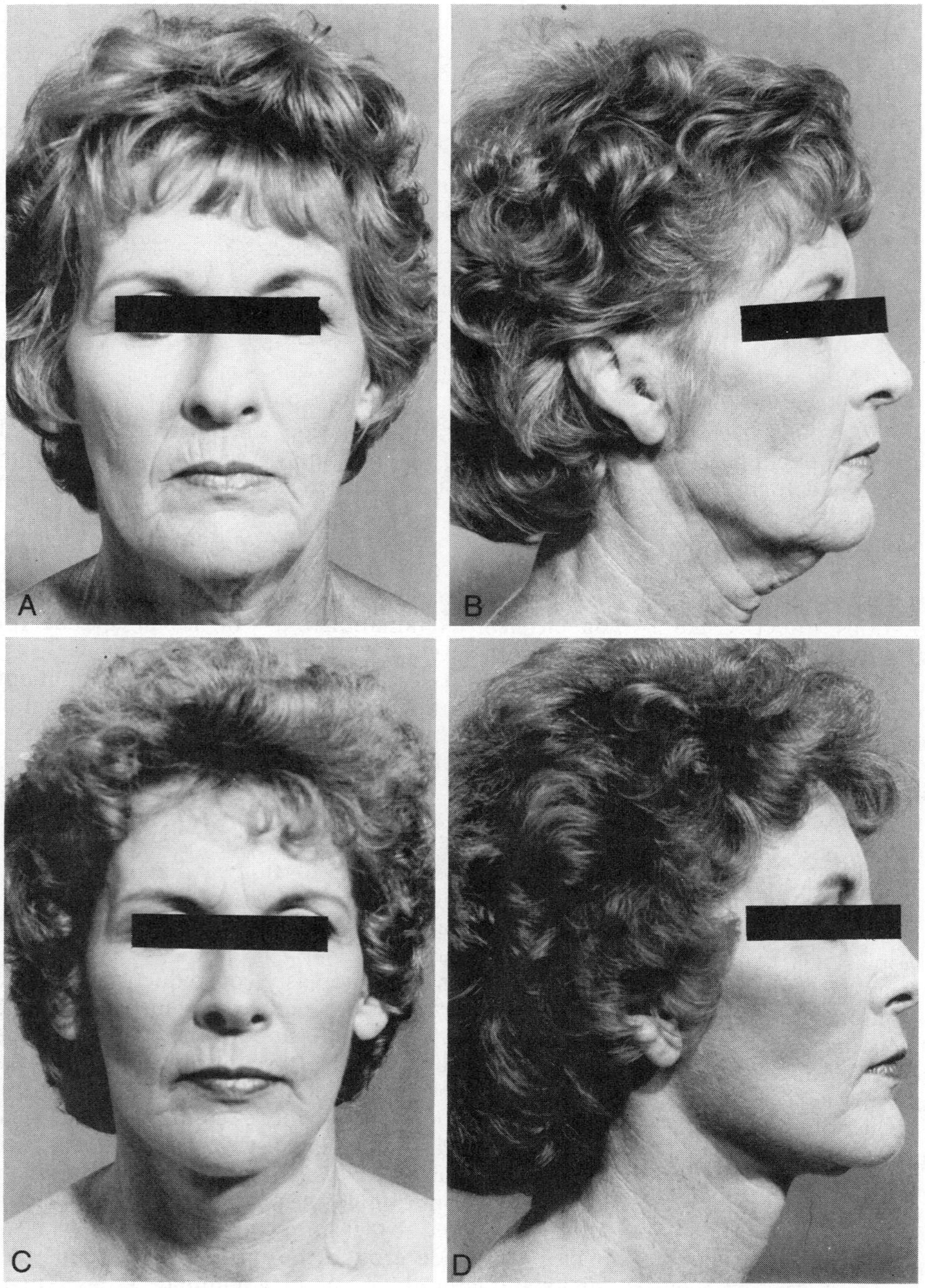

Figure 42–15. Preoperative photographs of patient desiring surgery for an aging face (*A* and *B*). Postoperative photographs of patient after rhytidectomy, blepharoplasty, and perioral peel (*C* and *D*). Note the change in the neck line in the lateral view.

to enlarge small or asymmetric breasts. A filled Silastic breast implant is placed between the breast tissue and the chest wall. An incision is made either in the skin fold under the breast or around the areola (Fig. 42–18).

There is no evidence of increased likelihood of breast cancer after breast augmentation. Continued physician follow-up for potential breast disease, regular mammography, and encouragement of self–breast examination is needed. Research and clinical series indicate that mammography and physical examination can accurately detect lesions in the augmented breast.

In rare circumstances an implant must be removed due to rejection by the patient or unforeseen complications, with replacement 3 to 6 months later. Occasionally, a scar capsule forms deeply around the implant, resulting in a very firm breast. A second operation may be advised to soften the breast by incising the capsule contracture.

Breast augmentation may be performed on an inpatient or outpatient basis, usually under general anesthesia.

A mastopexy, or breast lift, is designed to reshape the sagging breast. Most operations are performed in older patients who may or may not have

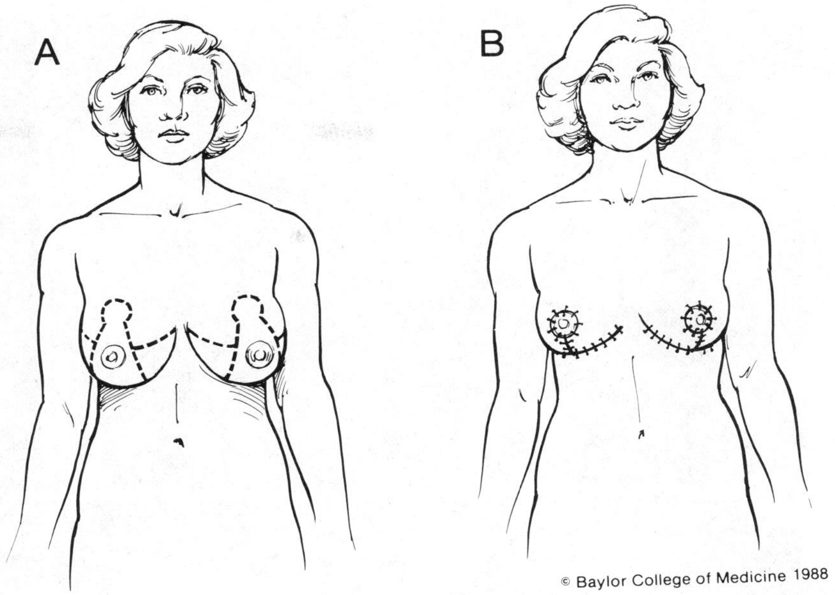

Figure 42–16. Pattern of skin excision (*A*), and resulting skin incision scars for a reduction mammoplasty and mastopexy (*B*)

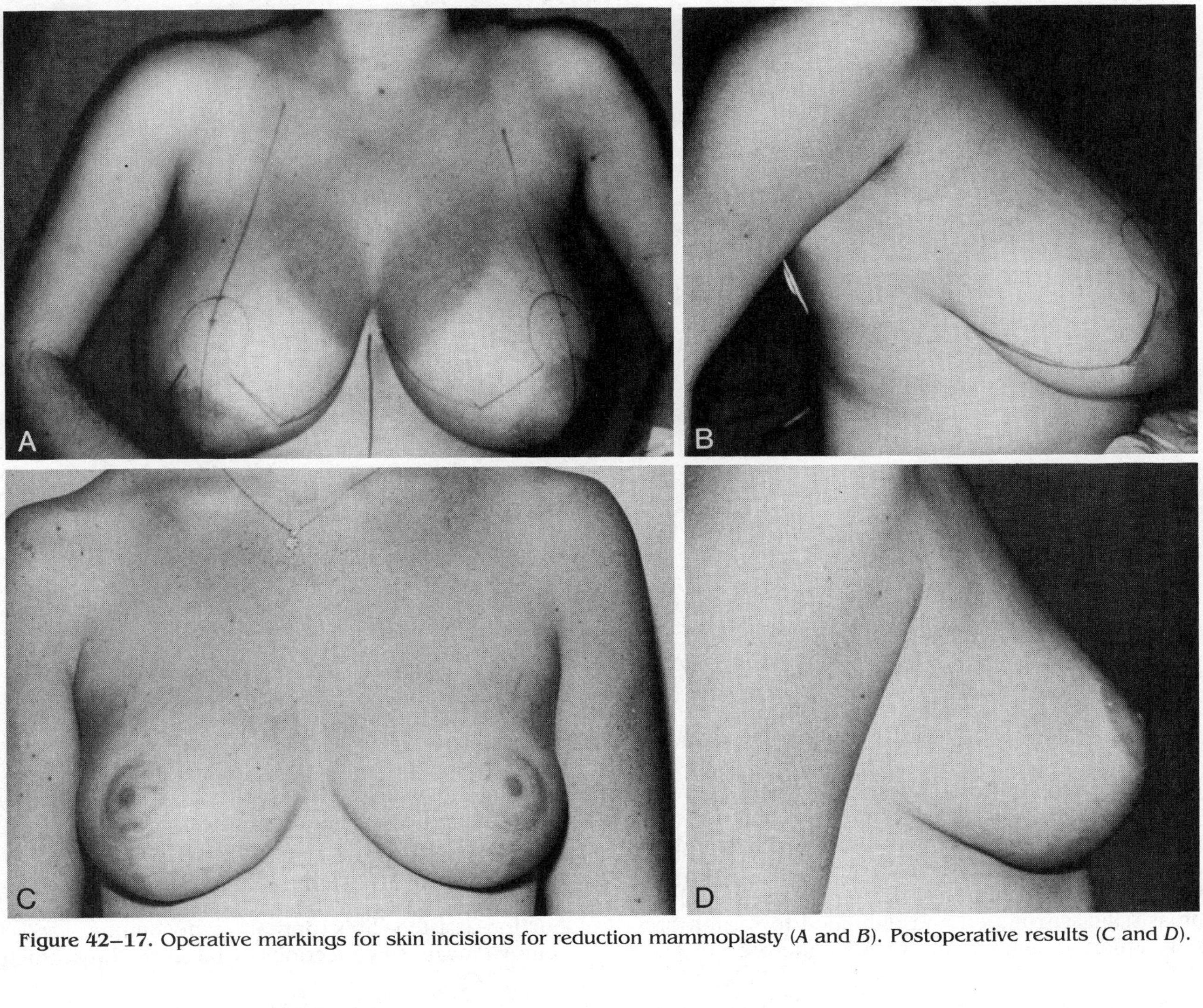

Figure 42–17. Operative markings for skin incisions for reduction mammoplasty (*A* and *B*). Postoperative results (*C* and *D*).

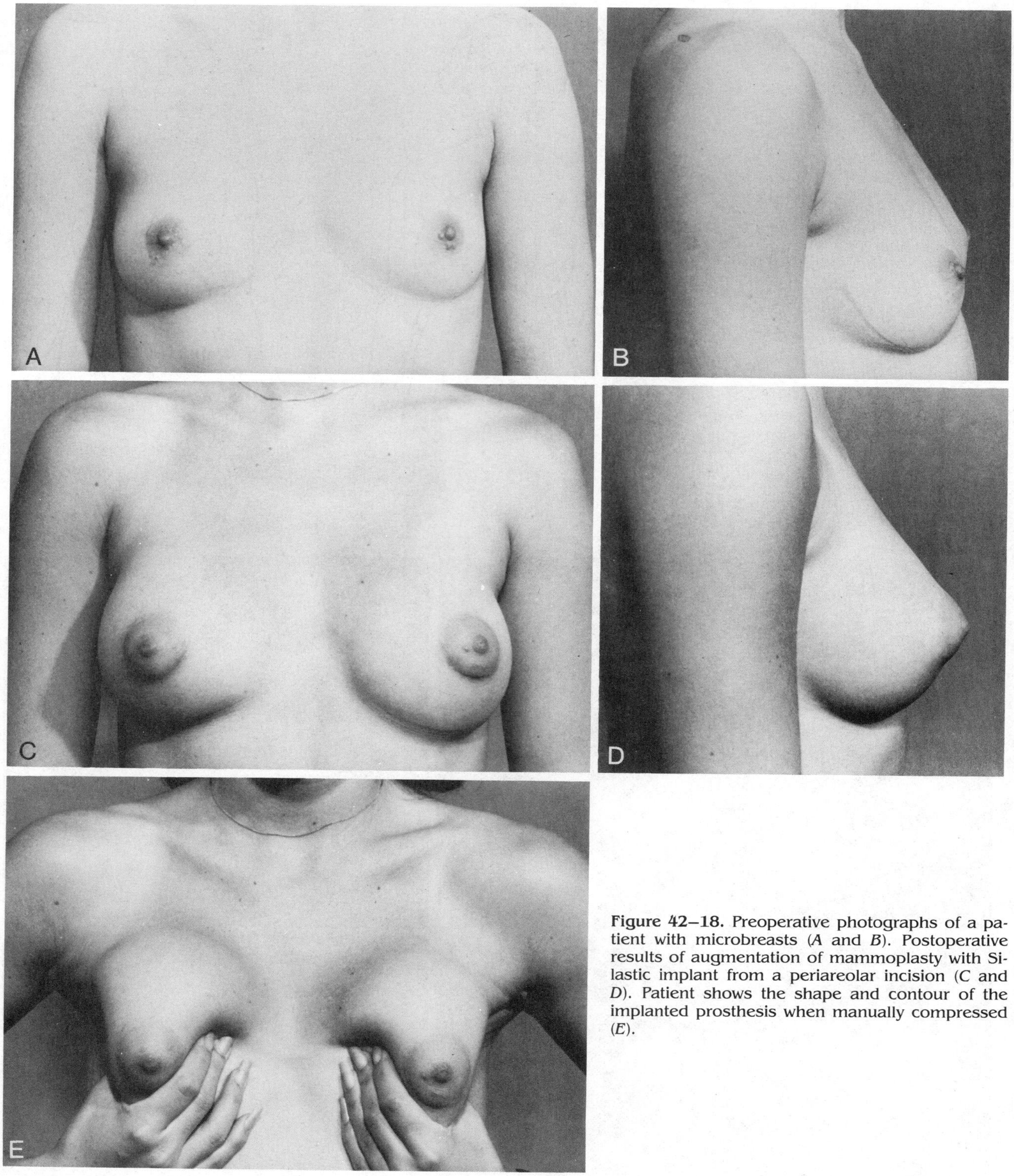

Figure 42–18. Preoperative photographs of a patient with microbreasts (*A* and *B*). Postoperative results of augmentation of mammoplasty with Silastic implant from a periareolar incision (*C* and *D*). Patient shows the shape and contour of the implanted prosthesis when manually compressed (*E*).

had large breasts when they were younger, but whose breasts now have sagged and have diminished in volume. This may accompany breast augmentation. An incision is made above the nipple and across the lower breast. The nipple is elevated, and excess lower breast skin is trimmed and tightened to form a brassiere effect to support and reshape the breast.

The hospital stay is usually 2 days, with surgery performed under general anesthesia.

BODY FAT REDUCTION

Suction-assisted lipectomy is a technique used to remove localized collections of fat in the hips, thighs, buttocks and abdomen, as well as on arms, knees, calves, neck, and under the chin. It is performed on a patient of relatively normal body build and weight to reduce disproportionately large areas of adipose tissue. Patients with young, healthy, and elastic skin of normal weight are the best candidates. Older individuals with less resilient skin may be advised to consider surgical lipectomy, where excess skin and adipose tissue are excised not suctioned. One- or two-cm. incisions are made in the areas to be suctioned to introduce the blunt suction device. Following the procedure, these small incisions are closed and a snug dressing is placed. Depending on the extent of surgery, the procedure is performed under general or local anesthetic, on an inpatient or outpatient basis.

The above aesthetic procedures are performed in a sterile operating room environment, with careful patient monitoring. Although relatively safe for most patients, these surgical therapies are operative techniques with attendant risks. The most serious complication of infection with sepsis is prevented by attention to a completely sterile procedure environment. Intraoperative blood loss may necessitate a blood transfusion.

Aesthetic surgery, after careful planning between an individual and the plastic surgeon, can offer improved appearance and function for the patient.

References

Allman, R. M., Laprade, C. A., Noel, L. B., et al.: Pressure sores among hospitalized patients. Ann. Intern. Med., *105*(9):337–341, 1986.

Bennett, L., Kavner, D., Lee, B. K., and Trainor, F. A.: Shear vs. pressure as causative factors in skin blood flow occlusion. Arch. Phys. Med. Rehabil., *60*:309–314, 1969.

Borges, A. F.: Elective Incisions and Scar Revisions. Boston, Little, Brown & Co., Inc., 1973.

Grabb, W. C., and Smith, J. W.: Plastic Surgery. Boston: Little, Brown & Co., Inc., 1979, pp. 1–16.

Husain, T.: An experimental study of some pressure effects on tissues, with reference to the bedsore problem. J. Pathol. Bacteriol., *66*:347–358, 1953.

Krouskop, T. A., Noble, P. C., Garber, S. L., et al.: The effectiveness of preventative management in reducing the occurrence of pressure sores. J. Rehab. Res. Dev., *20*(1):74–83, 1983. *A comprehensive program in pressure sore care, emphasizing patient education about skin care and utilizing periodic pressure evaluation of the wheelchair cushion, which resulted in a decrease of pressure sore recurrence rate from 32 per cent in 1975 to 4 per cent in 1981.*

Linder, R. M., and Upton J.: The prevention of pressure sores. Med. Times, *112*(11):52–63, 1984.

Longe, R. L.: Current concepts in clinical therapeutics: Pressure sores. Clin. Pharm., *5*:669–681, 1986.

Lowthcan, P. T.: Underpads in the prevention of decubiti. *In* Kenedi, R. M., Cowden, J. M., and Scales, J. T. (Eds.): Bedsore Biomechanics: Proceedings of a Seminar on Tissue Viability & Clinical Applications. Baltimore, University Park Press, 1976, pp. 141–145.

Mayhew, H. E., and Rodgers, L. A.: Basic Procedures in Family Practice. New York, John Wiley & Sons, 1984.

McGregor, I. A.: Fundamental Techniques of Plastic Surgery. London, Longman, 1975.

Robinson, J. K.: Fundamentals of Skin Biopsy. Chicago, Year Book Medical Publishers, Inc., 1986.

Shea, J. D.: Pressure sores: Classification and management. Clin. Orthop., *112*:89–100, 1975. *A classification system is outlined for pressure sores that aids in clearly recording the diagnosis and treatment progress of decubitus ulcers.*

Spicer, T. E.: Techniques of facial lesions, excision and closure. J. Dermatol. Surg. Oncol., *8*(7):551–556, 1982. *This article is a concise discussion of basic techniques of closure of facial incisions.*

Staas, W. E., and LaMantia, J. G.: Decubitus ulcers and rehabilitation medicine. Int. J. Dermatol., *21*:439–441, 1982.

Sugarman, B., Hawes, S., Musher, D. M., et al.: Osteomyelitis underneath pressure sores. Arch. Int. Med., *143*:683–688, 1983.

Taylor, T. V., Rimmer, S., Day, B., et al.: Ascorbic acid supplementation in the treatment of pressure sores. Lancet, *2*:544–546, 1974.

43

Office Gynecology

John Sutherland
Victoria Nichols-Johnson

The anatomy and physiology of the reproductive tract is one of the most dynamic processes in human beings. There is a need for clinicians to be knowledgeable, appropriately thorough, and sensitive in regard to history-taking and physical examination at all ages. Too often, review of a medical history and physical examination reveals the notations "deferred" or "referred," when it should be considered as integral and relevant to a comprehensive evaluation of a patient, as with any other organ system.

Reproductive Physiology and Anatomy

Reproduction requires a complex sequence of integrated events. The mechanisms of ovulation, fertilization, implementation, and maintenance of pregnancy necessary for female reproduction are interrelated between the central nervous system, ovary, and uterus as depicted in Figure 43–1 (Takizawa and Mattison, 1983).

The ovary is essential for female reproduction, because it controls the hypothalamus, the pituitary, and the uterus and allows conception and the maintenance of pregnancy. The endocrine physiology involves both pituitary and ovarian hormones. The requirements for a normal fertile cycle are normal estrogen feedback, with a rise in follicle-stimulating hormone as estrogen and progesterone fall at the end of the cycle; a positive estrogen response or a surge in luteinizing hormone (LH) after estradiol is released into circulation by the dominant follicle; and the life cycle of the corpus luteum (Fig. 43–2) (Speroff, 1989).

At the start of each menstrual cycle, several of the primordial follicles enlarge. Visually, only one of the developing follicles usually continues its differentiation into a mature follicle. When the distended follicle ruptures, the ovum is extruded into the ab-

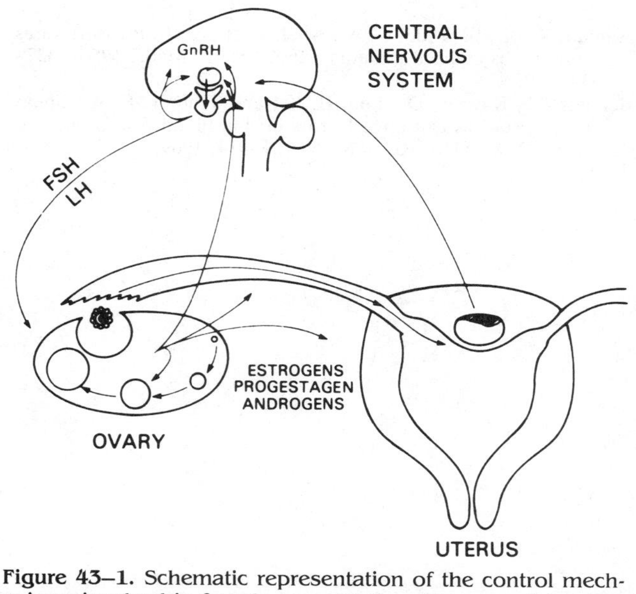

Figure 43–1. Schematic representation of the control mechanisms involved in female reproduction. The gonadotropins, follicle-stimulating hormone (FSH), and luteinizing hormone (LH) are released from the pituitary into the circulation in a pulsatile pattern by pulsatile release of gonadotropin-releasing hormone (Gn-RH). FSH supports the growth of the dominant follicle, which produces increasing quantities of estrogen. Ovulation occurs after the LH surge and is followed by luteinization of the dominant follicle and increasing production of progesterone. (Reproduced with permission from Mattison, D. R.: Reproductive and Developmental Toxicity of Metals. New York, Plenum Press, 1983.)

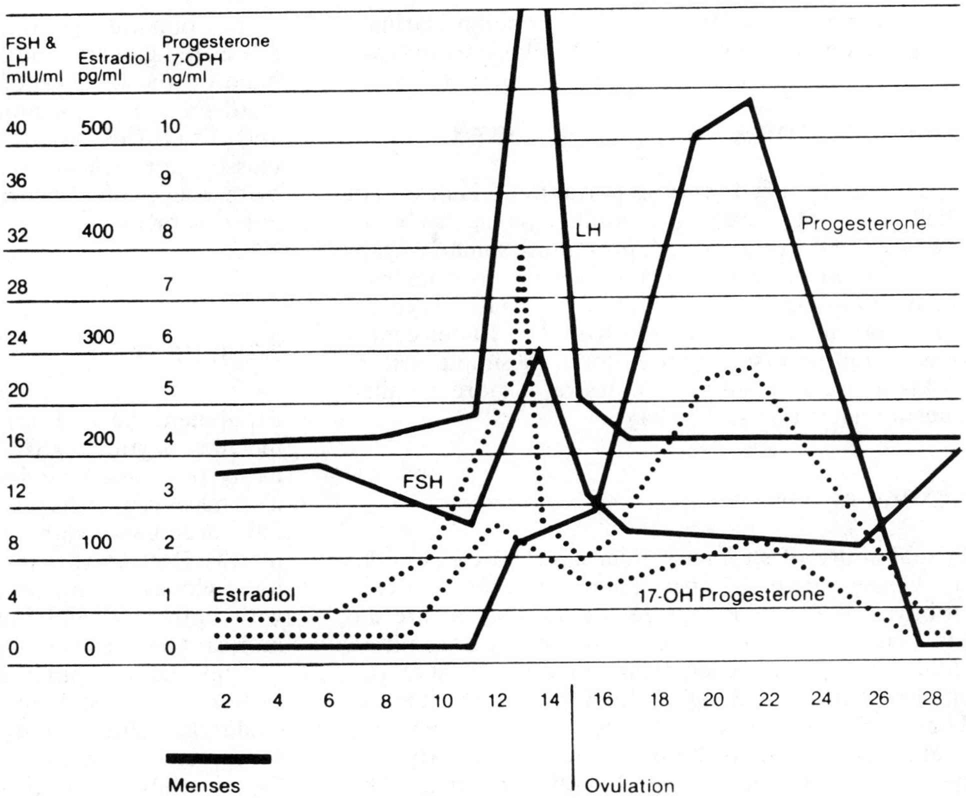

Figure 43–2. Hormone levels during menstrual cycle. (Reproduced with permission from Speroff, L.: Clinical Gynecologic Endocrinology and Infertility. Baltimore, Williams & Wilkins, 1989.)

dominal cavity during the process of ovulation. The granulosa cells of the ruptured follicle undergo luteinization, or yellowing. These cells proliferate into the corpus luteum, which produces all three classes of sex steroids—androgens, estrogens, and, most importantly, progestins.

The normal life span of a corpus luteum is 14 days, after which it regresses unless pregnancy has occurred. Luteal phases of 12 to 17 days may be considered normal, however.

The corpus luteum becomes vascularized by capillaries in the granulosa layer. This sometimes leads to bleeding into the central cavity, which further leads to a "hemorrhagic" corpus luteal cyst. This type of cyst may prolong the luteal phase also. This condition is discussed more fully under the section on benign neoplasms.

The fallopian tube is anatomically separated into fimbria, ampulla, ampullary-isthmic junction, and isthmus, each segment of which has a morphologically characteristic appearance.

The uterus can be divided into the corpus (body) and cervix. The corpus is divided into endometrium and myometrium histologically. The endometrium has the capacity to be a receptive environment for implantation, whereas the myometrium has the capacity for either quiescence or contractability.

The average menstrual cycle lasts 28 days (+ or − 4 days). The first day of the menstrual cycle is the first day of the menstrual period, which lasts 4 days (+ or − 2 days). The average amount of menstrual fluid per month varies from 30 to 80 ml. (Franz, 1988).

Menarche, the time of the first menstrual period, heralds the onset of reproductive function. The average age of menarche in the United States is 12.7 years old, with a normal range of between 10 and 15 years old. During the first 2 years after menarche, only about 50 per cent of menstrual cycles are ovulatory and intervals of 3 to 6 months between menses can be normal (Simmons, 1988).

Menopause is the event of a woman's last menstrual period. It is diagnosed when no menses have occurred for 12 consecutive months. The perimenopause is the time span prior to and after the menopause. The average age of menopause is 51 years, with a normal range of between 41 and 59 years. Premature menopause, which occurs before the age of 40, occurs in less than 1 per cent of women and its cause is usually unknown (Barbo, 1987).

History

GENERAL

The scope of the gynecologic history varies with the age of the patient. It includes, but is not limited to, the menstrual cycle, pregnancy (gravidity and parity), vaginal discharge, perimenstrual symptoms, sexually transmitted diseases, pelvic infections, pelvic pain, and cutaneous symptoms of the perineum. Urinary tract signs and symptoms are also helpful to review.

SEXUAL HISTORY

The sexual history is very important and is often not elicited without direct questioning. Sexual concerns are often expressed through presenting somatic symptoms. When physicians include sexual histories routinely, about 35 to 50 per cent of their patients reveal sexual problems as compared with 2 to 10 per cent if only a routine assessment is done. A simple history yields as many positive findings as a more detailed questionnaire (Driscoll, 1986).

SEXUAL ABUSE

Sexual abuse often must be considered as a possibility. Conservatively, 25 per cent of girls and 9 per cent of boys are abused by age 18. Preadolescents are the most vulnerable. The presence of sexually transmitted disease in children is most likely due to sexual abuse. It is estimated that 336,000 children are abused in the United States per year (Enos, 1986). A physical examination needs to be done, even though only 40 per cent of patients have definitive findings. The language used must be modified and phrased to suit the age of the alleged victim and the circumstances of the abuse. Necessary information requires extensive questioning of both the victim and complainant, if different (Ladson et al., 1987).

Physical Examination

The pelvic examination frequently induces anxiety in the patient, so it is essential that the examiner be calm, sensitive, reassuring, and communicative during the procedure. Rapport needs to be established or re-established with all patients. Contact should initially be with gentle touch of the perineum after the patient is in the dorsal lithotomy position. When possible, an examining table should be used with stirrups adjusted to patient comfort and with buttocks positioned at the very end of the table.

The examination should start with inspection of the external genitalia (vulva) for skin lesions and hair distribution. The vaginal introitus should then be inspected including assessment of the size of hymenal ring by introduction of one to two fingers into the vagina. An appropriately sized speculum should be warmed and moistened (not lubricated), with introduction into the vaginal canal at a 45-degree angle with a gentle downward pressure on the perineal body. It is then turned horizontally, opened, and secured so that the cervix and vaginal walls can be visualized and cytologic specimens taken, if appropriate.

A bimanual examination is done with one well-lubricated gloved hand in the vagina and the opposite hand on the lower abdomen, exerting gentle, downward pressure. The uterus and adnexa's size, shape, and position are noted, as is the presence of abnormal masses, tenderness, or pain with cervical motion. With the patient bearing down, relaxation of the anterior or posterior vaginal wall is assessed (Bates, 1983).

EQUIPMENT

Equipment needed for a basic pelvic examination includes a good light source, which is flexible and easily positioned for individual lighting needs. It is also necessary to have several different sizes of vaginal speculums, with stainless steel preferred over plastic. Both sterile and nonsterile disposable examining gloves should be available. A convenient sink with both cold and hot water is essential, as is a lubricant such as water-soluble jelly.

Special equipment needed is discussed in the section on gynecologic procedures. Basic needs include glass slides, cover slips, normal saline, 10 per cent potassium hydroxide, pH paper, cytologic fixative solution or aerosol, culture capability, and a cervical-endocervical spatula. These should be easily accessible to the examiner for every examination.

APPROACH TO THE PEDIATRIC PATIENT

The gynecologic evaluation of the female patient should be part of every general examination and is necessary when specific gynecologic indications arise. This is first done during the newborn period to assess the patient for congenital anomalies, prominent hymen, physiologic leukorrhea, and breast buds. Simple visualization of the external genitalia can be done through infancy and childhood with the child reclining with knees flexed and hips abducted. Infants and small children may feel more comfortable reclining in the lap of the parent who is also reclining on the exam table. Reassurance by the physician is essential. The otoscope is a helpful light source for viewing the vagina. The knee-chest position may be also helpful for perineal relaxation in early childhood. Pubertal development should be assessed by routine breast examination and observation of hair growth (Simmons, 1988).

Instrumentation and specimen procurement are needed only for special circumstances. A pediatric speculum, as well as other special techniques, may be carefully used by an experienced examiner. Tubing from a butterfly catheter attached to a saline-filled syringe can be used to obtain specimens through vaginal washings. Rarely is general anesthesia needed.

Periodic Health Examinations

In another chapter of this book this subject is covered in great detail. Screening for disease is an integral part of disease prevention and health maintenance and has long been associated with routine office gynecologic examinations.

Cancer of the cervix is the only cancer for which there has been long-term, widespread screening. Invasive cervical cancer has an incidence of 16,000 cases per year, with an additional 45,000 new cases of carcinoma in situ (CIS). The incidence is 13 per 100,000 population. There has been a dramatic reduction in the occurrence of invasive cancer because preinvasive neoplastic changes are recognized by the Papanicolaou (PAP) smear. Such neoplastic changes have now been widely accepted and labeled as cervical intraepithelial neoplasia [CIN]. This is subdivided into Grades I, II, and III, depending on how mild to severe the changes, as described in Figure 43–3. Figure 43–4 shows moderate dysplasia (Jones et al., 1988). CIN III is synonymous with CIS, for which the 5-year survival rate is almost 100 per cent.

The PAP smear is relatively inexpensive, painless, and accurate. A 30 per cent average false negative rate is substantially offset by the long duration of preinvasive stages. The frequency of this testing is still debated, with recommendations from various authorities ranging from 1 to 3 years.

Screening for ovarian cancer is very difficult because classic symptoms and signs do not occur in early disease. It is common with 18,000 new cases and 12,000 deaths each year, with a survival rate of only 35 per cent. An annual pelvic examination makes sense, since it provides the best opportunity for early diagnosis. Because symptoms are insidious, the disease is usually detected at an advanced stage (Brunton and Sutherland, 1988).

Screening for endometrial cancer is still done primarily through obtaining a history of abnormal bleeding, which is present in 80 to 90 per cent of the women who have the disease (American Cancer Society, 1980). It is a disease of perimenopausal and postmenopausal women, with an incidence of 30 cases per 100,000 women (Koss et al., 1982). Routine endometrial sampling is reserved for those with high-risk conditions, including obesity, nulliparity, pelvic irradiation, prolonged unopposed estrogen replacement, diabetes mellitus, hypothyroidism, and a history of endometrial hyperplasia.

Procedures

PAPANICOLAOU'S (PAP) SMEAR

This cytologic sampling technique was introduced into clinical medicine by Papanicolaou and Traut in 1943. Superficial cells are scraped from the cervix and endocervix and represent deeper processes accurately if taken optimally. Ideally, both the ectocervix and endocervix should be sampled. A reliable, experienced cytopathologist is essential, and that individual should be given accurate gynecologic medical history on the patients, including age, last menstrual period, parity, and significant previous cervical pathology (Havelock, 1974).

The techniques used vary but always include adequate exposure and lighting and gentle removal of excessive discharge from the cervix. The endocervical canal can be wiped with a cotton-tipped applicator or a cytobrush. The ectocervix should be scraped in a

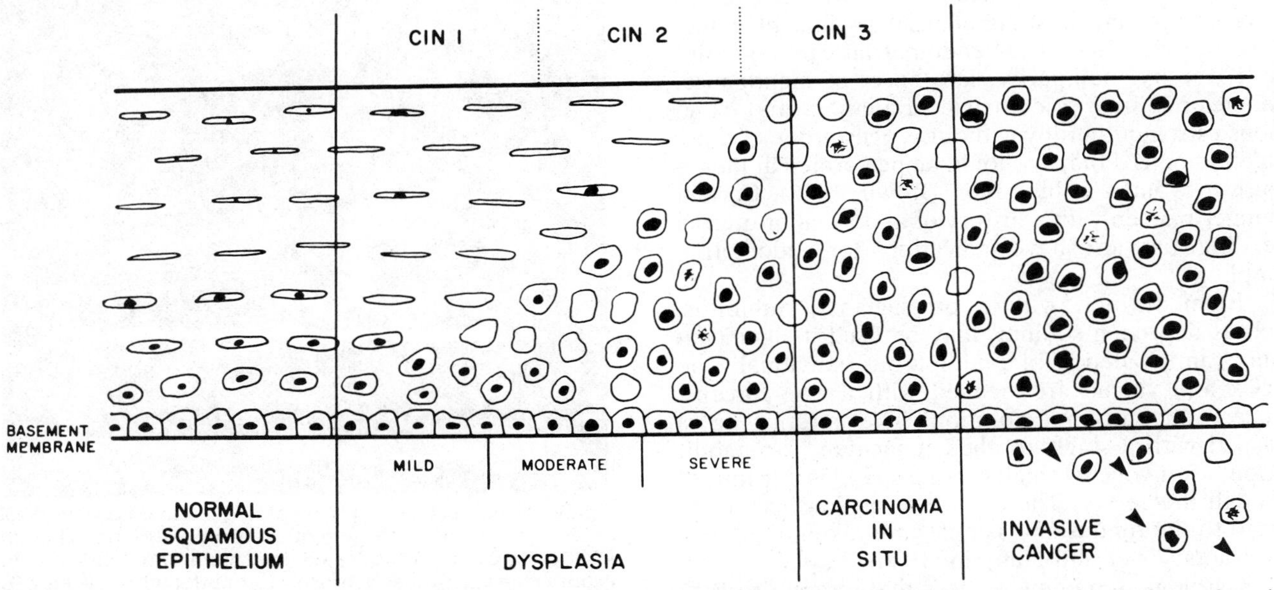

Figure 43–3. Diagram of cervical epithelium showing the varying terminology used to characterize progressive degrees of cervical neoplasia. *CIN 1, 2,* and *3* are the same as CIN I, II, and III. (Modified from Richart RM: Cervical intraepithelial neoplasia and the gynecologist. Can. J. Med. Tech., *38*:117, 1976.)

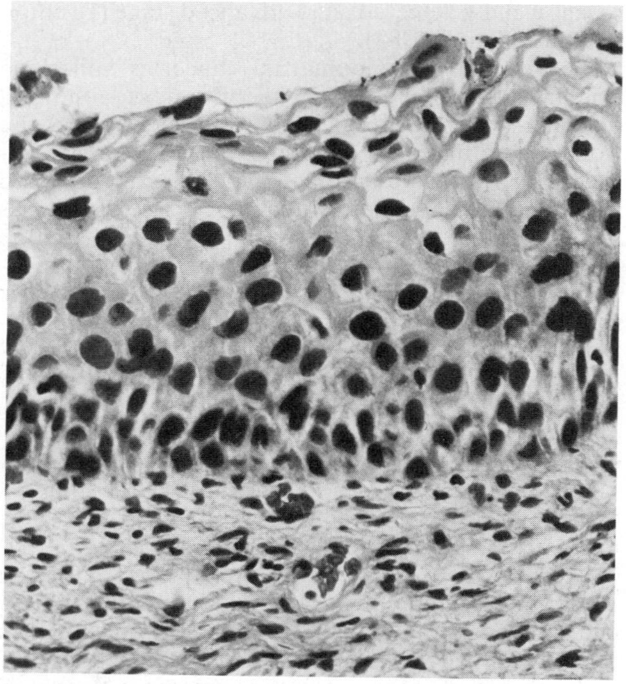

Figure 43–4. Definite line of demarcation between normal squamous epithelium *(right)* and moderate dysplasia *(left)*.

360-degree area with a protruding lip, wooden, plastic or metal spatula (Fig. 43–5). The specimens should be placed on marked slides and immediately fixed.

ENDOMETRIAL BIOPSY

Endometrial sampling has become increasingly important as a method of screening for endometrial hyperplasia and carcinoma. The primary indications are irregular menstrual bleeding in women over 40 years of age and postmenopausal vaginal bleeding. Increased risk factors for endometrial carcinoma include obesity, nulliparity, late onset of menopause, diabetes mellitus, prior pelvic irradiation, and exogenous estrogen therapy without progesterone cycling. An endometrial biopsy should be performed at menopause in women at high risk (Brown, 1986). Certain younger women with a history of abnormal or uterine bleeding may also have indications for endometrial sampling.

Premedication with a prostaglandin inhibitor, such as naproxen sodium, may be used if significant pain is anticipated as in a nulliparous individual. The cervix and vagina are cleaned with a ring forceps, gauze, and antiseptic solution. The anterior lip is grasped with a single-toothed tenaculum for stabilization, after which a small uterine sound is introduced through the cervix. The curette or aspirator is introduced to the fundus and samples are taken in all four quadrants (Oyer and Hanjuni, 1986).

Cytologic screening devices that scrape or brush the endometrium include the Endocyte, the Accurette, and the Mi-Mark sampler. Histologic sampling is more reliable and accurate via the Kevarkian curette, self-contained Vakutage, Pipelle, or the Vabra suction curettage (Fig. 43–6). These latter methods are 95 per cent accurate when successful. The Pipelle and other similar small devices have the advantage of being almost painless. The Vabra aspirator is a 21-cm.–long plastic curette that is 3 mm. in diameter and is connected to a separate suction device.

Although one should avoid biopsy of the endometrium in pregnancy, early conceptions are rarely disturbed by such sampling (Speroff et al., 1989).

CERVICAL BIOPSY

Cervical biopsy should always be done when there is a grossly visible lesion on the cervix. Colposcopic technique may be needed to determine a specific preferential location when a visible lesion is not present (Figure 43–7). Multiple biopsy instruments are available. Selection will depend on the size and depth needed for accurate diagnosis. The location of biopsy sites may be assisted by painting the cervix with an iodine solution [Schiller's solution 0.3 per cent or Lugol's solution 5 per cent], which is not taken up by dysplastic cells that do not contain glycogen.

COLPOSCOPY

Colposcopy has become the preferred method for investigating abnormal PAP smears (Benedet et al., 1982). It has reduced significantly the need for diag-

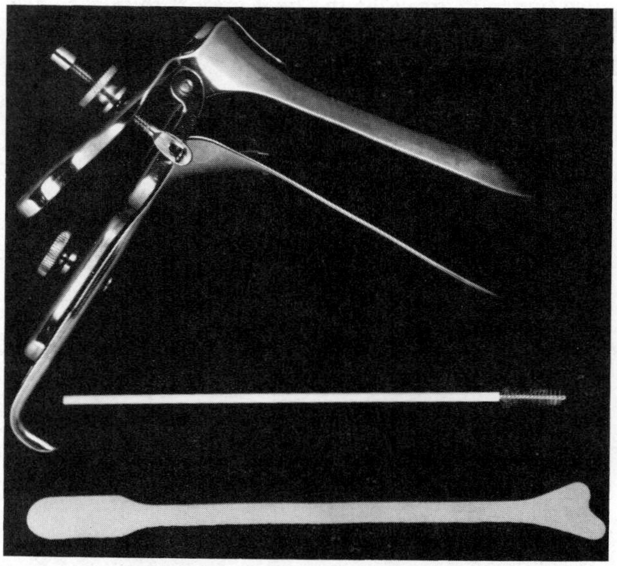

Figure 43–5. Technique for obtaining routine cervical cytology: (1) complete cytology request forms; (2) label slide; (3) insert dry or water-lubricated speculum—no lubricant; (4) expose cervix; (5) insert brush, cotton-tipped applicator, or aspirator in cervical os and twirl or aspirate *(A)*; (6) scrape external os area with cytology spatula *(B)*; (7) smear slide *(C)*; (8) fix immediately.

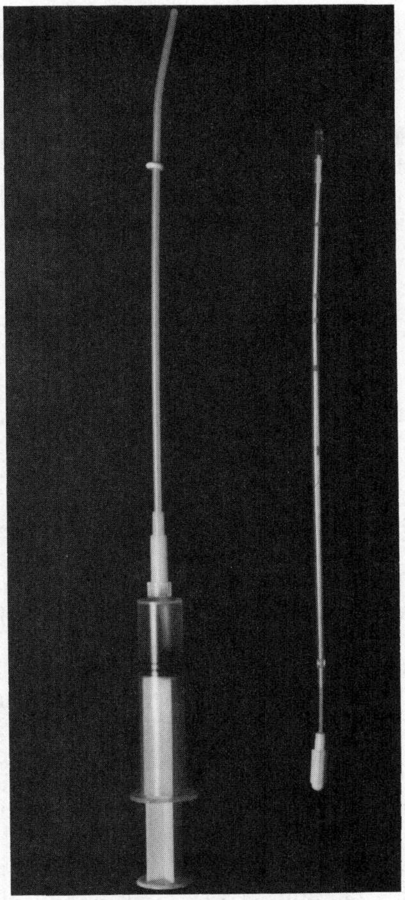

Figure 43–6. A Pipelle endometrial biopsy instrument.

nostic cold conization; only 15 per cent of patients with abnormal cytology that undergo colposcopy will still need conization. This simple diagnostic method provides a flexible means for assessment and diagnoses, which can be performed by a skilled and reliable colposcopist (Rodney et al., 1987). The colposcope is essentially a magnifying glass with a light source that illuminates the cervix, which allows definition of the size, site, and quality of cervical lesions (Goode et al., 1986). It is important that the entire transformation zone is visualized, which often necessitates the use of an endocervical speculum. Identified significant lesions need to be biopsied with study by an experienced histopathologist.

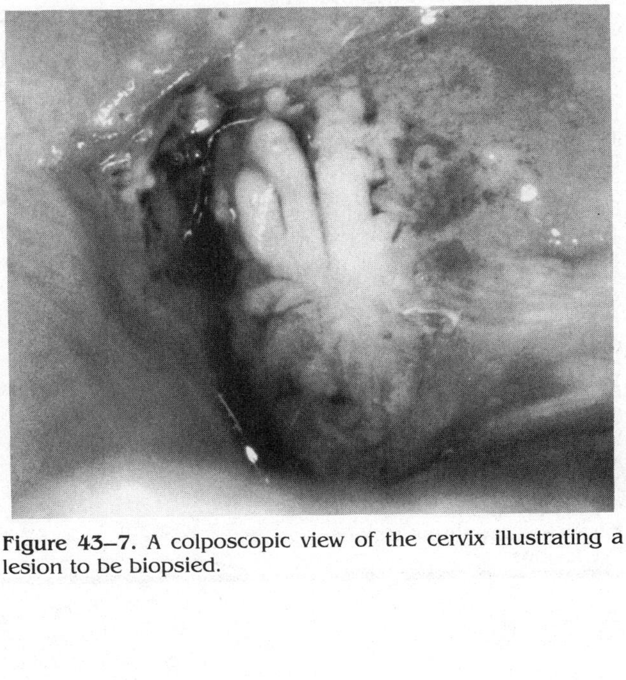

Figure 43–7. A colposcopic view of the cervix illustrating a lesion to be biopsied.

CRYOSURGERY

Cryosurgery has been used progressively in destructive treatment of cervical lesions, and has almost completely replaced hot cauterization. Indications include chronic benign cervicitis, dysplasia, koilocytotic atypia, and condyloma acuminata. This technique requires controlled subfreezing temperatures to as low as −20° C. (−68° F.), which produce tissue necrosis. Gas under high pressure is released for 10 to 15 seconds through a small hole inside the hollow tip of the cryosurgical probes into an area of lower pressure for 4 to 5 minutes. The probe, through direct contact after water soluble gel has been applied to the tip, creates dehydration that leads to denaturation of liquid and protein molecules (Brown and Kammeyer, 1986; Fray and Sims, 1982).

The cervix needs to be well exposed with a speculum, and excess mucus should be removed with cotton swabs. Freezing is continued until the iceball extends 3 to 5 mm. beyond the border of the tissue to be destroyed. Defrosting must be allowed sufficiently before the probe is pulled away from the cervix to prevent extensive tissue damage. Freezing after a 3-minute thaw reduces the probability of failure. Careful patient follow-up is very important (Rodney et al., 1987).

Menstrual Disorders

Menstruation is the last in a series of events of puberty, which includes axillary and pubic hair growth and breast development. Vaginal bleeding that occurs in the absence of other secondary sex characteristics should be considered highly unusual. Possible reasons for such bleeding could include sexual abuse, genital tumors, or infection. The first few menstrual periods may be irregular in frequency, length, and amount of flow. A patient who has not started her menstrual periods by age 16 should also be investigated to determine whether there are anatomic, genetic, or endocrine abnormalities.

AMENORRHEA

Amenorrhea is defined as the absence of menstrual bleeding at the expected time. Amenorrhea may be primary, indicating that the patient has not experienced menses by the age of 16 years, or secondary, indicating that menses were present for a time and then ceased. It is important to know whether a patient with primary amenorrhea has noticed development of secondary sexual characteristics or has experienced increasing cyclic pelvic pain. A careful pelvic examination will help determine anatomic abnormalities, such as absent internal genitalia, imperforate hymen, or vaginal atresia. Other causes are hormonal or chromosomal abnormalities.

The most common cause of secondary amenorrhea in the woman who is of reproductive age is pregnancy, and this cause should be ruled out in any woman with the complaint of a "missed period." Other causes of amenorrhea include oral contraceptive use; high prolactin levels, leading to pituitary suppression; polycystic ovarian syndrome; psychologic stress; rapid changes in weight; anorexia nervosa; neurotropic drugs; and chronic diseases.

DYSMENORRHEA

Primary dysmenorrhea is pain that occurs at the onset of the menses and is not associated with any anatomic abnormality. It is a common complaint during the teenage years and usually begins with the onset of ovulation, generally 1 to 2 years after menarche. Primary dysmenorrhea typically begins with the onset of flow and subsides over the next 24 hours. In the past, primary dysmenorrhea was frequently considered a psychologic disorder, but it is now accepted as due to uterine contractions that occur as prostaglandins rise at the onset of menses (Dawood, 1988).

Most patients with dysmenorrhea can do well with prostaglandin synthetase inhibitors (nonsteroidal anti-inflammatory drugs), or by just staying busy. Oral contraceptives usually provide excellent relief by stopping ovulation. Many patients with primary dysmenorrhea have significant relief after childbirth.

Secondary dysmenorrhea, or dysmenorrhea associated with an anatomic cause, is more prevalent in the late third and into the fourth and fifth decades. With benign disease, treatment can often be conservative using nonsteroidal anti-inflammatory drugs or oral contraceptives in the properly selected patient. Laparoscopic examination is recommended for cases that respond poorly to treatment. Small implants of endometriosis, adhesions, fibroids, or other abnormalities may be evident (Kresch, 1984). Hysterectomy should be discussed with those women who have disabling dysmenorrhea and who have completed their childbearing.

DYSFUNCTIONAL UTERINE BLEEDING

Dysfunctional uterine bleeding is defined as that bleeding that is unassociated with normal menses. Shortly after menarche and before menopause dysfunctional bleeding is most often due to anovulation or irregular ovulation. During the active childbearing years, dysfunctional bleeding is most commonly due to pregnancy or oral contraceptive use. A thorough pelvic examination should determine whether the bleeding is coming from the uterus, cervix, or vagina. Polycystic ovarian disease, endometrial neoplasia, and polyps are important causes of dysfunctional uterine bleeding.

PREMENSTRUAL SYNDROME

Premenstrual syndrome is defined as "the recurrence of symptoms in the premenstruum with absence of symptoms in the postmenstruum." Because such a diversity of symptoms is associated with premenstrual syndrome, many physicians had trouble accepting it as a valid diagnosis in the past. Depression, irritability, and fatigue are just three of the more common symptoms seen in the condition (Table 43–1) (Dalton, 1984).

Several causes have been proposed, including excess prostaglandin production, hormonal imbalance, pyridoxine hydrochloride deficiency, and increased aldosterone production in the luteal phase (Smith, 1986). Having the patient keep a menstrual diary is the best way to verify the recurrence of whatever symptoms become manifest.

Treatment of premenstrual syndrome is often a matter of trial and error. Diet modification (low intake of refined sugar and caffeine), exercise, rest, and social support are all nonmedical therapies worth trying. Hormones, vitamins, diuretics, and tranquilizers have all been used with success in some patients, with very little relief in others.

Table 43–1. SYMPTOMS OF PMS (PERCENTAGE OF FIRST VISIT)

	N = 160 n=	Per Cent
Depression	435	71
Irritability	343	56
Tiredness	212	35
Headaches	202	33
Bloatedness	188	31
Breast tenderness	129	21
Tension	115	19
Violence	80	13
Suicidal tendencies	36	6
Anxiety or panic attacks	33	5
Food cravings	30	5
Criminal acts	22	4
Epilepsy	19	3
Psychotic episodes	17	3
Skin lesions	17	3
Vertigo	16	3
Alcoholic urges	13	2
Asthma	9	1.5
Urinary symptoms	6	1
Ear, nose, and throat lesions	4	0.7
Eye lesions	4	0.7

CYCLIC INTERMENSTRUAL PAIN AND BLEEDING

Intermenstrual pain, or mittleschmerz, is due to ovulation, but the exact relationship is not known. The pain may vary in duration from a few hours to 2 to 3 days. Some patients also have accompanying uterine spotting or bleeding, most likely due to the drop in estrogen that occurs just prior to ovulation (Wentz, 1988).

If the pain is mild and definitely cyclic, reassurance or mild analgesics may suffice. In more severe cases, diagnostic measures such as a dilatation and curettage or laparoscopy may be needed. Treatment in these cases usually consists of hormonal suppression of the ovary with an oral contraceptive.

POSTMENOPAUSAL BLEEDING

Any bleeding that occurs after the menopause should be of concern. Endometrial neoplasia and bleeding from atrophic tissues of the vagina are frequent causes and need to be differentiated.

Infections

SEXUALLY TRANSMITTED DISEASES

The incidence of sexually transmitted diseases has increased as couples have decreased their use of barrier contraception. At the same time, we have seen increasing sexual activity in the teenage population during the last 30 years. It is often difficult to get these young people to recognize the importance of birth control, let alone the importance of using a barrier method or abstinence for contraception and to prevent the spread of sexually transmitted diseases. Nonoxynol 9, which is the active ingredient in most spermicides, also provides protection against sexually transmitted disease by inhibiting the various organisms. Condoms are a physical barrier, some of which contain nonoxynol 9 (Jones, 1988).

The most common sexually transmitted disease is *Chlamydia trachomatis.* Chlamydial cervicitis has now become easier to diagnose by rapid enzyme tests and immunofluorescent antibody tests. Results can be available in less than 24 hours. The false positive rate becomes acceptable when large volumes of patients are screened. Because *Chlamydia* is dependent on the cell for growth, it requires tissue medium for culture. Although there are inherent difficulties with this culture, it is still considered the "gold standard" for diagnosis. Because of interference of other organisms with the reaction of the rapid tests, these tests should not be used for detecting *Chlamydia* in the throat or in premenarchal girls owing to the number of false positives that may result.

In 80 per cent of cases, *Chlamydia* is asymptomatic (Glenney, 1988). Therefore, patients from high-risk groups, such as teenagers and patients with multiple partners, should be screened periodically. When taking a history, it is important to ask a patient whether or not there are any symptoms in her partner(s), such as dysuria or penile discharge. Most asymptomatic cases can be easily treated with tetracycline, or erythromycin if tetracycline is contraindicated. The treatment of chlamydial pelvic inflammatory disease is described later. Sexual partners of the patient also need to be treated. A test of cure should be done 10 to 14 days later.

Neisseria gonorrhoeae is the next most frequently diagnosed sexually transmitted disease. Gonorrhea is asymptomatic in 80 per cent of female patients and in 20 per cent of male patients. The organism requires chocolate agar medium, incubated in a carbon dioxide–rich atmosphere. Gram stain will reveal intracellular gram-negative diplococci.

If gonorrhea is suspected or diagnosed, treatment consists of 1 gram of probenicid followed one half hour later with a single dose of 3.5 mg. of ampicillin. Because concomitant infection with *Chlamydia* is so common, patients should also be given a prescription for 10 days of tetracycline or doxycycline (Glenney, 1988).

Since the Vietnam war, penicillinase-producing *Neisseria gonorrhoeae* (PPNG) has proved to be a treatment problem, particularly in large cities. PPNG is responsive to spectinomycin, but this antibiotic is not effective against syphilis. Spectinomycin should not be used routinely for the treatment of gonorrhea. A treatment option now available is ceftriaxone, a broad-spectrum cephalosporin, 250 mg. of which is effective against penicillinase and nonpenicillinase-producing strains of gonoccocus as well as *Chlamydia.*

Syphilis, which is caused by the spirochete *Treponema pallidum,* when left untreated, progresses through three stages. Primary syphilis occurs about 3 weeks after exposure and becomes manifest by a painless chancre on the vulva. This stage may be missed by the patient and routine serum tests may be negative because detectable serum levels of antibody may not be present for 4 to 6 weeks.

During the development of secondary syphilis, one can observe an evanescent maculopapular rash. This can progress to condyloma lata with an accompanying lymphadenitis. These oval, plateau-like lesions may appear both genitally and nongenitally and are highly infectious. Tertiary syphilis is rarely seen today but becomes manifest by the syphilitic ulcer or gumma often seen on the vulva. Because of accompanying necrosis and ulceration, it can cause rectovaginal fistulae. It may have the appearance of carcinoma.

Fortunately, syphilis responds well to penicillin (Table 43–2) (M.M.W.R., 1985). Pregnant patients can transmit the spirochete to the fetus, particularly after the fifth month. Prevention of congenital syphilis necessitates prenatal testing.

Less frequently seen granulomatous sexually

Table 43–2. RECOMMENDED TREATMENT FOR SYPHILIS

Early syphilis: Primary, secondary, or latent syphilis of less than 1 year duration
- Benzathine penicillin G, 2.4 million units I.M. in a single dose
- Penicillin-allergic patients:
  - Tetracycline HCl, 500 mg. p.o. four times daily for 15 days

Late syphilis: More than 1 year duration
- Benzathine penicillin (G., 2.4 million units I.M. once a week for 3 consecutive weeks [7.2 million units total])
- Penicillin-allergic patients:
  - Tetracycline HCl, 500 mg. p.o. four times daily for 30 days

Syphilis during pregnancy
- Benzathine penicillin in the appropriate dose schedule
- Penicillin-allergic patients
  - Erythromycin, 500 mg. p.o. four times daily for 15–30 days (tetracycline is not recommended during pregnancy)

transmitted diseases are chancroid, caused by *Haemophilus ducreyi;* granuloma inguinale, caused by *Calymmatobacterium granulomatis*; and lymphogranuloma venereum, a chlamydial infection. Biopsy of the lesions will help distinguish these infections from carcinoma. Carcinoma of the vulva has been known to be associated with granulomatous disease.

CONDYLOMATA ACUMINATA

Condyloma acuminata (venereal warts) are caused by the human papillomavirus (HPV). Several types have now been defined. The oncogenic potential of various serotypes of HPV has been demonstrated by Schneider and associates and others.

Condyloma acuminata appear as white, verrucous lesions. They may appear singly or in clusters about the labia, perineum, vagina, or cervix. The colposcope may be necessary to see flat lesions on the cervix. Large cauliflower-like lesions can be seen, especially in pregnant patients and in those who may be immunocompromised. Laryngeal condylomata can be found in newborns of patients with HPV. There is a possibility that fetal infection can occur through passage through the vagina, although intrauterine infection can apparently occur also. Patients with huge lesions filling the vagina will need to be delivered by cesarean section because of mechanical obstruction.

Condyloma acuminata must be treated carefully because of frequent relapses and the risk of malignancy. Destruction of the warts is most commonly done with topical podophyllin solution or trichloroacetic acid which is applied and then washed off after 4 to 6 hours. The variable success rate is evident in 3 to 4 days, and weekly reapplication is indicated when necessary. Other measures such as surgical removal, electrocautery, cryosurgery, or laser treatment can be used for resistant cases or when contraindications are present. Sexual partners should be treated, and both should be followed for 8 months after treatment because HPV is a major health concern.

HERPES SIMPLEX VIRUS

Herpes simplex virus type II becomes manifest by vesicles appearing on the vulva, perineum, and introitus, often within 3 to 7 days of exposure. The vagina and cervix may be involved alone or with external lesions. The external lesions, especially with a primary infection, are often very painful, probably owing to infection by secondary organisms. Systemic symptoms of fever and malaise may also be present. The best specimen for culture comes from fluid obtained from an unruptured vesicle. Diagnosis can also be made by seeing multinucleated inclusion bodies on the PAP smear.

After several days, the vesicles become painful ulcerations. Total healing in primary infections takes about 2 to 3 weeks. Recurrent infections often last less than a week. Virus can sometimes be cultured from the ulcers in their early stages.

The development of acyclovir has been of great benefit to patients in the treatment of herpes (Mertz, 1988). Acylovir oral tablets can be taken continuously to reduce the recurrence rate for those patients with frequent outbreaks. For patients with rare recurrences, the tablets can be taken at the time of a recurrence to reduce its length and severity. The I.V. medication is useful when there are severe systemic symptoms or if the patient is immunocompromised.

Vulvovaginitis

Leukorrhea, perineal pruritus, and external dysuria are common symptoms of the patient with vulvovaginitis. Taking time to make a specific diagnosis will help prevent recurrence. To preserve testing sensitivity, it is helpful to examine the patient when she has not used any medication in the vagina for 24 to 48 hours. The necessary basic diagnostic materials are isotonic saline and 10 per cent potassium hydroxide for wet mounts, a microscope, nitrazene paper for determination of pH level, slides, and a vaginal speculum (Table 43–3) (Sutherland, 1984).

TRICHOMONIASIS

Common complaints with *Trichomonas* vaginitis include foul-smelling leukorrhea (which is the most common complaint), often accompanied by burning, soreness, pruritus, and dysuria. On speculum examination, there is often a pool of greenish yellow discharge in the vagina that is bubbly. The vagina

Table 43–3. DIFFERENTIAL DIAGNOSIS OF VULVOVAGINITIS

Diagnosis	History	Physical Features	Laboratory Findings and Diagnostic Methods	Treatment
Gardnerella vaginalis vaginitis	Mildly odorous discharge	Gray, mucoid, pasty discharge; pH 5 to 6	Saline preparation—studded with "clue cells;" culture as needed	Metronidazole, 500 mg. t.i.d. for 7 days
Candidiasis	Recurrent pruritic discharge	Creamy, curdly discharge; ph 4 to 5	Potassium hydroxide preparation—mycelia, buds; culture as needed	Clotrimazole, miconazole, nystatin, or another antifungal agent
Trichomonal vaginitis	Odorous leukorrhea; dysuria	Greenish yellow discharge; pH 5–6.6; friable hyperemic cervix	Saline preparation—motile flagellate protozoa; culture as needed	Metronidazole, 2 grams in a single dose
Reactive vaginitis	Use of hygienic sprays and douches; odorous discharge	Foreign bodies; erythema	None	Elimination of offensive agent, corticosteroids
Atrophic vaginitis	Dyspareunia; burning	Sticky brown discharge; thin vaginal tissue	None	Topical estrogen
Normal cervical or vaginal discharge vaginitis	Minimal discharge	Clear mucoid discharge, pH 4.5; ectropion	Saline preparation—a few leukocytes and epithelial cells	None or povidone-iodine

and cervix may have small petechiae that give them a "strawberry" appearance.

Diagnosis is made by observing motile, pear-shaped parasites with flagella seen on the normal saline wet smear (Fig. 43–8). The leukorrhea pH is 5 to 6.5. Sperm are much smaller and should not be confused with trichomonads. A single 2-gram dose of metronidazole provides treatment with an acceptable failure rate and good patient compliance. Other dose regimens of metronidazole, such as 250 mg. t.i.d. for 7 days or 500 mg. b.i.d. for 5 days, have the advantages of fewer gastrointestinal complaints (Lossick, 1986). Because trichomoniasis is a sexually transmitted disease, it is essential that the partner be treated. Furazolidone (Tricofuron suppositories) or povidone-iodine (Betadine gel) may be useful when metronidazole is contraindicated (Spencer et al., 1987).

MONILIASIS

Yeast is part of the normal flora of the vagina. Under conditions that may increase the pH of the vagina or disturb its normal flora, yeast will flourish and cause

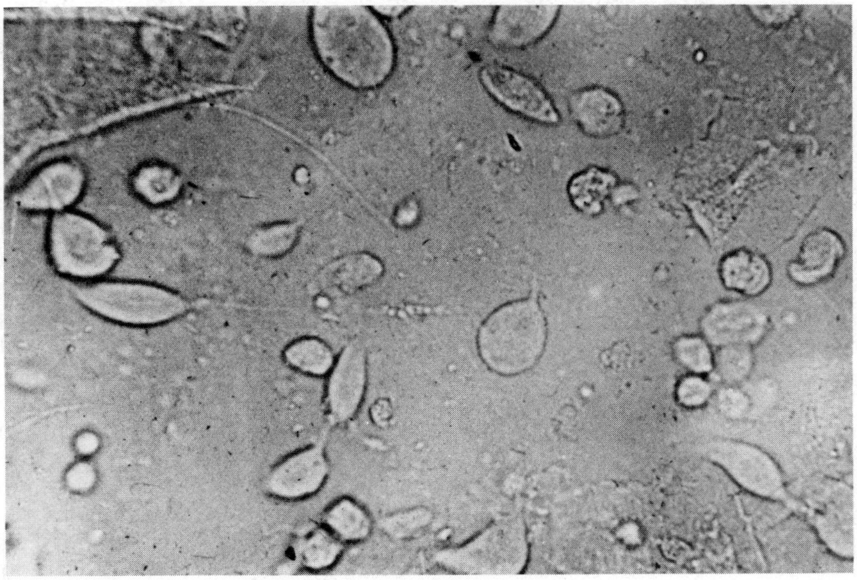

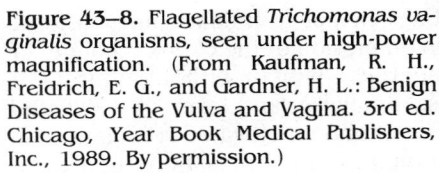

Figure 43–8. Flagellated *Trichomonas vaginalis* organisms, seen under high-power magnification. (From Kaufman, R. H., Freidrich, E. G., and Gardner, H. L.: Benign Diseases of the Vulva and Vagina. 3rd ed. Chicago, Year Book Medical Publishers, Inc., 1989. By permission.)

a vulvovaginitis. Pregnancy, diabetes mellitus, antibiotics, and oral contraceptives may be at fault. Candida albicans is the most frequent pathogenic strain. The most common complaints are intense pruritus and a white, curdly discharge with a pH of 4 to 5. When tested, discharge prepared with potassium hydroxide shows branching mycelia, pseudohyphae, and yeast buds (Fig. 43–9) (Sutherland, 1984).

Yeast infections are most commonly symptomatic in the premenstrual period. Several antimonilial agents include miconazole, clotrimazole, buconazole, terconazole, and gentian violet. When yeast vaginitis is recurrent, one needs to make sure of the diagnosis by re-examining the patient to confirm the diagnosis. One should rule out diabetes or immunocompromising disorders. Allergy to *Candida* has been described (Witkin, 1987). Absolute hygiene is essential, not only by keeping the area clean and dry, but also by always wiping from front to back when cleaning the perineum. Furthermore, tight-fitting clothing and synthetic underwear should be avoided so the perineum can "breathe" and not remain moist. In some persistent cases, a 500 mg. suppository of clotrimazole can be used once a month as prophylaxis.

GARDNERELLA VAGINITIS

Gardnerella is a common bacteria that causes a profuse, foul smelling discharge. Patients may complain of a "fishy" odor. Often there is no pruritus or burning sensation accompanying the discharge. Whether or not *Gardnerella* is sexually transmitted is a matter of debate. Certainly, it is found in virginal women. On the other hand, sexually active women may acquire it recurrently unless their sexual partners are treated concurrently. If it is found in prepubertal girls, one should be suspicious of sexual abuse.

Diagnosis of *Gardnerella* is made by wet preparation of the vaginal secretions with normal saline. One will see bacteria imbedded in the epithelial cells, so-called "clue cells" (Fig. 43–10) (Sutherland, 1984). One may also perform a "whiff test" by adding a drop of potassium hydroxide to a slide with a sample of vaginal discharge on it. A characteristic fishy odor will be emitted. The pH of the leukorrhea is 5 to 6.

The use of condoms and treatment of the sexual partner is also recommended. Metronidazole is the treatment of choice for infection with *Gardnerella*, with the most common current dosage regimen being 500 mg. three times daily for 7 days. Other antibiotics including ampicillin, cephalosporins, and tetracycline are also effective (Jones et al., 1988).

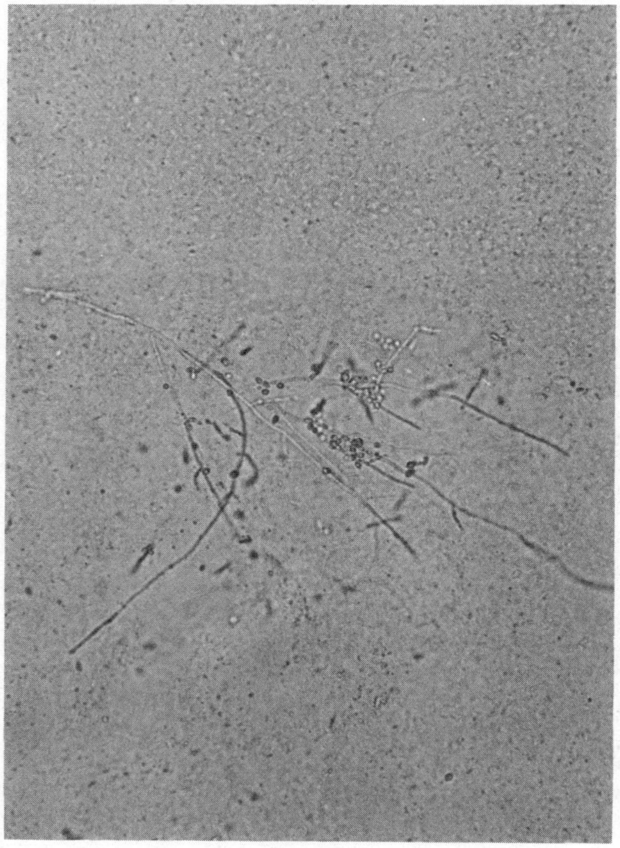

Figure 43–9. Yeast and mycelia, seen in potassium hydroxide preparation of candidiasis discharge.

PELVIC INFLAMMATORY DISEASE

Today, pelvic inflammatory disease is often defined as venereally acquired salpingitis. Approximately one million women per year are affected (Sweet, 1986). Infection in the pelvis, however, can result from appendicitis, infected diverticuli and fistulae, or postoperative or postpartum infections. Cartwright believes that a better name for this syndrome would be endometritis-salpingitis-peritonitis. Most commonly, pelvic inflammatory disease is an infection that ascends either along the mucosa or through the lymphatics. Rare exceptions to this pattern are direct spread of infection from other organs or hematogenous spread of tuberculosis bacilli or mumps virus.

The most common cause of acute salpingitis is *Chlamydia*, which usually begins with cervicitis before ascending to the upper genital tract. Since the cervicitis may be asymptomatic, routine culturing of high-risk groups is essential.

Clinical findings in pelvic inflammatory disease will consist of pain on motion of the cervix (chandelier sign); adnexal tenderness, with or without induration; and adnexal masses, malaise, and fever. An elevated white blood cell count and an elevated sedimentation rate may be additional useful information but are not universally present (Cartwright, 1988).

Patients with chlamydial pelvic inflammatory disease often present with vague abdominal pain, dyspareunia, or abnormal uterine bleeding. Mild cases are treated by tetracycline or doxycycline. Patients with gonorrheal pelvic inflammatory disease may present with a more acute condition. Patients are often quite ill and require hospitalization. Because pelvic inflammatory disease usually involves multiple organ-

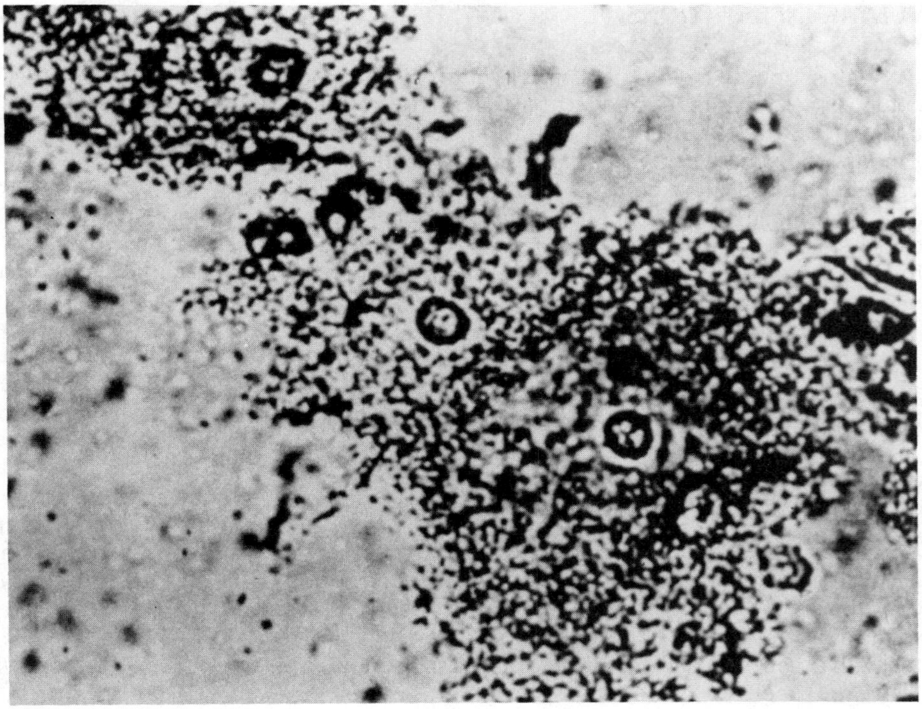

Figure 43–10. Microscopic appearance of "clue cells" (vaginal epithelial cells coated with bacteria) seen in *Gardnerella vaginalis* vaginitis.

isms, adequate treatment of severe cases requires combination therapy. Doxycycline and cefoxitin, and clindamycin and gentamicin are two successful combinations.

TOXIC SHOCK SYNDROME

Although toxic shock syndrome was first described in 1978 in children, its relationship to the use of tampons, especially highly absorbable ones during the menstrual period, has gained the most prominence. It is also seen in women who do not use tampons, those who use the contraceptive sponge and diaphragm, and in postoperative and postpartum patients. Toxic shock syndrome is usually associated with an exotoxin produced by *Staphylococcus aureus* (Baker, 1987; Berkley, 1987).

Toxic shock syndrome is characterized by the sudden onset of fever of at least 39° C. (102.2° F.), headache, vomiting, diarrhea, lethargy, and diffuse hyperemia of the skin and mucous membranes. Hypotension and shock soon follow. If the patient survives, desquamation of the palms and soles occurs in a few days.

Prompt treatment and hospitalization is essential because the mortality rate can be as high as 15 per cent. The physician should remove the tampon immediately, if it is present, and obtain cultures from the cervix, vagina, nasopharynx, and blood. Fluid and electrolyte support should be instituted with initiation of a beta-lactamase resistant antibiotic. Women who have been diagnosed with toxic shock syndrome probably should avoid using tampons in the future. To prevent toxic shock syndrome, women should be advised to use tampons only during the times of heavy flow during their menses and to avoid prolonged use of tampons. Contraceptive sponges and diaphragms should be used strictly according to directions and should not remain in the vagina for more than 24 hours. There has been significant decrease in the incidence of toxic shock syndrome since the public has become aware of the problem and the factors associated with it (Greenman and Immerman, 1987).

BARTHOLIN'S GLAND ABSCESS

Acute infection of Bartholin's gland has been attributed to gonococcus in the past, but there are many organisms that could be responsible. The entire labium can become swollen as abscess formation becomes evident in the gland. The patient complains of excruciating pain, and purulent material can be expressed from the gland, or it may spontaneously begin to drain.

Initial treatment consists of rest, analgesics, hot sitz baths or ice packs, and the administration of an antibiotic. When the abscess is fluctuant enough, incision and drainage on the vaginal side of the abscess should be accomplished. Insertion of a Word catheter, which has an inflatable balloon to keep it in place, will keep the abscess open and draining while healing progresses. This usually requires only local anesthesia. Recurrent cases sometimes require marsupialization for definitive treatment.

VULVAR INFESTATIONS

Pediculosis pubis (crabs, lice, nits), pulicosis (fleas), cimicosis (bed bugs), and scabies are infestations associated with pruritus and irritation of the vulva. Lindane is effective in treating most infestations of the vulva, but it must be used carefully. Because it is absorbed through the skin and is a neurotoxin, it can cause seizures, especially in large doses. Therefore, it should not be used in pregnant or lactating women or infants (Wynn, 1988).

Benign and Malignant Neoplasms

VULVA

Too often in performing the pelvic examination, there is so much interest in the cervix and uterus that one can bypass the vulva without inspecting it carefully, since many lesions can be asymptomatic. Biopsy of the vulva can be easily undertaken when needed to distinguish between benign and malignant lesions. A 3- or 4-mm Keyes skin punch biopsy instrument can be used with local anesthesia, obtains a good sample of tissue, and bleeding can be controlled with pressure or silver nitrate (Fig. 43–11).

Epithelial tissues in the vulva are subject to intraepithelial neoplasia as are those elsewhere in the lower genital tract. The average age of patients with cancer of the vulva is 62, but vulvar neoplasias associated with HPV are being found in adolescents and young adults (Carson, 1988; Downey, 1988).

The patient with vulvar carcinoma or carcinoma in situ (CIS) typically presents as an elderly woman with chronic vulvar pruritus. Ulceration, bleeding, and a mass may also be present. Surgery is the treatment of choice for vulvar carcinoma and is highly successful if the diagnosis is made before widespread lymphatic involvement occurs (Podratz, 1982).

Carcinoma in situ is present when malignant cells do not invade below the level of epithelium. Careful examination of the vulva is essential, particularly when intraepithelial neoplasia is present elsewhere in the genital tract. Approximately 20 to 30 per cent of vulvar neoplasia is associated with cervical CIS (Schneider, 1987).

CIS may appear white, red, pigmented or warty, and biopsy will reveal hyperkeratosis or parakeratosis with abnormal proliferation of basal cells with mitotic activity. CIS is often multifocal, and multiple biopsies should be done if necessary. Because it can be widespread on the vulva, CIS is a treatment challenge. However, surgery, laser ablation, and topical 5-fluorouracil are successful treatment modalities.

Nevi are important findings in the vulva because 3 to 4 per cent of malignant melanomas in women occur on the external genitalia. Any suspicious pigmented lesion of the vulva should be biopsied to rule out malignancy (DiSaia and Creasman, 1989).

Other rare, but important, malignancies of the vulva include basal cell carcinoma and malignant melanoma. Cancer of Bartholin's gland is rare but extends locally and metastasizes late in the course of the disease. Treatment consists of wide, local excision, sometimes including the rectum and surrounding tissues.

VAGINA

Benign and malignant neoplasms of the vagina are rare. Most are asymptomatic, such as vaginal polyps and rhabdomyomas. Local excision suffices as treatment. Asymptomatic Gartner's duct cysts, which are remnants of the mesonephric duct, and inclusion cysts, which can be mistaken for tumors, do not require treatment.

Ninety per cent of malignancies in the vagina are squamous cell carcinoma. If the patient has a cervix, this is usually considered to be the origin. Intraepithelial neoplasia, including CIS of the vagina, is increased after hysterectomy for cervical intraepithelial neoplasia or invasive neoplasia (Schneider, 1987). Because dysplastic and in situ lesions can be multifocal, the colposcope is useful for pinpointing the sources of abnormal cytology.

The average age of patients with invasive squamous cell carcinoma of the vagina is 60. The tumor may appear as an exophytic or ulcerative lesion, typically in the upper third of the vagina on the posterior wall. These lesions can be missed if the

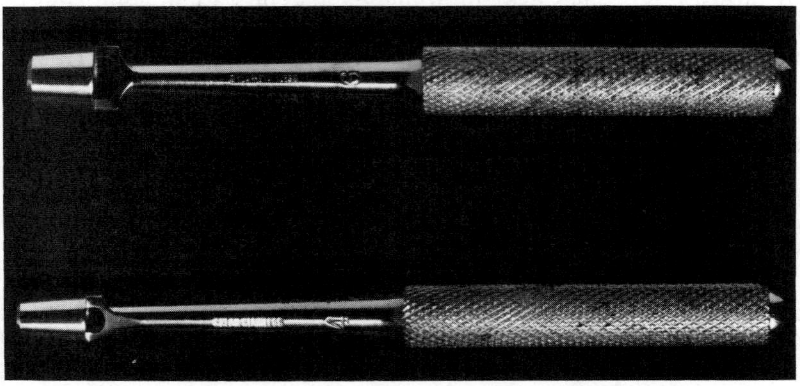

Figure 43–11. Keyes' skin punch.

vagina is not adequately inspected during the speculum examination. As long as the carcinoma is confined to the vagina, bleeding is the only symptom. Advanced disease can result in rectal or bladder fistulas and distant metastases. Radical surgery and radiation therapy provide the best modalities of treatment.

In 1971, Herbst and associates reported six cases at their institution of clear cell adenocarcinoma of the vagina in young women. Prior to this time, this rare tumor was found most often in the cervix and usually in postmenopausal women. Subsequent studies have established a relationship between the prenatal administration of diethylstilbestrol, commonly used around 1950 with vaginal adenosis and clear cell adenocarcinoma in female offspring. (Robboy, 1984). Although clear cell adenocarcinoma appears to arise from vaginal adenosis, when it is diagnosed it can be observed over time because the adenosis appears to regress. By the third decade, the risk of clear cell adenocarcinoma is extremely low.

Other important malignancies of the vagina include malignant melanoma, sarcoma botryoides, endodermal sinus tumor, and metastatic tumors from other sites. Malignant melanoma behaves in the vagina as elsewhere in the body—growing rapidly and metastasizing early. Radical surgery is the treatment of choice, but the prognosis is generally poor. Sarcoma botryoides (embryonal rhabdomyosarcoma), a grape-like tumor, is mentioned often but rarely seen. This tumor usually presents with vaginal bleeding in patients less than 5 years of age.

CERVIX

The most common benign lesions of the cervix are nabothian cysts and endocervical polyps. Nabothian cysts are created by the inclusion of endocervical glands by normal metaplastic change or by scarring, often from childbirth. These are interesting findings and do not require treatment.

Endocervical polyps may produce abnormal uterine bleeding, and one should be certain to rule out findings such as a pedunculated leiomyoma. Cervical polyps can be removed by grasping them at their base with a uterine forceps and twisting them off. Malignancy is rare, but they should be sent to the pathologist for examination.

The development and widespread use of the PAP smear to screen for preinvasive malignant changes in the cervix has led to a dramatic decrease in the incidence of invasive cancer. It has become evident that the etiology of preinvasive neoplasia is multifactorial. Two of the most important causal factors appear to be having more than one sexual partner and starting intercourse before the age of 20 (DiSaia, 1989). Women whose husbands were previously married to women with cervical cancer or whose husbands reported a history of multiple sexual partners have been found to have an increased risk of cervical neoplasia.

The factors mentioned earlier point to cervical intraepithelial neoplasia behaving as a sexually transmitted disease. Also along these lines is the fact that herpes simplex virus and most recently HPV have been associated with CIN. Furthermore, the finding of mild dysplasia or CIN I on the PAP smear sometimes reveals spontaneous regression to normal cytology on repeated tests.

CIN occurs in the "transformation zone" or the junction of the squamous epithelium of the exocervix and columnar epithelium of the endocervix. Therefore, it is important to get both ectocervical and endocervical swabs for the PAP smear. The length of time it takes to progress from CIN I to CIN III and then on to frank invasive cancer of the cervix varies but usually takes years (Watts, 1987). However, rapid progression in terms of months has been seen in a few women whose CIN was associated with HPV.

Present standards of treatment require the use of colposcopy to confirm the diagnosis of CIN, given that CIN is asymptomatic and usually offers no visual evidence. Random biopsies of the cervix are no longer acceptable. If a specific suspicious lesion is seen, biopsy is indicated, because tumor necrosis may lead to a negative PAP smear.

Treatment of CIN I to CIN III is usually an office procedure in patients who wish to retain their childbearing capacity and in whom good visualization of the transformation zone is seen with colposcopy. Excellent results have been obtained with cryocautery and laser ablation. Other patients will require either cold knife or laser conization to be sure all of the transformation can be examined by the pathologist. In patients who are no longer interested in childbearing, hysterectomy is a reasonable consideration (Fray and Sims, 1982).

Once cervical cancer has extended beyond the basement membrane, lymph node metastasis and direct spread throughout the pelvis becomes life-threatening. Surgery, radiation therapy, and chemotherapy have increased the chances for survival, particularly for stage I and II disease.

Other important malignancies of the cervix include adenocarcinoma and sarcoma. Adenocarcinomas account for about 10 per cent of cervical malignancies. Because they arise within the cervix, they may generally be diagnosed somewhat later than squamous cell cancers (DiSaia and Creasman, 1989).

UTERUS

The most common benign lesion in the uterus is the leiomyoma, especially in women in the third to the fifth decade. These are classified as subserosal, intramural, or submucosal, depending on their location in the uterus. They may occur singly or in large numbers in any given patient. They are also found occasionally in the broad ligament and at more distant sites in the abdomen. They are apparently estrogen dependent, since pregnancy and high-dose estrogen oral contraceptives stimulate growth, whereas menopause brings on the cessation of growth and regression in size.

Subserosal and intramural leiomyomas are often asymptomatic and usually require only observation. Surgical treatment should be reserved for those leiomyomas that are causing symptoms such as abnormal uterine bleeding, abdominal pain, reproductive loss, and dysmenorrhea. Surgery is also advised if the uterus is more than 12 to 14 weeks in size, if there is unexplained rapid growth, or if there is uncertainty as to whether the tumor might be ovarian in origin. Leiomyomata rarely undergo sarcomatous changes.

Endometrial polyps and simple hyperplasia (cystic hyperplasia) are benign lesions that may be incidental findings at dilatation and curettage or hysterectomy. Endometrial polyps can cause abnormal uterine bleeding and occasionally can cause uterine cramping by blocking the cervix. Simple or cystic hyperplasia is a misnomer that refers to the cystic changes that can occur in the inactive endometrium of postmenopausal patients. There is no premalignant potential.

Adenomatous hyperplasia, atypical adenomatous hyperplasia, and endometrial carcinoma are steps in a progression along the same continuum most often associated with those conditions that are associated with unopposed estrogen stimulation. These include polycystic ovarian syndrome, granulosa cell tumors, ovarian thecomas, and adrenocortical hyperplasia. They are also observed with unopposed exogenous estrogen administration. These patients will complain of irregular bleeding interspersed with long periods of amenorrhea. Postmenopausal bleeding is seen in the older patient.

Hyperplasia and endometrial carcinoma are diagnosed by endometrial sampling, dilatation and curettage, or both. Treatment of hyperplasia depends on the age of the patient and the patient's desire for childbearing. Medroxyprogesterone, oral contraceptives, and ovulation induction are all beneficial treatments. Surgery and radiation are used for the treatment of endometrial carcinomas and are highly successful in the early stages.

FALLOPIAN TUBE

Diagnosis of a fallopian tube mass usually occurs in the course of surgery for another reason. Paraovarian and paratubular cysts are usually small embryonic remnants that are interesting to observe. Occasionally, paraovarian cysts become large and require surgery. Preoperative diagnosis is most often an "ovarian mass." Carcinoma of the fallopian tube is very rare and usually is suspected to be an adnexal mass or ovarian cancer prior to surgery.

OVARY

The pelvic examination is helpful in distinguishing between benign and neoplastic masses in the adnexa (Table 43–4). The finding of a smooth, cystic, unilateral, mobile mass that is less than 8 cm. in diameter in a woman of reproductive age should lead one to think of a functional cyst and benign disease. These women can usually be observed for 4 to 6 weeks (one menstrual cycle) or given oral contraceptives to aid resolution of the cyst. Cysts that have not regressed during this time should be surgically investigated by laparoscopy or laparotomy (see Table 43–3) (DiSaia and Creasman, 1989).

Solid, irregular, bilateral, and fixed masses are suggestive of malignancy. Also, any mass found in a premenarchal or postmenopausal patient should be investigated surgically. An ultrasound study may provide additional information but should never replace the pelvic examination.

Serous cystadenomas, which are the most common benign neoplasms of the ovary in the patient of reproductive age, are epithelial in origin. Mucinous cystadenomas are less common but can become much larger and on occasion are bilateral. Both have malignant counterparts that result in good survival rates when the patient is promptly treated with surgery and chemotherapy.

Benign cystic teratomas are generally found in patients in the third decade. They may contain any variety of epithelial elements such as hair, teeth, or neurologic tissue. They are rarely bilateral and rarely undergo malignant change.

Ovarian malignancy is often called the "silent disease" because it does not become symptomatic until metastasis to other organs makes it evident. Gastrointestinal complaints often precede the diagnosis and should not be ignored, especially if the patient is between 40 and 70 years of age. A variety of germ cell and stromal malignancies, some of which have hormonal effects, are also found in the ovary.

Dermatologic Conditions

Common vulvar dermatoses are somewhat modified because the lax tissues of the vulva encourage edema

Table 43–4. BENIGN OVARIAN TUMORS

- I. Non-neoplastic tumors
  - A. Germinal inclusion cyst
  - B. Follicle cyst
  - C. Corpus luteum cyst
  - D. Pregnancy luteoma
  - E. Theca lutein cysts
  - F. Sclerocystic ovaries
- II. Neoplastic tumors derived from coelomic epithelium
  - A. Cystic tumors
    - 1. Serous cystoma
    - 2. Endometrioma
    - 3. Mucinous cystoma
    - 4. Mixed forms
  - B. Tumors with stromal overgrowth
    - 1. Fibroma, adenofibroma
    - 2. Brenner's tumor
- III. Tumors derived from germ cells
  - A. Dermoid (benign cystic teratoma)

rather than vesiculation. Lichenification is also common. Contact dermatitis is frequently seen, both because of skin susceptibility and irritation from cleansing, medications, and hygiene products. Impetigo, psoriasis, eczema, and other dermatologic conditions can occur in the vulvar area (Ive and Wilkinson, 1986).

ATROPHIC VAGINITIS

Atrophic vaginitis occurs as part of normal menopause and diminished estrogen supply. The vaginal epithelium becomes thinner and susceptible to inflammation. Symptoms of burning and soreness may occur. The vagina appears dry and pale, and a urethral caruncle, representing prolapsed epithelium, may occur. Treatment is very effective with local estrogen cream or suppositories applied daily or monthly (Rice et al., 1987).

PRURITUS VULVAE

Pruritus vulvae can occur secondary to an underlying disease, such as vaginitis, particularly candidiasis and trichomoniasis, or in an idiopathic primary form. It can also be caused by chemical reactions to cleansers, douches, contraceptive preparations, and perfume spray. Dermatologic abnormalities to consider include lichen sclerosis atrophicus, premalignant leukoplastic vulvae, and lichen planus (Jorizzo, 1983).

Primary pruritus vulvae occurs during the reproductive years or after menopause and often leads to lichen simplex vulvae, with thickening of the skin. The itch-scratch-itch cycle is implicated and a depressive disorder may be associated. Therapy includes hydration, bland creams or ointments, and dilute hydrocortisone.

CONDYLOMA ACUMINATA

Genital condylomata (warts), cauliflower-like exophytic small tumors, are an infectious condition caused by HPV. There are now 42 different types that have been defined, most commonly HPV6 and 11, whereas types 16, 18, and 31 have the greatest potential to generate squamous cell cancer. The flat type of condylomata acuminata is found on the cervix, often only visible with magnification with the colposcope. Subclinical HPV infection accounts for the frequent recurrence of warts (Eskelinen and Mashkilleyson, 1987).

Condylomata acuminata must be treated carefully because they frequently relapse and because of the risk of malignancy. Destruction of the warts is most commonly done with topical podophyllin, using a 20 (5 to 25) per cent solution in ethanol or benzoin, which is applied and then washed off after 4 to 6 hours. The variable success rate is evident in 3 to 4 days, and weekly reapplication is indicated when needed. Other measures, such as surgical removal, electrocautery, cryosurgery, or laser treatment can be used for resistant cases or contraindications, such as pregnancy. Sexual partners should be treated, and both should be followed for 8 months after treatment because HPV is a major health concern (Berman and Berman, 1988; Clark, 1987).

VULVAR DYSTROPHIES

Close inspection of the vulva must be carried out on all women complaining of vulvar symptoms, because 3 to 5 per cent have invasive carcinoma and 4 to 8 per cent have epithelial atypia. These disorders are most common in the postmenopausal age group. Biopsies are very important and are accomplished under local anesthesia through an excision or a dermatologic punch.

Hyperplastic dystrophy without atypia is the end result of the itch-scratch cycle, lichen simplex chronicus (neurodermatitis). Lichen sclerosis lesions are white to pale pink, flat-thickened macules that often coalesce into plaques. They are often symmetrical on any part of the perineum and medial thighs.

Vulvar epithelial hyperplasia with atypia (leukoplakia) is common and mandates biopsy at the onset of therapy and during interval follow-up. Therapy centers around good vulvar hygiene. Hypertrophic dystrophy is treated with corticosteroids. Lichen sclerosis is best treated with topical testosterone proprionate. Lesions with cytologic atypia demand wide local excisions with adequate skin margins (Soper and Creasman, 1986).

MOLLUSCUM CONTAGIOSUM

This is a common benign viral disease in which the skin lesion is a pearl white umbilicated papule, and most patients have multiple lesions of 3 to 6 mm. The incubation period is 14 days to 6 months. Pruritus is the most common symptom, and treatment is optional. Removal of lesions can be done with a sharp curette, liquid nitrogen, or cryotherapy. A typical case lasts for 6 to 9 months. It is associated with swimming, communal bathing, and sexual transmission (Lowy, 1979).

MISCELLANEOUS LESIONS

Sebaceous cysts containing cheesy material with duct blockage are usually relatively asymptomatic. Like other areas of the skin, if the cysts are large or inflamed, they may need excision or incision and drainage.

Mucinous cysts come from the minor vestibular glands and are located on the mucosal surface of the labia minora or by the urethra. They generally require no treatment.

Fibromas arising from fibrous tissue of the vulva are generally small but can become large and pedunculated. Surgical treatment is applied selectively.

Varicoceles and angiomas are also occasionally seen on the vulva. Most of the time no treatment is needed. Lipomas can arise from the subcutaneous fat and occasionally are large enough to warrant surgical excision.

Hidradenitis Suppurativa

This is a chronic suppurative and cicatricial disease of the apocrine gland–bearing skin areas, including the anogenital skin. The etiology is unclear, and individual predisposition is likely. The changes progress from keratinous plugging to dilatation to severe inflammation. Local extension occurs in the densely glandular area. Initial presentation may resemble a singular sebaceous cyst and speed of progression is variable. Staphylococci, streptococci, or *Escherichia coli* can be the causative organism. Systemic antibiotic treatment for 10 to 14 days with penicillin, erythromycin, or a cephalosporin is indicated. Limited local management with intralesional steroids is helpful sometimes, as is surgical treatment in extensive, recurrent cases. Local hygiene with cleansing, moist dressing, or topical antibiotics may be helpful (Hurley, 1979).

Pelvic Pain

In taking the history of a patient with pelvic pain it is important to determine the duration of pain, its character and location, and its relationship to the menstrual cycle. Because several etiologies of pelvic pain are life-threatening, they require prompt diagnosis.

ECTOPIC PREGNANCY

An ectopic pregnancy is any pregnancy that implants outside the mucous membrane lining the uterus. Ninety-eight per cent of ectopic pregnancies are tubal pregnancies (Jones, 1988). These now represent about 1 per cent of all pregnancies. Recent increases in incidence may be due to increases in pelvic inflammatory disease, tubal ligations, and reparative tubal surgery.

Frequent symptoms are abnormal uterine bleeding or amenorrhea, unilateral pelvic pain, and complaints of early pregnancy such as nausea and breast tenderness. An adnexal mass on the pelvic examination is not universally present, and in one study only 35 per cent of patients had such a mass (Easley et al., 1987). Tenderness with cervical motion and abdominal tenderness are more consistent findings. With the development of accurate tests for the measurement of serum human chorionic gonadotropin and ultrasound, it is now possible to diagnose ectopic pregnancy long before potential lethal rupture of the tube occurs. If serum beta human chorionic gonadotropin reaches a level of 6000 mIU./ml. and there is no evidence of an intrauterine pregnancy on ultrasound, laparoscopic investigation should be undertaken. A patient presenting with a ruptured ectopic pregnancy is in acute pain, often is hypotensive, and represents a true surgical emergency.

With early diagnosis and advances in laparoscopy, conservative management of an unruptured ectopic pregnancy is possible. Tubal salvage can be attempted in some cases of ruptured ectopic pregnancy (Easley et al., 1987).

OVARIAN CYST AND OVARIAN TORSION

Ovarian cysts, both functional and neoplastic, can cause pelvic pain of varying degrees, which usually results from hemorrhage into the cyst or necrosis. The size of the cyst is not related to the degree of pain. The severity and persistence of the pain will determine the need for clinical investigation. Unfortunately, malignant ovarian cysts are usually asymptomatic in the early stages. In late stages, pain may result from hemorrhage into the cyst or extension to other tissues.

Torsion can occur with ovarian enlargement from cysts or with pedunculated tumors on the ovary at any age. Patients present with an acute abdomen because of the ischemia and necrosis that develop distal to the point of torsion. Occasionally, torsion can occur in the normal ovary. Torsion of the fallopian tube can be a complication of tubal sterilization (Bernardus, 1984). Patients with these conditions require prompt surgical intervention.

PELVIC INFLAMMATORY DISEASE (PID)

PID is an important cause of pelvic pain and is covered in more detail under the section on infections in this chapter. It should always be considered in the differential diagnosis of pelvic pain, whether acute or chronic.

ENDOMETRIOSIS AND ADENOMYOSIS

Endometriosis, which is the development of ectopic endometrial tissue outside the uterus, has been described since the 1800's. Although endometriosis can be asymptomatic, many patients complain of increasing dysmenorrhea beginning in the third decade. It can occur at any age after menarche and in all socioeconomic groups. Most frequently, it is found throughout the pelvis. Implants on the ovary may give rise to large endometrioma and "chocolate cysts."

Several etiologies of endometriosis seem likely, including retrograde flow of the endometrial tissue through the fallopian tubes into the abdominal cavity and vascular and lymphatic dissemination of endometrial tissue. Endometriosis is asymptomatic in some patients and causes only mild dysmenorrhea in others. Still other women will experience low back pain, pelvic pain 1 to 2 weeks before menses, and severe dyspareunia. Symptoms may arise from involvement of the rectum, urethra, and bladder (Speroff, 1988). Endometriosis is usually not associated with dysfunctional uterine bleeding. As noted below, it can be a significant factor in infertility.

Examination may reveal a fixed uterus, tender nodularity along the uterosacral ligaments, or ovarian enlargement. Treatment may consist of medical suppression of the ovary or conservative surgery or hysterectomy, depending on the extent of the disease and the patient's desire for childbearing.

Adenomyosis or internal endometriosis is the deposition of endometrial tissue in the myometrium, usually seen in the fourth or fifth decade. Adenomyosis is a histologic diagnosis; however, such a diagnosis is suggested by a history of heavy menstrual bleeding or dysmenorrhea. The uterus is diffusely enlarged but is usually not over 12 weeks in size (Entman, 1988).

Nonsteroidal anti-inflammatory drugs may be sufficient for symptomatic relief, especially since menopause brings permanent relief. Otherwise, hysterectomy is the treatment of choice for disabling symptoms.

PELVIC PAIN OF UNKNOWN ETIOLOGY

Pelvic pain without any known pathology may have an underlying psychologic or psychiatric cause. Since the 1970's, laparoscopy has spared many of these women multiple laparotomies. Several studies have demonstrated a relationship of chronic pain with sexual abuse (Gross et al., 1981; Gidros-Frank et al., 1960). In addition, Harrop-Griffiths and associates (1988) showed a significantly greater prevalence of major depression, substance abuse, sexual dysfunction, and somatization. Once pathology has been ruled out as a cause of pelvic pain, one should investigate the etiologic possibilities mentioned earlier and institute counseling or psychotherapy when appropriate.

Infertility

Infertility is defined as 1 year of unprotected coitus without conception (Speroff et al., 1989). Approximately 15 per cent of couples are affected. Primary infertility refers to couples who have never conceived, whereas secondary infertility indicates one or both partners has had at least one conception. Investigation of the infertile couple must be directed equally toward both members, because 40 per cent of infertility is due to male factors and 40 per cent is due to female factors. Male and female factors are jointly responsible in 10 per cent of cases and no cause is ever demonstrated in another 10 per cent.

A careful history of both partners should include ages; marital and reproductive history; past and current medical history, especially chronic disease, pelvic pain, and previous infection history; and information about drug use and abuse and exposure to toxins. A detailed sexual history is essential. The physical examination will help delineate any physical barriers to conception and rule out current infections. The remainder of the investigation should be directed toward several factors:

1. Central or ovulation factor
2. Male factor
3. Mucous or cervical factor
4. Endometrial or uterine factor
5. Tubal factor
6. Peritoneal factors

A biphasic temperature curve of the menstruating female (Fig. 43–12) (Wentz, 1988) and semen analysis of the male should be done in the early stages of this investigation. Over a 3-month period, the temperature should be taken and recorded in the morning before getting out of bed. The semen samples should be collected after at least 48 hours of abstinence from sexual intercourse and transported to the lab within 2 hours of collection.

After reviewing the temperature charts, a midcycle postcoital test can be performed within 2 to 8 hours of intercourse to determine the receptivity of cervical mucus and the ability of the sperm to reach and survive in the mucus. The mucus should demonstrate a spinnbarkeit (stretchability) of 8 to 10 cm. and "ferning" when dried on a slide (Fig. 43–13). Further evidence of ovulation and adequacy of the luteal phase can be obtained by measurement of serum progesterone around day 20 of the cycle and by endometrial sampling for dating 2 to 3 days before the next expected menses.

Endometriosis deserves special mention as a cause of infertility. Its exact role in infertility is not always evident. Some women with very little endometriosis do not conceive, whereas other women with extensive disease have had several children without difficulty. Adhesions with interference of tubal motility are obvious causes of infertility in some patients with endometriosis.

Less extensive disease might still cause significant dyspareunia, which may decrease the frequency of intercourse. Prostaglandins produced by the endometriotic implants may be a factor. Information on mild endometriosis as a cause of infertility remains controversial.

Treatment of infertility may be complex, expen-

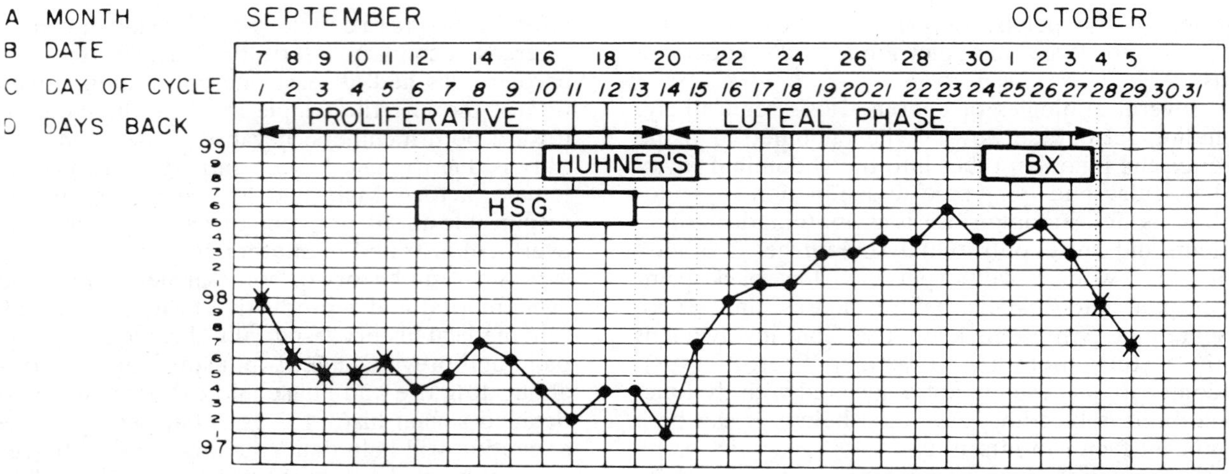

Figure 43–12. Typical ovulatory basal temperature record, showing the appropriate times during the cycle for the performance of tests to evaluate fertility potential. (Reproduced with permission from Jones, H. W., Wentz, A. C., and Burnett, L. S.: Novak's Textbook of Gynecology, Boston, Williams & Wilkins, 1988.)

sive, and time consuming. If the couple is referred to a specialist, the family physician should be prepared to provide continued emotional support.

Pelvic Relaxation

Pelvic relaxation describes a variety of structural abnormalities that are associated with a loss of fascial and ligamentous support. The etiology of this condition includes the trauma of vaginal delivery, prolonged lifting or coughing, and the physiologic process of aging.

The functional effect of pelvic relaxation needs to be assessed in order to determine the appropriate medical or surgical treatment. Symptoms of urinary incontinence or urgency, pelvic pressure, tissue prolapse, and tenesmus are commonly present in advanced stages. Mild degrees of relaxation are asymptomatic.

URETHROCELE AND CYSTOCELE

A urethrocele refers to the posterior anatomic displacement of the urethra into the vagina, which can be demonstrated through the patient's straining to produce increased intra-abdominal pressure. A cystocele refers to the protrusion of the bladder into the vagina, which involves most of the anterior wall. A second-degree cystocele or urethrocele denotes that the sagging reaches the vaginal introitus, whereas a third-degree cystocele or urethrocele extends beyond that.

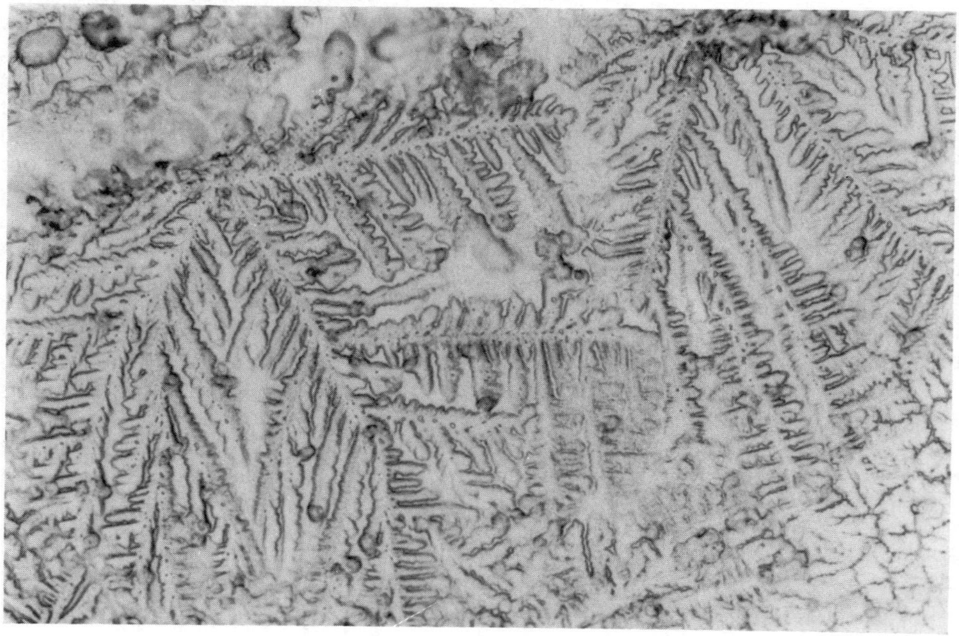

Figure 43–13. Presumptive ovulation determined by cervical mucus changes. Ovulation occurs at the time when fern formation is strongly positive.

UTEROVAGINAL PROLAPSE

Ureterovaginal prolapse refers to the descent of the cervix and uterus into the vaginal canal to various degrees. If the cervix comes to the introitus when straining, the prolapse is called second degree. Third-degree prolapse refers to a more significant extension, and complete prolapse (procidentia) means that the entire vaginal wall is inverted. The degree of symptoms varies with the associated forms of relaxation but symptoms are always present beyond second degree.

ENTEROCELE AND RECTOCELE

An enterocele refers to varying degrees of protrusion of intra-abdominal contents within the posterior vaginal cul-de-sac. A rectocele is related to weakness of the posterior vaginal wall, which becomes thin. The degrees of these conditions determine whether or not symptoms of pressure and difficulty with bowel movements will occur.

URINARY INCONTINENCE

Incontinence of urine is a common and frequently incapacitating condition that particularly affects the elderly. It is a difficult problem that is disruptive enough to often precipitate nursing home admission. Patients are reluctant to report this "embarrassing" problem while still independent. Between 28 and 50 per cent of the elderly in nursing homes are incontinent (Ouslander, 1981).

Types of incontinence include stress, urge, overflow, or total. Stress incontinence is caused by the anatomic disorders of pelvic relaxation and sphincter weakness, which makes the outlet resistance low. Leakage will occur with increases in intra-abdominal pressure. Urge incontinence is caused by bladder detrusor hyperreflexia because of suppression failure in central nervous system disease, such as stroke, or because of infection. The leakage of urine occurs owing to the patient's inability to delay voiding long enough after the urge is perceived. Overflow incontinence occurs with either anatomic obstruction or a hypotonic bladder such as in a spinal cord injury. Leakage of urine occurs because there is no way to empty the bladder when it is full. Total incontinence means there is no control, and it may be caused from severe sphincter damage or dementia (Bent and Ostergard, 1988).

The diagnostic approach requires a thorough history and physical examination, including ruling out systemic disease. In the majority of women, the source of leakage is urethral. It is important to identify the type as outlined earlier. Routine tests should include urine analysis and culture and postvoid residual determination (Walzer, 1988). Sometimes radiographic studies, cystoscopy, and urodynamic tests are indicated (Hadley, 1986). Medical therapy ranges from bladder training exercises to estrogen creams to anticholinergic drugs. Surgical therapy includes numerous vaginal and retropubic procedures, combined with vaginal hysterectomy after childbearing is over.

References

American Cancer Society: Report on cancer-related health checkup. Cancer Society, *30*:1–37, 1980.

Baker, D. A.: Gynecologic infections. *In* Rosenwaks, Z., Benjamin, F., Stone, M. L., et al. (Eds.): Gynecology, Principles and Practice. New York, MacMillan Publishing Company, 1987, pp. 383–384.

Barbo, D. M.: The physiology of the menopause. Med. Clin. North Am. *71*:11–22, 1987.

Bates, B.: A Guide to Physical Examination. Philadelphia, J. B. Lippincott Company, 1983, pp. 277–285. *This textbook is a comprehensive resource for appropriate examination of every system. Its segment on gynecology is basic.*

Benedet, J. L., et al.: Colposcopy, conization, and hysterectomy practices: A current perspective. Obstet. Gynecol., *60*:539–545, 1982.

Bent, A. E., and Ostergard, D. R.: Recurrent stress incontinence. Postgrad. Med., *83*:113–117, 1988.

Berkley, S. F., Hightower, A. W., Broome, C. V., et al.: The relationship of tampon characteristics to menstrual toxic shock syndrome. J.A.M.A., *258*:917–920, 1987.

Berman, A., and Berman, J. E.: New concepts in viral wart infection. Compr. Ther., *14*:19–24, 1988.

Bernardus, R. E., et al.: Torsion of the fallopian tube: Some considerations on its etiology. *64*:675–678, 1984.

Brown, F. H., and Kammeyer, S. E.: Office gynecologic procedures. Primary Care, *13*:493–511, 1986. *This article is a very practical summary of some of the most common office procedures, complete with pictures and descriptions of the techniques used.*

Brunton, S., and Sutherland, J.: Disease prevention and health maintenance. *In* Taylor, R. B. (Ed.): Family Medicine: Principles and Practice. New York, Springer-Verlag, 1988, pp. 81–93.

Carson, L. F., Twiggs, L. P., Okagaki, T., et al.: Human papillomavirus DNA in adenosquamous carcinoma and squamous carcinoma of the vulva. Obstet. Gynecol., *72*:63–67, 1988.

Cartwright, P. S.: Pelvic inflammatory disease. *In* Jones, H. W., Wentz, A. C., Burnett, L. S. et al. (Eds.): Novak's Textbook of Gynecology. Baltimore, MD, Williams & Wilkins, 1988, pp. 507–524.

Clark, D. P.: Condyloma acuminatum. Dermatol. Clin., *5*:779–788, 1987.

Dalton, K.: The Premenstrual Syndrome and Progesterone Therapy. London, William Heinemann Medical Books Ltd., 1984, p. 3. *Good overall discussion of symptomatology associated with premenstrual syndrome. Stresses progesterone as primary treatment.*

Dawood, M. Y.: Nonsteroidal anti-inflammatory drugs and changing attitudes toward dysmenorrhea. Am. J. Med., *84*:23–29, 1988.

DiSaia, P. J., and Creasman, W. T.: Clinical Gynecologic Oncology. St. Louis, MO, The C. V. Mosby Company, 1989, pp. 1–48, 67–132, 303.

Downey, G. O., Okagaki, T., Ostrow, R. S. et al.: Condylomatous carcinoma of the vulva with special reference to human papillomavirus DNA. Obstet. Gynecol., *72*:68–73, 1988.

Driscoll, C. E., Garner, E. G., and House, J. D.: The effect of taking a sexual history on the notation of sexually related diagnoses. Fam. Med., *18*:293–295, 1986. *This is a very relevant specific small study that sheds light on sexual history taking.*

Easley, H. A., Olive, D. L., and Holman, J. F.: Contemporary evaluation of suspected ectopic pregnancy. J. Reprod. Med., *32*:901–906, 1987. *One hundred and nineteen patients with suspected ectopic pregnancy were evaluated. Ectopic and nonectopic patients could present with the same signs and symptoms. A combination of culdocentesis and quantitative human chorionic gonadotropin maximized discriminative capacity.*

Enos, W. F., Conrath, T. B., and Byer, J. C.: Forensic evaluation of the sexually abused child. Pediatrics, *78*:385–398, 1986.

Entman, S. S.: Uterine leiomyoma and adenomyosis. *In* Jones, H. W., Wentz, A. C., Burnett, L. S., et al.: Novak's Textbook of Gynecology. Baltimore, MD, Williams & Wilkins, 1988, pp. 450–453.

Eskelinen, A., and Mashkilleyson, N.: Optimum treatment of genital warts. Drugs, *34*:599–603, 1987. *This review article sheds relevant light on the very important and evolving focus on therapy for this common condition.*

Franz, W. B.: Endocrinology of the normal menstrual cycle. Primary Care, *15*:607–616, 1988.

Fray, R. E., and Sims, C. D.: Cryosurgical treatment of cervical intraepithelial neoplasia. SA Med. J., *62*:469–470, 1982.

Gidros-Frank, L., et al.: Pelvic pain and female identity. Am. J. Obstet. Gynecol., *79*:1184, 1960.

Glenney, K. F., et al.: The prevalence of positive test results for *Chlamydia trachomatis* by direct smear for fluorescent antibodies in a south Texas family planning population. J. Reprod. Med., *33*:457–462, 1988. *Ten and one half per cent of a largely asymptomatic population were found to have chlamydial infection, which was determined by using the MicroTrak collection kit. Several variables were associated with positive results, including age, marital status, and positive gonorrhea tests.*

Goode, R. L., Degraw, J. R., and Hildebrand, W. L.: Abnormal pap smear: Colposcopy and cryosurgery. Am. Fam. Physician, *34*:99–105, 1986.

Greenman, R. L., and Immerman, R. P.: Toxic shock syndrome. What have we learned? Postgrad. Med., *81*:147–148, 153–154, 157–160, 1987.

Gross, R., Doerr, H., Caldirola, D., et al.: Borderline syndrome and incest in chronic pelvic pain patients. Int. J. Psychiatry. Med., *10*:79, 1980.

Hadley, E. C.: Bladder training and related therapies for urinary incontinence in older people. J.A.M.A., *256*:372–379, 1986.

Harrop-Griffiths, J., Katon, W., Walker, E., et al.: The association between chronic pelvic pain, psychiatric diagnoses, and childhood sexual abuse. Obstet. Gynecol., *71*:589–593, 1988. *Psychologic testing was performed on 25 women undergoing laparoscopy for chronic pelvic pain and on 30 women undergoing laparoscopy for tubal sterilization or infertility investigation. A significant number of psychologic disorders was found in the patients with chronic pelvic pain even though there was no difference in the quality or quantity of pathology present.*

Havelock, C. M.: The cervical smear test. Practitioner, *231*:74–80, 1982.

Hurley, H. J.: Apocrine gland. *In* Fitzpatrick T. B., Eisen, A. Z., Wolff, K., et al. (Eds.): Dermatology in General Medicine, New York, McGraw-Hill Book Company, 1979, pp. 1625–1628.

Ive, F. A., and Wilkinson, D. S.: Diseases of the Umbilical, Perineal, and Genital Regions. *In* Rook, A., et al. (Eds.): Textbook of Dermatology. Boston, MA, Blackwell Scientific Publications, 1986, pp. 2201–2228.

Jones, H. W., Wentz, A. C., and Burnett, L. S.: Novak's Textbook of Gynecology. Baltimore, MD, Williams & Wilkins, 1988, pp. 570–596, 643–675. *This standard gynecologic text is in its 11th edition. Its quality and comprehensiveness is outstanding, and its illustrations are very realistic. It is a necessity for a reference library in family practice.*

Jorizzo, J. L.: The itchy patient: A practical approach. Symposium on Office Dermatology, Primary Care *10*:339–353, 1983.

Koss, L. G., Schrieber, K., Moussouris, H., et al.: Endometrial carcinoma and its precursors: Detection and screening. Clin. Obstet. Gynecol., *25*:49–61, 1982.

Kresch, A. J., et al.: Laparoscopy in 100 women with chronic pelvic pain. Obstet. Gynecol., *64*:672–674, 1984. *Laparoscopic findings in 100 women with chronic pelvic pain in the same location were compared to findings in 50 women undergoing laparoscopy for tubal sterilization. Eighty-three per cent of the women with chronic pelvic pain had a pathologic condition as compared with 29 per cent of asymptomatic women.*

Ladson, S., Johnson, C. F., and Doty, R. E.: Do physicians recognize sexual abuse? A J. Dis. Child., *141*:411–415, 1987.

Lossick, J. G., Muller, M., Gorrell, T. E., et al.: In vitro drug susceptibility and doses of metronidazole required for cure in cases of refractory vaginal trichomoniasis. J. Infect. Dis., *153*:148–155, 1986.

Lowy, D. R.: Milker's nodules; molluscum contagiosum. *In* Fitzpatrick, T. B., Eisen, A. Z., Wolff, K., et al., Dermatology in General Medicine. New York, McGraw-Hill Book Company, 1979, pp. 1625–1628.

Mertz, G. J., Jones, C. C., Mills, J., et al.: Long-term acyclovir suppression of frequently recurring genital herpes simplex virus infection. J.A.M.A., *260*:201–206, 1988. *This is the first study to demonstrate the safety and efficacy of suppressive acyclovir therapy for more than 4 to 6 months. Acyclovir was compared with a placebo, and therapy was continued for 1 year.*

Ouslander, J. G.: Urinary incontinence in the elderly. West. J. Med., *135*(6):482–491, 1981. *This reference succinctly and comprehensively outlines the scope, complexity, and organized approach to this common problem.*

Oyer, R., and Hanjani, P.: Endocervical currettage: Does it contribute to the management of patients with abnormal cervical cytology? Gynecol. Oncol., *25*:204–211, 1986.

Podratz, K.: Carcinoma of vulva: Analysis of treatment failures. Am. J. Obstet. Gynecol., *143*:340–351, 1982.

Recommended treatment for syphilis. M.M.W.R., *345*:945, 1985.

Rice, P. A., Vayo, H. E., and Libman, H.: Sexually transmitted disease. *In* Noble, J. (Ed.): Textbook of General Medicine and Primary Care. Boston, Massachusetts, Little, Brown & Co., Inc., 1987, pp. 1723–1755.

Robboy, S. J., Noller, K. L., O'Brien, P., et al.: Increased incidence of cervical and vaginal dysplasia in 3,980 diethylstilbestrol-exposed young women. J.A.M.A., *252*:2979–2993, 1984.

Rodney, W. M., Felman, E., Morrison, T., et al.: Colposcopy and cervical cryotherapy. Postgrad. Med., *81*:79–86, 1987.

Rosenwaks, Z., Benjamin, F., and Stone, M. L.: Gynecology, Principles and Practice. New York, Macmillan Publishing Company, 1987.

Schneider, A., de Villiers, E., and Schneider, V.: Multifocal squamous neoplasia of the female genital tract: Significance of human papillomavirus infection of the vagina after hysterectomy. Obstet. Gynecol., *70*:294–298, 1987. *Six hundred and sixteen women who had had hysterectomy for cervical neoplasia, noncervical anogenital neoplasia, or benign disease were examined for the presence of human papillomavirus DNA. A history of cervical neoplasia and the presence of vaginal intraepithelial neoplasia was associated with human papillomavirus infection types 16 and 18.*

Siegel, A. L., and Raz, S.: Female urinary incontinence. Postgrad. Med., *83*:97–110, 1988.

Simmons, P. S.: Office pediatric gynecology. Prim. Care, *15*:617–628, 1988.

Simmons, P. S.: Common gynecologic problems in adolescents. Prim. Care, *15*:629–642, 1988. *This is part of a special issue of this journal that presents a broad range of topics relevant to this chapter in office gynecology. It treats this subject, which is often undervalued, comprehensively.*

Smith, M. A., and Yongkin, E. Q.: Managing the premenstrual syndrome. Clin. Pharm., *5*:788–797, 1986.

Soper, J. T., and Creasman, W. T.: Vulvar dystrophies. Clin. Obstet. Gynecol., *29*:431–439, 1986.

Spencer, M. R., and Adler, J.: Vaginitis and vaginal discharge in gynecology. *In* Rosenwaks, Z., Benjamin, F., Stone, M., et al. (Eds.): Gynecology, Principles and Practice. New York, Macmillan Publishing Company, 1987, pp. 579–585.

Speroff, L., Glass, R. H., and Kase, N. G.: Clinical Gynecologic Endocrinology and Infertility. Baltimore, MD, Williams & Wilkins, 1989, pp. 91–119, 513–563. *Reference text that is considered "must" reading for those who want a good basic understanding of the subjects discussed.*

Sutherland, J. E.: Vaginitis: Diagnostic specificity is important. The Female Patient, *9*:103–110, 1984.

Sweet, R. L.: Pelvic inflammatory disease. Sex. Transm. Dis.,

13:192–198, 1986. *Excellent review article on diagnosis and treatment of pelvic inflammatory disease. The clinician is reminded to provide coverage for* Chlamydia trachomatis, *gonorrhea, and anaerobes.*

Takizawa, K., and Mattison, D. R.: Female reproduction. Am. J. Ind. Med., *4*:17–30, 1983.

Townsend, D. E., and Marks, E. J.: Cryosurgery and the CO_2 laser. Cancer, *48*:632–637, 1981.

Walzer, Y.: Female urinary incontinence. Postgrad. Med., *83*:78–88, 1988.

Watts, K. C., Campion, M. J., Butler, E. B., et al.: Quantitative deoxyribonucleic acid analysis of patients with mild cervical atypia: A potentially malignant lesion? Obstet. Gynecol., *70*:205–207, 1987.

Wentz, A. C.: Dysmenorrhea, premenstrual syndrome, and related disorders. *In* Jones, H. W., Wentz, A. C., Burnett, L. S., et al. (Eds.): Novak's Textbook of Gynecology, Boston, MA, Williams & Wilkins, 1988, pp. 240–262.

Wentz, A. C.: Infertility. *In* Jones, H. W., Wentz, A. C., Burnett, L. S., et al. (Eds.): Novak's Textbook of Gynecology. Boston, MA, Williams & Wilkins, 1988, pp. 263–302.

Witkin, S. S.: Immunology of recurrent vaginitis. Am. J. Reprod. Immunol. Microbiol., *15*:34–37, 1987. *Inhibition of cell-mediated immunity to* Candida albicans *appears to be due to increased production by the patients' macrophages of prostaglandin E_2, which blocks lymphocyte proliferation by inhibiting interleukin-2 production.*

Wynn, R. M.: Obstetrics and Gynecology: The Clinical Core. Philadelphia, Lea & Febiger, 1988, pp. 192–193.

44

Contraception

Janet P. Realini
John H. Leversee

Control of reproductive capacity is extremely important to individuals and families. With available contraceptives, men and women can choose whether they will or will not have children and when and how many. They can choose childbearing at a time and under circumstances that are optimal for their physical, emotional, social, and economic well-being. Family physicians are in a unique position to help their patients in this important area with education and counseling about the available methods of contraception.

Current contraceptive technology offers a variety of safe and effective methods from which to choose. No method is perfect; each has its risks, benefits, advantages, and disadvantages. The effectiveness of contraceptive methods is a primary concern of patients and may be described in several ways. Two measures of effectiveness are listed in Table 44–1. Since use of a contraceptive method is an elective therapy and since the choice of the contraceptive method is a very personal and individual one, the family physician's task is to help patients make an informed choice of a suitable method.

Obviously, the technology available often exceeds the application and actual use of contraceptive methods. Over half of the pregnancies in the United States are unplanned. Teenagers account for over a million unintended pregnancies each year. Family physicians have an opportunity and an obligation to educate their patients, regardless of age, about decision-making regarding sexual activity and contraception. Further, a family physician can be a leader in the community in these matters.

The frightening specter of acquired immune deficiency syndrome (AIDS) is changing sexual mores and practices throughout the United States. To avoid transmission of human immunodeficiency virus, more couples are using condoms or maintaining mutually monogamous relationships, or both. More persons are practicing abstinence until establishing a lasting relationship, and women are more often buying con-

Table 44–1. EFFECTIVENESS OF CONTRACEPTIVE METHODS*

	Failure Rate (%)†	
Method	***Lowest Expected***	***Typical***
Chance	89	89
Spermicides	3	21
Periodic abstinence	2–10‡	20
Withdrawal	4	18
Cap (with spermicide)	5	18
Sponge	5 nulliparous >8 parous	18 nulliparous >28 parous
Diaphragm (with spermicide)	3	18
Condom (without spermicide)	2	12
Intrauterine device		6§
Progesterone-T	2.0	
Copper T 380A	0.8	
Oral contraceptives		3
Combined	0.1	
Progestin only	0.5	
Depot medroxyprogesterone acetate	0.3	0.3
Implants (rods)	0.2	0.2
Female sterilization	0.2	0.4
Male sterilization	0.1	0.15

*Adapted from Trussell, J., and Kost, K.: Stud. Fam. Plann., 18:237–283, 1987.

†Percent of couples experiencing an accidental pregnancy during the first year of use.

‡Rate varies with type of method used.

§Reflects experience in the United States with devices used in the late 1970's. Typical failure rates for currently marketed devices are not yet available.

doms in order to have them available. For the foreseeable future, contraception and AIDS protection will be clearly interrelated.

Oral Contraceptives

Oral contraceptives (OCs) are the most popular form of reversible contraception in the United States. It is estimated that about 10 million American women are currently taking OCs and that over 150 million women worldwide have taken OCs in the nearly 30 years since they have been available.

OCs have been studied more extensively and more has been written about them than any other medication in history. Unfortunately, OCs are misunderstood by the general public. A 1985 Gallup poll revealed that three fourths of women felt that OC use involves substantial risks. Nearly one third of women incorrectly thought that OCs caused cancer, and over two thirds incorrectly stated that the risk of dying from taking OCs was equal to or greater than dying from childbearing. It is thus important that family physicians offer their patients a balanced view of the benefits—as well as the risks—of OCs.

EFFECTIVENESS

The popularity of the pill may be attributed in part to its high effectiveness (see Table 44–1). Theoretically, OCs have a pregnancy rate that is close to zero. However, the effectiveness of OCs in actual use is less than perfect and depends a great deal on patient motivation and ability to remember to take the pill.

Oral contraceptives prevent pregnancy primarily by inhibiting ovulation through a negative feedback mechanism on the hypothalamus or anterior pituitary, or both. The midcycle gonadotropin surge is inhibited, and ovulation does not occur. Additional contraceptive mechanisms probably include alterations of cervical mucus, endometrial metabolism, and fallopian tube motility.

PRODUCTS AVAILABLE

There are many products commercially available (Table 44–2). Several pills contain only a small dose of progestin; these "mini-pills" will be discussed separately later. Each of the rest of the preparations contains both an estrogen and progestin. These combined OC preparations are grouped in the table according to the dosage of estrogen in the pill.

Since the introduction of OCs in the early 1960's, the dosages of estrogen and progestin have been gradually reduced. In 1988, OCs with estrogen doses over 50 μg. were withdrawn from the market.

The two estrogens that have been used in OCs, ethinyl estradiol and mestranol, are synthetic estrogens that are well absorbed orally. For all practical purposes, they are considered to be roughly equipotent. Ethinyl estradiol is the only estrogen used in low-dose OCs.

All the progestins used in OCs are chemically derived from nortestosterone. The relative potencies of these progestins are difficult to ascertain because different assays yield different results. In general, however, norgestrel is considered to be the most potent of the compounds: smaller milligram amounts are equivalent to larger amounts of the other progestins. (It should be noted that levonorgestrel is the active compound. Norgestrel is DL-norgestrel, a 50/50 mixture of the dextro- and levo-isomers.) The three other progestins, norethindrone, norethindrone acetate, and ethynodiol diacetate, are probably roughly equipotent.

Predicting the estrogenicity and progestogenicity of OC products is difficult. Many variables are involved, including the types and dosages of the progestins and estrogens; the estrogenic, antiestrogenic, and androgenic effects of the progestins; and the variability of the individuals taking the medication. Moreover, the relative estrogenicity and progestogenicity of various OC combinations have never been adequately studied in humans.

INSTRUCTIONS FOR USE

Several different methods of starting the first pack of OCs have been recommended. Traditionally, the patient takes the first pill either on day 5 of her menstrual cycle (day 1 is the day her period starts) or on the first Sunday after her period starts.

However, in many parts of the world, patients are instructed to begin their first pill on day 1 of the cycle; this technique is felt to reduce the incidence of ovulation and accidental pregnancy during the first cycle. If the first pill of the first cycle is taken later than day 5, a backup method of contraception should be used for at least 10 days.

Combined OCs are taken daily for 21 days, followed by a seven-day hiatus, during which withdrawal bleeding of the endometrium occurs. The number of pills that can be missed in one cycle without risking pregnancy is unknown. Patients are usually advised to take the forgotten pill as soon as it is remembered, without postponing the next pill. Two or more missed pills are "made up" by taking two pills a day. Most practitioners advise a backup method of contraception if two or more pills are missed in one cycle. There is no evidence of a need to periodically temporarily discontinue OCs. The risks associated with OC use do not appear to be related to the length of time a woman is on the pill.

RISKS AND SIDE EFFECTS

The adverse effects associated with OCs have received a great deal of attention in both the medical

Table 44–2. ORAL CONTRACEPTIVES: PREPARATIONS AVAILABLE

Brand Name	Estrogen (μg)	Progestin (mg)
High-Dose (Withdrawn 1988)		
Enovid 5 mg	Mestranol 75	Norethynodrel 5
Enovid 10 mg.	Mestranol 75	Norethynodrel 9.85
Enovid-E	Mestranol 100	Norethynodrel 2.5
Ovulen	Mestranol 100	Ethynodiol diacetate 1
Ortho-Novum 2 mg., Norinyl 2 mg.	Mestranol 100	Norethindrone 2
Ortho-Novum 1/80, Norinyl 1 + 80	Mestranol 80	Norethindrone 1
50 μg. Pills		
Ortho-Novum 1/50, Norinyl 1 + 50, Norethin 1/50, Nelova 1/50, Genora 1/50	Mestranol 50	Norethindrone 1
Demulen 1/50	Ethinyl estradiol 50	Ethynodiol diacetate 1
Norlestrin 1/50	Ethinyl estradiol 50	Norethindrone acetate 1
Norlestrin 2.5/50	Ethinyl estradiol 50	Norethindrone acetate 2.5
Ovcon-50	Ethinyl estradiol 50	Norethindrone 1
Ovral	Ethinyl estradiol 50	Norgestrel 0.5
Low-Dose Monophasics:		
Demulen 1/35	Ethinyl estradiol 35	Ethynodiol diacetate 1
Ortho-Novum 1/35, Norinyl 1 + 35, Norethin 1/35, Nelova 1/35, Genora 1/35	Ethinyl estradiol 35	Norethindrone 1
Modicon, Brevicon, Genora 0.5/35, Nelova 0.5/35	Ethinyl estradiol 35	Norethindrone 0.5
Ovcon-35	Ethinyl estradiol 35	Norethindrone 0.4
Lo-Ovral	Ethinyl estradiol 30	Norgestrel 0.3
Nordette, Levlen	Ethinyl estradiol 30	Levonorgestrel 0.15
Loestrin 1.5/30	Ethinyl estradiol 30	Norethindrone acetate 1.5
Loestrin 1/20	Ethinyl estradiol 20	Norethindrone acetate 1
Low-Dose Multiphasics:		
Ortho-Novum 10/11	Ethinyl estradiol 35	Norethindrone 0.5 × 10 days
	Ethinyl estradiol 35	Norethindrone 1.0 × 11 days
Ortho-Novum 7/7/7	Ethinyl estradiol 35	Norethindrone 0.5 × 7 days
		Norethindrone 0.75 × 7 days
		Norethindrone 1.0 × 7 days
Tri-Norinyl	Ethinyl estradiol 35	Norethindrone 0.5 × 7 days
		Norethindrone 1.0 × 9 days
		Norethindrone 0.5 × 5 days
Triphasil, Tri-Levlen	Ethinyl estradiol 30	Levonorgestrel 0.05 × 6 days
	Ethinyl estradiol 40	Levonorgestrel 0.075 × 5 days
	Ethinyl estradiol 30	Levonorgestrel 0.125 × 10 days
Mini-Pills:		
Micronor	None	Norethindrone 0.35
Nor-Q.D.	None	Norethindrone 0.35
Ovrette	None	Norgestrel 0.075

literature and the lay press. Serious complications due to OCs are relatively rare, and large-scale epidemiologic studies are required to demonstrate their associations with oral contraception. Much of the data we have on side effects is based on studies of women taking the older, higher-dose preparations (i.e., 50 μg. or more of estrogen). We may observe the side effects and risks begin to decline in frequency and severity as populations shift to using lower-dose OCs.

Cardiovascular Risks

Several serious and potentially fatal events have been associated with the use of OCs. Venous thromboembolism, i.e., deep vein thrombosis or pulmonary embolism, or both, has been consistently found to be associated with OC use. The relative risk is estimated to be 2 to 11 times that of women who do not use OCs, and the risk may be related to the estrogen dosage of the pill. Both thrombotic and hemorrhagic strokes, including subarachnoid hemorrhage, have been associated with OC use as well. Myocardial infarction has been found to be associated with OC use in a large number of retrospective studies, and the risks seem to be concentrated in older women who smoke and have other coronary risk factors.

Reversible hypertension develops in a few patients who are taking OCs, and the condition may be severe. In addition, small elevations in the mean systolic and diastolic blood pressure levels—to levels within the normal range—have been documented in some populations of women taking OCs, although not in others (Blumenstein, et al., 1980).

The mortality risks associated with OCs are primarily due to the risk of cardiovascular diseases (Fig. 44–1). In the Royal College of General Practitioners (RCGP) Study, these risks appear to be concentrated in women over 35 years of age who smoke (RCGP 1981). The risk of dying from taking OCs for younger women (including smokers) is quite low. The cardiovascular risks associated with OCs are presumably related to other cardiovascular risk factors as well, e.g., levels of cholesterol and blood pressure and the presence of diabetes mellitus. For older nonsmokers, the risks of OCs are comparable to using no contraception, although they appear substantially higher than the risks of using other methods of birth control.

Because of the RCGP findings, being over 40 years of age, even if the woman is a nonsmoker, was considered to be a contraindication to OC use. However, the RCGP study experience was based on women who were not selected for low cardiovascular risk. In addition, these women were taking higher doses of both estrogen and progestin than are currently used. More recent studies (Porter et al., 1985, 1987) have detected no increase in stroke or myocardial infarction in healthy women on OCs. Additionally, increased attention has been paid to the noncontraceptive benefits of OCs in women of all ages. Current recommendations allow for prescribing OCs to women over 40 when they are carefully screened for cardiovascular risk factors.

OCs and Cancer

OCs have not been shown to cause cancer of any kind. In fact, OC use appears to substantially protect against carcinoma of the endometrium and of the ovary. The risks of these tumors are about half those of nonusers of OCs. The reduction in risk is related to the duration of use of OCs and persists for years after OC use is discontinued.

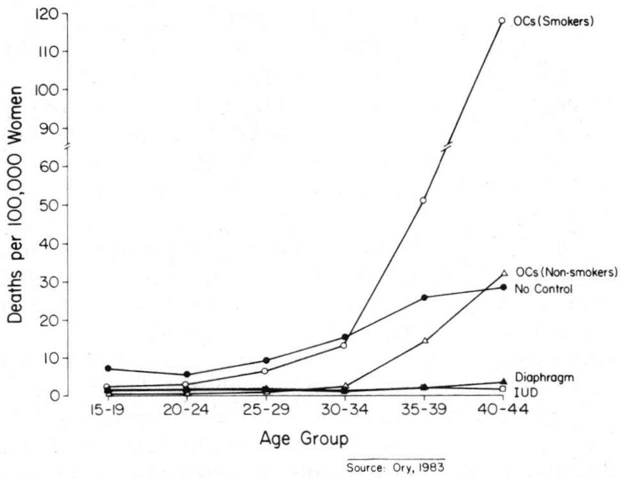

Figure 44–1. Computer projection of mortality risks associated with various methods of fertility control (after Ory, 1983). Rates of death include both method-related and birth-related deaths.

Concern that breast cancer might be caused by exogenous hormones has led to many studies and intense surveillance. Most of the studies have found no change in the risk of breast cancer with OC use. Some studies have suggested increased risks of breast cancer in some subgroups of younger women, but each tends to find elevated risks in a different subgroup. These inconsistent data are of uncertain significance (Wharton and Blackburn, 1988). Further epidemiologic studies of breast cancer and OC use are continuing.

Cancer of the cervix is particularly difficult to study from an epidemiologic standpoint, and its relationship to OC use is not clear. Several studies suggest an increased risk of cervical dysplasia or cervical carcinoma, whereas many do not. Performance of Papanicolaou smears at least yearly is recommended for women on OCs so that cervical dysplasia may be detected and treated early.

Since melanocytes in the skin respond to female sex hormones, the question of whether OC use might predispose a woman to malignant melanoma is an important one. An increase in risk was suggested by the Walnut Creek Study (Ramcharan, et al., 1981), but other studies have not confirmed this finding.

Rarely, benign hepatic tumors (hepatocellular adenomas) occur in association with long-term OC use. These tumors may present with hypovolemic shock due to rupture and intra-abdominal hemorrhage. Recent case-control studies from the United Kingdom suggest that the even rarer hepatocellular carcinoma may be associated with long-term OC use. These tumors are so rare that they are not considered a significant risk. Moreover, further study is needed before such an association is substantiated.

Metabolic Effects

There is concern that OC use may accelerate atherogenesis by affecting blood lipid concentrations. In general, estrogens tend to increase high-density lipoprotein (HDL) cholesterol, which is inversely related to coronary risk, and to reduce low-density lipoprotein (LDL) cholesterol, which has a direct relationship to coronary risk. The progestins used in OCs tend to lower HDL and increase LDL cholesterol. The effects of the various combinations of estrogens and progestins in OCs on these and other complex components of plasma lipids are under study. There are not yet randomized controlled trials that adequately compare various preparations of OCs. Available evidence suggests that minimizing the total progestin dose, as accomplished in low-dose multiphasic OCs, minimizes adverse effects on serum lipids. However, the clinical importance of lipid changes associated with various OC formulations has not been demonstrated.

Oral contraceptive use does not cause diabetes mellitus per se, although it may uncover diabetes in susceptible women. Even when fasting glucose levels are normal, however, use of many types of OCs is associated with glucose intolerance and relative insulin resistance. These effects appear to be due to the progestin component of the pill. However, studies of lower-dose OCs, including triphasic preparations and Ovcon-35R, demonstrate no abnormalities in glucose metabolism.

Minor Side Effects

Low-dose combination OCs are generally well tolerated, and side effects associated with their use are few. However, because so many women take OCs, physicians encounter patients with bothersome, but not serious, side effects. Nausea, breakthrough bleeding, and amenorrhea (i.e., failure to experience withdrawal bleeding) are relatively common. If these symptoms occur in the first three cycles of use, reassurance is usually all that is needed. No changes need to be made, since these symptoms usually subside spontaneously while the patient continues the initial regimen. When bothersome symptoms persist after the first 3 months, the following suggestions for management may be helpful (Hatcher et al., 1988; Speroff et al., 1983).

If *breakthrough bleeding* occurs just before the end of the cycle, the patient may stop her pills, wait 7 days, and then restart the next pill cycle. If bleeding or spotting begins after many months on the pill, the patient should be examined for chlamydial infection and treated, if appropriate.

If bleeding persists, some changes may be advisable. Breakthrough bleeding that occurs during the first half of the cycle may result from a relative estrogen deficiency. Usually it is not necessary to switch to a higher-estrogen formulation. Small daily doses of supplemental estrogen (e.g., conjugated estrogen, 0.625 mg., or ethinyl estradiol, 0.02 mg., each day, taken 12 hours after the OC) for one cycle often allows the patient to remain on the low-estrogen dose pill. Taking two or three of the patient's OCs each day is not helpful in controlling this type of bleeding, because the estrogen-progestin balance is not altered by doubling up on pill dosage.

Spotting in the second half of the cycle is said to be due to a relative progestin deficiency. This can be corrected by changing to a low-dose pill containing a relatively strong progestin (e.g., Nordette, Lo/Ovral, or Triphasil).

If *amenorrhea*, or lack of withdrawal bleeding, occurs, pregnancy must be excluded. The amenorrhea may result from a relative lack of either estrogen or progestin. It is usually advisable first to try increasing the progestin component by switching to a formulation with a relatively strong progestin, such as norgestrel or levonorgestrel. Changing to a pill with 50 μg. of estrogen for several cycles may also be effective.

If excessive *nausea* persists after several cycles, the patient may try taking her pill with food or at bedtime so that the nausea occurs during sleep. Nausea is generally attributed to the estrogen component of the pill and may be minimized by prescribing OCs with low estrogen content—35 μg. or less. One formulation (Loestrin) contains only 20 μg. of estrogen and may be useful for unusually sensitive women.

Authorities disagree about the effect of OCs on *acne*. Patients with acne are usually advised to avoid pills containing the relatively androgenic progestins norgestrel and levonorgestrel. The other progestins used in OCs, such as norethindrone, are believed to have minimal androgenic activity. Demulen 1/35, containing the progestin ethynodiol diacetate, is often recommended by dermatologists for women with acne.

Water retention symptoms such as breast tenderness, a bloated feeling, weight gain, some types of headache, and symptoms similar to premenstrual tension are often attributed to the estrogen component of the pill. These symptoms may be minimized or eliminated by prescribing an OC with a low estrogen content.

Other Adverse Effects

An increased risk of symptomatic gallstone disease has been noted in young women in the early years of OC use. OC use appears not to affect the overall risk of gallbladder disease, however (RCGP, 1982; Layde et al., 1982). It may be that OC use precipitates the development of symptoms in susceptible women.

Because of experience with high-dose progestins and diethylstilbestrol taken early in pregnancy, there was concern that OCs might cause congenital anomalies. However, careful study has failed to reveal convincing evidence that taking OCs early in pregnancy is teratogenic (Simpson, 1985). Similarly, pregnancies conceived shortly after discontinuing OCs are *not* at increased risk of congenital anomalies.

A short delay in the return of fertility is common after discontinuing birth control pills, but "post-pill amenorrhea" is not considered to be a distinct entity. Women who fail to menstruate within 6 months of discontinuing OCs have diverse underlying problems and should undergo careful evaluation for the cause of the amenorrhea.

Chlamydia trachomatis is more frequently cultured from the cervix of women on OCs than in nonusers. Whether this is a result of increased ability to culture the organism or due to an actual increased risk of chlamydial infection is not clear. The risk of clinical pelvic infection appears to be reduced by OC use.

Drug interactions may occur in women on OCs (Table 44–3). OC use may affect other drugs taken. Antibiotics and anticonvulsants may reduce OC effectiveness; some cases of accidental pregnancy have been reported. With the exception of rifampin, however, the risk of pregnancy appears to be only mildly elevated. Many physicians recommend use of a

Table 44–3. ORAL CONTRACEPTIVES: DRUG INTERACTIONS

I. Drugs Reported to Cause OC Failure

Antibiotics:
- Rifampin (best documented)
- Penicillins, especially ampicillin
- Tetracyclines
- Griseofulvin
- Others: chloramphenicol, erythromycin, metronidazole, sulfonamides

Anticonvulsants:
- Phenobarbital and other barbiturates
- Phenytoin
- Most others, except valproic acid

Mineral Oil: Theoretically, in large amounts

Any drug or condition that decreases intestinal transit time

II. Drugs Reported to be Affected by Oral Contraceptive Use

Drug	*Effect*
Acetaminophen	Metabolism may be increased
Anticoagulants (warfarin)	May increase or decrease anticoagulant effect
Antipyrine	Decreased metabolism
Benzodiazepines:	
Chlordiazepoxide (Librium), Clonazepam (Klonopin), Clorazepate (Tranxene), Diazepam (Valium), Flurazepam (Dalmane), Halazepam (Paxipam), Midazolam (Versed), Prazepam (Centrax), Triazolam (Halcion)	Decreased metabolism
Lorazepam (Ativan), Oxazepam (Serax), Temazepam (Restoril)	Enhanced metabolism
Corticosteroids	May enhance corticosteroid effects
Metoprolol (Lopressor) (may also apply to propranolol, timolol)	Possible decreased metabolism
Phenytoin	Possible altered metabolism
Salicylates	Possible increased metabolic clearance
Theophyllines	Probable decreased metabolism
Thyroid hormone	Possible increased T4 requirement
Tricyclic antidepressants	Possible increase in oral bioavailability
Troleandomycin	Combination may increase risk of cholestasis

backup method of contraception during short-term antibiotic therapy. Patients on long-term therapy with antibiotics or anticonvulsants should be informed of their slightly higher pregnancy risk with OCs. Some investigators recommend that these patients use other forms of contraception.

NONCONTRACEPTIVE BENEFITS

Table 44–4 lists conditions for which OC use confers protection. Ovarian and endometrial carcinoma are reduced by about half among OC users. Because OCs prevent ovulation, ectopic pregnancy is less likely to occur and primary dysmenorrhea is often relieved.

OC users have a reduced risk of pelvic inflammatory disease when compared to women using no contraception. Ovarian activity is inhibited, and functional ovarian cysts are reduced in frequency. Because women on OCs tend to lose less blood each month, iron deficiency anemia is less common with OC use than among nonusers. Benign breast disease is less common among OC users than among nonusers. Menstrual irregularities are less likely, and some women have relief of premenstrual symptoms on OCs. In addition, some evidence suggests that rheumatoid arthritis and toxic shock syndrome occur less frequently among OC users than among users of other forms of contraception. Ory (1982) estimated that 50,000 hospitalizations are prevented by OC use annually in the United States and that one user in 750 is spared a hospitalization.

CONTRAINDICATIONS

The absolute contraindications to OC use are straightforward and are listed in Table 44–5. The relative contraindications are less uniform in the literature. The use of OCs under these conditions is not recommended, but it may be considered if the indications are strong. The woman with a relative contraindication must be informed of her additional risks and should share in the decision of whether or not to use OCs.

Hypertension, diabetes mellitus, and hyperlipidemias are listed as relative contraindications because they may be worsened by OC use. In addition, these factors, as well as smoking cigarettes, are risk factors for cardiovascular disease and thus may increase the risks of oral contraception. Leiomyomata and varicose veins are no longer considered contraindications.

Active liver disease is a contraindication. Most authors recommend avoiding OCs after acute hepatitis until the liver enzymes have remained normal for several months. Women with a history of cholestasis in pregnancy may experience a recurrence on OCs. Gallbladder disease is listed as a relative contraindication. However, once stones have become

Table 44–4. NONCONTRACEPTIVE BENEFITS: CONDITIONS FOR WHICH OC USE OFFERS PROTECTION

- Ovarian carcinoma
- Endometrial carcinoma
- Ectopic pregnancy
- Pelvic inflammatory disease
- Functional ovarian cysts
- Menstrual irregularities
- Dysmenorrhea
- Iron deficiency anemia
- Benign breast disease
- Premenstrual syndrome

Table 44–5. ORAL CONTRACEPTIVES: CONTRAINDICATIONS

Absolute
Thromboembolism
Cerebrovascular disease
Coronary artery disease
Breast cancer, known or suspected
Estrogen-dependent malignancy, known or suspected (including endometrial carcinoma and melanoma)
Pregnancy, known or suspected
Undiagnosed abnormal genital bleeding
Liver neoplasm, benign or malignant
Relative
Hypertension
Diabetes mellitus
Hyperlipidemia
Chronic liver disease
Cholestatic jaundice of pregnancy
Smokers, especially if over 35 years old
Over 40 years old (now controversial)
Gallbladder disease
Migraine
Other Conditions That May Contraindicate OC Use
Sickle-cell disease, SC disease, or sickle-thalassemia (controversial)
Neurofibromatosis
Hereditary hemorrhagic telangiectasia
Psoriasis
Systemic lupus erythematosus (controversial)
Renal disease
Porphyria
Lactation (controversial)
Seizure disorder
Elective surgery (controversial)
Morbid obesity
History of serious depression
Chloasma
Vasomotor rhinitis
Congenital or rheumatic heart disease
Active inflammatory bowel disease

apparent and are treated, it is not clear that OCs can cause further harm. Age over 40 is felt to be less of a relative contraindication than in the past—assuming the woman has no other cardiovascular risk factors. Migraine headache is felt to be a strong contraindication by some authors and only a relative contraindication by others. Authors agree that headaches that develop or worsen on OCs require prompt discontinuation of the pill.

Although they are not mentioned in most lists of contraindications, a number of other conditions make OCs a less desirable contraceptive choice. Hemoglobinopathies that involve sickling of red blood cells are controversial contraindications. Case reports of pulmonary infarctions inhibit many practitioners from prescribing these drugs for patients with these conditions. However, in many parts of the world, OCs are prescribed for patients with sickling diseases without apparent problems. Sickle trait is not a contraindication to OC use. Patients with neurofibromatosis are known to experience worsening of their symptoms at puberty; therefore, the administration of exogenous steroids may pose a risk. Patients with hereditary hemorrhagic telangiectasia and psoriasis have been reported to have exacerbations with OC use. The relationship of the activity of systemic lupus erythematosus to pregnancy and oral contraceptive use is controversial. Some types of renal disease, especially those that involve hypertension, may contraindicate OC use. Patients with porphyria may have exacerbations of skin lesions or abdominal pain with OC use.

Breast-feeding has generally been considered a contraindication to the use of combined OCs because of the inhibitory effect of estrogens on breast milk formation. However, in many parts of the world, combined OCs are commonly prescribed for women whose supply of milk is well established. A seizure disorder is unlikely to worsen on OCs but is a relative contraindication, because most anticonvulsants speed the metabolic degradation of OC steroids and may render them less effective. Elective surgery is debated as a contraindication to OC use. Some authors recommend stopping OCs 6 weeks prior to surgery; others believe that the risk of pregnancy may be greater than the risk of thromboembolism. Since morbid obesity predisposes a woman to venous thromboembolism, it may be viewed as a contraindication to OC use.

Women with a history of serious depression could have a recurrence or worsening of symptoms on OCs. Women with melasma or chloasma may have worsening of skin lesions with the use of oral contraceptives. Pregnancy and exogenous hormones have been known to cause vasomotor rhinitis. A woman with these symptoms would thus have a mild relative contraindication to OC use. There have been reports of pulmonary hypertension in patients with congenital or rheumatic heart disease who have taken oral contraceptives. Because of a possible association of inflammatory bowel disease with OC use, some authors caution against OC use among women with these disorders.

CHOOSING A PILL

There is a large selection of effective and well-tolerated OC products (see Table 44–2). Most authors recommend beginning with a preparation containing 30 to 35 μg. of estrogen. Lower doses of estrogen (i.e., 20 μg.) are associated with a slightly higher pregnancy rate.

Recent literature suggests that the progestin dose should be minimized as well. The potency of the progestin must be taken into account as well as the milligram amount. The triphasic preparations allow a lower total monthly progestin dose and thus may be less likely to cause adverse changes in lipoproteins. Theoretically, these triphasic OCs may minimize any tendency toward atherosclerosis. Many practitioners now prescribe a triphasic preparation as their first choice. However, the effect of using these preparations on the noncontraceptive benefits of OC use—specifically the protection from endometrial carcinoma—is not known.

MINI-PILLS

Several OCs on the market contain no estrogen, only a small dose of progestin. These mini-pills are not as widely used as combination OCs. Their effectiveness is somewhat lower than that of combination OCs (see Table 44–1). Mini-pills prevent pregnancy by affecting cervical mucus viscosity, fallopian tube mobility, and endometrial suitability for implantation. Ovulation is sometimes inhibited, but much less consistently than with combined OCs.

Mini-pills are taken every day of the month, with no 7-day hiatus. They require excellent patient compliance to maintain their effectiveness; even one missed pill may result in pregnancy.

The side effects of progestin-only pills are primarily problems with menstrual irregularities. As many as two thirds of users experience menstrual irregularities, especially breakthrough bleeding and amenorrhea.

Because of their lower effectiveness, requirement for meticulous compliance, and frequent menstrual irregularities, the use of mini-pills is generally reserved for selected women whose choices of contraceptive methods are limited. They are most commonly used in lactating women. Mini-pills do not inhibit milk production as may combined OCs. Because the progestin enters the breast milk in small quantities, there is a theoretical risk of affecting the nursing infant, but most authorities consider this risk to be insignificant.

The systemic effects of the small doses of progestin in mini-pills are presumed to be less significant than those of combined OCs. The actual risks of mini-pills, however, are largely unknown. Some of the adverse effects of the combined OCs may be progestin-related. The effects of mini-pills, because they are used by much smaller numbers of women, have been studied much less than those of combined oral contraceptives.

Mini-pills prevent ectopic pregnancy less well than they do intrauterine pregnancy. Thus, if a pregnancy occurs while the patient is taking mini-pills, it is more likely to be an ectopic one than if she were using no contraception. Most authorities do not consider mini-pills to *cause* ectopic pregnancies, however.

Long-Acting Hormonal Methods

Injectable long-acting progestins are a popular form of contraception in other countries, but they are not approved for contraceptive use in the United States. Although several different preparations have been used and are being tested, the most popular and well-tested preparation is depot medroxyprogesterone acetate (Depo-Provera), given in a dose of 150 mg. intramuscularly every 3 months. This regimen is as highly effective as combined OCs (see Table 44–1).

Injectable progestins consistently inhibit ovulation. The first injection should be given during the first week of the menstrual cycle for optimal effectiveness.

The side effects associated with injectable progestins include weight gain and menstrual irregularities. Breakthrough bleeding, altered cycle length, and amenorrhea are common; heavy bleeding, however, is rare. The return of fertility after the use of intramuscular progestins is delayed for at least 3 months after the last injection, but there is no evidence that these medications cause permanent infertility. Injectable progestins may be used during lactation. The small amounts of the hormone in breast milk appear to have no adverse effects on nursing infants. Like OCs, long-acting progestins may have noncontraceptive benefits, including prevention of both iron deficiency anemia and pelvic inflammatory disease. Injectable progestins may reduce sickling in sickle cell anemia patients.

No changes in blood pressure or in the coagulation system have been observed in patients taking long-acting injectable progestins. Although extensive epidemiologic studies have not been conducted, these drugs have not been reported to cause thromboembolic or other cardiovascular events. Depo-Provera's effects on lipid metabolism are under study.

The United States Food and Drug Administration's (FDA) controversial decision not to approve Depo-Provera for contraceptive use is based on concerns about cancer risks. High doses of injectable progestins have been associated with increased risks of breast and endometrial cancer in laboratory animals. Epidemiologic studies in women have generally found no association with cancer. In spite of the lack of FDA approval, some physicians use Depo-Provera for contraception in exceptional cases. The American Academy of Pediatrics has acknowledged the usefulness of long-acting injectable progestins in the management of selected mentally retarded adolescents (American Academy of Pediatrics Committee on Drugs, 1980).

Several new and highly effective long-acting hormonal methods of contraception are being developed and tested. Norplant is a system of six capsules inserted under the skin on the inside of a woman's arm. The capsules slowly release norgestrel for 5 years, and then they must be surgically removed. Norplant-2 is a similar 2-rod system that lasts 3 years. In addition, work is proceeding on biodegradable implants of progestins, injectable microspheres and microcapsules, vaginal rings impregnated with progestin, and monthly injections of estrogen and progestin.

Intrauterine Devices

Intrauterine devices (IUDs) are used by millions of women throughout the world. IUDs cause a local inflammatory effect on the endometrium, which has been theorized to interfere with implantation of the fertilized ovum. However, recent evidence suggests that IUDs prevent pregnancy by preventing fertilization of the ovum by spermatozoa.

Several types of medicated and unmedicated IUDs are used around the world. In general, the addition of copper or other medication in the newer IUDs allows improved effectiveness with fewer side effects. In the United States, only two IUDs are commercially available: the TCu-380A (Paragard; GynoPharma) and the progesterone-T (Progestasert; Alza). IUD manufacturers in the United States have withdrawn other IUDs for a number of reasons. The Dalkon Shield was taken off the market during the 1970's owing to infectious complications related to its particular design. The unmedicated devices Saf-T-Coil and Lippes Loop were withdrawn because of declining usage. The Copper-7 and the Tatum-T were withdrawn owing to the cost of defending against liability lawsuits, even though the manufacturer won most of the cases.

The lowest expected pregnancy rates of IUDs are somewhat higher than those of oral contraceptives (see Table 44–1). However, because little patient compliance is required to use the method properly, the typically observed pregnancy rate of IUDs are comparable to those of OCs. In fact, the observed effectiveness of the TCu-380A (Paragard) is superior to that of OCs in many populations (Treiman and Liskin, 1988).

Proper insertion of the IUD with sterile technique high in the uterine fundus is essential to ensure optimal contraceptive function. Insertion has been conventionally performed during the menstrual period, but IUDs can be safely inserted at any time of the menstrual cycle, as long as pregnancy is excluded. Although immediate postpartum IUD insertion is safe, it is recommended that insertion be delayed until 6 to 8 weeks postpartum because of high expulsion rates after earlier insertions.

Although its copper may be effective for several years longer, the Paragard is approved for 4 years of use. It should be removed and another device inserted after this time. The Progestasert must be changed yearly.

There are several problems associated with the use of IUDs. Perforation of the uterus is an uncommon complication. Most perforations occur at the time the IUD is inserted, and some of these perforations are undetected for some time. Medicated IUDs may cause peritoneal inflammation and adhesions and should be removed if they perforate the uterus. Cervical perforations occasionally occur with T- or 7-shaped devices. In addition, an IUD may become embedded in the uterine wall without perforating it.

The risk of pelvic inflammatory disease appears to be increased by using an IUD. The risk of this complication is concentrated in the first few months after insertion and in women at risk of exposure to sexually transmitted diseases. Also, use of one particular type of IUD—the Dalkon Shield—was associated with a high risk of pelvic inflammatory disease. Tubal infertility, a possible complication of pelvic infection, has been associated with IUD use. The risk of infertility is related to having used a Dalkon Shield, and to the number of sexual partners of the woman. Copper devices carry only a slightly increased risk of tubal infertility. Because of the risks of pelvic infection, proper selection of candidates for IUD use is extremely important. Young, nulliparous women and those who are at high risk of sexually transmitted diseases are poor candidates for IUD use. Parous women with long-term, mutually monogamous sexual relationships are relatively good candidates.

Bleeding is the most common problem associated with IUD use. A small amount of bleeding often occurs at the time of IUD insertion. Intermenstrual bleeding due to the inflammation caused by an IUD may occur at any time but must be differentiated from other causes of bleeding. Menstrual blood loss is typically increased with all types of IUDs, except with the Progestasert, which may actually reduce the amount of menstrual blood flow.

Pain and cramping are common with the insertion of an IUD but usually resolve within several days. Dysmenorrhea is a frequent problem with IUDs and sometimes requires removal of the device.

Expulsion seems to be related to IUDs that are too large or too small for the particular patient's endometrial cavity. Expulsion is most common in the first month or two following insertion and may go unnoticed by the patient. In addition to instructing patients to check the string, many practitioners advise a pelvic examination after the first menstrual period with an IUD in place. Some even advise the use of a second form of contraception during the first cycle of IUD use.

If a pregnancy occurs with an IUD in place, it is likely to be complicated. More than half will end in spontaneous abortion, and a few of these may be complicated by maternal sepsis and death. If the string is visible, the IUD should be removed; the risk of miscarriage is less if the device is removed. If a pregnancy has occurred and the IUD string is not visible, sonography or roentgenography is necessary to determine the presence of the IUD. A pregnant woman with an IUD-in-situ that cannot be removed should be counseled about the risk of septic midtrimester abortion. If she declines therapeutic abortion, she should be followed extremely closely. If she carries to term, an increased risk of certain third trimester complications (e.g., chorioamnionitis and premature labor) may be expected. IUDs do not appear to cause congenital anomalies, however.

IUDs do not cause ectopic pregnancy. However, they prevent ectopic pregnancy less well than they do intrauterine pregnancy. Thus, a woman who becomes pregnant with an IUD in place has a greater chance of the pregnancy being ectopic than does a non-IUD user. The Progestasert appears to be associated with a higher rate of ectopic pregnancy than other IUDs.

The contraindications to IUD use are listed in Table 44–6. The possibilities of pregnancy and malignancy are strong contraindications. Any infection of the upper genital tract should be considered a contraindication, as well. Congenital uterine anomalies and submucous myomas may distort the endometrial cavity so that an IUD's effectiveness would be reduced. Cervical stenosis may interfere with the insertion of an IUD; the endocervical canal may have to be dilated under anesthesia to allow insertion. A history of ectopic pregnancy is a risk factor for the occurrence of another ectopic gestation; some authors feel this history should contraindicate IUD use.

Barrier Methods

Barrier methods of contraception are mechanical and chemical devices used at the time of intercourse that prevent spermatozoa from reaching the upper female genital tract. Their effectiveness varies considerably depending on the ability and willingness of the couple to use the method with each coitus (see Table 44–1). The failure rates tend to be lower for older, more highly motivated couples (Hatcher et al., 1988).

The barrier methods offer the advantage of local contact only and freedom from systemic effects. The risks associated with these methods are primarily those of pregnancy, if the method should fail. Notably, these methods provide protection against some forms of sexually transmitted diseases.

DIAPHRAGM

The diaphragm was first introduced in 1880 and has remained an important method of contraception. Patients who want to avoid OCs for medical reasons or because of personal preference often choose this method.

Table 44–6. INTRAUTERINE DEVICES: CONTRAINDICATIONS

Absolute
Pregnancy, known or suspected
Undiagnosed abnormal uterine bleeding
Gynecologic malignancy, known or suspected (including unresolved abnormal Papanicolaou's smear)
Acute cervicitis
Previous major pelvic surgery
Abnormalities of the uterus resulting in distorted uterine cavity
Presence or history of pelvic infection
Presence or history of sexually transmitted disease
Presence or history of postpartum endometritis or infected abortion
History of ectopic pregnancy
Relative
Dysmenorrhea
Hypermenorrhea
Multiple sexual partners
Nulliparity
Anemia
Coagulopathy
Congenital or rheumatic heart disease
Corticosteroid therapy

The diaphragm is a thin, shallow latex cup with a circular firm flexible rim to hold it in place in the vagina. The diaphragm covers the cervix and holds spermicidal cream or jelly at the cervical os. The spermicide placed inside the cup of the diaphragm and along the rim ensures a chemical barrier. When fitting a diaphragm, one should use the largest size that fits comfortably into the posterior vaginal fornix behind the cervix, with the anterior edge of the rim snugly above and behind the symphysis pubis. Sizes range from 55 to 90 mm. in diameter, increasing in 5 mm. increments. A diaphragm that is too small may not completely cover the cervix or may be easily dislodged during intercourse. A diaphragm that is too large may buckle in the vagina and feel uncomfortable or may lie vertically and ineffectively cover the cervix. When proper fit is obtained, the patient will not feel the presence of the diaphragm. After the fitting, the patient is instructed to insert and remove the diaphragm while still in the examination room, so that it is clear she understands these techniques.

The diaphragm is inserted prior to intercourse and left in place for at least 6 hours after coitus. For each additional act of coitus, additional vaginal spermicide is used without removing the diaphragm. Some couples incorporate insertion of the diaphragm into their sexual foreplay.

The diaphragm should be removed within 24 hours to avoid any risk of vaginal infection or toxic shock syndrome. After each use, the diaphragm should be washed with mild soap and water, rinsed, dried, and dusted with cornstarch or unscented talcum powder.

The flexible rim contains one of three types of springs: arcing, coiled, or flat. The arcing spring allows for easier insertion and is the most popular. Some patients report discomfort or urinary tract infections with the firm arcing spring; these problems may be overcome by switching to the less rigid coil or flat spring. A plastic introducer is available for flat or coil spring diaphragms.

Contraindications to diaphragm use include a history of toxic shock syndrome, sensitivity to latex or spermicide, inability of the patient to learn the proper insertion technique, or the presence of anatomic abnormalities such as prolapse, vaginal septum, or recent childbirth.

CERVICAL CAP

Cervical caps have been used in other countries and have now been approved for use in the United States. The Prentif Cavity Rim cap, the first to receive FDA approval, is a small cup-shaped latex rubber device with a firm flexible rim that fits tightly over the cervix. It is held in place by its close fit, producing suction.

The use of spermicide inside the cap enhances the seal and ensures a chemical barrier to spermatozoa.

The cap is left in place for at least 8 hours after coitus and may be left in place for up to 48 hours. Compared with the diaphragm, caps allow separation of contraceptive and sexual activity to some extent because coitus can occur multiple times without adding spermicide. Contraindications are the same as for the diaphragm; in addition, a normal Papanicolaou smear must be obtained before prescribing a cap. Cervical cytology should be repeated after 3 months of cap use.

Caps come in several sizes and must be fitted to an individual patient. Special training is required in order to fit caps.

CONDOMS

The use of condoms has increased in the past few years due to the threat of transmission of human immunodeficiency virus. In addition to preventing unintended pregnancy, condoms significantly reduce the risk of transmission of a number of sexually transmitted diseases. The marketing of condoms is now aimed at women as well as men.

Most condoms are made of latex; only 1 per cent are made from lamb intestine. Only the latex condoms have been shown to effectively prevent transmission of human immunodeficiency virus. There is some variation in size, shape, color, and thickness of condoms in order to appeal to personal preference. Lubricated condoms are generally more popular. Those with reservoir tips break less readily. Condoms lubricated with spermicide are available.

The typically observed failure rate of condoms is in the range of 12 per cent in the first year of use. With ideal use, the failure rate may be as low as 2 per cent.

The condom is placed on the erect penis prior to any entry into the vagina. The rim of the condom is rolled all the way to the base of the penis. If there is not a reservoir on the tip of the penis, about half an inch of empty condom should be left at the end of the penis to catch the semen. This is accomplished by pinching the end of the condom as it is rolled on. Oily lubricants should not be used because they may weaken the condom. If lubrication is needed, K-Y jelly, water, saliva, or contraceptive foam may be used. After coitus, the penis must be removed from the vagina prior to loss of erection to avoid the condom coming off and allowing semen to enter the vagina. As the penis is removed, the rim of the condom should be held at the base of the penis. The condom should be inspected to be sure it is intact, and then it is discarded. Condoms should not be reused.

A small number of people are sensitive to the latex material or to the spermicide. The most common complaints of male condom users are of a reduction in sensitivity of the glans and disliking the interruption of foreplay to put on the condom. The loss of sensitivity can be overcome by using textured, ultra-thin, or lubricated condoms, but greater care is needed to prevent breakage of the thinner condom. The objection to the interruption of foreplay can be overcome by having the partner put on the condom as part of the foreplay.

A "female condom" has been developed and will soon be marketed. This is a latex sheath about 2 1/2 inches in diameter and 6 inches long. There is a delicate flexible ring at the open end that fits up against the vulva and introitus and prevents the entire device from being pushed into the vagina. The sheath is placed into the vagina and is held inside by an elastic ring. The penis then penetrates into the vagina inside this sheath and has no contact with the vagina. There is also rather complete coverage of the external genitalia near the introitus, thus affording protection against human immunodeficiency virus, herpes simplex, and other sexually transmitted diseases.

VAGINAL SPERMICIDES

Vaginal spermicidal preparations include foams, jellies, creams, suppositories, sponges, and films. Each consists of an inert base and a spermicide, either nonoxynol-9 or octoxynol-9. These spermicides effectively kill sexually transmitted disease organisms, such as gonococcus, *Trichomonas vaginalis*, herpes simplex, and *Chlamydia trachomatis* as well as spermatozoa. Spermicides may be used alone or in combination with a diaphragm, cervical cap, or condom. Typical failure rates of 15 to 21 per cent are observed when spermicides are used alone.

Spermicides have the advantage of being available without a physician's examination or prescription. A contraindication is a sensitivity reaction. Spermicide use has not been shown to cause congenital anomalies.

Foam preparations have the best dispersal in the vagina and thus may best cover the cervix. Foam is also less slippery than cream or jelly and eliminates the problem of too little friction.

Creams and jellies are primarily used in conjunction with the diaphragm or cervical cap but can be used alone. These preparations are forced into an applicator tube, which is then placed into the vagina. The plunger is depressed and about a tablespoon of material is deposited. Convenient single-use applicators are available.

The vaginal contraceptive sponge was approved in 1983. The Today sponge is a small pillow-shaped sponge containing 1 gram of nonoxynol-9 spermicide. One side has a concave dimple that fits against the cervix, and the other side has a fabric tape to facilitate removal. The sponge is moistened with tap water and inserted into the vagina to fit up against the cervix. It may be left in place up to 24 hours, and is more effective in nulliparous women.

Spermicidal suppositories such as Encare Oval,

Semicid, and Intercept have the disadvantage that they require 10 to 30 minutes to dissolve and may not dissolve completely. The packages may be difficult to open and the tablets erroneously used rectally or orally. The Japanese suppository, Neo-Sampoon, with the spermicide menfegol, is popular around the world and will likely be approved for use in the U.S.

A contraceptive film, VCFR (C-film in England), has been approved by the FDA. This is a paper-thin, 2-by-2–inch film that contains nonoxynol-9. It is pushed deeply into the vagina, no less than 5 minutes before coitus, and remains effective for 2 hours. Its small size is an advantage.

Periodic Abstinence

Natural family planning, or rhythm, methods are based on the fact that a woman is fertile for only a few days each cycle, near the time of ovulation. Patients practice abstinence during the fertile period and confine intercourse to the "safe days." Charting materials are available to aid in the record-keeping and calculations in each of these techniques.

Effectiveness rates depend on motivation and self-control and are highly variable (see Table 44–1). Failure rates of about 20 per cent in the first year are typical. These methods are inexpensive and free of side effects. In addition, this type of contraception is the only method approved by some religions. The method is unsuitable for women with irregular cycles or for couples with a low level of self-discipline.

The calendar method requires keeping a record of at least eight menstrual cycles. The earliest day a woman is likely to be fertile is determined by subtracting 18 from the number of days in the shortest cycle. The latest day of likely fertility is determined by subtracting 11 from the number of days in the longest cycle. Abstinence is then practiced on these "likely" fertile days.

The basal body temperature method for predicting ovulation has a woman measure her temperature each morning before arising. A rise of about 1° F. occurs following ovulation. Pregnancy may be avoided by avoiding coitus until the temperature rise has been present for 3 days.

The cervical mucus, or Billings, method of natural family planning relies on an awareness of changes in the cervical mucus during the menstrual cycle. The woman checks the character of mucus daily by inserting a finger into the vagina. Around the time of ovulation, the discharge becomes abundant, thin, slippery, clear, and elastic. Intercourse is avoided until at least 4 days after the "peak" mucus symptom.

The sympto-thermal method combines checking the cervical mucus (symptoms) and the basal body temperature to determine the likely time of ovulation.

Typical failure rates for periodic abstinence are high. Rates as low as 2 per cent have been observed only for methods restricting intercourse to the postovulatory portion of the cycle. The lowest expected failure rates are higher for the other methods of periodic abstinence.

Sterilization

When a couple has completed its family and desires no further children, sterilization becomes an option. Although progress has been made in techniques to reverse both female sterilization and vasectomy, these operations should be considered permanent. Sterilization is inappropriate for individuals or couples with uncertainty about wanting more children.

Both female tubal sterilization and vasectomy of the male are safe and highly effective methods of contraception. Because of the intraperitoneal location of the female internal genitalia, female sterilization involves slightly higher rates of serious complications than does vasectomy.

TUBAL STERILIZATION

Obliteration or interruption of the fallopian tube prevents pregnancy by preventing the ovum from reaching the uterus and the sperm from reaching the ovum. Methods of tubal sterilization in use include minilaparotomy with tying of the tubes (the Pomeroy technique, and others); and laparoscopy with banding, clipping, or electrocoagulation of the tubes. The minilaparotomy can be performed in the immediate postpartum period, or 6 weeks or more after delivery. Laparoscopic procedures are not done until at least 6 weeks postpartum.

The effectiveness of tubal sterilization is high—but not 100 per cent effective. Failures can occur because of inadequate surgical technique, recanalization, and undetected early pregnancy at the time of the procedure. A high percentage of pregnancies after tubal occlusion are ectopic when compared with women using no birth control.

Operative complications are unusual but include bowel and vascular injuries and mesosalpingeal injury with bleeding. Fatalities are rare. Laparoscopic tubal sterilization has been associated with an increased risk for subsequent dysfunctional uterine bleeding and pelvic pain in some studies.

VASECTOMY

Interruption of the vas deferens, or vasectomy, prevents spermatozoa from becoming part of the ejaculate. Vasectomy is a relatively simple and safe office procedure because of the accessibility of the vas in the scrotum. Several techniques of interrupting the vas have been employed, including ligation, electrocoagulation, and placement of clips (see p. 1368). Most surgeons divide the vas and remove a segment of vas, which is sent for pathologic confirmation. Several techniques are available to prevent the severed ends of the vas from rejoining. Local anesthesia *without* epinephrine is used.

Proper preoperative evaluation and counseling is essential and should include a description of other methods of contraception available and explanation of the permanence of vasectomy. Side effects and failure rates should also be discussed.

Contraindications include current infection of the genital tract or scrotal skin, as well as marital or psychologic instability, or the expectation that the procedure will cure a sexual dysfunction.

Patients with varicocele, hydrocele, inguinal hernia, filariasis, or previous scrotal surgery may need to be referred to a specialist for their procedure. Patients with bleeding disorders or other medical conditions may require special measures or consultation, or both.

Vasectomy failures are uncommon but can occur because of faulty surgical technique, recanalization, or failure of the couple to protect themselves just after the procedure. Azoospermia is not immediate; 12 to 24 ejaculations may be required to clear the genital tract of viable sperm. Patients should be counseled before the procedure that another form of contraception should be used until the semen analysis demonstrates the complete absence of sperm.

Ecchymosis, swelling, and discomfort are common after the procedure and subside within 1 to 2 weeks. Less common complications of the procedure include infection, hematoma, and epididymitis. Spermatic granulomas may form at the site of the vasectomy or in the epididymis. Most granulomas are not symptomatic, but they may be responsible for pain, recanalization, or for preventing successful reversal of the vasectomy. Serious complications are rare. Vasectomy has been associated with accelerated atherogenesis in certain monkeys, but no acceleration of atherogenesis has been observed in vasectomized men. Although antibodies to sperm develop in many men after vasectomy, no increased risk of autoimmune disease has been observed. Vasectomy causes no serious long-term changes in testicular endocrine function nor does it cause sexual dysfunction.

Vasectomy reversal is an expensive microsurgical procedure. Vas patency is restored in over half of patients, but pregnancy rates vary widely.

OTHER METHODS

Coitus interruptus, or withdrawal, in which the penis is withdrawn from the vagina prior to ejaculation, has a failure rate of approximately 18 per cent in actual use (see Table 44–1). With ideal use, the failure rate may be as low as 4 per cent. Pregnancy can occur even when the method is used properly because the seminal fluid present prior to ejaculation may contain sperm. This method is inexpensive and always available, but requires a high degree of self-control during sexual activity.

Douching is not an effective method of contraception. Sperm penetration of the cervical canal can occur within 15 seconds of ejaculation. If a spermicide preparation has been used, a douche may wash out the spermicide and leave active sperm.

Noncoital sex can be an important option for some couples, especially adolescents. Many couples use this as an adjunct to periodic abstinence. Care must be taken to avoid semen being spilled near the vagina, or motile sperm may find their way to the cervix, even without penile penetration.

Abstinence from sexual activity may be a viable option for some individuals. While theoretically effective, typical failure rates of 20 per cent are observed.

Lactation reduces fertility, but not reliably so. To be effective in preventing ovulation, breast-feeding must occur frequently and around the clock, a practice that is uncommon in the United States. Pregnancy may even occur before menstruation is resumed. Thus, an additional method of contraception is recommended if pregnancy is to be reliably avoided.

POSTCOITAL FERTILITY CONTROL

All too often, situations arise in which coitus occurs without protection from pregnancy. Several measures are available that will prevent or interrupt pregnancy after unprotected intercourse. These methods are inappropriate for ongoing contraception.

"Morning-after-pills" are not approved as such by the FDA, but are nevertheless used by many practitioners for selected patients. Two Ovral tablets (see Table 44–2) are taken as soon as possible after the exposure, and two more tablets are taken 12 hours later. Preferably, treatment begins within 24 hours of unprotected intercourse—certainly no later than 72 hours after exposure. Nausea is common and may be prevented by concomitant use of an antiemetic. The risk of pregnancy after a single unprotected coitus at midcycle is estimated to be about 14 per cent; use of Ovral reduces the risk to about 2 per cent. Informed consent is essential; a theoretical (but probably not actual) risk of congenital anomalies exists should pregnancy continue.

High-dose estrogens are also effective as postcoital agents but are seldom used because of their toxicity. High-dose progestins are being considered for approval as postcoital agents.

Early pregnancy termination with progesterone antagonists (RU 486) and inhibitors of progesterone synthesis (epostane) is under study. These agents interfere with hormonal support of the endometrium and thus of any implanted ovum. When administered early after a missed menstrual period, bleeding may be induced and an early pregnancy interrupted.

Several procedures are available to terminate pregnancy once it is established. The type of procedure and the risks of having a legal abortion are directly related to the duration of the gestation. Early abortions—those up until 12 to 13 weeks from the beginning of the last menstrual period—are usually accomplished by cervical dilation followed by suction curettage. The procedure may be done on an outpatient basis, under general or paracervical anesthesia. After 14 weeks' gestation, the technique of amnioinfusion has been used. Dilatation with laminaria followed by mechanical evacuation of the products of conception appears to be the safer procedure but requires special training and expertise.

Menstrual extraction can be done within the first few weeks following a missed menstrual period and is sometimes performed without confirming the diagnosis of pregnancy. This office procedure is done with suction curettage using a 5- or 6-mm. cannula, usually without the need to dilate the cervical canal. This early in pregnancy, there is a higher incidence of failure to interrupt the pregnancy than by waiting until later in the first trimester.

Counseling of the patient both before and after a therapeutic abortion is extremely important. A woman with an unplanned pregnancy often has difficulty deciding on a course of action. The family physician's task is to apprise her of her options, and assist her in making an informed decision. If she elects to terminate the pregnancy, future contraception should be discussed.

Choosing a Method

In choosing a method of contraception, there are a number of factors to be considered. Patients or couples may have personal preferences, concerns, and previous experiences that influence their options. The importance of high effectiveness varies. Some people have difficulty complying with methods that require daily pill-taking; others may find it difficult to use a method at the time of intercourse. Some couples seek permanent contraception, whereas others need temporary measures. Options may be limited by method contraindications or health risks.

Age and parity affect the options available. Younger women have low cardiovascular risks with OCs, but young, nulliparous women are poor candidates for IUD use. Older parous women in mutually monogamous relationships are more appropriate candidates for IUD use. Older parous women who wish to have no more children also tend to be able to use barrier methods quite effectively.

Women over 40 years of age may consider using OCs if they do not smoke and have no other risk factors for cardiovascular disease. OC use should be considered only for nonsmoking older women with a serum cholesterol level under 200, normal blood pressure, no family history of premature coronary disease, and no reason to suspect diabetes mellitus. Other contraceptive methods, most often sterilization, are more commonly employed by older women, even if no cardiovascular risk factors are present.

The number of sexual partners that a woman (and her partner) has may influence the choice of contraceptive. Persons at high risk for sexually transmitted diseases may benefit from condom (and spermicide) use; certainly an IUD would be a poor choice. Persons at significant risk of exposure to human immunodeficiency virus should use condoms whether or not another contraceptive method is employed. They should also receive counseling about other ways of changing their behavior to reduce their risk of exposure to human immunodeficiency virus.

The expected frequency of intercourse may influence the choice of method. A woman who anticipates intercourse to occur only occasionally may find barrier methods particularly appropriate.

Postpartum patients should have received counseling about contraceptive methods during their prenatal care. If OCs are chosen, they are generally begun 1 to 3 weeks after delivery. Barrier methods, such as condoms and spermicides, are options for most postpartum patients. These may also be used until 6 to 8 weeks postpartum, when a diaphragm or cap may be fitted or when an IUD may be inserted, if appropriate. Planning for tubal sterilization should occur during the pregnancy. The procedure may be performed during the first few days after delivery or as an "interval" procedure at least 6 weeks postpartum. If sterilization is considered, vasectomy may be an option.

If a woman chooses to breast-feed her baby, an additional method of contraception should be recommended to reliably avoid pregnancy. Many breast-feeding women elect to use barrier methods until the baby is weaned. Mini-pills that contain only progestin may be prescribed; if combination OCs are chosen, they should be low-dose and should not be begun until after the milk supply has been well-established. IUD use, tubal sterilization, or vasectomy are other options to consider.

Adolescents form a group with special contraceptive needs. Abstinence is not a reliable alternative for many teenagers, and teens often fail to use contraception. Family physicians can play important roles by discussing contraception and responsible decision-making with teenagers frankly—and confidentially—*before* their needs become apparent. OCs and barrier methods are appropriate choices for teens to consider.

Patients and couples should be counseled and educated about the contraceptive methods that are available to them. Family physicians should present the advantages, disadvantages, risks, and benefits of the various methods and assist their patients in making an informed choice of an appropriate method.

References

American Academy of Pediatrics Committee on Drugs: Medroxyprogesterone acetate (Depo-Provera). Pediatrics, *65*:648, 1980.

American Academy of Pediatrics: Breast feeding and contraception. Pediatrics, *67*:1, 1981.

American College of Obstetricians and Gynecologists: Oral Contraception. ACOG Technical Bulletin, Number 106, July, 1987 (Washington DC: ACOG). *A concise summary of current knowledge, with recommendations.*

Blumenstein, B. A., Douglas, M. B., and Hall, W. D.: Blood pressure changes and oral contraceptive use: A study of 2676 black women in the southeastern United States. Am. J. Epidemiol., *112*:539–552, 1980.

Fischl, M.: Heterosexual AIDS transmission. Proceedings of conference: Condoms in prevention of sexually transmitted diseases. Atlanta, GA, February 20, 1987.

Grimes, D. A.: Reversible contraception for the 1980's. J.A.M.A., *255*:69–75, 1986. *A brief, well-written review by a leader in the field of contraception.*

Hatcher, R. A., Kowal, D., Guest, F., et al.: Contraceptive Technology, 1988–1989. 14th ed. New York, Irvington, 1988. *A useful handbook containing much information and practical advice.*

Layde, P. M., Vessey, M. P., and Yeates, D.: Risk factors for gallbladder disease: A cohort study of young women attending family planning clinics. J. Epidemiol. Comm. Health, *36*:274–278, 1982.

Liskin, L., Blackburn, R., and Ghani, R.: Hormonal contraception: New long-acting methods. Popul. Rep., Series K, Number 3, 1987.

Liskin, L., Pile, J. M., and Quillin, W. F.: Vasectomy—Safe and simple. Popul. Rep., Series D, Number 4, 1983.

Neinstein, L. S., and Katz, B.: Contraceptive use in the chronically ill adolescent female. Part I. J. Adolesc. Health Care, *7*:123–133, 1986. *Excellent discussion of contraceptive issues for women with chronic diseases.*

Neinstein, L. S., and Katz, B.: Contraceptive use in the chronically ill adolescent female. Part II. J Adolesc. Health Care, *7*:350–360, 1986. *Continuation of Part I, listed earlier.*

Ory, H. W.: The noncontraceptive health benefits from oral contraceptives. Fam. Plann. Perspect., *14*:182–184, 1982.

Ory, H. W.: Mortality associated with fertility and fertility control: 1983. Fam. Plann. Perspect., *15*:57–63, 1983. *A computer projection of risks associated with various contraceptive methods.*

Porter, J. B., Hunter, J. R., Jick, H., and Stergachis, A.: Oral contraceptives and nonfatal vascular disease. Obstet. Gynecol., *66*:1–4, 1985.

Porter, J. B., Jick, H., and Walker, A. M.: Mortality among oral contraceptive users. Obstet. Gynecol., *70*:29–32, 1987.

Ramcharan, S., Pellegrin, F. A., Ray, R., and Hsu, J. P.: The Walnut Creek contraceptive drug study. Vol. III. Bethesda, MD, Center for Population Research, 1981.

Realini, J. P., and Goldzieher, J. W.: Oral contraceptives and cardiovascular disease: A critique of the epidemiologic studies. Am. J. Obstet. Gynecol., *152*:729–798, 1985.

Royal College of General Practitioners: Oral contraceptives and health: An interim report. London, Pitman, 1974.

Royal College of General Practitioners Oral Contraception Study: Further analysis of mortality in oral contraceptive users. Lancet, *1*:541–546, 1981.

Royal College of General Practitioners Oral Contraception Study: Oral contraceptives and gallbladder disease. Lancet, *2*:957–959, 1982.

Simpson, J. L.: Do contraceptive methods pose fetal risks? Research Frontiers in Fertility Regulation, *3*(6):1–11, 1985. *A critical review of the evidence.*

Speroff, L., Glass, R. H., and Kase, N. G.: Clinical Gynecologic Endocrinology and Fertility. 3rd ed, Baltimore, MD, Williams & Wilkins, 1983, pp. 409–450.

Treiman, K., and Liskin, L.: IUDs—A new look. Population Reports, Series B, Number 5, 1988. *A comprehensive review of current issues regarding IUDs.*

Trussell, J., Kost, K.: Contraceptive failure in the United States: A critical review of the literature. Stud. Fam. Plann. *18*:237–283, 1987. *An authoritative evaluation and summary of what is known about the effectiveness of many methods.*

Wharton, C., and Blackburn, R.: Lower-dose pills. Popul. Rep., Series A, Number 7, 1988.

45

Interpretation of the Electrocardiogram

Carlos Vallbona

The electrocardiogram (ECG) is a simple test that family physicians can use effectively to analyze the electrical activity of the heart. The analysis can yield important information about cardiac function and may lead to the diagnosis of specific cardiovascular disorders.

Steps in the Analysis of the ECG

Analyzing the ECG includes the following steps. (1) determination of the average heart rate; (2) analysis of the predominant rhythm and detection of arrhythmias; (3) computation of the QRS axis in the frontal plane; (4) analysis of P, QRS, and T waves in the frontal and horizontal planes. If there is a deviation of the ST segment, it should be analyzed also; (5) measurement of the standard time intervals; and (6) assessment of the extent to which the ECG is normal or abnormal and, in the latter case, diagnosis of the specific abnormalities and their clinical significance.

Basic Concepts

THE ELECTRICAL FIELD GENERATED BY THE HEART

We may consider the heart as a dipole. The transmembrane action potentials (TAPs) generated during the cardiac cycle create an electrical field. Its center is the electrical center of the heart. At various locations in the electrical field it is possible to record whatever changes in potential (electromotive forces [EMFs]) occur during the cardiac cycle. The positive and negative portions of the field are separated by an isoelectric plane (Fig. 45–1).

Electrodes placed below the isoelectric plane will record positive potentials. Electrodes set above the plane will record negative potentials. Electrodes placed at the plane will record zero (isoelectric) potentials. Thus, in the example of Figure 45–1, an exploring electrode in the right arm will be above the plane and record negative potentials. An electrode in the left foot will be below the plane and record positive potentials. An electrode in the chest at the edge of the plane will record isoelectric potential.

The electrical field is three dimensional, but its projection in a frontal plane can be assessed by analyzing the standard limb leads (I, II, III, aVR, aVL, and aVF) and its projection in a horizontal plane by analyzing the precordial or chest leads (V_1–V_6).

The following basic assumptions are made in the analysis of the frontal and horizontal plane projections. (1) The body is a uniform conductor; (2) the heart is at the center of the body and functions as a dipole; and (3) all electrodes placed on the body surface are equidistant from the electrical center of the heart. Of course, these assumptions are not quite valid because the heart is not at the center of the body, and the electrodes, especially those placed in

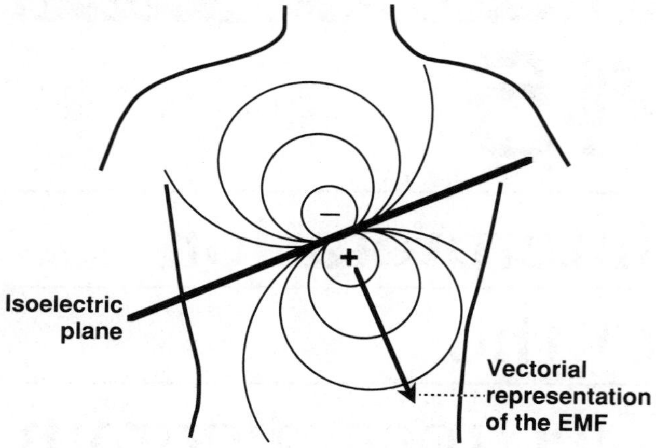

Figure 45–1. Electrical field generated by a transmembrane action potential of the heart.

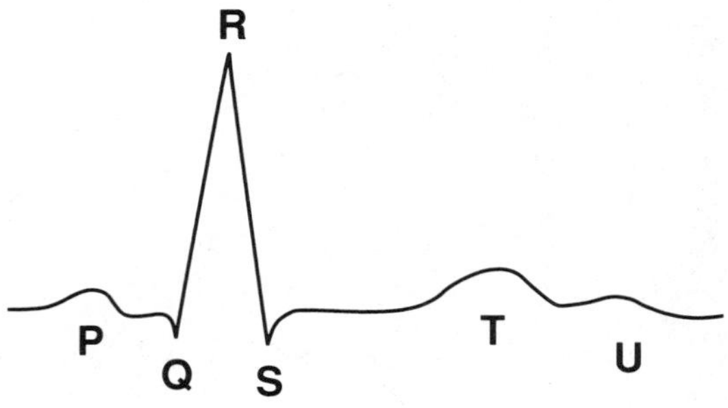

Figure 45–2. The normal components of the electrocardiogram.

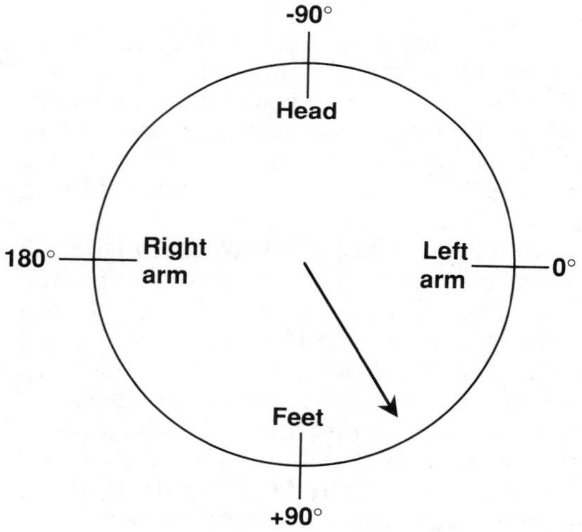

Figure 45–3. Reference points for measurements of the direction of the electrical axis of the heart.

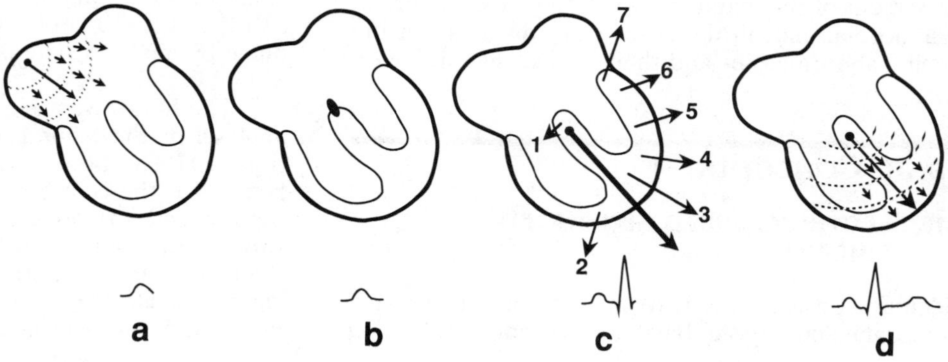

Figure 45–4. Sequence of depolarization and repolarization of atria and ventricles.

the precordial area, are not equidistant from the electrical center.

COMPONENTS OF THE ECG

The electromotive forces generated by the heart during systole are recorded as (1) P wave caused by depolarization of the atria, (2) QRS wave of depolarization of the ventricles, and (3) T wave due to repolarization of the ventricles (Fig. 45–2).

The U wave is an afterwave of repolarization. It may occur always, but, in general, it has a very small magnitude and can be detected only in those precordial leads where the electrodes are close to the myocardial mass. Certain electrolyte disturbances, e.g., hypokalemia, produce a large U wave in practically all leads.

MEASUREMENT OF ECG COMPONENTS

The ECG components may be analyzed as follows.

1. Pattern analysis—assessment of the shape and amplitude of the ECG waves in various leads
2. Vector analysis—determination of the vector values (direction in degrees and magnitude in millivolts [mV])
3. Scalar analysis—measurement of the duration of various ECG components (in 0.01 seconds). The measurement of voltages in various leads is a scalar analysis also, but it is necessary for the pattern or vector analysis.

THE ELECTRICAL AXIS

It is easy and useful to analyze the QRS complex from the standpoint of the direction of its mean vector in the frontal plane (electrical axis). Figure 45–3 shows the reference points that are used to compute the QRS electrical axis. It is equally feasible to compute the axis of the P and T waves although this cannot be done as accurately as the computation of QRS.

Sequence of Depolarization and Repolarization

During atrial depolarization, there is a slow progression of more or less parallel EMFs from the sinoatrial (SA) to the atrioventricular (AV) node. The resultant P vector has the following characteristics in the frontal plane: mean axis +45 degrees, magnitude ≤ 0.25 mV. (Fig. 45–4*A*). The atrial repolarization is seldom recorded because it takes place during the QRS complex, which is of greater magnitude and therefore cancels out the atrial repolarization forces.

There is no recorded electrical activity for a period of time (0.06 to 0.10 seconds) when the impulses are detained at the AV node before transmission to the bundle of His (Fig. 45–4*B*).

During ventricular depolarization, there is a rapid generation of nonparallel EMFs in a sequence that can be arbitrarily described in terms of seven vectors distributed as shown in Figure 45–4*C*. The resultant vector of QRS has the following characteristics in the frontal plane: mean axis +60 degrees, magnitude ≤ 1.5 mV. (Fig. 45–4*C*).

The ventricular repolarization occurs as a slow wave of more or less parallel EMFs that when summated, can be expressed as a vector almost parallel to that of QRS and with the following characteristics in the frontal plane: mean axis +60 degrees, magnitude ≤ 0.5 mV. (Fig. 45–4*D*).

ECG Lead System for the Frontal Plane

Traditionally, electrodes are placed on each one of the four limbs. The potential measured by an electrode on the right arm is expressed as VR, that on the left arm as VL, and that on the left foot as VF. Potentials measured on the right foot are almost identical to those on the left; therefore, the electrode placed on the right foot is for grounding purposes only.

Einthoven's law states that VR + VL + VF = 0. Lead I = VL − VR, when the potential recorded by the electrode in the right arm, R, is negative in relation to that of the left arm, L. Lead II = VF − VR, when the electrode in R is negative in relation to the foot electrode, F. Lead III = VF − VL when the electrode in L is negative in relation to F. The standard limb leads I, II, and III constitute the Einthoven's triangle (Fig. 45–5*A*). A triaxial system may be constructed by placing the three standard leads at the center of the triangle (Fig. 45–5*B*).

The mean QRS vector projects itself in all leads. From these projections, it is possible to compute the direction and magnitude of the QRS axis. Similarly, the axis of P, T (and even ST) may be computed. The Einthoven's triangle and its equivalent triaxial coordinate system provide a useful but cumbersome model to compute the QRS axis. Assume an ECG with the QRS tracings shown in Figure 45–6. These tracings can be expressed as the vector projections in each lead and from these projections it is possible to measure the directions and magnitude of the QRS vector fairly accurately in the frontal plane (Fig. 45–6*A*).

In addition to leads I, II, and III derived from the Einthoven's triangle, we have leads aVR, aVL, and aVF, which when superimposed with leads I, II, and III constitute a hexaxial system. Lead aVR records the difference in potential between the electrical

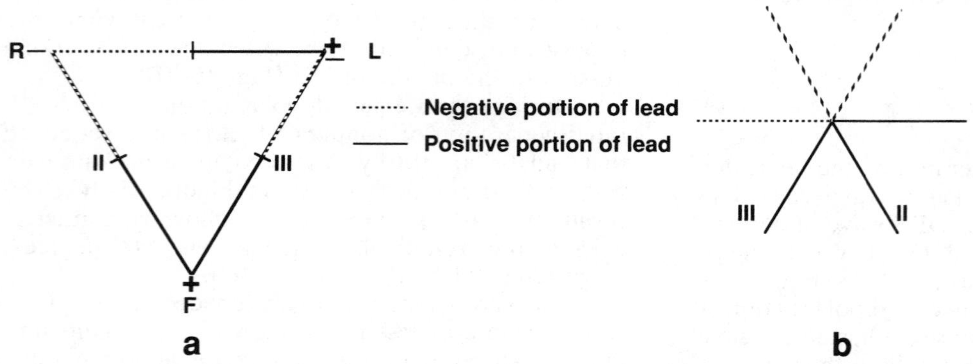

Figure 45–5. ECG system for the frontal plane.

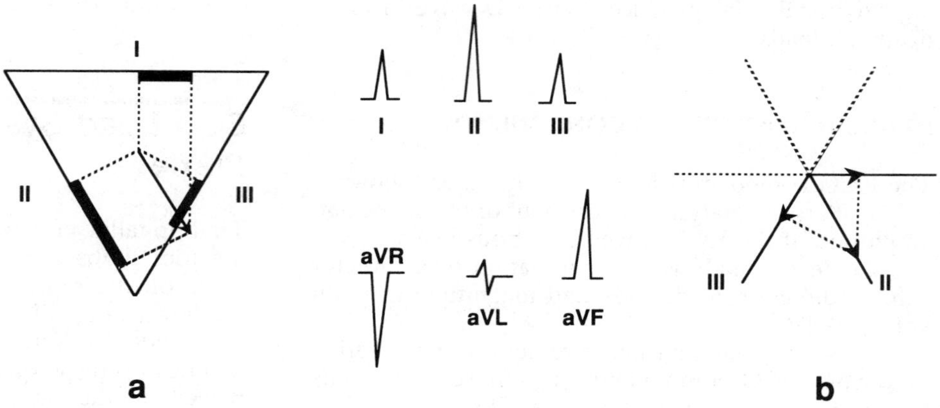

Figure 45–6. Example of determination of the axis of QRS.

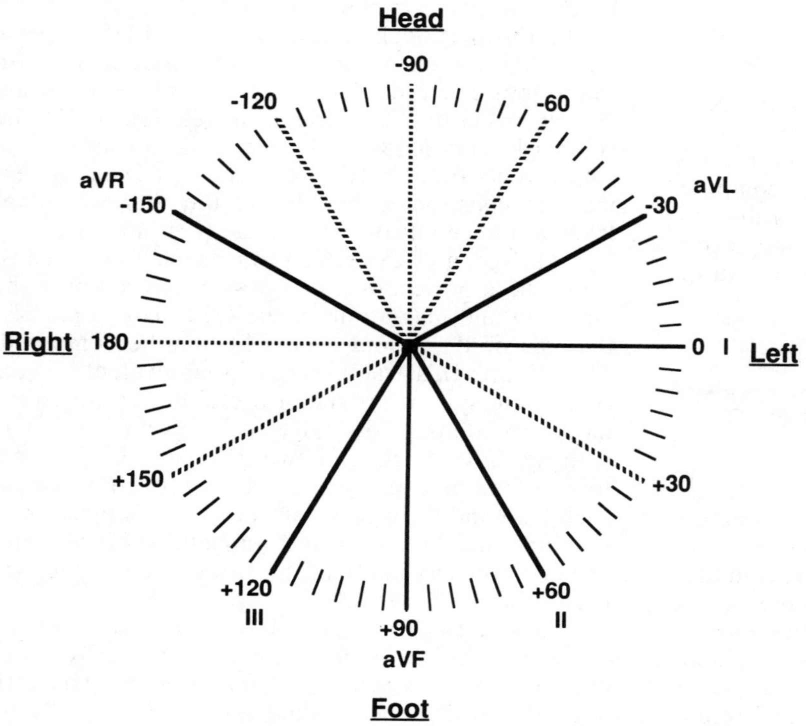

Figure 45–7. Diagram for the computation of the electrical axis and magnitude of vectors in the frontal plane.

center of the heart and a positive electrode in the right arm, R. Similarly, aVL and aVF record the difference in potential between the electrical center and the left arm electrode, L, or the left foot electrode, F, respectively. We can then plot the amplitudes of QRS in each one of the six leads and obtain the direction and magnitude of the projection of the mean axis of QRS in the frontal plane. This method offers the advantage of allowing for greater accuracy than the Einthoven's triangle method, but it is still cumbersome (Fig. 45–6*B*).

A simplified approach consists of finding the lead with an isoelectric complex. The axis is perpendicular to that lead and falls in the same direction as a lead that would be ideal to measure the direction and magnitude of the QRS vector.

The diagram of Figure 45–7 is very useful in computing the electrical axis and magnitude in the frontal plane.

An example of this can be seen in the tracing shown in Figure 45–6, which has an isoelectric aVL (whose direction is from −30 degrees to +150 degrees). This means that the axis direction is either −120 or +60 degrees. The lead parallel to the axis is II (from −120 to +60 degrees). Since II is positive, the axis direction is +60 degrees. The amplitude of QRS in lead II is 14 mm. Since the standard calibration is 10 mm. = 1 mV., the axis magnitude is 1.4 mV.

Normal Values in the Frontal Plane

QRS AXIS

Adults. The *direction* of QRS is normally between 0 and +90 degrees although some textbooks indicate that the normal range is from −20 to +110 degrees. The *magnitude* is equal to or less than 1.5 mV.

If the direction of QRS is between 0 and +90 degrees, it is considered within normal limits (WNL). If the direction is between +90 and 180 degrees, it is considered to be a right axis deviation (RAD). Extreme RAD occurs if the axis falls between 180 and −90 degrees. If the direction is between 0 and −90 degrees, there is a left axis deviation (LAD) (Fig. 45–8). An undifferentiated axis occurs whenever all leads are nearly isoelectric.

It is clear from this figure that normally the axis of QRS is projected in the positive part of leads I and aVF, whereas a RAD will cause a negative QRS in I and a LAD will cause a negative QRS in aVF. In the rare case of extreme RAD, QRS will be negative in both lead I and aVF. Thus, a very simplified pattern analysis of the QRS axis can be done by assessing leads I and aVF. The diagrams and QRS patterns in these two leads (Fig. 45–9) show the most common locations of the QRS axis in normal and abnormal conditions.

Newborn and Infants. There is RAD because of the relative preponderance of right ventricular forces in the neonatal period.

Elderly. There is a horizontal axis or slight LAD because of the preponderance of left ventricular forces in the majority of persons beyond the sixth decade of life.

P AXIS

The P axis has almost the same *direction* as that of QRS, but the range of normal is from +20 to +70 degrees. The *magnitude* is less than 0.25 mV.

In a pattern analysis, P is considered normal if it is positive in lead II. If P is negative in aVF, it suggests a marked left atrial enlargement or a nodal rhythm. If P is very small, isoelectric, or negative in lead I, it is likely due to right atrial enlargement.

T AXIS

In adults, the *direction* of the T axis is within 60 degrees counterclockwise of the QRS axis or within 45 degrees clockwise of the QRS axis. The *magnitude* is less than 0.5 mV. (Fig. 45–10).

Whenever the angle between the QRS and T axis exceeds 60 degrees counterclockwise (ccw) or 45 degrees clockwise (cw), the diagnosis of electrical strain is warranted. A T axis of strain points *away* from the ventricle where the strain occurs. Usual causes of strain are hypertrophy, bundle branch block, ischemia, digitalis, epinephrine effect, metabolic disturbances, and cerebral hemorrhage.

A simple pattern analysis of the T wave can be made by looking at the T wave in the lead of highest QRS positivity. If T is also positive, it is considered normal. The condition referred to as ventricular strain occurs when the T is negative in the lead of highest QRS positivity or, vice versa, when it is positive in the lead of highest QRS negativity.

Example tracings 1–5 show various locations of QRS axis. Example tracing 6 shows a case of left ventricular strain (LVS).

The Horizontal or Transverse Plane Leads

The precordial leads, in spite of their staggered placement across the chest, may be considered to lie on a horizontal plane whose center is the electrical center of the heart. Their location on the chest wall is shown in Figure 45–11*A* and their approximate direction in a hexaxial system is shown in Figure 45–11*B*. V_1 is placed in the fourth intercostal space at the right

Text continued on page 843

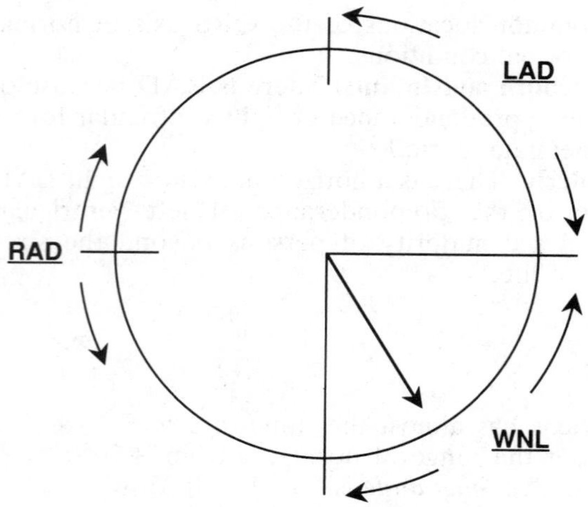

Figure 45–8. Normal values of QRS axis in the frontal plane.

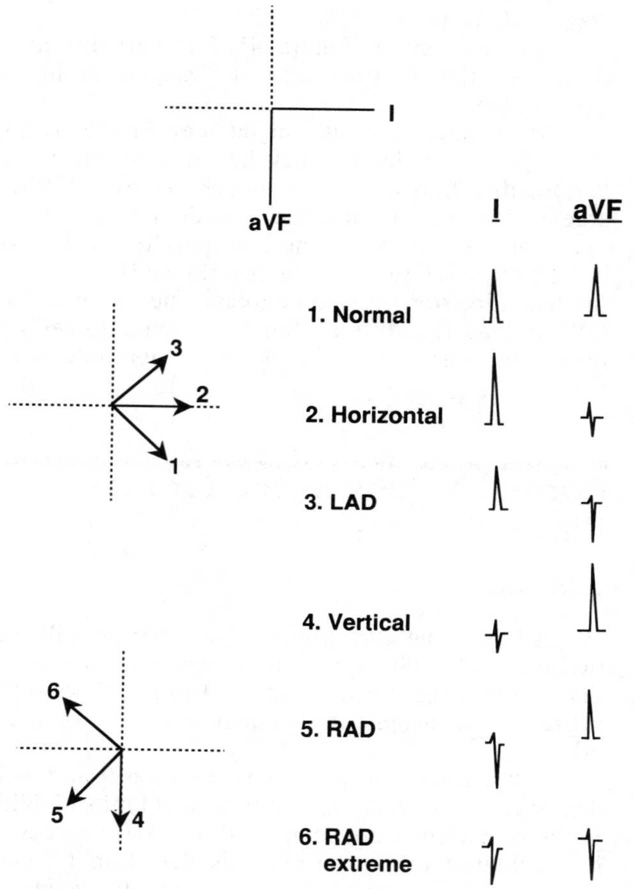

Figure 45–9. Pattern analysis of the electrical axis using leads I and aVF as references.

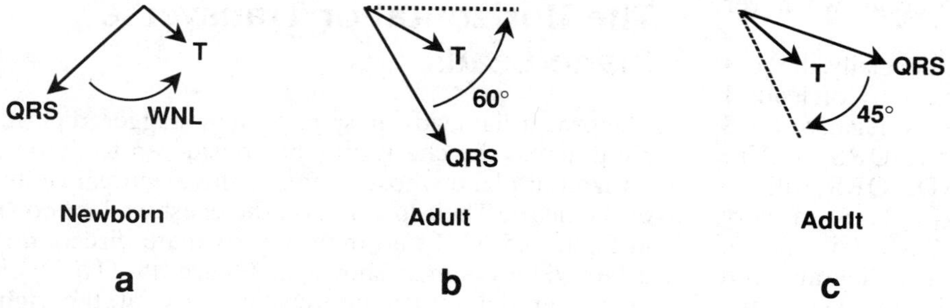

Figure 45–10. The normal relationship between the QRS and T axis.

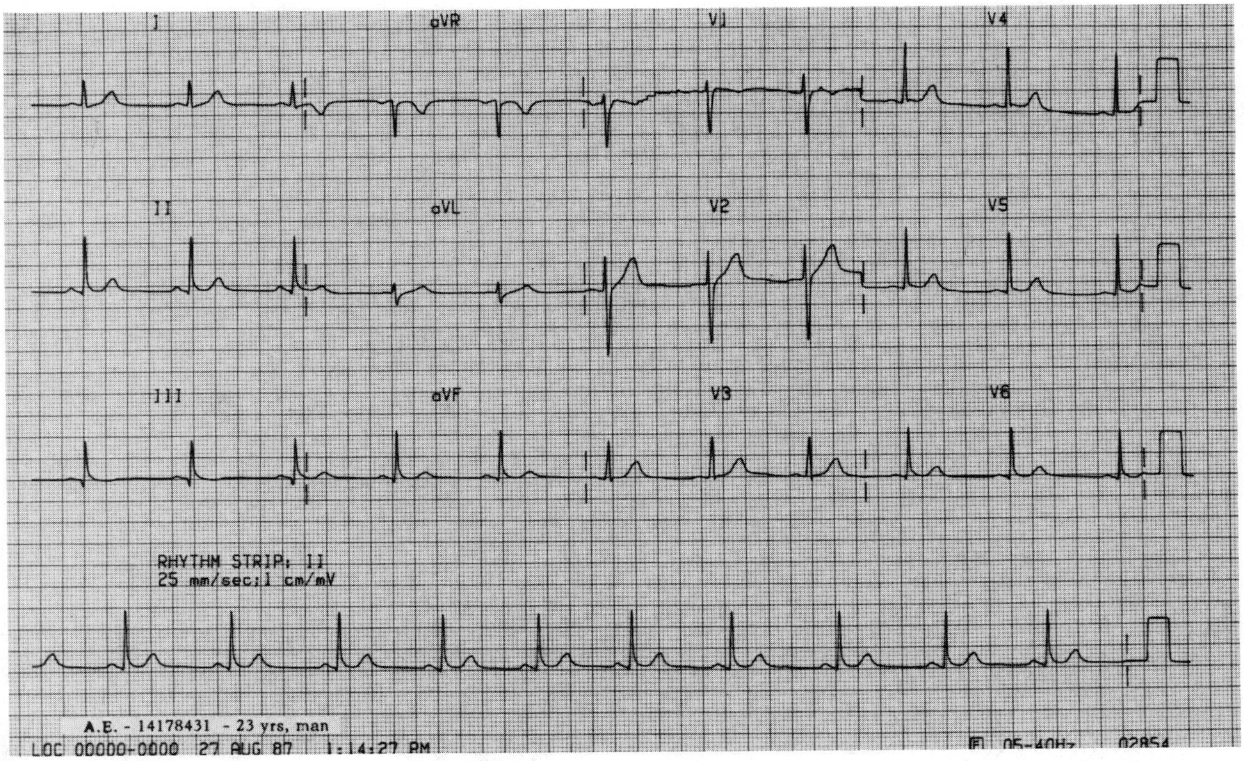

Tracing 1. Example of a normal ECG. Axis of QRS +60 degrees. Axis of T +30 degrees. P, QRS, and T normal in the precordial leads.

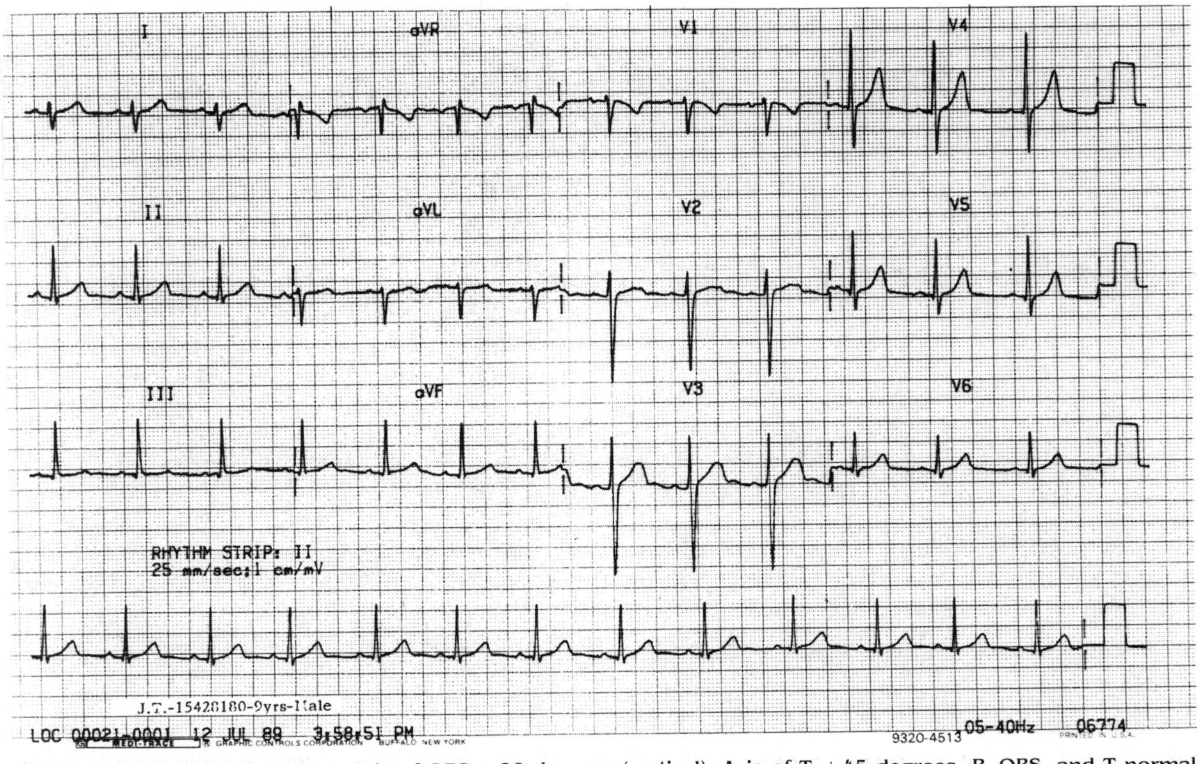

Tracing 2. Example of a normal ECG. Axis of QRS +90 degrees (vertical). Axis of T +45 degrees. P, QRS, and T normal in the precordial leads.

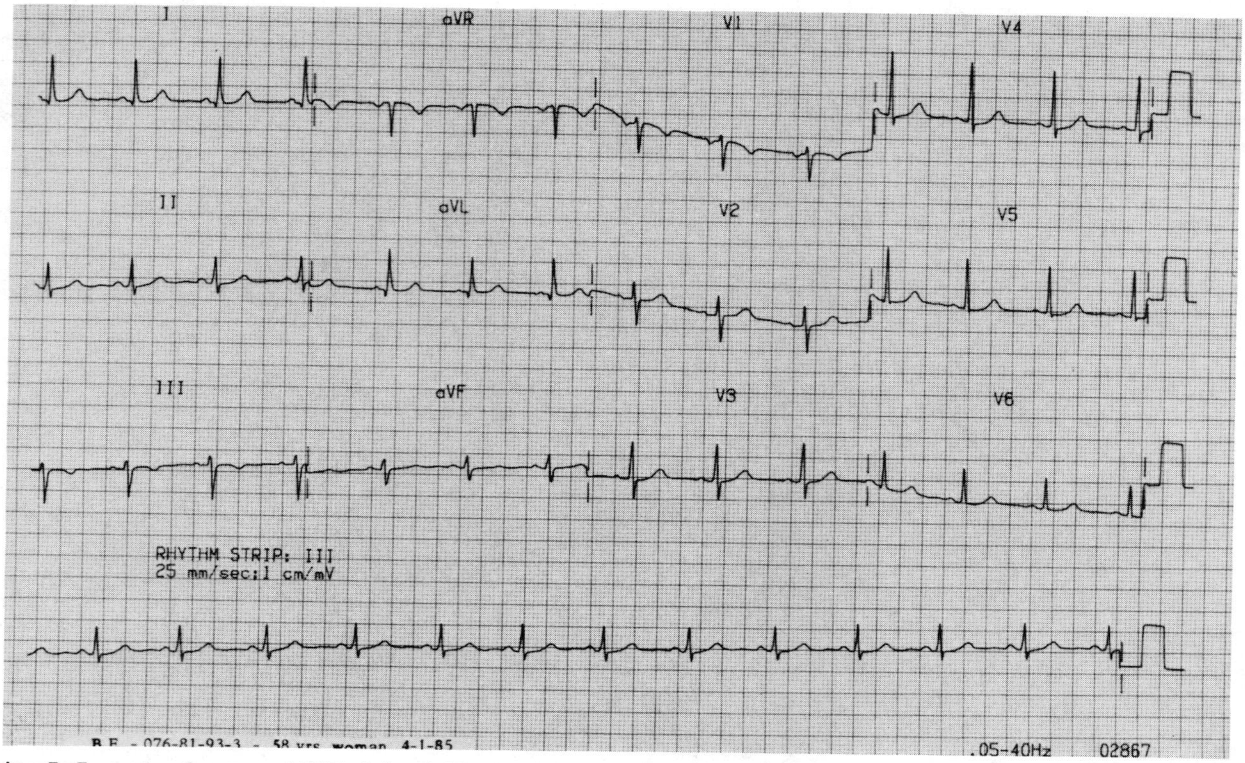

Tracing 3. Example of a normal ECG. Axis of QRS 0 degrees (horizontal). Axis of T +5 degrees. P, QRS, and T normal in the precordial leads.

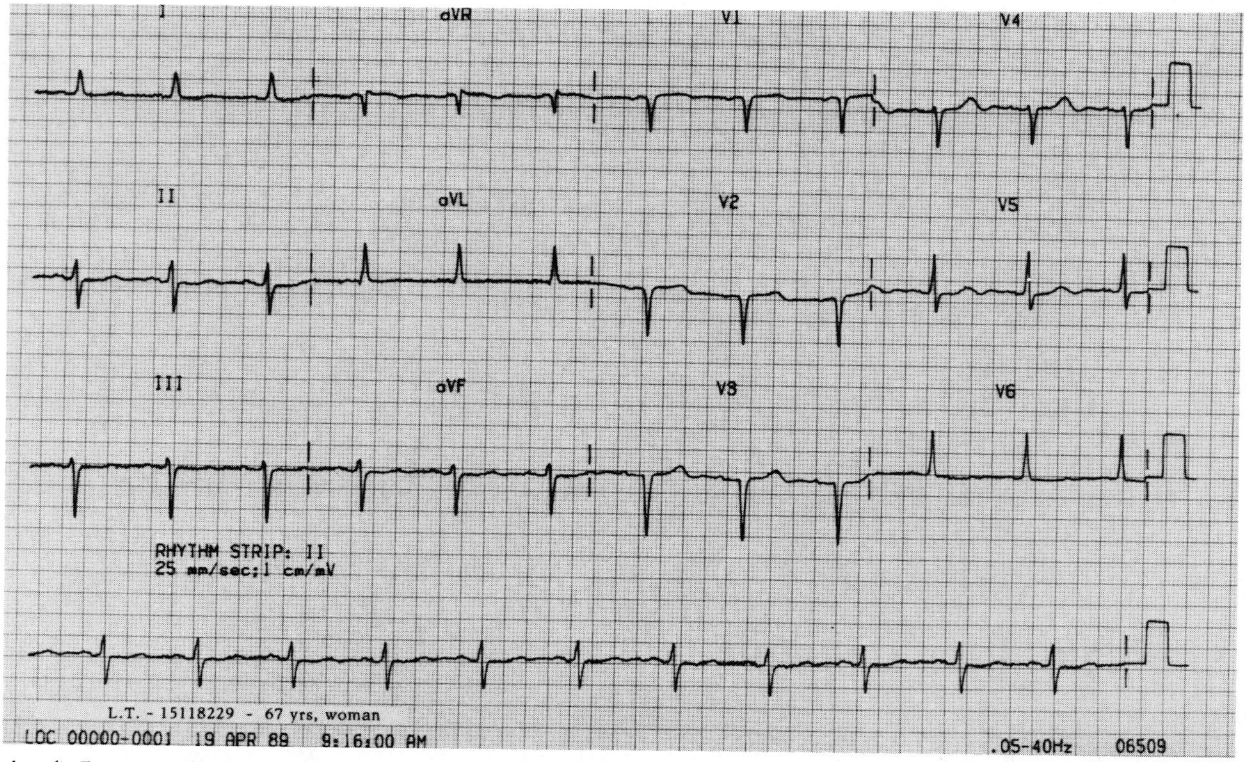

Tracing 4. Example of a left axis deviation. Axis of QRS −40 degrees. Axis of T 0 degrees. Poor R progression in the precordial leads due to an old anterior wall MI.

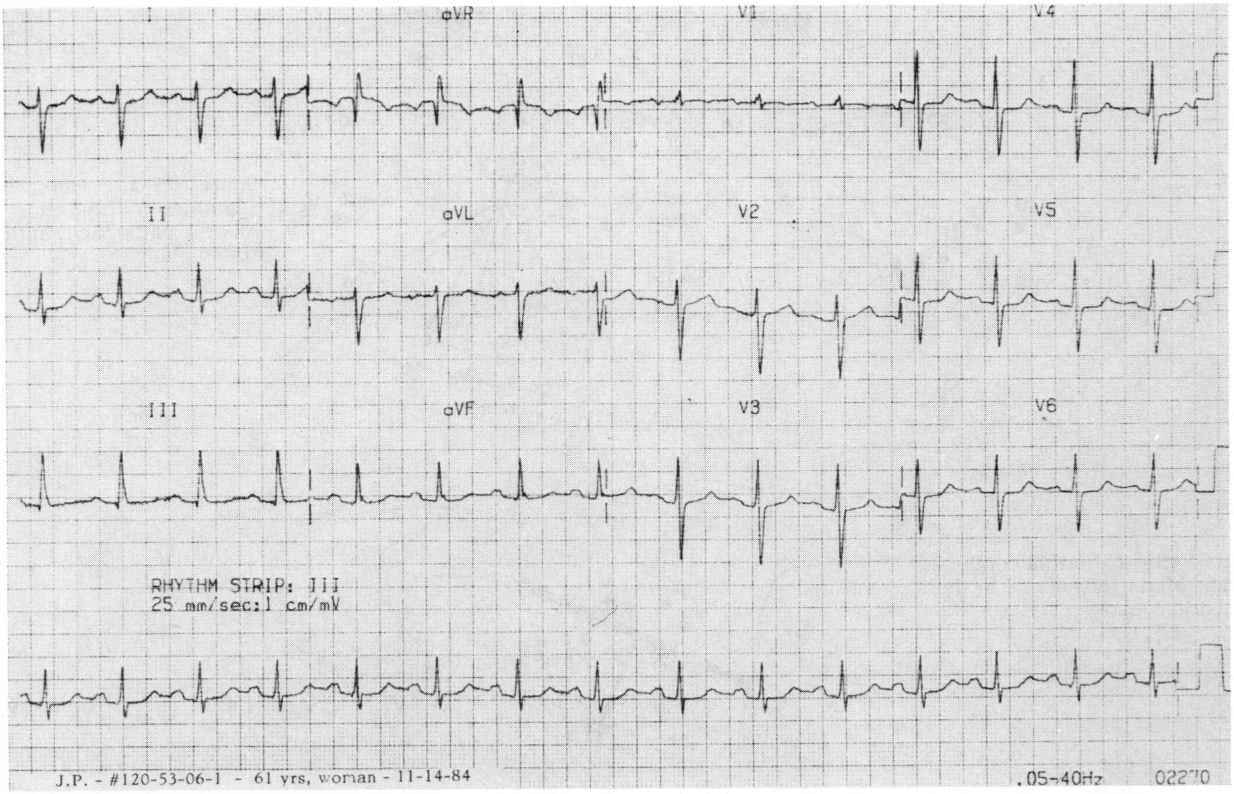

Tracing 5. Example of a right axis deviation. Axis of QRS +125 degrees. Axis of T +30 degrees. The almost isoelectric QRS complexes in the precordial leads are due to the fact that the chest electrodes lie in an isoelectric plane, which is perpendicular to the QRS axis.

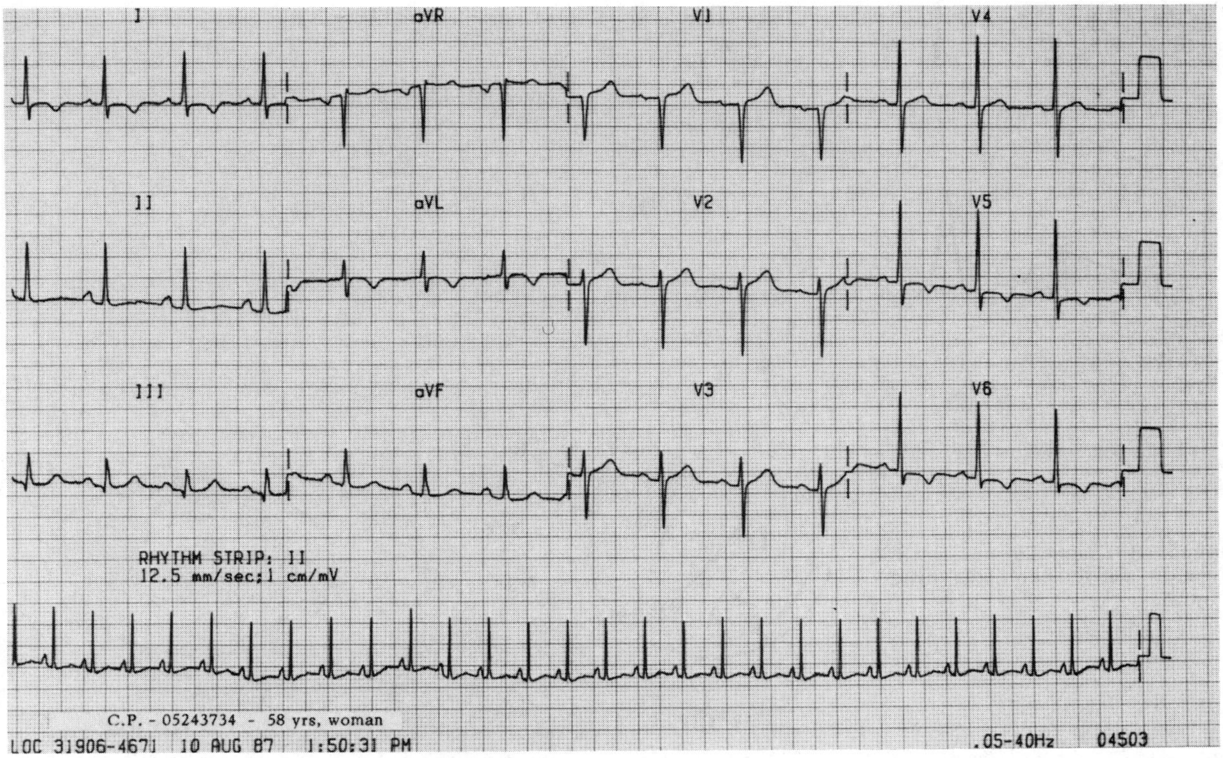

Tracing 6. Example of left ventricular strain. Axis of QRS +60 degrees. Axis of T +150 degrees. P and QRS within normal limits in the precordial leads, but there are negative T waves in V_5 and V_6.

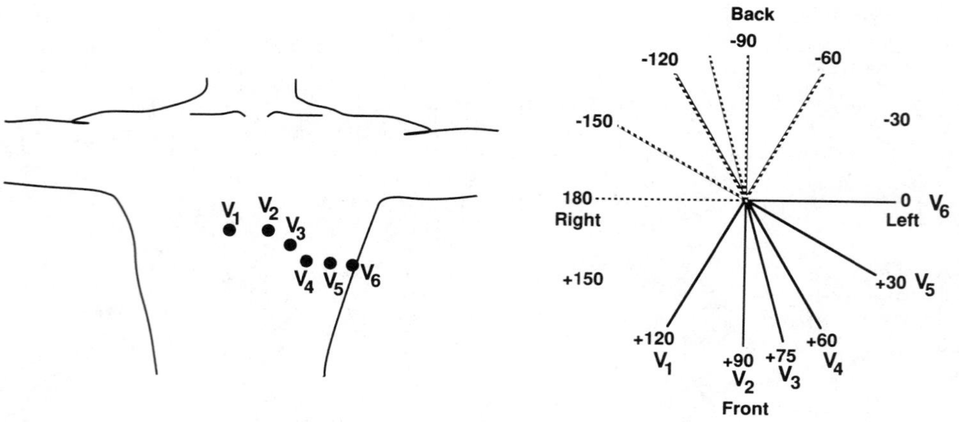

Figure 45–11. Placement of electrodes for the chest leads *(A)*, and lead system in the horizontal plane *(B)*.

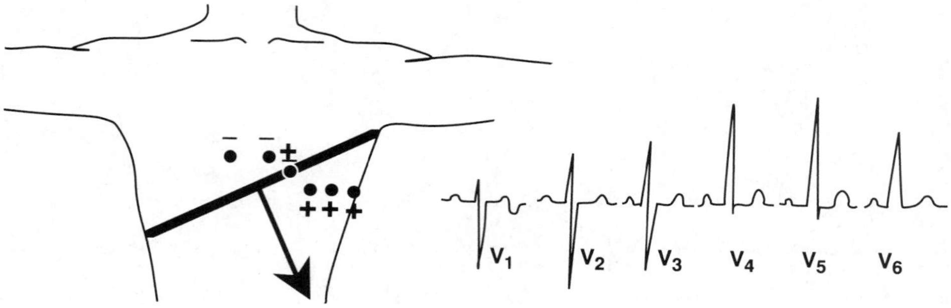

Figure 45–12. Normal configuration of P, QRS, and T in the precordial leads.

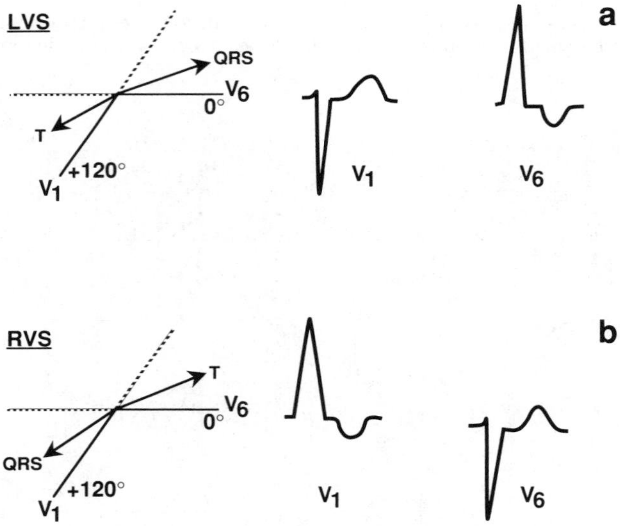

Figure 45–13. Abnormal T wave patterns in the precordial leads.

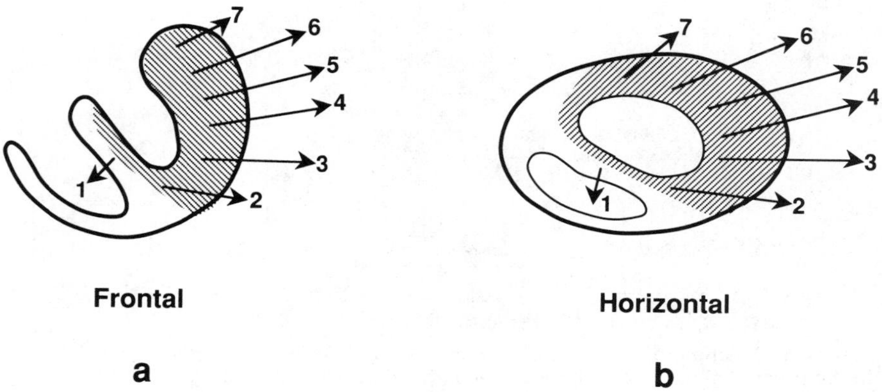

Figure 45–14. Genesis and electromotive forces in left ventricular hypertrophy.

sternal border, V_2 at the fourth intercostal space in the left sternal border, V_3 at the fifth intercostal space in the midclavicular line, V_5 at the same plane as V_4 but at the anterior axillary line, and V_6 in the same plane of V_4 at the midaxillary line.

There are several problems with the V leads that preclude accurate computations of the P, QRS, T axis in the horizontal plane.

1. Their positive side is toward the front of all leads (except V_6) and toward the left (except V_1 and V_2). Yet, the horizontal projection of the QRS axis is usually oriented toward the back and to the left, so in general the QRS axis does not lie parallel to any lead.

2. The electrical center of the heart is actually displaced to the left and to the front of the center of the transverse plane. This precludes accurate measurements of the amplitude and direction of the QRS axis.

3. Lung impedance causes decreased amplitudes in V_1, V_2, and V_6, which actually record approximately 60 per cent of the true amplitudes that would be recorded in these leads if there was no lung impedance.

4. The close proximity of the electrodes to the heart causes the amplitudes on V_3, V_4, and V_5 to be approximately 150 per cent larger than the true amplitudes that would be recorded if the electrical center of the heart coincided with the center of the transverse plane. Thus, high voltages of QRS, T, and upward ST displacement in these leads may not necessarily indicate the presence of pathology.

5. The staggered disposition of the electrodes on different planes (as shown in Figure 45–11 *A*) precludes computation of the transverse plane axis in the case of a vertical axis in the frontal plane.

PATTERN ANALYSIS OF PRECORDIAL LEADS

P Wave. Practically all V leads show a positive P (Fig. 45–12).

QRS Wave. There is a gradual increase in voltage of the R wave as it progresses from V_1 to V_5. In a normal R progression, V_2 or V_3 becomes the transitional lead (i.e., the lead that is isoelectric with a RS pattern), V_1 has a rS pattern (i.e., a small R and a large S), and V_6 has a Rs pattern (i.e., a large R and a small S) (Fig. 45–12).

T Wave. Practically all V leads show a positive T with the exception of V_1, which may be isoelectric or negative (Fig. 45–12). Negative T waves in V_1–V_3 indicate strain in the right (anterior) ventricle or in the anterior wall of the left ventricle (Fig. 45–13*A*). Negative T waves in V_4–V_6 indicate strain in the left (posterior) ventricle. This pattern is referred to as flipped Ts because normally the T waves are positive in these leads (Fig. 45–13*B*).

Left Ventricular Hypertrophy (LVH)

AXIS CHANGES

As a result of the large size of the left ventricle, there is an increased number of EMFs originating from the left (posterior) ventricle. As a result, most instantaneous EMFs point to the left and to the back (Fig. 45–14).

CRITERIA FOR DIAGNOSIS OF LVH

Frontal Plane

1. LAD or horizontal axis (except when the heart is displaced downward)

2. Magnitude of QRS in the lead of the mean axis: > 1.5 mV.

3. LVS very often present (reflecting a delay in the sequence of repolarization). The changes in the sequence of repolarization account not only for the changes in the T axis but also for the usual presence of ST displacement (opposite in direction to QRS).

- LVH + LVS—systolic overloading (as in aortic stenosis or in hypertension)
- LVH without LVS—diastolic overloading (as in aortic insufficiency or ventricular septal defect)

4. Duration of QRS: > 0.08 seconds < 0.12 seconds

Horizontal Plane

1. Posterior axis (i.e., transitional lead in V_3 or V_4). The axis may not be posterior when the heart is displaced forward.

2. High magnitude: $S_1 + R_5 > 3.5$ mV. (index of Sokolow and Lyon). This empirical index states that when the negative portion of QRS in V_1 (S_1) added to the positive portion of QRS (R) in V_5 exceeds 35 mm., the diagnosis of LVH should be considered.

3. LV strain very often (i.e., flipped T waves in V_4, V_5, and V_6). An example of LVH with left ventricular strain is shown in Tracing 7.

Right Ventricular Hypertrophy (RVH)

AXIS CHANGES

The ECG changes are quite different in infants and adults. In early infancy, the normal heart shows a relative preponderance of the right ventricle with a greater number of EMFs generated by the right ventricular mass than later on in life. As a result, the majority of QRS instantaneous forces point to the

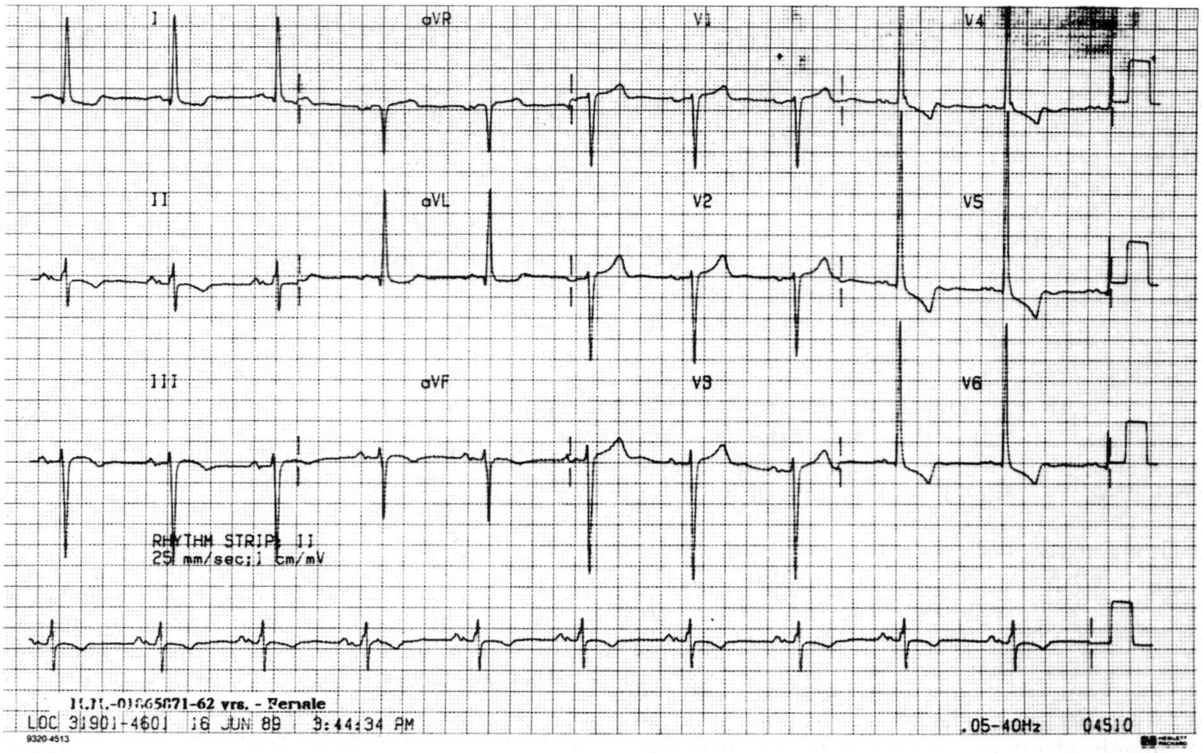

Tracing 7. Example of left ventricular hypertrophy with left ventricular strain. Axis of QRS −30 degrees in the frontal plane. Axis of T −120 degrees. The precordial leads show S1 + R5 equal 5.5 mV. Abnormal negative T waves on V_4, V_5, and V_6.

right and to the front. In the frontal plane, there is a right axis deviation. In the horizontal plane, the axis of QRS points to the right and to the front. In cases of congenital right ventricular hypertrophy, this infantile pattern persists for a long time (Fig. 45–15).

In acquired right ventricular hypertrophy, the sequence of depolarization begins in the right ventricle with preponderance of early forces pointing to the front. Subsequently, the forces point to the left because in spite of the right ventricular hypertrophy there is still a relative preponderance of the left ventricle. The terminal forces point to the right and to the front because of the late depolarization of the upper part of an enlarged right ventricle (Fig. 45–16).

CRITERIA FOR DIAGNOSIS OF RVH

Frontal Plane

1. RAD or vertical axis
2. Magnitude of QRS normal in the lead parallel to the QRS axis (exceptionally ≥ 1.5 mV.)
3. Right ventricular strain (RVS) often (especially in infants and/or with systolic overloading)
4. Normal duration of QRS

Horizontal Plane

1. Initial forces very anterior (tall R wave in V_1, i.e., $R_1 \geq 0.7$ mV.) or ($R_1/S_1 \geq 1$) and/or
2. Terminal forces to the right (deep S wave in V_6, i.e., $S_6 \geq 0.3$ mV. or greater S than R in V_6) or ($R_1 + S_5 \geq 1.0$ mV.). These terminal forces may also be displaced to the front (showing a nonslurred R′ in V_1)
3. RV strain often—i.e., negative T waves in V_1, V_2, and V_3 (especially in infants and/or with systolic overloading)
4. Normal duration of QRS

Tracing 8 shows an example of congenital RVH. An example of acquired RVH can be seen in Tracing 9.

Left Bundle Branch Block (LBBB)

AXIS CHANGES

The depolarization of the septal area proceeds from right to left, but subsequently most EMFs are generated rather slowly from the left ventricle. The right ventricle depolarizes early and rapidly, but the forces generated in the right ventricle are relatively small and counteracted by the more predominant left ventricular forces (Fig. 45–17).

CRITERIA FOR DIAGNOSIS OF LBBB

Frontal Plane

1. LAD
2. Magnitude of QRS within normal limits in the lead of mean axis (except where there is LVH also)

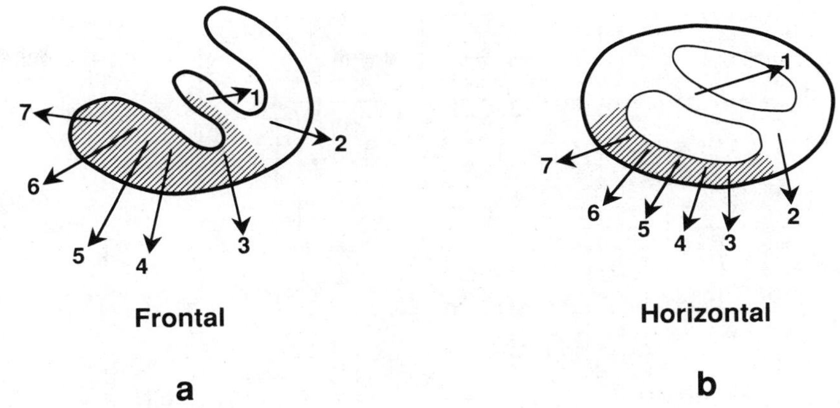

Figure 45–15. Genesis and sequence of electromotive forces of congenital right ventricular hypertrophy.

3. Left ventricular strain (LVS) very often (due to a change in the sequence of repolarization)
4. Duration of QRS > 0.12 seconds
5. Slurring of QRS in several leads

Horizontal Plane

1. Posterior axis (transitional lead at V_3 or V_4)
2. Magnitude within normal limits (except when there is LVH also)
3. LVS very often present (i.e., flipped T waves in V_4, V_5, and V_6)
4. Duration of QRS > 0.12 seconds
5. Slurring of QRS in several leads

An example of LBBB appears in Tracing 10.

Right Bundle Branch Block (RBBB)

AXIS CHANGES

The sequence of depolarization is similar to that in RVH. However, the anterior displacement of the initial forces is not as marked as in RVH and the terminal portion of depolarization occurs very slowly (Fig. 45–18).

CRITERIA FOR DIAGNOSIS OF RBBB

Frontal Plane

1. Normal or near vertical axis; horizontal axis or LAD if there is also a left anterior hemiblock
2. Low magnitude of QRS in lead parallel to mean axis (usually < 1.0 mV.)
3. RVS (may not be present)
4. Duration ≤ 0.10 seconds
5. Slurred S in lead I

Horizontal Plane

1. Posterior or undifferentiated axis
2. Low magnitude
3. RVS (may not be present)
4. Terminal forces of depolarization to the right (showing a slurred S in V_6). These terminal forces may be also displaced to the front (showing a RR′ pattern with a slurred R′ in V_1)
5. Slow speed in terminal forces (slurring of S_6 and of R′ if present)
6. Duration ≤ 0.10 seconds

An RBBB example can be seen Tracing 11.

Hemiblocks

GENERAL CONCEPTS

Normally, the conduction of impulses and the generation of QRS electromotive forces through the

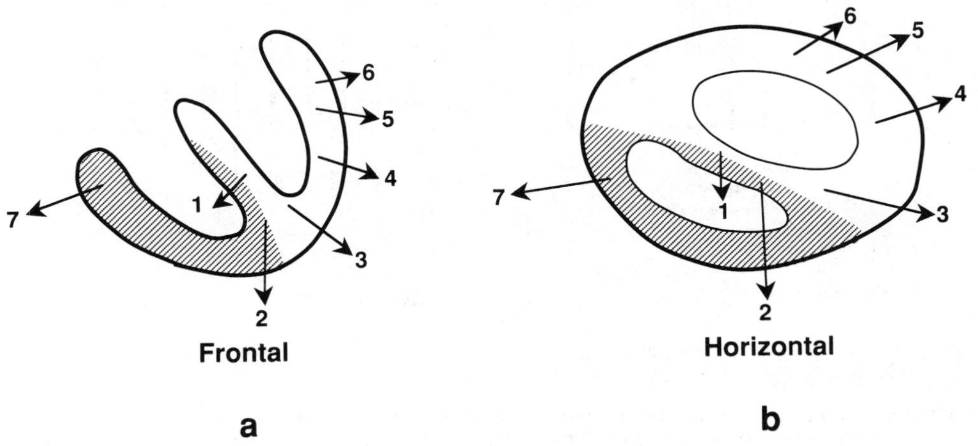

Figure 45–16. Genesis and sequence of electromotive forces in acquired right ventricular hypertrophy.

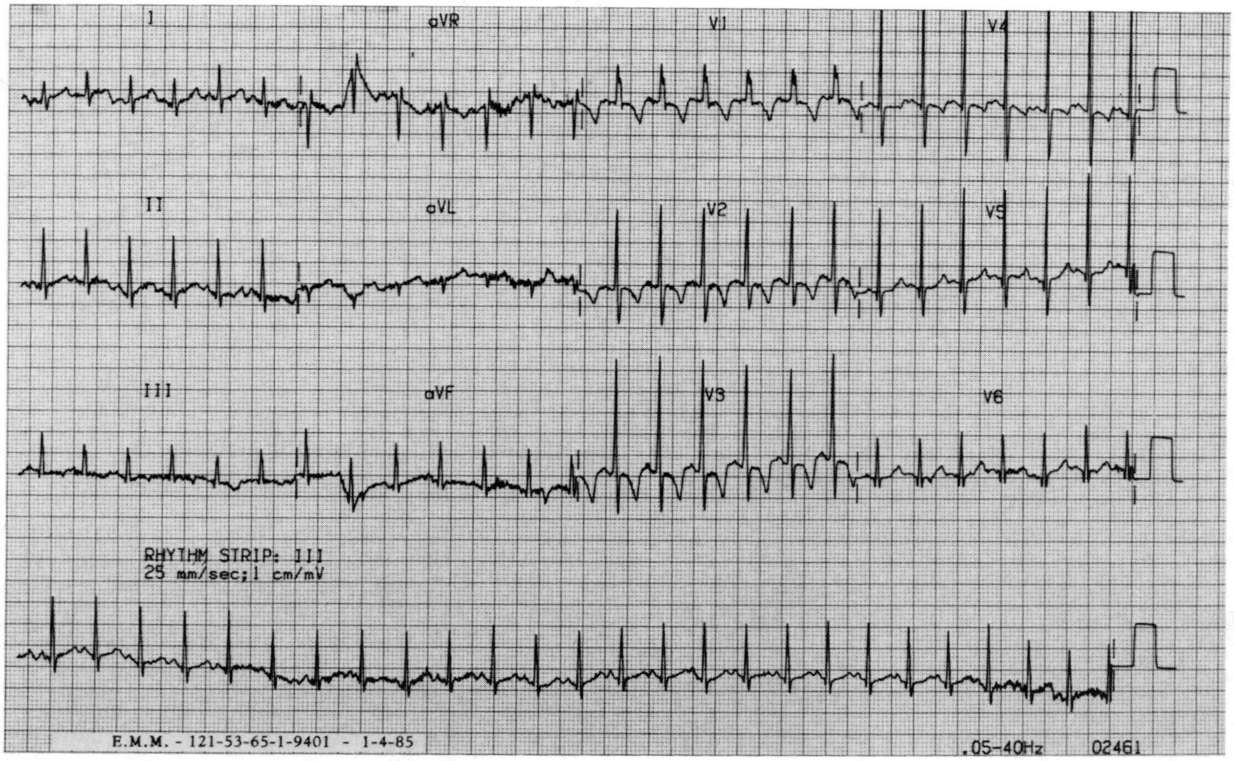

Tracing 8. Example of congenital right ventricular hypertrophy with right ventricular strain. Axis of QRS in the frontal plane +150 degrees. Axis of T +60 degrees. High voltage of R wave in V_1, V_2, and V_3. Negative T waves in V_1 to V_3.

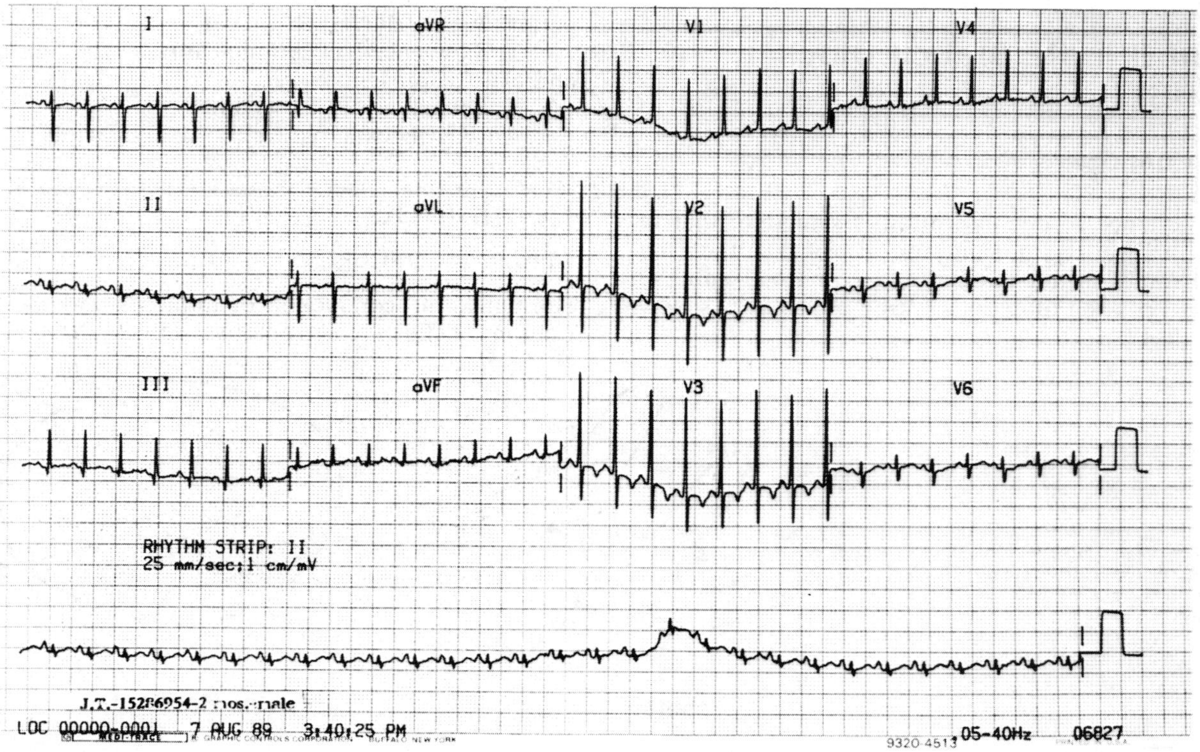

Tracing 9. Example of acquired right ventricular hypertrophy without ventricular strain. Axis of QRS +60 degrees. Axis of T +45 degrees. High voltage of R wave and V_1 to V_3. The electrode for V_4 was placed on the right side of the chest.

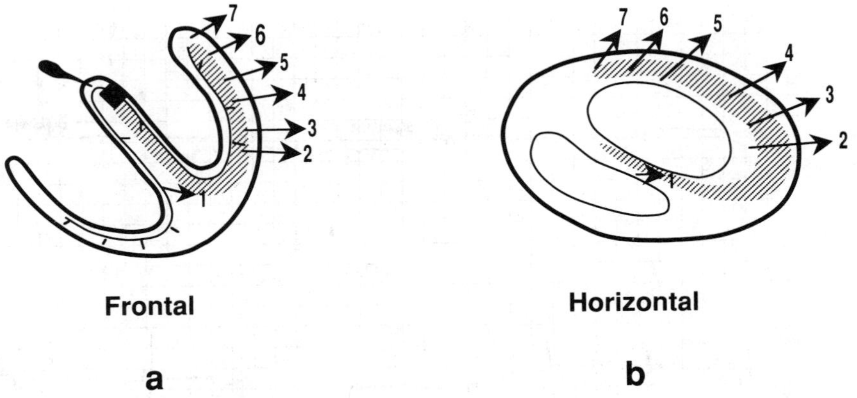

Figure 45–17. Genesis and sequence of electromotive forces in left bundle branch block.

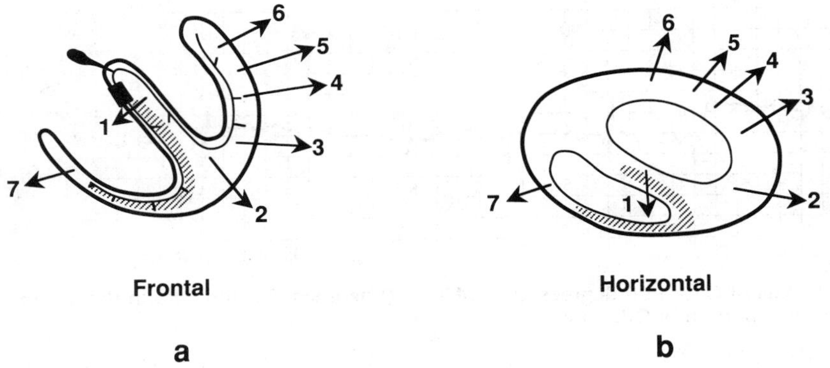

Figure 45–18. Genesis and sequence of electromotive forces in right bundle branch block.

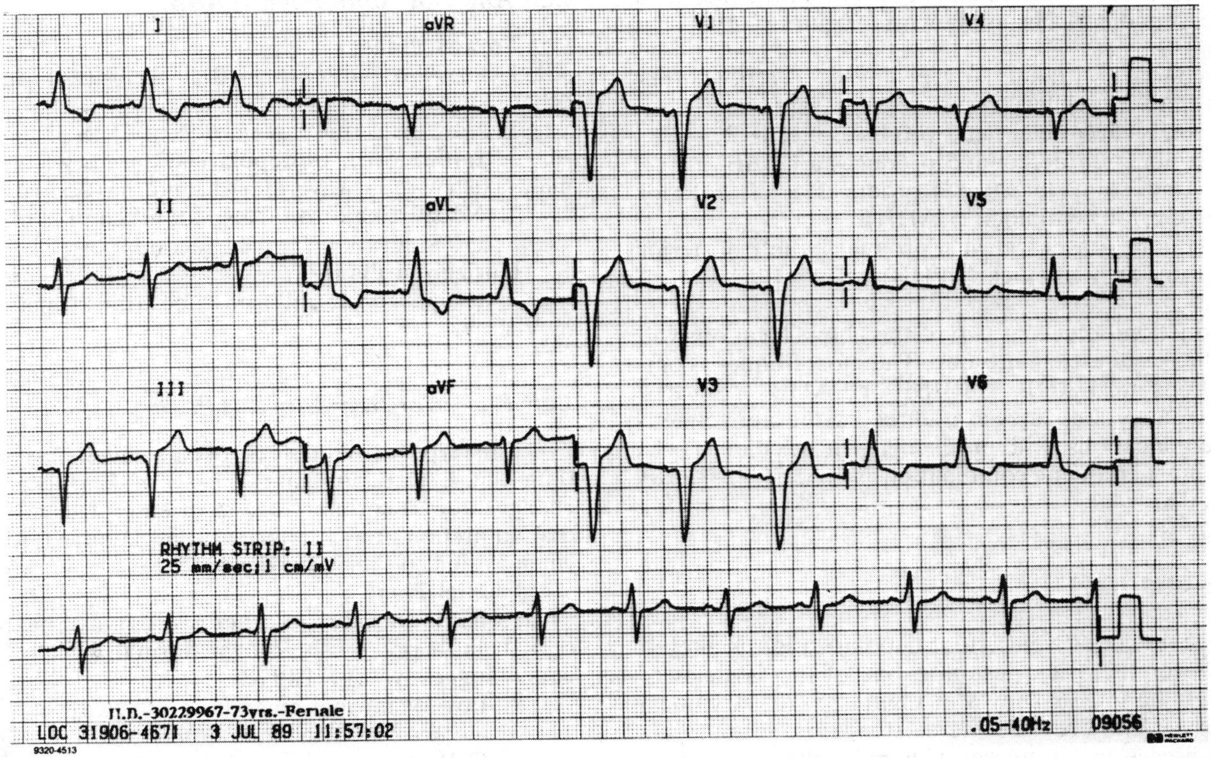

Tracing 10. Example of left bundle branch block. Axis of QRS in the frontal plane −30 degrees. Axis of T −140 degrees (left ventricular strain). Poor R progression in the horizontal plane. There are slurred and wide QRS complexes in all leads.

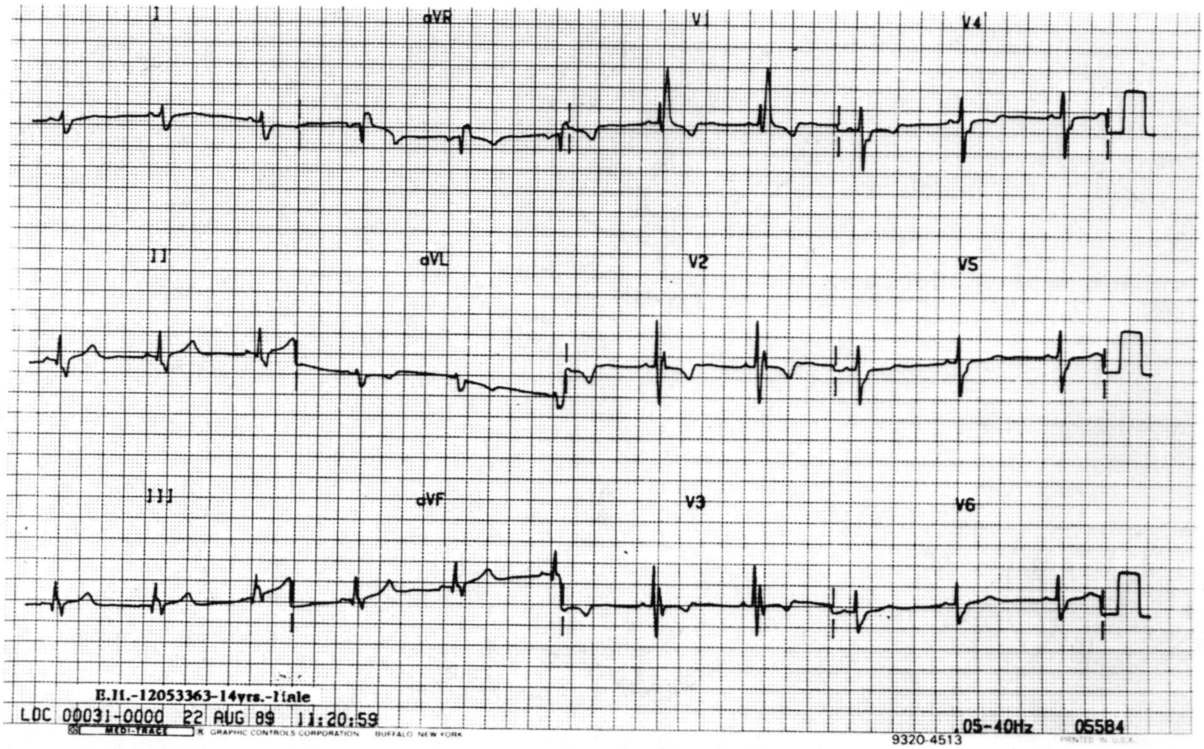

Tracing 11. Example of right bundle branch block. Axis of QRS +90 degrees. Axis of T +70 degrees. Slurred QRS in the frontal plane. There is a R-R′ in V_1 and slurring of the terminal portion of QRS in V_6.

bundle of His and its branches occur as shown in Figure 45–19*A*. Conduction disturbances may occur as a result of a lesion in one or several of the locations of the bundle of His as shown in Figure 45–19*B*.

- A conduction defect at 1 produces an atrioventricular block (AVB).
- A conduction defect at 2 produces a RBBB.
- A conduction defect at 3 produces a LBBB.
- A conduction defect at 4 produces a left anterior or superior hemiblock (LAHB).
- A conduction defect at 5 produces a left posterior or inferior hemiblock (LPHB).

Conduction defects at two of the above locations will produce a bifascicular block. The most frequent combinations are LAHB + RBBB or LAHB + AVB.

Conduction defects at three of the above-mentioned locations will produce a trifascicular block. The most frequent combination is LAHB + RBBB + AVB.

AXIS CHANGES

The sequence of ventricular depolarization is altered whenever there is a lesion in one of the fascicles of the left bundle as shown in Figure 45–20. A clinical history usually reveals the existence of coronary artery disease in most cases of hemiblock.

CRITERIA FOR DIAGNOSIS

Left Anterior Hemiblock (LAHB)

Frontal Plane

1. LAD of at least −30 degrees (not due to other causes)
2. Low or normal magnitude of QRS
3. Initial forces of depolarization away from the main axis (with Q wave in aVL and maybe in I)
4. No slurring or only a small notch in lead aVL
5. QRS duration: ≤ 0.12 seconds

Horizontal Plane

1. Usually posterior axis (i.e., transitional lead in V_3)

Left Posterior Hemiblock (LPHB)

This type of hemiblock occurs much less often than the LAHB. As in the case of LAHB, ECG changes due to coronary artery disease or to myocardial infarction may be present in addition to the changes due to the fascicular block.

Frontal Plane

1. RAD (not due to other causes); a shift to the right from a previously known normal direction (or LAD) suggestive of a LPHB
2. Low or normal magnitude of QRS
3. No slurring or a small notch
4. QRS duration: ≤ 0.12 seconds

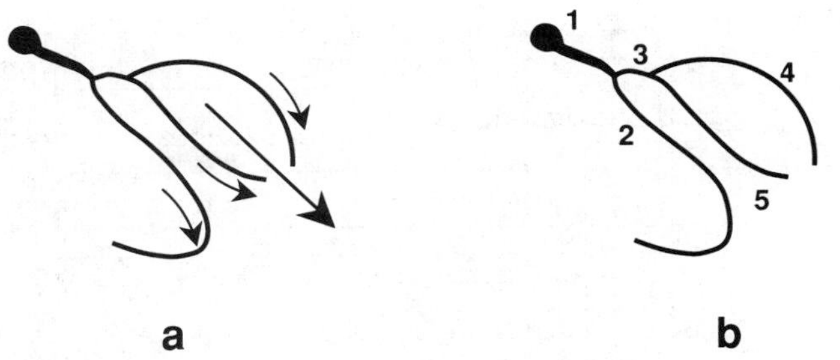

Figure 45–19. Normal conduction of electromotive forces in the ventricles and subdivision of the bundle of His (1, AV junction; 2, right bundle branch; 3, left bundle branch; 4, left anterior fascicle; 5, left posterior fascicle).

Horizontal Plane

1. ECG changes typical of the coronary artery disease or myocardial infarction that produced the hemiblock

Tracings 12–15 show examples of LAHB, LPHB, bifascicular block, and trifascicular block, respectively.

Right Atrial Enlargement (P-Pulmonale or RAE)

AXIS CHANGES

As a result of the increased size of the right atrium, most EMFs originate in that atrium and proceed in a slightly more rightward direction than normal (Fig. 45–21).

CRITERIA FOR DIAGNOSIS OF RAE

1. Direction of the axis of P is vertical, almost vertical, or deviated to the right (small P in I and negative P in aVL)
2. Magnitude ≥ 0.25 mV. (peaked P wave in II)
3. Duration of P < 0.08 seconds

Criteria based on the relative duration of P/PR are not reliable.

Tracing 16 shows an example of RAE (P-pulmonale) and chronic obstructive pulmonary disease.

Left Atrial Enlargement (P Mitrale or LAE)

AXIS CHANGES

The increased size of the left atrium causes a shift of late EMFs to the left, but the normal forces of depolarization of the right atrium occur earlier and in the normal direction. This explains the existence of two P waves. The first is due to depolarization of the right atrium and the second to depolarization of the left atrium. The P wave in several of the standard limb leads shows a double hump pattern (Fig. 45–22).

In patients with diffuse myocardial damage of the left atrium (as in atherosclerotic cardiovascular disease), the depolarization progresses slowly, first to the right atrium and then to the left. As a result, the P wave is broad, small, and has a double hump resembling a P mitrale. Since the problem here is not hypertrophy but delayed depolarization through a damaged myocardium, the preferred term is left atrial abnormality (LAA).

CRITERIA FOR DIAGNOSIS OF LAE OR LAA

1. There are usually two small axes of P, the first in the normal direction of about +60 degrees and the second (and often smaller) 30 to 60 degrees to the left of the first. This causes a double-humped P wave in lead II. In the horizontal plane, the two axes of P may produce a biphasic P wave in V_1.
2. The highest magnitude of either one of the two P waves is 2.5 mm. (0.25 mV.). In cases of LAA, the magnitude is very small.
3. Duration of P is usually > 0.08 seconds

A LAE (P-mitrale) example can be found in Tracing 17.

Changes Due to Chronic Obstructive Pulmonary Disease (COPD)

As a result of COPD, there is an increase in the volume of air contained in the lungs. This creates a

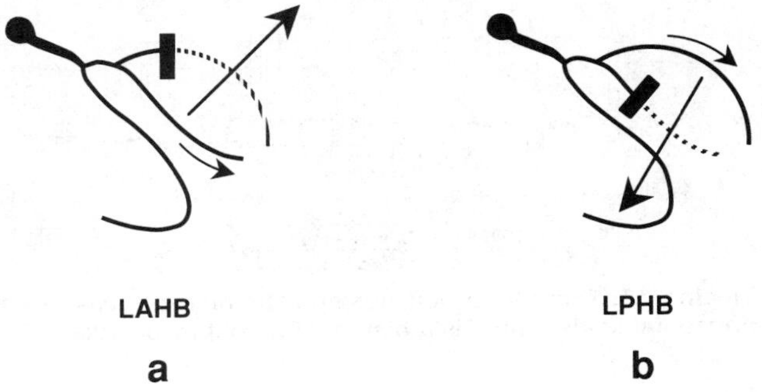

Figure 45–20. Axis deviation in hemiblocks.

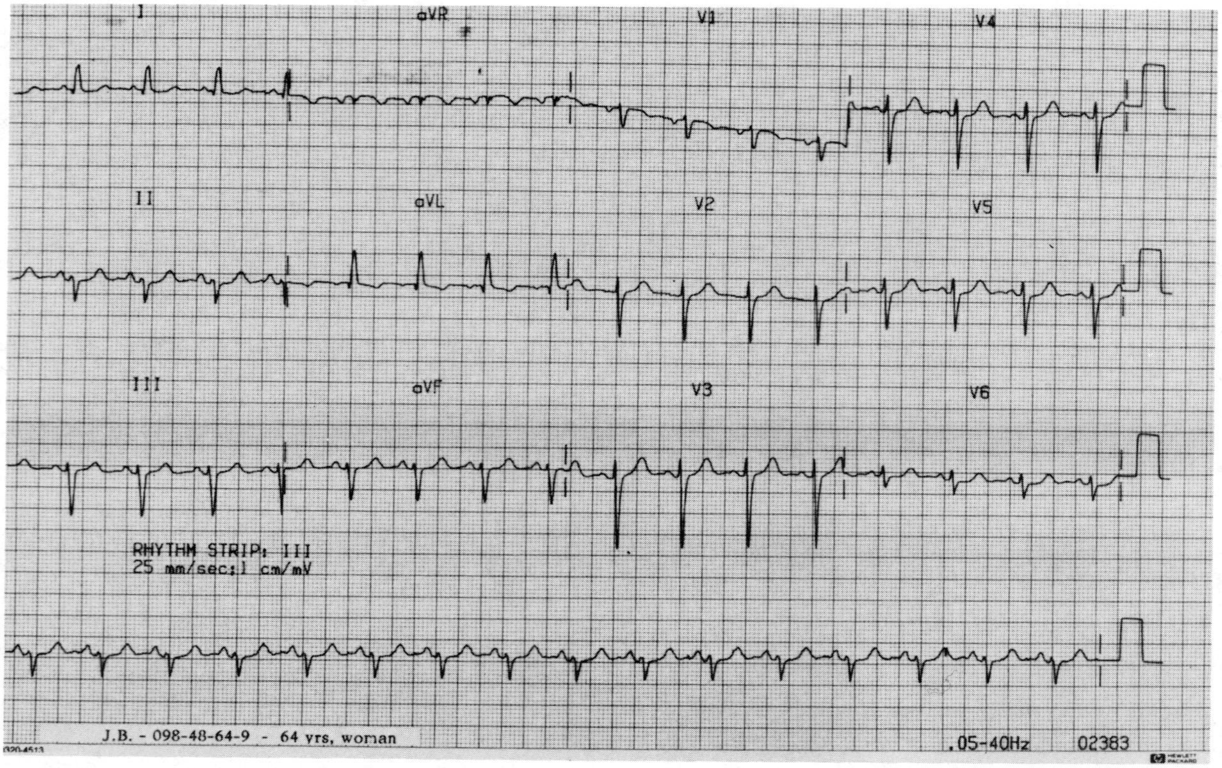

Tracing 12. Example of left anterior hemiblock. Axis of QRS in the frontal plane −50 degrees. Axis of T +65 degrees. The QRS complexes are not wide. There is a small Q and leads I and aVL.

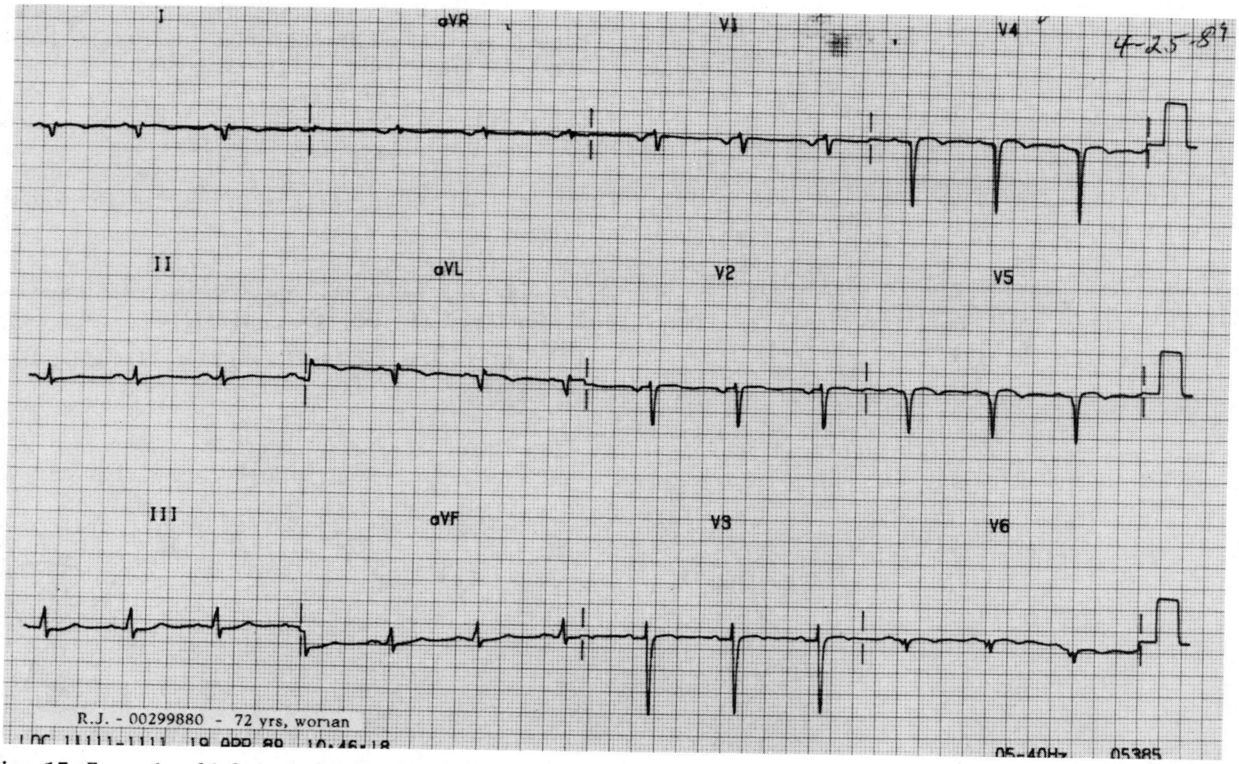

Tracing 13. Example of left posterior hemiblock. Axis of QRS +120 degrees. Axis of T +120 degrees. Poor R progression in horizontal leads. There is a history of an old myocardial infarction that affected the left posterior fascicle.

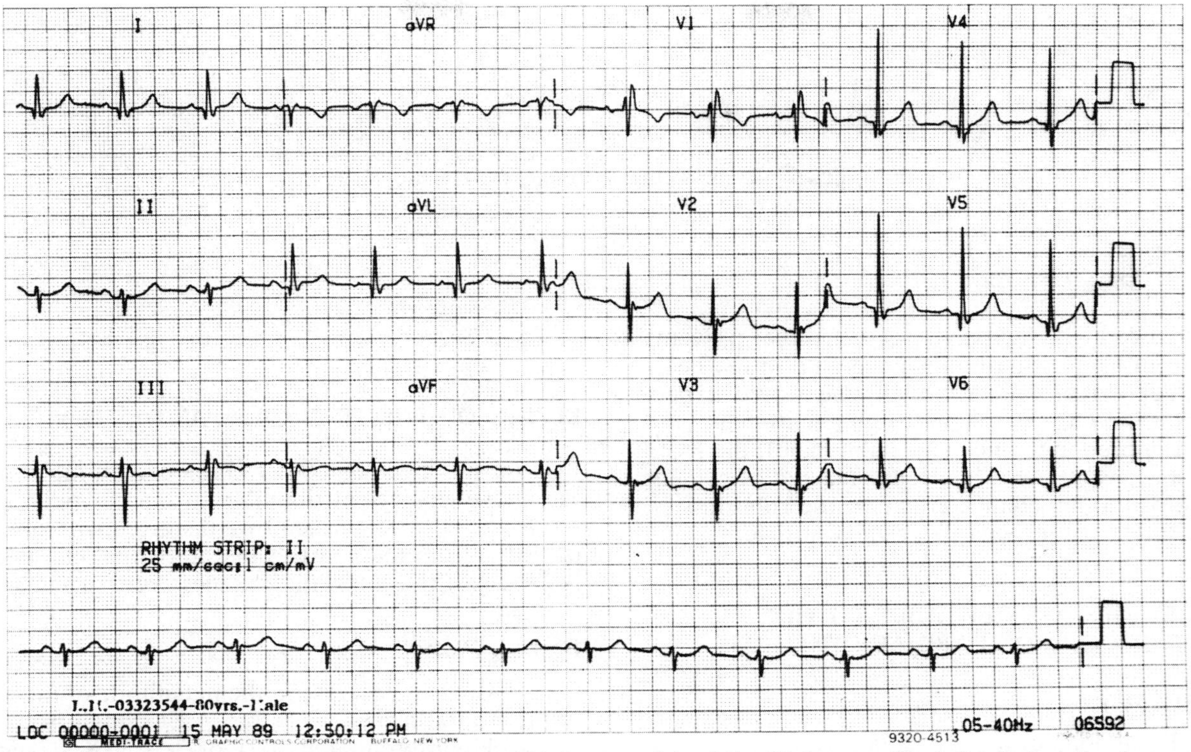

Tracing 14. Example of bifascicular block. Axis of QRS −40 degrees. Axis of T +15 degrees. The left axis deviation is suggestive of left anterior hemiblock. The R-R′ on V_1 and the slurring of QRS in V_6 are indicative of a right bundle branch block.

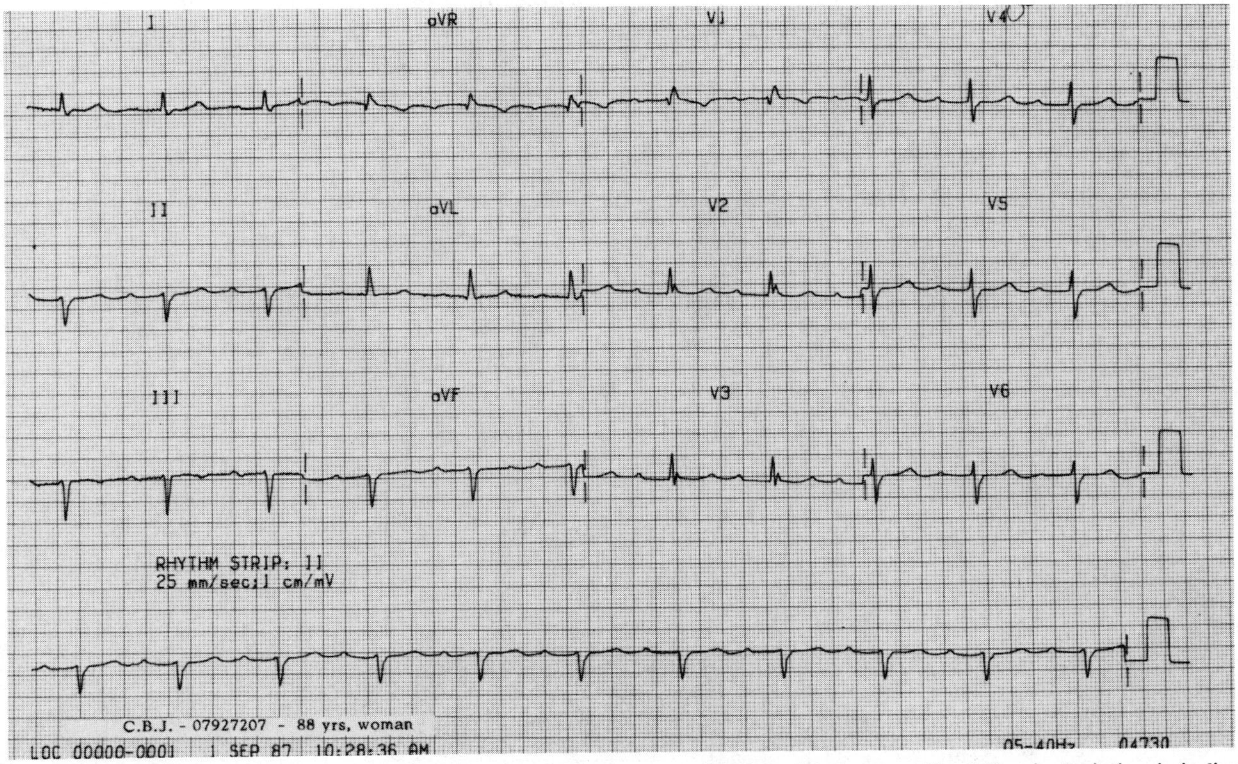

Tracing 15. Example of trifascicular block. Axis of QRS −70 degrees. Axis of T +30 degrees. The left axis deviation is indicative of a left anterior hemiblock. The precordial leads show right bundle branch block. The rhythm strip shows a PR interval of 0.36 seconds, indicative of a first-degree AV block.

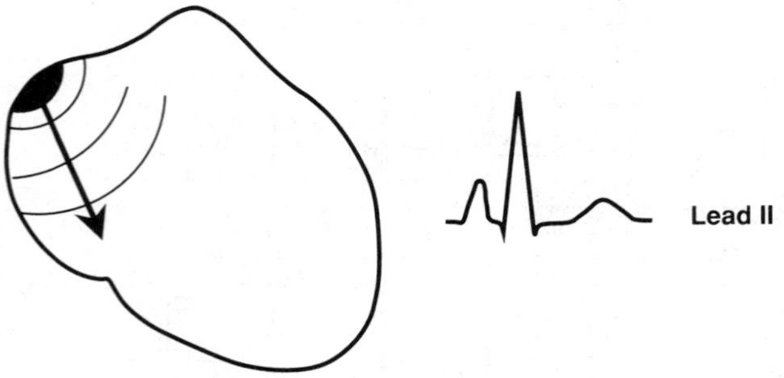

Figure 45–21. Genesis and sequence of electromotive forces in right atrial enlargement.

large area of high electrical impedance that prevents the transmission of the EMFs generated in the heart during depolarization. Although one would expect patients with COPD to have right ventricular and right atrial preponderance (cor pulmonale), the ECG manifestations of such a syndrome may not be evident because of the impedance effect on the transmission of the EMF from an enlarged right ventricle.

ECG CHANGES ATTRIBUTABLE TO THE EFFECT OF COPD ON CARDIAC DYNAMICS

Frontal Plane

1. P-pulmonale
2. Vertical axis deviation or RAD
3. RVS

Horizontal Plane

1. Usually undifferentiated axis
2. The late forces of depolarization point to the right (i.e., a deep S wave on V_6, not slurred)

See Tracing 16 for an example.

EFFECT ON THE TRANSMISSION OF EMFs

Due to the effect of COPD on electrical impedance, the above changes attributable to the cor pulmonale syndrome may be masked by a distorted transmission of EMFs from the heart to the precordial electrodes. As a result, the following changes are noticeable.

Frontal Plane

1. Overall decrease in the magnitude of the QRS in the frontal plane
2. Undifferentiated axis or left axis deviation that mimics a LAHB

The presence of a P-pulmonale and the clinical history help to establish the diagnosis of COPD.

Horizontal Plane

1. Decrease in the magnitude of QRS
2. Absence of the anteriorly displaced initial

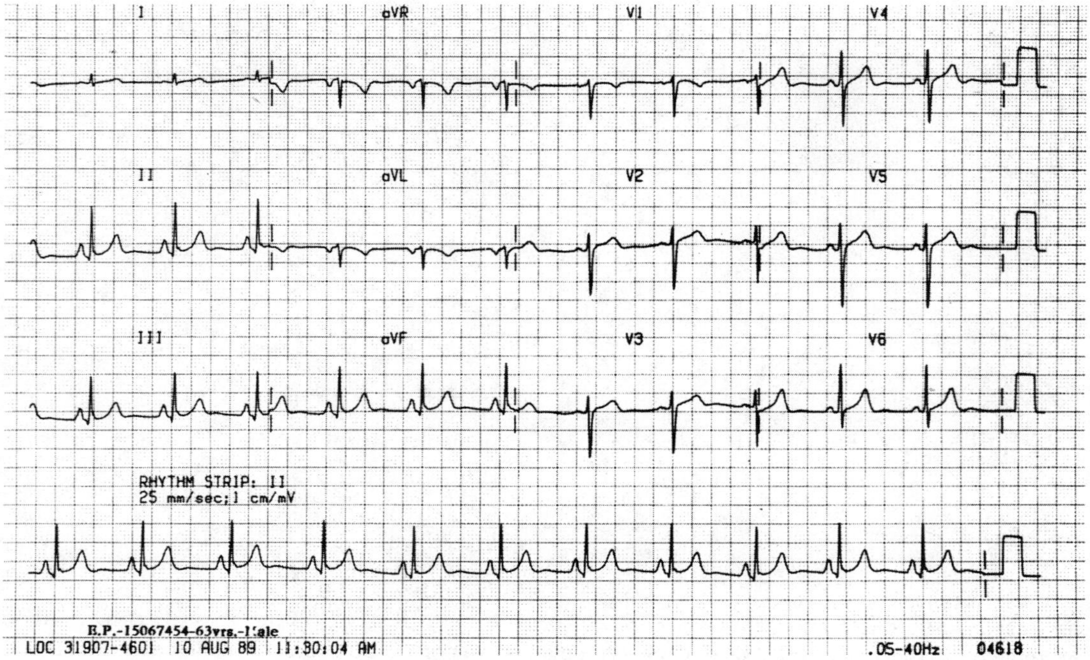

Tracing 16. Example of right atrial enlargement (P-pulmonale) and COPD. Very tall P wave on lead II, and vertical axis. Axis of QRS +85 degrees. Axis of T +75 degrees. The poor R progression in the precordial leads mimics an old anterior wall MI.

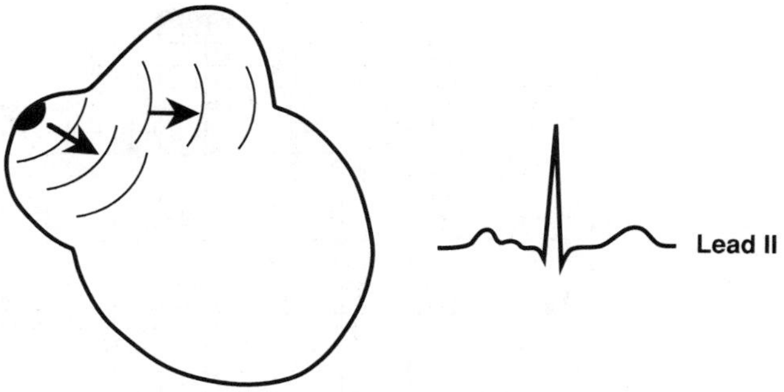

Figure 45–22. Genesis and sequence of electromotive forces in left atrial enlargement.

forces of depolarization (poor R progression). This situation mimics an old anterior wall myocardial infarction, but the presence of a P-pulmonale and the clinical history help to establish the diagnosis of COPD.

Tracing 18 shows an example of COPD LAD mimicking a LAH.

Changes Due to Myocardial Infarction (MI)

AXIS CHANGES

The pathologic changes that occur in the myocardium as a result of a MI produce characteristic changes in the QRS, ST, and T waves. The following are the important ECG components that help to diagnose MI.

1. *Initial forces of QRS* (first 0.04 seconds of the QRS complex). These forces point *away* from the *dead zone* because no EMFs are generated in the dead area. The presence of significant Q waves provides information on the direction of the initial QRS forces.

2. *Axis of ST.* This axis can be determined in the same way as other axes, i.e., by finding a lead with an isoelectric ST. Its axis points *toward* the area of *injury*.

3. *Axis of T.* This axis points *away* from the area of *ischemia* (ECG pattern of strain).

Figure 45–23 shows the effect of the three basic types of pathology on the QRS, ST, and T components of ventricular electrical activity.

Clinical information is essential for an accurate diagnosis.

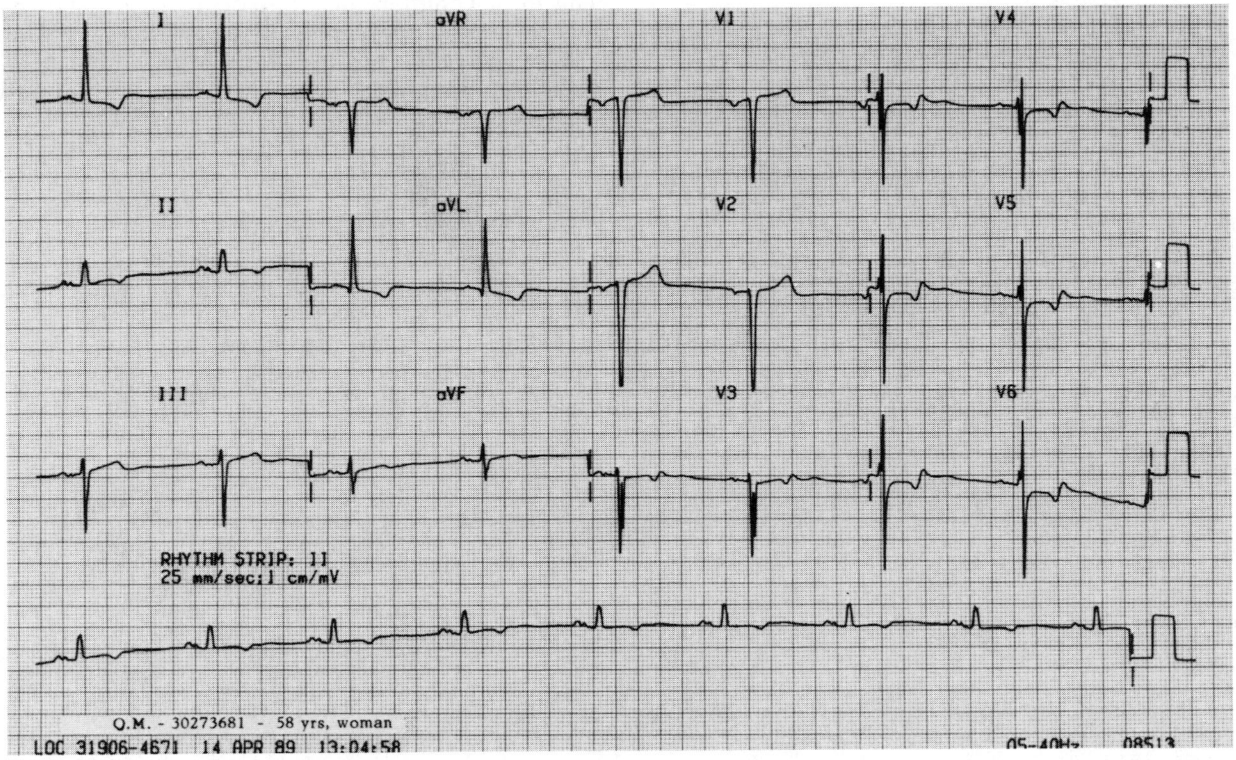

Tracing 17. Example of left atrial enlargement (P-mitrale). Axis of QRS 0 degrees. Axis of T +180 degrees. Double humped P wave in leads II and III. Poor R progression in the precordial leads with conduction defect (notches on V_3 and V_4).

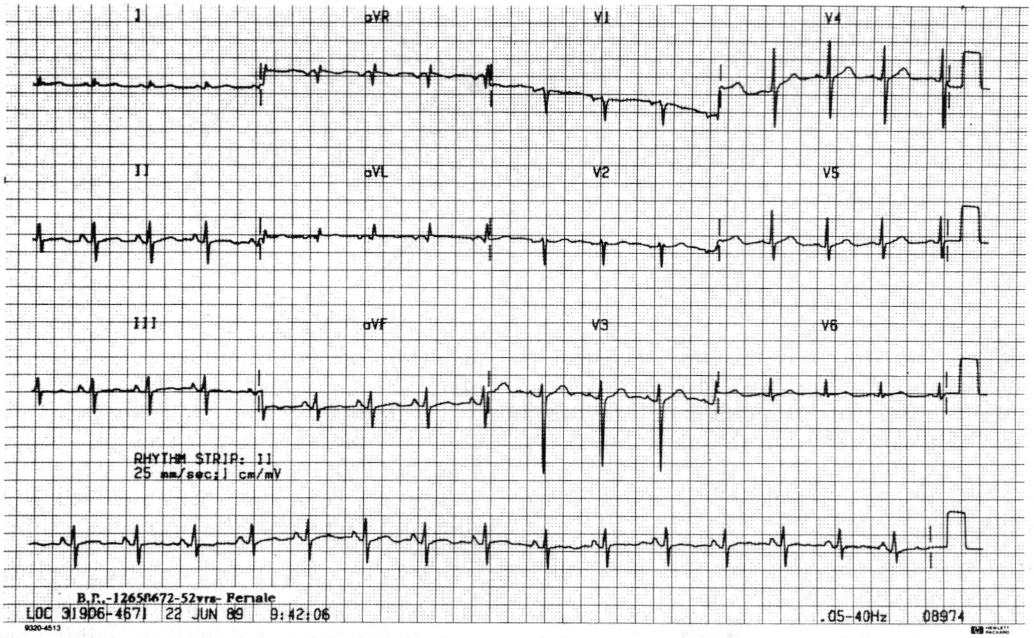

Tracing 18. Example of a COPD with left axis deviation mimicking a left anterior hemiblock. There is a P-pulmonale. The poor R progression in the precordial leads mimicks an old anterior wall MI but is due to the impedance produced by the expanded lungs.

EVOLUTION OF THE AXIS CHANGES

At each stage in the evolution of an infarction (acute, subacute, and post or old MI), there are prominent ECG changes that are characteristic. The diagram of Figure 45–24 indicates the relative prevalence of changes in each stage.

CRITERIA FOR THE DIAGNOSIS OF THE STAGE OF MI

Acute stage (0–4 weeks)

1. A prominent ST displacement (up or down) is noted.
2. Deep and wide Q waves may be present in leads that do not normally have Q waves.

Subacute stage (5–8 weeks)

1. A prominent negative T is present in the leads with a positive QRS (strain pattern).
2. Deep and wide Q waves may be present.

Old MI (> 8 weeks)

1. Deep and wide Q waves are noted.
2. Slurring in S waves may be noted.

COMMON LOCATIONS OF MI

The most common locations of a MI are shown in Figure 45–25. In this figure, the ventricles are drawn like a cone with a single chamber whose anterior wall includes the septum. The free anterior portion of the right ventricular wall is seldom the site of a localized infarction.

1. Anterior or anteroseptal—due to an occlusion of the left anterior descending artery
2. Anterolateral or anterobasal or superior—due to an occlusion of the circumflex artery
3. Apical—due to an occlusion of the terminal portion of the left anterior descending artery
4. Posterior—due to an occlusion of the right coronary artery (or one of its branches); may affect the SA and AV nodes and cause dysrhythmia

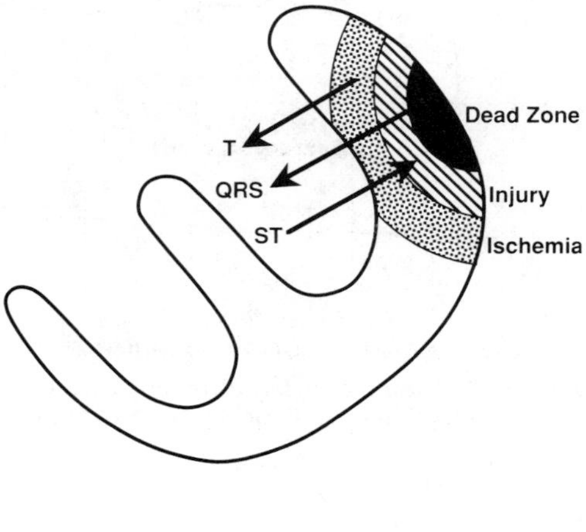

Figure 45–23. Relationship between the ECG and pathologic changes in myocardial infarction.

Stage of M.I.		Initial QRS	ST	T
Acute	(0-4 wks)	±	++	±
Subacute	(4-8 wks)	±	±	++
Post M.I.	(> 8 wks)	++	−−	±

(-) not present (±) may be present (+) apparent (++) very apparent

Figure 45–24. Evolution of ECG changes at various stages of myocardial infarction.

5. Inferior or diaphragmatic—due to an occlusion of the dominant right coronary artery or dominant left. If it results from an occlusion of the right, it may affect the SA and AV nodes and cause dysrhythmia.

CRITERIA FOR DIAGNOSIS OF THE LOCATION OF MI

General

- Significant Q: ≥ 0.04 seconds in duration *and* one-third height of QRS
- Significant ST: ≥ 2 mm. (0.2 mV.)
- Significant T—inverted in leads with positive QRS (ventricular strain), with a deep symmetrical shape of the inversion

Anterior or Anteroseptal

- ST positive in the first or anterior V leads (acute)
- T negative in the first V leads (subacute)
- QS pattern in V_1 and V_2, i.e., poor R progression (old)

See Tracings 19 and 20 for examples of acute and subacute anterior wall MI.

Anterolateral or Superior

- ST negative in the inferior lead aVF (acute)
- T positive in III and possibly in aVL (subacute)
- Q in the lateral leads I and aVL (old)

An example of an acute anterolateral MI is shown in Tracing 21.

Apical

- ST positive in I (acute)
- T negative in I (subacute)
- Q in I (old)

Posterior

- ST negative in the first or anterior V leads (acute)
- T positive in the first V leads (subacute)
- R prominent in the first or anterior V leads (old)

An example of an acute posterior wall MI is shown in Tracing 22.

Inferior or Diaphragmatic

- ST positive in the so-called inferior leads, II, III, and aVF (acute)
- T negative in II, III, and aVF (subacute)
- Q in II, III, and aVF (old)

Tracings 23 and 24 show examples of an old inferior wall MI.

Causes of ST Displacement

In addition to myocardial infarction, there are other conditions that may produce a measurable ST displacement.

PERICARDITIS

As a result of the inflammation of the pericardial sac, there is a small current of injury in the subepicardial

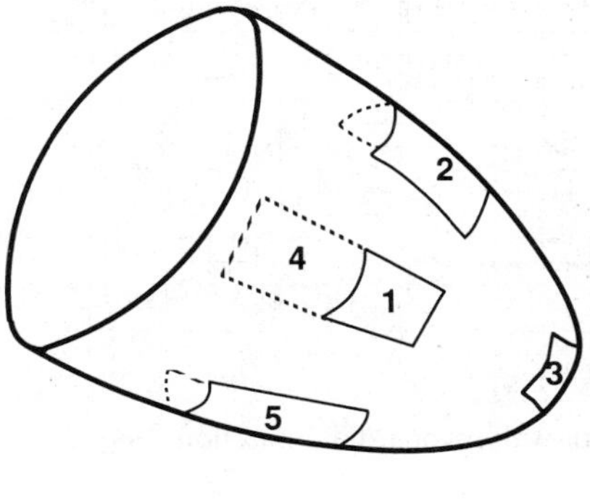

1. Anterior or Anteroseptal
2. Anterolateral or Anterobasal or Superior
3. Apical
4. Posterior
5. Inferior--Diaphragmatic

Figure 45–25. Common locations of myocardial infarction.

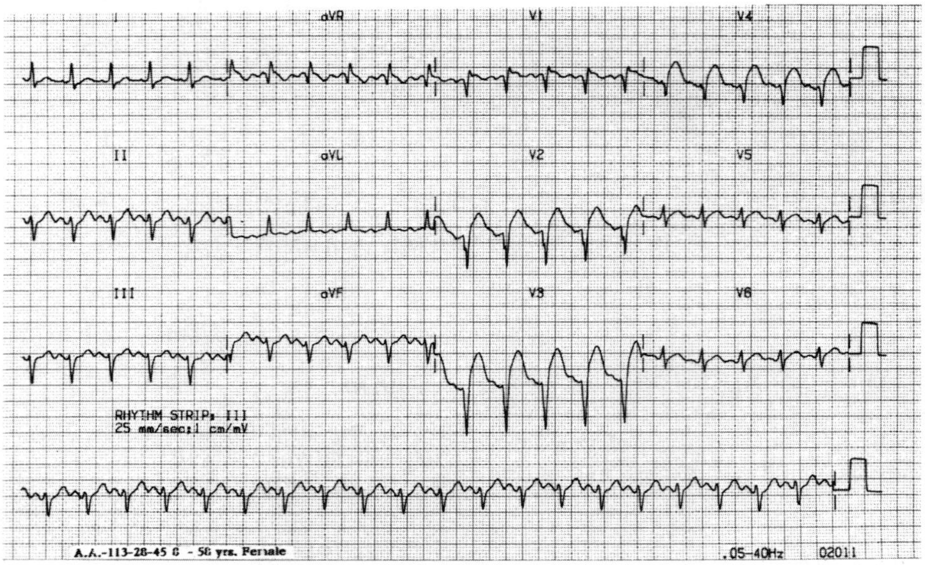

Tracing 19. Example of an acute anterior wall myocardial infarction. ST elevated in V_1–V_4. Poor R progression.

area that is oriented toward the front. This current causes a ST displacement with an axis that points downward and forward (i.e., toward the anterior wall of the ventricles).

Criteria for Diagnosis

1. Displacement of ST ≥ 2 mm. (0.2 mV.)
2. Axis of ST almost in the same direction of the QRS axis in the frontal plane (ST elevated in leads where QRS is positive)
3. Axis of ST anterior in the horizontal plane (ST elevated in anterior V leads)
4. Age of patient—often younger than in cases of MI
5. Evolution:

- ST displacement disappears within 1 to 2 weeks from onset of illness
- Usually there is no vector of ischemia (strain)
- There is no vector of dead zone (Q waves)

An acute pericarditis example can be seen in Tracing 25.

ISCHEMIA OF EXERCISE AND SUBENDOCARDIAL ISCHEMIA

During exercise, patients with coronary artery disease may develop acute insufficiency of coronary blood flow (ischemia), and this is reflected in a significant ST displacement. The mechanism for this displacement may be a difference in the sequence of repolar-

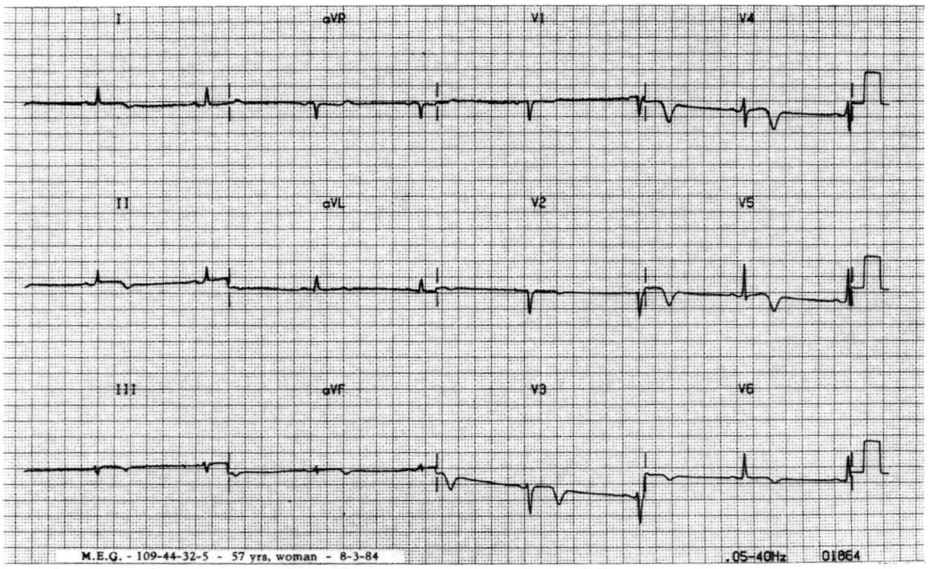

Tracing 20. Example of a subacute anterior wall myocardial infarction. Negative T waves. Poor R progression.

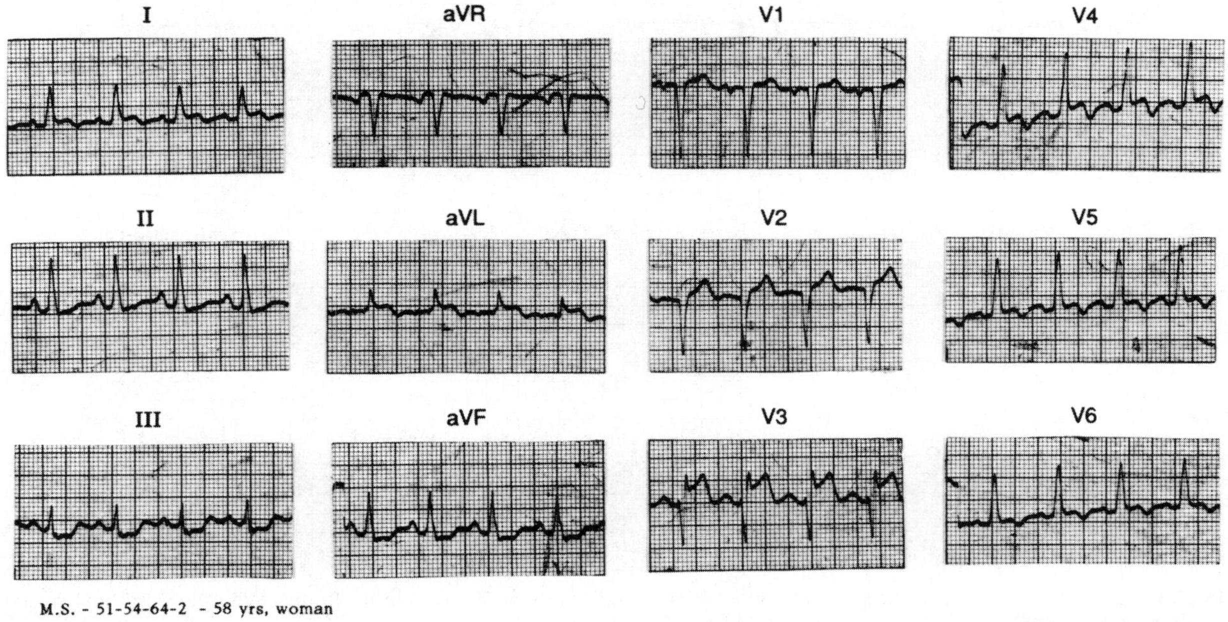

Tracing 21. Example of an acute anterolateral (superior) myocardial infarction. ST is elevated in leads I, aVL, and in the precordial leads. Poor R progression.

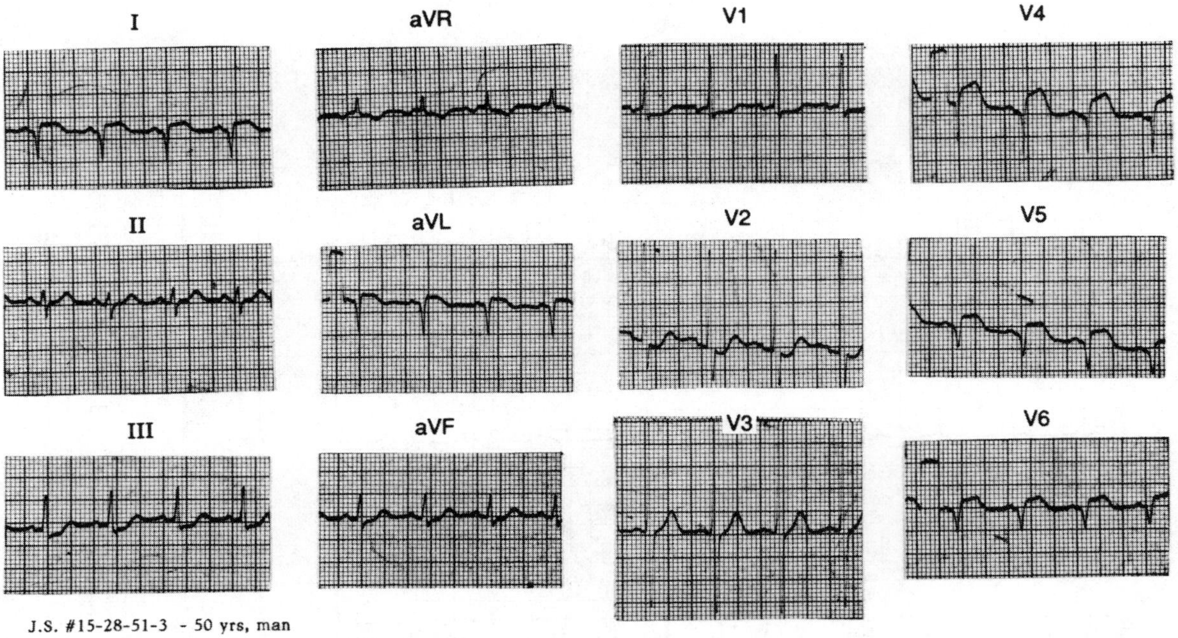

Tracing 22. Example of posterior wall myocardial infarction. Tall R wave and ST depression is shown in V_1 and V_2. QS waves and ST elevation are shown in V_3 to V_6.

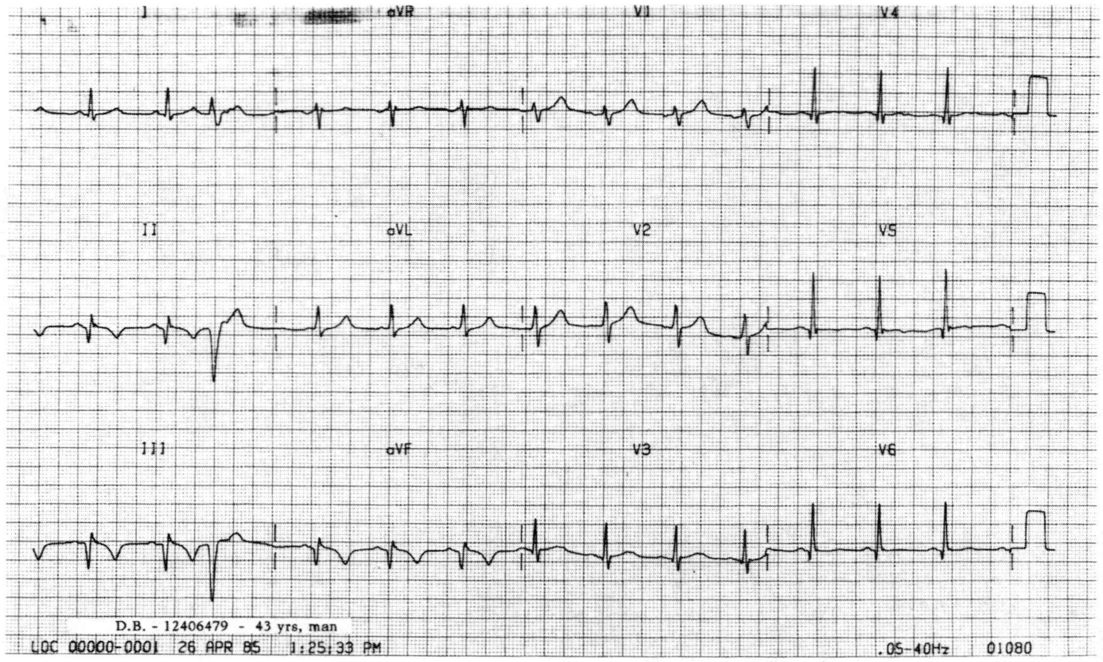

Tracing 23. Example of a subacute inferior wall myocardial infarction. Deep Q waves in II, III, and aVF. The third beat on leads I, II, and III is a VPB. Negative T waves in II, III, and aVF.

ization between the subendocardial and the subepicardial area. The diagram of Figure 45–26 shows the nonischemic and ischemic patterns of ST displacement during exercise.

The presence of a ST ischemic pattern in an ECG obtained at rest suggests the existence of subendocardial ischemia. LVH or LBBB may cause a ST displacement not due to ischemia.

Criteria for Diagnosis

1. Displacement of ST ≥ 2 mm. (0.2 mV.) lasting ≥ 0.08 seconds

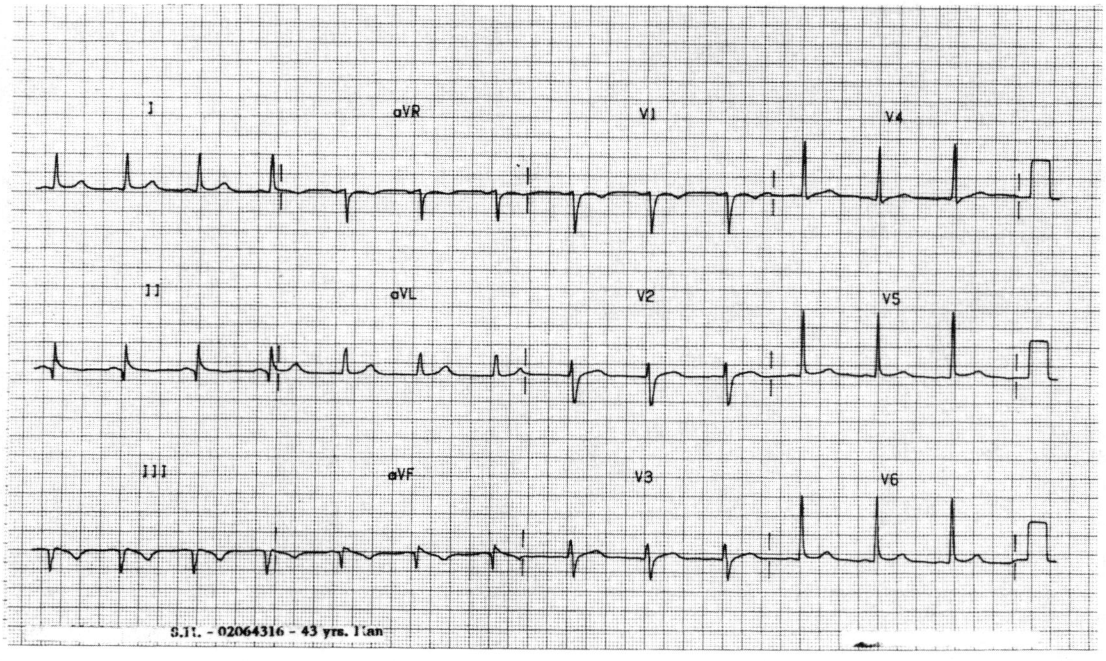

Tracing 24. Example of an old inferior wall myocardial infarction. Deep Q waves in II, III, and aVF.

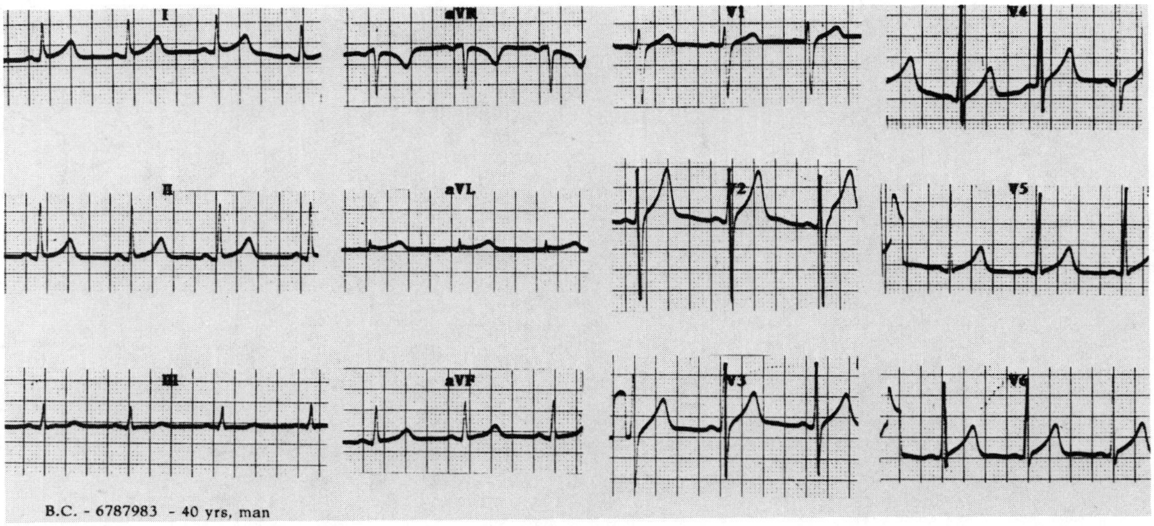

Tracing 25. Example of acute pericarditis. Small ST elevation is shown in all leads except in aVR and III.

2. Axis of ST in opposite direction of the QRS axis in the frontal plane (ST depressed in the leads where QRS is positive)

3. Axis of ST in opposite direction of QRS in the horizontal plane (ST depressed in V_4–V_6)

EARLY REPOLARIZATION

In some healthy persons, there may be a difference in the sequence of repolarization between the subepicardial and subendocardial areas. As a result, there is a ST displacement that apparently does not have any clinical significance.

Criteria for Diagnosis

1. Small elevation of ST < 2 mm. (0.2 mV.)
2. Axis of ST in almost the same direction of QRS in the frontal plane (ST elevated in the leads where QRS is positive)
3. ST elevated in anterior V leads (V_1–V_3)
4. Age—often young persons with a slow heart rate
5. No clinical manifestations of pericarditis

An example of early repolarization syndrome is shown in Tracing 26.

DIGITALIS

Digitalis usually speeds up the repolarization process (short QT time), but the effect is slightly different in the subepicardial and in the subendocardial areas. The difference accounts for the ST displacement.

Criteria for Diagnosis

1. Small ST depression usually ≤ 2 mm. (0.2 mV.) with downsloping and coving in leads with a positive QRS
2. QT shorter than normal
3. History of digitalis treatment

Digitalis effect can be seen in Tracing 27.

LEFT VENTRICULAR HYPERTROPHY

There is a ST displacement that is small and usually is negative in the leads where T is negative also. It is due to differences in the repolarization process between the subendocardial and subepicardial areas. See Tracing 7 for an example.

LEFT BUNDLE BRANCH BLOCK

The ST displacement is small and usually negative in the leads where T is negative. It is also due to differences in the repolarization process between the subendocardial and subepicardial areas. See Tracing 10 for an example.

Scalar Values of ECG

By scalar values, it is meant the measurements of time intervals between ECG events as well as the

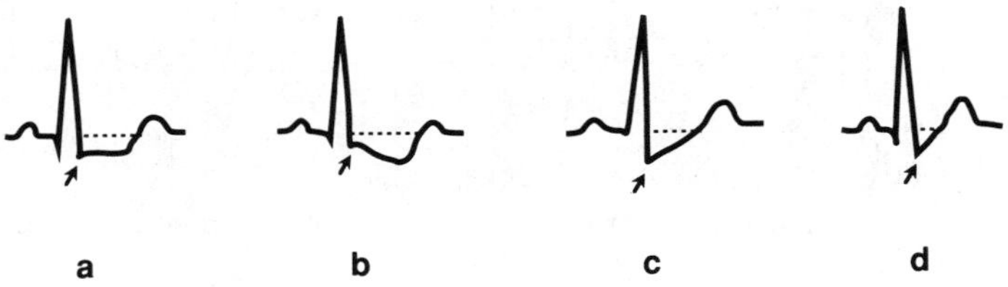

Figure 45–26. Ischemic and nonischemic changes during exercise.

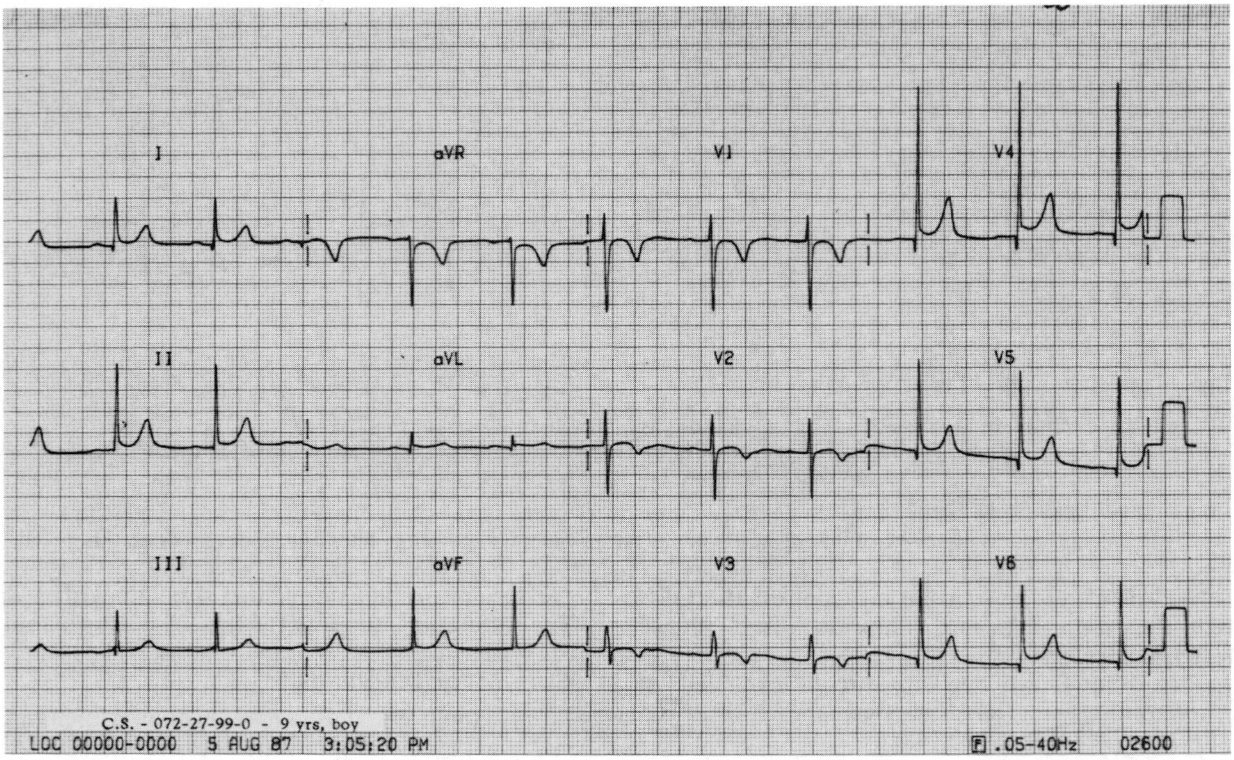

Tracing 26. Example of early repolarization syndrome. Small ST elevation is shown in all leads except in aVR and in V_1 to V_3. Inverted T is shown in V_1 to V_3 (juvenile pattern).

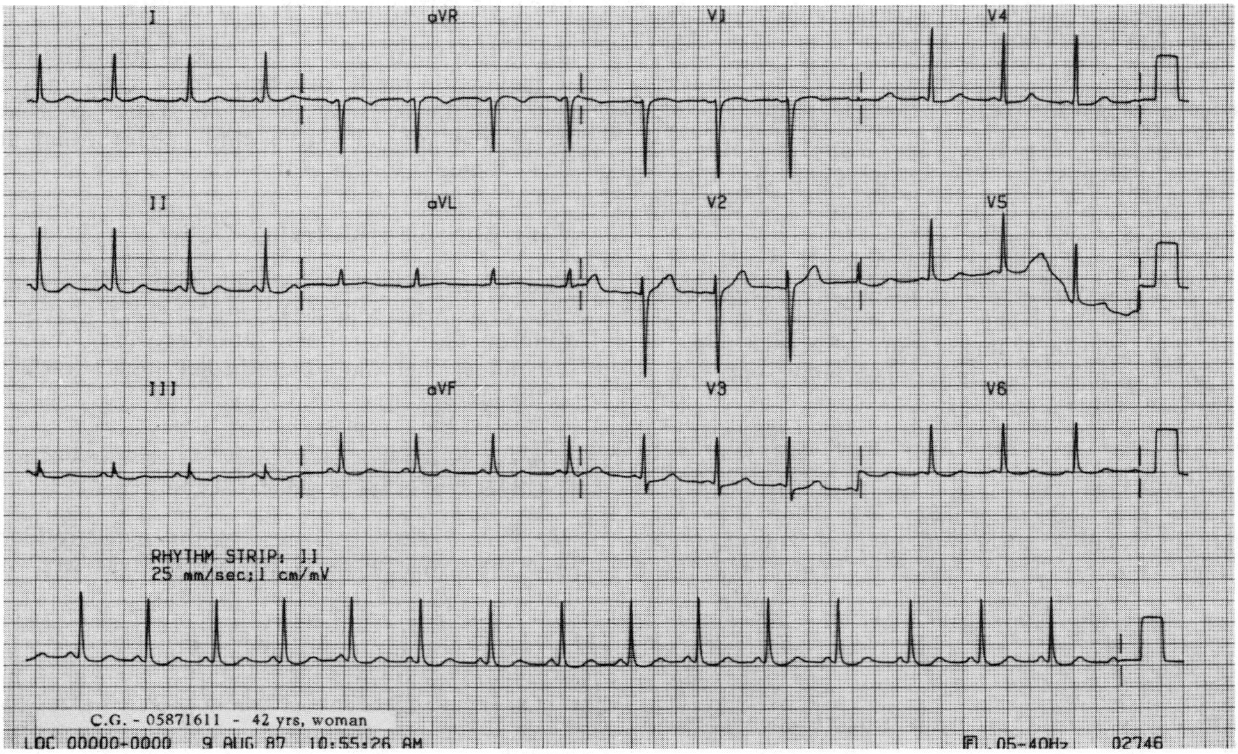

Tracing 27. Example of digitalis effect. Small and coved ST depression is shown in most leads except aVR.

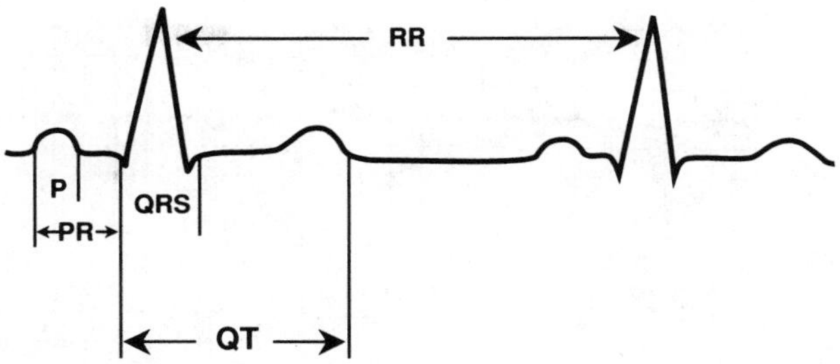

Figure 45–27. The standard time intervals of the ECG in the cardiac cycle.

P: Atrial depolarization time
PR: Atrial depolarization + AV conduction time
QRS: Ventricular depolarization time
QT: Electrical systole time
RR-QT: Electrical diastole time
RR: Cardiac cycle time

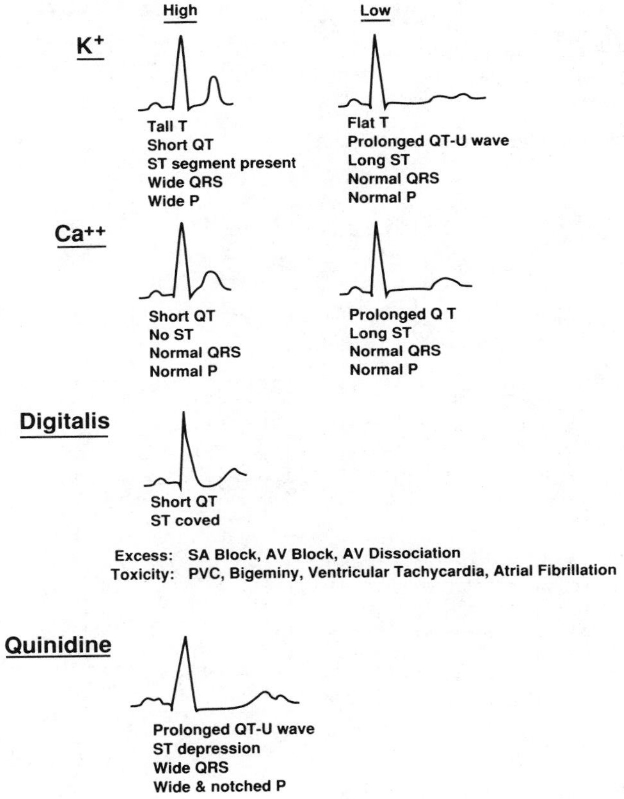

Figure 45–28. Typical patterns of electrocardiographic changes due to electrolyte disturbance and drugs.

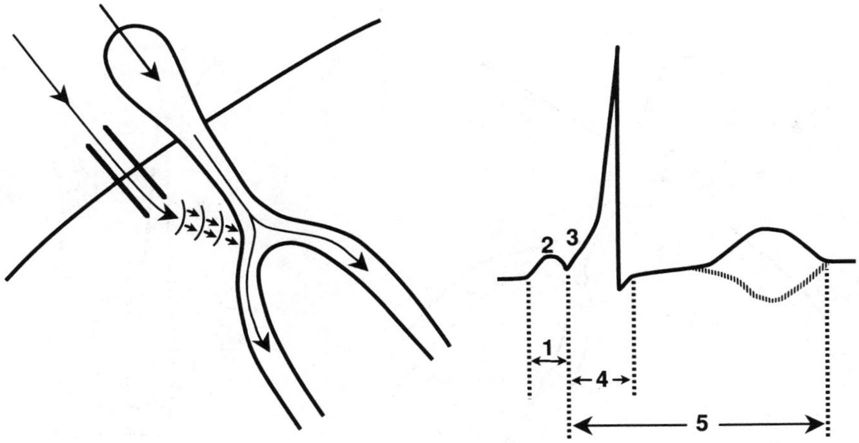

Figure 45–29. Transmission of electromotive forces in Wolff-Parkinson-White syndrome. 1, short PR; 2, normal P; 3, Δ wave; 4, prolonged QRS; 5, prolonged QT (there may be an inverted T).

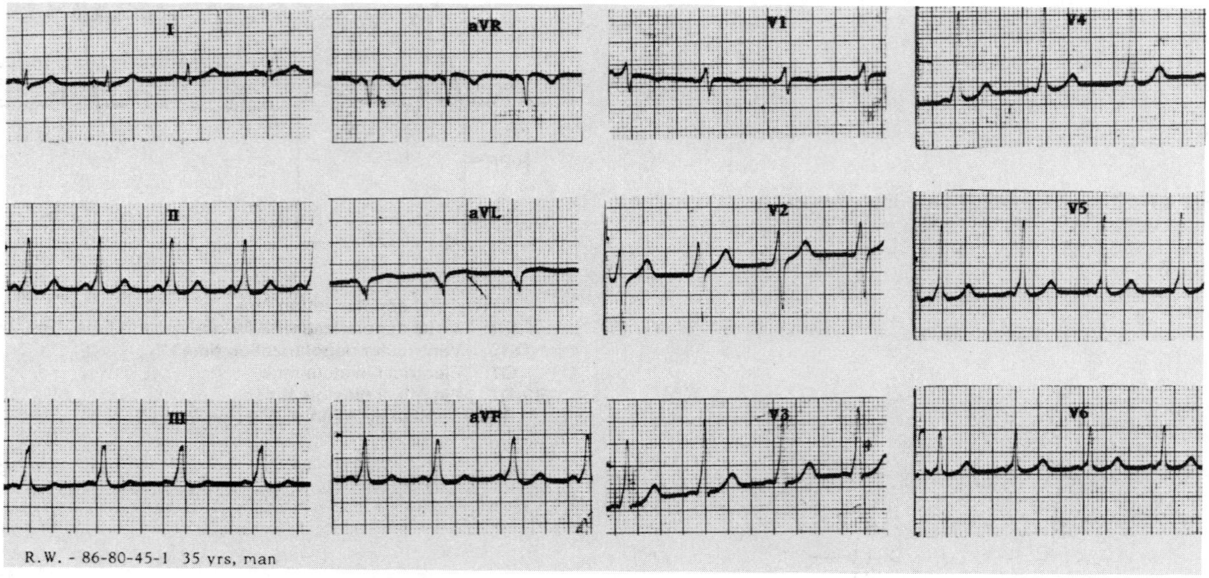

Tracing 28. Example of Wolff-Parkinson-White syndrome, type A.

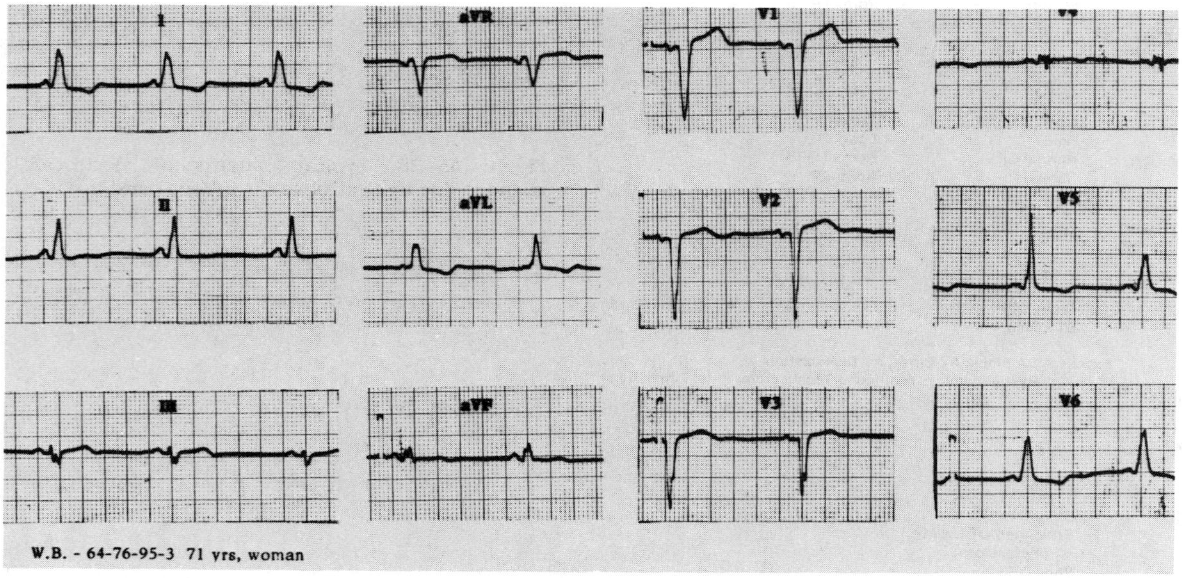

Tracing 29. Example of Wolff-Parkinson-White syndrome, type B.

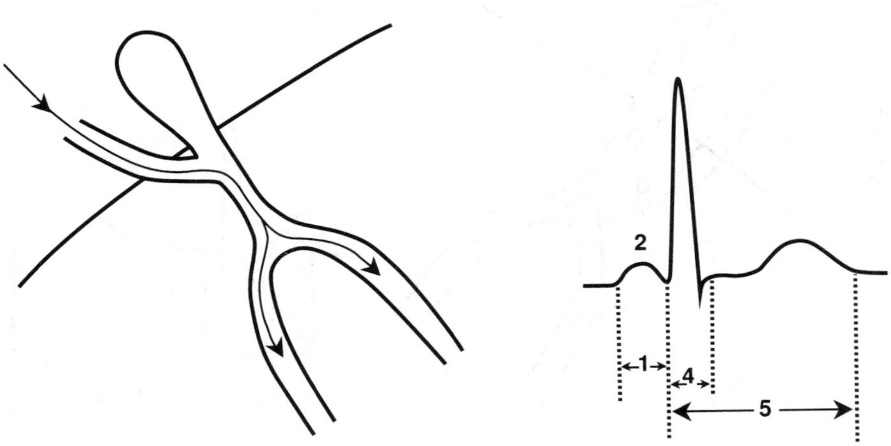

Figure 45–30. Transmission of electromotive forces in Lown-Ganong-Levine (short PR) syndrome. 1, short PR; 2, normal P; 3, no Δ wave; 4, normal QRS; 5, normal QT.

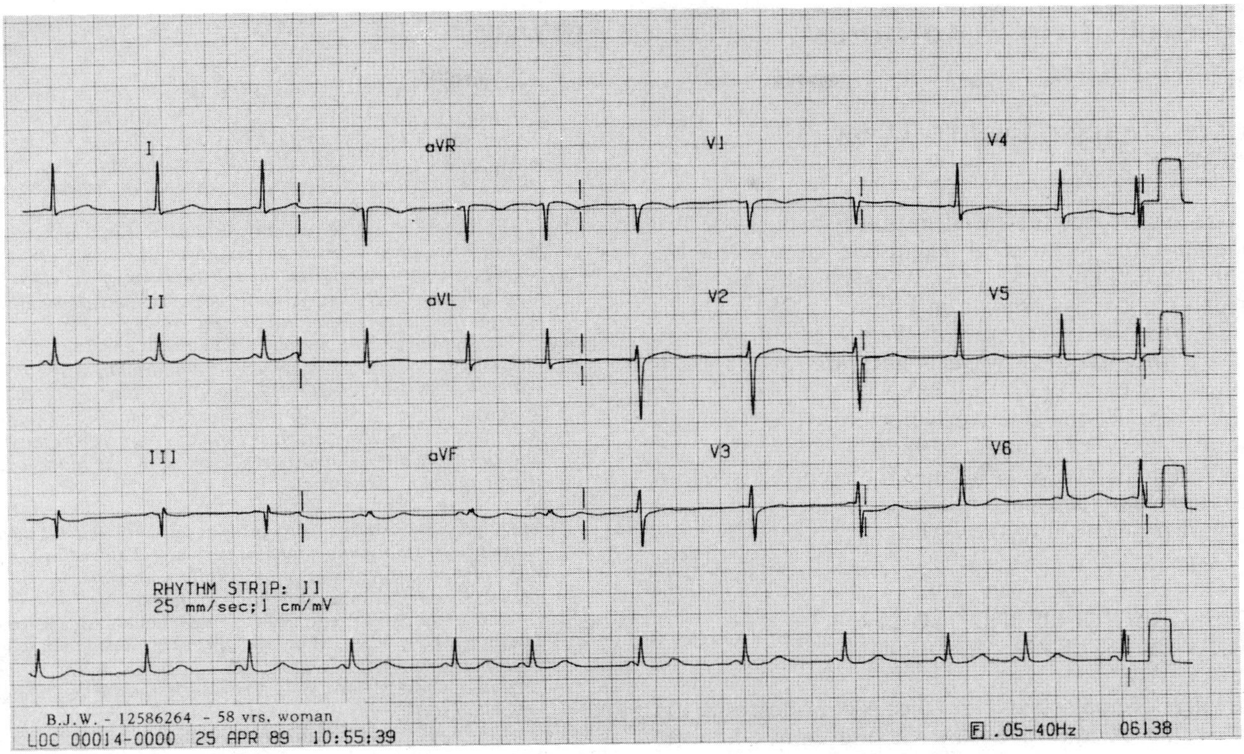

Tracing 30. Example of Lown-Ganong-Levine syndrome (short P-R interval syndrome).

measurements of voltages of P, QRS, and T in various leads. The time intervals shown in Figure 45–27 may convey very useful information. Since the usual paper speed is 2.5 cm./second the interval between two thin vertical lines is 0.04 seconds. The interval between two heavy vertical lines is 0.20 seconds.

NORMAL VALUES FOR ADULTS

P Wave. The P wave value is 0.08 seconds. It is prolonged in P-mitrale and in diffuse atrial damage but shorter in children. Usually, it is not affected by the heart rate.

PR Wave. This interval is affected by the heart rate and age so that a sustained increase in rate produces a shorter PR interval. The upper limit of normal at a rate of 60/minute is 0.20 seconds. Causes of prolonged PR interval include (1) 1 degree AV block due to coronary artery disease, rheumatic fever, or diphtheria (infrequent in the United States); (2) digitalis; and (3) increased vagal tone. Causes of short(ened) PR interval include (1) Wolff-Parkinson-White syndrome, (2) other pre-excitation syndromes, (3) wandering pacemaker, (4) nodal rhythm, and (5) PACs.

QRS Wave. This interval is 0.08 seconds. It is prolonged in bundle branch block, shorter in children, and usually not affected by the heart rate.

QT Wave. This interval is also affected by the heart rate. There are several regression equations to predict the normal value of QT for a given rate. A commonly used formula is as follows:

$$QT = 0.39 \sqrt{R\text{-}R} \pm 0.04 \text{ seconds}$$

At 60/minute, the upper limit of normal for QT is 0.40 seconds in men and 0.44 seconds in women. It is shorter than predicted in hypercalcemia and hyperkalemia and in the early stages of digitalization. It is longer than predicted in hypocalcemia, hypokalemia, and under the influence of some psychotropic drugs (especially tricyclic antidepressants and thioridazine). There are two rare congenital syndromes of prolonged QT that may occur in families and may cause episodes of syncope with a special pattern of ventricular tachycardia *(torsade de pointes)* and sometimes death. The congenital Jerwell-Lange-Nielsen syndrome is associated with deafness while the Romano-Ward syndrome is not.

RR Wave. This wave measures the length of the cardiac cycle and is inversely proportional to the heart rate. If the interval measures one division or 0.20 seconds, the heart rate is 300/minute. If it measures three divisions or 0.60 seconds, the rate is 100/minute. If it measures six divisions or 1.20 seconds, the rate is 50/minute.

Electrolyte and Drug Effects

The typical changes brought about by electrolyte disturbances or by drugs are shown in Figure 45–28.

Pre-excitation Syndromes (Short PR)

WOLFF-PARKINSON-WHITE (W-P-W) SYNDROME

In this syndrome, the atrial impulses bypass the AV node and the ventricular excitation occurs via the Kent bundle. The genesis of W-P-W and the criteria for its diagnosis are shown in Figure 45–29.

There are two types of W-P-W Syndrome. In type A, the delta (Δ) wave is anterior (i.e., there is a slurred R in V_1) (Tracing 28).

In type B, the Δ wave is posterior (i.e., there is a slurred Q in V_1) (Tracing 29).

Patients with W-P-W may have episodes of supraventricular tachycardia brought about by fast reentry of impulses into the atria.

LOWN-GANONG-LEVINE (L-G-L) OR SHORT PR INTERVAL SYNDROME

The atrial impulses bypass the AV node, and the ventricular excitation occurs via the James bundle. The genesis of L-G-L and the criteria for its diagnosis are shown in Figure 45–30. The original description of this syndrome indicated the occurrence of episodes of supraventricular tachycardia. Subsequently, the diagnosis of L-G-L syndrome has been made on the basis of the above criteria, regardless of supraventricular tachycardia. The World Health Organization recommends the term short PR interval syndrome rather than L-G-L (Tracing 30).

Disturbances of the Rhythm

Normally, the rhythm of cardiac activity is determined by the regular activation of the sinoatrial node with rapid transmission of impulses to the atria and to the ventricle as described earlier. It is common, however, to detect abnormalities of the rhythm, which are referred to as dysrhythmias or arrhythmias. Chapter 46, pp. 892–908, includes a discussion of the most common patterns of arrhythmia and their pathogenesis and treatment.

References

Beckwith, J. R.: Grant's Clinical Electrocardiogram: The Spatial Vector Approach. New York, McGraw-Hill, 1970. *This small book presents in very simple terms the vector approach to the analysis of the ECG. Robert Grant was the author of the first edition, and one of his pupils, Dr. Beckwith, wrote the second edition after Dr. Grant's death.*

Chung, E. K.: Electrocardiography: Practical Applications With Vector Principles. Norwalk, Appleton and Lange, 1985. *This is an excellent book with detailed discussions of the electrocardiographic changes that occur in various states of health and disease. It contains abundant example tracings.*

Dubin, D.: Rapid Interpretation of EKG's. 2nd ed. Tampa, Cover Publishing Co., 1988. *This is an important, easy to read textbook with very simple explanations of the ECG changes produced by a variety of pathologic conditions. The book contains excellent diagrams and provides numerous mnemonic rules to assist the unsophisticated person in obtaining a rapid interpretation of the ECG.*

Halhuber, M. J., Gunther, R., and Ciresa, M.: ECG: An Introductory Course. Berlin, Springer-Verlag, 1979. *This is a good, rather brief textbook that contains very useful diagrams in black and white and in red, which are helpful in the interpretation of the ECG using vectorcardiographic principles.*

Hurst, J. W., and Myerburg, R. J.: Introduction to Electrocardiography. New York, McGraw-Hill, 1973. *This is a very good book that is useful to cardiologists and other physicians interested in the analysis of the vectors of QRS and T and the QRS vector loop. It contains numerous example tracings.*

Marriott, H. J. L.: ECG. Baltimore, Williams & Wilkins, 1987. *This is a very popular textbook that emphasizes the pattern analysis of ECGs. It contains numerous examples of typical tracings.*

Rosenbaum, M. B., Erlizari, M. V., Lazzari, J. O.: The Hemiblocks. Tampa, Tampa Tracings, 1970. *This is the first monograph written on the topic of hemiblocks. Rosenbaum and coworkers described the genesis of axis deviations due to conduction disturbances in the anterior or posterior fascicles of the left bundle branch. This is a complicated book, but it is of major historical interest.*

Scheidt, S.: Basic Electrocardiography. West Caldwell, CIBA-GEIGY, 1986. *This is an excellent textbook that has been assembled for the purpose of assisting primary care physicians in the analysis and interpretation of the ECG. It is based on a previous monograph of the CIBA collection prepared by the author with superb illustrations made by Dr. Netter. It contains an excellent atlas of representative ECG tracings obtained with modern three-channel electrocardiographs.*

Sandöe, E., and Sigurd, B.: Arrhythmia—Diagnosis and Management: A Clinical Electrocardiographic Guide. Fachmed AG, Verlag für Fachmedien, St. Gallen, 1984. *This book, authored by two Danish electrocardiographers, was written on behalf of the European Society of Cardiology under a grant from Boehringer Ingelheim Company. Its English version has been widely distributed in the United States. Although the emphasis of this excellent book is on the description of arrhythmias and their genesis, it devotes several chapters to the fundamentals of electrocardiography and to the patterns of change produced by a variety of conditions.*

46

Cardiovascular Disease

Preventive Cardiology

Allan V. Abbott
David H. Blankenhorn

Preventive Cardiology

The number of Americans dying from cardiovascular diseases climbed throughout most of this century, peaked in 1973 at 1,037,000, and has been decreasing since (Walker, 1977). It now seems clear that the major credit for this recent reduction in deaths and decreased risk of cardiovascular diseases is the result of behavioral changes adopted by the public. Still today, cardiovascular diseases account for nearly one half of all deaths in the United States. Nearly three fourths of these deaths are the result of the major and most lethal manifestation of cardiovascular disease, coronary heart disease (CHD).

Atherosclerosis, or the development of atheromatous plaques in large and medium arteries, sets the stage for the onset of CHD. A great deal has been learned recently about the formation of atherosclerotic plaques. However, regardless of their pathology, clinical and epidemiologic evidence indicates that many risk factors are associated with acceleration of atherosclerosis. Americans have learned about the dangers of CHD risk factors and have made efforts to alter their risk by changing their life styles. Many adults have stopped smoking and have taken up exercise programs. The average consumption of dietary saturated fat has declined, as has the mean serum cholesterol level. In the 1970's and 1980's, detection and control of hypertension became the rule rather than the exception. Family physicians have played a critical role in these changes, both in educating the public and in identifying and treating the risk factors themselves.

Immutable Risk Factors

CHD risk factors are commonly divided into those that can be modified and those that cannot. Increasing age, male sex, and a family history of CHD are generally considered to be immutable (Table 46–1). Of all risk factors, the two most important are age and male sex. CHD is already the leading cause of death in men over the age of 35, and between the ages of 55 and 64, 40 per cent of all deaths are due to this single cause. CHD is not common in young women, yet after menopause there is a dramatic increase in both the incidence and severity of CHD.

The risk of CHD in individuals with a family history of heart disease is increased two- to sevenfold. However, most of this risk is the result of familial aggregation of CHD risk factors. A family history of CHD identifies those individuals who should be most carefully screened for the presence of other risk factors. Not only do modifiable risk factors tend to run in families, but individuals with a family history of CHD also seem to be especially susceptible to the detrimental effects of these factors, especially to smoking. This information may be helpful in convincing patients with a family history of CHD to make efforts to change their other risk factors (Khaw and Barrett-Connor, 1986).

Modifiable Risk Factors

CIGARETTE SMOKING

The United States Surgeon General's report on the health consequences of smoking states that cigarette smoking is the most important of the modifiable risk factors for CHD. A physician can do more to reduce a patient's CHD risk by successfully motivating him or her to stop smoking than through any other single intervention.

The greatest relative risk occurs in younger age groups, and smoking is particularly dangerous for women, for whom smoking is responsible for about one half of all clinical coronary events. Heavy smokers are at higher risk than light smokers, but smoking only one to four cigarettes daily doubled the risk of CHD in one group of young women (Willett et al., 1987). Even passive smoking may significantly increase the risk of CHD (Svendsen et al., 1987).

Smoking is particularly dangerous when accompanied by other risk factors. The American Heart Association urges every physician to develop techniques to encourage patients to reduce or stop smoking. The physician can greatly influence some patients by taking a firm stance against smoking and by showing concern at every visit for those patients who do smoke. The American Academy of Family Physicians has developed a Stop Smoking Kit (patient education pamphlets, history forms, information manuals, flow charts, and patient-education audiocassettes) that provides the family physician with the various tools needed to teach patients how to stop smoking in the context of the routine office visit.

Table 46–1. CORONARY HEART DISEASE RISK FACTORS

Immutable	Modifiable
Age	Cigarette smoking
Male sex	Hypertension
Family history of CHD	Hypercholesterolemia
	Diabetes mellitus
	Obesity
	Physical inactivity
	Type A behavior

HYPERTENSION

As both systolic and diastolic blood pressures rise, the risk of cardiovascular disease increases. In the 1988 report of the Joint National Committee on Detection, Evaluation, and Treatment of High Blood Pressure, diastolic pressure less than 85 mm. Hg and systolic pressure less than 140 mm. Hg were considered normal for all adults. It is significant that higher pressures are still accepted by some as "normal" despite the fact that they are associated with increased risk. A diastolic pressure of 89 to 94 mm. Hg has 1.6 times the risk of a diastolic pressure of less than 80 mm. Hg.

The risk imparted by hypertension is also affected by other risk factors. Impaired glucose tolerance, elevated low-density lipoproteins, and decreased high-density lipoproteins greatly increase the risk of CHD in the presence of hypertension. Also, there are additive risks imposed by a diet excessive in fat, calories, and salt; sedentary habits; unrestrained weight gain; and smoking. Thus, once the diagnosis of hypertension is made, the physician should not only look for other causes of hypertension but for other CHD risk factors as well. The physician should consider these factors in addition to returning blood pressure to the normal range when planning therapy.

The effects of blood pressure lability are now well recognized, and it is important for the physician to measure blood pressure correctly. It is not safe to record only the lowest of several blood pressure readings. Two or more measurements should be averaged at each visit. Blood pressure should be obtained using the properly sized cuff after the patient has been seated quietly for at least 5 minutes.

HYPERCHOLESTEROLEMIA

There is strong evidence that supports a causal relationship between high plasma cholesterol and CHD. Accelerated atherosclerosis has been primarily associated with elevation of the low-density lipoprotein fraction of total cholesterol (LDL-C), and reduced risk is associated with increases in the high-density lipoprotein fraction (HDL-C). Evidence from several major clinical trials has shown that lowering total cholesterol and LDL-C levels by diet and drugs reduces CHD. Thus, there is now strong justification for treatment of high plasma cholesterol for the purpose of reducing the risk of CHD (Blankenhorn et al., 1987).

The ratio of total cholesterol to HDL-C is a better indicator of CHD risk in population groups than either parameter alone. However, LDL-C is the single measure of choice for individuals. When a total cholesterol to HDL-C ratio of 4.4:1 is given a risk ratio of 1.0, a ratio of 3.0:1 imparts half the baseline risk, and a ratio of 6.2:1 increases the risk two-fold. The HDL-C level should be determined in any person whose total cholesterol exceeds 240 mg. per dl.; total plasma cholesterol, HDL-C, and triglycerides are measured together to estimate LDL-C by most laboratories. For individuals whose total cholesterol levels are between 200 and 240 mg. per dl. in the presence of one or more other risk factors, HDL-C, LDL-C, and triglycerides should be determined. Several environmental factors, obesity, lack of exercise, and smoking contribute to lowering HDL-C levels. Also, HDL-C levels can be lowered by severely fat-restricted diets and several drugs, including beta-adrenergic blockers, thiazides, and progestational agents.

Details of the relationship between triglyceride levels and the risk of CHD remain disputed. The upper limit of normal plasma triglycerides is about 150 mg. per dl. The first step in estimating risk in patients with elevated triglycerides is to determine the total cholesterol, HDL-C cholesterol, and the total cholesterol to HDL-C ratio. Whether elevated triglycerides alone impart risk beyond the standard risk factors is unresolved. Determination of the cause of hypertriglyceridemia is required for appropriate management. Obesity is a common cause, and weight reduction lowers triglyceride levels in many obese patients.

Treatment

In 1988, an expert panel of the National Cholesterol Education Program provided physicians with guidelines for detecting, evaluating, and treating elevated cholesterol levels. The risk of CHD increases with increasing levels of total cholesterol, beginning at 180 mg. per dl. The expert panel defined desirable total cholesterol levels as less than 200 mg. per dl., borderline high as 200 to 239 mg. per dl., and high as 240 mg. per dl. or greater. Patients with high levels of total cholesterol or with borderline levels and two or more other risk factors are advised to have LDL-C levels measured. LDL-C levels are then determined to be borderline risk at 130 to 159 mg. per dl. and high risk at 160 mg. per dl. or greater. Management in patients with high risk levels of LDL-C and in those with borderline risk levels in the presence of two or more additional risk factors is through diet. Treatment with drugs and a diet is suggested for patients with LDL-C levels of 190 mg. per dl. or greater and for those with LDL-C levels of 159 to 189 mg. per dl. who have two or more additional risk factors.

Dietary treatment is managed in steps. The initial step-one diet reduces total dietary fat to less than 30 per cent and saturated fats to less than 10 per cent of total calories. The step-two diet further reduces the saturated fat to less than 7 per cent of total calories and the dietary cholesterol to less than 200 mg. HDL-C levels can be improved through exercise, smoking cessation, and use of estrogens and by weight reduction in obese patients. The consumption of moderate amounts of alcohol can also raise HDL-C levels but should not be recommended for this purpose.

If high total plasma cholesterol levels persist beyond 3 months of the step-two diet, drug treatment is recommended. Many drugs have been used to lower plasma cholesterol (Table 46–2). The bile acid–binding resins cholestyramine and colestipol have been proven safe and effective for lowering plasma cholesterol concentrations. Niacin is effective in decreasing triglycerides, total plasma cholesterol, and LDL-C, and increasing HDL-C. Gemfibrozil, a fibric acid derivative, lowers triglycerides and very low density lipoproteins and increases HDL-C but may cause an increase in gallstones. Lovastatin inhibits the enzyme that catalyzes the rate-limiting step in cholesterol synthesis and appears to be more effective than any other currently used drug in lowering LDL-C levels; however, the long-term safety and effectiveness in preventing or reversing atherosclerosis has not been established.

DIABETES MELLITUS

Among persons with insulin-dependent and noninsulin-dependent diabetes mellitus, the risk of CHD is at least twice that in nondiabetics. The risk of CHD and the progression of diabetic retinopathy have been shown to be reduced but not eliminated by control of hyperglycemia. However, weight reduction and increased exercise can delay the progression of glucose intolerance when detected early. Thus, the American Heart Association recommends that fasting glucose levels be determined in normal healthy adults every 5 years until age 60, then every 2½ years until age 75. In patients with mild to moderate obesity (110 to 130 per cent of desired body weight), fasting glucose level checks should be twice as frequent after age 45, and yearly measurements are appropriate in markedly obese patients after age 50 (Grundy et al., 1987).

OBESITY

Many overweight patients have hypertension, elevated plasma cholesterol levels, lowered HDL-C levels, and diabetes mellitus, all of which increase the risk of CHD. The role of excess body fat (obesity) in the risk of CHD may differ in various forms of obesity and locations of fat deposits. The risk of CHD is greater for obese patients with large amounts of visceral fat accumulations, as opposed to those with more peripheral fat deposits. Until more sophisticated methods of determining fat distribution are available, measurements of waist (widest part of the abdomen) and hip (widest part of the gluteal area) circumferences are most useful. A waist-to-hips ratio greater than 1:1 in men and 0.8:1 in women indicates a significantly increased risk of CHD and cerebrovascular disease (Krotkiewski et al., 1983). Weight-reduction programs should emphasize physical exercise in addition to dietary restrictions.

Table 46–2. DRUGS USED IN THE TREATMENT OF HYPERCHOLESTEROLEMIA

		Drugs of First Choice			Other Drugs	
		Bile Acid Binders	***Nicotinic Acid***	***Lovastatin***	***Gemfibrozil***	***Probucol***
Average effect	LDL-C	↓	↓	↓	↔ ⇅	↓
	HDL-C	↔ (or slight ↑)	↑	↑ ↔	↑ (slight)	↓
	Triglycerides	↔ ↑	↓	↓ ↔	↓	↔
CHD risk reduction		Proven	Proven	Not proven, new drug	Proven	Not proven
Side effects		GI* effects; constipation; malabsorption of digitalis, thyroid, and vitamins	Flushing, LFT† ↑, arrhythmia, gout, glucose intolerance, GI effects	Minimal side effects LFT ↑, fatigue, headaches	Increased gallstones, LFT ↑, myopathy (rare)	GI effects, mild diarrhea, possible heart conduction disturbances
Contraindications		GI disease, peptic ulcer disease, severe hemorrhoids	Peptic ulcer disease, liver disease, gout, cardiac arrhythmias, bundle-branch block	Liver disease	Biliary obstruction, gallstones, liver disease	Ventricular irritability, prolonged QT interval
Dosage		Cholestyramine: 8 to 24 grams per day; Colestipol: 10 to 30 grams per day; taper on slowly	500 mg. to 2 grams t.i.d., taper on slowly and take with food	10 to 40 mg. b.i.d.	300 to 600 mg. b.i.d.	250 to 500 mg. b.i.d.

*GI = gastrointestinal
†LFT = liver function tests

PHYSICAL INACTIVITY

Many epidemiologic studies have suggested a beneficial association between physical activity and the prevention of CHD; others have shown no such association. A recent extensive review indicates that physical activity helps prevent CHD, and physical inactivity is a CHD risk factor of importance equal to or greater than other major risk factors (Powell et al., 1987).

When the results of this review were compared with the results of the Coronary Pooling Project (The Pooling Project Research Group, 1978), the strength of the association between lack of physical activity and CHD appeared to be similar to that found for high plasma cholesterol, high systolic blood pressure, and cigarette smoking and CHD. This is especially noteworthy considering the prevalence of these risk factors in the United States. Using current standards, about 36 per cent of Americans are at risk because of high blood pressure (>140/90 mm. Hg); approximately 25 per cent to 40 per cent are at risk because of high plasma cholesterol (>200 mg. per dl.); and about 30 per cent are believed to be current smokers and thus at risk. Approximately 59 per cent of Americans do not perform physical activity regularly (at least three times per week for more than 20 minutes at a time). Thus, it was concluded that more Americans are at risk of CHD because of physical inactivity than because of any one of the other three main risk factors (Centers for Disease Control, 1987).

Recent studies have suggested that moderate activity such as walking and working around the house helps prevent CHD, as does a moderate amount of more vigorous activity. Brisk walking is the most reasonable activity when the physician prescribes exercise for sedentary, middle-aged patients who have not maintained their fitness. The risk of sudden death during and shortly after intense exercise such as jogging or running is significant, especially among men over age 45. Physicians should recommend exercise stress tests for these individuals before they begin vigorous exercise programs, especially if they have other CHD risk factors.

Overall, however, there is a lower risk of both CHD and sudden coronary death in persons who are habitually active. The greatest CHD protection is associated with a life long program of regular physical activity at least three times per week. Rather than stressing the duration of exercise activities, the physician should emphasize the total energy expenditure of the regular exercise. A reasonable goal is for individuals to expend in physical activity at least 1500 to 2000 kcal. per week. As a general guide, the average person walking briskly expends about 5 kcal. per minute, or roughly 100 kcal. in walking a mile. For example, each week a businessperson might walk a total of 2 miles to and from the car (200 kcal.) and 2 miles around the office and to and from lunch (200 kcal.); thus, this individual would need an additional 1600 kcal. of leisure activity, or the equivalent of 16 miles of walking, to reach the goal of 2000 kcal. per week.

PSYCHOSOCIAL STRESS AND TYPE A BEHAVIOR

Many stressful situations have been shown to increase the risk of CHD; low socioeconomic status, demanding work conditions with poor control, and poor social support systems have been implicated. Poor family and social support can exacerbate the acutely stressful effects of life events such as the death of a spouse, job loss, divorce, and relocation.

In the 1970's, Type A behavior became a popular topic of discussion after it was identified as a risk factor for CHD. Type A behavior is thought to be a manifestation of chronic psychosocial stress. It is characterized by a chronic sense of time urgency (haste, impatience, tension, competitiveness) and by easily aroused hostility (Abbott and Peters, 1988).

Although the majority of early studies support the association of Type A behavior and CHD, several more recent studies have found no association between Type A behavior and CHD. This has left many physicians wondering whether Type A behavior is truly unhealthy. The bulk of the evidence still supports the link between Type A behavior and CHD. A recent critical review of the accumulating research suggests that Type A behavior is associated with the risk of CHD in otherwise healthy men, particularly in white-collar workers (Matthews and Haynes, 1986).

There is no simple test that can be used in the physician's office to easily and adequately assess Type A behavior. When the physician does recognize a patient with overt Type A behavior, this should be noted as a CHD risk factor that may add to the risk from other risk factors for that individual. Just as the physician should indicate the risk of smoking cigarettes to a smoker, the physician should point out the risk of Type A behavior to a high-risk patient with overt Type A behavior and other CHD risk factors. However, until more supportive evidence is gathered, efforts by physicians to alter Type A behavior are not usually warranted. Instead, it is reasonable to suggest to patients that efforts to increase their social network (family, friends, organizations) and to maintain high levels of interaction with that network during periods of adverse life events will improve the quality of their lives and may have as yet undocumented beneficial effects on survival (Hartley et al., 1987).

MISCELLANEOUS RISK FACTORS

Some studies have associated light to moderate alcohol consumption with decreased risk of CHD. Alcohol consumption, however, increases body weight, impairs glucose tolerance, and increases blood pressure, and anything that encourages consumption of alcohol is likely to increase social costs, traffic accidents, and other problems. The World Health Organization has stated that "increased alcohol intake is not recommended as a preventive measure in CHD, either in populations or in individuals."

Menopause induced by total hysterectomy and oophorectomy is a risk factor in women. It has been suggested that hysterectomy in premenopausal women probably increases the risk of cardiovascular disease more than it decreases the risk of uterine cancer. Estrogen therapy may reduce the risk of CHD in postmenopausal women, but in premenopausal women, estrogens such as those used in oral contraceptives increase the risk, especially in smokers over the age of 35. Estrogens do not decrease the risk of CHD in men.

A Comprehensive Approach for Family Physicians

Family physicians are strategically positioned to identify children, adults, and families at risk of atherosclerotic cardiovascular disease and to make crucial interventions in preventing CHD. Risk factors are best identified through periodic examinations beginning in early childhood and continuing through the geriatric years. American Heart Association recommendations for adult periodic health examinations appear in Figure 46–1.

Annual blood pressure measurements in children should begin at 3 years of age and continue from 6 years of age through adolescence at least every other year. Habits that maintain low cholesterol should be initiated in childhood when life style patterns are

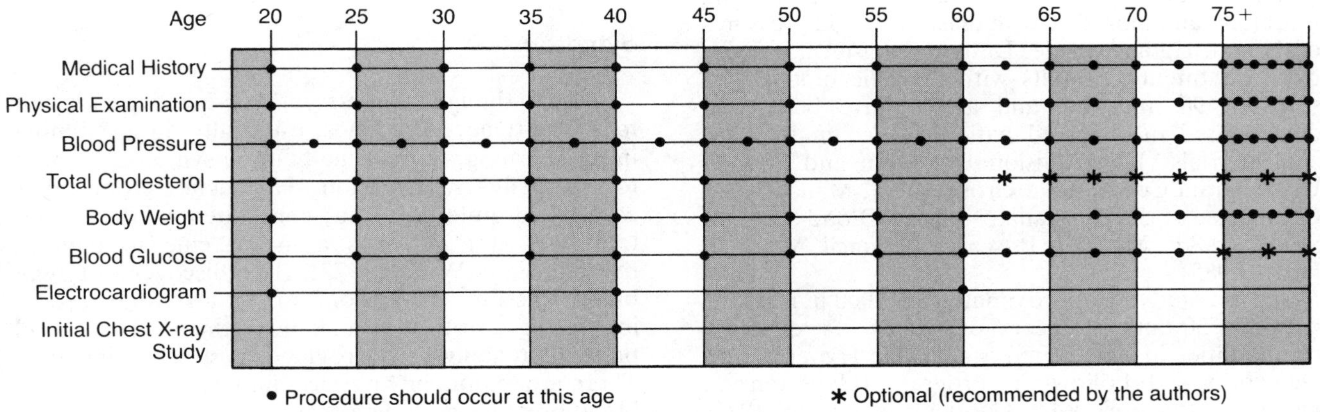

Figure 46–1. Periodic health examinations, as recommended by the American Heart Association.

established (National Institutes of Health Consensus Development Panel, 1985). Children should be screened for hypercholesterolemia by the taking of a careful family history, focusing on evidence of hypercholesterolemia or CHD before the age of 60 in first-degree relatives. If either of these risk factors is present, at least two blood cholesterol determinations should be obtained. Children whose total cholesterol levels are above the 90th percentile (approximately 185 mg. per dl.) should receive dietary counseling, evaluation of other risk factors, and close follow-up. When risk factors are identified, other family members should be screened and risk behaviors in the family modified.

When multiple risk factors are present in any one patient, they are interdependent and assume a strongly additive relationship. The risk of developing CHD at any given level of total plasma cholesterol, for example, is exacerbated by the addition of other risk factors. Thus, in patients and families with multiple risk factors, it is easy to underestimate the overall risk and it is important to evaluate each patient's risk factor status as a whole. In this respect, the family physician is in a better position than any other specialist to conduct therapy of multiple risk factors in individual patients of all ages and to promote new health behaviors with the support of patients' families.

Hypertension

Hilmon Castle

Blood pressure is controlled by the continuous interaction of the sympathetic nervous system, the extracellular fluid volume and sodium stores, the renin-angiotensin mechanism, salt-retaining steroids such as aldosterone, and other yet undiscovered mechanisms. Increased activity in any of these regulatory mechanisms may elevate blood pressure, which, in turn, provokes changes in the other interactive mechanisms to bring the blood pressure back toward the normal range. Eventually, however, these compensatory responses fail and blood pressure above the normal range becomes established. The time of day, the preceding activity, and the emotional state of an individual result in marked variation in blood pressure recordings.

Data reported from epidemiologic studies over the past 3 decades have established conclusively that blood pressure is a graded risk factor, with increasing morbidity and mortality with diastolic blood pressures of 84 mm. Hg and above. Definite long-term benefits from treatment of adults with diastolic blood pressures of 90 mm. Hg and above have been well documented in repeated national large multicenter clinical trials (Hypertension Detection and Follow-Up Program Cooperative Group, 1979; Management Committee of the Australian National Blood Pressure Study, 1980; Medical Research Council Working Party, 1985).

After studying approximately 150,000 individuals between 30 and 69 years of age in 14 different communities in the United States, the Hypertension Detection and Follow-Up Program (Hypertension Detection and Follow-Up Cooperative Group, 1977) revealed a prevalence of hypertension of 18 per cent among whites and 38 per cent among blacks, using 95 mm. Hg and above as the cutoff point to define hypertension as measured in the home.

Also, the Virginia Study of the type of medical problems presented in primary care office practice showed that 20 per cent of all adults have sufficiently elevated blood pressure to deserve follow-up and treatment (Marsland et al., 1976). Hypertension among adults is common, especially among blacks and people 50 years of age and older. Currently available drugs make control of blood pressure feasible in almost all patients who are aware of high blood pressure and who adhere to a treatment regimen. Classification of blood pressure levels and recommendations for follow-up are outlined in Table 46–3.

Symptoms

Even though patients with severe hypertension may experience headaches, especially on awakening in the morning, this is usually not a symptom of mild to moderate hypertension. Headaches from other causes are quite common; consequently, this symptom does not serve as a useful clue to identify hypertension (Weiss, 1972). The discovery of high blood pressure usually comes from a routine recording during an office visit or in settings where blood pressure readings are provided as a screening test. There are seldom any physical findings other than the blood pressure recording that indicates hypertension. Accurate blood pressure recordings should be ob-

Table 46–3. CLASSIFICATION OF BLOOD PRESSURE LEVELS AND FOLLOW-UP RECOMMENDATIONS

Classification of BP* in Adults Aged 18 Years or Older†		Follow-up Criteria for Initial BP Measurement For Adults Aged 18 Years or Older†	
BP Range in mm. Hg	*Category*	*BP Range in mm. Hg*	*Recommended Follow-up*
DBP‡		*DBP*	
<85	Normal BP	<85	Recheck within 2 years
85–89	High normal BP	85–89	Recheck within 1 year
90–104	Mild hypertension	90–104	Confirm within 2 months
105–114	Moderate hypertension	105–114	Evaluate or refer promptly to source of care within 2 weeks
≥115	Severe hypertension	>115	Evaluate or refer immediately to source of care
SBP§ when DBP <90 mm. Hg			
<140	Normal BP		
140–159	Borderline isolated systolic hypertension		
		SBP when DBP <90 mm. Hg	
≥160	Isolated systolic hypertension	<140	Recheck within 2 years
		140–199	Confirm within 2 months
		≥200	Evaluate or refer promptly to source of care within 2 weeks

*BP = blood pressure.
†Classification based on the average of two or more readings to two or more occasions.
‡DBP = diastolic blood pressure.
§SBP = systolic blood pressure.

tained routinely in all patient care settings with the patient comfortably seated and relaxed; a minimum of two recordings with a blood pressure cuff of the appropriate size fitted snugly and high around the upper arm should be taken. Systolic blood pressure is taken at the first appearance of Korotkoff's sound and diastolic blood pressure at the disappearance of sound. If the average of blood pressure readings recorded on two separate occasions remains above normal limits, then the patient should be considered hypertensive and of such risk as to warrant efforts to evaluate for adverse effects of high blood pressure and potential contributing factors. On physical examination, particular attention should be given to the patient's height and weight, optic fundi, heart, amplitude of peripheral arterial pulses and the presence of bruits over the neck and abdomen, size of the kidneys, and blood pressure in the lower extremities. Inquiries should be made into whether or not there is a family history of high blood pressure, diabetes mellitus, or cardiovascular diseases. The patient's diet, including salt intake, and the presence of other cardiovascular risk factors as well as symptoms that may suggest cardiovascular disease should be examined. Consideration should be given to any use of medication that might be associated with elevated blood pressure, e.g., oral contraceptives, decongestants, and stimulants. In addition, the history or symptoms of renal disease, pheochromocytoma, Cushing's syndrome, and hyperaldosteronism should be routinely explored. If there are clues that any of these exist, then special tests are appropriate.

Laboratory Studies

Routine laboratory studies should include a urinalysis; blood sugar, uric acid, and serum creatinine levels; electrolytes; and a lipid profile. The chest x-ray and ECG are desirable not only for establishing a baseline for follow-up but also for detecting evidence of organ damage that may have come from previously elevated blood pressure. All of these tests are relatively inexpensive and can be justified as screening tests for all patients with hypertension (Table 46–4). Special studies such as I.V. pyelogram, renal arteriography, plasma renin activity, and aldosterone and catecholamine levels should be performed only if there are specific clues or indicators that suggest the presence of one of these known causes of high blood pressure (Table 46–5). The purposes of initial evaluation of patients who have hypertension are to identify adverse effects of high

Table 46–4. EVALUATION OF PATIENTS WITH HIGH BLOOD PRESSURE

Recommended Routine Work-up:	Special Biochemical Tests:*
Mid to moderate high blood pressure:	If diastolic blood pressure >115, consider the following:
History and physical examination	Plasma renin activity
Urinalysis	Plasma aldosterone
Blood chemistries	Serum calcium
Glucose	Captopril test
Creatinine	Urinary metanephrine
Electrolytes	Renal arteriogram
Uric acid	
Lipids	
Controversial	
Chest X-ray	
ECG	

*If symptoms suggest a specific disease, i.e., renal disease, hyperaldosteronism, pheochromocytoma, hyperparathyroidism, then do specific diagnostic tests.

Table 46–5. CAUSES OF SECONDARY HYPERTENSION

Defects	Screening Tests
Renal parenchyma disease	History
Glomerulonephritis	Urinalysis
Chronic pyelonephritis	Serum creatinine levels
Interstitial nephropathy	
Diabetic nephropathy	
Polycystic disease	
Obstructive nephropathy	
Renovascular obstructions	Abdominal examination for bruits
	Timed IVP
	Suppressed PRA
Coarctation of the aorta	Blood pressure in legs
	Chest x-ray
Drugs	History
Oral contraceptives	
Steroids	
Thyroid hormones	
Vasopressor drugs	
Cushing's syndrome	Dexamethasone suppression test
Pheochromocytoma	Urinary metanephrine
Primary aldosteronism	Serum potassium
	Urinary or serum aldosterone levels
	Stimulated PRA

blood pressure, concomitant diseases that may complicate hypertension or its treatment, and potential correctable causes and to establish the baseline for treatment and follow-up.

The infrequency of correctable causes of hypertension makes the routine search for correctable causes expensive and unproductive. There are reports of secondary causes for 5 per cent of hypertension, but these reports are all in selected populations. When other populations have been studied, the frequency of secondary causes has been in the range of 1 per cent or less. Berglund and coworkers (1976) studied a randomly selected group of men between the ages of 47 and 54 with moderate to severe hypertension and found that 5 per cent had a suggestion of a secondary cause but only 0.3 per cent were found to have surgically correctable causes. Tucker and Labarthe (1977) reported on individuals admitted to the Mayo clinic with high blood pressure and found that only 0.23 per cent had surgically remediable causes for their high blood pressure. The Hypertension Detection and Follow-Up Program had over 11,000 participants with high blood pressure, ranging in ages from 30 to 69 years, in whom there was an even lower frequency of secondary causes (Lewin et al., 1985). The most frequent secondary cause identified in the Hypertension Detection and Follow-Up Program study was the use of oral contraceptives.

In view of the low prevalence of correctable causes, especially among those with mild or moderate hypertension, special diagnostic procedures should be reserved for those patients who have severe hypertension or blood pressure that responds inadequately to medication and individuals in whom some sign or symptom is present to suggest a disease process known to produce high blood pressure (see Table 46–4).

Treatment

The general purpose of treatment of hypertension is to lower blood pressure to the normal range with minimum adverse effects. Some patients with mild hypertension can control the disorder with behavioral measures, such as salt restriction, weight reduction if they are obese, regular aerobic exercise, and use of relaxation techniques. If these interventions do not satisfactorily control blood pressure, then drug therapy should be considered. The abundance and variety of drugs that are available and effective in lowering blood pressure plus the myriad of potential adverse effects of these drugs challenge physicians to select the proper drug or combination of drugs for treatment of individual patients.

The Joint National Committee on Detection, Evaluation, and Treatment of High Blood Pressure has held four consensus conferences over the past 15 years and issued reports and guidelines that have

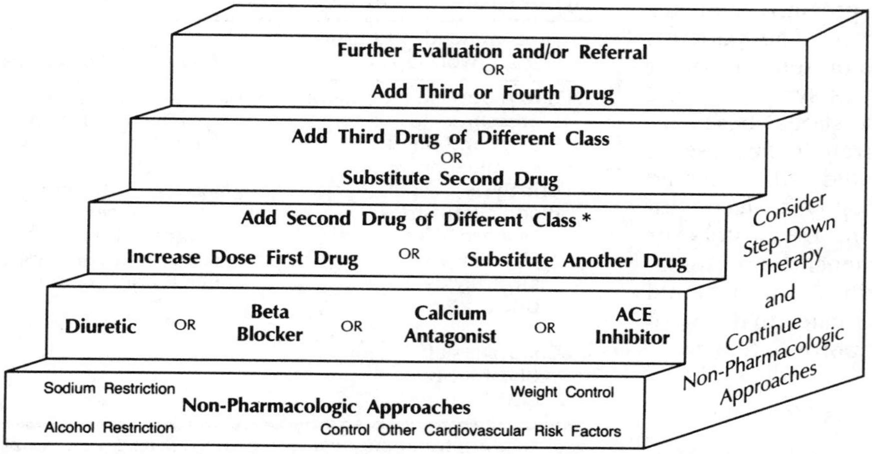

Individualized step-care therapy for hypertension. For some patients, nonpharmacologic therapy should be tried first. If blood pressure goal is not achieved, add pharmacologic therapy. Other patients may require pharmacologic therapy initially. In these instances, nonpharmacologic therapy may be helpful adjunct. ACE indicates angiotensin-converting enzyme; asterisk, drugs such as diuretics, β-blockers, calcium antagonists, ACE inhibitors, α-blockers, centrally acting α_2-agonists, rauwolfia serpentina, and vasodilators.

Figure 46–2. Stepped care. (From 1988 Report of the Joint National Committee on Detection, Evaluation, and Treatment of High Blood Pressure. Arch. Intern. Med. 148:1023–1038, 1988.)

Table 46–6. DRUGS AVAILABLE FOR TREATMENT OF HIGH BLOOD PRESSURE: THEIR POTENTIAL ADVERSE EFFECTS

Drugs	Selected Adverse Effects	Precautions and Special Considerations
Diuretics		
Thiazides	Hypokalemia, hyperuricemia, glucose intolerance	May be ineffective in renal failure; hypokalemia increases digitalis toxicity; may precipitate acute gout; increases blood levels of lithium
Potassium-sparing agents		
Amiloride		
Spironolactone		
Triamterene		
Loop diuretics	Same as for thiazides	Effective in chronic renal failure
Adrenergic inhibitors		
Beta-adrenergic blockers Acebutolol Atenolol Labetalol Metoprolol Nadolol Penbutolol sulfate Pindolol Propranolol hydrochloride Timolol	Bronchospasm, peripheral arterial insufficiency, fatigue, insomnia, sexual dysfunction, exacerbation of congestive heart failure, masking of symptoms of hypoglycemia, hypertriglyceridemia, decreased high-density lipoprotein cholesterol (except for pindolol and acebutolol)	Should not be used in patients with asthma, chronic obstructive pulmonary disease, congestive heart failure, heart block and sick sinus syndrome; use cautiously in insulin-treated diabetics and patients with peripheral vascular disease; should not be discontinued abruptly in patients with IHD
Centrally acting adrenergic inhibitors Clonidine Guanabenz Guanfacine hydrochloride Methyldopa Clonidine patch (Catapres-TTS) (patch)	Drowsiness, sedation, dry mouth, fatigue, sexual dysfunction Localized skin reaction to patch	Rebound hypertension may occur with abrupt discontinuance, particularly with prior administration of high doses or with continuation of concomitant beta-blocker therapy; may cause liver damage, Coombs-positive, hemolytic anemia, and orthostatic hypotension in elderly
Peripheral acting adrenergic inhibitors		
Alpha, adrenergic blockers Prazosin hydrochloride Terazosin hydrochloride	First-dose syncope, orthostatic hypotension, weakness, palpitations	Orthostatic hypotension in elderly
Vasodilators Hydralazine Minoxidil	Headache, tachycardia, fluid retention; positive antinuclear antibody test; hypertrichosis	
ACE inhibitors Captopril Enalapril Lisinopril	Rash, cough, angioneurotic edema, hyperkalemia, dysgeusia	Can cause reversible acute renal failure in patients with bilateral renal arterial stenosis or unilateral stenosis in a solitary kidney; proteinuria may occur; hyperkelamia can develop
Calcium antagonists Diltiazem Nicardipine Nifedipine Nitrendipine Verapamil	Edema, headache, tachycardia (all patients); constipation, flushing	May cause liver dysfunction

been extraordinarily helpful in bringing orderly and rational treatment to high blood pressure (1988 Joint National Committee on Detection, Evaluation, and Treatment of High Blood Pressure, 1988). The major focus of the first conference in 1973 was recognizing the large number of people with high blood pressure and clarifying that only about 12 per cent have their blood pressure under satisfactory control. The second conference of the Joint National Committee in 1980 emphasized the stepped care approach to blood pressure control. It was recognized that treatment of even mild hypertension, i.e., diastolic pressure of 90 to 104 mm. Hg, had a significant impact on reducing cardiovascular mortality and morbidity. In 1984, the Joint National Committee focused on methods for profiling and categorizing patients so that treatment could be individualized. The effectiveness of new drugs such as the angiotensin-converting enzyme (ACE) inhibitors and calcium channel blockers was emphasized. In 1988, the concept of stepped care was broadened. Greater concern was given to the quality of life, the adverse effects and costs of medication used, the degree to which patients became involved in monitoring their own blood pressure, and adjusting therapy to gain maximum blood pressure control while at the same time avoiding adverse effects.

Modern day stepped care provides the option of one of four classes of drugs to be used in the first step, depending upon the clinical profile of the patient. The second step suggested is either to increase the dosage of the first drug or to substitute another drug systematically until blood pressure control is obtained. Recommendations from the fourth Joint National Committee in 1988 are outlined in Figure 46–2. The drugs currently available for treatment of high blood pressure and their potential adverse effects are shown in Table 46–6.

The four profiles to consider are organized under demography—age, race, and socioeconomic class; hemodynamics—high cardiac output or increased peripheral resistance; biochemical information—high or low renin or high or low aldosterone; and presence of concomitant conditions—ischemic heart disease (IHD), chronic obstructive lung disease, or peripheral vascular disease. Elderly patients with increased peripheral resistance often respond better to diuretics and calcium antagonists than to beta-blockers or ACE inhibitors. Young people, especially those with hyperdynamic circulation, respond better to beta-blockers than ACE inhibitors. Concomitant diseases should always be considered when prescribing antihypertensive drugs. For example, beta-blockers may worsen asthma, obstructive pulmonary disease, and peripheral arterial diseases, but they may have added benefits for angina, arrhythmias, and migraine headaches. Adverse interactions with other drugs must always be taken into account when selecting an antihypertensive. The cost of therapy may be a barrier to patients and should be taken into account.

The objective is to keep blood pressure below 140/90 mm. Hg with the fewest side effects at the lowest cost. If blood pressure cannot be controlled satisfactorily with the previously described approach, then reconsideration of special tests to search for secondary causes is in order.

Chest Pain

Hilmon Castle

Among adults, chest pain is a common symptom that is frequently presented to the primary care physician. A detailed description of chest pain, including its location, frequency, and intensity and its duration and relationship to movement, deep inspiration, position, eating, and activity, is important in distinguishing benign causes from those that reflect serious disorders. Physical findings are usually absent or not helpful. Laboratory studies may be essential in arriving at the correct diagnosis. Anterior chest pain is often transient, without a specific cause ever being identified. The most common causes are chest wall pain and anxiety, which require observation and reassurance, but the most serious causes can include esophageal disease, pericarditis, dissecting aortic aneurysm, pulmonary emboli, herpes zoster, and myocardial ischemia and require specific laboratory testing.

CHEST WALL PAIN

Anterior chest wall pain occurs frequently and may last anywhere from a few seconds to several hours. It is usually of mild to moderate intensity. Movement of the chest or palpation often produces or accentuates the pain. Costochondral junctions on either side of the sternum may be inflamed and may produce generalized anterior chest pain. If this is present, localized tenderness can almost always be elicited by palpation over the area. The left second costochondral junction is the site most commonly inflamed. Injections of local anesthetics provide relief and serve to confirm the diagnosis of Tietze's syndrome.

Chest pain from compression of nerves and vascular structures exiting the superior portion of the thoracic cage can often be produced by elevation of the arms over the head; brachial arterial pulses can be diminished by pressing the arms along the patient's side. Palpation over the supraclavicular area is often tender. There may be evidence of nerve compression manifested by hypoesthesia, muscle weakness, and atrophy in the arm. Also, a deep inspiration may diminish or even obliterate the arterial pulses in the arm, especially if the neck is fully extended and rotated toward the side of the symptom. Aching in the arm may be more notable than anterior chest pain.

ANXIETY

Anterior chest pain that is due to anxiety may be sharp or stabbing and often is intermittent and located over the left anterior side of the chest. The pain is quite variable, and the patient often has difficulty describing the characteristics of the pain and distinguishing the pain from a feeling of a lump in the throat or transient shortness of breath. The pain may be chronic, and if unaltered by position, eating, or activity, palpitations are often described and hyperventilation is sometimes associated with the pain. Physical examination and the ECG usually show nothing abnormal.

HERPES ZOSTER

Chest pain from herpes zoster may be severe and present for several days without abnormal physical or laboratory findings. A careful history may disclose that the discomfort is distributed over a well-circumscribed area of the chest conforming to a specific dermatome and may include not only the anterior aspect of the chest but also the lateral and posterior aspects. The skin may be sensitive to touch. If a skin rash or blisters are present, then the diagnosis becomes apparent.

ESOPHAGITIS AND HIATAL HERNIA

Chest discomfort associated with esophagitis or hiatal hernia is usually described as burning in character and located in the low retrosternal area. Antacids often provide prompt relief. The discomfort is frequently prominent after meals or coffee ingestion and on assuming the supine position. The patient may be awakened at night with discomfort resulting from reflux through the inflamed esophagus, which occurs more easily when the patient is in the recumbent position. If the ECG is normal and stress testing does not suggest myocardial ischemia, then acid infusion of the esophagus (Bernstein's test) will test esophageal sensitivity to acid and often reproduce the symptoms found in reflux esophagitis. Esophagoscopy and further special tests may be necessary for a correct diagnosis. Relief of esophageal pain from nitroglycerin is common and thus may mislead one into thinking that myocardial ischemia is the cause of the chest pain.

ACUTE PERICARDITIS

Pain from pericarditis is usually sharp and persistent and is aggravated by deep inspiration or change of body position. The presence of a pericardial friction rub on auscultation of the heart will confirm the diagnosis. Unfortunately a friction rub is not audible more than 50 per cent of the time. The ECG may show characteristic S-T segment elevations in the standard leads. An echocardiogram helps confirm the diagnosis by demonstrating a pericardial effusion and sometimes increased reflectance from the pericardium. Pericarditis may be secondary to viral or bacterial infection, a generalized systemic disease, or a previous myocardial infarction (MI) or cardiac surgery (Dressler's syndrome). A history of any of these conditions is helpful in diagnosing pericarditis.

AORTIC DISSECTION

Aortic dissection is uncommon, but it produces chest pain that may be confused with that caused by myocardial ischemia. Chest pain from aortic dissection usually begins quite suddenly and is very severe and may be all but unbearable. Vagovagal reactions manifested as sweating, nausea, vomiting, and faintness are common. In addition, there may be signs of cerebral ischemia, syncope, or loss of carotid or arterial pulses in the arms. Not infrequently patients describe their pain as tearing, ripping, or stabbing. Often the chest pain migrates from its place of origin through the path of the dissection, which, if it goes distal, produces posterior interscapular pain. There is no relief with nitroglycerin or oxygen. Blood pressure may be elevated and aortic regurgitation may be audible if the dissection is in the ascending aorta. The intensity of the murmur may wax and wane because of factors such as blood pressure fluctuations, which will increase the murmur if blood pressure is high and diminish it if blood pressure is low. Other peripheral signs of aortic regurgitation may also be present. The ECG may show left ventricular enlargement that is a consequence of previously prolonged elevation of blood pressure. Ultrasound studies are very helpful in detecting an aortic dissection. A computed tomography scan with contrast material is quite accurate in detecting aortic dissection. The most definitive study, however, is the aortic angiogram, which is often required to define the full extent of the dissection.

PULMONARY EMBOLI

Chest pain and dyspnea are the most frequent symptoms of a pulmonary embolism, and the pain is often pleuritic. Apprehension and coughing are common signs and symptoms, whereas hemoptysis, although very helpful in diagnosing, is infrequent. Tachypnea is quite common, and an accentuated pulmonic second sound may be present on careful examination. The classic triad of chest pain, dyspnea, and hemoptysis is uncommon. The ECG is highly variable and is usually nondiagnostic. Ventilation perfusion scanning has high sensitivity and even greater specificity. If the ventilation perfusion scan is entirely normal, then the diagnosis of pulmonary emboli can usually be excluded. On the other hand, selective pulmonary arteriography remains the most dependable test available for inclusion and exclusion of the diagnosis of pulmonary emboli and may be necessary for a definitive diagnosis.

ANGINA PECTORIS

The term angina pectoris is used when the substernal pain has the characteristic of being provoked by activity, eating, emotion, or exposure to cold and is relieved by rest, relaxation, or nitroglycerin. William Heberden in 1768 described the characteristics of chest pain resulting from myocardial ischemia and called it angina pectoris.

Those who are affected with it are seized, while they are walking and more particularly when they walk soon after eating, with painful and most disagreeable sensation in the breast which seems as if it would take their life away if it were to increase or to continue. The moment they stand still, all this uneasiness vanishes. In all other respects, patients who are at the beginning of this disorder are perfectly well and in particular have no shortness of breath, from which it is totally different.

This description of angina pectoris is remarkably accurate and lucid. No one has claimed credit for describing it more concisely or accurately than Heberden.

Unfortunately, myocardial ischemia is not always painful, and when it is, patients do not describe their symptoms in such lucid terms. Chest pain with any of the characteristics described above should be a clue for further evaluation for heart disease. The resting ECG in patients with angina pectoris is usually normal or has only minor, nonspecific abnormalities. The ECG may be normal even while myocardial ischemia is present. On the other hand, a well-controlled exercise stress test usually shows S-T segment changes that support the diagnosis of ischemia. If pain is induced simultaneously, there is a high probability of myocardial ischemia and further evaluation and treatment for angina should be pursued.

Many patients describe vague symptoms, such as fatigue, shortness of breath, or pressure in their chest, but deny that they have pain. On the other hand, many patients describe chest pain typical of angina pectoris yet, after extensive testing, have no evidence of coronary disease or myocardial ischemia. Another factor that may confound the problem of accurate diagnosis is that some interviewers ask leading questions and solicit a description of chest pain indistinguishable from that of angina.

Caution in diagnosing is appropriate if the only positive evidence available to support a diagnosis of myocardial ischemia is the patient's history. The seriousness of coronary artery disease mandates that suspected episodes of myocardial ischemia should be confirmed by special testing.

Signs and Symptoms

The history is a critical element in the evaluation of patients with chest pain. If a clear description is not provided spontaneously by the patient, then the physician should probe for specific details of what provokes and relieves the chest pain. Angina is frequently described as a constricting feeling, tightness, or a deep pressure in the anterior chest. On occasion, the pain may be described as burning or aching and even sharp, although this is uncommon. The chest pain is retrosternal and may radiate to the neck, jaw, shoulders, arms, interscapular area, or epigastrium or may occur in only one of these radiation locations. Most often, myocardial ischemic pain is provoked by physical or emotional stress and it usually lasts for several minutes, but rest or relaxation is often followed within a few minutes by relief of pain. Chest pain lasting more than 30 minutes is usually not angina pectoris; rather, the possibility of injury and necrosis to the myocardium is likely. Patients may minimize their chest discomfort, leading physicians to consider the pain trivial or insignificant. Among patients with risk factors such as a family history of chest pain, high blood pressure, elevated serum lipids, cigarette smoking, diabetes mellitus, obesity, or a sedentary life style, a strong suspicion of myocardial ischemia should always prevail. Exercise treadmill ECG tests and thallium scans are available to most physicians and should be performed when there is a suspicion of significant coronary artery disease.

Symptoms other than chest pain may be the only manifestations of myocardial ischemia. Dyspnea, fatigue, or palpitations provoked by exercise and relieved by rest should alert patients as well as their physicians to the possibility of myocardial ischemia. Any significant ECG changes at rest or during exercise should enhance the suspicion of heart disease.

Physical Examination and Laboratory Findings

Palpating the chest for areas of tenderness or trigger points for induction of pain or having the patient move his or her arms and chest wall may be helpful in identifying a localized musculoskeletal cause for chest pain. Even if these localized causes are present, they do not exclude myocardial ischemia. Arrhythmias or a fourth heart sound raises the suspicion of heart disease and justifies special testing.

Criteria for Diagnosis

If other explanations for chest pain are not apparent, then special tests for myocardial ischemia should be done. As mentioned before, the ECG is often normal, as is the chest x-ray. On the other hand, any abnormality of the heart evident on the chest x-ray or ECG is helpful. Treadmill or bicycle ergometer exercise frequently produces objective ECG changes that confirm the presence of myocardial ischemia. An entirely normal ECG after intense exercise and achievement of the target heart rate considerably reduces the probability of myocardial ischemia as a cause of chest pain. If these tests are not revealing and both the patient and physician agree that a definite diagnosis should be established, then coronary arteriography is likely to be definitive in identifying the presence or absence of significant coronary disease. Provocative tests for coronary artery spasm may be necessary if the suspicion of myocardial ischemia is strong yet the coronary arteries fail to show significant obstructive lesions.

For the purpose of defining the patient's condition and establishing a baseline for treatment and follow-up, it is important to grade the symptom and limitation of the patient's physical activity. Several schemes have been recommended. One that is useful is recommended by the Canadian Cardiovascular Society and is condensed and simplified below.

- *Grade I:* Angina is provoked only by strenuous exertion; there is no limitation of ordinary activity such as walking or climbing stairs.
- *Grade II:* Patient is comfortable at rest, but ordinary activity such as walking more than two blocks or climbing more than one flight of stairs provokes symptoms; there is a slight limitation of physical activity.
- *Grade III:* Less than ordinary activity, such as walking two blocks or climbing one flight of stairs under normal relaxed conditions, provokes symptoms; there is moderate limitation of activity.
- *Grade IV:* Any physical activity may provoke symptoms, and symptoms may even be present at rest.

Treatment

The patient with stable angina pectoris should stop smoking and achieve ideal body weight and normal blood pressure and serum lipids. Regular exercise is appropriate for many patients, although the severity of coronary artery disease and the patient's exercise tolerance on a well-controlled exercise stress test must be known for a safe and proper recommendation for exercise. Clarity about the severity of coronary artery disease is important for any treatment of angina but is essential when exercise is being recommended as a part of the treatment. Most patients benefit from one half or one aspirin (160 to 325 mg.) daily, sublingual nitroglycerin for prompt relief of intermittent pain, and long-acting nitrates to reduce the frequency and severity of symptoms. Beta-adrenergic blocking agents are frequently recommended, and there are a large number of agents available and suitable for use. The advantages and disadvantages of each should be reviewed in detail. Specific objectives as to end-points or purposes for their use should be clear. Calcium channel blockers are also used in patients with angina pectoris. Those with greater vasodilator effect such as nifedipine and nicardipine are more likely to be helpful in the relief of symptoms. The role of beta-blockers as well as calcium channel antagonists can be best determined if the coronary artery anatomy is known and if left ventricular function and the degree of myocardial ischemia have been defined.

Coronary arteriography for all patients with stable angina pectoris or a history of previous MI remains controversial because of the risk and cost of this special procedure. There is general agreement, however, that patients who respond poorly to medical treatment or have progression or instability of symptoms should have this special invasive study. Obviously, each patient must be considered individually, and consultation with a cardiologist usually leads to a satisfactory recommendation as to appropriate testing and treatment of patients with IHD. Progression or instability of symptoms among patients with previously stable angina pectoris should provoke a prompt consultation.

VARIANT (PRINZMETAL'S) ANGINA

In variant angina, chest pain characteristically occurs at rest and often at about the same time each day. Emotional stress is more likely to provoke pain than is exercise. The patient may be able to exercise vigorously without symptoms or changes in the ECG. Nitroglycerin usually provides prompt relief, and long-term treatment with nitrates and calcium channel blockers such as nifedipine and nicardipine usually prevents episodes of pain secondary to variant angina. An ECG recorded during an episode of pain usually shows the distinctive abnormalities of elevation of S-T segments and increased amplitude of T waves. In contrast with the increased heart rate that usually occurs with coronary artery obstructions, coronary spasm often produces slowing of the heart rate. Arrhythmias during coronary artery spasm are common. Ventricular ectopy occurs about 50 per cent of the time, and, occasionally, transient atrioventricular (AV) heart block occurs. As soon as the spasm and chest pain disappear, the ECG usually reverts promptly to its previous status.

Proper treatment of variant angina is directed at preventing or relieving coronary spasm. Abstinence from smoking is essential, as is learning to avoid the conditions that provoke spasm. The calcium channel blockers are very helpful in variant angina, but beta-blockers often make the condition worse.

SILENT MYOCARDIAL ISCHEMIA

In the past, chest pain has been the bellwether of the diagnosis and treatment of patients with coronary artery disease. However, severe myocardial ischemia and even acute MI have been repeatedly documented without occurrence of pain. Silent ischemia is defined as the objective evidence of myocardial ischemia that is not associated with angina or angina equivalent such as acute dyspnea or arrhythmia. With increasing applications of diagnostic tests and monitoring by ECG and radioisotopes for myocardial contraction and left ventricular function, we have discovered that painless myocardial ischemia among patients with significant coronary artery disease occurs more frequently than painful myocardial ischemia. Balloon occlusion of coronary arteries has shown that the usual sequence of changes is decreased myocardial contractility, followed by ECG changes, and then later chest pain. In many subjects, decreased contractility and ECG changes were not followed by pain. Some have argued that the distinction between painless and painful ischemia is merely one of duration, but this does not explain how prolonged ischemia that leads to MI can be without pain. There may be detectable differences in pain perception and pain thresholds between individuals with silent ischemia compared with those who have painful ischemia. Adaptive or inherent differences in pain thresholds among individuals or in the same individual at different times may account for how often ischemia is associated with pain. Despite the various mechanisms for silent ischemia, it is unclear whether any one has more significance for the severity of the underlying disease or patient outcome.

Ambulatory ECG recordings have been used frequently for detection of silent ischemia, but recordings reveal that ECG changes of ischemia without pain occur in an average of 80 per cent of patients with stable and exertional angina. In patients observed with stable angina who have episodes of S-T segment depressions, at least 75 per cent of the episodes are silent. On exercise ECG testing, significant S-T segment changes occur without pain. Localized changes in myocardial contractility due to ischemia have also been demonstrated repeatedly with exercise radionuclide ventriculography and exercise echocardiography.

Unfortunately, there are no studies to demonstrate that control or elimination of silent ischemia has a significant beneficial effect on morbidity or mortality. Neither has it been confirmed that it is possible to eliminate silent myocardial ischemia with treatment.

Although it has become clear that silent myocardial ischemia is quite frequent among patients with coronary artery disease, it is not clear what should be done about it. The motivation for treating angina is usually relief of discomfort and restoration of a normal life style free of pain. Since silent ischemia may not result in symptoms, the justification for the cost and potential side effects of treatment has been improved survival and reduced morbidity. Elimination of silent ischemia seems to be a desirable goal, but no studies demonstrate that this can be done nor that it is clinically practical to treat such patients. However, risk-factor control may have a beneficial effect on patients with silent ischemia as well as those with angina.

Acute Myocardial Infarction

Irreversible cellular necrosis results from prolonged ischemia secondary to occlusion of a coronary artery, major reduction in blood flow to regions of the heart muscles, or inadequate blood flow relative to the oxygen demand in an area of the heart muscle. Coronary atherosclerosis is usually the primary underlying pathologic process in IHD, but other mechanisms such as platelet aggregation, fibrin formation, coronary artery spasm, and thrombosis may precipitate the acute event. Currently, the most commonly held view of the pathogenesis of an acute MI is rupture or split of an existing atherosclerotic plaque, which then stimulates further platelet aggregation, thrombus formation, and coronary vasospasm and ischemia that is sufficiently prolonged so as to result in necrosis of heart muscle. The sudden onset and rapid progression of manifestations of acute infarction supports the concept that thrombosis or spasm or a combination acting in the presence of atherosclerosis is the final event that produces MI. These mechanisms are also most likely responsible for the spectrum of presentation of unstable angina, non-Q wave infarction, and sudden cardiac death.

The current theory of atherogenesis is that endothelial injury is the primary stimulus for atherosclerosis, which is followed by a cellular proliferative process encompassing endothelial cells, monocytes, platelets, and smooth-muscle cells from the arterial media. Macrophages engulf lipids from the plasma and initiate yellow streaks, which eventually become internal plaques. Hormonal factors released from cells that accumulate in and around a plaque contribute to vasoconstriction and thrombosis. After acute MI, coronary arteriography almost always demonstrates coronary atherosclerosis. A primary decrease in blood supply to the myocardium rather than increased demand is the usual precipitating cause in acute MI, although increased demand by the myocardium can play a significant role.

Symptoms

Chest pain is considered the most frequent specific symptom of an acute MI. Pain may vary in intensity but is usually severe and lasts for more than 30 minutes and frequently for several hours. Usually the pain is in the anterior aspect of the chest and is described as pressing, squeezing, constricting, crushing, or as though someone were standing on the chest. The pain may radiate to the neck, shoulders, and arms but has a predilection for the left side. Pain may also be felt in the epigastrium or jaw. Patients who have previously experienced angina pectoris indicate that the pain of MI is similar to angina but more severe, longer lasting, and wider in distribution and is unrelieved by rest or nitroglycerin. Nausea, sweating, and generalized weakness are common. Unfortunately, a significant number of patients with acute MI have vague symptoms that may not be recognized as related to the heart, and only a high index of suspicion and testing with the ECG and cardiac enzymes lead to the correct diagnosis. The fact that other conditions, such as esophageal disease, pericarditis, and aortic aneurism, may produce pain indistinguishable from that provoked by myocardial ischemia necessitates confirmation of the diagnosis by ECG or other laboratory tests.

Physical and Laboratory Findings

Even though patients may appear in distress and exhibit restlessness, there are few other physical findings that are helpful in the diagnosis. The patient most likely will appear anxious and exhibit tachypnea, especially if a large infarction has occurred. The skin may be moist and feel cool. Blood pressure is often elevated during pain. Heart sounds may be diminished, and an S_4 heart sound may be audible at the apex. If complications have developed, then rhythm disturbances are audible as well as recordable on the ECG. Rales may be heard in the lungs.

Usually the ECG will be abnormal, especially if it is recorded during chest pain, but the changes may be only minor S-T segment deviations or T wave inversions. Serial changes in T waves, S-T segments, and QRS complexes over time may be diagnostic. These ECG changes are usually the most helpful if the patient is seen within minutes to a few hours of onset of myocardial ischemia. If cardiac enzymes are instead drawn within a few hours of onset, most likely they will be reported within the normal range. In emergency departments, cardiac enzymes are often inappropriately used to rule out acute MI when insufficient time has elapsed for one to reasonably expect that they would be elevated. Although creatine phosphokinase (CPK) may become elevated within the first few hours of onset, it usually reaches its peak approximately 18 to 24 hours after onset of myocardial necrosis.

Criteria for Diagnosis

The presence of substernal chest pain for 30 minutes and S-T segment elevation, T wave inversion, and the appearance of Q waves on the ECG usually prompt the diagnosis of an acute MI. Cardiac enzyme elevations that peak within 24 hours and return to normal in 3 days confirm the diagnosis and convey a general impression of the extent of the myocardial damage. If the diagnosis is uncertain or other potential causes of CPK elevation such as intramuscular injections or other trauma to skeletal muscle are possible, a myocardial band fractionation of the CPK is helpful. The degree of myocardial damage is the major determinant of prognosis. Morbidity and mortality correlate highly with the amount of myocardial loss. The following bedside clinical classification suggested by Killip and Kimball (1967) is useful in determining a prognosis:

- *Class I:* Clear lungs and normal heart sounds without an S_3.
- *Class II:* Rales present but over less than 50 per cent of the lung field and an audible S_3.
- *Class III:* Rales audible over more than 50 per cent of the lung field.
- *Class IV:* Shock.

Fortunately, the majority of patients admitted to the hospital with an acute MI are in Class I or II. In addition, if the correct diagnosis can be made within 6 hours of onset of symptoms, a significant reduction in the myocardial damage can be effected if reperfusion by lysis of the coronary artery clot by I.V. thrombolytic drugs occurs. Balloon angioplasty in the cardiac catheterization laboratory is also an effective means of reperfusion if this treatment can be applied promptly.

Treatment of Acute Myocardial Infarction

Traditional treatment of acute MI in the coronary care unit since the first reports of continuous rhythm monitoring in 1962 has included relief of pain with I.V. analgesics; oxygen by mask or nasal cannula; nitroglycerin administered sublingually, dermally, or I.V.; and I.V. lidocaine for control of ventricular arrhythmias. Emphasis has been placed on monitoring for early signs of complications and treating arrhythmias, hypotension, and heart failure as they appear. I.V. lidocaine is very effective in suppressing as well as preventing ventricular tachyarrhythmias. It remains controversial whether I.V. lidocaine should be given prophylactically in all patients suspected of an acute MI or just selectively in those who exhibit warning ventricular ectopy.

In the late 1960's, Lown and colleagues (1967) reported that primary ventricular fibrillation is responsible for most of the early deaths in acute MI. The frequency of ventricular fibrillation in acute MI in the hospital has been variously reported as being from 3 per cent to 15 per cent. Now that patients are arriving at hospitals earlier in the process of their acute illness, this number may be even higher. Lown and colleagues concluded that patients who experience ventricular fibrillation or life-threatening ventricular tachycardia have "warning arrhythmias," such as premature ventricular beats, R on T premature beats, and couplets or multiform ventricular ectopy. In addition, they reported that prompt recognition of warning arrhythmias and treatment with I.V. lidocaine prevented primary ventricular fibrillation. In their experience, use of lidocaine in 130 consecutive patients with acute MI and warning arrhythmias prevented ventricular fibrillation.

A major impetus for the prophylactic use of I.V. lidocaine came from the study reported by Lie and associates (1974), who demonstrated that prophylactic use of lidocaine eliminated primary ventricular tachycardia and ventricular fibrillation in 212 patients treated within 6 hours of onset of their symptoms (Table 46–7). Although most episodes of ventricular fibrillation may be preceded by warning arrhythmias, approximately 25 per cent of the patients in the coronary care unit failed to have warning arrhythmias

Table 46–7. LIDOCAINE ADMINISTRATION IN ACUTE MYOCARDIAL INFARCTION

Normal Cardiac and Hepatic Function	Evidence of Cardiac or Hepatic Failure
Loading dose: 100 mg. given I.V. over 2–3 minutes	Loading dose: same as for normal function
Continuous I.V. infusion at 3 mg. per minute	Continuous I.V. infusion at 1.5 mg. per minute
Second bolus of 50–75 mg. given I.V. over 2–3 minutes 30 minutes after loading dose	Second bolus of 50–75 mg. given I.V. over 2–3 minutes 30 minutes after loading dose
Maintain I.V. infusion of 3 mg. per minute for 24 hours after no ventricular ectopy	Maintain I.V. infusion of 1.5 mg. per minute for 24 hours after no ventricular ectopy
Monitor for side effects	Monitor for side effects
If there is uncertainty regarding efficacy or toxicity, measure lidocaine plasma levels	If there is uncertainty regarding efficacy or toxicity, measure lidocaine plasma levels

detected before their first episode of ventricular fibrillation; thus, warning arrhythmias appear to have a low sensitivity for predicting primary ventricular fibrillation. On the other hand, if I.V. lidocaine is given prophylactically to all patients suspected of acute MI, a large number of patients will be treated with lidocaine who eventually prove not to have MI. In a recent study by Wyse and colleagues (1988), a total of 333 patients who arrived within 6 hours of onset of suspected MI were randomized into either prophylactic or selected lidocaine treatment. Patients received a 100-mg. I.V. loading bolus over a 3- to 5-minute period and then an infusion of 3 mg. per minute continuously. A second 100-mg. I.V. bolus was given 30 minutes after the loading dose. Only 60 per cent of these patients were eventually confirmed as suffering from acute MI. The rate of lidocaine toxicity was 2.4 per cent in the prophylactic group and 0 per cent in the selective group. The rate of sustained ventricular tachycardia or fibrillation was not significantly different, nor were the toxicity endpoints different between the two groups. Based on an overview of 14 randomized control trials of prophylactic lidocaine use, MacMahon and associates (1988) found there was no apparent beneficial effect on early mortality. Wyse and colleagues (1988) suggested that in management of a definite MI in which rhythm monitoring and capabilities for resuscitation are uncertain, prophylactic lidocaine is the preferred strategy. They suggested that either strategy, i.e., prophylactic versus selective use after warning arrhythmias, can be supported depending on circumstances. There should be reasonable certainty that an acute MI is present before embarking on prophylactic use of lidocaine, and if dependable monitoring for pending arrhythmias is not present, then prophylactic lidocaine is preferred. If the patient is to be transported or if treatment can be initiated within the first few hours, then prophylactic use of lidocaine may be most desirable. If, however, there is uncertainty about the diagnosis or if the patient is in a setting in which warning arrhythmias can be dependably recognized, then the selected use strategy may be preferred. Clinical judgment appears to be as critical in the use of lidocaine for ventricular arrhythmias as in treatment of other aspects of acute MIs. Refer to Table 46–7 for the dosage and method of administration of lidocaine in the treatment of acute MI. If there are no ventricular arrhythmias after 24 hours, then lidocaine infusion may be discontinued.

Numerous clinical studies have demonstrated the beneficial impact of opening the occluded coronary artery producing the MI, especially if this can be accomplished within 6 hours of onset of symptoms. The myocardium can be preserved and mortality impressively reduced. Thrombolytic drugs, i.e., streptokinase, tissue plasminogen activator, urokinase, or anisolated plasminogen streptokinase activator complex, infused I.V., dissolve the coronary clot 65 per cent to 85 per cent of the time, depending upon the interval since onset and the drug used. The downside of this treatment is bleeding during thrombolysis, but if patients with previous strokes, significant hypertension (systolic blood pressure >180 or diastolic blood pressure >110), recent surgery, or trauma or diseases that are likely to produce bleeding are excluded, then serious bleeding complications are infrequent. For example, cerebral hemorrhage may occur in only 0.5 per cent.

Balloon angioplasty performed during the acute phase of an emergency is efficacious in opening the occluded artery and has the added benefit of improving the coronary artery stenosis that precipitated the final clot. The obvious disadvantage of balloon angioplasty is its unavailability in most hospitals, and even where it is available, there are often significant delays from the diagnosis of an acute MI until this procedure can be accomplished. Only a few of the 10 per cent to 15 per cent of the hospitals in the United States that have emergency angioplasty capabilities prefer emergency balloon angioplasty to prompt I.V. thrombolysis plus later reassessment for continuing myocardial ischemia. Coronary angiography and angioplasty can be done later under stable conditions, if appropriate.

Since the most critical factor in salvaging the myocardium is the time from onset of ischemia to reperfusion, I.V. thrombolysis in appropriately selected candidates is the preferred approach. Unfortunately, only 25 per cent to 30 per cent of patients with acute MIs qualify for I.V. thrombolysis based on currently recommended inclusion and exclusion criteria. The vast majority of patients with acute MI are treated with conventional therapy and are not considered candidates for thrombolysis.

If myocardial ischemia is suspected and symptoms persist for at least 30 minutes and are unrelieved by nitroglycerin and the ECG shows S-T segment elevations of 1 mm. or more in at least two leads, then thrombolytic therapy should be considered (Fig. 46–3). If this therapy can be applied within 6 hours

Criteria for Diagnosis

—Chest pain > 30 minutes

—ECG–S-T segment and T wave abnormalities, i.e., 1 mm. elevation in two or more leads

—Cardiac enzymes–unlikely to be helpful within the first 12 hours

→

Conventional Treatment:

- Bed rest
- Nasal O_2, 4 to 6 l. per minute
- Nitroglycerine, 0.4 mg. Administer two times if no relief
- Pain relief–morphine sulfate, 2 to 5 mg. I.V. titrate; alternative, Demerol, 25 to 30 mg. I.V.
- Treat arrhythmias promptly. Options–prophylactic drugs. Treat warning arrhythmias
- Treat complications as they emerge
- Control risk factors for thrombosis

→

Strategy for Active Salvage of Myocardium

Reperfusion via intravenous thrombolysis, if no contraindications

—tPA 100 mg. i.V. over 3 hours
10 mg. bolus
50 mg. bolus first hour
20 mg. bolus second hour
20 mg. bolus third hour
or
—Streptokinase, 1.5 million units over 60 to 90 minutes
or
—Urokinase* or APSAC*

Reduction in myocardial O_2 demand. Beta blocker I.V., e.g., metoprolol, 50 mg. b.i.d.

Unstable or recurrent ischemia–coronary arteriography and angioplasty, if appropriate

*Not approved for I.V. use as of 4/1/89.

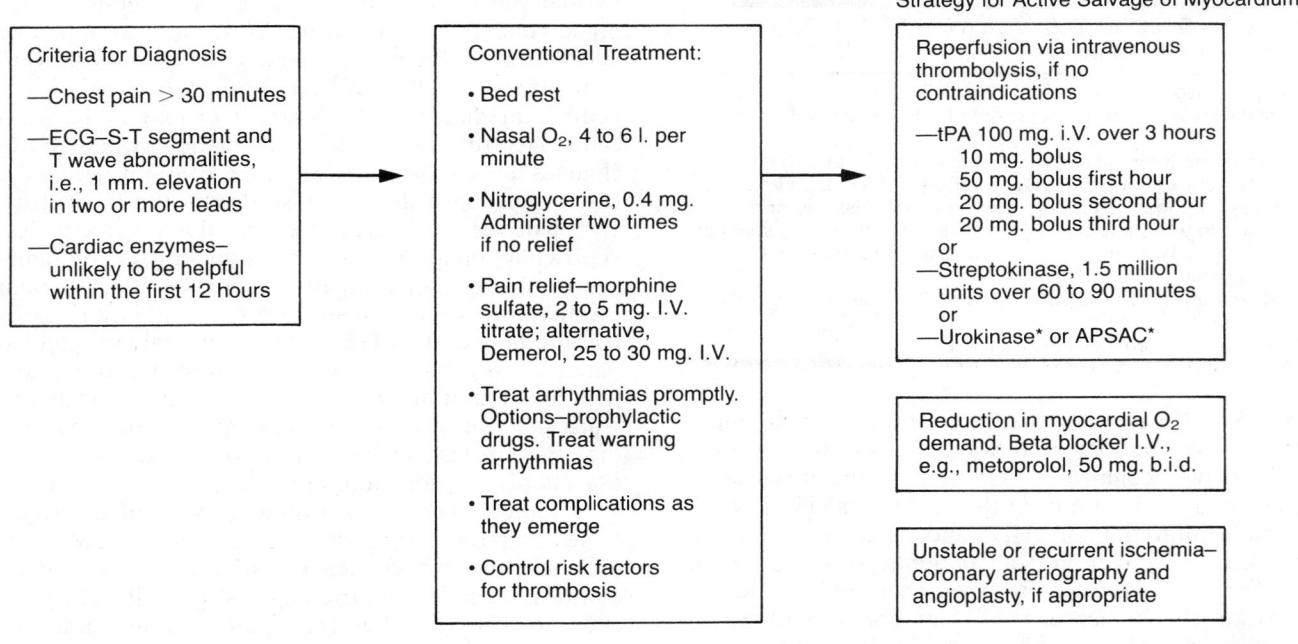

Figure 46–3. Acute myocardial infarction.

of onset of symptoms, there is potential for significant benefit. Since the major complications of this therapy are bleeding during thrombolysis, potential causes for bleeding, e.g., surgery or trauma, previous strokes, high blood pressure (systolic blood pressure >180 or diastolic blood pressure >110), an active or known source for internal bleeding or aneurysm, pericarditis, or cancer, are considered contraindications.

Bedside clues suggesting reperfusion are the disappearance of chest pain and resolution of S-T segment elevation. Ventricular arrhythmias occur frequently in acute MIs with or without reperfusion and are not useful signs (Califf et al., 1988). If there is no evidence of reperfusion and the patient is unstable, emergency coronary angiography should be done. If, however, there are signs of reperfusion and the patient is stable, coronary angiography can be delayed and performed later when there is evidence of spontaneous myocardial ischemia or ischemia induced by various stress-testing methods.

Since knowledge of coronary artery anatomy and left ventricular function is essential for determining prognosis and optimum long-term treatment of IHD, many recommend that coronary angiography be considered in all patients during hospitalization for acute MI, especially in those who have received thrombolytic therapy and have manifested evidence of reperfusion. The artery defect that precipitated the clot and produced the acute MI is most likely still present and places the patient in jeopardy for recurrent coronary thrombosis. If, however, the patient had a completed MI without evidence of recurrent spontaneous myocardial ischemia or ischemia after stress testing, then the cost and risk of coronary angiography may justify conservative and conventional treatment until there is evidence of recurrent myocardial ischemia.

An addition to conventional therapy recommended during the acute phase is the use of I.V. beta-blockers given as early as possible in the acute infarction. In a subset of patients in the TIMI-2-B study (The TIMI Study Group, 1989), there was a significant reduction in mortality among those given 5 mg. of metoprolol every 2 to 3 minutes for three doses followed by 50 mg. given orally twice daily for 1 day and then 100 mg. twice daily thereafter. This treatment should not be used if heart block or hypotension contraindicates the use of beta-blockers. Other I.V. beta-blockers will likely produce results similar to those found with metoprolol.

Long-term treatment following discharge from the hospital should consist of nitrates administered either orally or transdermally, 160 to 325 mg. of aspirin taken daily, administration of an oral beta-blocker for at least 1 year, and a structured exercise and education program concurrent with the control of risk factors to minimize progression of atherosclerosis (Table 46–8).

SPECIAL TESTS FOR DETECTING ISCHEMIC HEART DISEASE

A *resting ECG* should be obtained on all patients suspected of having ischemic heart disease (IHD). The vast majority of patients with angina as the only manifestation of IHD have a normal ECG while they are free of chest pain. Sequential changes of S-T

Table 46–8. LONG-TERM TREATMENT AFTER HOSPITAL DISCHARGE

Prescribe aspirin, 160 to 325 mg. daily
Prescribe nitrates, e.g., isosorbide dinitrate (Isordil), 10–20 mg. t.i.d.
Prescribe beta-blockers for at least 1 year, if tolerated
Help patient to control risk factors, e.g., decrease elevated lipids, eliminate smoking, lower blood pressure, and maintain adequate activity; provide education and specific drugs, if indicated, and help patient with behavioral changes
Perform submaximal ECG stress test 2–3 weeks after onset of acute MI
Provide structured exercise training

segment, T wave abnormalities, and the development of Q waves or loss of R waves typical of acute MI are easily recognizable. Obviously, the absence of such changes even during the acute episode does not exclude infarction or IHD, and other tests may be needed. Moreover, not all patients with transmural infarction develop Q waves on their ECG, and approximately 30 per cent of patients with Q waves during their MI lose them within 18 months. The sensitivity of the resting ECG for IHD is quite low. Even though the specificity of Q waves and absent R waves is much higher, there are many other diseases of the heart, e.g., myocarditis, that produce Q waves on the ECG and mimic MI.

Chest x-ray in patients with chest pain often identifies abnormalities not apparent on physical examination. Among patients with heart disease, the chest x-ray is of greatest help in determining heart size and the presence of congestive heart failure. For conditions that may mimic acute IHD, e.g., aortic dissection or pulmonary emboli, a chest x-ray is essential. Even though some of the complications of MI are identifiable, the vast majority of patients with IHD have normal chest x-rays.

The cardiac enzyme most helpful in diagnosing acute MI is CPK. This enzyme is a sensitive indicator of myocardial necrosis, but it is not specific because skeletal muscle as well as other tissues contain CPK. Fractionation for the per cent of CPK that is myocardial band enhances the specificity of elevated CPK for acute MI considerably when the clinical history and ECG are not typical. A normal serum CPK does not exclude recent MI, since the sample may not coincide with the brief period of elevation and laboratory errors are always a potential problem. Usually CPK increases in the serum within 6 hours of onset of myocardial necrosis, reaches a peak within 24 hours, and returns to the normal range within 3 days.

Stress tests with ECG monitoring usually result in ECG changes during and immediately after the procedure in patients with IHD. Treadmill exercise is the most frequently used stress test, but bicycle exercise and I.V. pharmacologic agents such as dipyridamole and dobutamine have been used to induce myocardial ischemia during ECG monitoring. The addition of thallium 201 injected in a peripheral vein at peak stress followed by radionuclide scans of the heart immediately and 4 hours later may add significantly to the diagnostic information when ECG changes are equivocal or when ECG abnormalities at rest compromise the response during the stress test, e.g., when there is hypokalemia, digitalis effect, left ventricular enlargement, or conduction or repolarization abnormalities on the resting ECG. Although the thallium scan may add information, it also adds considerable cost and should be done only in selected patients for whom the usual exercise treadmill test with ECG monitoring proves inadequate. Thallium scans are not always available, and when they are, they require meticulous attention to the technical aspects of the procedure and are time-consuming.

Radionuclide angiocardiography coupled with bicycle exercise testing is available in a few large hospitals and reflects segmental wall motion abnormalities of the left ventricle at rest as well as at peak exercise. This test has the additional advantage of reflecting left ventricular function through accurate measurement of ejection fractions.

Two-dimensional echocardiography and visualization of segmental contraction defects in the left ventricle following exercise on a treadmill or bicycle or during I.V. infusion of drugs, e.g., dobutamine, has sensitivity and specificity comparable to the use of radionuclide imaging for myocardial ischemia. Special equipment and experienced technical assistance are needed for this procedure, which is currently available in only a few medical centers.

Coronary arteriography is the "gold standard" for identifying anatomic abnormalities of the coronary arteries. This procedure provides a detailed and accurate visualization of coronary arteries and the degree of narrowing in various segments as well as the size of the artery below the stenosis, the presence of collateral circulation, and the status of the left ventricle as a contracting muscle. The value of coronary angiography for a specific patient depends on the clinical problem and circumstances. Certainly patients with unstable angina, that is, progression of angina with less and less physical exertion, occurrence of angina at rest, and episodes of prolonged pain without evidence of infarction, stand to benefit considerably from coronary arteriography. Even though arteriography may not be urgent in individuals with stable angina, there are still specific reasons why the coronary anatomy should be visualized. For example, we know that a large per cent of men with stable angina have either a left main coronary artery or three-vessel disease. Patients with a completed MI who continue to have bouts of chest pain secondary to ischemia despite good medical treatment will also benefit from coronary arteriography.

Rehabilitation After Myocardial Infarction

Allan V. Abbott
John C. Camp

The family physician should ensure the initiation and coordination of rehabilitation for the patient hospitalized with acute MI. This rehabilitation requires the use of consultants and other health professionals as well as knowledge of and access to community resources. Probably the most effective cardiac rehabilitation is through the coordinated team approach that has been developed by many hospitals. Because patients should avoid vigorous physical activities too soon after MI, medically supervised physical exercise is the central focus of this rehabilitation. The goals of this rehabilitation are (1) to enable the patient to achieve his or her optimal functional capacity and (2) to help the patient acquire the knowledge and confidence to maximize physical, social, and emotional functioning upon the return home (Greenland and Chu, 1988a).

Randomized trials of cardiac rehabilitation programs have documented their safety and have shown nonsignificant decreases in mortality in rehabilitation patients as compared with usual care. It has been concluded, however, that cardiac rehabilitation exercise probably helps prevent postinfarction deaths from cardiovascular causes as well as all other causes (Blackburn and Jacobs, 1988).

Patients who have had an MI commonly suffer a reduction in work capacity due to both the cardiac disease or injury and to the bed rest in the hospital. Fear and depression are also significant problems that affect work capacity. Most patients recover functional capacity without formal cardiac rehabilitation, but physical training can augment the recovery process and can enable many patients to reach levels of exertion that might not have been possible otherwise. Three conditions indicate the need for a supervised exercise program: a demonstrated limitation in the patient's functional capacity, the expectation that supervised exercise will significantly improve functional capacity, and concern regarding the safety of unsupervised exercise. Depressed patients may also respond favorably to a cardiac rehabilitation program because of the supportive environment.

IN-HOSPITAL REHABILITATION

Patients with uncomplicated MI should begin mild leg exercises immediately. Within the first 24 hours, they should begin feeding and grooming themselves, sitting up in a chair for 15 minutes, and using a bedside commode. This level of activity requires about 1 to 2 METs. An MET is defined as a multiple of resting energy expenditure (1 MET is about 3.5 ml. of oxygen per kg. of body weight per minute). Contraindications to participation in a supervised rehabilitation program include unstable angina, resting systolic blood pressure greater than 200 mm. Hg, resting diastolic blood pressure greater than 100 mm. Hg, severe aortic stenosis, active pericarditis or myocarditis, debilitating noncardiac disease such as renal failure or anemia, symptomatic or exertional hypotension, uncontrolled atrial or ventricular arrhythmias, uncontrolled tachycardia, symptomatic congestive heart failure, untreated third-degree heart block, recent pulmonary embolism, thrombophlebitis, resting S-T segment displacement greater than 3 mm., or uncontrolled diabetes (Greenland and Chu, 1988b).

The goal of exercise during hospitalization is to achieve a functional level that permits home-bound activities immediately after discharge. Household tasks require 2 to 3 METs. This is achieved in the hospital through walking, with stepwise increases in distance and speed as tolerated. This exercise begins with walking 50 feet on the level and progresses to 500 feet and up one flight of stairs. Counseling in the hospital should also address the reduction of other risk factors such as the elimination of smoking, control of diet and hypercholesterolemia, reduction of stress, and control of any associated diseases such as diabetes and hypertension. The patient without complications can usually be discharged within 5 to 10 days.

Predischarge low-intensity treadmill exercise testing can safely be performed at 1 to 3 weeks following uncomplicated MI. This identifies patients who are well suited for early discharge; helps define safely tolerated activity level; and helps identify patients at increased risk who develop ischemic ECG abnormalities, angina, or hypotension. Exercise testing can be conducted to a workload of 3 to 3.5 METs, or to 60 per cent of age-predicted maximum heart rate. The presence of the spouse during this test may lend psychologic support and can demonstrate to both persons the extent of exercise that can be safely achieved. Abnormal exercise tests, with ischemia or inability to raise blood pressure, indicate increased risk and the need for consultation, possible coronary angiography, and further treatment.

POSTHOSPITALIZATION REHABILITATION

Ideally, all patients should participate in medically supervised progressive exercise with the goal of returning to optimal function. However, economic constraints and logistics may limit access to supervised exercise in many cases. Medically supervised exercise with ECG monitoring is most important for patients with low functional capacity, severely depressed left ventricular function, complex ventricular arrhythmias, exercise-induced hypotension, and inability to self-monitor heart rate.

Rehabilitation exercise should be based on individual assessment and prescription for each patient. The usual procedure is to offer three 45- to 60-minute supervised exercise sessions per week beginning just after hospital discharge. This commonly involves walking on a treadmill or riding a stationary bicycle. Patients without complications can exercise at home on alternate days. The supervised activity may be discontinued when the patient is able to exercise at 8 or more METS without cardiac symptoms and when he or she has acquired the skills necessary to self-monitor unsupervised exercise at home. Physical work capacity typically plateaus at 8 to 12 weeks after starting exercise. Work capacity is usually determined by serial maximal exercise testing. Some patients may not be able to achieve a functional capacity level equal to 8 METS and may discontinue supervised exercise in the absence of improvement on serial exercise tests.

Selected patients without complications who have learned to self-monitor their heart rates can proceed with progressive exercise after discharge without direct supervision. Usually, a daily walking program arranged to suit the patient's particular circumstances is sufficient. Sexual activity can be resumed after the patient has become normally ambulatory, usually 3 to 4 weeks after uncomplicated infarction.

Additional measures may help prevent recurrence of MI. Smoking cessation is probably the most important. Control of hypertension, diabetes, and hypercholesterolemia is also essential. Beta-blocking drugs, when they are not contraindicated, may help reduce mortality during the first 3 years after infarction in high-risk patients. Long-term anticoagulant therapy with warfarin (Coumadin) is not generally recommended for survivors of MI. Aspirin has been shown to reduce the risk of reinfarction and can be given according to individual clinical judgment.

The long-term maintenance phase of cardiac rehabilitation includes continued regular medical care, education and counseling to minimize CHD risk factors, and exercise. The family physician should facilitate the maintenance of a healthy life style and a lifetime pattern of enjoyable regular exercise.

Heart Sounds and Murmurs

Hilmon Castle

Advances over the past 2 decades in invasive as well as noninvasive imaging of the heart have made it possible to confirm the presence of cardiac defects. This has enhanced rather than diminished the importance and usefulness of physical examination of the heart.

Careful physical examination can be the most cost-effective means of detecting defects in the heart valves or between the heart chambers. Helpful clues that indicate ventricular dysfunction are also detectable. For best results, all patients should have their heart examined in the sitting, supine, and left lateral positions. With the patient in the sitting position, it is important to examine the heart during normal respiration and during deep inspiration and exhalation. Systematic listening over the chest with both the diaphragm and bell of the stethoscope is essential for eliciting all the information that is available. Selective listening for the first sound (S_1) and then the second sound (S_2) and other sounds and murmurs is important. Any abnormalities identified through a systematic examination of the heart should then be re-examined with special maneuvers to assess the impact of respiration and position or the impact of maneuvers and pharmacologic agents.

Heart Sounds

Usually S_1 and S_2 are easily recognized and distinguished without difficulty. The second sound is louder when detected at the base of the heart, and it follows the shorter interval between the two prominent heart sounds. When the heart rate is fast (120 beats per minute or faster), systole and diastole become so similar in length that the interval is no longer useful as a marker to identify S_2. Another marker that distinguishes S_1 from S_2 is its slightly lower pitch, which occurs with the onset of the apical impulse and at the beginning of the carotid pulse. Also, S_1 is much softer than S_2.

The first sound is produced primarily by a combination of the closure of the mitral and tricuspid valves, abrupt tensing of the chordae tendineae and papillary muscles, and a sudden change in the direction of flow of the mass of blood in the ventricle. Usually, two components are heard as the first sound; mitral valve closure coincides with the first component and tricuspid closure with the second component. The first sound may seem slurred as the two components occur close together or distinctly split as they are more widely separated, as is present in complete right bundle-branch block.

The intensity of S_1 correlates with the position of the mitral and tricuspid valves at the moment the ventricle contracts. If these valves are widely opened at the onset of ventricular contraction, they will close with greater force; thus, a loud S_1 will be heard. If the valves have had time to float back near closure, as occurs with a prolonged interval from atrial to ventricular contraction (first-degree AV block), then S_1 is soft. If ventricular contraction is weak, then less sound is generated and a soft S_1 is heard. Arrhythmias that result in variation in heart rate or in an interval between atrial and ventricular contraction, e.g., complete AV heart block or atrial fibrillation, have variations in loudness of S_1 from beat to beat.

Defects in the mitral valve leaflets also alter the intensity of S_1. For example, in rheumatic mitral stenosis, in which the valve is often held open in an optimum position for closure under a pressure gradient between the left atrium and ventricle, an accentuated S_1 is produced. However, deformity in the valve leaflet that prevents complete closure at the time of ventricular contraction, as in mitral regurgitation, results in a soft S_1. Also, conditions that dampen the transmission of sound through the chest, such as a thick or obese chest wall, emphysema, or pericardial effusion, result in a soft S_1.

In summary, a soft S_1 suggests the following: a hypodyamic left ventricle, a prolonged interval between atrial and ventricular contraction, mitral regurgitation, or a condition that dampens sound transmission. An accentuated S_1 suggests mitral stenosis or hyperdynamic ventricular contraction, such as that which occurs in hyperthyroidism or in normal young individuals with a hyperdynamic circulation.

The second heart sound coincides with closure of the aortic and pulmonic valves. Upon exhalation, the aortic and pulmonic valves close almost simultaneously and only a single component is usually heard. On the other hand, deep inspiration produces a synchrony of closure with delay in pulmonic valve closure, and the aortic closure occurs slightly earlier than usual, so that two distinct components are easily heard. Events that prolong right ventricle contraction, e.g., increased volume in the right ventricle that occurs with deep inspiration or increased pulmonary artery pressure, delay pulmonic valve closure and split the two components of the second sound. Increased pulmonary artery pressure also produces a louder S_2. Conditions that overload the left ventricle or a left bundle-branch block delays completion of a left ventricular contraction and thus result in a paradoxical splitting, i.e., a narrow or single component of S_2 on deep inspiration and a more widely split S_2 on exhalation. Systemic hypertension accentuates the aortic component of S_2. whereas pulmonary hypertension accentuates the pulmonic component and results in wider splitting of the two components of S_2. Stenosis of either valve may restrict motion sufficiently to diminish or obliterate the sound generated by the defective valve, and thus only one component of S_2 may be heard.

In summary, a widely split S_2 that increases further with deep inspiration suggests a complete right bundle-branch block, right ventricular volume overload, or pulmonary hypertension. Hearing two components of the second sound more widely split on exhalation than on inspiration suggests a paradoxical splitting that is due to left bundle-branch block, left ventricular volume overload, or systemic hypertension.

A third heart sound (S_3) occurs shortly after S_2, is low pitched and soft in intensity, and is not normally heard but can be recorded frequently with a phonocardiograph. Under ideal conditions, S_3 may be heard in children or young adults in the area just medial to the apical impulse, especially if the patient is exhaling and has a thin chest or hyperdynamic circulation. There is uncertainty about what produces an S_3, but it occurs at the point of maximum filling rate and distention in early diastole when rapid flow of blood into the left ventricle suddenly strikes the wall and the mitral valve apparatus. These events most likely generate the low-pitched sound that occurs in the early part of diastole. Conditions that accentuate S_3 and make it audible in adults are high left atrial pressure or an abnormal left ventricle with decreased compliance. Left ventricular failure and mitral regurgitation with increased pressure and blood volume in the left atrium at onset of diastole are clinical conditions in which S_3 is often heard. An S_3 produced by the left ventricle usually is heard better on exhalation, and one from the right ventricle is accentuated by deep inspiration.

A fourth sound (S_4) is best heard at the apex and may be generated by an abrupt increase in distention and volume in late diastole coincident with atrial contraction, just prior to S_1. A seemingly wide split of S_1 should provoke consideration of S_4 that is occurring just prior to S_1. It is often difficult to distinguish a widely split S_1 from an S_4, but the S_4 precedes the apical impulse and is slightly lower in pitch than S_1. Exhalation accentuates S_4 if the sound is generated by the left side of the heart, which it so often is. Unfortunately, S_1 is also slightly accentuated on exhalation by virtue of better transmission of sound when there is less air in the chest.

Pathologic conditions with increased resistance to distention of the ventricle and more forceful atrial contractions result in an audible S_4. Patients with elevated systemic blood pressure commonly have an audible S_4, especially if careful and selected listening is done with the patient exhaling and in the left lateral position. Ventricular enlargement, either hypertrophy or dilatation, often produces an S_4. A dilated left ventricle that occurs with heart failure or congestive cardiomyopathy commonly has an S_3. An audible S_3 or S_4 suggests left ventricular dysfunction and justifies further noninvasive diagnostic studies, such as chest x-rays, ECG, and echocardiography, with Doppler flow studies performed for clarification.

The term gallop rhythm has been used frequently when an extra sound in addition to S_1 and S_2 is heard. The extra sound may be in systole or diastole, as described above. The implications of each of these may be very different and thus the common and inconsistent use of the term gallop is not very helpful and may actually be misleading. Various observers use the term quite differently. Some use it only when the sound is in diastole, tachycardia is present, and a gallop cadence is heard, whereas others use it even when an extra sound is heard in systole and even when heart rates are slow. To use the term gallop as a general and generic term without implications of a specific sound or pathophysiologic process, i.e., defining a gallop rhythm as one in which the heart sounds are going at such a cadence that they sound like a gallop, is acceptable, since this simply means that an extra sound is present along with tachycardia. To be more specific about whether the extra sound occurs in systole or in early or late diastole and whether or not tachycardia is present seems far more helpful than the usual inconsistent use of the term. A gallop produced by an S_3 and tachycardia strongly suggests heart failure or ventricular dysfunction, whereas a midsystolic click is more likely to be secondary to mitral valve prolapse and normal ventricular function.

Extra sounds in systole can be early or ejection sounds (clicks) or middle to late systolic sounds (clicks). Opening of the aortic and pulmonic valves at the onset of systole produces vibrations that, under normal conditions, are merged with S_1 and are of sufficiently low intensity to be inaudible. Certain defects that produce hemodynamic changes may increase the intensity of and delay these sounds, so that they can be heard immediately after S_1 as a relatively high-pitched, brief clicking sound.

Pathologic states associated with ejection clicks include stenotic but mobile aortic and pulmonic valves, ejection of a larger than usual volume of blood from the ventricles into major arteries, or more forceful ventricular ejection in the aorta or pulmonary artery because of hypertension. Ejection clicks may come from left-sided conditions, e.g., aortic stenosis or systemic hypertension, or from right-sided ones, e.g., pulmonic stenosis or pulmonary artery hypertension. Ejection clicks that originate from the right-sided heart structures are heard best along the left sternal border, especially in the left second and third interspaces. Ordinarily, they are not audible at the apex but are quite prominent at the base and leave the impression of marked splitting of S_1. Audible splitting of S_1 at the base serves as a clue that the sound is an ejection click. The quality of the clicking sound from pulmonic valve stenosis is markedly affected by respiration; it is louder on exhalation and much softer or absent on deeper inspiration. Ejection clicks from left-sided structures are also best heard at the base, but can also be heard along the left sternal border and at the apex. Unlike pulmonary ejection clicks, aortic clicks are not affected by respiration.

By far the most commonly occurring midsystolic sound is simply called a systolic click and is frequently associated with the click-murmur syndrome (prolapse of the mitral or tricuspid valve). Often, a late systolic murmur begins at the time of a midsystolic click and continues to the second sound in mitral prolapse syndrome. In addition, systolic clicks occur without other evidence of abnormality of the heart and are considered innocent. The presence of a systolic click justifies an echocardiogram to assess the dynamics of the mitral and tricuspid valves or other abnormalities that might produce this extra sound.

A snapping sound heard in early diastole close to the second sound may be produced by mitral or tricuspid stenosis. Even though the snapping sound is medium to high pitched and is of a different quality than an S_3, the only way to confirm by auscultation that this extra sound is an opening snap is its association with other signs of mitral valve disease. A phonocardiogram or an echocardiogram is helpful in clarifying the origin of this extra sound.

Heart Murmurs

There is uncertainty as to the precise mechanism responsible for the sounds of short duration in the heart that are called murmurs. Some hemodynamic events occur coincidentally with murmurs and must play a role, but multiple hemodynamic events occur simultaneously and perhaps some important events have still not been demonstrated. This makes it difficult to know which mechanisms generate murmurs in the heart. It is sufficient to say that turbulence occurs with systolic ejection murmurs, and the severity of turbulence correlates well with the intensity of the murmur recorded. The evidence that turbulence of blood flow is at least one mechanism for producing murmurs is convincing.

Another mechanism that may play a role in murmur production is the vibration of the valve leaflet that occurs when blood passes through the valve under pressure. Association of such murmurs with reflux of blood across incompetent valves has led to the term regurgitant murmur.

Murmurs are usually divided into *systolic, diastolic*, and *continuous* (Tables 46–9 and 46–10). Systolic murmurs are usually heard either during midsystolic ejection or are present throughout systole and thus called holosystolic. Some murmurs may be heard only in late systole, and, if they extend into S_2, they usually have the same significance as a holosystolic murmur and are referred to as regurgitant murmurs. An ejection systolic murmur does not begin until left ventricular pressure exceeds the aortic pressure and then ends as the pressure gradient diminishes in late systole, most noticeably before the second heart sound occurs. The gradient in aortic and pulmonic stenosis between the ventricles and the major blood vessels is at its maximum in the middle of systole; thus, the velocity of flow and turbulence are greatest, and the intensity of the murmur is loudest, at this point. Holosystolic murmurs that occur in ventricular septal defect and mitral and tricuspid regurgitation are produced by the flow of blood from a high-pressure chamber to a lower pressure. Since this pressure gradient occurs early in systole and actually persists into the second sound, regurgitation often produces murmurs throughout systole. When the valve is competent in early systole but prolapses or becomes incompetent in late systole, then the regurgitant murmur is heard only during this late period. The most critical dimension that aids in distinguishing the ejection from the regurgitant murmur is the presence of a silent interval from the end of the murmur to the second sound in the former and continuation of the murmur into the second sound at its usual intensity in the latter.

This emphasis on timing of systolic murmurs has called attention to the mechanisms of murmur production, but, unfortunately, all murmurs from the same type of valve defect do not conform to the anticipated timing characteristics. Thus, other characteristics are needed for describing and understanding murmurs. The pitch and quality of murmurs and their location are also helpful in distinguishing regurgitant murmurs from those produced by stenosis of aortic and pulmonic valves. If the interval from one beat to another varies, then the murmur intensity varies accordingly. Following a long diastolic filling phase, there is a larger volume to be ejected in the next cycle and, thus, murmurs from aortic and pulmonic stenosis are louder in the cycle following a long diastolic interval. For example, the beat that occurs after the pause from premature ventricular contractions produces a loud murmur. Also, in atrial fibrillation in which there is a marked variation in the interval from beat to beat, an aortic stenosis ejection murmur is louder after a long interval. A regurgitant systolic murmur from an incompetent mitral valve shows little, if any, variation in intensity or pitch following variation in the interval from beat to beat.

A uniform system for grading the intensity of murmurs should be employed. The one recommended by Freeman and Levine in 1933 is probably most

Table 46–9. CLASSIFICATION OF CARDIAC MURMURS

Systolic
- Ejection systolic murmurs
  - Innocent
  - Functional—due to degenerative changes in aortic valve
  - Pathologic
    - Left-sided
      - Aortic stenosis
      - Subaortic stenosis that is due to hypertrophic obstructive cardiomyopathy
    - Right-sided
      - Pulmonic stenosis
      - Atrial septal defect
- **Holosystolic regurgitant murmurs**
  - Left-sided
    - Mitral regurgitation
      - Prolapse of mitral valve
      - Rheumatic valve disease
      - Calcification of mitral valve anulus
      - Papillary muscle dysfunction
      - Dilatation of mitral ring
  - Right-sided
    - Tricuspid regurgitation
      - Prolapse of tricuspid valve
      - Rheumatic valve disease
      - Dilatation of tricuspid ring

Diastolic
- Regurgitant type
  - Left-sided
    - Aortic regurgitation
  - Right-sided
    - Pulmonic regurgitation
- Flow type
  - Left-sided
    - Large volume flow through mitral valve (ventricular septal defect and patent ductus arteriosus with large volume flow)
  - Right-sided
    - Tricuspid stenosis (rheumatic)
    - Atrial septal defect and ventricular septal defect with large volume flows

Continuous
- Left-sided
  - Patent ductus arteriosus
- Right-sided
  - Venous hum

Table 46–10. AUSCULTATION ASSESSMENT SYSTEM FOR EVALUATING HEART SOUNDS AND MURMURS

Timing: systolic, diastolic, continuous
Duration: midsystolic (ejection), holosystolic, late systolic (regurgitant)
Location: base (left or right of sternum)
Pitch: High, medium, low
Intensity: grades 1 through 6

frequently used and has served well to grade murmurs.

- *Grade 1:* The softest murmur that can be heard only under quiet conditions by a skilled examiner (1 out of 6).
- *Grade 2:* A slightly louder murmur that can be consistently heard by all examiners (2 out of 6).
- *Grade 3:* An even louder murmur but not loud enough to produce a palpable thrill (3 out of 6).
- *Grade 4:* A loud murmur accompanied by a palpable thrill (4 out of 6).
- *Grade 5:* A murmur sufficiently loud to be heard even if the stethoscope and piece is tipped on its edge but is still touching the chest (5 out of 6).
- *Grade 6:* A murmur loud enough to be heard with the stethoscope removed from the chest (6 out of 6).

SYSTOLIC MURMURS

Ejection systolic murmurs are commonly innocent and come from normal hearts, especially among children and adolescents. Innocent ejection murmurs are soft, usually Grade 1 or 2, rarely Grade 3, and are heard maximally over the base and just left of the sternum. They are softer when the patient is sitting rather than supine, decrease on deep inspiration, and increase slightly following exercise. Brief midsystolic murmurs are commonly heard over the base of the neck in children and adolescents. Hyperabduction of the shoulders and compression of the arteries as they exit the chest wall often obliterate this innocent murmur. An innocent murmur is usually the only auscultatory finding of note. The first and second sounds are normal, and there are no extra sounds or diastolic murmurs. If other findings, such as an ejection click, wide splitting of S_2, or diastolic murmur, accompany the ejection systolic murmur, then further diagnostic tests, such as chest x-ray, ECG, and echocardiogram with Doppler flow studies, are indicated.

Ejection systolic murmurs are heard commonly among older patients and usually are due to thickening and sclerosis of the aortic valve leaflets and aorta but are of no hemodynamic consequence. These degenerative changes in the aortic area can be confirmed by echocardiography. Bicuspid aortic valve, aortic valvular stenosis, hypertrophic cardiomyopathy, and other defects that produce ejection systolic murmurs can also be identified with echocardiography.

Other defects that produce ejection systolic murmurs include pulmonic stenosis and atrial septal defect. This murmur may be quite similar to those generated by the above defects, but the presence of a left parasternal heave, ejection click, or wide splitting of S_2 suggests the possibility of pulmonic stenosis or atrial septal defect. Deep inspiration often accentuates this murmur (see Table 46–13). A chest x-ray, ECG, and echocardiogram with Doppler flow studies usually suffice to identify these defects as the cause of the murmur.

Systolic regurgitant murmurs can be produced by defects in the valve leaflets, annulus, chorda tendineae, or papillary muscle of the mitral and tricuspid valve mechanism when regurgitation of blood into the atria occurs during systole. Also, ventricular septal defect results in blood flowing from left to right throughout systole because of a marked pressure gradient from the left to right ventricle. The murmur is usually holosystolic, harsh, and moderately loud along the left sternal border in the third and fourth interspaces. Transmission of this murmur depends mainly on its intensity. If it is loud, it is often accompanied by a thrill and heard over the entire precordium but poorly in the neck.

The most common defects that produce mitral or tricuspid regurgitation are prolapse of the valve (click-murmur syndrome), dysfunction of the papillary muscle, rheumatic valve disease, or calcification of the mitral anulus. Accentuation of the murmur on deep inspiration indicates that it is being generated by the tricuspid valve, whereas a slight decrease upon deep inspiration suggests a mitral origin (see Fig. 46–12). This type of murmur, regardless of whether it is mitral or tricuspid, justifies an echocardiogram and Doppler flow studies, which are usually definitive in diagnosis.

Bedside examination utilizing deep inspiration and exhalation and Valsalva's maneuver is helpful in confirming the cause of systolic murmurs. The sensitivity, specificity, and predictive value of these bedside techniques have had only limited testing, but Lembo and colleagues (1988), in evaluating 50 patients with systolic murmurs, found a high sensitivity, specificity, and predictive value for the various maneuvers recommended for distinguishing systolic murmurs from the right versus the left side of the heart and for distinguishing aortic from mitral murmurs. The simple maneuvers of auscultation of the patient's heart during deep inspiration and exhalation, Valsalva's maneuver while the patient moves from standing to squatting and back, and during isometric handgrip exercise are highly accurate in distinguishing systolic murmurs resulting from a pathologic defect from the far more common functional or innocent systolic murmurs.

The most helpful maneuvers used in the study by Lembo and colleagues are briefly paraphrased below. They are to be used after systolic murmur intensity with quiet respiration has been established (Tables 46–11 and 46–12).

1. *Inspiration and exhalation with the patient lying supine.* The observer listens while raising his or her hand to guide the patient during inspiration and then lowering it to indicate to the patient when to exhale. When slow cycles of inspiration and exhalation are established, changes in the intensity of the murmur at the peaks of inspiration and exhalation should be noted.

2. *Valsalva's maneuver.* Following a deep inspi-

Table 46–11. HELPFUL MANEUVERS FOR EVALUATING HEART SOUNDS AND MURMURS

Respiratory variation
Valsalva's maneuver
Standing to squatting
Squatting to standing
Elevation of legs with patient supine
Exercise
Sustained handgrip
Following a premature heartbeat
Administration of pharmacologic agents, e.g., amyl nitrite

ration, the patient closes the glottis and strains to exhale for 20 to 30 seconds. The murmur intensity is noted before the maneuver and near the end of the strain phase.

3. *Squatting to standing*. The patient squats for at least 30 seconds and then rapidly assumes the standing position. The murmur intensity is noted during the first 20 seconds of standing.

4. *Standing to squatting*. The patient is instructed to breathe normally and to avoid performing Valsalva's maneuver as he or she squats. The murmur intensity is noted before and immediately after squatting.

5. *Passive leg elevation*. With the patient supine and the legs straight, the legs are elevated 45 degrees and the change in murmur intensity during the 20 seconds after leg elevation is noted.

6. *Isometric handgrip exercise*. After 1 minute of maximum contraction of the hand around some suitably sized object, the murmur intensity is noted.

7. *Transient arterial occlusion*. Blood pressure cuffs are placed in the usual upper-arm positions for blood pressure recordings on both arms, and both cuffs are inflated simultaneously to 20 to 30 mm. Hg above previously recorded blood pressure levels. Twenty seconds after the cuff inflation, the change in murmur intensity is noted.

8. *Amyl nitrite inhalation*. A 0.3-ml. amyl nitrite ampule is broken into a 4 × 4 gauze pad; the patient is then instructed to take three rapid deep breaths of the amyl nitrite. The change in murmur intensity should be noted 15 to 30 seconds after inhalation.

Using these maneuvers as described, Lembo and colleagues reported that all right-sided murmurs increased in intensity with inspiration, whereas the majority of murmurs from the left side of the heart decreased or did not change. Murmurs coming from the right side of the heart increased in intensity in 100 per cent of patients upon inspiration, whereas in 100 per cent of patients with right-sided systolic murmurs, there was a decrease in intensity during exhalation. The majority of left-sided murmurs increased slightly or did not change with exhalation. Valsalva's maneuver was helpful in distinguishing hypertrophic subaortic stenosis from all other murmurs by an increase in intensity of the systolic murmur during the strain phase of Valsalva's maneuver. Also, the murmur of hypertrophic subaortic stenosis increased in 95 per cent of cases during rapid standing from squatting, and rapid squatting from standing consistently produced a decrease in the murmur intensity. Passive leg elevation decreased the murmur intensity of hypertrophic subaortic stenosis. Isometric handgrip exercise decreased the murmur from hypertrophic subaortic stenosis but accentuated the systolic murmur of mitral regurgitation and ventricular septal defect. Transient arterial occlusion by blood pressure cuff inflation augmented the murmur from mitral regurgitation and ventricular septal defect; these murmurs never decreased with this maneuver. The vast majority of other systolic murmurs did not change with this maneuver. Inhalation of amyl nitrite decreased the intensity of the systolic murmur from mitral regurgitation and ventricular septal defect, but murmurs from aortic stenosis and hypertrophic subaortic stenosis were accentuated by amyl nitrite. The sensitivity, specificity, and predictive positive and negative value of the various recommended maneuvers as reported by Lembo and colleagues are summarized in Table 46–13. Müller's maneuver is not included because it is not only difficult to perform, but it is also the least helpful of all the maneuvers.

DIASTOLIC MURMURS

Practically all diastolic murmurs can be divided into two types. One is a regurgitant type, which is a high-pitched, decrescendo murmur that begins immediately after S_2 and ends before S_1 and is heard maximally at the base and along the left sternal border. It is almost always due to either aortic or pulmonic valve regurgitation. Deep inspiration accentuates the regurgitant murmur that is due to pulmonic valve defect, whereas the aortic regurgitant murmur decreases slightly with deep inspiration. There may be signs of increased pulse pressure in the systemic circulation in aortic regurgitation. Diastolic regurgitant murmurs can be heard best with the patient sitting, exhaling, and leaning forward and with the examiner pressing firmly with the diaphragm of the stethoscope over the base of the heart or left sternal border.

The second type of diastolic murmur is a diastolic flow murmur, which is low pitched and sometimes rumbling and occurs in middle to late diastole, corresponding with the rate of blood flow from the atria to the ventricles through the mitral and tricuspid valves. With a large blood flow, this murmur can be generated by a normal valve, but usually such a diastolic murmur indicates pathologic narrowing of either the mitral or tricuspid valve. A long diastolic murmur that begins with the opening snap close to S_2 and persists throughout diastole with a presystolic accentuation occurring during atrial contraction usually means there is significant mitral or tricuspid stenosis. Increasing blood flow caused by exercise accentuates diastolic flow murmurs.

Murmurs from mitral and tricuspid defects can

Table 46–12. EFFECTS OF MANEUVERS AND EVENTS ON HEART MURMURS

Defect Producing the Murmur	Control	Deep Inspiration	During Valsalva's Maneuver	Sustained Handgrip	Following Premature Ventricular Contraction	Amyl Nitrite	Standing to Squatting	Squatting to Standing	Elevation of Legs	Transient Arterial Occlusion
					Maneuver					
Systolic Ejection										
Innocent	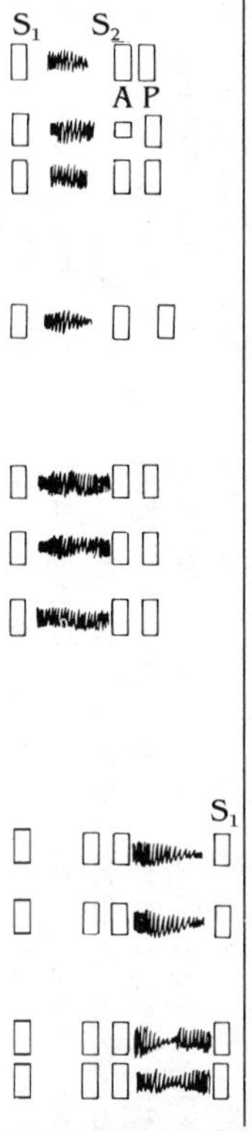	↓	→	→	→	→	→	→	→	→
Aortic Stenosis		↓	→	↓	↑	↑	↑	↓	→	→
Subaortic Obstructive Myopathy		↓	↑	↓	↑	↑	↓	↑	↓	→
Pulmonic Stenosis		↑	→	→	↑	→	→	→	→	→
Atrial Septal Defect		↑ ↓	→	→	→	→	→	→	→	→
Systolic Regurgitation										
Mitral Regurgitation		↓	↓	↑	→	↓	→	→	→	↑
Tricuspid Regurgitation		↑	↓	→	→	↓	↑	↓	→	→
Ventricular Septal Defect (Without Pulmonary Hypertension)		→	↓	↑	→	↓	→	→	→	↑
Diastolic Regurgitation										
Aortic Regurgitation		↓	↓	↑	→	↓	→	→	→	↑
Pulmonic Regurgitation		↑	↓	→	→	↓	→	→	→	→
Diastolic Flow										
Mitral Stenosis		↓	↓	↓	→	↑	→	→	↑	→
Tricuspid Stenosis		↑	↓ after release ↑	↓	→	↑	→	→	↑	→

Table 46–13. BEDSIDE MANEUVERS THAT AID IDENTIFICATION OF ORIGIN OF MURMUR

Origin of Murmur	Maneuver	Response	Sensitivity (in per cent)	Specificity (in per cent)	Predictive Value *Positive (in per cent)*	Predictive Value *Negative (in per cent)*
Right side	Inspiration	Increase	100	88	67	100
Right side	Exhalation	Decrease	100	88	67	100
HSS*	Valsalva's	Increase	65	96	81	92
HSS	Squatting to standing	Increase	95	84	59	98
HSS	Standing to squatting	Decrease	95	85	61	99
HSS	Leg elevation	Decrease	85	91	71	96
HSS	Handgrip	Decrease	85	75	46	95
MR† or VSD‡	Handgrip	Increase	68	92	84	81
MR or VSD	Transient arterial occlusion	Increase	78	100	100	87
MR or VSD	Amyl nitrite inhalation	Decrease	80	90	84	87

In summary, response of systolic murmur intensity to various maneuvers allows localization of most classes. For example, inspiration and exhalation response of the murmur is dependable and results in a high level of confidence. HSS increases with Valsalva's maneuver and squatting to standing and decreases with standing to squatting, leg elevation, and sustained handgrip, whereas MR and VSD increase with handgrip and leg elevation and decrease after amyl nitrite inhalation.

*HSS = Hypertrophic subaortic stenosis.

†MR = Mitral regurgitation.

‡VSD = Ventricular septal defect.

be distinguished by their location. Tricuspid diastolic murmur is heard maximally over the inferior portion of the sternum and slightly to the left, whereas murmurs from the mitral valve are heard maximally at the apex and with the patient turned in the left lateral position. Since both murmurs are of relatively low pitch, they can be more easily heard with the bell pressed lightly to the chest. A more helpful maneuver in distinguishing mitral from tricuspid murmurs is deep inspiration; tricuspid stenosis murmur is accentuated on deep inspiration, and mitral valve murmur decreases slightly. Alteration in the position of the mitral valve leaflet resulting from aortic regurgitation may generate a murmur indistinguishable from mitral stenosis.

Diastolic murmurs are usually pathologic and indicate defects in the aortic or pulmonic valve when a regurgitant type of murmur is heard or mitral or tricuspid stenosis when a flow type of diastolic murmur is heard. Deep inspiration accentuates right-sided murmurs, and exhalation increases the intensity of left-sided diastolic murmurs. Use of other physical findings, such as chamber size and arterial pulse, aids in clarifying the origin of murmurs. Echocardiography with color Doppler flow studies are the most sensitive and specific studies to use to clarify the origin of diastolic murmurs.

CONTINUOUS MURMURS

A continuous murmur heard over the upper chest is usually due to patent ductus arteriosus or venous hum. The patent ductus arteriosus murmur is heard maximally along the upper left sternal border and is usually machine-like in quality and peaks in intensity around S_2. This murmur is usually not significantly altered by changes in position or respiration. If there is a large defect, there may be signs of left ventricular enlargement and hyperdynamic circulation with increased pulse pressure. Venous hum is usually heard best in the upper right chest or supraclavicular area. It is louder when the patient is in a sitting position and may disappear when the patient is supine. Compression over the jugular veins above the point of auscultation obliterates the murmur. These maneuvers are sufficient to identify a venous hum, and further diagnostic tests are not indicated. The continuous murmur that suggests a patent ductus arteriosus requires cardiac catheterization and angiography.

Arrhythmias

Carlos Vallbona

Electrophysiology

Automaticity, conductivity, contractility, and rhythmicity are four basic properties of all cardiac cells. The fact that the atria and the ventricles contract rhythmically at a certain rate is due to the *automaticity* or periodic occurrence of transmembrane action potentials (TAPs) in a special group of cells more susceptible than others to becoming depolarized. These cells become the cardiac pacemaker because they produce an electrical stimulus, which is then conducted to other parts of the heart. The most common pacemaker is located at the sinoatrial (SA) node, although the atrioventricular (AV) junction and, to a lesser extent, the bundle of His and Purkinje's fibers may also act as pacemakers. The usual rate of automatic depolarization of the SA node is 60 to 100 beats per minute, whereas it is 40 to 60 beats per minute at the AV junction, and less than 40 beats per minute at the bundle of His and Purkinje's fibers. This difference in rates accounts for the predominance of the SA node as the normal cardiac pacemaker.

The typical ventricular TAP occurs when an impulse arriving through Purkinje's network finds the ventricular cell with a transmembrane resting potential of −90 mV. At that threshold level, the impulse opens up the fast sodium channel and sodium (Na^+) ions enter the cell, which becomes rapidly depolarized with a rebound reverse polarity of about +20 mV. (phase 0). At that time, the sudden influx of Na^+ stops, and there is a rapid drop of the potential (phase 1). The opening of a slow calcium channel allows for an influx of calcium (Ca^{++}) ions, which maintain the cell in a relatively depolarized state for a while (phase 2). At the end of this phase, there is an efflux of potassium (K^+) ions to the outside of the cell, with rapid return to the resting potential to −90 mV. (phase 3). However, this new state of repolarization is different from that before the onset of the TAP. The changes in intracellular Na^+ and K^+ concentration that have occurred in phases 0 to 3 must be restored to previous levels. This occurs during phase 4, thanks to a special pump mechanism that transports Na^+ ions from inside to outside of the cell and brings K^+ ions into the cell. The ionic flux during phase 4 does not alter significantly the transmembrane resting potential (Fig. 46–4*A*).

In the SA node, the ionic concentrations throughout the cardiac cycle are different. During diastole, there is a gradual influx of Ca^{++} and Na^+ ions across the membrane, which causes the transmembrane resting potential during diastole to be less negative than in other cells. At the threshold level of −60 mV., there is a faster influx of Ca^{++} and Na^+, causing a TAP whose rise and fall are not as steep as in the ventricular cells. Indeed, phase 0 is gradual, phase 1 is not noticeable, and phases 2 and 3 are also gradual and merged into one (Fig. 46–4*B*).

The ionic conditions across the cell membrane are critical determinants of the automaticity of all myocardial cells. This is the reason why arrhythmias may occur whenever the local extracellular or intracellular concentrations of Na^+, Ca^{++}, or K^+ are different from normal. Sympathetic or parasympathetic tone, hypoxia, and certain drugs affect the rate of rise of the transmembrane resting potential during diastole, thus changing considerably the normal electrical conditions and eventually causing cardiac arrhythmias.

The *conductivity* of electrical impulses depends on the state of refractoriness of the conduction system. During phases 0, 1, 2, and the early part of 3, the cells cannot respond to any stimulus (absolute refractory period). However, in the latter stage of phase 3, the arrival of a strong impulse may produce a new TAP (relative refractory period). Thus, changes in conductivity may occur under pathologic circumstances if an impulse arrives at a portion of the conduction system earlier than normal in the cardiac cycle. If the cells are in the relative refractory period, the impulse may be transmitted, but if they are in the absolute refractory period, the impulse may be blocked.

Another important phenomenon that explains the genesis of some arrhythmias is the *re-entry* mechanism. Conduction through Purkinje's branches usually proceeds in anterograde fashion (Fig. 46–5*A*). Should an increase in refractoriness occur in one branch (because of hypoxia or electrolyte changes), the anterograde conduction through that branch may be blocked, but an impulse may arrive later and retrogradely via a connecting branch. The previously blocked area may then no longer be refractory, and thus allows repeated re-entry impulses in the conducting circuit (Fig. 46–5*B*). This re-entry phenomenon explains the ventricular tachycardias in myocardial infarction and the episodes of supraventricular tachycardia that are common in the pre-excitation syndromes of Wolff-Parkinson-White or Lown-Ganong-Levine.

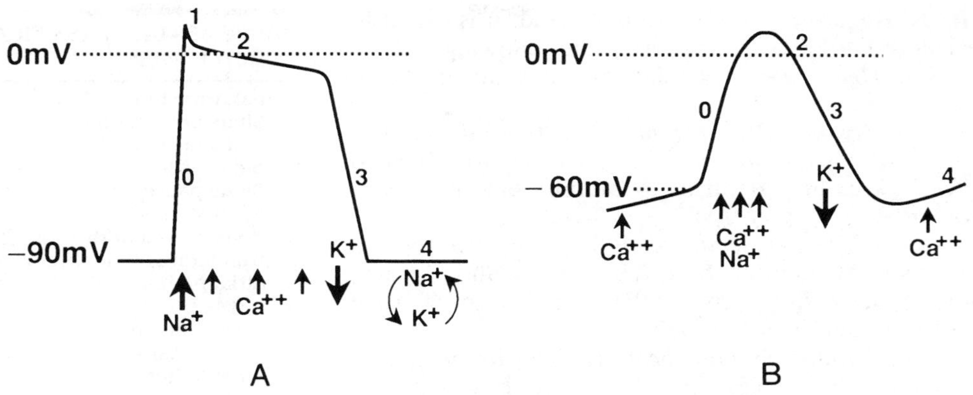

Figure 46–4. Transmembrane action potentials of the ventricle *(A)* and of the SA node *(B)*.

Etiology

Cardiac arrhythmias may result from disturbances in (1) automaticity; (2) conductivity, including re-entry; and (3) both automaticity and conductivity. The following are common causes of arrhythmia:

1. *Changes in autonomic nervous tone*. The sympathetic system increases automaticity and conductivity. The parasympathetic system has opposite effects, but an increased vagal tone may slow down the SA node so much that a secondary pacemaker (in the AV node or even in the ventricle) may take over.

2. *Organic or functional lesions of the central nervous system*. They may affect the normal activity of the cardiac regulatory centers, disturb the balance between sympathetic and parasympathetic tone, and produce arrhythmias.

3. *Electrolyte disturbances*. Hyperkalemia, hypokalemia, hypomagnesemia, and hypocalcemia are the most common electrolyte disturbances that significantly alter the ionic conditions across the cell membrane and therefore enhance or suppress cardiac automaticity or conductivity or both.

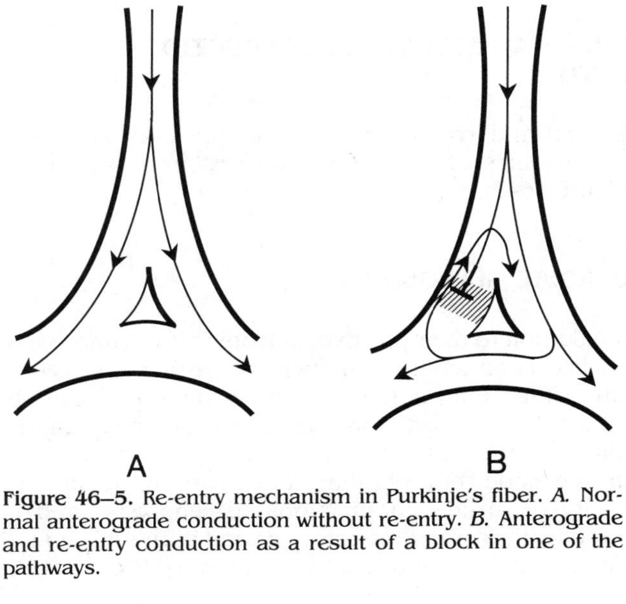

Figure 46–5. Re-entry mechanism in Purkinje's fiber. *A*. Normal anterograde conduction without re-entry. *B*. Anterograde and re-entry conduction as a result of a block in one of the pathways.

4. *Myocardial disturbances*. Ischemia, hypoxia, injury, and inflammation may change automaticity, conductivity, or both. Since these lesions are not evenly distributed throughout the heart, ectopic foci may produce TAPs unsynchronized with the pacemaker. Also, there may be localized areas of anterograde block, a condition which facilitates an abnormal re-entry process and subsequent tachycardia.

5. *Congestive heart failure*. In this condition, there are profound changes in oxygen concentration, pH, and electrolytes that alter the transmembrane resting potentials.

6. *Drugs*. Digitalis, antiarrhythmic agents, and sympathomimetic and psychotropic drugs cause changes in automaticity or conductivity or both. Excessive blood levels of these drugs may disturb the cardiac rhythm and cause undesirable arrhythmias.

7. *Endocrine disorders*. Thyrotoxicosis, myxedema, hyperparathyroidism, and pheochromocytoma are well-known causes of arrhythmia secondary to the extracellular metabolic changes that occur in these diseases.

8. *Miscellaneous causes*. Pulmonary embolism, hypertension, shock, anoxemia, anemia, and other conditions frequently cause arrhythmias because of secondary metabolic changes at the extracellular level. Also, the irritation of vagal receptors in the throat or in the tracheobronchial tree may explain the frequent occurrence of arrhythmias during bronchoscopy, gastroscopy, or nasopharyngeal suction in unanesthetized persons.

Steps in the Recognition of Arrhythmias

Whenever an ECG is obtained under usual circumstances, a strip of lead II is available for analysis of the rate and rhythm. In the case of patients who are monitored continuously in an intensive care unit or during regular activities by means of a Holter monitor, a beat-by-beat analysis of the cardiac rate and rhythm may be done from one of the selected chest leads. Regardless of the available lead, it is useful to analyze the ECG by answering the following:

1. *Heart rate*. Is it relatively constant or irregular?

2. *PP and RR intervals*. Are the PP and RR intervals consistently equal or variable from beat to beat? Are they identical to or different from each other?

3. *P–QRS–T sequence*. Is it normal? Is there a P wave not followed by QRS complex and T wave, or, conversely, is there a QRS complex and T wave not preceded by a P wave?

4. *Atrial premature beats (APBs) or premature atrial complexes (PACs)*. Are there P waves that occur earlier than normal, and, if so, are they followed by the usual QRS complex and T wave or by an aberrantly conducted ventricular activation? Are they occurring at random or periodically?

5. *Ventricular premature beats (VPBs), premature ventricular complexes (PVCs), or extrasystoles*. Are there QRS complexes and T waves that occur earlier than normal in the cardiac cycle, are not preceded by a P wave, and that have a configuration or duration that is different from the preceding or following beats? Are they occurring at random or periodically?

6. *Configuration of P waves, QRS complexes, and T waves*. Is the configuration of each one normal for the lead that is being monitored?

7. *Duration of the time intervals*. Are the standard time intervals normal for the prevailing heart rate?

Special analysis of arrhythmias with electrophysiologic stimulation (EPS) may be necessary in complex cases.

Table 46–14. CLASSIFICATION OF ARRHYTHMIAS

Atrial Arrhythmias
Sinus bradycardia
Sinus tachycardia
Sinus arrhythmia
Sinus pause
Atrial standstill
Nonsinus atrial rhythm
Wandering atrial pacemaker
Atrial premature beats or premature atrial contractions (PACs)
Multifocal atrial tachycardia
Paroxysmal atrial tachycardia (PAT)
Atrial flutter
Atrial fibrillation
Junctional Arrhythmias
Junctional premature beats (JPBs) or premature junctional contractions (PJCs)
Junctional or nodal rhythm
Ventricular arrhythmias
Ventricular premature beats (VBPs), or premature ventricular contractions (PVCs), or extrasystoles
Ventricular tachycardia
Ventricular fibrillation
Arrhythmias Due to Atrioventricular (AV) Conduction Defects
First-degree AV block
Second-degree AV block
Mobitz I (Wenckebach)
Mobitz II (Non-Wenckebach)
Third-degree AV block (complete) with AV dissociation
Rhythms Produced by Artificial Pacemakers
Special Clinical Syndromes that Predispose Patients to Arrhythmias
Pre-excitation syndromes: Wolff-Parkinson-White and Lown-Ganong-Levine
Sick sinus syndrome
Mitral valve prolapse syndrome
Prolonged QT interval syndrome

Classification

Table 46–14 shows a classification of the typical patterns of arrhythmia.

Antiarrhythmic Drugs

Several pharmacologic agents are useful in the treatment of arrhythmias because they have a favorable influence on the slope or duration of the various phases of the TAP. They may also have a favorable influence on the refractory period of the conduction system.

DRUGS AFFECTING AUTOMATICITY

There are four basic classes of drugs classified according to their specific mode of action. Figure 46–6 shows the Vaughn-Williams classification system and presents the specific effect of each drug class on the TAP at the SA node, AV junction, or ventricular cells. The drugs currently approved for use in the United States are listed.

DRUGS AFFECTING THE CONDUCTION SYSTEM

Several antiarrhythmic drugs may have an effect on various sites of the conduction system as shown in Figure 46–7.

CARDIAC GLYCOSIDES

In addition to their positive inotropic effect (improved cardiac contractility), digitalis and other glycosides have important antiarrhythmic properties because they increase vagal tone and decrease sympathetic tone. As a result, there is a slow discharge rate of the SA node (bradycardia), a decrease in the automaticity of atrial and junctional pacemakers, and a prolongation of the refractory period at the AV node. This is usually manifested by a prolonged PR interval.

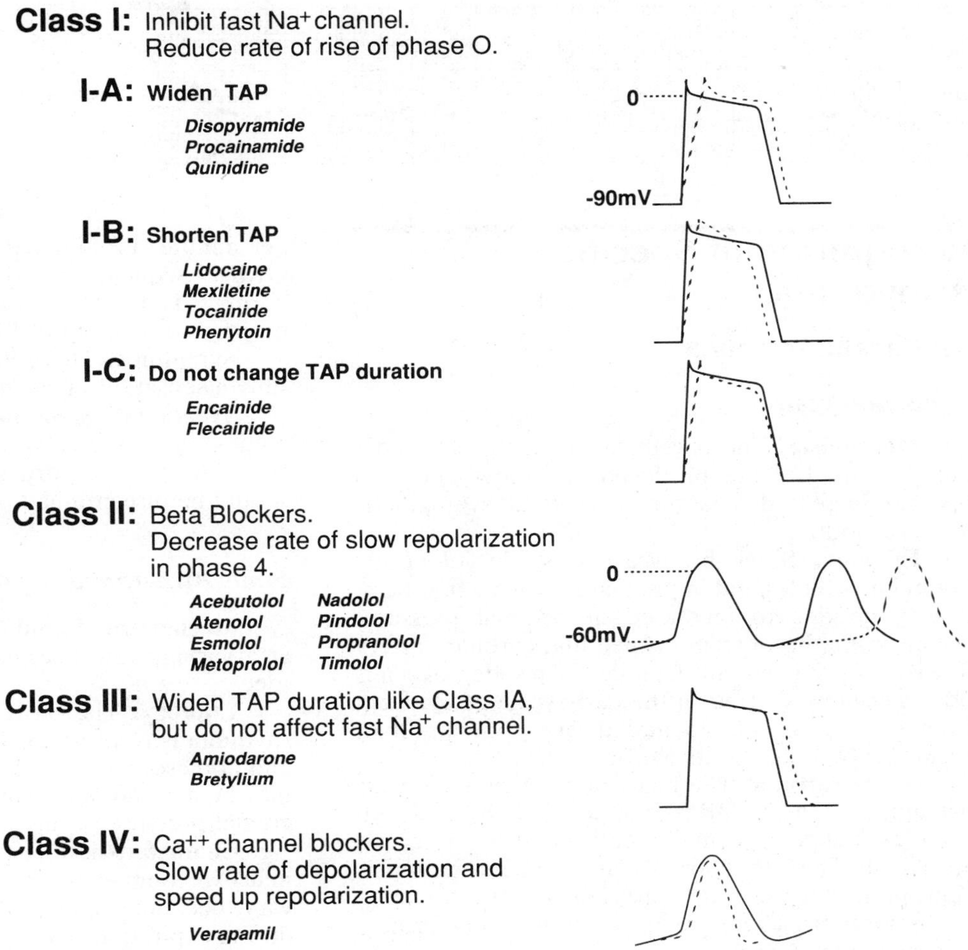
Class I: Inhibit fast Na+ channel.
Reduce rate of rise of phase O.
I-A: Widen TAP
Disopyramide
Procainamide
Quinidine
0
-90mV
I-B: Shorten TAP
Lidocaine
Mexiletine
Tocainide
Phenytoin
I-C: Do not change TAP duration
Encainide
Flecainide
Class II: Beta Blockers.
Decrease rate of slow repolarization
in phase 4.
Acebutolol
Atenolol
Esmolol
Metoprolol
Nadolol
Pindolol
Propranolol
Timolol
0
-60mV
Class III: Widen TAP duration like Class IA,
but do not affect fast Na+ channel.
Amiodarone
Bretylium
Class IV: Ca++ channel blockers.
Slow rate of depolarization and
speed up repolarization.
Verapamil

Figure 46–6. Vaughn-Williams classification of antiarrhythmic drugs and mechanism of action. (From Vaughn-Williams, V. E. M.: Classification of antidysrhythmic drugs. Pharmacol. Ther. Bull., *1*:115–138, 1975; modified from Sandóe, E., and Sigurd, B.: Arrhythmia. Diagnosis and Management. A Clinical Electrocardiographic Guide. St. Galen, Verlag für Fachmedien, 1984.)

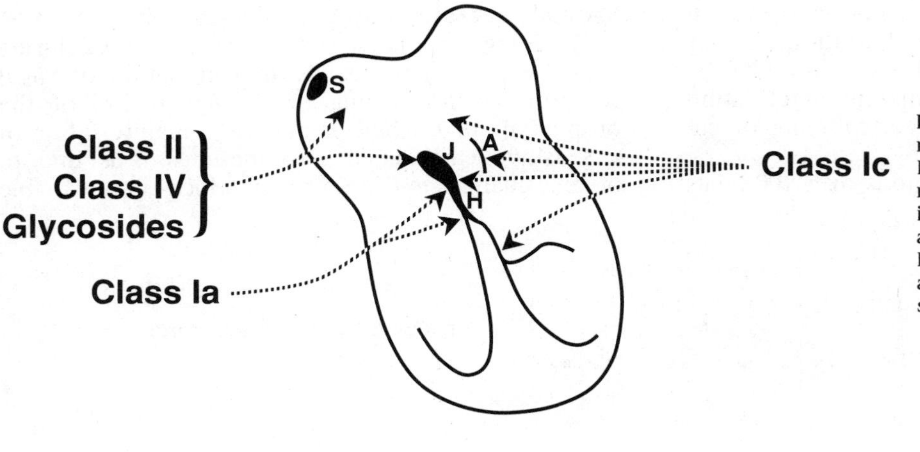

Figure 46–7. Site of action of antiarrhythmic drugs on conductivity. Class Ic drugs are also effective in blocking re-entry through the aberrant pathway in pre-excitation syndromes. S: Sinoatrial node; J: atrioventricular junction; H: bundle of His and its branches; A: aberrant pathway in pre-excitation syndrome.

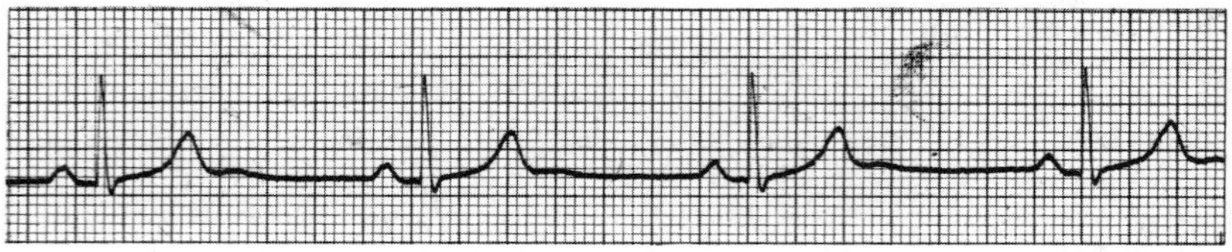

Figure 46–8. Sinus bradycardia.

Recognition of Specific Arrhythmias

ATRIAL ARRHYTHMIAS

Sinus Bradycardia

Mechanism. The pacemaker is at the SA node, but the impulses are produced at a slow rate as a result of increased vagal tone, decreased sympathetic tone, or both.

Etiology. Sinus bradycardia is physiologically normal in athletes and in pregnant women. In others, it may be due to increased intracranial pressure, lesions in the brain stem or medulla, coronary artery disease, myxedema, or jaundice. Episodes of sinus bradycardia may occur in the early stage of recovery from general anesthesia and during stimulation of vagal receptors of the throat or trachea.

Characteristics. The heart rate is below 60 beats per minute. The P–QRS–T sequence is normal. All complexes appear normal. The PP and RR intervals are equal. The PR interval may be increased but is appropriate for the heart rate (Fig. 46–8).

Symptoms. There are no symptoms, but dizziness or syncope may occur.

Treatment. If severe, sinus bradycardia may require atropine, isoproterenol, or even pacing.

Sinus Tachycardia

Mechanism. The impulses originate at the node at a rapid rate because of increased sympathetic tone, decreased vagal tone, or both.

Etiology. Sinus tachycardia occurs physiologically under the influence of exercise or emotion. It may be produced voluntarily by some persons. It occurs in febrile states, anemia, thyrotoxicosis, shock, congestive heart failure, hypoglycemia, and the adrenergic state of prolonged immobilization. It may also be a reaction to drugs such as atropine, nitrites, or quinidine, to alcohol, or to sympathomimetic stimulative substances such as tobacco, caffeine, or cocaine.

Characteristics. The heart rate is over 100 beats per minute. PP and RR intervals are equal. The P–QRS–T sequence is normal. All complexes appear normal. The PR interval may be shortened but appropriate for the rate (Fig. 46–9).

Symptoms. There are no symptoms except possibly a sensation of racing of the heart.

Treatment. Sinus tachycardia is treated by correcting the underlying cause. For example, use of sympathomimetic drugs or irritating substances should be discontinued.

Sinus Arrhythmia

Mechanism. Impulses originate at the SA node at a varying rate because of cyclic changes in vagal tone.

Etiology. The most common cause of sinus arrhythmia is respiration. It may be normal in children and adolescents, as well as in adults during sleep. It may be a pathologic manifestation of increased intracranial pressure or digitalis effect.

Characteristics. The P–QRS–T sequence is normal. All complexes are normal. PP and RR intervals vary, becoming shorter during inspiration and longer during expiration. However, the PP and RR intervals of the same cardiac cycle are identical (Fig. 46–10).

Symptoms. There are usually no symptoms. Physicians often unnecessarily request an ECG in a young, healthy person because of arrhythmic heart sounds. The respiratory origin of this arrhythmia may be easily detected by determining if the sounds speed up and slow down synchronously with respirations.

Treatment. No treatment is required.

Sinus Pause

Mechanism. There is a transient inhibition of the SA node because of a sudden increase in vagal tone.

Etiology. Sinus pause may be noticeable during deep sleep. It may be due to stimulation of vagal receptors while gagging or during suction of the oropharynx or trachea. It may be a manifestation of a sensitive carotid sinus. Sometimes it is due to organic changes in the SA node, which is not capable

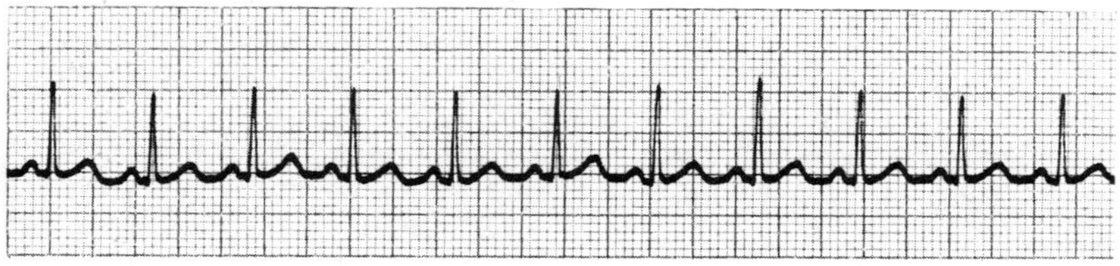

Figure 46–9. Sinus tachycardia.

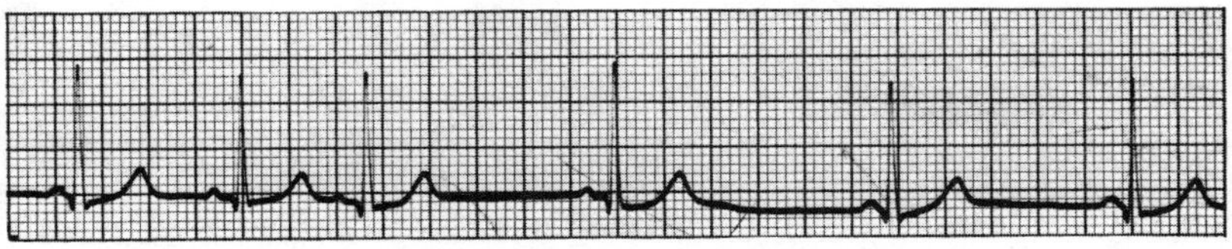

Figure 46–10. Sinus arrhythmia due to respiration. Beats 1 to 3 coincide with inspiration. Beats 4 to 6 coincide with expiration.

of producing regular TAPs as it occurs in the sick sinus syndrome.

Characteristics. There are random episodes of prolonged PP interval. The prevalent rhythm is of sinus origin, or there is a slight sinus arrhythmia (Fig. 46–11).

Symptoms. Symptoms are frequently unnoticed by the patient, but there may be dizziness if the pause is long.

Treatment. No treatment is required if the pause occurs infrequently and is not long. If the pause is long, it may be treated in the same way as an atrial standstill.

Atrial Standstill

Mechanism. In cases of sinus arrest because of vagal stimulation or an organic SA block, a nodal or ventricular pacemaker may take over and produce escaped beats. Sometimes the escaped beats occur at an accelerated rate.

Etiology. Atrial standstill is usually due to fibrosis of the SA node or to digitalis or quinidine intoxication. It may be a manifestation of sick sinus syndrome.

Characteristics. There are randomly occurring periods of absent P waves with junctional or ventricular escaped beats (Fig. 46–12).

Symptoms. There are usually no symptoms, although dizziness or blackout spells may occur.

Treatment. The patient may eventually require pacing. In case of sinus arrest, atropine or isoproterenol may be effective in restoring pacemaker activity.

Nonsinus Atrial Rhythm

Mechanism. There is a regularly activated low atrial pacemaker that is not at the SA node but is somewhat remote from the AV node. A common location is the coronary sinus.

Etiology. There is no specific cause, but nonsinus atrial rhythm may reflect an inability of the SA node to produce TAPs.

Characteristics. The heart rate is normal. P waves in leads II, III, and often in aV_F are inverted. The PR interval is usually normal. The QRS complexes and T waves are normal (Fig. 46–13).

Symptoms. There are usually no symptoms.

Treatment. There is no treatment required.

Wandering Atrial Pacemaker

Mechanism. The pacemaker shifts from one atrial location to the other, sometimes in a cyclic pattern.

Etiology. Wandering atrial pacemaker may occur physiologically as a result of changes in vagal tone. It is more frequent in young people.

Characteristics. The P waves change in configuration. The PR intervals vary from beat to beat. The PP and RR intervals vary also. The QRS complexes and T waves are normal (Fig. 46–14).

Symptoms. There are usually no symptoms.

Treatment. No treatment is required.

Atrial Premature Beats or Premature Atrial Complexes

Mechanism. Random impulses are generated by one or more irritable atrial foci, sometimes with a reentry phenomenon.

Etiology. Atrial premature beats may be benign if they are due to emotion, fatigue, or central nervous system excitation. They may be due to the effects of alcohol, tobacco, caffeine, sympathomimetic drugs, or other stimulating substances. They may also indicate digitalis effect or the existence of foci of hypoxic myocardial cells.

Characteristics. There is a random occurrence of abnormal P waves. The PR interval in the premature beats is usually long. The QRS complexes are usually normal except when there is aberrant conduction to the ventricles. A compensatory pause (prolonged PP interval) follows the atrial premature beat (Fig. 46–15).

Symptoms. There are usually no symptoms, although the patient may feel a thump in the chest.

Treatment. No treatment is required if atrial premature beats are benign. If they are not, the cause of ectopic excitation should be eliminated. Occasion-

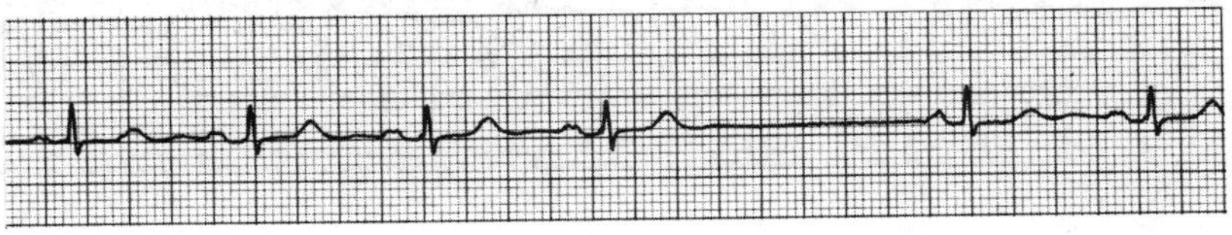

Figure 46–11. Sinus pause. The fourth beat is followed by a long pause before a return of the normal sinus rhythm.

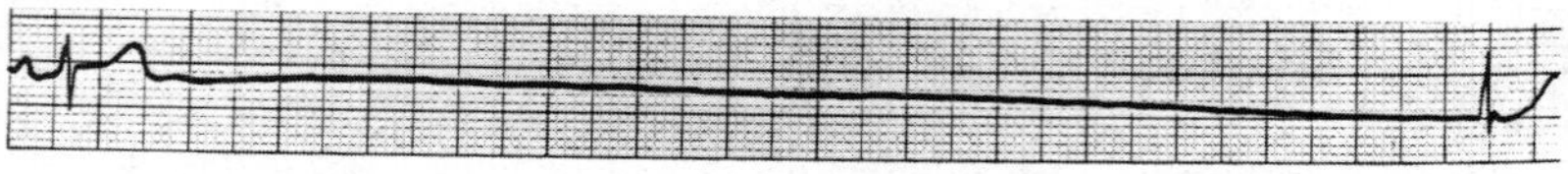

Figure 46–12. Sinus arrest followed by a junctional escape. (Reproduced with permission from Sandóe, E., and Sigurd, B.: Arrhythmia. Diagnosis and Management. An Electrocardiographic Guide. St. Galen, Verlag für Fachmedien, 1984.)

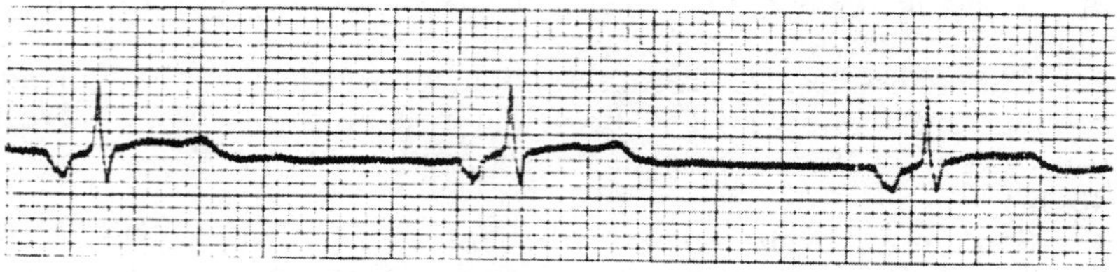

Figure 46–13. Nonsinus atrial rhythm. The pacemaker is located at the coronary sinus, causing the P waves on lead II to be negative.

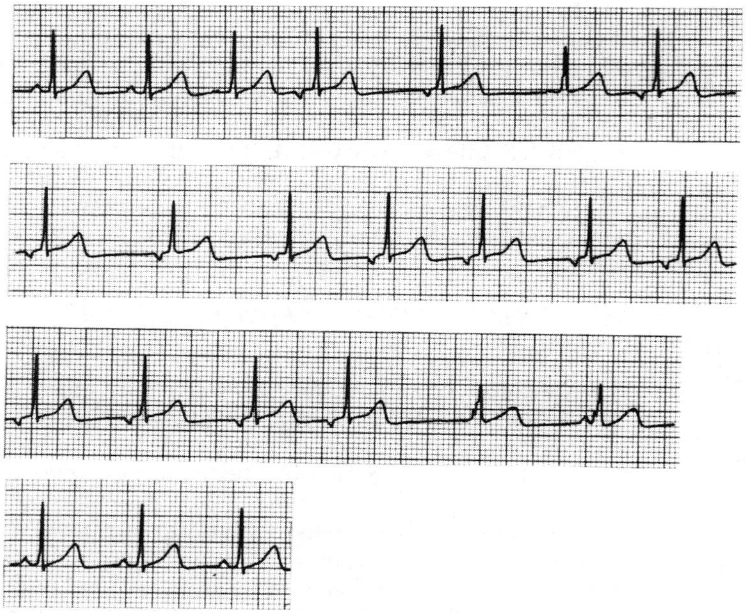

Figure 46–14. Wandering pacemaker. Consecutive rhythm strip of a tracing that shows the wandering of an atrial pacemaker.

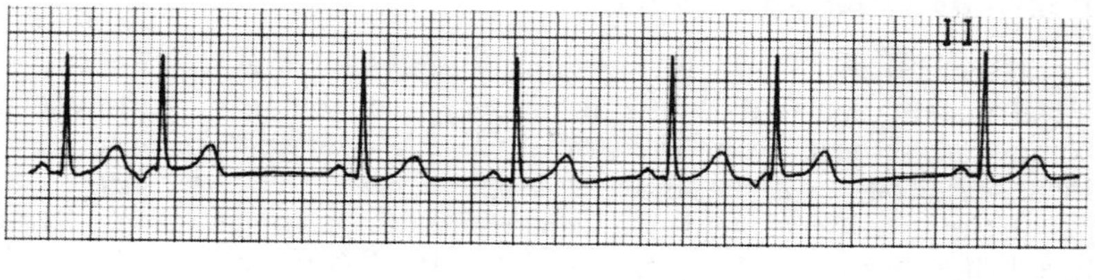

Figure 46–15. Atrial premature beats. The second and the sixth beats are produced by an ectopic atrial focus and are followed by a compensatory pause.

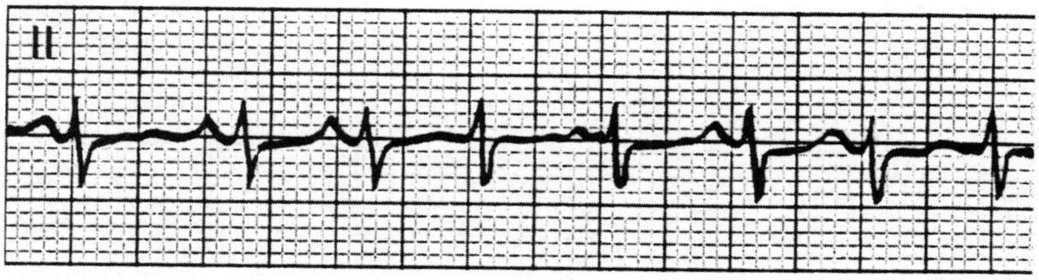

Figure 46–16. Multifocal atrial tachycardia. (Reproduced with permission from Sandóe, E., and Sigurd, B.: Arrhythmia. Diagnosis and Management. An Electrocardiographic Guide. St. Galen, Verlag für Fachmedien, 1984.)

ally there may be a need for treatment with a Class I or III drug.

Multifocal Atrial Tachycardia

Mechanism. Random impulses originate irregularly and at a high rate in different points of the atria.

Etiology. This arrhythmia occurs frequently in severe pulmonary disease.

Characteristics. There is a rapidly changing P wave configuration. The pattern resembles that of a wandering pacemaker, but the changes in P wave occur more randomly. The PR, PP, and RR intervals are variable. The prevalent heart rate is fast (Fig. 46–16).

Symptoms. Symptoms of pulmonary disease are clinically evident.

Treatment. It is necessary to correct the pulmonary condition. Digitalis may be tried cautiously. Other antiarrhythmic drugs are seldom effective, but a therapeutic trial with verapamil may be warranted.

Paroxysmal Atrial Tachycardia

Mechanism. TAPs are generated regularly and repeatedly in an ectopic focus at or near the AV node. They occur as a result of the re-entry phenomenon. Within the AV node, there is a longitudinal division of conduction fibers into alpha and beta pathways. A block in the latter pathway causes re-entry of impulses within the node, with retrograde depolarization of the atria and antegrade depolarization of the ventricles through the normal conduction system.

Etiology. This condition is usually pathologic. It may be congenital. Digitalis intoxication should be suspected if there is a block.

Characteristics. The atrial rate is 160 to 220 beats per minute. The P waves are regular and often inverted. The QRS complexes are normal. The PP and RR intervals are equal but short (Fig. 46–17*A* and *B*).

Symptoms. The patient notices thumping, fluttering, or palpitations that are sometimes associated with precordial pain, shortness of breath, or anxiety. Congestive heart failure precedes or follows the onset of paroxysmal atrial tachycardia.

Treatment. Treatment consists of vagal stimulation and sedation. Calcium channel blockers (verapamil) or beta-blockers may be useful as first-line drugs because of their inhibition of AV node conduction. Some cardiologists prefer Class IC drugs (encainide and flecainide) as the first-line drugs, but they should not be used for long-term maintenance. Quinidine, procainamide and disopyramide have been effectively used. Phenylephrine hydrochloride (Neo-Synephrine) may be useful because of its reflex vagal stimulation. If there is no evidence of digitalis intoxication, digitalis may be indicated in cases of congestive heart failure or shock. If there is an acute MI, cardioversion may be necessary.

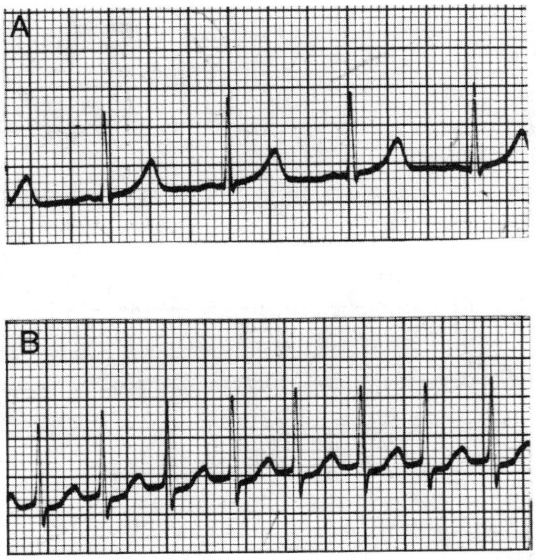

Figure 46–17. Paroxysmal atrial tachycardia. Tracing *A* was obtained just before the patient went into a witnessed episode of paroxysmal atrial tachycardia. Tracing *B* was obtained a few minutes after the episode started.

Atrial Flutter

Mechanism. An ectopic atrial focus produces rapid stimuli, which travel in circles in the atria. Only at the end of every second, third, or fourth atrial depolarization may the AV node be capable of conducting the impulse to the ventricles in a regular fashion.

Etiology. The process is usually pathologic and reflects organic heart disease.

Characteristics. The atrial rate is fast (250 to 350 beats per minute). The P waves are clearly visible, almost identical, and often produce the typical saw-tooth pattern (F waves). The QRS complexes are normal. The PP interval is very short, whereas the RR interval is longer and regular (Fig. 46–18*A*) except when the ratio P:QRS varies between 4:1, 3:1, or 2:1 (Fig. 46–18*B*).

Symptoms. There are usually no symptoms. If there are, they resemble those of paroxysmal atrial tachycardia if the ventricular rate is fast.

Treatment. The objective is to slow down the ventricular rate and convert to normal sinus rhythm or atrial fibrillation, which is more benign than flutter. This may be done with digitalis therapy, especially when there is congestive heart failure. Verapamil, quinidine, or procainamide may be added to digitalis. If there is no change in 12 to 24 hours, cardioversion with a small energy current may be useful.

Atrial Fibrillation

Mechanism. The atria depolarize from a variety of foci, which transmit impulses in a chaotic motion through random circular pathways.

Etiology. Atrial fibrillation is frequently associated with organic heart disease, but it may occur as

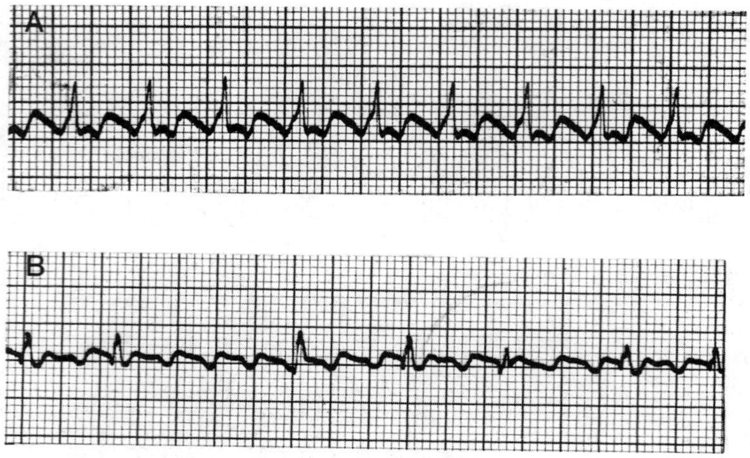

Figure 46–18. Atrial flutter. Tracing *A* shows a 2:1 atrial flutter with a fast ventricular rate. Tracing *B* shows a variable atrial flutter 4:1 or 3:1, which accounts for the variable RR interval.

an occasional episode in young adults without demonstrated coronary artery disease.

Characteristics. The P waves are not clearly identified, and the baseline is irregular. The QRS complexes are normal, but sometimes there are randomly occurring abnormal QRS complexes resulting from transmission of atrial impulses through aberrant pathways. PP intervals are not measurable. RR intervals are unequal. The predominant ventricular rate may be fast (Fig. 46–19*A*) or slow (Fig. 46–19*B*).

Symptoms. Although sometimes the patient does not notice any symptoms, there may be a sensation of palpitations and, occasionally, dizziness and collapse. If there is associated congestive heart failure, the symptoms of this condition are obvious.

Treatment. The primary aim of treatment is to slow down the ventricular response. This may be accomplished with digitalis alone or digitalis combined with either beta-blockers or calcium channel blockers. Class IA or IC drugs may be also used in combination with digitalis to re-establish a sinus rhythm. Cardioversion in a digitalized patient may be necessary to treat chronic fibrillation. It is important to administer anticoagulants to prevent the occurrence of emboli.

JUNCTIONAL ARRHYTHMIAS

Junctional Premature Beats or Premature Junctional Contractions

Mechanism. On a random basis, a premature beat arises from the junctional (AV node) area. The location of the ectopic focus may be in the upper, middle, or lower portion of the junction.

Etiology. These arrhythmias may be either benign or early manifestation of organic disease. They

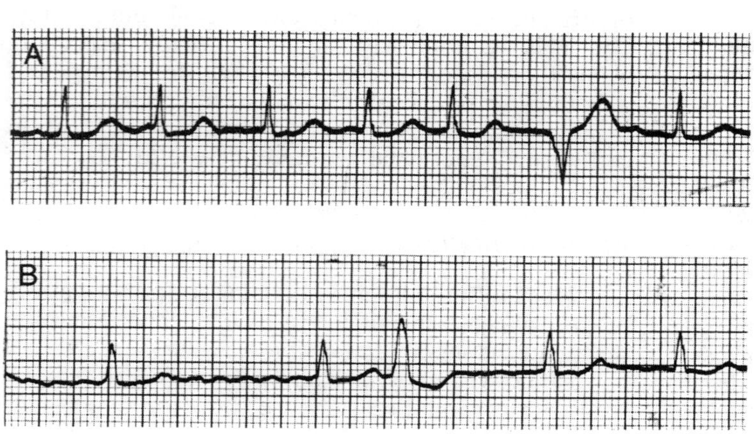

Figure 46–19. Atrial fibrillation. Tracing *A* shows atrial fibrillation with a fast ventricular response and one VPB (sixth beat). Tracing *B* shows atrial fibrillation with a slower ventricular response and one VPB (third beat).

may be secondary to excitation or use of drugs or stimulating substances.

Characteristics. An apparently normal or slightly abnormal QRS complex occurs earlier than usual in the cardiac cycle. The P wave is often inverted and precedes, is incorporated in, or follows the QRS complex, depending on the location of the ectopic focus. The PP and RR intervals are equal except in the prematurely occurring beat (Fig. 46–20*A* and *B*).

Symptoms. Symptoms are usually not noticeable except for a sensation of skipped beat.

Treatment. No treatment is required if the arrhythmias are benign.

Junctional or Nodal Rhythm

Mechanism. The pacemaker is consistently at the AV junction with retrograde conduction to the atria and antegrade transmission to the ventricles. The normal idiopathic junctional rhythm is slow, with a rate of 35 to 60 beats per minute (junctional bradycardia). This rhythm may occur as an escape mechanism because of extremely slow or absent SA node activity. In some instances, there is an accelerated junctional rhythm of 60 to 100 beats per minute because of enhanced junctional automaticity. In other instances, there is junctional tachycardia with a rate of 100 to 150 beats per minute. If the latter instance, then it may be difficult to distinguish it from atrial tachycardia because the P waves are not clearly seen in either case. Because of this, it may be preferable to use the nonspecific term of supraventricular tachycardia.

Etiology. This rhythm is usually benign and may occur as a result of excitation.

Characteristics. The rate may be slow, slightly accelerated, or tachycardic. All QRS complexes are normal. The P waves are negative and may precede, be incorporated in, or follow the QRS complex, depending on the location of the pacemaker within the junction. The PP and RR intervals are equal (Fig. 46–21*A* and *B*).

Symptoms. Symptoms are the same as those of bradycardia or tachycardia, depending on the predominant rate.

Treatment. No treatment is required except when there is tachycardia, in which case the treatment is similar to that of atrial tachycardia.

VENTRICULAR ARRHYTHMIAS

Ventricular Premature Beats or Premature Ventricular Contractions or Extrasystoles

Mechanism. An ectopic focus may randomly produce a TAP, which is then transmitted throughout the ventricle outside of the regular conduction system. The so-called R on T phenomenon occurs when a VPB starts just before the preceding T wave has returned to baseline. Sometimes two VPBs may occur in couplets or triplets, and it used to be thought that they heralded the imminent onset of ventricular tachycardia and fibrillation. However, there is no correlation between the so-called "warning VPBs" and the subsequent development of fibrillation.

Etiology. These arrhythmias may occur in otherwise healthy persons or during exercise. VPBs are considered benign if they are unifocal and occur at a rate of less than one per minute and 30 per hour. If they are more frequent or if they are multifocal, occurring in couplets or triplets, they are considered to be potentially lethal. They may actually be produced by some antiarrhythmic drugs, which have a proarrhythmia adverse effect in some patients (especially Class IC drugs and digitalis).

Characteristics. The QRS is wide, notched, and slurred. There is no preceding P wave, but sometimes the P wave is seen following the QRS complex as a result of retrograde conduction. The T wave is usually opposite in direction to the QRS complex. The PP

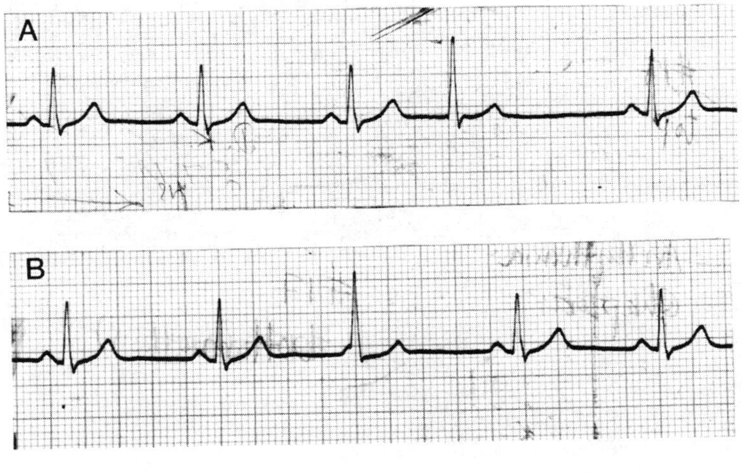

Figure 46–20. Junctional premature beat. In tracing *A*, the fourth beat originates at a middle nodal ectopic focus and it is followed by a compensatory pause. In tracing *B*, the third beat originates at a high ectopic nodal focus (it occurs almost simultaneously with the P wave) and it is also followed by a compensatory pause.

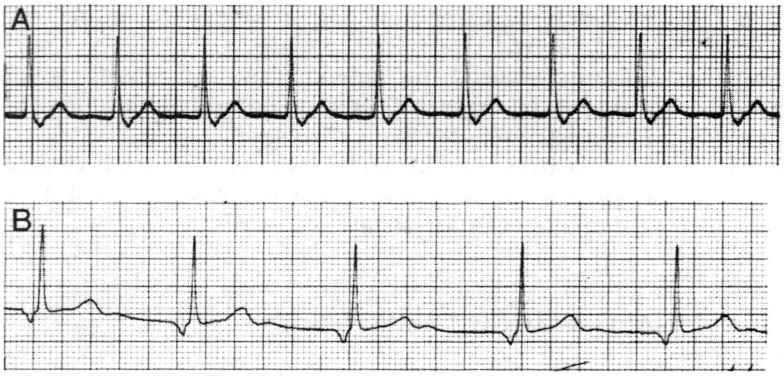

Figure 46–21. Junctional rhythm. Tracing *A* shows that the QRS complex has originated at the AV junction and the P wave is produced in a retrograde fashion after the QRS complex. Tracing *B* shows a junctional rhythm at a slower rate.

and RR intervals are equal and regular except at the prematurely occurring beat because of a compensatory pause. This pause is not seen when there is an underlying bradycardia, and the VPB may be interpolated within the regular cardiac cycle. Unifocal VPBs always have the same QRS configuration (Fig. 46–22*A*). Multifocal VPBs have varying configurations (Fig. 46–22*B*). In digitalis intoxication, the existence of a recurring pattern of a normal QRS complex followed by a VPB is referred to as *bigeminy* (Fig. 46–22*C*). Two consecutive VPBs occurring without compensatory pause are referred to as *couplets* (Fig. 46–22*D*).

Symptoms. Symptoms are the same as in other premature beats.

Treatment. Treatment is the same as for atrial or junctional premature beats. If treatment is indicated, the administration of a beta-blocker or one of the class IB, C, or A type drugs should be considered (in that order of priority).

Ventricular Tachycardia

Mechanism. Ventricular tachycardia occurs when at least three rapid consecutive beats are produced by TAPs that originate at a ventricular ectopic focus. The ectopy may occur because of enhanced ventricular automaticity or a re-entry phenomenon through an area of Purkinje's network affected by a focal injury.

Etiology. Ventricular tachycardia is commonly associated with MI, but it is also associated with other serious heart disease, ventricular aneurysm, and digitalis intoxication.

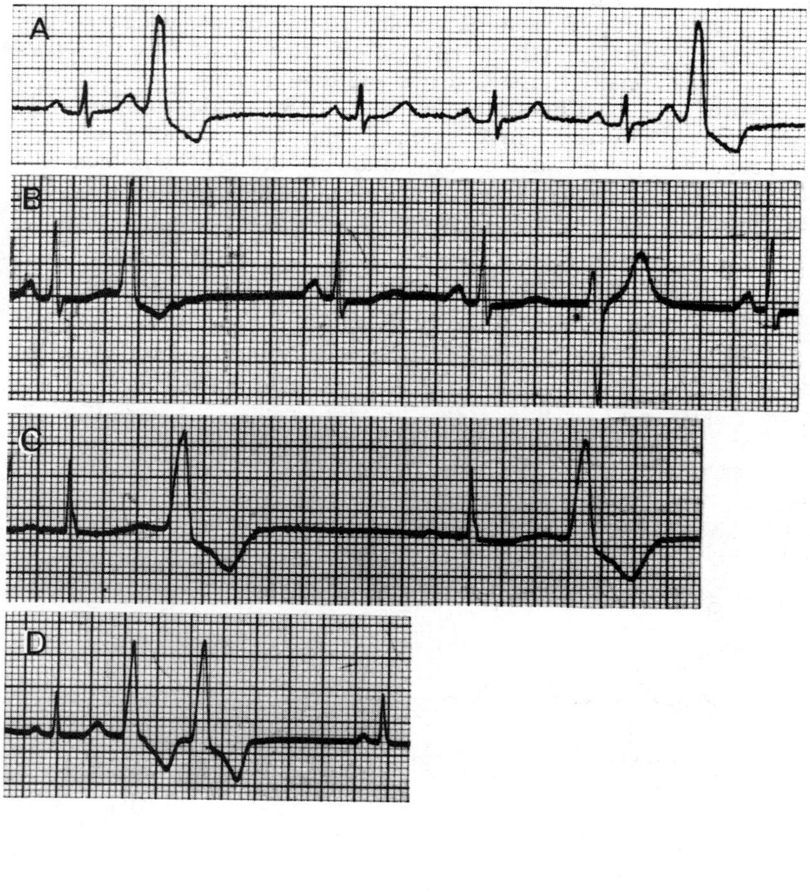

Figure 46–22. Ventricular premature beats. Tracing *A* shows two unifocal VPBs with a compensatory pause. Tracing *B* shows two VPBs that originate at different foci. Tracing *C* shows a bigeminal pattern, with a normal QRS complex followed by a VPB (the prolonged PR interval is probably due to digitalis). Tracing *D* shows a couplet of VPBs.

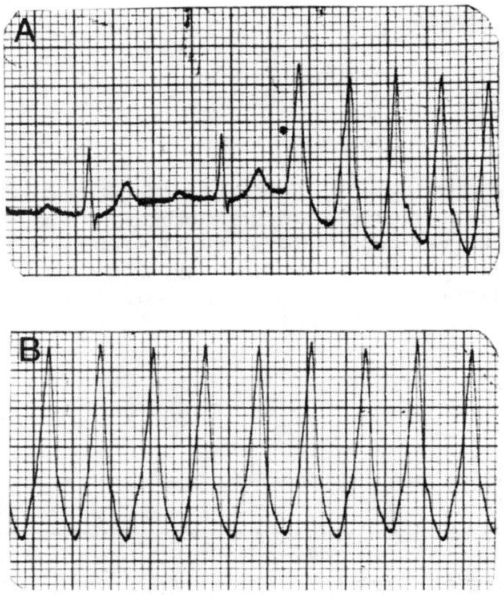

Figure 46–23. Ventricular tachycardia. Tracing *A* shows a normal sinus rhythm with a first-degree AV block followed by supraventricular tachycardia. Tracing *B*, obtained 1 minute later, shows sustained ventricular tachycardia.

Characteristics. There are regularly occurring, broad QRS complexes, with T waves moving in the opposite direction from QRS complexes. There are no visible P waves. The rate is faster than 120 beats per minute, usually 160 to 250 beats per minute (Fig. 46–23).

A special type of ventricular tachycardia is referred to as *torsade de pointes*, which is characterized by cyclic changes in the polarity of the QRS complexes (Fig. 46–24). This ventricular tachycardia may occur in MI or in patients with a congenital or acquired prolonged QT interval. Electrolyte disturbances or antiarrhythmic (Class IA) or psychotropic drugs may cause severe prolongation of the QT intervals.

Symptoms. The main symptom is a sensation of racing of the heart. There may be manifestations of unstable cardiac function.

Treatment. If the tachycardia is sustained and the patient is stable, an I.V. bolus of 60 to 100 mg. of lidocaine, followed by a drip of 0.1 per cent to 0.2 per cent lidocaine solution at 100 ml. per hour may be required. Thereafter, prevention with a Class IB drug or a beta-blocker may be indicated. In the unstable patient, cardioversion may be necessary after appropriate sedation. The combination of a temporary pacemaker with an I.V. lidocaine drip may be necessary.

Ventricular Fibrillation

Mechanism. A chaotic ventricular depolarization produced by multiple ectopic foci depolarizes the surrounding areas in a random fashion in ventricular fibrillation. There is no emptying of the ventricles, and ventricular fibrillation is invariably fatal unless it is corrected by immediate defibrillation. Appropriately applied cardiopulmonary resuscitation maneuvers may effectively empty the ventricles and allow for survival until a countershock may be applied.

Etiology. Ventricular fibrillation occurs in severe myocardial disease. When it develops more than 48 hours after MI, it has a very poor prognosis.

Characteristics. There are erratic voltages without discernible P waves or QRS complexes. Whenever the voltage changes are of appreciable magnitude, the condition is referred to as coarse fibrillation (Fig. 46–25*A*), but when the voltage changes are small, the condition is referred to as fine fibrillation (Fig. 46–25*B*).

Symptoms. The patient is in a state of cardiogenic shock.

Treatment. Cardiopulmonary resuscitation and defibrillation with DC countershocks are immediately needed. A precordial thump may be an effective defibrillating maneuver in the case of a witnessed arrest. Lidocaine or bretylium or both may be useful pharmacologic adjuvants to DC countershocks.

ARRHYTHMIAS RESULTING FROM ATRIOVENTRICULAR CONDUCTION DEFECTS

First-Degree AV Block

Mechanism. A partial block at the AV junction delays transmission of impulses to the ventricles.

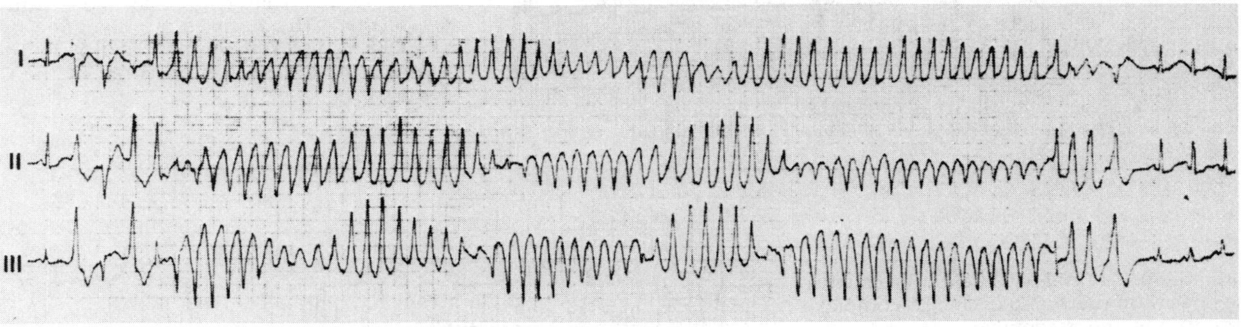

Figure 46–24. Ventricular tachycardia, *torsade de pointes*. At the beginning of this simultaneous recording of leads I, II, and III, several ectopic ventricular beats occur. Ventricular tachycardia follows until the last few beats, which are of sinus origin. (Reproduced with permission from Krikler, D. M., and Curry, P. V. L.: *Torsade de pointes*, an atypical ventricular tachycardia. Br. Heart J., 38:18, 1976.)

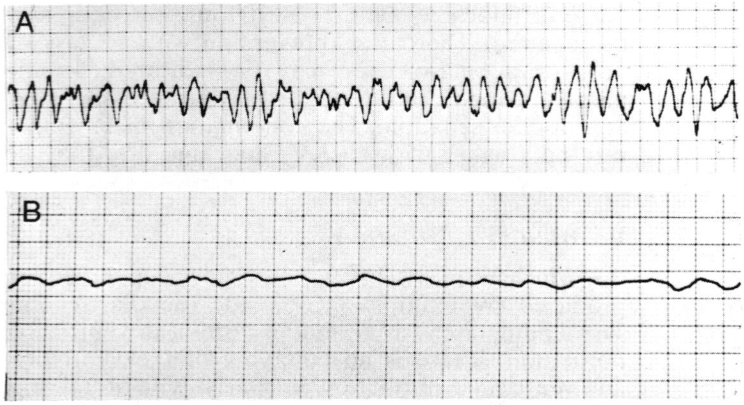

Figure 46–25. Ventricular fibrillation. Tracing *A* shows coarse ventricular fibrillation. Tracing *B* shows fine ventricular fibrillation. (Reproduced with permission. Textbook of Advanced Cardiac Life Support. Dallas, TX, American Heart Association, 1987.)

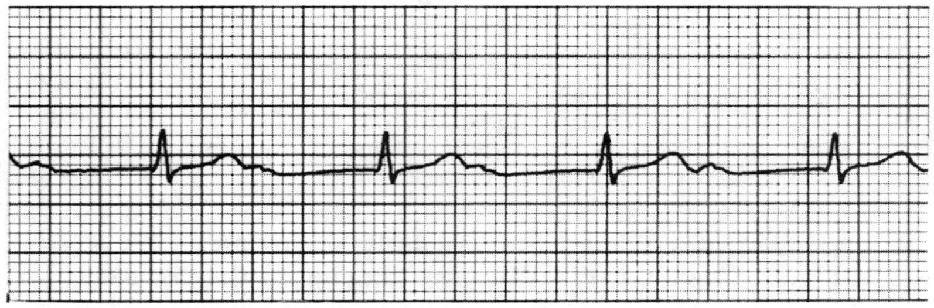

Figure 46–26. First-degree AV block. The PR interval measures 0.42 second.

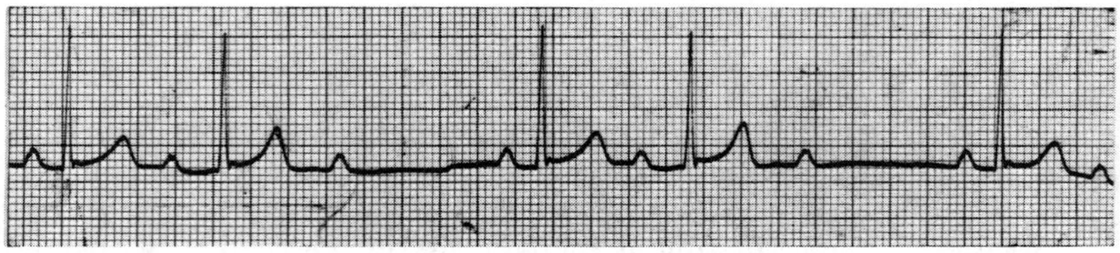

Figure 46–27. Second-degree AV block. Mobitz I. The first beat shows a PR interval of 0.18 second. The second beat shows a PR interval of 0.28 second. The third beat shows a blocked P wave. After a pause, the PR interval begins at 0.18 second.

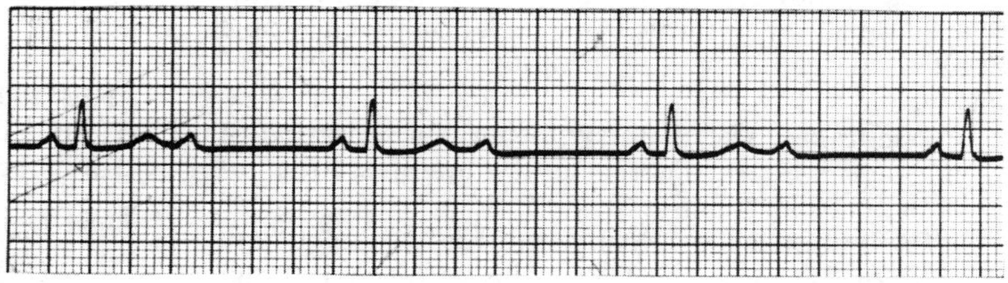

Figure 46–28. Second-degree AV block. Mobitz II. The P wave is blocked every second beat (2:1 AV block).

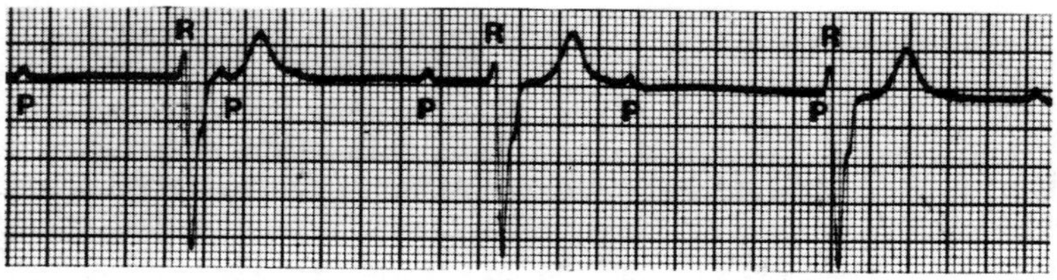

Figure 46–29. Third-degree AV block with AV dissociation. The P waves are identified by P. The QRS complexes are identified by R. The P wave on the last beat is obscured by the QRS complex.

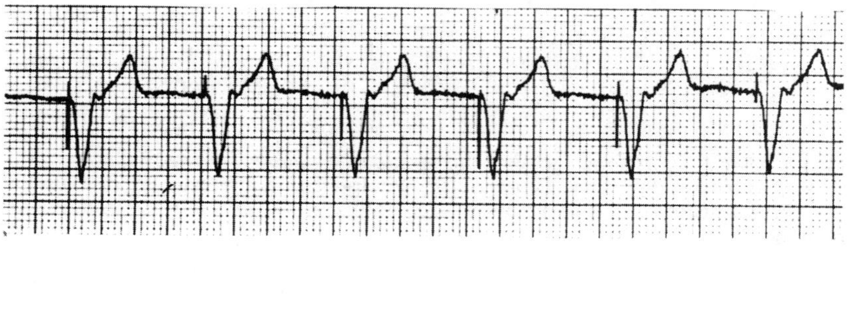

Figure 46–30. Artificial pacemaker. The sharp spike downward preceding each QRS complex is produced by the pacemaker.

However, all atrial impulses are eventually conducted through the normal pathways.

Etiology. Increased vagal tone may be the cause of a first-degree AV block in young persons. In the elderly, first-degree AV block may indicate digitalis effect or an organic lesion such as stenosis of a small branch of the right coronary artery that irrigates the AV node.

Characteristics. There are normally occurring P waves of SA origin. QRS complexes are normal. The PR interval is longer than would normally be expected for the heart rate. A PR interval greater than 0.20 second is indicative of first-degree AV block, unless the heart rate is very slow, in which case a PR interval of up to 0.24 second is considered normal. The PP and RR intervals are equal (Fig. 46–26).

Symptoms. There are usually no symptoms.

Treatment. Usually no treatment is required. The physician may consider stopping digitalis if the patient is being treated with this drug.

Second-Degree AV Block, Mobitz I (Wenckebach Heart Block)

Mechanism. In a cyclic fashion, there is a progressively increasing PR interval until eventually a normal atrial impulse is completely blocked at the AV junction.

Etiology. Second-degree AV block may occur in adolescents as a result of autonomic lability. In older persons, it is not as severe as a second-degree AV block of the Mobitz II type.

Characteristics. The PR interval may start within normal limits, but it becomes progressively longer in the next few beats until there is a dropped QRS complex. The PP intervals are equal. The RR intervals become progressively shorter, but when the complete block occurs, there is a long RR interval (Fig. 46–27).

Symptoms. There are usually no symptoms, although the blocked P wave may cause a thumping sensation and slight dizziness.

Treatment. No treatment may be required.

Second-Degree AV Block, Mobitz II (Non-Wenckebach Heart Block)

Mechanism. A complete AV block occurs at the AV junction or at the early portion of the bundle of His. This block occurs intermittently every other atrial beat or every two or three beats.

Etiology. Second-degree AV block is practically always a manifestation of organic heart disease.

Characteristics. The P waves occur regularly and are followed by normal QRS complexes, except when there is a dropped P wave. The PP intervals are equal. The RR intervals are equal, except in the blocked beat (Fig. 46–28).

Symptoms. There are no symptoms if the ventricular rate is normal. The patient may experience dizziness or collapse if the ventricular rate is very slow.

Treatment. When this heart block occurs every other beat, it can lead to serious consequences and may require pacing.

Third-Degree AV Block (Complete) with AV Dissociation

Mechanism. Impulses originate independently at the SA node and at the junction or ventricles.

Etiology. Third-degree AV block indicates serious cardiac disease, usually coronary stenosis affecting the branch of the right coronary artery that irrigates the AV node.

Characteristics. The PP intervals are regular and equal. The RR intervals are also regular and equal but usually longer than the PP intervals because the ventricular rhythm is out of sequence with the atrial rhythm. If the ventricular impulses originate at the AV junction, the QRS complexes are narrow and the T waves are usually in the same direction as the QRS complexes. If the ventricular beats originate at the ventricle, the QRS complexes are wide and slurred, and the T waves are in the opposite direction (Fig. 46–29).

Symptoms. Symptoms are usually those of either bradycardia or tachycardia.

Treatment. If the block is proximal (i.e., high in the junction) and accompanied by bradycardia or hypotension, it may be necessary to administer atropine or isoproterenol. If the block is distal (i.e., low in the junction or in the bundle of His), it may be necessary to insert a transvenous pacemaker.

RHYTHMS PRODUCED BY ARTIFICIAL PACEMAKERS

All well-functioning artificial pacemakers may be recognized by a sharp spike of voltage change that occurs just before a P wave or a QRS complex, depending on the location of the stimulating electrode. The permanent demand pacemakers are activated only when the patient's rate is lower than a pre-established threshold (Fig. 46–30).

Special Clinical Syndromes that Predispose Patients to Arrhythmias

Pre-excitation Syndromes

Both Wolff-Parkinson-White and Lown-Ganong-Levine syndromes may cause recurrent supraventricular rhythms with very rapid ventricular rates. The tachycardia is due to re-entry of impulses from the conducting tissue to the atria via the aberrant pathway

Table 46–15. INDICATIONS, ROUTE OF ADMINISTRATION, AND DOSAGES OF ANTIARRHYTHMIC DRUGS

Type of Drug	Primary Indication	Secondary Indication	Initial Dose	Maintenance Dose	Plasma Level (μg./ml.)	Contraindications and Complications
CLASS IA						
Disopyramide	VPB, VT	Prophylaxis VBP	p.o.: 100–200 mg. q. 6h.	p.o.: 100–200 mg. q. 6h.	3–6	Congestive failure Conduction defects Prolonged QT-proarrhythmia Atropine effect
Procainamide	VPB, VT	Prophylaxis AT, VT, AT in W-P-W*	I.V.: 50 mg. q. 6h. Max 1000 mg. or when QRS 50 per cent wider	p.o.: 500–1000 mg. q. 4–6h.	4–10	Prolonged QRS-proarrhythmia Hypotension Lupus syndrome
Quinidine	APB,† AF, VPB, VT	Prophylaxis AF	I.V.: 10 mg. per kg. p.o.: 250–400 mg. q. 4–6h.	p.o.: 300–600 mg. q. 12h.	2–4	Conduction defects Prolonged QT-proarrhythmia Idiosyncrasy Myasthenia
CLASS IB						
Lidocaine	VPB, VT, VF	Prophylaxis VPB, VT, VF	I.V.: 1 mg. per kg. bolus + 0.5 mg. per kg. q 8 min. Max: 3 mg. per kg.	I.V.: 1–4 mg. per minute	2–5	CNS‡ effects and seizures
Mexiletine	VPB, VT	Prophylaxis VPB, AT in W-P-W	p.o.: 400 mg. once p.o.: 100–300 mg. q. 8h.	p.o.: 200–300 mg. q. 12h.	0.5–2	CNS effects Liver dysfunction
Phenytoin	VPB, VT (digitalis induced)	Prophylaxis VPB	I.V.: 50–100 mg. q. 5 min. Max: 1000 mg.	p.o.: 100 mg. q. 8h.	10–18	CNS effects
Tocainide	VPB, VT	Prophylaxis VPB	p.o.: 200–400 mg. q. 8h.	p.o.: 200–600 mg. q. 12h.	4–10	CNS effects Blood dyscrasias
CLASS IC						
Encainide	VPB, VT	AT in W-P-W	p.o.: 25–35 mg. q. 8h. Max: 50 mg. q. 8h.			Avoid long-term use Proarrhythmia effect Aggravates congestive heart failure
Flecainide	VPB, VT	AT in W-P-W	p.o.: 100–200 mg. q. 12h. Max: 200 mg. q. 12h.		0.2–1.0	Avoid long-term use Proarrhythmia effect Aggravates congestive heart failure Interaction with Class II drugs
CLASS II						
Acebutolol		Prophylaxis ST, AT, VPB		p.o.: 200–400 mg. per day		
Atenolol		Prophylaxis ST, AT, VPB		p.o.: 50–100 mg. q. 12h.		
Esmolol	AT, AF, VT		I.V.: 0.025 mg. per kg. slowly + 0.025 mg. per kg. per minute			
Metoprolol		Prophylaxis ST, AT, VPB		p.o.: 50–100 mg. q. 8–12h.		
Nadolol		Prophylaxis ST, AT, VPB		p.o.: 40–80 mg. q. 8h.		

Table 46–15. INDICATIONS, ROUTE OF ADMINISTRATION, AND DOSAGES OF ANTIARRHYTHMIC DRUGS *Continued*

Type of Drug	Primary Indication	Secondary Indication	Initial Dose	Maintenance Dose	Plasma Level (μg./ml.)	Contraindications and Complications
Pindolol		Prophylaxis ST, AT, VPB		p.o.: 5–10 mg. q. 8h.		
Propranolol	VPB, VT	Prophylaxis ST, AT, VPB	I.V.: 1 mg. slowly + 1 mg. q. 2 min. Max: 7 mg.	p.o.: 10–80 mg. q. 6h.	40–85	
Timolol		Prophylaxis ST, AT, VPB		p.o.: 5–10 mg. q. 12h.		
CLASS III						
Amiodarone	Recurrent VT and VF	AT in W-P-W	p.o.: 800–1600 mg. per day for up to 3 weeks	p.o.: 100–400 mg. per day	1–2.5	Not first-line drug Bradycardia Conduction defects Other severe side effects
Bretylium	VF		I.V.: 5 mg. per kg. bolus + 10 mg. per kg. q. 15–30 min. Max: 30 mg. per kg.			Digitalis intoxication Hypotension
CLASS IV						
Verapamil	AT, AF with digitalis		I.V.: 5–10 mg. slowly + 5 mg. in 30 min.	p.o.: 40–120 mg. q. 6–8h.		Pre-excitation syndromes 2° AV block VT Hypotension
GLYCOSIDES						
Digoxin	AT, AF	Congestive failure	I.V.: 0.5 mg. slowly + 0.25 mg. q. 4–6h. Max: 1–1.5 mg.	p.o.: 0.125–0.5 mg. per day	0.001–0.002	AF pre-excitation syndromes in adults Proarrhythmia effect

INDICATIONS: ST = sinus tachycardia; AT = supraventricular tachycardia; AF = atrial flutter or fibrillation; VPB = potentially lethal ventricular premature beats; VT = sustained ventricular tachycardia; VF = ventricular fibrillation.

DOSE: I.V. = intravenous; p.o. = oral; Max = maximum dose.

CHILDREN: Dose should be calculated by body weight or body surface area.

ELDERLY OR RENAL FAILURE PATIENTS: Usually will require 50–70 per cent of adult doses.

*W-P-W = Wolff-Parkinson-White syndrome.

†APB = atrial premature beats.

‡CNS = central nervous system.

(Kent's bundle in Wolff-Parkinson-White syndrome or bundle of James in Lown-Ganong-Levine syndrome). The required treatment is the same as that for supraventricular tachycardia, but verapamil, digoxin, and beta-blockers should be used with great caution or not used at all because, although they block conduction through the AV node, they facilitate re-entry through the aberrant pathway. In children, digoxin seems to be effective. In some cases, surgical ablation of the aberrant pathway is effective.

Sick Sinus Syndrome

This syndrome occurs whenever there is an organic lesion of the SA node. In this condition, there are periods of irregular sinus pause with recurrent episodes of supraventricular tachycardia, bradycardia, or VPBs. Usually, this syndrome requires the establishment of a permanent demand pacemaker together with the administration of an antiarrhythmic drug.

Mitral Valve Prolapse Syndrome

In this condition, there is a myxoid change in the mitral valve with prolapse of one of the leaflets. In this syndrome, atrial premature beats, VPBs, or episodes of supraventricular tachycardia may be present. With rare exceptions, these arrhythmias are of benign course and usually respond well to beta-blockers.

Prolonged QT Syndrome

A prolonged QT interval may be congenital or acquired. There are two congenital syndromes that occur in families. One of them (Jervell and Lange-Nielsen syndrome) is accompanied by deafness, whereas the other (Romano-Ward syndrome) is not. An acquired prolonged QT interval may be due to electrolyte disturbances or drugs (especially tricyclic antidepressants and thioridazine). Regardless of the cause, a prolonged QT interval is dangerous because it can lead to *torsade de pointes* tachycardia.

Antiarrhythmic Drug Dosage and Administration

Table 46–15 presents a summary of the drugs currently approved for the treatment of arrhythmias in the United States. Only the most common indications and recommended dosages are listed. Some drugs, especially those of Class IC and III, should be used with great caution by physicians who have little experience with them. The administration of drugs for the treatment of severe arrhythmias should be done in a hospital under careful monitoring and ready access to countershock or pacing equipment.

Valvular Heart Disease

Hilmon Castle

AORTIC STENOSIS

Ejection systolic murmurs that are pathologic are most likely due to aortic stenosis or subaortic obstructive cardiomyopathy. Occasionally, the cause will be pulmonic stenosis or an atrial septal defect.

Bicuspid aortic valve is the most common cause of aortic stenosis and results from either a congenital fusion in young people or fusion of the leaflets from the fibrotic process produced by rheumatic endocarditis or calcification of the aortic valve in the elderly. Even though rheumatic fever is still an important cause of aortic stenosis, usually it is not the cause when aortic stenosis is the only lesion present. When aortic stenosis is accompanied by signs of mitral valve disease, then a rheumatic cause is much more likely. Both congenital bicuspid valves and rheumatic valves have a propensity for acquiring calcification, and,

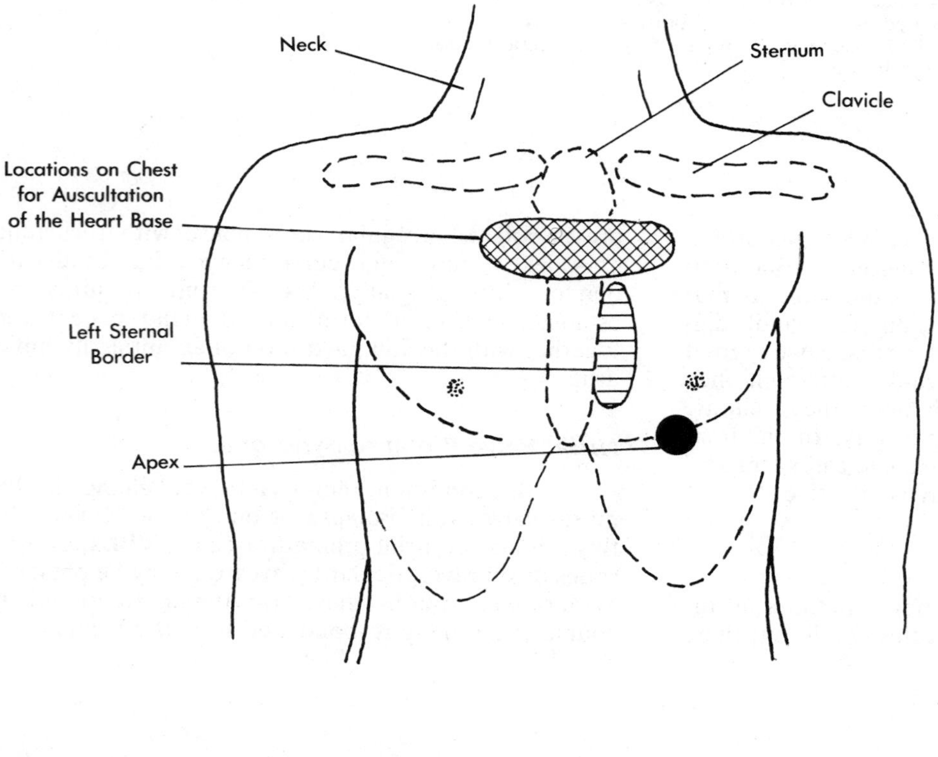

Figure 46–31. Chest location for anatomic structures.

after a significant amount accumulates, it is difficult, if not impossible, to determine the original stimulus for the valve disease.

The physiologic abnormalities that occur with aortic stenosis are an increased pressure in the left ventricular chamber and a pressure gradient across the obstruction that hinders the ejection of blood from the left ventricle to the aorta. These abnormalities result in an ejection systolic murmur and concentric hypertrophy of the left ventricle. If the condition is severe, then changes in the pulse may occur, i.e., a diminished palpable carotid pulse and a low pulse pressure on blood pressure recordings.

Subaortic Stenosis. Subaortic stenosis secondary to hypertrophic obstructive cardiomyopathy is mentioned in this section because the symptoms may be similar to and the ejection systolic murmur on initial examination consistent with that of aortic valvular stenosis. The asymmetrical hypertrophy of the ventricular septum and the anterior movement of the mitral valve mechanism in systole result in obstruction to outflow of blood from the left ventricle; thus, pressure gradients are produced within the left ventricular chamber. The clinical course, treatment, and prognosis of this condition are quite different from aortic valvular stenosis.

Symptoms

Patients with mild aortic stenosis usually have no symptoms. With severe stenosis or late in the course of a gradually developing stenosis, when the aortic valve orifice has reached a critical point of narrowing, chest pain, syncope, and symptoms of heart failure occur. The first clue to aortic stenosis usually comes when an ejection systolic murmur is detected on physical examination.

Physical and Laboratory Findings

An ejection systolic murmur, heard maximally at the base of the heart and to the right of the sternum (second interspace) with extension into the right side of the neck, is the most frequent and prominent finding (Figs. 46–31 and 46–32). The murmur is accentuated in the beat immediately following a premature ventricular contraction as well as following amyl nitrite inhalation. In hypertrophic obstructive cardiomyopathy, the murmur increases in intensity during Valsalva's maneuver and on standing from a squatting position. If the aortic stenosis is severe, the pulse pressure may be diminished in amplitude, as demonstrated by blood pressure recordings and palpation of carotid arteries with the fingertips. Chest x-rays may reveal calcification in the aortic valve, but unless there are other defects, the heart size and configuration usually appears normal. The ECG may show increased amplitude in QRS complexes consistent with left ventricular hypertrophy.

The echocardiogram is diagnostic in identifying aortic valve disease and impaired movement of the aortic valve as well as in identifying the presence of hypertrophic subaortic stenosis. The echocardiogram and Doppler flow studies using continuous wave recordings can establish the pressure gradient across the obstruction and allow the calculation of the valve area, left ventricular wall thickness, and chamber size.

Criteria for Diagnosis

An ejection systolic murmur with the characteristics described previously for aortic stenosis or subaortic stenosis is almost always present. Other signs, such as ejection clicks, calcification in the aortic valve (identified by x-ray), and left ventricular hypertrophy (identified by ECG) if present, are also helpful in diagnosis. The alternative diagnoses to be considered include innocent and functional murmurs, pulmonic stenosis, and atrial septal defect. The two-dimensional echocardiogram can be definitive in diagnosing the presence of aortic valve disease or hypertrophic obstructive cardiomyopathy, and Doppler flow studies can quantitate hemodynamic alterations. In order to determine the patient's prognosis, potential benefit from treatment, and the concomitant presence or absence of coronary artery disease, cardiac catheterization is usually needed.

Treatment

The treatment of aortic stenosis depends on the severity of stenosis, the stage of the disease, and the presence of other medical problems. If there are no symptoms secondary to the aortic valve disease and if none of the diagnostic tests indicate a critical degree of stenosis, then follow-up and observation for change may be the most appropriate course of action. When significant symptoms and evidence of critical narrowing of the aortic valve are present, then cardiac consultation to consider the potential value of cardiac catheterization and possibly surgical treatment is appropriate. Under proper circumstances, severe aortic stenosis that has not resulted in left ventricular failure may have excellent results from replacement of the aortic valve with a prosthetic one. Prophylactic antibiotics to prevent infective endocarditis should be administered any time there is increased risk of infections, i.e., during dental and surgical procedures and when there is the possibility of exposure to infections.

AORTIC REGURGITATION

Regurgitation through the aortic valve usually results from rheumatic or bacterial endocarditis on the aortic leaflets. Distortion of the valve may come from calcific aortic stenosis, which may also produce regurgitation. Systemic hypertension, if severe, occasionally causes incompetence of the aortic valve, which disappears when blood pressure is controlled. Syphilitic aortitis as a cause of aortic regurgitation was consid-

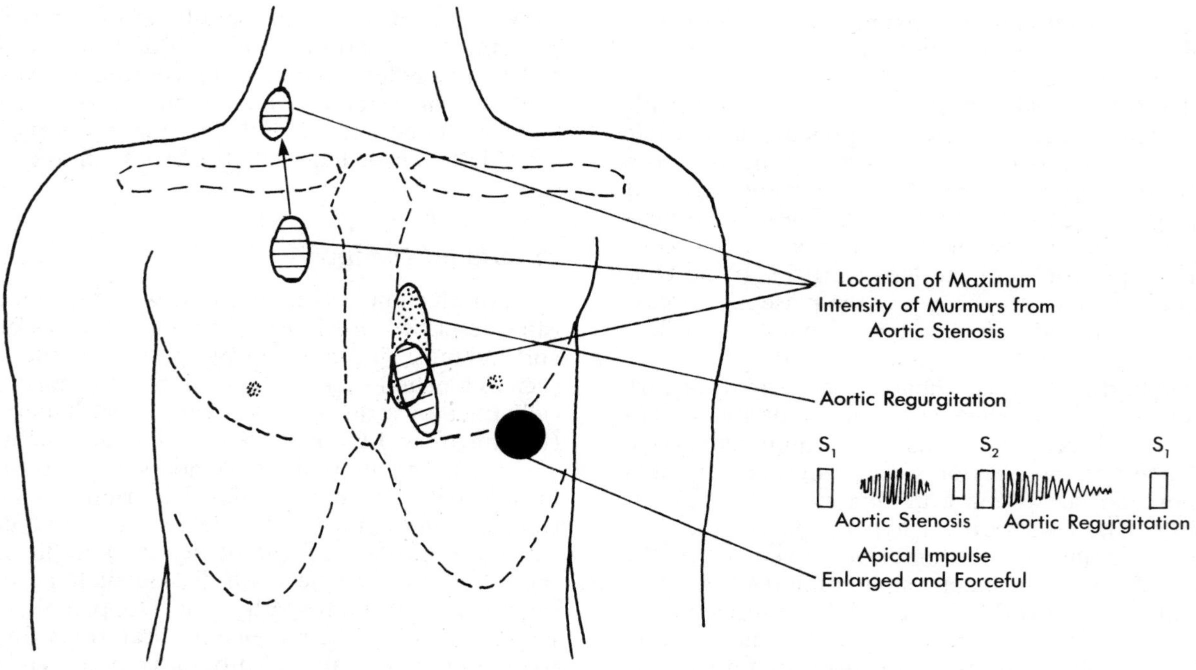

Figure 46–32. Chest location for maximum presentation of cardiac signs of aortic stenosis and regurgitation.

ered common in the past but is now rare. Primary diseases of the aorta with resulting medial necrosis, Marfan's syndrome, or dissecting aneurysm produce aortic regurgitation and should be considered as possible causes when the cause of aortic regurgitation is being sought.

Symptoms

Patients are usually asymptomatic until late in the course of severe aortic regurgitation. An increased pulse pressure may be noted as a prominent neck pulsation and by the patient's awareness of heartbeats, particularly when lying on the left side. Only after aortic regurgitation results in marked left ventricular dilatation and heart failure are symptoms of dyspnea, chest pain, and occasionally syncope present.

Physical and Laboratory Findings

The physical examination reveals an early, high-pitched, decrescendo diastolic murmur heard at the base of the heart and along the left sternal border with the patient sitting and leaning forward on exhalation. This murmur may be soft and difficult to hear. The usual maneuvers to clarify murmurs do not help very much, although inhalation of amyl nitrite decreases the intensity of the murmur and sustained handgrip increases it. When the aortic regurgitation is moderate to severe, the physical findings, in addition to the diastolic murmur, are usually an increased pulse pressure recorded on the blood pressure cuff and bounding peripheral arterial pulses. Chest x-rays may show increased cardiac size because of the increased diastolic volume and dilatation of the left ventricle. An ECG may show left ventricular enlargement.

Criteria for Diagnosis

The characteristic high-pitched, decrescendo diastolic murmur, heard maximally at the base of the heart and along the left sternal border, provides the clue that provokes the consideration of aortic regurgitation. When the murmur is soft, it is often overlooked. Pulmonic regurgitation may produce a similar murmur but will not be accompanied by signs of increased pulse pressure or signs of left ventricular enlargement by ECG, chest x-ray, or echocardiogram. The two-dimensional echocardiogram is critical to identifying abnormalities in the aorta or aortic valve that may cause aortic regurgitation, and Doppler color flow studies can provide a gross estimate of the degree of regurgitation. Assessment of the size of the left ventricular chamber, especially at end systole, is probably the most important determinant of prognosis and the potential benefit from surgery. If cardiac enlargement as determined by chest x-ray, ECG, or echocardiogram is present, then cardiac consultation is indicated. Consideration should be given to cardiac catheterization and to the potential benefit of surgical treatment.

Treatment

Effective treatment consists of correction of the defect causing aortic regurgitation at the critical time in the natural course of this condition. Cardiac consultation is especially important for this problem. Excellent results have been reported in the treatment of aortic valve regurgitation if it is corrected before the left ventricle dilates and heart failure occurs. As in aortic stenosis, prophylactic antibiotics to prevent infective endocarditis as recommended by the American Heart Association are in order before, during, and after dental or surgical procedures or whenever there is increased risk of infection.

MITRAL REGURGITATION

Even though rheumatic involvement of the mitral valve is still an important cause of mitral regurgitation, it is no longer the most common cause. When regurgitation is accompanied by signs of mitral stenosis or aortic valve disease, however, rheumatic origin is very likely. Prolapse of the mitral valve due to myxomatous degeneration of the valves and chordal structures is now considered the most common cause of mitral regurgitation. Patients with mitral valve defects that are due to either myxomatous degeneration or rheumatic disease have an increased incidence of infective endocarditis and cardiac arrhythmias. Sudden death has been reported to occur with the click-murmur syndrome, but in view of the large number of patients now identified with mitral valve prolapse, sudden death appears to be quite rare.

The prevalence of mitral valve prolapse observed in office practice is unknown, and the reported frequency varies considerably, depending on the population studied, the diagnostic methods used, and the criteria for diagnosis. Screening by physical examination of all children in a black South African school, using auscultatory findings of a mitral regurgitant murmur and a systolic click, revealed a prevalence of 1.4 per cent (McLaren et al., 1976). There are no reports of the per cent of people with mitral valve prolapse in the total community populations studied among North Americans, but the prevalence of a significant defect in the mitral valve among adults is probably closer to 4 to 5 per cent rather than the higher per cent reported in selected patient groups.

Among older patients, papillary muscle dysfunction resulting from ischemic heart disease is a cause of mitral regurgitation. Less commonly, calcification of the mitral annulus, dilatation of the left ventricle due to diffuse myocardial disease, and connective tissue disorder such as that which occurs in Marfan's syndrome result in mitral regurgitation. Acute causes of mitral regurgitation, such as rupture of a chorda tendineae or a papillary muscle or perforation of a valve leaflet from endocarditis, are rare.

Symptoms

Most patients are asymptomatic, but palpitations, fatigue, dyspnea, chest pain, and syncope have been associated with mitral regurgitation. Occasionally, patients with the click-murmur syndrome indicate that other family members have this disorder. Other patients with mitral regurgitation have angina and prior MI. The cause of their regurgitation is most likely papillary muscle dysfunction.

Physical and Laboratory Findings

A holosystolic murmur or a midsystolic click followed by a late systolic murmur that diminishes on deep inspiration and is accentuated on exhalation are the most characteristic physical findings of mitral valve prolapse (Fig. 46–33). Enlargement of the left atrium and left ventricle may be present on the chest x-ray, but unless the regurgitation is moderate to severe, the heart appears normal in size. The ECG may show evidence of left ventricular and left atrial enlargement, as well as nonspecific T wave and S-T segment abnormalities. However, the ECG usually is not very helpful.

In some patients with mitral valve prolapse, only the midsystolic click or a late systolic murmur may be heard at the apex of the heart. The presence of either is sufficient to suspect mitral valve prolapse, but when the physical findings are minimal or equivocal, then special maneuvers or noninvasive tests are needed to confirm the diagnosis. Maneuvers such as standing and inhaling amyl nitrite result in decreased venous return and arterial peripheral resistance, thus decreasing the size of the left ventricular chamber and in turn moving the click to earlier in systole and increasing the systolic murmur. Handgrip or transient occlusion of arteries in the extremities with inflated blood pressure cuffs increases the size of the left ventricle and in turn enlarges the left ventricular chamber and diminishes the degree of mitral valve prolapse, thus decreasing the intensity of the click and murmur and moving them to later in systole. In contrast, the murmur from rheumatic scarring and deformity of the mitral valve will increase in intensity when the left ventricular volume is increased and will decrease when the left ventricular volume decreases. These changes are helpful in distinguishing the causes of mitral regurgitation at the bedside.

Individuals with mitral valve defects that produce mitral regurgitation are at increased risk for development of infective endocarditis; this justifies the administration of antibiotics prophylactically for dental and invasive procedures. Whether or not the billowing of redundant mitral leaflets that may produce a systolic click but no regurgitation is associated with a risk of endocarditis is unclear but considered less likely. The use of prophylactic antibiotics when there is no murmur is controversial, but if mitral valve prolapse is unequivocal on two-dimensional echocardiography, most authorities on this subject recommend their use.

Criteria for Diagnosis

The presence of a systolic, regurgitant type of murmur that responds as discussed earlier serves as

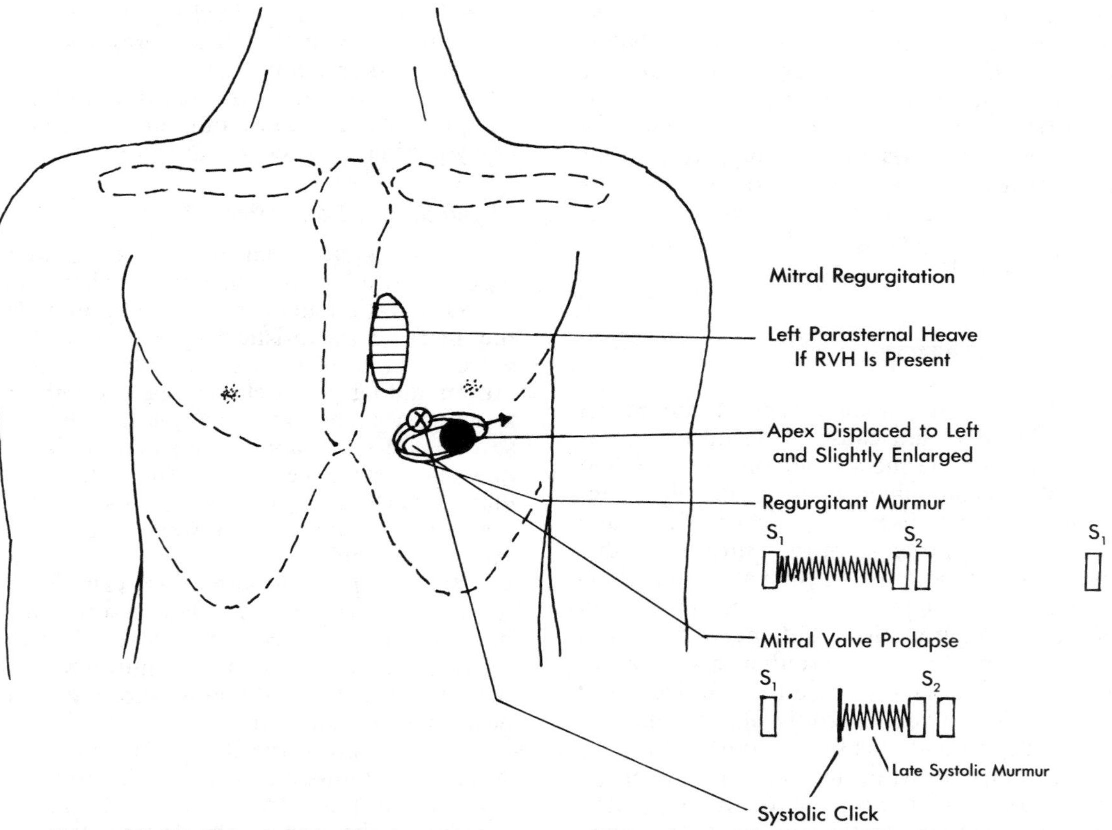

Figure 46–33. Chest location for maximum presentation of cardiac signs of mitral regurgitation.

strong clinical evidence for mitral regurgitation. The presence of a midsystolic click lends support to a diagnosis of mitral valve prolapse; a history of rheumatic fever and accompanying mitral stenosis or defects in other valves makes rheumatic endocarditis most likely. Signs or symptoms of myocardial ischemia suggest papillary muscle dysfunction as the cause of mitral regurgitation. The two-dimensional echocardiogram and Doppler flow studies are usually definitive in the diagnosis of mitral regurgitation. On occasion, cardiac catheterization is required to confirm the diagnosis and identify the cause. Catheterization may also be required to determine the severity of hemodynamic consequences and whether or not symptoms or cardiac function can be improved through surgical repair or replacement with a prosthetic valve. If surgical treatment is considered the preferred treatment, then coronary arteriography is needed in most patients to assess the risk and extent of the surgical intervention. If there are symptoms or changes in the cardiac chambers considered to be secondary to mitral regurgitation, then cardiac consultation should be obtained.

Treatment

Definitive treatment of mitral regurgitation requires open heart surgery. Symptoms of heart failure in patients with mitral regurgitation should be treated early and with afterload reduction. Evidence of mitral valve defects, whether they are due to myxomatous degeneration or rheumatic endocarditis, deserves the use of prophylactic antibiotics whenever there is increased risk of infective endocarditis, i.e., in the cases of dental or surgical procedures, use of immunosuppressive drugs, or exposure to infections (Table 46–16).

MITRAL STENOSIS

Mitral stenosis is usually secondary to recurrent rheumatic endocarditis, which produces scarring and contraction of the valve leaflets and chordal structures. As adhesions occur between the two major cusps of the mitral valve with concomitant shortening of their chordae, a funnel-shaped structure is formed with gradual stenosis of the orifice. Other conditions that impair blood flow from the left atrium to the left ventricle are unusual but include atrial myxomas, thrombosis, and bacterial vegetations.

The pathophysiology of mitral stenosis is a pressure gradient between the left atrium and ventricle in diastole that depends upon the size of the orifice and cardiac output. Indirectly, mitral stenosis imposes a pressure load on the left atrium, the pulmonary vasculature, and the right ventricle.

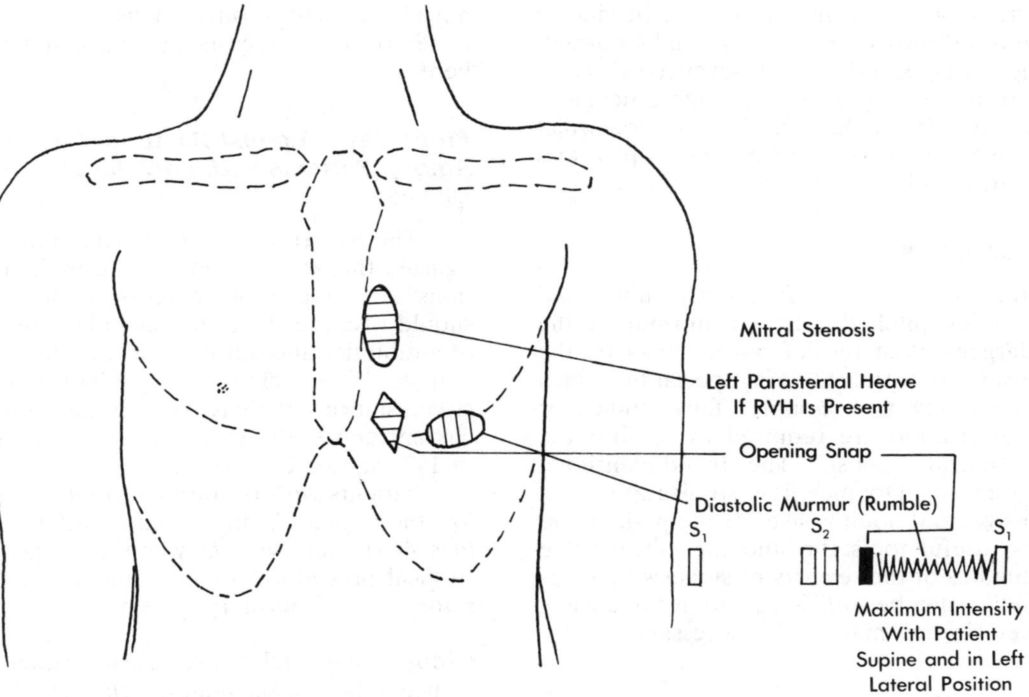

Figure 46–34. Chest location for maximum presentation of cardiac signs of mitral stenosis.

Symptoms

The most frequent signs and symptoms secondary to mitral stenosis are dyspnea, fatigue, palpitations, and hemoptysis. These symptoms progress slowly over the years.

Physical and Laboratory Findings

Findings on physical examination include an accentuated S_1, an opening snap along the left sternal border in the third or fourth interspace, a low-pitched diastolic murmur, and an accentuated S_2 (Fig. 46–34). If the process has advanced to severe mitral stenosis, the pulmonary artery pressure increases and the right ventricle becomes enlarged. A chest x-ray is usually not very helpful in diagnosis unless the process is advanced, in which case the left atrium may appear enlarged. The likelihood of atrial fibrillation increases with the age of the patient, along

Table 46–16. PROPHYLAXIS TO PREVENT BACTERIAL ENDOCARDITIS

Adults and Children Over 60 lb.	Children Less Than 60 lb.
Oral	*Oral*
Penicillin V 0.2 gram p.o. 30–60 minutes prior to procedure, then 500 mg. p.o. q. 6 h. × eight doses	Penicillin V 1.0 gram p.o. 30–60 minutes prior to procedure, then 250 mg. p.o. q. 6 h. × eight doses.
For patients allergic to penicillin, use:	*For patients allergic to penicillin, use:*
Erythromycin 1 gram 2 hours prior to procedure and then 500 mg. p.o. q. 6 h. × eight doses	Erythromycin 20 mg per kg. p.o. 2 hours prior to procedure, and then 10 mg. per kg. q. 6 h. × eight doses
or	*or*
Parenteral-Oral Combined	**Parenteral-Oral Combined**
Aqueous penicillin G 1 ml units mixed with procaine penicillin G 0.6 ml units I.M.* 30–60 minutes prior to procedure, then penicillin V 500 mg. p.o. q. 6 h. × eight doses	Aqueous penicillin G 30,000 units per kg. mixed with procaine penicillin G 600,000 units I.M., then penicillin V 250 mg. q. 6 h. × eight doses

*I.M. = intramuscularly.

Table 46–17. PROPHYLAXIS FOR INVASIVE PROCEDURES IN THE GENITOURINARY TRACT

Adults and Children Over 60 lb.	Children Less Than 60 lb.
	Same plan except for lower drug doses
Aqueous penicillin G 2 million units I.V. or I.M.*	Aqueous penicillin G 30,000 units per kg. I.V. or I.M.
or	*or*
Ampicillin 1 gram I.V. or I.M.	Ampicillin 50 mg per kg. I.V. or I.M.
plus	*plus*
Gentamicin 1.5 mg. per kg. (not to exceed 80 mg.) I.V. or I.M.	Gentamicin 2 mg. per kg. I.V. or I.M.
For patients allergic to penicillin, use:	*For patients allergic to penicillin, use:*
Vancomycin 1 gram I.V. over 30–60 minutes	Vancomycin 20 mg. per kg. I.V. over 30–60 minutes
plus	*plus*
Streptomycin 1 gram I.M. 30–60 minutes prior to procedure—same dose may be repeated in 12 hours	Streptomycin 20 mg per kg. I.M. 30–60 minutes prior to procedure—same dose may be repeated in 12 hours

*I.M. = intramuscularly.

with the increasing size of the left atrium. In mild to moderate mitral stenosis, the ECG is usually normal, but with more long-standing and advanced disease, there is a shift of the QRS axis to the right, increased amplitude of the QRS complex in the right precordial leads suggestive of right ventricular hypertrophy, and signs of left atrial enlargement.

Criteria for Diagnosis

Since the symptoms are frequently subtle and nonspecific, a low-pitched diastolic murmur at the apex or enlargement of the left atrium may be the only clue to suggest mitral stenosis. Special tests such as echocardiography and Doppler flow studies or cardiac catheterization are required to confirm the presence of mitral stenosis. The two-dimensional echocardiogram and Doppler flow studies are reliable, inexpensive, and noninvasive for the patient and are the most useful tools for studying mitral valve disease. Estimates of the severity of stenosis by Doppler flow studies may be sufficient, and in some cases cardiac catheterization may not be necessary.

Treatment

Quantitation of the hemodynamic changes by two-dimensional echocardiography and Doppler flow studies are essential, and in the majority of cases, cardiac catheterization and coronary arteriography are in order to determine the potential benefit of surgical correction of mitral stenosis. The choice of mitral commissurotomy versus valve replacement depends on many factors that have not been covered here.

Prophylaxis Against Bacterial Endocarditis Among Patients with Valvular Heart Disease

The American Heart Association Committee recognized that it is not possible to make recommendations for all possible clinical situations. Physicians should exercise their clinical judgment in the choice of antibiotics and duration of their use. Tables 46–16 and 46–17 are simplified guidelines for the usual circumstances. If there are any questions or unusual circumstances, the details of the Committee Report of 1977 should be reviewed.

Patients with conditions listed below should follow the outlined plans for antibiotic prophylaxis (Tables 46–16 and 46–17) when undergoing dental or surgical procedures or instrumentation of the respiratory or genitourinary system.

- Most congenital heart disease (does not include uncomplicated secundum atrial septal defect)
- Rheumatic or other acquired valvular heart disease
- Hypertrophic subaortic stenosis
- Mitral valve prolapse with mitral regurgitation

For instrumentation (invasive and surgery of the genitourinary and gastrointestinal tracts), antibiotic prophylaxis is directed primarily against enterococci.

Myocardial Diseases

Roland A. Goertz
Michael H. Crawford

CARDIOMYOPATHY

The cardiomyopathies are diseases that affect the intrinsic heart muscle cells. Although there are numerous identifiable etiologies, in many cases no underlying cause can be found. Dilated, restrictive, and hypertrophic are functional terms used to group patients according to pathophysiology and clinical presentation.

Dilated Cardiomyopathy

The common presentation is that of systolic heart failure discussed later in this chapter. The heart is enlarged, "floppy," and functions poorly. Cardiac output is depressed. Middle-aged men are more commonly affected, but dilated cardiomyopathy may occur in any population. Many cases have no discernible cause. It is believed that dilated cardiomyopathy is probably the end result of heart damage produced by a variety of toxic, metabolic, or infectious agents (Wynne and Braunwald, 1987).

Signs and symptoms include dyspnea on exertion, fatigue, paroxysmal nocturnal dyspnea, orthopnea, edema, and palpitations. The process may occur insidiously, and the heart may be significantly affected before findings are noted by the patient or physician. Angina is uncommon and, if found, suggests the possibility of coronary artery disease. Physical findings are those of systolic heart failure. Hypertension and diastolic murmurs are not characteristic. The most common chest x-ray, ECG, and echocardiogram findings are listed in Table 46–18. A transvenous heart muscle biopsy is sometimes helpful in identifying underlying causes that might be treatable.

Examples of dilated cardiomyopathies of known cause are alcoholic, prepartum or postpartum, diabetic, drug-induced (e.g., doxorubicin hydrochloride [Adriamycin], high-dose cyclophosphamide), and those related to neuromuscular disease (Duchenne's progressive muscular dystrophy, myotonic dystrophy, and Friedreich's ataxia). Heavy, continuous alcohol intake can directly affect the myocardial cells and can result in the most common form of dilated cardiomyopathy seen in the western world. Prognosis is dependent upon stopping alcohol intake prior to the development of advanced cardiac dysfunction. Peripartum dilated cardiomyopathy has no known cause and usually develops in the last month of pregnancy or in the first few months following delivery. The patient at high risk is typically multiparous, black, and over 30 years old. Persistent cardiomegaly after the first episode of heart failure is a poor prognostic sign. Future pregnancies should be discouraged.

Treatment of patients with dilated cardiomyopathies includes therapy for the underlying cause when it can be identified and treatment of the heart failure. The majority of patients enter a progressive downhill course and die within 2 years of onset of symptoms. Early consultation to eliminate the possibility of treatable underlying causes is warranted. Arrhythmias, refractory to usual therapy, often require surgical ablation of the arrhythmic focus or cardioverter-defibrillator implantation. These patients appear to be more sensitive to digitalis, and a high incidence of toxicity is noted. Cardiac transplantation should be considered in acceptable patients with advanced disease.

Restrictive Cardiomyopathy

A rigid ventricular wall that impairs ventricular filling and results in diastolic dysfunction is the functional abnormality common to the restrictive cardiomyopathies. A wide variety of diseases may result in fibrosis, hypertrophy, or infiltration of the myocardium. Examples include amyloidosis, hemochromatosis, glycogen deposition diseases, endomyocardial fibrosis, fibroelastosis, eosinophilia, and neoplastic infiltration.

Increased venous pressure results in the common findings of dependent edema; ascites; abdominal enlargement; and a tender, enlarged liver. Heart sounds may be distant; a third or fourth heart sound may be present. The jugular venous pressure does not fluctuate normally and may rise with inspiration (Kussmaul's sign). Laboratory findings are listed in Table 46–18. Echocardiography is helpful in aiding the clinician in differentiating this disease from the potentially surgically curable constrictive pericarditis. Transvenous heart biopsy is useful in differentiating the infiltrative causes.

Treatment of restrictive cardiomyopathies has limited success and is mostly palliative. Digitalis has little effect and diuretics do not significantly alter symptoms. If primary treatment of an infiltrative cause is available, then attenuation of heart involvement may be possible.

Hypertrophic Cardiomyopathy

This disease has also been known as idiopathic hypertrophic subaortic stenosis and hypertrophic obstructive cardiomyopathy. However, it is now recognized that the most common abnormality is diastolic dysfunction and that many patients do not have outflow tract obstruction (Wynne and Braunwald, 1987). Hypertrophic cardiomyopathy is characterized by an asymmetrical hypertrophy of the left ventricle that is not in response to a hemodynamic burden and is without identifiable cause. In most patients, the ventricular septum is hypertrophied more significantly than the remaining ventricular wall. Half of all cases appear to be transmitted in an autosomal dominant pattern, with variable but high penetrance.

Dyspnea, fatigue, chest pain, and syncope or near syncope are frequently noted symptoms, with dyspnea being the most common. Those patients with ventricular outflow obstruction demonstrate the classic murmur of hypertrophic cardiomyopathy: a harsh, diamond-shaped murmur that typically begins well after the first heart sound. The murmur is best heard at the lower left sternal border. When heard at the apex, the murmur may seem more holosystolic because of an element of mitral regurgitation that is often present. Any procedure that increases venous return, such as squatting or lifting of the legs while supine, reduces or eliminates the murmur. The mur-

Table 46–18. LABORATORY EVALUATION OF THE CARDIOMYOPATHIES

	Dilated	Restrictive	Hypertrophic
Chest x-ray	Moderate to marked cardiac enlargement Pulmonary venous engorgement	Mild cardiac enlargement	Mild to moderate cardiac enlargement
ECG	S-T segment and T wave abnormalities Left bundle-branch block	Low voltage conduction defects	S-T segment and T wave abnormalities Left ventricular hypertrophy Abnormal Q waves
Echocardiogram	Left ventricular dilatation and systolic dysfunction	Increased left ventricular wall thickness; normal systolic function	Asymmetrical septal hypertrophy; systolic anterior motion of the mitral valve

mur increases with the use of drugs or with maneuvers that reduce diastolic volume or increase contractility. Many patients have a double or triple apical impulse, a rapid upstroke and bisferious carotid pulse, and a fourth heart sound. The finding of hypertrophic cardiomyopathy at autopsy has a correlation with sudden death after physical exertion in children and young adults. Chest x-ray, ECG, and echocardiogram findings are summarized in Table 46–18. The echocardiogram is the diagnostic tool of choice and typically identifies the ventricular hypertrophy that is characteristic of the disease.

Beta-adrenergic blockers are commonly used for therapy, but there is no evidence of protection against sudden death. The calcium channel blockers, nifedipine and verapamil, have shown promising results in a number of patients. Digitalis, diuretics, nitrates, and beta-adrenergic agonists are not useful. Patients refractory to medical management and who have severe outflow obstruction may be helped by surgical myotomy and myectomy of the hypertrophied ventricular septum.

The prognosis for patients with hypertrophic cardiomyopathy is variable, with a number of patients improving over time. Sustained atrial fibrillation is associated with a poor prognosis. Patients should avoid strenuous exercise because of its relationship to sudden death. Endocarditis prophylaxis is recommended.

MYOCARDITIS

Virtually any agent that causes inflammation may affect the heart and cause myocarditis. Bacterial or viral infections, hypersensitivity states, chemicals, radiation, and drugs are all possible etiologies. Viruses are the most likely cause of acute myocarditis in the United States, with Coxsackie virus B being the most common. Coxsackie virus A, poliomyelitis, influenza, adenovirus, echovirus, and rubeola and rubella viruses are also causes. There is a frequent association of myocarditis with pericarditis.

Most cases of myocarditis are asymptomatic and are detected only by chance ECG findings of S-T segment and T wave abnormalities during a viral illness. More severe cases may present with heart failure or cardiac arrhythmias several weeks after a viral illness.

Appropriate treatment of the causal agent, when available, is indicated. Patients who develop heart failure respond to usual medications but exhibit increased sensitivity to digitalis. Arrhythmias commonly occur during acute illness and should be treated if indicated. The utility of immunosuppression is not proven except in rheumatic myocarditis. Viral myocarditis is usually self-limited and terminates without sequelae. An occasional patient may relapse or develop a chronic form. It is believed that numerous patients with idiopathic dilated cardiomyopathy had previous subclinical myocarditis.

CARDIAC TUMORS

Cardiac tumors are commonly divided into primary and secondary types. Primary tumors arise from the heart. Secondary tumors are metastatic to the heart and are more common than primary tumors. About 80 per cent of primary tumors are benign, most commonly myxomas in adults and rhabdomyomas in children. Malignant primary tumors occur predominantly on the right side of the heart and rarely develop in children. Secondary cardiac tumors usually occur as the result of metastases from lung cancer, breast cancer, or malignant melanoma.

Cardiac tumors are capable of producing any hemodynamic symptom or finding. Presentation is often dependent upon the size and location of the tumor. The most common finding is arrhythmias, most frequently atrial fibrillation. Myxomas are primarily found in the left atrium and are pedunculated. They usually present with mitral valve dysfunction or embolic phenomena. Secondary cardiac tumors result in clinical manifestations only about 10 per cent of the time and are usually not a cause of death. Echocardiography is the most useful diagnostic tool when a cardiac tumor is suspected. Surgical excision of benign tumors is indicated and is usually curative.

Heart Failure

Roland A. Goertz
Michael H. Crawford

Research over the past fifteen years has clarified many areas of cardiovascular physiology and has provided new treatment modalities. However, heart failure remains an enormous community and public health problem. Congestive heart failure has exponentially increased as a hospital discharge diagnosis during the 1970's and 1980's. Heart failure mortality rates have failed to decline despite decreases in deaths from

IHD and marked improvement in the treatment of hypertension (Smith, 1985). Approximately 200,000 patients die from the syndrome annually. Between 2 and 3 million Americans are affected, and approximately 400,000 new cases are diagnosed each year (Francis, 1988). Over 4 million office visits were made in 1981 for heart failure (Gillum, 1987). Family physicians care for over one third of the total patients seen in the office for heart failure, and a majority of these family physicians initiate and continue treatment after diagnosis (National Disease and Therapeutics Index, 1988).

Heart failure may be defined as the state in which an abnormality of cardiac function is responsible for the failure of the heart to pump blood at a rate commensurate with the requirements of the metabolizing tissues or can do so only from an abnormally elevated filling pressure (Braunwald, 1988). Clinically, heart failure may be described as a syndrome that causes limitation of a patient's activity because of the heart's inability to function successfully. Cardiac dysfunction can be due to a complex array of disease states. Primary abnormalities of the myocardium, such as the cardiomyopathies or extramyocardial disorders that result in myocardial damage such as hypertension or coronary artery disease, may result in heart failure. High output states such as hyperthyroidism, sepsis, or valvular heart disease and any form of left ventricular outflow obstruction are also causes.

In the 1970's, the Framingham study identified hypertension as the most common cause of heart failure, followed by a combination of hypertension and coronary artery disease, coronary artery disease alone, and valvular disease. Hypertension is a less frequent cause because of increased detection and improved treatment. Coronary artery disease is now the more common causal factor (Franciosa et al., 1983). The newly diagnosed heart failure patient must be thoroughly evaluated to detect reversible causes. A precipitating cause, when appropriately diagnosed, is more successfully treated than an underlying cause that has progressed to the point of heart failure (Braunwald, 1988). A systematic evaluation for both underlying and precipitating causes is essential to prescribe appropriate treatment (Tables 46–19 and 46–20).

The common pathway of the multiple etiologies of heart failure is eventual myocardial damage and subsequent ventricular dysfunction. A fall in cardiac output and a rise in pulmonary and systemic venous pressures soon result in the classic findings of dyspnea on exertion, paroxysmal nocturnal dyspnea, orthopnea, fluid retention, unexplained weight gain, or easy fatigability or some combination of these findings.

PATHOPHYSIOLOGY

Preload, afterload, and *contractility* are the major determinants of cardiac performance.

Table 46–19. COMMON CAUSES OF HEART FAILURE

Coronary artery disease
Left ventricular failure
Mitral regurgitation
Left ventricular aneurysm
Ruptured ventricular septum
Hypertension
Valvular disease
Mitral stenosis
regurgitation
Aortic stenosis
regurgitation
Prosthetic valve malfunction
Infective endocarditis
Cardiomyopathy
Dilated
Restrictive
Hypertrophic
Constrictive pericarditis

Preload may be defined as the tension placed on the myocardium prior to the onset of contraction. The Frank-Starling mechanism describes the phenomenon of enhancement of strength of a contracting muscle, within defined limits, by increasing the muscle's resting length. Resting heart muscle length is largely determined by end-diastolic volume, which is closely related to end-diastolic filling pressure. Therefore, an increase in end-diastolic volume or pressure enhances cardiac performance.

Afterload may be defined as the force the ventricle works against during contraction. An alternate definition is the tension or stress that the ventricle must develop to open the aortic or pulmonic valves and deliver blood to the aorta. Afterload is related to aortic pressure. Peripheral resistance and blood volume are significant determinants of aortic pressure, and increasing or decreasing these factors has an inverse effect on the velocity and volume of ejected blood from the ventricles during systole.

Contractility may be defined as the inherent strength or speed of contraction of the heart muscle (Strobeck and Sonnenblick, 1988). A failing heart with fewer or poorer functioning muscle fibers has less contractility and can do less work than a normally functioning heart (Fig. 46–35).

When the heart begins to fail, the body activates

Table 46–20. COMMON PRECIPITATING CAUSES OF HEART FAILURE

Medical noncompliance
Physical, dietary, or emotional excess
Infection
Anemia
Alcohol abuse
MI
Pulmonary embolism
Thyrotoxicosis
Infective endocarditis
Malignant hypertension
Myocarditis
Pregnancy
Arrhythmias

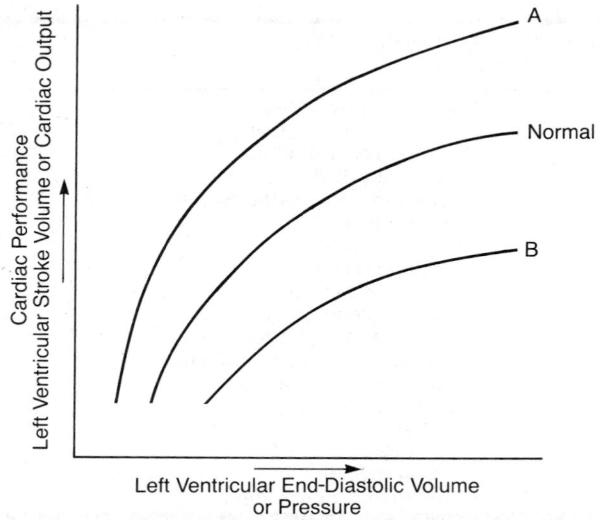

Figure 46–35. The Frank-Starling mechanism describes the enhancement of cardiac performance by an increase in length of resting muscle fibers (reflected here by an increase in left ventricular end-diastolic volume or pressure). Curve A represents a hyperdynamic heart, possibly resulting from enhanced contractility or decreased afterload. Curve B represents a failing heart ventricle, possibly resulting from reduced contractility or increased afterload.

compensatory mechanisms in an effort to improve cardiac function. Sympathetic tone increases, causing venous constriction, which augments preload. Myocardial hypertrophy begins so that the heart may cope with the increasing load. These early compensatory mechanisms have limited capacity to preserve heart function. The initial activation of compensatory mechanisms usually results in subtle signs such as tachycardia and ventricular dilatation, before signs and symptoms of heart failure are obvious.

Multiple central and peripheral compensatory mechanisms are activated to sustain cardiac output and preserve adequate perfusion of vital tissues and organs as heart failure worsens. Neurohumoral axes are stimulated to maintain arterial pressure; these include the sympathetic nervous system, the renin-angiotensin-aldosterone system, and the arginine-vasopressin system (Francis et al., 1984). The stimulated sympathetic nervous system causes vasoconstriction and increased systemic vascular resistance. The kidneys, sensing a fall in perfusion and increased sympathetic drive, stimulate the renin-angiotensin-aldosterone system. Activated angiotensin II and arginine-vasopressin, both potent vasoconstrictors, further increase systemic vascular resistance. Salt retention and fluid overload are worsened by an increase in aldosterone. Progressive stimulation of compensatory mechanisms leads to ever-increasing afterload and preload. Without therapeutic intervention, a vicious cycle of heart failure may develop (Fig. 46–36).

Numerous categorizations of heart failure have been used to simplify comprehension. Forward or backward, right-sided or left-sided, acute or chronic, and systolic or diastolic are all recognized descriptive forms. The concept of systolic versus diastolic heart failure is useful in the selection of optimal therapies (Moe and Armstrong, 1988).

Systolic failure is characterized by a decrease in contractility and is the traditionally recognized form in which the heart cannot adequately contract and expel its contents. The heart is generally dilated, and the ejection fraction (the percentage of blood ejected from the ventricle during a contraction) is usually less than 40 per cent. Systolic failure is characterized by inadequate cardiac output, with symptoms such as weakness and fatigue resulting from decreased tissue perfusion. Idiopathic dilated cardiomyopathy is an example of primarily systolic failure.

Diastolic failure describes a problem of relaxation and filling of the ventricle. The heart is usually of normal size or slightly hypertrophied, and the ejection fraction is normal. There is an increase in ventricular diastolic filling pressure without an increase in blood volume. Pulmonic or systemic congestive findings such as peripheral or pulmonary edema occur secondary to high venous pressures. Constrictive pericarditis results in primarily diastolic failure. Most patients probably have a combination of both systolic and diastolic failure. Heart failure from coronary artery disease is a form of both, systolic failure results from ischemic contractile depression, and diastolic failure results from fibrous replacement of destroyed myocardium.

DIAGNOSIS

Pulmonary Symptoms

Dyspnea (breathlessness) *on exertion* is often the earliest symptom of heart failure. As failure worsens, progressively less activity is required to produce dyspnea. The degree of activity needed to produce dyspnea in heart failure patients usually differentiates them from sedentary, obese, or anxious patients who experience breathlessness. Dyspnea is produced by a complex process that involves increased pulmonary venous pressure, decreased pulmonary compliance, and increased airway resistance resulting in increased work of breathing.

Paroxysmal nocturnal dyspnea is severe shortness of breath with feelings of suffocation that occurs several hours into the night and awakens the patient from sleep. Coughing and wheezing are common. The episodes are usually frightening, and bad dreams are often mentioned by patients. Sitting upright or walking around for 30 minutes or more usually provides relief. Maintaining an upright posture during waking hours tends to pool blood in the lower extremities. When the patient assumes the recumbent posture at night, this fluid is returned to the heart after a period of hours. If the heart is too weak to handle this increased load, fluid accumulates in the lungs, causing paroxysmal nocturnal dyspnea.

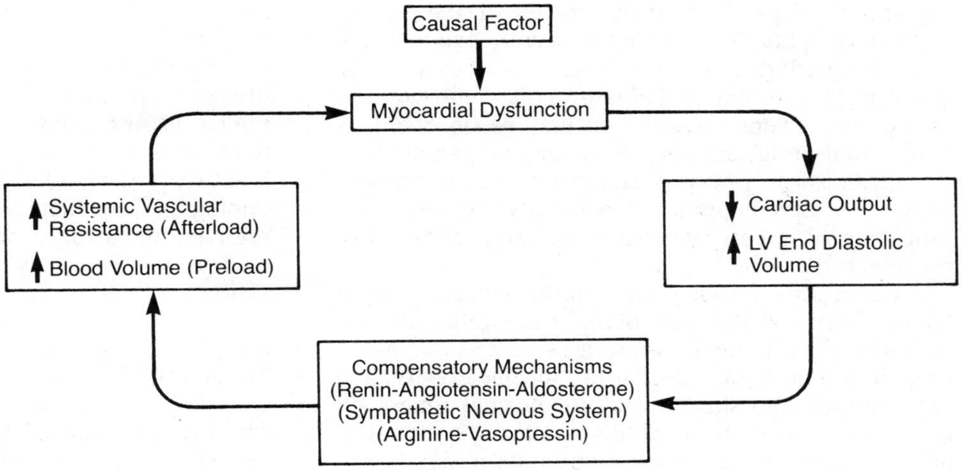

Figure 46–36. Vicious circle of heart failure. (Modified from Faxon, D. P.: ACE inhibition for the failing heart: Experience with captopril. Am. Heart J., *115*:1085, 1988.)

Orthopnea is dyspnea occurring immediately upon assuming the recumbent position. Redistribution of blood volume normally located in the legs and abdomen during upright posture quickly increases pulmonary capillary hydrostatic pressure in patients with severe heart failure, causing immediate dyspnea. Orthopnea is often quickly relieved by resuming an upright position or sleeping on a number of pillows. Sleeping in a sitting position may be necessary to provide relief in patients who have severe heart failure. A nonproductive cough that is more prominent at night and when the patient lies down is frequently observed.

Prior to diagnosing heart failure, there should be a careful search for other causes of pulmonary symptoms. Other causes include chronic obstructive lung disease, asthma, obesity, carcinoma, pneumonitis, hyperventilation, pneumothorax, pulmonary embolism, and pulmonary fibrosis.

Systemic Symptoms

These include weight gain, anorexia, and abdominal distention or discomfort. Weight gain is a result of fluid accumulation and edema. The kidneys, sensing decreased perfusion, attempt to restore it by retaining salt and water, which increases blood volume, preload, and systemic venous congestion. Initial changes may be subtle; patients may note swelling of the feet during the day or normally well-fitting shoes becoming unwearable. Systemic venous congestion may result in distention of the liver and ensuing right upper quadrant abdominal discomfort. Frank ascites is often seen in severe heart failure. Anorexia from splanchnic engorgement is frequent.

Miscellaneous Symptoms

These include fatigue, weakness, thought impairment, emotional disorders, nocturia, and insomnia. Nonspecific fatigue and weakness are common early findings related to a reduction in perfusion of skeletal muscle. Reduced cerebral perfusion and arterial hypoxia may produce confusion, impaired concentration, memory difficulties, headache, insomnia, anxiety, or even psychosis. These symptoms are more commonly seen in elderly patients with moderate to severe heart failure and associated cerebral arteriosclerosis. Nocturia occurs when renal blood flow improves at night in the supine position, decreasing renal vascular constriction and subsequently increasing urine production. Insomnia, commonly noted in heart failure patients, may be aggravated by nocturia.

Physical findings may be absent in patients who have mild heart failure. Diagnosis may be possible only when symptoms occur with exercise or increased activity. Worsening failure produces multiple findings, including rales, pleural effusion, edema, third heart sound, jugular venous distention, hepatomegaly, cardiomegaly, cyanosis, pulsus alternans, and Cheyne-Stokes breathing.

A continuum of pulmonary findings occurs as heart failure progresses. Moist, inspiratory, crepitant rales heard in the posterior lung bases are common in mild to moderate failure. With worsening pulmonary congestion, rales are heard throughout the lung fields and pleural effusions may develop. Effusions are more frequently seen in the right pleural cavity than in the left. Severe ventricular failure causes respiratory distress when the patient is sitting upright. Cheyne-Stokes breathing (cyclic episodes of hyperventilation followed by apnea) may develop if the respiratory center is depressed by drugs such as morphine or because of the prolonged circulation time from the lungs to the brain that is seen in heart failure patients.

A third or fourth heart sound may be found on cardiac examination but is not specific for heart failure. The apical impulse of the heart may be enlarged (>3 cm.), indicating cardiomegaly (Eilen et al., 1983). Pulsus alternans (a regular rhythm in which there are alternating strong and weak heart contractions with at least 5 to 15 mm. Hg variation in systolic arterial pressure) occurs in severe left ventricular failure.

Systemic venous congestion produces numerous

physical findings. Dependent edema of the legs in ambulatory patients and of the sacral region in patients on bed rest is often noted. Ascites may be found in severe failure. Hepatojugular reflux or elevated jugular venous distention may be observed. A tender, pulsating, enlarged liver may be palpated.

Cyanosis may occur secondary to a large amount of reduced hemoglobin in the blood. Oxygen offers little improvement because peripheral blood flow remains reduced.

Laboratory findings are minimal in early heart failure. An elevation in blood urea nitrogen and creatinine levels may be present as well as decreased urine production, increased urine specific gravity, and proteinuria. Potassium levels are normal unless diuretics have been given. Mild anemia and hyponatremia are common. If hepatic congestion is significant, liver enzymes may be elevated. Heart failure does not produce a specific ECG abnormality. The ECG may show abnormalities related to underlying cardiac disease.

Chest x-rays may show generalized cardiomegaly (transverse cardiac diameter divided by the thoracic diameter >0.50, Fig. 46–37) or specific chamber enlargement indicative of a particular cardiac process. However, normal heart size is present in patients with diastolic heart failure. Pulmonary artery enlargement, interstitial edema, Kerley's B lines, increased vascularity of the lung apices, and pleural effusions may be seen.

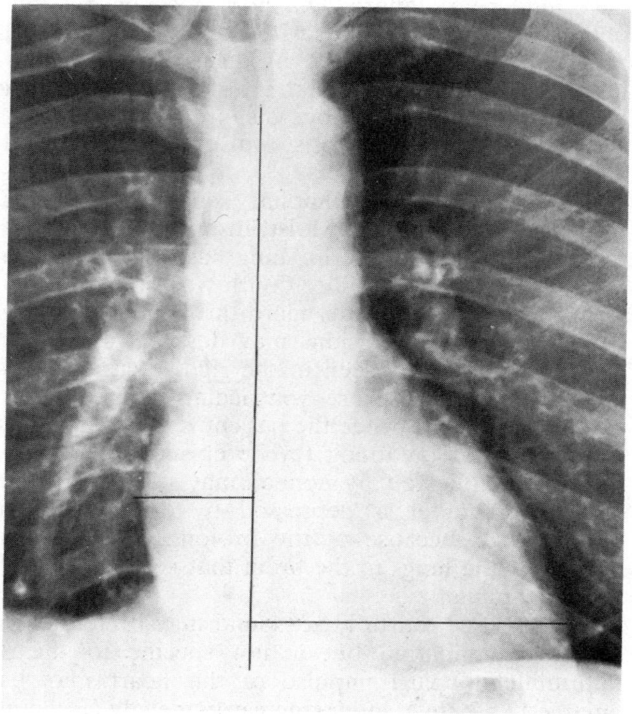

Figure 46–37. Measurement of the transverse cardiac diameter. A vertical reference line is first drawn through the spinous processes of the vertebrae. The greatest distances from this line to the right and to the left margins of the cardiac silhouette are then measured. Their sum constitutes the transverse cardiac diameter. (From Braunwald, E. (Ed.): Heart Disease. 3rd ed. Philadelphia, W. B. Saunders Co., 1988, p. 150.)

The family physician can establish the diagnosis of heart failure by balancing findings from the patient's history, physical examination, and laboratory tests. Prognosis and therapy are dependent upon identifying the underlying or precipitating causes. If etiology is not determined, the patient should be referred for further testing such as echocardiography, nuclear cardiology evaluations, or cardiac catheterization.

TREATMENT

The ultimate aim of therapy for heart failure is to alleviate symptoms, minimize complications, and prolong survival. There are three general approaches: correction of the underlying cause (the most desirable approach), removal of the precipitating cause, and control of the heart failure state (Braunwald, 1988). The first two approaches are self-explanatory and require identification and treatment of specific diseases. Controlling the failure state involves regulating excessive salt and water retention, improving contractility, and reducing cardiac workload. The aggressiveness of therapy is dependent upon the severity of clinical manifestations. Initial measures include restriction of physical activity to a level below stimulation of symptoms and limitation of salt intake to 3 or 4 grams per day. Ensuring adequate sleep and relieving anxiety are important adjuncts. For most patients, these efforts are insufficient to prevent symptoms or delay progression of failure and pharmacologic therapy is indicated.

It has been suggested that early treatment of asymptomatic left ventricular dysfunction prevents the onset of clinical heart failure and thereby improves survival (Furberg et al., 1985). Reports from large-scale, long-term clinical trials currently under way are needed to provide answers. The most salient advice is to base decisions about therapy upon established protocols, personal experience, and patient response and to remain acutely aware of the evolving literature. Representative drugs are summarized in Table 46–21.

Diuretics

Diuretics are a key first-line therapeutic option. Most act by inhibiting solute reabsorption in the kidneys, thereby enhancing excretion of salt and water. Reduced blood volume and atrial pressures decrease preload. This corrects pulmonary and systemic congestion and improves symptoms and edema. Diuretics do not affect myocardial contractility and usually do not improve cardiac output. A combination thiazide (e.g., hydrochlorothiazide) and potassium-sparing diuretic (e.g., spironolactone) may be effectively used in mild heart failure to lessen the risk of hypokalemia. More severe failure requires a loop

Table 46–21. REPRESENTATIVE DRUGS FROM EACH PHARMACOLOGIC CLASS FOR TREATMENT OF HEART FAILURE

Drug	Usual Dosage (oral)	Adverse Effects and Comments
Diuretics		
Hydrochlorothiazide	25–100 mg. per day	Hypokalemia
Furosemide (Lasix)	20–320 mg. per day	Hypotension or hypokalemia
Spironolactone (Aldactone)	25–100 mg. per day	Weak diuretic that spares K potassium
Metolazone (Zaroxolyn)	5–10 mg. per day	Potent diuretic even in renal failure
Positive inotropes		
Digoxin (Lanoxin)	0.125–0.5 mg. per day	Digoxin toxicity
Vasodilators		
Hydralazine (Apresoline)	25–150 mg. q. 8h.	Efficacy only in combination use
Isosorbide dinitrate (Isordil)	10–40 mg. t.i.d. (extended-release form)	Frequent tolerance
ACE inhibitors		
Captopril (Capoten)	6.25–50 mg. q 8h.	Initial hypotension
Enalapril (Vasotec)	2.5–20 mg. b.i.d.	Initial hypotension

diuretic such as furosemide. Combining a loop diuretic with a thiazide may maximize diuresis by acting on different sites within the kidneys. Refractory cases may require high doses of furosemide or use of metolazone, which can induce a potent diuresis even in the face of compromised renal function. Episodic use of metolazone for several days has been successful in returning decompensated patients to dry weight. The taking of daily weights provides an effective way of monitoring diuretic efficacy. Overzealous use of diuretics may cause hypovolemia or hypokalemia and must be avoided. Hypovolemia decreases cardiac output and renal blood flow, stimulating the renin-angiotensin-aldosterone system. Activation of the renin-angiotensin-aldosterone system can attenuate a diuretic response and increase the degree of failure. Hypokalemia may increase the patient's risk of ventricular tachycardia and associated sudden death. Combining an ACE inhibitor with a diuretic may reduce renin-angiotensin-aldosterone stimulation. Potassium-sparing agents should generally be avoided in patients taking ACE inhibitors in order to prevent hyperkalemia.

Inotropic Drugs

The traditional treatment of heart failure adds a cardiac glycoside to a diuretic to increase myocardial contractility. Digitalis works at the cellular level to increase calcium entry. Digoxin is probably the most frequently used digitalis preparation. Controversy exists as to which patient group should receive digitalis and whether or not ACE inhibitors should be used first. Clinical benefits from digitalis have been shown in patients with a large left ventricle and an S_3 gallop. It appears to be the drug of choice for patients with atrial fibrillation, and, in this group, ventricular response is a better measure of adequate dosage than are serum levels. Efficacy in heart failure patients with sinus rhythm is controversial. Digitalis has not been shown to be beneficial in patients with pure diastolic failure. Digitalis has a narrow therapeutic range, and toxicity is frequent. Toxicity is enhanced by abnormal serum electrolyte levels (especially decreased potassium levels), acid-base imbalance, hypothyroidism, and respiratory disease. Concomitant drug use (e.g., erythromycin, quinidine) and reduced renal function may increase digoxin levels into the toxic range.

Other inotropic drugs such as beta-adrenergic agents (e.g., dopamine and dobutamine) and phosphodiesterase inhibitors may be useful but, because of limited oral availability, have little place in primary care practice. These drugs are used primarily on hospitalized patients with severe or acutely decompensated heart failure. The long-term effect of inotropic agents on survival is not known. Some investigators have linked phosphodiesterase inhibitors with increased mortality because of increased life-threatening arrhythmias and accelerated left ventricular dysfunction (Packer et al., 1984).

Vasodilators

The management of heart failure has improved markedly since it was recognized that vasoconstriction is a major component in progression of the disease. Vasodilators relax smooth muscle, which alters the loading of the heart and improves cardiac performance. Vasodilators have been used effectively for many years in severe heart failure patients. A growing body of information indicates the efficacy of vasodilators in mild to moderate failure. Available drugs include hydralazine; prazosin; isosorbide dinitrate; and captopril and enalapril, the two ACE inhibitors. Hydralazine directly dilates arterioles and increases cardiac output. Problems have been noted with dosage adjustment, tolerance, palpitations, the development of a lupus-like syndrome, and possibly worsened myocardial ischemia. When combined with nitrates, a lower dose of hydralazine may be used, and side effects and difficulties with tolerance are lessened. Nitrates dilate veins and reduce ventricular size. They may be useful in patients with predominantly diastolic failure, especially if ischemia and angina are present. Tolerance is a major concern; however, use of nitrates in combination with hydralazine, which mostly affects arterioles, has been shown to improve survival in one large study (Cohn et al., 1986). Other vasodilators such as clonidine, minoxidil, and prazosin have not shown sustained clinical benefit in heart failure.

The ACE inhibitors are a group of vasodilators that primarily inhibit the renin-angiotensin-aldosterone system and thereby decrease vasoconstriction and fluid retention. These drugs may herald a new era in the treatment of heart failure. A study using pooled data from a number of randomized, controlled trials of vasodilators (Furberg et al., 1985) suggests that patients receiving the ACE inhibitor captopril have significant clinical improvement and decreased mortality. Also, the CONSENSUS study demonstrated improved survival in patients with moderate to severe heart failure treated with enalapril (The CONSENSUS Trial Study Group, 1987). ACE inhibitors are generally well tolerated by patients. Hypotension is the most frequent side effect, especially with the first dose. The risk of this occurring can be lessened by reducing or interrupting diuretic dosage when initiating the drug. In addition, skin rash, taste disturbance, or a nonproductive cough may occur and be severe enough to terminate usage. Renal function should be followed.

Other drugs such as calcium channel blockers and beta-adrenergic blockers have been used for heart failure, but the therapeutic role of each in patients without symptomatic myocardial ischemia remains unclear.

Selection of the appropriate therapeutic agent or agents depends on multiple factors. A reasonable strategy for treating classic systolic failure is to begin with a loop diuretic. If this is not sufficient, an ACE inhibitor should be added at a low dose or digoxin should be begun. Either approach can be efficacious. If worsening occurs, all three classes of drugs should be used: diuretics, vasodilators, and digoxin. Various combinations have merit and benefits. Acute pulmonary edema requires aggressive inpatient therapy with multiple modalities including morphine. In severely affected patients, short-term infusions of dobutamine over 72 hours may produce a clinical improvement for several weeks; then the infusion may be repeated.

Diastolic failure is not helped by inotropic medicines. Mild diuretics and salt restriction are the most useful treatments. Vasodilators may be helpful in patients who have diastolic heart failure and hypertension. Patients with diastolic heart failure often respond unpredictably to usual heart failure therapy, and early consultation is recommended if the patient is suspected of having diastolic failure. Consultation is also appropriate when the underlying or precipitating cause of heart failure is not identifiable or when the patient is not responding to therapy as expected.

The overall 1-year survival rate of patients with symptomatic heart failure is approximately 60 per cent. Once heart failure has become severe, transplantation becomes the only treatment likely to prolong survival and relieve symptoms. The hope is that ongoing, long-term, large-scale clinical trials will corroborate the suggestive findings that early treatment of left ventricular dysfunction prior to overt heart failure improves life and decreases mortality. If proven, primary care physicians will play a most important role in early identification of the syndrome.

Acute Pericarditis

Roland A. Goertz
Michael H. Crawford

Acute idiopathic pericarditis and acute pericarditis after MI are the most common pericardial diseases. Viruses are the presumed, but unproven, causal agent of many of the idiopathic group. Other common causes are uremia, neoplastic disease, rheumatologic diseases, and other infections (bacterial, fungal, tuberculous).

The diagnosis of acute pericarditis is primarily clinical and depends upon the identification of a characteristic precordial friction rub with accompanying chest pain, dyspnea, and serial ECG findings. The friction rub is often described as a scratching or grating sound during auscultation. There may be two or three components, with a two-component rub more commonly heard. The rub may be intermittent, may vary in intensity with respirations, or may only be heard with the patient sitting in an upright position with a slight forward lean. A paradoxical pulse may be present if tamponade ensues. Chest pain is usually acute at onset, may vary with body position, and is severe and constant over the precordial area. The pain commonly worsens with inspiration, differentiating it from the chest pain of MI. Dyspnea is more frequently noted when pericardial effusions are also present. A mild temperature elevation and sinus tachycardia often occur. ECG findings of diffuse S-T segment elevation in all leads except aV_R and sometimes lead III or lead V_1 are commonly noted during the first few days of illness. The absence of reciprocal S-T segment depression in opposite leads and the diffuseness of S-T segment elevation distinguish the pattern noted in acute pericarditis from that seen in MI. Echocardiography is useful for detecting the presence of an associated pericardial effusion.

Initial therapy should be directed at treatment of an underlying cause when present. Pain can be reduced by bed rest and decreased activity. Analgesics such as codeine, 15 to 30 mg. orally every 4 to 6 hours, may be used. Nonsteroidal anti-inflammatory drugs are the mainstay of treatment. Aspirin, 4 to 6 grams per day in divided doses, or indomethacin, 25 to 50 mg. four times daily, usually produces marked improvement in 24 to 48 hours. Prednisone, 60 to 80 mg. per day in divided doses with tapering after 1 week, is indicated in cases refractory to usual therapy, but rebound symptoms occur after withdrawal of the drug in 25 per cent of patients. Intrapericardial instillation of the corticosteroid triamcinolone has been effective in cases of acute pericarditis secondary to uremia. Recurrent acute pericarditis may require pericardiectomy. Systemic anticoagulation should be avoided in the patient with acute pericarditis because of the risk of bleeding into the pericardial space and possible development of tamponade.

Acute pericarditis normally resolves without sequelae, but a small number of patients develop a recurrent or chronic relapsing course. Progression to constrictive pericarditis occasionally occurs but is an uncommon complication.

Peripheral Arterial Disease

Roland A. Goertz
Michael H. Crawford

Arteriosclerosis is by far the most common cause of peripheral arterial disease. Smoking, hypertension, diabetes mellitus, and hyperlipidemia are risk factors for peripheral disease as well as for coronary artery arteriosclerosis. A significant number of patients with peripheral disease also have arteriosclerotic heart involvement. Patients under the age of 50 with advanced peripheral artery disease should be evaluated for the presence of heterozygosity for homocystinuria, a rare but potentially treatable cause.

A common presentation of peripheral arterial disease is intermittent pain in the lower leg upon walking (intermittent claudication) that readily responds to rest. The pain may be characterized as a dullness, aching, or numbness. A feeling of fatigue in the legs is also common. Self-curtailment of activity in response to early mild symptoms may lead to insidious advancement of the disease and delayed presentation of the patient to the physician. As obstruction advances, ulceration of the skin may develop secondary to minor trauma and the feet or lower legs may become cold and cyanotic. Gangrenous changes may be noted on the toes. A male patient may complain of impotence if the arteriosclerosis is severe in the aortoiliac region.

Peripheral pulses are often decreased and in severe cases may be detectable only with a Doppler instrument. A decreased systolic blood pressure in the lower leg measured just above the ankle following exercise compared with the systolic pressure in the arm may be a helpful clue to diagnosis. Measuring for differential blood pressures of arms and legs (with leg pressures lower than arm pressures) or performing Doppler flow studies may aid in diagnosis. An arteriogram of the involved extremity is usually necessary if surgery is being considered.

Therapy includes control or treatment of all arteriosclerosis risk factors. Smoking should be stopped completely, not only to reduce the risk of arteriosclerosis but also to prevent smoking-induced peripheral vasoconstriction. Significant occlusive disease is rare in nonsmokers unless they are diabetic. Daily exercise is the most effective treatment for intermittent claudication. Walking daily to the point of pain and then pressing on until pain prohibits further walking will, with time, significantly increase pain-free walking distance. Careful attention to foot care is vital in order to prevent the loss of a limb to amputation. The precipitating cause of most severe ulcerated or gangrenous extremities is mechanical, chemical, or thermal trauma. Foot care includes wearing proper footwear, inspecting feet daily, avoiding heat or cold, and caring for nails and skin properly. Drug therapy has not been as successful as anticipated, and vasodilating agents are generally not effective in occlusive vascular disease. Patients given pentoxifylline (Trental, an agent that affects the flexibility of red blood cells), 400 mg. orally three times daily, experienced a modest increase in walking distance in controlled trials. The effectiveness of the use of antiplatelet agents or prostaglandins is unclear. Anticoagulants have no role in the treatment of peripheral arterial disease. Any drug (e.g., ergot derivatives) that constricts peripheral vasculature should be avoided.

A number of surgical procedures are potentially helpful. Preliminary usage of catheter balloon angioplasty, the atherectomy catheter, and lasers have been promising but with some limitation depending on the location of the obstruction. Surgical consultation should be considered in patients who have resting pain, nonhealing ulcers, or early gangrene, for they are at risk for amputation. In patients who only have intermittent leg pain, surgical referral is indicated if their livelihood is threatened or their life style is severely impaired by the pain. Severe disease or gangrene requires prompt hospitalization. The possibility of coexisting coronary artery arteriosclerosis must be kept in mind if surgery is considered.

Surgery for Patients with Heart Disease

Roland A. Goertz
Michael H. Crawford

The presence of underlying cardiovascular disease presents unique evaluation challenges before surgery can occur. A multifactorial index to evaluate such patients has been devised (Goldman, 1980). The index assigns risk points to certain variables such as age, current cardiovascular and metabolic status, and site of proposed surgery. The eventual decision is clinical and must be framed with full consideration of the potential need for and benefits of the surgery versus the risk.

The evaluation of the patient should include a complete history and physical examination, current chest x-rays and electrolyte studies, baseline ECG, and any essential tests that may aid in assessing the patient's current physical status. An assessment of the emotional readiness of the patient for surgery should not be forgotten in elective situations. The objective is to have the patient in as stable a condition as possible prior to the procedure. Cardiac conditions that preclude elective surgery are unstable angina, recent MI, severe aortic stenosis, a high degree of heart block, decompensated heart failure, and severe hypertension.

ISCHEMIC HEART DISEASE

Stable coronary artery disease has a relatively low risk during surgery. If there are no signs of heart failure and at least 6 months have elapsed since MI, the surgeon may proceed with surgery if indications for surgery are clear. Emergency surgery in the face of recent infarction carries a high risk of death. If possible, delaying surgery for at least 3 weeks is recommended. Purely elective surgery should be postponed for 6 months after MI.

HYPERTENSION

Controlled hypertension without significant complications does not put the patient at significant added risk of death during surgery. Discontinuing medication for a week prior to surgery in hypertensive patients who have diastolic blood pressure measurements of less than 110 mm. Hg has been recommended by some authorities. However, patients receiving beta-adrenergic blockers on a continuing basis should not be abruptly withdrawn from the drug. Most hypertensives should continue therapy up to the night prior to surgery and resume therapy as soon as possible after the procedure.

HEART FAILURE

Patients whose heart failure is under control have a slightly increased risk during surgery. Increasing severity of failure increases the risk during surgery. Heart failure should be controlled for at least a month prior to surgery. Patients experiencing digitalis toxicity or hypokalemia secondary to the use of diuretics are poor candidates for surgery. There is controversy as to whether or not digitalis should be stopped prior to surgery.

ARRHYTHMIAS

Chronic atrial fibrillation with a controlled ventricular rate does not usually increase the risk during surgery. Isolated right or left bundle-branch blocks do not increase surgical risk significantly. However, advanced forms of heart block are serious warning signs, and a preoperative pacemaker may be warranted.

VALVULAR HEART DISEASE

Increased risk during surgery is noted with severe aortic stenosis and advanced mitral stenosis. Other valvular defects must be evaluated individually. Prophylactics against infective endocarditis should be given.

Generally, drugs that are required to control cardiovascular problems should not be withdrawn for surgery. The risks of the uncontrolled problem usually exceed the risks of the drug. Oral anticoagulants are an exception and should be stopped if possible or the patient switched to I.V. anticoagulants that can be reversed. For example, patients with prosthetic heart valves should never have oral anticoagulants stopped abruptly without heparin coverage, since acute valve thrombosis has been described in association with abrupt withdrawal of oral anticoagulants. The effects of heparin can be reversed temporarily for surgery by the administration of protamine. A complete medication list and full health history should be known by both the individual giving anesthesia and the surgeon. The family physician should not only consider disease implications for surgery but should also determine the patient's emotional readiness and help the patient and family to understand the disease process. Clinical assessment of risks and benefits remains the cornerstone of evaluation.

References

Abbott, A. V., and Peters, R. K.: Type A behavior and coronary heart disease: An update. Am. Famil. Phys. *38*:105, 1988. *A review of the current status of Type A behavior research and of the recent studies that have questioned the relationship between Type A behavior and CHD. Basic recognition of Type A behavior in the physician's office is discussed.*

Berglund, G., Andersson, O., and Wilhelmsen, L.: Prevalence of primary and secondary hypertension: Studies in random population sample. J. Br. Med., *2*:554, 1976.

Blackburn, H., and Jacobs, D. R.: Physical activity and the risk of coronary heart disease. N. Engl. J. Med., *319*:1217, 1988.

Blankenhorn, D. H., et al.: Beneficial effects of combined colestipol-niacin therapy on coronary atherosclerosis and coronary venous bypass grafts. J.A.M.A., *257*:3233, 1987.

Braunwald, E. (Ed.): Heart Disease: A Textbook of Cardiovascular Medicine. 3rd ed. Philadelphia, W. B. Saunders Co., 1988, p. 426, p. 474, and p. 1412. *An excellent comprehensive text on cardiovascular medicine with an extensive bibliography.*

Califf, R., et al.: Failure of simple clinical measurements to predict perfusion status after intravenous thrombolysis. Ann. Int. Med., *108*:658, 1988.

Centers for Disease Control: Protective effect of physical activity on coronary heart disease. M.M.W.R., *36*:426, 1987.

Chung, E. K.: Clinical Electrocardiography. Part III: Complex Cardiac Arrhythmias. New York, MEDCOM Learning Systems, 1972. *This is a self-instruction package containing a collection of slides that show typical patterns of arrhythmia.*

Chung, E. K.: Electrocardiography: Practical applications with vectorial principles. Norwalk, Conn. Appleton and Lange, 1985. *Although the emphasis of this book is on the ECG changes in a variety of diseases, there are several chapters devoted to an explanation of various types of arrhythmias.*

Cohn, J. N., Archibald, D. G., and Ziesche, S.: Effects of vasodilator therapy on mortality in chronic congestive heart failure: Results of Veterans Administration Cooperative Study. N. Engl. J. Med., *314*:1547, 1986. *One of the first studies suggesting that treatment with a vasodilator alters the mortality of heart failure.*

The CONSENSUS Trial Study Group: Effects of enalapril on mortality in severe congestive heart failure: Results of the Cooperative North Scandinavian Enalapril Survival Study (CONSENSUS). N. Engl. J. Med., *316*:1429, 1987. *A landmark study suggesting that usage of enalapril alters mortality of heart failure patients.*

Eilen, S. D., Crawford, M. H., and O'Rourke, R. A.: Accuracy of precordial palpation for detecting increased left ventricular volume. Ann. Int. Med., *99*:628, 1983. *A study indicating that the size of the apical impulse is a more accurate indicator of increased left ventricular volume than the amount of lateral displacement of the apical impulse.*

Erb, B. D., Fletcher, G. F., and Sheffield, T. L.: Standards for cardiovascular exercise in treatment programs. American Heart Association subcommittee on rehabilitation target activity group. Circulation, *59*:1084A, 1979.

Faxon, D. P.: ACE inhibition for the failing heart: Experience with captopril. Am. Heart J., *115*:1085, 1988.

Franciosa, J. A., et al.: Survival in men with severe chronic left ventricular failure due to either coronary heart disease or idiopathic dilated cardiomyopathy. Am. J. Cardiol., *51*:831, 1983.

Francis, G. S., et al.: The neurohormonal axis in congestive heart failure. Ann. Int. Med., *101*:370, 1984.

Francis, G. S.: Heart failure management: The impact of drug therapy on survival. Am. Heart J., *115*:699, 1988.

Furberg, C. D., Yusuf, S., and Thom, T.: Potential for altering the natural history of congestive heart failure: Need for large clinical trials. Am. J. Cardiol., *55*:45A, 1985.

Gillum, R. F.: Heart failure in the United States: 1970–1985. Am. Heart J., *113*:1043, 1987. *A comprehensive statistical review of heart failure during the indicated years.*

Goldman, L.: Guidelines for evaluating and preparing the cardiac patient for general surgery. J. Cardiovasc. Med., *5*:637, 1980.

Greenland, P., and Chu, J.: Efficacy of cardiac rehabilitation services, with emphasis on patients after myocardial infarction. Ann. Int. Med., *109*:650, 1988a. *This comprehensive review examines the evidence in the medical literature for the conclusions concerning the efficacy of cardiac rehabilitation.*

Greenland, P., and Chu, J.: Cardiac rehabilitation services. Health and Public Policy Committee, American College of Physicians. Ann. Int. Med., *109*:671, 1988b. *This concise position paper states the rationale for cardiac rehabilitation services. It lists recommendations, duration, and contraindications for low-, intermediate-, and high-risk patients.*

Grundy, S. M., et al.: Cardiovascular and risk factor evaluation of healthy American adults: A statement for physicians by an ad hoc committee appointed by the steering committee. American Heart Association, *75*:1340A, 1987. *A valuable comprehensive position statement by experts appointed by the American Heart Association. Detection of CHD risk factors is recommended through periodic health examinations. Relative risks and evaluation methods are described for cigarette smoking, blood pressure, cholesterol, glucose, body weight and fat, and exercise.*

Hartley, L. H., et al.: Secondary prevention of coronary heart disease. Circulation, *76*:I169, 1987.

The Health Consequences of Smoking: Cardiovascular Diseases: A Report of the Surgeon General. United States Department of Health, Education, and Welfare, Public Health Service. Washington, D.C., Government Printing Office, 1979.

Hypertension Detection and Follow-Up Program Cooperative Group: Blood pressure studies in 14 communities: A two-stage screen for hypertension. J.A.M.A., *237*:2385, 1977.

Hypertension Detection and Follow-Up Program Cooperative Group: Five-year findings of the Hypertension Detection and Follow-Up Program: I. Reduction in mortality of persons with high blood pressure, including mild hypertension. J.A.M.A., *242*:2562, 1979.

Killip, T., III, and Kimball, J. T.: Treatment of myocardial infarction in a coronary unit: A two-year experience with 250 patients. Am. J. Cardiol., *20*:457, 1967.

Khaw, K., and Barrett-Connor, E.: Family history of heart attack: A modifiable risk factor? Circulation, *74*:239, 1986.

Krotkiewski, M., et al.: Impact of obesity on metabolism in men and women: Importance of regional adipose tissue distribution. J. Clin. Invest., *72*:1150, 1983.

Lembo, N. J., et al.: Bedside diagnosis of systolic murmurs. N. Engl. J. Med., *318*:1572, 1988.

Lewin, A., et al.: Apparent prevalence of curable hypertension in the HDFP. Arch. Int. Med., *145*:424, 1985.

Lie, K. I., et al.: Lidocaine in the prevention of primary ventricular fibrillation. N. Engl. J. Med., *291*:1324, 1974.

Lown, B., et al.: The coronary care unit: New perspectives and directions. J.A.M.A., *199*:188, 1967.

MacMahon, S., et al.: Effect of prophylactic lidocaine in suspected acute myocardial infarction: An overview of results from the randomized, controlled trials. J.A.M.A., *260*:1910, 1988.

Management Committee of the Australian National Blood Pressure Study: The Australian therapeutic trial in mild hypertension. Lancet, *1*:1261, 1980.

Marsland, D. W., Wood, M., and Mayo, F.: A data bank for patient care curriculum and research in family practice: 526 patient problems. J. Fam. Prac., *3*:25, 1976.

Matthews, K. A., and Haynes, S. G.: Type A behavior pattern and coronary disease risk. Update and critical evaluation. Am. J. Epidemiol., *123*:923, 1986.

McLaren, J. J., et al.: Non-ejection systolic clicks and mitral systolic murmurs in black schoolchildren in Sowetto, Johannesburg. Br. Heart J., *38*:318, 1976.

Medical Research Council Working Party: MRC trial of treatment of mild hypertension: Principal results. Br. Med. J. Clin. Res., *291*:97, 1985.

Moe, G. W., and Armstrong, P. W.: Congestive heart failure. C.M.A.J., *138*:689, 1988.

National Disease and Therapeutics Index, IMS. Courtesy of The Heart Failure: Early Intervention Education Program, 1988.

National Institutes of Health Consensus Development Panel: Summary and recommendations of the consensus conference: Lowering blood cholesterol to prevent heart disease. J.A.M.A., *253*:2080, 1985.

The 1988 report of the Joint National Committee on Detection, Evaluation, and Treatment of High Blood Pressure. Arch. Intern. Med., *148*:1023, 1988. *A committee of experts presents a comprehensive new set of recommendations for the detection, evaluation, and treatment of hypertension. This information is essential for all physicians who manage hypertension.*

Packer, M., Medina, N., and Yushak, M.: Hemodynamic and clinical limitations of long-term inotropic therapy with amrinone in patients with severe chronic heart failure. Circulation, *70*:1038, 1984.

Parmley, W. W.: Position report on cardiac rehabilitation: Recommendations of the American College of Cardiology. J. Am. Coll. Cardiol., *7*:451, 1986.

Perkins, K. A.: Family history of coronary heart disease: Is it an independent risk factor? Am. J. Epidemiol., *124*:182, 1986.

The Pooling Project Research Group: Relationship of blood pressure, serum cholesterol, smoking habit, relative weight and ECG abnormalities to incidence of major coronary events: Final report of the Pooling Project. J. Chron. Dis., *31*:202, 1978.

Powell, K. E., et al.: Physical activity and the incidence of coronary heart disease. Annu. Rev. Public Health, *8*:253, 1987.

Report of the National Cholesterol Education Program Expert Panel on Detection, Evaluation, and Treatment of High Blood Cholesterol in Adults. Arch. Intern. Med., *148*:36, 1988. *This comprehensive report by experts on hypercholesterolemia provides the family physician with up-to-date guidelines that are essential for the management of a large number of patients.*

Sandöe, E., and Sigurd, B.: Arrhythmia: Diagnosis and Management. A Clinical Electrocardiographic Guide. Fachmed AG, Verlag für Fachmedien, 1984. St. Gallen, Switzerland. *This book, authored by two outstanding Danish electrocardiographers, was written on behalf of the European Society of Cardiology under a grant from Boehringer Ingelheim Company. The English version has been widely distributed in the United States. The emphasis of this excellent book is on the description of arrhythmias: their genesis, symptoms, management, and long-term prophylaxis.*

Scheidt, S.: Basic Electrocardiography. West Caldwell, N.J., CIBA-GEIGY, 1986. *This is an excellent textbook based on a previous CIBA monograph on the most typical patterns of arrhythmia prepared by the author with superb illustrations by Dr. Netter. There is an excellent discussion on cardiac pacemakers.*

Smith, W. M.: Epidemiology of congestive heart failure. Am. J. Cardiol., *55*:3A, 1985.

Strobeck, J. E., and Sonnenblick, E. H.: Deficiency in cardiac contraction. *In* Cohn, J. N. (Ed.): Drug Treatment of Heart Failure. 2nd ed. Secaucus, N.J., Advanced Therapeutics Communications, 1988, p. 13.

Svendsen, K. H., et al.: Effects of passive smoking in the Multiple Risk Factor Intervention Trial. Am. J. Epidemiol., *126*:783, 1987.

A Textbook of Advanced Cardiac Life Support. Dallas, American Heart Association, 1987. *This is a textbook that is used by all health care providers who wish to be certified as experts in advanced cardiac life support. Several chapters discuss the topic of acute arrhythmias and their management.*

The TIMI Study Group: Comparison of invasive and conservative strategies after treatment with intravenous tissue plasminogen activator in acute myocardial infarction. N. Engl. J. Med., *320*:618, 1989.

Tucker, R. M., and Labarthe, D. R.: Frequency of surgical treatment for hypertension in adults at the Mayo Clinic from 1973 through 1975. Mayo Clinic Proc., *52*:549, 1977.

Walker, W. J.: Changing United States life-styles and declining vascular mortality: Cause or coincidence? N. Engl. J. Med., *297*:163, 1977.

Weiss, N. S.: Relation of high blood pressure to headache, epistaxis, and selected other symptoms. The United States health examination survey of adults. N. Engl. J. Med., *287*:631, 1972.

Willett, W. C., et al.: Relative and absolute risk of coronary heart disease among women who smoke cigarettes. N. Engl. J. Med., *317*:1303, 1987.

Wynne, J., and Braunwald, E.: The cardiomyopathies and myocarditides. *In* Harrison's Principles of Internal Medicine. 11th ed. New York, McGraw-Hill Book Co., 1987, pp. 998–1005. *A concise presentation of myocardial diseases.*

Wyse, D. G., Kellen, J., and Rodemaker, A. W.: Prophylactic versus selective lidocaine for early ventricular arrhythmias of myocardial infarction. J. Am. Coll. Cardiol., *12*:507, 1988.

47

Emergency Medicine

Steven D. Morse
William Y. Rial

Evaluating the Seriously Injured Patient

Assess the patient's airway and ventilatory efforts. Consider the need for cardiopulmonary resuscitation, intubation, or, if the neck is injured or uncertain, cricothyrotomy. Check the pulse and pressure and begin chest compression if necessary. Control external blood loss with pressure. Rapidly establish large-bore intravenous access (16-gauge catheters or larger should be used, at least two in number). Intravenous lines below the diaphragm are potentially useless in the abdominal trauma victim owing to possible vascular disruption and should be avoided if at all possible. If concomitant chest trauma exists, with the possibility of intrathoracic vascular disruption, place lines on the side of the least traumatized hemithorax. Central venous cannulation in this context is perhaps best performed using an internal jugular approach, if the neck is cleared, to avoid pneumothorax. Otherwise, supraclavicular or infraclavicular subclavian access may be necessary, keeping in mind the attendant risk of iatrogenic pneumothorax. Follow central venous pressure and obtain blood for type and crossmatch. Infuse saline or Ringer's lactate.

The cervical spine requires stabilization with sandbags or a collar. The chest is next assessed, as discussed above, and then the abdomen (see below). The skeletal system is rapidly assessed, including the bony pelvis (by compression and visual assessment of leg length discrepancy), searching for crepitus or tenderness, deformity, or distal neurovascular compromise. Fractures should be splinted; dislocations or fractures with neurovascular compromise require emergency reduction. Quick neurologic assessment should follow, including pupillary size and reactivity and best ocular and motor responses to verbal or noxious stimuli. Evidence of coma, head trauma, or asymmetric pupils or motor response (including posturing) suggests intracranial injury and the need for rapid neurosurgical consultation and intervention.

Genitourinary trauma must not be overlooked in the general evaluation; a gentle attempt should be made to place a Foley catheter for diagnosis and monitoring of volume status, unless there is bleeding evident at the patient's urethral meatus. In that case a urologic consultation is rapidly obtained. Partial urethral injuries due to anterior pelvic fracture are readily converted to complete tears with false passage production by attempts at catheterization in this context.

Palpate the back (without necessarily rolling the patient) to check for spinal injury or other trauma. This area is often forgotten in the general evaluation. Also check for rectal-sphincter tone as a warning of neurologic injury and evaluate the face. Insert a nasogastric tube as well.

Significant injuries are unlikely to be missed if a complete evaluation is undertaken in the multiply injured patient. The final point to be made is that one's general surgical consultant should be called as rapidly as possible, while evaluation is still proceeding, to minimize the delay until definitive therapy is undertaken.

In the seriously injured patient in need of volume

repletion, up to 4 units of type O packed cells or whole blood (Rh-negative in the female of child-bearing age) may be given rapidly in most cases without subsequent complication arising when typed blood is given. Type O transfusions of larger magnitude require all subsequent blood to be type O in the acute context to avoid major reactions. Type-specific blood (without crossmatch) can also be utilized within a few minutes of patient arrival at most centers; if there is external bleeding, a clot placed in a blood tube may be immediately sent for this purpose, saving valuable time.

Cardiopulmonary Cerebral Resuscitation (CPCR)

BASIC LIFE SUPPORT

Outlining the basic steps in initiating CPCR makes the response to this emergency appear deceptively simple. In practice, it requires great familiarity for these techniques to be maximally effective. All physicians should be trained as providers of basic and advanced life support; opportunities for such training are available through the American Heart Association or other affiliated health organizations. Ample data demonstrate that even physicians need directed training and repeated review of these techniques.

The sequence of steps in CPCR includes the following:

1. Establish unresponsiveness (shake and shout)
2. Call for assistance
3. Adjust victim's position to allow further resuscitation
4. Airway establishment (A)
   a. Open the airway
   b. Establish breathlessness (look, listen, and feel)
5. Breathing (B)
   a. Rescue breathing (mouth to mouth or mouth to nose and mouth)
   b. Foreign body removal and/or dislodgement
6. Circulation (C)
   a. Establish pulselessness
   b. Activate prehospital emergency medical services (EMS)
   c. If pulseless, begin closed-chest compressions

MANAGEMENT OF THE AIRWAY

Opening the airway is the most important immediate action for successful resuscitation. In the unconscious victim, the tongue is the most common source of obstruction. Consequently, moving the jaw anteriorly will often unobstruct the airway. This may be achieved with head tilt alone or by a combination of head tilt and neck lift or jaw lift. Place one hand on the patient's forehead and push backward with the palm; use the other hand either to lift the neck from behind or to lift the chin by placing fingertips submentally, taking care not to occlude the airway by pushing on the submental soft tissues. The thumb can be used to keep the lower lip from occluding the airway, or to secure dentures, which should be left in place if they are manageable in order to afford a more secure seal for rescue breathing.

If these maneuvers do not open the airway, a jaw thrust may be helpful. Place one hand on each side of the victim's jaw at the angle of the mandible, and using the tips of your fingers while resting your elbows on the surface on which the patient is lying, lift the jaw forward. Again the thumbs may be used to open the lower lip. This can be done with head tilt or without a tilt if there is any question of injury to the cervical spine. Should rescue ventilation be required, the victim's nose can be occluded with your cheek.

Once the airway is open, establish breathlessness: look for chest excursions, listen for air flow, use your cheek to feel for airflow.

The initial ventilatory maneuver in the breathless patient involves four quick full breaths in sequence without permitting full deflation of the lungs between breaths, to minimize atelectasis.

If a single person is undertaking a complete, basic resuscitation, 15 chest compressions are followed by two quick breaths without allowing lung deflation between them. During two-person CPCR, a breath is interposed on the upstroke of each fifth compression (see below). Mouth-to-nose or mouth-to-stoma breathing may be needed in special circumstances and is quite effective if thoughtfully performed.

Frequently, artificial ventilation will lead to gastric distention, particularly when excessive inflation pressure is used. This is hazardous because of the risk of aspiration and because of impairment of lung inflation. In the field, the airway should be repositioned, and every effort should be made to avoid inducing further distention or aspiration. If regurgitation occurs, the victim should be rolled on his or her side, the mouth evacuated, and then CPCR continued.

Foreign Bodies in the Airway. Airway obstruction may be caused by foreign bodies or by derangement of normal anatomy. The lax tongue is the most common source of airway obstruction; swollen tissues due to trauma, infection, burns, and allergic reactions are also to blame as are such diverse entities as bilateral vocal cord paralysis, strangulation, and drowning.

Foreign body obstruction most commonly occurs during eating, particularly in the adult with a high blood alcohol level or with dentures or who is swallowing large and poorly chewed pieces of food.

Upper airway obstruction may be complete or partial. Partial obstruction with poor air exchange, as manifest by an ineffective cough, inspiratory crowing, and perhaps obvious retractions of respiratory muscles and cyanosis, should be managed as complete airway obstruction. Ask the victim, "Can you speak?" to delineate complete obstruction. The patient with good air exchange should be encouraged to cough forcefully, should be observed for deterioration, and should be transported to an emergency facility or a source of more advanced care if improvement is not evident.

Three simple maneuvers are recommended by the American Heart Association for relief of foreign body airway obstruction at a basic level: back blows, manual thrusts, and finger sweeps.

Back blows are delivered in sets of four blows between the scapulae, delivered in rapid succession. Support patients if they are conscious and standing. Place your other hand against the sternum and stand to one side. If unconscious, roll the patient on his or her side and support the sternum with one thigh.

If back blows do not relieve the obstruction, they may be alternated with sets of manual abdominal or chest thrusts to create a positive pressure gradient or artificial cough to expel impacted bodies from the glottis. The abdominal thrust sequence, an elaboration of the Heimlich maneuver, is generally performed. Airflow rates, airway pressure generated, and volume of gas moved do not differ substantially between the two methods. The chest thrust is performed in advanced pregnancy and marked obesity. The rescuer must always keep in mind the possibility of intrathoracic and intra-abdominal visceral injury; the hands should never be placed directly over the xiphoid process or rib margins.

If conscious, stand behind the victim and place your arms around the waist. Place the radial aspect of one fist on the abdomen, midway between the umbilicus and xiphoid process. The remaining hand grasps this fist. Press four times into the abdomen in the midline, pushing upward and inward. Chest thrusts utilize the same position, but the hands are placed at midsternum.

In the unconscious victim, if the rescuer places him- or herself alongside or astride the victim, the same maneuvers can be performed. One can retain speed and maneuverability more easily by working alongside the victim. However, if thrusts are not directly in the midline, the risk of visceral injury is much higher.

Back blows and manual thrusts should alternate in the rescuer's attempts to dislodge a foreign body. There is no evidence that either maneuver is superior and should be tried first. There is evidence that the combined maneuvers may be more effective than either one alone. Figure 47–1 demonstrates the use of chest compression, back blow, and abdominal thrust.

Finger sweeps are the final recommended maneuver. The airway is opened by taking the tongue and chin between the thumb and fingers and lifting up. The index finger is placed against the inner cheek and, sliding into the throat to the base of the tongue, probes for a foreign body. Care is taken not to force any foreign body back deeper into the airway. Obviously, this will only be tolerated by the unconscious patient.

In performing these basic maneuvers, it should be kept in mind that with progressive hypoxia, muscle relaxation may turn complete obstruction into partial obstruction, and improve the maneuvers' success or allow slow and full respirations to sustain life while help is obtained. Accordingly, after each set of maneuvers the airway is opened again and ventilation attempted.

Devices for extraction of foreign bodies will be discussed under advanced techniques of life support (see below).

CIRCULATION

After an airway and ventilation have been established, the presence or absence of cardiac output must be ascertained. After initially ventilating with four rapid breaths as described, search for a carotid pulse. After this check, if possible, another individual should activate the prehospital phase of EMS giving the dispatcher of such services full information as to location and condition of the victim. Time is of the essence; it is clear that the shorter the time between cardiopulmonary arrest and the institution of advanced techniques of life support, the more likely is high-quality survival for the victim.

Many areas of the country currently use a 911 telephone system for the activation of EMS. Information should be obtained from municipal authorities or police and fire departments regarding activation of EMS well in advance of the need for it.

If central pulses are absent, external cardiac compression must be started. By increasing intrathoracic pressure such compressions produce blood flow to compensate for the absence of cardiac output; the heart appears to act as a passive conduit. Because these compressions are of short duration and because the intracardiac valves remain open during CPCR, mean arterial pressure seldom exceeds 40 mm. Hg., and cardiac output is at best about one third of normal healthy values for age. However, when combined with ventilation efforts, properly performed compressions provide enough oxygenation to sustain cerebral metabolism for prolonged periods in many patients.

To initiate external cardiac compression, the victim is placed supine on as firm a surface as possible. Positioning himself close to the victim's chest on one side, the rescuer locates the lower margin of the victim's costal cartilages using the fingers of the hand closest to the feet of the victim. Running the hand toward the midline, the xiphoid process is easily located. The heel of the rescuer's other hand should be placed on the lower half of the sternum, two finger breadths above the xiphoid, in the long axis of the sternum, to decrease the chance of rib fractures or costal cartilage separations.

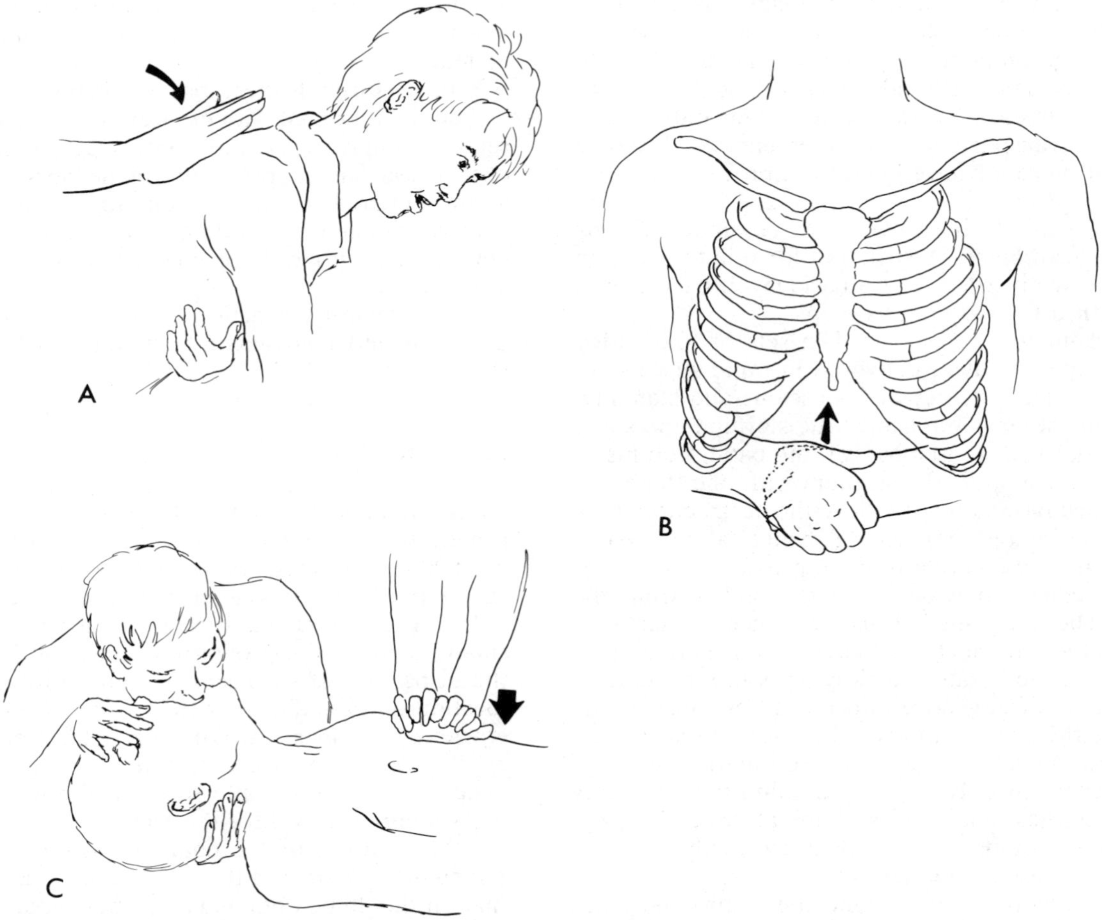

Figure 47–1. The correct positions to perform adult (*A*) back blows, (*B*) abdominal thrusts, and (*C*) CPR (single rescuer technique is shown; the compression-to-ventilation ratio is 15:2).

The heel of the rescuer's second hand is placed atop the first hand. Fingers should be kept off the chest wall to avoid lateral forces that may cause thoracic damage.

The use of straight elbows, with one's weight positioned directly over the patient, maximizes efficiency of compression and minimizes fatigue. The sternum should be smoothly compressed 4 to 5 cm. in the adult, and subsequently the compression should be smoothly terminated.

A single rescuer should perform chest compressions at a rate of 80 per minute, to allow for adequate cardiac output in the face of time lost when rescue breathing (2 breaths after each 15 compressions) is interposed. When two rescuers are present, compressions can be performed at a rate of 60 per minute, with a breath interposed after each 5 compressions.

The carotid pulse should be rechecked after the first 60 seconds of CPCR and every few minutes thereafter.

When a second rescuer arrives to aid a lone rescuer, he should identify himself as qualified in CPCR if this is the case; he checks the carotid pulse with and then without compression, and if the patient remains pulseless, gives the directive to "resume CPCR" and initiates it by delivering a breath to the victim.

Two rescuers can alternate their positions in prolonged CPCR; the switch of roles should be verbally initiated by the rescuer doing compressions, using any agreeable mnemonic based on the sets of five compressions, such as "next-time-switch-on-five." At the end of the designated sequence, this rescuer moves to the victim's head and performs a pulse check. The second rescuer moves to the victim's chest after a ventilation, and if the patient is still pulseless or apneic, appropriate CPCR continues. Pulse checks should take no more than 5 seconds.

Basic resuscitation should not be stopped for more than 5 seconds for procedures or checks, except for endotracheal intubation or problems with transportation, and then it should not cease for more than 30 seconds.

Basic resuscitation is not risk free; despite proper technique, many complications have occurred, including rib fracture, sternal fracture, pneumothorax, costochondral separations, hemothorax, pulmonary contusion, liver and spleen laceration, and fat emboli. Nevertheless, the alternative to the institution of basic resuscitative technique is death, so awareness of complications should not impede the performance of these techniques when needed.

Once basic resuscitation has begun, it should only be stopped in one of three situations:

1. Responsibility for the patient has been assumed by another, qualified individual
2. Respiration and circulation are restored
3. A rescuer suffers exhaustion and cannot continue

BASIC PEDIATRIC RESUSCITATION TECHNIQUE

The basic resuscitation principles do not change when infants and children are considered; some alterations are needed in techniques and in priorities because of the smaller size of the pediatric victim and because most cases of arrest in children are primary respiratory arrest with secondary cardiac arrest due to hypoxia. The preterminal arrhythmia in many such cases is profound bradycardia, culminating in asystole, rather than ventricular fibrillation. Such a bradyarrhythmia in a previously healthy heart is readily reversed by improving oxygenation, so even greater attention to airway patency is deserved in the pediatric arrest victim.

Although many etiologies may lead to respiratory arrest in the pediatric population (Table 47–1), it is important to note that many entities are remediable by control of the environment, such as attention to poisons around the home and sources of fire, and attention to minimizing trauma, such as use of car seats in motor vehicles. In this age group, a little prevention is worth a pound of cure.

For the purpose of resuscitation technique, children under 1 year of age are called infants and those aged 1 to 8 are called children. The child of average size over 8 years old may have basic adult techniques applied, as described above.

Positioning the victim is important for two additional reasons in this patient group. Because the head and neck are proportionately larger in the child than the adult, in relation to total body size, they require closer attention to handling as a unit in positioning and ventilation, to avoid inadvertent airway closure. Also, overly exuberant extension of the neck can occlude the pliant upper airway of the infant. An appropriate degree of neck extension can often be obtained by placing one hand under an infant to support its shoulders; this also often provides firm support for chest compression. Beyond these caveats, the techniques of establishing unresponsiveness, opening the airway, and checking for breathlessness are not significantly different from the adult.

Four staircase ventilations are delivered to the infant initially; to avoid overexpansion or gastric distention the infant should be ventilated using puffing respirations, allowing one's cheeks to bulge, and using volumes restricted to those that cause the chest to *begin* to rise. In the infant and young child, mouth seal may be applied over both the nose and mouth of the victim.

If no airflow is obtainable, airway obstruction must be suspected. Airway obstruction due to a foreign body in the infant is managed by sets of four back blows followed by four chest thrusts (abdominal thrusts are of greater risk in the infant, inducing liver or splenic injury), with the infant straddled over the rescuer's arm, the head and neck secured as a unit, and with the head lower than the trunk (Fig. 47–2). The heel of the hand is used between the scapulae, then the infant is turned as a unit, sandwiched between the rescuer's hands, and the chest thrusts are delivered, using two fingers over the midsternum, compressing ½ to 1 inch, and again carefully supporting the infant and using gravity as an aid (Fig. 47–2).

In the larger child, adult technique may be used, or back blows can be given with the child draped over a rescuer's knees.

Blind sweeps of the mouth are contraindicated in the pediatric patient. Foreign bodies may be further

Table 47–1. ETIOLOGIES OF PEDIATRIC AIRWAY OBSTRUCTION OR APNEA

Sudden infant death syndrome
Near-drowning
Trauma
Poisoning
Smoke inhalation
Foreign bodies
Croup
Epiglottitis

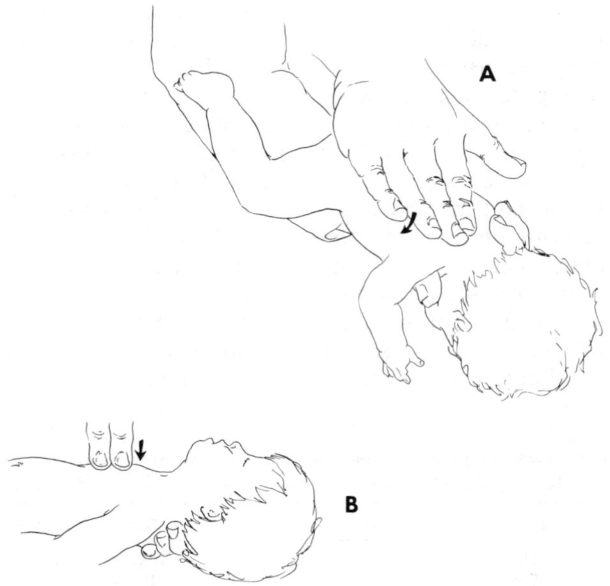

Figure 47–2. Position for back blows (*A*) and chest thrusts (*B*) in the infant. When chest thrusts are performed for an obstructed airway, the infant should be supported by the rescuer in a position analogous to that in (*A*), supported on the forearm with head lower than feet and the face up. The hand position in (*B*) is also utilized for infant CPR.

impacted by such a maneuver. Visualization of a foreign body should precede careful removal. Attempts at ventilation should follow each set of back blow and chest thrust maneuvers.

After delivering four staircase ventilations, circulation must be assessed. The carotid and precordial pulses are unreliable in the infant, and the brachial pulse is currently recommended for palpation, at the midpoint of the medial upper arm.

Because of a higher position in the chest of the infant's and child's heart, the position for compression in the infant is midsternal, at the midpoint of a line drawn between the nipples. The child's sternum should be compressed at a point midway between that suggested for the infant and the adult. Sternal compression of ½ to 1 inch is adequate in the infant and may be achieved with two or three fingers. Children may require the heel of one hand, with 1 to 1½ inch of compression.

Compression rate should be 100 per minute in infants and 80 per minute in children.

The ratio of ventilation to compression in infants and children, irrespective of whether one or two rescuers are present, should be 1:5.

Ratios, rates, depths, and hand usage are summarized in Table 47–2.

ADVANCED RESUSCITATION TECHNIQUES

Ventilation

Oxygen supplementation should be given to patients as soon as possible during resuscitation. Basic rescue breathing into previously normal lungs will produce a maximal alveolar oxygen tension of 80 torr (because the air used is only about 16 per cent oxygen). This oxygen tension is reduced still further in arterial blood owing to poor cardiac output and intrapulmonary shunting from atelectasis and uneven ventilation and perfusion. If the oxygen tension falls, metabolic acidosis supervenes and both disorders accentuate cerebral and myocardial dysfunction. The hypoxic and acidotic heart is resistant to drug and electrical therapy, so the need for maintenance of tissue oxygenation is readily apparent.

Rigid oropharyngeal airways and flexible nasopharyngeal airways should be used in patients being ventilated with the aid of a mask and bag (see below). An oropharyngeal airway is of proper size if it extends from the corner of the victim's mouth to the lobule of the ipsilateral ear. These airways should be inserted with care to avoid pushing the tongue into the pharynx and occluding the airway.

Masks, and bag-valve-mask assemblies, are useful adjuncts in ventilation. Higher tidal volumes can be provided to patients when using a mouth-to-mask technique than when using a full assembly. A full bag-valve-mask assembly is more difficult to use in general unless one has frequent need of it or practices often.

Transparent masks are best. A mask with a side inlet for oxygen, such as the Laerdal Pocket Mask, can provide 50 per cent oxygen during mouth-to-mask breathing with a flow rate of 10 liters/minute.

Intubation Devices and Techniques

Esophageal Obturator and Esophageal Gastric Tube Airways. For use only in the unconscious patient, these airways consist of a face mask through which passes a cuffed tube accommodating 30 cc. of air, for insertion into the esophagus. The obturator airway is blocked distally to occlude the esophagus. Several side holes open into the pharynx of the patient. When this tube is inserted, ventilation may be accomplished via the side holes, while the obturator prevents gastric distention and regurgitation. Insertion is rapid and relatively easy, utilizing jaw lift and some flexion of the neck.

The esophageal gastric airway, inserted into the esophagus in the same manner, is open at its distal tip. This permits passage of a nasogastric tube into the stomach if needed and avoids a major complication of the obturator airway, which is inadvertent tracheal intubation and subsequent inability to ventilate the patient because the obturator is occluded distally. The esophageal gastric airway may be used as an endotracheal tube in the event of a need for such an intubation.

Although rarely reported, the esophagus has been lacerated and even ruptured by the use of these tubes. There is also no experience using airway adjuncts in children.

Once these airways have been placed, they should not be removed until consciousness and respiratory stability have returned or an endotracheal tube is placed.

Table 47–2. RATES AND RATIOS IN BASIC RESUSCITATION

	Infant (<1 year old)	Child (1–8 years old)	Adult (>8 years old)
Hands	2 to 3 fingers	Heel of one hand	Heels of both hands
Position	Midsternal	Intermediate	Lower sternal
Rate of Compression	100/minute	80/minute	80/min., one rescuer 60/min., two rescuers
Depth of Compression	½ to 1 inch	1 to 1½ inches	1½ to 2 inches
Ventilation:Compression Ratio	1:5	1:5	2:15, one rescuer 1:5, two rescuers

Endotracheal Intubation. Intubation with a cuffed endotracheal tube (uncuffed for the infant and small child) prevents aspiration and ensures the delivery of high concentrations of oxygen to a patent airway with great ease during resuscitation. Tracheal intubation should generally be performed whenever patients cannot protect their own airways, when they cannot be ventilated with more conventional methods, or when there will clearly be a need for prolonged ventilatory management. A flexible stylet should be available, and endotracheal tube cuffs should be inflated to test integrity prior to use. Sterile lubrication jelly facilitates passage of the tube into the glottis.

Modern laryngoscopes contain a battery in the handle and a powerful light on the blade. Laryngoscope blades, straight or curved, are available in a variety of sizes to accommodate all ages and sizes of patients (Fig. 47–3). Battery and light function of all such equipment should be checked and recorded frequently to avoid frustration and confusion when the equipment is needed.

Formulas or tables (Table 47–3) can be consulted in the choice of endotracheal tube size. In the infant, a tube the size of the patient's fifth finger can be used. Alternatively, the following simple and quite approximate formula can be used:

$$\text{Tube Diameter (mm.)} = \frac{\text{Age in years} + 18}{4}$$

Tubes one size larger or smaller may be needed owing to individual variation in patient characteristics.

Equipment for suctioning the pharynx and airway

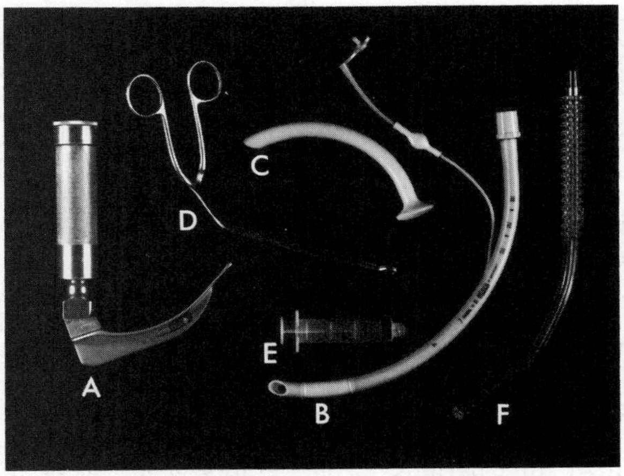

Figure 47–3. Laryngoscope (*A*) and endotracheal tube (*B*) in common use. Always check the light source and the endotracheal tube balloon before using the equipment. Suction and ancillary airways must be available. A flexible stylet (not shown) is useful in difficult situations. A nasopharyngeal airway (*C*) is a helpful adjunct for opening the upper airway in some patients.

Also shown are Magill's forceps (*D*) for directed endotracheal tube placement, a syringe (*E*) to test endotracheal tube balloon, and a Yankauer suction attachment (*F*), which is used in conjunction with wall suction equipment for airway toilet.

Table 47–3. ENDOTRACHEAL TUBE SELECTION

Patient Age	Internal Diameter (mm.) of Endotracheal Tube
Neonatal	3.0
6 months	3.5
18 months	4.0
3 years	4.5
5 years	5.0
6 years	5.5
8 years	6.0
12 years	6.5
16 years	7.0
Adult male	8.0–9.0
Adult female	7.0–8.5

should be available before intubation commences. After the pharynx is clear of debris and dentures are removed, the laryngoscope blade is inserted into the mouth, over the tongue and to the right. Curved blades should have their tips positioned in the vallecula, just anterior to the epiglottis. Straight blades are laid over the epiglottis itself (Fig. 47–4). The neck should be extended at this point with the occiput tucked in firmly (the sniffing position). The glottis is visualized by lifting upward and forward on the laryngoscope, taking care not to injure the teeth or soft tissues. Rocking motions are ineffective and hazardous. When the vocal cords are finally visualized and any foreign body extraction performed, the endotracheal tube may be passed down the right side of the laryngoscope blade into the glottis, and the cuff subsequently inflated. The tube should be taped securely in place to prevent dislodgement.

With the tube connected to a bag-valve device, both lung fields must be auscultated; inadvertent intubation of the right mainstem bronchus, seen particularly often in children but also in adults, impairs oxygenation and leads to progressive atelectasis of the unventilated lung. As soon as possible after resuscitation has been successful, a chest x-ray should be taken to verify tube position.

The endotracheal route is a highly effective way of administering many essential or useful resuscitative drugs (see below).

Blind *nasotracheal intubation* can be a useful technique in the resuscitation of many adult patients, such as the trauma victim in whom there is some question of cervical spine stability or the drug overdose victim who is obtunded and requires intubation to guard against aspiration during gastric lavage (see below).

The nares should be inspected and the more patent side chosen to receive the nasotracheal tube. The same type of tubes are utilized; a tube may be chosen of the same or slightly smaller inner diameter for nasotracheal use. If time permits, the naris may be anesthetized and vasoconstricted with a pledget of 10 per cent cocaine solution. Viscous xylocaine is also used. The lubricated tube is inserted over the inferior turbinate, with its bevel directed toward the nasal septum, and advanced into the nasopharynx. Entry

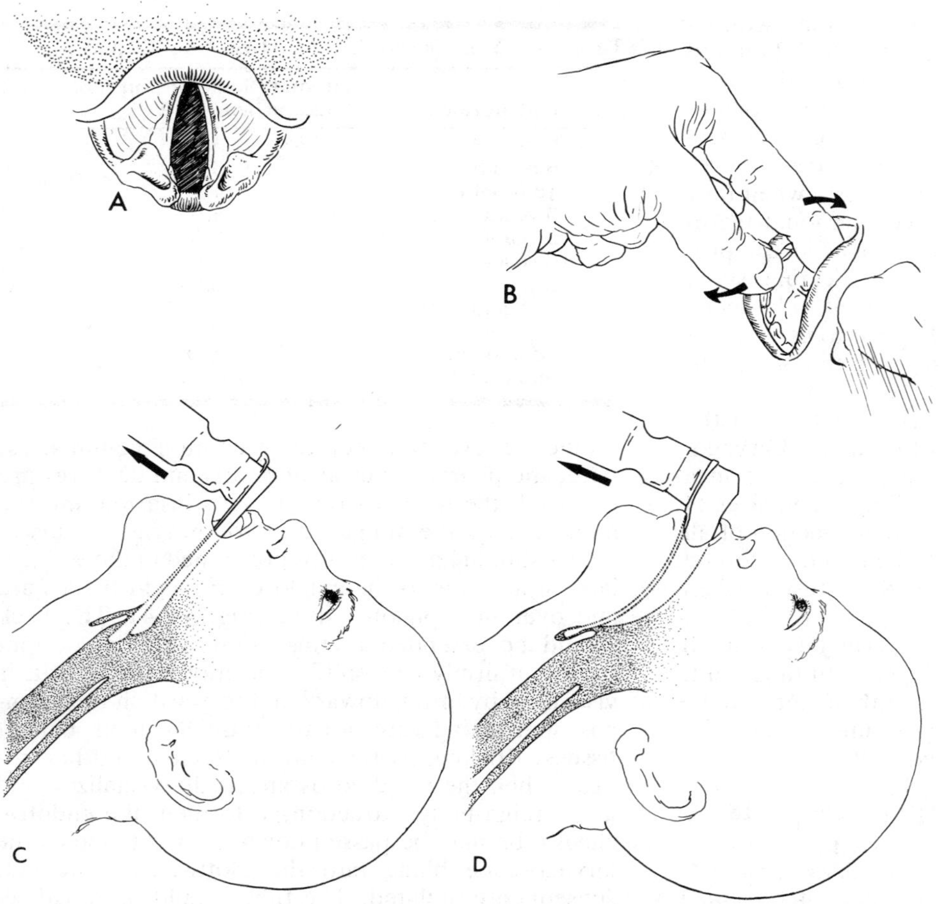

Figure 47–4. Technique of endotracheal intubation. The glottic orifice as viewed with the laryngoscope is seen (*A*). Open the jaws using a crossed thumb and index finger (*B*). Note that the head is in the "sniffing" position (neck extended and occiput tucked in). The straight blade lifts the epiglottis (*C*), and the curved blade enters the vallecula (*D*). Lift up and forward. *NEVER* use the teeth as a fulcrum.

into the nasopharynx is discernible as a give. The tube is then rotated into a midline position and slowly advanced, listening to breath sounds at the distal end of the tube. This can be facilitated by holding the patient's mouth and alternate naris closed. Advance the tube during inspiration. In many patients, some degree of coughing will signal entry into the glottis, as will absence of phonation. Again, when feasible, position must be checked with a radiograph.

Patients whose airway cannot be secured in any other way and who drastically need ventilation can be salvaged by additional procedures, including transtracheal catheter ventilation and emergency cricothyrotomy. This may be of particular use in the victim of trauma whose cervical spine is suspected to be unstable and in whom more conservative measures, including blind nasotracheal intubation, fail.

In *transtracheal catheter ventilation,* the cartilaginous landmarks of the anterior neck are palpated, and the notch of the thyroid cartilage is identified superiorly. The cricoid cartilage is identified several centimeters caudad, the gap between the two cartilages is identified. This gap is the location of the superficially placed and relatively avascular cricothyroid membrane. This membrane is perforated in the midline by a large-bore intravenous catheter-needle assembly, and the catheter is directed caudally, into the tracheal lumen. The catheter is secured in place with a stay suture and connected to a commercial system that allows rapid ventilation by jets of oxygen. Extremely rapid flow rates can be utilized, with volumes smaller than a patient's dead space, and this system will temporarily provide adequate oxygenation, through mechanisms that are still under scrutiny. The system becomes limited by progressive hypercarbia, however, as bulk flow of gas, necessary to wash carbon dioxide from the lungs, is not present. If this method is used to secure the airway, rapid preparation must be made for alternative means of ventilation.

Surgical *cricothyrotomy* can provide an emergency airway in a very short time. When the anterior cartilaginous landmarks of the neck have been identified, an incision is made through the cricothyroid membrane, into the tracheal lumen. This incision can be a single transverse one through all tissue layers, but if time permits, a better approach is a midline vertical incision through skin and soft tissues, followed by blunt dissection to assure that the strap muscles of the neck are retracted and that the membrane is well identified. A transverse incision is then made into the airway. Close control of the scalpel blade is needed to assure the safety of the posterior wall of the trachea. Once the lumen is entered, the scalpel handle can be placed in the incision and rotated 90 degrees to open the airway further. A cuffed plastic tracheotomy tube or, if necessary, an endotracheal tube can then be introduced and secured and the patient ventilated. The skin and soft tissues should be loosely approximated when time permits with interrupted sutures (Fig. 47–5). Bag-valve ventilation can be carried out immediately.

The complications of cricothyrotomy include hemorrhage, secondary infection, laryngeal stenosis, recurrent laryngeal nerve palsy, injury to the posterior tracheal wall, anterior or posterior false passages, and others. But if the alternative is death, the physician must not be deterred.

Circulation

Because chest compression is most efficacious when a victim is on a firm surface, bedboards that extend from shoulder to waist and across the full width of a hospital bed are in wide use. If available, they should always be utilized.

Cardiac, pulmonary, and cerebral perfusions are improved by an increase in mean arterial perfusion pressure. Particularly in the hypovolemic patient, such a central increase can be rapidly instituted by the use of the military antishock trousers, or MAST, suit. This appliance is constructed of a one-piece double-layered fabric and can maintain varying levels of internal pressure. It has separate sections, allowing individual inflation of each leg and the abdomen. Legs are inflated first, and abdomen is inflated last.

The mechanism by which this device improves perfusion pressure is at present uncertain; data exist to show no significant increase in intrapleural pressure when the garment is inflated during chest compression and ventilation, and the actual augmentation of central blood volume is probably not adequate to explain the effects seen. Nonetheless, the device is often helpful. Preliminary data in animals suggest that in cardiac arrest with external cardiac massage both perfusion pressure and central flow are increased substantially with MAST inflation. These garments should not be inflated above the patient's measured diastolic blood pressure, to avoid increasing peripheral hypoxemia and acidosis. MAST trousers clearly work best in states of collapse in which hypovolemia plays a major role. In cardiogenic shock or other states of high pulmonary wedge pressure, they may actually worsen the patient's condition.

With hemodynamic improvement, the MAST garment can be gradually deflated once adequate intravenous fluids have been given; one chamber at a time should be deflated, beginning with the abdomen. Blood pressure should be followed closely. Release 5 to 10 torr of MAST pressure and recheck arterial pressure before going further. A drop in arterial pressure mandates more intravenous fluids before the garment is further deflated.

Less commonly used devices, such as automatic chest compressors and intra-aortic balloon pumps, are highly experimental.

Cardiac Monitoring and Arrhythmia Correction

Monitoring cardiac rhythm during resuscitation efforts is of critical importance in the successful restoration of normal cardiac action (Fig. 47–6).

Attention should be briefly directed to the use of the precordial thump for arrhythmia conversion. It is recommended for use exclusively in the electrocardiographically monitored patient. In the adult, the thump is delivered as a sharp, quick, single blow over the midsternum, hitting with the ulnar side of the fist from 20 to 30 cm. above the chest wall.

The precordial thump has been effective in producing ventricular contraction in asystole and even in restoring sinus rhythm when delivered early after the onset of ventricular tachycardia or fibrillation. However, it is not risk free; it has been reported to cause ventricular fibrillation or asystole in cases of ventricular tachycardia, and it can cause chest injury if improperly done.

Repeated precordial thumps or a related technique, repeated coughing by an awake patient who has just become asystolic, may maintain adequate cardiac output and consciousness while other meas-

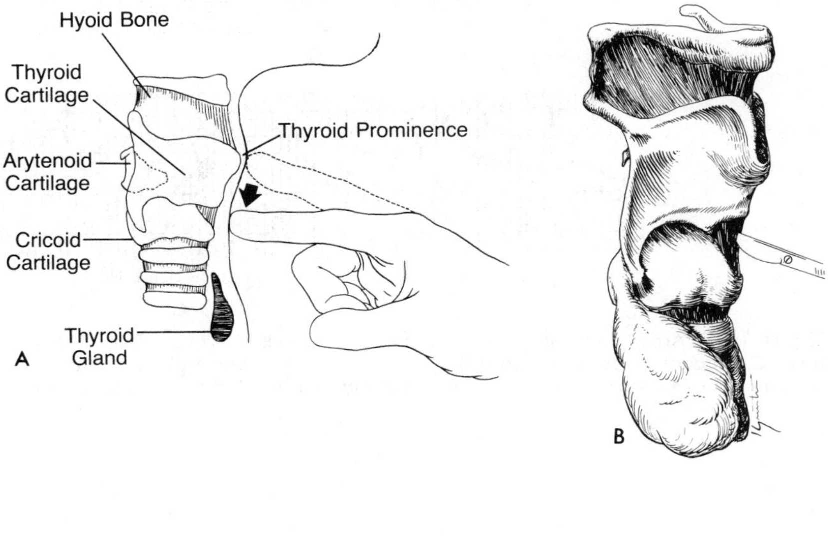

Figure 47–5. Cricothyrotomy. The cartilaginous landmarks of the larynx (*A*) and site of final incision through the cricothyroid membrane (*B*) are shown.

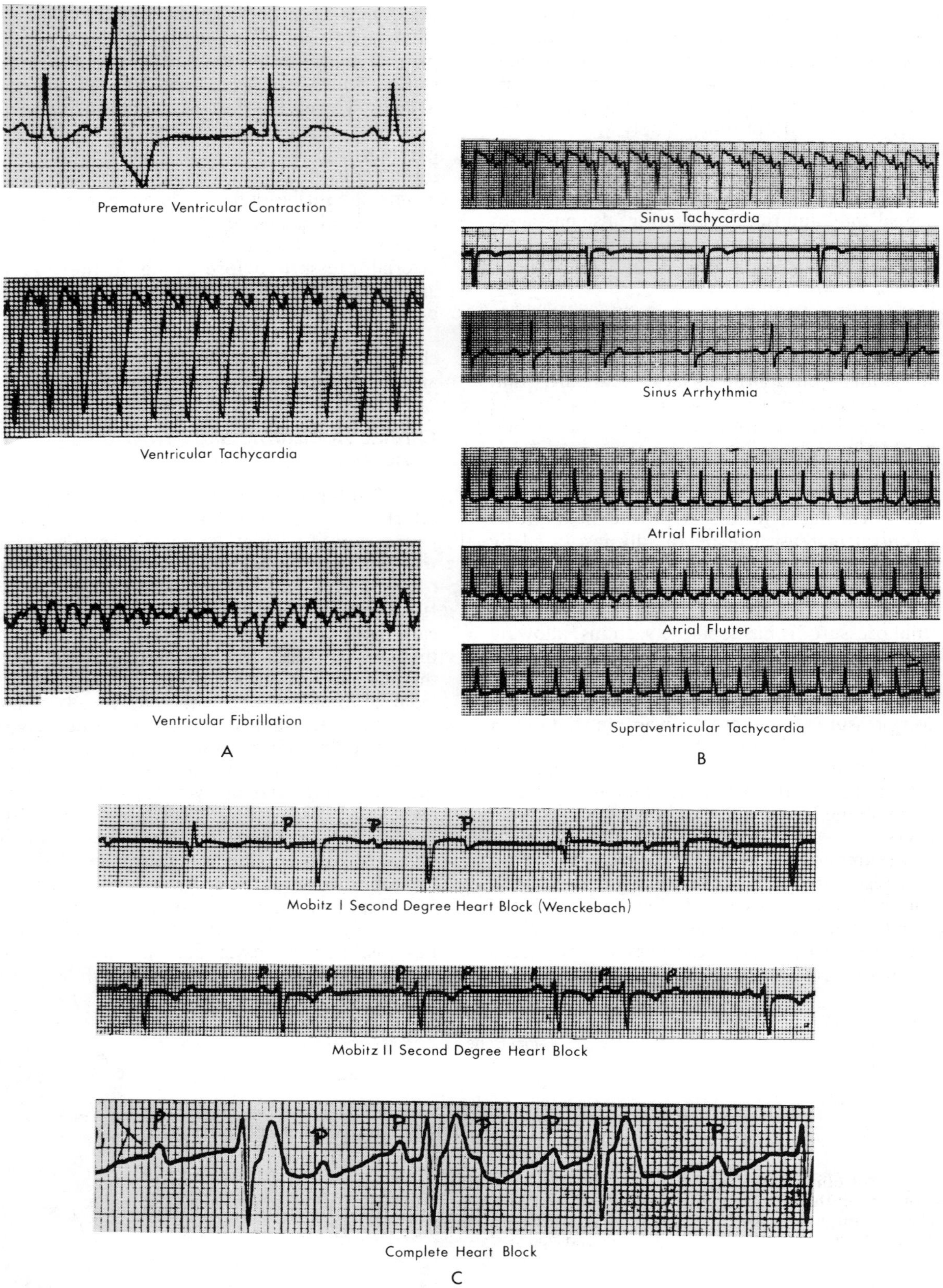

Figure 47–6. Arrhythmias and conduction disturbances. *A*, Ventricular; *B*, atrial: sinus rhythm variations and atrial tachyarrhythmias: *C*, junctional. (Adapted from Bigger, J. T.: Mechanisms and diagnosis of arrhythmias. *In* Braunwald, E. (Ed.): Heart Disease: A Textbook of Cardiovascular Medicine. Philadelphia, W. B. Saunders Co., 1980.)

ures are instituted. The latter maneuver—cough CPR—probably works in a manner analogous to external cardiac compression to produce flow, that is, the generation of intrathoracic to extrathoracic pressure gradients.

Ideally, cardiac monitoring can be performed utilizing adhesive-backed precordial electrodes, which feed their signal into a portable defibrillator. Oscilloscopic representation of the electrocardiogram (ECG) is then available for rapid interpretation and for use to trigger synchronized cardioversion.

Defibrillators that use direct current (DC) countershock are superior to older types that used alternating current (AC) in risk to operating personnel and potential damage to the patient. Only DC defibrillators should be used.

One defibrillating electrode is placed to the right of the victim's upper sternum, the other at the site of the cardiac apex. Electrode paste or colloidal pads are placed under these to enhance conduction of current, as the skin has a high impedance. Saline-soaked pads should be avoided, because they may burst into flame. Avoid smearing paste or gel between electrodes and press down firmly; otherwise, arcing of current may occur across the body surface, with subsequent burns to the patient.

Many portable defibrillators will transmit an oscilloscopic ECG signal when the defibrillator paddles are placed on the chest; this is useful when time is of the essence.

Most arrhythmias should be cardioverted with the defibrillator in the synchronized mode; that is, the instrument senses the QRS complex of the ECG and delivers a countershock on the downslope of the R wave. This avoids inadvertent countershock during the T wave of a beat, the so-called vulnerable period during which ventricular fibrillation is readily precipitated. However, ventricular fibrillation must be cardioverted in the asynchronized mode; occasionally, atrial fibrillation, if quite rapid and irregular, also requires such action.

There must be no contact with the patient or the patient's bed during cardioversion, to avoid accidental electrical injury to personnel (including ventricular fibrillation).

Progressive myocardial damage is seen with increasing voltages and multiple attempts at defibrillation. Accordingly, acceptable ranges of defibrillation energies are tabulated (Table 47–4) by arrhythmia; the lowest levels should usually be tried first, increasing voltages used progressively. It should be noted that if digitalis intoxication is suspected as an etiology for a tachyarrhythmia that is about to be cardioverted, the patient should receive 1 mg./kg. of intravenous lidocaine, and minimal energies to obtain defibrillation should be used to try to avoid precipitating further arrhythmias.

Intravenous Access and Infusions

Securing intravenous access is essential early in resuscitation. Access to the venous system may be secured peripherally, centrally, or via a cutdown technique, which is more often of use in infants and children.

Peripheral venipuncture is most often done in the upper extremities after obtaining venous distention with a tourniquet and securing the vein proximally and distally with digital pressure. In the volume-depleted patient, large-bore catheters, such as 14-gauge or 16-gauge, should be inserted, followed by saline or Ringer's lactate solution or, if appropriate, by blood. Otherwise, 5 per cent dextrose in water should be used to keep access open. Other sites for venipuncture include scalp veins, the saphenous vein anterior to the medial malleolus, and the external jugular vein. The femoral vein may also be cannulated and is useful for rapid volume repletion; however, aseptic technique is difficult to achieve, and infection, phlebitis, and arterial injury may occur. Femoral cannulation is contraindicated in abdominal trauma as it may be of no use. In cardiac arrest, central circulating levels of intravenously administered drugs are higher when given through a central venous cannulation than when given peripherally. Furthermore, femoral cannulation, even with very long catheters, does not assure intrathoracic placement during cardiac arrest, so that optimal drug delivery is not assured. For this reason, alternate means of cannulation of the central circulation are preferable in cardiac arrest.

Three additional methods of cannulation of the circulation are available: supraclavicular subclavian, infraclavicular subclavian, and internal jugular cannulation. Infraclavicular subclavian cannulation requires cessation of resuscitative efforts and has the highest incidence of pneumothorax complicating its performance. It will not be discussed further here.

Table 47–4. ENERGY RANGE FOR D.C. CARDIOVERSION OF ARRHYTHMIAS

Arrhythmia	Energy Level	Mode
Atrial fibrillation	50–200 watt-seconds	Synchronized
Atrial flutter	50–100 watt-seconds	Synchronized
Supraventricular tachycardia	50–100 watt-seconds	Synchronized
Ventricular tachycardia	10–20 watt-seconds	Synchronized
Ventricular fibrillation	200–400 watt-seconds	Unsynchronized
Infants and children	2 watt-seconds/kg.	
Open chest defibrillation	5–20 watt-seconds	

In supraclavicular subclavian catheter placement (see Fig. 47–7), after the skin is cleansed and the patient's head turned away and torso draped (if time permits), the catheter needle is inserted just lateral and deep to the lateral head of the sternocleidomastoid muscle, along a line bisecting the angle between this muscular head and the clavicle. The needle is advanced from below the coronal plane at an angle of 5 to 10 degrees, aspirating with advancement.

Pneumothorax or subclavian artery injury occasionally complicates this technique. The thoracic duct can be torn if placement is attempted on the left. The phrenic nerve is susceptible to injury bilaterally.

Internal jugular cannulation carries less risk of pneumothorax. The posterior approach to cannulation will be described. After prepping the skin and turning the head, the posterior border of the sternocleidomastoid muscle is palpated. A point two finger breadths above the junction of the posterior head and the clavicle is used for cannulation, the needle entering just posterior to the muscle. At an angle 5 to 10 degrees to the coronal plane, directed posteriorly, the needle is advanced toward the suprasternal notch, aspirating as it proceeds. The approach is shown in Figure 47–7.

Although this technique has the least interference with chest compression and the least risk of pneumothorax, it has the risks of carotid artery injury, vagus or phrenic nerve injury, and thoracic duct injury on the left. It is contraindicated in neck injuries and does restrict neck motion somewhat.

The central circulation should not be cannulated with catheters that pass through a needle. Pulling back on such a catheter while holding the needle stationary carries with it the risk of shearing the catheter and producing an embolus. Over-the-needle catheter set-ups are superior.

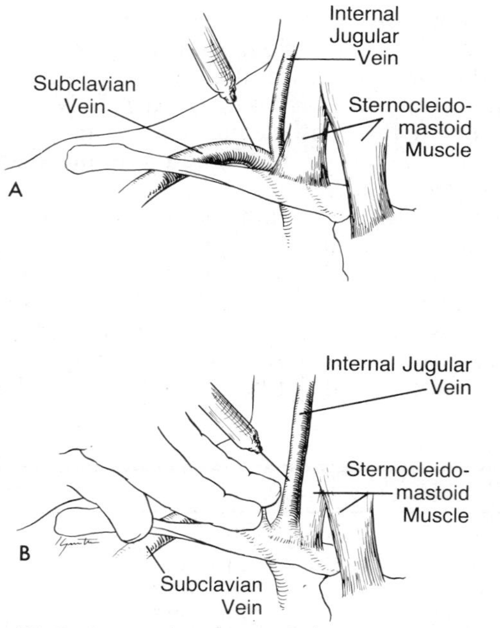

Figure 47–7. Approach to cannulating the central venous system via supraclavicular (*A*) and internal jugular (*B*) approaches. See text for details. (From Hedges, J.: Vascular access. Current Topics II in Emergency Medicine, *2*(1). Philadelphia, Medical College of Pennsylvania, 1982.)

Drug Therapy in Advanced Resuscitation

In addition to oxygen and fluid therapy, discussed above, there is a wide armamentarium available for resuscitative efforts, which is delineated in Table 47–5.

Morphine is a useful agent for the relief of pain and anxiety in the patient with a cardiac emergency. Because of a direct effect on venous capacitance vessels, causing peripheral pooling of blood, it decreases venous return to the heart, thereby decreasing ventricular preload, wall stress, and subsequent myocardial oxygen demand. This may improve myocardial performance and lower pulmonary capillary wedge pressure, affording relief in pulmonary edema. It also has a direct effect on systemic vascular resistance, giving some decrease in afterload to the myocardium.

Adverse consequences of morphine administration include respiratory depression (unlikely with small doses and readily reversible with naloxone) and hypotension, especially in volume-depleted patients. The hemodynamic effects of morphine are readily reversed with naloxone, a pure narcotic antagonist, in patients with otherwise normal cardiovascular systems; while this may not be true in patients presenting with cardiovascular disease, naloxone should still be tried if hypotension occurs. Small intravenous doses of morphine should be used, such as 2 to 5 mg. intravenously every 5 to 30 minutes.

Multiple drugs are available for the management of cardiac arrhythmias. Lidocaine, an extremely useful agent, is indicated (in the context of myocardial infarction or ischemia) for more than five unifocal Premature Ventricular Contractions (PVCs) per minute, multifocal PVCs, and PVCs occurring on the T wave of the prior beat and for bursts of two or more PVCs in succession. It is also indicated in defibrillation-resistant ventricular fibrillation.

Most lidocaine toxicity is related to the central nervous system, with obtundation, seizures, and other problems occurring. The drug is also a myocardial depressant and may intensify hypotension. In the presence of reduced cardiac output (shock, congestive heart failure), maintenance doses (see Table 47–5) should be reduced, but loading doses should remain the same. Repetitive boluses of 50 mg. may be given every 5 minutes for resistant ectopy to a total dose of 225 mg. in the 70 kg. adult.

Procainamide hydrochloride is efficacious in ventricular and supraventricular ectopy. Like lidocaine, it may induce hypotension and should be used cautiously. Dosage should be reduced in patients with renal failure. The drug may be given at a rate of 20 mg./minute, until a total of 1 gm. has been given, hypotension occurs, QRS widening by 50 per cent of

Table 47–5. DRUGS FOR USE IN RESUSCITATION

Drug	Adult Dose	Pediatric Dose
Atropine sulfate	0.5–2.0 mg.	0.01–0.03 mg./kg.
Bretylium tosylate	5 mg./kg.	5 mg./kg.
Calcium chloride	5 ml. 10% solution	25 mg./kg.
Calcium gluconate	10 ml. 10% solution	25 mg./kg.
Dexamethasone sodium phosphate	See specific indication	See specific indication
Dopamine hydrochloride	2–10 μg./kg./min.	2–10 μg./kg./min.
Dobutamine hydrochloride	2.5–10 μg./kg./min.	2.5–10 μg./kg./min.
Epinephrine hydrochloride	1 mg.	0.01 mg./kg.
Furosemide	20–80 mg.	1 mg./kg.
Isoproterenol hydrochloride	2–20 μg./min.	Greater than or equal to 0.1 μg./kg./
Lidocaine	75 mg. initial dose	min.
Lidocaine infusion	1–4 mg./minute	1 mg./kg./dose
Methylprednisolone sodium succinate	See specific indication for dose	30 μg./kg./min.
Norepinephrine hydrochloride	Greater than or equal to 0.1 μg./kg./	See specific indication for dose
Naloxone hydrochloride	min.	Greater than or equal to 0.1 μg./kg./
Naloxone infusion	0.8–2 mg. initial dose	min.
Sodium bicarbonate	Greater than or equal to 400 μg./hr.	0.01 mg./kg. initial dose
	1–2 mEq./kg./dose	
	or	1–2 mEq./kg./dose
	0.3 mEq. × kg. × base deficit	or
		0.3 × kg. × base deficit (dilute 1:1 with 5% dextrose in infants to avoid intraventricular hemorrhage)

original width develops, or arrhythmia control supervenes.

Bretylium tosylate, a quaternary amine, is effective against ventricular tachycardia and fibrillation. It has a delayed adrenergic-blocking action on the myocardium and a mildly positive inotropic effect (it initially liberates norepinephrine). It is recommended when more conventional agents do not convert the arrhythmia, but because a bolus of the drug may require up to 20 minutes to exert full antiarrhythmic effect particularly in ventricular tachycardia, it should probably be used quite early in resuscitation. The drug is initially given as a bolus of 5 mg./kg., followed by defibrillation. If not successful, 10 mg./kg. is given every 15 to 30 minutes to a maximal dose of 30 mg./kg. Use a continuous infusion of 1 to 2 mg./minute following conversion to normal rhythm.

Propranolol hydrochloride, the prototypical beta-adrenergic blocking agent, is useful for treating ventricular and atrial tachyarrhythmias. Given in 1 to 2 mg. increments every 5 minutes, it is contraindicated in the patient with bronchospasm, cardiac failure, hypotension, or bradycardia.

The parasympatholytic agent—atropine—improves sinoatrial and atrioventricular conduction. Uses include sinus bradycardia with hypotension or ventricular escape beats, high-grade atrioventricular block, and asystole. One half to 1 mg. is given every 5 minutes to a maximum of 2 mg. Smaller doses may have a paradoxical parasympathomimetic action to slow heart rate. Caveats in the use of atropine include the increase in myocardial oxygen consumption associated with increasing cardiac rate, and the occasional precipitation of ventricular arrhythmias with atropine use.

Isoproterenol hydrochloride is a beta-selective inotropic and chronotropic catecholamine that raises heat rate and myocardial oxygen consumption and causes peripheral vasodilatation. It is often of use in low-cardiac output states but may also cause ventricular ectopy. If cardiac rate fails to respond, vasodilatation may actually worsen hypotension, so use of this drug should be cautiously undertaken.

Verapamil hydrochloride, available for intravenous use in the management of supraventricular tachyarrhythmias (unassociated with the Wolfe-Parkinson-White syndrome), is a calcium channel blocker with vagotonic and myocardial depressant action, capable of rapidly slowing or converting arrhythmias in a dosage of 0.075 to 0.15 mg./kg. in adults and 0.1 to 0.2 mg./kg. in children, given as an intravenous bolus. Verapamil may be the drug of choice in initial management of supraventricular tachycardia. It is also extremely useful in rapid ventricular rate control in atrial fibrillation or atrial flutter. The drug has no effect on ventricular ectopic activity. Prior use of parenteral Inderal is a contraindication to use of this drug as severe myocardial depression has been reported in such cases. Caution should be exercised in its use with patients on oral beta-blocking agents as well.

A wide variety of drugs are available to effect changes in vascular tone and cardiac inotropy and chronotropy.

Epinephrine hydrochloride has both alpha-adrenergic (vasoconstrictor) and beta-adrenergic (vasodilating and cardiac-stimulating) properties. During chest compression, epinephrine elevates perfusion pressure. It also stimulates cardiac contraction in the asystolic heart and converts fine ventricular fibrillation into a coarser pattern that is more easily defibrillated.

The drug should be given in an intravenous bolus and repeated at short intervals because of its rapid catabolism and dispersion. The average adult dose is 1.0 mg.

Alternate routes of administration of epinephrine exist. In circulatory collapse states, such as anaphylaxis, the drug may be injected into the rich sublingual vascular plexus to allow absorption and benefit before an intravenous line is established.

Epinephrine, lidocaine, atropine, and naloxone (and probably several benzodiazepines) can all be administered endotracheally, if necessary, with excellent therapeutic effect comparable to intravenous use and with minimal effect on the tracheobronchial mucosa or on pulmonary function.

The intracardiac route for medications should be mentioned at this point to caution in favor of avoiding it whenever possible. Not only does resuscitation have to stop to allow the procedure, but the risks of coronary artery laceration, pneumothorax, cardiac tamponade, and intramyocardial injection (which in the case of epinephrine can lead to refractory ventricular fibrillation) are all substantial. This route of therapy should be used in extremely rare cases and with the greatest caution, when all other routes attempted have failed to allow circulatory access or therapeutic effect.

Norepinephrine (Levophed, Levarterenol) is a powerful vasoconstrictor and cardiac stimulant, and its vasoconstrictive properties are so pronounced that it may actually lead to a decrease in cardiac output if ventricular function is poor or vagally mediated bradycardia occurs with its use. Because it is free of vasodilating properties, it is the drug of choice for hypotension associated with the ingestion of drugs that cause pathologic vasodilation and blockage of sympathetic vasoconstriction, such as tricyclic antidepressants.

Norepinephrine enhances myocardial oxygen consumption and, if it extravasates, can cause local tissue necrosis. As other catecholamines, it is arrhythmogenic. Used as an infusion, it should be made up in a concentration of 16 μg./ml.

Dopamine hydrochloride (Intropin) has complex actions. In low doses of 2 to 5 μg./kg./minute, it dilates renal and mesenteric vessels to augment flow (so-called delta receptor effect). In doses of 5 to 15 μg./kg./minute, cardiac output is increased. At greater than 10 μg./kg./minute, vasoconstriction becomes significant (alpha effect) and by 15 to 20 μg./kg./minute, renal and splanchnic flows have fallen off substantially (at such high doses dopamine is effectively the same drug as norepinephrine).

Infusion concentrations are usually 400 μg./ml. or 800 μg./ml., with initial flow rates of 2 to 5 μg./kg./minute.

Dobutamine hydrochloride (Dobutrex) is a synthetic catecholamine. It is an excellent inotropic agent, increasing cardiac output, but it has minimal effect on heart rate or vascular tone. It is less arrhythmogenic than dopamine. Its greatest utility is clearly in the patient with hypotension due to impaired ventricular performance alone. The usual dose ranges from 2.5 to 10 μg./kg./minute.

The use of all these agents in a constant infusion mandates constant patient observation in an intensive care unit as rapidly as possible. Invasive monitoring will often be required, such as Swan-Ganz catheterization and intra-arterial monitoring, to best manage these patients' physiologic derangements and maintain systolic blood pressure at 90 mm. Hg. or above.

Calcium salts are of limited utility in resuscitation. They may increase cerebrovascular resistance and worsen neurologic prognosis in most cases of cardiac arrest. They potentiate the actions and toxicity of digitalis glycosides. Calcium preparations have a role in resuscitation, for treatment of hyperkalemia, hypocalcemia, and overdosage with calcium channel blockers. Any other use in resuscitation is controversial.

Sodium bicarbonate is less pivotal to resuscitation than in the past. It is now felt to be of little help in reversing acidemia in core circulation during cardiopulmonary resuscitation (CPR). Further, it may lead to hypernatremia, hyperosmolality, and volume overload with pulmonary edema, and by producing carbon dioxide in the patient it adds to the burden of gas exchange. Ventilation is more pivotal in acid-base balance in cardiac arrest, correcting much of the acidosis these patients manifest. Ventricular fibrillation is more appropriately managed initially with ventilation and defibrillation. If and when sodium bicarbonate is employed in resuscitative efforts, the initial empiric dose is 1 mEq./kg.; subsequent doses should be guided by arterial blood gas determinations. When this is not possible, half the original dose may be repeated every 10 minutes as resuscitative efforts continue.

Diuretic agents have a place in cardiopulmonary-cerebral resuscitation. Furosemide (Lasix), in an intravenous dosage of 0.5 to 2.0 mg./kg., has a direct vasodilatory effect on venous capacitance vessels to improve hemodynamics in acute pulmonary edema. It thereafter induces brisk diuresis, beginning 20 to 30 minutes after its administration. In addition, its use may decrease the incidence and severity of cerebral edema after resuscitation, by inducing free water loss, leading to fluid and electrolyte shifts out of brain tissue into the intravascular and extracellular spaces.

The role of steroids in resuscitation has been explored in recent years, and the indications for steroid use are now felt to be limited. These agents are now felt to be inefficacious, and possibly harmful, in states for which they were once recommended, including shock (with the exception of adrenal crisis states), aspiration of gastric contents, and various cardiac arrhythmias.

For cerebral edema (prevention and therapy after resuscitation from arrest), methylprednisolone sodium succinate in doses of 60 to 100 mg. intravenously, or dexamethasone sodium phosphate, 12 to 20 mg., every 6 hours, has been recommended. These agents may activate sodium-potassium adenosine triphosphatase (ATPase), hastening recovery of cerebral osmotic balance, but their value is not unequivocal except for tumor-related edema. Other adjuncts to control edema can be used as well and are probably more important, including controlled ventilation to PCO_2 of 25 to 35 torr, hypothermia, and mannitol osmotherapy, as well as invasive monitoring techniques to quantify intracranial pressure and cerebral perfusion pressure.

Ten seconds after cerebral blood flow ceases, available stores of cerebral oxygen are exhausted; coma and EEG silence follow abruptly. After 2 to 4 minutes, any glycogen and glucose present in brain tissue (very little is stored, and the brain requires glucose exclusively for metabolism) is also exhausted, and by 4 minutes of circulatory and respiratory arrest, all adenosine triphosphate is degraded; cell death will follow. With no energy source, membrane ATPase ceases to work; neurons and glial cells absorb sodium and cannot excrete it. Brain swelling begins. Vascular permeability also rises and vasogenic and interstitial brain edema occur. Vasospasm also develops.

During normal conditions, cerebral blood flow is constant over wide ranges of perfusion pressure. It also increases with hypoxia, hypercarbia, and hyperpyrexia. This autoregulation of blood flow is critical to cerebral metabolic needs. This property is lost after extended hypoxemia or hypercarbia. At this point (postarrest), cerebral blood flow is dependent on cerebral perfusion pressure, the difference between mean arterial pressure and intracranial pressure. Mean systemic arterial pressure may be calculated by taking the diastolic pressure and adding to it one third the difference between systolic and diastolic readings.

Cerebral perfusion pressure ideally should remain in the range of 80 to 100 mm. Hg. If the patient strains with tracheal toilet or against a ventilator, this will raise intracranial pressure; muscular paralysis may be needed. The patient's head should be elevated to promote venous drainage; positive-pressure ventilation will impair venous return.

Osmotherapy may be useful to reduce cerebral edema, but careful monitoring of urine output, volume status, and serum osmolarity is absolutely required. Mannitol, in a dose of 1 gm./kg., may be given intravenously initially, followed by 0.3 gm./kg./hr. in a constant infusion, keeping osmolarity in the range of 290 to 310 mOsm./kg. There is not universal agreement on the utility of osmotherapy with mannitol or other agents (such as urea or glycerol), although its use is most accepted in states of posttraumatic edema and tumor-induced severe edema with incipient herniation. The risks of osmotherapy are not inconsequential, including intracranial bleeding and rebound cerebral edema with recurrent cerebral dysfunction and herniation. Rebound cerebral edema occurs most probably because osmotherapy does not remove sodium from deranged cells where it has accumulated. Thus, the stimulus to edema remains.

There is agreement that shivering, hyperthermia, and seizure activity are all deleterious to cerebral recovery. The first raises intracranial pressure, and the other factors cause marked increases in cerebral metabolic needs and, thereby, derange function further.

Other postresuscitation complications must be aggressively watched for and, in some cases, actively avoided, such as neurogenic pulmonary edema, gastrointestinal bleeding due to stress, ulcerations of the gastric mucosa, and aspiration of gastric contents.

More complex modes of cerebral resuscitation, including hypertensive brain flushing, hypothermia, invasive intracranial pressure monitoring, and barbiturate loading, have been advanced in recent years for selected patients. Such modalities require extremely sophisticated centers and are in many cases of questionable efficacy, requiring continued study to delineate their range of indications and effectiveness.

When medical modes of therapy fail to restore cardiac action, emergency pacemaker insertion may be lifesaving.

Transthoracic pacemaker insertion is a rapid and fairly easy technique, especially useful in patients with asystole or profound bradycardia with severe hypotension that is medically unresponsive. It should be utilized rapidly in such situations, as prolonged anoxia and acidosis render the myocardium progressively refractory to such intervention.

The equipment for transthoracic pacemaker insertion is readily obtained and easily used. After chest compression and ventilation are briefly stopped, the transthoracic needle with pointed trocar is inserted subxiphoidally at a 30-degree to 45-degree angle to the skin, at the junction of the xiphoid and the left costal margin. The needle is advanced toward the suprasternal notch, and the right ventricle readily entered. Proper position is verified by aspiration of blood from the ventricular cavity. At this point, resuscitation can be resumed. The pacing wire is then introduced through the lumen of the cannula and attached to a plastic connector whose electrodes enter terminals on a pacemaker unit. The external pacemaker should be set on the asynchronous mode at a rate of 70 to 100 per minute. Current output should be turned to maximal milliamperage to facilitate capture of the ventricle.

When capture has been achieved and the patient stabilized, the position of the pacing wire should be verified with anterior-posterior and lateral chest x-rays. This study is also mandatory to rule out iatrogenic pneumothorax requiring therapy.

A complete 12-lead ECG should be obtained after capture has occurred. Placement of the pacing wire in the right ventricle is confirmed by paced beats, which have a left bundle-branch block pattern, while left ventricular placement results in beats with a right bundle-branch block configuration.

The entire pacemaker apparatus should be securely taped to the patient to avoid accidental dislodgement of the transmyocardial wire. The pacing catheter may be removed once a transvenous pacemaker has been placed and is functioning and secure (Fig. 47–8).

It is appropriate to consider the technique of pericardiocentesis at this time for it occasionally has utility in advanced resuscitation if a patient's cardiac state is one of electromechanical dissociation, and pericardial blood or fluid is suspected to be impairing cardiac filling (pericardial tamponade). A long spinal needle attached to a 50 cc. syringe is inserted into the chest in the same fashion as for transthoracic pacing. An alligator clamp is used to record from this needle on ECG lead V_1. When ST-segment elevation or premature ventricular beats are seen, indicative of ventricular irritation, the needle is withdrawn a few millimeters and aspiration attempted. The aspiration of nonclotting blood or other fluid with the resumption of perfusion is indicative of cardiac tamponade. A plastic catheter may be inserted to continually drain such fluid, and definitive therapy rapidly undertaken (Fig. 47–9).

The sequential steps in advanced management of ventricular fibrillation, asystole, and electromechanical dissociation may be diagrammatically listed for easier reference (Fig. 47–10).

Although resuscitation, with neurologically intact long-term survival from all causes of cardiac arrest, is successful in only about 15 to 30 per cent of cases, with a lower success rate in patients who arrest in asystole, the alternative to these techniques is certain death. Only after all the above techniques have been utilized, or the attending physician is convinced of irreversible severe cerebral damage making recovery impossible, is cessation of resuscitation efforts acceptable.

Poisoning

Modern technology has joined hands with nature to provide a seemingly endless list of substances for ingestion, inhalation, or cutaneous exposure by patients. Nearly any substance taken in excess may exert some toxic effect, and substances prescribed with the best of intent may be harmfully synergistic or antagonistic when taken closely together.

Poisonings may occur because of suicidal intent, manipulative behavior, accidental occurrence, homicidal intent, or, in children, out of sheer curiosity. The workplace, the home, and the hobbyist's bench are all sources for acute or chronic exposure to toxic agents.

Thousands of pharmaceutical products are available for use. However, fewer than 20 of these agents are responsible for 90 per cent of accidental toxic ingestions. Thus, some syndromes are common, and others, while uncommon, can be considered classic enough to merit some discussion.

Eighty-five per cent of all poisoning cases involve children, and more than 70 per cent are under 5 years of age. Thus, prevention should be paramount in poisoning management, and education by family physicians plays a major role.

Federal law requires that hazardous household products be safely packaged, and be labeled so as to bear information to protect and warn users against accidental ingestion by children. Labeling must include the common, usual, or chemical names of hazardous ingredients and a single word, such as poison, danger, warning, or caution—dependent on the ingredient's degree of toxicity. Also required is some statement of principal hazard, such as "causes burns on contact," precautionary measures to be taken, first aid instructions, and finally some state-

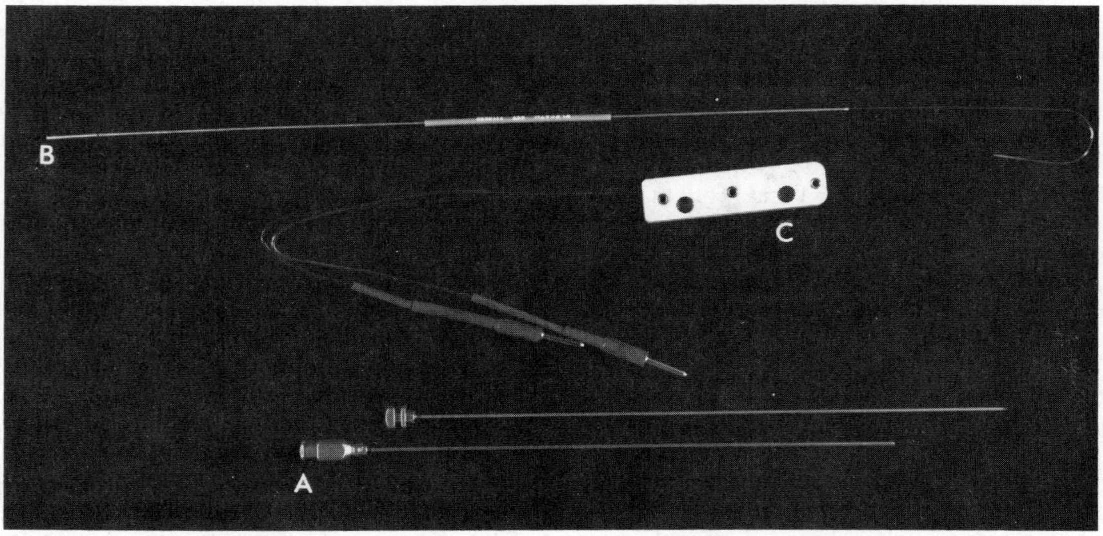

Figure 47–8. Equipment for transthoracic pacing. *A*, Steel cannula with inner trocar; *B*, Bipolar wire with sleeve; *C*, Electrical connector. Energy source not shown.

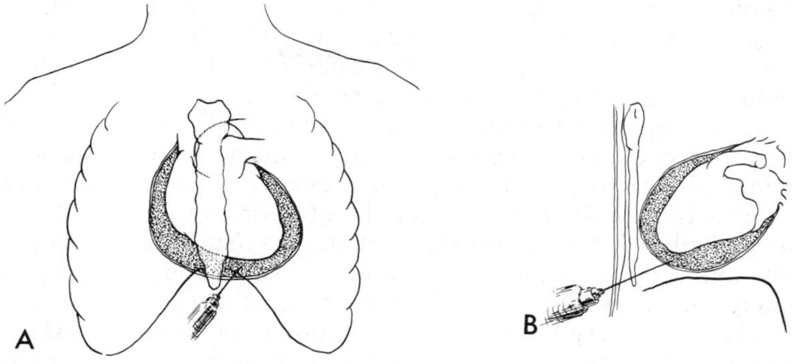

Figure 47–9. Technique of pericardiocentesis. See text for full description. (From Clarke, J. R.: Blunt and penetrating chest trauma. Current Topics II in Emergency Medicine, 2(9). Philadelphia, Medical College of Pennsylvania, 1982.)

ment to reinforce the warning that the product must be kept out of the reach of children.

Childproof containers should be used for medications (such as vials with grip-tight caps), and drugs should not be put in inappropriate or unlabeled containers. Hazardous products should be kept in a designated storage area, locked or securely out of reach of children, and out of sight.

Drugs should be administered seriously to children, never as a game. Drugs should never be referred to as candy (this includes vitamins). Adults should take their own medication out of sight so as to minimize risk of imitation by young children.

One of every two children who have ingested poison will do so again within a year. If this occurs in spite of preventive attempts, families should have a bottle of syrup of ipecac available to induce emesis en route to the hospital. Individuals should be educated in the use of ipecac as well as in the uselessness of the touted universal antidote of burned toast (charcoal), tea (tannates), and milk of magnesia (magnesium hydroxide).

The measures in poisoning management that are most responsible for patient survival are usually nonspecific and supportive. Maintenance of airway patency, breathing, and circulation are of main concern. Advanced resuscitative techniques, as well as control of body temperature and seizure activity, and prevention of infection and skin breakdown should be instituted when indicated.

Once vital functions are secure, further absorption of toxic substances should be prevented. If ingested, poisons can be removed by inducing emesis if the patient is awake and the airway protected by good cough and gag reflexes. Substances that slow gastric emptying, such as opiates, tricyclic antidepressants, or other anticholinergic substances, may be retrieved in sufficient quantity (by lavage or emesis) even many hours after ingestion.

Syrup of ipecac, containing emesis-inducing al-

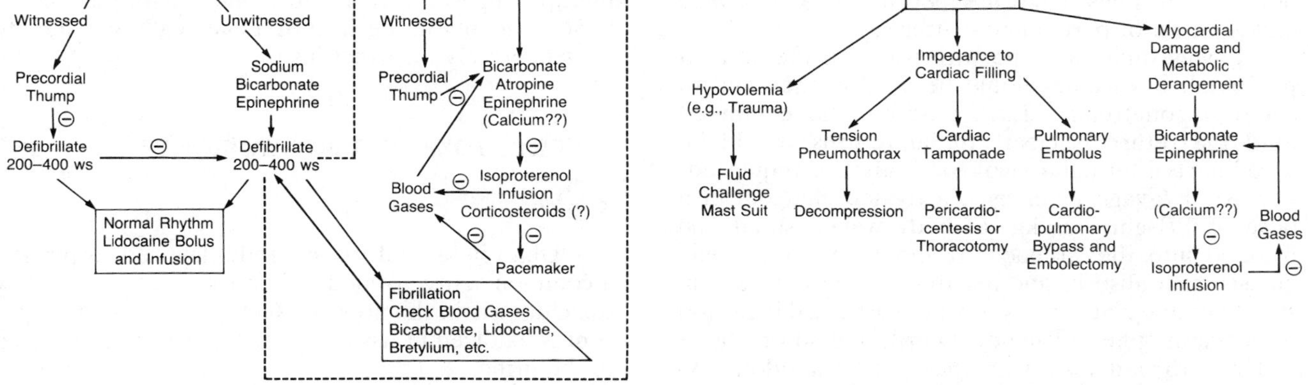

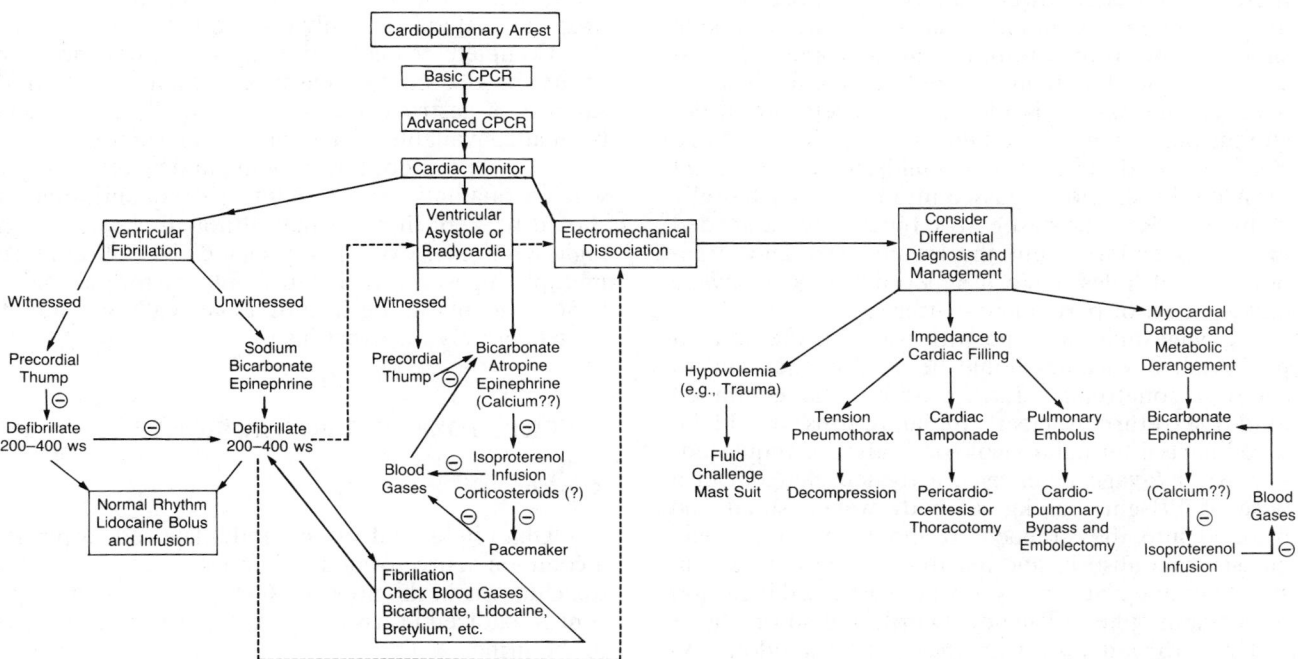

Figure 47–10. Schematic representation of arrhythmia management in cardiac arrest. The symbol ⊖ indicates that the preceding step was not effective.

kaloids, is the emetic of choice. It is given orally in dosages of 15 ml. for small children and 30 to 60 ml. for adults, followed by several glasses of water to induce gastric distention. Patients may need to walk around if possible to induce emesis. The initial dose may be repeated if there is no emesis in 20 to 30 minutes. This approach will induce emesis in most cases within an hour. Ipecac may be of poor efficacy in patients who have ingested antiemetics (such as phenothiazines). It may be contraindicated to some degree in ingestions in which vagal tone is already markedly increased and in which vomiting may lead to severe bradyarrhythmia, such as digitalis ingestion with intoxication.

Some studies demonstrate that induced emesis only removes 30 to 40 per cent of gastric contents, and some authorities recommend that gastric lavage follow emesis in all significant ingestions. The side effects of ipecac are minor save for cardiotoxicity and arrhythmias; if emesis does not occur, the drug must be removed by lavage.

Apomorphine hydrochloride can be used in a subcutaneous dose of 6 mg. for adults and 0.06 mg./kg. for children. It induces vomiting within 5 minutes, and although it has narcotic-like depressant effects on the central nervous system (CNS), these are readily reversed with naloxone hydrochloride, as are its emetic effects. The drug must be dissolved just before use and is highly labile.

Other emetics (including mechanical induction) are of little use and greater risk.

Gastric lavage should be performed if the patient meets several criteria. The airway should be protected by a good gag reflex or an endotracheal tube. Patients seen within 4 to 6 hours of large ingestions (longer if there is decreased bowel motility) with no emesis or incomplete emesis should be lavaged. The technique should be performed routinely in the comatose (possible ingestion) patient without a clearly negative history. The patient is placed in the left lateral decubitus position with head down. In adults a 30 to 36 French Ewald tube and in children at least a 24 French tube should be passed into the stomach orally or nasally. Routine nasogastric tubes may be needed in smaller children, but the Ewald's size and large-bore lateral holes make it superior for rapid lavage and removal of particulate matter (Fig. 47–11).

Lavage may be done with water in the adult if preferred, but saline should be used in the child to avoid hyponatremia. Lavage should be continued until the return is clear. Initial returns should be saved in case formal toxicologic analysis is requested.

After lavage or emesis, activated charcoal in a dose of 1.0 gm. per kg. of body weight should be instilled into the stomach. It should never precede emesis, as it absorbs and inactivates ipecac. Charcoal should not be given in a known or suspected ingestion of acetaminophen (Tylenol, Datril, and so on), as it will absorb and inactivate the specific antidote, *N*-acetylcysteine (Mucomyst).

In many cases, saline cathartics, such as Fleet's Phospho-Soda or magnesium sulfate or citrate, should be instilled with charcoal to enhance transit time of ingested materials. The dose of magnesium sulfate is 250 mg./kg. body weight.

If inhalation is the route of poisoning, it is axiomatic that the victim be removed from the environment and given fresh air or oxygen.

Absorption due to skin contamination can be stopped by removing contaminated clothing, washing copiously with soap and water or even with oils for lipid-soluble substances. Brush dry chemicals off. Absorption due to envenomation can be minimized as discussed below.

Patients may hide substances in bodily orifices (rectum, vagina, and so on) to avoid their detection, and the suicidal patient may insert drugs or toxins into these areas with self-destructive intent. This possibility must always be kept in mind in evaluating the poisoned or intoxicated patient, for an oversight may have disastrous consequences due to continued absorption that was easily avoidable.

It is axiomatic that the patient who deliberately poisons him- or herself deserves psychiatric intervention as soon as medically stable. The psychiatrist may be vital in setting up supports to aid the patient in avoiding recurrent ingestions. Further, if the self-poisoned patient refuses medical treatment, psychiatric evaluation may be pivotal in deciding whether the patient is mentally competent. Determining that the patient is incompetent to make such a decision will allow for medically indicated involuntary therapy.

The well-being of the vast majority of poisoned patients depends on these relatively simple interventions, along with highly skilled nursing care and close observation to avoid complications in their course. More sophisticated procedures, such as forced diuresis or dialysis, are only occasionally needed.

Complete toxicologic analysis is often not necessary in the mildly poisoned patient. If desired, samples of gastric contents, urine, and serum should be made available. Each practitioner should know what the lab can do, how rapidly, and whether results will be qualitative (less helpful) or quantitative. It should be kept in mind that although classic toxicologic syndromes exist, many such cases will represent multiple ingestion, delineated only by formal toxicologic screening in the face of a classically incomplete or deliberately incorrect history.

SPECIFIC TOXICOLOGIC SYNDROMES

Aspirin

Ubiquitous and often candy-flavored, aspirin is a common source of pediatric poisoning. The acutely toxic dose is in the area of 160 mg./kg. About 20 per cent is oxidized in tissues, and 70 per cent is excreted in the urine.

The first manifestation of salicylate toxicity may be respiratory alkalosis. In adults and older children,

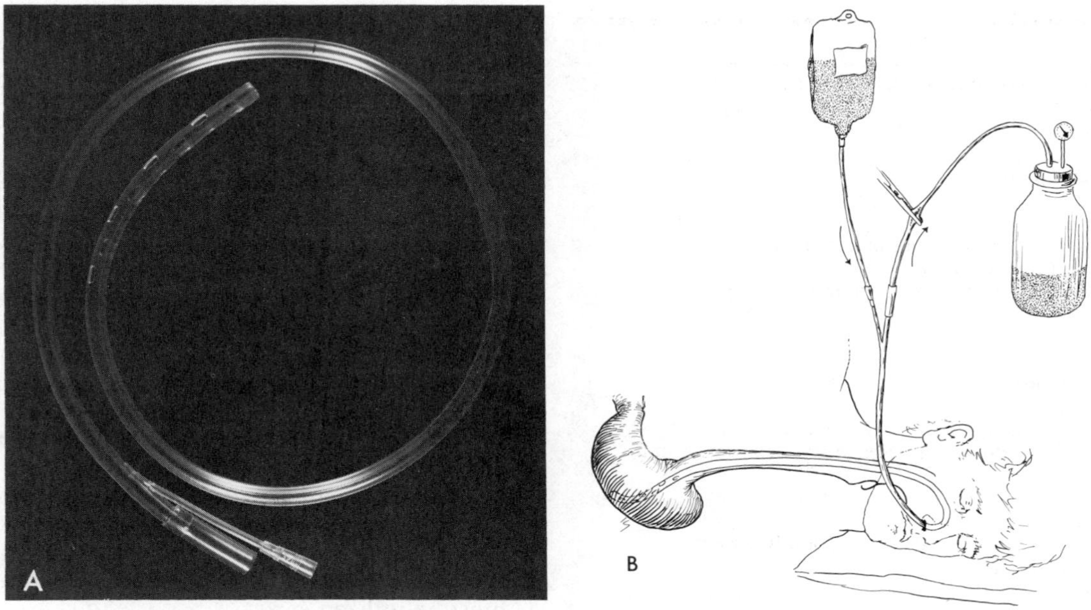

Figure 47–11. Perform nasogastric or orogastric lavage with an Ewald tube (*A*); its large caliber and multiple side-holes allow rapid, copious lavage and recovery of large pill fragments. Put the patient in the left lateral decubitus position (*B*); this minimizes loss of lavage through the pylorus. Drain the lavage by either wall suction or gravity.

no other derangement may occur. In infants and in older patients ingesting very large doses, a metabolic acidosis supervenes, probably due to an incompletely defined interference with intermediary metabolism. Metabolic acidosis may be the sole disturbance in children under 3 years of age. Hypoglycemia may be seen in salicylate poisoning. Salicylates cause reduction in liver glycogen and deplete ATP, leading to impairment of glucose production. Depression of synthesis of vitamin K-dependent clotting factors may lead to prolongation of the prothrombin time; inhibition of platelet function (ADP release) may add to this to produce a bleeding diathesis. In severe intoxication, noncardiogenic pulmonary edema may occur.

Acetaminophen

A dose of acetaminophen (Tylenol, Datril, and others) of 150 mg./kg. or greater should be considered toxic. Lower doses may be toxic if alcohol has been taken concomitantly. Gastric emptying should be undertaken within 8 to 12 hours after ingestion. Cathartics may be useful, but charcoal should probably be avoided, as it may decrease the efficacy of antidotal therapy. A plasma level of the drug should be obtained, but not earlier than 4 hours after ingestion, and a nomogram consulted.

Antidotal therapy given within 16 hours reduces hepatic damage, and fatality is prevented if therapy is given within 24 hours. *N*-acetylcysteine (Mucomyst) given orally is the most effective agent. It is given in a loading dose of 140 mg./kg. followed by maintenance doses of 70 mg./kg. every 4 hours for 17 doses. Nausea and vomiting, necessitating redosing, are the only side effects.

Early symptoms and signs of acetaminophen overdosage include anorexia, nausea, vomiting, pallor, and diaphoresis. These resolve, and in untreated patients an elevation of liver enzymes occurs in 1 to 4 days, followed eventually by hepatic failure. Mortality rate without antidotal therapy is 2 to 4 per cent.

Iron

Each year about 2000 cases of iron toxicity are reported in children in the United States. Ferrous sulfate, the cheapest and most common preparation, is most frequently involved in overdoses. Any patient who has ingested excessive iron should be hospitalized and observed for at least 24 hours.

The average human lethal dose of ferrous elemental iron is about 200 to 250 mg./kg. of weight. Elemental iron is equivalent to 20 per cent of the sulfate salt, 33 per cent of the fumarate, and 10 per cent of the gluconate. Serum iron concentrations are usually maximal by 4 hours after ingestion. In general, toxicity is expected when the serum iron level is over 500 μg./dl. or exceeds the total iron binding capacity.

There are four clinical stages in the evolution of iron toxicity (Table 47–6). Iron salts are directly corrosive to mucosal surfaces and hepatotoxic. Derangement of normal hepatocellular oxidative mechanisms by free iron leads to buildup of organic acid moieties and acidosis. Additionally, release of hepatic ferritin into circulation may reflexly cause shock and lactic acidosis. Healing of ulcerated gastrointestinal lesions leads to late complications of cicatrix.

Gastric lavage in iron ingestion should be performed with 5 per cent bicarbonate or Fleet's Phos-

Table 47–6. STAGES IN IRON TOXICITY

First Stage (1 to 6 hours): Local Toxicity
Nausea
Vomiting
Hematemesis
Abdominal pain
Diarrhea
Melena
Second Stage (10 to 14 hours): Latent Period
Deceptive Improvement
Third Stage (4 to 40 hours): Systemic Toxicity
Fever
Bleeding diathesis
Hyperglycemia
Hepatic failure
Hematochezia
Myocardial toxicity with T-wave inversion
CNS toxicity—lethargy, restlessness, seizures, coma
Shock
Acidosis
Death
Fourth Stage (2 to 5 weeks): Late Complications
Pyloric obstruction
High small bowel obstruction

pho-Soda diluted 1:4 with saline, since this produces insoluble carbonate or phosphate iron salts.

Estimates of the magnitude of recent iron ingestion can be made using an abdominal flat plate. Undissolved tablets of iron or other heavy metals, chloral hydrate, iodides, and phenothiazines are radiopaque (the mnemonic CHIPs is helpful).

Deferoxamine mesylate (Desferal), an iron-chelating agent, can be instilled into the stomach to inhibit absorption of retained iron.

Parenteral deferoxamine therapy (I.M. or I.V.) should be used in patients with any severe clinical signs or those who have ingested more than 500 mg. of elemental iron. Patients with shock or acidosis should receive 40 mg./kg. intravenously over 4 hours, then 20 mg./kg. intramuscularly every 3 to 12 hours, depending on the clinical picture, serum Fe level, and response to dose. The drug increases urinary iron excretion 100-fold, and a vin-rosé color will be imparted to the urine in the presence of excess serum iron.

Properly treated, most patients without shock or coma survive iron ingestion. The overall mortality is 2 to 3 per cent, but with shock or coma it rises to 10 per cent.

Caustics

A caustic is any chemical causing tissue injury to the gastrointestinal tract when it is ingested. Caustics may be divided into alkalis and acids. Common sources of caustic agents are listed in Table 47–7.

Acids produce coagulation necrosis of the gut mucosa; because of the eschar formed, damage is limited to superficial tissue layers unless the agent is unusually strong or contact quite prolonged. Alkalis produce liquefaction necrosis, with saponification of tissues and deep penetration, so that injury is often extensive and ongoing. Solid agents produce their greatest damage in the oropharynx and upper esophagus, while damage from liquids is more extensive. The esophagus is damaged more readily by alkali than acids (the squamous epithelium is relatively acid-resistant); the reverse is true for the stomach.

The pH of the caustic ingested is of importance. The higher or lower the pH, the greater the chance of harm. Ingestion of an alkali of pH under 12.5 will not cause esophageal ulceration.

Once the patient is stabilized, determine the substance taken, interval since ingestion, quantity taken, whether vomiting has occurred, and the pH. Ascertain whether there is pain, dysphagia, dyspnea, or hematemesis.

Physical examination should center on evidence of respiratory distress and signs of gastrointestinal perforation. Look for oral burns and drooling. One third of patients with oral burns have associated esophageal burns, but 15 per cent of esophageal burn patients will have no oral lesions. Thus, endoscopy must be utilized early.

The induction of emesis, gastric lavage, charcoal, and saline cathartics are all contraindicated in these patients. The caustic agent should be diluted with water or sterile saline, and the patient should be provided with potent analgesia, volume repletion, transfusion and definitive therapy for bleeding or perforation, hydration, and early endoscopy. Do not allow anything by mouth other than the diluent used acutely. Alkali should never be neutralized with acids, or vice versa, as further caustic damage, and generation of heat and gases, may rupture an already weakened viscus. The damage initially done is instantaneous, and neutralization efforts are useless.

Fiberoptic endoscopy is vital to direct therapy and delineate prognosis; its risk is low if the procedure is stopped at the first area of third-degree burn. No esophageal stricture occurs from first-degree burns. When second-degree burns are found, the risk rises to 15 to 30 per cent, and with third-degree burns the risk rises to 100 per cent.

Although efficacy of steroid therapy in caustic burns is unproven, they are currently used when

Table 47–7. SOURCES OF DIGESTED CAUSTICS

Acids
Toilet bowl cleaners
Swimming pool cleaners
Disinfectants
Battery acid
Metal cleaners
Permanent wave neutralizers
Alkalis
Bleaches
Disinfectants
Drain cleaners
Toilet bowl cleaners
Clinitest tablets
Paint removers
Electric dishwashing detergent
Hair dyes

patients are too unstable for endoscopy or have demonstrated circumferential esophageal burns, and there are no definite contraindications present to their use. Recommended dosage is 40 mg. of methylprednisolone every 8 hours in adults and children over 2, and 20 mg. per dose in children under 2.

Antibiotic therapy in this setting is controversial. It is clearly indicated in the presence of perforation, and many authorities recommend prophylactic use of a broad-spectrum agent effective against gram-positive organisms if steroid therapy is to be utilized.

Hydrocarbons

Commercially available hydrocarbons are usually a mixture of organic compounds. The risk of toxicity and complications from exposure to these agents correlates with their physical properties. Of these properties, viscosity is most important, as it directly relates to risk of pulmonary aspiration. Volatility and the presence of nonhydrocarbon additives also impact dramatically on toxicity.

Viscosity is quantified using the Saybolt Seconds Universal (SSU) unit, which measures the seconds it takes for a quantity of liquid to flow through a standard aperture (Table 47–8). Low-viscosity hydrocarbons possess the greatest risk of aspiration (most commonly at the time of initial ingestion) due to their ease of spread over mucous membranes. Volatile hydrocarbons, such as gasoline, pose a special aspiration risk, because they fume when in contact with the warm environment of the pharynx.

Additives and contaminants impart their other special toxicities to ingested hydrocarbons. The general classes of additives may be recalled by using the mnemonic CHAMP, for camphor, halogenated hydrocarbons, aromatics (e.g., benzene), metals (heavy), and pesticides. A comprehensive text of toxicology, a poison control center, or a Poisindex should be consulted on such additives.

The larger the volume of hydrocarbon ingested, the higher the risk of vomiting and aspiration. Patients who do not vomit have the lowest risk of pneumonitis. Symptoms of aspiration may be delayed for up to 6 hours after the event, but usually there is some immediate distress.

Most hydrocarbons are extremely irritating to the gut, causing nausea, vomiting, diarrhea, and pain in many cases. Contaminated skin and clothing must not be overlooked in order to protect skin, avoid further systemic absorption, and protect staff.

Table 47–8. VISCOSITY LEVELS OF VARIOUS HYDROCARBONS

Low (<60 SSU)	High (>100 SSU)
Gasoline	Diesel oil
Kerosene	Fuel oil
Lighter fluid	Grease
Turpentine	Petroleum jelly
Benzene	
Carbon tetrachloride	

Fever is common after hydrocarbon ingestion and usually resolves in a day or two. Marked central nervous system dysfunction or cardiac dysfunction in hydrocarbon ingestion is probably due either to toxic additives or to pulmonary aspiration with resultant hypoxia and acidosis.

The treatment of hydrocarbon ingestion is controversial in several respects, and only general and somewhat arbitrary guidelines can be presented.

Hydrocarbons of low viscosity should be removed from the gastrointestinal tract only if the patient is severely symptomatic in terms of gastrointestinal or central nervous system distress. If a hydrocarbon contains a toxic additive, it should be removed from the stomach, unless the amount ingested is extremely trivial. Induced emesis should be used for the conscious stable patient; lavage with airway protection (endotracheal tube) should be used for others.

Activated charcoal is probably not helpful in these patients unless a toxic additive is present. Saline cathartics may be of help if very large quantities of hydrocarbon have been ingested. Most hydrocarbons possess intrinsic cathartic properties.

Oil demulcents (e.g., mineral oil) are contraindicated; their use increases the frequency of pulmonary complications. Steroids and antibiotics in the management of hydrocarbon aspiration have to date been shown to be of no benefit and should not be used because of their inherent risks.

Patients ingesting hydrocarbons should be admitted to the hospital if respiratory distress, hypoxemia, or an abnormal chest x-ray exists or if any severe nonpulmonary symptoms supervene. Any significant ingestion containing a toxic additive also deserves admission.

Opiates

All narcotic agents, whether natural (morphine and codeine), semisynthetic, or synthetic, have similar effects, potential for addiction, and cross-tolerance.

The central nervous system contains stereospecific opiate receptors, concentrated in areas concerned with either pain transmission or pain perception. In these areas, high concentrations of biologically active peptides (enkephalins) have been found. The pituitary contains high concentrations of other peptides, the beta-endorphins. These peptides function as neurotransmitters at areas of opiate receptors, inhibiting neuronal activity. Thus, they behave in some manner as endogenous narcotics and are known as opioid neurotransmitters.

Narcotics may have pure agonist, pure antagonist, or mixed agonist-antagonist properties (Table 47–9). Agonist narcotics work like opioid neurotransmitters, binding to receptor sites to decrease sodium permeability and inhibit neuronal activity. Antagonist binding produces opposite actions and also probably

Table 47–9. NARCOTIC AGENTS

Drug	Dose	CNS Respiratory Depressant
Pure Antagonist		
Naloxone (Narcan)	0.8–2.0 mg.	No
Naltrexone		No
Mixed Agonist/Antagonists		
Nalorphine (Nalline)	10–15 mg.	Yes
Levallorphan (Lorfan)	5–10 mg.	Yes
Pentazocine (Talwin)	30–50 mg.	Yes
Pure Agonists		
Morphine		Yes
Codeine		Yes
Heroin		Yes
Others		Yes

alters receptor structure so that fewer receptors are available for agonist binding.

Agonist-induced inhibition of enkephalin production (a loss of endogenous sedation) may explain the hyperexcitability seen in sudden narcotic withdrawal, when neither endogenous nor exogenous opioids are present.

The physiologic effects of narcotic agents are listed in Table 47–10. Table 47–11 records the clinical signs of opiate withdrawal.

Emergency management of the comatose patient who has taken an overdose of opiates begins with assessment of airway patency, respiratory activity,

Table 47–10. SYMPTOMS OF NARCOTIC INJECTION OR INGESTION

Organ System	Effect
Central nervous system	Analgesia
	Progressive obtundation
	Respiratory depression
	Vomiting
	Hypothermia
	Impaired cough reflex
	Seizures (high doses)
Gastrointestinal tract	Ileus and constipation
	Increases sphincter tone
	Biliary spasm
	Risk of hepatitis
Cardiovascular system	Infectious risks; endocarditis, valve disease, embolization
	Orthostatic hypotension
Lungs	Bronchospasm
	Pulmonary edema
	Emboli
Genitourinary system	Urinary retention
	Glomerular disease
Eyes	Miosis
Skin	Cellulitis
	Ulcers
	Abscesses
	Lymphedema
Musculoskeletal system	Rhabdomyolysis
	Osteomyelitis
	Septic arthritis
Endocrine system	Hypoglycemia
	Amenorrhea
	Sterility (↓ testosterone)

Table 47–11. NARCOTIC WITHDRAWAL

Mild	Moderate	Severe*
Mydriasis	Agitation	Insomnia
Rhinorrhea	Hypertension	Diarrhea
Yawning	Tachycardia	Vomiting
Piloerection		Hypotension
Cramps		Seizures
Tearing		

*Emergency treatment should only be undertaken in a patient when severe manifestations are present.

and circulatory status. Intubation and mechanical ventilation, and establishment of a vascular access, are necessary. Other etiologies for the comatose state, as discussed later in this chapter, should not be overlooked, and trauma and infection, common in these patients, must be sought aggressively.

When venous blood has been obtained for appropriate toxicologic analysis, electrolytes, sugar, and blood counts, the patient should receive one or two ampules of 50 per cent dextrose in water followed by 0.8 to 2.0 mg. of naloxone intravenously or by endotracheal tube. This can be repeated in 5 minutes. If a response is achieved, 4 mg. (10 ampules) of the naloxone can be placed in 1 liter of intravenous solution and infused at 100 to 200 ml./hour. Additionally, 2 mg. of naloxone can be given intramuscularly, to avoid problems if the intravenous access is accidentally removed.

Because of their effect on gastric motility, opiates can often be recovered from the stomach by lavage many hours after their ingestion. Thus, the usual removal procedures should be followed even many hours postingestion.

Ninety per cent of opiate overdoses involve concomitant abuse of some other agent; most often barbiturates, benzodiazepines, tricyclic antidepressants, and alcohol are involved. This is one reason why an incomplete response to naloxone may be seen, and another good reason for gastric lavage. There is no cross-tolerance between these central nervous system depressants and narcotics and in subsequent management, simultaneous or sequential withdrawal syndromes may require medical management.

Because of the high rate of recidivism and repeated overdose in these patients, management is highly frustrating. The general approach to acute management is similar in patients who ingest other central nervous system depressants (barbiturates and so on).

Tricyclic Antidepressants (Elavil, Tofranil, and Others)

The tricyclic antidepressants possess three major pharmacologic activities—sedation, mood elevation, and, most important toxicologically, peripheral and central anticholinergic actions. They share this last property with the phenothiazines and the belladonna alkaloids (scopolamine, hyoscyamine, and so on) found in many sleeping preparations and naturally occurring plant sources. Anticholinergic signs and symptoms are listed in Table 47–12.

Tricyclic agents are metabolized almost exclusively in the liver, and there are many active intermediary metabolites. Most of the circulating drug (90 per cent) is protein bound. Because of lipid solubility, their volume of distribution in the body is very large. In overdose patients the half-life of these agents is generally greater than 24 hours. Thus, after overdose, high levels of active drug will remain at tissue sites for days. Tissue levels may have no relation to measured blood levels. Finally, a small change in the percentage of drug bound to protein will represent a huge change in unbound (and hence active) drug.

In initially evaluating these patients, history is not reliable in determining the true magnitude of ingestion. Further, the initial presence of peripheral anticholinergic signs does not correlate with the later development of major toxic symptoms.

Initial emergency management of the patient who ingests these agents includes the usual stabilization of airway and circulation, blood gas and venous blood samples for analysis, including toxicologic evaluation, and an electrocardiogram to look for widening of the QRS complex. Widening to a duration of 0.10 second or more is a significant toxic manifestation. In the presence of CNS signs, naloxone and 50 per cent dextrose are indicated.

Acute plasma levels of tricyclic antidepressants greater than 1000 nanograms per milliliter clearly correlate with high risks of coma, seizures, hypotension, cardiac arrhythmia, and respiratory embarrassment, although lower plasma levels are no guarantee of lack of tissue toxicity. Little data is available on toxic levels in children. One authority (Guzzardi, 1981) suggests that ingestion of one tablet by a 1-year-old child or two or more 25 mg. tablets by a 2-year-old child be treated aggressively, including intensive cardiac monitoring.

Definitive management includes the usual measures of gastric lavage, which should be performed up to 24 hours after ingestion because of delayed gastric emptying and activated charcoal/cathartic instillation. Hypotension is treated with saline. If a pressor is needed, norepinephrine is used.

Table 47–12. SIGNS AND SYMPTOMS OF CENTRAL ANTICHOLINERGIC SYNDROME

Central	Peripheral
Agitation	Mydriasis
Disorientation	Tachycardia/hypertension
Hallucinations	Vasodilatation
Seizures	Fever
Coma	Urinary retention
Respiratory failure	Ileus
Circulatory collapse	Saliva production
	Sweat production
	Bronchial secretion
	Lacrimation

Physostigmine, an anticholinesterase that can penetrate the blood-brain barrier, is quite useful for many aspects of tricyclic (and other anticholinergic) ingestion. The drug may be given in a dose of 1 to 4 mg. over 60 seconds, every 20 to 30 minutes, as needed. In children (over 6 months old), 0.5 mg. can be given every 5 minutes, to a maximal dose of 2 mg. or toxicity. The effects of this drug can be rapidly reversed with atropine.

Physostigmine can be used as a diagnostic tool in coma from an unknown ingestion or to treat cardiac depression and hypotension. It is not risk free, as it can itself induce bradycardia and seizures. The drug should be reserved for acute management of life-threatening symptomatology resistant to other measures.

Alkalinization of the blood with sodium bicarbonate, in an initial bolus of 0.5 to 3.0 mEq./kg. body weight, and subsequent dosage to keep arterial pH at 7.45 to 7.50, is the treatment of choice for arrhythmias induced by tricyclic antidepressants (and phenothiazine). It is also useful to acutely manage conduction blocks while obtaining a transvenous pacemaker. It is not of use in the CNS manifestations of toxicity, nor has it been proved of use in the prophylaxis of cardiotoxicity in tricyclic poisoning. The mechanism of action of bicarbonate is presently controversial.

Phenytoin, in low-dose aliquots, may improve cardiac arrhythmias and myocardial toxicity when physostigmine and bicarbonate have failed. While monitoring blood pressure and the ECG, doses of 50 to 100 mg. may be given slowly, not to exceed 50 mg./minute. Phenytoin itself can precipitate heart block and hypotension.

Propranolol has been utilized in the management of tricyclic-induced arrhythmias, and it is efficacious. Because of its depression of atrioventricular conduction and its myocardial depressant and beta-blockade characteristics, however, it is a third-line drug. When used, careful monitoring is essential, and small doses must be given (0.5 to 1.0 mg. every 5 minutes, not to exceed 5 mg.).

Hemodialysis is not efficacious in treating tricyclic antidepressant ingestion, due to the large volume of distribution of these drugs and their high degree of protein binding.

All patients with signs of toxicity (including only QT prolongation on ECG) or with an uncertain magnitude of ingestion should be hospitalized in an intensive care setting and monitored until signs of toxicity have been absent for 24 hours.

With aggressive supportive and specific therapy, the central anticholinergic syndrome and the cardiotoxicity of the tricyclic agents can be markedly ameliorated.

Phencyclidine

Phencyclidine, a powerful, easily synthesized low-cost agent, is one of the most widely available and abused drugs at the present time. It has many colloquial names (angel dust, elephant, magic mist) and is often used with other agents to enforce their potency. The drug is closely related to the anesthetic agent ketamine.

Phencyclidine's primary effects are on the cardiovascular and central nervous systems. They are dose related. The drug has mixed stimulant and depressant properties, which correlate with its complex action on receptors and membranes at various sites in the brain.

The major subjective effects of phencyclidine include difficulty in thinking, depersonalization, altered sensory perceptions, and derangement of body image. The user becomes inattentive and emotionally labile, and in most cases the major toxic behavioral effect is induction of a wildly agitated state with aggressive, even violent, behavior. Additional side effects of the drug include fever, hypertension, seizures, rhabdomyolysis and myoglobinuria, and respiratory depression with very large doses, along with hypotension from myocardial depression and vasodilation.

Overdose patients present with a confusional state or coma, often with associated aggressive behavior, and sometimes with an acute schizophreniform psychosis. There is often both vertical and horizontal nystagmus (the former nearly pathognomonic in the conscious intoxicated patient) and a sensory gait ataxia. The face stares blankly. There is increased muscle tone, and the heart rate and blood pressure are elevated. Subsequently, as the drug is hepatically metabolized and cleared in bile and urine, symptoms clear.

In higher dosage, the drug induces immobile coma of variable duration, in association with seizures in very high dose. Hypertension may give way to cardiovascular collapse and apnea.

Chronic abuse of phencyclidine can lead to a paranoid schizophrenia-like illness with auditory hallucination and violent behavior. In this respect, as well as in its production acutely of agitation, hypertension, fever, tachycardia, and seizures, the drug shares many characteristics with cocaine and amphetamines.

Specific evaluation and therapy for phencyclidine intoxication begins by obtaining a blood and urine sample for toxicologic analysis; the drug is heavily concentrated in the urine and most easily found there. The usual stabilization and lavage methods are appropriate.

Phencyclidine is a weak base, and acidification of the urine may markedly enhance its excretion. Confused patients who can nonetheless swallow may be given cranberry juice to drink and 2 gm. of ascorbic acid by mouth every 6 hours. The comatose patient can be given the ascorbic acid in intravenous fluids, and furosemide diuresis can also be used to enhance clearance of the drug. The urinary pH should ideally be less than 5.0.

Because of controversy regarding more aggressive acidification with agents such as ammonium chloride, and the significant risks involved, particularly in patients who may develop rhabdomyolysis and acute renal failure, such an approach should not be routinely used, but it may be helpful in more severe cases.

There is no specific antagonist for phencyclidine. Presently, symptomatic therapy is probably best. As with amphetamines, diazepam and haloperidol have been used most often for sedation. Psychosis, seizures, and hypertensive crisis respond to the usual pharmacologic agents.

Usually, mild cases of phencyclidine ingestion are behaving normally within 6 hours and may be discharged after 1 to 2 hours of normal behavior and after suicidal risk has been assessed. Occasionally, a confused patient will not clear for 24 to 72 hours and requires psychiatric hospitalization (such patients may be poor metabolizers of the drug).

Organophosphates and Carbamates

The organophosphates and carbamates, two distinct chemical compound groups, are both found in insecticides and other commercial products. Both produce inhibition of acetylcholinesterase, accounting for their toxicity due to a buildup of acetylcholine at cholinergic synapses. Organophosphate compounds may be absorbed by virtually any route: skin, conjunctiva, lung, or gastrointestinal tract.

The signs and symptoms of organophosphate poisoning may be classified into three categories (Table 47–13). Miosis is found in almost all patients with moderately severe poisoning, but its absence should

Table 47–13. SIGNS OF ORGANOPHOSPHATE POISONING

CNS Manifestations	
Agitation	
Emotional lability	
Headache	
Tremor	
Slurred speech	
Generalized weakness	
Ataxia	
Seizures	
Coma	
Respiratory and cardiovascular depression	
Nicotinic (Sympathetic and Somatic Motor) Symptoms	
Fasciculations	
Cramps	
Weakness	
Areflexia	
Hypertension	
Tachycardia	
Pallor	
Muscarinic (Parasympathetic) Manifestations	
*S*alivation	SLUD syndrome
*L*acrimation	SLUD syndrome
*U*rination	SLUD syndrome
*D*efecation	SLUD syndrome
Miosis	
Bronchospasm	

not delay treatment following exposure. Most organophosphate insecticides have a garlicky odor, which the patient may exhibit.

Onset of symptoms of organophosphate poisoning is most rapid following inhalation and least rapid after percutaneous absorption. Symptoms always begin within 24 hours of exposure, however. Carbamate compounds do not effectively penetrate the CNS and, thus, have a more limited toxicity. In all other respects, symptoms are the same as organophosphate poisonings.

Laboratory confirmation of exposure to organophosphates should be sought by measuring red cell cholinesterase or plasma pseudocholinesterase levels and by screening bodily fluids for organophosphates and their metabolites. The urine can be tested for paranitrophenol in the case of exposure to parathion, chlorothion, and EPN.

In acute poisoning, clinical manifestations generally occur only after more than 50 per cent of serum cholinesterase is inhibited. In mild poisoning, cholinesterase activity is 20 to 50 per cent of normal. It is 10 to 20 per cent of normal in moderate poisoning and less than 10 per cent of normal in severe cases.

If depression of cholinesterase activity occurs quite slowly and gradually, minimal symptoms may be present, even with very low levels of cholinesterase.

Specific pharmacologic intervention should not be delayed pending cholinesterase levels when there is strong suspicion of exposure to these agents.

Pharmacologic management is one portion of total management (Table 47–14) and involves two complementary drugs: atropine for muscarinic and CNS manifestations and pralidoxime (PAM) for nicotinic manifestations.

Cyanosis should be corrected before atropine is given to avoid hypoxia-related ventricular arrhythmias. If atropine is given, observation for at least 24 hours is mandatory.

Table 47–14. MANAGEMENT OF ORGANOPHOSPHATE POISONING

General Support
- Especially respiratory, with good toilet

Decontaminate
- Removal of contaminated clothing
- Copious skin washing
- Emesis/lavage/charcoal/cathartic

Pharmacologic Management
- Atropine—slowly I.V., every 15 minutes until atropinization (dry mucous membranes, dilated pupils, tachycardia)
  - 2–4 mg. in adults/dose
  - 0.05 mg./kg. in children/dose
  - Adjust subsequent doses to maintain therapeutic effect for next 24 hours
- Pralidoxime (PAM)—only for organophosphates—must give within 24 hours of exposure, given slowly I.V.
  - 1 gm. for adult
  - 10–12 mg./kg. for children
  - Repeat dose in 1–2 hours for persistent weakness or tremors

Pralidoxime is a specific antidote that restores acetylcholinesterase activity by prevention and reversal of phosphorylation of this enzyme but only before the complex undergoes a gradual change to an irreversibly bound state. Thus, the drug should be used as early as possible and is useless after 24 hours have elapsed. Improvement in muscle weakness usually occurs over 10 to 40 minutes. Giving PAM in the presence of atropine may increase the side effects of the latter drug, so close observation is required.

Carbamate inhibition of acetylcholinesterase is reversed spontaneously and rapidly by hydrolysis, so PAM is not required. PAM may even increase cholinesterase inhibition in this context by actions of its own, and it may reduce the efficacy of atropine as well. Thus, it is contraindicated in carbamate poisoning.

CNS depressants may worsen coma in these patients and should not be used. Phenothiazines and theophylline derivatives have anticholinesterase activity and are also contraindicated, as are succinylcholine, physostigmine, and any parasympathomimetic agent.

Death from organophosphates usually occurs from respiratory failure within 24 hours in untreated cases. With good treatment, complete recovery can be expected within 10 days. Following exposure, patients should not return to contact with these agents until cholinesterase levels have returned to at least 75 per cent of normal.

Occasionally, long-term sequelae may occur, lasting weeks to months. These include peripheral neuropathy, personality changes, memory impairment, confusion, depression, and thought disorders.

Carbon Monoxide

Carbon monoxide (CO) is a tasteless, odorless, colorless, nonirritating gas produced by incomplete combustion of carbonaceous materials. The most common sources are automobile exhausts, most illuminating and heating gases (except natural gas), cigarettes, insufficiently vented furnaces, stoves and chimneys, and the indoor use of charcoal grills.

The major toxic properties of carbon monoxide result from its propensity to combine with hemoglobin to form carboxyhemoglobin, which is unable to transport oxygen to tissues. Carbon monoxide has an affinity for hemoglobin that is 250 times that of oxygen. The gas may also bind to enzymes in the respiratory chair of mitochondria and to myoglobin, producing direct muscle hypoxia.

Although the reduction in the oxygen-carrying capacity of blood is proportional to the amount of carboxyhemoglobin, oxygen delivery to tissues is further reduced by a leftward shift of the oxyhemoglobin dissociation curve. Symptomatology correlates with carboxyhemoglobin level (Table 47–15).

Cerebral and myocardial hypoxia accounts for the major toxicity of carbon monoxide. Cerebral edema and increased intracranial pressure may occur

Table 47–15. SYMPTOMS OF CARBON MONOXIDE POISONING

Carboxyhemoglobin Concentration (%)	Symptoms and Signs
0–10	None
10–30	Progressively severe headache
30–40	Headache Nausea and vomiting Weakness Visual complaints
40–50	Syncope Tachycardia Tachypnea
50–60	Coma* Seizures Cheyne-Stokes breathing
60–70	Severe compromise of cardiopulmonary function
70–80	Death

*If carboxyhemoglobin level rises extremely rapidly, coma may occur before other symptoms become manifest.

due to hypoxia-induced capillary leak. In CO poisoning, the globus pallidus is often profoundly affected.

Myocardial toxicity, which does not correlate well with the carboxyhemoglobin level, may be apparent immediately, or require several days to evolve. ECG findings include ischemic ST-segment and T-wave changes, arrhythmias, and conduction blocks. Congestive heart failure may supervene.

A variety of skin changes have been reported, including edema (with or without pressure necrosis), erythema (cherry red skin), and bulla formation.

Therapy for CO poisoning requires immediate removal from the contaminated environment, followed by high-flow 100 per cent oxygen therapy, via endotracheal tube if necessary.

When room air is being inspired, the half-life of CO in the blood is 240 minutes. This decreases to 40 to 90 minutes when 100 per cent oxygen is used. Hyperbaric oxygen reduces the half-life still further, but it is not generally available.

Clinical instability is characteristic of CO intoxication. Severe clinical relapse may occur after apparently full recovery, correlating with extensive demyelination of cerebral hemispheric tissue. Deterioration is often noted after increased physical activity, so at least 10 days of bed rest are indicated following CO poisoning with neurologic manifestations.

The only long-term sequelae widely recognized from CO poisoning are parkinsonism and mental status changes of varying severity.

Although simple qualitative tests exist for use in the emergency unit to suggest CO poisoning, such as heating whole blood or adding sodium hydroxide to a blood and water mix (Goldfrank and Kirstein, 1978), it is best to ask the arterial blood gas lab to quantitate carboxyhemoglobin levels, as it can be done quickly and accurately.

Noxious Gases

Carbon monoxide may be considered an example of the noxious gases, which may be categorized by their pathophysiology, which in turn determines patient symptoms.

Noxious gases are of three types: biologically inert gases, which harm by hypoxia due to oxygen displacement; systemic toxins with specific (usually CNS) actions; and agents that act as mucosal irritants. Some noxious agents are both systemic toxins and local irritants.

Local irritants produce injury proportional to concentration, duration of exposure, water content of exposed tissue, and water solubility of the gas.

Table 47–16 lists some common gases by type and the common symptom complexes seen with each. Table 47–17 lists some specific treatments available for a variety of systemic gaseous poisons. The production of methemoglobinemia, in which a portion of the circulating hemoglobin iron is in the ferric (+3) state, is certainly of utility in cyanide poisoning, for methemoglobin binds the cyanide ion very tightly. The hepatic enzyme rhodanese subsequently utilizes thiosulfate as a cofactor to degrade the cyanide moiety and detoxify it. In the United States, the only available cyanide antidote is the Lilly cyanide kit. The instructions for dosage of amyl nitrate pearls, sodium nitrite, and sodium thiosulfate must be explicitly followed.

This therapy must be stopped if hypotension supervenes or the methemoglobin level exceeds 40 per cent. As in the case of nitrite poisoning, it is possible to reverse excessive levels of methemoglobinemia, if necessary, by the use of methylene blue, which acts to generate reducing equivalents in the

Table 47–16. NOXIOUS GASES

Gas	Symptom Complex Mechanism
Biologically Inert	
Carbon dioxide	Hypoxia/narcosis
Hydrocarbons	Hypoxia/narcosis
Systemic Poisons	
Carbon disulfide	CNS stimulation then depression
Carbon monoxide	Tissue hypoxia due to COHgB
Hydrogen cyanide	Inhibition cytochrome oxidase
Mucosal Irritants	
Ammonia* Halogens* Hydrogen halides* (symptoms may be delayed) Oxides of nitrogen Phosgene Sulfur dioxide	*All may produce the following:* Keratoconjunctivitis Pharyngitis/rhinitis Laryngeal edema Tracheobronchitis Bronchospasm Pulmonary edema Nausea/vomiting
Combined Irritant/ Toxin	
Hydrogen sulfide	Blocks cellular oxidations
Methylated halogens	CNS depression Organ injury by blocking oxidation pathways in lung, heart, liver, kidney

*Skin injury

Table 47–17. SPECIFIC THERAPY FOR SYSTEMIC POISONS

Poison	Therapy
Carbon disulfide	Sedation ?Methemoglobinemia*
Carbon monoxide	100% oxygen
Hydrogen cyanide	100% oxygen Methemoglobinemia* ?Hydroxocobalamin
Hydrogen sulfide	100% oxygen ?Methemoglobinemia*
Methylated halogens	Wash skin/clothing Sedation Bicarbonate for acidosis Dialysis for renal failure ?Penicillamine Observe for delayed symptoms

*Production of methemoglobinemia (prepackaged kits may be obtained from Eli Lilly Co. [Lilly cyanide kit]).
1. Inhalation of 1 ampule amyl nitrate every 5 minutes until I.V. is established.
2. Three per cent nitrate intravenously: adult, 10 ml. over 2 to 4 minutes; children 0.33 ml./kg. (10 mg./kg.) then 5 mg./kg. every 30 minutes to maintain 30 per cent methemoglobin.
3. Sodium thiosulfate, 25 per cent solution, 50 ml. I.V. over 15 minutes.

red cell, which reconvert the methemoglobin iron to its reduced or ferrous (+2) state, thus permitting oxygen transport once again. Methylene blue is given in a dose of 1 to 2 mg./kg. of a 1 per cent solution over 5 to 15 minutes. It may be repeated once in 30 to 45 minutes if no improvement is evident.

Methemoglobin levels are easily followed spectrophotometrically, by most blood gas laboratory machines. The clinical correlate of methemoglobinemia is cyanosis unresponsive to supplemental oxygen and chocolate-brown arterial blood that does not change on exposure to air, with normal oxygen tension on arterial blood gases. The patient is often more blue than sick.

The irritant effect of noxious gases can usually be treated symptomatically on an outpatient basis. However, no patient who is dyspneic while breathing room air should be discharged.

Pulmonary edema is usually not delayed in exposure to noxious gases, except in the case of phosgene gas. These patients should be admitted for 24-hour observation after significant exposure even in the absence of symptoms.

If therapy is prompt and vigorous, the prognosis after inert or local irritant gas exposure is often good for complete recovery. Patients exposed to systemic poisons have a more guarded prognosis, and persistent mental changes or neurologic deficits are not uncommon.

POISON CONTROL CENTERS

A network of poison control centers exists across the United States, most of which are located in hospital emergency departments. The majority of these centers offer a variety of services, including product identification, toxicity information, telephone consultation in management, record keeping for data collections, professional education, and poison prevention information.

All practicing physicians should have ready access to their center's phone number; many comprehensive lists are available (see Arena, 1979, pp. 662–692).

Bites and Envenomation

HUMAN AND ANIMAL BITES

Animal bites, mostly dog bites, are common occurrences in the United States. National estimates range from 300 to 700 bites yearly per 100,000 population. Dog and cat bites involve laceration, avulsion, and crush injuries to tissue and the introduction into various tissue planes of a variety of bacterial organisms, with potential for infection.

Cat bites may contain anaerobic flora, streptococci, and coagulase-positive staphylococci. Very often, *Pasteurella multocida,* a highly penicillin-sensitive gram-negative rod, will cause early local wound infection in cat bite injury. This organism can occur in dog bite flora as well but is less characteristically seen.

Treatment of dog and cat bites includes acute wound management, possible tetanus prophylaxis, possible rabies prophylaxis, and surveillance for wound infection.

Acute wound management does not differ from any other complicated, contaminated laceration. The wound should be copiously irrigated with sterile saline under pressure (a large syringe with a 19-gauge needle is useful for this) until 200 to 300 ml. has been used. Debridement of devitalized tissue can be undertaken if necessary, unless it would produce difficulty with cosmesis or function. Dog and cat bite wounds, if deep or extensive or cosmetically deforming, may be sutured using routine techniques (see below). There are no data that prove antibiotic therapy decreases the infection rate of sutured cat or dog bites as long as they have been well cleansed and debrided. The patient should be closely followed for infection and should be given antibiotics should it supervene. Sutures should also be removed at this time if cosmetically feasible.

If infection supervenes, cat bites may be initially treated with oral penicillin, assuming that *P. multocida* plays a major role. Dog bites are probably better managed initially with a cephalosporin, for its broad gram-positive and gram-negative activity. All wounds or pus should be cultured first. Infection at this point may also be attacked with debridement, drainage, elevation, warm compresses, and splinting. Evidence of septicemia or severe infection in vital areas (such as the hand) mandate inpatient intensive surgical and antibiotic therapy.

If a bite is seen several hours after its occurrence, it may be treated as an old (greater than 6 to 8 hours) laceration, with cleansing, splinting, antibiotics, and reinspection at 48 to 72 hours to consider delayed primary closure.

Human bites often are more virulent than animal bites. The mixed aerobic-anaerobic flora of the human may be more virulent, but, in addition, many of these injuries occur when patients punch opponents in the teeth, causing deep inoculation of organisms into the soft tissues about the metacarpal heads, and even occasionally into the extensor tendons or the metacarpophalangeal joints, with resultant tenosynovitis, septic arthritis, or osteomyelitis. Human bites in these locations must be examined with the joint in extension and flexion, to reproduce the position of injury. Otherwise, deep penetration may be missed, with a subsequently deforming infection of tendon or joint space.

Human bites of the hand should never be closed primarily. After good wound cleansing and debridement, the hand should be splinted in the position of safe immobilization (Fig. 47–12), elevated, and watched closely for infection. If delayed closure is anticipated, oral antibiotics may be given.

If infection occurs in a human bite, antibiotic therapy following cultures can be initiated with an agent with broad-spectrum activity against gram-positive organisms, such as a cephalosporin. Coverage against anaerobes and gram-negative rods may need to be added. One of the second- or third-generation cephalosporins may be particularly useful for its added gram-negative and anaerobic spectra. Augmentin (amoxicillin-clavulanic acid) and clindamycin are also reasonable alternatives as is the use of multiple agents as dictated by initial clinical impression, followed as soon as possible by culture and sensitivity data. These considerations hold for infected animal bites as well.

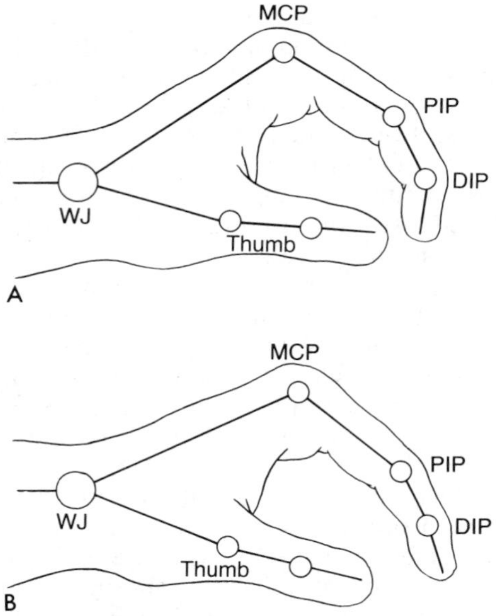

Figure 47–12. Splinting the injured hand. The two most common positions are those of function (*A*) and safe immobilization (*B*). See text. (WJ = wrist joint, MCP = metacarpophalangeal joint, PIP = proximal interphalangeal joint.)

Tetanus Prophylaxis

Tetanus has become rare with the routine use of tetanus toxoid in pediatric immunization and with subsequent injuries violating the integument. However, there are still about 100 cases reported yearly (95 reported in 1980), occurring almost exclusively in patients of unknown or inadequate immunization status.

In 10 to 20 per cent of tetanus cases, no wounds or chronic skin lesions are present.

Neonatal tetanus occurs in infants born to mothers not adequately immunized, who cannot confer passive immunity transplacentally.

Narcotic addicts are at particularly high risk of tetanus.

Spores of the anaerobic gram-positive rod *Clostridium tetani* are ubiquitous in nature. There is no natural immunity to tetanus toxin. Appropriately timed toxoid injections are mandatory to protect all age groups. The toxoid is highly effective, promoting active immunity that persists at least 10 years after adequate immunization.

Boosters, even for wound management, need to be given only every 10 years unless a wound is tetanus prone (for example, a deep puncture wound, a wound with devitalized, crushed tissue, or a significantly contaminated wound). In that case, a toxoid injection should be given if the patient has not received one in 5 years. Patients who have never had a full primary series of immunizations may require toxoid and passive immunization with tetanus immune globulin (TIG) at initial management.

Patients 7 years and older should receive active immunization with so-called Td, containing diphtheria toxoid in reduced dose (to decrease local and systemic reactions). This is for enhancement of diphtheria protection, as many adults are susceptible. Patients under age 7 should receive routine DPT (diphtheria-pertussis-tetanus) vaccine. In all cases in which inadequate primary immunization is documented or probable (the required regimen is four primary injections and a preschool booster at age 4 to 6), a primary immunization sequence should be completed (Table 47–18).

If passive immunization is needed, human TIG

Table 47–18. Td IMMUNIZATION SEQUENCE

Dose 1	First management (0.5 ml. each dose)
Dose 2	1 to 2 months later
Dose 3	6 to 12 months after dose 1
Booster	Every 10 years

Table 47–19. Td/TIG USE IN WOUND MANAGEMENT

Past Doses of Toxoid	Clear, Tiny Wound		All Other Wounds	
	Td	*TIG*	*Td*	*TIG*
0	Yes	No	Yes	Yes
1	Yes	No	Yes	Yes
2	Yes	No	Yes	If wound is greater than 24 hours old
3+	If none in 10 years	No	If none in 5 years	No
unknown	Yes	No	Yes	Yes

is used, in a dose of 250 units intramuscularly for average wounds. This must be injected at a site distant to the toxoid site to avoid neutralizing the toxoid. Because this is human globulin, the risk of adverse reactions is minimized.

Table 47–19 provides a summary of the use of Td and TIG in wound management.

Rabies Prophylaxis

Rabies is a rare but dreaded disease, and animal bites prompt consideration of prophylaxis, which is now easy and relatively risk free since the development of a vaccine derived from human cells in tissue culture, which has supplanted the old duck-embryo vaccine. Six doses of this vaccine are given, on days 1, 3, 7, 14, 30, and 90 after exposure. Human rabies globulin (RIG) is also used on day 1, for passive immunity, in a dose of 20 units/kg. body weight. Half the RIG is injected into and about the bite in question; the remainder is given at other sites intramuscularly.

The difficult question in rabies prophylaxis is when to treat. Bites from wild skunks, foxes, racoons, and bats should be treated as presumptively rabid unless the animal's brain is available for study. Dogs and cats should only be considered presumptively rabid if rabies has been reported in the area and the animal is not available for observation. If available, the animal should be observed for 10 days. Most animals cannot transmit rabies virus in saliva more than a few days before development of clinical illness (although bats, an important exception, may do so for months). If the animal becomes ill, the brain should be tested by fluorescent antibody technique to confirm rabies. If positive, treatment must commence at once.

SNAKEBITE (OPHIDISM)

Forty thousand persons die from snakebite each year around the world. In the United States, about 6000 to 7000 victims of poisonous snakebites are treated annually, and deaths average about 15 per year. There are about 19 venomous species of snake in the United States.

In the spring, when the snakes first emerge from hibernation with full poison glands, snakebite is generally more severe (and more common). The fangs of poisonous snakes produce two distinct fang puncture marks, while the teeth of nonpoisonous snakes only produce two rows of similar scratches. Poisonous snakes that are pit vipers (rattlesnakes, copperheads, and water moccasins) cause nearly all poisonous bites in the United States and are easily distinguished from nonpoisonous snakes by several features (Fig. 47–13). The secretive coral snake on rare occasions can produce a poisonous bite, but generally it prefers to retreat.

Table 47–20 lists major poisonous species, their geographic location, and the major venomous syndrome they produce.

The coral snake is a small banded snake with bands of black, yellow, and red; its snout is blunt, flat, and always black. A yellow band follows this, then a second black ring. Several harmless species of snake resemble the coral snake, but their snouts are usually red or gray. In the coral snake also, the red and black body rings never touch. This is not so in masquerading nonpoisonous snakes. This coloration method of identification is not infallible, however.

The bite of the coral snake may be more difficult to distinguish from benign bites by pattern, as it does not leave the prominent fang marks left by pit vipers.

Snakebite Syndromes

Marked local symptoms appear rapidly following a poisonous bite. Pain is prominent, followed by

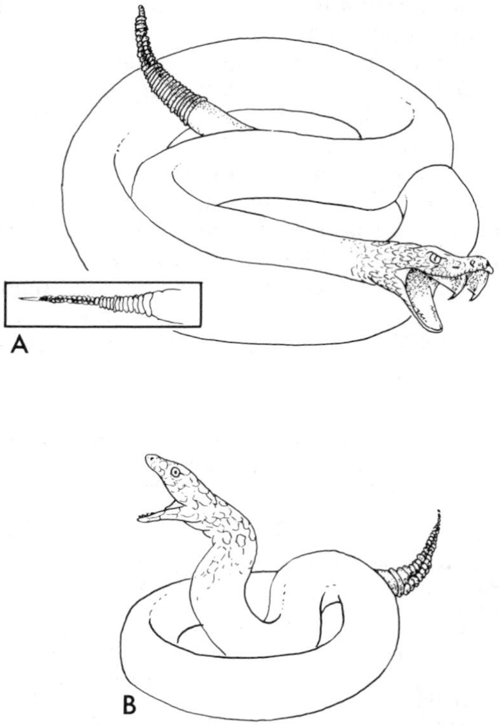

Figure 47–13. Distinguishing features of (most) poisonous (*A*) and nonpoisonous (*B*) snakes of the United States.

Table 47–20. MAJOR POISONOUS SNAKES IN UNITED STATES

Snake	Geographic Location	Syndrome
Florida diamond back rattler (*Crotalus adamanteus*)	North Carolina south, west to the Mississippi	Hemotoxic
Texas diamond back rattler (*C. atrox*)	Arkansas to Southern California	Hemotoxic
Timber rattler (*C. horridus*)	Entire East Coast, west to Minnesota through Texas	Hemotoxic
Prairie rattler (*C. viridis*)	Great Plains to Rockies	Hemotoxic
Pacific rattler (*C. oreganus*)	Pacific Coast, Idaho, Arizona	Hemotoxic
Pigmy rattler (*Sistrurus miliarius*)	Carolinas south, west to Texas	Hemotoxic
Massasauga (*S. catenatus*)	New York through Great Plains to Texas and Arizona	Hemotoxic
Copperhead (*Agkistrodon moreson*)	Massachusetts to Florida, Great Plains, south to Texas	Hemotoxic
Water moccasin (*A. piscivorus*)	Virginia to Florida, Gulf States, Midwest, and Texas	Hemotoxic
Coral, or Harlequin, snake (*Micrurus fulvius*)	Southeastern United States	Neurotoxic

edema, which progresses proximally from the bite. An entire extremity may become massively swollen within 1 hour. Local hemorrhage with bloody ooze and tissue necrosis may both be prominent, particularly with hemotoxic venom.

Systemic symptoms, including nausea, vomiting, hemorrhage, cardiorespiratory distress, coma, and collapse, will follow with significant envenomation in the absence of therapy.

Snake venoms are complex proteinaceous mixtures; the most toxic components are peptides and proteins of low molecular weight. Most venoms are both neurotoxic and hemotoxic, but what syndrome predominates is dependent on relative enzymatic activities.

Table 47–21 delineates the clinical signs of the two major syndromes.

Table 47–21. MAJOR SNAKEBITE SYNDROMES

Neurotoxic	Hemotoxic
Drowsiness	Local hemorrhagic necrosis
Bradycardia/hypotension	Petechiae due to thrombocytopenia
Muscle weakness	Parenchymal hemorrhages
Ptosis	Fibrinolysis
Difficulty swallowing	Disseminated intravascular coagulation (DIC)
Respiratory failure	Hemolysis
Trimus	
Nausea/vomiting	
Coma/seizures	
Cardiorespiratory collapse	

A variety of recommendations exist in the medical and lay literature for the initial management of snakebite. These include tourniquet techniques to decrease lymphatic drainage, immobilization, mobilization, ice, incision and suction, and a variety of other measures. Recently, these measures have come into question regarding efficacy following literature review (Steward et al., 1981). No large cooperative case studies of first-aid techniques in snakebite have been performed; the data collection and stratification obstacles are massive.

Some current procedures, such as incision and suction, tourniquet, and ice packing, may be harmful in common situations, increasing local damage. Splinting the bitten area, nonoral suction at the bite without incision, and avoiding unnecessary exertion may have some benefit as first-aid measures and certainly do no harm; at this point they are the only first-aid measures rigorous analysis allows the emergency physician to support. Parenthetically, rescuers should not orally suction a snakebite if they have mucosal lesions, as they may absorb toxin or infect the wound.

The single, undisputed, vital course of action following poisonous snakebite is rapid transport to an emergency facility capable of administering antivenin for definitive therapy. Intravenous administration is preferable, if possible, as it allows titration of antivenin dose while observing symptom progression or regression. The antivenin can also be given intramuscularly or subcutaneously.

Polyvalent antivenin for the treatment of pit viper bites is available from numerous sources and prevents death, relieves pain, aborts serious effects, and shortens convalescence. The initial dose is 10 to 50 ml. of reconstituted serum depending on severity of symptoms, lapse of time since the bite, size of patient, and size of snake. Antivenins are heterologous sera (horse) and use should be preceded by conjunctival and skin testing for allergy. When sera are given, equipment to manage anaphylaxis and cardiopulmonary collapse should be on hand.

If the victim is seen within 2 hours of envenomation, a small quantity of antivenin may be injected around the bite, except for bites on the digits.

Additional doses of antivenin may be given every 30 minutes to 2 hours as needed. Hospitalization and early cross-matching of blood are mandatory, since snake venom may interfere with cross-matching if it is delayed.

Coral snake antivenin can be obtained from the Centers for Disease Control.*

An antivenin index center† exists in Oklahoma, providing emergency information 24 hours daily on antivenins available for all snakes that are stocked in zoos, labs, and other institutions in North America. The scientific and common names of the snake involved should be ascertained.

SPIDER BITES

All spiders inject venom when they bite, but only two species of spider in the United States routinely cause serious envenomation syndromes: the black widow spider (*Latrodectus mactans* or *curacaviensis*) and the brown recluse spider (*Loxosceles* species, especially *L. reclusa*).

The black widow spider is found in nearly all states of the continental United States. The adult female has a globular black body about ½-inch long with an orange-red hour-glass figure on its ventral surface. The male is about ½ the size of the female. The web usually looks disordered and is out of doors or in outhouses, and the spider is often not visible during the day.

The initial sharp pain of the black widow spider's bite usually fades rapidly. The patient develops local muscle cramps 15 minutes to 2 hours later. The neurotoxic venom causes muscle pain, contraction, and ascending motor paralysis. The abdomen may become boardlike. Serious systemic symptoms may follow, including delirium, seizures, shock, cyanosis, and, in occasional cases, death. In nonfatal cases, symptoms peak in 3 to 24 hours and then gradually resolve over several days.

When the diagnosis is made, the patient should receive one ampule of Lyovac antivenin (Merck, Sharp & Dohme) intramuscularly after conjunctival and skin testing for horse-serum sensitivity. Lyovac antivenin is a horse-derived heterologous antiserum produced using black widow spider venom. It is specific for the management of black widow spider bites and has no utility in managing brown recluse spider bites or snakebite. One or two doses of Lyovac usually resolve symptoms in 1 to 3 hours, counteracting the neurotoxic venom.

Victims of black widow spider envenomation should be admitted to a hospital for good nursing care and ancillary therapy. Muscle pain responds to heat and infusion of 10 per cent calcium gluconate. Sedatives, muscle relaxants, and adrenocorticoids are also efficacious in managing muscular symptoms. Respiratory status must be carefully observed. Local therapy at the bite site is of no value nor are tourniquets or suction.

The brown recluse spider's venom is cytotoxic and hemotoxic, causing both local progressive tissue necrosis and systemic syndromes including DIC (disseminated intravascular coagulation).

The spider is brown, with a violin-shaped dark area on its dorsal thorax. Its body is about 1 centimeter in size. The spider lives indoors, in cellars and other areas, and is even found in shoes or bedding. It cannot live at temperatures less than 40°F. and is generally found in the southern states.

On initial envenomation, the spider injects a venom rich in protease, hyaluronidase, and esterase. Mild pain becomes progressively more severe. A blister forms and then escharifies by the end of the first week postbite. In 2 to 5 weeks, the eschar is loose, leaving a necrotic ulcer that heals poorly.

In severe cases, arthralgia, rash, and prolonged high fever may occur, with weakness and prostration. Hemolysis and hemoglobinuria may be seen, with shock and renal derangement.

There is no specific antidote for the brown recluse's bite. Local infiltration of phentolamine (Regitine) may decrease ischemia from the norepinephrine present in the venom. Antihistamines and steroids often help more systemic symptoms.

The best early therapy is total excision of all involved tissue with primary closure. Once necrosis and ulceration are present, tissue excision may need to extend to muscle fascia with subsequent skin grafting.

HYMENOPTERA STINGS (BEES AND WASPS)

Stings from bees and wasps are common occurrences requiring acute care. These insects kill more Americans annually than snakes, due to anaphylactic reactions.

Bees' stingers are hooked and remain in tissue after their insertion. This leads to evisceration and death of the stinging bee and continued pumping of venom into the wound. Wasps, lacking a hook on their stinger, can sting multiple times and are potentially more dangerous. Their stings are also more

*Centers for Disease Control can be reached at 404-633-3311.
†Antivenin Index Center can be reached at 405-271-5454.

Table 47–22. ANAPHYLAXIS MANAGEMENT

Epinephrine: 0.3 to 0.5 ml. of 1:1000 solution S.Q., I.M., or sublingual injection I.V. more cautiously
Corticosteroids: 100 mg. hydrocortisone I.V.
Antihistamines: 25 to 50 mg. diphenhydramine I.V.
Oxygen
Trendelenburg, fluids, pressors, CPR as needed

tetanus prone than those of bees, as many species of wasp or hornet are saprophytic and even feed on excrement.

Hymenoptera venom resembles mild snake venom, having both hemotoxic and neurotoxic properties. It has a strong histamine-like action on tissue. A local pruritic wheal is the most common reaction, requiring only cold compresses and occasionally antihistamines, wound toilet, and tetanus prophylaxis.

A delayed syndrome of local hymenoptera allergy is not uncommon, with progressive localized heat, redness, and swelling of tissue around the sting, often with low-grade fever. This may be difficult to differentiate from infection when it occurs 1 or more days after the sting. The presence of intense pruritus and absence of lymphangitis or adenopathy suggest an allergic reaction. These patients are best treated initially with antihistamines, ice, elevation, splinting, and careful observation, with antibiotic use reserved for further progression of signs.

The anaphylactic response to hymenoptera stings, including cardiovascular collapse, bronchospasm, diarrhea, and urticaria, is dramatic and life threatening. It requires the use of such agents as epinephrine (which may be injected sublingually in profound collapse if no intravenous or endotracheal route is available), antihistamines, corticosteroids, oxygen, intravenous fluids, and on occasion complete cardiopulmonary resuscitation. This response always mandates hospitalization, if only for observation (Table 47–22).

Recovery from anaphylaxis due to stings is usually complete within 48 hours. All patients should subsequently carry a kit with them containing epinephrine (such as the ANA-kit from Hollister-Stier Labs, which is dispensed by prescription), wear a bracelet documenting their sensitivity, and consider undergoing desensitization therapy.

Trauma

PRINCIPLES OF WOUND CARE

The fundamental principles of wound care necessary to prepare and suture lacerations adequately are relatively few and straightforward but of great importance. Adherence to basic principles invariably leads to an optimal result.

All wounds must be cleansed. Initially, scrubbing with a sponge or soft brush and antiseptic solution will provide debridement. This should be followed by copious irrigation with saline solution for large lacerations, for which 150 to 300 ml. should be used in a high-pressure irrigation using a syringe and a 19-gauge needle. High-pressure irrigation with sterile saline alone reduces bacterial counts in wounds and decreases the risk of infection.

Within the limits imposed by cosmesis or function, tissue that is crushed or devitalized should be excised prior to wound closure.

Once the wound is irrigated, the patient draped and anesthetized and debridement completed, the wound may be closed. For optimal scar formation, wound margins must be free of undue tension. A layered closure of lacerations is helpful to achieve reduction of tension for skin closure in deep lacerations.

Ideally, each layer of subcutaneous tissue should be separately sutured, but, in practice, all that is often needed is to assure eversion of wound edges and release of surface tension by sutures placed at the dermal-fatty junction of subcutaneous tissues.

Initial sutures should divide a laceration evenly in half, then into quarters, and so forth. Entry and exit of sutures should be equally distant from wound margins. Usually sutures placed every 5 mm. will allow approximation without tension. Sutures must not be placed so tightly that subsequent swelling of wound edges (which always occurs) leads to train-tracking and increased scar formation.

The factors involved in permanent scar formation are listed in Table 47–23. The larger the bite taken by a suture and the longer a suture remains in place, the more prominent will be scar formation.

Eversion of wound edges produces a better scar. This can be accomplished by making sutures that are deeper than they are wide. Angle the needle back away from the wound edge, making a bottle-shaped entry and scrape the needle under the skin on the way out to ensure everted edges. Vertical mattress sutures may also be used to the same purpose (Fig. 47–14).

Sutures are divided into absorbable and nonabsorbable materials. A 3–0 or 4–0 suture of chromic catgut is a good general purpose absorbable suture for deep layer closure. Polyglycolic acid (Dexon) sutures can be alternatively used; they are somewhat easier to handle, are less reactive, and last longer.

For skin closure, practical differences between nonabsorbable sutures are slight. Synthetics are

Table 47–23. FACTORS IN SCAR FORMATION IN SUTURED WOUNDS

Tension on sutures
Length of time sutures in place
Amount of tissue held by suture (bite)
Region of body (face, hands, soles of feet less likely to railroad-track)
Infection
Keloid formation

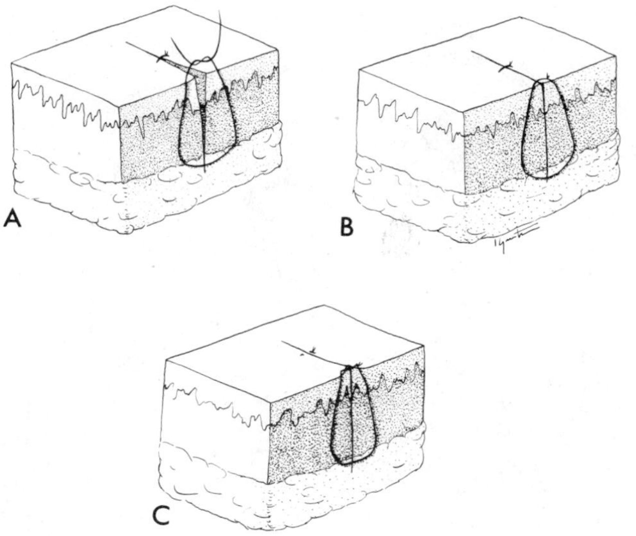

Figure 47–14. Good eversion of wound edges is crucial to subsequent cosmetic results. Make sutures deeper than they are wide, and wider at bottom than top to produce this result (*A, B*). A vertical mattress suture (*C*) is a simple variation that achieves good eversion and assures minimal tension on wound edges.

stronger but harder to manipulate (nylon or Dermalon, polypropylene or Surgilene, and so on) than silk or cotton. The braided structure of silk sutures makes them prone to infection, in theory, in comparison to monofilament synthetic sutures.

For routine wound closure, 4–0 suture will usually be adequate. Cosmetic repair requires 6–0 suture material. Sutures of 3–0 material may be required at sites, such as the scalp or over major joints, to provide additional strength.

A useful schedule for suture removal is listed in Table 47–24; these represent general guidelines to be tempered by experience and individual preference.

Several areas of the body require attention to a few special principles. The scalp is very vascular and bleeds profusely; shock due to extensive blood loss may be seen with large lacerations, and rapid closure may be advisable. Clamping of vessels is usually an inappropriate maneuver unless a major proximal artery has been transected and is identifiable. Hemostasis can otherwise be obtained first by direct pressure and then by either interrupted, vertical mattress, or running lock-stitch sutures. It is wise after anesthetizing the wound to probe with the gloved finger and rule out an associated skull fracture (usually skull x-rays will not be required). Do not mistake the torn edges of the galea aponeurotica of the scalp for a bony defect; this is a common error. If at all possible, the edges of the torn galea should be reapproximated.

Table 47–24. SUTURE REMOVAL

Face	3 to 5 days (subsequent reinforcement with benzoin tincture and microporous adhesive tape [Steri-strips] advised)
Scalp	7 to 10 days
Extremity	
Not over joint	7 days
Over joint	10 to 14 days (augment with splinting)
Feet	10 to 14 days (only sew feet if absolutely necessary)
Trunk	
Anterior	7 days
Back	10 to 14 days

Use large sutures, such as 3–0, on a large strong needle for scalp closure. If oozing persists, apply direct pressure. The patient can wash the area normally in 24 to 48 hours, as with any other uncomplicated laceration.

Eyebrow lacerations should be managed without shaving the brow; it may not grow back, and shaving it causes loss of a landmark to judge the cosmetic results of the repair.

The vermilion border of the lip requires special attention in closure of lacerations; the first suture placed should exactly reapproximate the edges at this border for a defect of only 1 to 2 mm. is obvious (Fig. 47–15). In through-and-through lip lacerations, close the muscular tissues first with 4–0 or 5–0 chromic sutures, then the vermilion and external tissues with synthetic sutures. Some authorities close mucosal lacerations in the mouth with silk sutures, arguing for less hypertrophic scar formation and morbidity with this approach. However, doing so raises the potential for infection in the wound, particularly if tissue is contused, since the mouth is never sterile. If closure is performed, oral penicillin coverage is advisable while the sutures are in place. Careful attention to oral hygiene is mandatory during healing in either event. Remove the sutures in 5 days.

Lacerations of the tongue rarely require suturing. However, a laceration of the tip longer than 1 cm. will heal with a forked tongue deformity unless reapproximated.

Intra-oral lacerations in children can be closed with absorbable suture material. This will obviate the need for subsequent removal and lessen the child's ordeal.

Lacerations seen more than 8 to 12 hours after injury, not due to bite wounds, may be cleaned, dressed, and followed. If no infection is present by

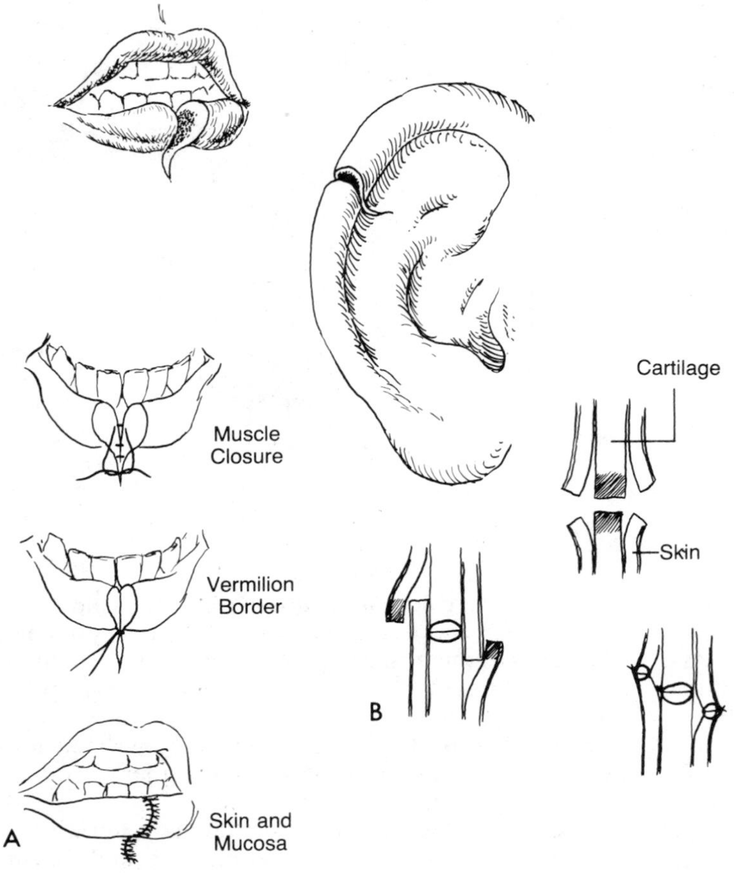

Figure 47–15. Ear and lip repairs require some special care. Close through-and-through lip lacerations in a layered fashion (*A*); the first surface suture must *exactly* reapproximate the torn vermilion border. The ear (*B*) requires closure of cartilage and *perichondrium* with absorbable sutures; stagger the skin suture closure as shown to avoid a "pitting" deformity when the pinna heals; anesthetize the pinna using plain lidocaine and injecting all the way around the base of the ear a full 360 degrees subcutaneously.

the third to fifth day after injury and closure is mandatory, secondary closure can be done.

Ear lacerations require closure of the perichondrium over any exposed cartilage to avoid necrosis from devascularization. The skin may be closed thereafter, and a pressure dressing may be applied to prevent hematoma and a cauliflower-ear deformity. Anesthesia is obtained by intradermal and subcutaneous injection of agents free of epinephrine around the base of the pinna for a full 360 degrees.

Anesthesia Techniques

In general, whichever anesthetic is used, "use the smallest effective amount of the least toxic substance in the safest possible manner" (Ervin, 1978).

Local anesthetics in common use are the -caine substances, which may be grouped into several chemical classes. In general, allergic responses to one chemical class do not occur to another, but specific patients may not follow such a rule. Always be prepared to treat major allergic responses and perform resuscitation in such a situation. Table 47–25 lists representative drugs for local anesthesia.

A solution of lidocaine, 1 to 2 per cent, is most often used in local anesthesia. When working in vascular areas, such as the face, solutions containing 1:100,000 epinephrine will aid in hemostasis as well as help to prolong duration and minimize toxicity of anesthetics. However, epinephrine must never be used in anesthetizing end organs (digits, nose, ears, or penis) as it can cause ischemic gangrene.

A wound should be approached from its cut margin, placing a sufficient quantity of anesthetic into the dermal layer to provide the desired result. Introducing the needle into the wound is less painful than placing it through intact skin. Anesthesia should be provided before any vigorous cleansing or debridement; this has not been shown to increase rate of wound infection.

A 25-gauge needle should be used, raising a skin wheal and then advancing, aspirating each time before injection to avoid an inadvertent intravascular injection. In an adult, up to a maximum of 300 mg. of lidocaine may be used in one local application; this must be scaled down appropriate to body weight in children.

Sedation of children before suturing is occasionally helpful, although a restraining papoose board or blanket is often equally useful. If sedation is used, one useful regimen is meperidine (Demerol) 0.5 to 1.0 mg./kg. and promethazine (Phenergan) 0.2 to 0.5

Table 47–25. LOCAL ANESTHETIC AGENTS

Chemical Class	Agent Commonly Used	Comment
	Procaine (Novocain)	
Para-aminobenzoic acid (ester)	Tetracaine (Pontocain)	
	Chloroprocaine (Nesacaine)	
Diethylamino-2′,6′-acetoxylidide (amide)	Lidocaine (Xylocaine)	
dl-N-methylpipecolic acid 2,6-dimethylanilide (amide)	Mepivacaine (Carbocaine)	
	Bupivacaine (Marcaine)	Marcaine is very long acting (up to 24 hours) Useful in toothache analgesia
Benzoic acid (ester)	Cocaine	Cocaine approved only for use in epistaxis Cocaine is the only local anesthetic that is a vasoconstrictor Appears useful for wounds topically with tetracaine and adrenaline (topical TAC therapy)

mg./kg. intramuscularly (the addition of chlorpromazine [Thorazine] in doses of 0.1 to 0.2 mg./kg. produces even more profound sedation).

Nerve Block Techniques

Regional anesthetic techniques are many and varied. The most useful for laceration repair are digital blocks and regional facial blocks.

Digital nerves in the hand may be anesthetized before they divide at the metacarpal heads or selectively at the base of a finger.

To perform transmetacarpal block, a 25-gauge needle is inserted perpendicular to the skin of the dorsum of the hand at the level of the metacarpal head (distal palmar crease) and advanced laterally to the same depth as the middle of the metacarpal head. Two or three milliliters of anesthetic is placed and the needle withdrawn. This is repeated on the other side of the digit. Anesthesia is obtained in less than 5 minutes.

More selective digital nerve block again uses a 25-gauge needle, placing anesthesia at the base of the proximal phalanx on both sides both dorsal and ventral. A quantity of local anesthetic that is too large can induce vascular compression with this technique and resultant gangrene, so care is required (Fig. 47–16).

Facial sensation may be blocked selectively at the foraminal exits of each of the three trigeminal nerve divisions. The foramina for the supraorbital, infraorbital, and mental nerves lie in a nearly vertical line that lies just medial to the patient's cornea in the position of forward gaze (Fig. 47–16).

Infiltration over the eyebrow and glabella blocks the supratrochlear and supraorbital nerves, to anesthetize the forehead and anterior scalp. Injection around the infraorbital foramen blocks the infraorbital area and the upper lip. Infiltration at the mental foramen blocks the lower lip and chin.

TENDON REPAIR

If primary repair of an extensor tendon is to be attempted, superb wound toilet is vital to prevent the disaster of a serious hand infection. At minimum, even if tendon repair is not carried out, irrigation, debridement, loose primary skin closure, and splinting are mandatory.

Monofilament nylon suture material or wire is most favorable for tendon repair. Reactive materials like catgut are contraindicated. For wrist tendons 3–0 suture is used, but in most cases 4–0 suture will be adequate. In children a 6–0 suture may be adequate.

In general, to minimize scar formation preserve paratendinous tissue cautiously. The tendon ends, if macerated or ragged, must be carefully trimmed back to fresh, even fibers and sutured accurately.

The capacity for severed tendons to heal primarily end to end is quite limited; it appears that ingrowth of cells from surrounding connective tissue is required for restoration of tendon continuity. The tendon is made up of longitudinal fibers. Thus, simple through-and-through sutures do not hold, and criss-cross sutures collapse. For thin, flat, extensor tendons, it is best to use horizontal mattress sutures, and for thick and round flexor tendons, a locking mattress suture (Fig. 47–17), supplemented by continuous fine marginal sutures of nonabsorbable material such as 6–0 nylon.

Close follow-up and aftercare is vital after tendon repair. A padded plaster splint immobilizes the sutured tendon in a relaxed position, for a minimum of 3 weeks. On splint removal, a graded exercise program is started to repair function.

THORACIC TRAUMA

Trauma is the leading cause of death in this country in patients 1 to 44 years of age. Chest and abdominal trauma will be considered below as to emergency stabilization and diagnosis.

Trauma to the chest may be blunt or penetrating. Penetrating thoracic injury is a common entity in metropolitan hospital emergency departments. Blunt injury, most commonly from motor vehicle accidents but seen in many other contexts, is common and frequently lethal. One fourth of motor vehicle deaths

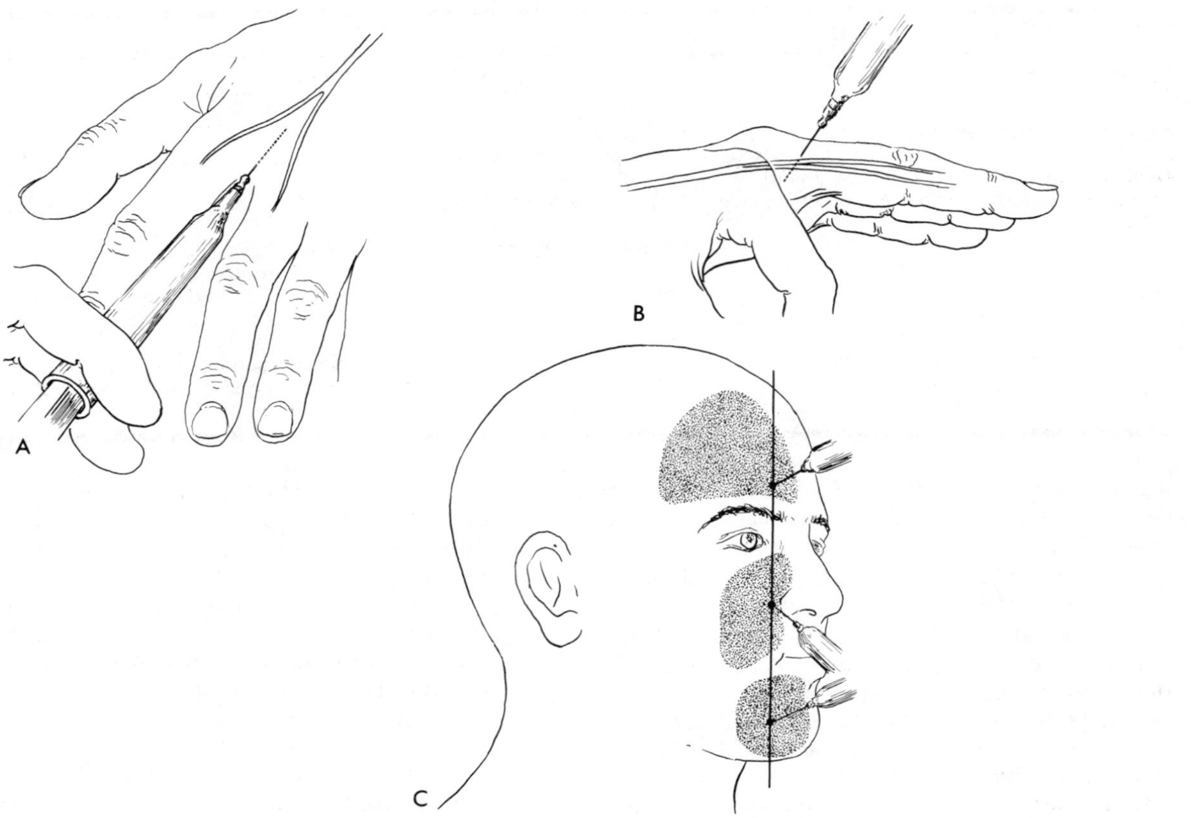

Figure 47–16. Regional blocks. Dorsal fingerweb entry is used for transmetacarpal block (*A*). A more distal site and arclike pattern of injection provide a digital block (*B*). The branches of the trigeminal nerve, blocked in facial blocks, enter the face through foramina that lie in a straight line (*C*).

each year are caused by or in some way related to chest trauma.

The morbidity and mortality of blunt chest trauma are high for several reasons: there is a high frequency of associated injury to the abdominal viscera, head and neck, and musculoskeletal system, which must not be missed; the injuries intrathoracically are often multiple and severe; and finally very severe intrathoracic injury may initially be silent clinically, leading to serious deterioration later in the patient.

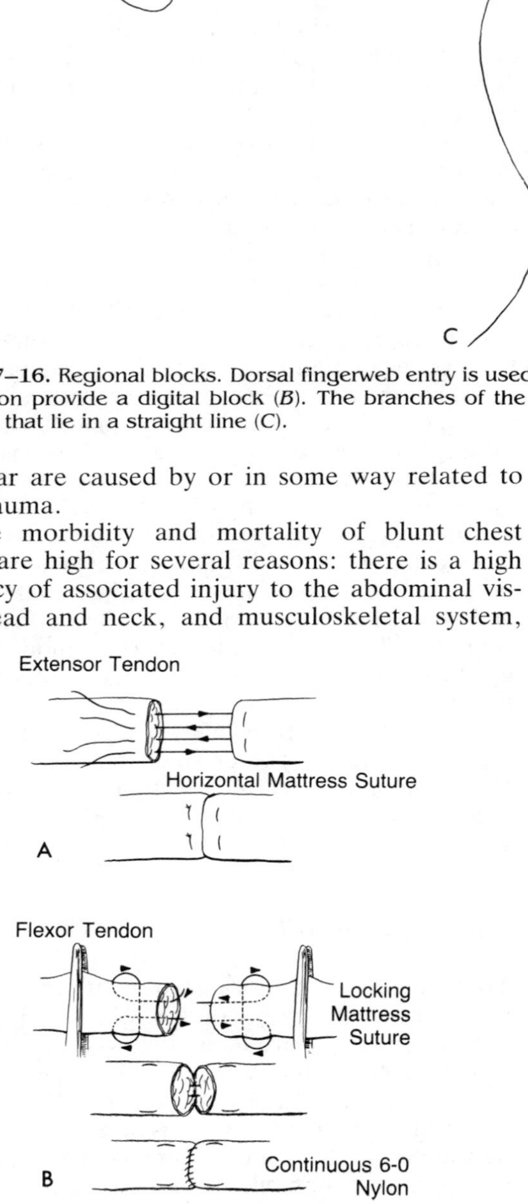

Figure 47–17. *A*, Extensor tendon repair; *B*, Flexor tendon repair.

The forces experienced in blunt chest trauma are of two sorts: shearing forces due to tethering on intrathoracic structures and blunt impact forces. Shearing forces may lead to tissue disruption affecting the heart, aorta, tracheobronchial tree, and esophagus. Direct forces affect ribs, lungs, and diaphragm.

Initial evaluation of the chest-injured patient often proceeds simultaneously with resuscitative therapy. Adequate respiration must be assured; large-bore intravenous access, including central venous pressure determinations begun; blood sent for type and cross-match and other studies; and a thorough systematic examination completed. Blood gases, ECG, and chest x-rays are minimum required studies.

Color, chest wall motion, and nature of respiration are vital. Note the patient's neck veins. Shock with distended neck veins suggests tension pneumothorax or cardiac tamponade as an etiology. Flat-neck-vein shock suggests hemothorax or an extrathoracic cause for hypovolemia.

Paradoxical chest wall motion represents a flail chest, common after steering wheel injury, due to multiple two-point rib fractures. Large flail segments make adequate gas exchange impossible and mandate intubation and positive-pressure ventilation.

Absent breath sounds represent pneumothorax or hemothorax. The amount of respiratory distress seen with pneumothorax is a function of pulmonary reserve, and young healthy patients may have no distress with a complete unilateral pneumothorax. Tracheal deviation suggests tension pneumothorax: progressive mediastinal displacement acutely leads to compression of the great veins with loss of venous return to the right heart and eventual cardiovascular collapse. The patient with tension pneumothorax and cardiopulmonary compromise should receive immediate decompression with a large-bore needle in the second intercostal space, midclavicular line. This usually affords enough improvement that tube thoracostomy (see below) can proceed at a reasonably comfortable pace.

Respiratory distress without absent breath sounds or tracheal deviation may represent a ruptured diaphragm, an often missed serious injury that requires a high index of suspicion for diagnosis. Look for fuzziness of the hemidiaphragm on portable chest film. (Usually the left hemidiaphragm is involved. If a nasogastric tube is in the stomach, it may be seen in the hemithorax.) Endotracheal intubation and nasogastric intubation may be helpful.

Tracheobronchial disruption may present in several ways, of which the most subtle may be a mediastinal crunch or subcutaneous emphysema. This injury may also present as complete unilateral atelectasis, mediastinal emphysema, pneumothorax with or without tension but with persistent air leak on chest tube drainage, or bronchiectasis. Hemoptysis varies from absent to massive; if present, it must not be ignored.

The clinical relevance of a hemothorax depends upon its magnitude and continued accumulation sufficient to cause signs of blood loss and often upon some degree of respiratory embarrassment due to compression atelectasis. Lacerations of the heart and great vessels that cause hemothorax lead to death rapidly. Injuries to pulmonary parenchyma are less rapidly lethal, however, because the low pressure pulmonary circulation tends to bleed more slowly, and the high thromboplastin levels in pulmonary tissue promote clot formation. Clinically significant hemothorax usually is due to disrupted intercostal or internal mammary arteries. The unclotted blood in a hemothorax may be drained via chest tube into an autotransfusion apparatus (see below) and returned to the patient.

Pulmonary contusion occurs commonly in the patient with blunt chest trauma and should be suspected particularly in patients with rib fractures or flail chest. Damage to tissue causes interstitial pulmonary hemorrhage with impairment of gas exchange. Blood gases and portable chest x-ray are vital to diagnosis but may be unrevealing soon after the injury. Assisted ventilation may be required if contusion is severe or reserve marginal.

There are three types of cardiac injury in blunt chest trauma: myocardial contusion, pericardial tamponade, and cardiac rupture. The mechanism of injury is a swinging disruptive force. The heart is tethered at its base, and there is a direct impact of the heart against the sternum.

Myocardial contusion may mimic infarction on an electrocardiogram, and enzyme elevations, arrhythmias, and congestive heart failure or shock may be seen. These should be treated in the usual fashion. The clinical course of myocardial contusion is generally more benign than that of infarction; histologically, a contusion resolves into tiny areas of fibrosis, which are scattered among normal parenchyma, rather than a single focal scar.

If pericardial tamponade is suspected after blunt trauma (narrow pulse pressure, high central venous pressure, and distant heart sounds with low voltage on the electrocardiogram, possibly with electrical alternans of the QRS complex), pericardiocentesis may be a useful temporizing measure (see Fig. 47–9). Emergency thoracotomy is mandatory.

Cardiac rupture from blunt trauma is usually rapidly lethal; only the rare patient will survive the trip to hospital to undergo emergency thoracotomy.

Aortic disruption most often occurs at the ligamentum arteriosum, just distal to the left subclavian artery. A wide mediastinum on chest x-ray, blood pressure differential between the upper extremities, and a positive aortogram mandate surgical repair.

Esophageal rupture, although rare in blunt chest trauma, must not be missed, as fatal mediastinitis will ensue within hours while diagnosis is delayed. Unexplained mediastinal air requires a Gastrografin swallow and/or endoscopy. Surgery is mandatory to avoid a fatal outcome.

Associated injuries must not be missed. Stabilize the trauma victim's neck with a collar or sandbags at the start if a neck injury is suspected. If intubation or cricothyrotomy is necessary, the possibility of cervical spine instability must be considered. The abdomen must be carefully evaluated, and if there is any sign of serious injury, the general surgeon must be made aware of this also. Peritoneal lavage may be required in questionable cases (see below). Foley catheterization may be diagnostic of urinary tract injury (hematuria) in these patients or may be required to relieve bladder distention, especially in the patient with a spinal injury.

Simple rib fractures, probably the most common injury with blunt chest trauma, are managed with analgesia, rest, and careful outpatient follow-up. Fractures of the lower left ribs, however, may be associated with splenic injury, and liver-spleen scan or inpatient observation may be wise. Further, fractures of any of the first four ribs should make one highly suspicious of associated visceral or vascular injury requiring observation and possibly aortography. In spite of optimal therapy of blunt chest trauma, complications are not infrequent, including adult respiratory distress syndrome, due to diffuse pulmonary contusion or associated injuries.

PENETRATING CHEST TRAUMA

The general resuscitative considerations of blunt chest trauma apply to penetrating chest trauma as well, and such wounds to the chest can produce pneumothorax, hemothorax, cardiac laceration, and many of the injuries discussed previously. Also, open pneumothorax (a sucking chest wound) can be produced.

When respiration and circulation are assured, the chest wound should be covered with an occlusive dressing, such as Vaseline gauze, to prevent ingress of air. In general, these wounds should never be probed; one can convert an innocuous injury to a dangerous one by injudicious probing. An open pneumothorax, with the lack of effective ventilation that accompanies it, must at minimum be treated with an occlusive dressing and a chest tube in rapid succession. Usually, emergency intubation of the patient is also required.

As in blunt chest trauma, penetrating trauma to the chest may be accompanied by abdominal and/or renal injury, and these must be ruled out by examination and laboratory data, possibly including peritoneal lavage (see below).

Tube Thoracostomy Drainage (Chest Tube Drainage)

Pneumothorax is the commonest entity managed by chest tube drainage (Fig. 47–18). It is relatively common; one out of each 1000 general hospital admissions is for pneumothorax. The etiology of the atraumatic, spontaneous pneumothorax is probably rupture of a subpleural bleb in the lung apex. It is most often seen in patients 20 to 40 years old, with no underlying disease. Men outnumber women five to one. While there is no association with exertion, there is with cigarette smoking, smokers being the victims of spontaneous pneumothorax more often.

Catamenial pneumothorax is a rare form of the disease, of unknown etiology, associated with menses. Some of the patients do have pulmonary endometriosis but not all.

Iatrogenic pneumothorax, due to central line placement, CPR, ventilator mechanics, liver biopsies, and so on are not uncommon in the hospitalized patient.

Radiographic diagnosis of pneumothorax ideally requires posterior-anterior (PA), lateral, and expiratory views of the chest. From the PA chest film, the percentage of the pneumothorax may be estimated (Fig. 47–19) as the area of the hemithorax minus the area of collapsed lung divided by the area of the hemithorax.

The ECG in the patient with pneumothorax may demonstrate many changes due to intrathoracic air, cardiac rotation, right ventricular dilatation, and altered coronary blood flow: the QRS axis shifts rightward, R-wave voltage may decrease, the overall amplitude of the QRS complex may decrease, and the precordial T waves may become inverted, simulating ischemia.

Spontaneous pneumothorax rarely develops intrathoracic tension; only about 15 per cent of all pneumothoraces are tension pneumothoraces. Bilateral spontaneous pneumothorax occurs in less than 5 per cent of cases; it must always be rapidly considered in the trauma patient, however. Hemothorax is only present in 15 per cent of spontaneous pneumothoraces, while it occurs in up to 75 per cent of traumatic pneumothorax.

The recurrence rate of spontaneous pneumothorax is one third of patients after a first episode, and at least one half of patients after a second

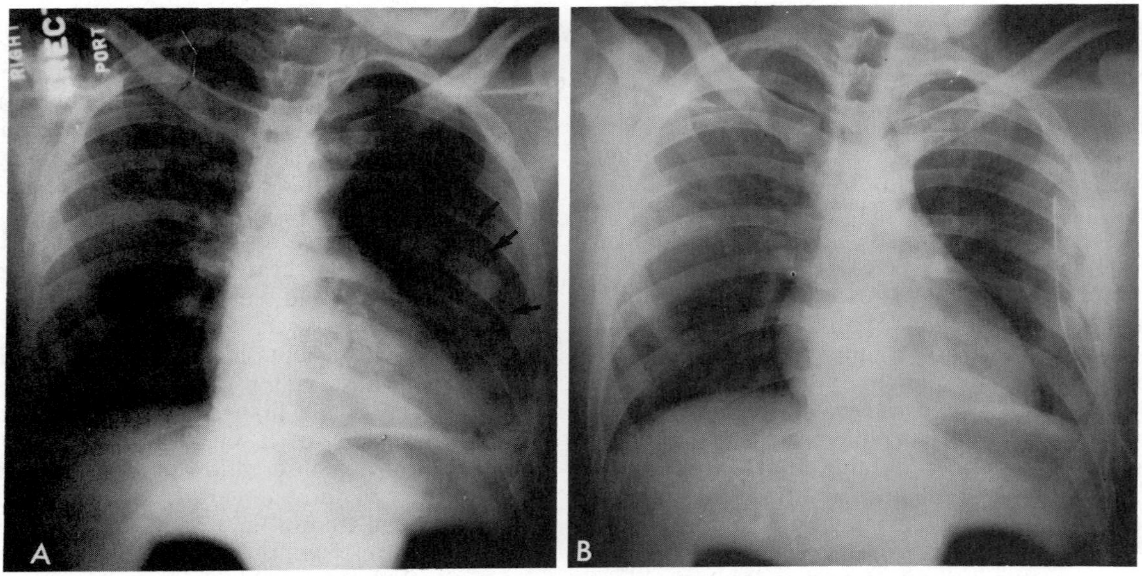

Figure 47–18. Pneumothorax (*A*) with subsequent chest tube re-expansion (*B*).

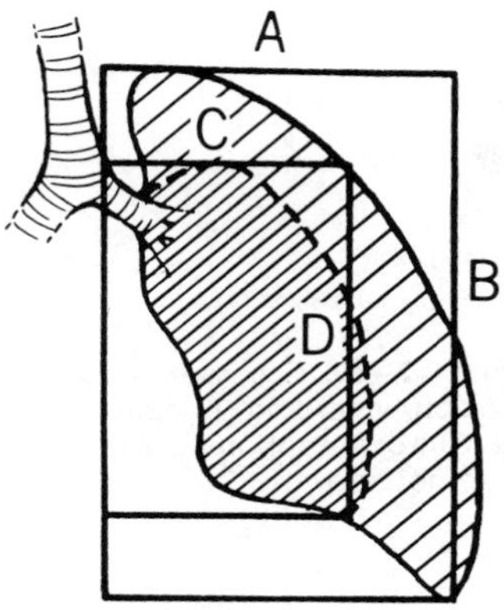

Figure 47–19. Method of calculating percentage of pneumothorax. AB = area of hemithorax:
CD = area of collapsed lung;

$$\frac{(AB - CD)}{AB} = \text{per cent pneumothorax.}$$

(From Donovan, J. W.: Pneumothorax. Current Topics II in Emergency Medicine, 2(7). Philadelphia, Medical College of Pennsylvania, 1982.)

episode. Such patients may require pleural abrasion and bleb resection procedures.

There is fairly general agreement on the need for tube drainage of any traumatic pneumothorax. Controversy exists, however, over the management of spontaneous pneumothorax.

Chest tube insertion is not a benign procedure. In order of frequency, its complications are the following (Curtis, 1978): hemothorax, pulmonary edema, bronchopleural fistula, pleural leaks, subcutaneous emphysema, and contralateral pneumothorax. These complications, in addition to arguments about the low risk of tension development in spontaneous pneumothorax, the pain of a chest tube, and the cost of hospital stay, are raised by proponents of less aggressive chest tube insertion.

The percentage of pneumothoraces mandating chest tube insertion is similarly variable; estimates range from less than 10 per cent and minimal or no symptoms (Donovan 1978) to 30 per cent (Curtis 1978). Suggestions on management without a chest tube vary from outpatient follow-up to hospitalization and observation, with a repeat chest film in 4 to 6 hours to assure no progression. The latter is certainly the more prudent course. Ambulatory outpatient chest tube management, while uniquely provocative, cannot be widely recommended at present.

Several techniques are available for chest tube insertion; one may use a trocar, finger dissection or a large Kelly clamp or hemostat to enter the pleural space. The Kelly is a personal favorite and carries less chance of extrapleural insertion than a finger method. For spontaneous pneumothorax a 22 French chest tube is adequate. For draining hemothorax, use a 32 French tube. Figure 47–20 demonstrates the main equipment for tube thoracostomy.

The tube may be inserted in the fifth intercostal space, anterior axillary line, for all indications. The patient is supine. The skin is prepped and draped, and the skin over the sixth rib is anesthetized down to periosteum. A 3-cm. horizontal incision is made down to fat, and a clamp is used to extend a tract to the next interspace above (never below, as the neurovascular bundle runs under the rib). The clamp is then pushed into the pleural space, and the hole is dilated. Check for adherent lung with the gloved finger. Grasp the chest tube with the Kelly clamp. Measure skin-to-lung apex distance on the chest tube and mark this end point on the chest tube with a small clamp. Place the tube in the chest with the Kelly, directing it posterior and cephalad.

Secure the tube with 0 wire or silk, apply a petrolatum gauze dressing, connect to suction, and remove the small clamp. Verify tube placement with a chest film (Fig. 47–21).

Large hemothoraces, if unclotted, can be salvaged via chest tube drainage and returned to the unstable patient's blood volume using an autotransfusion technique (Davidson, 1979, 1981). The apparatus is simple, readily obtainable, functions in place of the water-seal Pleurevac unit, and accommodates a 32 French chest tube.

Emergency Thoracotomy

In rare cases, it may be necessary to do an emergency thoracotomy to resuscitate the chest-injured (or abdomen-injured) patient, but only if the patient is moribund, will not respond to other forms of therapy, and has had tension pneumothorax ruled out. There should be a reasonable chance of helping the patient specifically, such as releasing cardiac tamponade unresponsive to pericardiocentesis attempts, controlling a bleeding point, or cross-clamping the descending thoracic aorta in cases of exsanguinating hemorrhage below the diaphragm.

Generally, emergency thoracotomy is only of utility in penetrating thoracic injury. It is most helpful in myocardial stab wounds with cardiac tamponade in which the tamponade is readily released with pericardial incision and the myocardial lacerations oversewn with silk sutures. Gunshot wounds of the heart are generally less salvageable.

Since thoracotomy is required in only 10 per cent of major thoracic trauma overall, emergency department thoracotomy is not a common procedure in most centers. Intubation and intravenous access are mandatory prior to actual thoracotomy.

ABDOMINAL TRAUMA

Abdominal examination, which must be repeated at intervals, focuses on signs of peritoneal irritation. Absent bowel sounds, progressive distention, the presence of severe tenderness on palpation, rebound tenderness, and guarding are all suggestive of intra-abdominal injury. (However, these are initially absent

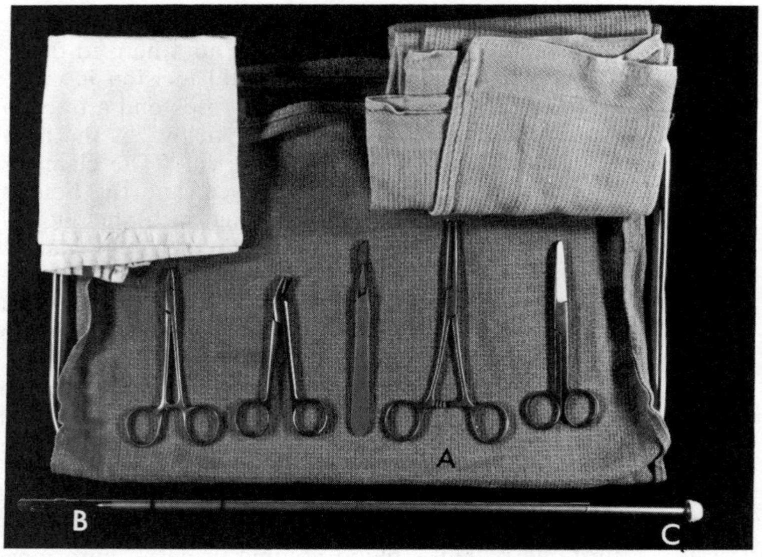

Figure 47–20. Necessary equipment for chest tube insertion, including (*A*) Kelly's clamp, (*B*) chest tube, and (*C*) trocar (optional). Wire suture and petrolatum gauze not shown.

in up to one third of patients with visceral injury.) Abdominal rigidity, involuntary on the part of the patient, is unequivocal evidence of peritoneal irritation, and the presence of rigidity or progressive development of other listed signs mandates laparotomy in the blunt or penetrating trauma victim.

A high index of suspicion is necessary to find abdominal trauma in many patients. The peritoneal cavity can extend up to the fourth intercostal space anteriorly on expiration, and the seventh intercostal space posteriorly, so that blunt or penetrating chest trauma may easily have concomitant abdominal injury. Abdominal visceral injury occurs in stab wounds of the back 7 to 14 per cent of the time and in flank wounds 21 to 44 per cent of the time (Peck and Berne, 1981; Jackson and Thal, 1979).

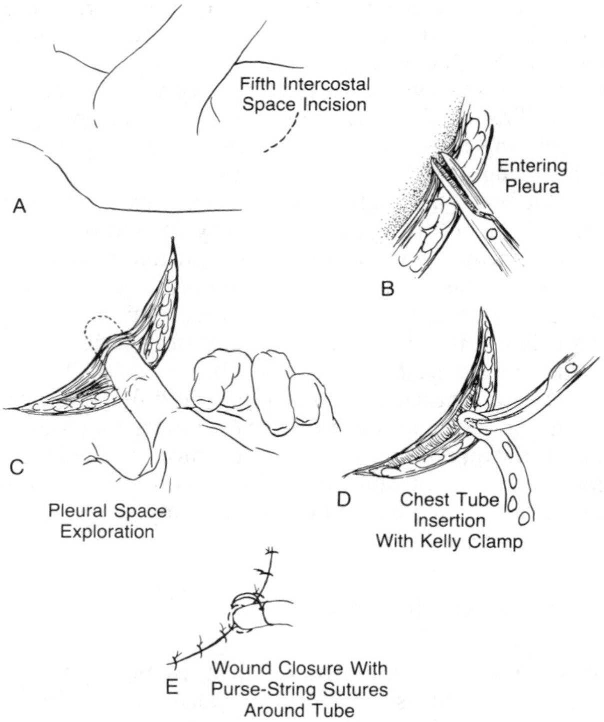

Figure 47–21. The major steps in chest tube insertion. See text for details. After the tube is sutured securely, wrap the wound with petrolatum gauze to decrease air leakage.

Whether the abdomen is penetrated by stab or gunshot wounds (the major etiologies of penetrating trauma) affects the rate of visceral injury. Stab wounds enter the peritoneum in two thirds of victims but cause visceral damage in less than half of these cases. In contrast, gunshot wounds penetrate the peritoneal cavity over 80 per cent of the time and, in those cases, cause an almost 100 per cent rate of visceral injury due both to direct injury and a blast effect (Moore, 1981). Because of these data, there has been little controversy regarding mandatory exploratory laparotomy for a gunshot wound to the abdomen, although if the patient is stable there is an increasing tendency to consider abdominal computerized tomographic scanning (CT scan) prior to surgery to delineate the injuries and any associated retroperitoneal trauma. A negative scan does not rule out hollow visceral injury however; thus, most surgeons would still explore all such patients.

Stab wounds to the abdomen have been managed in a wider variety of ways. Perhaps the commonest means of managing these wounds is by selective observation (often accompanied by CT scan). In the patient with no signs of instability or peritoneal irritation on physical examination, many surgical authors have recommended either local wound exploration under local anesthesia to exclude peritoneal entry or even a stabogram using radiologic contrast media (although this has fallen into a large measure of disuse). To perform a stabogram, contrast medium such as Gastrografin is injected into the stab wound tract under moderate pressure and radiographs taken. Documentation of communication of the wound tract with the peritoneal cavity mandates laparotomy. As mentioned, the approach based on local exploration under anesthesia has more advocates.

Most surgeons, at centers where CT scanning is available, would currently recommend abdominal scans for most abdominal stab wound victims, especially those without instability or local findings suggesting visceral injury, which would mandate rapid laparotomy. CT scanning would demonstrate occult or tamponaded solid visceral trauma or intraperitoneal fluid or blood. Injury to hollow organs might be missed and thus admission and observation, supplemented with lavage, other studies, and even exploration, as appropriate, would still be required, even in the face of a negative scan.

PERITONEAL LAVAGE

If local exploration, CT scanning, or other techniques cannot exclude peritoneal entry or if other indications exist, peritoneal lavage should be performed. Lavage is also useful in instances of blunt trauma in which abdominal findings are equivocal and radiographic studies unrevealing or contraindicated (such as early pregnancy).

Peritoneal lavage is an extremely sensitive technique for the detection of intra-abdominal injury; its overall accuracy is reported to range from 90 to 100 per cent. Prepackaged lavage kits containing anesthetic, drapes, tubing, and multiple-holed trocar-catheters are available commercially.

There are many possible indications for lavage. A trauma victim with an equivocal abdominal exam and hypotension or signs of blood loss not otherwise explained should be considered for lavage. The patient with multiple injuries with altered mental status from any source (including alcohol), the patient with an injured spinal cord, and patients with fractures of the lower ribs or pelvis deserve consideration for lavage. Further indications include the presence of discontiguous injuries or cases in which emergency surgery under general anesthesia is required for nonabdominal injuries to avoid deterioration in the operating suite from unsuspected intraperitoneal injury.

The contraindications to lavage are few. Absolute contraindications include a prior decision to perform laparotomy and a full bladder (always insert a Foley catheter first). Relative contraindications include prior abdominal surgery and midline scars and abdominal wall hematomas (may give a false positive). The presence of a gravid uterus requires using a higher site than usual for lavage but does not absolutely contraindicate the procedure. Some authorities also suggest a higher lavage site in patients with pelvic fracture or hematoma to attempt to decrease false positives.

The increased availability and use of CT scanning in abdominal trauma has led to a more thoughtful and selective approach to peritoneal lavage in recent years but not rendered the procedure obsolete. CT scanning and lavage are best regarded as complimentary techniques in the evaluation of these patients. If CT scanning is performed after lavage, the presence of intra-abdominal fluid from the procedure may suggest hemorrhage and confuse the clinician, thus CT scanning is best performed first if it is readily available and the patient is stable. Prior lavage will not obscure occult solid visceral intraperitoneal injury in the face of a negative lavage. The scan may in addition demonstrate unsuspected retroperitoneal damage that the lavage fails to show or demonstrate intact solid intraperitoneal viscera and the presence of pelvic fracture or hematoma causing falsely positive lavage results. It is important to emphasize that the scan may not reveal injury to hollow organs, such as the gut or bladder, hence positive lavage results of any sort (see below) not explained by the scan will require further study (cystogram, GI studies) or laparotomy, dependent upon clinical context and patient condition.

The reported rates of complication from lavage range from 0.9 to 6.0 per cent (Lazarus and Nelson, 1980). Possible complications include hematomas, separation or infection of the abdominal incision, incisional hernia, vascular lacerations, omental lacerations, and bowel perforations.

The technique of peritoneal lavage (Fig. 47–22) begins with Foley catheterization of the bladder and nasogastric intubation. The area between the umbilicus and pubic symphysis is shaved, prepped with Betadine, and draped. A site in the midline, one third the distance from the umbilicus to the pubis, is anesthetized using lidocaine with epinephrine for hemostasis. A scalpel (no. 11 blade) is used to make a vertical incision several millimeters long through the skin and subcutaneous tissue. The trocar-catheter assembly is introduced into this incision. If awake and cooperative, the patient is asked to tense his or her abdominal musculature. Using two-hand control of the trocar (with one hand at the skin surface to avoid overpenetration of the catheter into the abdomen), pressure is applied until the trocar is felt to pop into the peritoneal cavity. The catheter should slide easily into the cavity; if it does not, extraperitoneal insertion is a possibility. Remove the catheter in this case and re-insert it. Slide the catheter toward the right colic gutter. Once it is in place, gently aspirate with a syringe. A return of 10 ml. of nonclotting blood is a positive test and mandates laparotomy.

If no blood is aspirated, infuse Ringer's lactate through the catheter (20 ml./kg. in children and 1 L in the adult), gently move the patient from side to side, and then allow the fluid to drain by gravity. Pink fluid through which newsprint cannot be read is a positive lavage; there is a 94 per cent chance of finding lesions requiring surgical correction (Parvin et al., 1975).

Aliquots of lavage fluid should be sent for red cell count (RBC), white cell count (WBC), amylase level, and Gram's stain. Greater than 100,000 RBC/

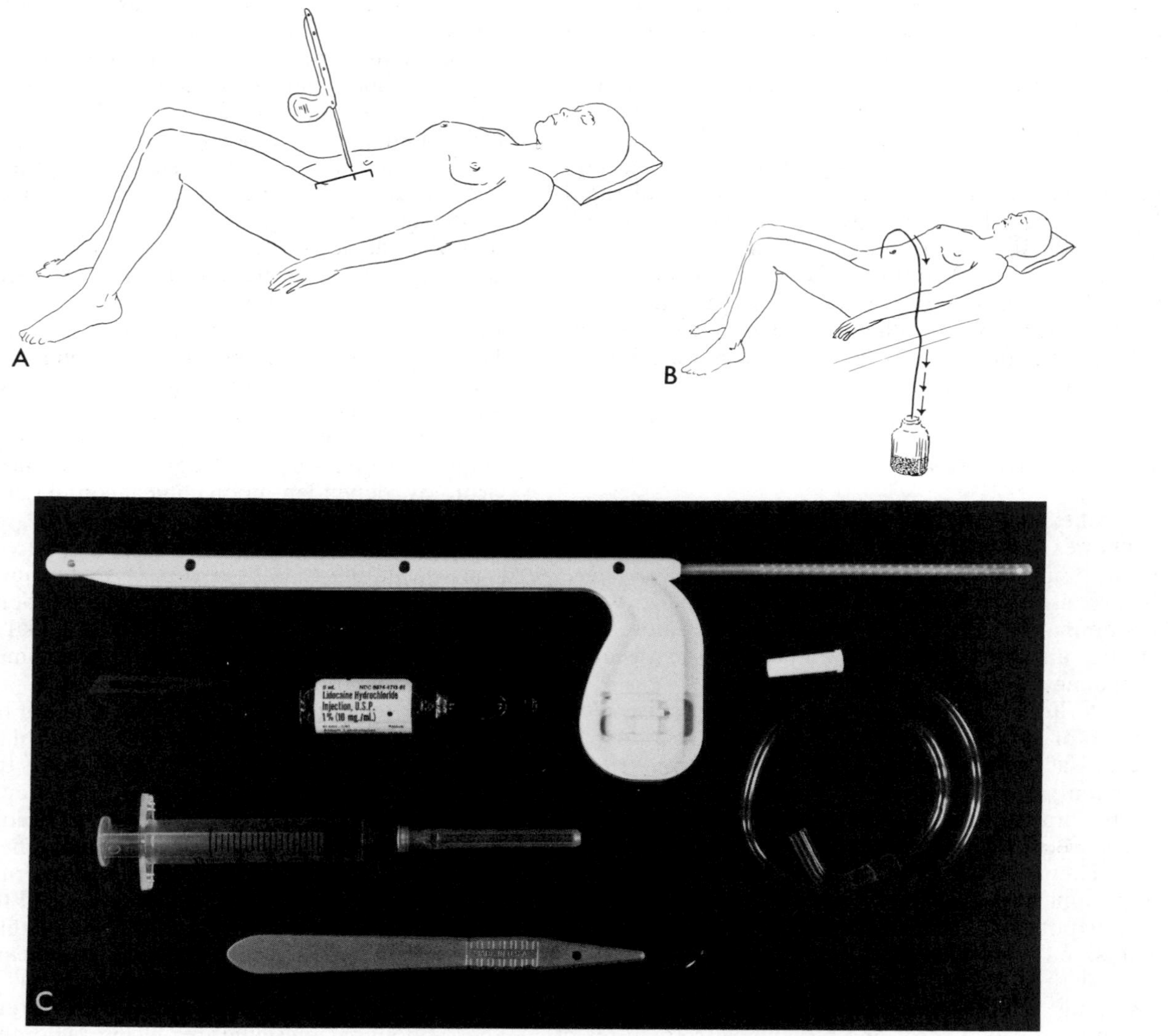

Figure 47–22. Peritoneal lavage. An infraumbilical entry (*A*) with a twisting or cautious pushing motion (if a trocar technique is used) is preferred. After fluid instillation and after the patient is gently shaken, drain the fluid by gravity (*B*). Representative equipment for catheter instillation is shown (*C*).

cubic millimeter in the lavage fluid is an absolute indication for surgical exploration, and it provides an overall diagnostic accuracy of 93 per cent, sensitivity of 91 per cent, specificity of 94 per cent, and a false negative rate of only 4 per cent for stab wounds of the anterior abdominal wall (Thompson et al., 1980). Red cell counts of 50,000 to 100,000 are equivocal, and the decision for laparotomy is individualized and often aided by other studies, such as CT scan. Less than 50,000 red cells requires immediate observation only, unless chest wounds are present. In such patients, as few as 5000 RBCs require surgical intervention. At minimum, a diaphragmatic rent requiring repair will be found (Kessler and Stein, 1971). If tangential gunshot wounds are lavaged, an RBC count of 5000 or more also warrants laparotomy to assess damage to a hollow viscus. Such patients, it should be emphasized, are often helpfully studied by thoracoabdominal CT scanning preoperatively to delineate trauma as fully as possible prior to exploration and repair.

A lavage fluid WBC count of 500/cubic millimeter or higher in blunt abdominal trauma suggests significant intra-abdominal injury; this is not the case in penetrating injury, in which the WBC count is far less useful (Mueller et al., 1981).

A lavage fluid amylase of over 400 units or the presence of bacteria, feces, or bile in the fluid also indicates a positive lavage and mandates laparotomy, with or without further radiographic study as appropriate to the individual case.

Retroperitoneal injury may not be diagnosed by lavage, as already mentioned, including genitourinary tract damage, colon injury, or pancreaticoduodenal trauma. Accordingly, many authorities have suggested aggressive exploration of all back or flank gunshot wounds unless obviously superficial, and a more selective policy is used in stab wound management in these areas. The potential use of CT scanning techniques in both these patient groups is now widely recognized and this modality is used in most stable patients if available. If there is any question as to genitourinary injury, an injected CT scan will be of great utility. If this is unavailable or not desired, or the patient may not be moved to the radiology suite, an infusion urogram may be performed in the emergency department with portable technique, using 1 to 2 ml./kg. of 50 per cent Renografin dye given rapidly intravenously followed by an abdominal flat plate after 5 minutes to see the upper urinary tracts in any case of trauma (even with hypotension this technique is efficacious and usually not associated with subsequent renal failure). Renografin diluted with sterile saline (to a total volume of 250 to 300 ml. in the adult) may also be placed in the bladder via Foley catheter to rule out bladder rupture via flat plate. This will not diagnose urethral injury, however. Urethrography will do so but should be performed in concert with urological consultants. Note that peritoneal lavage fluid may be recovered by Foley catheter in large quantity during the lavage in the face of bladder disruption, and this may be the first or only clue to lower GU injury.

After peritoneal lavage is completed, the catheter is removed, and the abdominal wall is closed with interrupted sutures. Patients with negative lavage may be discharged (rarely), subjected to further study (including CT scanning) as appropriate, and (in most cases) admitted for observation.

SPECIAL SITUATIONS

Falls from Heights

Falls from heights, while not common, are an interesting source of morbidity in the pediatric age group, and in the adult who is intoxicated, suicidal, fleeing the law, or simply unfortunate. Falls are most common in the first three decades of life; males outnumber females at all ages.

In children, the majority of falls occur before age 5, usually from rooftops or windows. Correlates of childhood falls include prior accidents, mental retardation, seizure disorders, minimal brain dysfunction with hyperactivity, low socioeconomic status, and parental neglect. Because of the relatively large size of the young child's head compared to the adult, a child's center of mass is quite high; children tend to land on their heads, and there is a high incidence of skull and upper extremity fracture. In falls over three stories, 70 per cent of children will suffer skull fracture (Smith et al., 1975). Despite this, in large series of falls in children, cervical spine injury is quite rare, as is spinal cord damage, although this must always be ruled out. Also uncommon are lower extremity or pelvic fracture, rib fracture, or pulmonary contusion.

Falls from heights in adults carry about a 20 per cent mortality rate overall. Lower extremity fractures are common; all bones may be fractured. Upper extremity fractures are next most common, followed by skull, face, vertebral, and lastly pelvic (usually pubic ramus) fracture. Vertebral fractures occur at the thoracolumbar junction 85 to 90 per cent of the time due to the lordosis-to-kyphosis transition and subsequently concentrated forces at this point. Lumbar fractures occur in 60 per cent of cases. Neurologic dysfunction is rare, however.

Associated visceral injury occurs in about 20 per cent of fall victims. Thoracic injury is more frequent than abdominal or genitourinary injury; all must be excluded. Visceral, skull, or pelvic trauma increases mortality rate; with six skeletal injuries or more, plus a visceral injury, the mortality approaches 100 per cent.

Classically, adults who fall are said to land on their heels, bend over, and brace themselves with their hands, leading to a classic fracture triad: calcanei, thoracolumbar spine, and radii. Like most classic patterns, this is quite uncommon, but all these sites must be evaluated.

Bicycle Injury

Bicycle-related injury is usually a pediatric entity; in most cases, motor vehicles are not involved. Often these injuries occur in the context of misuse of the vehicle, including doubling up to ride. Frequently injuries occur on the first ride, when ignorance of risk is greatest.

Bicycle-spoke-induced injuries are seen in very young children (predominantly 2½ to 4 years old) most often. Usually the child sits behind an older sibling or parent and the foot and ankle are caught in between the spokes. This induces a variety of injuries, ranging from contusions and lacerations to hematomas and fractures.

As the child adducts his thighs, the foot is caught in a slight inversion between the spokes, and pulled forward until the lateral side of the foot reaches the vertical rod of the cycle frame. The ankle is crushed against the rod. If wheel motion continues, the ankle is angulated into varus against the rod, resulting in fracture of the distal tibia and fibula, oblique in nature with a varus deformation. Other spoke fractures have been reported, including phalangeal fractures of toes and spiral tibia fractures.

The soft tissue injury to the ankle has a high incidence of necrosis with the need for subsequent skin grafting, especially if parents delay seeking treatment.

Of all injuries to bicyclists, 70 per cent are caused by falls (Graz, 1979). If the cyclist stops short, he may be thrown forward, and bicycle handlebars are an important source of blunt trauma inflicted in the pediatric age groups.

Wringer Injury

Wringer-type injury may be seen in children who put their hands between the rollers of older washing machines still in use. More commonly, adults will present with such an injury from an industrial accident, since mechanical devices using rollers or other rotating surfaces produce a similar shearing and compressive injury.

The initial appearance of a wringer injury may be very benign. However, three major types of force have injured tissue, and injuries may be clinically manifest after some delay: compressive force leads to soft tissue edema with potential loss of vascular supply due to a compartment syndrome; frictional force generates heat and may lead to full-thickness burns; shearing force can separate the dermis from deeper tissue and cause a delayed necrosis. Severe injury to hands and fingers with permanent functional loss or amputation is not uncommon.

About half the wringer-type injuries seen will have some significant complication. Commonest are soft-tissue injuries, ranging from abrasion to full-thickness skin loss. Fractures or dislocations of phalanges may be present, but long bones are usually spared. Peripheral nerve injuries are common but usually incomplete and temporary.

The wringer injury's severity is classically difficult to assess in its early stage. Edema may not be maximal for a day, deep burns may not be clinically obvious for 48 hours, and devascularization may be relatively inapparent for up to a week.

Initial evaluation of wringer injury includes determination of presence of edema and neurovascular status. Search for fractures and dislocations. Good wound care should be performed but lacerations should not be primarily closed until it is clear from history and examination that the injury is trivial, as these are really burst and crush injuries of uncertain viability.

Treatment is expectant in these injuries: elevate and follow neurovascular status; a soft compression dressing and elevation using stockinette and an I.V. pole are good maneuvers. Most physicians advise that all patients with wringer injury, regardless of initial physical examination, be admitted to the hospital for 24 hours for elevation and observation, unless the duration and extent of injury are clearly trivial by history. Evidence of progressive neurovascular deterioration mandates fasciotomy.

Grease-Gun Injury (High-Pressure Injections)

High-pressure injection injuries generally occur in young people in the workplace. Typically, a worker's paint gun malfunctions, and he wipes it with the nondominant hand, usually the index finger. He presents, after receiving an inadvertent injection, with a pinpoint injection site and a digit that is not especially swollen or painful. A nearly normal range of motion will be present. If an aggressive approach is not undertaken immediately, within several hours the digit, hand, and even the arm, will become dramatically swollen, tender, and exquisitely painful. Skin and subcutaneous tissue necrosis are well established at 4 hours, and considerable functional loss may be expected due to the delay if more than 12 hours have passed.

The commonest substances injected are grease, paint, and solvents. The last is the most inflammatory, while the first has a higher frequency of delayed hand abscesses and residual fibrosis.

The etiology of necrosis and gangrene of digits in these injuries involves the direct toxic effects of solvents and the associated thrombosis of arteries and/or veins in digits. Neurovascular compression due to the injection into a closed space also occurs. Many solvents have a directly toxic effect on digital nerves, causing hypesthesia and making the early wound deceptively pain free. Thus, the surgical management involves extensive tissue decompression and debridement of all foreign material and necrotic debris as rapidly as possible.

The spread of injected material is a function of injection pressure, the tissues struck, and the viscosity of the substance injected. While thick greases are usually stopped at the retinacula of the wrist, solvents may track up even into the proximal forearm, requiring extensive surgery.

The initial history obtained from these patients should include hand dominance, occupation, material injected, time and pressure of injection, any previous therapy, and circumstances of the injury. Determine the motor and sensory status of the injured extremity, and the vascular status. Do not at any time give local anesthesia for pain relief. At best this wastes time, and by increasing tissue pressure it may worsen necrosis.

Many injected materials will be radiopaque. Obtain x-ray studies of the injured extremity to assess extent of spread of the injection. These patients must be told of the serious nature of their innocuous-looking injury at once and rapidly referred to a hand surgeon. Wide decompression and debridement are usually required, and often the wounds must be left open for copious irrigation and further debridement. Elevation, antibiotics, steroids, and tetanus toxoid are important adjuncts. Prolonged disability and slow healing are common with these injuries, which require prolonged follow-up and intense rehabilitative efforts.

Fishhooks (and Other Impalements)

Impalement, especially of the hand, by fishhooks is common in warm months. If the hook is caught in the soft fleshy part of the skin, with the point tenting up, the area should be anesthetized (either locally or by digital block in the finger), the hook pushed gently through and the barb cut off; the shaft may be withdrawn then without further tissue damage. Antibiotics, tetanus toxoid, and observation thereafter are appropriate.

If the hook is pointing toward deeper structures, one can insert an 18-gauge needle adjacent to the barb so its bevelled open end fits over the barb; the needle and hook are then backed out together (Fig. 47–23).

Thermal Injury and Exposure

BURNS AND SMOKE INHALATION

Most burn injuries are minor and manageable by the family physician with no need for consultation. About 90 per cent of burns are due to thermal injuries (flame, scalds, and so on). Chemical burns and electrical burns, while uncommon, deserve special attention regarding management.

Burns are extremely common injuries; between 2 and 3 million people per year are burned in the United States seriously enough to need medical attention. About 12,000 people per year die from their burns or their complications; scores of thousands are partially or totally disabled for various periods and require expensive, extensive care, usually in highly specialized regional burn centers.

The epidermis, or outer layer of the skin, acts as a barrier to entry of bacteria and egress of moisture and electrolytes; these functions are lost in the area of a burn wound. The stratum germinativum, or germinal layer of the epidermis, provides cellular replacement for elements that are constantly being shed during normal skin growth.

Below the epidermis lies the dermis, the deeper layer of skin within which lay nerve endings, blood vessels, collagen, elastin fibers, and other elements, of which hair follicles and sweat glands are of particular importance in burn repair. Hair follicles and sweat glands have epidermal linings, which permit regeneration of epithelium for resurfacing of second-degree burns (see below).

Burns are either first-, second-, or third-degree at any point. First-degree burns are red, hypersensitive, warm, tender, painful, and often swollen. There is no blistering. Usually, healing is spontaneous within

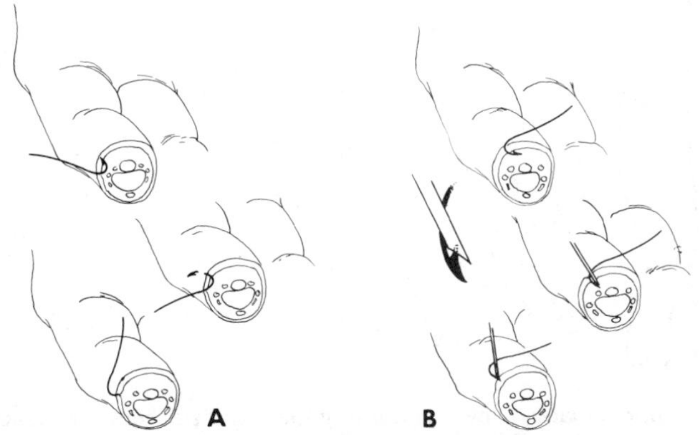

Figure 47–23. Techniques of fishhook extraction. Either push the barb through and cut it off (*A*) or cover the barb with the bevel of a hypodermic needle and extract the two together (*B*).

about 1 week, with some measure of desquamation of damaged skin. The classical sunburn is an example of such a burn.

Second-degree burns have some measure of blister formation. The entire epidermis is destroyed, but the dermis with its follicles, sweat glands, and other structures remains intact, permitting spontaneous repair. Healing usually requires 2 to 3 weeks, unless secondary trauma and/or invasive infection cause further tissue destruction.

Third-degree burns cause total skin necrosis. Since the dermal structures (including nerves) are destroyed, this burn is hard, thick, and entirely anesthetic. No spontaneous regeneration is possible; skin grafts will be needed for eventual repair except in the most trivial cases.

The Rule of Nines is used to estimate the surface area of a cutaneous burn. In the adult, the surface of the body is divided into areas that are a multiple of 9 per cent; this is altered somewhat in the child because of the large size of the head in relation to the lower extremities so that percentages in these areas are age dependent (Fig. 47–24).

Another useful guideline is to note the area of the patient's palm; this represents about 1 per cent of the bodily surface area and can be used to estimate (very roughly) the extent of irregular burns in a hurried situation.

Second-degree burns of greater than 15 per cent or third-degree burns of more than 5 per cent in the adult should initially be treated in the hospital. Much more liberal policies should be followed in small children because of the added difficulty of burn toilet and protection. In addition, the possibility of child abuse should be kept in mind in examining all burned children. Punctate burns, such as those inflicted by cigarettes, burns of the diaper area or genitalia, or any situation in which parental attitude or history do not seem to fit clinical circumstance should prompt the consideration of protective admission to the hospital.

Small burns can be effectively treated on an outpatient basis with analgesics and topical therapy. When seen initially, the burn should be treated with cold compresses for 15 to 20 minutes to stop further destruction of tissue. Bullae should be left intact, but any loose dead tissue or debris should be gently but thoroughly debrided.

There is no place for butter, petroleum jelly, or other creams in the initial therapy of the burned patient, at home or in the office. After cooling and debridement, a topical antibiotic preparation is applied to second- or third-degree burns (not necessary in first-degree cases). Silvadene (silver sulfadiazene) cream is most commonly used; it is quite efficacious in the prevention of early burn wound sepsis. Early burn wound infection is most often due to streptococci; sebum is streptococcicidal, but this property is lost when serum leaks into the burn wound (Robson et al., 1979). Other antibiotics in use include sulfamylon (mafenide acetate), betadine ointment, silver nitrate, and other newer agents.

Area	Age — Years					% 2°	% 3°	% Total
	0-1	1-4	5-9	10-15	Adults			
Head	19	17	13	10	7			
Neck	2	2	2	2	2			
Ant. Trunk	13	17	13	13	13			
Post. Trunk	13	13	13	13	13			
R. Buttock	2½	2½	2½	2½	2½			
L. Buttock	2½	2½	2½	2½	2½			
Genitallia	1	1	1	1	1			
R. U. Arm	4	4	4	4	4			
L. U. Arm	4	4	4	4	4			
R. L. Arm	3	3	3	3	3			
L. L. Arm	3	3	3	3	3			
R. Hand	2½	2½	2½	2½	2½			
L. Hand	2½	2½	2½	2½	2½			
R. Thigh	5½	6½	8½	8½	9½			
L. Thigh	5½	6½	8½	8½	9½			
R. Leg	5	5	5½	6	7			
L. Leg	5	5	5½	6	7			
R. Foot	3½	3½	3½	3½	3½			
L. Foot	3½	3½	3½	3½	3½			
				Total				

Rule of Nines

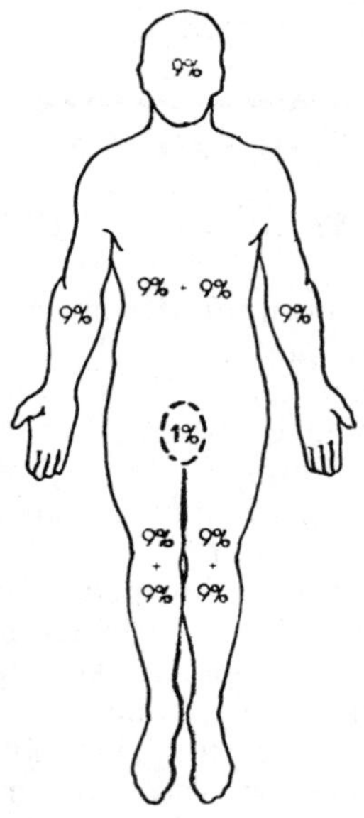

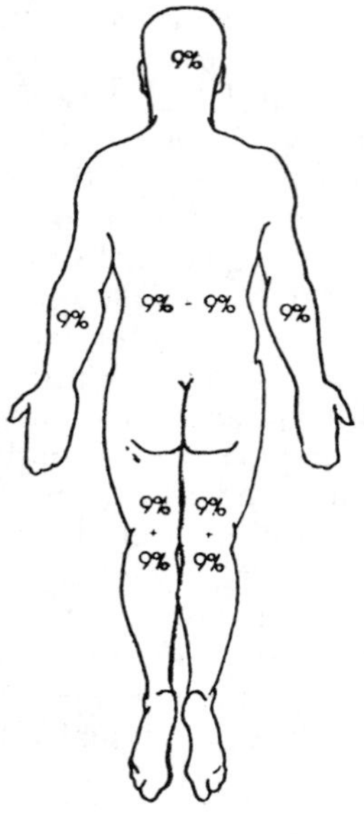

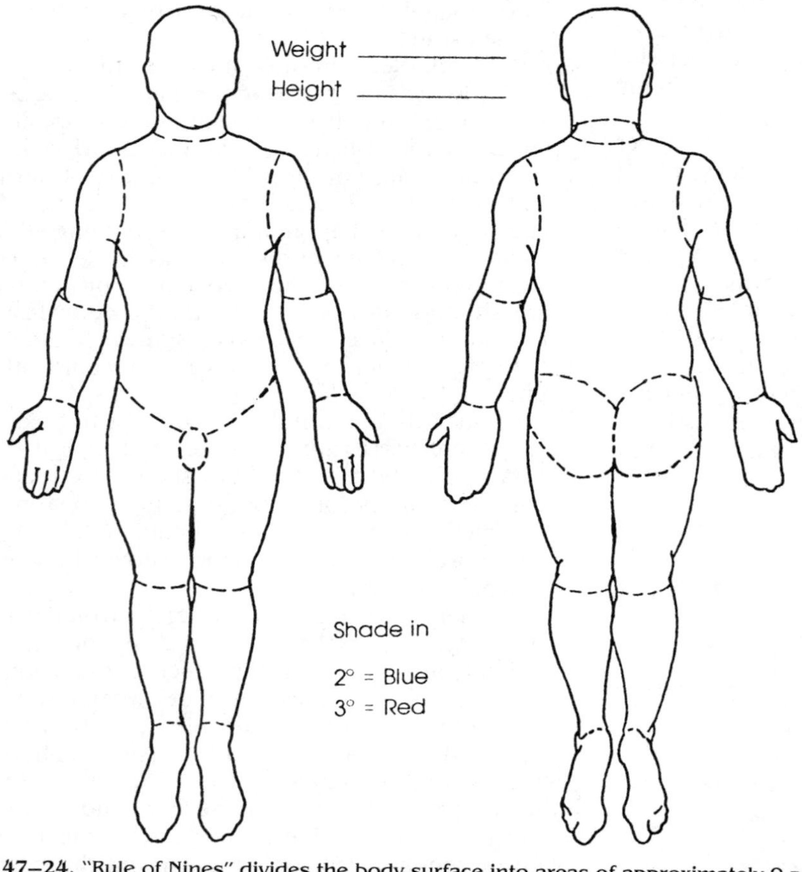

Figure 47–24. "Rule of Nines" divides the body surface into areas of approximately 9 per cent or multiples of 9 per cent; the head and neck and an upper extremity each represents 9 per cent; a lower extremity and the front and back of the torso represents 18 per cent; the perineum 1 per cent. This method of estimation is sufficiently accurate for emergency situations. It is modified in children from birth to 1 year of age to allow 19 per cent for the head and neck and 13 per cent for each lower extremity. One per cent is subtracted from the head and neck and added to the lower extremities for each year from ages 1 to 10. (From Dimick, A. R.: Emergency treatment of extensive burns. Current Topics II in Emergency Medicine, *1*(7). Philadelphia, Medical College of Pennsylvania, 1982.)

Even if burns are not extensive in terms of body surface involvement, admission to the hospital is still advisable if extensive involvement of highly functional or dirty areas is present. This includes the hands, feet, perineal area and genitalia, face and neck, eyes, and ears. Burn toilet in all these areas is of paramount importance.

After topical antibiotic therapy is applied, a nonadherent dressing is applied, using either Telfa or petrolatum gauze followed by a gauze wrap. Dressings are usually changed daily; it is wise for the physician to observe the burn daily at the start even with the most motivated patients. Further debridement or whirlpool treatments may be needed for good toilet, and early infection must be aborted. Analgesia and elevation and tetanus immunization will complete the outpatient regimen. When the physician feels comfortable with it, home care is entirely plausible with the motivated patient.

A systematic and thorough regimen is required to deal with more extensively burned patients. In severely burned patients, there is a generalized increase in capillary permeability throughout the body, leading to fluid loss into extravascular spaces and a state of hypovolemia, possibly with shock. This lasts about 24 hours and must be aggressively managed with fluid resuscitation.

Generally, central venous pressure and urinary output should be closely monitored. Intravenous lines may be started through burned skin but only if absolutely necessary. One useful formula to estimate volume requirements is: 2 to 4 ml. Ringer's lactate × percentage of burn × weight in kilograms, to be infused over 24 hours. The first half of this volume should be given in the first 8 hours postburn; the remainder, in the next 16 hours.

Seriously burned patients may incur a variety of other problems, including respiratory injury (see below), chest or extremity constriction from circumferential burns, myoglobinuria or hemoglobinuria with secondary renal failure, ileus with vomiting and aspiration, and fractures or other trauma if the burn occurred in association with an explosion or fall (the history must search for associated sources of injury). Table 47–26 summarizes the management of the more extensively burned patient.

Chemical burns occur from strong acids or alkalis. The thrust of therapy is removal of the caustic, usually by diluting with water, as quickly and thoroughly as possible. All contaminated clothing must be removed. In general, chemical neutralization is contraindicated. The heat generated only increases tissue damage, and searching for antidotes wastes valuable time.

Acids cause coagulative necrosis, and the damage they produce is generally more superficial than that produced by strong bases, which produce a liquefaction necrosis. Base burns can be quite deep and progressive if all the offending material is not adequately removed.

Eye exposure to caustics demands extensive irrigation with water, beginning immediately and continuing en route to the hospital. An ophthalmologist should be consulted.

TABLE 47–26. MANAGING EXTENSIVE BURNS

1. Assure airway control. Intubate for suspected or definite airway edema. Provide supplemental oxygen.
2. Apply dry sterile dressings. Insulate with blankets to minimize heat loss. Avoid cold compresses with attendant risk of hypothermia and frostbite.
3. Aggressive volume resuscitation is necessary, owing to increased capillary permeability over the first 24 to 48 hours. Ringer's lactate may be given, in a dose of 4 ml./kg. body weight/burn percentage. Follow central venous pressure and urinary output.
4. Paralytic ileus is common. Decompress the stomach via nasogastric tube.
5. Give tetanus toxoid and hyperimmune globulin for prophylaxis.
6. Don't miss other injuries, particularly if the history suggests blunt trauma, a fall, smoke inhalation, and so on.
7. Analgesia should be given intravenously in small doses. Morphine in small aliquots is the drug of choice.
8. Avoid topical creams prior to transfer to a burn facility.
9. Perform escharotomy for respiratory or neurovascular extremity compromise.

Do not irrigate dry chemicals off the body surface with water; they should be brushed off.

Exposure to hydrofluoric acid requires subcutaneous injection of calcium salts into the affected area in addition to irrigation, to minimize the deep progressive necrosis that otherwise results.

Smoke inhalation produces most of the morbidity and mortality in fires. Heated gases can lead to direct upper airway damage with edema and airway obstruction. In addition, smoke is a poisonous, noxious mixture of variable composition, dependent upon the material burning. Wood fires produce a large amount of carbon monoxide. The plastic polymers in many homes, when burned, can liberate a variety of noxious gases, including hydrochloric acid, nitric acid, sulfuric acid, and hydrogen cyanide. These agents can produce severe airway and alveolar damage and systemic poisoning.

Pulmonary damage due to smoke inhalation seems to evolve in three distinct stages. During the first 24 hours, bronchospasm, alveolar damage, and disrupted alveolocapillary membranes cause acute ventilatory insufficiency. This leads to a second stage of noncardiogenic pulmonary edema. After about 72 hours, with loss of local defenses, a final pneumonitis due to secondary infection may occur. Often these patients succumb.

The diagnosis of smoke inhalation requires a high index of suspicion. Was the patient exposed to smoke or flames in a confined space? Did the patient lose consciousness? Was the victim in an electrical fire, a steam explosion, or a natural gas explosion? All these historical factors increase the patient's risk.

Several findings on physical examination are presumptive of smoke inhalation. Note should be made of cyanosis, respiratory distress, obtundation, singed nasal or facial hair, burns of the face or pharynx, rales or rhonchi, wheezes, and production of soot-stained sputum.

Victims of smoke inhalation require intensive management. Oxygen should be provided, with adequate humidification. Intubation may be needed in victims with upper airway burns and to facilitate good pulmonary toilet with suctioning. Bronchospasm will respond to aminophylline in the usual dose range. Serial blood gases, including carboxyhemoglobin levels, are required for optimal management.

Chest x-rays are often normal in the early phases of smoke inhalation, and roentgen findings may lag behind the clinical picture by 24 to 48 hours.

All victims of smoke inhalation require an electrocardiogram; myocardial infarction and arrhythmias are not uncommon, especially in the older patient, owing to hypoxia.

Severely affected patients uniformly deserve admission to either an intensive care setting or a burn unit.

At this time, there is no role for steroids or prophylactic antibiotics in the smoke inhalation victim.

HEAT-INDUCED ILLNESS

Three forms of systemic heat-induced illness are generally recognized: heat cramps, heat exhaustion, and heat stroke.

Heat cramps are the most benign and easily treated form of heat illness. After a period of exertion, patients experience painful cramps of utilized muscles, due either to a transmembrane imbalance of sodium and potassium or to the unopposed effect of calcium in the presence of salt depletion. The cramps respond to rest in a cool environment and to salt replacement orally.

Heat exhaustion is a more profound clinical syndrome, occurring in either a salt-depletion form (in which the patients have ingested free water) or a water-depletion form (Table 47–27). Both types of patients complain of weakness, fatigue, nausea, and lightheadedness. The water-depletion form of heat exhaustion is more likely to present with fever and more profound alterations of sensorium. This subset of patients may proceed to frank heat stroke.

TABLE 47–27. HEAT EXHAUSTION

	Salt-Depletion Type	Water-Depletion Type
Sweat losses	+ + + +	+ + + +
Water repletion	+	−
Still sweating	+	+
Hypotension	+	+ + +
Cramps	+	−
Neurologic symptoms	+	+ + +
Temperature	Normal	100–103° F.
Leads to heat stroke	+/−	+ +
Nausea/vomiting	+	+
Serum sodium	+/−	+/−
Respiratory alkalosis	+	+

TABLE 47–28. HEAT STROKE

	Exertional Type	Sedentary Type
Core temperature	105+°F.	105+°F.
Neurologic symptoms	+ + + +	+ + + +
Anhidrosis	+	+/−
Patient type	Young healthy athlete	Old; complicating drugs or diseases; rarely infants

Patients with either form of heat exhaustion usually respond rapidly to removal from the hot environment and to appropriate salt and water replacement as dictated by their mental status. There are no sequelae.

Heat stroke is a true medical emergency, with a mortality rate reported in the literature varying from 10 to 80 per cent. Two forms of heat stroke exist (Table 47–28), but both are characterized by a core temperature of 105°F. or greater, profound neuropsychiatric symptoms, and, in most cases, anhidrosis. The exertional type of heat stroke usually involves the young, healthy athlete, while the sedentary form involves older, usually chronically ill patients, or, on rare occasions, the swaddled infant with a cold and fever.

The development of heat stroke is more likely on hot, still, humid days, when heat dissipation to the environment is limited to losses via sweating. Increased metabolic rate or increased mechanical work will increase heat generation and further predispose to a marked rise in core temperature.

Many organ systems are deranged in acute heat stroke, but the cardiovascular consequences are often the most profound. Acute circulatory failure causes death in over 80 per cent of heat stroke fatalities. Elderly patients are often hypovolemic, with hypotension and a low central venous pressure. The young patient is usually hyperdynamic, with a high cardiac output and low or normal CVP. On rare occasions, a hypodynamic response occurs, with hypotension, low cardiac output, and an elevated CVP. This may be due to direct thermal toxicity to the myocardium and/or increased pulmonary vascular resistance with right ventricular overload. Intravenous isoproterenol (1 to 4 μg./minute) dramatically improves the hemodynamic picture in this subset of patients. Myocardial ischemia or infarction must be ruled out in most of these patients, particularly when they are elderly.

The pulmonary effects of heat stroke include respiratory alkalosis, a high incidence of pneumonia due to aspiration, and a spurious effect on arterial blood gases (Table 47–29).

Mental status changes, seizures, ataxia, and residual mental retardation in children are common central nervous system effects of heat stroke.

Acute renal failure occurs in up to 30 per cent

TABLE 47–29. VARIANCE OF BLOOD GASES WITH BODY TEMPERATURE*

	↑ 1°C.	↓ 1°C.
pH	↓ .015	↑ .015
Pco_2 (mm. Hg)	↑ 4.4%	↓ 4.4%
Po_2 (mm. Hg)	↑ 7.2%	↓ 7.2%

*Departures from values at 37° C.

of cases of heat stroke. Rhabdomyolysis with myoglobinuria is not uncommon, owing to pressure necrosis of muscles, hypokalemia, relative hypoxia, and direct thermal toxicity to muscle. Intravascular hemolysis and hemoglobinuria may also lead to acute tubular necrosis. Hypoxia, thrombosis, parenchymal hemorrhage, vasoconstriction, direct thermal injury, and hyperuricemia have all been postulated as contributing factors to acute renal failure in heat stroke patients. Urinary output and renal function must be closely followed.

Bleeding diatheses, while rare, can occur in the patient with heat stroke and should be sought by appropriate studies.

The thrust of managing heat stroke involves use of standard techniques of CPCR, rapid cooling, and CVP monitoring. Table 47–30 summarizes management concepts.

Many rapid cooling techniques have been used in heat stroke patients (Table 47–31). Monitor the core temperature (rectal or esophageal probe) continuously. Ice packs placed in pivotal spots of arterial flow are probably the method of choice for temperature reduction. Ice baths are inconvenient and hinder resuscitative efforts. Core temperature should be lowered to nearly normal within 1 hour. Stop actively cooling the patient when the core temperature reaches 102°F. to avoid an overshoot into systemic hypothermia.

Education of the public in avoiding unnecessary heat stress, use of appropriate clothing and fluid intake, and awareness of the effects of alcohol and various drugs on heat dissipation will markedly decrease the risk of systemic heat illness.

Table 47–30. MANAGEMENT OF HEAT STROKE

ABC still applies
Rapid cooling
Oxygen
CVP monitoring
Volume challenge for hypotension
Isuprel (1 μg./min.) for hypodynamic state
Foley catheterization
Steroids, antibiotics, anticonvulsants only for specific indications
Search for organ dysfunction, bleeding diathesis, precipitating illness
Prophylaxis for G.I. bleeding

TABLE 47–31. RAPID COOLING TECHNIQUES IN HEAT STROKE

Ice bath or hypothermia blanket
  Both can raise core temperature, cause shivering, discomfort
  Bath hinders CPR
Ice packs to pivotal spots
  Neck, axillae, groin, perhaps trunk with or without massage
Ice gastric lavage
Cool water/breeze/exposure method (used in Middle East)
Hypothermic fluids (like I.V. infusions at room temperature)
Thorazine, aspirin, Tylenol—not useful
Stop at core temperature (continuously monitored) of 102° F. to avoid overshoot
Get core temperature to near normal within 1 hour

COLD-INDUCED ILLNESS

Cold-induced injury may be local in nature (frostbite, chilblains, immersion injury) or systemic (hypothermia).

Frostbite injury may be thought of as superficial or deep. Superficially, frostbitten tissue appears white and waxy acutely and with thawing becomes mildly edematous and vesiculated. Eventually, the damaged area peels to reveal pink, somewhat cold-sensitive skin. Deep frostbite, a more severe injury, also looks white, waxy, and hard prior to thawing. With thawing, either the part remains cold and hard (an ominous sign of possible full-thickness tissue death), or massive swelling, large hemorrhagic bullae, and later a black dry eschar will form. Healing or mummification follows over subsequent weeks. In general, the depth of tissue injury, and tissue viability, cannot be determined acutely in frostbite injury. This mandates a conservative approach to therapy, surgery being reserved only for uncontrolled secondary infection of injured tissue.

Frostbite generally affects areas of end-arterial flow, especially the hands, face, and feet. Cold exposure produces reflex arteriolar spasm with cessation of capillary blood flow. Ice crystallization in the intercellular extravascular space causes osmotic changes in interstitial fluid. Movement of water out of cells to maintain osmotic equilibrium is felt to produce intracellular dehydration and enzymatic dysfunction and lead to cell death. Only in the most severe cases does actual freezing of deep tissue occur. Nerves, blood vessels, and muscles are the most easily damaged tissues.

Table 47–32 summarizes the treatment of frostbite. The affected part should never be rubbed. This only adds mechanical damage to thermal damage. The part should never be rewarmed in the cold. Hikers have walked to safety on frozen feet but have been incapacitated by pain when rewarmed in the cold. Subsequent refreezing is even more damaging.

Rapid rewarming is the method of choice in treating a frostbitten part, but a point source of heat

TABLE 47–32. TREATMENT OF FROSTBITE

Never rewarm outdoors or away from medical aid
No tobacco or alcohol
Rapid rewarming method of choice
Never rub
Keep warm, dry, open, or loosely dressed
Gentle cleansing, whirlpools, P.T., no early surgery
Leave bullae intact
Tetanus prophylaxis
Prevention with education and awareness of symptoms
Most cases heal without surgery, the worst in 6 to 12 months

should never be used, as anesthesia of the part may predispose to superimposed thermal burns. The part should be immersed for 20 minutes in a large vessel of water kept at 108 to 112°F. (42 to 44°C.). As thawing occurs, potent analgesia will usually be needed.

After rewarming, frostbitten digits should be left open to the air or loosely dressed, and physical therapy and gentle cleansing utilized. Tetanus prophylaxis is mandatory. Bullae should not be debrided. Most cases of frostbite either heal or mummify without surgery, although the worst cases can require 6 to 12 months for healing.

Patient education regarding exposure protection and the early symptoms of frostbite (loss of discomfort in the cold, hardness and coldness of a distal part) is of paramount importance. Patients who have been frostbitten in the past are more prone to recurrent cold injury in the affected part.

The sequelae of frostbite include paresthesias, vasospasm on exposure to cold, periarticular osteoporosis in adults, and loss of epiphyseal growth centers in children. Thin skin, hyperhidrosis, loss of skin appendages, and chronic pain may also be seen.

Systemic hypothermia is defined as a core temperature less than 95°F. (35°C.). This definition is utilized because metabolic heat production in response to cold stress peaks at a core temperature of 95°F. and falls off at lower temperatures, leading to a progressive clinical syndrome.

A variety of clinical settings predisposes individuals to hypothermia (Table 47–33). Elderly patients, neonates, patients who are obtunded or physically immobile, those who are intoxicated or on agents that impair heat generation, and those who become exhausted and glycogen-depleted in the cold are all at increased risk for developing hypothermia if cold stressed.

The major determinant of mortality in hypothermia is the presence and severity of associated disease states. Reported mortality rates in large series of patients range from 10 to 80 per cent. Only in myxedema coma is the depression of core temperature related per se to mortality.

Cardiovascular and neurologic consequences of hypothermia are often profound. Progressive bradycardia develops, and all intervals lengthen on the electrocardiogram. Diffuse T-wave inversion may occur. Distension of the atria may lead to atrial flutter or fibrillation. Although gross shivering may have ceased, fine muscular tremor may be apparent on the cardiogram. Osborne waves (Fig. 47–25) are pathognomonic.

By a core temperature of 77°F. (25°C.), hypotension develops. At 82°F. (28°C.) the ventricular myocardium becomes irritable, and minimal stimulation of the patient can induce ventricular fibrillation. This sensitivity peaks at 77 to 70°F. (25 to 21°C.). Below 70°F., asystole may supervene.

There is a 7 per cent decrease in cerebral blood flow for each 1°C. decrease in core temperature. Mentation progressively deteriorates. The pupils are dilated and fixed at 84°F. (30°C.) and below. The electroencephalogram is flat at 66°F. (20°C.) and below.

Clearly, profound hypothermia may simulate death. However, the severely hypothermic patient is relatively protected from hypoxia, hypotension, and circulatory arrest, and prolonged resuscitative efforts are justified as complete neurologic and medical recovery can occur, particularly in the young and previously healthy patient. Therefore, "NO ONE IS DEAD UNTIL HE OR SHE IS WARM AND DEAD."

A variety of other organ dysfunctions occur in the hypothermic patient. Respiration may be compromised by aspiration and a cold-induced bronchorrhea with markedly increased tracheobronchial secretions. Hemoconcentration occurs, owing to fluid shifts into interstitial spaces. Ileus is common below 93°F. (34°C.). Hepatic function decreases progressively, producing more pronounced and/or prolonged effects from administered drugs dependent on hepatic degradation. In some patients, pancreatitis with pancreatic necrosis has been reported.

Renal blood flow and glomerular filtration rate fall with decreasing core temperature. However, in

TABLE 47–33. CLINICAL SETTINGS FOR HYPOTHERMIA

1. Exposure
2. Drugs
   a. Alcohol
   b. Barbiturates
   c. Phenothiazines
3. Endocrinopathies
   a. Hypoglycemia
   b. Diabetic ketoacidosis
   c. Myxedema
   d. Hypoadrenalism
   e. Panhypopituitarism
4. Central nervous system dysfunction
   a. Wernicke's encephalopathy
   b. Anorexia nervosa
   c. Cerebrovascular disease
   d. Head trauma
   e. Spinal cord transection
5. Sepsis
6. Malnutrition
7. Skin dysfunction—burns, erythrodermas

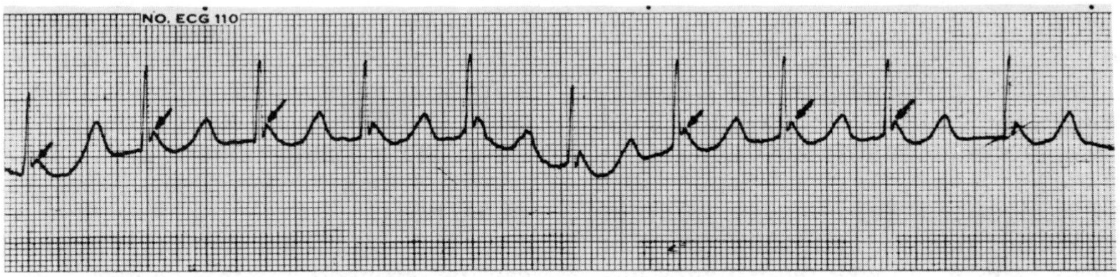

Figure 47–25. Osborne waves (←) in an 80-year-old male with core temperature 86° F. (30° C.). These waves disappeared with rewarming.

patients who become hypothermic over days, volume depletion may occur, because a temperature-dependent decrease in enzymatic function in the distal renal tubules can lead to salt and water loss, a so-called cold diuresis.

Glucose utilization is impaired in hypothermic patients, and hyperglycemia is not uncommon. The potent nature of insulin in the presence of decreased hepatic function and the possibility of hypovolemia should be kept in mind, however. Only extreme hyperglycemia should be actively treated.

Table 47–34 summarizes the therapeutic approach to systemic hypothermia. Passive rewarming by removal from cold stress and the application of blankets is safe and efficacious in the mildly hypothermic patient. In extreme cases, core rewarming via such methods as gastrointestinal irrigation with hot fluids, dialysis, extracorporeal blood rewarming, and even thoracotomy with mediastinal lavage (if intractable ventricular fibrillation occurs) have been advocated.

Some controversy exists regarding active external rewarming methods such as immersion in hot water, electric blanket use, and so on. These methods are probably safest in young, mildly hypothermic cases (where they are least needed). In more severe cases, they may make the patient inaccessible for CPCR, cause vasodilatation and shock in volume-depleted patients, burn the patient, and even suppress endogenous heat production by neural reflexes. In addition, in theory, vasodilation may shunt cold peripheral blood back to the body's core suddenly, causing core temperature afterdrop. The use of active external rewarming methods should not be undertaken lightly, owing to their theoretical risks, and active core rewarming should be reserved for severe cases.

TABLE 47–34. THERAPY IN HYPOTHERMIA

1. Don't miss head trauma, frostbite, injection sites (e.g., insulin, opiates, and so on)
2. Hospitalize and monitor if temperature is less than 91°F. (33°C.)
3. Use glass thermometer that reads into *low* range, or electronic probe
4. Usual ABCs of CPR; handle cautiously to avoid cardiac arrest
5. Minimize drug use; avoid insulin when possible
6. Atrial arrhythmias revert with rewarming
7. PVCs—check Po_2, check pH, use lidocaine if needed, check electrolytes
8. Warm intravenous fluids with blood coils to 99°F. to 112°F. (37–43°C.)
9. Heated oxygen, good pulmonary toilet
10. Thyroxine (400 μg.) and steroids (300 mg. hydrocortisone) for myxedema coma
11. Warm oral fluids if awake
12. Rewarming—active or passive
13. Prolong CPR—no one is dead until warm and dead

ELECTRICAL INJURY

Each year in the United States, about 1000 people are killed in electrical accidents and about 200 are killed by lightning. Injuries may be classified as low voltage (less than 1000 volts) or high voltage (greater than 1000 volts). The latter, while uncommon, produce devastating tissue damage.

Heat generation is responsible for the burns seen with electrical injuries, being proportional to the square of the current amperage and the tissue resistance. Tissue resistance falls dramatically with prolonged current exposure.

Direct current is less devastating than alternating current. The former often produces a repelling muscle contraction that separates the victim from the current, while the latter induces tetany and involuntary clenching of the hands, freezing the patient to the current source.

The pathway of the current also determines the severity of tissue damage. Burn damage is proportional to current density. Hence, a finger will be more damaged than a trunk, all other factors being equal.

Heat damage is proportional to tissue resistance. Bone is a poor conductor and holds heat a long time, often causing severe damage to deep tissues while superficial layers are spared. Skin, when dry, is of very high resistance, but when wet, it is markedly more conductive, leading to increased electrical injury.

Neurovascular and muscle bundles are much more sensitive to current injuries than would be expected from their electrical properties. Thrombosis, neural damage, and myoedema with ischemia are all seen in a delayed fashion after electrical injury.

Several types of burns are seen with electrical injury, including thermal burns from direct contact with current, deep electrical arc burns, flash burns, and flame burns from ignited clothing. Always undress the patient fully and look for both an entry and an exit wound.

Electrical injuries can be deceptive in their early appearance; they should all be admitted to hospital for neurovascular checks of the extremities and other monitoring as needed.

When electrical current traverses the body, it may obliterate recent memory and cause transient neurologic deficits. This may make the patient's history unreliable. Always evaluate such a patient for associated craniospinal or other trauma and initially treat the neck as unstable.

All victims of electrical injury deserve an electrocardiogram to rule out myocardial damage and monitoring for 24 hours if the path of the current traversed the heart.

All patients should be evaluated for the presence of myoglobinuria or hemoglobinuria. Aggressive volume resuscitation is needed owing to pigmenturia and third space losses. Urinary output should be between 0.5 and 1.5 ml./kg./hour.

Frequent neurovascular checks of all extremities involved are required for the early detection of edema-caused compartment syndromes necessitating fasciotomy.

The remainder of electrical burn management, when burns are severe, is similar to thermal burn management. If the current traversed the head and neck, ophthalmologic evaluation is necessary, as cataracts may form up to 2 years after the incident.

Toddlers chewing on electrical cords may suffer lip burns, usually at the commissure. These patients should be hospitalized and surgical consultation obtained. In up to 20 per cent of cases, the labial artery will produce delayed, profuse bleeding, and surgical revision may be necessary.

Lightning is a massive, instantaneous direct current countershock. It seldom causes more than second-degree burns. Asystole occurs, but the automaticity of the heart causes a resumption of sinus rhythm. However, respiratory paralysis leads to death in these victims from hypoxia. The triage rule in multiple lightning casualties is to resuscitate the dead (Cooper, 1982). The victims require neurologic and cardiac monitoring; many have tympanic membrane rupture, which is treated conservatively. Cataract formation is not uncommon, and ophthalmologic consultation should be sought.

Foreign Bodies

Inquisitive children, perverse or retarded adults, and seriously suicidal patients may use any bodily orifice for the insertion of a wide variety of foreign materials. In initial evaluation, there are two questions of major importance. First, what is the chemical and physical nature of the object? Second, exactly what is it? An answer to these questions allows an appropriate clinical response for management.

Hydrocarbons, caustics, contaminated objects, wood, and organic fibers are highly reactive, inducing a marked foreign body reaction. Metal, glass, and uncontaminated inert objects, on the other hand, are rather nonirritating unless their physical shape is jagged or their location is an already irritated region of the body.

Regions of the body where foreign objects lodge can be grouped by the danger level the foreign object's presence produces. Tracheobronchial, intravascular, and intraocular foreign bodies are all highly dangerous threats to life or organ function. Objects lodged in solid viscera, bodily orifices, the esophagus, and joints and cavities are potentially dangerous. Obstruction to drainage or tissue contamination may lead to sepsis, and erosion or perforation of structures may occur with jagged objects. Minimal danger is present when objects lodge in skin, subcutaneous tissue, muscle, or enter the stomach and intestines. Specific situations will be examined below. Figure 47–26 demonstrates some representative radiopaque foreign bodies.

Tracheobronchial foreign bodies may be radiopaque or radiolucent. Coughing, choking, transient cyanosis, and an inspiratory wheeze over the involved bronchus should suggest this entity. If the object is made of organic vegetable material, it may absorb water and enlarge, producing progressive obstruction. Proximal migration may lead to acute subglottic obstruction and respiratory arrest if therapy is not rapidly undertaken.

Inspiratory and expiratory films of the chest or bilateral decubitus films should be obtained. Patients with radiolucent foreign bodies show the following:

1. Early hyperaeration on the involved side
2. No loss of volume when the involved side is dependent
3. Mediastinal shift away from the involved side
4. Delayed atelectasis and pneumonia

Bronchoscopy is indicated as quickly as possible for removal.

Esophageal foreign bodies are common, and three locations are characteristic. Most commonly, the ingested object rests at the esophageal inlet due to the actions of the cricopharyngeus muscle sphincter, and if it is smooth and flat, it rests in the coronal plane (Fig. 47–26).

Smooth, nonreactive objects can be removed at this area by use of a Foley catheter, if the patient is cooperative or easily restrained. The procedure should be done under fluoroscopy with the patient in the semiprone Trendelenburg's position to avoid aspiration and with contrast material instilled in the Foley balloon. The catheter is advanced beyond the object, the balloon inflated, and the catheter withdrawn. Sharp objects should be removed endoscopically to avoid perforation and its sequelae.

Esophageal foreign bodies also occur at the middle third of the esophagus where it abuts mediastinal structures and at the gastroesophageal junction.

Glucagon (1 mg. I.V. or I.M.) and other agents

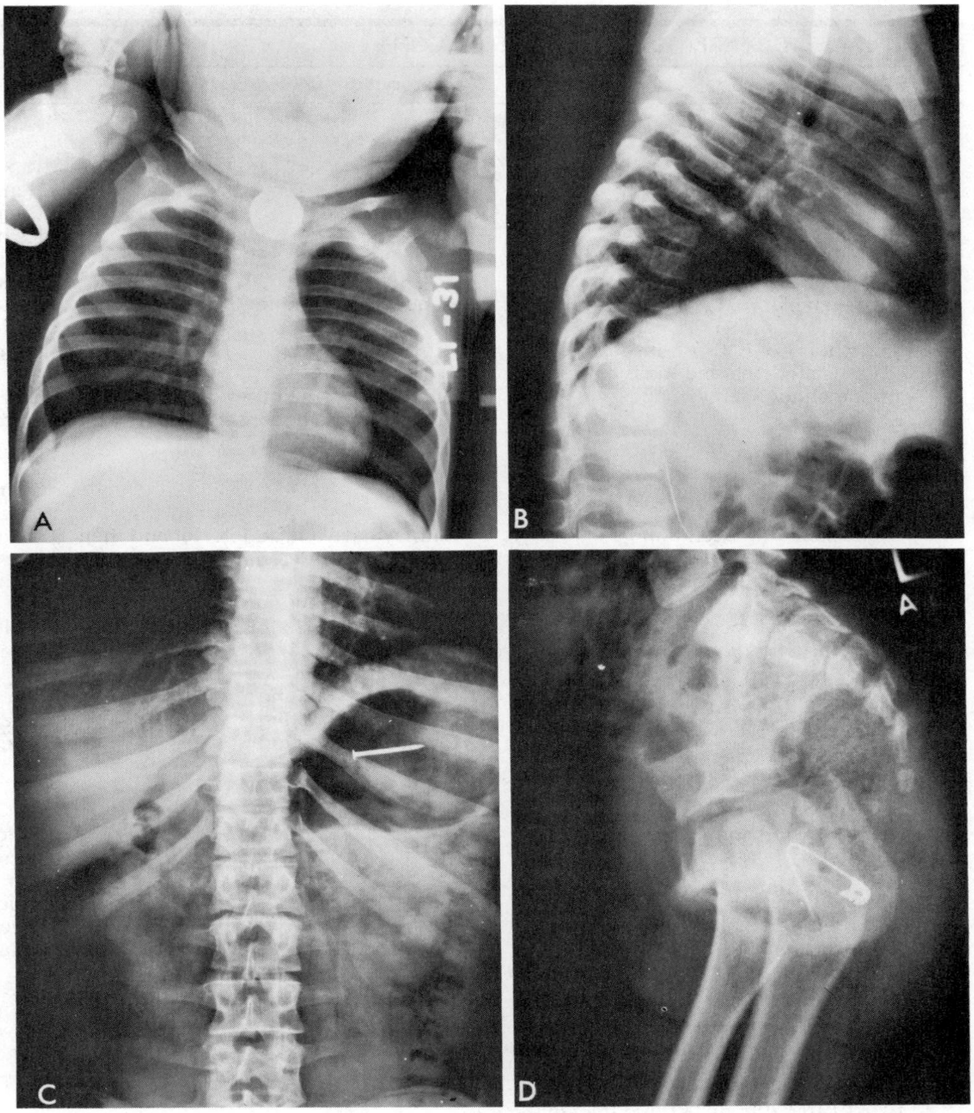

Figure 47–26. Multiple examples of foreign bodies. The swallowed coin (*A*) is classically caught at the thoracic inlet and is in the coronal plane. Even very sharp objects (*C*) usually pass once the stomach is entered and should be expelled from the rectum *blunt end first*. Thus the safety pin (*D*) is atypical and may have been inserted via the anus; consider child abuse. (From Wagner, D. K.: Ingestions and foreign bodies. Current Topics II in Emergency Medicine, 4(2). Philadelphia, Medical College of Pennsylvania, 1982.)

have been suggested for esophageal relaxation to promote passage of foreign objects.

Nonreactive objects that enter the stomach will be spontaneously passed 95 per cent of the time, including sharp objects (Fig. 47–26). Owing to peristaltic activity, these objects invariably pass through the anus blunt end first. Follow-up examination and roentgenograms are required to document passage.

Rectal foreign bodies are of concern because if perforation occurs invasive infection will occur. Attempts to remove large objects from the rectum produce a suction effect. A 30 cc. Foley catheter passed proximal to the object will aid in extraction and break the vacuum. Occasionally, general anesthesia may be necessary. A sharp object in the rectum, which has its point directed toward the anal verge was probably instilled through the anus. In the child, consider abuse (Fig. 47–26).

Nasal foreign bodies may present as a malodorous discharge with obstruction. After cocainizing the nostril, the child can be laid supine and mouth-to-mouth breathing used with a single forceful breath, closing the unobstructed nostril. The foreign object will usually be expelled. Alligator forceps may also be used for extraction.

Aural foreign bodies are not uncommon in children. It is best to extract these with fine forceps or spoons, under anesthesia if necessary. Objects beyond the isthmus of the auditory canal often cannot be reclaimed by irrigation. Vegetable matter may expand and become painful if irrigation is attempted. Insects should be killed prior to removal, using mineral oil or ether (ether is preferable as it dehydrates the insect).

Foul vaginal discharge in a child means foreign body until proved otherwise. Rectal examination usually allows palpation of the object through the rectovaginal septum. Extraction can be carried out using a nasal speculum and a fine forceps, or under anesthesia if necessary. Foreign bodies in the rectum or

TABLE 47–35. DIFFERENTIAL DIAGNOSIS OF COMA

Entity	History	Physical Findings
Intracranial Processes		
1. Vascular disease		
a. Intracerebral bleeding		
1) Lateral to basal ganglia	Headache	Hemiplegia Conjugate eye deviation toward lesion
2) Thalamic		Downward convergence of eyes
3) Pontine		Loss of lateral eye movements
4) Cerebellar	Headache, vomiting	Ataxia, eye palsy, respiratory irregularities
b. Infarction—of RAS or with severe cortical edema and mass effect		Appropriate focal findings
c. Subarachnoid hemorrhage	Headache, vomiting	Fever, meningismus, ± focal deficit
2. Trauma	Transient loss of consciousness	No focal deficit
a. Concussion	Rapid improvement	
b. Mass lesion		Signs of head injury (treat the neck as unstable)
1) Contusion—laceration	All may have a lucid interval and then progressive deterioration	
2) Epidural hematoma		
3) Subdural hematoma		
3. Tumor		
a. Secondary hydrocephalus	Usually tumor is already diagnosed	Papilledema
b. Sudden hemorrhage		Focal findings
4. Infection		
a. Meningitis	Headache, vomiting	Fever, meningismus, nonfocal
b. Encephalitis	Headache, vomiting	Fever, ± focal findings
c. Brain abscess	Headache, vomiting	Fever, papilledema, focal findings
5. Epilepsy—status epilepticus or postictal state		
Extracranial Processes		
1. Metabolic encephalopathy		No focal findings unless a prior brain lesion existed that is now unmasked
a. Respiratory failure (↑ P_{CO_2}, ↓ P_{O_2})		
b. Uremia		Myoclonic jerks
c. Hepatic failure		Specific signs of associated disease state
d. Hypo- or hypernatremia		
e. Hypercalcemia		
f. Myxedema, addisonian crisis, hypopituitarism		
g. Hyperviscosity (hyperproteinemias or polycythemia/leukemia)		
h. Nutritional deficiency (thiamine, and so on)		
i. Hyperosmolarity (hyperglycemia, and so on)		
j. Severe hypertension or hypotension		
k. Hyperthermia or hypothermia		
2. Toxic encephalopathy		Nonfocal neurologic exam—pinpoint pupils, track marks
a. Narcotic		
b. Sedative-hypnotics		Pupils dilated with barbiturates and Doriden
c. Ethanol		
d. Salicylates		
e. Many other agents (anticholinergics, carbon monoxide, and so on)		
3. Psychiatric pseudo-coma (recent stress history)		Fluttering lashes Patient's hand, when dropped over the face, will swerve to avoid impact

vagina of children should always raise the issue of child abuse in the mind of the examining physician.

Ocular foreign bodies are usually conjunctival, corneal, or intraocular.

Conjunctival foreign bodies usually lodge under the upper lid beneath the tarsal plate. Pulling the upper lid over the lower will usually sweep the plate clean and clear the object. The lid can be everted for direct inspection. Whenever a foreign body is found, the cornea must be stained with fluorescein to look for an abrasion.

Corneal foreign bodies are removed using topical anesthesia, irrigation, and if necessary a moist swab or a spud. Small children may require anesthesia. Associated abrasions must be closely followed and should be at least 50 per cent healed in 24 hours and totally healed in 48 hours. Mydriatics, topical antibiotics, patching, and systemic analgesia are often employed.

If any possibility exists that an ocular injury has occurred while high-velocity fragments were generated (such as during grinding or hammering) or if slit-lamp examination reveals scleral laceration, an intraocular foreign body must be suspected. This demands orbital ultrasound and ophthalmologic consultation.

The hands and feet are prone to receive implanted foreign bodies. If visible or palpable, extraction can be immediate. Otherwise, allow the object 3 to 5 days to encyst in the soft tissues. Removal can then be easily carried out (under fluoroscopy if necessary) with local anesthesia.

Approach to the Unconscious Patient

The emergency management of the comatose patient is challenging, requiring simultaneous diagnostic and therapeutic maneuvers in most instances for optimal outcome.

Normal consciousness requires intact cerebral hemispheric function and normal function of the ascending reticular activating system (RAS), a complex set of neurons in the upper brainstem responsible for normal cortical arousal. Dysfunction of either the RAS (which is quite sensitive to both toxins and mass lesions) or both cerebral hemispheres may lead therefore to the comatose state.

Coma may be viewed as either intracranial or extracranial in primary etiology, for the purpose of differential diagnosis and management. Table 47–35 summarizes the etiologies in both classes of coma. A careful physical examination should be done with emphasis on signs of trauma, track marks, and signs of shock or elevated intracranial pressure (hypertension, bradycardia, and irregular respiratory effort). Pupillary size and responsiveness, fundoscopic exam, respiratory pattern and adequacy, and the presence of any focal neurologic findings are of great help. As diagnosis and therapy proceed, repeated directed exams should be done to delineate changes in the patient's status.

After an adequate airway is assured, an intravenous line should be placed, and blood drawn for electrolytes, urea nitrogen, glucose, calcium, blood counts, and a possible toxic screen. Patients suspected of being alcoholic or malnourished should receive 100 mg. of thiamine I.V., to avoid producing or worsening Wernicke's encephalopathy, followed in all patients by 50 ml. of 50 per cent dextrose in water. All patients should probably also receive 2 ampules (0.8 mg.) of naloxone hydrochloride (Narcan) intravenously. Stabilize the neck if necessary and treat shock or malignant hypertension aggressively.

Arterial blood gases should be obtained and supplemental oxygen of appropriate route and degree supplied to the patient. Other useful data include chest film, urinalysis, electrocardiogram, and in cases in which trauma is suspected, skull and cervical spine x-rays with other studies as appropriate.

Associated medical illness should be sought and aggressively managed. If an intracranial mass lesion is suspected, emergent neurosurgical consultation and computed tomography should be requested. Progressive rapid deterioration in the neurologic status may require the placement of burr holes by a neurosurgeon without any further diagnostic studies.

All comatose patients who do not have a mass lesion should undergo lumbar puncture with cerebrospinal fluid analysis of protein, glucose, cell count and differential, and appropriate bacteriologic stains and cultures, and other tests as necessary.

The general approach to the comatose patient, coupled with attention to pulmonary toilet, constant attendance by nursing staff, frequent reassessment by the physician, and prompt neurologic or surgical consultation, will sustain the patient's life and minimize neuronal damage prior to more definitive therapies being carried out for intracranial or extracranial etiologies of coma. Pseudocoma, due to hysteria or psychosis, requires compassion, and psychiatric intervention in many cases.

References

CPCR

Gadzinski, D. S., White, B. C., Hoehner, P. J., et al.: Canine cerebral cortical blood flow and vascular resistance post cardiac arrest. Ann. Emerg. Med., *11*:58, 1982. *Elegant demonstration of postarrest increase in cerebrovascular arteriolar resistance, raising the issue of therapy with the new calcium channel blockers.*

Jaffe, A. S., et al.: Textbook of Advanced Cardiac Life Support. 2nd ed. Dallas, TX, American Heart Association, 1987. *Exhaustive treatise on advanced cardiac life support. Required reading.*

National Conference on Cardiopulmonary Resuscitation and Emergency Cardiac Care: Standards and Guidelines for CPR and ECC. J.A.M.A., *244*:453, 1980. *The bible for techniques and dosages in basic and advanced CPR. Available from the American Heart Association and elsewhere.*

Roberts, J. R., and Greenberg, M. I.: Emergency transthoracic pacemaker. Ann. Emerg. Med., *10*:600, 1981. *Excellently written review. The historical perspective and mechanical instruction are both well done.*

Safar, P.: Pathophysiology of Acute Central Nervous System Failure. *In* Schwartz, G. R., Safar, P., Stone, J. H. (Eds.): Principles and Practices of Emergency Medicine. Philadelphia, W. B. Saunders, 1978. *Thorough discussion of the basics of cerebral dysfunction and resuscitation in cardiac arrest.*

Sung, R. J., Elser, B., and McAllister, R. G.: Intravenous verapamil for termination of re-entrant supraventricular tachycardias. Ann. Intern. Med., *93*:682, 1980. *Lucid study of the efficacy of verapamil in this re-entrant arrhythmia; a valuable new therapeutic addition.*

Poisoning

Arena, J. M.: Poisoning. Springfield, Illinois, Charles C Thomas, 1979. *An excellent and comprehensive review of all aspects of toxicology.*

Arena, J. M.: Hydrocarbon poisoning—current management. Pediatr. Ann., *16*(11):879–883, 1987.

Burns, R. S., Lerner, S. E., and Linder, R. L.: The clinical picture of phencyclidine intoxication. Current Topics II in Emergency Medicine, *3*(10), 1981.

Crome, P.: Poisoning due to tricyclic antidepressant overdosage. Clinical presentation and treatment. Med. Toxicol., *1*(4):261–285, 1986. *Thorough and authoritative, detailed review.*

Done, A. K.: Salicylate poisoning. Current Topics II in Emergency Medicine, *3*(2), 1981. *A concise definitive review from the recognized authority on salicylate ingestion.*

Doweiko, H.: Identifying street names of drugs. J. Emerg. Nur., *5*:44, 1979. *A useful compendium of jargon.*

Goldfrank, L. R., and Kirstein, R.: Toxicologic Emergencies: A Handbook in Problem Solving. New York, Appleton-Century-Crofts, 1978.

Goldfrank, L., Bresnitz, E., and Weissman, R.: Opioids and opiates. Current Topics II in Emergency Medicine, *3*(8), 1981. *A superb review of all aspects of narcotic addiction.*

Goldfrank, L., Bresnitz, E., Kirstein, R., and Weissman, R. S.: Organophosphates (SLUD). Hospital Physician, December 1981, p. 56.

Guzzardi, L. J.: Tricyclic antidepressant overdose. Current Topics II in Emergency Medicine, *3*(7), 1981. *Comprehensive review of cardiotoxicity and central anticholinergic symptomatology.*

Haddad, L. M.: Iron poisoning. J.A.C.E.P., *5*:691, 1976.

Hedges, J. R.: Acute noxious gas exposure. Current Topics in Emergency Medicine, *2*(10), 1978.

Howell, J. M.: Alkaline ingestions. Ann. Emerg. Med., *15*(7):820–825, 1986. *Thorough and detailed review of the problem.*

Kulig, K., and Rumack, B. H.: Hydrocarbon ingestion. Current Topics II in Emergency Medicine, *3*(4), 1981. *Exhaustive review of all aspects of management, pathophysiology, and physicochemical peculiarities of hydrocarbons.*

Kunkel, D. B.: Principles of toxicology. Current Topics II in Emergency Medicine, *3*, 1981.

Lanphear, W. F.: Gastric lavage. J. Emerg. Med., *4*(1):43–47, 1986. *A review of when, why, why not, and how to.*

McClain, C. J., Holtzman, J., Allen, J., et al.: Clinical features of acetaminophen toxicity. J. Clin. Gastroenterol., *10*(1):76–80, 1988.

Mozingo, D. W., Smith, A. A., McManus, W. F., et al.: Chemical burns. J. Trauma, *28*(5):642–647, 1988.

Norkool, D. M., and Kirkpatrick, J. N.: Treatment of acute carbon monoxide poisoning with hyperbaric oxygen: A review of 115 cases. Ann. Emerg. Med., *14*(12):1168–1171, 1985. *Good review of physiology, clinical scenarios, and sequelae.*

Proudfoot, A. T., Simpson, D., and Dyson, E. H.: Management of acute iron poisoning. Med. Toxicol., *1*(2):83–100, 1986.

Roberts, J.: Drug overdose in the emergency room. Current Topics in Emergency Medicine, *3*, 1979. *Incisive basic review of general principles of evaluation and management of drug overdose.*

Schimelman, M.: Nitrate/nitrite poisoning. Current Topics II in Emergency Medicine, *3*, 1981. *Useful discussion of methemoglobinema production.*

Temple, A. R.: Emergency treatment of acetaminophen overdose. Current Topics II in Emergency Medicine, *3*, 1981.

Ulin, L. S.: Caustic ingestions. Current Topics II in Emergency Medicine, *3*, 1981.

Zwiener, R. J., and Ginsburg, C. M.: Organophosphate and carbamate poisoning in infants and children. Pediatrics, *81*(1):121–126, 1988.

Bites and Envenomation

Arena, J. M.: Poisoning. Springfield, Illinois, Charles C Thomas, 1979, pp. 558–580. *A delightful but in-depth discussion of envenomation.*

Callahan, M. L.: Treatment of common dog bites: infectious risk factors. J.A.C.E.P., *7*:83, 1978.

Connolly, W. B., and Kilgore, E. S.: Hand Injuries and Infections. Chicago, Year Book Medical Publishers, 1979, pp. 17–18. *A short, well-illustrated guide to hand infection and splinting.*

Corey, L.: Rabies and other rhabdoviruses. *In* Isselbacher, K. J. et al. (Eds.): Harrison's Principles of Internal Medicine. New York, McGraw-Hill, 1980, pp. 818–821.

Goldstein, E. J. C., Citron, D. M., and Finegold, S. M.: Dogbite wounds and infection: a prospective clinical study. Ann. Emerg. Med., *9*:508, 1980.

Goldstein, E. J. C., Citron, D. M., Wield, B., et al.: Bacteriology of human and animal bite wounds. J. Clin. Microbiol., *8*:667, 1978. *A study done with the best culture techniques to delineate aerobic and anaerobic flora in bite wounds.*

Immunization Practices Advisory Committee, Centers for Disease Control: Diphtheria, tetanus, and pertussis. Ann. Intern. Med., *95*:723, 1981.

Malinowski, R. W., Strate, R. G., Perry, J. F., Jr., and Fischer, R. P.: The management of human bite injuries of the hand. J. Trauma, *19*:655, 1979.

Martin, L. T.: Human bites: Guidelines for practical management. Postgrad. Med., *81*(6):221–224, 1987.

Maun, R. J., Hoffeld, T. A., and Farmer, C. B.: Human bites of the hand: twenty years of experience. J. Hand Surg., *2*:97, 1977. *A well-illustrated and comprehensive report of a long-term experience.*

Pennell, T. C., Babu, S. S., and Meredith, J. W.: The management of snake and spider bites in the southeastern United States. Ann. Surg., *53*(4):198–204, 1987.

Russell, F. E.: Snake venom poisoning in the United States. Ann. Rev. Med., *31*:241, 1980. *An excellent review with clinical emphasis.*

Snyder, C. C., and Knowles, R. P.: Snakebites: Guidelines for practical management. Postgrad. Med., *83*(6):52–60, 65–68, 71–75, 1988.

Stewart, M. E., Greenland, S., and Hoffman, J. R.: First-aid treatment of poisonous snakebite: are currently recommended procedures justified? Ann. Emerg. Med., *10*:331, 1981. *Engagingly reviews the myriad of suggestions for snakebite management. Convincingly casts doubt on them all.*

Strassburg, M. A., et al.: Animal bites: patterns of treatment. Ann. Emerg. Med., *10*:193, 1981.

Toewe, C. H.: Bug bites and stings. Am. Fam. Phys., *21*:90, 1980. *Excellent review of spider, tick, and more exotic insect bites.*

Trauma Wound Care

Connolly, W. B., and Kilgore, E. S.: Hand Injuries and Infections. Chicago, Year Book Medical Publishers, 1979, pp. 67–71.

Dushoff, I. M.: A stitch in time. Emerg. Med., Jan., 1973; Feb., 1974. *Engagingly written review of basics of suturing.*

Dushoff, I. M.: About face. Emerg. Med., vol. 6, no. 11, November 1974.

Dushoff, I. M.: Handling the hand. Emerg. Med., vol. 8, no. 10, October 1976.

Ervin, M. E.: Minor surgical procedures. *In* Schwartz, G. R., Safar, P., Stone, J. H. (Eds.): Principles and Practice of Emergency Medicine. Philadelphia, W. B. Saunders Co., 1978, pp. 386–398.

Chest Trauma and Thoracostomy Tubes, Autotransfusion, Thoracotomy

Baker, C. C., Thomas, H. N., and Tranhey, D. D.: The role of emergency room thoracotomy in trauma. J. Trauma, *20*:848, 1980.

Bricker, D. L.: Safe, effective tube thoracostomy I & II. ER Reports, *2*:45, 1981. *Clear, how-to presentation on chest tube techniques.*

Clarke, J. R.: Blunt and penetrating chest trauma. Current Topics in Emergency Medicine, *2*(9), 1978. *Review of pathophysiology and mechanisms of injury.*

Curtis, P.: Spontaneous pneumothorax: a dilemma of management. J. Fam. Prac., *6*:367, 1978. *Excellent discussion of chest tube pros and cons.*

Davidson, S. J.: Autotransfusion from hemothorax. Current Concepts in Trauma Care, *2*:2, 1979.

Davidson, S. J.: Correct use of autotransfusion in the emergency patient. ER Reports, *2*:73, 1981. *A very clear and how-to presentation on a powerful new technique.*

Davis, Z., and Kuracina, M. J.: Acute response to blunt chest trauma. ER Reports, *1*:97, 1980.

Donovan, J. W.: Pneumothorax. Current Topics in Emergency Medicine, *2*, 1978.

Oparah, S. S., and Mandal, A. K.: Operative management of penetrating wounds of the chest in civilian practice. J. Thorac. Cardiovasc. Surg., *77*:162, 1979.

Oparah, S. S., and Mandal, A. K.: Penetrating stab wounds of the chest: experience with 200 consecutive cases. J. Trauma, *16*:868, 1976.

Rutherford, R. B.: The pathophysiology of trauma and shock. *In* Zuidema, G. D., Rutherford, R. B., and Ballinger, W. F. (Eds.): The Management of Trauma. Philadelphia, W. B. Saunders Co., 1979.

Abdominal Trauma and Peritoneal Lavage

Anderson, C. B., and Ballinger, W. F.: Abdominal Injuries. *In* Zuidema, G. D., Rutherford, R. B., and Ballinger, W. F. (Eds.): The Management of Trauma. Philadelphia, W. B. Saunders Co., 1979, pp. 429–482.

Galbraith, T. A., Oreskovich, M. R., Heimbach, D. M., et al.: The role of peritoneal lavage in the management of stab wounds to the abdomen. Am. J. Surg., *140*:60, 1980. *A lucid discussion of the indications for lavage.*

Hawkins, M. L., Scofield, W. M., Carraway, R. P., et al.: Diagnostic peritoneal lavage in blunt trauma. South. Med. J., *81*(3):293–296, 1988.

Kane, N. M., Dorfman, G. S., and Cronan, J. J.: Efficacy of CT following peritoneal lavage in abdominal trauma. J. Comput. Assist. Tomogr., *11*(6):998–1002, 1987. *Abdominal fluid post-lavage can mask hemorrhage on CT but does not render CT useless in all cases.*

Kessler, E., and Stein, A.: Diaphragmatic hernia as a long-term complication of stab wounds of the chest. Am. J. Surg., *132*:34, 1976.

Lazarus, H. M., and Nelson, J. A.: Refining the technique of diagnostic peritoneal lavage. ER Reports, *1*:111, 1980. *Good discussion of technique is contained in this article.*

Merlotti, G. J., Dillon, B. C., Lange, D. A., et al.: Peritoneal lavage in penetrating thoraco-abdominal trauma. J. Trauma, *28*(1):17–23, 1988.

Moore, E. E.: Evaluating and managing penetrating abdominal injuries. ER Reports, *2*:85, 1981.

Mueller, G. L., Burney, R. E, and Mackenzie, J. R.: Sequential peritoneal lavage and early diagnosis of colon perforation. Ann. Emerg. Med., *10*:131, 1981.

Parvin, W., Smith, D. E., Asher, W. M., and Virgilio, R. W.: Effectiveness of peritoneal lavage in blunt abdominal trauma. Ann. Surg., *181*:255, 1975.

Pedi, J. J., and Berne, T. V.: Posterior abdominal stab wounds. J. Trauma, *21*:298, 1981. *Discussion of a special situation, which should not allow false security.*

Powell, R. W., Smith, D. E., Zarins, C. K., et al.: Peritoneal lavage in children with blunt abdominal trauma. J. Ped. Surg., *11*:973, 1976. *Attention is directed here to the traumatized child in a lucid account.*

Sigel, B., and Baker, R. J.: Blunt and penetrating abdominal trauma. Current Topics in Emergency Medicine, *1*, 1979.

Thal, E. R., May, R. A., and Beesinger, D.: Peritoneal lavage. Arch. Surg., *115*:430, 1980.

Thompson, J. S., Moore, J. E., Van Duzer-Moore, S., et al.: The evolution of abdominal stab wound management. J. Trauma, *20*:478, 1980. *A review with well-done historical emphasis on procedures and management.*

Walters, H. L., Hupp, J., McCabe, C. J., et al.: Peritoneal lavage and the surgical resident. Surg.-Gynecol.-Obstet., *165*(6):496–502, 1987. *Suggests that CT will avoid false positives due to pelvic fractures and so on seen in lavage.*

Wilder, J. R., and Kudchadker, A.: Stab wounds of the abdomen: Observe or explore? J.A.M.A., *243*:2503, 1980.

Special Topics in Trauma

Bergquist, D., Hedelin, H., Lindblad, B., et al.: Abdominal injuries in children: an analysis of 348 cases. Injury, *16*(4):217–220, 1985. *Most frequent cause—a bike accident.*

Booth, C. M.: High pressure paint gun injuries. Br. Med. J., *2*:1333, 1977. *Contains illustrative case reports and a useful discussion.*

Gouski, C., Southcombe, W., and Cohen, D.: Bicycle accidents in childhood. Med. J. Aust., *2*:270, 1979.

Gratz, R. R.: Accidental injury in childhood: a literature review on pediatric trauma. J. Trauma, *19*:551, 1979. *An epidemiologic approach yields additional understanding.*

Justis, E. J.: Trauma to the hand. *In* Schwartz, G. R., Safer, P., Stone, J. H., et al. (Eds.): Principles and Practice of Emergency Medicine. Philadelphia, W. B. Saunders Co., 1979, pp. 728–729.

Palmaccio, A. J., and Greenberg, M. O.: Wringer injury. *In* Greenberg, M. I., and Roberts, J. R. (Eds.): Emergency Medicine: A Clinical Approach to Challenging Problems. Philadelphia, F. A. Davis Co., 1982, pp. 11–15. *A superb little text addressing complex and often unusual issues in our field.*

Roffman, M., Moshel, M., and Mendes, D. G.: Bicycle spoke injuries. J. Trauma, *20*:325, 1980.

Silsby, J. J.: Pressure gun injection injuries of the hand. West. J. Med., *125*:271, 1976. *Superb review of high-pressure injection injury.*

Sparnon, A. L., and Ford, W. D.: Bicycle handlebar injuries in children. J. Pediatr. Surg., *21*(2):118–119, 1986. *Long hospital stays were common, due to abdominal injury.*

Tucci, J. J., and Barone, J. E.: A study of urban bicycling accidents. Am. J. Sports Med., *16*(2):181–184, 1988.

Burns and Smoke Inhalation

Dimick, A. R.: Emergency treatment of extensive burns. Current Topics II in Emergency Medicine, *1*, 1981. *A useful summary of the points of burn management.*

Herndon, D. N., Langner, F., Thompson, P., et al.: Pulmonary injury in burned patients. Surg. Clin. N. Am., *67*(1):31–46, 1987.

Jelenko, C.: Chemicals that burn. J. Trauma, *14*:65, 1971. *Caustic and esoteric agents causing burns and their management.*

Navar, P. D., Saffle, J. R., and Warden, G. D.: Effect of inhalation injury on fluid resuscitation requirements after thermal injury. Am. J. Surg., *150*(6):716–720, 1985. *Fluid requirements per per cent surface burned increased almost 50 per cent when lung injury was also present.*

Robson, M. C., Krizek, T. J., and Wray, R. C.: Care of the thermally injured patient. *In* Zuidema, G. D., Rutherford, R. B., and Ballinger, W. F. (Eds.): The Management of Trauma. Philadelphia, W. B. Saunders Co., 1979, pp. 666–730. *An exhaustive review of burns large and small and other local thermal injuries. Exceedingly complete and well written.*

Heat Trauma

Clowes, G. H. A., and O'Donnell, T. F.: Current concepts: heat stroke. N. Engl. J. Med., *291*:564, 1974.

Danzl, D. F.: Hyperthermic syndromes. Am. Fam. Physician, *37*(6):157–162, 1988. *Good review encompassing differential diagnosis and management.*

O'Donnell, T. F., and Clowes, G. H. A.: The circulatory abnormalities of heat stroke. N. Engl. J. Med., *287*:734, 1972. *An elegant summary of clinical data describing hemodynamic subsets of victims of heatstroke.*

Tucker, L. E., Stanford, J., Graves, B., et al.: Classical heatstroke: clinical and laboratory assessment. South. Med. J., *78*(1):20–25, 1985. *Detailed breakdown on risk factors, prognostic indices, lab phenomena.*

Sine, R. J.: Heat illness. J.A.C.E.P., *8*:154, 1979. *An exhaustively referenced review of all forms of heat illness and their pathophysiology and management.*

Vicario, S. J., Okabajue, R., and Haltom, T.: Rapid cooling in classic heatstroke: effect on mortality rates. Am. J. Emerg. Med., *4*(5):394–398, 1986. *The faster the cooling, the better the outcome.*

Frostbite and Hypothermia

Kyosola, K.: Clinical experience in management of cold injuries: a study of 110 cases. J. Trauma, *14*:32, 1974.

O'Keefe, K.: Accidental hypothermia: a review of 62 cases. J.A.C.E.P., *6*:491, 1977.

Orr, K., and Fainer, D.: Cold injuries in Korea during winter of

1950–51. Medicine, *31*:177, 1952. *An exhaustive clinical review. Epidemiologic data and pictures are outstanding.*

Reuler, J.: Hypothermia: pathophysiology, clinical settings, and management. Ann. Intern. Med., *89*:519, 1978. *Excellent review both for clinical data and physiologic basis for abnormalities in hypothermia.*

Washburn, B.: Frostbite. N. Engl. J. Med., *266*:974, 1962. *More good discussion and superb photographs of frostbite.*

Electrical Injuries

Cooper, M. A.: Electrical injuries. Current Topics II in Emergency Medicine, *1*, 1981. *A superb review of the physics, physiology, and clinical management of all forms of electrical insult. Short and to the point.*

Cooper, M. A.: Lightning injuries: prognostic signs of death. Ann. Emerg. Med., *9*:134, 1980.

Foreign Bodies

Blazer, S., Navek, Y., and Friedman, A.: Foreign body in the airway: a review of 200 cases. Am. J. Dis. Child., *134*:168, 1980.

Fox, J. R.: Fogarty catheter removal of nasal foreign bodies. Ann. Emerg. Med., *9*:61, 1980. *An alternative how-to approach.*

Koloshe, A. M.: Tracheobronchial foreign bodies in children: back to the bronchoscope and a balloon. Pediatrics, *66*:321, 1980.

Wagner, D. K.: Ingestions and foreign bodies. Current Topics II in Emergency Medicine, *4*, 1982. *A lucidly written, entertaining, and complete clinical review of this fascinating topic.*

The Unconscious Patient

Plum, F., and Posner, J. B.: The Diagnosis of Stupor and Coma. 2nd ed. Philadelphia, F. A. Davis Co., 1972. *The best short text available on the subject. Well written with lucid discussion of rostral-caudal degeneration in the comatose patient.*

Sabin, T. D.: Coma and the acute confusional state in the emergency room. Med. Clin. North Am., *65*:15, 1981. *A complete discussion of acute diagnosis and management of a comatose or confused patient.*

Sabin, T. D.: Evaluation of coma in the emergency room. Current Topics in Emergency Medicine, *3*, 1979. *A more compact but extremely useful discussion of rostral-caudal degeneration, the RAS, and coma diagnosis.*

48

Sports Medicine

David C. Campbell
John T. Yetter

The association between sports and medicine has been noted throughout history. The duality of that relationship was also recognized by the earliest of sports physicians. Herodicus, who lived during the 5th century B.C., not only treated the injuries of athletes but also used therapeutic exercises and diet in the treatment of other patients. His most famous student, Hippocrates, verified this approach through his writing of the value of exercise in the treatment of many illnesses.

Galen became the first of what would be analogous to today's team physician when he was appointed physician to the gladiators in the 2nd century A.D.

The 20th century has witnessed significant expansion in the field of sports medicine. The first American work in sports medicine is credited to Walter Meanwell, who, in 1931, collaborated with Knute Rockne in discussing the role of team physicians and athletic trainers in the care of the athlete. In 1938, Augustus Thorndike published the first American text on athletic injuries emphasizing prevention of injuries, as well as diagnosis and treatment.

In the last three decades, growth in the field of sports medicine has paralleled the increasing interest of society in sport and fitness. Major milestones in the development of sports medicine occurred in 1950 with the establishment of the National Athletic Trainers Association in Kansas City and, in 1954, with the founding of the American College of Sports Medicine.

Today, 52 per cent of the American public participate in some sporting endeavor, and 5 to 7 per cent of the American public will injure themselves sometime during their sporting activity.

Table 48–1 from the National Safety Council shows estimates of numbers of participants and injuries associated with various sports. (It should be noted the methods of reporting vary among sources and therefore comparisons among sports may be flawed and no inference can be made regarding relative hazards).

Football fatalities. Four fatalities directly attributable to football injuries occurred in 1987, according to a report covering professional, college, high school, and sand lot actiities. All the fatalities occurred in high school play, with three occurring during games and one in practice. Two of the fatalities resulted from injuries to the head and two from neck injuries. Three of the fatalities occurred while tackling, and for one the activity was unknown.

In addition, there were five indirect fatalities recorded in 1987 (those fatalities which are caused by systemic failure as a result of exertion while participating in football activity or by a complication). Three of the indirect fatalities were associated with high school football and two with college football.

The 1987 rate of direct fatalities per 100,000 participants was 0.30 for high school football (Mueller and Schindler, 1988).

Sports Medicine as a Field of Medicine

Despite its ancient roots and traditions, and its recent growth, sports medicine as a discipline awaits clarification. As of this writing, there is no certifying board of sports medicine, and there is considerable debate within family medicine as to whether or not it should be an area for Certification of Added Qualifications (as has been done in the field of geriatric medicine).

The differentiation must also be made between

Table 48–1. SPORTS INJURIES*†

Sport	Participants	Injuries	Fatalities
Archery	5,100,000	3,366	([a])
Baseball	13,900,000	348,539	0
Basketball	21,200,000	467,160	4
Bicycle riding	49,700,000	561,764	([a])
Boating	38,200,000	3,501[b]	1,036[b] t
Bowling	34,200,000	17,152	([a])
Boxing	500,000	5,671	([a])
Fishing	47,500,000	65,021	([a])
Football	12,000,000	329,987	4[c]
Golf	20,000,000	22,648	([a])
Gymnastics	4,800,000	34,217	([a])
Handball	1,700,000	4,113	([a])
Hang gliding	7,000[d]	([a])	8[d]
Hockey	1,900,000	23,679	0
Ice skating	4,400,000	12,270	([a])
Lacrosse	400,000	([a])	0
Parachuting	115,000[e]	([a])	28[c]
Racquetball	7,800,000	19,761	([a])
Rugby	300,000	6,943	([a])
Scuba diving	2,600,000[f]	([a])	76[f]
Soccer	8,200,000	86,409	3
Softball	20,900,000	([a])	0
Snow skiing	14,400,000	49,483	1
Snowmobiling	3,600,000	10,289	([a])
Swimming	72,600,000	94,053	2,000[g]
Tennis	18,000,000	19,627	0
Volleyball	20,700,000	91,639	([a])
Water skiing	11,900,000	22,583	36[b]
Wrestling	1,300,000	35,585	1

*From National Safety Council. Accident Facts, 1988 Edition. Chicago, National Safety Council, 1988.

†Source: Participants—National Sporting Goods Association (1986), except where noted; figures include those who participate more than one time per year except for bicycle riding and swimming, which include only those who participate more than six times per year. Injuries—Consumer Product Safety Commission (1987), except where noted; figures include only hospital emergency room treated injuries. Fatalities—National Collegiate Athletic Association (NCAA) (1986–1987 school year), except where noted; figures include school or college sponsored sports. [a]Estimate not available. [b]U.S. Coast Guard (1987), [c]NCAA (1987), [d]U.S. Hang Gliding Association (1987), [e]U.S. Parachute Association (1987), [f]National Underwater Accident Data Center (1987), [g]National Safety Council (1987).

sports medicine and sports traumatology. Sports traumatology is the diagnosis and treatment of sports injuries. Sports medicine includes this and also addresses the assessment of the athlete, nutritional concerns, and other factors contributing not only to the treatment but also to the prevention of injuries.

Few medical schools offer a structured curriculum in sports medicine. The American Academy of Family Physicians has issued Recommended Core Curriculum Guidelines on Sports and Recreational Medicine for Family Practice Residencies (see Table 48–2), but programs are required only to provide orthopedic training, and many residents do not receive a true sports medicine experience.

Sports Medicine Liability

In several states, the health care provider, acting as a volunteer team physician rendering emergency care to participants in athletic activities, is excused from claims of ordinary negligence. Despite these statutes, the assessment of the players' ability to play after an injury is not protected. When providing nonemergency care, the team physician can expect to be held to the standard of care of reasonable, prudent team physicians, knowledgeable in accepted sports medicine techniques.

A complete discussion of the civil liability issues associated with volunteering as a team physician is included in Todaro (1986). He offers the following guidelines: Find out if the Good Samaritan law in your state includes a qualified immunity statute for volunteer team physicians and obtain a copy of it. From this, identify the limits of your coverage and notify the school in writing that your services are limited. Check with your own malpractice insurance carrier to assure that you are covered when acting in a volunteer capacity as team physician. Be sure you are current on managing emergency and life-threatening conditions including head and spinal cord trauma. Any reimbursement you receive, including cost-based reimbursement for x-ray studies, dressings, or medication, may disqualify you as a volunteer under the law (Todaro, 1986).

Preparticipation Assessment

CHILD AND YOUTH EXAMINATION

"Johnny needs a physical before he can play football." This is one of the most common sports medicine scenarios facing the practicing family physician. Usually, this request is accompanied by a basic history and physical form to be completed and signed. What opportunity does this afford the practicing physician to thoroughly examine this patient and truly assess his or her suitability for participation in sports, particularly contact sports? The preparticipation examination should be a rigorous and thorough assessment of the potential athlete's ability to participate in the chosen sport without unnecessary risk. As such, the exam should be sport specific. It should be carried out to accomplish the following: (1) determination of general health, (2) assessment of cardiovascular fitness, (3) evaluation of pre-existing injuries, (4) assessment of size and maturation, and (5) determination of whether restriction or disqualification is indicated by the presence of disease or physical limitation that would preclude safe participation. If participation is restricted, appropriate alternative activities should be suggested (Mellion, 1988).

The health history is the most important part of the examination. Attention must be focused on prior

Table 48–2. RECOMMENDED CORE CURRICULUM GUIDELINES ON SPORTS AND RECREATIONAL MEDICINE FOR FAMILY PRACTICE RESIDENTS*

As the population of the United States becomes more conscious of health and exercise related activities, family physicians and family practice residencies should develop knowledge, skills and attitudes appropriate to sports and recreational medicine. Family physicians often function as the "team physician" to the communities in which they practice. This often involves the provision of physical examinations appropriate to the age of the athlete as well as assessment of and care for the injured athlete. Attention to principles of exercise physiology and the relationship of exercise to optimal functioning of many organ systems is important in the training of family practice residents.

The teaching of recreation to the family unit should also be included in the sports medicine system of family practice residency training. The rationale for extending education in recreation to the family unit is that of promotion of personal and family well-being. Structured family recreational activities promote pleasant exercise, family togetherness, attention to nutrition and increased awareness of general health issues. Family practice residencies should encourage their residents to engage in regular exercise and, in particular, to engage in exercise with members of their families. If residents learn to develop structured educational and scheduled recreational activities with their individual families, it is easier for them to teach recreational principles to the family units of their patients.

When incorporating these curricular guidelines into a family practice residency, it is stressed that attention be given to the basic principles of family practice including continuity and comprehensiveness of care.

Core of Knowledge

I. General Considerations
   A. Integration of family practice philosophy
   B. Ethical, social, economical and medical-legal issues
   C. Interaction with all the sports medicine team
   D. Basic science
   E. Exercise physiology
   F. Biomechanics and kinesiology
   G. Nutrition, fluid and electrolyte
   H. Research

II. Health Promotion and Prevention
   A. Role of exercise in health promotion
   B. Pre-participation evaluation by a qualified physician
   C. Injury prevention
      1. Equipment
      2. Taping techniques
      3. Coaching techniques
      4. Environment
   D. Conditioning and training techniques
   E. Exercise prescription
      1. Age related
      2. Chronic illness
      3. Handicapped
      4. Cardiac rehabilitation
   F. Community programs and facilities, e.g., YMCA
   G. Establishing a community sports medicine system (network)
   H. Epidemiology of exercise and injury
   I. Promotion of patient education

III. Patient Care Aspects
   A. The role as a team family physician including on-site supervision
   B. Assessment and care of acutely injured athlete including transportation
   C. Medical management of the athlete including sports specific injuries
   D. Rehabilitation of ill and injured athletes
   E. Exercise as treatment—physical and psychological problems
   F. Medical care considerations for special athlete groups
      1. Prepubescent
      2. Female
      3. Geriatric
      4. Impaired (diabetic, epileptic, hypertensive)
      5. Recreational
      6. Professional
   G.
   H. Medical decision making involving interaction with athlete, coach, parents, significant others and consultants

Skills

I. History and Physical
II. Promotion of Preventive Techniques Including Physical Training and Safety
III. Medical Management of an Athletic Event
IV. Comprehensive Management of the Athlete
   A. Assessment and care of the acutely injured
   B. Ill athlete
   C. Sports specific injuries
V. Rehabilitation
VI. Exercise Prescription
VII. Use of Medical Equipment and Supplies Including Taping and Strapping Techniques

Implementation

The implementation of this core curriculum should be longitudinal, throughout the resident's experience. The residents library should have reference material available which amplifies the topics in the curricular guidelines. The core curricular guidelines should be integrated into the schedule of conferences and other teaching modalities such as film and live demonstrations. The resident should gain hands-on experience as a team physician and be involved in on-site medical management of recreational and sporting events. Evaluation of the effectiveness of the program is desirable.

Physicians who have demonstrated enthusiasm and skills in caring for the athlete should be available to act as role models to the residents. They should be available to give support and advice to individual residents in the management of their patients. A multidisciplinary approach, coordinated by the family physician, is an appropriate way of structuring teaching experiences in this area. Individual attention and small group discussion will help promote appropriate attitudes. Each family practice resident should be able to demonstrate the ability to work with various individuals involved in the total treatment of the athlete. This will include an understanding of relationships with athletes, parents, coaches, trainers, officials, medical consultants and the various medical and paramedical personnel available in the community.

The resident must have responsibility for patients, and be active as the decision maker. This educational program should provide the resident with an appreciation of the needs of the recreational athlete and enable the resident to prescribe appropriate programs.

Precise details of the implementation will depend on locally available facilities, faculty, pre-existing programs, goals of the residency, and the attitudes and level of interest of the existing residents.

*This document was developed by representatives of, and has been endorsed by, the American Academy of Family Physicians.

diseases or injuries, as well as on the cardiovascular and musculoskeletal systems. Most disqualifying conditions are determined from the health history (Goldberg et al., 1980). The major cause of cardiac sudden death in young athletes is outflow tract obstruction. A positive response to the question "Have you ever felt dizzy, fainted, nearly or actually passed out while exercising?" should prompt a more detailed cardiovascular evaluation, including electrocardiogram, echocardiogram, and graded exercise testing.

The physical examination should give particular attention to the cardiovascular and musculoskeletal systems, including an assessment of physical maturation in the young athlete. The cardiovascular examination should include blood pressure evaluation with the upper limits (not requiring further evaluation) for individuals up to the age of 11 being 130/75, and for children 12 and above being 140/85. The presence of a murmur, while not disqualifying, should be investigated. A systolic murmur that is accentuated by Valsalva's maneuver raises suspicion of the possibility of asymmetric septal hypertrophy and obstructive hypertrophic cardiomyopathy. Any diastolic murmur requires investigation.

Maturation should be assessed and whenever possible compared with others in the group with which the young athlete will be competing. This is of particular importance in contact sports, to protect the preadolescent from a physical mismatch. Standards for rating pubertal development have been established by Tanner (Tanner, 1962). The musculoskeletal examination outlined in Table 48–3 is considered an excellent screening tool and should take the average physician not more than 2 minutes to administer.

The remainder of a complete physical examination should reveal evidence of any infections, visceromegaly, or other limiting or disqualifying abnormalities. See Table 48–4 for a listing of disqualifying abnormalities.

ADULT EXAMINATION

A somewhat different challenge faces the family physician when an adult presents for approval to participate in a new sport or exercise program. In addition to a lengthier history, a more thorough evaluation of cardiovascular risk is indicated. A maximal exercise test is recommended for all individuals over the age of 45 and for individuals over the age of 35 who have either symptoms suggestive of coronary disease or one or more of the major coronary risk factors: (1) history of high blood pressure (above 145/95), (2) elevated total cholesterol to high-density lipoprotein (HDL) ratio (over 5), (3) cigarette smoking, (4) abnormal resting electrocardiogram, (5) family history of coronary disease with onset prior to age 50, and (6) diabetes mellitus (American College of Sports Medicine, 1986).

Table 48–3. ORTHOPEDIC SCREENING EXAMINATION*†

The orthopedic screening examination requires about 90 seconds. Time studies indicate it is most efficiently done one athlete at a time rather than in small groups. It is designed to reveal previous inadequately rehabilitated injuries or those few previously unrecognized orthopedic conditions that might be adversely affected by participation in a sports activity. Positive findings require a more extensive examination and/or history. A more detailed examination **should not** be attempted at the screening examination.

Athletic Activity (Instructions)	Observation
Stand facing examiner	Acromioclavicular joints; general habitus
Look at ceiling, floor, over both shoulders; touch ears to shoulders	Cervical spine motion
Shrug shoulders (examiner resists)	Trapezius strength
Abduct shoulders 90° (examiner resists at 90°)	Deltoid strength
Full external rotation of arms	Shoulder motion
Flex and extend elbows	Elbow motion
Arms at sides, elbows 90° flexed; pronate and supinate wrists	Elbow and wrist motion
Spread fingers; make fist	Hand or finger motion and deformities
Tighten (contract) quadriceps; relax quadriceps	Symmetry and knee effusion; ankle effusion
"Duck walk" four steps (away from examiner with buttocks on heels)	Hip, knee, and ankle motion
Back to examiner	Shoulder symmetry; scoliosis
Knees straight, touch toes	Scoliosis, hip motion, hamstring tightness
Raise up on toes, raise heels	Calf symmetry, leg strength

*From Smith, N. J. (Ed.). Sports Medicine: Health Care for Young Adults. Evanston, IL., American Academy of Pediatrics, 1983.

†May require reflex hammer, tape measure, pin, and examination table.

While ancillary tests are not routinely needed in the child or young athlete, in adults a urine analysis, lipid profile, glucose, and complete blood count are indicated. If office spirometry is available, assessment of vital capacity and forced expiratory flow is helpful.

When this evaluation has been completed, the physician should discuss the type of exercise the patient wishes to begin and give instruction regarding the frequency and intensity of the exercise as well as planned follow-up. The type of exercise should be one that is enjoyable to the patient and should be one that is maintained continuously and is aerobic in nature. While a frequency of even 1 day a week may result in some improvement in fitness, the ideal is three to four times a week. Exercising on nonconsecutive days allows the body to recover between sessions.

Intensity of exercise is a key factor in fitness exercising. Training intensity will vary according to age and the baseline physical condition. It is most conveniently measured by pulse rate, and cardiovascular endurance is most positively affected when exercise results in a pulse of between 60 and 90 per cent of maximal heart rate. An estimate of maximal heart rate is calculated as:

220 minus the patient's age

The exercise program should be begun at an intensity to achieve 60 per cent and gradually build toward 90 per cent.

The duration of activity is also important. Some improvement can be seen with sessions as short as 10 minutes, but the general recommendation is 15 to 60 minutes of continuous exercise. Patients should be cautioned that it will likely take 4 to 6 weeks to produce measurable effects (Kirkendall, 1984), and the physician should be available for periodic follow-up.

FITNESS TESTING FOR THE COMPETITIVE ATHLETE

A more comprehensive evaluation includes assessment of (1) cardiovascular fitness—aerobic and anaerobic, (2) agility, (3) balance, (4) flexibility, and (5) strength. This type of testing would be undertaken by the team physician and could be best accomplished through mass testing, with various stations set up at the school, and manned with the assistance of allied health personnel including physical therapists and

Table 48–4. DISQUALIFYING CONDITIONS FOR SPORTS PARTICIPATION*

Conditions	Collision†	Contact‡	Noncontact§	Other‖
General				
Acute infections	X	X	X	X
Respiratory, genitourinary, infectious mononucleosis, hepatitis, active rheumatic fever, active tuberculosis				
Obvious physical immaturity in comparison with other competitors	X	X		
Hemorrhagic disease	X	X	X	
Hemophilia, purpura, and other serious bleeding tendencies				
Diabetes, inadequately controlled	X	X	X	X
Diabetes, controlled	X	X	X	X
Jaundice				
Eyes				
Absence or loss of function of one eye	X	X		
Respiratory				
Tuberculosis (active or symptomatic)	X	X	X	X
Severe pulmonary insufficiency	X	X	X	X
Cardiovascular				
Mitral stenosis, aortic stenosis, aortic insufficiency, coarctation of aorta, cyanotic heart disease, recent carditis of any etiology	X	X	X	X
Hypertension on organic basis	X	X	X	X
Previous heart surgery for congenital or acquired heart disease¶				
Liver				
Enlarged liver	X	X		
Skin				
Boils, impetigo, and herpes simplex gladiatorum	X	X		
Spleen				
Enlarged spleen	X	X		
Hernia				
Inguinal or femoral hernia	X	X	X	
Musculoskeletal				
Symptomatic abnormalities or inflammations	X	X	X	X
Functional inadequacy of the musculoskeletal system, congenital or acquired, incompatible with the contact or skill demands of the sport	X	X	X	
Neurologic				
History or symptoms of previous serious head trauma, or repeated concussions	X			
Controlled convulsive disorder**				
Convulsive disorder not moderately well controlled by medication	X			
Previous surgery on head	X	X		
Renal				
Absence of one kidney	X	X		
Renal disease	X	X	X	X
Genitalia††				
Absence of one testicle				
Undescended testicle				

**From* American Medical Association, Committee on the Medical Aspects of Sports. Medical Evaluation of the Athlete—A Guide. Chicago, American Medical Association, 1966, pp. 7–8.

†Includes football, rugby, hockey, lacrosse.

‡Includes baseball, soccer, basketball, wrestling.

§Includes cross-country track, track, tennis, crew, swimming.

‖Includes bowling, golf, archery, field events.

¶Each patient should be judged on an individual basis in conjunction with his cardiologist and operating surgeon.

**Each patient should be judged on an individual basis. All things being equal, it is probably better to encourage a young boy or girl to participate in a noncontact sport rather than a contact sport. However, if a particular patient has a great desire to play a contact sport, and this is deemed a major ameliorating factor in his/her adjustment to school, associates, and the seizure disorder, serious consideration should be given to letting him or her participate if the seizures are moderately well controlled or the athlete is under good medical management.

††The Committee approves the concept of contact sports participation for youths with only one testicle or with an undescended testicle(s), except in specific cases such as an inguinal canal undescended testicle(s), following appropriate medical evaluation to rule out unusual injury risk. However, the athlete, parents, and school authorities should be fully informed that participation in contact sports for such youths with only one testicle does carry a slight injury risk to the remaining healthy testicle. Following such an injury, fertility may be adversely affected. However, the chances of an injury to a descended testicle are rare, and the injury risk can be further substantially minimized with an athletic supporter and protective device.

athletic trainers. While such an endeavor is personnel intensive, it can be accomplished with very little equipment. Sport-specific norms are not available for all age groups and hence athletes may serve as their own control with the testing repeated twice per year.

Cardiovascular fitness is tested using some standard stress, such as bench step maneuver, stationary cycle, or preferably a 1½ mile run. In the case of the latter, the time needed to complete the run, as well as the pre- and postexercise pulse and blood pressures, and the postexercise time to return to normal readings are measured.

Agility, defined as the ability to change directions rapidly while moving at a high rate of speed, is dependent on elements of strength, reaction time, speed of movement, and specific coordinations (Gould et al., 1985). A relatively simple general test of agility is the shuttle run, which involves the athlete running from a starting point to a point about 30 feet away, picking up a small object, returning to the start and then repeating this once. Norms have been established (Gould, 1985).

Balance can be affected by injury and, if not recognized, may lead to reinjury, even if strength has been restored. This can be screened by having the athlete stand on one foot and close both eyes. One measures the length of time before movement of the nonweight-bearing extremity is required to maintain balance. Comparisons between sides should not vary by more than 5 seconds, although more specific norms are not available (Gould, 1985).

Posture is evaluated by having the athlete stand behind a plumb line while deviations from normal erect posture are noted (Kendal et al., 1983). Abnormal neck posture, such as a forward head, should be noted since it may predispose to injury. A check on upper extremity mobility includes active movement of the shoulders in all planes. Deviation from the normal 1 degree scapular motion for each 2 degrees of humeral motion should be noted. Elbows, wrists, and hands are assessed for normal range of motion.

Trunk flexibility should include checking for full range of motion of the neck. Scoliosis screening should be included. Low back range-of-motion assessment includes knee-to-chest and prone-press-up tests. Lower extremity flexibility screen of the hamstrings involves passive straight leg raises. A more specific lower extremity flexibility assessment consists of the Thomas test described by Daniel and Worthingham (1977).

Quadriceps strength should be tested against the examiner's resistance. Gastrocnemius/soleus strength can be measured by 7 to 10 repetitive heel rises while standing on one foot. Athletes should be tested bilaterally and used as their own controls.

Computerized isokinetic testing devices are available at physical therapy and sports assessment facilities and should be considered if questionable results are obtained on these screenings.

EVALUATION OF BIOMECHANICS

Later in this chapter, various soft tissue and overuse syndromes will be discussed. In order to effectively address the underlying causative factors in many of these problems, it is important to have some understanding of the arthokinematics of the involved segments. A discussion of each functional unit is beyond the scope of this chapter. Since the foot is the base of support for all upright activity, a basic understanding of static and dynamic foot mechanics will aid the clinician in recognizing the predisposing cause of many lower extremity abnormalities.

During the evaluation, the patient should first be screened for leg length discrepancy. The toes and soles of the feet should be examined for calluses, hammer toes, and hallus valgus, all of which are signs of abnormal foot mechanics. The patient's footwear should be evaluated for excessive wear patterns consistent with one of the common pathomechanical syndromes. A quick check for abnormal pronation in the static foot is assessment of Feiss' line. In the normal foot, Feiss' line is a *straight* line drawn from the tip of the medial malleolus to the first metatarsal-phalangeal joint (Fig. 48–1). If the navicular tubercle lies *below* the line in the weight-bearing patient, this represents abnormal pronation, and further evaluation is indicated.

To aid in further evaluation of the static and dynamic foot mechanics, draw two lines on the patient's leg, one bisecting the heel and the other bisecting the calf (Fig. 48–2). In order to perform a thorough gait evaluation, an understanding of the gait cycle is necessary. The gait cycle is divided into two phases, swing phase and stance phase. The majority of time is spent in the weight-bearing stance phase, and this discussion will be limited to it.

Just prior to heel strike, the foot is supinated and the calcaneus should appear slightly inverted. (Fig. 48–2—normal heel strike.) As the foot makes contact with the ground and weight is beginning to be accepted onto the foot, the subtalar joint pronates rapidly until the foot is flat on the ground. This acts to significantly dampen the shock incurred at initial weight bearing. The midfoot then unlocks to allow mobile adaptation of the forefoot to accommodate to

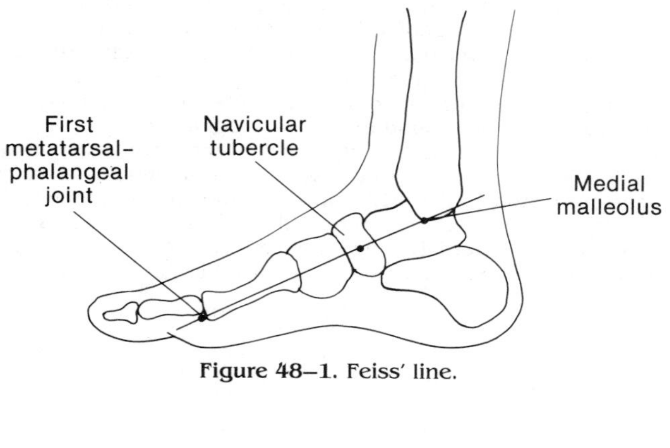

Figure 48–1. Feiss' line.

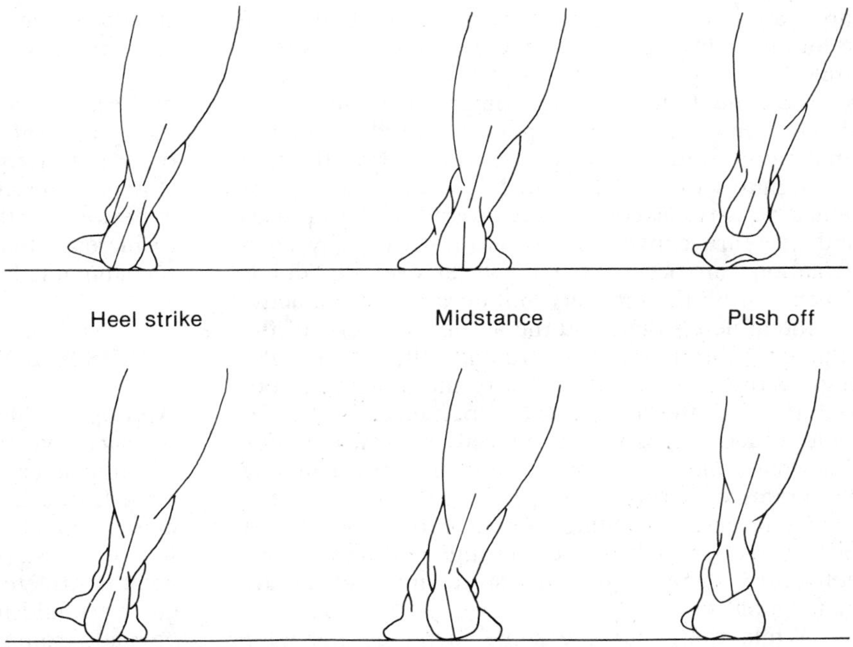

Figure 48–2. Stance phase of gait (posterior view of right foot), demonstrating normal and excessive pronation.

uneven terrain. By this time, the body weight is transferred fully onto the stance foot. (Fig. 45–2—normal midstance). As the heel begins to rise, the foot supinates to convert it into a rigid lever. Weight is then transferred to the first ray and great toe for push-off (Fig. 48–2—normal push-off).

The two most common mechanical problems are excessive pronation and supination. Evidence of these are noted in static observation, gait evaluation and examination of footwear, and callus formation on the soles of the feet. Supination is characterized by inversion of the calcaneus at midstance, and push-off from the lateral forefoot. Affected patients will frequently have calluses over the lateral aspect of the foot and are prone to proximal stress phenomena, such as tibial stress fracture, because of the loss of the shock-absorbing function normally provided by pronation.

The much more common foot abnormality is excessive pronation (Fig. 48–2—excessive pronation). Affected patients often stand in some calcaneal eversion that will become more evident during ambulation at heel strike or midstance. Since the patient pronates excessively and usually long after supination should have begun to lock the foot (converting it into a rigid lever), the foot is less stable. Push-off is shifted onto the second and third metatarsals. These bones do not tolerate full weight bearing like the first ray and great toe and are, therefore, more prone to stress fractures in these patients. Tibial rotation is also associated with hyperpronation and can lead to malalignment syndromes in the proximal segments, especially patellar-femoral dysfunction syndrome and tendinitis of the musculature around the ankle and knee. Examination of the feet in these patients usually reveals callus formation over the second and third metatarsal heads to help reduce stress. The patient will frequently have some degree of hallux valgus. Abnormal shoe wear is evident as excessive wear in the center of the forefoot, indicating push-off shifting to the middle metatarsal heads.

If findings suggest excessive pronation in one foot and supination in the other, suspect a leg length discrepancy. This is a compensatory mechanism for the leg length discrepancy and can be a source of chronic low back pain. (Functionally, supination lengthens a limb and pronation shortens it.)

If this screening raises suspicion of abnormal foot mechanics, consider referral to a physical therapist specializing in foot mechanics for a more thorough evaluation and fabrication of corrective orthotics. Over-the-counter arch supports are *not* adequate substitutes since they are neither biomechanically corrective nor patient specific.

Inflammatory conditions are frequently a result of abnormal biomechanics, and, unless treatment is directed both at the acute inflammation and at correcting the underlying problem, recurrences can be expected.

Nutritional Considerations

Good nutrition is essential to achieving a healthy and fit body and to optimal athletic performance. The amount of protein an athlete in training requires is under study, but most recent recommendations suggest that 1.0 to 1.5 gm./kg. body weight per day is appropriate (compared with the average adult recommendation of 0.8 gm./kg. body weight per day (A.D.A., 1986). The total calories from protein sources in the diet should be approximately 15 per cent of the total daily calories. While protein provides the same fuel value as carbohydrate (i.e., 4 kcal./gm.), it is a less efficient fuel source. In addition, large amounts of ingested protein can stress the kidney's ability to handle the resultant amount of urea.

Carbohydrates are the primary fuel source and should comprise 55 to 60 per cent of the athlete's total caloric intake. Glucose is used during the first few minutes of moderate to heavy activity. In sustained activity, glycogen stores found in the muscles and liver are converted back to glucose. Glycogen depletion can occur as a result of exercise and is dependent on the intensity and duration of the activity, the athlete's diet, and the aerobic capacity of the athlete. If during intensive training, the athletes glycogen stores are depleted as a result of a low carbohydrate diet, the athlete will experience chronic fatigue, reduced speed, and reduced endurance. While a normal athlete's diet would contain approximately 350 grams of carbohydrate, it is recommended that during intensive training a high carbohydrate diet (550 to 600 grams/day) be consumed. Complex carbohydrates increase glycogen stores more efficiently than simple sugars.

While there may be some increased need for certain vitamins (thiamine, riboflavin, pyridoxine, folacin, and iron) in training athletes, there is no need for supplementation and no evidence that supplementation has a beneficial effect. Since caloric expenditure is high and dietary intake is increased over the average population, the nutrients provided by food alone are two to three times the Recommended Daily Allowance.

EVENT NUTRITION

The major function of the pre-event meal is to maximize liver glycogen stores. Timing of the meal is very important. It should be consumed 2 to 5 hours before competition. If consumed less than 1 hour prior to competition, hypoglycemia may result secondary to postprandial hyperinsulinemia. If consumed more than 5 hours prior to the event, this may result in less than maximal glycogen stores.

The pre-event meals should be: (1) high in carbohydrate (60 to 70 per cent of the total calories); (2) relatively low in fat, which slows gastric emptying; (3) relatively low in protein, which increases urination and, hence, is a threat to hydration; (4) minimal in bulk; and (5) adequate in fluid intake. In the 2 hours immediately preceding the event, no solid food should be eaten, but low-caloric fluid can be ingested in amounts depending on the anticipated fluid loss during the event.

During the event, fluid losses should be replaced with water. The exception is endurance events (e.g., marathons), when fluid, glucose, and electrolyte replacement is indicated. (See section on fluid and electrolytes.)

Within the first 2 hours after the exercise event, 2 grams of carbohydrate per kilogram of body weight should be ingested. This will decrease muscle fatigue and soreness.

In regard to postcompetition nutrition, a study by Castill (1981) indicated that consumption of up to 650 grams of carbohydrate per day resulted in a proportionately greater amount of muscle glycogen storage. The average dietary intake of carbohydrate is between 250 and 450 grams per day, so an effort to increase that intake to about 600 grams a day is recommended.

FLUIDS AND ELECTROLYTES

Appropriate fluid replacement and an understanding of electrolyte needs as they relate to exercise and sporting events are essential. If fluids are not replaced, dehydration results, which can have a detrimental effect on the athlete's performance and, in severe cases, poses an obvious threat to his or her health. Athletes should not rely on thirst as their only guide to fluid needs. Some estimate of fluid loss can be made from pre- and postevent weighings in certain sporting endeavors. (This will be discussed further in the section on heat-related illness.) Electrolytes must also be considered but historically too much emphasis has been placed on the role of salt loss through perspiration. In the well-trained athlete, only trace amounts of salt are lost, and the kidneys become proficient at excreting little salt in the urine. A normal diet will replace most, perhaps all, salt needs. For most people, three daily meals easily replace the salt lost in up to 10 pounds of exercise-induced sweat (Cantu, 1982).

Water serves, therefore, as an excellent source of fluid replacement. If commercial exercise drinks are to be used, it must be remembered that they are generally too hypertonic. Dilution, according to Table 48–5, should be considered.

Fluid absorption must also be considered. Volume and fluid temperature have an effect on absorption. Fluids ingested in relatively small amounts at regular intervals are most effective. Pre-event anticipatory hydration has been recommended, with approximately 20 ounces consumed 1 to 2 hours before the event and another 12 to 16 ounces consumed 15 to 20 minutes before the event. During the event, 3 to 6 ounces every 10 to 20 minutes may be consumed, depending on the apparent fluid loss. Drinks cooled to 40 to 50° F. are recommended for maximal absorption.

Drug Use in Sports

The issue of drug use in sports dates back with the history of sports itself, and the reports of probable use of mushrooms and herbs in the athletes of the ancient Greek Olympiads. The messages sent to athletes have at times been unclear, with substances

Table 48–5. BEVERAGES FOR EVENT FLUID REPLACEMENT*

Beverages that can be used as is (without dilution):	
Water	
Exceed	
Club soda†	
Perrier†	
Seltzer†	
Beverages recommended for dilution with water:	
One Part	***Diluted with Water***
Gatorade‡	2¼ parts
ERG‡	1 part
Sportade‡	3 parts
Sugar-free soda†	1 part
Regular soda†	3 parts
Fruit juices	7 parts
Take 5‡	7 parts
Quick Kick‡	2½ parts

*Information adapted in part from Costill, D. L., Track and Field News, 1979, and American College of Sports Medicine, Med. Sci. Sports, 7:vii, 1975.

†Recommended to defizz carbonated drinks if used before or during the activity.

‡Dilutions apply when products made according to manufacturer's directions.

banned but punishments inconsistent. The dilemma and controversy for today's athletes involves the use of anabolic steroids. The use of these substances is not limited to the professional or olympic level athlete. Use among high school and even preadolescent athletes is on an alarming rise. The physician working with athletes must be knowledgeable about the dangerous effects of anabolic steroid use (Table 48–6). The physician's responsibility is not only to recognize and treat these problems but to be a resource to the community to alert athletes, parents, and coaches alike to the danger and inappropriateness of the use of these substance. As has been found in other areas of substance abuse, one of the most effective means of addressing the issue is through motivated and informed peer support groups.

Table 48–6. REPORTED SIDE EFFECTS OF ANABOLIC STEROIDS

Affective syndrome	Pope and Katz, 1988
Psychotic symptoms	Pope and Katz, 1988
Elevated transaminases	Lenders et al., 1988
Elevated systolic blood pressure	Lenders et al., 1988
Lower HDH cholesterol	Lenders et al., 1988
Elevated LDL cholesterol	Lenders et al., 1988
Enlargement of sebaceous glands	Kiraly et al., 1987
Diminished glucose tolerance	Cohen and Hickman, 1987
Case Reports:	
Stroke	Frankle et al., 1988
Acute myocardial infarction	McNutt et al., 1988
Hepatic tumors	Creagh, 1988
Cholestasis	Everly, 1987
Tendon rupture	Kramhft, 1986
Addiction: physiologic and psychologic	Black, 1988

Catastrophic Injury in Sports

The National Center for Catastrophic Sports Injury Research, located in Chapel Hill, North Carolina, collects data from around the country on high school and collegiate athletes suffering catastrophic injury or death as a result of participation in sports sponsored by high schools or colleges. The purpose of such data collection is directed toward identifying the areas of greatest danger, which should lead to appropriate rule changes and safety measures to reduce such catastrophic injuries. A success story is exemplified by the 1976 rules change by the National Collegiate Athletic Association and high schools to make it illegal to spear block in football. This has led to a demonstrable decrease in the catastrophic injury rate in football (Mueller, 1986). All physicians serving as team physicians should understand the appropriate reporting mechanism in their state.

Psychologic Aspects of Sports

Much attention has been given of late to psychologic aids to enhance performance in sports. Professional teams having a slump or unproductive season have hired psychologists to work with the team.

For the family physician working with athletes, the recognition of the individual athlete with sports-related psychologic problems is the more relevant issue. These issues include the counseling of parents and children in competitive level and sport selection, as well as the recognition of burnout among some of the most gifted athletes in their sport.

Feigley (1984) characterizes burnout among elite athletes as a condition caused by working too hard for too long in a high-pressured situation. In addition, the athlete displays feelings of being locked in a routine and may show loss of purpose. In the earliest stages, the athlete may present with fatigue, minor body complaints, headaches, etc. and on further questioning may relate a history of increased irritability and loss of enthusiasm. Progression is usually associated with some withdrawal, significant self-doubt, and more physical symptoms that occasionally manifest as eating disorders. Overachievers and athletes with perfectionist traits are more susceptible. Early recognition is key to successful intervention.

Diagnosis and Treatment of Common Sports-Related Injuries

APPROACH TO THE DOWNED ATHLETE

Before discussing the approach to the downed athlete, it is appropriate to remind anyone providing event medical coverage of what should be done BEFORE the event begins. Plan for initiating the emergency medical system: (1) who will make the call and where is the radio or phone, (2) how will the emergency vehicle enter and exit the playing field, and (3) how close is the nearest hospital or ambulance service? Also make sure the players and coaches know that a fellow athlete who goes down is to be left alone and not moved or rolled over.

Anytime the health care professional is called to evaluate the downed athlete, one must consider the possibility that this is a catastrophic, life-threatening situation. As with all basic life support, assure the ABCs of airway, breathing, and circulation first. Identify the level of consciousness. If the athlete is conscious, there may be splinting of the neck with muscle spasm. Immobilize the neck, reassure the athlete, inquire for the painful area, and perform a brief neurologic exam. If the athlete is unconscious, assume the worst, i.e. that a possible head or neck injury is present, and proceed with establishing an airway, check for breathing and circulation, and immobilize the neck. In the case of a sport with head gear, leave the helmet on, unless doing so precludes establishing an airway. Today's equipment is designed to provide emergency access (i.e., removal of the face guard in the case of football helmets), and it is imperative that the health care provider be familiar with this equipment prior to the event. One piece of equipment that should be included in the medical bag for event coverage is a pocket mirror. This can help establish that breathing is taking place when the athlete is face down (place the mirror in front of the nose and mouth to look for fogging).

For assessing the downed athlete with a possible concussion, Cantu (1986) has developed a useful and practical, on-the-field grading scheme for identifying concussion in contact sports and making recommendations for return to sport. A grade 1 concussion is a situation where the athlete does not lose consciousness but suffers impaired intellectual function, particularly in memory of recent events and interpreting new information. This is sometimes difficult to diagnose, because the athlete is able to walk and talk; but, since he is not at peak cognitive ability and agility, he is at risk for more serious injury.

Grade 2 is considered a moderate concussion and is associated with unconsciousness of 5 minutes or less. Grade 3 is defined as unconsciousness of more than 5 minutes or posttraumatic amnesia of approximately 24 hours. The athlete will need to be removed from the playing field on a fracture board and observed closely at a hospital with neurosurgical treatment facilities and monitored for possible intracranial bleeding.

The physician is then faced with the decision of when the athlete can return to sport (Table 48–7). In the case of a grade 1 mild concussion with no loss of consciousness, if the athlete has no headache, dizziness, or impaired concentration after 15 to 20 minutes of observation, and can demonstrate normal agility, clinical judgment may allow this athlete to return to the game.

When evaluating the athlete on the playing field with a musculoskeletal injury, check for circulation, neurologic deficit, and deformity. Ask the athlete about motor and sensory function. Follow the acronym "PRICES"—protect, rest, ice, compression, elevation, and support.

In approaching the downed athlete, particularly where trauma did not appear to be involved, one must consider heat illness or a cardiovascular event. While cardiovascular events in athletes over 30 years of age are most commonly a result of coronary artery disease, in athletes under 30 years of age one must consider structural deformities, hypertrophic cardiomyopathy, and anomalous coronary arteries.

Environmental Illness

HEAT-RELATED ILLNESS

Prevention of heat-related illness by recognition of environmental and individual risk factors for heat-related illness is the first responsibility of the family physician. The physician should be familiar with the heat stress index available from the National Weather Service. The index takes into account both air temperature and relative humidity. Table 48–8 charts the heat stress index. Individuals with a febrile or gastrointestinal illness, as well as those with previous heat-related illness, should be considered at high risk. A child sweats only 40 per cent as efficiently as an adult and is therefore at greater risk. Similarly, the impaired thermoregulatory system of the elderly places them at increased risk. Obesity, sleep deprivation, uncontrolled diabetes, uncontrolled hypertension, cystic fibrosis, alcoholism or substance abuse, and cardiac disease are additional risk factors for heat-related illness. Athletes taking diuretics, neuroleptics, beta blockers, anticholinergics, or antihistamines are at risk as well (Mellion, 1988). It must be remembered that heat acclimatization requires four to seven bouts of exercise in the hot environment for 1 to 4 hours each. The sessions should be of gradually increasing intensity over a 7 to 10 day period. Athletes should be observed daily for evidence of dehydration. Body weight is the most logical measure. Weigh-ins before and after the workout should be considered, and particular attention must be given to athletes showing a practice weight loss of 3 per cent or more. If they have not regained the weight by the next practice session, activity should be restricted.

Heat-related illness is usually divided into three syndromes, which represent stages along a continuum of clinical conditions caused by dehydration, electrolyte imbalances, and disruption of the body's normal heat-dissipating mechanisms. These are identified as heat cramps, heat exhaustion, and heat stroke. One may also encounter the mild heat-related entity of heat syncope, which generally occurs when the athlete abruptly stops exercising, as at the end of an endur-

Table 48–7. GUIDELINES FOR RETURN TO PLAY AFTER CONCUSSION*

	1st Concussion	2nd Concussion	3rd Concussion
Grade 1 (mild)	May return to play if asymptomatic† for 1 wk	Return to play in 2 wk if asymptomatic at that time for 1 wk	Terminate season; may return to play next season if asymptomatic
Grade 2 (moderate)	Return to play after asymptomatic for 1 wk	Minimum of 1 mo; may return to play then if asymptomatic for 1 wk; consider terminating season	Terminate season; may return to play next season if asymptomatic
Grade 3 (severe)	Minimum of 1 mo; may then return to play if asymptomatic for 1 wk	Terminate season; may return to play next season if asymptomatic	

*From Cantu, R. C. Physc. Sportsmed., *14*(10):75, 1986. Reprinted by permission of the Physician and Sportsmedicine. Copyright McGraw-Hill, Inc.

†No headache, dizziness, or impaired orientation, concentration, or memory during rest or exertion.

ance race. It is secondary to pooling in the dilated vessels of the lower extremities and is treated by having the patient lie down with legs elevated.

Heat cramps, or heat stress, is characterized by involuntary and sometimes painful muscle cramps and spasms, mild dehydration, and diminished response time, though the patient remains oriented. Treatment consists of rest, rehydration, and cooling of the skin.

Heat exhaustion is characterized by marked fatigue and weakness, as well as lightheadedness, profuse sweating, and nausea. The patient is usually tachycardic and may exhibit temperature elevation though, by definition, it is less than 105°F. rectally. The sweating mechanism is intact, and the treatment is rest, rehydration, and cooling of the skin. Cooling can be accomplished by removing the clothes and sponging or misting with tepid or cool water. For transportation, consider packing ice around the victim. In the hospital, a large fan or other means to enhance evaporation is beneficial.

Heat stroke is a serious and life-threatening entity with rectal temperatures over 105°F. There is severe central nervous system disturbance and circulatory collapse. Often the sweating mechanism will have failed, and the patient will be hot and flushed but dry. Treatment must be prompt and foremost must involve external cooling of the body. Intensive care treatment and monitoring is necessary to assure airway management and careful fluid and electrolyte administration.

HYPOTHERMIC INJURY

Hypothermia is defined as occurring when the core body temperature drops below 35°C. (95°F.) (Table 48–9). Symptoms include mental deterioration, anxiety, irritability and apathy, shivering, motor difficulty, clumsiness, muscle weakness, and cramps. The patient should be kept from continued exposure to the cold (i.e., wrapped in blankets), but rapid warming, such as immersion in hot water, is not recommended. Applying heat primarily to the trunk and sparingly to the extremities is recommended, since the initial vasodilatation could lead to an influx of cold blood from the extremities, resulting in a further drop of the core temperature (afterdrop effect). Avoid rough handling of the patient during transport, which could precipitate ventricular fibrillation. Severe cases (core temperature less than 90°F.) will require

Table 48–8. HEAT STRESS* (APPARENT TEMPERATURES IN ° F.)

		Air Temperature (°F)										
		70	75	80	85	90	95	100	105	110	115	120
Relative Humidity (%)	0%	64	69	73	78	83	87	91	95	99	103	107
	10%	65	70	75	80	85	90	95	100	105	111	116
	20%	66	72	77	82	87	93	99	105	112	120	130
	30%	67	73	78	84	90	96	104	113	123	135	148
	40%	68	74	79	86	93	101	110	123	137	151	
	50%	69	75	81	88	96	107	120	135	150		
	60%	70	76	82	90	100	114	132	144			
	70%	70	77	85	93	106	124	144				
	80%	71	78	86	97	113	136					
	90%	71	79	88	102	122						
	100%	72	80	91	108							

DANGER ZONE = +90° F. (temperatures in bold-faced type, above)

*From Mellion, M. B.: Sports Medicine—Prevention of Athletic Injuries. Philadelphia, Hanley & Belfus, 1988; and The National Weather Service.

Table 48–9. WINDCHILL INDEX (EQUIVALENT IN COOLING POWER ON EXPOSED FLESH)*

Wind Speed† (mph)	Air Temperature (°F)																
	35	30	25	20	15	10	5	0	−5	−10	−15	−20	−25	−30	−35	−40	−45
4	35	30	25	20	15	10	5	0	−5	−10	−15	−20	−25	−30	−35	−40	−45
5	32	27	22	16	11	6	0	−5	−10	−15	−21	−26	−31	−36	−42	−47	−52
10	22	16	10	3	−3	−9	−15	−22	−27	−34	−40	−46	−52	−58	−64	−71	−77
15	16	9	2	−5	−11	−18	−25	−31	−38	−45	−51	−58	−65	−72	−78	−85	−92
20	12	4	−3	−10	−17	−24	−31	−39	−46	−53	−60	−67	−74	−81	−88	−95	−103
25	8	1	−7	−15	−22	−29	−36	−44	−51	−59	−66	−74	−81	−88	−96	−103	−110
30	6	−2	−10	−18	−25	−33	−41	−49	−56	−64	−71	−79	−86	−93	−101	−109	−116
35	4	−4	−12	−20	−27	−35	−43	−52	−58	−67	−74	−82	−89	−97	−105	−113	−120
40	3	−5	−13	−21	−29	−37	−45	−53	−60	−69	−76	−84	−92	−100	−107	−115	−123
45*	2	−6	−14	−22	−30	−38	−46	−54	−62	−70	−78	−85	−93	−102	−109	−117	−125

*From U.S. Department of Commerce. National Oceanic and Atmospheric Administration.
†Wind speeds greater than 40 mph have little additional cooling effect.
Example—A 30 mph wind, combined with a temperature of 30 degrees F (−1 degree Celsius), can have the same chilling effect as a temperature of −2 degrees F (−19 degrees Celsius) when it is calm.

hospitalization for monitored rewarming and volume expansion.

ALTITUDE ILLNESS

Athletes are neither unique nor immune to the development of altitude sickness. Physiologically, the decreased barometric pressure results in a decreased inspired oxygen pressure. Symptoms include headache, insomnia, nausea, vomiting, ataxia, and possibly impaired consciousness. These symptoms are accentuated by exercise. Acclimatization through gradual ascent is the best prevention. Maintaining adequate hydration, avoidance of sedation and use of acetazolamide (Diamox) 250 mg. three times a day beginning 16 hours prior to the ascent are also recommended. Treatment is to return to a lower altitude.

AIR POLLUTION

At lunchtime, downtown in any large metropolitan area in this country, the streets are filled with joggers, and the air is filled with pollutants. How well do those things coexist? The air pollution is made up of two types of substances: (1) reductive, consisting primarily of carbon monoxide and sulfur oxides, and (2) oxidant, including ozone. Carbon monoxide in levels up to 50 parts per million (ppm) has not been shown to have a significant effect on healthy, noncardiovascularly compromised people, though more study is needed. Ozone in levels above 0.2 ppm has been shown to decrease performance and compromise lung function. The sulfur dioxide threshold for affecting lung function appears to lie between 1 and 2 ppm (Raven, 1988).

Soft Tissue Injury

Whether actively involved in sports medicine or not, two of the most common types of injuries seen by the family physician are the sprain and the strain. The sprain is a disruption of the connective tissue that connects bone to bone (ligamentous injury). The strain is a disruption of the connective tissue that connects muscle to bone (muscle-tendon unit injury). For the purpose of both assessment and treatment plans, these injuries are graded according to severity.

Grade 1, or first-degree injury, is a mild disruption of the fibers with minimal swelling, minimal tenderness, and minimal loss of function. The joint is stable in this case. Grade 2, or second-degree injury, shows swelling with some limited range of motion, but here also, the joint integrity is intact. Grade 1 and 2 injuries are treated acutely with ice and compression and, subsequently, by protecting the involved area with a splint or air cast. The involved muscle groups should be subjected to isometric, progressive resistance and isokinetic exercise during healing. Therapy should be continued not only until symptoms subside but also until rehabilitation of the associated muscle groups is assured and the athlete is prepared for return to sport.

Grade 3, or third-degree injury, is associated with pain, swelling, limited range of motion and *instability* of the joint. These injuries may require surgery for repair of the ligaments. Referral for possible surgery should be considered as soon as the diagnosis is made so surgery can be carried out before the development of atrophy and increasing instability.

A contusion is the disruption of the blood vessels causing bleeding into soft tissue (skin or muscle). Initial management includes ice and compression. Early initiation of electrical stimulation and ultrasound is also helpful. The amount of bleeding is important, since heavy bleeding into a muscle may lead to the development of myositis ossificans.

Overuse Syndromes

Overuse syndromes represent, by definition, excessive distribution of load over an anatomical site, leading to pain, inflammation, and reduction of function. The following is a discussion of some of the most common overuse syndromes seen by the primary care physician caring for the competitive or recreational athlete.

Shin splints is not a medical term but rather a layperson terminology commonly used to describe any pain below the knee and above the ankle. The differential can include a tendinitis/periostitis syndrome due to inflammation of the attachment of the posterior tibialis tendon and/or to soleus dysfunction leading to a periostitis at the site of attachment. Treatment is directed toward the reduction of inflammation and correction of the biomechanical factors that led to the symptoms. Return to activity is gradual and based on symptom resolution.

Another consideration in the differential of lower leg pain is *compartment syndrome.* The muscles of the lower leg are enveloped in fascial compartments, which are relatively unyielding. Muscle swelling within the compartment can result in excessive pressure on the neural and vascular elements of the lower leg. This can occur acutely and may require surgical intervention through fasciotomy (see chapter on orthopedics). This syndrome can also present with a slow, insidious onset, with pain primarily with activity. This is usually a result of inappropriate training techniques and should be managed with rest and gradual reinstitution of training at a more gradual pace.

Stress fracture of the tibia or fibula must also be considered in the differential of lower leg pain. Stress fractures are the result of repetitive activity. They may present with pain alone or be associated with some swelling. Initial radiographs may be nondiagnostic so the level of suspicion must continue to be present on the part of the family physician. Inappropriate training techniques (too much, too fast) is usually the cause. Recognition is the key. Once the diagnosis is made, the involved extremity should be rested for 8 to 12 weeks (splinted or casted for 2 to 3 weeks depending on the reliability of the patient), with gradual return to activity once any biomechanical problems have been corrected.

Another lay term, *runner's knee,* is most likely the result of patellar chondromalacia or patellar-femoral dysarrangement syndrome. It is characterized by pain brought on by activity, such as climbing stairs, squatting, kneeling, or sitting for prolonged periods with the knee bent. The patient complains of mild-to-moderate swelling with a history of the knee giving way with no locking. On physical exam, there may be minimal effusion with a positive apprehension test of lateral deviation of the knee cap. Further evaluation of the biomechanics of the lower extremity and foot mechanism is indicated, with determination of the Q angle and the patellar tendon insertion. (The Q angle, which should be measured in the standing position, is that angle formed by a line from the anterior superior iliac spine, to the center of the patella, and the line from the center of the patella to the center of the tibial tubercle.) If radiographs are normal, treatment should include correction of the biomechanical problems with quadriceps and hamstring strengthening (with attention to the vastus medialis oblicus). Full arc quadriceps contractions and heavy weight lifting during exercise should be avoided.

Plantar fasciitis is inflammation and micro tears of the plantar fascia at the attachment to the calcaneus. It is caused by poor foot mechanics and trauma (overuse) of the calcaneal fat pad. The patient complains of heel pain on arising, with the pain diminishing after some walking (hence stretching of the soft tissue). There is no numbness or tingling, and pain should not increase with activity. The differential includes tarsal tunnel syndrome and stress fracture of the calcaneus. Treatment is addressed to treating the inflammation, increasing the flexibility of the plantar fascia and Achilles tendon with an appropriate gastrocnemius and soleus strengthening program, and gradual return to activity after the biomechanical problems have been corrected. Injection and surgery should be reserved for persistent and chronic symptoms. Radiographs are obtained to assure that there are no other structural defects.

Lateral epicondylitis of the elbow (*tennis elbow*) presents as chronic pain. It is caused by overuse of the wrist *extensors* (and abnormal mechanics of the radiohumeral, as well as radiocarpal, joints causing abnormal transmission of forces). The patient complains of gradual onset of lateral elbow pain that increases with repeated wrist use. On physical examination, there is tenderness of the lateral epicondyle (at the site of attachment of the wrist extensors) with pain on locking the wrist in the neutral position and resisted extension of the middle digit. The differential diagnosis must rule out either nerve entrapment within the upper extremity or bony abnormality. Treatment is directed toward reducing the inflammation and increasing wrist extensor strength. Physical therapy referral for phonophoresis and mobilization to treat the abnormal mechanics should be considered. A tennis forearm band can be used to help reduce inflammation.

Medial epicondylitis represents an overuse of the wrist *flexors.* On physical examination, there is tenderness of the medial epicondyle at the site of the wrist conjoint tendon attachment with tenderness over the ulnar groove. The physician should consider instability of the medial oblique ligament and entrapment of the interosseous nerve as part of the differential, and radiographs should be obtained to rule out loose bodies or a chronic avulsion fracture in the skeletally immature athlete. Treatment consists of rest, with gradual rehabilitation of the wrist flexors, and consideration of a medial epicondylar brace. Sometimes casting or use of an ulnar gutter splint is needed to rest the elbow.

Bursitis is inflammation of the bursal sacs, which are located anatomically to reduce friction where the gliding of tendons is near bony structures. It is frequently caused by abnormal biomechanics leading to excessive stress on adjacent structures, resulting in the inflammatory condition. The most common sites are the olecranon surface of the elbow, the acromial bursa of the shoulder, the prepatellar bursa of the knee, and the trochanteric bursa of the hip. Treatment is directed toward rest and treatment of the inflammation and evaluation and treatment of the underlying mechanical problem.

Tendinitis represents inflammation and/or micro tears of the tendon (attachment of muscle to bone). A detailed discussion of all possible tendinitides is beyond the scope of this work, but some of the most commonly noted in sports medicine are discussed here. Consideration of supraspinatus tendinitis is age related. In the young throwing athlete, this really represents an anterior subluxation of the humerus due to weakness of the posterior rotator cuff. In the older athlete, there is narrowing of the subacromial space leading to an actual impingement of the supraspinatus muscle. Diagnosis is made by evaluation of the rotator cuff looking for the strength of both the anterior and posterior cuff, as well as for capsular instability.

Patellar tendinitis, also known as *jumper's knee,* is commonly seen in jumping sports. The patient complains of peripatellar pain, increasing with jumping. On physical examination, there is tenderness either at the site of origin of the patellar tendon or in the body of the patellar tendon itself. In the skeletally immature athlete, tenderness of the insertion with a tender knob is Osgood-Schlatter disease. Evaluation should include radiographs to rule out skeletal abnormality. Treatment includes rest, nonsteroidal anti-inflammatory drugs, quadriceps and hamstring strengthening, and a stretching program with a correction of any biomechanical problems.

Iliotibial band syndrome represents about 14 per cent of all overuse syndromes. The patient complains of lateral knee pain distal to the joint line (distal to Gerdy's turbercle). The pain comes on with going up or down stairs. Treatment should include physical therapy for stretching of the iliotibial band and correction of the biomechanical problems, which may include foot orthosis. If symptoms are unresponsive to these measures, consider steroid injection.

Persistent medial joint line pain of the knee with a snapping fibrous band noted on physical exam is *plica syndrome.* On examination, the physician will note point tenderness one finger breadth above the medial joint line, and, with palpation, can actually roll over the painful band (O'Connor's sign). Surgical release is usually indicated in symptomatic patients.

Achilles tendinitis, which is actually a peritendinitis, is due to significant biomechanical problems of the lower extremity and lack of flexibility in the Achilles tendon. The patient complains of pain specifically on initiating activity (especially when first arising in the morning) located 4 to 5 cm. above the attachment of the Achilles tendon. On exam, one finds tenderness 4 to 5 cm. above the attachment of the Achilles tendon, with pain on compression. The Thompson test (squeezing the gastrocnemius muscle with resulting dorsiflexion of the foot) is used to assure that the Achilles tendon is intact. The examiner should feel along the tendon to check for thickening or defect in the Achilles tendon. To investigate for possible causes, check for leg length discrepancy as well as hyperpronation, forefoot varus, subtalar varum, femoral torsion, or external tibial torsion. Treatment should be directed toward addressing any biomechanical problem noted, as well as to improve the flexibility of the Achilles tendon and the strength of the gastrocnemius and soleus muscle groups. A heel cup may be used to reduce the pull on the tendon, and weight-bearing sports should be restricted until pain has subsided and flexibility is improved.

ATHLETIC TAPING

Taping is a method of both supporting tissues and limiting their function. Taping does not, however, completely immobilize the joint. The use of protective taping and bandaging to support weak or injured limbs dates back to the recorded use by the early Greeks of a paste that was made of lead oxide, olive oil, and water. Controversy exists today, though, regarding what has become the routine use of ankle taping.

Arguments against routine ankle taping are (Arnheim, 1985):

1. Tape is applied over movable skin.
2. Moisture collects under the tape, increasing its looseness.
3. Constant taping weakens supporting tendons.
4. Tape supports reduce 40 per cent after approximately 10 minutes of activity.
5. Ankle wrap loses 34 to 77 per cent support during exercise.
6. Taping replaces thorough rehabilitation of the joint.
7. Taping gives the athlete a false sense of security and can become a psychologic crutch.
8. Because taping does not significantly reduce ankle torque, it does not decrease the athlete's potential to injury to his lower leg.

Arguments in favor of routine ankle taping include:

1. Taping the ankle does not significantly hinder motor performance.
2. Properly applied tapings, even though they loosen during activity, provide critical support at the limits of ankle movement.
3. Because tapings do loosen in the initial period of activity, the mid range of ankle movement is allowed, thus removing adverse stress from the knee joint.
4. Athletes with recent injury or chronically weak ankles should be given all protection against further injury.

5. Statistics show that athletes that wear tape as a prophylaxis have fewer injuries.

The family physician's role here includes assuring that definitive treatment is not delayed and thorough rehabilitation is completed (i.e., so that taping does not take the place of appropriate medical treatment).

A complete guide to athletic taping is beyond the scope of this work, and the reader is referred to Arnheim (1985) and Cerney (1972).

REHABILITATION

Whether an injury is the result of acute trauma or a chronic overuse syndrome, once bony abnormalities and instabilities have been ruled out, the patient should be referred for physical therapy and rehabilitation. Through application of modalities such as ice, intermittent compression, heat, massage, electrical stimulation, and ultrasound, the healing process can be enhanced, returning the athlete to sport. The rehabilitation process should also include appropriate strengthening, proprioception, and flexibility exercises to the affected area. Correction of any underlying biomechanical problems by foot orthosis or specific joint mobilization and by muscle stretching and strengthening should be done to maximize safe athletic performance and minimize the risk of recurrence.

Caring for Special Groups of Athletes

ATHLETES WITH CHRONIC DISEASE

Asthma. While the possible precipitation of an asthma attack by exercise has been recognized since at least the 2nd century A.D., the exact mechanism of exercise-induced asthma remains under study today. Theories have focused on histamine release, respiratory heat loss, and respiratory water loss, but no one theory has shown the single conclusive cause. What is known is that with proper management, the patient suffering from exercise-induced asthma can be active and participate in competitive and recreational sports.

Exercise-Induced Asthma. Exercise-induced asthma is common, occurring in 80 to 90 per cent of asthmatics. It has also been found to occur in 40 to 50 per cent of persons with allergic rhinitis but no previous history of asthma (Mellion, 1988). The clinical entity is described as a transient increase in airway resistance (15 per cent or more decrease in FEV1 or PEFR) following vigorous exercise. Factors that influence the severity of the exercise-induced asthma attack are the type, intensity, and duration of the exercise, as well as the conditions under which exercise took place (e.g., temperature, humidity, air pollutants, etc.). Simply performing office pulmonary function tests before and after exercise (6 to 8 minutes, attaining 80 per cent of maximal predicted heart rate) will give the physician some idea of the role of exercise-induced asthma in a given patient.

Management of the condition includes both pharmacologic and nonpharmacologic measures. Exercising in warm, humid environments reduces the likelihood of attack. Breathing through the nose maximizes the benefit of the air warming and humidifying the nasal passages. Occasionally, wearing a face mask has proved useful. Exercising in short bursts may help, particularly in the conditioning phase. Pharmacologic treatment has centered on four groups of medications: (1) beta-adrenergic agents, (2) theophylline, (3) cromolyn sodium, and (4) anticholinergics. When considering the beta-adrenergic agents in competitive athletes, only the beta-2 specific agents in inhaler form have been approved by the International Olympic Committee. Albuterol administered by aerosol 10 to 20 minutes before exercise has been shown to be effective for 4 to 6 hours.

Theophylline has been shown to have a more useful prophylactic effect when used chronically, rather than as a single dose prior to exercise. Cromolyn given within 20 minutes of exercise is useful in up to 70 per cent of exercise-induced asthma patients but does not cause bronchodilation and, hence, does not improve baseline pulmonary function tests. The anticholinergic agents are only moderately effective and require near normal baseline pulmonary function tests.

Diabetes. Exercise in diabetic patients not only is recognized as a useful part of therapy but also is an important aspect of leading a normal life. Young diabetics, in particular, receive the cardiovascular benefit of exercise including development of endurance and improvement of the lipid profile. Several precautions must be observed. Good diabetic control should be obtained before a vigorous exercise program is begun. In diabetic patients over 40 years of age (or if the duration of their diabetes is more than 25 years), an exercise tolerance test should be performed before the exercise program is begun. Patients with diabetic retinopathy should avoid strenuous activity that could result in hemorrhage, and those with peripheral neuropathy must guard against foot trauma.

Often the diabetic patient on insulin will be concerned about having an insulin reaction as a result of exercise. This should be addressed through education of the patient. Generally, it is best to begin exercise about 1 hour after eating. This will reduce the likelihood of hypoglycemia. If this is not possible, a snack may be taken. It is appropriate for the patient to measure his or her glucose before beginning. If the blood glucose is less than 130 mg./dl., he or she should be instructed to consume one carbohydrate equivalent before beginning and one every 20 to 30 minutes of exercise. In prolonged exercise, carbohydrates should be consumed every 20 to 30 minutes.

It is of educational value for the patient to measure accurate blood sugar both before and after exercise as a baseline to show just how much the sugar will drop. If the exercise program is to be ongoing, the insulin (or oral hypoglycemic) will typically need to be reduced by 20 to 40 per cent over the first several months. The site of insulin injection may need to be adjusted. Injection in an area that will be significantly influenced by the subsequent exercise (increased blood flow to the area) may result in too rapid absorption of the insulin. Abdominal sites are recommended. The diabetic patient should also be cautioned about possible hypoglycemia the day after excessive exercise since muscle glycogen stores may be depleted.

Hypertension. Hypertensive patients who have previously been sedentary should be screened with a graded exercise tolerance test before initiating an exercise program. The hypertensive patient on medication presents a challenge for the family physician. Thiazides may exacerbate fluid and electrolyte loss particularly in endurance activities or exercising in heat and humidity. Exercise in the heat, when the patient has a low serum potassium, has been shown to lead to rhabdomyolysis (Knochel, 1972). Thiazides have been felt to be associated with a syndrome of muscular cramping even in the absence of potassium depletion (Mellion, 1988).

Beta blockers can be used in exercising hypertensive patients if the level of exercise is moderate or the sport has periodic interruptions. Central alpha-antagonists permit a normal but mildly attenuated hemodynamic response to exercise, and are unlikely to affect performance (Mellion, 1988). Alpha-1 blockade appears to normalize blood pressure at rest and during exercise and is very appropriate for use in mild and moderate hypertensives who exercise. Caution still must be given to the possibility of a first-dose hypotensive episode. Angiotensin-converting enzyme inhibitors work by decreasing total peripheral resistance with virtually no effect on heart rate and an increase in stroke volume. This would appear to make them a useful agent for the exercising hypertensive patient.

Epilepsy. Studies have shown that vigorous aerobic exercise does not produce seizures (AMA, 1974), and the family physician is likely to be faced with questions from his epileptic patients regarding exercise and sports. Any decision must be an individual one based on the level of control and patient compliance. Sports involving heights, including diving, are not recommended. Contact sports need not be universally excluded, but the frequency, time, and type of seizures, and the level of control must be considered. Children or adolescents with frequent daytime seizures, petit mal seizures, or psychomotor seizures should not participate in contact sports. Children or adolescents with generalized seizures that are well controlled may participate (American Academy of Pediatrics, 1983).

There is much debate regarding swimming, and an individual decision must be based on level of supervision. The effects of vigorous exercise on seizure medication is not well understood, and it is recommended that levels be checked to assure they remain in a normal range.

HANDICAPPED ATHLETES

The injury rate for the disabled appears to be in the same range as the general population; however, the types of injuries seen in the physically handicapped athlete are quite different. Disabled athletes should be advised of the importance of warm-up and cool-down exercise, just as the nondisabled athlete. In wheelchair athletes, upper extremity injuries are common. The physician should be aware of the increased incidence of carpal tunnel syndrome caused by nerve compression from the continual pressure of the heel of the hand against the rims of the wheelchair wheel. Bloomquist (1986) has summarized several safety measures that can be considered for the handicapped athlete's wheelchair. As participation of the wheelchair athletes increases in endurance events, the physician must be aware of their increased susceptibility to hyper- and hypothermic stress. Their relative lack of muscle mass reduces their ability to shiver and generate heat and makes them more susceptible to cold stress. Wet clothing will lead to further cooling through evaporation, and wrapping the wheelchair marathoner in plastic has been suggested. In hot climates, the disabled athlete is at greater risk because the sweating mechanism may be deficient below the level of a spinal cord injury. Adequate hydration should be maintained in both hot and cold environments.

A special note must be made about patients with Down's syndrome. Atlantoaxial instability is present in 17 per cent of patients with Down's syndrome (Cooke, 1984). As a result, it is recommended that these patients be prohibited from participation in gymnastics, diving, swimming the butterfly stroke, high jump, pentathalon, soccer, and any warm-up placing pressure on the head and neck muscles, until an examination including radiographs has ruled out this condition.

PREADOLESCENT ATHLETE

Reference has been made throughout this chapter regarding the child and adolescent athlete including preparticipation assessment and increased susceptibility to heat stress. Injuries unique to prepubescent athletes are generally related to the growth plate. Twelve to thirteen years of age is the peak incidence of epiphyseal fractures, when it has been shown that the ligaments are two to three times stronger than the epiphyses. Radiographs may not demonstrate these injuries, and the key to recognition is the exquisite tenderness over the epiphyses. Apophyseal

Table 48–10. AMERICAN COLLEGE OF OBSTETRICIANS AND GYNECOLOGISTS GUIDELINES FOR EXERCISE DURING PREGNANCY AND POSTPARTUM*

EXERCISE GUIDELINES. The following guidelines are based on the unique physical and physiological conditions that exist during pregnancy and the postpartum period. They outline general criteria for safety to provide direction to patients in the development of home exercise programs.

Pregnancy and Postpartum

1. Regular exercise (at least three times per week) is preferable to intermittent activity. Competitive activities should be discouraged.
2. Vigorous exercise should not be performed in hot, humid weather or during a period of febrile illness.
3. Ballistic movements (jerky, bouncy motions) should be avoided. Exercise should be done on a wooden floor or a tightly carpeted surface to reduce shock and provide a sure footing.
4. Deep flexion or extension of joints should be avoided because of connective tissue laxity. Activities that require jumping, jarring motions or rapid changes in direction should be avoided because of joint instability.
5. Vigorous exercise should be preceded by a 5-minute period of muscle warm-up. This can be accomplished by slow walking or stationary cycling with low resistance.
6. Vigorous exercise should be followed by a period of gradually declining activity that includes gentle stationary stretching. Because connective tissue laxity increases the risk of joint injury, stretches should not be taken to the point of maximum resistance.
7. Heart rate should be measured at times of peak activity. Target heart rates and limits established in consultation with the physician should not be exceeded.
8. Care should be taken to gradually rise from the floor to avoid orthostatic hypotension. Some form of activity involving the legs should be continued for a brief period.
9. Liquids should be taken liberally before and after exercise to prevent dehydration. If necessary, activity should be interrupted to replenish fluids.
10. Women who have led sedentary lifestyles should begin with physical activity of very low intensity and advance activity levels very gradually.
11. Activity should be stopped and the physician consulted if any unusual symptoms appear.

Pregnancy Only

1. Maternal heart rate should not exceed 140 beats per minute.
2. Strenuous activities should not exceed 15 minutes in duration.
3. No exercise should be performed in the supine position after the fourth month of gestation is completed.
4. Exercises that employ the Valsalva maneuver should be avoided.
5. Caloric intake should be adequate to meet not only the extra energy needs of pregnancy but also of the exercise performed.
6. Maternal core temperature should not exceed 38°C.

*From American College of Obstetricians and Gynecologists. Exercise During Pregnancy and the Postnatal Period (ACOG Home Exercise Programs). Washington, D.C., ACOG, 1985, p. 4.

injuries must also be considered. The apophyseal centers are the tubercles or protuberances on bones at the point where major muscle tendons attach. They have separate areas of growth much as the epiphyseal plate. Whereas, a tendon injury might occur in the adult, an apophyseal injury will occur in the prepubescent athlete. Sites to consider this injury include the ischial tuberosity, proximal femur, iliac crest, and the lesser and greater trochanters. Ligaments and tendons are more flexible and hence the physician sees fewer strains in the young athlete. However, several diseases are related to microtears and hemorrhage into the tendons, including Sinding-Larson's (inferior pole of the patella), Osgood-Schlatter's (tibial tubercle), and Sever's (calcaneus).

The psychologic immaturity of this age group poses other challenges. Young athletes are less likely to be compliant in regard to injury rehabilitation that involves activity restriction. They will be more likely to be indifferent to proper fitting of protective equipment. The family physician may also need to counsel parents to watch for problems with self-esteem, psychologic stress, mismatching of child to sport or competitive level, and inappropriate coaching philosophy that stresses negative reinforcement and in general takes the fun out of the sport.

SENIOR ATHLETE

The family physician will be confronted with a wide spectrum of senior athletes from those who have been sedentary and now wish to begin a walking program, to the competitive athlete participating in swimming or track events in local Senior Olympic competitions. Guidelines for the consideration of exercise tolerance testing are given earlier in this chapter. It has also been pointed out that the senior athlete is more susceptible to environmental extremes, owing in part to the diminished thermoregulatory control. An assessment of bone density, particularly in the senior female athlete, is recommended before initiation of a high impact endeavor.

FEMALE ATHLETE

The effects of strenuous exercise on the menstrual cycle have long been debated and while there is evidence that participation in certain sports is associated with amenorrhea and oligomenorrhea, studies defining the cause-and-effect relationship are lacking. Regular exercise has been found to reduce menstrual symptoms in most women, but increases symptoms in a few (Appenzeller, 1981).

Regarding the athletic patient who becomes pregnant, Lotgering and colleagues (1985) concluded that "although the increased demands of pregnancy might compete with those of exercise, under most circumstances the maternal organism can meet the combined demands of gestation and exercise through a remarkable reserve of physiological adjustments." The issues in advising the pregnant patient regarding strenuous exercise are heat stress, uterine oxygen consumption, and infant size. In regard to heat stress, a definitive answer is not available. Contributing data indicate that while heat stress to the infant causes deleterious effects, the relationship between exercise and heat stress to the infant is not established. It is known that fetal temperature does not rise as rapidly as maternal temperature with exercise (Lotgering, 1984), and some believe that the increased intravascular volume of the mother during pregnancy enhances the fetal maternal heat transfer and dissipation (Jones, 1985).

Clapp (1984) found that women who continued endurance exercise throughout pregnancy (at or above minimum conditioning levels) had less weight gain, earlier deliveries, and infants with lower birth weight for gestational age, but no increased infant morbidity. Infants born to women who exercised only through 28 weeks did not show the reduction in birth weight.

Table 48–10 shows the recommendations of the American College of Obstetricians and Gynecologists for exercise during pregnancy and postpartum.

Many breast problems in female athletes are reduced or eliminated by the use of a proper sports bra. Women with medium-sized breasts usually prefer a compressive sports bra that is like a wide elastic bandage and binds the breast to the chest wall. Women with larger breasts can select a sports bra with good upward support with nonelastic material. These usually have wide bands under the breasts and wide shoulder straps. Traumatic injuries to the breast should be treated with ice and compression and reassurance that there is no relationship between trauma and tumors (Haycock, 1987).

Certain musculoskeletal injuries are felt to be more common in female athletes. The wider female pelvis may lead to increased vulnerability to patellar syndromes. In general, the recommendation is to assess the female athlete for biomechanical abnormalities and encourage appropriate training for the chosen sport.

Acknowledgments

Our thanks to Jennifer Andersen, R.D., Julie Hereford, P.T., and Thomas Nash, A.T., for their assistance in the preparation of this material.

References

American Academy of Orthopedic Surgeons. Athletic Training and Sports Medicine, Chicago, IL, American Academy of Orthopedic Surgeons, 1984.

American Academy of Pediatrics. Sports Medicine: Health Care for Young Athletes. Evanston, IL, American Academy of Pediatrics, 1983. *An excellent reference volume for the physician dealing with young athletes, with chapters detailing injury considerations in both the healthy child and those with chronic illnesses.*

American College of Obstetricians and Gynecologists. Exercise During Pregnancy and the Postnatal Period (ACOG Home Exercise Program). Washington, D.C., American College of Obstetricians and Gynecologists, 1985.

American College of Sports Medicine. Guidelines for Exercise Testing and Prescription. Philadelphia, PA., Lea & Febiger, 1986. *Provides detailed guidelines for exercise testing and exercise prescription including recommendations for patients with chronic illnesses.*

American College of Sports Medicine. Position Statement on Heat Injuries. Med. Sci. Sports, 7:vii, 1975.

American Dietetic Association. Sports Nutrition—A guide for the Professional Working with Active People. American Dietetics Association, 1986.

American Medical Association. Should epileptics be barred from contact sports? Med. World News., *15*:62, 1974.

Appenzeller, O., and Atkinson, R. Sports Medicine. Baltimore, MD., Urban & Schwarsenberg, 1981.

Arnheim, D. Modern Principles of Athletic Training. 6th ed. St. Louis, MO., Times Mirror/Mosby College Publishing, 1985.

Black, D. L. Anabolic-androgenic steroid addiction (clinical note). Physc. Sportsmed., *16*(12):27, 1988.

Blackett, P. R. Child and adolescent athletes with diabetes. Physc. Sportsmed., *16*(3):133, 1988. *Represents a thorough review of handling the young diabetic athlete including various insulin regimens and proper laboratory follow-up.*

Bloomquist, L. E. Injuries to athletes with physical disabilities: prevention implications. Physc. Sportsmed., *14*(9):96, 1986. *Participation in sports by disabled athletes is increasing. With this, injuries are increasing also. Prevention techniques for injuries specific to disabled weight lifters, wheeler, and Down's syndrome athletes.*

Braden, D. S., and Strong, W. B. Preparticipation screening for sudden cardiac death in young athletes. Physc. Sportsmed., *16*(10):128, 1988. *Gives guidelines for screening for young athletes at risk for sudden cardiac death and recommendations regarding the indication for echocardiogram.*

Brunnstrom, S. Clinical Kinesiology. 3rd ed. Philadelphia, PA, F.A. Davis Co. 1980.

Cailliet, R. Pain Series. 2nd ed., Philadelphia, PA., F.A. Davis, 1981.

Caine, D. J., and Broekhoff, J. Maturity assessment: a viable preventive measure against physical and psychological insult to the young athlete? Physc. Sportsmed., *15*(3):67, 1987. *Reduction of the risk of physical and psychological injury to adolescent athletes may be facilitated through maturity assessment. This aspect of young athlete assessment appears under recognized.*

Cantu, R. C. Sports Medicine in Primary Care. Lexington, MA., The Collarmore Press, 1982. *Includes a section to assist the new team physician in preparing a sports-medicine bag.*

Cantu, R. C. Clinical Sports Medicine. Lexington, MA., The Collarmore Press, 1984. *Several chapters deal with the handicapped athlete and with psychologic considerations of sports medicine.*

Cantu, R. C., and Gillespie, W. J. Sports Medicine, Sports Science—Bridging the Gap. Lexington, MA., The Collarmore Press, 1982.

Cantu, R. C. Guidelines for return to contact sports after a cerebral concussion. Physc. Sportsmed., *14*(10):75, 1986. *This article presents guidelines for recognizing, classifying, and managing concussion as well as for determining when an athlete may safely return to play.*

Cerney, J. V. Complete Book of Athletic Taping Techniques. West Nyack, N.Y., Parker Publishing, 1972. *As the title relates, a thorough work on taping for those who wish to learn techniques.*

Clapp, J. F., and Dickstein, S. Endurance exercise and pregnancy outcome. Med. Sci. Sports Exerc. *16*:556, 1984.

Cohen, J. C., and Hickman, R. Insulin resistance and diminished glucose tolerance in powerlifters ingesting anabolic steroids. J. Clin. Endocrinol. Metab., *64*(5):960, 1987.

Cook, R. E. Atlantoaxial instability in individuals with Down's syndrome. Adapted Physical Activity Quarterly, *1*(3):194, 1984.

Costill, D. L. A scientific approach to distance running. Track and Field News, 1979.

Costill, D. L., Sherman, W. M., Fink, W. J., et al.: The role of dietary carbohydrate in muscle glycogen resynthesis after strenuous running. Am. J. Clin. Nutr., *34*:1831, 1981.

Council on Scientific Affairs. Drug abuse in athletes, anabolic steroids and human growth hormone. J.A.M.A., *259*(11):1703, 1988. *This represents the first in a three part series on drug abuse by athletes. Specifically covers AMA resolutions regarding the use of human growth hormone.*

Cowart, V. S. Should epileptic exercise? Physc. Sportsmed., *14*(9):183, 1986.

Creagh, T. M., Rubin, A., and Evans, D. J.: Hepatic tumours induced by anabolic steroids in an athlete. J. Clin. Pathol., *41*(4):441, 1988.

Daniels, L., and Worthingham, C.: Therapeutic Exercise for Body Alignment and Function. 2nd ed. Philadelphia, PA., W.B. Saunders, 1977.

Everly, R. S., Triger, D. R., Milnes, J. P., et al.: Severe cholestasis associated with stanozolol. Br. Med. J., *294*(6572):612, 1987.

Feigley, D. Psychological burnout in high level athletes. Physc. Sportsmed., *12*(10):109, 1984. *Addresses problems seen with some of the most gifted athletes, indicating the gradual onset and pointing out signs to watch for.*

Ferguson, A. B. The case against ankle taping. J. Sports Med., *1*:8, 1973.

Fischer, R. D. The measured effect of taping, joint range of motion, and their interaction upon the production of isometric ankle torques. Athletic Training, *17*:218, 1982.

Frankle, M. A., Eichberg, R., and Zachariah, S.: Anabolic androgenic steroids and a stroke in an athlete, case report. Arch. Phys. Med. Rehabil., *69*(8):632, 1988.

Glick, J. M.: The prevention and treatment of ankle injuries. Am. J. Sports Med., *4*:4, 1976.

Goldberg, B., Saraniti, A., Witman, P., et al.: Preparticipation sports assessment—an objective evaluation. Pediatrics, *66*:736, 1980.

Gould, J. A., and Davies, G. J. Orthopaedic and Sports Physical Therapy. St. Louis, MO., The C.V. Mosby Co., 1985. *While this book is designed for the physical therapist, it is an excellent reference for assessing biomechanical abnormalities, as well as diagnosing sports injuries.*

Haycock, C. E. How I manage breast problems in athletes. Physc. Sportsmed., *15*(3):89, 1987. *Discusses breast problems in both men and women athletes, with recommendations for recognition and prevention.*

Hellstedt, J. C.: Kids, parents, and sports: some questions and answers. Physc. Sportsmed., *16*(4):59, 1988. *Suggests ways physicians and parents can be more attuned to the psychologic problems affecting children in sports. Helpful reproducible handout included.*

Hudson, P. B. Preparticipation screening of special olympics athletes. Physc. Sportsmed., *16*(4):97, 1988. *Handicapped athletes participating in the growing special olympics present unique problems. Suggestions to the physicians asked to clear the athlete for competition are included.*

Jones, R. L., Botti, J. J., Anderson, W. M., et al. Thermoregulation during aerobic exercise in pregnancy. Obstet. Gynecol., *65*:340, 1985.

Kapandji, I. A. Physiology of the Joints. Vol. 1–3. 2nd ed. New York, Churchill Livingstone, 1974.

Katz, R. M. Coping with exercise-induced asthma in sports. Physc. Sportsmed., *15*(7):100, 1987. *Reviews the physiology of EIA (exercise-induced asthma) and makes suggestions for dealing with it.*

Kendal, M. O., and McCreary, E. K.: Muscles, Testing and Function, 4th ed., Baltimore, Md., Williams and Wilkins, 1983.

Kiraly, C. L., Collan, Y., and Alen, M.: Effect of testosterone and anabolic steroids on the size of sebaceous glands in power athletes. Am. J. Dermatopathol., *9*(6):515, 1987.

Kirkendall, D. T. Exercise prescription for the healthy adult. Primary Care, *11*(1):23, 1984.

Kisner, C., and Colby, L. A. Therapeutic Exercise, Foundations and Techniques. Philadelphia, PA., F.A. Davis Co., 1985.

Knochel, J. P., et al. Pathophysiology of intense physical conditioning in a hot climate. I. Mechanism of potassium depletion. J. Clin. Invest., *51*:242, 1972.

Kozak, B. Effects of ankle taping upon dynamic balance. Athlet. Tr., *9*:94, 1974.

Kramhft, M., and Solgaard, S. Spontaneous rupture of the extensor pollicis longus tendon after anabolic steroids. J. Hand Surg. [Br.], *11*(1):87, 1986.

Kulund, D. The Injured Athlete. Philadelphia, PA., J.B. Lippincott, 1982.

Kuprian, W. Physical Therapy for Sports. Philadelphia, PA., W.B. Saunders, 1982.

Lenders, J. W., Demacker, P. N., Vos, J. A., et al.: Deleterious effects of anabolic steroids on serum lipoproteins, blood pressure, and liver function in amateur body builders. Int. J. Sports Med., *9*(1):19, 1988.

Lombardo, J. A.: Pre-participation physical evaluation. Primary Care, *11*(1):3, 1984.

Lotgering, F. K., Gilbert, R. D., and Longo, L. D.: Maternal and fetal responses to exercise during pregnancy. Physio. Rev., *65*:1, 1985.

Lotgering, R. K., Gilbert, R. D., and Longo, L. D.: The interaction of exercise and pregnancy: a review. Am. J. Obstet Gynecol, *July 1*:560, 1984.

Marcus, J. B. Sports Nutrition—A Guide for the Professional Working with Active People. American Dietetic Association, 1986.

McNutt, R. A., Ferenchick, G. S., Kirlin, P. C., et al. Acute myocardial infarction in a 22 year old world class weight lifter using anabolic steroids. Am. J. Cardiol., *62*(1):164, 1988.

Mellion, M. B. Office Management of Sports Injuries and Athletic Problems. Philadelphia, PA., Hanley & Belfus, 1988. *An excellent text for the practicing primary care physician. Has sections on special populations.*

Monahan, T. Wheelchair athletes need special treatment but only for injuries. Physc. Sportsmed., *14*(7):121, 1986.

Morris, A. F. Sport Medicine—Prevention of Athletic Injuries. Dubuque, IO., Wm. C. Brown Publishers, 1984. *Contains section dealing with athletic training and conditioning for sports but is really directed at the physical educator.*

Morton, A. R. Physical activity and the asthmatic. Physc. Sportsmed., *9*(3):50, 1981.

Mueller, F. O., and Blyth, C. S. An update on football deaths and catastrophic injuries. Physc. Sportsmed., *14*(10):139, 1986.

Mueller, F. O., and Schindler, R. D.: Annual Survey of Football Research, 1931–1987. National Collegiate Athletic Association, 1988.

Pope, H. G., and Katz, D. L. Affective and psychotic symptoms associated with anabolic steroid use. Am. J. Psychiatry, *145*(4):487, 1988.

Rarick, L. The measurable support of the ankle joint by conventional methods of taping. J. Bone Joint Surg., *44A*:1183, 1962.

Raven, P. B. Clinical and physiological consideration of air pollution. American College of Sport Medicine Clinical Conference, 1988 Syllabus, 1988, p. 17.

Rowland, T. W. Exercise fatigue in adolescents: diagnosis of athlete burnout. Physc. Sportsmed., *14*(9):69, 1986.

Roy, S., and Irvin, R. Sports Medicine: Prevention, Evaluation, Management and Rehabilitation. Englewood Cliffs, N.J., Prentice-Hall Inc., 1983.

Schneider, R. C., Kennedy, J. C., and Plant, M. L. (eds.): Sports Injuries—Mechanisms, Prevention and Treatment. Baltimore,

MD., Williams & Wilkins, 1985. *This text is organized by sport-specific injuries, including chapters on auto racing, scuba diving, and lacrosse, as well as the more common sports.*

Scott, W. N., Nisonson, B., and Nicholas, J. A.: Principles of Sports Medicine. Baltimore, MD., Williams & Wilkins, 1984. *Deals with sports injuries by system and contains a valuable section on preventative sports medicine, dealing with equipment considerations.*

Smikstein, G. Health evaluation of high school athletes. Physc. Sportsmed., *9*(8):73, 1981.

Strauss, R. H. Drugs and Performance in Sports. Philadelphia, PA., W.B. Saunders Co., 1987. *Offers an excellent overview of the problem of performance and therapeutic drugs in sports.*

Sutton, J. R. Altitude Sickness. American College of Sports Medicine Clinical Conference, 1988 Syllabus, 1988, p. 1.

Tanner, J. M. Growth at Adolescence. 2nd ed. Springfield, IL., Charles C Thomas, 1962.

Todaro, G. J. The volunteer team physician—when are you exempt from civil liability? Physc. Sportsmed., *14*(2):147, 1986. *While some details will vary from state to state, this article guides the would-be team physician through the legal considerations.*

VanCamp, S. P. Exercise-related sudden death: risk and causes, part I. Physc. Sportsmed., *16*(5):96, 1988.

VanCamp, S. P. Exercise-related sudden death: cardiovascular evaluation of exercisers. Physc. Sportsmed., *16*(6):47, 1988.

Williams, J. G. P., and Sperryn, P. N. Sports Medicine. London, England, Edward Arnold Ltd., 1979. *Presents a systems approach to sports injuries.*

49

Orthopedics

John F. Connolly
O. Max Jardon

Acute or chronic pain is the most common reason for a patient to consult a physician. The physician's charge is to identify the cause of complaint and, when possible, to relieve it. The diagnostic skills of the family physician can be readily applied to musculoskeletal causes of pain, and diagnosis depends in the main on an accurate historical and physical assessment, accompanied by minimal laboratory aids.

Lacerations, Contusions, and Amputations

LACERATIONS

Lacerations are the leading musculoskeletal cause of a visit to the family physician. Management by cleansing and irrigation with antibiotic solution and primary suture usually gives a satisfactorily healed wound with minimal scar and few complications. There are, however, some types of wounds in which primary closure is fraught with hazard and may even be contraindicated. Some types of lacerations frequently involve deep structures and are noted for frequent complication.

Wounds Near Joints

These wounds should be considered a major hazard and closed only after ascertaining that the joint space or underlying major tendinous and ligamentous structures have not been violated.

A 6-year-old boy who sustained a nail puncture near the left patella was treated by superficial cleansing and primary closure. He subsequently developed signs of joint sepsis from the undiagnosed penetration. (Some studies report an incidence of 70 per cent infection from untreated or unrecognized penetration). He was further treated with antibiotics and no drainage. The end result was an osteomyelitis with arrest of the growth center about the knee, a fused knee, and a six-inch shortening of the limb at maturity (Fig. 49–1*A*).

This was later corrected to one inch by multiple operations (Fig. 49–1*B, C, D, E*). These operations occurred over 20 hospitalizations, and there was a liability settlement.

Management by the Family Physician. Any wound adjacent to a joint must be assessed for penetration and contamination of the joint space. Penetration can sometimes be detected by injecting 30 to 40 ml. of sterile saline into the joint and observing flow from the puncture. However, when in doubt the best course is to explore to the depth of the wound under sterile conditions.

If there is an indication of penetration, the joint must be explored and thoroughly irrigated. Reliance on antibiotics "coverage" is a fool's game and is no substitute for exploration and drainage. Signs of infection in a joint demand surgical exploration and cleansing, not a mere change in antibiotics.

Lacerations about the knuckles of the hand are prone to major complications such as infection and tendon laceration. One should suspect tendon involvement in any wound or fracture over the proximal or distal interphalangeal joints. These may cause mallet finger or boutonnière deformity, which are discussed in the section on finger sprains.

Human Bite Injury

This is the most serious and complication-prone laceration about the knuckles of the hand. Several

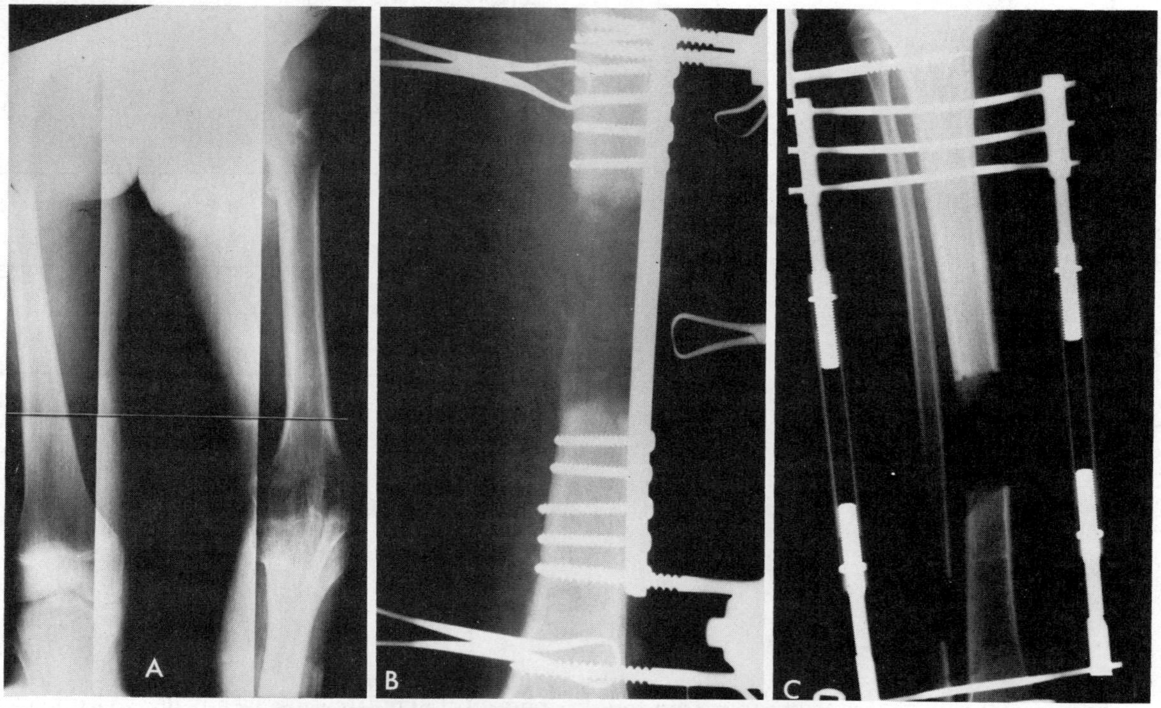

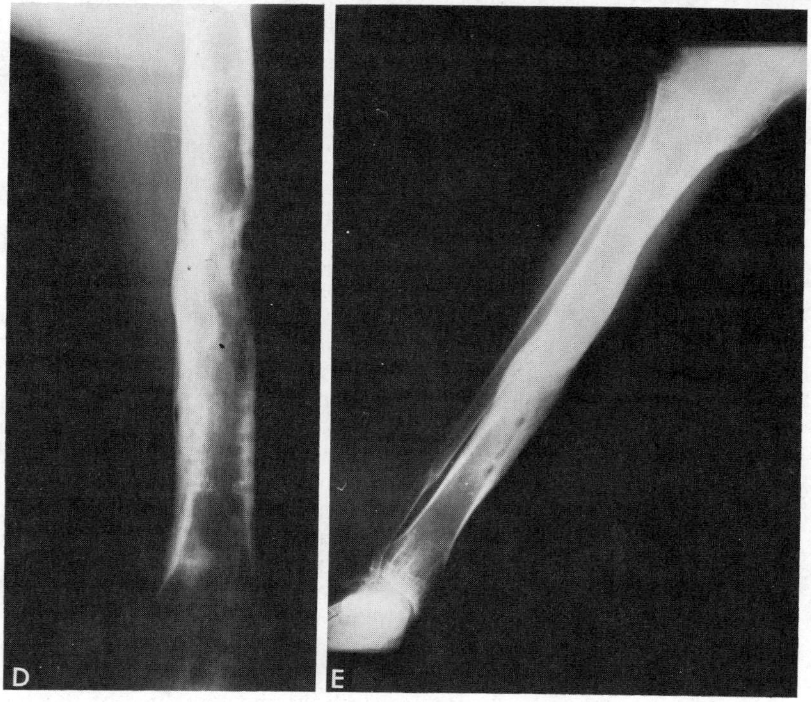

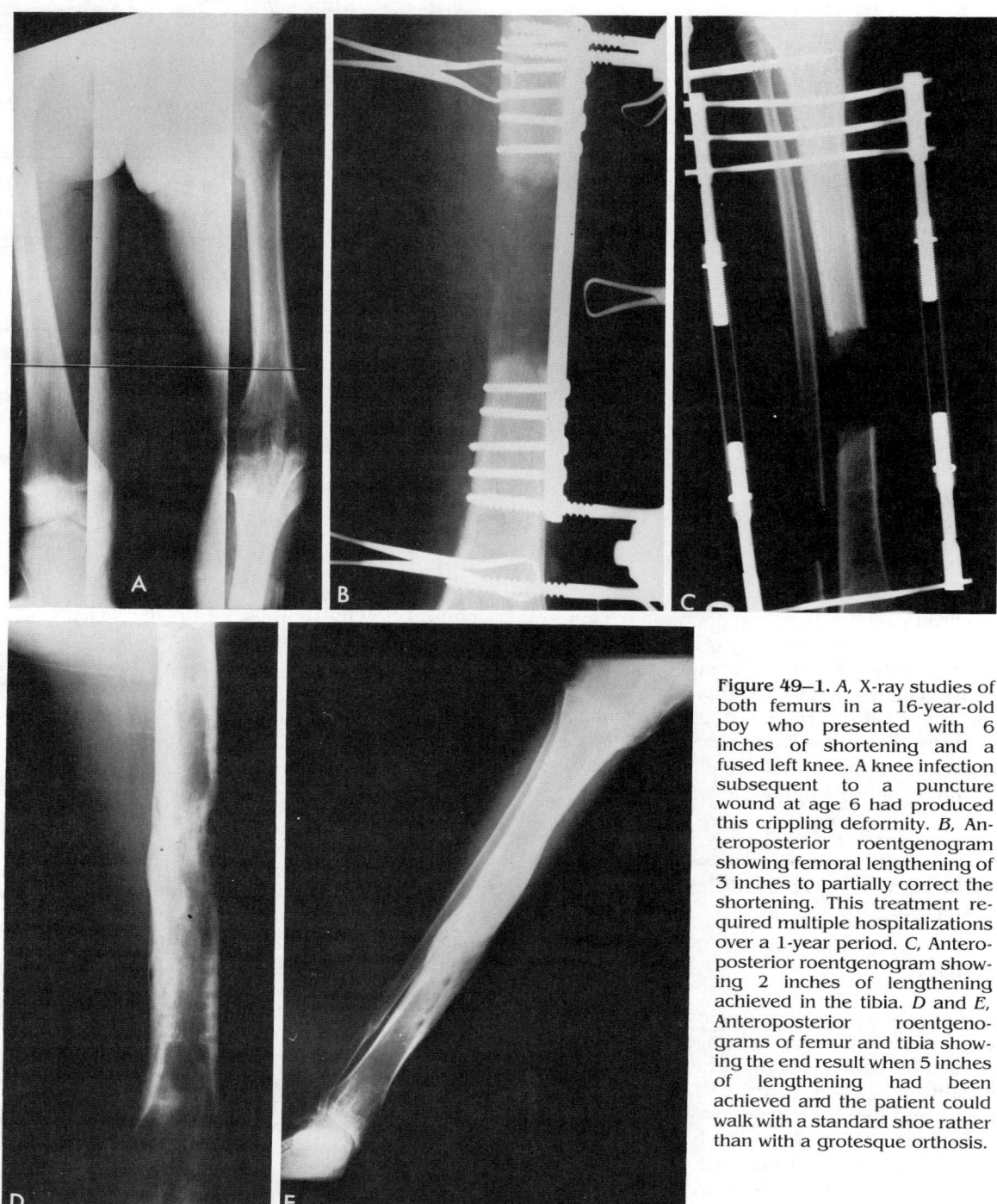

Figure 49–1. *A,* X-ray studies of both femurs in a 16-year-old boy who presented with 6 inches of shortening and a fused left knee. A knee infection subsequent to a puncture wound at age 6 had produced this crippling deformity. *B,* Anteroposterior roentgenogram showing femoral lengthening of 3 inches to partially correct the shortening. This treatment required multiple hospitalizations over a 1-year period. *C,* Anteroposterior roentgenogram showing 2 inches of lengthening achieved in the tibia. *D* and *E,* Anteroposterior roentgenograms of femur and tibia showing the end result when 5 inches of lengthening had been achieved and the patient could walk with a standard shoe rather than with a grotesque orthosis.

serious complications can result from a seemingly innocuous laceration caused by human teeth in contact with the hand. When the fist is clenched and strikes the teeth of an opponent (fight bites), the joint is especially prone to penetration.

Often treatment is delayed as the problem appears benign and the patient is reluctant to seek early care. Human saliva contains in excess of 1,000,000 organisms per milliliter of about 42 species of both aerobic and anaerobic types. Mann (1981) and others reported complications in over 50 per cent of human bite injuries. These included permanent stiffness of joints, amputation of one or more fingers (Fig. 49–2*A*, *B*), and rapidly spreading infections requiring high amputation. At least eight deaths have been reported as caused by human bites. This is never a trivial injury.

Management by the Family Physician. Primary care of such wounds includes high suspicion of this injury even when denied by the patient. Human bites behave in a unique fashion, as contrasted to other wounds, especially in the hand. Wound material must

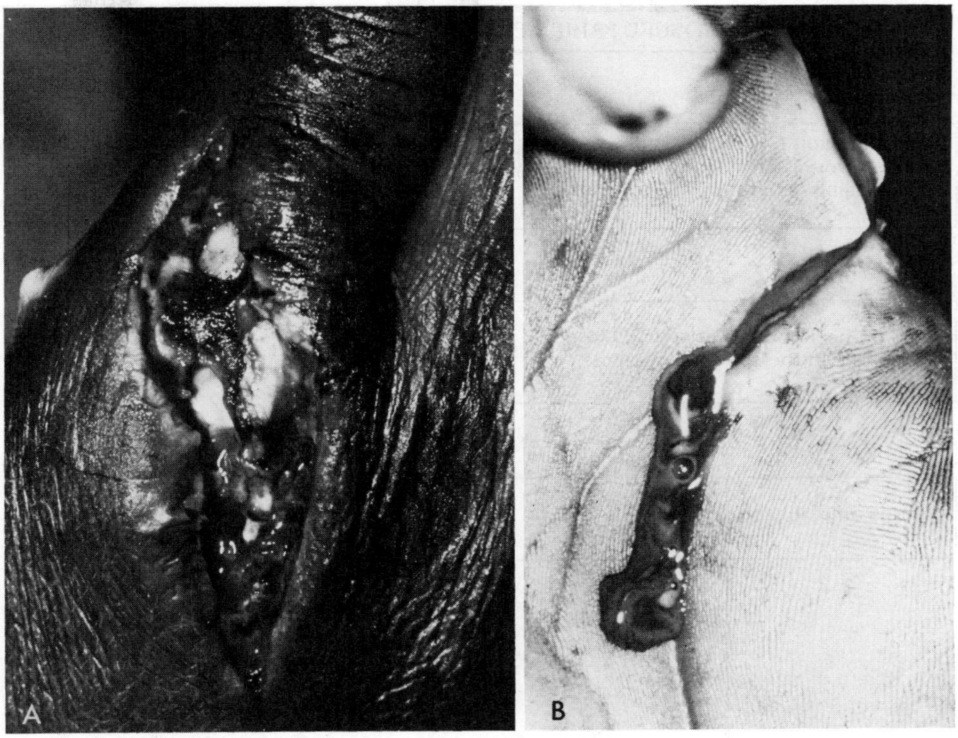

Figure 49–2. *A,* Dorsal view of a neglected human bite to the index finger. *B,* Palmar view showing deep palmar space infection. This eventually resulted in amputation of the digit.

be cultured for both anaerobic and aerobic bacteria. No culture can be considered negative unless both cultures are done. An x-ray should be obtained to help rule out osteomyelitis, fractures, retained teeth, or bone abscesses.

Mann has frequently demonstrated that these wounds must be surgically debrided and irrigated thoroughly. Broad-spectrum antibiotics such as gentamicin sulfate (Garamycin) are used, and the patient is hospitalized. Debridement is needed to convert the anaerobic environment to an aerobic one. All necrotic tissue is removed, and all infected spaces are drained.

The wounds are never closed primarily but left open for drainage. This wound is best managed by a surgeon skilled in serious hand infections.

After drainage, the hand is splinted for 24 hours, then active motion is encouraged. Intravenous antibiotics are continued for about 5 days, and if all is well, the patient is discharged on oral antibiotics and followed until healing by secondary intention is complete.

Dog and Cat Bites

Over 2,000,000 bites per year cause about one per cent of all emergency room admissions. Large dogs tend to lacerate while small dogs avulse pieces of tissue. Cats cause puncture-type wounds. Twenty per cent of bites are caused by German shepherds, 63 per cent from a family or neighbor's dog. The average age is 5 years, with 92 per cent under 21 years of age (Zook et al., 1980).

Management by the Family Physician. Zook and associates (1980) showed that meticulous debridement, irrigation, and antibiotic treatment reduced the complications of infection, scarring, and systemic symptoms for dog bites. Cat bites need only cleansing and antibiotics effective against hemophilus-type organisms.

When rabies is a concern, follow the guidelines of the Public Health Service Advisory Committee as described by Corey and Hattwick (1975) (Table 49–1) for most dog bite lacerations: start ampicillin or a cephalosporin intravenously and hospitalize for 48 hours of further therapy.

Small lacerations and minor avulsions can be managed under local anaesthetic in the emergency room. More severe cases need a general anesthetic in an operating room.

The wound is copiously irrigated with a water pic or other lavage system. The wound edges are sharply excised with a scalpel, and loose fat and foreign matter are removed. Subcutaneous sutures should be avoided and wound edges closed with minimal tension.

A pressure dressing will obliterate the dead space. Small 5–0 nylon sutures are best. The sutures are removed at 5 days, and Steri-strips can support the wound for a few more days.

This approach decreases the incidence of infection; however, the wound should be closely monitored for 3 to 5 days in case infection develops.

Lacerations Prone to Clostridial or Other Life-Threatening Infections

Clostridial or life- and limb-threatening infections are particularly prone to occur in certain types

Table 49–1. POSTEXPOSURE RABIES PROPHYLAXIS ALGORITHM*

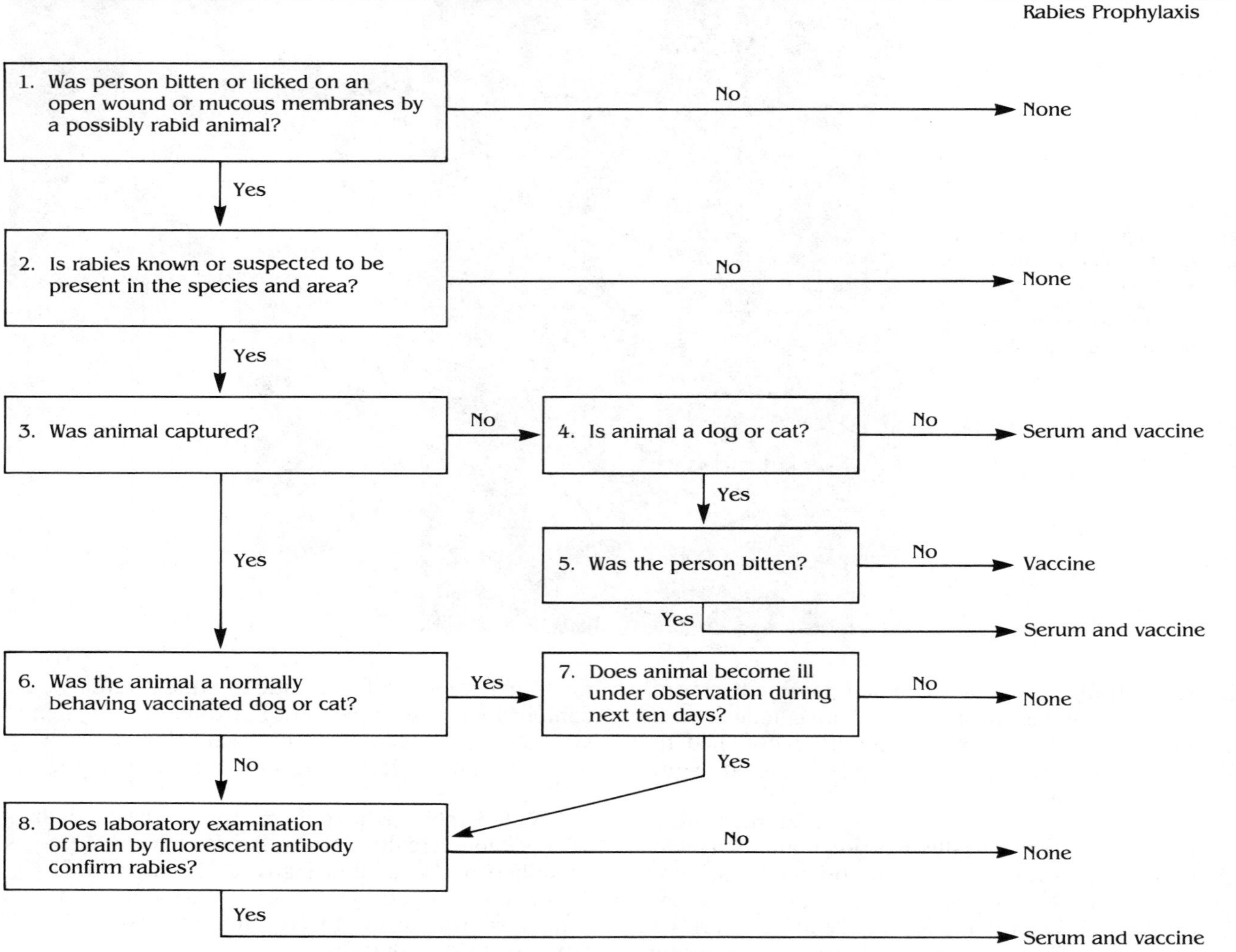

*From Corey, L., and Hattwick M.: J.A.M.A., 232:272, 1975. (With permission).

of wounds, e.g., small punctures over open fractures; wounds sustained in water; wounds about the buttocks; and mass casualty wounds.

Small Puncture Over Open Fracture. The wound size belies the extent of contamination. Bone ends can carry dirt and debris back under the skin. Superficial irrigation cannot cleanse these tissues, and serious infection is the consequence. Amputation of the limb is not an uncommon result of superficial debridement or cleansing of an open fracture. Youngsters are especially prone to this complication.

Management by the Family Physician. Undertreatment must be avoided. All open fractures require surgical exploration and thorough cleansing, regardless of a benign appearance. Referral for appropriate management is essential.

Wounding in Water. Lacerations incurred in water are most deceptive. They look clean, but contamination and soft tissue damage can be extensive. Boat propeller injuries often cause extensive muscle necrosis.

Closure of such wounds creates an abscess as damaged tissue dies. Brown and Kinman (1974) discussed 10 cases of gas gangrene in survivors of a Miami Everglades plane crash. These authors point out that primary closure of wounds incurred in water is inexcusable.

Management by the Family Physician. Care is based primarily upon prompt and complete debridement and cleansing of the wound. Wound closure is avoided because the amount and kind of contamination is uncertain.

Wounds about the Buttocks. Although infrequent, these wounds cause a disproportional number of septic complications. They are often contaminated with feces or may represent an open pelvic fracture.

Open pelvic fractures or those communicating with vagina or rectum are lethal injuries. The risk of death from sepsis or hemorrhage exceeds 50 per cent. Many cases will require colostomy with rectal disimpaction and irrigation. All such severe wounds require specialized surgical management.

Management by the Family Physician. This class of severe injuries requires prompt referral to specialty surgical care.

Wounds in Mass Casualties. Many of these wounds are prone to clostridial and other overwhelming infection. For example, the Texas City explosion and the Worcester and Flint tornadoes had an incidence of gas gangrene of 3 to 5 per cent of wounds. This is the frequency experienced in World War I. Military surgery has improved, and in Viet Nam, the incidence of gas gangrene was only 0.016 per cent (22 cases). During this same period, Brown and Kinman (1974) reported 29 cases in a single metropolitan area.

Management by the Family Physician. Military surgeons have repeatedly urged that all wounds be promptly and thoroughly debrided, irrigated, dressed, and not closed (Trueta and Orr) (Connolly, 1981). No contaminated wound should be closed primarily, especially in the mass casualty scenario, as debridement and cleansing are often marginal.

Debridement and irrigation should not be delayed in musculoskeletal wounds or open fractures because of some imagined need to observe for head or abdominal wounds.

Scanning techniques are such that head and abdominal injuries can be assessed accurately and wound care in the extremities can proceed. Poor debridement of open fractures often produces the most severe complications in the multiply injured patient.

Management of Contaminated Open Fractures. The poem of Sir James Learmouth summarizes debridement very well:

On the edge of the skin take a piece very thin.
The tensor the fascia, the more you should slash'er.
Of muscles much more 'til you see fresh gore,
And the bundles contract at the least impact.
Hardly any of bone only bits quite alone.

The etymology of "debridement" is "debridlement," meaning unleashing all tight restrictions about a wound. In debridement, conserve skin, bone, and neurovascular structures while excising all damaged muscle, leaving only that which is contractile and viable. Copious irrigation is mandatory using around 10 to 12 liters of antibiotic solution or 50 per cent Betadine solution.

All contaminated wounds are left open and never tightly packed to allow egress of wound drainage and contaminated material. Close only enough soft tissue to cover vascular or neural structures, no more.

Wounds can be closed in 5 to 10 days when clean or allowed to close secondarily (Fig. 49–3).

The ancients knew of the ability of wounds to close and never closed wounds. We moderns often forget (Figs. 49–4 and 49–5).

Secondary closure should be delayed until swelling and risk of infection are eliminated and the wound is clean.

A contaminated wound after debridement and irrigation is best put at rest with splintage or a plaster cast. When needed, unstable fractures can be stabilized with external fixation or pin and plaster for 3 or 4 weeks. Pins and plaster are best as they support the soft tissues and allow good wound drainage. The most a physician can do in wound management is clean up, prevent sepsis or hemorrhage, and produce a wound capable of healing. Antibiotics are a mere adjunct; the priority is to follow good surgical practice.

Lacerations Endangering Neurovascular Structures

Certain lacerations should be suspected of nerve or arterial injury. Deep forearm lacerations are notorious for such complications.

The physician must assess motor function and sensation, but it can be most unreliable in the acutely injured or inebriated patient. The only certain way to assess nerve laceration is wound exploration in an operating room. When the physician suspects nerve damage, the patient should be referred to an experienced surgeon.

Arterial Damage

Major damage to arteries can go unrecognized unless the physician is acutely aware of the possibility of such damage. Deep laceration of the knee and elbow, supracondylar humeral fractures, dislocation of the knee, shoulder dislocation in the elderly, or multiple shoulder dislocation all put a patient at risk (Connolly and Brooks, 1973) (Jardon, 1973).

Puncture wounds in the vicinity of major vessels need assessment. The presence or absence of a distal pulse can be an unreliable sign. Pulsatile swelling as a consequence of penetrating or blunt trauma is the most reliable.

Management by the Family Physician. Evaluation of lacerations, fracture, or dislocation about joints requires alertness to possible vessel damage. Any doubts as to the integrity of distal circulation require arteriographic study.

If injury is demonstrated, repair is indicated. Too often in years past ligation of the artery was done. This frequently led to ischemic contracture, severe sepsis, or amputation. Arterial repair even with grafting is preferable.

Appropriate, rapid (1 to 4 hours) referral to a competent vascular surgeon is mandatory.

SOFT TISSUE INJURY AND CONTUSIONS

The contusions most apt to cause problems and raise questions with regard to management are those as-

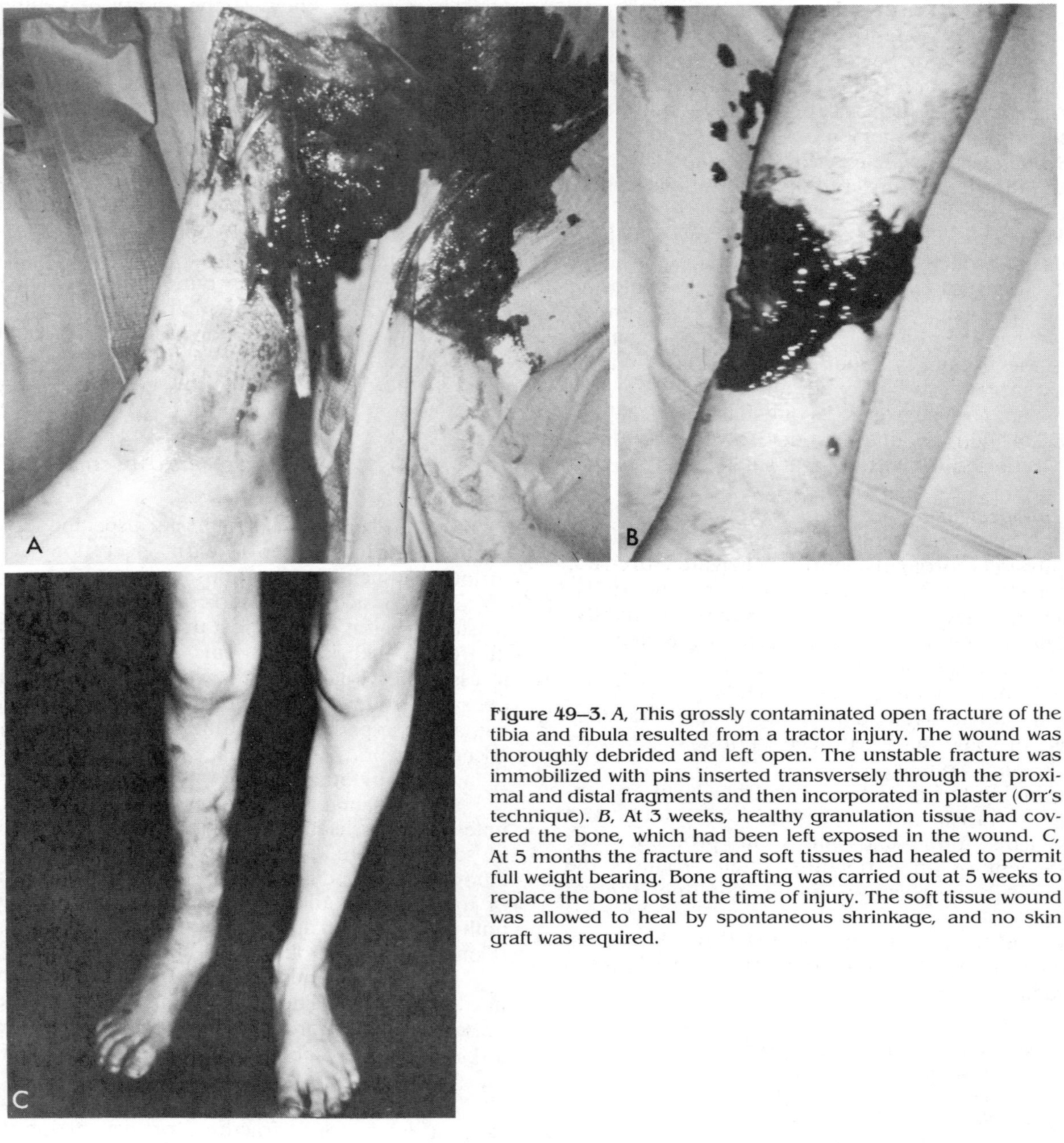

Figure 49–3. *A,* This grossly contaminated open fracture of the tibia and fibula resulted from a tractor injury. The wound was thoroughly debrided and left open. The unstable fracture was immobilized with pins inserted transversely through the proximal and distal fragments and then incorporated in plaster (Orr's technique). *B,* At 3 weeks, healthy granulation tissue had covered the bone, which had been left exposed in the wound. *C,* At 5 months the fracture and soft tissues had healed to permit full weight bearing. Bone grafting was carried out at 5 weeks to replace the bone lost at the time of injury. The soft tissue wound was allowed to heal by spontaneous shrinkage, and no skin graft was required.

sociated with gunshot wounds, severe contusions of the hand and wrist, contusions of the foot and ankle, and compartment syndromes.

Gunshot Wounds

These wounds are endemic in every life setting—rural, urban, civilian, and military. No legislation can eliminate them; however, mandatory sentencing and increased penalties for felonious gun use can reduce the problem as has happened in Detroit.

Treatment over the centuries has been modified as we understand more about physics, inflammation, infection, and surgical technology. Ballistic studies have shown that low velocity wounds (under 1000 feet per second) will produce a wound of entry and exit of about the same size and will do minimal damage along the bullet tract. Minimal skin debridement and thorough irrigation with antibiotic coverage is all that is needed unless some vital structure such as nerve, vessel, or bone has been injured. Once a bullet stops moving, damage eases. Removal of a bullet is necessary only if the location is likely to produce symptoms, for instance, in or near a joint or a superficial location in a hand or foot.

Forensic and legal considerations must be kept in mind; bullets and fragments must be labeled as to locations, and witnesses to removal should be noted for legal reasons.

Wounding from high velocity rifles (over 3000 feet per second) may exhibit a smaller entry wound with very large exit wound and considerable cavita-

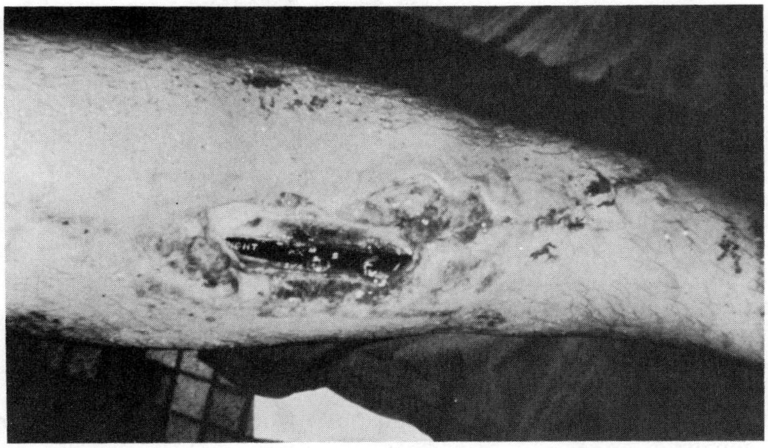

Figure 49–4. Tight fixation and tight wound closure after an open fracture produced extensive necrosis of the soft tissues and bone. This photo was taken 2 weeks after injury.

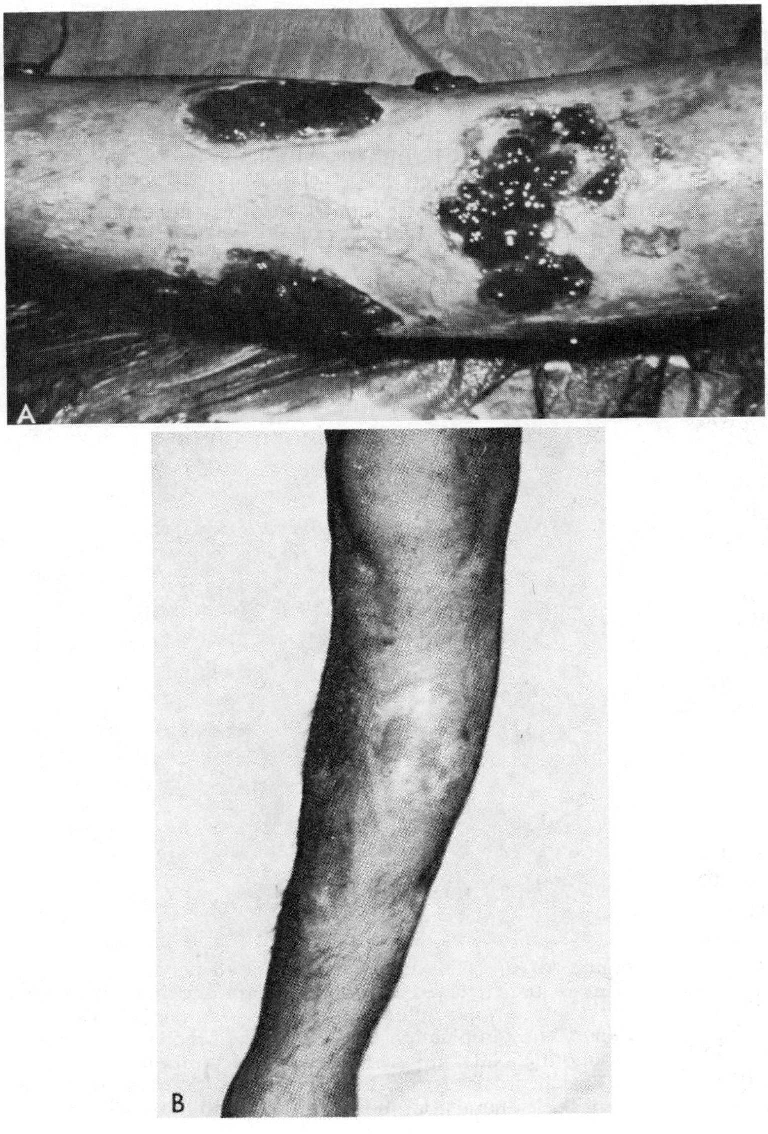

Figure 49–5. *A,* This open tibial fracture was left open after thorough debridement. Note the granulation tissues that are enveloping the exposed bone at 2 weeks after injury. *B,* At 6 months, the soft tissue and fracture healing were well advanced. No skin grafting procedure was required. Continuous cast immobilization allowed the wound to heal by intussusception. (From Connolly, J.: Perils and pitfalls of open tibial fractures. Am. Fam. Physician, *11*;64, 1975.)

tion and tumbling. Some secondary missile damage can result from bone fragments when bone is struck (Fackler and O'Benar, 1987).

Cavitation is the process in which a cavity develops around the bullet tract which may be many times the diameter of the projectile. Pressure within this cavity is below the atmospheric pressure, and consequently, debris and clothing are sucked into the wound. This necessitates open debridement of the bullet tract by the surgeon to evaluate damage to skin, bone, vessels, and nerves.

Very high velocity wounds (5000 feet per second) cause greater cavitation and secondary missile damage. The tissue death is greater and requires even more extensive debridement and open wound management.

Shotgun wounds have most of the characteristics of high velocity missile wounds. These blow tissue away and carry dirt into the wound. In addition, wadding frequently follows behind the shotgun pellets and is left to contaminate the depths of the wound. Shotgun injuries, therefore, need thorough debridement and open treatment to remove foreign material. The shotgun pellets themselves may be left in the soft tissues.

Management by the Family Physician. Fractures and other injuries associated with gunshot wounds are treated for the most part by thorough debridement and open wound management. The only exception is a fracture produced by a low caliber handgun, which can be managed by local wound care and external cast immobilization without exploring the fracture site.

All wounds from either high or low velocity missiles that involve a joint require exploration of that joint to remove any potential foreign material. Any penetrating wound near a large vessel requires arteriography to demonstrate the integrity of the vessel. The only gunshot wounds requiring minimal care are those produced by low velocity pistol and standard .22 rifle wounds. The remainder are specialized surgical problems of varied complexity.

All gunshot wounds should have appropriate antibiotic coverage. The usual clean low velocity wounds to the limbs that are seen in civilian practice can sometimes be handled without such coverage. The interested reader is referred to the Swans' monograph on gunshot wounds.

Severe Contusions of the Hand and Wrist

Contusions and crush injuries of the hand are more disruptive to the soft tissue structures than to the bone. Of major concern is the swelling subsequent to any injury, which can compromise circulation to the intrinsic muscles of the hand. Edema should be considered much like a glue that restricts soft tissue motion and stiffens the joints. Swelling is the arch-enemy of the physician who attempts to restore the patient's hand function after injury. In many fractures of the hand and wrist, the contusion and swelling can be of far greater significance than the skeletal injury itself.

The problem of edema and the complications that can develop when soft tissue swelling is ignored is illustrated by the following patient:

A 55-year-old state highway worker sustained a Colles' fracture of his left wrist, which was reduced and immobilized in a snugly applied cast. The patient complained of painful swelling and stiffness in the hand following cast application. Unfortunately, his complaints were not taken seriously, and his physician insisted that the cast should stay on for 8 weeks until the fracture healed. When the cast was finally removed, the patient was unable to move his painful stiff fingers, and this stiffness persisted despite encouragement for many months from numerous individuals.

When he was seen in consultation 2 years post injury, he had lost all motion of the metacarpophalangeal (MP) joints of the fingers and had a permanent 50 per cent functional loss of the hand (Fig. 49–6).

Management by the Family Physician. Do not concentrate solely on reducing the fracture. In cases such as those illustrated here, the physician should treat the edematous hand to eliminate swelling as promptly as possible. The swollen hand should be wrapped in a compressive dressing and elevated in a comfortable position continuously (see Fig. 49–8). Failure to eliminate swelling can produce ischemic necrosis of the intrinsic muscles and cause permanent contractures of the hand (Fig. 49–7*A*, *B*, *C*).

The position for immobilizing the swollen hand should be one that maintains joint ligaments at their maximum length. Ligaments that tighten when they are out to full length are far less likely to restrict motion subsequently than are ligaments that tighten in the shortened position.

To determine the position for immobilization,

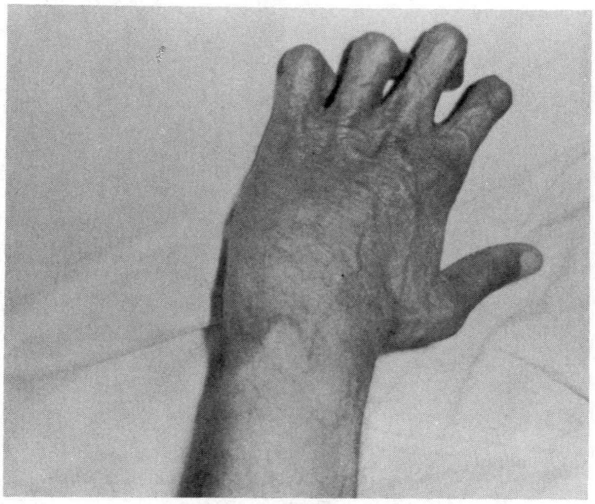

Figure 49–6. This patient demonstrated persistent contractures of the metacarpophalangeal (MP) and interphalangeal (IP) joints 2 years after sustaining a fracture of this distal radius. The combination of hand edema, which acted like glue around the joints and the tight cast, which produced ischemic muscle necrosis, led to this deformity. (Courtesy of Mr. R. James, Sir Charles Gardner Hospital, Perth, Australia.)

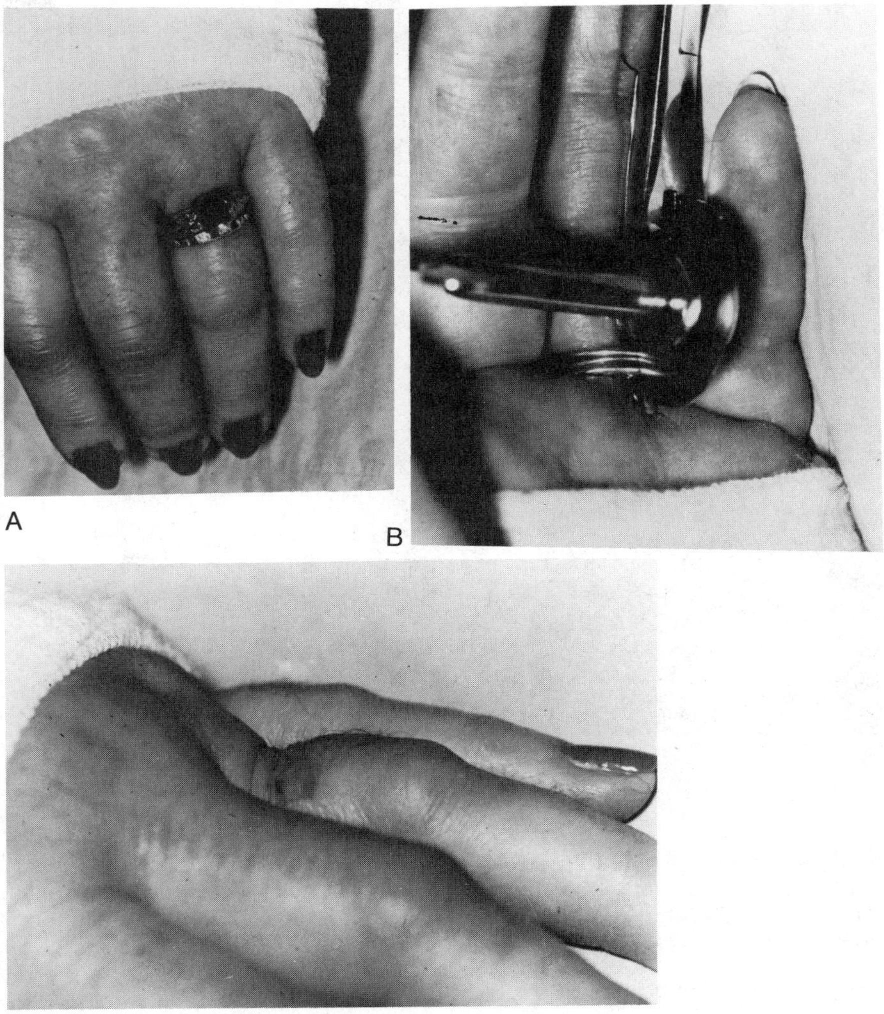

A B C

Figure 49–7. *A, B,* and *C,* All restricting objects should be removed prior to cast or splint application. Otherwise rings will have to be sawed off *(B)* to avoid strangulation of fingers *(C).* (Courtesy of Mr. R. James, Sir Charles Gardner Hospital, Perth, Australia.)

test your own MP joint motion. It is evident that the ligaments of the joint are most resistent to abduction and adduction stress and out to full length in maximum flexion of approximately 80 degrees. Interphalangeal (IP) joint ligaments reach maximal length at about 10 to 15 degrees of flexion. Consequently, any swollen hand should be immobilized with the MP joints flexed maximally and the IP joints flexed slightly. The thumb should be abducted out of the palm. The wrist should be extended. This position can be maintained best by a "boxing glove" type bandage, which is illustrated in Figure 49–8.

Splint the hand in this position, with elevation for 2 to 3 days until swelling subsides. When the edema has diminished, encourage active motion of all joints.

Keep in mind that adjacent joints, particularly the shoulder, must be exercised to avoid stiffening. Avoid the use of a sling with wrist or hand injury, since this encourages stiffening of the shoulder and inhibits active shoulder motion exercises.

By emphasizing this program to combat the complications of contusions and edema, the physician facilitates the patient's recovery and avoids the unsatisfactory complications illustrated in Figure 49–6.

Contusions of the Foot and Ankle

Blunt injury without fracture can produce serious and permanent damage, as illustrated by the following case. Soft tissue swelling was the main culprit.

While playing softball, a 16-year-old girl twisted and severely bruised her ankle. She was seen several hours afterward by her family physician, who wrapped her ankle with a rigid Unna cast-type dressing. The girl used crutches but did not elevate the leg, and the cast dressing became progressively tighter as the ankle continued to swell. For some reason her dressing was not removed for several weeks, and by that time the patient suffered from a fixed equinovarus deformity of the foot and ankle.

The edema of the leg and the rigid dressing applied to the swollen limb combined to produce permanent damage to the important inverting muscles of the foot. We saw her with this persistent problem one year later. Fixed contraction of the posterior tibial and other muscles of the deep posterior compartment had left this girl with a permanent functional impairment (Fig. 49–9).

Management by the Family Physician. The disability subsequent to contusions and swelling about the ankle can be prevented if the potential problems from the swelling are recognized promptly. Avoid

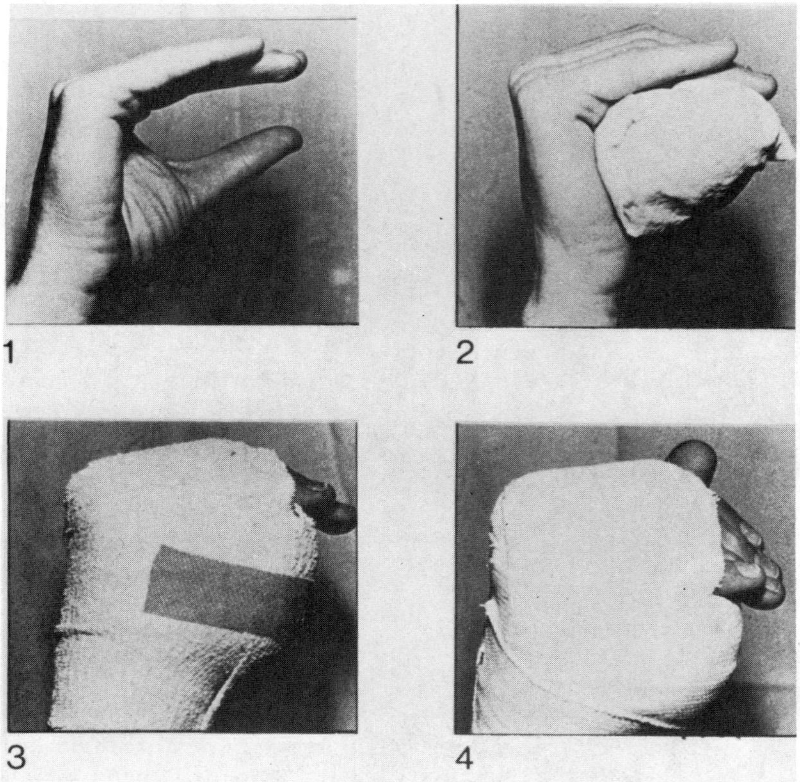

Figure 49–8. Position of immobilization of the hand after injury as it should be, with MP joints flexed maximally and the IP joints slightly flexed. Thumb is abducted and opposed to the other fingers. Maintain this position by a firm ball dressing inserted into the palm to produce a "boxing glove bandage." (Courtesy Mr. J. Sikorski, Department of Surgery-Orthopaedics, University of Western Australia.)

rigid dressings for a patient with any such injury. Understanding the pathophysiology of compartment syndrome is essential to avoid unfortunate complications from these relatively minor injuries.

Compartment Syndromes from Contusions and Swelling

A compartment syndrome results from increased pressure within a closed osteofascial space, compromising the circulation within that space. It can result from many causes, as Table 49–2 indicates. The basic pathophysiology has been found to be a decrease in local blood flow to a level insufficient to meet metabolic needs of muscles and nerves.

Local blood flow (LBF) to a muscle compartment is determined by arterial (PA) and venous (PV) pressure difference as well as by the local resistance to flow within the compartment. The formula

$$\text{LBF} = \frac{\text{PA} - \text{PV}}{\text{R}}$$

shows these relationships between local blood flow, arterial pressure, venous pressure, and resistance.

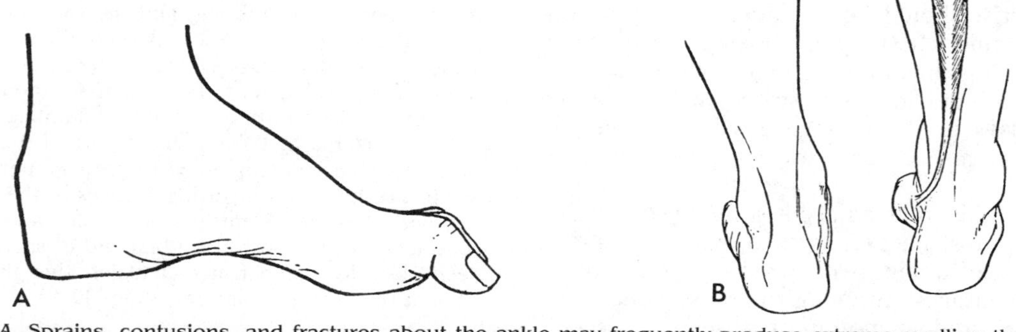

Figure 49–9. *A*, Sprains, contusions, and fractures about the ankle may frequently produce extreme swelling that can develop into compartment syndromes, particularly if a rigid dressing is applied. *B*, Ischemic contractures of the posterior compartment muscles leave the patient with a fixed inverted deformity of the ankle with a painful high arch and clawtoes. (From Connolly, J. F.: DePalma's The Management of Fractures and Dislocations: An Atlas. 3rd ed. Philadelphia. W. B. Saunders Co., 1981, with permission.)

Table 49–2. ETIOLOGIES OF COMPARTMENTAL SYNDROMES*

Decreased Compartmental Volume	Closure of fascial defects Application of excessive traction to fractured limbs

Increased Compartmental Content	Bleeding
	  Major vascular injury
	  Coagulation defect
	    Bleeding disorder
	    Anticoagulant therapy
	Increased capillary filtration
	  Reperfusion after ischemia
	    Arterial bypass grafting
	    Embolectomy
	    Ergotamine ingestion
	    Cardiac catheterization
	    Lying on limb
	  Trauma
	    Fracture
	    Contusion
	  Intensive use of muscles
	    Exercise
	    Seizures
	    Eclampsia
	    Tetany
	  Burns
	    Thermal
	    Electric
	  Intra-arterial drug injection
	  Cold
	  Orthopedic surgery
	    Tibial osteotomy
	    Hauser procedure
	    Reduction and internal fixation of fractures
	    Snakebite
	Increased capillary pressure
	  Intensive use of muscles
	  Venous obstruction
	    Phlegmasia cerulea dolens
	    Ill-fitting leg brace
	    Venous ligation
	  Diminished serum osmolarity—nephrotic syndrome
	  Other causes of increased compartmental content
	  Infiltrated infusion
	  Pressure transfusion
	  Leaky dialysis cannula
	  Muscle hypertrophy
	  Popliteal cyst

Externally Applied Pressure	Tight casts, deressings, or air splints Lying on limb

*From Matsen, F. A.: Compartmental Syndromes. New York, Grune & Stratton, 1980, with permission.

The precipitating cause is usually increased resistance within the compartment as the result of swelling after injury. However, decreased arterial blood flow in shock, decreased venous flow after injury or ligation, or increased metabolic needs in the athlete may all affect this formula as illustrated in Table 49–2.

Recognizing the multiple factors in the compartmental syndrome formula has helped to explain some of the puzzling clinical findings associated with this syndrome.

Compartment syndrome does not result primarily from arterial injury, so the distal pulses are usually palpable despite significant muscle ischemia. Increased metabolic demands during exercise may also cause intermittent compartment syndromes of the leg. These can be confused with stress fractures or shin splints.

The compartment syndrome has been confused most often with arterial occlusion, phlebitis, and nerve injury. The differential diagnosis of these conditions can, for the most part, be made on the basis of physical findings, as outlined in Table 49–3.

The most reliable signs and symptoms include:

- *Pain out of proportion to the injury or clinical situation.* This pain is due to the fact that ischemic skeletal muscle causes the same persistently intense pain as does ischemic cardiac muscle. Increasing muscle ischemia causes a type of pain that is unaffected by even the strongest analgesics.
- *Pain on passive extension of the fingers or toes.* This finding is due to the fact that ischemic muscle contracts. Any sudden stretching of the contracted muscle exacerbates the intense deep muscle pain.
- *Hypesthesia in the distribution of nerves coursing through the compartment.* Ischemia rapidly affects nerve conduction. Within 5 minutes of complete ischemia, e.g., after tourniquet application, all nerve conduction ceases. Careful assessment of skin sensation supplied by the nerves that are typically involved in the compartment syndrome will consistently indicate some loss of sensation. Motor paralysis follows sensory loss.
- *Muscle weakness.* Ischemic muscle weakens rapidly. The patient with an anterior compartment syndrome loses dorsiflexion of his toes. However, this muscle weakness should be assessed carefully, since toe flexion may still be possible and can be confused with active toe extension. The patient's ability to "wiggle" the toes or fingers should not assure the physician that muscle function is normal.

Table 49–3. CLINICAL FINDINGS OF COMPARTMENT SYNDROME, ARTERIAL OCCLUSION, PHLEBITIS, AND NERVE INJURY*

	Compartment Syndrome	Arterial Occlusion	Phlebitis	Nerve Injury
Compartment pressure increased above 50 mm. Hg	+	−	−	−
Pain on passive stretching	+	+	+	−
Paresthesia or anesthesia	+	+	−	+
Paresis or paralysis	+	+	−	+
Intact distal pulse	+	−	+	+

*Modified from Mubarak, S. J., and Hargens, A. R.: Compartment Syndromes and Volkmann's Contracture. Philadelphia, W. B. Saunders Co., 1981.

- *Tenseness of involved muscle compartments.* This physical finding may be evident when the patient complains of tightness or pressure in the area of the muscle compartment. The physician can usually find compartment tightness by direct palpation. The compartmental pressure should be measured directly when the diagnosis cannot be established or excluded by the signs and symptoms. Compartmental pressure can be measured by direct insertion of a needle, wick, or split catheter inserted into the muscle. This has been described by Whitesides and coworkers (1975) as well as by Matsen (1980) and Mubarak and Hargens (1981). The reader is referred to these authors for further discussion of the simple methodologies.
- Clinical experiences with accurate compartmental pressure measurements indicate that pressures under 30 mm. Hg are compatible with muscle viability. Persistent pressures above 30 or 40 mm. Hg are associated with muscle ischemia and permanent neuromuscular damage unless the pressure is relieved.

Management by the Family Physician. The compartment syndrome has been known to develop anywhere from 2 hours to 7 days post injury; therefore, continued surveillance must be the rule with any limb swelling. Six hours of ischemia is sufficient to produce permanent muscle and nerve degeneration. Surgical decompression by complete fasciotomy is emergent once the correct diagnosis is made. Any delay increases the damage inflicted on the intracompartmental tissues and the incidence of complications.

Awareness of the three most common compartmental syndromes will allow the physician to move quickly in preventing permanent damage (Fig. 49–10).

The technique of fasciotomy is relatively straightforward and should be considered much like a tracheostomy. It must be done promptly once the physician recognizes its indication. Parafibular decompression of all four compartments of the leg, as well as techniques for decompression of forearm muscle compartments, has been graphically demonstrated by Matsen and coworkers.

Prompt orthopedic consultation is essential when fasciotomy is deemed necessary. Significant muscle loss and even limb loss, as well as other problems such as renal damage, may follow these severe injuries despite prompt fasciotomy.

AMPUTATIONS

The frequency of amputation is about 1:10,000 population per year (Hansson, 1964). Consequently, the family physician sees a good number of amputee patients with a variety of problems.

Rehabilitation Management of the Amputee

Before 1952, the most common cause of amputation was trauma; subsequently, peripheral vascular disease, particularly diabetic in origin, became the most common indication for amputation (Hansson, 1964). Gangrene from vascular disease causes 85 per cent of the lower limb amputations. This change in etiology reflects not only increasing life span but more active treatment of peripheral vascular diseases and improved management of fractures and vascular injuries.

The treatment of elderly amputees has changed considerably over the past three decades. An amputation was considered an admission of defeat by the surgeon and was carried out with little thought to rehabilitation. More recently, an amputation has come to be recognized as an effective rehabilitative procedure. If planned to maximize the patient's chance for prosthetic use, good function is restored.

Management of the unilateral foot problem for diabetic or nondiabetic peripheral vascular disease should anticipate that more than half will in time develop problems in the opposite limb (McCollough et al., 1972).

The initial amputation in the diabetic patient should be as conservative as possible. Understand the difference between a hot and cold foot (see Table 49–5). Sixty per cent of diabetic gangrene occurs in a hot foot with an intact major vascular flow. Here, resection of an infected or gangrenous toe or ray preserves a satisfactory weight-bearing foot (Fig. 49–11).

When a higher level amputation is necessary because of major vessel disease (gangrene in a cold foot), the knee joint should be preserved if at all possible. The major criterion for the level of amputation should be vascularity of the skin flaps evident at the time of surgery. By using the evidence from skin flap bleeding, Sarmiento and Warren (1969) were able to increase the percentage of successful below-knee (BK) amputations from 30.7 to 83 per cent. The BK amputation allowed 64 per cent of their elderly patients to become active prosthetic users as opposed to only 24 per cent who underwent above-knee amputations.

Prosthetic rehabilitation can provide the patient with considerably better function than can a persistently infected or painfully ischemic limb. Figure 49–12 shows the tibial roentgenograms of a patient who had suffered from chronic osteomyelitis for 30 years and had undergone 27 operations during that time. The most effective rehabilitative procedure proved to be a below-knee amputation. This gave him improved function and also eliminated the need for constant treatment. Had amputation been done 20 years earlier, conceivably it would have been of even greater rehabilitative benefit to this hard-working man.

Management by the Family Physician. The family physician should appreciate the importance of conserving knee function for any amputee, particu-

ANTERIOR COMPARTMENTAL SYNDROME OF THE LEG

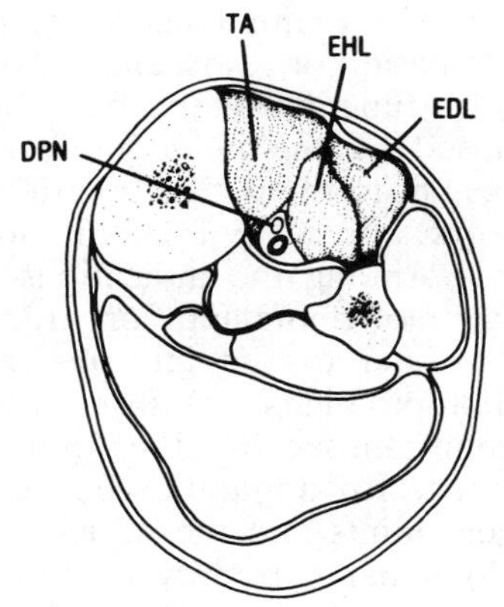

Symptoms and signs

- Weakness of toe extension and foot dorsiflexion
- Pain on passive toe flexion and foot plantar flexion
- Hypesthesia in the dorsal first web space
- Tenseness of the anterior compartmental fascia

A

VOLAR COMPARTMENTAL SYNDROME OF THE FOREARM

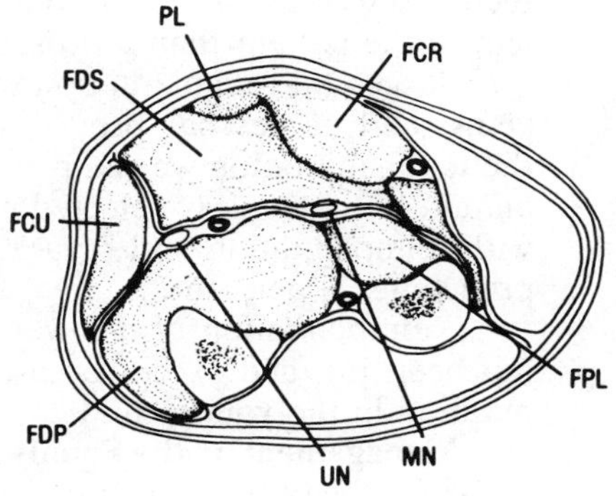

Symptoms and signs

- Weakness of finger and wrist flexion
- Pain on finger and wrist extension
- Hypesthesia of the volar aspect of the fingers
- Tenseness of the volar forearm fascia

B

DEEP POSTERIOR COMPARTMENTAL SYNDROME OF THE LEG

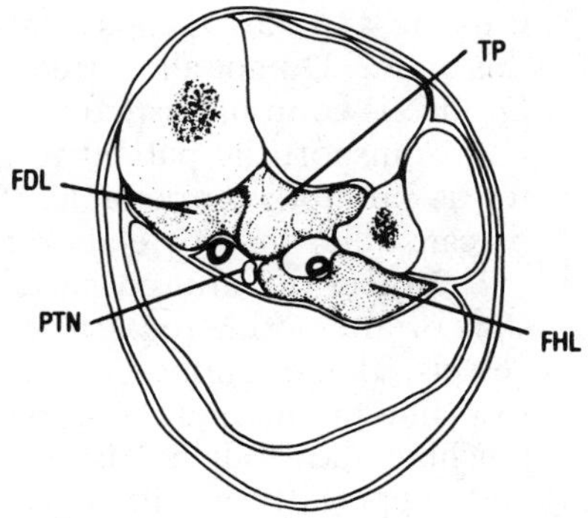

Symptoms and signs

- Weakness of toe flexion and foot inversion
- Pain on passive toe extension and foot eversion
- Hypesthesia of the plantar aspect of the foot and toes
- Tenseness of the deep posterior compartmental fascia (between the tibia and Achilles tendon)

C

Figure 49–10. *A, B,* and *C,* Summary of symptoms and signs as well as a schematic of the anatomic lesion associated with the most common compartment syndromes. (From Matsen, F. A.: Compartmental Syndrome. New York, Grune & Stratton, 1981, with permission.)

larly for the elderly. Keep in mind the important difference between hot and cold gangrene in the diabetic foot (Table 49–4). Use conservative drainage or ablative procedures whenever indicated rather than below-knee amputation (see Fig. 49–11). (Consult also the section in this chapter on diabetic problems.)

Refer the patient who requires amputation to a surgeon who appreciates the important rehabilitative

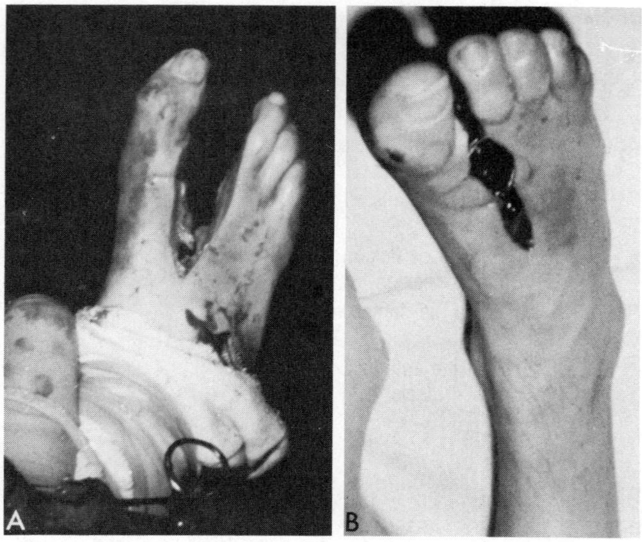

Figure 49–11. *A,* This patient suffered diabetic gangrene of the second toe with a warm foot. Resection of the ray proved to be the treatment of choice, since circulation to the remaining foot was normal. *B,* Two weeks following ray resection, the wound site was granulating satisfactorily. The patient had the benefit of a normally functioning and useful foot.

implications and is not solely interested in the surgical or technical aspects.

Reimplantations

Although amputation with prosthetic fitting improves function in the lower limb, it provides less satisfactory rehabilitation for the injured upper limb. Increasingly, the answer for traumatic amputation of the upper limb is sought in reimplantation.

Microvascular techniques have resulted in successful salvage of amputated thumbs, multiple fingers, hands, and forearms. Inappropriate reimplantation of a single digit or of a badly damaged upper limb can sometimes impair function; hence, it is not always indicated.

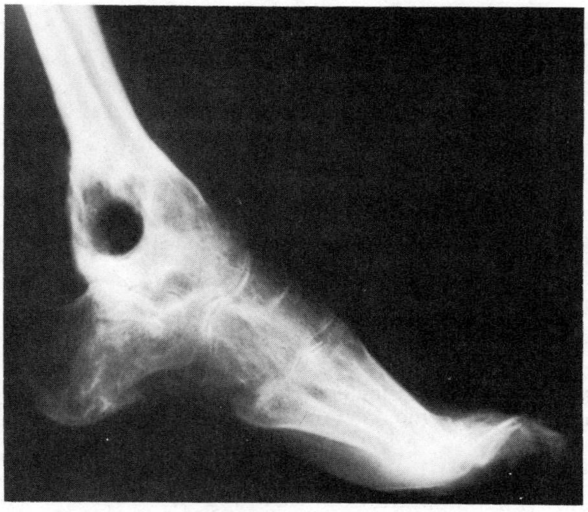

Figure 49–12. Lateral roentgenogram of a patient with a 30-year history of osteomyelitis and multiple operations. A below-knee amputation with prompt prosthetic fitting provided better function for the patient than did his chronically infected limb.

The major considerations in deciding on reimplantation or revascularization are: (1) Will the long-term function of the hand be improved or compromised by the procedure? and (2) Is the potential benefit to the patient worth the risk, expense, loss of work, and costly rehabilitation?

Among the indications shifting the decision in favor of reimplantation are: (1) thumb amputations proximal to the interphalangeal joint; (2) loss of multiple digits; (3) a one-digit amputation in a hand compromised by other injuries or prior injuries; (4) transverse amputation between the metacarpophalangeal joints and the midportion of the forearm; and (5) upper extremity amputations at more proximal levels in children (Phelps et al., 1978).

A major determinant of the rehabilitative potential after complete or partial amputation of the upper limb is the extent of damage to the peripheral nerves. The upper limb that survives without effective protective sensation or motor control is more of a problem to the patient than a prosthesis.

Successful reimplantation with repair of arteries, veins, and nerves has proved superior to any prosthetic rehabilitation we can provide to the upper limb amputee. In properly selected cases, the success rate with reimplantation and revascularization is now approaching 90 per cent.

Reimplantation of a lower limb amputation has not been justified except occasionally for a foot amputation in the young child.

Management by the Family Physician. Reimplantation can be offered to almost any patient who meets the listed indications and who can be transported promptly. Bear in mind some of the common traps, however.

To decrease their metabolic demand, cool the devascularized tissues with a sterile saline-soaked dressing and seal the part in a plastic bag and cool this on ice. Do not allow freezing of the part to occur. Dry ice is contraindicated.

Transport the patient to the reimplantation center as promptly as possible. This may best be done by car rather than by elaborate air transportation.

Protect the injured part. Avoid applying hemostats or attempting to perfuse the ends of the severed vessels. If the amputation is incomplete, be careful to maintain anatomic positioning without twisting or pinching the bridging tissue. Reposition the tissues and support them with loose dressings and a well-padded splint.

Avoid unnecessary medications. Intravenous fluids and antibiotics such as cephalothin, 2 grams, in one liter of Ringer's can be instituted prior to transportation. Avoid anticoagulants or vasopressor agents.

Do not tell the patient that reimplantation will be successful or even attempted. Tell the patient and his family that he is being sent merely for evaluation.

Table 49–4. ETIOLOGIES OF DIABETIC GANGRENE

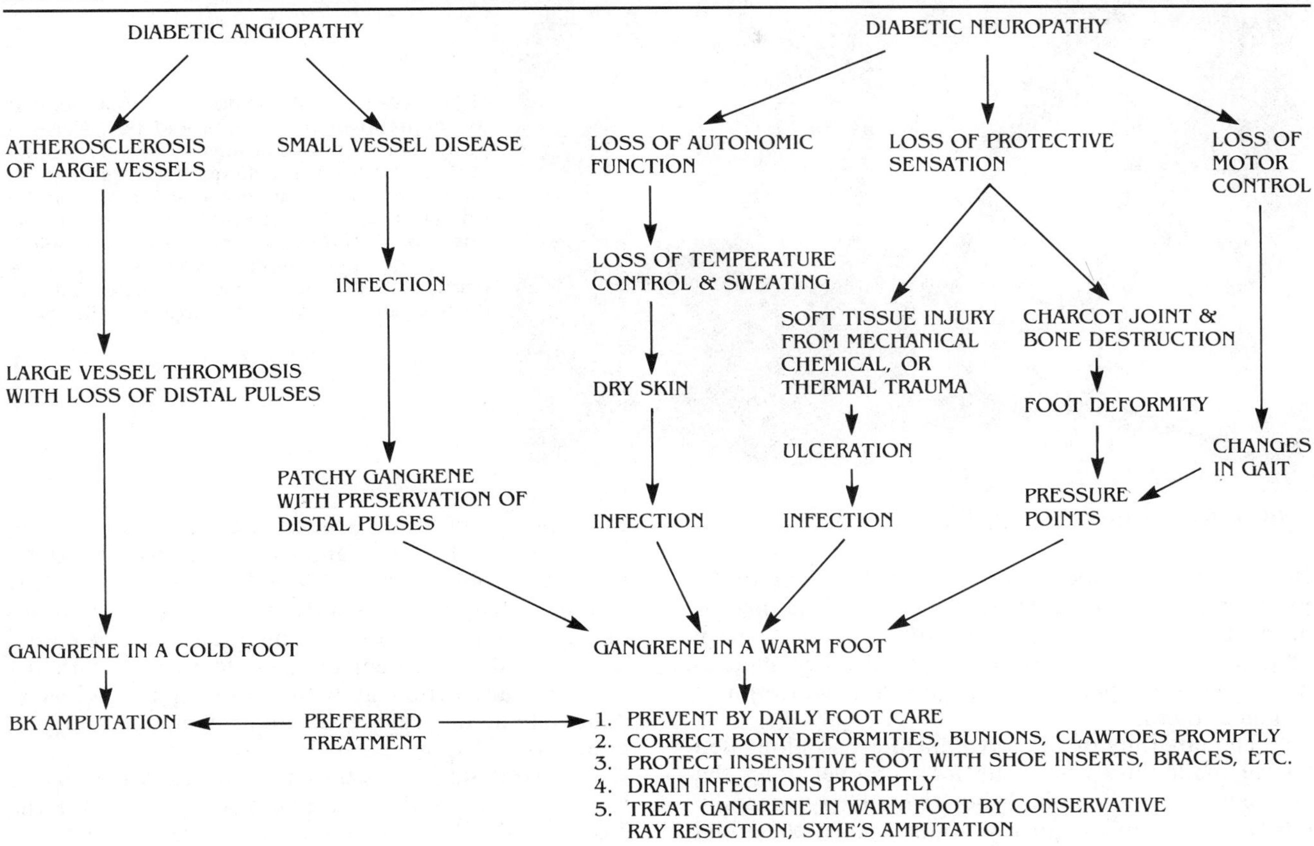

Fingertip Amputations

Usually, a fingertip amputation occurs in the young child who catches a fingertip in a car door. The amputation goes through the nailbed and the pulp of the fingertip. The distal phalanx may or may not be involved.

Many elaborate skin grafts and flaps have been described, but the simplest and most effective technique depends on using natural wound shrinkage and secondary healing. Healing by secondary intention provides a smaller, less sensitive scar than can be obtained from surgical procedures, including full-thickness skin grafts or cross finger flaps.

Management by the Family Physician. Fingertip amputations represent one type of injury that frequently can be more effectively managed by the family physician using the process of wound intussusception than by the surgeon using elaborate technical procedures. Under sedation and local anesthetic, gently cleanse the injured fingertip, leaving the nail in situ to act as a splint. In the adult, any exposed bone can be rongeured, but this is unnecessary in the child's injury. After cleansing the wound, apply an occlusive cast dressing over sterile gauze. Give tetanus toxoid and antibiotics as appropriate. Elevate the hand in a sling support for 2 to 3 days post treatment. The cast dressing can be soaked off at approximately 10 to 14 days. The wound will usually be completely epithelialized. If bone was exposed in the fingertip, 3 weeks of cast immobilization is preferable.

This technique is especially gratifying in a young child, who has impressive regenerative capabilities after fingertip amputations (Fig. 49–13). The method maintains the maximum finger length possible. It is simple and minimizes unnecessary disability from these common injuries. It is considered the treatment of choice in most instances.

Sprains, Strains, and Differential Conditions

The common problems we shall discuss here are those involving (a) ankle sprains, both acute and recurrent; (b) finger sprains, or the jammed finger; (c) wrist sprains and differential conditions; (d) elbow sprains; (e) shoulder sprains, pain, and stiffening; and (f) knee sprains and differential conditions.

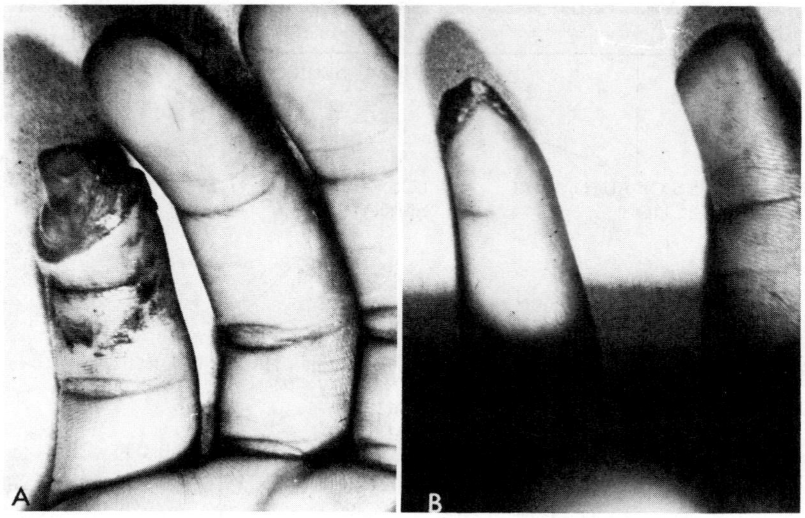

Figure 49–13. *A*, A car door injury amputated the fingertip in this 10-year-old boy. The exposed bone was not removed but was cleaned and immobilized in a finger cast dressing. *B*, After 3 weeks of continuous cast treatment the wound edges had completely covered the exposed bone and the wound was well-epithelialized. Fingertip amputations treated in this manner give better, less sensitive scars than do those treated by elaborate surgical methods.

ANKLE SPRAINS: GRADES I, II, AND III

Injuries to the ankle produce the most common of joint instability problems. Depending on the mechanism of injury, the ankle may suffer either a sprain or a fracture. Sprains result from inversion mechanisms, while eversion and external torsional injuries produce fractures.

The anatomy of the ankle includes an elongated lateral malleolus, which sits in a groove along the lateral aspect of the tibia. When the ankle is forcefully inverted, the fibula quickly abuts against the tibial tubercle in the anterior aspect of its groove. The resultant strain is absorbed primarily by the weak anterior talofibular ligament (Fig. 49–14). Continued inversion overloading disrupts the calcaneofibular and talocalcaneal ligaments.

It has been estimated that one significant ankle sprain occurs daily per 10,000 population. This injury represents one of the most frequent musculoskeletal problems treated by the family physician. The majority of ankle sprains are minor disruptions of the anterior talofibular ligament, which are best managed with minimal external support and early mobilization.

About one in four patients with acute ankle sprains have recurrent episodes of instability. These should not be ignored or undertreated, as instability can prove significantly disabling. Untreated recurrent instability can lead to significant degenerative arthritis. Such problems can be avoided and corrected by reconstructive procedures. In contrast to ligamentous injuries about the knee, which are best repaired acutely, ankle ligament injuries do as well with delayed reconstruction as with acute repair. When in doubt about the degree of ankle ligament injury, a nonoperative approach is the best course.

In your initial evaluation, consider whether the patient has suffered any similar ankle problems in the past and also keep in mind the future demands the individual will make on the ankle.

A history of popping or a painful snap at the time of ankle injury is usually indicative of significant ligament tear or fracture.

Physical examination should include direct palpation for the areas of maximal tenderness anterolaterally, posterolaterally, and occasionally anteromedially. Palpate particularly for a tender sulcus in the anterolateral aspect on inversion of the ankle.

The degree of pain bears no relationship to the amount of anatomic disruption. Complete ligamentous tears may be relatively pain free on stressing despite considerable instability of the ankle.

Always x-ray the sprained ankle, as some will be confused with fractures of the facets or of the osteo-

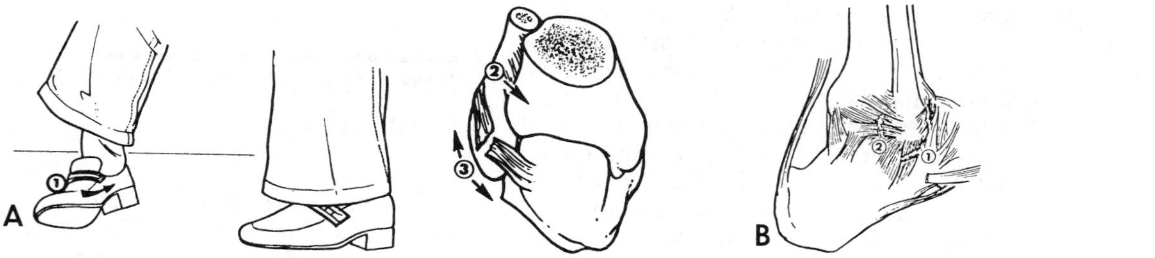

Figure 49–14. *A*, Ankle sprain characteristically results from inversion injuries *(1)*. This causes the fibula to abut against the anterior aspect of its groove in the tibia *(2)*. The strain is absorbed by the anterior tibiofibular ligament, which ruptures *(3)*. *B*, Most common sites of ankle sprains are the anterior fibulotalar ligament *(1)* and the posterior fibulotalar and calcaneofibular ligaments *(2)*. (From Connolly, J. F.: DePalma's The Management of Fractures and Dislocations: An Atlas. 3rd ed. Philadelphia, W. B. Saunders Co., 1981, with permission.)

chondral surfaces of the talus. Take care, also, that the x-ray is not coned so diligently on the ankle that a fracture of the proximal tibia or fibula is missed. Stress x-rays taken with the ankle in forced inversion are helpful to demonstrate instability, but ankle instability can be present with a normal stress x-ray.

Management by the Family Physician. Most ankle sprains can be treated with minimal external support and elevation to eliminate the swelling which follows these injuries. Allow the patient to bear partial weight with crutches, since non-weight-bearing tightens the heel cord and calf muscles.

A simple and effective method of supporting the ankle is to wrap an Ace bandage from the toes to above the malleoli. Then reinforce the support with a full roll of 2.5 cm. tape applied medially and laterally (Fig. 49–15). The air cast or splint (Fig. 49–16) can give good support and be fitted with ease. The strips are adjusted for heel width. The splint is placed and the bottom straps tightened. The shoe is then put on. The top strap is then placed and the splint pressurized. The straps can be readjusted in turn until comfortable pressure is felt.

The ankle is wrapped mainly for the patient's comfort. If the patient experiences swelling or irritation, the wrapping or support should be relieved. Advise the patient to elevate the ankle for 2 to 3 days and apply ice to the painful areas.

Encourage functional rehabilitation of the injured proprioceptive and ligamentous structures about the ankle. Use a series of exercises on a balance board to develop coordination of the calf muscles as well as inversion and eversion balance (Fig. 49–17). A period of ankle rehabilitation for 7 to 10 days is the minimum needed to help the patient avoid recurrent problems of instability.

By assessing the patient's history and the degree

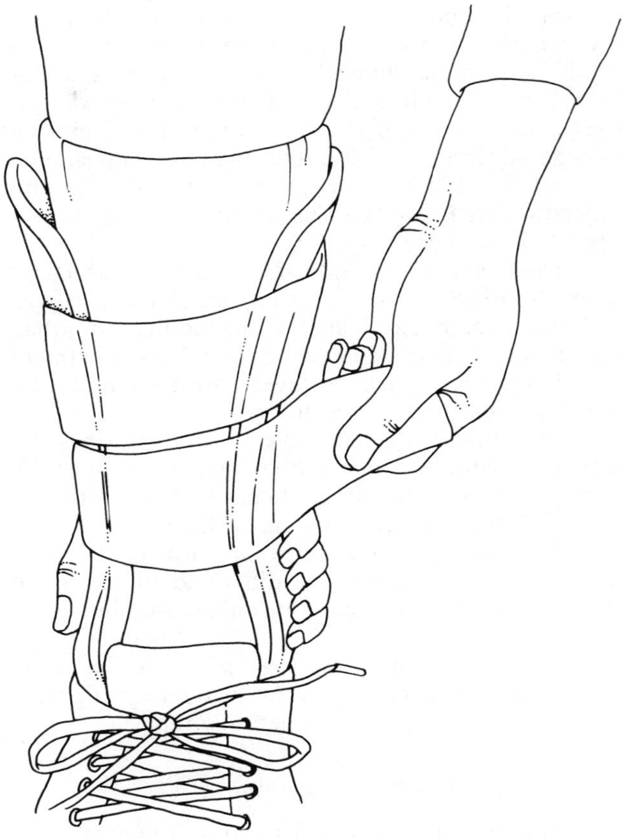

Figure 49–16. Diagram of an air splint. Straps are adjusted to heel size and the lower straps wrapped about ankle and the side extensions are centered. The splint is then pressurized and straps adjusted until a comfortable support and pressure is attained.

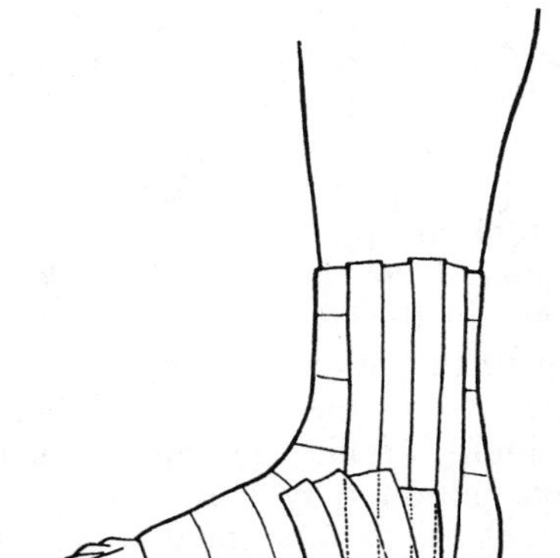

Figure 49–15. The most effective method of supporting most acute ankle sprains is by using an Ace wrap reinforced with 1-inch medial and lateral tape strips. Leave the anterior and posterior aspects of the ankle free to allow the patient to flex and extend the ankle. Encourage the patient to bear weight with crutches. (From Connolly, J. F.: DePalma's The Management of Fractures and Dislocations: An Atlas. 3rd ed. Philadelphia, W. B. Saunders Co., 1981.)

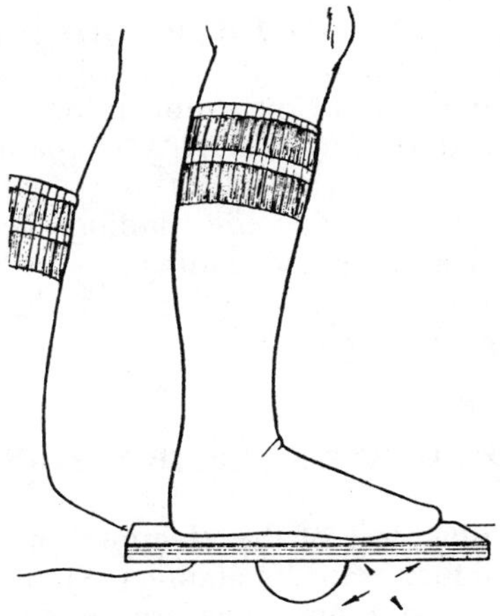

Figure 49–17. As the ankle pain subsides, about the third to the fifth day, begin balancing exercises to allow the patient to regain ankle proprioception and to avoid recurrent instability problems. (From Connolly, J. F.: DePalma's The Management of Fractures and Dislocations: An Atlas. 3rd ed. Philadelphia, W. B. Saunders Co., 1981.)

of instability and pain on stressing and palpating for any localized defects in the capsule, the physician can usually determine clinically if the sprain is a minor Type I or a complete Type III injury. In between is a gray zone, or Type II injury, where the degree of damage is difficult to ascertain acutely. This should be treated initially as a Type I or minor sprain, understanding that if later instability occurs, operative repair may be necessary.

Management of Grade III Injury. Grade III or complete injuries of the anterior talofibular and posterior calcaneofibular ligament may require more than taping and elevation. In general, avoid cast treatment of ankle sprains because severe stiffness and prolonged disability often result.

If the ankle is so unstable that taping does not provide adequate support, the ligament is best repaired acutely. This is particularly true with the unstable ankles of active young athletes.

The individual with recurrent problems of instability and an acute Grade III injury should be offered operative repair. Long-standing ankle instability leads to degenerative arthritis.

Avulsion fractures seen on x-ray of the acute injury usually indicate significant ligamentous damage and often warrant primary operative repair.

Recurrent Instability of the Ankle

Persistent ankle instability is a well-known problem in athletes as well as in active adults. The ankle is assessed for instability problems by inversion stress x-rays. The significance of these x-rays should be considered much like myelography in the diagnosis of a ruptured intervertebral disc. The results are not always reliable but can be used as an adjunct to careful history and physical examination. In general, more than 10 degrees of tilt in comparison with the opposite ankle is considered evidence of significant lateral instability.

Management by the Family Physician. More important than the radiographic signs of recurrent instability are the history of recurrent sprain or giving way of the ankle during mild activity. A palpable sulcus in the anterolateral aspect of the ankle joint on inversion stressing is a positive finding. Refer patients with these symptoms and findings for reconstruction of the lateral ligaments by one of the variety of methods now available.

"JAMMED FINGER" OR FINGER SPRAINS

Within the diagnosis of the "jammed finger" lurks a number of hidden traps, including (1) tendon avulsion (mallet finger, boutonniere deformity, and flexor profundus avulsion); (2) phalangeal fractures; and (3) dislocations. The jammed finger usually results from an unimpressive injury, which can produce disproportionate disability. To detect, treat, and prevent potential problems physicians should systematically evaluate all of these injuries, no matter how unimpressive they appear.

Such an evaluation should include (1) thorough palpation for areas of tenderness; (2) active and passive range of motion and stress testing to detect joint instability or loss of tendon function; and (3) adequate anteroposterior and lateral x-rays centered on the finger to detect fracture deformity.

Tendon Avulsions

Mallet Finger. A mallet finger deformity is the most common injury to the tendon of a digit. It results generally from a blow to the end of the finger, producing pain, swelling, and some deformity. The degree of deformity varies, but the patient cannot extend the distal phalanx actively. If the tendon continues to retract, the deformity increases (Fig. 49–18*A, B*).

Management by the Family Physician. Prompt recognition of the extensor tendon avulsion allows closed treatment with a dorsal splint for 5 to 6 weeks (Fig. 49–18*C*). Mallet finger deformities associated with fractures that cannot be reduced anatomically require open reduction and internal fixation.

Flexor Tendon Avulsion. Another unrecognized tendon injury confused with a "jammed finger" is avulsion of the flexor profundus insertion. This occurs most often in the ring or small finger when the patient forcefully grasps the shirt of someone like a football player as he lunges forward (Fig. 49–19). Flexor profundus avulsion also occurs in older patients who avulse the tendon while lifting heavy objects. Too often, the significance of the flexor tendon injury goes unrecognized. The profundus tendon then retracts proximally into its sheath or completely up into the palm (Fig. 49–19).

Physical examination will show the tenderness to be localized either over the proximal interphalangeal joint or in the palm, but not at the usual site of tendon insertion. The diagnosis is made readily by observing the patient's inability to flex the distal interphalangeal joint. The sublimis function is undisturbed; hence, the patient still has the ability to flex at the proximal interphalangeal joint.

Management by the Family Physician. The prompt repair of the avulsed flexor tendon restores normal grip to the injured finger. To avoid missing these injuries, assess the patient's ability to flex and extend all joints of his "jammed" finger actively. Delayed recognition may leave the patient with a permanent degree of functional impairment. Refer the patient with this injury promptly to a hand surgeon for tendon repair. Extensor tendon lacerations proximal to the IP joint can often be repaired by the experienced family physician. Lacerations of tendons distal to the IP joint pose problems in repair because these tendons are in reality a series of bands that function in a complex manner.

Proximally, where the extensor is a single unit, cleansing and simple suture with a double right angle

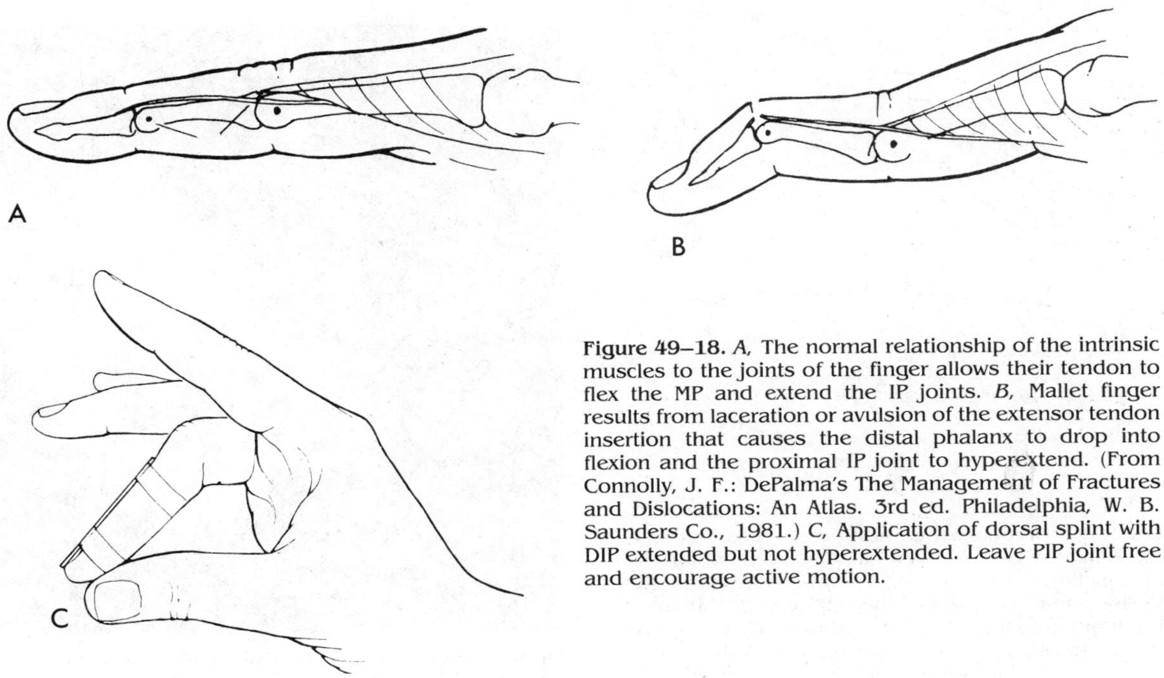

Figure 49–18. *A*, The normal relationship of the intrinsic muscles to the joints of the finger allows their tendon to flex the MP and extend the IP joints. *B*, Mallet finger results from laceration or avulsion of the extensor tendon insertion that causes the distal phalanx to drop into flexion and the proximal IP joint to hyperextend. (From Connolly, J. F.: DePalma's The Management of Fractures and Dislocations: An Atlas. 3rd ed. Philadelphia, W. B. Saunders Co., 1981.) C, Application of dorsal splint with DIP extended but not hyperextended. Leave PIP joint free and encourage active motion.

stitch (Fig. 49–20) will suffice. The thumb extensor should probably be handled by a surgeon trained in hand work.

Boutonniere Deformity. This can be a treacherous injury. Usually it results from a direct laceration over the proximal interphalangeal joint which involves the extensor slip attachment to the middle phalanx, and this permits a progressive flexion contracture to develop. Another mechanism is a closed, crushing injury that avulses the central slip.

Since the flexion deformity may not be initially evident, the significance of the injury to the extensor mechanism frequently goes unrecognized. Progressive disruption of the central slip occurs, and the proximal phalanx then "buttonholes" through the disrupted tendon (Fig. 49–21*A*). The result is a flexion contracture of the proximal interphalangeal (PIP) joint and an extensor contracture of the distal interphalangeal (DIP) joint, which develop only weeks or months after injury.

Management by the Family Physician. To avoid

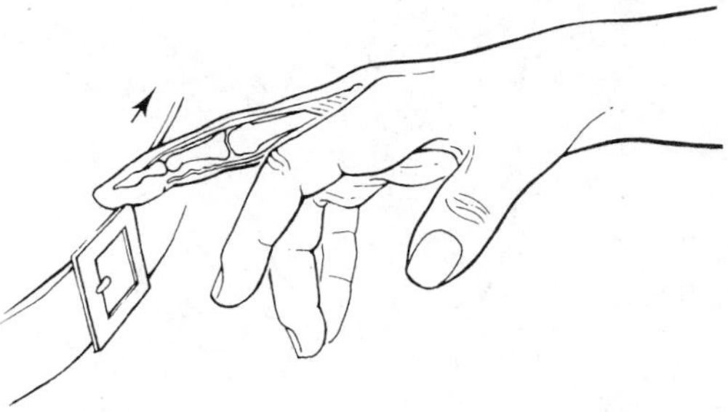

Figure 49–19. Flexor profundus tendon is avulsed during forceful flexion of the finger. The injury tends to pass unrecognized or will be dismissed as a "jammed" finger unless the patient's inability to flex his distal phalanx is recognized. The diagnosis becomes obvious once the patient is asked to move the distal phalanx. (From Connolly, J. F.: DePalma's The Management of Fractures and Dislocations: An Atlas. 3rd ed. Philadelphia, W. B. Saunders Co., 1981.)

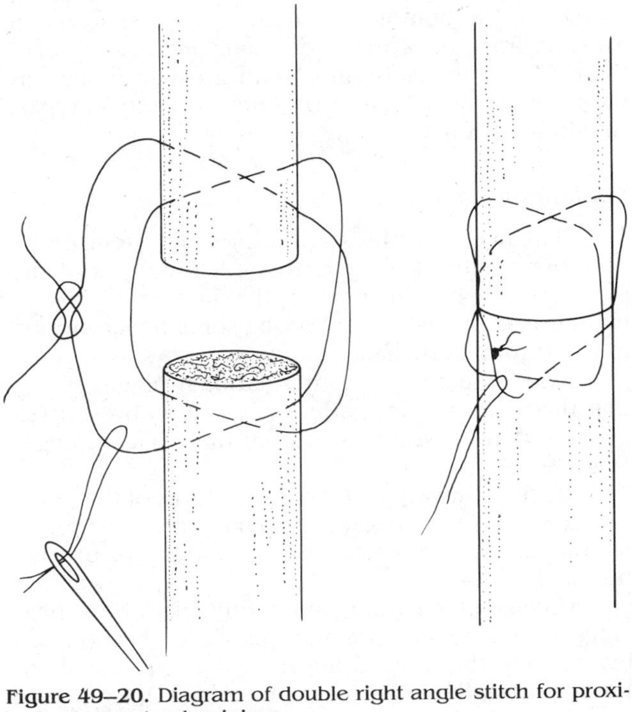

Figure 49–20. Diagram of double right angle stitch for proximal extensor tendon injury.

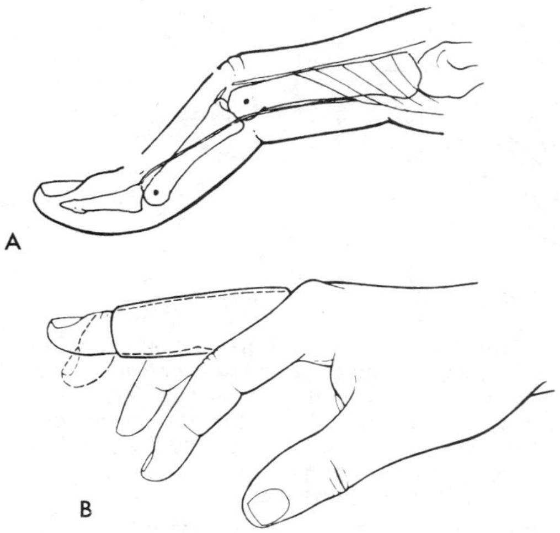

Figure 49–21. *A,* Disruption of the central slip insertion onto the middle phalanx leads to gradual displacement of the proximal phalanx dorsally, with flexion contracture of the PIP joint and extension contracture of the DIP joint. *B,* If there is any suspicion of boutonniere deformity, immobilize the proximal interphalangeal joint in an extension splint. This is one of the rare indications for immobilization of a finger injury in extension. (From Connolly, J. F.: DePalma's The Management of Fractures and Dislocations: An Atlas. 3rd ed. Philadelphia, W. B. Saunders Co., 1981.)

chronic problems of this nature evaluate all lacerations and direct injuries to the PIP joint carefully. If you have any doubt about the integrity of the tendon, immobilize the joint in an extension cast for 3 to 6 weeks to ensure adequate healing and to prevent flexion contracture of the joint (Fig. 49–21*B*).

Even in the patient seen 6 to 12 weeks after the initial injury, cast treatment may be effective in correcting the boutonniere deformity. If there is an avulsion fracture of the middle phalanx evident or if there is anterior dislocation with gross instability as the patient moves the PIP joint, operative repair should be recommended.

Phalangeal Fractures

Phalangeal fractures are injuries that tend to be both overtreated and undertreated. Fractures of the phalangeal bones heal promptly, and most can be treated best by methods allowing some finger motion to avoid joint stiffness.

Take care to maintain rotational alignment so that the fractured finger does not heal in a distorted position that causes it to overlap the adjacent finger (Fig. 49–22).

Fractures involving articular surfaces of the joints or fractures of the proximal phalanges are most prone to complications either of joint instability or of fracture malunion.

Management by the Family Physician. Most phalangeal fractures that are undisplaced are best treated by splinting the injured finger to the adjacent uninjured finger ("buddy taping," Fig. 49–23).

Avoid splinting the fractured phalanx in extension, since this tends to allow the fracture to rotate and produce overlapping, such as illustrated in Figure 49–22.

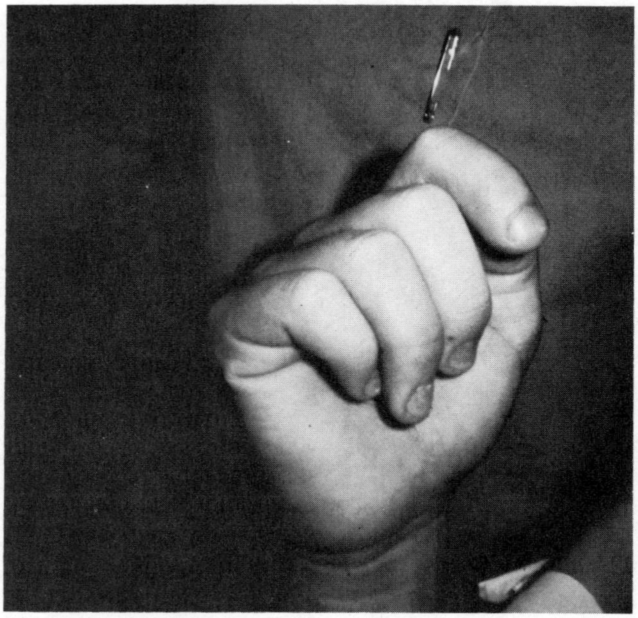

Figure 49–22. After this patient's middle phalangeal fracture had been treated with an extension splint, he noted that his injured ring finger overlapped his small finger when he made a fist. Derotational osteotomy was necessary to correct the overlapping finger deformity. Such torsional deformities can be avoided by using "buddy" taping.

Fractures involving articular surfaces are best referred for orthopedic evaluation of joint instability. Fracture of the proximal phalanx can be a problem. Inadequate reduction or inadequate x-ray of the hand rather than a true lateral x-ray of the finger may result in a fracture that heals with unacceptable angulation.

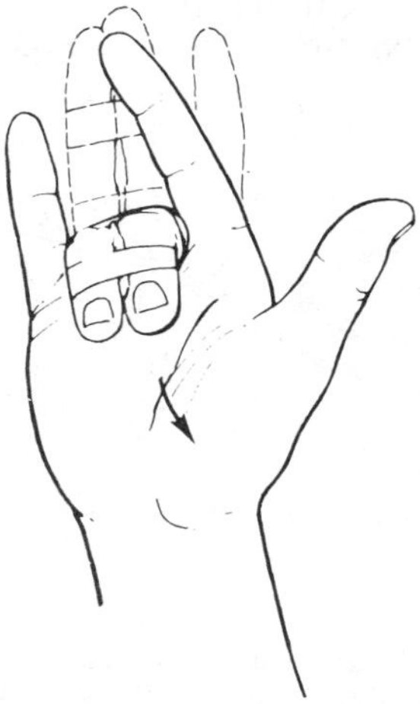

Figure 49–23. Most phalangeal fractures can be effectively aligned and held by "buddy" taping to the adjacent, uninjured finger. This allows the patient to move the joint and ensures correct rotational reduction (From Connolly, J. F.: DePalma's The Management of Fractures and Dislocations: An Atlas. 3rd ed. Philadelphia, W. B. Saunders Co., 1981.)

Dislocations of the Interphalangeal Joints

Lateral dislocations of the interphalangeal joints are usually considered minor injuries. In fact, the dislocation is frequently reduced by the patient or bystander soon after the injury. Be very wary of the joint that is unusually swollen or tender after a dislocation. This may indicate more than usual damage to the ligaments.

Management by the Family Physician. In most areas if the dislocation is still present, it can be reduced by direct traction on the distal phalanx. Subsequent to reduction, evaluate the functional stability of the joint by having the patient move the finger. Use digital nerve block if necessary. Dislocation of the interphalangeal joints can be manipulated as illustrated in Figures 49–24 and 49–25 (Connolly, 1981). Most often the dislocated joint requires only a brief period of support by "buddy taping" the finger to the adjacent uninjured finger (see Fig. 49–23). Buddy taping should continue until there is clinical stability (usually 2 to 3 weeks) but slightly longer when the joint will be subjected to heavy use (Connolly, 1981). Avoid prolonging immobilization of a dislocation for more than 3 to 5 days. By far the most common complication of injury to the PIP joint is not instability but stiffness.

Any instability in hyperextension or hyperflexion on active or passive stress testing is most likely to occur when the dislocation is associated with an articular fracture. Any question about the functional stability of the joint after reducing the dislocation calls for referral to an orthopedic consultant.

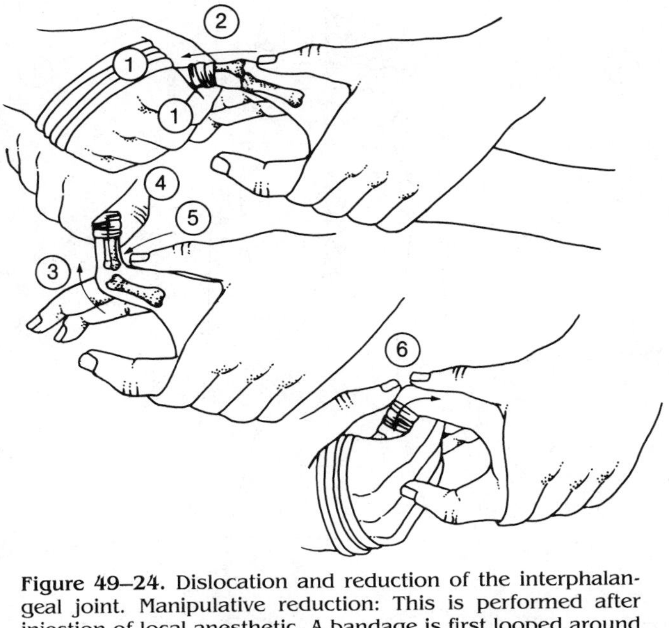

Figure 49–24. Dislocation and reduction of the interphalangeal joint. Manipulative reduction: This is performed after injection of local anesthetic. A bandage is first looped around the end of the injured figure and then around the operator's hand. Bring the phalanx into the hyperextended position. While traction is being maintained, slide the base of the phalanx distalward to a position opposite the head of the proximal phalanx; then flex the interphalangeal joint and immobilize the plaster splint.

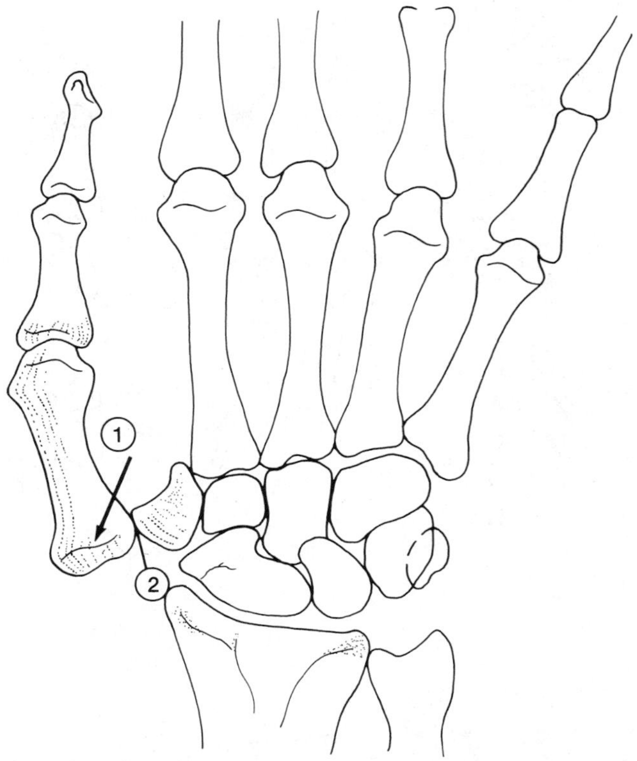

Figure 49–25. Reduction of dislocation of thumb metacarpal. Prereduction x-ray film: The metacarpal is displaced upward and backward. Traction is made in the long axis of the thumb, the thumb is gradually abducted and, at the same time, direct pressure is exerted against the head of the metacarpal bone. As the thumb is pulled downward and outward, the head of the metacarpal is pushed forward and inward.

Displaced fractures of the distal phalanx can usually be manually reduced with finger manipulation or towel clip traction as shown in the Figures 49–26 and 49–27 (Connolly, 1981).

Fractures of the mid (Figs. 49–28 to 49–30) and proximal phalanx can be manipulated by traction and immobilized as in Figures 49–24 and 49–31. Immobilization is usually necessary for 3 to 4 weeks, followed by active physical therapy (Connolly, 1981).

Nondisplaced fractures of the bases of the metacarpals can be immobilized for 3 weeks in a short arm cast as illustrated in Figures 49–32 and 49–33 (Connolly, 1981).

WRIST SPRAINS AND DIFFERENTIAL CONDITIONS

Wrist or carpal bone injuries are among the most likely to be misdiagnosed or subject to delayed diagnoses. Fractures of the carpal scaphoid are notorious for their tendency to pass unrecognized or to be dismissed as a "wrist sprain."

Other conditions that the family physician should consider in this complex include (1) dorsal ganglia; (2) synovial ganglion of the hand; (3) scapholunate separations; (4) fractures of the hamate or other

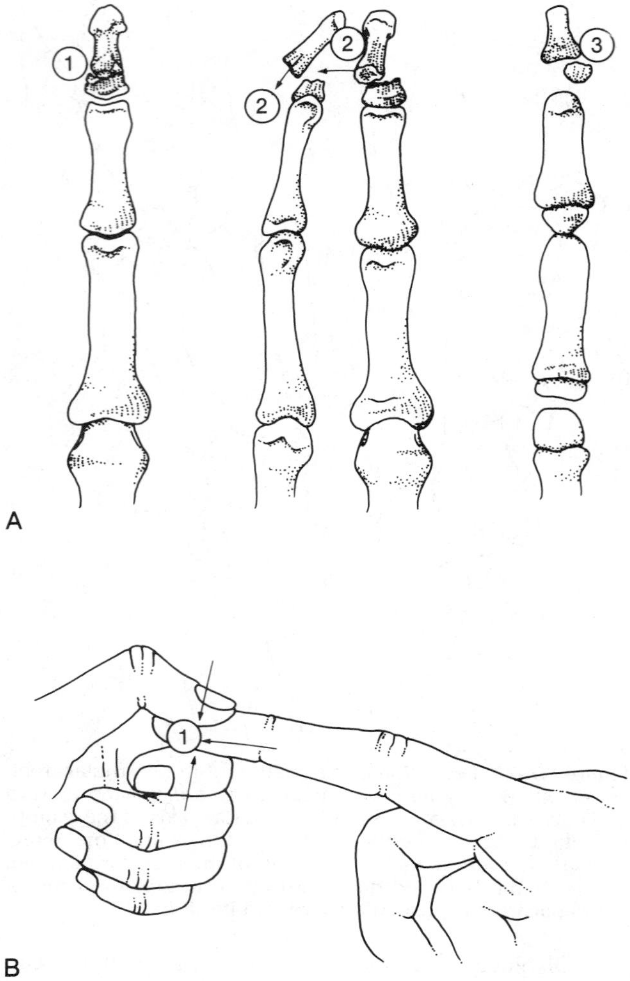

Figure 49–26. *A,* Comminuted fracture of distal phalanx. Appearance on x-ray film: *(1)* This fracture requires no reduction; *(2)* fracture of the terminal phalanx with upward, backward, and lateral displacement of the distal fragment; *(3)* this epiphyseal fracture should be reduced. The nail bed serves as a very effective splint after the fracture is reduced. *B,* Method of reduction. The physician applies traction and molds the fragments between the thumb and index finger.

carpal bones; (5) de Quervain's stenosing tenosynovitis; (6) osteoarthritis of the first carpometacarpal joint; and (7) carpal tunnel syndrome. All of these produce symptoms that can be confused with a "wrist sprain."

X-ray Evaluation of the Wrist Sprain

One reason for misdiagnosis of wrist injuries is inadequate x-ray. The usual anteroposterior and oblique views may not detect even complete dislocation of the carpus.

In evaluating any seriously injured wrist radiographically, be sure to include anteroposterior x-rays with the wrist in maximum radial and ulnar deviation, particularly to detect scaphoid fractures.

Obtain a lateral view of the wrist in flexion and extension to assess for carpal instability.

A supinated wrist view with the fist clenched should demonstrate mild carpal subluxations.

Last, a tunnel view may be necessary to detect fractures in the volar aspect of the wrist, particularly fractures of the hook of the hamate.

Scaphoid Fractures

The scaphoid fracture is the most frequent and most frequently overlooked fracture in the carpus. Suspect a fractured scaphoid in every case of an "acutely sprained wrist." Insist that x-rays include a view taken in maximum ulnar deviation to show a scaphoid fracture.

Management by the Family Physician. Even when x-ray fails to demonstrate a fracture, if the pain is localized to the snuffbox region, treat the injury as a fracture and apply a cast that immobilizes the thumb

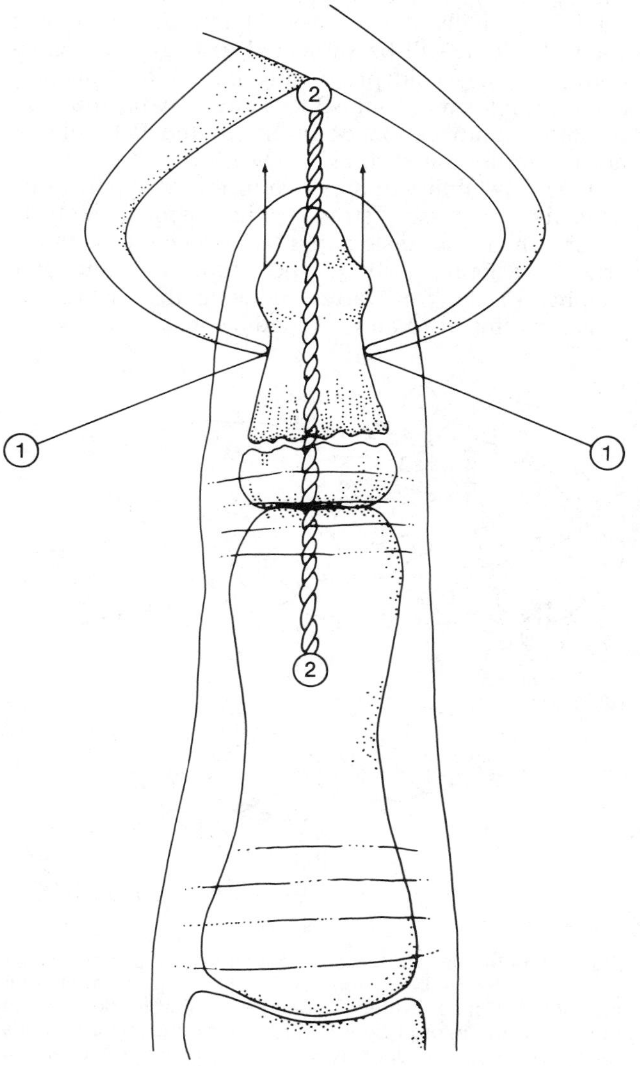

Figure 49–27. Fracture of the distal phalanx. Grasp the distal fragment with a towel clip and use straight traction. Pass a threaded wire through both fragments, across the distal joint, and into the middle phalanx.

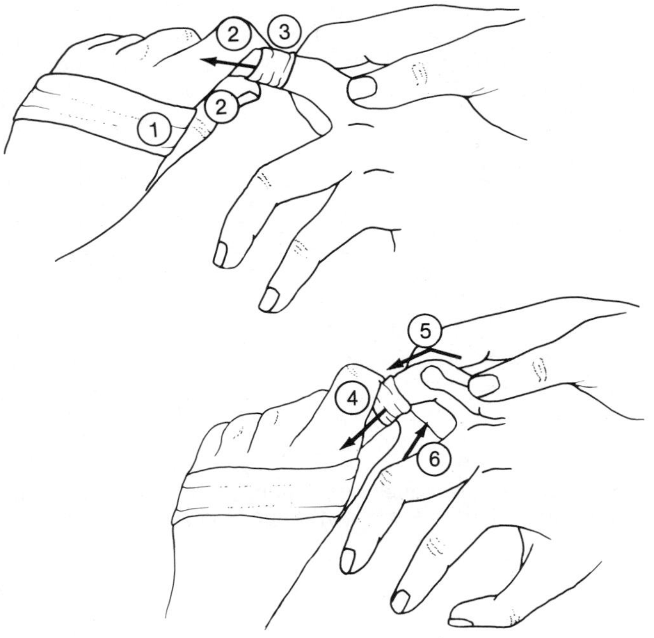

Figure 49–28. Reduction of phalanx fracture. Manipulative reduction: Loop a gauze bandage around the end of the finger and your hand. Grasp the finger between your thumb and index finger and use steady traction in the line of the finger. While traction is maintained, flex the finger over the index finger of your other hand. This pushes upward at the apex of the angular deformity.

and wrist. Remove the cast after 2 weeks and repeat the wrist x-ray. At this time, the vascular response should demonstrate a fracture line if one is present. If none is evident after 2 weeks and the patient still has pain, consider the possibility of a scapholunate subluxation.

If a scaphoid fracture is evident, immobilize the wrist with a cast that includes the thumb and carpal bones. Eighty-five to 95 per cent of acute scaphoid fractures heal if treated by adequate immobilization. The 10 to 15 per cent of scaphoid fractures that are unstable or displaced need referral for early operative fixation.

If the patient is pain free at the end of 8 to 10 weeks of cast immobilization, discontinue the cast. The scaphoid fracture should be treated on the basis of the patient's symptoms rather than the radiographic appearance. Clinical union precedes x-ray union sometimes by several months.

Dorsal Ganglion of the Wrist

Disruption of the strong scapholunate or perilunate ligaments in the wrist on the dorsal surface may allow the synovial lining to produce a cystlike herniation or ganglion cyst. This characteristically causes discomfort on the dorsal surface of the wrist as the firm mass develops and enlarges.

Management by the Family Physician. Treat the usual ganglion cyst by aspirating the fluid content and then immobilizing the wrist in a cast for 3 weeks. Holding the wrist dorsiflexed encourages scar formation sufficient to heal the area of capsular damage. If the ganglion recurs after this treatment, surgical excision should be advised. Keep in mind that the wrist ganglia and synovitis from rheumatoid arthritis can be confused. Any progressively enlarging lump or bump belongs in the pathologist's bottle, not in the patient's body.

Synovial Ganglion of the Hand

These are small ganglia in the fingers, similar to those that develop in the wrist. They should be kept in mind as they are quite common. They usually result from an injury that bends the finger backward. They are about 5 mm. in diameter, are quite tender, and may be disabling in grasping.

These small synovial ganglia herniate through the tendon sheath of the finger. They may disappear as suddenly as they came. This is due to spontaneous rupture. On the other hand, treatment by needle rupture is quite simple and should be tried in preference to surgical excision.

Management by the Family Physician. Palpate the pea-sized ganglion at the base of the finger. This usually can be ruptured with a 2-gauge needle introduced through a small skin wheal raised by injection of 2 per cent Novocain. Try not to merely puncture the ganglion but to tear its walls so as to simulate a rupture. Relief is usually immediate and complete (Bruner, 1963).

The appearance of these lesions following trauma and the response to the needle aspiration suggest that they are produced by a small bit of synovial membrane pushing through the flexor tendon sheath. These small sensitive ganglia need not be operated on; they can be readily managed by the family physician.

Acute and Chronic Scapholunate Subluxation (Dissociation)

Disruption of the carpal ligaments on both the dorsal and volar surfaces will allow dissociation between the scaphoid and lunate. Widening of the joint space between the scaphoid and lunate is evident on x-ray (Fig. 49–34*A*). Do not dismiss it as simply a wrist sprain.

Chronic dissociation of the scaphoid and lunate allows proximal migration of the capitate and rapid progressive arthritis of the wrist joint. In the acutely sprained wrist, if you do not demonstrate fracture of the carpal scaphoid, rule out subluxation of the scapholunate joint with adequate x-rays. Obtain a true lateral view of the wrist and a posteroanterior view with the fist clenched and the wrist supinated.

On the lateral x-ray, the axes of the radius, lunate, and capitate should form a straight line. The axis of the scaphoid should intersect the radio-lunate-capitate axes at an angle between 30 and 60 degrees. When the scapholunate subluxation occurs, the scaph-

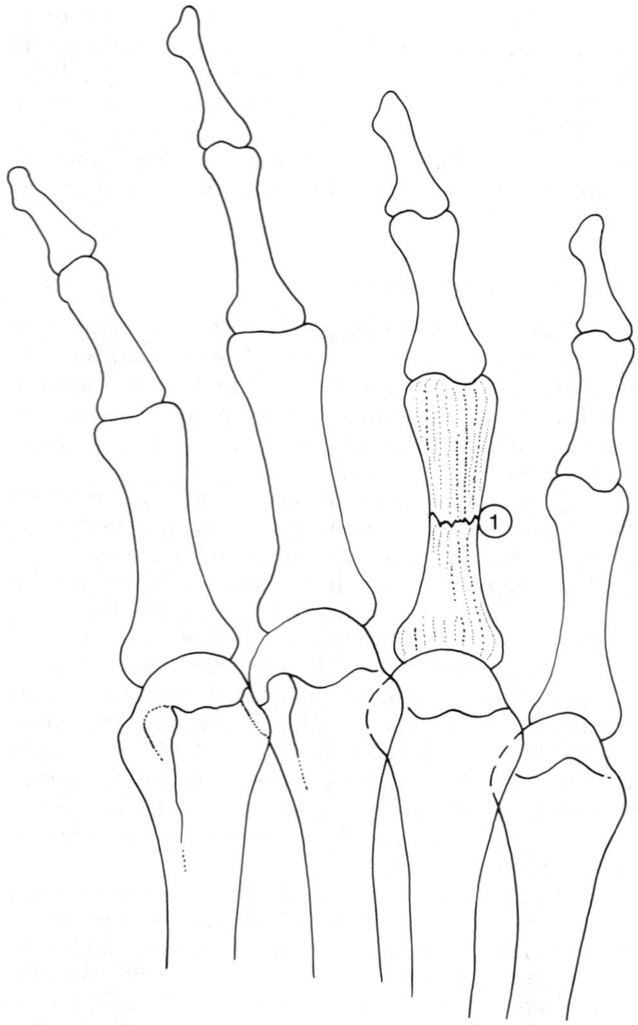

Figure 49–29. Postreduction position. *(1)* The fragments of the proximal phalanx are engaged and in normal alignment.

oid rotates downward and the lunate tilts upward so that this angle exceeds 70 degrees (Fig. 49–34*B*).

In the posteroanterior view, the space between the scaphoid and lunate normally does not exceed 2 mm. Greater spacing than this indicates that separation between the scaphoid and lunate has occurred with imminent collapse of the distal carpal row and capitate on the proximal row (Fig. 49–34*C*).

Scapholunate subluxation can also occur in individuals such as carpenters who subject their wrists to repetitive heavy loading. The diagnosis can be recognized by (1) characteristic pain in the radioscaphoid region, particularly on wrist extension; (2) a palpable click on extension of the wrist; and (3) loss of grip strength and decreased wrist motion.

Management by the Family Physician. This is not an uncommon injury and must be suspected in any patient with persistent pain mimicking a carpal scaphoid fracture but without x-ray evidence of fracture after several weeks. If the snuffbox pain persists despite a trial cast immobilization, assess the wrist carefully for scapholunate dissociation using the supinated wrist view as previously described.

In the acute injury, refer the patient for reduction of the scapholunate subluxation under fluoroscopy with percutaneous Kirschner wire fixation. For chronic pain secondary to scapholunate subluxation, operative fusion of the carpal bones may be necessary.

Fractures of the Hamate

Isolated fractures of the carpal bones may lead to frequent failures of diagnosis. Typical of these are fractures of the hamate, which are notorious for going unrecognized.

The fracture results from a direct blow against the hamate produced by the handle of the tennis racket, golf club, or bat during an unbalanced swing. Hamate fractures can produce persistent pain symptoms, particularly in athletes or other individuals requiring strong grip.

Typically, the patient suffers from pain localized to the dorsal ulnar aspect of the wrist rather than the palmar area. This is due to the fracture's occurring at the base of the hamate rather than at its tip.

The diagnosis depends on the physician's suspi-

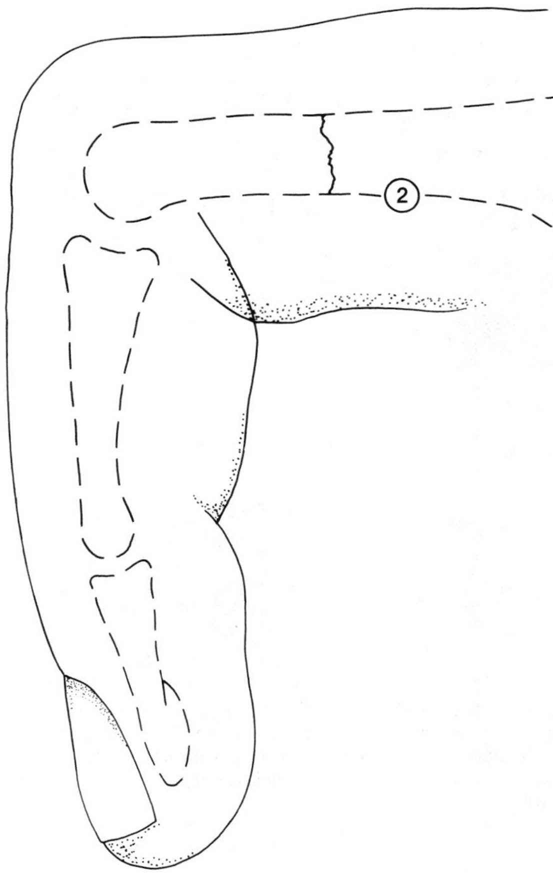

Figure 49–30. A true lateral x-ray film shows the volar angulation has been completely corrected.

cion from the history and physical examination and particularly on adequate carpal tunnel x-rays. The standard x-rays of the wrist do not demonstrate this lesion, whereas a carpal tunnel and oblique view will show a fracture of the base of the hamate (Fig. 49–35).

Management by the Family Physician. Although this fracture may unite if the hand and wrist are immobilized in plaster after an acute injury, in most cases the patient should be referred for excision of the fracture fragment. This is particularly true when the diagnosis has been delayed.

de Quervain's Stenosing Tenosynovitis

Tenosynovitis at the base of the thumb (de Quervain's syndrome) may be misdiagnosed as an acute wrist sprain. This characteristic tendinitis of the abductor longus and extensor pollicis brevis tendons around the distal end of the radius above the wrist can be readily diagnosed by history and physical examination. The pain of de Quervain's tenosynovitis is usually felt radiating down the thumb and up into the forearm.

Tenderness may be evident at the level of the carpal bones or at the insertion of the abductor longus into the base of the first metacarpal. Occasionally, the condition produces pain at the styloid process that has been called radial styloiditis. This is a misnomer since the pain results from the tendon and not from any bony involvement. Crepitus may also be evident. Wrist swelling or thickening may be palpable on the radial side of the wrist.

The diagnosis of tenosynovitis of the thumb extensor and abductor tendon is made by testing for pain on resisted extension and abduction of the thumb. This necessitates gliding of the inflamed tendons and, therefore, constantly reproduces the pain.

Management by the Family Physician. Treat the tenosynovitis by injecting 1 to 2 cc. of Depo-Medrol or similar cortisone solution and bupivacaine hydrochloride (Marcaine) or similar long-acting anesthetic. This can be done using a very fine 25-gauge needle. Take care that the medication is injected between the tendon and the sheath and not directly into the tendon itself. Begin the injection at the base of the first metacarpal and continue upward toward the radial styloid.

The patient should be relieved of symptoms within 7 to 10 days after injection. If there is still some persistence of pain, reinject the tendon sheath. Operative release of the tendon is rarely necessary since response to appropriate injection is quite prompt and predictable.

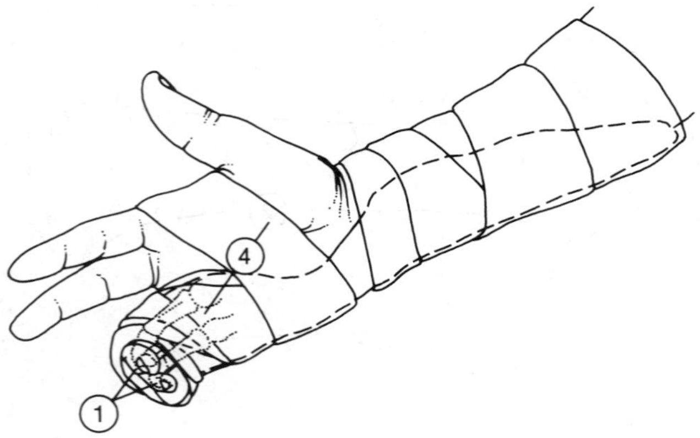

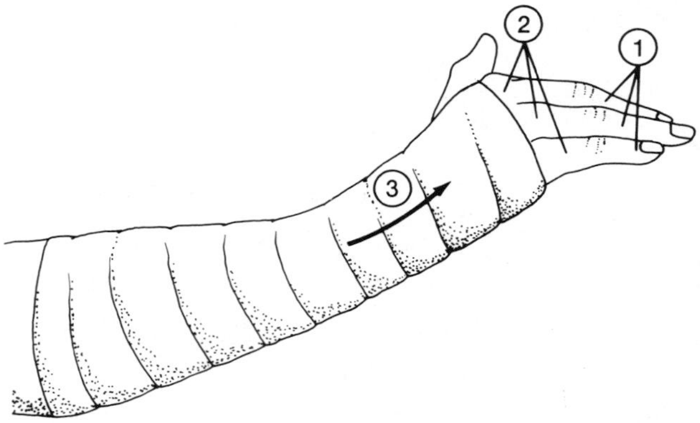

Figure 49–33. Method of immobilization of an undisplaced fracture. Most of these displaced fractures can be treated by immobilization in a short arm cast for 2 or 3 weeks. The fingers are free. The patient is able to actively exercise the MP joints. The wrist is slightly dorsiflexed.

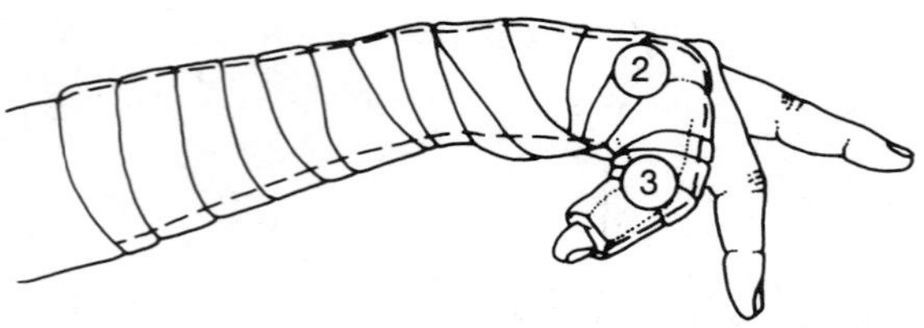

Figure 49–31. Immobilization of fractures of proximal phalanx. Apply a plaster cast splint as shown. The MP joint is placed in 70 degrees of flexion. The rotational realignment is controlled by the fingertips pointing toward the tuberosity of the scaphoid.

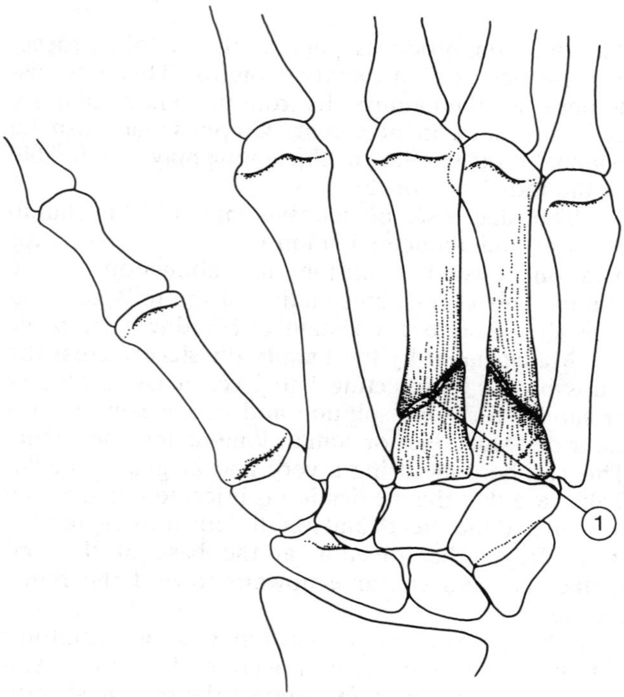

Figure 49–32. Undisplaced fractures of the third and fourth metacarpals. Evaluate these fractures carefully on the x-ray film for any dissociation of the carpometacarpal joint. Volar displacement of the fracture may involve the motor branch of the ulnar nerve and may require open reduction with internal fixation.

Osteoarthritis of the First Carpometacarpal Joint

This is a common source of wrist pain that tends to be misdiagnosed as a sprain or tendinitis. In contrast to de Quervain's stenosing tenosynovitis, arthritis of the first carpometacarpal joint is characterized by pain on passive as well as active extension of the joint. The anterior capsule of the joint is most affected by the arthritic process and is the source of the pain. Abduction of the thumb may be limited.

X-rays show characteristic changes in the joint that are most often seen in middle-aged women. Traumatic arthritis of this joint may occur with relatively minor injury and may pass unrecognized by superficial examination.

Management by the Family Physician. Treatment for symptomatic osteoarthritis of the carpometacarpal joint begins with local cortisone injection. For persistent problems with this joint, operative arthroplasty should be recommended.

Carpal Tunnel Syndrome

The causes of this compression syndrome may vary from overuse of the wrist by a heavy laborer to rheumatoid synovitis or a Colles' fracture deformity in the less active patient. Compression of the median nerve in its narrow passageway through the wrist produces common and remarkably consistent symptoms.

The initial symptoms include numbness, with characteristic paresthesias or pins and needles in the radial three and one-half digits of the hand. Using the hand, particularly in the dependent position, increases the pins and needles symptom. Frequently these paresthesias awaken the patient at night. Rest and elevation or shaking the wrist gives some relief.

Paresthesias such as these represent the peripheral nerve's signals that partial, but significant compression is being applied to the axons. The pins and needles symptom of carpal tunnel syndrome has been related by Flatt (1974) and others to anoxia of the

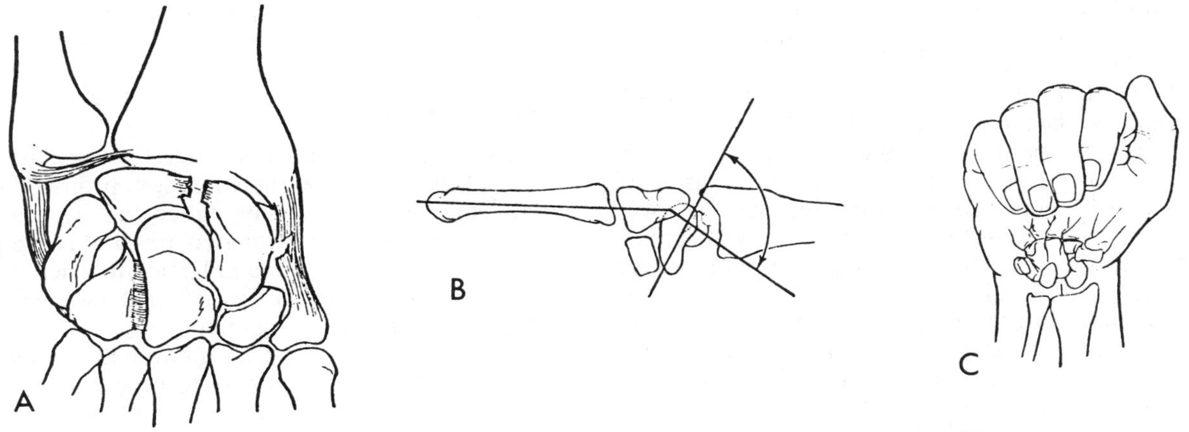

Figure 49–34. *A,* Disruption of the scapholunate and radiocarpal ligament leads to progressive dissociation between the scaphoid and the rest of the carpal bones. This injury is frequently mistaken for a persistent wrist sprain. *B,* Chronic dissociation of the scapholunate joint allows the scaphoid to rotate downward toward the palm. This increases the angle between the scaphoid axis and the radio-lunate-capitate axis. The capitate then slowly migrates toward the radius, and osteoarthritis rapidly develops. *C,* A space greater than 2 mm. between the scaphoid and the lunate indicates scapholunate subluxation. This view is best obtained with the wrist in a supinated position and the fist clenched. (Connolly, J. F.: DePalma's The Management of Fractures and Dislocations. An Atlas. 3rd ed. Philadelphia, W. B. Saunders Co., 1981.)

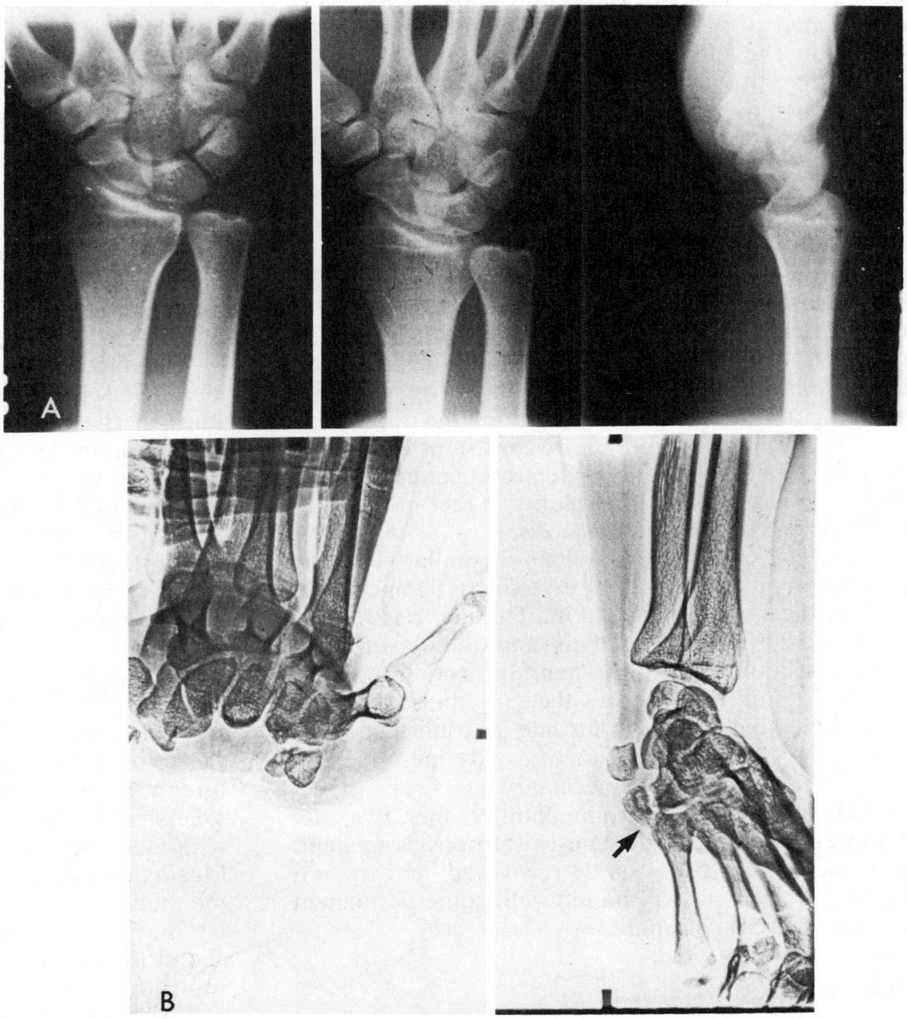

Figure 49–35. *A,* This patient had persistent wrist pain after a blow to the palm from the handle of a baseball bat. Standard x-ray films of the wrist showed no fractures. *B,* His physician wisely suspected that the hamate was fractured. This could be demonstrated only on special carpal tunnel and oblique views of the hamate. He was treated by excision of the fractured process.

nerve produced by venous stasis. Nighttime inactivity eliminates the muscle pumping that prevents venous stasis. When the patient awakens with paresthesias, moving or shaking the hand eliminates the venous stasis and the paresthesias are relieved.

Cyriax has pointed out the clinical significance of pins and needles, which are sensed only distal to the site of the nerve compression and may be used to localize the site. Aching symptoms may be noted proximal to the site of compression, but paresthesias always proceed distally.

The major differentials of carpal tunnel syndrome include cervical lesions and thoracic outlet compression. Cervical disc lesions produce paresthesias in one or two digits and not just the radial three and one-half. Also, cervical disc paresthesias are not necessarily related to wrist function, in contrast to the carpal tunnel syndrome, in which flexion of the wrist for a minute followed by sudden extension will produce the symptoms. Periscapular pain is often associated with a cervical disc.

The thoracic outlet syndrome may also awaken the patient at night. Here again, the paresthesias are not related to wrist activity and are also commonly noted on the ulnar side of the forearm and hand rather than the radial side.

Electromyographic study of nerve conduction is important for differentiating these three conditions and should be obtained prior to compression of the carpal tunnel.

Management by the Family Physician. When electromyographic testing shows impaired conduction of the median nerve at the wrist, operative decompression is advisable. The only exception is the carpal tunnel syndrome that develops in the last trimester of pregnancy. This usually subsides after delivery and can be managed adequately by protective splinting of the wrist and nerve during the pregnancy.

If the clinical symptoms are consistent with carpal tunnel syndrome, but the electromyogram demonstrates no conduction abnormality, a therapeutic trial will help to confirm the diagnosis.

Inject 2 cc. of triamcinolone or similar cortisone preparation under the transverse carpal ligament parallel to the nerves and tendon. The nerve is located between the palmaris longus and the flexor carpi radialis tendon. Avoid intraneural injection.

If the injection relieves the symptoms, the diagnosis of carpal tunnel syndrome is confirmed. The relief may not be permanent, and operative decompression may still be necessary.

Do not delay recommending operative decompression until thenar muscle atrophy is evident. Intrinsic muscle loss is rarely recovered, and when it occurs, the patient will be left with some permanent weakness of grip strength.

ELBOW SPRAINS

As with other joint problems, the pain from the elbow can arise either from intra-articular structures or from adjacent musculotendinous and nerve structures.

Nursemaid's Elbow

Nursemaid's elbow is so called because it results from a forceful pull on the extended, pronated elbow of a child who is usually under the age of four. Traction on the child's pronated arm in this age group produces a tear in the annular ligament. The pronated position then allows the overshaped radial head to slip partially under the ligament.

The characteristic presentation is a child who refuses to move the elbow from the flexed, pronated position.

X-rays of the nursemaid's elbow or subluxed radial head show no abnormality at the elbow. The diagnosis is purely clinical.

Take care, however, to rule out undisplaced supracondylar fracture of the humerus prior to diagnosing a nursemaid's elbow. Sometimes supracondylar fracture lines may not be initially evident and can only be detected by an elevated fat pad sign. This is seen best on a lateral roentgenogram as a radiolucent line posterior to the distal humerus and indicates hematoma from the fracture elevating the fat behind the elbow.

Management by the Family Physician. Treatment of the nursemaid's elbow consists of gentle but firm supination of the child's forearm. Flex the child's elbow gently to 90 degrees with one hand on the forearm. With the other hand, hold the humerus and place your thumb over the radial head, then rapidly and firmly rotate the child's forearm into full supination.

Reduction is achieved usually with a palpable click. This promptly relieves the child's pain symptoms in the acute injury. For the injury of longer than 12 hours in duration the relief of pain may not be as prompt.

Immobilize the elbow with a sling for 5 to 7 days and caution the parents about pulling on the child's forearm. If report of the symptoms has been delayed for more than 12 hours or the problem is a recurrent one, immobilize the elbow in a splint for 2 weeks.

Little Leaguer's Elbow

Little Leaguer's elbow results from fatigue injuries to the adolescent athlete's throwing elbow. Most often it is seen in boys who practice baseball pitching excessively. The adolescent's bone structure cannot withstand the loading from repetitive hard throwing. Most commonly, the injury is an avulsion fracture of the medial humeral epicondyle (Fig. 49–36).

Fatigue fractures of the radial head or osteochondritis of the lateral humeral condyle may also result from radiohumeral compression.

Management by the Family Physician. The most effective treatment is preventive. The adolescent athlete should be warned to avoid overusing his throwing

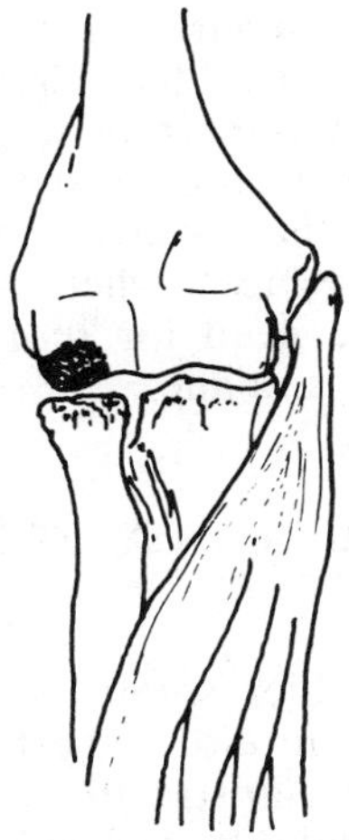

Figure 49–36. Little Leaguer's elbow results from overuse of an adolescent's pitching elbow. Lesions may include fatigue fractures of the medial epicondyle, radial head, or capitate. (From Connolly, J. F.: DePalma's The Management of Fractures and Dislocations: An Atlas. 3rd ed. Philadelphia, W. B. Saunders Co., 1981.)

elbow, particularly by excessive practice pitching. If necessary, a cast can ensure that this warning is heeded. Skeletal fatigue injuries may also occur in the adolescent's shoulder. Most, however, develop in the elbow.

Tennis Elbow

This very common entity results most often from small tears in the origin of the wrist extensor muscles from the lateral humeral condyle. The injury occurs most often in the part-time or nonathlete in the fourth decade. Only 5 per cent of Coonrad and Hooper's (1973) 1000 patients actually played tennis or golf. Many other individuals with tennis elbow are never seen by a physician and recover without treatment.

When the patient does come to the physician, the usual complaint is pain down the back of the forearm and into the wrist and dorsum of the hand. Pain also will move upward from the elbow toward the shoulder. This pain is worsened by any attempt to lift objects of any weight. Twinges of pain may become so severe that the patient has to drop even relatively lightweight objects such as a cup.

Consistently, the patient will recall no injury to the arm, only progressively increasing pain on exertion. The history and course support the conclusions of Cyriax, as well as those of Coonrad and Hooper, that the condition results from a scar's forming in a partial tendon tear. Repeated irritation of this scar from muscle pull prevents adequate healing. The scar itself then becomes the source of pain.

Physical examination of the passive and active range of motion in the elbow is usually painless. As with any tendinitis, the physical finding essential for the diagnosis is to reproduce the pain by stressing the involved tendon. For tennis elbow, this is accomplished by having the patient extend the wrist against resistance. The elbow simultaneously must be kept in extension so that the resultant stress is applied directly to the wrist extensor origin. Wrist extension against resistance reproduces the patient's pain symptoms in the lateral condyle and forearm. The specific muscle most often at fault is the extensor carpi radialis brevis arising off the epicondyle.

Management by the Family Physician. The primary treatment for tennis elbow is rest. If the symptoms have been present for less than 6 weeks, this may suffice for treatment. This is best accomplished with a dorsal plaster splint, maintaining the wrist in extension for 2 to 3 weeks while the tendon heals.

If this period of rest is not sufficient, inject the point of maximum tenderness over the extensor origin with 1 ml. of triamcinolone mixed with 5 cc. of bupivacaine. First spray the region with ethylchloride and then use a 25-gauge needle to minimize discomfort during the injection. The medication is then massaged directly into the tendon.

Following the injection, the wrist is kept at rest with a dorsal splint (see Fig. 49–33) for approximately 7 days to allow the anti-inflammatory action of the medication to take effect. Permanent cure after one or two injections is the rule.

Occasionally, painful symptoms persist despite repeated injections. For patients with symptoms of more than a year's duration, surgical treatment is advised. The approach is to release the extensor origin and remove any bursa or synovitis that might be the source of the symptomatology.

Our experience has been that this is one of the more predictable and successful orthopedic procedures and well worth recommending for the patient with a persistent and frustrating pain problem.

Golfer's Elbow

Tendinitis in the medial aspect of the elbow from tear in the common origin of the wrist flexors occurs far less frequently than tendinitis on the lateral side of the elbow. It is also usually less disabling and less persistent than tennis elbow.

Characteristically, having the patient flex the wrist against resistance produces the pain. The maneuver rarely, however, produces the sharp incapacitating twinges associated with lateral tendinitis, or tennis elbow.

Management by the Family Physician. Treatment of this condition, once again, is with local infiltration of the tendon using triamcinolone in conjunction with resting the wrist flexors. Persistence of symptoms for more than 2 weeks warrants a second injection.

An important consideration is to differentiate the relatively mild tendinitis at the flexor origin from the more serious problems with which it might be confused. Particularly, take care to rule out angina, Pancoast's tumor in the pulmonary apex, and ulnar nerve entrapment at the elbow. All of these conditions can produce pain along the medial aspect of the elbow and forearm.

Ulnar Nerve Entrapment at the Elbow—Cubital Tunnel Syndrome

As the ulnar nerve runs behind the medial humeral condyle, it passes from a fixed position at the medial epicondyle to a movable one adjacent to the olecranon. The arcuate ligament holds the nerve in its groove and also subjects it to compression with prolonged flexion. This results in the common complaint of pins and needles in the fourth and fifth fingers after minor but prolonged activities requiring elbow flexion. Such actions as holding a telephone receiver or sleeping with the elbow flexed and the hand behind the head may readily bring on these usually temporary symptoms of ulnar entrapment.

Permanent neuropathy can result from cast application holding the elbow in an excessively flexed position. The ulnar nerve is extremely sensitive to pressure and ischemic injury. These seemingly minor accidents may produce permanent functional loss of the intrinsic muscles of the hand. One should avoid immobilizing the elbow in 90 degrees or more of flexion for even brief periods of time during surgical procedures or in casts. Iatrogenic nerve injury is a serious and preventable cause of cubital tunnel syndrome.

A second common cause of ulnar nerve entrapment at the elbow is a cubitus valgus deformity following childhood fracture. Most often, the cause of ulnar nerve symptoms is unknown.

Before diagnosing a cubital tunnel syndrome, take care to rule out causes of ulnar compression proximal or distal to the elbow. This would include conditions such as the thoracic outlet syndrome proximally or ganglia or other impingement on the nerve distally at the wrist joint.

Cyriax's rule that the pins and needles always begin at the site of nerve entrapment and move distal to it is helpful in differentiating the locus. Nerve conduction studies by a competent electromyographer are the most specific help in pinpointing the source of the symptomatology.

Management by the Family Physician. If electromyograms show persistent impaired conduction at the elbow, anterior transposition of the nerve should be recommended promptly.

If signs of impaired nerve conduction are not demonstrable by EMG, a therapeutic injection of triamcinolone may be diagnostic. The nerve sheath, not the nerve, should be injected with 1 to 2 cc. of triamcinolone. Take care to pass the small 25-gauge needle deep into the condylar groove between the nerve and bone. Avoid repeated injections.

Pancoast's Tumor

Consider Pancoast's tumor in the pulmonary apex of any patient suffering from shoulder, arm, or forearm pain. Severe weakness of the intrinsic muscles of the hand may develop quite rapidly.

This rapidly progressive lesion has frequently been mistaken for ulnar neuropathy, cervical disc lesions, or a frozen shoulder (Fig. 49–37).

Horner's syndrome (ptosis, miosis, anhidrosis, enophthalmos, narrowing of the palpebral fissure, slight elevation of the lower lid, and flushing of the affected side of the face), when associated with arm pain, indicates the need for thorough radiographic studies of the lung and apex.

SHOULDER SPRAINS, PAIN, STIFFNESS, AND INSTABILITY

Symptoms of shoulder sprain and pain most commonly originate from either the tendons enveloping the joint or the articular structures. Since the shoulder is designed for mobility rather than stability, any stiffness of this joint can cause considerable functional impairment. The mobility of the glenohumeral joint can be excessive; consequently this joint is most susceptible to dislocation and subluxation.

Chronic and Acute Tendinitis and Bursitis

Almost any tendon about the shoulder is subject to tearing and painful scarring, depending on the activities of the patient. Young athletic individuals suffer commonly from acute and chronic wear injuries. The baseball pitcher may experience tendinitis at the origin of the triceps off the inferior glenoid. The swimmer is subject to small avulsions of the teres major and other internal rotators of the shoulder.

Tendon degeneration in most individuals occurs from a gradual wear process that involves the rotator cuff structures. The supraspinatus and the long head of the biceps are especially susceptible. This is due to the fact that the mechanism of shoulder abduction requires that the humeral head externally rotate at 70 to 80 degrees of elevation to clear underneath the anterior acromion and particularly under the coracoacromial ligament (Fig. 49–38). When these structures impinge on the supraspinatus tendon and biceps, they produce irritation, attrition, and eventual rupture of these tendons.

The symptom of tendon attrition is generally a nondescript, painful, aching shoulder. The pain from a supraspinatus tendinitis is not necessarily localized to the tendon but is generalized throughout the whole deltoid region. The aching from tendinitis frequently extends down the forearm to the wrist and consequently is quite nonspecific.

This lack of specificity in shoulder pain is due to our primitive interpretation of the source of pain as coming from the C-5 dermatome rather than from any structure of the shoulder itself. The same type of generalized aching can be associated with glenohumeral arthritis, bursitis, adhesive capsulitis, or lesions in the apex of the lung.

Physical examination alone can differentiate these lesions by demonstrating whether or not the pain is aggravated when the tendon is stressed. Shoul-

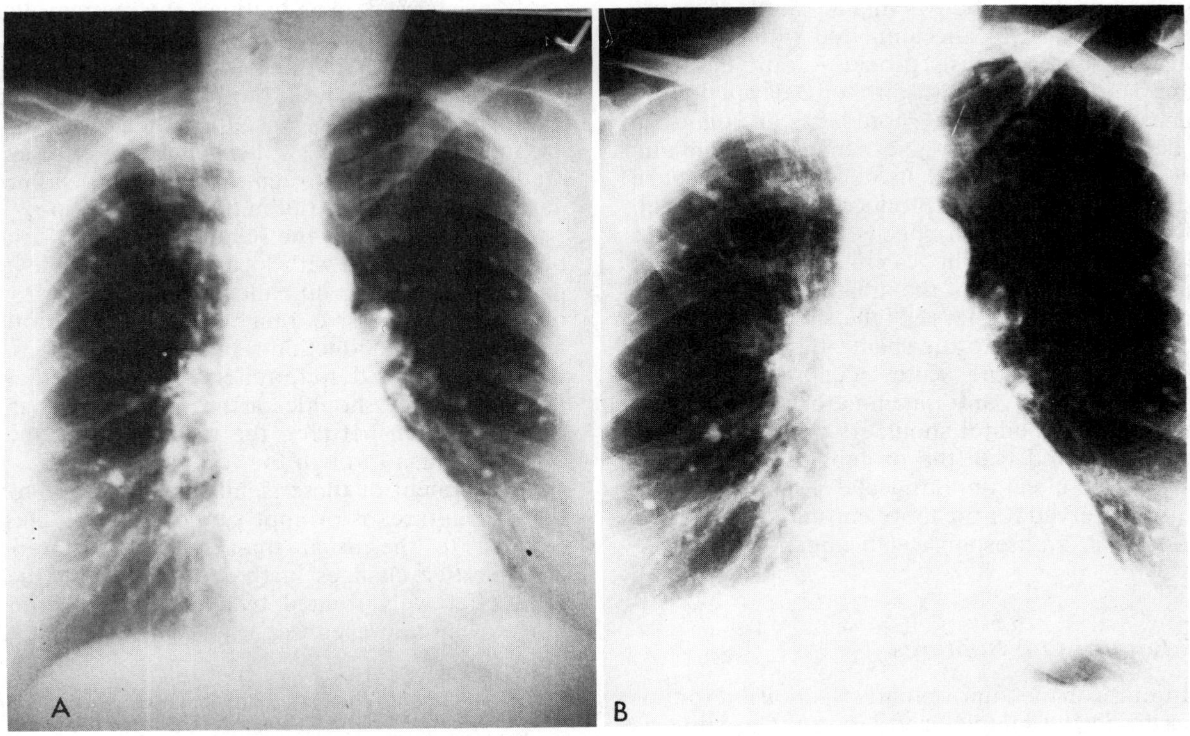

Figure 49–37. *A*, This patient was hospitalized with a diagnosis of cubital tunnel syndrome because of pain radiating down the medial aspect of her right arm. The chest x-ray film at the time of admission for ulnar nerve transfer is shown here and was interpreted as normal. *B*, The patient's pain in the elbow and forearm persisted after nerve transfer. She also noted shoulder pain on the same side. Chest x-ray films 4 months after initial evaluation showed a massive apial lung tumor (Pancoast's tumor), which was evident on retrospective review of the initial x-ray films.

der examination should not consist of merely poking the patient to find the site or "trigger point." To diagnose supraspinatus tendinitis, the patient's pain should be aggravated when he abducts the shoulder and externally rotates it against resistance.

With bicipital tendinitis the pain is aggravated when the patient flexes his shoulder forward and adducts it against resistance. Ask the patient to work the shoulder as if he were shooting a bow and arrow.

Tendon lesions will demonstrate a full range of passive motion and only active resisted motion is impaired. The other differential conditions of shoulder pain such as arthritis or adhesive capsulitis usually impair passive as well as active resisted motion.

X-ray of the shoulder with painful tendinitis is usually unrevealing but must be obtained to rule out other conditions, including chronic posterior shoulder dislocation, infections, and tumor. In 10 to 15 per cent of these painful shoulders, the x-ray may demonstrate some calcification in the supraspinatus tendon insertion into the greater tuberosity of the humerus. These calcifications are usually inert but become sufficiently large to require surgical removal (Fig. 49–38).

Management by the Family Physician. The majority of these conditions can be effectively relieved by injecting one per cent bupivacaine into the subacromial bursa or tendon region and then applying ice. This therapy should also help to distinguish the differential conditions such as subluxation and glenohumeral arthritis.

Avoid injecting directly into the tendon of the athlete, since this weakens the structure and can lead to rupture.

Treat the overuse syndrome in the athlete's shoulder by rest and anti-inflammatory medication for 5 to 7 days.

Advise the baseball pitcher to avoid throwing overhead, the swimmer to alter his breathing style and avoid breathing from one side, the tennis player to rotate the side of his body toward the net as he raises his arm above the horizontal. All of these simple steps are designed to avoid pinching the supraspinatus and biceps between the coracoacromial ligament and humeral head during arm elevation.

For the acute calcific bursitis in the more usual patient, i.e., the middle-aged individual, more intense therapy may be necessary. Frequently these patients are in a good deal of pain and are unable to sleep comfortably. X-rays may show calcific deposits in the bursa or inflamed tendon.

Acute symptoms of tendinitis with or without calcification usually diminish by 3 weeks, but the pain can be considerably mitigated by local injection of triamcinolone or similar cortisone preparation. Mechanically needling the tendon and subacromial bursa gives the sensation of dispersing calcium or cartilaginous substances. This mechanical dispersal of the deposit speeds up the body's inflammatory response to the material that has accumulated within the tendon. It also simultaneously provides gratifying relief to these patients, usually within 1 or 2 days.

Calcification about the shoulder is analogous to urate deposits in the gouty joint. Invasion by inflammatory cells and the resultant degenerative enzyme released from these cells produce the severe pain. Injection into the sheath speeds up this resorptive process and disperses the calcium. Cortisone also diminishes the intensity of the inflammatory response and, consequently, the level of the shoulder pain.

Local injection into the sheath then is the treatment of choice for the acute calcific inflammatory condition. Systemic anti-inflammatory medications for these acutely painful shoulders are relatively ineffective compared with the prompt response to accurately placed injection. Surgical excision of calcium deposits is reserved for the more chronic symptomatic condition that is unresponsive to injection (Fig. 49–38).

Acute Rotator Cuff Ruptures

Rupture of the supraspinatus tendon or rotator cuff occurs in the middle-aged laborer who subjects the shoulder to a sudden load. The typical example is the individual who catches his body weight with one arm when falling from a height (Fig. 49–39). A sudden pull on the support muscles of the shoulder causes massive rupture of their tendinous attachment to the tuberosity of the humerus. The patient feels or hears a sudden pop in the shoulder and then suffers severe pain. Subsequently, he is unable to elevate his arm.

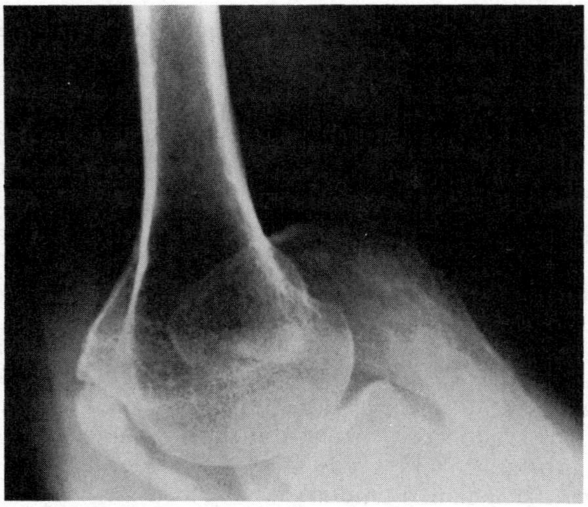

Figure 49–38. This chronic calcium deposit seen on axillary view of the shoulder caused the supraspinatus tendon to be pinched between the coracoacromial ligament and the humerus during elevation of the arm. We removed the calcium and released the coracoacromial ligament to restore shoulder elevation and relieve the patient's painful impingement. Ordinarily, calcium deposits need not be removed unless they are causing mechanical impingement syndromes.

On physical examination, the patient demonstrates a painful arc in that he can passively abduct the shoulder to 40 degrees without pain but has pain from a range of about 40 to 100 degrees and has no pain when the arm is raised overhead. This painful arc indicates that the swollen, avulsed, and sensitive tendon is pinched between the humeral head and the anterior acromion in the midrange of motion.

Management by the Family Physician. Injection of the painful area with local anesthetic relieves the patient's discomfort and allows the examiner to demonstrate that passive range of shoulder motion is normal. Active abduction remains limited to less than 60 to 90 degrees despite relief of pain. The diagnosis is confirmed by shoulder arthrogram, demonstrating communication between the glenohumeral and subacromial bursa through the torn rotator cuff.

Treatment of these significant acute rotator cuff tendon ruptures is prompt surgical repair. This is in contrast to the usual small tears associated with degenerative changes in the rotator cuff, which are most effectively treated by cortisone injection and range of motion exercises.

Rupture of the Biceps Tendon

Rupture of the long head of the biceps occurs also as the result of chronic degenerative changes or sometimes from repeated cortisone injections into the tendon. The patient notices a mass developing when he flexes the elbow. This may or may not cause pain. The stress test of biceps function with the "bow and arrow" maneuver as previously described confirms the diagnosis.

Management by the Family Physician. Biceps ruptures are frequently asymptomatic in the older patient and may not require operative repair. Refer younger, more active individuals or heavy laborers who rupture the tendon for prompt surgical repair. Repair may be impossible if not done within a week or two. Chronic rupture of the long head of the biceps proximally decreases shoulder strength and increases symptoms in the patient who must use the shoulder actively.

Operative repair of the acute bicipital tendon rupture is even more imperative if the tear occurs at the distal insertion into the radius.

Frozen Shoulder (Adhesive Capsulitis)

Adhesive capsulitis restricts shoulder motion in all directions. The chronically painful, stiff or "frozen shoulder" generally begins without any trauma in middle age. The duration of symptoms may range from 6 months to several years. In a study of 154 patients with frozen shoulders, we found that the average duration of symptoms prior to our treatment was 8 months (Connolly et al., 1972). Only 7 per cent of patients demonstrated any calcification on shoulder x-ray. Eight per cent of patients developed symptoms bilaterally.

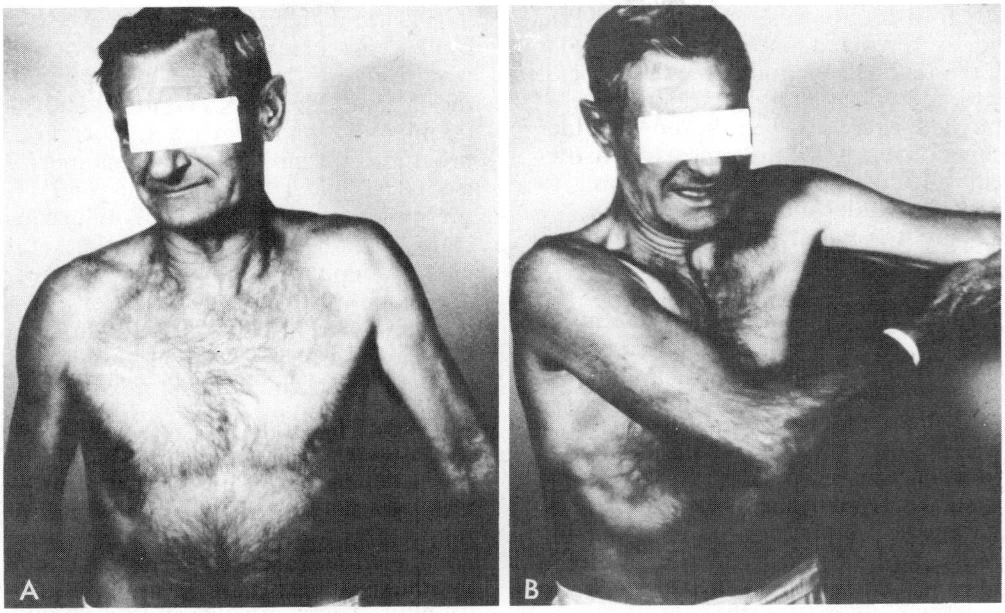

Figure 49–39. *A,* This 45-year-old house painter in falling from a scaffolding hung the weight of his entire body on his left shoulder. He felt a sudden "pop" and giving way of the shoulder. On examination 1 month later, as shown here, he had considerable deltoid atrophy and could only abduct to approximately 30 degrees without pain. *B,* Passive elevation of the shoulder between 30 and 90 degrees produces a painful arc. The pain comes from the torn rotator cuff being pinched between the anterior coracoacromial ligament and the head of the humerus. Prompt repair of this acute tendon injury is essential in the working man before permanent muscle atrophy complicates restoration of shoulder function. Chronic tendon degeneration, however, in the elderly patient does not usually require operative repair.

Major differentials to consider in evaluating patients with frozen shoulders include low-grade infections, chronic posterior dislocations, severe degenerative arthritis, and Pancoast's tumor (see Fig. 49–37). Infection can be particularly deceptive in diabetics who have received cortisone injections and should always be kept in mind in these patients. A chronically locked posterior shoulder dislocation must be ruled out by axillary roentgenograms. Finally, two patients in our observation were found to have a tumor of the scapula and the lung as the source of what was considered initially to be a nondescript frozen shoulder. The diagnosis of a frozen shoulder is common but should be considered only after these other serious problems have been excluded.

The etiology of the frozen shoulder appears to be an alteration in the normally mobile axillary fold of the shoulder capsule. The shoulder capsule, which ordinarily permits considerable mobility, shrinks in these middle-aged patients and becomes a "checkrein" restricting shoulder motion. Motion is limited, not only in abduction and external rotation but in flexion, extension, and internal rotation as well. Arthrogram of a frozen shoulder demonstrates loss of redundant folds in the axilla causing a "checkrein" (Fig. 49–40).

Biopsy of the capsule from frozen shoulders shows morphologic changes of fibrosis and fibroplasia without evidence of inflammation (Lundberg, 1969); consequently, the term "capsulitis" should be abandoned. These microscopic as well as biochemical changes are similar to those found in the fibroplasia of Dupuytren's contracture. The chronic frozen shoulder, therefore, results from fibroplasia or alteration in middle age associated with changes in the characteristics of the collagen content of the joint capsule.

The frozen shoulder condition is entirely unrelated to any inflammatory or traumatic process. It is particularly not related to tendinitis or injury to the rotator cuff. The frozen shoulder presents with passive as well as active limitation of range of motion in

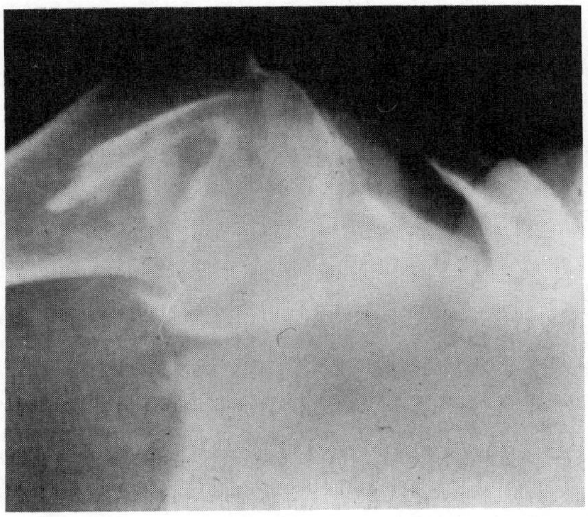

Figure 49–40. An arthrogram of a frozen shoulder demonstrates loss of normal redundancy in the axillary folds and complete obliteration of the space in the axillary region. This restricts the shoulder motion and acts as a checkrein on movement in all directions.

all directions. A torn rotator cuff or a tendinitis, on the other hand, is restricted only in the particular range in which the tendon functions. The rotator cuff symptoms described above generally respond to cortisone injection and exercise. The frozen shoulder requires stretching or release of the capsular constriction in the axillary fold, using passive stretching to regain full range of shoulder motion.

Management by the Family Physician. Management of the frozen shoulder has varied from nugatory neglect to intrepid intervention. Symptoms from the frozen shoulder seem sometimes to last forever and respond minimally to standard physical therapy modalities. This is because the capsular checkrein must be passively stretched out to regain the necessary external rotation and abduction. With proper recognition the pathophysiology of this condition should not be so frustrating for either the patient or the physician.

Overcoming the capsular restraint to motion is best achieved by an exercise program in which the patient brings clasped hands behind the head (Fig. 49–41). While standing with the back against a wall to immobilize the scapula, the patient forces the elbows back toward the wall. This may require a good deal of push and frequent encouragement from another determined individual, such as the patient's husband. Persistence in this exercise program on an hourly basis is usually rewarded by improvement in motion and diminution of pain over a 3- to 4-week period.

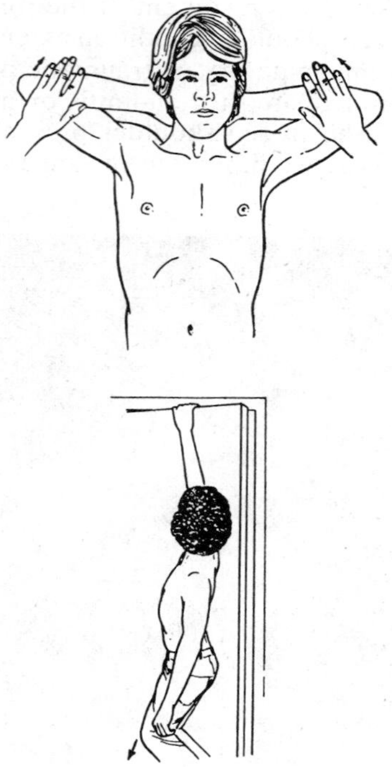

Figure 49–41. Abduction-external rotation exercises for the frozen shoulder will overcome the restriction by the axillary fold to shoulder motion. (From Connolly, J. F.: DePalma's The Management of Fractures and Dislocations: An Atlas. 3rd ed. Philadelphia, W. B. Saunders Co., 1981.)

If the patient has not improved symptomatically by 6 weeks of exercise, refer her to an orthopedist who can perform shoulder manipulation under anesthesia. This allows abduction beyond 100 degrees and permits the patient to continue with the exercise program in a more effective manner. Carefully controlled shoulder manipulation under general anesthesia is a useful adjunct to relieve patients of this common and commonly frustrating source of shoulder pain. Manipulation, however, must be done carefully with good control of the shoulder and without excessive torsion or force so as not to inflict further damage (Connolly et al., 1972). The shoulder, the knee, and the spine are the joints for which we have found careful manipulation to be of considerable value.

Anterior Glenohumeral Dislocation

The glenohumeral joint, because of its great mobility, is the joint most subject to dislocation. The usual mechanism is forceful abduction and external rotation. The complete anterior shoulder dislocation is usually obvious to all observers and demands prompt reduction.

Management by the Family Physician. The standard methods of reduction, such as the Stimson maneuver or Hippocratic technique, have been described by Connolly (1981). However, avoid overvigorous attempts at manipulative reduction without adequate anesthetic, since fractures of the humeral head or avulsion of the axillary artery may occur, particularly in the older patient (Jardon, 1973). Use adequate anesthetic and muscle relaxants to avoid these serious complications.

Recurrent Glenohumeral Subluxation

Occasionally, patients do not completely dislocate but rather subluxate the humeral head in and out of the glenoid. This results in repeated episodes of sharp shoulder pain without grossly evident dislocation.

The mechanism of subluxation is a forceful external rotation and abduction which is sufficient to tear the capsule anteriorly. This allows the head to slide briefly over the rim of the glenoid without completely dislocating out of socket. The humeral head sliding in and out over the glenoid may cause pain without overt signs of instability.

The diagnosis of the subluxation is based on the mechanism of external rotation and abduction associated with this sudden sharp and brief symptomatology. X-ray may or may not show a small avulsion of the anterior rim of the glenoid.

Management by the Family Physician. These symptoms, which impair the patient's function considerably, can sometimes be relieved by circumduction shoulder exercises. If these exercises fail, refer the patient for operative repair of the shoulder capsule and anterior support structures. These are generally the same procedures that are performed for chronic recurrent shoulder dislocation. The patient's symptoms of shoulder instability should not be dismissed merely because of lack of immediate evidence of dislocation.

Posterior Glenohumeral Dislocation

Anterior dislocations and subluxations occur characteristically in the young athletic individual and represent the majority of shoulder luxations. Five to 10 per cent of shoulder dislocations are posterior. The victim most often is an older person who falls directly on the front of the shoulder or is an epileptic who dislocates the shoulder from violent internal rotation and adduction during a seizure.

The dislocation may pass unrecognized, or it may be treated as an unusually painful stiff shoulder.

The posterior displacement of the humeral head may not be evident clinically or by standard anteroposterior roentgenograms. An axillary view of the shoulder should and can always be obtained to rule out posterior dislocation after an injury causing shoulder stiffness.

Recurrent posterior dislocation is a rare cause of shoulder symptoms. These patients complain of shoulder instability with any loading on the shoulder in the internally rotated and adducted position (Fig. 49–42). Commonly, this instability comes on in the push-up position or when the patient is lifting up from a chair.

Management by the Family Physician. Patients with symptomatology of posterior shoulder dislocation or of a shoulder that is locked in internal rotation and adduction should not be subjected to delayed or missed diagnosis. Remain attuned to the wide variations on the theme of shoulder instability. Assess all shoulder injuries and stiff shoulders with axillary x-rays, especially when the shoulder is fixed in adduction and internal rotation.

Reduction of the acute posterior shoulder dislocation is carried out as described by Connolly (1981). For chronic or recurrent posterior shoulder dislocations refer the patient to a surgeon capable of performing the fairly unusual operative repair.

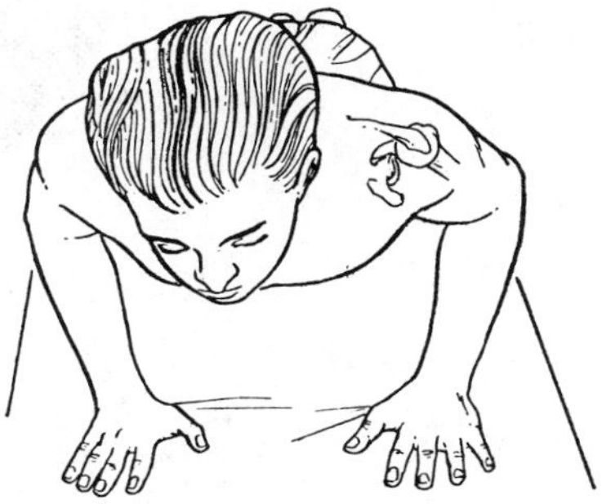

Figure 49–42. A posterior glenohumeral dislocation occurs usually with the shoulder adducted and internally rotated. The patient will frequently complain of shoulder instability in the push-up position or when arising from a chair. (From Connolly, J. F.: DePalma's The Management of Fractures and Dislocations: An Atlas. 3rd ed. Philadelphia, W. B. Saunders Co., 1981.)

Acromioclavicular Dislocations

Injury to the acromioclavicular (AC) joint causes shoulder disability of widely varying degrees. This injury occurs as a result of force directly on the tip of the shoulder or arm. The force tears the acromioclavicular and frequently the coracoacromial ligaments, allowing varying degrees of upward clavicular displacement.

The completely displaced clavicle in an individual with heavy shoulders frequently causes minimal acute symptoms and no long-term functional impairment (Fig. 49–43). A prominently displaced clavicle in a slender person with torn trapezius and deltoid muscle fibers usually has a good deal of symptomatology and operative repair (Fig. 49–44*A*, *B*).

Management by the Family Physician. Attempted treatment with harnesses or braces to hold the acromioclavicular separation has proven uncomfortable for the patient and ineffective in our experience. Except for the widely displaced separation, we prefer to treat the acute injury symptomatically. Apply ice to the shoulder and support the shoulder with an arm sling for 3 to 5 days. During this time the patient is actively contracting the deltoid and trapezius muscles around the shoulder. Subsequently, the patient begins circumduction and then active elevation of the shoulder. By the second week he should regain normal shoulder function and be able to return to work or athletic competition considerably earlier than with any other treatment.

The completely dislocated AC joint frequently produces fewer symptoms than does a partially subluxated one. Should the patient be bothered by the displacement, partial resection of the distal clavicle and repair of the coracoacromial ligament can be done electively. In slender patients with complete AC separations, the prominence of the clavicle may require that this procedure be done soon after the injury (Fig. 49–44).

This approach to acromioclavicular joint separation allows the patient to test the shoulder through a period of trial mobilization to determine whether symptoms warrant operative repair. We feel this is an excellent example of management tailored according to the symptoms and needs of the patient rather than the converse.

Tietze's Syndrome

In 1921 Tietze described recurrent painful attacks of pain at the costochondral junction. These recurrent attacks of pain can last for a minute or so. A painful swelling at the costochondral junction is often palpable or visible and coarse crepitation may be present with a scapulothoracic excursion.

Management by the Family Physician. This is a slowly self-limiting condition of vague etiology (likely

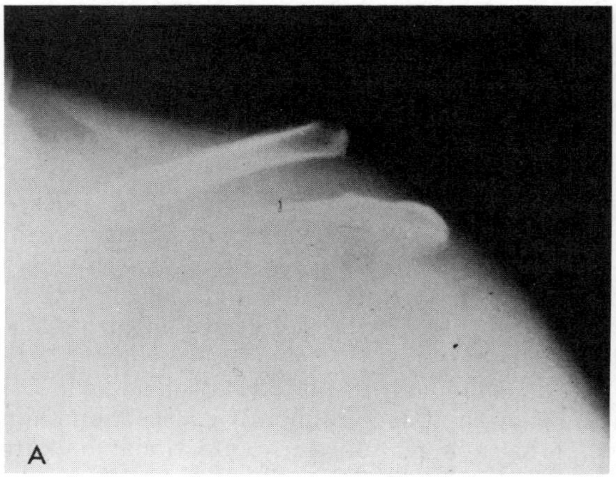

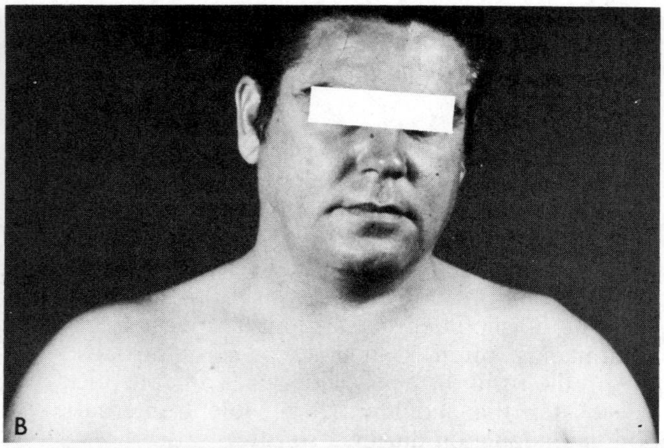

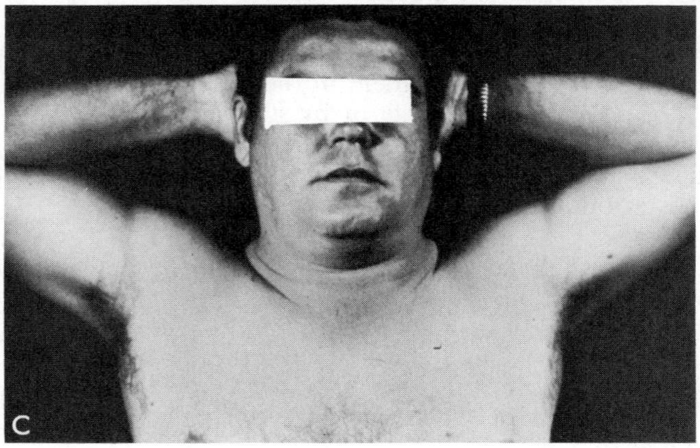

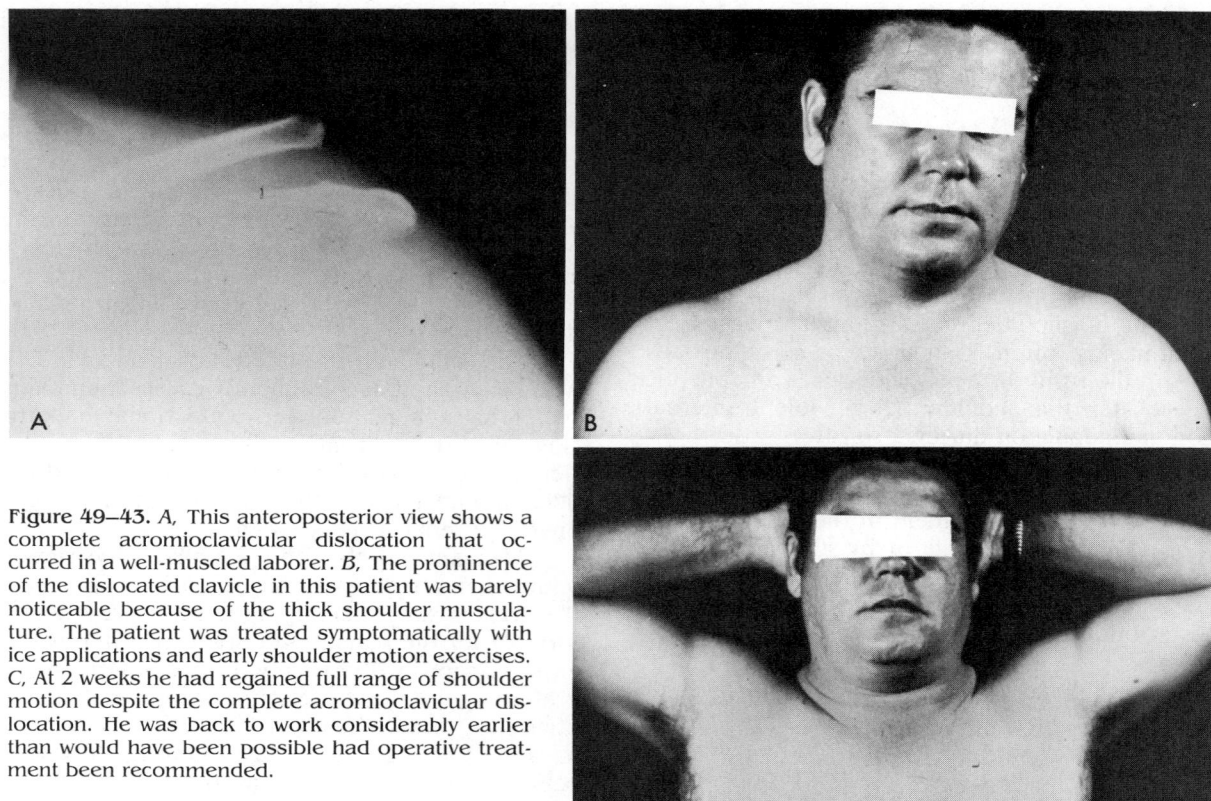

Figure 49–43. *A,* This anteroposterior view shows a complete acromioclavicular dislocation that occurred in a well-muscled laborer. *B,* The prominence of the dislocated clavicle in this patient was barely noticeable because of the thick shoulder musculature. The patient was treated symptomatically with ice applications and early shoulder motion exercises. *C,* At 2 weeks he had regained full range of shoulder motion despite the complete acromioclavicular dislocation. He was back to work considerably earlier than would have been possible had operative treatment been recommended.

trauma or stress upon the junction). Treatment is supportive. Injection of triamcinolone and local anesthetic mixed together in the area of maximal tenderness is often helpful. Heat and analgesics are useful (Connolly, 1981).

KNEE SPRAINS AND INJURIES

Only the ankle is more vulnerable than the knee to both ligamentous and bony injury. The unstable knee produces even more functional impairment than does

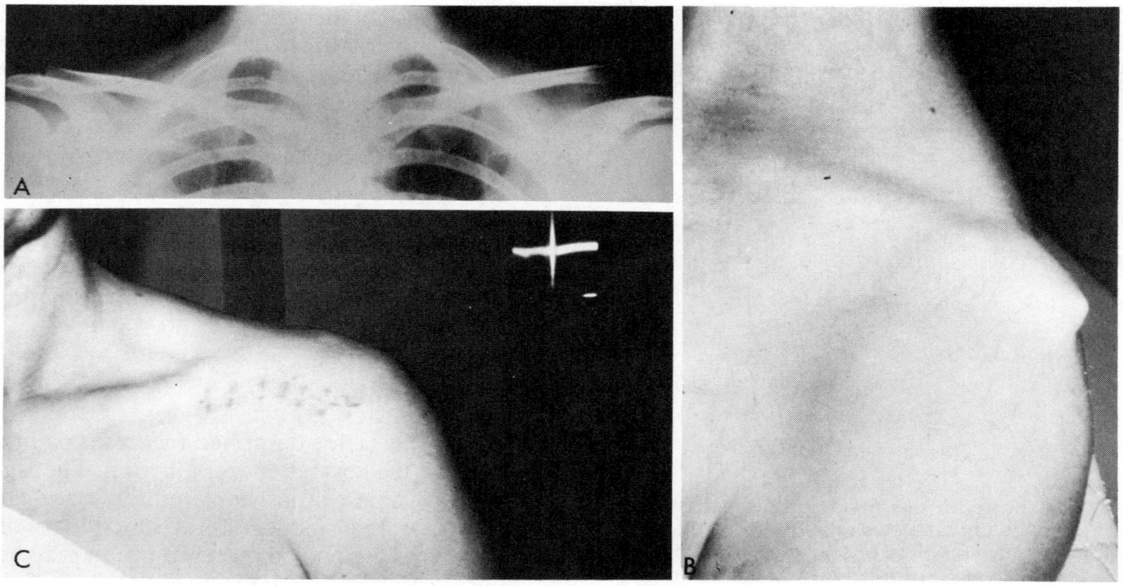

Figure 49–44. *A,* Anteroposterior x-ray film showing complete dislocation of an acromioclavicular joint in a relatively asthenic woman. *B,* In contrast to the patient shown in Figure 49–43, this woman had little shoulder musculature and the upward displaced clavicle produced pain. *C,* The deformity was corrected by an elective repair of the coracoclavicular ligaments with resection of the distal 1 cm. of the clavicle.

an unstable ankle. Effective reconstructive procedures are available for the unstable ankle. The chronically unstable knee is more difficult to correct. Early recognition and repair of the acute damage offers the best chance of retaining normal function.

Ligamentous Injuries

The family physician who first evaluates the patient with a knee injury has the best opportunity to determine the need for operative repair. Train yourself to separate the major, or Grade III, injury from the minor, or Grade I. There are also Grade II injuries, but these are in a gray zone which may or may not prove to be of major significance. These Grade II injuries require a judicious period of observation to determine the degree to which they will impair joint function. Understanding the mechanisms of injuries and the anatomic structures likely to be involved helps one to sort out those injuries.

Mechanisms of Injury. Most ligamentous injuries result characteristically from twisting the knee with the foot fixed to the ground. Either a valgus-external rotational injury or a varus-internal rotational twist may be applied to the joint. Depending on the mechanism, the support structures on either the medial or lateral side of the joint are then injured (Fig. 49–45).

Hyperextension or hyperflexion mechanisms can also disrupt knee ligaments. Most often the anterior cruciate ligament is torn with hyperextension over-

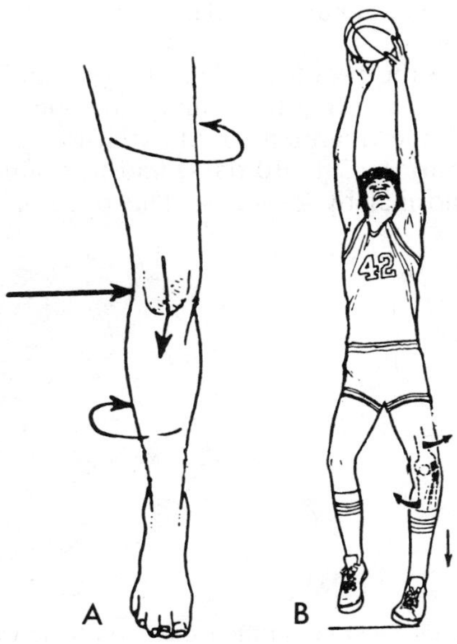

Figure 49–45. *A*, A valgus-external rotational injury to the knee disrupts the medial joint structures. *B*, A varus-internal rotational, torsion injury to the knee disrupts the lateral joint structures. Characteristically, this occurs as an individual lands off balance and applies a varus stress to the knee joint. (From Connolly, J. F.: DePalma's The Management of Fractures and Dislocations: An Atlas. 3rd ed. Philadelphia, W. B. Saunders Co., 1981.)

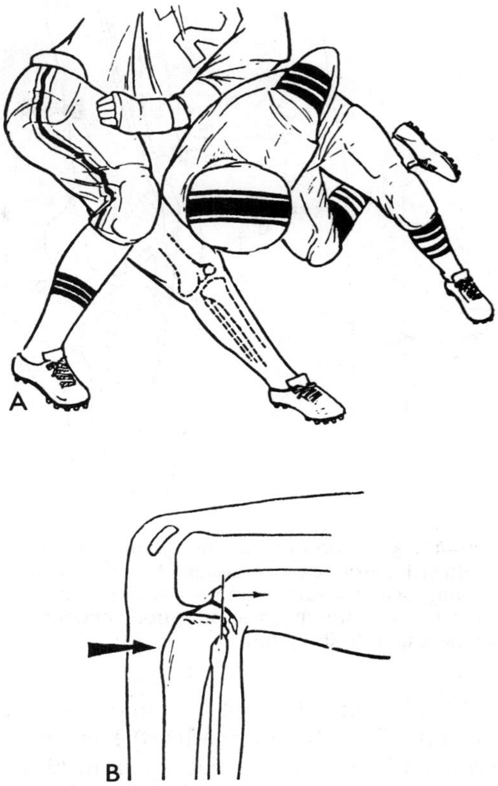

Figure 49–46. *A*, A hyperextension injury to the internally rotated knee frequently causes disruption of the anterior cruciate ligament. *B*, A hyperflexion injury to the flexed knee jars the tibia's posterior relationship to the femur and disrupts the posterior cruciate ligament. (From Connolly, J. F.: DePalma's The Management of Fractures and Dislocations: An Atlas. 3rd ed. Philadelphia, W. B. Saunders Co., 1981.)

load, and the posterior cruciate is injured most commonly by hyperflexion (Fig. 49–46*A*, *B*).

History and Physical. The history usually is that the patient felt a "pop" at the time the knee was twisted and gave way. This always indicates significant structural disruption. It remains up to the physician to identify the anatomic area and the degree of involvement.

Inspect the knee carefully for ecchymosis or localized swelling and watch how the patient moves the knee actively. Particularly determine if there is any limitation of motion from a mechanical obstruction or locking or loss of quadriceps function. Quadriceps tendon rupture and patellar dislocation are among the more commonly overlooked conditions presenting as common "knee sprains."

Feel carefully for areas of tenderness that indicate the site of torn muscle, ligament, or cartilage.

One of the more specific signs of meniscal injury is point tenderness along the anteromedial and posteromedial joint line.

If an effusion is palpable, try to pin down precisely its source. Fluid that accumulates within 2 hours after injury indicates intra-articular bleeding. Marked effusion can be aspirated from the joint as shown in

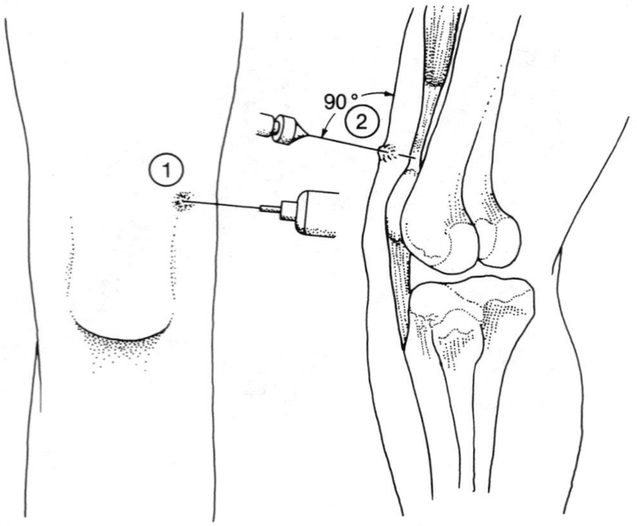

Figure 49–47. Aspiration of the knee joint. Perform the procedure with strict aseptic precautions. *(1)* Raise an intradermal wheal, using local anesthetic and a fine hypodermic needle. *(2)* After a few minutes pass a large-bore needle at a right angle to the skin into the joint.

Figure 49–47 (Connolly, 1981). Fluid that becomes evident only 12 to 24 hours after the injury usually represents an irritative synovial reaction. One of the more common causes of hemarthrosis identified by arthroscopy is a tear of the anterior cruciate ligament.

Integrity of the knee ligaments can be cited early (30 minutes) with no anesthetic. After this period anesthetic is needed. Evaluate for both medial and lateral instability as well as for anterior and posterior drawer signs (Fig. 49–48). Such an assessment particularly depends on the examiner's tactile sense, which one should develop in order to assess the ligamentous injury with confidence.

Grades of Injury. The family physician who evaluates knee injuries should be capable of separating a Grade I from a Grade III type of injury. Grade I, or incomplete injuries, have a few fibers of the ligaments injured. There is usually no history of functional instability, of "giving way." The swelling and tenderness about the knee are minimal. On abducting the knee at both 0 and 30 degrees of flexion, the injured joint opens up no greater than the uninjured side. X-ray studies show no fracture about the joint and no opening of the joint line on stressing.

With Grade III injuries there is complete rupture of capsular ligaments, either within the substance of the ligament or at its bony attachments. The patient usually gives a history of popping and gross functional instability after the injury. Some individuals may be able to lock the knee with the quadriceps and be fully weight-bearing in spite of their significant injury.

Pain with complete ligament injuries tends to be less than incomplete injuries. That is because the blood from the completely torn ligament extravasates outside the joint. Partial ligament tears tend to bleed into the joint and produce painful capsular distention. Consider the injury to be a Grade III if you feel the joint open more than 5 mm. compared with the uninjured side with the knee in 30 degrees of flexion.

Management by the Family Physician. Grade III injuries in most patients should be referred for prompt operative repair of the medial capsular or lateral capsular structures.

Lesser injuries should be treated nonoperatively. Treat these more common partial ligament injuries by applying a compression dressing. The patient can walk with partial weight-bearing using crutches and must immediately begin quadriceps strengthening exercises. Apply ice to the area of swelling and tenderness to help eliminate any painful inhibiting function of the knee.

Follow the progress of the patient and his knee closely to be sure that the injury is responding appropriately to the treatment. Full extension of the knee should return by 7 to 10 days, and flexion should be close to normal by 2 weeks. The patient may then

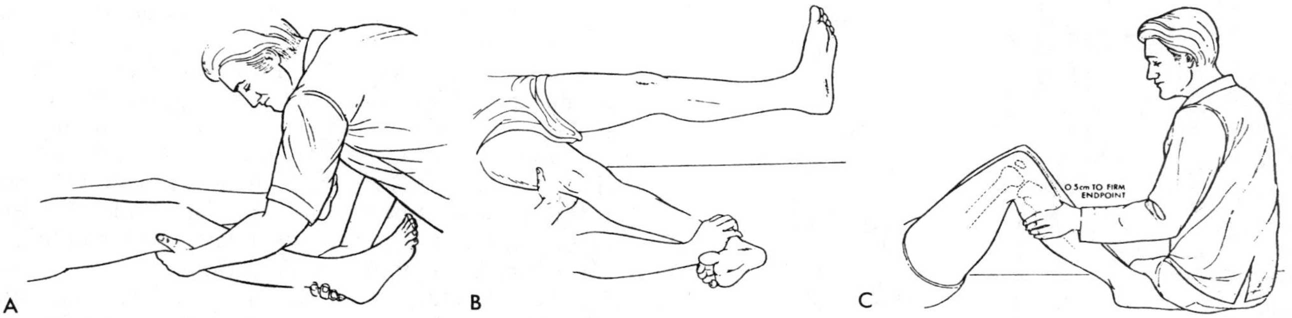

Figure 49–48. *A,* Abduction-adduction stress test of knee ligaments. The patient must lie on the examining table with the hip extended over the edge to relax the hamstrings. The examiner places one hand on the lateral side of the thigh and one hand above the ankle. Test the uninjured side first. *B,* The test should be done on the injured side with the knee in 30 degrees of flexion and in full extension. Instability of the knee in full extension is indicative of a serious ligamentous disruption (Grade III injury). *C,* Anterior-posterior drawer testing for cruciate ligament injury. The patient lies with the hips flexed 45 degrees and the knees flexed 90 degrees. The examiner rests gently on the patient's feet and checks the uninjured side first. The tibia is drawn forward in external rotation, neutral rotation, and internal rotation. Forward displacement of 0.5 cm. more than on the uninjured side and without a firm endpoint is a positive result. (From Connolly, J. F.: DePalma's The Management of Fractures and Dislocations: An Atlas. 3rd ed. Philadelphia, W. B. Saunders Co., 1981.)

gradually resume activities such as running and participation in sports in a few weeks.

The major criteria showing that the knee is returning to normal are diminished swelling and tenderness in the knee ligaments and progressive recovery of full motion.

Any patient who does not demonstrate this expected pattern of recovery within 7 to 10 days should be referred for examination of the joint instability under anesthetic.

Quadriceps Rupture

Other conditions are frequently confused with ligamentous injuries of the knee. One of the more common is disruption of the extensor apparatus, either from patellar dislocation or from tearing of the quadriceps.

Quadriceps rupture occurs most often in middle-aged and elderly patients who sustain a sudden hyperextension or flexion twist to the knee. This can be confused with ligamentous tears but should not be difficult to diagnose. These patients cannot extend the knee actively. Never forget the importance of inspection. Always have the patient actively move the joint before you palpate or move it passively.

Unlike the locked knee from a torn meniscus, passive extension with the torn quadriceps is full. However, a palpable gap is evident above the patella when the patient is asked to contract the quadriceps forcefully.

Management by the Family Physician. The disrupted quadriceps tendon apparatus should be repaired promptly.

Patellar Instability

Patellar instability is more common than is quadriceps rupture. It is seen most often in active young individuals, particularly teenage girls with knock knees. It can occur from any injury to the knee that tears the medial patellar retinaculum and allows the patella to slide laterally over the femoral condyle.

Typically, the patient gives a history of coming down rapidly with the knee extended. A valgus and external rotatory strain then causes the patella to shift laterally; the patella quickly dislocates and causes the whole extensor support to give way. The patient falls to the ground and the patella may or may not then reduce spontaneously.

The diagnosis of patellar instability should be suspected by this somewhat bizarre history of a "drop attack." The suspicion is confirmed by a "fear" sign on physical testing. This apprehension sign is elicited with the patient's knee relaxed in a flexed position. The examiner then presses the patient's patella laterally and provokes the patient's fear of impending instability or patellar dislocation proving there is pathologic laxity.

Management by the Family Physician. An acute patellar dislocation can be managed by supporting the patella with a knee cylinder for 3 to 4 weeks to allow the medial patellar retinaculum to heal. The patient has about a 50 per cent chance of avoiding future recurrences of the dislocation if this technique is used (Fig. 49–49).

Recurrent episodes of patellar instability require operative repair before chondromalacia or patellofemoral arthritis develops.

Meniscal Tears

Medial meniscus tears are the most common cause of knee joint pain or sprain. The medial joint cartilage is torn by a twisting injury with the knee partially flexed. The meniscus in this position is forced toward the center of the joint and becomes caught between the femur and tibia. It is then torn longitudinally by shearing forces when the joint is suddenly extended. If the tear extends sufficiently anteriorly, the detached segment may catch in the intercondylar notch like the handle of a bucket. This obstructs normal articular gliding of the femur on the tibia and thereby locks the knee or prevents it from completely extending.

The medial meniscus is five to seven times more susceptible to such tears than is the lateral meniscus. Both medial and lateral meniscal tears produce the common medial joint line pain and the sensation of locking.

The clinical diagnosis of meniscal tears may be difficult for even an experienced orthopedic surgeon. The most consistent physical finding of meniscal tear is tenderness to palpation along the joint line anterior and posterior to the collateral ligament.

Reproducing a painful click during McMurray's test is diagnostic. Have the patient lie supine with the

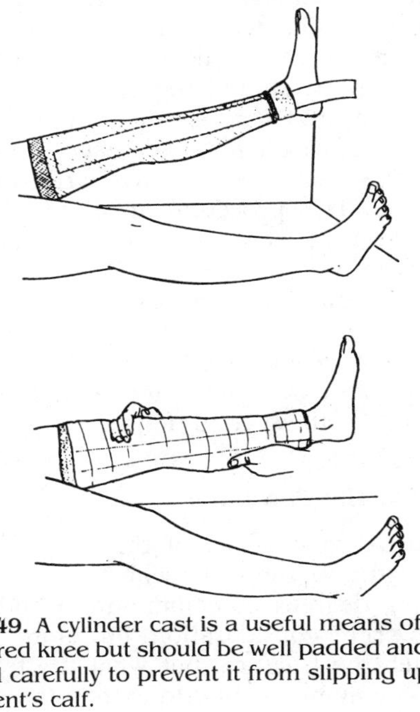

Figure 49–49. A cylinder cast is a useful means of immobilizing the injured knee but should be well padded and supported and applied carefully to prevent it from slipping up and down on the patient's calf.

hip and knee flexed acutely and maximally. McMurray's test cannot be done in the acutely tender knee. Palpate the posterior medial joint line with one hand and then externally rotate the foot and leg with the other as far as possible. Slowly extend the externally rotated and flexed knee. As the torn meniscus is caught between the femur and tibia, a click is felt which the patient describes as painful. Most often this results from posterior meniscal tears and consequently occurs with the knee going from complete flexion to approximately 90 degrees.

To examine for lateral meniscal tear, flex the knee and internally rotate the leg. Then slowly extend the leg while trying to produce the painful click.

A dynamic method of testing for meniscal injury is to have the patient walk in a duck waddle or squatting position. This maneuver applies an extreme compression load on the joint and is never possible when the patient has a torn meniscus. However, other conditions, including a ligamentous tear and patellofemoral arthritis, will produce pain on squatting and prevent the patient from carrying out this test. Nevertheless, if the patient is able to duck-waddle without pain, the likelihood of internal derangement of the knee is extremely low.

Management by the Family Physician. The family physician can serve his patient best by identifying the individual with possible meniscal tear before further damage is inflicted on the knee. The patient who persists with a locked knee is particularly likely to damage the anterior cruciate ligament adjacent to the torn meniscus. Abrasions of the femoral condyle and chondromalacia of the patella also occur with altered knee mechanics from meniscal injury. The sooner the pathology is recognized and corrected, the better is the long-term prognosis for the knee to remain free of arthritis.

If there is any diagnostic doubt, refer the patient for arthroscopy. This technique, which visualizes the meniscus directly, has considerably improved diagnostic accuracy. It should be employed liberally to evaluate the injured knee, particularly when there is any suspicion of cartilaginous damage. Removal of a torn meniscus, via the operative arthroscopy, has become a standard procedure in many areas of the country. It appears to reduce morbidity and recovery time significantly.

Other injuries affecting extension of the knee include patellar fractures and Osgood-Schlatter disease. Both can be managed by the family physician who distinguishes the significant from the insignificant consequences of these conditions.

Fractures of the Patella

The usual mechanism of this injury is a direct blow to the front of the knee, which produces fracture with varying degrees of comminution and displacement. The prime consideration, therefore, should be not so much the fracture, but what the fracture has done to the patient's ability to extend the knee.

Occasionally, the patella retinaculum which surrounds the patella fracture maintains the integrity of the extensor apparatus and allows the patient to extend his knee fully despite the fracture. Knee flexion may then be possible to 45 degrees without evidence of fracture distraction. Such an obvious stable fracture requires only symptomatic treatment to relieve pain and temporary protective splinting to prevent further damage to the extensor mechanism.

Displacement of the fractured patella with knee flexion or inability of the patient to extend the knee actively indicates disruption of the extensor apparatus and the need for operative repair.

Management by the Family Physician. The major component of the patient's pain symptoms comes not from the fracture but from the hemarthrosis distending the sensitive joint capsule. The hemarthrosis can be aspirated and the patient's range of motion can be better evaluated.

If the patient can actively extend the knee with no lag, and flexion to 30 to 40 degrees causes no palpable opening of the fracture, the patella retinaculum has not been disrupted. These stable fractures require protective support.

Apply a cylinder cast with the patient's knee fully extended. First use long strips of 2-inch tape with adhesive sprayed onto the skin. Apply a stockinette over the tape. Pad the malleoli well. Wrap 4-inch plaster rolls and incorporate tape strips to suspend the cast and prevent it from abrading the malleoli (Fig. 49–49). Encourage the patient to bear weight on the injured limb as tolerated.

By the end of 5 to 7 days the patient will experience sufficient pain relief and regain confidence in the knee so that the cylinder can be bivalved and active knee exercises can be allowed.

When the patient is walking, the splint should also be reapplied to protect against sudden flexion. Also, if the patient will not follow directions and will not exercise due caution, it is prudent to wait 6 weeks before removing the splint. This allows time for the fracture to consolidate but also assures a stiff knee when the cast is removed. This stiffness requires about twice as long (12 weeks) to work out as it took to produce it.

An alternative treatment is internal fixation of the patellar fracture followed by an active exercise program supervised in the hospital. Either a stable patellar fracture in an unstable patient or, more usually, a displaced or comminuted patellar fracture in any patient is best referred for adequate internal fixation and early immobilization of the extensor apparatus.

Osgood-Schlatter Disease

Osgood-Schlatter disease results from repetitive hyperextension strain produced by the pull of the patellar tendon on the tibial tuberosity. The usual teenage patient presents with a chief complaint of a painful knob just below the knee. This prevents the young boy or girl from participating in vigorous sports. It is tender to direct palpation, and frequently, a small mobile fragment can be felt or seen on x-ray of the tibial tuberosity (Fig. 49–50).

Generally, the pain symptoms subside with rest but tend to return as the individual resumes sports or does much stair climbing.

We physicians tend to dismiss the symptoms as "growing pains" or undertreat the lesions of the patellar tendon insertion. The young person usually learns to avoid sports and activities that bring on the symptoms. The result is that he tends to be labeled as a laggard.

Symptoms can persist and flare up in the active adult with a history of Osgood-Schlatter disease who attempts to participate in sports or is forced to do much marching during military training (Fig. 49–50).

A more specific treatment of this common disability in adolescence could avoid much of the recurring problems in the active individual.

Management by the Family Physician. The most effective way to relieve acute symptoms of Osgood-Schlatter disease is to protect the knee with a splint in full extension. Apply a cylinder cast as previously described in the section on patellar fractures (see Fig. 49–49). This eliminates a good deal of the loading on the bone fragments and allows any freshly avulsed fractures to heal.

The cast should be removed after 3 to 4 weeks. In most instances, the tibial tuberosity is no longer painful. The patient may then resume range of motion exercises and slowly return to active sports.

For recurrent symptoms in the skeletally mature girl over 15 or the boy over 16, advise removal of any loose bone fragments. This is only necessary in approximately 10 to 15 per cent of patients with Osgood-Schlatter disease, but when indicated, surgical treatment can effectively relieve symptoms and allow the young individual to return to sports and other vigorous activities.

Although one should wait to recommend removal of bone fragments associated with Osgood-Schlatter disease until the individual is skeletally mature, most of us tend to be overly conservative (Fig. 49–50).

Morton's Neuroma

Morton (1876) described a type of severe pain in the forefoot. The history is that of a patient seized with pain necessitating standing still on the good foot and perhaps removing the shoe to rub the painful area. In a short time the pain will abate. Between bouts of pain the patient has no symptoms. The disorder is usually seen between ages 15 and 55 and is more common in females. The etiology may be mechanical irritation of the digital proper nerve between adjacent metatarsal heads (Betts, 1940).

Most commonly affected is the nerve between the third and fourth toes, although it can be seen between others. Direct compression of the interspace will elicit or reproduce the pain.

Management by the Family Physician. Resection of the nerve is curative, although less severe cases can benefit from placement of a small metatarsal pad in the shoe.

Diabetic Problems

Minor foot problems such as bunions or claw toes can become limb-threatening or even life-threatening for the diabetic patient. Diabetes produces the ma-

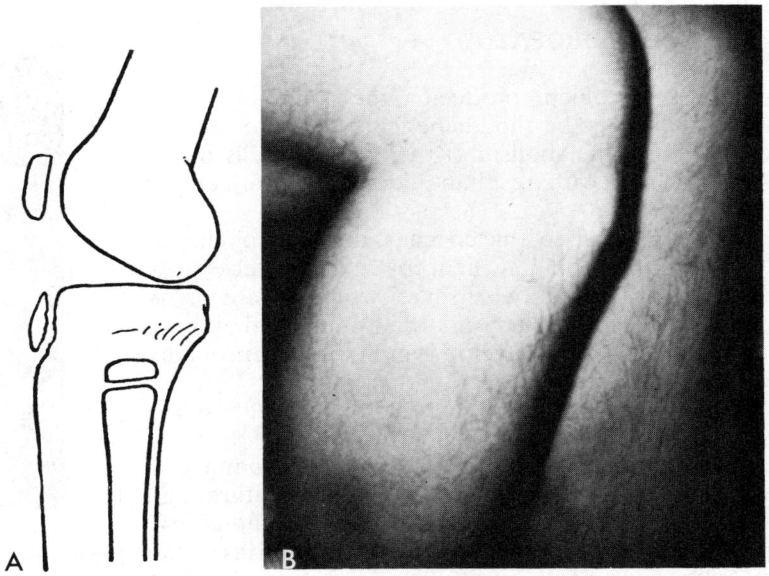

Figure 49–50. *A,* Osgood-Schlatter disease frequently produces a loose ossicle on the superior aspect of the tibial tuberosity, pulled loose by the patellar tendon. *B,* Persistent Osgood-Schlatter disease in a 25-year-old man prevented this patient from participating actively in sports for 10 years. The symptoms were relieved by simple excision of the loose ossicle in the tibial tuberosity.

jority of adult amputees today. This contrasts with the statistics prior to 1951 when most amputations followed trauma.

The major orthopedic problems from diabetes that will be discussed in this section are diabetic vascular disease and diabetic neuropathy.

DIABETIC VASCULAR DISEASE

The major difference between diabetic and nondiabetic peripheral vascular disease is that in diabetes, the basement membrane of the capillaries and small vessels becomes pathologically thickened, thereby preventing profusion across the capillary wall. This thickening, at least in the mature diabetic patient, is a segmental lesion. It does not obstruct flow, but it does limit exchange across the vessel wall. This produces edema, local lymphatic obstruction, and an interstitial backwash, which makes an ideal medium for infection. Consequently, infection and subsequent gangrene is 40 times more common in the diabetic patient than in the nondiabetic patient with atherosclerosis. Diabetic infection with gangrene occurs in either a foot that is cold owing to proximal obstruction without collateral distal flow or a foot that is warm or even hot, indicating adequate small vessel flow but impaired perfusion.

Approximately one third of diabetic gangrene occurs in the cold foot, and this is managed like any other atherosclerotic occlusion, either with arterial grafting or with amputation. The remaining two thirds of patients with diabetic gangrene usually have palpable major pulses and adequate peripheral flow. For these patients, drainage of infection, debridement of necrotic tissue, and conservative amputation are most successful (see Table 49–4). Distinguishing between the two types of diabetic gangrene is usually not difficult.

DIABETIC NEUROPATHY

The basic problem producing the common neuropathic changes in the diabetic appears to be the alteration in metabolism of the Schwann cells in the nerve sheath with resultant demyelinization of the nerve.

As with angiopathic changes, the onset of clinical symptoms from diabetic neuropathy is not necessarily related to the duration or severity of the diabetes. A number of patients may first find out that they have diabetes when they develop symptoms of neuropathy or distal gangrene.

Anatomic, sensory, and motor nerve fibers are all involved in the neuropathic process.

The diabetic patient's loss of autonomic function causes inability to control body temperature and inadequate sweating mechanism. The result is dry, scaly skin, which makes wounds and abrasions of the patient's foot most susceptible to infection. The loss of autonomic control may cause the patient's skin temperature in the foot to be 4° to 5° less than the body's core temperature and results in the characteristic diabetic "cold foot." The unwary individual then may sustain burns from keeping hot water bottles or other heating aids on the cold foot while asleep.

Sensory neuropathy in diabetics can produce extremely painful paresthesias, which are sometimes described as dartlike or tabetic in nature. The paresthesias are worse at night and frequently are aggravated by cold and are generally associated with decreased ankle jerk reflexes. This pain of neuropathy is generally relieved by walking as opposed to the pain of angiopathy, which is made worse by walking. Diabetic "tabes" can be confused with disc disease.

The most devastating neuropathy of diabetes is that which results in the loss of protective sensation and causes the patient to walk on pressure points such as a pebble or a tack, literally walking the protective skin off the sole (Fig. 49–51). The loss of protective sensation can break down the skeletal support of the foot from repetitive fatigue fractures. This neuropathic destruction of the bones and the diabetic foot is now the most common cause of Charcot's joint. Quite frequently, in our observation, the radiographic changes of this neuropathic bone destruction are confused with those of osteomyelitis (Fig. 49–52*A*). This is completely unnecessary and avoidable, since the differential between osteomyelitis and Charcot's changes can be made by simple clinical observations. Bone scans are no help, as circulation is increased in both conditions.

Osteomyelitis is most often associated with abscess formation or draining infection. Charcot's changes characteristically produce swelling, deformity, and sometimes redness, but not drainage or other signs of acute infection (Fig. 49–52*B*).

Involvement of motor nerve fibers may result in paralysis, including foot drop or wrist drop. This does tend to improve with time and with control of the

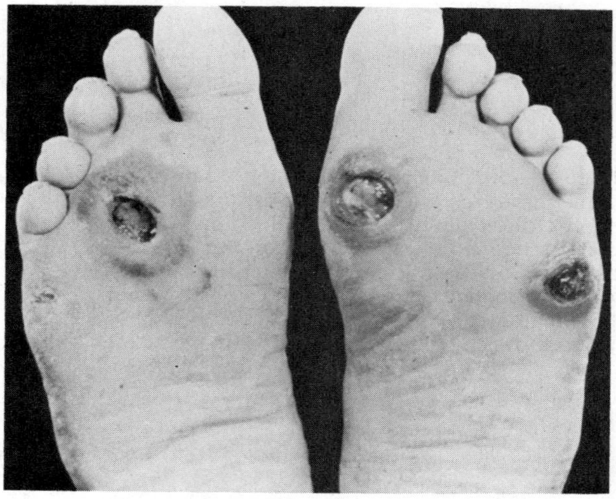

Figure 49–51. Typical multiple neurotrophic ulcers have developed in this diabetic patient owing to loss of protective sensation over pressure areas.

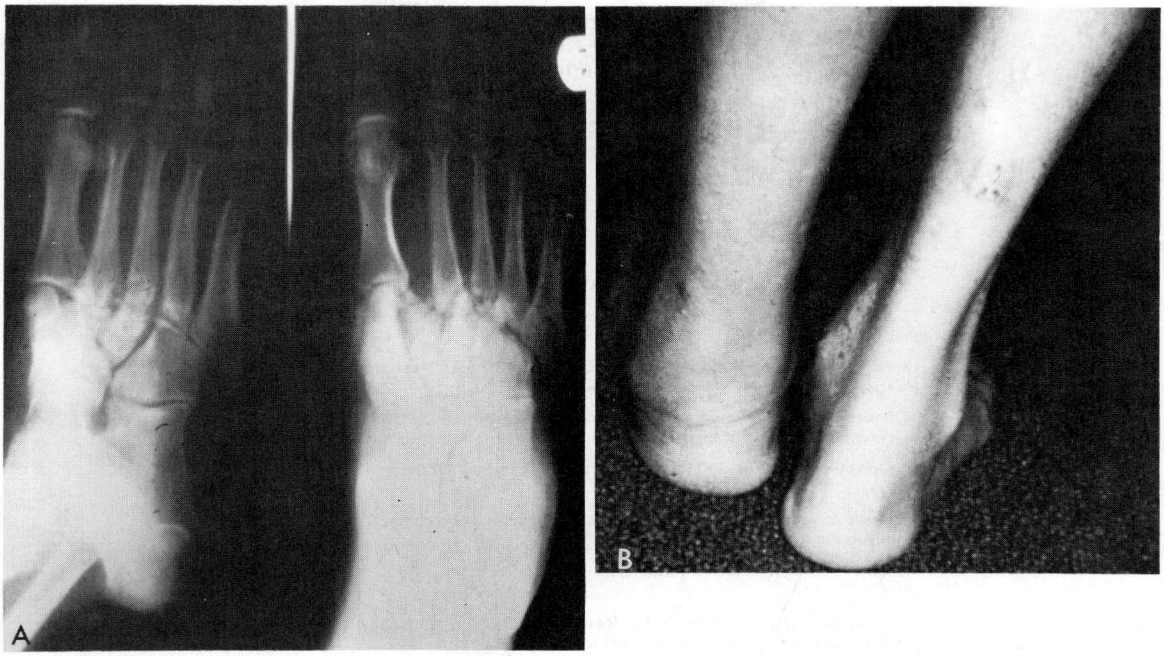

Figure 49–52. *A*, Neurotrophic changes led to this bone destruction (Charcot's joints), as seen on these x-ray films of a diabetic patient. This should not be confused with osteomyelitis if the physician examines the foot as well as the x-ray film. *B*, A patient with neurotrophic foot and ankle demonstrates swelling and warmth but no drainage or ulceration.

blood sugar. Weakness of the intrinsic muscles of the foot produce gait alteration and adds to the development of pressure points, abrasion, infection, and ultimate gangrene.

Management by the Family Physician. The disconcerting fact is that no single therapy, including control of blood sugar, can prevent these complications of angiopathy and neuropathy, which ultimately lead to gangrene. At present, therapeutic, environmental, and dietary factors play some role and make some contribution to the prevention or provocation of diabetic complications. Of primary importance, however, is the luck of the genetic draw and particularly the host response.

Host response may be altered with education. We have developed a self-evaluation program to remind the diabetic patient of the high likelihood of having vascular and neurologic disease. The patient must be reminded to pay proper attention to the care of feet and with each visit is encouraged to do so. (The patient information form used at the University of Nebraska Medical Center is shown on page 1048).

The diabetic foot must be inspected either by the patient or, if the patient has poor vision, by a family member every day. Nails should be trimmed evenly so as to prevent ingrowth and infection of the nail edges.

The diabetic patient should wash and carefully dry the feet each day and particularly avoid walking barefooted, hot water applications, and chemical treatment of calluses. Inadequate attention to foot care invariably leads to trouble (Fig. 49–53).

Bony prominences that cause calluses, bunions, or clawtoes are likely to produce pressure necrosis and infection of the skin. These should be corrected promptly by surgical procedures before the infection supervenes. Rather than being a contraindication to foot surgery, the diabetic state should be considered a prime indication for early surgical correction of foot deformities.

Shoes are extremely important and must be chosen carefully. We prefer thick-soled shoes or ripple soles to relieve pressure points and absorb weight-bearing forces. If necessary, a pressure area can be relieved by paring down the ripple of the sole over either the first or fifth metatarsal head.

Neuropathic bone destruction or Charcot's deformities have been particular therapeutic problems in our observation with juvenile diabetics who sometimes try to ignore their condition. These impressively damaged skeletal structures do heal when adequately protected with cast and weight-bearing orthoses. A very effective orthosis is the "patellar-tendon-bearing" type, which includes a rigid ankle and transfers the weight-bearing load to a custom-made socket contacting the proximal tibia and patellar tendon.

Surgical Management of Diabetic Gangrene. The source of most therapeutic indecision about diabetic care is the infected foot that has not responded to the usual modalities of bed rest, elevation, and antibiotics.

In managing such a problem, do not delay more than 2 to 3 days in deciding about surgical drainage. To persevere determinedly with antibiotic treatment of an abscessed foot will only convert a salvageable limb to a below-knee amputation.

The amputation, should it become necessary, must be as conservative as possible in the diabetic

University of Nebraska Medical Center

Patient Information

Date: ____________

For (Patient's Name): ____________

Things you can do to help your feet

1. Don't use tobacco in any form. It hurts the circulation to the feet.

2. Keep warm. Letting your feet get cold reduces the amount of blood that can reach them.

3. Protect your feet. Avoid walking in crowds, and select level ground for your exercise.

4. Shoes make a difference! Wear wide-toed shoes that have good arch support and feel comfortable on your feet. Choose thick, warm, loose-fitting socks.

5. Don't wear elastic garters that encircle the leg. These cut off blood flow to the legs and feet.

6. Don't sit with your knees crossed. This position has a tendency to shut off blood supply to the foot.

7. If the bedding feels uncomfortable, place a pillow to hold it off your feet while you sleep.

8. Don't apply any heat to the feet or legs without checking with a physician. Even a small amount of heat might cause a sore to form on your foot.

9. Don't put any medicine on your feet unless a physician tells you to do so. Even nonprescription medicine may be too strong for a foot with poor circulation.

10. Wash the feet at least every other day. Use warm water and soap. Dry your feet thoroughly, especially between the toes. Use the towel to mop, not rub, the water away.

11. Apply lanolin if your feet are dry and scaly.

12. Apply powder if your feet are moist.

13. Cut your toenails properly. First, soak your feet in warm water for 10 minutes to soften the nails. Cut straight across. NEVER CUT DOWN INTO THE CORNERS, AND DON'T CUT THE NAILS CLOSE TO THE FLESH! If you are treated by a podiatrist, tell him that the blood flow to your feet is reduced.

14. Consult your physician promptly when you notice redness, blistering, pain, or swelling of the feet. Any break in the skin may become an ulcer or even lead to gangrene unless it is properly treated by your physician.

15. Seek medical help for athlete's foot. The infection starts as peeling and itching between the toes, and calls for treatment by a physician.

16. Don't swim in cold water or in the ocean.

17. Avoid sunburn.

18. Walk slower, but walk often. Walking actually helps your legs and feet. By stimulating the growth of blood vessels, it improves the circulation.

19. If the toes rub each other, apply lamb's wool between them.

foot with warm gangrene (Table 49–4). Soft tissue drainage (Fig. 49–54), a partial ray resection (see Fig. 49–11), or Syme's amputation work well in the foot with small vessel disease but adequate major arterial flow. If a complicating infection extends close to the site of amputation, the wound can be left open and closed secondarily.

There is very little justification today for automatically selecting an above-knee level for diabetic gangrene, especially when one considers that 20 to 30 per cent of diabetic amputees will eventually require amputation of the opposite limb. Studies over the past 10 years have shown that in the elderly diabetic patient, below-knee amputation heals quite well. Since the rehabilitation potential is so much greater when the patient's knee is preserved, the lower level should be employed in almost every instance of diabetic gangrene.

Radiographic or bone scan changes in the foot are not reliable indices of infection. Areas of bone destruction and dislocation seen on x-ray are frequently indicative of neuropathic rather than infectious destruction.

Effective management of the diabetic's foot problems starts with patient education and training in self-surveillance. It aims at correcting mechanical deformities such as bunions and clawtoes early before they produce significant problems. It uses early surgical drainage of soft tissue infections and minimal amputation at the lowest possible level.

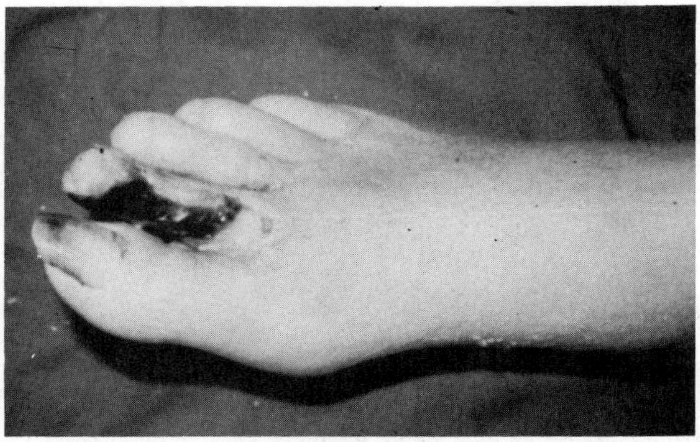

Figure 49–53. Failure of this patient to attend to proper nail and foot hygiene produced this infection and eventual diabetic gangrene.

A Potentially Fatal Complication of Trauma—Malignant Hyperthermia

This is a life-threatening complication of injury or surgery in patients suffering from this inherited muscular disorder. Death can come from stress of injury alone or from anesthesia and surgery. The stress of injury need not be major in degree.

The condition may resemble heat stroke or overwhelming sepsis in some cases. Typically, cases with high heart rate and rapidly rising temperature will exhibit a marked acidosis and high potassium levels. Often there is associated muscle rigidity, especially of the masseter muscle. The disease probably is a consequence of increased calcium levels in the myoplasm, resulting in continued contracture.

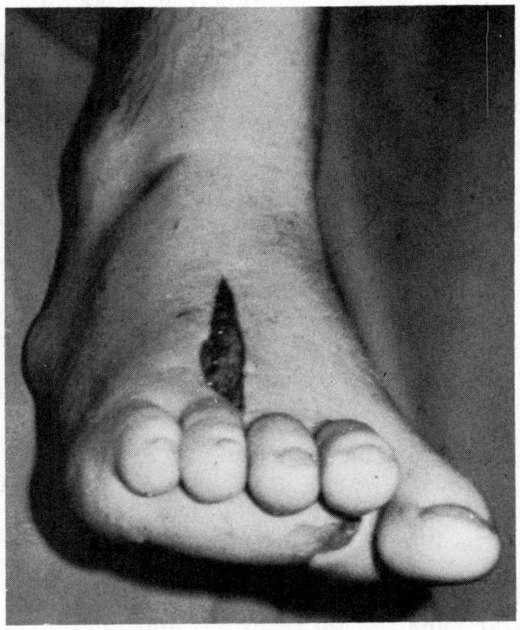

Figure 49–54. Prompt drainage of the dorsal and plantar abscesses of this diabetic patient's foot salvaged a useful weight-bearing extremity. Do not expect antibiotic treatment to cure diabetic foot abscesses.

Typical signs in order of occurrence are tachycardia, rise in core body temperature, muscle rigidity in 60 per cent of patients, and often a mottled, cyanotic appearance to the skin.

Untreated, the patient usually dies of acidosis, electrolyte-induced dysrhythmia, renal failure, or coma. Patients are very acidotic and have high serum potassium levels, dysrhythmia of the heart (tachycardia followed by fibrillation), myoglobinuria, and shocklike appearance with unexplained high core temperature.

There is no reliable screening test. Most reliable is obtaining a family history of sudden death from surgery or injury. Patients with a history of acrocyanosis of feet and hands, intolerance to exercise in heat with muscle cramping, kyphosis, scoliosis, ptosis, or club feet are particularly suspect.

Typically, a tachycardia is noted with a rapid rise in core temperature of 1° to 2° C. each 5 minutes up to temperatures of 47.5° C. prior to death. All have severe acidosis and tachypnea with high CO_2 and potassium levels.

The treatment and prophylaxis are cooling, intravenous recarbonate, and dantrolene sodium intravenously.

The disease is well described with regard to onset and treatment by Jardon (1979 and 1980).

Management by the Family Physician. The major safeguard in this condition is awareness of its existence and its early signs. During any surgical or trauma problems, temperature and heart rate should be monitored for signs of this rather rare, but extremely life-threatening condition.

Dantrolene sodium intravenously at 1 or 2 mg. per kg. body weight every 10 to 15 minutes is specific treatment (usual effective total dose 2.5 to 3.5 mg. per kg., but occasionally 10 to 12 mg. per kg. may be needed). Sodium bicarbonate, cooling in ice, and osmotic diuretics are helpful. Most anesthesiologists are treatment experts and should be consulted at the first sign of a problem.

Arthritis

In this section, rather than skipping superficially through the arthritides, which are well covered elsewhere, we shall focus on them from an orthopedic perspective. We shall discuss fundamental concepts that have been useful for us to maximize the effect of both medical and surgical treatment. We shall also present a few common problems that both the family physician and we orthopedists tend to overlook or undertreat.

TRAUMATIC ARTHRITIS

Traumatic arthritis represents a common, but only casually understood disease that is particularly likely to afflict young, active individuals subject to injury. Arthritis secondary to trauma should be distinguished from osteoarthritis resulting from biochemical breakdown of cartilage matrix. The boundary between traumatic arthritis and osteoarthritis has been obscured by the tendency of patients to relate most joint diseases to a traumatic episode, either real or imagined.

Trauma sufficient to fracture the joint surface may or may not induce arthritis. This is beyond the control of the physician. Other factors, particularly the severity of joint stiffening and the degree of joint instability, are to a significant extent related to initial treatment.

Upper Limb Problems

In the upper limb, the major complication to avoid is a stiff joint. In the lower limb, joint instability as well as stiffening is of prime concern. In the upper limb, we tend to overtreat the fracture by imposing unnecessary immobilization and inducing a stiff joint. In the lower limb, we are prone to undertreat articular fractures and accept joint instability, which could and should be avoided.

Techniques that are most likely to minimize traumatic arthritis include both appropriate fracture stabilization and emphasis on early restoration of joint motion. At one time, rest was considered essential for healing a disease or injured joint. Despite occasional benefits in the past from prolonged and uninterrupted rest of diseased joints, the detrimental results of prolonged joint immobilization and the importance of motion for articular cartilage healing have been demonstrated repeatedly (Salter et al., 1980).

Avascular cartilage must be nourished by synovial fluid, which is "pumped" into the cartilage during motion. Complete immobilization of joints for only a few weeks produces measurable changes in the cartilage matrix and eventual breakdown of usually smooth articular joint surfaces.

Immobilization also weakens the tensile strength of the ligaments supporting joints. Frequently the result is ligamentous laxity, induced by even brief periods of joint immobilization.

Examples of upper limb articular fractures in which joint motion should be emphasized over fracture reduction include fractures of the radial head and fractures of the surgical neck of the humerus. Radial head or neck fractures are best managed by aspirating the hemarthrosis and then encouraging the patient to move the elbow promptly. The major portion of pain after injuries to joints results from distention of the joint capsule. Aspirating the hemarthrosis, which may amount to only a few cubic centimeters in the elbow, does much to relieve the patient's acute discomfort (Fig. 49–55).

Avoid immobilizing the elbow in flexion for more than 2 or 3 days. The usual motion limited after radial head fractures is elbow extension. If necessary for

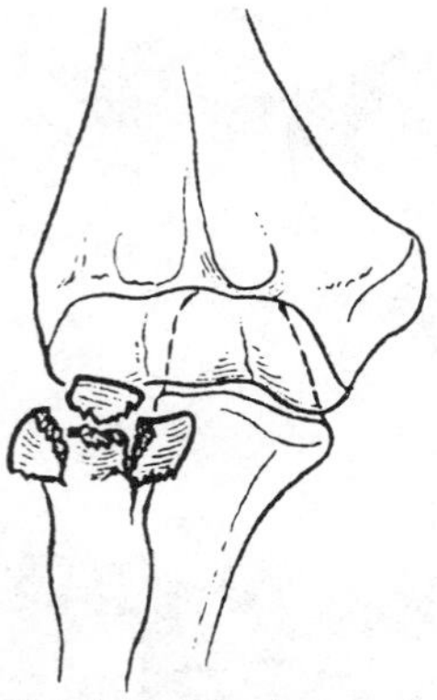

Figure 49–55. Radial head fractures should be treated by aspirating the elbow joint to relieve the pain from capsular distention. Then inject local anesthetic and check the range of elbow motion to determine whether any of the fracture fragments block flexion or extension. Surgical excision is necessary only if there is blockage of joint motion; otherwise, encourage active range of motion of the elbow.

patient comfort, apply a plaster-of-Paris splint to maintain the elbow in maximum extension at night. However, encourage active elbow flexion during daytime activities.

If on moving the elbow the radial head fracture fragment is found to block flexion, it can be removed surgically. This is best determined first by a trial of motion. Such an approach allows the patient to return to most activities in 2 or 3 weeks. This contrasts with the 3 or 4 months of recovery induced by prolonged immobilization or inordinately aggressive surgical treatment.

Another common fracture of the upper limb for which treatment is likely to impair joint function is a fracture of the surgical neck of the humerus. Prolonged immobilization until there is radiographic evidence of fracture union neglects the rapid and detrimental effect of immobilization on joint function. The supraspinatus muscle, an important suspensory muscle of the shoulder, is particularly prone to rapid atrophy with disuse. The result is that the humeral head will subluxate or partially dislocate inferiorly and the shoulder will tighten in a "frozen" position (Fig. 49–56). The consequence is an injury that requires 6 months for recovery rather than 6 weeks as it should.

To avoid this unnecessary sequence of joint maladies, treat the patient with a humeral neck fracture symptomatically and ignore the x-ray. These are usually stable injuries and invariably heal despite some shoulder motion.

As soon as the patient's acute pain symptoms subside, usually within 3 to 7 days, begin a range of motion program starting with circumduction. Advance over the subsequent weeks to external rotation and abduction exercises as illustrated in Figure 49–41.

Our emphasis on restoring joint motion, however, depends on the initially adequate assessment that the articulation is stable. That is, we should be

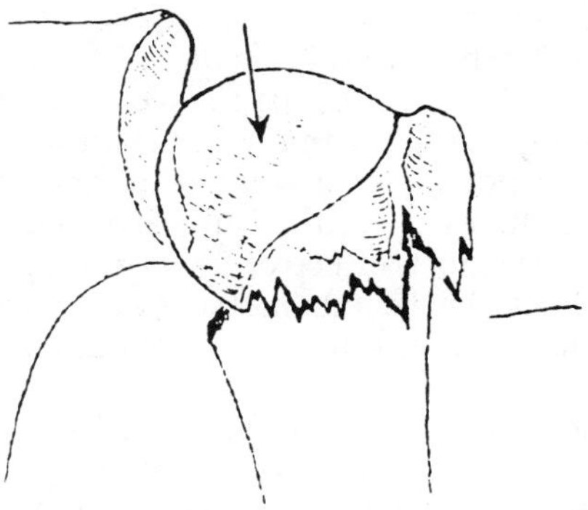

Figure 49–56. Prolonged immobilization of a surgical neck fracture of the humerus frequently causes inferior subluxation of the humeral head due to atrophy of the supraspinatus muscle. This can be combated by early range of motion exercises.

sure we are not dealing with a dislocation as well as a fracture.

A fracture that has caused joint instability mandates internal fixation prior to allowing the joint motion so necessary for articular healing. This is particularly true with articular fractures in the lower limb that alter weight-bearing mechanics of the joint.

Lower Limb Problems

Bear in mind that not all articular fractures involve weight-bearing portions of joints. Consequently, not all interarticular fractures are invariably followed by traumatic arthritis. The most common fracture of the acetabulum, the fracture of the central portion (Fig. 49–57*A*), rarely produces traumatic arthritis. However, fractures involving the superior weight-bearing portion of the acetabulum are very likely to impair hip function (Fig. 49–57*B*).

Although fractures of the lateral tibial plateau may be comminuted, incomplete reduction can be accepted without risking residual arthritis (Fig. 49–58*A*). This is due to the fact that a good portion of weight is borne in the lateral compartment of the knee by the lateral meniscus rather than the fractured articular surface. In contrast, fractures of the medial tibial condyle carry a high risk of joint instability and subsequent arthritis when treated closed. Internal fixation with relatively simple percutaneous pins stabilizes these joint fractures and permits early restoration of motion (Fig. 49–58*B*).

Fractures of the ankle are among the most problematic for the family physician to treat. These have been indicated as a common source of medical liability settlements among nonorthopedists who treat fractures. Ankle fractures may seem relatively innocuous, but slight displacement of the talus and the ankle mortise can lead to an unsatisfactory result.

Internal fixation and early mobilization of the ankle joint provides the most satisfactory answer to the bimalleolar fracture, which commonly causes ankle instability (Fig. 49–59).

Management by the Family Physician. The optimum treatment of traumatic arthritis is preventive. Management of fractures about joints must incorporate methods of relieving pain immediately by joint aspiration and should be directed at restoring joint

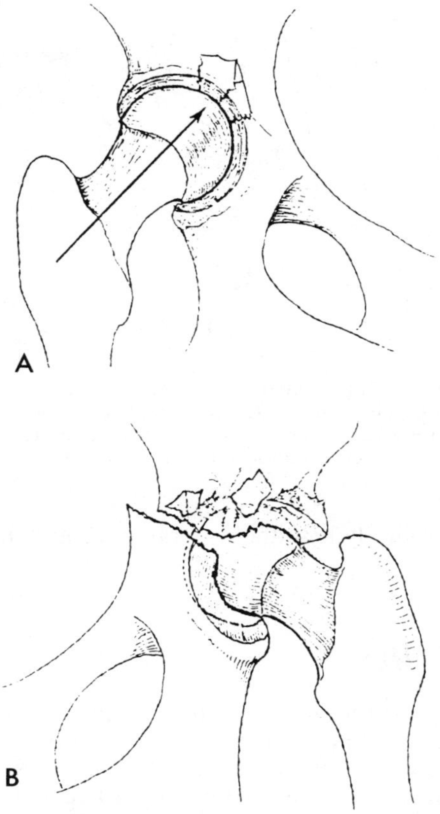

Figure 49–57. *A,* The most common acetabular fracture involves the central non-weight-bearing portion and can be treated symptomatically unless there was central protrusion. *B,* An acetabular fracture involving the weight-bearing portion commonly leads to traumatic arthritis.

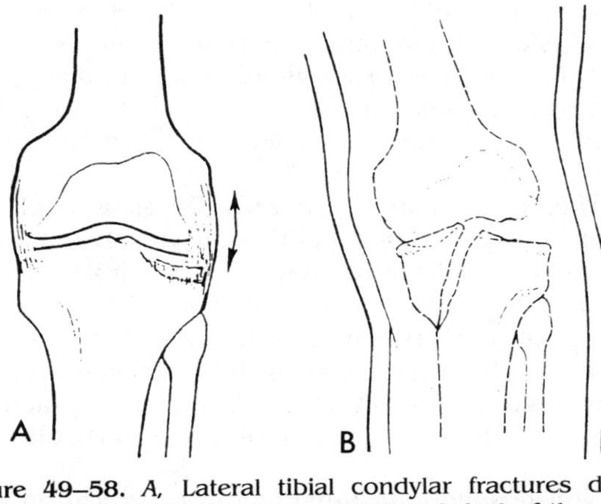

Figure 49–58. *A,* Lateral tibial condylar fractures do not require anatomic reduction, since a good deal of the weight in the lateral portion is carried by the lateral meniscus. *B,* Medial tibial condylar fractures require anatomic reduction if progressive varus deformity and traumatic arthritis are to be avoided.

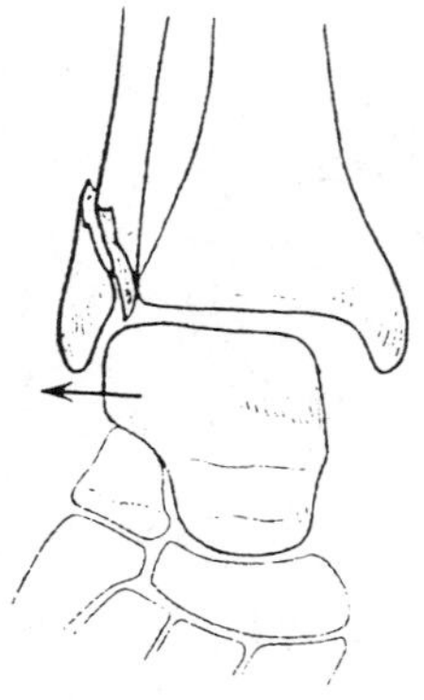

Figure 49–59. Ankle fractures are sometimes treacherous, since the degree of lateral displacement may not be evident without careful assessment of x-ray films. Generally, internal fixation is necessary to allow early mobilization of the ankle joint.

motion promptly by either operative or nonoperative techniques.

OSTEOARTHRITIS

This is by far the most common form of arthritis we treat either as family physicians or orthopedists. The disease results from a combination of biochemical and biomechanical breakdown of articular cartilage frequently superimposed on collapse of the subchondral joint support. Wear and tear is not the only factor producing osteoarthritis. Many patients also have genetically governed susceptibility to joint breakdown as manifested by Heberden's nodes, the pathognomonic finding in osteoarthritis.

The symptoms from this disease may range from painless stiffening or crepitance of the joint to a constant joint ache which severely handicaps the patient. The degree of x-ray changes does not necessarily correlate with the severity of pain symptoms. McCarty (1976) and others have pointed out that only 30 per cent of patients with radiographic evidence of osteoarthritis actually are symptomatic. Analogous to gout, it is the inflammatory response within the joint, which, by releasing prostaglandins and inflammatory lysozymes, causes much of the pain. Our major objective in treating the osteoarthritic patient is to relieve pain.

Management by the Family Physician. A basic approach to providing pain relief in most patients with osteoarthritis is to decrease the inflammatory intra-articular response. This may merely require rest and aspirin, our first line of treatment. Simmons and Chrisman (1965) have shown the beneficial effect of sodium salicylate in inhibiting cartilage degradation and promoting reconstitution of injured articular surfaces.

Nonsteroidal anti-inflammatory medication such as indomethacin and ibuprofen are well-known to the family physician as the second line of defense against disabling joint pain. Steroidal treatment has a definite place as well in managing osteoarthritis. Intra-articular injections of triamcinolone or similar steroidal preparations, when used judiciously, can provide significant relief of arthritic pain. We continue to use this joint injection technique intermittently. However, we do not inject a weight-bearing joint more than three times a year. Intra-articular cortisone injections are most effective in non-weight-bearing joints such as the thumb metacarpal or carpometacarpal joints, the elbow, or the shoulder (Fig. 49–60).

Physical modalities are frequently overlooked in the medical management of early symptomatic arthritis. They can effectively diminish joint loading by using walking aids at night or on weekends. This is particularly ideal for relief of acute arthritic flare-ups.

Orthoses or braces offer another mechanical means for unloading painful weight-bearing joints. The patellar-tendon-bearing orthosis (PTB), which we have mentioned in the treatment of diabetic joint disease, has been particularly helpful for unloading symptomatic arthritic ankles (Fig. 49–61). Knee braces may also be useful, particularly for the patient whose pain results from ligamentous stretching of the unstable knee.

One of the most common areas where bracing can relieve arthritic pain symptoms is in the spine. Older patients whose spine has become unstable because of arthritic degeneration of the intravertebral and facet joints frequently experience symptoms of spinal claudication. This is due to the fact that the back hurts with any prolonged standing or walking as a result of dural impingement by the narrowed lumbar spine. Frequently, these patients obtain relief only by lying down with the lumbar spine flexed. This contrasts with claudication symptoms from ischemia, which can be relieved by sitting or standing still. Lumbar arthritic symptoms can frequently be improved by flexion jackets made of light plastic material. These jackets maintain lumbar flexion and allow the patient to walk comfortably without impingement on the sensitive dura.

Exercise can be of definite therapeutic benefit if done to relieve joint contracture. For example, the patient who walks with his knee flexed because of a 15-degree flexion contracture at least doubles the load he must carry on the knee. This is due to muscles constantly firing and loading the joint to prevent the knee from buckling. Effective therapy of an arthritic knee must work to eliminate such flexion contractures. Advise the patient not to sleep with a pillow under the knee, since this only adds to the flexion deformity. When the patient sits, recommend that he sit with the leg out on another chair and the knee maximally extended. He can then use gravity to work for further extension and also actively contract the quadriceps in the extended position to stretch the posterior capsule and hamstrings.

In the hip, the common deformity to deal with is adduction and flexion. Such contractures concentrate loading on a narrow area of articular cartilage and accelerate joint breakdown.

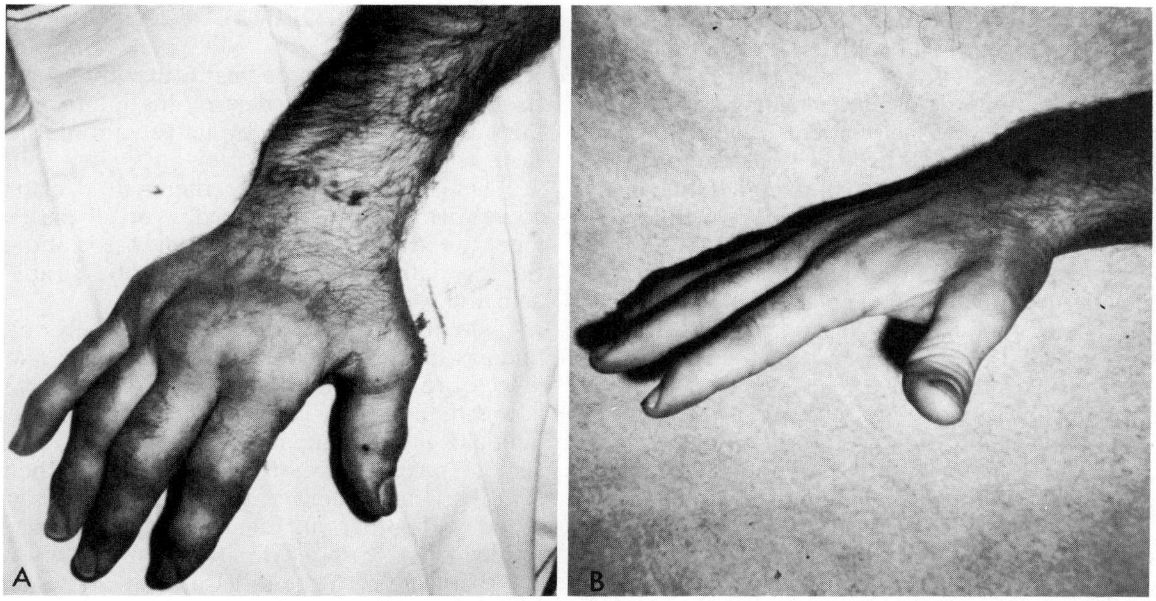

Figure 49–60. *A*, This patient had considerable pain and stiffening in the small MP joints of his hand as a result of early synovitis. The synovitis was treated with a series of three intra-articular injections into all of the joints using cortisone preparations as described in the text. *B*, Synovitis cleared rapidly after a series of three cortisone injections, and mobility returned to near normal.

Exercises that range the hip passively using a skateboard or a stationary bicycle help distribute loading across the articular surfaces. Swimming is another excellent form of exercise therapy that can be prescribed for the arthritic patient without fear of overloading the diseased joints. By employing these well-proven therapies, the family physician can help the arthritic patient maximize the use of his own joint systems for many months or years prior to the need for any surgical treatment.

Indications for Reconstructive Joint Surgery. The ultimate mechanical solution to the arthritic problem is total joint replacement. Although this has proved to be a very useful technique, it is only a halfway solution to the problem of arthritis. The main indication is to relieve pain unresponsive to other therapies. Artificial joints, like any mechanical device, carry a risk of mechanical failure. The present estimate is that at least 20 per cent of total hips can be expected to produce symptoms from loosening within 5 years after operation. Newer methods and techniques are being developed to diminish this complication rate, but mechanical failure will be intrinsic to any mechanistic approach.

Joint replacements offer dramatic relief in many patients so they tend to be recommended too freely. A total joint arthroplasty should not be recommended for a person who is grossly overweight. The active young individual who is apt to abuse the joint once he is relieved of the pain should also be considered a poor candidate for total joint replacement. The middle-aged man with mild genu varum and a knee ache,

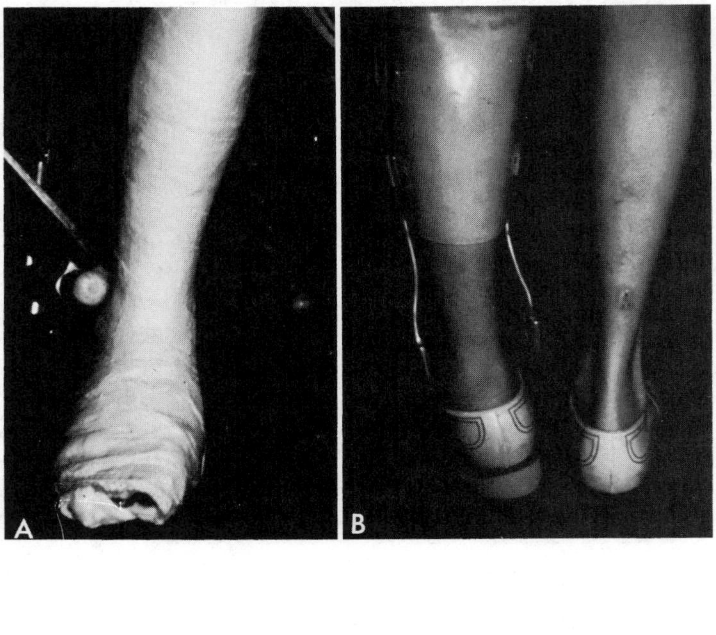

Figure 49–61. *A*, This diabetic patient with neurotrophic fractures of her foot and ankle can be treated by well-padded, protective casts until the acute fractures subside. *B*, A weight-bearing orthosis can then be used to shift the weight off the neurotrophic foot and ankle to the proximal tibia.

moderately symptomatic after 18 holes of golf or 2 hours of racquetball, should also not be considered for joint replacement. Other simple treatment modalities such as swimming or bicycle riding should be given a complete trial by such patients.

Other procedures such as high tibial osteotomy can be recommended for the active patient with early arthritic symptoms. In our experience, when employed for a limited arthritis of the joint, this can provide good pain relief in 80 per cent or more of patients without artificial joint replacement (Fig. 49–62*A*, *B*). The technique shifts the weight load from the diseased medial joint space over toward the more lateral side of the joint.

A previous history of joint infection is no longer considered an absolute contraindication to arthroplasty. A history of gram-negative sepsis does provide a caution light. Careful assessment of the joint for active infection based on sedimentation rate, bone scanning, and joint biopsy or aspiration can determine whether a total joint arthroplasty is likely to become infected. New techniques, such as biologic fixation and those incorporating an antibiotic into the cement, can permit reconstructive arthroplasty despite a previous but inactive joint infection.

The family physician can aid his patients with osteoarthritis quite effectively by selecting and timing the appropriate medical, physical, and surgical therapies. He should be cognizant of the indications and contraindications for various modalities of treatment, including surgery, and should keep in mind that total joint replacement is not the only, nor always the most effective, solution to arthritic pain symptoms.

RHEUMATOID ARTHRITIS

Rheumatoid arthritis begins in the joint's synovium. Its ultimate effect is to destroy the joint surfaces and the supporting ligaments by actively proliferating synovitis.

Diagnostic criteria for rheumatoid arthritis are constantly being re-evaluated. Not all patients who meet the American Rheumatism Association's criteria for definite rheumatoid arthritis (Table 49–5) actually prove to have the disease.

Do not hinge the diagnosis on merely one or two findings, particularly laboratory findings. The prevalence of rheumatoid arthritis in adults under 35 years is less than 0.3 per cent. This figure increases exponentially in subsequent decades and exceeds 10 per cent in patients over 65 years of age. Rheumatoid arthritis is infrequent in young adult males, as compared with other inflammatory arthritides, particularly ankylosing spondylitis.

The course of the disease is always variable and difficult to predict at its onset. A positive serum rheumatoid factor and bone erosive changes on x-ray imply poor prognosis. As a general rule, one third will have some functional limitation, and one third will become severely handicapped (see Tables 49–6 and 49–7). These statistics may not be entirely comforting to the patient, but they indicate that a majority of patients with rheumatoid arthritis do not, in fact, become severely crippled. The possibility of severe crippling should not be passed over lightly. Chronic rheumatoid arthritis is a very disabling and debilitating disease and needs constant care.

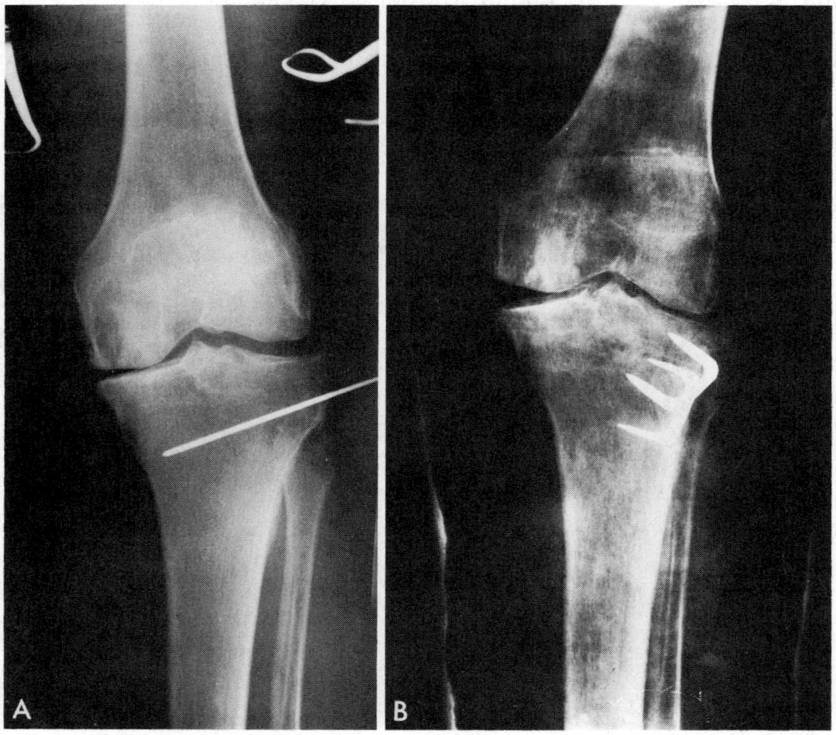

Figure 49–62. *A,* This is an intraoperative roentgenogram showing typical arthritic changes in the medial joint space but relative preservation of the lateral joint space of the knee. *B,* The high tibial osteotomy corrected the weight-bearing alignment and shifted the load of the knee toward the lateral side of the joint.

Table 49–5. RHEUMATOID ARTHRITIS DIAGNOSTIC CRITERIA (A.R.A. 1958 REVISION)

1. Morning stiffness
2. Pain on motion or tenderness in at least one joint
3. Swelling (soft tissue thickening of fluid, not bony overgrowth alone) in at least one joint
4. Swelling of at least one other joint
5. Symmetrical joint swelling with simultaneous involvement of the same joint on both sides of the body; terminal phalangeal joint involvement will not satisfy the criterion
6. Subcutaneous nodules over bony prominences, on extensor surfaces, or in juxta-articular regions
7. Roentgenographic changes typical of rheumatoid arthritis (which must include at least bony decalcification localized to or greatest around the involved joints and not just degenerative changes)
8. Positive agglutination (anti-gammaglobulin) test
9. Poor mucin precipitate from synovial fluid (with shreds and cloudy solution)
10. Characteristic histologic changes in synovial membrane
11. Characteristic histologic changes in nodules

Categories	Number of Criteria Required	Minimum Duration of Continuous Symptoms
Classic	7 of 11	Six weeks (Nos. 1–5)
Definite	5 of 11	Six weeks (Nos. 1–5)
Probable	3 of 11	Six weeks (one of Nos. 1–5)

Management by the Family Physician. The following is a brief outline of therapy based particularly on the American Rheumatism Association's Functional Class and Anatomic Stages of Disease (Tables 49–6 and 49–7). These serve as helpful comparative tools for the family practitioner to select therapy and to evaluate response.

The aims of treatment are to (a) educate the patient and his family; (b) relieve pain; (c) suppress inflammation; and (d) prevent or correct deformities promptly.

Treatment should be problem oriented, and the physician should know the patient, the past treatment and response to therapy, and any complications or coexisting disease, including allergies, gastrointestinal diseases, renal diseases, hepatic diseases, infection, and altered immunities.

Stage I, Class I Patients. The single most important element in the management of rheumatoid arthritis is patient education. Remind the patient that symptoms do remit and fluctuate from day to day. Help with the patient's psychologic adjustment. Advise reasonable rest and salicylates to control pain and encourage moderate, simple exercise therapy for these patients. Carefully observe for progressive deformities of the hands and feet.

Rheumatoid arthritis is primarily a disease of the small joints of the hands and feet. Intrinsic muscle tightness in the hands produces an unbalanced pull, which eventually dislocates the MP joints and subsequently stiffens the PIP joints (Fig. 49–63).

Table 49–6. AMERICAN RHEUMATISM ASSOCIATION FUNCTIONAL CLASS

Class	Function
I	Complete ability to carry on all usual duties without handicaps
II	Adequate for normal activities despite handicap of discomfort or limited motion at one or more joints
III	Limited only to little or none of duties of usual occupation or self-care
IV	Incapacitated, largely or wholly bedridden or confined to wheelchair; little or no self-care

Table 49–7. AMERICAN RHEUMATISM ASSOCIATION ANATOMIC STAGES

Stage I, Early
- *1. No destructive changes roentgenologically
- 2. Roentgenologic evidence of osteoporosis may be present

Stage II, Moderate
- *1. Roentgenologic evidence of osteoporosis, with or without slight bone destruction; slight cartilage destruction may be present
- *2. No joint deformities, although limitation of joint mobility may be present
- 3. Adjacent muscle atrophy
- 4. Extra-articular soft tissue lesions, such as nodules and tenovaginitis, may be present

Stage III, Severe
- *1. Roentgenologic evidence of cartilage and bone destruction, in addition to osteoporosis
- *2. Joint deformity, such as subluxation, ulnar deviation, or hyperextension, without fibrous or bony ankylosis
- 3. Extensive muscle atrophy
- 4. Extra-articular soft tissue lesions, such as nodules and tenovaginitis, may be present

Stage IV, Terminal
- *1. Fibrous or bony ankylosis
- 2. Criteria of Stage III

*The criteria prefaced by an asterisk are those that must be present to permit classification of a patient in any particular stage or grade.

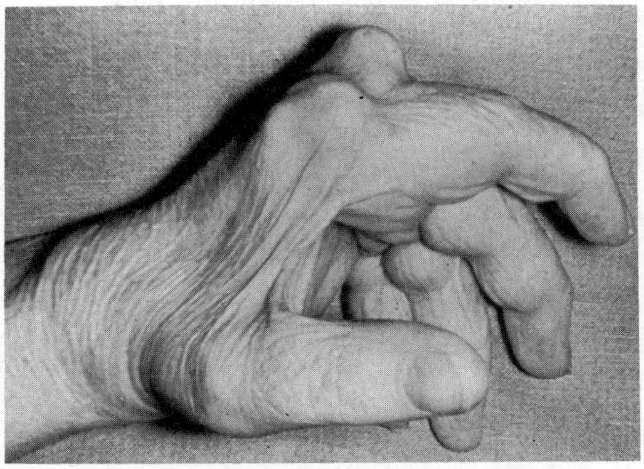

Figure 49–63. Long-standing rheumatoid arthritis destroys the metacarpophalangeal joints and produces volar subluxation of the MP joints and stiffening of the PIP joints. Of major concern is progressive deformity of the thumb, which may become superimposed on the severe finger deformities.

Test for tightness and intrinsic muscles that are the flexors of the MP joints and extensors of the IP joints by reversing the position of these joints. That is, if you hold the MP joint extended in a normal finger, the patient should still have the ability to flex the distal interphalangeal (DIP) joint. If the patient's intrinsic muscles are tight, however, the stretching of the tendons of the MP joint prevents any flexion of the DIP joint.

A useful exercise when intrinsic muscle tightness first becomes evident is to have the patient hold a block in his hand to keep the MP joints extended. By trying to grip around the block the patient stretches out the tight intrinsics by active function of the extrinsic flexors, particularly the profundi, which tend not to be as severely involved as the intrinsic muscles.

Always carefully evaluate the feet of your rheumatoid patient just as you would for your diabetic patient. Simple methods such as metatarsal bars and appropriately placed pads in shoes can afford the rheumatoid patient considerable relief from common foot symptoms. Surgical correction should be recommended promptly for symptomatic bunions, clawtoes, or arthritis of the hindfoot. Do not allow concern for the large joints of the body to overshadow real problems in the small joints.

Stage II, Class II Patients. These patients require the same basic regimen of therapy and anti-inflammatory drugs as do the patients in the early stages and classes. Our observation has been that gold therapy should be introduced at this level. It need not be reserved because of excessive concern about side effects.

Gold is our present treatment of choice for rheumatoid arthritis. One should not wait for severe deformities before using this in a rheumatoid patient, any more than one would wait for permanent joint destruction before using penicillin to treat gonococcal arthritis. Between 60 to 70 per cent of patients treated with gold experience suppression of their inflammatory symptoms without significant side effects.

The few contraindications to gold therapy include previous toxicity or allergies to gold as well as kidney or liver disease. Leukopenia has been recognized as a complication, but this and the anemia of rheumatoid arthritis may improve on gold therapy.

Other therapeutic agents, including antimalarial and penicillamines, may be used if the patient cannot be given gold.

However, we as orthopedic surgeons strongly encourage the family physician and rheumatologist to use the most effective medication for the rheumatoid patient before the disease progresses to destruction of the joints, necessitating orthopedic reconstruction.

Stage III, Class III Patients. These patients demand continued vigorous therapy. We have found particularly that steroids can be of value here, not so much when given systemically but when injected intra-articularly (Fig. 49–60). These intra-articular injections should be given over a month's time at biweekly intervals. Each inflamed joint should be injected separately with a small 25-gauge needle. In essence, this provides a chemical synovectomy, which we have found particularly valuable in the small joints of the hand.

If synovitis persists and remains unresponsive to chemical synovectomy and to systemic medical treatment for more than 6 months, advise surgical synovectomy. Stage III and Stage IV disease particularly demands contributions by the orthopedic surgeon in cooperation with the family physician or rheumatologist before the patient advances unnecessarily to a functional Class IV. Most family physicians are quite familiar with the frequently dramatic pain relief following total hip replacement in the rheumatoid patient. Many are unaware of or inattentive to problems in the small joints, particularly the hand and foot, that are equally amenable to appropriate treatment.

Some deformities in particular may be allowed to pass without adequate correction. The patient then progresses rapidly to a state at which she must hold cups or glasses with both hands in order to drink (Fig. 49–63). Correction of the deformities in the thumb joints, although seemingly a minor undertaking to offer your patients, can provide significant functional improvement.

Deformities of the thumb rank with foot problems as causes of persistent symptoms that can be readily alleviated by your prompt attention.

A final area that tends to be undertreated or underrecognized in the rheumatoid patient is the cervical spine. This may frequently become of life-threatening significance. Synovitis attacks ligaments in the first and second cervical vertebrae (Fig. 49–64). About 5 per cent of these rheumatoid patients actually go on to cord injury and myelopathy as a result of the cervical spine instability. Keep this possibility in mind when your rheumatoid patient suddenly complains of weakness in the arms or legs. Generalized weakness is usually due to neurologic complications rather than to worsening of the rheumatoid process.

Be careful to evaluate by flexion-extension x-ray any rheumatoid patient who is to undergo surgical procedures. We were consulted on two patients in whom the unfortunate complication of quadriparesis could have been avoided if the rheumatoid disease of the cervical spine had been recognized and the cervical instability anticipated before induction of anesthesia.

Rheumatoid arthritis then is a long-term problem that can be effectively managed by the family physician, particularly one who perceives the progressive functional and anatomic nature of the disease, is aware of appropriate therapies for each stage, and appreciates indications as well as contraindications for surgical management.

SEPTIC ARTHRITIS

The unfortunate end result illustrated in Figure 49–1, which introduced this chapter, was, in the prean-

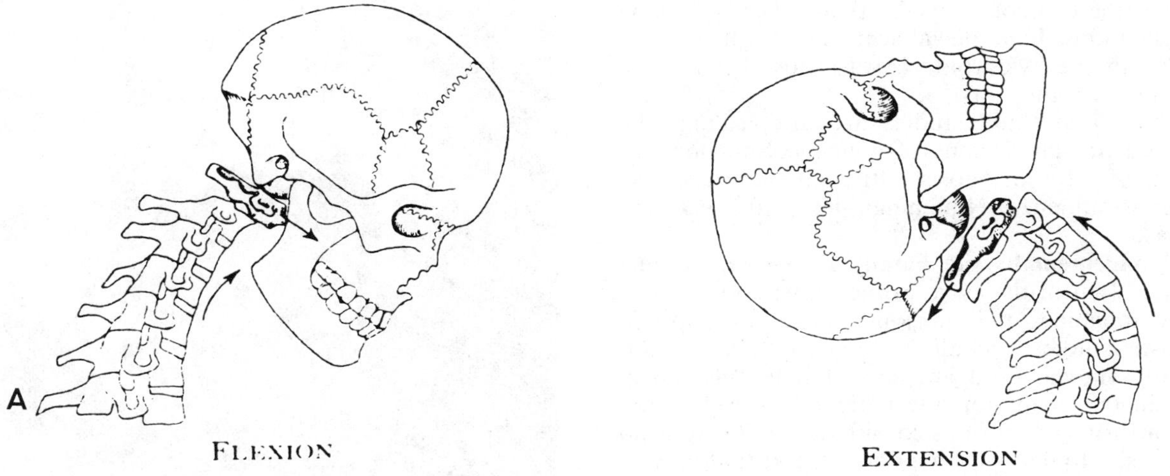

Figure 49–64. *A,* Rheumatoid arthritis commonly causes anteroposterior C1-C2 instability in the chronic patient. This should be evaluated by flexion-extension x-ray films prior to endotracheal intubation. *B,* A less frequent complication is upward migration of the odontoid through the base of the skull, producing cranial nerve symptoms.

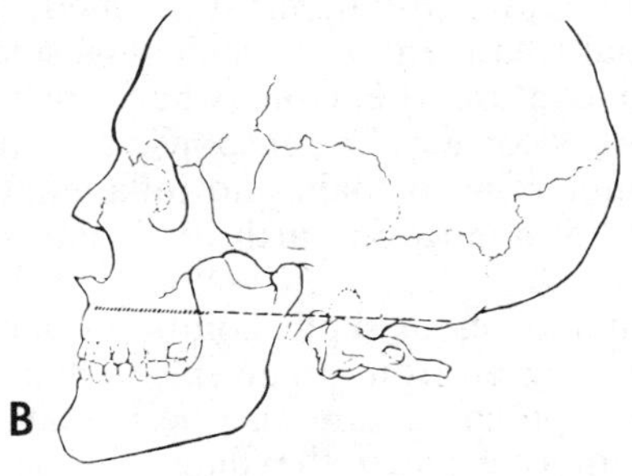

tibiotic era, the norm following joint infection. Mortality from acute osteomyelitis and joint infections frequently exceeded 30 per cent in the 1930's and 1940's.

No development in orthopedics has produced more significant benefit to patients than has the effective treatment of septic arthritis and osteomyelitis. Many senior physicians can well remember orthopedic wards filled with patients suffering both acute and chronic symptoms of bone and joint infections.

Septic arthritis and associated osteomyelitis as we see them today usually develop from direct penetration of the joint, as illustrated by Figure 40–1, from an open fracture, or by spread from contiguous infection such as a diabetic foot or a pressure sore in a paralyzed patient. The source of septic joint from hematogenous spread that we see most commonly today is gonococcal arthritis.

It is essential that the family physician appreciate these different etiologies of septic arthritis. Some infections, such as those produced by direct penetration of the joint or associated with an open fracture or spread from a contiguous infection, require prompt surgical drainage. Others, particularly those produced by hematogenous spread as from gonococcal infection, do not usually require surgical drainage.

Gonococcal Arthritis and Other Joint Infections Not Requiring Surgical Drainage

The gonococcus appears to have an unusually strong affinity for synovial tissue when gonococcemia occurs. Most patients are in the second or third decades, but newborn infants as well as elderly patients have been infected. The joint infection usually occurs 1 to 2 weeks after the urethritis, but as long as the individual is carrying the gonococcus in the genitourinary tract or rectal mucosa, spread to the joints is possible.

With gonococcemia characteristic skin lesions also develop. These are small hemorrhagelike spots 5 to 6 mm. in diameter with 1 to 2 mm. central necrosis.

Erythematous inflammation around tendon sheaths, particularly in the heel, is characteristic of the condition. The individual with gonococcal arthritis usually presents with severe discomfort and a good deal more local pain to touch than do other patients with inflamed joints, except those with gout.

The major differentials when there is multiple joint involvement include acute rheumatic fever, infectious hepatitis B, and systemic lupus. In male patients, Reiter's syndrome must also be considered. Monoarticular involvement brings gout and pseudogout into the differential conditions.

The diagnosis depends on blood or joint fluid cultures of gonococcus. A positive culture from the genitourinary tract does not necessarily make the diagnosis of gonococcal arthritis in the absence of a positive blood or joint culture. The organism is relatively fastidious, and the joint fluid should be cultured immediately after aspiration.

Most synovial fluid cell counts with gonococcal arthritis are over 50,000 per mm.[3] However, take care that the cell count on the synovial fluid is done properly and without glacial acetic acid, which, when mixed with the hyaluronidase of synovial fluid, will precipitate out the cells.

When joint fluid studies are unrevealing, the characteristic skin lesions of gonococcemia may be quite helpful for diagnosis, although these are also seen in H-influenza, N-meningitides, and other septicemias.

Management by the Family Physician. Suspect gonococcal arthritis as a prime possibility in any acutely inflamed, painful joint. After appropriate diagnostic studies, including blood cultures and cultures of synovial fluid and any skin lesions, begin penicillin treatment for any patient in whom gonococcal arthritis is a serious consideration. There is no good reason to delay for a culture report that may or may not be positive.

Withhold anti-inflammatory medications during the initial treatment with penicillin, since these only tend to confuse the issue when your presumptive diagnosis is correct. The response to penicillin should be prompt relief of pain and inflammation. Surgical drainage of gonococcal arthritis is almost always unnecessary.

Other types of septic joints produced by hematogenous spread from organisms such as staphylococcus or streptococcus are also best treated by intravenous antibiotic when the diagnosis has been made promptly. The antibiotics should be administered in high doses and by intravenous route to ensure adequate blood and synovial fluid levels. Surgical drainage is not ordinarily necessary for the usual septic knee, in a child, which has been recognized and treated promptly and monitored closely. Knee aspiration should be performed repeatedly to determine the response to therapy as indicated by diminution in synovial fluid cell count. The synovial fluid represents dialysate of blood, and in most instances, antibiotic levels in the joint approach those in the blood. However, if the septic joint does not respond within 48 hours of adequate parenteral therapy, advise prompt surgical drainage.

Joint Infections Requiring Surgical Drainage

Although certain joint infections such as gonococcal arthritis and staphylococcus and streptococcus infections in the knee can be treated successfully by high-dose parenteral antibiotics, other infections, owing to their notorious effect on joints, demand surgical drainage.

Septic arthritis of the hip is one such joint infection for which prompt surgical drainage is essential (Fig. 49–65). Pus accumulating in the hip joint space rapidly displaces and then dislocates the young infant's hip. The common result is permanent deformity after the childhood infection resolves.

Diagnosis of the septic hip joint should be made first by aspirating pus from the hip. When a positive hip aspirate is obtained, surgical drainage should be carried out as soon as the patient can tolerate anesthetic. The capsule should be opened widely for adequate decompression and the hip maintained in extended position until the infection has been controlled.

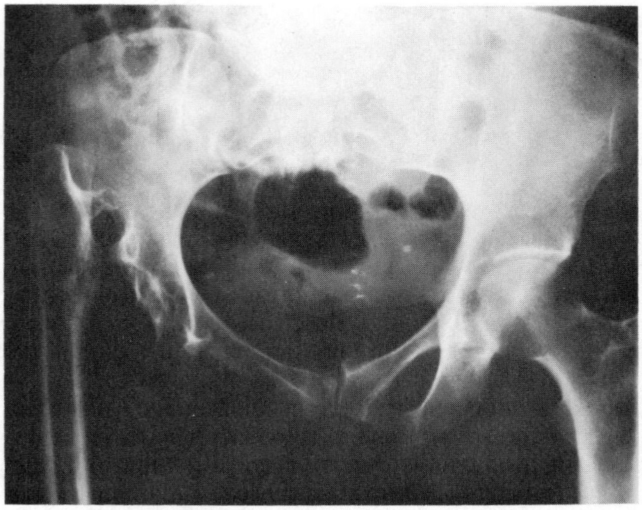

Figure 49–65. The residual effect of a septic joint in infancy resulted in this severely destroyed hip joint in the adult. (Courtesy of Dr. Walter W. Huurman, Department of Orthopaedic Surgery, University of Nebraska Medical Center, Omaha, Nebraska.)

Other infected joints that mandate prompt surgical drainage include those with a pre-existing chronic synovitis that prevents adequate antibiotic penetration. This is particularly true in the rheumatoid patient or the patient with chronic arthritis of the joint. Although virtually all antibiotics penetrate synovial membranes and reach therapeutic levels in joints equivalent to blood levels, if a tense, undrained effusion limits antibiotic access, the joint then becomes essentially a walled-off abscess rather than a true joint. This should be treated like an abscess anywhere in the body.

Certain gram-negative infections such as those seen in drug addicts or in patients with poor circulation owing to sicklemia require open drainage more promptly than do the more usual gram-positive infections.

Joints that become infected postoperatively or even many years after arthroplasty require prompt drainage if the artificial joint is to be salvaged. Hematogenous spread from the genitourinary tract to a previously satisfactorily functioning joint has occurred 2 or more years postoperatively in our observation.

Consequently, prophylactic antibiotics should be administered during any manipulative procedure, such as a tooth extraction or cystoscopy, that might cause bacterial septicemia and risk hematogenous infection of the prosthetic joint.

Back Problems

Back pain is responsible for vast numbers of patient visits, lost time, a large number of operations, and great amounts of litigation. About 120,000 discectomies are done per year, and many of these could be prevented by a knowledgeable primary care physician.

The spinal column is a chain of vertebrae stacked upon one another and held together by a ligamentous and muscular complex. There are essentially 24 vertebrae and the sacrum and coccyx of fused elements with interposed discs, two facet joints with interposed ligaments, and a neural foramen between the vertebrae.

A number of the concepts presented in this section were gleaned from the thoughtful contribution of James Cyriax. He has been generous in teaching his concepts and techniques at the University of Nebraska as well as other North American centers.

We strongly recommend careful study of Cyriax's publications to all physicians who treat problems of the spine. Lower back pain can be caused by disorders of any of the structures making up the spinal column complex as well as problems remote to the spine (see Table 49–8).

A fairly large percentage of back pain results from degenerative disc disease particularly at the L4-L5-S1 levels. Only a small percentage is noted above this level. Thus, when making a diagnosis of disc pain at higher levels, we must look hard for other causes such as malignancy, disc space infection, or trauma.

The cervical and lumbar spine are highly mobile and hence are prone to disc herniation at the C7, T1, and L4-L5-S1 levels where flexion-extension loads are concentrated. Most vertical (up and down) loading is absorbed by the annulus fibrosus, the casing of the disc (Fig. 49–66).

Table 49–8. DIFFERENTIAL OF ETIOLOGIC FACTORS IN BACK PAIN

1. Tumors
   a. Benign (such as meningiomas, neuromas, osteoid osteomas, Paget's disease)
   b. Malignant—primary bone or neural tumors and metastatic
2. Trauma
   a. Acute sprain or strain
   b. Chronic sprain or strain
   c. Fractures
   d. Subluxed facet (facet syndrome)
   e. Spondylolisthesis with strain
3. Toxicities from heavy metals
4. Congenital asymmetries of facets or transitional vertebrae
5. Metabolic disorders—osteoporosis or osteomalacia
6. Inflammatory arthritis—rheumatoid and Marie-Strümpell's disease
7. Infections, acute and chronic
8. Degenerative disc or facet disease
9. Mechanical disturbance
   a. Poor muscle tone
   b. Poor posture
   c. Unstable vertebrae
   d. Scoliosis (severe)
10. Extrinsic disease such as aortic aneurysm, uterine fibroids, prostate disease, hip disease, etc.
11. Psychologic to include hysteria, malingering, and acute remunerative spinal pain (Green-Poultice disease)

When this structure is torn it may allow the degenerated content of the nucleus pulposus to impinge on sensitive adjacent structures. This will result in back pain of lumbago or low back pain without radiation down the legs.

Rupture of the annulus may also allow the central pulpy material to work out and impinge on the nerve structures located lateral to the disc. The result is a neurogenic pain or sciatica radiating down the leg. (This should be distinguished from the lumbago produced by the central protrusion.) The roots usually involved in sciatica are those that exit below the level of the disc herniation, i.e., L5 root with L4-L5 disc herniation and S1 root with the L5-S1 herniation (Fig. 49–67).

The mechanism of disc rupture, either from a tear of the annulus or from nuclear displacement, is quite consistently a twist with the lumbar spine flexed. This may result as the patient simply bends forward over a sink to brush his teeth. Flexion makes the lumbar spine vulnerable because it produces lumbar kyphosis with subsequent gap in the posterior aspect of the intervertebral joint (Fig. 49–68*A*).

The body weight in the flexed position forces the intervertebral joint contents posteriorly. This contrasts with the normal position of lumbar lordosis, which narrows down the posterior aspect of the disc space (Fig. 49–68*B*).

Pain is produced by pressure on the sensitive dural sleeve that surrounds the root for about 2 cm. as it exits the canal. A peripheral nerve itself is quite insensitive to pressure as anyone knows who has sat on a hard theater seat for a few hours. Compression of the peripheral nerve characteristically produces paresthesias, or pins and needles, distal to the compression (see also the section on Carpal Tunnel Syndrome).

Any stretching of an entrapped dural sleeve with peripheral disc herniation produces a sharp radiating pain down the leg, frequently to the foot or ankle. In the absence of such positive nerve stretch symptoms, the diagnosis of disc herniation is not likely.

The other type of dural pain, i.e., lumbago, is associated with a central herniation, which also causes pain by stretching the dura. This dural pain may not follow any consistent pattern of reference in contrast with that associated with the peripheral dural and nerve root entrapment. Pain from central entrapment of the dura can be referred anywhere in the body between the waist and the feet. These sites include the anterior abdominal wall, where the pain can be mistaken for appendicitis or an ovarian cyst. Entrapment may produce pain radiating into the groin, much like a hernia, or up the trunk toward the thorax, or down in the perineum toward the testicles or the coccyx. Pain from a central disc protrusion stretching dura is a great mimic and must always be considered with the diagnosis of atypical abdominal, perineal, or thigh symptoms.

A useful technique for identifying nondescript dural pain is an epidural anesthetic, which distin-

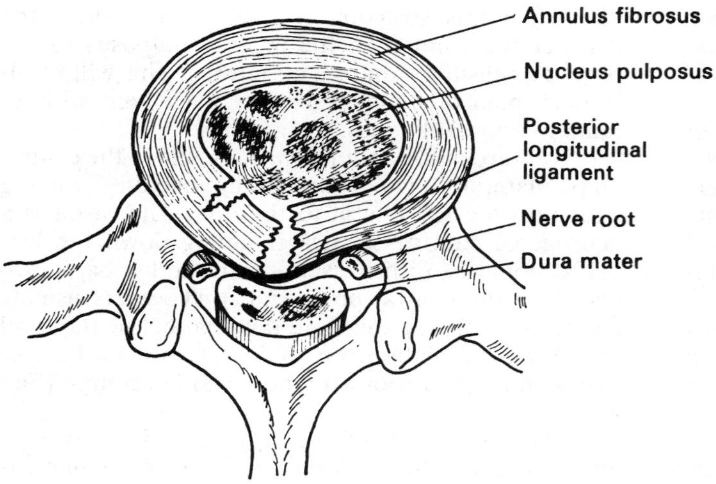

Figure 49–66. The disc structure includes an outer fibrocartilaginous annulus fibrosus and an inner, more fluid nucleus pulposus. Either of these structures may rupture and produce either lumbago or sciatica. (Cyriax, J.: Orthopaedic Medicine. Vol. 1. London, Cassell Ltd., 1978.)

guishes the discogenic pain from its numerous differentials. We will discuss this technique more fully toward the end of this section.

MISLEADING CONCEPTS OF BACK PAIN

Unfortunately the diagnosis of disc disease has been considerably confused by terms such as myofascial strain, trigger points, and muscle spasm. The terms trigger points and myofascial syndrome have been manufactured because of poor appreciation of the unpredictable radiation of dural pain.

Muscle spasm or guarding, although characteristically evident with acute disc herniation, represents the body's response to the deep source of its pain, i.e., the dural stretch. The patient must rigidly position himself to prevent inadvertently stretching the nerve sheath or dura. Consequently he will list to one side or the other so that the paraspinal muscles become tight. These tight muscles no more deserve treatment than do the tight abdominal muscles found with acute appendicitis. It is the deep source of the patient's pain from the impingement that requires treatment.

DIAGNOSTIC CONSIDERATIONS

History of Onset

Other causes of backache can literally range from "A" (ankylosing spondylitis) to "Z" (herpes zoster). Tumors, both primary and secondary; infections; and vascular disorders are particularly important differentials to be considered. To diagnose the common cause of back problems, ie., disc disease, effectively and with reasonable assurance of not overlooking other causes, a systematic approach is absolutely essential. We must listen to and examine the backache patient as carefully as we would the patient with chest pain.

The patient's presenting history of symptoms may vary considerably because of the nature of the disc lesion, which can be either a cartilaginous loose body or a fluid gelatinous leak. The first type of lesion, the loose cartilage from the annulus, produces a sensation of the back's suddenly going out. This usually occurs with a "click" as the patient moves into a flexed position and experiences a sharp pain. However, the annulus may also slowly bulge out and cause backache only after the patient stands for long

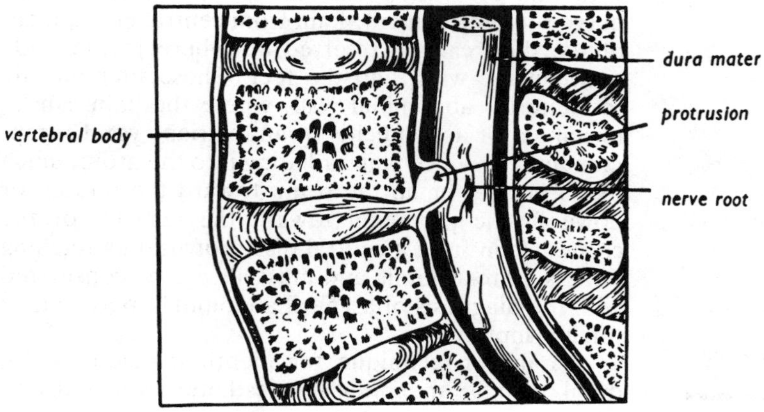

Figure 49–67. Herniation of the nucleus pulposus through the tear in the annulus produces a collar stud abscess type of herniation that does not reduce spontaneously the way a moveable cartilaginous displacement reduces. (Cyriax, J.: Orthopaedic Medicine. Vol. 1. London, Cassell Ltd., 1978.)

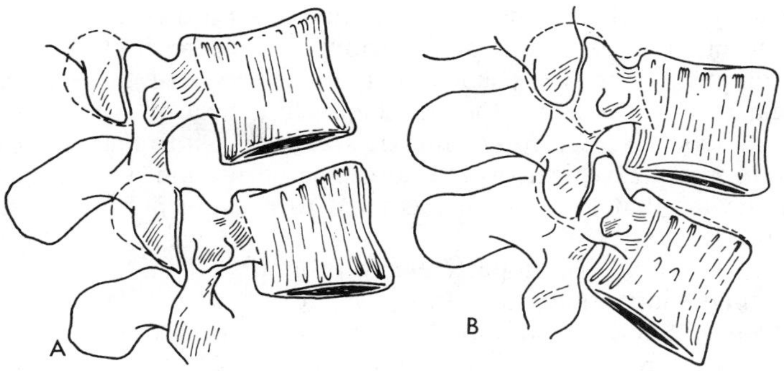

Figure 49–68. *A*, Flexion of the lumbar spine produces most disc protrusions and herniations. When the spine is flexed forward in the standing position, the disc space is opened posteriorly and the cartilaginous portion of the annulus is pushed back toward the spinal canal. This may cause the lumbago associated with prolonged standing in this flexed position. *B*, With the lumbar spine in lordotic position, the disc space closes posteriorly. Treatment for lumbago should be directed, therefore, at increasing lumbar lordosis. (Cyriax, J.: Orthopaedic Medicine. Vol. 1. London, Cassell Ltd., 1978.)

periods in a slightly flexed position. Individuals who stand during work are quite familiar with this particular pain, which can be generally relieved by hyperextending the lumbar spine.

The second type of lesion, the slow leak of the nuclear material, alters the patient's history considerably. Leakage of the nucleus pulposus past the annulus results in a large mass that slowly pushes out through its narrow tract to impinge on the dura, much like a collar-stud abscess (see Fig. 49–67). For example, the patient may give a history of working in the garden, following which he experiences a slight backache. The next day, however, he cannot get out of bed because of severe pain down the leg rather than in the back. This indicates that the nucleus pulposus has pushed through the torn annulus and is impinging on the dural sleeve around the nerve root rather than the central part of the canal.

The persistent location of this type of herniated pulpy nucleus is in the posterolateral aspect of the intervertebral joint, the weakest part of the system. This is due to the strong posterior longitudinal ligament, which is centrally located and turns the disc to one side or the other. The dural sleeve is most exposed to entrapment by the disc at this location. The universal symptoms of pain down the leg then are from stretching of the dural sleeve. Such a peripheral herniation may not initially be sufficiently large to affect nerve conduction, and no neurologic deficit may be evident.

The motor and sensory components of the root emerge separately. Impingement from above impairs sensory conduction. As the disc material moves farther laterally on the peripheral nerve, it moves away from the sensitive dural sleeve and consequently the pain diminishes as the neurologic deficit worsens. Frequently the patient notices that when foot drop occurs the sharp pain down the leg goes away.

Factors Affecting History. Comprehending the variations and permutations in pathology is essential to appreciate the possible variations in the patient's history. A common symptom indicating dural irritation is pain on coughing or sneezing; this, however, is not pathognomonic for disc disease. Neural tumors and occasionally sacroiliac joint disease may also be aggravated by sudden changes induced by coughing.

The position that brings on the back symptoms also reflects disc pathology. Nachemson and Morris (1964) directly measured pressures in the disc space of volunteers and found that the greatest load occurs in the seated position. Pressures measured while seated were 30 per cent higher than those measured in the standing position and 50 per cent over those with the subject lying down. The detrimental effect of inadequate sitting posture without lumbar lordosis (Fig. 49–68) is quite understandable. The increased load of sitting and the inadequate lumbar lordosis push disc material posteriorly in the disc space. Simultaneously, the space itself is open posteriorly, encouraging protrusion.

Older patients suffering from disc disease associated with asymmetric narrowing of the spinal canal characteristically develop back symptoms during walking. This has been called "spinal claudication" but differs from the claudication of vascular origin in that the patient must lie down to relieve the pain. Vascular claudication, on the contrary, is relieved by any kind of rest in any position. The back pain produced by walking in the elderly patient only remits when the sensitive dura is no longer stretched by the stenotic canal. The discogenic pain can be aggravated or even produced by sitting and is relieved only by the supine position.

Considerations in Physical Assessment

Observe the patient's entry, undressing, and movement to the exam table as well as body habitus, posture, and obvious deformities.

Proceed with examination of leg length, ability to walk on heel and toe, pelvic obliquity, and any listing or flexion. Check also the site of pain and extent of pain radiation as well as active flexion, extension, rotation, and side-to-side motion. With the patient supine proceed to examine the true leg length (anterior superior spine to medial malleolus). Check all hip movements to see if hip disease is present as well as the straight-leg-raising test. Examine the abdomen for tumor, aneurysm, gall bladder tenderness, and such. While the patient is sitting do a brief neurologic examination of motor power reflexes and sensory changes. Measure calf and thigh for atrophy. Last, do a rectal on both sexes and a pelvic examination on female patients.

The combination of a good history before examination and then an examination as outlined will usually give the diagnosis. Additional laboratory data and plain x-rays in anteroposterior, lateral, and both oblique planes will usually sort out the rest of the diagnostic problems. Inspect the architecture of the patient's spine carefully while he stands. A list to one side is quite typical of an acute disc herniation and indicates that the patient has tried to prevent nerve and dural stretch.

A sciatic list is particularly pronounced in the younger individual with any L4-L5 disc lesion (Fig. 49–69). Such a list may be confused with lumbar scoliosis. Keep in mind that idiopathic scoliosis is never acutely painful by itself.

The best estimate of leg length discrepancy is made with the patient standing evenly on both legs while the physician palpates the top of the iliac crest. This allows direct visual and tactile estimation of the pelvic tilt. If one iliac crest is lower than the other, place one-quarter-inch blocks under the shorter limb until you and the patient feel the crests to be even. This technique provides the most significant information regarding leg lengths, i.e., do both legs reach the ground without causing the pelvis to tilt?

Always test muscle plantar flexion and dorsiflexion strength by having the patient balance on the tiptoes and heels.

Then proceed to test spine motion. Begin with spine extension, then lateral bending, and last, flexion, which is most likely to aggravate the patient's pain. Keep in mind that the patient leans in the direction in which the nerve root is being pushed by the disc. The disc that protrudes lateral to the nerve root, for example on the patient's right, will cause him to lean to the left. A disc that protrudes central to the nerve root on the right side will cause the patient to lean toward the side of the lesion, i.e., the right side.

A frequently observed phenomenon during spine motion is a sudden deviation to one side as the patient reaches a half-flexed position. This is a significant manifestation of a painful arc whereby the patient experiences the dura's suddenly being stretched over a protruded disc in that particular part of the flexion arc (Fig. 49–69). The patient deviates suddenly laterally in this half-flexed position and may not even be aware that he does so.

This visible alteration in spine motion occurs as a loose disc fragment suddenly shifts position when the lumbar spine passes from a lordotic to a kyphotic shape. The painful arc, therefore, is pathognomonic of a disc lesion. The other differential conditions do not produce evidence so consistently of a loose body shifting within the intervertebral joint and altering motion. Test for sensory loss by simply touching lightly and simultaneously over the patient's feet and inquiring about any differences in sensation to this slight touch stimulus. This sensory testing entirely depends on the patient's subjective response as well as his ability to answer accurately. Attempts at other sensory testing, such as pin prick or vibratory testing, equally rely on the patient's responses and are unnecessary for the usual disc evaluation.

After testing for the patterns of cutaneous dysesthesia, the next step is careful assessment of motor function, beginning with the hip and working to the toes. A useful guide to the relationship of the nerve roots to muscle function is listed in Table 49–9.

All these tests must be carried out against resistance and compared with the opposite limb function in order to detect subtle diminution of muscle strength. Careful motor testing, however, is a very useful diagnostic aid in localizing the site of the disc lesion.

A common finding may be a weakness of the big

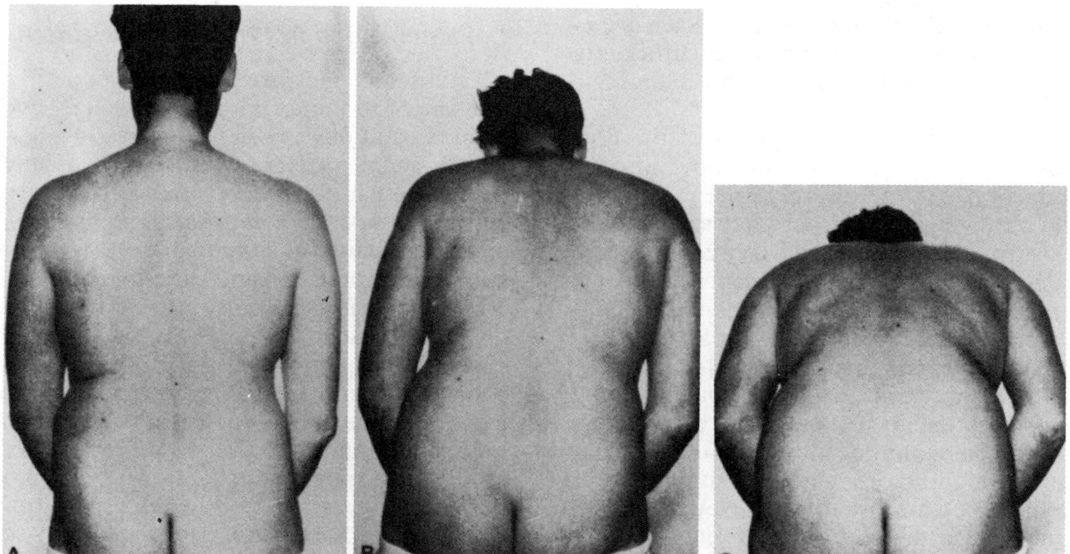

Figure 49–69. The sciatic list or a painful arc is characteristic of a herniated disc. The painful arc particularly is evident as a brief jog during certain ranges of flexion. (From Cyriax, J.: Orthopaedic Medicine. Vol. 1. London, Cassell Ltd., 1978.)

Table 49–9. LEVELS OF INNERVATION FOR MOTOR FUNCTION IN LOWER LIMBS

Nerve Level	Motor Function
L2,3	Hip Flexion
L4,5	Hip Extension
L3,4	Knee Extension
L5-S1	Knee Flexion
L4,5	Ankle Dorsiflexion
S1-S2	Ankle Plantar Flexion
L4	Foot Inversion
L5-S1	Foot Eversion

toe extensor. This should be checked for carefully, as it may indicate an L4 or L5 nerve root lesion. If the peroneal everting muscles are also weak in conjunction with a weak toe extensor, the lesion then would be at L5. If peroneal weakness is accompanied by a weak calf muscle, as seen on plantar flexion, the conclusion would then be an S1 nerve root lesion is involved. Weakness of the anterior tibial muscle most often indicates an L4 root lesion.

Palpate for arterial pulse from the femoral artery downward. Claudication from iliac artery thrombosis can mimic sciatica and must always be ruled out, and not only in the elderly. We have seen several young patients referred with back and buttock symptoms produced by a Marfan-like disease of the aortoiliac arteries.

A diminished ankle jerk may be apparent only as a decreased push against the examiner's hand when the Achilles tendon is tapped. This most often indicates an S1 nerve root lesion.

Check the Babinski reflexes, particularly when the symptoms arise in the upper lumbar spine or are associated with diffuse muscle weakness or bilateral involvement. Keep in mind that a common cause of an upper motor neuron lesion in the elderly patient is a central protrusion of a disc in the cervical spine (see section on Cervical Disc Disease).

Evaluate for sacroiliac pathology by pressing down and out on the anterior superior iliac spine with the patient resting on the firm examining table. Advise the patient that the object of this maneuver is not so much to produce pain localized to the sacroiliac joint as it is to determine whether this aggravates his lumbago or sciatica.

The final and most important test of the physical examination is the nerve stretch test. This is done with the patient's pelvis supported on the firm examining table. Begin with the uninvolved side first. Lift the limb with the knee extended in order to demonstrate the test. Then raise the limb on the symptomatic side, again with the knee extended. At the point at which the patient first notices pain beginning in the back, buttock, or leg, hold the leg steady. Then ask the patient to flex his neck. This should reproduce pain down the involved buttock and leg if there is disc impingement that prevents gliding of the dura.

This test is specific for dural entrapment and eliminates other diagnoses such as sacroiliac strain or facet syndromes, which may confuse the clinical picture. There is no other structure between the head and the leg, besides the dura, which could be stretched by this maneuver. This test is as specific for disc disease as Kernig's sign is for meningitis. Always test carefully for this dural stretch sign and suspect a diagnosis other than disc herniation if this test is negative. Children and older patients do sometimes prove exceptions to this rule.

The straight-leg-raising test may be positive without neurologic signs if there is only a small protrusion sufficient to interfere with dural gliding but not yet large enough to affect nerve conduction. Conversely, with severe sciatica, the disc may compress the nerve so firmly that it becomes insensitive. Muscle weakness and foot drop then develop. The ankle jerk is lost, and the skin in the foot becomes insensitive. The straight-leg-raising test then will become normal as the patient gains relief of the pain symptoms but at the expense of neurologic impairment.

Other Diagnostic Tests: X-rays, Myelogram, and CT and MRI Scans

The initial diagnosis of disc disease should be entirely a clinical one. Standard x-rays are of no value other than to rule out differential conditions such as fracture, spondylolisthesis, tumor, or occasionally a disc space infection.

Myelography or computerized tomographic (CT) or magnetic resonance scan should not be done at the time of initial diagnostic evaluation. These are necessary only if the patient has not responded to the described treatment as expected. Computerized tomographic scans are particularly useful in defining conditions such as arachnoidal adhesions, extradural infections, congenital anomalies, trauma to the spine, or degenerative joint or disc disease. Metastatic disease to the spine is also found earlier with the scanning technique.

Intraspinal tumors are best demonstrated by myelography, although the CT scan can assist in defining the exact extent of the lesion. Tethered cord, diastematomyelia, and meningocele are other conditions well defined by CT scan. The shape and the size of the canal are also best determined by this newer diagnostic method. In fact, assessment of back pain and back conditions has become the most widely accepted indication for body scanners since the introduction of this technology (Fig. 49–70). This technology should not be allowed to supplant careful physical assessment supplemented by diagnostic methods such as epidural and facet injections, which we will discuss later in this section.

Management by the Family Physician. The prime objective in treating disc disease is pain relief. Only infrequently is the neurologic deficit sufficient to be of concern. Occasional massive central defects that cause bilateral symptoms, weakness, and numbness, as well as bladder or bowel paralysis are major exceptions. Always be alert to the infrequent patient

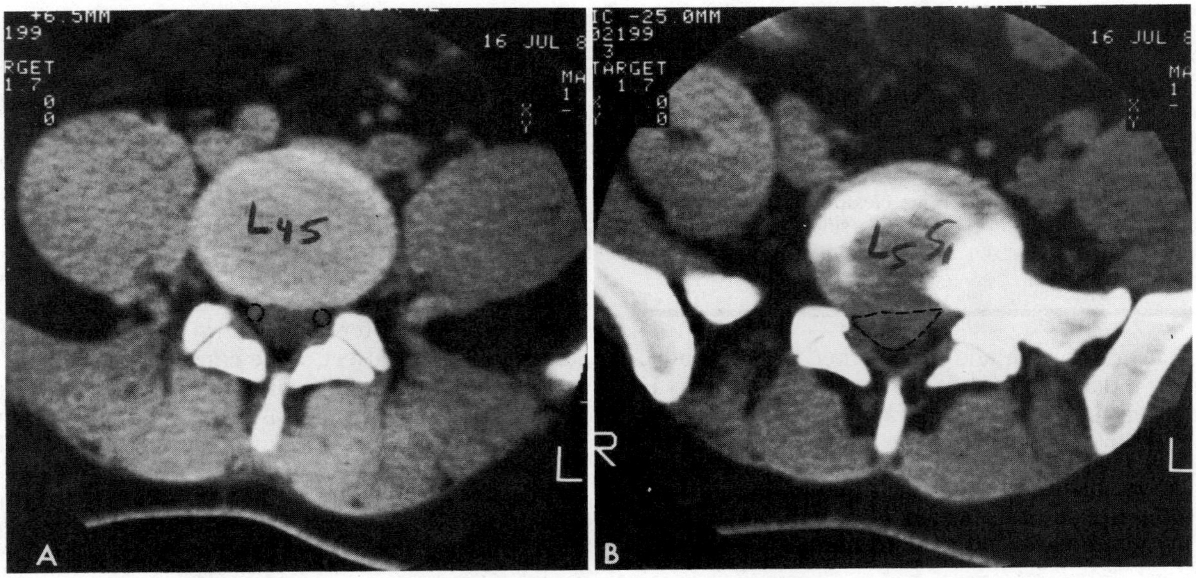

Figure 49–70. *A*, L4-5 interspace showing no compression and no bulging. *B*, Same patient showing L5-S1 interspace with central to right herniation of nucleus pulposus into the canal, displacing the right nerve root posteriorly and laterally with some evidence of lateral movement of the dural contents to the left. At the time of surgical exploration, this patient was found to have a very large herniation onto the axilla of the S1 nerve on the right.

with loss of sphincter control, which indicates a midline defect requiring immediate surgical decompression.

For most patients treatment should be directed at relieving the mechanical obstruction to the dura and nerve sheath, thereby eliminating the source of the pain. Bed rest helps, since it minimizes disc pressure, but it does not ordinarily bring about a reduction of the cartilage or pulpy disc herniation. This is ultimately what is necessary to relieve the dural impingement. Bed rest merely makes the patient as comfortable as possible while the disc either reduces spontaneously; erodes by pressure into the posterior inferior aspect of the vertebral body, thereby forming a bony ridge; causes the compressed nerve root to atrophy while the pain subsides but the neurologic deficit worsens; or shrinks spontaneously.

Systemic analgesics do not get to the basic mechanical problem of disc protrusion. Analgesics should be used for a very brief period until the specific therapy directed at the mechanical back derangement becomes effective.

Muscle relaxants make little sense at all in the treatment of disc lesions, just as they would not be rational for acute appendicitis. The objective must be to correct the underlying pathology producing the protective muscle guarding.

Local heat or ice applications provide temporary analgesic effect for pain symptoms. They are less complicated by side effects than are systemic analgesics and therefore are preferable.

Mechanical correction of a disc protrusion must constitute the main treatment. This can be done in several ways. For the mild discogenic or lumbago pain, treatment may simply require postural correction; educate the patient regarding habitual acts likely to bring on the disc symptomatology (Fig. 49–71). Particularly emphasize the importance of maintaining the proper lumbar lordosis.

For a significant acute cartilaginous displacement causing lumbago, reduce the cartilage promptly by extension manipulation. These techniques are quite fully described in Cyriax's book and should be referred to before attempting the maneuver. An alter-

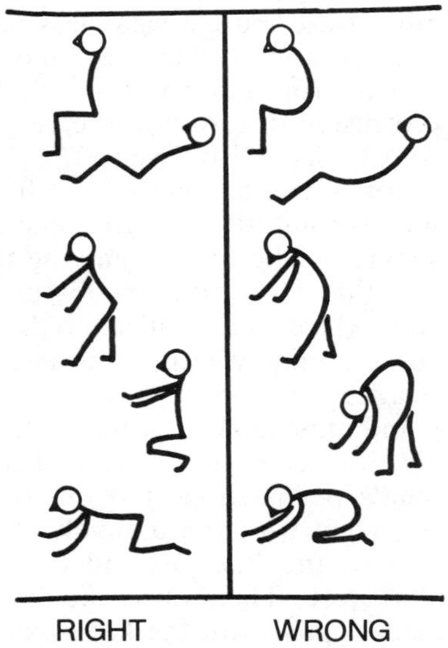

Figure 49–71. Patient education is important and particularly should emphasize ways in which the patient can improve habitual actions that lead to back symptoms. On the left are schematic illustrations of the correct ways to sit, stand, lift, or bend, which maintain lumbar lordosis. On the right are the incorrect ways for carrying out these activities, which flex the lumbar spine, eliminate lumbar lordosis, and produce lumbago. (From Cyriax, J.: Orthopaedic Medicine. Vol. 1. London, Cassell Ltd., 1978.)

native is to refer the individual to a therapist familiar with the techniques, indications, and contraindications, as described by Cyriax and other authors. Manipulation of the spine does have a definite place in the treatment of a lumbago produced by acute cartilaginous disc displacement. For acute nuclear protrusions with neurogenic symptoms or paresthesias in the leg (sciatica), the treatment of choice is heavy traction or flexion exercises. These methods are designed to open up the disc space posteriorly and gradually allow the nuclear material to recede back into the disc space.

Traction and Flexion Exercises for Sciatica. The traditional method of managing sciatica by applying 10 to 15 pounds of traction via a pelvic sling is entirely ineffective. This is because the force necessary to distract the lumbar disc space must be as strong as possible, i.e., 100 pounds or greater. As heavy traction is applied, the disc space can be increased and the disc encouraged to recede (Fig. 49–72). Tightening the posterior longitudinal ligament by traction also helps push this material back into the space and creates a vacuum effect, which may further draw the protrusion toward the center of the disc space. To accomplish all of this, we use a traction apparatus that stabilizes the patient's trunk wall. Heavy traction

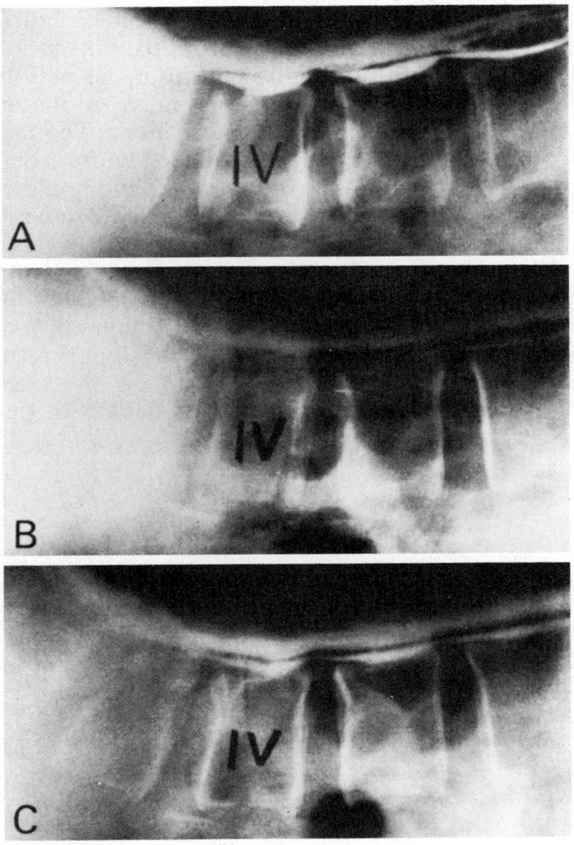

Figure 49–72. Heavy lumbar traction on the pelvis does affect disc protrusion as seen on this air myelogram before *(A)*, during *(B)*, and after *(C)* traction. (From Cyriax, J.: Orthopaedic Medicine. Vol. 1. London, Cassell Ltd., 1978.)

can then be applied to the pelvis in order to affect the involved lumbar disc space (Fig. 41–73).

In conjunction with traction we also employ a series of flexion exercises. These have been standard techniques in a number of hospitals in the United States, but their application has sometimes been inappropriate. They should be used primarily to make the patient comfortable and should not aggravate the symptoms of sciatica. The patient should be shown the exercises carefully and the reason for each position explained (Fig. 49–74).

If the patient complains that a certain type of exercise aggravates the nerve stretch pain down the leg, this particular activity is eliminated.

In our experience with a combination of traction and exercise therapy, more than 80 per cent of patients with disc lesions can be relieved of pain symptoms and returned to work activities within 4 to 6 weeks. To accomplish this, however, patient education is essential.

Educate the patient, particularly in the mechanics of disc protrusion and the importance of lumbar lordosis in maintaining the disc space. Illustrative guides such as those shown in Figure 49–71 are helpful. Be sure that this is discussed with the patient, rather than merely handed to him like a political flyer as he goes out the door.

Reassure the patient that this is not a crippling disease. Discuss seating posture in detail, since this is the major culprit causing backache in today's sedentary age. Encourage the patient to participate in a regular sport that maintains lumbar lordosis, such as swimming, golf, or even horseback riding. Discourage activities that require a good deal of lumbar flexion, such as gardening, racquetball, or tennis.

A return to a full range of vocational or avocational activities without pain and without surgical intervention should be the norm in most patients with back pain of lumbar disc origin.

If the described therapies, including manipulation, traction, and exercises, do not relieve the patient's symptoms, the next step should be epidural injection. This technique can be valuable both diagnostically and therapeutically. Epidural injections help to ensure that the back pain is dural and not coming from articular facets or the sacroiliac joint. It helps isolate pain referred from some other unusual condition such as chronic appendicitis or an ovarian cyst. It also differentiates the myelopathy associated with a disc at a higher level, particularly the cervical spine.

The technique of epidural injection may be helpful in the backache developing in the last trimester of pregnancy. It can also be helpful in distinguishing cases of coccyodynia resulting from sacral nerve root involvement. Epidural injection is indicated for root pain of sciatica with or without neurologic signs. It should be tried before advising laminectomy, since it does not work well after laminectomy.

The technique is simple and is suitable for outpatients. It should be thoroughly described to the

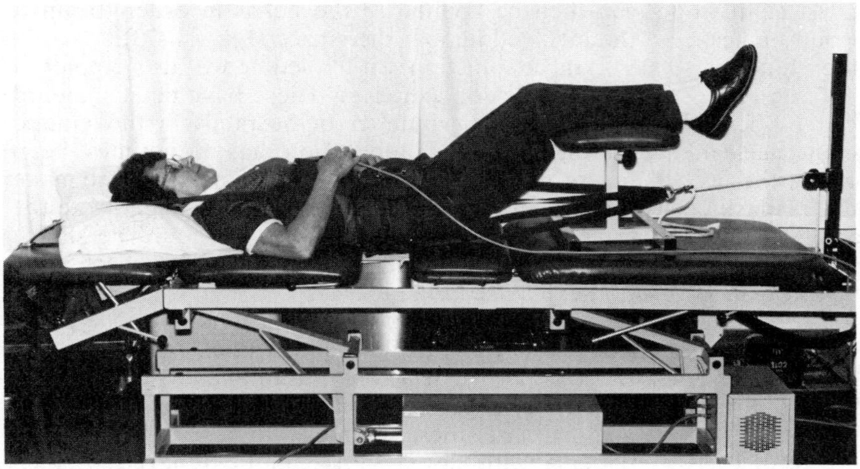

Figure 49–73. A pelvic traction apparatus must be sufficiently strong to support the patient and apply several hundred pounds of traction across the pelvis. Ordinary sling traction in bed does nothing more for the patient than enforce immobilization.

patient and distinguished from a lumbar puncture, which many patients fear.

The method has been well described by Cyriax and others and will not be presented in-depth here. The objective is to place a needle or cannula into the sacral canal. This can be done with the patient quite comfortable in the prone position (Figs. 49–75*A* and 49–75*B*). The technique of the injection, as described by its advocates, must be carefully followed so that the solution remains epidural and is not intrathecal.

The response to the epidural injection may be variable. Some patients experience increased pain for 1 to 2 days and then improve. Others relapse. The dural stretch test, i.e., straight leg raising with neck flexion, is a useful index of response. If pain symptoms improve but the patient does not return to normal after the injection, repeat the injection one or two times. Many patients may require two to three epidurals over a 4- to 7-day interval to relieve symptoms.

If the pain and dural stretch signs persist, laminectomy or intradiscal chymopapain should be advised.

Indications for Laminectomy. The main indication for laminectomy and disc excision is to relieve leg and back pain. The worst results from laminectomy are those done for pain in the patient without definite neurologic or myelographic findings. Myelogram or CT scan is now always performed preoperatively to confirm the clinical diagnosis of a disc herniation and to define the level.

The second indication for laminectomy is persistence of a gross lumbar list despite adequate therapy. This generally indicates a disc sufficiently large to be resistant to closed methods.

A relative indication is limited neurologic deficit, such as weakness of the foot. If the patient notices progressive inability to control the foot, he may be suffering from involvement of two nerve roots and the foot weakness can become permanent. The pain may be relieved as the neurologic deficit worsens, but complete paralysis is likely to persist. This should be explained to the patient and disc removal advised promptly if a foot drop develops.

Weakness of the foot is not an absolute indication for laminectomy while weakness of the bladder with incontinence or retention of urine is a definite indication for early laminectomy. This is usually the result of a massive midline herniation involving the sacral nerve roots, which can leave the patient with per-

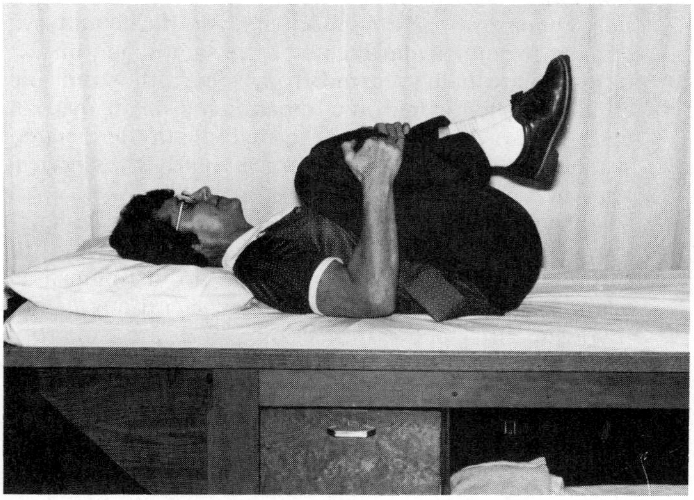

Figure 49–74. Flexion exercises, as illustrated here, are very useful to open the space in the posterior portion of the spine and relieve entrapment of the dura from herniated disc material.

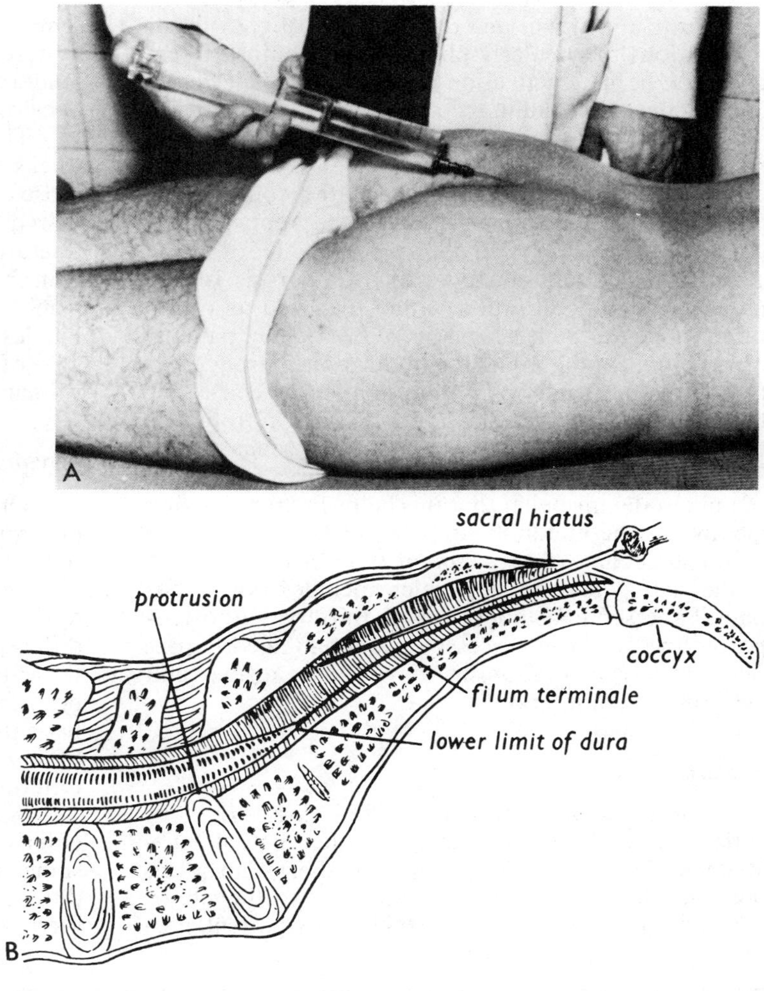

Figure 49–75. *A* and *B*, Epidural injection, as described by Cyriax, can be a useful diagnostic and therapeutic tool in managing acute disc herniations. The method should be considered prior to recommending surgical intervention. (From Cyriax, J.: Orthopaedic Medicine. Vol. 1. London, Cassell Ltd., 1978.)

manent loss of sphincter control. Such an acute paresis is fortunately quite infrequent from disc lesions, occurring in less than 2 per cent of disc herniations in our experience.

Discectomy, when advised for the proper indications, can be a very effective and gratifying operation. However, it is employed far too often, in our opinion, as a quick but inadequate solution to disc problems. The patient with severely disabling symptoms after laminectomy is far more common than is the patient with a disabling result or intermittent backache after conservative treatment.

By appreciating the mechanisms of backache as well as the rationale of treatment, the interested family physician can serve the patient with common low back problems quite effectively. He may even help the individual avoid induction into the growing army whose insignia is the laminectomy scar.

One must certainly avoid cynicism but also recognize the great difficulties that compensation and medical insurance create by their rewards for staying ill rather than healthy. Nevertheless, most patients avoid coming to the physician without real concerns. Despite a system that can and has been readily abused, the true malingerer is still rare.

OSTEOPOROSIS CAUSING BACKACHE

Osteoporosis is a major skeletal disorder produced by too little or too porous bone, leading to a pathologic weakening and fracture deformity. In 26 per cent of women surveyed over the age of 60 (Urist et al., 1970) bone had progressed to this pathologic state.

The most common presentation is back pain from a compression fracture of the vertebral body. The most frequently compressed body is T12, which is also the most subject to flexion-extension overloading. Any fracture above T7 should generally be considered as resulting from trauma, electroconvulsive therapy, epilepsy, or metastatic tumor rather than a failure from osteoporosis.

Other fractures related to pathologic failures in osteoporotic bone include Colles' fracture, femoral neck fractures, and proximal humeral fractures.

Osteoporosis can be confused with osteomalacia, in which the adult bone is not adequately mineralized. The osteomalacia that we see today is most often the result of intestinal malabsorption or kidney disease, particularly associated with renal dialysis. In younger epileptic patients, a frequent cause of osteomalacia is long-term anticonvulsant treatment. Anticonvulsant medications, particularly phenytoin (Dilantin), interfere with hepatic activation of vitamin D. The result is a decreased calcium absorption from the gut, hypocalcemia, and osteomalacia with secondary hyperparathyroidism. Osteoporosis may be associated with osteomalacia, but the etiology and the contrast between these two conditions should be kept in mind (Table 49–10).

The most common type of osteoporosis is that induced by immobilization, either localized to a fractured bone or generalized in a bedridden patient. This complication from immobilization is frequently forgotten, particularly in young patients. The result may be massive mobilization of calcium from the bone and hypercalcemia complicated by renal stones. The tendency of young patients to drink a great deal of milk in the misbelief that this helps fracture healing aggravates the metabolic imbalance.

The second most common type of osteoporosis is the hypogonadal type, which includes postmenopausal and senile osteoporosis. A third type of osteoporosis results from excessive catabolic agents, particularly hypercortisonism, hyperthyroidism, and cytotoxic chemotherapy.

History

The usual presentation of a pathologic osteoporotic fracture is typically in a postmenopausal, fair-skinned, lightweight woman of Northern European descent who experiences pain localized to the site of a recent thoracic fracture. Usually this patient presents 10 years after menopause or 3 to 4 years after hysterectomy and oophorectomy. Generalized bone tenderness is not characteristic of osteoporosis but does occur with osteomalacia and myeloma.

The acute fracture pain should subside in a few weeks. Persistence or worsening of the pain should cause one to suspect an underlying malignancy rather than osteoporosis. Also, bone pain from osteoporotic fracture should be relieved by rest in contrast with pain from malignancy. Not all compression fractures from pathologic osteoporosis produce symptoms. Painless vertebral compression can cause considerable loss of height, particularly in the postmenopausal woman or in a patient with Cushing's syndrome.

Physical Examination

On physical assessment of the patient with back pain suspected of being due to an osteoporotic fracture, look for stigmata of Graves' and Cushing's diseases as well as of renal, gastrointestinal, and liver dysfunction. Most important, consider the common differentials of carcinomatosis and myeloma. Suspect these possibilities in patients with too much osteoporosis too soon after menopause. Five per cent of patients initially diagnosed as having osteoporotic fractures prove to have these more serious underlying differential conditions (Gordon and Vaughan, 1976).

Another consideration is the possibility that the elderly patient's pain results from arthritis of the spine rather than from osteoporosis. These two conditions are mutually exclusive. The bone mass that increases in osteoarthritis prevents the diminution of

Table 49–10. CONTRAST BETWEEN OSTEOPOROSIS AND OSTEOMALACIA*

	Osteoporosis	Osteomalacia
Definition	Too little bone	Abundant uncalcified osteoid
Mineralization	Normally calcified	Insufficiently calcified
Physical properties	Brittle Leads to fracture	Soft Leads to bowing
Bone tenderness	Local at fracture site	Generalized
Serum calcium	Normal (upper limit)	Low or normal
Serum phosphate	Elevated (except in Cushing's disease)	Low or normal
Serum (Ca^{++} phosphate)	Normal	Low
Alkaline phosphatase	Normal	High
Parathyroid hormone	Normal	High
X-ray	Loss of spongiosa Thin but intact cortex Vertebral deformities Biconcave Wedge Collapsed	Loss of cortex, often eroded
Biopsy	Sparse, thin trabeculae	Osteoid seams and secondary hyperparathyroidism
Candidate	Postmenopausal women, not black Immobilized person Corticoid excess Thyroid excess Chronic alcoholic (?)	Intestinal malabsorption Uremia Tubular effects Familial vitamin D–resistant rickets Anticonvulsant therapy Cirrhosis
Reversibility	Usually *not*	Yes

*From Gordon, G., and Vaughan, C.: Clinical Management of the Osteoporoses. Bucks, England, HM & M Publishers, 1976, p. 10.

bone associated with osteoporosis. The presence of osteophytes, particularly the pathognomonic Heberden's nodes on the distal interphalangeal joints, shifts the diagnosis to osteoarthritis.

Careful assessment of the patient with symptomatic osteoporosis should also include accurate measurement of the individual's height. Osteoporotic compression fractures invariably lead to thoracic kyphosis and loss of height. The best indicator of the patient's response to treatment is whether or not the height is stabilizing. Measure the standing height accurately at each visit and compare with baseline measurements to evaluate the course of the pathologic osteoporosis as well as the response to treatment. A loss in height of 6 mm. or more indicates a new fracture and failure of treatment for some reason.

Laboratory Findings

The initial laboratory assessment of the patient suspected of having pathologic osteoporosis, i.e., symptomatic fracture, should include serum calcium, phosphate, alkaline phosphatase, and electrophoretic protein pattern. All of these studies should be normal or in the normal range with osteoporosis. Abnormal levels in these studies help to detect the most common differentials, including osteomalacia, metastatic malignancy, myeloma, and osteitis fibrosa.

Hypercalcemia occurs in most conditions of rapid bone turnover, i.e., malignancy, hyperparathyroidism, thyrotoxicosis, acromegaly, and acute disuse osteoporosis in children but not in adults. Consequently, hypercalcemia in an osteoporotic patient should cause the physician to consider conditions other than the garden-variety postmenopausal osteoporosis.

An elevated serum phosphate level is also usually a good indicator of osteolysis. However, it may be lowered if the condition responsible for the bone lysis also decreases tubular reabsorption of phosphate. The conditions most likely to cause this include hyperparathyroidism, hypercorticism, and myeloma producing an acquired Fanconi's syndrome.

Serum alkaline phosphatase is of particular importance in the differential diagnosis of osteoporosis. In the absence of liver disease or pregnancy, alkaline phosphatase reflects osteoblastic activity. The most marked elevations occur in osteitis fibrosa (Paget's disease), osteomalacia, polyostotic fibrous dysplasia, and metastases. Long bone fractures only elevate the alkaline phosphatase transiently, and vertebral body fractures have no effect at all. Consequently, an elevated alkaline phosphatase level on repeated careful determinations indicates an underlying cause other than the usual hypogonadal osteoporosis.

Roentgenographic Findings

X-rays of the osteoporotic spine show the characteristic loss of bone tissue with disproportionate loss of trabecular bone relative to cortical bone. However, by the time these changes become evident on standard x-ray, the pathologic process is far advanced.

The pathognomonic x-ray finding is eburnation or thickening of the superior-inferior end plates. This gives a false appearance of increased cortical density which is relative because of excessive loss of trabecular bone, which is the primary bone that becomes porotic. In using x-rays, take care that overpenetration has not produced artifactual osteoporosis.

Compression of the vertebral body in the osteoporotic spine occurs most often at the T12 level (Saville, 1970). A single fracture at T7 or above should always be evaluated for causes other than osteoporosis. Any osteoporotic atraumatic-type compression fracture in a man under 60 should also prompt a search among the differential conditions, particularly myeloma.

Differential Diagnosis

Myeloma, the most common of all malignancies of bone, radiographically mimics osteoporosis. Chemically it simulates hyperparathyroidism. Myeloma may present in its early states as painless vertebral fractures. Most typically, however, the patient suffers a generalized and persistent bone tenderness and malaise. The alkaline phosphatase level tends to be low owing to crowding out of osteoblasts by myeloma cells in the marrow. Although a myeloma spike on the serum electrophoresis pattern can be demonstrated in 70 to 80 per cent of cases, the diagnosis depends on bone marrow histology. This can usually be done by sternal aspiration.

Waldenstrom's macroglobulinemia closely resembles osteoporosis and multiple myeloma. Metastatic breast carcinoma is another cause of back pain that must be distinguished from osteoporosis. Lung, kidney, ovary, thyroid, and gastrointestinal tract must also be considered as primary sources for metastases to the spine. A careful history, particularly of a primary tumor elsewhere and persistent back pain unrelieved by rest, is most helpful in the differential diagnosis.

Alkaline phosphatase is elevated with metastases in contrast with the normal levels in osteoporosis. X-rays may show cortical erosion with progressive destruction of the vertebrae, which would be more consistent with metastases than with osteoporosis. Bone scans can be particularly helpful in differentiating between these two conditions, particularly when done sequentially (Galasco and Sylvester, 1978). Needle biopsy is rarely indicated for this differential. When in doubt about the cause of an isolated compression fracture of a vertebral body, procrastination is in order. Metastasis, particularly from the breast, soon becomes evident elsewhere. In contrast, the pain from an osteoporotic fracture improves within 3 to 4 weeks.

If the patient manifests any neurologic changes, the differential diagnostic consideration should not delay the urgently needed treatment. Operative biopsy and stabilization of the spine become mandatory.

Management by the Family Physician. Treatment of the symptomatic osteoporosis of the spine should be based on what we know at present about its etiology. The underlying cause, i.e., increased bone absorption relative to bone formation, ultimately results in an overall decrease in bone mass in the postmenopausal woman (Heaney and Recker, 1975).

This sudden loss of bone tissue appears directly related to the abrupt depletion of gonadal hormones at menopause. Estrogen therapy can prevent these changes and can restore normal premenopausal values for calcium balance and bone turnover. This is well worth considering, not only because of an overall fracture rate in osteoporotic patients of 5 per cent per annum more than nonosteoporotic patients. The technique of cyclic estrogen administration was introduced originally by Albright and remains relevant as elucidated by Gordon and Vaughan (1976).

The regimen is to give conjugated estrogens, 1.25 mg. daily, but have the patient omit the pill for the first 5 days of each calendar month. This period may be extended for 7 to 10 days each month if necessary to complete endometrial sloughing and to avoid mastodynia. The variability of withdrawal bleeding should be discussed with the patient; however, the major problem is breakthrough bleeding. Such bleeding is unrelated to estrogen withdrawal and requires gynecologic dilatation and curettage. Endometrial carcinoma does not appear to be of significantly greater frequency in patients on estrogen maintenance. In fact, surveillance with estrogen treatment usually allows early detection of any endometrial carcinoma and decreases already low mortality.

Many women will prefer to put up with the osteoporosis rather than with continued estrogen maintenance. Newer modalities of treatment include vitamin D metabolites or calcium supplemented with phosphorus. These have been shown to decrease the frequency of fractures, which is really the only objective assessment of therapy. If compression fractures continue to shorten the patient's height by 6 mm. or more on careful follow-up measurements, the regimen is not working. For the majority of patients at this time, however, estrogen maintenance therapy remains the first line of treatment for symptomatic osteoporosis.

Besides medical treatment of the osteoporosis, do not overlook the local pain problem in the back. The acute back pain after an osteoporotic compression fracture should subside in 2 to 3 weeks with symptomatic treatment. Avoid prolonged bed rest or strong analgesics. Local application of ice or ice massage relieves a good deal of the patient's pain and is generally preferable to heat application, but try both. Corsets or external casts should be avoided in all but the extremely symptomatic patient.

Most of our patients are made more uncomfortable by orthoses that are heavy enough to support the spine. Instead, we concentrate on active extension exercise, particularly wall push-ups and swimming (Fig. 49–76). Stationary bicycle riding is also an excellent exercise quite suitable for most patients with osteoporotic problems.

Dietary and familial factors that contribute to any physical and mental problems of the patient should be addressed, particularly prior to instituting any long-term estrogen therapy. Dietary counseling must also be integrated into the overall management. No single therapeutic modality but rather a combination of treatments will best aid patients suffering with this common and perplexing disease of bone.

FACET SYNDROME

Localization of pain in the low back, buttock, and leg may be referred from the lumbar facet joint. This has been demonstrated by Mooney and Robertson (1976), among others, who injected hypertonic saline into the lumbar facets and caused pain referred to the buttocks and legs in patients with and without prior symptoms of lumbago and sciatica (Fig. 49–77). In patients with back pain, but no nerve stretch or neurologic symptoms, i.e., a motor or sensory deficit, local infiltration of the lower lumbar facet joints with 1 ml. methylprednisolone acetate (Depo-Medrol) and 5 ml. local anesthetic can be a valuable diagnostic and therapeutic tool. The method is relatively simple and well described by Mooney and Robertson (1976). It can be combined with epidural injection and computerized tomography to evaluate the vast majority of known anatomic causes of low back pain in your patients. About 50 per cent of patients treated by facet injection for back pain may experience sufficient

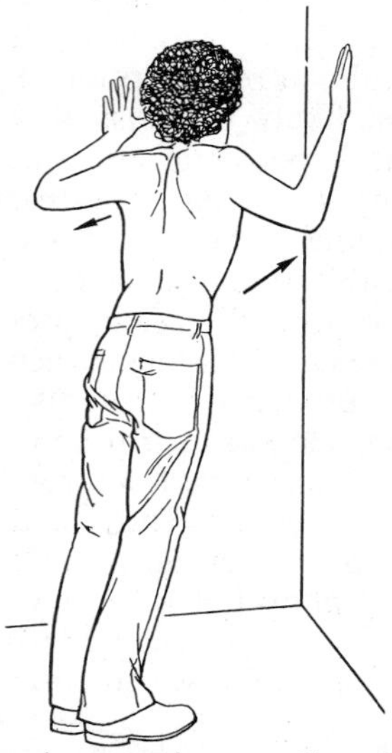

Figure 49–76. Extension exercise or wall push-ups are particularly helpful for patients with osteoporotic thoracic spine fractures and ankylosing spondylitis. Even elderly patients can become quite adept at this particular form of exercise. (From Connolly, J. F.: DePalma's The Management of Fractures and Dislocations. 3rd ed. Philadelphia, W. B. Saunders Co., 1981.)

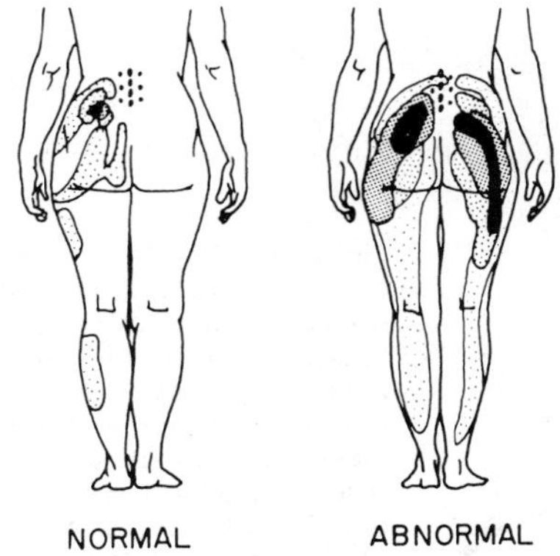

Figure 49–77. Injection of lumbar facet joints in both asymptomatic (normal) and symptomatic (abnormal) subjects produced pain referred into the buttock and down the thigh. This study confirmed that a referral pattern from the facet joint may mimic lumbago and sciatica. (From Mooney, V., and Robertson, J.: The facet syndrome. Clin. Orthop., *115*:152, 1976.)

relief of symptoms to return to most daily activities. This, of course, depends on appropriate selection and limitation of this method to patients without definite disc disease.

The technique of facet joint injection can be incorporated into the family physician's diagnostic and therapeutic approaches to help the patients with low back pain.

NECK PAIN AND CERVICAL DISC PROTRUSION

Neck pain is secondary only to backache in the list of universal musculoskeletal afflictions. Not everyone with a "pain in his neck" consults his physician, but those who do should receive the benefit of effective therapy from an interested physician. Unfortunately, too often all that we physicians offer is merely reassurance that symptoms will subside with passive resignation.

As in the lumbar spine, the vast majority of cervical spine pain results from disc disease. Very often much of the mechanical derangement from cervical disc disease persists or progresses. As mentioned previously, cervical myelopathy from chronic disc disease is among the most common of spinal cord disease in middle-aged and elderly patients (Wilkinson, 1964). This disease can and does progress to the point of cord damage and frequently is mistaken for amyotrophic lateral sclerosis or progressive muscle atrophy, both of which are much less common conditions.

Although management of cervical disc disease is controversial and sometimes marked by unprofessional casuistry, the pathophysiology is fairly well understood, thanks particularly to the work of James Cyriax, among others. The family physician who sees patients with neck problems should review Cyriax's publications, which have been the primary source for this presentation.

History of Neck Pain

Cervical disc protrusion generally progresses in easily recognized stages throughout life. A young person in his teens or 20's may wake up once or twice a year with severe unilateral neck pain, wryneck, or acute torticollis. This pain lasts for 2 or 3 days but recovers spontaneously in 7 to 10 days. Such acute torticollis, or "cervicago," is quite analogous to the acute lumbago described previously. It represents a sudden displacement of a cartilaginous fragment of the disc with spontaneous repositioning back into the disc space (Fig. 49–78).

Subsequently, the patient in his late 20's or 30's will begin to experience intermittent attacks of scapular pain. These attacks last 2 to 4 weeks and are usually unilateral. However, they may involve alternating sides of the neck. These, once again, represent a loose disc fragment, which eventually returns to its intervertebral position. However, the symptoms may at any time become much worse and progress to severe unilateral pain from compression on the dural sleeve of the root (Fig. 49–79). Such root pain is characterized by brachial or arm radiation which is much worse at night and may or may not be associated with "pins and needles" in the hands. Such nerve root symptomatology remains severe for 2 to 3 months and then usually subsides.

If the disc continues to protrude centrally, it eventually will push out the posterior longitudinal ligament and compress the dura. The result is a constant aching that the patient experiences from the occiput down to the scapula. This is particularly common in the older patient with chronic disc disease. Chronic compression of the spinal cord from central protrusion will produce paresthesias in the patient's hands or feet and can eventually progress to paresis or total paraplegia. This cervical myelopathy has been mentioned previously in the section on low back pain as an important differential in evaluating a patient for lumbar as well as cervical disc disease.

Other Considerations in the History of Cervical Disc Pain. The usual pain from a cervical disc lesion locates in the scapular region and is referred upward toward the ear (see Fig. 49–78). It is generally not aggravated by coughing. This contrasts with the pain from thoracic and lumbar disc lesions, which are characteristically worsened by increased intradural pressure during coughing.

In the elderly patient the disc pain will frequently persist as a severe occipital/cervical headache. This is particularly likely to awaken the individual from sleep in the morning. It is resistant to most analgesics.

Differential considerations are numerous, but they particularly should exclude metastatic lesions to the spine. Symptoms from metastases come on much more rapidly and are associated with more marked

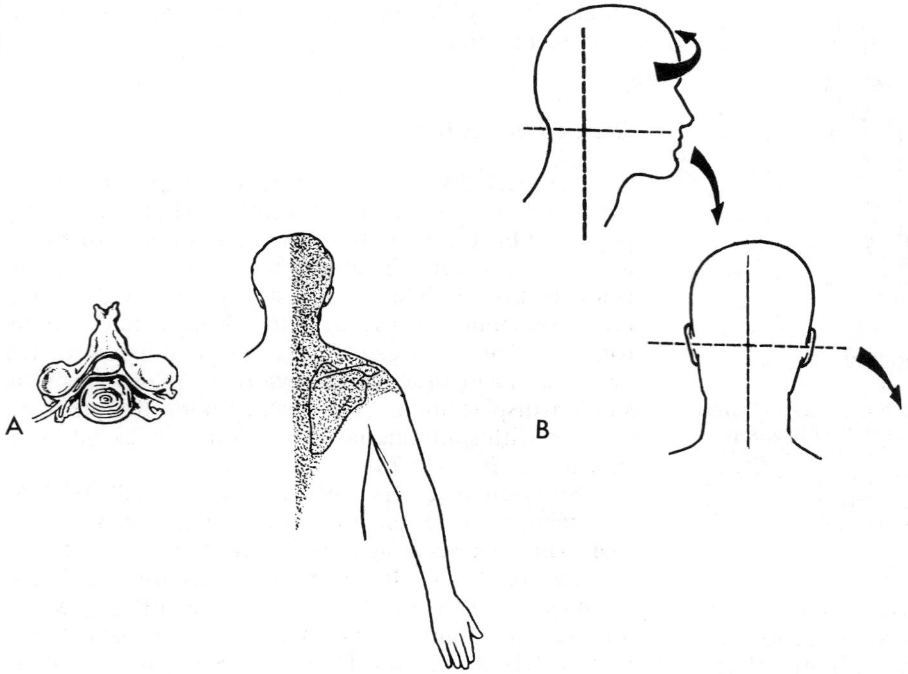

Figure 49–78. *A,* "Cervicago," analogous to lumbago, is the result of disc impingement on dura. Characteristically, the pain radiates to the neck, trapezius, and occipital and interscapular areas without radiation down the arm. *B,* With a protruded disc sensitizing the dura, flexion, extension rotation, or lateral bending of the neck will worsen pain symptoms. This relationship to neck motion is as important for the diagnosis of the cervical disc disease as is positive straight leg raising for lumbar disc disease.

limitation of neck motion than is seen in cervical spine disease.

In the younger patient consider the possibility of ankylosing spondylitis as the cause of neck pain and stiffness. Cervical stiffness may sometimes present as a first complaint of this condition. However, further evaluation will always demonstrate diminished chest expansion and lumbosacral as well as cervical spine stiffness.

Physical Examination

Inspection. To evaluate your patient with neck pain adequately, your physical examination should be as systematic as it would be for any patient with chest pain.

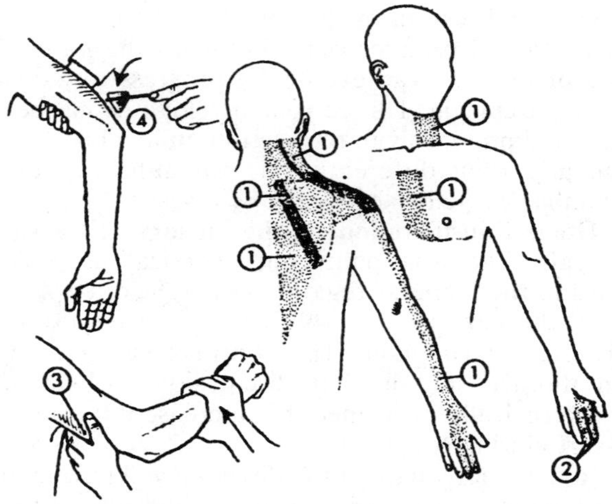

Figure 49–79. Should the disc cause entrapment of the 7th cervical nerve root, pain will radiate into the neck, trapezius region, vertebral border of the scapula, anterior chest wall, outer aspects of the arm, and index and middle finger *(1)*. The patient will experience paresthesias of the index and middle fingers particularly *(2)*. There will be diminished muscle power evident, particularly in the triceps *(3)*. The triceps reflex tends to be diminished *(4)*.

Full examination of a patient with neck and scapular pain begins with inspection for any asymmetric posture or torticollis. Acute torticollis in children generally results from a minor injury that causes a rotatory subluxation of C1 on C2. This differs from torticollis of the disc lesions in the young adult (Fig. 49–80). This traumatic torticollis usually resolves with brief head halter traction; however, it may require manipulative reduction. The other possibility to keep in mind as causing torticollis in children is a retropharyngeal infection.

In the teenager and younger adult acute torticollis generally results from sleeping with the neck in an awkward side flexion. Young people who sleep on their stomachs are "prone" to this complication. As the patient lies with the neck twisted sideways the disc fragment displaces and then partially blocks cervical joint motion. Such a situation, which might be termed "cervicago," is analogous to lumbago from acute displacement of the cartilaginous disc fragments fixing the lumbar spine in flexion. However, with the cervical spine the position is that of lateral flexion and rotation. Acute cervical torticollis of this type in the young adult or adolescent will subside in 7 to 10 days. However, effective treatment, as described later in this section, can improve symptoms more rapidly than this.

Range of Motion Testing

With the patient sitting on an examining stool, evaluate neck motion, including flexion, extension, rotation, and lateral flexion to both sides (see Fig. 49–78). Note particularly the motion that reproduces the pain. Have the patient move the neck actively.

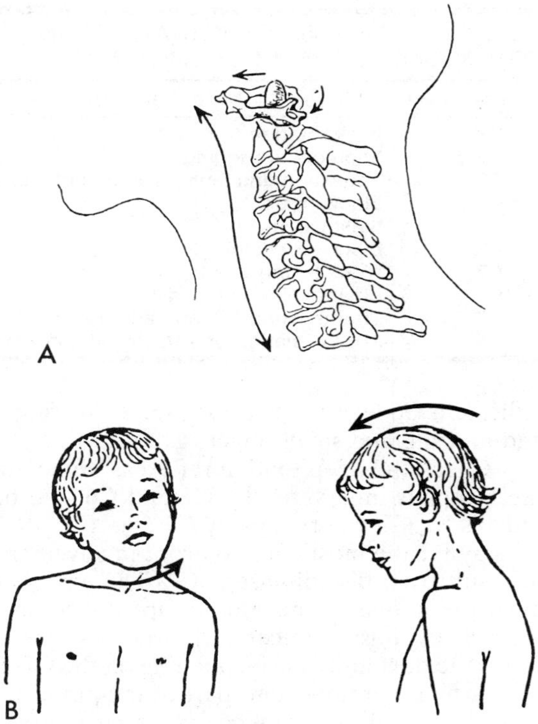

Figure 49–80. *A,* Traumatic torticollis occurs in the young individual owing to subluxation of C1 and C2. *B,* Characteristically, the head is rotated forward and the child assumes a "cock robin" position. This is due to the anteriorly rotated displacement of the atlas on the axis. It can usually be corrected by cervical traction.

Then move the patient's neck passively through all six motions. Be sure to evaluate for scapular motion, which includes shoulder elevation and forward and backward movement. Check for scapular winging by having the patient press against a wall with arms held forward.

Interpretation. Your interpretation of range of motion tests should be based on the fact that neck flexion stretches the dura in the cervical and thoracic regions. Typical findings in a patient with cervical disc disease include gross limitation of side flexion and rotation toward one side. Motion on flexion and rotation to the other side is usually full, although it may be slightly painful.

If side flexion of the neck away from the painful side produces pain, be wary of a tumor in the apex of the lung. Here pain results from passive stretching of the lung apex. Also, if pain is produced by scapular approximation, the thoracic region rather than the cervical region is implicated.

Arthritis in the cervical spine of an older patient generally causes painless stiffening. Pain caused by motion of the arthritic neck would indicate disc disease as well as arthritis. Marked limitation of motion coming on quickly and associated with steadily increasing severity of pain suggests metastases.

Gross limitation of passive motion in a young person is characteristic of ankylosing spondylitis. Also, symptoms of a cervical disc lesion with radiating pain down the arm usually do not present under the age of 30 to 35. Any patient in his 20's with severe neck and arm or brachial pain should be considered as having a neuroma or tumor in the neural foramen. If the patient complains of pain on coughing, if the nerve root pain lasts for more than 3 to 4 months, if there is unusual weakness, or if long track signs are evident in the young person, a neuroma is a very likely diagnosis.

Testing for Nerve Function

Following your assessment of neck and scapular motion, evaluate the patient for muscle strength in the neck, shoulder, and arm to detect any evidence of nerve root paresis.

Most patients with cervical disc protrusions do not present with root paralysis. Rather, as mentioned above, the major presentation from the disc is neck and shoulder pain reproduced in testing of neck motions (see Fig. 49–78). One should not wait for neck movements to produce pain radiating down the arm or for clear root palsy to appear in order to diagnose a cervical disc. By the time these occur and make the diagnosis obvious, the chance for simple, effective treatment has passed.

Motor function must be tested against resistance. This can be done expeditiously by the same systematic manner in which you test for neck motion. Weakness of motor function reflects certain root levels as outlined in Table 49–11.

Also examine carefully for cutaneous analgesia. Numbness in the thumb and index finger would

Table 49–11. LEVELS OF INNERVATION FOR MOTOR FUNCTION IN THE UPPER LIMB

Nerve Level	Motor Function
C1	Neck rotation
C2,3,4	Shoulder shrugging
C5	Abduction and lateral rotation of shoulders
C5,6	Elbow flexion
C6	Wrist extension
C7	Elbow extension
C7	Wrist flexion
C8	Ulnar deviation at wrist
C8	Thumb extension and adduction
T1	Approximation of 4th and 5th fingers

indicate a C6 level; index, long, and ring fingers, C7; and midring and small finger, C8.

Check the deep tendon reflexes. Remember that the biceps is innervated by C5 and C6; the brachioradialis by C5; the triceps by C7 (see Fig. 49–79).

By far the most common root involvement likely to result from disc disease is C7. The explanation is, as in the lumbar spine, the abrupt transition from a thoracic kyphosis to a cervical lordosis which concentrates the flexion-extension loading on the C7-T1 disc.

A final but important part of the physical assessment is to look for evidence of upper motor neuron lesions. No examination of the cervical spine is complete without checking for this. Similarly, no assessment of myelopathy is adequate unless the possibility of a central disc protrusion at the cervical level is considered. Examine the patient for spasticity, hyperactive reflexes, and positive Babinski reflexes in the lower limb as a final part of your cervical spine evaluation.

Other Considerations: Whiplash Injuries

This term carries with it a certain opprobrium in the minds of physicians, but we should not forget that real pathology may be present. Invariably, the neck is injured in a rear-end collision in which the occupant in the front seat receives an unexpected hyperextension-hyperflexion overload to the cervical spine.

The result may rarely cause rupture of the anterior longitudinal ligament and backward subluxation of one vertebra on the other, producing quadriplegia and sudden death; or it may produce the usual lesion, which is a cervical disc protrusion with symptoms causing progressive pain and aching from dural stretch.

Because the emphasis too often is placed on x-ray rather than physical examination, the problem becomes a frustrating one for physicians, patients, attorneys, and insurance carriers alike.

Quite frequently, the compensation aspects overshadow the patient-physician relationship and cloud the issue. The pain symptoms are real and are frequently amenable to treatment, as with any other disc lesion.

Most patients prefer prompt treatment of the disc lesion even though this might diminish their insurance settlement. Treatment should be based on the pathology and in particular derived from adequate physical examination. It should not be merely an overly optimistic hope, based on a "negative" x-ray, that strained muscle and ligaments will heal provided the patient is given a cervical collar and enough time.

X-ray Evaluation of Cervical Disc Lesions

The expense of x-rays far exceeds any benefit they are likely to provide in the diagnosis of cervical disc disease. The only real help from x-ray is a negative one—that is, an x-ray should be taken to rule out conditions such as fractures or bone-destroying processes such as tumor or infection.

Keep in mind that narrowing of a disc space is commonly seen in painless necks. Osteophytes are virtually universal in cervical spines after the age of 30. Usually, disc lesions occur in joints where the space has not decreased in size. It is essential to remember that the x-ray diagnosis must always be subject to the findings of our physical examination and not the converse.

Management by the Family Physician. Prophylactic treatment is the first consideration in this common source of progressive spinal and neurologic disease. It should begin in the young individual who is bothered by "cervicago." As indicated by the fact that many such patients awaken with acute torticollis, sleeping posture is an important contributing factor. Advise these patients to avoid sleeping prone, since this necessitates twisting the head to one side. It is particularly helpful to sleep without a pillow or with a very low one.

Before the patient goes to bed, a hot shower relieves some of the neck ache. A simple cervical collar can be made out of a bath towel folded on itself and then wrapped around the neck as a comfortable aid for sleeping and to avoid twisting the neck during sleep.

If the patient works at a desk, requiring long periods of neck flexion, the cervical posture should be corrected (Fig. 49–81). A few simple techniques can help typists and others avoid this common source of cervical disc disease.

The protruding disc that recurs and causes repeated neck problems eventually may not reduce spontaneously. After the age of 35 a protruding disc may well incapacitate the patient and cause severe nerve root symptoms. Osteophytes then develop as the bulging disc lifts up ligament and periosteum. Nerve root or cord signs may then well follow.

This sequence is not inevitable and should not be accepted with passive resignation. Early manipulative treatment can reduce disc fragments quite readily and should be considered the treatment of choice for acutely symptomatic patients. This holds true despite reports of occasional complications, particularly cerebral vascular accidents, occurring from inappropriate chiropractic manipulation. Manipulation

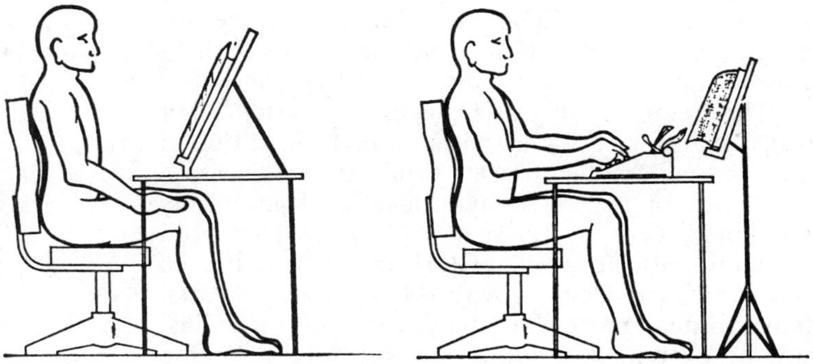

Figure 49–81. Habitual positioning of the neck in certain occupations is a great cause of cervical disc problems, e.g., working at a desk with the neck flexed can produce "cervicago." Educate the patient about the need to improve neck posture and use simple supports to avoid neck flexion as illustrated here. (Cyriax, J.: Orthopaedic Medicine. Vol. 1. London, Cassell Ltd., 1978.)

must be done by individuals who are knowledgeable about the cervical lesions as well as about the technique described by Cyriax and others.

During manipulation the patient should be fully awake and cooperative so as to be able to inform the manipulator regarding any change for better or for worse after each maneuver. Manipulation done in this safe manner can be effective in relieving neck pain of years' duration as well as of recent onset.

Cervical manipulation by an expert proves safer by far than most surgical procedures such as discectomy or fusion, which are well known to produce their share of death and quadriplegia. The patient may need a series of such manipulations but usually leaves the physician's office considerably improved following this technique.

Subsequent Follow-up. The patient should be advised that recurrent attacks may be expected unless he is careful about the posture of his neck, particularly at night. If the disc displaces again it should be reduced as promptly as possible.

A soft cervical collar can be useful in protecting the neck against postural strain. The patient should be reminded about sleeping posture and avoiding the use of a pillow. A bath-towel type of collar should be recommended for support at night. Exercises are inadvisable for cervical discs. They may actually produce recurrent displacement of the disc cartilage.

If a patient is subject to frequent recurrence of the disc protrusion, advise him to use a home traction apparatus. This allows the individual to exert heavy traction on his neck via a pulley system that can be extended over a door. It is important that the individual apply sufficient traction to the neck to lift the buttocks off the seat of a chair (Fig. 49–82). While traction is applied and the disc space is open, the patient can find a position of lateral flexion or rotation that is corrective of the disc displacement.

Failure to respond to this approach should prompt you to look diligently for destructive processes in the cervical spine, particularly if there are nerve root problems. Discogenic pain that fails to respond to manipulation should be referred for consideration of an anterior cervical fusion or possibly for removal of an osteophyte stretching adjacent nerve roots.

Once again the physician who appreciates the pathomechanics of disc disease and the simple but important mechanical methods of therapy can best serve patients.

Childhood Orthopedic Problems—Limp and Clumsiness

CONGENITAL DISLOCATION OF THE HIP

Congenital hip dislocation remains a common cause of limp in childhood. Despite the well-documented advantages of early detection in routine perinatal examinations, a large portion of initial diagnoses are still made by the mother or grandmother. The parent's suspicion is usually aroused by a previous history of congenital dislocated hip (CDH) in a relative or by the observation that the infant's hip has become stiff when the diapers are changed.

A family physician can do much to improve the

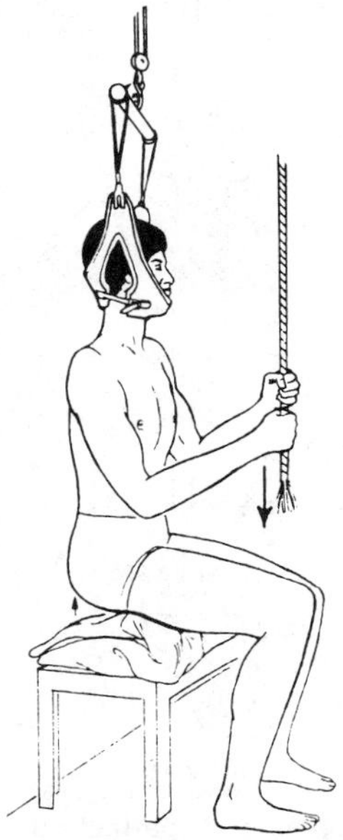

Figure 49–82. A cervical traction apparatus can be quite helpful for the patient with recurrent disc symptoms and can be used at home. The patient should apply traction with sufficient vigor to lift the buttocks from the stool. (Connolly, J. F.: DePalma's The Management of Fractures and Dislocations. 3rd ed. Philadelphia, W. B. Saunders Co., 1981.)

outcome in treating CDH by understanding the differing modes of presentation and the pitfalls in diagnosis, particularly over-reliance on x-ray.

The frequency of CDH ranges from 4 to 15 per 1000 live births, but this varies greatly in different races and geographic areas. Certain factors increase the chance of a congenital dislocation significantly and should alert the physician. Firstborn girls born to a family with a history of CDH, infants with breech presentation, and babies with other musculoskeletal abnormalities, particularly clubfeet and torticollis, must be examined carefully and repeatedly for hip instability.

Congenital hip dislocation is not an all-or-none phenomenon. That is, instability may develop subsequent to, as well as prior to, birth. Postnatal factors, particularly the position in which the child's hip is maintained, can encourage a dysplastic or subluxated hip to dislocate completely. Conversely, by positioning the hip in flexion and abduction, one can encourage normal development of the acetabulum and a stable hip (Fig. 49–83). Since congenital hip dislocation can evolve after birth, the infant must be evaluated not only in the newborn nursery but at each well-baby check-up to detect postnatal instability. The longer the delay in diagnosis, the longer and more complex is the treatment. The unstable hip detected in the newborn nursery usually requires only 3 to 4 months of splinting in a simple harness to stabilize the hip (Fig. 49–84). Teratogenic dislocations that occur in utero are much more resistant to treatment. The unstable hip detected at 6 months requires a year or more of treatment. The advantages of effective and early treatment are obvious.

The key to diagnosis is the physical finding of either hip instability or hip stiffness (Fig. 49–85).

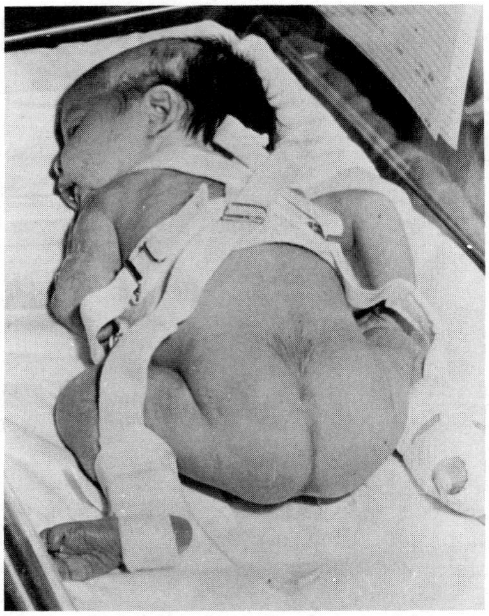

Figure 49–84. Any unstable hip in the newborn should be positioned with hips flexed maximally and in slight abduction (the human position). Double or triple diapers are ineffective for this purpose. A simple harness (Pavlik's harness) works quite well.

Any palpable sensation of the hip clunking or dislocating during flexion and abduction and then clunking again as it reduces in abduction (Ortolani's maneuver) is diagnostic. Treatment without further delay or debate is mandatory.

The other suspicious finding is hip stiffness. Ordinarily the newborn's hip can be abducted to lie flat on the examining table. Asymmetric limitation of abduction is diagnostic of a unilateral CDH. How-

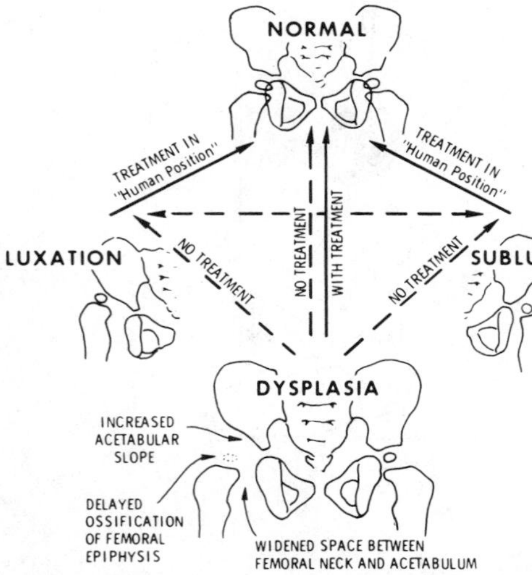

Figure 49–83. A dysplastic or partially developed hip in the newborn can evolve to a luxated, subluxated, or normal joint. This evolution depends particularly on whether the infant's hip is positioned to encourage molding of an adequate acetabulum (the human position). (Connolly, J.: The easy diagnosis and misdiagnosis of congenital hip dislocation. Nebraska Med. J., *60*:471, 1975, with permission.)

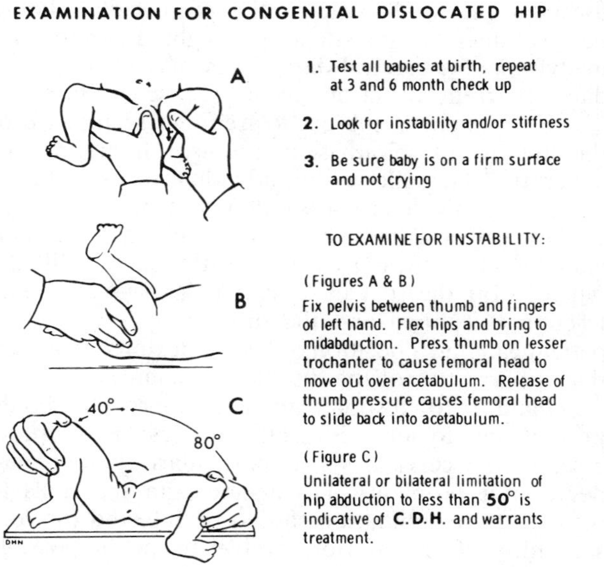
EXAMINATION FOR CONGENITAL DISLOCATED HIP
A
B
C
40°
80°
1. Test all babies at birth, repeat at 3 and 6 month check up
2. Look for instability and/or stiffness
3. Be sure baby is on a firm surface and not crying
TO EXAMINE FOR INSTABILITY:
(Figures A & B)
Fix pelvis between thumb and fingers of left hand. Flex hips and bring to midabduction. Press thumb on lesser trochanter to cause femoral head to move out over acetabulum. Release of thumb pressure causes femoral head to slide back into acetabulum.
(Figure C)
Unilateral or bilateral limitation of hip abduction to less than 50° is indicative of C.D.H. and warrants treatment.

Figure 49–85. The diagnosis of congenital hip dislocation in the newborn is entirely clinical. The tests for hip dislocation include palpable instability of the hip or limitation of abduction.

ever, approximately 35 per cent of congenital hip dislocations occur bilaterally. Therefore, any abduction limitation to less than 60 degrees should be considered abnormal (Fig. 49–85).

A major trap is the tendency of the physician to rely on x-ray rather than physical findings of congenital dislocation. Because of a lack of ephiphyseal ossification, roentgenograms are extremely unreliable at birth. This was exemplified by two patients whom we have treated over the years.

The first patient was a female and the product of a breech delivery. Two maternal cousins had a history of CDH. The physician examining the newborn was suspicious of instability in the left hip. X-rays were taken in the newborn nursery and were interpreted as normal (Fig. 49–86*A*). Orthopedic consultation recommended that the instability be treated, and the parents were advised to keep the child in triple diapers. However, because of parental conflict and eventual divorce, follow-up was sporadic, and when the child began walking at 14 months, a limp was noted. X-rays at that time (Fig. 49–86*B*) demonstrated dislocation of the left hip that required operative treatment for reduction.

The second patient was initially seen by a visiting nurse during a well-baby check-up when the girl child was 2 months of age. She had been the product of a normal delivery and in good health.

The nurse felt stiffness of the infant's right hip and suspected dislocation. The child was taken to her family physician, but he inappropriately advised that since the x-ray would not be helpful at 2 months, the child should be returned at 6 months to obtain adequate x-rays of the hip. When these were finally taken, the hip was indeed dislocated, but treatment was not instituted until the child was 9 months of age. After several operations and 2 years of therapy, the child was still under active treatment. This might have been mitigated by treatment at the first physical sign.

Management by the Family Physician. Congenital dislocated hip must be considered a physical and not a radiographic diagnosis. Treatment should be instituted early enough to improve long-term prognosis. Any suspicion of instability or stiffness in the neonate's hip warrants treatment by positioning in a Pavlik harness. This device allows the hip to be maintained in the fetal position necessary to induce normal development of the joint structures (see Fig. 49–84).

Triple diaper therapy should not be recommended for the unstable hip, as it does not achieve

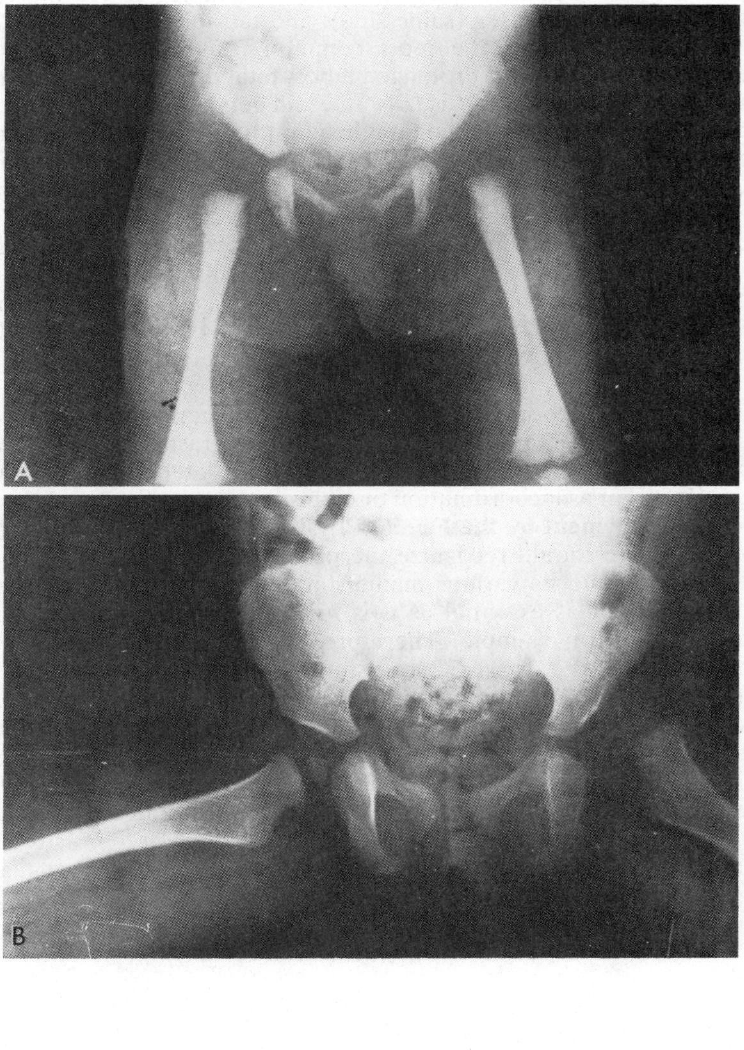

Figure 49–86. *A*, X-ray films taken in the newborn baby girl were interpreted as normal. Actually, the x-ray films are completely unreliable at this age, and the diagnosis must be entirely clinical. *B*, X-ray films at 14 months showed a completely dislocated hip in a child whose initial x-ray films were interpreted as normal.

the desired degree of flexion. It tends to be more expensive than the harness and de-emphasizes the importance of proper hip positioning during the critical first months after birth. Parental failure to follow through with triple diaper therapy is common.

The physician should evaluate the child repeatedly on well-baby check-ups for range of hip motion and evidence of any instability. Systematic screening and follow-up evaluation for congenital hip deformities are essential components of effective preventive care.

CEREBRAL PALSY

This diagnosis represents a spectrum of all nonprogressive conditions in which damage occurs to the upper motor neurons in the prenatal or neonatal period. Cerebral palsy is a nonprogressive abnormality in motor function which may also affect intellect, emotional behavior, speech, sight, hearing, and touch.

The main types are spastic and athetoid palsy. The degree of affliction can vary from the barely perceptible to the vegetative, immobile, and institutionally dependent. The severity can be described in part by the term monoplegic, diplegic (both legs), hemiplegic arm and leg (same side), and tetraplegic.

Birth trauma is the most common cause and includes precipitous or prolonged labor, fetal distress, asphyxia, or kernicterus (usually athetoid in type from basal ganglia damage). Neonatal head injury, anoxia, or viral encephalitis can be a cause. Such damage results in spasticity incoordination and muscle agonist-antagonist imbalance. These imbalanced forces can lead to fixed and severe orthopedic deformities.

The athetoid type has a writhing or continuous abnormal movement pattern with speech difficulty in the presence of a fully functional intellect. Severely affected children can be detected in the neonatal period as floppy children, spastic children with a feeble cry or poor sucking reflex, an exaggerated startle reflex, or an abnormally persistant grasping reflex. Milder cases may not be noted until later in development as incoordination or clumsiness is noted.

Management by the Family Physician. The family physician should recognize the prevalence of cerebral palsy and its various manifestations. Early detection is not as essential as it is for congenital hip dislocation, for example. Therefore, when in doubt about the nature of a gait or posture abnormality in an infant or child, it is usually prudent to wait and see. As the child matures, the true nature of any neurologic deficit will become evident.

Keep in mind that cerebral palsy is a nonprogressive disease of childhood. Paraparesis without involvement of the upper limb or progressive worsening of the neurologic deficit should cause one to look for treatable conditions, particularly spinal cord lesions.

The aims of treatment are to maximize function through prevention or correction of fixed deformities and the teaching of compensatory skills. Orthotics and bracing have, in our experience, been very useful in conjunction with therapy and surgery in the prevention and correction of gross deformity. Programmed approaches to the problem which preclude the judicious use of surgical procedures or orthotics are not realistic in practice. Many of these youngsters are surprisingly independent, bright, and communicative after an effective multidisciplinary approach to therapy.

MUSCULAR DYSTROPHIES

The dystrophies are a group of rather rare hereditary myopathies of a progressive nature. Several types are described and have variable ages of onset, sex-linked character, hereditary patterns, and different rates of progression, and patterns of afflicted muscle may vary.

Duchenne's, or pseudohypertrophic, dystrophy is inherited most often as a sex-linked recessive pattern. Hence it afflicts males. Age at onset is about 3 to 5 years, presenting as a weakness of the calf muscles with an apparent hypertrophy of the muscles.

Characteristically the boy's calves become enlarged and doughy to palpation. However, the characteristic physical test is the child's inability to raise himself from the floor without bracing his knees with his hands (Fig. 49–87). This is due to weakness beginning primarily in the quadriceps and hip extensor muscles.

Other conditions of myopathy that involve the limb girdle regions or the shoulder and pelvic muscles come on slowly and progress less rapidly than does the most common pseudohypertrophic form.

The diagnostic laboratory findings include elevated creatinine phosphokinase and aldolase. Any male child seen because of a complaint of clumsiness, leg weakness, or easy fatigability should be screened by these laboratory tests.

Management by the Family Physician. Suspect the possibility of muscular dystrophy in any "clumsy boy." Obtain a creatinine phosphokinase (CPK) promptly in any such child. In some areas CPK studies are recommended in newborn boys routinely, much in the way that phenylketonuria screening has been accepted.

Female members of the family should also be evaluated with CPK studies when an individual boy is detected. Carriers of the condition should be so informed and given genetic counseling.

Treatment of the condition can be only supportive, not curative. Therapy should concentrate on stretching tight muscles and strengthening whatever remains in the diseased muscles. Lightweight orthotic support of ankles is particularly useful in preventing equinovarus deformity. Surgery should be recommended with extreme caution, since it may occasion-

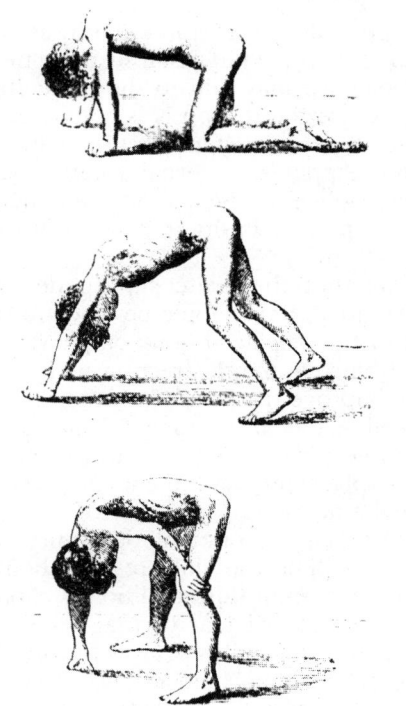

Figure 49–87. Illustration of Gower's sign from Gower's original text shows the process by which the boy with muscular dystrophy must raise himself from a crouched position using his arms and hands rather than the weakened thigh muscles. (Gower, W. R.: Pseudohypertrophic Muscular Paralysis. Churchill, 1879. Courtesy of B. Kakulas, Professor of Neuropathology, U. of Western Australia.)

ally aggravate the child's problem rather than help if it is not appropriately timed.

As the disease progresses, the spine tends to collapse and requires constant adjustment of wheelchairs and spinal orthoses. The spinal deformity contributes significantly to the young man's ultimate demise from respiratory insufficiency.

To manage the multiple problems of these severely handicapped individuals, a well-run rehabilitative facility or clinic is quite essential. As these boys grow into young adulthood, they become progressively weaker and are more difficult to care for at home.

Unfortunately, our present attempts to treat this progressive disease can be considered only halfway solutions, and we anxiously await developments from fundamental research studies.

Limb Girdle Types

This type may be inherited as a dominant or recessive gene. Presentation is usually during adolescence or early adulthood with weakness and wasting of the shoulder pectoral muscles. Usually the presentation is weakness in reaching above the head.

The progression is one of slow progression which can cripple in 10 to 20 years and is not often fatal.

Fascioscapulohumeral Type

This disease is an autosomal dominant inherited genetic myopathy of incomplete penetrance. The onset is during adolescence with facial muscle weakness (can't whistle). Soon, wasting of the shoulder girdle muscles is noted (can't get arms over head). The malady is slowly progressive with years of mild involvement, and life expectancy is normal.

Management by the Family Physician. The family physician should be aware of all of the dystrophies and their inheritance patterns. Referral should be made early for definitive diagnosis and effective counseling and treatment.

LEGG-CALVÉ-PERTHES' DISEASE

Legg-Calvé-Perthes' disease (avascular necrosis of the capital femoral epiphysis) is another condition that should be high on the list of the differential diagnoses in childhood limp. This condition of impaired vascularity to the femoral epiphyseal growth center generally occurs between the ages of 3 and 10 years when the capital femoral epiphysis is most susceptible to vascular insult.

Eventually mechanical collapse occurs in the subchondral bone of the weight-bearing portion of the head. The result can be considerable anatomic distortion of the proximal femoral epiphysis. Children at this age are capable of reconstituting the shape of their proximal femur, and the prognosis is not as poor as it is with avascular necrosis in the adult.

The characteristic presentation is a history of a limp and some pain in the knee for 1 to 2 months. If the family physician overlooks the referred pattern of pain from the hip to the knee, the hip condition may go unrecognized or be dismissed as "growing pains."

The most effective means of detecting the early stages of Legg-Calvé-Perthes' disease is by physical examination. The patient is usually a boy around 6 years of age who, although he points to the knee as a source of his problem, has tenderness to palpation in the anterior and posterior aspects of the hip. The first sign of hip pathology is limitation of joint rotation. This can be elicited as the child lies supine with the hips extended. Gently rotate the hip internally and feel firm soft tissue resistance. Observe the child for signs of pain during hip rotation. Abduction of the hip also elicits a similar feeling of resistance and pain in the hip which may be only mild.

X-rays in the early stages of Legg-Calvé-Perthes' disease must be carefully evaluated primarily for signs of capsular swelling, widening of the joint space, and demineralization in the femoral metaphysis or femoral neck immediately subjacent to the growth line. Only in the later stages does the femoral epiphysis develop increased density in whole or in part as the changes progress.

Management by the Family Physician. The childhood limp or knee pain should always be taken seriously. If you cannot find an underlying cause, refer the patient for other ideas and full assessment.

Usually the clinical and roentgenographic diagnosis is straightforward. Occasionally the possibility of tuberculosis or pyogenic hip infection must be ruled out by hip aspiration.

About 10 to 15 per cent of Legg-Calvé-Perthes' patients develop bilateral symptoms. This must be kept in mind in any child under treatment for a unilateral condition. In addition, patients with bilateral involvement should also be evaluated for conditions such as multiple epiphyseal dysplasia or hypothyroidism, both of which cause fragmentary epiphyseal ossification confused with avascular necrosis.

The disease is a long-term management problem, usually requiring orthoses and occasionally surgical osteotomy to maintain normal articulation between the femoral head and acetabulum. This needs continuing orthopedic consultation and evaluation of the child's response to treatment.

SLIPPED CAPITAL FEMORAL EPIPHYSIS

Another cause of childhood limp that frequently may be painless is slippage of the capital femoral epiphysis. This results from a gradual fatigue failure occurring through the growth plate of the proximal femur during the preadolescent period of rapid growth. This slip occurs most often in the overweight boy or in the tall, lanky, rapidly growing individual. It is about five times more common in boys and occurs in the age range of 10 to 17 years, a slightly older group than for Legg-Calvé-Perthes' disease.

The slip may come on as an acute failure, much like a femoral neck fracture in 10 to 15 per cent of cases. About 20 per cent of patients develop a similar slip on the opposite side. This should always be of concern when the individual is walking with crutches while recovering from the original slip.

The diagnosis of slipped femoral epiphysis may be overlooked for two reasons. The first is that the problem once again presents initially as knee pain rather than hip pain. The source of the problem coming from the hip should be readily apparent if that joint is only examined in any patient with knee pain. With the displaced articular surface of the femoral head, the younger patient cannot flex his hip without externally rotating it (Fig. 49–88*A,B*).

The second pitfall of the diagnosis is incomplete x-ray. A standard anteroposterior view of the hip may not visualize the displacement of the femoral epiphysis in a posterior and inferior direction. Widening of the epiphyseal line and demineralization of the metaphysis may be evident. However, to recognize the early slip, a lateral view is usually necessary. This will demonstrate the step-off between the femoral neck and the bony epiphysis (Fig. 49–88*C*).

Management by the Family Physician. Treatment of the slipped capital femoral epiphysis should commence as soon as the physician suspects the diagnosis. Further slippage may add to the difficulties in management. Once the diagnosis is confirmed by x-rays, place the patient in skin traction with the hip in abduction. Apply an internal rotation strap to the thigh (Fig. 49–89). The patient can then be safely referred for pinning in situ to prevent further slippage (see Fig. 49–88*D*).

For all but the acute slip (under one week's duration), no attempt should be made to improve the position of the displaced bony epiphysis. If an acute slip has occurred, gentle traction with internal rotation may improve the position of the proximal epiphysis as well as the child's range of motion.

Multiple pins are preferable to a single nail to prevent displacement and to encourage closure of the epiphyseal plate.

A surprising amount of deformity can be corrected by the time the child reaches bony maturity. Of major concern in this condition is chondrolysis or complete loss of articular cartilage and residual osteoarthritis. This usually requires fusion of the young adult's hip. An important additional concern is the 20 per cent chance of bilateral involvement. This should always be kept in mind until the patient reaches skeletal maturity.

SPINAL CORD TUMORS AND OTHER CAUSES OF CHILDHOOD LIMP

Limps can result from neurologic conditions, particularly developmental defects, diastematomyelia, Friedreich's ataxia, von Recklinghausen's neurofibromatosis, syringomyelia, and polio.

Frequently overlooked, however, is spinal cord tumor. A progressive neurologic deficit in a child, particularly with scoliosis or other structural deformities, needs investigation for the possibility of a tumor. Usually there is a triad of symptoms: (1) a history of early, often transient neurologic deficit (this frequently is considered to be cerebral palsy or even polio); (2) development of progressive scoliosis; and (3) progressive paraparesis resulting from mechanical compression of the spinal cord (Curtiss and Collins, 1961).

The 4-year-old boy illustrated in Figure 49–90*A* was seen in our department after a history of intermittent limping for approximately 6 months. He was noted to have bilateral weakness of the extensors of his feet and also pronounced lumbar scoliosis and lordosis (Fig. 49–90*B*). The spaces between the pedicles in the L2-L3 region were abruptly widened as seen on anteroposterior view of the spine. The myelogram demonstrated complete obstruction from an intraspinal astrocytoma (Fig. 49–90*C*).

Usually scoliosis is not painful nor associated with neurologic deficit. Spinal cord tumors do characteristically produce scoliosis with neurologic deficit. Extradural tumors such as osteoid osteoma or osteo-

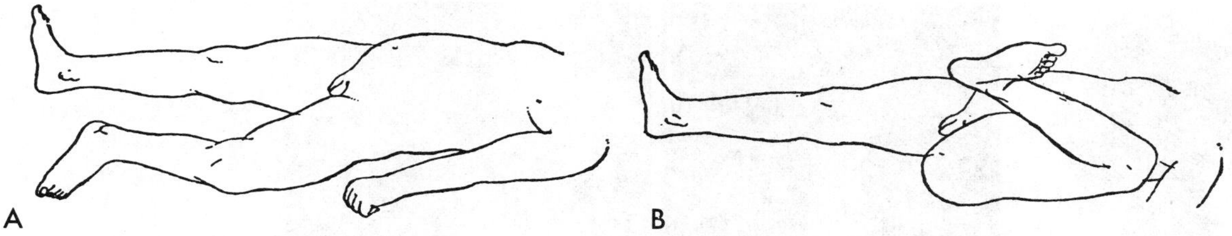

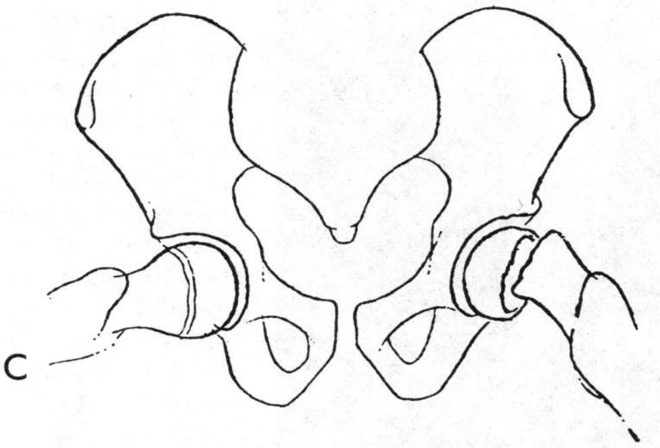

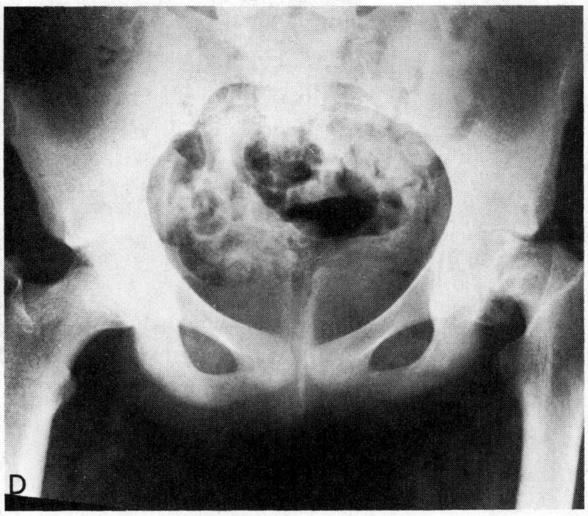

Figure 49–88. *A*, Characteristically, the adolescent with acute slipped capital femoral epiphysis maintains the leg in a shortened, abducted, externally rotated position like an adult with a femoral neck fracture. *B*, The characteristic sign of a chronic slipped capital femoral epiphysis is the tendency of the hip to externally rotate markedly during flexion. *C*, A roentgenogram, in particular a frog-leg lateral view, shows widening of the epiphyseal line and displacement of the bony epiphysis. *D*, A chronic slip may progress to a severe deformity as shown here. This can be prevented by prompt recognition and early pinning in situ. (Illustrative case courtesy of Professor J. Glancy, Queen Elizabeth II Medical Center, Perth, Australia.)

blastoma, on the other hand, produce scoliosis that is painful but usually without neurologic symptoms.

Management by the Family Physician. The family physician, in evaluating these conditions, can contribute much to the overall management of the limping or clumsy child. By his careful follow-up and observation of patients with these conditions, he may be the first to detect signs and symptoms indicating the need to look beyond the ordinary.

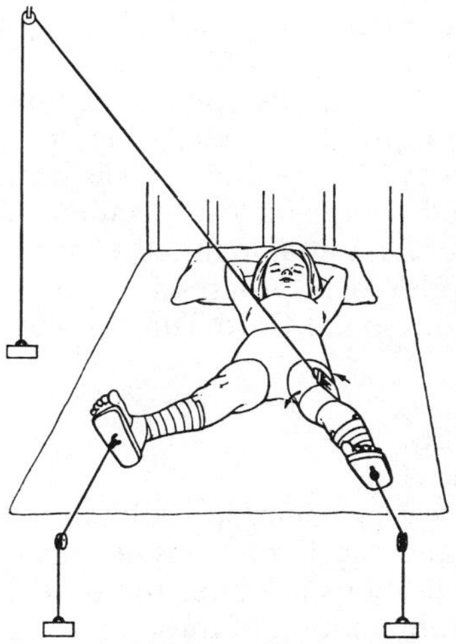

Figure 49–89. The acute slipped capital femoral epiphysis should be protected in skin traction with an internal rotation strap applied to the thigh.

Common Foot Problems

The two most common foot problems in children are pigeon toes and flat feet. A number of these feet are merely variants within the range of normal development which will correct with time. Overtreatment of these normal variants can be worse than the disorder. A percentage of these deformities do persist into adulthood and cause disability that might have been prevented by a more vigorous treatment.

The family physician should be alert to the pathomechanics of these problems in order to determine whether treatment by reassurance of the parents, by corrective splints and exercise, or by referral for more vigorous orthopedic management is indicated.

EXAMINATION OF THE INFANT'S FOOT

The thing to remember when examining the foot of an infant or child is that your examination should not be restricted to the foot. Look carefully for any signs indicating a more serious problem, particularly muscle weakness or spasticity as the child stands or lies.

Examine the child unencumbered by diapers or clothing. Particularly inspect the undersurface of the foot to evaluate for deformities in either the forefoot or hindfoot.

Move the foot in inversion and eversion to detect rigidity or limitation of motion. Continue examining

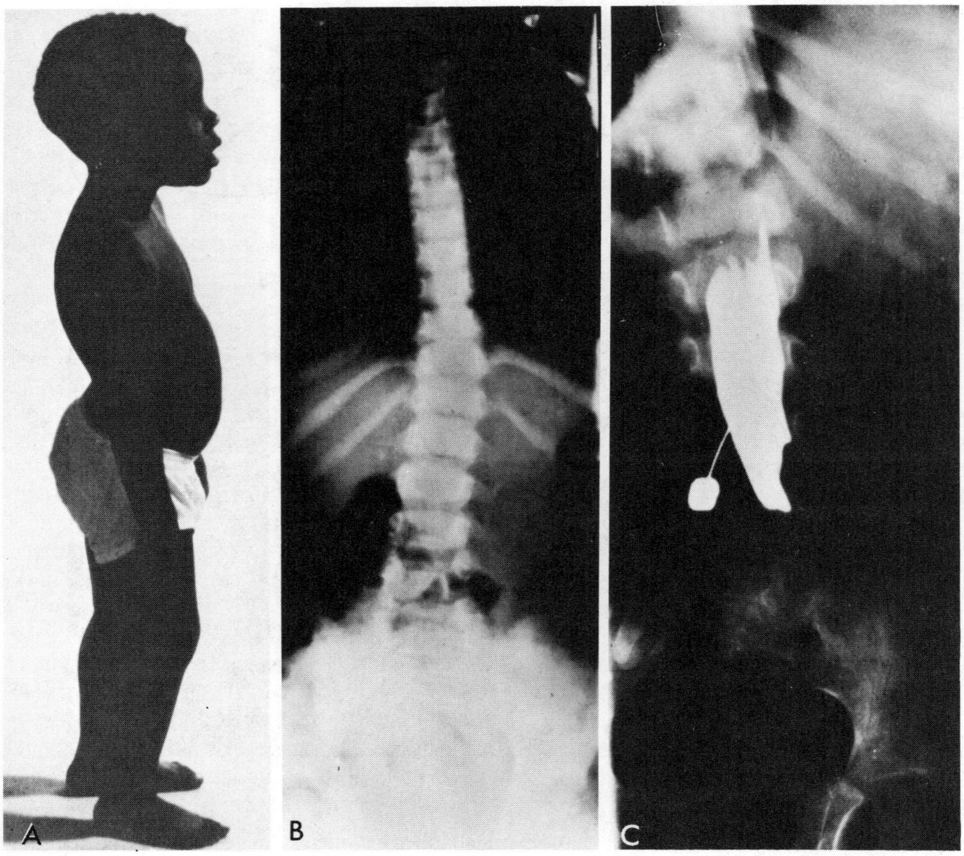

Figure 49–90. *A*, This 4-year-old boy presented with a limp and a progressively increasing lumbar lordosis. He also had detectable motor weakness of the foot dorsiflexors. *B*, Roentgenogram showed lumbar scoliosis with abrupt widening of the interpedicular spaces at L-2 and L-3. *C*, A myelogram demonstrated an obstruction from an intraspinal tumor, which proved to be an astrocytoma. (Illustrative case courtesy of Charles Emerson, M.D.)

up the legs to note torsion or bowing of the tibia or knee motion and particularly check for hip abnormalities.

Any examination of an infant or young child, orthopedic or otherwise, should include testing the hip for congenital dislocation. The earliest reliable sign of hip instability is Ortolani's "click" or "clunk," which is present in the infant at the newborn stage. This test should be done on the newborn baby as well as on follow-up well-baby examination. (See section on Congenital Dislocation of the Hip and Fig. 49–84).

After the hip examination, inspect the spine for curvature, dimpling, or evidence of intraspinal abnormalities. Neurologic deficits can be causes of foot deformities.

A similar complete examination should be carried out in the older child whom you see for the first time for foot problems. Observe walking with the shoes on and off. Inspect the shoes for abnormal wear. Normal heel/toe gait wears the shoes more on the outer border of the heel and inner border of the toes. Abnormal wear may indicate a spasticity or some mechanical deformity in the foot. Check the child's feet carefully for blisters or calluses reflecting abnormal gait or poorly fitting shoes.

Check the arches of the feet while standing and sitting. The common flexible flat foot appears to have a normal arch when the patient does not bear weight. Flattening becomes evident only with weight-bearing. Rigid flat feet, in contrast, are flat and everted whether or not the patient is bearing weight. Check the range of both eversion and inversion of both feet to determine any rigid limitation. Also look for heel cord tightness by holding the foot inverted to control motion of the subtalar joint and then maximally dorsiflexing the ankle with the knee extended.

Palpate for peroneal muscle tightness around the lateral malleolus as the foot is inverted. This is frequently secondary to conditions such as congenital coalitions of joints. Peroneal muscle spasm may also indicate early rheumatoid arthritis of the hindfoot joints.

Evaluate the child's spine and hips. Quite frequently major problems, including scoliosis, diastematomyelia, and congenital hip dislocation, present only an initial complaint of "peculiar gait." One of the most common initial manifestations of spinal cord tumors in children is progressive gait abnormalities (see section on Spinal Cord Tumors and Fig. 49–90).

PIGEON TOES

Toeing-in is a very common problem which both the orthopedist and the family physician manage. It results from conditions in either the foot, the tibia, the femur, or a combination of these three. These include (1) metatarsus adductus; (2) tibial torsion; and (3) femoral anteversion.

Metatarsus Adductus

The characteristics of this deformity are (1) adduction of the tarsometatarsal joint, causing the individual to walk on the lateral side of the foot (adductovarus); (2) an increase in the height of the longitudinal arch; and (3) an increase in the space between the first and second toes (see Figs. 49–91 and 49–93).

Metatarsus adductus has been described as "one third of a clubfoot." This deformity of the forefoot is also seen in the clubfoot, but in true clubfoot, a heel varus and equinus of the ankle is noted (Fig. 49–92). Metatarsus adductus produces, if anything, a valgus position of the heel. Recent experience has indicated that metatarsus adductus is diagnosed approximately 30 times more commonly than clubfoot.

Infants normally tend to turn their forefoot inward in response to any plantar stimulus.

The most reliable method to decide whether the forefoot is fixed in adduction is to inspect that lateral border of the foot from the undersurface (see Fig. 49–91*A*). In the normal infant's foot there is a definite concavity felt and seen along the lateral border at the base of the fifth metatarsal. If the forefoot is adducted, this concavity becomes a convexity associated with a prominent base of the fifth metatarsal.

Management by the Family Physician. The majority of pigeon toes from forefoot adduction will correct spontaneously by 2 to 3 years of age, provided the child's foot is flexible. You can demonstrate this flexibility by stroking along the lateral border of the child's foot and ankle so as to stimulate the peroneal musculature. If the child is able to straighten out the forefoot adduction, generally the problem will correct spontaneously. Further treatment is not required.

If there is a question about the flexibility of the foot, refer the child for treatment as soon as possible. Do not advise the parents to apply a regular shoe to the opposite foot, that is, the right shoe on the left foot. This is actually harmful, since it tends to flatten the longitudinal arch of the child's foot.

The treatment for the inflexible metatarsus adductus or one that does not completely correct with peroneal muscle action is a series of casts applied over a 2- to 4-month period. These can be molded firmly around the lateral border of the foot to restore the natural concavity and eliminate the convexity. The result is usually a satisfactory correction with two to three cast changes.

Failure to correct metatarsus adductus does not cause a great deal of disability for the patient, although it can result in discomfort and painful calluses. These are most likely to occur under the first and fifth metatarsals in association with a structurally inefficient high arch or cavus foot (Fig. 49–93).

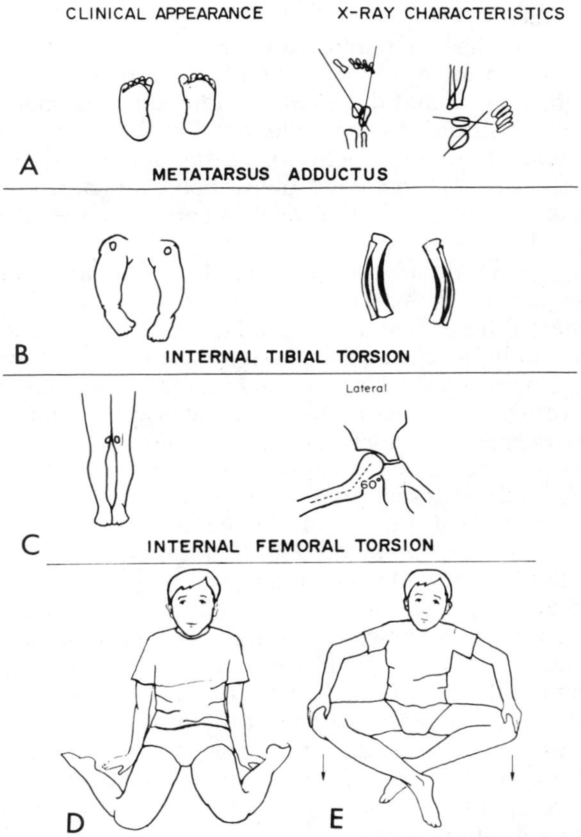

Figure 49–91. *A*, Pigeon toes due to metatarsus adductus are characterized by a convex lateral border of the foot and prominent base of the fifth metatarsal. Anteroposterior x-ray films show adduction of the forefoot and widening of the space between the first and second metatarsals. The talocalcaneal angle is increased as the calcaneus is turned out from under the talus, while the talus remains relatively fixed by the ankle. On lateral x-ray films the metatarsals appear to be stacked on one another owing to the turned in position of the forefoot (adductovarus). *B*, Toeing-in from tibial torsion is characterized by a posterior position of the medical malleolus relative to the lateral malleolus. X-ray films frequently show bowing of the tibia, which magnifies the apparent internal rotation. Increased medial cortical density seen as bowed tibia and fibula is due to compressive stress. *C*, Femoral torsion is characterized by an inward turning of the patellas with the hips in full extension. Lateral x-ray views show an increased angle of anteversion between the femoral neck and shaft. *D*, Children with excessive internal femoral torsion tend to sit with legs tucked under thighs and hips rotated inward. *E*, An effective method of decreasing internal femoral rotation is to have the child regularly sit "Indian style." While sitting in this position, he can then push his thighs and hips out into external rotation, stretching out the iliofemoral ligament.

Tibial Torsion

In a normal fetus the tibia is internally rotated so that the medial malleolus is posterior relative to the lateral malleolus. At birth the malleoli become even. When the child starts walking, the medial malleolus is about 20 degrees anterior to the lateral one. The habit of laying the infant prone with the feet turned in slows this normal external rotational process of the ankle. However, the need to externally rotate the feet becomes inevitable as the child starts walking and needs a stable base of support.

Clinical assessment is made by inspecting the alignment of the knee and ankle with the knees flexed (see Fig. 49–91*B*). Invariably, tibial torsion is evident

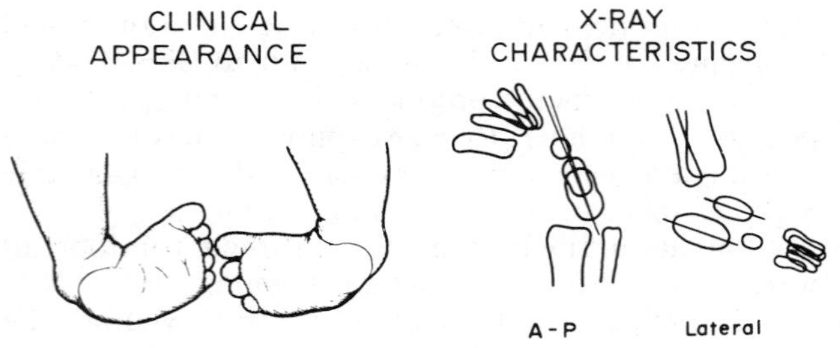

Figure 49–92. Clubfoot, in addition to adduction of the forefoot, includes varus of the hindfoot and equinus of the ankle. This is characterized on anteroposterior x-ray films by adduction of the forefoot and narrowing of the talocalcaneal angle as the calcaneus is turned under the talus and into varus position. On lateral x-ray views, both the talus and the calcaneus are in equinus and their axes are almost parallel. (Connolly, J., Regen, E., and Hillman, J. W.: Pigeon-toes and flat feet. Pediatr. Clin. North Am., *17*:295, 1970.)

in any child who first starts walking. This will correct spontaneously in a normal child who is not overweight or rachitic. The fact remains that mother and grandmother are concerned about the child's bowlegs and tendency to turn the feet inward. Our usual approach is to correct the in-turning by simple splintage. This can be done effectively with a device such as an extra shoelace or key chain run through the holes at the back of the infant's shoes (Fig. 49–94). This maintains the child's legs externally rotated during sleep. If a more rigid device is needed, a bar attached to the shoes will hold the feet externally rotated. In addition, the bar stimulates the everting muscles of the child's foot as he tries to kick off the splint.

Femoral Torsion

Another common cause of in-toeing evident in the older child who has been walking is internal femoral torsion or anteversion. Femoral anteversion is the degree to which the head of the femur lies anterior to the transcondylar axis of the shaft (see Fig. 49–91*C*).

At the 30th week in utero this angle is about 60 degrees and results from the fetus positioned with the lower limbs fully flexed onto the abdomen. After birth the neck-shaft angle decreases to 40 degrees as limbs are brought down into extension, although full hip extension is not possible in the newborn. As the hips continue to extend, the neck angle is remolded from the force of the tight anterior hip capsule ligament and the response of growing bone to applied forces. The anterior angle of the femoral neck continues to decrease until in the adult it is only about 12 degrees.

Physical Examination. Femoral anteversion causes in-toeing as a result of the forces from the tight capsule and the anterior iliofemoral ligament in full extension. As the child walks with the hip fully extended, this ligament forces the femur to rotate internally. The patient's knees then characteristically face one another in the weight-bearing phases of gait (see Fig. 49–91*C*).

A simple method for detection of femoral anteversion is to measure the range of external and internal hip rotation with the hip both fully extended and fully flexed. If there is significant femoral anteversion when the hip is extended, external rotation is zero while internal rotation may measure as much as 60 degrees or more. As the hip flexes toward 90 degrees, the anterior capsule becomes relaxed. Consequently, external rotation and internal rotation then become equal, i.e., about 60 degrees.

Management by the Family Physician. The child with femoral anteversion generally is more comfortable sitting with the hips internally rotated. Consequently, he assumes a position with the legs tucked under his thighs and his hips turned in while doing things like watching television (see Fig. 49–91*D*). This adds to the tightening of the hip capsule and its tendency to perpetuate the torsional deformity. Persistent anteversion of the femur may cause the child to compensate by turning his tibia externally, producing a flat-footed gait.

To avoid this problem it is best to treat femoral anteversion by simple external rotational exercises. Have the child sit with the legs externally rotated and

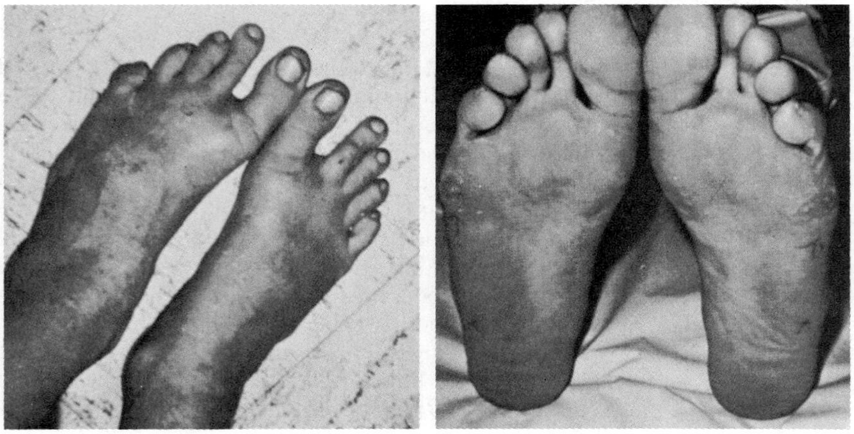

Figure 49–93. Persistent metatarsus adductus in the 21-year-old man has resulted in painful calluses under the first and fifth metatarsals. (Connolly, J., Regen, E., and Hillman, J. W.: Pigeon-toes and flat feet. Pediatr. Clin. North Am., *17*:295, 1970.)

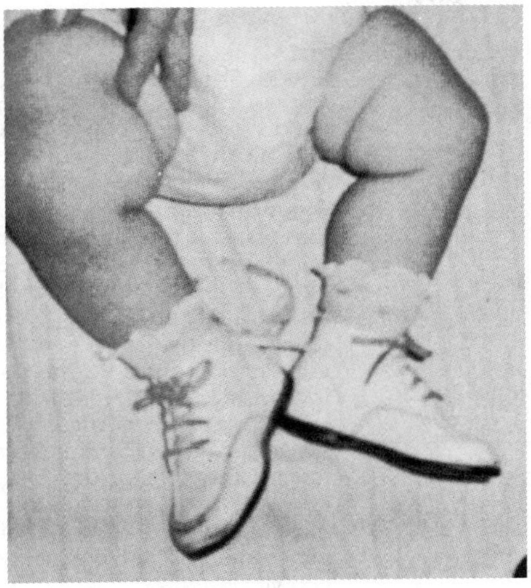

Figure 49–94. A simple inexpensive method of maintaining a child's legs externally rotated for treating "tibial torsion" is to run an extra lace between slits in the backs of the shoes. (Connolly, J., Regen, E., and Hillman, J. W.: Pigeon-toes and flat feet. Pediatr. Clin. North Am., *17*:291, 1970.)

encourage him to force his knees downward toward the floor (see Fig. 49–91*E*).

Attempted correction by twister cables or bars is worse than the disease. These devices tend to rotate the limb at the knee rather than at the hip. This is particularly a problem if there is any spasticity of the muscles, producing the internal femoral torsion.

Operative correction by derotational osteotomy is not indicated for femoral torsion in the otherwise normal child. Derotational osteotomy may prove a useful procedure if the child has cerebral palsy with muscle spasticity. If you suspect spasticity as a cause of this gait abnormality or femoral anteversion, refer the child for orthopedic evaluation.

FLAT FEET

The majority of flat feet are the flexible type. That is, flattening is evident only as the individual loads the arch during standing. Approximately 2 per cent of flat feet are classified as rigid due to severe bony alterations. In these rigid flat feet, the foot remains flat whether or not the patient is bearing weight.

Common causes of rigid flat feet include congenital vertical talus or talonavicular dislocation, congenital coalitions or bars between the bones of the hindfoot, and accessory navicular bones (Figs. 49–95 and 49–96).

Flexible Flat Feet

Flattening of the arch of the foot occurs when the talus loses its base of support and is depressed medially. The result is a grossly evident, prominent medial talus with weight-bearing (Figs. 49–95*B* and 49–96*B*).

Most of the support for the talus is provided by the anterior end of the calcaneus or the sustentaculum talus. It is actually the loss of support as the calcaneus drifts into a valgus or turned-out position that is the basic problem in the flexible flat foot.

Adding to the valgus tendency of the heel is a tight Achilles tendon. The Achilles normally is a weak foot inverter as well as a plantar flexor. However, as it displaces laterally with the calcaneus, it tends to pull the heel further out from under the talus.

The valgus position of the heel causes the forefoot to twist out into abducted position. Consequently, the bones on the medial side of the foot become separated, while those on the lateral side of the flat foot are compressed. The medial border becomes convex and elongated. The lateral border appears concave and shortened. The intrinsic plantar muscles become stretched and lose their strength reducing the contribution these muscles make to normal foot architecture.

The result of these mechanical alterations is that the talus must be supported by ligaments rather than bone. The normally strong ligaments of the foot are stretched and ultimately become lax. The muscles of the foot and calf then must support the talus and the other components of the longitudinal arch. Consequently, symptoms from flat feet in the older child or adolescent begin with aching of the calf muscles with prolonged standing. The arch of the foot also hurts from overstretching the ligaments.

Conditions that should be differentiated from the usual flexible flat foot include congenital vertical talus, congenital coalitions, and accessory navicular problems (Figs. 49–95 and 49–96).

Not infrequently, flattening of the foot may result from muscle imbalance either as a result of paralysis or injury to the posterior tibial muscle or as a result of peroneal spasticity in cerebral palsy (Fig. 49–96*D*). The everting peroneal muscles overpull in relation to the inverting muscles. The result is that the heel, or calcaneus, is pulled out from under the talus, causing an unstable, severe flat foot.

All of these conditions should be kept in mind as one evaluates the individual patient's symptoms and physical findings as previously described in this section.

Management by the Family Physician. Most infants are flat footed when they first start to walk. They develop an arch by around the second or third year of life as they gain balance and muscle control of the foot. The status of the infant's arch can be determined on physical examination by palpating the medial border of the foot and feeling the relationship of the talus and the calcaneus. The stability of the talus is the key physical finding in judging the need for active treatment of the infant's flat foot. In general no corrective treatment is necessary for the usual infant's flat foot. Special shoes are usually more of a detriment than a value in this age group.

Rarely, if there is evidence of talocalcaneal instability or a possibility of a congenital rigid flat foot,

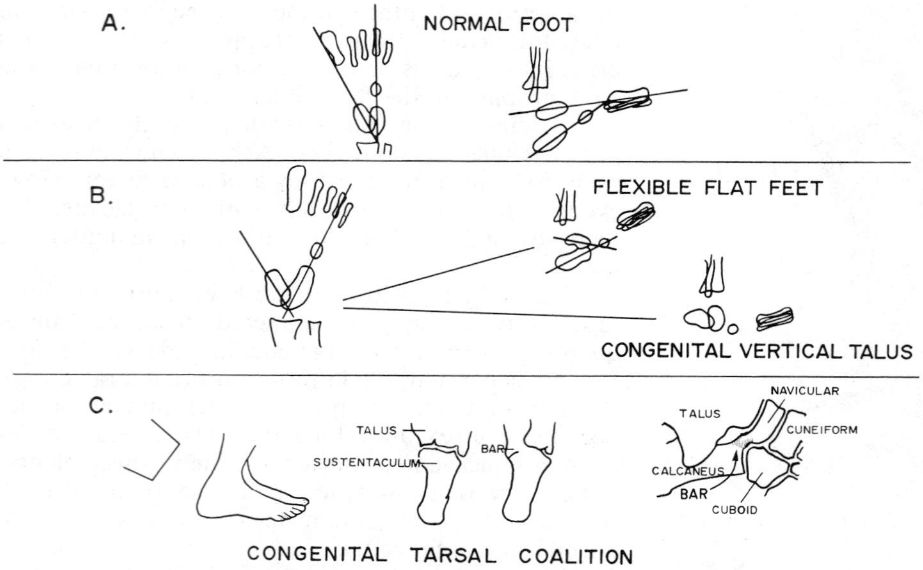

Figure 49–95. X-ray findings in flat feet. *A*, X-ray films of the normal child's foot are characterized by a talocalcaneal angle between 30 and 50 degrees in anteroposterior and in weight-bearing lateral views. *B*, X-ray films of flat feet show an increased talocalcaneal angle as the calcaneal support is lost and the calcaneus turns out from under the talus. In the weight-bearing lateral view, the talus is pointing into the sole of the foot in the flexible flat foot, while in true congenital vertical talus, both the talus and calcaneus are directed toward the sole of the foot and the talus no longer articulates with the navicular. *C*, Calcaneonavicular bars are frequently detected only on special views.

treatment with a Denis Browne bar may be indicated. This is worth trying, particularly if there is a family history of symptomatic flat feet.

The Denis Browne bar is applied with the severe flat foot inverted (Fig. 49–97). The splint in essence is a dynamic correction and stimulates development of a normal arch. As the child is required to walk on this device, one foot works against the other, requiring muscle activity on both sides during both inversion and eversion. The splint should be kept on the child when he is walking and should be continued for approximately 6 to 10 months. As might be imagined, the method is sometimes a nuisance to parents who are not willing to put in the time and effort, but it does help encourage development of a normally arched foot in the toddler with significant flattening. If the mother cannot accept this, an alternative is to have her practice inversion exercises with the child by encouraging dancing or walking on the outer border of the foot.

"Corrective shoes" are of no value in actually correcting foot deformities. They offer only static support to the foot, and they do little to alter any architectural instability. When a child reaches adolescence and becomes symptomatic from flat feet, arch supports or inserts may be useful to relieve mild

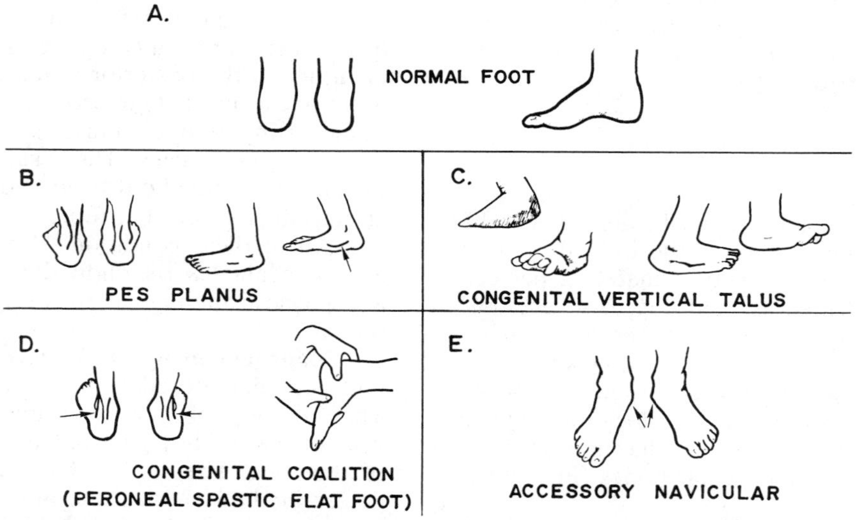

Figure 49–96. Clinical appearance of flat feet. *A*, In the normal foot, weight is borne slightly on the medial side of the heel, as seen from the rear. On side view, the normal arch has adequate talar support from the calcaneus, and weight is transmitted to the os calcis and metatarsal heads. *B*, Flat feet are characterized by a turning out of the calcaneus from under the talus as seen from the rear. On side view, the loss of talar support *(arrow)* is evident as weight is borne on the entire medial side of the foot. *C*, Congenital vertical talus in infancy appears as a rigid calcaneovalgus foot but characteristically has a concavity on the dorsolateral border of the foot. If the deformity is untreated, with weight bearing the foot takes on a "rocker bottom" appearance as the heel goes into equinus and the forefoot dorsiflexes. *D*, Congenital coalitions are associated with a valgus heel position and a tendency to symptomatic muscle spasm *(arrows)*. These rigid flat feet have limitation of subtalar motion due to the bony block. *E*, Accessory navicular bones *(arrows)* may occasionally become sufficiently symptomatic in the older child or adult to benefit from surgical removal. (Connolly, J., Regens, E., and Hillman, J. W.: Pigeon-toes and flat feet. Pediatr. Clin. North Am., *17*:291, 1970.)

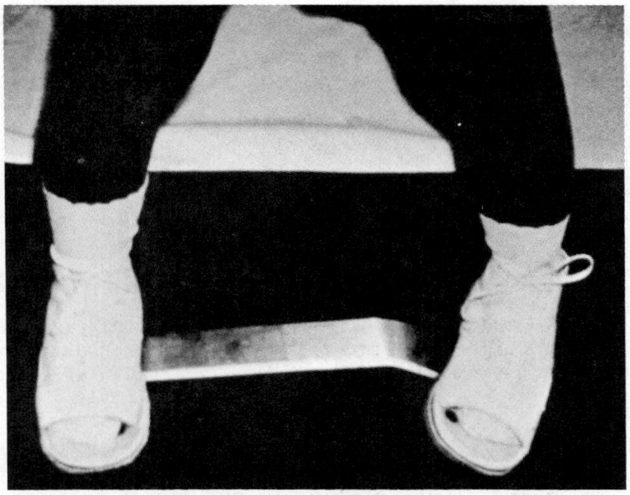

Figure 49–97. Method of utilizing a Denis Browne bar for correcting severe flat feet in a young child. The toes are cut out of the shoe and the foot or feet are held inverted by bending the bar. (Connolly, J., Regens, E., and Hillman, J. W.: Pigeon-toes and flat feet. Pediatr. Clin. North Am., *17*:291, 1970.)

aching. When the main problem is a defect in the bony architectural support of the foot, the most effective treatment is surgical correction of the bony defect at about age 14 or 15. The timing and the indication for surgical correction vary with each individual's symptoms. Only 5 to 10 per cent of young people with symptomatic relaxed flat feet are sufficiently disabled to need surgical correction.

Flat foot conditions that require orthopedic correction are those producing a rigid flattening, particularly congenital vertical talus or congenital tarsal coalition.

Congenital Vertical Talus

This might be better described as congenital talonavicular dislocation. It results from a dorsal displacement of the navicular to the superior aspect of the talus. This forces the talus vertically down into the medial aspect of the sole. The condition is found in approximately one per cent of flat feet treated by orthopedic surgeons.

The deformity should be particularly suspected in a severe calcaneal valgus foot in the newborn. Inspect these feet along the outer border. The congenital talonavicular dislocation is evident from a dorsal concavity rather than a lateral concavity as in the normal foot (see Fig. 49–96*C*). The head of the talus can be felt in the foot as the examiner traces the child's arch with his thumb.

Most calcaneovalgus feet in the newborn correct spontaneously. This is in contrast to the exact opposite deformity, equinovarus or clubfoot, which requires early active treatment. The calcaneovalgus foot that fails to correct in the first few months must be suspected of actually being a talonavicular dislocation.

Walking is usually not delayed with congenital vertical talus, but as the child stands to walk, the deformity is worsened and the foot then develops a "rocker bottom" appearance, with the midfoot resting on the ground. The heel and forefoot become suspended off the ground (see Fig. 49–96*C*).

Early diagnosis depends on clinical assessment. X-rays of the congenital talonavicular dislocation show a downward displacement of the talus and a downward displacement of the anterior end of the calcaneus (see Fig. 49–98). The problem with x-ray diagnosis is that the navicular does not ossify in the infant's foot until about the age of 3 to 5 years, and therefore, the relationship between the talus and navicular must be implied.

In the congenital talonavicular dislocation, the long axis of the talus is markedly displaced in the plantar direction even with the foot held in plantar flexion. This indicates that the navicular dislocation is not corrected merely by plantar flexion of the foot. In contrast with congenital vertical talus, any apparent dorsal displacement of a navicular associated with the flexible flat foot can be corrected by plantar flexion (Fig. 49–98).

Other conditions must be considered as a cause of deformity. These include polio, cerebral palsy, spina bifida, trisomy 13-15, and trisomy 18. The condition most frequently associated with congenital vertical talus is arthrogryposis, which tends to involve multiple joints, particularly the knees and hips.

Management by the Family Physician. The usual congenital calcaneovalgus, or reverse clubfoot, deformity can be treated by a Denis Browne bar as previously described for the flexible flat foot (see Fig. 49–97). Be sure that the problem is not that of a congenital vertical talus or talonavicular dislocation, as these conditions require more vigorous therapy. Too often congenital talonavicular dislocation persists undetected into early childhood and then will require extensive surgical correction to relieve symptoms.

Congenital Tarsal Coalition

The most frequent congenital coalitions, or fusions, are those between the talus and calcaneus and between the navicular and calcaneus. All varieties of single or multiple coalitions have been noted in the foot. There have been several familial reports indicating that multiple tarsal coalitions run in families (Fig. 49–99).

Congenital coalitions can cause rigid flat feet that may be completely asymptomatic. Pain usually develops if the congenital bar fractures as the child becomes active in preadolescence. The result then is symptomatic strain and spasm in the peroneal and extensor muscles of the foot.

Rigid flat feet from congenital coalitions remain flat whether or not the patient remains weight-bearing. There is considerable limitation of motion, particularly inversion and eversion, owing to the bony block of the subtalar joint.

The patient will usually have no complaints until

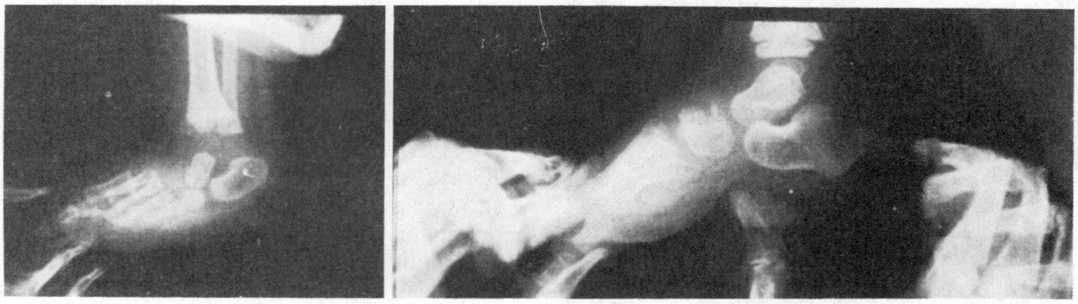

Figure 49–98. Congenital vertical talus deformity in a 1-year-old girl. The talus does not line up with the forefoot on plantar flexion. After 2 years of treatment with Denis Browne splints, the vertical talus has been corrected and the talonavicular relationship is normal. (Connolly, J., Regens, E., and Hillman, J. W.: Pigeon-toes and flat feet. Pediatr. Clin. North Am., *17*:291, 1970.)

near adolescence when he begins to stand for prolonged periods. He may be bothered by aching in the medial aspect of the foot and ankle and note pain in the lateral peroneal and calf region from muscle overstrain.

To add to his predicament, the x-rays of the foot may appear normal unless the possibility of congenital coalition is considered. An oblique view of the subtalar joint must be obtained to visualize the more subtle coalitions. Tomograms or CT scan may also be necessary.

A frequent finding in a more mature foot is lipping of the superior margin of the head of the talus. This is due to the alterations imposed by the congenital coalition on the gliding motion in the talonavicular joint (Fig. 49–99).

If the coalition such as a calcaneal or navicular bar is recognized early, the symptoms may be relieved by excision of the bar. Alternatively, if the symptoms are allowed to persist and develop structural changes of the talus, a triple arthrodesis may be required.

Management by the Family Physician. The majority of patients with coalitions do not require treatment. If a well-defined calcaneonavicular bar is evident on x-ray and is causing peroneal spastic flat foot, surgical excision of the bar should be recommended.

Ideally, early detection by the family physician may allow treatment by less extensive methods than triple arthrodesis. However, the possibility of triple arthrodesis should not be excluded for patients with recurring, persisting symptoms of a rigid flat foot.

Accessory Navicular Bones Causing Symptomatic Flat Foot or "Double Ankle"

A common and undertreated cause of flat foot, particularly seen in the preadolescent, is a sesamoid bone situated along the medial arch. This accessory navicular bone, the most frequent sesamoid in the foot, is located on the medial side of the navicular in close proximity to the posterior tibial tendon. It may cause enough of a prominence to be termed as a "double ankle" (Fig. 49–96*F*).

Symptoms, like symptoms from congenital coalitions, may not be noticeable until adolescence or young adulthood. The bony prominences then become quite tender, especially along the medial arch.

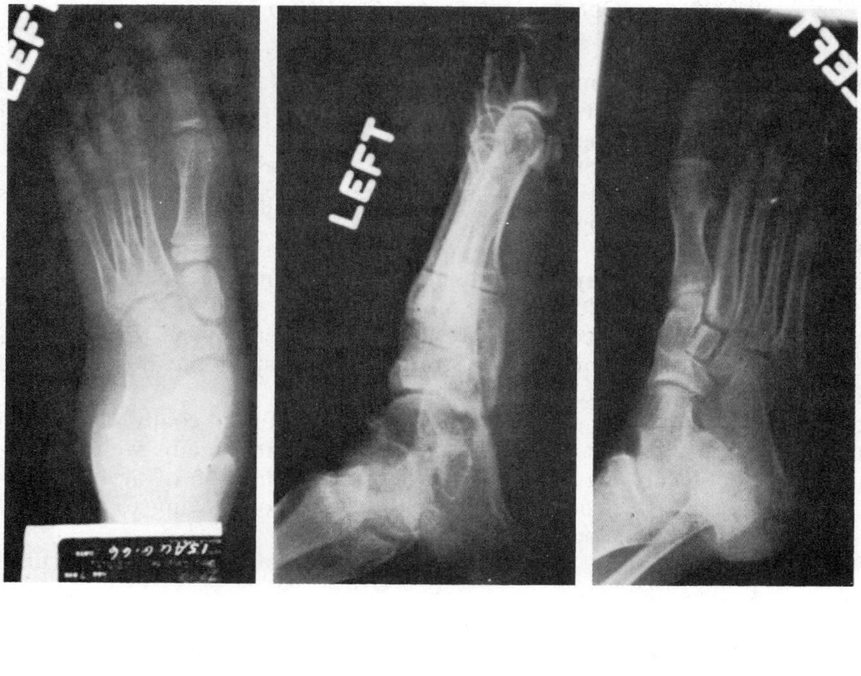

Figure 49–99. Multiple similar tarsal coalitions in a 7-year-old girl *(left)*, her 35-year-old father *(center)*, and her 5-year-old sister *(right)*. These include the calcaneocuboid, the talocalcaneal, and the naviculocuneiform joints. The break seen on the dorsal surface of the talus in the father's foot is frequently associated with talocalcaneal and calcaneonavicular fusions due to alternations in the normal gliding of the navicular on the talus. (Connolly, J., Regens, E., and Hillman, J. W.: Pigeon-toes and flat feet. Pediatr. Clin. North Am., *17*:291, 1970.)

There may also be associated muscle contracture and pain with prolonged standing.

The pain is the result of several factors, including a bursitis developing over the bony prominence. There is also a tendency for the accessory bones to overcrowd the soft tissues and tendons on the medial side of the foot. The altered pull of the posterior tibial tendon impairs the mechanics of the foot.

Management by the Family Physician. Mild symptoms may be relieved by inversion exercises and longitudinal arch support in the young individual. However, do not persist in these methods if they are not completely successful. Refer the patient for removal of the accessory bone or the navicular prominence, a procedure that is quite successful in relieving the annoying and persisting symptoms of these conditions.

Geriatric Considerations in Orthopedics

GERIATRIC OSTEOPENIA

Recent research points to some association of vitamin D deficit and geriatric osteopenia, and metabolic problems resulting from aging can complicate supplementation of vitamin D. Geriatric osteopenia can be treated or prevented. (See discussion of Osteoporosis in Back Pain.)

Management by the Family Physician. When poor vitamin D status is shown to contribute to geriatric osteopenia, vitamin D supplementation is useful. This can be accomplished by a single oral dose of 100,000 units of vitamin D about every 5 or 6 months (Goldray et al., 1988). Further, calcium intake is often faulty in the elderly, and supplemental calcium in doses of 750 to 1000 mg. per day should be given.

HIP FRACTURE IN THE ELDERLY

About 250,000 hip fractures per year are seen in the United States. The incidence doubles each decade after age 50 so that by the ninth decade about 30 per cent of women and 16 per cent of men will have had at least one hip fracture.

The major cause of these fractures is decreased strength of the femur secondary to senile osteopenia. Other factors are contributory such as poor balance, poor motor control, impaired reflexes and mentation, and sometimes drug use in this age group.

Fractures can be intracapsular or extracapsular and hence will require different treatments. A few intracapsular fractures can be handled conservatively if stable and in good position. Most will require orthopedic intervention.

Patient Evaluation

The best means of evaluation is the use of standard x-rays. Clinically, most will be in pain and unable to ambulate. Inspection usually shows an externally rotated, shortened extremity with pain on motion.

Management by the Family Physician. When it is established that hip fracture is present, the patient must be hospitalized and, in general, prepared for surgical intervention by an orthopedic surgeon. During the preoperative period the patient should have Buck's traction of 4 to 5 pounds applied and sand bags medially and laterally to immobilize the limb.

The patient should be well hydrated and evaluated by an anesthesiologist as well as the orthopedic surgeon in preparation for operative treatment.

In general, the patient is in the best condition for intervention hours after the incident. Delays for "tuning up" and unneeded detailed evaluation can be disastrous. Even 2 or 3 days can lead to thromboembolic problems, urinary problems, skin breakdown, and pulmonary and cardiac problems which would be less likely in a patient operatively stabilized. Early operative stabilization allows an easier and safer postoperative care with fewer complications than in the long-delayed case.

Prevention of senile osteopenia can reduce the incidence of hip fracture in the elderly.

References

Allen, M. J.: Conservative management in fingertip injuries in adults. The Hand, *12*:250, 1980.

Brown, P., and Kinman, P.: Gas gangrene in a metropolitan community. J. Bone Joint Surg., *56*A:1445, 1974. *This classic article shows that the incidence of serious life-threatening wound infections in at least one metropolitan community was significantly higher when compared with results from the Viet Nam military experience. The principles of wound management outlined in this article should not be ignored by civilian physicians.*

Bruner, J.: Treatment of sesamoid synovial ganglia of the hand by needle rupture. J. Bone Joint Surg., *45*A:1689, 1963.

Connolly, J. F., Regen, E., and Hillman, J.: Pigeon-toes and flat feet. Pediatr. Clin. North Am., *17*:291, 1970.

Connolly, J. F., Regen, E., and Evans, O. B.: The management of the painful stiff shoulder. Clin. Orthop., *84*:97, 1972. *We have reviewed the commonest cause of shoulder pain and stiffening in this article. A three-pronged approach is described, which includes injection, passive stretching exercises, and occasional shoulder manipulation for chronically stiff shoulder problems.*

Connolly, J. F., and Brooks, A. L.: Vascular problems in orthopaedics. American Academy of Orthopaedic Surgeons Instructional Course Lectures, *22*:12–27. St. Louis, C. V. Mosby, 1973.

Connolly, J. F.: Early diagnosis and mis-diagnosis of congenital dislocated hip. Nebr. Med. J., *60*:471, 1975a.

Connolly, J. F.: Perils and pitfalls of open tibial fractures. Am. Fam. Phys., *11*:64, 1975b.

Connolly, J. F.: Depalma's The Management of Fractures and Dislocations: An Atlas. 3rd ed. Philadelphia, W. B. Saunders Co., 1981. *The reader should refer to this illustrated atlas for clarification of any techniques of fracture management mentioned in this chapter.*

Connolly, J. F.: Wound management and the legacy of H. Winnett Orr. Nebr. Med. J., March 1982.

Coonrad, R. W., and Hooper, W.: Tennis elbow: Its course, natural history, conservative and surgical management. J. Bone Joint Surg., *55*A:1177, 1973.

Corey, L., and Hattwick, M.: Treatment of persons exposed to rabies. J.A.M.A., *232*:272, 1975. *The authors describe the U.S. Centers for Disease Control's clinical and epidemiological criteria for treatment of persons exposed to rabid animals. This is an important reference and is lucidly and logically presented.*

Curtiss, P., and Collins, W.: Spinal cord tumor—A cause of progressive neurological changes in children with scoliosis. J. Bone Joint Surg., *43*A:517, 1961.

Cyriax, J.: Orthopaedic Medicine. Volumes I and II. London, Cassell, Ltd., 1978. *This classic and comprehensive text is recommended for further reading, particularly sections on the diagnosis and nonoperative management of musculoskeletal problems.*

Einhorn, T. A.: Hip fractures in the elderly. Resident and Staff Physician, *34*(9):97–113, Sept. 1988.

Fackler, M. L., and O'Benar, J. D.: Letter to the editor on ballistics. Milit. Med., *192*:531–534, Oct. 1987.

Flatt, A.: The Care of the Rheumatoid Hand. St. Louis, C. V. Mosby, 1974.

Galasko, G., and Sylvester, B.: Back pain in patients treated for malignant tumors. Clin. Oncol., *41*:273, 1978.

Goldray, D., Merdler, C., and Weisman, Y.: Vitamin D deficiency and osteopenia in the elderly. Geriatr. Med. Today, *7*(7):49–53, July 1988.

Gordon, G., and Vaughan, C.: Clinical Management of the Osteoporoses. Bucks, England, H M & M Publishers, 1976. *This well-written and illustrated text presents many useful concepts pertaining to the diagnosis and management of osteoporosis.*

Hansson, J.: The leg amputee. Acta Orthop. Scand., Supplement 69, 1964.

Heaney, R. P., and Recker, R. R.: Estrogen effects on bone remodeling at menopause. Clin. Res., *23*:535, 1975.

Heyse-Moore, G.: A rational approach to the use of epidural medication in the treatment for sciatic pain. Acta Orthop. Scand., *49*:366, 1978. *Wide variations in the results of this treatment are found. These can be explained in part by the variation in severity of scarring and changes around the nerve root in cases of sciatica. The authors show that treatment is more successful in cases of acute onset, particularly when epidural medication is used within six months of the onset of symptoms.*

Hoehler, F. K., Tobias, J. S., and Buerger, A. A.: Spinal manipulation for low back pain. J.A.M.A., *245*:1835, 1981.

Jardon, O. M., et al.: Complete avulsion of axillary artery as a consequence of anterior shoulder dislocation. J. Bone Joint Surg., *55*A:189–192, Jan. 1973.

Jardon, O. M., Wingard, D., Barak, A. J., et al.: Malignant hyperthermia. J. Bone Joint Surg., *61*A:1064, 1979.

Jardon, O. M.: Physiologic stress, heat stroke, malignant hyperthermia—A perspective. Milit. Med., *147*:8 1982.

Larsson, U., et al.: Auto-traction for treatment of lumbago-sciatica: A multicentre controlled investigation. Acta Orthop. Scand., *51*:791, 1980. *Traction is shown in this study to give prompt relief of pain from acute sciatica more often than does treatment with only rest or a corset.*

Levin, M. E., and O'Neal, L. W.: The Diabetic Foot. St. Louis, C. V. Mosby, 1973. *This is a very useful and practical monograph. It is recommended for the library of any physician who treats diabetic patients.*

Lundberg, B. J.: The frozen shoulder. Acta Orthop. Scand. Suppl., *119*:5–50, 1969.

Mann, R. J.: Human bites of the hand. Am. Fam. Phys., *23*:110, 1981. *This impressively illustrated article reviews the significance of human bite wounds to the hand. Principles of treatment are clearly outlined and should be reviewed by all family physicians, who invariably will manage this common injury.*

Matsen, F. A., III: Compartmental Syndromes. New York, Grune & Stratton, 1980. *This very thorough text presents important clinical and basic research information which should be available to any physician treating injuries.*

McCarty, D. J.: Arthritis and Allied Conditions. Philadelphia, Lea & Febiger, 1979.

McCullough, N., Jennings, J., and Sarmiento, A.: Bilateral below-the-knee amputation in patients over fifty years of age. J. Bone Joint Surg., *54*A:1217, 1972. *The authors show that a high degree of successful rehabilitation is possible in an older patient despite bilateral below-knee amputations. This is a compelling reason for making every effort to amputate below the knee in the dysvascular patient.*

Miller, R. G., and Burton, R.: Stroke following chiropractic manipulation of the spine. J.A.M.A., *229*:189, 1974.

Mooney, V., and Robertson, J.: The facet syndrome. Clin. Orthop., *115*:149, 1976. *The authors present convincing information to suggest that structures related to the facet joint can be a persistent cause of chronic pain in the low back and leg.*

Mubarak, S. J., and Hargens, A. R.: Compartment Syndromes and Volkmann's Contracture. Philadelphia, W. B. Saunders, 1981.

Nachemson, A., and Morris, J.: In vivo measurements of intradiscal pressure. J. Bone Joint Surg., *46*A:1077, 1964. *This is a classic article that contains information about the mechanics of lumbar discs and the production of low back pain.*

Newman, J.: Non-infective disease of the diabetic foot. J. Bone Joint Surg., *63*B:593, 1981.

Phelps, D., Lilla, J., and Boswick, J.: Common problems in clinical replantation and revascularization in the upper extremity. Clin Orthop., *133*:11, 1978. *This is a useful article that reviews the indications and problems in attempting replantation and revascularization.*

Salter, R., Bell, R., and Keely, F.: The protective effect of continuous passive motion on living articular cartilage in acute septic arthritis. Clin. Orthop., *159*:223, 1981.

Salter, R., et al.: The biological effect of continuous passive motion on the healing of full-thickness defects in articular cartilage. J. Bone Joint Surg., *62*A:1232, 1980.

Sarmiento, A., and Warren, D.: A re-evaluation of lower extremity amputations. Surg. Gynecol. Obstet., *129*:799, 1969. *This important review demonstrates the feasibility of below-knee amputations for the majority of such operations involving the lower extremity.*

Saville, P.: Observations on 80 women with osteoporotic spine fractures. *In* Barzel, U. (Ed.): Osteoporosis. New York, Grune & Stratton, 1970, p. 3.

Simmons, D., and Chrisman, D.: Salicylate inhibition of cartilage degeneration. Arthritis Rheum., *8*:960, 1965.

Swan, K. G., and Swan, R. C.: Gunshot Wounds: Pathophysiology and Management. Littleton, Mass., P.S.G. Publishing Co., 1980.

Urist, M., Gurvey, M., and Fareed, D.: Long-term observations on aged women with pathologic osteoporoses. *In* Barzel, U. (Ed.): Osteoporosis. New York, Grune & Stratton, 1970.

Whitesides, T. E., et al.: Tissue pressure measurements as a determinant for the need of fasciotomy. Clin. Orthop., *113*:43, 1975.

Wilkinson, M.: Anatomy and pathology of cervical spondylosis. Proc. R. Soc. Med., *57*:159, 1964. *This is a review of the common problems of cervical disc disease and a discussion of the advantages and disadvantages of cervical traction. This article should be read in conjunction with Cyriax's discussion.*

Zook, E., Miller, M., Van Beek, A., and Wavak, P.: Successful treatment protocol for canine fang injuries. J. Trauma, *20*:243, 1980. *This is a useful discussion of the most common bite injury in the United States, including its social and economic problems. A method of management is proposed which includes copious saline pressure irrigation, meticulous wound edge debridement, adequate antibiotic coverage, and careful postoperative monitoring. The result is an impressively low wound infection rate for this frequently complicated injury.*

50

Rheumatic Disease

Charles M. Plotz

The Arthritis Foundation estimates that there are well over 30,000,000 people in the United States suffering from one or another form of arthritis or one of its related diseases. The family physician numbers musculoskeletal and rheumatic complaints well up in the top 10 reasons for patient office visits. It is, therefore, of major importance to be able to recognize and treat the various forms of musculoskeletal disease.

Unfortunately, unlike many other clinical entities, musculoskeletal complaints can represent diseases unto themselves, can be part of other clinical conditions, and can be psychosomatic in nature. The clinical acumen of the family physician is of great importance, and knowledge of the patient's background and family situation places the family physician in a better position than the consultant to establish the definitive diagnosis. It is the aim of this chapter to enable the attending physician to establish a clear diagnosis in over 90 per cent of patients, to start and carry out a program of treatment that should benefit the patient, and to recognize when it is necessary to call in a consultant either to help establish a diagnosis or to carry forward a difficult and hazardous program of therapy.

Definitions

A few simple definitions will be useful. First, one should recognize that a *joint* is a *joining*, and wherever two bones in the body meet, they are connected by a joint that may be diarthrodial or fibrous or, as in the case of the sacroiliac joint, a combination of the two. The joint is a complex mechanism, since it consists of the two ends of bone (periarticular bone); the joint cartilage, which includes both the cartilage at the ends of the bone and cartilage within the joint as in the case of the knee joint; a joint capsule, which consists of fibrous tissue often deriving from the ends of tendons and investing the joint to give it strength and stability; and, within the joint, a lining or synovium that is normally thin but becomes thickened and inflamed in the course of many rheumatic diseases. It is from the synovium that joint fluid or synovial fluid originates; when the synovium is inflamed, excess fluid is secreted, giving rise to the characteristic joint swelling.

Evaluation of Musculoskeletal Disease

Despite the fact that the rheumatologic literature is replete with extremely complex matters related to immunology chemistry and genetics, the vast majority of musculoskeletal complaints and musculoskeletal disease can be resolved by the simple old-fashioned technique of history and physical examination.

HISTORY

It is almost always musculoskeletal *pain* that brings the patient to the family physician's office. Pain is obviously something that is subject to a good deal of individual variation, and here again the skill of the family physician in evaluating a patient's complaint can be most helpful in establishing a diagnosis. In considering musculoskeletal pain, it is obviously important to know whether this is acute or chronic, whether there was previous trauma or infection, whether this is a recurrent phenomenon as might be expected in gouty arthritis, whether single or multiple areas are affected, and whether it is really the joints that hurt or whether the problem primarily involves muscles and tendons as in polymyalgia rheumatica or fibromyalgia. The pain can radiate, as in the case of sciatic syndrome. It is vitally important to remember that musculoskeletal pain can be the first manifestation of underlying visceral disease, as when pain in the right trapezius muscle is due to gallbladder disease, or pain in the left shoulder and arm is related to coronary artery disease.

The examining physician should also inquire about whether tingling or burning is present, which would indicate possible nerve entrapment or impingement, and whether swelling has been noted.

It is extremely important in the evaluation of musculoskeletal disease to inquire about *stiffness.* Next to pain, stiffness is the single factor that is most likely to bring a patient to a physician. It is well known that morning stiffness is a characteristic of rheumatoid arthritis, and indeed the inability to get going in the morning is sometimes extremely troublesome. In addition to this inquiry, the patient should be asked the usual questions relative to general health.

PHYSICAL EXAMINATION

Once the history has been taken, a physical examination can be performed relatively easily. The attending physician can use his or her own presumably normal joints as a frame of reference so that impairment of range of motion can be readily detected. One should observe how the patient has walked into the room, sat down in the chair, risen from the chair, climbed onto the examining table, and laid down. Does the patient hold himself rigid, or wince when certain motions are undertaken? All of this can be easily detected in a brief period. The examination of specific joints involves observation, palpation, and to a certain extent auscultation since crepitus is a manifestation of some rheumatic diseases and the leathery sound of a thickened synovium that occurs in chronic rheumatoid arthritis is characteristic.

Much of the history can be taken while the patient is undressing, and it is important to have the patient undress sufficiently so that not only can a complete physical examination be performed, but as many of the joints in the body as possible can be seen accurately. It is essential to have the shoes and stockings removed. Since back pain is such a common rheumatic complaint, it is important to take a good look at the spine and pay attention to the presence or absence of kyphosis, lordosis, scoliosis, or other spinal abnormality. Have the patient bend forward and see if a nice rounding of the back occurs. Have the patient bend backward to see whether the normal concavity of the spine is present. Is there muscle spasm? Do the ribs move normally when the patient inhales? Expansion of the chest is impossible in advanced ankylosing spondylitis.

Is there a positive straight-leg raising test? If the patient cannot achieve at least 90 degrees of straight leg raising when lying flat on the back, is it possible when sitting and the legs are straightened in front? If you are in any doubt as to whether a complaint is genuine, try to distract the patient and test it during the time of distraction.

Simple light pounding of the spine with the fist can detect vertebral abnormalities, including neoplasm, which might not otherwise be obvious on inspection. If the fibromyalgia syndrome is suspected, feel carefully for trigger points, particularly in the trapezius muscles and paraspinally.

Neck. The neck is a special area of the spine that is particularly vulnerable to rheumatic problems. In almost every adult past middle age there is some osteoarthritis of the cervical spine. This is most likely due to the prolonged effort of maintaining the erect position and moving the head over the course of a lifetime. There are specific problems, however, that can aggravate symptoms connected with the neck. These include the so-called whiplash injury that occurs when a vehicle is struck from the rear and the head suddenly snaps back. The same kind of injury can occur during the course of athletic endeavors. The fact is that most "whiplash" injuries are transitory in nature, and many persist only because of litigation that is sometimes associated with the aggravating incident. The family physician must be on the lookout for this and not succumb to the blandishments of a patient who is looking for a report that would look good in the courtroom. The family physician also must be careful not to misinterpret radiographs of the cervical spine, ascribing all symptoms to the underlying arthritis that probably was there long before the pain occurred and which probably would be present in half of patients of age 50 and over.

Nevertheless, many cervical root syndromes do have their origin in rheumatic problems. It must be remembered that most of the innervation of the head, arms, and upper torso comes from nerve roots located in the neck. It should be easy, therefore, to trace radicular patterns and to determine whether a complaint follows such a logical pattern.

Other cervical rheumatic problems include the neck-shoulder-hand syndrome. This can result in a puffy hand that is sometimes painful. Not all neck problems are necessarily nerve-root in origin. For example, neck-shoulder-hand syndrome can occur following myocardial infarction when there is referred pain to the neck and the autonomic nervous system is activated, producing edema of the hand.

The neck is also a favorite place for the pain of

fibromyalgia (see later). So-called trigger areas are common in the neck and trapezius muscles. These can sometimes be treated by spraying with ethyl chloride or injection with Novocain.

Shoulders. The shoulders are particularly susceptible to rheumatic complaints. As can easily be determined by going through a range of motion yourself, the shoulder has perhaps the widest range of motion of any joint in the body and therefore is subject to rheumatic problems that can affect one or another of these various motions. It is wise to review the anatomy of the shoulder, particularly the origins and insertions of the muscles of the shoulder, the tendons and their location, and the presence of the rotator cuff. One of the best ways of assessing shoulder range of motion is to have the patient go through the maneuvers that he or she would encounter in hooking a bra in the back. Those with considerable pathologic changes of the shoulder joint or disorders of the rotator cuff will find this almost impossible to do.

Elbow. The elbow is not commonly involved in rheumatic complaints except in people who are active in sports. Tennis elbow or lateral epicondylitis occurs not only in tennis players but may occur in people who use their arm for such mundane purposes as carrying heavy luggage and similar occupations. The major problem in tennis elbow is pain at the insertion of the tendon at the lateral epicondyle of the elbow, and there is usually exquisite tenderness at that area. Far less common is medial epicondylitis or golfer's elbow. The management of both of these is discussed later.

Wrists and Hands. The wrists and hands are common sites for rheumatic complaints. In rheumatoid arthritis, the wrists may be the most commonly involved joints although it is not always so recognized by the patient. The range of motion of the wrist can be simply determined by using the so-called "prayer" sign, which consists of clasping the hands palm to palm and raising both elbows as if one were praying. The maximum angle between the hand and forearm can be measured in a semiobjective technique to determine the range of motion of the wrist. A special form of arthritis of the wrist is Jaccoud's arthritis, which produces over a period of years relatively painless ulnar deviation of the wrist and can be associated with systemic lupus, rheumatic fever, or rheumatoid arthritis. Another somewhat more common condition at the wrist is de Quervain's disease, a stenosing tenosynovitis of the tendon sheath around the abductor pollicis longus and extensor pollicis brevis at the base of the thumb. This is usually treated with rest or local steroids. Perhaps the most common rheumatic involvement of the wrist is the carpal tunnel syndrome, an entrapment neuropathy of the median nerve at the wrist producing pain or tingling of the first three fingers of the hand often associated with atrophy of the thenar eminence. There are many potential causes for carpal tunnel syndrome and in many instances the causes can never be determined. Local injections may sometimes help as may splinting, but in many instances surgery becomes necessary.

The hands are extremely commonly involved in arthritis. So-called Heberden's nodes are familial and possibly hormonal, since they occur around the time of menopause and involve the distal interphalangeal joints of the fingers with some deformity but very little pain or interference with function. Bouchard's nodes are similar osteoarthritic changes involving proximal interphalangeal joints, and these likewise are not inflammatory and produce bony deformity but little functional damage. By far the most serious rheumatic disease affecting the hands is rheumatoid arthritis that involves the proximal interphalangeal and metacarpophalangeal joints of the hands as well as the wrists; since the disease is inflammatory and destructive, it can cause severe crippling. Another form of inflammatory arthritis involving the hands is psoriatic arthritis; when the fingernails are affected by the psoriasis, it is not uncommon for distal interphalangeal joints to be affected and even destroyed by the psoriatic arthritic process.

Sternoclavicular Joints. The sternoclavicular joints are not commonly affected and usually are not painful when they are affected. There can be swelling and enlargement of these joints in rheumatoid arthritis and also in the course of infectious processes such as tuberculosis. A particular rheumatic complaint that is very troublesome to the patient and to the family physician is Tietze's syndrome. This is a costochondritis involving the attachments of the anterior ribs to the sternum and can cause considerable pain that is often misdiagnosed as being cardiac in origin. The usual clue is that even light pressure over the costochondral junction can reproduce the pain, which is often exquisite.

Hip, Knee, and Ankle. Until recent years, involvement of the hip was a devastating rheumatic problem. The hip, like the shoulder, has a very wide range of motion; since it bears the brunt of the weight of the body and is involved in all walking activities, it is subject to a good deal of trauma. As a result, and also because of familial factors, osteoarthritis of the hip is not uncommon and can gradually lead to severe dysfunction.

Rheumatoid arthritis likewise can involve the hips; in patients given steroids over a long period of time, aseptic necrosis of the head of the femur can occur. One of the most important advances in arthritis over recent decades has been the development of joint replacement, and nowhere is this better exemplified than in the hip. Many patients who would otherwise have severe loss of function and even confinement to a chair are now able to lead active and productive lives thanks to this remarkable operation.

The knee is commonly involved, particularly by osteoarthritis but also by rheumatoid arthritis. The range of motion of the knee is far less than that of the hip, but it also carries with it the full weight of the body. The knee has an active bursa both anteriorly and posteriorly, and these bursae can swell and become painful. The swelling of the anterior bursa is sometimes known as "housemaid's" knee, and the swelling of the posterior bursa behind the knee is known as Baker's cyst. The most important feature of this problem is its tendency to rupture and have the fluid gravitate downward, producing a syndrome that superficially resembles acute thrombophlebitis. Joint replacement has revolutionized the therapy of knee arthritis as well as that of the hip.

Involvement of the ankles, surprisingly, is not as common as involvement of other major joints, and involvement of the foot is very similar to involvement of the hands.

All in all, a reasonably careful examination of all of the joints of the body can be undertaken once the patient is undressed and while you are talking with the patient about any of the other things you wish to talk about in under 10 minutes.

Laboratory Data

Many of the tests done in rheumatic disease are relatively simple and can be performed in the office of the family physician. It goes without saying that patients should have a routine complete blood count including differential count and urinalysis. An elevated white blood cell count should make one suspicious of the possibility of infection, although there is often a mild elevation in rheumatoid arthritis. A suspiciously low white blood cell count should put one on the alert for the possibility of systemic lupus. Whereas a refractory moderate anemia is present in active rheumatoid arthritis, significant anemia should always be viewed with a certain amount of alarm and thorough testing should be done to rule out causes of severe anemia.

Perhaps the simplest of all tests in rheumatic disease and one that is often not performed is the erythrocyte sedimentation rate. This is the best way to distinguish between inflammatory and noninflammatory disease. It would be very unusual indeed to have active rheumatoid arthritis in the presence of a normal sedimentation rate. Likewise a markedly elevated sedimentation rate should ring a bell and alert the family physician to the possibility of other underlying disease or the presence of either polymyalgia rheumatica or multiple myeloma. The best technique for the sedimentation rate is the Westergren method, which involves the use of a 200 mm. tube and anticoagulated blood and the wait of 1 hour to see how long it takes for the red blood cells to settle. No special technique is necessary and this is easily done in the physician's office. With the growing use of commercial laboratories, sedimentation rates can sometimes become unreliable, since they are done on blood that has been standing around for many hours. It should be recognized that there are rare but significant conditions that can prevent an elevation of sedimentation rate. These include sickle cell disease and polycythemia.

Serum uric acid level is of importance in the diagnosis of acute gout. It should always be done in conjunction with the determination of urea nitrogen to make sure that an elevation of uric acid is not simply an indicator of kidney disease with an elevation of all nitrogenous elements. Elevated uric acid levels can occur in patients taking thiazide diuretics and in the presence of diseases with unusually rapid cell turnover such as psoriasis and leukemia. One should beware of the trap of assuming that any rheumatic complaint plus an elevated serum uric acid level equals gout. Gout is a very specific disease; more will be mentioned of this in the discussion of the various rheumatic syndromes. In general, it is rare to have true acute gout in the absence of an elevated serum uric acid level, and therefore this test is of some differential diagnostic significance.

The two serologic tests most commonly used by the family physician in the differential diagnosis of rheumatic disease are the latex fixation test for rheumatoid factor and the antinuclear antibody (ANA) test for systemic lupus. The latex fixation test is significantly positive (greater than 1:160) in about 70 per cent of patients with active peripheral rheumatoid arthritis in the absence of psoriasis. This still leaves some 30 per cent who will have rheumatoid arthritis with a negative latex test. The incidence of positive reactions drops to around 30 per cent in children and may be negative in very early disease. Significantly positive latex titers are seen in many conditions other than rheumatoid arthritis. These include chronic liver disease, chronic infectious disease, and disorders of gamma globulin.

The antinuclear antibody test is almost always positive in patients with systemic lupus and generally produces a homogeneous speckled pattern. However, positive antinuclear antibody tests of this sort are seen with the chronic administration of certain drugs, in rheumatoid arthritis, and in the course of some infectious diseases.

The antinuclear antibody test therefore is of most differential diagnostic significance if it is negative, since it would be very unusual to have systemic lupus with a negative ANA.

Synovial fluid analysis is of great importance in the fine differential diagnosis of rheumatic disease and is not very difficult to perform. Obviously, it is important to have a significantly swollen joint so that there is a source of synovial fluid. The technique of obtaining this fluid is very simple. Under sterile precautions, one inserts a number 20 or larger needle attached to a syringe or collecting tube and selects the point of maximum fluctuation to get the fluid. After the fluid has been obtained, the first thing that one must do is to look at it and see whether it is clear or turbid. If it is clear, it is unlikely that we are dealing either with infection or with significant crystal disease. On the other hand, if it is turbulent, we must be much more careful in our analysis. All fluid should have a total white blood cell and differential count. Ordinary joint fluid has a white blood cell count of under 1000 per cu. mm., whereas infected fluid may have counts as high as 100,000 per cu. mm. or greater. The differential count in these instances shows a marked shift to the left. The presence of marked inflammatory fluid always indicates the necessity for smear and culture. Culturing synovial fluid in those instances can actually be a lifesaving procedure since severe infection can be detected.

In the absence of infection one should examine the fluid for crystals. These can often be seen under an ordinary microscope using a coverslip, although urate crystals require the use of polarization. It takes a certain amount of experience to be able to recognize urate crystals; it would probably be a good idea, therefore, to send such fluid out to an adequate laboratory with a polarizing microscope for analysis.

One of the simplest tests of synovial fluid is the "string" test, which simply involves taking a drop of the fluid between thumb and forefinger and slowly separating them to see whether a short or long stringing phenomenon takes place. A long string implies a very viscous fluid, and this in turn means that the hyaluronic acid complexes of the synovial fluid are intact and the fluid is probably not inflammatory. On the other hand, a short string or no string at all indicates depolymerization of the hyaluronate, and this is indicative of an inflammatory synovial fluid. Obviously one should use a plastic glove for this test since one does not wish to expose one's own flesh to fluid that might contain disease contaminants.

Other tests such as the determination of glucose protein and serologic studies are generally not very helpful. These will probably be reported if the fluid is sent to a laboratory, but they really do not tell very much that is not easily available from other sources.

Radiology

Radiology in rheumatic disease is helpful in advanced stages, but not very helpful in early stages. In fact, even in advanced stages, radiographs mostly only confirm what you already know, namely, that a joint is deformed, ankylosed, or swollen. Areas in which radiology is likely to be helpful are the determination of erosions in rheumatoid arthritis, the detection of "punched out" areas in gout, and the possible early detection of infection. Radiology is helpful in the detection of the presence of calcium pyrophosphate dihydrate (CPPD) crystals, which commonly affect the articular cartilage. Urate crystals are not detectable on x-ray examination except insofar as they have induced "punched out" areas. Early ankylosing spondylitis can usually be detected by careful x-ray examination of the sacroiliac joints, which are almost invariably the first affected in this condition. Indeed, the presence of normal sacroiliac joints is a powerful argument against ankylosing spondylitis. Later x-ray changes only confirm what you really know, namely, that the spine is virtually fused because of the calcification of the intervertebral ligaments. Occasionally, the spine in severe osteoarthritis will produce a picture similar to that of ankylosing spondylitis, but usually in those instances the sacroiliac joints are not affected. Psoriatic arthritis can be extremely destructive and indeed can lead to complete absorption of terminal phalanges (Fig. 50–1).

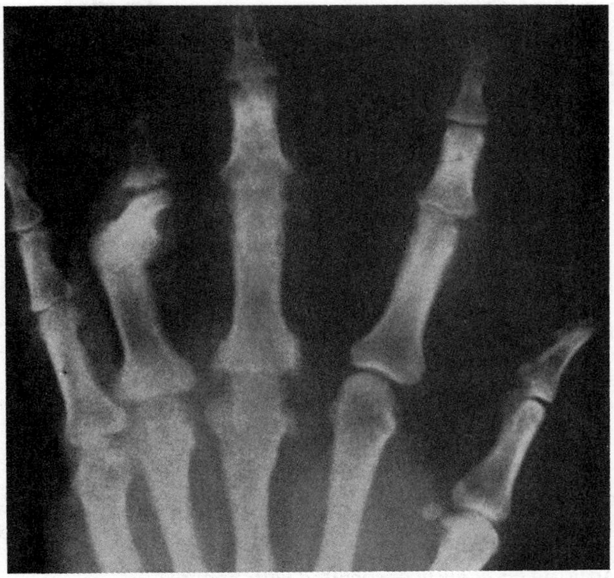

Figure 50–1. Psoriatic arthritis. The joints affected are primarily those of the middle and ring fingers, including terminal joints. Note the irregular bone apposition at sites of involvement and absence of osteoporosis. (Reprinted from Schumacher, R. H., Jr., Klippel, J. H., and Robinson, D. R. [Eds.]: Primer on the Rheumatic Diseases. 9th ed. Atlanta, GA, Arthritis Foundation, 1988, p. 68. Used by permission of the Arthritis Foundation.)

Charcot joints or neuropathic joints are very uncommon now in syphilis since tertiary syphilis is very rarely seen. The most common cause of Charcot joints is diabetes mellitus, and one must always be on guard for this.

Computed tomography (CT) and magnetic resonance imaging (MRI) are seldom of very significant help in most of the rheumatic conditions seen by the family physician. This is also true of joint and bone scintigraphy.

If arthroscopy and synovial biopsy become necessary, the rheumatologist or orthopedic surgeon should be consulted. These tests require not only excellent technique but the experience of knowing what you are looking at; for this reason, they are generally beyond the scope of the family doctor.

Management of Rheumatic Disease

The classification of rheumatic disease is presented in Table 50–1.

Table 50–1. CLASSIFICATION OF THE RHEUMATIC DISEASES

Diffuse Connective Tissue Diseases
- Rheumatoid arthritis
- Juvenile arthritis
  - Systemic onset
  - Polyarticular onset
  - Oligoarticular onset
- Systemic lupus erythematosus
- Progressive systemic sclerosis
- Diffuse fasciitis
- Polymyositis–dermatomyositis
- Necrotizing vasculitis and other vasculopathies
  - Polyarteritis nodosa group (includes hepatitis B–associated arteritis)
  - Hypersensitivity vasculitis (includes Henoch-Schönlein purpura and others)
  - Granulomatous arteritis
    - Wegener's granulomatosis
    - Giant cell arteritis
    - Takayasu's arteritis
  - Mucocutaneous lymph node syndrome (Kawasaki's disease)
  - Behçet's disease
- Overlap syndromes (includes mixed connective tissue disease. Sjögren's syndrome, and others)
- Others (includes polymyalgia rheumatica, panniculitis (Weber-Christian disease), erythema nodosum, relapsing polychondritis, and others)

Arthritis Frequently Associated with Spondylitis
- Ankylosing spondylitis
- Reiter's syndrome
- Psoriatic arthritis
- Arthritis associated with chronic inflammatory bowel disease

Degenerative Joint Disease (Osteoarthritis, Osteoarthrosis)
- Primary (includes erosive osteoarthritis)
- Secondary

Arthritis, Tenosynovitis, and Bursitis Associated with Infectious Agents
- Direct
  - Bacterial
  - Viral
  - Fungal
  - Parasitic
  - Unknown, suspected (Whipple's disease, Lyme disease)
- Indirect (reactive)
  - Bacterial (includes acute rheumatic fever, intestinal bypass, post-dysenteric [shigella, yersinia] and others)
  - Viral (hepatitis B)

Metabolic and Endocrine Diseases Associated with Rheumatic States
- Crystal-induced conditions
  - Monosodium urate (gout)
  - Calcium pyrophosphate dihydrate (pseudogout, chondrocalcinosis)
  - Hydroxyapatite
- Biochemical abnormalities
  - Vitamin C deficiency (scurvy)
  - Specific enzyme deficiency states (includes Fabry's, Faber's, alkaptonuria, Lesch-Nyhan, and others)
  - Hyperlipidemias (types II, IIa, IV)
  - Mucopolysaccharidoses
  - Hemoglobinopathies (SS disease and others)
  - Amyloidosis
  - Biochemical disorders of connective tissue (Ehlers-Danlos, Marfan's pseudoxanthoma elasticum, and others)
  - Others
- Endocrine diseases
  - Diabetes mellitus
  - Acromegaly
  - Hyperparathyroidism
  - Thyroid disease (hyperthyroidism, hypothyroidism)
- Immunodeficiency diseases
- Other hereditary disorders
  - Arthrogryposis multiplex congenita
  - Hypermobility syndromes
  - Myositis ossificans progressiva

Neoplasms
- Primary (includes synovioma, synoviosarcoma)
- Metastatic

Neuropathic Disorders
- Charcot joints
- Compression neuropathies
  - Peripheral entrapment (carpal tunnel syndrome and others)
  - Radiculopathy
  - Spinal stenosis
- Reflex sympathetic dystrophy
- Others

Table 50–1. CLASSIFICATION OF THE RHEUMATIC DISEASES *Continued*

Bone and Cartilage Disorders Associated with Articular Manifestations
Osteoporosis
Generalized
Localized (regional)
Osteomalacia
Hypertrophic osteoarthropathy
Diffuse idiopathic skeletal hyperostosis (includes ankylosing vertebral hyperostosis [Forrestier's disease])
Osteitis
Generalized (osteitis deformans [Paget's disease])
Localized (osteitis condensans ilii, osteitis pubis)
Avascular necrosis
Osteochondritis (osteochondritis dissecans)
Congenital dysplasia of the hip
Slipped capital femoral epiphysis
Costochondritis (includes Tietze's syndrome)
Osteolysis and chondrolysis
Nonarticular Rheumatism
Myofascial pain syndromes
Generalized (fibrositis, fibromyalgia)
Regional
Low back pain and intervertebral disc disorders
Juxta-articular lesions
Bursitis
Tendon lesions (includes tendinitis, tenosynovitis, nodules)
Enthesopathy
Ganglions, cysts, geodes
Vasomotor disorders
Erythromelalgia
Raynaud's disease or phenomenon
Miscellaneous pain syndromes
Benign arthralgia and/or myalgia (e.g., coccydynia, metatarsalgia, growing pains)
Psychogenic rheumatism

OSTEOARTHRITIS

Perhaps the most common rheumatic condition seen in medical practice is osteoarthritis (OA), which is also known as osteoarthrosis, hypertrophic arthritis, or degenerative joint disease (this term should almost never be used, since its connotations to the patient are often significantly bad). While almost everyone will eventually develop at least x-ray evidence of osteoarthritis, we now realize that this condition is not simply an inexorable process of aging. There are many factors—genetic, serologic, inflammatory, and others—that enter into the picture, and of course the question of trauma is always of concern, particularly in young athletes. It is always of importance to realize that radiologic evidence of OA is not necessarily indicative of the association of rheumatic symptoms with the radiologic findings. Severe pain and disability can occur in the presence of relatively normal x-ray films, whereas quite severe x-ray changes can have no symptoms at all.

Whereas almost any joint in the body can be affected by OA, certain areas are more commonly involved. Heberden's and Bouchard's nodes involving the fingers have been mentioned; these, while sometimes unsightly, rarely produce much in the way of functional disability. On the other hand, hip and knee involvement as well as severe neck involvement can be very symptomatic and indeed disabling.

Osteoarthritis of the dorsal spine, although common, rarely produces any significant symptoms.

The management of osteoarthritis of the fingers basically is symptomatic (Fig. 50–2). First, reassure the patient that this is OA and not rheumatoid arthritis (RA). This can be very reassuring to patients who have the ugly spectre of functional deformity in their minds. Aside from this, mild analgesics when necessary are indicated as well as the use of some local heat such as is provided with paraffin baths or even hot water, along with simple exercises for flexibility.

Involvement of the neck is a special situation. Many times, patients will complain of severe neck pain—often radiating to the arms—in the presence of cervical osteoarthritis. They will note that this neck pain is particularly severe on arising from bed. Very likely this is due to the fact that while during the day the head is held in a position that causes the least discomfort, during the night the patient may allow the head to fall into positions that produce nerve impingement and be entirely unconscious of this. A very simple method of combating this is the use of a soft rubber collar to be worn while in bed, or one can easily improvise a soft collar using a large bath towel rolled lengthwise and wrapped around the neck and pinned. Patients soon learn to use this during the night and find that their symptoms are far less in the morning. The use of a more rigid collar during the day is sometimes necessary, and of course patients should be warned against any activity that causes sudden motion of the neck. Special neck pillows may also be helpful.

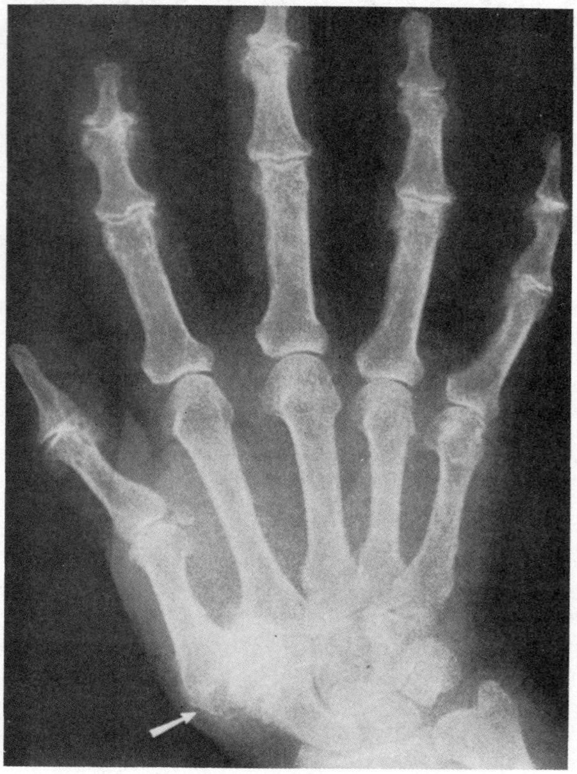

Figure 50–2. Osteoarthritis. Interphalangeal joints are primarily affected, but there is also severe involvement of the trapeziometacarpal and trapezionavicular joints. There is osteophyte formation, subchondral sclerosis, and nonuniform narrowing of the interphalangeal interosseous spaces. (Reprinted from Schumacher, R. H., Jr., Klippel, J. H., and Robinson, D. R. [Eds.]: Primer on the Rheumatic Diseases. 9th ed. Atlanta, GA, Arthritis Foundation, 1988, p. 64. Used by permission of the Arthritis Foundation.)

The lower back is a particularly troublesome area. Osteoarthritis of the lumbosacral spine is common, and once again we must be careful not to ascribe all symptoms to the radiographic findings that are almost invariably found in older patients.

The problem of the hip is more troublesome (Fig. 50–3). This disease, which is often familial, is usually associated at the beginning only with relatively mild pain and mild limitation of motion so that patients frequently do not consult their family physician until later in the disease. Generally speaking, the progress is very slow, and only in more advanced cases do patients find themselves sufficiently disabled to seek medical advice. One of the cardinal symptoms in OA of the hip is the inability to put on shoes and stockings in the normal fashion because of the inability to rotate the hip properly so as to bring the foot up close enough to the body to slip on the footwear. Patients will have all kinds of improvised ways of trying to help themselves with this, but eventually they will come to the doctor and the diagnosis is quite easy.

The management of OA of the hip is generally symptomatic at first and consists of the use of analgesic and anti-inflammatory medications, which are discussed in the following section.

It seems likely that the minor trauma of trying to use a hip that in essence is a square peg in a round hole produces some local inflammation, and thus the use of anti-inflammatory agents seems justified. In any event, many patients are materially relieved for many months or years, and operation can therefore be delayed. Along with these medications, range of motion exercises up to tolerance are generally indicated. Even with these, however, the range of motion slowly diminishes. Local injections of the hip are rarely indicated or necessary, and in some instances may actually be detrimental. It goes without saying that weight reduction in obese patients is important for all osteoarthritis occurring from the waist down. One of the best ways of convincing patients to lose this weight is to tell them that while it may be that their overweight did not cause the arthritis, if they were of normal weight would it make any sense to carry 20, 30, or 50 pounds in weight every time they walk around? Patients soon realize that the excess weight is causing a burden on an already troubled joint. In any event, many patients with OA of the hip come to surgery, and one should always offer this to the patient early on as a possibility so that his or her mental set will be such that he or she will welcome joint replacement rather than fight against it. Since

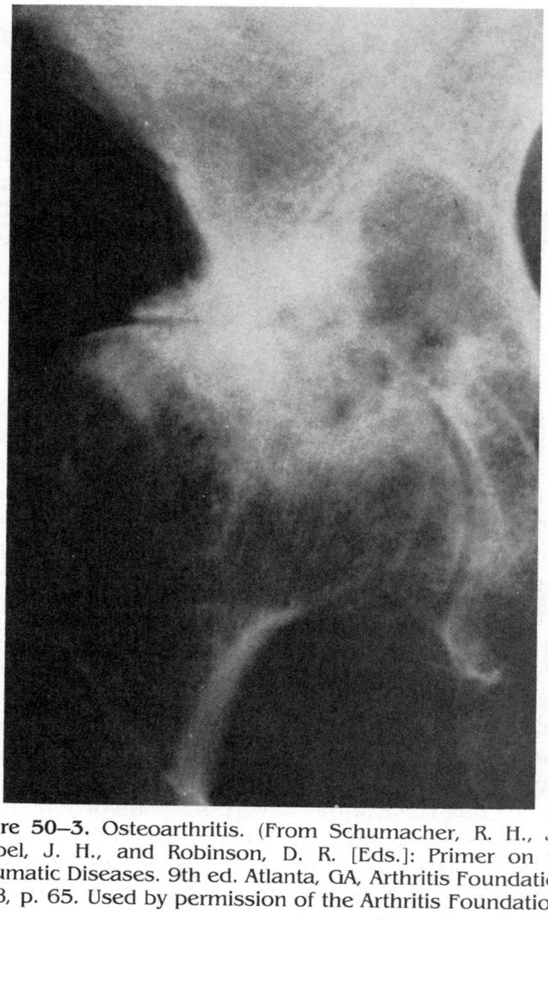

Figure 50–3. Osteoarthritis. (From Schumacher, R. H., Jr., Klippel, J. H., and Robinson, D. R. [Eds.]: Primer on the Rheumatic Diseases. 9th ed. Atlanta, GA, Arthritis Foundation, 1988, p. 65. Used by permission of the Arthritis Foundation.)

the operation is usually over 95 per cent successful, it is rare for patients not to be extremely grateful to the family physician for recommending them to a hip surgeon early in the course of the disease. The usual period of morbidity following surgery has been greatly decreased in recent years, and patients are frequently out of the hospital within 10 days after surgery and are walking with only a cane or nothing at all within 3 months.

Osteoarthritis of the knee is particularly common in overweight elderly patients, and most of the time the medial compartment of the knee is significantly narrowed and associated with localized osteoarthritis. On examination there may be tenderness, crepitus, and genu varus or valgus; swelling may also be present. The management of this condition is sometimes difficult. When it is associated with instability of the knee, a hinged elastic knee support may be supplied, or a more elaborate knee cage with straps going at least from midcalf to midthigh. Local steroid injections are useful for temporary flare-ups as long as it is completely certain that no bacterial infection is present. In general a good rule to follow is never to inject a weight-bearing joint more than three times in a calendar year. As with the hip, analgesics and nonsteroidal anti-inflammatory agents are indicated with knee OA; these often provide considerable relief. Although not as uniformly successful as hip replacement, knee replacements have become more and more common and they can be advised in patients with particularly troublesome knee OA.

RHEUMATOID ARTHRITIS

Rheumatoid arthritis (RA) is a far less common condition than osteoarthritis, but it is so devastating in its potential morbidity that the family physician must pay special attention to it. It is far more common in adults than in children, but may occur at any age.

Diagnosis

For the family physician there are some key words to remember when considering the diagnosis of rheumatoid arthritis. These are *symmetrical, inflammatory, systemic,* and *diurnal.* First let us consider *symmetrical.* For reasons that are certainly not clear, the joints affected by rheumatoid arthritis tend to be symmetrical. That is, if the proximal interphalangeal joint of the middle finger of the right hand is affected, the corresponding joint on the left hand is likely to be affected. If one knee is affected, the other one is likely to be. The major exception to this is in the presence of hemiplegia, in which case the paretic side is usually not affected by the arthritic process. This has led some people to believe that there is an autonomic nervous system etiology to rheumatoid arthritis, and it may well be that this is at least a factor.

The next word is *inflammatory.* Rheumatoid arthritis, in contrast to OA, is an inflammatory disease. It carries with it all of the cardinal manifestations of inflammation, namely, heat, redness, and swelling. As a result of the inflammatory process, lysosomal enzymes are released that are proteolytic in nature, and these cause erosions and eventually destruction of cartilage, periarticular bone, and surrounding joint structures. This leads to joint instability and deformity and the crippling phenomenon that is the dread end stage of rheumatoid arthritis. In fact, the crippling is caused by the healing process, namely, the formation of that peculiar scar tissue within the joint called pannus which eventually contracts and leads to the typical flexion contracture of the disease. The attending physician, then, must try insofar as possible to counteract the effects of inflammation and in a strange sense to counteract the effects of healing.

The next word to remember is *systemic.* Rheumatoid arthritis is usually a systemic disease in which the joints are the most dramatic manifestation. It is usual in RA to have a patient feel fatigue and weakness and to be somewhat anemic. Specific organ systems of the body can be involved; these include the heart, lungs, kidneys, small blood vessels, skin, and eyes, although almost any part of the body has the potential to be affected. It is sometimes difficult to distinguish the systemic effects of the disease from the systemic effects of the medications that are used in the treatment of the disease. Perhaps it is for this reason that life insurance companies frequently either refuse to accept patients with RA or give them a significantly higher rating. The lungs are affected mainly by involvement of the pleura with deposits similar to subcutaneous nodules. These can cause a pleuritis. Less commonly, an actual interstitial pneumonitis can occur. It is rare for pericarditis to occur but it has been described, as has myocarditis, which is likewise a rare manifestation. Kidneys are far more commonly involved in systemic lupus and as a result of some of the nonsteroidal anti-inflammatory agents. Rheumatoid vasculitis is a dread complication of RA and usually occurs in the presence of subcutaneous nodules and high titers of rheumatoid factor. It is frequently associated with a peripheral neuropathy that can cause wrist drop and other neuropathic manifestations. In severe cases, actual gangrene can occur with loss of digits. The eye is uncommonly involved in contrast to ankylosing spondylitis, which is discussed later. Occasionally a subcutaneous nodule-like deposit will occur in the sclera and can actually cause scleral perforation and blindness. This is a very rare phenomenon, however. Involvement of the skin is usually a manifestation of small vessel vasculitis, and a rash, of course, can occur as a result of almost any of the commonly used medications.

In making the diagnosis of RA, *diurnal variation* is an important factor. In contrast to OA, in which patients feel better after rest and worse when using the affected joint, RA patients feel at their worst after a period of rest. Thus, morning stiffness is a cardinal manifestation of RA and progress of the disease is frequently measured in terms of duration of morning stiffness. The same can occur after sitting for a long period of time.

There are many other clues to help the family physician in the diagnosis of RA, such as the "rheumatoid flop"; owing to instability about the knee joints, a person will upon sitting get about halfway down to the chair and then fall or flop into the sitting position. It is usual for the diagnosis to be made strictly on clinical grounds, and laboratory and x-ray studies are not especially useful except for the sedimentation rate.

The sedimentation rate, preferably done by the Westergren method, is an important measure of inflammatory disease. This should always be done in any work-up of a rheumatic patient, and it is very rare indeed for a person with active RA to have a normal sedimentation rate. The latex fixation test is positive 1:160 or greater in about 60 to 70 per cent of patients, but it is a relatively nonspecific test and is not necessary for the diagnosis of the disease. Frequently it is normal in early stages and is usually normal in rheumatoid arthritis of children (Still's disease).

The subcutaneous nodule occurs in about 20 per cent of patients with RA and is usually indicative of a serious and potentially crippling condition. These nodules, which are firm, somewhat rubbery, and not tender, tend to occur at extensor surfaces of joints, particularly the elbows, fingers, and sometimes back of the neck. No one is very sure of what the cause or the meaning of these nodules is, but it has been suggested by some that perhaps they should be studied further as more refined techniques for detection of viruses are developed, since it is possible that they bear a similar relationship to RA as the tubercle does to tuberculosis. This is, of course, entirely theoretical. It is sometimes difficult to distinguish the subcutaneous nodule of RA from the tophus of gout; but the tophus of gout is whitish, since it is composed of urate crystals, and the disease of gout is clinically quite different from that of RA.

Other laboratory tests tend to be confusing. The antinuclear antibody test (ANA) is sometimes positive in rather low titer, and therefore the diagnosis of systemic lupus is made incorrectly. The ANA, which in RA is usually diffuse and homogeneous, is a rather nonspecific test. Other tests are not particularly helpful. Determination of immunoglobulins is a refined technique that usually adds very little to your knowledge and it is seldom necessary to analyze synovial fluid unless the possibility of crystalline disease such as gout is suspected.

Radiology is of minimal use in rheumatoid arthritis since it rarely helps the family physician. In early disease there may be bony erosions, and of course in late disease the destruction and subluxation that occurs is almost equally well detected with the naked eye.

Treatment

The treatment of RA is difficult, since without good knowledge of etiology it is almost impossible to have rational treatment. One is, therefore, faced with symptomatic treatment and, it is hoped, prevention of destruction. It is a good general rule to realize that when a diagnosis of RA is made initially, the 5-year outlook is approximately 25 per cent for complete remission, 50 per cent for continuing disease activity, and 25 per cent for severe disease with deformity and crippling. The first thing the family physician must do when the diagnosis of RA has been made is to spend a little extra time at the beginning with the patient and the patient's family to establish the fact that it is a chronic disease and that improvement, if any, comes slowly and patience is required. This will put the patient and the people close to the patient in a frame of mind that is aware of the fact that slow and steady is preferable to spectacular and risky. A little extra time involved in the beginning is a worthwhile investment.

It is usual to consider the treatment of RA as a pyramid (Fig. 50–4). The base of the pyramid consists of the use of analgesic and anti-inflammatory medications and simple home physiotherapy. The usual analgesic and anti-inflammatory medication is aspirin in full dosage, which for an adult is about 3 to 4 grams daily. This dose of aspirin suppresses prostaglandins and therefore reduces inflammation and of course is an analgesic as well. For those patients who are able to take it, it is a very satisfactory treatment. Unfortunately, as with all prostaglandin inhibitors,

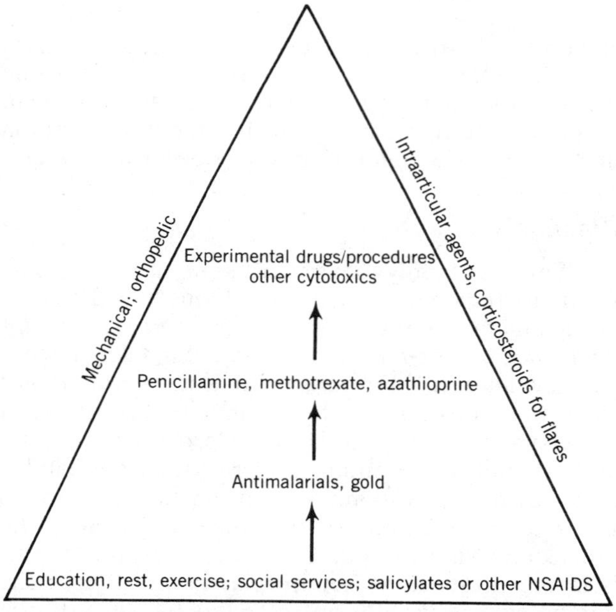

Figure 50–4. Treatment pyramid for rheumatoid arthritis. (From Schumacher, R. H., Jr., Klippel, J. H., and Robinson, D. R. [Eds.]: Primer on the Rheumatic Diseases. 9th ed. Atlanta, GA, Arthritis Foundation, 1988, p. 93. Used by permission of the Arthritis Foundation.)

the stomach is frequently upset and indeed erosions and bleeding can occur. This has been, until relatively recently, a very significant and difficult problem to cope with, but the development of oral synthetic prostaglandins such as misoprostol (Cytotec) may help prevent the gastric erosions and bleeding, although it is less effective in preventing the dyspepsia that frequently accompanies prostaglandin inhibitors.

Simple home physiotherapy consists of the use of range of motion exercises to maintain, insofar as possible, a normal range of motion for every joint in the body. It is easy for the family physician to devise such exercises since he or she has his or her own joints to use as a control. The important thing is to strengthen extensor muscles in order to combat flexion deformity. This does involve a certain amount of training since the rest position for most joints is in flexion, and many people consider good exercise to be exercise that maintains joints in the position of flexion such as knitting or crocheting for women. A far better exercise for the fingers is the flicking of crumpled up paper balls or similar objects into a basket. This forced extension can do more for prevention of flexion deformity than a day's worth of knitting. Good lists of specific exercises can be obtained from the Arthritis Foundation or any of its local chapters (see Table 50–2). They also have excellent booklets on many different rheumatic conditions and a particularly good one on self-help directed primarily at the patient with rheumatoid arthritis. Lists of helpful gadgets can also be obtained.

The next step on the pyramid is the use of more potent or at least different nonsteroidal anti-inflammatory drugs (NSAIDs). The list of available NSAIDs keeps growing almost weekly. They vary in their activity and there seems to be much individual variation so that it may be necessary to try two or three NSAIDs before one finds a drug that both is helpful to the patient and does not have major side effects. Do not believe the blandishments of the pharmaceutical companies, which would have you believe that *their* drug is stronger and has fewer side effects. That is generally not true. The use of the NSAIDs is helpful to perhaps another 10 or 15 per cent of patients who are not helped by the base treatment. The family physician will become familiar with two or three NSAIDs, and it is generally wise to stick to them. As new drugs are developed they can be tried with some caution, but it should be recalled that a number of NSAIDs have been removed from the market because of side effects that developed some time after their introduction.

Moving upward on the pyramid, we now come to the use of what is known as disease-modifying antirheumatic drugs or DMARDs. There are many people who do not believe that these drugs truly modify disease, but in any event they are longer acting than the NSAID. These agents differ from the nonsteroidal anti-inflammatory drugs mainly in the fact that they take longer to work and seem to exert their beneficial influence, when it does occur, in different ways. The most commonly used such drugs, and the ones most within the realm of therapy for the family physician, are gold and penicillamine.

The use of gold salts for rheumatoid arthritis has been available for over 50 years. There have been varying fashions in the use of gold salts, but by and large they have achieved a definite place. In former years they could be given only by weekly injection, and the incidence of side effects particularly involving the blood and urine was formidable. More recently, oral gold, Auranofin (Ridaura), has become available, and although there is a somewhat higher incidence of diarrhea with this medication, the incidence of the more dread side effects seems to be lower. In any event it is far easier for the patient to take than weekly intramuscular injections. In general the aim is for the use of approximately 50 mg. of gold weekly until a total of 1000 mg. has been reached. When the injectable gold is used, this means gradually increasing intramuscular doses to a maximum of 50 mg. per week; with the oral gold, it means the use of 6 mg. per day. It takes about 6 months for this initial course of gold to have been accomplished. Frequent testing of blood count, platelets, and urine—particularly examination for protein and red blood cells—is necessary, and gold should be discontinued at any sign of leukopenia, thrombocytopenia, hematuria, or significant proteinuria. Assuming none of these occurrences, at the end of 1000 mg. the patient should be evaluated; if a beneficial effect has occurred, the gold should be continued for at least 2 years although at reduced levels with injections every 2 to 4 weeks and oral gold reduced to 3 mg. daily. If no beneficial effect has been achieved after the initial 6-month period, it is usually not fruitful to proceed further. About 20 per cent of patients with active rheumatoid arthritis can be reasonably well controlled with gold.

The use of penicillamine was introduced by Jaffe in the early 1960's, but the dose used was so high that formidable toxic effects occurred. In recent years, it has become apparent that smaller doses of the order of 250 to 500 mg. of penicillamine daily are just about as effective and with a far lower risk of toxic effects. Many feel that penicillamine is preferable to gold, but in any event it is an alternative and can be used if gold has failed. Patients of course must be watched at approximately 2- to 4-week intervals with complete blood count, platelet count, and urinalysis.

Another drug that should be mentioned at this stage is chloroquine or its analogue hydroxychloroquine. These antimalarial drugs suppress inflammation in a small number of patients with active rheumatoid arthritis, and although their use is more beneficial in general in systemic lupus, they have a small place in the armamentarium for rheumatoid arthritis. In any patient in whom these drugs are used, a baseline ophthalmologic examination should be obtained and should be repeated at approximately 3-month intervals because of the risk of irreversible chloroquine retinopathy.

Table 50–2. ARTHRITIS FOUNDATION CHAPTERS

Alabama Chapter
Birmingham, AL
(205) 870-4700

South Alabama Chapter
Mobile, AL
(205) 434-3589

Alaska Unit
Anchorage, AK
(907) 274-2393

Central Arizona Chapter
Phoenix, AZ
(602) 264-7679

Southern Arizona Chapter
Tucson, AZ
(602) 326-2811

Arkansas Chapter
Little Rock, AR
(501) 664-7242

Northeastern California Chapter
Sacramento, CA
(916) 921-5533

Northern California Chapter
San Francisco, CA
(415) 673-6882

San Diego Area Chapter
San Diego, CA
(619) 492-1094

Southern California Chapter
Los Angeles, CA
(213) 938-6111

Rocky Mountain Chapter
Denver, CO
(303) 756-8622

Connecticut Chapter
Rocky Hill, CT
(203) 563-1177

Delaware Chapter
Wilmington, DE
(302) 764-8254

Florida Chapter
Bradenton, FL
(813) 795-3010

Georgia Chapter
Atlanta, GA
(404) 873-3240

Hawaii Chapter
Honolulu, HI
(808) 523-7561

Idaho Chapter
Boise, ID
(208) 344-7102

Central Illinois Chapter
Peoria, IL
(309) 672-6337

Illinois Chapter
Chicago, IL
(312) 782-1367

Indiana Chapter
Indianapolis, IN
(317) 844-3341

Iowa Chapter
Des Moines, IA
(515) 278-0636

Kansas Chapter
Wichita, KS
(316) 263-0116

Kentucky Chapter
Louisville, KY
(502) 459-6460

Louisiana Chapter
New Orleans, LA
(504) 897-1338

Maine Chapter
Brunswick, ME
(207) 729-4453

Maryland Chapter
Lutherville, MD
(301) 561-8090

Massachusetts Chapter
Watertown, MA
(617) 926-2900

Michigan Chapter
Southfield, MI
(313) 350-3030

Minnesota Chapter
Minneapolis, MN
(612) 874-1201

Mississippi Chapter
Jackson, MS
(601) 956-3371

Eastern Missouri Chapter
St. Louis, MO
(314) 644-3488

Western Missouri–Greater Kansas City Chapter
Kansas City, MO
(816) 361-7002

Montana Chapter
Billings, MT
(406) 248-7602

Nebraska Chapter
Omaha, NB
(402) 391-8000

Nevada Chapter
Las Vegas, NV
(702) 367-1626

New Hampshire Chapter
Concord, NH
(603) 224-9322

New Jersey Chapter
Iselin, NJ
(201) 388-0744

New Mexico Chapter
Albuquerque, NM
(505) 265-1545

Central New York Chapter
Syracuse, NY
(315) 455-8553

Genesee Valley Chapter
Rochester, NY
(716) 423-9490

Long Island Chapter
Melville, NY
(516) 427-8272

New York Chapter
New York, NY
(212) 477-8310

Northeastern New York Chapter
Albany, NY
(518) 459-5082

Western New York Chapter
Buffalo, NY
(716) 837-8600

North Carolina Chapter
Durham, NC
(919) 477-0286

Dakota Chapter
Fargo, ND
(701) 282-3653

Central Ohio Chapter
Columbus, OH
(614) 488-0777

Northeastern Ohio Chapter
Cleveland, OH
(216) 791-1310

Northwestern Ohio Chapter
Toledo, OH
(419) 473-3349

Southwestern Ohio Chapter
Cincinnati, OH
(513) 271-4545

Eastern Oklahoma Chapter
Tulsa, OK
(918) 743-4526

Oklahoma Chapter
Oklahoma City, OK
(405) 521-0066

Oregon Chapter
Portland, OR
(503) 222-7246

Central Pennsylvania Chapter
Camp Hill, PA
(717)763-0900

Eastern Pennsylvania Chapter
Philadelphia, PA
(215) 574-9480

Western Pennsylvania Chapter
Pittsburgh, PA
(412) 566-1645

Rhode Island Chapter
East Providence, RI
(401) 434-5792

South Carolina Chapter
Columbia, SC
(803) 254-6702

Middle-East Tennessee Chapter
Nashville, TN
(615) 329-3431

West Tennessee Chapter
Memphis, TN
(901) 365-7080

North Texas Chapter
Dallas, TX
(214) 826-4361

Northwest Texas Chapter
Forth Worth, TX
(817) 926-7733

South Central Texas Chapter
San Antonio, TX
(512) 224-4857

Texas Gulf Coast Chapter
Houston, TX
(713) 579-1700

Utah Chapter
Salt Lake City, UT
(801) 486-4993

Vermont & Northern New York Chapter
Burlington, VT
(802) 864-4988

Virginia Chapter
Richmond, VA
(804) 270-1229

Metropolitan Washington Chapter
Arlington, VA
(703) 276-7555

Washington State Chapter
Seattle, WA
(206) 622-1378

West Virginia Chapter
Dunbar, WV
(304) 768-3667

Wisconsin Chapter
West Allis, WI
(414) 321-3933

Once we get past these drugs, we are approaching the tip of the pyramid and the pyramid is becoming a volcano. We are now at the point at which truly risky and dangerous drugs must be used. One of these—and one that many physicians would have used long before this—is corticosteroids. The problem of corticosteroids in rheumatoid arthritis has been evolving over 40 years. The initial wave of tremendous enthusiasm gave way to dismay as the expected side effects occurred, and we are now approaching a somewhat middle ground on the swing of the pendulum. There is no drug as dramatic in its effect as the steroids, but nevertheless their use should be confined to specific situations. First of all, large doses of corticosteroids (15 mg. daily of prednisone or greater) should be reserved for very serious or life-threatening complications of rheumatoid arthritis, since these large doses are almost invariably associated with serious and significant side effects. Smaller doses of steroids (up to 10 mg. daily of prednisone) can be used when other agents have failed and when social situations require that a patient get more immediate and dramatic relief than can otherwise be obtained. The truly difficult problem, as every experienced family physician knows, is stopping the steroids once they have been started; therefore, one should never start them without realizing that while starting is easy, stopping is difficult. The adrenal glands are suppressed by the use of steroids, and this can be a serious and even life-threatening situation in the event of trauma, surgery, and so forth. In any patient who has received corticosteroids within the year previous to surgery, the surgeon and anesthetist should be alerted; usually the use of intravenous corticosteroids at time of surgery is indicated. When corticosteroids are used, they should be given as a single dose usually in the morning. Alternate-day therapy in rheumatoid arthritis is rarely successful. When very serious disease occurs and pulse therapy with very large intravenous doses of steroids is indicated, this should usually be done in the hospital and under the supervision of an experienced rheumatologist. The use of intra-articular corticosteroids is sometimes beneficial, but one must realize that no single joint should be injected more than three times in a calendar year—and this is particularly true of weight-bearing joints. The risk of infection is serious and in rheumatoid arthritis we are dealing with continuing inflammatory disease so that the best that one can hope for is a temporary remission.

We are now at the very tip of the volcano where the lava is hottest. This is the point at which one must consider the use of both approved and nonapproved drugs that are immunosuppressive and cytotoxic. Such drugs as methotrexate, cyclophosphamide, azathioprine, and others of these families are extremely dangerous and potent and generally beyond the scope of the family physician. When the use of these drugs is contemplated, consultation with an experienced rheumatologist should be obtained.

SPECIAL SITUATIONS IN RHEUMATOID ARTHRITIS

Juvenile Rheumatoid Arthritis (Still's Disease)

The very rare condition known as juvenile rheumatoid arthritis or Still's disease generally falls into three main categories. These are *pauciarticular arthritis* in which only one or very few joints are affected in a chronic, usually not very serious way, and aside from the more frequent occurrence of uveitis it frequently burns out at puberty. *Polyarthritis* resembles adult rheumatoid arthritis, and the *systemic variety* presents as a fever of unknown origin often associated with a rash or dermatographia and lymphadenopathy. The diagnosis is therefore frequently extremely difficult, especially since both spleen and liver can be enlarged. The rash is probably the best clue to the diagnosis of the systemic form of Still's disease. The treatment of juvenile RA is about the same as the adult form with generally good prognosis, although the rare occasional patient may become devastated with the disease. As with any condition involving the growing point or epiphysis of the bone, premature closure may occur, and as a result both microdactyly and micrognathia are common. Thus, an adult who no longer has active arthritis but who had juvenile rheumatoid arthritis can sometimes be recognized by the so-called "Andy Gump" syndrome, which is basically a very small jaw.

Arthritis of Psoriasis

Peripheral psoriatic arthritis is very similar to ordinary rheumatoid arthritis except for the fact that it can involve distal interphalangeal joints, particularly when the fingernails and toenails are involved, and can be extremely destructive. What is perhaps more significant is that psoriasis is not infrequently associated with ankylosing spondylitis and thus falls within the group of conditions known as seronegative spondylarthropathies. This refers to the fact that their latex fixation tests are almost uniformly negative and that the genetic factor HLA-B27 is almost always positive. Other seronegative spondylarthropathies include the arthritis of ulcerative colitis and Reiter's syndrome. The management of peripheral psoriatic arthritis is very much the same as that of rheumatoid arthritis except that gold and penicillamine are usually ineffective. Methotrexate is now an approved drug for use in psoriatic arthritis and in many instances has proved to be quite effective.

Ankylosing Spondylitis

The arthritis that much more commonly affects men than women is ankylosing spondylitis, also

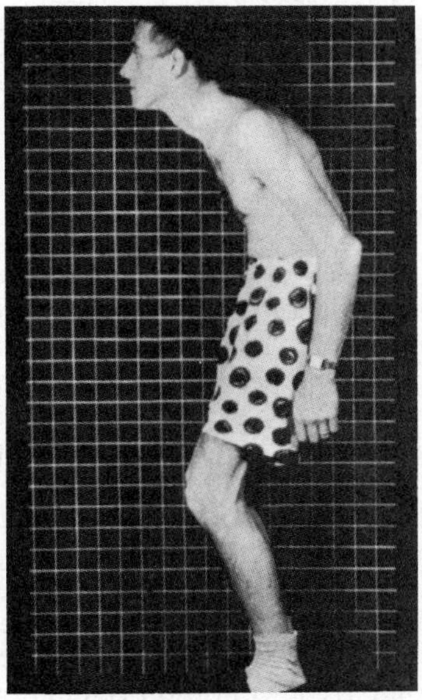

Figure 50–5. Severe ankylosing spondylitis with lumbar, hip, and knee flexion deformities. (From Schumacher, R. H., Jr., Klippel, J. H., and Robinson, D. R. [Eds.]: Primer on the Rheumatic Diseases. 9th ed. Atlanta, GA, Arthritis Foundation, 1988, p. 145. Used by permission of the Arthritis Foundation.)

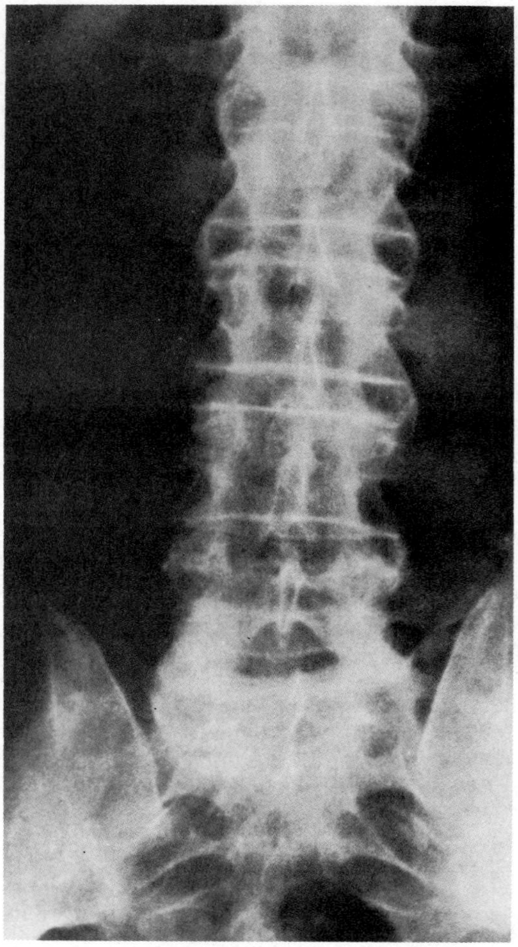

Figure 50–6. Ankylosing spondylitis, frontal view, illustrating well-developed syndesmophytes involving the discovertebral joints of the lumbar spine, giving a "bamboo spine" appearance. (From Schumacher, R. H., Jr., Klippel, J. H., and Robinson, D. R. [Eds.]: Primer on the Rheumatic Diseases. 9th ed. Atlanta, GA, Arthritis, Foundation, 1988, p. 67. Used by permission of the Arthritis Foundation.)

known as Marie-Strümpell or von Bechterew's disease. This condition usually begins rather indolently with some vague backache and is often not diagnosed early in the disease. Indeed the patient may well not realize there is a problem. As the disease progresses, it defies the law of gravity and migrates upward from the sacroiliac joints to the lumbosacral spine, the dorsal spine, the cervical spine, and in rare but often devastating instances to the large peripheral joints such as the hips and shoulders (Figs. 50–5 and 50–6). The first changes are almost always in the sacroiliac joints; if one suspects ankylosing spondylitis, a good radiograph of these joints should reveal clouding, narrowing, or even fusion. It is very rare for ankylosing spondylitis to occur in the presence of normal sacroiliac joints. The condition is manifested more by stiffness than by pain, and as the disease progresses, the usual flexion deformity of active inflammatory arthritis occurs with the patient assuming a forwardly bent position. Movement in the spine is slowly lost, and when the disease affects the dorsal spine, the costovertebral joints become fused so that the ribs cannot rock properly and breathing becomes abdominal as the patient is forced to expand the lungs by lowering the diaphragm. This is a characteristic finding, and indeed one of the measures of progression of ankylosing spondylitis is to measure chest expansion, which instead of the usual 3 to 4 inches will be reduced to 1 inch or less. The patient will often not consult the physician until the cervical spine becomes affected, because it is really only at that time that the disease presents as a serious disability. Not being able to turn one's head can be a real problem when driving a motor vehicle and of course in many other instances of daily living. By the time the neck has been affected, however, the disease is far advanced.

The management of ankylosing spondylitis consists of the use of anti-inflammatory drugs, particularly indomethacin, diclofenac, and naproxen. As these anti-inflammatory drugs are given, a series of exercises and instructions for daily living should be given to the patient. These include the use of a thin, firm mattress placed on a bed board so that the spine is maintained as much as possible in a straight position; the use of a small or no pillow so that the neck is not forward flexed; and a series of exercises, particularly breathing exercises, to maintain insofar

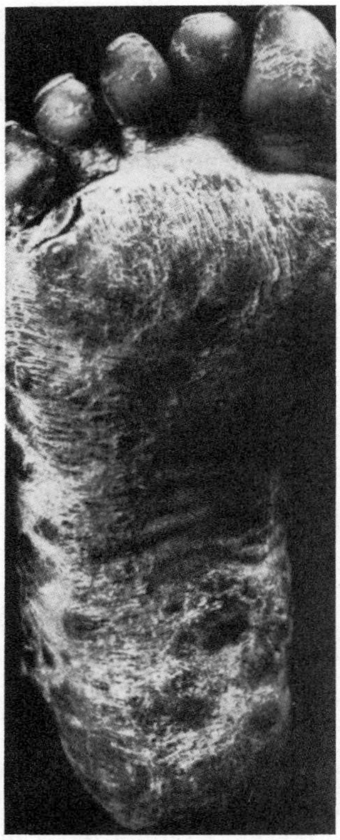

Figure 50–7. Keratoderma blennorrhagica in a 49-year-old man with Reiter's syndrome. These lesions healed without scarring. (Schumacher, R. H., Jr., Klippel, J. H., and Robinson, D. R. [Eds.]: Primer on the Rheumatic Diseases. 9th ed. Atlanta, GA, Arthritis Foundation, 1988, p. 148. Used by permission of the Arthritis Foundation.)

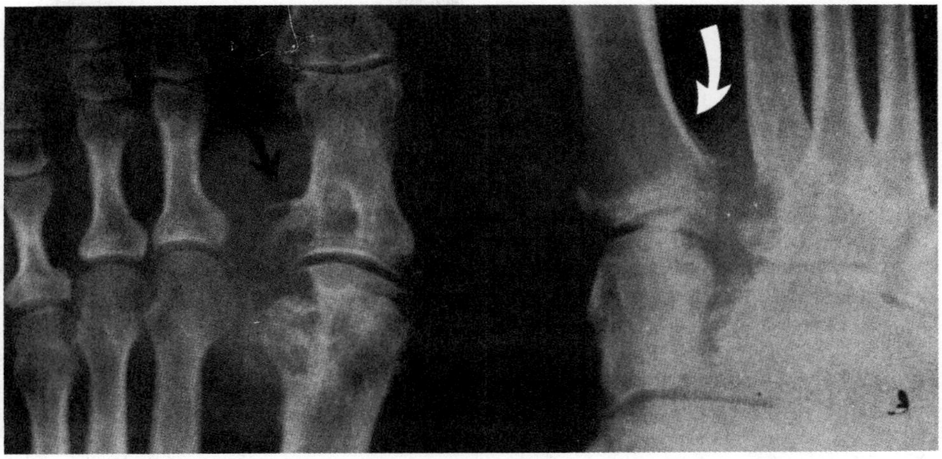

Figure 50–8. Gout. Left, the left first metatarsophalangeal joint exhibits sharply marginated erosions with overhanging margins *(straight arrow)*. Right, there is a large destructive lesion in the right metatarsus with minimal adjacent new bone formation *(curved arrow)*; this was associated with a large soft tissue tophus on the dorsum that was apparent in the lateral projection. (From Schumacher, R. H., Jr., Klippel, J. H., and Robinson, D. R. [Eds.]: Primer on the Rheumatic Diseases. 9th ed. Atlanta, GA, Arthritis Foundation, 1988, p. 63. Used by permission of the Arthritis Foundation.)

as possible normal posture and pulmonary function. Despite all of this, however, there are significant concomitant effects, the most common of which are aortic insufficiency and uveitis and iritis. One should always be aware of these possibilities and particularly in the event of eye complications begin treatment at once.

Arthritis of Ulcerative Colitis and Ileitis

The arthritis of ulcerative colitis and ileitis is basically that of ankylosing spondylitis and the management is one that should be instituted as with the other conditions. It is of some interest that patients with ulcerative colitis have not infrequently been treated with sulfasalazine, and there has recently been a flurry of interest in the use of this drug for other kinds of arthritis. There is no convincing evidence that it is effective, and a very significant number of patients develop severe side effects including rash, blood dyscrasias, and gastrointestinal complications.

Reiter's Syndrome

Reiter's syndrome is a fairly uncommon form of seronegative polyarthritis again particularly affecting men. It is characterized by an inflammatory arthritis mainly involving fingers, toes, and large joints, occasionally by nonspecific urethritis or conjunctivitis, and most commonly by a somewhat psoriatic skin rash known as keratodermia blennorrhagica (Fig. 50–7). This rash occurs primarily on the soles of the feet, the genital organs, and sometimes the palms and is typical of Reiter's syndrome. The nonarthritic components of this syndrome sometimes respond to the use of antibiotics such as tetracycline or erythromycin and the arthritic components frequently respond to potent NSAIDs. If drugs stronger than these are necessary, rheumatologic consultation should be obtained.

CRYSTAL DISEASE

Gout

The most notable crystal disease is acute and chronic gout (Figs. 50–8 and 50–9). Gout has become a much more common disease since the use of thiazide diuretics. These diuretics have the potential of raising uric acid levels and inducing attacks of gout. Acute gout is a characteristic condition. It is an explosive, usually monoarticular arthritis associated with intense redness, heat and swelling, and exquisite pain. This occurs over a 12- to 24-hour period and the attack can last as long as 2 weeks if untreated. The patient then usually remains quite well until the next attack. What happens if treatment is not instituted is that the attacks become more and more frequent and closer together so that they sometimes run into each other, a condition known as chronic gout that is rarely confused with chronic rheumatoid arthritis. The diagnosis of acute gout is made definitively by the detection of needle-shaped, birefringent urate crystals in joint fluid under the polarizing microscope. This may necessitate having the fluid examined by someone who possesses the proper equipment and can recognize urate crystals. It is extremely rare to have an attack of acute gout in the presence of a normal serum uric acid level, but one must beware of making the diagnosis of gout in every patient who has the combination of arthritis and an elevated uric acid, since this can occur in many conditions other than gout. The management of the initial attack of acute gout is with colchicine given in a dose of 0.6 mg. every hour to a maximum of 10 doses, stopping when gastrointestinal side effects occur. Almost the only acute arthritis that responds dramatically to this use of colchicine is gout, and the therapeutic regimen in this instance is therefore also diagnostic. After the initial attack, it is not necessary to give colchicine, which can produce quite severe gastrointestinal side effects; the use of a potent NSAID such as indomethacin or naproxen is quite sufficient. The attack usually subsides within 24 hours. The preventive aspects consist of managing the patient between attacks. During this intercritical period, the use of an agent to lower uric acid such as allopurinol 300 mg. daily is advisable if the uric acid level remains over 9 mg. daily. In addition to this, colchicine 0.6 mg. once or twice daily should also be given, since minor attacks can occur while the uric acid level is being mobilized from places in the body in which it is stored and finally excreted. The use of Colbenemid is less popular than it used to be. Unfortunately skin eruptions occur in about one person in 30 receiving allopurinol, and this may require discontinuance.

Pseudogout

Pseudogout is a misnomer. It is a synovitis somewhat similar to gout but produced by calcium pyrophosphate dihydrate (CPPD) crystals (Fig. 50–10). These crystals are very different from urate crystals and again can be recognized sometimes on direct microscopy but certainly on polarizing microscopy.

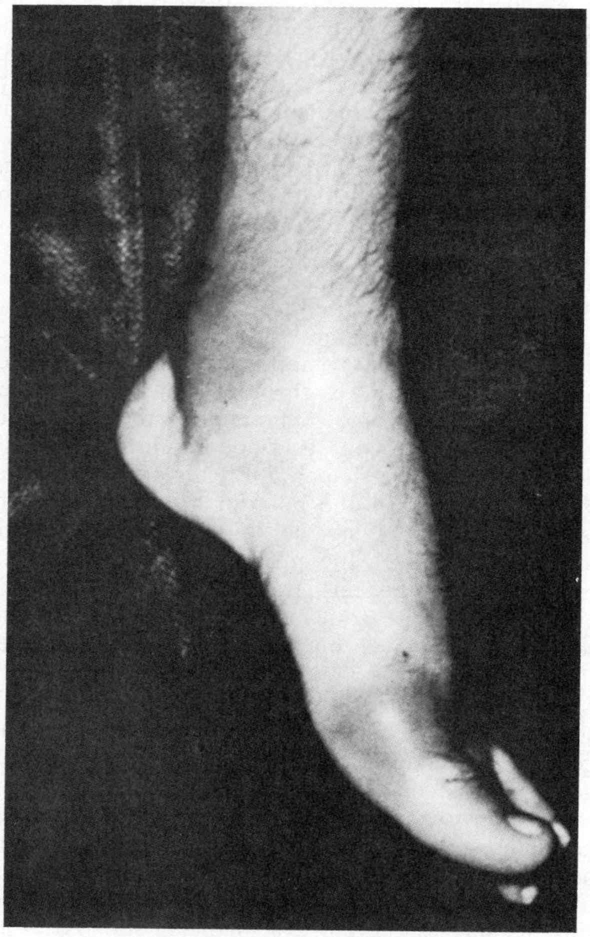

Figure 50–9. Acute gouty arthritis at first metatarsophalangeal and ankle joints. (From Schumacher, R. H., Jr., Klippel, J. H. and Robinson, D. R. [Eds.]: Primer on the Rheumatic Diseases. 9th ed. Atlanta, GA, Arthritis Foundation, 1988, p. 199. Used by permission of the Arthritis Foundation.)

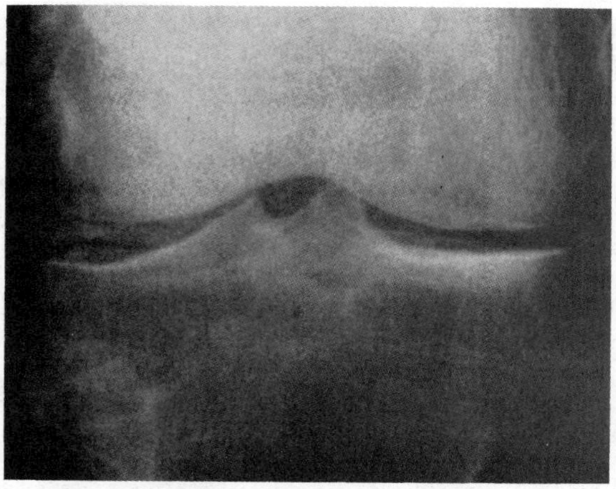

Figure 50–10. Chondrocalcinosis. Calcification is present in both menisci but more evident in the lateral meniscus *(arrow)*. There is slight narrowing of the interosseous space medially with subchondral sclerosis, reflecting degenerative change in the cartilage. Hyaline cartilage calcification was evident in the lateral view but, as is common, was obscured by the fibrocartilaginous calcification in this projection. (From Schumacher, R. H., Jr., Klippel, J. H., and Robinson, D. R. [Eds.]: Primer on the Rheumatic Diseases. 9th ed. Atlanta, GA, Arthritis Foundation, 1988, p. 63. Used by permission of the Arthritis Foundation.)

The acute attack of pseudogout is seldom as severe as acute gout, and the underlying disease is much more that of osteoarthritis with which it is usually associated. The best way of making the diagnosis is by taking an x-ray film of the affected joint and noting the typical calcified line in the cartilage about the affected joint, which represents deposit of CPPD crystals. The treatment of pseudogout is basically of the underlying osteoarthritis.

Hydroxyapatite

Occasionally other crystals such as hydroxyapatite are deposited in or about the joint; when this occurs about the shoulder associated with osteoarthritis, the condition is known as Milwaukee shoulder. The deposition of hydroxyapatite crystals can occur in tendons and soft tissues and is most common in elderly patients and those with severe renal impairment. The management is again that of the underlying osteoarthritis.

INFECTIOUS ARTHRITIS

Lyme Disease

The most important new infectious arthritis is Lyme disease. This was originally known as Lyme arthritis, but it is now recognized to be a true systemic disease with particular predilection for the nervous system and the heart as well as the joints. Lyme disease has been described in almost every part of the world but is most characteristic in those areas having a high population of deer ticks, particularly

Ixodes dammini, although other variations of Ixodes can occur in other parts of the world. The causative agent following the tick bite is *Borrelia burgdorferi*, which is a spirochete and can therefore be treated in ways similar to other spirochetal diseases.

The usual natural history of Lyme disease starts with the tick bite and the characteristic reddish area that can surround the area of the bite for several centimeters. Unfortunately many patients do not recall being bitten by a tick, and it is only in rare instances that one can see this typical rash; this is truly unfortunate, since it is at this stage that the causative agent is most susceptible to antibiotic therapy. About a month after this tick bite, although the period is variable, a variety of systemic conditions occur including headache, muscle aches, arthralgias, malaise, fatigue, stiffness, and in severe instances fever and chills. Other systemic symptoms can occur, and in general particularly during tick season and shortly thereafter the diagnosis of influenza should be made only after one has seriously considered the possibility of Lyme disease. Roughly 60 per cent of patients who develop frank arthritis usually develop it in the knees, although generalized polyarthritis can occur. The arthritis can be chronic and can actually result in erosion of cartilage and bone and crippling. More serious are the neurologic abnormalities, which include facial palsy, optic atrophy, and various other neuritic complaints including central nervous system syndromes resembling encephalitis or even multiple sclerosis. A small number of patients can develop cardiac involvement with heart block and both myocarditis and pericarditis. Morbidity can be severe. Mortality is rare.

The diagnosis of Lyme disease is sometimes difficult, although if one is fortunate enough to know about the tick bite it is easy. The important thing for the family physician is to maintain a high index of suspicion, particularly if in one of the coastal areas, where Lyme disease is especially prevalent. Laboratory findings consist of the determination of antibody titers, but unfortunately serial tests are usually necessary to see if titers are rising or if one is simply detecting an old condition or a natural variation. The treatment of early Lyme disease is the use of tetracycline 250 mg. four times daily or erythromycin in the same dosage or penicillin 500 mg. four times daily, each for a period of three weeks. If the diagnosis is not made until later in the disease, the treatment should be somewhat similar to that given for syphilis, namely, intravenous penicillin 20 million units daily for 10 days. Once arthritis has been clearly established, large doses of penicillin are likewise indicated along with sufficient NSAIDs to control symptoms. The use of corticosteroids is contraindicated, and the use of other drugs used in rheumatoid arthritis is of no benefit.

Gonococcal Arthritis

Of the other forms of infectious arthritis, clearly the most common in many areas is gonococcal arthritis. This is a dramatic condition usually starting as a polyarticular disease and frequently settling into a single joint. It is usually associated with a rash that is sometimes pustular. The organisms can sometimes be confirmed by cultivation from the blood, the joint fluid, or one of the vesicles. In establishing the diagnosis of gonococcal arthritis, one must consider that it is far more likely to occur in a sexually active 21-year-old girl than in an 83-year-old man. Common sense is helpful.

Staphylococcal Arthritis

The most dreaded form of infectious arthritis is staphylococcal involvement. This usually occurs when the joint is penetrated from the outside or rarely during the course of systemic staphylococcal infection. In the event that staphylococcal arthritis occurs, hospitalization and large doses of intravenous penicillin or one of its variants is indicated. If drainage of the infected joint becomes necessary, as it often does, competent orthopedic consultation should be obtained.

Viral Arthritis

Many viral infections are associated with arthritis, but particularly rubella, which in adults can produce arthritis in about 10 per cent. This is also true of adults who are vaccinated against rubella, but the arthritis is usually transitory and subsides spontaneously.

Hepatitis B frequently produces an arthritis, and one is seeing more and more of this condition. The arthritis involves large joints and is often associated with a skin rash and, of course, the characteristic tests indicating liver involvement. The management of the condition is that of the underlying disease and consequently is quite difficult. Prednisone is sometimes the drug of choice.

Other Forms of Infectious Arthritis

Tuberculous arthritis and fungal arthritis are both uncommon and the management is that of the underlying disease.

SYSTEMIC CONDITIONS

Sarcoidosis

Rheumatic complaints are a feature of many systemic conditions, but one of the more common is sarcoidosis. This systemic condition is characterized by the presence of noncaseating granulomas somewhat similar to tuberculomas, hilar adenopathy, some pulmonary infiltration, skin and eye complications, and in about 10 to 15 per cent an acute arthritis or a chronic arthralgia. This acute arthritis is sometimes the first manifestation that brings the patient to the

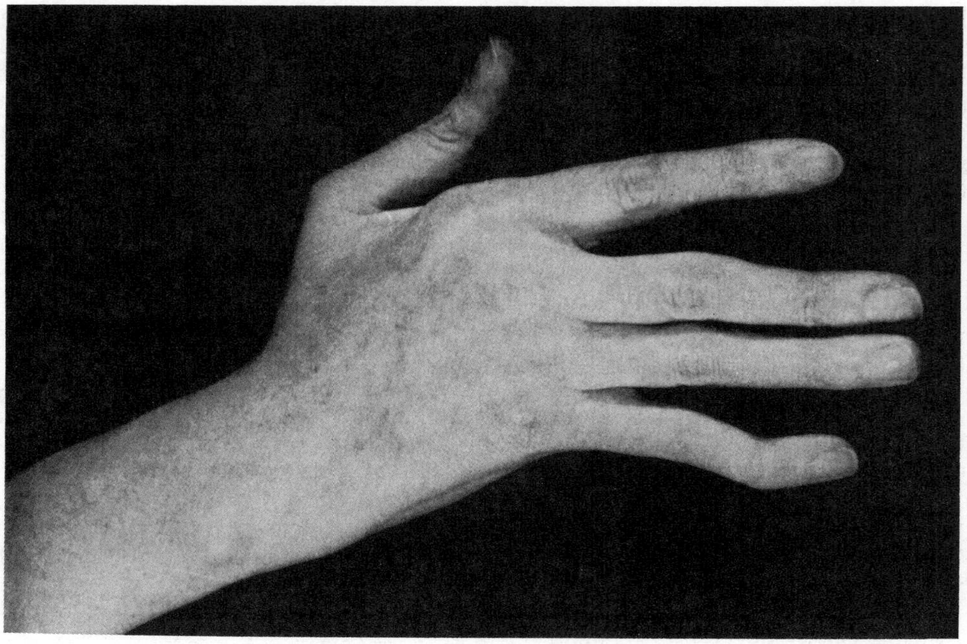

Figure 50–11. Hand deformities in SLE vary from isolated flexion contractures to severe Jaccoud's deformity as shown in this figure. (From Schumacher, R. H., Jr., Klippel, J. H., and Robinson, D. R. [Eds.]: Primer on the Rheumatic Diseases. 9th ed. Atlanta, GA, Arthritis Foundation, 1988, p. 100. Used by permission of the Arthritis Foundation.)

family physician. A chest film is usually indicated if sarcoidosis is suspected as it should be in any patient with a rather vague and unspecific arthritis particularly involving the ankles and knees, although occasionally involving the hands in a somewhat atypical rheumatoid way. The presence of involvement of skin and eye should make one particularly suspicious. A word of caution: hyperuricemia is common in sarcoidosis, and since there are occasionally multiple punched out bony lesions particularly involving the hands, one should be on guard against making the diagnosis of gout. In general, patients with the arthritis of sarcoidosis do well with nothing but symptomatic treatment. Only rarely is the use of steroids necessary; when they are used, the disease responds extremely well.

Familial Mediterranean Fever

Familial Mediterranean fever (FMF) is an unusual condition, most commonly seen in people whose genetic origins lie in those areas around the Mediterranean, particularly Arabs, Israelis, Greeks, Italians, and Turks. This unusual condition can be very severe, and arthritis, while common, is a relatively minor part of the syndrome. Diagnosis is made on the basis of family history; treatment is with colchicine, to which most patients respond well.

Behçet's Syndrome

Behçet's syndrome is another condition seen in people of Mediterranean origin although it is very common in Japan and Korea. This syndrome consists of mucous membrane and skin lesions particularly involving the inside of the mouth and the genitalia. These lesions can become deep ulcerations and be very painful indeed. Many other systemic involvements occur as well as arthralgia and low-grade arthritis; the treatment, again, is that of the underlying disease. However, treatment is usually extremely difficult. In the rare instance of a family physician suspecting this condition, consultation is usually advisable mainly for confirmation of the diagnosis.

Systemic Lupus Erythematosus

Systemic lupus erythematosus (SLE) is a condition marked more by arthralgia than by true arthritis (Fig. 50–11). It is a systemic disease that can involve almost any organ system of the body; commonly the skin (typical butterfly rash) (Fig. 50–12), the blood (leukopenia and thrombocytopenia), the heart, lungs, and brain, and most particularly the kidneys are involved. Raynaud's phenomenon is very common, and the combination of arthralgias and Raynaud's phenomenon should be considered lupus until proven otherwise. Lymphadenopathy and splenomegaly can also occur. Whereas lupus occurs at any age, it is most common in young adults and more common in young women than in young men. The almost invariable finding of positive tests for antinuclear antibodies (ANA) provides a way of excluding lupus rather than diagnosing it. That is, the presence of a negative test should make one view the diagnosis with great suspicion, whereas a positive test is not diagnostic. The patterns of antinuclear antibodies are important. The common pattern in SLE is homogeneous and diffuse. A speckled pattern can also occur as can a nucleolar pattern, but these are less common and should make one suspect one of the other connective tissue diseases.

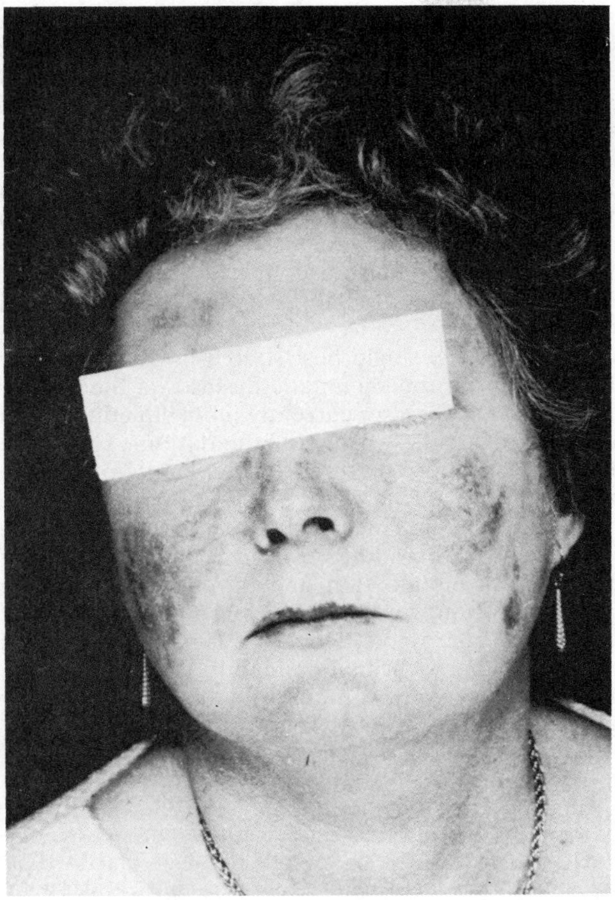

Figure 50–12. Typical malar butterfly rash of SLE. (From Schumacher, R. H., Jr., Klippel, J. H., and Robinson, D. R. [Eds.]: Primer on Rheumatic Diseases. 9th ed. Atlanta, GA, Arthritis Foundation, 1988, p. 101. Used by permission of the Arthritis Foundation.)

The treatment of SLE requires considerable clinical judgment. Generally one should treat the disease and not the diagnosis. In other words, it is not necessary to hit the patient with everything in the book, particularly the corticosteroids. If a patient is getting along reasonably well, symptomatic therapy is usually indicated along with the sensible regimen one would impose in any chronic disease. NSAIDs are useful and the management of anemia is appropriate. Corticosteroids should be given only when the disease is becoming progressive or when major disease activity such as involvement of heart, kidney, or central nervous system is present. Even at that time, the dose should be kept as low as possible. The antimalarials, particularly hydroxychloroquine, are most useful in the management of SLE and should generally be tried before corticosteroids are introduced.

In the unlikely event of serious renal or central nervous system disease, the various immunosuppressive agents and cytotoxic agents can be used as well as pulse therapy; but if these are contemplated, consultation with the rheumatologist is advised. The prognosis of SLE is far more favorable than it has been previously, and mortality is around the 5 per cent level at this writing. One of the best ways of following patients with lupus is by the determination of serum complement. A sudden fall in complement is usually a precursor of the dread renal complications and should be treated in a most aggressive way.

Drug-induced lupus is usually mild and responds to withdrawal of the offending drug.

Scleroderma

Scleroderma is a systemic disease primarily of the dermis with thickening of the skin, deposition of calcium, and not infrequently involvement of the heart, lungs, and kidneys. Arthritis is not really a part of this condition although the flexion of the fingers that commonly occurs as a result of the thickening and tightening of the skin can sometimes be confusing. There is no effective treatment at this time for scleroderma, but the disease progresses very slowly and thus the long-term outlook is not as unfavorable as might be imagined.

Polymyositis and Dermatomyositis

Polymyositis and dermatomyositis are conditions primarily affecting muscles, and weakness rather than severe pain is the predominant feature. The diagnosis can be established by muscle biopsy as well as determination of muscle enzymes in the blood. In the event of the diagnosis of dermatomyositis, a strong search should be instituted for underlying malignancy. It is generally advisable when faced with conditions such as scleroderma or polymyositis that consultation be obtained with guidance from someone who sees a good deal of these conditions, such as a rheumatologist, to help the family physician best manage the patient.

Polymyalgia Rheumatica

The condition frequently best treated by the family physician and that is becoming increasingly recognized is polymyalgia rheumatica and the associated syndrome of giant cell arteritis. This is a disease of older people typically associated with severe muscular pain about the shoulder muscles and less commonly the pelvic girdle muscles without any true limitation of motion due to the involvement of the joints, although joint scintigraphy has frequently detected synovitis in the shoulders. The condition usually has a reasonably abrupt onset and the disease tends to cluster so that if one patient is seen, two or three others may be seen within a 2- or 3-week period. Polymyalgia rheumatica should be suspected in every patient over 60 years of age who suddenly develops muscle pains about the shoulders. The diagnosis is relatively easy and the treatment extremely effective. The single test that makes the diagnosis is the sedimentation rate, which is unusually elevated in patients with polymyalgia rheumatica (PMR). In fact, in any patient over the age of 60 who has pain in the muscles about the vertebrae and has a sedimentation rate of 100 or greater, one should always assume that the diagnosis is either PMR or multiple myeloma, the diagnosis of which is relatively easy with appropriate blood analysis, urine tests, and radiographs. PMR responds dramatically to the use of small (10 mg. a day of prednisone or less) doses of corticosteroids; it is generally not necessary to start with large doses, although that is a popular regimen in some circles. The usual beginning dose is 15 mg. a day of prednisone, and this can rapidly be reduced to approximately 7.5 mg. daily given as a single morning dose. This can slowly be reduced so that over a period of 6 months to 2 years, which is the natural history of most patients with PMR, the dose can eventually be eliminated. The single dread complication of PMR is the development of giant cell arteritis, which is manifested to the patient as temporal arteritis and can lead to partial or total blindness. This is an unusual complication occurring in fewer than 2 per cent of patients, but it must be treated immediately with large doses of corticosteroids (60 mg. of prednisone a day) and urgent ophthalmologic consultation. The examination of the temporal arteries should always be instituted; involvement consists of tenderness, thickening, and swelling of these arteries. The arteries themselves have very little function, and if one is suspicious of temporal arteritis, a biopsy of 2 cm. or so of the artery is indicated. The importance, of course, is that it is an indicator of what is going on behind the eye, and treatment can be instituted on the basis of the relatively benign procedure of temporal artery biopsy. Most patients with polymyalgia rheumatica will never need to see any physician beyond the family physician and treatment is enormously effective. Fibromyalgia has a normal ESR, trigger areas, and, usually, a good deal of tension and anxiety.

Perhaps the single best source book for further information on the rheumatic diseases is the *Primer on Rheumatic Diseases* currently in its 9th edition and available from the Arthritis Foundation. There are also many textbooks written for the family physician, but the *Primer* is one of the best and least expensive sources for the guidance of the treating doctor. Table 50–2 includes the addresses and phone numbers of the Arthritis Foundation and its chapters, and the family physician would do well to obtain not only the *Primer* but a copy of each of the small monographs put out by the Arthritis Foundation for the guidance of patients since they contain a good deal of important material and it is always wise for the doctor to know at least as much as the patient!

51

Dermatology

Shelley Roaten, Jr.
Walker A. Lea, Jr.

Evaluation of Skin Lesions

HISTORY AND EXAMINATION

Patients often begin the visit by pointing out their skin lesions, tempting the physician to omit the history in favor of examination. Unfortunately, the current lesions are like a single frame from a movie and may make little sense in the absence of a history. Some clinicians find it helpful to consciously follow the sequence of cursory examination, history, and detailed skin examination, a simple plan that satisfies the urge to look, while avoiding omission of important data.

The complaints of a dermatologic patient are rather limited; he or she itches, has a rash, or may occasionally have pain. Our task is to discover the temporal characteristics, precipitating or palliative factors, and related personal or family history. Most of this information is obtained with a few simple questions:

- How long has the rash or itching been present?
- How has the appearance changed?
- Is it constant or recurrent?
- Are there factors that seem to make it better or worse?
- Has a similar problem occurred in a family member?
- Has it been treated at home or by another physician?
- Are any drugs being taken, either prescription or nonprescription?

If not already known, questions regarding the patient's age, occupation, habits, and physiologic state (menses, pregnancy) may also be indicated. The history or examination may lead to specific additional questions, but generally the history obtained with these few questions is complete. Most errors occur by omission of the general drug history and the previous treatment of the skin condition.

We should not, of course, allow the ease of the dermatologic history to divert our attention from the patient as a whole. In the first place, the complaint may be only a means of entry into the office, with a more important agenda awaiting discovery. Secondly, the skin may be one of several organs affected by an underlying disease or condition. Either of these situations indicate the need for a more general medical history.

Although there are many reasonable exceptions for dermatoses of limited distribution, the most thorough skin examination is accomplished with the patient disrobed and then covered with appropriate gown or drapes. The examiner must seek both specific individual lesions and an overview of patterns and distribution. Visual inspection and palpation are the most important methods. The individual lesions sought are traditionally referred to as *primary* and *secondary*. Although they are not well standardized, these descriptive categories of lesions facilitate our ability to diagnose and to communicate our findings to other physicians.

Primary Lesions

Primary lesions (Fig. 51–1) are defined as those arising de novo in the skin, without an antecedent visible lesion. *Macules* and *patches* are flat areas of skin that differ in color from the surrounding skin; patches are larger areas. *Papules, nodules*, and *tumors* are solid elevated lesions of respectively larger sizes, and *plaques* are only slightly elevated relative to their large surface area. *Vesicles, bullae*, and *pustules* are

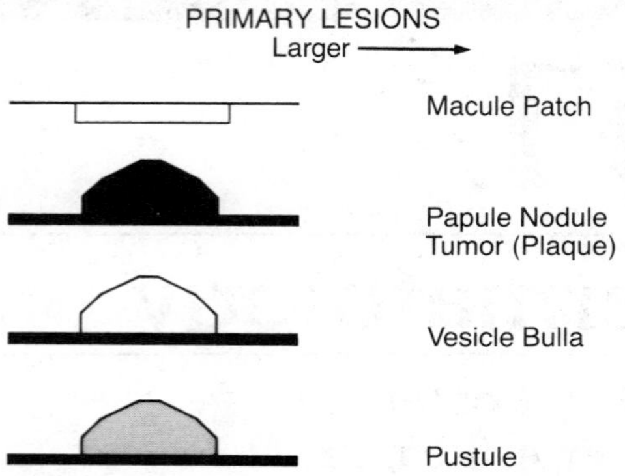

Figure 51–1. Morphology of lesions.

raised, fluid-filled lesions that differ in size and fluid composition. *Wheals* are elevated lesions that are edematous and transitory. *Petechiae* and *purpura* are circumscribed deposits of blood or blood pigments, the latter-mentioned lesion being larger.

Some authorities also recognize a subcategory of special primary lesions that are particularly characteristic of a few diseases. Acne, for example, is easily recognized by its open and closed *comedones*. Typical *burrows* help identify scabies and cutaneous larva migrans. A discrete, globular, *umbilicated papule* is virtually diagnostic of molluscum contagiosum.

Secondary Lesions

Secondary lesions evolve from a preceding visible lesion. *Scales* and *crusts* are actually superficial to the skin; the former are flakes composed of aggregates of shedding epidermal cells, and the latter are masses that result from the drying of exudates. *Excavations* of the skin are areas where superficial skin layers are interrupted, including *ulcers, fissures*, and *excoriations*.

Lichenification is an area of skin that is thickened with increased prominence of skin lines indicating connective tissue repair. If scars are hypertrophic, they are called *keloids*. *Atrophy* of the epidermis or dermis may produce several appearances, most often areas depressed below the level of surrounding skin.

Often, primary and secondary lesions are intermingled on the skin of a single patient, requiring "selective vision" or attention to each type of lesion. Each patient may have all the lesions that occur during the natural evolution of his or her disease, for which the history can establish the appropriate sequence of events.

Arrangement and Distribution of Lesions

Attention is then refocused to determine arrangement and distribution of the lesions. Helpful groupings or arrangements include the following examples:

linear:	contact dermatitis; occasionally psoriasis, lichen planus, vitiligo, and some nevi
annular:	erythema multiforme (iris lesions), pityriasis rosea, superficial fungi, and, occasionally, mycosis fungoides
grouped:	herpesvirus, plantar warts, urticaria

The distribution of the lesions, or groups of lesions, may also be an important diagnostic observation. With some risk of oversimplification, skin diseases may be described as localized, regional, or generalized. In most cases, the reason for a given distribution is unknown, but these examples point out how some factors influence the sites of predilection:

Sunlight exposure:	Photosensitive reactions in sun-exposed areas
Contact:	Contact dermatitis in areas exposed to jewelry, perfumes, skin cleaners, and so on
Local minor trauma:	Vitiligo, psoriasis
Warm, moist areas:	*Candida albicans*
Dermatomal involvement:	Varicella/zoster virus
Bilateral symmetrical:	Suggests "endogenous" causes, such as allergy, drug hypersensitivity, virus infection, and so on

Just as a knowledgeable botanist might identify a geographical area from a description of its forest and trees, the observant physician can often identify a rash from an accurate description of its lesions and their distribution. It is important to remember that only differential diagnoses may be possible at the initial visit, which are then clarified by later visits. Physicians must also accept an occasional condition that resolves spontaneously without an accurate label or treatment.

Effects of Lighting on Examination

Some of the dilemmas in diagnosis are resolved with the use of appropriate diagnostic procedures. One of the simplest manipulations available is changing the lighting for examination. Using natural sunlight may accent distinctive hues, side-lighting confirms elevation, subdued lighting may increase contrast of pigmented lesions, and ultraviolet light causes some lesions to fluoresce.

The use of filtered ultraviolet light from an inexpensive Wood's lamp in a darkened room aids in presumptive diagnosis of certain conditions. It is most often used for confirmation of the dermatophytoses, superficial fungus infections of the skin and its appendages. Hairs infected with *Microsporum audouini* or *M. canis* fluoresce brilliant green, aiding in the confirmation of scalp ringworm. Since other scalp fungi do not fluoresce (especially *Trichophyton* species), the absence of fluorescence does not rule out tinea capitis and microscopic examination of the hairs is indicated. Upon exposure to Wood's light, the lesions of tinea versicolor exhibit a dull brown color. If the ova of pediculosis capitis are difficult to locate, their grayish fluorescence can be helpful in diagnosis.

Microscopic Examinations

Microscopic examinations are also most often used to support the diagnosis of common dermatophytes. Scale, hair, vesicles, and nail scrapings can be examined by this method. Slide preparation time limits usefulness in a busy office, but knowledge of the techniques is valuable for unusual lesions; other patients can be examined while slides macerate for the appropriate period of time.

Specimens from scaly lesions or from fingernails are most easily obtained by scraping the material onto the center of a microscope slide. A vesicle roof can be removed with a scalpel, whereas hairs are removed by plucking them with tweezers or similar instrument. A drop or two of 10 to 20 per cent potassium hydroxide and a coverslip are added, and light pressure is applied to the coverslip to "flatten" the scales. Gentle heating of the slide hastens maceration. Scales and hair are generally readable within 10 to 15 minutes, but nail scrapings may take several hours. Solutions of potassium hydroxide with dimethyl sulfoxide are available and greatly reduce maceration time. Microscopic examination reveals characteristic spores and hyphae or budding yeast forms. The key maneuver is moving the microscope condenser up and down under a likely-looking fragment until the light causes maximum contrast between fungus and its surroundings. Usually, the low-power objective is the best choice for detection, with the medium-power objective used for confirmation.

Sometimes the examiner finds a lesion that "looks fungal," but the potassium hydroxide preparation appears to be negative. For superficial fungi, no harm will result if the examination is repeated after the patient applies 1 per cent hydrocortisone cream to the lesion for 1 week. This maneuver is particularly helpful if lesions have been partially treated prior to the first examination; hyphae will be more evident at the next visit.

Examination of smears prepared with Gram's stain is occasionally indicated to distinguish bacterial and fungal skin infections or to establish tentative identity of a bacterium. Staining is also helpful to confirm herpesvirus. For that purpose, the base of a vesicle is scraped with a scalpel and the material is placed on a slide and stained with Wright's or Giemsa's stain (referred to as a Tzanck preparation). Multinucleate giant cells are characteristic of herpes infection.

Microscopic examination can sometimes confirm a resistant or atypical case of scabies, by scraping the mite onto a slide with mineral oil or microscope immersion oil. Admittedly, the examination is almost superfluous if the burrow is typical.

Biopsy

Biopsy is most often indicated for lesions that may be malignant (exhibiting a change in color or growth) and for chronic lesions in which the diagnosis is imprecise or unknown.

Immunofluorescent techniques are valuable for identification of bullous disease and suspected lupus erythematosus. The most popular methods for obtaining tissue are excisional biopsy, shave biopsy, and punch biopsy, all of which can ordinarily be accomplished with simple local anesthesia.

Excisional biopsy is indicated for the best cosmetic result and when removal of the entire lesion is desired. Full-thickness excisional biopsy also is necessary for the most accurate histologic diagnosis. Shave biopsy easily removes small elevated lesions and the bleeding is stopped with light electrocautery. Shaving is quick and simple, and is useful in areas where the cosmetic result is not too important. Punch biopsy also yields excellent tissue specimens quite easily. Both reusable and disposable punches are available. The punch instrument is rotated into the skin to the desired depth, the cylinder of skin excised, and the bleeding stopped with pressure, sutures, or Monsel's solution (ferrous subsulfate). A specimen obtained by any of these biopsy methods should be placed immediately in a labeled specimen container with formalin or another suitable preservative.

If excisional biopsy is indicated, an ellipse of skin is ordinarily removed. For best closure, the length of the ellipse should be at least 2.5 to 3 times its width. The long axis is oriented parallel to natural skin lines, so that a less noticeable scar results (see Figs. 42–1 and 42–2, Ch. 42). Punch biopsy can also result in a small ellipse, if the skin is stretched *perpendicular* to skin lines while the instrument is being inserted.

Cultures

Practically speaking, bacterial and fungal cultures are neither necessary nor cost effective for the majority of typical skin infections encountered in the family physician's office. For lesions that are uncommon, clinically atypical, or fail to respond to standard therapy, accurate identification of the organism is indicated. Initial cultures for bacteria are usually performed on blood agar or a reliable transport medium, and suspected fungal organisms are inoculated in Sabouraud's agar or similar media.

Other Diagnostic Tests

Obviously, a wide variety of blood or radiologic examinations are appropriate when skin disease is potentially related to abnormalities of other organ systems, such as for cutaneous lupus, sarcoidosis, or suspected secondary syphilis. Cytologic imprints, viral cultures, and cell cultures are helpful in some special situations.

General Management

HYDRATION

Probably the oldest rule of dermatology is "if it's wet, dry it, and if it's dry, wet it." Wet dressings and soaks paradoxically cause drying of the skin by their application and, therefore, are considered useful for moist, weeping, or encrusted lesions. Although water is probably the active ingredient, a mild astringent or antibacterial agent is often included to perform those respective additional functions. Useful astringents include *Burow's solution* (one Domeboro tablet per pint of water) and weak solutions of white *vinegar* (an ounce or two per pint of water), applied as dressings or soaks several times daily. Two per cent hydrogen peroxide may be used if there is an infection present. Powders might seem to be useful for their drying effect, but they have disadvantages. Talc, for example, serves fairly well as a dry lubricant but is totally nonabsorbent. Starch absorbs moisture well, but tends to aggregate into irritating clumps and can serve as a nutrient for bacteria and yeast.

The moistening of dry, scaling lesions is usually accomplished through the occlusive effect of ointments or pastes, which increase relative hydration of the skin by reducing water loss. If the area is soaked in water for a few minutes immediately before application, considerable moisture is retained. Frequently used preparations are *zinc oxide ointment* and plain white *petrolatum*.

MANAGEMENT OF ITCHING

Itching alone or in association with various visible lesions often responds to nonspecific antipruritic measures. Orally administered antihistamines can be given two to four times daily, using a slightly larger dose at bedtime to promote sleep. *Diphenhydramine* (Benadryl) is safe and reliable; some authorities prefer *hydroxyzine* (Atarax, Vistaril) for the itching associated with urticaria and similar lesions of presumed allergic etiology. Newer antihistamines such as terfenadine (Seldane) offer reduced sedation. Several proprietary topical preparations containing camphor and phenol are useful for relief of itching confined to small areas. Calamine lotion is popular and safe, but many physicians avoid Caladryl because of the risk of sensitization to the additional antihistamine. If the itching is more widespread, some patients obtain temporary relief from cool or tepid baths without soap. Others find the addition of Aveeno colloidal oatmeal to the bath water very soothing, suggest the addition of one cup to the water, and caution patients or their parents that the tub becomes slippery.

The itching associated with dry skin (xerosis) deserves special emphasis because it is so common. It is easily the most common cause of itching seen in a primary care office and must be considered before a complicated work-up is begun for the differential diagnosis of itching. Xerosis responds to simple hydration and to the avoidance of various factors that result in dehydration of the skin. In particular, patients should use mild soaps (Ivory, Dove, Basis) sparingly, and should avoid excessively hot water. For some reason, a few people try to treat itching with alcohol rubdowns, which actually exacerbates the problem of dry skin by removing protective lipids.

Pruritus ani, itching of perianal skin, is probably just a puzzling symptom rather than a distinct clinical or pathologic entity. No lesion is customarily seen, but there may be localized chronic lichenification, redness, edema, or fissures. There is no clear etiology, but there are associations with emotional stress, diabetes mellitus, and other conditions. The most important task is to discover and treat any of the specific diseases that are accompanied by perianal itching, such as pinworms, fungal infections, contact dermatitis, colitis, and Hodgkin's disease. If no cause can be found, local application of nonhalogenated topical steroid cream or lotion will help control the itching.

AVOIDANCE OF CAUSATIVE AGENTS

Perhaps because the principle seems obvious, physicians may spend too little time explaining the avoidance of causative factors or suspected causes. Allergic contact dermatitis is a particularly good example, and its cause should be discussed with the patient. Appropriate avoidance may follow easily from identification of the allergen, or may require more complicated general advice about clothing, gloves, jewelry, cosmetics, and other environmental factors. It may be necessary to sequentially eliminate possible causes.

Skin lesions associated with the ingestion of medications often pose a greater problem. Should the offending drug be discontinued, continued with close observation, or exchanged for another drug of similar purpose? These questions usually yield to common sense, with the answer derived from the importance of the drug relative to the severity of the skin reaction. Although the skin reactions and drugs are too numerous for discussion here, the authors must point out that any drug should be suspected when its ingestion precedes a rash.

CORTICOSTEROIDS

Dermatoses generally responsive to topical corticosteroids are:

1. Eczema (contact and irritant dermatitis, neu-

rodermatitis, atopic dermatitis, some photosensitivity reactions)

2. Psoriasis
3. Seborrheic dermatitis
4. Types of pruritus ani, especially in association with psoriasis

A few other dermatoses that respond less predictably include lichen planus, granuloma annulare, pemphigus, and some lesions that respond to intralesional steroid injections.

These lists are limited, and the clinician's first obligation is to be reasonably certain that he or she is treating a lesion likely to respond. The second step is the selection of the appropriate steroid from a staggering list of commercially prepared alternatives. That selection depends upon relative steroid potency, side effects, vehicle, and cost.

Clinical potency and potential side effects of topical steroids are directly related; no steroid preparation offers greater strength without a parallel increase in the probability of side effects and cost. Systemic side effects are rare, but can occur with widespread application to abnormal skin, especially in children. Local effects include striae, skin atrophy, hypopigmentation, and acneiform eruptions. Both potency and side effects are greater for fluorinated steroids than for nonfluorinated steroids. The correct steroid is the *least* potent one that can reasonably be expected to achieve results. Results can often be predicted from a knowledge of the usual natural history of the disease or from the patient's previous response to steroids used for the condition. As a general rule, no fluorinated steroid should be applied to the face or to the axillary, vaginal, or anal areas; hydrocortisone is a safer alternative.

The vehicle in which the steroid is incorporated affects potency and convenience of application. Vehicles vary in their ability to cause percutaneous absorption; more steroid absorption into the skin means more clinical potency (and more side effects). With some unavoidable oversimplification, vehicles can be ranked in order of their ability to promote absorption as follows, from greatest to least: gels and ointments, creams, lotions, and sprays.

Naturally, the ease of application is represented approximately in reverse order, which probably helps explain why creams are a popular compromise. The rank also suggests, for example, that an inadequate response to a steroid cream might improve with a change to an ointment formulation of the same steroid. Ointments are usually undesirable on the face and in intertriginous areas, but may be useful elsewhere. Gels and lotions are usually most desirable on the scalp.

Apart from the effect of vehicles, steroids vary in their inherent potency *as formulated*. They also differ drastically in cost. The information in Table 51–1 is adapted from the *Medical Letter*, and is intended as a guide to the selection of corticosteroids based on potency groups. The examples were selected as relatively low-cost representative choices in their groups. Note that knowledge of very few alternatives covers the entire spectrum of potency, and that generic preparations are available for most strengths (Table 51–1).

Although Table 51–1 was prepared with attention to low cost, wholesale costs vary substantially. The *Drug Topics Red Book* or a similar source is suggested. Patients should be told that hydrocortisone for topical use is available without a prescription for treatment of relatively mild skin conditions (e.g., Cort-Aid).

The use of occlusive materials, such as plastic wrap, over areas of topical steroid application is a method of dramatically increasing absorption and potency. Disadvantages are the inconvenience and the higher risk of adverse effects. Occlusion may be best tolerated with nighttime use and should be used for only resistant conditions for a few days at a time. Often, the change from a cream to an ointment or gel provides sufficient "occlusion." Although intralesional steroid injections are indicated for some diseases, cautious use is in order due to the atrophy and other complications that may result.

APPLICATION OF MEDICATIONS

As for other medications, writing a prescription for the appropriate amount of a topical medication requires attention to the area of coverage, frequency and expected duration of treatment, and appointment schedule. As a rough rule of thumb, approximately 30 grams of a cream or ointment are required to cover the skin of an average adult. By estimating surface areas in a manner similar to estimating the area of skin burns, one can roughly predict the amount required per application. Coverage of an entire arm, for example, requires about 3 grams (9 to 10 per cent of 30 grams). An expected treatment course of 20 applications over 10 days for one arm would, therefore require, about 60 grams.

The pharmacokinetics of topical application are not well established; it has been empirically determined that application two or three times daily is sufficient for most medicines. Recent evidence suggests that a single application each day may be just as effective for most topical steroids. A good general rule is to attempt to reduce the frequency after a beneficial effect is achieved.

TREATING THE WHOLE PERSON

A methodical scientific approach to the treatment of specific diseases is desirable but not to the extent that we ignore the impact of disease on the patient and his or her social environment. The physical disabilities and the emotional or social consequences of skin diseases vary depending upon the individual and the disease involved. Each patient has his or her own perception of the problem, and to the extent that

Table 51–1. TOPICAL CORTICOSTEROIDS*

Potency Class	Steroid/Strength	Trade Names
Lowest	Hydrocortisone 0.25 to 0.5 per cent	several, non-prescription
	Hydrocortisone 1 per cent	Penecort, Cort-Dome
	Methylprednisolone acetate 1 per cent	Medrol
Low	Desonide 0.05 per cent	DesOwen, Tridesilon
	Fluocinolone acetonide 0.1 per cent	Synalar
	Triamcinolone acetonide 0.025 per cent	Aristocort, Kenalog
Intermediate	Betamethasone valerate 0.1 per cent	Valisone
	Halcinonide 0.025 per cent	Halog
	Triamcinolone acetonide 0.1 per cent	Aristocort, Kenalog
High	Betamethasone diproprionate 0.05 per cent	Diprosone, Alphatrex
	Desoximetasone 0.25 per cent	Topicort
	Triamcinolone acetonide 0.5 per cent	Aristicort, Kenalog
Highest	Betamethasone diproprionate 0.05 per cent	Diprolene
	Clobetasol proprionate 0.05 per cent	Temovate

*Compiled from the Medical Letter.

skin is a "public organ," those around the patient may have reactions that range from curiosity to actual fear. Obviously, skin diseases can impair health, job performance, and relationships with family and friends.

The mere fact that a knowledgeable physician can touch, critically inspect, and discuss the lesions without evidence of avoidance is reassuring to the patient. An important early step is to explore the patient's understanding of his or her disease briefly and to dispel myths associated with such conditions as acne, warts, and leprosy. A perceptive physician not only helps the patient understand the disease and its management but also helps the patient deal with the confusion, anger, frustration, helplessness, and withdrawal that may accompany severe skin disorders. Finally, a positive approach includes methods of reducing the physician's own potential frustration during management of difficult problems.

Specific Skin Lesions and Disorders

ECZEMAS

Contact Dermatitis

Allergic eczematous contact dermatitis is a cutaneous immune response that lends itself to interesting diagnostic exercises and that responds dramatically to appropriate therapy. It is primarily a cell-mediated hypersensitivity but may involve other immune responses. The eruption is characterized by papules, vesicles, excoriation, erythema, and sometimes edema (Fig. 51–2). Especially in its early stages, the rash involves mainly the skin sites contacted by the allergen (hapten). If exposure is chronic, the skin may become lichenified, hyperpigmented or hypopigmented, and erythematous, with only occasional vesicles (Fig. 51–3).

The classical "acute" reactions occur most often following contact with the oleoresins of poison ivy (see Fig. 51–2), poison oak, and poison sumac, after which linear streaks of vesicles are especially characteristic. Contact dermatitis can be caused by numerous natural and synthetic substances such as dyes, metals, cosmetics, bandage materials (Fig. 51–3), and several topical medications. Diagnosis is accomplished by careful assessment of the distribution of lesions and the history of exposure to likely contactants in those areas. Confirmation occasionally requires systematic avoidance of suspected materials.

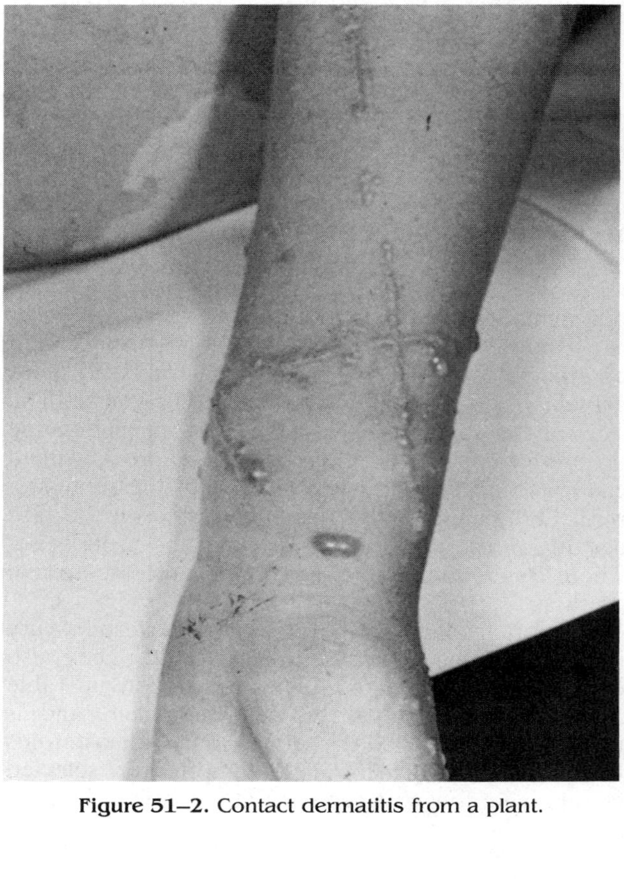

Figure 51–2. Contact dermatitis from a plant.

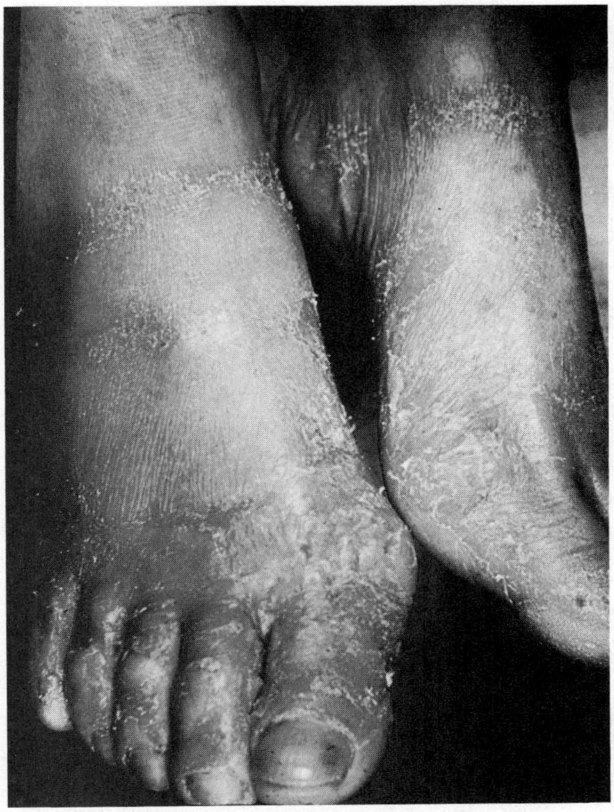

Figure 51–3. Contact dermatitis from shoe dye.

Physicians should be alert to the contact dermatitis that can occur with topical medications. Notable examples are reactions to topical antibiotics, anesthetics, antiseptics, antihistamines, and even corticosteroids. If the original rash being treated fails to respond or changes in character, contact dermatitis should be considered.

Patch tests are occasionally helpful for the diagnosis of a mystifying case, subject to the limitations of examiner experience, cost, and the risk of further sensitization to the testing materials.

Treatment

The treatment of contact dermatitis naturally includes cessation of contact. Victims of poison ivy contact, for example, should learn what the plant looks like and where it grows. The relationship of skin lesions to other contactants should be explained in enough detail so that patients can eliminate contact in the future.

In its early weeping stages, the typical papulovesicular eruption responds to wet dressings or soaks. Patients may also obtain some minimal relief from itching by using oral antihistamines, especially at bedtime. After the weeping subsides, topical steroids are applied at a strength consistent with the estimated severity of the rash. Particularly severe reactions can be treated with a brief course of a steroid, such as prednisone, given orally in the appropriate dosage. A typical regimen for an adult is prednisone 60 mg., administered orally daily in divided doses, then tapered very gradually. Exacerbation may occur if the steroid is discontinued too quickly, and tapering the dosage for two or three weeks is customary. A parenteral steroid such as triamcinolone (Kenalog) can be administered intramuscularly for sustained effect; adult dosage is 40 mg., repeatable once weekly.

Neurodermatitis (Lichen Simplex Chronicus)

The term neurodermatitis can lead to some confusing searches through textbook indices. Some authors use the term neurodermatitis, or disseminated neurodermatitis, in reference to the adult form of atopic dermatitis. Others are referring to circumscribed neurodermatitis, or lichen simplex chronicus, which is the usage intended here.

Lesions of neurodermatitis appear as poorly circumscribed patches of excoriation and lichenification that may be chronic (Fig. 51–4). The lesions are thought to be the skin's response to repeated scratching; because they itch, the lesions are self-perpetuating. The initial event may have been a minor irritant, but chronicity and recurrence are due to scratching. Patients with xerosis often have associated neurodermatitis. Lesions are most often seen in adults on the posterior neck, wrists, ankles, ears, and perianal areas.

Treatment

Effective treatment of neurodermatitis logically includes an explanation to the patient of the probable etiology and a request that scratching be avoided. An Unna boot or similar protective dressing may be useful for lesions on the extremities. In the anal or genital area, hydrocortisone cream is safe and effective; the more potent fluorinated steroids can be used for other areas. It is sometimes clear that the lesions

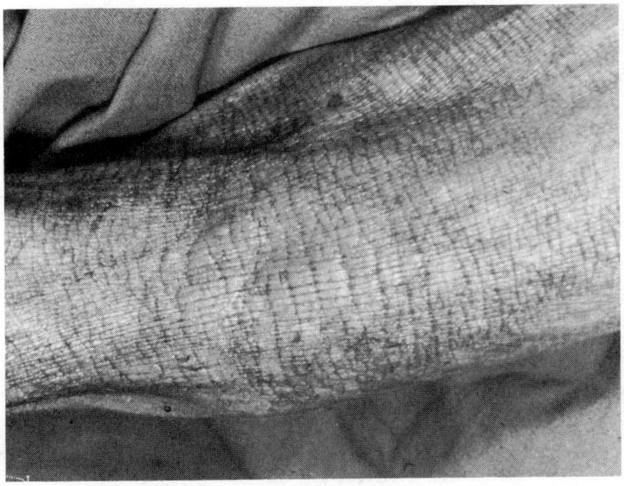

Figure 51–4. Neurodermatitis.

are at least partly related to emotional stress, for which counseling and short-term psychotropic medication might be indicated. Hydroxyzine (Atarax) is a popular choice.

Atopic Dermatitis (Atopic Eczema)

Eczema is a rather vague morphologic term that describes a clinical picture of scaling, serous exudates, excoriation, erythema, and fissures. Atopic dermatitis is often expressed as an eczematous eruption but tends to vary according to the patient's age. Itching is a common feature. In infants, eczematous lesions tend to appear on the face, scalp, and extensor aspects of the extremities. In childhood, papules, erythema, and lichenification tend to predominate on flexor surfaces, wrists, and neck. In adults, flexor surfaces, neck, scalp, and chest frequently have scaly, lichenified, and erythematous lesions (Fig. 51–5). Especially for infants and children, the history often reveals hay fever, asthma, or allergic rhinitis in the patient or a family member.

Treatment

Patients with atopic eczema should use a mild bath soap, such as Dove or Ivory. Treatment consists primarily of symptomatic relief, usually with antihistamines for the itching, and topical corticosteroids. Weeping, moist lesions should be treated first with Burow's or vinegar soak solution. Efforts to discover a particular food, inhalant, or other factor that leads to exacerbations should be attempted, even though success is uncommon. General reduction of common allergens in the household may be helpful, but immunotherapy by desensitization has no proven benefits. Patients with atopic eczema should probably maintain a small amount of low-potency topical steroids in the home medicine cabinet, to initiate therapy for exacerbations. Do not prescribe the more potent steroids on a long-term basis.

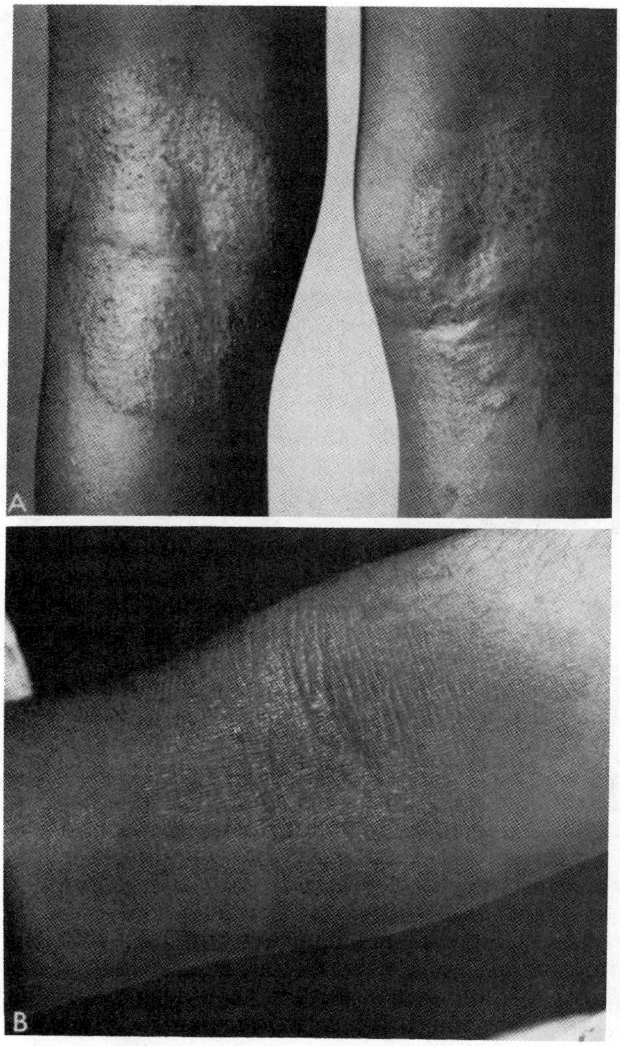

Figure 51–5. *A* and *B*, Atopic dermatitis. (From Larsen, W. G., and Maibach, H. I.: Dermatitis and eczema. *In* Moschella, S. L., and Hurley, H. J. (Eds.): Dermatology. 2nd ed. Philadelphia, W. B. Saunders Company, 1985, p. 337.)

DISEASES OF SWEAT AND SEBACEOUS GLANDS

Acne Vulgaris

Acne vulgaris is a common disease usually seen in adolescents, consisting of a variety of lesions including comedones, papules, pustules, cysts, and subsequent scars. The lesions occur primarily on the face but may involve the upper trunk and shoulders (Fig. 51–6). The condition is self-limited but can last for years and may have significant social consequences for the patient. Diagnosis is usually quite simple, but some thought should be given to acne variants. Acne or similar lesions may occur, for example, with drug ingestions (corticosteroids, iodides, bromides, isoniazid, phenytoin, lithium), occupational exposures (coal tar derivatives, some oils), and possibly some cosmetics and detergents.

Ordinary acne is a multifactorial disease of the sebaceous follicles; its occurrence is probably most dependent upon genetic predisposition and the influence of androgens on the follicles. The most useful pathophysiologic model states that comedones begin with increased sebum production and altered keratinization. Keratinized cells sloughed into the follicular lumen are abnormally adherent to each other, thereby mechanically limiting the extrusion of lumen contents. The bacterial flora of the follicle, principally *Propionibacterium acnes*, cause breakdown of the sebaceous lipids to more inflammatory products, initiating the familiar sequence of papules, pustules, cysts, and scars. Diet, surface dirt, and sexual habits have generally been discredited as etiologic factors.

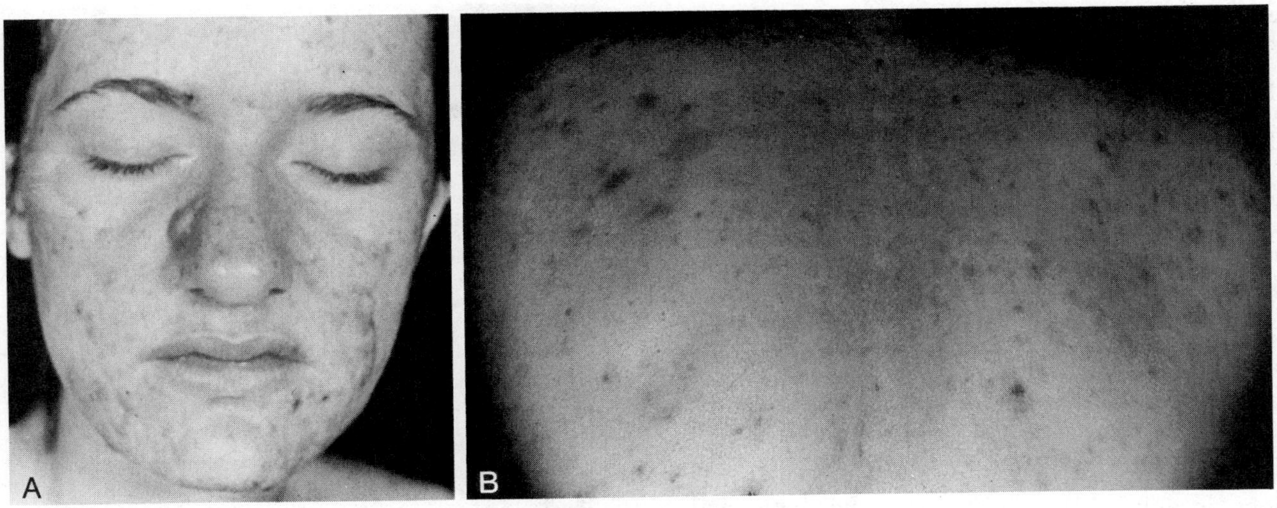

Figure 51–6. Acne vulgaris.

TREATMENT

Rational therapy can be based on the pathophysiologic model described earlier, keeping in mind that many patients with acne get along nicely with no medical therapy at all. Table 51–2 summarizes a reasonable approach.

Retinoic acid (vitamin A acid, Retin-A) is available in a cream (0.05 per cent, 0.1 per cent), a gel (0.025 per cent, 0.01 per cent), and a less desirable liquid form. Its chief action is to reduce adherence of keratinized cells, thereby discouraging comedogenesis, but it also has keratolytic properties. Since skin irritation causes some patients to abandon therapy, it is suggested that application of retinoic acid be started slowly, with a low strength preparation applied once daily.

Significant irritation need not be incurred with retinoic acid for improvement of acne. Many patients tolerate application of a cream or a gel twice daily. Explanation of use should include the following:

1. Improvement will be noticed only after several weeks, and an *exacerbation* of acne may occur during early therapy.
2. The eyes, mouth, and angles of the nose should be avoided during application.
3. Exposure to sunlight should be reduced.
4. Abrasive soaps and cleansers should not be used.

Table 51–2. ACNE THERAPY GUIDE

Lesion/Stage	Therapy
Primarily comedones	Retinoic acid cream or gel
Mildly inflammatory: comedones and papules	Topical antibiotic *or* benzoyl peroxide lotion or gel (sometimes retinoic acid)
Moderately or severely inflammatory: many papules and pustules, some cysts	Benzoyl peroxide *and* oral or topical antibiotic (sometimes retinoic acid). Referral of treatment failures
Conglobate abscesses, severe scarring	Referral

Benzoyl peroxide is available in several strengths of cream, gel, or lotion. It acts primarily as an antibacterial agent to reduce the population of *Propionibacterium acnes*, and it has a keratolytic effect. As for retinoic acid, the therapeutic response and the potential skin irritation can be modified by the choice of formula and frequency of application. Application usually begins once daily, and some patients tolerate twice daily use. If irritation can be avoided, combined therapy with retinoic acid and benzoyl peroxide is rational, provided that they are applied at different times of the day. The precautions about irritation, abrasive soaps, and avoidance of mucous membranes are similar to those for retinoic acid.

Some antibiotics are also useful in the control of inflammatory acne. Tetracycline is the one most often administered orally, with minocycline (Minocin) a popular choice for resistant cases. Tetracycline should not be prescribed for children or for pregnant women because of its staining effect on developing teeth.

Topical antibiotics are also gaining popularity in acne therapy, including tetracycline (Topicycline), erythromycin (T-Stat, EryDerm), and clindamycin (Cleocin T) preparations. Erythromycin and clindamycin are probably most desirable; tetracycline may cause yellow staining.

Routine acne is an inappropriate indication for estrogen therapy. Patients who are already taking an oral contraceptive pill for another indication will often have improvement of acne with a more estrogenic pill, but that approach incurs the risk of other side effects due to estrogen. The potential benefits and risks must be weighed carefully.

Cis-retinoic acid (isotretinoin, Accutane) can be given orally for severe cystic acne; it has serious potential side effects and should be prescribed only by those who are experienced with its use.

Rosacea

Rosacea is a chronic condition of insidious onset that affects the facial skin of adults, particularly around the nose. It becomes manifest by hyperemia and telangiectases (Fig. 51–7), sometimes with papules, pustules, or nodules. Rosacea occurs most often between the ages of 30 and 50 years; women are affected more frequently, but men typically have the more severe cases. It may ultimately lead to rhinophyma (Fig. 51–8), a hyperplasia of the nasal soft tissues with enlargement and deformity. The red-nosed appearance, reminiscent of W. C. Fields, is a significant cosmetic and social problem.

The etiology of rosacea is unknown but probably is related to dysfunction of the sebaceous glands. Seborrheic dermatitis is commonly coexistent. Associations are also known to exist with some ocular lesions, including blepharitis and conjunctivitis, and with migraine headache. In addition to the cosmetic consequences, patients may also be stigmatized by the presumed relationship of "rum nose" to alcohol consumption and dietary indiscretions. No causative relationships have been established, and the disease occurs in nondrinkers.

The differential diagnosis includes seborrheic dermatitis, acne vulgaris, cutaneous tuberculosis, halogen acne, and eczema. Inappropriate use of fluorinated topical steroids on the area can also lead to a similar appearance; questions about steroids must be a part of the initial history.

TREATMENT

Treatment of the acne-like component of the condition is similar to that for acne vulgaris. Tetracycline is reported to control the acneiform lesions as well as to reduce the hyperemia or erythema by unknown mechanisms. Other treatments include electrodesiccation of the telangiectases and surgical repair of the nasal hyperplasia. It also seems logical to avoid stimuli that may increase the cutaneous vasodilation, such as heat, cold, excessive sunlight, alcohol, highly seasoned foods, and avoidable emotional stress.

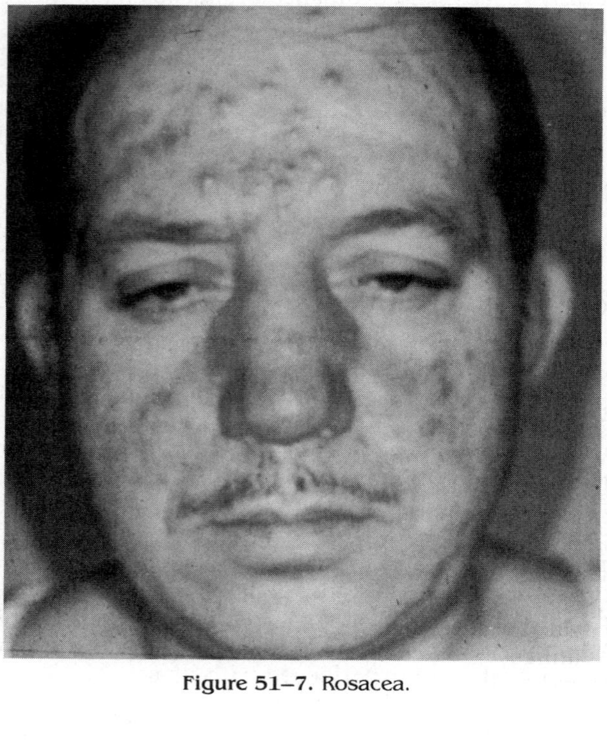

Figure 51–7. Rosacea.

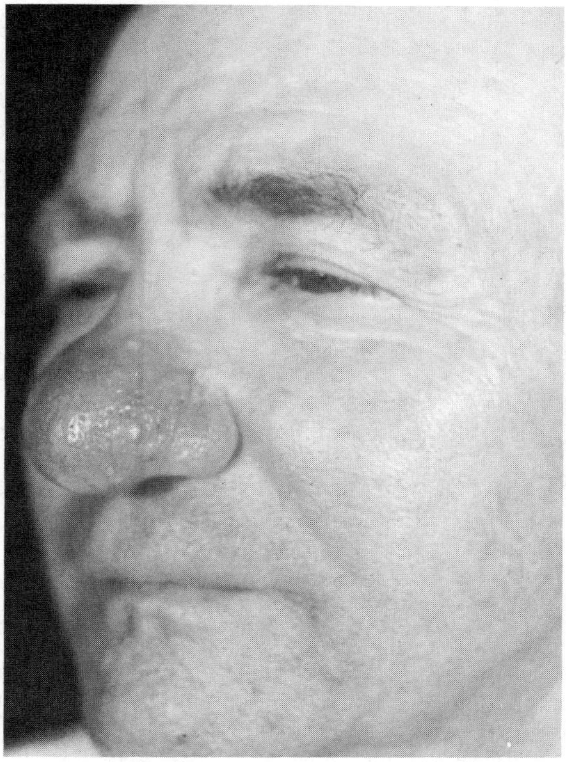

Figure 51–8. Rosacea.

Seborrheic Dermatitis

Seborrhea and seborrheic dermatitis are the major clinical expressions of an ill-defined disorder of the sebaceous glands. The conditions are typically chronic or intermittent, and all ages are affected. In infants, it appears as "cradle cap," diaper-area dermatitis, and sometimes as a generalized erythematous eruption. Adults may suffer only from occasional dandruff or may have associated scaly, red skin lesions in hairy areas of the body. Typical locations are around the ears and eyebrows, in the nasolabial folds (Fig. 51–9), along the sternum, and near the pubis. The distribution is bilaterally symmetrical. Individually, the lesions are poorly circumscribed patches of erythema with yellowish, greasy-looking scales. Facial seborrheic dermatitis is the most common cause of a "butterfly rash," and should be considered before systemic lupus erythematosus.

TREATMENT

Seborrhea of the scalp (dandruff) usually responds to selenium sulfide (Selsun) or tar shampoos

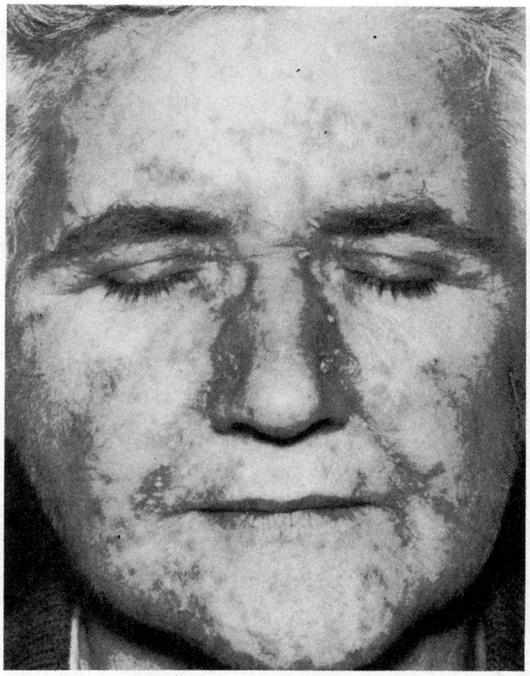

Figure 51–9. Seborrheic dermatitis. (From Fitzpatrick, T. B., et al. [Eds.]: Dermatology in General Practice. 3rd ed. New York, McGraw-Hill, 1987, p. 980.)

(e.g., Pentrax) used two or three times weekly. Daily use may sometimes be necessary at the beginning of therapy. Severe cases will benefit from an occasional application of hydrocortisone, Kenalog, or Valisone lotion to the scalp. Patience and regular use of standard baby shampoos usually suffice for cradle cap.

Seborrheic skin lesions in adults respond to topical steroids applied sparingly to the affected area. Hydrocortisone is often effective and is probably the only reasonable choice for facial lesions but may require application several times daily.

The infantile forms of seborrhea are usually self-limited and, therefore, best "treated" with nonmedical measures such as dry diapers and clean skin. In severe cases, short-term application of hydrocortisone produces a dramatic response. In infants, seborrheic dermatitis can be confused with atopic eczema or with early manifestations of Letterer-Siwe disease.

Miliaria (Heat Rash)

Miliaria is a common skin condition in infants, and almost half of adults retain the tendency. It results from obstruction of the sweat pores, rupture of the duct wall, and retention of sweat within the skin. Recognized subtypes are called crystallina, rubra, and profunda when sweat retention occurs at successively greater depths. Miliaria crystallina is characterized by tiny vesicles on normal looking skin without inflammation, usually in the intertriginous areas. Miliaria rubra is the most common type, often known as "prickly heat," consisting of small erythematous papules with a minute central vesicle. Pustules may develop in chronic cases. Miliaria rubra occurs most often on the trunk and neck and consistently spares the face and volar surfaces. Itching or burning in the affected areas is common. Miliaria profunda produces papular lesions without itching or burning.

Patients are predisposed to miliaria in a hot, humid environment, especially when clothing is occlusive. Infants and the bedridden elderly are most susceptible. Miliaria is the most prevalent form of anhidrosis, since the normal functions of sweat production are lost in the affected areas. Patients with extensive miliaria rubra can suffer hyperpyrexia or heat exhaustion if they remain in the environment.

The only effective treatment is to place the patient in a cooler environment, where the obstructions will gradually resolve over several days. No topical therapy has proven value, and many medications will exacerbate the problem.

Dyshidrosis (Pompholyx, Dyshidrotic Eczematous Dermatitis)

This condition of unknown etiology usually is found in areas of hyperhidrosis. It is probably a simple eczema promoted by the moist conditions. The lesions are small, tense vesicles seen on the palms and soles, lateral surface of digits, and the interdigital spaces (Fig. 51–10). There is itching and sometimes a burning sensation. Secondary bacterial infection may ensue.

The principal conditions to be distinguished from dyshidrosis are fungal infections and contact dermatitis, both of which can produce vesicles in a similar distribution. Some authorities believe that the disease can be a precursor of psoriasis.

Treatment

Management starts with attempts to control the hyperhidrosis or secondary infections, as necessary. Topical steroids are used as for other kinds of eczema.

Hyperhidrosis

To a large extent, the existence of hyperhidrosis is in the eye of the beholder; if the patient perceives excessive sweating, he or she has it. Typical locations for hyperhidrosis are the palms and soles or the axillae, but it may occur almost anywhere on the body and may even be unilateral. The clearest association is with anxiety and stress, exacerbated by hot weather. Areas of excessive perspiration may be observed during the examination (Fig. 51–11). If palms and soles are involved, the skin may appear pink, soft, and waterlogged. Tenderness of the feet may be found.

Causes of secondary hyperhidrosis should be sought during the initial evaluation, especially if the sweating is generalized, the onset is relatively sudden, or anxiety does not seem to be a factor. The primary diseases include hyperthyroidism, hypothalamic disorders, exposure to cholinergic agents, lymphomas, defervescence of fever, hypoglycemia, syncopal episodes, pheochromocytoma, Horner's syndrome, drug withdrawal, tuberculosis, and others.

TREATMENT

The treatment of primary hyperhidrosis requires attention to the underlying anxiety as well as localized therapy for the affected areas. Several options are available for the hands and feet, and different ones for the axillae. No treatment is uniformly successful, but the most popular is topical application of aluminum preparations. For hands, feet, or axillae, use a solution of aluminum chloride in anhydrous ethanol (Xerac A.C., Drysol). The solution is applied to *thoroughly dry* skin at bedtime, and occlusion with plastic wrap increases effectiveness. The frequency of application may be decreased for maintenance after the first few days. Sensible advice about selection of clothing and absorbent socks is also in order.

An additional option for sweating of hands and feet is topical applications of glutaraldehyde solution. A 2 per cent glutaraldehyde solution (Cidex) can be used for the hands. It is applied daily for a week or two, then less often for maintenance. A stronger solution of about 10 per cent is desirable for the feet, which must be prepared by dilution of the 50 per cent solution available commercially. Other alternatives used for hands and feet include systemic anticholinergic agents, topical methenamine, and iontophoresis with anticholinergic agents.

When aluminum compounds are not successful in the axillary areas, other options or adjunctive methods include systemic anticholinergic agents, topical scopolamine hydrobromide, and surgical intervention for the most severe cases.

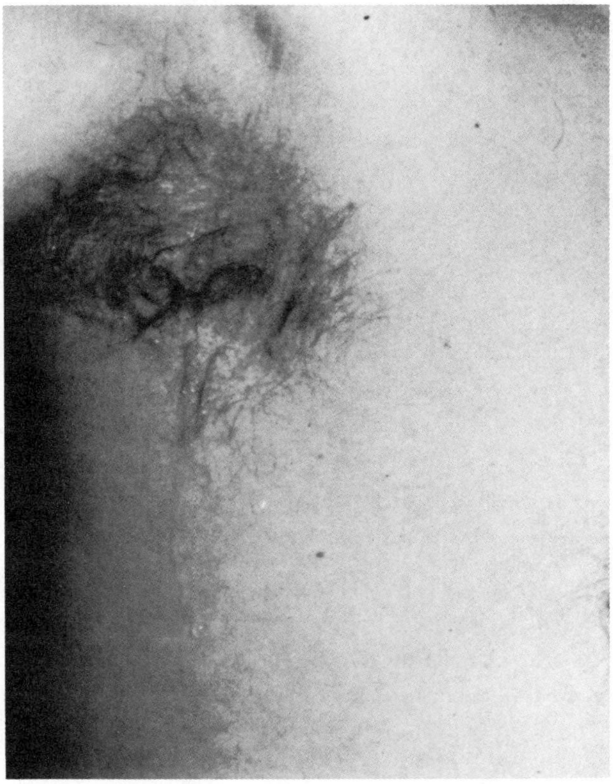

Figure 51–11. Hyperhidrosis. (From Hurley, H. J.: Diseases of the apocrine and eccrine sweat glands. *In* Moschella, S. L., and Hurley, H. J. [Eds.]: Dermatology. 2nd ed. Philadelphia, W. B. Saunders Company, 1985, p. 1346.)

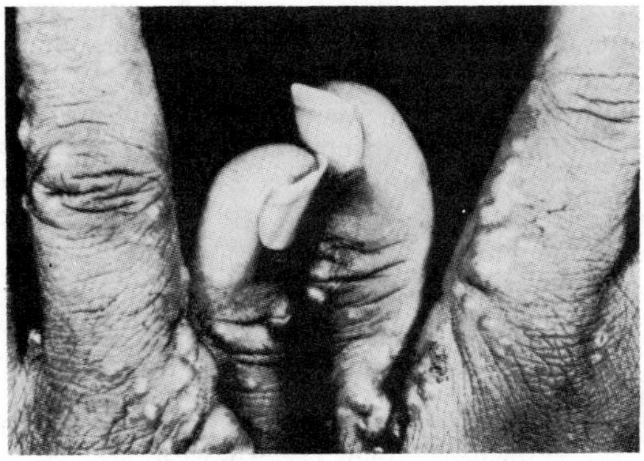

A

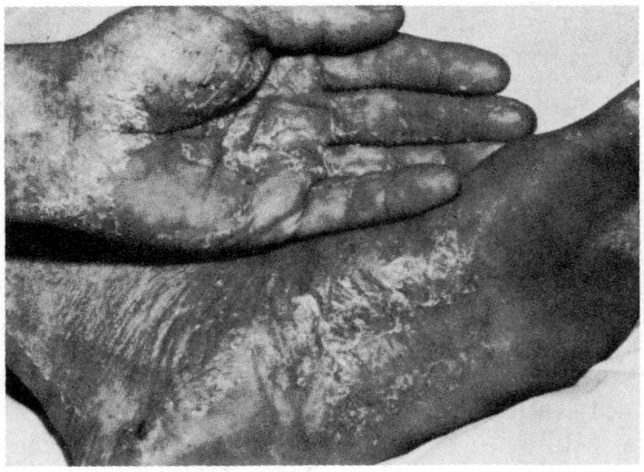

B

Figure 51–10. Dyshidrosis. (From Fitzpatrick, T. B., et al. [Eds.]: Dermatology in General Medicine. 3rd ed. New York, McGraw-Hill, 1987, p. 1371.)

Perioral Dermatitis

Perioral dermatitis is a descriptive term applied to a papular, erythematous eruption around the mouth. It occurs most often in young women but is also occasionally described in men. Some regard the condition as a clinical variant of rosacea or seborrheic dermatitis. Associations have been suggested with oral contraceptives, hormonal factors, and particularly with the use of potent topical steroids on the face. Contact dermatitis (from toothpaste or mouthwash) must also be considered.

TREATMENT

Successful treatments have been reported with oral tetracycline, 250 mg. two to four times daily, and somewhat paradoxically, with 1 per cent hydrocortisone cream. The more potent steroids should not be used.

Hidradenitis Suppurativa

Hidradenitis suppurativa is a chronic disease of the apocrine sweat gland areas, characterized by infection, abscess formation, and scarring. It occurs most often in the axillae but, at times, involves the anogenital area or areolae of the breasts. It results from occlusion of the apocrine duct and bacterial colonization, principally by staphylococci, streptococci, or some gram-negative organisms. There may be an antecedent history of local trauma or irritation, and the condition is commonly associated with obesity.

Clinically, the established condition is seen as recurrent abscess formation with purulent drainage and the formation of sinus tracts and scars. The areas are painful and tender. The incidence is slightly higher in women, and exacerbations may be related to menses. Although the presentation is characteristic, early occurrences may be confused with carbuncles. The differential diagnosis of anogenital lesions includes lymphogranuloma venereum, granuloma inguinale, and ulcerative colitis.

Treatment

Early recognition is important, and systemic antibiotics are the principle method of therapy. Antibiotic selection should be based on culture and sensitivity tests. Incision and drainage of the fluctuant nodules is tempting but promotes the development of sinus tracts. Oral penicillin, erythromycin, or tetracycline is most often indicated, with other antibiotics administered for the less typical organisms. Some clinicians add systemic or intralesional injections of corticosteroids for the more severe cases. Adjunctive therapy includes the use of soothing compresses of Burow's solution and the avoidance of depilatories, commercial deodorants, shaving, and constrictive clothing. Bedtime applications of aluminum chloride in anhydrous ethanol (Xerac A.C.) can be used for its antiperspirant and antibacterial properties. Gentle cleansing of the area with an antibacterial soap is also reasonable (Betadine, Hibiclens). Failure of conservative management requires surgical excision of the areas involved. The uncontrolled disease can lead to limited limb mobility and disseminated infection.

NONFUNGAL INFECTIONS

Impetigo

Impetigo Contagiosa

Impetigo contagiosa is a type of superficial pyoderma with transient vesicular lesions followed by a characteristic "honey-colored," thick crust that appears to sit on normal skin (Fig. 51–12). Bacterial cultures yield mixtures of group A streptococcus and *Staphylococcus aureus*. Typical impetigo occurs mostly in children, especially those of preschool ages, and is highly communicable. Spread to new areas of the body occurs by autoinoculation due to scratching. The peak seasonal incidence is summer, and lesions may occur and spread for weeks if untreated. The main risk for untreated patients is poststreptococcal glomerulonephritis.

Treatment. Appropriate management of impetigo requires the use of antibiotics. Penicillin is the traditional choice; benzathine penicillin may be given intramuscularly, or penicillin V may be given orally four times daily for 10 days. Erythromycin may be used four times daily for 10 days in patients allergic to penicillin. More recently, a topical mupirocin ointment (Bactroban) has been introduced, and should be applied to the lesions three times daily. Increased attention to skin hygiene is indicated, with gentle soap and water cleansing; vigorous scrubbing is unnecessary. Although antibiotics have not been proved to prevent glomerulonephritis in the patient, they do hasten resolution of skin lesions and reduce transmission to contacts.

Bullous Impetigo

Bullous impetigo, in contrast, is caused by group 2 staphylococci in infants and children. It is characterized by rapid evolution of flaccid bullae without surrounding erythema, which rupture and leave a

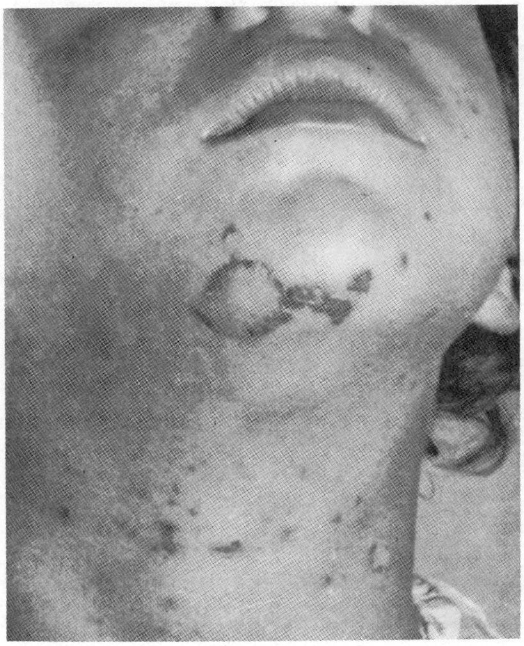

Figure 51–12. Impetigo. (From Marples, R. R., and Leyden, J. J.: Bacterial infections. Section I. Fundamental cutaneous microbiology. *In* Moschella, S. L., and Hurley, H. J. [Eds.]: Dermatology. 2nd ed. Philadelphia, W. B. Saunders Company, 1985, p. 603.)

thin, light brown crust. The scattered, round lesions are thought by some observers to resemble cigarette burns, which must, therefore, be included in the differential diagnosis.

Treatment. Oral penicillin is usually effective, but penicillinase-resistant penicillins, such as dicloxacillin, should be considered if the initial response is not prompt. Other expressions of staphylococcal skin infection include the scalded skin syndrome and scarlatiniform eruptions.

Ecthyma

Ecthyma is very similar to impetigo contagiosa, and is probably best thought of as "deep impetigo." It is caused by group A streptococci, sometimes with *S. aureus*, and may result from poor hygiene or minor trauma. Children and neglected elderly patients are the usual victims, with occurring lesions on the lower extremities, buttocks, hands, or vulva. There is an initial transient vesicle or pustule, followed by a deep ulcer extending into the dermis, covered by an adherent brown or yellowish crust (Fig. 51–13). The lesion is best distinguished clinically from impetigo by a surrounding halo of erythema. Relationships to poststreptococcal glomerulonephritis and autoinoculation are the same as for impetigo.

Treatment. Treatment requires the same antibiotics as those used for impetigo, but they usually are given for a longer time due to the depth or extent of infection.

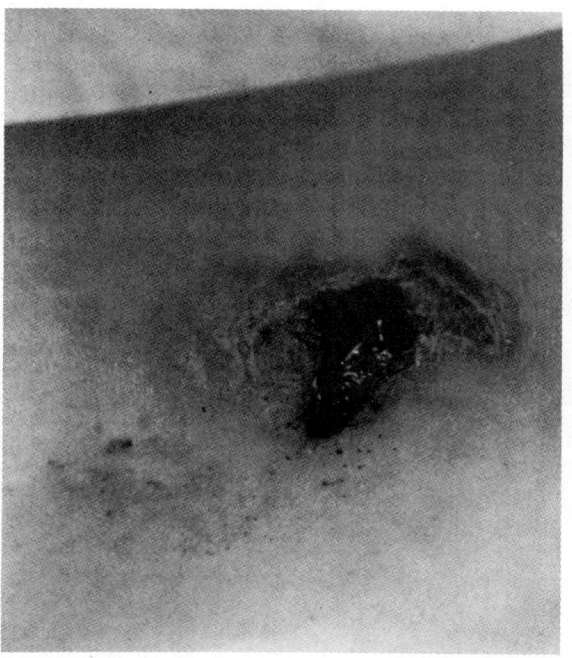

Figure 51–13. Ecthyma. (From Maibach, H. I., Aly, R., and Noble, W.: Bacterial infections. Section II. Bacterial infections of the skin. *In* Moschella, S. L., and Hurley, H. J. [Eds.]: Dermatology. 2nd ed. Philadelphia, W. B. Saunders Company, 1985, p. 617.)

Erysipelas (St. Anthony's Fire, Streptococcal Cellulitis)

Erysipelas is a superficial cellulitis due to group A streptococci, with marked involvement of the lymphatics. It occurs most often in infants, toddlers, and the elderly. The portal of entry for the organism may be a site of minor trauma, but this is seldom recognized at the time of diagnosis. In adults, there is a predilection for the face and head; in infants, the umbilical stump and anterior abdomen may be infected, with rapid progression to bacteremia. In addition to bacteremia, subsequent myocarditis, otitis media, and glomerulonephritis have been described. Patients with nephrotic syndrome are thought to be particularly susceptible to erysipelas.

The infection evolves rapidly, and the patient is generally acutely ill and febrile. The area is brawny red, edematous, tender, and warm, with a distinct slightly elevated margin. There may be vesicles or bullae within the area of redness, and, occasionally, petechiae or ecchymoses. Local desquamation occurs with healing. Significant differential diagnoses include herpes zoster, osteomyelitis of the facial bones, contact dermatitis, and erysipeloid (an infection of seafood handlers).

Treatment. The infection can be self-limited but is also lethal for some patients and thus demands antibiotic therapy, most often with appropriate dosages of penicillin or erythromycin. There is a tendency for the condition to recur in the same area, which can be attributed to damaged lymphatics.

VERRUCAE (WARTS)

Verrucae Vulgaris (Common Warts)

Warts are benign tumors of the skin caused by several DNA viruses of the papova group. The typical common wart is a rounded nodule or tumor with a velvety, vegetative surface. Warts receive several descriptive names, depending on appearance and location.

Wart Types

1. Filiform warts, usually found on the face and the neck, have an exaggerated velvety surface.
2. Flat warts, found on the face, the arms, and the knees, do not have a velvety surface.
3. Common warts, usually found on the hands, appear as described earlier (Fig. 51–14).
4. Anogenital warts (condylomata acuminata), found on the external genitalia or perianal area, have an exaggerated velvety surface (Fig. 51–15).
5. Plantar warts, found on the soles of feet, have a hyperkeratotic surface (Fig. 51–16).

Treatment

A brief explanation is required for the following descriptions of preferred therapy. Generally speak-

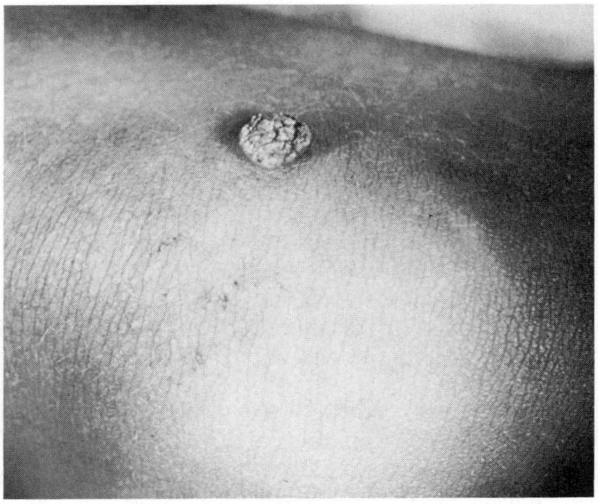

Figure 51–14. Common wart.

ing, wart therapy is based on an attempt to destroy the lesion, for which a variety of methods have been employed. A theory of "immune recognition" has been invoked with some support, but the basic fact is that warts tend to come and go without much explanation, and their disappearance sometimes follows treatment.

Flat warts on the face can be treated with keratolytic agents such as benzoyl peroxide or 2 per cent salicylic acid, with topical 5-fluorouracil or with liquid nitrogen. Filiform warts are probably best treated by excision. Depending upon location, common warts can be treated with liquid nitrogen or carbon dioxide cryotherapy, or a variety of noxious chemicals. Patients may try proprietary medications such as Compound W with some success. Chemicals for office use include trichloracetic acid. Because of the discomfort of freezing, periungual common warts are usually treated by painting lesions with cantharidin or 20 to 50 per cent salicylic acid. Anogenital warts are painted with 20 per cent podophyllin in tincture of benzoin. Because podophyllin can cause severe local and systemic toxicity, it should be applied only to lesions of limited size and number and washed from the skin within 2 to 6 hours. It should not be used for treatment in pregnant women. Never prescribe or dispense podophyllin for use at home. Cryotherapy is a reasonable alternative, and surgical excision or carbon dioxide laser excision are preferred for extensive anogenital lesions. Weekly follow-up is often desirable during wart therapy, especially for anogenital warts. Anoscopy is also advised when perianal warts are seen. Plantar warts may be painful, and their removal difficult. Cautious treatment is necessary, since plantar scars are also painful in some cases. Various combinations of freezing or topical chemotherapy with gentle debridement are indicated. The topical agents include 50 per cent salicylic acid in vaseline, other products with salicylic acid in vaseline, or other products with salicylic acid (e.g., Duofilm).

Molluscum Contagiosum (Water Wart)

Molluscum contagiosum is a viral disease seen most often in children as umbilicated, discrete, flesh-colored papules (Fig. 51–17); most patients have multiple lesions. It can be transmitted sexually and is

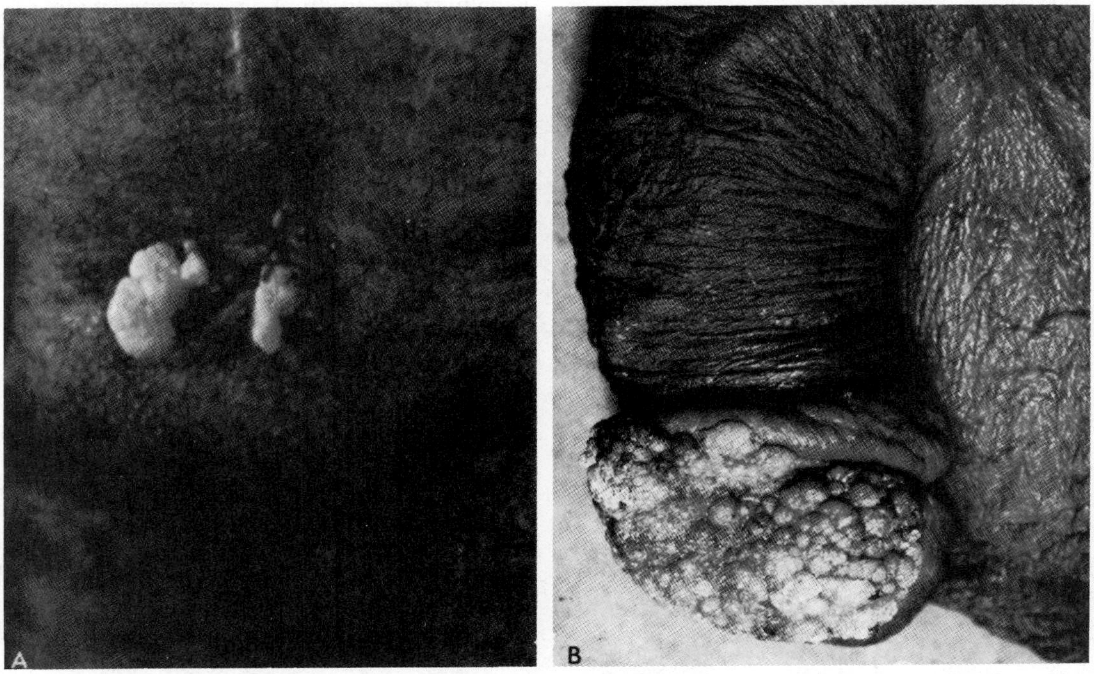

Figure 51–15. *A* and *B*, Anogenital warts. (From Burnett, J. W., and Crutcher, W. A.: Viral and rickettsial infections. *In* Moschella, S. L., and Hurley, H. J. [Eds.]: Dermatology. 2nd ed. Philadelphia, W. B. Saunders Company, 1985, p. 693.)

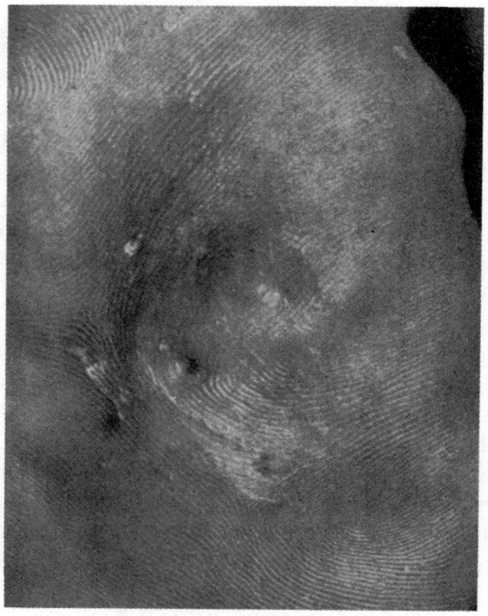

Figure 51–16. Plantar warts. (From Burnett, J. W., and Crutcher, W. A.: Viral and rickettsial infections. *In* Moschella, S. L., and Hurley, H. J. [Eds.]: Dermatology. 2nd ed. Philadelphia, W. B. Saunders Company, 1985, p. 691.)

seen in adults. The papules are dome-shaped with a central depression from which a curd-like material can be expressed. The head, eyelids, trunk, and genitalia are most often affected.

The lesions of molluscum contagiosum must be distinguished from warts, varicella, papillomas, and epitheliomas. If necessary, laboratory studies may be done. Stained smears of the central material show eosinophilic inclusion bodies. Also, biopsy is diagnostic.

TREATMENT

Individual lesions are self-limited, lasting about 2 to 4 months, but autoinoculation occurs and crops of lesions may recur for years. Removal can be accomplished with a sharp curette or liquid nitrogen.

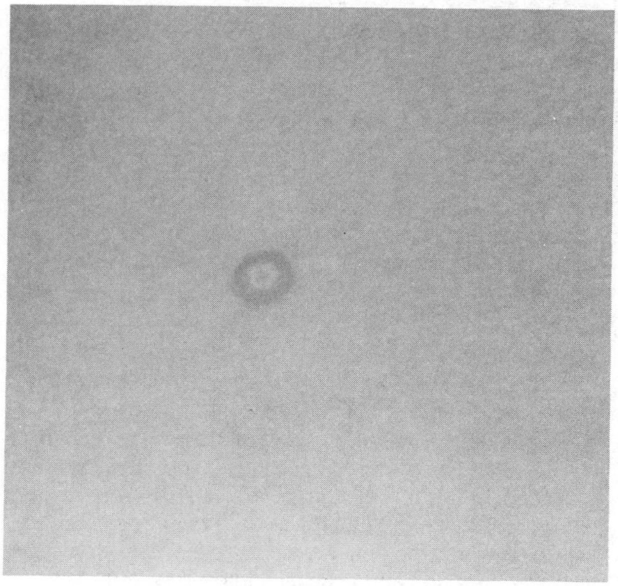

Figure 51–17. Molluscum contagiosum.

HERPES VIRUS INFECTIONS

Herpes Simplex

The herpes simplex virus causes a variety of disorders including lesions of the skin and mucous membranes, keratoconjunctivitis, and encephalitis. Complete discussion of the mucocutaneous lesions alone could fill a book, but some key clinical points deserve emphasis.

There are two types of virus labeled HSV-I and HSV-II. Generally, but not exclusively, type I produces lesions "above the belt," and type II infections are primarily genital. The primary lesion from first infection is more severe than lesions that appear during recurrences. After the primary infection, the virus lies dormant in neural cells until it is reawakened spontaneously or by a precipitating factor. The usual precipitating factors are emotional stress, sunlight, fever, and surgical manipulation of the nerve ganglia. Most transmission occurs through direct mucocutaneous contact.

Clinical syndromes include primary herpes gingivostomatitis, recurrent herpes labialis, and herpetic whitlow.

Primary herpes gingivostomatitis favors children and young adults, especially those aged 1 through 5 years. Manifestations are fever and sore throat, with painful vesicles on the tongue, palate, gingiva, buccal mucosa, or lips. The vesicles tend to be found in clusters, in contrast with aphthous ulcers, which are usually fewer in number and more widely scattered. The vesicles coalesce into plaques covered with a gray exudate. Diagnostic maneuvers may be needed to differentiate herpes from the other causes of sore throat pain. Treatment is symptomatic. Acetaminophen or aspirin can be given for fever and discomfort. Some practitioners use mouth rinses made from extemporaneous blends of acetaminophen syrup, liquid antacids, viscous lidocaine, and Benadryl.

Recurrent herpes labialis (cold sore) occurs at the junction of lip and contiguous skin (Fig. 51–18). About one third of the population of the United States have recurrent cold sores; the factors determining individual susceptibility are unknown. Ulcers found entirely on the oral mucosa are more likely to be aphthous ulcers or erythema multiforme than herpes. Symptomatic remedies are used.

Primary genital herpes erupts as a patch of grouped vesicles, followed by ulcers, 3 to 14 days after contact (Fig. 51–19). Tender inguinal lymph nodes, malaise, and dysuria are common, and aseptic meningitis is seen more often among infected women. Cervical herpes may be seen without external herpetic lesions; features are mucopurulent discharge, friability, and ulceration. Recurrences are more frequent after type II infection; approximately 20 per cent of

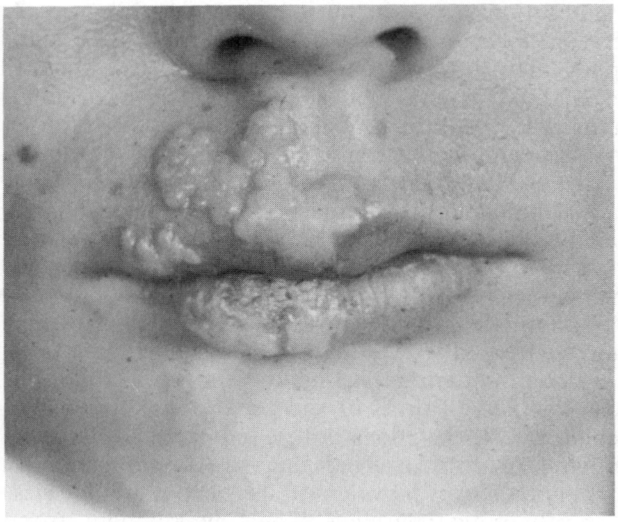

Figure 51–18. Herpes simplex of the lip.

primary infections are due to type I. The differential diagnosis includes syphilis, chancroid, lymphogranuloma venereum, and granuloma inguinale. Recurrences are described as more likely to be painful in women but more frequent in men. Many patients report a prodrome of burning, itching, or dysesthesia. See the discussion of acyclovir, which is given later.

Herpetic whitlow is a primary or recurrent herpes infection of fingers and hands. Those at greatest risk are dentists, physicians, and dental technicians. The infection causes localized vesicles, erythema, edema, and pain, and may last from 2 to 6 weeks. It is essential to differentiate herpetic whitlow from a bacterial infection, and microscopic identification of multinucleated giant cells is helpful (see the section on Tzanck preparation, later).

Other important factors to note in herpes infections include the following:

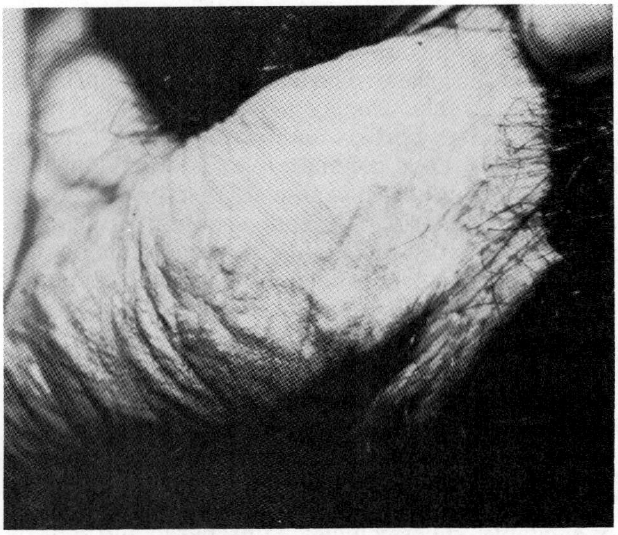

Figure 51–19. Herpes simplex of the penis. (From Fitzpatrick, T. B., et al. [Eds.]: Dermatology in General Medicine. 3rd ed. New York, McGraw-Hill, 1987, p. 2306.)

1. Herpes keratoconjunctivitis is a leading cause of infectious blindness in the United States. The superficial corneal ulcer is characteristic. Ophthalmologic evaluation and early treatment are essential.

2. Eczema herpeticum is widely disseminated herpetic lesions associated with other skin disorders, such as atopic or seborrheic dermatitis.

3. Herpes simplex encephalitis is a highly lethal sporadic disease, which is unrelated to previous herpes infection.

Diagnostic Tests

A Tzanck preparation or a Tzanck smear is a relatively obscure name for a simple technique, the examination of tissue fluid smears for the multinucleated giant cells characteristic of herpes simplex. The smear is prepared in the usual manner from vesicle fluid, with gentle heat fixation and staining with Wright's or Giemsa's stain. Any staining material used for routine blood smears should work.

Treatment

Acyclovir (Zovirax) is the first relatively nontoxic and effective agent for treatment of herpes simplex, but clinical results are still limited. If used for facial or oral lesions, acyclovir has been shown to hasten negative results on viral cultures, but produces no significant change in clinical course or recurrences. The picture is slightly more promising for genital lesions. There is more rapid healing of primary lesions when acyclovir is applied topically, but no change occurs in recurrence rates. Topical acyclovir has very little benefit when used for a recurrent eruption. The long-term use of oral acyclovir to suppress recurrence is investigational. The use of intravenous acyclovir for herpes encephalitis has improved survival, but mortality is still 20 to 30 per cent.

Herpes Zoster (Shingles, Zoster)

The varicella/zoster virus produces a primary infection called varicella (chickenpox) and recurrent skin eruptions called herpes zoster or shingles. Like its cousin herpes simplex, the virus resides in nerve cells until reawakened. The time between the onset of chickenpox and the onset of herpes zoster is ordinarily many years, but primary infection at a very early age is thought to shorten the average time for recurrence.

Chickenpox is characterized by a generalized rash with successive crops of lesions beginning on the face and spreading to the trunk with relatively few lesions on the extremities. Individual lesions progress rapidly from macules and papules to vesicles, pustules, and crusts. Vesicles and shallow ulcers are seen on the oral mucosa. Pruritus is often intense, and older children and adults with the disease may have fever, chills, headache, and other constitutional symptoms.

Herpes zoster (shingles) is a delayed expression of the same virus that originally caused chickenpox, although the original infection may have been quite mild or even unnoticed. The dormant virus resides in sensory nerve ganglia for a variable period of time. Some reversions of the latent virus to an active and infective state are halted by immune responses. When a reversion overcomes the immune reaction, the virus first multiplies within the ganglion, leading to neuritis and neuralgia. Then viral particles are released into skin at the nerve endings, yielding characteristic clusters of vesicles (Fig. 51–20). A syndrome of radicular pain without cutaneous lesions has been reported, when immune mechanisms are able to recover in the middle of the process.

Clinically, patients with herpes zoster experience segmental pain and paresthesia, followed in hours or days by the appearance of grouped vesicles on an erythematous base. The rash is typically unilateral and does not cross the midline, but patients may occasionally have some hematogenous spread resulting in lesions occurring at other locations. Crusting occurs as the vesicles resolve. There is some historical correlation between the site of lesions and the site where the primary eruption was most intense.

Herpes zoster is more common in patients with cancer and other immunosuppressed states, but the converse relationship is not established; i.e., the occurrence of herpes zoster, in itself, does not justify a search for malignancy or immune defects.

The most common complication is persistent pain (postherpetic neuralgia), particularly in older patients. Other complications include localized hypesthesia or anesthesia, secondary bacterial infections, ophthalmic zoster, and disseminated zoster. Immunocompromised hosts are at much greater risk for complications.

TREATMENT

Treatment for most cases of varicella is symptomatic, with more specific treatments reserved for the complications. Aspirin must be avoided because of the association with Reye's syndrome, but acetaminophen may be used for fever. Pruritus will usually respond to cool compresses, calamine lotion, or tepid baths with 1/4 cup of baking soda added. Simple antihistamine medications, given orally, also appear to be safe. Another popular alternative is to give the patient baths with colloidal oatmeal, but make sure that parents or patients know that the bathtub becomes very slippery and potentially dangerous with this method.

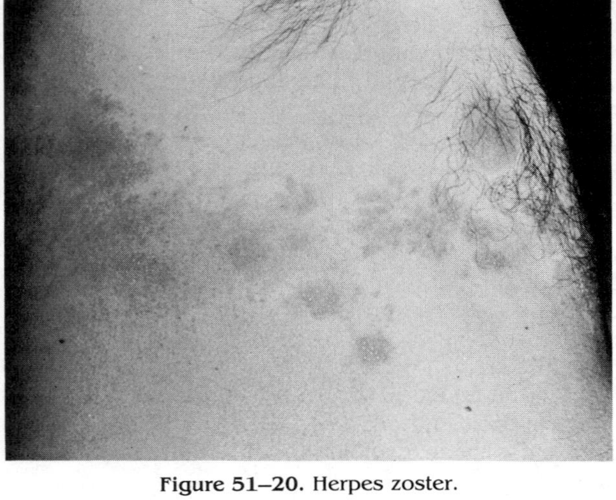

Figure 51–20. Herpes zoster.

Immunocompromised patients with herpes zoster may be treated with antiviral agents, including acyclovir and vidarabine. Immunocompetent patients younger than 50 years of age generally experience a benign course that does not justify the use of either antiviral or corticosteroid therapy. Immunocompetent patients over 50 years of age have a greater risk of postherpetic neuralgia. They may benefit from antiviral therapy, but the merits of this treatment have not yet been established conclusively. Some authorities advocate systemic corticosteroids, for which the benefits are also unproved. When postherpetic neuralgia occurs, it may persist for months and may be difficult to control effectively. Analgesics are fairly helpful, but they must be used with care to avoid habituation or addiction. Tricyclic antidepressants or chlorprothixene (Taractan) in small doses reduce pain for some patients. Sublesional corticosteroid injections, transcutaneous nerve stimulation, and other methods have proponents. An occasional patient with intractable pain is treated with neurosurgery.

SYPHILIS AND OTHER SEXUALLY TRANSMITTED DISEASES

Syphilis

PRIMARY SYPHILIS

Syphilis results from infection with *Treponema pallidum*, a spirochete. The classical lesion of primary infection is the chancre, a single, painless ulcer with raised, indurated borders and a scant serous exudate (Fig. 51–21). Less common presentations include multiple erosions and ulcers, exudative balanitis, and edematous phimosis. There is usually a painless regional adenopathy. Though ordinarily seen on the genitalia, chancres have been found around the anus, mouth, lips, tonsils, tongue, fingers, toes, axillae, umbilicus, eyelids, breasts, and even colostomy sites.

Particularly when there are multiple ulcers, the differential diagnosis includes genital herpes, chancroid, granuloma inguinale, lymphogranuloma venereum, and other causes of balanitis or vulvitis. The diagnosis of primary syphilis is best established by dark-field microscopy. If dark-field examination is not available, slides can also be prepared and sent by mail for direct immunofluorescent examination. Serology (Venereal Disease Research Laboratory test

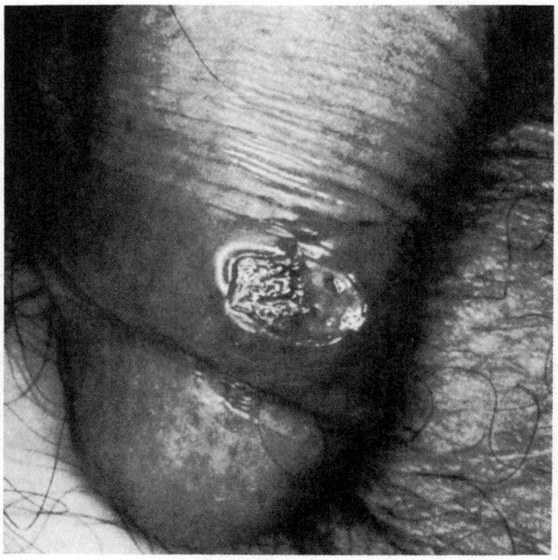

Figure 51–21. Primary syphilis. (From Fuimara, N. J.: The treponematoses. *In* Moschella, S. L., and Hurley, H. J. [Eds.]: Dermatology. 2nd ed. Phildelphia, W. B. Saunders Company, 1985, p. 824.)

or rapid plasma reagin test) may be positive on initial presentation, but conversion may not occur until 2 or 3 months after the chancre appears. With the appropriate risk factors and clinical presentation, a serology test that had negative results must be repeated to exclude syphilis.

Secondary Syphilis

Secondary syphilis develops 2 to 6 months after infection occurs or within 6 to 8 weeks after the chancre is seen. The chancre may still be present when secondary lesions erupt. With the onset of lesions, the Venereal Disease Research Laboratory test or rapid plasma reagin test is reliably positive. The more specific fluorescent treponemal antibody absorption test is then used for verification. The lesions reflect dissemination via blood or lymph circulation, and each of them is loaded with spirochetes.

The rash of secondary syphilis is a great mimic, and may resemble a wide variety of other skin diseases. The classical lesions are papulosquamous, with a predilection for the head, the neck, the palms (Fig. 51–22), and the soles. Most of these lesions do not itch, but itching does not eliminate the possibility of secondary syphilis. Even this characteristic presentation requires differentiation from other common papulosquamous eruptions, including superficial fungi, pityriasis rosea, drug eruptions, and psoriasis. In addition to the typical lesions, secondary syphilis may also produce macules, papules, follicular lesions, pustules, nail changes, nodules, mucous membrane lesions, and "moth-eaten alopecia" of the scalp. There may also be systemic signs or symptoms reflecting involvement of other organ systems, harbingers of the consequences of late syphilis. The multiple complications and delayed consequences of untreated syphilis are beyond the scope of this summary.

Treatment

The treatment of primary or secondary syphilis is two intramuscular injections of 2.4 million units benzathine penicillin, 1 week apart. An alternative regimen is available for aqueous procaine penicillin. Patients sensitive to penicillin may be treated with tetracycline or erythromycin, 500 mg. four times daily for 15 days.

Chancroid

Chancroid is an infectious, autoinoculable disease caused by *Haemophilus ducreyi*, a gram-negative bacillus. It is characterized by a small, soft, round ulcer with an erythematous halo. In contrast to the chancre of syphilis, lesions are usually tender and usually multiple (two to six lesions). Typical locations are genital and perianal. About half of the patients have tender, enlarged regional lymph nodes that may form inguinal abscesses with spontaneous drainage. Confirmation of the clinical diagnosis is aided by stained smears or cultures of exudates, but exclusion of syphilis and other etiologies is essential.

Treatment

Chancroid was formerly treated with tetracycline or sulfonamides prior to the emergence of resistant

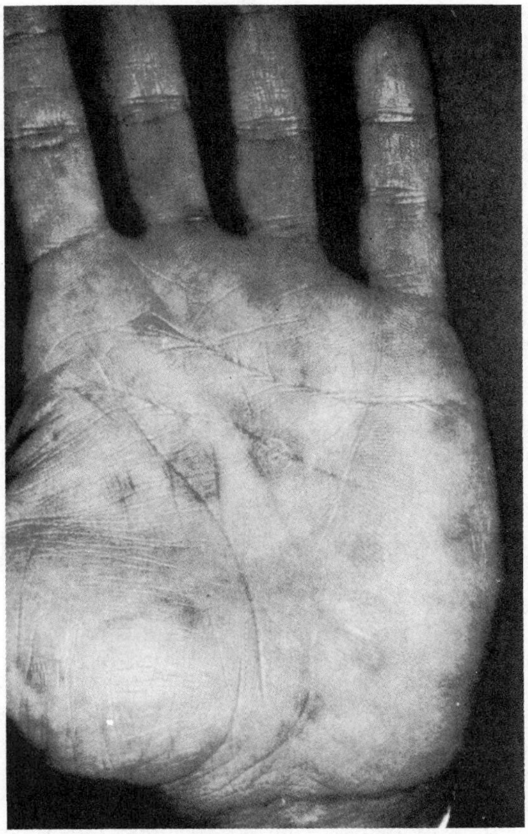

Figure 51–22. Secondary syphilis. (From Fuimara, N. J.: The treponematoses. *In* Moschella, S. L., and Hurley, H. J. [Eds.]: Dermatology. 2nd ed. Philadelphia, W. B. Saunders Company, 1985, p. 828.)

strains. The current recommendations are trimethoprim/sulfamethoxazole, 320/1600 mg. daily, or erythromycin, 2 grams daily, for 1 week. Some effectiveness has been demonstrated for single-dose regimens.

Lymphogranuloma Venereum

Lymphogranuloma venereum is caused by *Chlamydia trachomatis*. The primary lesion is a soft, painless genital ulceration, followed in 1 or 2 weeks by tender inguinal lymph nodes. The nodes tend to coalesce into a fixed inguinal mass and may lead to drainage and chronic sinus formation. Red or purple discoloration of the skin develops over the mass of lymph nodes. The diagnosis is accomplished by a complement-fixation test or by culture.

Treatment

Standard treatment is oral tetracycline, 500 mg. four times daily for 3 weeks; minocycline (Minocin) is an alternative.

Granuloma Inguinale

Granuloma inguinale results from infection by *Calymmatobacterium granulomatis*, a gram-negative rod. The primary lesion may be a papule, subcutaneous nodule, or ulcer on the genitalia or other locations. The subcutaneous nodule may be mistaken for a lymph node, but true adenopathy is rare. A smear prepared with Wright's or Giemsa's stain is examined for characteristic Donovan's bodies, which are the safety pin–shaped dark bacilli in the cytoplasm of macrophages. The infection responds to tetracycline, 500 mg. four times daily for 3 to 4 weeks. Some resistance occurs, and alternative regimens include ampicillin and other choices.

KERATOSES

Keratoses are tumors of the epidermis, of which the two seen most often in the family physician's office are the actinic and seborrheic types. Each of the two types has a distinct prognosis and preferred treatment; neither should be treated by excision.

Seborrheic keratoses are benign lesions of purely cosmetic significance that tend to occur after the 4th decade of life and are unrelated to seborrheic dermatitis. There are often multiple lesions, each one of which starts as a flat tan or brown lesion and grows very slowly to produce a raised, thick superficial brown or black scale. Each keratosis is from 2 mm. to 2 cm. in size, with a surface characterized by tiny pits and furrows (Fig. 51–23). Reassurance may be the only management required, but lesions can be removed easily by electrodesiccation and curettage or with liquid nitrogen cryotherapy.

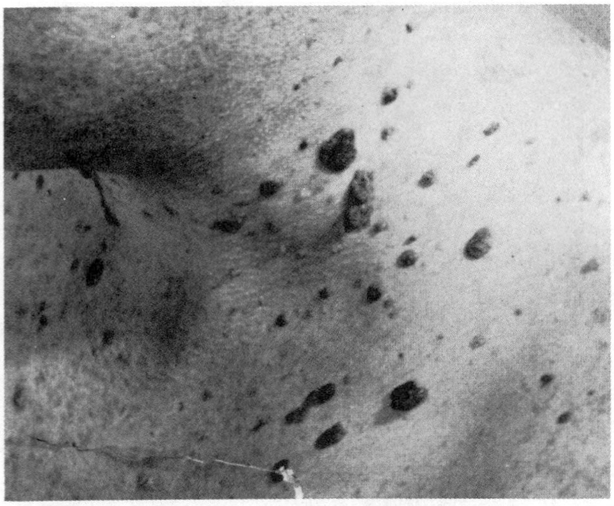

Figure 51–23. Seborrheic keratosis. (From Caro, W. A., and Bronstein, B. R.: Tumors of the skin. *In* Moschella, S. L., and Hurley, H. J. [Eds.]: Dermatology. 2nd ed. Philadelphia, W. B. Saunders Company, 1985, p. 1535.)

Actinic keratoses in contrast, are premalignant lesions related to excessive sunlight exposure. They may be single but are more often multiple, occurring primarily in the same age group as seborrheic keratoses but favoring sun-exposed areas of fair-skinned individuals (Fig. 51–24). Individual lesions of 2 mm. to 1 cm. diameter appear as flat, gray tan, or brown spots, with an adherent scale and mild surrounding erythema. If the scale is scraped away, the lesion usually bleeds. Because of potential transformation to squamous cell carcinoma, the lesions should be treated. If only a few are present, liquid nitrogen application is very effective or electrodesiccation and curettage may be used. A more practical treatment for multiple lesions is topical 5-fluorouracil cream or solution (Efudex). This treatment causes a violent inflammatory response, which must be explained carefully to the patient. Some authorities recommend application to separate areas sequentially or alternative applications of a topical steroid to control the inflammation. For resistant lesions on the back of the hands, some add nightly application of retinoic acid cream to the usual regimen of 5-fluorouracil. Patients

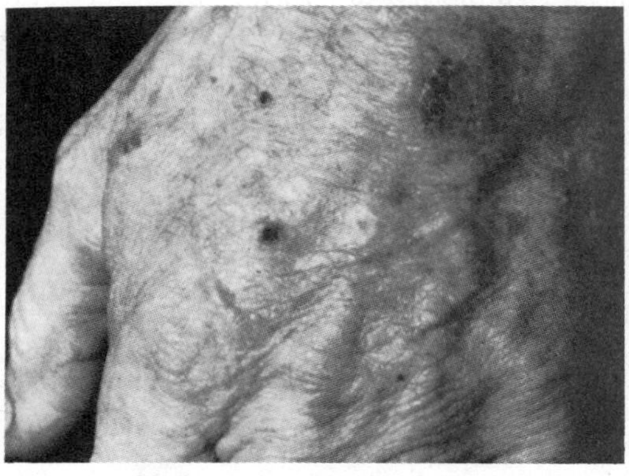

Figure 51–24. Actinic keratosis. (From Caro, W. A., and Bronstein, B. R.: Tumors of the skin. *In* Moschella, S. L., and Hurley, H. J. [Eds.]: Dermatology. 2nd ed. Philadelphia, W. B. Saunders Company, 1985, p. 1547.)

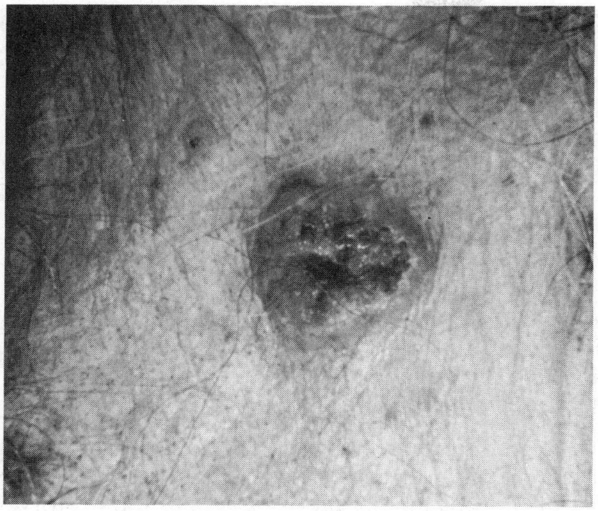

Figure 51–25. Basal cell carcinoma.

with actinic keratoses obviously should limit subsequent exposure to sunlight by avoidance, with appropriate clothing, and with sunscreen preparations.

COMMON MALIGNANCIES

Certain malignancies merit description by virtue of their frequency of occurrence and their potential seriousness. With few exceptions, the basic message is that any skin lesion with features suggestive of malignancy deserves a biopsy. General features of malignancy include rate and type of growth, color change, ulceration, bleeding, and loss of skin markings within the lesion. If malignancy is suspected, the best biopsy technique is usually excision. New evidence of patient concern about an old lesion should arouse suspicion that the lesion is changing.

Basal Cell Carcinoma (Basal Cell Epithelioma)

Basal cell carcinoma is a serious disease. Although it rarely metastasizes, untreated local spread can be extremely destructive. Morphologically, the most common basal cell carcinoma is the noduloulcerative type. It begins as a whitish or pinkish nodule with telangiectasia, then evolves into a sessile tumor with a raised, pearl-colored, telangiectatic border, with central ulceration and crusts (Fig. 51–25). The center often bleeds when crusts are removed. Occasionally, basal cell carcinoma is flat, resembling a persistent plaque of neurodermatitis or eczema.

TREATMENT

All suspected lesions should be biopsied before treatment; small lesions may be easily excised, but incisional biopsy is sufficient for diagnosis of larger ones. Excision is a standard method of therapy by family physicians, but some physicians are also experienced in electrodesiccation and curettage. The need for plastic surgery or for more extensive chemosurgery or x-ray therapy usually indicates consultation with someone experienced in these techniques.

Squamous Cell Carcinoma

Squamous cell carcinoma is a more treacherous lesion than basal cell carcinoma because of its faster growth rate, greater tendency for metastasis, and its variability of appearance. It may arise from actinic keratoses, leukoplakia, or chronic ulcers and may first look like a benign nodule or papilloma. An important diagnostic feature is the increase in size. Lesions may have a raised border and a central ulcer like basal cell carcinoma (Fig. 51–26), or may be fungoid in appearance. The most common locations are the lips, ears, tongue, and dorsal surface of the hands, and the incidence increases with the patient's age.

TREATMENT

The preferred treatment is excision or radiation therapy, or both, provided by an experienced professional.

Melanoma (Malignant Melanoma; see Color Plate Illustrations)

Melanoma is the most feared of cutaneous malignancies, but early recognition can save the patient's life. Metastasis is erratic but is fairly common and very lethal. The four recognized histopathologic types of melanoma are called lentigo maligna melanoma, superficial spreading melanoma, nodular melanoma, and acral-lentiginous melanoma.

Features of pigmented lesions that should prompt biopsy are given in the following list:

1. Variegation of color is probably the single most important feature. Besides brown and tan, look

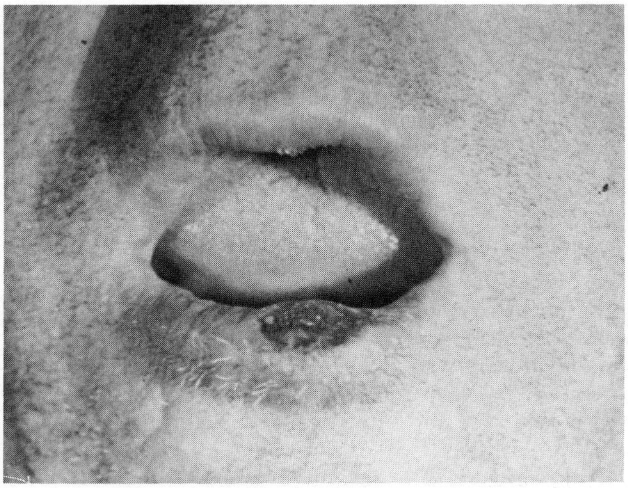

Figure 51–26. Squamous cell carcinoma.

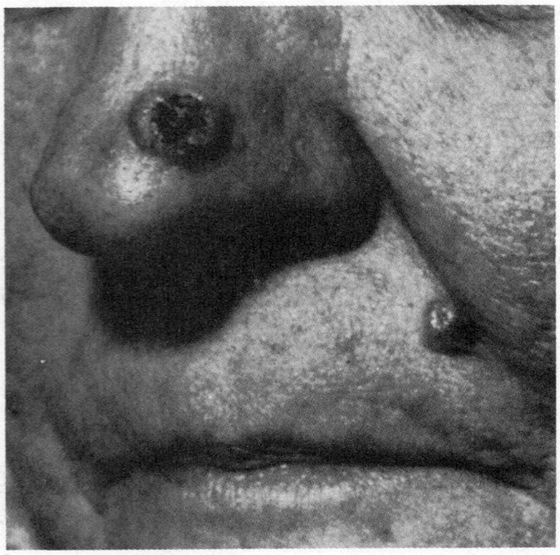

Figure 51–27. Keratoacanthoma. (From Caro, W. A., and Bronstein, B. R.: Tumors of the skin. *In* Moschella, S. L., and Hurley, H. J. [Eds.]: Dermatology. 2nd ed. Philadelphia, W. B. Saunders Company, p. 1543.)

for admixtures of blue, red, white, pink, purple, and gray.

2. Irregularity or notching of the tumor border is also characteristic of melanoma.

3. Rapid growth is commonly observed.

4. Loss of skin markings within the lesion is a common finding, but this characteristic also is seen in benign lesions.

TREATMENT

Since there is no substantial evidence that biopsy increases the risk of metastasis, either incisional or excisional biopsy is acceptable. Of the two extremes, reluctance to biopsy a lesion has more serious consequences than does performing unwarranted biopsy. Reluctance is particularly common when pigmented lesions are under the nail; such lesions must be biopsied or referred for biopsy. Definitive treatment includes wide excision and other measures, which are beyond the scope of this discussion.

Keratoacanthoma

Keratoacanthoma is a common, benign tumor that is thought to arise from hair follicles. It occurs primarily on the face and hands as a solitary, dome-shaped flesh-colored or red growth with a depressed central crust (Fig. 51–27). There may be fine blood vessels just beneath the surface. The central keratotic plug may grow into a horn, or it may disintegrate to leave a lesion that resembles a dry ulcer crater with an elevated border. Size ranges from 2 mm. to 1 cm. or more at diagnosis, and the growth rate is rapid. Both clinically and histologically, a keratoacanthoma can be confused with squamous cell carcinoma and its appearance can resemble basal cell carcinoma. The rapid growth adds to fear of malignancy.

TREATMENT

Since the lesion is considered benign and usually resolves spontaneously over several weeks or months, the experienced and courageous clinician might advocate only observation at frequent intervals. Because of the differential diagnoses and cosmetic considerations, however, complete excision is advised, with histologic examination performed to exclude the possibility of malignancy.

Squamous Cell Carcinoma In Situ (Paget's Disease, Squamous Cell Carcinoma In Situ, Erythroplasia of Queyrat, Intraepithelial Epithelioma)

Bowen's disease is the eponym for squamous cell carcinoma in situ, usually seen as a single lesion of skin or mucous membrane. It serves as the prototype for this discussion of a group of lesions that share a similar histology but have acquired separate names before the relationship was understood. Considering all of them as variations of the same fundamental process probably obscures details, but it leaves us free to move on to more pressing matters. The usual descriptive nomenclature is as follows:

Bowen's disease:	trunk and extremities
Paget's disease:	areola and nipple, vulva
Erythroplasia of Queyrat:	glans penis

The skin lesion of Bowen's disease is a sharply demarcated maculopapule or plaque with fissures or thick scales (Fig. 51–28). The color is red or brown and may resemble melanoma clinically. The surface may also be verrucous, causing confusion with an inflamed wart or seborrheic keratosis. Clinical fea-

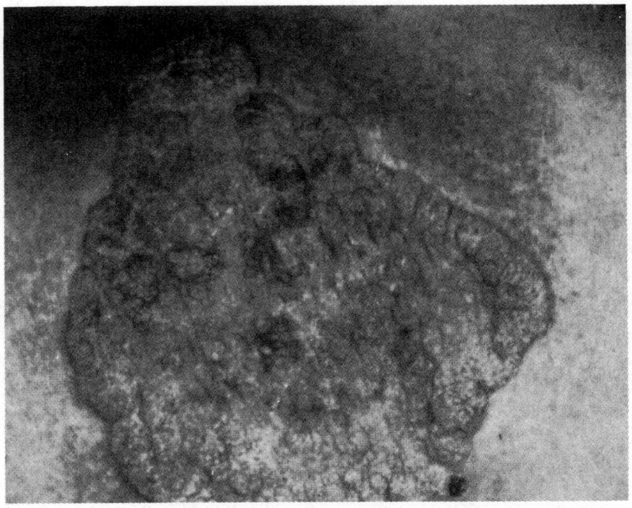

Figure 51–28. Bowen's disease. (From Caro, W. A., and Bronstein, B. R.: Tumors of the skin. *In* Moschella, S. L., and Hurley, H. J. [Eds.]: Dermatology. 2nd ed. Philadelphia, W. B. Saunders Company, 1985, p. 1550.)

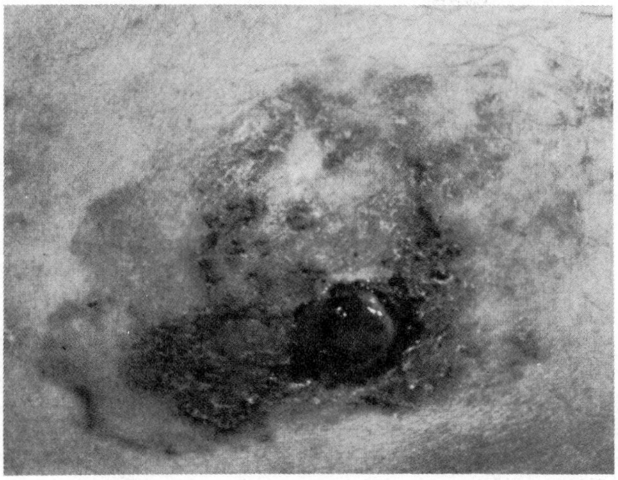

Figure 51–29. Paget's disease. (From Caro, W. A., and Bronstein, B. R.: Tumors of the skin. *In* Moschella, S. L., and Hurley, H. J. [Eds.]: Dermatology. 2nd ed. Philadelphia, W. B. Saunders Company, 1985, p. 1551.)

tures vary in the intertriginous regions and on mucosal surfaces.

Erythroplasia of Queyrat is histologically similar to Bowen's disease, and the characteristic morphology is a well-circumscribed, red, velvet-like plaque, sometimes with a slight amount of scale or crust. It is found most often on the glans penis of uncircumsized men. Clinically, it must be distinguished from a variety of lesions, including syphilis, basal cell carcinoma, and others. To add to the confusion, this diagnostic term has been applied to lesions of similar appearance at other sites, where other specialists would use the terms erythroplasia or erythroplakia.

Paget's disease is another variant that compounds the confusion of names. The characteristic lesion is a unilateral, well-defined, scaly red macule on the areola or nipple, more commonly found in women (Fig. 51–29). Some exudate or crust may be present. Differential diagnoses include eczema, contact dermatitis, and neurodermatitis. The basic pathology is considered to be intraepithelial neoplasia, but some cases appear to represent cutaneous extension of an underlying intraductal carcinoma. Finally, the term extramammary Paget's disease has been applied to erythroplasias of the vulva, lips, penis, nose, trunk, and extremities.

Treatment

Therapeutic decisions about these entities requires biopsy and consideration of other conditions that may be related to the visible lesions. Bowen's disease can coexist with visceral malignancies when there is a history of arsenic exposure, and the occurrence of anogenital lesions in women warrants investigation for uterine, vaginal, or cervical malignancies. Paget's disease of the breast often indicates breast carcinoma.

When the diagnosis is clearly established, therapeutic options include excision, topical chemotherapy with 5-fluorouracil, or destruction of the lesion with liquid nitrogen or electrodesiccation and curettage. The choice of the specific technique must be individualized.

SUPERFICIAL FUNGUS INFECTIONS

The common superficial fungi of skin are *Candida albicans*, tinea versicolor, and the dermatophytes called "tinea." Except for *Candida*, these fungi affect only the skin and its appendages. Recall that identification is aided by Wood's lamp and microscopic examination.

Tinea Versicolor

Tinea versicolor is caused by *Malassezia furfur*, a fungus that is resistant to griseofulvin. It occurs as scattered hypopigmented or hyperpigmented discrete plaques covered with very fine scales, located primarily on the trunk but also seen on the extremities. The plaques may coalesce over large areas (Fig. 51–30). The condition tends to be chronic and occurs in both children and adults; itching is unusual. The lesions often appear hypopigmented in warm months and darker than surrounding skin in cool months, hence the name "versicolor."

The abnormalities of pigmentation probably occur because the transportation of melanin from its site of manufacture is altered by the fungus. If necessary, a potassium hydroxide preparation confirms

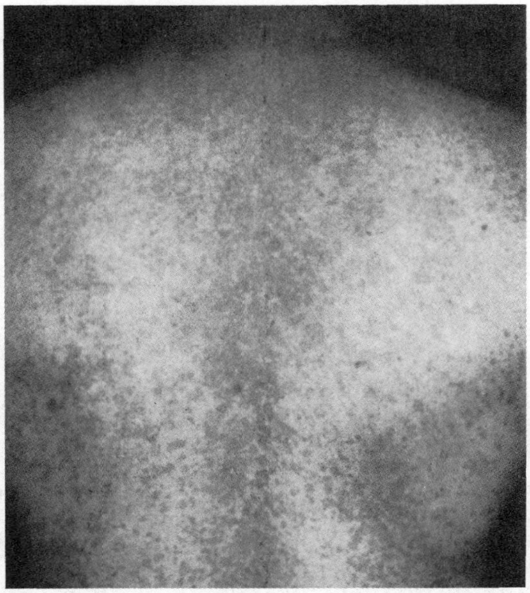

Figure 51–30. Tinea versicolor. (From Allen, H. B., and Rippon, J. W.: Superficial and deep mycoses. Section I. Superficial mycoses. *In* Moschella, S. L., and Hurley, H. J. [Eds.]: Dermatology. 2nd ed. Philadelphia, W. B. Saunders Company, 1985, p. 740.)

the thin hyphae and clusters of spores, often described as "spaghetti and meatballs."

TREATMENT

The lesions respond gradually to application of selenium sulfide shampoo (Selsun) to the affected areas; many authorities recommend daily application for 1 week, followed by weekly application for about 6 weeks. A 25 per cent solution of sodium thiosulfate (Tinver) can also be used, applied twice daily. The newer antifungal agents, such as clotrimazole and miconazole, are effective but ultimately very expensive for the large areas involved. Probably the most important feature of management is to tell the patient that pigmentation normalizes very slowly, recurrence is common, and that lesions are solely a cosmetic problem.

Infection with Candida Albicans

This yeast-like fungus is an opportunist that causes lesions in a susceptible host, involving mucous membranes or moist areas of skin. Growth is encouraged by diabetes mellitus, oral contraceptives, broad-spectrum antibiotics, and immunosuppression. Potassium hydroxide preparations confirm budding yeast-like cells. The major clinical syndromes associated with *Candida albicans* are oral moniliasis, monilial vaginitis, monilial paronychia, and monilial intertrigo.

Oral moniliasis (thrush) occurs most often in infants. When it occurs in an adult, some thought must be given to the possibility of immunosuppression. It is seen as white, curd-like plaques on the oral mucosa or tongue (Fig. 51–31), sometimes accompanied by fissures at the corners of the lips (perlèche). Thrush is treated most often with nystatin oral suspension (Mycostatin, Nilstat), placed in the mouth four times daily. A dosage of 2 ml. for infants is used or 4 to 6 ml. for children and adults. Treatment is continued until 48 hours after the visible lesions are gone.

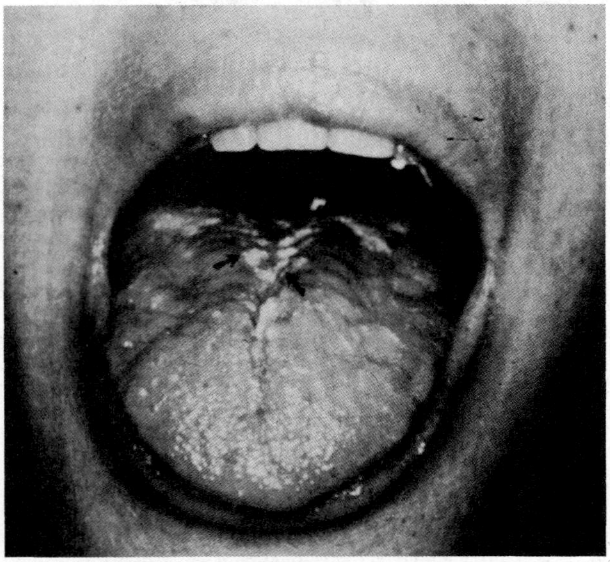

Figure 51–31. Thrush. (From Fitzpatrick, T. B., et al. [Eds.]: Dermatology in General Practice. 3rd ed. New York, McGraw-Hill, 1987, p. 2233.)

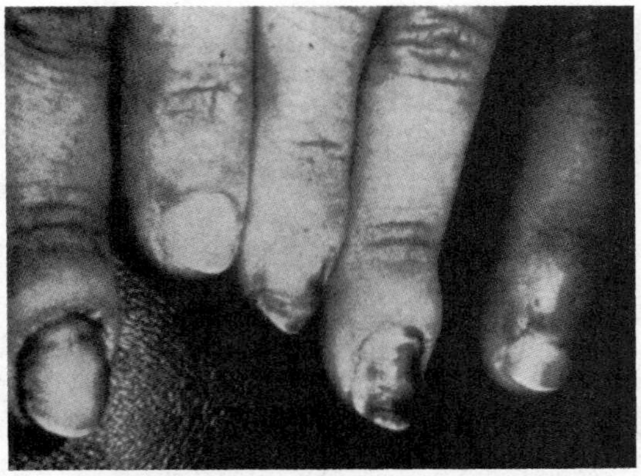

Figure 51–32. Paronychia. (From Norton, L. A.: Disorders of the nails. *In* Moschella, S. L., and Hurley, H. J. [Eds.]: Dermatology. 2nd ed. Philadelphia, W. B. Saunders Company, 1985, p. 1409.)

Monilial vaginitis is seen as white, curd-like plaques on a red base in the vagina, occasionally accompanied by lesions of the perineal skin. Nystatin vaginal tablets may be inserted once daily for 14 days. Clotrimazole (Gyne-Lotrimin) and miconazole (Monistat) are also effective and offer a shorter duration of therapy. The vaginal cream formulations are especially helpful if there are skin lesions outside the vagina, since creams can be applied to both mucosa and skin.

Monilial paronychia involves the nail folds; there is chronic but relatively painless redness and swelling, from which a cheesy material can often be expressed (Fig. 51–32). The condition should be distinguished from bacterial paronychia, which is more acute, painful, and purulent. Potassium hydroxide preparation of the cheesy material confirms budding yeast-like cells. The most effective therapy consists of rubbing an antifungal agent such as clotrimazole solution (Lotrimin) or econazole (Spectazole) cream into the nail area twice daily, often for several months. Patients should also make a special effort to keep the hands dry.

Monilial intertrigo consists of beefy red, fairly well-circumscribed patches with satellite pustules in moist areas of the groin, perineum, axillae, and under the breasts. A topical antifungal agent, such as clotrimazole or econazole, may be used successfully, and the area should be kept dry.

Dermatophytes

Lesions caused by these fungi are most often referred to by the name tinea, followed by a word that denotes the area of the body affected. In this section, the word "topicals" refers to clotrimazole, econazole, miconazole, or ketoconazole, unless otherwise specified.

Tinea capitis is characterized by circular patches of hair loss with fine scales on the scalp, usually seen in prepubertal children (Fig. 51–33). The lesions in some patients exhibit greenish fluorescence when examined with a Wood's lamp; those that do not fluoresce can be confirmed with a potassium hydroxide preparation. The topical antifungal preparations are not ordinarily effective, and treatment with oral griseofulvin (Grifulvin V, Grisactin, Gris-PEG) is required. The dosage should be determined with care, since "microsize" and "ultramicrosize" formulas are available, with considerable variation in strength. For adults, a daily dose of 500 mg. of the microsize type is effective, or 5 mg. per pound for children. The ultramicrosize preparations, such as Gris-PEG, require only about two thirds of that dosage. The medication should be taken *with* food. Treatment of tinea capitis takes about 4 to 6 weeks.

Tinea corporis (ringworm) results in persistent oval or round lesions with central clearing and a red, scaly or vesicular border (Fig. 51–34), usually seen in children. In adults, it may be associated with diabetes mellitus or immunosuppression. The lesions may be single or multiple, with no particular grouping or pattern. They can be distinguished from other papulosquamous eruptions by scraping a few scales onto a microscope slide and performing a potassium hydroxide preparation to observe the characteristic hyphae. Lesions in reasonable numbers respond to a topical antifungal agent, such as clotrimazole or miconazole, in 2 to 4 weeks. Widespread or resistant lesions are treated with oral griseofulvin for the same period of time. Treatment should be continued for a few days after clinical resolution.

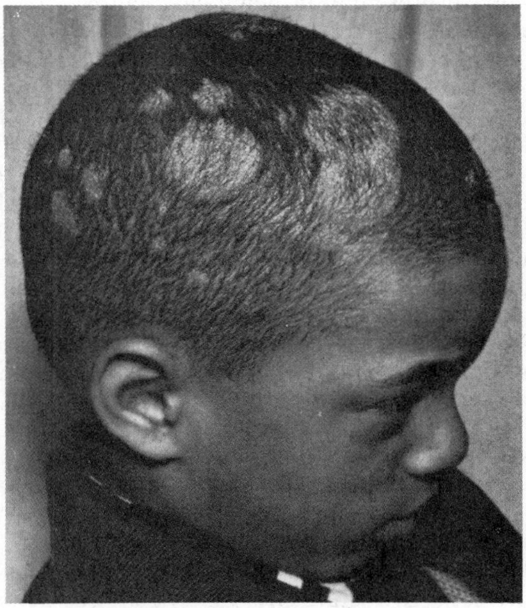

Figure 51–33. Tinea capitis. (From Allen, H. B., and Rippon, J. W.: Superficial and deep mycoses. Section I. Superficial mycoses. *In* Moschella, S. L., and Hurley, H. J. [Eds.]: Dermatology. 2nd ed. Philadelphia, W. B. Saunders Company, 1985, p. 744.)

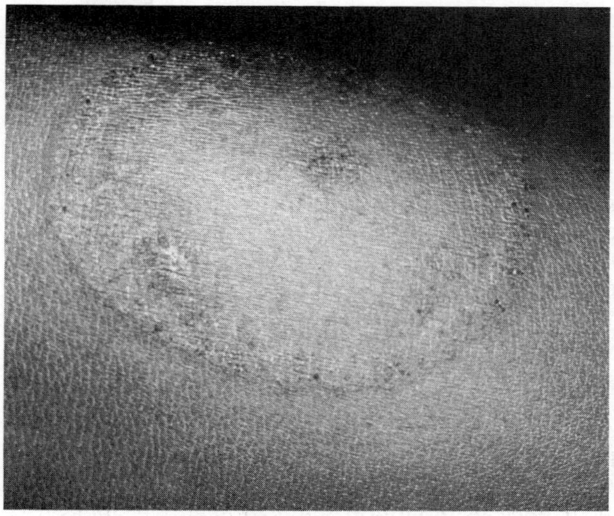

Figure 51–34. Tinea corporis.

Tinea Cruris

Tinea cruris (jock itch) occurs in the genital intertriginous areas, with similar morphology and treatment as described for tinea corporis. Rather than discrete small lesions, there tends to be a large area of coalescent rash (Fig. 51–35), with the characteristic central clearing and distinct scaly or vesicular border. In contrast, erythrasma is a brownish red rash that can be distinguished by its red fluorescence under a Wood's lamp. Monilial intertrigo is associated with satellite pustules and causes more involvement of the scrotum than is seen with tinea cruris.

Treatment. Topical antifungal agents work well for tinea cruris, and have the additional advantage that they are effective for *Candida*.

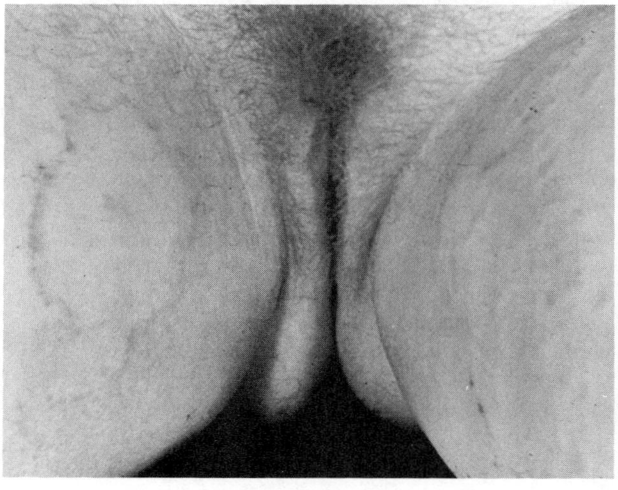

Figure 51–35. Tinea cruris.

Tinea Pedis

Tinea pedis (athlete's foot) most often causes cracking and maceration between the toes (Fig. 51–36) but may also become manifest as an acute vesiculobullous eruption of the plantar surface. Lesions are often secondarily infected by bacteria, and tinea infection of the toenails also may be present. A peculiar variation is the "one hand, two feet syndrome" associated with *Trichophyton rubrum*. Tinea pedis can usually be distinguished clinically from contact dermatitis, psoriasis, and other foot conditions with a potassium hydroxide preparation as needed.

Treatment. Topical antifungal agents are often used, with adjunctive soaks or antimicrobials used as indicated by the presentation. Oral griseofulvin is sometimes necessary, often for as long as 3 months. Recurrence is common, and preventive measures include absorbent socks and the use of antifungal powders (e.g., Tinactin, undecylenic acid). Hyperhidrosis may also be present and should be treated concurrently.

Tinea Manum

Tinea manum is fungal infection of the hand (Fig. 51–37) often found in association with tinea pedis. *T. rubrum* causes the "one hand, two feet" variant, where one palm is spared. There is scaling and slight redness, particularly along skin lines.

Treatment. Griseofulvin is usually necessary for several weeks until the lesions clear.

Tinea Unguium

Tinea unguium is the more specific term, referring to dermatophyte (tinea, superficial fungi) infection of

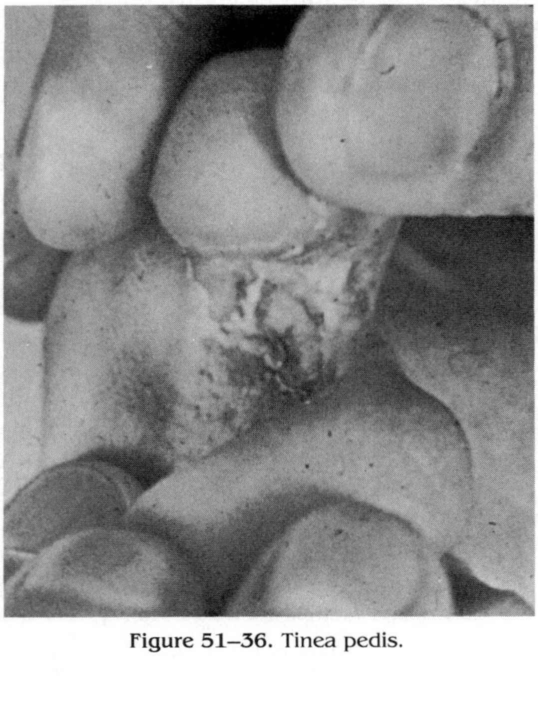

Figure 51–36. Tinea pedis.

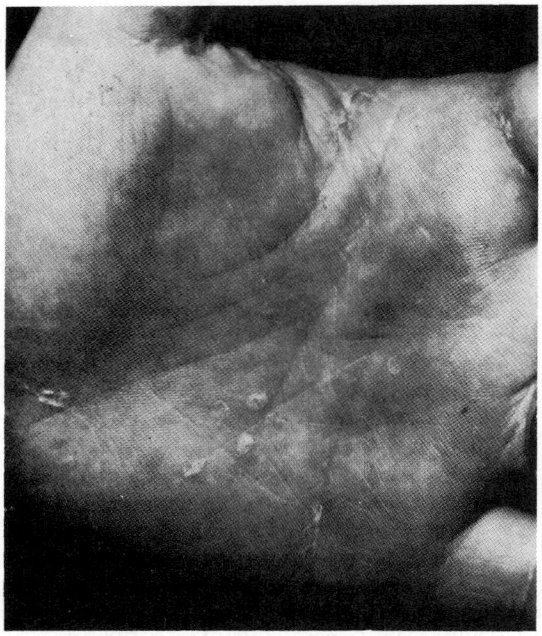

Figure 51–37. Tinea manum. (From Allen, H. B., and Rippon, J. W.: Superficial and deep mycoses. Section I. Superficial mycoses. *In* Moschella, S. L., and Hurley, H. J. [Eds.]: Dermatology. 2nd ed. Philadelphia, W. B. Saunders Company, 1985, p. 758.)

the nail plate, whereas the term onychomycosis includes nail infection by any fungus or yeast. Onychomycosis is the most common disorder of nails and is frequently associated with fungus infection elsewhere on the body.

There is a rather complicated system for clinical classification of onychomycosis into subtypes, with each clinical presentation being characteristic of certain organisms. Specific diagnosis by means of potassium hydroxide preparations and fungal or mold cultures is problematic and probably useful only as an academic exercise, since therapy is essentially identical for all common types. It is important, however, to distinguish these infections from some other nonfungal causes of nail destruction. Ordinarily, clinical distinction is possible, since the associated skin lesions will be characteristic (i.e., distorted nails associated with psoriasis, hand eczema, Darier's disease, and lichen planus).

Probably the most characteristic clinical presentation of tinea unguium is a process of insidious onset that results in a discolored nail (white, brown, yellow), with a ragged edge and accumulated keratotic debris under the end of the nail (Fig. 51–38). The process may involve some or all of the fingernails and toenails. There are no other symptoms unless secondary infection occurs.

Treatment. Systemic therapy with griseofulvin (Grifulvin-V, Grisactin, Gris-PEG) requires at least 4 to 6 months for fingernails and 12 to 18 months for toenails; recurrences are very common, especially for toenail infections. Many clinicians are reluctant to recommend griseofulvin for toenail infections. Since

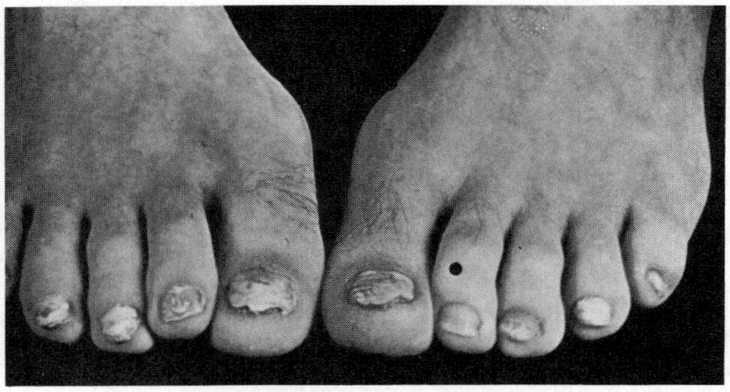

Figure 51–38. Tinea unguium.

griseofulvin is not free of cost or side effects, patients should be well informed and may choose to live with ugly nails until secondary infection or ingrown nails force treatment. Surgical avulsion of the nail may be necessary, sometimes in combination with the use of griseofulvin or a topical agent. Some authorities report success with nail destruction using 40 per cent urea preparations, with or without antifungal agents. Use of topical antifungal agents alone is not very effective, but a trial may be justified if the other methods are inappropriate or contraindicated.

Other Nail Conditions

Other conditions worthy of brief mention include:

Photo onycholysis:	nail discoloration related to photosensitizing drugs (e.g., tetracycline)
Psoriasis:	changes associated with psoriatic arthropathy
Spoon nails:	thin, concave nails with an everted free edge
Transverse ridges (Beau's lines):	follow febrile illness

Tinea Barbae

Tinea barbae (tinea sycosis) is a fungal infection of the beard and mustache areas in men. It is seen most often in rural areas, associated with exposure to cattle and dogs. *Microsporum* or *Trichophyton* species are common causes. Clinical presentations include circinate lesions similar to tinea corporis, superficial ones resembling folliculitis, and an inflammatory type similar to kerion of the scalp (Fig. 51–39). Majocchi's granuloma is another name for a solitary kerion-like lesion.

Wood's lamp examination is helpful with *M. canis* infections, whereas potassium hydroxide examination or culture on Sabouraud's medium is required to confirm other types of infection. The differential diagnosis includes bacterial folliculitis, perioral dermatitis, contact dermatitis, *Candida* infection, and herpes simplex; additional diagnostic aids include bacterial or viral cultures, Tzanck's smear, and contact allergy testing.

Treatment. Although most lesions of tinea barbae resolve spontaneously in weeks or months, oral griseofulvin hastens resolution. Warm compresses with Burow's or saline solution may provide some symptomatic relief, and systemic antibiotics are indicated for bacterial superinfection.

Sporotrichosis

The cutaneous form of sporotrichosis is a chronic, progressive disease resulting from implantation of *Sporothrix schenkii*, a fungal saprophyte found on thorns, splinters, or other plant materials. It is commonly associated with occupational exposure or cultivation of rose bushes. The disease is spread by lymphatics from the original site, and the same fungus can invade the viscera. The characteristic appearance is a roughly linear spread of lesions along the lymphatics from a primary lesion on the hand (Fig. 51–40). Individual lesions are indurated papules or nodules with central ulceration; they are painless unless secondarily infected.

Differential diagnoses include tularemia, staphylococcal lymphangitis, and mycobacterial infection.

Treatment

Treatment of the localized disease is with a saturated solution of potassium iodide, administered orally at a daily dosage of 2 to 6 grams. A typical starting dosage is 10 drops, 3 times daily after meals. Intravenous sodium iodide is an alternative. Patients intolerant to the iodides or with disseminated disease are treated with intravenous amphotericin B.

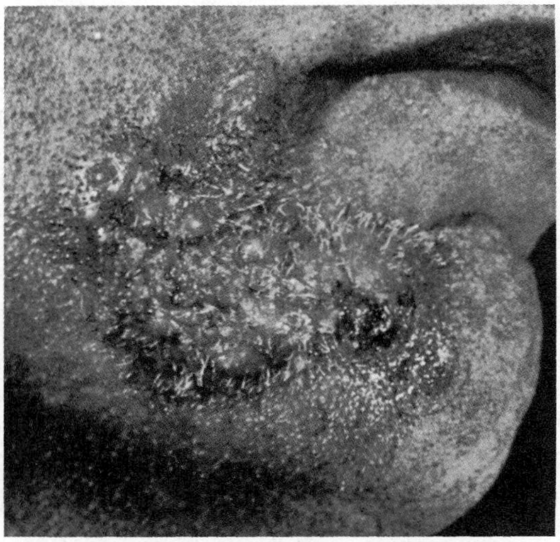

Figure 51–39. Tinea barbae. (From Allen, H. B., and Rippon, J. W.: Superficial and deep mycoses. Section I. Superficial mycoses. *In* Moschella, S. L., and Hurley, H. J. [Eds.]: Dermatology. 2nd ed. Philadelphia, W. B. Saunders Company, 1985, p. 748.)

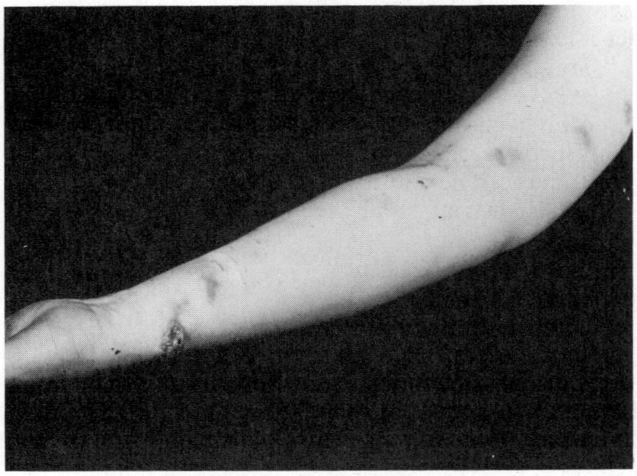

Figure 51–40. Sporotrichosis.

PITYRIASIS ALBA AND ROSEA

Pityriasis Alba

Pityriasis alba is a mild, chronic, self-limited disease of prepubescent children and teenagers. It appears as irregular, well-circumscribed ovoid patches on the face with extremely fine scales and hypopigmentation.

TREATMENT

Some authorities believe the condition may be a minor form of atopic dermatitis, and advocate use of a skin lubricant such as petrolatum. Others recommend 0.5 per cent or 1 per cent hydrocortisone and additional sun exposure to repigment the areas. It should be differentiated from tinea versicolor, and an explanation may be sufficient treatment.

Pityriasis Rosea

Pityriasis rosea is a self-limited papulosquamous eruption that occurs in all ages but is most common among young adults. An initial single plaque, called the "herald patch," is usually seen somewhere on the body days or weeks before the generalized eruption. The subsequent rash consists of multiple tan or "fawn-colored" oval plaques covered with fine scales, arranged with their long axes along skin cleavage lines (Fig. 51–41). Lesions are commonly confined to the trunk and proximal extremities but may be seen on the face, especially in children. New lesions may appear for a week or two, but the rash usually disappears entirely within 5 or 6 weeks.

TREATMENT

Itching is sometimes an associated feature, requiring only symptomatic therapy. The most important aspect of the management of pityriasis rosea is consideration of the differential diagnoses. Because the lesions are morphologically similar to those of some cases of secondary syphilis, serologic examination is prudent, especially if a herald patch was not seen. Drug eruptions, psoriasis, and lichen planus should be considered. The herald patch may suggest tinea corporis, which may be confirmed by a potassium hydroxide preparation.

PSORIASIS

Psoriasis is a chronic or recurrent papulosquamous eruption in which discrete areas of skin develop an increased mitotic rate and increased capillary blood supply. Clinically, the result is multiple irregular plaques with a red base and superimposed silvery-white thick scales. Psoriasis is most often recognized in adults, although it also occurs in children. A familial predisposition to the disease is known. The lesions of psoriasis commonly appear on the scalp, elbows, and knees, but may be seen anywhere on the skin (Fig. 51–42). They exhibit the Koebner phenomenon, since they tend to appear in scar tissue following injury.

Another clue to diagnosis is Auspitz' sign, which means that a punctate bleeding site appears when a scale is plucked from the lesion. Ridges or pits may be seen in the nails. Psoriasis tends to be worse in

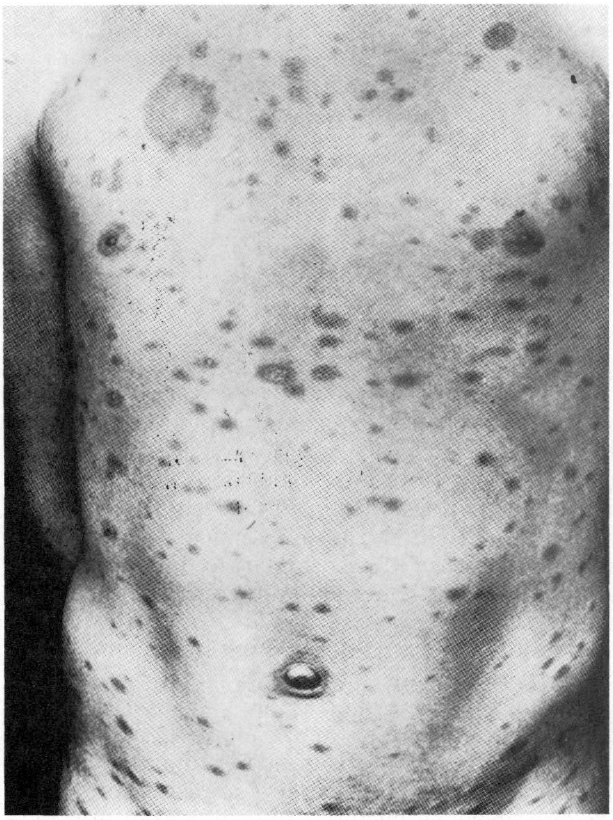

Figure 51–41. Pityriasis. (From Fitzpatrick, T. B., et al. [Eds.]: Dermatology in General Practice. 3rd ed. New York, McGraw-Hill, 1987, p. 984.)

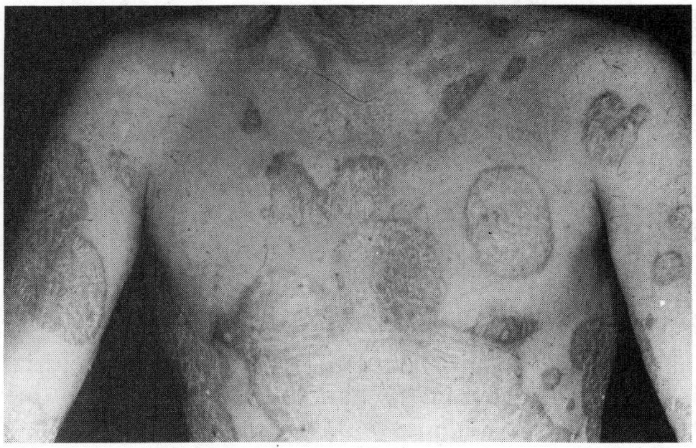

Figure 51–42. Psoriasis.

the winter. Only a minority of patients have itching, but the cosmetic impairment can be quite severe.

Psoriasis can occasionally cause confusion with other skin diseases, including tinea corporis, seborrheic dermatitis, pityriasis rosea, secondary syphilis, and lichen planus. In the appropriate circumstances, biopsy, potassium hydroxide preparation, blood serology, or dermatologic consultation may be indicated.

Treatment

Multiple therapies have been used for psoriasis. Topical steroid applications are by far the most often used and are usually effective. Many patients respond best to the potent ointment or gel steroid preparations and may need occlusion intermittently. Coal tar shampoos are useful for scalp lesions, and new gel forms of coal tar derivatives are less messy for use on the skin. Recalcitrant scalp lesions may also be treated with a topical steroid lotion (triamcinolone acetonide [Kenalog] and betamethasone valerate [Valisone] are popular). Intralesional steroid injections are helpful for small, highly visible lesions if one has experience with the technique. The general rules for steroid use are especially important for patients with chronic, widespread lesions. Recall that fluorinated steroids should not be used for facial lesions; a second prescription for 1 per cent hydrocortisone cream may be given for use on the face. Patients generally benefit from the use of skin lubricants or bath oils, and often respond to moderate sunlight exposure and exposure to ultraviolet light.

Methotrexate can be administered orally for control of resistant cases when the physician is thoroughly familiar with its use; most family physicians would initiate this therapy through consultation. Many authorities recommend that a liver biopsy must be obtained and be proved normal before methotrexate therapy is begun. Another method of therapy available by referral is superficial x-ray (Grenz ray) therapy. Treatments that employ controlled exposure to ultraviolet radiation include the Goeckerman regimen and oral psoralens combined with long-wave ultraviolet A (PUVA).

URTICARIA AND ERYTHEMA MULTIFORME

Urticaria

Urticaria is an eruption of skin characterized by a typical primary lesion called a wheal. The wheal is a circumscribed, raised, edematous, red lesion that itches. Individual lesions are transitory but may last minutes, hours, or days. There may be pallor of the surrounding skin. Multiple lesions are the rule (Fig. 51–43).

Wheals are an end result of a variety of immunologic and nonimmunologic processes that lead to localized release of histamine and other vasoactive substances from mast cells of the skin. An abbreviated list of precipitating factors includes food, venoms, drugs, pollens, heat, cold, light, blood products, radiocontrast agents, helminths, pressure, emotional stress, and chronic infections.

It should be apparent that recognition of urticaria is simple, but the etiologic diagnosis can be very difficult or impossible. A thorough history and examination are indicated when urticaria is persistent or chronic (arbitrarily, longer than 4 to 6 weeks). If etiology is still totally unknown, reasonable evaluation could include a complete blood cell count with differential count, urinalysis, chest x-ray study, and stool examination for parasites. Special cases may require immunologic investigation, which is beyond the scope of this summary.

TREATMENT

Parenteral epinephrine is indicated for acute urticaria associated with anaphylaxis or angioedema. Ordinarily acute urticaria or chronic urticaria is treated with an antihistamine, the most effective of which is hydroxyzine (Atarax, Vistaril). A brief

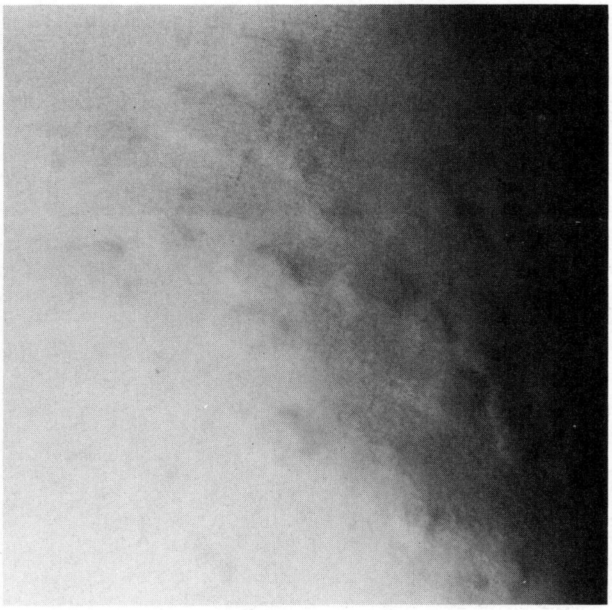

Figure 51–43. Urticaria.

course of oral steroids is used occasionally for persistent cases.

Erythema Multiforme

Erythema multiforme is an acute or recurrent rash that occurs through immune mechanisms, either in response to known precipitating factors or of idiopathic cause. The most convincing causative associations have been established with herpes simplex and mycoplasma infections and with sulfa drugs, particularly the sulfonamides. In about half the cases, no precipitating factor can be identified. More cases are seen in the spring and fall than in other seasons. The erythema marginatum observed in rheumatic fever is a variant of erythema multiforme.

The lesions may be widespread on skin and mucous membranes and are occasionally accompanied by itching or burning. Some patients have fever, with or without an associated infection or source of inflammation. Typically, there are multiple, symmetrically distributed target (iris) lesions that have a predisposition for acral areas (Fig. 51–44). There may also be urticarial plaques, which are more persistent than the wheals seen in urticaria. Favored locations include flexor surfaces of the extremities, palms and soles, genitalia, and lips. The development of vesicles or bullae in pre-existing lesions signals a more severe course. The most severe form of the disease is known as the Stevens-Johnson syndrome, which is characterized by significant constitutional signs and symptoms and by multiple inflammatory bullae on the mucous membranes.

Although typical cases are rather easily identified, the differential diagnosis of atypical cases includes urticaria, necrotizing vasculitis, secondary syphilis, septicemia, Rocky Mountain spotted fever, viral exanthems, lichen planus, and bullous impetigo.

Treatment

Treatment of milder cases is generally symptomatic, with antihistamines, salicylates, and other anti-inflammatory agents employed resulting in varying degrees of success. More severe cases require additional supportive care and attention to the metabolic consequences and specific organs affected. Probably the most difficult task is judging the appropriate methods and extent of a search for occult causes. As for urticaria, the search is most often dependent on a thorough history and examination. A typical eruption subsides in 2 or 3 weeks, but recurrences are fairly common.

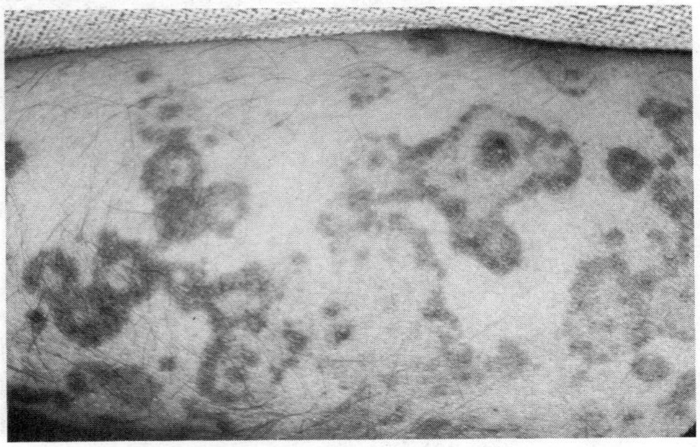

Figure 51–44. Hemorrhagic erythema multiforme.

FOLLICULITIS

The term folliculitis generally refers to a bacterial infection localized to the hair follicle, most often due to *Staphylococcus aureus*. The everyday form of folliculitis is found in a hot, humid environment with the use of occlusive clothing. The lesions are small papules or pustules at the openings of hair follicles, identified by the protruding hair. Individual lesions are transient, but new ones tend to appear as long as the particular environmental conditions exist.

Similar lesions are observed following exposure to some hydrocarbons in industrial settings or following ingestion of certain foods or medications containing halogens (iodide, bromide, chloride). Prominence of the hair follicles, with or without mild inflammation, is seen in malnourished adults.

Not unexpectedly, there are variations on the name:

Follicular impetigo (Bockhart's impetigo):	Pustules of scalp hair follicles in children
Perifolliculitis capitis:	Follicular pustules, abscesses, and scars with resultant scalp alopecia
Folliculitis rubra (many synonyms):	Probably a variant of keratosis pilaris, an inflammatory condition of unknown etiology
Folliculitis decalvans:	Scarring and alopecia of unknown cause

Treatment

This kind of folliculitis responds best to cooler surroundings and lighter clothing. Individual lesions can be touched with a drop of benzoyl peroxide lotion (Benoxyl, Desquam-X), and oral antibiotics may occasionally be indicated for the more severe cases. If needed, synthetic penicillins or erythromycin are appropriate choices.

SELECTED ALOPECIAS*

Androgenetic Alopecia ("Male-Pattern" Baldness)

In androgenetic alopecia, men are affected more often than women, and the hair loss in women is

*See "tinea" descriptions for hair loss due to fungi.

more diffuse. In men, the typical pattern is recession in the parietal areas and on the crown, leaving behind scalp of normal appearance. In women, diffuse loss on the crown is typical. If the process occurs in a woman under 50 or 60 years of age, endocrinologic evaluation should be considered to seek a source of excessive androgens, especially if there are other signs of virilization.

TREATMENT

Hair transplantation and cosmetic remedies (hair styling and wigs) have been the mainstays of legitimate therapy. Topical minoxidil (Rogaine) is the first medication approved by the Food and Drug Administration for the treatment of male baldness, although it is not recommended for everyone. The best candidates are men under 40 years of age whose balding has progressed for less than 10 years. The presence of remaining "peach fuzz" hairs seems to be the most important single factor predictive of success. The treatment is fairly expensive and requires a long-term commitment; the hair growth is lost a few months after the applications are stopped.

Telogen Effluvium (Febrile Alopecia, Toxic Alopecia)

A large number of hair follicles enter the telogen (resting) phase in unison, with resultant hair loss. The loss is usually diffuse rather than patchy, and follows a stressful event by 2 to 4 months. Postpartum telogen effluvium is a common example, and others include occurrences following a severe infection, a fever, and an adverse drug reaction.

TREATMENT

Hair regrowth usually occurs within a year, and no specific treatment speeds recovery.

Traumatic Alopecia (Traction Alopecia, Trichotillomania)

Trichotillomania results from repetitive, often subconscious, manipulation of hair by the patient. The typical presentation is a well-circumscribed area of absent and broken hairs, without evidence of scalp involvement (Fig. 51–45); the diagnosis is confirmed primarily by history. A similar pattern of traumatic hair loss results from damage by rollers and some other hair styling methods.

TREATMENT

Treatment consists of management of the underlying psychopathology or avoidance of the hair styling methods that cause damage.

Alopecia Areata

This general term refers to single or multiple patches of well-demarcated hair loss from the scalp (Fig. 51–46). Alopecia totalis is the total or near-total loss of scalp hair, and alopecia universalis is generalized loss of body hair. The sexes are affected about equally, with the peak incidence occurring at ages 40 through 60. The underlying skin appears normal. If present, "exclamation point hairs" are pathognomonic; they are short, stubby hairs tapered at the proximal end. Spontaneous regrowth usually begins at the periphery and spreads centrally, but recurrences are common. Although the etiology is unknown, suggested contributing factors include genetic predisposition, stress, and disorders of immune regulation. Associated findings are nail dystrophies, cataracts, atopy, and pernicious anemia.

Diagnosis on clinical grounds is the rule, but biopsy may be necessary. Fungal tests are appropriate if there are signs of inflammation, and serologic tests for syphilis may be in order.

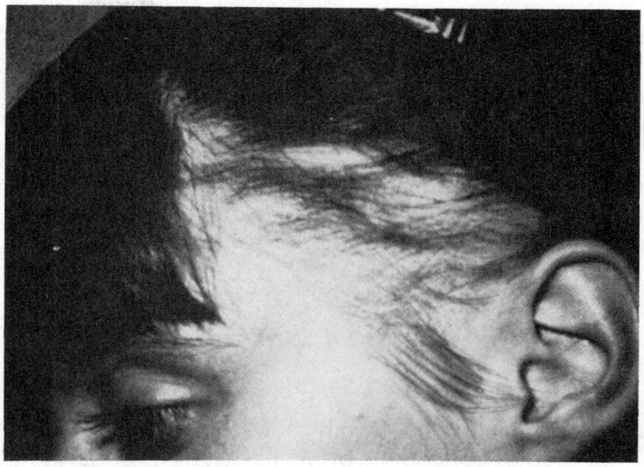

Figure 51–45. Trichotillomania. (From Maguire, H. C., Jr., and Hanno, R.: Diseases of the hair. *In* Moschella, S. L., and Hurley, H. J. [Eds.]: Dermatology. 2nd ed. Philadelphia, W. B. Saunders Company, 1985, p. 1381.)

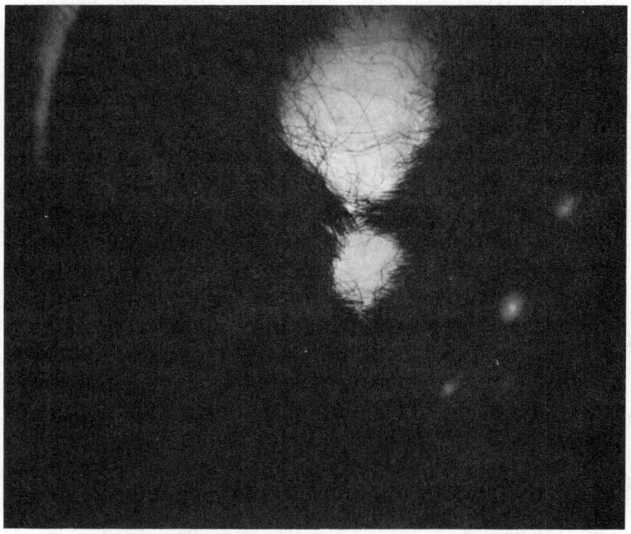

Figure 51–46. Alopecia areata.

Treatment

No treatment is entirely satisfactory, and these efforts should probably be left to physicians with considerable experience with the condition. Alternatives include systemic and local injections of steroids, topical irritants, and PUVA therapy. Topical minoxidil (Rogaine) may also prove useful for this condition.

PIGMENTED NEVUS (MOLE; SEE COLOR PLATE)

Moles are very common, benign lesions of skin, composed of collections of nevus cells within the skin. The nevus cells are of neuroectodermal origin, some resembling melanocytes and some similar to Schwann cells. The traditional histologic classification is junctional, intradermal, or compound, depending on whether the predominant location of the cells is in the epidermis or dermis, or both sites, respectively. The lesions first appear in early childhood, increase in number through early adulthood, then usually resolve with advancing age. Pigmented nevi may be flat, dome-shaped, pedunculated, or verrucoid, with great variation in size and surface characteristics. Some are hairy, and others are hairless. For the experienced examiner, there are some correlations between appearance and histologic type.

If moles are benign and virtually ubiquitous, why pay much attention to them? Moles earn most of their importance from relationships to cutaneous melanoma. Many melanomas arise from pre-existing nevi, so there is some degree of malignant potential, and the appearance of melanoma and nevi can be quite similar. The assessment of malignant potential or the differentiation of melanoma from atypical mole on clinical grounds can be very difficult. There are not enough physicians, time, or money to remove all the moles from mankind, but there are some reasonable guidelines for excision that have met the test of time:

1. Removal for cosmetic reasons or due to irritation: Patients may desire removal for cosmetic reasons or when contact by clothing causes chronic irritation of the mole.

2. Atypical appearance or change in appearance: Worrisome features include very dark pigmentation, irregular distribution of pigment, irregular borders, "satellite" lesions, asymmetry, and large size (5 mm. or more). Inflammation, infection, bleeding, and sudden onset of growth in a stable mole are also cause for excision and biopsy.

3. Specific lesions with increased malignant potential: These lesions include dysplastic nevi, some nevi present from birth, and those on acral and mucosal surfaces.

4. Removal from sites that are difficult to monitor: Patients are advised to observe pigmented nevi for change, particularly when there is a personal or family history of melanoma. It is probably wise to offer excision of lesions that are difficult to see, such as those on the scalp or perianal areas.

Complete removal by some method of excision is the acceptable treatment; destructive methods should not be employed. The safest course is pathologic examination of *every* specimen, regardless of its benign appearance. Preliminary incisional biopsy is justified for lesions in difficult locations.

PARASITIC INFESTATIONS

Scabies

Scabies results from parasitic infestation of the skin. The disease is highly contagious on close contact and is seen more often in crowded conditions, such as nursery schools and in large families in one household. It also occurs as a contemporary form of venereal disease. The cause is the bite of a mite called *Sarcoptes scabiei,* the female of which burrows into the skin and lays her eggs.

The primary lesion of scabies is a tiny burrow of 2 to 3 mm. in length, but it is frequently hidden within the secondary eruption, and very few mites are actually present in a single patient. Secondary lesions are minute reddish papules and excoriations of the finger webs, forearms, axillae, lower abdomen, and genitalia, which probably represent a hypersensitivity reaction to a small number of bites (Fig. 51–47). The face is rarely involved, except in infants. Itching is intense and is particularly noticeable at night. With some skill and luck, the mite can be recovered from a burrow for confirmation of the diagnosis under a microscope. Burrows are most often found on the forearms and finger webs.

Treatment

For adults and for children older than 3 years of age, a single topical application of 1 per cent lindane (gamma benzene hexachloride, Kwell) is probably sufficient treatment. The lotion is applied to the entire body surface from the neck down and washed off after 24 hours. If the patient washes his or her hands, the lotion must be reapplied to that area. A second treatment in 3 to 7 days may be necessary in a few cases. Because of the association of lindane with seizures in children, 5 to 10 per cent precipitated sulfur in petrolatum is the preferred treatment for patients younger than 3 years of age. It is messy but has an established record of safety and effectiveness when applied each night for three consecutive nights from the neck down. Benzyl benzoate and 10 per cent crotamiton (Eurax) are alternative topical agents for adults and older children. Preparations based on pyrethrin insecticides (Rid, A-200) are alternatives available without a prescription order. Concurrently with treatment, clothing and bed linens should be laundered and dried with heat.

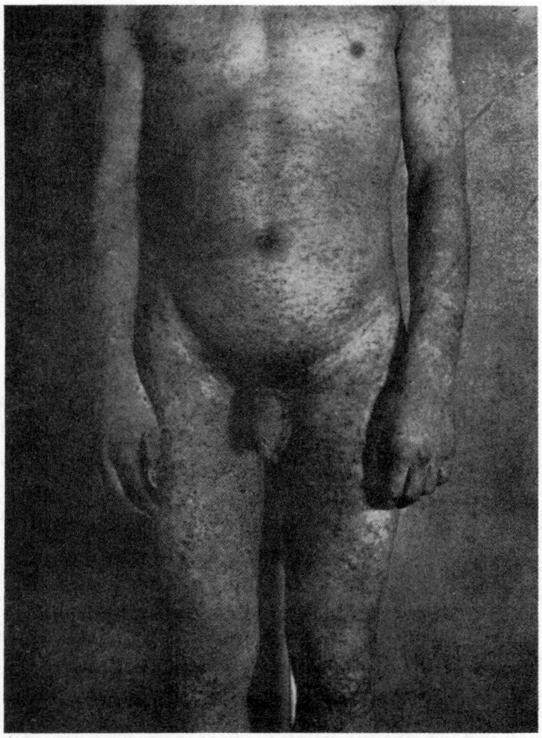

Figure 51–47. Scabies. (From McKay, K. C., and Moschella, S. L.: Parasites, arthropods, hazardous animals, and tropical dermatology. *In* Moschella, S. L., and Hurley, H. J. [Eds.]: Dermatology. 2nd ed. Philadelphia, W. B. Saunders Company, 1985, p. 1781.)

Pediculosis (Lice)

Pediculosis Capitis

Pediculosis capitis (head lice) is a condition associated with crowded living conditions and longer hair, often seen among children in schools or day care centers. It is transmitted by shared combs, hats, and pillows. The lice are sometimes seen, but diagnosis is usually made by observation of the tiny, pearl-colored nits (ova) attached to hair shafts. Grayish fluorescence under a Wood's light will accentuate the nits, if necessary, and they are more evident when the hair is wet. In fact, the diagnosis is frequently made by the patient's mother, barber, or teacher or as an incidental finding by the physician.

Treatment. The usual treatment is gamma benzene hexachloride (lindane, Kwell); agents containing pyrethrins (e.g., A-200) are probably safer for children under 5 years of age. Kwell is used as a shampoo, then it is reapplied after the hair is dry as an overnight lotion. Ordinarily only one application is necessary, but it may be repeated in a week or so as needed. Although it is not necessary to remove all the nits to achieve a cure, removal can usually be accomplished with a fine-toothed comb as desired for aesthetic reasons. Removal is made easier if the hair is covered for a few hours with a towel soaked in white vinegar to soften the cement that holds nit to hair shaft.

Pediculosis Corporis

The body louse, pediculosis corporis, is seen less often than head lice. Lice and ova may be seen on skin or hair, but are found most easily in the seams of clothing. Itching and scattered erythematous macules are typical.

Treatment. The customary treatment is lindane (Kwell) applied as a body lotion, followed by improved hygiene. Clothing should be washed and dried, since dry heat is effective against the lice and eggs.

Phthiriasis Pubis

Phthiriasis pubis (crab louse) is often transmitted by sexual contact, but also by shared clothing. In spite of its name, the louse may be found in hair-bearing areas elsewhere on the body. Itching is common, and the diagnosis may be obscured by secondary infection of the excoriations. There may be a scattered macular rash, and occasionally other allergic responses.

Treatment. Lindane (Kwell) is used as for pediculosis corporis, with attention given to secondary infections or allergic sequelae as needed.

PARONYCHIA

Fungal Paronychia

Paronychia results from infection of the nail fold with bacteria or yeast. Some clinical features help distinguish the cause, with bacterial or yeast cultures for confirmation. Paronychia due to *Candida* (monilia) is characterized by a relatively insidious onset, with redness, some tenderness, and swelling of the skin just proximal to the nail and along its lateral margins. Thick cheese-like material may be expressed in some cases, and there may be some green or brown discoloration of the nail. Chronic cases lead to distortion and discoloration of the nail. The condition is more likely to occur in those who frequently immerse their hands in water, particularly if detergents are used. Involvement of multiple fingers or toes is common. Diagnosis is confirmed by culture on Sabouraud's agar.

Treatment

Treatment includes avoidance or protection from water and detergents, and topical applications of antifungal agents such as clotrimazole (Lotrimin) or nystatin (Mycostatin). If nail damage occurs, it resolves slowly or incompletely.

Bacterial Paronychia

Bacterial paronychia, in contrast with fungal paronychia, ordinarily has a more acute onset, more pain and tenderness, and may be accompanied by localized vesicles or pustules. If material can be expressed from beneath the edge of the skin, it is frankly purulent. Involvement of only one finger is typical. The introduction of bacteria into the nail fold often results from traumatic removal of a hangnail. Diagnosis is confirmed and antibiotic sensitivity is determined from the exudate.

TREATMENT

Treatment includes administration of a systemic antibiotic and may require incision and drainage; lack of treatment can result in a closed-space infection or osteomyelitis.

Because the paronychias may lead to some destruction or distortion of the nail, they may be confused with other causes of nail dystrophy, such as tinea (onychomycosis). The other causes of nail changes are not accompanied by the tenderness, redness, or edema unless there is coexistent paronychia.

SUNLIGHT AND ITS CONSEQUENCES

Acute Reactions to Sunlight (Sunburn and Photosensitivity Reactions)

The most common reaction to acute sunlight exposure is sunburn, characterized by erythema in the exposed areas and sometimes accompanied by pain, swelling, and the formation of vesicles or bullae as occurs with first and second degree burns from other causes. The injury results from ultraviolet radiation from any source, especially the ultraviolet B and C spectrums. Relative susceptibility is in part determined by genetic factors, and some additional protection from sunburn is afforded by induced pigmentation, or tanning. Particularly when the sunburn does not fit the previous pattern for an individual, some thought should be given to the possibility of porphyria, phototoxicity, and photoallergy.

TREATMENT

In view of the self-limited nature of simple sunburn, it is essential that treatments cause no additional harm. Many commercial remedies fail that requirement due to their high cost and the potential for sensitization. Reasonable therapy for mild cases of sunburn includes avoidance of further acute exposure, soothing compresses with tap water or Burow's solution, and emollients for dry skin. Steroid lotions or sprays may also be used when justified by the symptoms present. Protection from recurrence depends on reduced exposure, controlled exposure to induced tanning, and the use of sunscreens or other barriers.

Phototoxic Reactions and Photoallergy

Phototoxic reactions refer to the hastening or exacerbation of sunburn due to the combined action of sunlight and a chemical applied to the skin or ingested. These reactions are said to be reproducible in almost anyone if the dosage of chemical and sunlight is sufficient. Phototoxic reactions are also called photoallergic contact dermatitis in some sources. Examples of the offending substances include certain plants, tetracycline, psoralens, hexachlorophene (used in some bath soaps), and unfortunately, the para-aminobenzoic acid esters found in some sunscreens.

Photoallergy is an immune-mediated process requiring sensitization to the causative agent. Sulfonamides, thiazides, and chlorpromazine (Thorazine) are examples. The resulting rash may have eczematous and papular components and may involve areas of the skin not exposed to sunlight. For clinical purposes, the distinction between photoallergy and phototoxicity is not critical.

TREATMENT

Therapy is based on avoidance of the offending agent and treatment of the eczematous component.

Porphyria Cutanea Tarda

Porphyria cutanea tarda might be considered a photoallergy to endogenous agents, i.e., the circulating porphyrins that lead to a bullous eruption and characteristic urine findings (dark discoloration and red fluorescence under Wood's light).

Repeated or Chronic Sunlight Exposure

Prolonged exposure to sunlight or to ultraviolet radiation from artificial sources can produce skin damage, which is ameliorated to some extent by the natural protection of skin pigments. The damage falls into two broad categories, carcinogenesis and the conditions called dermatoheliosis:

Skin Cancer	Dermatoheliosis
Basal cell cancer	Solar keratoses
Squamous cell cancer	Solar lentigo
Melanoma	Aging, wrinkles, telangiectasia

The cumulative effects of ultraviolet exposure to ultraviolet light are *directly* related to the intensity and duration of the exposure and *inversely* related to the effectiveness of natural protection due to skin color, tanning ability, and mechanisms of skin repair.

TREATMENT

Logical measures to reduce the lifetime burden of radiation include avoidance of midday sun, use of protective clothing, and controlled exposure to increase protective tanning. Consistent use of sunscreens is also helpful. The simplest agents are the physical barriers, including combinations of titanium oxide, zinc oxide, iron oxide, or red veterinary petrolatum. They offer effective protection for small areas but are usually less acceptable cosmetically than the transparent sunscreens. The new commercial preparations in bright colors may help solve the problem with cosmetic appearance and acceptance.

The chemical sunscreens are colorless or invisible on the skin and reduce the penetration of ultraviolet radiation. Relative effectiveness of these preparations is stated numerically as a "sun protection factor," which have been adopted for comparisons by the Food and Drug Administration; a higher number means greater protection. The sun protection factor for a given product is determined by comparing the dosage of sunlight required to produce erythema both with the product and without it. In addition, other properties of importance for the sunscreens include resistance to sweating and water immersion, ease of application, and propensity to cause phototoxicity or other adverse reactions. As a rule of thumb, fair-skinned individuals should probably use a product with a high number (15 to 30), whereas those with darker skin who tan more easily can use a lower number (4 to 10). Adverse reactions should prompt change to another agent with different ingredients. Table 51–3 shows a representative sample of sunscreen formulas.

AIDS-ASSOCIATED CONDITIONS

Acquired immune deficiency syndrome (AIDS) can cause a variety of immunologic defects, which in turn can result in several kinds of abnormalities of the skin and the mucous membranes. Most of these are infectious, but some other dermatoses are promoted by AIDS. The following discussion emphasizes key clinical features and recognition of the more common manifestations, which indeed may be early clues that the syndrome exists.

Table 51–3. SUNSCREENS

Category/Trade Name	SPF
Para-Aminobenzoic Acid	
Pre-Sun 15	15
Pabanol	15
Para-Aminobenzoic Acid ester:	
Block out	6 to 8
PABAFILM	6 to 8
Sundown	8 to 10
Para-Aminobenzoic Acid combinations:	
Total Eclipse-15	15 to 18
Sundown-15	15 to 20
Bain de Soleil	15 to 18
Non-Para-Aminobenzoic Acid	
Piz Buin-8	15 to 20
UVAL	10 to 12

Kaposi's Sarcoma

Kaposi's sarcoma (idiopathic hemorrhagic sarcoma) is a multifocal neoplasm with vascular tumors in the skin and other organs. The variety associated with AIDS is sometimes called "epidemic" Kaposi's sarcoma to distinguish it from the classical form described in elderly patients of eastern European, Jewish, or African origin. It begins as a violaceous or reddish pink macule that develops quickly into a nodule or plaquelike tumor of 1 to 3 cm. in diameter. There are usually multiple lesions located on the extremities (Fig. 51–48), and they sometimes become confluent and may ulcerate. Discomfort is uncommon unless there is irritation by clothing. The affected extremity may be enlarged due to edema. Biopsy will distinguish the lesions from other tumor-like growths on the extremities. Several treatment methods are used, depending on the clinical circumstances, but recurrences are common.

Although melanoma and some other tumors have been found in AIDS patients, no pathophysiologic relationships are established.

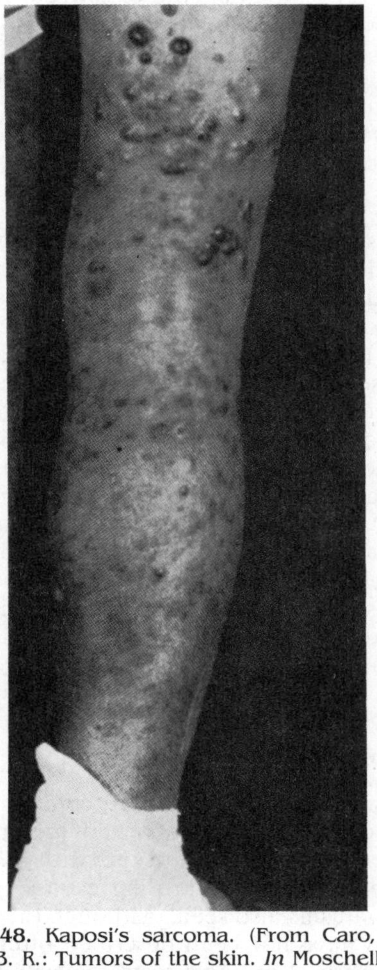

Figure 51–48. Kaposi's sarcoma. (From Caro, W. A., and Bronstein, B. R.: Tumors of the skin. *In* Moschella, S. L., and Hurley, H. J. [Eds.]: Dermatology. 2nd ed. Philadelphia, W. B. Saunders Company, 1985, p. 1612.)

Dermatoses

Seborrheic dermatitis is found in more than three fourths of patients with AIDS late in the course of disease, and it is frequently severe and generalized. Generalized redness of the skin and xerosis are also common. Psoriasis, pityriasis rosea, and ichthyosis have been reported less often. Reported vascular manifestations include angiomas, petechiae, telangiectasis, purpura, and splinter hemorrhages of the nail beds.

Fungal Infections

Candida infections may be found in multiple locations, the most common of which is the mouth, descending into the esophagus. Typical white plaques are seen on the tongue and oral mucosa, with sore throat and dysphagia. If necessary, esophagoscopy confirms the esophageal component. As the number of T helper cells drops, *Candida* lesions increase in severity. Treatment with topical agents such as miconazole or nystatin is effective for the milder cases, with systemic ketoconazole used for the difficult cases.

Tinea versicolor and the superficial fungi commonly affect AIDS patients, and may be relatively resistant to standard therapy.

Cryptococcosis, histoplasmosis, sporotrichosis, and other fungi have also been identified, fairly often in disseminated form or with atypical presentations.

Viral Infections

Herpes simplex infections are present in most patients with AIDS. The lesions tend to exhibit erosion and ulceration rather than the classical vesicular eruption and are more widespread. Lesions are commonly located in the perirectal and oral areas.

Molluscum contagiosum is also very common in the oral, genital, and rectal areas. Confirmation by culture and biopsy is probably appropriate, since similar lesions have been reported due to histoplasmosis and cryptococcosis. Anogenital warts are often a problem, but the specific role of immunodeficiency states is not known.

Both chickenpox and herpes zoster are common occurrences, with relative severity paralleling the decreasing number of T helper cells. The onset of herpes zoster in an unusually young patient justifies at least a thorough history of AIDS risk factors.

Bacterial Infections

Bacterial skin infections are common, particularly in those AIDS patients who are intravenous drug abusers. Localized infections with *Staphylococcus* or *Streptococcus* are leading causes, with some unusual organisms also seen. Although the associated skin lesions have not been described often in AIDS patients, positive serologic tests for syphilis are not unusual.

OTHER COMMON LESIONS

Xerosis (Dry Skin)

Xerosis is really a rather simple condition of the skin that has some features that suggest disease. A patient with dry skin commonly presents with a chief complaint of itching. It occurs most often in the elderly but may be seen in patients of all ages, depending upon their environment and bathing habits. Occurrence increases during cold, dry weather. The history may include excessive bathing (sometimes as a misdirected treatment for itching) and the use of strong detergent bath soaps. Upon close inspection, the skin appears dry, with excoriations and fine fissures or scales. Occasionally, patches of eczema develop.

TREATMENT

In the right setting of history and examination, dry skin should be considered *first* as the cause of generalized itching, before the more exotic differential diagnoses. Treatment is logical and consists entirely of efforts to preserve skin moisture. Patients should limit bathing to reasonable frequency in water that is not too hot. They should use bland soap, such as Ivory or Basic, or a soap that includes a lubricating base, such as Dove. The application of skin lubricants immediately after bathing is helpful, such as Aquacare HP, Neutraplus, or others. Short term therapy with oral antihistamines may be indicated.

Skin Tag (Acrochordon)

Most people develop at least a few skin tags during middle or late adulthood. Most lesions are small, pedunculated, flesh-colored, and soft, but some can be several centimeters in size and a few are darkly pigmented. They are commonly located on the face, upper chest, and intertriginous areas. The tags are completely asymptomatic unless they become irritated by clothing or when the pedicle twists and causes infarction. Sometimes, they fall off spontaneously or may be accidentally removed by the patient during shaving or some other activity.

Although the diagnosis is usually evident, the pigmented skin tags may cause some concern, and biopsy will confirm the diagnosis and reassure the patient. Patients may also request removal of the skin tag due to repeated irritation or for cosmetic reasons; options include simple amputation at the base, excision, and destruction by liquid nitrogen.

Dermatofibroma (Histiocytoma)

Dermatofibroma is a benign nodule usually found on the leg and is more common in women. The lesion is usually firm, round, less than 1 cm. in diameter, and ranges in color from pink to red or purple. It is fixed to the skin but not to underlying tissues. The lesions tend to be stable for many years and are often mentioned by patients as an afterthought. Occasionally confusion might occur with a mole, wart, or keloid, which is easily resolved by excisional biopsy.

Senile Hemangioma (Senile Angioma, Cherry Angioma, Cherry Spot)

Senile hemangiomas are small (2 to 4 mm.), raised, red or purple lesions that occur primarily on the trunk of middle-aged and older adults. They are usually multiple and may be associated with tiny petechia-like spots. They persist indefinitely, but they are completely benign and do not require treatment. If removal is desired for cosmetic reasons, desiccation and curettage is used or destruction with liquid nitrogen may be effective.

Pyogenic Granuloma

Pyogenic granuloma is a pedunculated or sessile, red or purple, polypoid benign tumor composed of highly vascular granulation tissue. It often occurs at sites of trauma or infection, but in spite of the name, no infectious etiology is proved. Although it is benign, pyogenic granuloma grows rapidly and bleeds easily with minor trauma. Clinically, it may be confused with Kaposi's sarcoma, metastatic renal cell carcinoma, or malignant melanoma. Surgical excision is the treatment of choice.

Lipoma

A lipoma is a benign tumor composed of mature adipose cells. It is flesh-colored, soft or rubbery in consistency, and sometimes lobulated. Lesions may be single or multiple. A neurofibroma may have similar appearance but is usually distinguished by other clinical features of Von Recklinghausen's disease. If removal is justified due to sudden enlargement or for cosmetic reasons, excision is used. If the tissue does not look like normal fat on gross examination, it should be submitted for histologic examination.

Diaper Rash

There are four common causes of diaper rash, but an individual patient may have combinations of causative factors. Most rashes in the area are due to irritant or contact dermatitis, *Candida* infection, or bacterial infection. A few are due to seborrheic dermatitis, which is usually recognized by its coexistence in other typical areas such as the scalp (cradle cap) and face.

Irritant or contact dermatitis appears as simple redness in the area, with distinct borders at the diaper edges and sparing of the skin folds. *Candida* infections are characterized by a dark red rash including satellite papules and pustules, with the skin folds more likely to be involved. The differentiation of *Candida* infections from atypical cases of seborrheic dermatitis may require fungal cultures. Bacterial infections are often a complication secondary to other causes but also may represent a localized occurrence of impetigo contagiosa or bullous impetigo.

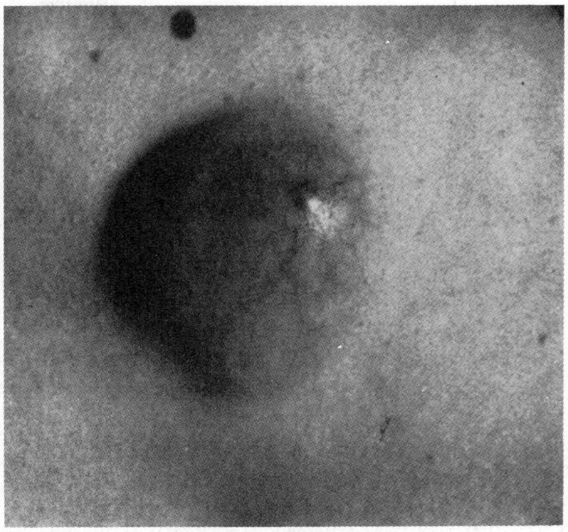

Figure 51–49. Sebaceous cyst. (From Caro, W. A., and Bronstein, B. R.: Tumors of the skin. *In* Moschella, S. L., and Hurley, H. J. [Eds.]: Dermatology. 2nd ed. Philadelphia, W. B. Saunders Company, 1985, p. 1540.)

Treatment

In general, the treatment of diaper rash should include frequent diaper changes, careful cleansing to remove urine and feces, and the avoidance of plastic pants or other occlusive clothing. For irritant or contact dermatitis, those simple measures may suffice. Though true contact dermatitis is probably uncommon, a change in the type of diapers or laundering method is worthwhile for resistant or recurrent episodes. Some physicians would recommend a brief course of hydrocortisone cream, 0.5 per cent or 1 per cent, or a protective agent like zinc oxide ointment, Desitin, or A & D Ointment. Those with bacterial infections should also receive an appropriate systemic antibiotic such as penicillin or erythromycin. Those with *Candida* infection are treated with topical nystatin (Mycostatin) cream. If irritation and *Candida* infection both appear to be involved, nystatin cream and hydrocortisone cream 1 per cent can be combined in equal parts, or nystatin with triamcinolone (Mycolog) may be useful.

Sebaceous Cyst (Epidermoid Cyst, Epidermal Cyst)

A sebaceous or epidermal cyst (Fig. 51–49) is a fairly firm, smooth, flesh-colored nodule with a small central pore. The cyst may be found almost anywhere on the body but most often on the face, scalp, neck and back. The size ranges from a few millimeters to about 5 cm. The cyst is filled by a foul-smelling, semisolid keratin material, surrounded by a cyst wall.

The lesion is normally asymptomatic but may become red and tender with infection.

Treatment

Treatment is incision and removal of the entire cyst and its contents. All of the cyst wall must be removed to ensure a cure. Depending on the degree of past and present inflammation, that feat may not be as easy as it sounds. One suggested method is to use a narrow skin ellipse that includes the pore, followed by sharp and blunt dissection to remove the cyst and its contents en bloc. Others favor the use of a 4-mm. skin punch to remove a plug of skin containing the pore, expression of the contents, and then sharp curettage to remove the cyst wall. If the cyst is obviously infected, it may be more prudent to incise and drain it, pack it temporarily with Iodoform gauze, and consider definitive removal after the inflammation subsides.

References

Abramowicz, M.: Clobetasol—a potent new topical corticosteroid. Med. Lett., *28*(715), 1986. *Contains a succinct list of topical steroids, organized into sections by relative potency, with representative costs.*

Abramowicz, M.: Sunscreens. Med. Lett., *30*:768, 1988.

Arndt, K. A.: Manual of Dermatologic Therapeutics. Boston, Little, Brown, & Company, Inc. 1978. *An easily readable, practical approach to dermatologic therapy, with limited information about diagnosis.*

Burnett, J. W., and Robinson, H. M., Jr.: Clinical Dermatology for Students and Practitioners. New York, Yorke Medical Books, 1978. *Well-organized, brief summaries of common conditions and a section that summarizes general principles of diagnosis and management.*

Fitzpatrick, Thomas B. et al.: Dermatology in General Medicine. New York, McGraw-Hill, 1987. *A comprehensive reference text; more detailed information than is needed for typical daily use.*

Lazarus, G. S., and Goldsmith, L. A.: Diagnosis of Skin Disease. Philadelphia, F. A. Davis, 1980. *An effort to simplify differential diagnosis; organization of the text is based on descriptions of lesions rather than clinical entities. No therapy is discussed; no color photographs.*

Lookingbill, D. P.: Principles of Dermatology. Philadelphia, W. B. Saunders, 1986.

Moschella, S., and Hurley, H.: Dermatology. Philadelphia, W. B. Saunders, 1985. *A well-balanced presentation of both photographs and text.*

Reeves, J. R. T., and Maibach, H.: Clinical Dermatology Illustrated. Baltimore, Williams & Wilkins, 1986. *Superb color photographs accompanied by summaries of clinical features and treatment. Also includes a series of patient guides and a formulary of common treatments.*

Sauer, G. C.: Manual of Skin Diseases. Philadelphia, J. B. Lippincott, 1985.

52

Endocrinology

Collin Baker
Kay F. McFarland

Diabetes Mellitus

Diabetes mellitus, a metabolic disorder characterized by hyperglycemia, results from a deficiency or ineffectiveness of insulin. Eventually, diabetes affects most organ systems, the most significant changes taking place in the eyes, kidneys, blood vessels, and nerves. There is an unresolved controversy as to whether the pathologic changes seen in diabetes are due solely to abnormally high blood glucose levels or whether other unknown factors contribute to the development of the long-term complications. It is generally agreed, however, that the control of hyperglycemia is of great importance in diabetes management.

CLASSIFICATION

Diabetes mellitus may be divided into at least three categories that differ in both etiology and pathogenesis. Even within each category the natural history, clinical manifestations, and biochemical changes of the disease may show great variability. Distinction is made between Type I, insulin-dependent diabetes; Type II, non–insulin-dependent diabetes; and other types of diabetes.

Ten to twenty per cent of diabetic patients have Type I diabetes, characterized by absolute insulin deficiency and dependence on injected insulin to prevent ketosis and sustain life. The inability of the pancreas to produce insulin is believed to be due to direct damage of the islet cells by viral infection or other exogenous factors or to autoimmune destruction in genetically susceptible individuals. Type I diabetes also has been called juvenile-onset or brittle diabetes.

Type II diabetes, previously referred to as maturity-onset or stable diabetes, accounts for about 85 per cent of all cases. The abnormality in these patients is an ineffectiveness of insulin action rather than a total lack of insulin. Many cases can be controlled by diet, but some may require oral hypoglycemic agents or insulin for correction of persistent hyperglycemia. There is a greater familial occurrence of Type II diabetes than of Type I; in at least some patients with Type II diabetes, there is an autosomal dominant pattern of inheritance. Other types of diabetes, previously known as secondary diabetes, include cases of pancreatic disease, hormonal disorders, drug and chemically induced abnormalities, insulin receptor defects, and genetic syndromes that produce hyperglycemia.

CLINICAL MANIFESTATIONS

Type I diabetes may begin at any age, although the onset is usually before age 40. These patients present with signs of hyperglycemia, including the classic symptoms of polyuria, polydipsia, and recent weight loss in spite of increased intake of food. There also may be complaints of recent onset of headaches, blurred vision, fatigue, and malaise. Signs of recent weight loss and hepatomegaly frequently are the only significant physical findings. It is now rare for patients to present in frank ketoacidosis with dry mucous membranes, fruity breath, rapid deep respirations (Kussmaul breathing), and alterations of consciousness.

Type II, non–insulin-dependent diabetes mellitus

is frequently insidious in onset, lacking the classic triad of increased thirst, frequent urination, and weight loss. These patients, many of whom are quite obese and have a strong family history of diabetes, may present initially with blurred vision, vaginal and perineal pruritus, impotence, and paresthesias. Rapid weight loss is uncommon. The onset of Type II diabetes is often so subtle that it is discovered only in the course of examination for other, totally unrelated illnesses. The most frequent physical findings are retinopathy (microaneurysms, hemorrhages, exudates, proliferation of new vessels), neuromuscular changes (absent ankle reflexes, loss of vibratory sensation), and peripheral vascular disease (rubor on dependency, pallor on elevation, absent pedal pulses, gangrene). Because the signs may be subtle, evidence of target organ damage must be carefully searched for in every patient who is at high risk for developing Type II diabetes.

DIAGNOSIS

There is no clear line of demarcation between normal and abnormal glucose levels. This makes the definition of inappropriate hyperglycemia rather arbitrary and based primarily on statistical data. For example, the elderly commonly have blood sugar levels that are appreciably higher than those of young adults, yet in any age group the diagnosis of diabetes may be made on the basis of any one of the following:

1. A glucose level of greater than 250 mg./dl. in the presence of classic symptoms of diabetes (polyuria, polydipsia, and weight loss despite a good appetite)
2. A fasting blood sugar greater than 140 mg./dl. on more than one occasion
3. Following a 75-gram oral glucose load, a serum glucose level that equals or exceeds 200 mg./dl. twice within a 2-hour period

For the diagnosis of diabetes in pregnancy, the fasting blood sugar must exceed 105 mg./dl. on two occasions, or two of the following three values must be exceeded after a 100-gram oral glucose load: 190 mg./dl. at 1 hour; 165 mg./dl. at 2 hours; and 145 mg./dl. at 3 hours.

The Glucose Tolerance Test

The glucose tolerance test is greatly overused in the diagnosis of diabetes. If either the first or second criterion mentioned above is met, there is no need to do a glucose tolerance test. The most commonly accepted indications for the oral glucose tolerance test are the following:

1. Glycosuria in the absence of diagnostic hyperglycemia
2. Identification of unrecognized hyperglycemia in a patient with unexplained neuropathy, retinopathy, nephropathy, or skin lesions suggestive of diabetes
3. Abnormal screening glucose during pregnancy

A flat glucose tolerance curve, or one in which the peak glucose level rises less than 20 mg./dl. above the fasting level, is not, as is sometimes thought, abnormal and does not signify impending diabetes. Low curves of this type are observed in a significant number of young healthy adults. An individual's response to an oral glucose load may vary considerably on different days under identical conditions.

Two other categories of abnormal glucose tolerance should be mentioned. First, individuals whose glucose levels are between normal and those diagnostic of diabetes may be classified as having impaired glucose tolerance; this condition is frequently seen in obese people. Glucose tolerance may improve, especially if they lose weight, may remain unchanged on repeated testing, or may progress to frank diabetes.

Care must be used in interpreting the significance of an abnormal glucose level. Vigorous dieting or numerous drugs may render glucose levels abnormally low or impair glucose tolerance. Some of these drugs are listed in Table 52–1.

There are few data to indicate exactly how frequently screening glucose levels should be done. For patients at risk, such as those with obesity or a strong family history of non–insulin-dependent diabetes, a dipstick urine for glucose at each office visit and a postprandial or fasting glucose might be done at yearly intervals.

TREATMENT

The treatment plan for diabetes must be adapted to the needs and lifestyle of each individual in order to minimize the impact of the disease. Listening to the patient's concerns is the starting point, and a great deal of flexibility is necessary in planning a treatment regimen that is practical. In the absence of complications, emphasis is placed on achieving the best possible glucose levels with the least possible change in the patient's life style. With these factors in mind, the objectives of therapy in the rough order of their importance are:

1. Prevention of ketosis
2. Avoidance of severe hypoglycemic reactions
3. Maintenance of optimal body weight in adults and normal growth in children

Table 52–1. DRUGS ADVERSELY AFFECTING GLUCOSE TOLERANCE

Cimetidine	Indomethacin
Clonidine	Marijuana
Corticosteroids	Medroxyprogesterone
Ethanol	Morphine
Diuretics	Oral contraceptives
Haloperidol	Phenothiazines
Isoniazid	Phenytoin
Heparin	Propranolol
Lithium	Tricyclic antidepressants

4. Maintenance of glucose levels near normal at all times

Patients rarely need to be hospitalized in order to achieve better control. Treatment regimens are best initiated in the normal home setting where patients are active and where they manage their own dietary intake. Rarely, a patient may need to be hospitalized to discover the factors that contribute to hyperglycemia. The exception to the general rule of ambulatory management is made during pregnancy when normalization of the blood sugar should be achieved quickly in order to reduce the likelihood of complications in the infant.

Patient Education

The purpose of diabetes education is to encourage each patient to assume primary responsibility in the management of the disease, with the physician being solely a supportive consultant and supervisor. Patients must understand the basic principles of a healthy diet, the rational use of insulin or oral hypoglycemic agents, the effects of exercise and illness on glucose levels, home monitoring of blood sugar and urine ketone levels, and appropriate foot care. They must be able to recognize the symptoms and appropriate treatment of hyperglycemia and hypoglycemia. Smoking and excessive use of alcohol should definitely be discouraged. These basic principles of diabetic care should be explained in detail at the time of diagnosis and reviewed regularly thereafter. It is important that the level of instruction and the recommended regimen be individually tailored to each patient's specific needs, as this is essential to promote optimal psychologic and social adaptation.

Diet

The goals of the diabetic diet can best be achieved by making the dietary prescription as simple as possible and adapting it to the individual patient. The typical American diet is not nutritionally balanced, as it is high in both fat and sugar. However, eating habits are changing, owing to an increased awareness of the need to limit the intake of red meat, fried foods, and sugar-containing snacks, and to increase the amount of fiber in the form of bran, vegetables, and fruit. Dietary counseling that takes these factors into account from the first, patiently and gradually modifying the patient's eating habits, is much more likely to achieve success than an approach that hurriedly explains a rigid, restrictive dietary program.

When the major goals of the diabetic diet are kept in mind, the diabetic meal plan can be viewed as a healthy, nutritionally balanced diet rather than one that is restrictive. The emphasis should be placed on achieving and maintaining normal weight, regular timing of meals, avoidance of refined carbohydrates and saturated fats, and relative consistency of meal proportions from day to day. The regimen should be based on the following principles:

1. The total caloric intake should achieve and maintain optimal body weight based on the estimated ideal weight and the anticipated activity level of that individual. This may be calculated roughly as follows:

Males: 106 lb. for 5 feet plus 6 lb. for each additional inch

Females: 100 lb. for 5 feet plus 5 lb. for each additional inch

Using the calculated ideal weight, the total caloric requirement for 24 hours may be estimated as follows:

For inactive or overweight adult: ideal weight in pounds × 10

For adult engaged in average activity: ideal weight in pounds × 15

For very active adult: ideal weight in pounds × 20

The American Diabetes Association publishes a series of exchange diets that provide a way to regulate day to day consistency of caloric intake, while allowing considerable food variability. For those patients who are able to use them intelligently by adapting their dietary habits to the foods listed, they are of considerable value; they are not, however, a substitute for individual counseling. The services of a dietician or nurse who has been specially trained in dietary counseling are invaluable. Many patients with non–insulin-dependent diabetes who need to lose considerable weight may find joining Weight Watchers helpful. Such a program provides a well-balanced, structured dietary plan and increases motivation through weekly meetings.

2. To avoid hypoglycemic episodes, patients with insulin-dependent diabetes should normally eat their meals within a half hour of the same time each day. For patients who are particularly prone to hypoglycemic reactions, midafternoon and bedtime snacks should be added. The content of the meal is not as important as its timing in patients with widely fluctuating blood sugars.

3. In addition to avoiding candy, cake, pie, and other foods obviously high in sugar content, patients should be advised of the high sugar content of soft drinks, cookies, sherbet, ice milk, beer, wine, and canned fruits. Elimination of fried foods, limiting the intake of red meat and eggs to twice weekly, substituting skim milk for whole milk, and limiting the amount of cheese eaten will help reduce dietary fat. The use of a food diary may help discover unsuspected misconceptions that patients have about nutrition and the use of special diet foods that are expensive and are not needed.

However, unsweetened or artificially sweetened

canned foods, carbonated beverages, chewing gum, and desserts should be recommended in the place of those containing sugar. Alcohol does not directly require insulin for its metabolism and may be permitted in moderation in selected patients. Patients who are on weight reduction diets should remember that one ounce of liquor contains roughly 100 calories; sweet wines and beer contain a considerable number of calories in addition to sugar and should be avoided.

For insulin-dependent, Type I diabetic patients the emphasis is on regular timing and consistency of meals, rather than on the exact caloric content of the meals. The appetite is a more reliable indicator of caloric requirements than any technique of calculation, especially in diabetic children and adolescents, in whom activity levels vary widely. It is not uncommon for teenagers to consume more than 3000 calories a day without gaining weight.

On the other hand, obese non–insulin-dependent diabetic patients need to carefully restrict the total caloric content of their meals, with less importance being attached to the timing of meals unless hypoglycemic agents are being used. Consistent reduction of caloric intake is difficult for anyone, whether or not they have diabetes, and persistent encouragement and nonjudgmental acceptance are essential to maintaining a satisfactory physician-patient relationship.

Oral Hypoglycemic Agents

Few areas in medicine have been the subject of greater controversy than the role of the sulfonylurea drugs in the treatment of diabetes. The oral agents should be reserved for patients who are not ketosis-prone and in whom dietary management has failed in controlling symptoms related to hyperglycemia. Risk and benefits of insulin versus oral hypoglycemic agents should be thoroughly discussed with the patient before a decision of whether insulin or an oral agent is used.

Although there is no doubt that oral agents lower blood sugar, there is great variability in the consistency with which they do so. In addition to a significant primary failure rate, there is also a high secondary failure rate. Periodic monitoring of the blood sugar in all patients on sulfonylurea agents is necessary in order to discover possible loss of metabolic control as early as possible. When this occurs, the use of these drugs should be discontinued and insulin therapy instituted. In most cases, the combination of insulin and a sulfonylurea drug is not more effective than insulin alone.

The most commonly used oral agents are the sulfonylureas listed in Table 52–2. There are several mechanisms by which these drugs lower glucose levels, including augmenting endogenous insulin release, increasing insulin receptor sites, and enhancing glucose utilization within the cell. Most sulfonylureas are metabolized in the liver and are excreted by the kidney and liver. For this reason, their use is contraindicated in patients with liver disease, renal impairment, and heart failure and in patients with erratic or inadequate caloric intake. Serious prolonged hypoglycemia may occur with any of these agents and is particularly threatening in elderly patients. Other side effects of the sulfonylurea drugs are uncommon but include gastrointestinal symptoms, skin eruptions, cholestatic jaundice, hematologic reactions, and an occasional disulfiram-like reaction. Several oral agents, particularly chlorpropamide, may potentiate the effect of antidiuretic hormone on the distal renal tubule, resulting in hyponatremia and edema. Again, this may be more common and devastating in elderly patients. Drugs that affect the action or dosage of the oral hypoglycemic agents include chlorpromazine, thiazides, phenytoin, sulfonamides, propranolol, phenylbutazones, dicumarol, monoamine oxidase inhibitors, guanethidine, clofibrate, salicylates, and anabolic steroids. The newer sulfonylurea drugs, glyburide and glipizide, are no less effective and have slightly fewer side effects than the older or first-generation hypoglycemic agents.

Table 52–2. ORAL HYPOGLYCEMIC AGENTS

Drug	Dose Size	Therapeutic Range
Tolbutamide	500 mg.	500–2000 mg.
Chlorpropamide	100/250 mg.	100–500 mg.
Acetohexamide	250/500 mg.	250–1500 mg.
Tolazamide	100/250 mg.	100–500 mg.
Glyburide	25/2.5/5 mg.	2.5–20 mg.
Glipizide	5/10 mg.	5–30 mg.

Insulin

The goal of insulin therapy is to normalize blood glucose levels with the simplest possible regimen while avoiding the complications of therapy. If normal blood levels cannot be achieved through diet alone, the use of insulin is indicated in patients who (1) have symptomatic hyperglycemia; (2) develop hyperglycemia owing to infection, trauma, surgery, or the use of medications such as steroids; (3) are pregnant, whether or not they are symptomatic; (4) have ever had ketoacidosis.

Most patients may be started on insulin without hospitalization and certainly fine adjustments of the dose must be made when patients are eating their usual diet and participating in their normal activities. There may be considerable variability in the response to different insulin preparations, and doses should be modified based on the blood sugar, the patient's life style, work and exercise habits, situational and emotional stress, and general health. A list of the most commonly used types of insulin and their duration of action is found in Table 52–3.

Insulins having an intermediate range of action, such as NPH or lente, are usually used initially as maintenance therapy. A reasonable starting dose is a single dose of 0.5 unit per kg. body weight for children or 20 to 30 units for adults given before breakfast.

Table 52–3. DIFFERENCES IN ACTION OF THE INSULINS

Class	Preparation	Peak Activity	Duration of Activity
Rapid	Regular	2–4 hours	5–7 hours
	Semilente	2–8 hours	10–16 hours
Intermediate	NPH	6–14 hours	18–28 hours
	Lente	6–14 hours	18–28 hours
Prolonged	Ultralente	18–24 hours	30–36 hours

Since most patients with Type I diabetes will require at least two injections daily, some physicians initiate therapy with divided doses to avoid having patients feel that they are getting worse if a second dose is added later. Regardless of the type of insulin used, the total insulin requirement rarely exceeds 1.2 units per kg. per day. Doses in excess of this amount may actually lead to wider fluctuations or brittleness in Type I diabetic patients and steady weight gain in those with Type II diabetes. Guidelines for initial and maintenance doses of insulin are contained in Table 52–4.

Urine sugars are seldom used now to regulate insulin dosage. Changes in the dose of insulin are governed by the pattern of variation in glucose levels throughout the day. For example, if the blood sugar becomes elevated after breakfast, it may be necessary to add regular or semilente insulin before breakfast to control this early rise. If both early morning and evening blood sugars are high, two doses of intermediate-acting insulin may be recommended.

Changes in the doses of intermediate-acting insulin generally are not made more than once or twice weekly and then are made in increments of about 10 per cent. The major objective is to prevent hyperglycemia from occurring, rather than to treat an already elevated blood sugar (Table 52–5). The goal is to keep fasting levels below 140 mg./dl. and postprandial blood sugars below 200 mg./dl. while avoiding hypoglycemia at any time. Adding or subtracting 2 to 4 units of regular insulin before meals often is effective in modifying the effect of stress and diet changes on blood glucose levels.

It is usually easier to modify the diet by increasing snacks or the portions taken at meals than to alter insulin prior to anticipated strenuous exercise. Even during times of illness when the diabetic patient is not eating as much as usual, the dose of intermediate-acting insulin should not be decreased, as insulin need frequently is increased by infectious illnesses. However, if the patient is nauseated and vomiting and blood sugar levels are normal, the dose of regular insulin given before meals may need to be decreased.

Table 52–4. GUIDELINES FOR INSULIN DOSAGE*

	One Dose Daily	Two Doses Daily
Average starting dose	0.5 U./kg. before breakfast	0.7 U./kg. ⅔ before breakfast ⅓ before breakfast
Average maintenance dose	0.5 to 1.0 U./kg.	0.5 to 1 U./kg.
Ratio NPH or lente/regular	(NPH or lente)	NPH plus regular 2 NPH:1 regular before breakfast 1 NPH:1 regular before supper

*These dosages may be altered by 10 per cent every 3 to 4 days for nonhospitalized patients.

Urine acetone should also be checked when glucose levels are high or nausea and vomiting occur. Four or more units of regular insulin may be added before meals when there is significant hyperglycemia and ketonuria. If the urine acetone does not clear after one or two doses of additional regular insulin, the physician should be called for advice.

Patients who exhibit widely fluctuating blood sugar levels are almost always those with insulin-dependent, ketosis-prone diabetes. Although an insufficient amount of insulin is usually the cause of persistently elevated glucose levels, it is important to recognize that paradoxical hyperglycemia and ketonuria may follow the hypoglycemia caused by excessive insulin administration. This phenomenon, the Somogyi effect, is caused by the release of catecholamines, cortisol, growth hormone, glucagon, and other counter-regulatory hormones. The importance and frequency of the Somogyi effect are questioned, because it is impossible to determine whether hyperglycemia following an insulin reaction is due to the food eaten during the hyperglycemic reaction, the Somogyi effect, or both of these.

Clinical clues that the insulin dose may be too high are:

1. Hypoglycemia followed within a few hours by marked hyperglycemia
2. Onset of weight gain in an insulin-dependent patient who has significant hyperglycemia
3. Development of extreme brittleness unrelated to meals or activity
4. Significant glycosuria in the early morning with a history of nocturnal sweating or headache
5. Significant ketonuria without glycosuria
6. Unexplained increase in insulin requirements
7. Insulin requirements exceeding 1.2 units per kg. per day

Rather than continually increasing insulin doses in patients with widely fluctuating blood sugar levels, the proportion of short-, intermediate-, and long-acting insulin may need to be altered and the total dose decreased. Frequent blood sugar determinations are critical in determining whether hyperglycemia is a result of a previous hypoglycemic episode, requiring a decrease in the insulin dose, or the result of insulin deficiency, which is treated by increasing the insulin dose.

Mild local reactions to insulin are a common occurrence at the beginning of insulin therapy. Some patients will experience some redness and itching at the site of the injection for the first few days or

Table 52–5. GUIDELINES FOR MODIFYING DOSAGE*

Time of Hyperglycemia or Glycosuria	One Dose Daily A.M.	Two Doses Daily A.M. and P.M.
Fasting	Increase A.M. NPH† OR Change to ultralente OR Split dose to b.i.d.	Increase P.M. NPH
Between breakfast and lunch	Add or increase A.M. dose of regular	Add or increase A.M. dose of regular
Between lunch and supper	Increase regular or NPH	Increase regular or NPH in A.M. or add regular before lunch
After supper or at bedtime	Increase dose of NPH If both hyperglycemia and hypoglycemia occur, split dose to b.i.d.	Increase regular in P.M.

*These dosages may be altered by 10 per cent every 3 to 4 days for nonhospitalized patients.
†May use lente instead of NPH.

weeks; usually these local reactions cease to occur with continued use of insulin. If local reactions persist or become more severe, several strategems may be tried. First, if beef or pork insulin is being used, the patient may be switched to human insulin. If this is not effective, then lente insulin may be substituted for NPH insulin, thus avoiding the modifying protein protamine, another possible irritant.

Another option is to switch to an insulin manufactured by another company, as the diluent used may be slightly different and less irritating to that particular patient.

Systemic reactions, such as generalized urticaria and dyspnea, are signs of sensitivity to some component in the insulin preparation and should be treated like all other allergic reactions with epinephrine and steroids, depending on the severity of the reaction. Patients showing such sensitivity should be re-evaluated to consider whether the use of insulin is mandatory or whether it is possible for them to be treated with oral hypoglycemic agents. Obviously, in the ketoacidosis-prone diabetic patient, insulin therapy is essential and desensitization must be carried out, following which these patients should be given their insulin in divided doses at least twice daily.

The frequency of both local and systemic insulin allergy is much less common, now that highly purified forms of insulin are available. This is also true of lipoatrophy, a loss of subcutaneous tissue at the site of injection. This condition usually develops several months after the initiation of insulin therapy. Injection of human insulin into the areas of lipoatrophy frequently results in marked improvement or complete disappearance of the lesions within 2 or 3 months. Insulin hypertrophy causes lumps or mounds of fat to accumulate in the subcutaneous tissue. The current recommendation for this condition is the use of human insulin with rotation of injection sites and avoidance of the hypertrophied areas.

Finally, a rare and frequently unrecognized complication of insulin therapy is fluid retention or insulin edema. This most commonly occurs in patients who have had prolonged hyperglycemia and ketonuria followed by restoration of normal blood sugar levels with insulin therapy. Most cases clear spontaneously after a few days with no specific treatment.

Hypoglycemic Reactions

Hypoglycemia is a major complication of treatment with insulin as well as with oral hypoglycemic agents. The most common causes of hypoglycemia are omission or delay of meals and unusually heavy exercise; other common causes are chronic insulin overdose and errors in measuring and injecting insulin. Even changing the site of insulin administration from the legs to the arms, administering insulin after a hot shower, and massaging the injection site may increase the rate of absorption and lead to hypoglycemic reactions. Most of these causes can be discovered by taking a careful history and can be eliminated by proper education. Frequent hypoglycemic reactions that continue without explanation should suggest the possibility of renal insufficiency, hypothyroidism, adrenal insufficiency, or early pregnancy.

Insulin-dependent diabetic patients should be instructed always to have immediate access to sugar in some form and to wear a bracelet or necklace identifying them as having diabetes. They should be taught the symptoms of hypoglycemia and instructed to eat immediately if there is any possibility that they may be having an insulin reaction. The patient's family and friends should also be instructed regarding the symptoms that may occur during hypoglycemia, such as sweating, abnormal behavior, and impaired thinking.

Symptoms of hypoglycemia, especially in children, may be difficult to recognize. For example, the child may become irritable and cry without provocation or may be difficult to arouse in the morning or from a nap. A sudden change in behavior in any diabetic individual should be considered to be a sign of a hypoglycemic reaction until proven otherwise. Bizarre behavior may be mistaken for alcoholic intoxication, when actually it is the characteristic behavior of that individual when hypoglycemic. Excessive sweating, anxiety, headache, hunger, and sudden mood changes are also commonly seen during hypoglycemic reactions. Mild insulin reactions that respond quickly to oral administration of sugar are not thought to produce permanent brain damage.

Many patients become extremely uncooperative when they are hypoglycemic and must actually be forced to eat or drink a sweetened beverage. If the patient is able to swallow, commercially available glucose solutions or thick corn syrup may be placed in the patient's mouth. Liquids by mouth should not be given if the patient is unconscious, because of the danger of aspiration. If the patient is comatose, intravenous glucose or intramuscular glucagon should be given.

Monitoring Control

Blood sugar testing methods applicable to home use now offer the most accurate means of monitoring diabetic control and are of special value in patients who have insulin-dependent or gestational diabetes mellitus. A number of reflectance colorimeters for home glucose monitoring are available for less than $200 and are quite accurate when proper technique is used. Many of the newer instruments eliminate several steps in which errors could be made, making test results more reliable. The procedure for measuring blood glucose at home is further simplified by the use of automatic lancets that reduce the pain of a fingerstick. Usually, there is very good correlation between the capillary blood sugar obtained using home glucose monitoring and the values reported using automated instruments in a pathology laboratory.

Insulin-dependent diabetic patients should be encouraged to measure and record their blood sugar levels several times per week and more frequently during times of stress, such as during an illness or a change in daily routine (Fig. 52–1). During pregnancy, four or more blood sugar checks daily may be needed to insure the best possible glucose control. Type II non–insulin-dependent diabetic patients often find it reassuring to check their urine for sugar two or more times per week. When glycosuria occurs, they should be encouraged to monitor their blood sugar at home either by visibly reading the glucose test strip or by using a glucose meter. If problems, such as polyuria or weight gain, are noted, daily blood glucose monitoring should be encouraged.

Although the renal threshold for glucose increases with age and may change with impairment in renal function, most of the time when the urine sugar is negative, the blood sugar is under 200 mg./dl. Urine ketones should be checked if glycosuria is 2 per cent or over or if the blood sugar is greater than 250 mg./dl. A physician should be contacted if ketonuria persists for more than a few hours. Even when all urines are negative for both sugar and ketones, periodic monitoring of the blood sugar is necessary to assure that the levels remain close to normal, the goal being less than 140 mg./dl. fasting and 200 mg./dl. after meals at least 80 per cent of the time.

Glycated hemoglobin (also called glycohemoglobin, hemoglobin A1c, and glycosylated hemoglobin) is used as a measure of long-term control. The rate of attachment of glucose to hemoglobin is proportional to the degree and duration of hyperglycemia, and a single determination of glycated hemoglobin reflects roughly the mean glucose levels during the previous 8 weeks. This test is most valuable in insulin-dependent patients who have significant daily changes in glucose levels. Generally, the level of glycated hemoglobin in diabetic individuals can be kept within two percentage points of the upper limit of normal. Glycated hemoglobin levels are not of great value in non–insulin-dependent diabetic subjects, as fasting glucose determinations do not vary greatly from day to day and are an inexpensive and accurate measure of control. In addition to blood and urine glucose measurements and acetone determinations, careful records of the insulin dose administered, weight, changes in diet and exercise, intercurrent illness, menstruation, medications, and reactions should be kept to provide a profile of the response to therapy. Such records are the key to skillful management of diabetes. A sample form for use by the patient is shown in Figure 52–1.

Physicians will want to follow a number of additional parameters, as well as certain physical findings, in their diabetic patients. The physician's record should include headings for weight, blood pressure, insulin dosage, other medications taken, number or per cent of high and low home glucose values reported, frequency in timing of hypoglycemic reactions, and records of the office glucose and glycated hemoglobin measurements. Patients who are monitoring their own blood sugar at home should bring their instrument to the office at each visit in order to check their meter results against those obtained in the physician's office or a pathology laboratory. Also, provision should be made by the physician to record the results of periodic examination of the fundi, peripheral pulses, and vibratory sensation in the lower extremities.

Patients may need to be seen weekly or biweekly until blood sugar levels are reasonably stable and then the interval between visits may be extended. Both insulin–dependent and non—insulin-dependent diabetic patients who have no other problems may be seen as infrequently as twice per year. Overweight patients may need to be seen more often to encourage them to continue to lose weight or reinforce the need for more stringent dietary restriction.

KETOACIDOSIS

Patients with diabetic ketoacidosis usually present with nausea, vomiting, polyuria, and tachypnea; in

PATIENT'S DIABETIC RECORD

Name ____________________ Doctor ____________________

			BLOOD TESTS								BLOOD SUGAR		EVENTS AND COMMENTS
Month	Insulin/OHA		Brkfs		Lunch		Dinner		Bdtime		Time	Result	
Date	Time	Dose	S	A	S	A	S	A	S	A			

S = blood sugar; A = acetone.

Figure 52–1. Patient's diabetic record.

more severe cases, alterations of consciousness are seen. Frank coma is seen only rarely now but mild impairment of consciousness and lethargy are common. Children and young adults may present with a confusing picture of severe abdominal pain and may be misdiagnosed as having an acute abdomen if diabetes is not suspected. In patients who present with abdominal pain, tenderness with guarding and decreased bowel sounds may be present, but rebound tenderness is usually absent. On physical examination, the most striking abnormality is evidence of dehydration with dryness of the mucous membranes, poor skin turgor, rapid respiration with a fruity odor of the breath, hypotension, and increased pulse rate.

The diagnosis of ketoacidosis is established by finding a plasma glucose above 300 mg./dl., a strongly positive reaction for ketones in the urine, and acidosis with a pH less than 7.3 or a CO_2 below 18 mEq./dl. Initial laboratory studies should include a blood sugar, CO_2, potassium, blood urea nitrogen (BUN) or creatinine, and urinalysis. Blood gases may be helpful but are not essential. When the patient initially presents, a large indwelling needle or intravenous catheter should be placed first to obtain blood and then to infuse fluids rapidly.

Treatment

Therapy must be initiated immediately when the diagnosis is established. Basic therapy consists of administration of insulin, intravenous fluids, and potassium with close monitoring of the laboratory parameters. Initially 10 or more units of regular insulin are given via intravenous (I.V.) push, and regular insulin is continued in the I.V. fluids at a rate of 10 units per hour until the CO_2 rises to 18 mEq./dl. or more. Blood sugar levels are expected to fall at least 75 mg./dl. per hour. If the blood sugar does not fall this rapidly, the rate of insulin infusion should be doubled to assure a more rapid reduction in glucose levels. When the blood sugar reaches 250 mg./dl. or less, the intravenous rate of insulin administered should be slowed to try to keep the blood sugar in the range of 100 to 200 mg./dl (Table 52–6).

The use of intermediate-acting insulin may be begun when the patient is alert and ready to eat, the blood sugar is less than 250 mg./dl., and the CO_2 is 18 mg./dl. or more. Additional regular insulin still may need to be given every 4 hours in order to maintain the blood sugar within an acceptable range.

Most patients are quite dehydrated, and intravenous fluids should be given rapidly. The first liter usually is infused within the first 2 hours and then the rate is slowed to 150 to 300 ml. per hour until the patient is adequately rehydrated. Normal saline is used initially, but as soon as the blood sugar falls to 250 mg./dl. or below, the solution should be changed to 5 per cent dextrose/water at 150 to 200 ml. per hour. The high infusion rate is needed to help clear the serum of ketones. Intravenous glucose may be discontinued when the patient is alert and able to eat and drink.

Table 52–6. TREATMENT SCHEDULE FOR DIABETIC KETOACIDOSIS

Insulin	Fluids and Electrolytes
1. Regular insulin, 10 U. I.V. bolus, then 10 U./h. continuous infusion, or 10 U./h. I.M.	1. 0.9% NaCl IV—1 L. at 300–500 ml./hr., then 150–300 ml./hr. until blood sugar is below 250 mg./dl.
2. Double insulin dose if blood sugar fails to fall 75 mg./hr. during the first 3 hours	2. Potassium chloride—20 mEq./hr. until patient is eating; exclude hyperkalemia and check that urine output is adequate before starting KCl
3. Discontinue I.V. insulin when blood sugar 250 mg./dl, then	3. Glucose—D_5W at 150–300 ml./hr. after blood sugar is below 250 mg./dl.; discontinue when patient is eating and drinking well
4. Start regular insulin 10 U.S.Q. initially, and adjust dose q. 3–4 h., as needed	4. Bicarbonate not usually needed unless pH is below 6.9
5. Begin NPH or lente insulin after breakfast and after supper when patient is alert and eating and blood sugar is less than 250 mg./dl. and CO_2 is above 18 mg./dl.	5. Phosphate is not needed unless serum phosphorus is less than 1 mg./dl.

It is undesirable to administer bicarbonate unless the arterial pH is below 6.9 or coma and shock are present. In most cases of diabetic ketoacidosis, the acidosis will correct simply with adequate fluids and insulin. Bicarbonate when administered rapidly may decrease respiratory drive in a severely acidotic patient and may necessitate more rapid replacement of potassium.

Potassium should be given as soon as it is established that the urine output is adequate and hyperkalemia has been excluded. As much as 20 mEq. of potassium chloride may be given each hour to maintain the serum potassium in the normal range. Potassium phosphate salts theoretically are of value, as phosphorus is also depleted in patients with ketoacidosis; however, the use of phosphates should be reserved for patients with a serum phosphorus level of less than 1 mg./dl. and who have normal renal function.

As soon as the patient's condition is stable, a search should be made for the precipitating causes of ketoacidosis. The most common causes are the omission of insulin, infection, or other illnesses or trauma. The reasons for omission of insulin are quite varied. Some patients simply deny that they have diabetes and stop taking insulin; others are afraid that they may become hypoglycemic if they take their insulin when they are not eating regularly. The cost of insulin may be a problem in a small number, and many patients have emotional factors that lead them to omit the required insulin.

Sore throat and urinary tract infections are the most common infections precipitating ketoacidosis. Blood and urine cultures should be obtained in any patient with fever who does not have an obvious site of infection. Leukocytosis is not a reliable sign of infection, for it may normally occur in diabetic ketoacidosis. Fever, however, is almost always a sign of infection, and antibiotics should be used empirically in diabetic patients presenting with fever and ketoacidosis, even if the source of the elevated temperature is obscure.

Early diagnosis and close monitoring of the patient are the most critical factors influencing the successful outcome of diabetic ketoacidosis. Blood sugar levels are usually checked every 1 to 2 hours by a fingerstick method and more precise glucose measurements, CO_2, and potassium levels monitored every 3 hours or so. Catheterization of the bladder is rarely needed, even in severely ill patients, and should be avoided if possible because of the risk of infection. When the CO_2 rises to 18 mEq./dl. and the patient is eating, the CO_2, blood sugar, and potassium may be monitored every 4 to 6 hours until the patient is completely stable.

Ketoacidosis may also recur rapidly in patients who have high circulating levels of organic acids, and, therefore, ketogenesis must be suppressed by the administration of fairly large doses of insulin. This, of course, may mean that the infusion rate of glucose may need to be increased to prevent hypoglycemia. Almost all patients in ketoacidosis will require replacement of potassium, for as the acidosis is corrected, hypokalemia may be accentuated. Therefore, potassium should be started early in the treatment course.

Other Causes of Acidosis

Metabolic acidosis with an increased anion gap is not always due to diabetic ketoacidosis. It may be due to the failure of excretion of inorganic acids, as in renal failure, or the presence of excess organic acids caused by increased production of lactate, ingestion of alcohol, salicylates, paraldehyde, methanol, or ethylene glycol or in starvation. A simple formula for calculating the anion gap is as follows:

$$\text{anion gap} = \text{Na} \pm (\text{CL} \pm \text{HCO}_3-)$$

$$(\text{normal} = \text{less than 12 mEq./l.})$$

Alcoholic ketoacidosis generally occurs in patients with a long history of excessive alcohol use, a recent history of binge drinking with little or no food intake, and recurrent vomiting. The fluid and electrolyte therapy outlined for the treatment of diabetic ketoacidosis can also be applied to patients with hyperglycemia and alcoholic ketoacidosis. When the blood sugar is normal, as in starvation or alcoholic ketoacidosis, exogenous insulin is not needed, as insulin release is induced by administration of intravenous glucose solutions. Bicarbonate therapy should not be used in alcoholic ketoacidosis unless the metabolic acidosis is life-threatening and then should be instituted only after calcium and magnesium are replaced to near-normal levels. Raising the pH rapidly with bicarbonate alters the binding of calcium by serum proteins and may precipitate tetany in patients with low calcium or magnesium levels.

Lactic acidosis is suspected when there is evidence of decreased tissue perfusion and no other obvious cause of acidosis. The diagnosis is verified by finding a plasma lactate level greater than 4 mEq./l. There is no specific therapy for lactic acidosis; therefore, attention is paid to trying to correct the suspected underlying cause. In the diabetic patient, myocardial infarction with decreased tissue perfusion is the most common cause of lactic acidosis and may not be initially suspected because of the absence of chest pain.

HYPEROSMOLAR HYPERGLYCEMIA

Hyperosmolar, nonketotic hyperglycemia usually occurs in elderly patients. It is characterized by marked elevation of the blood sugar, dehydration with prerenal azotemia, alterations of consciousness, and the absence of ketoacidosis. Blood sugar levels are usually over 600 mg./dl. and frequently exceed 1000 mg./dl.; serum or plasma osmolality is often elevated to more than 350 mOsm./kg. of water. About half of the patients with this life-threatening syndrome are not known to have diabetes, but many are on medications that impair glucose tolerance or predispose to dehydration. These drugs include glucocorticoids, diuretics, phenytoin, and beta blockers. Intravenous hyperalimentation and renal dialysis may also precipitate hyperosmolar hyperglycemia. Some patients develop the classic manifestations of symptomatic hyperglycemia, including polyuria and polydipsia, days to weeks before their significance is appreciated. Physicians should be alert to the possibility of hyperosmolar hyperglycemia whenever changes in consciousness occur in elderly patients.

Treatment

The therapy of hyperosmolar coma is nearly identical to that of diabetic ketoacidosis, with emphasis on correction of dehydration and the prevention of shock and hypokalemia. Isotonic solutions, such as normal saline, should be used initially, as they are more effective in rapidly expanding intravascular volume than hypotonic solutions. Insulin may be given by intermittent intravenous push or slowly by continuous infusion. Potassium chloride may be needed to prevent hypokalemia, but frequent monitoring of the serum potassium is necessary, especially if renal function is impaired. The prognosis is primarily dependent on the nature of the underlying cause and is also related to the duration and severity of the hyperosmolar state.

NEUROPATHY

Diabetic neuropathy may develop in either insulin-dependent or non–insulin-dependent diabetic patients, particularly in those who have had the disease for 10 years or more. The most common form of diabetic neuropathy is characterized by a symmetrical, slowly progressive sensory loss affecting the distal portion of the lower extremity or, paradoxically, by hyperesthesia and pain with nocturnal intensification. In the latter case, the patient complains of pain that begins after retiring and that is relieved somewhat by walking around. Ulcers may develop on the feet owing to repeated minor trauma, but these may go unrecognized and untreated because they are not usually painful. Sensation in the fingertips may be slightly diminished in patients who have had diabetes for a long time, but usually there is no pain or paresthesias in the hands.

Another form of neuropathy, mononeuropathy, is characterized by the sudden onset of unilateral pain, most often in an extraocular or thigh muscle. The etiology is thought to be ischemic infarction of the involved nerve; spontaneous recovery within 6 to 12 weeks is the rule. In some patients, the autonomic nervous system may be affected, resulting in orthostatic hypotension, vasomotor instability, anhydrosis, impotence, urinary retention, or gastrointestinal symptoms, such as diarrhea, constipation, or a malabsorption syndrome.

The diagnosis of symmetrical peripheral diabetic neuropathy may be verified by noting the absence of ankle reflexes and decreased vibratory sensation in the ankles and toes. Atrophy of the first dorsal interosseous muscles of the hands may be prominent, even in the absence of any history of sensory or motor loss involving the hands. Although the diagnosis is not difficult in the presence of the typical history and physical findings, certain important differential points should be noted. Almost all ulcers due to neuropathy will be over a pressure point and surrounded by callus; pain will be minimal, if present at all. Ulcers due to arterial occlusive disease, on the other hand, are usually very painful and the pain is not chiefly nocturnal as is the rule in neuropathy.

Treatment of symmetrical peripheral neuropathy is not very satisfactory. There is some evidence that normalization of the blood sugar is associated with increased nerve conduction velocity; however, the symptoms may actually get worse early during normalization of the blood sugar. Treatment is, therefore, chiefly symptomatic. A number of drugs have been used in an attempt to relieve pain and dysesthesias, but their efficacy is difficult to evaluate. Amitriptyline may be effective in promoting sleep and reducing symptoms; phenytoin and fluphenazine have also been found to be helpful in some patients.

Probably the most important aspect of treatment is education of the patient in proper foot care. The patient should be taught to examine the feet carefully for evidence of trauma, since the reduction in sensation may result in small lesions being overlooked. The patient must wear shoes at all times and avoid open-toed shoes and sandals. The temperature of bath water should be checked with the hand before placing the feet into it. Heating pads are definitely contraindicated, and patients should be instructed never to cut calluses on their feet but to leave this to the physician or podiatrist.

Treatment of autonomic involvement is empiric, symptomatic, and supportive. The best treatment for bladder neuropathy, for example, is to encourage frequent urination with the application of suprapubic pressure. Repeated catheterization should be avoided unless other methods are ineffective.

Gastric retention may be relieved with metoclopramide hydrochloride given before meals. Diabetic diarrhea, which may be due to altered gastrointestinal motility with development of a blind loop syndrome, occasionally will respond to a 10 to 14 day course of a broad-spectrum antibiotic. Treatment of impotence due to autonomic dysfunction is usually disappointing, but repeated penile injections of papaverine or the use of a surgically placed penile implant may produce satisfactory results. The need for education and counseling of the patient, of course, should not be overlooked.

NEPHROPATHY

Renal disease is a significant source of morbidity and mortality in patients with longstanding diabetes. Asymptomatic proteinuria is often the first manifestation of diabetic renal involvement. Impairment of creatinine clearance follows after a variable period of time—generally within 5 years of the appearance of proteinuria. Patients with diabetic neuropathy almost invariably show retinopathy also; in the absence of retinal changes, another explanation of the renal dysfunction should be sought.

The treatment of chronic renal disease due to diabetic neuropathy is similar to the management of other forms of chronic renal disease. Hypertension should be treated vigorously and urinary tract infections managed appropriately. It should be remembered that the development of renal disease may be associated with a marked reduction in exogenous insulin requirements. As in all cases of severe renal failure, chronic dialysis and renal transplant may be considered. It has been found that the survival rate of diabetic patients who receive a kidney is only slightly less than that of the non-diabetic patient and is superior to that of diabetic individuals undergoing chronic dialysis.

RETINOPATHY

Impaired vision in patients with diabetes may be caused by cataracts, glaucoma, retinal edema, refractive changes, or retinopathy. There is evidence that cataracts and refractive changes are directly related to changes in the blood sugar. Accumulation of sorbitol, a nondiffusible sugar alcohol, causes alteration in the shape of the lens and blurred vision in some patients with hyperglycemia. The abnormality may be accentuated for the first few days after the blood sugar is lowered owing to alteration of the osmotic gradient between the blood and the lens. Newly diagnosed diabetic patients should be assured that the blurred vision will resolve in a month or less, but refraction for glasses should be delayed for 6 weeks or more until control is stable.

Retinopathy is common in patients who have had diabetes for 10 or more years. Microaneurysms, which are minute aneurysmal dilatations of the retinal capillaries, are among the earliest lesions of diabetic retinopathy (Fig. 52–2). Hard, waxy exudates appear as yellow splotches on the retina due to extravasation of protein and lipid material from the retinal capillaries. The course of background or nonproliferative retinopathy is quite unpredictable, and, at present, there is no specific therapy for the condition. Tight control of the blood sugar is advocated, although it is hard to prove that there is a direct relationship between the blood sugar and the course of retinopathy. Proliferative retinopathy, on the other hand, is characterized by the appearance of a network of new vessels (Fig. 52–2*B*). These vessels are very friable and bleed easily. Hemorrhage from these capillaries into the vitreous results in marked visual impairment, and traction of fibrous tissue surrounding the new vessels may cause retinal detachment and result in permanent blindness.

There is substantial evidence that early treatment of proliferative retinopathy is beneficial. Treatment by photocoagulation tends to prevent the growth of new vessels and regression of those already present. All diabetic patients, therefore, should have a careful direct funduscopic examination at the time of the original diagnosis of diabetes and at intervals of 1 to 2 years thereafter. The appearance of any of the signs of retinopathy—hemorrhage, microaneurysms, or exudates—is an indication for referral for ophthalmologic consultation. Photocoagulation is advocated for new vessel formation on the disk or if there is neovascularization elsewhere with an associated vitreous hemorrhage. Expert ophthalmologic consultation and follow-up is essential to the management of diabetic retinopathy.

OTHER VASCULAR COMPLICATIONS

Gangrene involving the toes and feet is 50 to 70 times more frequent in diabetic patients than in those without diabetes. Rapidly progressive infection may threaten the life of the patient who has severe vascular insufficiency of the lower extremities, whether it is due to large vessel or small vessel disease. Erythema, heat, and exudate are signs of infection that must be

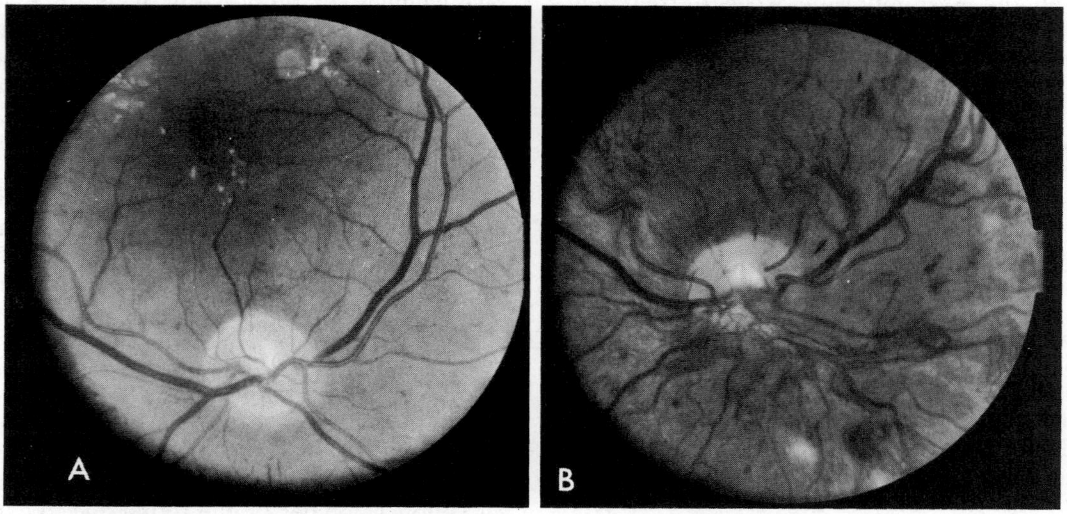

Figure 52–2. *A*, Background diabetic retinopathy with dot hemorrhages, microaneurysms, and early exudates. *B*, Proliferative diabetic retinopathy with neovascularization extending from the disc.

treated aggressively with antibiotics. Patients with ulceration, pain, and vascular insufficiency of the lower extremities should be hospitalized and treated vigorously.

The presence of gas in the tissues of the feet is not necessarily due to clostridial infection. In fact, it is more often due to infection with anaerobic streptococci, *Escherichia coli,* or *Bacteroides.* Whatever the causative agent, because of the poor vascular supply, the rate of healing is slow and the risk of recurrence is high. Frequently, extensive surgery is required and amputation may be necessary.

The clinical manifestations and pathologic findings associated with arteriosclerotic heart disease do not differ greatly in diabetic and non-diabetic patients; but the onset of arteriosclerotic changes may occur somewhat earlier. It is also important to note that myocardial ischemia and infarction are more often asymptomatic in diabetic individuals, particularly in diabetic women. Diabetic patients who have had a myocardial infarction have a higher incidence of heart failure and a higher mortality rate than those without diabetes.

DIABETES AND PREGNANCY

Maternal mortality and the development of long-term complications of diabetes are not appreciably altered by pregnancy. However, the perinatal mortality for infants of diabetic mothers remains three to four times that of other infants, and morbidity in the infant is common. The three factors that are considered to be most important in influencing the outcome of diabetic pregnancies are (1) maintenance of normoglycemia, (2) careful prenatal fetal assessment, and (3) expert care of the neonate. Close attention must be paid to maintenance of normal blood sugars from the time of conception until delivery.

Most pregnant patients are quite willing to accept regimentation of their eating habits and frequent monitoring of their blood sugar at home if they are counseled on the importance of these activities. The majority of patients can be taught to monitor their own blood sugars by the use of glucose-sensitive strips and a reflectance meter. When the accuracy of the home glucose measurements is verified, these values are used to regulate the insulin dose. Blood sugar measurements have completely replaced urine sugar levels as a means of monitoring control during pregnancy.

Insulin resistance increases as pregnancy advances, and, therefore, very high doses of insulin may be needed during the third trimester of pregnancy. Generally, during the first trimester of pregnancy there is little change in insulin need, and often the insulin dose must be decreased slightly to prevent insulin reactions. However, during the second trimester, and particularly early in the third trimester, there is an increase in the insulin need, and frequently the dose of insulin at the time of delivery is two or more times that required prior to the onset of pregnancy. Prenatal fetal assessment should begin at about 34 weeks of gestation, using nonstress tests. All deliveries of diabetic women should be done in a hospital that can provide intensive care for the newborn to assure the best possible outcome.

In view of the current successful outcome in most diabetic pregnancies, patients with long-standing diabetes should not be advised against having a baby. They should, however, be cautioned of the risk, ordeal, and additional expense that management of a diabetic pregnancy may entail. A summary of the approach to diagnosis and management of diabetes during pregnancy is given in Table 52–7.

Table 52–7. MANAGEMENT OF DIABETES DURING PREGNANCY

Screening
All obstetric patients except those with diabetes should have a screening blood sugar level 1 hour after 50 grams of glucose solution at 24 to 30 weeks of gestation.

Diagnosis
A 3-hour glucose tolerance (100 grams of glucose) should be obtained if
1. 50-gram screen exceeds 150 mg./dl.
2. Fasting glycosuria is present.
3. There is a past history of gestational diabetes.
4. There is a past history of a stillbirth.

Gestational diabetes is diagnosed when: fasting blood sugar is greater than 105 mg./dl. on two occasions or after a 100-gram oral glucose load; two glucose levels exceed: 190 mg./dl. at 1 hour, 165 mg./dl. at 2 hours, or 125 mg./dl. at 3 hours.

Diet
Should contain adequate calories to achieve a 25- to 30-pound weight gain, with emphasis on nutritionally balanced meals, regularity of meals and snacks, and avoidance of refined carbohydrates.

Insulin
Start insulin if
1. Fasting glucose exceeds 105 mg./dl.
2. Two-hour postprandial glucose exceeds 150 mg./dl.

Follow usual guidelines of insulin dosage, remembering that in the latter half of pregnancy large doses of insulin may be required. Most patients are controlled better on divided doses.

Fetal Assessment
1. Ultrasonography between 16 to 30 weeks to estimate fetal age
2. Nonstress test weekly starting at 34 weeks
3. Oxytocin challenge test if nonstress test is nonreactive

Delivery
Deliver at term if:
1. L/S ratio—3/1
2. Nonstress test reactive
3. Oxytocin challenge test negative
4. No history of stillbirth, evidence of pre-eclampsia, or other suspicion of increased fetal risk

Deliver as soon as L/S ratio is greater than 2/1 in high-risk infants.

Genetic Counseling

There is now much evidence that diabetes is a genetically heterogeneous group of disorders that share the common feature of glucose intolerance. This makes genetic counseling very difficult, because there are several different modes of inheritance. Overall, there is about a 10 per cent risk that the offspring of a diabetic individual will develop diabetes before age 65. The risk increases slightly when more than one person in the family is affected.

DIABETES AND SURGERY

The best possible diabetic control should be obtained in all patients prior to surgery except in the most urgent emergencies. Ideally, the fasting blood sugar should be below 140 mg./dl., and the postprandial level below 200 mg./dl. On the day of surgery and for the first 2 or 3 postoperative days, slightly higher blood sugar levels are acceptable, with the therapeutic range extending from 100 to 250 mg./dl. Since breakfast is withheld, an intravenous infusion of 5 per cent dextrose in water may be begun 2 to 4 hours before surgery and half the dose of intermediate-acting insulin given. A blood sugar is obtained in the recovery room and the other half of the insulin dose is given if the blood sugar is within the desired range. This dose may be adjusted up or down by perhaps 10 per cent, depending on the blood sugar level. Regular insulin is used for any additional insulin requirements.

Even though they may miss regular meals, patients rarely need less insulin on the day of surgery, and it is best to give insulin as outlined above rather than to wait until the blood sugar is elevated and use a sliding scale. Blood sugar determinations should be done periodically and extra regular insulin given if the levels are elevated. If, on the other hand, the levels are a bit lower than optimal, more intravenous glucose should be given. Approximately 150 to 200 grams of glucose is required every 24 hours to supply the tissues that preferentially use glucose, such as the brain, kidney, and red blood cells. Most commonly, 150 grams of dextrose is given in 3 liters of fluid intravenously during a 24-hour interval.

Serum glucose measurements, rather than urine glucose levels, are used to maintain control and adjust insulin dose. However, the urine should be tested at intervals for the presence of acetone, which would indicate the need for additional carbohydrate intake. The patient may be considered to be in satisfactory control when blood sugar is under 200 mg./dl., most urine sugars are negative, the patient is having no insulin reactions, and there is no acetone in the urine. The full preoperative dose of insulin will usually be needed even before the patient is eating regularly, because of the additional stress imposed by surgery.

Patients who are taking oral hypoglycemic agents before surgery need receive no hypoglycemic medications as long as their blood sugar remains below 250 mg./dl. An intermediate-acting insulin may be given in a dose of 25 units/24 hours, with extra regular insulin added if needed. Since insulin probably will be used only for a short period of time, it is recommended that human insulin be used as it causes less antibody response than beef or pork insulin.

A detailed flow sheet that accurately records fluid intake, insulin given, urine checks, and blood sugar determinations is essential to the postoperative management of the diabetic patient. The now deeply entrenched sliding scale method should be abandoned, and the blood sugar levels kept as normal as possible throughout the perioperative period.

Hypoglycemia

The frequency of occurrence of hypoglycemia has been greatly exaggerated in recent years by articles in lay magazines and books. It has become popular to employ the diagnosis of hypoglycemia to explain a wide variety of complaints ranging from depression to general malaise when, in fact, symptomatic hypoglycemia is uncommon. Plasma glucose concentrations normally are closely regulated between 60 and 120 mg./dl.

Hypoglycemia results when more glucose is extracted from the blood by the peripheral tissues than is absorbed from the diet or delivered from the liver. Hypoglycemia is most frequent during the neonatal period, when blood sugar levels may fall as low as 30 mg./dl. without serious consequences. In the adult, however, glucose levels in this range are uncommon and levels below 50 mg./dl. with symptoms establish the diagnosis of hypoglycemia.

ETIOLOGY

In certain circumstances, such as in normal athletes after strenuous exertion, a low blood sugar may be normal. Up to a third of healthy athletes who exercise to exhaustion have a glucose level of 45 mg./dl. or lower. This apparently does not impair athletic performance or endurance. Moderate degrees of exercise do not produce abnormal glucose levels (Table 52–8).

Some individuals produce too much insulin in response to meals. The classic method of diagnosis of this condition was formerly the 5-hour glucose tolerance test; the critical value usually was taken to be about 45 mg./dl. However, the glucose tolerance test is not reliable in the diagnosis of hypoglycemia because the differences in glucose levels reached between symptomatic and asymptomatic patients are not significantly different.

The majority of hypoglycemic reactions occur inadvertently in the patient receiving insulin, especially if the patient's diabetes is under tight control. The intentional production of hypoglycemia is uncommon, but it does occur, especially in hospital personnel and others in health-related fields. Oral hypoglycemic agents may also produce hypoglycemia, and their use is contraindicated in patients who have irregular eating habits or who suffer from renal insufficiency. Other drugs that rarely may cause or aggravate hypoglycemia are listed in Table 52–9.

Hypoglycemia resulting from heavy alcohol use with little or no food intake is the most common cause of secondary hypoglycemia. Chronic renal failure is another common cause of secondary hypoglycemia in hospitalized patients. Patients with chronic renal failure are prone to hypoglycemic attacks because they often have nausea, vomiting, and anorexia with depletion of glycogen stores and reduced gluconeogenesis. This state may be aggravated by several drugs, especially the beta blockers. Severely ill patients who have one or more glucose levels below 50 mg./dl. have a high mortality rate.

Pituitary or adrenal insufficiency and insulinoma can cause hypoglycemia. Since their occurrence is rare, the other factors described above should first be excluded. Patients with insulinoma, however, often have symptoms for weeks or months before the diagnosis is considered, and the bizarre behavior resulting from severe hypoglycemia is often attributed to a psychiatric disorder.

Table 52–8. CAUSES OF HYPOGLYCEMIA

Physiologic/reactive
Drug/alcohol-induced
Renal failure
Starvation
Adrenal/pituitary insufficiency
Infection
Insulin-secreting tumor
Extrapancreatic tumors
Neonate of diabetic mother
Erythroblastosis fetalis

Table 52–9. DRUGS THAT MAY MASK OR BLOCK RESPONSE TO HYPOGLYCEMIA

Psychotropics
Haloperidol
Lithium
Monoamine oxidase inhibitors
Anti-inflammatories
Phenylbutazone
Salicylates
Antibiotics
Chloramphenicol
Oxytetracycline
Trimethoprim-sulfamethoxazole
Miscellaneous
Dextropropoxyphene
Disopyramide
Pentamidine
Probenecid
Quinidine

CLINICAL MANIFESTATIONS

The symptoms of hypoglycemia are tremulousness, sweating, palpitations, anxiety, weakness, and hunger. These are nonspecific, as similar symptoms may occur in the absence of hypoglycemia. Likewise, low glucose levels may occur without any symptoms whatsoever—a fact that complicates the diagnostic process. A severe drop in glucose levels may produce headache, blurred vision, diplopia, lethargy, inappropriate affect, motor incoordination, bizarre behavior, seizures, and loss of consciousness (Table 52–10).

DIAGNOSIS

It must be emphasized that a low blood glucose does not in itself establish the diagnosis of hypoglycemia unless the onset of symptoms is coincident with a fall in the glucose level and the symptoms resolve when

Table 52–10. SIGNS AND SYMPTOMS OF HYPOGLYCEMIA*

Adrenergic	Cerebral
Tremulousness	Headache
Anxiety	Blurred vision/diplopia
Sweating	Incoherent speech
Hunger	Confusion
Palpitations	Inappropriate affect
Faintness	Incoordination
Weakness	Seizures
	Coma

*Signs in infants are nonspecific and include: tremors, cyanosis, apnea, irritability, and lethargy.

the blood sugar is restored to normal. If no sustained decrease in blood sugar can be demonstrated in the presence of symptoms, the symptoms are undoubtedly due to another cause. When both symptoms and a low glucose level are documented, further diagnostic evaluation to determine the etiology is warranted. Patients who are suspected of having hypoglycemia can be asked to check their own glucose levels at home whenever they develop symptoms. Even patients who are not accustomed to this procedure can be taught to read test strips visually with reasonable accuracy in one office visit. If the patient obtains low values at home, results should be confirmed by a reliable laboratory before the diagnosis is made. The normal range of fasting plasma glucose levels is 70 to 115 mg./dl. The diagnosis of hypoglycemia is confirmed by a laboratory report of below 50 and then only if typical symptoms were present.

Renal insufficiency and other systemic diseases that may produce low glucose levels should be ruled out by history and/or appropriate tests. Alcohol dependency should be considered in all cases and every drug that the patient is taking should be suspect, even if none are known to cause hypoglycemia. If all these studies are inconclusive, investigation of a possible pituitary or adrenal insufficiency is the next step. A computed tomography (CT) scan of the sella and luteinizing hormone (LH), follicle-stimulating hormone (FSH), thyroid-stimulating hormone (TSH), and T_4 levels is useful in evaluating the pituitary. Adrenal insufficiency may be excluded by means of the cosyntropin stimulation test, in which a baseline cortisol level is obtained and compared with another obtained after the injection of 0.25 mg. of cosyntropin, a synthetic adrenocorticotropic hormone (ACTH) preparation. The serum cortisol should rise to 21 μg./dl., or at least 11 μg./dl. over the baseline level, within 60 minutes after the injection.

If the adrenal and pituitary tests are normal, the possibility of hyperinsulinism becomes more likely. To evaluate this possibility, the glucose, insulin, and C-peptide levels should be determined every 12 hours during a 72-hour fast. An insulin-glucose ratio greater than 0.3 suggests the presence of an insulinoma. Self-induced hypoglycemia should also be considered, especially if the patient is a health worker or is taking insulin or an oral hypoglycemic agent. Intentional overdose of insulin is likely if C-peptide determinations are undetectable in the presence of high insulin levels. C-peptide that is not present in commercial insulin preparations is present in equimolar amounts in endogenously produced insulin. Use of oral hypoglycemic agents may be detected by urinary assays for sulfonylureas.

THE NONHYPOGLYCEMIC SYNDROME

Hypoglycemia is believed by many to be a common cause of chronic fatigue and depression. This belief leads to the prescription of low-carbohydrate diets without adequate evidence of true hypoglycemia. Surprisingly, some patients are improved by such a diet, even when no glucose abnormality can be demonstrated by rigid criteria. This is possibly because the rigid diet encourages regular meals and a degree of self-discipline that gives the patient a sense of stability and control.

Hypoglycemia is very uncommon in healthy children and adults. Its symptoms last for minutes or, at most, hours; chronic symptoms of increased heart rate, tremor, hunger, and anxiety are not due to hypoglycemia and are produced by the same sympathetic mechanism as that in true hypoglycemia.

Such patients may benefit from a dietary plan consisting of regular meals and snacks, but they should be reassured of the normality of their glucose metabolism—by repeated tests, if necessary. Most of all, they need empathy and understanding from the physician, which may encourage insight and lead the patient to obtain the counseling needed to reduce stress and conflict.

Thyroid Disorders

Abnormalities of thyroid size and function are among the most common disorders encountered in practice. These include (1) goiter—generalized enlargement of the gland, (2) nodular goiter—focal enlargement of glandular elements, (3) hyperthyroidism—excessive thyroid hormone production, and (4) hypothyroidism—decreased production of thyroid hormone. An irregular, firm (but not hard) enlargement of the thyroid without symptoms of hyperthyroidism or hypothyroidism is usually due to a nontoxic nodular goiter. A single, hard nodule raises the possibility of carcinoma, whereas a less firm nodule that is smooth and has a rubbery feel is likely to be a fluid-filled cyst. A symmetrical soft enlargement of the gland may be due to a colloid goiter, but a firmer, symmetrically enlarged gland is more likely to be caused by Hashimoto's thyroiditis. Pain associated with thyroid enlargement, often with a very firm gland, may be due to subacute thyroiditis or hemorrhage into a nodule.

THYROID FUNCTION TESTS

Generally, a history, physical examination, T_4 (serum thyroxine) level, and T_3 (triiodothyronine) uptake can establish with reasonable certainty the diagnosis when an abnormality of the thyroid is suspected. Occasionally, one of the other tests mentioned below will be needed either to establish the diagnosis, to identify the etiology of the thyroid dysfunction, or to follow the course of a patient who already has an identified thyroid abnormality. In cases of suspected hyperthyroidism in which the screening T_4 and T_3 are within normal limits, a T_3-radioimmunoassay may be the only abnormal thyroid test. The TSH level is useful in differentiating between hypothyroidism due to failure of the thyroid gland from that secondary to pituitary failure.

Fine needle aspiration of the thyroid is being used with increasing frequency to establish a diagnosis, particularly to exclude thyroid carcinoma in patients with thyroid enlargement. A technetium scan is of help in determining whether there is a cold nodule present and is generally used in patients in whom there is a suspicion of thyroid carcinoma. Thyroglobulin levels, although seldom used, may be helpful in following some patients who have been treated for thyroid carcinoma. Thyroid antibodies are helpful in establishing the diagnosis of Hashimoto's thyroiditis.

Serum Thyroxine (T_4)

The T_4, a measure of circulating thyroxine, in conjunction with the T_3 uptake is the most frequently used test to diagnose abnormalities in thyroid function. The most common causes of a high T_4 are hyperthyroidism and high levels of serum-binding proteins due to estrogen administration or pregnancy. Low serum thyroxine levels are most commonly due to hypothyroidism or to low serum-binding proteins caused by liver disease, malnutrition, severe illness, or administration of steroids or testosterone. Occasionally, low or elevated levels of serum-binding proteins are due to hereditary factors. The T_4, T_3 uptake, and free thyroxine index, which is calculated from the T_4 and T_3 uptake, are generally the only tests needed to assess thyroid function in patients who are felt to be euthyroid and in whom there is no suspicion of carcinoma.

Triiodothyronine (T_3) Uptake

T_3 red cell or resin uptake is not actually a test of thyroid function per se but is a relatively inexpensive method of estimating the level of thyroid-binding globulins (TBGs). The amount of T_3 that is bound to TBG depends on two factors, the amount of T_3 produced by the gland and the level of protein available to bind the hormone. As the level of TBG rises, the amount of bound T_3 also increases. TBG increases in patients who are on thyroid supplementation, as well as in pregnant patients. On the other hand, if there is a decrease in TBG, the amount of bound T_3 will decrease. This occurs in patients with chronic liver disease and those on androgens and other anabolic steroids.

There are a number of drugs that compete with the binding of T_3 to serum proteins; among the most common are phenytoin, heparin, salicylates, and clofibrate. The measurements of the T_4 and T_3 levels give an accurate assessment of the level of thyroid function only if the serum protein levels are normal. Therefore, the free thyroxine index (FTI) derived mathematically from the T_4 and the T_3 uptake provides a number that adjusts the measured T_4 for the circulating TBG. The T_4 or the T_3 uptake is seldom used alone as a measure of thyroid function, but they are used together to calculate the free thyroxine index, which reflects most accurately the level of thyroid function.

Thyroid-Stimulating Hormone

The measurement of TSH is of value in determining the etiology of hypothyroidism and detecting thyroid hormone failure prior to the development of clinically detectable hypothyroidism. As the thyroid begins to decompensate, serum thyroxine levels decrease slightly, causing the pituitary to secrete more TSH. In primary hypothyroidism from any cause, TSH elevation occurs in response to a subtle change in circulating thyroxine, and this effect may be noted prior to any change in the free thyroxine index. Very low or undetectable levels of TSH are found in patients with hypothalamic/pituitary disorders, but this does not differentiate these patients from normal, for the levels of TSH may be very low in euthyroid patients. The TSH is often low in patients with hyperthyroidism but really has very little diagnostic significance and is rarely helpful in delineating its cause.

Thyroid Antibodies

The finding of high levels of thyroid antibodies, specifically thyroglobulin and microsomal antibodies, aids in the diagnosis of autoimmune thyroiditis; low levels may occur in many other types of thyroid disease and are not of diagnostic value. Generally, thyroid antibodies are ordered when the diagnosis of Hashimoto's thyroiditis or transient painless thyroiditis is suspected.

Thyroglobulin Levels

Thyroglobulin is present in small amounts in euthyroid patients and at higher levels in those with hyperthyroidism and other thyroid abnormalities. Thyroglobulin levels are chiefly useful in following patients who have been treated for thyroid carcinoma. A rise in the thyroglobulin level is indicative of tumor recurrence or metastasis. Serial determinations are needed in following these patients.

Radioactive Iodine (^{131}I) Uptake

The ^{131}I uptake generally is not used as a test for thyroid function. Rather, it is helpful in establishing the etiology of hyperthyroidism or for choosing the dose of ^{131}I needed for therapy. The ^{131}I uptake is usually greatly increased in patients with Graves' disease and usually slightly elevated in those with toxic nodular goiter. Patients with hyperthyroidism due to subacute thyroiditis, autoimmune thyroiditis, or factitious hyperthyroidism have a low ^{131}I uptake. The test is not of value in diagnosing hypothyroidism because the uptake is influenced by the amount of iodine in the diet. This test should not be used in pregnant women, because ^{131}I will cross the placental barrier.

The ^{131}I uptake is determined by administering a tracer dose of the isotope and measuring its uptake by the thyroid gland at 6 and 24 hours. The uptake of the isotope is inversely proportional to the amount of iodine in the serum and the gland and is also dependent on the rate of iodine utilization by the thyroid gland. In most areas of the United States, the normal radioactive iodine uptake is below 25 per cent. Elevation of the ^{131}I uptake is most commonly due to hyperthyroidism and iodine deficiency. A low uptake is most frequently due to increased iodine in the diet, although it may also be found in hypothyroidism.

Thyroid Scan

A thyroid scan, using technetium 99, is useful in the investigation of patients in whom there is some question about the uniformity of the thyroid gland. The most common use is in determining whether a palpable nodule is a single nodule and, if so, whether it concentrates technetium (Fig. 52–3) or fails to take up the isotope and is cold. Functional nodules are very seldom malignant, whereas cold nodules have an incidence of carcinoma of between 10 and 20 per cent.

HYPERTHYROIDISM

Thyrotoxicosis or hyperthyroidism is a relatively common disorder with a prevalence rate of 19 per 1000 women and 1.6 per 1000 men. There is an annual incidence of 2 to 3 per 1000 women. Differentiation of the possible causes is important, because they differ not only in their natural history but also in the therapy required (Table 52–11). For example, hyperthyroidism associated with a diffuse goiter is usually caused by Graves' disease, subacute thyroiditis, or autoimmune thyroiditis. A single hyperfunctioning adenoma or a multinodular goiter may also produce hyperthyroidism. Less commonly, a small or normal-sized thyroid may be associated with hyperthyroidism caused by an excess exogenous thyroid or by painless thyroiditis. Other rare causes of hyperthyroidism are radiation thyroiditis, thyroid carcinoma, excessive TSH or TSH-like substances, and struma ovarii.

Clinical Manifestations

Some patients with hyperthyroidism initially present with subtle, nonspecific complaints, such as nervousness and fatigue, while others have an unmistakable constellation of symptoms, such as fullness in the throat, heat intolerance, increased sweating, and weight loss in spite of a good appetite. Other common complaints include tremulousness, insomnia, headache, palpitation, dyspnea, itching, burning, and excessive tearing of the eyes. Diarrhea is uncommon, but an increase in the number of bowel movements is frequent. Abdominal pain occasionally is a problem. Although the menstrual flow may be decreased in quantity, menstrual periods usually are regular or are just slightly irregular. Symptoms associated with hyperthyroidism are listed in order of relative frequency in Table 52–12.

Occasionally, patients with hyperthyroidism appear to be asymptomatic, but careful questioning usually reveals that the patient has some emotional lability, mild muscle weakness, or dyspnea on exertion. For example, many patients when specifically questioned will admit to using the handrail to pull themselves up the stairs because of weakness of their legs, and about three fourths will have some dyspnea on exertion. The inability to concentrate, forgetfulness, and lability in mood may negatively affect their job performance and interpersonal relationships, as well as interfere with therapy. Some patients will not be able to remember to take pills on a regular basis but become upset when a member of the family or a friend is asked to supervise the therapeutic program. Marital discord is very common, as patients are often emotionally labile, one minute completely agreeable and the next crying and despondent. Depression and withdrawal are more commonly seen in older patients, in contrast to mood lability and hyperkinesis in younger patients.

Physical Findings

The most characteristic physical findings of hyperthyroidism are enlargement of the thyroid gland, persistent tachycardia, and hyperkinesis. Lid lag and retraction, with a crescent of sclera visible over the iris, may be present in patients with hyperthyroidism of any etiology, whereas the classic eye signs of Graves' disease—periorbital edema, exophthalmos, conjunctivitis with tearing, and ocular muscle palsies—may occur with or without hyperthyroidism (Fig. 52–4).

The skin is as smooth as silk, and the hair is fine and brittle. Thinning of the hair, especially in the temporal regions, is common. Typical nail changes

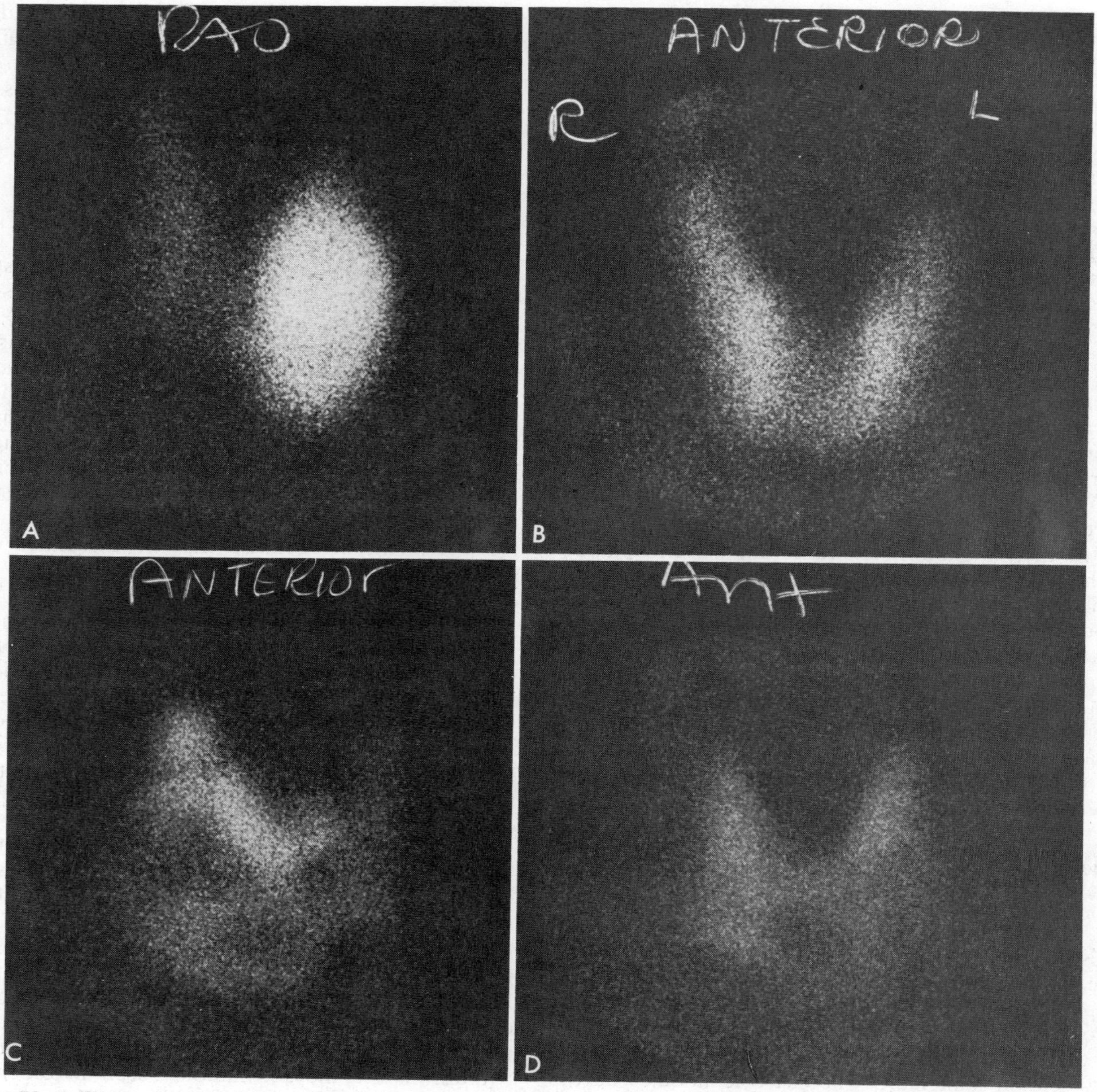

Figure 52–3. ^{131}I thyroid scan. *A,* Hyperfunctioning adenoma. *B,* Diffusely enlarged gland due to Graves' disease. *C,* Patchy uptake of a multinodular gland. *D,* Cold nodule, suspicious for malignancy.

involve separation of the distal nail from its bed, making it difficult to keep the fingernails clean. This change, called onycholysis or Plummer's nails (Fig. 52–5), is most commonly found on the fourth digit. The palms are red, warm, and moist. Sometimes the examiner can even feel heat radiating from the patient's hands without actually touching them. Other changes in the skin include vitiligo and hyperpigmentation. Vitiligo is present in about 7 per cent of patients with Graves' disease and is located primarily on the hands and feet.

Cardiac manifestations of hyperthyroidism are especially common in the older age groups. Tachycardia, a third heart sound, edema, and dyspnea may all be present with or without congestive heart failure. Atrial fibrillation, although present in only a small percentage of patients with hyperthyroidism, should always suggest the diagnosis. The arterial pulses are bounding, and the difference between the systolic and diastolic blood pressures is often greater than 70 mm. of mercury, with the systolic blood pressure being slightly elevated. One often detects a systolic ejection murmur and sometimes a more scratchy murmur in the left second intercostal space. The presence of a bruit over the thyroid is considered to be diagnostic of hyperthyroidism. Even in the absence of congestive heart failure, an increased respiratory rate is a very common finding.

Tremor may be striking, or, if not obvious, can often be demonstrated by having the patient extend

Table 52–11. ETIOLOGY OF HYPERTHYROIDISM

Disorder	Condition of Gland
Graves' disease	Diffusely enlarged
Toxic multinodular goiter	Nodular enlargement
Hyperfunctioning adenoma	Solitary nodule
Subacute thyroiditis	Tender enlargement
Autoimmune thyroiditis	Normal size or enlarged
Exogenous thyroid	Normal or small
Rare Causes	
Radiation thyroiditis	Normal
Thyroid carcinoma	Solitary nodule
Excessive TSH stimulation	Diffusely enlarged
Excessive iodine intake	Normal or enlarged
Struma ovarii	Normal or small
Trophoblastic disese	Normal or enlarged

the arm and spread the fingers. Myasthenia may be demonstrated even when patients are unaware of any weakness. Older patients, especially, may not be able to rise from an ordinary chair without assisting with their hands, and younger patients may not be able to stand up from a deep kneebend without assistance.

Diagnosis

A T_4 level, T_3 uptake, and the resultant free thyroxine index are the only tests needed in most cases to establish the diagnosis of hyperthyroidism. If the clinical impression is not substantiated by these tests, they should be repeated and a serum T_3 level by radioimmunoassay ordered. In the absence of obvious signs of Graves' disease, such as ophthalmopathy or pretibial myxedema, a radioiodine uptake may be helpful in ruling out transient or autoimmune thyroiditis. Thyroid antibodies also should be obtained if it is felt that the patient has thyrotoxicosis due to autoimmune thyroiditis, although this is relatively rare.

The typical patient with hyperthyroidism has several characteristic signs and symptoms including goiter and tachycardia, but the findings may vary considerably. Most of those in the younger age group have the typical findings of Graves' disease with ophthalmopathy, whereas patients in the older age group may appear less hyperkinetic but show signs of cardiac decompensation. The feel of the gland may be helpful in determining the etiology: a diffusely enlarged gland suggests Graves' disease or autoimmune thyroiditis; an irregular gland, toxic multinodular goiter; and a small gland with a single nodule, a hyperfunctioning adenoma.

Table 52–12. SIGNS AND SYMPTOMS OF HYPERTHYROIDISM*

Subjective Findings	Objective Findings
Nervousness	Goiter
Heat intolerance	Tachycardia
Palpitation	Tremor
Dyspnea	Hyperkinesis
Fatigue/weakness	Warm, moist hands
Weight loss	Thyroid bruit
Eye symptoms	Lid lag

*In relative order of frequency.

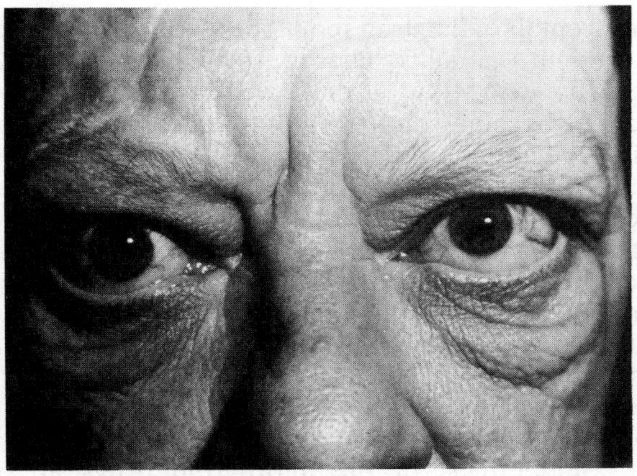

Figure 52–4. Ophthalmopathy of Graves' disease with periorbital edema, conjunctival injection, and extraocular muscle enlargement but little proptosis.

Treatment

Propylthiouracil and methimazole are the two most widely used drugs that inhibit thyroid hormone synthesis. The choice between these drugs is largely a matter of individual preference. Propylthiouracil inhibits extrathyroidal T_4 conversion to T_3 and because of this action may be the preferred drug when a rapid response to therapy is desired. Methimazole, on the other hand, has the advantage of coming in two dosage strengths, whereas propylthiouracil comes in only one. This, and the fact that methimazole has a longer half-life, may lead to better patient compliance, since fewer tablets are taken less frequently.

The basic drug regimen is to start with propylthiouracil, 400 mg. per day, or methimazole, 30 mg. per day. Often propylthiouracil is given four times daily and methimazole twice daily, but now there is evidence that propylthiouracil is effective given twice daily and methimazole given once daily. If there is any reaction to the antithyroid drug or if the patient finds that taking medication on a regular basis is

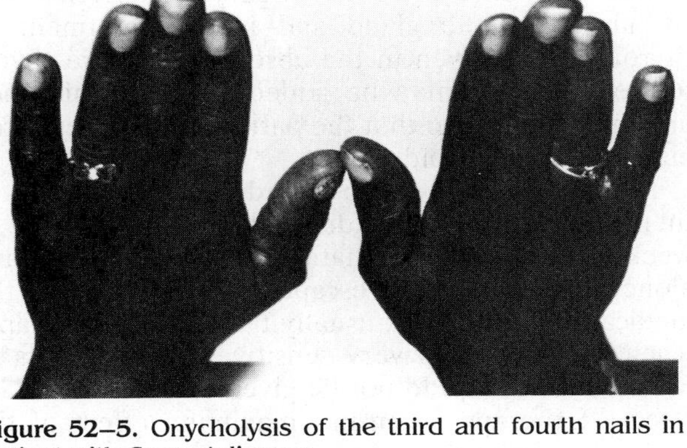

Figure 52–5. Onycholysis of the third and fourth nails in a patient with Graves' disease.

unacceptable, the drug should be stopped and another treatment modality chosen. Clinical improvement may be evident in 1 or 2 weeks, and usually the patient becomes euthyroid between 2 and 3 months after the initiation of therapy. If the antithyroid drugs fail to control the hyperthyroidism, one should suspect inadequate dose or noncompliance. Once the patient is euthyroid, the dose of antithyroid medication may be reduced by one third every couple of months as long as the hyperthyroidism is controlled. There is no clear indication of how long the drug should be continued after the patient has been rendered completely euthyroid, but commonly the drugs are continued for 6 months to a year.

Side effects of the antithyroid drugs are not uncommon, but fortunately most are mild and reversible. Rashes are common and may subside without treatment. More serious reactions include agranulocytosis, thrombocytopenia, anemia, hepatitis, arthritis, and fever.

Generally, a white blood cell count and liver enzymes are obtained at the start of therapy; these are repeated after that only if the patient develops new symptoms or signs suggestive of a toxic reaction. Continued periodic monitoring of the white count and liver function is not often helpful, because adverse reactions may develop rapidly even when these tests are normal. Patients should be instructed to contact their physician if they develop any new symptoms, particularly fever and sores on their lips or in the mouth, while on these drugs. When a severe reaction occurs, the medication should be stopped. It is then generally wise to give ^{131}I rather than to change to another antithyroid drug.

Inorganic iodine is rapidly effective in controlling hyperthyroidism, for it not only inhibits hormone synthesis but also prevents the release of thyroid hormone from the gland. Very small doses are needed, and two drops of saturated solution of potassium iodide in juice daily is more than adequate except during thyroid storm, when larger doses usually are required. Lithium carbonate acts like iodine in inhibiting thyroid synthesis and release, but because of its toxic effects should not be used routinely.

There are several well-accepted indications for iodine therapy. The most common is a 7 to 10 day course of iodine prior to surgery to decrease the vascularity of the gland and in the treatment of thyroid storm. Even in the absence of severe thyrotoxicosis, iodine may be added to propylthiouracil and methimazole so that the patient may be rendered euthyroid more rapidly.

Iodine should not be used as a sole form of therapy for hyperthyroidism, however, because a week or two after the initiation of therapy with iodine alone, there may be an escape from the effect of the medication. This is not usually true after ^{131}I therapy, when the thyroid is very sensitive to the effects of iodine. Iodine should not be given for at least 3 days after ^{131}I therapy to ensure maximum effect of the radioactive isotope.

Propranolol, the beta blocker that has been the most widely used in the treatment of hyperthyroidism, is effective in reducing the associated tachycardia, palpitations, heat intolerance, and nervousness. This drug does not normalize the metabolic rate, however, and should not be used alone in the treatment of hyperthyroidism except in cases of transient hyperthyroidism due to autoimmune thyroiditis. The usual dose is 40 to 200 mg. per day in divided doses.

Administration of radioactive iodine (^{131}I) is the simplest method of treatment of hyperthyroidism and is not only effective but relatively inexpensive. Antithyroid therapy often is used prior to and following ^{131}I treatment in severely symptomatic patients, because several months may elapse before the patient becomes euthyroid after treatment with the isotope alone. Another disadvantage of ^{131}I is that hypothyroidism is almost an invariable consequence of its use. Past concerns regarding a high risk of carcinoma of the thyroid, leukemia, or genetic damage to the offspring of a woman in child-bearing years have not been substantiated by follow-up of treated patients for more than 30 years. The amount of radiation to the ovaries from a therapeutic dose of ^{131}I is about the same or less than the radiation associated with an intravenous pyelogram or barium enema.

Several methods are used for calculating the ideal dose of ^{131}I, none of which produce predictable results. Most patients are given between 5 and 15 Ci of ^{131}I, the lower dose being given to patients with small glands and high uptakes, and higher doses to those with large glands and relatively low ^{131}I uptake. Most patients will be euthyroid within 3 to 6 months after therapy; a sizable number will become hypothyroid during the first year. As many as 3 per cent of the remaining patients will become hypothyroid each year for the next 20 years. Eventually, most patients treated with ^{131}I will become hypothyroid. Therefore, every patient who receives ^{131}I must understand that hypothyroidism is the expected consequence of therapy and that replacement therapy with thyroxine may be necessary for life.

Allergy to iodine does not preclude the use of ^{131}I because the amount of iodine used is very small. Pregnancy, however, is an absolute contraindication to ^{131}I therapy. Therefore, all women in the reproductive age group should be questioned about pregnancy, and a pregnancy test should be done if there is any possibility of pregnancy.

Surgical treatment of hyperthyroidism is used principally in the treatment of children and young adults who are unwilling or are unable to be treated with antithyroid drugs. Subtotal thyroidectomy may be the treatment of choice in patients with very large multinodular glands, particularly those whose iodine uptake is low, which makes treatment with ^{131}I ineffective. The advantage of surgery is that it is a definitive form of therapy that renders the patient euthyroid quickly. On the other hand, the risks are numerous, including the risk of general anesthesia possible injury to the recurrent laryngeal nerve with vocal cord paralysis, and the possibility of permanent hypothyroidism and/or hypoparathyroidism.

Patients who undergo thyroidectomy should first be rendered euthyroid with antithyroid medications and should receive a 7 to 10 day course of iodine preoperatively. Hyperthyroidism recurs in a small number of patients postoperatively; radioiodine should be used to treat these patients. In addition to the patients who are rendered hypothyroid immediately following surgery, 1 to 2 per cent will become hypothyroid each succeeding year and will require thyroid replacement therapy.

THYROID STORM

Thyroid storm is a severe form of hyperthyroidism and is life-threatening. The disease usually is precipitated in patients with hyperthyroidism by trauma or illness, although it also may occur in patients who have abruptly discontinued antithyroid medication. Although hyperthyroidism may not have been diagnosed previously, in most cases it will have been present for months.

Most of the usual signs of hyperthyroidism are present in patients with storm, but the clue to the diagnosis is the presence of fever in a patient with severe hyperthyroidism. Other striking features are tachycardia and marked agitation, even to the point of psychosis. It may be very difficult to determine whether the hyperthyroid patient with fever has thyroid storm, infection with fever, or both infection and thyroid storm. Patients with fever and significant hyperthyroidism, therefore, should be treated as if they were in thyroid storm. Institution of treatment should not await verification with thyroid function tests. Blood should be drawn for the necessary tests and the patient treated on clinical grounds as soon as thyroid storm is suspected. The diagnosis is confirmed if the T_4 and T_3 are found to be elevated and the patient rapidly responds to therapy.

Treatment of thyroid storm should begin with propylthiouracil 200 mg., every 4 hours. If the patient is unable to swallow the tablets, they may be crushed and put down a nasogastric tube; a parenteral form of the medication is not available. Iodine is subsequently given, preferably orally but intravenously if necessary. Five drops of saturated solution of potassium iodine are given orally four times daily; the intravenous dose is 10 to 20 mg./day. Propranolol, 20 to 40 mg. every 4 hours, may also be given orally.

Other important supportive measures include fluid and electrolyte replacement, temperature control with acetaminophen, and possibly a cooling blanket. Adrenocorticosteroids are commonly given, but their effectiveness is questioned. If their use is elected, 100 mg. of hydrocortisone intravenously may be given initially, followed by tapering doses over the next 24 hours.

The response to therapy is often dramatic, with lysis of the fever within hours. A number of days may be needed for clearing of the sensorium and improvement of the other signs of hyperthyroidism, however. Treatment with antibiotics should be started if there is evidence of infection or on empiric grounds if there is not a prompt drop in the temperature after antithyroid drugs and iodine have been given.

GRAVES' DISEASE

Graves' disease is the most common cause of hyperthyroidism in the third and fourth decades of life. The diagnosis is straightforward in patients with diffuse goiter and the classic infiltrative ophthalmopathy, but easily recognized eye signs are present in only about half of these patients. In the absence of the classic eye signs or pretibial myxedema, the diagnosis should be suspected in patients with hyperthyroidism and diffuse goiter, especially those in the younger age group. The thyroid in Graves' disease is usually symmetrically enlarged, to two to four times normal size, and is normal to slightly soft in consistency.

Graves' disease may be characterized clinically by hyperthyroidism, but typical eye signs may be present in the absence of hyperthyroidism. Also, the ophthalmopathy and the hyperthyroidism may follow entirely independent clinical courses. The most frequent example of this occurs when control of hyperthyroidism has no effect on the accompanying infiltrative ophthalmopathy.

Treatment

Antithyroid drugs, ^{131}I ablation, and subtotal thyroidectomy are all effective in treating the hyperthyroidism of Graves' disease. The chief advantage of antithyroid drug therapy is that it does not cause permanent thyroid damage, and a significant number of patients experience permanent remission of hyperthyroidism following several months of treatment with propylthiouracil or methimazole. As many as 10 per cent of patients, however, have reactions to the medication and require some other method of therapy.

The major advantage of ^{131}I therapy is that it is simple and effective. It takes several weeks to be effective, however, and it permanently damages the thyroid gland. Hypothyroidism is such a common sequel that it should be anticipated after ^{131}I treatment in all patients.

The risks and expense of subtotal thyroidectomy are greater than those of ^{131}I and antithyroid drugs, and this method generally should be reserved for those patients who are noncompliant, for those in whom other methods are unacceptable, and for children. Surgery is also suitable for patients who insist on a rapid cure, because there is a lag of several weeks between treatment with ^{131}I and restoration of the euthyroid state. If hyperthyroidism recurs after surgery, ^{131}I should be recommended because the incidence of complications after a second operation is greatly increased.

Ophthalmopathy

There is no really satisfactory treatment for the ophthalmopathy of Graves' disease, but the disorder is usually self-limiting. Improvement in the metabolic status of the patient with treatment will decrease the lid retraction and ameliorate the stare, but it may not affect the course of true infiltrative ophthalmopathy. Symptomatic treatment may help, however. Liquiform tears of methylcellulose drops may be used as needed for the burning, itching, and tearing of the eyes. Raising the head of the bed on 8-inch blocks and the use of diuretics may reduce periorbital swelling. Sunglasses should always be worn in bright light to reduce tearing and irritation of the eyes. Cold, wet compresses may be used to cover the eyes at night, particularly if the proptosis is severe. Occasionally, surgery may be indicated but should not be undertaken until all inflammatory signs have subsided.

TOXIC MULTINODULAR GOITER

Hyperthyroidism caused by a multinodular goiter may be difficult to recognize. These glands, generally asymmetrical with distinct nodularity, may be extremely large and cannot be differentiated from nontoxic nodular goiter by palpation. It is impossible to determine prospectively which patients with multinodular goiter will become thyrotoxic in the future, and periodic evaluation of patients with multinodular glands is necessary to avoid overlooking the insidious development of hyperthyroidism (Fig. 52–6).

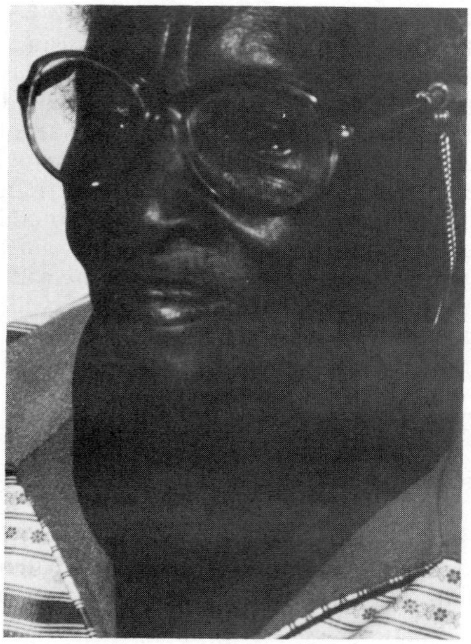

Figure 52–6. Large nodular goiter present for over 40 years before chemical evidence of hyperthyroidism could be demonstrated.

Diagnosis

Cardiac symptoms are often the patient's presenting problem. The diagnosis is established by finding a multinodular thyroid in a patient with hyperthyroidism who does not have extrathyroidal manifestations of Graves' disease. A thyroid scan may be useful in cases in which it is difficult to decide by examination whether the thyroid is multinodular or simply irregular.

Treatment

The treatment of toxic nodular goiter is definitive therapy with either ^{131}I or surgery. The hyperthyroidism may be controlled with antithyroid drugs, but these drugs will not induce a permanent remission and therefore should not be used except as interim therapy. The decision between treatment with ^{131}I and surgery is often made on nonclinical grounds, such as the availability of skilled surgeons and the patient's preference. Occasionally, the size of the goiter may be a factor, because large multinodular glands do not respond well to ^{131}I.

Generally, the dose of ^{131}I used for treatment of a multinodular goiter is larger than that used for treatment of a patient with Graves' disease. Hypothyroidism rarely occurs after ^{131}I therapy of a multinodular gland, because the normal thyroid tissue is suppressed and does not take up the radioactive iodine. Special consideration must be given to patients with coexistent heart disease, for both ^{131}I therapy and surgery may exacerbate congestive heart failure.

SOLITARY HYPERFUNCTIONING ADENOMA

Solitary hyperfunctioning adenomas usually arise during the fourth and fifth decades, in contrast to the later occurrence of hyperthyroidism due to multinodular goiter. The female to male ratio is about 4 to 1. Almost all nodules that become hyperfunctioning measure at least 3 cm. in diameter. These patients usually do not appear quite as toxic as those with hyperthyroidism due to Graves' disease, and eye signs and pretibial myxedema are absent.

Diagnosis

On examination, the nodule is smooth, well defined, and soft to firm in consistency, and moves when the patient swallows. The scan shows intense radioactive uptake in the nodule with absence of uptake in the rest of the gland. If TSH is given to the patient, the adjacent thyroid tissue will also take up the isotope.

Most patients with a solitary adenoma will not become thyrotoxic. This realization has dispelled the belief that a single hot nodule on scan means that the patient is hyperthyroid or will become hyperthyroid in the future. Incidentally, a bruit is not heard in this form of hyperthyroidism.

Treatment

Hyperthyroidism produced by a hyperfunctioning adenoma does not respond to drug therapy with permanent remission, so definitive ablative therapy with ^{131}I or surgery is indicated. Here again, large doses of ^{131}I must be used if the nodule is to be effectively destroyed. The risk of hypothyroidism after ^{131}I is minimal, as the suppressed thyroid tissue does not take up the radioactive iodine in appreciable amounts.

TRANSIENT HYPERTHYROIDISM

Autoimmune thyroiditis, sometimes also referred to as lymphocytic thyroiditis, painless thyroiditis, or postpartum thyroiditis, may be characterized by one or more brief episodes of hyperthyroidism followed by normal thyroid function or hypothyroidism. Although many of these patients have a small, nontender goiter with elevated thyroid function tests, most of them surprisingly show a suppressed or zero radioactive iodine uptake. A 24-hour ^{131}I uptake is of value in differentiating this transient form of hyperthyroidism from Graves' disease. Thyroid antibodies may or may not be present; when present, the titer is usually high. The condition improves spontaneously, but recurrences are common. Many of these cases occur following pregnancy—thus, the name postpartum thyroiditis. On biopsy, many of these glands have lymphocytic infiltration.

The hyperthyroidism associated with most forms of thyroiditis is transient and as a rule does not require definitive therapy. Exceptions to this are patients who have recurrent transient hyperthyroidism or symptoms of hyperthyroidism superimposed upon another concurrent disease. Antithyroid drugs may be needed temporarily in some patients; propranolol may be used alone if the patient is only mildly symptomatic.

EXCESSIVE EXOGENOUS THYROID

Occasionally, patients are seen who are hyperthyroid owing to administration of exogenous thyroid compounds. Some patients take large amounts of thyroid medication in the hope of losing weight or of gaining more energy. Actually, neither of these effects results from normal replacement doses. Weight loss may result, however, from the ingestion of sufficient thyroid hormone to cause hyperthyroidism. Many patients who develop this problem work in a medical setting or are closely related to someone who does.

A patient will occasionally be rendered hyperthyroid because doses of T_3 have been increased by their physician in order to bring a low T_4 to normal levels. If the thyroid taken has been primarily in the form of triiodothyronine, the T_4 will be low in spite of the presence of clinical hyperthyroidism. The diagnosis is usually made by taking a careful drug history in a patient with a normal or small thyroid gland. The diagnosis may be confirmed by finding a suppressed radioiodine uptake.

HYPERTHYROIDISM IN PREGNANCY

It is difficult to evaluate a patient's metabolic state during pregnancy, for many normal women have a mild tachycardia, slight enlargement of the thyroid, and other symptoms suggestive of hyperthyroidism. The presence of a goiter or an elevated resting pulse should make one consider the possibility of a thyroid disorder. The diagnosis can be confirmed by using the free thyroxine index. It is normal in pregnancy for the T_4 to be elevated, due to an increase in TBG, but the free thyroxine index should be within normal limits. Hyperthyroidism in pregnancy is usually due to Graves' disease and should be treated with an antithyroid drug. The dose of propylthiouracil or methimazole should be the minimum needed to control the hyperthyroidism; usually, the dose required is lower than that used in the nonpregnant state. The antithyroid drugs do cross the placenta and may produce a goiter in the fetus, although this is rare. It is usually recommended that patients not breast-feed while taking antithyroid medications.

Surgery offers no advantages and may be associated with increased fetal loss. Radioactive iodine is contraindicated. Inorganic iodine should not be used, since the fetal thyroid is especially sensitive to the effects of iodine, and the infant may be rendered hypothyroid in utero. Patients with hyperthyroidism in pregnancy should be seen frequently, to be certain the patient is complying with the medical regimen and for periodic follow-up with thyroid function tests.

NEONATAL HYPERTHYROIDISM

Occasionally, infants of mothers who have Graves' disease are hyperthyroid at birth or develop hyperthyroidism after delivery. The mothers of these infants may or may not have been euthyroid during pregnancy. The diagnosis of hyperthyroidism in the infant may be difficult, but the symptoms are similar to those of adults and include tremulousness, tachycardia, hyperactivity, and heart failure. Thyroid enlargement is present, and exophthalmos may be striking. The duration of neonatal hyperthyroidism is dependent on the amount of thyroid stimulator from the mother that crosses to the infant. The half-life of thyroid-stimulating immunoglobulins is 14 days.

Levels of T_4 and T_3 in infants are higher than in adults, but neonates with hyperthyroidism have even higher serum T_4 and T_3 levels than normal infants. Normal T_4 cord concentrations are 6 to 12 mg./dl. with an increase in the neonate up to 18 mg. within 2 days after delivery. Several weeks after delivery the values are similar to those found in the adult. Although neonatal hyperthyroidism subsides spontaneously within a few weeks, when the disease is severe it should be treated with antithyroid drugs and propranolol. The neonate usually is not given iodine.

NONTOXIC DIFFUSE GOITER

Goiter is simply an enlargement of the thyroid gland. Unselected autopsy series in the United States indicate a prevalence of approximately 5 per cent. The condition is much more common in females. Sporadic cases of goiter usually occur after puberty; in endemic regions, the highest incidence is in the second through the sixth decades of life. Causes of diffuse goiter include iodine deficiency, iodine excess, congenital defects in thyroid hormone synthesis, and the effects of pharmacologic agents such as lithium. Goiter due to iodine deficiency is much less common now that iodine is routinely added to salt and other foods.

Most goiters do not cause any symptoms and may be discovered on a routine physical examination. Symptoms, such as hoarseness and obstruction of the trachea, are rare in benign thyroid enlargement. The presence of pain is also quite uncommon, usually occurring only in patients with subacute thyroiditis or as a result of hemorrhage into a cyst or adenoma.

NONTOXIC MULTINODULAR GOITER

Multinodular enlargement of the thyroid is common, but the cause is not known with certainty. The enlargement is usually noted by the patient or is found on routine physical examination. Occasionally, a patient is first seen because an asymptomatic superior mediastinal mass was noted on chest x-ray.

Rarely, patients present with rapid enlargement and tenderness in the neck due to hemorrhage into a cyst. Coughing or choking related to tracheal compression is rare. Not uncommonly, patients with goiter complain of a lump in the throat; the fullness in the throat may suggest globus hystericus precipitated or heightened by awareness of the enlarged thyroid gland. Patients may report periodic fluctuation in the size of the thyroid, but this generally is difficult to document.

Diagnosis

The diagnosis of a multinodular gland can usually be made simply by physical examination. Many nodules are commonly found, some barely palpable, others several centimeters in diameter. Routine thyroid function tests are indicated to rule out toxicity; they usually reveal a normal T_4, T_3 uptake and free thyroxine index. A scan and radioactive iodine uptake are not indicated unless there is some question about the uniformity of the gland and coexistent malignancy. At times, it may be difficult to differentiate a multinodular gland from autoimmune thyroiditis, since the typical Hashimoto's gland has a lobulated, irregular surface.

The thyroid scan or ultrasound will be helpful only if the diagnosis of a multinodular gland cannot be made by physical examination. Typically, the scan shows a patchy distribution of the radioisotope within the gland. Although the possibility of malignancy within a multinodular gland may be of concern to the patient, it is rare, and unless the gland is enlarging rapidly or hoarseness is present, the patient can be reassured and simply followed. Surgery is rarely indicated. In cases in which there is enlargement of the thyroid despite adequate thyroid replacement therapy, a needle biopsy and/or subtotal thyroidectomy may be considered.

Treatment

In the past, thyroid replacement therapy was routinely given to patients with a multinodular gland with the assumption that suppression of TSH with exogenous hormone would prevent further growth of the enlarged gland and could actually cause the normal elements in the gland to decrease in size. More recent evidence indicates that treatment with thyroid hormone for as much as 6 months will not cause any reduction at all in the size of thyroid nodules. Some authorities, however, still believe that suppression with exogenous thyroid is warranted in patients with multinodular goiters, unless there is a history of angina or other known heart disease. Periodic monitoring of the thyroid function is indicated in patients with multinodular goiters, including those on thyroid replacement, as a small number of them will develop hyperthyroidism.

SOLITARY NODULES

Solitary nodules in the thyroid gland are more likely to be benign than malignant, but the incidence of malignancy is substantially higher in single nodules than in multinodular glands and the question of whether a solitary nodule might be malignant always troubles the physician. Signs that increase the likelihood of malignancy are a history of radiation exposure, rapid enlargement, and a solid nodule that is cold on scan. Enlargement sufficient to cause hoarseness or obstruction is particularly disturbing. Only 10 to 20 per cent of solitary nodules, even those cold on scan, are malignant; most of these are very slow-growing and of low-grade malignancy. On scan or at surgery, at least half of the glands thought to contain solitary nodules will be found to be multinodular; most are benign.

Patients with solitary nodules should have a T_4,

T_3 uptake, free thyroxine index, and a thyroid scan or aspiration biopsy of the thyroid. Most are euthyroid. If the nodule is hot with suppression of the rest of the gland, one can be assured with 99 per cent certainty that the lesion is benign. In euthyroid cases, no therapy is indicated except for follow-up. Patients with a solitary adenoma who are hyperthyroid may be satisfactorily treated with radioiodine or surgery. Since most glands show little change over a 10-year period, prophylactic surgery to prevent hyperthyroidism or malignancy is not indicated.

Ultrasonography to determine whether the mass is solid or cystic may be helpful. If it is cystic, aspiration with review of the cytology may be done as a diagnostic procedure in lieu of surgical excision. If the cytology is normal, no therapy is indicated.

Fine-needle biopsy of the thyroid is probably the procedure of choice in patients with a cold nodule on thyroid scan. However, in most regions of the country there are few physicians with experience in this technique and the small amount of tissue obtained is frequently difficult to interpret, even by well-trained pathologists. For this reason, surgical excision is usually selected for these patients. If fine-needle biopsy is normal, the patient should be given thyroid suppression therapy.

Another option is to give a 3-month course of thyroid suppression therapy without biopsy. If the nodule continues to enlarge after 3 months of thyroid suppression therapy, surgery is indicated. If the nodule disappears or at least decreases in size, continuous suppression therapy may be undertaken.

SUBACUTE THYROIDITIS

This condition is one of the two most common causes of a painful thyroid; the other is hemorrhage into a thyroid adenoma. Patients with subacute thyroiditis give a history of gradual onset of pain and tenderness of the gland; they may or may not notice that the thyroid is enlarged. The tenderness begins in one part of the thyroid and may slowly move to encompass a larger area, perhaps involving the opposite lobe.

Often the patient will complain of a sore throat or pain in the neck around the ear and is unaware that the thyroid gland is actually tender or that it is enlarged. Systemic symptoms, such as a low-grade fever, malaise, and fatigue, are very common, and there is often a history of a preceding viral illness.

The course may be protracted, lasting several months. Many times, the patient has waited 1 or 2 weeks prior to seeking medical attention and will improve spontaneously without treatment. Diagnostically, an elevated sedimentation rate, a depressed ^{131}I uptake, and a normal or elevated plasma T_4 are characteristic.

In mild cases, aspirin, 600 mg. four times a day, is sufficient to relieve symptoms. In others, glucocorticoid therapy, starting with prednisone, 40 mg. daily and tapering to 10 mg. over a period of 2 weeks, may be necessary. If glucocorticoids are used, they should be continued for about a month after the patient is asymptomatic. Relapse is common.

In general, about a third of patients will be asymptomatic after 1 month and another third after 2 months; the remainder may take as long as 6 months to become asymptomatic. Hyperthyroidism may occur early in the course of the disorder and hypothyroidism may be a late development. It is unusual, however, for thyroid function to be permanently impaired.

THYROID CARCINOMA

Thyroid carcinoma is rare, but it is clinically important because of the frequency with which it is considered in the differential diagnosis of goiter. Carcinoma of the thyroid is three times more common in women than in men and occurs at all ages, peaking in the sixth decade. Occult thyroid carcinoma has been found in 5 to 10 per cent of autopsies and is therefore much more common than is recognized clinically. As many as one third of patients who receive radiation to the head and neck as children develop thyroid carcinoma 10 or so years later.

The majority of thyroid malignancies are papillary or follicular in type. They grow slowly, whereas undifferentiated tumors spread rapidly and often have metastasized at the time of diagnosis. Medullary carcinoma has a familial occurrence and may be associated with the other endocrine abnormalities, especially pheochromocytoma.

Diagnosis

A history of radiation exposure is the single most important question that should be asked of patients who are suspected of harboring a thyroid carcinoma. In these patients, the presence of a single cold nodule in the thyroid is an indication for surgical removal. Other characteristics that make one suspicious of carcinoma are a recent history of hoarseness or obstructive symptoms, a family history of thyroid malignancy, or a rapidly enlarging, indurated thyroid gland. Pain is rarely associated with thyroid carcinoma.

On physical examination, fixation of the thyroid to the surrounding structures and firmness or hardness of the gland are suspicious findings. The neck should be palpated to exclude lymphadenopathy. A single cold nodule on scan and a solid nodule on ultrasonography are suggestive of carcinoma.

Any patient who has a neck mass that is thought to be malignant should have it removed. The cure rate for anaplastic tumors is very poor, but papillary carcinomas have a 99 per cent 10-year survival rate and may be cured by resection even after long delays.

Treatment depends on the type and extent of local spread of the tumor. Most commonly, a simple lobectomy is done, but in patients with lymph node involvement more extensive dissection of the involved side is carried out. In the presence of bilateral involvement or extrathyroidal disease, a bilateral lobectomy and neck dissection are usually performed. Total thyroidectomy generally is not necessary; it carries the risk of hypoparathyroidism and vocal cord paralysis. Thyroid hormone suppressive therapy prior to surgery is effective in preventing the growth of most papillary carcinomas and also diminishes the risk of distant metastases. The use of the hormone after surgery also greatly improves the prognosis.

In cases with definitive evidence of lymph node involvement, the patient should receive one or more doses of ^{131}I after subtotal thyroidectomy to ablate the residual thyroid tissue. Additional ^{131}I is given if metastases are later demonstrated by scan. Patients who are euthyroid should receive stimulating doses of TSH prior to the scan; hypothyroid patients have their own endogenous TSH. Except when receiving ^{131}I therapy, all of these patients should receive thyroid hormone in doses sufficient to completely suppress TSH, as many tumors are TSH-dependent, and exogenous hormone therapy will prevent further growth or may actually produce involution of the tumor.

Serum calcitonin levels should be followed in patients with medullary carcinoma; a rise indicates tumor recurrence or metastasis. Serum thyroglobulin levels are used for the same purpose in differentiated thyroid carcinoma.

HYPOTHYROIDISM

Hypothyroidism, the result of a deficiency of thyroid hormone, is relatively common. Approximately 1 per cent of the population has symptomatic hypothyroidism; an elevated TSH may be present in another 5 per cent. Hypothyroidism is considered to be primary if the hormone deficiency results from a disorder within the thyroid gland. Secondary and tertiary hypothyroidism are caused by a lack of TSH and of thyrotropin-releasing hormone (TRH) secretion by the pituitary and hypothalamus, respectively.

The major cause of hypothyroidism in this country is definitive therapy for hyperthyroidism, by either thyroidectomy or ^{131}I therapy. In patients with a goiter, Hashimoto's thyroiditis is by far the most common cause of hypothyroidism. Other causes of hypothyroidism occurring in a patient without thyroid enlargement include pituitary/hypothalamic disorders, developmental defects, and, most common, idiopathic hypothyroidism. Rarely, drugs, iodine deficiency, or inherited defects in thyroid hormone synthesis may cause hypothyroidism (Table 52–13).

Table 52–13. CAUSES OF HYPOTHYROIDISM

Without Goiter	With Goiter
Posttreatment ^{131}I	Autoimmune thyroiditis
Postthyroidectomy	Drug-induced
Idiopathic	Iodine deficiency
Pituitary/hypothalamic disorder	Inherited defect in synthesis of thyroid hormone
Developmental defect	

Clinical Manifestations

Hypothyroidism may be a very difficult diagnosis to make because often the symptoms are nonspecific and the onset is insidious. Early symptoms include easy fatigability, weakness, and lethargy. Frequently, patients are more forgetful and are slow both mentally and physically; in older patients, this is often wrongly attributed to aging. Constipation, diminished hearing, and paresthesias of the hands due to the carpal tunnel syndrome are common. Menorrhagia is one of the more common presenting complaints in women; galactorrhea may also be seen. Some patients complain of intermittent or persistent hoarseness, and, occasionally, swelling of the hands, face, and feet may be a presenting symptom. Although still nonspecific, the symptoms most suggestive of hypothyroidism are hoarseness, cold intolerance, paresthesias, dry skin, and decreased sweating (Table 52–14).

There is a false impression that obesity may be a sign of hypothyroidism. This is not true, although patients with hypothyroidism frequently gain 10 to 15 pounds owing to accumulation of fluid.

In children, impairment of mental and physical activity may also be present. For example, the neonate with hypothyroidism rarely cries and may have to be awakened to be fed. If hypothyroidism is not promptly recognized and treated in a newborn, mental retardation is a common sequel. Mental retardation does not occur, however, unless hypothyroidism becomes manifest within the first few years of life. Growth retardation and delayed puberty so often result that if a child is of normal size, hypothyroidism can virtually be excluded. Galactorrhea and breast development have been described in some girls with hypothyroidism, but other accompanying signs of precocious maturation usually are not present. As in adults, dry skin, cold intolerance, hoarseness, and diminished hearing are clues to the diagnosis.

There may be slight differences in the clinical manifestations of hypothyroidism, depending on the etiology. Muscle pain, cramps, and paresthesias are more commonly seen in patients who become hypothyroid after treatment with ^{131}I. Patients with peri-

Table 52–14. SIGNS AND SYMPTOMS OF HYPOTHYROIDISM*

Lethargy/weakness	Slow reflex relaxation
Slow movement and speech	Dry, coarse, pale skin
Cold intolerance	Edema, especially facial
Constipation	Impaired memory
Hair loss	Weight gain
Menorrhagia	Deafness
Paresthesia	Bradycardia
	Decreased sweating

*In relative order of frequency.

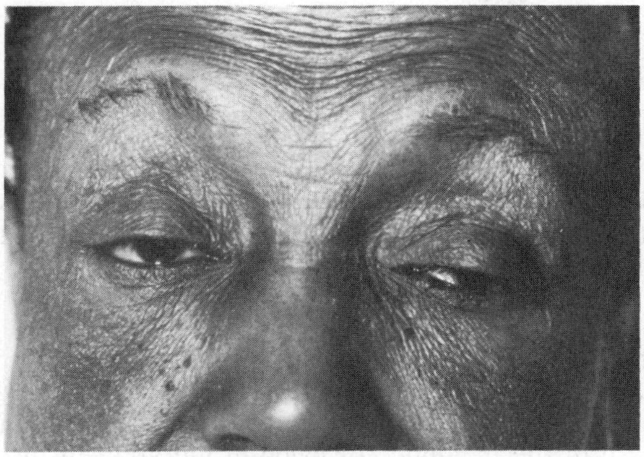

Figure 52–7. Sleepy appearance of eyes in a patient with profound hypothyroidism.

orbital and peripheral edema, hoarseness, and coarse skin are more likely to have primary hypothyroidism, whereas those with weight loss without edema more often have secondary hypothyroidism due to pituitary insufficiency.

Characteristically, hypothyroid patients talk very slowly, look sleepy, and move slowly (Fig. 52–7). They typically have coarse, cool, dry skin and dry hair, which may lose its natural curl; generalized hair loss may be apparent (Fig. 52–8). Periorbital puffiness and peripheral edema are frequent findings, and the tongue may be thick and smooth. Bradycardia occurs only in a small percentage of patients. Sparse eyebrows with loss of the lateral half are common, but this sign is nonspecific and occurs in many euthyroid patients as well.

The thyroid may be enlarged, normal in size, or not palpable. The heart rate is slow, and the diastolic blood pressure is elevated. Occasionally, pericardial effusion and ascites will be detected. A very specific finding is the delay in relaxation of the deep tendon reflexes, particularly the ankle reflexes. Occasionally, other neurologic signs, including ataxia and confusion, may be prominent. Psychosis may develop if the hypothyroidism is long-standing, and its onset actually may be precipitated by therapy with thyroid hormone. Hypothermia should always raise the possibility of hypothyroidism, especially in the absence of the other common causes of hypothermia, which include exposure, sepsis, and diseases of the central nervous system, such as cerebrovascular accidents.

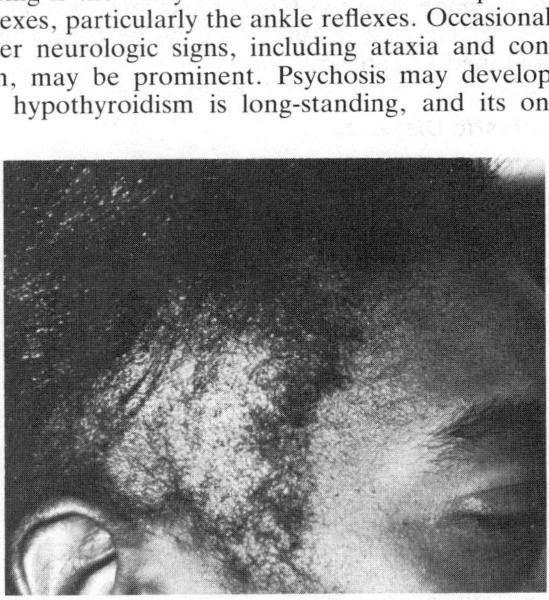

Figure 52–8. Hair loss, more marked in the temporal region, in a patient with hypothyroidism.

In infants, hypotonia, umbilical hernia, and delayed mental and physical development are the most striking findings. Children or infants with this disorder often appear younger than their chronologic age, as they are both small in stature and immature in facies. The skin is dry with a yellowish tinge, and it is sometimes mottled. Bradycardia and a large tongue also may be noted.

Diagnosis

The diagnosis of hypothyroidism is confirmed by the finding of a low serum thyroxine and free thyroxine index. A TSH level will differentiate primary from secondary hypothyroidism. A low TSH in a patient with a low T_4 is indicative of hypothyroidism of pituitary or hypothalamic origin, and a high TSH confirms the diagnosis of primary thyroid failure. The ^{131}I uptake is usually not helpful in assessing a patient with hypothyroidism, as a low uptake not only may be secondary to other thyroid disorders but most often is simply related to ingestion of large amounts of dietary iodine.

Other laboratory findings that may be abnormal in hypothyroidism include the serum transaminase (aspartate amino transferase [AST]), which may be high; sodium, which may be low; blood sugar, which may be low even without coexistent pituitary failure; and the creatine phosphokinase, which may be considerably elevated. Triglycerides and cholesterol may be high. In fact, since hypercholesterolemia is so common in hypothyroidism, the presence of an elevated cholesterol in any patient should raise the possibility of hypothyroidism.

The electrocardiogram may show flat and inverted T-waves, minor ST-segment depression, and low amplitude. There may be abnormalities in the blood arterial gases reflecting hypoventilation. The urinary 17-hydroxysteroids and 17-ketosteroids may be low, reflecting the low metabolic rate. Plasma prolactin may be elevated owing to high thyroid-releasing hormone levels. Mild anemia is common and may be hypochromic or normochromic, macrocytic or microcytic.

A wide variety of symptoms should raise the possibility of hypothyroidism. This diagnosis should be considered in children with growth retardation and in adults with menorrhagia, galactorrhea, carpal tunnel syndrome, hypothermia, periorbital edema, or hypercholesterolemia.

Treatment

Treatment of hypothyroidism is simple and effective. In patients under the age of 40 with no complicating medical problems, full replacement therapy may be started immediately. The serum TSH will return to normal range within a few weeks in most patients who receive levothyroxine 0.15 mg. or desiccated thyroid 120 mg. daily. Patients with pre-existing heart disease or angina and those over the age of 40 should be started on one fourth to one third of these amounts, with increases every 2 weeks until the maintenance dose is reached. The use of T_3 as standard replacement therapy has the disadvantage that it is more expensive and the adequacy of replacement cannot be monitored by T_4 determinations, as the T_4 will remain low on adequate T_3 replacement therapy.

The time required for a patient to become euthyroid after the institution of therapy varies, but several weeks may elapse before the patient is asymptomatic. Once the diagnosis of hypothyroidism is established, particularly after ablative doses of ^{131}I or thyroidectomy, the patient should be instructed to take the exogenous thyroid indefinitely. The dosage of thyroid replacement for children is approximately 0.1 mg. daily for infants up to age 2 and 0.15 to 0.2 mg. for older children. In patients with pituitary hypothyroidism, it is important to replace adrenal steroids prior to thyroid hormone replacement.

Patients who are hypothyroid should not undergo elective surgery. If surgery cannot be avoided, the respiratory status of the patient should be monitored closely, as respiratory depression is very frequent. Caution should be used in prescribing narcotics and hypnotics as these drugs may precipitate myxedema coma in the severely hypothyroid patient.

The family physician frequently must decide whether a patient who is on thyroid medication needs to continue it. The simplest course is to discontinue the use of the thyroid medication and to obtain a T_4 and TSH in 4 to 6 weeks. By then, most patients with true hypothyroidism will have become symptomatic, and the T_4 will be low or low normal. The TSH will be elevated in patients with primary hypothyroidism.

Myxedema Coma

Occasionally, a patient with severe long-standing hypothyroidism will develop myxedema coma, which is a life-threatening emergency. This disorder most often occurs during the winter months and may be precipitated by exposure to the cold. It may also be precipitated by infection, hypoglycemia, narcotics, or an allergic reaction. Hyponatremia and hypoglycemia may contribute to the obtundation. If there is any possibility that coma is related to hypothyroidism, the patient should be treated vigorously without waiting for laboratory confirmation, as delay in treatment may be fatal.

Heat loss should be prevented by wrapping the patient in blankets, and electrolytes must be monitored closely because of the tendency to develop hyponatremia and hypoglycemia. Fluid restriction may be necessary if the patient becomes hyponatremic; hypertonic saline is rarely needed. Traditionally, myxedema coma or severe hypothyroidism with coma is treated with intravenous doses of thyroxine in the range of 0.2 mg. followed by an oral dose of 0.10 mg. daily.

Disorders of Calcium Metabolism

HYPERCALCEMIA

Parathyroid hormone, calcitonin, and vitamin D maintain the serum calcium within a very narrow range, normally 9 to 10.5 mg./dl. The apparent increase in the incidence of calcium metabolism disorders, previously considered relatively rare, is largely due to the introduction of automated multiphasic testing.

Hypercalcemia is produced by increased bone resorption, increased intestinal absorption, or decreased renal excretion of calcium and is caused by many different clinical disorders. Changes in the serum albumin significantly affect serum calcium levels, and alterations in acid-base balance may affect the amount of calcium that is ionized and thereby the total serum calcium measured. For each gram per deciliter decrease or increase in the serum albumin, there is a 0.8 mg./dl. change of the serum calcium in the same direction.

Generally, 99 per cent of body calcium is contained within the bones, and only 0.1 per cent of the total body calcium is contained in the extracellular fluid; approximately half of this is in ionized form and half is bound to albumin. The ionized fraction is decreased by alkalosis and increased by acidosis.

Primary hyperparathyroidism, neoplastic diseases, renal failure with secondary hyperparathyroidism, sarcoidosis, and vitamin D excess are among the most common causes of hypercalcemia (Table 52–15). Characteristic features of each of their causes are outlined in Table 52–16.

Neoplastic Diseases

Neoplastic diseases may cause hypercalcemia depending on both the type of malignancy and the stage

Table 52–15. CAUSES OF HYPERCALCEMIA

Neoplastic disease
Primary hyperparathyroidism
Renal failure with hyperparathyroidism
Vitamin D excess
Endocrine disorders
Hyperthyroidism
Adrenal insufficiency
Pheochromocytoma
Acromegaly
Granulomatous diseases
Sarcoidosis
Tuberculosis
Immobilization
Idiopathic hypercalcemia of childhood

Table 52–16. DIFFERENTIAL DIAGNOSIS OF HYPERCALCEMIA: MAJOR CONSIDERATIONS

	Malignancy	Hyperparathyroidism
Duration	Acute (recent onset)	Chronic (long history)
Serum calcium	Frequently > 14 mg./dl.	Usually < 14 mg./dl.
Serum chloride	Usually < 103 mEq/dl.	Usually > 103 mEq./dl.
Anemia	Frequent	Unusual
Serum PTH	Slightly high for calcium level	Quite high for calcium level
Urinary calcium	> 400 mg./day	< 400 mg./day
Sedimentation rate	Increased	Normal
Alkaline phosphatase	Increased	Usually normal
Weight loss	Marked	Minimal
Serum phosphate	Low, normal, or high	Usually low
Renal stones	Uncommon	Common
Response to steroids	Sometimes effective	Not responsive
X-ray study	Soft tissue lesions, metastatic lesions	Subperiosteal bone resorption
HCO_3	Normal, high	Normal, low

of the disease. The neoplasms most commonly associated with hypercalcemia are lung tumors, multiple myeloma, renal cell carcinoma, and hematologic malignancies. Hypercalcemia most often occurs as a late manifestation of malignant disease, and its appearance usually denotes a very poor prognosis. In cases where there is no obvious cause for hypercalcemia, it may be very difficult to exclude the possibility of an occult malignancy, for there are no clinical signs or laboratory findings specific for the hypercalcemia due to malignancy.

Neoplasms may cause hypercalcemia by bone metastasis or by production of parathyroid hormone, prostaglandins, osteoclastic activating factors, or possibly a vitamin D-like sterol. The variety of the substances produced by malignancies is at least partially responsible for the great variability noted in the effectiveness of specific types of therapy.

Hyperparathyroidism

Hyperparathyroidism is estimated to occur in 28 persons per 100,000; it affects females more commonly than males. A solitary parathyroid adenoma is responsible in the majority of cases, and about 15 per cent of cases are due to hyperplasia; carcinoma is rarely seen. Because most cases are detected by routine multichannel screening, many patients have no symptoms. Symptomatic bone disease, once one of the most common manifestations of hyperparathyroidism, is now quite rare. Renal stones are the presenting symptom in nearly a third to a half of the patients with hyperparathyroidism. The occurrence of renal stones does not have great diagnostic value in differentiating the etiology of hypercalcemia, although it is more often seen in primary hyperparathyroidism. This may be due to the fact that the disease is chronic, with mild to moderate hypercalcemia often going undetected for months to years.

Hyperparathyroidism occurs in association with other disorders and is seen in multiple endocrine adenomatosis, both Type I and Type II. Familial hyperparathyroidism may also be seen without the coexistence of the other endocrine disorders.

There is considerable debate over whether the incidence of peptic ulcer disease and that of pancreatitis are increased in patients with primary hyperparathyroidism. There appears to be some relationship between hypertension and hyperparathyroidism, even though the elevation of blood pressure may persist after successful surgical removal of a parathyroid adenoma and normalization of the serum calcium. Secondary hyperparathyroidism refers to the hypercalcemia that occurs in patients with renal failure and is usually due to parathyroid hyperplasia rather than an adenoma.

Other Causes

Vitamin D intoxication is another cause of hypercalcemia and is caused by the enhancement of intestinal calcium absorption and bone reabsorption. Vitamin D intoxication usually occurs in patients who are given the drug therapeutically for the treatment of rickets or hypoparathyroidism. It occasionally occurs in individuals taking large doses of vitamins or other over-the-counter preparations having a high vitamin D content, such as cod liver oil. Patients with granulomatous diseases, such as sarcoidosis and tuberculosis, may easily become vitamin D-intoxicated, even on small doses. Inexplicably, hypercalcemia may suddenly develop in a patient who has been maintained on a particular dose of vitamin D for a long time, and the hypercalcemia may persist for weeks owing to the storage of large quantities of the vitamin in fat.

Large doses of vitamin A may also cause hypercalcemia, but this occurs much less frequently. The combination of milk and absorbable antacids, such as sodium bicarbonate or calcium carbonate, may cause hypercalcemia in patients with impaired renal function. The hypercalcemia of the milk-alkali syndrome responds promptly to discontinuance of milk and antacid, but the renal failure usually persists.

Hypercalcemia occurs in about 10 per cent of patients with sarcoidosis and in a few patients with other granulomatous diseases, such as tuberculosis and coccidioidomycosis. In sarcoidosis, the increased conversion of 25-hydroxy-D to 1,25-dihydroxy-D is responsible for increased gastrointestinal calcium absorption and bone resorption, thereby producing hypercalcemia.

Prolonged immobilization, particularly in children and young adults, is another cause of hypercalcemia. Management may be particularly difficult in chronically bedridden patients.

As many as 20 per cent of patients with hyperthyroidism have mild to moderate hypercalcemia owing to an increased rate of bone turnover. Acute adrenal insufficiency may also produce hypercalcemia owing to the loss of cortisol, which normally opposes the effect of vitamin D on bone resorption and intestinal calcium absorption. A vast number of drugs may cause hypercalcemia, the thiazides being the most common. Idiopathic hypercalcemia of infancy, a very rare disorder, is mentioned only because it is associated with very distinctive features, including supravalvular aortic stenosis, mental retardation, peculiar facies, and a variety of other somatic abnormalities.

Clinical Manifestations

Those patients with hypercalcemia usually have nonspecific symptoms such as malaise, fatigue, weakness, anxiety, depression, constipation, or abdominal bloating. Muscle weakness, particularly involving the proximal muscles, is another frequent symptom, and one that is often overlooked. Nausea is another common complaint, and with very high calcium levels, anorexia with persistent vomiting may occur. Lethargy, followed by confusion, stupor, and finally coma, occurs frequently if the levels are very high; this is due, at least in part, to the accompanying dehydration. Many of the nonspecific symptoms will be relieved with parathyroidectomy, although many of these complaints are found in the absence of hypercalcemia, and one cannot be certain, prospectively, which symptoms will be relieved with normalization of the serum calcium.

A number of abnormal physical findings may be apparent on examination, although they are often not noted unless specifically sought. Those most commonly noted are elevation in blood pressure, weakness of the proximal muscles, particularly in the legs, and tenderness on pressure of the pretibial areas. Band keratopathy, a grayish ring around the iris, may be more easily seen with the use of a slit lamp. The presence of these abnormalities, however, usually is of little help in determining the etiology of the hypercalcemia.

The presence of hypercalcemia is documented by finding the serum calcium to be greater than 10.5 mg./dl. on two or more occasions. Other laboratory data may be helpful in establishing the etiology of hypercalcemia but usually are not diagnostic. The routine tests that are the most helpful are the chloride, hemoglobin, hematocrit, serum phosphate, and alkaline phosphatase.

Diagnosis

When a patient is found to have hypercalcemia on routine testing or the diagnosis is suspected from the history, one must exclude drugs and diseases that are associated with hypercalcemia. If none of these is apparent, the differential diagnosis lies primarily between malignancy and primary hyperparathyroidism. The historical finding that may be of greatest value is the duration of the hypercalcemia. The presence of an elevated calcium for more than 1 year is strong evidence for primary hyperparathyroidism, as an occult malignancy is seldom present for a year without obvious signs or symptoms. A history of renal stones is also suggestive of chronicity, favoring the diagnosis of hyperparathyroidism.

Serum calcium levels greater than 14 mg./dl. occur much more commonly in patients with malignancy than in those with hyperparathyroidism. The alkaline phosphatase is more commonly elevated in patients with malignancy but may be high in as many as 25 per cent of patients with primary hyperparathyroidism. The sedimentation rate is usually elevated in patients with a malignancy, but half the patients with hyperparathyroidism will also have an elevated sedimentation rate. The serum phosphate is low in most patients with primary hyperparathyroidism and may be anywhere from low to high in those with malignancy. An elevated serum chloride is a strong point in support of the diagnosis of primary hyperparathyroidism, for most patients with a malignancy have a value of less than 103 mg./dl. Metabolic acidosis is frequent with hyperparathyroidism, whereas those with a malignancy more often have a metabolic alkalosis. Anemia is very common in association with neoplastic disease but also may occur in 20 per cent or so of patients with primary hyperparathyroidism. Finally, the parathyroid hormone level is higher in relation to the level of serum calcium in patients with hyperparathyroidism than in those with a malignancy.

Treatment

The choice of therapy is dependent upon the etiology of the hypercalcemia. Patients with a neoplasm are usually treated with surgery, irradiation, or chemotherapy. Some malignancies, especially multiple myeloma and breast carcinoma, are responsive to steroids. The treatment of primary hyperparathyroidism is surgical removal of a parathyroid adenoma, or three and a half glands if hyperplasia is present. Patients with vitamin D or vitamin A intoxication are responsive to steroids, as are those with sarcoidosis, tuberculosis, or Addison's disease. Obviously, if the hypercalcemia is related to drug ingestion, the offending drug should be stopped. To correct the milk-alkali syndrome, the patient should be switched to nonabsorbable antacids.

Medical therapy is indicated for patients with severe hypercalcemia and for those in whom treatment of the underlying disease has not been effective. Table 52–17 lists medications commonly used in treatment, with their indications and dosages.

Fluids should be given in all cases of hypercalcemia, even in those with mild elevation of serum calcium. Usually 3000 ml. a day orally is effective in mild cases. In acutely ill patients with dehydration, intravenous fluids must be given rapidly, and the cardiac status and electrolytes should be monitored closely. Furosemide may be added, either orally or intravenously, in doses of 40 mg. every 6 to 8 hours.

Oral phosphate, which is occasionally used for treatment of chronic hypercalcemia, is often poorly tolerated, with diarrhea developing even on fairly low doses. It may take several days for the serum calcium to normalize during treatment with phosphate, and there may be a further decrease in the serum calcium for a day or more after the phosphate has been discontinued. In severely ill patients, I.V. phosphates may be given very slowly, but they are contraindicated in patients with abnormal renal function. Phosphates should be discontinued when the serum phosphorus exceeds 5.5 mEq./L.

Prednisone, in a dose of 10 to 60 mg./day, is very effective in the treatment of hypercalcemia due to sarcoidosis and in some cases of tumor-associated hypercalcemia. The reduction of calcium may take days to weeks after the initiation of therapy, and steroids are therefore not effective in the treatment of acute hypercalcemic crisis. Indomethacin, 25 mg. four times a day, may be helpful in tumors that secrete prostaglandins. Again, it may take several days to produce a significant response.

Calcitonin, 2 mg./kg. every 6 hours, may be given intramuscularly (I.M.) for acute hypercalcemia. It is effective within hours. Tolerance to the medication may develop after the initial dose, however, and therefore the drug cannot be relied upon for long-term therapy.

Mithramycin has been used in all types of hypercalcemia that are unresponsive to other methods of therapy. This very potent drug is used in a dose of 25 mg./kg. I.V., and hematologic, renal, and liver functions must be monitored periodically. Hemodialysis is occasionally indicated in patients with renal failure and hypercalcemia.

HYPOCALCEMIA

Hypocalcemia usually results from deficiency or ineffectiveness of either vitamin D or parathyroid hormone. The most common form is neonatal hypocalcemia, which is seen in a third of premature infants, in a similar proportion of infants with birth asphyxia, and even more often in children born to diabetic mothers. Serum calcium levels below 7.0 mg./dl. frequently are noted within the first 3 days of life in these infants. The disorder usually resolves within the first week; therefore, I.V. calcium to correct the hypocalcemia is only needed temporarily. The etiology appears to be transient hypoparathyroidism.

The pathogenesis of neonatal hypocalcemia occurring about 1 week or so after birth is slightly different. In all likelihood, it is due to a high intake of phosphorus in the formula; this type frequently occurs in full-term infants. A third type of hypocalcemia in the neonate is known as DiGeorge's syndrome, which is due to agenesis of the parathyroid, a very rare congenital abnormality.

In adults, probably the most common cause of mild hypocalcemia is hypoalbuminemia. Ionized calcium levels remain normal in these patients. Hypocalcemia and hypomagnesemia are very common

Table 52–17. TREATMENT OF HYPERCALCEMIA

Therapy	Usual Dose	Indication	Comment
Fluids	3000 ml./day or more	Serum calcium greater than 12.0 mg./dl.; give rapidly I.V. if stuporous	Use 0.9 per cent NaCl if given I.V.; monitor cardiac status and electrolytes, especially serum K
Furosemide	80 mg. q. 2 h.	Add when fluids given rapidly	
Phosphate	Oral: Neutraphos 2 caps q.i.d. IV: 1500 mg. P. over 6–8 hr.	Serum calcium greater than 12 mg./dl. in symptomatic patient with normal renal function and serum P less than 5 mg./dl.	Keep P greater than 5.5 mg./dl. May take several days to show maximum effect: poor gastrointestinal tolerance
Prednisone	10–60 mg./day	Responsive tumor or sarcoidosis	May take a week for response
Indomethacin	25 mg./q.i.d.	Responsive tumor	Effective in 8 hours. May be ineffective after 2 or more doses
Calcitonin	2 μg./kg. S.Q.	Acute hypercalcemia	Effective within 8 hours
Mithramycin	25 μg./kg. I.V.	Failure of or contraindication to other therapies	Effect may last for days Effective in 48 hours Monitor renal and liver function, WBC, BUN, SGOT, platelets
Hemodialysis		Renal failure	

findings in hospitalized alcoholics, occurring in approximately 50 per cent.

Although the pathogenesis of the abnormality is not entirely clear, hypomagnesemia may result in a decrease in parathyroid synthesis and/or secretion, as well as resistance to the action of parathyroid hormone. Hypocalcemia may also be induced by a number of drugs other than alcohol; these include phosphate, calcitonin, mithramycin, and gentamicin.

Another common cause of hypoparathyroidism is surgical removal or injury of the parathyroid glands during subtotal thyroidectomy. Idiopathic hypoparathyroidism, a rare disorder, may occur alone or with other autoimmune endocrine disorders. Hypoparathyroidism may be associated with cutaneous candidiasis, hypothyroidism, ovarian failure, pernicious anemia, alopecia, vitiligo, myasthenia gravis, and Addison's disease.

Pseudohypoparathyroidism, characterized by hypocalcemia and high levels of parathyroid hormone, is a familial disorder caused by unresponsiveness to parathyroid hormone. These patients are frequently mentally retarded and have round faces, short stature, and short metacarpals. They present with the classic signs and symptoms of hypocalcemia and often have diarrhea.

Hypocalcemia also characterizes vitamin D resistance or deficiency, the cause of osteomalacia in adults and rickets in children. Vitamin D deficiency is an extremely rare disorder, now that many foods are supplemented with vitamin D. Patients who develop vitamin D deficiency not only may have a diet deficient in vitamin D or malabsorption of the vitamin but also may have inadequate exposure to ultraviolet light. Either vitamin deficiency or resistance may cause osteomalacia in adults and hypocalcemia sometimes may be seen in acute pancreatitis, especially between the third and the tenth day. The lower the calcium level, the poorer the prognosis for recovery.

Clinical Manifestations

The classic clinical manifestation of hypocalcemia is tetany. The earliest signs of tetany are paresthesias of the hands, toes, and perioral region. This is followed by muscle cramps and carpopedal spasm, which produces abduction of the thumb into the palm of the hand, followed by flexion of the fingers, which are tightly pressed together. Spasms may also be seen in other muscle groups, such as those of the forearm. Laryngeal stridor and generalized seizures are less frequent. Nevertheless, because seizures may occur with hypocalcemia even in the absence of frank tetany, the serum calcium should be checked in any patient with an idiopathic seizure disorder. A wide variety of mental symptoms may occur with hypocalcemia, including irritability, emotional lability, anxiety, and even frank psychosis. Tremor, ataxia, and choricathetosis are rare.

The clinical signs of hypocalcemia are usually not observed unless the serum calcium drops below 7.5 mg./dl. In the absence of overt tetany, the most specific indication of hypocalcemia is Trousseau's sign, which is elicited by inflating a blood pressure cuff on the arm to slightly higher than the systolic blood pressure. A positive response is the demonstration of carpal spasm within 2 or 3 minutes (Fig. 52–9). Chvostek's sign is less specific, as it may also occur in normal patients. A positive Chvostek's sign is muscular twitching at the corner of the mouth when the facial nerve is tapped about an inch in front of the ear.

Other physical findings that may be noted are dry, scaly skin, cutaneous candidiasis, alopecia, dental hypoplasia, and delayed eruption of the teeth. Cataracts are frequent and are correlated with the duration of the hypocalcemia. Congestive heart failure, if present, may be reversed by calcium replacement. Mental and physical retardation are common.

Diagnosis

The presence of true hypoparathyroidism can be verified by finding a low parathyroid hormone level, and pseudohyperparathyroidism can be verified by an elevated parathyroid hormone level in the presence of hypocalcemia and a normal serum magnesium. A low calcium with a high phosphorus level is seen in hypoparathyroidism, pseudohyperparathyroidism, and renal failure; in rickets and osteomalacia the phosphorus level will be low. Magnesium levels should also be checked routinely, as hypocalcemia may be secondary to hypomagnesemia.

Treatment

Acute hypocalcemia with tetany is treated with intravenous calcium, initially 10 to 20 ml. of calcium gluconate given slowly intravenously, followed by a constant infusion, the dose determined by the amount needed to maintain normal serum calcium levels. When it is clear that long-term therapy will be needed, vitamin D, with or without oral calcium, should be prescribed. Mild hypocalcemia, particularly

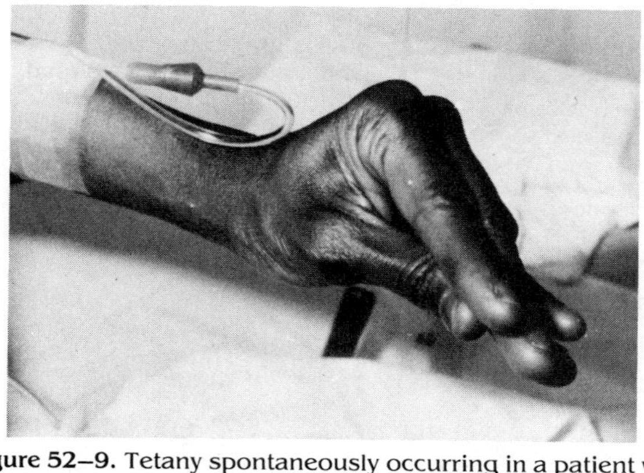

Figure 52–9. Tetany spontaneously occurring in a patient with hypomagnesemia and hypocalcemia. In latent tetany, this hand position may be induced by compression of the upper arm with a blood pressure cuff (Trousseau's sign).

that seen postoperatively, may be treated with oral calcium supplementation alone, but moderate to severe hypocalcemia requires the use of vitamin D. Oral calcium is usually prescribed as calcium gluconate tablets (four 1000 mg. tablets four times daily), calcium lactate (8 gm. dissolved in water), or calcium gluconate (11 gm. given as the syrup or two tablespoons four times a day). Vitamin D is given as ergocalciferol (50 to 100 thousand units per day); 1,25-dihydroxy-D-3 (0.5 to 2.0 μg. per day) may be substituted but is expensive. Vitamin D may be used without calcium supplementation if the intake of dietary calcium is normal.

The goal of therapy is to maintain the serum calcium at the lower range of normal. Serum levels of calcium and phosphorus should be checked daily initially and then weekly until serum calcium and phosphorus levels are stable. Thereafter, calcium and phosphorus levels should be checked at 3-month intervals indefinitely, as vitamin D intoxication may occur in a completely unpredictable manner months or years after a stable regimen has been instituted. If the serum magnesium is low, magnesium may be given intravenously or intramuscularly. Correction of a low magnesium will often correct associated hypocalcemia, even without calcium supplementation. It is important to avoid giving bicarbonate or other alkalizing solutions to patients with hypocalcemia, because these will alter the percentage of calcium that is bound and may induce tetany and seizures.

Pituitary Disorders

HYPOPITUITARISM

Hypopituitarism results from a deficiency in anterior pituitary function; the function of the posterior pituitary may be normal or abnormal. Pituitary failure may be secondary to a wide variety of disorders, including ischemic necrosis, pituitary tumors, surgery, effects of irradiation of the head and neck, starvation, or granulomatous disease, such as tuberculosis and sarcoidosis, or it may be the result of trauma (Table 52–18). The pituitary gland itself may be totally or partially destroyed or the disorder may result from inadequate stimulation of the intact pituitary by the releasing factors. The clinical manifestations of hypopituitarism vary, depending on age and sex, the type of hormone involved, and the extent of impairment of hormonal secretion. Generally, three fourths or more of the gland must be destroyed before hypopituitarism is clinically apparent.

Clinical Manifestations

Signs and symptoms of anterior pituitary insufficiency cover a wide spectrum. Mild cases may be undetected for years, while near-total loss of hormonal secretion may be life-threatening. Prolactin and growth hormone are often the first to be affected. Disruption of the pituitary-hypothalamic connections results in a fall in prolactin-inhibiting factors and a rise in serum prolactin levels. This leads to galactorrhea, a very common presenting manifestation of hyperprolactinemia due to pituitary tumors. Near-total destruction of the anterior pituitary, on the other hand, results in low prolactin levels. This is most commonly due to postpartum pituitary necrosis, a condition known as Sheehan's syndrome, which usually occurs following severe postpartum hemorrhage and hypotension.

Table 52–18. CAUSES OF HYPOPITUITARISM

Vascular	**Nutritional**
Postpartum ischemic necrosis	Starvation
Diabetic ketoacidosis	Anorexia nervosa
Pituitary Tumors	**Granulomatous**
Adenoma	Sarcoidosis
Craniopharyngioma	Tuberculosis
Meningioma	**Traumatic**
Metastatic	
Iatrogenic	
Surgery	
Radiation	
Glucocorticoids	

Impaired growth hormone secretion does not produce any significant symptomatology in the adult but is associated with growth retardation and delayed sexual development in children and adolescents. Symptoms of fasting hypoglycemia are frequent in children deficient in growth hormone. A deficiency of LH and FSH occurring prior to puberty results in failure of normal sexual development; the deficiency is manifested in women by amenorrhea and in men by testicular atrophy and loss of libido.

Hypothyroidism resulting from lack of TSH has features almost identical to those seen in primary hypothyroidism. Growth retardation is seen in children, as are the other classic features of hypothyroidism, including cold intolerance, mental and physical slowness, constipation, dry skin, and hoarseness. Lack of ACTH is manifested by typical signs of cortisol deficiency, including weakness and fatigue, weight loss, hypotension, dehydration, nausea, vomiting, and hyperthermia. A feature that helps to distinguish primary from secondary adrenal insufficiency is lack of the pigmentation found when the disorder is caused by ACTH deficiency.

Diagnosis

Nearly any of the physical findings associated with deficiency of thyroid, adrenal, or gonadal hormones may be seen in patients with hypopituitarism. A rather distinctive feature in patients with anterior pituitary deficiency is the pallor of the skin, which also tends to be dry and wrinkled, particularly around the mouth and eyes. This causes patients to appear older than their chronologic age. Blood pressure, heart rate, and body temperature all tend to be on the low side, and generalized muscle weakness may be demonstrable. Mental apathy, confusion, or frank psychosis often is apparent. Children tend to be small for their age, with fairly normal body proportions. The testes are small and very soft. There is often failure of development of pubic hair, and other body hair may be greatly decreased.

Diagnostic Tests

A large number of tests, many of which require expert interpretation, is used to evaluate anterior pituitary function. Most patients, however, can be adequately assessed by routine tests that evaluate the function of the thyroid gland, gonads, and adrenal gland (Table 52–19). The existence of a pituitary tumor should be excluded in every patient suspected of impairment of anterior pituitary function. This can be done quite satisfactorily with an x-ray study or computed tomography (CT) scan of the sella and a prolactin level. Generally, a lateral skull x-ray for estimation of sella size will detect a tumor that is large enough to cause anterior pituitary insufficiency, and the prolactin is elevated in 75 per cent or more of patients with pituitary tumors.

Thyroid function can be readily assessed with a T_4, T_3 uptake, and TSH. As a rule, there will be a decrease in the T_4 level and free thyroxine index. Deficiency of gonadotropin release is demonstrated by low to normal levels of FSH and LH in patients who show evidence of ovarian or testicular failure, such as amenorrhea, poor estrogen effect on vaginal smear, testicular atrophy, or decreased testosterone secretion.

Table 52–19. EVALUATION OF SUSPECTED ANTERIOR PITUITARY DYSFUNCTION

Exclude tumor	
Lateral skull x-ray for sella size	May not detect microadenoma
Prolactin level	Elevated 75 per cent of the time if tumor present
Evaluate end organ function if above tests positive or if abnormality of thyroid, adrenal, and/or gonadal function suspected:	
T_3, T_4, TSH	If all values low = pituitary deficiency
LH, FSH if amenorrhea or testicular atrophy present	
Maturation index	For evidence of estrogen effect
Plasma cortisol before and after I.V. ACTH	Failure to rise at least 11 µg./dl. indicates adrenal insufficiency
Stimulation Tests	
Insulin-induced hypoglycemia	
Metyrapone stimulation test	
L-dopa stimulation test	

Adrenal function is usually evaluated by measuring serum cortisol rather than ACTH levels. Baseline early morning cortisol levels are low, and usually there is an inadequate increase in plasma cortisol after a single injection of ACTH. The serum cortisol will return to normal after prolonged stimulation with ACTH.

Other commonly used stimulation tests are insulin-induced hypoglycemia, L-dopa stimulation, and the metapyrone test. Numerous factors must be considered in interpreting these tests, and endocrinologic consultation is advisable if these tests are to be undertaken.

Treatment

Acutely ill patients with panhypopituitarism should be managed in the same way as for a patient with acute adrenal insufficiency. Hydrocortisone, 100 mg., is given intravenously every 6 hours; dehydration and electrolyte disturbances are treated with I.V. fluids. Glucose should also be given, as many of these patients are hypoglycemic.

Treatment of chronic hypopituitarism involves replacement of each of the individual hormones that are deficient, in addition to treatment of the cause of the hypopituitarism. Treatment of ACTH deficiency requires glucocorticoids, usually in slightly lower doses than those used for replacement therapy in patients with primary adrenal insufficiency. The usual daily doses of glucocorticoids used in patients with pituitary failure are cortisone acetate, 25 mg.; hydrocortisone, 20 mg.; prednisone, 5 mg.; and dexamethasone, 0.5 mg.

Large doses of glucocorticoids may precipitate psychosis in patients who have had long-standing hypopituitarism. Therefore, therapy often is begun with doses lower than those needed for maintenance, with a gradual increase to customary doses. Mineralocorticoids are seldom needed in patients with pituitary insufficiency, as aldosterone secretion is only partially dependent upon ACTH secretion, and adequate secretion is usually maintained in the absence of pituitary ACTH. Preoperatively, these hydrocortisone patients should be given 100 mg. of hydrocortisone intravenously, just as if they had primary adrenal insufficiency. Hydrocortisone is given every 6 hours, the dose being halved every 24 hours until maintenance doses are reached. If the patient develops complications or a fever after surgery, the dose should be increased again.

Patients with pituitary insufficiency should wear a bracelet or carry identification with a diagnosis of secondary adrenal insufficiency, rather than pituitary insufficiency, so that it will be clear that the patient needs glucocorticoid replacement in the event of trauma or illness. Likewise, patients should be given 100 mg. of injectable hydrocortisone in a prefilled syringe to use if vomiting occurs and access to medical care is delayed.

Patients with secondary hypothyroidism due to TSH deficiency should be treated with standard maintenance doses of thyroid hormone. It is important that these patients receive glucocorticoids before thyroid hormone is given if both deficiencies are present, as thyroid replacement may aggravate or precipitate an adrenal crisis in patients in whom glucocorticoids have not been replaced. Initially, thyroxine, 0.05 mg., or triiodothyronine, 10 μg., is given orally. If triiodothyronine is used, the dose may be increased every few days until the maintenance dose is reached, but the dose of thyroxine should be increased only every 2 weeks.

Triiodothyronine is not recommended for long-term maintenance, and when a dose of 50 to 75 μg. is reached, the patient should be switched to thyroxine. The maintenance dose of thyroxine is about 0.15 mg. per day. In women over the age of 50, estrogen replacement is optional. In younger women, ethinyl estradiol, 0.02 mg., or conjugated estrogens, 0.6 to 1.25 mg., may be given daily for 25 days each month with 10 mg. of medroxyprogesterone daily added for the last 10 days.

In men, testosterone enanthate or cypionate 100 to 300 mg. may be given every 2 to 3 weeks to restore libido and sexual function. Infertility is treated with clomiphene citrate, FSH-LH preparations, and human chorionic gonadotropin; success is limited even with combination therapy. Growth hormone replacement is not needed in adults, but growth hormone should be administered to children to promote normal growth and development.

DIABETES INSIPIDUS

Diabetes insipidus, a disorder characterized by the excretion of large volumes of dilute urine and secondary polydipsia, is caused by deficiency of, or unresponsiveness to, vasopressin. This rare disorder may be due to trauma, tumors, granulomatous diseases, meningitis, Sheehan's syndrome, or surgery. At times, it occurs without any identifiable cause.

Clinical Manifestations

The major symptoms of diabetes insipidus are polyuria and polydipsia. Most patients excrete more than 3 liters of urine per day. The onset of symptoms is often acute, the patient being able to name the exact hour when the polyuria and polydipsia began. Frequent nocturia is the rule, and patients nearly always drink water several times during the night. They may have a very strong preference for ice cold water. As long as the patient has an intact thirst mechanism and is able to drink at will, there are usually no other specific symptoms. Irritability and depression attributed to interrupted sleep caused by the polyuria may be seen.

There are no specific physical findings of diabetes insipidus. Since anterior pituitary failure is often seen in conjunction with diabetes insipidus, the abnormalities noted on physical examination may result from deficiency of the anterior pituitary trophic hormones. The classic laboratory findings suggestive of diabetes insipidus are excretion of 3 or more liters of urine per day with a specific gravity of less than 1.010 and osmolality of less than 300 mOsm./kg.

Diagnosis

Diabetes insipidus must be differentiated from other causes of polyuria and polydipsia, such as glycosuria due to diabetes mellitus, hypercalcemia, sickle cell disease or trait, lithium or meclocycline ingestion, pyelonephritis, and postobstructive uropathy. The diagnosis can be established by a water deprivation test, which will distinguish between primary polyuria due to compulsive water drinking, true diabetes insipidus, and nephrogenic diabetes insipidus. The test is done by discontinuing all fluids for at least 6 to 8 hours or until three consecutive specimens of urine and plasma collected at half-hour intervals show no change in osmolality. A serum vasopressin level is drawn just before giving aqueous pitressin subcutaneously and urine is collected 1 hour later. Patients with nephrogenic diabetes insipidus will not be able to concentrate their urine, whereas those with central diabetes insipidus will have a urine osmolality considerably higher than the plasma osmolality. Patients with a total deficiency of antidiuretic hormone will be found to have a very low serum osmolality prior to the injection of antidiuretic hormone, and the urine osmolality will increase by 50 per cent after aqueous pitressin. Those with partial diabetes insipidus will have intermediate levels of serum vasopressin, and their urine osmolality will increase by 10 to 30 per cent. Patients with primary polydipsia will have normal serum vasopressin levels, and the urine osmolality will not change significantly after the injection of vasopressin.

Nephrogenic diabetes insipidus, which results from the failure of the renal tubule to respond to antidiuretic hormone, may be difficult to distinguish from compulsive water drinking. Serum antidiuretic hormone levels will be low in patients with diabetes insipidus and high in those with primary polyuria or nephrogenic diabetes insipidus.

Treatment

Diabetes insipidus may be treated with pitressin tannate in oil or synthetic vasopressin (DDAVP) and one of several oral drugs that may potentiate antidiuresis. Five units of pitressin tannate in oil is usually given two or three times a week intramuscularly. A synthetic analog of vasopressin (DDAVP) can be administered by nasal insufflation two to three times daily; in the absence of rhinitis or sinusitis, it is very effective. Its greatest disadvantage is its high cost.

Chlorpropamide, 100 to 250 mg./day, is quite effective in potentiating the action of vasopressin on the renal tubule, thus greatly reducing the polyuria and polydipsia. An unwanted pharmacologic action of the drug is hypoglycemia, which is particularly worrisome in patients with anterior pituitary insufficiency, who already have a tendency to develop hypoglycemia spontaneously.

Clofibrate also may be used to decrease polyuria. It probably acts by augmenting the release of antidiuretic hormone from the posterior pituitary. Thiazide diuretics, such as hydrochlorothiazide 50 mg./day, may reduce the urine volume as much as 50 per cent by inhibiting sodium reabsorption and thus interfering with maximum urinary dilution.

ACROMEGALY

Excessive growth hormone production by a pituitary tumor is responsible for the development of acromegaly in adults and gigantism in children. The clinical features of acromegaly are due to the mass effect of the tumor, the effects of excessive growth hormone secretion, or deficiency of one or more of the other pituitary hormones.

Clinical Manifestations

The most frequent presenting complaints are amenorrhea, headache, arthralgia, paresthesias, and galactorrhea. Patients may be aware of deepening of their voice but usually will not volunteer this information unless specifically asked. The presence of headache and increased sweating indicates active disease.

Other characteristic features of growth hormone excess are enlargement of the hands and feet and coarsening of the facial features. Both soft tissue and bony structures may be involved, with an increase of the soft tissues around the eyes, nose, and mouth and enlargement of the mandible leading to prognathism. The onset of the disorder is so insidious that many patients and their families are unaware of the striking changes that occur over the years. Old photographs may be helpful in assessing the progression of the disorder. It is helpful to inquire about changes in shoe and ring size and whether dentures have been replaced owing to poor fit.

Often, the most striking findings are the very large hands and feet. The facial features are coarse, with thickening of the nose and periorbital region and prominence of the nasolabial folds. There may be prominence of the forehead and enlargement of the lower jaw, with a significant underbite. The skin is thickened and oily, with an increased incidence of fibroma molluscum. There is often a wide space between the front teeth. Thyromegaly and cardiac enlargement also may be detected on physical examination.

Routine laboratory findings are of little help. The serum inorganic phosphorus may be elevated and the glucose tolerance test abnormal. The electrocardiogram commonly shows left ventricular hypertrophy and premature ventricular beats.

Diagnosis

In advanced cases, acromegaly is not a difficult diagnosis to make on clinical grounds, as the patient's facial features are very characteristic. The problem usually arises in excluding acromegaly in patients with very coarse facial features and large hands and feet or in simply overlooking insidious changes that have occurred over a period of years.

Basal levels of growth hormone are elevated in acromegaly. A number of other chronic diseases will cause growth hormone elevation, but they should pose no problem in the differential diagnosis, as other signs of acromegaly are lacking. If the basal growth hormone level is elevated, the diagnosis of acromegaly may be established by demonstrating lack of growth hormone suppression by glucose. Hyperglycemia decreases growth hormone in normal individuals but does not change growth hormone levels in acromegalic patients. Glucose, 50 to 100 grams, may be ingested and a growth hormone level obtained 1 to 2 hours later. If the levels remain elevated after glucose administration, the presence of acromegaly is confirmed.

Treatment

The standard methods of treatment of acromegaly are surgery and irradiation, although medical therapy is used when surgery and radiation have not restored growth hormones to normal. The most common surgical procedure used is transsphenoidal removal of the tumor, which results in rapid lowering of growth hormone levels. Conventional x-ray doses of 5000 rads as well as proton beam irradiation have been used.

The disadvantage of radiation therapy is the time interval between treatment and normalization of the growth hormone levels. It may be several years before satisfactory results are obtained. Bromocriptine, medroxyprogesterone, chlorpromazine, and antiserotonin drugs have all been used, but they are not considered definitive therapy.

PITUITARY TUMORS

Pituitary tumors account for about 10 per cent of intracranial tumors. They often do not manifest themselves clinically; in one autopsy series, there was a 22 per cent incidence of clinically unrecognized pituitary adenomas. In another series, over 50 per cent of pituitary microadenomas were first discovered at autopsy. The peak incidence for recognition of pituitary adenomas is the fifth decade, while craniopharyngiomas are more common in children. Most patients with pituitary tumors present with endocrine disorders or neurologic manifestations; occasionally, an enlarged sella due to a pituitary tumor is discovered on a skull x-ray that was obtained for some other purpose.

Clinical Manifestations

Any of the symptoms related to hyperfunction or hypofunction of the gland may be the presenting complaint of patients with pituitary tumors. Amenorrhea, galactorrhea, and infertility are particularly common presenting symptoms, as are headaches and visual disturbances, which may be the earliest manifestations, caused by the increased size of the pituitary and its pressure on the overlying dura or optic chiasm.

A wide range of physical findings may be found in patients with pituitary tumors. These may be due to hypofunction of the anterior pituitary with decreased secretion of gonadal, adrenal, or thyroid hormones or to excess secretion of growth hormone, prolactin, ACTH, or, very rarely, TSH or FSH. Diabetes insipidus caused by lack of vasopressin occurs frequently in patients with craniopharyngioma, but it is rare in those with pituitary adenomas.

Occasionally, an abnormality in the visual fields can be demonstrated in the examination room, but most of the time the detection of these defects requires careful perimetric studies. Gallman visual fields are particularly useful in following patients with pituitary tumors. Temporal field defects are common in tumors that extend above the sella and produce chiasmal compression.

The most useful single study is a lateral skull x-ray to estimate the size of the sella turcica. Normally, it is smaller than a dime and the cross-sectional area does not exceed 120 mm^2. An anterior-posterior view of the skull may assist in determining sella size.

An enlarged sella turcica, however, is not pathognomonic of pituitary tumor, for similar enlargements may be caused by the empty sella syndrome, by tumors above the sella that invade the pituitary fossa, by granulomatous disease, and by increased intracranial pressure. More rare, but of importance from the standpoint of surgical treatment, is an arterial aneurysm. Calcification in the suprasellar region is highly suggestive of a craniopharyngioma.

When there is a high clinical index of suspicion of an intrasellar lesion and findings on the standard lateral skull film are normal or questionable, magnetic resonance imaging or computed tomography may be of value in demonstrating supersellar extension of pituitary tumors or in helping establish the diagnosis of empty sella syndrome.

Endocrine evaluation is an important part of the diagnosis of pituitary tumors. The history and physical examination should help to delineate exactly what tests will be most helpful. Generally, measurements of serum prolactin, TSH with concurrent determinations of T_4 and T_3 uptake, and FSH are the most helpful tests of endocrine function.

Tumors of the pituitary, whether primary or metastatic, are usually quite large by the time the diagnosis is made. Extrasellar tumors occasionally grow into the pituitary fossa, and rarely carcinomas metastasize to the pituitary. The clinical clue to diagnosis of the empty sella syndrome is the finding of an enlarged sella turcica in a young woman with increased intracranial pressure. Endocrine function is usually normal.

Sarcoidosis involving the hypothalamus may cause diabetes insipidus. In addition, there may be other evidence of endocrine dysfunction or optic atrophy due to involvement of the optic nerve. There is no feature diagnostic of an intrasellar aneurysm, but throbbing headaches with vomiting and visual disturbances are frequently noted. Primary hypothyroidism and hypogonadism may also be associated with an enlarged sella.

Treatment

Replacement of glucocorticoids and thyroid hormone is the first step in treating patients who have hypopituitarism. Disorders associated with hyperfunction, such as acromegaly and Cushing's disease, may be treated by surgery, radiation, or drugs. Specific aspects of therapy are discussed more completely under each of these disease headings.

Many pituitary tumors do not require any therapy, and transsphenoidal removal of the tumor is usually recommended only to limit loss of pituitary function or loss of vision from suprasellar extension of the tumor. The intracranial operative route is indicated only rarely. External irradiation, using 4000 to 5000 rads given over a 6-week period, is an alternative method of therapy. Bromocriptine has been shown to reduce the size of prolactin-producing tumors; its use for treatment of other pituitary tumors is questionable.

Adrenal Disorders

Diseases of the adrenal gland are relatively uncommon but are of importance because they mimic many other conditions that are seen commonly in clinical practice. Although the adrenal gland secretes more than 50 different steroids, there are only three major classes: glucocorticoids, mineralocorticoids, and androgens. Clinically, the most important hormones of the adrenal cortex are cortisol, the major glucocorticoid, and aldosterone, a mineralocorticoid.

The production of cortisol is controlled by ACTH, which is in turn modified by the levels of serum cortisol and the hypothalamic hormone, corticotropin-releasing hormone. Glucocorticoids have diverse functions, including regulation of both protein and carbohydrate metabolism, suppression of inflammation, and regulation of calcium absorption. Aldosterone is regulated primarily by the renin-angiotensin system, although potassium and ACTH levels also affect its secretion. The major effect of aldosterone is the conservation of sodium and the excretion of potassium. Several other hormones produced by the adrenal cortex will not be considered, as they are of less clinical importance.

In contrast to the steroid hormones produced by the adrenal cortex, the adrenal medulla produces catecholamines and is thereby linked with the sympathetic nervous system. The major hormones produced by the medulla are norepinephrine, which is an alpha agonist, and epinephrine, which has both alpha- and beta-adrenergic effects. Norepinephrine produces both arterial and venous constriction, whereas epinephrine causes an increase in heart rate and myocardial contractility and also peripheral vasodilatation.

Disorders of the adrenal result from decreased or increased secretion of one or more of these hormones. There is such wide variation in the normal rate of hormone production that determinations done in the basal state alone are rarely diagnostic. Suppression tests are usually indicated if hyperfunction of the gland is suspected, and stimulation tests if hypofunction is suspected.

PRIMARY ALDOSTERONISM

Excessive production of aldosterone by the adrenal gland may be due to an aldosterone-producing adenoma, bilateral adrenocortical hyperplasia, or, very rarely, adrenocortical carcinoma. The significance of hyperaldosteronism lies not in its frequency, as it is quite uncommon, but rather in the fact that it mimics essential hypertension. Only about 1 per cent of patients with high blood pressure have primary aldosteronism. Primary aldosteronism occurs in all age groups, with peak incidence during the third to fifth decades; more women are affected than men.

Clinical Manifestations

Almost all of the features of primary aldosteronism result from the fact that high levels of aldosterone production promote excessive sodium conservation and potassium excretion by the kidney. This produces the classic clinical findings of the disorder, hypertension and hypokalemia. Many patients are completely asymptomatic, whereas others have nonspecific complaints of tiredness, fatigue, nocturia, and weakness. With severe potassium depletion, polyuria, nocturia, visual disturbances, muscle cramps, paresthesias, and frank tetany may occur.

There are no specific physical findings in primary aldosteronism. Findings characteristic of hypertension may be noted, although retinopathy and cardiac enlargement usually are milder than would be expected for the level of blood pressure. Although aldosterone causes sodium retention and expansion of the vascular volume, clinical edema is not seen. A positive Trousseau's or Chvostek's sign, resulting from decreased levels of ionized calcium associated with the hypokalemic alkalosis, may be noted. Latent tetany may be precipitated under these circumstances by even brief hyperventilation.

Hypokalemia is a hallmark of the disease, and the presence of a low potassium in a hypertensive patient who is not on diuretics should immediately raise the possibility of primary aldosteronism. Other manifestations of potassium deficiency may be evident, such as impaired urine-concentrating ability and prominent U waves on the electrocardiogram. The serum sodium is usually normal or elevated, but is almost always above 139 mEq./l.

Diagnosis

The diagnosis of primary aldosteronism rests on the demonstration of hypertension, hypokalemia, and excessive excretion of aldosterone. The best screening test for primary aldosteronism is measurement of the serum potassium. Hypokalemia may not be evident in patients on a low salt intake or in those taking spironolactone, which blocks the effects of aldosterone on the distal tubule.

The most common cause of hypokalemia is diuretic therapy. Even with potassium supplementation, many patients on diuretic therapy will have a low serum potassium. Therefore, in the evaluation of primary aldosteronism, diuretics must be stopped for 3 to 4 weeks before hypokalemia is considered to be inappropriate. Other common causes of hypokalemia that must be excluded include diarrhea, chronic laxative use, excessive licorice ingestion, and Cushing's disease.

In the absence of evidence of these conditions, plasma renin activity should be measured. Levels will be low in patients with primary aldosteronism, as excessive rates of aldosterone secretion suppress plasma renin. Initially, a random plasma renin level should be determined. If it is low, a stimulated renin level should be obtained by placing the patient on a low salt diet for 5 days prior to measurement of the plasma renin activity or by giving furosemide 40 mg. by mouth 3 hours before the blood is drawn for plasma renin activity. A normal or elevated plasma renin excludes primary aldosteronism and suggests prior diuretic therapy, renovascular hypertension, drug therapy such as estrogen administration, or some other cause of high blood pressure. The diagnosis of primary aldosteronism is confirmed by finding a high aldosterone level (greater than 20 ng./dl.) 5 days after the patient has been on a high salt diet.

Treatment

It is important to distinguish between a solitary adenoma and bilateral adrenal hyperplasia as the source of excessive amounts of aldosterone, for removal of a solitary adenoma results in cure of the hypertension in more than 50 per cent of patients.

Surgery is not indicated for bilateral hyperplasia, as only a minority of patients are benefited, even with bilateral adrenalectomy. Spironolactone 25 mg. four times a day usually controls the blood pressure if surgery is not indicated.

CUSHING'S SYNDROME

Cushing's syndrome refers to the metabolic disorder that results from high levels of glucocorticoids. It may be due to excessive pituitary production of ACTH with resultant adrenal hyperplasia, autonomous function of an adrenal adenoma or carcinoma, ectopic production of ACTH from a nonadrenal tumor with chronic stimulation of the adrenal, or sustained excessive administration of glucocorticoids of ACTH. Hypothalamic or pituitary dysfunction accounts for 70 per cent or more of the cases of Cushing's syndrome, and the majority occur in women between the ages of 20 and 40. Most are due to microadenomas.

Ectopic production of ACTH is responsible for only 15 per cent of reported cases of Cushing's syndrome, but this undoubtedly underestimates the true incidence, since many of these patients, predominantly males over the age of 50, lack many of the classic features of the disorder. Tumors from more than 20 different tissues have been demonstrated to secrete ACTH or its precursors. Carcinoma of the lung is responsible for most cases of ectopic production of ACTH. Thymomas, pancreatic islet cell carcinoma, medullary carcinoma of the thyroid, and neural crest tumors are others that commonly produce ACTH.

Glucocorticoid excess produced by the autonomous function of an adrenal adenoma or carcinoma produces a clinical picture that is indistinguishable from that of pituitary/hypothalamic ACTH excess. Cushing's syndrome in childhood is most often due to adrenal carcinoma, with fewer than half the cases due to pituitary/hypothalamic disease. Both adrenal adenomas and carcinomas occur predominantly in women.

Clinical Manifestations

Patients with Cushing's disease usually present with weight gain, easy bruising, severe acne, and/or menstrual irregularity. Back pain is a common symptom and is related to the development of osteoporosis. Muscle weakness is often noted, and emotional lability with depression may be marked. Hirsutism is less common but may be a presenting manifestation of the disease (Table 52–20).

Table 52–20. CLINICAL MANIFESTATIONS OF CUSHING'S SYNDROME*

Obesity	Striae
Plethoric facies	Muscular weakness
Hypertension	Backache
Glucose intolerance	Easy bruising
Mental disorders	Hirsutism

*In relative order of occurrence.

Most of these patients have truncal obesity, with a round, plethoric face and thickening of the fat pads in the supraclavicular areas and at the base of the neck. The arms are relatively small. The blood pressure is almost always elevated. The skin is thin, with wide, purplish-red striae present in over half the patients. Growth retardation is a common feature in children; and if a child follows a normal growth pattern, Cushing's syndrome can be virtually excluded on that basis alone.

Glucose intolerance is usually found in Cushing's disease, and markedly elevated blood glucose levels may be present. Hypokalemic, hypochloremic alkalosis is found in a small number of patients, particularly those with severe clinical manifestations of Cushing's disease. Hypercholesterolemia is common. Some patients have an elevated hemoglobin and hematocrit, and granulocytosis with a relative decrease in eosinophils.

Diagnosis

The diagnosis of Cushing's disease is frequently entertained but rarely substantiated. In patients in whom the diagnosis cannot be dismissed with confidence, a screening test should be done. The easiest and simplest method is for the patient to take dexamethasone, 1 mg. at midnight, and to have a plasma cortisol level drawn at 8 A.M. the next morning. If the plasma cortisol level is suppressed to 5.0 mg./dl. or less, the diagnosis of Cushing's syndrome can be excluded.

If the cortisol level is higher than 5.0 mg., the next step is to place the patient on low-dose dexamethasone, 0.5 mg. every 6 hours, for 2 days. A 24-hour urine is collected on the second day and tested for 17-hydroxysteroids, free cortisol, and creatinine. A positive test is indicated by failure of the 17-hydroxysteroids to be decreased to less than 4 mg./24 hours, or the urinary-free cortisol to less than 25 mg./24 hours. If there is any question about the completeness of the urine collection, a creatinine determination may be done on the same sample. The ratio of hydroxysteroids to creatinine should be less than 8 to 1. As a further check, a plasma cortisol level drawn at the end of the test period that exceeds 5 mg./dl. substantiates the urinary findings and supports the diagnosis of Cushing's syndrome.

False-positive dexamethasone suppression tests are very rare, but they have been reported in the presence of acute severe emotional or physical stress, malnutrition, diabetes mellitus, intrasellar tumors that do not produce ACTH, and pregnancy, and with the ingestion of drugs including alcohol, estrogen, diphenylhydantoin, and phenobarbital.

Once the diagnosis of Cushing's syndrome is established, the etiology must be ascertained. Pituitary ACTH hypersecretion must be differentiated from ectopic ACTH excess and from primary adrenal tumors. The tests that are most helpful in determining the cause of the overproduction of cortisol are the high-dose dexamethasone suppression test, basal ACTH levels, and CT scans of the sella turcica and the adrenals (Table 52–21). The head CT scan will be abnormal in the majority of patients with pituitary Cushing's syndrome, and a CT scan of the adrenals will show bilateral hyperplasia in patients who have excess ACTH from any source. The CT scan may also identify an adrenal tumor.

Characteristically, patients with pituitary Cushing's disease will have suppression of urinary and plasma cortisol levels to less than half the baseline levels after 2 days of high-dose dexamethasone—2.0 mg. every 6 hours for eight doses. Those with adrenal tumors and ectopic ACTH production show no such suppression. Basal ACTH levels are low or nondetectable in patients with adrenal tumors but are normal or elevated in cases of pituitary Cushing's disease. Very high levels of ACTH may be found in patients with ectopic ACTH production, but there is considerable overlap of these values with those found in pituitary Cushing's disease. Most of the time, the etiology of Cushing's syndrome can be established with reasonable certainty, but there are enough false positives and false negatives for each test that establishing the diagnosis may be difficult in some patients.

Treatment

Patients with pituitary Cushing's disease are usually treated with transsphenoidal surgery to remove the pituitary adenoma. Pituitary irradiation may be beneficial, but there is a delay before the treatment has its full effect in adults; children often respond favorably to irradiation, however. Medical therapy, using cyproheptadine and bromocriptine, is effective in controlling the syndrome in many cases but does not produce a permanent cure. Aminoglutethimide and metyrapone have been used in the treatment of patients with fulminant Cushing's disease prior to surgery, but long-term therapy with these agents has not been adequately studied.

Cushing's syndrome due to ectopic ACTH production is treated by removal of the secreting tumor. In the case of inoperable tumors, the patient may respond to mitotane (O,P′-DDD). Total adrenalectomy will cure the hypercortisolism but is seldom performed. Surgical removal is the treatment of choice in patients with a solitary adenoma.

Table 52–21. DIAGNOSTIC TESTS FOR CUSHING'S SYNDROME AND ADRENAL INSUFFICIENCY

Suppression Tests for Cushing's Syndrome	Stimulation Tests for Adrenal Insufficiency
Office Screening Tests	
8 A.M. plasma cortisol after dexamethasone 1 mg. at midnight	Plasma cortisol before and 1 hour after ACTH 250 mg. I.V.
Abnormal if cortisol >5 μg./dl. at 8 A.M.	Abnormal if cortisol increase <11 μg./dl.
If Abnormal	
Dexamethasone 0.5 mg. q. 6 hr. × 8, then: 24-hr. urine hydroxysteroids second day	8 A.M. ACTH and plasma cortisol
Plasma cortisol at 48 hr.	
Indicative of Cushing's if:	Adrenal insufficiency Primary if:
Urine hydroxysteroids > 4 μmg./dl.	ACTH > 250 pg./dl.
Plasma cortisol > 5 mg/24 hour	Cortisol < 10 pg./dl.
	Secondary if:
	ACTH < 50 pg./dl.
	Cortisol < 10 pg./dl.

ADRENAL INSUFFICIENCY

Adrenocortical insufficiency, the result of deficient production of glucocorticoids, is due to either failure of the adrenal gland (primary) or deficient production of pituitary ACTH (secondary). Although an uncommon disorder, it often is considered in the differential diagnosis of severely ill patients with hypotension or electrolyte abnormalities and in outpatients with nonspecific complaints of weakness and fatigue. In most cases, Addison's disease, or primary adrenal cortical insufficiency, results from idiopathic atrophy or tuberculosis of the adrenal glands. All the other identifiable causes, including hemorrhagic disorders, neoplasia, and other infections, account for only about 1 per cent of cases.

Idiopathic adrenal failure, in which autoimmune factors play the major role, is more frequent in females, whereas Addison's disease due to tuberculosis is more common in males. Most cases are diagnosed between the third and fifth decades. A number of other disorders are associated with the idiopathic or autoimmune type of adrenal cortical insufficiency. These include primary ovarian failure, thyroiditis with hypothyroidism, diabetes mellitus, vitiligo, hyperparathyroidism, and pernicious anemia.

Clinical Manifestations

Weakness, easy fatigability, and weight loss are almost universally seen in patients with Addison's disease. Depression, irritability, and, in more advanced cases, confusion may also be seen. Hyperpigmentation and darkening of the hair are common. Postural dizziness is present in a minority of patients. Menstrual disturbances and amenorrhea are less common.

Many of the other symptoms of Addison's disease are nonspecific. These include nausea, vomiting, vague abdominal bloating or pain, and, rarely, diarrhea. A history of salt craving, if it can be elicited, is very helpful, although it occurs only in a minority of patients.

The most characteristic physical finding in Addison's disease is hyperpigmentation, which is especially pronounced over the knees, elbows, and knuckles. The hair darkens in color, and there may be a bluish-black discoloration of the lips, gums, and mucous membranes. Axillary and pubic hair is sparse. In patients with adrenal insufficiency due to pituitary failure, the skin may be pale. One cannot always distinguish between primary and secondary adrenal insufficiency by the presence or absence of pigmentation, as occasionally patients with primary adrenal failure do not have a striking increase in pigmentation. The blood pressure is characteristically low but may be normal; however, the presence of hypertension virtually excludes the diagnosis. An unusual but diagnostically important finding is calcification of ear cartilage.

In the absence of renal disease, hyponatremia and hyperkalemia should suggest the possibility of Addison's disease. Mild acetonuria is common. Slight anemia, with an elevated white count, eosinophilia, and relative or absolute lymphocytosis, also is found. Elevated serum calcium has been reported in a small percentage of patients. About half the patients with adrenal insufficiency due to tuberculosis will have adrenal calcification visible on a flat plate of the abdomen.

Diagnosis

The diagnosis of Addison's disease is confirmed by the demonstration of an inadequate glucocorticoid response to ACTH. The test is done by first drawing a baseline plasma cortisol and then injecting synthetic ACTH 0.25 mg. slowly intravenously, followed by measurement of plasma cortisol 60 minutes later. If plasma cortisol rises by an increment of more than 10 μg./dl., or if any value exceeds 25 μg./dl., adrenal insufficiency is excluded. This test does not differentiate between primary and secondary insufficiency, however, because atrophic adrenals seldom will be stimulated adequately by this rapid test.

In patients who are acutely ill or hypotensive, steroid therapy must be given prior to laboratory confirmation of the diagnosis. In this instance, synthetic ACTH 0.25 mg. may be placed in 1000 ml. of normal saline with 4 mg. of dexamethasone and infused over 1 hour. If plasma cortisol levels drawn before and after the infusion are below 15 mg./dl., the diagnosis is established. Hydrocortisone is not used in this procedure for it will elevate the plasma cortisol levels.

In patients in whom the diagnosis has been established, primary and secondary adrenal failure should be differentiated. In untreated patients, this can be done by means of ACTH and cortisol determinations drawn at 8 A.M. The plasma cortisol will be less than 10 μg./dl. and the ACTH greater than 250 pg./ml. in patients with primary adrenal insufficiency. Those with secondary adrenal insufficiency will have cortisol levels that are also low, but the ACTH level will be less than 50 pg./ml. Other tests for hypopituitarism are outlined in Table 52–18. In addition, there are a number of other methods for verifying the diagnosis of primary and secondary adrenal insufficiency, most of them involving ACTH stimulation over 1 to 5 days.

Treatment

Acute adrenal insufficiency is treated with large doses of intravenous glucocorticoids, and the associated dehydration is treated with rapid infusion of saline to expand the vascular volume and correct the electrolyte abnormalities. As soon as the diagnosis is established, hydrocortisone may be given in a dose of 100 mg. intravenously every 6 hours. As the patient improves, the dose of hydrocortisone may be tapered and the rate of fluid infusion decreased. Generally, hydrocortisone is tapered over a 3- to 5-day period to oral maintenance doses of 30 mg./day. An equivalent dose of another glucocorticoid may be used for maintenance. Most commonly, cortisone acetate, 37.5 mg., or prednisone, 7.5 mg., is used, with approximately two thirds of the dose being given in the morning and one third at night. Prednisone is satisfactory for maintenance therapy at a considerably lower cost than cortisone. It should be noted that cortisone acetate must not be used intramuscularly for it has been demonstrated that adequate blood levels are not achieved by administration of this preparation by that route.

Patients with adrenal failure secondary to pituitary insufficiency do not need mineralocorticoid replacement, but most patients with primary adrenal insufficiency will require the use of a mineralocorticoid. The one most commonly used is fludrocortisone acetate, 0.05 to 0.1 mg./day. Evaluation of the efficacy of replacement therapy is based on clinical symptoms rather than on laboratory tests. The dosage of the mineralocorticoid should be decreased in patients who develop edema or hypertension, and the addition of a mineralocorticoid or an increase in the glucocorticoid dose will be required in those who continue to have postural hypotension.

Education is extremely important in patients with adrenal insufficiency. They should be urged to wear an identification bracelet and to carry a card in their wallet bearing the diagnosis and the medications that they normally take. In addition, they should be instructed to double their dose of medication in the event of minor illness, triple the dose if fever occurs, and to promptly call their physician if they begin vomiting or are otherwise unable to take oral steroid replacement therapy. To emphasize this point, patients should be given a prescription for hydrocortisone 100 mg. contained in a preloaded syringe for use in the event that they are unable to take oral medications and medical care is not readily available. It is also helpful to give patients a copy of their medical records or a letter detailing how the diagnosis of adrenal insufficiency was established, in case another physician is consulted. This is particularly valuable if the patient ever undergoes surgery or if there is any question about the diagnosis in the future.

Patients with adrenal insufficiency from any cause who must undergo surgery should be given steroids preoperatively and in large doses for at least 24 hours after surgery. A commonly used dose of hydrocortisone is 100 mg. I.V. or I.M. just prior to surgery and every 6 hours for 24 hours thereafter, tapering by half each day until the maintenance dose is reached. It is important to prescribe this regimen for any patient who has taken steroids for more than a week within 6 months prior to surgery. High doses of hydrocortisone should be continued if fever or other complications occur.

CONGENITAL ADRENAL HYPERPLASIA

Congenital adrenal hyperplasia is rare, occurring only once in every 5000 births. The significance of this condition lies in the severity of the clinical manifestations and the problems associated with diagnosis and management. The signs and symptoms depend on the degree and type of enzyme deficiency.

The most common cause of congenital adrenal hyperplasia is 21-hydroxylase deficiency. In this disorder, cortisol synthesis is decreased and androgens are produced in excess, resulting in signs of adrenal insufficiency as well as precocious puberty in males and virilism in females. Deficiency of the 11-hydroxylase enzyme, the second most common cause of congenital adrenal hyperplasia, results in a similar picture except that hypertension is present, secondary to the accumulation of large amounts of deoxycorticosterone. Patients with 17-hydroxylase deficiency present with hypertension and sexual infantilism. Deficiency of 3-beta-ol-dehydrogenase is usually fatal in the neonatal period.

Diagnosis

The diagnosis of congenital adrenal hyperplasia should be suspected in any infant with ambiguous genitalia, in infants who develop signs suggestive of adrenal insufficiency, in children who have had rapid growth with the development of pubic hair at a very early age, and in young women exhibiting sexual infantilism and hypertension. Signs of adrenal insufficiency include vomiting, dehydration, hyperkalemia, and shock. Plasma cortisol and urinary hydroxysteroid levels both are low.

Treatment

Treatment of 21-hydroxylase or 11-hydroxylase deficiency is similar to that of adrenal insufficiency. The aim of therapy is to increase plasma cortisol levels sufficiently to decrease ACTH production and thereby lower the production of androgens. This will prevent the development of adrenal insufficiency and result in a normal rate of growth and normal levels of 17-ketosteroid secretion.

PHEOCHROMOCYTOMA

Pheochromocytomas are tumors derived from embryonic chromogen cells, about 90 per cent of which are located in the adrenal medulla. Of the remaining 10 per cent, at least three fourths are found in the abdomen. Approximately 10 per cent are bilateral. Many of the tumors are functional, producing catecholamines that cause hypertension. Pheochromocytoma is a very rare cause of high blood pressure, however, accounting for less than 0.5 per cent of all cases of hypertension. The importance of detecting a pheochromocytoma lies in the fact that the hypertension it produces is surgically curable, and the presence of a pheochromocytoma may be a clue to the coexistence of other endocrine disorders.

Clinical Manifestations

Blood pressure elevation, usually indistinguishable from essential hypertension, is the most common symptom leading to the diagnosis of a pheochromocytoma. Often a history of paroxysmal headache, palpitations, increased sweating, nervousness, dyspnea, and chest or abdominal pain can be elicited. Characteristically, the patient will be noted to be quite pale during the paroxysms. Paroxysms may be precipitated by micturition if the tumor is in the bladder wall, or during induction of anesthesia, or occasionally by abdominal palpation. Weight loss and heat intolerance suggesting hyperthyroidism are common. Congestive heart failure, arrhythmias, and fever, all due to catecholamine excess, may occur but are rare.

The only really specific physical finding is the presence of intermittent hypertension. Orthostatic hypotension is common, and rarely patients will present with paradoxical recumbent hypotension as the chief manifestation of an epinephrine-producing tumor. Neurofibromas and cafe-au-lait spots are also associated. The thyroid gland should be examined carefully, as there is an association of pheochromocytoma with medullary carcinoma of the thyroid. Most patients are of normal weight or slender.

Diagnosis

The diagnosis of pheochromocytoma should be suspected in hypertensive patients, especially young patients in whom there is a history of paroxysms of headache, sweating, and nervousness. Even in this very narrow category of patients, the discovery of a pheochromocytoma as the cause of the hypertension is rare. The initial screening test should be the measurement of the 24-hour urinary excretion of vanillylmandelic acid (VMA) and metanephrines. If these tests are normal and there is still a strong suspicion of pheochromocytoma, a second 24-hour urine should be collected immediately after a spontaneous paroxysm, and two or three tests done: VMA, metanephrines, and urinary catecholamines.

Both drugs and foods may cause false positives and false negatives. For example, most sympathomimetic drugs, including nasal vasoconstrictors, bronchodilators, theophylline, and amphetamines, may elevate the level of urinary catecholamines, but they usually do not have an appreciable effect on the VMA and metanephrine determinations. Drugs with high fluorescence may interfere with the determination of the catecholamines; examples of these are tetracycline, erythromycin, and chloral hydrate. Monoamine oxidase inhibitors are also offenders, as they will lower the metanephrines and increase VMA levels. Clofibrate may decrease VMA levels, and nalidixic acid may produce a false positive. Therefore, as a general rule, it is best to discontinue all nonessential medications.

A question frequently arises regarding the continuation of antihypertensive medications during testing. Although clonidine and other antihypertensives may depress urinary catecholamines, it is unlikely that they will produce a false negative finding in a patient with a pheochromocytoma. Long-term administration of reserpine or hydralazine usually does not significantly affect excretion of either VMA or metanephrine. Thiazides should not pose a problem; alpha-methyldopa may interfere with the determination of metanephrines but will not alter the excretion of VMA.

Provocative pharmacologic tests are rarely warranted and carry an appreciable risk. If a provocative agent is to be used, pretreatment of the patient with phenoxybenzamine may decrease the severity of the response and make the test safer.

After the diagnosis has been established, localization of the tumor is important. Computed tomography of the abdomen is the most helpful procedure. Ultrasonography and tomograms of the suprarenal area may also be helpful.

Treatment

Patients should be treated with an alpha-adrenergic blocker, such as phenoxybenzamine, prior to surgery. The usual starting dose is 10 mg. twice daily, with the dose being increased by 10 mg. per day until hypotension occurs or the paroxysms are controlled. Tachycardia is a frequent complication, and a beta blocker, such as propranolol, may be added to the regimen if needed. Orthostatic hypotension may be aggravated or precipitated as the dose of phenoxybenzamine is increased and may limit its dose. Prazosin, also an adrenergic blocker, has both diagnostic and therapeutic value in the treatment of the hypertension produced by a pheochromocytoma. Standard doses of the drug are used, starting with 1 mg. three times daily.

Reproductive Endocrinology

Alteration in the normal sequence of sexual maturation may result from (1) abnormalities of the chromosomes, (2) exposure of the female fetus to excess androgens, (3) decreased androgen production or effect in a male fetus, (4) a wide variety of disorders of the ovaries and testes, or (5) dysfunction of the hypothalamic/pituitary/gonadal axis. The most complex problem in this field is infertility, as it may involve one of the above abnormalities or any of a host of other disorders in either partner.

Normal Sexual Development

Under chromosomal influence, the cortical portion of the gonad differentiates into ovaries or the medullary portion into testes. The fetal testis produces two substances, a müllerian-inhibiting factor, which causes regression of the female ducts, and testosterone, which promotes development of the wolffian duct and masculinization of the external genitalia. In the absence of dihydrotestosterone, the external genitalia will be female. The fetal ovary is not responsible for development or regression of either wolffian or müllerian ducts.

It is still not known exactly what triggers the increased gonadotropin production that produces maturation of the ovaries and testes and the onset of puberty. However, understanding the normal sequence and range of sexual maturation is essential when one is dealing with problems involving early sexual development or a delay in normal sexual maturation. In boys, the first sign of puberty is pigmentation and wrinkling of the scrotum with enlargement of the testes. This occurs around age 12. Pubic hair appears around age 14, owing to increasing levels of testosterone. Axillary hair is usually noted soon thereafter, but the development of facial hair is often delayed until after age 16. There is great variability in the age at which these events occur, but the sequence is usually orderly, with steady progression from one stage to another.

In girls, the earliest sign of sexual development is breast buds, which are apparent around age 11; pubic hair is usually noted at the same age. Maximum linear growth occurs about a year later at age 12. Girls usually grow 5 to 10 cm. per year and boys considerably more during the year of maximum growth. In the United States, the mean age of menarche is 12½ to 13 years; axillary hair appears shortly thereafter. This means that menarche usually occurs 1½ to 2 years after the onset of breast development. It is not uncommon for ovulation to be delayed for 1 or more years after the onset of menses (Table 52–22).

As a general rule of thumb, the normal range for each stage of development can be estimated by adding or subtracting 3 years from the mean. If one

Table 52–22. PATTERN OF PUBERTAL DEVELOPMENT

Sign	Mean Age (years) Girls	Boys
Breast buds	11	
Testicular enlargement		11
Pubic hair	11	13
Maximum linear growth rate	12	14
Menses	12	
Axillary hair	13	15
Facial hair		16+

applies this rule, the normal range for menarche would be 9 to 16 years. There is a tendency for sexual development to occur later in thin female adolescents as compared with those who are of normal weight.

PRECOCIOUS PUBERTY

Precocious puberty, or the premature development of secondary sex characteristics, occurs much more commonly in girls than in boys (about 10:1). The cause can be identified in only 20 per cent of girls, but in over half of boys an underlying organic disorder will be found. The diagnosis of constitutional or idiopathic precocious puberty is made only after exclusion of all other known causes of early sexual development, such as drug ingestion or excessive hormone production by adrenal, ovarian, or testicular tumors. Precocious puberty may also be caused by head trauma, tumors near the hypothalamus, meningitis, encephalitis, and hydrocephalus.

Girls who develop breast buds and boys who have an increase in testicular size before age 8½, or who have other evidence of sexual development more than 3 years earlier than the mean, should have a very thorough and systematic evaluation to establish the cause. The skin should be carefully assessed for the presence of cafe-au-lait spots, which are part of a syndrome characterized by polyosteotic fibrous dysplasia and precocious puberty. Dark pigmentation of the nipples in girls suggests estrogen ingestion. Studies that may be of help in assessing the problem are x-ray studies of the hands for bone age, urinary 17-ketosteroids, a computed tomography scan of the sella, an electroencephalogram, and an ultrasonogram of the pelvis in girls. Even when an extensive evaluation fails to reveal an underlying cause, close follow-up is necessary to exclude an organic lesion, which may later become identifiable.

In girls, medroxyprogesterone and, more recently, danazol have been used in treatment of constitutional precocious sexual development; therapy is continued until the chronologic age is equal to the bone age. However, treatment should not be instituted until the patient has been carefully evaluated and serious organic causes of precocious puberty have been excluded.

KLINEFELTER'S SYNDROME

One of the most common abnormalities of sex chromosomes leading to abnormal testicular development is Klinefelter's syndrome. Approximately one in 500 newborn males will be found to be chromatin-positive, meaning that instead of the usual 46 XY chromosomal constitution, one or more extra X chromosomes are present, with 47 XXY being the most common associated karyotype. These patients frequently present initially for evaluation of infertility or gynecomastia. The classic finding on physical examination is the presence of small, firm testes that measure less than 2 cm. in the greatest diameter. Most patients are tall, but there is considerable variability in the body habitus and the degree of virilization. Gynecomastia occurs in a significant proportion, and mental retardation is not uncommon. Histologically, the testes show hyalinization of the seminiferous tubules, which accounts for the azoospermia and infertility. Testosterone production by the Leydig cells is usually normal or low.

In a male with small testes, the diagnosis may be confirmed by the presence of a Barr body on buccal smear or the demonstration of a 47 XXY karyotype. FSH and LH levels are elevated, but there is no need to measure the gonadotropins, as they have no diagnostic or prognostic usefulness. There is no treatment for the infertility; testosterone treatment is indicated only in those who have evidence of androgen deficiency. Mastectomy may be done for cosmetic reasons.

TURNER'S SYNDROME

Turner's syndrome is due to a chromosomal abnormality, with 45 XO the most commonly associated karyotype. It is rare, affecting one in every 2000 to 3000 female infants. Clinically, the syndrome is characterized by short stature (mean height of 54 inches), lack of breast development, amenorrhea, and a number of other somatic abnormalities. These include a low hairline, strabismus, webbed neck, widely spaced nipples, short fourth metacarpal, coarctation of the aorta with absence of the femoral pulses, and lymphedema in the newborn. The diagnosis is confirmed by demonstrating the absence of the Barr body on a buccal smear or by a 45 XO karyotype. There is no treatment for the infertility, but cyclic estrogen/progesterone replacement should be started at the usual age of puberty to promote breast development.

DELAYED PUBERTY

The failure of appearance of breast buds in girls and testicular enlargement in boys by age 14 is an indication that puberty is delayed. A delay in the normal sequence of events of puberty also may be important. For example, if breast buds appear but menarche does not follow within 2 to 3 years, or if testicular enlargement occurs but pubic hair does not develop, investigation for delayed puberty is warranted. The history may be particularly significant, as both systemic diseases and severe emotional disorders may retard sexual development. Attention should be paid to the previous growth pattern as well as to the current height and weight. Noting whether the patient has a sense of smell is important, for anosmia may be associated with hypogonadism.

Laboratory data that may help are a lateral x-ray of the skull for sella size, thyroid function tests, and bone age. (See Amenorrhea—Primary for more detailed discussion of delayed puberty in females.) In contrast to precocious puberty, delayed puberty is more common in boys than in girls and is more likely to be due to organic disease in girls than in boys. Therapy is dependent primarily on the underlying cause. Human chorionic gonadotropin has been used in boys, but it is reserved for use only after a very careful evaluation has failed to reveal a treatable organic lesion.

HYPOGONADISM

Male hypogonadism, due to a primary defect in the testes or secondary to abnormal hypothalamic/pituitary function, may affect spermatogenesis and production of testosterone. In primary hypogonadism, FSH and LH levels are elevated, whereas in hypothalamic/pituitary disorders, the gonadotropins are low. Primary hypogonadism may result from genetic disorders, such as Klinefelter's syndrome, trauma, orchitis, chemotherapy, sickle cell anemia, or surgical castration. Spinal cord damage is especially prone to produce primary hypogonadism. Over half of males with spinal cord injury will have impotence, inability to ejaculate, and impaired spermatogenesis. A number of other systemic diseases are associated with abnormalities in testicular function, either by direct testicular damage or through hypothalamic/pituitary dysfunction. Among these are liver disease, alcoholism, hemochromatosis, adrenocorticoid tumors, Addison's disease, Cushing's disease, hyperthyroidism, and hypothyroidism.

The clinical manifestations of hypogonadism are dependent largely on the age at which the disorder occurs. Androgen deficiency occurring early in utero results in ambiguity of the external genitalia. Prepubertal hypopituitarism, on the other hand, usually is associated with growth retardation, a youthful appearance, eunuchoid habitus, and sexual infantilism. Decreased libido and infertility are the main features of postpubertal hypogonadism.

When there is a deficiency of testosterone during puberty, in addition to sexual infantilism, there is a delay in epiphyseal closure with continued long bone growth, resulting in excessively long extremities. Usually, the span of the arms exceeds the height by 2 or more inches, and the distance from the floor to the pubic symphysis is 55 per cent or more of the height. Most patients are tall, but this is not always seen. The shoulders tend to be narrow, and frequently there is an excess of fat deposition in the hips and lower abdomen. Acne and baldness are not present. Other clinical signs are a small prostate, diminished body and facial hair, fine wrinkles around the eyes and mouth, and a sallow complexion.

Diagnosis

The diagnostic investigation is guided by the clinical manifestations. T_4, prolactin, testosterone, FSH, and LH determinations and a search for Barr bodies or karyotyping may be indicated.

Treatment

The primary aim of therapy is to replace testosterone and, when possible, to restore fertility. In patients with pituitary failure producing secondary hypogonadism, fertility sometimes may be restored by the combined use of human chorionic gonadotropin and human menopausal gonadotropin. Patients with high FSH and LH levels and low androgen levels, indicating that the primary abnormality is in the testes, may benefit from treatment with testosterone, but their infertility is not amenable to therapy. Long-acting preparations of testosterone, such as testosterone enanthate or testosterone cyclopropionate, 100 to 200 mg. I.M., are given every 2 to 4 weeks. Oral testosterone is not as potent as injectable preparations, and methyl testosterone may cause cholestatic jaundice, though recovery is usually rapid and complete after cessation of therapy.

Any discussion of the use of androgens would be incomplete without a mention of the interest in the use of androgens by athletes. The side effects, which include a reduction in the sperm count sometimes resulting in infertility, contraindicate their use except in patients who are actually androgen-deficient.

AMENORRHEA—PRIMARY

The mean age of menarche in the United States is about 12½ to 13 years but the normal range is usually considered to extend from 9 to 16 years. Primary amenorrhea is defined as failure to menstruate by the age of 16 and may be due to a number of causes, genetic, anatomic, physiologic, or endocrinologic (Table 52–23).

Clinical Manifestations

Failure to begin menstruating when expected is a matter of great concern to most adolescent girls and their parents, and this anxiety is the motivation for consulting the physician. Although most cases will prove to be due to physiologic delay, the problem should be taken seriously and a detailed history taken. It is especially important to obtain a record of the

Table 52–23. CAUSES OF PRIMARY AMENORRHEA

Physiologic	**Anatomic**
Delayed puberty	Genital tract obstruction
Pregnancy	Failure of müllerian development
Genetic	**Ovarian**
Turner's syndrome	Ovarian agenesis
Testicular feminization	Polycystic disease
Thyroid	**Pituitary/Hypothalamic**
Hypothyroidism	Pituitary tumor
Adrenal	Hyperprolactinemia
Congenital adrenal hyperplasia	Hypothalamic dysfunction
Iatrogenic	Sarcoidosis
Oral contraceptives	Low body weight

growth pattern and history regarding the timing of the onset of breast development and pubic hair.

Body weight is a significant factor influencing the time of menarche. Thin girls tend to menstruate at an older age than heavy girls. Most girls weigh over 90 pounds before the onset of menses. A thorough physical examination will rule out most of the common organic causes. Observation of the body habitus and of secondary sex characteristics is especially important. Although many physicians are hesitant to perform a pelvic examination on adolescents, it is necessary to assure that there is no anatomic barrier to the menstrual flow by visualizing or palpating the cervix. If the cervix cannot be visualized, an abnormality of the müllerian system should be searched for through x-ray examination, ultrasonography, or laparoscopy.

Diagnosis

If there is evidence of breast development and/or pubic hair by age 14 and the physical findings are normal, the patient and her parents may be reassured and any further investigation delayed for 6 months. A more thorough evaluation should be begun earlier if the findings suggest a genetic or anatomic abnormality. The initial steps in such an investigation consist of determination of T_4 and prolactin levels, x-ray studies of the hands for bone age, and a buccal smear or karyotype. The final step in evaluation is to obtain FSH and LH levels. A complete outline of the evaluation of primary amenorrhea is contained in Table 52–24.

Table 52–24. EVALUATION OF PRIMARY AMENORRHEA

History and physical	Exclusion of pregnancy
Prolactin level	T_4, T_3 uptake
Bone age	Buccal smear or karyotype

If prolactin elevated, get computed tomography scan of sella.
If hirsutism present, get 11-hydroxysteroids and 17-ketosteroids.
If all above normal, get FSH and LH.

Treatment

The plan for treatment is dependent on the nature of the abnormality. Surgery may be required for an imperforate hymen. Endocrine problems are to be treated in the manner described in the appropriate section of this chapter.

AMENORRHEA—SECONDARY

Although pregnancy is the most common cause of secondary amenorrhea, omission of an expected menstrual period may occasionally occur in otherwise normal women as the result of emotional or physical stress or the effect of drugs. The causes of secondary amenorrhea are listed in Table 52–25. Investigation of the cause for a single missed period may require no more than a thorough history, a pelvic examination, and a pregnancy test. More extensive tests need not be undertaken until the third period is missed, for in the majority of cases the normal menstrual cycle will be resumed without treatment.

The historical inquiry should include a detailed record of the length and duration of menses, the chronology of sexual exposure, the method of contraception used, and a careful drug history. One should also ask about changes in the breasts and abdominal or pelvic discomfort.

Diagnosis

The initial step to be taken is to rule out pregnancy, and it is advisable to repeat both the urine pregnancy test and the pelvic examination in 2 to 4 weeks if they are initially negative. When the decision is made to look further, the first step is to consider the possibility of hypothyroidism or an abnormality of the pituitary by means of a thorough physical examination, serum thyroxine, and serum prolactin levels. If these are normal, medroxyprogesterone, 10 mg. daily, may be given by mouth for 5 days to try to induce withdrawal bleeding (Table 52–26).

Another method for evaluating estrogen effect is examination of a smear of vaginal mucosal cells. Estrogen is required in the maturation of parabasal cells through the intermediate stage to the cornified

Table 52–25. CAUSES OF SECONDARY AMENORRHEA

Physiologic	**Anatomic**
Pregnancy	Endometrial destruction
Menopause	**Thyroid**
Lactation	Hypothyroidism
Ovarian	**Iatrogenic**
Polycystic disease	Progesterone injections
Pituitary/Hypothalamic	Oral contraceptives
Weight loss	
Pituitary tumor	
Sheehan's syndrome	
Hyperprolactinemia	
Sarcoidosis	

Table 52–26. EVALUATION OF SECONDARY AMENORRHEA

1. History and physical examination
2. Exclude pregnancy
3. T_4 level
4. Prolactin level

If these are all normal, institute trial of progesterone: medroxyprogesterone, 10 mg./day orally for 5 days.
If this does not produce menstruation:
Get: FSH and LH levels
Give: Ethinyl estradiol 0.02 mg./day for 28 days
Medroxyprogesterone 10 mg./day last 5 days
If hirsutism present, get 17-hydroxysteroids and 17-ketosteroids.

state. The relative degree of estrogen deficiency may be gauged by the Maturation Index as the percentage of parabasal, intermediate, and cornified cells in the smear. Very few parabasal cells are present if estrogen levels are adequate and the majority of cells are cornified.

If the physical and laboratory findings are normal and withdrawal bleeding occurs after progesterone, one can assume that there is adequate estrogen and that the amenorrhea is due to anovulation. If withdrawal bleeding does not occur, a pregnancy test should be repeated before a course of estrogen and progesterone is given in an attempt to induce bleeding. If withdrawal bleeding occurs after the combined use of estrogen and progesterone but not after progesterone alone, the cause of the amenorrhea is estrogen deficiency. A CT scan of the sella and FSH and LH determinations will help determine whether the deficiency is due to primary ovarian failure or hypopituitarism. In the presence of hirsutism, 17-ketosteroid and 17-hydroxysteroid levels should be obtained to establish or exclude the diagnosis of polycystic ovarian disease and other ovarian or adrenal disorders (Table 52–26).

Treatment

Amenorrhea due to anovulation may be treated with cyclic progesterone therapy. Medroxyprogesterone, 10 mg. daily for 10 days every 2 to 3 months, is given to convert the proliferative endometrium produced by endogenous estrogen to the secretory phase with subsequent bleeding within 1 week after stopping the progesterone. The treatment of the endocrine causes of amenorrhea are discussed in other sections of this chapter under the specific disorder.

GALACTORRHEA

Secretion of fluid from the breasts is considered to be nonphysiologic if it occurs more than 12 months after the last pregnancy or after discontinuation of nursing. This discharge, which is usually clear or white, can also be yellowish or greenish and may be either unilateral or bilateral. Galactorrhea may occur with or without hyperprolactinemia or amenorrhea. The disorder usually results from a reduction in the production or delivery of the prolactin-inhibiting factor to the pituitary, with a resultant increase in prolactin secretion, or from autonomous production of prolactin by a pituitary tumor. Hypothyroidism may also produce galactorrhea because of an increase in thyrotropin-releasing hormone, which in turn directly stimulates prolactin release from the pituitary. An important but rare cause of galactorrhea is ectopic production of prolactin by nonendocrine neoplasms.

Probably the most common cause of galactorrhea is drug ingestion, especially estrogen or contraceptive pills. Phenothiazines, tricyclic antidepressants, antihypertensives such as methyldopa and reserpine, and a wide variety of other drugs may cause galactorrhea. Less frequently, galactorrhea may occur because of stimulation of the efferent sensory neural arc by chest wall scars or herpes zoster. Stress, trauma, surgery, or medication may be associated with galactorrhea (Table 52–27).

Diagnosis

Secretion of any quantity of fluid from the breast in nulliparous women or more than 12 months after termination of pregnancy or nursing deserves evaluation. A very thorough drug history should be taken. It is important to note that galactorrhea may persist for up to 6 months after stopping a drug, so it is important to determine what drugs have been taken in the recent past as well as the ones the patient is presently taking. If there is no drug history to account for the galactorrhea, a serum prolactin and CT scan of the sella are done. Visual fields should be obtained on any patient with an abnormal head CT scan, headaches, or visual symptoms. If these are normal, then the patient should be reassured. A repeat prolactin level may be done in a year for follow-up.

If the prolactin level is elevated but the sella is completely normal, no further study is mandatory. Patients with either an elevated prolactin or an abnormal sella should have yearly follow-up examinations, usually with repeat prolactin levels and periodically with a lateral skull x-ray or CT scan, for

Table 52–27. CAUSES OF GALACTORRHEA

Drugs	**Endocrine/Hypothalamic**
Estrogens	Pituitary tumors
Phenothiazines	Hypothalamic tumors
Tricyclic antidepressants	Hypothalamic sarcoid
Methyldopa	Hypothyroidism
Reserpine	**Stress**
Amphetamines	Trauma
Diazepines	Surgery
Butyrophenones	Emotional stress
Neurogenic	
Suckling	
Chest wall scars	
Herpes zoster	
Spinal cord lesions	

hyperprolactinemia may antedate the detection of intrasellar tumors by many years.

Treatment

If the galactorrhea is disturbing, producing pain and tenderness in the breasts, treatment may be started with bromocriptine, 2.5 mg. daily. Generally, when the drug is stopped, the galactorrhea will recur. Some patients will find that the side effects of bromocriptine, usually nausea, dizziness, and weakness, are more undesirable than the galactorrhea. Surgery for a pituitary adenoma is indicated if there is evidence of visual field abnormalities or a deficiency of any anterior pituitary hormone. The reason for surgical removal is to preserve vision and to prevent loss of other pituitary hormones.

Many pituitary tumors, both macro- and microadenomas, may be followed for years without showing any enlargement. Patients who desire to be pregnant should be warned, however, that microadenomas or any pituitary tumor may enlarge during pregnancy. Even during pregnancy, treatment with bromocriptine may obviate the need for surgery.

MENOPAUSE

Menopause, the cessation of menses, occurs at a mean age of 51 years. For 10 years or more prior to menopause, ovarian function wanes, ovulation occurs less frequently, and estrogen production by the ovarian follicles progressively decreases. As estrogen levels decrease, FSH levels rise; after menopause, FSH levels usually exceed 40 mI.U./ml. As ovarian function decreases, the percentage of estrogen derived from adrenal androstenedione increases. The rate of extragonadal estrogen production increases with increasing body weight; postmenopausal women who are overweight tend to have higher estrogen levels than thin women.

Clinical Manifestations

One of the earliest symptoms related to waning estrogen production is menstrual irregularity with either an increased or decreased amount of flow. Vasomotor instability with hot flashes and sweats occurs in most women; these often are severe after abrupt castration by surgery or irradiation. The hot flashes are wavelike sensations that move up the chest to the head and are associated with profuse perspiration and flushing. They may last anywhere from a few seconds to an hour. They occur more frequently at night and as many as ten hot flashes in a 24-hour period is not uncommon. Anxiety, depression, and irritability are also frequent in the perimenopausal years, as are nonspecific complaints, such as headache, insomnia, and fatigue.

Atrophy of the vulva and vagina occurs frequently, causing dyspareunia and pruritus. Osteoporosis, a reduction in the quantity of bone, is a significant postmenopausal problem, particularly in thin Caucasian women. Its significance lies in its associated morbidity and mortality due to vertebral compression fractures and hip fracture.

Family physicians who must make a subjective judgment regarding the severity of symptoms associated with estrogen deficiency will be influenced by their own attitudes toward the menopause as a problem, as well by the patient's complaints. Some physicians who regard the menopause and its consequences as something that all women must endure offer minimal treatment for as short a time as possible. Others believe that the complications of estrogen deficiency, especially the osteoporosis, are significant enough to warrant long-term therapy.

Treatment

There is considerable controversy regarding postmenopausal estrogen replacement therapy, particularly who should receive estrogen and for how long. It is generally agreed, however, that if estrogen replacement is undertaken, the lowest dose of estrogen that reverses the deficiency should be used and that any woman who receives estrogen therapy in the postmenopausal years should be followed closely. Vasomotor reactions, such as hot flashes and perspiration, usually will be relieved by conjugated estrogen, 0.625 mg., or ethinyl estradiol, 20 μg., given daily for 25 days during the month with medroxyprogesterone, 10 mg., added daily during the last 10 days. This will, produce an interruption of the growth of the endometrium in patients who have a uterus, preventing endometrial hyperplasia and carcinoma. Since the effect of the different schedules for estrogen administration on the breast is not well known, it is probably best to maintain the same cyclic schedule with estrogen and progesterone, even in women who have had a hysterectomy.

The use of estrogen postmenopausally for the treatment of emotional lability, anxiety, depression, and headaches is more controversial. A number of studies suggest that estrogen retards the development of osteoporosis and the resultant incidence of fractures by decreasing the rate of bone loss. Also, there is considerable evidence that postmenopausal estrogens protect against coronary artery disease.

Estrogen therapy is contraindicated in patients who have a previous history of endometrial carcinoma, estrogen-dependent breast tumors, or thromboembolic disease. Combined therapy with cortisone must be used in women who have hypertension. Certainly, continued support and understanding by the physician is essential, for symptoms of the climacteric occur in virtually all women, although their severity is dependent not only on the rate of estrogen withdrawal but also on genetic and acquired factors that affect the overall aging process.

HIRSUTISM

The exact amount of hair growth that may be considered excessive is difficult to define, but if the patient is concerned about increased hair growth, the problem deserves evaluation. Hypertrichosis refers to the excessive growth of hair on the extremities, head, and back. Hirsutism, on the other hand, refers to an increase in growth of sexual or hormone-dependent hair, which is located primarily in the pubic, axillary, abdominal, chest, and facial areas.

Hair follicles are found over most of the body except for the palms and soles and have a similar distribution and concentration in both men and women. The differences in hair growth in men and women result primarily from differences in levels of circulating androgens. Although routine laboratory studies, including testosterone or 17-ketosteroids, often do not demonstrate abnormally high levels of circulating androgens, the relative production rate of the androgens or sensitivity to the androgens is higher in hirsute women than in women with normal amounts of body hair.

The aim of medical evaluation is to exclude serious abnormalities associated with increased androgen production. There are numerous causes of hirsutism, the most common being genetic, drug-induced, and endocrine-related; other causes include anorexia nervosa, head injury, or rare congenital abnormalities. Genetic factors determine not only the number of hair follicles but also the sensitivity of the follicles to the androgens. For example, Mediterranean women have more hair than Scandinavian women, who in turn have more hair growth than Oriental women. Drugs most commonly associated with increased hair growth are phenytoin, diazoxide, and androgens. There are a number of adrenal causes of increased hair growth, with Cushing's syndrome being the most common. Congenital adrenal hyperplasia is a very rare cause of hirsutism. The most common ovarian cause of hirsutism is polycystic ovarian disease; ovarian tumors are very rare.

Clinical Manifestations

Hirsutism usually develops very slowly, beginning shortly after the onset of menses, and often becomes of enough concern to the patient for her to seek medical attention in her early twenties. The most important aspect of the history relates to the regularity of menses. Women who have regular menstrual periods usually have a genetic cause for the increased hair growth. If menses are irregular, however, it becomes necessary to rule out a serious cause of excess androgen effect.

It is important to note the blood pressure, as elevated blood pressure is a common feature of Cushing's syndrome. Acne and obesity are commonly associated with increased hair growth but do not have any particular diagnostic significance. Most women with high androgen production will have normal or large muscles, and the presence of muscular wasting or weakness immediately raises the possibility of Cushing's syndrome. It is important to note the presence or absence of other signs of virilism, such as an enlarged clitoris, deepening of the voice, balding, or a change in the body habitus.

Diagnosis

Excessive hair growth in women who have normal menses can be attributed to genetic causes, and laboratory evaluation is unnecessary. However, in the majority there will be some irregularity of menses, and testosterone and 17-ketosteroids should be determined. If there is any suspicion of Cushing's syndrome, such as an elevated blood pressure, glucose intolerance, centripetal obesity, or elevated urinary ketosteroids, a dexamethasone suppression test described under Cushing's Syndrome should be done. Testosterone levels are frequently above the upper limits of normal in hirsute women, but levels more than three times normal warrant more extensive evaluation for a possible androgen-producing tumor. Very high levels of ketosteroids are seen in congenital adrenal hyperplasia, a very rare cause of hirsutism.

Treatment

The basic treatment depends on the etiology; when there is no surgically treatable ovarian or adrenal cause, as is the case in most women, the local removal of hair is indicated. Medical therapy with oral contraceptives or spironolactone may be tried, but it must be emphasized to the patient that there is really no single drug or drug combination that will quickly eliminate the excess hair or even retard its growth. It usually takes at least 3 to 6 months to notice any decrease in the rate of hair growth after beginning oral contraceptives or spironolactone. By 6 months, plasma testosterone levels should have decreased significantly on medical therapy, but a decrease in hair growth may or may not be evident. Patients who are unable to take the oral contraceptives may be tried on medroxyprogesterone in a dose of 150 mg. I.M. every 3 months.

Electrolysis is the only permanent method of locally removing hair. It is expensive, time-consuming, uncomfortable, and not a realistic way to remove a great quantity of hair. Generally, only 20 or so hairs are removed at a sitting. Bleaching the hair is one of the most acceptable methods of dealing with the hair cosmetically. Wax depilatories are better than plucking, but they require repeated application. Chemical depilatories should be avoided, as they usually cause skin irritation.

Shaving remains the single most effective simple, inexpensive way of removing hair. Shaving the face, however, seems to be unacceptable to most women. It is difficult to convince patients that shaving will not increase the rate of hair growth on their face or change the consistency of the hair. The obvious difficulty with shaving is that it needs to be done very frequently—at least daily if hair is heavy and occasionally more often. If the patient can be convinced that this is the major objection to shaving, and that there is no evidence to suggest there is any change in the quality or quantity of hair in the area shaved, it may become an acceptable method of hair removal in women who previously felt that shaving would only compound their problem.

INFERTILITY

Infertility is defined as the failure of conception to occur after 1 year of unprotected coitus. More than 10 per cent of couples in the United States have difficulty in conceiving. The problem may involve only a single factor in male or female, but multiple factors are involved in a substantial number of couples. The evaluation of infertility should be systematic and rapid. All possible sources of the problem should be evaluated, and any abnormalities discovered should be treated as the evaluation proceeds. The expectations of both the physician and the couple must be realistic, with the understanding that in spite of a thorough evaluation a cause will not be found in as many as 20 per cent of infertile couples.

Clinical Manifestations

It is important to inquire about previous fertility, methods of contraception, and the duration of infertility. The frequency and timing of intercourse should be noted, as well as whether lubricants and douches that may interfere with sperm survival are used. Information regarding the regularity of menses helps to determine whether or not ovulation is occurring. A history of medical problems, pelvic inflammatory disease, and surgical procedures also may give clues to the cause of infertility.

Although a complete physical examination should be done on both partners, the evaluation of the testes and pelvic examination need to be particularly detailed. Normally, the testes measure at least 4 cm. in the long diameter. A varicocele of the left internal spermatic vein or the presence of thickened adnexae with palpable tubes, especially if there is a history of pelvic inflammatory disease, may indicate the source of the problem.

Diagnosis

If the history and physical examination are completely unrevealing, the next step in the evaluation is a semen analysis and documentation of ovulation. Regular menses that occur every 26 to 32 days—especially if accompanied by premenstrual tension, headaches, or cramps—are almost invariably associated with ovulation. Ovulation also may be verified by showing a basal body temperature rise of at least 0.4°F. from the first half of the menstrual cycle (luteal or secretory phase). The infertility evaluation should not be delayed by obtaining several months of basal body temperature charts, for the presence of regular menses alone is excellent evidence of ovulation. Other methods of documenting ovulation are the demonstration of a progesterone level of greater than 3 ng./ml. on day 21 to 24 of the menstrual cycle or an endometrial biopsy between day 22 and 24 that demonstrates secretory endometrium.

In a normal semen analysis, there are at least 20 million sperm per ml., with a volume of 2 to 5 mg. More than 60 per cent of the sperm are motile 2 hours after ejaculation, and more than 60 per cent have a normal morphology (Table 52–28). If an abnormality, such as poor motility, is found on semen analysis and a varicocele is noted on physical examination, the patient should be referred for surgical correction while evaluation of the female partner continues.

If these tests are normal, the next step in evaluation is usually the postcoital test, which is done by aspirating cervical mucus from the cervical os 2 to 8 hours after coitus on day 12 to 14 of the menstrual cycle. If the cervical mucus is of good quality, stretchable to 5 inches, copious, and clear, with at least five or more motile sperm per high-power field, the postcoital test can be considered adequate. If all of these tests are normal, evaluation of the female genital tract by hysterosalpingogram or laparoscopy is indicated.

The evaluation to this point should take less than 6 months in most cases. Many general physicians will refer patients to a specialist if they are unable to detect a treatable abnormality on history and physical examination, or they may elect to institute medical treatment for induction of ovulation if there is a problem in this area.

Treatment

Most of the agents used for medical treatment of male infertility are of questionable, or at least unproven, efficacy. Clomiphene citrate, 25 mg./day for 25 days with 5-day rest periods, has been used.

Table 52–28. EVALUATION OF INFERTILITY

History and physical examination	
Semen analysis: (normals)	Count over 20 million/ml. Volume 2–5 ml. Motility over 60 per cent Morphology normal in over 60 per cent
Documentation of ovulation:	Regular menses Elevation of basal temperature Progesterone level above 3 ng./ml. Endometrial biopsy
Postcoital test	
Evaluation of female genital tract:	Hysterosalpingogram Laparoscopy

Cortisone acetate, 5 mg. twice daily for 25 days with 5-day rest periods, also has been used with clomiphene. Both of these regimens produce questionable results.

In the male, testosterone enanthate, 200 mg. every 2 weeks, or depotestosterone cyprionate, 100 mg., or delalestrol, 200 mg. weekly, may be given I.M. until azoospermia is produced. This is a last-resort therapy used in the hope that when the drug is stopped there will be a rebound spermatogenesis. Tetracycline, 250 mg. three times daily, also has been advocated for empiric treatment to eradicate mycoplasma, since this organism has been implicated in some cases of infertility in the male.

If retrograde ejaculation is a problem, sympathomimetic drugs, such as Ornade, one capsule twice daily, or ephedrine, 15 mg. 1 to 2 hours before coitus, may be used in an attempt to correct it. Thyroid, low-dose androgens, human menopausal gonadotropin, and human chorionic gonadotropin are all outmoded, or at least unproven, therapeutic agents.

The medical management of female infertility has been slightly more successful, as there are several agents that may induce ovulation. Clomiphene citrate 50 mg. may be given by mouth for 5 days, beginning on day 5 of the cycle. If ovulation does not occur with this dose, then the dose may be increased every month by 50 mg. until a dose of 200 mg./day has been reached. Clomiphene induces ovulation by stimulating hypothalamic secretion of the gonadotropins. Use of human menopausal gonadotropin and human chorionic gonadotropin may be used to stimulate or substitute for LH action but usually a great deal of expertise is required for their proper use. Bromocriptine, 2.5 mg. one to three times daily, is very effective in inducing ovulation in patients with hyperprolactinemia. Danazol, 500 mg. twice daily, has been used to suppress gonadotropins and to treat endometriosis.

Conjugated estrogens, 0.625 mg., or estinyl estradiol, 0.02 mg., from day 5 through 12 may improve the quality of the cervical mucus. Dexamethasone, 0.5 mg./day, has been used to decrease ACTH-mediated androgen secretion. Tetracycline, 250 mg. four times a day, is also used in females for empirical treatment to eradicate mycoplasma.

If, after a very thorough evaluation, no cause for infertility can be ascertained, the physician should be candid with the couple, letting them know that there is no known cause for their infertility and that further testing and treatment will offer little chance for improving fertility. The physician should encourage adoption for couples with infertility of 3 or more years for which no cause can be found.

GYNECOMASTIA

Gynecomastia, the enlargement of male breasts, may occur during normal puberty or may result from a wide range of disorders or drugs. In most instances, there is a relative increase in estrogen and decrease in androgen production or an increase in prolactin. Fifty per cent or more of adolescent boys will have some kind of gynecomastia during puberty. Breast enlargement may also be familial. The most common drugs associated with gynecomastia are estrogens, testosterone, phenothiazines, spironolactone, marijuana, digitalis, and reserpine. Cirrhosis is a common cause of male breast enlargement. Refeeding after starvation may cause gynecomastia. A host of other disorders, including Hodgkin's disease, bronchogenic carcinoma, testicular tumors, and tumors of the adrenal, may cause gynecomastia as well.

In the adolescent male, if the physical examination is completely within normal limits except for the presence of gynecomastia, the patient may be reassured. Additional laboratory tests are not warranted. In adults or young children, however, the occurrence of breast enlargement warrants a careful evaluation to establish the underlying cause. A chest x-ray, skull films, liver and renal function tests, and LH, human chorionic gonadotropin (HCG), estradiol, and plasma testosterone levels should be obtained in selected cases. Mastectomy may be recommended for cosmetic purposes in patients with Klinefelter's syndrome or other causes of permanent breast enlargement.

CRYPTORCHIDISM

Cryptorchidism, more commonly known as undescended testis, is present in less than 0.5 per cent of adult men but is considerably more frequent in newborn male infants. The great majority of undescended testicles are in the inguinal canal, and unilateral cryptorchidism is more common than bilateral undescended testes. Cryptorchidism may occur with or without other gonadal abnormalities or disorders of sexual development.

The most important aspect of the examination is to be sure that the testis is truly undescended and not simply a retractile testis. It may be necessary to examine the patient on several occasions to be certain of the diagnosis. It is generally agreed that surgical correction, or administration of human chorionic gonadotropin followed by orchiopexy, is indicated before adolescence, although the age at which it should be undertaken is not agreed upon. Some advocate surgical intervention before the age of 3; others would delay surgery in the hope that the testis will descend spontaneously.

These patients have an increased incidence of hypogonadism even if only one testicle is involved and even if orchiopexy is done at an early age. Therefore, the patient should be examined yearly to be sure that sexual maturation is occurring normally. Even after surgery, the testes should be palpated at least yearly, as there is an increased incidence of testicular carcinoma in men who have a history of an undescended testicle.

Other Endocrine Metabolic Disorders

ECTOPIC HORMONE PRODUCTION

A wide variety of tumors secrete one or more hormones that may produce systemic metabolic effects. The cost and complexity of the procedures involved in their detection, however, limit the clinical utility of hormone panels as a means of detecting tumors. Detection of hormonal secretion by tumors may also have prognostic value, but experience in this area is limited. There are a number of excellent reviews dealing with the subject of ectopic hormone production. Table 52–29 lists some tumors associated more frequently with hormone production.

Table 52–29. TUMORS ASSOCIATED WITH ECTOPIC HORMONES

1. **ACTH**
   - Carcinoma of lung
   - Thymoma
   - Pancreatic tumors
   - Bronchial carcinoid
   - Medullary carcinoma of the thyroid
   - Pheochromocytoma
2. **Antidiuretic Hormones**
   - Carcinoma of lung
   - Thymoma
   - Lymphomas
   - Bronchial carcinoid
3. **Calcitonin**
   - Lung carcinoma
   - Breast carcinoma
   - Pancreatic carcinoma
   - Pheochromocytoma
4. **Erythropoietin**
   - Renal cell carcinoma
   - Pheochromocytoma
   - Cerebellar hemangioblastoma
5. **Gastrin**
   - Pancreatic carcinoma
   - Ovarian carcinoma
6. **Glucagon**
   - Lung carcinoma
7. **Gonadotropin**
   - Lung carcinoma
   - Pancreatic islet cell tumors
   - Melanoma
8. **Growth Hormone**
   - Lung carcinoma
   - Bronchial carcinoid
9. **Human Chorionic Gonadotropin**
   - Lung carcinoma
   - Hydatidiform mole
   - Choriocarcinoma
   - Testicular tumors
10. **Insulin-like Activity**
    - Mesenchymal tumors
    - Hepatomas
    - Gastrointestinal carcinoma
    - Adrenocortical carcinoma
    - Lung carcinoma
11. **Osteoclastic Activating Factor**
    - Multiple myeloma
    - Chronic lymphocytic leukemia
    - Burkitt's lymphoma
12. **Parathyroid Hormone**
    - Lung carcinoma
    - Renal carcinoma
13. **Placental Lactogen**
    - Lung carcinoma
    - Thyroid carcinoma
    - Breast carcinoma
    - Gastric carcinoma
14. **Prostaglandin**
    - Renal carcinoma
    - Lung carcinoma
15. **Serotonin and 5-Hydroxytryptophan**
    - Lung carcinoma
    - Pancreatic tumors
16. **Renin**
    - Lung carcinoma
    - Renal carcinoma
17. **Pseudothyroid Stimulating Hormone**
    - Hydatidiform mole
    - Choriocarcinoma
18. **Vasoactive Polypeptide/Gastric Inhibition Peptide**
    - Lung carcinoma
    - Pancreatic tumors
    - Pheochromocytoma

MULTIPLE ENDOCRINE ADENOMATOSIS (MEA)

Hyperfunction of two or more endocrine glands occurs with such frequency that several well-defined syndromes known as multiple endocrine adenomatosis or multiple endocrine neoplasia have been described. The most common combination of abnormalities in the multiple endocrine adenomatosis Type I syndrome is hyperparathyroidism associated with either pancreatic or pituitary tumors or both. MEA-II syndromes most commonly involve medullary carcinoma of the thyroid, hyperparathyroidism, and pheochromocytomas (Table 52–30). The finding of any one of these conditions warrants evaluation for the others as well as screening of other immediate family members. Members of the family of a patient with MEA-I syndrome should be screened with a serum calcium to exclude hyperparathyroidism. In the case of MEA-II syndromes, family members should be screened by means of a stimulated calcitonin level, which will be elevated if medullary carcinoma of the thyroid is present. Yearly urinary metanephrine and vanillylmandelic acid determinations should also be done to exclude the possibility of pheochromocytoma.

AUTOIMMUNE ENDOCRINE DISORDERS

Endocrine disorders thought to be caused by autoimmune mechanisms include Addison's disease, diabetes mellitus Type I, Hashimoto's thyroiditis, and ovarian failure. Autoimmunity may affect several glands at the same time, resulting in hypofunction of the affected glands. Graves' disease with hyperthyroidism is one of the few autoimmune disorders causing hyperfunction of a gland. Nonendocrine autoimmune diseases, such as pernicious anemia, vitiligo, and rheumatoid arthritis, also occur with increased frequency in these patients.

SYNDROME OF INAPPROPRIATE ANTIDIURETIC HORMONE (SIADH)

This syndrome is caused by secretion of antidiuretic hormone (ADH) in the absence of an osmotic or volumetric stimulus. Normally, ADH is secreted when a slight increase in the serum sodium raises the osmotic pressure. The hormone promotes retention of water and restores normal serum osmolality and volume. Conversely, a decrease in the serum sodium inhibits the release of the hormone and thereby permits excess water to be excreted. Many conditions that are characterized clinically by hyponatremia have been associated with the inappropriate release of ADH (Table 52–31). In addition, tumors of the lung, gastrointestinal tract, pancreas, and thymus may cause ectopic production of ADH. A number of drugs, including chlorpropamide, clofibrate, thia-

Table 52–30. SYNDROMES DUE TO MULTIPLE ENDOCRINE ADENOMATOSIS

Gland	Hormone	Clinical Manifestations
	MEA I	
Parathyroid adenomas	Parathyroid hormone	Hypercalcemia
Pancreatic tumors	Insulin	Hypoglycemia
	Gastrin	Peptic ulcer disease
	Growth hormone	Acromegaly
Pituitary tumors	ACTH	Cushing's syndrome
	Prolactin	Galactorrhea
	Nonfunctioning	Asymptomatic
		Headache
		Visual disturbances
Carcinoid		Carcinoid syndrome
Adrenocortical adenoma	ACTH	Rarely functioning
Thyroid adenoma	Nonfunctioning	
	MEA II	
	A	
	Medullary carcinoma of the thyroid	
	Pheochromocytoma	
	Parathyroid adenoma	
	B	
	Medullary carcinoma of the thyroid	
	Pheochromocytoma	
	Multiple mucosal neuromas	

zides, and vincristine, enhance the secretion of antidiuretic hormone or the effectiveness of its action on the renal tubule. Inappropriate secretion of ADH may also result from head trauma, endocrine disorders such as hypothyroidism and Addison's disease, and certain central nervous system disorders such as viral infections, subarachnoid hemorrhage, brain abscess, and meningitis.

Clinical Manifestations

In mild cases, patients manifest only the signs and symptoms of the disease process responsible for the inappropriate secretion of ADH. However, when the serum sodium concentration falls below 120 mEq. per liter, the patient may become lethargic or confused or complain of a headache. With continued water retention and severe hyponatremia, the patient may become comatose and develop seizures. There are no specific physical findings suggestive of inappropriate secretion of ADH, although abnormalities associated with the underlying disease process may be obvious.

Table 52–31. CAUSES OF SIADH

Tumors/Malignancy	**Drugs**
Bronchogenic carcinoma	Vasopressin
Pancreatic carcinoma	Oxytocin
Gastrointestinal malignancies	Chlorpropamide
	Thiazide
	Vincristine
Central Nervous System	Phenothiazines
Head injury	
Viral infections	**Endocrine Disorders**
Subarachnoid hemorrhage	Hypothyroidism
	Addison's disease
Brain abscess	Hypopituitarism
Meningitis	
Pulmonary Disease	
Tuberculosis	
Pneumonia	

Diagnosis

The diagnosis of SIADH is made by demonstrating (1) hyponatremia with renal salt wasting, (2) an inappropriately high urine osmolality for the serum osmolality, (3) the absence of dehydration, (4) normal renal function, and (5) normal adrenal function. The usual problem facing the physician is distinguishing between inappropriate secretion of ADH and other causes of hyponatremia. Once the serum sodium is determined to be low, pseudohyponatremia, which may be caused by hyperlipidemia, hyperglycemia, or hyperproteinemia, should be excluded. This is done simply by measuring the serum glucose and proteins and examining the serum for the presence of turbidity indicative of high levels of triglycerides. Most of the time other causes of hyponatremia can be excluded by a careful history and physical examination.

Nevertheless, documentation of normal renal function by means of a blood urea nitrogen or creatinine and liver function tests to exclude cirrhosis should be considered. A normal T_4, T_3 uptake, and TSH will exclude hypothyroidism. A cosyntropin stimulation test may be necessary in order to exclude the possibility of adrenal insufficiency.

Treatment

Restriction of water to less than 1500 ml. per day is the primary method of treatment. In patients with central nervous system manifestations, infusion of 3 per cent sodium chloride to raise the serum sodium is indicated. Demeclocycline, which decreases the sensitivity of the renal tubule to antidiuretic hormone, may be used for long-term therapy. Lithium carbonate may be used as an alternate drug, but it is associated with more side effects, including nephrogenic diabetes insipidus.

OBESITY

Obesity, one of the most common problems seen in family practice, and also the most common disorder of metabolism, is fully discussed in Chapter 54.

References

American Diabetes Association: Position statement: Nutritional recommendations and principles for individuals with diabetes mellitus, 1986. Diabetes Care, *10:*126, 1987.

DeGroot, L.J., Besser, G.M., Cahill, G.F., Jr., et al. (Eds.): Endocrinology. Philadelphia, W.B. Saunders Co., 1989. A three-volume encyclopedic text covering the pathophysiology of endocrinology. The clinical aspects of endocrinology are covered but are not emphasized.

Ellenberg, M., and Rifkin, H. (Eds.): Diabetes Mellitus, Theory and Practice. New York, Medical Examination Publishing Co., Inc., 1983. An 1105-page text covering all aspects of diabetes. It is very readable, clinically oriented, and comprehensive.

Ewing, D.J., and Clark, B.F.: Diabetes autonomic neuropathy: present insights and future prospects. Diabetes Care, *9:*648, 1986.

Felig, P., Baxter, J.D., Broadus, A.E., et al. (Eds.): Endocrinology and Metabolism. New York, McGraw-Hill Book Company, 1987. An excellent text containing discussions and diagrams summarizing the pathophysiology, clinical manifestations, and diagnostic approach to endocrine disorders.

Hirsch, J., and Leibel, R.L.: New light on obesity. N. Engl. J. Med., *8:*509, 1988.

Ingbar, S.H., and Braverman, L.E.: Werner's The Thyroid. Philadelphia, J.B. Lippincott Co., 1986. The standard text used by thyroidologists and endocrinologists as well as others who are involved in the management of thyroid disorders.

Kohler, P.O.: Treatment of pituitary adenomas. N. Engl. J. Med., *1:*45, 1987.

Marble, A., Kroll, L.P., Bradley, R.F., et al. (Eds.): Joslin's Diabetes Mellitus. Philadelphia, Lea and Febiger, 1985.

McFarland, K.F., Baker, C., and Ferguson, S.D.: Demystifying hypoglycemia. Postgrad. Med., *82:*54, 1987. A review of the clinical evaluation of hypoglycemia.

Morley, J.E., Mooradion, A.D., Rosenthal, M.J., and Kaiser, T.E.: Diabetes mellitus in elderly patients. Is it different? Am. J. Med., *83:*533, 1987.

Mundy, G.R.: Hypercalcemia of malignancy revisited. J. Clin. Invest., *82:*1, 1988. Excellent, sophisticated review of the mechanisms involved in the hypercalcemia of malignancy.

Rittmaster, R.S., and Loriaux, D.L.: Hirsutism: a clinical review. Ann. Intern. Med., *106:*95, 1987. A comprehensive paper with 246 references.

Rotter, J.I., and Rimoin, D.L.: The genetics of diabetics. Hosp. Pract., *22:*79, 1987. A detailed discussion of a complicated subject.

Speroff, L., Glass, R.H., and Kase, N.G.: Clinical Gynecologic Endocrinology and Infertility. Baltimore, William & Wilkins, 1989. An excellent, easy-to-read text with exceptionally clear diagrams covering the pathophysiology and clinical aspects of reproductive endocrinology.

Stunkard, A.J., Sorensen, I.A., Harris, C., et al.: An adaption study of human obesity. N. Engl. J. Med., *314:*193, 1986. A study that concludes that genetic factors influence the development of obesity more than environmental ones.

Williams, R.H.: Textbook of Endocrinology. Philadelphia, W.B. Saunders Co., 1985. This has been a standard reference textbook for endocrinology since the first edition in 1950. It has extensive references and contributions by 52 authorities in the field. It contains much basic information regarding pathophysiology of endocrine diseases and is well referenced.

53

Nutrition

Patrick J. Fahey
Charlette Gallagher-Allred

Introduction

Family physicians are in an excellent position to impact the nutrition status of their patients. This includes not only assessing nutrition well-being but also advising patients about nutrition throughout the life cycle and treating specific diseases and disorders from a dietary perspective when appropriate.

Nutrition Assessment of the Adult Patient

SCREENING AND ASSESSMENT

Malnutrition has reached alarming proportions particularly among patients in hospitals and nursing homes where it is estimated that up to 50 per cent may show clinical or laboratory evidence of malnutrition (Bistrian, et al., 1976). Patients recovering at home are also at risk for malnutrition. Don't be fooled by patients who look good. Family physicians should think about nutrition when examining patients, especially during stages of their life cycle when poor nutrition intake can result in serious medical problems, such as during periods of rapid growth (infancy, childhood, and adolescence), during pregnancy or lactation, and during the elderly years. Patients at high risk for malnutrition include those with obesity who are always dieting, those who are underweight, and those who report changes in appetite or food tolerance. Patients with food faddist ideas; those who have acquired immune deficiency syndrome (AIDS), cancer, liver disease, pulmonary disease, or gastrointestinal problems; and those who take numerous prescriptions or over-the-counter medications that affect nutrition status are also at high risk for malnutrition.

If a nutrition problem is suspected in any patient, it should be confirmed with a nutrition screen, which gathers nutrition-related information through the medical history and physical examination. The nutrition screen includes the measurement of weight and height at every visit in children and adolescents and periodically in adults. Questions related to appetite, dentition, and chronic gastrointestinal disturbances will further identify patients at risk. The screen may also include simple, appropriate laboratory tests, but often laboratory tests are best reserved for a more in-depth nutrition assessment. Observation of the patient's fat and muscle mass may indicate limited calorie and protein intake and be a clue to food faddism or signal the potential for anorexia nervosa, bulimia, or malignancy.

A nutrition screen includes the following four basic questions regarding food intake:

1. How many meals and snacks a day do you eat? If the patient says one, suspicion should be raised.

2. What foods do you eat? This will determine whether the patient is eating a varied diet, including foods from the four basic food groups. Children,

adolescents, and adults should daily consume at a minimum:

- 2 to 3 servings of dairy products, such as milk, cheese, or yogurt
- 4 to 6 ounces of meat, including fish, poultry, dried beans, peas, seeds, or nuts
- 4 servings of fruits or vegetables, including a citrus fruit daily and a leafy green or deep yellow vegetable every other day
- 4 or more servings of grain products including breads and cereals

These four basic food group recommendations will supply 100 per cent of the Recommended Dietary Allowances (R.D.A.) (Table 53–1) for protein, vitamins, and minerals (except iron for premenopausal women).

3. Do you take vitamin or mineral supplements or health foods of any kind and why? This can often be a trigger as to what someone has been told or suspects as a deficit in their diet.

4. What foods do you avoid? Your concern should be raised if patients avoid all dairy products or all breads and cereals, for example.

Patients hospitalized for elective surgery in whom a nutrition deficit is suspected should have a serum albumin and total lymphocyte count as part of the preadmission work-up (Gray and Kaminski, 1983).

	Degree of Deficiency		
	Mild	Moderate	Severe
Albumin (gram per cent)	3.0–3.5	2.5–3.0	<2.5
Total lymphocyte count	1500–1800	900–1500	<900

This information will provide good evidence of the patient's nutrition status. If the test results are low, or the patient has experienced recent weight loss, renourishment should be given at home prior to hospitalization.

Table 53–1. RECOMMENDED DIETARY ALLOWANCES PER DAY OF SELECTED VITAMINS AND MINERALS*

	Infants (0–1 yr)	Children (1–10 yrs)	Males (11 yrs +)	Females (11 yrs +)	Pregnant Women	Lactating Women	Best Food Sources
Vitamin							
A (μg.)	375	400–700	1000	800	800	1200–1300	Butter, fortified margarine, yellow vegetables, liver, egg yolk
D (μg.)	7.5–10	10	5–10	5–10	10	10	Butter, egg yolk, ultraviolet radiation, fortified milk
E (mg.)	3–4	6–7	10	8	10	11–12	Vegetable oils, green vegetables
C (mg.)	30–35	40–45	50–60	50–60	70	90–95	Citrus fruits, tomatoes, potatoes, green leafy vegetables, cabbage
Thiamin (mg.)	0.3–0.4	0.7–1.0	1.2–1.5	1.0–1.1	1.5	1.6	Wheat germ, enriched breads and cereals, pork, nuts, legumes
Riboflavin (mg.)	0.4–0.5	0.8–1.2	1.4–1.8	1.2–1.3	1.6	1.7–1.8	Milk, liver, green leafy vegetables, enriched breads and cereals
Niacin (mg.)	5–6	9–13	17–18	13–14	17	20	Liver, meats, legumes, nuts
Pyridoxine (mg.)	0.3–0.6	1.0–1.4	1.7–2.0	1.4–1.6	2.2	2.1	Organ meats, fish, cereals, legumes
Folacin (μg.)	25–35	50–100	150–200	150–180	400	260–280	Green vegetables, liver, nuts
B_{12} (μg.)	0.3–0.5	0.7–1.4	2.0	2.0	2.2	2.6	Animal foods
Minerals							
Calcium (mg.)	400–600	800	800–1200	800–1200	1200	1200	Milk and milk products, cheeses
Iron (mg.)	6–10	10	10–12	10–15	30	15	Liver, meat, egg yolks, wheat germ, enriched breads and cereals, dried fruits, leafy green vegetables
Magnesium (mg.)	40–60	80–170	170–400	280–300	320	340–355	Green leafy vegetables, nuts, soybeans
Zinc (mg.)	5	10	15	12	15	16–19	Seafood, meats, nuts, green leafy vegetables

*Adapted from Recommended Dietary Allowances, 10th ed. Washington, DC, National Academy of Sciences, 1989.

NUTRITION SUPPORT OPTIONS

Traditional foods may be augmented by commercial medical nutrition products taken orally or administered via an enteral tube feeding. More costly parenteral supplementation and total parenteral nutrition (T.P.N.) are also available alternatives. Significant financial savings can occur by providing nutrition support in a home setting when feasible (Becker, 1988).

Medical nutrition products are designed to provide optimal nutrition in a convenient form. Most are liquid and can be consumed orally or administered through a tube leading into the stomach or small intestine. Medical nutrition products for oral consumption are also available in a pudding form or powdered for reconstitution as liquid. Most products meet the R.D.A. for vitamins and minerals in 1500 to 3000 ml. volumes. They differ in their source and content of carbohydrate, protein, fat, and calories.

Medical nutrition products that provide 1 kilocalorie (kcal.) per ml. are usually appropriate for patients needing 2000 to 3000 kcal. per day, such as patients who have cancer and loss of appetite, or those undergoing oral surgery, diagnostic testing, and cancer therapy. These products can contain varying amounts of lactose, fiber, and residue (Table 53–2).

Many older or bedfast patients require fewer calories (less than 2000 kcal. per day) but not a reduction of protein, vitamins, and minerals. Nutrient-dense products that provide higher levels of protein are often appropriate for these patients and for those who have undergone surgery or who have fractures or infections. To meet these patients' needs, products should be selected that provide increased protein levels.

Some patients have very elevated needs (3000 kcal. or more). Burn patients or multiple trauma and sepsis patients need high-calorie (1.5 to 2.0 kcal./ml.), nutrient-packed products often in small volume. These products are also appropriate for cardiac and renal patients on fluid restriction and for anorectic patients.

Special medical nutrition products and modular products have been developed. For example, predigested or hydrolyzed formulas that enhance nutrient availability and may decrease diarrhea are available for patients with pancreatic insufficiency or regional enteritis. Pulmocare, a low-carbohydrate, high-fat product has been shown to be helpful for pulmonary failure patients by reducing carbon dioxide production. Patients with renal failure or liver failure patients may benefit from products low in protein and fluid. PediaSure, the only enteral nutrition product designed for children 1 to 6 years of age, can be used for total nutrition support by tube feeding or oral feeding; it supplies 100 per cent of the R.D.A. in 1100 kcal. Modular products that supply protein, carbohydrate, fat, and flavors can be combined with existing formulas or normal foods to augment specific nutrients. Table 53–2 identifies several commercial medical nutrition formulas and modular products.

COST EFFECTIVENESS OF NUTRITION SUPPORT

As with any disease state or condition, the best time to detect a nutrition deficit is early through screening and assessment. When detected early, a deficit can be corrected more easily and more cost effectively. Malnutrition is expensive. Malnourished patients stay in the hospital two thirds longer than do adequately nourished patients (Weinsier, et al., 1979). Hospital bills for the average malnourished patient with major complications are at least three times higher than the charges for a well-nourished patient with no complications (Reilly, et al., 1988). Maintaining good nutrition status reduces postoperative complications by two and a halffold, major postoperative sepsis by sixfold, and mortality from 28 to 4 per cent (Mullen, et al., 1980). If the patient is hospitalized, the services of an available nutrition support team can be of invaluable assistance in nourishing the patient in a cost-effective manner (Driscoll, 1986).

Nutrition During Pregnancy and Lactation

The period during a woman's life when she is pregnant or breast-feeding is critical in terms of adequate dietary intake for both the woman and fetus or infant. Especially critical are the last two trimesters of pregnancy when rapid growth and development of the fetus and supporting tissues occur. Studies have demonstrated that little weight gain during pregnancy is strongly associated with intrauterine growth retardation and prematurity—the major birth problems in North America. The family physician can play a vital role in advising female patients regarding healthy diets well before pregnancy occurs. Failing that, especially in light of the high number of unexpected pregnancies, the physician can still perform a nutrition assessment and provide sound nutrition information for patients throughout pregnancy.

NUTRIENT NEEDS

Body weight remains the easiest practical tool in assessing caloric needs in everyday practice. The requirement for kilocalories during pregnancy is based on preconceptional weight and weight gain throughout the pregnancy. Caloric needs prior to conception range from 30 kcal. per kg. body weight per day (14 kcal. per pound per day) for the mature female to double that for the young adolescent. An additional 300 kcal. per day are necessary to achieve

Table 53–2. SELECTED COMMERCIAL MEDICAL NUTRITION PRODUCTS

Requirement for 2000 to 3000 kcal. Per Day
(Useful for patients with cancer, loss of appetite, undergoing oral surgery, diagnostic testing, and cancer therapy)

Lactose-free, low-residue products
- Ensure[1]
- Sustacal[2]
- Resource[3]
- Travasorb[4]

Milk-based products
- Forta milkshake[1]
- Carnation Instant Breakfast[5]
- Complete B[3]
- Meritene Liquid and Powder[3]

Isotonic, low-residue products
- Osmolite[1]
- Isocal[2]

Lactose-free, fiber-containing products
- Enrich[1]
- Sustacal with fiber[2]

Requirement for Less Than 2000 kcal. Per Day With Increased Protein, Vitamins, and Minerals
(Useful with older or bedfast patients who require nutrient-dense products with fewer calories, patients who have undergone surgery, or patients who have fractures or infection)

- Ensure HN[1]
- Jevity[1]
- Osmolite HN[1]
- Sustacal HC[2]
- Precision HN[3]

Requirement for More Than 3000 kcal. Per Day, With High Protein, Vitamin, and Mineral Needs and Possibly Volume Restriction
(Useful for burn, multiple trauma, sepsis, and anorectic patients)

- Ensure Plus[1]
- Ensure Plus HN[1]
- TwoCal HN[1]
- Sustacal HC[2]
- TraumaCal[2]
- Isocal HCN[2]
- Isotein HN[3]
- Magnacal[6]

Special Requirements Products

Clear liquid diet
- Ross SLD[1]
- Citrotein[3]

Pancreatic insufficiency or regional enteritis (predigested or hydrolyzed formulas)
- Vital HN[1]
- Criticare HN[2]
- Travasorb HN[4]
- Vivonex HN[7] and T.E.N.[7]

Pulmonary disease
- Pulmocare[1]

Renal failure
- Travasorb Renal[4]
- Amin-Aid[8]

Liver failure
- Travasorb Hepatic[4]
- Hepatic-Aid[8]

Child formula
- *PediaSure*[1]

Modular products

Carbohydrate sources
- Polycose[1]
- Moducal[2]
- Sumacal[6]

Protein sources
- ProMod[1]
- Casec[2]
- Propac[6]
- Promix[9]

Fat sources
- MCT Oil[2]
- Microlipid[6]

Flavor source
- Vari-Flavors[1]

[1]Ross Laboratories, Columbus, Ohio
[2]Mead Johnson, Evansville, Indiana
[3]Sandoz, Minneapolis, Minnesota
[4]Baxter-Travenol (Clintec Division), Deerfield, Illinois
[5]Carnation, Los Angeles, California and Baxter-Travenol (Clintec Division)
[6]Sherwood, St. Louis, Missouri
[7]Norwich-Eaton, Norwich, New York
[8]Kendall, Irvine, California
[9]Corpak, Wheeling, Illinois

Table 53–3. DAILY KILOCALORIE REQUIREMENTS DURING PREGNANCY AND LACTATION FOR THE MATURE FEMALE*

Preconceptional Weight		Preconceptional Caloric Need	Total Caloric Need During Pregnancy	Total Caloric Need During Lactation† (kcal.)	
(kg.)	(lb.)	(kcal.)	(kcal.)	*1 Month*	*6 Months*
50	110	1500	1800	1800	2200
55	120	1650	1950	1950	2350
60	132	1800	2100	2100	2500
65	143	1950	2250	2250	2650
70	154	2100	2400	2400	2800

*From Cox, J. H., and Gallagher-Allred, C. R.: Normal diet: pregnancy and lactation. *In* Nutrition and Health Promotion in Primary Care Series. Columbus, Department of Family Medicine, The Ohio State University, 1980, p. 3.

†Assuming normal weight gain during pregnancy to provide maternal caloric stores; if weight gain is inadequate, increase kilocalorie allowance by 200 kilocalories. These kilocalorie levels are based on infant growth at the 50th percentile.

an ideal weight gain of 10 to 12 kg. (22 to 27 pounds) during pregnancy (Table 53–3).

Weight gain greater than 10 to 12 kg. may be desirable if the female is more than 10 per cent underweight at the time of conception. Weight loss is not recommended during pregnancy. Because the incidence of maternal morbidity increases when the weight gain exceeds 18 kg. (40 pounds), control of weight gain is highly desirable.

There is a national dilemma caused by large numbers of pregnancies in the early teenage years, (Naeye, 1981). Maximal height and weight are not achieved until 4 to 7 years after menarche, with the most significant growth in the first 2 years after menarche. Unfortunately, teenage girls often have poor dietary habits with nutrient-poor and irregular intake. Surveys of pregnant teenagers frequently show poor intake of calcium, iron, zinc, folic acid, vitamin A, vitamin C, and vitamin B_6.

The caloric intake of a pregnant teenage girl who is at normal weight for height should support a gestational weight gain of 10 to 12 kg. plus the amount normally expected during the teenager's year of growth. Overweight teenage patients should experience a weight gain of about 9 kg. (20 pounds), and underweight patients would need to pick up the gestational gain of 10 to 12 kg. plus the weight gains for both normal postmenarcheal growth and normalization of weight.

Rate of weight gain during pregnancy is also important. Weight-gain goals for older teenagers and adults should be in the vicinity of 2 to 3 pounds in the entire first trimester and a pound per week in the last two trimesters. The younger teenager, especially if underweight, needs to be carefully monitored and counseled early in the pregnancy to ensure more significant gains *throughout* the pregnancy, not simply at the end.

A discussion of protein is important, especially in growing teenage patients and in patients with limited financial resources in whom problems often revolve around inadequate intake of meats and dairy products. The recommended protein intake during pregnancy for the purpose of building fetal and accessory tissue is based on the age and preconceptional weight of the pregnant female. Recommended protein intake during pregnancy varies as can be seen in Table 53–4.

COUNSELING TIPS

Practical recommendations that can help pregnant patients increase both their energy intake and their protein intake include:

1. Increasing servings of protein-rich meats and meat substitutes by one or more per day, emphasizing the leaner cuts if extra calories are not needed; a meat serving should be 2 to 3 ounces, supplying about 15 to 20 grams of protein.
2. Increasing consumption of dairy products by two servings per day, from the usual two (three in teenagers) to four and even five per day in growing teenagers; the usual 8-ounce serving of milk or its equivalent provides 8 grams of protein.

Increases in both of these food groups provide other essential nutrients including iron, calcium, and vitamins that are needed in larger amounts during preg-

Table 53–4. RECOMMENDED PROTEIN INTAKE FOR VARIOUS-AGED PREGNANT WOMEN*

Age	Recommended Protein Intake: *Grams Per kg. ideal body weight*	*Grams Per lb. ideal body weight*
Adolescent female		
Age 11–14 yrs	1.7	0.77
Age 15–18 yrs	1.5	0.68
Mature female	1.3	0.59

*From Cox J. H., and Gallagher-Allred C. R.: Normal diet: pregnancy and lactation. *In* Nutrition and Health Promotion in Primary Care Series. Columbus, Department of Family Medicine, The Ohio State University, 1980, p. 2.

nancy. If a patient's calorie and protein needs are met, it is probable that vitamin and mineral needs will also be met.

Patients need to be advised to increase fruits and vegetables to five servings daily, including one serving of leafy green or deep orange vegetables and two servings of a vitamin C rich fruit (oranges, grapefruits) or vegetables (greens, tomatoes, potatoes) instead of the usual one. Although this food group may not have the same percentage increase in requirement as does the dairy group, it does need special emphasis since many females do not get the four recommended servings of this particular group in the first place. Besides providing a generous amount of vitamin A, the orange vegetables and fruits and the leafy green vegetables also provide several other vitamins and minerals, especially vitamin C, folic acid, magnesium, and iron.

The grain group does not need to be increased during pregnancy, remaining at four servings per day. The physician needs to emphasize the importance of this group, however, because enriched products make it a valuable source of iron, phosphorus, B-complex vitamins, and fiber.

The fifth food group—"others"—includes foods such as sugar, salad dressings, soft drinks, pies, cakes, and alcoholic beverages. Patients should be cautioned not to consume alcohol-containing products during pregnancy. A useful role that this food group may serve is as a source of extra calories for growing teenagers and others who may have increased caloric needs. This should only be advised if the patient is consuming adequate amounts of the other four food groups that provide nutrients in addition to calories.

For some patients, added calories from the increases in the meat, milk, and fruit-vegetable groups may result in too many calories. If this is the case, or if the patient is gaining weight too quickly, suggest elimination of one or more servings from the "other" category. Specifically:

1. Substitute a fruit serving for a piece of pie for dessert.
2. Choose milk instead of a soft drink for lunch.
3. Snack on a grain product or a fruit or vegetable instead of a high-calorie "other" product.
4. Eat three regularly scheduled meals plus an evening snack instead of only one or two full meals daily.

If patients do not like specific foods, suggest alternatives in each group. For example, if they do not like milk, suggest cottage cheese, yogurt, or ice cream. Those who don't like meat may be surprised to find out that substitutes can include eggs, peanut butter, and cheese.

Although debate continues about whether a sufficiently balanced diet during pregnancy requires supplementation with vitamins and minerals, two important concepts remain.

1. There are increased vitamin and mineral needs during pregnancy.
2. Deficiencies during pregnancy do occur, especially of iron and folic acid.

Iron-deficiency anemia is not uncommon during pregnancy, and low folic acid levels have been found in nearly half of low-income patients. Thus, it seems reasonable to recommend that all patients take a prenatal multiple vitamin and mineral supplement with at least 60 mg. of iron and at least 400 micrograms of folic acid daily. Special circumstances, such as iron-deficiency anemia, may require additional supplementation. Since iron can be constipating, ensure consumption of adequate fluid and fiber. Since water-soluble vitamins are stored to only a limited degree in the body, this daily prenatal vitamin will also help meet increased needs of the B vitamins and vitamin C. Caution patients not to take more than one prenatal vitamin per day to avoid the potential toxicity of excessive fat-soluble vitamins.

Sodium and Calcium. Since sodium is important in fetal and infant tissues and increased maternal blood volume requires sodium, there does not appear to be a role for the routine restriction of sodium during pregnancy. If sodium is restricted because of hypertension or heart disease, it makes sense to still allow for at least 3 grams of sodium per day. Calcium needs are definitely increased during pregnancy and lactation. The pregnant or lactating patient needs about 1200 mg. per day of calcium, and the growing adolescent needs about 1600 mg. daily. The recommended increase in the milk group and the daily intake of a prenatal vitamin and mineral supplement containing calcium will enable the patient to meet these calcium needs.

Breast-Feeding. Women who are breast-feeding should be counseled regarding appropriate dietary intake. Postpartum mothers are often eager to lose weight quickly in order to return to their former weight, yet lactation clearly requires increased nutrients, especially energy (700 to 800 kcal. per day), protein, and calcium. These increased needs should not hinder the mother's goal to lose weight slowly. The new mother will likely be able to achieve a balance by increasing intake from the food groups needed during pregnancy. One multiple vitamin and mineral tablet daily continues to be a reasonable suggestion. The patient who has trouble losing weight may need to be reminded that regular exercise is an important part of the energy intake-output equation.

If the patient was anemic during pregnancy or immediately postpartum, measuring the hemoglobin several weeks later can assist the physician in determining if additional supplemental iron is necessary. At least 2 liters per day of fluid should be encouraged, most of it as milk. If the infant seems to be adversely affected by certain foods consumed by the mother, the mother should avoid those foods. Caffeine and alcohol should be limited, and most drugs avoided, such as antimetabolites, tetracycline, iodides, lithium, anticoagulants, propylthiouracil, sedatives, diuretics, anticonvulsants, and oral contraceptives.

Nutrition in Geriatrics

SPECIAL NUTRIENT NEEDS

The geriatric population is particularly vulnerable to nutrition problems, and because this is a highly heterogeneous group, generalizations concerning their nutrition status are frequently erroneous. However, common physiologic changes occur with aging that affect nutrient needs.

1. Dental problems, including ill-fitting dentures, are common. Therefore, food selection is often self-restricted to liquids or soft foods that may not be nutritionally adequate.
2. There is a shift in body composition, including a decrease in total body water and lean muscle mass, an increase in body fat, resulting in changes in drug metabolism, and an increase in storage of fat-soluble drugs and nutrients.
3. Hepatic and renal functions gradually decline with age, impairing metabolism and excretion of drugs and increasing the likelihood of drug-nutrient interactions.
4. Sensitivity to thirst decreases, thereby putting elderly patients at risk for dehydration unless they make an effort to consume adequate liquids.
5. The senses of taste and smell gradually become less acute with age. Foods may seem relatively tasteless, and off-tastes or off-odors that are warnings of spoilage often go unnoticed. While flavors can be safely enhanced by adding spices or sharper-tasting ingredients, many older persons compensate instead with a hand on the salt shaker, which may aggravate pre-existing hypertension.
6. Decreased secretion of gastric acid and digestive enzymes occurs that impairs the absorption of some nutrients, particularly iron and calcium.
7. Gastric and intestinal motility slow with age, and chronic constipation becomes a frequent complaint. Constipation may be exacerbated by poor dentition that makes some fiber-rich foods difficult or unpleasant to chew.
8. Glucose tolerance decreases with age, possibly owing to increased insulin resistance and increased body weight. Frank diabetes is different from this entity; rigid dietary restrictions are not demanded for what is likely to be typically elevated postprandial glucose levels.

Additionally, financial limitations and decreased ability to shop and prepare food make elderly patients good candidates for malnutrition. Individuals over the age of 60 who live below the poverty level frequently eat less than 1000 kcal. per day.

DIETARY CONSIDERATIONS

Except for a lower total calorie requirement, nutrient needs of healthy elderly patients may not be much different than those of younger adults. Dietary restrictions should be minimal. Elderly patients need to be encouraged to eat a well-balanced and varied diet, and the family physician should show interest in the patient's eating patterns by asking questions about food intake at regularly scheduled office appointments.

Moderate overweight (10 to 15 per cent above ideal) is not a proven risk factor for patients over 60 years of age. The grossly obese elderly patient who also suffers from diabetes, hypertension, or hyperlipidemia, however, is at greater risk of chronic hyperglycemia, stroke, and pancreatitis, respectively. Weight loss is the safest intervention to reduce each of these risks. Elderly patients who need to lose weight should:

- Eat smaller portions
- Eat less food, more often, and more slowly (thereby helping them feel less hungry and keeping them from overindulging)
- Limit alcohol, fats, and sugars
- Use low-fat dairy products
- Substitute fruits and whole grain breads or cereals for rich pastries and sweets
- Go easy on sauces and gravies
- Choose lean meats and remove skin and excess fat
- Avoid fatty and fried foods
- Avoid fad or miracle diets

Patients with hypertension should be advised to substitute herbs and spices for the salt shaker. Mild to moderate hypercholesterolemia in normal weight elderly patients rarely merit dietary intervention (Taylor, et al., 1987).

Undernutrition and unintentional weight loss are more common than obesity in elderly patients. Underweight patients are subject to marginal or even overt malnutrition as a result of chronic illness, multiple drug therapy, and general apathy toward maintaining a healthy life style. Pressure sores occur frequently in underweight, apathetic elderly patients who spend considerable time in bed or a chair. Pressure sores increase calorie, protein, vitamin C, and zinc needs. Patients with pressure sores should boost calories and other nutrients by:

- Increasing portion sizes and eating more frequently, especially before bedtime
- Selecting higher-calorie fruit juices instead of coffee or tea
- Substituting higher-calorie dairy products and fried foods for lower-calorie and broiled foods
- Fortifying casseroles, soups, or meat dishes with cheese, nonfat dry milk, cream, or Half-and-Half
- Supplementing meals and evening snacks with commercial medical nutrition products

If the patient is unable or unwilling to eat a varied and well-balanced diet, the consumption of a multiple vitamin and mineral supplement (with or without iron) may be advisable. Discourage the intake of individual vitamins or minerals because self-medication frequently results in a megadose intake of nutrients that can result in toxicity, cause liver damage, antagonize medications, and provide a false sense of nutrition security. When choosing a multiple vitamin and mineral supplement, advise patients to look for one that contains 100 per cent of the RDA for at least the following 11 vitamins and minerals: thiamin, riboflavin, niacin, pyridoxine, vitamin C, vitamin B_{12}, folic acid, vitamin A, zinc, calcium, and iron.

In the absence of blood loss, iron deficiency may result from either inadequate iron ingestion or impaired absorption. If iron supplementation is required, ferrous sulfate, 300 mg. three times a day with meals, will usually correct an iron deficiency within a few months if the cause of iron deficiency is also corrected. Patients taking iron supplementation should be cautioned that it may be constipating, and they should be encouraged to consume adequate fiber (whole grains, legumes, fruits, and vegetables) and fluids (6 to 8 cups) daily. The physician may still need to compromise and only give the iron preparation twice daily if constipation persists.

NUTRIENT-DRUG INTERACTIONS

Although persons over age 65 constitute only 11 per cent of the population, they consume 25 per cent of all prescription and nonprescription drugs (Fisher, 1980), many of which interact with nutrients. In addition, drugs can alter nutrition status by influencing appetite and metabolism. If elderly patients are regularly taking antacids, antimicrobials, aspirin, barbiturates, L-dopa, anticonvulsants, hypocholesterolemic agents, or laxatives, recommend that they take a multiple vitamin and mineral supplement. Foods high in tyramine that should be avoided while patients are taking monoamine oxidase inhibitors are identified in Table 53–5. Be sure patients taking diuretics and digitalis consume high-potassium foods. Caution patients taking anticoagulants to avoid self-prescribed vitamin K supplements.

Table 53–5. FOODS TO AVOID ON A TYRAMINE-RESTRICTED DIET

Hard cheeses: especially Cheddar, Gruyere, Stilton, Ementhal, Brie, Camembert
Chianti wine
Broad beans
Smoked or cured meats; especially bologna, pepperoni, salami, sausage
Dried, pickled, or kippered foods; especially herring
Liver and pâtés
Figs, raisins, dates
Soy sauce and meat tenderizers
Caffeine-containing beverages, including chocolate

Nutrition-Related Disorders and Dietary Modifications

OBESITY

Prevention of obesity should be of primary importance to the family physician (N.I.H. Consensus Development Conference, 1985) (also see chapter on obesity). Obesity prevention in infancy and childhood begins with careful supervision of the feeding of infants and children. Accurate weights and lengths of infants and children should be plotted in a timely manner on growth charts. Dietary interviews with mothers should be conducted. An abnormal weight status of a child may reflect a problem of mother-child interaction. Because obesity often develops in school-aged children, especially those who are not involved in daily sports, children should be encouraged to participate in physical education programs in elementary and secondary schools. During adolescence, food plays a primary role in socialization and may be abused owing to fads. It is during this impressionable age that overweight-conscious girls are prone to try crash dieting to control their weight, even to the extreme condition of anorexia nervosa. Others may establish a life-long pattern of obesity during this period that can lead to the binge-purge activity of bulimia. The development of adult obesity in persons who have not been overweight in earlier life is less common than one might suspect. Yet, persons who have had an active life prior to age 30 to 50 may gain significant amounts of weight if physical activity is limited owing to demands of employment. An algorithm for evaluating an obese patient is shown in Figure 53–1.

The initial approach in the management of obesity should be medical and behavioral (Council on Scientific Affairs, 1988). Management should include a balanced, low-calorie diet, behavioral guidance in dieting, and an exercise program. The diet, individualized to the patient's needs and life-style patterns, should be developed through close interaction between patient and physician and may require the assistance of a registered dietitian. Characteristics of behavioral therapy that enhance an individualized weight-reduction program have been described by Stunkard (Stunkard, 1985). The exercise component should not only be effective and safe but should promote an increased activity level within the individual's life style that can last a lifetime. Anorectic medications (not amphetamines) may be useful for a few weeks in some instances as adjuncts to therapy, but the physician must remember their potential hazards plus the lack of data regarding their long-term efficacy.

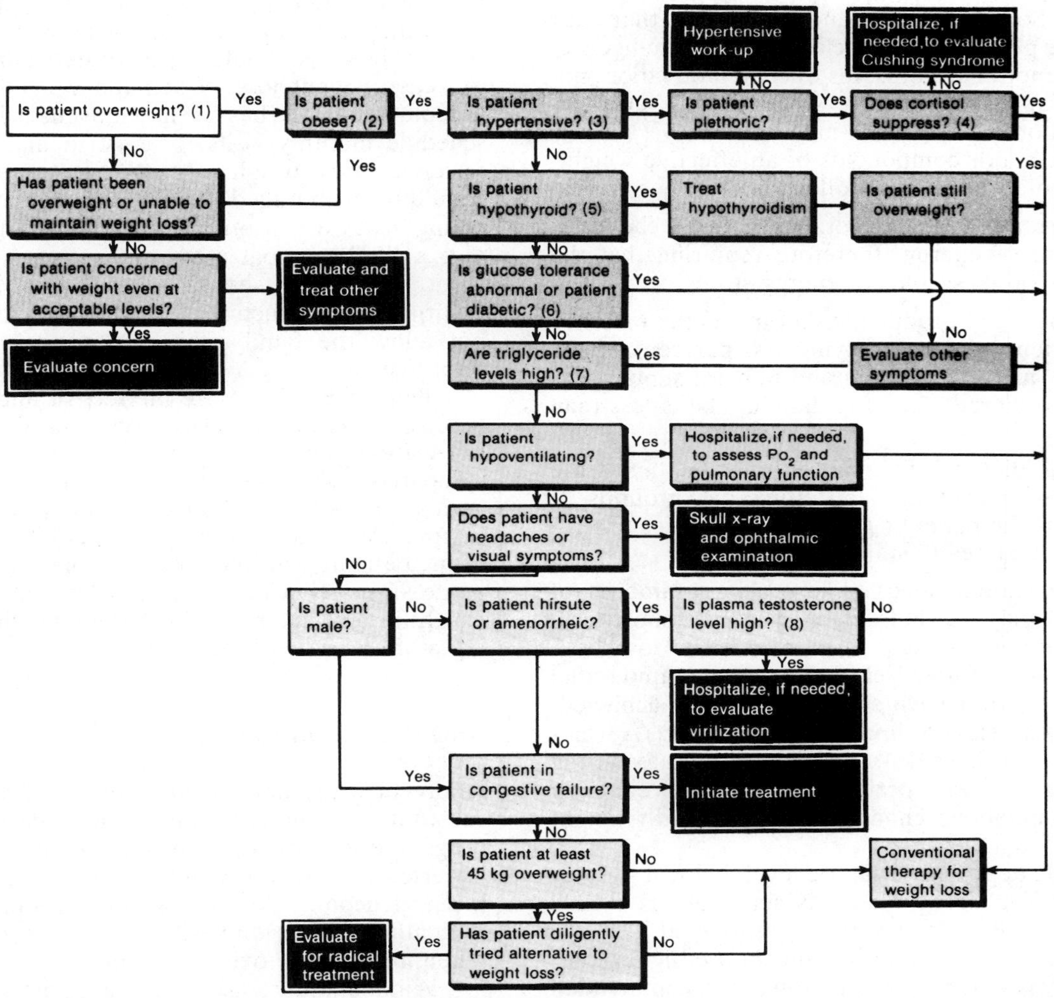

Figure 53–1. Algorithm for evaluating an obese patient. (From Bray, G. A., et al. Algorithm for evaluating an obese patient. J.A.M.A. 235:2009, 1976, copyright 1976, American Medical Association.)

WEIGHT-REDUCTION DIETS

To determine the patient's motivation to lose weight and goals for weight reduction, answers to the following questions should be sought:

- What does the patient want to weigh?
- How long does the patient expect it will take to achieve this weight?
- Why does the patient want to lose weight?

If the patient's attitude does not support weight loss, it may be best to postpone the weight-reduction program. Some attitudes and conditions that may necessitate postponement include limited intelligence, unstable emotional status, insufficient motivation, unrealistic expectations, the "you-cure-me" attitude, and the "nothing-works-for-me" attitude.

Three major components of an effective weight-reduction diet include the following:

1. The kilocalorie level is less than the daily expenditure of energy, therefore requiring that the body draw on its surplus of energy stores.

2. The weight-reduction diet meets the patient's basic nutrient needs, supplying 100 per cent of the R.D.A. A multiple vitamin and mineral supplement is usually required when the daily intake is less than 1200 kcal.

3. The diet is individualized to the patient's life style and socioeconomic and ethnic backgrounds. It also reflects the patient's goals and objectives regarding weight and health status.

If the patient needs to lose a large amount of weight, it may be helpful to establish short-term intermediate goals, such as a consistent loss of 1 pound per week for 4 weeks following the rapid initial weight loss. After each short-term goal is achieved, another goal should immediately be set. A "no-weight-gain-for-2-weeks" goal is appropriate during holidays or plateau periods that occur frequently owing to metabolic changes associated with weight loss.

A daily appropriate calorie level that will support weight loss for most moderately active adults is 1200 to 1500 kcal. for females and 1500 to 2000 kcal. for males. More active adults should choose higher kilocalorie levels. The consumption of recommended amounts of the basic food groups, when prepared without added sugar and fat, will provide 1000 to 1200 kcal. and meet the R.D.A. for protein, vitamins, and minerals with the exception of iron for premenopausal women. For many adult patients, the recommendation to follow the basic food group plan is the best advice that can be given. Table 53–6 identifies several meal patterns that are generally accepted by patients when specific kilocalorie recommendations are needed. These meal patterns can be used in conjunction with Exchange Lists for Meal Planning from the American Diabetes Association and the American Diabetic Association. Tables 53–6 and 53–7 identify the calorie and alcohol contents of common alcoholic beverages, and are useful in instructing patients on weight-reduction diets.

Community self-help groups for weight reduction are often helpful. Consider the merits and disadvantages of specific groups when recommending them to patients (Table 53–8).

Follow-up visits must be a part of the total weight-reduction program. During follow-up visits, discussion should center on the patient's progress and problems with the diet, behavior modification, and exercise program. Time should also be spent in changing the program as needed and in supporting and motivating the patient. Initial weekly visits and later bimonthly visits should be instituted during periods of active weight loss. When the weight goal or an acceptable weight has been achieved, it is helpful to schedule monthly visits to assist in maintaining the lowered body weight. Most importantly, patients should be encouraged to make permanent changes in eating behaviors. Motivating patients to make proper diet a life-long goal requires continuous reinforcement. The patient should be referred to a registered dietitian for instruction and follow-up if time does not allow the family physician to provide needed reinforcement.

Fad Diets. These are ineffective and often dangerous in treating obesity. While a well-balanced, low-calorie diet may seem dull to patients when compared with fad diets, a diet containing a wide variety of everyday foods can be practiced for a lifetime. Without a permanent change in eating patterns, patients will likely become one of the approximate 95 per cent of dieters who regain their former weight in 2 years. Table 53–9 identifies the disadvantages of a variety of fad diets.

ANORECTIC DRUGS

Anorectic drugs must be an adjunct to, rather than a substitute for, modification of eating patterns. These drugs are contraindicated in patients with severe hypertension, hyperthyroidism, advanced arteriosclerosis, glaucoma, extreme anxiety hypersensitivity to sympathomimetic amines, and in patients who have taken monoamine oxidase inhibitors recently.

Amphetamines are potent appetite suppressants but have a high potential for abuse and should not be used in the context of obesity management. Other drugs, such as diethylpropion (Tenuate) and mazindol (Mazanor) (useful in hypertensive patients), fenfluramine (Pondimin) (useful in diabetics but contraindicated in patients with a history of depression), and phentermine (Ionamin) appear to have a low potential for abuse. However, these products still have some stimulant properties and are controlled substances, usually Schedule III or IV. Physicians should be very cautious in using these agents. Over-the-counter anorectic drugs are effective only for a few days, if at all, and generally should be discouraged.

Table 53–6. FOOD PATTERNS FOR VARIOUS KILOCALORIE WEIGHT-REDUCTION DIETS*

Kilocalories	Total Daily Exchanges	Breakfast	Lunch	Dinner	Evening Snack
800	5 Meat	1 Meat	2 Meat	2 Meat	Meat
	4 Starch	1 Starch	1 Starch	1 Starch	1 Starch
	3 Fruit	1 Fruit	1 Fruit	1 Fruit	Fruit
	Any vegetables	0 Vegetables	Any vegetables	Any vegetables	Vegetables
	0 Fat	0 Fat	0 Fat	0 Fat	Fat
	0 Milk	0 Milk	0 Milk	0 Milk	Milk
1000	5 Meat	1 Meat	2 Meat	2 Meat	Meat
	5 Starch	1 Starch	1 Starch	2 Starch	1 Starch
	3 Fruit	1 Fruit	1 Fruit	1 Fruit	Fruit
	Any vegetables	0 Vegetables	Any vegetables	Any vegetables	Vegetables
	0 Fat	0 Fat	0 Fat	0 Fat	Fat
	1 Milk	1 Milk	0 Milk	0 Milk	Milk
1200	6 Meat	1 Meat	2 Meat	3 Meat	Meat
	6 Starch	1 Starch	2 Starch	2 Starch	1 Starch
	3 Fruit	1 Fruit	1 Fruit	1 Fruit	Fruit
	Any vegetables	0 Vegetables	Any vegetables	Any vegetables	Vegetables
	0 Fat	0 Fat	0 Fat	0 Fat	Fat
	2 Milk	1 Milk	0 Milk	0 Milk	1 Milk
1400	7 Meat	1 Meat	3 Meat	3 Meat	Meat
	7 Starch	2 Starch	2 Starch	2 Starch	1 Starch
	3 Fruit	1 Fruit	1 Fruit	1 Fruit	Fruit
	Any vegetables	0 Vegetables	Any vegetables	Any vegetables	Vegetables
	1 Fat	0 Fat	0 Fat	1 Fat	Fat
	2 Milk	1 Milk	0 Milk	0 Milk	1 Milk
1500	7 Meat	1 Meat	3 Meat	3 Meat	Meat
	7 Starch	2 Starch	2 Starch	2 Starch	1 Starch
	4 Fruit	1 Fruit	1 Fruit	1 Fruit	1 Fruit
	Any vegetables	0 Vegetables	Any vegetables	Any vegetables	Vegetables
	2 Fat	1 Fat	0 Fat	1 Fat	Fat
	2 Milk	1 Milk	0 Milk	1 Milk	Milk
1600	7 Meat	1 Meat	3 Meat	3 Meat	Meat
	8 Starch	2 Starch	2 Starch	2 Starch	2 Starch
	4 Fruit	1 Fruit	1 Fruit	1 Fruit	1 Fruit
	Any vegetables	0 Vegetables	Any vegetables	Any vegetables	Vegetables
	2 Fat	1 Fat	0 Fat	1 Fat	Fat
	2 Milk	1 Milk	0 Milk	1 Milk	Milk
1800	8 Meat	1 Meat	3 Meat	4 Meat	Meat
	8 Starch	2 Starch	2 Starch	2 Starch	2 Starch
	5 Fruit	2 Fruit	1 Fruit	1 Fruit	1 Fruit
	Any vegetables	0 Vegetables	Any vegetables	Any vegetables	Vegetables
	4 Fat	1 Fat	1 Fat	2 Fat	Fat
	2 Milk	1 Milk	0 Milk	1 Milk	Milk
2000	8 Meat	1 Meat	3 Meat	4 Meat	Meat
	8 Starch	2 Starch	2 Starch	2 Starch	2 Starch
	5 Fruit	2 Fruit	1 Fruit	1 Fruit	1 Fruit
	Any vegetables	0 Vegetables	Any vegetables	Any vegetables	Vegetables
	6 Fat	2 Fat	2 Fat	2 Fat	Fat
	3 Milk	1 Milk	1 Milk	1 Milk	Milk

*Adapted from Fahey, P. J., and Gallagher-Allred, C. R.: AAFP Home Study Self-Assessment Monograph #41: Obesity, 1982.

(Numbers in the table represent the number of exchanges from each of the listed food groups (meat, starch, fruit, vegetables, fat, and milk). Serving sizes vary according to food groups. The total number of daily exchanges have been divided into three meals (breakfast, lunch, dinner) and an evening snack and may not be appropriately designed for individual preferences. The total number of exchanges per day from each food group is the most important information. Patients may consume the total number of exchanges (but not over the total number) in any pattern they desire—one or more meals, small or large meals, etc. For diets with less than 1200 kilocalories, it is desirable to recommend a multivitamin and mineral supplement equal to 100 per cent of the U.S. Recommended Dietary Allowances.)

Phenylpropanolamine usually works for 3 days, then ceases to be effective and is contraindicated in those patients earlier identified. Fiber-containing drugs, sugar-containing drugs, and anesthetic-containing drugs are no better than a placebo when given under controlled conditions and should generally be discouraged.

DIABETES MELLITUS

General Diet Principles

Diet, with or without insulin, is the cornerstone of diabetic treatment. To permit the patient to lead a normal life in good health is the principal goal of therapy. The treatment program should be designed to achieve the following objectives:

1. Regulate blood sugar to as near normal as possible

2. Promote desirable weight in the adult and normal growth and development in the child and adolescent

3. Supply adequate amounts of all nutrients

4. Prevent or delay the long-term complications of diabetes

5. Satisfy the patient's desire for pleasurable meals and promote psychosocial adjustment

Because a patient with diabetes is committed to a life-long change in behavior, an extensive patient education program is essential, and a team approach, including a diabetes nurse educator and a diabetes nutrition educator (or registered dietitian), is important.

The nutrient requirements for the diabetic patient are basically the same as for nondiabetics. Protein, vitamin, mineral, and fluid needs are unaltered. The diabetic patient's reduced ability to deal with as high a simple sugar diet as the general population consumes is what distinguishes the low simple sugar diabetic diet from a diet not restricted in simple sugars.

The American Diabetes Association (A.D.A.), in collaboration with The American Dietetic Association and the Chronic Disease Program of the U.S. Public Health Service, has developed an A.D.A. exchange system that translates the diabetic dietary prescription into an easily understood meal plan that allows for variability and control by the patient. Working with a diabetes nutrition educator, the physician will need to write an appropriate dietary prescription for the patient. The following steps are suggested to accomplish this:

1. Determine an acceptable body weight and kilocalorie prescription, considering special needs such as pregnancy, exercise, planned surgery, and other disease conditions

2. Calculate the proportion of nutrients as carbohydrate, protein, and fat

3. Consider meal spacing depending on treatment such as type of insulin, oral agent, or diet alone

The diabetic diet has changed drastically over the past 30 years, beginning first as a low-carbohydrate, high-protein, and high-fat diet. During the 1970s, recommendations included increasing the carbohydrate portion of the diet to as high as 60 to 70 per cent of total calories. During this time, a high-fiber intake was also recommended by many researchers (Anderson, et al., 1980). The lower glycemic index of foods high in fiber and fat may reflect the effect of these nutrients on slowing gastric emptying time (Jenkins, et al., 1981). Recent research supports the benefits of a diet in which 55 to 60 per cent of calories come from carbohydrate, 15 to 20 per cent from protein, and up to 30 per cent from fat (A.D.A., 1987). Approximately 65 to 70 per cent of the total carbohydrate should come from starches and 25 to 30 per cent from lactose, fructose, and sucrose occurring in milk, fruits, and vegetables.

Protein needs increase during pregnancy and lactation, and 25 per cent of total calories from protein is recommended for the diabetic. For diabetic patients with chronic renal failure, protein intake must often be limited to what is tolerated with the extra kilocalories supplied by complex carbohydrates.

The fat portion of the diabetic diet should consist primarily of polyunsaturated fatty acids and the saturated fatty acids limited so as to potentially delay atherosclerosis, the incidence of which is increased in diabetics. One of the most important methods for decreasing the incidence of atherosclerosis or to delay its occurrence is to achieve an ideal body weight. In addition, when hyperlipidemia (usually type IV) is present in the diabetic, carbohydrate intake should be reduced to 40 to 50 per cent of the total kilocalorie intake. If blood cholesterol is elevated, a trial of limiting dietary cholesterol to approximately 300 mg. daily should be tried; if the cholesterol restriction does not decrease serum cholesterol, medications to lower cholesterol should be considered. The diabetic patient who is also hypertensive is at greater risk for both microvascular and macrovascular disease. Hypertension should be managed with weight loss if appropriate and a reduction in salt intake to 5 grams daily (2000 mg. sodium). If the patient does not respond to sodium restriction, prescription of medical antihypertensive therapy is preferable to imposing further dietary restrictions on an already restricted life style.

When counseling the insulin-dependent diabetic, special consideration must be given by the physician and diabetes nutrition educator to medication, meal timing, food intake, and exercise to prevent wide swings in blood glucose levels. Depending on the type of insulin used, intake of dietary carbohydrate should be planned so that carbohydrate absorption coincides with peak action time of insulin. Meals should be approximately 4 to 5 hours apart. A meal should be eaten within 30 minutes following the injection of insulin. The patient and family must be educated to include a bedtime snack with protein and starch to prevent early morning hypoglycemia. Acceptable evening snack combinations that are also appropriate for other snacks during the day include milk and graham crackers, a meat or cheese sandwich, cheese and crackers, plain yogurt and a hard-boiled egg, and cheese and fresh fruit. The meal patterns (see Table 53–6) and A.D.A. exchange system may be appropriate for the diabetic patient. Higher calorie levels can be planned for pregnant women, athletes, and growing adolescents. If a midmorning and midafternoon snack are also needed, a fruit, starch, milk serving, or half sandwich is usually appropriate.

Type II diabetes is primarily treated by diet with or without oral hypoglycemic agents. Patients with type II diabetes are frequently overweight and should be encouraged to lose weight. For a number of these patients, weight loss, through diet and exercise, significantly improves glycemic control (Wing, et al., 1987) and may result in a reduced need for oral hypoglycemic drugs (Cohen, et al., 1988). These patients should divide their food intake evenly throughout three meals per day.

Special Diet Considerations

Diabetics, whether receiving insulin or oral agents, should be taught to recognize and treat insulin reactions. If hypoglycemia occurs, patients should know to consume 10 to 20 grams of simple sugar, such as one-half roll of Life Savers candy, one-half cup sweetened carbonated beverage or fruit juice, or 2 tablespoons sugar dissolved in one-half cup water. If the symptoms remain after 10 to 15 minutes, patients should consume another serving of simple sugars. When insulin-dependent diabetics find themselves in the common situation where a meal will be delayed for 1 to 2 hours, patients should be instructed to ingest 15 to 30 grams of carbohydrate to prevent hypoglycemia. This could include 1 or 1 1/2 cups fruit juice, 1 to 2 slices bread, or 2 to 4 graham crackers. If the evening meal is to be delayed for several hours, patients should be instructed to eat their bedtime snack at the regular evening meal time and eat their evening meal at the snack hour.

Regular exercise should be recommended for all diabetic patients, especially those who need to lose weight. If exercise is anticipated by the diabetic, it is usually recommended that the patient consume extra food instead of changing the insulin dosage. This consists of 10 to 15 extra grams of carbohydrate per hour of exercise if engaging in moderate exercise (such as walking, sweeping, or cleaning). If the exercise is vigorous (such as running or playing basketball or tennis), an additional 20 to 30 grams of carbohydrate per hour should be consumed.

The diabetes nutrition educator can teach diabetic patients how to allow alcohol in moderation in their diet. When episodes of nausea, vomiting, or anorexia occur, sick-day meal plans need to be developed so that patients avoid dehydration, ketosis, or hypoglycemic episodes.

Text continued on page 1223

Table 53–7. ALCOHOL AND CALORIC CONTENT OF SELECTED BEVERAGES*

Beverage	Serving Size	Alcohol Content (grams)	Kilocalorie Content
Ale, mild	8 ounces	8.9	98
Beer, regular, average	8 ounces	8.9	114
Beer, average, light	8 ounces	9.6	66
Brandy, California	1 brandy glass = 30 cc.	10.5	73
Cream de Menthe	1 cordial glass = 20 cc.	7.0	67
Daiquiri	1 cocktail glass = 90 cc.	15.1	122
Eggnog, Christmas	4 ounces	15.0	335
Gin, dry	1 jigger = 45 cc.	15.1	105
Highball	8 ounces	24.0	166
Manhattan or martini	1 cocktail glass = 90 cc.	19.0	150
Mint julep	10 ounces	29.2	212
Rum	1 jigger = 45 cc.	15.1	105
Tom Collins	10 ounces	21.5	180
Whiskey, scotch	1 jigger = 45 cc.	15.1	105
Wine, champagne	1 wine glass = 4 ounces	11.0	84
Wine, sherry	1 sherry glass = 60 cc.	9.0	84

*From Hurley, R. S., and Gallagher-Allred, C. R.: Dietary management for alcoholic patients. *In* Nutrition and Health Promotion in Primary Care Series. Columbus, Department of Family Medicine, The Ohio State University, 1980, p. 11.

Table 53–8. INFORMATION PHYSICIANS CAN USE TO HELP PATIENTS EVALUATE DIET PROGRAMS*

Program	Critique
Diet Center	This program emphasizes quick weight loss. The diet provides approximately 1000 kcal. per day and is combined with daily counseling, if desired by the client. People are encouraged to take a Diet Center Supplement four times a day. The supplement contains B-vitamins (at megadose levels), protein, and sugar and is supposed to raise the blood sugar to a level that decreases appetite. No scientific evidence indicates that such a supplement is effective other than to provide a short-term placebo effect. The expense of the supplement is probably not justified. This type of program tends to teach people that weight control is a temporary effort rather than a life-long change in eating habits. This program is more expensive than weekly visits to a registered dietitian for weight-control counseling.
Nutri-System	Clients who follow this program eat Nutri-System's prepackaged meals to control their caloric intake. Food preparation and menu planning are done for clients, thus they do not learn how to make wise food choices. This is a major drawback that "sets the client up" for rebound weight gain once the program is discontinued. Weekly counseling is provided for an additional fee. This program is more expensive than weekly visits to a registered dietitian for weight-control counseling.
Overeaters Anonymous	People who belong to this organization view overeating as an addiction that cannot be cured. Meetings are modeled after Alcoholics Anonymous and may appeal only to those who see themselves as "compulsive eaters." Low-calorie diets may be given to members, but the majority of time is spent discussing ways to control eating behaviors. Members may not learn how to make wise food choices. There is no set fee.
TOPS (Taking Off Pounds Sensibly)	Members of this women's organization attend weekly meetings to receive group support and set weight-loss goals. Quality of group sessions varies depending upon the skills of the leader. People may be "turned off" by weekly weigh-ins, which are not kept confidential. Those who do not lose weight may be "put on the spot" and embarrassed. Members frequently admit that they avoid eating and drinking the day prior to a meeting so they lose weight. It is not uncommon for groups to go out for dessert after each meeting to celebrate by overeating! Unfortunately, this approach does not promote change in eating habits.
Weight Watchers, Inc.	This organization offers several diet plans that are based upon the diabetic diet exchange lists. Many health professionals recommend this program. Safe weight loss is encouraged. Members attend weekly meetings to obtain group support, recipes, and weight-loss tips. Weight maintenance diets are provided when weight goals are reached. The company sells a variety of lower calorie foods, cookbooks, and magazines, which members may be encouraged to buy. Cost of the program varies depending upon the number of products purchased by the client.

*From Crosser, G. H.: Decoding fad diets. *In* Nutrition and Health Promotion in Primary Care Series. Columbus, Department of Family Medicine, The Ohio State University, 1985, p. 11.

Table 53–9. WHAT THE PHYSICIAN SHOULD KNOW ABOUT FAD DIETS*

Diet Category	Name of Diet	How Diet Works	Advantages	Possible Problems	Fallacies
Fasting	Fasting: The Ultimate Diet Fasting is a Way of Life	Rapid weight loss due to loss of lean body mass and fat.	Dieter is encouraged by rapid weight loss of water, which may be mistaken for loss of fat.	Hypoglycemia, neutropenia, hyponatremia, hypokalemia, ketosis, dehydration, increased uric acid levels, nausea, dizziness, fatigue, alopecia, increased renal loss of phosphate and magnesium, negative nitrogen balance, loss of lean body mass, atrophy of organs such as the liver and heart, impaired cellular immunity, sudden death. Does not educate the dieter how to maintain weight. Return to initial pre-fasting weight is likely once fast is stopped. If used, must be carefully monitored in a hospital setting.	Fasting cleanses the body of impurities. Fasting normalizes metabolism.
Low-protein, low-fat, high-carbohydrate diets	Pritikin Diet	Calories are limited automatically since most of intake consists of vegetables, whole grains, and fruits. Meat and fish are limited to 16 oz. per week. Only 10% of calories come from fat.	Possible reduction of serum cholesterol, triglyceride, and uric acid levels. Promotes permanent changes in eating habits.	Unpalatable for those who enjoy, meat (allows 2–3 oz. meat per day). Extreme low fat level is difficult for most Americans to achieve, and is unpalatable for many. Nearly impossible to follow if one eats in restaurants. If protein intake is too low, it may increase risk of infection and result in poor wound healing. Possible negative nitrogen balance. Flatulence; possible iron-deficiency anemia since most iron is obtained from non-heme sources. Possible decreased absorption of trace minerals, calcium, and zinc owing to increased intake of phytates.	Claims that the diet prevents degenerative diseases.

Table continued on following page

Table 53–9. WHAT THE PHYSICIAN SHOULD KNOW ABOUT FAD DIETS* *Continued*

Diet Category	Name of Diet	How Diet Works	Advantages	Possible Problems	Fallacies
Ketogenic diets or low-carbohydrate (100 grams or less), high-protein, high-fat diets	Dr. Atkin's Diet Revolution Stillman's Diet DuPont Diet	Rapid initial weight loss followed by slower but substantial weight loss.	Reduced hunger, palatable, socially acceptable.	Elevated serum cholesterol and triglyceride levels, ketosis, hyponatremia, hypokalemia, hyperuricemia, dehydration.	Claims that the diet promotes production of "fat-mobilizing hormone," which mobilizes fat stores and reduces ketones.
	Air Force Diet Drinking Man's Diet Calories Don't Count Diet Dr. Charlton Frederick's Diet Beacon Hill Diet Scarsdale Diet	Highly effective diet owing to low carbohydrate intake and reduced serum insulin level, which inhibits lipogenesis.	Should be used only in conjunction with nutrition counseling and behavior modification.	Specific blood changes in calcium, thiamin, riboflavin, ascorbic acid, folate, and vitamin A. Dizziness, fatigue. Possible renal failure if inadequate fluid intake; bad breath. Does not educate the dieter on weight maintenance. Diuresis promotes loss of vitamins and minerals that may not be replaced by the diet.	Actually the caloric value of ketones produced and excreted in 24 hours rarely exceeds 100 kcal. Claims that unlimited calories can be eaten as long as ketosis is present. Actually caloric intake will probably be limited because of the appetite depressant effect of ketosis.
Liquid protein-sparing modified-fast diets	Last Chance Diet	Very low-calorie intake (600 kcal. per day), which uses a liquid protein drink, Prolinn.	Rapid weight loss during first few days. Patients like the fact that they do not have to make food choices or think about portion sizes.	Product contains low-quality protein that causes unacceptable danger. Protein-calorie malnutrition, cardiac muscle atrophy, arrhythmias, cellular immune deficiency, severe ketosis, gout, hypokalemia, dehydration, vomiting, dizziness, diarrhea, muscle cramps, hypotension, psychologic symptoms, alopecia, skin dryness, weakness, and fatigue have been reported. Reports of sudden death even though patient was receiving medical supervision. Product is deficient in many nutrients. Monotonous; high attrition rate. Refeeding after use of low-quality liquid protein formulas results in redistribution of nutrients, sodium and water retention, increased catecholamine production, arrhythmias, and the possibility of sudden death.	Claims that use of such weight-control products is "the answer" to being overweight and will solve future weight-control problems. Claims that if one needs to lose only a few pounds it is OK to use this or a similar product for a few days.

Table 53–9. WHAT THE PHYSICIAN SHOULD KNOW ABOUT FAD DIETS* *Continued*

Diet Category	Name of Diet	How Diet Works	Advantages	Possible Problems	Fallacies
	Cambridge Diet	Very low-calorie (330 kcal. per day) and very low-carbohydrate intake promotes rapid loss of water in addition to loss of fat and protein. Consists of a powdered mix that is added to water. Use of Cambridge Diet or any high-quality protein liquid diet should be undertaken only under medical supervision. Periodic biochemical and ECG monitoring is needed.	Patients like the fact that they do not have to make food choices or think about portion sizes. Product is easy to mix. Contains high-quality protein. Rapid weight loss during first few days. May decrease hunger, serum insulin, blood pressure, cholesterol, triglycerides, and serum glucose.	Nitrogen balance may not be attained until the 5th or 6th week of the diet or may not ever be attained in some individuals. Severe protein losses are possible in some people, even though protein is of high quality. Does not educate dieter on proper eating practices. Monotonous; high attrition rate. "Diet counselors" who sell the diet have not had formal nutrition training and may provide misinformation. Many diet participants do not seek medical supervision, as recommended by the company. Total compliance with the plan could result in moderate ketosis and fluid and electrolyte depletion. Constipation, diarrhea in lactose-intolerant people, and alterations in menstrual cycle are common.	Claims that use of such weight-control products is "the answer" to being overweight and will solve future weight-control problems. Claims that if one needs to lose only a few pounds it is OK to use this or a similar product for a few days.
One- or two-food diets	Skim Milk-Banana Diet Steak-Tomato Diet Egg-Wine Diet Fiber Diet Fruit Diet Kempner Rice Diet Zen Macrobiotic Diet Strawberry and Cream Diet	If weight loss occurs, it is probably due to reduced caloric intake as a result of boredom, monotony, and an unpalatable meal plan.	None	Nutritionally incomplete; usually low in protein, vitamins, and minerals. Boring, monotonous diet that does not educate the dieter on proper eating practices. Death by malnutrition if followed long-term. High attrition rate. Health food supplements recommended by some of the diets are expensive.	Claims that refined sugar and refined flour are unhealthy and should be avoided. Actually, these foods may be eaten as long as excessive amounts are not used. Some of these diets suggest that fiber lowers the number of calories one receives from food eaten. Claims that use of high-fiber supplement will promote early satiety by increasing gastric distention.

Table continued on following page

Table 53–9. WHAT THE PHYSICIAN SHOULD KNOW ABOUT FAD DIETS* *Continued*

Diet Category	Name of Diet	How Diet Works	Advantages	Possible Problems	Fallacies
	Pumpkin-Carrot Diet Hot Dog Diet Egg and Orange Diet				Claims that certain foods, nutrients, or health food supplements have newly discovered, magical properties that promote weight loss. Promotional materials often suggest that physicians are unaware of or unwilling to use these "breakthroughs." Kempner Rice Diet may be erroneously considered beneficial for the kidneys, blood pressure, and heart function.
Trick Your Body's Metabolism Diets or "Magic Ingredient" diets	Hilton Head Metabolism Diet Starch Blockers Fructose Diet Mannan Human Chorionic Gonadotropin (HCG) K-28 Powder I Love NY Diet Fat-Off Diet Grapefruit Diet or Magic Mayo Diet	If weight loss occurs, it is due to reduced calorie intake. Health food supplements have no effect on promoting weight loss other than a short-term placebo effect.	None	Nutritionally incomplete resulting in possible protein, vitamin, and mineral deficiencies. Some are "crash diets." Such diets are usually ineffective. If effective, would be hazardous to health because of nutrient inadequacy, nausea, vomiting, or diarrhea. Attrition rate is high. Does not educate dieter on eating properly for life-long weight maintenance. Any weight loss is usually temporary.	Implies that a particular food combination and/or health food supplement or enzyme will "melt off" or "emulsify" unwanted fat. Frequently uses the meaningless term "cellulite" for unwanted fat. Claims that the diet and/or supplement will inhibit food intake, remove toxic substances from the body and increase the metabolic rate, resulting in large amounts of quick weight loss. Promotional materials often suggest that physicians are unaware of or unwilling to use these "breakthroughs." Claims that grapefruit is a catalyst for burning fat.

Table 53–9. WHAT THE PHYSICIAN SHOULD KNOW ABOUT FAD DIETS* *Continued*

Diet Category	Name of Diet	How Diet Works	Advantages	Possible Problems	Fallacies
	Enzyme Catalyst Diet	Same as above	None	Save as above	Claims that raw fruits, vegetables, seeds, and plant juices provide the dieter with enzymes which trigger mitochondrial function, "melt accumulated fat," and allow fat to be washed out of the body. Actually, any enzymes in foods are digested to amino acids and play no enzymatic role once absorbed.
	Lecithin, B_6, Vinegar, Kelp	Same as above	None	Same as above	Claims that lecithin emulsifies fat. B_6 metabolizes fat, and that vinegar flushes fat out of the body. Claims that vinegar is a good potassium source. Actually, there are only 5 mg of potassium in 1 tsp of vinegar. Claims that iodine in kelp causes the thyroid gland to produce more thyroxin and speed up metabolism.
	Lipogene-GH Diet	Same as above	None	Same as above	Growth hormone dissolves fat and "cellulite" while you sleep. Actually the lipogene-GH tablets are amino acids. The body would have no way of knowing the difference between Lipogen-GH amino acids and those from steak or tofu.
	Body Clock Diet	Same as above	None	Same as above	Claims that people can lose weight while continuing to eat their usual foods if they eat earlier in the day.
	Dolly Parton Diet	Same as above	None	Same as above	Claims that food combinations recommended by this diet require more calories to digest than they actually contain. This is impossible!

Table continued on following page

Table 53–9. WHAT THE PHYSICIAN SHOULD KNOW ABOUT FAD DIETS* *Continued*

Diet Category	Name of Diet	How Diet Works	Advantages	Possible Problems	Fallacies
	Beverly Hill's Diet	Same as above	None	In addition to the problems listed above, adherence to this diet could result in severe diarrhea, weakness, shock, hypotension, gout, and renal stones. Strenuous exercise could result in dehydration, and cardiac arrhythmias.	Claims that undigested food gets stuck to the body and causes fat to be made. Claims that sesame seeds are good source of calcium and that fruit requires no digestive enzymes because they contain all enzymes needed for digestion. Claims that being overweight is caused by the combination of foods eaten. This is based on Shelton's 30-year-old food-combining theories. Claims that digestive enzymes for protein and carbohydrate cannot work at the same time, therefore carbohydrate and protein should not be eaten in the same meal. Claims that unlimited intake of french fries will not produce weight gain as long as fresh pineapple is eaten the next day.

*From Crosser, G. H.: Decoding Fad Diets. *In* Nutrition and Health Promotion in Primary Care. Columbus, Department of Family Medicine, The Ohio State University, 1985, p. 5–9.

Osteoporosis

Although it appears that relatively little can be done from a dietary standpoint to reverse osteoporosis once there is the onset of fractures, a great deal can be accomplished by focusing on the preventive measures against this debilitating disease. Measures such as adequate daily calcium intake, exercise, and rational drug use need to be instituted as a matter of daily habit early in life rather than as a short-term treatment once a problem has been diagnosed. The family physician is in a pivotal position to help patients begin good habits early in life.

PREVENTION

Methods to prevent osteoporosis are controversial. Many, but not all, studies indicate that a life-long pattern of less-than-adequate calcium intake is one factor in the development of osteoporosis; therefore, adequate consumption of calcium throughout life, and especially prior to development of peak bone mass at approximately age 35, is recommended (N.I.H. Consensus Conference, 1984).

Intake of calcium is a function of several factors. Because foods that contain the largest amount of calcium tend to be those that are more expensive, calcium intake can be an economic factor. Ethnic eating patterns and lactose intolerance can also affect calcium intake; however, lactose intolerance is found most often in oriental and black populations, who are not at particular risk for osteoporosis. Older persons often avoid milk and dairy products believing that milk is needed only by children or that it contains too much cholesterol; others find cheese and dairy products constipating. Table 53–10 identifies foods highest in calcium that can be recommended for improving calcium intake.

Excess phosphorus, or low amounts of dietary calcium relative to phosphorus, results in skeletal defects in animals. In humans, however, there is little evidence that this is the case. Instead, a Ca/P ratio of 1 or a little greater appears to be ideal for humans (Food and Nutrition Board, 1980). Because most major food groups are higher in phosphorus than calcium and because our dietary intake of phosphorus is high, owing in part to the large amount of colas consumed, it is difficult to obtain this ratio.

Dietary components, such as fiber, oxalate (found in fiber-containing green leafy vegetables), and phytate (found in fiber-containing whole grain products) bind dietary calcium and decrease its absorption. Therefore, excessive fiber intakes (greater than 20 grams daily) should not be recommended. Total vegetarians have lowered bone mass compared with lacto-ovo vegetarians and should be counseled about the short- and long-term hazards of these dietary practices, for themselves and especially for their children (Marsh, et al., 1983).

Table 53–10. CALCIUM CONTENT OF COMMON FOODS*

Item	Serving Size	Calcium Content (mg.)
Milk, skim, whole, 2 per cent	8 oz	300
Milkshake, homemade	8 oz.	360
Milk, malted	8 oz.	345
Milk, chocolate or buttermilk	8 oz.	285
Swiss cheese	2 oz.	550
Cheddar cheese	2 oz.	410
Colby cheese	2 oz.	390
Processed American cheese	2 oz.	350
Cottage cheese	½ cup	75
Yogurt, plain, lowfat	8 oz.	415
Ice cream	1 cup	170
Pudding	½ cup	135
Pizza, with cheese	1 medium piece	145
Macaroni and cheese	1 cup	360
Sardines, canned	2 oz.	170
Salmon, canned, with bones	2 oz.	150
Oysters, raw	7–9	115
Collards, raw	½ cup	180
Mustard greens or kale, raw	½ cup	100
Blackstrap molasses	1 Tbsp.	135
Dried beans, cooked	1 cup	90

*From Roehrig, K. L.: Protecting bone and teeth. *In* Nutrition and Health Promotion in Primary Care Series. Columbus, Department of Family Medicine, The Ohio State University, 1985, p. 13.

Aluminum-containing antacid abuse can lead to phosphorus depletion, which, in turn, could precipitate osteomalacia. Likewise, cellulose phosphate and cholestyramine bind dietary calcium and could possibly contribute to the development of osteoporosis. Laxative abuse decreases calcium absorption.

TREATMENT

The easiest way to ingest adequate calcium, besides rational food choices, is by exogenous supplementation. Not all supplements, however, provide the same amount of calcium by weight. Calcium carbonate is higher in calcium than calcium phosphate, calcium lactate, and calcium gluconate and is generally the best supplement to suggest to patients. Bone meal and dolomite preparations should be avoided because they may be contaminated with toxic metals. Calcium supplements can be taken with a small amount of milk or yogurt, both of which contain vitamin D and lactose that promote the absorption of calcium. Encourage patients to take calcium supplements at mealtimes when gastric acid is higher because calcium generally requires an acid environment for optimal absorption. Research is currently underway to evaluate the bioavailability of various calcium salts.

The NIH Consensus Conference on Osteoporosis (N.I.H. Consensus Conference, 1984) recommended that calcium intake prior to menopause be 1000 to

1500 mg. and after menopause should be 1500 mg. unless the patient is taking estrogen. These recommendations have yet to be fully substantiated, but it is known that consumption greater than 2000 to 2500 mg. daily can result in calcification of soft tissues, hypercalciuria, hypercalcemia, and formation of urinary calculi. Supplemental fluoride is currently recommended only in the treatment of osteoporosis, not in its prevention. Sodium fluoride (40 mg. daily) has been shown to decrease the fracture rate in women (Riggs, et al., 1980). Because vitamin D is toxic in small amounts, vitamin D supplementation is not recommended for prevention or treatment of osteoporosis unless it is prescribed in an amount equal to (or twice) the R.D.A. for those patients who are not exposed to sunlight and who consume no dairy products, fish, or eggs.

Estrogen replacement for postmenopausal women should be used with caution (Ryan, 1982) but is effective in decreasing bone resorption if started soon after the onset of menopause (Saville, 1984). Its side effects can be minimized with a scientific and logical approach such as in combination with cyclical progesterone (Glowacki, 1988). Exercise is an important part of the maintenance of healthy bones, and patients should be encouraged to participate in moderate exercise throughout their lives.

Hypertension and Congestive Heart Failure

The objectives in treating the hypertensive patient include:

1. Providing a well-balanced diet with sufficient protein, kilocalories, vitamins, minerals, and fluids to ensure optimum health
2. Achieving an ideal body weight using a safe, balanced-diet approach
3. Ensuring appropriate sodium restriction
4. Preventing potassium deficiency in patients on diuretics that deplete potassium and prevent potassium overload in patients with chronic renal failure or those using potassium-retaining drugs like spironolactone or ACE inhibitors (captopril, enalapril, etc.)
5. Treating hyperlipidemia if present

Patients with hypertension will often benefit from a low-salt diet. The best rule-of-thumb for an uncomplicated hypertensive patient is a diet with no added salt (5 grams salt or 2000 mg. sodium). The patient with severe chronic congestive heart failure probably needs a more severe salt restriction, such as 1.5 to 2.0 grams (600 to 800 mg. sodium) per day if there is associated pulmonary congestion or ascites. The grossly edematous (3+ to 4+) patient without heart failure should also be more restricted, perhaps to a 2.5 to 4 gram salt diet (1000 to 1600 mg. sodium). The presence of renal failure will also require tighter restrictions. Diets under 4 to 5 grams of salt daily are difficult to maintain, and referral to a registered dietitian for counseling is prudent.

Most physicians and patients are aware of the high salt content (Table 53–11) of potato chips and cured meats, but the silent giants in sodium content are bread and many cultured dairy products, especially cheese and buttermilk. There are also high quantities of sodium in oriental, creole, Italian, and "soul" foods. Frequent restaurant visitors need special guidance to escape the facility without a sodium bolus. More sodium is often added to the diet via food processing, food preparation, food additives, and over-the-counter medications, such as antacids, than may be in food itself.

Prior to counseling patients on a low-sodium diet, estimate the sodium content of the patient's usual foods and the amounts added in preparation. Patients need to know that one teaspoonful of table salt contains 2 grams of sodium. Since water in certain areas of the country is relatively high in sodium, tap water and soft drinks made in these areas may provide

Table 53–11. HIGH-SODIUM FOODS TO BE AVOIDED ON LOW-SODIUM DIETS*
(2 grams sodium or less)

Milk	***Breads and Cereals***
Buttermilk	Instant oatmeal and Cream of Wheat
Meat	Dry cereals
Ham	Quick-cooking rice
Bacon	Instant mashed potatoes
Salt pork	Potato chips, salted
Chipped beef	Popcorn, salted
Corned beef	Snack crackers
Smoked tongue	Salted-top crackers
Smoked fish	***Convenience Foods***
Luncheon meats	TV dinners
Frankfurters	Frozen vegetables in seasoned sauce
Sausage	Biscuit, muffin, pancake, cake, and cookie mixes
Canned meats	Self-rising flour
Anchovies	Seasoned rice
Caviar	Packaged potato dishes
Meat extracts	Hamburger extenders
Bouillon cubes	Seasoned bread stuffings
Meat sauces	Canned soups
Meat substitutes (soy protein)	Salted nuts
Vegetables	Prepared condiments, relishes, Worchestershire sauce, pickles, olives
Frozen peas and lima beans	Seasoning salts
Celery	
Sauerkraut	
Watercress	
Beets	
Turnips	

*From Molleson, A. L., and Gallagher-Allred, C. R.: Dietary management in hypertension. *In* Nutrition and Health Promotion in Primary Care Series. Columbus, Department of Family Medicine, The Ohio State University, 1980, p. 23.

an additional sodium burden. Use of a diuretic does not obviate the need for salt restriction.

Preliminary results from the intersalt study in the late 1980's, the largest international cooperative study ever undertaken that involves life-style links to hypertension, not only reaffirms the need for restricting salt in some populations but also demonstrates the benefits of three other dietary therapies in the treatment of hypertension: (1) increasing daily potassium intake from 40 mEq. to 70 mEq., (2) reducing body mass, and (3) reducing daily alcohol intake to approximately 25 grams per day (Phillip, 1988). To put alcohol into perspective, one 12 oz. can of beer provides 13 grams alcohol; 4 oz. white wine contains 10 to 15 grams alcohol; and one jigger hard alcohol averages 15 grams alcohol (see Table 53–7).

Table 53–12. FOODS HIGH IN POTASSIUM*

Food	Amount Description	mEq.
Juices		
Prune	4 oz.	8.0
Tomato	4 oz.	7.0
V-8	4 oz.	7.0
Orange	4 oz.	6.5
Grapefruit	4 oz.	5.5
Pineapple	4 oz.	5.0
Fruits		
Avocado	1 cup	27.0
Prunes	5 whole	15.0
Raisins	½ cup	14.0
Banana	1 large	13.0
Canteloupe	1 cup	13.0
Dates	10	12.5
Apricots	5 whole dried	12.0
Honeydew	1 cup	11.0
Nectarine	2½ inches	10.5
Peach	2½ inches	8.0
Apricots	3 fresh	8.0
Orange	1 medium	7.0
Strawberries	1 cup	6.5
Cherries	¾ cup	6.0
Pear	1 medium	5.5
Watermelon	1 cup	5.0
Vegetables		
Acorn squash	½ cup	21.5
Yams	½ cup	19.0
Winter squash	½ cup	14.0
Potatoes	1 medium	14.0
	10 fries	13.0
	½ cup baked/mashed	10.0
Spinach	½ cup	9.0
Sweet potatoes	½ cup	8.0
Parsnips	½ cup	8.0
Pumpkin	½ cup	7.5
Tomatoes	½ cup	7.0
Dill pickle	1 large	7.0
Brussels sprouts	½ cup	5.5
Succotash	½ cup	5.5
Turnips	½ cup	5.5

Food	Amount Description	mEq.
Vegetables		
Broccoli	½ cup	5.0
Cauliflower	½ cup	5.0
Carrots	½ cup	4.0
Corn	½ cup	4.0
Peas	⅔ cup	3.5
Bread-Cereal		
Bran, 100 per cent	1 cup	12.0
Bran muffin	1 medium	4.5
Bran flakes, 40 per cent	1 cup	3.5
Whole wheat bread	1 slice	2.0
Dairy Products		
Eggnog	1 cup	15.0
Milkshake	1 cup	10.0
Milk	1 cup	9.0
Yogurt, plain	1 cup	8.5
Custard	½ cup	5.0
Pudding	½ cup	5.0
Ice cream	½ cup	3.0
Cottage cheese	½ cup	3.0
Cheese, American	1 oz.	1.0
Meat and Meat Substitutes		
Lasagne	3 inch square	12.0
Navy beans	½ cup	10.0
Lima beans	½ cup	9.0
Kidney beans	½ cup	8.0
Almonds	¼ cup	6.5
Peanuts	¼ cup	6.5
Walnuts	10 large	6.0
Macaroni and cheese	1 cup	6.0
Peanut butter		
Fish	2 Tbsp.	5.0
Pecans	1 oz.	5.0
Beef	¼ cup	4.5
Egg	1 oz.	3.0
Tuna	1	2.5
Ham	1 oz.	2.0
Chicken	1 oz	2.0
Others	1 oz.	2.0
Cream soup		
Chocolate	⅔ cup	5.0
	6 kisses	3.0

*From Koehrig, K. L.: Risk Factors and Disease Prevention. *In* Nutrition and Health Promotion in Primary Care Series. Columbus, Department of Family Medicine, The Ohio State University, 1985, p. 13. (By permission.)

Potassium intake can be increased by eating fruits and vegetables, including fruit juices, bananas, dried apricots, peaches, or potatoes at each meal (Table 53–12). Salt substitutes are a rich source of potassium and thus serve two purposes. Owing to their bad taste in large amounts, however, they can be consumed in only small amounts. Morton's Lite Salt contains only half the potassium content of most true substitutes; the other half is sodium chloride. Studies are currently underway to evaluate the therapeutic value of increased calcium intake in hypertension (McCarron, et al., 1984).

Hyperlipidemia and Coronary Heart Disease

The relationship of diet in the causation and prevention of coronary heart disease and in the etiology and therapy of the various hyperlipidemias has been the most studied of all disease-diet interrelationships; Grundy (1982) provides an in-depth review of this literature. Several large dietary intervention studies have demonstrated that a low cholesterol diet (300 mg. or less daily) reduces blood cholesterol an average of 5 to 10 per cent. Other population studies show that a diet high in polyunsaturated fat and low in saturated fat can decrease blood cholesterol by an equal amount.

Even with the lack of firm cause-and-effect data on dietary changes affecting morbidity and mortality, dietary therapy is still the first step in therapy of hyperlipidemias since we do know that dietary modifications can lower elevated lipids to some extent in many patients (Table 53–13). In patients with hyperlipidemia, the total cholesterol level and the low-density lipoprotein cholesterol (LDL-C) level appear to be raised by dietary saturated fat. Dietary steps that tend to decrease these levels include certain water-soluble fibers, such as oat bran and psyllium hydrophilic mucilloid (Metamucil) and polyunsaturated fatty acids (Anderson, et al., 1988).

When the family physician determines that dietary intervention is warranted for elevated cholesterol, the National Cholesterol Education Program recommends a two-step approach. The Step-One Diet restricts total fat to less than 30 per cent of calories, saturated fatty acids to less than 10 per cent of calories, and cholesterol to under 300 mg. per day. If necessary, the Step-Two Diet is employed, which restricts saturated fats to less than 7 per cent of calories and total cholesterol to less than 200 mg. per day. When the goal is to reduce blood cholesterol, the key element of the diet is the reduction of the saturated fat intake. Follow-up cholesterol levels should be measured at about 6- and 12-week intervals, with a goal of perhaps a 10 to 15 per cent reduction.

Cholesterol is present in the fat and tissue of animal products only and is not found in foods of plant origin, such as fruits, vegetables, cereals, grains, legumes, and nuts. Egg yolk, organ meats, and high-fat cheeses are high in cholesterol. Highly saturated fats especially are restricted on a modified-fat diet for hypercholesterolemic patients. Foods listed according to fatty acid composition are given in Table 53–14. Harmful oils (more than 30 per cent saturated fats) include coconut oil and palm kernal oil. Better oils (less than 20 per cent saturated fats) include peanut, olive, soybean, corn, sunflower, and canola oil. Monounsaturated fats appear to be as effective in reducing cholesterol as polyunsaturated fats when substituted for saturated fats.

Many foods that are available in supermarkets are good choices for use in treating hyperlipidemia. Owing to the continual addition and removal of processed foods in the marketplace, a listing of brand names soon becomes out of date. Egg substitutes, low-fat cheese, soybean vegetable protein, polyunsaturated margarines, low-fat frozen desserts, and soybean nondairy creamers are current examples. Patients must learn to read and interpret labels, purchasing products labeled low fat and selecting skimmed milk and products made with skimmed milk instead of whole milk. For patients who also need to restrict dietary sodium, highly processed and convenience foods are usually higher in sodium than less processed foods. Owing to the sodium and fat contents of most processed foods, the patient on a diet for the control of hyperlipidemia will often need to prepare foods at home, using allowed ingredients (Table 53–15). A number of helpful cookbooks with recipes for fat-controlled, low-cholesterol meals have been published.

Table 53–13. DIETARY AND DRUG TREATMENT BASED ON LDL-CHOLESTEROL

LDL-Cholesterol Level	Patient Description Classification
< 130 mg./dl.	Desirable LDL-Cholesterol
130–159 mg./dl.	Borderline High-Risk LDL-Cholesterol
≥ 160 mg./dl.	High-Risk LDL-Cholesterol

LDL-Cholesterol Level to Initiate Diet Therapy to Lower Cholesterol

Risk Factor Status	*Initiation Level*	*Goal*
No CHD or less than two other risk factors	≥ 160 mg./dl.	< 160 mg./dl.
With CHD or two other risk factors	≥ 130 mg./dl.	< 130 mg./dl.
Drug Treatment Plus Dietary Treatment		
No CHD or less than two other risk factors	≥ 190 mg./dl.	< 160 mg./dl.
With CHD or two other risk factors	≥ 160 mg./dl.	< 130 mg./dl.

Risk factors include family history, cigarette smoking, HDL-C < 35 mg./dl., hypertension, diabetes, and male sex.

Table 53–14. FOODS DIVIDED INTO FATTY ACID COMPOSITION GROUPS*

More Than 30 Per Cent Saturated Fatty Acids	20 to 30 Per Cent Saturated Fatty Acids	Less than 20 Per cent Saturated Fatty Acids
Butterfat	Poultry	Fish
Beef, lamb, pork, veal	Margarine†	Margarine†
Butter	Shortening	Oils, including peanut, corn, olive, safflower, sesame
Margarine†	Cottonseed oil	Nuts
Shortening		
Coconut, palm oils		

*From Gallagher-Allred, C. R., and Townley, N. A.: Dietary management in hyperlipidemia. *In* Nutrition and Health Promotion in Primary Care Series. Columbus, Department of Family Medicine, The Ohio State University, 1980, p. 10.

†The kind of fat and composition of fat in margarine vary considerably.

Table 53–15. LOW-CHOLESTEROL, LOW-SATURATED FAT, LOW-SIMPLE SUGAR DIET*

Foods	Foods Allowed	Foods Omitted
Beverages	Coffee (regular and decaffeinated), tea, unsweetened carbonated beverages, skim milk, products made with skim milk, such as low-fat yogurt, cheeses, cottage cheese	Low-fat and whole milk, and products made with these milks, sweetened cocoa, sweetened drinks, and fruitades. Imitation milk
Breads/Cereals	Any except those that should be omitted	Sugar-coated cereals, sweet rolls, other pastries
Desserts	Fruits, sugar-free gelatin desserts	All containing sugar, cream, whole and low-fat milk, eggs, butter, coconut, and pies, cakes, pastries, sherbet, ice cream, cookies
Eggs	Three eggs per week, prepared without fat	More than three eggs weekly including eggs used in cooking
Fats	Margarine made with vegetable oils (corn, safflower, soybean, cottonseed, olive, peanut, sesame); salad dressings made with allowed oil; nuts	Commercial mayonnaise, coconut oil, butter, lard, margarine made with hydrogenated shortening, bacon
Fruits	Three daily	Avocado
Soups and Sauces	Broth based or those made with skim milk	All made with whole and low-fat milk or cream
Sweets	None	All candy, jelly, honey, molasses, marshmallows, syrups
Vegetables	Any, prepared without whole or low-fat milk or cream	None
Meat, fish, fowl, cheese	Lean beef, poultry without skin, fish, lean fresh pork, low-fat cheeses, dry curd (farmer's) cottage cheese	Frankfurters, ham, luncheon meats, sugar-cured meats, cheeses made with whole milk, liver, kidney, sweetbreads, and shrimp; lamb and beef should be limited to three servings per week

*From Gallagher-Allred, C. R., and Townley, N. A.: Dietary management in hyperlipidemia. *In* Nutrition and Health Promotion in Primary Care Series. Columbus, Department of Family Medicine, The Ohio State University, 1980, p. 19.

Steps that lower triglyceride levels include reduction of calorie intake, weight loss, reduction of carbohydrates and alcohol, and increased intake of omega-3 fatty acids found in fish. The triglyceride-lowering diet, which in many respects is a good diabetic diet, often has a dramatic effect on serum triglycerides, lowering them as much as 30 to 50 per cent. Deep-water ocean fish appear to have a greater effect on triglycerides than fresh-water fish. Patients should be advised to eat fish two to three times a week and avoid fish oil supplements. Fish oil capsules contain some cholesterol and may contain toxic amounts of vitamins A and D and an inadequate amount of vitamin E. Because omega-3 fatty acids reduce platelet aggregation, they are usually contraindicated in patients taking aspirin and other drugs that inhibit blood coagulation.

Fiber in various forms has been widely studied in recent years in relationship to serum cholesterol. Although wheat-based fiber sources, such as dark wheat bread, have been disappointing in terms of cholesterol-lowering effects, certain fibers are proving to have a more beneficial effect. Water-soluble fibers, such as the fiber in oat bran, appear to decrease not only total cholesterol by modest amounts, but more importantly, it appears that this reduction is in the harmful LDL-C component only, not the HDL-C component, and thus improves the total cholesterol/HDL-C ratio. New oat bran products are appearing in the bread and cereal industry that may be useful. The amount of oat bran needed to affect serum cholesterol is the equivalent of less than two-thirds cup of cooked oat bran per day according to some and two servings per day according to others. Patients should be watchful via the label that the cereal manufacturers haven't added saturated fats like coconut oil to make oat bran taste better.

Another important issue for the family physician is whether to prescribe the American Heart Association's "prudent diet" for everyone as that Association urges. This approach may deprive the large number of Americans who do not have a cholesterol problem of desirable, tasty foods and may lead to dietary insufficiencies in certain pediatric, pregnant, and geriatric populations. Whether the physician opts for the broad-based attack with a lipid-lowering diet for everyone or the more selective approach, it would seem more imperative that each and every patient, regardless of family history and other risks, have a lipid profile determination just as they have a blood pressure determination. Rational dietary counseling depends upon an adequate databank of clinical information.

The worse the LDL-C, the greater the need for lowering fat intake to 30 per cent of calories with a 10:10:10 ratio of saturated:monounsaturated:polyunsaturated fatty acids and testing the effect of lowering dietary cholesterol; the worse the triglyceride level, using perhaps 150 to 170 as an upper limit of normal, the more aggressive the need for restricting calories, sweets, and alcohol, and achieving weight loss.

Peptic Ulcer Disease

The term *peptic ulcer disease* is used to describe any localized erosion of the mucosal lining of those portions of the alimentary tract that come into contact with gastric juice. The majority of ulcers occur in the first part of the duodenum; gastric ulcers also often occur along the lesser curvature of the stomach near the pylorus. Although the etiology of peptic ulcer disease is unclear and under investigation, there appear to be three factors involved in its development. These factors include:

1. Large amounts of gastric acid and pepsin secretion

2. Decreased mucosal resistance to gastric acid and pepsin

3. High degree of anxiety and internalization of emotional stress

The principal goals in the management of peptic ulcer disease include the reduction of the secretion of gastric acid and pepsin, neutralization of the acid that is secreted, protection of the ulcerated region, and the promotion of healing. Thus, medical therapy includes agents such as the histamine H_2 receptor antagonists, antacids, and the locally protective sucralfate. The no-gastric-stimulant diet in the treatment of ulcer disease is simple and not highly restrictive:

1. Omit known gastric stimulants—regular and decaffeinated coffee, tea, cocoa, chocolate, meat extracts, alcohol, black pepper, chili powder, mustard seed, and nutmeg.

2. Provide frequent, small feedings during the acute stage.

3. Individualize the diet as the patient prefers, but make certain that it supports a well-balanced nutrient intake.

Several dietary treatments have been used in the past, varying from a strict milk and cream regimen (the Sippy diet) to a liberal diet as tolerated. The American Dietetic Association recognizes that the historic bland diet is not supported by scientific evidence. Many seasoned foods do not, in fact, irritate the gastric mucosa. Known irritants should be omitted only if they are not tolerated by the patient. Milk has minimal buffering action against acid and indeed may increase acid secretion (American Dietetic Association, 1971).

Although the products of protein digestion stimulate gastric acid secretion, protein still needs to be consumed in an amount equal to the R.D.A. (0.8 gram per kg. of body weight). Although roughage and citrus fruits may adversely affect some patients, they are not proven mucosal irritants and should be eliminated only on an individual basis. For a patient handout on the no-gastric-stimulant diet, see Table 53–16. The newer drug therapies for peptic ulcer

Table 53–16. ACCEPTABLE AND NONACCEPTABLE FOODS ON A NO-GASTRIC-STIMULANT DIET*

Food Types	Acceptable Foods	Foods to Avoid
Milk and Milk Products	Use as desired	Chocolate milk
Meats, Fish, Poultry, Eggs	Beef, veal, pork, ham, lamb, poultry, liver, fish, eggs, and peanut butter	Highly seasoned meats, such as bratwurst and lunchmeats, should be avoided if there is discomfort associated with their ingestion (some contain black pepper)
Fruits and Vegetables	Use as desired. Fresh, frozen, canned as well as all juices	None, unless citrus juices cause pain to individual patients
Breads and Cereals	Use as desired. Enriched breads and cereals, crackers, rice, noodles, and macaroni	None
Fats	Use as desired. Butter, margarine, cream, salad dressings, sour cream, bacon, and cooking oils	Spicy salad dressings, such as Italian. (some may contain black pepper, mustard seed, chili powder, nutmeg)
Beverages	Cereal beverages and carbonated beverages except cola beverages	Coffee (regular and decaffeinated), tea, cola beverages, cocoa, chocolate drinks, alcoholic beverages
Desserts and Sweets	Cakes, pies, pastries, cookies, and others (restrict only when kilocalorie restriction is indicated)	Desserts using chocolate or cocoa as an ingredient
Miscellaneous Foods	Soups, spices, and condiments as tolerated	Gravies, bouillon, black pepper, chili powder, mustard seed, and nutmeg if not tolerated by the patient

*From Stein, J. Z., and Gallagher-Allred, C. R.: Dietary managment in gastrointestinal diseases. *In* Nutrition and Health Promotion in Primary Care Series. Columbus, Department of Family Medicine, The Ohio State University, 1980, p. 4.

disease may enable patients to be less circumspect in their approach to the dining table; individualization is critical.

Reflux Esophagitis

Reflux esophagitis, popularly labeled heartburn, is another important component of acid-peptic disease. The problem here is an incompetent lower esophageal sphincter. Patients with reflux esophagitis may be quite sensitive to certain foods and gastric acid that reflux into the esophagus when the lower esophageal sphincter is weak. Thus, these patients may need to avoid citrus juices and spicy foods. Although fatty foods may actually inhibit gastric acid secretion, they may also make the lower esophageal sphincter weaker and thereby increase reflux. Protein increases sphincter pressure, thereby decreasing reflux.

Some restrictions for treating reflux esophagitis are similar to peptic ulcer disease: omit regular and decaffeinated coffee, chocolates, tea, and alcohol. These foods appear to decrease the esophageal sphincter pressure, in addition to being direct irritants. Patients may benefit from antacids before meals or immediately afterward, rather than waiting an hour as in peptic ulcer disease, since the symptoms often occur much sooner in reflux esophagitis. Weight loss in overweight patients also appears to be a helpful dietary tool. Pharmacotherapy, such as histamine H_2 receptor antagonists and metoclopramide, may also prove helpful.

Gallbladder Disease

The trend of more patients with gallbladder disease being seen in the family practice setting is possibly due to the increased incidence of obesity, the reluctance of some surgeons to operate in very obese patients, and the reluctance of patients to choose elective surgery. Regardless of the reasons, the family physician should be able to provide increased comfort for the patient with gallbladder disease who is not planning cholecystectomy by recommending a diet similar to that used for reflux esophagitis; it should be low in fat, include small, frequent meals, and lead to weight loss if the patient is overweight. For reasons not well understood, avoiding gastric irritants and spices seems to allow some of these patients to do better, although these restrictions need to be individualized. Dietary guidelines for a low-fat, no-gastric-stimulant diet are shown in Table 53–17, which may be used as a guide for patients with both cholelithiasis and reflux esophagitis. Following gallbladder removal, many patients have no trouble tolerating fats, and the diet should be liberalized as tolerated.

Lactose Intolerance

Lactose intolerance is a significant problem for large numbers of blacks, Asians, and those with Mediterranean basin roots. Additionally, many patients, especially young children, may have a temporary prob-

Table 53–17. ACCEPTABLE AND NONACCEPTABLE FOODS ON A LOW-FAT NO-GASTRIC STIMULANT DIET*

Food Types	Foods Allowed	Foods to Avoid
Beverages	Cereal beverages, and carbonated beverages except colas	Coffee, tea, cocoa, cola beverages, alcohol
Milk	Skim milk, buttermilk, low-fat yogurt	Whole milk, 2 per cent milk, buttermilk made from whole milk, cream
Eggs	No more than 1 egg per day	Fried eggs
Cereals	Enriched, cooked, and dry cereals	None
Meat and Substitutes	Baked, broiled, roasted, or stewed lean beef, veal, lamb, poultry. Meat must have all visible fat removed; poultry must have skin removed. Fresh and frozen fish, canned tuna, salmon, crab, and lobster (water packed or rinsed and drained), low-fat cottage cheese, mozzarella cheese, Parmesan cheese, or other low-fat cheeses	Fatty fish, fatty meats, ham, pork, bacon, duck, goose, highly seasoned meats such as bratwurst, lunchmeats, and sausages, frankfurters, corned beef, fried meats or fish, all other cheeses, and peanut butter
Potatoes and Substitutes	Boiled, mashed, baked, or escalloped white potatoes, baked or mashed sweet potatoes, noodles, rice, spaghetti, macaroni	Fried potatoes
Soups	Clear or skimmed broth, soups with vegetables added. Creamed soups made with skim milk	All others
Vegetables	All vegetables fresh, frozen, or canned	None. Some patients may complain of dyspepsia or discomfort after eating vegetables such as cabbage, broccoli, Brussels sprouts, cauliflower, and onions. If so, these as any other foods should be avoided
Fat	One to three teaspoons daily of butter, margarine, oils, and low-calorie salad dressing. Gravies made with skim milk or with clear fat-free broths and thickened with cornstarch or flour	Gravy, bacon, sour cream, regular commercial salad dressings, mayonnaise, salad oil

*From Stein, J. Z., and Gallagher-Allred, C. R.: Dietary management in gastrointestinal diseases. *In* Nutrition and Health Promotion in Primary Care Series. Columbus, Department of Family Medicine, The Ohio State University, 1980, p. 8.

lem tolerating a lactose load after a gastrointestinal infection. When the body has deficient lactase in the jejunum, lactose is not hydrolyzed and remains in the gut lumen exerting a hyperosmolar effect. Water is drawn into the lumen, and discomfort begins. When lactose is finally metabolized to lactic acid by colonic bacteria, an increased osmolar load leads to more cramping, bloating, flatulence, and loose stools.

Patients who have a severe deficiency of lactase can tolerate little lactose in the diet. Patients who cannot handle milk should be encouraged to consume fermented dairy products, such as buttermilk, yogurt, cottage cheese, and other cheeses. If fermented dairy products are not consumed, the diet should be supplemented with a multiple vitamin and mineral supplement. Many patients may be able to drink milk by purchasing over-the-counter lactase tablets or by purchasing the more expensive milk with less lactose. Table 53–18 identifies foods that contain lactose.

Diverticulosis, Irritable Colon Syndrome, and Constipation

Three additional problems relative to the lower gastrointestinal tract—diverticulosis, irritable colon syndrome, and constipation—all appear to have a central theme in their dietary management: the need for increased dietary fiber.

Diverticula of the colon are quite common in the elderly and are usually asymptomatic; thus, diverticulosis is not a true disease but simply the outpouching of the mucosa through the walls of the colon. However, the complications of bleeding, infection, and perforation are clearly pathologic and need to be treated and prevented if possible. The formation of diverticula with muscle hypertrophy seems to be related to colonic muscle spasm with increased luminal pressure and is thus related to the irritable colon syndrome. Diverticula without hypertrophy have an unknown etiology.

Symptoms of irritable colon syndrome include abdominal pain, loose stools, or constipation. The colonic musculature of these patients is more sensitive to stress, meals, and other factors than unaffected individuals. Comprehensive evaluation is needed to rule out other disorders.

Constipation is often seen in the geriatric population as well as people who decrease their activity levels, alter their diet, or otherwise modify their daily routine. Prior to considering a dietary approach to this symptom, the physician needs to rule out causes of constipation, such as colonic neoplasm, hypothyroidism, depression, drug side effects, and rectal disorders. Discussing the need for regular bowel habits and the avoidance of bowel stimulants is important.

A high-fiber diet is helpful treatment for diverticulosis, irritable colon syndrome, and constipation. Because a large fecal mass in the sigmoid prevents the close approximation of the colonic walls, dietary treatment for diverticula is aimed at increasing fecal mass, decreasing intraluminal pressure, and decreasing the accumulation of luminal residue inside the diverticula. On a high-fiber diet, a large stool forms owing to the water-holding capacity of the fiber, and the large luminal mass passes quickly through the bowel. Such a diet should also be helpful for patients with chronic constipation and constipation secondary to the irritable colon syndrome. Bulking the stool with fiber and fluids may also be useful in slowing the hyperactive bowel of these same patients and in diminishing pain, since the colonic musculature should not be able to spasm as much if the lumen is filled with soft stool. When initiating fiber therapy, start gradually and warn the patient about the possibility of increased bowel sounds and flatulence.

In patients with diverticulosis, a dietary restriction of nuts, seeds, hulls (such as popcorn), and berries (particularly strawberries, blueberries, raspberries, and blackberries) may be warranted. The rationale for this is that such items may become trapped in the diverticula and become painful. With a high-fiber diet and fast colon transit, the incidence of trapping of these items in the diverticula is diminished, and therefore, these products may not always need to be eliminated from the diet of the patient with diverticulosis. Patient tolerance should be the deciding factor.

DIETARY FIBER

The two terms, *fiber* and *roughage*, are used synonymously. These terms describe the polysaccharide and lignin components of plant cell walls and the sap component that is responsible for cell structure. Fiber consists of cellulose, hemicellulose, lignin, pectin, and gums that are sugar polymers and are not enzymatically digestible by the human digestive system. The term *crude fiber* refers to the fibrous residue left after laboratory extraction with a strong acid and base. Crude fiber measures only cellulose and lignin and, therefore, greatly underestimates total dietary fiber. Published fiber figures are usually crude fiber values.

Unprocessed wheat bran, unrefined breakfast cereals, and whole wheat and rye flours are the most significant food sources of dietary fiber. Fruits (except bananas), vegetables (except potatoes), nuts, and legumes are also major contributors of dietary fiber. When consuming bran, it is advisable to start with small doses (1 teaspoon a day) and gradually increase (as tolerated by teaspoons) up to 3 to 4 tablespoons (9 to 12 teaspoons) and increase fluid intake. Six teaspoons a day is generally effective in relieving pain associated with various gastrointestinal diseases treatable with a moderate- to high-fiber diet. Starting with large amounts of bran may give rise to considerable

Table 53–18. ACCEPTABLE AND NONACCEPTABLE FOODS ON A LACTOSE-RESTRICTED DIET*

Food Group	Acceptable Foods	Foods to Avoid
Beverages	Coffee, tea, carbonated beverages, whiskey, gin, rum, Scotch, vodka, ale, beer, cordials, liquors, pure cocoa or chocolate	Instant coffee and powdered soft drinks (e.g., Koolaid), cocoa beverages, and Ovaltine because lactose is added frequently in small amounts as an anticaking compound
Dairy Products	Soybean milk and other milk-free supplements, lactose-free non-dairy creamer, fermented cheeses, yogurt, buttermilk, cottage cheese (dry curd), sour cream	Milk, malted milk, evaporated or sweetened condensed milk, cocoa powders, curds, whey, milk chocolate, instant chocolate, infant formulas and supplements containing milk or milk products, powdered coffee creamer
Vegetables and Fruit Juices	All except those listed to avoid as they contain some added lactose in processing	Canned or frozen vegetables and dietetic fruit if milk or milk products have been added as cream sauces
Meat and Meat Substitutes	All meats, poultry, fish, and eggs prepared without breading, gravies, or sauces containing no milk or milk products, dried beans and peas, peanut butter and soybeans, yogurt-made gravies and sauces	Processed cheeses (American spreads), canned fish or meat, weiner, sausage, luncheon and breaded meat products if milk or a milk product has been added
Starches	Potatoes, spaghetti, noodles, rice, macaroni, dry cereal if no milk added, milk-based bread products if tolerated up to 3 servings per day, water-based bread products such as French or Italian bread and bagels as desired	Instant mashed potatoes and prepared instant cereal if milk is added (Total, Special K, Cocoa Krispies, Fortified Oat Flakes), zwieback, waffles, corn curls, commercial French fried potatoes, commercial sweet rolls, regular bread made with nonfat dry milk
Fats	Butter, margarine, salad dressings (if they do not contain milk or milk products), pure mayonnaise, shortening and vegetable oils, bacon, olives, meat gravy without milk	Cream and cream substitutes, mayonnaise containing milk or milk products, milk-based gravies, whipped toppings
Desserts and Sweets	Fruit ices made with water (slushes), gelatin, angel food cake, homemade cakes, pies, and cookies (if made without milk), pure chocolate or cocoa, sugar, honey, jam, candies made without milk (gumdrops, hard candy, jelly beans, colored mints), marshmallows	Commercial desserts and prepared mixes with milk or milk products, ice cream, sherbert, milk chocolate, puddings, custard, malted milk candies, chocolate cream candy, caramels, fudge
Condiments and Seasonings	Salt, pepper, pure spices, herbs	Any spice blend with a milk-based filler, monosodium glutamate, citric acid
Miscellaneous	Pretzels, potato chips, corn chips, popcorn, nuts, Melba toast	Cheese-flavored chips, commercial party dips, ascorbic acid tablets, and other medications with a milk product filler

*From Stein, J. Z., and Gallagher-Allred, C. R.: Dietary management in gastrointestinal diseases. *In* Nutrition and Health Promotion in Primary Care Series. Columbus, Department of Family Medicine, The Ohio State University, 1980, p. 12–13.

abdominal discomfort and flatus. Wheat bran can be purchased and added to milk, cereal, yogurt, and other foodstuffs, or it can be added to flour when cooking.

When helping patients increase the quantity of fiber in their diet, the following suggestions should be helpful:

- Use unprocessed wheat bran and unrefined breakfast cereals.
- Substitute rye or whole wheat flour for white flour when baking.
- Use whole wheat, rye, or pumpernickel bread instead of white bread for toast, bread dressing, French toast, sandwiches, and croutons.
- Consume raw or cooked vegetables and salads.
- Consume cooked legumes, such as chick peas, baked beans, lima beans, and soybeans.
- Use fresh, dried, and canned fruits, such as orange sections, fresh grapefruit, raisins, or prunes, for breakfast and snacks.
- Use fruits for desserts; if cakes or cookies are consumed, they could be made with whole wheat flour and flavored with nuts, coconut, dates, and other dried fruits.
- When snacking, include foods such as fruits, vegetables, and whole grain breads and cereals.

A table showing the fiber content of some common foods is presented in Table 53–19.

Table 53–19. FOODS HIGH IN FIBER

Food	Serving Size	Dietary Fiber (grams)
Baked beans	1 cup	18.6
All bran cereal	½ cup	9.9
Beans, white	½ cup	9.3
Currants	¼ cup	8.8
Raspberries	½ cup	8.0
Apricots, dried	¼ cup	7.8
Bran, 100 per cent	½ cup	7.5
Dried dates	10	7.0
Peas	½ cup	6.6
Peanuts	½ cup	6.6
Figs	2 small	6.4
Dried figs	2	6.4
Squash, winter	½ cup	6.3
Spinach	½ cup	5.7
Pumpkin	½ cup	5.4
Parsnips	½ cup	5.0
Prunes	3	4.8
Corn	½ cup	4.7
Orange	1 medium	4.5
Bran, unprocessed	2 Tbsp.	4.4
Pear	1 medium	4.1
Whole wheat bread	2 slices	4.0
Sunflower seeds	¼ cup	4.0
Carrots	½ cup	3.7
Dates	4	3.6
Peach	1 large	3.4
Apple	1 medium	3.2
Tomato	1 medium	3.0
Oatmeal	1 cup	3.0
Pineapple, canned	3 slices	3.0
Potato	1 medium	3.0
Broccoli tops	½ cup	3.0

Inflammatory Bowel Disease

Dietary advice for patients with inflammatory bowel disease may well be best done with the help of a registered dietitian and should be individualized to each patient's specific problems. Dietary management for the patient with Crohn's disease should include foods that are nutritionally balanced, high in protein and kilocalories, and easily tolerated. Six small feedings per day, use of medium-chain triglycerides, administration of a multiple vitamin and mineral preparation, and a diet low in fat and high in dairy products may be indicated.

Ulcerative Colitis

Dietary management for the patient with ulcerative colitis is supportive rather than curative. The diet is usually high in protein and kilocalories (and may be high in medium-chain triglycerides) and low in fiber and fat. It generally consists of small feedings and may need to be low in lactose and oxalate and high in dairy products if renal oxalate stones develop from increased bowel absorption of oxalate and malabsorption of calcium.

Liver Disease

Patients with primarily biliary cirrhosis may experience decreased steatorrhea by reducing dietary fat and substituting medium-chain triglycerides. The osteomalacia in these patients can be helped by extra vitamin D and calcium. Patients with alcoholic cirrhosis usually benefit from a daily multiple vitamin and mineral tablet. Signs of hepatic encephalopathy warrant protein restriction, and ascites merits a severe sodium restriction. Since alcohol is a known hepatotoxin, this should of course be excluded in patients with chronic liver disease of any etiology.

Pancreatic Disease

Acute pancreatitis occurs from several causes, and a N.P.O. (nothing by mouth) diet order is recommended in the initial hospital management. In patients with chronic pancreatitis, most often secondary to alcoholism, a low-fat diet is needed. Diet rarely helps the pain, but malabsorption resulting from deficient pancreatic enzymes can be controlled by five to eight capsules of a pancreatic enzyme mixture at mealtimes, maybe with sodium bicarbonate if needed to increase their effectiveness.

Renal Disease and Kidney Stones

Chronic renal failure requires dietary modifications to augment medical therapy. The chronic renal failure patient is frequently unable to handle potassium, protein, and sodium loads owing to reduced creatinine clearance. Loop diuretics are generally used in chronic renal failure patients (thiazide diuretics are not very effective), and a dietary salt restriction of 2.5 to 4.0 grams (1000 to 1600 mg. sodium) is usually required. Instead of emphasizing the need for potassium-rich foods, which is done for hypertensive patients using diuretics, chronic renal failure patients need to avoid high potassium foods if their serum potassium is elevated. Patients with a creatinine clearance of 30 (using furosemide twice daily) may not need to be as concerned about potassium intake. Regular monitoring of electrolytes, including calcium and phosphorus, is essential. The extent of the protein restriction depends on creatinine clearance. Consultation with a registered dietitian is warranted for these patients.

Prevention and treatment of kidney stones may involve diet. Urine citrate normally forms a soluble salt with calcium. Since women excrete more citrate and less calcium, they tend to form fewer calcium stones than men. Low urine citrate from bowel disease, renal tubular acidosis, or genetics can raise calcium oxalate supersaturation and lead to stone formation. Seventy to eighty per cent of stones are primarily calcium oxalate. Low urine pH promotes uric acid stones; high urine pH increases calcium phosphate supersaturation.

Dietary management of renal stones is based on the type of stone and etiology of its presence. Calcium oxalate stone forms from enteric hyperoxaluria, i.e., poor ileal absorption of calcium, and patients may need citrate administration in addition to a diet low in oxalate and moderate to high in calcium owing to significant calcium excretion in this particular entity. These patients must also be advised against taking vitamin C supplements because vitamin C is metabolized to oxalate before final excretion.

Patients with idiopathic calcium oxalate stones (less than 10 per cent have other causes such as hyperparathyroidism or renal tubular acidosis) usually have one or more metabolic abnormalities, such as hypercalciuria, hyperoxaluria, or decreased urine citrate. The most common abnormality is hypercalciuria, and patients should be advised against an intake of more than 1 gram of calcium per day. They should also be advised against a high salt intake, which increases calcium excretion and decreases the therapeutic effect of thiazide diuretics. Hyperuricosuria may be a contributor to calcium oxalate stones; thus, restriction of excessive intake of animal protein and purines may be helpful for this condition. Hypocitraturia is becoming a more recognized clinical entity and can be treated with citrate supplementation. The clinical significance of the mild hyperoxaluria seen in these patients and the benefits of a low-oxalate diet are both unclear; 24-hour urine testing for all these chemicals should be considered for recurrent stone formers and a therapeutic diet should be retested to see if the diet is making any actual difference (N.I.H. Consensus Development Conference Statement, 1988).

Patients with uric acid stones will need to limit dietary purines and may benefit from alkalinization of the urine. Patients with cystinuria will need counseling from a registered dietitian in addition to alkalinization of the urine. All renal stone formers will benefit from increased fluid intake. One guideline for adequate hydration is to consume enough fluid to allow for 2 liters of urine daily.

Oncology

PREVENTION

Recently, there has been increasing pressure to use dietary means to prevent cancer as well as to support the patient who already has cancer. The National Cancer Institute has recommended that individuals drink alcohol only in moderation, if at all, reduce dietary fat from 40 to 30 per cent of total calories, include whole grains and vegetables high in carotenoids in the diet, limit ingestion of smoked, pickled and cured meats, increase fiber consumption, increase vitamin C consumption, and limit consumption of nitrates and nitrites (Washington Post, 1984). The National Research Council recommends a reduction of dietary fat from 40 to 30 per cent of calories; inclusion of whole grains and vegetables high in carotenoids; limitation of cured, pickled, or smoked meats; and limitation of alcohol (Committee on Diet, Nutrition, and Cancer, 1982). The American Cancer Society recommends that people avoid obesity, reduce total fat intake, eat more high-fiber foods, include foods rich in vitamins A and C, include cruciferous vegetables such as cabbage, consume moderate alcohol if at all, and consume moderate amounts of salted, smoked, or nitrate-cured foods (American Cancer Society, 1984). The Council on Agricultural Science and Technology (CAST), on the other hand, has suggested that there is insufficient evidence to warrant specific dietary guidelines or to mandate changes in our patterns of eating (Pariza, 1984); the American Council on Science and Health (1985) and the Food and Nutrition Board of the National Academy of Sciences (1980) concur (Pariza, 1986).

At this time, there is inadequate scientific knowledge to recommend dietary modifications to the general public for the purpose of reducing the risk of developing cancer. On the other hand, dietary modification may be warranted in patients at high risk for developing cancer, such as breast cancer in women who have a history of breast cancer in the family and who consume a high-fat diet. There is a strong epidemiological association between a high-fat diet and the development of breast cancer in women.

There is very little evidence that a low-fat and high-fiber diet will prevent the development of colon cancer in males or females or that vitamin A and vitamin C supplementation will reduce the chance of lung or epithelial cell cancer. Until further evidence is available, patients should be encouraged to eat a variety of foods, cautioned not to overconsume any particular food or category of foods (such as fruits and vegetables including cruciferous plants), and cautioned against taking vitamin or mineral supplements (especially vitamins C, E, and A including beta-carotene), in hopes that such practices will reduce their risks for developing cancer.

The Committee on Diet, Nutrition, and Cancer of the National Academy of Sciences states, "The data are not sufficient to quantitate the contribution of diet to the overall cancer risk or to determine the percent reduction in risk that might be achieved by dietary modifications. . . . It is not now possible, and may never be possible, to specify a diet that would protect everyone against all forms of cancer" (Committee on Diet, Nutrition, and Cancer, 1982). Patients, therefore, should be encouraged to eat a well-balanced and varied diet. Family physicians can be of invaluable benefit to cancer patients and their families by reassuring them (based on the most current scientific evidence) that the patients' cancer was not caused, nor could it have been prevented, by what was or was not eaten.

TREATMENT

Cancer can exert a profound effect on a patient's nutrition needs, both by increasing caloric demands and by interfering with the patient's ability to meet those demands. Cancer cachexia is a major cause of death in patients with neoplastic disease. Although its causes are unknown, cachexia is not an obligatory consequence of neoplasia.

Family physicians who are aggressively treating patients with malignancy should consider aggressive nutrition support, including oral, enteral, and parenteral feedings, when lack of such support could decrease the effectivenss of medical therapy. Inadequate intake, diarrhea, vomiting, stomatitis, enteritis, early satiety, and taste acuity changes, due to the presence of a tumor or effects of chemotherapy, radiotherapy, or surgery, can be significantly reduced with appropriate nutrition support. And, on occasion, it may be advisable to delay potentially debilitating therapy until the patient's nutrition status is improved, especially if the patient is malnourished prior to therapy.

The following general guidelines are helpful for most patients with difficulties consuming adequate intake:

1. Increase calorie intake by encouraging high-calorie foods, such as eggnogs, milkshakes, nonfat

dry milk, sour cream, mayonnaise and salad dressings, cream or Half-and-Half, gravies, and sauces. Use high-fat cheeses. Keep snack foods available. Suggest that commercial medical nutrition products be consumed as part of therapy.

2. Serve foods when the patient's appetite is the best, often early in the day. Several small meals may be preferred to fewer large meals. Indulge the patient's preferences. Eliminate food odors if they cause nausea. Serve foods attractively. A small alcoholic appetizer prior to a meal may stimulate the appetite. Socialize and relax prior to and during meals.

3. If foods taste bitter, avoid red meats, coffee, tea, chocolate, tomatoes, sour citrus juices, and foods cooked or served in metal pans. Try fish, poultry, eggs, and dairy products. Use plastic utensils and glass pots and pans.

4. If foods taste too sweet, avoid highly sweetened foods or dilute the flavor with lemon, other sour juices, mayonnaise, vinegar, or soy sauce. Cold or frozen foods usually taste less sweet than warm or room temperature foods.

5. If foods have little or no taste, add herbs and spices, salt, sugar, and sauces. Serve foods warm.

6. If the patient has trouble chewing or swallowing, serve soft, ground, pureed, or liquid foods at room temperature, never hot or frozen. Avoid alcohol and extremely salty or sour foods.

7. If nausea and vomiting occur, advise patients not to eat when nauseated. Encourage them to slowly eat small meals in a relaxed atmosphere. Limit fluids during a meal of solid foods. Don't combine cold and hot foods at the same meal. Clear, cool beverages including carbonated beverages, popsicles, jello, sherbet, cereal, toast, crackers, potatoes, and soups are usually well tolerated. Advise the patient not to lie flat for 2 hours after eating.

8. When diarrhea occurs, foods high in fiber may need to be avoided; encourage foods such as applesauce and other fruits that contain pectin. Avoid dehydration.

Chronic Obstructive Pulmonary Disease

Chronic obstructive pulmonary disease (COPD) patients are frequently anergic and protein-calorie malnourished (exhibiting marasmus-type malnutrition with weight loss, poor lean muscle mass, and limited adipose tissue stores) because of poor nutrient intake and increased caloric requirements due to respiratory distress (Brown and Light, 1983). Additionally, poor nutrition status results in compromised respiratory muscle structure and function (Rochester and Esau, 1984) and lowered resistance to infection (Law, et al., 1973).

Recognition of the common occurrence of anergy and protein-calorie malnutrition should alert the family physician to the need for the development and initiation of aggressive nutrition support therapies for patients with COPD. Caloric intake should approximate energy needs, limit weight loss, or promote slow weight gain. Excessive caloric intake should be discouraged because it can lead to increased carbon dioxide production (Bartlett, et al., 1984). Increased protein and calorie needs can be met by liberally adding fats, sugars, and nonfat dry milk to foods. A disease-specific product, Pulmocare, is a medical nutrition product that can be taken orally or tube fed in patients who have difficulty with ventilation or who are on ventilators. This high-fat, low-carbohydrate formula has been shown to reduce carbon dioxide production and respiratory quotient, thereby making it easier to wean patients from ventilators and decreasing the workload of the respiratory system (Goldstein, et. al., 1986).

Acquired Immune Deficiency Syndrome (AIDS)

Complications of AIDS often have a negative impact on nutrition status (Kotler, et al., 1985). Weight loss, protein depletion, and malabsorption are common (O'Sullivan, et al., 1985; Kotler, et al., 1984). AIDS patients often exhibit increased nutrient needs, decreased nutrient intake, and impaired nutrient absorption that contribute to malnutrition. Causes of decreased nutrient intake and absorption may be poor appetite, oral and esophageal pain, mechanical problems with eating, gastrointestinal complications, such as diarrhea and malabsorption (Dworkin, et al., 1985), and emotional response to the diagnosis of a life-threatening illness (Dilley, et al., 1985). Although the relationship between disease development and disease progression with nutrition status has not been established, maintaining good nutrition status may support response to treatment of opportunistic infections and improve patient strength and comfort (Resler, 1988).

For the patient with decreased appetite, small frequent feedings may be better tolerated than larger meals. Individual tolerance to foods should be determined. Highly seasoned foods or acidic foods may increase oral and esophageal pain. Extremes in temperatures also may be poorly tolerated. Fluids and blenderized foods minimize chewing and are easier to swallow. Nutritionally complete medical nutrition products taken by mouth or nasogastric tube may be needed if eating is greatly impeded. A low-lactose, low-fat diet and formula may be helpful if steatorrhea is present. A low-fiber diet may help if ulcerative lesions are present in the gastrointestinal tract. If bacterial overgrowth is present, the addition of fermented dairy products should be considered. If a readily treatable cause for diarrhea and malabsorption is found, bowel rest and total parenteral nutrition may be indicated. Above all, patients should play an active role in making decisions regarding the nutrition care they receive. Describing the pros and cons of unorthodox nutrition therapies, including the macrobiotic diet, immune-system-stimulating diets, and megadoses of vitamins (A, C, E, and B_{12}) and minerals (selenium and zinc) is essential (Dwyer, et al., 1988). A registered dietitian can be of benefit to the patient who needs dietary assistance and who asks questions about unproven nutrition therapies.

Anorexia Nervosa and Bulimia

The personal physician plays an important role in the diagnosis and treatment of anorexia nervosa and bulimia (American College of Physicians, 1986). The rate of eating disorders among adolescent athletes has skyrocketed in recent years, and the family physician has an important responsibility to educate coaches and athletes about the dangers of eating disorders. If a patient is suspected of having an eating disorder, immediate and aggressive treatment is indicated. Nutrition rehabilitation and psychologic counseling are the cornerstones of treatment. Large communities, colleges, and universities often have eating disorder societies or support groups that can be of assistance to patients and their families. Information about centers that offer individual and group therapy can be obtained from the American Anorexia/Bulimia Association, 133 Cedar Lane, Teaneck, NJ 07666 (Telephone, 201–836–1800). The following tips can help the physician recognize anorexia nervosa and bulimia (Crawshaw, 1985):

1. Maintain a healthy skepticism toward epidemiologic findings that point to narrowly defined, predisposing factors for anorexia nervosa and bulimia.

2. Screen all female patients ages 13 to 50 for early signs of eating disorders. Ascertain the patient's weight history and medical history, self-image, and sensitivity to weight.

3. Be alert for the symptom clusters and common complaints that may flag an incipient eating disorder, such as a gastrointestinal disorder, menstrual or reproductive dysfunction, compulsive exercise, hyperactivity, and sports-related injury, laxative abuse, hypokalemia, fatigue, irritability, and depression.

4. Keep a few key physical signs of anorexia nervosa and bulimia in mind to help identify these disorders in the early stages, including weight loss, anorexia, carotenemia, cardiac arrhythmia, parotid enlargement, and erosion of teeth.

5. Interview the parents or spouse of a patient in whom you suspect an eating disorder to help assess the patient's frankness, uncover abnormal eating behaviors in other family members, and get an impression of family members' attitudes toward one another.

6. The initial history, physical, and laboratory evaluation will define the severity of an eating disorder. A weekly weight check and regularly scheduled discussions with the patient will determine the need for other intervention.

ANOREXIA NERVOSA

Treatment of anorexia nervosa can occur on an outpatient or inpatient basis. The decision to hospitalize the patient depends upon (1) the severity of weight loss (below 25 per cent of ideal body weight), (2) the lack of success of outpatient therapy, (3) the presence of metabolic abnormalities, such as hypokalemia, alkalosis, severe depression, or suicidal ideation, and (4) the ability of the family to cope with the patient's problems. The recommended sequence of treatment consists of:

1. *Nutrition rehabilitation*. A gradual increase in caloric intake is recommended, not to exceed 200 to 300 kcal. at a time. Weight stabilization is the first goal, followed by very gradual weight gain. A 1400 to 1600 kcal., low-fat, lactose-free, low-simple sugar diet may be tried initially. Behavior modification programs can be successful.

2. *Psychotherapy*. Psychotherapy (individual, group, and family as appropriate) is individualized to the patient and must address the patient's personal fears so that the patient can learn to deal directly with feelings instead of indirectly through use of food.

3. *Maintenance period and follow-up*. Once the patient has returned to a more normal body weight and accomplished what is possible in counseling, the responsibility for choosing foods and exercise should be gradually returned to the patient. Encouragement and guidance are often needed for a lifetime.

BULIMIA

The family physician should be sensitive to the possibility of bulimia (binge-purge syndrome) in any patient who is dieting and is excessively concerned about body weight, particularly the younger or middle-aged female. As with anorexia nervosa, hospitalization may be required. Treatment is still in the developmental stages, but it appears that dietary restrictions should be minimal. Treatment instead should emphasize self-acceptance and more effective coping skills. Cognitive restructuring, combined with behavioral techniques to avoid overrestraint and binging, has been beneficial in controlling bulimic behavior (Russell, 1979). Registered dietitians in private practice and clinical psychologists who specialize in eating disorders can jointly implement an effective treatment program.

Counseling the Patient

The family physician must be ready to tackle the issue of fad diets. Patients cannot help but be exposed to erroneous exposés about dietary cures for numerous problems. Physicians must be willing to listen to their patients and offer pros and cons of diets as appropriate. If the physician doesn't demonstrate a willingness to listen to the patient, the patient is not likely to listen in reply to the physician's advice. Unfortunately, a 1-hour talk-show guest on television has a much better chance to make a case for a new diet than does a physician in the 2-minute wrap-up of a brief office call. The physician may well need to schedule a special appointment regarding diet with the patient.

Some guidelines for physicians that might be useful include:

1. Be wary if the diet does not have the usual balance of intake from each of the food groups.

2. Keep articles from reputable lay and medical educators concerning popular diets in your office and reception area; many patients are more likely to believe what they see in a reputable consumer magazine such as *Consumer Reports* than in a reputable medical journal.

3. For weight-reduction diets, be wary if they promise too-rapid weight loss, suggest the patient can eat anything and a magic potion will melt off the weight, require laxatives or diuretics, require that the patient buy certain supplements, recommend periods of fasting, and ignore behavioral and exercise considerations.

4. Have a series of questions regarding each new diet and its promoters. The following tips will help you and your patients spot food and nutrition quacks (Herbert, 1980):

- Advises you to go out and buy something that you would not otherwise have bought
- A fake specialist with imposing "front" titles
- Says that most disease is due to a bad or faulty diet
- Says that most people are poorly nourished
- Tells you that soil depletion and the use of chemical fertilizers cause malnutrition
- Alleges that modern processing methods and storage remove all nutritive value from our food
- Tells you that under stress, and in certain diseases, your need for nutrients is increased
- Says that you are in danger of being poisoned by food additives and preservatives
- Tells you that if you eat badly, you'll be OK if you take a vitamin or vitamin and mineral supplement
- Recommends that everybody take vitamins or health foods or both
- Recommends a wide variety of substances similar to those found in your body
- Claims that natural vitamins are better than synthetic ones
- Promises quick, dramatic, miraculous cures
- Uses testimonials and case histories to support claims
- Offers a "vitamin" that isn't a vitamin
- Claims that he or she is being persecuted by orthodox medicine and that his or her work is being suppressed
- Is legally belligerent

References

American Cancer Society: Eating the right stuff (Editorial). Cancer News, American Cancer Society, Spring/Summer, 1984, pp. 4–6.

American College of Physicians, Health and Public Policy Committee: Eating disorders: anorexia nervosa and bulimia. Ann. Intern. Med., *105*:790, 1986. *This American College of Physicians position paper identifies four major positions: (1) need for increased physician awareness of the problem of eating disorders, (2) need for increased physician sensitivity to patients' emotional insecurities, (3) need for expansion of medical education in eating disorders, and (4) need for increased public education regarding these disorders.*

American Diabetes Association: Position statement: nutritional recommendations and principles for individuals with diabetes mellitus: 1986. Diabetes Care, *10*:126, 1987. *This position statement provides an in-depth overview of the principles and dietary recommendations in treating insulin and noninsulin dependent patients. Although prepared by an impressive panel of physicians and nutritionists, no bibliography is included and some recommendations are exceedingly difficult to follow and may be unrealistic to a majority of diabetic patients.*

American Dietetic Association: Position paper on the bland diet in the treatment of chronic duodenal ulcer disease. J. Am. Dietet. Assoc., *59*:3, 1971.

Anderson, J. W., Zettwoch, N., Feldman, T., et al.: Cholesterol-lowering effects of psyllium hydrophilic-mucilloid for hypercholesterolemic men. Arch. Intern. Med., *148*:292, 1988. *This is not only an impressive study of a familiar product but also a scholarly review of soluble fiber in therapy of high serum cholesterol.*

Anderson, J. W., Chen, W. L., and Sieling, B.: Hypolipidemic effects of high-carbohydrate, high-fiber diets. Metabolism, *29*:551, 1980.

Bartlett, R. H., Deckert, R. E., Mault, J. R., et al.: Metabolic studies in chest trauma. J. Thorac. Cardiovasc. Surg., *87*:503, 1984.

Becker, R. J.: The hidden costs of malnutrition. Business and Health, *5*(7):32, 1988. *This article encourages health care payers to consider the cost savings that can be accrued by performing a timely nutrition screen and assessment and by providing nutrition support when indicated. Costs of nutrition support (oral vs. enteral vs. parenteral) are compared in the hospital and home settings.*

Bistrian, B. R., Blackburn, G. L., Vitale, J., et al.: Prevalence of malnutrition in general medical patients. J.A.M.A., *235*:1567, 1976. *A simple, practical, and inexpensive method to assess the nutrition status of hospitalized patients is defined in this article.*

Brown, S. E., and Light, R. W.: When COPD patients are malnourished: what is now known about protein-energy depletion. J. Respir. Dis., *4*:36, 1983.

Cohen, M. P., Field, J. F., Krosnick, A., et al.: Diet and exercise in type II diabetes. Patient Care, *22*(16):117, 1988.

Committee on Diet, Nutrition, and Cancer: Diet, Nutrition, and Cancer. Washington, D.C., National Research Council, National Academy Press, 1982. *This document is an excellent, in-*

depth review of hundreds of epidemiologic and laboratory studies on nutrition and cancer. It can be obtained for free or at a nominal cost and is a must for physicians' and dietitians' personal libraries.

Council on Scientific Affairs: Treatment of obesity in adults. J.A.M.A., *260*:2547, 1988. *A concise review of the standard accepted practice in the management of patients with obesity.*

Crawshaw, J. P.: Anorexia and bulimia: the earliest clues. Patient Care, *19*(18):80, 1985. *This very readable article provides the physician with skills needed to diagnose and treat patients with the eating disorders of anorexia nervosa and bulimia. The practical approach of the authors is adaptable to a broad range of family practice settings.*

Department of Family Medicine, The Ohio State University: Nutrition and Health Promotion in Primary Care Series, Columbus, 1985. *A practical series of 26 self-study modules, written for family physicians, and emphasizing management of common nutrition problems seen in family medicine. Several patient handouts and tables, and a few paragraphs of text, have been used in this chapter.*

Dilley, J. W., Ochitill, H. N., Perl, M., et al.: Findings in psychiatric consultations with patients with acquired immune deficiency syndrome. Am. J. Psych., *142*:82, 1985.

Driscoll, D. F., Galvin, M., Blackburn, G. L., et al.: Nutritional support teams and services. Hosp. Material Manage. Quart., *7*:16, 1986. *The formation of a nutrition support team, the responsibilities of its team members (physician, nurse, pharmacist, dietitian, and coordinator), and the benefits of a nutrition support service to patient care are discussed.*

Dworkin, B., Wormser, G. P., Rosenthal, W. S., et al.: Gastrointestinal manifestations of the acquired immunodeficiency syndrome: a review of 22 cases. Am. J. Gastroenterol., *80*:774, 1985.

Dwyer, J. T., Bye, R. L., Hoh, P. L., et al.: Unproven nutrition therapies for AIDS: what is the evidence? Nutr. Today, *23*:25, 1988. *AIDS patients or their families may request unorthodox diets proposed to treat AIDS. The information presented in this article will provide the physician with scientific concepts to refute megadose vitamin and mineral therapy, macrobiotic diets, and immune-stimulating diets.*

Fisher, C. R.: Differences by age group in health care spending. Health Care Finance Rev., *1*:65, 1980.

Food and Nutrition Board, National Research Council: Recommended Dietary Allowances. 10th ed. Washington, D.C., National Academy of Sciences, 1989. *The standard text documents the nutrient needs of healthy persons at all ages and is an update of the 1980 version. The R.D.A. are the standards by which menus and meal plans for groups of people are judged for nutrient adequacy. The values identified for each nutrient will meet the needs for over 95 per cent of healthy persons. This text is recommended for inclusion in a physician's personal library.*

Glowacki, G. A.: A new look at osteoporosis and estrogen replacement therapy. Comp. Therapy, *14*(2):49, 1988.

Goldstein, S. A., Thomashow, B., and Askanazi, J.: Functional changes during nutritional repletion in patients with lung disease. Clin. Chest Med., *7*(1):141, 1986.

Gray, D. S., and Kaminski, M. V.: Nutrition support of the hospitalized patient. Am. Fam. Phys., *18*:143, 1983.

Grundy, S. M., Bilheimer, D., Blackburn, H., et al.: Rationale of the diet—heart statement of the American Heart Association, report of the Nutrition Committee. Circulation, *65*:839A, 1982. *This paper is a review of the diet-heart issue from the perspective of the A.H.A. It presents a highly affirmative view of the controversy between diet and disease.*

Herbert, V.: The health hustlers. *In* Barrett, S. (Ed.): The Health Robbers. 2nd ed. Philadelphia, George F. Stickley Company, 1980. *This book, edited by a physician, reveals the truth about nutrition-medicine-health quackery. It is a book that the discerning public should read to learn how to tell if someone has a legitimate treatment or is simply out to make money. It also explains how quackery is being fought, how it persists, and how the public can get the best possible health care from their physicians.*

Jenkins, D. J. A., Woliver, T. M., Taylor, S. H., et al.: Glycemic index of foods: a physiologic basis for carbohydrate exchange. Am. J. Clin. Nutr., *34*:362, 1981.

Kotler, D. P., Goetz, H. P., Lange, M., et al.: Enteropathy associated with the acquired immunodeficiency syndrome. Ann. Intern. Med., *101*:421, 1984.

Kotler, D. P., Wang, J., and Pierson, R. N.: Body composition studies in patients with the acquired immunodeficiency syndrome. Am. J. Clin. Nutr., *42*:1255, 1985. *The authors report body composition data for 38 immunodeficient patients (33 with AIDS and 5 with ARC). A group of 58 adult men and women was used as the laboratory control group as were 5 homosexual controls. Another control group consisted of 9 patients with anorexia nervosa or bulimia. The authors suggest that nutritional status is probably not related to the early pathogenesis of AIDS but that the later course might be influenced by the development of malnutrition. The authors further suggest that the time of death is possibly as related to the body's energy reserve as it is to the disease process itself.*

Law, D. K., Dudrick, S. J., Abdou, N. I., et al.: Immunocompetence of patients with protein-calorie malnutrition: the effects of nutritional repletion. Ann. Intern. Med., *79*:545, 1973.

Lipid Research Clinics: Coronary primary prevention trial report. J.A.M.A., *251*:351, 1984.

Lovastatin Study Group II: Therapeutic response to lovastatin in nonfamilial hypercholesterolemia: a multicenter study. J.A.M.A., *256*:2829, 1986.

Manual of Clinical Dietetics. 3rd ed. Chicago, American Dietetic Association, 1988. *This updated diet manual of the Association is an excellent reference book for the family physician's library and an appropriate choice as a diet manual for nursing homes. It includes information sections on pediatrics, modified consistency, gastrointestinal diets, protein, calories, and sodium-controlled diets as well as fat-modified diets.*

Marsh, A., Sanchez, T. V., Chafee, F. L., et al.: Bone mineral mass in adult lacto-ovo vegetarian and omnivorous males. Am. J. Clin. Nutr., *37*:453, 1983.

McCarron, D. A., Morris, C. P., and Henry, H. J., et al.: Blood pressure and nutrient intake in the United States. Science, *224*:1392, 1984. *This was the first significant report of an association between inadequate dietary intake of calcium and the development of hypertension. Although not widely accepted as dogma, this noteworthy article should be familiar to physicians who care for hypertensive patients.*

Mullen, J. L., Buzby, G. P., Matthews, D. O., et al.: Reduction of operative morbidity and mortality by combined preoperative and postoperative nutritional support. Ann. Surg., *192*:604, 1980.

Naeye, R. L.: Teenaged and pre-teenaged pregnancies: consequences of fetal-maternal competition for nutrients. Pediatrics, *17*:146, 1981. *This is an excellent review of the battle for nutrients between the growing adolescent and the developing fetus.*

National Cholesterol Education Program: Report of the expert panel on the detection, evaluation, and treatment of high blood cholesterol in adults. Arch. Intern. Med., *148*:36, 1988. *This landmark report defines hypercholesterolemia primarily in terms of LDL-C levels and provides guidelines on screening and confirming the diagnosis. The report also describes a step-care approach, including dietary and pharmacologic guidelines.*

National Institutes of Health Consensus Development Conference Statement: Prevention and treatment of kidney stones. Vol. 7(1), March 30, 1988. *The guidelines discussed in the text were drawn from this comprehensive overview of renal stones.*

National Institutes of Health Consensus Development Conference Statement: Health implications of obesity. Ann. Intern. Med., *103*(6, pt. 2):1073, 1985. *This well-referenced review article provides the physician with up-to-date research on obesity, diet-exercise-behavior modifications in treating obesity, and health complications of obesity.*

National Institutes of Health Consensus Development Conference: Osteoporosis. J.A.M.A., *252*:799, 1984. *This Consensus Development Conference provided dietary recommendations for pre- and postmenopausal women when sufficient scientific lit-*

erature support such recommendations. The Conference concluded that diet is only one factor, albeit important, in the causation and treatment of osteoporosis.

O'Sullivan, P., Linke, R. A., and Dalton, S.: Evaluation of body weight and nutritional status among AIDS patients. J. Am. Diet. Assoc., *85*:1483, 1985. *The purpose in this study was to gather nutrition assessment data on 50 AIDS patients in several New York City hospitals. Fifty-nine per cent of patients were significantly underweight, 62 per cent had experienced a greater than 10 per cent weight loss, and weight loss during hospitalization was common. Data on serum albumin and nutrient intake were collected but not reported.*

Pariza, M.: A perspective on diet, nutrition, and cancer. J.A.M.A., *251*:1455, 1984.

Pariza, M. W.: Analyzing current recommendations on diet, nutrition and cancer. Food & Nutr. News, *58*(1):1, 1986. *Dr. Pariza provides a comparison and critique of the dietary guidelines suggested by various groups, such as the American Cancer Society, National Cancer Institute, National Academy of Sciences, and CAST. It is his belief that the public does not want our speculation about nutrition and cancer, preferring recommendations only when scientific support for their efficacy exist.*

Phillip, P.: Salt intake leads lifestyle links to hypertension in global study. Medical World News, *29*(16):10, August 22, 1988.

Reilly, J. J., Hull, S. F., Albert, N., et al.: The economic impact of malnutrition: a model system for hospitalized patients. J. Parent. Enter. Nutr., *12*(4):371, 1988. *This study provides excellent data on cost-effectiveness of nutrition support and the economic impact of malnutrition. The average hospital charge, billed to insurance companies or other payers for a well-nourished patient having no complications in 1985 was $6,858; the charge for a malnourished patient with a major complication was $26,369.*

Resler, S. S.: Nutrition care of AIDS patients. J. Am. Diet. Assoc., *88*:828, 1988. *Causes of malnutrition in AIDS are identified in this article, written for the dietitian or other caregivers. Nutrition problems (anorexia, oral and esophageal pain, mechanical problems with eating, and gastrointestinal complications) and treatment options are discussed. The author contends that supportive and nonjudgmental care is the most important factor in the care of AIDS patients.*

Rifkind, B. M., and Segal, P.: Lipid research clinic's program reference values for hyperlipidemia and hypolipidemia. J.A.M.A., *250*:1869, 1983.

Riggs, B. L., Hodgson, S. F., Hoffman, D. L., et al.: Treatment of primary osteoporosis with fluoride and calcium: clinical tolerance and fracture occurrence. J.A.M.A., *243*:446, 1980.

Rochester, D. F., and Esau, S. A.: Malnutrition and the respiratory system. Chest, *85*:411, 1984.

Russell, G.: Bulimia nervosa: an ominous variant of anorexia nervosa. Psycholog. Med., *9*:429, 1979.

Ryan, K.: Postmenopausal estrogen use. Ann. Rev. Med., *33*:171, 1982.

Saville, P.: Postmenopausal osteoporosis and estrogens. Postgrad. Med., *75*(2):135, 1984.

Stunkard, A. J.: Behavioral management of obesity. Med. J. Aust., *142*:S13, 1985.

Taylor, W. C., Pass, T. M., Shepard, D. S. et al.: Cholesterol reduction and life expectancy. Ann. Intern. Med., *106*:605, 1987. *The controversial concepts in this article merit the physician's review.*

Washington Post: Anti-cancer diet gets big federal push. Columbus Dispatch, March 7, 1984, p. 1.

Weinsier, R. L., Hunker, E. M., Krumdieck, C. L., et al.: Hospital malnutrition: a prospective evaluation of general medical patients during the course of hospitalization. Am. J. Clin. Nutr., *32*:418, 1979.

Wing, R. R., Koeske, R., Epstein, L. H., et al.: Long-term effects of modest weight loss in type II diabetic patients. Arch. Intern. Med., *147*:1749, 1987.

54

Obesity

Jeffery Sobal
Herbert L. Muncie, Jr.

Obesity is an excess amount of body fat and is very prevalent in the United States. The 1976–1980 National Health and Nutrition Examination Survey reported that 34 million adults were obese and 13 million were severely obese (Van Itallie, 1985). Obesity increases with age but declines in prevalence among the elderly. Obesity is more frequent among women of lower socioeconomic status (Sobal and Stunkard, 1989).

Obesity is less frequent as a patient complaint than as a diagnosis, with young adult women most often seeking medical help because of weight gain or obesity. In the Virginia Study of half a million family physician–patient encounters, obesity was the tenth most frequent diagnosis, and other investigations also report that patients who see family physicians are frequently obese (Rosenblatt et al., 1982).

Obesity is associated with many of the common diseases encountered by physicians, including hypertension, diabetes mellitus, coronary artery disease, and skeletal system diseases (Bray, 1976; Van Itallie, 1985). In addition to its role in morbidity and mortality, obesity leads to a variety of psychosocial problems. People who are obese suffer from stigmatization and discrimination because of their body shape, and often feel shame and guilt about their weight (Powers, 1980).

Many theories exist about the causes of obesity, and they may be useful in understanding weight loss interventions (Brownell, 1982). Obesity is a multifactorial condition, with no single cause or theory completely determining obesity. The biopsychosocial model provides a framework for examining the entire scope of obesity as well as theories about obesity (Engel, 1977).

Biological theories have predominated in the analysis of obesity. Genetic factors are important, with polygenic inheritance playing a role in obesity for many patients. Metabolic theories include several factors. Endocrinologic disturbances such as thyroid, adrenal, or hypothalamic disorders may lead to obesity, but such cases are relatively rare. An important metabolic theory is the set point theory, which proposes that body weight is regulated in a homeostatic manner (Newsholme, 1980). The set point for a person's body weight is influenced by genetics and environmental factors and can be reset by diet, exercise, and medications. Developmental theories have included the fat cell theory, which hypothesized that only at the critical growth periods of infancy and puberty did fat cells increase in number, with increases only in fat cell size at other stages of life (Bjorntorp, 1984). Although this theory received much media attention, it was later demonstrated that fat cells can develop at any age. Satiety and hunger theories focus on somatic cues for eating and stopping eating, with problems in perception of cues and feedback rates leading to overeating.

Psychological theories of obesity have taken several forms (Powers, 1980). Personality theories considered food addiction, problems in motivation, and excessive susceptibility to the sight of food as an external cue to eating. Learning theories have emphasized the learning of maladaptive eating styles. Perceptual theories have examined such things as body image distortion.

Sociocultural theories examine the socialization of people into unhealthy eating and activity, such as in the context of the family (Sobal, 1984). Other social perspectives about obesity consider the norms and values of a community, society, or culture about appropriate body shapes and the need to gain or lose weight.

As a common condition with physiologic and

psychosocial consequences, obesity is a problematic issue for physicians. Many patients desire weight reduction and seek physician assistance in losing weight. Other patients would benefit from weight loss because of disease risk, but do not seek physician input or adhere to physician advice.

Assessing and Monitoring Obesity

Defining obesity as an excess amount of body fat requires an interpretation of excess and a method of assessing the amount of fat. Because levels of fatness are distributed in a normal curve in the population, any specific cutoff determining "excess" is arbitrary. Several methods for assessing obesity provide cutoff levels that can be used as guidelines (1) for determining whether weight loss is appropriate and (2) as goals in losing weight. These cutoff points are based on inflection points in mortality curves, where higher rates of mortality begin to occur at an increasing level of overweight.

Simple observation is often sufficient for determining that a patient is obese. However, determination of obesity through observation alone is only a first step because it does not allow more precise assessment of the level of obesity or the monitoring of progress in weight loss. Therefore, quantitative techniques for assessing obesity are important for assessing obese patients and setting goals for interventions.

The assessment of weight in relationship to height is the most fundamental way to assess obesity. Comparisons with established standards of weight and height can be performed, and weight and height relationships can be used to monitor weight loss progress by the physician and patient. The two major weight-height assessments are ideal body weight (IBW) and body mass index (BMI).

Ideal body weight (IBW) standards were developed by the Metropolitan Life Insurance Company and published in the form of tables that indicate weights associated with the lowest mortality rates for healthy men and women (Table 54–1). These tables present interpretation problems because of the need to determine frame size, which can be assessed using wrist diameter or elbow breadth (Table 54–2). The Metropolitan tables have been criticized because they represent only individuals with insurance, and weights and heights were only reported and not measured. However, they remain the most widely used standards for determining obesity and setting goals for weight loss. Obesity is defined as greater than 120 per cent of the midpoint of the range of ideal weights in the tables. Patients who exceed 120 per cent of IBW can benefit from weight loss and can use that level as a goal for the amount of weight to lose.

Body mass index (BMI) gives a more exact assessment of the amount of body fat than do IBW estimates and also offers the advantage of not needing tables to evaluate. BMI is calculated as weight (in kilograms) divided by height (in meters) squared:

Table 54–1. HEIGHT AND WEIGHT TABLES FOR IDEAL BODY WEIGHT (IBW)

Height		Weight (in pounds)		
ft.	*in.*	*Small Frame*	*Medium Frame*	*Large Frame*
		MEN		
5	2	128–134	131–141	138–150
5	3	130–136	133–143	140–153
5	4	132–138	135–145	142–156
5	5	134–140	137–148	144–160
5	6	136–142	139–151	146–164
5	7	138–145	142–154	149–168
5	8	140–148	145–157	152–172
5	9	142–151	148–160	155–176
5	10	144–154	151–163	158–180
5	11	146–157	154–166	161–184
6	0	149–160	157–170	164–188
6	1	152–164	160–174	168–192
6	2	155–168	164–178	172–197
6	3	158–172	167–182	176–202
6	4	162–176	171–187	181–207
		WOMEN		
4	10	102–111	109–121	118–131
4	11	103–113	111–123	120–134
5	0	104–115	113–126	122–137
5	1	106–118	115–129	125–140
5	2	108–121	118–132	128–143
5	3	111–124	121–135	131–147
5	4	114–127	124–138	134–151
5	5	117–130	127–141	137–155
5	6	120–133	130–144	140–159
5	7	123–136	133–147	143–163
5	8	126–139	136–150	146–167
5	9	129–142	139–153	149–170
5	10	132–145	142–156	152–173
5	11	135–148	145–159	155–176
6	0	138–151	148–162	158–179

Source of basic data: 1979 Build Study, Society of Actuaries and Association of Life Insurance Medical Directors of America, 1980.

Source: Statistical Bulletin, Metropolitan Life Insurance Company.

$$\text{BMI} = \text{WT (kg.)} / \text{HT}^2 \text{ (m.)}$$

An easy formula for estimating BMI using nonmetric units of measurement is 705 times weight in pounds divided by height in inches squared (Stensland and Margolis, 1990):

$$\text{BMI} = 705 \times \text{WT (lb.)}/\text{HT}^2 \text{ (inches)}$$

A BMI of 27 or greater corresponds to 20 per cent above ideal body weight (National Institutes of Health Consensus Development Panel, 1985). Rapid calculation of BMI can also be done using the nomogram presented in Figure 54–1. A patient's target weight could be set to correspond to a BMI below 27, which is a realistic goal for the severely obese.

Skinfold thickness, a more direct assessment of body fat than weight-height indices, is useful for physicians who want a precise estimate of obesity and

Table 54–2. METHODS FOR DETERMINATION OF FRAME SIZE

Method 1: Wrist Circumference

Height is recorded without shoes on.
Wrist circumference is measured just distal to the styloid process at the wrist crease on the right arm using a tape measure.
The following formula is used:

$$r = \frac{\text{Height (cm.)}}{\text{Wrist circumference (cm.)}}$$

Frame size can be determined as follows:

Males	*Females*
r > 10.4 small	r > 11.0 small
r = 9.6–10.4 medium	r = 10.1–11.0 medium
r < 9.6 large	r < 10.1 large

Source: Grant, J. P.: Handbook of Total Parenteral Nutrition. Philadelphia, W. B. Saunders Co., 1980, p. 15.

Method 2: Elbow Breadth

The patient's right arm is extended forward perpendicular to the body, with the arm bent so the angle at the elbow forms 90 degrees with the fingers pointing up and the palm turned away from the body. The greatest breadth across the elbow joint is measured with a sliding caliper along the axis of the upper arm, on the two prominent bones on either side of the elbow. This is recorded as the elbow breadth. The following tables give the elbow breadth measurements for medium-framed men and women of various heights. Measurements lower than those listed indicate a small frame size; higher measurements indicate a large frame size.

Men		*Women*	
Height in 1″ Heels	Elbow Breadth	Height in 1″ Heels	Elbow Breadth
5′2″–5′3″	2½″–2⅞″	4′10″–4′11″	2¼″–2½″
5′4″–5′7″	2⅝″–2⅞″	5′0″ –5′3″	2¼″–2½″
5′8″–5′11″	2¾″–3″	5′4″ –5′7″	2⅜″–2⅝″
5′0″–6′3″	2¾″–3⅛″	5′8″ –5′11″	2⅜″–2⅝″
6′4″	2⅞″–3¼″	6′0″	2½″–2¾″

Source: Metropolitan Life Insurance Company, 1983.

for calculation of percentage of body fat. Overweight and overfat are not always interchangeable. The use of skinfolds helps the physician detect patients who are overweight because of large muscle mass but have little fat, and patients who are within ideal weight but have excessive fat and little muscle mass. Skinfolds can be taken at a number of sites, with triceps the most common (Jackson and Pollock, 1985).

Other fatness assessment methods used for clinical assessment include underwater weighing, ultrasound, bioelectric impedance, and radiography (Powers, 1980). Underwater weighing has been the standard against which other techniques are assessed but requires equipment usually available only in research settings. Other mechanical techniques were also previously limited to research settings, but advances in equipment have made them available for physicians who deal frequently with obese patients. They are rapid, calculate percentage of body fat, and appear "scientific" to patients. However, the equipment is relatively expensive.

The distribution of body fat deposits allows differentiation between two body types of obesity. Android obesity occurs where most excess fat is in the upper body and abdomen, producing an "apple" body shape. Android obesity is more common in men and is associated with an increased risk of diabetes, hypertension, and coronary heart disease (Selby et al., 1989). Gynoid obesity occurs where most excess fat deposits are around the hips and femoral region, is more common among women, and is more benign in disease outcome. Waist-to-hip (abdominal-to-gluteal) ratios of less than 1 are associated with decreased morbidity and mortality based on the differentiation of these two types of fat patterns (Kissebah et al., 1982).

In evaluating an obese patient, the physician should obtain a complete medical history and conduct a thorough physical examination with appropriate laboratory tests. Physicians need to assess the patient's risk for developing complications associated with obesity. A family history of hypertension, diabetes mellitus, or atherosclerosis suggests a more aggressive approach toward a patient's obesity. The history and physical examination can exclude many secondary causes of obesity, and selected laboratory studies can prove to be helpful. The evaluation of glucose, liver function, and thyroid function would be appropriate.

Patient evaluation should also include a dietary history, which can assess specific food intake with a 24-hour food recall and examine patterns in food consumption with a food frequency assessment for major foods. An exercise/activity history will indicate the caloric expenditure of the patient. The physician should always inquire about past attempts to lose weight. Diet and activity can be assessed in detail by having the patient keep a diary of all foods and beverages consumed and all activities for a period of 1 to 7 days. However, compliance with a diary request requires a highly motivated patient.

Once the physician has established that a patient is obese and how far the patient is from an appropriate body weight, specific medical problems may need to be addressed before beginning treatment with a weight loss program. Secondary causes of obesity would include hypothyroidism, medication side effects (steroids), hypopituitarism, and psychogenic causes. Such conditions should be considered as causes of obesity but constitute only a small proportion of obesity in the population.

Weight Loss Techniques

A variety of techniques for losing weight are available. This chapter reviews weight loss techniques by grouping them into methods frequently used by the public without medical advice, and techniques physicians can offer to their patients. All weight loss techniques are limited in their success, with a 1959 review by Stunkard and McLaren-Hume concluding

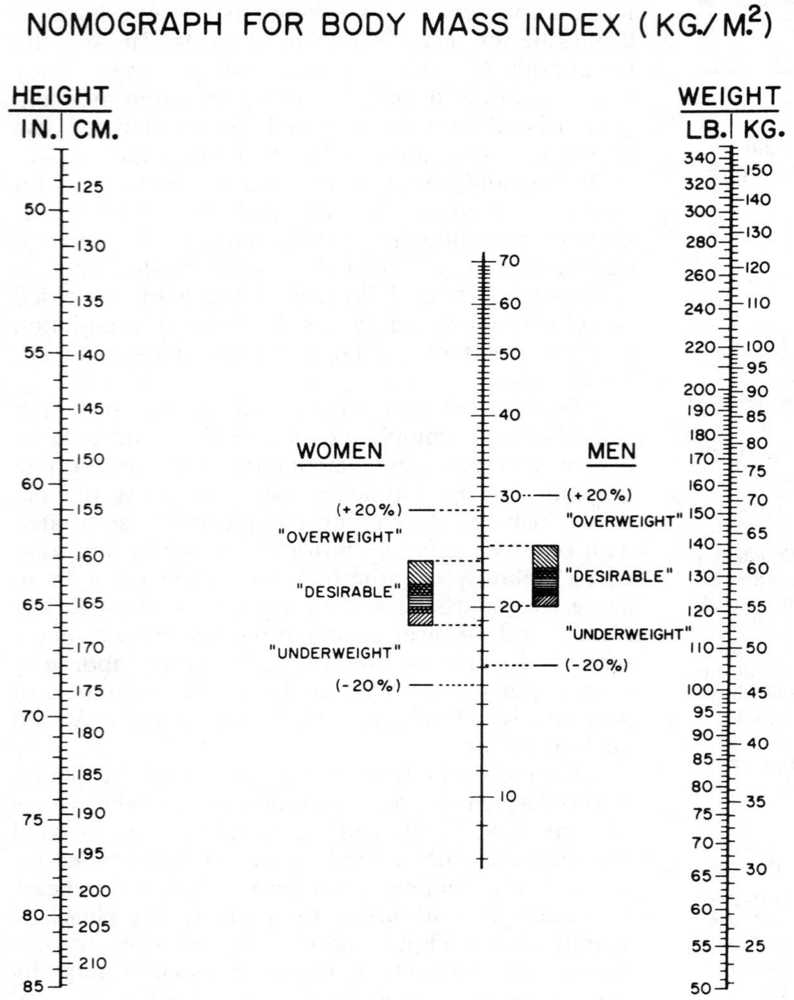

Figure 54–1. The ratio weight/height² is read from the central scale. The ranges suggested as "desirable" from life insurance data must be interpreted with clinical judgment regarding relative skeletal and muscle mass, as explained in the text. (From Thomas, A. E., McKay, D. A., and Cutlip, M. B.: A nomograph for assessing body weight. Am. J. Clin. Nutr., *29*:302, 1976.)

Most obese persons will not enter treatment for obesity, of those who enter treatment, most will not lose weight, and of those who lose weight, most will regain it.

More recent reviews by Wing and Jeffery (1979) and Holmes et al. (1989) are similarly pessimistic, with attrition rates of over 50 per cent in many clinical studies of weight loss attempts. Most of these studies have evaluated specific interventions. More optimistic population data show that "the obese do not necessarily stay obese" (Garn and Cole, 1980). Jeffery et al. (1984) found that many people, especially men, were formerly overweight but not currently overweight, and Schacter (1982) found that over half of obese people who tried to lose weight were eventually successful.

POPULAR WEIGHT LOSS METHODS USED BY THE PUBLIC

Patients may attempt to lose weight using a variety of individual methods, with some popular and fad diets being harmful (see Table 53–10). Patients also participate in commercial weight loss groups as well as organized community or worksite weight loss programs.

Popular and Fad Diets. Thousands of diets have been touted as weight loss methods. These diets appear so rapidly and frequently that it is difficult for a physician to keep informed about currently popular diets. Although popular diets are occasionally reviewed in the medical literature, up-to-date compendiums produced by consumer organizations can be used by physicians to learn about current diets (Berland, 1986).

If a physician is not familiar with a popular diet, it is important to ask patients to describe the practices specified in a diet. This includes the rules for types of food eaten, limitations on the amount of foods consumed, use of special preparations instead of foods, inclusion of exercise, and changes in eating patterns. This information, along with an assessment of the patient's dietary practices, can be used to advise patients about prudent involvement in popular diets. Diets that do not include foods from the four food groups (grains, dairy, fruits/vegetables, meat/protein), severely restrict calories, or fail to include an exercise component should be discouraged.

Obesity must be viewed as a chronic, noncurable condition, with all treatments evaluated for their long-term continued use and effectiveness. When working with obese patients, the physician must stress this long-term perspective and indicate that slow and sustained changes will be more beneficial and more likely to be ultimately successful in achieving and maintaining a desired weight.

Several classes of popular diets exist, including fasting, very-low-calorie diets, unbalanced low-energy diets, balanced low-energy diets, and novelty/fad diets (Newmark and Williamson, 1983a; 1983b; Council on Scientific Affairs, American Medical Association, 1988).

Fasting. Short fasts do not result in major changes in body fat, and long fasts can be hazardous. Total fasting can produce ketosis, hyperuricemia, hyponatremia, hypokalemia, hypoglycemia, and increased renal loss of phosphate and magnesium. Because fasting has significant risks and offers no long-term benefits in energy intake and expenditure, it should be discouraged.

Very Low Calorie Diets. Two major types of very-low-calorie diets exist: (1) protein-sparing modified fasts, and (2) liquid formula diets. Protein-sparing modified fasts focus on consumption of high-protein foods such as meat, fish, and poultry and eliminate almost all carbohydrates from the diet. The source of fat is through the protein sources. These diets are often deficient in many vitamins and minerals. Whereas they can provide impressive and rapid weight loss, they do not provide healthy eating patterns that can be sustained to maintain weight loss.

Liquid formula diets provide formulas based on milk or egg substrates that are consumed instead of foods. They are often high in protein but also contain carbohydrates and fat. Early versions of liquid protein diets did not contain all necessary nutrients and resulted in a number of deaths. More recent versions have remedied this problem. However, by providing a substitute for foods rather than helping people choose foods wisely, these diets do not offer long-term strategies for healthy eating to maintain desirable body weight.

Balanced Low-Energy Diets. Low-energy diets range from 1000 to 1500 kcal. per day and can produce weight loss in many patients. Ideally, this caloric intake will come from a balanced nutrient intake that contains about 10 to 20 per cent of kilocalories as protein, 30 per cent as fat, and 50 per cent or more from carbohydrates, plus consumption of adequate vitamins and minerals. These diets are the most useful for achieving weight loss because they are nutritionally adequate but simply include lower caloric intake.

Unbalanced Low-Energy Diets. In contrast to the balanced low-energy diets, many popular diets are unbalanced because they overemphasize one nutrient. Low-carbohydrate diets are the most frequent and often lead to rapid initial weight loss because of diuresis. Loss of water weight makes patients believe they are losing fat, but weight is rapidly regained once usual carbohydrate intake is reinstated. Fatigue, nausea, orthostatic hypotension, dehydration, and electrolyte imbalance may occur on these diets. Other unbalanced low-energy diets may lead to weight loss by emphasizing only one or two types of foods, leading to boredom with eating and consequent weight loss.

Novelty/Fad Diets. Many novelty diets are produced every year for public consumption (Newmark and Williamson, 1983a). They often play on public ignorance with almost magical claims about how they operate. In the evaluation of any popular diet, specific questions need to be asked to determine its safety and efficacy. Table 54–3 presents some questions easily asked by the physician about popular diets. If the diet does not prove acceptable on these issues, then patients should be discouraged from continuing with that diet or followed if they do proceed on that regimen.

Commercial Weight Loss Groups. Patients seeking to lose weight often enter weight loss programs run by commercial organizations. Unfortunately, insufficient evaluation of most of these programs has been published to make clear recommendations about the programs. The high dropout rate and reliance on testimonial evidence about long-term outcomes makes them difficult for a physician to evaluate. However, weight loss groups are effective for some patients and may be safe and effective methods to lose weight. For motivated patients who can afford the cost of entering these programs, the peer pressure and social support provided by these groups can be useful in weight loss.

Some groups may be useful as adjuncts to physician care (Rosenblatt, 1988). *TOPS (Take Off Pounds Sensibly)* is a nonprofit group that is relatively inexpensive, meets weekly, and combines exchange system diets with behavior modification. *Weight Watchers* provides an eating plan, group support, self-awareness, and optional exercise program through weekly meetings and weigh-ins accompanied by relatively small fees. *Diet Center* provides private counseling and frequent weighings with relatively restric-

Table 54–3. QUESTIONS FOR ASSESSMENT OF POPULAR DIETS

What physiologic principle is involved in the diet?
Is the diet safe in the short and long term?
How difficult is it for the patient to adhere to the diet?
Are the foods inexpensive and easy to obtain?
Can the whole family eat the food recommended by this diet?
Will the diet contribute to good long-term eating habits?
Is the diet balanced with foods from all four food groups?
Is the purchase of special foods, devices, or pills required?
Is the weight loss excessively rapid (over 2 to 3 pounds per week)?
Are there sensational claims made in advertisements for the diet?
Are drugs included?
Is the focus on diet alone, excluding exercise and behavior?

tive diets of 1000 kcal. or less combined with special supplements and behavior modification and is moderately expensive. *Nutri/System* and *Optifast* provide special foods for participants that are expensive and do not change everyday eating patterns. *Overeaters Anonymous* is patterned closely after Alcoholics Anonymous, seeing compulsive eating as a problem that can be overcome through inner changes. Physicians should become aware of regional and local commercial weight loss groups that exist in their communities.

Community and Worksite Programs. Health promotion campaigns have established community-wide and worksite programs to try to change behavioral risk factors in the general population. Community programs may encourage residents to lose weight, and provide general guidelines for weight loss. Physicians should be aware of community-wide programs for two reasons. First, physicians can build on community support in motivating their patients to lose weight. Second, as patients attempt to lose weight on their own, physicians can provide advice about safe and reasonable weight loss methods.

Many companies recognize that a healthy work force is more productive and therefore provide wellness programs to their employees. One component of a wellness program may include weight loss (Brownell et al., 1985). After assessing whether such plans are reasonable, physicians may encourage use of such plans as resources to supplement their own weight loss guidance.

WEIGHT LOSS METHODS PHYSICIANS CAN OFFER TO PATIENTS

Several weight loss methods can be used by physicians assisting their patients in losing weight. Every patient presents a unique case for weight loss therapy, with many possible causes of obesity and various options for treatment. Three major treatment modalities (dietary intervention, physical activity, and behavior modification) are most effective and should be used in conjunction to achieve weight loss. The combination of these three methods leads to greater weight loss and maintenance of lower weight than any one method alone. Two other modalities (drugs and surgery) have many problems and should be avoided in routine weight loss programs.

Dietary Intervention. Dietary interventions include education about healthy eating patterns and programs of lower caloric intake. Because the purposes of weight loss are improved health, prevention of new disease, and treatment of existing disease, patients need to learn to maintain sound eating patterns for their entire lives.

Nutrition education for obese patients should include instruction both about weight loss and about healthy eating patterns. Patients need to be taught that the secret to weight loss is that there is no secret, only that caloric intake needs to be less than caloric expenditure. Explaining that foods contain energy and this energy is measured by calories is necessary for some patients. Education about the role of energy balance in weight loss reinforces the combination of dietary restriction and increased exercise in a sound program.

Nutrition education for patients losing weight should include emphasis on eating from the four food groups. Two servings of dairy products, two servings of meat/protein products, four servings of fruits/vegetables, and four servings of grains can provide a healthy diet that includes only 1200 to 1500 kcal., depending on the types of foods chosen. Patients need to learn about choosing lower calorie foods within a food group, such as skim milk rather than whole milk. Patients should be reminded that alcoholic beverages contain calories, and alcohol consumption should be considered when losing weight. Such a basic eating plan provides essential nutrients for most patients and also can be a basis for gradual weight loss.

Gradual weight loss is the best strategy, with a goal of losing only one or two pounds per week. More specific dietary restriction should emphasize a balanced variety of foods without overly restricting calories. Because a pound of fat contains 3500 kcal., losing a pound a week requires creating a negative energy balance of 500 kcal. per day. Both reduced food intake and increased energy expenditure should be used to create this 500 kcal. daily deficit.

Each patient must have individualized dietary restrictions. Daily meal plans for reduced kilocalories (e.g., 800, 1000, 1200, and 1500 kcal.) are available, but these do not take into account food preferences, ethnic and cultural food patterns, coordination of food intake with other family members, and other factors that can lead to very poor adherence to such weight loss plans.

Highly motivated patients can use a food diary, writing down all the foods they consume and counting calories to assist in weight loss. Such close monitoring can prove effective, and the very act of having to write down a food can increase prudent food choice. Other patients can do well by simply increasing their awareness of the caloric content of foods and avoiding foods with high caloric density (i.e., many kilocalories per serving compared with other food choices). This can be as simple as avoiding desserts and snacks, or as complex as looking up caloric values in tables.

Weight loss using only caloric restriction is difficult because of several physiologic factors. The body's metabolic rate adapts to energy restriction within a day or two, becoming more efficient and requiring less energy to maintain current weight. This slowing down of metabolism makes continued weight loss through caloric restriction alone difficult. However, exercising while restricting calories can help to lessen this metabolic slowdown. Also, once caloric restriction is ended, the metabolic rate slowly returns to its previous level, often lagging behind increased food intake. Such a continuing low metabolic rate after caloric restriction often leads to weight gains once a diet is ended.

Physicians often see patients who have engaged in weight cycling, or "yo-yo" dieting, where repeated cycles of weight loss and gain occur. Weight cycling makes each subsequent attempt to lose weight increasingly difficult, leading to frustration by patients and physicians. A patient involved in this pattern often uses unsound nutritional practices, puts increased stress on the body, and develops negative experiences and beliefs about weight loss. Weight cycling may alter body composition, increasing the proportion of fat by replacing lean tissue. Because of the problems associated with weight cycling, slow steady weight loss is the most important strategy. Patients may even be advised that they should not attempt to lose weight for short-term goals if they do not seriously intend to maintain the loss afterward through a life style of healthy eating and exercise.

Physical Activity. Exercise is an important modality for a weight loss program. Used alone, it generally does not have a dramatic effect on body weight, but it is a valuable adjunct to dietary restriction. Most important, exercise improves the general health of a patient, preventing diseases for which obesity is a risk factor. Exercise also contributes to the long-term maintenance of ideal body weight. Combining exercise with caloric limitation preserves lean body tissue. With exercise, weight loss will consist primarily of fat, whereas without exercise, caloric restriction leads to the loss of some lean tissue.

Increasing physical activity should be tailored to the patient's needs, preferences, and life style. Walking is one of the easiest and most convenient activities that an obese patient can begin to practice and offers a very low risk of complications or athletic injuries. Swimming is an especially good activity for obese patients who have developed arthritis complications in weight-bearing joints.

The amount of caloric expenditure per minute of various recreational activities is presented in Table 54–4. These values vary greatly by how actively a person engages in exercise. Many people prefer to gauge their activity and set goals by the duration of time they participate in an activity. Time is the most appropriate measure of energy expenditure for many activities, such as volleyball. However, for propulsion sports in which a person travels over a distance for exercise, distance may be a more appropriate yardstick than time. A 150-pound person expends about 100 kcal. per mile walking or running, irrespective of the pace. Expending 100 kcal. requires roughly 440 yards of swimming or 2.5 miles of bicycling.

Poor adherence to regular exercise programs is a problem for many patients (Bjorntorp, 1978). Physicians are well advised not to prescribe a particular exercise, but to assist patients in picking an exercise program they enjoy and that fits their life style so that they can continue it for a long period of time. Physicians and patients also learn from a negotiating process exactly which dietary and exercise patterns patients are able and willing to follow.

Table 54–4. AVERAGE CALORIC EXPENDITURE PER MINUTE FOR VARIOUS RECREATIONAL ACTIVITIES

Activity		Kcal. per Minute*
Ping pong–table tennis		4.9–7.0
Calisthenics		5.0
Rowing: pleasure-vigorous		5.0–15.0
Cycling: 5–15 mph (10-speed)		5.0–12.0
Skating: recreational-vigorous		5.0–15.0
Archery		5.2
Badminton: recreational-competitive		5.2–10.0
Basketball: half-full court (more for fast break)		6.0– 9.0
Bowling (while active)		7.0
Tennis: recreational-competitive		7.0–11.0
Water skiing		8.0
Soccer		9.0
Snowshoeing (2.5 mph)		9.0
Handball and squash		10.0
Mountain climbing		10.0
Skipping rope		10.0–15.0
Judo and karate		13.0
Football (while active)		13.3
Wrestling		14.4
Skiing:	moderate to steep	8.0–12.0
	downhill racing	16.5
	cross-country: 3–8 mph	9.0–17.0
Swimming:	pleasure	6.0
	crawl: 25–50 yd./min.	6.0–12.5
	butterfly: 50 yd./min.	14.0
	backstroke: 25–50 yd./min.	6.0–12.5
	breaststroke: 25–50 yd./min.	11.0
	sidestroke: 40 yd./min.	
Dancing:	modern: moderate-vigorous	4.2– 5.7
	ballroom: waltz-rhumba	5.7– 7.0
	square	7.7
Walking:	road-field (3.5 (mph)	5.6– 7.0
	snow: hard-soft (2.5–3.5 mph)	10.0–20.0
	uphill: 5–10–15% (3.5 mph)	8.0–11.0–15.0
	downhill: 5–10% (2.5 mph)	3.6–3.5
	15–20% (2.5 mph)	3.7–4.3
Hiking:	40-lb. pack (3.0 mph)	6.8
Running:	12-min. mile (5 mph)	10.0
	8-min. mile (7.5 mph)	15.0
	6-min. mile (10 mph)	20.0
	5-min. mile (12 mph)	25.0

*Estimate depends on efficiency and body size: add 10 per cent for each 15 lb. over 150 lb. weight. Subtract 10 per cent for each 15 lb. under 150 lb. weight.

From Sharkey, B. J.: Physiology of Fitness. Champaign, IL, Human Kinetics Publishers, 1979.

Behavior Modification. Behavior modification is the systematic change of eating behaviors or cues for eating to control food intake (Stunkard and Wadden, 1983). The advantage of behavior modification is that it establishes long-term changes in eating that permit immediate weight loss and also maintenance of lower weight.

The first step in behavior modification is to determine current eating behaviors. This begins with keeping a dietary log, in which the patient records everything eaten, along with the setting where it was eaten, and how the patient felt when eating. The information in the log may be enough to identify problem eating behaviors, such as excessive snacking in a particular setting (such as when driving) or associated with specific feelings (such as loneliness). Counseling about these issues is then necessary.

Another step in behavior modification is the establishment of goals and rewards for achieving the goals. The goals can be the modification of behaviors or the achievement of lower weight levels. When specific goals are met, appropriate rewards established in advance are made, such as going to a play.

Cognitive restructuring, learning to think about events in a different way, also plays a part in the goals and rewards. Relapses need to be seen as learning events rather than examples of self-worthlessness or badness. Cognitive restructuring includes eliminating negativism and pessimism and reinforcement of positive behaviors.

Pharmacotherapy. A wide variety of prescription and nonprescription drugs are available for weight control. Physicians and patients use appetite suppressants or anorectic drugs frequently. However, pharmacotherapy alone is an inappropriate method of weight loss. Drugs do not lead to long-term changes in eating or activity patterns, and therefore weight gain occurs once they are discontinued. Physicians may want to use drugs for very short periods in conjunction with other weight loss methods. Development of tolerance, abuse through development of dependence or addiction, and adverse side effects are hazards of pharmacotherapy for weight loss. Some nonanorexiant drugs, such as bulking agents like methyl cellulose or psyllium, may be more safely used in weight loss. However, consumption of high-fiber foods is preferred, and bulking agents also do not lead to long-term changes in eating behavior.

Surgery. Surgical treatment of obesity is a last resort for the most morbidly obese patients (100 per cent over their ideal body weight) who have life-threatening conditions complicated by their obesity and for whom all other techniques have failed (Task Force of the American Society for Clinical Nutrition, 1985). Four major types of surgical interventions exist, including those that (1) interfere with ingestion of food, (2) decrease stomach volume, (3) decrease intestinal absorption, and (4) remove subcutaneous fat.

Jaw wiring or dental fixation, which permits only liquids to be consumed, interferes with ingestion of food. This method still permits unlimited caloric intake of high-calorie liquids and offers no long-term solution once the jaws are unwired.

Many types of surgery as well as the implantation of devices such as balloons in the stomach reduce gastric volume. Surgical techniques have procedural risks to patients and in themselves do not change behavioral aspects of eating or activity.

Intestinal bypass surgery decreases intestinal absorption by shortening the small intestine to minimize absorption of foods. Complications and deaths from this procedure have led to a decline in its use.

Liposuction, the cosmetic removal of existing adipose tissue, has increased in popularity. Subcutaneous fat is removed with suction tubes through small incisions, and often accompanying surgery is performed to tighten up loose skin. This procedure carries infectious and other complications and only improves appearance in certain places.

Family physicians may be called on to refer patients for surgical interventions and to perform preoperative assessments of obese patients before surgery. The complications and side effects of surgical interventions for obesity recommend against them except in the most extreme cases of obesity.

Prevention of Obesity

Prevention is the intervention of choice for obesity. As a malleable condition, adult obesity can be prevented or delayed with health promotion activities such as balanced nutritional practices and participation in exercise. Physicians should encourage good dietary and exercise habits in childhood and continue that emphasis at all ages.

Patients and physicians should regularly monitor weight. Regular self-weighing (at least weekly) with a scale in the home provides patients with early detection of weight gain and motivation to prevent weight gain. Physicians should weigh patients at every visit, and this weight should be recorded in the medical record. In providing continuous care, physicians can note weight gains and intervene to prevent obesity from developing in their patients.

Physicians can provide anticipatory guidance about weight gain. For events such as holidays, vacations, and pregnancy, physicians need to provide patients with advice about not gaining excess weight and losing any weight gained. Patients who are gaining weight because of entry into a more sedentary life style need more general guidance.

Family screening can also occur for obesity, with the physician inquiring into the weight status of the other members of an obese patient's family. If other family members are obese, the intervention should be directed toward the entire family unit. Thus the whole family can change eating patterns, develop exercise activities, or engage in behavior modification.

It is inappropriate to place growing children on calorie-restricted diets. Obese children respond well to increased activity and a balanced intake of usual amounts of food. Adolescents often gain extra weight just prior to the onset of puberty and may not require intervention for this weight gain. The family is the most appropriate treatment unit for obesity, involving all members in healthy diets and increased activity throughout their lives.

References

Berland, T.: Rating the Diets. New York, Signet Press, 1986. *A useful description and assessment of popular diets which has been updated regularly.*

Bjorntorp, P.: Exercise and obesity. Psychiatr. Clin. North Am., *1*:691–696, 1978.

Bjorntorp, P.: Adipose tissues in obesity. *In* Hirsch, J., and Van Itallie, T. (Eds.): Recent Advances in Obesity Research IV. London, John Libbey and Co., 1984.

Bray, G. A.: The Obese Patient. Philadelphia, W. B. Saunders Co., 1976. *An excellent and complete overview of obesity.*

Brownell, K. D.: Obesity: Understanding and treating a serious, prevalent, and refractory disorder. J. Consult. Clin. Psychol., *50*:820–840, 1982.

Brownell, K. D., Stunkard, A. J., and McKeon, P. E.: Weight reduction at the worksite: A promise partially fulfilled. Am. J. Psychiatry, *142*:47–52, 1985.

Council on Scientific Affairs, American Medical Association: Treatment of obesity in adults. J.A.M.A., *260*:2547–2551, 1988.

Engel, G. L.: The need for a new medical model: A challenge for biomedicine. Science, *196*:129–136, 1977.

Garn, S. M., and Cole, P. E.: Do the obese remain obese and the lean remain lean? Am. J. Public Health, *70*:351–355, 1980.

Holmes, M. D., Zysow, B., and Delbanco, T. L.: An analytic review of current therapies for obesity. J. Fam. Pract., *28*:610–616, 1989. *A brief but very useful review of weight loss techniques geared toward practicing family physicians.*

Jackson, A. S., and Pollock, M. L.: Practical assessment of body composition. Physician Sportsmedicine, *13*:76–89, 1985.

Jeffery, R. W., Folsom, A. R., Luepker, R. V., et al.: Prevalence of overweight and weight loss behavior in a metropolitan adult population: The Minnesota Heart Survey experience. Am. J. Public Health, *74*:349–352, 1984.

Kissebah, A. H., Vydelingum, N., Murray, R., et al.: Relation of body fat distribution to metabolic complications of obesity. J. Clin. Endocrinol. Metab., *54*:254–260, 1982.

National Institutes of Health Consensus Development Panel: Health implications of obesity. Ann. Intern. Med., *103*:147, 1985.

Newmark, S. R., and Williamson, B.: Survey of very-low-calorie weight reduction diets. I. Novelty diets. Arch. Intern. Med., *143*:1195–1198, 1983a.

Newmark, S. R., and Williamson, B.: Survey of very-low-calorie weight reduction diets. II. Total fasting, protein sparing modified fasts, chemically defined diets. Arch. Intern. Med., *143*:1423–1427, 1983b.

Newsholme, E. A.: A possible metabolic basis for the control of body weight. N. Engl. J. Med., *302*:400–405, 1980.

Powers, P. S.: Obesity: The Regulation of Weight. Baltimore, Williams & Wilkins, 1980. *A practical overview of the scope of issues surrounding obesity.*

Rosenblatt, E.: Weight-loss programs. Postgrad. Med., *83*:137–180, 1988.

Rosenblatt, R. A., et al.: The structure and content of Family Practice: Current status and future trends. J. Fam. Pract., *15*:681–722, 1982.

Schacter, S.: Recidivism and self-cure of smoking and obesity. Am. J. Psychol., *37*:436–444, 1982.

Selby, J. V., Frideman, G. D., and Queensberry, C. P.: Precursors of essential hypertension: The role of body fat distribution pattern. Am. J. Epidemiol., *129*:43–53, 1989.

Sobal, J.: Marriage, obesity and dieting. Marriage Family Rev., *7*:115–140, 1984.

Sobal, J., and Stunkard, A. J.: Socioeconomic status and obesity: A review of the literature. Psychol. Bull., *105*:260–275, 1989.

Stensland, S., and Margolis, S.: A formula for calculating Body Mass Index using English units. J. Am. Diet. Assoc., 1990 (in press).

Stunkard, A. J.: Obesity. Philadelphia, W. B. Saunders Co., 1980. *A series of chapters provide expert insights into most of the key issues surrounding obesity and its treatment.*

Stunkard, A. J., and McLaren-Hume, M.: The results of treatments of obesity. Arch. Intern. Med., *103*:79–85, 1959.

Stunkard, A. J., and Wadden, T. A.: Behavior therapy and obesity. *In* Conn, H. L., Defelice, E. A., and Kuo, P. (Eds.): Health and Obesity. New York, Raven Press, 1983, pp. 105–130. *An overview of behavior modification.*

Task Force of the American Society for Clinical Nutrition: Guidelines for surgery for morbid obesity. Am. J. Clin. Nutr., *42*:904–905, 1985.

Van Itallie, T. B.: Health implications of overweight and obesity in the United States. Ann. Intern. Med., *103*:983–988, 1985.

Wing, R. R., and Jeffery, R. W.: Outpatient treatments of obesity: A comparison of methodology and clinical results. Int. J. Obesity, *3*:261–279, 1979.

55

Gastroenterology

Wm. MacMillan Rodney
Marvin Derezin

Study the past, diagnose the present, foretell the future. Practice these acts. As to disease, first of all, do no harm.

HIPPOCRATES

In the adult office practice experience of many family physicians, gastrointestinal (GI) illnesses rank among the top ten most common complaints. Questions relating to the gastrointestinal system occur each and every practice day. Furthermore, repeated surveys have documented the high prevalence of gastrointestinal complaints that frequently go unreported (Table 55–1).

This high prevalence of GI illness is becoming more and more important as the percentage of patients over age 50 increases. These prevalence studies identify only a minority of patients as truly asymptomatic. For example, this factor causes confusion as family physicians attempt to implement the early detection and prevention of colorectal cancer. Among patients 65 years of age and older, hiatal hernia, constipation, and diverticulosis exist in 50 per cent of patients or more. This factor causes uncertainty for the family physician who must integrate those findings into the context of chief complaint, present illness, primary diagnosis, secondary diagnoses, therapy, and prognosis.

Table 55–1. ADULT PREVALENCE OF GI CONDITIONS*

	Per Cent
Hemorrhoids	50 to 80
Dyspepsia	50 to 80
Abdominal Pain	30 to 70
Diverticulosis	30 to 50
Hiatal Hernia	20 to 50
Symptoms of IBS†	14 to 17
Gallstones	10 to 32
Constipation	9 to 30
Colonic Polyps	8 to 20

*Utilizing questionnaires, interviews, autopsy data, and symptom diaries, multiple studies have documented substantial numbers of illnesses in a variety of populations. As age increases, the prevalence increases.

†IBS, Irritable bowel syndrome.

This chapter proposes that the family physician can greatly benefit from an integrated overview of common GI symptoms, signs, and disorders. Powerful new tools are emerging for use within the office setting. The development of flexible sigmoidoscopy in the 1970's has created a generation of office-based primary care endoscopists in the 1980's. These physicians are examining, photographing, obtaining biopsies, and videorecording gastrointestinal pathophysiology on a daily basis. In addition to improved early detection of colorectal cancer, these tools enhance high quality patient care via improved information management and more accurate diagnosis in the office. Remote and real-time consultation similar to that seen by remote computer-assisted electrocardiogram interpretation will become available. Family physicians in the 1990's will routinely apply office-based diagnostic methods that were available only in university medical centers during the 1970's (Rodney, 1986).

This chapter begins with an examination of emergency conditions, which are less common but absolutely necessary to identify immediately, followed by the less urgent, although more common, chronic disorders.

Acute Abdominal Pain

In 1921, Sir Zachary Cope published the first edition of his classic text *Early Diagnosis of the Acute Abdomen.* Using only the history and physical examination, the author sought to assist readers so that disease requiring surgery could be identified rapidly and accurately. "The general rule can be laid down that the majority of severe abdominal pains which ensue in patients who have been previously fairly well, and which last as long as 6 hours, are caused by conditions of surgical import" (Cope, 1972).

Abdominal pain is the fifth most common presenting complaint of adult medical patients. Although renal colic and pelvic inflammatory disease are examples of nongastrointestinal illness that may be exhibited as abdominal pain, most abdominal pain results from a gastrointestinal disorder. In Adelman's recent study of family practice patients presenting with abdominal pain, 9 per cent were admitted to the hospital for evaluation or surgery (Adelman, 1987). The final diagnoses of 556 ambulatory patients presenting over 2 years (Table 55–2) suggested that a large percentage of these patients have a self-limited illness that eludes a definitive diagnosis.

Since the identification of illnesses requiring urgent intervention is paramount, this chapter begins with descriptions and definitions of the acute abdominal pain syndromes. These disorders are used as "learning examples." Mastery of these approaches is useful for the diagnosis and management of the disorders that follow. Usually, it is the patient who defines his or her pain as being "acute." One working definition for acute abdominal pain is when the patient cannot wait until tomorrow or next week for an appointment.

The history, the physical examination, the laboratory, and the radiology suite form the basic foundation for the diagnostic process. First and foremost, the diagnosis is best served by a rigorous history. In 85 per cent of patients, the experienced physician can make the correct diagnosis in this fashion by systematically using the "attributes of pain" mnemonic $(PQR)^2ST^3$ (Table 55–3) and a uniform review of systems (DeGowin, 1981). The diagnosis can be missed simply by underrating this first important step. Therefore, this diagnostic tool bears repeating. An accurate, systematic, and thoughtful description of the presenting complaint is the hallmark of excellence in differential diagnosis.

APPENDICITIS

Background Comments

Identification of appendicitis was one of the first benefits of a revolution that transformed all of medicine. This revolution was the application of the scientific method. It allowed the pathologist-physician R. H. Fitz to propose in 1886 that the common and usually fatal disease of perityphlitis was actually appendicitis. In a controversial paper, Dr. Fitz advocated that surgery could cure appendicitis (Fitz, 1886). One hundred years have passed, but much remains unexamined by this special new tool—the scientific method.

Clinical Epidemiology

Appendicitis occurs most frequently between 10 and 30 years of age. However, 7 per cent of patients are under age 5, and 5 per cent are over age 60. Appendicitis, diverticulosis, hemorrhoids, hiatal hernia, and irritable bowel syndromes have been described as diseases of western civilization. An asso-

Table 55–2. FINAL DIAGNOSIS FOR THE PRESENTING SYMPTOM OF ABDOMINAL PAIN (ACUTE AND CHRONIC) IN FAMILY PHYSICIANS' OFFICES*

Diagnosis	Frequency	Per Cent‡	Cumulative Per Cent
Abdominal pain, etiology undocumented	280	50.4	50.4
Acute gastroenteritis	51	9.2	59.5
Urinary tract infection	37	6.7	66.2
Irritable bowel syndrome	32	5.8	71.9
Pelvic inflammatory disease	21	3.8	75.7
Hiatal hernia or reflux	13	2.3	78.1
Diverticulosis	12	2.2	80.2
Diarrhea, cause undetermined	9	1.6	81.8
Cholelithiasis	9	1.6	83.5
Tumor, benign	8	1.4	84.9
Duodenal ulcer	8	1.4	86.3
Urolithiasis	7	1.3	87.6
Appendicitis	6	1.1	88.7
Ulcerative colitis	5	.9	89.6
Muscular strain	5	.9	90.5
Other†	53	9.5	100.0

*Adapted from Adelman, A.: Abdominal pain in the primary care setting. J. Fam. Pract., *25*(1):27–32, 1987.
†Includes pyelonephritis, endometriosis, malignant tumors, esophagitis, gastritis, gastric ulcer, hepatitis, spontaneous abortion, anxiety, depression.
‡Does not total 100 per cent because of round-off error.

Table 55–3. ANALYSIS OF A SYMPTOM ABDOMINAL PAIN [(PQR)²ST³]*

Provoking—What makes your pain worse? Does it hurt more when you move, take a deep breath, or cough?
Palliating—What makes your pain improve?
Quantity—On a scale of 1 to 10, how bad is the pain?
Quality—Could you describe what this pain feels like?
Region—Where is the pain located?
Radiation—Does the pain radiate (to the back, shoulders, genitals)?
Severity—Is the pain sufficiently severe to disrupt activities of daily living?

Temporal issues
1. Was the onset sudden or gradual?
2. Does the pain come and go or is it constant?
3. Is this the first time you have had this pain?

*These 11 questions are the foundation of rational inquiry regarding the etiology of abdominal pain. Although there are variations and disease-specific augmentations, these data should be obtained during the diagnostic process.

ciation with low-fiber and high-fat diets exists for all of these diseases. Although the lifetime risk of appendicitis is projected at 7 per cent, appendectomy is no longer among the ten most frequent operations in the United States. In centers utilizing sensitivity and specificity theory to derive improved predictive value from physical findings and laboratory values, negative surgical exploration rates have dropped without a corresponding increase in the frequency of perforation (Schwartz, 1987; Malt, 1986).

Present Illness

Since the bowel is mobile and anatomy varies, the location of the appendix is not constant. This explains the number of signs and symptoms that have been associated with acute appendicitis. In particular, this variability explains the fact that less than 50 per cent of patients with the disease follow a so-called textbook clinical course. Nevertheless, the textbook description is useful in emphasizing another traditional strong point of clinical medicine, i.e., the practice of serial observations of the patient is an important diagnostic tool. Generally, patients initially report a malaise that may be attributed to indigestion. Common initial symptoms include mild epigastric pain, colicky periumbilical pain, and some irregularity of bowel habit. This symptom may be exhibited as constipation or diarrhea. During the initial stages, anorexia, nausea, and vomiting are common. Within hours or during the course of the day, the pain may shift to the right lower quadrant (McBurney's point). If not reported, tenderness on deep palpation may be elicited. A low-grade fever may be reported by the patient. When the condition is untreated, perforation may occur. This complication leads to generalized peritonitis, and in some cases, a tender mass may develop in the right lower quadrant (a periappendiceal abscess).

Since careful clinicians formulate the differential diagnosis on the basis of the history alone, it is appropriate to itemize considerations in the differential diagnosis of acute abdominal pain (Table 55–4). At this point, items in the differential diagnosis are reinforced, excluded, or de-emphasized depending on the results of the physical examination, laboratory studies, and further observations. Since the differential diagnosis list is comprehensive, the consideration of acute appendicitis serves as a useful clinical model for the analysis of many of the gastrointestinal disorders.

Review of Systems

In addition to a rigorous analysis of symptoms (see Table 55–3), the family physician must deal with the entire constellation of personal, family, and community issues associated with each case. Common errors of omission include the past medical history such as information on allergies, medications, previous surgeries, previous hospitalizations, family history, social history, and the use of social drugs. For women, the obstetric history and the date of the last normal menstrual period are critical. The temporal sequence of positive items within the review of systems should be described in detail. This sequence is important in isolating appendicitis from the other possible conditions within the differential diagnosis.

Physical Examination

The diagnostic process cannot succeed without the attainment of vital signs, a chest examination, an abdominal examination, a pelvic examination, and a rectal examination. The principles of inspection, aus-

Table 55–4. STRUCTURAL APPROACH TO THE DIFFERENTIAL DIAGNOSIS OF ACUTE ABDOMINAL PAIN

Thoracic Structures
- Cardiac, e.g., myocardial infarction
- Pulmonary, e.g., pneumonia
- Esophageal
- Vascular, e.g., aneurysm

Abdominal Structures
- Liver
- Gallbladder
- Pancreas
- Stomach
- Small intestine
- Large intestine
- Kidneys, ureters, bladder
- Female reproductive organs
- Blood vessels
- Rectum
- Musculoskeletal
- Vascular, e.g., aneurysm

Miscellaneous
- Psychogenic
- Metabolic, e.g., diabetes
- Abscess
- Infections
- Neoplastic
- Trauma or obstruction

cultation, palpation, and percussion are particularly important in the examination of abdomen. At this point, some of the confirmatory special examinations can be utilized when appropriate. Tenderness of the right lower quadrant is frequently over a small area, and rebound tenderness can be elicited. Confirmatory signs such as the iliopsoas sign, the obturator sign, and Hoover's sign, are beyond the scope of this chapter. The digital rectal examination may be valuable in diagnosing acute appendicitis. Some examiners have noted the tenderness on the right side as the single most useful diagnostic sign in acute appendicitis. In the consideration of a rigid abdomen with no bowel sounds, one may assume that generalized peritonitis is present and surgical consultation is urgently needed.

The Diagnostic Plan

Although hemograms, urinalyses, and x-ray studies have generally been ordered in the investigation of acute abdominal pain, none of these items are diagnostic. A negative laboratory examination in conjunction with of a strongly suggestive clinical history merits serial observation. White blood cell counts above 15,000 per μl. should raise the suspicion of a perforated appendix, but this finding would also be consistent with mesenteric adenitis. The finding of some white blood cells and red blood cells in the urine is entirely consistent with appendicitis. On the other hand, it is nonspecific. The finding of more than 30 red blood cells and/or more than 20 white blood cells in the urine would suggest a primary lesion in the urinary tract. In selected instances, chest and abdominal x-ray studies may be helpful. But the same may be said for intravenous pyelograms, culdocenteses, barium enemas, and ultrasound examinations. Physicians who consider these examinations realize that each case must be individualized. These additional laboratory studies, however, are not routine studies to be ordered in every case.

Psychosocial Aspects and Special Considerations

Since the vast majority of patients who present with acute abdominal pain do not have an abdominal problem requiring surgery, the negative predictors of appendicitis are frequently more helpful than the textbook descriptors of classic appendicitis. Symptoms lasting more than 72 hours, with pain in locations other than those stipulated, suggest that appendicitis is not the diagnosis. If the patient has no anorexia and the temperature is below 37.5° C. (99.5° F.) or above 38.6° C. (101.5° F.), the clinician is advised to consider other conditions.

Recent Literature and New Information

1. Women who survive a perforated appendix have a five-fold increased risk of infertility (Mueller et al., 1986).

2. Ultrasonography is a relatively inexpensive, noninvasive, nonirradiating modality that has been added to the nonspecific diagnostic armamentarium but adds little at this time (Puylaert et al., 1987).

3. Laparoscopy, which is rarely indicated, may evolve as a useful tool with which to confirm diagnosis or prevent unnecessary surgery in patients with suspected appendicitis (Paterson-Brown et al., 1988).

4. Amylase is elevated in at least 10 per cent of cases of appendicitis, but this finding does not help with diagnosis. Therefore, amylase, electrolytes, glucose, creatinine, and calcium are examples of biochemical tests that should be carefully individualized in each situation.

In conclusion, if the family physician suspects appendicitis after the initial evaluation, consultation with a colleague in general surgery is frequently very helpful.

CHOLECYSTITIS AND CHOLELITHIASIS

Background Comments and Important Definitions

Since cholecystectomy is one of the four most frequently performed operations in the United States, family physicians are frequently involved in the initial care of patients with acute cholecystitis. The advent of potential medical therapy and the understanding that most gallstones exist asymptomatically have been major developments in the 1980's. Although gallstone dissolution is a promising and FDA-approved therapy, cholecystectomy remains the definitive treatment, except for a few patients who could be candidates for dissolution. The dissolution drug, ursodiol (Actigall), has some side effects. Additionally, the drug would need to be taken daily for years, and possibly indefinitely, for dissolution to occur. Diagnostically, new additions to therapy have been ultrasound, cholescintigraphy, endoscopic retrograde cholangiopancreatography, and others. Each development has yielded useful new knowledge but at the cost of increased complexity. Although diagnostic yield (sensitivity) has improved, controversy over elective cholecystectomy in asymptomatic gallstone patients reflects the unresolved predictive value of early diagnosis (Gracie and Ransohoff, 1982; Donaldson, 1982). Our bias is against elective surgery unless there are individual mitigating circumstances.

The differential diagnosis of acute cholecystitis is straightforward most the time. Chronic cholecystitis is a histologic disease. There are no symptoms unless a stone blocks the cystic duct. Once blockage occurs, then acute biliary colic occurs.

Clinical Epidemiology

The prevalence of gallstones between the ages of 55 and 65 is 23 per cent for females and 10 per cent for males. The majority of gallstones are derived from cholesterol. A traditional clinical picture of a patient likely to have gallstones relied heavily on the four "F's" (female, fat, forty, and fertile). Autopsy studies have demonstrated that the prevalence of cholelithiasis increases with age. Females predominate. The prevalence in the age group 60 to 79 is 23 per cent, with a prevalence of 32 per cent over the age of 80. Groups with a high prevalence of gallbladder disease are women who have been pregnant, diabetics, American Indians, and women who are overweight. Rare causes of pigmented stones include hemolytic disease, long-standing cirrhosis, and disorders of the ileum (e.g., regional enteritis, obesity bypass surgery, and others). Although birth control pills have been linked to a higher prevalence of gallstones, this association is not clinically important. The clinician should also consider this entity among low-risk patients. Since cholecystitis is so common, many patients really do not fall into the high-risk groups.

Present Illness

Among the group treated with a placebo in the national cooperative gallstone study, 305 patients were followed for 2 years. The chief conclusions were

1. Most patients without a history of biliary tract pain remain asymptomatic.
2. A history of biliary tract pain is highly predictive of future episodes of pain.
3. Gallstones do not grow rapidly, but they rarely dissolve or pass spontaneously. Family physicians frequently encounter patients with biliary tract pain. A stone blocking the cystic duct results in acute biliary colic that, if it continues for a prolonged period, can evolve into acute suppurative cholecystitis.

The pain is abrupt, frequently causing the patient to double over with a 10/10 severity. (The patient reports the pain to be a 10 on a scale of 1 to 10, where 1 is mild and 10 is most severe or terrible). Much of the time, the colic is steady and the pain is most commonly epigastric. It may radiate along the right upper quadrant around to the back, straight through to the back, or even up to the shoulder.

The patient frequently rolls around to get relief, whereas a patient with coronary ischemia will not. Patients are nauseated, and they sometimes vomit. The attacks commonly awaken people from their sleep between 1 and 3 A.M.. The pain may resolve in a few hours or within 8 to 12 hours, or not until the patient receives a narcotic. Usually an injection of narcotic relieves the pain. When the pain does subside, it does so rapidly. Attacks of biliary colic rarely lead to cholecystitis and urgent surgery. When a stone is not blocking the cystic duct, chronic cholecystitis and cholelithiasis are asymptomatic entities. They are *not* responsible for flatulence or indigestion.

Review of Systems

The onset of pain is rarely related to meals or to the type of food eaten. Many patients with postprandial abdominal pain believe they have gallbladder disease, but many of these patients suffer from one of the dyspepsia syndromes or chronic abdominal pain syndromes that are described later. Acute surgical cholecystitis becomes a consideration when pain persists or worsens. Surgical consultation may be considered when the pain is associated with fever, there is increasing leukocytosis, and there is a worsening response on physical examination. Most patients with acute cholecystitis have had abdominal pain that has persisted for at least 4 to 6 hours and was unrelieved by narcotic injections.

Physical Findings of Value

The gallbladder is rarely palpable in severe acute cholecystitis. As biliary colic leads to acute cholecystitis, there is increasing localized tenderness that spreads and is associated with muscle guarding or rigidity, or both, in the right upper quadrant. Right-sided pain, which worsens with deep inspiration, may appear. Murphy's sign has been defined as an right upper quadrant tenderness in the midclavicular line that worsens during deep inspiration. This finding suggests acute cholecystitis. Mild jaundice has been found in up to 20 per cent of patients.

The Diagnostic Plan

A hemogram usually reveals an increased white blood cell count. Although serum amylase and lipase values are usually normal, they may be elevated if there is associated pancreatitis. Serum alkaline phosphatase and bilirubin levels are rarely elevated. Sometimes the transaminases (serum glutamic-oxaloacetic transaminase and serum glutamic-pyruvic transaminase) can be in the low 100's, whereas the bilirubin level may increase as high as 4 mg. per dl. in an uncomplicated attack of acute cholecystitis. Unless the white blood cell count is high, laboratory tests frequently lack any predictive value.

Only 10 to 15 per cent of gallstones are visible on plain x-ray studies, thus abdominal films are rarely helpful. Ultrasound imaging has evolved as the procedure of first choice. When calculi, gallbladder wall thickening, and gallbladder sludge are found, the diagnosis of acute cholecystitis is reinforced. But the presence of stones by themselves do not ensure the diagnosis of acute cholecystitis. To make this diagnosis, technetium-99m image display and analysis scans have been invaluable. After I.V. injection, images are obtained within the first 60 minutes and repeated at 3 to 6 hours. The isotope is excreted with the bile and fills all ducts as well as the gallbladder unless the cystic duct is obstructed. When the gallbladder does not appear on the image, it is presumed that gallbladder duct obstruction is present. Oral cholecystography is not indicated as a test for acute cholecystitis; however, it is still extremely valuable in regions where ultrasound is not available. There is no longer any need for intravenous cholangiography.

Ultrasonography can be used in acute situations because it takes very little time. It is noninvasive, emits no radiation, and is not obstructed by high bilirubin levels. It can also be used for pediatric and pregnant patients. At the same time, other abdominal contents can be visualized, such as the kidney, liver, and pancreas. Technical difficulties can occur in very obese patients, and occasionally, overlying bowel gas interferes with the image. Nevertheless, the overall sensitivity of sonography has been calculated at 85 to 94 per cent, with a positive predictive value of over 90 per cent. As late as 1987, some continue to favor the oral cholecystogram as the initial diagnostic study (Robles et al., 1987). This may be true only in regions where ultrasound is not available.

Management and Therapy

Upon hospitalization or in the emergency room, an intravenous line is established and patients are given nothing by mouth. Hydration and electrolyte balance are maintained. Nasogastric suction is rarely necessary, although sometimes it is helpful if the patient is vomiting. Meperidine can be used every 2 to 3 hours in a dosage of 75 to 100 mg. intramuscularly for pain. Morphine-type drugs are generally avoided because of the theoretical spasm in the sphincter of Oddi, which is believed to worsen the pain. If the pain does not resolve after several hours, an emergency operation may be indicated. Furthermore, if the physical findings are worsening and the white blood cell count is increasing, an emergency operation may be needed in this case also. If an initial dose of meperidine does not relieve the pain, surgical consultation should be sought. If too much time is allowed to elapse, gangrene and perforation or abscess may occur. Thus, in the routine course of events, the diagnosis of acute cholecystitis provides sufficient indication for emergency cholecysectomy. Under emergency circumstances, cholecysectomy can be a life-saving measure.

Summary and Special Considerations

The guidelines for the management of gallbladder disease are fairly discrete when the condition is exhibited asymptomatically as biliary colic or acute cholecystitis. However, it is less clear how to manage patients with "asymptomatic" gallstones that have been found coincidentally (Laupacis et al., 1988). The fear that future attacks of biliary colic may occur have led to a large number of elective cholecystectomies. Most patients with asymptomatic gallstones remain asymptomatic, whereas those with attacks are likely to continue with attacks. Therefore, surgery is generally indicated for symptomatic patients, but surgery is generally not performed in asymptomatic patients.

New treatments are emerging with some promise, i.e., ursodiol (Actigall). This agent is an oral stone dissolution drug. However, the patient must have cholesterol gallstones and a functioning gallbladder to be a candidate for this therapy. Furthermore, the patient may need to take the drug daily for 2 years with full knowledge of a 40 per cent failure rate. The drug is costly. Shockwave lithotripsy and ultrasonic fragmentation of gallstones are now being used in a large national study.

The phenomenon of phantom pain after cholecystectomy is a particularly difficult one. Usually, the authors obtain a second opinion and consider psychometric evaluation for a somatomization disorder if no other organic causes can be found. Among women of reproductive age with negative imaging studies but with clinical syndromes similar to acute and chronic cholecystitis, treatment for anterior perihepatitis, also known as Curtis-Fitz-Hugh syndrome, resulted in a cure (Shanahan et al., 1988). These authors suggested that all sexually active patients with suspected acute cholecystitis and a normal ultrasound should be screened for *Chlamydia trachomatis*.

DIVERTICULOSIS AND DIVERTICULITIS

Background Comments and Important Definitions

Diverticulosis is the presence of saccular outpouchings from the large intestine. These occur most commonly in the sigmoid colon. Once regarded as a pathologic curiosity, the low-fiber and high-fat dietary environment of the civilized 20th century has been associated with an autopsy-confirmed prevalence of up to 60 per cent of patients over the age of 60. The hypothesis of the relationship between dietary fiber and diverticulosis has been supported by multiple studies, including a prevalence study of Oxford vegetarians (12 per cent) and matched controls (33 per cent) (Gear et al., 1979). The widespread diagnosis of diverticulosis and the frequent application of accurate imaging studies (x-ray studies an endoscopy) among the large number of family practice patients presenting with symptoms of abdominal pain reflects the high prevalence of the condition.

As with gallstones and hiatal hernia, the presence of the condition does not necessarily mean it is the cause of the patient's pain. The vast majority of patients with diverticuli do not have symptoms. A minority of patients experience diverticulitis, perforation, hemorrhage, and subsequent complications. In a tertiary care setting, where more patients with more complicated conditions are seen, 294 selected patients were prospectively followed over 15 years. During the follow-up period, clinical diverticulitis developed in 25 per cent, perforation in 5 per cent, substantial hemorrhage in 5 per cent, and obstruction in 5 per cent of the patients (Boles and Gordon, 1958). Having come under medical observation for one reason or another, these patients probably represent a select group. This phenomenon is also known as referral bias. Therefore, in most patients, diverticulosis is an incidental finding that may reflect many years of a Western diet and life style. At this point, it is only speculation on our part whether or not life-style modifications can prevent the development of diverticulosis-associated morbidity.

Diverticulitis begins with the inflammation of one or more diverticuli, but it is not known why the inflammation occurs. Clinical pain arises from inflammation of the colon wall and the adjacent peritoneal surface. Most of the time, the inflammation is confined to the bowel wall, resulting in the most common entity, i.e., diverticulitis. If the inflammation continues, an abscess may arise and perforation or obstruction may follow. These are uncommon complications.

Diverticular hemorrhage is emerging as a probable cause in 20 to 40 per cent of adults who present with lower GI bleeding. It should be noted that diverticular hemorrhage does not occur as part of the clinical syndrome of diverticulitis. Most often, diverticular hemorrhage appears suddenly in an asymptomatic patient (Casarella et al., 1972).

Present Illness

A syndrome attributed to diverticuli has been called "painful diverticular disease." This syndrome may be exhibited as generally constant left lower quadrant pain. Sometimes, the pain may be perceived in the right lower quadrant or in the suprapubic area. Patients may complain of associated constipation or diarrhea, or both, but it is difficult to know whether or not this finding represents a coincidental event or a true association. Sometimes, the pain is made worse by the passage of a bowel movement. The pain may be intense with localized tenderness, but the white blood cell count is normal. Acute diverticulitis could be suspected in these cases, but it is not likely when pain has been present for weeks to months without signs of inflammation.

Acutely ill patients who present with the rapid development of fever and an acute, severe abdominal pain in the left lower quadrant merit immediate attention. Depending on the severity of the findings, an outpatient or a hospital setting is chosen.

The Review of Systems

At one time, diverticulitis was described as a "left-sided appendicitis," because patients can present with pain in the left lower abdomen. There is historical merit for this concept (Orebaugh, 1978). A previously documented attack of diverticulitis is historically helpful. The patient with diverticulitis usually reports a severe and steady left lower quadrant pain that is frequently associated with urinary frequency. The pain becomes worse when the patient walks, coughs, or moves around.

Physical Findings of Value

The most common finding is abdominal tenderness that localizes to the left lower quadrant. Sometimes, a palpable mass is found. Even if the palpable mass is not present, there usually is exquisite tenderness in the left lower quadrant. Bowel sounds are usually present. Rectal examination may reveal tenderness high on the left side. If the severity of the inflammation worsens, a tender mass may be palpable, the abdominal signs may worse, and the bowel sounds may disappear. With extreme cases, peritoneal signs are evident and sepsis may be the presenting syndrome. With acute diverticulitis, the oral temperature is usually 38.0° C. (100.4° F.) or lower. As the inflammation spreads, the fever and the white blood cell count increase.

The Diagnostic Plan

The history and physical examination usually establish the diagnosis. Laboratory tests are generally of little value unless the white blood cell count goes above 15,000. If the white blood cell count and the temperature are elevated and abdominal findings are present, surgical consultation should be requested without delay. Most patients with acute diverticulitis may be managed as outpatients. Some cases of diverticulitis with more advanced findings require hospitalization.

In one series of hospitalized patients with severe diverticulitis, physical findings were tabulated to reveal the following: abdominal tenderness, 67 per cent; palpable pelvic mass, 27 per cent; palpable abdominal mass, 26 per cent; signs of generalized peritonitis, 14 per cent; and shock, 4 per cent. Eighteen per cent of the patients had negative physical findings (Walker et al., 1977). Flexible sigmoidoscopy or colonoscopy and barium enema cannot be used in these cases, because there is considerable risk of perforation with instrumentation if diverticulitis is present. Therefore, a period of observation during medical therapy is preferred prior to any invasive studies. In those cases in which the differential diagnosis includes ischemia or colitis, or both, a very gentle and limited sigmoidoscopy can be performed. Excessive air insufflation and forceful manipulation should be avoided while performing this procedure. Once the patient is identified as possibly having a severe case of diverticulitis, hospitalization, intravenous antibiotics, and consultation rapidly ensue. Management is individualized at that point.

Differential Diagnosis and Therapy

For those who are hospitalized, the family physician and consultant team usually work through the clinical course. If the patient deteriorates (i.e., has more pain, an increasing fever, and worsening findings on physical examination despite antibiotic therapy), surgery should be considered to avoid perforation or a full blown peritonitis, or both. For those patients who have had previous attacks of diverticulitis, surgery should be considered earlier because they are more likely to have attacks in the future.

Usually, the sigmoid colon alone is removed. Patients who must be emergently decompressed may require a colostomy with resection. If the attack of diverticulitis can be stabilized medically, an elective sigmoid resection is preferred. An elective resection is performed only if the patient is repeatedly symptomatic or develops a fistula to the bladder (or other organs).

For those patients who are not hospitalized, there are many management issues. The differential diagnosis for the mild left lower quadrant abdominal pain includes, but is not limited to, irritable bowel syndrome, inflammatory bowel disease, carcinoma, ischemic colitis, radiation colitis, and infectious colitis. More information follows in specific sections dealing with each of the common entities.

Psychosocial Aspects and Special Considerations

Although hospital services and surgical operations for diverticulitis and its complications are reported commonly in the literature, the necessity for operative intervention has been measured at 0.4 per cent (Horner, 1958). Many cases that were previously described as "diverticulitis" may actually have been irritable bowel syndrome, self-limited gastroenteritis, and other conditions. There seems to have been a high natural remission rate, and it should be noted that the vast majority of patients with incidentally noted diverticulosis are free from acute diverticulitis and the severe complications described earlier. These individuals can be safely managed as outpatients. Since abdominal pain that is not associated with any anatomic or inflammatory abnormality is so common, previous associations between diverticular disorders and the various other irritable bowel syndromes have been difficult to sort out (Drossman et al., 1982).

Treatment of Acute Diverticulitis

The patient with localized left lower quadrant pain and a temperature below 38.9° C. (102° F.) (who does not have abdominal distention) can be managed as an outpatient with the concurrence of the surgical consultant.

These patients should receive liquids only for diet. Bed rest and antibiotics such as the oral cephalosporins can be prescribed. Oral codeine may be used for pain. While at home, the patient should be advised to report worsening pain, spreading pain, abdominal distention, vomiting, or temperature spikes. These features would reflect a worsening course. The physician must be notified and hospitalization considered urgently.

Diet and Drug Therapy

Previously recommended bland low-fiber, "low-seed" diets are no longer indicated for diverticulosis. After the acute attack, recommendations now include a high-fiber, low-fat diet. Anticholinergic drugs, antispasmodic drugs, sedatives, and tranquilizers may be used for those patients who have concurrent irritable bowel syndrome or unspecified colonic spasm, or both.

There are no direct clinical data indicating that a high-fiber diet prevents the formation of diverticuli or prevents the development of diverticulitis. However, the epidemiologic data are convincing in the minds of some but not all experts. A study of 100 patients who had been discharged with confirmed diverticular disease compared those patients who complied with the recommendation of 40 grams of fiber per day with those who did not comply with the diet. The high-fiber diet was associated with a 91 per cent probability of the patient being symptom free. Only 80 per cent of the patients who did not follow the high-fiber diet were symptom free, and all major complications occurred in this group as well (Hyland and Taylor, 1980). In any case, it seems reasonable to recommend high-fiber diets, since they are healthy. For those patients who dislike raw dietary bulk, hydrophilic colloids (Metamucil, Konsyl, Modane bulk, and others) may be prescribed, recommending use of one heaping tablespoon once or twice a day. Rapid initiation of large amounts of fiber can cause flatulence, distention, and discomfort. Therefore, a gradual build-up to the desired amount is recommended. Anticipatory guidance regarding the side effects should also be given.

Clinical Suggestions

As in the irritable bowel syndrome, the opportunity to explore life-style issues and dietary considerations is very important here. It may be useful to create a kind of "grocery store" quiz regarding equivalent weights of dietary products that are required for an intake of 20 grams of fiber per day. This amount of fiber intake will approximately double the daily fecal weight. For example, this would require 22 oz. of whole carrots, 49 oz. of fresh apples, 13 oz. of whole meal bread, or 4½ oz. of commercial bran cereal. The equivalent amount of unprocessed bran would be 1½ oz. Another equivalent would be approximately two bowls of commercial cereals such as Allbran or Bran Buds. There are many choices. Any of the many good diet books available make the above calculations and food choices as simple as looking at a table. Although data are incomplete, diet seems to help alleviate some symptoms of the condition (Brodribb, 1977).

ACUTE PANCREATITIS

Background Comments and Important Definitions

Acute pancreatitis seems a logical fourth element in this overview of acute abdominal pain syndromes (Blake, 1988) in which early identification is the key to appropriate hospital therapy and consultation. Appendicitis, cholecystitis, diverticulitis, and pancreatitis are diseases with degrees of clinical severity ranging from mild to severe. When severe, each condition may be exhibited as a potential acute surgical abdomen. The family physician must be aware of these life-threatening illnesses, even though most patients with abdominal pain do not require hospitalization.

Since the clinical presentation of acute pancreatitis may vary from acute abdominal pain to episodes of excruciating abdominal pain and vascular collapse, pancreatitis is included within the broad differential diagnosis of abdominal pain. Regardless of the underlying cause, the common pathway in the pathogenesis of pancreatitis is the liberation of corrosive pancreatic enzymes. Local pancreatic digestion and possible hemorrhage ensue. There is massive third spacing of intravascular fluid with subsequent hypovolemia. When severe massive tissue destruction adjacent to the pancreas occurs, organs that are distant to the pancreas can be affected as well.

Clinical Epidemiology

The majority (65 to 90 per cent) of patients with acute pancreatitis have either chronic alcoholism or gallstones. Perforated peptic ulcer disease, trauma, neoplasms, hypercalcemia, hyperlipidemia, drugs, viral infections, and other conditions account for a small percentage of cases. The condition may be idiopathic in as many as 25 per cent of cases. The disease may occur at any age but most frequently occurs between the ages 40 and 60. Acute pancreatitis typically occurs in males in the 30's or 40's who have been drinking heavily for 6 to 10 years. For alcohol abuse of this degree, the estimated risk of pancreatitis is 5 to 10 per cent. Gallstone pancreatitis, the more dangerous of the two types, occurs at a later age.

Chronic pancreatitis indicates that there has been some permanent and progressive damage to the pancreas. In some cases, this damage leads to diabetes or malabsorption, or both. Patients with chronic pancreatitis present with repeated attacks of abdominal pain.

Present Illness and Review of Systems

The patient presents with a history of deep, gnawing, constant epigastric pain that radiates to the back in 50 per cent of patients. In some patients, the pain is substernal, generalized to the left upper quadrant or right upper quadrant, or even to the lower abdomen. Most often, the pain has been present for greater than 24 hours. This pain is worsened by the ingestion of food or alcohol and, in an alcoholic, may be precipitated by binge drinking. Sometimes, the pain is less severe when the patient leans forward. In advanced stages, movement worsens the pain, as it does in any of the previously discussed acute abdominal pain syndromes. The onset of pain is usually gradual, with a plateau being reached in several hours.

Physical Findings of Value

A low-grade fever of 37.8° to 38.9° C. (100° to 102° F.) may be present, but temperature in excess of 38.9° C. (102° F.) suggests another diagnosis or complication. Since hypovolemia is usually a complication, orthostatic vital signs should be obtained. Regulation of an appropriate fluid intake is essential. Urinary output must be monitored carefully. Even when blood pressure is normal, mild tachycardia may reflect worsening hypovolemia.

The patient with pancreatitis is in severe distress from abdominal pain. A stoic acceptance of discomfort suggests other diagnoses. The abdomen is tender but not rigid. Distention and decreased bowel sounds may be evident when ileus results from the diffusion of inflammatory fluid around the pancreas. The purplish discoloration of extravasated pancreatic hemorrhages (i.e., Grey Turner's sign in the flanks and Cullen's sign in the periumbilical area) are rarely seen.

The Diagnostic Plan

An elevated serum amylase level continues to be the sine qua non of acute pancreatitis. However, a perforated viscus or bowel obstruction can cause elevated amylase levels. Other causes of high amylase levels include tubal pregnancy and parotitis. Serum amylase levels return to normal in 1 to 3 days and, thus, abnormal values are rarely missed. The serum lipase level remains elevated for 7 to 14 days or more, and this finding is occasionally helpful. Although amylase-creatinine clearance ratios were widely acclaimed in the late 1970's (and continue to have some advocates in the 1980's), their usefulness has not survived the test of time (Lumeng, 1978, Moosa, 1984).

The hematocrit temporarily may be high as a secondary effect of hypovolemia. When rehydrated, patients with a low hematocrit may be suffering from acute hemorrhagic pancreatitis. If the bilirubin, serum glutamic-oxaloacetic transaminase, serum glutamic-pyruvic transominase, and alkaline phosphatase levels rise, a common duct stone may exist. This possibility could be further explored with an abdominal ultrasound and possibly with endoscopic retrograde cholangiopancreatography. Hypocalcemia, hypoalbuminemia, hyperglycemia, and leukocytosis in the range of 15,000 to 20,000 white blood cells per μl. are frequently found. Leukocytosis above 20,000 suggests a more severe disease. Since "shock lung" may ensue, chest x-ray studies and blood gas measurements should be considered. In severe cases, renal failure may appear despite adequate fluid intake. Urinary output should be monitored with care.

There have been a variety of promising laboratory assays directed at the improvement of the clinical diagnosis of pancreatitis, but none have established a clear advantage over the serum amylase test (and clinical evaluation). In addition to the amylase and creatinine clearance ratio, experimental and/or discarded tests include serum levels of trypsin, elastase, serum isoenzymes, and others. Most recently, a 5-minute agglutination assay that detects a serum concentration of lipase has been reported (Mayer et al., 1985). Lipase is believed to be an extremely sensitive and specific assay for pancreatic disorders, although this has been questioned. Using a cutoff for amylase of about 1.5 times the upper limit of normal, a sensitivity of 99.9 per cent and a specificity of 98.4 per cent were found. Some authors concluded that total serum amylase is the initial assay of choice in acute pancreatitis (Steinberg et al., 1985). Peritoneal lavage and methemalbumin are no longer recommended in the diagnostic work-up (White et al., 1988).

Although other abdominal diseases can elevate the amylase level, a patient with an acute attack of abdominal pain and an elevated serum amylase level probably has acute pancreatitis. Hospitalization and consultation would be justifiable even under the most stringent criteria. Although some have questioned the acquisition of routine chest and abdominal films for these patients, the absence of free air in the abdomen remains one reassuring sign that a large perforated viscus is not likely. Furthermore, some x-ray findings help to reinforce the diagnosis. These findings include an absent left psoas shadow, calcifications in the region of the pancreas, and an isolated air-filled loop of small bowel that cuts off in the area of the transverse colon (i.e., the sentinel loop). There have been dramatic improvements with the utilization of ultrasound, endoscopic retrograde cholangiopancreatography, and computerized tomography. Nevertheless, with the laboratory tests and evaluations discussed to this point, the family physician should have sufficient diagnostic information to warrant an appropriate disposition for the acutely ill patient.

Differential Diagnosis

Since the presentation of acute pancreatitis can be similar to many other entities that present with diffuse upper abdominal pain, all of the other causes of acute abdominal must be considered. The other diseases that commonly can be confused with pancreatitis include acute cholecystitis, choledocholithiasis, perforated peptic ulcer, and ruptured abdominal aneurysm. Pancreatitis can be exhibited with diffuse upper abdominal pain, back pain, left upper quadrant pain, and right upper quadrant pain. Therefore, all of the causes of acute abdominal pain should be considered.

Psychosocial Aspects and Special Considerations

Prognostically, a 10 per cent mortality rate continues to exist for acute pancreatitis. Almost all cases resulting in death are associated with acute necrotizing or hemorrhagic pancreatitis. Another 40 per cent of patients are quite ill but survive their attack. The remainder have a relatively mild and self-limited disease. Medical therapy is primarily supportive, with the major objective being stabilization.

Permanent pathologic damage to the pancreas results in chronic pancreatitis. In addition to exocrine deficiency (with malabsorption or diabetes, or both), a chronic pain syndrome may be present that is difficult to manage. Many of these patients suffer from substance abuse and other behavioral problems that require time, patience, compassion, and skill to resolve. Those patients who continue drinking are more likely to have recurrent attacks. In those patients who can stop drinking, the frequency of attacks may decrease. This is an area in which the family physician can apply basic preventive principles to counsel his or her patients with the hope of reducing the number future attacks. Exocrine deficiency may be treated with supplementation of pancreatic enzyme preparations with each meal. Chronic pancreatitis also leads to the need for diabetic management, which is discussed in Chapter 52.

These patients with chronic pancreatitis frequently have complex symptoms, and it is best for them to be referred to a gastroenterologist for evaluation. Depending on the results from the consultation, some of these patients can be successfully followed by their family physician.

Special Clinical Questions

When biliary tract disease is believed to be the cause of pancreatitis and the pancreatitis is stabilized, surgery (cholecystectomy) should be scheduled in the next several weeks if no other contraindications exist. Presumably, additional gallstones will migrate, causing additional episodes of pancreatitis. Therefore, surgery usually should be performed quickly.

Diabetes associated with chronic pancreatitis is usually very brittle. In these instances, the follow-up is most helpful using daily monitoring to the extent that the patient will comply. Hypoglycemia is a very real risk, and frequently, tight control is not possible.

Pancreatic enzymes can be administered clinically, with the physician determining the dose by monitoring the steatorrhea and the patient's weight. Tablets must be given before, during, and after eating until the stool volume and stool fat visibly decrease.

OBSTRUCTION AND DISTENTION SYNDROMES

The family physician cannot proceed to diagnose and manage the remainder of gastrointestinal disorders without a working knowledge of these acute conditions that require hospitalization and urgent consultation. It is not essential to achieve an instantly accurate diagnosis in each case; however, the key is

Table 55–5. CAUSES OF BOWEL OBSTRUCTION AND ABDOMINAL DISTENTION SYNDROMES

Cardiovascular Conditions
- Cardiac low output—congestive heart failure
- Thromboembolism
- Mesenteric ischemia

Medication
- Anesthetics
- Narcotics
- Anticholinergics

Neuromuscular Conditions
- Multiple sclerosis
- Parkinson's disease
- Paraplegia
- Others

Endocrine Conditions
- Diabetes
- Hypothyroidism
- Others

Abdominal Inflammatory Conditions
- Appendicitis
- Cholecystitis
- Diverticulitis
- Pancreatitis
- Pelvic inflammatory disease
- Crohn's Disease
- Ulcerative colitis
- Toxic megacolon

Miscellaneous Conditions
- Ascites
- Aerophagia

Mechanical Obstruction (see Table 55–6)

generic recognition of the cases in which delay would be harmful in the patient. Thus, a final tabular classification of intestinal obstruction and distention syndrome etiologies should assist in completing this section (Tables 55–5 and 55–6). Furthermore, approaches to these conditions may be considered as building blocks for approaches in sections to follow on gastroenteritis, GI bleeding, and inflammatory bowel disease.

William Silen compiled the overall causes of intestinal obstruction from 13 reported series, comprising a total of 12,731 patients. The differences in the distribution of causes between adults and children are seen in Table 55–7.

Table 55–6. MECHANICAL CONSIDERATIONS IN THE DIFFERENTIAL DIAGNOSIS OF BOWEL OBSTRUCTION AND ABDOMINAL DISTENTION SYNDROMES

Luminal Lesions	Extrinsic Lesions
Cancer	Adhesions
Foreign bodies	Abscess
Bezoars, gallstones	Extrinsic tumors
Intussusception	**Strangulating Lesions**
Fecal impaction	Adhesions
Inflammation	Hernias
	Volvulus

Table 55–7. CAUSES OF MECHANICAL INTESTINAL OBSTRUCTION IN ADULTS AND CHILDREN*

Adults	Per Cent	Children	Per Cent
Hernia	41	Hernia	38
Adhesions	29	Pyloric stenosis	15
Intussusception	12	Ileocecal intussusception	15
Cancer	10	Atresias	14
Volvulus	4	Annular pancreas	14
Miscellaneous	4	Adhesions	7
		Miscellaneous	4

*Adapted from Silen, W. (Ed.): Cope's Early Diagnosis of the Acute Abdomen. 15th ed. New York, Oxford University Press, 1979.

Acute Diarrheal Syndromes

BACKGROUND COMMENTS AND IMPORTANT DEFINITIONS

Diarrhea has been defined in many ways. Some believe it means more frequent bowel movements, whereas others have defined it as being the passage of formless stools. More pathophysiologic investigators believe that stool weight per day is the most reliable definition. A good working definition of diarrhea is having more and looser bowel movements than usual.

The clinical questions in office practice may include but not necessarily be limited to the following: How sick is this patient? Is he or she febrile? Is the patient toxic with dehydration or hypotension, or both? Is this an illness requiring hospitalization or consultation, or both? If it is an illness suitable for ambulatory management, is it self-limited? Should an antibiotic be prescribed, or is the best treatment supportive?

Acute gastroenteritis frequently occurs among adults and children. The likelihood of dehydration sufficiently severe to merit hospitalization is more likely among children of developing countries. Several family physicians (such as Mull and Smilkstein) are internationally prominent for their work in oral rehydration therapy and international health. In the United States, the vast majority of the diarrheal illnesses are self-limited and merely require reassurance, dietary counseling, occasional antibiotics, and observation for complications. Rehydration solutions are not commonly required.

CLINICAL EPIDEMIOLOGY AND DIFFERENTIAL DIAGNOSIS

Exceeded in frequency only by upper respiratory infections, gastroenteritis is the second most common illness in the United States. Viral infection is the most common cause of gastroenteritis. Acute diarrheal syndromes are generally defined as those of abrupt onset. These syndromes usually last less than 2 to 3 weeks. Some physicians believe that pediatric acute diarrheal syndromes may last up to 4 weeks or more (Bruckstein, 1988). This section focuses on the infectious causes, which include viruses, bacteria, and parasites. Rotavirus, Norwalk-like agents, other small viruses, and enteric adenoviruses cause many of the viral gastroenteritis syndromes. Stool viral cultures are not indicated. Virus identification does not make a clinical difference, and the tests themselves are difficult and expensive. These viral illnesses are self-limited, and an aggressive diagnostic work-up is not indicated.

Special situations include traveler's diarrhea, food poisoning, diarrhea in the elderly and in children in day care centers, and antibiotic-associated colitis. New office laboratory methods, such as an enzyme-linked immunoassay for rotavirus (Rotazyme) and latex agglutination for *Clostridium difficile* (Marion Labs) will continue to emerge. Decision analysis is combining probability theory with clinical observations to produce a new set of management strategies by which physicians can learn and teach. For example, stool cultures represent the gold standard for the diagnosis of bacterial infection. Since the likelihood of bacterial infection is less than 50 per cent, and since stool cultures require time and expense, it is not clear when the physician should order stool cultures, particularly among infants who are at highest risk for severe complications.

Using regression analysis techniques, the clinical history, and a stool smear for leukocytes, the presence of five or more leukocytes per high-powered field provides a positive predictive value of 59 per cent and a negative predictive value of 97 per cent for bacterial etiology in acute childhood diarrhea. Three historical questions emerge as being helpful:

1. Was the onset abrupt?
2. Were there more than four stools per day?
3. Did the diarrhea start before the vomiting?

Positive answers to all of these three questions provide a more powerful predictor (7 to 1) of a bacterial cause of diarrhea than when only one of the questions was answered negatively (DeWitt et al., 1985). This type of study should be modified to suit various family practice questions and should be replicated.

A reasonable work-up can be better understood if the diarrhea syndromes are schematically classified into inflammatory and noninflammatory causes (Table 55–8). Other diarrheal classifications have been based on osmotic, malabsorptive, and structural factors. For family physicians, Table 55–8 demonstrates that most (but not all) of the diseases that are treatable with antibiotics are inflammatory. Since clinical findings in the different types of inflammation are similar, a set of simple steps should quickly answer the major questions.

Table 55–8. COMMON ACUTE DIARRHEA SYNDROMES* AND BACTERIAL AGENTS

Inflammatory (Fecal Leukocytes Usually Present)	Noninflammatory (Fecal Leukocytes Usually Absent)
Salmonella	Viral infections
Shigella	*Giardia lamblia*
Campylobacter	*Cryptosporidium*
C. difficile	*Vibrio cholerae*
Invasive *E. coli*	Toxigenic *E. coli*
Entamoeba histolytica	Lactose intolerance
Yersinia	Sprue
Crohn's disease†	Staphylococcal food poisoning
Ulcerative colitis†	

*In the correct setting, the addition of a methylene blue stain to a liquid stool specimen can provide strong, but not pathognomic, presumptive evidence for a bacterial infection. Note that some parasitic and idiopathic inflammatory conditions may also produce fecal leukocytosis.

†Does not commonly present as acute diarrhea

PRESENT ILLNESS

Most of these disorders induce some combination of abdominal pain, diarrhea, nausea, vomiting, fever, and tenesmus. Rotavirus is exhibited most frequently in infants and children. After an incubation period of several days, the affected children present with an initial temperature of 37.8° to 38.9° C. (100° to 102° F.). There is associated respiratory distress, vomiting, and some degree of dehydration. The syndrome usually lasts 7 to 10 days, and the stools are generally watery without blood, pus, or mucus. Some clinicians have found it useful to initially investigate these cases via an enzyme-linked immunoassay, which is 97 per cent accurate in identifying rotavirus (Rotazyme) (Kovacs et al., 1987).

The Norwalk agents are the most common causes of diarrhea among adults, whereas rotavirus effects mainly infants and children. The Norwalk virus usually causes a low-grade fever with malaise, which arrives abruptly and lasts for 1 to 3 days. The patient may feel terrible, and the white blood cell count may be extremely variable. Nevertheless, resolution can be expected within 3 days in most cases. The rotavirus illness usually lasts 5 to 6 days and is accompanied by more extensive vomiting and diarrhea. These distinctions are useful only in a retrospective manner. The physician who advises the patient that viral gastroenteritis is likely may suggest that the course can last up to and beyond 7 days. In those cases that last longer, further evaluation is usually necessary.

When the present illness is characterized by diarrhea that contains blood, the probability of such agents as *Shigella, Salmonella, Escherichia coli, Campylobacter,* and *Yersinia* is increased. *Entamoeba histolytica* can produce symptoms ranging from mild to severe dysentery, but it is rare in most parts of the United States. *Yersinia* has been known to mimic acute appendicitis, but fortunately it is uncommon. Nevertheless, *Yersinia*, which can mimic appendicitis, highlights the variability of the syndromes and the need for ongoing observation of patients with severe acute diarrheal syndromes.

PHYSICAL FINDINGS OF VALUE

The pediatric literature has reinforced the value of "soft data" (i.e. the observational gestalt) acquired by the experienced clinician as he or she scans the general appearance of the patient and creates an impression regarding the patient's toxicity. Hydration is assessed by observing the mucus membranes and estimating volume depletion. Orthostatic blood pressure and pulses should be noted. Weight is the most important measurement in children, and it is particularly useful for the family physician who has continuity of care. The intensity of fever indicates the need for hydration.

The abdominal examination generally reveals diffuse tenderness, with normal or increased bowel sounds. Findings of focal tenderness, rigidity, and peritoneal signs are not consistent with viral gastroenteritis. These factors are covered in more detail in the section of acute abdominal pain syndromes. Digital rectal examinations are generally not helpful in adults or children. Abnormal orthostatic hemodynamic measurements may be more prevalent than previously believed. Among 281 adult patients discharged with the diagnosis of acute gastroenteritis, 27 per cent had positive orthostatic vital sign changes (defined as a pulse increase of 30 on standing) (Olshaker and Mason, 1988).

THE DIAGNOSTIC PLAN

The initial work-up requires few studies. A hemogram is usually not necessary. A methylene blue stain of the stool should be obtained and cultures obtained when the stain reveals positive results. Occasionally, the clinician may wish to obtain stool cultures despite the absence of fecal leukocytes. This is rare. Although many diarrhea algorithms exist, excessive laboratory tests are not necessary. Some of the information that follows may be useful in those rare cases in which additional studies have been obtained. For example, eosinophilia on a hemogram is rarely found with a protozoan infestation such a *E. histolytica* or *Giardia*. Peripheral eosinophilia usually indicates the presence of a helminthic infestation such as *Ascaris lumbricoides*, for example. An appropriate travel history may suggest the need for stool samples for ova and parasites. In suspected cases of ambebiasis, a positive indirect hemagglutination titer of greater than 1:256 is helpful.

Recently, *Cryptosporidium* has been implicated as a human pathogen (Scully, 1985). The diarrhea produced by this agent is usually self-limited but may persist for a month. Since no therapy has been effective in immunocompromised patients (who are at greatest risk) and no treatment is necessary in immunocompetent individuals, testing is not advised.

Dehydration and toxicity are the critical criteria for hospitalization. Most frequently, these complications occur at the extremes of age, i.e., among infants and the elderly. For example, patients presenting with delirium clearly should be admitted for further work-up and management. Findings consistent with acute surgical abdomen should be admitted. Patients with serious underlying illness such as severe organic heart disease, malignancy, and vascular diseases may be special cases in which the threshold for hospital admission is lower. As a general rule, the clinician should otherwise accept the wide margin safety associated with these self-limited illnesses.

DIET AND THERAPY

Therapeutic considerations for viral illnesses generally focus on patient comfort and dietary therapy. Even in those cases in which a bacterial agent is strongly suspected, culture results do not arrive until 2 days later. Initial oral fluid and electrolyte replacement may include carbonated beverages and commercially available drinks such as Gatorade. When nausea and vomiting continue to prohibit adequate replacement therapy, hospitalization and intravenous therapy should be considered. Once the appropriate rehydration therapy is tolerated, dietary considerations include food selection, feeding intervals, and meal quantity. It is not necessary to completely rest the bowel, and, as far as possible, the patient should be allowed to select his or her own foods. Since a transient secondary lactase deficiency is common in diarrheal states, milk products are generally avoided. Among infants, reintroduction of lactose-containing substances such as milk may be monitored by testing for stool pH. The presence of a reducing substance or the lowering of stool pH to 4 or 5, as found by using Clinitest tablets or Nitrazine sticks, suggests a continuing disaccharidase deficiency.

In developing countries, diarrhea is a major cause of death and malnutrition in children. The World Health Organization has stated, "Oral rehydration therapy (ORT) is the keystone of all diarrheal disease control programs because it is simple, highly effective, inexpensive, and technologically appropriate. A solution prepared from oral rehydration salts is used both to treat clinically evident dehydration and to prevent dehydration by replacing losses early in the course of disease." The solution recommended by the World Health Organization contains in grams per liter: NACl 3.5; KC1 1.5; trisodium citrate 2.9 (or $NaHCO_3$ 2.5); and glucose 20. Home-based ORT therapy can be given at the onset of diarrhea to minimize dehydration (Mull, 1984; and Mull and Mull, 1988).

Although highly effective in treating dehydration, ORT does not diminish the amount of diarrhea. Appropriate drug therapies are useful adjuncts. Even without drugs, approximately 90 per cent of children with watery diarrhea who visit a health care facility can be successfully and optimally treated solely with ORT and continued feeding. In these developing world situations, antibiotic or antiparasitic therapy should be reserved for patients with dysentery, proved or presumed cholera, or proved infection with *Entamoeba histolytica* or *Giardia lamblia*.

"Currently available adjunct agents, including antimotility and antisecretory agents, exogenous aciduric flora, and adsorbents, have no practical value and increase both the cost of treatment and the risk of adverse reactions. The practice encountered in many countries of routinely treating episodes of diarrhea with multiple adjuncts and antibiotics, sometimes available as combination agents, is to be deplored." Oral rehydration therapy is the only proven cost-effective method of treating routine self-limited diarrhea, and the economic savings from treating the disease in this way can be considerable (World Health Organization, 1988).

In children, clear liquids do not include caffeinated colas. Increasing the number of small feedings may be more effective (i.e., 30 to 60 ounces every 60 minutes) in place of two or three large meals. Some have recommended that fruit juices be withheld because of high osmolality and inherent fruit juice malabsorption potential (Hayms, 1988). In that study, it was interesting to note that evidence of carbohydrate malabsorption was accompanied by symptoms in only 30 to 40 per cent of subjects. Therefore, diet therapy is extremely variable and must be individualized. Adequate caloric intake is important in all cases. Even adults can benefit from variations of the so-called BRAT (bananas, rice, cooked apple, and toast) diet for achieving a return to a regular diet as soon as possible. A return to nearly normal diet can be accomplished even though the stools may remain loose for several days to several weeks or more. Oral electrolyte solutions may also be used (Table 55–9). In some cases, children may have alterations of bowel habit persisting for the remainder of their toddlerhood. In these cases, appropriate growth and development should be monitored. Usually, the child continues to do well.

The most common indication for empiric antibiotic therapy is traveler's diarrhea. The treatment regimen usually consists of sulfamethoxazole-trimethoprin taken twice daily for three days or until symptoms resolve.

Although they are strongly tempted to empirically prescribe antibiotics and antidiarrheals, physicians should resist. Drugs that are effective for one disease may exacerbate another. Antibiotics effective for shigellosis may enhance the carrier state of salmonellosis. Opiate-containing agents such as diphenoxylate hydrochloride and atropine (Lomotil) may actually convert a nonbacteremic dysentery into sepsis or produce serious problems such as toxic megacolon. Opiates and anticholingergics also carry with them the risk of side effects, such as ileus dry mouth, blurred vision, drowsiness, urinary retention, and insomnia. The psychologic benefits for the patient of prescribing a medication are acknowledged. Compounds such as Kaopectate and Pepto-Bismol confer the psychologic benefits and are generally quite safe. The physician should wait for culture results before starting antibiotics (Table 55–10). Certain exceptions may exist, such as treating antibiotic-associated colitis when the history is appropriate. For example, antibiotics may be started in septic shock in an elderly patient with adherent yellowish plaques on the bowel wall, as seen on endoscopy.

There are many other causes of infectious diarrhea, such as *Clostridium perfringens, Listeria monocytogenes, Aeromonas, Hydrophilia,* and *Bacillus cereus*. Each family physician must decide the point at which consultation, hospitalization, or referral is indicated. Symptoms such as nocturnal diarrhea, weight loss of 10 to 20 per cent, and progressive abdominal pain may be important clues that indicate the need for further evaluation. It should be emphasized that the vast majority of the acute diarrhea syndromes are self-limited.

Gastrointestinal Bleeding Syndromes

BACKGROUND COMMENTS

Upper gastrointestinal hemorrhage most frequently presents as hematemesis, or the vomiting of blood or

Table 55–9. SOME ORAL ELECTROLYTE SOLUTIONS*

Product	Concentration When Diluted (mEq per l) *Na*	*K*	*Cl*	*Base*†	Glucose (grams per l)	Form	Cost per Quart‡	mOsm per l
WHO Oral Rehydration Salts	90	20	80	30	20	Powder	$0.35§	333
Rehydralyte (Ross)	75	20	65	30	25	Liquid	40.8	305
Infalyte (Pennwalt)	50	20	40	30	20	Powder	2.88	251
Lytren (Mead Johnson)	50	25	45	30	20	Liquid	3.35	220
Pedialyte (Ross)	45	20	35	30	25	Liquid	2.81	250
Resol (Wyeth)	50	20	50	34	20	Liquid‖	2.52	269
Gatorade	20	3						330

*Modified from Rakel, R. E. (Ed.): Conn's Current Therapy, 1988. Philadelphia, W. B. Saunders Company, 1988, p. 12.
†HCO_3 or derived from citrate.
‡Cost to the pharmacist, based on Average Wholesale Price, "Drug Topics Red Book" 1987 and June 1987 "Update."
§Available in the USA only from Jianas Brothers Packaging, 2533 SW Blvd., Kansas City, MO 64108.
‖Also contains 4 mEq each of Ca and Mg, and 5 mEq of PO_4.
Modified with permission from Conn's Current Therapy, 1988.

Table 55–10. ANTIBIOTICS FOR SPECIFIC DIARRHEA SYNDROMES

Specific Pathogen	Drug	Adult Dosage
Salmonella	Drugs are usually not indicated due to prolongation of carrier state. When absolutely needed, TMP-SMX (Bactrim DS, Septra DS) is given.	1 tablet b.i.d. 500 mg. b.i.d.
	Alternative drug, ciprofloxacin	
Shigella species	TMP-SMX	800/160 b.i.d.
	Alternative, ciprofloxacin	500 mg. b.i.d.
Campylobacter infections	Erythromycin	500 mg. q.i.d. × 5 to 10 days
C. difficile	Oral vancomycin	125 mg. q. 6 hours × 1 week
	Alternative, metronidazole	250 to 500 mg. t.i.d., × 7 days
	Adjunctive, cholestyramine (binds toxin)	4 grams q.i.d.
Food poisoning due to *Staphylococcus aureus*	No antibiotic	
Giardiasis	Atabrine-quinicrine	100 mg. t.i.d. × 7 days
	Alternative, metronidazole (Flagyl)	250 mg. t.i.d. × 7 days
Amebiasis	Metronidazole	750 mg. t.i.d. × 10 days
	For intraluminal phase, use iodoquinol (Yodoxin)	650 mg. t.i.d. × 20 days
	Pepto-Bismol	30/60 ml. q.i.d.
Yersinia enterocolitica	Sensitive to many drugs, but none alter the course	
Traveler's diarrhea	TMP-SMX	800/160 b.i.d.
	Doxycycline	100 mg. b.i.d.
	Alternative, ciprofloxacin	500 mg. b.i.d.

a darker coffee-ground material. Initially, it may or may not be associated with melena, a black-tarry sticky substance with a sickly sweet odor.

Hemorrhoidal bleeding is characterized by the passage of bright red blood after the bowel movement, with soiling of the toilet tissue and toilet water with blood and streaks of bright red blood on the stool. Hematochezia or lower gastrointestinal hemorrhage, on the other hand, becomes manifest by the passage of large amounts of bright red to burgundy-colored stool.

Since hematemesis, melena, or hematochezia due to any cause is associated with significant losses of blood, patients with this condition merit hospitalization. Unwitnessed or dubious self-reports of hematemesis should be evaluated on an urgent basis.

When patients with gastrointestinal hemorrhage are admitted to the hospital, within 24 hours, 90 per cent of them mysteriously stop bleeding. However, relatively rapid diagnosis is advisable in order to plan treatment and possibly to perform intervention endoscopy with coagulation of bleeding sites. Whereas most patients with upper gastrointestinal bleeding have hematemesis or melena, or both, about 15 per cent of these patients have only hematochezia with negative findings in the nasogastric aspirate.

False alarms that mimic melena can be caused by the ingestion of iron, bismuth preparations, and certain fruits such as blackberries and cherries. A fecal occult blood test quickly tells the story. For those patients who are found to be anemic, a stool guaiac test (the most popular of which is Hemoccult) may be positive when there is no physical evidence of GI bleeding. These tests are best obtained from a stool that has been passed rather than after a digital examination, since the digital examination may give false positive results (Longstreth, 1988).

The differential diagnosis of the most common causes of gastrointestinal bleeding is listed in Table 55–11.

CLINICAL EPIDEMIOLOGY

Over a 10-year period, 351 patients admitted with a diagnosis of acute GI hemorrhage were classified by bleeding location as follows: stomach and duodenum, 57 per cent; esophageal varices, 33 per cent; and lower gastrointestinal source, 10 per cent. Emergency surgery was required in almost one fourth of the cases (Greenberg, 1985). This report reflects the typical experience of hospitals serving patients with gastroin-

Table 55–11. DIFFERENTIAL DIAGNOSES FOR GI BLEEDING

Upper GI	Lower GI, Rectal
Esophageal	Diverticulosis
Hemorrhoids	
Varices	Angiodysplasia
Fissure	
Mallory-Weiss	Cancer
Cancer	IBD*
Polyp	
Erosive esophagitis	Ischemic disease
IBD*	
Gastric	Coagulopathy
Other	
Erosive gastritis	Radiation
Gastric ulcer	Colitis
Cancer	Polyps
Varices	Hemorrhoids
Duodenal ulcer	
Epistaxis	

*IBD = inflammatory bowel disease, including Crohn's disease, ulcerative colitis, and many of the infectious diseases such as *Shigella, Yersinia,* and *Campylobacter*.

testinal hemorrhage. However, the rate of emergency surgery is extremely high.

Once patients have been documented to be experiencing gastrointestinal hemorrhage, it is crucial that they be hospitalized as soon as possible. Immediately upon admission to the emergency facility, they should be assessed for evidence of hypovolemia, and at least two large-bore intravenous catheters should be placed. Blood should be tested for type and cross-match as well as coagulation factors. As soon as possible, surgical consultation should be requested.

According to the latest survey, 87 per cent of practicing family physicians maintain intensive care unit privileges and, therefore, remain involved in the management of hospitalized patients with acute GI bleeding (Ferentz et al., 1988). Although many university-based family practice training programs have been unable or unwilling to secure hospital privileges in these areas, the average patient continues to expect and value involvement by the family physician.

UPPER GI BLEEDING

In the office or over the phone, the guiding principle is urgent evaluation. The patient is usually directed to the emergency room if there is any suspicion in the physician's mind of upper GI bleeding. After vital signs have been recorded, the intravenous lines have been established, and blood has been sent for type and cross-match and coagulation tests, the history-taking process and thorough physical evaluation may begin. A nasogastric tube is placed to observe whether any blood is present in the stomach, and whether it can be cleared with cool saline. Testing nasogastric aspirate that has no visible evidence of blood seems to be a worthless endeavor. If hypotension continues before the blood transfusion is ready, the lower part of the body should be elevated, and in some instances, a MAST suit can be utilized.

The patient is asked whether he or she has ever had bleeding before and, if so, what kind. The patient is quizzed about the presence of symptoms of peptic ulcer disease or whether or not nonsteroidal anti-inflammatory drugs have been taken recently. The knowledge of a history of alcoholism is useful, as is a description of easy satiety and prolonged weight loss. These few simple questions cover the most common causes of upper gastrointestinal hemorrhage, namely esophageal varices, peptic ulcer disease, erosive gastritis, and tumor. Physical examination may reveal the stigmata of chronic liver disease, i.e. an abdominal mass, hepatosplenomegaly, and ascites. In most instances, once the patient has been stabilized, endoscopy is carried out. If lesions such as bleeding esophageal varices or a vessel in a peptic ulcer are seen, they are treated. It would seem that sclerotherapy of varices can stop bleeding but does not affect the patient's life course overall. The value of coagulation of bleeding ulcers is still unknown, but the vast literature already amassed on the subject seems to favor the procedure.

LOWER GI BLEEDING

Lower gastrointestinal bleeding can be roughly divided into two vastly different types—(1) hematochezia and massive lower gastrointestinal hemorrhage and (2) minimal lower GI bleeding seen with perianal disease, which is probably the most common cause of bright red blood per rectum. It is very rare for the bleeding of hemorrhoids to lead to anemia.

Patients presenting with large amounts of bright red blood per rectum or maroon stools must be stabilized as described in the previous section on upper gastrointestinal hemorrhage. When the patient is stable, a nasogastric tube should be placed to determine whether or not the source is the upper GI tract. The bleeding in 10 to 15 per cent of patients with hematochezia has an upper GI source.

Patients with lower GI bleeding frequently have no previous history of the condition. The most common causes are diverticulosis, angiodysplasia, carcinoma, and ischemic colitis. The list of less common causes is vast (Cello, 1985; Burakoff, 1985; Steer, 1983).

Not only do patients with lower GI bleeding have no previous history of the disorder, but many have no present symptoms other than GI hemorrhage. The most common causes, namely diverticular disease and angiodysplasia, are asymptomatic. Patients with colon cancer and ischemic colitis may have had a change in their bowel habits and cramping as well.

Once again, as soon as the patient has had two large-bore intravenous catheters inserted and blood has been sent for type and cross-match as well as measurement of coagulation factors, discussion with a consultant is helpful.

For those patients who have massive bleeding and who have been stabilized by blood transfusion, abdominal angiography is done to determine the site of bleeding. In the colon, sometimes embolization may stop or slow the bleeding. If the patient is bleeding at a rapid rate, he or she may also undergo a technetium-tagged red blood cell study that may show the bleeding site. This determination is very important because if emergency surgery is required, the part of the bowel that is affected must be known before it can be resected. Angiodysplasia and diverticuli predominantly bleed from the right side of the colon, but some actively bleeding lesions frequently stop bleeding when the patient is anesthetized and the abdomen is opened. At the time of surgery, it may be impossible to find the source of the hemorrhage. If the bleeding has slowed down or stopped, the patient may then be given a balanced electrolyte purge (GOLYTELY) and colonoscopy may be performed. The site of bleeding can be determined in many patients, and sometimes, treatment is definitive such as when an angiodysplastic lesion of the right colon is cauterized.

PERIANAL DISEASE AND HEMORRHOIDS

Hemorrhoids may defined as varicosities arising from the hemorrhoidal veins in the perianal area (Table 55–12). This affliction of civilization may occur in 50 per cent or more of the population in the United States. Many are fortunate enough not to suffer from hemorrhoids, but some suffer from hemorrhoids repeatedly.

External hemorrhoids originate distal to the dentate line and drain via the inferior hemorrhoidal plexis to the iliac veins. Internal hemorrhoids are located proximal to the dentate line. These vessels come from the superior hemorrhoidal venous plexus, and they drain through the inferior mesenteric veins. Both internal and external hemorrhoids communicate with one another.

Both internal and external hemorrhoids may be asymptomatic. Some patients have no other discomfort than soiling of their underclothing because the hemorrhoids do not allow a hermetic seal of the anus. This may lead to perianal itching and burning from the irritating fecal liquid. The most common presentation of hemorrhoids is asymptomatic bleeding. Most commonly, the person notices blood streaking the stool, and when they wipe themselves, they find blood on the toilet tissue. If the bleeding is significant enough, they see blood in the toilet bowl.

For unknown reasons, hemorrhoids thrombose periodically. If the hemorrhoids are internal, the patient may just notice the prolapsing of tissue with the bowel movement; whereas if the hemorrhoids are external, extreme pain is felt, especially when the patient moves the bowels or even touches the swollen perianal area.

If the patient has acutely thrombosed external hemorrhoids (that is, they are turgid blue and extremely tender), under the proper circumstances and with local anesthesia, the physician can make a nick over the hemorrhoid. Removal of the clot affords the patient some relief. However, if the hemorrhoid has been thrombosed for several days and is "not ripe," the procedure only increases the pain.

Table 55–12. DIAGNOSTIC GRADING SYSTEM FOR HEMORRHOIDS*†

First degree	No prolapse, usually asymptomatic
Second degree	Prolapse during defecation that later reduces spontaneously
Third degree	Prolapse that requires and allows simple manual reduction by the patient
Fourth degree	Prolapse that cannot be easily reduced by the patient

*Adapted from Bedell, A. W.: Thrombosed hemorrhoids. *In* Mayhew, H. E., and Rogers, L. A. (Eds.): Basic Procedures in Family Practice. New York, John Wiley & Sons, 1984.

†This hemorrhoidal classification system is based on the degree of prolapse.

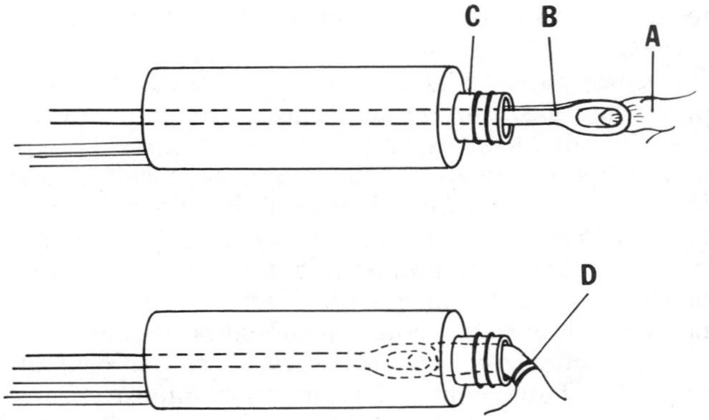

Figure 55–1. Rubber band ligation of an internal hemorrhoid. *A,* Hemorrhoid; *B,* ring forceps; *C,* double-banded ligator; and *D,* double bands. (See text for discussion of the procedure.) (From Mayhew, H. E.: Basic Procedures in Family Practice: An Illustrated Manual. New York, John Wiley & Sons, Inc., 1984, p. 247. By permission.)

When the patient has an acutely thrombosed external hemorrhoid, pain is the most difficult problem. Most salves and ointments really are not very helpful. Sometimes, treatment with an anesthetic ointment can be helpful. The most soothing treatment is for the patient to stay off of the feet as much as possible to decrease the pressure of gravity and also to take sitz baths throughout the day. In this instance, analgesics may be necessary. If a patient has recurring episodes of thrombosis that interfere with the quality of his or her life, local surgical treatments are available. Prior to surgery, these patients should avoid constipation by using bulk agents, and if they feel tissue prolapsing after a bowel movement, they should gently push the hemorrhoids back where they belong.

Ligation (or banding) is a simple and quick method used to relieve *internal* hemorrhoids in the office. It is not appropriate for external hemorrhoids due to the extremely painful nature of the procedure when squamous epithelium is entrapped by the rubber bands that are applied. Specific instruments such as the McGiveny Hemorrhoid Ligator are available from surgical supply houses.

The patient need not be in a knee-chest position. Using a slotted anoscope, the hemorrhoidal complex is visualized. The hemorrhoid is grasped with forceps (Fig. 55–1). Once stabilized, the barrel of the ligator is placed down over the hemorrhoidal complex and a rubber band is mechanically displaced. It is this band placement that ligates the blood supply to the hemorrhoidal complex. When the patient experiences immediate severe pain, this usually indicates that placement below the pectinate line has occurred. In these cases, the rubber band should be snipped off and reapplied. Removal of an inappropriately placed band should be attempted even though there may be difficulty in doing so.

The patient should be advised of a dull ache immediately after application of the ligation. Later in the day, the patient may have a feeling of fullness or an urge to defecate. The patient should resist this urge. The discomfort is rarely severe enough to cause the patient to be absent from work, but symptoms persist at a low level over the next 2 to 3 days. Stool softeners and analgesics are usually prescribed, depending on the individual judgment of the physician. It is not recommended to ligate more than one hemorrhoid every 3 weeks. Hundreds of thousands of these procedures have been performed in offices. Nevertheless, it should be noted that some specialists have stopped performing hemorrhoidal banding. In May of 1985, four case reports described death following rubber band ligation of internal hemorrhoids. These reports underline the fact that increasing pain following hemorrhoidal banding should not be ignored as an insignificant symptom. These reports emphasize that "the combination of urinary hesitancy, perianal pain, and systemic symptoms shortly after ligation of hemorrhoids should alert the physician to a potential life-death threatening condition requiring immediate evaluation and therapy" (Russell, 1985).

ANAL FISSURE

The anal fissure is closely related to the hemorrhoid. A fissure is a crack that occurs in the mucocutaneous line that is very painful, especially with defecation, and that can frequently lead to blood on the surface of the stool. Constipation results because of fear of pain with defecation. On the physical examination of the area, especially with a proctoscope, one may see the fissure, although many of these patients do not allow examination of the area because of discomfort. They may respond to analgesic ointments, but many who continue to have chronic symptoms, do well with a surgical consultation. With the patient under anesthesia, the surgeon stretches the muscles of the anal opening, and this method frequently results in healing of the fissure.

Colorectal Cancer

BACKGROUND COMMENTS

Colorectal cancers appear in 150,000 Americans each year. One half of those people die within 5 years. The majority of these patients have come to the physician after symptoms have occurred. It is now quite clear that for colon cancer, the earlier the stage and the more limited to the bowel wall, the higher the 5-year survival rate. Whereas, 50 per cent of patients who appear with symptoms have died within 5 years, 80 to 90 per cent of those patients with tumors detected with screening programs and found to have tumors localized to the bowel wall will survive. Since the main risk factor in the United States is age, the best way to save people from this disease is to detect it in its early stages by screening the asymptomatic individual over the age of 50.

Screening is especially valuable, since it appears that colon cancers take many years to grow and to become invasive and many of them, if not most, arise from colorectal polyps.

The American Cancer Society Guidelines of 1980 were established on the basis of sophisticated mathematical modeling techniques that have been endorsed by the American Academy of Family Physicians and other institutions. These recommendations include performing annual rectal examinations starting at age 40 and three fecal occult blood tests annually starting at age 50. Sigmoidoscopic examinations are recommended annually starting at age 50. After two negative examinations, the interval between sigmoidoscopic examinations may be extended to every 3 to 5 years.

In clinical practice, the major barriers to early detection have been patient and physician noncompliance. During the 1980's, fecal occult blood testing was widely encouraged as a low-cost, noninvasive method. Enthusiasm was sufficiently high to create television-sponsored mass mailings and supermarket distribution of hundreds of thousands of screening kits. Several published studies are now available. One author believes that these studies reflect the imperfection of mass screening by this method.

DIAGNOSTIC YIELD OF SCREENING

The diagnostic yield of the rectal examination for cancer is low (3 to 5 per cent). Compliance with fecal occult blood tests ranges from 22 to 80 per cent (Rodney, 1985). Elderly patients, with the greatest age-related risk, report a reluctance to lean down into a toilet bowl and attempt to retrieve, with a small wooden stick, a fresh stool specimen to be smeared on a small card. The card is then stored in their house, pending transport by them to their physician at a later time. Many of the recommendations regarding avoidance of false positives such as those that result from the ingestion of red meat, aspirin, and peroxidase-containing foods (beets, radishes, turnips) are usually ignored. The low sensitivity for polyps (5 to 20 per cent) and cancer (25 to 70 per cent) has raised serious doubts about the wisdom of mass screening for fecal occult blood. However, it is the best test physicians have at the present and should be offered to the patient with enthusiasm until we have something better to suggest. Only 3 to 5 per cent of patients over the age 50 are found to have positive fecal occult blood test. About 15 per cent of those patients have polyps, and 2 to 3 per cent of those patients have cancer, most often in a very early stage. It is very important that the fecal occult blood test card be developed as soon as possible after collection, since the true positive rate diminishes rapidly with time. If even one of the three specimens is positive for blood, the patient must be evaluated. A repeat examination is not indicated; it only takes one positive stool sample to be a beacon for carcinoma. Unless there are mitigating circumstances, positive results on the fecal occult blood test should lead to colonoscopy. There is a lot debate about whether or not the patients should have just a sigmoidoscopy and barium enema, since the yield is so low for treatable lesions such as polyps. Considering cost restraints, however, the performance of a barium enema and a sigmoidoscopy would suffice an 85 per cent of those patients with positive stool samples. The other 15 to 20 per cent of patients would require a repeat preparation, this time with a balanced electrolyte purge for colonoscopy and polypectomy.

Poor compliance for rigid sigmoidoscopy had been recorded in multiple studies. However, the 1980's witnessed the introduction of flexible endoscopy into the office of the family physician (Hocutt et al., 1982). Diagnostic yields were higher, patient comfort was improved, the increased capability of visualization was astounding, and the technique was teachable (Rodney, 1984). Sensitivity was 40 to 80 per cent, depending on the depth of insertion, and the predictive value of a positive result was nearly 100 per cent. Videoendoscopy and image processing allowed documentation, remote consultation, patient education, and a variety of powerful information management techniques that could be performed at relatively low cost in the office (Rodney, 1985). A 5-year longitudinal study suggested that flexible sigmoidoscopy in the office was associated with positive changes in the behavior of physicians and patients for all of the colorectal cancer screening tests (Rodney et al., 1985). In this series and most others, it should be pointed out that most procedures were performed in patients with two or more GI symptoms. Significant lesions have been detected among 10 to 20 per cent of family practice patients who are screened for the first time (prevalence yield). Follow-up examinations occurring after precancerous lesions have been harvested (incidence yield) detect lower percentage of significant lesions. These authors highly recommend flexible sigmoidoscopy as a basic diagnostic skill that should be obtained by all practicing family physicians.

Thus, patients over the age of 50 should have a yearly fecal occult blood test, and starting at age 50, patients should have at least two flexible sigmoidoscopic examinations a year apart and then every 3 years thereafter. If an adenomatous polyp is seen on fibersigmoidoscopy, colonoscopy is indicated because in 20 to 30 per cent of the patients, there are more polyps proximally. The battle against colorectal cancer, one of the most common cancers in this country, must be fought at the family physician's office where the physician must convince his or her asymptomatic patients, who are 50 years of age and older, to do uncomfortable things such as collect stools for blood and present themselves for sigmoidoscopy.

The Jaundice Syndromes

BACKGROUND COMMENTS

For purposes of clarity, the first topic presented in this section is neonatal jaundice. Again, for purposes of clarity, we can think of two general classifications of jaundice for clinical use. The first group represents those patients without any symptoms other than jaundice. The other group would include those patients who are symptomatic, usually with anorexia, nausea, fatigue, and are usually suffering from parenchymal liver damage. In contrast, the first group may have anything from cholestatic jaundice to carcinoma of the pancreas. In either of the two cases, jaundice is not a medical emergency. Patients may be jaundiced for as long as 6 months from an obstructed common bile duct before evidence of fibrosis appears. There are a few circumstances in which diagnosis and treatment are necessary, such as in ascending cholangitis with sepsis and acute pancreatitis caused by a stone in the common bile duct. Thus, for the most part, work-up can take place thoughtfully and in an unhurried manner.

NEONATAL JAUNDICE

Background Comments

In 1975, the purpose of identifying neonatal jaundice was to prevent kernicterus, a brain damage syndrome associated with a bilirubinemia of greater than or equal to 20 mg. per dl., leading to seizures and mental retardation. In the subsequent 15 years, millions of infants in the United States have been placed under "bilirubin lights" as prophylaxis for this serious disease. During this time, it has been apparent that we have overexercised the strategy of catastrophic expectations. The major problem has been in the definition of risk for kernicterus. The initial definitions were based on the study of a few infants, with little or no thought given to the effect of the baby's race, feeding habits, and basic principles associated with Bayes theorem (Kivlahan, 1984).

Clinical Epidemiology and Differential Diagnosis

Kernicterus is real, and the differential diagnosis of neonatal jaundice is substantial. Benign physiologic jaundice is the most common type of jaundice that is seen. There are clues that alert the physician to the possibility of abnormal jaundice when jaundice is evident in the first 24 hours. When these clues are present, infection or isoimmunization should be considered. Physiologic jaundice rarely increases by more than 5 mg. per dl. in any one day. Physiologic jaundice does not contain more than 1 or 2 mg. per dl. of direct bilirubin. Finally, physiologic jaundice usually resolves in 1 week in the full-term neonate or in 10 days in the premature infant. When neonatal jaundice exhibits unusual characteristics, a working differential diagnosis should include hemorrhage (such as cephalhematoma), isoimmunization (such as ABO incapability or Rh disease), infection, polycythemia, congenital liver damage, and others.

Useful historical items in assessing risk include the mother's gestational history and a description of the events surrounding birth. A normal comprehensive neonatal physical examination should be performed, but laboratory studies define the syndrome. In the United States, screening is now legislated for hypothyroidism, phenylketonuria, and galactosemia. In addition, most hospitals have a protocol for the acquisition of cord blood while the mother and child are in the delivery room. All infants born to O positive women have a blood type done. If the infant is type A, B, or AB, a Coombs' test is done. When the Coombs' test is positive, additional tests include cord blood for direct and total bilirubin, a hemogram with peripheral smear, and a reticulocyte count. When the cord bilirubin is greater than or equal to 4 mg. per dl., levels are drawn at 4, 8, 12, 18, and 24 hours of age. Further levels are drawn as indicated. If the bilirubin is rising rapidly or phototherapy has been instituted, levels will be drawn more frequently. For the term infant, phototherapy rarely begins unless the bilirubin rises to 10 mg. per dl. before 12 hours of age, 12 mg. per dl. before 18 hours of age, and 14 mg. per dl. before 24 hours of age. Exchange transfusions are rarely initiated unless the bilirubin rises to 20 mg. per dl. or more. In Great Britain, with certain age- and maturity-adjusted guidelines, phototherapy is rarely instituted before the bilirubin rises to 18 mg. per dl. and exchange transfusions usually do not start until the bilirubin rises to 23 mg. per dl. It should be noted that Oriental, Indian, and Hispanic infants have a higher level of bilirubinemia. Among breast-fed infants, 63 per cent demonstrate a serum bilirubin level of 12 mg. per dl. or more at some time. Hospitalization treatment strategies have led to a significant decline in the ability of some mothers to continue breast-feeding their infants. This factor is of concern, since breast-feeding has tangibly documented benefits and the benefits of zealously applied hospital phototherapy have not been documented. Furthermore, the financial costs of phototherapy are significant.

By 1981, a number of investigators were pointing out the need to redefine physiologic jaundice and more closely study the natural history of neonatal jaundice in a variety of settings and ethnic phenotypes (Kivlahan, 1984). Other investigators have pointed out that contemporary definitions of normal serum bilirubin have falsely labeled a group of healthy jaundiced babies with no disease (Maisels et al., 1988). Most frequently, a review of the mother's history, the mother's blood type, and a careful physical examination of the newborn are sufficient to rule out disease and to act on significant data. Repeat serum bilirubin determinations, when indicated, can easily be obtained in the office or during a home visit. Occasionally, hospitalization or consultation, or both, are required. These are rare occurrences. Jaundice that lasts beyond 1 week and a bilirubin level increasing beyond 17 mg. per dl. in the outpatient setting may merit consultation and serial observations on a day-to-day basis.

JAUNDICE IN THE ADULT

For the purposes of clinical discussion, the topic of jaundice may be divided into two types—(1) jaundice with very few other symptoms and (2) jaundice with marked constitutional symptoms. The patients with few symptoms frequently present with obstructive jaundice or complicated parenchymal disease. The family physician should complete a full history and physical examination. The usual liver tests include a bilirubin, serum glumatic-oxaloacetic tramsaminase and serum glutamic-pyruvic transaminase, alkaline phosphatase, and prothrombin time. These tests are followed by an ultrasound examination of the liver to demonstrate if obstruction is present. With this baseline information, the patient with a clearly complicated case may be referred for consultation. The consultant recommends or engages in invasive studies. Most of the time, the patient presenting with constitutional symptoms and jaundice is suffering from hepatitis.

Viral Hepatitis

In the United States, the most common causes of hepatitis are hepatitis A, hepatitis B, and hepatitis non-A and non-B. There are tiny percentages of mononucleosis, toxoplasmosis, and cytomegalovirus, but they are very rare. Very rarely, toxic poisoning, such as with carbon tetrachloride, or an allergic reaction to drugs may mimic hepatitis. It is most important to ask about drug exposure with any patient presenting with hepatitis, since certain drugs such as isoniazid (INH) may destroy the liver if not stopped immediately.

Most patients with hepatitis present with lethargy, fatigue, anorexia, and possibly nausea and vomiting. Some have right upper quadrant pain and discomfort as well as yellow skin and very dark urine. The presence of a high fever above 38.3° C. (101° F.) is not uncommon.

Hepatitis A is very common in industrialized populations and is spread readily where there is a breakdown in hygiene, such as in the less developed countries. This illness, after an incubation period of 2 to 6 weeks, may result in a severe viral hepatitis syndrome, but the vast majority of patients recover within several weeks. There is no chronic carrier state of hepatitis A, so that once the patient acquires the disease, immunity follows. Unfortunately, a very small percentage of patients go on to develop fulminant hepatic necrosis. At the present, there is no way to identify these patients nor is there any way to prevent their downhill course. The antibody that develops after infection is the anti-HAV IgG. Table 55–13 describes the current serologic markers for hepatitis. It is important to do some investigating to find the patient's contacts so that those exposed in the 2 weeks prior to the discovery of the patient's illness may be passively immunized with immune globulin.

Table 55–13. VIRAL HEPATITIS SEROLOGIC TESTS AND KEY DEFINITIONS

Hepatitis A	
Anti-HAV IgM	IgM antibody to hepatitis antigen. The antibody of the IgM class signifies a recent acute infection. This develops at the onset of symptoms and resolves in less than 1 year.
Anti-HAV IgG	IgG antibody to hepatitis A antigen. In the face of a negative Anti-HAV IgM, this indicates a past HAV infection. This indicates the patient is immune and appears 1 to 2 weeks after the IgM antibody.
Hepatitis B	
HB_sAg	Hepatitis B surface antigen is the earliest indicator of the presence of acute hepatitis B infection. It can be present for several months before symptoms and may remain detectable for up to 6 months. Persistence past 6 months may indicate a chronic carrier state.
Anti-HB_s	Antibody to hepatitis B surface antigen is an indicator of clinical recovery and subsequent immunity. It appears 1 to 2 months after HB_sAg disappears, and it may be present for life.
HB_cAg	No clinical significance, not readily available.
Anti-HB_c IgG	Antibody to hepatitis B core antigen is an early indicator of acute infection. It is also a life-long marker that represents past exposure. It may precede the detection of HB_sAg. This persists for years, but does not necessrily confer immunity.
IgM Anti-HB_c	This is an early indicator of acute active infection and is usually short lived (3 to 6 weeks). Persistence of e antigen may suggest the progression to a chronic carrier state.
HB_eAg	Active infection is present and the patient is highly contagious.
Anti-HB_e	Seroconversion from antigen to antibody is prognostic for resolution of infection and, in a carrier, means very low infectivity.
IgM Anti-HB_c	IgM fraction of antibody to hepatitis B core antigen is the test of choice to rule out acute hepatitis B infection. The IgM fraction disappears within the first few months.
Hepatitis Non-A, Non-B	No markers available, epidemiology parallels hepatitis B.
Hepatitis D (Delta Agent)	Markers not commercially available.

Hepatitis B is a tremendous burden in our society. Ten per cent of those who are infected have evidence of chronic infection. This disease has been spread by sexual contact, especially among gays, and by sharing of needles by drug users. In the hospital environment, the virus may be transmitted by needle stick. Prior to screening transfusions for hepatitis B markers, it was the most common cause of post-transfusion hepatitis. Now it accounts for less than 10 per cent. See Figure 55–2 for the schematic course of acute hepatitis B.

Non-A and non-B hepatitis usually follows transfusion up to 6 months later, or it can be a sporadic infection. Research studies now underway are isolating the actual virus particles, and soon more will be known about this disease that, up until now, has defied intensive epidemiologic investigation.

Acute hepatitis A, B, or non-A and non-B frequently is exhibited with anorexia, malaise, nausea, vomiting, and the appearance of jaundice and dark urine. Some patients may have a rash, and some patients may have arthralgias and myalgias. Physical examination usually reveals an unhappy individual who appears jaundiced. The abdomen may be tender, especially in the right upper quadrant where the liver is tender. Gentle percussion tenderness may be elicited as well.

Elevations in the bilirubin, serum glutamic-oxaloacetic transminase, serum glutamic-pyruvic transaminase and alkaline phosphatase levels occur. The level of bilirubin in an attack of acute viral hepatitis may rise as high as 30 mg. per dl. Patients have been identified with acute viral hepatitis who have had serum enzymes in the thousands. An elevation of the alkaline phosphatase level usually suggests a cholestatic phase. If the patient has a high-grade fever and an alkaline phosphatase level ten to twenty times the normal level, a common duct stone with cholangitis must be suspected. The levels of the serum enzymes cannot be used to prognosticate. In other words, the patients with extremely high levels of serum glutamic-oxaloacetic transaminase, serum glutamic-pyruvic transaminase, and bilirubin are not less likely to have total resolution than other patients. Therefore, the liver tests need to be repeated only as a means of determining a general resolution of the illness. The danger symptom of severe parenchymal destruction is an altered sensorium in the form of hepatic encephalopathy. Liver flap as well as prolongation of the prothrombin time is seen.

Since most all of these diseases resolve without complications the patient can be managed as an outpatient, which gives him or her an opportunity to rest when fatigued and to eat hungry. However, the patient must keep utensils and glassware separate and clean and away from other family members. The liver disease is improving when the patient notices a return

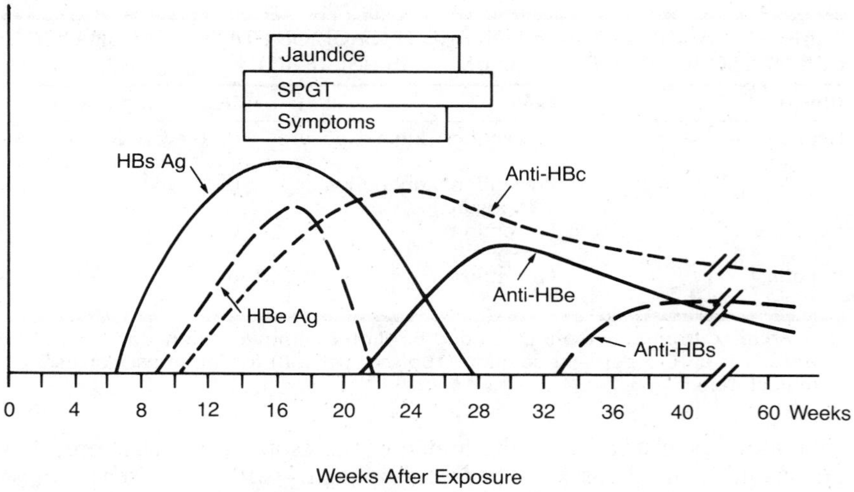

Figure 55–2. The course of acute hepatitis B.

of appetite and a lessening of fatigue. These signs appear before evidence of improvement of the liver on laboratory tests. Should the patient become confused and not be able to eat, hospitalization is indicated and consultation is sought. If possible, it is much more beneficial to allow the patient to recover at home. Not only is this recommended for the patient's good, but when the patient admitted to the hospital, he or she becomes a potential infective source for hospital employees. See Tables 55–14 and 55–15 for the public health services recommendations for immunization for hepatitis.

The clinical course of hepatitis is usually one of recovery over a period of weeks to months. The patient may return to physical activity when he or she feels ready. There is no evidence that premature exercising or physical activity prolongs or worsens acute viral hepatitis. However, if a patient becomes physically active before being ready, he or she feels fatigued and worn out after exercise, sometimes becoming nauseated. Thus, the best approach is to allow the patient to resume his or her life when ready. If a patient with hepatitis does not recover as expected (i.e., exhibits persistent elevation on liver tests and the continuation of symptoms), referral to a gastroenterologist would be indicated.

In many areas, subspecialists, such as gastroenterologists, are ready and willing to be consulted by telephone about a troublesome case that a family physician may be following. This contact is frequently helpful and sometimes may make a referral unnecessary. It may be mentioned parenthetically that no treatment will shorten the course of acute hepatitis or prevent chronicity, including corticosteroids. These medications may make the patient feel better, but they have no effect on improving the disease. Steroids may even lead to chronicity.

The Dysphagia Syndromes

ESOPHAGEAL DISORDERS

Important Definitions and the Differential Diagnosis

Dysphagia describes the subjective report of difficulty in swallowing. Dysphagia is almost always due

Table 55–14. RECOMMENDATIONS FOR HEPATITIS B PROPHYLAXIS FOLLOWING PERCUTANEOUS EXPOSURE*

Source	Unvaccinated	Exposed Person Has Been Vaccinated
HB$_s$Ag-positive	1. HBIG* × 1 immediately† 2. Initiate HB vaccine‡ series	1. Test exposed person for anti-HB$_s$§ 2. If inadequate antibody, HBIG‖ (× 1) immediately plus HB vaccine booster dose
Known source		
High risk	1. Initiate HB vaccine series 2. Test source for HB$_s$Ag if positive, HBIG × 1	1. Test source for HB$_s$Ag only if exposed person is vaccine nonresponder; if source is HB$_s$Ag-positive, give HBIG × 1 immediately plus HB vaccine booster dose
Low risk HB$_s$Ag-positive	Initiate HB vaccine series	Nothing required
Unknown source	Initiate HB vaccine series	Nothing required

*Adapted from MMWR 1985; 34(22):313–334

†HBIG dose 0.06 ml. per kg. I.M.

‡HB vaccine dose 20 μg. I.M. for adults; 10 μg. I.M. for infants or children under 10 years of age. First dose within 1 week; second and third doses, 1 and 6 months later

§Unless the person has been tested within the last 12 months. If the exposed person has adequate antibody, no additional treatment is indicated.

‖Less than 10 SRU by RIA, negative by EIA

Table 55–15. INDICATIONS FOR AND DOSAGE OF STANDARD HUMAN IMMUNE SERUM GLOBULIN FOR INTRAMUSCULAR USE (IGIM)*†

Illness	Goal	Dose (ml. per kg.)†	Comments
Hepatitis A	Prevention, single exposure	0.70 every 2 to 4 weeks	Use higher dose in adults or those persons heavy exposure
	Prevention, continuous exposure	0.02–0.40	Repeat every 4 to 5 months if exposure continues
Hepatitis B	Prevention	0.06 to 0.12	Use if hepatitis B immune globulin unavailable or exposure uncertain
Hepatitis non-A, non-B	Prevention	0.12	Use with transfusions under special circumstances

*Adapted from Anderson, D. C., and Strohm, R.: Immunization. J.A.M.A., *258*:3001–3304, 1987.
†IGIM is a 16.5 per cent solution (165 mg. per ml.) for intramuscular use, available only in 2- or 10-ml. vials from several manufacturers.

to anatomic constriction of the lumen of the esophagus from such diseases as peptic esophagitis with stricture, lower esophageal ring, and neoplasia. These lesions account for the vast majority of patients who present with dysphagia. Much rarer diseases that cause difficulty in swallowing are achalasia, scleroderma, and a vast number of systemic neurologic diseases, including pseudobulbar palsy from stroke. Even rarer causes include extrinsic compression upon the esophagus by an enlarged atrium, aortic arch, aortic aneurysm, mediastinal tumors, or pulmonary cancer. Dysphagia should not be confused with odynophagia, which is pain on swallowing.

The site of obstruction can usually be described easily by the patient by putting a finger over the area. The only exception is that some patients feel a blockage at the gastroesophageal junction in their neck. A sense of obstruction in the neck may indicate globus hystericus. Patients with globus hystericus describe a lump or fullness in the throat that is present all of the time, and yet it does not impede swallowing. Globus hystericus is easily differentiated from dysphagia, and family physicians are aware of its frequent occurrence in response to psychosocial problems. When a patient presents with a description of dysphagia and globus hystericus cannot be easily be ruled out, a full evaluation is necessary, which must begin with upper endoscopy. One author believes that radiography may be an appropriate initial test.

The terms chalasia and achalasia are related to the dysphagia syndromes, since they describe mechanical problems of anatomy relating to the function of the lower esophageal sphincter. Achalasia is a rare cause of infant and adult regurgitation in which the lower esophageal sphincter remains closed and does not relax to permit passage of food. Chalasia is seen in the more frequently observed infant regurgitation syndrome in which the lower esophageal sphincter does not close and feedings are allowed to pass in a retrograde fashion from the stomach.

Clinical Epidemiology

The dysphagia syndromes are not frequently seen, but the family physician encounters several cases in the course of 1 year. Peptic esophageal stricture, lower esophageal rings, and cancer are diseases most prevalent in the middle-aged adult (40 to 60 years). Stroke patients and those with neurologically derived dysphagia represent a group of severely afflicted patients for whom pharyngeal dysphagia represents a special problem. Aspiration, chronic coughing, and decreased food intake are especially difficult problems for these patients. Consultation with specialists in rehabilitation medicine and nursing can be helpful (Gaffne and Campbel, 1974). The geriatric literature points out that these stroke patients can rapidly develop nutritional depletion, aspiration pneumonia, and death. Since there is no effective treatment for most patients with this condition, the recent use of percutaneous endoscopic gastrotomies has increased.

Useful Eponyms

1. Plummer-Vinson syndrome is characterized by iron deficiency anemia, atrophic gastritis, spoon nails, and upper esophageal webs. This condition is extremely rare in the United States.

2. Barrett's esophagus describes the finding of columnar epithelium extending up into the esophagus, displacing the normal squamous epithelial covering. This condition results from chronic gastrointestinal reflux and is frequently associated with esophagitis and stricture. The primary concern is that the metaplastic epithelium of the Barrett's esophagus may be premalignant. Adenocarcinoma within the columnar line segment of the esophagus develops in 3 to 10 per cent of these patients over several years. Some physicians recommend repeated endoscopic evaluations with biopsies every 1 to 2 years to identify the dysplasia that is a forerunner of carcinoma.

3. Schatzki's ring is an circumferential band located at the squamocolumnar junction (lower esophageal ring), and is characterized by the abrupt onset of food sticking in the esophagus. Eventually, the food is regurgitated or passes on, and the patient can complete the meal without difficulty. As the ring gets narrower, the attacks occur more often and the bolus of food that causes the obstruction is smaller. Endoscopic dilatation of these rings preclude the need for surgery. The beneficial effects of this procedure are

permanent, but some patients require additional dilatations several years later.

4. Zenker's diverticulum is located in the proximal (pharyngoesophageal) portion of the esophagus. It is an outpouching that retains undigested food, thereby compressing the true esophagus and producing dysphagia through external compression. Regurgitation of undigested food may follow in a variable period of time, ranging from hours to days. This condition is also a very rare cause of dysphagia.

Present Illness and Review of Systems

The history is very helpful to determine causes of dysphagia. However, once the diagnosis of the symptom is established, all of these patients require upper endoscopy. One author notes that many physicians recommend an initial investigation with barium swallow x-ray studies.

A benign narrowing, such as Schatzki's ring, may be exhibited with acute distal esophageal obstruction when a large piece of food that has not been chewed thoroughly is swallowed. The patient suddenly feels as though he or she is going to choke. The person may salivate and tear and move around rapidly to obtain relief and sometimes tries to drink a carbonated beverage. Eventually, the regurgitation of the food results in complete relief. When these patients do not have an acute obstruction from a large bolus of food, they rarely have any dysphagia whatsoever. This used to be called the "steak house syndrome" (Goyal et al., 1977).

A constant, progressive, and rapidly evolving dysphagia without previous esophageal symptoms suggests carcinoma of the esophagus or cardia of the stomach. Intermittent dysphagia, similar to that occurring with the lower esophageal ring, may be seen in a less dramatic form in the patient suffering from motility disorders of the esophagus. Chronic dysphagia, which is described as waxing and waning in intensity but sustained over the years, is more consistent with some of the neurologic motor disorders or with peptic esophagitis with stricture. If a long history of heartburn (pyrosis) has preceded the development of dysphagia, a benign esophageal stricture is likely to be the cause.

Regurgitation of undigested food, with postprandial gurgling in the neck, several hours after eating is suggestive of a Zenker's diverticulum, but this is a rare problem. In the patient who has sustained a stroke and who has difficulty with speech as well as coughing after eating, oral pharyngeal dysphagia must be suspected.

Physical Findings of Value

For most patients with dysphagia, three physical findings confirm the diagnosis. The most common finding is evidence of weight loss if the dysphagia is especially severe. Patients with carcinoma may have palpable supraclavicular nodes from metastatic disease or upper abdominal masses. Other than these few exceptions, the physical examination is not very helpful. For those very few patients who have neuromuscular dysphagia, usually glaring neurologic abnormalities are evident or the patients have presented with dysphagia after the diagnosis of a disabling neurologic disease. For patients who have sustained large strokes and who have difficulty swallowing, having the patient drink a glass of water is helpful. If the patient starts coughing and liquid comes through the nose, the diagnosis is almost certain. Also, if the patient does not have a gag reflex when a tongue blade is inserted deeply, the diagnosis of pseudobulbar palsy is likely.

The Diagnostic Plan

Initially, the best test is esophagoscopy, which is used to uncover any evidence of luminal obstruction. The only exception to the use of this test is a patient who has a severe neurologic disorder and in whom an oropharyngeal dysphagia is suspected. In these patients, a cine-esophogram with Gastrografin is most helpful.

At the time of endoscopy, if an esophageal stricture or a lower esophageal ring is seen, it could be immediately treated with endoscopic dilation. Any tumors should be biopsied. Achalasia has a typical endoscopic appearance. The esophageal lumen is widely distended, with few or no contractions. The lower esophageal sphincter is tight, but once intubated, the sphincter pops open.

If the results of endoscopy are negative, the next step is to obtain a cine-esophagram, with or without the patient swallowing a bolus of food. From that point, decisions can be made by the consultant for further work-up. Esophageal manometry can be a very helpful test, but it is not available in all areas. Also, it requires a great deal of care and interpretation. The manometric study confirms the diagnosis in achalasia and scleroderma as well as many of the neurologic disorders.

Psychosocial Aspects and Special Considerations

In office practice, the evaluation of dysphagia is frequently straightforward. Most patients with this condition have lower esophageal rings or peptic esophageal strictures that can be treated by endoscopic dilatation.

Less frequently, this common complaint is the tragic precursor to terminal esophageal carcinoma or metastatic carcinoma, or both. With the appropriate consultation for definitive treatment of the primary cancer, the family physician becomes the provider of care and the manager of resources during the terminal phase of these illnesses. This is equally true regarding care and management for those patients with irreversible neuromuscular disorders.

Chest Pain of Noncardiac Cause

Some patients present with chest pain that suggests coronary ischemia, and yet results from a cardiac work-up are negative. Some of these patients are thought to have esophageal spasm. Frequently, they are very difficult to evaluate. For these cases, consultation with a gastroenterologist or a cardiologist for diagnostic evaluation may be helpful.

The Dyspepsia Syndromes

BACKGROUND COMMENTS AND DIFFERENTIAL DIAGNOSIS

This section deals with the most common causes of dyspepsia that are encountered in a family physician's outpatient practice. These include nonulcer dyspepsia, peptic ulcer disease, and reflux esophagitis. All of these conditions cause symptoms that are usually localized in the upper abdomen and lower mid-chest area.

NONULCER DYSPEPSIA

Definitions

Most agree that nonulcer dyspepsia is a variable and frequently vaguely described upper abdominal discomfort that is related to the ingestion of food or drink. During the 1800's, it was viewed as a symptom of overindulgence and sometimes still is viewed in this way. The patient usually complains that immediately after eating, they notice bloating, distention and belching, flatulence, heartburn, and most often, just a mild upset in the upper abdomen. This condition can be described as upset stomach, nausea, or even as pain. Some may emphasize one symptom or all of the aforementioned symptoms. Many of these patients describe their discomfort as "my ulcer," although peptic ulcer disease has not been diagnosed. Only a tiny number of these patients actually have organic disease, and among those who do have organic disease, it is frequently from a peptic ulcer or from nonsteroidal anti-inflammatory drugs.

Clinical Epidemiology

The extraordinary frequency of this generally noninfectious, non-neoplastic disorder is a benchmark tribute to the dietary excesses and physical deconditioning of the 20th century. In addition to adiposity, this condition is associated with tobacco and alcohol. Stress is most often closely related to the symptoms. In the vast majority of patients, these symptoms represent some of the manifestations of the irritable bowel syndrome that affects 20 per cent of the population. Although stress plays a dominant role, a reduction of fatty, greasy foods and spices in the diet, sometimes in conjunction with an antispasmodic or antispasmodic sedative combination, may result in marked relief. When these patients undergo extensive diagnostic evaluations, no organic disease is found. Indeed, they never go on to develop organic disease such as peptic ulcer. This information is very valuable to the patient, since the worry about their abdominal symptoms frequently adds to their overall stresses.

Nonulcer dyspepsia may also be caused by medications that lower the pressure of the lower esophageal sphincter, such as nitrites, anticholinergics, some tranquilizers, and beta-adrenergic agents (e.g., theophylline). Common dyspepsia-producing drugs include the nonsteroidal anti-inflammatory drugs (e.g., aspirin and ibuprofen).

Pregnancy is a self-limited condition that has been associated with lowered pressure of the lower esophageal sphincter. In any female of child-bearing age with the recent onset of dyspepsia, the absence of pregnancy should be confirmed before any medication is prescribed.

In practice, less than 1 per cent of patients who present dyspepsia have organic disease. However, it is the fear of organic disease that frequently causes the patient to seek an appointment. This fear may invoke the ordering of multiple radiologic and endoscopic investigations to rule out cancer. Yet, the vast majority of dyspepsia problems remain idiopathic and self-limited.

Since the symptoms of nonulcer dyspepsia and peptic ulcer disease may be very similar, most physicians suggest that the patients should be placed on a 2-week course of H_2 blockers. If the patient does not improve, endoscopy should then be performed. One author has modified this program in that if the patient does not respond to H_2 blockers after 7 to 10 days, a trial of sedative antispasmodic drugs for another week to 10 days may confirm nonulcer dyspepsia. If these patients have resolution of their symptoms while on H_2 blockers, they should be continued for a total of 6 weeks without further diagnostic studies, since the diagnosis of peptic ulcer disease is very likely. If the symptoms return when the H_2 blockers are stopped at the end of the 6-week period, an endoscopic evaluation is in order.

PEPTIC ULCER DISEASE

Benign gastric ulcers, pyloric channel ulcers, and duodenal ulcers are considered in this section. Esophageal ulcers are dealt with in the section on reflux esophagitis.

Peptic ulcer disease is a very frequent problem that is seen in the family physician's office. Most patients with this condition, unlike the patients with nonulcer dyspepsia, have a fairly straight-forward history. They describe epigastric discomfort as covering a small area or a large area and describe the pain with varying adjectives such as emptiness, burn-

Table 55–16. A RISK-SCORING SYSTEM FOR SERIOUS PATHOLOGY AS THE CAUSE FOR DYSPEPSIA*†

	Risk Multiplier
Age	
50 to 59 years	2×
60 to 69 years	3×
>70 years	4×
Vomiting	2×
Male sex	2×
Smoking	3×
Previous ulcer	3×
Hiatal hernia present	3×

*From Holdstock, G., Harmon, M., Machin, D., et al.: Perspective testing of a scoring system designed to improve case selection for upper gastrointestinal investigation. Gastroenterology, *90*:1164–1169, 1986.

†These six historical items created a weighted score which correctly identified all referral center in the UK.

ing, heaviness, and bloating. The finding that is diagnostic for peptic ulcer disease, however, is that the onset of discomfort occurs half an hour to 2 hours after a meal and is relieved by eating. Some patients also are awakened at 2:00 to 3:00 in the morning and, likewise, are relieved by eating or drinking. The reoccurring postprandial nature of the symptoms, with complete relief or almost complete relief by eating or drinking, is almost as good as a diagnostic study. When asked, many of these patients describe previous episodes that lasted for weeks or months, interspersed with periods that were totally symptom free. This is another classic symptom of peptic ulcer disease that does not occur with nonulcer dyspepsia.

The only positive physical finding may be mild epigastric tenderness. Carcinoma of the stomach is suspected when a patient in their late 40's or 50's presents for the first time with dyspepsia, anorexia, and co-existing weight loss. Table 55–16 depicts a risk-scoring system for malignancy.

Therapeutic Considerations

The American College of Physicians created a formal policy statement in response to the perceived overapplication of diagnostic testing for the dyspepsia syndromes (Kahn, 1985). Physicians were urged to use clinical judgment, technologic restraint, and, where appropriate, empiric therapy (Read et al., 1982). Thus with dyspepsia or suspected peptic ulcer disease, therapy would precede laboratory investigations. This plan of action would not hold for those patients who were suspected of having organic disease other than a peptic ulcer. The following statement is a useful rule of thumb for sequencing most diagnostic strategies of the isolated dyspepsia syndromes. *Endoscopy is reserved for two subsets of patients: for those who have no response or minimal response to empiric therapy after 7 to 10 days; and for approximately 30 per cent of patients whose symptoms persist (improved, but not resolved) after a 6 to 8 week period of empirical therapy. If all dyspeptic patients are treated empirically, considerable diagnostic resources will be saved* (Kahn, 1985). One of the authors elects to treat dyspeptic patients who seem to have the irritable bowel syndrome with a 2-week trial of sedative antispasmodics rather than H_2 blockers.

A wide variety of therapeutic agents are available (Table 55–17). Note that most of the agents have received FDA approval on the basis of proven effectiveness for documented dyspepsia due to peptic ulcer disease. It is acknowledged that many of these drugs have been prescribed for nonulcer dyspepsia, even though these agents have not proved helpful in clinical trials in nonulcer dyspepsia (Nyren et al., 1986). The most helpful recent changes have been the effectiveness of the once-a-day bedtime regimens, replacing the initially recommended four-times-a-day protocols. Furthermore, there has been evidence supporting maintenance therapy at reduced dosages (cimetidine, 400 mg. every hour of sleep; ranitidine, 150 mg. every hour of sleep; famotidine, 20 mg. every hour of sleep). Antacids continue to be an approved modality (Goodson et al., 1986), but patients usually prefer the ease and convenience of pills. When antacids are used, special attention should be given to selecting an agent with high neutralizing ability (Maalox TC, Gelusil II, Mylanta II), the right amount (30 ml., *not* a tablespoon), and the correct schedule (1 hour after meals; at bedtime, repeat the dosage 3 hours after meals if not eating; attempt to take seven dosages a day) (Drake and Hollander, 1981). Not only is this program almost impossible to follow, but also guarantees the development of diarrhea as well as noncompliance. The H_2 blockers are the treatment of

Table 55–17. COMMONLY PRESCRIBED AGENTS FOR THE EMPIRICAL THERAPY OF PRESUMED DYSPEPSIA DUE TO PEPTIC ULCER DISEASE*

Agents	Dosage Schedule
H_2 receptor antagonists	
Cimetidine (Tagamet)	300 mg. a.c. and h.s. or 400 mg. b.i.d. or 800 grams q.h.s.
Ranitidine (Zantac)	150 mg. b.i.d. or 300 mg. q.h.s.
Famotidine (Pepcid)	20 mg. b.i.d. or 40 mg. b.i.d. or 40 mg. q.h.s.
Nizatidine (Axid)	300 mg. q.h.s.
Sucralfate (Carafate)	1 gram q.i.d. or 2 grams b.i.d.
Antacids	
Liquid	140 mEq. (usually 30 ml.); 1 h and 3 h.p.c. and q.h.s. or
Tablet	120 mEq. tablet q.i.d.
Omeprazole† (Losec)	Use indicated only under special circumstances

*A variety of other drugs such as anticholinergics, tricyclic antidepressants, bismuth preparations, and prostaglandin analogues have been tried overseas but have not been proved to be as effective as H_2 blockers for the treatment of peptic ulcer disease. There is little evidence that combined therapy accomplishes more than the administration of individual agents.

†Not released in the United States.

choice because of their ease of administration, patient compliance, and clinical response.

Generally, the H_2 receptor antagonists have overshadowed all other drugs. Although side effects exist, they are rare. The margin of safety is judged by some to be so large as to merit over-the-counter (OTC) status for cimetidine by the 1990's. Although there is much discussion regarding the relative advantages and disadvantages of the three widely available H_2 receptor antagonists, the effectiveness of these agents are probably equivalent for most noncomplicated cases. Patients frequently notice some improvement in 1 to 3 days, which is in contrast to sucralfate and antacids that take a longer amount of time to work.

A problem arises in pregnant patients who have peptic ulcer disease. None of these drugs has been shown to be free of teratogenic effects in humans. Thus, these patients must tolerate antacid programs or use sucralfate, which has no systemic effects.

For those patients taking many drugs, such as the elderly, ranitidine is probably better than cimetidine (Tagamet), since it is less likely to cause drug interactions.

Once a therapeutic agent is selected, it seems reasonable to treat the patient for a period of 6 to 8 weeks and then to stop. Ninety per cent of ulcers have healed by that time. If the symptoms do not return, no further investigation or treatment is necessary. More than half of such successfully treated patients have a recurrence of the condition. It seems reasonable to reinitiate therapy when a recurrence is brought to the attention of the physician. A reevaluation at that time would be necessary to determine whether or not aggressive invasive diagnostic studies should be carried out. Once again, there are well-respected experts on both sides of this decision. A recent study followed a group of patients with duodenal ulceration for 5 years. Half of the patients were randomized to receive cimetidine continuously, whereas the others received it intermittently (i.e., for symptoms only). At the end of 5 years, the patients receiving continuous therapy had a 24-per cent probability of remaining symptom free, whereas none of the patients receiving intermittent therapy had remained symptom free (Wade and Roley-Jones, 1988). This study points out that any patient who has two or more relapses within 2 years probably is a candidate to be maintained on continuous H_2 receptor antagonist (or an equivalent) therapy. Some patients would still rather wait for symptoms to appear and then initiate a full therapeutic program. This is quite acceptable, since symptoms are usually obliterated in 2 to 5 days and, in the early stages, are not severe. The optimum duration and the long-term effects of these treatment strategies are unknown.

If a patient fails the trial period of H_2 blockers and a gastric ulcer is found through endoscopy, multiple biopsies around the rim are obtained to determine whether the lesion is benign or malignant. It would appear that waiting 2 to 4 weeks on an empiric H_2-blocker regimen would not affect the outcome of a patient with gastric carcinoma.

Patients with nonulcer dyspepsia and peptic ulcer disease are best cared for by the family physician. Thus, by seeing the patient in continuity with a full understanding of the patient's family history, life style, personal values, and medical history, the physician is uniquely helpful. In selected cases, the family physician may ask consultants to evaluate the patient, and when the assessment is completed, the patient returns to the care of the family physician.

GASTROESOPHAGEAL REFLUX

Gastroesophageal reflux is an extremely common symptom. It is almost always associated with a large or small hiatal hernia. The most common symptom is substernal burning after eating, with the patient describing the sensation as rising up from the epigastric area to the neck. It is made worse by fatty foods, spicy foods, and large meals, especially if accompanied by alcohol or caffeine. When these patients do heavy lifting or bending, they may actually feel food or liquid rising into their throat, and some are awakened at night with a suffocating cough, as acid and gastric contents rise up into the throat. The substernal burning is frequently relieved by drinking fluids, especially antacids. When the pain is intense, it may mimic coronary heart disease and may even radiate up into the jaws and down both arms.

Most of the patients with reflux esophagitis do not have visible abnormalities on endoscopy. But if they are biopsied, it will be noted that the superficial layers of squamous epithelium are thinned and the rete pegs of the sensory nerve endings are close to the surface. The physician cannot tell by history alone whether the patient has ulcerative esophagitis with peptic ulcerations or just acid reflux symptoms. The main complication of reflux esophagitis is peptic ulceration and stricture, which is very uncommon. An increased risk of cancer appears only when a Barrett's esophagus develops as a result of chronic reflux.

It is unclear why gastrointestinal reflux is symptomatic in some patients and not in others. Common findings in the symptomatic group are obesity and dietary indiscretion, possibly combined with smoking.

Diagnosis

When patients present with typical symptoms of reflux esophagitis, a therapeutic trial is in order. Endoscopy is not necessary at this stage, nor is an upper gastrointestinal series. First, the patient is instructed carefully about his or her diet. The patient is told avoid greasy foods, fatty foods, and spicy foods because they enhance reflux. The size of the patient's meals should be diminished, and the patient should have nothing to eat for at least 3 to 4 hours before bedtime. Caffeinated beverages may be allowed in moderation and are not harmful. Decaffeinated beverages frequently produce more symptoms because of the way they are prepared. It is known that spicy foods cause symptoms but do not physically harm the mucosa. The reaction is similar to pouring alcohol over a cut. It hurts, but the cut is not made larger and healing is not affected. If the patient smokes, he or she is encouraged to stop. If the patient is unable to stop, he or she should at least cut down. Also the patient should be asked carefully about the use of any irritant drugs such as nonsteroidal anti-inflammatory drugs.

If the patient is overweight, he or she is encouraged to lose, since loss of weight of even 5 to 10 per cent may result in tightening of the lower esophageal sphincter and a decrease in reflux. The patient is also advised to place a 3- to 4-inch block under the bedpost at the head of the bed, so that when sleeping at night, there is encouragement for the acid and reflux material to stay below the sphincter. For those patients with milder symptoms, antacid tablets and antacid liquid may be used. For those patients who have very severe symptoms, H_2 blockers are prescribed and sometimes continued for many months. If the patient does not experience improvement or has any symptoms of dysphagia whatsoever, the physician should seek a consultation from a gastroenterologist for further evaluation.

Gastropathy Due to Intake of Nonsteroidal Anti-Inflammatory Drugs

This topic is added to the discussion of dyspesia because so many people take these compounds for various aches and pains. Although cited as having fewer side effects than aspirin, they are associated with gastric ulceration and hemorrhage in a small number of patients. Some patients who have symptoms when taking the drugs have no ulcers on endoscopy. Other patients who have gastrointestinal hemorrhage without prior symptoms are found to have ulcerations in the stomach or duodenum, or both. Thus, the endoscopic appearance may be totally unrelated to the symptoms.

If the patient who is taking these drugs develops symptoms, the drug is suspended and the administration of an H_2 blocker is started. Depending on the severity of the condition, enteric coated aspirin (Ecotrin) may be used or the physician may choose one of the nonacetylated salicylates such as Trilisate, Salsalate, or Dilazid. If symptoms reccur or continue despite the administration of H_2 blockers and the drug must be continued, consultation may be requested for evaluation and possible endoscopy at this time.

It is important to note that a patient who has a history of an ulcer while taking aspirin in the past should be taking H_2 blockers while they are taking nonsteroidal anti-inflammatory drugs, even if the administration takes place over a prolonged period of time.

Chronic Abdominal Pain and Diarrhea

Background Comments

Many patients who come to the family physician complain of chronic abdominal pain and diarrhea. The task is to differentiate functional from organic disease and then to be able to apply the proper therapy. The vast majority of these patients are suffering from irritable bowel syndrome. The following discussion should help the physician arriving at the correct diagnosis.

INFLAMMATORY BOWEL DISEASE

History of Present Illness and Pathophysiologic Correlations

Of the two major categories of inflammatory bowel disease, ulcerative colitis and Crohn's disease have several unique pathologic features and some distinct clinical differences that help to distinguish them.

There is no known cause for these diseases. Ulcerative colitis is limited to the colon and rectum. Crohn's disease may involve any part of the gastrointestinal tract from the mouth to the anus. Five per cent of patients with either of these disorders may have extraintestinal manifestations. Ulcerative colitis, which also includes proctitis and proctosigmoiditis, involves the rectum in over 95 per cent of the cases, and if there is proximal spread, the involvement is continuous and symmetric. Crohn's disease, on the other hand, involves the rectum in less than 50 per cent of the cases, and the mucosal abnormalities are discontinuous, asymmetric, and patchy. In ulcerative colitis, the mucosa is primarily involved, whereas in Crohn's disease, the entire thickness of the bowel wall is affected by the inflammatory reaction. This explains the predominance of obstruction, abscesses, and fistulas in Crohn's disease. These lesions are rarely seen in ulcerative colitis. Multiple granulomas can be found in diseased tissue in 60 per cent of patients with Crohn's disease, whereas there are none in ulcerative colitis. In irritable bowel syndrome, the mucosa and biopsies of the wall of the bowel are normal. The finding of a severe perianal fistula with burrowing and abscesses are hallmarks of Crohn's disease.

Clinical Epidemiology

The incidence of idiopathic inflammatory bowel diseases crosses racial and ethnic barriers. In the United States, irritable bowel disease seems to be a much more common among whites than blacks and among females than males. The median age of presentation is approximately 30 years of age, with about 25 per cent of patients presenting in their teens.

Although there are no genetic markers, disease clusters in families have been noted in approximately 30 per cent of the cases. Although some have speculated that there is a male predominance in Crohn's disease and a female predominance in ulcerative colitis, these distinctions are not useful in clinical practice. It should be noted that there have been secondary peaks in the incidence of ulcerative colitis and Crohn's disease during or beyond the 6th decade (Kirsner and Shorter, 1982). Utilizing data from the Mayo Clinic Epidemiology Project, the prevalence of chronic ulcerative colitis among residents of Rochester, Minnesota during the 19-year period from 1960 to 1979 was 225 per 1,000,000 population (Treacher et al., 1986).

History of Present Illness and Review of Systems

Most patients with inflammatory bowel disease present with chronic diarrhea that may not be different in any way from the diarrhea of patients with irritable bowel syndrome. However, when diarrhea is bloody, inflammatory bowel disease is more likely. Weight loss and awakening in the middle of the night because of diarrhea almost guarantees the diagnosis of organic disease. In youth, retarded growth or delayed puberty is common with Crohn's disease. Other symptoms such as fever, anorexia, and weight loss are common with inflammatory bowel disease. Extraintestinal manifestations such as iritis, nondeforming arthritis, ankylosing spondylitis, erythema nodosum, pyodermic gangrenosum, and aphthous ulcers can occur in 2 to 5 per cent of patients with inflammatory bowel disease but never in patients with the irritable bowel syndrome.

Most patients with ulcerative colitis present with diarrhea that is mild to moderate and without constitutional symptoms. The more severe the illness, the greater the number of stools and the more likely they are accompanied by constitutional symptoms such as fever, fatigue, and weight loss. The course of ulcerative colitis can be intermittent with flare ups, and remission can occur without therapy. A minority of patients with ulcerative colitis present with severe or fulminant panniculitis, ranging from an acute abdomen to toxic megacolon, and there is little doubt that these patients need urgent hospitalization. During an exacerbation, patients with ulcerative colitis and Crohn's disease may look and feel very ill, yet if the disease is mild, they may appear normal except for the complaint of diarrhea.

When Crohn's disease primarily involves the colon, the condition may be indistinguishable from ulcerative colitis. Since Crohn's disease frequently affects the terminal ileum or the terminal ileum and the right side of the colon, patients with this condition may have steady right lower quadrant pain due to transmural inflammation. The pain may worsen with movement. Sometimes abscesses may develop because of the microperforations in the area of disease, and sometimes acute small bowel obstruction appears because of cicatricial narrowing and the injudicious ingestion of high-residue food. Some of these people develop painful perianal fissures and fistulas that are diagnostic of Crohn's disease.

Physical Findings

The patient with ulcerative colitis or Crohn's disease may exhibit weight loss and anemia. Oral aphthous ulcers may be present. Less frequent findings are erythema nodosum, iritis, and asymmetric nondeforming arthritis. In Crohn's disease, a tender mass may be felt in the right lower quadrant. During the illness, the abdominal examination may reveal mild to severe tenderness. However, during remissions, the results of the physical examination may be entirely negative. When a mass is palpated, the possibilities raised are matted inflamed loops of small bowel versus an abscess. Bowel sounds are not helpful unless the patient presents with severe cramping abdominal pain and distention. In this severe setting, a lack of bowel sounds suggests obstruction. Positive fecal occult blood in a patient with chronic diarrhea changes the diagnosis from functional to organic disease, requiring a full evaluation. Pelvic examination should be performed in all females. At the bedside of patients with irritable bowel syndrome, the tenderness of muscle spasm–related pain tends to diminish with persistent palpatory pressure, whereas the inflamed bowel causes a pain response that does not diminish and frequently becomes more uncomfortable.

Endoscopic Examination

Sigmoidoscopic examination and fecal occult blood testing should be part of the examination in all patients presenting with chronic diarrhea. Colonoscopy of the cecum is not always required, but flexible sigmoidoscopy, widely available in many offices, is essential for the initial evaluation.

Endoscopically, the findings of confluent erythematous inflammation of the rectum is most consistent with ulcerative colitis and infectious colitis. Pseudopolyp formations indicate chronic inflammatory colitis. Solitary aphthous ulcers, rake-like lesions, strictures, and rectal sparing are very consistent with Crohn's disease. In cases in which dense inflammation is seen, the physician should only perform a biopsy, since the risk of iatrogenic perforation is high. Once the endoscope is already inserted, it remains appropriate to obtain biopsies beneath the peritoneal reflection, even if no abnormalities are seen. Frequently, neutrophilic infiltration may be seen in a mucosa that appeared normal to the observer's eye. Thus, biopsies of normal mucosa may be helpful if the clinical history is strongly suggestive.

The finding of anal or perianal lesions, such as sinus tracts, rectovaginal fistulas, and abscesses, is consistent with Crohn's disease, but not with ulcerative colitis. The mucosa in a patient with Crohn's disease may appear cobblestoned or nodular. Pseudopolyps may appear in Crohn's disease and ulcerative colitis. Loss of haustra or distortion of normal architecture, or both, may be found. Light reflection patterns and subtle signs of edema (loss of vascularity) may be helpful in directing the clinician to biopsy certain affected areas.

The Diagnostic Plan

Among patients presenting with diarrhea, fecal occult blood testing and leukocyte smears are obtained. Positive results merit stool cultures for pathogens and smears for ova and parasites when applicable. A fibersigmoidoscopy could be done with biopsies. When inflammatory bowel disease is suspected, consultation is usually sought from a gastroenterologist.

Among patients presenting with diarrhea, fatigue, anemia, loss of skin turgor, weight loss, and positive orthostatic measurements, hospitalization is ordered and a consultation is requested. The majority of patients with inflammatory bowel disease initially consult their family physician and are documented as outpatients. Very few patients have clear-cut cases of inflammatory bowel disease, and it is up to the family physician to distinguish them from the multitudes with the irritable bowel syndrome.

In patients with chronic intermittent abdominal pain, altering diarrhea with constipation, and those with chronic diarrhea who lack any constitutional symptoms, it may be entirely appropriate to order no studies and simply advise them to maintain a low-fat, low-residue diet with the addition of a bulk agent or sedative antispasmodic, or both. If the patient has irritable bowel disease, he or she usually is markedly improved within a 2-week period, whereas the patient with inflammatory bowel disease has no significant recovery. Patients who experience prolonged diarrhea for the first time at the age of 40 or older require sigmoidoscopy and barium enema to rule out colorectal cancer.

Endoscopic biopsy results that are consistent with nonspecific inflammation mean absolutely nothing. The patient's presentation determines the need for consultation. When the endoscopic findings are clearly abnormal or if biopsies of normal tissue demonstrate significant polymorphonuclear inflammation, consultation may be useful.

Because of the increasing risk of cancer in ulcerative colitis over time, when patients have had ulcerative colitis for 8 years or more they should receive colonoscopic surveillance (Lashner, 1988).

THE IRRITABLE BOWEL SYNDROME

Introduction

This common malady exists in 14 to 17 per cent of the population, most of whom do not seek medical care. By far, irritable bowel syndrome is the most common cause of chronic abdominal pain, diarrhea, and constipation. It is second only to the common cold in causing loss of time from work, and patients with this condition account for 50 per cent of the patients seen by gastroenterologists.

Irritable bowel syndrome is a functional disorder that does not have any evidence of structural abnormalities, and it never becomes an organic disease, although many patients who have it are concerned about the development of carcinoma or colitis. The syndrome appears in the late 20's, although it may occur in the teens and in patients as old as age 40. Beyond that time, the physician must suspect organic disease. In the United States, females with the condition predominate over males, whereas in India, the opposite is the case, so there must be some type of culturally dictated difference relating to the cause of irritable bowel syndrome.

The syndrome can be roughly broken down into four types, although many patients have mixtures of one or more.

1. Alternating diarrhea with constipation. These patients may continue for several days without any bowel movements, and then they awaken early in the morning and pass a formed stool. They may need to return several more times to pass increasingly soft stools. Then they may continue through the entire day without bowel activity, or they may move their bowels once or twice after a meal. The onset of diarrhea may occur after severe lower abdominal cramping in the midline or left or right lower quadrant.

2. Nervous diarrhea. These patients have diarrhea frequently after meals as well as following stress. The onset of diarrhea may occur suddenly and with little cramping pain.

3. Constipation is a very common malady in our country, and patients complain of an inability to move their bowels and have difficulty moving their bowels when the delayed urge arises. This does not relate to those patients who have the wrong conception about bowel activity, namely, that they should have a bowel movement every day.

4. Upper gastrointestinal distress with bloating, distention, and discomfort after eating. This has been described with the upper gastrointestinal dyspeptic syndromes and is known as nonulcer dyspepsia.

Pathophysiology

Patients with irritable bowel syndrome are hypersensitive to bowel stimulation. Many studies have been done to demonstrate this hyperreaction. When their bowel is distended with the nasogastric tube patients with the irritable bowel syndrome tube experience discomfort and pain long before a control patient with no irritable syndrome. These patients are most sensitive to food and emotional distress. If these patients are given spicy foods or large amounts of roughage, they will frequently complain of abdominal distention, cramping, and sometimes, diarrhea. If the patients are under stress, their symptoms may become markedly intensified and they will become even more sensitive to food. An analogy that may be pointed out to them is the albino person, for whom normal sunlight can cause skin burning, whereas normal sunlight has no effect on someone else without the problem.

There is an increased incidence of the condition in families of patients with the irritable bowel syndrome, and that information may be helpful.

On physical examination, the only findings may be a tender left lower quadrant, sometimes with a rope-like loop of tender colon. Results of diagnostic studies such as sigmoidoscopy, barium enema, stool cultures, and occult blood are negative. Sometimes, sigmoidoscopy with air insufflation reproduces the patient's pain and discomfort. This reaction may help the family physician determine the patient's response to noxious stimuli.

Differential Diagnosis

The differential diagnosis of irritable bowel syndrome includes the inflammatory bowel diseases, as described in the previous section. Lactose intolerance may mimic the irritable bowel syndrome and can easily be discovered by having the patient avoid milk completely for a period of 3 to 5 days. If the symptoms markedly improve or cease altogether, the diagnosis is established.

Treatment

It must be emphasized that patients with irritable bowel syndrome are not malingering. They do have true pain and discomfort secondary to the hypersensitivity. Similarly, some people blush and sweat more easily than others. The patient must understand that the family physician is aware that the condition is a true physical problem and not an imaginary illness. In these patients, acute or chronic emotional stresses may bring on or enhance the irritable bowel syndrome. Thus, one of the first issues that must be addressed is the possibility of any stresses that occurred at the time that the disease appeared or intensified. It is at this point that the family physician must explain to the patient that he or she is looking for a cause of increased sensitivity of the bowel, and that the patient's conscious mind has no control over the condition. If the physician is able to identify psychosocial issues, these should be addressed on an individual basis. However, the patient should not be probed aggressively for causes of stress, since this will make them more stressed. At this point, treatment of the physical symptoms should be attempted. With time, the patient may be willing to talk about stresses or may become aware of them. The patient's diet should not include spicy foods, fried foods, and fatty foods. Likewise, the patient should not eat very large meals at one time or raw roughage in large quantities, such as fruits, vegetables, or salads. Certainly, a salad and a fruit a day is fine. The patient is then advised to take a bulk agent. Usually, psyllium seeds are recommended because this bulk agent seems to be tolerated much better by these patients. The dosage can start out as 1 heaping tablespoon a day in a glass of juice or water, which can be taken at any time. If no improvement occurs after 1 or 2 weeks, then an antispasmodic agent may be added, and if the patient is exceptionally stressed or anxious, a sedative antispasmodic may be used. Table 55–18 describes various medical therapies that have been recommended. If the patient does not get better with this regimen, consultation with a gastroenterologist would be appropriate.

If the patient is amenable, some form of psychotherapy may be very beneficial. A study showed that even a short course of ten psychotherapy sessions improved the treated group when compared with a control group who received no psychotherapy (Svedlund et al., 1983).

Patient Education

It should be pointed out that excellent patient education materials are available from the National Foundation for Ileitis and Colitis, which has an office in New York City. Two excellent resource books include *The Crohn's Disease and Ulcerative Colitis Fact Book* and *People Not Patients.* An excellent four-page handout entitled "Coping with Irritable Bowel Syndrome" was published in the August 1982 issue of *Drug Therapy* (Freedman, 1986; Schuster, 1987). Additionally, some excellent dietary tips are available in the literature (Freedman, 1986; Schuster, 1987) and from commercial sources, such as the Patient Information Library.* Some family physicians believe that the use of videoendoscopy may be an important patient education technique that allows the patient and the families to actually visualize the intestinal mucosa (Rodney, 1987).

Endoscopic Diagnosis and the Role of Biopsy in the Office

During the past 10 years, new perspectives on colorectal disease have developed from multiple studies describing office-based flexible sigmoidoscopy. Relatively low-priced video and computer enhancement techniques allow physicians to recognize and understand colorectal lesions in an improved way. In particular, videoendoscopy has provided a new dimension—information management. This dimension of image processing can be manipulated by the physician to improve diagnostic skill. Case management, patient education, and compliance issues also appear to

*Patient Information Library, 345-G Serramonte Plaza, Daily City, CA 94015, phone number 415-994-1150.

Table 55–18. ORAL THERAPY FOR SYMPTOMS OF IRRITABLE BOWEL SYNDROME*

Agent	Dosage	Comments
For Constipation-Predominant Irritable Bowel Syndrome—Cathartic Agents		
Psyllium agents, e.g., Metamucil, Konsyl, Modane	1 tablespoon daily t.i.d.	Usually with meals or in juice, start dosage low to avoid gas, encourage at least eight glasses H_2O daily, avoid other cathartics
Lactulose	15 to 30 ml. daily t.i.d.	Individually titrated to desired bowel pattern
Others		
For Diarrhea-Predominant Irritable Bowel Syndrome—Constipating Agents		
Psyllium agents	As above	As above
Loperamide	4 mg. initial dose, followed by 2 gm. for q. unformed stool	Average daily dose 4 to 8 mg., now available over-the-counter
Diphenoxylate HCl (Lomotil)	2.5 to 5.0 mg. after each unformed stool	Maximum daily dose 20 mg., average dose 2.5 to 5.0 mg. b.i.d.
Codeine phosphate	7.5 to 30 mg. daily b.i.d.	Not recommended, risk of addiction
Aluminum hydroxidigel (Alugel)	30 ml. of 3 to 4 hrs. p.r.n.	Use with caution in patients with chronic renal failure
Anticholinergic-Antispasmodic Agents		
Dicyclomine (Bentyl)	10 to 20 mg. b.i.d. or q.i.d.	No clinical trials, have established benefit
Clidinium (Quarzan)	2.5 to 5.0 mg. a.c. and q.h.s.	Not proven by clinical trials
Propantheline bromide (Probanthine)	15 mg. a.c., q.h.s.	Not proven by clinical trials
Glycopyrrolate (Robinul)	1 to 2 mg. a.c.	Not proven by clinical trials
Anisotropine (Valpin)	50 mg. a.c., q.h.s.	Not proven by clinical trials
Tincture of belladonna	4 to 20 grams a.c., q.h.s.	Not proven by clinical trials
Anticholinergic/Antispasmodic Drugs with Sedatives		
Librax	1 to 2 days a.c., q.h.s.	No proven clinical benefit
Donnatal	1 to 2 tablets a.c., q.h.s.	No proven clinical benefit
Combid spansules	1 capsule b.i.d.	No proven clinical benefit
Pathibamate	1 to 2 tablets a.c., q.h.s.	No proven clinical benefit
Low dose antidepressants	q.h.s.	
Miscellaneous Agents		
Simethicone (Mylicon, Silain)	2 to 4 tablets p.c., q.h.s.	For gas No proven clinical benefit
Activated charcoal	2 to 4 tablets p.c., q.h.s.	No proven clinical fenefit

*The multitude of options reflect the poorly understood multifactorial pathophysiology of irritable bowel syndrome. These medications usually represent only one aspect of a coordinated therapeutic approach, which should include patient education, diet, counseling, and regularly scheduled follow-up visits. A therapeutic trial should last at least 3 weeks before being labeled unsuccessful. The antidyspepsia agents are helpful in selected patients.

be improved with the use of this increasingly available office procedure.

With office-based physicians increasing their expertise in these endoscopic techniques, larger amounts of colorectal mucosa will be visualized by newly trained endoscopists (Rodney, 1986). These physicians will encounter a wide variety of lesions including, but not limited to, malignant cancers (Plate XXI), benign polyps (Plate XXII), hemorrhoids, varices, and foreign objects (Plates XXIII and XXIV). Normal anatomic variants as well as anomalous structures can be observed. This section presents clinical cases from a family practice.

Examples include vascular variation (Plate XXV), squamous metaplasia of the anal canal (Plate XXVI), hypertrophied papillae and (Plate XXVII) fibrous internal skin tags. A variety of these lesions, as noted in this office-based primary care practice, are displayed and discussed in the color plate section.

Tissue diagnosis remains the gold standard, but not all lesions can be biopsied or excised with equally low morbidity. This factor remains true despite the improved design of biopsy equipment used with the newer flexible endoscopes. These flexible biopsy forceps operate with a biting mechanism that penetrates less deeply into the mucosa. This lowers both the risk of perforation and the risk of hemorrhage after the procedure. Tissue specimens obtained with newer biopsy forceps appear miniscule compared with those taken with methods used previously. These tissue amounts remain sufficient for histologic analysis. Specimens returned as being inadequate in amount should be discussed individually with the pathologist. Specimens of this nature were not common in pathology training programs prior to 1973. Some pathologists have fixative preferences, others accept the standard 10 per cent formalin preservative.

As with previously used biopsy techniques, tissue obtained from a fibrinous plaque or a necrotic ulcer base rarely yields an acceptable diagnosis. Biopsy of vascular structures is contraindicated (Plate XXVIII). Relatively contraindicated is the biopsy of lesions for which management is obvious. Polyps on a stalk, in most cases, would be an example (Plate XXIX). On the other hand, newly trained endoscopists should be encouraged to biopsy abnormal lesions for which the diagnosis is not clear. With experience, the need for biopsy should diminish. Hypertrophied papillae, skin tags, scope trauma, and fecal debris variants may be biopsied by the neophyte. With experience, these items are noted and left alone.

Hyperplastic polyps are a special problem. Large numbers of these lesions are found. The diagnosis of hyperplastic polyps should not be made without some tissue analysis. Hyperplastic polyps are not neoplastic, and they do not carry an increased risk of cancer for their bearer (Fenoglio-Preiser and Hutter, 1985). Unfortunately, sampling is not perfect and multiple biopsies are time consuming. Some physicians initially biopsy several of these lesions and return to the others only if the biopsy results indicate that the lesions are neoplastic (adenoma or carcinoma). Other physicians compulsively remove all lesions and perform annual surveillance colonoscopies. This method remains controversial, with the current trend favoring a less invasive and more conservative approach. On this issue, Hippocrates' axiom regarding the difficulty of decision ("Life is short and the art long . . . ") timelessly applies to the need for individualized clinical judgment by the managing physician.

Not all anorectal lesions are apparent to the naked eye, and biopsy is helpful for many nonvascular lesions. Although some specialists have advocated against the biopsy of obviously malignant lesions, biopsy can be helpful even in these cases. Immediate biopsy greatly assisted in the diagnosis and management of a specific case of anorectal melanoma. A metastatic work-up was performed prior to referral. Tragically, metastasis had occurred, but this information obviated further invasive procedures. Health care fragmentation was minimized and family support was mobilized in a timely fashion.

SUGGESTIONS FOR THE ACQUISITION AND MAINTENANCE OF ENDOSCOPIC SKILLS

Skills in gastrointestinal endoscopy have at least six major dimensions. The first of these dimensions is demonstration of the mechanical skills in manipulating and relating to the equipment. This should include the ability to maintain and disinfect the equipment.

Second, the physician must have the ability to obtain and record diagnostic information. Skills in recognition, documentation, and tissue confirmation of pathology are desirable. Appropriate use of other sources of diagnostic assistance and consultation deserve mention and further study.

Third, the ability to effectively manage the diagnostic information obtained should be demonstrated.

Fourth, there should be a commitment to an ongoing analysis of outcomes. Continued professional growth is not possible without continuing study and self-inspection. A data base that systematically records the indications, diagnoses, and outcomes of the first 100 endoscopic procedures is an example.

It is not necessary to perform 10 procedures a day to remain capable. Large volumes of endoscopies are not necessary as long as there is rational thought, prudent judgment, and good management.

The fifth component would be the incorporation of new knowledge or the synthesis of new knowledge as the physician gains experience. It is the professional responsibility of a physician to follow and contribute to the progress of medical knowledge.

Finally, a teacher learns twice. Meaningful participation in ongoing educational programs can help a good physician to become even better.

References*

Adelman, A.: Abdominal pain in the primary care setting. J. Fam. Pract., 25:27–32, 1987. *This is one of the first published studies to use sound epidemiologic principles in describing the true nature of abdominal pain as it presents to the family physician's office. This allows our specialty to describe the reality which may be very different from that of the hospital or the emergency room.*

Adelman, A. M.: Management of dyspepsia. Am. Fam. Physician, 35(4):222–229, 1987. *An excellent and comprehensive review written for family physicians by a family physician. One of the authors would agree with the suggestion that relief of pain with food occurs as often in nonulcer dyspepsia as in patients with peptic ulcer disease. This review provides the literary basis for this observation.*

Almy, T. P., and Howell, D. A.: Diverticular disease of the colon. N. Engl. J. Med., 302:324–331, 1980. *A review that is still current by one of the most respected physician-educators who devoted his career to the study of gastrointestinal illness.*

Bedell, A. W.: Thrombosed hemorrhoids. *In* Mayhew, H. E., and Rodgers, L. A. (Eds.): Basic Procedures in Family Practice. New York, John Wiley & Sons, 1984, p. 243.

Blake, R. L.: Acute pancreatitis. Prim. Care, 15(1):187–199, 1988.

Boles, R. S., and Gordon, S. M.: The clinical significance of diverticulosis. Gastroenterology, 35:579–582, 1958.

Brodribb, A. J.: Treatment of symptomatic diverticular disease with a high-fiber diet. Lancet, 1:664–666, 1977.

Bruckstein, A. H.: Acute diarrhea. Am. Fam. Physician, 38(4):217–228, 1988.

Burakoff, R.: Case records of the Massachusetts general hospital: Weekly clinical pathological exercises. N. Engl. J. Med., 312:427–435, 1985.

Casarella, W. J., Kantor, I. E., and Seman, W. B.: Right-sided colonic diverticula as a cause of acute rectal hemorrhage. N. Engl. J. Med., 286:450–453, 1972.

Cello, J. P.: Diagnosis and management of lower gastrointestinal tract hemorrhage—medical staff conference, University of California, San Francisco. West. J. Med., 143:80–87, 1985. *A concise and extremely useful paper that deals with most of the diagnostic and management issues necessary for the family physician.*

Coleman, W. H.: Gastroscopy: A primary care diagnostic procedure. Prim. Care, 15:1–12, 1988. *One of the real pioneers in family medicine describes his use of diagnostic endoscopy in practice. One of the authors disagrees with the desirability of family physicians performing this procedure.*

Cope, Z.: The Early Diagnosis of the Acute Abdomen. London, Oxford University Press, 1972, p. 3.

*Space limitations prohibit a comprehensive listing of all the worthwhile publications on this topic. Nevertheless, I have created a comprehensive bibliography of the resource material upon which this chapter was based. It is available upon request.

Crouch, M. A.: Irritable bowel syndrome: Toward a biopsychosocial systems understanding. Prim. Care, *15*:99–110, 1988. *Dr. Crouch is a fellowship-trained family physician-educator who provides one of the most comprehensive reviews of this common problem in family medicine. There are many excellent references on this topic. Anything written by Dr. Thomas Almy or Dr. Marvin M. Schuster are recommended.*

DeGowin, E. L., and DeGowin, R. L.: Bedside Diagnostic Examination. New York, Macmillan Publishing Co., 1981, p. 32.

DeWitt, T. G., McCarthy, P. L., and Humphrey, K. F.: Who should have stool cultures? Pediatrics, *76*:551–556, 1985.

Donaldson, R. M.: Advice for the patient with "silent gallstones." N. Engl. J. Med., *307*:815–816, 1982.

Dooley, C. P., Larson, A. W., Stace, N. H., et al.: Double-contrast barium meal and upper gastrointestinal endoscopy: A comparative study. Ann. Intern. Med., *101*:538–545, 1984. *A landmark study describing the overwhelming advantages of endoscopy when compared with radiology. Generic principles from this article can be applied widely in practice.*

Drake, D., and Hollander, D.: Neutralizing capacity and cost effectiveness of antacids. Ann. Intern. Med., *94*:215–217, 1981.

Drossman, D. A., Sandler, R. S., McKee, D. C., et al.: Bowel patterns among subjects not seeking health care: Use of a questionnaire to identify a population with bowel dysfunction. Gastroenterology, *83*:529–534, 1982.

Fenoglio-Preiser, C. M., and Hutter, R. V. P.: Colorectal polyps: Pathologic diagnosis and clinical significance. Cancer, *35*:322–344, 1985.

Ferentz, K. S., Sobal, J., and Colgan, R.: Hospital privileges for family physicians: Patterns of recent residency graduates, residency director perceptions, and resident expectations. J. Fam. Pract., *3*:297–301, 1988.

Fitz, R. H.: Perforating inflammation of the vermaform appendix: With special reference to its early diagnosis and treatment. Am. J. Med. Sci., *92*:321–346, 1886.

Freedman, G.: The role of fiber and other dietary factors in IBS. Pract. Gastroenterol., *10*(2):51–56, 1986.

Gaffne, T. W., and Campbel, R. P.: Feeding techniques for dysphagic patients. Am. J. Nurs., *74*:2194–2195, 1974.

Gear, J. S. S., Ware, A., Fursdon, P., et al.: Symptomless diverticular disease and intake of dietary fibre. Lancet, *1*:511–514, 1979.

Goldsmith, G., and Patterson, M.: Irritable bowel syndrome: Treatment update. Am. Fam. Physician, *31*:191–195, 1985. *Dr. Goldsmith is emerging as an important family physician-investigator working in this area. This article cites some important sources for patient education materials.*

Goodson, J. D., Richter, J. M., Lane, R. S., et al.: Empiric antacids and reassurance for acute dyspepsia. J. Intern. Med. *1*:90–93, 1986.

Goyal, R. K., Glancy, J. J., and Spiro, H. M.: Lower esophageal ring. N. Engl. J. Med., *282*:1298–1305, 1977.

Gracie, W. A., and Ransohoff, D. F.: The natural history of silent gallstones. The innocent gallstone is not a myth. N. Engl. J. Med., *307*:798–800, 1982.

Greenburg, H. I.: Changing patterns of gastrointestinal bleeding. Arch. Surg., March 1985, p. 341.

Hayms, J. S.: Carbohydrate malabsorption following fruit ingestion in young children. Pediatrics, *82*:64–68, 1988.

Hocutt, J. E., Hainer, B. L., and Jackson, M. G.: Flexible fiberoptic sigmoidoscopy: Its use in family medicine. J. Am. Bd. Fam. Pract., *1*:189–193, 1988. *The most comprehensive prospective published study to date on flexible lower GI endoscopy performed by family physicians. The results of this study support a significant advantage in pathology detection for the 65-cm. scope compared with the 35-cm. scope. In addition to this important study, Dr. Hocutt has been an important advocate for the advancement of our specialty in the 1980's.*

Hocutt, J. E., Jaffe, R., Owens, G. M., et al.: Flexible fiberoptic sigmoidoscopy. Am. Fam. Physician, *26*(5):133–141, 1982.

Holdstock, G., Harmon, M., Machin, D., et al.: Perspective testing of a scoring system designed to improve case selection for upper gastrointestinal investigation. Gastroenterology, *90*: 1164–1169, 1986.

Horner, J. L.: Natural history of diverticulosis of the colon. Am. J. Dig. Dis., *3*:343–350.

Hyland, J. M. P., and Taylor, I.: Does a high fibre diet prevent the complications of diverticular disease? Br. J. Surg., *67*:77–79, 1980.

Jones, R.: Self-care in primary care of dyspepsia: A review. Fam. Pract., *4*:68–77, 1987. *An excellent scholarly review of dyspepsia and its management from a British point of view.*

Kahn, H., and Greenfield, S.: Position paper: Endoscopy in the evaluation of dyspesia from the Health and Public Policy of the American College of Physicians. Ann. Intern. Med., *102*:266–269, 1985. *In 1989, this paper continues to be the definitive statement that outlines the dilemma of early investigation versus empirical therapy.*

Kirsner, J. B., and Shorter, R. G.: Recent developments in "non specific" inflammatory bowel disease. N. Engl. J. Med., *306*:775–785, 1982.

Kivlahan, C. S., and James, R. H.: Natural history of neonatal jaundice. Pediatrics, Sept 1984, p. 364.

Kovacs, A., Chan, L., Hotrakita, C., et al.: Rotavirus gastroenteritis, clinical and laboratory features and use of the Rotazyme test. Am. J. Dis. Child., *141*:161–166, 1987.

Lashner, B. A., Silverstein, M. D., Hanauer, S. B., et al.: Cancer surveillance in patients with ulcerative colitis. N. Engl. J. Med., *318*:51–52, 1988.

Laupacis, A., Sackett, D. L., and Roberts, R. S.: An assessment of clinically useful measures of the consequences of treatment. N. Engl. J. Med., *318*:1728–1733, 1988.

Leonard, M. H., and Schrebier, M. H.: Is a gastrointestinal series necessary in patients with gallstones? J.A.M.A., *240*:146–147, 1978.

Longstreth, G. F.: Checking for "the occult" with a finger: A procedure of little value. J. Clin. Gastroenterol., *10*:133–134, 1988.

Lumeng, J.: Amylase-creatinine clearance ratio. Arch. Intern. Med., *138*:1750, 1978.

MacLeod, J. H.: A Method of Proctology. Hagerstown, MD, Harper and Row, 1979. *This is a book on the practical issues necessary for diagnosis and care of anorectal problems. Quoting from the New England Journal of Medicine, February 14, 1980, "It is a delightful book that serves the purpose that the author has intended." This statement remains true in 1989.*

Maisels, M. J., Gifford, K., Antle, C. E., and Leib, G. R.: Jaundice in the healthy newborn infant: A new approach to an old problem. Pediatrics, *81*:505–511, 1988.

Malt, R. A.: The perforated appendix. N. Engl. J. Med., *315*:1546–1547, 1986.

Mayer, A. D., McMahon, M. J., Holdsworth, P. J., et al.: Screening for acute pancreatitis: A rapid assay for plasma lipase. Br. J. Surg., *72*:346–348, 1985.

Moosa, A. R.: Diagnostic tests and procedures in acute pancreatitis. N. Engl. J. Med., *311*:639–643, 1984.

Mueller, B. A., Daling, J. R., Moore, D. E., et al.: Appendectomy and the risk of tubal infertility. N. Engl. J. Med., *315*:1506–1508, 1986.

Mull, J. D.: Oral rehydration therapy: an oasis of hope in the developing world. J. Fam. Pract., *18*:485–487, 1984.

Mull, J. D., Mull, D. S.: Mothers' concepts of childhood diarrhea in rural Pakistan: What ORT program planners should know. Soc. Sci. Med., *27*(1):53–67, 1988. *This is the synopsis of what is known regarding oral replacement therapy for childhood diarrhea in the third world. Dr. Mull is an internationally respected family physician-educator who has selflessly dedicated himself to this important global public health problem.*

Nyren, O., Adami, H. O., Bates, S., et al.: Absence of therapeutic benefit from antacids or Cimetidine in non-ulcer dyspepsia. N. Engl. J. Med., *314*:339–343, 1986.

Olshaker, J. S., and Mason, J. D.: The usefulness of serum electrolytes in the evaluation and treatment of acute adult gastroenteritis. Ann. Emerg. Med., *17*:423, 1988.

Orebaugh, C. R.: Diverticular disease of the colon. Am. Surg. Nov, 1978, p. 12.

Paterson-Brown, S., Thompson, J. N., Eckersley, J. R. T., et al.: Which patients with suspected appendicitis should undergo laparoscopy? Br. Med. J., *296*:1363–1364, 1988.

Puylaert, J. B. C. M., Rutgers, P. H., Lalising, R. A., et al.: A prospective study of ultrasonography in the diagnosis of appendicitis. N. Engl. J. Med., *317*:666–669, 1987.

Read, L., Pass, T. M., and Komaroff, A. L.: Diagnosis and treatment of dyspepsia: A cost-effective analysis. Med. Decision Making, *2*:415–438, 1982.

Robles, A., Devore, D., Wang, H., and Warren, C.: Oral cholecystography and sonography of gallbladder in cholecystectomy patients. West. J. Med., *147*:342–344, 1987.

Rodney, W. M.: Flexible Sigmoidoscopy and the despecialization of endoscopy. J. Fam. Pract., *23*:279–280, 1986.

Rodney, W. M.: Videosigmoidoscopy in a family medicine residency. Pri. Care Cancer, *5*(6):41–46, 1985.

Rodney, W. M. (Ed.): Flexible Sigmoidoscopy for the Family Physician. Kansas City, MO, American Academy of Family Physicians and the American Society for Gastrointestinal Endoscopy, 1985.

Rodney, W. M.: New uses for videoendoscopy in the office: Patient Education. Diagnosis, *9*(5):52–57, 1987.

Rodney, W. M.: Procedural skills in flexible sigmoidoscopy and colonoscopy for the family physician. Prim. Care, *15*:79–91, 1988. *This article explains my approach to the technique of flexible sigmoidoscopy. In addition, I outline my vision of the impending information management revolution currently available through videoendoscopy. The process of credentials and privileges is discussed.*

Rodney, W. M., and Albers, G.: Flexible sigmoidoscopy: Primary care outcomes after two types of continuing medical education. Am. J. Gastroenterol., *81*:133–137, 1986.

Rodney, W. M., Beaber, R. J., Johnson, R. A., and Quan, M.: Physician compliance with colorectal cancer screening (1978–1983): The impact of flexible sigmoidosopy. J. Fam. Pract., *20*:265–269, 1985.

Rodney, W. M., and Felmar, E.: Why flexible sigmoidoscopy instead of rigid sigmoidoscopy? J. Fam. Pract., *19*:471–476, 1984.

Rodney, W. M., and Ruggiero, C.: The Coloscreen self-test for detection of fecal occult blood. J. Fam. Pract., *21*:200–204, 1985.

Rogers, A. I.: Inflammatory bowel disease: Diagnosing with confidence. Pract. Gastroenterol., *11*(1):17–30, 1987. *Dr. Rogers is a gastroenterologist who has written quite clearly over the years on a wide variety of gastrointestinal illnesses. This is an example of his work. Furthermore, this journal is a very useful one for the practicing family physician with an interest in gastroenterology.*

Russell, T. R., and Donahue, J. H.: Hemorrhoidal banding: A warning. Dis. Colon Rectum, *28*:291–293, 1985.

Scharschmidt, B. F.: Peptic ulcer disease—pathophysiology and current medical management (medical staff conference). West. J. Med., *146*:724–733, 1987. *A scholarly, but brief review of the drugs and the underlying pathophysiology. This author also notes the dissociation between the presence of an ulcer and the presence of pain.*

Schuster, M. M.: What to feed the patient with irritable bowel syndrome. Pract. Gastroenterol., *11*(1):13–14, 1987.

Schwartz, S. I.: Tempering the technological diagnosis of appendicitis. N. Engl. J. Med., *3127*:703–704, 1987.

Scully, R. E. (Ed.): Weekly clinicopathological exercises. N. Engl. J. Med., *313*:805–815, 1985. *A case of a six-year-old girl admitted to the hospital because of vomiting and diarrhea, who was ultimately diagnosed as having infectious diarrhea due to* Cryptosporidium.

Shanahan, D., Lord, P. H., Grogono, J., et al.: Clinical acute cholecystitis and the Curtis-Fitz-Hugh syndrome. Ann. Roy. Coll. Surg., *70*:44–48, 1988.

Silen, W.: Cope's Early Diagnosis of the Acute Abdomen. 15th ed. New York, Oxford University Press, 1979. *A timeless classic on acute abdominal pain. It has been brought up to date and remains useful. The use of this book dates back three generations in my family.*

Silverstein, F. E., and Tytgat, G. N. J.: Atlas of Gastrointestinal Endoscopy. Philadelphia, W. B. Saunders Company, 1987. *An excellent atlas of the endoscopic views of various gastrointestinal illness.*

Slater, L., Brewer M. F.: Home versus hospital phototherapy for term infants with hyperbilirubinemia: A comparative study. Pediatrics, *73*:515–519, 1984.

Smith, C. W. (Ed.): Primary Care Clinics in Office Practice-Gastrointestinal Diseases. Philadelphia, W. B. Saunders Company, 1988.*This is an excellent scholarly review of most of the major gastrointestinal illnesses seen in office practice. It is written especially for family physicians and cannot be recommended too highly.*

Spiro, H. M. (Ed.): Clinical Gastroenterology. 3rd ed. New York, MacMillan, 1985. *Dr. Spiro is an internationally known gastroenterologist with a laudable penchant for humanism. Dr. Spiro also edits the Journal of Clinical Gastroenterology. This is one several excellent comprehensive textbooks on gastroenterology.*

Steer, M. L., and Silen, W.: Current concepts: Diagnostic procedures in gastrointestinal hemorrhage. N. Engl. J. Med., *309*:646–650, 1983.

Steinberg, W. M., Stafford, G. S., Davis, N. D., et al.: Diagnostic assays in acute pancreatitis. Ann. Intern. Med., *102*:576–580, 1985.

Svedlund, J., Ottson, J., Sjodin, I., and Dotevall, G.: Controlled study of psychotherapy in the irritable bowel syndrome. Lancet, *1*:589–592, 1983.

Treacher, D. F., Barkes, D. J. P., Hutton, J. P., et al.: Irritable bowel syndrome: Is a barium enema necessary? Clin. Radiol., *37*:87–88, 1986.

Wade, A. J., and Roley-Jones, D.: Long-term management of duodenal ulcer in general practice: How best to use Cimetidine? Br. Med. J., *296*:971–974, 1988.

Walker, J. D., Gray, L. A., and Polk, H. C.: Diverticulitis in women: An unappreciated clinical presentation. Ann. Surg., *185*:402–405, 1977.

White, J. D., and Gagzzi, K., Petruska, D., and Slotkoff, A.: Clinical and cost effectiveness of serum amylase in acutely ill adults. (Abstract.) Ann. Emerg. Med., *17*:423, 1988.

World Health Organization: Diarrhoeal Disease Control Programme: Drugs in the Management of Acute Diarrhoea in Infants and Young Children. World Health Organization, Geneva, Switzerland, 1988.

56

Oncology

L. Martin Jerry
E. Bruce Challis

The term cancer describes more than 100 different diseases characterized by the common property of abnormal cell growth. Cancer is the second leading cause of death in the United States, and excluding accidents, it is the leading cause of death in children between the ages of 3 and 14 years. One in three Americans will develop cancer, and one in five will die from the disease. Improvements in early diagnosis and therapy have pushed the 5-year survival rate to nearly 50 per cent. Since cancer is a chronic disease, the term "cure" relates to the natural history of each tumor. Thus, patients carry the diagnosis for life and are declared "cured" with acceptable levels of probability at variable intervals of 1, 3, 5, or 10 years or longer, depending on the type of neoplasm.

The American Cancer Society provides yearly information summarizing the incidence and mortality rates for the common varieties of cancer. Some cancers have increased in incidence since the 1940's (e.g., lung cancer), some have maintained a steady incidence (e.g., breast cancer in women), and others have decreased in incidence (e.g., carcinomas of the stomach and uterus, and of the bladder and rectum in women). Lung cancer is the leading cause of death among all cancer patients. Because of smoking, its incidence is rising rapidly in young women and has exceeded breast cancer. Colorectal cancer is the second leading cause of death from cancer. Diet is thought to play a significant role in its causation, and two thirds of the deaths are preventable by early diagnosis. Breast cancer is the third leading cause of cancer deaths and the most common cause in women. Early diagnosis of localized disease gives a 5-year survival of 85 per cent. Other tumors, in order of frequency, include prostatic, uterine, urologic, oral, and pancreatic cancers, followed by leukemia and cancers of the ovary and skin.

Comprehensive Cancer Care

Cancer management is complex and multidisciplinary in nature. The past decade has seen the organization of cancer services into regional comprehensive cancer centers, which integrate the sophisticated technology needed for diagnosis and treatment and provide educational and consultative resources to surrounding communities. Excellence in service to patients is assured by up-to-date clinical and basic research programs. Educational endeavors continuously translate rapid advances in diagnosis and therapy to the bedside and to the community physicians. Today, cancer patients are managed more and more as outpatients, even in the terminal phase of illness. Thus, the family physician is involved at all stages of the natural history of the disease in continuing consultative interactions with specialists at a cancer center in various aspects of cancer medicine (surgical and medical and pediatric and radiation oncology) as well as with supportive care and rehabilitation experts.

In 1980, it was estimated that 131,000 patients would die who might have been saved by early diagnosis of their disease and by proper initial expert management during the controllable stage of disease. Thus, early referral of all cancer patients for multidisciplinary management by specialists is of utmost importance. Often the only chance for cure is the first attempt at treatment.

The Biology of Neoplasia

Neoplasms are abnormal cell growths, which may be benign or malignant. Malignant tumors invade normal tissues or spread to distant organs (metastasis). The degree of malignancy depends on the propensity for invasion and distant spread. Separation of malignant cells from the primary tumor is an essential part of the metastatic process. The propensity of new growths for local, regional, and distant spread gives rise to all major clinical problems of cancer, including death.

Cancer is characterized by an increase in the number of abnormal cells derived from a normal tissue, by invasion of adjacent tissues by these abnormal cells, and by lymphatic or blood-borne spread of the malignant cells to regional lymph nodes and to distant sites as metastases. An interplay of environmental and genetic factors is thought to give rise to neoplasia. Although environmental factors may predominate in some situations and genetic influences in others, it is the interaction of these elements that determines the development of neoplasia. This interplay first induces changes in the genetic material of somatic cells by such mechanisms as oncogene activation or gene deletion. These changes then lead to the synthesis of gene products that appear to promote the formation of preneoplastic lesions. Then comes the progression from preneoplasia to neoplasia and finally to clonally evolved, heterogeneous neoplasia.

Several lines of evidence confirm that the fundamental molecular event or events that cause cells to become malignant occur at the level of the DNA. For example, when a normal cell is experimentally transformed to a neoplastic cell, all daughter cells carry the neoplastic phenotype, which indicates that the defect is inherited. Certain diseases like xeroderma pigmentosa are characterized by defective DNA repair mechanisms and are associated with a high instance of epithelial carcinoma and melanoma of the skin exposed to ultraviolet light. The prime event in chemical carcinogenesis is the interaction of a chemical agent with DNA. Most carcinogens are mutagens. The demonstration that DNA isolates from tumor cells can transfect normal cells and render them neoplastic provides direct proof that an alteration of the DNA is responsible for cancer.

The words **cancer, neoplasia,** and **malignancy** are often used as synonyms. Cancer is a disease process which involves abnormal growth and differentiation. Cancer cells behave differently from normal cells in terms of four characteristics: (1) clonality: tumors originate from a single stem cell which proliferates to form a clone of malignant cells; (2) autonomy: the growth of tumor cells is not properly regulated by normal biochemical and physical influences in the microenvironment; (3) anaplasia: there is lack of normal coordinated cell differentiation, i.e., tumors differ from normal cells, not only in quantity (cell proliferation) but also quality (abnormal differentiation); and (4) metastasis: the capacity for local invasion, discontinuous growth, and subsequent dissemination to other parts of the body. This property is primarily responsible for death. It should be noted that normal cells can express these properties at certain appropriate times, such as in embryogenesis or wound repair. In cancer, however, these characteristics are either inappropriate or excessive. **Malignant transformation** describes the process by which a normal cell is converted into one which exhibits these characteristic traits.

As relatively autonomous growths of cells in tissues, neoplasms may be benign or malignant. Benign tumors tend to be encapsulated, noninvasive, highly differentiated, showing rare mitoses and slow growth with little or no anaplasia and no tendency to metastasize. Malignant tumors, on the other hand, are invasive and nonencapsulated. Their cells appear poorly differentiated. Mitoses are common and growth is rapid. Anaplasia is variable and metastases are the rule. Tumors arising in epithelial tissues derived from embryonic ectoderm or endoderm are called carcinomas. Tumors arising in connective tissue derivatives of the embryonic mesoderm are called sarcomas. Any cell type which is capable of proliferation can give rise to cancer. Tumors may have a variable resemblance to the tissue of origin and appear clinically late in the natural history of the disease after a long latency period. Hyperplasia and dysplasia tend to precede neoplasia by months or years as a preneoplastic lesion. Even after locoregional recurrence, tumors can remain dormant, sometimes for decades, before recurring. Spontaneous remission is occasionally seen in particular tumor types. There is no essential distinctive structural or biochemical difference between malignant and normal cells.

Pathobiology of Cancer

In 1981, Doll and Peto estimated the influence of life-style and environmental factors as causes of cancer. Diet that is high in fat and low in fiber figured in 35 per cent of cancer deaths, with smoking in 30 per cent. Viruses and occupational exposures provided 5 per cent and 4 per cent, respectively, while alcohol consumption and excessive sunlight exposure provided 3 per cent each. Environmental pollution and food additives provided 2 per cent and 1 per cent, respectively. Thus, a total of 83 per cent of cancer deaths could be attributed to life-style and environmental factors.

Traditionally, viruses, chemicals, and radiation have been considered the three major causes of cancer. They are thought to act through the production of mutations in the host genome with activation of oncogenes that, in turn, result in a clonal growth advantage. The subsequent activation of additional oncogenes results in malignant transformation with escape from growth control, invasiveness, and metastasis.

THE ONCOGENE HYPOTHESIS

Oncogenes are genes that can cause cancer. They were first described in viruses. In 1911, Rous described a sarcoma in chickens and later in mice, rats, and hamsters, which could be transferred from host to host by both tumor cells and cell-free filtrates. This Rous sarcoma virus was the first of the RNA tumor viruses that are now so well studied. The oncogene hypothesis was developed in 1969 by Huebner and Todaro, and the current revolution in genetic engineering has brought us a long way in our understanding of the role of these genes in cancer production. There are more than 20 homologues called proto-oncogenes in the normal genome which are highly conserved in evolution, appearing in yeast, fruit flies, mice, rodents, and humans. The proto-oncogenes appeared in evolution before they were picked up by viruses and appear to play an important normal role in growth and development of cells. Proto-oncogenes present in cells are designated *C-onc*, and oncogenes in viruses, *V-onc*.

There appear to be three ways by which proto-oncogenes are activated to give oncogenes. The first is through point mutation. The *ras* oncogenes were described in bladder tumors and found to be activated by a single base pair alteration in codon 12, which results in a glycine to valine switch. The p21 protein product that results has a reduced GTPase activity. Other members of the *ras* family have had single mutations described in positions 13 or 61. It is interesting that in the nitrosomethylurea mammary carcinoma model in rats, this chemical carcinogen can produce a similar point mutation in the *ras* family. Through O^6 methylation of guanine, DNA undergoes faulty replication with a GC pair switched to an AT pair in the 12th codon, and a similar abnormality in the p21 product results.

A second mode of activation involves amplification or increase in gene dosage. Four kinds of chromosomal abnormalities have been described in tumors, including breaks, translocations, homogeneously staining regions, and double minutes. The latter two represent cytogenetic markers for chain amplification. This has been described with the *ras* family, the *C-myc* in small cell lung carcinoma, with *N-myc* in neuroblastoma, and with *C-myc* in the HL-60 cell line derived from a promyelocytic leukemia. The resulting gene amplification produces increased amounts of the protein product which leads to malignant transformation. The presence of these amplified genes can be used as markers for adverse prognosis, such as *N-myc* in neuroblastoma. The mechanism of amplification is unknown. The process occurs in the silkworm and in the frog as an important step in development; however, it is not usually seen in higher animals except in drug resistance to methotrexate and colchecine.

The third mode of activation involves translocation. The oncogenes are activated at the break points. In chronic myelogenous leukemia, the Philadelphia chromosome is formed through a 9:22 translocation. The *abl* oncogene is translocated to chromosome 22 from chromosome 9, and the *sis* oncogene is translocated from chromosome 22 to chromosome 9. The *abl* proto-oncogene now becomes fused with a second previously unlinked gene (BCR) on chromosome 22. The resulting hybrid gene specifies a hybrid BCG-ABL protein which acts differently from normal ABL protein and which may have a role in the pathogenesis of this leukemia. The abnormal product is a p210 protein instead of the usual p120 protein and has an enhanced protein kinase activity. Besides the production of a new or altered protein, translocations can also alter the regulation of a proto-oncogene. In Burkitt's lymphoma a reciprocal translocation between chromosomes 8 and 14 occurs with a movement of the *myc* oncogene from chromosome 8 to a location near the constant region of the immunoglobulin heavy chain gene on chromosome 14. The variable region of the immunoglobulin gene in turn is transferred from chromosome 14 to chromosome 8. The restructured gene or chromosome 22 specifies a normal protein, but the amounts of this protein are no longer appropriately regulated since the oncogenes are adjacent to promoter or enhancing sequences from the immunoglobulin genes which increase oncogene transcription. This constitutive expression of the *myc* protein alters the control of proliferation and differentiation.

At least two or more genetic changes are required for malignancy. It is found that oncogenes may act in a form of complementation. One class of oncogenes tends to produce immortalization of cells through activity in the nucleus. These include oncogenes such as *myc* and *myb*. A second class of oncogenes produces morphologic transformation through action in the cytoplasm. These include the *ras*, *src*, and *abl* families. Members from each of the two families can complement each other to produce a full malignant transformation.

Proto-oncogenes affect growth and development by means of the pathway of growth factors. Growth factors are small molecules that signal activation, replication, and differentiation of cells by binding to receptors on the surface of their target cells. The signal to proliferation is external, with the growth factor interacting with a membrane receptor which, in turn, activates a second messenger system within the cytoplasm to turn on DNA synthesis in the nucleus. Cell activation, growth, and development are the result. Oncogenes produce constitutive unregulated signals for cell growth from particular positions within this pathway. Some do so by mimicking growth factors. The *sis* oncogene produces an abnormal beta chain homologue for platelet-derived growth factor (PDGF). PDGF is required for the growth of fibroblasts through interaction with a tyrosine kinase receptor. The *sis* product produces a constitutive growth signal by bypassing this receptor. A second site of action involves membrane receptors for growth factors which have tyrosine protein kinase activity. Protein activation is more usual through phosphorylation of serine and threonine residues than tyrosine. Phosphatases tend to remove these phosphate groups. Transmembrane receptors with protein kinase activity include receptors for epidermal growth factor, platelet derived growth factor, and colony stimulating factor-1, as well as the insulin receptors. Their activation involves an autophosphorylation of tyrosine on the receptor as well as other proteins. The kinase activity of the receptor is at its C-terminus which projects into the cytoplasm. The *V-erb-B* oncogene produces a homologue of the epithelial growth factor receptor with deleted sections. This abnormal receptor is unable to bind to epithelial growth factor itself so that the growth factor receptor complex can be internalized. The abnormal receptor stays on the membrane, functioning as a constitutive protein kinase giving unregulated signal for cell growth. The oncogene *V-fms* is a homologue of the colony stimulating factor-1 receptor.

A third mechanism of action of oncogenes involves second messengers within the cytoplasm. Some tyrosine protein kinases are cytoplasmic proteins associated with cytoplasmic membranes, such as *src*, *abl*, and *fes*. The N-terminal portion of the kinase is hooked to cytoplasmic membranes, and the C terminal tyrosine kinase extends into the cytoplasm and is activated by autophosphorylation of tyrosine 416. An alternative second messenger system involves the G proteins, which characterize the *ras* family which shows GTP binding and GTPase activity. The altered p21 proteins, through point mutation at positions 12 or 13 or 16 as described above, show either poor binding or reduced GTPase activity. The result is a stimulation of the adenylcyclase system and further protein kinases. It has been suggested that oncogenes *mil* and *mos* may activate cells by phosphorylation of serine and threonine in the cytoplasm.

Yet another mechanism of action involves oncogenes such as *myc*, *myb*, and *fos*. These act in the nucleus, and their overproduction results in constitutive formation of their messenger RNAs and uncontrolled cell proliferation.

The oncogenes considered so far are growth promoting or stimulatory oncogenes which act through cell growth and differentiation in a dominant fashion to stimulate growth and proliferation. They are the central regulators of growth in normal cells. These are the classic oncogenes like *ras*, which were identified first through studies with oncogenic viruses. They have homologues in our own cells called proto-oncogenes, and their normal growth regulatory functions can be altered by the several mechanisms described above of chromosomal translocation, gene amplification, and point mutation. A second group of oncogenes has been postulated which are tumor suppressor or growth suppression genes or antioncogenes. These function to inhibit tumor growth by suppressing proliferation. Loss of these genes and their function in a cell by inherited or somatic deletions or other mechanisms will allow abnormal proliferation. This second class of oncogenes may turn out to be as important as the stimulatory oncogenes. Deletions have been described on chromosomes 5, 17, and 18 in colonic carcinoma. But the best example is the Rb gene in retinoblastoma which is a rare inherited tumor of the retina, occurring in 1 in 20,000 infants and children. The Rb gene is on chromosome 13. In familial retinoblastoma, infants are born with one normal Rb gene and one which is mutant and inactive. Thus, the first of the minimum two steps has been taken for oncogene activation so that the infant is at risk. The normal Rb gene is dominant, but if it is lost, the Rb influence is lost and retinoblastoma occurs. The same phenomenon occurs with the osteosarcomas that these children also develop. In the sporadic form of the disease the infant may be born with two normal Rb genes and both have to be lost for retinoblastoma to occur. The Rb gene makes a p105 protein in the nucleus which probably regulates gene expression. If this regulatory protein is missing, the regulation of gene expression does not occur properly. The E1A oncoprotein of the adenovirus transforms infected cells by binding to a host p105 protein whose functional absence results in the tumor, and this is likely the same p105 protein that is specified by the Rb gene.

Genetic Instability

With tumor progression, a neoplasm tends to become more aggressive in clinical and biologic activities over time. Tumors are clonal, arising from a single cell. They acquire genetic changes in the clone which give rise to subpopulations of tumor cells with increasing aggressive characteristics. The genetic apparatus of tumor cells is abnormally unstable, and progressive chromosomal breaks and translocations appear in a multistep fashion which is characteristic at each step. It is unknown why tumor cells are more genetically labile than comparable normal cells. Possibilities include the presence of mutator genes, chromosomal rearrangements, and inherited genetic defects that characterize diseases that have chromosomal fragility as part of their syndrome such as Fanconi syndrome, Bloom syndrome, and ataxia telangiectasia, all of which have an increased incidence of cancer. The basis of the inherited susceptibility to cancer that is found in the usual family history is unknown, as, for example, in colorectal cancer. It is presumed that there is an inheritance of a clinical defect which produces a tissue-specific genetic instability.

The above discussion describes the genetic basis of tumor progression. Little is known about the genetic basis for invasion and metastasis. Introduction of the activated *ras* gene into fibroblasts confers a capacity on these cells to metastasize. It is unknown whether this is an effect of *ras* itself or whether the oncogene destabilizes the rest of the genome, letting other genes be responsible.

We are only beginning to see the outline of the series of genetic events occurring in the development of cancer. They are very complex, and the patterns are not uniform. Perhaps only 15 to 20 per cent of human tumors can be shown to have these kinds of abnormalities. Some individuals feel that all of this is an epiphenomenon and irrelevant, resulting from the neoplastic state rather than being the cause. The weight of opinion, however, is that these changes are in fact causal. They have significant implications for both diagnosis and prognosis, since cDNAs for oncogenes can be used to identify their presence in a tumor to make prognostic and diagnostic correlations.

The oncogene hypothesis allows for an understanding of the action of viruses, chemicals, and radiation in carcinogenesis. When oncogenic DNA viruses infect their host cells, the viral DNA is integrated into the host DNA. If the viral DNA is replicated and assembled into a new virus, cancer does not result. If the integrated viral genome is transcribed with the host enzymes, viral proteins of the T variety result, which transform the host cell to a cancer cell. The RNA viruses, on the other hand, carry their genetic information as an RNA chromosome in the virus. Upon invasion of the host cell, a reverse transcriptase synthesizes viral DNA on the virus RNA template. The result eventually is a DNA copy of the original viral RNA chromosome which is then integrated into the host chromosome. If viral proteins are translated with host enzymes, a malignant transformation occurs. Oncogenes in RNA viruses have been found to have been picked up and integrated into the viral genome. They thus represent human passenger proto-oncogenes which have been activated to oncogenes and are carried by the virus. Viruses are associated only with about 5 per cent of human cancer. The Epstein-Barr virus is associated with Burkitt's lymphoma and nasopharyngeal carcinoma. Human retroviruses have been described in T cell leukemia and in Kaposi's sarcoma as a significant complication of acquired immune deficiency syndrome. Hepatitis B virus infection results in hepatocellular carcinoma, and the papilloma viruses are important in the causation of warts and some varieties of cervical cancer. Chemical carcinogenesis operates through the production of point mutations. An initiator-promotor model describes the process. Initiation is a genetic event, and most chemical carcinogens are activated by metabolism, often through the cytochrome P450 system. Their activation results in the appearance of electrophilic activity from highly reactive sites on the carcinogens so that they are capable of reacting with cellular DNA as the primary carcinogenic event. This DNA alteration produces an oncogene from a proto-oncogene through point mutation. Promoter action, on the other hand, is nongenetic and depends on the presence of previous initiation. Promoters are not electrophiles and require no metabolism. They are capable of producing a reversible phenocopy of the transformed state. They appear to be analogs of physiologic signaling substances, and typical examples are phorbol esters which are analogues of diacyl glycerol and work through activation of protein kinase C.

Two types of radiation can modify DNA. Ultraviolet radiation does so through the formation of thymine dimers. Ionizing radiation, such as atomic particles or x-rays, produces breaks in DNA strands. Surprisingly, the primary lesions in DNA are not mutagenic. Mutagenesis is caused instead indirectly by DNA repair or lack of repair. The repair of double-strand breaks can result in translocation of pieces of DNA from one chromosome to another with occasional activation of oncogenes. Xeroderma pigmentosa has loss of the ultraviolet repair pathway, and ataxia telangiectasia has loss of the x-ray repair pathway.

The net effect of malignant transformation results in changes in a large constellation of cellular properties. These include aspects of growth control, morphology, cell-to-cell interactions, membrane properties, cytoskeletal structure, protein secretion, and gene expression. Some of the changes are probably interrelated, and others seem independent of one another. Not all transformed cells show all the changes, and we know little about the molecular basis that underlies these phenomena. Whatever the causal linkage is, transformation appears to result from a small number of independent events with far reaching consequences. Some types of cell transformation are known to result from the synthesis of one or two new proteins.

Monoclonal Expansion

Preneoplastic lesions may eventually take the final step of malignancy after a long latent period. For most cancers this event is monoclonal. A single cell from either normal or preneoplastic tissue becomes neoplastic in expansion if that clone ultimately produces cancer. The evidence for monoclonal origin of human tumors comes from study of idiotypes of immunoglobulins produced by tumors of B cells or unique rearrangements of T cell receptor genes described in T cell lymphoma and leukemia. Such a study demonstrates the presence of a single isoenzyme of glucose-6-phosphate dehydrogenase in heterozygous women in chronic myelogenous leukemia and various solid tumors and identifies unique restriction fragments coding for X-linked enzymes in heterozygous women in acute myelogenous leukemia, leiomyoma, and Wilms' tumor. Thus, malignancy can be perceived as an aberration of cell renewal. The developmental pathways for renewal of cells for specific tissues from stem cells have been worked out, particularly in the case of the bone marrow. Studies of T cell malignancies have revealed that the neoplastic event is not only monoclonal, but monoclonal at a specific level of differentiation. In T cell acute lymphocytic leukemia, the neoplastic event and monoclonal expansion occur at a very immature stage of T cell development, whereas in the T cell cutaneous lymphoma these changes occur at the level of mature helper T cells. Thus, the major molecular event in cancer may be arrest of differentiation, leaving proliferation as the only remaining option for the cell. At least in the leukemias and lymphomas, each tumor then represents a clonal proliferation frozen at a particular step in the normal lineage of parent cell differentiation.

Tumors then undergo clonal evolution as they develop. They tend to show significant heterogeneity with respect to appearance, the degree of differentiation, and other factors. Tumor cells are kinetically unstable to varying degrees compared with normal cells, and this instability leads to phenotypic heterogeneity. For example, chronic myelogenous leukemia can transform to acute leukemia, and clonal evolution to a more highly malignant state probably occurs in most clinical tumors. The follicular non-Hodgkin's lymphomas may evolve into a more aggressive diffuse lymphoma; chronic lymphocytic leukemia to an aggressive diffuse non-Hodgkin's lymphoma; low-grade sarcomas to higher grade, more aggressive tumors; and preneoplasia to neoplasia, as in squamous cell carcinoma of the cervix. This clonal evolution also appears to involve a sequence of oncogene activation. Oncogene activation by either gene amplification or increased transcription independently and adversely correlates with prognosis. Thus, cancers are heterogeneous histopathologically, in terms of estrogen or other hormone receptor distribution, human tumor antigen production, cytogenetics, blood supply and supply of oxygen to metabolites, and in variations in growth fraction and response to radiotherapy and chemotherapy. Heterogeneity plays a major role in the development and selection of drug resistent tumor cells.

Invasion

The first evidence of tumor invasion is destruction of the underlying basement membrane which is generally composed of collagen Type IV. Once through the basement membrane, the tumor gains access to adjacent stroma where it can interact with structural glycoproteins such as laminin and fibronectin. The number of laminin receptors on tumor cells is positively correlated with the invasiveness and number of lymph node metastases. These receptors provide malignant cells with a lattice for anchorage and advancement. Tumor cells also produce several proteases which can destroy the adjacent stroma. Tumor cells also synthesize autocrine motility factors. Tumors rarely invade resistant tissues such as fascia, bone, or thick-walled arteries or arterioles, but they readily penetrate single-cell walled capillaries, venules, and lymphatics. Lymphatics lack a basement membrane. As they increase in size, tumor angiogenesis is required above 150 micrometers in diameter. Eventually mechanical pressure may compromise intratumor vascularity, causing hemorrhage and necrosis in hypovascular areas.

The capillary and lymphatic systems are interconnected so that regional lymph node involvement implies that hemotogenous dissemination has occurred. Removal of positive regional nodes has regional therapeutic potential, but increasingly it is a staging step to determine the risk for disseminated metastasis and the need for systemic treatment. Regional nodes are often hyperplastic, suggesting host response. The regional spread of tumors is influenced by the anatomy of the regional lymphatics and the lymph nodes, which significantly influences the approach to surgical and radiation treatment of local regional tumor.

Metastasis results from a spread of cells from a primary cancer to a noncontiguous site, usually by way of the blood stream or lymphatics and sometimes through implantation of serous membranes. A secondary growth is established. Release of tumor cells from the primary tumor into the blood is a critical step and, ultimately, the major cause of cancer death. It is not a random process in that it selects a subpopulation of cells in the primary tumor, which has high metastatic potential. When small clumps of tumor cells are trapped in capillaries, the initial event probably involves an interaction between the tumor cell membrane and the capillary endothelium. Platelet adherence occurs, the capillary endothelial junctions retract, and the underlying basement membrane is exposed. The cells invade the adjacent tissue and form a secondary focus from which further showers of metastases can occur. Some tumor cells produce procoagulants that have thromboplastinlike activities. They may form a protective fibrin cocoon around themselves. Tumor procoagulant production may partly account for the hypercoagulable state commonly seen in patients with disseminated cancer.

These micrometastases enlarge to approximately 1 mm. in diameter, about one million cells, before growth is halted by the limitation of metabolites. Further growth requires vascularization produced by the tumor's secretion of tumor angiogenesis factor, which stimulates and directs nearby endothelium in such a way as to bring the capillaries toward and finally into the micrometastasis. Once vascularization occurs, exponential tumor growth becomes possible. As tumors enlarge, they become increasingly hypovascular, leading to necrosis and low growth fractions. Capillaries supply adequate nourishment to the subjacent first, second, and perhaps third layers of tumor cells, but oxygen and nutrient diffusion is compromised below this level, leading to hypoxia, low growth fraction, and eventually necrosis. Hypoxia significantly impairs the biologic effect of radiotherapy, which is oxygen dependent.

When tumors are small the volume doubling time progressively lengthens. This is due to diminished blood supply, competition for metabolites, and related factors that lead to a decrease in growth fractions and an increase in cell dropout owing to cell death or differentiation. As tumors enlarge, an increasing proportion of cells drop out of the mitotic cycle and enter either a prolonged G1 period or a G0 resting stage. These mitotically inactive cells can reenter the cycle and serve as tumor stem cells and are not necessarily end-stage cells. The exponential growth means that the rates of cell production and loss are proportional to the number of cells in the population. Thus, clinical disease appears only after a latency because of our relative inability to detect disease by imaging procedures until about two thirds of the natural history has elapsed. The first detection of the disease on x-ray occurs at about 27 doublings when the tumor is 1/2 cm. in size and contains about one million cells. First clinical detection occurs when a tumor is about 1 cm. in size, weighs a gram, and contains one billion cell at 32 doublings. This period through to death at about 1 kg. of tumor mass or 10^{12} cells represents the final third of the tumor's natural history. Thus, cancer is diagnosed at a relatively late stage in its natural history. Advances in tumor markers, early diagnosis, and screening are essential for further progress. Diagnosis occurs at the point when the tumor has outstripped natural host defense, since the immune system is thought not to operate above a tumor burden of 10^5 cells. This limitation in detection results in the necessity for long-term follow-up with cancer patients, since one can never tell whether a patient has been cured or only partially responsive when tumor disappears clinically after therapy. One must wait 2 to 3 years or longer to see whether recurrence develops. Thus, the measurement of disease-free interval as well as survival becomes important in clinical trials. These properties of cell kinetics are essential in the design of the clinical trials of chemotherapy and radiation therapy. This natural progression through the metastatic cascade from primary site to local regional disease to systemic disease forms the basis of cancer staging and, when combined with size of the initial tumor, of prognosis.

HISTOLOGIC DIAGNOSIS

The absence of a specific marker for malignancy means that histologic examination of tissues or exfoliated cells remains the principal method of diagnosis. Characteristic histologic aberrations can predict malignant disease with high accuracy. Besides disordered tissue architecture, malignant cells may have large, irregular nuclei with enlarged and more than the usual number of nucleoli. Polyploidy is common. Mitotic figures are increased, especially in rapidly growing tumors, with abnormal mitosis and macronucleated cells. The cytoplasm may be scanty with increased basophilia owing to an increased content of RNA. The greater the lack of differentiation (anaplasia), the easier the diagnosis of malignancy, but the more difficult it is to identify the tumor of origin. For example, false positive interpretations can occur with lymph node abnormalities associated with insect bites, phenytoin administration, or systemic lupus erythematosus being mistaken for malignant lymphoma. Conversely, the malignant nature of thyroid follicular carcinoma or chondrosarcoma may not be reflected in its microscopic appearance.

Etiologic Factors of Clinical Significance

Several acquired nonneoplastic disorders are associated with an increased incidence of cancers. These tumors arise from tissues showing increased cellular proliferation during prolonged regeneration. Actinic dermatitis from chronic exposure to sunlight, as well as keratoses and thermal burns, may be associated with squamous skin cancer. Leukoplakia may precede squamous cancer of mucous membranes of the mouth, vagina, and bladder. Paget's disease of the nipple may signal the presence of adenocarcinoma of the breast. Bowen's disease, a cutaneous carcinoma in situ sometimes associated with ingestion of arsenic or exposure to ionizing radiation, tends to evolve into squamous cancer. It may be associated also with respiratory, gastrointestinal, or genitourinary cancers. Both aplastic anemia and paroxysmal nocturnal hemoglobinuria may develop into acute leukemia. Sideropenic dysphagia may be associated with squamous cancer of the oropharynx and proximal esophagus (Plummer-Vinson and Patterson-Brown-Kelly syndromes). Adenocarcinoma of the liver may develop with postnecrotic or alcoholic cirrhosis. Protein deficiency and parasitism are additional factors in some geographic areas. Adenocarcinoma of the colon may develop at multiple sites in relation to pseudopolyps in chronic ulcerative colitis. Chronic cervicitis is associated with squamous cancer of the cervix, especially with multiparity and lower socioeconomic status, but is rare in Jews. Similarly, chronic balanitis is associated with squamous cancer of the penis but is rare in men who have had neonatal circumcision. Osteogenic sarcoma may complicate Paget's disease of bone, and squamous metaplasia of the bronchial epithelium correlates with an increased incidence of squamous cancer. Colonic polyps that develop in older age groups are regarded by many as premalignant lesions but with much lower potential than the familial polyposes. Chondromas of bone occasionally develop into sarcomas.

OCCUPATIONAL AND ENVIRONMENTAL CARCINOGENS

Hundreds of chemicals from industry, farms, and homes, and in foods as additives and preservatives have been implicated. Forty per cent of all cancers are thought to be related directly or in part to cigarette smoking. More than 15 carcinogens, such as hydrocarbons and aromatic amines, have been isolated from tobacco smoke. Smokers have an increased risk not only of lung cancer but also of cancers of the head and neck, esophagus, and bladder. Asbestos, uranium, and alcohol exposure synergistically increase the risk.

Different populations vary widely in susceptibility to the same carcinogen because of hereditary differences in levels of enzymes that activate or degrade carcinogens. For example, elevated levels of aryl hydrocarbon hydroxylase activity may predispose smokers to lung cancer. The long latency of years between exposure to a carcinogen and the development of neoplasia obscures detection of the association and makes screening programs in animals difficult.

Epidemiologic techniques are also used. Mapping cancer mortality by small geographic areas within a country reveals patterns of etiologic significance. Japanese migrating to Hawaii or the continental United States have a decreasing risk of stomach cancer, implicating environmental factors. Changes in the incidence of particular cancers with time is helpful. The increase in colon cancer is associated with a high-fat, low-fiber diet, and bile salts have been implicated as cocarcinogens.

Occupational cancers appear at the site of the most intense and prolonged exposure. The characteristics of the tumor and its subsequent course differ little from the spontaneous counterpart.

Radiation and various drugs may be associated with the induction of cancer. The survivors of Hiroshima and Nagasaki had an increased incidence of acute and chronic myelogenous leukemia, peaking 7 years after exposure, as well as myelofibrosis with myeloid metaplasia. A similar latent period is seen with acute leukemia developing after radiation therapy for enlarged tonsils and thymus and for ankylosing spondylitis. Patients who have had radiotherapy for tonsillar and thymic enlargement are also at increased risk for thyroid carcinoma. Fetal irradiation markedly increases the risk of a fatal malignant disease before 10 years of age. There is a dose-response relationship to a plateau, and an acceptable safe dose of radiation has not been determined. Even very low exposures, such as repeated chest fluoroscopy for follow-up of tuberculosis, may increase breast cancer risk in women. Radioisotopes are also hazardous. Radioactive phosphorous has been associated with acute leukemia, radium or mesothorium with osteosarcoma and sinus carcinoma, and thorotrast with hepatic hemangioendothelioma.

Immunosuppressive regimens for renal transplantation are associated with a hundred-fold increased risk of cancer, particularly of primary central nervous system lymphomas. The treatment of cancer by radiation and regimens containing alkylating agents capable of interacting with DNA has been associated with a one to five per cent incidence of acute myelogenous leukemia or its variants in patients with Hodgkin's disease, non-Hodgkin's lymphoma, multiple myeloma, and ovarian cancer. This complication may relate to immunosuppressive or carcinogenic effects of the treatment. Secondary leukemia, on the average, develops 5 to 7 years after treatment of the primary tumor and is relatively refractory to induction of remission with combination chemotherapy.

Hormones may also cause neoplasms in man. Prenatal exposure to synthetic estrogens has been associated with vaginal adenosis as well as vaginal and cervical adenocarcinomas of the clear cell type. Daughters of women who received diethylstilbestrol (DES) during pregnancy have been found especially prone to this disorder. Postnatal exposure leads to a five-fold risk for endometrial carcinoma of the adenosquamous type. Estrogens in birth control pills may be associated with bleeding hepatic adenomas as well as liver cancers. Androgenic anabolic steroids may predispose to benign liver tumors and to hepatocellular carcinoma.

Viruses are known to be oncogenic in several animal species, including mammals, chickens, fish, and frogs. The Epstein-Barr virus (EBV) is the best example in man. This DNA herpes virus causes infectious mononucleosis and is associated with Burkitt's lymphoma, mainly in children in Central Africa and New Guinea and sporadically elsewhere. The peculiar geographic distribution can be explained if the virus acts as a cocarcinogen in concert with other factors such as immunosuppression from malaria. EBV is also associated with nasopharyngeal carcinoma in the Orient, where genetic factors also determine susceptibility. Herpes simplex virus has been associated with cancer of the cervix. The C-type RNA viruses produce leukemia or sarcomas in other species, and their presence has been detected in tumor tissues from patients with acute leukemia and lymphoma. B-type RNA viruses resembling the murine mammary tumor (Bittner) agents have been found in cultured cell lines derived from human breast cancers.

The Host-Tumor Interrelationship

A tumor does not grow freely in its human host as it would in a tissue culture. The host puts up a defense to counter the inherent aggressiveness of the tumor as it proliferates, invades, and metastasizes. It is a common belief that once a diagnosis of cancer is made, the patient is helpless before the relentless onslaught of his disease. This misconception fuels that excessive sense of hopelessness and despair that invests the word cancer. Current research is evolving a biology of host resistance to neoplasia, having mechanisms similar to those already known to operate in infections. In addition to age and sex, immunologic, endocrine, nutritional, psychologic, growth factors, and, likely, other as yet undefined factors condition host resistance to determine favorable or unfavorable outcomes, responses to treatment, and occasionally periods of long remission (dormant, residual tumor), or even spontaneous regression. Until recently, it has been difficult to explain and hence to accept how host resistance might operate in cancer and, particularly, how psychologic and behavioral variables might influence clinical outcomes. The recent elaboration of the psychoneuroimmunology hypothesis now provides a paradigm to understand the mechanism of these host influences. The immune, endocrine, and autonomic and central nervous systems share reciprocal innervation and mutual hormonal and peptide messengers to allow integrated responses. Through perceptions based on belief systems (for example, stress) mind may set the level and quality of responsiveness in this network. The effectiveness of host resistance as well as the relative significance of its components varies greatly from tumor to tumor. Moreover, current therapies for destroying cancer cells (surgery, chemotherapy, radiotherapy) do so at the expense not only of some normal body tissues, but also with some associated, usually transient, depression of host resistance.

HORMONES

A number of tumors are sensitive to the hormonal milieux of the body. Breast cancer is the outstanding example, where a number of therapeutically effective hormonal manipulations have been devised. Estrogens, progesterones, adrenal steroids, prolactin, and other hormones are all involved. In the first two, sensitivity to hormonal action depends on the presence of estrogen or progesterone receptors in the tumor cell cytoplasm to bind the hormones. The presence of receptors is related to the degree of differentiation of the tumor. Prostatic and endometrial cancers are other examples of hormone-sensitive tumors.

TUMOR IMMUNOLOGY

Participation of the immune response requires the host to be able to recognize foreign or "nonself" chemical configurations called tumor-associated antigens (TAA) on the surface membranes of malignant cells. In animals these configurations are clearly demonstrable through the end point of specific rejection of a transplantable tumor (tumor-specific transplantations antigens, TSTA) in syngeneic hosts in which general histoincompatibility is excluded. Distinctive antigenicity has been shown in spontaneous animal tumors as well as in those induced by chemicals, physical agents, or viruses. TSTA are individually specific for each chemically induced tumor. Tumors caused by the same DNA virus share common neoantigens but lack virion antigens, while tumors caused by the same RNA virus share both common TSTA and virion antigens. In addition, fetal or embryonic cytoplasmic and membrane antigens inappropriately reappear during malignant transformation through gene derepression by mechanisms similar to those leading to ectopic hormone production.

Analogous principles apply in man, but the antigens are termed tumor-associated (TAA) rather than tumor-specific (TSA), since the end point of a tumor transplant rejection cannot be used for definition. Fetal antigens have been demonstrated in cancers of the bowel, pancreas, and lung (carcinoembryonic antigen), in hepatoma and embryonal cancers (-fetoprotein), and in a wide variety of other tumors (-fetoprotein and others). TAA of both the individually specific and cross-reactive as well as cytoplasmic and membrane types has been described in Burkitt's lymphoma and nasopharyngeal cancer (some related to EBV), cervical cancer, melanoma, osteogenic sarcomas, soft tissue sarcomas, neuroblastoma, leukemias, and others. There is suggestive evidence only that some TAA may relate chemically to altered HLA antigens (recognition of altered self).

In animals and in some human tumors it is clear that the host mounts both humoral and cellular specific antitumor immune responses. The potential significance of such responses is shown by the markedly increased incidence of neoplasms in immunodeficient or immunosuppressed individuals and by the ease with which immunotherapy can control the growth of experimental tumors in animals. Many cancer patients resist the progress of their disease. Long-term dormancy of multiple metastases may be seen after removal of the primary tumor. Spontaneous regressions are occasionally seen in neuroblastoma, hypernephroma, choriocarcinoma, and melanoma. Genetic factors as well as the integrity of the immune system as altered by anticancer therapy will determine the ability to mount an immune response. The response is "compartmentalized" and plays varying roles during tumor progression.

On the humoral side, multiple antibody systems are mounted, each of which may have a different biologic role. In melanoma, for example, the disappearance from the circulation of IgG, complement-fixing, individually specific tumor antimembrane antibodies correlates within a few months with the appearance of visceral metastases from blood-borne spread. The role of secretory IgA on mucous membrane surfaces is just being explored.

As tumors progress, patients develop profound suppression of immunity, especially cellular (anergy), with systemic spread of tumor through the blood stream. The old concept that tumors are rejected like transplants by cellular immunity and that humoral immunity interferes (blocking) has been replaced by regulation models. Rather than immunosuppression, an imbalance between the B and T arms of the immune response is present.

The mechanisms that interfere with immune responsiveness as the tumor progresses are only beginning to be understood. In some instances tumor cells themselves secrete inhibitory factors such as prostaglandins. Tumor cells also shed surface antigens into the lymphatics and blood stream. These materials alone, or in combination with antibody as immune complexes, can react with and block receptors on immune lymphoid cells at a distance from the tumor (central blockade). Antibody may also coat tumor cells and block recognition of tumor-associated antigens by immune cells (peripheral blockade), but this mechanism appears to be of more importance in the laboratory. Circulating immune complexes (CIC) are extremely heterogeneous clinically and can be detected with increasing frequency and in increasing amounts with advancing disease. Assays for CIC in individual patients, however, do not predict well for either tumor burden, prognosis, or recurrence. Immune complex-mediated nephrotic syndrome is a rare complication of malignancy. Fever and systemic symptoms in Hodgkin's disease may relate to CIC. It is not understood why CIC so rarely produce symptoms. Excessive suppressor cell activity is also thought to play an important role in immunosuppression. The hypogammaglobulinemia seen in thymoma, multiple myeloma, and rare leukemias is mediated by circulating suppressor T-cells and monocytes. Similar mechanisms underlie the severe anergy of Hodgkin's disease and advanced solid tumors. One can even have tumors of helper cells (Sezary's syndrome) or suppressor cells (rare T-cell acute lymphocytic leukemias with hypogammaglobulinemia).

Clinical Manifestations of Cancer

EVALUATION OF THE CANCER PATIENT

Early Diagnosis

Particularly for the more common cancers, early detection and prompt treatment are essential for cure and prolonged survival. The Papanicolaou smear has reduced the incidence of invasive cervical cancer and lowered mortality by 50 per cent. Population-based screening for other tumors at present is controversial in terms of cost effectiveness. The family physician should identify and monitor individuals at high risk for cancer based on genetic, family, occupational, and social history. Patients participate actively in detection of their cancer. Over 90 per cent of new breast cancers are discovered each year by the patient, so education on thorough, frequent self-examination is necessary. Between 35 and 40 a baseline mammogram is recommended for asymptomatic women. Between the age of 39 and 49, women at high risk should have a mammogram yearly, while those of average risk a 2-year interval is recommended. Starting at age 50, an annual mammogram is suggested regardless of the risk factors. The "seven warning signals of early cancer" (American Cancer Society) are designed to encourage people to seek medical help for the early detection of cancers of the skin, breast, larynx, lung, and genitourinary and gastrointestinal tracts: (1) change in bowel and bladder habits; (2) a sore that does not heal; (3) unusual bleeding or discharge; (4) thickening or lump in the breast or elsewhere; (5) indigestion or difficulty in swallowing; (6) obvious change in a wart or mole; and (7) nagging cough or hoarseness.

History and Physical Examination

Careful observation of the patient can give many clues as to the presence of malignant disease. A few are illustrated in Table 56–1. Nonspecific symptoms suggestive of a systemic disease, such as infection, can also indicate the presence of a malignant tumor. An orderly history with thorough review of systems is important.

Clinical Signs. The skin frequently provides clues to the presence of malignancy internally. Painless, hard, nonhealing ulcers in sun-exposed areas may represent squamous or basal cell carcinoma. Careful palpation of the oropharyngeal cavity is important. Four per cent of patients with lung cancer may present with superior vena caval obstruction. The neck, face, and upper extremities swell, especially after a night of recumbency, and veins in the upper half of the body are dilated with downward venous flow. Superior sulcus tumors of the lung can produce Horner's syndrome with ptosis, miosis, and decreased facial sweating on the affected side owing to involvement of the stellate ganglion.

Malignancy is one cause for accumulation of fluid in pleural and peritoneal spaces. Tumor masses, in the breast, for example, are usually hard, painless, and circumscribed, do not move freely in the soft tissues, and are clearly felt with the flat surface of the fingers. Such a lesion is almost certainly malignant in the breast if it is fixed to the skin or if nipple retraction, skin edema, or deep fixation is present.

Enlarged lymph nodes from tumor are usually firm and painless and may be matted. Enlarged femoral lymph nodes are considered malignant until proven otherwise. Rectal examination is extremely important. An adnexal mass detected by pelvic examination in a premenopausal woman is usually a benign cyst if less than 6 cm. in diameter. Any adnexal mass in a postmenopausal woman needs investigation.

Diagnosis

Given the risks of staging procedures and therapy, histopathologic proof of malignancy must be obtained. There are rare exceptions, such as a glioma located in a critical area of the brain. Often the biopsy is easily obtained, such as in a subcutaneous nodule or enlarged lymph node, but occasionally it is difficult, as for example in the case of an inaccessible peripheral lung lesion requiring thoracotomy. An experienced pathologic opinion is essential, and if there is any doubt, the histologic material should receive expert review. Ancillary aids such as cytochemistry electron microscopy and tumor markers of various types may be needed for full classification.

Table 56–1. HISTORY AND PHYSICAL EXAMINATION IN CANCER DETECTION

Finding	Significance
History	
Fever, weight loss, night sweats	Tumor vs. Infection
Persistent cough ± hemoptysis	Tracheobronchial tree
Hoarseness	Recurrent laryngeal nerve or vocal cords
Hematemesis, jaundice, melena, increasing constipation ± abdominal pain	Gastrointestinal tract
Painless, recurrent hematuria	Urinary tract
Enlarging, firm, fixed mass	Breast or lymph node
Thyroid nodule	Thyroid
Sudden onset of intestinal obstruction in previously asymptomatic patient ≥ 50 years	Gastrointestinal tract
Petechiae, ecchymoses, uncontrolled bleeding, and persistent infections	Replacement of normal bone marrow by malignant cells
Physical Examination	
Skin	
Subcutaneous or dermal metastatic nodule	Breast, GI, lung, ovary, uterus
Pulsatile nodule	Hypernephroma, thyroid
Erythema multiforme, dermatomyositis, superficial migratory thrombophlebitis, necrotizing vasculitis, bullous dermatoses, acanthosis nigrans	Internal malignancy
Herpes zoster; unusual fungus infection	Impaired immunity in cancer
Head and Neck	
Tongue ulcer; unilateral enlarged tonsil	Oropharyngeal tumor
Superior vena cava obstruction	Lung cancer
Horner's syndrome	Superior sulcus lung tumor
Enlarged left supraclavicular lymph node (Virchow)	Abdominal malignancy
Breasts	
Mass	Breast tumor
Abdomen	
Umbilical mass	Peritoneal carcinomatosis
Abdominal mass, hepatomegaly	Abdominal tumor
Splenomegaly	Lymphoid or myeloid tumor (melanoma)
Genitals	
Unilateral or scrotal edema	Lymphatic obstruction by tumor
Ulcerating nodule of anus	Squamous cell carcinoma
Rectal exam	
Luminal mass	Rectal adenocarcinoma
Prostatic nodule	Prostatic carcinoma
Testicular mass	Tumor vs. epididymitis
Pelvic exam—adnexal mass	Tumor vs. cyst
Vaginal ulcer or nodule	Vaginal tumor
Lymphatic	
Lymphadenopathy	Primary or metastic cancer

Invasion of normal tissues, especially lymphatic channels and blood vessels, and extension through natural barriers such as a lymph node capsule are all important hallmarks of malignancy and are part of some histologic staging systems.

Staging

The outcome of any treatment regimen will relate to the interaction of the disease, the patient, and the therapy. A general scheme of systematic patient evaluation is needed to make a precise diagnosis and to delineate associated physiologic abnormalities and additional degenerative diseases, such as myocardial and respiratory insufficiency, which may limit therapy. A precise anatomic formulation includes the neoplasm's location, site of origin, and tissue type. The anatomic extent of the disease locally and regionally and the extent of its spread throughout the body influence the choice of a potentially curative or palliative therapy.

Staging systems are based on the known pathophysiology of a tumor. No two tumors have the same natural history so that a variety of systems is used. Some are based on biologic staging. The International Union Against Cancer uses a system based on the volume or size of the primary tumor, the degree of local spread to regional lymph nodes, and the distant spread as metastases. The clinical TNM (Tumor, Nodes, Metastasis) classification applies to patients not previously treated (Table 56–2). Most staging classifications assess tumor volume poorly. They do provide guidance for clinicians for the selection of treatment and the assessment of prognosis. They assume comparability of cases in various institutions and permit communication of data among treatment centers for clinical studies.

Pathologic staging using a staging operation may also be needed to find the extent or stage of disease so that appropriate definitive treatment can be selected. For example, mediastinoscopy will detect regional spread in lung cancer preoperatively; 35 per cent of such patients will have mediastinal lymph node metastases, a contraindication to thoracotomy. Bone marrow biopsy can establish the presence of tumor spread to the bone marrow. Regional lymph node dissections in melanoma or breast cancer are essentially staging procedures to determine occult regional spread (prognosis) and the need for adjuvant systemic therapy in breast cancer. The staging laparotomy in Hodgkin's disease attempts to assess exact disease extent to avoid undertreatment with risk of early relapse or overtreatment with risk of excessive morbidity and mortality. The procedure includes splenectomy, since splenic involvement can be determined only through pathologic serial sectioning, as well as biopsies of the liver and various retroperitoneal and mesenteric lymph nodes. Areas of biopsy and masses are marked with metal clips to allow the radiotherapist subsequently to plan therapy. A staging laparotomy is a meticulous procedure that should be done by an experienced surgeon.

Table 56–2. TNM PRETREATMENT CLINICAL CLASSIFICATION*

Primary Tumor (T)	
T0	No evidence of primary tumor
TIS	Preinvasive carcinoma (carcinoma in situ)
T1, T2, T3, T4	Progressive increase in tumor size and local extent
TX	Minimum requirements to assess the regional lymph nodes cannot be met
Regional Lymph Nodes (N)	
N0	No evidence of regional lymph node involvement
N1, N2, N3	Progressive involvement of regional lymph nodes
N4	Involvement of juxtaregional lymph nodes
NX	Minimum requirements to assess the regional lymph nodes cannot be met
Distant Metastases (M)	
M0	No evidence of distant metastases
M1	Evidence of distant metastases
PUL: Pulmonary	MAR: Bone Marrow
OSS: Osseous	PLE: Pleura
HEP: Hepatic	SKI: Skin
BRA: Brain	EYE: Eye
LYM: Lymph nodes	OTH: Other
MX	Minimum requirements to assess the presence of distant metastases cannot be met.

*From Harmer, M. H. (ed): TNM Classfication of Malignant Tumors. 3rd ed. Geneva, UICC, 1978.

Tumor markers are needed to guide the duration and intensity of further therapy by measuring the small amounts of residual disease presumed to be present after surgical resection or drug-induced remission. Undetected residual disease is a major obstacle to curative therapy. A distinctive diagnostic test for cancer applicable to blood or urine remains elusive. In a sense, the measurement of liver enzymes, acid phosphatase, or serum calcium, for example, represents tumor markers of host origin that are useful in monitoring disease. Other markers exist at the cellular level. Hormone receptors in breast cancer and lymphocyte surface markers or oncogene probes in leukemia are examples. Ectopic hormones and oncofetal antigens produced by tumor cells are most commonly thought of as tumor markers. They are all limited in usefulness by being present in detectable amounts in normal adults if sensitive enough assays are used.

Many tumors produce excessive amounts of hormones or proteins normally produced by the cell of origin, which can also be used as markers. Hypersecretion of insulin or gastrin by islet cell tumors, the M spike in multiple myeloma, and the elevated serum acid phosphatase in prostate cancer are all examples.

Other tumors secrete markers ectopically that are foreign to the cell of origin. All somatic cells contain a full genetic complement. Ectopic hormone production after malignant transformation is due to selective derepression of dormant genes as part of disordered differentiation. Small cell lung cancers secrete adrenocorticotropic hormone (ACTH), antidiuretic hormone (ADH), and calcitonin. Islet cell carcinomas secrete ACTH, vasoactive intestinal polypeptide (VIP), serotonin, and HCG. Nonseminomatous testicular cancers may secrete chronic gonadotrophic as well as alpha-fetoprotein. Medullary thyroid carcinomas secrete ACTH and serotonin. Often the peptide hormones exist in precursor forms (proinsulin, pro- or "big" ACTH), which may have little or no bioactivity when compared with the derived circulating hormones.

Clinical Presentation of Cancer

Neoplastic diseases present varied and inconstant clinical profiles. Onset is difficult to date, but where there has been known carcinogenic exposure (atom bomb survivors, thymic irradiation, chromate exposure), a prolonged latency or induction period may be seen. A decade or more may pass before detectable disease evolves so that clinical manifestations represent the end-stage of natural history.

The earliest recognizable stage of clinical cancer, bordering on premalignancy, is carcinoma in situ. It is seen not only on the uterine cervix but at many tissue sites. A significant proportion may never evolve into clinical cancer.

Malignant neoplasms may persist for months or years and produce few symptoms, being discovered by chance or pursuing a chronic course with multiple recurrences over decades, as in melanoma. Of men over age 40, 15 per cent will have pathologic evidence of prostatic cancer at autopsy (death from any cause), but only 2 per cent will develop clinically progressive disease. Chronic lymphocytic leukemia may persist for long periods with few symptoms and require no definitive therapy.

Advancing tumors cause symptoms of two types: masses or growths including the properties of invasion and metastasis and physiologic derangements. Solid primary tumors grow as masses and produce physical alterations in adjacent organ systems, including pressure, destruction, perforation, and invasion with replacement. Nonhealing ulcerative lesions may lead to chronic infection and bleeding. In liquid tumors such as the leukemias, the disease is disseminated, with replacement of the bone marrow by malignant cells, resulting in fever from infection as well as bleeding.

Disseminated or metastatic tumors can also cause mass-related symptoms. Tumor cells spread principally by vascular and lymphatic routes and occasionally along serous surfaces (peritoneal, pleural, or pericardial) with the formation of effusions. The most common sites for metastatic disease are the lungs (osteogenic sarcoma, renal carcinoma) and the liver (gastric and colon cancers). Malignant cells are thought to be present but not detectable in these sites initially. Thus, cancer is frequently a systemic disease at presentation.

The more frequent sites of presentation of metastatic neoplasms include cervical and supraclavicular lymph nodes, lungs, liver, bones, and brain. Melanoma and primary tumors of breast, bronchus, stomach, and kidney may present with widespread nodular and infiltrative skin and subcutaneous deposits. Stomach, colon, and ovarian cancers may present with metastatic masses in the umbilicus. Tumors of the nasopharynx, pharynx, oral cavity, and thyroid may present with involvement of cervical lymph nodes but rarely with more distant metastases. The supraclavicular lymph nodes may be involved at presentation by tumors of the bronchus, breast, stomach, esophagus, pancreas, colon, testes, ovary, and uterine cervix. Nonpalpable scalene nodes rarely yield a diagnosis of metastatic cancer. Tumors of the genitalia and rectum may present with inguinal lymph node involvement, but inflammatory disease is a frequently encountered alternative. Several neoplasms (breast, colon, kidney, testes, stomach, skin, thyroid) may present in the lungs, usually with multiple nodules, and rarely as a solitary lesion or as lymphangitic spread. Hepatomegaly, usually with hepatic insufficiency, may be the presenting manifestation of tumors of the colon, breast, bronchus, stomach, and pancreas. The lactate dehydrogenase isoenzymes may be elevated early, and disproportionate elevations of hepatic alkaline phosphatase are seen later. Tumors of the colon and stomach may spread to the ovary (Krukenberg's tumor) and exceed the size of the primary tumor several times. Several tumors may present with lesions in marrow-bearing bones (breast, bronchus, kidney, prostate, thyroid). Most lesions are lytic, occasionally sclerotic, and produce pain, local tenderness, and occasionally a mass or fracture and deformity. In 70 per cent of instances, metastases to the central nervous system are usually multiple and may be the mode of presentation of tumors of the bronchus, breast, colon, and kidney. Seizures, pain, localizing symptoms such as paresis, and increased intracranial pressure can all result. Tumors of the bronchus, breast, and ovary, and lymphoma can present in serous cavities with effusions. Cytologic studies should be interpreted cautiously.

Many physiologic abnormalities associated with tumors may not relate to the physical consequences of their presence yet may be the primary determinants of prognosis and therapy in some patients (Table 56–3). Tumors may arise in organs that normally produce physiologically active products such as hormones. These tumors may escape normal feedback controls and produce excessive amounts of these substances. Such is the case, for example, with functional adenomas of the pituitary, parathyroid, thyroid, pancreatic islets, and adrenal cortex and medulla. Usually tumors arise from organs that normally do not elaborate hormones, yet certain of these tumors produce polypeptides with hormonal activity. Bronchogenic neoplasms may produce an ACTH-like substance that induces hyperadrenocorticism or a parathormonelike material that induces hypercalcemia. Some bronchogenic tumors may inappropriately secrete antidiuretic hormone or substances responsible for disproportionate anorexia and wasting or hypertrophic pulmonary osteoarthropathy.

These ectopic hormone-producing tumors are classified into two groups. Those arising from neural crest cells, which have migrated to the foregut and branchial arches, include small cell lung cancer, medullary thyroid cancer, thymoma, pancreatic islet cell tumors, and carcinoids. These tumor cells may contain large neurosecretory granules and active aromatic amines (Pearse's APUD cells). They may secrete calcitonin, ACTH, MSH, vasopressin, insulin, gastrin, secretin, glucagon, serotonin, histamine, and other biogenic amines. The second group of tumors originate in endoderm or mesoderm. They include cancers of the bronchus, gastrointestinal tract, and kidney, sarcomas of connective tissue and blood vessels, lymphoreticular tumors, non-germ-cell gonadal tumors, and adrenal cortical tumors. They may secrete parathormone, erythropoietin, gonadotrophins, prolactin, growth hormone, renin, or thyrotrophin.

Table 56–3. PARANEOPLASTIC SYNDROMES: ECTOPIC HORMONE PRODUCTION

Mechanism	Syndrome	Tumor Type
Pituitary Hormones		
ACTH	Cushing's Syndrome	Oat cell carcinoma, thymoma, pancreatic islet cell tumors bronchial carcinoids, thyroid medullary carcinoid
ADH	Inappropriate ADH	Oat cell carcinoma, other lung tumors, duodenum, pancreas, thymoma, lymphoma
MSH	Hyperpigmentation	Oat cell carcinoma, lung tumors
LTH, FSH, STH	Clubbing, hypertrophic pulmonary osteoarthropathy	Adenocarcinoma and epidermoid carcinoma of lung, esophagus, colon
HCG, LTH	Gynecomastia	Lung carcinoma; rarely cancers of liver, adrenal, and dysgerminoma of ovary
TSH	Hyperthyroidism	Choriocarcinoma, hydatidiform mole, embryonal carcinoma of testis
Parathyroid Hormones		
PTH	Hyperparathyroidism	Kidney, lung (squamous), pancreatic, and ovarian tumors
(also prostaglandin E2)	Hypercalcemia	
Calcitonin	Hypocalcemia	Thyroid medullary carcinoma, breast cancer, oat cell carcinoma
Gastrointestinal Hormones		
Pancreas-islets of Langerhans		
Insulin, Insulinlike activity	Hypoglycemia	Retroperitoneal sarcomas and liver tumors, mesothelioma, lymphoma
glucagon	Hyperglycemia	Islet cell tumors
gastrin	Zollinger-Ellison syndrome	Islet cell tumors, multiple endocrine adenomatosis Type I
Intestine		
vasoactive intestinal peptide	Pancreatic cholera	Islet cell tumors
gastrin	Zollinger-Ellison syndrome	
Renal Hormones		
Renin	Hypertension	Renal tumors
Erythropoietin	Erythrocytosis	Cerebellar hemangioma, renal cell, liver, and uterine tumors
Angiotensin	Hypertension	Renal tumors

The production of ectopic hormones, as well as proteins ordinarily synthesized at or around fetal life, is a useful marker for neoplastic growth and an important biologic indicator of the defective gene regulation and deranged differentation operative in oncogenesis with inappropriate activation of latent genes.

Principles of Therapy

In treating cancer it is assumed that all malignant cells should be destroyed, removed, or neutralized to achieve cure, since experimentally the control of tumors requires eradication of the last neoplastic cell. It is not known at present whether successful treatment must eradicate all neoplastic cells or merely reduce the cell number to a level that the host's own defenses can control. Four modalities of therapy exist today: surgery, radiotherapy, endocrine therapy, and chemotherapy. Immunotherapy has experienced a resurgence of interest in the 1980's within a broader context of biologic therapies, which promise to become a fifth modality for treating cancer. Because cancer is not one but 100 or more different diseases, many therapeutic strategies are needed. For some tumors a specific therapy may exist; for others there may be several satisfactory alternatives. Thus, optimal therapy depends not only on the nature and extent of the disease but also on the experience of the treating physician and the treatment facilities available.

For solid tumors, surgery and radiotherapy are traditionally chosen first to deal with the early locoregional presentation of the disease. Once the disease has disseminated, a systemic therapy such as chemotherapy is needed for secondary or tertiary treatment. Hematologic malignancies are frequently disseminated from the start, so chemotherapy may be the treatment of choice initially.

The multiplicity of diseases and therapies requires a multidisciplinary input from surgical oncologists, radiation oncologists, medical oncologists, and pathologists. The pediatric oncologist has demonstrated the value of a multimodal therapeutic attack on cancer, as shown by advances in the treatment of Wilms' tumor, embryonal rhabdomyosarcoma, and

Ewing's sarcoma. More recently, adult oncologists have appreciated the combined modality approach in adult solid tumor therapy.

Many tumors that are apparently localized at the time of diagnosis are in fact microscopically disseminated, as subsequent recurrences after attempts at curative locoregional therapy prove. Groups of patients in whom dissemination can be assumed to have occurred at diagnosis in a large percentage of instances include breast cancer with positive axillary lymph nodes, colon cancer with penetration through the entire bowel wall or involving regional lymph nodes, and all gastric, pancreatic, and lung cancers after "curative" resection. Current diagnostic tools fail to identify these patients. Thus, a systemic therapy, such as chemotherapy, is added as an adjuvant to local therapy to reduce recurrences and prolong survival. In this case, "cure" means a life expectancy the same as "normal" life expectancy of a matched cohort in the general population.

Experimentally, chemotherapy is more effective with smaller tumor cell burdens, since drugs kill by first order kinetics (each dose kills a fixed percentage rather than a fixed number of cells). Thus, adequate cell kill can be achieved with a small tumor burden using a reasonable number of repetitive doses. With a large tumor cell burden the same doses would still leave residual cells, resulting in regrowth of resistant cell populations. For adjuvant regimens, drugs are chosen that can give objective regressions (greater than 50 per cent tumor shrinkage) frequently in advanced disease. It is then assumed that they will achieve total cell kill of the microscopic residual disease remaining after surgical removal of the great mass of tumor bulk. Recent results in the adjuvant therapy of breast cancer and osteogenic sarcoma suggest that this assumption is valid.

The use of immunotherapy as an adjuvant to surgery and radiotherapy has a similar rationale. However, the modality kills a fixed number of cells per application of treatment and is able to control only small cell numbers. Therefore, regression of advanced disease cannot be used to predict success, and there is no correlation yet established between tumor cell control and the various tests of immune function. The lack of effective monitoring and the empirical approach necessary for design of therapy make immunotherapy an experimental modality at present.

The rapid technologic developments in the delivery of these various modalities have made the bulk of cancer therapy deliverable in the outpatient and office setting. This is a significant development for patients who must cope, often for months or years, with their cancer therapy in addition to their normal daily activities.

LOCOREGIONAL THERAPY

Optimally, antitumor treatment should eradicate all manifestation of the disease completely and permanently. The cancer cell is regarded as an offending foreign "organism" to be removed or destroyed by various therapeutic modalities.

Surgery

Historically cancer has been a surgical disease. Surgical excision is still the current principal curative therapy, especially for cancers at accessible sites that can be detected early and excised completely. The location and extent of the tumor rather than its type limit the surgeon. The operative risks of anesthesia and surgery and the morbidity after the procedure must all be taken into account.

With some tumors systemic speed is thought to occur early with micrometastatic deposits beyond the tumor field. Regional lymph node involvement becomes an indicator of metastatic activity with adverse survival. Stage II breast cancer or Duke's C colon cancer are examples. Here surgery of the primary tumor is becoming less radical, with, for example, a lumpectomy with breast radiotherapy producing results as good as with radical or modified radical mastectomy in breast cancer. In this setting regional node dissection is a staging procedure in addition to providing regional control. Nontherapeutic staging procedures are also used, such as laparotomy for Hodgkin's disease and other lymphomas and second-look procedures for ovarian and colon cancer.

Laser surgery, often with an operating microscope, is becoming a useful approach in certain settings. Blood dyscrasias, seriously ill patients, and palliation of obstructing esophageal and tracheobronchial lesions through a rigid endoscope are examples of its use. The tissue is vaporized and small blood vessels and lymphatics are sealed with a fine incision and minimal damage to adjacent tissue. The controlled depth of penetration helps avoid perforation in surgery of the head and neck and tracheobronchial tree. Laser surgery through a colposcope can provide control of early uterine cervical neoplasms, as can cryosurgery.

Radical surgery in the head and neck region, pelvic exenteration, and hemicorporectomy are less often used as a last resort for locally advanced primary or recurrent tumors. Advances in prosthetics and reconstructive surgery of the head and neck and pelvis may make these radical procedures more acceptable.

Radiotherapy

Ionizing radiations of various types and energies are used to destroy localized populations of cancer cells. The location and anatomic extent of the lesion limit the procedure. As with surgery, results are best with relatively small lesions detected before they produce dysfunction of major organs or spread beyond the limits of feasible treatment fields. The tolerance of adjacent normal tissue limits the amount of radiation that can be given.

X-rays are nonparticulate, electromagnetic ionizing radiations (photons) produced by machine; gamma rays are emitted by natural or artificially produced radioisotopes, such as radium or cobalt-60. These radiations have high energy and short wavelengths with extremely high penetrating power in materials of low atomic number (e.g., water and tissue) but are stopped by materials of high atomic number like lead. Through ionization of water molecules the radiation produces free radicals and oxidants within the target cells. These chemically reactive agents break and damage DNA molecules. Although the exact mechanism is undefined, irradiation through altering nucleotide sequences seems to produce a change in transcription and defective repair, which leads to cell death.

Cobalt irradiation units are the workhorse of radiation oncology, and linear (electron) accelerators are photon generators that are becoming widely employed. Because of reduced skin doses and lesser internal scatter, high doses of radiation can be delivered to tumors at any depth in the body by megavoltage irradiation. Linear accelerators deliver sharper beam margins than cobalt units and can also provide electrons that are particulate and penetrate in a tighter range with an abrupt fall off in tissues (Bragg effect), sparing deeper normal tissues from irradiation. Linear accelerators can also provide electrons. Their low penetrance spares deeper tissues so that they are useful for skin lesions, such as myosis fungoides, and for intraoperative radiotherapy. Other forms of particulate irradiation that are more penetrating than electrons are under experiment. These include fast neutrons and charged particles such as protons, helium ions, and negative pi mesons. These particles produce a more intense deposition of energy per unit path in the tissue (high linear energy transfer, or LET) than ordinary photons. They also have, theoretically, a greater relative biologic effectiveness because hypoxic areas of tumors respond better to them than to conventional photons. Early and promising studies are in progress with ocular melanomas, head and neck and salivary gland cancers, and gastric and pancreatic cancers with intraoperative radiotherapy.

Radiation dosage is expressed in units called grays (Gy), which measure the amount of energy absorbed per unit volume of tissue. One gray equals 100 rad. The effects of radiation depend on the time over which it is delivered and the dose per fraction. Usual dose fractionation is about 10 Gy (1000 rads) per week delivered in 1.5 to 2.5 Gy (150 to 250 rad fractions). Megavoltage equipment now allows experimentation with shorter and more intense dose fractionation.

Whole body irradiation is used infrequently in clinical practice. Most radiation therapy is directed toward specific anatomic sites or regions, and the patient may experience a systemic reaction as well as effects produced on normal tissues within the treatment field. Radiation sickness is characterized by general debility, anorexia, and vomiting that begins soon after the onset of treatment and subsides promptly when therapy is stopped or the dose reduced. Occurrence relates to dose and to volume and type of tissue treated.

The early regional toxic effects of radiation produced within days result from acute cell injury and death, sometimes with tissue necrosis complicated by infection. Within weeks tissue regenerates, but with scarring and fibrosis. Severe late radiation effects, occurring after months, arise chiefly from vascular damage that produces tissue atrophy and necrosis and ulceration in the skin or delayed development of organ dysfunction as in radiation nephritis or myelitis. Neoplastic changes may occur years later.

Radiosensitizer Drugs. As a tumor mass enlarges, it outgrows its blood supply. The peripheral edge of the tumor remains well vascularized, but the center becomes hypoxic and may infarct or undergo necrosis. Irradiation is less effective to hypoxic tissues than to well-oxygenated ones, since the free radical state of molecular oxygen is needed to interact with the ionization products created by the radiation beam for its effect. In experimental tumor systems, the size of the hypoxic fraction is directly proportional to the failure rate of local treatment. Hyperbaric oxygen, high LET radiation, and hypoxic cell sensitizer drugs have all been used to improve the destruction of hypoxic cells. The nitroimidazoles have the greatest potential as radiosensitizers since they penetrate to hypoxic centers of tumors in spite of poor blood supply. Examples are metronidazole or misonidazole. Their use in clinical trials to date has been limited owing to neurotoxicity. Thiol-depleting agents like N-ethylmaleimide or buthionine sulfoxime render cells radiosensitive, as do certain cytotoxic drugs such as bromodeoxyuridine and idoxuridine in noncytotoxic doses. The toxic effects of doxorubicin, dactinomycin, and bleomycin are enhanced on normal tissues such as skin, heart, and lungs when used with radiotherapy. Some chemicals are also radioprotectors, but ethiofos, for example, protects normal and tumor tissue equally.

Hyperthermia. The means to produce safe and effective deep internal hyperthermia in humans in the range of 43° to 45° C. is only now being developed with radiofrequency, microwave, ultrasound, and other sources, so that most investigation has centered on superficial lesions. Experiments show that for the roughly one third of tumors that can be heated, hyperthermia alone may be beneficial as a single agent. Its greatest potential may be in combination with other therapies. A synergistic or additive effect may exist between heating and both chemotherapy and radiotherapy, leading to the hope of reducing doses of both to provide effective treatment with fewer side effects. Heat kills cells in the S phase, the most radioresistant phase of the cell cycle, and tumor cells are more sensitive than normal cells. Sensitivity to heat is increased in the interior of tumors under low pH, hypoxia, poor perfusion, and nutrient supply where radiation is poorly effective. Current emphasis is on the use of microwave hyperthermia to potentiate photon radiotherapy.

Photodynamic Therapy

Light-absorbing substances like hematoporphyrin derivatives are selectively retained by tumor cells which are then killed when exposed to laser beams of appropriate wavelengths. Superficial and localized lesions of the skin or intrabronchial tumors now respond to laser beams through an endoscope. The approach is new and still experimental.

SYSTEMIC THERAPY

Chemotherapy

The introduction of the polyfunctional alkylating agents in the early 1940's ushered in the modern era of chemotherapy. Now several classes of these agents are in common use (Table 56–4), and many more are under continual development.

Most agents work by affecting enzymes or substrates acted upon by enzyme systems (Table 56–5). Usually these effects relate to DNA synthesis or function. Drugs interfering with DNA synthesis or mitosis are active against proliferating cells rather than resting cells. They are most effective during the S phase (DNA synthesis) of the cell cycle or when the mitotic spindle is forming. These drugs are most active against tumors with a high rate of cellular proliferation and relatively ineffective against tumors with a small growth fraction.

Agents that are mainly effective during a particular phase of the cell cycle are called cell cycle specific or phase specific. Drugs whose action is prolonged and independent of DNA synthesis are called cell cycle nonspecific or phase nonspecific and will be effective against tumors with relatively low proliferative activity. This distinction between specific and nonspecific agents is relative rather than absolute.

An undesirable consequence of these drug actions is that normal tissues that have a high rate of cellular proliferation suffer toxic side effects. These include normal bone marrow elements (anemia, leukopenia with infection, thrombocytopenia with bleeding), the gastrointestinal tract (anorexia, nausea, vomiting, diarrhea, surface ulceration), and the hair follicles (alopecia).

The major toxicities for individual drugs are listed in Table 56–4. Because of the seriousness of potential side effects, the narrow therapeutic range separating toxicity from therapeutic efficacy, and the necessity to use maximum tolerated doses for effective tumor cell kill, it is essential that cancer chemotherapy be given in consultation with an experienced oncologist. Specific written protocols for particular disease regimens should be consulted and carefully followed for details of drug dose and scheduling as well as indications and contraindications defining patient eligibility. Drug doses are frequently modified for specific toxicities as well as for concomitant hepatic or renal dysfunction.

In addition to the development of sensitive methods to measure the active portion of both drugs and their cellular targets within the therapeutic range, the advent of infusion devices to provide continuous infusion chemotherapy has been a significant advance. This strategy can overcome pharmacokinetic problems with drugs that have short half-lives by exposing tumor cells to effective drug levels for periods in excess of the cell cycle of the tumor. In the liver one can use drugs that are metabolically inactivated by normal liver to reduce systemic toxicity. Totally implantable access ports and infusion pumps allow outpatient therapy with flexible scheduling and greater convenience and comfort for the patient. Treatment of hepatic metastases from colon carcinoma by this approach is promising and can be combined with external radiation therapy with or without the use of vasoconstrictors or drugs trapped in starch granules which are subsequently dissolved by amylase. Experimental approaches to ovarian cancer uses intraperitoneal therapy with dialysis. Intra-arterial infusion therapy is used for gliomas, hepatic metastasis, and malignant melanoma in extremities combined with hyperthermia by warming the infusate.

Combination Chemotherapy. Drug combinations are used principally to try to circumvent the development of drug resistance (Tables 56–6 to 56–8). Various mechanisms have been proposed for the development of resistance, chiefly on the basis of experimental systems. Unlike animal tumors, human tumors have a very small percentage of cells in the proliferating pool so that single drugs used over a short time will not guarantee maximum tumor cell kill. Repeated therapy over long time periods not only increases the risk of toxicity but also leads to clinical resistance to the drugs. Tumor cells regrow between cycles of therapy (which must be separated by intervals long enough to let normal tissues recover), and few tumor cells are killed with each successive treatment cycle because of the evolution of resistant cell lines. Human tumors are heterogeneous, so resistance may relate to the preferential selection of a pre-existing population of neoplastic cells in the tumor inherently resistant to the drug used. Alternatively, drug resistance can result from a stepwise induction of resistance by analogy with bacterial populations. Thus, additional effective drugs are needed to treat each resistant cell line. The success of drug treatment will thus depend both on the number of resistant lines in the tumor and on the number of available drugs for use in effective combinations.

The biochemical approach to designing drug combinations selects agents that produce multiple, different biochemical lesions in biosynthetic pathways or inhibit several processes needed to maintain the function of essential macromolecules. Both of these strategies reduce the production and availability of a

Table 56–4. COMMON CANCER CHEMOTHERAPEUTIC DRUGS

Drug	Acute Toxicity	Delayed Toxicity
Alkylating Agents		
Mechlorethamine (Nitrogen mustard)	*GI (N, V);* phlebitis	*M(L, T):* skin vesicant
Busulfan (Myleran)	*GI (N, V);* rare diarrhea	*M(L, T);* anemia; pulmonary fibrosis; pigmentation; amenorrhea; gynecomastia; wasting syndrome
Chlorambucil (Leukeran)	None	*M(L, T);* anemia; pancytopenia with long-term use
Cyclophosphamide (Cytoxan)	*GI (N, V);* anaphylaxis	*M(L);* alopecia; anemia; hemorrhagic cystitis; thrombocytopenia less severe; pigmentation
Ifosfamide	*GI (N, V);* confusion	*M(L);* hemorrhagic cystitis; alopecia; sterility; nephrotoxicity; inappropriate ADH
Melphalan (Phenylalanine mustard)	*Nausea,* hypersensitivity	*M(L, T);* anemia; thrombocytopenia persistent after long use
Thiotepa	*GI (N, V);* local pain	*M(L, T);* anemia
Antimetabolites		
Methotrexate (Amethopterin)	*GI (N, V);* diarrhea; fever; anaphylaxis	*M(L, T);* anemia; oral and GI ulceration, perforation; hepatic (necrosis, cirrhosis) and renal toxicity; alopecia, dermatitis and osteoporosis
6-Mercaptopurine	*GI (N, V);* diarrhea	*M(L, T); cholestasis and hepatic necrosis; oral and intestinal ulcers;* anemia; reduce dose to 26% with allopurinol
6-Thioguanine (Lanvis)	*GI (N, V);* occasional	*M(L, T);* anemia; stomatitis; hepatotoxicity; no dose adjustment with allopurinol
5-Fluorouracil	*GI (N, V);* diarrhea	*Oral and GI ulcers; M(L, T);* anemia; lacrimination; cerebellar ataxia; pigmentation, alopecia; dermatitis
Floxuridine (FUDR)	*GI (N, V);* diarrhea; hypersensitivity	M; oral and GI ulcers; alopecia; dermatitis
Deoxycoformycin	*GI (N, V)*	*M(L, T);* nephroxicity; CNS depression
Cytosine arabinoside (Cytosar)	*GI (N, V);* diarrhea; anaphylaxis	*M(L, T);* megaloblastosis; oral ulcers; hepatic toxicity; alopecia
Azacytidine	*GI (N, V);* diarrhea; fever; drowsiness	*M(L, T);* liver and heart damage; muscle pain and weakness
Plant Alkaloids		
Vinblastine (Velban)	*GI (N, V);* phlebitis	*M(L);* anemia, thrombocytopenia uncommon; alopecia; stomatitis, peripheral neuropathy; jaw pain, paralytic ileus
Vincristine (Oncovin)	Local necrosis with extravasation	*Peripheral neuropathy;* alopecia; M(L) mild; obstipation
Etoposide (VP16)	*GI (N, V);* diarrhea; fever; hypotension	M; alopecia, peripheral neuropathy allergic reactions; liver toxicity
Vindesine sulfate	Local reaction with extravasation; fever; GI (N, V); diarrhea	M; alopecia; peripheral neuropathy; jaw pain
Teniposide (VM-26)	GI (N, V); diarrhea; phlebitis anaphylaxis	M; alopecia; peripheral neuropathy
Antibiotics		
Actinomycin D (Dactinomycin)	*GI (N, V);* diarrhea; phlebitis	*Mucositis; oral ulcers; M(L, T),* anemia; alopecia, acne; severe dermatitis in irradiated areas
Adriamycin (Doxorubicin)	*GI (N, V);* diarrhea, red urine; local necrosis with extravasation; transient ECG changes, ventricular arrhythmia; hypertensive encephalopathy	*M(L);* anemia and thrombocytopenia less common, *cardiotoxicity;* alopecia, stomatitis not to exceed total dose of 550 mg. per m^2
Bleomycin (Blenoxane)	*GI (N, V);* fever; anaphylaxis	*Pneumonitis, pulmonary fibrosis; dermatitis;* stomatitis; alopecia; pigmentation, maximum dose 400 units
Daunorubicin (Rubidomycin)	*GI (N, V);* red urine, necrosis on local extravasation, transient ECG changes, fever	*M(L, T); anemia cardiotoxicity, alopecia* stomatitis; dermatitis; maximum dose 600 mg. per m^2
Mithramycin (Mithracin Plicamycin)	*GI (N, V);* diarrhea; fever	*Coagulation defects;* M(T), leukopenia; thrombocytopenia, hepatic toxicity, stomatitis; skin flushing
Mitomycin C (Mutamycin)	*GI (N, V);* local necrosis with extravasation; fever	*M(L, T* cumulative); anemia; stomatitis; renal toxicity; alopecia; pulmonary fibrosis; hepatotoxicity
Mitoxantrone HCl	*GI (N, V);* blue-green sclerae	M; stomatitis; alopecia; white hair; cardiotoxicity
Nitrosoureas		
BCNU (Carmustine)	*GI (N, V);* phlebitis	*M(L, T* delayed 4–6 weeks and prolonged); pulmonary fibrosis; pigmentation
CCNU (Lomustine)	*GI (N, V)*	*M(L, T* delayed 4–6 weeks and prolonged) stomatitis; alopecia

Table 56–4. COMMON CANCER CHEMOTHERAPEUTIC DRUGS *Continued*

Drug	Acute Toxicity	Delayed Toxicity
Methyl-CCNU (Semustine)	*GI (N,V)*	M(*L,T* delayed 4–6 weeks); thrombocytopenia severe; anemia; alopecia; myelosuppression cumulative
Streptozotocin	*GI (N,V);* local pain; chills	Renal damage; hyperglycemia; hepatotoxicity; M(LT), anemia; diarrhea
Enzymes		
L-Asparaginase (Elspar)	*GI (N,V); fever, hypersensitivity* chills, headache; anaphylaxis; abdominal pain; hyperglycemia leading to coma	Pancreatitis; CNS toxicity; coagulation defects; renal and hepatic damage; hypofibrinogenemia
Miscellaneous		
cis-Platinum	*GI (N,V);* anaphylactoid reactions; fever	*Renal damage;* M(L,T), anemia; high frequency ototoxicity; hydration and mannitol to prevent renal toxicity
Carboplatin	*GI (N,V)*	M; rare peripheral neuropathy
Estramustine phosphate sodium	*GI (N,V);* diarrhea	Gynecomastia; rare M; increased vascular accidents; edema; dyspnea; pulmonary infiltrate, fibrosis, leukemia
Amsacrine (AMSA)	*GI (N,V);* diarrhea; anaphylaxis	M; hepatic injury; convulsions; stomatitis; alopecia; ventricular fibrillation
Dacarbazine (Imidazole carboxamide)	*GI (N,V);* pain; anaphylaxis	*M(L,T* cumulative); flulike reaction; alopecia, renal and hepatic toxicity
Procarbazine	*GI (N,V);* CNS depression	*M(L,T*-delayed); stomatitis, dermatitis, pigmentation; CNS toxicity; side effects with monoamine oxidase inhibitors
o,p′-DDD (Mitotane)	*GI (N,V);* diarrhea	*CNS depression,* dermatitis; adrenal insufficiency
Hexamethylmelamine	*GI (N,V)*	*M(L,T),* anemia; peripheral neuritis
Hydroxyurea	*GI (N,V);* allergy to tartrazine dye	*M(L,T),* megaloblastosis; stomatitis; rash; alopecia
Biologics		
Interferon (alpha)	Fever; chills, myalgia; fatigue headache; arthralgia; hypotension	M; anorexia; renal and hepatic damage
Interleukin-2	GI (N,V); diarrhea; fluid retention; hypotension; rash	M(T); anemia; capillary leak syndrome; nephromyocardial and hepatotoxicity

Major dose limiting toxicities are italicized. Only usual toxicities are listed.
Abbreviations: GI (N,V): Nausea and vomiting; M(L,T): Bone marrow depressions (leukopenia).

specific end product vital for tumor cell growth and replication. In sequential blockade different enzymatic steps are inhibited in a biochemical pathway that produces an essential metabolite. In concurrent blockade there is simultaneous inhibition of parallel metabolic pathways that synthesize a common end product. Complementary inhibition occurs when one selects agents that produce biochemical lesions at different sites in the synthesis of polymeric macromolecules. Although intellectually satisfying, none of the successful drug combinations used today have been developed purely by this approach but may owe some of their effectiveness to such synergistic mechanisms.

Table 56–5. CHARACTERISTICS OF COMMON ANTICANCER DRUGS

Drugs	Cell Cycle	Mechanism
Alkylating Agents Nitrosoureas	Nonspecific (G2 arrest) Cyclophosphamide is cycle active	Alkylation of nucleic acids, especially bases in DNA with cross-linking of strands
Antimetabolites Hydroxyurea	Specific S-phase most sensitive	Interfere with critical enzyme functions; drugs are structural analogues of normal enzyme substrates
Antibiotics cis-Platinum DNA	Specific S-phase most sensitive ADR is cycle nonspecific	Intercalate in minor groove of DNA to interfere with transcription; cause breaks in strands
Plant Alkaloids	Specific Metaphase arrest	Mitotic inhibitors: interact with microtubular proteins to prevent assembly of mitotic spindle
Miscellaneous	Nonspecific	Procarbazine: reacts with DNA to fragment strands o,p′-DDD: impairs 17 O-H corticosteroid synthesis with damage to adrenal cortex L-Asparaginase: depletes asparagine to deprive asparagine-dependent tumor cells

Table 56–6. DRUGS CURRENTLY PREFERRED FOR DISEASES IN WHICH CHEMOTHERAPY HAS MAJOR ACTIVITY

Acute lymphocytic leukemia (ALL)	Induction: vincristine and prednisone ± asparaginase ± doxorubicin or daunorubicin
	CNS prophylaxis: intrathecal methotrexate ± radiotherapy
	Maintenance: combination chemotherapy with methotrexate and mercaptopurine or other combinations
	Bone marrow transplant for chemotherapy failures
Acute myelocytic leukemia (AML)	Daunorubicin and cytarabine ± thioguanine
	Marrow transplantation with cyclophosphamide and total body irradiation
Breast cancer*	Tamoxifen, progestins
	CMF or CMFP: Cyclophosphamide and methotrexate and fluorouracil ± prednisone
	AC or CAF: Cyclophosphamide and doxorubicin ± fluorouracil
Choriocarcinoma	Methotrexate ± dactinomycin
Embryonal rhabdomyosarcoma*	VAC: Vincristine and dactinomycin and cyclophosphamide ± doxorubicin
	Vincristine and doxorubicin and cyclophosphamide
Ewing's sarcoma*	CAV: Cyclophosphamide and doxorubicin and vincristine
Hairy cell leukemia	Interferon or deoxycoformycin*
Hodgkin's disease	MOPP: Mechlorethamine and vincristine and procarbazine and prednisone.
	ABVD: Doxorubicin and bleomycin and vinblastine and dacarbazine ± cyclophosphamide
	MOPP: alternated with ABVD
	CVPP: Chlorambucil and vinblastine and procarbazine and prednisone ± carmustine
	MOP/ABV: Mechlorethamine and vincristine and procarbazine and doxorubicin and bleomycin and vinblastine
Lung	
small cell (oat cell)	CAV: Cyclophosphamide and doxorubicin and vincristine
	Etoposide and cisplatin ± vincristine
	CAE: Cyclophosphamide and doxorubicin and etoposide
	MACC: Methotrexate and doxorubicin and cyclophosphamide and lomustine
Non-Hodgkin's lymphoma	
Burkitt's lymphoma	Cyclophosphamide
	Cyclophosphamide, vincristines, methotrexate
	Cyclophosphamide and high dose cytarabine ± methotrexate with leucovorin
Diffuse histolytic lymphoma	CHOP: Cyclophosphamide and doxorubicin and vincristine and prednisone
	BACOP: Bleomycin and doxorubicin and cyclophosphamide and vincristine and prednisone
	M-BACOP: Bleomycin and doxorubicin and cyclophosphamide and vincristine and prednisone and methotrexate with leucovorin rescue
	ProMACE-MOPP: Prednisone and methotrexate-leucovorin and doxorubicin and cyclophosphamide and etoposide-mechlorethamine and vincristine and procarbazine and prednisone
	COP-BLAM: Bleomycin and doxorubicin and cyclophosphamide and vincristine and prednisone and procarbazine
	MACOP-B: Methotrexate with leucovorin and doxorubicin and cyclophosphamide and vincristine and prednisone and bleomycin
	COMLA: Cyclophosphamide and vincristine and methotrexate-leucovorin and cytarabine
Osteogenic sarcoma*	Doxorubicin and/or high-dose methotrexate and leucovorin rescue ± cisplatin ± bleomycin ± cyclophosphamide ± dactinomycin
Testicular	PVB: Cisplatin and vinblastine and bleomycin
	BEP: Bleomycin and etoposide and cisplatin
	VAB-6: Vinblastine and dactinomycin and bleomycin and cyclophosphamide and cisplatin
Wilms' tumor*	Dactinomycin and vincristine ± doxorubicin

*Adjuvant chemotherapy to surgery, radiotherapy, or both.
**Investigational use only
Adapted from the Medical Letter *29*: 29–36, March 27, 1987. Refer to original publication for alternative drug combinations.

The second approach is empirical and uses drugs that are active as single agents in the specific tumor. Such tumors are usually "drug sensitive" so that several effective drugs having differing mechanisms of action are available. Drug selection is also guided by the type of dose-limiting toxicity likely to be produced by the other agents to be used in the combination. This allows each agent to be given in full clinical dosage.

Successful combinations use intermittent treatment schedules in full doses rather than continuous daily administration. If the combination selectively kills tumor over bone marrow, an interval of 2 to 4 weeks between courses allows recovery of the marrow

Table 56–7. DRUGS CURRENTLY PREFERRED FOR DISEASES IN WHICH CHEMOTHERAPY HAS MODERATE ACTIVITY

Adrenocortical carcinoma	Mitotane
	Cisplatin
Bladder	M-VAC: Cisplatin and/or doxorubicin ± methotrexate ± vinblastine
	Instillation of thiotepa or doxorubicin or BCG* or mitomycin
Brain	
glioblastoma	Carmustine or lomustine
medulloblastoma	Vincristine and carmustine ± mechlorethamine ± methotrexate
	MOPP: Mechlorethamine and vincristine and procarbazine and prednisone
	Vincristine and cisplatin
Cervix	Cisplatin and bleomycin ± methotrexate
	Bleomycin and mitomycin and vincristine ± cisplatin
Chronic lymphocytic leukemia	Chlorambucil ± prednisone
Chronic myelocytic leukemia (CML)	
Chronic phase	Busulfan
	Hydroxyurea
	Bone marrow transplantation with cyclophosphamide and total body irradiation
Acute phase	Daunorubicin and cytarabine and vincristine and prednisone ± thioguanine
	Vincristine and prednisone for lymphoid variant
Endometrial	Megestrol acetate or hydroxyprogesterone caproate or medroxyprogesterone acetate
	Doxorubicin ± cyclophosphamide ± cisplatin
Gastric	FAM: Fluorouracil and doxorubicin and mitomycin.
	Fluorouracil and doxorubicin and semustine*
Head and neck, squamous cell	Bleomycin and cisplatin ± methotrexate
	Cisplatin and fluorouracil
Kaposi's sarcoma (epidemic)	Etoposide or interferon
Islet cell carcinoma	Streptozocin ± fluorouracil
Mycosis fungoides	Combination chemotherapy as in Hodgkin's disease or non-Hodgkin's lymphoma
	Mechlorethamine (topical)
Myeloma	Melphalan (or cyclophosphamide) and prednisone
	Melphalan and carmustine and cyclophosphamide and prednisone
	Dexamethasone and doxorubicin and vincristine
Neuroblastoma	Doxorubicin and cyclophosphamide and cisplatin and teniposide*
	Doxorubicin and cyclophosphamide
	Cisplatin and cyclophosphamide
Non-Hodgkin's lymphoma	
Follicular lymphoma	Cyclophosphamide or chlorambucil ± vincristine and prednisone or etoposide (combinations not demonstrably superior to single agents)
Ovary	CP, CAP: Melphalan (or cyclophosphamide) ± cisplatin ± doxorubicin
	CHAP: Cyclophosphamide and hexamethylmelamine* and doxorubicin and cisplatin
Prostate	Diethylstilbestrol, other estrogens, leuprolide or depot-formulation of LHRH analogues
	Cisplatin ± cyclophosphamide ± doxorubicin ± fluorouracil
Retinoblastoma	Doxorubicin and cyclophosphamide
	Doxorubicin and cyclophosphamide and cisplatin and teniposide*
Sarcomas (soft tissue, adult)	Doxorubicin and dacarbazine and cyclophosphamide ± vincristine
	Doxorubicin and dacarbazine
	Doxorubicin and dacarbazine and ifosfamide*

*Investigative use only
Adapted from the Medical Letter *29*:29–36, March 27, 1987. Refer to the original publication for alternative drug combinations.

TABLE 56–8. DRUGS CURRENTLY PREFERRED FOR DISEASES IN WHICH CHEMOTHERAPY HAS ONLY MINOR ACTIVITY

Colorectal	Fluorouracil
	Intra-arterial floxuridine (hepatic metastases)
Liver	Doxorubicin
	Fluorouracil ± methotrexate ± semustine*
Lung	
nonsmall cell	CAP: Cyclophosphamide and doxorubicin and cisplatin
	Vindesine* and cisplatin ± mitomycin
	Vinblastine and cisplatin ± mitomycin
	FAM: Fluorouracil and doxorubicin and mitomycin
	MACC: Methotrexate and doxorubicin and cyclophosphamide and lomustine
Melanoma	Dacarbazine or semustine*
Pancreatic	FAM: Fluorouracil and doxorubicin and mitomycin
	SMF: Streptozocin and mitomycin and fluorouracil
Renal	Interferon

*Investigational use only
Adapted from the Medical Letter *29*:29–36, March 27, 1987. Refer to the original publication for alternative drug combinations.

TABLE 56–9. HORMONES USED TO TREAT CANCER

Drugs	Acute Toxicity	Delayed Toxicity
Androgens		
Testosterone propionate (Oreton)		*Fluid retention; masculinization;* hypercalcemia
Fluoxymesterone (Halotestin)		*Fluid retention; masculinization;* hypercalcemia cholestatic jaundice; hirsutism; painful clitoral hypertrophy
Testolactone (Teslac)	Local pain, inflammation at injection site	Hypercalcemia; nonhepatotoxic; alopecia rare
Dromostanolone (Drolban)		*Fluid retention; masculinization;* hypercalcemia; nonhepatotoxic
Anti-Androgens		
Flutamide	Nausea	Gynecomastia; hepatotoxicity
Pituitary Releasing Factors		
Leuprolide (LH-releasing hormone analogue)	Transient increased bone pain; hot flashes	Impotence; amenorrhea; testicular atrophy
Progestins		
Hydroxyprogesterone caproate (Delalutin)	Local pain, abscess	Hypercalcemia; cholestatic jaundice
Megestrol acetate (Megace)	Allergy to tartrazine dye	Fluid retention; thromboembolism
Medroxyprogesterone acetate (Provera) (Depo-Provera)	Rarely, nausea P.O. Local pain, abscess I.M.	Fluid retention; hypercalcemia
Estrogens		
Diethylstilbestrol (DES)	*Nausea, vomiting;* cramps; urinary incontinence	*Fluid retention;* hypercalcemia; feminization; uterine bleeding; vaginal carcinoma in offspring if given during pregnancy; increased frequency of vascular accidents; increased mortality from heart disease in males
Ethinyl estradiol (Estinyl)		*Fluid retention;* hypercalcemia; feminization; uterine bleeding; increased incidence of vascular accidents
Antiestrogens		
Tamoxifen (Nolvadex)	Nausea, vomiting, hot flashes transient increased tumor or bone pain	Vaginal bleeding and discharge; rash; hypercalcemia; retinopathy; keratopathy; decreased visual acuity; peripheral edema; depression; dizziness; headache, fluid retention; rare thrombocytopenia and leukopenia
Thyroid Hormones		
Thyroxin		Hyperthyroidism; arrhythmias; angina
Adrenocorticosteroids		
Prednisone Dexamethasone Methylprednisone Hydrocortisone	As a group, hyperglycemia; euphoria; fluid retention	Gastrointestinal bleeding; increased risk of infection; immunosuppression; osteoporosis; hypertension; hypokalemic alkalosis; cataracts; glucose intolerance; mental aberration
Aminoglutethamide	Drowsiness; nausea; dizziness; rash	Bone marrow depression; fever; hypotension; masculinization; hypothyroidism

Major dose-limiting toxicities are italicized

to pretreatment levels without significant regrowth of the tumor. Intermittent scheduling also may permit recovery of the patient's immune system, often with rebound and overshoot, between the cycles of chemotherapy.

Useful or disadvantageous pharmacologic interactions between drugs in a combination may also occur. The action of some antitumor drugs can be enhanced by other drugs with no antitumor effect by preventing the metabolic degradation of the active agent. For example, allopurinol enhances the activity of 6-mercaptopurine by preventing its conversion into the inactive thiouric acid. Tetrahydrouridine and 2-deoxycoformycin prevent deamination of cytarabine by the ubiquitous deaminases present in serum and tissue. Cyclophosphamide is activated to the 4-OH metabolite by oxidative microsomal enzymes. Thus drugs that induce or inhibit these enzymes will enhance or depress cyclophosphamide activity.

Endocrine Therapy

Tumors arising from the breast, prostate, and uterine endometrium may respond to hormonal manipulation (Table 56–9). Steroid hormones act by binding to receptors in the tumor cell cytoplasm and sterically altering the shape of the receptor protein. The receptor is transported to the cell nucleus, where it interacts with cellular DNA to initiate specific messenger RNA and protein synthesis. After this interaction the cytoplasmic receptor concentration is restored and the cycle can be repeated. Receptors are known to exist for estrogens (ER), progesterones (PR), androgens, and adrenocorticosteroids. The latter also uniquely exert some antitumor effect on nonendocrine targets such as acute lymphocytic leukemic cells.

Estrogens. Breast and prostate cancers may be treated by removing sources of circulating hormones (ablation of endocrine organs) that stimulate or support tumor growth or by giving pharmacologic doses of estrogens, androgens, progesterones, or glucocorticoids to suppress tumor growth. Until recently, hormonal therapy has been empirical and based on menopausal status, disease-free interval, site of dominant disease, and response to prior endocrine therapy. The discovery of estrogen (ER) and progesterone (PR) receptors has placed such therapy on a more rational basis. In the case of breast cancer, 65 per cent of ER (+) patients respond to hormonal manipulation. The responses increase to 75 per cent if PR is also positive. In contrast, less than five per cent of patients who are ER (−) will respond to hormonal manipulation. Both ER and PR may be needed for optimum response, since nearly 40 per cent of ER (+) women still fail to respond to hormonal manipulation. Premenopausal women with breast cancer have a lower incidence of ER positivity and lower levels of binding protein in their tumor cell cytosol. In contrast, postmenopausal women have a higher incidence of ER positivity and quantitatively higher levels of ER protein in their tumor cell cytosol. Indeed, responsiveness to antiestrogens is directly related to the quantitative levels of hormone receptors in the tumor. ER (−) tumor cells may either be less well differentiated or have an increased growth (drug sensitive) fraction, so that ER (−) patients may respond better to cancer chemotherapy than ER (+) patients. Similar conditions of response to hormonal manipulation with the frequency and quantity of binding proteins have yet to be made for prostate and endometrial cancers.

Ablative surgery has been used in breast cancer. Chemotherapy is preferred for patients with ER (−) recurrent tumor, a short disease-free interval, hepatic metastases, lymphangitic spread to the lung, or refractoriness to prior hormone therapy. However, castration may benefit over 50 per cent of premenopausal women with ER (+) tumors that are slowly growing (long disease-free interval) or who have mainly osseous and soft tissue metastases. Patients not responding to castration are unlikely to respond to further endocrine manipulation and should be given chemotherapy. However, 50 per cent of ER (+) women who again relapse after a response to castration may again respond to adrenalectomy or hypophysectomy. Since the procedures are equally effective, the choice depends on the patient's condition and the available surgical expertise. Postmenopausal women who have responded to estrogen may also benefit. Responses last, on the average, 16 to 18 months.

Some 70 per cent of men with breast cancer also respond to castration, and 50 per cent of those who have recurrences will then respond to adrenalectomy or hypophysectomy.

Many men with prostatic cancer respond for 2 to 3 years after orchiectomy, which should be reserved for those requiring rapid response, since estrogens are equally effective. Estrogens provide an added benefit when castration is used.

Antiestrogens are estrogen analogues that antagonize estrogen stimulation of target tissues. They bind competitively to the estrogen receptor, translocate with it into the nucleus, and initiate early estrogenic responses. A complete response does not develop, the antiestrogen retains the receptor in the nucleus for prolonged periods, and the genome remains refractory to the action of estrogens for a time. Up to 60 per cent of ER (+) patients with breast cancer respond to antiestrogens such as Tamoxifen, which help to avoid the need for so many ablative procedures.

Androgens may help postmenopausal women with breast cancer, particularly those with osseous metastases and ER (+) tumors. Response to therapy, including stimulation of erythropoiesis, may require 6 to 12 weeks; all androgen preparations are equally useful. Aside from bony metastases, however, androgens are less effective than estrogens for postmenopausal women.

Progestins may produce responses in 30 per cent of women with metastatic endometrial cancer which can last several years. Progestins are related to progesterone produced by the corpus luteum and the placenta. Older women with slow growing, well-differentiated tumors respond best. About 10 per cent of patients with metastatic renal cell and ovarian cancers may also respond.

Thyroid nodules presumed to be cancer and 70 per cent of thyroid papillary adenocarcinomas, even when metastatic to the neck, can be suppressed for over 10 years with thyroid hormone given to tolerance.

Adrenal corticosteroids may produce complete remission in 60 per cent of patients with lymphoblastic leukemia and partial responses in 70 per cent of patients with chronic lymphocytic leukemia. These hormones are active in 10 per cent of women with breast cancer and against lymphomas and myeloma. Responses correlate with the presence of a corticosteroid receptor in the tumor, and the hormones also suppress mitosis and lyse normal and neoplastic lymphoid cells by inhibiting synthesis of cellular proteins. Their activity in breast cancer partly relates to suppression of estrogen production by the adrenal cortex.

Medical adrenalectomy can be achieved by the use of aminoglutethamide, which inhibits the conversion of cholesterol to pregnanelone in the adrenal cortex. It is given orally at 250 mg. four times daily along with 40 mg. of hydrocortisone daily. This regimen produces a response rate in patients with breast cancer that is as good as adrenalectomy. The regimen is helpful in women with widespread bony metastases who are too debilitated for surgery. Skin rash and lethargy occur acutely and subside spontaneously with continued therapy. Occasional hypothyroidism is managed by replacement therapy.

Analogues of luteinizing hormone-releasing hormone (LHRH) in the form of an analogue called leuprolide has been found to be therapeutically equivalent to diethyistilbestol (DES) with fewer side effects in the treatment of prostate cancer. LHRH is a hypothalmic decapeptide with a paradoxical action. Short-term administration stimulates release of pituitary LH, which results in a concomitant increase in serum testosterone and a transient flare in symptoms of prostate cancer, such as bone pain or ureteral obstruction. Chronic administration causes a complete depression of LH and serum testosterone, in part owing to receptor inhibition at the pituitary. Antiandrogens may also be used in prostatic cancer to block the physiologic action of dihydrotestosterone at the cellular level. Flutamide and cyproterone acetate can be used in newly diagnosed or untreated patients with advanced prostate cancer, but they are of no benefit once resistance to alternative hormone therapy occurs. Ketoconazole, an antifungal agent, profoundly impairs advanced testicular androgen production to castrate levels with few side effects and is under investigation.

Biologic Therapies

For over 20 years, there have been many attempts to use chemicals and biologic substances to modulate biologic responses in patients with cancer. Any nonspecific immunomodulaters such as a variety of chemicals and extracts of bacteria and viruses will modulate immune responses in experimental animals as well as humans, but these nonspecific immunomodulators have not been highly effective in clinical trials to date. Immunotherapy at the end of the 1970's failed to establish itself as a major mode of cancer treatment. The recent resurgence of interest in this area comes in part from advances in genetic engineering which allow the availability to the clinician of numerous natural biologic response modifiers and also to a broadening of our perspective beyond the immune system of the potential components making up host resistance in patients with cancer.

Tumor biotherapy refers to the use of any biologic substance and more specifically products of the mammalian genome. Biologicals and biologic response modifiers may (1) augment host defenses providing effectors or direct or indirect mediators of an antitumor response through the administration of cells, the natural mediator, or synthetic derivatives of it; (2) enhance antitumor response by augmenting or restoring effector mechanisms or reducing a portion of host reaction that is harmful; (3) use modified tumor cells or vaccines to stimulate an antitumor response or increase tumor cell sensitivity to an existing response; (4) reduce transformation or increase differentiation or maturation of tumor cells; (5) block growth factors produced by tumor cells; (6) interfere with tumor metastasis; (7) enhance the ability of a patient to tolerate damage by cytotoxic cancer therapies. Table 56–10 summarizes the various varieties of biologicals and biologic response modifiers. In the opinion of some, biotherapy is now considered the fourth major modality of cancer therapy which can be effective alone or in association with surgery, radiotherapy, and chemotherapy, including hormones. Biotherapy can have activity on clinically apparent disease and is not restricted to situations in which the tumor cell mass is imperceptible.

Nonspecific immunomodulators (Table 56–11) have been tested under immunotherapy since the early part of this century as bacterial and viral products which would nonspecifically stimulate host immune responses. They have been useful adjuvants and nonspecific stimulants in animal tumor models but success in clinical trials in man has been disappointing. BCG and its derivatives have been the

Table 56–10. BIOLOGICALS AND BIOLOGIC RESPONSE MODIFIERS

IMMUNOMODULATORS	
Chemicals: e.g., Azimexon, Bestatin, Cimetidine, Glucan, Lentinan, Levamisole, Prostaglandin inhibitors (aspirin, indomethacin)	
Bacteria and extracts: e.g., BCG, *B. abortus*, *C. parvum*, endotoxin, muramyldipeptide (MDP), mixed bacterial vaccines, Detox, cell wall skeleton (cws)	
Viruses	
Immune RNA	
Biologicals: Tuftsin	
LYMPHOKINES AND CYTOKINES	
Colony-stimulating factors	
Erythropoietin	
Interferons - alpha, beta, gamma interferon inducers	
Interleukins - IL-1, 2, 3, 4, etc.	
Lymphotoxins - (TNF)	
Macrophage - activating factors	
Thymosins - alpha-1, fraction 5	
Transfer factors	
GROWTH AND MATURATION FACTORS	
Colony stimulating factors	
Interleukins	
EFFECTOR CELLS	
Macrophages	NK cells
Cytotoxic T-cells	LAK cells
Helper cells	
TUMOR-ASSOCIATED ANTIGENS	
Antigens	
Vaccines—cells, viral oncolysates, purified antigens, synthetic antigens, and peptides	
—idiotope vaccines	
MONOCLONAL ANTIBODIES	
Alone	
Immunoconjugates with—chemotherapeutic agents	
—radionuclides	
—toxins (ricin, Pseudomonas)	
OTHER APPROACHES	
Liposome—encapsulated biologics	
Bone marrow transplantation	
Plasmapheresis	
Ex vivo use of activation columns, immunoadsorbents	

Table 56–11. CANCER BIOTHERAPY

Solid Tumors	
Melanoma	Immunostimulation — BCG, cell wall skeleton — Allogenic melanoma cell vaccines (responses but no improved survival) Interferon — IFN 20% RR; ⅓ of CR enduring — Under study: and — IFN Combinations with chemotherapy: DTIC, BCNU IL-2 and LAK cells - Transient partial responses of 50% Antibodies — Mabs alone only minor clinical effects — Some responses seen to IgG3 Mabs specific for GD2 and GD3 membrane gangliosides — Immunotoxin with ricin A chain—low level responsiveness
Genitourinary Cancers	
Renal cell carcinoma	Immunostimulation — Tumor vaccines with bacterial adjuvants—15–25% RR — Immune RNA: Response in 3/6 patients — Thymosin fraction V: 15% RR — Renal artery embolization augments NK activation Interferon—IFN: 15–20% RR lasting 3 to 4 months —IFN under study —IFN little activity IL-2 and LAK cells: transient partial responses of 50–75%
Bladder cancer	Intravesical BCG for superficial Stage A: Prolonged objective responses Interferon: Intravesical for superficial Stage A: prolonged objective responses Systemic in papillomas of bladder: prolonged objective responses
Prostate cancer	Mabs against prostatic acid phosphatase and prostate-specific antigen under test for toxicity and imaging
Gastrointestinal cancer	Immunostimulation: Irradiated autologous tumor cell vaccines with BCG—reduced recurrences in Dukes B and C colon cancer Interferon: IFN — No effect in colorectal or gastric cancer Antibodies: Mabs to CEA and 17-1A antigens - no responses in colorectal cancer Pabs to ferritin—responses in hepatocellular cancer IL-2 and LAK cells: only minor occasional responses
Breast cancer	Immunostimulation: BCG, Levamisole, Poly A: (IFN inducer) all show some benefit in early adjuvant studies Immunoadsorption: Response in a few patients with advanced disease when their serum was passed over Protein A columns, perhaps removing circulating immune complexes Interferon: IFN—only marginal effects Antibodies: Several varieties of Mabs under study for imaging and therapy as immunoconjugates to drugs and toxins (ricin)
Lung cancer	Immunomodulation: Intrapleural BCG - may be deleterious in NSCLC Thymosin fraction IV - ineffective in SCLC Interferon: IFN — no effect in NSCLC — may delay metastasis in SCLC, but enhances radiation toxicity IL-2 and LAK cells: modest activity with NSCLC Antibodies: Mabs and drug immunoconjugates ineffective in NSCLC Mabs to bombesin under trial in SCLC
Gynecologic Cancer	
Ovarian cancer	Immunomodulation; i.p. *C. parvum* enhances chemotherapy in minimal residual disease Interferon: IFN and IFN systemically promising in advanced cancer i.p. administration augments NK activity IL-2 and LAK cells: systemic and i.p. administration under study
Cancer of uterine cervix	Interferon: IFN—no responses
Endocrine Tumors	
Carcinoid tumors	Interferon: 17 responses in 36 patients with median duration 2.5 years
Tumors of the Nervous System	Interferon: Partial responses in 6 of 19 patients with recurrent glioma IL-2 and LAK cells: Phase I intralesional trials in progress Antibodies: Mabs conjugated to daunorubicin or chlorambucil gave 9 responses in 12 children with neuroblastoma Mabs to GD2 - C & PR in neuroblastoma

Table continued on following page

Table 56–11. CANCER BIOTHERAPY *Continued*

Sarcomas	Interferon: Only minimal activity Kaposi's sarcoma - 30% RR with no improvement in the immune deficiency or opportunistic infections or survival IL-2 and LAK cells: No responses Antibodies: Under study using antigens shared with melanoma
Hematopoietic Tumors	
Lymphoma and leukemia	Immunomodulation: Early reports of prolonged survival of ALL (with BCG) and AML (with leukemia Pseudomonas) not substantiated. BCG may give 6 months' survival advantage after first relapse Interferon: Leukemia: transient partial responses IFN induces terminal differentiation of leukemic cells Lymphoma: transient 50% RR in well-differentiated NHL Antibodies: Mabs such as T-101, Leu-1, anti-CALLA, and anti-TAC show transient reductions in counts but no prolonged effects Cutaneous T-cell lymphoma the most promising anti-idiotypic antibodies initially promising in lymphomas Pabs to ferritin under study for refractory Hodgkin's disease Mabs to T cells being used to purge bone marrow to tumor cells and of T cells to reduce GVH IL-2 and LAK cells: anecdotal positive reports in HD and NHL
Myeloproliferative syndromes	Interferon: Normalization of peripheral counts in chronic phase of CML
Hairy cell leukemia	Interferon: IFN—80% RR which can be prolonged Not curative
Multiple myeloma	Interferon: IFN—20% RR. May be synergistic with cytotoxic drugs

Adapted from Oldham, R. K. (ed.): Principles of Cancer Biotherapy. New York, Raven Press, 1987.

Abbreviations:

ALL	Acute lymphocytic leukemia	IL-2	Interleukin-2
AML	Acute myelogenous leukemia	i.p.	Intraperitoneal
BCG	Bacillus Calmette-Guérin	LAK	Lymphokine-activated killer cells
CEA	Carcinoembryonic antigen	Mab	Monoclonal antibody
CML	Chronic myelogenous leukemia	NHL	Non-Hodgkin's lymphoma
C. parvum	*Corynebacterium parvum*	NK	Natural killer cells
CR	Complete response	NSCLC	Non-small-cell lung cancer
GD2, GD3	Gangliosides	Pab	Polyclonal Antibody
GVH	Graft-versus host disease	PR	Partial response
HD	Hodgkin's disease	RR	Response rate
IFN	Interferon	SCLC	Small cell lung cancer

prototype. Many others represent bacterial extracts, prostoglandin, and inhibitors such as aspirin or indomethacin, mediators such as tuftsin, immune regulators such as Levamisole, and inhibitors of suppressor cells such as Cimetidine.

Active specific immunotherapy has used irradiated or chemically modified autochronous or allogeneic tumor cells in an attempt to produce host immunity to tumors. A major limitation of this approach has been the availability of purified tumor-associated antigens, but the advent of synthesized and genetically engineered antigens, not to mention the use of idiotope vaccines, is generating new interest in the area. The thymosins have immunologic activity; and thymosin alpha-1 and thymosin fraction 5 have had the most study. They can correct selected immunodeficiency states and can augment suppressed T-cell responses in patients with cancer. Clinical studies are ongoing. The lymphokines and the cytokines provide more than 20 categories of natural mediators that are now being made available through genetic engineering techniques. These are molecules secreted by a variety of cells, and they are one way by which immune cells communicate with one another and control the overall immune response. The possibility of using these in the future to manipulate the immune response in favor of the host is exciting. To date, the agents are used pharmacologically in high doses for their antiproliferative action rather than their immunomodulatory abilities. Use for the pharmacologic treatment of tumors of the lymphoid system is an important possibility. They include the interleukins, of which at least seven are now described and four are receiving clinical attention. Several subclasses of colony-stimulating factors are being examined along with factors that control the proliferation and maturation of B-cells and macrophages.

Purified interleukin-2 (IL-2) has been used to activate a population of lymphocytes referred to as LAK cells (lymphokine activated killer cells). These differ from natural killer cells and, when used combined with IL-2, have been found to produce complete and partial remissions in patients with advanced metastatic melanoma and renal cancers, particularly. Lymphotoxin, a product of antigen- or mitigen-stimulated leukocytes and a principal effector of the delayed hypersensitivity, is also under study. Tumor necrosis factor (TNF; alpha-lymphotoxin) is in early phase trials. Various forms of colony-stimulating factor are being examined for their ability to correct cytopenias related to myelodysplastic syndromes, leukemias, and treatments with chemotherapy. Many of these cytokines such as TNF, interferon, and IL-2 are also being examined in combinations for complementary effects.

The interferons are small proteins with antiviral, antiproliferative, and immunomodulatory activity. Over 20 varieties have been described. Alpha inteferon has shown activity in hairy cell leukemia, renal cell cancer, and several other tumors, especially hematologic malignancies. It is still unclear whether interferons work primarily by their antiproliferative activity or through alterations of immune responses. The beta and gamma interferons are also under study, with gamma interferon showing particular interest. Combining interferons with chemotherapeutic agents and with other lymphokines and cytokines is just beginning. The side effects of cytokines and lymphokines are considerable and require a highly specialized expertise to administer effectively, particularly if they are given with cellular therapy such as LAK cells.

Monoclonal antibodies have become available in large quantities since the development of the hybridoma methodology in 1975. Monoclonals react to tumor-associated antigens for tumors of the colon, lung, pancreas, and melanoma, and for leukemia and lymphomas. They are being studied clinically alone and as immunoconjugates coupled with chemotherapeutic agents, toxins such as ricin or Pseudomonas toxin, or with radionuclides, especially alpha particle emitters. Temporary regressions have been seen in leukemia, lymphoma, melanoma, and hepatocellular carcinoma. Such antibodies are useful for radioimmunoimaging of tumor cell masses and for the removal of T-cells and tumor cells from bone marrow to improve bone marrow transplantation techniques. The heterogenalty of tumors and the vascular access of these agents to tumors still present major obstacles to be overcome. Cocktails of antibodies sufficient to cover the heterogeneity of the different tumor cell types, chosen by typing the tumor from each patient, may require an individualized approach to be effective.

The Role of Surgery and Radiotherapy in Advanced Disease

Resection of solitary brain metastases, especially in a young patient, will lengthen survival, reduce later intracranial complications from the tumor, and occasionally give long-term control. Resection of pulmonary metastases may be helpful if solitary, but even if multiple, it may yield long-term control with some sarcomas and testicular tumors. Resection of localized hepatic metastases may produce long-term remissions in 25 per cent of patients. In general, however, debulking surgery prior to chemotherapy does not seem to improve the ultimate results of chemotherapy, except in ovarian cancer.

Useful palliation can be achieved with surgery for intestinal obstruction (ovarian, bowel, and pancreatic cancers), for gastrointestinal bleeding, and for urinary or hepatobiliary diversions. Surgery may also relieve pain with neurosurgical procedures.

With lymphomas, radiotherapy can reduce tumor load to enhance cure rates with drugs and can be used for sanctuary sites such as the brain and meninges as an auxillary to drug treatment for leukemia and small cell lung cancer. In combination with drugs radiotherapy will relieve superior mediastinal obstruction, as well as ureteral obstruction in drug-resistent lymphoma and testicular tumors. It will relieve bone pain and may prevent fractures. Prophylactic internal fixation of the bone may be required. Radiation of the brain and spinal cord may reduce neurologic incapacitation in terminal disease. Radiation can also be used to reduce soft tissue lesions, relieve bleeding and discomfort in massive hepatic metastases, and arrest gastrointestinal hemorrhage.

ADJUVANT THERAPY

Multimodal primary (or adjuvant) therapy combines systemic modalities with the locoregional approaches of surgery and radiotherapy to try to prevent recurrence of minimum residual disease, rather than waiting for the tumor to recur before using systemic treatment. This approach has improved survival and altered the approach to local control for a number of tumors. The effect is best where drugs can produce significant response rates, even cures, in patients with advanced disease. Chemotherapy has replaced hysterectomy in choriocarcinoma; chemotherapy has also altered or even replaced radiotherapy in the management of Stage II and Stage III Hodgkin's disease, Wilms' tumor, Stage I and Stage II diffuse large cell lymphoma, nonseminomatous testicular cancer with sensitive biologic markers, and small cell lung cancer. Even for tumors where drug cure of advanced disease is not possible, adjuvant therapies have improved survival and altered local therapy in breast cancer, sarcomas of the limbs, and anorectal cancer. Trials are now being carried out of drugs and radiation used in the preoperative and intraoperative setting and in the neoadjuvant situation where the systemic therapy is given prior to surgery of the primary lesion.

SUPPORTIVE CARE AND MANAGEMENT OF COMPLICATIONS

Vigorous therapy with surgery, radiation, and chemotherapy can improve the results of cancer treatment. A favorable outcome also depends on sustaining patients through periods of major physiologic impairment. Intensive alimentation, reconstructive surgery, restorative devices and prosthetics, blood component transfusion, and control of infection are all essential. Rehabilitation and psychosocial support are needed from the start. This intestive multidisciplinary support often requires the integrated services of a comprehensive cancer center.

Anemia occurs in 60 per cent of patients with disseminated cancer and may be its first manifestation. Usually it is an anemia of chronic disease with low serum iron and iron-binding capacity but normal iron stores. Both increased destruction of red cells and inadequate compensatory erythropoiesis are seen. There is no specific therapy and most patients remain asymptomatic if their hemoglobin is maintained above 8 grams per dl. with transfusion. Less often, blood loss, vitamin deficiencies, hemolysis, or myelophthisis are responsible. Both warm and cold autoimmune hemolytic anemias are seen in lymphomas and chronic leukemias, and adrenal corticosteroids may control the warm variety. Splenectomy may be beneficial if treatment of the primary tumor is ineffective, but splenic irradiation is rarely effective.

Hemorrhage results usually from tumor invasion of blood vessels, thrombocytopenia, or disseminated intravascular coagulation. Defective platelet function with normal or increased counts is occasionally responsible. In thrombocytopenia, life-threatening hemorrhage is unusual unless the platelet count falls below 20,000 per ml. or unless additional coagulation defects are present. Platelet transfusions used routinely in severe thrombocytopenia reduce the risk of fatal hemorrhage by more than 50 per cent. Fresh histocompatible platelets obtained by pheresis from a pool of normal HLA-typed donors are optimum when prolonged support is required since antiplatelet antibodies soon develop when random donors are used. Disseminated intravascular coagulation occurs with several tumors, probably initiated by release of thromboplastins from cancer cells directly into the blood. Increased levels of fibrin degradation products without hemorrhage are frequently seen. Heparin is rarely indicated except in patients with acute promyelocytic leukemia who often bleed after treatment is initiated.

Infection is the most frequent serious complication and cause of death in cancer patients. Fever occurs in 70 per cent of hospitalized cancer patients and is usually due to infection. Nearly 90 per cent of deaths due to infection are caused by bacteria. Seven major defects in host defense account for this predisposition. Immunosuppression, both humoral and cellular, may be caused by the tumor itself or be induced by radiation or chemotherapy. Neutropenia, malnutrition, splenectomy, surgery, foreign bodies (catheters, shunts), and adverse drug reactions all contribute. Patients with B-cell neoplasms such as chronic lymphocytic leukemia or multiple myeloma have defective B-cell function (humoral immunity) with hypogammaglobulinemia. They are susceptible to infections with pyogenic encapsulated bacteria such as *Streptococcus pneumoniae*. Gamma globulin is of little benefit in the prophylaxis or treatment of cancer patients with hypogammaglobulinemia. Patients with Hodgkin's disease have predominant deficit in cellular immunity with susceptibility to infections by intracellular parasites, fungi *(Cryptococcus)*, and viruses (herpes zoster). Splenectomy increases susceptibility to sepsis with encapsulated cocci, and prophylaxis with penicillin and bacterial vaccines may be helpful, especially in children.

Most infections are caused by gram-negative bacilli such as *Escherichia coli, Klebsiella, Pseudomonas aeruginosa,* and *Bacteroides*. Organisms of low pathogenicity, such as *Bacillus* species or *Staphylococcus epidermidis,* can be fatal in the presence of neutropenia. Fungal infections with *Candida* and *Aspergillus* are important in hematologic malignancies. Pneumocystis pneumonia may occur in a variety of cancers and respond to prophylaxis with trimethoprim-sulfamethoxazole.

Severe neutropenia should be considered a medical emergency since infection is frequent and can be rapidly fatal. Classic signs and symptoms of infection such as erythema, tenderness, and pus may be diminished or absent because of suppressed inflammatory response or lack of neutrophils. The risk of infection is 12 per cent at a neutrophil count of 1500 per mm^3 but rises to nearly 100 per cent below the count of 100 per mm^3.

Infection can occur in almost any site and be caused by any organism. A thorough physical examination should emphasize even minimal tenderness or erythema, since cellulitis may be subtle and abscesses rarely become fluctuant. The pharynx, ears, esophagus, respiratory tract, skin, soft tissues, and perianal area should all be examined. Bacterial and fungal cultures of blood (both aerobic and anaerobic), sputum, and urine should be obtained along with cultures from any other suspicious sites, such as the throat, or intravenous sites, including cerebrospinal fluid. A chest x-ray may detect "silent" pulmonary infiltrates. Serologic tests for viral, fungal, or protozoan infections may be useful. The nitroblue tetrazolium (NBT) and limulus tests will not exclude infection.

Prompt antimicrobial therapy should be instituted in the febrile neutropenic patient unless a bacterial etiology can be categorically excluded (e.g., reaction to drug or blood product). Antibiotics should be bacteriocidal, given intravenously, and be broad-spectrum drugs to cover both gram-negative and gram-positive organisms. Initiate empirical treatment immediately after appropriate cultures on the presumption that bacteremia exists rather than waiting several days to document it. A cephalosporin (cephalothin or cephazolin) with carbenicillin or gentamicin, or carbenicillin plus gentamicin, or all three drugs may be used. Nephrotoxicity (4 per cent incidence), especially with cephalothin plus gentamicin (12 per cent incidence), is of concern. Antibiotic therapy can be adjusted according to drug sensitivity once the causative organism is identified. Granulocyte transfusions may improve survival in septic patients with prolonged neutropenia (longer than 2 weeks). Adverse reactions are frequent and may be reduced by using histocompatible granulocytes. Granulocytes may be obtained by cytopheresis of patients with chronic myelogenous leukopheresis. A minimum daily dose of 10^{10} white blood cells is required until infection clears. Circulatory shock will develop in 20 per cent of patients with bacteremia and is usually associated with endotoxins released by gram-negative organisms; mortality is more than 70 per cent.

Neurologic emergencies such as intracerebral metastases arise most frequently from melanoma, breast, and lung cancers. About half present with headache; motor weakness and altered mental status occur in a third. On examination, about 75 per cent of these patients show impaired cognition, two thirds have involvement of the motor system, and only one fourth will have papilledema. Radionuclide brain scan and computed tomography are the most valuable tests. A lumbar puncture is unhelpful and potentially dangerous if increased intracranial pressure is present. Rarely, solitary metastases can be removed, with long periods free of symptoms, but usually cerebral metastases are multiple. Stable patients are treated with 4 mg. of dexamethasone orally every 4 hours to reduce inflammation and edema around the tumor, followed by whole brain radiation to 3000 to 4000 rads over 3 to 4 weeks; then steroids are tapered over 10 to 14 days as tolerated. Anticonvulsants are used only when seizures are present, and phenytoin will reduce corticosteroid effectiveness by enhancing its hepatic metabolism. Acute cerebral herniation may require the addition of osmotic agents such as mannitol or glycerol. Systemic or intrathecal chemotherapy, even with highly lipid-soluble nitrosureas, is usually ineffective. Whole brain radiotherapy is the most beneficial therapy, increasing survival from 1 month to 6 months.

Epidural spinal cord compression may complicate breast, lung, prostate, and kidney cancers as well as lymphomas and multiple myeloma. Local or radicular pain is the most common and earliest symptom and is followed by weakness and dysfunction of bladder and bowel, as well as numbness and paresthesias. A myelogram is diagnostic. The spinal tap is done at the time of the myelogram since herniation of the spinal cord can occur. Cerebrospinal fluid pressure is reduced distal to the compression, the protein is increased, and malignant cells are not usually found. Radiotherapy is used for patients with radiosensitive tumors and slowly progressing neurologic deficits; surgical decompression is employed when neurologic signs are progressing rapidly, especially if the tumor is radioresistant. Systemic chemotherapy may benefit responsive tumors, and corticosteroids are often used empirically, but neither is a substitute for radiation or surgery. Recovery from complete paralysis is rare.

Superior vena caval obstruction occurs most frequently with lymphomas and small cell lung cancers. This is the major vessel most commonly obstructed by tumor. The diagnosis is based on the presence of a mediastinal mass and a distinctive clinical syndrome that includes facial swelling, distention of the veins of the neck and upper chest wall, loss of venous pulsations, conjunctival injection, and edema, headache, and convulsions. Corticosteroids and diuretics allow time for histologic diagnosis when necessary, and definitive management includes chemotherapy if the tumor is susceptible and full-dose radiotherapy to the site of obstruction along with corticosteroids.

Malignant effusion may result from one or a combination of two mechanisms. Fluid may form directly from the presence of tumor on serous surfaces (peripheral effusions). Increased fluid formation may result from decreased fluid resorption owing to impaired venous or lymphatic drainage from tumor obstruction (central effusions). Coexisting infection or congestive heart failure may also cause effusions in cancer patients. Exudates are usually seen with peripheral effusions and transudates with central effusions. In the absence of trauma, true chyle indicates obstruction of the thoracic duct by tumor or infection.

Pleural effusions develop in nearly 50 per cent of patients with disseminated breast or lung cancer and less frequently with lymphoma, mesothelioma, sarcoma, ovarian, and gastric cancer. Tetracycline is the best drug for the management of recurrent malignant effusions; 500 mg. is dissolved in 30 ml. saline and instilled into the chest during thoracentesis, followed by 50 ml. of saline. A chest tube is inserted and attached to water-sealing drainage, which is continued for 12 hours or longer until less than 60 ml. of fluid is drained in 24 hours. Intrapleural nitrogen mustard, fluorouracil, bleomycin, and quinacrine are used less frequently. Alkylating agents are unpredictably absorbed and may compromise bone marrow function in the face of systemic chemotherapy. Pleurectomy is rarely required and is associated with significant morbidity.

Ascites usually results from implantation of tumor cells on the peritoneum, most frequently from ovarian carcinoma and lymphoma. Malignant ascites is best controlled by treating the underlying disease, but severe distention and abdominal discomfort may require paracentesis. Refractory cases receive abdominal irradiation and drug instillation. Nitrogen mustard and tetracycline frequently cause adhesions with bowel obstruction. Bleomycin (60 to 120 mg.) may prove beneficial with minimal side effects.

Pericardial effusions may result from neoplastic infiltration of the pericardial sac or from mediastinal irradiation. As little as 200 ml. can produce cardiac tamponade. Breast and lung cancer, acute leukemias, and lymphomas are usually responsible. Tumor implantation on the serosal surface with fluid exudation and lymphatic obstruction by hilar or mediastinal neoplastic infiltration with fluid transudation can both occur. In addition to systemic therapy for responsive tumors, local radiotherapy is the initial treatment of choice. Intracavitary therapy with fluorouracil or nitrogen mustard is infrequently used because of frequent transient cardiac arrhythmias and worsened cardiac output from the initial reactive effusion from the sclerosing agent. Pericardiectomy or a pleural-pericardial window is used for refractory cases or for severe radiation-induced pericarditis.

Hypercalcemia may develop in up to 25 per cent of patients with metastatic breast cancer or squamous lung cancer, and less often with tumors of the kidney, head and neck, cervix, and prostate, and neuroblastoma and hematologic malignancies. Extensive bone involvement (seen in 80 per cent of cancer patients with hypercalcemia) may result in hypercalcemia as well as immobilization with or without bony metastases. Prostaglandins E1 and E2 secreted by tumor cells enhance bone resorption. High levels of prostaglandin metabolites have been found in the urine of cancer patients with hypercalcemia, and in those patients without demonstrable bony metastases, indomethacin may reverse the hypercalcemia. Ectopic production of parathyroid hormone accounts for most instances of hypercalcemia without demonstrable bone metastases (most commonly renal cell, lung, and head and neck cancers). In hematologic malignancies the osteoclastic resorption of bone may be mediated by a small, soluble polypeptide, osteoclast-activating factor (OAF), produced locally by tumor cells.

Acute hypercalcemia presents with anorexia, nausea, constipation, polydipsia, and polyuria and requires prompt attention. Chronic hypercalcemia may lead to nephrocalcinosis and irreversible impairment of renal function. Hypercalcemia may be aggravated by immobilization and by estrogens, androgens, or progestins used to treat breast cancer.

Hydration with saline will manage calcium levels of less than 13 mg. per dl.; for levels of 13 to 15 mg. per dl., vigorous saline hydration and intermittent intravenous furosemide will produce calcium diuresis. Corticosteroids may be added, especially with myeloma, breast cancer, and lymphomas, but may predispose to infection. Sodium sulfate and sodium phosphates facilitate renal excretion of calcium. They act slowly and cannot be used in renal failure, and phosphates may produce metastatic soft tissue calcification. Unresponsive calcium levels of 13 to 15 mg. per dl. or levels above 15 mg. per dl. will respond to a single intravenous dose of mithramycin (25 micrograms per kg.) within 24 to 48 hours and then can be maintained at normal levels with similar doses repeated weekly.

Hyperuricemia results from increased formation and destruction of tumor cells and accompanying breakdown of nucleoproteins. It is most common in acute leukemia and is aggravated by both chemotherapy and radiotherapy. Uric acid is actively secreted by the kidney and is most soluble in alkaline urine. When concentration exceeds solubility, uric acid precipitates in the tubules, causing obstruction and reduced glomerular filtration leading to anuria. Allopurinol blocks the formation of uric acid from xanthine and hypoxanthine and is used prophylactically to prevent urate nephropathy. Urate nephropathy can also be prevented with a water diuresis and administration of sodium bicarbonate to maintain urinary pH above 7.0.

Malnutrition and cachexia can be profound and debilitating in malignancy. It may relate to anorexia and distorted taste sensation, with aversion to specific foods such as meat, but often has a more complex and ill-understood basis. There is loss of adipose tissue and protein stores with insulin resistance, augmented hepatic and renal gluconeogenesis, and excessive consumption of fatty acids for metabolic fuel. All contribute to a net energy loss of normal tissue far in excess of calories consumed. Hyperalimentation to 3000 calories per day, employing total parenteral nutrition (TPN) through a catheter in the superior vena cava, may be used in patients with painful swallowing or intestinal obstruction or to restore debilitated patients who have a chance for tumor control by surgery, chemotherapy, or radiotherapy. Oral hyperalimentation is preferred and effective. TPN does not enhance tumor growth and may reverse immunologic anergy.

Psychosocial Aspects

Much has been written about the psychosocial dimensions of terminal cancer. The reader is also referred to Chapter 11 on The Dying Patient. The physician must remember, however, that cancer patients who survive also face severe psychologic adjustments to accepting the diagnosis of a chronic and potentially fatal disease. Particular stresses are seen at diagnosis, during intensive treatment, at the time treatment is stopped, at the time of recurrences, and in the terminal phase of the disease. From the moment of detection and diagnosis, both the patient and the medical team must face the certainty of their own mortality. Individuals involved in patient treatment and support need to examine their own attitudes toward cancer and death before attempting to care for others. Life with cancer may imply social unacceptability, including fear of painful suffering, disability, disfigurement, impaired body function, and loss of sexual attractiveness and self-esteem. Patients may be shunned by others because of unwarranted fears of "catching" cancer and may experience problems with their jobs.

Competent and compassionate care should be open, honest, and based on trust. Treatment goals should respect both quality and quantity of life. Neither the patient nor the family should be abandoned, and the patient should not be isolated from family or caregivers by a conspiracy of silence. Patients should be informed of both the benefits and the hazards of treatment. Communication, acceptance, accessibility, and consistent support lessen the patient's ambivalence—his anxiety to begin therapy and reluctance to suffer side effects. Physicians cannot predict with certainty the course of a given patient with cancer and should not hesitate to share this uncertainty honestly with the patient.

The Management of Terminal Illness

Few situations in medicine convey so dramatically and unambiguously the specter of death as does cancer. Death from cancer is perceived as failure of the patient's battle against his disease and of the medical team in providing effective treatment. As generally understood, terminal care refers to the management of patients in whom death is both certain and not far off. The medical team alters its focus from investigation and active treatment aimed at elimination or control of disease to the control and relief of symptoms of uncontrollable tumor, including assessment and relevant investigations, and the support of both patient and family. This philosophic distinction between active palliative care and terminal care should not be perceived as a sharp one. Rather, the process is one of overlapping phases in a spectrum of care designed to match the natural history of progressing tumor. Unhappily, the terminal stage is often still defined as beginning at the moment when the clinician says, "There is nothing more to be done," and then begins to withdraw from the patient. There is always something that can be done, and abandoning a patient and family at this critical time is inexcusable.

In the past few years hospice care has burgeoned like a grass roots movement. Fortunately, the family physician now has access to increasingly sophisticated techniques of symptom control as well as to the multidisciplinary services of the many hospice programs that are springing up all over the United States.

Of major concern to the family physician is the psychologic and spiritual support that must be given to the patient and family during the terminal illness. Suicide is not common in incurable cancer patients, who prefer their shortened existence so as to effect closure and resolution of their lives as long as physical and emotional comfort can be maintained.

Regardless of their importance, spiritual and psychologic issues can only be dealt with in the context of adequate control of physical symptoms. A patient in pain or lying uncomfortably in a wet bed is unlikely to care much about the spiritual issues of dying. Of the many discomforts faced by the terminal cancer patient, the most feared is pain. Moderate to severe pain is experienced by approximately 33 per cent of cancer patients with the intermediate stages of the disease and by 60 to 80 per cent of patients with advanced cancer.

Important parameters to evaluate are (1) the location of the pain; (2) the mechanism of the pain; (3) the nature of the cause of the disease; (4) the physical and mental condition of the patient; and (5) the availability and practicality of the various methods of pain relief available. A diagnosis of cancer does not always mean that the malignant process is responsible for the particular episode of pain. The etiology of cancer pain may fall into one of three categories: (1) pain associated with direct tumor involvement and infiltration of bone, nerve, and hollow viscus (75 per cent); (2) pain associated with cancer therapy, postsurgery, postchemotherapy, or postradiation (20 per cent); and (3) pain unrelated to cancer or cancer therapy (5 per cent). Cancer pain is usually caused directly or indirectly by one or more of the following mechanisms:

1. Neuralgia from radiculopathy or neuropathy from compression of nerve roots, trunks, or plexus by tumor or by pathologic fractures of adjacent bones. The pain is sharp, shooting, well localized, knifelike and aggravated by movement.
2. Sympathetic pain from irritation of sensory nerve endings from perivascular and perineural lymphangitis owing to infiltration of the nerves and blood vessels by tumor cells. The pain is diffuse and burning.
3. Visceral pain that is dull, diffuse, deep, and poorly localized may result from chronic obstruction of a viscus, particularly in the gastrointestinal and genitourinary tracts. Crampy pain of acute obstruction may also develop.
4. Partial or complete occlusion of blood vessels by adjacent tumor may cause painful venous engorgement, arterial ischemia, or both.
5. Infiltration and swelling in tissue enclosed snugly by fascia, periosteum, or other pain-sensitive structures.
6. Necrosis, infection, and inflammation of pain-sensitive structures produced by contiguous tumors can cause excruciating pain.

Cancer patients suffer "total pain," with physical, mental, social, and spiritual dimensions. Acute pain may be mild, moderate, or severe, but chronic pain is a continuum from aching to agony. The agony phase is the severe, chronic pain, affecting about 20 per cent of patients, that becomes the total focus of existence and destroys dignity. Continual physical pain produces anxiety, often mixed with reactive depression, which in turn, produces deviation from normal sleeping, eating, and social interactions. The patient grows hostile and is avoided, resulting in isolation, loneliness, increasing hostility, anxiety, and depression in a vicious cycle.

While analgesic drugs are a major modality used to manage cancer pain, good psychosocial support is needed. Nerve blocks, local irradiation of painful tumors, palliative antineoplastic drug therapy, and other treatment such as electrostimulation of nerve tissue, transcutaneous nerve stimulation, biofeedback and acupuncture all have their place in addition to drug therapy (Tables 56–12 and 56–13).

Aspirin is still the most effective drug for mild to moderate pain. Acetaminophen lacks gastrointestinal irritant and platelet-inhibitory effects and is a better substitute for aspirin for patients on cytotoxic chemotherapy. Weak narcotics like codeine, pentazocine, and oxycodone provide an additive, if not

Table 56–12. MANAGEMENT OF MILD TO MODERATE CHRONIC PAIN IN CANCER*

Aspirin 650 mg.
Acetaminophen 650 mg.
Codeine 65 mg. + aspirin 650 mg. or acetaminophen 650 mg.
Pentazocine HCl (Talwin) 25 mg. + aspirin 650 mg. or acetaminophen 650 mg.
Oxycodone (Percodan) 9 mg. + aspirin 650 mg. or acetaminophen 650 mg.

*Adjuncts
Pain with anxiety: Add phenothiazine or benzodiazepine
Pain with depression: Add antidepressant
Bone pain: Add nonsteroidal anti-inflammatory agent

synergistic effect, and numerous combinations with aspirin are commercially available. A mild laxative may be needed for constipation. Pentazocine is less useful because of more severe central nervous system side effects, such as confusion, hallucinations, and dysphoria. Nonsteroidal anti-inflammatory agents, alone or combined with the narcotics, assist with pain from bone metastases through inhibiting prostaglandin E2 production. Ibuprofen and naproxen are more potent prostaglandin inhibitors than indomethacin or phenylbutazone.

For severe chronic pain, narcotics are the analgesics of choice, and morphine is the standard of comparison. The various narcotics are similar in potency and side effects but differ significantly in duration of action. In equianalgesic doses each narcotic produces similar analgesia when administered at the appropriate dose and time interval. Drugs with a longer duration of action are preferred for chronic pain. Narcotics, especially the more lipophilic levorphanol and methadone, may produce accumulation several days to weeks after starting therapy, resulting in CNS depression and sedation, particularly in the elderly and the very young. It is therefore better to increase narcotic dosage by raising the amount of drug per dose than by shortening the dosage intervals.

While tolerance and dependence are sometimes seen in patients receiving narcotics for acute or psychosomatic pain, in chronic pain from cancer little tolerance to narcotics develops and dependence is not a problem, even over long periods of 50 to 100 weeks of therapy.

Three important principles must be followed in giving narcotic analgesics. First, the optimal dose should be determined by titration for effect. A comfort control chart displaying the patient's perceived level of comfort on an arbitrary scale of 0 to 10 against time (in 4-hour increments) over 24 hours is helpful. High doses may be needed for initial pain control and will not alter vital signs. Relatives should be instructed that for the first few days the patient will be drowsy and may sleep for extended periods to recover from the exhaustion induced by severe pain.

Second, start with a dose that is a little too high and titrate down. A low initial dose with the intent to titrate up or down will necessitate a higher dose for complete pain control because of the patient's increasing anxiety from lack of adequate initial analgesia.

Third, administer the narcotic on a regularly scheduled basis. Prevention of pain recurrence is the objective and requires less analgesic because of the lessened anxiety about the pain coming back. Once initial pain control is achieved, the dose can be lowered slightly every 2 to 3 days without loss of effectiveness, probably owing to a reduction in the patient's anxiety about pain. The optimal dose is the lowest dose that prevents pain recurrence and lies between the last effective dose and the insufficient one. With disease progression, the procedure is repeated, increasing for effective control and then re-establishing the lower optimal dose. Increasing narcotic requirements usually represents disease progression rather than narcotic tolerance.

Oral therapy is preferred, and some narcotics can be administered in rectal suppositories. Parenteral administration may be painful in the presence of marked muscle wasting and may create undue emotional dependence and intimations that heroic measures are being undertaken. Although morphine is only two thirds absorbed orally, it is still effective with proper dose adjustment: 15 mg. of oral morphine sulfate is as effective as a 10 mg. parenteral dose.

A number of analgesic drug cocktails have been advocated, but simple aqueous solutions of morphine are just as good. Oral morphine solution (OMS) may be made up in concentrations of 1, 2, 5, and 10 mg.

Table 56–13. MANAGEMENT OF SEVERE CHRONIC PAIN IN CANCER

Drug	Oral	Route and Dose (mg.) (Equal Analgesic Doses) *I.M.*	*Rectal*	Duration Action (hours)
Morphine sulfate	10	5	10	4
Levorphanol (LevoDromoran)	2	2	—	6
Hydromorphone (Dilaudid)	2	3	3	4
Methadone (Dolophine)	5	5	—	8
Meperidine (Demerol)	100	75	—	3
Pentazocine HCl (Talwin)	50	30	—	3
Oxycodone (Percodan)	5	—	—	4
Codeine	60	60	—	4

per dl. The availability of either morphine hydrochloride or sulphate in various strengths in the forms of syrup, drops, concentrate, tablets, liquid, and suppositories (MOS or Statex varieties), as well as sustained release tablets (MS-Contin), facilitates the ease and flexibility with which pain control can be achieved. Prochlorperazine (Compazine), 5 mg. orally or by suppository one half hour before the OMS, is given to a maximum of 25 mg. in 24 hours to help control mild nausea over the first 3 days. Haloperidol, 0.5 mg. two or three times daily as needed, may also be used but is sedating in older patients. All patients become constipated and should receive instructions on foods, laxatives, stool softeners, and bowel care.

Several adjunctive drugs may be used with narcotics. Phenothiazines not only control nausea but reduce anxiety and allow a lower dose of narcotic for effective pain control. The piperazine phenothiazines given in low doses are best to produce minimal sedation and maximum antiemetic activity. Prochlorperazine, 5 mg. every 8 hours, is effective. Piperidine phenothiazines, like thioridazine or mesoridazine, are anticholinergic and are not recommended because they are constipating and lead to fecal impaction when used with a narcotic. The alkylamine phenothiazines like chlorpromazine and promethazine are quite sedating but may be useful in an agitated patient. Benzodiazepines are also useful adjuncts for control of anxiety.

Reactive depression may resolve when anxiety diminishes with pain control and often does not require specific treatment unless it is a major problem in itself. Tricyclic antidepressants such as imipramine and amitriptyline have significant anticholinergic activity and are not optimally effective in exogenous depression.

In spite of all the treatment modalities outlined and the increasing number of "cured" patients, the stigma created by the word cancer cannot be ignored. The patient, as an individual human being, deserves the respect and dignity we all expect and cannot and must not become modern-day lepers. As physicians we must offer our skills, our optimism, our compassion, and our faith to our cancer patients. To withdraw behind the "I can do no more" philosophy is unacceptable. The physician facing defeat may be tempted to withdraw, become less available, and deny that the patient is indeed dying. It is imperative therefore that we, as physicians, assess our own mortality in order to overcome our patients' greatest fear, that of being abandoned. If we are not prepared to give, we should not accept the responsibility in the first place. To deny the patient of ourselves is to remove one of the finest medicines available. When the final treatment modality has lost its effect and death becomes inevitable, the art of medicine must be practiced to its fullest.

The physician cures rarely, relieves often, comforts always.

ANONYMOUS

References

Billings, J. A.: Outpatient Management of Advanced Cancer, Philadelphia, J. B. Lippincott Co., 1985. *A clinician's guide to the palliative care of advanced cancer patients in the office and home. Symptom control, psychosocial support, and hospice-in-the-home are emphasized.*

Cancer Chemotherapy. The Medical Letter *29* (736), 29–36, 1987. *This issue is devoted to cancer chemotherapy at roughly 2 year intervals.*

Casciato, D. A., and Lowitz, B. B.: Manual of Clinical Oncology. 2nd ed. Boston, Little, Brown, and Co., Inc., 1988. *An organized, concise handbook for the complete management of cancer patients at the bedside.*

DeVita, V. T., Hellman, S., and Rosenberg, S. A. (eds.): Cancer. Principles and Practice of Oncology. 3rd ed. Philadelphia, J. B. Lippincott Co., 1989. *A comprehensive multi-author text for the specialist. The first section covers principles of oncology. The second section on the practice of oncology presents integrated, multidisciplinary discussions of all modalities for each tumor.*

Dorr, R. T., and Fritz, W. L.: Cancer Chemotherapy Handbook. New York, Elsevier, 1980. *This reference, along with See-Lasley and Ignoffo, is a concise, soft-cover reference manual summarizing the technical details of chemotherapy and its complications.*

Dutcher, J. P., and Wiernik, P. H. (eds).: A Handbook of Hematologic and Oncologic Emergencies. New York, Plenum Medical Book Co., 1987.

Howland, W. S., and Carlon, G. C.: Critical Care of the Cancer Patient. Chicago, Yearbook Medical Publishers, 1985. *Multi-author text on managing the complications of malignancies.*

Leventhal, B. G., and Wittes, R. E.: Research Methods in Clinical Oncology. New York, Raven Press, 1988. *A concise text on clinical trial methodologies for cancer.*

Nealon, T. F., Jr.: Management of the Patient with Cancer. 3rd ed. Philadelphia, W. B. Saunders Co., 1986. *A medium-sized, multi-author text.*

Oldham, R. K. (ed.): Principles of Cancer Biotherapy. New York, Raven Press, 1987. *At the time of writing, the only comprehensive text on biological therapies for cancer.*

PDQ (Physician Data Query): *Provides easy access to state-of-the-art cancer treatment through an interactive computerized database maintained by the National Cancer Institute. The database contains interlinked files on cancer treatment, ongoing treatment methods, and a directory of physicians and organizations that provide cancer care. It is distributed online through the National Library of Medicine's (NLM) MEDLARS System, as well as through commercial database vendors. For information through NLM contact: MEDLARS Management Section, NLM, Bldg 38, Rm 4N421, 8600 Rockville Pike, Bethesda, MD 20894 (301)–496–6193, 1–(800)–638–8480.*

Saunders, C. M.: The Management of Terminal Disease. Chicago, Year Book Medical Publishers, 1978. *A multi-author, concise text on palliative care.*

See-Lasley, K., and Ignoffo, R. J.: Manual of Oncology Therapeutics. St. Louis, C. V. Mosby Co., 1981.

Wittes, R. E.: Manual of Oncologic Therapeutics, 1989/1990. Philadelphia, J. B. Lippincott Co., 1989. *A multi-author, concise handbook on diagnosis, staging, and treatment of cancer patients.*

57

Hematology

Joseph Hobbs
Troy H. Guthrie
Leonard H. Brubaker
Paul A. Bilodeau

General Approach to Patients With Elevated Cell Counts

ELEVATED WHITE COUNT

White cell count elevation (greater than 8000 per microliter depending on the laboratory) may be due to granulocytes (neutrophils, eosinophils, and basophils) or lymphocytes. The most common granulocyte elevation involves neutrophils and may be caused by a leukemoid reaction or a myeloproliferative disease, such as chronic myelogenous leukemia or myelofibrosis. A leukemoid reaction may be differentiated from the others because it is composed mostly of mature polys and does not have teardrop or nucleated red cells. Also, a leukemoid reaction usually has an identifiable cause, such as an infection or tumor.

An elevated lymphocyte count can be caused by a lymphocytic leukemoid reaction consisting of normal cells or a malignant transformation of lymphocytes. A lymphocytic leukemoid reaction occurring secondary to infection with a virus such as Epstein-Barr virus or cytomegalovirus or postviral syndromes (for example, mumps, varicella, or hepatitis B) requires no further investigation or treatment. Malignant transformation of lymphocytes may be secondary to a type of leukemia most often chronic and less frequently acute lymphoblastic leukemia or related diseases.

ELEVATED PLATELET COUNT

Platelet counts over 400,000 and up to about 800,000 per microliter may occur in iron deficiency and certain cancers, particularly lung cancer. This, in and of itself, represents no problem. When the platelet count rises to about 1 million per microliter, the patient may have idiopathic thrombocytosis or a myeloproliferative disease related to polycythemia vera. Isolated platelet elevation may occur in patients with polycythemia vera who have chronically bled down to a normal or even low hematocrit resulting in absence of iron in the marrow. This can be differentiated from idiopathic thrombocytosis (IT) because of the adequacy of bone marrow iron stores in IT.

ELEVATED RED BLOOD CELL COUNT

There are two main causes of an elevated red blood cell count: an absolute increase in the number of red cells or decreased plasma volume. Determination of this difference in many instances may be obvious but may require direct measurement of the red cell volume using radioactive chromium-labeled red cells for proper diagnoses of states of actual increase in numbers of red cells. However, hematocrits greater than 60 per cent suggest true erythrocytosis (excessive red cells). Direct determination of plasma volume is a much less reliable tool in evaluating the causes of elevated red blood cell counts. Volume contraction is an obvious cause of decreased plasma volume. Decreased plasma volume can also be produced by the losses of fluid from the intravascular space in edematous states, such as hepatic cirrhosis.

A more subtle problem involving decreased plasma volume as a cause of increased red cell count is *spurious erythrocytosis*, the precise cause of which is not understood. Patients with this disorder may be emotionally stressed, may smoke, or may be hypertensive. If the patient also uses diuretics, the elevated red cell count can be made worse. Although most of these patients have no complications and require no treatment, a few will develop an increased risk of thrombotic diseases since it is difficult to eliminate the hyperviscosity caused by the high hematocrit. Phlebotomy in this setting is not indicated because it exacerbates the already low blood volume. Use of a vasodilator, such as hydralazine, that can increase salt and water retention (thus increasing blood volume) may be of benefit. If the patient is a smoker, smoking cessation is much more beneficial. In fact, any patient with an elevated red cell count, regardless of the cause, should be advised to stop smoking.

Polycythemia Vera

When the red cell count is high because of an excessive production of red cells, the condition is called erythrocytosis. *Primary erythrocytosis,* or polycythemia vera, is a malignant overproduction of red cells. The spleen is enlarged in over half of the patients, and the arterial oxygen saturation is over 91 per cent as opposed to erythrocytosis secondary to hypoxic states. Overproduction of white cells and platelets is also common, leading to high blood counts in these cell lines. The excessive neutrophil production can lead to an elevated serum B_{12} binding protein level. Criteria for making the diagnosis have been published by the Polycythemia Vera Study Group.

The main aim of treatment of polycythemia vera is to get and keep the patient's hematocrit less than 45 per cent to avoid thromboembolism and hemorrhage. This normal hematocrit must be maintained for 4 months before any elective surgery to avoid a high risk of these complications postsurgically. If the patient is elderly or has already had a stroke or other thrombotic episode, radioactive phosphate intravenously is the best treatment. Hydroxyurea is also effective, and perhaps less leukemogenic, but it is difficult to monitor. The treatment of choice in the majority of patients, especially younger ones, is phlebotomy to the point of iron deficiency.

Secondary Erythrocytosis

This is caused by some problem outside of the marrow. Any cause of arterial desaturation, such as chronic obstructive pulmonary disease, cyanotic heart disease, and carboxyhemoglobinemia, will stimulate erythropoietin production, and the marrow responds appropriately by making increased amounts of red cells. In contrast to polycythemia vera, there is usually no need to lower the red cell count by phlebotomy or radioactive phosphate because the problem is a physiologic and beneficial response to hypoxia. In other causes of secondary erythrocytosis, there is an inappropriate production of erythropoietin, such as benign renal cysts, and large uterine fibroids. Phlebotomy represents a safe therapeutic option. Malignant kidney, liver, and cerebellar tumors also produce erythropoietin inappropriately.

General Approach to Patients With Low Blood Counts

LOW WHITE COUNT

There are many benign causes of leukopenia. Many viral diseases produce a transient leukopenia. The mean neutrophil count of the black population is some 500 per microliter less than that of the nonblack population. Some black persons have a chronically low neutrophil count, but when their marrows are stimulated, as during an infection, the neutrophil count rises to the same degree of elevation as the general population. In general, the neutrophil count may go as low as 0.8×10^3 per microliter (absolute count) without harm in the presence of a normal bone marrow. However, counts less than 800 to 1000 per cubic microliter may be associated with increased risk of infection. There are a variety of serious illnesses that may produce a low count of one or another of the white cell types. Usually, a bone marrow examination is required to help differentiate between these. Examples are B_{12} and folate deficiency, hypersplenism, aplastic anemia, agranulocytosis, acute leukemia, acquired immune deficiency syndrome (AIDS) (low lymphocyte count), some preleukemic conditions, and tumor invading the bone marrow.

LOW PLATELET COUNT

The number of circulating blood cells of any kind depends on the balance between production and destruction. Another factor that affects the platelet count is splenic sequestration, which can decrease the number of platelets available for peripheral circulation. Therefore, the causes of low platelet counts may be either low production, rapid destruction, excessive pooling in the spleen, or a combination of these.

Low production may be caused by a disease, such as aplastic anemia, or by drugs that produce marrow aplasia, e.g., most of the anticancer drugs. The marrow elements that produce platelets may be replaced by malignant cells, such as those of acute leukemia, breast cancer, or prostate cancer. In all of these cases, an aspirate or biopsy of the bone marrow will show decreased platelet precursors. A slightly different mechanism is at work in the ineffective production of platelets in megaloblastic anemias caused by folate or B_{12} deficiency or alcohol.

Rapid destruction of platelets is caused most commonly by the auto-immune disease, *idiopathic thrombocytopenic purpura (ITP).* A bone marrow aspiration will reveal a large number of the platelet-generating megakaryocytes in the marrow. The discrepancy between the clear evidence of marrow production of platelets and the low platelet count is the best diagnostic criterion routinely available. Special laboratories can show the presence of antibodies on platelets, but this test is difficult to obtain. Of course, the marrow must be free of other pathology, such as pronounced megaloblastic changes secondary to B_{12} or folate deficiency.

ITP may be divided into three types depending on age and sex of the patient, which determine the type of treatment and prognosis. ITP is not uncommon in children under 10 years and is usually short-lived and requires no treatment. ITP occurring in women under about age 40 usually does not remit spontaneously but usually responds to steroid administration or splenectomy. Older women and men after puberty who develop ITP are much more difficult groups. They may not respond to initial treatment, and, if they do, they often relapse quickly. They also require repeated changes of therapy because of transient, poor, or no response and suffer from major bleeding episodes, some fatal. Such patients need early referral to a specialized treatment center.

If a patient has a clinical picture of ITP with megakaryocytes in the marrow, it is very important to rule out drugs as the cause of platelet destruction. Some of the more common drugs implicated are quinidine, quinine, sulfonamides, and oral diuretics. Certainly, all nonessential drugs should be stopped in any patient with ITP. Also, aspirin, bismuth salicylate, and nonsteroidal anti-inflammatory drugs should not be given to patients with a low platelet count because they interfere with platelet function and may cause bleeding.

Patients with AIDS frequently develop the adult form of ITP. Their prognosis is especially poor.

Heavy consumption of ethanol may also cause a clinical picture consistent with ITP, but withdrawal of ethanol results in a normal platelet count in about a week without further therapy.

A patient who is acutely ill with thrombocytopenia, fever, central nervous system abnormalities, and hemolysis of red cells with fragmented red cells on the peripheral smear blood has findings consistent with *thrombotic thrombocytopenic purpura.* This is a life-threatening, but treatable, disease using plasma exchange therapy. Such a patient should be promptly referred to a center with the facilities for the plasma exchange or other similar recently developed therapeutic modalities.

Splenic sequestration of platelets can cause a decreased platelet count. Any cause of splenomegaly can cause splenic platelet sequestration. The larger the spleen, the greater the excessive platelet pooling. Platelets are tiny cell fragments that can easily become trapped temporarily in the sinuses of the large spleen. Splenic sequestration of platelets in and of itself does not lead to a bleeding diathesis, but the cause of the splenomegaly (for example, lymphoma) may also affect marrow production of platelets. Rarely, the spleen must be removed to allow a higher number of circulating platelets. More often, recognition of an enlarged spleen in association with a platelet count of about half the lower limit of normal in a patient with liver disease and portal hypertension will reassure the physician that no special therapy is needed for this cause of thrombocytopenia.

LOW RED BLOOD CELL COUNT (THE ANEMIAS)

Once dilutional causes of low red blood cell counts have been ruled out one must assume that there is an anemia—an absolute decreased quantity of red cells in the peripheral circulation. This anemia can be caused by bone marrow hypoproliferation, or accelerated destruction or loss of red cells in association with a hyperproliferative bone marrow. The bone marrow's response to an anemia is determined by the reticulocyte production index. This index (normal is 1) is a correction of the reticulocyte count (RC) as follows: RC × patient's hematocrit/45 divided by 2 (to account for early shift of reticulocytes out of the marrow and into the circulation). A reticulocyte index less than 1 means that the marrow is not producing red blood cells. A reticulocyte count greater than 3 suggests that the marrow is active. In this case, destruction of red blood cells or hemolysis may be occurring.

In hyperproliferative anemia, the bone marrow actively responds to the low red blood cell count but not at rates that can match the rate of red cell destruction and/or loss. These hyperproliferative states are characterized by an increased percentage of reticulocytes in the peripheral circulation and an increased reticulocyte production index. The causes of this type of anemia are hemolytic processes and acute hemorrhage. The increased reticulocyte index, however, in this setting depends on adequate essential nutrients for red blood production, such as folate, B_{12}, and iron. Without these nutrients, the reticulocyte response may be blocked, making diagnosis difficult. The mean cell volume in these hyperproliferative states tends to be increased because of the number of immature red blood cells in the peripheral circulation that are larger than mature red blood cells.

In hypoproliferative anemia, the bone marrow does not show any active response to the anemia. This is demonstrated by a reticulocyte production index of less than one. Under these circumstances, there is either a nuclear maturation arrest caused by B_{12} or folate deficiency, a cytoplasmic maturation arrest caused by a deficiency of a component of hemoglobin such as iron (iron deficiency anemia), globulin (thalassemia), heme (lead intoxication), or decreased marrow proliferation due to decreased erythropoietin (renal failure), metabolic blocks (anemia of chronic disease), or replacement of bone marrow by fat, fibrosis, or tumor.

An inspection of the peripheral blood smear will help to categorize the causes of hypoproliferative anemias. In the presence of hypochromic, microcytic cells, and a MCV less than 80, cytoplasmic arrest would appear to be the most likely cause of an anemia. If macrocytic cells with an MCV greater than 100 and hypersegmented polymorphonuclear leukocytes are seen on peripheral smear, the cause of the anemia is most likely an arrest of nuclear maturation. If neither of these characteristics can be found on the peripheral blood smear and the MCV is normal, the problem is most likely secondary to decreased marrow proliferation, secondary to metabolic blocks or actual replacement of marrow element. Also if the anemia does not fit either the criteria for a hypoproliferative or hyperproliferative type of bone marrow response, one must consider the presence of more than one cause of the anemia. If a hypoproliferative anemia is believed to be secondary to a cytoplasmic maturation arrest, the evaluation should include serum iron levels, iron-binding capacity, ferritin level, and a search for target cells. In iron deficiency anemia, the iron and ferritin levels are low and the iron-binding capacity is high. Target cells could be indicative of thalassemia.

If all evidence suggests a nuclear maturation arrest, the evaluation should include measurements of vitamin B_{12} and folate levels and red cell folate concentration. Consideration should also be given to therapeutic test doses using tiny doses of vitamin B_{12} or folate looking for bone marrow response as indicated by reticulocytosis. If it appears that there is some general depression of bone marrow proliferation, a bone marrow biopsy might be necessary in order to determine the presence of fibrosis and/or tumor or other findings suggestive of an anemia due to chronic disease. The bone marrow biopsy for the initial evaluation of most anemia can probably be avoided if the evaluation seeks to determine the physiologic response to decreased red blood cells.

If the evaluation shows that the anemia is associated with a hyperproliferative bone marrow and obvious bleeding has been ruled out, hemolytic anemia would be the most likely cause. In this setting, studies such as a Coombs' test, serum haptoglobin levels, and urine hemosiderin should be made.

Iron Deficiency Anemia

The most common anemia of all age groups is iron deficiency anemia. The deficiency of iron results in inadequate hemoglobin production, arrest of cytoplasmic maturation, and a hypoproliferative bone marrow response to the ensuing anemia. Although the classic red cell morphology of microcytosis and hypochromia are suggestive of iron deficiency anemia, these findings occur late in the sequence of worsening iron deficiency. The lack of precise morphologic changes early in the course of iron deficiency makes it necessary for the physician to anticipate its presence in situations where patients are prone to have a negative iron balance, such as blood loss, increased iron utilization (for example, pregnancy or growth spurts), inadequate dietary iron intake, and malabsorption.

IRON METABOLISM

Iron is complexed in the body to heme-containing substances, such as hemoglobin, myoglobin, and heme-containing enzymes. Hemoglobin contains the majority of the body's iron, representing at a minimum approximately 66 per cent of the body's total iron content. The remaining iron is found in myoglobin and storage sites consisting of ferritin and hemosiderin. The quantity of the iron stored in these sites is relatively stable in normal men but varies considerably in normal women because of menstrual (25 mg. of iron lost per normal menstrual period) and pregnancy-related blood losses (400 mg. of iron is transferred from mother to fetus and placenta, 300 mg. of iron is lost at a normal delivery, and 400 mg. of iron is required for maternal blood volume expansion). This variability of iron stores in women does not cause an anemia as long as the macrophage-derived iron, the remaining iron stores, and the increased intestinal absorption of iron are sufficient to permit normal red blood cell production.

Because the body's iron is efficiently reutilized as old red cells are physiologically destroyed and the loss of iron is only 1 mg. per day (total iron in a normal man is 3200 mg.), severe anemia caused solely by inadequate dietary iron rarely occurs. The exception, however, would be infants of iron deficient mothers and in states of increased physiologic iron demands caused by the rapidly increasing number of red blood cells that occurs in growth spurts of infants and young children.

Dietary iron in the ferric form (most common type of dietary iron) must be made soluble by gastric acidity in order for intestinal absorption to occur, whereas the solubility of the ferrous form (primary form of iron found in meats) and its absorption is not dependent on gastric acidity. Dietary iron is absorbed along most levels of the intestinal tract, but the absorption of the greatest quantity of iron occurs in the duodenum. Iron is transported from the intestinal absorption sites and iron storage sites bound to plasma transferrin. It is eventually delivered to hemopoietic tissue to be incorporated in developing red cells.

The process of intestinal iron absorption is enhanced in the states of iron deficiency prior to the development of anemia. The buffer between accelerated loss, hyperutilization, malabsorption, and/or dietary inadequacies of iron and the development of anemia is the storage pool of iron. Therefore, any process that reduces iron storage compartments increases vulnerability to iron deficiency anemia.

Iron is not an abundant part of the typical American diet, representing on an average only four to six times the daily requirements. This may be sufficient for persons with stable iron requirements but may be inadequate for those with enhanced requirements. Iron-rich foods, such as liver and legumes, represent greater sources of iron when compared to beef, pork, chicken, and fish. Iron-fortified foods may not provide absorbable iron since much of the iron may be irreversibly complexed to substances within the food.

Several pathologic processes occur during the development of iron deficiency before the classic picture of a hypochromic microcytic anemia is seen. First, there is continuous depletion of the iron stores that serve as a buffer to protect against the development of anemia. As long as these storage sites are present, red cell production remains normal. The rate of the decline of these iron storage sites can be slowed albeit minimally by increasing intestinal iron reabsorption. When the storage sites are depleted (as can be seen by bone marrow examination), serum iron and ferritin are also decreased, and the total iron-binding capacity and transferrin are increased. Anemia then ensues, which initially appears normochromic and normocytic. As the process of iron deficiency proceeds, microcytic normocytes predominate. Further progression of the iron deficiency leads to the typical microcytic hypochromic anemia. Severe anemia is marked by cytoplasmic maturation disturbance, leading to red cells of different sizes and shapes (poikilocytosis and anisocytosis) in the peripheral circulation.

Table 57–1. CAUSES OF IRON DEFICIENCY ANEMIA

I. Dietary Lack of Iron
   A. Decreased intake of iron (growth and developmental, economic, medical, or life style reasons)
   B. Diets low in iron or containing iron irreversibly bound to food stuffs
II. Blood Loss
   A. Gastrointestinal tract
   B. Urinary tract
      1. Hematuria
      2. Hemosiderinuria and hemoglobinuria associated with severe chronic intravascular hemolysis
   C. Gynecologic/Obstetric
      1. Functional uterine bleeding
      2. Dysfunctional uterine bleeding
      3. Blood loss at the time of delivery
   D. Pulmonary
      1. Chronic hemoptysis
   E. Surgical blood loss without replacement
III. Increase Iron Utilization
   A. Pregnancy
   B. Growth spurts (infancy, adolescence)
   C. Polycythemia
IV. Malabsorption of Iron
   A. Inflammatory bowel disease
   B. Surgical removal or bypass of iron absorptive sites
   C. Surgical removal of all or part of the stomach
   D. Atrophic gastritis
   E. Pica

ETIOLOGY OF IRON DEFICIENCY ANEMIA (TABLE 57–1)

Blood loss represents the most frequent cause of iron deficiency anemia. Iron deficiency anemia occurring in postmenopausal women and men is most frequently related to a loss of blood through the gastrointestinal (GI) tract. These GI bleeding sites include benign sources, such as peptic ulcers, gastritis, vascular anomalies, diverticulitis, polyps, and inflammatory bowel disease. A disruption of the integrity of the GI mucosa caused by substances such as ethanol, salicylates, and other nonsteroidal agents can cause bleeding. Intestinal infestation with parasites also can cause chronic GI blood loss. Malignant lesions of any level of the GI tract can result in both occult and obvious bleeding. Menstrual blood loss is an important source of iron loss especially when menstruation is superimposed on clinical situations, such as small iron stores, inadequate replacement of the iron losses/requirements of pregnancy and delivery, and/or inadequate daily ingestion of dietary iron. A less frequent site of blood loss is through the urinary tract caused by both benign and malignant lesions. Urinary tract iron loss occurs in severe and/or chronic hemolytic anemias because of hemosiderinuria and hemoglobinuria. Pulmonary blood loss caused by hemoptysis is an additional mechanism of blood loss albeit less frequent than those previously discussed.

Another cause of iron deficiency anemia is the increased iron requirements associated with pregnancy and certain stages of growth. Typically, the increased need is caused by the expanding red cell mass during these periods of accelerated growth that may not be matched by adequate dietary iron replacements, leading to depleted iron stores and ultimately anemia. Growing infants who do not have a diet that includes appropriate dietary iron will develop iron deficiency anemia within 1 to 2 years of life. The iron requirements also increase for those infants who are born prematurely. Pregnant patients who have obligate blood losses (i.e., transferents) to the fetus and placenta plus an additional expansion in blood volume run a significant risk of developing iron deficiency anemia without additional iron supplementation. Abnormal states, such as primary and secondary erythrocytosis, can also result in depleted iron stores.

Malabsorption of iron will occur if there is surgical removal or bypass of significant amounts of iron absorption sites or if those sites are rendered dysfunctional by inflammatory bowel disease. Decreased absorption of iron also occurs in atrophic gastritis where the ferric form of iron is more likely to remain insoluble because of an elevated gastric pH. Another cause of decreased iron absorption is the chronic ingestion of nondietary substances, such as clay and starch (pica), which can chelate dietary iron, making it unavailable for absorption. When pica is not the primary cause of iron deficiency anemia, but rather a symptom of the anemia caused by other factors, it still may contribute to the persistence of the anemia because of the potential of chelating therapeutic iron replacements.

Iron deficiency anemia caused solely by insufficient intake of dietary iron should only be considered when other causes of iron deficiency anemia have been ruled out. The deficiency of dietary iron is more likely to be a contributing factor to the development of iron deficiency anemia as opposed to the primary cause.

Historical Evaluation

The history of iron deficiency anemia is represented by nonspecific findings, such as chronic fatigue and shortness of breath. Often, the patient may not be aware of associated symptoms especially if the anemia has been developing slowly. Depending on the severity of the anemia, patients may have signs associated with high output cardiac failure, such as palpitations, postural dizziness, dyspnea on exertion, and exercise-related fatigue. Other symptoms include sore tongue and pica to include pagophagia (compulsive ice eating).

Since early iron deficiency anemia is asymptomatic, it is important to suspect its presence in certain situations such as in children (secondary to growth spurts), women (secondary to menstrual and pregnancy-related blood losses), indigent persons (secondary to a lack of access to foods containing adequate iron), frequent blood donors, and elderly persons (secondary to GI bleeding and in some settings lack of access to dietary iron). It should be noted that black Americans have a mean blood hemoglobin concentration that, on an average, is about 1 gram per deciliter less than the white population without any evidence of decrease in iron stores.

Physical Evaluation

Many of the physical findings of iron deficiency anemia are common to other types of anemia. They include pallor, glossitis, tachycardia, and signs of high output cardiac failure, such as systolic flow murmurs, tachycardia, postural blood pressure, and pulse changes. The magnitude of these findings depends on the severity of the anemia. Patients may also have koilonychia, cheilosis, and angular stomatitis. Rarely, in severe cases of iron deficiency anemia, there is association with Plummer-Vinson syndrome, which may be manifested historically by dysphagia. Splenomegaly is also a rare occurring physical finding in iron deficiency anemia.

Laboratory Evaluation

A hemoglobin and hematocrit should be performed, which may reveal low values. The examination of the peripheral smear in fully developed iron deficiency anemia will reveal microcytosis and a low MCV. Peripheral film in fully developed iron deficiency anemia will also show poikilocytosis and anisocytosis (Fig. 57–1). The red cell distribution width will be elevated. However, these characteristic findings of iron deficiency anemia are usually preceded by iron depletion in the face of no anemia or iron deficiency in the face of an anemia with morphologic characteristics inconsistent with full blown iron deficiency anemia. In iron deficiency, there is a hypoproliferative bone marrow response as manifested by a reticulocyte count that is less than 1 per cent and a low reticulocyte production index. A reduction in the serum ferritin level is the first parameter to reflect iron deficiency often when other measurable estimates (i.e., blood counts, endices, red cell morphology) are within normal limits. Usually, when morphologic evidence of iron deficiency is present, serum iron levels are low, total iron-binding capacity is elevated, and transferrin saturation is low. However, these measurements of iron status may be normal in the face of iron deficiency anemia. It should also be recognized that serum iron, total iron-binding capacity, transferrin saturation, and serum ferritin can be altered by chronic inflammation, which may result in values inconsistent with those typically found in iron deficiency anemia. If historical, physical, and laboratory evaluations discussed above do not reveal the likely cause of an anemia, further examination of a bone marrow aspiration should be performed. In the setting of iron deficiency anemia, there would be absence of both intracellular and extracellular iron.

Therapy

Once the primary cause of iron deficiency anemia has been determined, then replacement of the body's stores of iron can ensue. An acceptable regimen is ferrous sulfate 300 mg., which contains 60 mg. of elemental iron, given three times per day before, with, or after meals. There are those who would advocate giving ferrous sulfate only between meals because without food it is better absorbed. If the patient develops GI problems with ferrous sulfate, a decrease in the amount of iron provided is a more acceptable alternative than switching to enteric-coated pills or sustained-release pills, which do not consistently deliver the required therapeutic amounts of iron. If patients continue to have some intolerance to plain ferrous sulfate, then ferrous sulfate syrup may be used although this has the potential to discolor teeth. Patients should be advised that these iron preparations will cause black stools.

The first response to iron replacement therapy is reticulocytosis, which usually occurs within the first 7 days. The hematocrit will return to normal over the

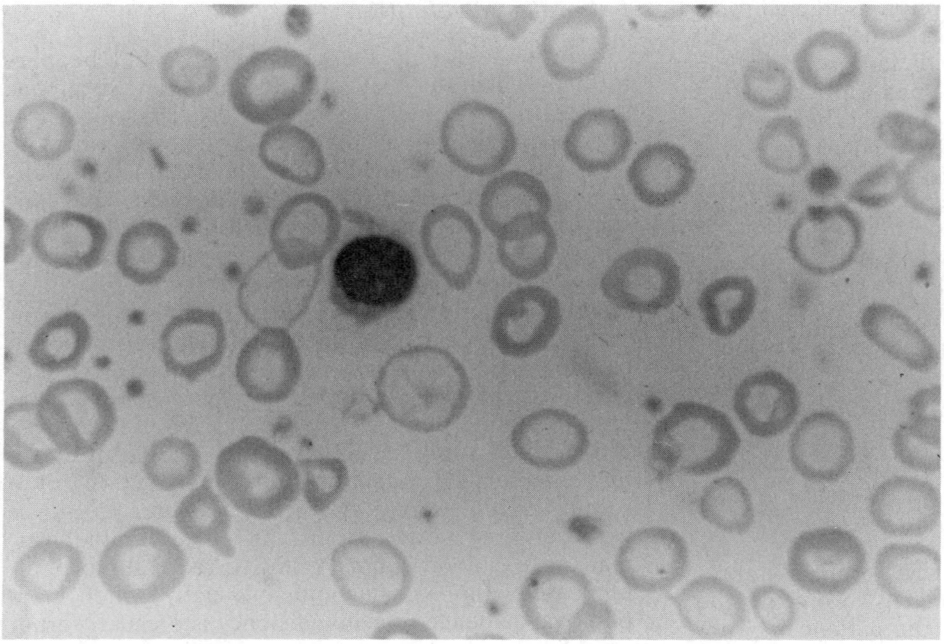

Figure 57–1. Severe iron deficiency anemia, showing hypochromia, microcytosis, central pallor, poikilocytosis, and anisocytosis.

course of 1½ to 2 months, but therapy should continue for approximately 4 months so that iron stores can be replenished. If the patient has a chronic source of blood loss (iron loss) that has not been controlled, iron therapy may be required for a longer period. If there is no response to therapy, one must consider chronic blood loss, noncompliance, the wrong diagnosis, presence of more than one cause of the anemia, or inability to absorb ferrous sulfate from the GI tract. There are a few situations in which parenteral iron therapy may be required. These include patients unable to take oral iron, inflammatory bowel disease that may affect iron absorption, and continuous bleeding that cannot be stopped. Transfusions in iron deficiency anemia should be avoided since in chronic anemias the patients usually are hypervolemic and the addition of more blood volume might cause patients to develop circulatory overload. If transfusions are used in iron deficiency anemia, they are used in the setting of cardiac decompensation, symptoms related to hypoprofusion of vital organs such as the brain, heart, and kidney, and it should be given extremely slowly to avoid further cardiac decompensation and pulmonary edema.

In children, the treatment of iron deficiency anemia should be continued for at least 6 months after a normal hemoglobin level has been reached. Oral therapy for children is 6 mg. per kg. of elemental iron given in three divided dosages with ferrous sulfate again being the most affective and least expensive agent. Although the oral iron is absorbed best when not given with foods, if decreasing the iron dose does not remove GI intolerance then iron given with meals may be an acceptable alternative. As in all cases of iron deficiency anemia, successful treatment cannot occur without adequate follow-up. If there is no reticulocytosis in 14 days or the hematocrit is not normalized over the course of 1½ to 2 months, then there is a treatment failure, and the patient needs to be reinvestigated.

Megaloblastic Anemias

Megaloblastic anemia is a hypoproliferative macrocytic anemia usually caused by a deficiency of folic acid and/or vitamin B_{12} that results in disturbed DNA synthesis resulting in nuclear maturation arrest. Other causes of megaloblastic anemia (e.g., erythroleukemia, lead arsenic) are rare, and the underlying mechanisms are not known. The morphologic changes of this disorder are usually found in rapidly proliferating cells, such as blood and mucosal cells. This nuclear defect causes the destruction of an increased number of blood cell precursors in the bone marrow and a decreased delivery of blood cells to the peripheral circulation, referred to as ineffective erythropoiesis, thrombopoiesis, or leukopoiesis.

Folic acid and vitamin B_{12} deficiencies can be caused by decreased intake, malabsorption or inadequate utilization of dietary sources, and body stores of the vitamins. Folic acid deficiency can also be caused by hyperutilization of folate.

BIOCHEMICAL BASIS OF MEGALOBLASTOSIS

Megaloblastic transformation is caused by deficient or defective conversion of deoxyuridine monophosphate (dUMP) to deoxythymidine monophosphate (dTMP), which requires the presence of 5,10-methylene tetrahydrofolate (5,10-methylene FH4), which is folate and B_{12} dependent (Fig. 57–2).

Physiology of Vitamin B_{12}

Vitamin B_{12} is a water-soluble cobalamin vitamin that is obtained by humans through ingestion of animal foodstuffs containing B_{12} of microbial origin. The chief dietary sources of B_{12} are meats and dairy products. The minimum daily requirement of B_{12} is approximately 2 μg. The total body stores of B_{12} range from 2 to 3 mg. Therefore, complete cessation of dietary B_{12} for 3 to 4 years would be required for B_{12} deficiency to become manifest assuming enterohepatic circulation of the vitamin was also impaired.

Dietary vitamin B_{12} complexed to proteins can be released by cooking, gastric acids, and intestinal enzymes. The free B_{12} then binds to a glycoprotein R binder in the stomach. The R binder-B_{12} complex is digested in the duodenum, and the released B_{12} binds to intrinsic factor. The intrinsic factor-B_{12} complex is resistant to enzymatic digestion in the small bowel. Intrinsic factor is produced by gastric parietal cells and parallels hydrochloric acid secretion. In the small bowel, the intrinsic factor-B_{12} complex is bound to specific ileal receptors, and B_{12} is transferred to the portal blood, leaving intrinsic factor behind.

Once in the portal blood, some B_{12} binds loosely to a transport protein, transcobalamin II, which rapidly delivers B_{12} to sites of utilization, such as the bone marrow and other dividing cells, and to sites of storage, such as the liver. The majority of B_{12} in the serum is bound tightly to another transport protein, transcobalamin I, and this complex represents the serum and intracellular storage pool of vitamin B_{12}.

In the liver, vitamin B_{12} is converted to two coenzymes—deoxyadenosyl B_{12} and methyl B_{12}. Deoxyadenosyl B_{12} is necessary for the catabolism of propionic acid, and therefore, abnormal fatty acid metabolism in B_{12} deficiency may be the cause of the neurologic findings that are a common complication. Methyl B_{12} is an important regulator in folate metabolism. Without methyl B_{12}, there would be an inability to convert the major form of plasma folate into forms that can be used in the metabolic steps necessary for DNA synthesis. This interaction between vitamin B_{12} and folate may explain why large dosages of folate may reverse the megaloblastic changes in the hematopoietic system caused by B_{12} deficiency. However, folate will not alter any of the neurologic findings associated with B_{12} deficiency.

Physiology of Folate

The major function of folate is the transfer of one-carbon fragments to organic compounds—an important step in the synthesis of purines. Humans are unable to synthesize their total daily requirement of folate and, therefore, must depend on a dietary source of this vitamin. The major dietary sources of folate are fruit and vegetables; other sources include liver, kidney, yeast, and mushrooms. The daily requirement of folate is 50 to 100 μg. The total body stores of folate range from 10 to 20 mg. Complete cessation of dietary folate would result in depletion of the body stores within a few months.

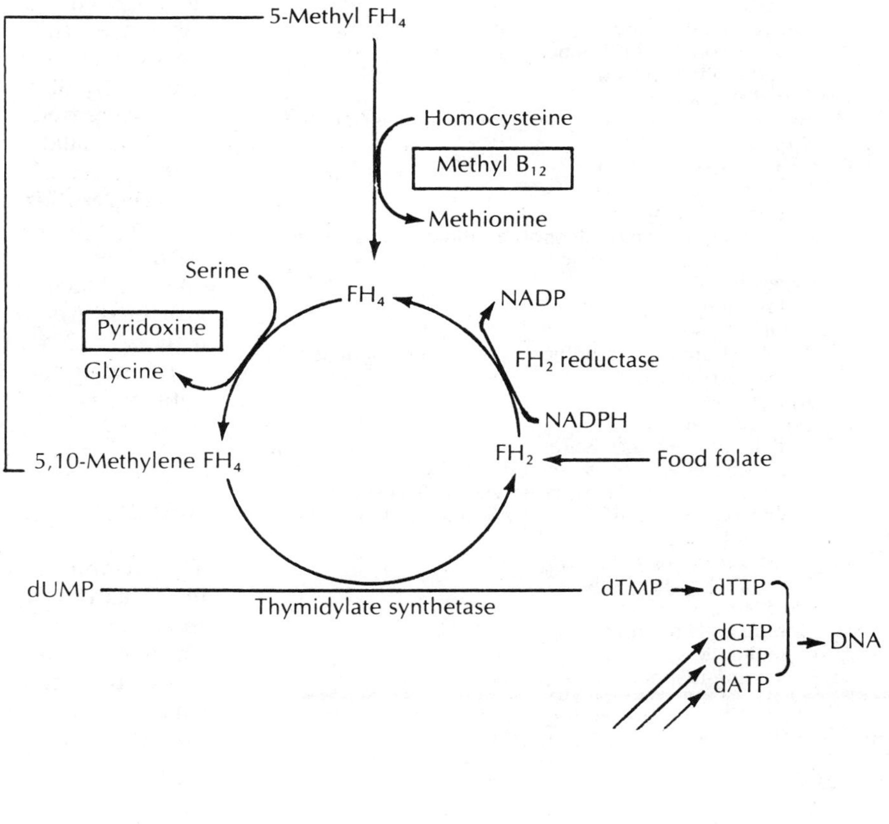

Figure 57–2. Relationship of B_{12} and folate in the process of DNA synthesis. (DNA = deoxyribonucleic acid; dTMP = deoxythymidine monophosphate; dTTP, dGTP, dCTP = nucleotide components of DNA; dUMP = deoxyuridine monophosphate; FH_4 = tetrahydrofolate; FH_2 = dihydrofolate; NADP = nicotinamide-adenine dinucleotide phosphate; NADPH = NADP in reduced form). (From Hobbs, J.: Megaloblastic anemias. Am. Fam. Physician 22(6):129, December, 1980. By permission.)

CAUSES OF MEGALOBLASTIC TRANSFORMATION (TABLE 57–2)

Vitamin B_{12} Deficiency

Inadequate Intake. Because of the large body stores of vitamin B_{12}, the enterohepatic circulation of B_{12}, and the ubiquity of B_{12} in meats and dairy products, insufficient dietary intake of B_{12} is a rare cause of megaloblastic transformation. Inadequate intake is most often found in strict vegetarians who stopped B_{12} intake for at least 10 to 20 years and in their breast-fed infants.

Table 57–2. CAUSES OF MEGALOBLASTIC ANEMIAS*

- I. Vitamin B_{12} Deficiency
  - A. Inadequate intake (rare; most often associated with strict vegetarianism)
  - B. Decreased absorption
    - 1. Intrinsic factor deficiency
      - a. Acquired pernicious anemia
      - b. Following gastrectomy
      - c. Corrosive damage to gastric mucosa
    - 2. Intrinsic factor dysfunction (congenital pernicious anemia)
    - 3. Disorders of ileal intrinsic factor-B_{12} (IF-B_{12}) receptor sites
      - a. Inflammatory bowel disease (tropical sprue, regional, enteritis, Crohn's disease)
      - b. Neoplastic diseases of IF-B_{12} receptor sites
    - 4. Surgical resection of If-B_{12} receptor sites
    - 5. Competition for B_{12}
      - a. Intestinal bacterial overgrowth (blind loop syndrome)
      - b. Fish tapeworm infestation
    - 6. Nondigestion of R binder-B_{12} complex (pancreatic insufficiency)
    - 7. Decreased bicarbonate production (pancreatic insufficiency)
  - C. Inadequate utilization
    - 1. Transcobalamin II deficiency
    - 2. Metabolic blocks (nitrous oxide)
- II. Folic Acid Deficiency
  - A. Inadequate intake (poor diet, chronic illness, alcohol abuse)
  - B. Decreased absorption
    - 1. Inflammatory bowel disease (tropical and nontropical sprue)
    - 2. Drugs (phenytoin, alcohol, barbiturates, isoniazid, estrogens, cycloserine)
  - C. Hyperutilization
    - 1. Pregnancy, lactation
    - 2. Growth spurts
    - 3. Accelerated hematopoiesis (hemolytic anemias, hemorrhagic states)
    - 4. Neoplasms
  - D. Inadequate utilization
    - 1. Folic acid antagonist (methotrexate, trimethoprim, triamterene, diamidine compounds)
    - 2. Incorporation of folate into ineffective cellular components (purine and pyrimidine antagonists)
- III. Mechanism Unknown
  - A. Hereditary orotic aciduria
  - B. Erythroleukemia
  - C. Lead, arsenic
  - D. Sideroblastic anemia
  - E. Preleukemic syndrome
  - F. Pyridoxine-responsive megaloblastic anemia

*From Hobbs, J., and Rodriguez, A.: Megaloblastic anemias. Am. Fam. Physician, *22*:131, 1980.

Decreased Absorption. In order for vitamin B_{12} to be absorbed, it must first survive the enzymatic activity of the small bowel and then bind to specific ileal receptor sites. This can be accomplished only when the vitamin is bound to intrinsic factor. Therefore, situations that decrease the availability of intrinsic factor decrease the amount of B_{12} available for binding and eventual absorption. Acquired pernicious anemia is due to the decreased production of intrinsic factor caused possibly by an autoimmune process with antibodies directed against gastric parietal cells. Decreased absorption of vitamin B_{12} can also occur if the stomach is removed or chemically damaged. Bacterial overgrowth or infestation of the bowel with organisms that utilize B_{12} can result in a decreased availability of the vitamin for human absorption. Intestinal resection or inflammatory bowel disease involving specific ileal receptor sites, where the intrinsic factor-B_{12} complex binds, can also result in decreased absorption of the vitamin B_{12}. Pancreatic insufficiency can also cause decreased B_{12} absorption because of inadequate bicarbonate production and enzymatic activity to release B_{12} from the R-Binder.

Inadequate Utilization. In transcobalamin II deficiency, there is an inability to transport B_{12} from serum to sites of utilization and storage. This results in a normal serum B_{12} level in the face of frank evidence of tissue B_{12} deficiency.

Folic Acid Deficiency

Inadequate Intake. Folic acid deficiency commonly occurs as a result of poor dietary intake of substances containing this vitamin. Folic acid deficiency is associated with poverty, alcohol abuse, and chronically ill or demented states.

Decreased Absorption. Folic acid deficiency can occur in malabsorption syndromes and in association with the use of certain drugs.

Hyperutilization. Folic acid deficiency can be caused by hyperutilization of body stores of folate in conditions involving an increased rate of cellular division, such as pregnancy, hemolytic anemia, and growth spurts in adolescence and infancy (especially if there is also a borderline daily intake of folate).

Inadequate Utilization. The use of folic acid antagonists and alkylating agents that disrupt DNA synthesis can lead to folate deficiency.

HISTORY

The symptoms of megaloblastic anemias have an insidious onset. However, there are certain clues in the history that may be helpful in establishing a cause for megaloblastic transformation as opposed to other causes of anemia. A history of chronic diarrhea may cause malabsorption due to changes in the epithelial lining of the small bowel. Diarrhea may also be associated with inflammatory bowel diseases, which can cause decreased absorption of both folate and B_{12}.

Indications of B_{12} Deficiency

The major difference between the presentation of folic acid deficiency and that of B_{12} deficiency is the association of B_{12} deficiency with neurologic manifestations of a subacute degeneration of the nervous system. The earliest neurologic manifestation of B_{12} deficiency is paresthesias of the hands and toes, which are secondary peripheral nerve dysfunctions. Symptoms of cerebral dysfunction associated with B_{12} deficiency are forgetfulness, irritability, and, in some situations, psychosis. A history of gastric or intestinal surgery in a patient with anemia should suggest the possibility of malabsorption of vitamin B_{12}, bacterial overgrowth, disordered bile salt metabolism, and loss of B_{12} absorption sites.

A history of conditions associated with increased folate demand, inadequate folate intake, and malabsorption of folate should be sought. A drug history may reveal the use of chemotherapeutic agents, such as direct inhibitors of DNA synthesis or folic acid antagonists. It is also important to determine whether the patient is taking drugs that can decrease the absorption of folate from the GI tract (e.g., phenytoin). Lack of dietary intake of folate might be difficult information to obtain from the elderly and abusers of alcohol and other addicting drugs.

PHYSICAL EVALUATION

Patients may show evidence of ineffective erythropoiesis, such as pallor and icterus, and those with chronic anemia may have extramedullary hematopoiesis (as manifested by hepatosplenomegaly). Depending on the severity of the disease, signs of anemia (such as tachycardia, wide pulse pressure, pale mucous membranes, and cardiac decompensation) may be present. The atrophic, tender, beefy red tongue is a common finding in both B_{12} and folic acid deficiencies. Patients with folic acid deficiency frequently present with generalized malnutrition. Neurologic examination in patients with B_{12} deficiency may reveal generalized weakness, ataxia, positive Romberg's and Babinski's signs, impaired vibratory and position sense, disturbed gait, and impaired urinary bladder function—all indicative of damage to the dorsal and lateral columns of the spinal cord.

LABORATORY EVALUATION

After a hypoproliferative anemia has been confirmed by decreased hematocrit and red blood cell count and an adequate elevation of the reticulocytes index, careful attention must be given to the red blood cell indices. If the mean corpuscular volume exceeds 100 cubic μ, a macrocytic hypoproliferative anemia exists. Macrocytic anemias not only result from defective DNA synthesis but also occur in reticulocytosis (e.g., in hemolytic anemia and hemorrhage), increased red blood cell surface area (e.g., target cells of hepatic disease and obstructive jaundice), and in hypoplastic, acquired sideroblastic and myelophthisic anemias. Evidence of a megaloblastic transformation in the peripheral blood is hypersegmentation of the nucleus of neutrophils. Megaloblastic anemia should be suspected if the average number of nuclear lobes in neutrophils is more than 3.4. Red cell morphology is characterized by significant anisocytosis and poikilocytosis, classically represented as macro-ovalocytes and teardrop forms (Fig. 57–3).

The bone marrow is hypercellular, with numerous mitotic figures and evidence of delayed nuclear maturation, because there is an inability to increase the amount of DNA necessary for cellular division, resulting in abnormally large cells. Many of these cells are destroyed before reaching the peripheral circulation because of associated cellular dysfunctions. The red cell precursors have a reticular nucleus that fails to condense and become pyknotic, even though cytoplasmic maturation progresses with normal hemoglobin production and many of these defective cells do not reach the circulating blood volume. This results in an inappropriately low reticulocyte count for the degree of anemia. Megakaryocytes are usually abnormally large, with an arrested nucleus. There are also giant band cells with horseshoe-shaped nuclei and other evidence of nuclear developmental disarray.

As a result of ineffective erythropoiesis, leukopoiesis, and thrombopoiesis, the amount of stainable bone marrow iron may be increased if the patient does not have concurrent iron deficiency anemia. In the serum, there are increased amounts of unconjugated bilirubin, lacate dehydrogenase, and iron, as well as increased saturation of transferrin.

The laboratory findings discussed so far are the same in both folic acid and B_{12} deficiencies. The precise determination of the etiologic mechanism of megaloblastic transformation lies in the actual measurement of serum levels of B_{12} and folate. Because of the biochemical relationship between B_{12} and the production of folate, the evaluation of all megaloblastic anemias should include determination of both serum B_{12} and serum folate levels.

The normal value of serum B_{12} ranges from 200 to 800 pg. per ml. However, measurement of serum B_{12} levels by radioimmunoassay method may at times reveal normal concentrations in the face of other evidence of overt B_{12} deficiency (megaloblastic transformation and low serum B_{12} levels by microbiologic assay). Apparently, radioimmunoassay measures not only vitamin B_{12} but also B_{12} analogues. B_{12} deficiency with its neurologic manifestation is now recognized as occurring in some instances without hematologic findings consistent with anemia or megaloblastosis. Low serum B_{12} levels with adequate tissue levels of

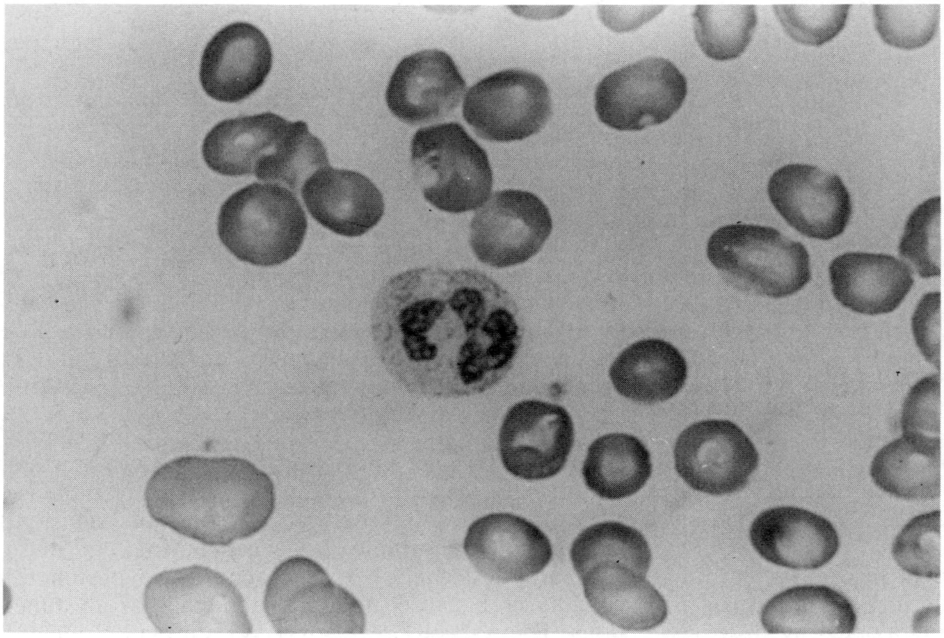

Figure 57–3. Macro-ovalocytosis and hypersegmented neutrophils of megaloblastic anemia caused by B_{12} deficiency.

B_{12} may be seen in folate deficiency, pregnancy, contraceptive use, and transcobalamin I deficiency.

Once vitamin B_{12} deficiency has been established, the *Schilling test* can be performed to determine whether the deficiency is due to a lack of intrinsic factor (pernicious anemia) or to an inability to bind the intrinsic factor-B_{12} complex at its ileal receptor site (inflammatory bowel disease or surgical absence of receptor sites). The test consists of two parts. The first part, which consists of the oral administration of radioactive B_{12} (after B_{12} storage sites have been saturated with nonradioactive B_{12}), should result in the urinary excretion of more than 5 per cent of radioactive B_{12} in the first 24 hours. Excretion of less than 5 per cent indicates either an intrinsic factor deficiency or an absence of disease of the ileal receptor sites that normally bind the intrinsic factor-B_{12} complex. In the second part of the test, the patient is given radioactive B_{12} bound to intrinsic factor to determine whether the defect is secondary to intrinsic factor deficiency. If the urinary excretion of radioactive B_{12} becomes normal in the second part, intrinsic factor deficiency exists. If the amount of radioactive B_{12} excreted remains low in the second part of the test, a malabsorption problem exists. In this case, a trial of antibiotics may be given if bacterial overgrowth is considered a possible cause; after the course of antibiotic, the Schilling test is repeated to determine whether radioactive B_{12} excretion returns to normal.

Radioimmunoassay is a reliable method of determining serum folate levels, which normally range from 6 to 20 ng. per ml. However, serum folate levels can be acutely altered by fluctuation in dietary folate, although tissue levels of folate are not acutely affected. Measurement of red blood cell folate is a more reliable means of determining tissue levels of folate. Serum folate levels generally fall within 12 to 14 days after dietary intake of folate has ceased, whereas red blood cell folate levels do not fall until 3 to 4 months after the cessation of dietary folate. The decline in red blood cell folate parallels the appearance of megaloblastic transformation. Although the serum folate determination is the more sensitive test for true folate deficiency, the microbiologic assay of red blood cell folate is by far the more specific test. A patient on antibiotics may have a false low red blood cell folate level on microbiologic assay.

TREATMENT OF MEGALOBLASTIC ANEMIA

Vitamin B_{12} Deficiency

The mainstay of treatment for vitamin B_{12} deficiency caused by a lack of intrinsic factor is chronic intramuscular injection of vitamin B_{12}. The body stores of B_{12} are first replenished by intramuscular injection of 100 μg. of B_{12} daily for 14 days or 1000 μg. every 7 days for 3 weeks. Maintenance therapy consisting of 100 μg of B_{12} monthly must be continued for life. Patients with B_{12} deficiency who present with neurologic symptoms are given the replenishing therapy, followed by 100 μg. of B_{12} intramuscularly every 2 weeks for at least 6 months and, finally, 100 μg. of B_{12} monthly for life. If a megaloblastic anemia of severe proportion is noted, therapy with both B_{12} and folate should ensue (after obtaining serum B_{12} and folate levels) until the laboratory results of serum B_{12} and folate levels become available.

Bone marrow response is usually complete in 2 days with the appearance of reticulocytosis. A normal red blood cell count is attained in approximately 1 to 1½ months. If this response does not occur, the diagnosis should be reconsidered, and the patient should be re-evaluated for concurrent iron deficiency anemia and/or folic acid deficiency.

Sodium retention and hypokalemia are potential side effects of B_{12} therapy. (They may also occur with therapy of folic acid deficiency.) These side effects could present problems in the patient with a compromised cardiovascular status secondary to the sudden increase in production of red cells (increased intravascular volume or K^+ update by newly formed cells). Occasionally, a patient has anemia that is severe enough to precipitate angina and congestive heart failure. In these circumstances, a small volume of packed red blood cells should be slowly given to alleviate only the patient's symptoms, thus avoiding further compromise of the cardiovascular status while awaiting the response to appropriate vitamin therapy.

If intestinal bacterial overgrowth is the cause of vitamin B_{12} deficiency, specific antibiotics are required to decrease the quantity of bacteria competing for B_{12}. During therapy, it may be necessary to provide parenteral sources of vitamin B_{12} until the bacterial overgrowth is eliminated or, as in inflammatory bowel diseases, until the acute phase of the inflammatory process subsides.

Folic Acid Deficiency

The aim of therapy in folic acid deficiency is to replace the depleted folate stores. A daily dose of 1 to 5 mg. of folic acid is given for as long as the deficiency persists. The response to therapy is similar to that seen in B_{12} deficiency, and the approach to cardiovascular problems is the same. Diets that are high in folate should be encouraged. Folic acid is almost always administered orally, even with malabsorption problems.

The Hemolytic Anemias

Hemolytic anemias are characterized by red cell destruction that overwhelms the compensatory response of a hyperproliferative bone marrow. This red cell destruction or hemolysis is premature, resulting in shortened red cell life span, and occurs at rates exceeding red cell production.

PATHOPHYSIOLOGY

Hemolysis, the process of red blood cell destruction, is the natural fate of each red cell after approximately 120 days in the peripheral circulation. This process is normally precipitated by a decrease in the aging red cell's ability to withstand the mechanical and chemical stresses of circulation (Fig. 57–4).

Normally, the rate of red cell destruction equals the rate of red cell production. The stimulus for red cell production is mediated through erythropoietin,

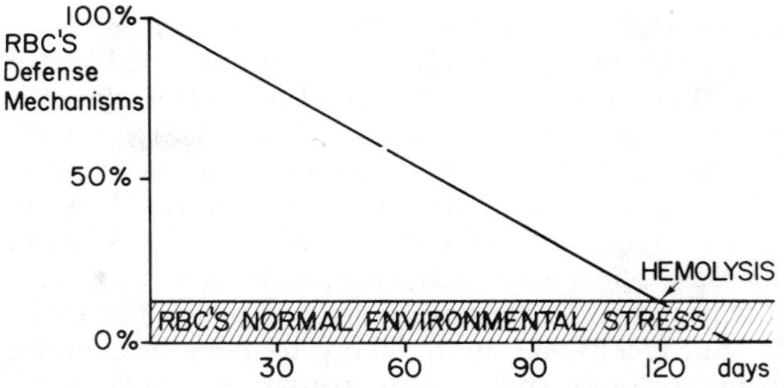

Figure 57–4. The fate of normal red blood cells exposed to normal red blood cell environment is hemolysis at approximately 120 days. (From Hobbs, J.: The hemolytic anemias. Am. Fam. Physician *20*(1):83, July, 1979. By permission.)

which increases in response to decreased oxygen transport. Over a period of 48 to 72 hours, the bone marrow can respond to the decreased oxygen transport caused by a hemolytic event by increasing erythropoietin stimulation that can double or triple the rate of erythropoiesis. The increased rate of erythropoiesis, which can be seen morphologically as erythroid hyperplasia, results in an increased number of immature red cells, such as reticulocytes and polychromatophilic and nucleated red blood cells, in the peripheral circulation. Approximately 1 per cent of the circulating red cell mass is produced daily, and, thus, the normal reticulocyte count is about 1 per cent. A rise in the number of reticulocytes—as would be the case in a hemolytic anemia—indicates an increase in the daily production of red cells. This response assumes that adequate substrates for red cell production, such as iron, vitamin B_{12}, and folate, are constantly available.

Red Blood Cell Metabolism in Hemolytic States

The biconcave shape of the red cell is characterized by a surface area that is greater than the volume it contains. This shape permits considerable cellular twisting and bending of the red cell thus permitting it to negotiate the microcirculation, where vessel diameter is at times smaller than the diameter of the nondeformed red cell.

The flexibility of the red cell is maintained by a properly functioning adenosine triphosphate (ATP) dependent red cell membrane. When this membrane does not function properly, there is increased sodium movement into the cell, resulting in increased intracellular volume that reduces the red cell's flexibility, making the cell more susceptible to entrapment, fragmentation, and/or osmotic lysis in the microcirculation.

Ninety per cent of ATP for red cell functions is obtained through the anaerobic metabolism of glucose to lactic acid, via the Embden-Meyerhof glycolytic pathway. About 5 to 10 per cent of glucose is metabolized through the hexosemonophosphate shunt (HMPS), where nicotinamide-adenine dinucleotide phosphate (NADP) in its reduced state (NADPH) is produced. NADPH maintains glutathione in its reduced state (GSH); in turn, GSH protects the globins and other intracellular proteins from irreversible oxidation. Therefore, any decrease in the quality or quantity of enzymes in the HMPS, as in glucose-6-phosphate dehydrogenase deficiency, results in red cells that have increased oxidant sensitivity. Such cells are more likely to hemolyze under normal or increased oxidant stress (Fig. 57–5).

Fate of Hemoglobin and Iron During Hemolysis

When excessive hemolysis occurs in extravascular sites (spleen, liver and other reticuloendothelial system sites), the unconjugated portion of bilirubin may increase, and urobilinogen may be found in the urine and feces.

Intravascular hemolysis results in the presence of free hemoglobin in the serum, which is rapidly bound by the serum protein haptoglobin. This hemoglobin-haptoglobin complex is then removed from circulation and metabolized in the liver. When hemolysis is rapid, free hemoglobin is bound to all of the available free haptoglobin, and the remaining free hemoglobin appears in the plasma and urine. Free plasma hemoglobin is oxidized further to methemoglobin, which can also bind to albumin.

The rate of reticulocytosis in hemolytic states is usually higher than that in hemorrhagic states. This difference occurs because hemorrhage causes a frank loss of iron from the body, whereas in hemolytic states the iron is available for reutilization in erythropoiesis.

ETIOLOGIC CLASSIFICATION OF THE HEMOLYTIC ANEMIAS

The hemolytic anemias can be grouped into two categories: those caused by inherent defects in the red cell (intrinsic defects) and those caused by increased environmental stress on the red cell (extrinsic defects). These categories are not absolute, because some inherent defects may cause premature hemolysis only when the red cells are exposed to increased environmental stress (Table 57–3).

Inherent Defects in the Red Cell

This group includes those hemolytic disorders in which the high susceptibility to hemolysis is due to a congenital or, occasionally, an acquired defect in the red cell. The inherent defects may result from alter-

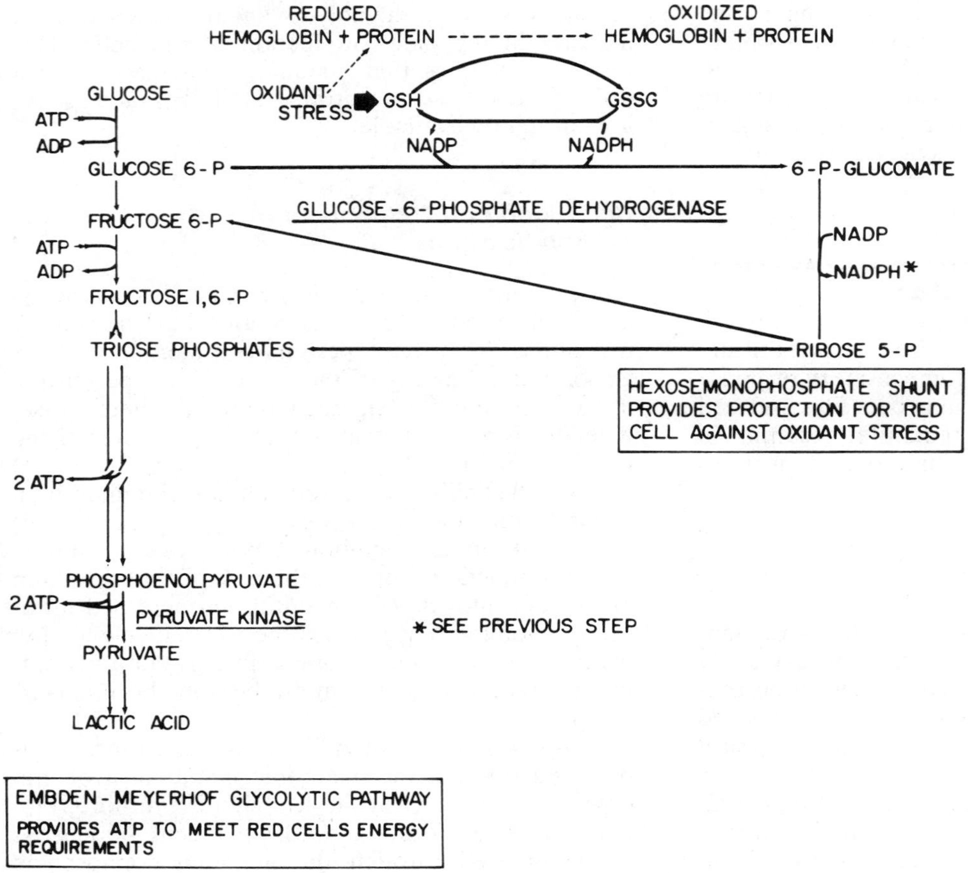

Figure 57–5. Normal red blood cell metabolism for energy production and protection against protein oxidation. (From Hobbs, J.: The hemolytic anemias. Am. Fam. Physician *20*(1):85, July, 1979. By permission.)

Table 57–3. CLASSIFICATION OF THE HEMOLYTIC ANEMIAS*

- I. Red Blood Cells' Inherent Defects
  - A. Membrane defects
    - 1. Hereditary spherocytosis
    - 2. Paroxysmal nocturnal hemoglobinuria
    - 3. Hereditary elliptocytosis
  - B. Enzyme deficiencies
    - 1. In the anaerobic pathway (e.g., pyruvate kinase deficiency)
    - 2. In the hexosemonophosphate shunt (e.g., G6PD deficiency, glutathione reductase deficiency)
  - C. Hemoglobinopathies
    - 1. Quantitative deficiencies (thalassemias)
    - 2. Qualitative deficiencies
      - a. Sickle cell anemia
      - b. Hemoglobin C disease, etc.
      - c. Unstable hemoglobins
  - D. Nutritional deficiencies (e.g., vitamin B_{12} folic acid) inducing ineffective erythropoiesis
- II. Red Blood Cells Exposed to Increased Environmental Stress
  - A. Immunohemolytic anemias
    - 1. Isoantibody formation and/or reaction
      - a. Transfunction with incompatible blood
      - b. Hemolytic disease of the newborn (erythroblastosis fetalis)
    - 2. Warm-antibody formation and reaction
      - a. Idiopathic
      - b. Hemopoietic cancer, autoimmune disease etc.
    - 3. Cold-antibody formation and reaction
      - a. Idiopathic
      - b. Mycoplasma, infectious mononucleosis
      - c. Paroxysmal cold hemoglobinuria
  - B. Chemical agents (e.g., phenacetin, lead)
  - C. Infectious agents (e.g., malaria, clostridial)
  - D. Physical factors
    - 1. Thermal injury
    - 2. Prosthetic heart valve
    - 3. External impact
    - 4. Increased circulatory resistance (disseminated intravascular coagulopathy and other microangiopathic anemias)
    - 5. Poisons (e.g., snake and brown recluse spider venoms)
  - E. Disease processes causing splenomegaly
  - F. Secondary to another disease process not involving immune reaction (e.g., liver disease)

*Adapted from Hobbs, J., and Wright, C. S.: Hemolytic anemias. Am. Fam. Physician, *22*:87, 1979.

ations in the red cell membrane, enzymes, or hemoglobin content (Fig. 57–6).

In *hereditary spherocytosis,* a membrane defect results in a reduced ratio of surface area to volume and in increased intracellular sodium and volume. This inherent defect is demonstrated in the laboratory as increased osmotic fragility. However, this defect is not the sole cause of hemolysis. Entrapment of the spherical cell in the spleen adds the critical environmental factor that causes hemolysis. This is demonstrated by the normal red cell life span in splenectomized patients with hereditary spherocytosis, although the inherent defects remain.

Another example of an inherent defect is an insufficient quantity and/or quality of the enzyme glucose-6-phosphate dehydrogenase (G6PD), which results in a cell that is more sensitive to oxidant stress (Fig. 57–7). There are two clinical variants of *G6PD deficiency,* the African and the Caucasian. The African variant does not present with hemolysis unless unusual oxidant stress (drugs, severe infection) is imposed. The Caucasian variant, however, presents with chronic hemolysis as a result of the normal physiologic oxidant stress of the body.

The type of hemoglobin is also an important consideration. In sickle cell disease, for example, red cells exposed to decreased oxygen content cause abnormal aggregation of hemoglobin, resulting in rigid cells that are prematurely destroyed by entrapment, fragmentation, and lysis in the microcirculation (Fig. 57–8).

Increased Red Cell Environmental Stress

Increased red cell environmental stresses that can cause premature hemolysis result from factors such as mechanical (e.g., turbulence or stagnation of flow), chemical (e.g., byproducts of metabolism drugs), and immunologic surveillance. An increase in these stresses or the addition of other stresses creates a more hostile environment in which the red cell must circulate (Fig. 57–9).

The immunohemolytic anemias are the most common forms of hemolytic anemia secondary to increased environmental stress. These anemias are characterized by the production of isoantibodies directed against red cells, as occur after blood transfusions with incompatible red cells or in maternal-fetal ABO or Rh incompatibility. Certain drugs are bound in various ways to the red cell membrane, resulting in antibody formation directed against the altered cell, complement fixation, and hemolysis.

Increased chemical stress can be caused by certain drugs that exert increased oxidant stress on the red cell. Red cells deficient in enzymes of the HMPS are highly sensitive to oxidant stress, but normal red cells are also potentially sensitive if sufficient dosage of an oxidant drug is given.

Physical trauma to the red cell can be caused by such factors as artificial heart valves and diseased arteriolar endothelium from disseminated intravas-

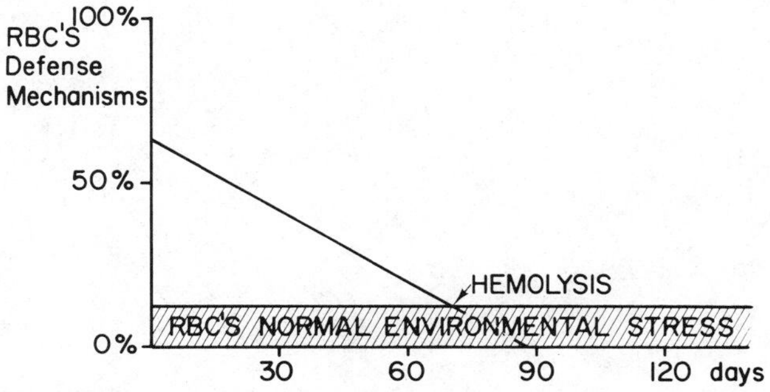

Figure 57–6. The fate of a red blood cell with an inherent membrane, enzyme, or hemoglobin defect exposed to a normal red blood cell environmental stress is premature hemolysis. (From Hobbs, J.: The hemolytic anemias. Am. Fam. Physician *20*(1):86, July, 1979. By permission.)

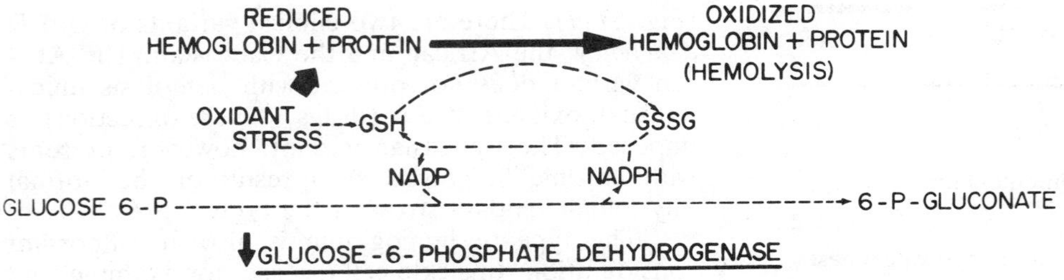

Figure 57–7. The altered metabolism in G6PD deficiency that results in decreased ability of red blood cells to withstand oxidant stress. (From Hobbs, J.: The hemolytic anemias. Am. Fam. Physician *20*(1):86, July 1979. By permission.)

cular coagulation, tumors, or diffuse atherosclerosis (Fig. 57–10). Direct disruption of the cell membrane may occur because of the lytic effects of clostridial toxins and the venoms of the brown recluse spider and certain snakes. Thermal injury can also alter red cell membrane function and result in hemolysis.

HISTORICAL EVALUATION

The patient's age at the onset of the hemolytic process helps in organizing a list of probable diagnoses. For example, a hemolytic process in a neonate may be due to maternal-fetal blood group incompatibility. A hemolytic process that begins in infancy and continues throughout life suggests an inherent (congenital) disorder. A hemolytic process beginning in adult life may indicate environmental stress on the red cell (e.g., drugs, infections, etc.). The patient's sex is an important factor in identifying the inherent defects that are genetically transmitted as sex-linked traits, such as G6PD deficiency. Ethnic background may point toward sickle cell disease in a patient of African descent or may implicate pyruvate kinase deficiency in a patient of Northern European descent.

The symptoms associated with the hemolytic event can be helpful diagnostic clues. For example, intermittent fever is characteristic of malaria, while bone pain is common in sickle cell disease. The history may reveal recent episodes of hemoglobinuria, suggesting intravascular hemolysis, or jaundice, indicating extravascular hemolysis. The severity of the presenting symptoms, such as shock, hypotension and prostration, may reflect the degree of intravascular hemolysis.

The patient's activity before the hemolytic event may include a history of long-distance running (march hemoglobinuria) or exposure to cold (paroxysmal cold hemoglobinuria). Hemoglobinuria noted after rising from sleep makes paroxysmal nocturnal hemoglobinuria an important consideration in the differential diagnosis. Other significant medical history may include placement of a prosthetic heart valve, transfusion, malignancy, or other information that may direct the clinician to the cause of the hemolytic process.

Careful attention must be given to the family history because the occurrence of similar hemolytic processes in other family members suggests not only a genetically transmitted inherent defect but also the pattern of that inheritance. By careful examination of the family history, the mendelian inheritance of

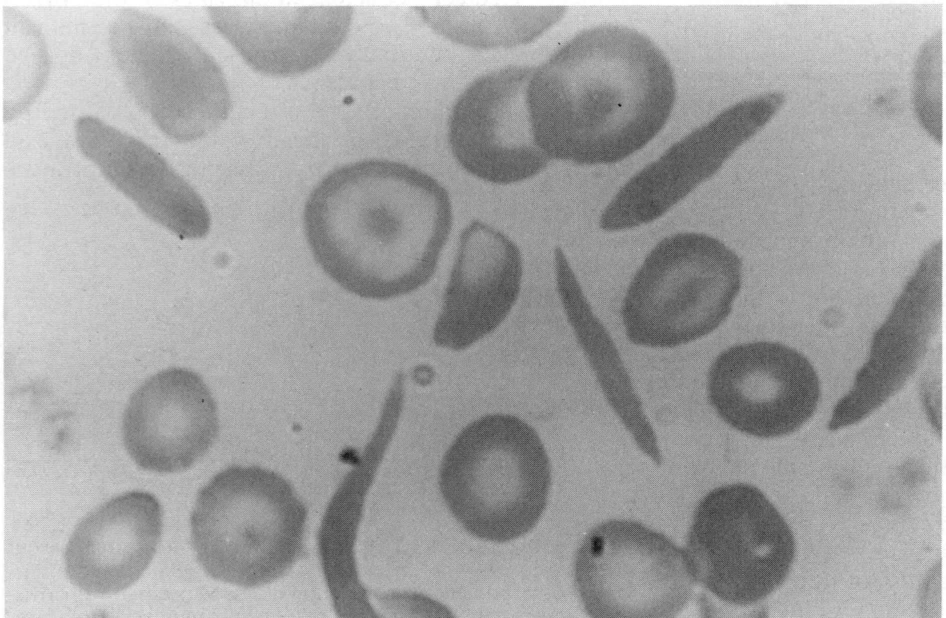

Figure 57–8. Distortion of the red blood cell shape caused by the hemoglobinopathy of sickle cell disease.

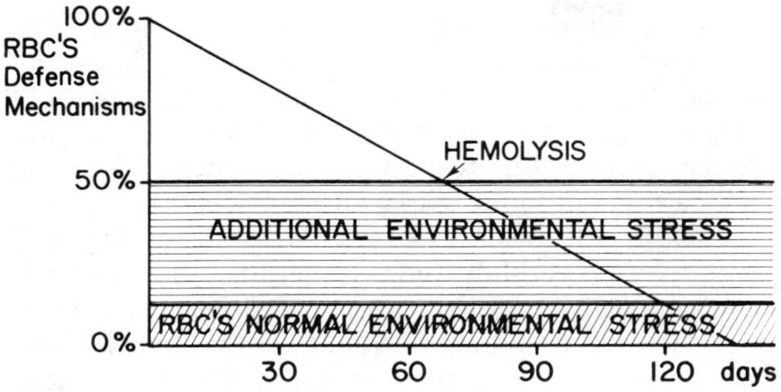

Figure 57–9. The fate of a normal red blood cell when exposed to abnormally high red blood cell (e.g., immunohemolytic anemia) environmental stress is premature hemolysis. (From Hobbs, J.: The hemolytic anemias. Am. Fam. Physician *20*(1):88, July 1979. By permission.)

sickle cell disease can be differentiated from the sex-linked inheritance of G6PD deficiency. A medical history of jaundice, splenomegaly, and biliary stones, plus a family history showing an autosomal-dominant inheritance pattern, places hereditary spherocytosis high on the list of diagnostic possibilities.

A complete drug history is of utmost importance when considering the oxidant injury of G6PD deficiency or the immunologic injury associated with drugs, such as quinidine and phenacetin. Occupational exposure to oxidant substances must also be investigated.

PHYSICAL EVALUATION

The severity of hemolysis may be detected by the presence of significant postural blood pressure and pulse changes or frank hypertension. Chronic hemolytic anemia may be associated with signs of high output heart failure. Special efforts should be made to detect scleral icterus or splenomegaly, which may represent evidence of increased red cell destruction. Evidence of compensatory mechanisms may be found, such as increased bone marrow volume in children with homozygous beta-thalassemia and in some patients with sickle cell anemia.

LABORATORY EVALUATION

The presence of anemia is established by the hematocrit and/or the hemoglobin level. (It should be noted that premature and accelerated hemolysis may occur without anemia if the rate of hemolysis does not exceed red cell production.) The smear may show polychromatophilic and nucleated red cells, signs of the bone marrow's attempt to compensate for the accelerated red cell destruction. Special stains reveal the presence of an elevated reticulocyte count, which represents increased production and earlier entry of red cells into the peripheral circulation (Plate XXX). Increased red cell production is documented by calculating the reticulocyte index. The bone marrow examination discloses erythroid hyperplasia. The quality and quantity of the bone marrow's compensatory response depends on the severity of the hemolytic process, the adequacy of red cell substrates, and the amount of erythropoietin.

Increased indirect bilirubin and the presence of urobilinogen in the urine and feces are associated with extravascular hemolysis. Intravascular hemolysis is characterized by hemoglobinemia, hemoglobinuria, depletion of free serum haptoglobin, methemoglobinemia, and methemalbuminemia. Prussian blue stain may reveal iron in the urine sediment (hemosiderinuria), representing chronic intravascular hemolysis.

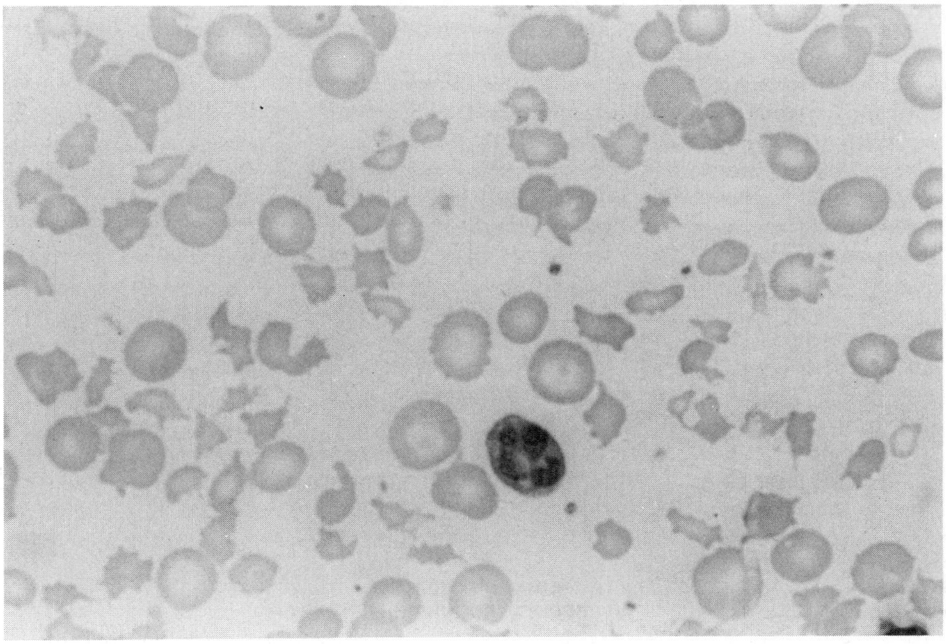

Figure 57–10. Microangiopathic hemolytic anemia.

Serum lactate dehydrogenase may also be moderately elevated but not as high as that seen in megaloblastic anemias.

Once a hemolytic anemia has been established, considerable etiologic information can be obtained merely by observing the red cell morphology on the peripheral smear. For example, an increased number of spherocytes is associated with hereditary spherocytosis or hemolysis resulting from factors such as immunologic injury or snake venom. Spur cells with large accumulations of cholesterol in their membranes are present in severe hepatocellular disease, while burr cells are found in uremic states. Target cells are noted in certain inherent defects, such as hemoglobin C disease and other hemoglobinopathies, Hb SS, and the thalassemias. Alteration in the red cell environment can also cause targeting, as in hepatocellular disease and obstructive jaundice. Sickle cells indicate the presence of either homozygous or heterozygous hemoglobin S. Fragmented red cells are associated with red cell disruption due to physical trauma, such as prosthetic heart valves, long-distance running, tumors, diffuse atherosclerosis, disseminated intravascular coagulation, or other microangiopathic disorders.

An early search for an immunologic basic is necessary because an immune mechanism is involved in a significant proportion of the acute hemolytic processes. Coombs' test differentiates immunologic and nonimmunologic causes of hemolytic anemia. The direct Coombs' test demonstrates the presence of incomplete antibodies on the red cell membrane, and the indirect Coombs' test reveals incomplete red cell antibodies free in the serum (Figs. 57–11 and 57–12).

Heinz bodies, which are precipitates of intracellular hemoglobin, are visible after special staining and are found in G6PD deficiency or excessive oxidant exposure (acute or chronic). Heinz bodies may also be present in a patient with unstable hemoglobins if the spleen has been removed or is nonfunctioning.

The detection of G6PD deficiency depends on the red cells' ability to reduce oxidant substances, such as methylene blue. Since G6PD-deficient red cells cannot reduce oxidants, the hemoglobin is oxidized to methemoglobin, which is identified by its dark brown color. However, this screening test and even a quantitative test are negative immediately after a hemolytic episode. The reason is that all of the enzyme-deficient cells are hemolyzed, leaving only younger cells with normal or near-normal enzyme activity. Hence, this test should be repeated several weeks after the hemolytic event.

Sickle cell disease and trait can be detected qualitatively by adding sodium metabisulfite (induces red blood cell deoxygenation) to a drop of blood to cause the sickling phenomenon. Since both sickle cell disease and trait give positive screening tests, these disorders must be differentiated by hemoglobin electrophoresis. Hemoglobin electrophoresis is also used in identifying hemoglobin C disease and in detecting elevation of Hb A_2 and Hb F in the thalassemia. Other laboratory procedures include test of red cell fragility in hypotonic saline to aid in the diagnosis of hereditary spherocytosis.

TREATMENT

Patients presenting with significant intravascular hemolysis require emergency measures. For those in shock, treatment is aimed at preventing end-organ damage by providing good circulatory support.

In the inherent disorders, since the defect cannot be removed, attempts should be made to minimize complications, such as infections, and to prevent the provocation of acute crisis. Patients with sickle cell anemia have an increased susceptibility to infectious agents, such as *Salmonella* and pneumococci because of decreased host defense, which is caused partly by autoinfarction of the spleen (hyposplenism). Similarly, susceptibility to infection is increased in hereditary spherocytosis patients who have been treated with splenectomy.

If the Coombs' test is positive, an immunohemolytic anemia is probable. The environmental substance eliciting the immune response must be identified and eliminated if possible. In drug-induced immunohemolytic anemia, discontinuing the drug may be all that is necessary. Excision of malignant tumors or treatment of a primary disease associated with an immunohemolytic anemia may bring about remission of hemolysis. If the acuteness and severity of the hemolytic process prevent identification and

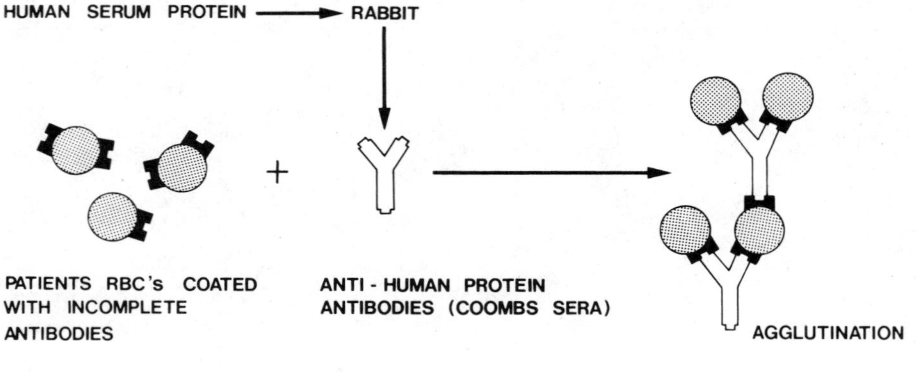

Figure 57–11. Direct Coombs' test detects the presence of antibodies attached to red blood cells. (From Hobbs, J.: The hemolytic anemias. Am. Fam. Physician *20*(1):93, July, 1979. By permission.)

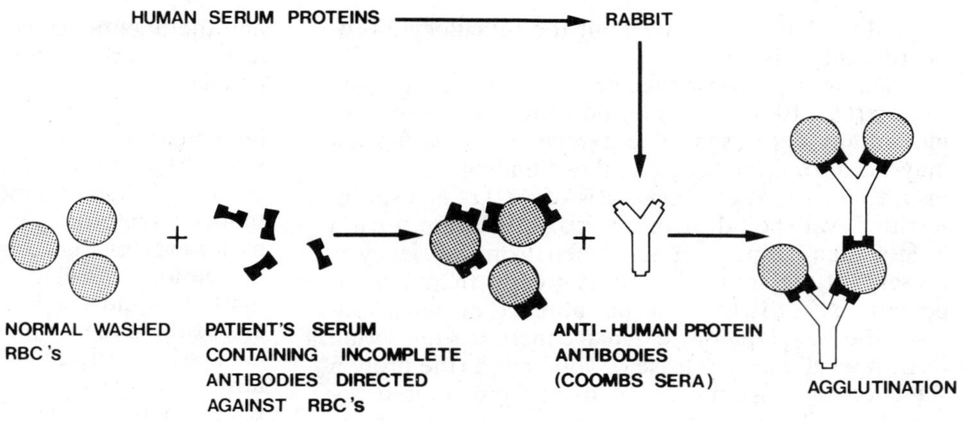

Figure 57–12. Indirect Coombs' test detects the presence of antibodies in serum that have the potential to attach to red blood cells. (From Hobbs, J.: The hemolytic anemias. Am. Fam. Physician *20*(1):93, July, 1979. By permission.)

removal of the offending agent, corticosteroid therapy is indicated. Blood transfusion may be required in emergency situations, but crossmatching and administration of donor blood are difficult because of numerous red cell antigens. If corticosteroids are ineffective, cause serious side effects, or are required in large dosage, splenectomy is indicated. Immunosuppressive therapy has been used with some success when corticosteroids and/or splenectomy have not stopped the hemolytic process.

Prevention of the hemolytic process is the mainstay of therapy in certain situations. For example, in erythroblastosis fetalis, Rh sensitization in a Rh-negative mother is prevented by giving Rh immunoglobulin after delivery of an Rh-positive infant. Patients with G6PD deficiency can prevent hemolytic anemia by avoiding over-the-counter products that contain oxidant substances.

Chronic Disease Anemias

The anemia of chronic disease (ACD) is a frequently encountered problem in clinical practice. Superficially, it resembles iron deficiency with microcytosis, hypochromia, hypoproliferation, and a low serum iron in many cases. Patients may have coexisting iron deficiency and ACD (as may be found in a patient with metastatic colon cancer who has secondary chronic GI bleeding).

ACD is found in association with chronic infections, other inflammatory processes, and cancer. The anemia is mild to moderate with a hemoglobin of 7 to 11 grams per deciliter. Early ACD is normochromic and normocytic, later progressing to microcytosis and hypochromia, but the mean corpuscular volume (MCV) is rarely less than 70 fl. Anemia of chronic disease is characterized by an anemia, an associated chronic disease, low serum iron, and adequate or, more often, increased macrophage iron stores. The mechanisms of ACD are multiple and include abnormal iron metabolism, shortened RBC survival, and reduced marrow production of RBCs. After an initial fall, the hemoglobin remains stable at 7 to 11 grams per dl. This occurs when RBC destruction and production become equal.

Iron reutilization is abnormal in these patients with ACD. When senescent ^{59}Fe-labeled RBCs are injected into patients with chronic disease, there is a marked reduction in the amount of ^{59}Fe incorporation, over time, into the RBC mass when compared with normal subjects. The mechanism is likely a defect in the release of monocyte/macrophage iron to circulating transferrin. It has been noted that there is a significant drop in the serum iron within hours after a stressful event, such as surgery or onset of an acute infection. When the underlying stressful event continues for 4 to 8 weeks, anemia develops. Often, this time frame appears to be accelerated when a previously ill patient is hospitalized, has his or her volume replenished with intravenous fluids, and is subjected to multiple phlebotomies for diagnostic purposes.

Reduced RBC production and shortened RBC survival are also factors in the pathogenesis of ACD. A functional hypothyroid state resulting from reduced T_4 to T_3 conversion may lead to decreased erythropoietin production thus resulting in a suboptimal marrow response to the anemia. RBC survival is shortened by approximately 30 per cent.

DIAGNOSIS

Typically in ACD, the hemoglobin is 7 to 11 grams per dl. with a mean corpuscular hemoglobin concentration (MCHC) less than 31 per cent and a mean corpuscular volume in the range of 70 to 80 fl. The red cell distribution width, a measure of variation in RBC size, is normal or slightly elevated. Examination of the peripheral smear reveals absence of marked poikilocytosis and markedly reduced or absent polychromatophilic macrocytes indicating reduced marrow production of RBCs. Abnormalities in the platelet count or morphology and white blood cells (WBCs) are variable and usually attributable to the underlying illness. The absolute reticulocyte count is normal to slightly elevated, but the reticulocyte production index is low.

The serum iron concentration is often reduced to less than 10 mg. per dl. and transferrin levels are moderately decreased. The percentage of saturation may be normal or low, but these findings alone are insufficient to make a diagnosis of ACD. The serum ferritin level should be measured. If a serum ferritin is less than 12 ng. per ml., then iron deficiency is present. If the serum ferritin is greater than 150 ng. per ml., ACD is likely in the absence of hepatocellular disease. Hepatocyte damage increases the serum ferritin level due to release of apoferritin (the protein shell, containing little or no iron) from injured hepatocytes. Between these values, uncertainty exists. An erythrocyte sedimentation rate is helpful when a bone marrow examination is not readily available. In general, the higher the erythrocyte sedimentation rate, the greater the degree of uncertainty in the accuracy of the serum ferritin as an indicator of marrow iron stores. For example, if the serum ferritin is 25 ng. per ml. and the erythrocyte sedimentation rate is markedly elevated (greater than 50 mm. per hr.), iron deficiency is still a major consideration.

Bone marrow examination is desirable in all questionable cases and may occasionally reveal an unsuspected underlying problem such as metastatic carcinoma or multiple myeloma. It is essential that the distinction between ACD and iron deficiency be made since the subsequent diagnostic and therapeutic modalities differ greatly. Unwarranted iron replacement is not only useless, it may delay further evaluation and is potentially harmful.

Therapy

The patient should be transfused only if symptomatic. Careful attention to the patient's volume status is warranted since patients with ACD have a normal volume and too rapid an infusion of RBCs may precipitate or aggravate congestive heart failure. Therapy with oral or intravenous iron, cobalt, androgenic steroids, or corticosteroids is not advisable. Therapy should be directed at the underlying disorder. The role of recombinant erythropoietin is yet to be defined.

General Approach to Lymphadenopathy

Primary care physicians are often confronted with patients who have lymph node enlargement of a localized or generalized nature. An *initial* historical and physical evaluation can separate most of those patients with benign or self-limiting problems from those who require a more comprehensive work-up. Knowledge of the anatomic distribution of the superficial lymphatics is important in making diagnostic and therapeutic decisions. Numerous anatomy, medical, and surgical texts provide this information in detail.

It is important to characterize lymph node enlargement by assessing the anatomic site(s) involved, size of the nodes and their characteristics (e.g., single or matted, hard, rubbery, fluctuant, inflamed, warm, tender, asymptomatic, etc.). As a general rule, lymph nodes greater than 2 cm. in diameter deserve further evaluation. Smaller nodes, if fixed, rock hard, or matted should also be investigated without delay. The age of the patient and the associated clinical problem also assists in determining the cause of lymphadenopathy. Under normal circumstances, the inguinal lymph nodes of both children and adults may be palpable without obvious cause. Children tend to have more pronounced lymphadenopathy as a response to infectious agents and a longer persistence of lymph node enlargement after the cessation of an infectious process. Lymph nodes that are enlarged, rubbery, firm, nontender, and matted together are consistent with lymphomas. Hard, fixed nodes should suggest the possibility of a metastatic cancerous process. Enlarged, tender nodes suggest an infectious process.

If a potential inflammatory or infectious cause is suspected, careful surveillance with treatment of the underlying cause is appropriate. If metastatic carcinoma is suspected, biopsy or fine-needle aspiration is indicated. This is particularly true if a hard scalene, cervical, or axillary mass is palpated.

Generalized lymph node enlargement may be encountered in chronic lymphocytic leukemia, non-Hodgkin's lymphoma, immunoblastic lymphadenopathy, collagen-vascular diseases, and drug reactions, such as to Dilantin. Infectious causes include AIDS, tuberculosis, secondary syphilis, infectious mononucleosis, toxoplasmosis, cytomegalovirus, histoplasmosis, brucellosis, infectious hepatitis, and coccidiodomycosis.

CERVICAL/AURICULAR LYMPHADENOPATHY

Acute, localized enlargement of cervical and auricular nodes associated with tenderness suggests pyogenic infection (e.g., staphylococcus, streptococcus, etc.), rubella, adenovirus, dental infection, trachoma, cat scratch fever, tularemia, or infectious mononucleosis. Chronic adenopathy can be caused by lymphoma, tuberculosis, or collagen-vascular diseases. Occasionally, syphilis may cause cervical/auricular lymph node enlargement.

Unilateral, painless cervical adenopathy in the absence of a thyroid mass suggests metastasis from an asymptomatic nasopharyngeal tumor, laryngeal cancer, or lymphoma. In this circumstance, examination of the upper aerodigestive tract is essential.

SUPRACLAVICULAR LYMPHADENOPATHY

Left-sided supraclavicular node enlargement is often related to intra-abdominal disease. Neoplasms of the stomach, kidney, ovary, and testes are potential causes of isolated left supraclavicular enlargement. Right supraclavicular masses are most often owing to lung cancer or esophageal cancer. Infections rarely cause supraclavicular adenopathy.

AXILLARY LYMPHADENOPATHY

Unilateral axillary nodes may be enlarged owing to inflammation from pyogenic infection in the arm and/or hand, cat scratch fever, or as a consequence of malignancy. Breast cancer, Hodgkin's and non-Hodgkin's lymphoma, melanoma, small cell lung cancer, and, occasionally, recurrent head and neck cancer are possible causes. In a female, unilateral axillary lymph node enlargement containing adenocarcinoma and with an occult primary should be treated as breast cancer.

EPITROCHLEAR LYMPHADENOPATHY

Epitrochlear nodes may be enlarged from chronic trauma or infection of the upper extremity or from secondary syphilis. While enlargement due to lymphoma is not rare, this is not often the primary site of the disease.

INGUINAL NODES

The inguinal nodes are located below the inguinal ligament and medial to the femoral artery. Due to recurrent or chronic infections of the lower extremities, the inguinal nodes are often easily palpable. Lymphogranuloma venereum, chancroid, herpes, pyogenic agents in the skin and other structures of the perineum, and syphilis are known infectious etiologies. If the prominent bilateral nodal enlargement or a unilateral node greater than 2 cm. in size is noted, histologic examination is warranted. Potential causes include malignancies of the lower extremity, cervix, vulva, anus, ovary, and penis.

OTHER CAUSES

Other causes of lymphadenopathy include serum sickness, sarcoidosis, connective tissue disease, dermatopathic lymphadenopathy, myeloproliferative syndromes, acute leukemias, lipid storage disease, angiofollicular lymph node hyperplasia, hyperthyroidism, and Addison's disease.

Overall, if an enlarged lymph node does not regress with appropriate therapy or under observation, then further investigation is indicated. It is important to note that nodal enlargement due to lymphoma may regress spontaneously. The best method for obtaining tissue—fine needle aspirate or excisional or wedge biopsies—depends on the clinical circumstances.

Screening for Hemostatic Defects

Screening for coagulopathies using a directed history coupled with selected coagulation studies should result in a rapid evaluation and initiation of treatment for all but the most complex bleeding problems. This process depends upon a recognition of important historical facts, adequate interpretation of routine coagulation studies, and, finally, a diagnostic approach to frequently occurring coagulation problems in the primary care setting.

SCREENING HISTORY

An appropriate history is the foundation of a coagulopathy work-up. The history should include past abnormal bleeding episodes, acquired diseases (such as uremia or cirrhosis likely to impair hemostasis), a drug history (consisting of coumadin, aspirin, or other agents capable of impairing coagulation, etc.), family history of abnormal bleeding, and past bleeding complications associated with surgery or dental extraction. A history of spontaneous bruises greater than 4 to 5 cm. bleeding 24 hours postsurgically or from dental extraction longer than 6 hours are of concern. Epistaxis provoked by aspirin is suggestive of thrombocytopenia or platelet dysfunction. Bleeding after surgery or lacerations on the second or third day suggest defects in the fibrin-clotting mechanism.

PHYSICAL EXAMINATION

If abnormal bleeding is suspected, the physical should include a search for excessive bruising around the venipuncture and intramuscular injection sites and spontaneous bruises particularly in low trauma areas, such as the trunk. Petechiae below a tourniquet or on the legs implies thrombocytopenia, platelet dysfunction, or increased capillary fragility. The physical should also include a search for signs of liver failure, such as jaundice, spider angiomas, palmar erythema, and splenomegaly.

INTERPRETATION OF SCREENING COAGULATION STUDIES

If the historical and/or physical evaluation suggests the presence of a coagulopathy, the integrity of the hemostatic system should be tested. The initial platelet plug is assessed by a platelet count, review of platelet morphology on the peripheral blood smear, a bleeding time to assess platelet function, and, occasionally, a bone marrow to assess megakaryocyte mass. The generation of thrombin and an intact fibrin clot can be measured using the activated partial thromboplastin time (APTT) that screens the intrinsic or contact activation of plasma. A protime (PT) screens for extrinsic or tissue factor activation of plasma. Finally, thrombinfibrinogen reactions and clot stability are measured by doing a thrombin time (TT) and clotting stability studies. Depending on the initial results of the screening laboratory, it may be necessary to evaluate for the presence of excessive fibrin degeneration products by a radioimmunologic assay or to test for the presence of procoagulation inhibitors by tube dilution studies in the APTT system.

The bleeding time measures the adequacy of platelets to form an initial platelet plug to a minimal incision in the skin. The test is influenced both by platelet number and platelet function. The Ivy Bleeding Time is the classic study and has a normal range of 3 to 11 minutes. Thrombocytopenia in the range of 100,000 or less produces variable prolongations of the bleeding time. Consumption thrombocytopenia, such as ITP, has better preservation of the bleeding time than marrow failure syndromes. The bleeding time also measures platelet overall function and will be prolonged in both congenital or acquired platelet dysfunction.

Platelet counts should range between 150,000 and 450,000 per microliter. If function is normal, platelet counts of 50,000 to 100,000 permit the performance of most surgical procedures without major risks of hemorrhage. At platelet counts of 20,000 to 50,000 per microliter, excessive bleeding occurs, and below 20,000, spontaneous bleeding without known trauma is common.

The APTT measures the integrity of intrinsic coagulation factors (XII, high molecular weight kininogen, XI, IX, and VIII) as well as the common pathway factors X, V, thrombin, and fibrinogen. Both common hemophilia diseases (factor VIII and IX deficiencies), as well as most patients with von Willebrand's disease, will have prolonged APTT and normal PT values. Patients receiving heparin and coumadin, patients with liver failure, and patients with disseminated intravascular coagulation (DIC) have both APTT and PT prolonged. An unexpected isolated APTT should be repeated to rule out artifactual prolongation. In patients with systemic lupus erythematous, taking certain drugs and, as an isolated finding, a prolonged APTT and normal PT may indicate the presence of the lupus anticoagulant, which is associated with thrombosis not bleeding.

The extrinsic activation pathway factors VII, X, and V are best measured with the PT of which factor VII is uniquely measured in the system. A prolonged PT and normal APTT and TT mean factor VII deficiency. Most commonly, both PT and APTT are prolonged meaning multiple deficiencies of clotting factors, such as DIC or liver failure.

The TT measures thrombin-fibrinogen interaction. It is prolonged in the presence of increased antithrombin activity (heparin), high levels of fibrin degeneration products, and severe hypofibrinogemia or dysfibrinogemia.

Inhibitor screens, which may be done in either the PT or APTT systems, are useful to separate an absolute clotting deficiency from the presence of an immune anticoagulant, such as a factor VIII antibody. In both the APTT-PT systems, values are normal until factor levels fall below 30 per cent. Thus, a 1:1 dilution of normal plasma to patient's plasma will give normal values if an absolute deficiency exists. However, a circulatory anticoagulant in a patient's plasma will inactivate the normal plasma coagulation factor, and the PT or APTT will not return to normal.

CLINICAL PATTERNS OF COAGULATION ABNORMALITIES

An isolated, prolonged bleeding time signifies moderate to severe thrombocytopenia or platelet dysfunction. If the platelet count is greater than 100,000 then the presence of uremia or drug ingestion affecting platelets should be evaluated. Otherwise, a congenital defect exists and will need a specialized coagulation center's attention. In patients with uremia who are bleeding or require an invasive procedure, a number of methods exist to normalize the bleeding time. Aggressive dialysis is the best if time permits. Otherwise, desmopressin or cryoprecipate can correct the abnormality in selected patients. If aspirin has caused the defect, it is present for the lifespan of the affected platelets, and elective surgery should be delayed 7 to 10 days.

In patients whose APTT is the only abnormal study, the first study should be an inhibitor screen. If an inhibitor is present and the patient is bleeding, prompt transfer to a center where expertise in coagulation, immunology, and blood banking exist should be made. In a patient with a negative inhibitor screen, factor VIII and IX deficiencies are the most common causes. If bleeding exists and the ability to obtain coagulation factors is not available, fresh frozen plasma may stabilize patients prior to transport to more specialized centers.

If both the bleeding time and APTT are prolonged, this is almost diagnostic for von Willebrand's disease. This can be confirmed by an immunologic assay for von Willebrand's factor or a ristocetin aggregation study. If von Willebrand's disease is confirmed, cryoprecipitate is the preparation of choice to treat bleeding.

Factor VII deficiency is the only coagulation deficiency that produces isolated prolongation of the protime. If abnormal bleeding is present, FFP will correct the protime. Occasionally, patients taking coumadin will have only the PT prolonged, but a drug history will reveal this etiology.

Prolongation of both the PT and APTT with normal platelet count and bleeding time is consistent with liver failure, vitamin K deficiency, heparin or coumadin usage. A careful history and physical will help to identify these entities. Heparin will prolong the TT, but coumadin will not. Severe hypofibrinogenemia will prolong the PT, APTT, and thrombin time.

Finally, the most common coagulation problem is one of multiple defects: prolongation of the PT, APTT, and lowered platelet count. The usual differentiation is between DIC and liver failure with cirrhosis. In cirrhosis, the PT and APTT can be prolonged owing to failure of the production of various coagulation factors. Thrombocytopenia occurs in the setting of portal hypertension and hypersplenism. Fibrin degradation products are primarily cleared by the liver and, in the setting of severe liver dysfunction, are often evaluated. Thus, both DIC and hepatic failure often have the same coagulation profile and, if fever is present, may be difficult to distinguish clinically. Two aids in differentiation are reviewing the peripheral blood smear for schistocytes and obtaining a factor VIII level. In DIC, fragmentation of red cells (schistocytes) occurs from traumatic shearing from fibrin strands in small vessels. This is lacking in liver failure. Likewise DIC consumes all coagulation factors including factor VIII. In liver failure, factor VIII levels will be normal since it is produced in endothelial cells unlike all other coagulation factors that come from hepatocytes.

The final point to cover is screening for abnormalities when the PT, APTT, bleeding time, and platelet count are all normal. In reality, the chance of missing a significant bleeding disorder is small but not absolute. Further testing should be directed by the history. First, if the patient's history suggests mucosal bleeding, then suspect platelet dysfunction. The bleeding time should be repeated and, if still normal, consider doing either platelet aggregation studies or an aspirin tolerance test. If no surgery is imminent, then aspirin will markedly increase the bleeding time of patients with mild platelet dysfunction. However, since the effect of aspirin lasts 5 to 7 days, this study is not safe preoperatively and more difficult platelet aggregation studies must be done in the setting of urgent surgery.

If the patient's history suggests increased bleeding after trauma or surgery, then levels of factor VIII and IX should be done. An occasional patient with mild hemophilia A or B will have a normal APTT. In addition, a clot stability test will detect the rare XIII deficiency.

Treatment With Blood Products

The use of blood and blood components has increased dramatically over the last 3 decades. For example, blood transfusions increased in the United States from 2.3 million units in 1978 to 8.2 million units in 1983 and fresh frozen plasma from 77 million units to 120 million units in the same time period. This intolerable demand for blood products coupled with the public's increasing concern about transfusional complications, such as HIV infection, behooves physicians to have clear-cut guidelines for usage of blood products in their patients. These transfusional blood products include red cell preparations, platelets, white cells, and coagulation factors.

RED BLOOD CELL TRANSFUSIONS

The indications for RBC transfusions vary with the rate of red cell mass loss. In patients with slowly developing anemias, a number of compensating developments occur that diminish symptoms and decrease the risks associated with a reduced number of circulating red cells. These compensatory factors include shifts in the oxygen dissociation curve in order to increase oxygen tissue delivery and increase cardiac output and plasma volume to maintain effective circulating volume. The patient with the slowly developing anemia who is asymptomatic should be rapidly evaluated for treatable causes and, in almost all cases, transfused only if symptoms are present as opposed to transfusions based on a specific hemoglobin level. Specific symptoms suggesting the need for transfusion (Table 57–4) include signs of cardiac or cerebral decompensation, extreme age, or the rare need to rapidly correct the anemia for other medical needs, such as radiation therapy or impending surgery.

RED BLOOD CELL TRANSFUSION PREPARATIONS

Red blood cell preparations include whole blood, packed red cells, frozen blood, leukocyte-depleted red cells, and irradiated blood.

Whole blood is a unit of blood with no component removed, although depending on storage time some loss of platelet function may occur and factor VIII and factor V levels may decrease. Because of the volume of a whole blood transfusion unit, its use is only indicated for active bleeding with signs of volume depletion.

Packed red blood cell transfusion units are prepared from fresh blood by removing plasma and platelet components, reducing the volume to approximately 250 cc. This is the preparation of choice for chronic or acute anemia in the absence of signs of significant uncompensated volume depletion and significant active bleeding. There are, however, an appreciable number of platelets, white cells, and some plasma components in packed red blood cells that may precipitate febrile or allergic reactions. In addition, the hematocrit of packed cells is about 70 per cent and may aggravate symptoms in patients with hyperviscosity syndromes.

Frozen blood is washed repeatedly and stored at −70°C. It has a long shelf life but is expensive and requires special refrigeration equipment. It is ideal

Table 57–4. INDICATIONS FOR RED BLOOD CELL TRANSFUSION

Type of Anemia	Factors Assessed	Indicators for Transfusion	Number of Units Needed	Comments
Acute	Orthostatic changes in blood pressure	Significant orthostatic blood pressure decrease or pulse increase	No set number; reverse orthostatic blood pressure and pulse changes, and blood loss should be matched	Remember even if colloids are administered, the hemoglobin or hematocrit will not readjust for blood loss faster than 24 hours
	Volume of blood loss	Estimated acute loss of 20 per cent of blood volume		
	Hazard of continued blood loss	High probability of continued blood loss		
Chronic	Cardiac function	Angina pectoris	Generally one unit will increase the average-sized adult hemoglobin level 102 grams per cent. Rarely should patient be transferred above Hgb 10 grams per cent.	Patients with chronic anemias have increased plasma volumes and rapid transfusion may precipitate congestive heart failure
	Cerebral function	Ischemic EDG changes		
	Socioeconomic factors	High output congestive heart failure		
	Age and other diseases			
		Transient ischemic attacks		
	Other medical factors			
		Organic brain syndrome		
		Geriatric age with other medical problems		
		Unable to remain sedentary		
		Need for surgery, radiation therapy, chemotherapy, etc.		

for autotransfusion for elective surgery in patients with rare blood types or religious convictions that preclude the use of donor blood. In addition, in this era of fear of HIV infections the use of autotransfusion has dramatically risen.

Leukocyte-depleted blood can be prepared in a number of ways. The most effective is the use of online filters that remove 99 per cent of white cells present. A more expensive and time-consuming method is repetitive washing or use of frozen blood. Leukocyte-depleted blood is indicated for patients with febrile reactions who have been transfused several times, and premature infants under 1000 grams (to avoid cytomegalovirus infections).

Irradiated blood is given to patients who are profoundly immunosuppressed to avoid graft versus host disease from engraftment of donor lymphocytes. This group includes congenital combined immune deficiency, bone marrow transplant patients, very small premature infants, and certain patients receiving very intensive chemotherapy.

RED CELL TRANSFUSION PROBLEMS

A number of potential dangers exist from red cell transfusions. Some of the more serious include bacterial contamination, volume overload, hepatitis, HIV infections, febrile reactions, and the rare true hemolytic reactions. Most are avoidable by proper blood preparation or decision for usage. Viral infections—including hepatitis B, non-A and non-B hepatitis, cytomegalic virus, and HIV-I and III virus—pose significant risks. Blood products are routinely screened for the HIV-III virus and, with current technology, pose approximately a 1:3 million transfusion risk to recipients. Unfortunately, in non-A and non-B hepatitis, the major viral risk will occur in 1 out of 10 transfusions in the United States with urban areas having a much higher incidence.

The real fear of most physicians about transfusions is of a transfusion reaction. Fortunately, the true hemolytic reaction is rare and occurs in less than 1 in 10,000 units transfused. On the other hand, febrile reactions are common and occur in 3 per cent of all transfused units. Rapid distinguishment (Table 57–5) is important. Hemolytic reactions are rapid in the outset, associated with vital organ dysfunction, hemoglobulinuria, and hemoglobinemia. All hospital blood banks have established protocols for manage-

Table 57–5. TRANSFUSION REACTIONS

	Hemolytic	Leukoagglutinin
Incidence	Rare (1 in 10,000 transfusions)	Common (3 per cent of all transfusions)
Classic clinical features	Arm pain, chest pain, back pain, shock, diaphoresis; may be only chills and fever	Chills and fever
Time of symptoms	Early in transfusion	Late in transfusion
Plasma/urine	Red (brown); free hemoglobin	Normal
Fatality	High fatality	Almost never fatal

ment of suspected hemolytic reactions. General principles include immediate cessation of blood infusion, rechecking patient and blood unit identification, drawing blood samples for recrossmatch, plasma-free hemoglobin, and free haptoglobin. The unit of blood, blood samples, and urine sample are then returned to the blood bank for evaluation. Meanwhile, a hematocrit tube is spun to examine the plasma for a reddish-brown tinge suggestive of free hemoglobulin. Patients who exhibit a high-risk profile for hemolytic reactions should have colloids and mannitol administered to produce high urine output in order to prevent renal damage from hemoglobinuria. Vital signs should be monitored and supported if necessary. Further transfusions, if possible, should be delayed until the patient is stable or laboratory results fail to support the presence of a hemolytic transfusion. If the patient is actively bleeding and blood must be given, all blood must be recrossmatched and cleared by the blood bank as being compatible.

Febrile reactions or leukoagglutinin reactions, while troublesome, represent no major risk to the patient's life. Once a patient has had one febrile reaction there is a 10 per cent risk that subsequent units will provoke similar reactions. In patients with a pattern of repeated febrile reactions, the use of leukocyte filters to deplete white cells is the most effective management technique; modern filters remove 99.9 per cent of all white cells. For patients with minor febrile reactions, prophylaxis with acetaminophen 650 mg. and diphenhydramine 50 mg. orally is effective.

PLATELET TRANSFUSIONS

Platelet transfusions are given for thrombocytopenic bleeding or as prophylaxis for patients with platelet counts less than 20,000 per microliter whose thrombocytopenia is expected to resolve. Generally, no significant risk of bleeding exists when the platelet count is greater than 50,000 unless platelet dysfunction coexists. As the platelet count falls progressively from 50,000 to 20,000, the risk of bleeding from minimal vascular trauma increases. When the platelet count is less than 20,000 per microliter, then spontaneous bleeding is frequent. Certain factors increase the risk of bleeding at any given platelet level. These include the presence of fever, older age, rapid falls in platelet counts, presence of primary marrow disorders, and exogenous factors, such as drugs or uremia, that adversely affect platelet function.

A unit of platelets is obtained from one unit of fresh whole blood by centrifugation by both RBCs and WBCs plus 10 cc. of plasma. Because of RBC contamination, platelets are given with ABO Rh matching. When forced to give platelets from a RH+ donor to a Rh− woman of child-bearing age, RhoGAM should be given. If platelet allosensituation is suspected, the HLA-matched single donor platelets should be given. If a patient is a possible bone marrow recipient, platelets should not be given from potential donors. If platelets are given to thrombocytopenic patients with bone marrow failure, a rise of 10,000 per ml. can be expected for each unit given. When active bleeding or fever exists, suboptimal rises in counts occur.

PLASMA COMPONENT THERAPY

The use of single donor fresh frozen plasma or cryoprecipitate has risen steadily over the last 2 decades. Fresh frozen plasma contains all clotting factors but because of its volume it is not the preparation of choice for the common congenital coagulation defects. On the other hand, cryoprecipitate contains only factors VIII, von Willebrand's factor, fibrinogen, and antithrombus VII. The indications for fresh frozen plasma include correction of warfarin overdosage, treatment of liver failure coagulopathy, treatment of thrombotic thrombocytopenia purpura, replacement in plasma-exchange procedures, and reversal of documented coagulopathy in the setting of massive blood transfusion. Cryoprecipitate is the preparation of choice for deficiencies of von Willebrand's factor, fibrinogen, and mild factor VIII deficiency. In addition, when given in large amounts (10 to 15 units), cryoprecipitate may overcome the platelet defect in uremia.

GRANULOCYTE TRANSFUSIONS

Granulocyte transfusions should be reserved for infected, severely neutropenic (less than 500 absolute neutrophils) patients. ABO matching is required, and HLA matching is preferred. Febrile reactions are common and occasional pulmonary leukoagglutinin reactions occur. If granulocyte transfusions are given, the rise in neutrophil counts is very transient lasting less than 24 hours. If transfusions are begun, then they must be continued until the patient is able to maintain an absolute granulocyte count of 500 or greater.

Multiple Myeloma

Multiple myeloma is an incurable malignancy in which a clone of neoplastic plasma cells infiltrates the bone marrow. In most patients, a monoclonal immunoglobulin is present in the serum. This is detected on the serum protein electrophoresis as a narrow band in the beta or gamma region.

These proteins are most often IgG or IgA, with occasional patients having IgM, IgD, or IgE myeloma. Complete immunoglobulin (Ig) is produced in most patients. There may be overproduction of light chains that, in the absence of renal failure, are excreted in the urine as Bence Jones protein. Thirty per cent of cases exhibit only light chain production in which case the serum protein electrophoresis will show hypogammaglobulinemia but no monoclonal protein. Light chains, particularly lambda chains, may be deposited in the tissues as amyloid or may lead to progressive renal insufficiency via deposition in the kidney with subsequent renal injury. Myeloma cells can produce osteoclast activating factor, which causes hypercalcemia via osteoclast activation and pathologic bone resorption and destruction. Consequences of progressive accumulation of myeloma cells include reduced humoral immunity due to hypogammaglobulinemia, pathologic fractures, hypercalcemia, progressive anemia, neutropenia, thrombocytopenia, and renal failure.

CLINICAL FEATURES

Most patients are over 50 years of age. Patients may come to medical attention with bone pain, often due to pathologic fractures, infections, renal insufficiency, symptoms of hypercalcemia or anemia, and, occasionally, symptoms of hyperviscosity syndrome. Hyperviscosity is particularly frequent in cases with IgM production, including Waldenstrom's macroglobulinemia, and with IgA, which polymerizes. Certain subtypes of IgG may also cause hyperviscosity syndrome. These patients exhibit mucosal bleeding, central nervous system symptoms, including altered mental status, convulsions, papilledema, and congestive heart failure secondary to increased blood volume.

Spinal cord compression and cauda equina syndrome may occur secondary to cord compression by extramedullary masses of myeloma cells. Multiple myeloma may cause a peripheral neuropathy secondary to amyloidosis.

LABORATORY AND RADIOGRAPHIC FEATURES

Abnormalities in the serum and urine proteins are as noted previously. A polyclonal increase in gammaglobulin on serum protein electrophoresis virtually rules out a diagnosis of multiple myeloma. Almost all patients have a normochromic, normocytic anemia. The WBC count may be normal but, more often, is reduced. Platelets are usually low except in early cases. The erythrocyte sedimentation rate is elevated. Serum uric acid may be elevated. The serum beta-2 macroglobulin is often elevated. In the absence of renal disease, this generally reflects overall tumor burden and can be serially measured to assess for response to therapy or predict relapse or progression. Rouleaux, and occasionally plasma cells, may be seen on the peripheral blood smear. Late, undiagnosed patients may present with large numbers of circulating plasma cells (plasma cell leukemia).

The bone marrow may be normal if involvement is patchy. In these cases, another site(s) should be sampled with both aspiration and biopsy. Increased numbers of plasma cells are diagnostic if these occur in sheets or if many bizarre cells are present with varying size, nucleoli, or are multinucleated. It is important to note that many chronic inflammatory and infectious processes stimulate production of increased numbers of plasma cells. However, these appear normal morphologically and are single rather than forming sheets. An important clue may be found on routine automated serum chemistry profiles in that a large gap between the total protein and albumin is noted. If the difference between the total protein and albumin exceeds 4.5 grams, a serum protein electrophoresis and appropriate urine studies are indicated.

Radiographic findings include osteoporosis, compression fractures, and lytic or punched out lesions in marrow-containing bones. These include the proximal long bones, central skeleton, and skull. Only rarely are osteoblastic or sclerotic changes noted. For this reason, bone scans are a poor diagnostic tool in assessing myeloma patients.

DIAGNOSIS AND STAGING

Typical bone marrow findings allow a diagnosis of multiple myeloma to be made. In their absence, one should assay for a monoclonal serum protein or Bence-Jones proteinuria. A skeletal radiographic survey searching for lytic lesions should be requested. Hypercalcemia and renal insufficiency, without other obvious cause, are suggestive but not diagnostic, as is the detection of amyloidosis. Soft tissue masses, often in the upper airway, and masses adjacent to marrow-containing bones can occur. On biopsy, these will show only plasma cells. The disease may be more likely to present in this fashion in younger patients.

If no diagnosis can be made, the patient is serially followed for the development of typical findings or rising monoclonal protein. Patients with benign monoclonal gammopathy will not have a progressive increase in their monoclonal protein.

THERAPY

All patients should be instructed to maintain an intake of 3 liters of fluid per day and remain as active as possible. Infection should be *promptly* evaluated and treated. For a myeloma patient with infection, the physician should be more liberal than usual in electing to hospitalize for intravenous hydration and parenteral antibiotic therapy.

Hypercalcemia should be treated with intravenous saline, furosemide steroids, and treatment of the underlying disease. Calcitonin or mithramycin may sometimes be required to control hypercalcemia. Radiation therapy to bone lesions is often necessary to control severe pain. *Impending* pathologic fractures of the weight-bearing bones should be pinned.

Chemotherapy is initiated with an alkylating

agent, usually intermittent oral doses of melphalan and prednisone. High-dose steroids alone are often successful if cytoxic drug therapy must be delayed or withheld. High-dose prednisone may be given on alternate days with reduction of steroid-induced complications. Cyclophosphamide is often effective when melphalan has not yielded a response. Infusions of vincristine and doxorubicin plus high-dose steroids are often used in patients who present with extensive disease or who have relapsed from prior therapy. Remissions occur with patients appearing stable for weeks or months off therapy. At the time of relapse, the initial therapy may be reinstituted with success in many patients. Good supportive care and adequate hydration are essential in minimizing morbidity and for prolonging patient survival in this disease.

Hodgkin's and Non-Hodgkin's Lymphoma

Patients with Hodgkin's disease are largely curable. Staging of the disease is based on the Ann Arbor classification scheme. Patients with localized disease are most often treated initially with radiation therapy. Many can be salvaged, after relapse, with combination chemotherapy regimens. Age, unfavorable histology, and extensive disease class adversely effect prognosis. The staging work-up and treatment for Hodgkin's disease is best supervised by the hematologist or medical oncologist.

Non-Hodgkin's lymphomas are classified by several different schemes. Overall, it is useful to divide the patients into indolent, intermediate, and high-grade lymphomas. Indolent lymphomas are, at present, incurable although progression to death usually takes years. Treatment with an alkylating agent and corticosteroids are offered to symptomatic patients. Intermediate and high-grade lymphomas are curable—in many cases, with combination chemotherapy and/or radiotherapy, where appropriate. Untreated or relapsing patients progress more rapidly than patients with less aggressive types of lymphoma. HTLV infection is known to be associated with certain types of aggressive lymphomas. This includes HTLV-I and HTLV-III (HIV) infected patients.

The role of the primary care physician is to recognize patients with lymphoma as early as possible and proceed with lymph node or other tissue biopsy in suspected cases. Consultation should be obtained when the diagnosis is made, and the results of diagnostic studies, including pathologic specimens, should be forwarded to the referral center. This facilitates initial evaluation and allows further review of the pathologic material. The latter is important since there may be disagreement among reviewers as to the exact classification. Correct classification is essential to the selection of therapy.

Additionally, many patients will be treated at centers remote from their homes. In these cases, the primary physician will often be called upon to monitor progress, supply posttreatment laboratory studies, and recognize and promptly treat sequelae of therapy. In the neutropenic patient, it is particularly important to recognize infection, drug reactions, symptomatic anemia, and bleeding secondary to thrombocytopenia. Patients in remission will also need periodic follow-up for evidence of disease recurrence.

Acute Lymphocytic Leukemia

Acute lymphocytic leukemia (ALL) is the most common malignant disease in childhood. Peak incidence is between 2 and 10 years of age with a second peak beginning in middle age. ALL results from the development of a malignant clone of early lymphoid precursors that has undergone malignant transformation in the early stages of processing from B to T lymphocytes. Most ALL appear to be of B-cell lineage.

Immune marker studies using monoclonal antibodies allow further classification of ALL patients. For example, CD-10 (CALLA or common ALL antigen) is present in common type ALL. These studies allow identification of early and differentitated B and T cells. This has prognostic significance and, with assessment of other prognostic factors, will effect the choice of therapy.

Histochemical staining of ALL cells is also done to help confirm lymphoid origin. Cytogenetic studies often reveal aneuploidy. Certain chromosomal abnormalities are associated with specific clinical syndromes and may, therefore, help predict prognosis.

As soon as a diagnosis of ALL is made or suspected, the patient should be referred to a center capable of providing the necessary diagnostic and support services. These patients require combination chemotherapy with close observation during induction therapy and often require frequent access to blood products not readily available in all hospitals.

CLINICAL FEATURES

The onset of ALL is almost always acute with a prodromal period of days or weeks. Malaise, anorexia, weight loss, and lethargy may occur. Petechiae or purpura secondary to thrombocytopenia may be seen. Low-grade fever may be present. High fever mandates a search for underlying infection. Bone and joint pain is particularly common in younger patients. Superficial lymph node enlargement, splenomegaly, and hepatomegaly are noted in many, but not all, cases. Focal neurologic signs and symptoms are evidence that leukemic meningitis may be present at the time of initial presentation. Problems related to defects in cellular or humoral immunity and autoimmune phenomenon are not common features of ALL.

LABORATORY FEATURES

A normochromic/normocytic anemia without poikilocytosis is usually present. Thrombocytopenia and a reduced absolute neutrophil count are present at diagnosis in most patients. The leukocyte count is usually elevated but may be normal or low. The bone marrow is hypercellular with marked infiltration by lymphoblasts. Normal marrow elements are usually strikingly reduced.

The circulating lymphoblasts are classified by their morphologic features. This is done according to criteria established by the French-American-British Co-operative Group. These classification criteria rely on the size of the blasts, features of the nuclear chromatin, presence or absence of nucleoli, vacuoles, and amount and characteristics of the cytoplasm.

A lumbar puncture is routinely obtained to rule out leukemic meningitis. A chest film is obtained in all cases. This is usually normal but may reveal a mediastinal mass in patients with acute T-cell lymphoblastic leukemia. The serum lactate dehydrogenase, uric acid, and plasma fibrinogen levels may be elevated at diagnosis or in relapse.

DIAGNOSIS

As discussed above, the complete diagnosis with subset classification requires a comprehensive evaluation by the hematologist with the support of the laboratory. At presentation to the primary care physician, other diagnoses may deserve consideration. Cytopenias may occur due to aplastic anemia or infection with cytomegalovirus, toxoplasmosis, and infectious mononucleosis. The latter three disorders may also cause lymph node enlargement, fever, splenomegaly, and hepatomegaly with circulating atypical lymphocytes.

In children, lymphocytic lymphomas with marrow involvement must be considered. These patients may present with overt leukemia. In older patients, marrow replacement by metastatic carcinoma must be excluded. In adults, chronic lymphocytic leukemia, hairy cell leukemia, prolymphocytic leukemia, or lymphomas may be initially confused with ALL.

TREATMENT

Remission induction with vincristine and prednisone plus a third drug, such as daunorubicin, doxorubicin, methotrexate, or L-asparaginase is standard. When remission is obtained, central nervous system prophylaxis with cranial irradiation and intrathecal methotrexate is begun. Consolidation and maintenance therapies are variable but usually include L-asparaginase, methotrexate, 6-mercaptopurine, vincristine, and prednisone. Treatment is continued for 2 to 3 years.

PROGNOSIS

Approximately 50 per cent of children and most adults die from the disease or due to complications of therapy. The best prognosis exists in children ages 2 to 10 years with common type (L1) ALL and low blast counts. Adverse prognostic factors include sex (male) and race (black); involvement of the central nervous system, mediastinum, and testes; and unfavorable histology (types L2 or L3).

The role of the primary care physician in caring for patients with ALL (and other hematologic malignancies) is most often to recognize treatment-related complications, particularly bleeding and infection. Prompt institution of appropriate therapy is essential when an unacceptable delay would result from transferring the patient to the referral center.

Chronic Lymphocytic Leukemia

Chronic lymphocytic leukemia (CLL) is the most common leukemia in the Western world. Most cases result from the expansion of a clone of differentiated, small, B-cell lymphocytes. The clonal nature of the disease is demonstrated by the fact that the malignant cells exhibit monoclonal staining for surface immunoglobulin and only a single light chain type.

The incidence of CLL does not appear to be affected by prior exposure to ionizing radiation or cytotoxic drug therapy. Most patients are older with 90 per cent being over 50 years of age. The male:female ratio is approximately 2 to 1. Family disease patterns support the possibility of genetic factors in the etiology of CLL.

DIAGNOSIS AND STAGING

Clinically, the disease manifests itself in numerous ways. The patient may be asymptomatic with the diagnosis suspected from a routine complete blood count. Patients may complain of fever, night sweats, anorexia, malaise, and fatigability. Upper and lower respiratory tract infections and skin infections are increased. Herpes zoster also occurs with increased frequency in CLL patients. Enlarged nodes may be absent early in the course of CLL but are present in most patients with high tumor burden. Early stage patients (stage A) may have only a lymphocytosis in excess of 15,000 per microliter of well-differentiated, small lymphocytes. No anemia or thrombocytopenia is present, and up to two sites of lymph node enlargement may be apparent. Stage B patients have more than three involved nodal areas and no thrombocytopenia or anemia. Stage C patients have anemia with a hemoglobin less than 10 grams per deciliter, platelets less than 100,000 per microliter, or both, regardless of the number of areas of lymphoid enlargement.

CLL is a disease characterized by a progressive

increase in total tumor burden. Untreated patients, with occasional exceptions, progress to a point of diffuse lymph node enlargement, hepatosplenomegaly, and virtual marrow replacement with lymphocytes. Early on, the marrow may be infiltrated with a small number of lymphocytes in a diffuse or patchy pattern. Survival is related to stage at the time of presentation and is also dependent on the growth rate of the abnormal clone in a given patient. Stage A patients survive approximately 8 to 10 years; stage B survival is approximately 7 years with expected survival of 2 to 3 years for stage C patients.

Serum protein electrophoresis is usually normal in early stage patients, but, with progression, many patients develop severe hypogammaglobulinemia secondary to reduced antibody synthesis. Cell surface marker studies may help confirm or rule out the diagnosis in questionable cases and allow identification of an abnormal clone in patients with lymphocyte counts above normal but less than 15,000 per microliter.

It should be noted that the same malignant cell is responsible for diffuse, small, well-differentiated lymphocytic lymphomas. A lymph node biopsy will not allow separation of the two diseases. The absence of striking marrow involvement and of a peripheral lymphocytosis helps distinguish this lymphoma from CLL. This is largely of academic interest as management is often the same in both cases.

THERAPY

Early stage patients are usually observed. This allows the clinician to make an estimate of the growth rate of the disease. Patients with rapidly progressive disease and advanced stage disease, and those with disease-related complaints or problems, are treated. These indications may include bulky node masses, aesthenia related to high tumor burden, ureteral obstruction by retroperitoneal node masses, or other localized problems due to lymphoid enlargement. Autoimmune hemolytic anemia and immune thrombocytopenia may develop suddenly and are treated with high doses of corticosteroids. Autoimmune thrombocytopenia may not respond well to therapy. The disease may transform into a more aggressive phase in the form of prolymphocytoid transformation (increased numbers of circulating larger lymphocytes with some features of prolymphocytes) or Ritcher's syndrome. This is characterized by a sudden increase in the growth rate of a localized node group or extra nodal site. Biopsy reveals a proliferation suggestive of large cell lymphomas. In both of these circumstances, the disease usually becomes refractory to further treatment, and death follows within a few weeks or months.

The usual initial therapy is with pulse doses of an alkylating agent, often chlorambucil, and prednisone every 2 to 4 weeks. When the disease becomes resistant to this combination, a second alkalating agent may be tried. Steroids alone may be tried in patients with severe cytopenias where alkalating agents might be hazardous. Fludarabine, an investigational agent, appears to offer promise in some CLL patients. Radiation of localized node groups causing obstruction or pain is a useful adjunctive therapy.

Acute Nonlymphocytic (Myeloid) Leukemia

Acute nonlymphocytic leukemia (ANLL) results from malignant transformation of a hematologic stem cell. The proliferation of this abnormal clone leads to marrow replacement with early myeloid forms. ANLL may arise de novo or in the setting of a pre-existing myeloproliferative or myelodysplastic syndrome. ANLL is also known to be a late complication of prior therapy with alkalating agents, such as cyclophosphamide, busulfan, etc. ANLL arising in this setting or in a patient with a pre-existing myelodysplastic syndrome carries a poor prognosis.

The myelodysplastic disorders include refractory anemia with or without ringed sideroblasts and may be accompanied by excess blasts in the marrow. They are characterized by a hematopoiesis with peripheral cytopenias. The widely used French-American-British classification scheme allows a diagnosis of ANLL to be made when blasts account for 30 per cent or more of nucleated marrow elements, thus separating ANLL from myelodysplastic disorders.

Since the pretreatment evaluation for suspected ANLL requires a bone marrow examination with special stains, cytogenetic analysis, and cell surface marker analysis, it is desirable to refer these patients to appropriate centers as soon as possible.

INITIAL EVALUATION AND CARE

Patients with ANLL usually consult a physician with symptoms due to marrow failure. These symptoms include bleeding, petechiae, or purpura from thrombocytopenia, weakness, or fatigue secondary to anemia or with infections due to reduced numbers of granulocytes. Lymph node enlargement is not common. The spleen may be enlarged in patients with acute monocytic leukemia and in those with prior myeloproliferative diseases. Skin lesions due to infiltration by blasts, oral ulcers, gum hypertrophy, evidence of central nervous system involvement, and perirectal ulcers/abscesses may be noted.

Pancytopenia is often present. The WBC count may be high, normal, or low. If high, circulating blasts will be easily found on the peripheral smear. If the WBC count exceeds 100,000 per microliter, the patient may experience central nervous system symptoms or pulmonary symptoms due to vascular plugging by masses of blasts (leukostasis). Immediate therapy with leukophoresis and/or hydroxyrea should be given if available. Patients with suspected infection should receive immediate broad-spectrum, intravenous antibiotic therapy after appropriate cultures have been obtained. The antibiotics selected should include two antipseudomonal drugs plus Gram-positive coverage. A typical regimen is gentamicin, piperacillin, and cephalothin.

Bleeding patients should be screened for DIC, which is especially common in patients with acute promyelocytic leukemia. If the initial clotting studies are prolonged, fibrin split products and the fibrinogen should be measured. The peripheral smear may reveal fragmented red cells (schistocytes). If DIC is present, therapy is begun with low-dose, continuous infusion heparin (500 units per hr.) and cryoprecipitate. Patients with life-threatening complications of anemia or bleeding secondary to thrombocytopenia should be given appropriate blood products. Patients less than 50 years of age may be candidates for bone marrow transplantation later. Blood products from relatives who may be potential marrow donors are best avoided to reduce the risk of sensitization to tissue antigens and the subsequent risk of allograft failure.

Often, patients with these and other complicating problems present to a physician in a rural setting. If transfer to a referral center will result in a significant delay in therapy, the primary physician is urged to contact a specialist at the referral institution for guidance in the optimal initial therapy and transfer procedures. Copies of all test results and radiographs should be sent with the patient as this will facilitate prompt care at the receiving institution.

INDUCTION THERAPY

Remission induction therapy for ANLL commonly consists of an infusion of cytosine arabinoside (ARA-C) at doses of 100 to 200 mg. per M^2 per day for 7 days and daunorubicin (Cerubidine), 45 mg. per M^2 per day for 3 consecutive days. Aplasia of the marrow results from this therapy, and many patients develop severe infections and require frequent support with blood products. With current therapy, a remission can be obtained in 60 per cent or more of patients. The risk of death as a consequence of induction therapy is higher in older patients and those with significant underlying medical illnesses. Duration of remission varies from several months to 2 or more years and increasing numbers of patients appear to be cured of their disease. Great improvements in the therapy for ANLL have occurred in the past 2 decades. It is suggested that patients be referred to a center participating in ongoing clinical trials whenever possible.

Chronic Myelogenous Leukemia

Chronic myelogenous leukemia (CML) is a disease resulting from malignant transformation of a hematopoietic stem cell. This is supported by demonstration of the Philadelphia chromosome (Ph^1) and a single isotype of G6PD in all of the patient's neutrophils, basophils, eosinophils, monocytes, megakaryocytes, erythroid precursors, and B-lymphocytes. The Ph^1 chromosome is present in approximately 90 per cent of cases. It results from loss of the long arm of chromosome 22, which is translocated to chromosome 9. The resulting chimeric gene produces a protein that promotes proliferation via uncontrolled cell activation.

CLINICAL FEATURES AND COURSE

CML is primarily a disease of middle age but may occur in other age groups from infants to the very elderly. Early cases may be asymptomatic. Almost all patients are found to have splenomegaly by the time the peripheral WBC count reaches 50,000 per microliter. With disease progression, the WBC count continues to rise, and development or worsening of anemia occurs. The spleen, and sometimes the liver, progressively enlarge. The patient may appear wasted and show signs of a hypermetabolic state. Lymph node enlargement does not occur commonly.

The median patient survival is 36 months after diagnosis. CML may terminate in an accelerated phase characterized by increasing anemia and thrombocytopenia and increasing WBC count with increased numbers of blast forms in the blood and bone marrow. In some patients, the terminal event is a blast crisis, which is the sudden appearance of large numbers of blasts in the blood and bone marrow. Standard induction chemotherapy for acute nonlymphocytic leukemia is largely ineffective. Some 20 to 30 per cent of CML blast crises are acute lymphoblastic leukemia and may briefly respond to therapy with vincristine and prednisone.

LABORATORY FEATURES

The WBC count is elevated. In early cases, it is less than 100,000 per microliter but may exceed 400,000 in patients with more advanced disease. Increased numbers of mature granulocytes, bands, and metamyelocytes are found on the peripheral smear. In addition, occasional myelocytes, promyelocytes, and blasts are also noted. Eosinophils, basophils, and macrophages may be increased.

Anemia is usually present. *Small* numbers of nucleated RBCs may be seen as CML progresses. Platelets may be increased in early CML, but thrombocytopenia ensues later. Anemia and thrombocytopenia may be aggravated by a component of hypersplenism and by the use of chemotherapy. As a result of increased cell turnover, the lactate dehydrogenase is elevated along with the uric acid, serum B_{12}, serum B_{12} binding proteins, and urine lysozyme.

The marrow is hypercellular with a markedly

increased myeloid to erythroid ratio. Increased numbers of granulocytic precursors of all stages are noted. Occasional late cases may demonstrate increased marrow fibrosis, which necessitates ruling out myelofibrosis with myeloid metaplasia.

The Ph^1 chromosome is present in approximately 90 per cent of cases. Patients without the Ph^2 chromosome either do not have CML or have similar but more subtle chromosomal rearrangements requiring more sophisticated techniques for detection. Other cytogenetic abnormalities may be found, especially in patients studied during the accelerated phase or blast crisis. The leukocyte alkaline phosphatase (LAP) score is very low, usually less than 10. This may help separate CML from patients with a leukemoid reaction in which that score is high. Splenomegaly is normally absent in leukemoid reactions, and promyelocytes and myeloblasts are not found on examination of the peripheral smear. In addition, the Ph^1 chromosome is absent.

CML must also be distinguished from myelofibrosis. In the latter case, the LAP score may be high or low, the peripheral blood contains numerous nucleated RBCs, the Ph^1 chromosome is absent, splenomegaly is massive, the WBC count is rarely greater than 50,000 per microliter, and a bone marrow biopsy reveals marked fibrosis with megakaryocytic hyperplasia.

THERAPY

Early, asymptomatic cases may be observed until symptoms develop. Therapy with busulfan, an alkalating agent, or hydroxyurea may be used. Busulfan may cause a syndrome of pulmonary fibrosis, GI symptoms, hyperpigmentation, and weight loss. Once initial control is achieved, busulfan may be given intermittently while hydroxyurea therapy must be continuous and requires closer patient monitoring to adjust the dose. Recently, treatment with recombinant alpha interferon has also proved effective. With initial therapy, the WBC count falls, symptoms and anemia improve, and splenomegaly may regress somewhat. Therapy does not appear to increase survival. Resistance emerges as clones of cells resistant to chemotherapy develop.

In patients under 40 years of age, with an identical twin, marrow transplantation offers the hope of cure. Patients under 40 are now being transplanted with marrow from human leukocyte antigen compatible siblings. Transplantation is best accomplished when the disease is in the chronic phase. About one third of these patients are lost to infection, graft versus host disease, or interstitial pneumonia. The remaining patients appear cured.

References

Bachmann, E. Diagnostic approach to mild bleeding disorders. Semin. Hematol., *17*(4):292–305, 1980. *Describes a differential approach to the assessment of patients with bleeding disorders based on historical, physical, and laboratory data. This approach helps to determine whether the etiology of the disorder is platelet, vascular, or a coagulation defect in origin. Is very applicable to primary care practice.*

Barton, J. C.: Nonhemolytic non-infectious transfusion reactions. Semin. Hematol., *18*(2):95–121, 1981.

Beck, W. S.: General considerations of megaloblastic anemias. *In* Williams, W. J., Rindles, R. W., Beutler, E., and Erslev, A. J. (Eds.): Hematology. 2nd ed. New York, McGraw-Hill, 1977, pp. 300–306. *Easily understood and well written. Although the reference chapter on megaloblastic anemias is old, most of the concepts are consistent with today's understanding of these anemias.*

Boye, J. R.: Transfusion-transmitted diseases: current problems and challenges. Prog. Hematol., *16*:123, 1986. *Concise update on problems confronting physicians when using blood products. Mechanisms to avoid transfusion-related AIDS; hepatitis is discussed in detail.*

Carmel, R.: Pernicious anemia: the expected findings of very low serum cobalamin levels, anemia, and macrocytosis are often lacking. Arch. Intern. Med., *148*(8):1712–1714, 1988. *One of several recent articles that relate the presence of significant B_{12} deficiency without the associated megaloblastic transformation. Supports the need to obtain B_{12} levels in any unexplained neuropsychiatric disorder even in the face of a normal hemogram.*

Carmel, R., and Karnaze, D. S.: Physician response to low serum cobalamin levels. Arch. Intern. Med., *146*(6):1161–1165, 1986.

De Vita, V. T., Jr., Jaffe, E. S., and Heilman, S.: Hodgkin's disease and the non-Hodgkin's lymphomas. *In* De Vita, V. T., Jr., Hellman, S., and Rosenberg, S. R. (Eds.): Cancer, Principles and Practice of Oncology. 2nd ed. Philadelphia, J. B. Lippincott Company, 1985, pp. 1623–1710.

Erslev, A. J.: Anemia of chronic disorders. *In* Williams, W. J., et al. (Eds.): Hematology. 3rd ed. New York, McGraw-Hill Book Company, 1983, pp. 522–528.

Hobbs, J., and Rodriguez, A. R.: Megaloblastic anemias. Am. Fam. Physician, *22*:128–136, 1980. *Concise review of pathophysiology and treatment of megaloblastic anemia with emphasis on diagnosis and treatment. A useful diagnostic approach for primary care practices.*

Hobbs, J., and Wright, C. S.: Hemolytic anemias. Am. Fam. Physician, *22*:82–93, June 1979. *A practical approach to the evaluation of hemolytic anemia is presented in this article that was prepared for a primary care audience. It described hemolytic anemia based on the source of the premature hemolysis, i.e., intrinsic or environmental.*

Kasper, C. K., and Dietrick, S. L.: Comprehensive management of hemophilia. Clin. Hematol., *14*(2):489–512, 1985.

Kolhouse, J. F., Kondo, H., Allen, N. C., et al.: Cobalamin analogues are present in human plasma and can mask cobalamin deficiency because current radioisotope dilution assays are not specific for true cobalamin. N. Engl. J. Med., *299*:785–792, 1978.

Lindenbaum, J., Healthon, E. B., Savage, D. G., et al.: Neuropsychiatric disorders caused by cobalamin deficiency in the absence of anemia or macrocytosis. N. Engl. J. Med., *318*(26):1720–1728, June 30, 1988. *Emphasizes the fact that B_{12} deficiency can and probably does occur frequently in the absence of anemia or other megaloblastic transformation. Emphasizes the need to routinely obtain B_{12} levels in patients evaluated for neurologic dysfunctions.*

Moake, J. L.: Hemostasis and thrombosis. *In* Reich, P. R. (Ed.): Hematology: Physiopathologic Basis for Clinical Practice. 2nd ed. Boston, Little, Brown and Company, 1984, pp. 439–494.

Mollison, P. L.: Transfusion in clinical medicine. 3rd ed. Boston, Blackwell Publishing Co., 1983.

Osteen, R., and Wilson, R.: Lymph nodes and subcutaneous masses. *In* Branch, W. T., Jr. (Ed.): Office Practice of Medicine. Philadelphia, W. B. Saunders Co., 1982, pp. 1097–1110. *A practical approach to the evaluation of lymphadenopathy in adult patients. Emphasis is placed on differential benign and malignant causes of lymphadenopathy. The chapter was prepared for use by primary care physicians and students receiving training in primary care.*

Pierce, H. L., and Hillman, R. S.: The value of the serum vitamin B_{12} level in diagnosing B_{12} deficiency. Blood, *43*:915–921, 1974.

Reich, P. R.: Hypochromic anemias. *In* Reich, P. R. (Ed.): Hematology: Physiopathologic Basis for Clinical Practice. 2nd ed. Boston, Little, Brown and Company, 1984, pp. 35–68. *This and other chapters of this textbook by Reich on hematology provide comprehensive yet concise discussions of the pathophysiology, diagnosis, and treatment of common hematologic disorders. Aspects of hematologic disorders are easily found because of the outline format used in this textbook.*

Reich, P. R.: Megaloblastic anemia. *In* Reich, P. R. (Ed.): Hematology: Physiopathologic Basis for Clinical Practice. 2nd ed. Boston, Little, Brown and Company, 1984, pp. 69–108.

Reich, P. R.: Hemolytic anemia. *In* Reich, P. R. (Ed.): Hematology: Physiopathologic Basis for Clinical Practice. 2nd ed. Boston, Little, Brown and Company, 1984, pp. 109–128.

Reich, P. R.: Coombs' test-positive hemolytic anemias. *In* Reich, P. R. (Ed.): Hematology: Physiopathologic Basis for Clinical Practice. 2nd ed. Little, Brown and Company, 1984, pp. 129–154.

Reich, P. R.: Coombs test-negative hemolytic anemias. *In* Reich, P. R. (Ed.): Hematology: Physiopathologic Basis for Clinical Practice. 2nd ed. Boston, Little, Brown and Company, 1984, pp. 155–216.

Saxena, S., Cramer, A. D., Weiner, J. M., and Carmel, R.: Platelet counts in three racial groups. Am. J. Clin. Pathol., *88*(1):106–109, July 1987.

Shohet, S. B., and Ness, P. M.: Hemolytic anemias: failure of the red cell membrane. Med. Clin. North Am., *60*(5):913–932, September 1976.

Silverstein, M.: Relative and absolute polycythemia: how to tell them apart. Postgrad. Med., *81*(5):285–288, April 1987. *Describes a good diagnostic approach to a problem that occasionally confronts the primary care physician. The article provides mechanisms to avoid expensive and time-consuming evaluation of elevated platelet counts that do not represent a primary hematologic disorder, i.e., relative polycythemia.*

Sinow, R. M., Johnson, C. S., Karnaze, D. S., et al.: Unsuspected pernicious anemia in a patient with sickle cell disease receiving routine folate supplementation. Arch. Intern. Med., *147*(10):1828–1829, October 1987. *Highlights the impact of therapeutic quantities of folate on development of anemia associated with B_{12} deficiency. Because patients receiving therapeutic amounts of B folate may not show the hematologic changes usually associated with B_{12} deficiency, it becomes necessary to suspect the vitamin deficiency based on other findings (e.g., neurologic).*

Tollefson, D. M.: Disorders of hemostasis. *In* Orland, M. J., and Saltman, R. J. (Eds.): Manual of Medical Therapeutics. Boston, Little, Brown and Company, 1987. *Easy-to-follow explanation of a diagnostic approach to bleeding disorders although the pathophysiology is discussed at a minimum, plus the description of laboratory evaluation is more than sufficient. Understood the rationale of the therapeutic consideration.*

Weinstein, I. M.: Lymph node enlargement and splenomegaly. *In* Williams, W. J., Beutler, E., Erslev, A. J., and Lichtman, M. A. (Eds.): Hematology. 3rd ed. New York, McGraw-Hill Book Company, 1983, pp. 937–943.

58

Urinary Tract Disorders

Urology

Steven H. Selman
Harry E. Mayhew
William Leon Heth

Diagnostic Evaluation

Evaluation of the genitourinary (GU) system begins with a focused history and physical examination. In addition, a urinalysis should be performed. There are a number of noninvasive techniques for imaging the GU system that complement the evaluation.

HISTORY

The urologic history is the first step in formulating a diagnostic plan. In addition to the general medical history, review of the GU systems should cover specific complaints.

Frequency

Patients should be questioned as to the frequency of voiding. Both daytime and nighttime voiding patterns are important. The patient should be asked to relate the amount of urine passed on voiding, the strength of the urinary stream, and whether each voiding is perceived as complete emptying.

Urgency

Urgency is the perceived need to void. Normally, a patient is not aware of bladder filling until a critical volume is reached. Most patients feel no urge to void until the bladder has filled to about 150 cc. (Wein and Stephenson, 1984). Inflammatory or infectious processes in or around the bladder and urethra irritate the sensory fibers from the bladder and will be perceived as a need to urinate.

Hematuria

Gross hematuria will be detected by the patient. The physician should note whether the hematuria is initial or terminal, painful or painless. Associated complaints or urgency and frequency should also be recorded. A history of trauma, including high-impact athletics, should be sought. It should be remembered that certain foodstuffs, such as beets, consumed in excess will give the urine a red appearance.

Hesitancy

As obstruction increases, there is increasing hesitancy in initiating the urine stream. This is a common complaint in men with benign prostatic hyperplasia or urethral stricture.

Pneumaturia

Patients with enterovesical fistulae may pass air while voiding.

Hematospermia

Blood in the ejaculate is called hematospermia. The patient may complain that the ejaculate has a dark brown appearance. Hematospermia is seen in men with inflammation of the prostate or seminal vesicals.

Pain

Pain arising from the kidneys may be located in the upper posterior flank (costovertebral angle). Pain of renal origin may radiate anteriorly along the $T_{11,12}$-L_1 dermatome. Ureteral pain also tends to radiate along the dermatomes. Pain arising from the upper ureter will follow the $T_{11,12}$-L_1-$_2$ dermatomes, whereas that arising from the mid or lower ureter typically follow the L_1-$_2S_2$ dermatomes (Fig. 58–1). Irritation of the bladder generally is perceived as suprapubic discomfort, and the pain is usually greatest after voiding. In the male, pain arising from the bladder may be referred to the tip of the penis. Prostatic pain is usually perceived as discomfort deep within the perineum.

PHYSICAL EXAMINATION

Kidney

Normal kidneys are not palpable transabdominally. In a very thin patient, the lower pole of the right kidney may be palpable with deep inspiration. Elevation of the flank with an examining hand will facilitate transabdominal palpation of the kidney. Mild percussion to the costovertebral angles with the hypothenar aspect of the clenched fist should be done to elicit costovertebral tenderness.

Bladder

The empty bladder should not be palpable transabdominally. A distended bladder presents as a firm midline suprapubic mass. In obese patients, this may not be detectable. Percussion can help in defining the outline of the bladder. If deep palpation in the suprapubic region elicits a sense of urinary urgency, a poorly emptying bladder should be suspected.

Penis

The penile skin should be carefully inspected for lesions. If the patient is uncircumcised, the foreskin should be retracted to examine the glans penis. The corpora of the phallus should be palpated for any irregularities.

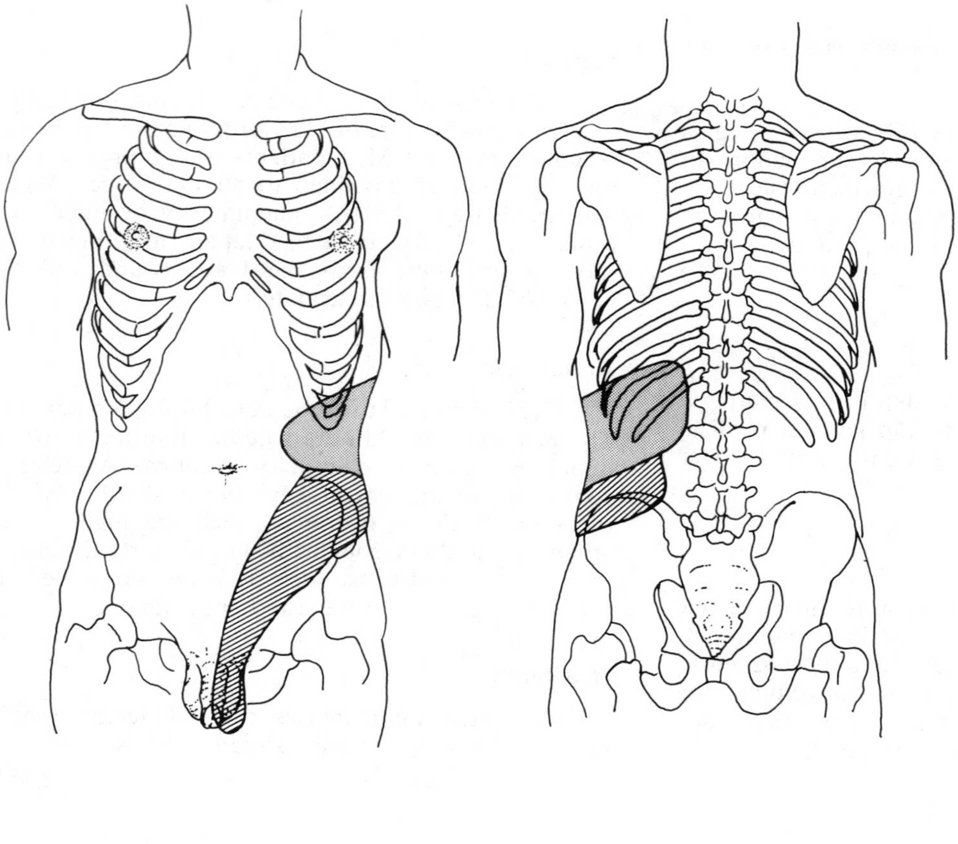

Figure 58–1. Referred pain from kidney (dotted areas) and ureter (shaded areas). (Reproduced with permission from Tanagho, E. A., and McAninch, J. W.: Smith's General Urology. 12th ed. Copyright Appleton & Lange, 1988.)

Urethra

The male urethra should be palpated from the perineum to the meatus. In patients complaining of a urethral discharge, the urethra should be milked from the proximal bulbous urethra to the meatus. In the female patient, examination of the external urethra is part of the pelvic exam. The urethra should be milked distally in order to detect and empty a urethral diverticulum when investigating recurrent urinary tract infections.

Scrotum and Testes

The physician should carefully inspect and examine the scrotum and its contents in both the supine and standing position. The testicles should be gently rolled between the examining fingers in an effort to detect any abnormalities of size and consistency. The epididymides, which are normally posterior, should be palpated from their most caudad aspect (globus minor) to the cephalad aspect (globus major). The cord structures should also be palpated. Every male patient should be encouraged to perform periodic self-examination of the testes.

Prostate

Examination of the prostate is best performed in the standing position with the patient bending over the examination table. The gloved examination finger should be liberally lubricated. Placing the examining digit on the anus and letting it remain there for a few seconds before entering the rectum allows for relaxation of the external anal sphincter and decreases patient discomfort. The prostate should be palpated by sweeping the finger from the lateral border to the median sulcus on each lobe. The entire gland from base to apex should be systematically examined. The normal prostate has the consistency of the thenar eminence of the clenched fist.

Prostatic nodules associated with early carcinoma often do not protrude from the surface of the gland but are felt for within the substance of the prostatic tissue. The seminal vesicles normally are not palpable.

URINALYSIS

Examination of the urine is an integral part of the urologic examination. The examining physician should perform the microscopic part of the urinalysis.

Collection

An improperly collected sample of urine contributes to inaccurate diagnoses and improper treatments. In the adult male, the glans penis should be cleansed with soap and water and initial and midstream specimens collected. In the female, a midstream sample is collected only after proper cleansing of the vulva. The labia need to be retracted during sample collection. Examination of the urine sample should be performed within 20 minutes of its collection. The first morning specimen is best for detecting bacteria, RBCs, WBCs, and casts.

Physical Characteristics

The color of the urine should be noted. The specific gravity should also be determined since very dilute urine will result in the lysis of cellular elements.

Chemical Analysis

The chemical analysis of urine has been simplified by commercially available cellulose strips impregnated with agents to detect RBCs, WBCs, and protein glucose and to determine pH.

Microscopic Examination

The microscopic examination should be performed on both the spun and unspun specimen. Examination should be performed at both the 4X and 40X magnification. The specimen should be examined with the diaphragm as small as possible since strong illumination obscures cellular outlines.

IMAGING

A variety of imaging techniques that permit visualization of the genitourinary system are available. These techniques complement the endoscopic techniques that are part of the urologist's diagnostic armamentarium.

Intravenous Urography

The intravenous urogram or pyelogram has been the cornerstone of urologic radiographic evaluation for many years. The examination is based on the concentration of radiopaque contrast material within the kidneys and the subsequent opacification of the renal outlines and collecting system.

Retrograde Pyelography

This examination entails the retrograde instillation of contrast into the ureters and renal pelvis. It is usually reserved for patients who are allergic to intravenous contrast.

Antegrade Pyelography

Relatively atraumatic puncture of the renal collecting system is possible with a fine (skinny) needle. Contrast material can then be instilled. The technique is most useful for obstructed renal units in which the retrograde pyelogram has been unsuccessful.

Cystography

In the static cystogram, contrast medium is instilled in the bladder and radiographs obtained. Its usefulness in delineating vesical pathology is limited. It is, however, the radiographic examination of choice in evaluating vesical injury.

The voiding cystourethrogram (VCUG) is a dynamic study in which instilled contrast is voided under flouroscopy. It is most useful in detecting vescioureteral reflux and detecting abnormalities of the urethra. Nuclide cystography can be used in children to minimize x-ray exposure.

Retrograde Urethrography

Contrast is injected in a retrograde manner into the urethra. This examination is most useful in cases of male stricture disease and in cases of suspected urethral trauma.

Coaxial Tomography

Computerized axial tomographic scanning has its greatest application in urology in providing a two-dimensional image of retroperitoneal structures. It is most helpful in determining the nature of a renal mass (Weyman, 1980).

Ultrasonography

Ultrasound offers noninvasive diagnostic imaging of the genitourinary system. It is well suited for differentiating between cystic and solid renal masses (Pollack, 1982) as well as for the detection of hydronephrosis. Residual bladder urine can be determined with transabdominal ultrasound. Scrotal ultrasound allows for the visualization of scrotal anatomy. Transrectal prostatic ultrasound can be used to detect and stage prostatic carcinoma (Lee, 1987).

Nuclear scanning can provide information as to renal function, architecture, perfusion, and obstruction. Bone scanning is an integral part of the evaluation of patients with urologic malignancies.

Magnetic Resonance Imaging

Another noninvasive technique for imaging genitourinary structures is magnetic resonance imaging. A cost-effective place in the diagnostic armamentarium has yet to be completely defined vis-à-vis other currently available technologies.

Genitourinary Infections

INTRODUCTION

Infections of the GU tract are common. They encompass a spectrum of clinical problems from asymptomatic infections of the normal bladder to fulminant sepsis associated with complicated genitourinary anomalies. Most infections are managed by the primary physician. Recurrent or complicated infections are best handled by referral to or consultation with a urologist.

Normally, urine is sterile. Urine obtained as a voided specimen, as opposed to direct puncture of the bladder, may be contaminated by organisms from the urethra or the introitus. The classic operational definition of significant bacteria is the presence of $> 10^5$ bacteria per cc. Using this guideline, the clinician can be assured of a 95 per cent confidence level in the diagnosis of a bacterial infection (Kass, 1956). However, bacterial infections warranting treatment can be present when smaller numbers of bacteria are present (Fowler, 1986; Mulholland, 1987). In addition, the GU tract can be infected with fungi or the tubercle bacillus.

The GU tract can be divided into the lower and the upper tract. In the male, the lower tract includes the bladder, prostate and seminal vesicles, urethra, and testes and epididymides. In the female, the bladder and urethra are included. The upper tract includes the kidneys and ureters. All of these sites are potential foci for infections. Usually, the family physician can accurately localize the site of infection by history and physical examination alone. Cystitis is a clinical syndrome associated with lower tract infections. Typically, the patient complains of urgency, hematuria, increased frequency, and dysuria. A high fever is uncommon. On the other hand, pyelonephritis—an upper tract infection—is associated with general malaise, high fever, and flank pain.

URINARY TRACT INFECTIONS IN CHILDREN

In the newborn period, the frequency of urinary tract infections is greater in the male than in the female infant (Abbott, 1972). After the first few months of life, the incidence of infections in females increases. The finding of bacteriuria in the newborn period should alert the primary physician to the possibility of an underlying congenital abnormality, such as an infected poorly draining duplicated renal segment, ureteral pelvic junction obstruction, or posterior urethral valves. A focused exam should be performed. Palpation of the flank area may delineate a mass while the suprapubic region should be examined for a distended bladder. Since urosepsis developing in the newborn period is usually associated with significant congenital abnormalities, a urologic consultation should be obtained.

In the preschool years, the incidence of bacteriuria (either symptomatic or asymptomatic) is higher in female patients. Since at this age vesicoureteral reflux caused by an incompetent antireflux mechanism at the ureterovesical junction can damage developing renal parenchyma, it is important that the child undergo a renal ultrasound and VCUG. An intravenous pyelogram (IVP) may be necessary to complement these studies. In some patients, a urodynamic evaluation of the lower tract may also be necessary. Evidence of parenchyma scarring on the IVP or ureterovesical reflux on the VCUG warrants urologic referral. Treatment of asymptomatic bacteriuria is indicated in this age group (Gillenwater, 1979). A urinary tract infection in the preschool male patient should be followed by a urologic referral. Any child presenting with a clinical syndrome associated with acute pyelonephritis needs evaluation of the GU tract. It is important to remember that in the preschool age group fever may be the only sign of a urinary tract infection.

In the school age population, urinary tract infections are most commonly encountered in girls. In a significant number of these patients (20 per cent) infection is associated with vesicoureteral reflux, a pathologic condition in which urine refluxes up to the kidney with each bladder contraction (Whitaker, 1984). However, during this period (> 5 years) further parenchymal damage associated with vesicoureteral reflux is unlikely to occur (Gillenwater, 1979). Infections should be treated even if asymptomatic. In addition, careful follow-up with repeat cultures after therapy is important to detect persistent or recurrent infection. The indications for surgical repair of vesicoureteral reflux have changed significantly over the last 15 years. Antireflux procedures, which were commonly performed, are now done only in patients with massive reflux or if breakthrough upper tract infections occur despite prophylactic antibiotic therapy. Most patients with lesser degrees of reflux will have spontaneous resolution of their problem by the onset of adolescence. Once reflux or other urologic abnormality is identified, urologic consultation should be obtained.

URINARY TRACT INFECTIONS IN THE ADULT

Urinary tract infections are common in the adult female while relatively uncommon in the adult male until the seventh decade of life. The short female urethra and its close anatomic relation with the perianal area may in part account for the high frequency of infection. Sexual intercourse probably contributes to the ascending route of infection from the introital area to the urethra and into the bladder. Most infections in the adult female are caused by aerobic coliform bacteria.

Acute Cystitis

Acute bacterial infections of the bladder are associated with urinary frequency, urgency, dysuria, and hematuria. The increased frequency is usually severe and associated with a sense of urgency and often urge incontinence. Dysuria is often described as knifelike in character. Hematuria at times may be heavy. The most common organism associated with the initial episode of bacterial cystitis is *E. coli*. During the first infection, treatment may be empiric. An uncomplicated, acute cystitis can be treated with a short 3-day course of oral antibiotics (Fair, 1980).

Recurrent Cystitis

Recurrent cystitis of the bladder is defined as recurrent infection occurring within 3 months of the initial episode. Recurrent infections may result from a new infecting organism or from an infected source that was not obliterated during the therapy. Culture of the urine is indicated. Organisms such as *Proteus mirablis* or *Staphlococcus aureus* should alert the primary physician to the possibility of an underlying anatomic abnormality. A thorough exam should be done including a pelvic exam. A urethral diverticulum may at times be the source of recurrent infections. An IVP and VCUG should be obtained in patients with recurrent infections. Treatment of recurrent infections is controversial. Classically, treatment consisted of a 7 to 10 day course of oral antibiotics (see chapter 31). In some patients with recurrent infections, chronic suppressive therapy is instituted. Guidelines for this form of therapy are sparse. A once-a-day bedtime dose of a sulfonamide or a furadantoin derivative for 3 months may prove useful. Another approach is intermittent, self-administered single-dose therapy such as nitrofurantoin (Furadantin), 100 mg, or trimethoprim/sulfamethoxazole (Bactrim DS), 1 tablet, at the first sign of an infection (Fowler, 1986). Patients on furadantoins must be monitored for pulmonary toxicity.

Chronic Cystitis

This term should be abandoned in favor of recurrent cystitis.

Acute Pyelonephritis

Acute pyelonephritis is a clinical term associated with an acute nonsuppurative infection of the renal parenchyma. Patients usually present with flank pain and fever. The urine shows white cells and bacteria. Hospitalization and systemic broad-spectrum antibiotics (an aminoglycoside and ampicillin) are indicated until culture and sensitivity results are available and should be continued until the patient is afebrile. Oral antibiotic therapy should be continued for at least 6 weeks. An IVP, VCUG, and repeat cultures should be obtained after the patient has convalesced. If an abnormality is found, referral to a urologist is indicated.

Chronic Pyelonephritis

This term is usually associated with the radiographic appearance of renal parenchymal scarring and loss of renal size. Since there are a large number of noninfectious problems (such as interstitial nephritis) that can lead to a similar radiographic appearance, the term should be abandoned.

Renal Abscess

The clinical presentation of a patient with a renal abscess may be similar to pyelonephritis. Renal abscesses are either hematogenous or ascending in origin. The diagnosis should be suspected in the patient who presents with the clinical picture of pyelonephritis but fails to respond to antibiotic therapy. A computerized tomography scan will usually make the diagnosis. Percutaneous drainage has been successful in selected cases (Costello, 1983).

INFECTIONS OF THE ELDERLY

The incidence of urinary tract infection increases in an aging population. This increase in part reflects the increased incidence of urinary tract infections in the male population. Prostatic enlargement causing obstruction and residual urine are factors that contribute to the problem in the male patient. In the elderly female, urethral prolapse and pelvic descendens may effectively shorten the urethra decreasing the barrier to bacterial ascent into the bladder. Associated diseases (such as diabetes and cerebral vascular accidents) may compromise the bladder's ability to empty. Urethral catheterization occurs more frequently in the older population and with it an increased chance for infection.

Urinary tract infections in the elderly are treated as those in the younger adult population. If infections are recurrent, further investigation is needed including (at the minimum) an IVP. In the elderly diabetic patient, an IVP should be performed only when the patient is well hydrated. In addition, an assessment of residual urine should be done preferably by transabdominal ultrasound or if necessary via urethral catheterization using strict aseptic technique. Referral to a urologist may be needed if the infection cannot be cleared with antibiotic therapy.

PROSTATITIS

Prostatic infection and inflammation are commonly encountered clinical problems.

Acute Bacterial Prostatitis

Acute bacterial prostatitis is a disease of the adult male. Culture of the urine will usually identify the infecting organism as an aerobic gram-negative bacillus. Perineal pain, dysuria, and fever are presenting complaints. The prostate is exquisitely tender on rectal exam. Prostatic massage should never be attempted in such a situation. Some patients are unable to void, in which case it is better to place a suprapubic tube percutaneously rather than manipulate the urethra.

Intravenous broad-spectrum antibiotics (an aminoglycoside and ampicillin) are indicated. Rarely, a prostatic abscess may develop. Care of the patient with acute bacterial prostatitis should be shared with a urologic colleague.

Chronic Bacterial Prostatitis

The hallmark of chronic bacterial prostatitis is recurrent urinary tract infections. Patients with chronic bacterial prostatitis are rarely as ill as those with acute bacterial prostatitis. Perineal discomfort (often described as an ache), dysuria, and urgency are common complaints. The prostate is often described as boggy, but this is an inconstant and subjective finding. Greater than 15 to 20 WBC per hpf. should be demonstrable in the expressed prostatic secretions in order to make the diagnosis. Treatment for 10 days is either with trimethoprim (Proloprim), 100 mg. every 12 hours, or carbenicillin (Geocillin), 1 to 2 tablets four times daily. Recurrences requiring treatment are common. In some patients, chronic low-dose suppressive therapy may be warranted with trimethoprim.

Nonbacterial Prostatitis

Men with nonbacterial prostatitis who have symptoms of chronic bacterial prostatitis without documented urinary tract infections are diagnosed as having nonbacterial prostatitis. Examination of expressed prostatic secretions shows greater than 15 to 20 WBC/hpf. A number of organisms, such as *Chlamydia* and *Ureaplasma*, have been suggested as causative agents. However, the cause of this common problem is unknown. Treatment is usually empiric. Antibiotics can be tried, but prolonged treatment is not justified.

Prostatosis/Prostadynia

Patients with symptoms of perineal discomfort, urgency, and dysuria in whom there is no objective evidence of prostatic inflammation or infection and in whom other pathologic conditions have been ruled out may be diagnosed as having prostatosis/prostadynia. Currently, there is neither good explanation for this symptom complex nor proof that the prostate is the source of the problem. These patients need symptomatic treatment, reassurance, and, when appropriate, an evaluation for a psychosocial dysfunction.

EPIDIDYMITIS

Epididymitis is an acute inflammatory process of the epididymis. The problem is seen in all age groups except for the very young. Patients complain of the rapid onset of scrotal pain and swelling frequently associated with fever and malaise. If untreated, symptoms will progress. On exam, the involved epididymis is swollen and exquisitely tender. If an inflammatory hydrocele has developed, it may be impossible to delineate the architecture of the scrotal contents. Scrotal erythema and fixation of the testicle to the scrotal wall are common findings especially in more advanced cases. Differentiation between epididymitis and testicular torsion is crucial. Scrotal ultrasound and testicular scanning are supportive but cannot be relied on solely for the diagnosis. Patients with epididymitis usually have fever, leukocytosis, and pyuria, findings which are not frequently seen in acute testicular torsion.

Once the diagnosis of epididymitis is established, antibiotic treatment should be instituted. Since the etiologic agent rarely can be established, treatment with broad-spectrum antibiotics (such as tetracycline) is indicated. Bed rest, scrotal support, and ice packs are general supportive measures that are usually employed. The use of NSAIDs can be added to the treatment regimen. In a small number of patients, the signs and symptoms of epididymitis do not resolve within 72 hours of therapy. Abscess formation may be responsible for the lack of a therapeutic response requiring urologic consultation.

Occasionally, patients will develop chronic pain in the epididymis. A 3-week course of either tetracycline or erythomycin may result in a satisfactory resolution of the problem. In some cases, an epididymectomy is necessary.

ORCHITIS

Isolated orchitis is most commonly seen as a result of a mumps infection. Treatment is symptomatic. The testicle may also become secondarily infected in cases of severe epididymitis. Treatment in the latter situation would follow the guidelines for epididymitis.

URETHRITIS

Infections of the male urethra are infectious diseases most commonly caused by sexually transmitted diseases (see chapter 31). An indwelling urethral catheter or other forms of urethral manipulation can also lead to urethral infection. Urethritis in these patients will usually be associated with the development of a thick urethral discharge. In the patient with catheter-associated urethritis, removal of the catheter should lead to prompt resolution of the problem. Delay in treatment in these cases can lead to periurethral abscess formation. Antibiotics should be administered until the purulent urethral discharge disappears.

In the female, isolated urethritis without cystitis is uncommon. Many female patients are encountered with acute symptoms of dysuria, frequency, and stranguria. If pyuria and bacteriuria are present, diagnosis and treatment is usually straightforward. However, if objective findings of infection or inflammation are absent, establishment of the correct diagnosis may be difficult. A careful pelvic exam should be done to exclude inflammatory problems of the vulva and reproductive organs. Cystoscopy should be performed in the patient over 50 to rule out carcinoma-in-situ of the bladder. If an infection or serious pathologic processes are excluded, a diagnosis of acute urethral syndrome is justified (George, 1986). As in the male with nonbacterial prostatitis, an etiologic agent responsible for the urethral syndrome has not been identified. A course of oral antibiotics may be successful. However, prolonged continuous antibiotic use is not indicated. The use of urethral dilatation for this condition is unwarranted.

OTHER INFECTIONS

Tuberculosis

GU tuberculosis is still encountered in many parts of the world. Patients with sterile pyuria should be suspected of infection. The first morning urine is best for isolating the tuberculous bacilli. At least three urine specimens should be obtained for culture. If GU tuberculosis is found, triple drug (rifampin, isoniazid, and pyrazinamide) therapy for 6 months is recommended (Fox, 1981; Gow, 1986).

Fungal Infections

Fungal infections are encountered principally in clinical situations in which there is immunosuppression, a foreign body within the urinary tract, or prolonged use of broad-spectrum antibiotics. Diabetics seem especially prone to these infections. *Candida albicans* is the most frequently encountered organism. Treatment should be aimed at removing those factors contributing to the infection. Systemic therapy may be necessary if the patient is symptomatic. In cases of fungal cystitis, local irrigation with amphotericin B may be successful in eradicating the infection (Wise and Kozinn, 1982).

SPECIAL PROBLEMS

Urethral Catheterization

Indwelling catheters dispose the bladder to bacterial colonization. Placement of catheters under strict sterile technique and the use of closed drainage systems lessen the short-term risk of infection. However, if left longer than 4 days, 50 per cent of bladders drained with a closed drainage system will become colonized with bacteria (Fowler and Marshall, 1983). Colonization in this situation results from the breakdown of the normal defense mechanism against bacterial growth. If catheterization is only temporary, then one is probably justified in administering a course of antibiotics after the catheter has been removed. Patients in whom long-term catheterization is planned should not be treated prophylactically with antibiotics. Antibiotic administration in this situation will only lead to emergence of resistant organisms. If the patient develops signs of infection, antibiotic administration based on sensitivities is indicated.

Pregnancy

Both asymptomatic and symptomatic urinary tract infections in the pregnant patient should be treated aggressively. Urinary tract infections in the pregnant patient have been associated with premature labor, pre-eclampsia, congenital anomalies, and postpartum renal disease (Norden and Kass, 1968). One should be cautious in administering antibiotics to make certain the antibiotics do not affect fetal development. Four antibiotics that have this potential are tetracycline, trimethoprim/sulfamethoxazole, chloramphenicol, and erythromycin estolate. Pyelonephritis of pregnancy should be treated with hospitalization and systemic intravenous antibiotics.

Dysfunctions of Micturition

Two functions of the urinary bladder are (1) storage and (2) elimination of urine. Changes, either perceived or real, in the bladder's ability to perform either of these tasks will usually lead to patient concern and consultation.

NEUROANATOMY

The urinary bladder is a muscular (the detrusor muscle) viscus. Urinary continence is maintained by the internal sphincter, a circular condensation of smooth muscle fibers at the bladder neck. These fibers contract as the bladder fills and relax when the bladder empties. In the male (and to a lesser extent in the female), another group of fibers arising from the levator ani muscles of the pelvic floor condense around the distal urethra to form a second sphincter, the so-called external sphincter. Urinary continence and elimination are dependent on the coordinated activity of these muscle groups.

Voiding and maintenance of continence is a complex process. The bladder and sphincter are controlled by several voiding centers. A simple but useful picture is that of the central nervous system connected to the bladder by afferent and efferent peripheral nerves. The voiding centers are located within the central nervous system. These consist of the cerebral cortex voiding center responsible for the social aspects of urinary elimination, a brainstem-cerebellar center acting as a coordination and balance center, and a spinal cord center located between spinal segments S_2-S_4 acting as a lower voiding center coordinating detrusor sphincter activity (Wein, 1981).

Both sympathetic and parasympathetic fibers enervate the bladder and sphincters. Bladder emptying is principally parasympathetic while storage activities are sympathetic. Sensory and motor peripheral fibers complete the circuit.

EVALUATION

A complete history is important in the evaluation of the patient with voiding complaints. The onset of symptoms, the rate of progression, the frequency of urination, and oral fluid intake (as well as the amount voided) should be recorded. Toilet bowl inserts are available to measure urinary volumes. In some patients, a voiding diary is helpful in providing this information. Medical problems, such as diabetes mellitus, multiple sclerosis, cerebrovascular accidents, and medications consumed should be documented. A history of stool incontinence or constipation should be recorded. In addition, the male patient should be questioned about problems with potency.

The physical exam should include neurologic evaluation. In addition to a standard neurologic evaluation, a careful sensory exam (including pinprick and light touch in the perineal region) is essential. Rectal sphincter tone should be noted, and the bulbocavernosus reflex provides valuable information about the integrity of the sacral cord. This reflex is initiated by applying noxious stimuli to the glans penis or clitoris and assessing the contractile response of the external anal sphincter.

While a urinalysis is part of the initial evaluation, a complete urodynamic evaluation requires urologic consultation. Usually, this will consist of uroflow in which the velocity of voiding is plotted against the time of voiding. Nomograms are available for the patient's age and sex. A cystometrogram, which documents the bladder's capacity for receptive relaxation and detrusor contraction, is a basic component of urodynamic evaluation. An electromyogram of the external sphincter can also be obtained that will evaluate the synergy between the sphincter and the detrusor. An IVP may be necessary to document changes in the upper tracts that have resulted from voiding dysfunction.

NEUROGENIC BLADDER

The neurogenic bladder is usually associated with pathologic problems of the brain–spinal cord axis or the peripheral nerves enervating the bladder. The Lapides classification system is commonly used (Lapides, 1970) (Fig. 58–2).

The Uninhibited Neurogenic Bladder

Patients with the uninhibited neurogenic bladder complain of frequency, urgency, and incontinence.

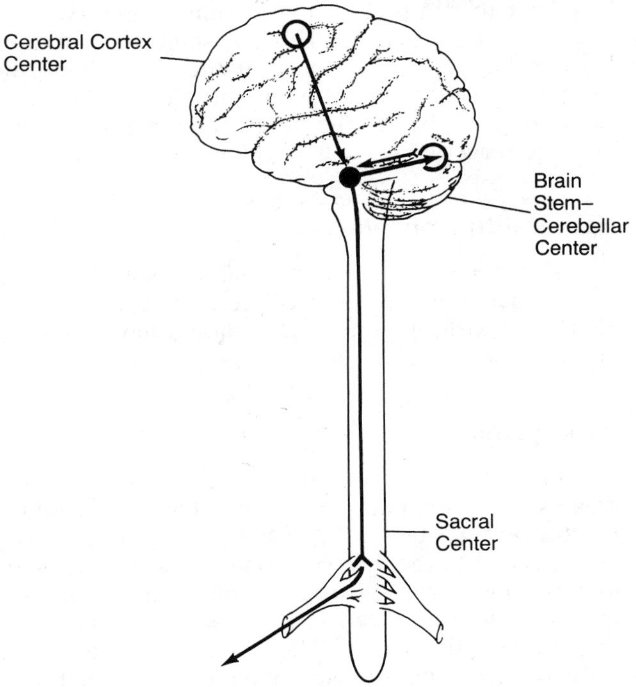

Figure 58–2. Central nervous system "voiding centers."

The primary cause is disruption of the corticoregulatory tracts. Pathologic lesions may be in either the frontal lobe area or spinal column. Cerebral vascular accidents and multiple sclerosis are two commonly encountered disease processess in which uninhibited bladder contractions are found. The cystometrogram typically shows a strong detrusor contraction at a relatively low volume. Treatment is usually with oral anticholinergic medication, such as oxybutynin (Ditropan), 5 mg. three times daily.

The Reflex Neurogenic Bladder

These patients usually have a severe neurologic deficit, such as trauma to the cord or transverse myelitis. Voiding is controlled by the sacral reflex center. The goals of therapy should be to keep the patient uninfected and develop a bladder that is neither chronically overdistended nor constantly emptying. These patients generally require long-term urologic management.

The Autonomous Neurogenic Bladder

In these patients, the sacral voiding center has been destroyed, leaving the bladder autonomous of higher centers. Patients can neither perceive bladder fullness nor initiate a detrusor contraction. Trauma or extensive pelvic surgery can create this problem. The bulbocavernosus reflex is absent. These patients usually are managed by clean intermittent catheterization.

The Sensory Neurogenic Bladder

Patients with a sensory neurogenic bladder have disruption of the afferent sensory fibers from the bladder. There is no sensation of bladder fullness and consequently of the adequacy of the bladder emptying. Diabetes mellitus and multiple sclerosis are diseases in which this type of problem may occur. Patients can be managed with timed voidings.

The Motor Neurogenic Bladder

These patients have adequate sensation of bladder filling but are unable to initiate a detrusor contraction. Tumor, trauma, or diabetes mellitus can cause this problem. Patients are best managed by clean intermittent catheterization.

It is possible, of course, for patients to have combinations of these problems or incomplete lesions. Some lesions are reversible while others remain stable over many years. In other cases, the voiding dysfunction worsens as the underlying disease process advances. The goal in any patient with a neurogenic bladder is to keep the genitourinary system uninfected and to preserve renal function. The use of chronic indwelling catheters in these patients invariably leads to infection, tissue damage of the bladder and kidney, stone formation, and eventually renal insufficiency. A number of pharmacologic agents, such as oxybutynin chloride, are available to improve the bladder's storage capabilities. If the patient has use of the hands, intermittent catheterization using clean technique is preferable to an indwelling catheter.

INCONTINENCE

Patients with urinary incontinence have problems in the storage phase of urinary bladder function. The general approach to the patient is the same as outlined above. Additional inquiries into the history serve to delineate the type of incontinence.

Stress Incontinence

Stress incontinence is the involuntary loss of urine associated with increased intra-abdominal pressure. It is most commonly found in women but may also be seen in men who have pelvic surgery. The usual history is one of loss of urine with coughing, sneezing, or lifting. Most women, at some time in their lives, will experience an occasional episode of stress incontinence. However, if incontinence is frequent and the patient is forced to wear pads to protect her clothing, urologic evaluation should be sought. It is important to differentiate stress incontinence from urge incontinence.

Urge Incontinence

Incontinence associated with an immediate need to urinate and not associated with stress is referred to as urge incontinence. It is a common complaint. Patients usually complain that they hardly have enough time to reach the commode. Most of the patients do not, in fact, have incontinence, only the feeling of impending incontinence. However, some women will, in this situation, have a bladder contraction with resultant loss of urine. These women may have unstable bladders that will contract with the slightest provocation (Mundy, 1985). A trial of an anticholinergic agent, such as dicyclomine (Bentyl), may be helpful. It is important to remember that neoplasms of the bladder as well as other intravesical pathology can also cause urge incontinence.

Overflow Incontinence

A greatly distended bladder will begin to overflow. This problem is most commonly encountered in male patients with silent prostatism and diabetics with neuropathy. The usual complaint is voiding in small amounts. The diagnosis becomes obvious when the distended bladder is palpated.

Pediatric Problems

The pediatric patient can present the primary care physician with urologic problems in diagnosis and management. The nature of these problems changes as the child matures.

NEONATAL PROBLEMS

Ambiguous Genitalia

It is usually easy to determine the gender of the newborn within the first few minutes of life. However, in some cases the sex of the newborn is uncertain. If a question of gender should arise, examination of the external genitalia will provide important clues. The scrotum or labioscrotal fold should be examined for the presence of gonads since ovaries almost never descend. The size of the phallus on stretch should be measured from base to tip, and the location of the urethral meatus should also be documented. Additional information can be obtained from an ultrasound examination of the pelvis and retroperitoneum, which will provide information as to the presence of a uterus. Chromosomal sex is determined with a buccal smear or karyotyping.

The most common cause of sexual ambiguity is congenital adrenal hyperplasia caused by a 21-OH deficiency (Walsh, 1978). In the female, this entity leads to fused labia and clitoral hypertrophy or both, while in the male the problem does not present problems in neonatal sex identification but rather in sexual precosity in infancy. In addition to the evaluation outlined above, serum electrolyte determination should be made to document salt loss that, if severe, may lead to death. Elevated serum 17-hydroxyprogesterone and urinary 17-keto are important in making the diagnosis. Treatment of the adrenal insufficiency is by steroid replacement and the masculinized external genitalia in the female by reconstructive urologic surgery.

Neonatal Hydronephrosis

The increased use of prenatal ultrasound has led to the increased detection of fetal hydronephrosis. Newborns with hydronephrosis should have immediate urologic consultation.

Hypospadias

Incomplete closure of the penile genital folds creates a hypospadiac urethra in which the urethral meatus fails to open in the distal portion of the glans penis. Distal to the urethral opening on the hypospadiac phallus fibrous bands are found in the urethra groove. These will lead to a chordee or bending of the phallus with erection. The foreskin is incompletely formed and is usually described as a dorsal hood. The degree of hypospadias varies from mild forms in which only the distal glandular urethra is absent to severe forms in which the urethra opens in the perineum. In severe hypospadias, sexual identity must be made before any attempts at reconstruction are made (Belman, 1985).

In the hypospadiac male, circumcision should never be performed in the newborn period since the foreskin is used for construction of the distal urethra. Surgical repair within the first year of life is usually successful in creating a normal appearing phallus.

Posterior Urethral Valves

The persistence of urethral folds distal to the prostate leads to obstruction of the normal flow of urine (King, 1985). These folds are referred to as urethral valves. It is important that the newborn male is observed in the first 24 hours of life for adequacy of the urinary stream. In any male with urosepsis, uremia, or a palpable distended bladder, posterior urethral valves should be suspected and urologic consultation obtained.

PREPUBESCENT PROBLEMS

Urethral Stenosis

The normal urethral meatus is an elliptically shaped opening located on the distal glans penis. Occasionally, irritation from diapers and powders will lead to narrowing of the urethral meatus. Overzealous diagnosis of this condition should be avoided. If a good urinary stream is observed, meatal stenosis does not exist.

Cryptorchidism

All infant males should be examined for normal testicular descent. Failure of the testicles to descend into the normal position in the scrotum is referred to as cryptorchidism. In full-term boys, the incidence is 3 to 6 per cent while in premature infants the incidence may be as high as 30 per cent (Frey, 1982). Patients should be referred to a urologist and treatment started by 10 months of age. There is increased fertility with early treatment. Patients with cryptorchidism have a 20 per cent increased risk of malignancy and thus need yearly follow-up and instructions in self-examination.

OTHER PEDIATRIC PROBLEMS

Scrotal Swelling

Normally, the palpable scrotal contents include the spermatic cord, testicle, and epididymis. The first step in determining the nature of an additional scrotal mass is transillumination. If the mass transilluminates, it is most likely benign (hydrocele). Nontransilluminable masses need further evaluation, such as ultrasound, to exclude a testicular neoplasm. The adolescent child, suspected of having a varicocele, should be examined in the supine and standing position. The varicocele should disappear when the patient is supine.

Urinary Tract Infections

Urinary tract infections are common in children. Children with urinary tract infections should be evaluated with a VCUG and ultrasound examination of the kidneys. If either shows an abnormality, such as vesicoureteral reflux or a renal anomaly, consultation is indicated.

Incontinence

Unsuppressible bladder contractions are common in children and lead to maneuvers to prevent incontinence, such as squirming, squatting, leg crossing and other sphincter-tightening techniques. This can lead to high intravesical pressure, vesicoureteral reflux, and urinary tract infections.

Enuresis

Nocturnal wetting is found in up to 15 per cent of 5 year olds and 1 per cent of 15 year olds. As suggested by these figures, most children eventually outgrow this problem. If the patient is uninfected, has no problems emptying the bladder, and has no daytime wetting, no further work-up is necessary. Noninvasive testing using ultrasound for assessment of postmicturition bladder residual and upper tract evaluation can be done if parents insist. Imipramine or alarm systems can be used in selected cases (Esperanca and Gerrurd, 1969; Koff, 1988) (see chapter 41).

Genitourinary Malignancies

The screening for and diagnosis of malignancies comprises a considerable proportion of the primary care physician's activities. As in solid tumors in other organ systems, those arising in the GU tract are treated best when detected early.

RENAL NEPHROBLASTOMA (WILMS' TUMOR)

Nephroblastoma is the most common renal malignancy of childhood. The median age of detection is about 3 years of age. In most patients, the presenting sign is a palpable mass discovered on routine physical exam. However, an abdominal mass palpated in the newborn is more likely to be a dysplastic kidney. Tumors may grow quite large before presenting systemic symptoms. IVP, CT scanning, and ultrasonography can aid in the preoperative evaluation, but the diagnosis is made principally by surgical intervention that allows for staging of the disease. In addition to surgery, adjuvant treatment includes radiation and chemotherapy (Green, 1985).

RENAL ADENOCARCINOMA

Carcinoma of the kidney, also known as nephrocarcinoma, clear cell carcinoma, or hypernephroma, is not easily detectable on physical exam. The retroperitoneal position makes the kidney accessible to the examining hand only possible in the thinnest of patients. Palpation of a kidney even in a very thin patient should make the examiner suspicious that there is underlying pathology. Adenocarcinoma of the kidney has often been called the clinician's tumor because of the multiple ways in which it can present. These include fever of unknown origin, unexplained weight loss, anemia, polycythemia, and paraneoplastic syndromes (e.g., ectopic adrenocorticotropic hormone production). The classic triad of pain, hematuria, and a mass is seen mainly when the disease is in an advanced stage. Tumors growing in close proximity to the collecting system may present early with hematuria when the tumor is still small.

Patients suspected of harboring a renal cell carcinoma require an expeditious evaluation. The intravenous urogram provides important information regarding the architecture of both renal units. However, it cannot definitively differentiate between a solid neoplasm or a simple renal cyst, the latter of which is extremely common. A renal ultrasound is sensitive in differentiating these two entities. If all the ultrasonographic signs for a cystic lesion exist in an asymptomatic patient, further work-up is usually not necessary (Pollack, 1982). However, if doubt exists or the patient has hematuria or other symptoms, then CT examination is indicated. In unusual cases, renal arteriography may be necessary to make the diagnosis. Once the diagnosis is suspected, a bone scan and chest x-ray are necessary in the preoperative work-up. Urinary cytology is not helpful in making the diagnosis since cells are not shed into the collecting system.

The primary treatment of renal cell carcinoma is surgical removal. Patients with metastatic disease at the time of diagnosis rarely benefit from nephrectomy. Currently, effective chemotherapy for renal cell carcinoma does not exist. Radiation therapy is ineffective against the primary disease. Immunotherapy does hold some promise for the future (deKernion, 1983).

CARCINOMA OF THE RENAL PELVIS

Carcinoma of the renal pelvis arises from the uroepithelial lining of the upper collecting system. Micro- or macroscopic hematuria is usually the presenting finding. An intravenous urogram will usually show a filling defect within the renal pelvis or calyceal system. Modern ureteroscopic instruments have improved the urologist's ability to differentiate these tumors from other nonopaque filling defects such as blood clots or noncalcified calculi. Voided urinary cytology may aid in the diagnosis, but the yield is usually low. The treatment is primarily surgical, nephroureterectomy being the standard surgical procedure.

CARCINOMA OF THE URETER

Carcinoma of the ureter also arises from the transitional cell uroepithelial layer lining the ureter. Hematuria is the most common initial finding and negative filling defects in the ureter on IVP are the characteristic radiographic findings. With larger tumors, the kidney may appear hydronephrotic or may be totally obstructed and nonfunctioning. Standard treatment is surgery, which usually consists of nephroureterectomy.

CARCINOMA OF THE BLADDER

Rare in patients under 40, the incidence of carcinoma of the bladder increases with age (Cutler and Henry, 1982). It is a disease with a wide spectrum of pathology from the small noninvasive papillomas to the fast-growing solid lesions that can rapidly lead to the patient's demise. The presenting complaint is often gross hematuria. With other patients, an unexplained microhematuria, either continuous or intermittent, requires evaluation. Patients with bladder tumors may present with bladder irritability, an especially dangerous situation when this symptom leads to a label of cystitis or urethral syndrome, and the patient is not referred for cystoscopy.

The evaluation of a patient with unexplained hematuria includes consultation with a urologist and cystoscopy, which usually can be done as an outpatient procedure under local anesthesia. At the time of cystoscopy, urinary cytology is usually obtained. If a bladder tumor is found, management will depend on the grade and stage of the tumor. Low-grade, low-stage tumors can almost always be handled with endoscopic techniques of removal or ablation either with fulguration, transurethral resection, or laser ablation. Up to 70 per cent of patients with superficial bladder tumors will develop recurrences or new occurrences from months to years after the initial onset (Cutler and Henry, 1982). Therefore, patients must be followed closely with frequent cystoscopies to ensure early detection and treatment of recurrences. There is some evidence that instillation of chemotherapeutic agents into the bladder will retard the onset of new tumors.

Tumors that are invasive into the bladder wall, in general, require a more aggressive therapy. Although small muscle-invading lesions may at times be handled endoscopically, the majority require major extirpative surgery with cystectomy and urinary diversion. Currently, there is accumulating evidence that cisplatin-based chemotherapy regimens are effective against metastatic uroepithelial cancers, but long-term evaluation of these chemotherapeutic regimens is still pending (Sternberg and Yugoda, 1985).

CARCINOMA OF THE URETHRA

Carcinoma of the urethra is relatively rare and is found more frequently in the male with a history of urethral stricture and venereal disease. In these patients, a rapid worsening of symptoms should raise suspicion of the possibility of a cancer arising in the area of stricture. Palpation of the entire urethra in both the male and female patient should be a routine part of the general medical exam. Treatment is principally surgical although in the female patient interstitial radiotherapy may be effective (Sullivan and Grabstald, 1978).

CARCINOMA OF THE PROSTATE

Carcinoma of the prostate is the second most common malignancy of the adult male in the United States. Unfortunately, since there is no good screening test for early disease, over 50 per cent of these malignancies are discovered after they have spread beyond the confines of the prostate. The presentation varies depending on the stage of disease. A small, hard nodule in the prostate does not give rise to symptoms and can only be detected by a thorough rectal exam of the prostate. Patients may present with urinary retention, but this occurs when the disease is advanced. However, patients may have concomitant prostatic hypertrophy, central gland disease producing disturbances of voiding, and prostatic carcinoma, peripheral gland disease. Low back or hip pain in the older patient may be the first sign of the disease, signaling metastases to the lumbar spine.

A prostatic nodule detected by the primary physician on rectal examination always requires further evaluation. Needle biopsy can be done either transrectally or transperineally and will usually establish the diagnosis. The biopsy can usually be done accurately under ultrasound guidance. Once the diagnosis is established, clinical staging is done: an IVP to document ureteral involvement, cystoscopy to assess bladder involvement, serum acid phosphatase to detect spread outside the prostatic capsule, and bone scan and chest x-ray to detect distant metastases. CT scanning has not proved helpful in clinical staging. Treatment of localized disease is usually surgery consisting of radical prostatectomy, although in some patients radiation therapy is an effective alternative, especially if other concurrent diseases are present. Recently, a prostatic specific antigen has proven useful in following the response to therapy (Stamey et al., 1987). The assay is not useful as a screen for the detection of carcinoma of the prostate since levels also are elevated with benign prostatic hypertrophy.

Patients with advanced disease present therapeutic challenges. Testosterone deprivation will result in significant symptomatic relief of pain and sense of well-being in patients with carcinoma of the prostate. However, hormonal manipulation either by orchiectomy or estrogen therapy has not been shown to increase patient survival, and, currently, this form of therapy is reserved for palliation of the symptomatic patient (Veterans Administration Cooperative Urological Research Group, 1968). Patients with significant bladder outlet obstruction can be managed with transurethral resection while those with localized bony metastasis can be treated with spot radiation for pain relief. There is no known effective chemotherapy for carcinoma of the prostate.

CARCINOMA OF THE TESTES

Carcinoma of the testes is a disease of the younger male and is most prevalent between 20 and 40 years of age. The most common presenting complaint is a painless mass in the scrotum. Usually, the diagnosis is not difficult to make although at times there is difficulty differentiating a mass in the epididymis from that in the testicle. Acute epididymitis is usually associated with pain, fever, leukocytosis, and pyuria. A transcrotal ultrasound may be helpful in differentiating a neoplasm of the testes from an inflamed epididymis. If considered epididymitis, it is important to follow the patient to confirm that the swelling resolves.

Once a testicular tumor is suspected, the patient must be referred to a urologist for rapid establishment of the diagnosis and treatment. Common testicular tumors are seminoma, teratoma, embryonal cell carcinoma, and choriocarcinomas. Preoperative evaluation should include serum markers, B-HCG and AFP, chest x-ray, and CT of the retroperitoneum. The diagnosis is established via inguinal orchiectomy. Transcrotal biopsy should never be done in a patient with a suspected carcinoma of the testicle since it will contaminate the scrotal lymphatics. Further treatment is determined by the cell type and stage of disease. In general, patients with seminoma (30 per cent of all testicular tumors) are treated with radial orchiectomy and radiotherapy with a 90 to 95 per cent cure rate. Patients with nonseminomatous tumors require further surgery with retroperitoneal node dissection and/or chemotherapy (Skinner and Lieskovsky, 1988). Patients with carcinoma of the testes require careful follow-up since there is an increased risk over the general population of developing a cancer in the contralateral testicle.

CARCINOMA OF THE PENIS

Carcinoma of the penis is rare in the circumcised male. These tumors are squamous cell in origin and present as firm, irregular lesions of the skin. As the lesion advances, the underlying structures are directly invaded. It is important for the physician of an uncircumcised male to teach good hygiene and to retract the foreskin on routine exam to search for such a lesion since tumors in the early stages are curable. Unfortunately, delay in patient presentation is frequent either from embarrassment or neglect. Tumors limited to the foreskin can usually be treated with circumcision while lesions of the shaft require either partial or total penectomy.

BENIGN PROSTATIC HYPERPLASIA

Prostate

The prostate of the younger male is a walnut-sized gland located above the urogenital diaphragm, surrounding the bladder neck. The muscle fibers of the trigone-bladder neck complex extend down the urethra and invest into the substance of the prostate. With such an intimate relationship between these two organs, it is apparent that pathologic processes in one will affect the other. The prostate can be thought of as consisting of glandular prostatic tissue located in the peripheral zone of the prostate and a central zone of periurethral glands immediately surrounding the urethra. The majority of the prostate is made of the peripheral glandular material but with advancing age there is gradual involution of the peripheral zone and hypertrophy and hyperplasia of the central glandular tissue. If there is sufficient enlargement of these centrally located glands, the prostate will encroach upon the lumen of the urethra, narrowing its diameter and elongating it resulting in an increased resistance to urinary flow.

Clinical Presentation

There is a wide spectrum of presenting complaints and problems for men with benign prostatic hyperplasia (BPH). Patients with very large prostates, as determined by rectal exam, that reveal an absence of median sulcus and an inability to reach the base of the prostate with an examining finger may have no symptoms. On the other hand, some patients with a palpably small gland may have the so-called median lobe hypertrophy in which the subtrigonal prostatic tissue enlarges and creates a ball valve–like obstruction of the urethra. In some patients with "silent prostatism," there is gradual prostatic enlargement leading to bladder decompensation from increasing outflow resistance, and they present eventually with urinary retention, hydronephrosis, and uremia. Most frequently, however, patients present with a symptom complex loosely referred to as prostatism. This term encompasses the symptom complex of urinary frequency, urgency, nocturia, hesitancy, and postmicturition dribbling. Symptoms may wax and wane over many years. Progression of symptoms does not always occur. It has been estimated that 20 to 25 per cent of the males will require operative intervention for BPH by the time they are 80 (Birkhoff, 1983). If the urinary symptoms progress, gross hematuria may also occur. This is usually attributed to rupture of dilated veins around the bladder neck. As residual urine increases, patients may develop urinary tract infections that are difficult to eradicate without improving bladder emptying.

Evaluation

Men are usually not reticent in describing their voiding problems, and often voiding complaints will initiate the office visit. However, some patients will not discuss their voiding patterns unless specifically asked. In the review of systems, the physician should specifically ask about changes in daytime and nocturnal voiding. Inquiry should also be directed to the caliber of the urinary stream, the presence of initial hesitancy or terminal dribbling, double voiding, urgency and urge incontinence, and hematuria. A history of recurrent urinary tract infections should also be investigated.

On physical exam, the lower abdomen should be inspected for a midline mass caused by a distended bladder. If gentle deep palpation in the midline elicits a strong urge to void, inadequate bladder emptying should be suspected. Percussion in the suprapubic region especially in the thin patient can outline a distended bladder.

The rectal exam allows some estimation of the size of the prostate and is an excellent screening exam for carcinoma of the prostate. The normal prostate has the consistency of the thenar eminence of a clenched fist. Carcinomas, on the other hand, are usually firm areas within the substance of the gland. Thus, on palpation of the prostate, it is important not only to sweep the examining finger over the surface of the gland to gain an estimation of size but also to detect areas of firmness within the gland. It is important to remember that an increased size of prostate alone is not an indication for either referral or surgical intervention. Urinalysis is an integral part of the exam. Blood urea nitrogen (BUN) and creatinine can be used as an index of renal function but may not be elevated if hydronephrosis has not developed. An acid phosphatase should be drawn before the prostatic exam since manipulation of the prostate may cause a spuriously high serum level of the enzyme (Pearson and Dombrouskis, 1983).

Management

The management of patients with BPH varies with the severity of presenting symptoms. Acute urinary retention should be treated with Foley catheter drainage and referral to a urologist. Cystitis may exacerbate symptoms and should be treated with appropriate antibiotics. Hematuria cannot be attributed solely to BPH in the older male and always requires a thorough evaluation. As mentioned above, many symptoms may remain constant over many years or may wax and wane. Surgery is usually reserved for those patients whose symptoms interfere with their life style or affect renal function.

The most commonly performed procedure for obstructive uropathy is the transurethral resection of the prostate. This endoscopic procedure can be performed with minimal morbidity. Hospitalization is short (3 to 5 days), and full recovery is usually rapid. The procedure is associated with a small risk of incontinence (< 1 per cent) and impotence (< 6 per cent) (Blandy, 1986). Patients with severely decompensated bladders may have very slow return of bladder function after relief of the obstruction.

BENIGN DISEASES OF MALE EXTERNAL GENITALIA

A variety of benign diseases can affect the male genitalia. Among the most common are the sexually transmitted diseases that are covered in chapter 31.

SKIN LESIONS

Phimosis

Phimosis in the adult male can be distressing. Patients may complain of pain on intercourse or develop recurrent episodes of balanitis. The problem seems to be especially common in diabetics who frequently present with *Candida balanitis*. Treatment consists of control of the infection and circumcision that, in the adult, can be done under local anesthesia.

Balanitis Xerotica Obliterans

This poorly understood process affects the glans penis of the older male. Typically, a nonpainful thickening of skin of the glans and urethral meatus occurs. This results in severe meatal stenosis that can be difficult to control.

Lichen Nitidus

This is a commonly encountered benign condition of the external genitalia. At the corona of the glans penis, the patient notices a circumferential row of pearly white papules. No treatment is necessary other than reassurance.

Condyloma Acuminatum

This is one of the most frequently encountered genital skin lesions of the sexually active population. Lesions may occur anywhere on the external genitalia and vary from pinpoint to large verrucous lesions. The lesions are typically multiple and appear as small cauliflower-like growths. Examination of the urethral meatus is important since these lesions can at times be found there. Treatment includes podophyllin application, fulguration, or laser ablation. Sexual partners also must be examined and treated. Recurrence rates may be as high as 70 per cent (Coldiron and Jacobson, 1988).

Angiokeratoma of Fordyce

This benign condition occurs on the scrotum of the older male. It appears as numerous small (1 to 2 mm.), slightly raised, cherry red lesions. No treatment is necessary.

BENIGN DISEASES OF THE SCROTAL CONTENTS

Epididymitis

The patient with acute epididymitis usually presents with an acutely swollen, exquisitely tender scrotum. The disease usually has a gradual onset over 12 to 24 hours. In the early stages of the disease, the testicle can be palpated anterior to the swollen epididymis. As time progresses, an inflammatory hydrocele may develop and make differentiation from the testicle difficult. In these situations, scrotal ultrasound may be helpful. In later stages of the disease process, fixation of the skin to the underlying inflammatory mass occurs. Pyuria, leukocytosis, and fever are frequently present although their absence does not rule out the diagnosis. Differentiating between testicular torsion and epididymitis can be very difficult. In some cases, surgical exploration is necessary to confirm the diagnosis.

Treatment consists of antibiotics, usually tetracycline (500 mg. four times a day × 10 days), or erythromycin. Supportive measures include ice, scrotal elevation, and bed rest. If patients appear toxic, hospitalization and intravenous broad-spectrum antibiotic coverage is warranted. If the symptoms fail to resolve within 72 hours, abscess formation should be suspected and surgical exploration is indicated.

Hydrocele

Hydrocele occurring in the pediatric patient is almost always associated with a developmental patent processus vaginalis. In the adult patient, the pathologic process consists of a gradual accumulation of fluid between the parietal and visceral layers of the tunica vaginalis investing the testicle. It is most important to differentiate this condition from an indirect inguinal hernia. The commonly occurring hydrocele usually feels as though it surrounds the testicle but not the cord structures. Additionally, there is no change in size in the supine position and a hydrocele is transilluminable. Definitive treatment consists of surgical excision if the patient is symptomatic. Asymptomatic patients require no therapy as long as the examining physician is certain there is no underlying pathology such as a testicular tumor causing the hydrocele.

Spermatocele

Literally a small body of sperm, a spermatocele arises as a fluid-filled cyst of the epididymis. These are usually discovered on self-examination or on routine physical exam. Spermatoceles are transilluminable. Treatment consists of patient reassurance and surgical removal undertaken only when size warrants.

Varicocele

A varicocele is an abnormal dilatation of the veins of the pampiniform plexus. Varicoceles are very common, being found in up to 15 to 20 per cent of the adult population. The cause and effect relationship between a varicocele and infertility is controversial (Greenberg and Lipshultz, 1978). On physical examination, the scrotal side containing the varix (usually the left) has a characteristic bag-of-worms consistency. This is pronounced when the patient is standing and usually diminishes or vanishes completely when the patient is supine. A varicocele causing scrotal discomfort may, if the discomfort is significant, require surgical treatment. This consists of division of the spermatic veins, usually done through an inguinal incision.

UROLITHIASIS

Stones can occur in the GU tract from the tip of the renal papilla to the tip of the external urethra meatus. Stones of the upper urinary tract are most commonly encountered in Western countries, while in lesser developed countries where nutrition is poor and untreated cystitis and parasites more common, bladder stones occur more frequently especially in children. The management of renal and ureteral lithiasis has been revolutionized by technologic advances in urologic instrumentation, radiographic imaging, and shock wave technology.

Pathogenesis

There has been considerable investigation into the pathogenesis of renal lithiasis in the last 20 years. Calcium oxalate and phosphate stones are the most commonly encountered stones in the United States. Hypercalcuria may be the underlying cause of recurrent stone disease resulting from excessive absorption of calcium from the gut (absorptive hypercalcuria) or from excessive renal leak of calcium from the renal tubule. The two can be differentiated by outpatient metabolic studies (Pak, 1987). Hypercalcuria may also result from resorptive hypercalcemia secondary to a parathyroid adenoma. Other causes of hypercalcuria include prolonged immobilization, sarcoidosis, drug ingestion (such as acetazolamide), type I renal tubular acidosis, and hypervitamintosis D. In some patients, calcium stones occur in the presence of normal 24-hour urinary calcium excretion levels ($<$ 300 mg. per day). Although excessive oxalate may lead to calcium stone formation, disease states where this occurs are rarely encountered. However, some patients with intestinal bypass procedures or inflammatory bowel disease may have hyperabsorption of dietary oxalate.

Uric acid stones account for approximately 5 to 10 per cent of the stone disease. Uric acid is poorly soluble in a solution below a pH of 5.75, and these patients typically have an acid urine. Hyperuricosuria and hyperuricemia are not always present in patients with uric acid stones.

Struvite or triple phosphate stones are associated with chronic urinary tract infections. These stones are associated with an alkaline urine (pH $>$ 7.0) created by urea-splitting organisms. Struvite stones are more common in women than in men.

Cystine stones develop in patients with an inborn error in the reabsorption of the amino acids: cystine, lysine, ornithine, and arginine. Only the relatively insoluble cystine forms stones. This type of stone is the most common stone encountered in children.

SIGNS AND SYMPTOMS

Stones in the GU tract may cause pain, hematuria, infection, or be entirely asymptomatic. Signs and symptoms are a function of the size and location of the stone. Calyceal stones may cause an intermittent dull back ache. Stones free in the renal pelvis can give intermittent flank pain when they occlude the ureteropelvic junction. Pain usually radiates around to the anterior abdominal wall and may simulate biliary colic. Stones moving down the ureter are usually associated with excruciating pain distributing from the flank down to the scrotum or inner thigh. Stones located near the bladder may cause severe urgency and frequency. Nausea and vomiting are frequently experienced when the stone is obstructing. Patients typically cannot find a comfortable position and are diaphoretic. Fever should be regarded with extreme concern since an obstructed and infected kidney may lead to sepsis and death.

On examination, the patient with a nonobstructing stone (e.g., in a calyx) will not have abnormal physical findings. Patients with high-grade obstruction of the ureter and kidney will usually have costovertebral tenderness. Tenderness to palpation in the lower quadrant may be found in patients with lower ureteral stones. Hypoactive bowel sounds can occur because of a reflex ileus. Patients with infection superimposed upon obstruction may appear toxic, with tachycardia and diaphoresis, and, if treatment is delayed, they may go into shock.

EVALUATION

The evaluation of the patient with urolithiasis may be done leisurely as an outpatient if the patient is asymptomatic or urgently if the patient presents with acute symptoms in the emergency department. Patients suspected of a stone need a rapid assessment including location of the stone, the degree of obstruction, and whether infection is present. A urinalysis usually shows microscopic hematuria, but the absence of hematuria does not rule out a calculus. A white blood cell count should be obtained as well as a BUN. A marked elevation in the white blood cell count is not common with a simple stone, and the BUN should not be elevated if the patient has two normal kidneys and one stone.

The intravenous urogram is the easiest way to establish the diagnosis of urolithiasis in a patient with normal renal function. Careful inspection of the abdominal film taken before the injection of a contrast agent may show the position and size of a radiopaque stone. Radiolucent stones cannot be seen on the plain abdominal film while opaque stones overlying a transverse process of a vertebral body or over the sacrum also will not be visualized. Delay in excretion of contrast will be seen in patients with significant obstruction. A delayed film 1 or more hours after injection is helpful in this situation to delineate the site of obstruction. It is important for patients with lower ureteral stones to empty their bladders and obtain a postvoid film in order that contrast in a full bladder does not obscure the stone's position.

Patients with a history of allergy to contrast media must be handled with caution. Intravenous Benadryl and steroids can be given prior to injection of the contrast medium, or newer hypoallergenic agents can be used. In some situations, retrograde pyelography is the safest route to establish the diagnosis. Ultrasound or nuclear renography may also be helpful in detecting obstruction in this situation.

A stone suspected in the pregnant patient also requires special consideration. Although irradiation is cumulative and should be minimized to the fetus, it is in the first 6 weeks of gestation that x-ray exposure is most dangerous. In the second and third trimester, one can obtain a limited IVP with a scout film followed by a film at 1 hour. This is usually sufficient to make the diagnosis as well as localize the stone.

In cases where a negative filling defect is found and the distinction between a radiolucent stone and a urothelial tumor cannot be made with standard radiographic techniques, a CT scan may differentiate between the two based on the detection of small amounts of calcium in the stone (Resnick and Kursh, 1984).

TREATMENT

Treatment, of course, depends on many factors, but the size of the stone, presence of significant pain or obstruction, and/or associated infection usually determine the need for and type of therapeutic intervention.

Size

As stone size increases, the likelihood of passage decreases. Stones greater than 6 mm. are unlikely to pass spontaneously through the ureter and into the bladder (Carstensen and Hansen, 1973).

Obstruction

As stone size increases, obstruction also increases. Ureteral stones that are totally obstructing on IVP usually require more aggressive intervention than nonobstructing stones.

Infection

The presence of infection behind a stone is a urologic emergency. With proper drainage of the involved renal unit, sepsis can usually be avoided.

Pain

Severe pain requires hospitalization and intramuscular narcotics. Moderate pain can be handled with oral analgesics, such as acetaminophen with codeine.

Stone Recovery

It is important that the urine is strained in order to capture a stone that passes. The stone can then be sent to one of several commercial labs for analysis.

Several treatment options are listed below. The optimum treatment of the small asymptomatic stone in the kidney is controversial. Careful consideration must be given to the potential for development of problems versus the risk of treatment. Stones ($<$ 5 mm.) located in the ureter can usually be managed expectantly with oral analgesics. However, as the stone size increases, some form of therapy is usually required.

Stone Dissolution

Uric acid stones can, at times, be managed without urologic manipulation. Uric acid is insoluble at a pH less than 5.5 but in alkaline urine the solubility dramatically increases. Patients with uric acid stones can usually be managed with systemic alkalinization either with sodium bicarbonate or oral citrate solution so that the urinary pH is greater than 6.0. Patients who are unable to take oral fluids can be managed with intravenous M/6 lactate solution (Kursh and Resnick, 1984). If the stone is totally obstructing, a percutaneous nephrostomy can be placed above the stone and $NaHCO_3$ instilled directly onto the stone's surface. Once the stone is dissolved, patients should be maintained on a urinary alkalinization program indefinitely.

Extracorporeal Shock Wave Lithotripsy (ESWL)

ESWL has revolutionized the treatment of urinary calculi (Chaussy and Fuchs, 1987). This technology employs focused shock waves to pulverize the stone. Stone fragments are then washed down the ureter into the bladder. Stones located in the renal pelvis and upper ureter are best treated by this method. As the stone size increases, however, morbidity from the procedure also increases. The most common problem is obstruction of the lower ureter by stone fragments. If these are numerous, they may fill the distal ureter and form a *Steinstrasse* or street of stone. A variety of urologic maneuvers are available to deal with this problem. Large stones often need more than one treatment session to adequately fragment the stone. Overall there is greater than a 90 per cent success rate with ESWL for stones located in the kidney or renal pelvis. ESWL has been used with somewhat less success in the treatment of stones of the mid and lower ureter.

Percutaneous Nephrolithostomy

This technique, developed in the late 1970's and early 1980's, involves percutaneous access to the kidney using standard Seldinger techniques (LeRoy and Segura, 1986). Once access to the collecting system is attained, the opening is gradually enlarged to allow the introduction of instruments capable of crushing and extracting the stone. Although usually successful, the technique is invasive and is not without morbidity, which includes pain, hemorrhage, and A-V fistula formation. Since the widespread availability of ESWL, this technique is now less frequently used.

Ureteroscopy

Advances in instrumentation have led to the development of rigid and flexible instruments for direct ureteral visualization. These instruments have fostered the development of a variety of graspers and baskets for the removal of ureteral stones under direct vision. Larger stones that cannot be removed in their entirety can be fragmented with an ultrasonic lithotrite or a pulsed laser and the fragments either removed directly or allowed to pass spontaneously.

Surgical Removal

Surgical removal of either renal or ureteral calculi is infrequently performed. However, there are situations where this is the best available method.

Bladder Calculi

Bladder calculi are almost exclusively found in patients with bladder outlet obstruction or indwelling catheters. Removal is relatively simple either by direct endoscopic manual crushing using a lithotrite or through the use of an endoscopically placed electrohydraulic lithotripsy probe. Once the stone is removed, bladder outlet obstruction should be treated.

Long-Term Management

The analysis of a recovered stone or stone fragment guides the long-term care. Patients should collect a 24-hour urine for measurement of calcium, phosphorus, uric acid, and creatinine excretion. If the patient forms more than one stone per year, a full metabolic work-up is indicated.

The foundation for stone prevention is adequate hydration. Patients should be encouraged to drink at least 10 to 12 glasses of water per day with a glass of water at bedtime, as well as one during the night. Patients should further increase their fluid intake during periods of hot weather and after strenuous exertion. Fluids high in oxalates, teas, and colas should probably be discouraged.

Patients found to have renal hypercalcuria can be treated with thiazides. The usual dose of hydrochlorothiazide is 50 mg. twice daily. Patients with absorptive hypercalcuria can be treated with a dietary restriction of calcium, oral calcium binders (such as cellulose phosphate), or orthophosphates.

Patients with renal tubular acidosis (type I) are treated with hydration and alkalinization. Those with hyperoxaluria should be treated by maintaining good hydration and restriction of foods rich in oxalates. Pyridoxine in large doses can reduce urinary oxalate levels. Patients with hyperuricuria can be treated with allopurinol and urinary alkalinization. Cystine stones are treated with alkalinization and hydration. Penicillamine is also often used to form a soluble complex with cystine. Patients with infection and stones should have a careful search for urologic abnormality to prevent recurrent infection and stone formation (Table 58–1).

UROLOGIC EMERGENCIES

Renal Trauma

Although protected by the lower ribs and thick muscles of the flank, the kidneys may be injured by either penetrating or blunt trauma. When the family physician is called to evaluate a patient with blunt trauma, a careful general and focused abdominal and flank exam should first be performed. A microscopic exam of the urine should be included. The absence of blood does not rule out renal injury since renal pedicle injury can occur without resulting hematuria. Fracture of the lumbar processes of L1 or L2 on a flat plate of the abdomen or chest x-ray revealing fracture of the eleventh or twelfth ribs should alert the physician to a possible renal injury. When there is concern of a renal injury, a consultation with a urologist and an IVP with tomography should be obtained if the patient's condition permits. Nonfunction of a renal unit may result from renovascular disruption, which should be confirmed by renal arteriography. Extravasation of contrast on an IVP usually means that a major renal laceration has occurred. Minor contusions of the kidney usually do not produce abnormalities in the IVP. If the intravenous pyelogram is abnormal, a CT scan is useful in staging the extent of the injury.

Treatment of the renal injuries is determined by the stability of the patient and the extent of associated injuries. Minor contusions are treated with bed rest. The treatment of patients with major renal lacerations is controversial. Conservative management consists of hospitalization and strict observation. Secondary hemorrhage can occur up to 2 weeks after the initial injury. Additionally, the presence of hematoma and urine around the kidney may lead to perirenal fibrosis and hypertension. Surgical exploration is mandatory if there is evidence of continued retroperitoneal hemorrhage. Immediate surgical exploration in cases of major renal trauma can be difficult, but the advantages are debridement of necrotic tissue, repair of renal parenchyma, and establishment of drainage. However, these must be weighed against the risk of loss of the renal unit if uncontrollable hemorrhage is encountered as well as the risks associated with a major surgical exploration.

Table 58–1. CLASSIFICATION OF URINARY TRACT STONES

Stone Type	Incidence	Causes	Treatment
Calcium oxalate	33 per cent	Renal leak of calcium; excess absorption of calcium; hyperparathyroidism; excess oxalate excretion (congenital oxaluria, inflammatory Buluel disease); idiopathic	Thiazide (renal leak); cellulose phosphate (excess absorption); parathyroidectomy; limit oxalate hydration
Calcium phosphate	6 per cent	Idiopathic; distal renal tubular acidosis	Hydration; potassium citrate (distal RTA)
Mixed calcium oxalate and phosphate	35 per cent	Above	Above
Magnesium ammonium phosphate	15 per cent	Infection	Antibiotics; acetohydroxamil acid
Uric acid	8 per cent	Persistent aciduria, hyperuricosuria, chronic dehydration	Allopurinol, potassium citrate, hydration
Cystine	3 per cent	Cystine excess (congenital defeltin amino acid reabsorption)	Potassium citrate, penicillamine, hydration

Ureteral Trauma

Isolated ureteral injury for nonpenetrating renal trauma is rare. Occasionally, the ureteral pelvic junction will be disrupted in a severe deacceleration injury or in a hyperextension injury in a child. Most ureteral injuries are iatrogenic, such as during difficult pelvic surgery. Patients with iatrogenic ureteral injury will often develop fever, ileus, and leukocytosis. A mass (urinoma) may develop in the area of injury if there is no mechanism for egress of urine. If suspected, an IVP and urologic consultation should be obtained.

Bladder Trauma

Injuries to the bladder may occur during pelvic crush injuries. The bladder may be ruptured by a direct blow, especially if it is distended, or may be punctured by a bony fragment from a disrupted pelvic skeletal ring. Injuries may be either intra- or extraperitoneal. Patients with bladder injury usually have grossly bloody urine. If the patient does not have blood at the tip of the urethra (the *sine qua non* of urethra rupture) then a Foley catheter should be passed into the bladder. In cases where bladder injury is suspected, a cystogram should be performed by instilling 200 cc. of a diluted contrast medium into the bladder using gravity drainage. An anterior-posterior and lateral film is taken with the bladder distended. The bladder is then emptied and a drainage film obtained. Usually, the cystogram differentiates between intra- and extraperitoneal rupture. The treatment of bladder injuries is usually surgical repair although small extraperitoneal ruptures have been treated successfully with bladder drainage alone (Corriere and Sandler, 1986).

Urethral Trauma

The majority of significant urethral injuries occur in males. Injuries are most often encountered in patients who have sustained blunt injuries. Major urethral injuries occur with either straddle injuries in which the bulbus urethrae is crushed or pelvic crush injuries in which the membranous urethra is sheared off at the pelvic floor. If urethral injury is suspected (either by the nature of the injury or the presence of blood at the meatus), a retrograde urethrogram should be obtained.

This is performed by injecting a water-soluble contrast medium into the urethra through a small (#12) Foley catheter placed just within the urethral meatus with the balloon slightly inflated. The patient should be positioned so that the pelvis is rotated 30 degrees to the horizontal plane and the penile urethra drawn parallel to the coronal plane. Urologic consultation should be sought if urethral injury is demonstrated by extravasation of the contrast medium. Passage of a Foley catheter should never be attempted in this situation.

The urethra can also be injured by attempts at difficult urethral catheterization. Usually, the prostatic urethra is injured when the catheter develops a false passage into the periurethral glandular substance. Blood appearing at the urethral meatus should alert the physician that a false passage has been created. Urologic consultation should be obtained before any further urethral manipulation is attempted.

Penile Trauma

Because of its mobility, the penis is not a common site of trauma. However, injury to the penis and scrotum may occur with degloving injuries associated with machinery injuries. The extent of injury should be assessed and the wound debrided and covered with a moist, sterile dressing. Urologic consultation should be obtained.

Rarely, the penis may be fractured during sexual activity. When this occurs, the patient develops pain, detumescence, and swelling of the penis as blood escapes from the ruptured tunica albuginea. Treatment is prompt surgical repair.

Testicular Trauma

A direct injury of a testicle is extremely painful. Severe trauma can cause a rupture of the tunic albuginea of the testicle and a hematoma develops rapidly. In cases in which the trauma appears to be minor, treatment is conservative with scrotal elevation and ice packs. If the integrity of the testicle cannot be assessed, urologic consultation should be obtained.

Testicular Torsion

Testicular torsion may occur at any age but it is most commonly seen in adolescence (Allen and Ransler, 1982). Torsion of the spermatic cord results in ischemia of the testicle with the rapid onset of pain. Scrotal swelling usually occurs. If the patient is seen early after the onset of the torsion, the testicle will be found to have an abnormal lie high in the scrotum with its longitudinal axis oriented parallel to the horizontal plane. Fever, leukocytosis, or pyuria are uncommon in patients with torsion. Testicular Doppler or technetium studies may be useful in differentiating between torsion and epididymitis. However, false negatives can occur with both and should not be relied upon solely for the diagnosis.

When the examining physician suspects testicular torsion, urologic consultation should be promptly obtained. Occasionally, the testicle can be detorsed by infiltrating the spermatic cord with 1 per cent xylocaine and then rotating the testicle in the direction opposite to the torsion. However, this is a temporary solution, since only surgical orchiopexy will prevent recurrence.

Torsion of the Appendix Testicle/Epididymis

Torsion of the vestigal appendages on the testicle or epididymis may cause acute scrotal pain. Characteristically, the patients are in the same group as those in whom torsion of the testicle occurs. A small painful (often blue) lump is felt on examination. If the primary physician and consultant are confident that the patient does not have a testicular torsion, then nonsurgical treatment can be instituted.

Paraphimosis

Paraphimosis results from failure to replace the retracted foreskin after manipulation. The foreskin becomes edematous and painful. Usually, the foreskin can be reduced by grasping it between the thumb and index finger of both hands while the thumbs simultaneously push on the glans penis. In situations where this is unsuccessful, the dorsal foreskin should be incised (dorsal slit) under regional anesthesia as discussed under circumcision. One or two chromic sutures may be needed to control bleeding and oversew the mucosa after the paraphimosis is reduced.

UROLOGIC SKILLS

Bladder Catheterization

Catheterization of the male urethra requires skillful and gentle technique. The meatus of the urethra should be carefully cleansed. In the uncircumcised male, this requires that the foreskin be fully retracted. The foreskin in patients with severe phimosis should be cleansed as well as possible with cotton swabs impregnated with an antimicrobial solution. The smallest Foley or straight catheter that can be easily passed, one that will drain the bladder contents, should be used. There is little rationale for using a large (> 16F) catheter if drainage of the bladder is all that is required. The catheter should be liberally lubricated with a water-soluble lubricant prior to passage. The patient should be supine and the bed adjusted to a comfortable height for the physician before catheterization is attempted. The penis should be straightened by grasping the glans and raising it 90 degrees to the horizontal plane. The catheter should be advanced slowly. There is usually slight resistance felt as the catheter encounters the distal urethral sphincter. Gentle steady pressure will usually allow the catheter to slip past this point. Once the catheter is in the bladder, a sample of urine should be collected and sent for culture and sensitivity. If the catheter is to remain in place, the balloon should then be inflated and the catheter taped to the abdominal wall. In situations where there is a history of urethral stricture, urologic consultation should be obtained. In those situations where a urologist is not available and a catheter cannot be passed, suprapubic catheterization of the bladder can be performed.

Long-term catheterization is needed in some situations. The smallest catheter should be used in this situation. The catheter should be changed every 4 to 6 weeks. Prophylactic antibiotics should not be used as they only lead to the development of resistant strains of bacteria.

Vasectomy

Family planning, postponing, or ending procreation is an integral part of family practice. Eighty per cent of American couples by the age of 30 state that they have all the children they want or can raise (Mayhew, 1981). With 20 years of reproductive life remaining, more and more are electing a permanent method to prevent reproduction.

A counseling session with the couple requesting a vasectomy is essential to determine their level of knowledge and commitment. The physician should also explore with the couple the other available options of contraception, the vasectomy procedure, and possible risks of the operation.

Vasectomy is usually performed as an outpatient procedure, either in the physician's office or in an ambulatory surgery area of a hospital. The penis is taped to the abdomen, scrotum shaved and cleansed, and the operative field draped. The vas deferens is isolated from the other cord structures and elevated toward the skin. After a local anesthetic agent has been infiltrated into the skin and the tissues surrounding the vas, a towel clamp is used to secure the vas. A small incision is made over the vas and it is delivered through the wound by sharp and blunt dissection freeing it from the investing areolar tissue. A segment is excised and sent to pathology for confirmation. The free ends of the severed vas are either ligated with a nonabsorbable suture, occluded with metal clips, or fulgurated by electrocautery. Every effort should be made to keep the cut ends of vas on separate tissue planes. This can usually be accomplished by enveloping one vas segment in a pursestring suture of the surrounding fascia. After hemostasis is assured, the dartos fascia and skin are closed.

The postoperative care is important to the prevention of complications. It is best to have the patient wear an athletic or postoperative hernia supporter for 3 days. The patient should stay recumbent for the first 2 hours after the operation with an ice bag applied to the scrotum and rest for the remainder of the day. Intercourse and strenuous work or activity should be avoided for at least 3 days after the operation.

It is important that the patient and his mate realize that sterility does not result immediately after the operation. At least 12 to 15 ejaculations are necessary for all sperm to be emptied from the seminal vesicles. An alternate form of contraception must be continued until sterilization is confirmed by the pathology report, which states that the specimens removed at the time of operation were vas deferens, and there are two ejaculate specimens absent of sperm.

There are major and minor complications of vasectomy. The minor include the pain caused by the procedure, scrotal swelling and ecchymosis, superficial wound infection, and small hematomas. The problems resolve with little active therapy other than time, reassurance, and avoiding drugs that encourage bleeding.

The major complications cause more concern to both patient and physician. Large hematomas may have to be surgically evacuated. Epididymitis should be treated with an anti-inflammatory medication and a broad-spectrum antibiotic. Deep abscesses may require incision and drainage in addition to appropriate antibiotic therapy. Sperm granuloma presenting as a nodular swelling may be a secondary response to leakage from the severed end of the proximal vas. If small and asymptomatic, it does not require treatment. Larger, symptomatic granulomas are treated with anti-inflammatory and antibiotic medication. If persistent, excision may be necessary. Patients with sperm granulomas may be at increased risk for recannulization and should have periodic semen analyses.

Pregnancy is reported in between 1 in 1000 and 1 in 2000 couples in whom the male partner has had a vasectomy. This is ascertained by the partner becoming pregnant and sperm being detected in the postvasectomy patient semen specimen. The physician cannot guarantee sterility but only that the segments of vas were removed as confirmed by pathology report and that follow-up ejaculate specimens did not contain sperm.

While most physicians accept vasectomy as a highly effective and simple method of permanent conception control with few apparent side effects, some physicians are concerned that antisperm immune complexes may cause late adverse effects in some patients. The body must develop a new mechanism for sperm disposal. As sperm degenerate and die, multiple antigens are released and absorbed into the body. Approximately 50 per cent of the men who have had a vasectomy develop autoantibodies to sperm. However, at the present time, there are no published studies of vasectomized men developing increased disease as compared to match controls.

Vasectomy, a simple and effective permanent contraceptive method, has a great appeal for those who are concerned about the long-term, personal, and social risk of unplanned procreation. At the present time, it is considered by most physicians to be a safe method, useful in the control of overpopulation and improving the quality of family life.

Neonatal Circumcision

Until recently, circumcision of the newborn was considered performed primarily for social or religious reasons although medical statements were given to support it. Although controversial, recent medical studies do support that the procedure decreases the risk of penile cancer, balanitis, urinary tract infection in the infant male, and sexually transmitted diseases (Wiswell and Metcalf, 1988). Contraindications to circumcision include the presence of neonatal illness, prematurity, bleeding disorder, and congenital anomaly such as hypospadias.

PREPARATION

The infant should be physically well and in stable condition. To lessen the chances of regurgitation and aspiration, the infant should not eat for several hours before the procedure. A suction bulb syringe must be readily available. The infant is restrained by a device or assistant. The operative area is prepped with an antiseptic solution and a perforated drape placed over the infant, exposing the penis. The drape should not cover the infant's face, allowing monitoring during the procedure.

PROCEDURE

Anesthesia

The dorsal nerves emerge on each side of the penis in an area corresponding to the ten and two o'clock positions at the root of the penis (Figure 58–3). It is at a point 0.5 cm. distal to these positions that the injection is made after stabilizing the penis with gentle traction. A tuberculin syringe is filled with 1 ml. of 1 per cent lidocaine without epinephrine. The 27-gauge needle is inserted at a 20 to 30 degree angle at either the ten or two o'clock position into the subcutaneous tissue to a depth of 0.25 to 0.50 cm. The needle tip should be freely movable, verifying that it is in the subcutaneous and not the erectile tissue. Infiltrate 0.3 to 0.4 ml. of anesthetic solution, taking care to aspirate the syringe before injection to prevent intravascular injection. The procedure is repeated on the opposite side, allowing 3 or 4 minutes for anesthesia to take effect.

METHODS

One of two methods for newborn circumcision is used by most family physicians. They are the plastic bell, marketed as Plastibel (Fig. 58–4), and the Gomco clamp (Fig. 58–5).

Plastibel

The Plastibel is a clear acrylic dome, marketed in a variety of sizes (1.1, 1.2, 1.3, and 1.5 cm. in diameter). It is flanged near the proximal opening of the dome to accept a ligature, and has a paddle-like handle over the distal opening facilitating manipulation of the device (see Fig. 58–4*A*) (Seeley, 1989).

To perform the circumcision, the skin is adequately prepared, and a penile dorsal nerve block is performed as previously described. The opening of the foreskin is dilated by inserting a closed, small hemostat and opening the jaws a few millimeters. It is essential that the meatus is identified to prevent the inadvertent insertion of hemostat or scissors.

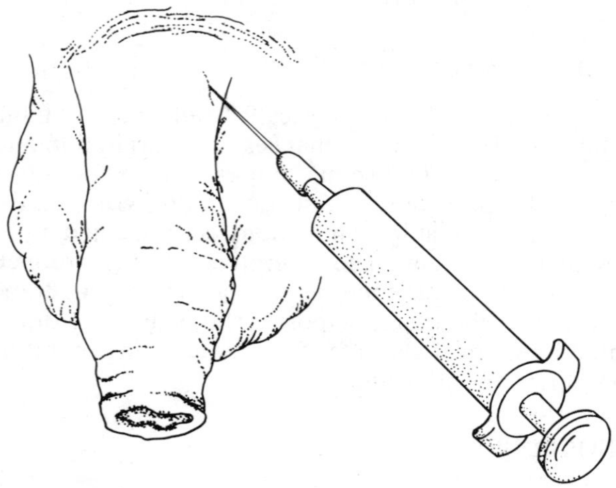

Figure 58–3. Penile dorsal nerve block at the 2-o'clock position. (From Kimmel, S. R.: Neonatal Circumcision. Basic Procedures in Family Practice, New York, Churchill Livingstone, 1984, pp. 100–106.)

After enlarging the opening of the foreskin, a flexible probe is inserted between the skin and the glans and the adhesions bluntly dissected. The dorsal skin is clamped with a hemostat for a distance of 5 to 6 mm. It is then removed and a scissors cut is made along the crushed line made by the clamp (see Fig. 58–4*B*). The prepuce is retracted, and the adhesions at the corona are lysed by blunt dissection (see Fig. 58–4*C*).

The plastic bell is inserted between the foreskin and the glans, avoiding the 6 o'clock position to prevent damage to the ventral blood vessels (see Fig. 58–5*D*). To facilitate inserting the bell, the corner of each side of the dorsal slit is grasped with mosquito clamps and, after inserting the bell, the clamps are crossed over one another. An alternative method of preventing displacement of the bell is placing a safety pin through the two corners of the slit after the bell is in place. It is essential to insure that the bell size is optimum and that the rim of the bell is not creating undue pressure on the frenulum at the ventral midline. Assured of correct position of the bell, the linen ligature packaged with the device is placed around the foreskin just proximal to the flange on the bell, which can be palpated through the foreskin (see Fig. 58–5*E*). The ligature is then tied very tightly with a square knot. The ligature must be secure enough to produce complete ischemia of the tissues underlying the ligature to insure hemostasis. The redundant tissue is removed by trimming with a scalpel, utilizing the distal groove of the flange as a guide. The handle is then broken off by flexing it back and forth until it separates and the broken edges may be smoothed by rubbing with a rough towel or with an emery board. No dressing is necessary. The tissue beneath the ligature sloughs in about 5 to 10 days, and the bell and ligature fall off.

The parents should be advised to report bleeding, marked swelling, or erythema that might indicate infection. They should be reassured that, although most often the sloughed bell is found free in the diaper, it may be retained by a thread of tissue for 2 to 3 days, much as is sometimes exhibited by the umbilical cord stump. Follow-up care is routinely planned 2 weeks after hospital discharge.

Follow-Up Care

The most common complications of circumcision are bleeding and infection. The operative site must be observed in the early postoperative period for bleeding. Oozing can usually be controlled by pressure or a gauze saturated with 1:100,000 epinephrine. Occasionally, interrupted chromic gut sutures will be required, particularly if the bleeding is in the area of the frenulum. Routine care includes placing a gauze on the operative site, which usually falls off after several diaper changes. Petroleum jelly may then be applied until the exposed edges and mucous membrane are sufficiently toughened to withstand irritation from the diapers. During this time, the child should be sponge bathed as usual until the circumci-

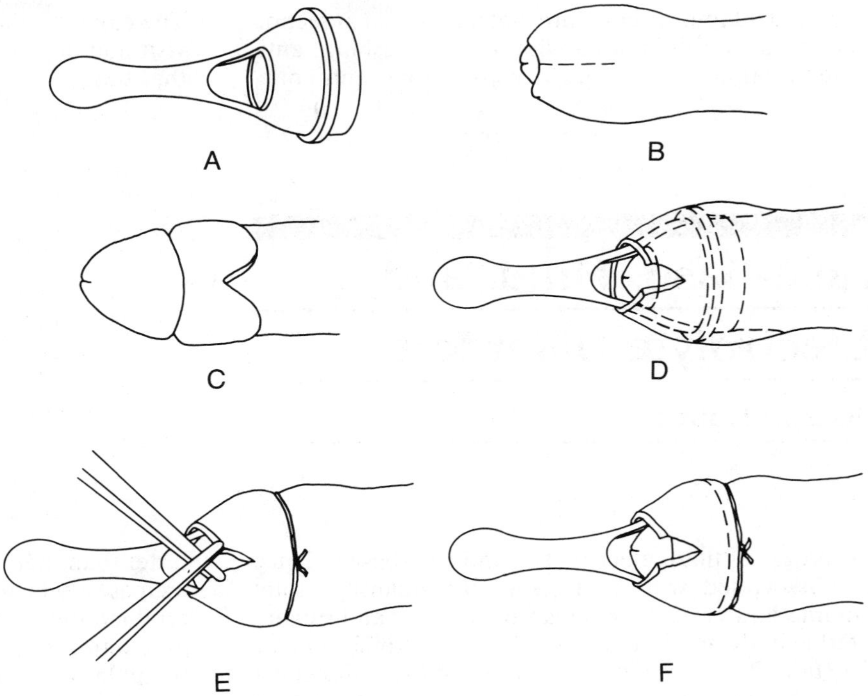

Figure 58–4. Circumcision using the Plastibel.

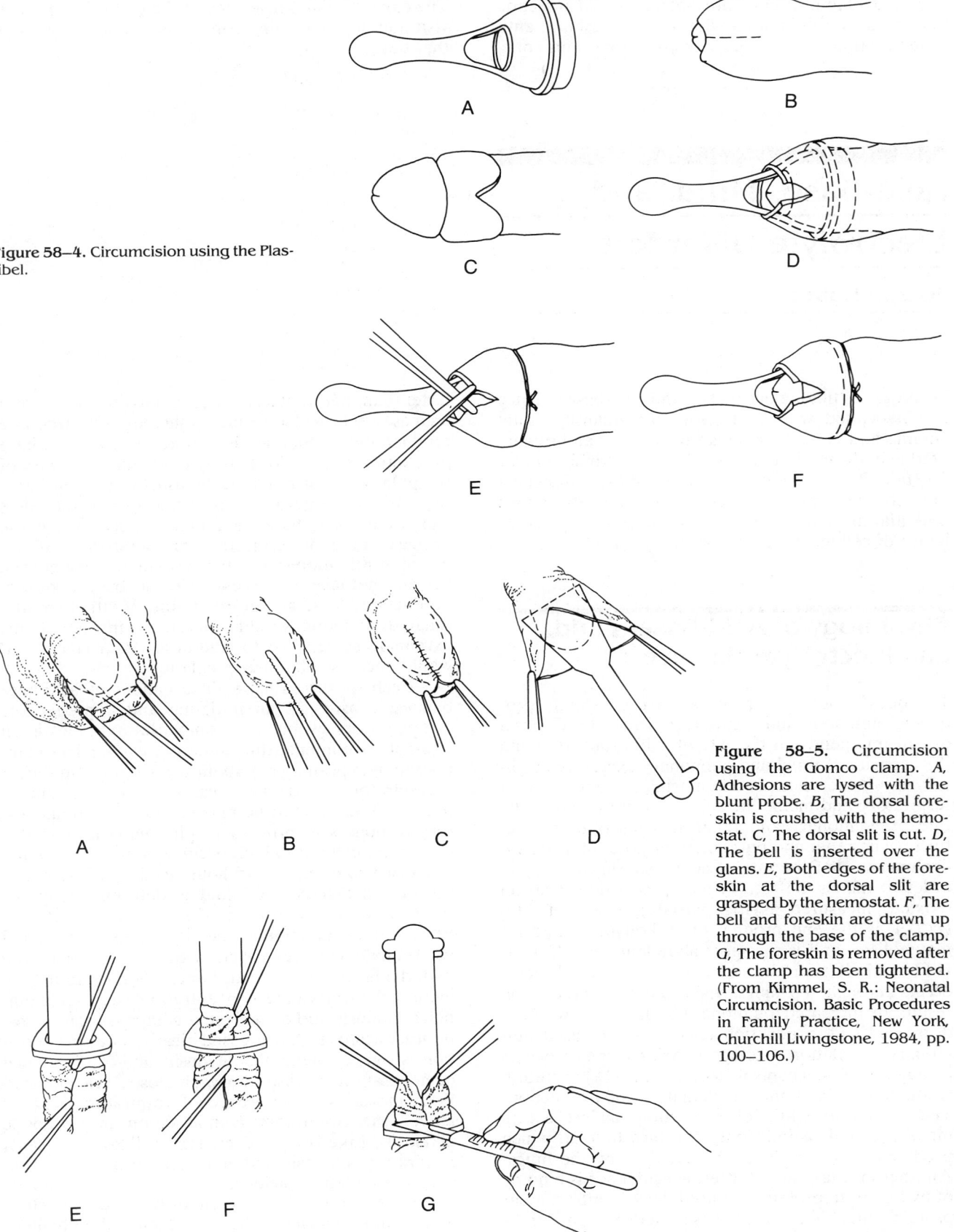

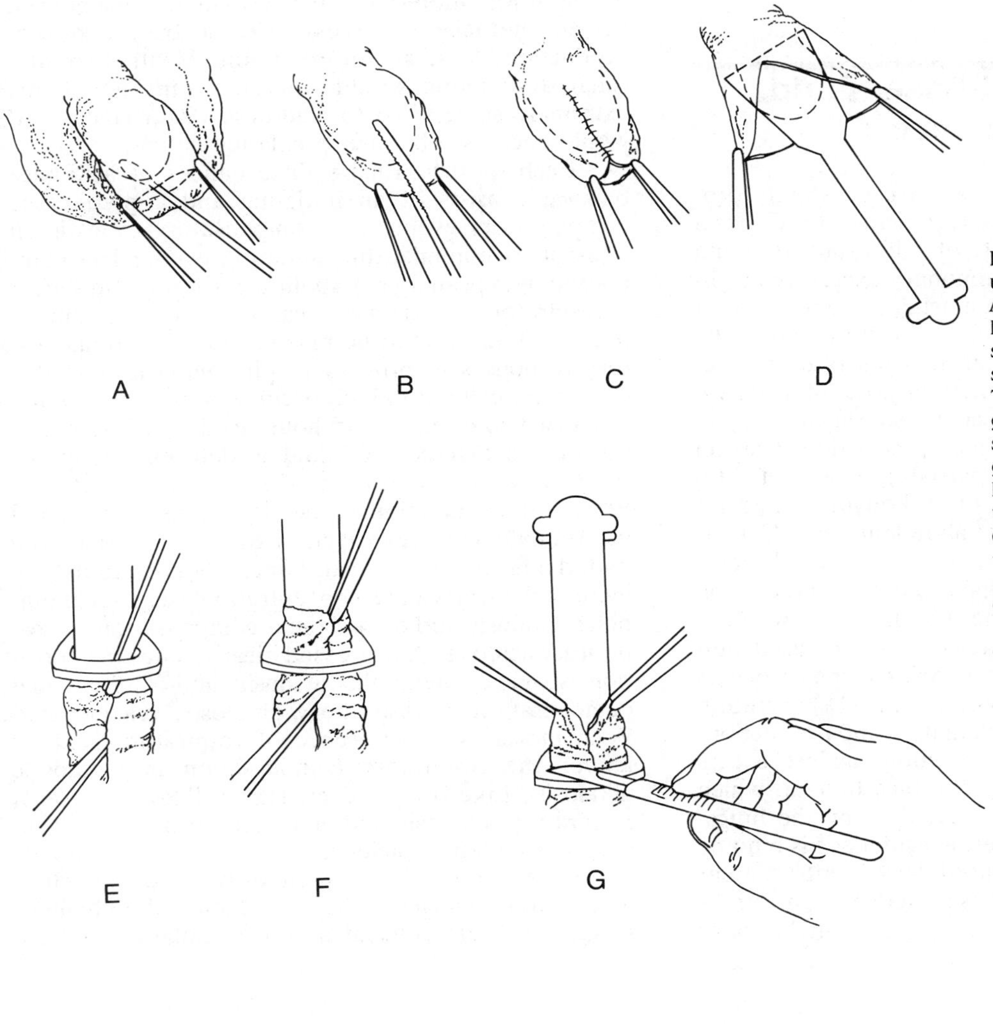

Figure 58–5. Circumcision using the Gomco clamp. *A*, Adhesions are lysed with the blunt probe. *B*, The dorsal foreskin is crushed with the hemostat. *C*, The dorsal slit is cut. *D*, The bell is inserted over the glans. *E*, Both edges of the foreskin at the dorsal slit are grasped by the hemostat. *F*, The bell and foreskin are drawn up through the base of the clamp. *G*, The foreskin is removed after the clamp has been tightened. (From Kimmel, S. R.: Neonatal Circumcision. Basic Procedures in Family Practice, New York, Churchill Livingstone, 1984, pp. 100–106.)

sion and umbilical cord are healed. Local infection may occur and is treated with a good washing, antibiotic ointment, and, rarely, a parenteral antibiotic. The circumcision is inspected at the first routine office visit and any remaining adhesions should be lysed at that time.

Acid-Base, Fluid, and Electrolyte Disorders

Joseph Hobbs

Disorders of fluid, electrolytes, and acid-base balance are associated with changes in the quantity (total volume and effective circulating volume) and quality of the body fluids that can disrupt normal cellular function. The detection, therefore, of these disorders must be prompt and specific in order to reduce potential morbidity and mortality imposed by disturbance of cellular functions of vital organs.

Physiology of Acid-Base, Fluid, and Electrolyte Balance

The body's metabolic processes are constantly producing metabolic and respiratory acids, the disposal of which depends on the rate of acid production and the capacity of renal and pulmonary excretory mechanisms. Under normal circumstances, the rate of respiratory and metabolic acid production equals the rate of pulmonary and renal acid disposal, respectively. The renal and pulmonary disposal of acids are dynamic so that the rate of acid disposal can vary in order to match the rate of acid production. Carbon dioxide, measured as the partial pressure of CO_2 (PCO_2), is the end product of carbohydrate and fat metabolism, and is the most abundant acid ($CO_2 + H_2O = H_2CO_3$) produced by the body. CO_2 disposal occurs through the lungs. Increased CO_2 production results in increased pulmonary ventilation, whereas decreased CO_2 production results in decreased pulmonary ventilation. Metabolic acids disposal occurs through renal mechanisms where acid (H^+) excretion is coupled to bicarbonate reclamation and production. The body's first line of protection against excess metabolic acids is buffering with bicarbonate, which produces CO_2, which can be excreted by the lungs. Another mechanism of buffering acid loads is binding of hydrogen to protein, extracellular and intracellular protein, and bone. Once these fixed concentrations of chemical and protein buffers are consumed at rates faster than their replacement, renal hydrogen disposal increases, which also results in increased bicarbonate production. As long as the variation in acid or base production or loss does not overwhelm the ability of the pulmonary or renal mechanisms to appropriately respond to these variations, no acid-base disorders will occur. Acid-base disturbances occur when the primary route of respiratory or metabolic acid removal or retention is insufficient to maintain a normal pH in the face of excess acid or base addition, production, loss, and/or retention. Ventilatory and renal dysfunction would, therefore, make patients extremely susceptible to acid-base disturbances and would decrease effective circulating volume.

Each of the primary disturbances of acid-base balance consists of an initiating and a predictable compensatory event. The compensatory event is an attempt to minimize the initiating event. The compensation in primary metabolic acid-base disturbances is respiratory in origin and can occur within minutes but may take days to be maximized. The compensatory responses in primary respiratory acid-base disorders are cellular (which occur within minutes) and renal (which occur within hours to days). The pH of the body's extracellular fluid is determined by the ratio of the concentration of serum bicarbonate to PCO_2. An examination of the alterations of PCO_2 and bicarbonate may reveal clues to the nature of the underlying acid-base disturbance. For example, an increased bicarbonate concentration suggests metabolic alkalosis and/or the renal compensation in respiratory acidosis. A decreased bicarbonate concentration suggests metabolic acidosis and/or the renal compensation in respiratory alkalosis. An elevated PCO_2 indicates the presence of respiratory acidosis and/or the respiratory compensation in metabolic alkalosis. Likewise, a decrease in PCO_2 represents respiratory alkalosis and/or the respiratory compensation in metabolic acidosis.

Other fluid and electrolyte disturbances are characterized by changes in the constituents of body fluids (e.g., potassium concentration), osmolality, and absolute and effective circulating volume. In order for body systems to function appropriately, there must be adequate amounts of volume in the intravascular, interstitial, and intracellular spaces. The amount of solutes in these spaces defines the appropriate amount of water in which they must be dissolved. Factors that are essential to maintain appropriate effective circulating volume include adequate vascular tone, oncotic and hydrostatic forces, and cardiac output as determined by preload, contractility, rate, and peripheral vascular resistance.

A General Approach to the Patients With Fluid, Electrolyte, and Acid-Base Disorders

HISTORICAL EVALUATION

Since, in primary care, the physician is frequently confronted with patients who have disorders of fluid, electrolyte, and acid-base balance, recognition of these disorders begins with an anticipation of their presence in patients who are at risk. These at-risk patients include those treated with thiazide and loop diuretics for hypertension and congestive heart failure, the patient with insulin-dependent diabetes, and children with viral gastroenteritis. Historical evaluation may reveal a patient who is at risk of development of two or more acid-base disturbances occurring concurrently (e.g., a patient with insulin-dependent diabetes mellitus and who has asthma). A history of acute weight loss or gain could be evidence of excess volume loss or retention, and a history of postural dizziness and syncope may suggest the presence of decreased effective circulating volume.

PHYSICAL EVALUATION

The physical examination should determine the level of consciousness, volume status as determined by the presence or absence of edema, postural blood pressure and pulse changes, urine output, and cardiac status (e.g., signs of congestive heart failure, dysrhythmia—rapid or slow rates). Further evaluation should determine the respiratory rate, pulmonary reserve and any impairment thereof, and abnormal growth patterns that may indicate congenital diseases that predispose to acid-base disturbances.

LABORATORY EVALUATION

Assessment of Acid-Base Balance

An elevated serum pH represents alkalemia, which could be the result of either metabolic or respiratory alkalosis or a combination of two acid-base disturbances whose resultant pH is alkalemic. A decreased serum pH indicates the presence of metabolic or respiratory acidosis causing acidemia or a combination of two acid-base disturbances, the resultant serum pH of which is acidemic. The presence of a normal pH in the presence of an abnormal bicarbonate concentration and P_{CO_2} indicates the presence of mixed acid-base disorders.

Effective Circulating Volume

The laboratory assessment of effective circulating volume can be obtained by measuring the urine sodium concentration. Urine sodium concentrations less than 10 mEq. per liter indicate avid renal sodium conservation, which is characteristic of decreased effective circulating volume. In metabolic alkalosis, the measurement of urine chloride is used to assess volume and chloride status. Urine chloride concentration less than 10 mEq per liter in the presence of metabolic alkalosis indicates volume concentration and chloride depletion as the cause of the disorder (chloride responsive metabolic alkalosis). A urine chloride concentration greater than 10 mEq. per liter in the presence of metabolic alkalosis indicates increased activity of the distal tubule independent of chloride or volume status (e.g., excess mineralocorticoid activity—chloride-resistant metabolic alkalosis). It should also be noted that urine sodium concentrations and/or chloride concentrations can be greater than 10 to 20 mEq. per liter in the setting of volume contraction if diuretics, which inhibit sodium and chloride reabsorption, are in use or if there is a tubular sodium reabsorption defect.

Anion Gap

The anion gap ($[Na^+]+[K^+]-[Cl^-]+[HCO_3^-]$) is a useful measurement to detect the presence of excess anions other than chloride or bicarbonate. These anions usually originate from metabolic acids. An elevated anion gap represents the presence of metabolic acidosis with increased unmeasured anions. This measurement is extremely useful when a large anion gap metabolic acidosis is combined with other acid-base disturbances, thus making the classic picture of decreased bicarbonate concentration with an appropriately decreased P_{CO_2} not readily apparent. A decreased anion gap is found in clinical situations that cause increased cations, such as polyclonal gammopathies, multiple myeloma, lithium intoxication, and polymyxin B administration. A decreased anion gap caused by unmeasured anions can occur in hypernatremia, hyponatremia, hypochloremic metabolic alkalosis, and errors of electrolyte measurements (overestimation of sodium bicarbonate concentration). In acid-base disturbances, possible toxin or drug consumation, which may alter level of consciousness, initiate or perpetuate organic acidosis, or cause central nervous system stimulation or depression, must be considered.

Osmolality

Although the plasma osmolality is $2(Na^+)$ + glucose/18 + BUN/2.8, the effective osmolality can be determined by $2 \times Na^+$ + glucose/18. (Note: BUN diffuses across the cell wall and, therefore, is an ineffective osmole.) If the calculated effective osmolality is decreased (hypo-osmolality or hyponatremia), water excess is present. If the effective osmolality is increased (hyperosmolality or hypernatremia), a water deficit is present.

Serum Electrolytes

The serum electrolytes are important diagnostic tools, for they often point to the primary cause of fluid, electrolyte, and acid-base disorders. As mentioned previously, alterations in the serum bicarbonate concentration implies the presence of metabolic acid-base disturbances or the renal compensation in respiratory acid-base disturbances. Serum potassium concentration elevation is more likely to indicate the presence of acidemia. It should be noted, however, that in states of acidemia, although the potassium level may be elevated, most patients (exceptions are patients with chronic renal failure) are usually total body potassium depleted. Decreased serum potassium concentration represents alkalemia, but it also can occur during the treatment of acidemic states and in profound states of potassium deficiency where the pH-induced increase in potassium is blunted. An elevated serum chloride concentration indicates hypochloremic metabolic acidosis or the renal compensation in respiratory alkalosis. Decreased serum chloride concentration represents metabolic alkalosis or the renal compensation in respiratory acidosis. The decreased sodium concentration represents hypo-osmolality or water excess. It should be noted that water excess must be interpreted in lieu of the presence of other solutes, such as glucose, lipids, and protein, that might give the false impression of water excess when actually the patient has either a water deficit or normal total body water. Elevated serum sodium indicates the presence of hyperosmolality or water deficit.

Urinalysis and Urine Potassium Concentration

The urinalysis provides important information concerning the etiologies of fluid, electrolyte, and acid-base disturbances. The urine specific gravity is elevated in the setting of overnight water restriction, hyperosmolality, decreased effective circulating volume, hyponatremia caused by volume contraction, syndromes of inappropriate ADH secretion, and excretion of osmotic agents (e.g., radiographic contrasts). Urine specific gravity is low in the setting of hypo-osmolality/hyponatremia not caused by volume contraction such as primary polydipsia, lack of ADH (nephrogenic and central diabetes insipidus), and diuretic-induced inhibition of sodium, chloride, water reabsorption, and ATN. Urine specific gravity has a direct relationship to urine osmolality, which defines, for the most part, the concentration and diluting responses of the kidney.

The presence of ketones in the urine indicates an increased use of fats as a fuel source, either because of starvation, insulin deficiency, or resistance. Urine pH is usually maximally acidic in systemic acidosis. Lack of an acid urine in the setting of systemic acidosis indicates the presence of renal tubular dysfunction. An alkaline diuresis is usually present in the setting of the recovery of metabolic alkalosis caused by volume contraction and can be present if the patient has a urinary tract infection caused by urease-containing micro-organisms. In metabolic alkalosis, urine is paradoxically acidic.

Urinary potassium concentration in the presence of hypokalemia can differentiate renal from other sources of potassium loss. Potassium loss causing hypokalemia via the GI tract and/or skin routes would result in a urinary potassium less than 10 mEq. per liter (exception is vomiting—see Hypokalemia), if there is no renal disease and if drugs that promote potassium excretion are not in use. Urinary potassium greater than 10 mEq. per liter with hypokalemia indicates inappropriate renal loss of potassium (e.g., diuretics or certain intrinsic renal defects).

Fractional Excretion of Sodium

Often it is necessary to differentiate prerenal azotemia from acute tubular necrosis. This differentiation can be determined by calculating the fractional excretion of sodium, which is the percentage of sodium filtered that eventually is excreted.* A fractional excretion of sodium less than 1 per cent indicates prerenal azotemia and those greater than 2 per cent represent acute tubular necrosis. This study becomes less helpful in the setting of chronic renal failure. The urine sediment would be free of renal tubular cells and cast in prerenal azotemia but may be present if tubular damage has occurred.

Arterial Blood Gases

Arterial blood gases are used to assess the acid-base status by measuring the pH and PCO_2 and reporting a calculated bicarbonate ion concentration. The numerical ratio of bicarbonate to PCO_2 determines the arterial pH or hydrogen ion concentration ($[H^+] = 24\ PCO_2/[HCO_3]$ or $pH = 6.1 + \log [HCO_3]/0.03PCO_2$. In all single acid-base disorders,

---

*Fraction excretion of Sodium (FE_{Na} %)

$$= \frac{U_{Na} \times P_{Cr}}{P_{Na} \quad U_{Cr}} \times 100$$

U_{Na} = Urine Sodium Concentration
U_{Cr} = Urine Creatinine Concentration
P_{Na} = Plasma Sodium Concentration
P_{Cr} = Plasma Creatinine Concentration

Table 58–2. PRIMARY ACID-BASE EVENTS

Disturbance	Primary Event	Compensatory Event	Average Rate of Compensation
Metabolic acidosis	↓ $[HCO_3^-]$	↓ P_{CO_2}	$P_{CO_2} = 1.2\ [HCO_3^-]$
Metabolic alkalosis	↑ $[HCO_3^-]$	↑ P_{CO_2}	$P_{CO_2} = 0.9\ [HCO_3^-]$
Respiratory acidosis	↑ P_{CO_2}	↑ $[HCO_3^-]$	Acute $[HCO_3^-] = 0.1\Delta P_{CO_2}$ Chronic $[HCO_3^-] = 0.35\Delta P_{CO_2}$
Respiratory alkalosis	↓ P_{CO_2}	↓ $[HCO_3^-]$	Acute $[HCO_3^-] = 0.2\Delta P_{CO_2}$ Chronic $[HCO_3^-] = 0.5\Delta P_{CO_2}$

Δ = changes in

an initial change in either bicarbonate concentration or P_{CO_2} will result in a predictable quantitative compensatory change in the corresponding factor, either P_{CO_2} or bicarbonate, respectively (Table 58–2). If that predicted compensation occurs, then the findings are consistent with a single acid-base disturbance. If the predicted compensation fails to occur, either the patient has not had time to fully compensate or more than one acid-base disturbance exists. The appropriateness of compensation in acid-base events can also be determined by the use of an acid-base map (Fig. 58–6). Data falling within the confidence bands of a particular acid-base disorder on an acid-base map are for the most part consistent with (not diagnostic of) a single acid-base disorder. The data falling outside of these confidence bands indicate inappropriate compensation for the same reasons noted above. The acid-base map does not predict the presence of three or more disturbances nor does it predict the presence of the combination of metabolic acidosis and metabolic alkalosis. Clinical correlation and/or inspection of electrolyte data (chloride concentration or anion gap) is required to appropriately interpret these more complex acid-base disturbances. All acid-base data must be correlated to the historical and physical assessment of the patient to insure appropriate interpretation.

It should be noted that none of the pH-altering effects of these primary events can be totally obliterated by the compensatory event with the exception of chronic respiratory alkalosis. Therefore, the presence of an abnormal bicarbonate concentration and P_{CO_2} when the pH is near normal would indicate the presence of two or more acid-base disturbances occurring concurrently. If two acid-base disturbances are occurring simultaneously, both of which produce either acidemia or alkalemia, the pH may be greatly deviated from normal. However, if two acid-base

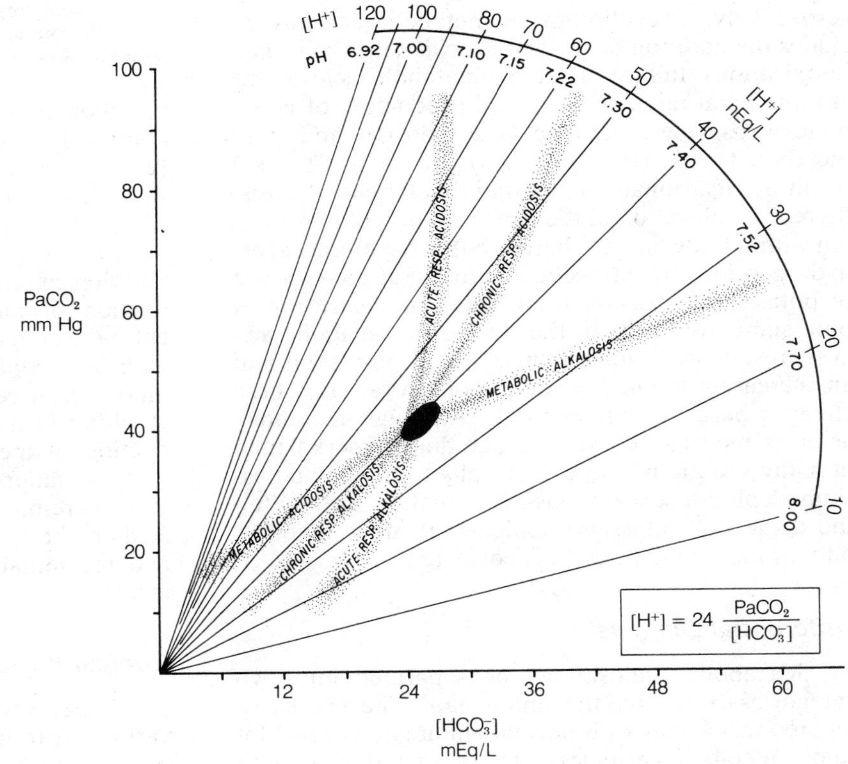

Figure 58–6. Acid-base map describing the relationships between the arterial pH, H^+ concentration, P_{CO_2}, and HCO_3^- concentration. The dark area in the center represents the range of normal values for these parameters; the stippled areas represent the different simple acid-base disturbances. Points A, B, and C indicate the three mixed acid-base disorders discussed in the text. (From Harrington, J. T. Cohen, J. J., and Kassirer, J. P.: Mixed acid-base disturbances. *In* Cohen, J. J., and Kassirer, J. P. (Eds.): Acid/Base. Boston, Little, Brown, 1982.)

disturbances occur with one producing alkalemia and the other producing acidemia, the resulting pH may be close to normal. In these mixed acid-base disturbances, the full potential of each event might be unmasked as one unknowingly corrects one acid-base disorder without anticipating the existence of the second disorder.

Primary Acid-Base Disturbances

METABOLIC ACIDOSIS

Pathophysiology

Metabolic acidosis occurs as a result of the primary depletion of bicarbonate—the body's most abundant chemical buffer. This depletion of bicarbonate is caused by either bicarbonate loss, which occurs in diarrhea, or the consumption of bicarbonate by titration with metabolic acids, which occurs in the setting of diabetic ketoacidosis. The resulting decreased bicarbonate ion concentration causes an increased ventilatory excretion of CO_2. This physiologic compensation in metabolic acidosis is such that for every one mEq. per liter decrease in bicarbonate concentration there is a 1.2 mm. Hg decrease in Pco_2. This compensation begins within minutes of the depletion of bicarbonate but may take up to 12 hours for completion. A reduction of the Pco_2 less than or greater than the appropriate compensation represents metabolic acidosis combined with primary respiratory acidosis or primary respiratory alkalosis, respectively. The etiology of metabolic acidosis includes the addition of metabolic acids (e.g., salicylate intoxication), failure to excrete metabolic acids (e.g., chronic renal failure), increased production of metabolic acids (e.g., diabetic ketoacidosis), and pure bicarbonate loss (e.g., diarrhea) (Table 58–3). As a result of bicarbonate depletion in metabolic acidosis, there is an elevation in the concentration of hydrogen ion within body fluids. There is buffering of the excess hydrogen ions by intracellular protein at the expense of potassium extrusion from cells. This extrusion of potassium from cells in the setting of metabolic acidosis results in an intracellular loss of potassium and an increased serum potassium concentration. These changes occur within minutes. Although metabolic acidosis may cause extracellular fluid hyperkalemia in many situations, there is actually total body potassium depletion except possibly renal failure. Often the degree of potassium depletion is made manifest only as metabolic acidosis is corrected.

Differential Diagnosis

Metabolic acidosis can be separated into two categories based on the anion gap. The causes of metabolic acidosis with normal anion gap (hypochloremic metabolic acidosis) are associated with pure bicarbonate loss from the body. This occurs most commonly with bicarbonate loss from the GI tract (e.g., diarrhea and ureterosigmoidostomy) and kidneys (types I, II, and IV renal tubular acidosis). Metabolic acidosis with increased anion gap (normochloremic metabolic acidosis) is caused by the addition of, failure to excrete, or the increased production of metabolic acids whose anions are not chloride or bicarbonate. As these acids are titrated with bicarbonate, they leave their negative ions behind, which results in increased unmeasured anions resulting in an increased anion gap. Increased production of metabolic acids occurs in lactic acidosis whereas failure to excrete these metabolic acids occurs in uremic renal failure. The addition of metabolic acids to body fluids occurs in salicylate intoxication and in methanol, paraldehyde, and ethylene glycol ingestion.

Table 58–3. CAUSES OF METABOLIC ACIDOSIS

- **High Anion Gap (Normochloremia)**
  - Increased Production of Organic Acids
    - Ketoacidosis
      - Alcoholic
      - Diabetic
      - Starvation
    - Lactic acidosis
    - Massive muscle necrosis
    - Decreased metabolic acid excretion
      - Renal failure
    - Ingestion of substances causing organic acidosis
      - Ethylene glycol
      - Methanol
      - Paraldehyde
      - Salicylates
- Normal Anion Gap (Hyperchloremic)
  - Bicarbonate wasting
    - Gastrointestinal tract bicarbonate loss
      - Diarrhea
      - Ureterosigmoidostomy
      - Loss of bicarbonate-containing fluid via fistulas or tubes
      - Cholestyramine
    - Renal bicarbonate loss
      - Proximal renal tubular acidosis (type II)
      - Early renal dysfunction
      - Correction of chronic hypocapnia
  - Renal hydrogen retention
    - Distal renal tubular acidosis (type I)
    - Hypoaldosteronism
    - Tubulointerstitial nephritis
  - Addition of HCl
    - Ammonium chloride
    - Some hyperalimentation fluids
  - Drugs
    - Amphotericin B
    - Acetozolamine (carbonic anhydrase inhibitors)
    - Amiloride (inhibits distal renal tubular Na^+ reabsorption)
    - Spironolactone (aldosterone antagonist)

Clinical Presentation

Patients with metabolic acidosis can present with various neurologic dysfunctions, such as alteration of consciousness or seizures, that can be a direct result of the metabolic toxins, volume contraction, or the severity of the acidosis. There may be signs of increased cardiac irritability secondary to the acidosis and the associated electrolyte disturbances. In most cases of metabolic acidosis, with the exception of uremic renal failure, there is usually evidence of decreased effective circulating volume.

If the compensatory ventilatory response in metabolic acidosis is impaired, a more significant rise in the hydrogen ion concentration will ensue; therefore, an assessment of the respiratory pattern and rate and the ability of the patient to maintain the physical effort required in the compensatory respiratory response must be made. Since most patients are volume contracted, evaluations of postural blood pressure and pulse change must be made to access the adequacy of the circulating volume. Cardiac functions should also be evaluated since in the setting of metabolic acidosis and the accompanying hypokalemia, impairment of the cardiac contractility and rhythm may occur. The history of decreased visual acuity along with the finding of retinal edema and/or papilledema strongly suggest methanol intoxication.

The electrolyte changes in metabolic acidosis are decreased pH secondary to increased hydrogen ion concentration, a decreased plasma bicarbonate, and a decreased P_{CO_2}. It should be noted that plasma chloride concentration would be increased in normal anion gap metabolic acidosis but would be normal in increased anion gap metabolic acidosis. In metabolic acidosis, for every 0.1 unit decrease in pH there should be an approximate 0.6 mEq. per liter increase in the potassium ion concentration. If this increase fails to occur, then one should consider profound potassium depletion that may be exacerbated by the correction of the acidosis. The blood urea nitrogen can be increased in many of these settings because of the associated volume contraction but may also represent the presence of intrinsic renal disease.

In metabolic acidosis, the presence of elevated glucose and ketosis can be indicative of diabetic ketoacidosis and alcoholic ketosis. Serum ketones. also can be found in the presence of starvation ketosis. Elevated serum lactate may indicate the hypoprofusion of organs that can occur in volume-contracted states. Patients with large anion gap metabolic acidosis who have a history of toxic ingestions require toxicologic screening. Urinalysis should be performed to determine urinary pH, which should be maximally acid unless there is a urinary acidification defect, such as distal renal tubular acidosis (type I RTA). Maximally urinary acidification occurs in proximal renal tubular acidosis (type 2 RTA) if the plasma bicarbonate concentration is less than 18 mEq. per liter (the depressed renal threshold for bicarbonate reabsorption in type 2 RTA). However, in proximal RTA, a plasma bicarbonate greater than approximately 18 mEq. per liter will result in a less than maximally acidic urine. Urinary sediment may reveal cast and crystals that occur in ingestions, such as ethylene glycol. Unexplained elevations in serum osmolality may also suggest methanol and ethylene glycol ingestion. The metabolic acidosis caused by salicylate intoxication may be proceeded by respiratory alkalosis caused by salicylate-induced central nervous system stimulations. A patient suspected of acute alcoholic intoxication because of breath odor and behavior who has a large anion gap should suggest ethylene glycol ingestion since alcoholic ketoacidosis is associated with a relatively small anion gap.

Treatment

The primary aim of treatment of metabolic acidosis is the cessation of acid production and retention and pure loss of bicarbonate. Another primary aim of treatment is to maintain and/or restore the effective circulating volume. The issue of when to use bicarbonate in metabolic acidosis remains controversial, and the decision should be made based on a total assessment of the patient's bicarbonate and respiratory reserves. If the pH is less than 7.2, and the bicarbonate ion concentration is less than 10 mEq. per liter and there is a persistent production of acids (organic acidosis) or a large uncontrolled loss of bicarbonate, the utilization of sodium bicarbonate is warranted. Impairment of the mechanism of compensatory hyperventilation would add support to the decision to use bicarbonate. The initial goal when using bicarbonate therapy in metabolic acidosis is to raise the pH only to 7.2 to avoid posttreatment metabolic alkalosis. In the setting of diabetic ketoacidosis, bicarbonate therapy is given only when the pH is less than 7.0 and the bicarbonate is less than 10 mEq. per liter. This assumes that the patient has the ability to sustain ventilatory compensation and the absence of other concurrent causes of acidosis. The need of sodium bicarbonate in the setting of diabetic ketoacidosis is minimized because this organic acidosis can be promptly terminated with the administration of insulin, and the complicated picture of lactate acidosis can be prevented with the administration of appropriate volume repletion. Bicarbonate is also used in the setting of salicylate intoxication to alkaline the urine, which promotes renal clearance of salicylate.

In the treatment of diabetic ketoacidosis, potassium is required once urinary output is established because treatment of hyperglycemia with insulin and the restoration of normal acid-base balance will exacerbate any underlying extracellular potassium deficits. Phosphate salts are used to treat underlying phosphate deficiency, which may predispose to muscle neurosis in diabetic ketoacidosis and in other causes of metabolic acidosis. If the patient has ingested a toxin, an increase in glomerular filtration rate may be helpful for rapid renal removal of the agent (salicylate and paraldehyde). In certain cases, hemodialysis (e.g., salicylates, methanol, ethylene glycol) and the use of ethanol to block enzymes that produce toxic substances from the ingested toxin (i.e., methanol and ethylene glycol) may be necessary.

METABOLIC ALKALOSIS

Pathophysiology

Metabolic alkalosis results when there is primary retention of bicarbonate. The retention of bicarbonate is caused by either hydrogen loss from body fluid (e.g., vomiting) or the excessive administration of bicarbonate to body fluids (e.g., milk alkali syndrome) (Table 58–4). The results of the excess bicarbonate administration and/or hydrogen loss are an increased pH (decreased hydrogen concentration) and elevated plasma bicarbonate concentration. In metabolic alkalosis, the compensation for the primary elevation of plasma bicarbonate is hypoventilation such that for every 1 mEq. per liter increase in bicarbonate concentration the P_{CO_2} rises by 0.9 mm. Hg. (increased P_{CO_2}). It should be noted that hypoxemia can blunt this compensatory response, therefore making metabolic alkalosis a poorly compensated acid-base disturbance especially in severe settings. The increased bicarbonate retention in metabolic alkalosis is caused by accelerated activity of the distal renal tubule. This accelerated activity results in increased sodium reabsorption in exchange for potassium and hydrogen loss, which is coupled to cellular production of bicarbonate that is added to the blood. The causes of increased sodium reabsorption in the distal tubule are primary mineralocorticoid excess or decreased effective circulating volume and chloride deficiency. One other setting where bicarbonate can be retained and cause metabolic alkalosis is when bicarbonate is administered at rates faster than the kidneys' excretory capacity, e.g., milk alkali syndrome. Metabolic alkalosis can also be caused by intracellular shifts of hydrogen ion as would occur in profound potassium depletion. One or more of these factors must be present in order for plasma bicarbonate levels to rise since the threshold of renal bicarbonate excretion is so low (24 mEq. per liter).

Metabolic alkalosis can be divided into two types based on whether the alkalosis is generated by decreased effective circulating volume and chloride deficiency (i.e., chloride responsive) or caused by either autonomous excessive activity of the distal tubule, intracellular sequestration of hydrogen, or excessive alkali administration (i.e., chloride resistant).

Table 58–4. CAUSES OF METABOLIC ALKALOSIS

Secondary mineralocorticoid excess resulting from volume and chloride depletion causing bicarbonate retention (chloride responsive; urine chloride less than 15 mEq. per liter)
Gastrointestinal H^+ loss
Vomiting/nasogastric suction
Congenital chloriduria
Renal H^+ loss
After or late in diuretic therapy
Correction of chronic hypercapnia
Primary mineralocorticoid excess causing volume expansion and bicarbonate retention (chloride resistant, urine chloride greater than 20 mEq. per liter)
Primary aldosteronism
Cushing's syndrome
Primary reninism
Excess ingestions of glycyrrhizic acid (licorice)
Bartter's syndrome
Other states of mineralocorticoid excess
Hydrogen-ion intracellular sequestration (chloride resistant, urine chloride greater than 20 mEq. per liter)
Profound hypokalemia
Refeeding alkalosis
Primary bicarbonate retention (chloride resistant, urine chloride greater than 20 mEq. per liter)
Large blood transfusion
Aggressive use of sodium bicarbonate (especially in renal insufficiency)
Milk alkali syndrome
Miscellaneous (chloride resistant, urine chloride greater than 20 mEq. per liter)
Hypercalcemia
Hyperparathyroidism

Clinical Presentation

The majority of symptoms in metabolic alkalosis are caused by volume contraction, hypokalemia, and the subsequent neurologic, gastrointestinal, and cardiovascular dysfunctions. Metabolic alkalosis should be suspected if there is evidence of volume contraction, hydrogen and chloride loss (e.g., vomiting, nasogastric suctioning, and diuretic use), ingestion of substances with mineralocorticoid activity (licorice), or excessive ingestion of alkali.

The physical examination should search for signs of volume contraction or volume excess. This can be done by assessing postural blood pressure and pulse changes and determining the presence or absence of edema. The hypokalemia in metabolic alkalosis may predispose to dysfunction of cardiac and other smooth (GI tract) as well as skeletal muscle. In chronic and profound states of hypokalemia, the patient might present with demonstrable decreased muscle strength.

Laboratory evaluation should reveal an increased plasma bicarbonate concentration, a predictable increased P_{CO_2}, decreased pH, hypochloremia, and hypokalemia. The P_{CO_2} and bicarbonate concentration, if plotted on an acid-base normogram, should fall within the expected band of compensation for metabolic alkalosis. Urine chloride concentration would be less than 10 mEq. per liter in metabolic alkalosis caused by volume and chloride depletion (except with loop and cortical diuretic use). Urine chloride is greater than 20 mEq. per liter in all other forms of metabolic alkalosis (by primary mineralocorticoid excess, intracellular sequestration of hydrogen ions, and in excessive ingestion of alkali). Compensation less than or greater than predicted represents metabolic alkalosis combined with respiratory alkalosis or acidosis, respectively.

Treatment

In patients with metabolic alkalosis caused by decreased effective circulating volume and chloride repletion, the aims of therapy are the restoration of effective circulating volume with sodium and chloride and repletion of potassium stores. All potassium deficits should be replaced with potassium chloride because of the accompanying chloride depletion. In patients with normal or increased effective circulating volume because of mineralocorticoid excess, therapy is aimed at stopping or blocking the mineralocorticoid activity and restoring potassium and chloride hemostasis. In these settings, potassium chloride is administered to force hydrogen out of cells, and spironolactone can be used to block the effects of aldosterone. Sometimes surgical removal of mineralocorticoid-producing tumors may be required.

RESPIRATORY ALKALOSIS

Respiratory alkalosis is caused by the depletion of CO_2 from the body, resulting in a decrease in P_{CO_2}. The compensation for this decreased P_{CO_2} is enhanced cellular extrusion of hydrogen and renal excretion of bicarbonate. The compensation in respiratory alkalosis is such that in the acute respiratory alkalosis there is a 2.0 mEq. per liter fall in the plasma bicarbonate concentration for each 10 mm. Hg decrease in P_{CO_2}. Usually, the bicarbonate concentration in the acute respiratory alkalosis will not fall less than 18 mEq. per liter and maximum compensation occurs within minutes. In chronic respiratory alkalosis, there is a 5.0 mEq. per liter decrease in the plasma bicarbonate concentration for each 10 mm. Hg fall in P_{CO_2}. The bicarbonate concentration in chronic respiratory alkalosis usually will not fall less than 14 mEq. per liter, and maximum compensation occurs within 2 to 3 days. Reductions in bicarbonate concentration less than or greater than those noted are consistent with the presence of respiratory alkalosis plus metabolic alkalosis or metabolic acidosis, respectively.

Respiratory alkalosis can be caused by hypoxemia (e.g., pulmonary disease), psychogenic hyperventilation, CNS disorders (e.g., CNS hemorrhage), salicylate intoxication, hypermetabolic states (e.g., thyrotoxicosis), cirrhosis, assisted ventilation, gram-negative sepsis, and postcorrection of metabolic acidosis. The treatment in respiratory alkalosis is aimed at the primary disorder that is responsible for the enhanced pulmonary ventilation.

RESPIRATORY ACIDOSIS

Respiratory acidosis is caused by the retention of CO_2 secondary to states of inadequate pulmonary ventilation. Respiratory acidosis is caused by an increase in the P_{CO_2}, which is associated with compensation in the acute stage by cellular and in the chronic stage by renal bicarbonate production and retention. In acute respiratory acidosis, there is a 1.0 mEq. per liter increase in the plasma bicarbonate concentration for every 10 mm. Hg rise in P_{CO_2} (cellular buffering). In chronic respiratory acidosis, there is a 4.0 mEq. per liter elevation in the plasma bicarbonate concentration for every 10 mm. Hg increase in P_{CO_2} (renal bicarbonate retention). Elevations of bicarbonate levels less than or greater than those noted above are consistent with respiratory acidosis plus metabolic acidosis or metabolic alkalosis, respectively. Compensation may also be inconsistent with that expected in a single acid-base disorder if there is a mixture of acute and chronic respiratory acidosis, which would be the case in a patient with chronic lung disease who acutely decompensates.

The causes of respiratory acidosis include inhibition of the respiratory centers (sedative overuse), disorders of respiratory muscles and chest wall (e.g., extreme obesity), and disorders of gas exchange across the alveolar membrane (e.g., diffuse intrinsic pulmonary disease). The treatment of respiratory acidosis is aimed at increasing the patient's pulmonary ventilation and treatment of the patient's primary disease process.

Disorders of Osmolality

HYPONATREMIA

Pathophysiology

True hyponatremia is usually indicative of a hyperosmolal state that occurs when water retention leads to an excess of water in relationship to solute. Factors that diminish renal water excretion can lead to hyponatremia. These include diminished renal excretion of free water secondary to decreased effective circulating volume, renal insufficiency, and the inhibition of chloride and sodium reabsorption by diuretics. Water retention can also be caused by appropriate or inappropriate presence of ADH. Water retention caused by an appropriate presence of ADH occurs in the setting of decreased effective circulating volume, adrenalin sufficiency or hypothyroidism, and in syndromes of inappropriate ADH secretion where water retention occurs without regard to volume or osmolality. It should be noted that volume, not osmolality, is the most potent stimulant to ADH secretion. In fact, water retention will persist even in the presence of profound hypo-osmolality in order to preserve circulating volume.

Those disorders that cause hyponatremia because of decreased effective circulating volume include gastrointestinal, renal, and skin volume loss and edematous states, such as heart failure, hepatic cirrhosis, and nephrotic syndrome (Table 58–5). Profound potassium depletion can also contribute to a hyponatremic state because of the intracellular movement of sodium to replace the loss of intracellular potassium. Renal disease that affects the collecting tubule may also result in an inability to excrete the unrestricted

Table 58–5. CAUSES OF HYPONATREMIA

- Hyponatremia with normal osmolality or pseudohyponatremia (280 to 295 mosm per kg.)
  - Hyperlipidemia
  - Hyperproteinemia
- Hyponatremia with hyperosmolality (greater than 295 mosm per kg.)
  - Hyperglycemia
  - Mannitol infusion
- Hyponatremia with hypo-osmolality (less than 280 mosm per kg.)
  - Decreased effective circulating volume causing ADH secretion and retention of ingested and endogeneously produced water
    - Total body hypovolemia by physical assessment
      - Gastrointestinal volume loss
        - Vomiting
        - Diarrhea
        - Enteral tube drainage
      - Renal volume loss
        - Diuretics
        - Hypoaldosteronism
        - Na^+ losing nephropathy
      - Skin volume loss (burns)
      - Third spacing
    - Total body hypervolemia (edematous) by physical assessment
      - Liver disease with hypoalbuminemia
      - Congestive heart failure
      - Nephrotic syndrome
    - Total body euvolemia by physical assessment
      - Hypothyroidism
      - Adrenal insufficiency
  - Secretion of ADH *not* caused by hyperosmolality or volume depletion
    - Syndrome of inappropriate ADH secretion
    - Severe pain and other psychophysiologic stress
  - Water ingestion at rates greater than renal excretory capabilities
    - Primary polydipsia
    - Normal water ingestion in advanced renal disease

daily water ingestion. Diuretics, such as thiazides, can cause volume contraction with ADH-induced water retention. They also can cause potassium depletion that can contribute to the hypo-osmolal state. Loop diuretics, such as furosemide and ethycrinic acid, can cause volume contraction with a resultant ADH-induced water retention, and they also disrupt the urinary-diluting mechanism, thereby decreasing the net amount of water that can be excreted. Cortical diuretics are more frequent causes of hyponatremia because of their frequent use and their ability to cause volume contraction without altering renal water conservation capacity.

Hyponatremia can also occur where there is no abnormality in renal water excretion, but the ability of the kidney to excrete water has been overwhelmed by excessive ingestions of water. This occurs in primary polydipsia (psychogenic water drinking). Prolonged hyponatremia can result in a reset of the body's osmostat thus causing ADH to be produced at lower levels of serum sodium concentration.

There are clinical settings where hyponatremia does not actually reflect hypo-osmolality, commonly called pseudohypernatremia. Hyponatremia with normal plasma osmolality occurs in the setting of severe hyperlipidemia, hyperproteinemia, and the use of isotonic glycine after transurethral resection of the prostate. Hyponatremia with elevated plasma osmolality occurs with hyperglycemia ($[Na^+]$ depressed by 1 mEq. per liter for every 62 mg. per dl. of glucose) and administration of hypertonic mannitol. It should be noted that the measured serum osmolality in chronic renal failure will be high because of the excess presence of BUN. However, BUN is not an effective osmole; therefore, calculation of the effective serum osmolality will reveal the actual osmolality affecting water balance in patients with azotemia.

Clinical Presentation

The symptoms associated with hyponatremia depend upon the rapidity of the reduction of serum sodium concentration. Patients can present with confusion, headache, lethargy, obtundation, seizures, and coma depending upon the degree and the rate of serum sodium reduction. Patients are at great risk to develop permanent neurologic damage if the changes are acute and severe. Since the most frequent causes of hyponatremia are associated with volume contraction, many patients present with signs of hypovolemia, such as weakness, postural dizziness, and hypotension.

When hyponatremia is present, the most important first study is the measurement of the plasma osmolality. If the plasma osmolality is low, then true hyponatremia is present. If the measured plasma osmolality is normal or elevated, then the patient has either pseudohyponatremia or renal failure. If in the setting of hypo-osmolality the urine osmolality is less than 100 mosm per liter, then primary polydipsia should be considered. If the urine osmolality is greater than 100 mosm per liter, consideration of appropriate or inappropriate presence of ADH as the cause of hyponatremia should be made. Measurements of urine sodium can help to determine whether or not the patient's circulating volume is depleted. If the urine sodium is less than 10 mEq. per liter then the patient has decreased effective circulating volume. This decreased effective circulating volume would stimulate the production of ADH and hence water retention. If the urine sodium concentration is greater than 20 mEq. per liter, one should consider those disorders where volume is relatively normal or increased (i.e., primary polydipsia), or the ability to conserve sodium is impaired (a volume-contracted patient who is taking diuretics).

Treatment

In hyponatremia caused by true volume contraction including adrenal insufficiency and those states caused by the overuse of diuretics, the infusion of normal saline to restore effective circulating volume is first required before one attempts to restore normal osmolality. In many situations, the restoration of effective circulating volume is sufficient to decrease

ADH production and hence permit a water diuresis and a return of normal osmolality. In the setting of hyponatremia, the potassium status should also be monitored because in many cases potassium depletion is present that requires potassium repletion as the hypo-osmolar state is corrected. In edematous states—the syndrome of inappropriate ADH secretion (SIADH), primary polydipsia, and renal failure—water restriction can be used in order to restore normal osmolality. The acute treatment of symptomatic SIADH where the serum sodium concentration has been reduced to extremely low levels may include water restriction plus an infusion of hypertonic saline plus the use of a loop diuretic. An approach used in less urgent cases is water restriction and/or increased sodium chloride intake and in some instances the utilization of loop diuretics to promote free water loss to normalize osmolality. If hyponatremia is caused by a drug with ADH-like activity, simple removal of the agent in mild cases may be the only treatment required. The use of hypertonic saline solution is determined by the degree of hyponatremia (levels less than 115 mEq. per liter) and the patient's symptoms. There has been controversy regarding the rate of the correction of the hypo-osmolality in symptomatic patients. Present evidence is conflicting regarding the rate of correction of hyponatremia and its impact upon the development of central pontine myelinolysis. Therefore, it is prudent to never attempt to raise the serum sodium concentration to normal ranges within the first 12 to 24 hours. If the patient has severe hyponatremia with symptoms, raising the serum sodium to approximately 120 mEq. per liter in the first 8 to 12 hours might be an appropriate objective. However, if the patient deteriorates during that period, re-evaluation of the rapidity of osmolality normalization should be reassessed.

HYPERNATREMIA

Pathophysiology and Differential Diagnosis

Hypernatremia results when there is a net loss of water or retention of excess sodium causing hyperosmolality. Pure water loss as a cause of hypernatremia occurs with insensible and urinary losses at rates greater than water replacement. Renal water losses occur in the setting of decreased renal sensitivity to ADH (i.e., nephrogenic diabetes insipidus), decreased production of ADH (i.e., central diabetes insipidus), osmotic diuresis (e.g., hyperglycemia), and hypothalamic disorders (Table 58–6). Sodium retention as the cause of hypernatremia usually occurs inside the hospital where patients receive isotonic or hypertonic infusions of sodium bicarbonate or other hypertonic sodium-containing compounds (e.g., enteral and parenteral feeding) without appropriate free water. Elderly persons are more likely to have a decreased sense of thirst and are at an increased risk

Table 58–6. CAUSES OF HYPERNATREMIA

- Hypotonic fluid loss with inadequate access to water replacement
  - Renal hypotonic volume loss
    - Osmotic diuresis
    - Diuretics
  - Gastrointestinal hypotonic volume loss
    - Diarrhea
    - Vomiting
  - Skin hypotonic volume loss
    - Sweating
    - Burns
  - Respiratory hypotonic volume loss
    - Chronic hyperventilation (e.g., infection)
- Pure water loss
  - Renal
    - Central diabetes insipidus
    - Nephrogen diabetes insipidus
- Decreased water intake secondary to diminished thirst response and inadequate access to water
  - Hypodipsia
    - Diminished thirst response of the elderly
    - Comatose patients
  - Lack of access to water
    - Infants with volume loss
    - Debilitated patients
- Hypertonic volume gain
  - Hypertonic saline
  - Hypertonic sodium bicarbonate

to develop water loss, especially in the setting of fever, where there is increased insensible loss. Osmotic agents, which include endogenously produced glucose or exogenously administered osmotic agents (such as mannitol), may cause hyperosmolality but present with hyponatremia (pseudohyponatremia). Hypercalcemia can result in a net water diuresis and hence lead to hypernatremia, which can be further exacerbated especially if the associated mental changes decrease the response to thirst or limit access to water. In sickle cell anemia, red blood cell sickling in the low oxygen environment of the renal medulla can result in disruption of the concentrating mechanisms of the kidney and hence conservation of water can be impaired. Both central and nephrogenic diabetes must be considered when the more common causes of hyponatremia have been eliminated or are inconsistent with the patient's presenting problems.

Hypernatremia can present with neurologic symptoms—the severity of which are directly based upon the rate of water loss and the advancing hypernatremia. Patients with hypernatremia (with the exception of those who have received hypertonic solutions) are invariably volume contracted and will have the signs associated with absolute hypovolemia.

The urine osmolality in hypernatremia less than 300 mosm per kg. (a specific gravity less than 1.010) suggests the presence of central or nephrogenic diabetes insipidus (diuretic use, intrinsic renal disease, partial diabetes insipidus, or osmotic diuresis). Urine osmolality greater than 800 mosm per kg. in hypernatremia is caused by insensible water loss, decreased water intake, or excess sodium intake.

Treatment

The rapid correction of hypernatremia with hypotonic fluids must be avoided to decrease the potential of permanent neurologic damage and death because of excess water movement into the brain. The resulting cerebral edema is caused by the presence of CNS iatrogenic osmoles. Therefore, the serum sodium should be decreased by no more than 2 mEq. per hour. In pure water loss, hypotonic solutions can be given by oral or intravenous routes unless hypotension or volume depletion is present, at which time normal saline is given to first restore effective circulating volume, after which attention can be directed to the restoration of normal osmolality.

If the patient has central diabetes insipidus, in most cases, vasopressin is used, but drugs that increase ADH secretion (i.e., clofibrate) and those that potentiate ADH activity (e.g., chlorpropamide) can also be used. Nephrogenic diabetes insipidus can be treated by eliminating the hypercalcemia, hypokalemia, or discontinuation of drugs that might cause the renal defect. However, if treatment is required because of symptomatic polyuria (small percentage), then a low sodium diet and thiazide diuretics can be used to enhance sodium chloride excretion and ensure a mild decrease in the effective circulating volume that will result in a net decrease in renal water loss. The use of nonsteroidal anti-inflammatory drugs that inhibit prostaglandin synthesis has also been shown to enhance water retention.

Table 58–7. CAUSES OF HYPOKALEMIA

- Hypokalemia without alterations in total body potassium depletion
  - Intracellular K^+ sequestration
    - Alkalemia (respiratory and metabolic origins)
    - Insulin activity
    - Beta-adrenergic agonists
    - Hypokalemic periodic paralysis
    - Prelude to delirium tremens
    - Treatment of severe anemias
    - Lab error (e.g., extremely high white count or aged blood sample)
- Hypokalemia with total body potassium depletion
  - Gastrointestinal potassium losses
    - Diarrhea
    - Vomiting
    - Villous adenoma
    - Laxative abuse
  - Decreased dietary potassium intake or absorption
    - Diets poor in potassium
    - Clay ingestion
  - Renal potassium losses
    - Metabolic alkalosis*
      - Chloride responsive (e.g., vomiting and diuretic use)
      - Chloride resistant (e.g., hyperaldosteronism and licorice ingestion)
    - Metabolic acidosis
      - Tubular acidosis (types I and II)
      - Carbonic anhydrase inhibition
      - Diabetic ketoacidosis (glucose-induced osmotic diuresis)
      - Ureterosigmoidostomy
    - Postobstructive uropathies
    - Diuretic phase of acute tubular necrosis
    - Salt-losing nephropathies
    - Hypomagnesemia
    - Increased sweating
- Total body potassium depletion without hypokalemia
  - Acidemia

*See Table 58–6.

Other Disorders of Electrolyte Concentration

HYPOKALEMIA

Pathophysiology and Differential Diagnosis

Hypokalemia, the most common electrolyte abnormality in ambulatory family medicine, can be caused by increased loss of potassium through GI, renal, and skin routes and decreased dietary potassium intake (Table 58–7). Hypokalemia can occur without alterations in the total body potassium content as a result of intracellular sequestration of potassium. The most frequent cause of this form of hypokalemia is alkalemia where potassium movement into cells is exchanged for hydrogen movement out of cells. This intracellular movement of potassium can result in extremely low serum potassium levels, especially if pre-existing total body potassium depletion was already present. The treatment of severe anemia can lead to hypokalemia as the newly formed red cells begin to sequester available extracellular potassium. An intracellular shift of potassium is also thought to be the cause of the hypokalemia that precedes the development of delirium tremens (respiratory alkalosis as a part of the electrolyte changes preceding delirium tremens may also add to the degree of hypokalemia). A falsely reduced serum potassium concentration can occur if a blood sample is permitted to stand as functioning blood cells continue to utilize available extracellular potassium.

Hypokalemia, as a reflection of total body potassium depletion, can be caused by the loss of potassium-containing GI fluids that occur with vomiting, diarrhea, intestinal fistulas, and removal of these fluids through tube drainage. Laxative abuse and villous adenoma are also modes of potassium-containing GI fluid loss. Skin volume loss through profuse sweating can also result in significant total body potassium loss. These extrarenal causes of hypokalemia result in renal conservation of potassium, which is manifested by a low urinary potassium concentration (less than 15 to 25 mEq. per liter, assuming the absence of renal dysfunction or diuretic use). The exception to the renal conservation of potassium with GI loss of fluid would occur in vomiting, which, because of the associated chloride deficiency, results in a net loss of urinary potassium that compounds the hypokalemia. Patients can consume diets that are deficient in potassium such that the obligate daily requirement of dietary potassium is not met. Ingestion of clay can nonspecifically bind dietary potassium and can result in hypokalemia.

All forms of metabolic alkalosis associated with either a primary mineralocorticoid excess (hyperaldosteronism) or a secondary mineralocorticoid excess (vomiting and volume contraction) will result in potassium depletion because of the excess activity of the distal renal tubular sites. Metabolic alkalosis caused by a primary retention of bicarbonate causes potassium depletion secondary to intracellular potassium shifts.

Certain forms of metabolic acidosis can also cause hypokalemia. Type II RTA causes urinary potassium wasting as a result of therapy with large doses of sodium bicarbonate. Type I RTA causes urinary potassium loss secondary to hyperaldosteronism, which is caused in part by associated volume contraction. Carbonic anhydrase inhibition results in metabolic acidosis and renal potassium wasting. Diabetic ketoacidosis with associated hyperglycemia causes an osmotic loss of potassium resulting in extreme potassium depletion. Postobstructive uropathy, the diuretic phase of acute tubular necrosis, salt-losing nephropathies, and hypomagnesemia can all cause hypokalemia because of an associated renal tubular dysfunction.

Clinical Presentation

Potassium depletion from any cause can present with many symptoms from generalized weakness and muscle cramps to frank paralysis. Polyuria and polydipsia may occur because of the impairment of renal concentration and diminished thirst that may be caused by profound potassium depletion. Constipation and, in some instances, signs of frank bowel obstruction may also occur. Hypokalemia makes muscles more vulnerable to the development of rhabdomyolysis. Cardiac manifestations of hypokalemia include predisposition to supraventricular and ventricular dysrhythmias and heart block especially in patients with coexisting myocardial disease. Hypokalemia also makes the manifestations of digitalis toxicity occur at lower serum levels of the drug. Electrocardiographic evidence of hypokalemia is manifested by flattening of the T waves and the presence of U waves.

Treatment

The treatment of hypokalemia includes the utilization of potassium chloride given either orally or intravenously if the GI tract cannot be used or if the patient needs rapid potassium replacement. Potassium replacement should be slow unless there is evidence of significant clinical complications that require rapid restoration of potassium homeostasis. Oral therapy can be given in dosages from 40 to 100 mEq. per day based on the degree of potassium depletion and the relative rates at which the potassium loss continues to occur. In those settings where intravenous use of potassium chloride is required, potassium administration should not exceed concentrations of 40 mEq. per liter and should not exceed an infusion rate of greater than 10 mEq. per hour unless there is an urgent necessity to give greater amounts—at which time as much as 40 mEq. per hour can be given. If reasonable amounts of potassium repletion are provided and the patient continues to remain hypokalemic, then one should reassess the possible routes of potassium loss to insure that an unsuspected route of depletion does not persist. A concurrent magnesium deficiency should also be considered because in the setting of hypomagnesemia often it is difficult to establish normal potassium homeostasis until the underlying magnesium depletion has been corrected. It should be anticipated that patients who are on hydrochlorathiazide at amounts greater than 25 mg. per day will invariably become hypokalemic and as such require constant monitoring of potassium levels. In patients who develop significant hypokalemia or who have a predisposition to the development of myocardial dysrhythmias, concurrent use of potassium replacement via potassium salts, the utilization of potassium-sparing diuretics, or slow-release potassium products present in a wax matrix formulation should be instituted. It should be noted that wax matrix preparations, although not producing as many GI symptoms as the enteric-coated ones, can cause endoscopically significant changes in the GI tract. It appears that these findings are common in all forms of slow-release potassium products, therefore making their use not suitable for all patients (e.g., pre-existing gastritis and active peptic ulcer disease).

HYPERKALEMIA

Pathophysiology and Differential Diagnosis

Hyperkalemia can be caused by excess potassium intake, decreased potassium excretion, and the movement of potassium from intracellular to extracellular sites (Table 58–8). Hyperkalemia caused by increased intake tends to occur most frequently in situations where there is underlying renal disease and/or the patient has received an inadvertent infusion of excess potassium through intravenous fluid administration. The extrusion of potassium from intracellular sites and/or the failure of cells to take up potassium can be caused by acidosis (e.g., diabetic ketoacidosis), excessive tissue catabolism, beta-adrenergic blockade, digitalis intoxication, and insulin deficiency. Shifts of potassium to extracellular sites can also occur with the utilization of the muscle relaxant succinylcholine and the catatonic amino acid arginine hydrochloride. Hyperkalemia caused by decreased urinary excretion occurs in acute and chronic renal failure and prerenal azotemia because of the associated, decreased glumerulofiltration rates. Hyperkalemia is also caused by an inability to excrete excess potassium

Table 58–8. CAUSES OF HYPERKALEMIA

Hyperkalemia with normal total body potassium
Laboratory measurement of old blood sample
Hemolysis of blood sample during collection
Increased blood cell counts
Drawing blood samples from an ischemic extremity
Extracellular shifts of K^+ with normal total body potassium
Acidosis
Insulin deficiency
Beta blockade
Hyperkalemic periodic paralysis
Digitalis intoxication
Excess tissue catabolism
Infectious mononucleosis (cell membrane dysfunction)
Excess potassium intake
Decreased potassium excretion
Renal insufficiency (acute and chronic)
Mineralocorticoid deficiency or the lack of mineralocorticoid effect
Hypoaldosteronism
Hyporeninemic hypoaldosteronism
Drugs (e.g., NSAIDs, ACE inhibitors)
Drugs that antagonize renal potassium excretion
Triamterene
Spironolactone
Amiloride
Miscellaneous
Sickle cell nephropathy
Obstructive uropathy

at the distal renal tubular as a result of hypoaldosteronism (decreased aldosterone or decreased aldosterone effect). Hyporeninism resulting in hypoaldosteronism and hyperkalemia (the most frequent cause of hypoaldosteronism) can be caused by nonsteroidal anti-inflammatory agents because of their antiprostaglandin inhibiting effects that inhibit renin release and is seen in patients with diabetes with mild renal failure. Angiotension converting enzyme (ACE) inhibitors (e.g., captopril) can also cause states similar to hyporeninemic hypoaldosteronism with the associated hyperkalemia because of the decreased production of angiotension II and the resultant decreased release of aldosterone. Although the clinical consequences of captopril-induced hypoaldosteronism is not unlike hyporeninemic hypoaldosteronism, renin levels are actually high because of the ACE inhibition. Drugs that directly antagonize renal potassium excretion and also result in hyperkalemia (i.e., triamterene, spironolactone, and amiloride) are most often found in combinations with thiazide-like diuretics to decrease the associated kaluresis of the thiazides. Other causes of hyporeninemic hypoaldosteronism can also be seen in the uropathy induced by sickle cell disease and postobstructive uropathy.

Clinical Presentation

Patients with hyperkalemia can present with general weakness, paresthesias, and frank flaccid paralysis, but these are usually preceded by the more life-threatening cardiac effects. Electrocardiographic evidence of hyperkalemia progresses with the severity of the potassium concentration elevation. These changes usually begin with peaking of the T waves, and as the hyperkalemia progresses, the T waves can become less prominent and the duration of the QRS complex can increase. There can also be an increase in the PR interval. Severe hyperkalemia can cause progression to ventricular fibrillation and cardiac standstill.

Treatment

Hyperkalemia should be aggressively treated because of the lethal effects it can have on the myocardium especially if the electrolyte abnormality is acute and/or the patient has underlying myocardial disease. The hypokalemic affect on the myocardium can be antagonized by the use of calcium gluconate which is given intravenously over 2 to 5 minutes (approximately 20 ml. of a 10 per cent solution). Alkalinization of the extracellular fluid with sodium bicarbonate will promote potassium movement into cells, thereby decreasing hyperkalemia. Potassium movement into cells can also be prompted by insulin administration along with glucose to prevent hypoglycemia. The removal of potassium from the body can be accomplished by the use of sodium polystirene sufonate, which is a potassium sodium exchange resin that can be given orally (usually with sorbitol to cause rapid GI transit) or as a retention enema. In severe cases not responsive to these measures, hemodialysis may be required.

MAGNESIUM DISORDERS

Magnesium disorders significant enough to affect physiologic function have only recently been recognized but are commonplace in primary care practice. Magnesium is essential to many cellular functions, such as energy production, and intracellular enzymatic processes. Magnesium is obtained from the diet and absorption occurs along the small bowel. As a result, hypomagnesemia can occur as a result of malabsorption and inadequate dietary intake. Hypomagnesemia can also occur in association with hyperparathyroidism, primary hyperaldosteronism, hyperthyroidism, and diabetes mellitus. The most common causes of hypomagnesemia are diuretic use and alcoholism. DKA with increased urinary excretion of potassium is also a common mechanism of potassium loss. Hypomagnesemia, along with hypokalemia, hypophosphatemia, and metabolic alkalosis, can also herald the onset of delirium tremens. Hypomagnesemia appears to occur in a mechanism similar to hypokalemia when diuretics are in use. However, potassium repletion is impaired as long as the magnesium deficiency persists. The symptoms of magnesium deficiency are nonspecific and include weakness, anorexia, and at times nausea and vomiting. The physical examination may reveal disorders of nerve conduction and muscle dysfunctions. In patients who have symptoms requiring immediate intervention, 8 to 12 grams of intramuscular magnesium sulfate may be required in the first 24 hours followed by 4 to 5 grams daily for 3 to 4 days. This large amount of magnesium is required since a significant amount will be excreted in the urine even in the presence of magnesium depletion. In situations where treatment of magnesium depletion is less urgent, magnesium oxide can be given orally 30 mEq. four to six times per day until appropriate levels are restored and stabilized.

Hypermagnesemia occurs usually in situations where patients have received excessive amounts of magnesium especially in the presence of renal insufficiency. This occurs commonly in situations where patients with renal insufficiency excessively consume magnesium-containing antacids. If levels are high enough to warrant therapy (more than just stopping the excess ingestion of magnesium), administration of calcium can result in a transient decreased magnesium concentration. In severe cases of symptomatic hypermagnesemia, hemodialysis may be required.

CALCIUM DISORDERS

Physiology

Calcium exists in the serum bound to protein, complexed to other small molecules, and in an ionized state. It is the ionized portion of calcium (45 to 50 per cent) that is responsible for the appropriate function of cells, especially those involved in neuromuscular functions. The body maintains calcium concentrations in limits of approximately 4 to 5 mg. per dl., which equates to a total calcium of 8.6 to 10.6 mg. per dl. If mechanisms to determine serum-ionized calcium are not available, estimations can be made by considering the amount of calcium-bound protein that can be determined using normograms for estimating protein-bound calcium. Factors regulating calcium balance include parathyroid hormone, which promotes bone calcium reabsorption, increases renal tubular reabsorption of calcium, and stimulates the production of 1,25-dihydroxyvitamin D. 1,25-dihydroxyvitamin D causes bone reabsorption and mobilization of calcium and enhances GI reabsorption of calcium. Calcitonin works in opposition to the parathyroid hormone, thereby inhibiting bone reabsorption and enhancing the renal excretion of calcium.

Hypercalcemia

In hypercalcemia, there is excess production of the parathyroid hormone (e.g., primary hyperparathyroidism and parathyroid producing tumors), or there is increased production of 1,25-dihydroxyvitamin D (e.g., sarcoidosis). Other causes of hypercalcemia include abnormal mobilization of excessive amounts of calcium as would occur in cancers, skeletal immobilization, and thyrotoxicosis. Excessive intestinal absorption of calcium leading to hypercalcemia can occur in the setting of vitamin D toxicity and milk alkali syndrome. Defective renal excretion of calcium leading to hypercalcemia can occur in the setting of decreased effective circulating volume and thiazide therapy. In order to complete the matrix for bone formation, phosphates are required and, therefore, hypophosphatemia can result in hypercalcemia because of reduced bone formation. If patients have become hypercalcemic and are symptomatic enough to necessitate emergency intervention, treatment consists of isotonic saline infusion with a loop diuretic (e.g., furosemide) to increase renal calcium excretion. Mithromycin and calcitonin can also be used in order to inhibit bone reabsorption. The treatment of hypercalcemia must be tempered by the presence of underlying heart disease, which may be exacerbated by the rapid infusion of isotonic volume. In situations where the hypercalcemia is not symptomatic and imposes no immediate threat to the patient, less urgent mechanisms for calcium control can be used. They include increased PO volume intake to avoid volume contraction, review of patient medications to avoid drugs that may inhibit the renal reabsorption of calcium (e.g., thiazides), regular exercise to impair bone reabsorption, diets low in calcium, and avoidance of the inadvertent ingestion of vitamin D and calcium-containing OTC preparations such as antacids.

Hypocalcemia

Hypocalcemia occurs in situations when there is inadequate production of the parathyroid hormone or decreased production of 1,25-dihydroxyvitamin D as would occur in the setting of chronic renal failure. Hypocalcemia also can occur when calcium cannot be mobilized from the bone (e.g., osteomalacia and hypomagnesemia) and when there is increased calcium utilization (e.g., osteoblastic activity of metastatic prostate cancer). Calcium sinks, which remove calcium rapidly from the extracellular fluid, can occur in rhabdomyolysis and pancreatitis. In emergency situations involving hypocalcemia, calcium gluconate intravenous infusion should be given along with the anticipated chronic treatment including oral calcium supplements and vitamin D. In general, oral calcium supplementation should be approximately 2 grams of elemental calcium given daily. If hyperphosphatemia is a part of the presenting picture, diets low in phosphates should be given. Phosphate lowering can also be accomplished by using aluminum-containing antacids to bind dietary phosphates. The administration of vitamin D preparation should be given with the understanding of the possibility of vitamin D toxicity and the potential of soft tissue calcification when given in the presence of hyperphosphatemia.

VOLUME CONTRACTION

Pathophysiology and Differential Diagnosis

Volume contraction occurs when there is real or absolute fluid loss through the GI and respiratory tract, the kidneys, and the skin at rates faster than fluid replacement. Volume contraction also occurs as a result of blood loss from the intravascular space (Table 58–9). This volume loss causes a reduction in intracellular water and potassium content and/or interstitial and intravascular sodium and water content. The results of volume contraction caused by renal or extrarenal volume loss are decreased effective circulating volume and decreased renal profusion. The decreased renal profusion causes an increased renin, angiotension II production, and aldosterone resulting in increased tubular reabsorption of sodium and decreased urinary sodium excretion. The decreased circulating volume will also activate the production of ADH, which leads to renal water retention and plasma osmolality decrease (e.g., hyponatremic volume contraction if there is access to hypotonic fluid replacement). A loss of volume from the intravascular space, as would occur with hemorrhage, results in a decrease in the intravascular hydrostatic pressure that permits a net movement of volume from the interstitial spaces to the intravascular space. This redistribution of fluids (internal volume infusion) provides the first line of defense that protects the effective circulating volume.

Table 58–9. VOLUME CONTRACTION

Absolute volume loss causing decreased effective circulating volume
Gastrointestinal volume loss
Gastric fluids via vomiting and tube suction
Intestinal fluids via diarrhea, fistular, or tube drainage
Gastrointestinal bleeding
Renal volume loss
Osmotic diuresis (e.g., hyperglycemia, radiographic contrast material)
Diuretics
Adrenal insufficiency
Sodium-losing nephropathies
Skin and respiratory volume loss
Insensible losses (e.g., sweating, fever, tachypnea)
Burns
Relative volume loss causing decreased effective circulating volume
Third space sequestration
Gastrointestinal
Bowel obstruction
Pancreatitis
Peritonitis
Vascular
Venous obstruction
Bleeding into internal spaces or tissue
Massive tissue injury
Removal of third space fluid that rapidly reaccumulates
Ascites
Pleural effusion
Decreased vascular tone
Overuse of vasodilating drugs
Septic shock
Decreased effective circulating volume as a cause of edematous states
Congestive heart failure (i.e., pump failure)
Hepatic cirrhosis (i.e., decreased oncotic pressure)
Nephrosis (i.e., decreased oncotic pressure)
Nonsteroidal anti-inflammatory drugs (i.e., decreased renal profusion)
Vasodilating drugs (i.e., decreased vascular tone)

There are circumstances where there is no actual loss of fluid from the body but significant quantities of fluid have become sequestered into spaces that cannot be immediately accessed to support the effective circulating volume. Examples of this sequestration into third spaces occur in situations such as pancreatitis, intestinal obstruction, intra-abdominal bleeding disorders, and peritonitis. Although evaluation may not show evidence of classic changes associated with patients who present with absolute volume contraction (e.g., decreased skin turgor and dry mucous membranes), they are at the same risk of developing significant compromises in the effective circulating volume as manifested by hypotension, postural blood pressure and pulse changes, and tachycardia. Another example of third space sequestration of fluids occurs in ascites that, if it develops slowly, may permit enough time for compensatory increases in salt and water retention, which can partially restore the effective circulating volume.

The edematous states of congestive heart failure, hepatic cirrhosis, and nephrosis, although appearing hypervolemic during physical assessment, truly represent settings where the effective circulating volume has been compromised because of decreased cardiac output, decreased protein production, and increased urinary protein loss, respectively, all of which result in renal salt and water retention and the development of edema. Although these edematous states are managed in part with diuretics to enhance renal salt and water loss, therapy is aimed primarily at the restoration of those factors that can enhance myocardial contractility and oncotic forces. It should be recognized that the treatment of edema in these settings with diuretics carries with it the potential of further decreasing the effective circulating volume, which can result in significant reduction in tissue profusion and hypovolemic shock.

Clinical Presentation

Absolute volume loss occurs with vomiting, diarrhea, fever, sweating, polyuria, bleeding, decreased salt and water intake, lack of access to fluids (e.g., infants and patients who are debilitated, confused, comatosed, or have CNS disease). A historical record of the time preceding the patient's presentation for volume contraction may reveal reports of thirst, weakness, postural dizziness, or diuretic use. The physical assessment of these patients with absolute volume loss may reveal dry mucous membranes and decreased skin turgor if the volume loss has occurred over time (i.e., days). Determination of volume loss sufficient to rob the vascular space of effective circulating volume is achieved by assessing postural changes in blood pressure and pulse. However, significant postural changes in blood pressure and pulse can also occur in settings not related to absolute volume loss, such as the neuropathy of diabetes, use of vasodilators, and diminished sympathetic tone found in some aging patients. A physical assessment of the central venous pressure may reveal values that may be undetectable by physical inspection. If the patient has been seen on a frequent basis, a sudden loss of weight may also give evidence of the presence of significant volume loss.

The laboratory evidence of absolute volume contraction includes an increase in both BUN and creatinine at a ratio greater than 20:1. Depending on the rate of volume loss, hemoconcentration may be present. However, if there is an acute volume loss involving the loss of red cells, the hematocrit may reflect the loss only if appropriate time for equilibration between fluid spaces has occurred (approximately 12 hours). Urine sodium concentration is usually less than 10 mEq. per liter except in the setting of an osmotic loss of volume, salt-losing nephropathies, or if diuretics are in use at the time of the urine sample collection. Urine osmolality will be greater than 450 mosm per kg., reflecting the volume-induced increase in ADH secretion (failure to concentrate may occur in the presence of loop diuretic use or intrinsic renal disease). Serum sodium determinations may reveal hyponatremia, hypernatremia, or normonatremia, depending on whether the patient has access to fluids or the osmolality of those fluids. The volume-contracted patient, who had the oral intake of water as partial replacement of isotonic volume loss, may become hyponatremic, especially as ADH secretion is maximally stimulated in this setting. If the patient has partially replenished his or her volume loss with isotonic fluid, it is more likely that the serum sodium concentration will be within normal limits. Failure to ingest fluid (e.g., hypothalamic dysfunction, unconsciousness, or confusion) may result in hypernatremia. If the hypovolemia has not caused tubular renal damage, the fractional excretion of sodium should be less than 1 and the examination of the urinary sediment should be free of renal tubular cells and casts, which implies acute renal tubular cell damage (ATN). If the volume contraction is acute, the risk for developing ATN is greater.

Impact of volume contraction on potassium and bicarbonate concentrations would be variable depending on the source of the volume loss and the presence of any concurrent acid-base abnormality. For example, the potassium concentration in volume contraction would usually be elevated in the setting of metabolic acidosis caused by renal azotemia but depressed in metabolic alkalosis caused by vomiting.

Treatment

In many instances of mild volume contraction, the restoration of normal volume can be accomplished through the oral route. However, with more profound volume contraction the administration of intravenous fluids may be required. In volume contraction where the effecting circulating volume has been significantly compromised, restoration of the effective circulating volume is the first priority, and the ideal solution for the initial treatment is an isotonic saline solution (e.g., normal saline). Changes in osmolality (e.g., hyponatremia and hypernatremia) can be managed once the patient's tissue profusion pressures have been restored. Correction of hyponatremia induced by volume contraction will occur with restoration of effective circulating volume, which will prompt a brisk water diuresis as the volume-dependent secretion of ADH ceases. In the setting of hypernatremia and hypovolemia, the administration of normal saline may restore the effective circulating volume but provides no free water for normalization of the osmolality. Once the effective circulating volume has been restored, solutions containing free water (hypotonic saline and/or dextrose solutions) can be administered. Depending on the nature of the volume loss, potassium chloride might be required when, along with the volume contraction, significant potassium depletion has also occurred. Potassium may also be required if large quantities of volume are required to maintain effective circulating volume. If the patient's hypovolemia is secondary to blood loss, then blood replacement is required. Since all of the lost volume in hemorrhage comes acutely from the intravascular space, volume replacement is most efficient using substances such as blood or other plasma expanders (plasma, albumin, and dextrose-transient effect), which remain intravascularly. In lieu of the immediate availability of blood, an isotonic infusion of normal saline can be given since each 1000 ml. results in an addition of 250 ml. to the intravascular space. The rate of volume replacement should be aggressive until the patient is stabilized with further repletion being gradual while observing parameters (such as input and output) and attempts are made to induce a positive balance. Indicators that suggest appropriate volume repletion include weight gain, loss of postural blood pressure and pulse changes, a urinary output that is dilute and has a sodium content consistent with sodium intake (greater than 20 mEq. per liter), return of normal BUN and creatinine at ratios of 10:1, and restoration of accompanying acid-base and osmolality disorders. In some settings where patients have underlying lung and/or cardiac disease, recognition and management of volume contraction can be complicated because of cardiac failure, peripheral and pulmonary edema, and increased or decreased peripheral vascular resistance. In these settings, volume repletion may require the use of monitoring via central venous lines or getting estimates of left atrial pressures by determining the pulmonary capillary wedge pressure.

VOLUME EXPANSION

Pathophysiology

In most instances, volume expansion occurs in the presence of decreased effective circulating volume, which results in renal hypoperfusion and increased aldosterone production (Table 58–10). The

Table 58–10. VOLUME EXPANSION

Absolute volume gain caused by decreased effective circulating volume and renal sodium and water retention
Edematous states
Increased hydrostatic pressure (e.g., CHF)
Decreased protein production (e.g., cirrhosis)
Increased protein loss (e.g., nephrosis)
Increased capillary permeability (e.g., burn, inflammation, trauma, malignant ascites)
Decreased vascular tone (e.g., vasodilator drugs)
Decreased renal prostaglandin synthesis (e.g., NSAIDs)
Local venous or lymphatic obstruction
Absolute volume gain causing increased effective circulating volume
Renal failure
Infusion/ingestion of hypertonic sodium solution

increased aldosterone production enhances renal sodium reabsorption in an effort to restore some portion of the effective circulating volume. If sodium retention is insufficient to restore effective circulating volume, chronic excessive sodium retention results in edema formation. Although there is total body volume expansion, the sodium retention is perpetuated by renal hypoprofusion. This renal hypoprofusion can be caused by decreased cardiac output, decreased oncotic forces (e.g., increased protein loss, decreased protein production), decreased vascular tone (e.g., vasodilator drugs), and increased vascular permeability. Excess sodium retention that forms edema because of increased venous pressure is immediately available to support the circulating volume when intravascular hydrostatic pressure is acutely lowered (e.g., diuretic use). However, edema caused by a disruption of capillary integrity (e.g., burns, inflammation, malignant ascites) or obstruction (e.g., lymphatic obstruction) is not in rapid equilibrium with the circulating volume and as a result cannot support acute intravascular volume losses. The preservation of renal blood flow is determined in part by renal prostaglandins that decrease vascular resistance in low-flow states. If prostaglandin synthesis is blocked by the use of nonsteroidal anti-inflammatory agents, vascular resistance may be high enough to compromise renal profusion that causes sodium retention. Sodium retention resulting in increased circulating volume occurs in renal failure where the kidneys are not able to excrete the excess amount of sodium, and similar increases in circulating volume can be seen in patients who are consuming hypertonic saline solutions.

Treatment

The edema produced by these disorders usually does not require urgent removal unless ventilation is impaired (e.g., pulmonary edema or laryngeal edema of anaphylaxis). The removal of edema caused by increased venous pressure can be accomplished by the use of diuretics. The diuresis can be brisk as long as edema is present. Once the edema is no longer detectable, the diuresis should be extremely slow to avoid hypotension and to prevent prerenal azotemia. The goal of therapy in these states of volume expansion is not, in every instance, to remove all edema fluid. A good example of this point would be in the setting of severe congestive cardiomyopathy where elevated left ventricular end diastolic pressures are required to support cardiac output. With these increased venous pressures, the development of edema may ensue (e.g., lower extremity edema and pulmonary edema). In this setting, aggressive diuresis may lead to a picture of prerenal azotemia and hypotension because cardiac preload has been lowered enough to affect the cardiac output. Therefore, diuresis should proceed with a full appreciation of the potential risk of compromising effective circulating volume.

Thiazides (e.g., hydrochlorathiazide) and medullary loop diuretics (e.g., furosemide) are frequently used to accomplish the removal of excess salt and water. Although diuresis produced by medullary loop diuretics is much greater than that of the thiazide, both share similar adverse effects. These consist of hypokalemia, hyponatremia, hypochloremia, hyperuricemia, hypomagnesemia, metabolic alkalosis, prerenal azotemia, and worsening glucose intolerance. In states in which the edema is refractory to the use of a single diuretic, the utilization of two diuretics working at different tubular sites can result in an increased rate of diuresis. Distal diuretics are most often in combination with more potent diuretics for their additive effects. Aldactone, which is an aldosterone antagonist, has a unique place in hepatic cirrhosis with ascites where a slow but sustained diuresis is required. Aldactone along with the other distal diuretics, amiloride and triamterene, all share the potential side effects of metabolic acidosis and hyperkalemia.

Renal Failure

Joseph Hobbs

Renal Failure

PATHOPHYSIOLOGY

Renal failure occurs when there is a decrease in the kidney's ability to excrete normally produced metabolic end products and to maintain acid-base, fluid, and electrolyte balance. This dysfunction can be caused by glomerular and/or tubular dysfunction in a variety of disease states. Glomerular lesions can be caused by certain nonimmunologic factors, such as diabetes mellitus and hypertension, but immunologic glomerular disease is the most frequent cause of renal disease of glomerular origin. Causes of tubulointerstitial disease include acute tubular necrosis (renal tubular toxins, hypovolemia, ischemia, and analgesic nephropathy), tubular obstruction (uric acid nephropathy, multiple myeloma, and hypercalcemia), polycystic kidney disease, and acute and chronic polynephritis.

The rate of renal excretion of nitrogenous products (blood urea nitrogen, creatinine, and uric acid), cations (magnesium, potassium, and sodium), and acid anions (phosphates and sulfates) in renal disease is decreased, resulting in an accumulation of these substances in body fluids. Since the maintenance of acid-base balance via hydrogen-ion secretion, excretion, and bicarbonate generation is a function of the renal tubules, renal tubular dysfunction can result in metabolic acid retention and acidemia. The mechanism of potassium excretion is part of a similar tubular function, and potassium retention is also seen as a part of advancing renal dysfunction.

Since both glomerular and tubular functions are dependent on adequate renal blood flow (even in normal kidneys), any evaluation of decreased renal function must start with an assessment of the appropriateness of the circulating volume. Reduced circulating volume can cause decreased renal excretory function in normal kidneys (i.e., prerenal azotemia) and make chronic renal failure appear worse than can be accounted for by the progressive loss of functional nephrons (e.g., prerenal azotemia in a patient with chronic renal disease). In both these settings, the renal function can be restored to premorbid levels by simply restoring appropriate circulating volume. Failure to restore effective circulating volume can cause intrinsic renal dysfunction in normal kidneys and exacerbate intrinsic renal dysfunction in abnormal kidneys, especially if the process of volume contraction has been rapid and sustained.

GENERAL EVALUATION

When patients present with elevated BUN and serum creatinine concentration, it may not be apparent whether the renal dysfunction is acute, chronic, or an acute process superimposed upon a chronic process. The importance of identifying the acute pre- and postrenal components of renal dysfunction is that their deleterious effects can be rapidly reversed when the participating causes, such as volume depletion and postrenal obstruction, are removed. However, intrinsic acute renal failure may require time and the removal of nephrotoxic agents before renal function returns to normal.

Patients with renal failure are characterized by decreased creatinine clearance and an increase in the serum concentration of BUN and creatinine. The creatinine clearance can be estimated by the following:

1. $$\text{Creatinine clearance (ml./minute) (males)} = \frac{(140 - \text{age}) \times (\text{weight in kg.})}{\text{Serum creatinine concentration (mg./dl.)} \times 72}$$
2. $$\text{Creatinine clearance (mg./dl.) (females)} = 0.85 \times \text{the above value}$$

These formulas are helpful in estimating creatinine clearance in patients with stable renal function ages 18 years and older.

Estimation of creatinine clearance in children ages 1 to 18 years is obtained by the following formula:

$$\text{Creatinine clearance (ml./minute) (children)} = \frac{0.48 \times \text{height (cm.)} \times \text{body surface area (m}^2\text{)}}{\text{Serum creatinine (mg./dl.)} \times 1.73\ (\text{m}^2)}$$

It should be noted that the results of these calculations can be affected significantly by changes in metabolic states, body habitus, and age. The actual measurement of creatinine clearance* eliminates the need to consider the effect of age on serum creatinine, and a steady state is not required for the measure-

*creatinine clearance (ml./minute) =

$$\frac{\text{Urine creatinine concentration (mg./dl.)} \times \text{Volume of urine (ml./minute)}}{\text{Plasma creatinine concentration (mg./dl.)}}$$

$$\text{or Cl creatinine} = \frac{[U]\,[V]}{[P]}$$

ments to be an accurate estimate of the glomerulofiltration rate (GFR). Since the GFR decreases by approximately 5 per cent per decade, patients without any history of renal disease who are elderly have decreased renal excretory capacity. This factor must be considered when prescribing drugs with potential nephrotoxicities and/or drugs that are renally excreted to older patients.

Urine sediment may be used in determining the origin of renal disease. Red blood cells and red cell casts indicate the presence of glomerulonephritis or vasculitis whereas white blood cells and white cell casts indicate possible tubulointerstitial disorder of which pyelonephritis is an example. Renal epithelial cells and casts are found in acute tubular necrosis. Fatty casts as well as oval fat bodies and free fat droplets are present in glomerular disorder associated with nephrotic syndrome (proteinuria greater than 3.5 grams per day). Crystals such as negatively birefringent urate may be present in a postrenal obstructive process. Hematuria can be present in many situations, such as bladder or urethra infections, coagulopathies, polycystic kidney disease, benign hematuria, trauma, stones, glomerulonephritis, and urinary tract tumor (e.g., transitional cell cancer of the bladder).

BUN is the best index of symptoms caused by renal failure (uremia). The more rapid the rise in BUN the more likely the patient is to be symptomatic. In the evaluation of patients with chronic renal disease, one should probably not attribute symptoms to uremia unless the BUN is greater than 100 mg. per dl. Symptoms of uremia would include nausea, vomiting, peripheral neuropathy, pericarditis, mental status changes, bleeding tendencies, and pruritus.

The BUN to creatinine ratio, which is normally 10:1 to 20:1, remains stable as these indices rise in intrinsic renal disease. If the BUN to creatinine ratio is elevated, a prerenal source of the dysfunction (such as absolute volume contraction—especially if urine specific gravity is greater than 450 mosm per kg. and urine sodium is less than 10 mEq. per liter—decreased effective circulating volume, postrenal obstructive component, or hypercatabolic states) must be considered. The evaluation of BUN and creatinine must take into account the clinical situation of the patient. For example, the patient with mildly reduced renal function (serum creatinine level approximately 2 mg. per cent) may become significantly uremic with a BUN of greater than 100 mg. per cent in the presence of GI bleeding. However, a patient with severe chronic renal disease with a serum creatinine greater than 8 mg. per cent may present without uremia (BUN less than 100 mg. per cent), in the presence of protein malnourishment or severe hepatic dysfunction. If the serum creatinine is greater than 2 mg. per cent, it usually implies dysfunction in both kidneys. (In patients with one normally functioning kidney, the serum creatinine is usually less than 1.5).

Renal size as estimated by renal ultrasound or plain x-ray study of the abdomen is extremely helpful in determining the origin of renal dysfunction. If both kidneys are small, chronic renal disease is most likely the cause. If both kidneys are large, it would suggest bilateral obstruction, polycystic renal disease, or infiltrative processes (e.g., amyloid). In the setting of renal failure, bilaterally small kidneys suggest a chronic process, whereas normal to increased renal size more likely suggests an acute process. If one of the kidneys is large, unilateral obstruction, tumor, and cystic disease of the kidney are probable causes. If one of the kidneys is small, unilateral renal artery stenosis and congenital small kidney are potential causes. IVP is used when it is necessary not only to ascertain renal size but also to visualize the collecting system and assess renal function. The benefits of an IVP must be weighed against the risk of complication in patients who have diabetes or known renal disease or are elderly. Renal function should be evaluated and effective circulatory volume restored prior to IVP studies.

Acute Renal Failure

Acute renal failure is characterized by a sudden and/or progressive decrease in renal function manifested by retention of BUN and serum creatinine over several days (Tables 58–11 and 58–12). Acute renal failure can be either oliguric (urine output less than 400 cc. per day) or nonoliguric (urine output greater than 400 cc. per day)—the most common presentation. No matter how severe the acute renal failure appears, most forms of acute renal failure are reversible.

Acute renal failure can be classified as either prerenal, postrenal, or renal in origin.

PRERENAL

Prerenal azotemia occurs when there is depression of renal excretory function secondary to decreased renal perfusion as would be the case in true volume depletion (e.g., diarrhea and vomiting), decreased effective circulating volume (e.g., congestive heart failure), loss of vascular integrity (e.g., septic shock), or third space sequestration of fluids (e.g., pancreatitis, intestinal obstruction, and peritonitis). Prerenal origins of acute renal failure are the most frequent cause of acute renal failure in community hospitals and ambulatory health care settings. Prerenal disease is most frequently caused by absolute volume contraction secondary to volume losses from the GI tract (e.g., diarrhea and vomiting), kidneys (e.g., osmotic diuresis, diuretic-induced inhibition of sodium reabsorption), and skin at rates greater than volume replacement.

Table 58–11. CAUSES OF ACUTE RENAL FAILURE

Prerenal azotemia
- Decrease effective circulating volume
  - Absolute volume loss*
    - Gastrointestinal volume losses (e.g., diarrhea, vomiting, and bleeding)
    - Renal volume losses (e.g., diuretics, diabetes insipidus, osmotic diuresis, and adrenal insufficiency)
    - Skin losses (e.g., profuse sweating, burns, and cystic fibrosis)
  - Total body hypervolemic states*
    - Congestive heart failure
    - Hepatic cirrhosis
    - Nephrotic syndrome
  - Third spacing
    - Peritonitis
    - Pancreatitis
    - Intestinal obstruction
  - Loss of vascular integrity
    - Shock (e.g., septic, neurogenic, and allergic)

Postrenal obstruction
- Prostatic*
- Renal calculi*
- Cancer impinging on lower urinary tract
- Injury and/or fibrosis of lower urinary tract

Intrinsic renal failure
- Tubular
  - Acute tubular necrosis (severe progression of all causes of I.A.1. above)*
  - Nephrotoxins (e.g., aminoglycosides,* radiocontrast dye, myoglobinuria, heavy metals, myeloma protein)
  - Uric acid nephropathy, hypercalcemia
- Glomerular (e.g., acute glomerulonephritis of multiple origins)
- Vascular (e.g., vasculitis, arterial thrombosis, venous occlusion)
- Interstitial (e.g., allergic interstitial nephritis)

*Frequent in the setting of primary care

POSTRENAL

Postrenal causes of acute renal failure and decreased renal excretory capacity occur in the setting of obstructive lesions of the lower urinary tract as would be the case in prostatic obstruction, renal stone, and papillary necrosis with urethral obstruction.

RENAL

Renal causes of acute renal failure include tubular, glomerular, vascular, or interstitial dysfunctions. The most common intrinsic cause of acute renal failure in primary care settings is acute tubular necrosis secondary to severe and rapid progression of all those causes of decreased effective circulating volume that can initially present as prerenal azotemia. The use of nephrotoxic agents (such as aminoglycosides, radiocontrast dyes, and the exposure of the renal tubules to myoglobin) are also frequent causes of acute tubular injury seen in primary care practices.

Acute nephrotoxicity can be caused by any nonsteroidal (nonsalicylate) anti-inflammatory drug, because these drugs reduce the production of renal prostaglandins, which results in renal vasoconstriction and decreased renal blood flow. This adverse effect of nonsteroidal anti-inflammatory drugs is made more likely in the setting of pre-existing decreased effective circulating volume (e.g., absolute volume depletion, congestive heart failure, cirrhosis, diuretic use, and pre-existing intrinsic renal disease). Since renal prostaglandins promote renin secretion, nonsteroidal anti-inflammatory drugs can cause decreased renin, angiotensin II, and aldosterone production that results in potassium and hydrogen retention (metabolic acidosis caused by hyporeninemic hypoaldosteronism). The increased incidences of nonsteroidal anti-inflammatory drug–induced nephrotoxicity are made manifest by the sheer number of persons who use these agents on a chronic basis.

The common pathway of renal injury in acute renal failure is either renal ischemia or nephrotoxicity. No matter what the cause of the acute intrinsic

Table 58–12. LABORATORY FINDINGS IN CAUSES OF ACUTE RENAL DISEASE

	Prerenal	Renal	Postrenal
Serum BUN/serum creatinine*†	> 10:1	10:1	> 10:1
Urine specific gravity*	High‡	Low§	Low
Urine osmolality*	> 500‡	< 350§	
Urine osmolality/plasma osmolality	> 1.3	< 1.1	
Urine creatinine/plasma creatinine	> 40	< 20 (ATN)	< 20
Urine urea/plasma creatinine	> 8	< 3 (ATN) 78 (GN)‖	< 3
Urine sodium*	<20‡	> 40§	
Fractional excretion of sodium*	< 1 per cent‡	> 2 per cent§	> 2 per cent
Urinary sediment*	Acellular hyaline cast	Renal epithelial cell and casts in ATN. RBCs and RBC casts in vasculitides and glomerulonephritis	

*Most frequently used assessment of acute renal failure in a family medicine hospital setting
†Assuming a steady state of nitrogenous waste production
‡Assuming no drug use (e.g., diuretics) or concomitant disease states (e.g., diabetes mellitus) that affect sodium reabsorption and/or urinary concentration
§Assuming that intrinsic renal disease affects sodium reabsorption and/or urinary concentration
‖GN = glomerulonephritis

renal failure, the clinical course follows a common path consisting of an oliguric phase, a diuretic phase, and a recovery phase. The oliguric phase typically follows a clinical event, e.g., severe hypotension, and is characterized by decreased urine flow in the face of appropriate volume repletion. This phase can last from 7 to 21 days. The oliguric stage is characterized by a progressive increase in BUN and serum creatinine. Patients may also develop hyperkalemia and hyperphosphatemia. The diuretic phase can begin anywhere from 5 to 30 days after the onset of the acute intrinsic renal injury. It is characterized by a gradual increase in urinary output that may, at times, increase to large volumes of urine being produced as newly recovering and generated renal tubular cells are not able to reabsorb an appropriate (e.g., physiologic) amount of the tubular filtrate. These newly functioning and recovering nephrons also may not be able to adequately retain salt, water, and potassium. These electrolyte problems tend to subside as the process of recovery continues. Often, the diuretic phase of acute tubular necrosis may not be clinically apparent if the primary renal insult left a large number of functioning nephrons or if volume intake was insufficient to match urinary output.

TREATMENT

Since, in the setting of primary care, the most common cause of acute renal failure is acute tubular necrosis caused by hypovolemic states and nephrotoxicity, treatment begins with the removal of all nephrotoxic agents (e.g., aminoglycosides, nonsteroidal anti-inflammatory agents) and the restoration of effective circulating volume. Patients should be managed closely to insure maintenance of fluid and electrolyte balance, provide appropriate nutrition, and continue the process of removing factors that precipitated the acute event (e.g., sepsis). Volume overload can be avoided by repleting only urinary and actual insensible loss (actual insensible loss equals calculated insensible loss minus endogenous water formation). In certain clinical settings (e.g., congestive heart failure and septic shock), maintenance of appropriate volume status may require intravascular pressure monitoring.

In order to avoid uremia and provide the necessary fuel substrates for renal recovery, a diet low in protein-containing essential amino acids, which also has high caloric content, should be used. Electrolytes should be given only as needed based on serial measurements. The development of hyponatremia signifies excessive water retention and can be avoided by tighter water restriction. However, calories in the form of carbohydrates at 100 or more grams per day are limited by the amount of water restriction. Essential amino acids and additional calories are indicated if dialysis therapy is instituted and continues for more than a week. If patients continue to retain renally excreted substances, such as phosphates (greater than 5 mg. per dl.), phosphate binders may be required. Calcium gluconate, glucose and insulin, sodium bicarbonate, and sodium polystyrene sulfonate (Kayexalate) can be used to treat hyperkalemia (greater than 5.5 to 6 mEq. per liter). Significant bicarbonate depletion leading to severe metabolic acidosis may require the administration of bicarbonate as sodium bicarbonate or sodium citrate plus citric acid (Shohl's solution). Hemodialysis would be indicated if the patient has symptomatic uremia, hyperkalemia uncontrolled with Kayexalate, excessive volume expansion, severe metabolic acidosis, or other metabolic derangements that cannot be managed through more conservative mechanisms. If hemodialysis is not immediately available and acute uremia ensues during the interim before the referral to a dialysis center, peritoneal dialysis can be used. The major problem involved with peritoneal dialysis is the potential to cause intra-abdominal infection if anything less than sterile technique is used.

In the treatment of acute intrinsic renal failure, one must still not forget the potential that persistent hypovolemia will lead to decreased renal perfusion and continue to complicate recovery. Patients who do not respond as expected should be re-evaluated to insure that their effective circulating volume has been restored. The patient also must be evaluated for a possible infectious source (e.g., pulmonary and urinary) as the cause complicating the recovery from acute tubular necrosis (ATN).

The management of postobstructive causes of acute renal failure is based principally on the removal of the cause of the obstruction and following the urine output, which can become considerable after the postrenal obstruction has been removed. The postobstructive diuresis can be significant enough to lead to significant hypovolemic hypotension. The patients are managed by appropriate fluid and electrolyte replacement, maintenance of body weight, and evaluation of the patients on a daily basis to determine whether or not postural blood pressure and pulse changes occur.

Chronic Renal Failure

Chronic renal failure is caused by decreased numbers of functioning nephrons that occur over the course of months and years. This decrease is progressive and in most cases represents a permanent loss of renal function. The diagnosis of chronic renal failure should only be made once the absence of acute renal failure has been confirmed. The date of onset of chronic renal failure is often not known and in many instances is detected as a result of routine health assessments in a patient with and without problems that might place them at risk (e.g., diabetes mellitus and hypertension). The more common causes of chronic renal failure include diabetic glomerulosclerosis, hypertensive nephrosclerosis, chronic glomerulonephritis, chronic interstitial nephritis, and polycystic kidney disease. The majority of patients (75 per cent) with chronic renal disease have glomerular lesions as an initiating factor of their renal pathology. Although many patients have tubulointerstitial dysfunction, it is usually secondary to a primary glomerular disorder. However, about 25 per cent of chronic renal disease is caused by primary renal tubulointerstitial dysfunction (e.g., chronic polynephritis). Nonimmunologic and, more frequently, immunologic lesions of the glomerulus can be focal and/or diffuse, with diffuse glomerulonephritis more likely resulting in nephrotic syndromes (hypoalbuminemia, edema, hyperlipidemia, and lipiduria).

A useful way to follow patients with chronic renal disease is to plot the creatinine clearance versus the time that predicts the progression of renal dysfunction. If the rate of renal function loss is more rapid than predicted by the above plot, an acute cause of the rapid deterioration of renal dysfunction (volume depletion, uncontrolled hypertension, urinary tract infection, urinary tract obstruction, and the use of a nephrotoxic drug) should be considered. If the rate of fall is less than the expected rate, it more than likely indicates that some aggravating factor causing the progression of renal dysfunction has been removed (e.g., controlled hypertension, improved volume status secondary to improvement of cardiac output). End-stage renal disease is a useful term to describe such severe renal failure that dialysis and/or renal transplantation are required for the patient to continue to survive. The plotting of the creatinine clearance versus time is useful in predicting when this stage will be reached.

Chronic renal failure that develops over a period of years characteristically is asymptomatic until the patient begins to develop signs associated with uremia. These signs typically do not appear until the patient has reached a creatinine clearance less than 20 mm. per minute. Also because the progression of renal failure is so insidious, patients may not realize that they are not feeling as well as they did months to years before.

Uremia

Uremia is a multisystemic process caused by the retention of substances normally excreted by the kidney, renally induced endocrine abnormalities, failure of volume regulation, and disturbance of the ability to maintain a stable acid-base balance. All these factors combine to present one with the symptoms typical of uremia. There are certain renal adaptations in chronic renal failure that minimize the impact of the loss of functioning renal mass, thus permitting a significant decrease in the GFR before retention of toxic waste products occurs.

FLUID, ELECTROLYTE, AND ACID-BASE DISORDERS

Urea and creatinine rise in direct proportion to the degree of fall in the GFR. Hydrogen ion, uric acid, phosphate, and calcium balance are usually maintained until the GFR has dropped less than 30 to 40 ml. per minute. Disorders of serum sodium (water), potassium, and volume regulation are usually maintained until the GFR falls below 10 to 15 ml. per minute. Although the balance of specific solutes can be maintained to extremely low GFRs, it should be noted that the kidney in chronic renal failure has less functional reserve and as a result will not be able to respond to extremes of solute or volume deprivation or excessive solute or volume administration (e.g., potassium). For example, patients with normal kidneys may be able to excrete in excess of 10 liters of ingested water per day. However, patients with severe renal disease may not be able to handle the ingestion of water in excess of 1.5 to 3.5 liters per day without the development of water intoxications (i.e., hyponatremia). Hyperkalemia, although occurring at an extremely low GFR, can occur at a high GFR if excessive potassium from dietary or medication sources is consumed because the impaired kidney is not able to excrete large amounts of potassium per unit time.

When the renal ability to secrete and excrete hydrogen ions becomes impaired (GFR less than 30 ml. per minute), a normal anion gap hyperchloremic metabolic acidosis ensues. As the process of renal failure progresses, the acidosis becomes a high anion gap metabolic acidosis because of the retention of phosphates and sulfates (GFR less than 15 ml. per liter).

CALCIUM AND PHOSPHATE DISORDERS

As the GFR falls in chronic renal failure, the phosphate retention causes hypocalcemia. The hypocalcemia stimulates increased parathyroid hormone and increased bone reabsorption, which releases additional free-ionized calcium in an attempt to normalize serum levels. However, this process eventually can result in osteitis fibrosa. The elevated parathyroid hormone causes the remaining intact nephrons of the failing kidney to increase the excretion of phosphorus, the reabsorption of calcium, and the formation of 1,25-dihydroxyvitamin D, which can result in increased intestinal reabsorption of calcium. However, because of the decreased amount of functional renal mass, there is a deficiency of 1,25-dihydroxyvitamin D, which impairs the mineralization of bone resulting in osteomalacia in adults and rickets in children. Because of the decreased functioning renal mass, renal phosphate excretion normally induced by parathyroid hormone is blunted as is calcium reabsorption.

MAGNESIUM DISORDERS

The inability to excrete magnesium in chronic renal failure is usually not clinically important unless the patient receives substances containing magnesium, such as magnesium-containing antacids. Because of the problem with the inability to excrete magnesium, the use of aluminum-containing antacids is indicated to decrease the intestinal absorption of phosphates. However, the excessive use of aluminum-containing phosphate binders is not without problems, since elevated aluminum levels are associated with the development of osteomalacia and the encephalopathy of chronic renal disease.

ANEMIA

The anemia of renal disease may be caused in part by the decreased production of erythropoietin, which stimulates red cell production in the bone marrow. The activity of erythropoietin, which is normally produced by the kidney, is reduced, resulting in a normochromic normocytic anemia. If the hemoglobin is less than 7 grams in chronic renal failure, a compounding cause, such as bleeding, must be sought. In addition to the anemia, patients may also manifest a platelet disorder that can lead to dysfunctional hemostasis. Again, this platelet dysfunction may lead to bleeding, which will exacerbate the degree of anemia. There also appears to be an indefinite environmental factor (extrinsic) that causes red blood cells to hemolyze prematurely. There are also associated white cell dysfunctions that are a part of the general depressed immune system function seen in uremia, thus predisposing patients to increased risk for infection.

HYPERURICEMIA

Hyperuricemia caused by chronic renal failure usually does not require treatment unless it is associated with gouty arthritis. Significant elevations of uric acid should not be blamed solely on chronic renal disease but should suggest the presence of other states that can increase uric acid production, such as volume depletion and increased cell lysis.

GLUCOSE INTOLERANCE

Patients with chronic renal disease have mild glucose intolerance that does not usually require therapy. Patients with diabetes may in fact have a decrease in insulin requirements as chronic renal failure progresses because of decreased insulin clearance.

CARDIOVASCULAR DISORDERS

Hypertension as a cause of advanced renal failure occurs because of extracellular volume expansion and hyperreninemia. Cardiopulmonary complications of severe uremia can include pericarditis, pleuritis, pulmonary edema, and cardiac tamponade. Chronic renal failure is associated with accelerated vascular disease, which is thought to be secondary to the presence of hyperlipidemia.

PATIENT PRESENTATION

The signs and symptoms of uremia are insidious and are usually associated with fatigue and generalized malaise. Growth rate can be impaired in children with chronic renal disease because of the associated hyperparathyroidism and the nutrition deficiency. Growth is also impaired by the utilization of corticosteroids that might be employed in the treatment of some of the glomerulonephropathies. Patients with uremia can develop encephalopathy and peripheral neuropathy involving both motor and sensory modalities.

TREATMENT

A very cautious and conservative approach to chronic renal failure should occur until the creatinine clearance has dropped to 5 to 10 ml. per minute. Diet becomes an important part of the treatment of chronic renal failure when the creatinine clearance is less than 30 mm. per minute. Protein restrictions (approximately 40 grams) with an adequate amount of calories (30 calories per kilogram) are indicated to prevent tissue catabolism and negative nitrogen balance. The first goal of therapy of the bone disease of chronic renal failure is the dietary restriction of phosphates plus the use of aluminum-containing phosphate binders that help to maintain and restore normal phosphate concentration. If hypocalcemia is present after the utilization of aluminum-containing, phosphate-binding antacids then calcium supplementation should be considered as well as vitamin D preparations.

The amount of salt that is given is determined by the presence of edema, hypertension, and pulmonary edema. Because there is an obligatory loss of sodium in patients with renal failure, the amount of salt taken in per unit time may exceed 10 grams, while others might require very severe salt restrictions (less than 2 grams per day). Usual salt restrictions for most patients should be maintained at approximately 4 to 6 grams of sodium per day since the renal excretory mechanisms continue, in most instances, to handle that dietary load in spite of advancing renal failure. In patients who are developing metabolic acidosis, administration of sodium bicarbonate may be required to maintain bicarbonate levels at greater than 20 mEq. per liter. Elimination of foodstuffs high in potassium is also required in patients who have creatinine clearance less than 10 mm. per minute in order to avoid severe hyperkalemia.

Hypertension, developing as a cause of chronic

renal disease, requires sodium restriction plus the utilization of loop diuretics since the etiology of the hypertension is volume expansion. Failure of diuretics alone to control hypertension is an indication for the use of a second class of antihypertensive agents.

Treatment for the anemia of chronic renal failure due to a lack of erythropoietin effect is under investigation at present. Human erythropoietin is presently being used to treat the anemia of chronic renal failure in selected patients on dialysis. However, it is important to eliminate other causes of anemia (such as iron deficiency), since human erythropoeitin may compound the anemia of renal failure and signal the presence of other serious underlying disease (e.g., GI bleeding from an occult GI cancer).

Infections in general as well as infections of the kidney should be considered as the cause of unexpected rapid progression of chronic renal disease and should be treated aggressively. Nephrotoxic agents should be avoided unless other acceptable agents are not available to treat underlying disease processes.

Management of diabetes is extremely important since hyperglycemia can cause osmotic diuresis and enhance hypoperfusion of the kidneys, causing acute or chronic renal failure.

Patients with chronic renal disease should always be evaluated in conjunction with a nephrologist so that preparations can be made for those candidates who will require chronic hemodialysis, intermittent perineal dialysis, and renal transplantation.

References

Abbott, G. D.: Neonatal bacteriuria: a prospective study in 1460 infants. Br. Med. J., *1*:267–269, 1972.

Allen, T. D., and Ransler, C. W.: Torsion of the spermatic cord. Urol. Clin. North Am., *9*:245–249, 1982.

Belman, B. A.: Urethra: Clinical Pediatric Urology. Philadelphia, W. B. Saunders Co., 1985, pp. 527–553. *Standard textbook of pediatric urology.*

Bia, M., and Thier, S. O.: Mixed acid-base disturbances: a clinical approach. Med. Clin. North Am., *65*(2):347–611, 1981. *Excellent discussion of a diagnostic approach to determine the presence of mixed acid-base disturbances. It discusses expected compensations and limits of compensation of primary acid-base disturbances as a basis to determine the presence of a mixed acid-base event.*

Bidani, A.: Electrolyte and acid-base disorders. Med. Clin. North Am., *70*(5):1013–1036, 1986. *An excellent review of the pathophysiology of acid-base disturbances with the presentation of a diagnostic approach to these disorders. The article makes a complex issue very understandable.*

Birkhoff, J. D.: Natural history of BPH. *In* Hinman, F. (Ed.): Benign prostatic hypertrophy. New York, Springer Verlag, 1983, p. 5.

Blandy, J.: Operative Urology. Boston, Blackwell Scientific Publications, 1986, pp. 162–163.

Carstensen, H. E., and Hansen, T. S.: Stones in the ureter. Actu. Chir. Scand. (Suppl.), *433*:66–71, 1973.

Chaussy, C. G., and Fuchs, G.: Extracorporeal shock wave lithotripsy (ESWL) for the treatment of upper urinary stones. *In* Gillenwater, J., et al. (Eds.): Adult and Pediatric Urology. Chicago, Year Book Medical Publishers Inc., 1987, pp. 605–619. *Short chapter in recently published textbook provides discussion of indications and complications of ESWL.*

Coldiron, B. M., and Jacobson, C.: Common penile lesions. Urol. Clin. North Am., *15*(4):671–674, 1988.

Corriere, J. N., Jr., and Sandler, C. M.: Management of the ruptured bladder: 7 year experience with ill cases. J. Trauma, *26*:830, 1986.

Costello, A. J.: Percutaneous aspiration of renal cortical abscess. Urology, *21*:201, 1983.

Cronin, R. E.: Magnesium disorders: fluids and electrolytes. Philadelphia, W. B. Saunders Co., 1986, pp. 502–512. *Excellent discussion of volume and chloride deficiency as a frequent cause of metabolic alkalosis. This type of metabolic alkalosis (saline responsive) is common in primary care because of the number of patients who are treated with diuretics.*

Cutler, S. J., and Henry, N. M.: Bladder cancer. AVA Monographs, *1*:35, 1982.

deKernion, J. B.: Treatment of advanced renal cell cancer-traditional methods and innovative approaches. J. Urol., *130*:2, 1983.

Emmett, M., and Narins, R. G.: Clinical use of the anion gap. Medicine, *56*(1):38–54, 1977. *Illustrates the important diagnostic potential of the often overlooked laboratory value. The implication of its use in the diagnosis of normochloremic metabolic acid alone and mixed with other acid-base disturbances is emphasized.*

Esperanca, M., and Gerrard, J. W.: Nocturnal enuresis: studies in bladder function in normal children and enuretics. Can. Med. Assoc. J., *101*:324, 1969. *Two hundred ninety seven normal children and 50 enuretic children were evaluated over 1 week with frequency and volumes of urine recorded. Standardized physiologic bladder capacity was measured. Enuretic children were found to have markedly smaller bladder capacities and were more frequent voiders both during the day and at night.*

Fair, W. R.: Three day treatment of urinary tract infection. J. Urol., *123*:717–721, 1980. *Women with documented cystitis were treated with either penicillin-G or trimethoprim-sulfamethoxazole at conventional dosages. Results of 3 days of therapy were found to be equal to 10 days of identical therapy. The patients were derived from an unselected general practice, and treatment was assigned without knowledge of in vitro susceptibilities.*

Felts, P. W.: Ketoacidosis. Med. Clin. North Am., *67*(4):831–843, 1983. *An excellent review of the pathophysiology of ketoacidosis and its impact on patient presentation and treatment.*

Fowler, J. E.: Urinary tract infections in women. Urol. Clin. North Am., *13*:4, 1986. *A review article summarizing data from several studies. In four separate reports with over 1100 patients, the risk of catheter-associated bacteriuria was clearly related to the duration of catheterization and ranged from 4 to 7.5 per cent per day.*

Fowler, J. E., Jr., and Marshall, V.: Nosocomial catheter associated urinary tract infection. Infect. Surg., *2*:43–53, 1983.

Fox, W.: Whether short course chemotherapy. Br. J. Dis. Chest, *75*:331, 1981. *Four hundred twenty two patients with tuberculosis were treated for 6 months and only 4 (1 per cent) relapsed. Patients received daily streptomycin, isoniazid, ritampicin, and pyrazinamide for the first 2 months followed either by isoniazid, ritampicin, and pyrazindmide or isoniazid and ritampicin alone for the next 4 months.*

Frey, H. L., and Rajter, J.: Incidence of cryptochidism. Urol. Clin. North Am., *9*:3, 327, 1982.

George, N. J. R.: Urethral syndrome—clinical features. *In* George, N. R., and Gosling, J. A. (Eds.): Sensory Disorders of the Bladder and Urethra. New York, Springer-Verlag, 1986, pp. 91–102.

Gillenwater, J. Y.: Natural history of bacteriuria in schoolgirls. N. Engl. J. Med., *30*:396, 1979.

Gow, J. G.: Genitourinary tuberculosis. *In* Walsh, P. C., and Stamey, T. A. (Eds.): Campbell's Urology. Philadelphia, W. B. Saunders Co., 1986, p. 1057.

Green, D. M.: The diagnosis and management of Wilms' tumor. Pediatr. Clin. North Am., *32*:3, 1985.

Greenberg, S. H., and Lipshultz, L. I.: Experience with 425 subfertile male patients. J. Urol., *119*:507, 1978.

Hamm, L., and Jacobson, H. R.: Mixed Acid-base Disorders: Fluids and Electrolytes. Philadelphia, W. B. Saunders Co., 1986.

Helfant, R. H.: Hypokalemia and arrhythmias. Am. J. Med., *8*(Suppl. 4A):13–22, 1986. *A good discussion of the detrimental effects of hypokalemia in the setting of patients with or without underlying cardiovascular disease. The article emphasizes the fact that diuretic-induced hypokalemia is not as benign as once was believed.*

Henry, J. B.: Todd, Sanford, Davidsohn Clinical Diagnosis and Management by Laboratory Methods. Vol. 1. 16th ed. Philadelphia, W. B. Saunders Co., 1979, pp. 616, 621, 626, 628.

Hobbs, J.: Disturbances in acid-base metabolism: recognition in the office setting. Postgrad. Med., *83*(2):121–130, 1988. *A comprehensive review of common acid-base disturbances seen in office practice with emphasis on appropriate recognition and diagnosis. A general therapeutic approach to acid-base problems is also discussed.*

Hobbs, J.: Office laboratory evaluation of fluid, electrolyte, and acid-base disorders. Prim. Care, *13*(4):761–782, 1986. *Illustrates the use of simple and inexpensive office laboratory studies in the preliminary evaluation of acid-base disorders. The use of office-based chemical analysis is also discussed.*

Hobbs, J., and Yens, D. P.: Characteristics of the anion gap in a family practice population. J. Med. Assoc. Ga., *71*:331–335, 1982.

Hollifield, J. W.: Potassium and magnesium abnormalities: diuretics and arrhythmias in hypertension. Am. J. Med., *77*(Suppl. 5A):28–46, 1986. *A good discussion of the relationship of potassium and magnesium deficiency secondary to diuretic therapy. The rate of the need to treat magnesium disorders in hypokalemic patients is also discussed.*

Humes, H. D., Narins, R. G., and Brenner, B. M.: Disorders of water balance. Hosp. Pract., *14*:133–145, 1979. *An easy to understand discussion of hyponatremia and hypernatremia. Pathophysiology is clearly outlined and diagnostic flow charts have been directed applicably to a practice setting.*

Kaehny, W. D.: Respiratory acid-base disorders. Med. Clin. North Am., *67*(4):915–928, 1983.

Kaplan, G. W.: Post infection reflux. Soc. Pediatr. Urol. Newsletter, April 9, 1980.

Kass, E. H.: Asymptomatic infections of the urinary tract. Trans. Assoc. Am. Physicians, *69*:57, 1956. *An often quoted classic study from Boston City Hospital. Asymptomatic women were randomly catheterized and a quantitative basis was established for diagnosing true (noncontaminant) bacteriuria (> 10^5 bacteria/ml.).*

Kimmel, S. R.: Neonatal Circumcision: Basic Procedures in Family Practice. New York, John Wiley Medical Publishing Co., 1984, pp. 100–106.

King, L. R.: Posterior Urethra: Clinical Pediatric Urology. Philadelphia, W. B. Saunders Co., 1985, pp. 527–553.

Koff, S. A.: Enuresis in office urology. Urol. Clin. North Am., *15*(4):769–775, 1988.

Kokko, J. P., and Tannen, R. L.: Fluids and Electrolytes. Philadelphia, W. B. Saunders Co., 1986, pp. 3–62.

Kursh, E. D., and Resnick, M. I.: Dissolution of uric acid calculi with systemic alkalization. J. Urol., *132*:286, 1984.

Lapides, J.: Neuromuscular, vesical and ureteral dysfunction. *In* Campbell, M. F., and Harrison, J. H. (Eds.): Urology. Philadelphia, W. B. Saunders Co., 1970, pp. 1343–1379. *The Lapides classification scheme for neurogenic vesical dysfunction.*

Lee, F.: Needle aspiration and core biopsy of prostate cancer: comparative evaluation with transrectal vs. guidance. Radiology, *163*(2):515–520, 1987.

LeRoy, A. J., and Segura, J. W.: Percutaneous removal of renal calculi: interventional uroradiology. Radiol. Clin. North Am., *24*(4):615–622, 1986.

Massey, F. J., Bernstein, G. S., O'Fallon, W. M., et al.: Vasectomy and health: results from a large cohort study. J.A.M.A., *252*(8):1023–1029, 1984.

Mayhew, H. E.: Vasectomy. Semin. Fam. Med., *2*(2):94–100, 1981.

Mulholland, S. G.: Uncomplicated adult urinary tract infections. AVA Update Series, Vol. VI, Lesson 14, 1987.

Mundy, A. R.: The unstable bladder. Urol. Clin. North Am., *12*(2):317–328, 1985.

Narins, R. G., and Cohen, J. J.: Bicarbonate therapy for organic acidosis: the case for its continued use. Ann. Intern. Med., *106*(4):615–618, 1987. *The controversy over the use of bicarbonation in organic acidosis continues, and this article argues for its use in clear and precise terms. Although one may support the opposing view, the argument of bicarbonate use in certain settings is clearly discussed.*

Norden, C. W., and Kass, E. H.: Bacteriuria of pregnancy: a critical appraisal. Ann. Rev. Med., *19*:432–470, 1968.

Pak, C. Y. C.: Medical management of nephrolithiasis in Dallas: update 1987. J. Urol., *140*:3, 1988. *A review of the pathophysiology, diagnosis, and medical management of nephrolithiasis. A protocol for evaluation is presented as well as indications and dosages for thiazide, potassium citrate, allopurinal, and dietary management.*

Pak, C. Y. C.: Calcium disorders: fluids and electrolytes. Philadelphia, W. B. Saunders Co., 1986, pp. 472–501.

Pearson, J. C., and Dombrouskis, S.: RIA of serum acid phosphatase after prostatic massage. Urology, *21*:37, 1983.

Phillips, P. A., Rolls, B. J., Ledingham, J. G., et al.: Reduced thirst after water deprivation in healthy elderly men. N. Engl. J. Med., *311*:753–759, 1984. *Emphasizes the risk that older patients confront when they are exposed to excess water loss and a lack of access to water—a greater tendency toward water depletion (hypernatremia).*

Pollack, H. M.: The accuracy of grey scale renal ultrasound in differentiating neoplasms from benign cysts. Radiology, *143*:741, 1982.

Raiffer, J., and Bennett, C. J.: Vasectomy. Urol. Clin. North Am., *15*(4):631, 1988. *This particular edition of the Urologic Clinics of North America is on office urology and contains discussions on several topics of interest to primary care physicians. Included are color plates of common penile lesions, vasectomy, circumcision, catheterization, and the management and evaluation of voiding disorders in children.*

Resnick, M., and Kursh, E. D.: Use of computerized tomography in the delineation of uric acid calculi. J. Urol., *131*:9–10, 1984.

Rose, B. D.: Glomerular Disease: Pathophysiology of Renal Disease. 1st ed. New York, McGraw-Hill, 1981a, pp. 98–197.

Rose, B. D.: Pathophysiology of Uremia: Pathophysiology of Renal Disease. 1st ed. New York, McGraw-Hill, 1981b, pp. 419–474.

Rose, B. D.: Acute Renal Failure: Pathophysiology of Renal Disease. 1st ed. New York, McGraw-Hill, 1981c, pp. 55–95.

Rose, B. D.: Tubulointerstitial Disease: Pathophysiology of Renal Disease. 1st ed. New York, McGraw-Hill, 1981d, pp. 295–323.

Rose, B. D.: Diagnostic Approach to Patients With Renal Disease: Pathophysiology of Renal Disease. 1st ed. New York, McGraw-Hill, 1981e, pp. 31–53. *A comprehensive yet easy to read discussion concerning the evaluation of patients with renal disease. The article discusses the diagnostic utility of urinalysis, urine sediment, urine electrolytes, creatinine clearance, and serum electrolytes as they relate to findings in renal disease. The additional chapters (1981a–1981d) are equally well written and easy to understand with good applicability to primary care practices.*

Rose, B. D.: Edematous States and the Use of Diuretics: Clinical Physiology of Acid-Base and Electrolyte Disorders. 2nd ed. New York, McGraw-Hill, 1984a, pp. 310–360. *An excellent review of the pathophysiology of edema formation and the use of diuretics. The pharmacotherapeutics of diuretics as they relate to certain edematous states, including indications for use and side effects, is also discussed.*

Rose, B. D.: Hyperkalemia: Clinical Physiology of Acid-Base and Electrolyte Disorders. 2nd ed. New York, McGraw-Hill, 1984b, pp. 617–645.

Rose, B. D.: Hyperosmolal States—Hypernatremia: Clinical Physiology of Acid-Base and Electrolyte Disorders. 2nd ed. New York, McGraw-Hill, 1984c, pp. 515–547.

Rose, B. D.: Hyperosmolal States—Hyperglycemia: Clinical Physiology of Acid-Base and Electrolyte Disorders. 2nd ed. New York, McGraw-Hill, 1984d, pp. 548–566.

Rose, B. D.: Hypoosmolal States—Hyponatremia: Clinical Physiology of Acid-Base and Electrolyte Disorders. 2nd ed. New York, McGraw-Hill, 1984e, pp. 482–514.

Rose, B. D.: Hypovolemic States: Clinical Physiology of Acid-

Base and Electrolyte Disorders. 2nd ed. New York, McGraw-Hill, 1984f, pp. 279–309.

Rose, B. D.: Introduction to Simple and Mixed Acid-base Disorders: Clinical Physiology of Acid-Base and Electrolyte Disorders. 2nd ed. New York, McGraw-Hill, 1984g, pp. 361–373. *One of the best explanations of mixed acid-base disturbances I have read. Author discusses expected rates of compensation of primary acid-base disturbances as the basis to detect mixed acid-base disturbances. He also discusses the use and limitation of the acid-base map in the diagnosis of these disorders.*

Rose, B. D.: Meaning and Application of Urine Chemistries: Clinical Physiology of Acid-Base and Electrolyte Disorders. 2nd ed. New York, McGraw-Hill, 1984h, pp. 271–278. *An excellent discussion of the diagnostic potential of urine chemistry to acid-base disturbances, hypovolemic states, hypokalemia, and disorders of osmolality. The limitation of the use of their measurements is also discussed.*

Rose, B. D.: Metabolic Acidosis: Clinical Physiology of Acid-Base and Electrolyte Disorders. 2nd ed. New York, McGraw-Hill, 1984i, pp. 394–439. *A chapter out of one of the most understandable books on acid-base and fluid and electrolyte disorders. This discussion of metabolic acidosis provides a clear description of the pathophysiology, diagnosis, and treatment without bogging down in nonessential detail what may or may not benefit the practitioner in primary care. The other chapters for this book (1981a–1981e; 1984a–1984m) are equally informative.*

Rose, B. D.: Metabolic Alkalosis: Clinical Physiology of Acid-Base and Electrolyte Disorders. 2nd ed. New York, McGraw-Hill, 1984j, pp. 374–393.

Rose, B. D.: Respiratory Alkalosis: Clinical Physiology of Acid-Base and Electrolyte Disorders. 2nd ed. New York, McGraw-Hill, 1984k, pp. 462–470.

Rose, B. D.: Hypokalemia: Clinical Physiology of Acid-Base and Electrolyte Disorders. 2nd ed. New York, McGraw-Hill, 1984l, pp. 579–616.

Rose, B. D.: Respiratory Acidosis: Clinical Physiology of Acid-Base and Electrolyte Disorders. 2nd ed. New York, McGraw-Hill, 1984m, pp. 440–461.

Saxton, C. R., and Seldin, D. W.: Clinical Interpretation of Laboratory Values: Fluids and Electrolytes. Philadelphia, W. B. Saunders Co., 1986, pp. 3–62. *An exploration of the diagnostic potential of commonly ordered laboratory studies as they relate to the use of bicarbonate therapy in organic acidosis is presented. The emphasis on the overuse of alkali and its consequences is made. A more conservative approach to the use of bicarbonate in DKA is also discussed.*

Seeley, E. C.: Department of Family Practice, University of Kentucky, Lexington, Kentucky. Personal communication and art work, 1989.

Skinner, D. G., and Lieskovsky, G.: Diagnosis of Management of Genitourinary Cancer. Philadelphia, W. B. Saunders Co., 1988, pp. 508–531.

Stacpoole, P. W.: Lactic acidosis: the case against bicarbonate therapy. Ann. Intern. Med., *105*(2):276–279, 1986. *An excellent discussion presenting a controversial point of view concerning the treatment of lactic acidosis with bicarbonate. The author cautions against the indiscriminate treatment of lactic acidosis with bicarbonate because of associated side effects of volume overload, posttreatment metabolic acidosis, and hypokalemia and increased hemoglobin O_2 affinity.*

Stamey, T. A., Norman, Y., Hay, A. R., et al.: Prostate-specific antigen as a serum human marker for adenocarcinoma of the prostate. N. Engl. J. Med., *317*(15):909–916, 1987. *Prostatic specific antigen (PSA) and prostatic acid phosphatase (PSP) were measured in 699 patients, 378 of whom had prostatic cancer. Both may be elevated in benign prostatic hyperplasia as well as in prostatic cancer and thus neither is specific enough for use in diagnosis. PSA is useful in monitoring response and recurrence after therapy.*

Sternberg, C. N., and Yugoda, A.: Preliminary results of M-VAC for transitional cell carcinoma of the urothelium. J. Urol., *133*:403–407, 1985.

Sullivan, D. G., and Grabstald, H.: Management of carcinoma of the urethra. *In* Skinner, D. G., and deKernion, J. B. (Eds.): Genitourinary Cancer. Philadelphia, W. B. Saunders Co., 1978, p. 419.

Toto, R. D.: Metabolic Acid-base Disorders: Fluids and Electrolytes. Philadelphia, W. B. Saunders Co., 1986, pp. 229–304.

Veterans Administration Cooperative Urological Research Group: Factors in prognosis of carcinoma of the prostate: a cooperative study. J. Urol., *100*:59, 1968. *The VA clinical trials with over 2200 patients are the most extensive studies of endocrine therapy for adenocarcinoma of the prostate. Survival data is presented by stage of disease, treatment, and cause of death. There have been three studies to date. Very briefly, delayed endocrine therapy does prolong survival in patients with state D disease. DES at 1 mg. daily was as effective as other endocrine agents but 5 mg. was associated with a higher cardiovascular death rate. Progression of Stage C and D cancer was restrained by orchiectomy or DES.*

Walsh, P. C.: The differential diagnosis of ambiguous genitalia in the newborn. Urol. Clin. North Am., *5*(1):213–221, 1978. *A concise review of ambiguous genitalia, including an easy to follow schedule for dealing with the family, relatives, and friends.*

Wein, A. J.: Classification of neurogenic voiding dysfunction. J. Urol., *125*:605–609, May 1981. Review article.

Wein, A. J., and Stephenson, T. P.: Urodynamics, Principles, Practice and Application. New York, Churchill Livingstone, 1984. *Excellent review of classification systems, used for neurogenic voiding dysfunctions.*

Weyman, P. J.: Comparison of CT and angiography in the evaluation of renal cell carcinoma. Radiology, *137*:417, 1980. *Forty-nine patients with renal cell carcinoma were preoperatively studied with both CT and angiography. The diagnostic accuracy of CT was 95 per cent, 89 per cent with angiography.*

Whitaker, R. H.: Another look at diagnostic pathways in children with urinary tract infections. Br. Med. J., *288*:839, 1984.

Wise, G. J., and Kozinn, P. J.: Amphotericin B as a urologic irrigant in the management of noninvasive candiduria. J. Urol., *128*:82, 1982.

Wiswell, T. E., and Metcalf, T.: Challenging opinions: routine neonatal circumcision. Postgrad. Med., *84*:5, 1988.

59

Ophthalmology

Earl R. Crouch, Jr.
Alexander Berger

Patients present to the family physician with a limited set of symptoms in which there may be subtle differences between nonserious and serious ocular conditions. In order to be able to decide when to treat patients and when to refer them to an ophthalmologist, the family physician must possess a complete appreciation of the subtle differences in presenting symptoms between serious and nonserious ophthalmologic diseases. Knowledge of the basic anatomy of the eye is essential in determining these diagnostic differences (Fig. 59–1).

The Red Eye

The family physician frequently encounters patients who complain of a red eye. Usually, the condition causing the red eye is a simple disorder such as conjunctivitis or subconjunctival hemorrhage. These conditions improve spontaneously or are readily treated. A red eye, however, may be a symptom of a more serious disorder, i.e. herpetic dendritic ulcer, iritis, acute angle closure glaucoma, ophthalmia neonatorum, and congenital glaucoma. These conditions must be clearly distinguished from the much more common conjunctivitis and subconjunctival hemorrhage because immediate referral to the ophthalmologist is paramount.

To evaluate the red eye, the family physician needs a penlight, a magnifying glass, a visual acuity chart, fluorescein dye, anesthetic drops, and a Schiotz tonometer.

SYMPTOMS AND SIGNS (SUMMARIZED IN TABLE 59–1)

Patients who complain of a red eye generally will be able to tell the physician whether the eye became very rapidly irritated or whether the irritation has progressed slowly. A small foreign body, such as a grain of sand, lodged in the conjunctival sac will produce a very rapid hyperemia whereas a viral or allergic conjunctivitis, or an iritis, will generally have a slowly progressive redness of the eye.

Ocular pain is an important symptom. Irritation of the superficial layer of the cornea, such as caused by a small foreign body, will be accompanied by a superficial grain-of-sand sensation in the eye. Deeper inflammatory processes, such as iritis or iridocyclitis or a deeper penetrating foreign body in the cornea, will present with a more severe dull pain in the eye that is often compared by patients to the pain felt when hit on the eye with a fist.

Abnormal light sensitivity (photophobia) is a third symptom that must be elicited by the family physician. It is a danger signal and occurs with corneal inflammation and iritis. Patients who have conjunctivitis usually do not have abnormal light sensitivity (Table 59–2).

Patients who complain of a red eye often complain of discharge from the eye (Table 59–3). If they do not complain of eye discharge spontaneously, the physician must inquire into the presence, type, and quantity of discharge. Purulent (creamy white or yellow watery) discharge suggests a bacterial etiology. A serous or clear discharge suggests a viral cause. Scanty, white, stringy exudate occurs most commonly in allergic conjunctivitis. The absence of discharge indicates an unusual cause for a red eye such as iridocyclitis, ultraviolet light keratitis (snow blindness), or acute angle closure glaucoma.

A complaint of diminished visual acuity is a serious danger signal and must be elicited in the history.

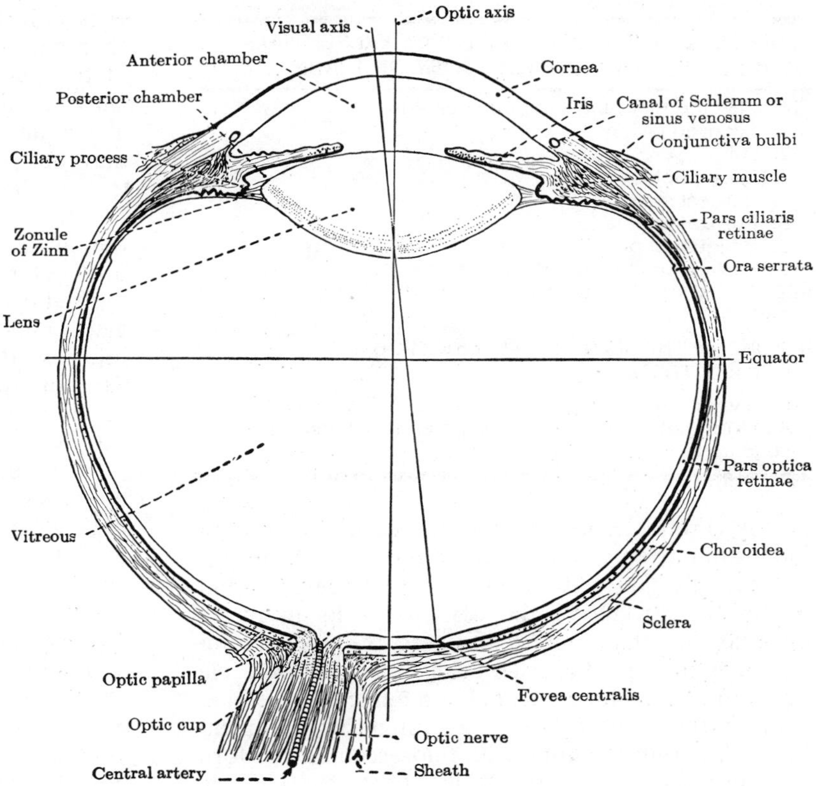

Figure 59–1. Anatomy of the right eyeball. (From Scheie, H. G., and Albert, D. M.: Textbook of Ophthalmology. 9th ed. Philadelphia, W. B. Saunders Company, 1977. By permission.)

PHYSICAL EXAMINATION

It is very important to examine both eyes since many of the patients with conjunctivitis in one eye will have clear signs of early conjunctivitis in the other. The type of injection must be closely inspected: conjunctival injection is characterized by clearly delineated, individually visible vessels in the conjunctiva that are branching from the corner of the eye towards the cornea. Ciliary injection (Plate XXXI), on the other hand, appears as a red ring surrounding the limbus of the cornea in which individual vessels are not clearly visible—and if they are visible, they appear parallel rather than branching. The significance of ciliary injection is that the deep ciliary vessels are involved. A ciliary injection signifies a much more serious inflammatory condition of the eye, such as a deep corneal infection, an iritis, and/or iridocyclitis. The palpebral conjunctiva should be inspected carefully with magnification to see whether a lymphoid hyperplasia (cobblestone appearance) exists. The type and quantity of discharge needs to be assessed by pulling down the lower lid. The appearance of the punctum—the entrance point of the tear duct—should be examined to demonstrate whether pus is coming out of the tear duct. Palpation of the tear sac on the upper portion of the nose (lacrimal crest) will demonstrate tenderness in cases of dacryocystitis.

Table 59–1. THE RED EYE—DIFFERENTIAL DIAGNOSIS

	Conjunctivitis Bacterial	Iritis	Keratitis	Acute Glaucoma
Vision	Normal	Blurred	Blurred	Marked blurring
Pain	None	Moderately severe; intermittent stabbing	Sharp, severe	Very severe; sometimes nausea and vomiting
Photophobia	None	Moderate	Moderate	Moderate
Discharge	Usually significant with crusting of lashes	None	None to mild	None
Conjunctival Injection	Diffuse	Circumcorneal (surrounding the cornea)	Circumcorneal	Diffuse
Appearance of Cornea	Clear	Clear	Cloudy	Cloudy
Pupil Size	Normal	Constricted	Normal	Dilated
Intraocular Pressure	Normal *Caution:* do not measure with discharge present	Normal or low	Normal	Elevated

From American Academy of Ophthalmology: *The Red Eye*, San Francisco, CA: Professional Information Committee, 1986.

Table 59–2. APPROACH TO PATIENT PRESENTING WITH RED EYE (WITHOUT HISTORY OF TRAUMA)

Check for the following symptoms or signs:

1. Reduced vision
2. Pain
3. Photophobia
4. Corneal staining
5. Corneal edema
6. Unequal pupils
7. Elevated intraocular pressure

REFER TO OPHTHALMOLOGIST IF ANY OF THESE SIGNALS ARE PRESENT.

IF NONE OF THE ABOVE IS PRESENT, PROBABLY CONJUNCTIVITIS.

The triad of a *red eye, pain,* and *loss of vision* should ALWAYS alert the examiner to a potentially blinding condition.

A careful examination of the cornea is of paramount importance in assessing a red eye. The cornea is normally perfectly transparent. Excessive fluid within the stroma of the cornea results in partial opacification that can be observed by direct illumination with a penlight. A diffuse corneal haze can occur in congenital glaucoma and angle closure glaucoma. After inspection with a penlight under magnification, corneal staining with fluorescein in the form of sterile filter paper strips should be performed. The stain part of the strip is moistened with water and touched to the conjunctiva away from the cornea. With blinking, the fluorescein spreads over the cornea. An ultraviolet light source enhances fluorescence (Plate XXXII). Areas of bright green staining denote absent or diseased epithelium. Corneal staining will readily demonstrate abrasions of the cornea and will help identify corneal foreign bodies and infectious epithelial defects such as herpetic, dendritic keratitis.

The pupils must be examined carefully for size and shape. In most people, the pupils are of equal size. In a small percentage of people, there is congenital variation in a size of the pupils (anisocoria). In these cases, the patients are often aware of the fact that their pupils are unequal. In patients with previously equal pupils, inequality of the pupil may indicate iritis in which the affected pupil is typically partially constricted. In acute angle closure glaucoma, the pupil is usually partially dilated and may not be quite round. Unequal pupils may be the only sign of significant ocular trauma.

Anterior chamber depth may be estimated by side illumination with a penlight. If the anterior chamber is normal or deep, the entire surface of the eyes will be well illuminated. When the anterior chamber is shallow, the iris on the more distant side of the pupil will be in shadow. A shallow anterior chamber in a red eye may indicate acute angle closure glaucoma or ocular trauma. The anterior chamber may be extremely deep in congenital glaucoma or trauma that results in a ruptured globe.

Table 59–3. CONJUNCTIVITIS CLUES

Discharge Type	Etiology
Purulent	Bacterial
Serous or Clear	Viral
Stringy, White	Allergic
Preauricular lymph node enlargement	Viral

If the red eye does not have an obvious infection, the intraocular pressure should be measured by a tonometer. The pressure is normal in most causes of the red eye with the exception of acute angle closure glaucoma. In iritis and traumatic perforating ocular injuries, the intraocular pressure is generally low. The tonometer should be sterilized before and after application to a red eye preferably by heat sterilization.

Preauricular lymph node enlargement is a frequent sign of viral conjunctivitis and usually is not present in acute bacterial conjunctivitis. (See Table 59–3.)

The Red Eye in Infants

Several conditions that occur specifically in the first year of life include ophthalmia neonatorum, acute and chronic dacryocystitis, and congenital glaucoma.

OPHTHALMIA NEONATORUM

Ophthalmia neonatorum is an inflammation of the conjunctiva that occurs during the first 4 weeks of life. Possible causes include chemical conjunctivitis, *Neisseria gonorrhoeae*, nongonococcal bacterial conjunctivitis, and *Chlamydia*. The increased incidence of venereal disease and shortcomings of silver nitrate prophylaxis are significant factors in the constantly evolving clinical picture of ophthalmia neonatorum. Frequently, cases of ophthalmia neonatorum are a manifestation of a systemic infection that indicates the need for precise etiologic diagnosis in all but the most transient cases. Table 59–4 lists types of management for ophthalmia neonatorum.

Chemical Conjunctivitis

Chemical conjunctivitis is a condition resulting from the use of silver nitrate prophylaxis. In recent years, the silver nitrate prophylaxis has been replaced by erythromycin prophylaxis so that the incidence of chemical conjunctivitis has decreased significantly. Silver nitrate is not active against *Chlamydia*.

Prior to the Credé form of prophylaxis, gonorrhea was the common cause of ophthalmia neonatorum. Half of the patients with gonococcal conjunctivitis developed corneal clouding—a major cause of blindness. Gonococcal conjunctivitis still occurs in spite of silver nitrate or erythromycin prophylaxis. Frequently, the infant with gonococcal conjunctivitis

Table 59–4. MANAGEMENT OF OPHTHALMIA NEONATORUM

Disease	Diagnosis	Treatment
Gonococcal conjunctivitis	Gram-negative intracellular diplococci + growth on chocolate agar or Thayer-Martin + fermentation glucose + maltose −	Topical tetracycline or erythromycin ointment q.i.d. × 2 weeks Systemic aqueous procaine penicillin, 50,000 units/kg. body weight/day intravenously × 7 days Ophthalmology consultation
Other causes of bacterial conjunctivitis	Gram stain + growth on blood agar or chocolate agar	Gram positive—erythromycin ointment (0.5 per cent) q.i.d. × 2 weeks Gram negative—gentamicin ophthalmic (0.3 per cent) solution q.i.d. × 2 weeks
Inclusion conjunctivitis *(Chlamydia)*	Giemsa stain—basophilic intracytoplasmic inclusion bodies Chlamydial culture	Tetracycline or sulfacetamide ointment q.i.d. × 4 weeks; with systemic involvement add systemic erythromycin × 3 weeks

presents with swollen lids, purulent exudates, beefy red conjunctiva, and conjunctival edema. The gonococcus organism can penetrate the intact corneal epithelium and produce corneal perforation if recognition and treatment are delayed. When gonoccoccal conjunctivitis is suspected, referral to an ophthalmologist is mandatory. Patients may also have systemic involvement with associated central nervous signs. Both parents should be examined for venereal disease and treated when indicated.

Bacterial Conjunctivitis

The most common gram-positive bacteria that are causative agents in conjunctivitis include: *Staphylococcus aureus, Streptococcus pneumonia*, and group A and B streptococcus (Fig. 59–2). Gram-negative organisms include *Haemophilus influenzae, Escherichia coli,* and *Pseudomonas aeruginosa*. Bacterial conjunctivitis can occur at any age from the first day of life. Chemosis (edema of the bulbar conjunctiva), purulent discharge, lid edema, and injection are common signs. An associated systemic septicemia can occur, especially with pseudomonas. Cultures should be taken on blood and chocolate agar. The best treatment prior to culture results is erythromycin ointment. Gram-negative organisms are best treated with gentamicin ophthalmic. Systemic antibiotics are recommended when there is evidence of systemic disease.

Chlamydia *Infection*

Chlamydia infections are a leading cause of ophthalmia neonatorum. There is a high incidence of this type of infection because of the frequent exposure of the newborn during delivery and the lack of effect of silver nitrate prophylaxis on *Chlamydia*. The onset of infection can occur at any time. The typical picture is a mild unilateral or bilateral mucopurulent conjunctivitis with moderate lid edema, chemosis, and conjunctival injection. Systemic involvement may include rhinitis, vaginitis, and otitis media. Treatment is either tetracycline ointment or sulfacetamide ointment four times daily for 4 weeks. In addition, both parents should be treated with oral erythromycin or sulfacetamide for 3 to 4 weeks. Systemic tetracycline should be avoided in breast-feeding women who might transmit this to the newborn.

ACUTE DACRYOCYSTITIS

Neonates may present with acute dacryocystitis, an inflammation of the lacrimal sac (Fig. 59–3). Pain, tearing, redness, and discharge may be present. If the child is febrile, cultures and gram stains should

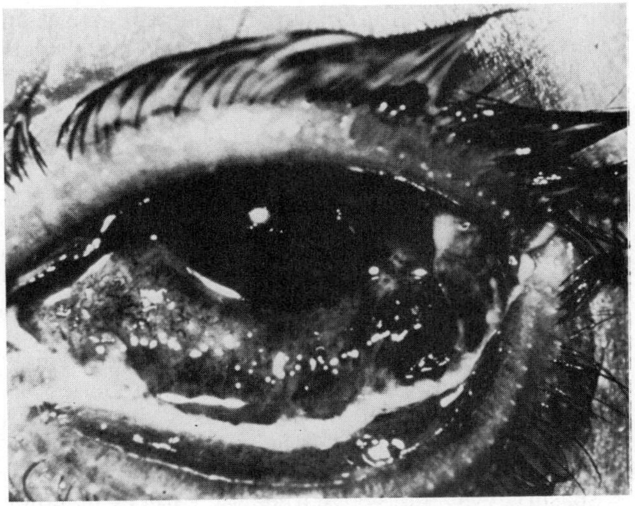

Figure 59–2. Purulent conjunctivitis can indicate infection with *Staphylococcus, Haemophilus influenzae, Streptococcus,* or *Pseudomonas.* (From *The Red Eye,* American Academy of Ophthalmology, Professional Information Committee, San Francisco, California.)

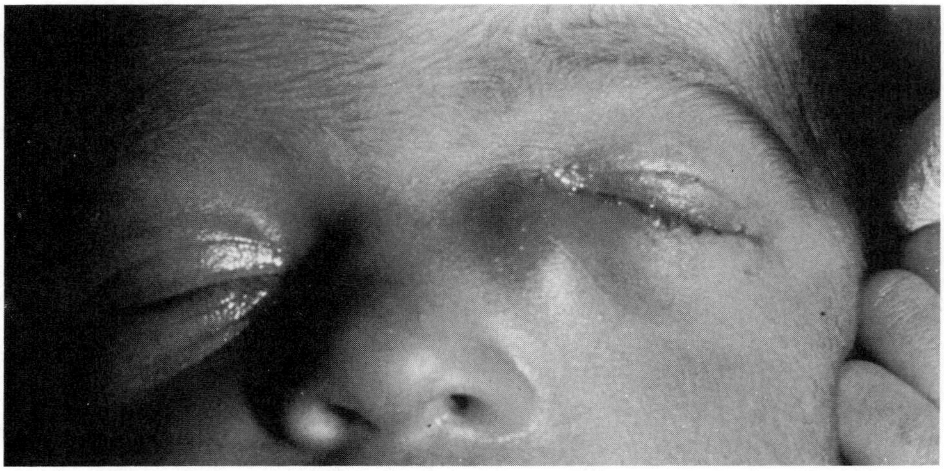

Figure 59–3. Acute dacryocystitis in a neonate with fever and malaise. Lacrimal sac massage and systemic antibiotics relieved the acute infection.

be performed. Pneumococcosis, *Staphylococcus aureus,* and *Streptococcus pneumonia* are the most common organisms. Systemic antibiotics are indicated in the acute stage. The ophthalmologist should be consulted immediately, because irrigation and probing may be necessary to establish drainage as quickly as possible.

CHRONIC DACRYOCYSTITIS (PARTIAL NASOLACRIMAL DUCT OBSTRUCTION)

These infants usually present to the physician with a chronic history of tearing and mattering with a chronic yellow discharge. Topical antibiotics such as sulfacetamide four times daily should be employed. The mother should be taught to compress or massage the lacrimal sac four to six times a day. Approximately 80 per cent of these inflammations will resolve spontaneously by 6 months of age. If treatment is not successful or when dacryocystitis persists, the patient should be referred for possible probing and irrigation of the nasolacrimal duct. Prior to age 1, a single probing is curative in the majority of cases.

CONGENITAL GLAUCOMA

Congenital glaucoma is a potentially blinding condition with an incidence of 1 per 10,000 births. It is often confused with chronic dacryocystitis. About two thirds of these cases are bilateral. These patients, like those with dacryocystitis, present with excessive tearing. In addition, the infants usually are extremely light sensitive (photophobic). The child buries his head in a blanket or pillow or uses the mother's shoulder to block out the light. These infants frequently have intense blinking or lid spasm (blepharospasm). An enlarged cornea or corneal clouding can be detected clinically (Fig. 59–4). The corneal edema is the result of elevated intraocular pressure, which causes breaks in the inner corneal layers and intrusion of anterior chamber fluid into the corneal stroma. The increased intraocular pressure causes significant optic nerve damage that can lead to blindness. Whenever glaucoma is suspected, immediate consultation is indicated. The surgical treatment of congenital glaucoma is successful in approximately 90 per cent of cases. However, these patients must be followed by an ophthalmologist for the rest of their lives as a precaution against recurrent elevations of intraocular pressure and amblyopia (lazy eye).

The Red Eye in Adults and Older Children

BLEPHARITIS

Blepharitis is a chronic lid inflammation involving abnormalities of the glands surrounding the eyelashes. The two most common types are (1) chronic staphylococcal infections of the lid and (2) seborrheic blepharitis (Fig. 59–5). Staphylococcal blepharitis is the most common inflammation of the external eye. It is frequently asymptomatic initially, but as the disease progresses, the patient complains of foreign body sensation, matting of the lashes, and burning. Lid crusting, discharge, redness, and loss of lashes are observed. Seborrheic blepharitis is associated with seborrhea of the scalp, lashes, eyebrows, and ears. It is characterized by greasy, dandruff-like scales on the lashes but no skin ulcerations. Treatment of both these conditions is long and laborious. Lid hygiene is recommended for both conditions. Topical antibiotics are prescribed for staphylococcal blepharitis. Both are recurrent conditions that require repeated therapy.

STYE (HORDEOLUM) (FIG. 59–6)

A stye is the most common localized infection of one of the glands of the eyelids. It is an acute, boil-like

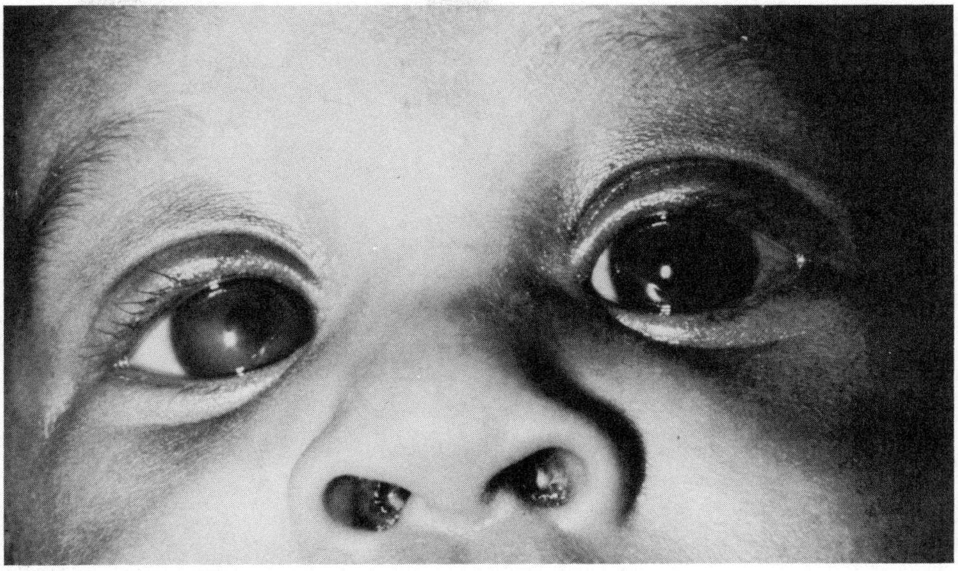

Figure 59–4. Congenital glaucoma in a two month old infant who presented with cloudy cornea involving the right eye. Intraocular pressure was elevated; the diagnosis was congenital glaucoma.

lesion, and the patient usually has a swollen, tender, red eyelid. There may be a moderate amount of conjunctival injection. Treatment is warm compresses for 15 minutes four times a day. Topical antibiotics may be given, but systemic antibiotics are not indicated. Generally, the stye spontaneously drains within several days. If resolution does not occur within 2 weeks, the patient should be referred.

CHALAZION (FIG. 59–7)

A chalazion is a chronic swelling of the eyelids that is not associated with conjunctivitis. The chalazion, a granulomatous inflammatory reaction, may persist for weeks or even months. Chalazia are usually rubbery, cystic, and nontender on palpation. When the upper lid is involved, vision is often temporarily blurred. If the chalazion persists for more than 3 months, it may require incision and curettage. Recurrent chalazia may be caused by an underlying sebaceous gland carcinoma and should be biopsied and sent to pathology.

BACTERIAL CONJUNCTIVITIS

All common bacteria may cause conjunctivitis. Presently, *staphylococcus aureus, Diplococcus pneumoniae, Haemophilus influenzae,* and *Pseudomonas* are the most common organisms. In the presence of a severe purulent discharge, culture of the conjunctiva

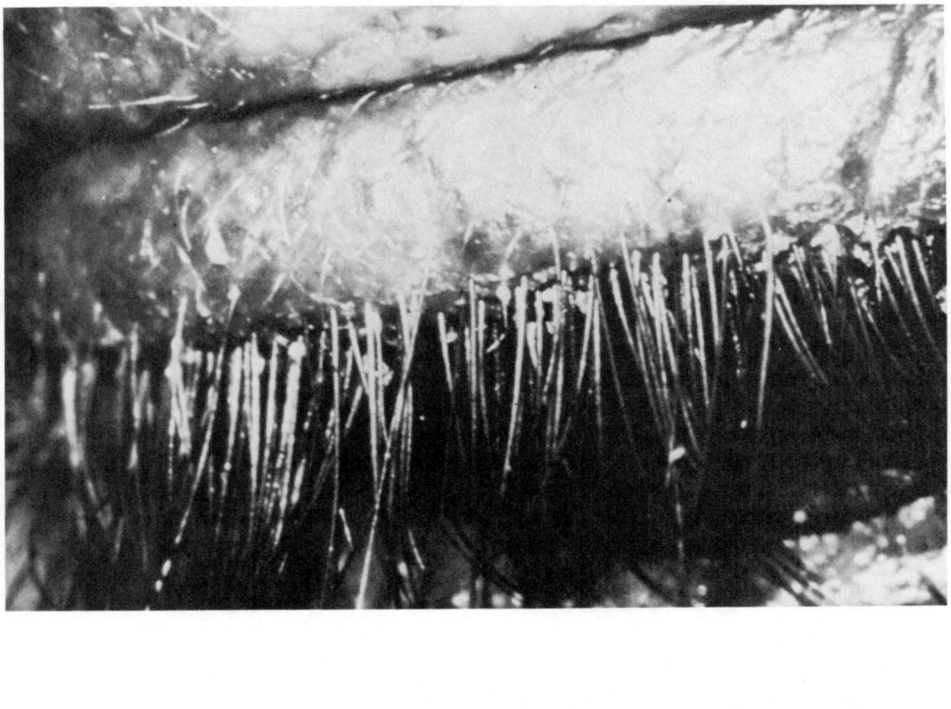

Figure 59–5. Seborrheic blepharitis is characterized by greasy, dandruff-like scales on the lashes. (From *The Red Eye,* American Academy of Ophthalmology, Professional Information Committee, San Francisco, California.)

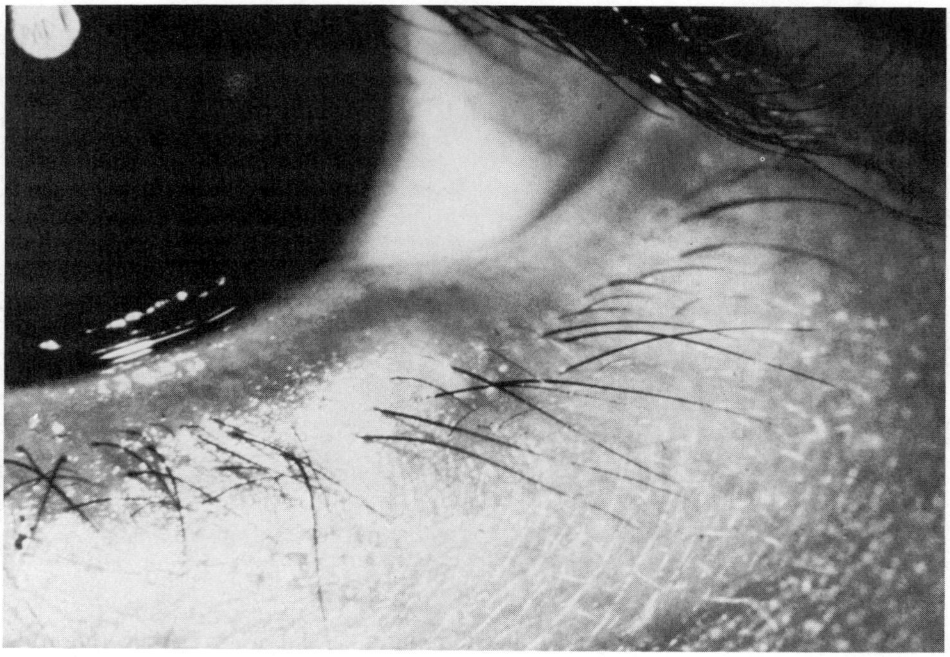

Figure 59–6. Acute hordeolum or stye. The swollen, tender, red eyelid includes acute, boil-like lesion. Treatment includes warm compresses and topical antibiotics. (From *The Red Eye,* American Academy of Ophthalmology, Professional Information Committee, San Francisco, California.)

is mandatory (see Fig. 59–2—bacterial conjunctivitis). Subconjunctival hemorrhage can occur with bacterial conjunctivitis and is especially common with *Haemophilus influenzae* conjunctivitis. Treatment of conjunctivitis includes a topical antibiotic, such as sulfacetamide, erythromycin, or neomycin-polymyxin B combination. Gentamicin or tobramycin ophthalmic should be reserved for unresponsive cases, especially pseudomonas and proteus. Gonococcal and *Haemophilus* conjunctivitis require both systemic and topical therapy.

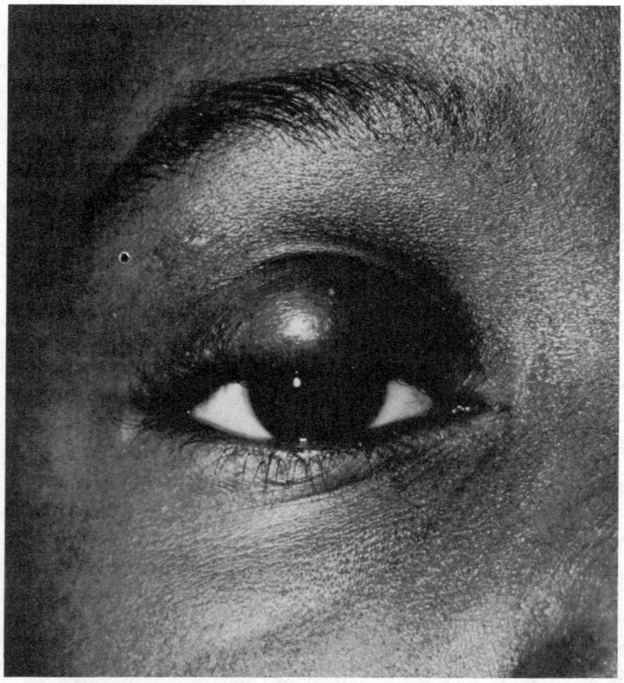

Figure 59–7. Chalazion of the right upper eyelid in a 10-year-old female. (From *The Red Eye,* American Academy of Ophthalmology, Professional Information Committee, San Francisco, California.)

If the conjunctivitis does not improve in 2 or 3 days or the patient develops pain or reduction in vision, referral is indicated.

Be certain *not* to use topical steroids or antibiotic-steroid combinations in conjunctivitis or other causes of the red eye.

Topical corticosteroids have four potentially serious ocular side effects and are contraindicated in conjunctivitis:

1. Steroids can facilitate penetration of an undetected corneal herpetic infection to the deeper corneal layers and cause corneal perforation.
2. Prolonged local use of the corticosteroids (usually longer than 2 weeks) can cause chronic open-angle glaucoma.
3. Prolonged use of topical corticosteroids can cause cataracts.
4. Topical corticosteroids are capable of potentiating the development of fungal corneal ulcers.

VIRAL CONJUNCTIVITIS

Viral conjunctivitis, in contrast to bacterial conjunctivitis, has a less prominent discharge that is usually watery. The condition is highly contagious, and hand washing is very important to avoid infection. Infected hospital personnel, day care workers, and others should avoid contact with others when infected. Palpable preauricular lymph nodes frequently are present in viral conjunctivitis and are an important sign to differentiate it from bacterial conjunctivitis. An associated upper respiratory infection may occur. In advanced cases, there may be true photophobia and blurred vision caused by corneal involvement that require consultation. However, most viral conjunctivitis is self-limiting, and no specific treatment is indicated. Topical steroids are contraindicated. Most viral infections resolve in 10 to 14 days and specific serologic diagnosis is not necessary. If the conjunctivitis persists or there is any pain or change in vision, the patient should be referred.

ALLERGIC CONJUNCTIVITIS

A number of antigens may give rise to superficial conjunctival reactions. Because of the elasticity of the conjunctival tissues, there may be considerable swelling. Allergic conjunctivitis patients have tearing and itching and present with redness and swelling of the conjunctiva and lids. A scanty, white, stringy discharge occurs with allergic conjunctivitis.

Allergic conjunctivitis frequently occurs in patients with hay fever, asthma, or eczema. The allergic condition of contact allergy commonly is associated with drugs, chemicals, or cosmetics coming in contact with the conjunctiva or eyelids. The offending drug or allergens should be discontinued. The treatment of most allergic conditions includes oral antihistamines and occasionally topical antihistamines and vasoconstricting drops such as naphazoline. Cromolyn has been found to be especially effective in treating allergic conjunctivitis, giant papillary conjunctivitis, and vernal keratoconjunctivitis.

SUBCONJUNCTIVAL HEMORRHAGE

A patient may present with a bright red eye, normal vision, and no pain. Usually, no obvious cause exists, but in some patients a history of coughing, sneezing, or straining prior to the hemorrhage is present. The patient should be reassured that it is nothing more than hemorrhage of the conjunctiva. There is no therapy, except reassurance that the blood will clear in 2 or 3 weeks. Hematologic or blood coagulation studies are usually of limited value in patients with subconjunctival hemorrhages unless there is a history of recurrence.

If trauma is suspected, the patient should be referred to an eye physician to rule out more serious injuries, such as perforation or severe contusion to the eye, causing damage to the intraocular structures. In a child, subconjunctival hemorrhage may indicate a battered child, and other signs of bodily trauma should be investigated.

CORNEAL HERPETIC INFECTIONS

Herpetic infections of the eye can produce conjunctivitis, corneal inflammation (keratitis), and uveitis (inflamed iris, ciliary body, and choroid). The herpes simplex virus is the most common cause of corneal opacification in countries in the temperate zone. The human is the only natural host for this DNA virus. Approximately 90 per cent of the population have systemic antibodies to the virus. Type 1 herpes simplex virus is the oral or labial type, and Type 2 is the genital type. The incubation period of simplex infection is from 2 to 12 days. Herpes type 1 is the most common cause of ocular infection, but transmission of herpes type 2 also can occur.

PRIMARY HERPES SIMPLEX INFECTION

Primary ocular infection in a nonimmune subject usually presents as a conjunctivitis with a clear, watery discharge, skin vesicles on the lids, and preauricular nodes. Associated vesicles and ulcers on the oral mucosa and skin are common. Corneal involvement also may occur with single or multiple dendrites. If dendrites are present, the patient should be referred for treatment.

RECURRENT CORNEAL HERPES (SEE PLATE XXXII)

At the time of the primary herpetic infection, the virus gains access to the central nervous system where it resides in a latent state in the trigeminal and other ganglia. Recurrent attacks occur when the latent state is reversed. The virus travels via the sensory nerves to target tissues, one of which is the eye. Recurrent corneal involvement also includes the development of single or multiple dendritic ulcers. After a brief period of time, the plaque of epithelial cells desquamates to form a linear branching ulcer (dendrite). When a corneal dendrite is detected by corneal staining with fluorescein, the patient should be referred.

ORBITAL CELLULITIS (FIG. 59–8)

Orbital cellulitis, most commonly caused by an extension of infection from the ethmoid sinus, can occur in both adults and children. It is the most common cause of exophthalmos (a protruding eye) in children. Sometimes it is difficult to differentiate a periorbital or anterior lid cellulitis from a true posterior orbital cellulitis. With a true orbital cellulitis, the child or adult will have pain on movement of the eye, conjunctival edema, and limited extraocular movements.

The most common causative organisms are *Staphylococcus aureus, Streptococcus,* and *Haemophilus influenzae.* Cultures should be obtained from the nasopharynx, conjunctiva, and blood. Immediate hospitalization and ophthalmologic consultation is necessary. Appropriate antibiotic treatment depends on the causative organism. Cavernous sinus throm-

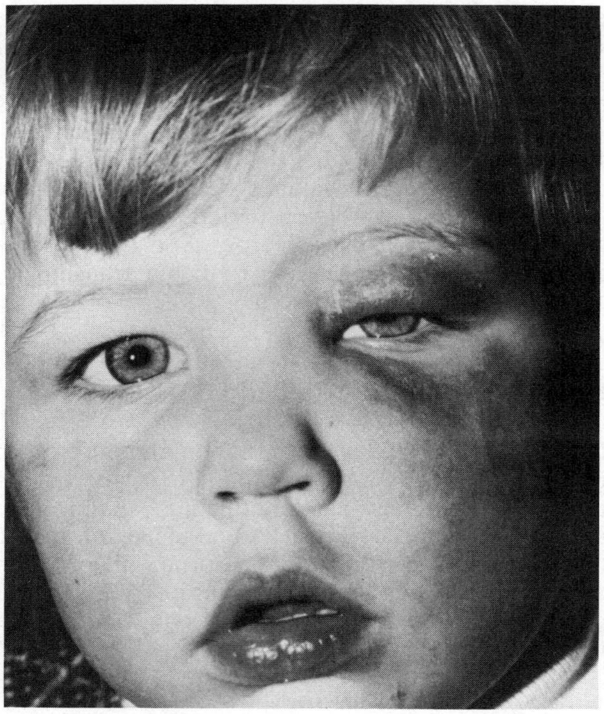

Figure 59–8. Orbital cellulitis in a 3-year-old patient. (From *The Red Eye*, American Academy of Ophthalmology, Professional Information Committee, San Francisco, California.)

bosis and meningitis and blindness are serious complications that still develop from orbital cellulitis.

IRITIS

An iritis patient may present with redness, pain, and photophobia. No discharge is seen and the pupil will be constricted. Circumcorneal (ciliary) injection may occur. Intraocular pressure will be normal or low. Consultation should be obtained on all such patients.

ANGLE-CLOSURE GLAUCOMA

Acute elevations in intraocular pressure can occur when the outflow of aqueous is suddenly blocked. An acute angle closure attack can follow an episode of emotional or physical stress, dilation of the pupil in dim lighting, or, rarely, after the instillation of dilating eyedrops. A patient who is having an acute attack usually will have symptoms including severe ocular pain, redness, blurred vision, rainbow-colored haloes around lights, and sometimes nausea and vomiting. On examination, the eye is usually red, the pupil in middilation and oval, the cornea cloudy, and the intraocular pressure markedly elevated. Generally, only one eye is affected at a time. An acute episode of angle closure glaucoma is an ocular emergency and requires immediate treatment to lower the intraocular pressure by medical treatment. Once the intraocular pressure is under control, YAG or ARGON laser peripheral iridectomy is performed.

Ocular Trauma and Other Emergencies

EMERGENCIES

True emergencies can be classified as those where therapy should be instituted within minutes. Two true emergencies in the eye include chemical burns of the cornea and central retinal artery occlusion.

Chemical Burns

Burns of the eye by acids or alkalis are true ocular emergencies. Alkali, such as lye, can cause permanent, irreversible blindness. The immediate treatment of chemical burns must be continual irrigation of the eyes with up to 1000 cc. normal saline or lactated Ringer's solution. If these are not available, a shower, spigot, bathtub, or drinking fountain is appropriate. After initial lavage, ophthalmologic consultation is immediate.

Central Retinal Artery Occlusion

Central retinal artery occlusion is generally not the result of trauma. However, prolonged intraorbital swelling can cause occlusion of the central retinal artery. This can occur particularly in patients who are having an operation in the face-down position. Characteristic fundus appearance with central retinal artery occlusion is narrow arterioles and a pale optic disc. In addition, there is a diffuse retinal whitening. A cherry-red spot only occurs several hours after the initial retinal artery occlusion. The treatment must be immediate, including breathing in a small paper bag as a means to increase the patient's carbon dioxide level. Emergency paracentesis is a rapid way to decompress the eye and may actually provide immediate restoration of vision. However, most physicians are reluctant to do paracentesis on a patient within a few minutes. Ocular massage is another means of decompressing the eye.

URGENCIES

Urgent situations include those where therapy should be instituted within several hours. These include penetrating injuries of the globe, acute narrow angle glaucoma, pupillary block glaucoma, orbital cellulitis, corneal ulcer, corneal foreign body, corneal abrasion, gonococcal conjunctivitis, ophthalmia neonatorum, and acute iritis. In addition, trauma with retinal tears, vitreous hemorrhage, retinal detachment, and hyphemas are urgent situations.

Ocular Foreign Body and Other Eye Injuries

The most common eye injury encountered in family practice is a foreign body in the eye. The most common causes of a foreign body in the conjunctival sac or one embedded in the cornea include particles blown in by the wind, occupational or work-related injuries, and metallic foreign bodies that may fly into the eye, such as after a person hits a metal object with a hammer. It is important to evaluate the location of the foreign body and, in the case of corneal foreign bodies, the depth of penetration. Symptoms may be helpful since superficial foreign bodies in the cornea generally present with the symptom of a dust particle in the eye. Foreign bodies that have penetrated deeper into the corneal stroma produce a dull, aching pain perceived in or behind the eye. On examination, it is important to look carefully at the inflammatory response of the eye. A purely localized conjunctival inflammation pattern is generally associated with superficial foreign bodies. Ciliary injection is a warning sign that a deep penetration may have taken place and an ophthalmologic consultation should be sought immediately. An examination of the eye should be carried out after the instillation of ophthalmic local anesthetic in order to avoid blepharospasm and evasive eye movements. The cornea should be inspected with a penlight or the ophthalmoscope in a darkened room. Use of the slit on the ophthalmoscope may help visualize irregularities in the corneal surface. Staining with fluorescein will demonstrate abrasions and help identify otherwise transparent foreign bodies.

Management. The family physician may elect to remove a foreign body in the conjunctival sac by irrigation with sterile solutions or after eversion of the upper lid with a moistened cotton swab. In the case of superficial corneal foreign bodies, an attempt at removal with a moist sterile swab may be undertaken.

Corneal Abrasions

Corneal abrasions are often due to foreign bodies underneath the upper lid. Lid eversion and inspection to remove these conjunctival foreign bodies is essential. To evert the lid, the patient is seated and asked to look downward. The upper lid is grasped by its central lashes and pulled downward and slightly outward. The examiner then depresses the upper lid with a cotton applicator proximal to the upper tarsus margin. Gentle pressure is maintained until the upper lid is flipped into the everted position. Frequently, the foreign body will then be observed and can be removed with a cotton applicator. If the conjunctival or corneal foreign body is not easily removed with a cotton applicator, ophthalmologic consultation should be obtained. Corneal abrasions generally can be treated with an antibiotic ointment and patching.

Metallic Foreign Bodies

Metallic foreign bodies, if allowed to stay in the eye for a number of hours, frequently leave a rust ring that is clearly visible after the removal of the foreign body. Rust rings are irritating to the cornea and result in long-lasting inflammatory changes in the eye. Follow-up should be at daily intervals with staining of the cornea to demonstrate the expected rapid healing. If healing does not take place over a period of 24 to 48 hours, one must suspect an infection in the corneal stroma and consultation obtained. Topical antibiotic ointments are used routinely after removal of foreign bodies in an attempt to prevent this complication.

Corneal and Scleral Lacerations

Corneal and scleral lacerations fall within the realm of the ophthalmologist and should be referred immediately after a shield is placed on the eye. Frequently, signs of corneal and scleral lacerations include unequal pupils, hypotony (low intraocular pressure) and/or hyphema. Frequently, with a corneal laceration the lens will also be involved. In addition, it is important to consider that there may be posterior injuries to the globe including retinal detachment, retinal tear, and vitreous hemorrhage (Fig. 59–9).

Blunt Eye Injuries

Blunt eye injuries are also quite common. They may be the result of relatively trivial injuries or high velocity serious impact on the eye.

An exact history of the trauma must be obtained in order to assess the velocity involved, which, in turn, may indicate the extent of ocular damage that may have occurred. Inquiry must be made as to visual acuity changes that occurred immediately after the injury. Flashing lights are often seen at the instant of injury and indicate irritation of the retina since any message to the brain from the retina is perceived as light. Persistent blurred vision is indicative of a more serious injury. It may indicate blood in the anterior chamber that is suspended in the aqueous humor refracting light and distorting the visual image. Free-floating blood in the anterior chamber cannot be appreciated by ophthalmoscopic examination and a slit-lamp is necessary in order to observe the suspended red blood cells.

The Black Eye (Bruised Eyelids)

This condition can be serious or relatively minor. If accompanied by severe pain, bleeding, or constant blurred vision, more serious eye trauma needs to be considered.

Red Eye

Almost all ocular trauma cases include bleeding or dilation of blood vessels on the surface of the eye

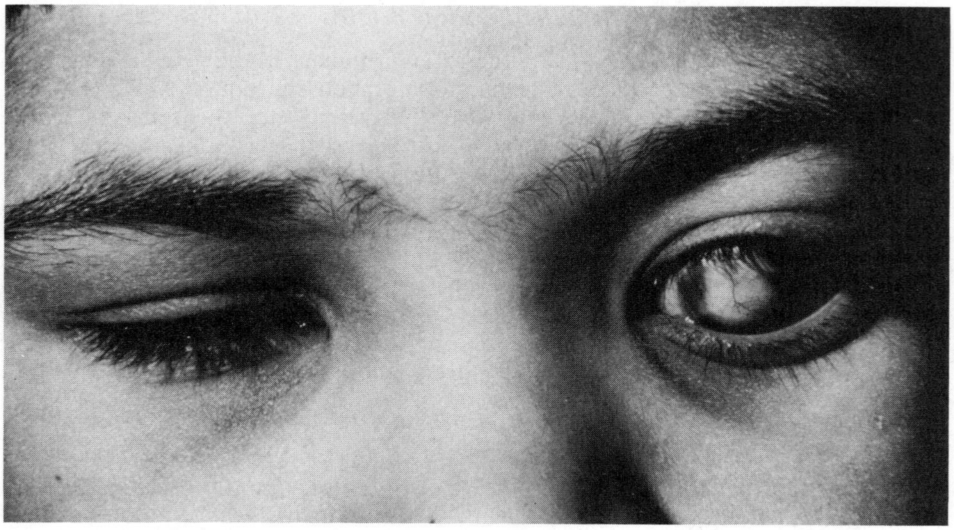

Figure 59–9. Corneal leukoma in a 6-year-old male. The diagnosis was ocular trauma and penetrating corneal laceration.

(subconjunctival hemorrhage). This sign can be observed with any degree of eye injury. For instance, a subconjunctival hemorrhage may be spontaneous or may indicate a mild or very serious injury.

Pupillary Change

Blunt trauma to the eye may result in lacerations of the sphincter muscle of the pupil. This will be manifested by a so-called traumatic mydriasis. Unlike the unequal pupils seen in congenital anisocoria, traumatic mydriasis is characterized by recent onset of unequal pupils and by the irregularity of the dilated pupil. While traumatic mydriasis by itself is not harmful, it suggests severe blunt trauma and is an indication for a careful assessment of other ocular structures, including the vitreous and retinal periphery.

Traumatic Hyphema

Blunt trauma to the eye can cause injury to the iris, angle structures, and other intraocular structures. Hemorrhage into the anterior chamber, or hyphema, is most often found in children. The agent producing this hyphema usually is a projectile that strikes the exposed portion of the eye. In child abuse, fists and belts frequently cause these injuries. Signs and symptoms include a red eye, decreased vision, and pain.

Hyphemas can be associated with devastating visual complications, including blood staining of the cornea and elevated intraocular pressure that may lead to atrophy of the optic nerve.

A hyphema is an ocular emergency and should be referred immediately (Plate XXXIII).

Retinal Detachment

Traumatic detachment of the retina can be observed after blunt eye injury especially in older individuals. The patient may complain of reduced overall brightness in the involved eye or may have continuous light flashes indicating retinal traction. Following eye trauma, it is imperative to inspect not just the central portions of the retina but as far as possible the peripheral portions as well. This examination should be performed in a darkened room and after instilling a short-acting mydriatic agent. Any questionable findings should be referred to an ophthalmologist immediately. Other serious post-traumatic injuries are: traumatic tears of the iris, subluxation or dislocation of the lens that occasionally displaces into the anterior chamber, and blowout fracture of the orbit that presents with impaired eye movement in the upward direction because of entrapment of the inferior rectus muscle. Fortunately, these extremely serious injuries are usually easy to recognize.

Pediatric Ophthalmology

A misalignment of the eye muscles results in strabismus. Adults who have strabismus frequently develop double vision, but children with strabismus quickly learn to ignore, or suppress, the image seen by the wandering eye. As a result of suppression, the straight eye takes over most of the work of seeing, and the crossed eye develops reduced central vision from lack of use. Loss of vision in the strabismic or crossed eye is called amblyopia. There are a number of conditions that can cause amblyopia, but the most common is strabismus (Fig. 59–10).

PSEUDOSTRABISMUS

A common misconception is that children with crossed eyes outgrow the condition. This belief stems from confusion between true strabismus and what is known as pseudostrabismus or false strabismus. A child with pseudostrabismus has broad folds of skin that partially cover the top of each eye and a flat

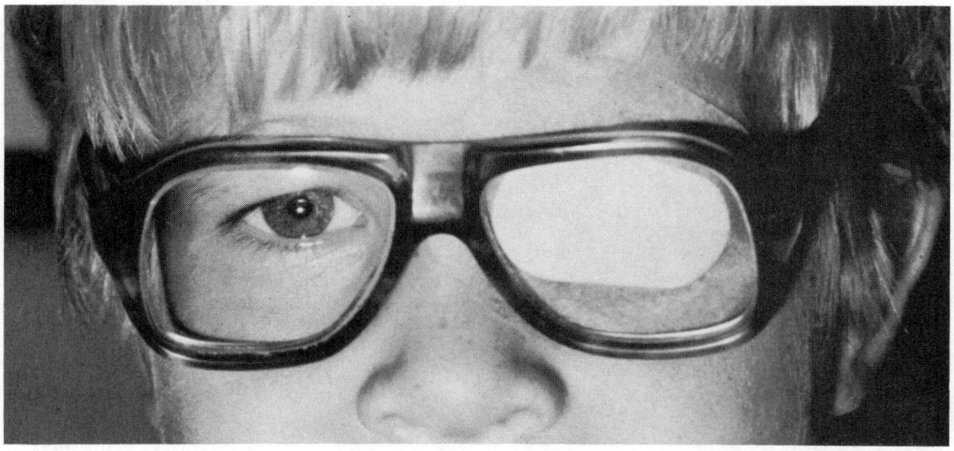

Figure 59–10. Amblyopia. This 5-year-old patient also required patching of the better-seeing eye to improve vision in the amblyopic eye.

nasal bridge that creates the illusion of crossed eyes. As the child gets older and the skin fold becomes less apparent, this condition will become less noticeable.

When a child's eyes are truly crossed, it is always a serious condition and requires the care of an ophthalmologist.

STRABISMUS AND AMBLYOPIA

There are several diagnostic tests used to detect strabismus and amblyopia. These include visual acuity, the corneal light reflex test, the cover-uncover test, extraocular rotations, simultaneous red reflexes test, and fundus examination.

The best way to test for possible visual loss due to amblyopia is to measure the visual acuity or fixation preference of both eyes. Visual acuity testing must be geared to the age of the patient. For children under 3½, the ability to observe and follow small moving objects is critical. When there is no apparent sign of strabismus, the only clue to poor vision may be an aversion to having the better eye occluded (fixation preference) when one eye is covered or demonstrates an inability to fix at distant objects. These are both common signs of amblyopia that may be due to a refractive error (optical), media opacities, and abnormality in the retina or optic nerve.

In testing children between 3½ and 4 years of age, symbols such as illiterate E's or Allen picture cards are appropriate. For children over 4, test with a line of Snellen letters, numbers, or E's. Titmus testing is particularly useful over age 5 years (Fig. 59–11). If visual acuity is worse than 20/40, or if there is a two-line difference between the eyes, i.e., 20/20 and 20/30, the child should be referred for further evaluation.

The Corneal Light Reflex Test, the Cover-Un-

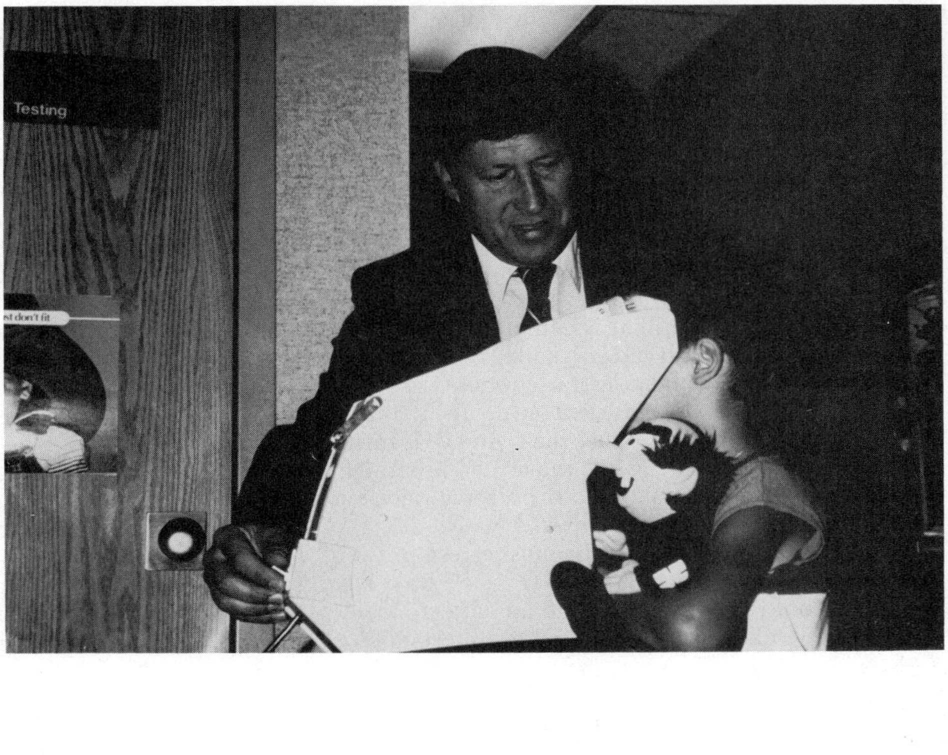

Figure 59–11. Titmus testing is an excellent way to screen children, particularly over the age of 5 years.

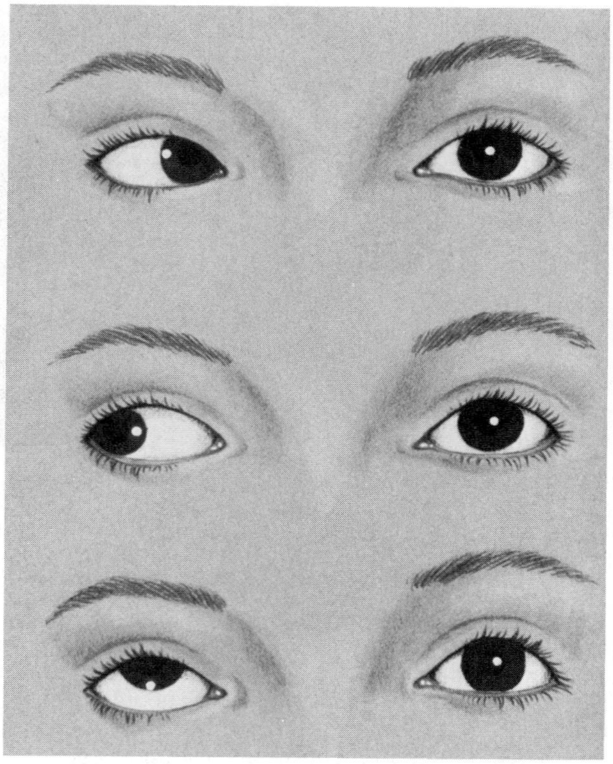

Figure 59–12. Strabismus diagram of *(top)* right esotropia, *(middle)* right exotropia, *(bottom)* right hypertropia. (From *The Child's Eye: Strabismus and Amblyopia*, American Academy of Ophthalmology, Professional Information Committee, San Francisco, California.)

cover Test, and extraocular rotations are three basic tests for strabismus. To perform the Corneal Light Test, project a penlight onto the cornea of both eyes simultaneously while the child looks straight ahead. Compare the placement of the two corneal reflections. When the eyes are straight, the light will appear at the same point on each cornea. If a muscle deviation is present, the reflected light will appear slightly off center in one eye.

The strabismus drawing (Fig. 59–12) illustrates the placement of corneal reflections as they would appear for each direction of deviation. In the top example, notice that the light is centered on the cornea of the left eye but is displaced laterally, or outward, on the right cornea. This indicates that the right eye is turned inward or is esotropic. In the second illustration, the light is centered again on the left cornea but is displaced medially, or inward, on the right cornea. This demonstrates an outward turning, or exotropia, of the right eye. In the third example, the light indicates that the right eye is turned upward or is hypertropic, while the left eye is straight. The bottom illustration shows a hypotropic right eye, that is, the eye is rotated downward.

To perform the second diagnostic test for strabismus, the Cover-Uncover Test (Fig. 59–13), have the child look straight ahead at an object 20 feet away. An eye chart is commonly used to test children over age 3. For younger children, it is helpful to use a colorful moving object, such as a noise-making toy. As the child looks at the distant object, cover the right eye and look for movement of the uncovered left eye. If the left eye does not move, there is no apparent misalignment of that eye. If the eye moves outward, as it does in this child, the eye is esotropic. If it moves inward, it is exotropic. After testing the left eye, repeat the same procedure with the right eye. A third test is to check extraocular movements in the cardinal positions of gaze (Fig. 59–14).

The results of the Corneal Light Test, Cover-Uncover Test, and extraocular rotations provide a good basis for determining whether or not a misalignment is present.

Once you have performed the basic diagnostic tests for strabismus and amblyopia, use an ophthalmoscope to examine the red reflexes. Simultaneous examination of both retinal red reflexes is useful both as a test of ocular alignment and to rule out abnormalities of the ocular media. This test is performed in a darkened room with the ophthalmoscope at maximum brightness. Once the child is properly positioned, the examiner should move back approximately 18 to 24 inches until both red reflexes are seen simultaneously through the ophthalmoscope. The two reflexes are compared. If an abnormality of the ocular media is present, such as a cataract or tumor, the red reflexes will be asymmetrical or a white reflex will be present.

After examining the red reflexes, observe the ocular fundus, noting the size, shape, color, and cupping of the optic disc. Ophthalmoscopy permits direct visual examination of the retina, optic disc, and retinal vessels and may detect an underlying organic problem or disease condition.

PEDIATRIC VISION SCREENING GUIDELINES

The American Academy of Pediatrics and the American Academy of Ophthalmology Vision Screening Statement emphasizes that vision screening on all infants in the newborn nursery should include:

1. Penlight examination to ascertain corneal clarity and absence of nystagmus
2. Simultaneous examination of both red reflexes

Vision screening at 6 months includes:

1. Fixation preference and following movements
2. Penlight examination to rule out lid and corneal abnormalities
3. The corneal light reflex test and the cover-uncover test
4. Simultaneous examination of the red reflexes.

Vision screening at age 3½ should include:

1. Visual acuity testing using the Snellen acuity, E-game, or Allen picture cards
2. Corneal light reflex test
3. Cover-uncover test
4. Fundus examination and red reflexes

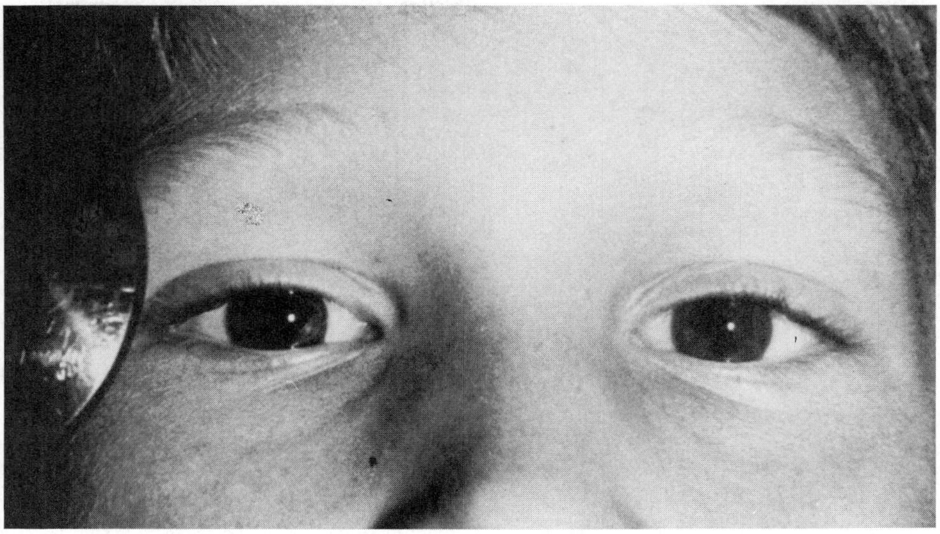

Figure 59–13. Cover-uncover test. Evaluate the unoccluded eye for strabismus. (From *The Child's Eye: Strabismus and Amblyopia*, American Academy of Ophthalmology, Professional Information Committee, San Francisco, California.)

Vision screening and eye examination after the age of 5 years include:

1. Visual acuity assessment with Snellen ABCs
2. Cornea light reflex test
3. Cover-uncover test
4. Fundus examination and red reflexes

The American Academy of Pediatrics and American Academy of Ophthalmology criteria for referral to the ophthalmologist from birth to 3½ years:

1. Reduced visual acuity or aversion to occlusion in one eye as compared to the other eye or reduced visual acuity in both eyes
2. Strabismus
3. Nystagmus
4. Any ocular pathology

Referral criteria from the age of 3½ to 5 years include:

1. Visual acuity worse than 20/40 in one or both eyes, or a two-line difference between the two eyes (such as 20/30 in the right eye and 20/20 in the left eye)
2. Strabismus
3. Any ocular abnormality

Over the age of 5 years referral is indicated for:

1. Visual acuity worse than 20/30 in one or both eyes
2. Strabismus
3. Any ocular pathology

Table 59–5 summarizes these findings.

Forms of Strabismus

Congenital esotropia accounts for nearly one fourth of all patients who present with strabismus. This is usually apparent shortly after birth or in the first 6 months of life. The deviation is generally constant and may be accompanied by a reduced ability to abduct (move the eyes outward). Babies with congenital esotropia usually do not have associated systemic

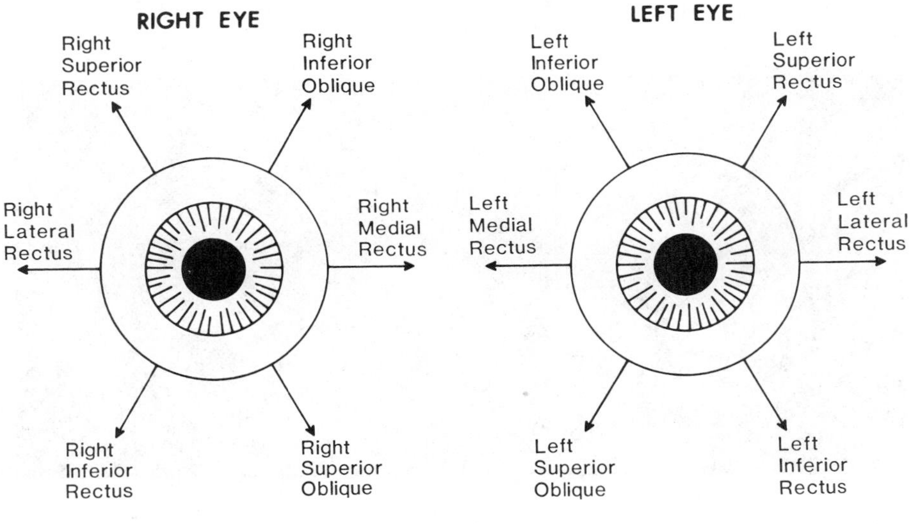

Figure 59–14. Ocular muscle movement in cardinal fields of gaze.

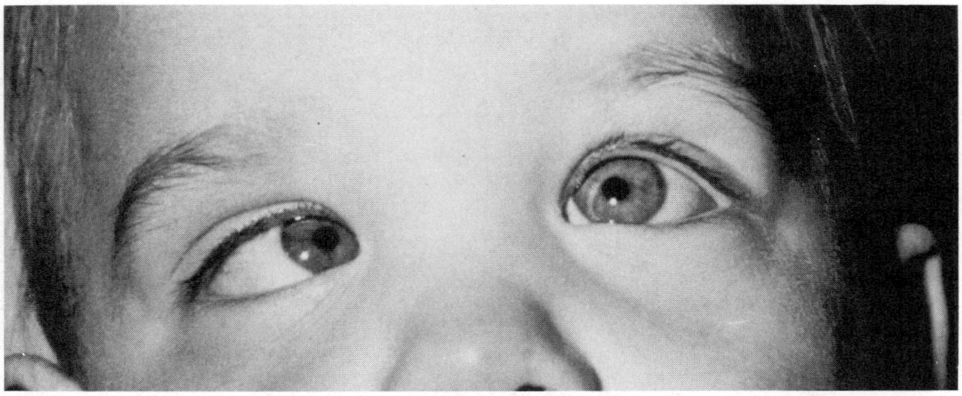

Figure 59–15. Congenital esotropia. With the right eye fixing, there is a left esotropia in this 12-month-old infant.

Table 59–5. VISION SCREENING BY FAMILY PHYSICIANS

Age	Examination	Referral
Newborn	Penlight exam of cornea and to rule out nystagmus Red reflexes	Any ocular pathology Abnormal red reflexes or white reflex Nystagmus
By age 6 months	Fixation to light or small toys Penlight exam Corneal light reflex test Cover-uncover test Red reflexes	Aversion to occlusion Strabismus Nystagmus Abnormal red reflexes or white reflex and ocular pathology
Age 3½ years	Visual acuity Corneal light reflex test Cover-uncover test Fundus exam Red reflexes	Visual acuity of 20/40 or less in one or both eyes Strabismus Any ocular pathology
Age 5 or older	Visual acuity Corneal light reflex test Cover-uncover test Fundus exam Red reflexes	Visual acuity of 20/30 or less in one or both eyes Strabismus Any ocular pathology

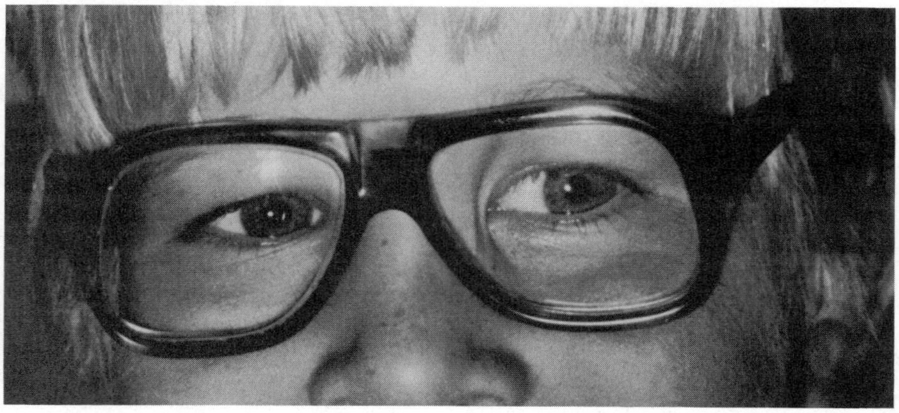

Figure 59–16. Accommodative esotropia and anisometropic amblyopia in a 5-year-old patient who has unequal refractive errors between the two eyes as well as accommodative esotropia.

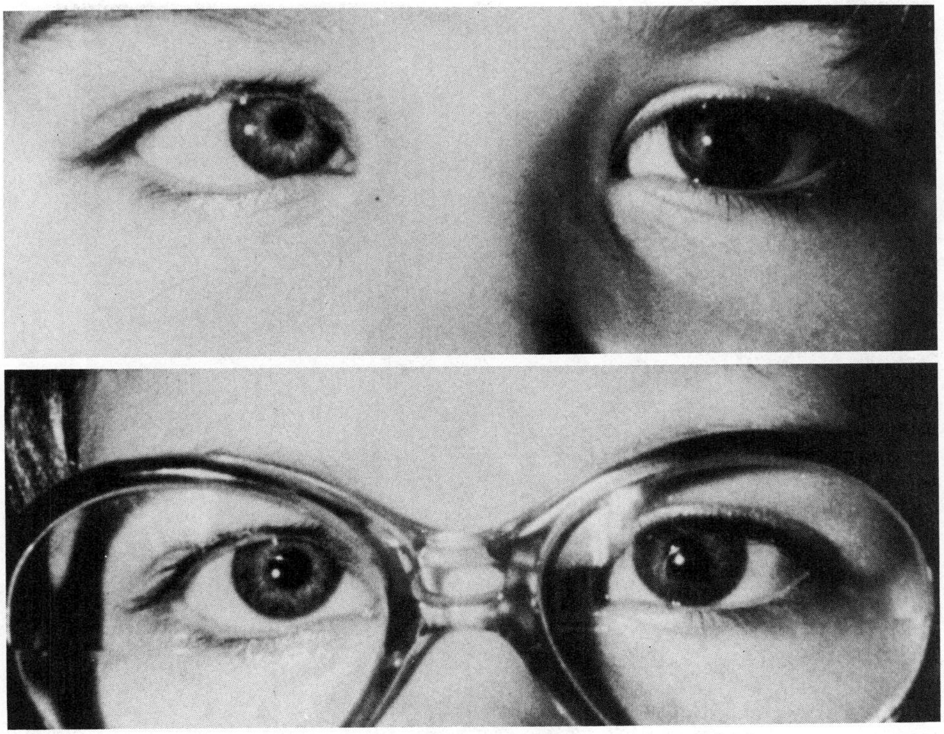

Figure 59–17. Accommodative esotropia in a 3-year-old patient uncorrected and corrected by hyperopic (farsighted) glasses. (From *The Child's Eye: Strabismus and Amblyopia*, American Academy of Ophthalmology, Professional Information Committee, San Francisco, California.)

findings. Generally, surgery is the primary treatment to correct this condition (Fig. 59–15).

Accommodative esotropia is the most common cause of esotropia and accounts for nearly one half of cases. This type of esotropia is because of excessive focusing or accommodation. Generally, accommodative esotropia is intermittent initially and gradually becomes constant. The age of onset is about 2 years, but it may occur as early as 6 months of age or as late as 7 years of age. Generally, patients with accommodative esotropia have a moderate amount of hyperopia (farsightedness). Glasses are commonly prescribed to relieve the eyes of the need to accommodate (Fig. 59–16). In this way, focusing is done by the glasses, enabling the eyes to straighten. Glasses are generally worn at all times to effectively straighten the eyes. If the inturning is greater at near than at distance, bifocals may also be required (Fig. 59–17).

Nonaccommodative esotropia or acquired esotropia is not caused by excessive accommodation. The most common causes of nonaccommodative esotropia include unequal refractive errors, cataracts, or corneal scars. Generally, the treatment is directed to the underlying condition, including the correction of amblyopia. Eye muscle surgery may be needed to correct the misalignment.

Exotropia accounts for approximately 20 per cent of cases of strabismus. Eighty per cent of cases of exotropia start out on an intermittent basis that may confuse or delay the diagnosis. Frequently, the parents notice the child closes one eye in bright sunlight or has an outturned eye when fatigued or sick. It is important to test patients with exotropia both at near and distant positions when this condition is suspected. Other causes of exotropia include third nerve palsy, neurologic disease, and abnormalities in the bony orbit. Patients with Apert-Crouzon syndrome frequently present with exotropia. (Figs. 59–18 to 59–20).

Vertical deviations account for less than 5 per cent of strabismus patients (Fig. 59–21). Vertical deviations are important because they can frequently occur in conjunction with serious conditions such as trauma, tumors of the brain and orbit, and thyroid disease. A vertical deviation is usually named for the higher eye, that is for a right or left hypertropia. Patients with vertical deviations may have a head tilt that must be differentiated from ocular torticollis (Fig. 59–22—Ocular Torticollis).

Paralytic and mechanical causes of strabismus occur with trauma and Duane's syndrome. In addition, neurologic trauma accounts for paralysis to the cranial nerves IV (innervates superior oblique), VI (innervates the lateral rectus), and III (innervates all other extraocular muscles) (Fig. 59–23).

The proper corrective treatment for strabismus includes nonsurgical treatment such as patching and eyeglasses. Eye muscle surgery is performed when it is clear that nonsurgical methods may not correct the misalignment. Four aspects of strabismus surgery should be stressed:

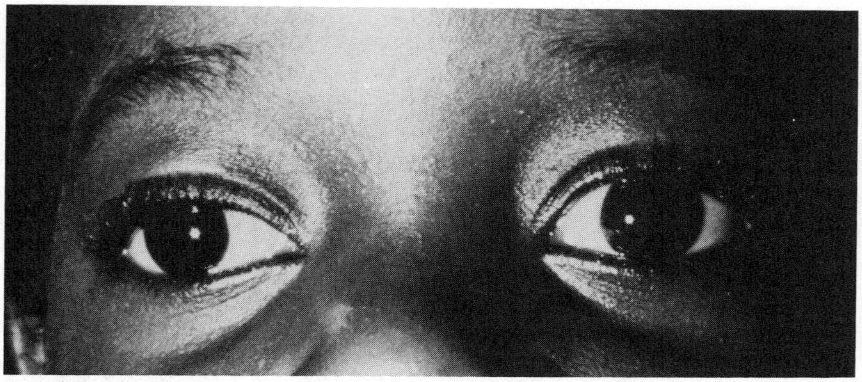

Figure 59–18. Exotropia in an 8-year-old patient with a right exotropia.

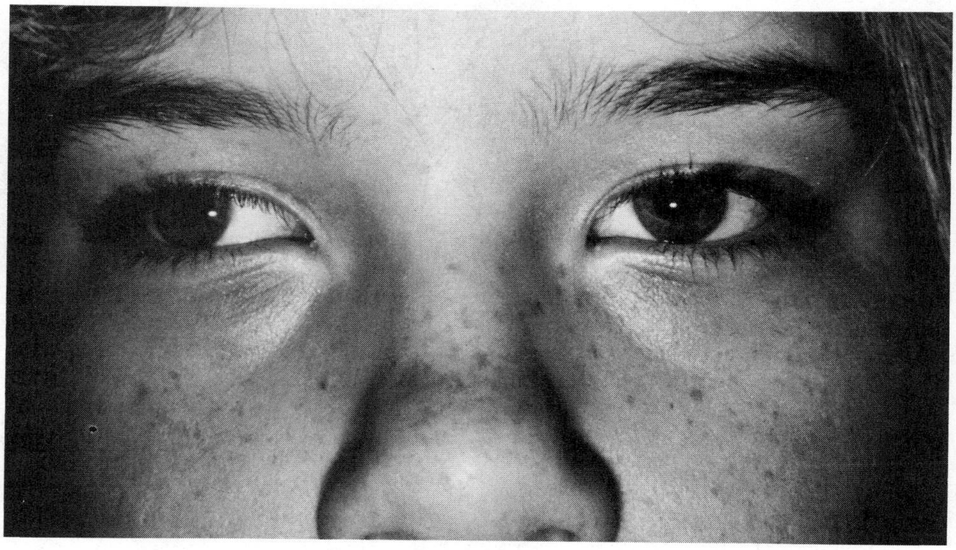

Figure 59–19. Positive angle kappa, which appears similar to exotropia, in an 8-year-old patient. Actually, this patient has retinopathy of prematurity with bilateral dragged maculae.

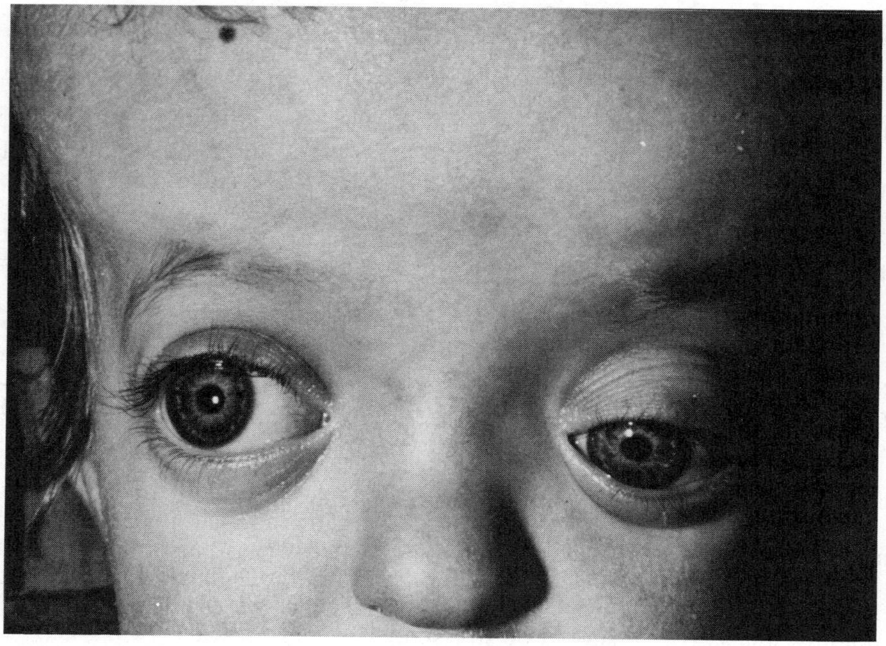

Figure 59–20. This patient presented with proptosis, amblyopia, and a left exotropia. This patient had the diagnosis of Crouzon's syndrome.

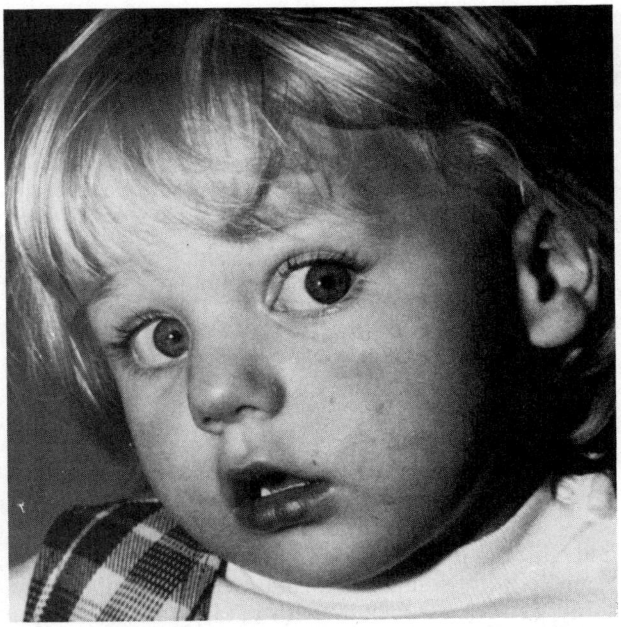

Figure 59–21. Positive head tilt in this 4-year-old child can indicate a vertical deviation, especially a superior oblique palsy. (From *The Child's Eye: Strabismus and Amblyopia*, American Academy of Ophthalmology, Professional Information Committee, San Francisco, California.)

1. The surgery is safe and effective.
2. The eyeball is never removed to perform the surgery.
3. More than one operation may be required to straighten the eyes.
4. Both eyes may require surgery to correct the muscle deviation.

The goals in treating strabismus include the ability to provide and maintain equal vision in both eyes, to enable the eyes to work together, and to improve depth perception when possible.

REFRACTIVE ERRORS AND COLOR VISION

Some eyes are either too long or too short and need help focusing light onto the retina. If an eye is too long, the light rays will focus in front of the retina and the image on the retina will be blurred. An individual with this condition can move things closer to see better or can wear glasses. This condition is called *nearsightedness* (myopia). In *farsightedness* (hyperopia), the light focuses behind the retina since the eye is too short and causes a blurred image. Both conditions are corrected by glasses or contact lenses. *Astigmatism* is another common error in the focusing abilities of the eye. It is caused by an unequal curvature of the front surface of the cornea. Corrective eyeglasses are necessary if it causes blurred vision or discomfort. Unless there is a marked amount of myopia (nearsightedness), hyperopia (farsightedness), or astigmatism, or a significant refractive difference between the eyes, eyeglasses will adequately compensate for these problems.

Refractive errors requiring eyeglasses exist in nearly 20 per cent of the pediatric population prior to the attainment of full growth.

Color vision defects rarely result in significant visual difficulties. Eight per cent of white males have some red-green color deficiency, whereas less than 1 per cent of females are affected. In isolation, this defect rarely results in any real drawback to normal function, especially in childhood. We think that no special emphasis should be placed on the diagnosis of color blindness at early childhood examination. Although the identification of such defects can be helpful in a classroom situation, too much emphasis should not be placed on these minor abnormalities at this age. Color vision testing may not be done unless a retinal dystrophy (abnormality) is suspected, the family history is positive, or the family specifically requests it.

HEADACHES

Headache is one of the most common conditions of human beings, but children do not seem to have as many complaints about headaches as do adults. Most headaches are not usually serious and frequently are caused by tension. Many people believe incorrectly that eyestrain and the need for glasses are common causes of headaches.

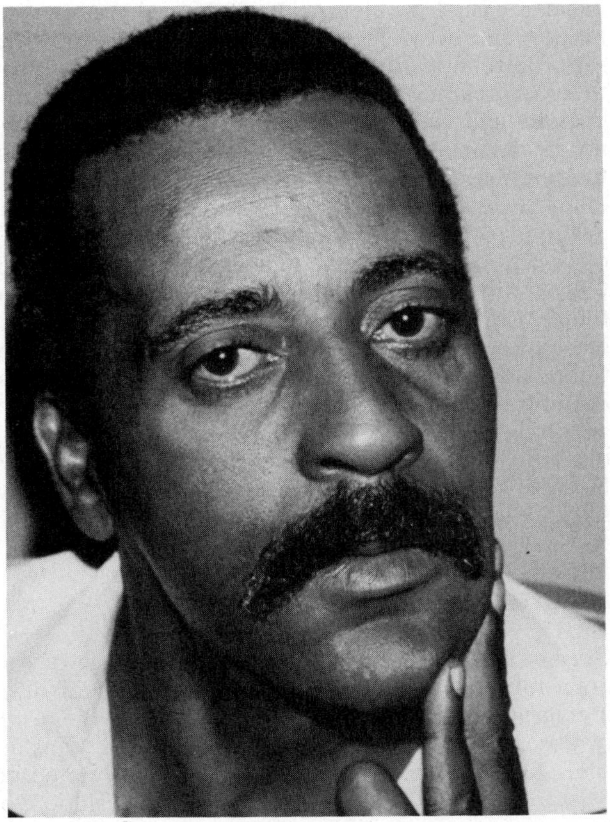

Figure 59–22. A 34-year-old patient with ocular torticollis. Notice abnormal head tilt.

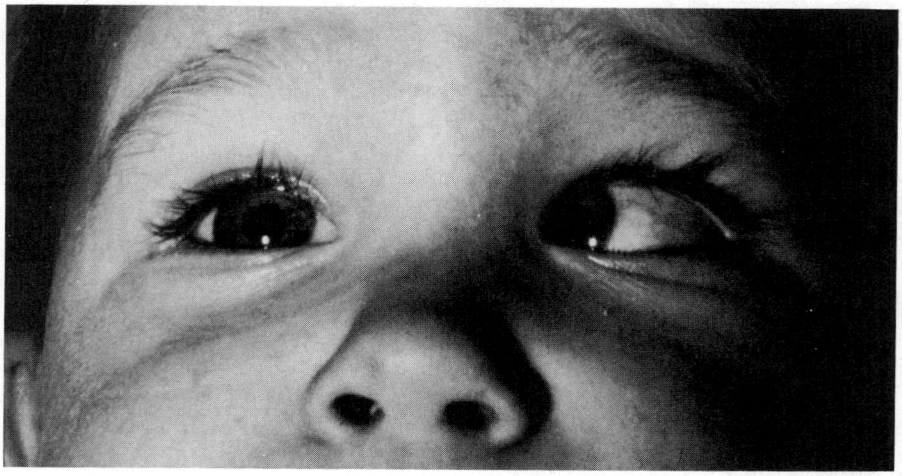

Figure 59–23. This 14-month-old patient presented with a chief complaint of an underaction of the left lateral rectus muscle and left esotropia after an upper respiratory infection. This patient actually had a VI nerve palsy related to the viral syndrome.

Headaches caused by eye disease are usually felt in the eye or in the brow on the same side as the involved eye. Frequently, these headaches are associated with some other symptom, such as blurred vision, haloes around lights, or extreme sensitivity to light. Most headaches are related to stress.

THE EYE AND LEARNING DISABILITIES

Although reading may be easier and faster when sight is clear, visual problems do not cause learning disabilities, and eye defects are not responsible for reversal of letters or other signs of reading disabilities. In the past, reading problems have been blamed on the eyes though children with a learning disability have no greater incidence of eye problems than the rest of the population.

It is important that a thorough medical eye examination be performed. The presence or absence of visual defects can be diagnosed and corrected. Once vision is corrected, no other examinations or therapy involving the eyes will diminish a learning disability. Visual training, muscle exercises, perceptual training, or hand-eye coordination exercises do *not* improve the child's learning abilities.

It is difficult to absolutely diagnose a learning disability before a child reaches the age of 6 or 7. However, once a diagnosis is made, educational assistance is needed promptly.

PEDIATRIC CATARACTS

Certain neonatal disorders have an incidence of cataract formation. Galactosemia is one inborn error of metabolism that may cause cataracts. This is the result of absence of galactose-1-phosphate uridyl transferase. A second form of galactosemia is related to galactokinase deficiency. The only manifestation of this deficiency is a childhood cataract.

Other disorders that cause cataracts in infants and children include hypoglycemia and hypocalcemia. Some chromosomal abnormalities, particularly Trisomy 21, are associated with cataracts. In addition, cataracts may occur with Trisomy 13 and Trisomy 18. Rubella cataracts may occur as a manifestation of the classic rubella syndrome, the triad of cardiac defects, hearing impairment, and cataracts.

Traumatic cataract is the most common cause of unilateral cataract in children from penetrating or blunt trauma. Posterior lenticonus cataracts are the second most common cause of unilateral acquired cataract in children. Posterior lenticonus is a circumscribed oval or round bulge in the infant's or child's posterior lens capsule and cortex restricted generally to a 2 x 7 mm. axial diameter. The bulge progressively increases and cataractous changes occur in the cortex surrounding the posterior lenticonus. Generally, there is a reduced red reflex initially with posterior lenticonus and traumatic cataracts. The condition may occur as early as 3 months of age or as late as 15 years of age. If the vision becomes worse than 20/70 to 20/80, the cataract should be removed by specialized instrumentation followed by contact lens fitting. If a contact lens is not successful, an epikeratophakia procedure may be required.

RETINOBLASTOMA

Retinoblastoma is the second most common primary intraocular malignancy in all age groups (melanoma is most common in adults) and is the most common intraocular malignancy of childhood. Its incidence is approximately one in every 14,000 births. Generally, between 250 and 300 new cases a year occur in the United States. There may be a viral or oncogenic factor related to the environment that may occur with this condition.

The tumor occurs bilaterally in up to one third of cases. It is generally diagnosed between 14 and 18 months of age, and over 90 per cent of the tumors are diagnosed by age 3 years. Familial cases of retinoblastoma account for 6 per cent of patients. The disease is inherited through an autosomal dominant gene with incomplete penetrance. The remaining 94 per cent of patients are sporadic cases that occur as a result of genetic mutation in 25 per cent and as a somatic mutation in about 75 per cent. It is difficult if not impossible to clinically differentiate the genetic mutations and to determine which tumors will be passed on to offspring. There are occasionally rare cases of retinoblastoma related to chromosomal abnormalities in the partial deletion of the long arm of the 13 chromosome. It has also been associated with trisomy 21.

The diagnosis is made by the patient presenting with a white pupil (leukocoria) in 61 per cent of cases, strabismus in 22 per cent of cases, and sometimes with a retinal detachment, red, painful eye, or spontaneous hyphema (Fig. 59–24). Generally, patients with small retinoblastomas present with problems with vision or strabismus. More advanced lesions present with leukocoria and sometimes a secondary glaucoma. The advanced lesions may metastasize to the orbit and produce proptosis through the orbital spread. In addition, patients with retinoblastoma may have systemic metastases to the central nervous system, skull bones, lymph nodes, and other organs.

The treatment of retinoblastoma is generally enucleation in the cases of advanced retinoblastoma involving over 50 per cent of the eye. If the second eye is involved, treatment depends on the size of tumor and whether or not there is extraocular extension. External beam irradiation treatment may be performed on the second eye and also in bilateral cases. Photocoagulation or cryotherapy are equally effective with small retinoblastomas confined to the retinal periphery. Systemic chemotherapy may be indicated following enucleation in advanced unilateral or bilateral cases.

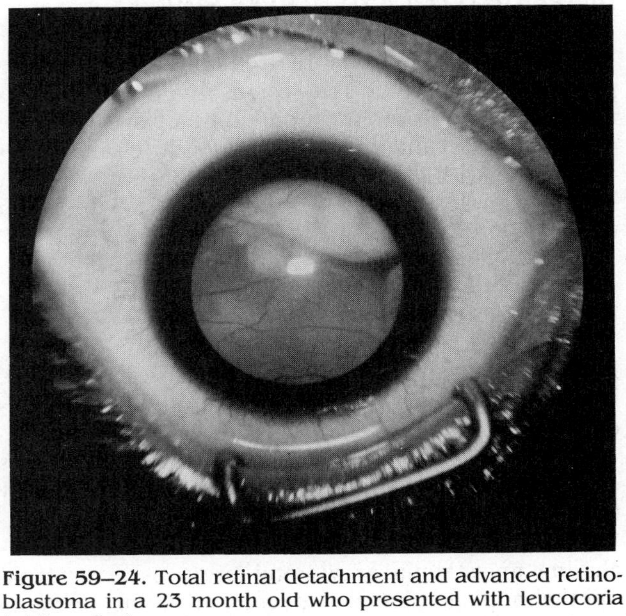

Figure 59–24. Total retinal detachment and advanced retinoblastoma in a 23 month old who presented with leucocoria (white reflex).

Contact Lenses

Major uses of contact lenses include the correction of myopia, aphakia, and astigmatism. It is critical to have a well-motivated patient in order to successfully fit contact lenses. Frequently, the patient is motivated by cosmetic appearance in contacts as compared to glasses. In addition, the aphakic patient may be motivated by improvement of visual quality possible with contact lenses. There are many types of contact lenses but they fall primarily into four groups:

1. Daily wear hard lenses
2. Daily wear soft lenses
3. Rigid, gas-permeable hard lenses (daily and extended wear)
4. Extended wear soft lenses

Hard lenses have generally been constructed of PMMA (polymethyl methacrylate). This material has minimal absorption of fluid as compared to soft lenses, which may be hydrated up to 80 per cent. The main problems with hard lenses include discomfort associated with the use of the lens for at least 2 weeks after initial fittings. However, these lenses last generally more than 3 years. New materials for both hard and soft lenses continue to be developed, including silicone lenses that are now available to the public. A major advantage of PMMA lenses includes the correction of corneal astigmatism up to 2 diopters.

Soft contact lenses do not require a prolonged adaptation period nor is a rigid wearing schedule essential for successful use. The primary disadvantage of soft lenses is that visual acuity is decreased if the patient has a corneal astigmatism of greater than 1 diopter. In addition, there are some fluctuations in visual acuity with blinking. The lens is easily damaged with handling, and the lenses have a short life span as compared to the conventional hard lenses. Generally, soft lenses last no longer than 1 year. The material used in soft lenses is generally hydrophilic material, such as hydroxyethylene methyl methacrylate (HEMA).

Rigid gas-permeable contact lenses are more comfortable than conventional PMMA hard contact lenses. In addition, they provide better visual acuity than soft lenses if astigmatism is present.

Extended wear hydrogel lenses are lenses that enable the eye to adapt to the lens for an indefinite period of time and provide stable visual correction if there is not a significant astigmatism. We are now in a third generation of extended wear hydrogel lenses. These extended wear lenses can be used for disease as well as for aphakic eyes. Complications of extended wear lenses include infection, ocular allergies including enlargement of the follicles, contact lens opacification due to calcium deposits or lipoprotein coatings, corneal edema, and corneal vascularization. Therefore, patients wearing extended wear lenses should be treated with caution. Corneal ulcers are more common with extended wear lenses as compared to daily wear lenses. Careful patient hygiene and lens cleaning of both hard and soft lenses and particularly extended wear lenses cannot be overemphasized.

Ocular Medications

Ocular medications may have significant systemic side effects. Miotic eye drops, such as pilocarpine, are used for the treatment of chronic open angle glaucoma, and may cause cholinergic effects on rare occasions with systemic absorption. Epinephrine eye drops can be absorbed in high enough concentrations to cause an acute elevation of blood pressure, headaches, and heart palpitations. Epinephrine should be used with caution in patients with systemic hypertension or coronary artery disease. Systemic absorption of timolol may exacerbate asthma. In addition, it may cause difficulties in breathing, brachycardia, and hypotension. This medication is contraindicated in patients with heart block, congestive heart failure, asthma, or obstructive lung disease. Other agents used in glaucoma include carbonic anhydrase inhibitors, oral medications to lower intraocular pressure and decrease aqueous production. Carbonic anhydrase inhibitors (Diamox or Neptazane) cause increased urination, decreased appetite, nausea, malaise, and kidney stones. Carbonic anhydrase inhibitors lower the serum potassium, particularly in patients taking diuretics. Potassium supplements should be prescribed to prevent hypokalemia.

Unfortunately, at times patients are given an antibiotic-steroid combination that may increase intraocular pressure, cause cataracts, or potentiate fungal ulcers. Steroid glaucoma is a form of open angle glaucoma. If the condition is undetected and the patient continues to refill the medication, damage may occur to the optic nerve including glaucomatous optic atrophy. Generally, the intraocular pressure is lowered once the steroids are discontinued. However, it may take several months for the pressures to return to normal levels. Vision loss that occurs during this period of time may be permanent. Because of the relative frequency of steroid glaucoma, cataracts and exacerbations of viral infections, topical corticosteroids should be avoided in minor ocular inflammations. It is important to emphasize that generally ocular conditions that warrant the use of topical steroids also warrant the consultation of an ophthalmologist.

Ophthalmic Conditions in the Adult

The most important causes of central and peripheral visual impairment in the elderly include glaucoma, cataract, diabetic retinopathy, and macular degeneration. Most of these conditions can be controlled or, as in the case of cataracts, vision can be restored to a significant level to improve the quality of life. Glaucoma and macular degeneration may be arrested with proper treatment. Regular eye examinations for the elderly can detect early signs of ocular abnormalities and ensure that proper treatment is initiated. Generally, adults after the age of 40 should have a complete exam at least every 3 years. After age 65, the exams should be at 2-year intervals.

DISEASES OF THE EYELIDS

Entropion is a turning in of the eyelid margin so that there is a rubbing of eyelashes or cilia with resultant ocular irritation. An ectropion is a turning out of the eyelid margin so that the eye builds up excessive tears and becomes inflamed. Both conditions are more common in the aging population. Entropion and ectropion can cause symptoms of irritation and corneal changes.

Basal cell carcinoma is much more common in the elderly. The carcinoma occurs more commonly on the lower lid. Generally, basal cell carcinomas have pearly edges and a central depression that becomes ulcerated.

Dermatochalasis, or baggy eyelids, may interfere with vision, covering part of the eye. This condition is caused by an atrophy of the skin of the lids, resulting in falling of the loose skin onto or over the eyelashes. Dermatochalasis does not cause any permanent damage to vision.

Blepharospasm is a chronic spasm of the eyelids in older adults. It may interfere with reading and driving. Botulinum injection in very small doses is presently the treatment of choice (Fig. 59–25).

HERPES ZOSTER AND HERPES SIMPLEX

Herpes zoster occurs more frequently in the aging population. When the skin lesions involve the eyelids and tip of the nose, the ophthalmologist should be consulted for evaluation. Corneal dendrites and ulcers can occur with herpes zoster and herpes simplex. Herpes simplex is more commonly associated with uveitis (Plate XXXIV).

PTOSIS

Ptosis can occur in a number of different forms, including congenital ptosis, pseudoptosis, and acquired ptosis (Fig. 59–26).

Congenital ptosis can occur as a bilateral ptosis or with a Marcus Gunn jaw winking ptosis secondary to misdirected third nerve.

Acquired forms of ptosis include myogenic, including myasthenia gravis and progressive external ophthalmoplegia, and neurogenic, including Horner's syndrome or third nerve palsy (Fig. 59–27).

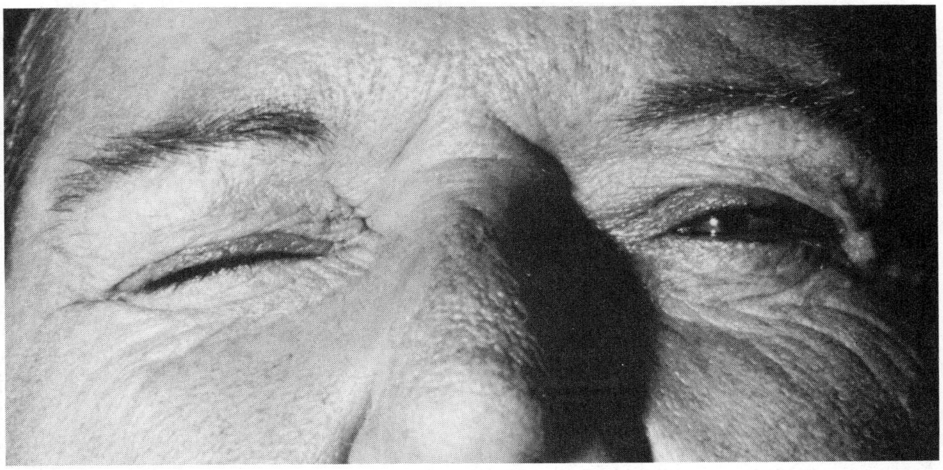

Figure 59–25. A 68-year-old female with history of lid spasm that was impossible to control. The blepharospasm was responsible for her inability to drive.

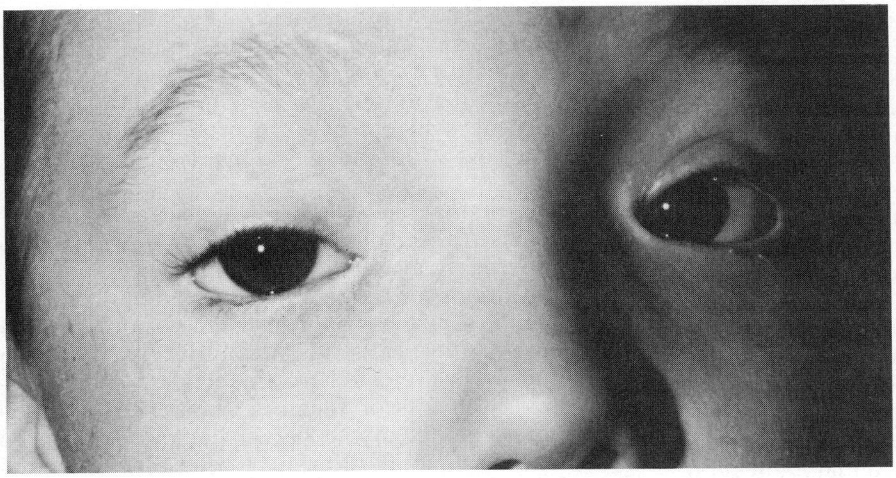

Figure 59–26. Congenital ptosis seen in a 4-year-old patient with bilateral ptosis of a congenital variety.

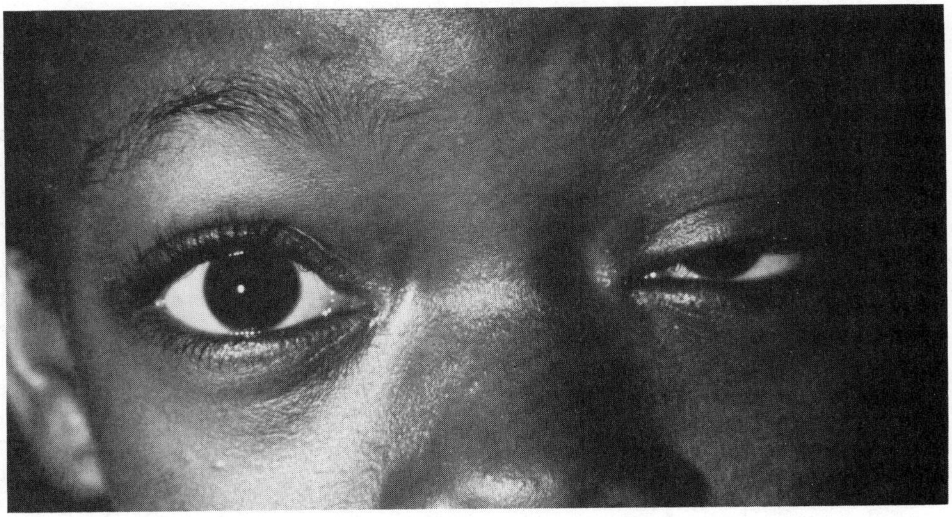

Figure 59–27. Ptosis of the left upper lid in an 8-year-old patient who had ocular myasthenia and subsequently developed a ptosis of the right upper lid and exotropia.

In addition, a traumatic ptosis or mechanical ptosis may occur.

Pseudoptosis is due to conditions giving the appearance of a ptosis but actually is more related generally to a small eye. This is particularly common with microphthalmia (small eye) or phthisis bulbi. It may also be secondary to a hypotropia.

Congenital ptosis generally is corrected with a bilateral fascia lata brow suspension or a levator resection in instances where there is good levator function. Adult forms of ptosis include correction with a tarsoconjunctival resection or a strengthening of the levator aponeurosis.

THE DRY EYE AND KERATITIS SICCA

Keratoconjunctivitis sicca is an acquired disorder seen frequently in the fifth decade of life. The sexual predilection is towards women. Initial symptoms include a foreign body sensation, dryness, and burning, which often worsens as this progresses.

Examination reveals a lack of corneal and conjunctival luster with some dry spots being seen. With a decrease in aqueous tears, an attempt to compensate by increase in mucin production occurs leading sometimes to a stringy, rope-like discharge. Some cases of keratoconjunctivitis sicca are related to an autoimmune etiology, particularly those with dryness of other mucous membranes. This also occurs commonly with such conditions as rheumatoid arthritis (Sjögren's syndrome).

Treatment of dry eyes includes artificial tears to replace the tear deficiency in symptomatic patients. At that time, the ophthalmologist is required to perform surgical closure of the punctum, tarsorrhaphy, and advocate goggles in severe cases. Topical antibiotics are only required if secondary infection occurs.

ARCUS SENILIS

Arcus senilis or corneal arcus is a hazy white or yellow arc or deposit in the peripheral cornea. There are many causes of arcus senilis, and it is more common in the aging population. The deposit is composed of cholesterol and other lipids and does not generally indicate an underlying systemic abnormality in the elderly. It does not interfere with vision or function of the eyes.

THYROID MYOPATHY

Hyperthyroidism is characterized by a diffuse hyperplasia of the thyroid and an infiltrative ophthalmopathy. The thyroid myopathy is seen in association with thyroid function. However, the thyroid function test may also be normal. In thyroid myopathy, the extraocular mechanism is unknown and the genetic predisposition is uncertain.

Graves' ophthalmopathy occurs in approximately 95 per cent of patients with Graves' thyroid disease but is only rarely seen in Hashimoto's thyroid disease. The diagnosis of euthyroid Graves' ophthalmopathy is primarily a clinical diagnosis with the assistance of computerized tomography.

Clinical characteristics include hypotropia, esotropia, or a combination of both a vertical and horizontal muscle deviation. Almost always there is a positive forced duction test on examination. Many patients are euthyroid at the time of diagnosis, but there may have been a previous history of thyroid abnormalities. Thyroid myopathy is a common cause of acquired vertical deviation in adults but relatively uncommon in children.

Werner has classified eye involvement in Graves' disease by a "NO-SPECS" phenomenon:

*N*o signs of symptoms
*O*nly signs of lid retraction or gaze palsy with or without lid lag and proptosis
*S*igns and symptoms of soft tissue involvement
*P*roptosis
*E*xtraocular muscle involvement
*C*orneal involvement with corneal drying
*S*ight loss with optic nerve involvement

The total muscle volume of the extraocular muscles increases as the disease worsens. The volume can be computed by averaging serial CT sections.

Indications for treatment of thyroid ophthalmopathy include diplopia, abnormal head position, a large horizontal or vertical strabismus, and loss of vision. Generally, the preferred treatment is an orbital decompression if loss of vision is threatened. Nonsurgical management of the patient includes prisms to alleviate the diplopia in primary position and/or surgery, generally on adjustable sutures.

CATARACTS

Cataract is a condition that affects a large percentage of the population (Plate XXXV). Generally, the normal aging and cataractous changes in the lens are related to its metabolic activity and changes in the concentration in various proteins and minerals. Developmental or congenital cataracts can be divided into those that are subcapsular opacities involving the capsule and the underlying cortex and those that are primarily in the lens substance itself. Anterior and posterior polar or capsular cataracts are discreet opacities in the axial capsule layer. Posterior subcapsular cataracts often interfere with vision, while the anterior cataracts may not interfere with vision.

Acquired cataracts may occur related to penetrating trauma or from irradiation, heat, or blunt trauma (Plate XXXVI). Metabolic cataracts may occur particularly in association with diabetes. Changes in the blood glucose may alter the refractive power of the lens. With hyperglycemia, there is an increased concentration of glucose in the anterior chamber aqueous humor. When the glucose enters the lens, water follows with resultant swelling.

Senile cataract (nuclear sclerosis) is the most common cause of lens opacity seen by the ophthalmologist. The most common type of cataract in older patients involves the lens nucleus. There is an increased density centrally in the lens that makes the lens focusing power stronger. As a result of this change in focusing power, frequent changes in glasses are required. This type of cataract develops slowly, and surgery may not be necessary for several months or even years.

Subcapsular cataract, particularly posterior subcapsular cataract, is an opacity just in front of the posterior capsule. This may be associated with reduced vision particularly with bright sunlight or night driving. The treatment for cataracts depends on whether or not vision is impaired or the patient's life style is limited because of the cataracts.

Should cataract surgery be decided upon, the operation involves removal of the cataract or cloudy lens material. Generally, this is performed under local anesthesia but may be performed under general anesthesia. Formerly, the primary procedure for cataract removal was an intracapsular cataract removal, i.e., a freezing of the entire lens, removing both the anterior and posterior capsule, the lens cortex, and lens nucleus. At the present time, the majority of ophthalmologists utilize an extracapsular cataract procedure. There are two forms of extracapsular cataract surgery. One is the aspiration technique and the other phacoemulsification.

The aspiration technique with instrumentation is utilized in adults as well as children. In children, the lens material is generally soft and can be removed by the aspiration technique. In the older patient, the hard nucleus is first removed, or expressed, and then the remaining soft cortex tissue is removed.

Phacoemulsification is an extracapsular technique utilizing sound waves in the form of ultrasonic energy to break up the lens material so that it may be withdrawn through a small needle. Unfortunately, phacoemulsification has been confused with a laser treatment for cataract removal. It is important to emphasize to patients that the laser is not used to remove the cataractous lens. Part of the confusion lies in the fact that secondary cataracts or opacification of the posterior capsule is eliminated with the use of the YAG laser. With the YAG laser, there is a photodisruption of the capsule that produces an opening and provides good visual acuity.

Cataract removal is one of the most successful operations performed. Generally, adult patients have intraocular lenses implanted at the time of surgery. Children are usually treated with extended wear or gas permeable hard contact lenses. If the patient has bilateral aphakia, then strong spectacle lenses or cataract glasses may be worn. However, there is a moderate amount of visual distortion that occurs with spectacle lenses as well as restriction of the peripheral field. Spectacles cannot be used when a cataract is removed from one eye only and the other eye is normal. An extended wear contact lens is an alternative if an intraocular lens is contraindicated.

GLAUCOMA

Glaucoma is responsible for at least 10 per cent of blindness in the United States. With increased intraocular pressure, damage to the optic nerve and visual field abnormalities can occur. The most common type of glaucoma is open angle glaucoma where there is a gradual increase in intraocular pressure causing a gradual loss of the peripheral (side) vision followed by reduction of the central field (Figs. 59–28 and 59–29). Unfortunately, the damage to the vision caused by glaucoma is irreversible. If the glaucoma can be detected early, in most instances it is controlled and curable by medical treatment, by laser surgery, by trabeculectomy, or by other filtering surgeries. It is important to emphasize that glaucoma may occur at any age. Causes include congenital glaucoma, chronic open angle glaucoma, narrow angle glaucoma, or other forms of glaucoma including pigmentary glaucoma. The number of people with glaucoma increases dramatically with age, particularly after age 40, and also is more severe in the black population. The incidence of glaucoma at the present time is 2 per cent of people in the United States. The family physician can measure the intraocular pressure by using tonometry to detect glaucoma. Tonometry can be used with a Schiotz tonometer held vertically or with a Goldman applanation tonometer horizontally. This test should be performed at least every 3 years beginning at age 35 years.

MELANOMA

Choroidal melanoma is the most common intraocular malignancy. It is a pigmented, elevated mass in the choroid. As the tumor spreads, it may produce a retinal detachment. In addition, retinal pigment epithelial alterations can occur in the form of drusen or as lipofuscin or orange pigment. The differential diagnosis of choroidal melanoma includes choroidal nevus, retinal detachment, and metastatic tumor to the choroid. All patients with intraocular tumors should have an extensive physical examination and laboratory testing to exclude metastatic spread of the neoplasm. Only 1 to 3 per cent of ocular melanomas have metastasis prior to the diagnosis of the eye lesion.

The management of melanomas of the choroid is presently controversial. Many ophthalmologists recommend enucleation for the treatment of intraocular melanomas. However, other studies have questioned the role of dissemination of the tumor and worsened morbidity from metastasis with enucleation. The ma-

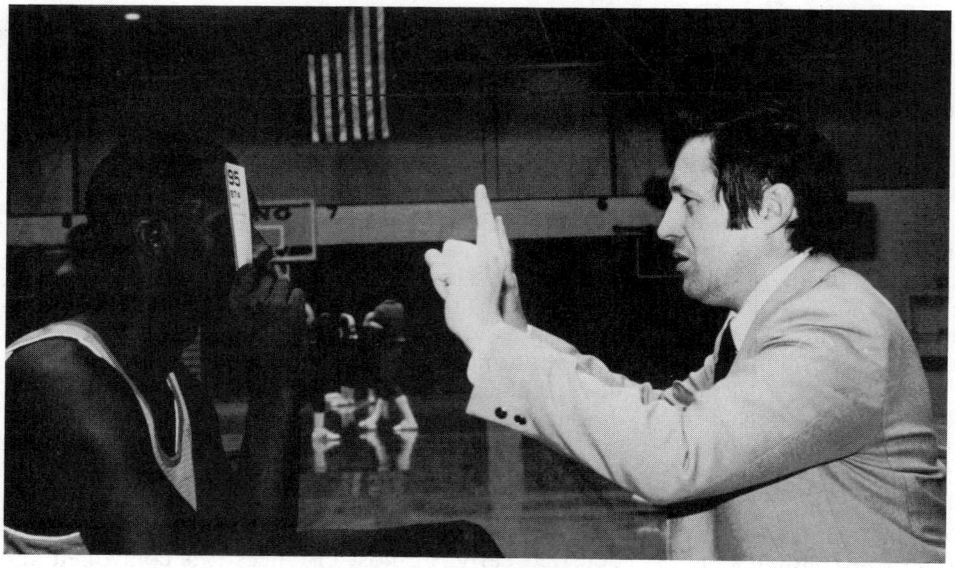

Figure 59–28. Testing of peripheral fields by confrontation. (From *The Athlete's Eye*, American Academy of Ophthalmology, Professional Information Committee, San Francisco, California.)

jority of ophthalmologists do feel that enucleation is the preferred treatment in the larger lesions. When a smaller melanotic lesion is detected, observation is generally indicated in older patients with slow growing lesions.

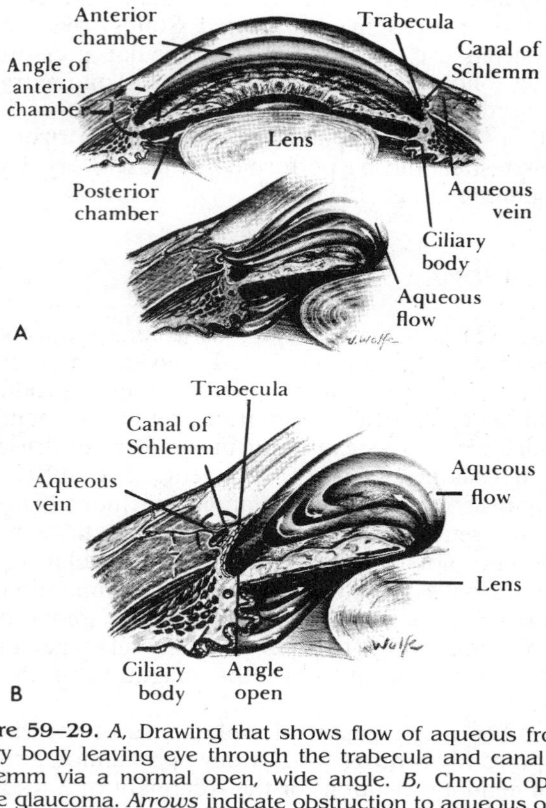

Figure 59–29. *A*, Drawing that shows flow of aqueous from ciliary body leaving eye through the trabecula and canal of Schlemm via a normal open, wide angle. *B*, Chronic open angle glaucoma. *Arrows* indicate obstruction to aqueous outflow in angle wall. (From Scheie, H. G., and Albert, D. M.: Textbook of Ophthalmology. 9th ed. Philadelphia, W. B. Saunders Company, 1977. By permission.)

UVEITIS

A red eye, pain, photophobia, and increased tearing are presenting symptoms of anterior uveitis. In addition, there may be decreased vision. The vascular injection is a circumcorneal injection involving the deep vessels of the conjunctiva and is one of the key signs in anterior uveitis. Generally, uveitis patients are light sensitive or photophobic. In addition, the inflammatory process may hinder the aqueous production and reduce intraocular pressure. Patients suspected of an anterior uveitis should be referred to an ophthalmologist for consultation and treatment.

Patients with posterior uveitis usually present with a reduction in vision as a definitive symptom. There are many causes of posterior uveitis that preclude an extensive discussion. However, the most common causes of uveitis include sarcoidosis, ankylosing spondylitis, Reiter's syndrome (a urethritis, polyarteritis, and ocular inflammation), juvenile rheumatoid arthritis, ulcerative colitis, and ileocolitis.

One of the most common causes of posterior uveitis is toxoplasmosis, which accounts for up to 30 per cent of these cases. Toxoplasmosis may destroy the macula or other important visual structures in the eye. Characteristically, there is an exudation with an inflammatory process in the retina. In addition, toxocara canis can also present as a uveitis.

Diseases of the Retina and Optic Nerve

Retinal diseases account for a large percentage of blindness. Included are conditions such as macular degeneration, diabetic retinopathy, retinal detachment, and retinal vascular disease.

AGE-RELATED MACULOPATHY

Age-related maculopathy (formerly macular degeneration) leads to loss of fine or central vision but not side vision (Plate XXXVII). Laser treatment may be of benefit in selected cases. However, most people with macular degeneration have an abnormality in size or position that precludes laser therapy from arresting progression. It is also important to emphasize that there is a 10 per cent chance of the condition occurring in the fellow eye within 1 year.

RETINAL CHANGES IN SYSTEMIC DISEASES

Routine ophthalmoscopy in hypertensive patients awards the physician a direct view of the arterioles and helps assess the long-term duration and severity of the hypertension as well as evidence of accelerated or malignant hypertension. In the vascular system, arterioles serve as the resistance vessels, and the overall cross section of the arteriolar bed determines peripheral resistance. In the eye ground, the physician has the ability of directly observing the degree of spasm in arterioles and the effects of long-term hypertension on the arteriolar wall.

The normal arteriolar wall is transparent, and the visible image is one of the blood column as it passes through the arteriolar lumen. An additional anatomic fact is that at the point of crossing of the arteriole and venule they share a common adventitial layer so that when arteriolar thickening occurs the venule is compressed resulting in AV (arteriolar-venous) nicking.

It is practical to divide the changes in the eye ground seen in hypertension into two scales: the hypertensive and an arteriole-sclerotic scale. The hypertensive scale reflects a degree of spasm within the arteriolar system. There is no universally accepted classification of fundus changes in hypertension. Scheie's classification considers arteriolar vascular leakage changes and arteriolar sclerosis separately. Hypertensive retinopathy is graded as follows:

- Grade 1—Generalized attenuation of retinal arterioles (particularly smaller branches)
- Grade 2—More pronounced attenuation and focal arteriolar attenuation
- Grade 3—Generalized and focal arteriolar attenuation with retinal exudates, cotton-wool spots, and hemorrhages (Plates XXXVIII and XXXIX)
- Grade 4—Grade 3 changes plus papilledema

Grading of the arteriolar changes include:

- Grade 1—Broadening of the arteriolar reflex, minimal AV crossing defects
- Grade 2—Increased arteriolar light reflex and AV crossing changes
- Grade 3—Copper-wire arterioles and marked AV crossing changes
- Grade 4—Silver-wire arterioles and severe AV crossing changes

DIABETIC RETINOPATHY

Diabetic retinopathy (DR) is the most common cause of blindness in Americans aged 20 to 74. Diabetics have 25 times greater incidence of becoming blind from diabetic retinopathy as compared to nondiabetics becoming blind from all other causes. Diabetic retinopathy is more common in women but men appear to develop a more complicated and severe proliferative retinopathy.

Findings indicate that in type I diabetics it is unusual to detect diabetic retinopathy before 5 years after onset of disease. At 15 years, most type I diabetics have some diabetic retinopathy, with the incidence of proliferative disease being greater than 40 per cent.

In type II diabetics, onset after age 30 years, diabetic retinopathy is often detectable at initial diagnosis. Diabetics requiring insulin have a higher incidence of diabetic retinopathy and proliferative disease.

The pathogenesis of diabetic retinopathy appears to be related to aldose reductase pathways and their inhibition. There is an increased retinal blood flow similar to the increased glomerular filtration in the kidneys. Following this, there is breakdown of the blood-retinal barrier allowing large molecules to enter the extracellular space of the retina, causing macular edema.

It is important to emphasize that a high percentage of diabetic retinopathy is a background retinopathy, including microaneurysms, dot and blot hemorrhages, hard lipid exudates, and intraretinal microvascular abnormalities (IRMA) (Plate XL). One of the major causes of visual loss in diabetic retinopathy is secondary to macular edema, which is much more common in type II diabetics. In addition, vitreous hemorrhage, retinal detachment, and neovascular glaucoma occur with proliferative diabetic retinopathy. A diabetic retinopathy study has proven that laser photocoagulation has reduced the rate of severe visual reduction and proliferative disease.

At the present time, yearly ophthalmologic examinations are recommended for type I diabetes, more often if the disease is active. Yearly exams are also recommended for type II disease.

RETINAL DETACHMENT

Retinal detachment is a separation of the retina from its blood supply, and it usually follows a tear or hole in the retina. Retinal tears may be caused by trauma or retinal diseases, but the cause of most tears is not clear. When the retina is detached, vision is lost from the involved area of the retina. If the macula detaches, irreversible loss of vision may occur unless the detachment is treated within 24 hours. Anatomical reattachment of the retina is successful in up to 90 per cent of cases.

GIANT CELL ARTERITIS—TEMPORAL ARTERITIS

Giant cell arteritis or temporal arteritis is a generalized inflammatory process of medium sized and large arteries. This generally occurs in patients over age 55, with no sex predilection. Involvement may occur in any organ system. Ocular involvement is generally associated with inflammation of the posterior ciliary arteries. Systemic features may include malaise, weight loss, fever, and a tenderness of the scalp. In addition, there may be pain and tenderness of the muscles and joints and over the temporal arteries, ear, or jaw. The patient may have only a few of these symptoms. One of the presenting symptoms includes sudden visual loss, either partial or complete, double vision, or amaurosis fugax. The visual loss is caused by an ischemic process in the optic nerve. Central retinal artery occlusion may also occur. Giant cell arteritis is important to diagnose as early as possible. Without corticosteroid treatment, patients may develop permanent visual loss bilaterally. When one eye is involved with the giant cell arteritis, the second eye loses vision in 65 per cent of untreated patients. Generally, involvement of the second eye may occur within 10 days. When the diagnosis is suspected on the basis of clinical symptoms and signs, temporal artery biopsy may be necessary to confirm the diagnosis. Erythrocyte sedimentation rate (ESR) is often markedly elevated, but it may be normal for age. Patients with ischemic optic neuritis without signs or symptoms suggesting giant cell arteritis and a normal sed rate may not need to be biopsied. However, when there is any question or doubt, temporal artery biopsy should be performed. Once the diagnosis is made, steroid therapy should be instituted immediately. Up to 100 mg. prednisone should be given orally as well as intravenous corticosteroid therapy for the first 48 hours in order for the oral steroids to take effect. The patient can be monitored by the symptoms that occur after the institution of treatment and by monitoring the sed rate. Because of the severe systemic effects of giant cell arteritis, the patient should be followed closely.

ISCHEMIC OPTIC NEUROPATHY

The clinical characteristics of ischemic optic neuropathy include onset generally over age 60, a painless vision loss, and an afferent pupillary defect (Marcus Gunn pupil). In addition, there is usually a visual field abnormality. Examination of the optic disc reveals disc edema in virtually all cases. Pathology appears to be related to a diseased ciliary circulation. It is generally difficult to determine whether the disc edema will result in a mild peripheral (side) visual field defect and good visual acuity or a reduced central acuity and significant large visual field defect.

It is important to emphasize that giant cell arteritis or temporal arteritis needs to be ruled out in these patients. Sedimentation rate and a general physical examination are indicated. No treatment prevents the progression of ischemic optic neuropathy including steroids and anticoagulants.

TRANSIENT ISCHEMIC ATTACKS IN CAROTID ARTERY DISEASE

Transient ischemic attacks (TIAs) are neurologic deficits lasting less than 24 hours. TIAs are reversible. The most common ophthalmologic TIA is amaurosis fugax, by definition a fleeting monocular blindness due to an embolic event. There is a sudden graying or reduction of vision often moving from the peripheral vision to the center to cover the entire visual field within a few seconds. After 1 to 5 minutes, the vision will return starting with central vision. Other causes of transient ischemic attacks include chronic disc edema, where vision loss lasts seconds but not minutes, chronic papilledema with bilateral blackouts based on optic nerve disease, often also lasting a few seconds and due to postural changes, and TIAs due to basilar artery insufficiency. Those related to basilar artery insufficiency are usually bilateral blackouts lasting seconds or minutes, often with changes in the posterior circulation.

The most important mechanism involving carotid TIAs in stroke are an embolization from the carotid artery or its branches, reduced perfusion due to carotid stenosis or occlusion, or a combination of both. In the majority of patients, up to 90 per cent, the sight of obstruction is the carotid sinus. Hollenhorst plaques are bright yellow cholesterol emboli that rarely occlude the retinal arterioles and may not produce visual symptoms. Fibrin platelet emboli can occur near retinal arterioles and produce visual symptoms. Either a cholesterol or fibrin platelet embolus is indicative of ulcerative disease in the carotid arteries and is associated with a high incidence of ischemic heart disease, peripheral vascular disease, and aortic abdominal aneurysms. A rarer form of carotid transient ischemic attacks (TIAs) is related to valvular heart disease, particularly with a prolapsed mitral valve or with cardiac arrhythmias. It is important to emphasize that approximately 50 per cent of patients with TIAs in the carotid will have a major stroke within a month of the first attack.

References

American Academy of Ophthalmology Interprofessional Education Committee: The Child's Eye: Strabismus and Amblyopia. San Francisco, American Academy of Ophthalmology, November, 1989.

American Academy of Ophthalmology Professional Information Committee: The Aging Eye. San Francisco, American Academy of Ophthalmology, November, 1984.

American Academy of Ophthalmology Professional Information Committee: The Athlete's Eye. San Francisco, American Academy of Ophthalmology, November, 1986.

American Academy of Ophthalmology Professional Information

Committee: The Red Eye. San Francisco, American Academy of Ophthalmology, November, 1986.
American Academy of Pediatrics Committee on Practice and Ambulatory Medicine: Vision Screening and Eye Examination in Children. Pediatrics, 77:918–919, 1986.
Apple, D. J.: Ocular Pathology: Clinical Applications and Self-assessment. 3rd ed. St. Louis, The C. V. Mosby Co., 1985.
Crouch, E. R., and Goodrich, K. A.: Practical aspects of pediatric vision screening. Am. Orthop. J., 38:62–72, 1988.
Duane, T. D. (Ed.): Clinical Ophthalmology. Hagerstown, MD, Harper & Row Publishers, 1983.
Ellis, P. P.: Ocular Therapeutics and Pharmacology. 6th ed. St. Louis, The C. V. Mosby Co., 1981.
Fraunfelder, F. T., and Roy, F. H. (Eds.): Current Ocular Therapy 2. Philadelphia, W. B. Saunders Co., 1985.
Grayson, M.: Diseases of the Cornea. St. Louis, The C. V. Mosby Co., 1979.
Harley, R. D. (Ed.): Pediatric Ophthalmology. 2nd ed. Philadelphia, W. B. Saunders Co., 1983.
Havener, W. H.: Synopsis of Ophthalmology. 5th ed. St. Louis, The C. V. Mosby Co., 1979.
Helveston, E. M., and Ellis, F. D.: Pediatric Ophthalmology Practice. St. Louis, The C. V. Mosby Co., 1980.
Henderson, J. W.: Orbital Tumors. Philadelphia, W. B. Saunders Co., 1973.
Jaffe, N. S.: Cataract Surgery and Its Complications. 4th ed. St. Louis, The C. V. Mosby Co., 1984.
Kolker, A. E., and Hetherington, J., Jr.: Becker-Schaffer's Diagnosis and Therapy of the Glaucomas. 4th ed. St. Louis, The C. V. Mosby Co., 1976.
Miller, D.: Ophthalmology: The Essentials. Boston, Houghton Mifflin, 1979.
Moses, R. A. (Ed.): Adler's Physiology of the Eye: Clinical Application. 7th Ed. St Louis, C.V. Mosby Co., 1981.
Newell, F. W.: Ophthalmology: Principles and Concepts. 6th ed. St. Louis, The C. V. Mosby Co., 1986.
Parks, M. M.: Ocular Motility and Strabismus. Hagerstown, Maryland, Harper & Row Publishers, 1976.
Paton, D., and Goldberg, M. F.: Management of Ocular Injuries. Philadelphia, W. B. Saunders Co., 1980.
Peyman, G. A., Sanders, D. R., and Goldberg, M. F.: Principles and Practice of Ophthalmology. 3 vols. Philadelphia, W. B. Saunders Co., 1980.
Read, J., and Crouch, E. R.: Trauma: Ruptures and bleeding. In Duane, T. D. (Ed.): Clinical Ophthalmology. Vol. 4. Philadelphia, Harper & Row, 1983, pp. 1–17.
Scheie, H. G., and Albert, D. M.: Textbook of Ophthalmology. 9th ed. Philadelphia, W. B. Saunders Co., 1977.
Shields, J. A.: Diagnosis and Management of Intraocular Tumors. St. Louis, The C. V. Mosby Co., 1983.
Vaughan, D., and Asbury, T.: General Ophthalmology. 9th ed. Los Altos, Lange Medical Publications, 1980.
Walsh, F. B., and Hoyt, W. F.: Clinical Neuro-Ophthalmology. 3rd ed. 3 vols. Baltimore, Williams & Wilkins, 1969.

60

Neurology

Disorders that affect the nervous system are frequently encountered in the practice of family medicine. Manifestations of neurologic disease include the development of new experiences and behaviors and the loss of previously existing capabilities. *Positive* signs of neurologic dysfunction include the presence of abnormal sensations or pain; involuntary motor events such as tremor, chorea, or convulsions; and the display of bizarre behavior or mental confusion. *Negative* signs are those that represent the loss of function, such as paralysis, imperception of external stimulation, lack of ability to speak, and loss of consciousness. The nature of the neurologic symptom or sign indicates the location of the pathologic change within the anatomic structures of the nervous system. Once localized by history and neurologic examination, the likely disease process can be diagnosed. It is not merely an intellectual exercise to localize the neurologic lesion; rather, with such clinicoanatomic information a proper differential diagnosis can be considered, specific therapeutic measures can be employed, and a reasonable prognosis based on pathophysiologic knowledge can be rendered.

This chapter offers a symptomatic approach to the diagnosis and treatment of neurologic disorders. The reader is referred to basic texts for more detail about the neurologic examination and neuroanatomy than might be found here.

---

*Contributors: Sanford Auerbach, M.D., Assistant Professor of Neurology; Viken Babikian, M.D., Assistant Professor of Neurology; Thomas R. Browne III, M.D., Professor of Neurology; David E. Burdette, M,D., Teaching Fellow in Neurology; Robert G. Feldman, M.D., Professor of Neurology; Jules Friedman, M.D., Assistant Professor of Neurology; Marc Kamin, M.D., Assistant Professor of Neurology; Jan Kucera, M.D., Professor of Neurology; Simmons Lessell, M.D., Professor of Neurology; Clifford Michaelson, M.D., Assistant Professor of Neurology; Jeannette Chirico-Post, M.D., Associate Professor of Neurology; Marie Saint-Hilaire, M.D., Assistant Professor of Neurology; Philip A. Wolf, M.D., Professor of Neurology.

Headache

Marc Kamin

The most common reason for visits to a primary care physician is headache. The major categories of headache encountered are outlined in Table 60–1. Pain described as "headache" may result from irritation of afferent nerve endings that supply certain structures inside and outside of the cranial vault, such as the dura mater, falx cerebri, or meninges (Table 60–2). Other headaches, such as muscle contraction and vascular headaches, have more obscure causes that have not been fully worked out.

Diagnostic Considerations

The diagnosis of headache depends primarily on a clinical history and neurologic examination. Careful analysis must be made of each patient's complaint of headache (Table 60–3). An initial goal of the evaluation is to differentiate the more benign forms of headache, such as muscle contraction and migraine, from potentially life-threatening types of headache.

Table 60–1. CLASSIFICATION OF COMMONLY ENCOUNTERED HEADACHE SYNDROMES

- Migraine or vascular headaches
  - Classic
  - Common
  - Cluster
- Tension or muscle contraction
  - Mixed
  - Temporomandibular joint dysfunction
- Headache of extracranial origin
  - Nasal sinusitis
  - Temporal arteritis
- Headache of intracranial origin
  - Meningeal
    - Infectious—bacterial, fungal, viral
    - Subarachnoid hemorrhage
  - Subdural
    - Hematoma
    - Empyema
  - Intraparenchymal
    - Hypertensive hemorrhage
    - Tumor
    - Encephalitis
    - Abscess
    - Ischemic vascular disease
  - Obstructive and nonobstructive hydrocephalus
  - Cerebral venous sinus occlusion
  - Positional
  - Toxic-metabolic
    - Anemia
    - Fever
    - Withdrawal—caffeine, aspirin, ergots

Table 60–2. HEADACHE: PAIN-SENSITIVE STRUCTURES

Intracranial
- Circle of Willis blood vessels
- Medium-sized arteries and major branches
- Large veins
- Dura
- Meninges

Extracranial
- Skin, scalp, fascia, muscles
- Mucosal linings of sinuses
- Arteries
- Temporomandibular joints
- Teeth

A *meningeal process* must be suspected when headache is of recent origin with a gradual onset accompanied by fever, with or without a stiff neck. Etiologic agents include bacterial, viral, or other chronic infections. Common bacterial organisms encountered are *Streptococcus pneumoniae, Haemophilus influenzae,* and *Neisseria meningitidis.* A variety of viral organisms are responsible for "aseptic" meningitis. Spirochetal infection may also cause an aseptic meningitis such as meningovascular syphilis or Lyme disease. Cryptococcal meningitis, the most common form of chronic meningitis, is encountered in situations of immunodeficiency, especially the acquired immune deficiency syndrome (AIDS) or chronic steroid usage. Viral organisms may also directly affect the brain, causing encephalitis. The treatable variety that clinicians should be aware of is herpes encephalitis, which presents as headache, fever, confusion, early seizures, and typically signs of temporal lobe dysfunction, such as aphasia.

The headache associated with *subarachnoid hemorrhage,* whether due to rupture of an aneurysm or to vascular malformation, is frequently described by the patient as explosive and accompanied by vomiting. Migraine not uncommonly presents as the abrupt onset of the "worst headache ever," but subarachnoid hemorrhage is always the first consideration. The headache may, or just as commonly may not, be

Table 60–3. HEADACHE: QUALITY OF PAIN

Quality of Pain	Possible Significance
Dull, constant ache	Increased intracranial pressure
Tight band, cramplike	Muscle tension
Throbbing, lateralized	Migraine, vascular
Pulsating, generalized	Meningeal irritation; subarachnoid hemorrhage

related to exertion. It is usually generalized, but may be lateralized or even focal. In almost half the cases a "sentinel" hemorrhage or leak of the aneurysm may precede the more catastrophic rupture by several days or weeks. This headache is of sudden onset, usually generalized but possibly focal, lasting from hours to days with few associated symptoms. The clinician must have a high index of suspicion in these instances.

Subdural hematoma is usually the result of obvious head injury, but its presence must also be suspected in patients describing mild chronic headache and subtle neurologic signs such as early dementia or mild hemiparesis with no history of head trauma. It may also present as a seizure or a transient ischemic attack (TIA) in an older individual. *Subdural empyema* causes focal neurologic signs, usually hemiparesis in individuals with headache and fever in the setting of an untreated sinusitis.

Cerebrovascular diseases may result in several varieties of headache. An ischemic cerebrovascular accident or TIA may be accompanied by severe headache, commonly unilateral in nature. A transient unilateral headache may be the only manifestation of a carotid artery TIA. Intraparenchymal cerebral hemorrhage from hypertension or bleeding diathesis results in severe headache if the patient remains conscious, in addition to prominent focal neurologic signs. Cerebellar hemorrhage can be particularly difficult to diagnose, but it is treatable. Anyone with acute onset of headache and dizziness or vertigo should be considered to have a cerebellar hemorrhage and not labyrinthitis.

An increasingly severe headache associated with nausea, vomiting, and transient visual obscurations suggests *increasing intracranial pressure.* These headaches intensify with sudden head movement, coughing, sneezing, or straining. They tend to be worse upon awakening and are accompanied by papilledema. Possible causes include brain tumor and brain abscess, which are commonly associated with focal neurologic signs or symptoms. Obstructive hydrocephalus and increased intracranial pressure may result from third or fourth ventricular tumors, acqueductal stenosis, or subarachnoid hemorrhage.

The headache of *benign intracranial hypertension* or "pseudotumor cerebri" has all of the characteristics of an increased intracranial pressure headache, but patients look surprisingly well except for an occasional sixth nerve palsy. This syndrome is of unknown cause but is commonly seen in overweight or pregnant young women or in association with hypervitaminosis A or outdated tetracycline usage. A major venous sinus thrombosis can cause a similar picture, but patients are typically sicker, with more extensive focal findings. There is a recurring headache associated with venous angiomas that has a sudden onset of pain with peak intensity reached within minutes. These headaches can easily be confused with migraines.

Disorders of *extracranial structures* commonly give rise to headache. Inspection of the scalp and palpation of the cranium may reveal skin infection or external masses. Percussion of the sinuses may reveal an inflammatory process. Individuals over the age of 55 years with persistent unilateral or bitemporal headache, particularly when associated with constitutional symptoms such as myalgias and arthralgias, tender temporal arteries, and jaw claudication, are assumed to have temporal arteritis until proven otherwise. Rapid diagnosis is imperative so that steroid treatment can be instituted in order to prevent the complication of blindness.

A common diagnostic dilemma is that of differentiating a *migraine headache* from a tension or *muscle contraction headache.* These headaches can be considered to be on a symptom spectrum. At one end is the classic muscle contraction headache and at the other is the classic migraine. Along this spectrum lie two other headache syndromes: the common migraine and a mixed headache pattern.

The most common cause of acute recurring headache is the result of a migrainous process. These headaches are commonly unilateral and throbbing in nature. The two main varieties of migraine headache are *classic migraine* and *common migraine.* Both types of headache have a variety of precipitating factors. The headache may be precipitated by the ingestion of foods containing tyramine (cheese, nuts), sodium nitrite (sausage, bologna), or phenylalanine (chocolate). More comprehensive food lists may be obtained from headache texts. Other precipitants are stress or the post-stress period, oral contraceptives, and hypoglycemia. A family history of migraine is common. Interestingly, these patients commonly have a history of motion sickness. In classic migraine, the headache begins with an aura of neurologic symptoms that evolves over 30 minutes. These include scotomas with scintillations (flashing lights) around them, unilateral paresthesias, hemiplegias, or aphasia. In some individuals the neurologic symptoms may occur without developing the headache; this may account for many unexplained transient neurologic episodes, but other, more serious conditions must be considered first. The headache that usually follows begins as a dull ache, becoming pulsatile, evolving over 1 hour and lasting up to 24 hours. Autonomic symptoms such as nausea, vomiting, photophobia, chills, or diarrhea may be prominent. Common migraine presents with more generalized throbbing head pain and no neurologic symptoms. Onset is frequently upon awakening. These headaches may be abrupt or gradual in onset and may last hours to days, but affected persons have days or weeks of pain-free intervals. It should be kept in mind that all headaches in a migraineur are not migraine, and more serious conditions may be overlooked.

In some patients vascular-type headaches occur in clusters over a period of several weeks. These *cluster headaches*, which affect males 95 per cent of the time, may recur on a seasonal basis. The pain of these headaches is unilateral, located in the temple or eye, is intensely knifelike, and lasts 15 to 30 minutes. Several acute episodes may recur during the day or awaken the patient from sleep. This form of headache is often associated with ipsilateral prominence of a temporal artery, conjunctival redness, lacrimation, and ipsilateral nasal stuffiness. Alcohol, nicotine, or other vasodilators are potent triggers for an attack.

Muscle contraction or tension headaches are characterized by a constant aching sensation throughout the head or in a classic hatband distribution. It is present "from the time I get up, to the time I go to sleep." Its intensity has little variability. Tenderness may be elicited over frontalis or cervical muscles. Patients are commonly chronically tense or anxious. They may display signs or symptoms of depression. A mixed or overlap headache pattern is very common, in which a common migraine headache of several hours or days is superimposed on a steady-state muscle contraction headache.

Related somewhat to tension headache is the headache associated with temporomandibular joint dysfunction. Aching pain in both temporal regions is classically present upon awakening and is aggravated by chewing.

An acute headache can develop in the presence of a systemic illness such as hypertensive crisis, hypoglycemia, severe dehydration, anemia, or uremia. Patients with chronic lung disease may complain of morning headaches due to significant carbon dioxide retention during the night and resulting increased intracranial pressure. Withdrawal from large amounts of caffeine can result in headache, which is then relieved by the next dose, setting up a significant addiction potential. Treatment is slow withdrawal of caffeine.

Positional headaches pose a challenging problem for the clinician. The most common headache aggravated by leaning forward is actually migraine, but sinusitis must always be considered. Headaches produced by intracranial tumors may be worsened by head movement. The neurologic syndrome of worsening headache aggravated by change in position raises the possibility of a lesion in the ventricular system behaving like a ball-valve and causing intermittent obstructive hydrocephalus, such as a colloid cyst of the third ventricle. A headache worsened by assuming the upright position and relieved promptly by lying down may be the classic lumbar puncture headache or be due to a congenital deformity at the base of the skull, the Arnold-Chiari malformation (Fig. 60–1).

Diagnostic Studies

Once a tentative diagnosis is made after analyzing the quality, location, and temporal profile of the pain, one turns to laboratory tests to confirm abnormalities or to eliminate life-threatening possibilities.

The *cerebrospinal fluid* (CSF) examination can be very helpful when looking for the cause of acute headache (Table 60–4). If meningitis, aseptic or otherwise, or a subarachnoid hemorrhage is suspected, a lumbar puncture must be performed. Contrary to popular thought, a computerized tomographic (CT) scan of the brain will detect only 90 to 95 per cent of subarachnoid hemorrhages and will not rule out the diagnosis. In the presence of focal neurologic signs or symptoms, evidence of increased intracranial pressure with papilledema and obtundation, a CT scan of the brain must be obtained prior to lumbar puncture. Posterior fossa mass lesions such as cerebellar hemorrhage or infarction can mimic labyrinthitis when the headache is accompanied by vertigo, or a meningeal process when it is accompanied by a stiff neck. CT scan must be performed before lumbar puncture in patients in whom a posterior fossa disorder is suspected. In the presence of a mass lesion causing headache and increased intracranial pressure, lumbar puncture carries a significant risk of cerebral and/or tonsillar herniation. Use of cell counts and appearance of the supernatant are well known in the diagnosis of bleeding or infection. A commonly encountered problem with lumbar puncture is that of traumatic tap. When a cell count is critical, it is best to measure the cells in the first and fourth tubes obtained. A progressively falling count suggests traumatic tap, whereas constant numbers support a subarachnoid hemorrhage. After centrifugation of the CSF, the supernatant should be crystal clear and colorless after a traumatic tap. Xanthochromia (orange tinge) to the supernatant suggests breakdown of red blood cells already present in the fluid. Early stages of a viral meningitis may be characterized by polymorphonuclear cells, but 24 to 48 hours later lymphocytes predominate. The CSF sugar is typically normal in viral meningitis but is reduced in bacterial and fungal meningitis. Interestingly, it can be very low in subarachnoid hemorrhage as well. Carcinomatous meningitis is usually associated with low CSF sugar and high protein as well as abnormal cytologic examination, which should be performed if the diagnosis is suspected. In cases of suspected fungal meningitis, both India ink stain and cryptococcal antigen as well as fungal culture should be obtained. Cases of cryptococcal meningitis associated with AIDS have been described with normal cell counts, protein, and sugar with only the cryptococcal antigen positive.

The widespread availability of *CT scanning* has made it possible to visualize the intracranial contents quickly. Using enhancement during a CT scan demonstrates vascular markings of an arteriovenous malformation, or vascular tumor, brain abscess, or subdural hematoma. CT scanning can rapidly diagnose intracerebral hemorrhages, infarctions, neoplasm, and hydrocephalus. A decision that is frequently faced by primary care physicians is when to obtain a CT scan. When structural disease is highly suspected in the face of clear-cut neurologic signs or symptoms, the decision is easy. However, one of the most

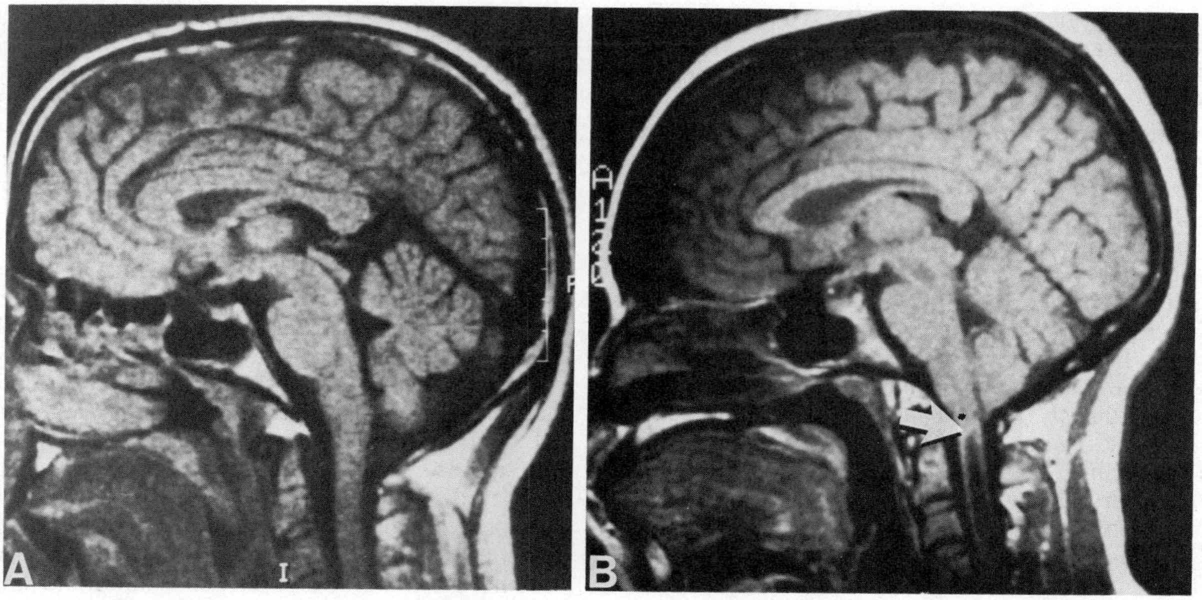

Figure 60–1. *A,* Normal MRI of the brain. *B,* MRI of an Arnold-Chiari malformation. Note herniation of cerebellar tonsils into the foramen magnum and the cervical spinal cord syrinx.

commonly encountered situations is when the complaint is only headache in an otherwise well patient. The current legal climate drives some clinicians to reflexively order scans on all patients. Certain guidelines may be helpful in this regard. Any patient with strictly unilateral headaches must have a CT scan with and without contrast enhancement. Progressive headache in a previously pain-free individual, positional headaches, and a change in a life-long pattern of headaches are also good standing indications for CT scan. Sometimes the decision is made only after a 1- to 2-week follow-up period when further historical or physical findings are obtained. A normal CT scan can be reassuring to some patients and even be therapeutic in that regard.

Magnetic resonance imaging (MRI) of the brain is rapidly becoming a valuable tool in the evaluation of certain types of headache and may someday become the standard imaging technique for brain disorders. For headache it is most helpful in evaluating lesions of the posterior fossa such as fourth ventricular tumors, aqueductal stenosis, and Arnold-Chiari malformation. Third ventricular tumors, venous angiomas, and subdural hematomas not seen on CT scanning may be imaged well with MRI scans. Because of its significant cost, MRI is not a routine part of the headache work-up. Although MRI produces exquisite pictures, their acquisition is more difficult and time-consuming, so CT scanning remains preferable for many conditions such as head trauma, acute hemorrhage, meningioma, and bony abnormalities as well as for the more difficult patient.

Radiographic studies of the skull are no longer a routine part of headache evaluation. They are still useful in assessing head trauma when an emergency CT is not available. They may demonstrate displacement of a calcified pineal gland, thus indicating shift of intracranial structures. Enlargement and erosion of the sella turcica indicate a local tumor or chronically increased intracranial pressure. Hyperostosis of the sphenoid wing may be the only finding to suggest a meningioma. Sinus x-ray films can confirm a clinical suspicion of sinusitis. Electroencephalograms (EEG's) may show focal slow waves in patients with brain tumor or abscess, and a particularly helpful focal periodic pattern in herpes encephalitis. The EEG of patients with migraines occasionally shows a paroxysmal pattern that can be helpful therapeutically.

Some routine laboratory tests can be very helpful in diagnosing headache. Utilizing a routine complete blood count for all headache patients is not unreasonable, to look for anemia or signs of infection. An erythrocyte sedimentation rate should be obtained immediately in all patients over the age of 50 years with new-onset or undiagnosed headache to rule out temporal arteritis. A normal result with a strong clinical suspicion should not deter one from obtaining a temporal artery biopsy. Clotting studies must be obtained when intracranial hemorrhage is suspected. A chest radiograph is always helpful if metastatic brain lesions are suspected.

If the headache problem is not solved promptly with these tests, a neurologic or neurosurgical consultation should be obtained.

Therapeutic Measures

When a structural cause is discovered for the headache, the therapy is usually straightforward. Controversy still exists about many aspects of neurologic

Table 60–4. CEREBROSPINAL FLUID FINDINGS

Condition	Appearance	Pressure (in mm water)	Cells (per liter)	Protein	Miscellaneous Findings
Normal lumbar tap	Clear and colorless	70–200	0–5	15–45 mg. per dl.	Glucose 50–70 mg. per dl.
Normal ventricular tap	Clear and colorless	70–190	0–5 (lymphocytes)	5–15 mg. per dl.	VDRL negative
Traumatic tap	Bloody; supernatant fluid clear	Normal	Red blood cells	4 mg. per dl. rise per 5000 red cells	Bloody; less blood in succeeding tubes
Cerebral hemorrhage, ventricular or subarachnoid	Bloody; supernatant fluid yellow (xanthochromia)	Slightly increased	Red blood cells	4 mg. per dl. rise per 5000 red cells	Blood equal in all three tubes
Meningitis, acute purulent	Clear, cloudy, milky, or xanthochromic; occasional clot formation	Greatly increased (250–700)	Polymorphonuclear cells, usually over 1000	Increased	Glucose decreased early; chlorides decreased late; organisms on smear and culture
Meningitis, acute tuberculous	Opalescent to turbid; faint fibrin web or pellicle formation	Moderately increased (200–400)	10–500 (lymphocytes)	Increased	Chlorides decreased early, often before decrease of glucose; smear, culture, and guinea pig inoculation for organisms
Meningoencephalitis	Clear and colorless	Normal	Normal or increased (mostly lymphocytes)	Normal or slightly increased	Serologic tests of value in viral infections
Brain abscess	Clear and colorless	Greatly increased	Polymorphonuclear cells normal or increased	Increased	Pressure may go as high as 600–700 mm water
Brain tumor	Usually clear and colorless	Increased	Normal or increased	Increased	Findings depend on location and type of tumor
Subdural hematoma	Classically yellow, but often clear and colorless	Usually increased	Normal	Normal or slightly increased	

Modified from Chusid, J. Q.: Correlative Neuroanatomy and Functional Neurology. 19th ed. Los Altos, CA, Lange Medical Publications, 1985.

therapy for, for instance, cerebrovascular accidents and subarachnoid hemorrhage, but discussion of these topics is beyond this section. Treatment of migraine and tension headache is a task facing primary care physicians on a daily basis and is dealt with in some detail.

MIGRAINES

The approaches to classic and common migraine are similar and consist of abortive and preventive measures. Abortive measures are directed at stopping or ameliorating the headache as it is starting or once it has begun. Preventive measures are daily therapies directed at reducing the frequency and intensity of headache. Preventive or daily therapy is usually instituted when headaches have reached a frequency of one per week or are significantly interfering with the patient's functional ability. Table 60–5 summarizes some frequently used drugs for migraine.

Patients should be instructed to lie in a dark room; frequently, cold compresses across the forehead will be of benefit. Several categories of drugs are available for abortive therapy. Mild analgesics such as aspirin or acetaminophen combined with caffeine and butalbital may be effective. Potential for abuse and addiction must be kept in mind with these drugs. Large doses of nonsteroidal anti-inflammatory drugs such as 500 to 750 mg. of naproxen (Naprosyn) can manage some acute migraines. Side effects of gastric distress are most common and nausea makes their administration difficult. A mild vasoconstrictor known as isometheptene (Midrin) is useful in some individuals. Two tablets are taken by mouth at the onset of the neurologic aura or headache and one tablet can be repeated hourly up to a total of five tablets within a 12-hour period. Midrin is contraindicated in patients with hypertension or ischemic heart disease.

The mainstay of acute migraine therapy remains the ergot derivatives. Ergotamine tartrate is the most commonly used preparation. The drug can be administered in a variety of ways. Oral preparations such

Table 60–5. THERAPY CHART* FOR CLASSIC AND COMMON VASCULAR MIGRAINE

Route	Drug	Dosage
Prophylactic		
Oral	Methysergide maleate (Sansert)	2 mg. t.i.d.
	Cyproheptadine (Periactin)	4–16 mg. daily as tolerated
	Propranolol (Inderal)	80–240 mg. as required in common migraine
	Amitriptyline (Elavil)	50–100 mg. at bedtime
	Clonidine (Catapres)	0.1 mg. t.i.d.
	Platelet inhibitors	
Abortive		
Oral	Ergotamine, caffeine, belladonna, pentobarbital (Cafergot-PB)	1 or 2 tablets at onset—may repeat 1 tablet every ½ hour if necessary, to a maximum of 6 per day, 10 per week
	Isometheptene mucate, dichloralphenazone, and acetaminophen (Midrin)	2 capsules at onset, followed by 1 capsule every hour until relieved, up to 5 capsules in 12-hour period
Sublingual	Ergotamine (Ergomar, Ergostat, Wigrettes)	1 tablet at onset, under the tongue—repeat at ½-hour intervals if necessary, but not more than 3 tablets in any 24-hour period
Inhalation	Ergotamine (Medihaler-Ergotamine)	1 dose immediately—repeat every 5 minutes to a maximum of 6 per day, if necessary
Intramuscular	Dihydroergotamine	1 ml at hourly intervals, up to 3 ml per day, if necessary
Rectal	Ergotamine and caffeine (Cafergot, Wigraine)	Insert 1 suppository in rectum immediately—repeat in 1 hour, if necessary
	Ergotamine, caffeine, belladonna, pentobarbital (Cafergot-PB, Wigraine-PB)	

*Recommended dosages of drugs do not conform with FDA-approved package circulars but have proved effective in the authors' management of headache patients with minimal side effects.

Modified from Diamond, S., and Dalessio, D. (Eds.): The Practicing Physician's Approach to Headache. 4th ed. Baltimore, Williams & Wilkins, 1986, p. 56.

as Cafergot, which contains 1 mg. ergotamine tartrate and 100 mg. caffeine, have an initial dose of two tablets by mouth, followed by one tablet at half-hour intervals to a total of no more than five to six per day or until the necessary effect has been obtained. If nausea precludes the oral route, ergotamine can be administered sublingually (Ergostat, Ergomar; 2 mg. at onset repeated every half hour for a total of three tablets), by suppository (Cafergot, one immediately, repeated hourly for a total of three), or by inhalation (Medihaler, 0.36 mg. per puff, one puff every 5 minutes up to three doses, not to exceed six per day). The minimum effective dosage of ergotamine has to be individualized to balance side effect against benefit. The maximum dosage of ergotamine that is typically tolerated is 6 to 8 mg. per day. Signs of overdosage or ergotism include pale or blue extremities, tingling of the hands and feet, muscle cramps, nausea and vomiting, and aggravation of angina pectoris. Ergot derivatives should not be used if the prodromal neurologic symptom is longer than 30 minutes. They are contraindicated in pregnancy, peripheral vascular diseases, ischemic heart disease, and impaired hepatic or renal function. Addiction to ergots can occur if they are abused, and subsequent withdrawal can result in severe rebound headaches. Rebound headaches can also result from abuse of milder analgesics or caffeine.

If the headache has been unresponsive to the milder abortive medications and is still evolving, a parenteral ergot, dihydroergotamine mesylate (DHE-45), has been found to be very effective. One mg is administered intramuscularly, usually with 10 mg. of metoclopramide (Reglan) intravenously. Acute dystonic reactions can occur with intravenous metoclopramide. If the headache is fully developed, 0.75 mg. DHE-45 is given intravenously with 10 mg. of metoclopramide. Another 0.5 mg. can be given in 30 minutes if the desired effect has not been obtained. The same precautions using ergots should be employed with the parenteral preparations, avoiding the contraindicated situations, being aware of recent total usage of other ergot derivatives, and not administering it in the presence of focal neurologic deficits. If a common migraine is already fully developed at the time of awakening, a trial of ergotamine tartrate via one of the previously described routes is still recommended. In-hospital treatment of unresponsive migraines, which should be with the aid of a neurologist, includes periodic injections of DHE-45 or parenteral corticosteroids.

There are various options for preventive therapy of classic and common migraine. It should be kept in mind that in some studies placebo alone will decrease the frequency of attacks by 50 per cent. Adequate relaxation, improvement in restful sleep, and stress reduction will reduce the frequency of migraine attacks. A good initial approach is to eliminate potentially precipitant foods from the diet. The drug of choice is propranolol (Inderal), administered in doses of 60 to 240 mg. daily. Bradycardia, fatigue, and depression are common side effects. Other commonly used prophylactic drugs include methysergide (Sansert) 3 to 6 mg. per day and amitriptyline (Elavil) 25 to 100 mg. at bedtime. Methysergide should not be used for longer than 6 months at a time because of the potential complication of retroperitoneal fibrosis. Daily use of nonsteroidal anti-inflammatory drugs such as naproxen 500 mg. two times a day may be helpful. Careful monitoring of renal function is necessary. Finally, daily use of calcium channel blockers such as verapamil in doses of 240 to 480 mg. per day has recently been found to be effective. Other less frequently used drugs include phenobarbital 60 to 120 mg. per day or phenytoin (Dilantin) 300 mg. daily, especially when there are paroxysmal EEG abnormalities. Prophylactic medications are typically administered for 12 to 18 months and then tapered if possible.

A variety of treatments are available for cluster headaches. Some feel calcium channel blockers for the duration of the cluster attack are most effective. More commonly used agents include sublingual ergotamine 2.0 mg. or one to three puffs of an aerosolized form at the onset of the attack. Oral ergotamine 1 to 2 mg. at bedtime may prevent nocturnal attacks. Instillation of lidocaine nose drops, 1 ml. of 4 per cent solution administered once or twice, can terminate the headache. Inhalation of 8 to 10 liters per minute of 100 per cent oxygen at the outset is occasionally helpful. Daily use of methysergide, 2 to 6 mg. per day, is an effective prophylactic treatment in many patients. A 2- to 3-week course of prednisone 60 mg. per day initially and then tapering can be very effective in breaking the cycle. Daily therapy with lithium or a calcium channel blocker is effective for chronic cluster headaches. The beta blockers and tricyclic antidepressants effective in migraine have little use in the therapy of cluster headaches.

MUSCLE CONTRACTION

It is necessary to break the cycle of anxiety and depression leading to headache and to identify the underlying psychological conflicts and precipitating emotional events. Biofeedback and other relaxation techniques are useful in the management of muscle tension headache. Sometimes a 2-week course of muscle relaxants such as diazepam 5 mg. three times a day, or cyclobenzaprine (Flexeril) 10 mg. three times a day, or nonsteroidal anti-inflammatories such as ibuprofen 400 to 600 mg. three times a day is necessary. Longer-term therapy with antidepressants is best administered in conjunction with behavioral consultation. More severe exacerbations can be treated with one or two doses of narcotic-containing preparations. For intermittent symptomatic relief, treatment may include two tablets of a combination of butalbital 50 mg and aspirin 325 mg, with or without caffeine 40 mg (Fiorinal), taken at onset of headache. This combined with two additional aspirin (650 mg) often provides relief of pain. Gastric irritation may occur in some patients. In these cases preparations containing acetaminophen instead of aspirin should be used. Potentially habituating medications such as barbiturates, caffeine-containing prescriptions, and benzodiazepines should not be prescribed for longer than 1 to 2 weeks. The mixed tension/migraine headache pattern previously described responds well to tricyclic antidepressants such as amitriptyline 25 to 200 mg. at bedtime. The most important aspect of therapy for all headache patients is good follow-up.

Dizziness

Jules Friedman

The vague complaint of dizziness is difficult to describe and is even more difficult to evaluate. Nevertheless, systematic application of well-established techniques of assessment usually leads to a proper diagnosis. Problems of the vestibular system are the most common cause of dizziness. Hyperventilation syndrome, cerebrovascular insufficiency, toxic and metabolic disturbances, cardiac diseases, multiple sclerosis, and epilepsy may cause dizziness. Some patients use the word "dizziness" to describe a sensation of lightheadedness, faintness, or even blurriness of vision. A minority of patients who complain of dizziness actually experience *vertigo,* the sensation of movement of self or surroundings with a feeling of unsteadiness, tilting, or pulsion. Vertigo is produced whenever the normal balance in the neural activity of the vestibular system is upset asymmetrically.

Nystagmus, the rhythmic eye movements that accompany vestibular disorders, can usually be observed in vertiginous patients (see the Visual Disturbances section for nonvestibular causes of nystagmus). Nystagmus consists of a slow tonic deviation of the eyes in one direction and a fast return. These slow and fast components alternate and together form the rhythmic oscillations of nystagmus. It should be noted that it is the *lesion* of the *vestibular system* that produces the *slow tonic ocular deviation;* the fast jerk return is merely a reflex compensatory reaction originating elsewhere in the central nervous system (CNS). By convention, however, the direction of nystagmus is described according to the fast component. Thus, *nystagmus with the slow component to the left and fast component to the right is described as "right-beating nystagmus."*

There may be associated symptoms secondary to excitation of the parasympathetic nervous system (vegetative symptoms). Nausea, vomiting, pallor, and diaphoresis are common. On occasion, diarrhea or even hypotension with syncope may occur. The extent of vegetative symptomatology in a given vestibular lesion varies greatly from patient to patient. Some patients complain of "dizziness" to describe lightheadedness or faintness. The sensation may be caused by hypotension resulting from vasovagal and orthostatic reflexes or more serious cardiovascular conditions. Metabolic dysfunction, especially hypoglycemia, may cause such symptoms. Hyperventilation syndrome, usually associated with anxiety or depression, produces lightheadedness, which may be followed by circumoral and distal extremity paresthesias, unsteadiness, precordial pain, and even tetany or syncope. Often, tightness or fullness in the head stemming from common tension-related cranial or cervical muscle spasm is described along with the dizziness. Visual disturbances, including blurred vision or diplopia, can be so described. Toxic agents, especially sedatives, tranquilizers, narcotics, and tobacco, can produce such symptoms. Patients with any combination of bilateral visual dysfunction, proprioceptive dysfunction, or vestibular dysfunction (multiple sensory deficits) may experience spatial disorientation and describe this as dizziness or unsteadiness. This is quite common in older age groups and especially in diabetics.

As in evaluation of disease of other parts of the nervous system, the differential diagnosis of dysfunction of the vestibular system depends on precise *localization* of the site of the lesion and determination of the *pathologic process* responsible for the lesion at that locus. The former is accomplished by the recognition of symptoms and physical findings characteristic of lesions at a given locus in the vestibular system and the latter by selecting from among those pathologic processes known to occur at a given locus according to their characteristic *clinical profiles.* Whether the vestibular symptoms are caused by disease of the vestibular nerves in the periphery or in the medullary brainstem connections, a careful neurologic examination and special confirmatory diagnostic tests are necessary.

Vestibular Causes of Dizziness

Dysfunction of the vestibular system can be separated into (1) acute paroxysmal, (2) acute onset with gradual resolution, (3) chronic, (4) motion-induced, and (5) position-induced types.

Acute Paroxysmal Vestibular Dysfunction. Symptoms occur suddenly and persist for several minutes to hours. Hearing loss and tinnitus may be aggravated during an attack of vertigo. Autonomic nervous system symptoms of nausea, vomiting, diaphoresis, hypotension, and even syncope are often concomitant problems. The ataxia associated with vestibular dysfunction is characterized by an unsureness of gait, tendency to veer off to one side, and increased awkwardness of walking when in the dark or when making sudden movements or turns in direction. The best example of an acute paroxysmal disturbance of the peripheral vestibular system is *Ménière's disease* (endolymphatic hydrops). This disease clinically involves both the vestibular and auditory end organs (labyrinth and cochlea). The clinical course can be marked by periods of remission, in which episodes of vestibular dysfunction and even hearing loss and tinnitus may significantly resolve for weeks or months. In approximately 10 to 20 per cent of cases, the involvement becomes bilateral by 10 years after onset.

Another peripheral lesion that has an acute paroxysmal profile is the syndrome of the *perilymphatic fistula.* The perilymphatic fistula is formed after a rupture of either the round or oval labyrinthine window. This lesion, which commonly follows head trauma or barotrauma or occurs as a known complication of stapedectomy, frequently occurs spontaneously, characterized by hearing loss that may be slowly progressive or of sudden onset. The loss of hearing may, as in Ménière's disease, have significant fluctuations. Tinnitus and a "blocking" feeling of the ear are common. The vestibular manifestations of perilymphatic fistula include episodes of acute paroxysmal vertigo, ataxia, and vegetative symptoms lasting minutes to hours. In addition, episodes of positional vertigo, sometimes lasting nearly a minute, may occur with changes in position. Sensorineural and conductive hearing loss (as documented by audiometry), positional nystagmus of the peripheral type (Table 60–6), ataxia (often independent of ver-

Table 60–6. POSITIONAL NYSTAGMUS

Peripheral Vestibular Lesions	Central Vestibular Lesions
Begins after a latency of several seconds	Begins immediately without a latency period
Mixture of horizontal, vertical and/or rotary movements	Purely horizontal or vertical movements
Vertigo is prominent	Vertigo is absent or minimal
Resolves within 60 seconds	Persists beyond 60 seconds
Recurs with change in position	No further response with change in position
Repetitive testing results in progressive diminution of nystagmus (accommodation)	No accommodation occurs
Intensity varies from examination to examination	Consistently reproducible

tigo and exaggerated when the eyes are closed), and a positive *fistula test* are the diagnostic features. The fistula test is performed by compressing a column of air in the ear canal with a pneumatic otoscope. A positive response consists of forced deviation of eyes and head away from the stimulated side, followed by brief nystagmus and accompanied by momentary vertigo.

Infectious processes involving the middle or the inner ear, or both, uncommonly cause paroxysmal vestibular manifestations. When secondary *cholesteatoma* develops, an acute paroxysmal profile is common, with eventual development of a fistula into the lateral semicircular canal. This finding can be documented with adequate otoscopic or microscopic examination of the ear, with the fistula test, and with adequate radiography. Syphilitic involvement of the peripheral vestibular system can also exhibit a clinical picture similar to those described earlier.

Of those lesions of the *central vestibular system* exhibiting an acute paroxysmal profile, transient ischemia in the distribution of the vertebrobasilar arterial system is not common. *Transient* vertebrobasilar insufficiency is a diagnosis that should be made with great hesitancy when the sole manifestation is vertigo. However, the diagnosis becomes much more likely when vertigo is accompanied by any other manifestation of brainstem ischemia (e.g., diplopia, dysarthria, facial paresthesias, obscured vision). On rare occasions, vertebrobasilar insufficiency may be secondary to compression in one vertebral artery by spondylotic spurs on one or more cervical vertebrae and may occur with rotation and hyperextension of the neck. *Demyelinating disease* (multiple sclerosis) involving the central vestibular connections may have symptoms of the acute paroxysmal type. *Seizure disorders* may become manifested by acute paroxysmal episodes of well-defined vertigo if the cortical representation of the vestibular system in superior temporal and inferior parietal lobes is involved. Less well-defined dizziness may be one of the manifestations of mesial temporal lobe seizures. Often manifestations of seizure activity in other cortical areas will precede or follow the vertigo. Loss of consciousness following vertigo or dizziness is suggestive of a seizure disorder.

Acute Onset with Gradual Resolution. In this second clinical group of symptoms and signs of vestibular dysfunction, compensation occurs at the level of the vestibular nuclei for the most part. In cases of vestibular dysfunction of acute onset with gradual resolution, central nervous system mechanisms reestablish the balance of neural activity between both sides of the vestibular system, which had been disrupted by the causative lesion. Spontaneous nystagmus resolves in 3 to 7 days, although vigorous head movements may provoke momentary recurrences (Table 60–7). Ataxia subsides gradually over several weeks, although it may present a persistent problem in darkness or when the eyes are closed. Of the illnesses of the peripheral vestibular system associated with acute onset and gradual resolution, viral and bacterial infections are quite common. *Viral inflammations* may involve the labyrinth (labyrinthitis) or the nerve (neuritis), but these entities are difficult to distinguish clinically, although labyrinthitis is more likely to extend to involve cochlear and auditory functions. Commonly, a viral upper respiratory infection prodrome occurs within 1 or 2 weeks of the acute onset. *Bacterial labyrinthitis* occurs as an extension of acute or chronic otitis media on otoscopic examination.

Table 60–7. SPONTANEOUS NYSTAGMUS IN VESTIBULAR DISORDERS

Central Vestibular
Not increased with reduced ocular fixation
Intensity out of proportion to vertigo or ataxia
Horizontal, vertical, or rotary movements
Peripheral Vestibular
Increases with eyes closed or in darkness (reduced ocular fixation)
Intensity in proportion to degree of vertigo and ataxia
Mixed rotary and oblique movements
Resolves within 3 to 7 days
Central or Peripheral Vestibular
Not altered by position of gaze
Intensity increases with gaze in the direction of the fast component

Head trauma results in symptoms with acute onset and gradual resolution through labyrinth involvement in temporal bone fracture. Almost invariably, the cochlea is also involved, with concurrent impairment of auditory function.

Chronic Vestibular Disturbances. *Chronic dysfunction* may follow as an unremitting, fluctuant, subjective feeling of "dizziness," unsteadiness of gait, or blurring vision in cases of central lesions, which produce symptoms and signs of vestibular dysfunction and also disrupt the process of compensation at its site of action within the central vestibular system.

Motion-Induced Dysfunction. Motion-induced dysfunction is present if symptoms of vertigo and ataxia occur only when there is a *sudden rapid movement* of the head or body in relation to gravity or a fixed point. When the process of impairment is slowly progressive, accommodation is able to reduce the symptoms. In cases of slowly progressive impairment of vestibular function, accommodation keeps pace and minimizes acute symptoms. However, the lesion becomes sufficiently disabling when accommodation can no longer minimize the symptoms. The most common such lesion is acoustic neurinoma in the cerebellopontine angle. This benign tumor initially causes progressive sensorineural hearing loss. Its most common presenting symptom is tinnitus. Its vestibular manifestations are usually confined to brief episodes of motion-induced vertigo and unsteadiness together with ataxia, which may appear when the patient is walking in darkness or has his or her eyes closed. When the tumor becomes larger, other cranial nerves (i.e., fifth, seventh), the cerebellum, and the brainstem may be compromised.

Position-Induced Dysfunction. Position-induced dysfunction is characterized by vertigo, ataxia, and vegetative symptoms reproduced only *with major change in position*, such as lying back, sitting up, turning over, stooping over, or hyperextending and rotating the neck.

In such cases, positional nystagmus may be induced by performing special positional testing. In this useful maneuver (Nylen-Bárány maneuver), the patient, who is seated near the end of a table, is rapidly placed in the supine position with the head extended over the edge of the table, and is rotated to one side. The patient fixes his eyes at a point several feet ahead. Observations are made for 60 seconds, and the patient is rapidly returned to the sitting position, in which he again fixes his gaze. The maneuver is repeated in the same fashion with the head rotated to the opposite side and once again with the head straight. Two patterns of pathologic response can be identified—one due to lesions of the labyrinth and the other due to lesions of central vestibular connections or other brainstem or cerebellar connections, or both (see Table 60–6).

There are two lesions of the labyrinth that produce position-induced dysfunction. Cupulolithiasis results from the release of particles or debris into the posterior semicircular canal of one labyrinth. This can occur spontaneously or as the end result of almost any type of significant insult to the labyrinth, be it traumatic, infectious, or vascular. In all cases, positional nystagmus is of the peripheral type. The clinical course is usually one of ongoing remissions and exacerbations over months to years. Perilymphatic fistula (described earlier) is another lesion of the labyrinth that can produce this profile. Central lesions may produce position-induced dysfunction. In such cases, positional testing indicates a central lesion. The cause may be a vascular or a demyelinating disorder or a mass lesion involving the brainstem or cerebellum. The physician should evaluate the associated symptoms and signs together with the clinical course to localize the lesion further and narrow down the list of the possible diagnoses.

Diagnostic Approach

The neurologic examination shows objective signs of abnormal station and gait, which include past pointing, a positive Romberg test, and gait ataxia. *Past pointing* is determined by having the patient extend both arms forward. He places the index finger of each hand on the examiner's palms. With eyes closed, the patient then raises both arms over his head and then slowly returns them to the original position. This is repeated several times and past pointing is said to be present if the position of the arms deviates laterally upon return to the original position. The patient may be unable to stand with both feet together, first with eyes opened and then with eyes closed (Romberg's sign). Patients in the acute phase of unilateral vestibular lesions and patients with cerebellar lesions have a definite tendency to fall, both with eyes opened and with eyes closed. Cerebellar lesions can often be distinguished from vestibular lesions by testing of the extremities (heel to shin test, finger to nose test, rapid alternating movements), with resultant intention tremor or dysmetria. Lesions of the proprioceptive system can be documented by direct testing of position sense in the distal extremities. *Gait ataxia* may be present. Patients with acute unilateral lesions of the vestibular system have a staggering gait, usually with a predilection to fall to a particular side. With less acute or mild lesions, gait is usually wide based, with occasional staggering and a tendency to drift toward a particular side. Ataxia due to cerebellar lesions is often difficult to distinguish from that due to vestibular lesions, but the latter are characterized by striking enhancement of gait difficulties with eyes closed or when the patient is in darkness.

Central vestibular lesions may produce only a portion of the potential symptom complex of vertigo, ataxia, and nystagmus. This is due to the fact that the lesion may be so situated as to interfere with neural transmission in only one of the central vestibular connections. Transmission between the intact peripheral systems and all remaining central connections, however, remains unimpaired. There may, for instance, be nystagmus alone with no vertigo or ataxia in lesions that affect only vestibulo-ocular pathways. Central lesions may be so situated as to interfere with the process of accommodation, thus resulting in a duration of clinical manifestations much greater than that expected with peripheral lesions.

Specific testing of the function of each side of the vestibular system can be performed. The minimal ice water caloric test can be performed easily at the bedside or in an office setting. With the patient's head tilted to one side, 0.4 to 2 ml of ice water is instilled by syringe against the tympanic membrane of the uppermost ear. After 20 seconds, all the water is decanted out by tilting the head in the opposite direction. The head is then immediately extended back 60 degrees (if the patient is seated) or flexed forward 30 degrees (if the patient is supine). This position produces observable horizontal nystagmus beating away from the stimulated ear. After a 5-minute rest, an identical stimulus can then be applied to the contralateral ear and the duration of the two responses compared. If one ear responds with a nystagmus duration 20 to 30 seconds less than the other, vestibular dysfunction on that side is to be suspected.

Sensitive testing of vestibular function can be performed with electronystagmography (ENG), a method for recording eye movement using surface electrodes applied at the corner of each orbit. This type of testing provides a means of documenting caloric responses with much greater accuracy than the minimal caloric test. Further, it provides a means of recording and evaluating spontaneous and positional nystagmus under conditions in which the patient's eyes are closed (which enhances all forms of vestibular nystagmus).

Documentation of associated auditory dysfunction provides valuable localizing and etiologic information in the evaluation of vestibular dysfunction. A sophisticated *audiogram* is thus a necessary part of any such evaluation and should always be included in the preliminary battery of tests. Modern audiometry can often differentiate lesions of the cochlea from those of nerves and thus helps to localize more precisely the underlying lesion.

X-ray studies of the skull, with special attention to *temporal* and *mastoid* portions, are invaluable in the evaluation of traumatic, infectious, and mass processes. In cases of suspected acoustic neurinoma, plain and tomographic views of the *internal auditory canal* are essential. Should these be positive, *posterior fossa myelography* is the study of choice for documentation of this lesion. For this and other posterior fossa vascular or mass lesions, *CT scans, arteriography*, and *pneumoencephalography* may be indicated.

The electroencephalogram is invaluable in documenting and localizing seizure disorders. In cases of suspected temporal lobe epilepsy, the use of special nasopharyngeal leads is often diagnostic.

Therapeutic Measures

Vertigo and associated vegetative symptoms are often treated symptomatically with agents such as meclizine (Antivert) or dimenhydrinate (Dramamine) with varying degrees of success. Since drowsiness is a common side effect, patients should be duly cautioned. Scopolamine patches applied behind the ear have been useful in controlling vertigo, especially that associated with travel sickness.

Bacterial labyrinthitis requires appropriate antibiotic and, if necessary, surgical intervention. Secondary *cholesteatoma* requires surgery. Viral labyrinthitis or neuritis is self-limited and requires at most symptomatic treatment.

Ménière's disease is often treated only symptomatically with sedatives and antihistamines, with rather poor results. Attempts at specific therapy such as oral diuretic or salt restriction, or both, are far from definitive. Corrective surgical procedures such as endolymphatic shunts are also less than definitive treatment. Destructive labyrinthectomy, if complete, permanently halts episodes of vestibular dysfunction in that ear. This entails sacrifice of hearing in that ear and should be entertained only in cases of severe, prolonged incapacitation. Since 10 to 20 per cent of cases eventually involve the contralateral ear, even this radical therapy may not give permanent relief. Fortunately, significant spontaneous remissions in the disease are common, and efforts should be directed at providing patients with symptomatic treatment and encouragement until such remissions occur.

Perilymphatic fistulas can be definitively diagnosed and treated with exploratory tympanotomy with repair of the fistula. However, many fistulas heal spontaneously and a trial of several weeks should be given, especially if auditory function appears stable.

The syndrome of *benign positional vertigo* can best be treated by utilizing the vestibular system's intrinsic process of accommodation. Patients should be encouraged to assume the precipitating position several times each day in order to hasten this process and thus limit the duration of the clinical course.

Episodes of *transient vertebral basilar* ischemia may require anticoagulation, with due consideration of the many contraindications of the potentially dangerous therapy.

Acoustic neurinomas must be resected surgically. Early diagnosis significantly reduces morbidity.

Seizure disorders can be managed with anticonvulsant therapy once it has been determined that no progressive structural lesion underlies the seizure focus.

Visual Disturbances

Clifford Michaelson
Simmons Lessell

Although most problems of visual disturbance encountered in family practice are related to changes in refractive error, cataracts, or intraocular pressure, visual symptoms and signs are frequently present in patients with diseases of the nervous system. Complaints of blurred vision, loss of vision, or double vision may have valuable localizing significance in neurologic disease (Table 60–8).

Alterations in Vision

Amaurosis. Transient blurring or loss of vision is frequently due to atherosclerosis of the carotid or vertebral arteries. Transient unilateral visual loss (amaurosis fugax), lasting minutes in typical cases, suggests the presence of a lesion of the ipsilateral internal carotid artery. A bruit may be auscultated over the ipsilateral carotid artery. A variety of noninvasive tests including ophthalmodynamometry, carotid ultrasound, directional Doppler ultrasound, and digital angiography are available to assess the patency of the carotid system, but angiography (arterial) remains the definitive test. Less commonly, transient monocular blurring may be secondary to emboli of cardiac origin. Momentary monocular or binocular visual loss may be seen in chronic papilledema, as is reported in pseudotumor cerebri. Transient bilateral visual blurring may also implicate the vertebrobasilar arterial system and suggests ischemia of both occipital lobes.

Visual Hallucinations. Visual symptoms in patients with migraine headache include hallucinations in the form of scintillating colored lights, swirls, or patterns; transient hemianopias; scotomas; and monocular amaurosis. In classic migraine, the visual symptoms precede the onset of headache and may reflect cerebral or retinal vasoconstriction. Visual hallucinations can result from lesions of the eye or brain. Some patients develop hallucinations when there is loss of visual function. This can occur when the loss is partial or complete, monocular or binocular, or hemianopic. These hallucinations presumably result from release of visual areas of the brain from the modulating effect of normal visual input. Brain lesions can generate ictal (epileptic) visual hallucinations. Temporal lobe lesions produce formed images such as scenes, people, and animals. Similar visual hallucinations of occipital origin are usually simple photisms—flashes of light or color. These may occur as isolated phenomena in focal seizures or form part of the symptom complex in occipital lobe or temporal lobe tumors or vascular accidents.

Cortical Blindness. Geniculocalcarine (cortical or cerebral) blindness refers to bilateral loss of vision from disease of the visual system "behind" the optic tract. The pupils react normally to light, and the optic discs do not show atrophy. Such blindness can result from any bilateral geniculate or retrogeniculate lesion. Bilateral occipital lobe infarction from vertebrobasilar occlusive disease is the most common cause in adults. Trauma, anoxia, Schilder's disease, angiography, mercury intoxication, Jakob-Creutzfeldt disease, and tumors can all produce geniculocalcarine blindness.

Table 60–8. LOCALIZATION VALUE OF EYE FINDINGS

Feature	Clinical Significance
Pupil size	Third nerve
Mydriasis (dilated)	Pons
Miosis (constricted)	Iritis
	Horner's syndrome
Optic nerve	
Papilledema	Increased cerebral pressure
	Pseudotumor cerebri
Inflammation	Optic neuritis
Ischemia	Hypertension
	Vascular occlusion
	Arteritis
Atrophy	Glaucoma
	Traumatic
	Secondary to chronic compression
Visual field defects	
Unilateral (monocular)	Cornea, retina, optic nerve
Central scotoma	Optic neuritis, retina
Superior temporal field in contralateral eye	Optic nerve adjacent to chiasm
Altitudinal field defect	Infarction, retina, optic nerve, glaucoma, retinal detachment
Bitemporal field defects	Chiasm
Homonymous field defects	Posterior to chiasm
Superior quadrantanopia	Temporal lobe
Inferior quadrantanopia	Parietal lobe
Hallucinations	
Unformed	Occipital
Formed	Temporal

Visual Fields

When a specific loss of vision is limited to one eye, the responsible lesion must be situated somewhere between the cornea and the optic chiasm. Central scotomas (areas of depressed vision located at the patient's point of fixation) are most characteristic of optic neuritis, but they also occur in diseases of the retina. Lesions of the optic nerve *adjacent* to the chiasm may produce a central scotoma or blindness in the *ipsilateral eye* and a *superior temporal field defect* in the *contralateral eye*. This occurs because the inferior nasal retinal fibers from each eye dip into the opposite optic nerve after crossing at the anterior angle of the chiasm. Altitudinal field defects (upper or lower) are usually caused by infarction of the retina or optic nerve, glaucoma, or retinal detachment.

Lesions of the chiasm usually produce some degree of *bitemporal field loss*, but these defects are rarely symmetrical. The most common cause of bitemporal field defects is pituitary tumors, in which the defects typically start in the superior temporal fields.

Lesions posterior to the chiasm produce *homonymous field defects* (i.e., the defect is on the same side in both eyes). The closer the lesion is to the occipital pole, the more likely it is for the defect to be congruous (of similar size, shape, and density in both eyes). Even in complete homonymous hemianopias (with splitting of fixation) the visual acuity is normal. Superior quadrantanopias are characteristic of temporal lobe lesions, and inferior quadrantanopias are most characteristic of parietal lesions (see Table 60–8).

Disorders Involving the Optic Nerve

Papilledema. Papilledema is swelling of the optic nerve due to increased intracranial pressure. Any condition that produces increased intracranial pressure can produce papilledema. It is most pronounced and occurs earliest with tumors of the posterior fossa, which produce obstructive hydrocephalus and increased intracranial pressure. It is also seen in pseudotumor cerebri, hypertensive encephalopathy, carbon dioxide retention, meningitis, and subarachnoid hemorrhage. Occasionally, it is encountered in Guillain-Barré syndrome, and in other conditions when the spinal fluid protein is markedly elevated.

It is important to differentiate papilledema from pseudopapilledema (nonpathologic disc elevation), which may be secondary to disc drusen (calcific deposits), congenital disc anomalies (hypoplasia, tilting), myelinated nerve fibers, or high hyperopia. Concurrent findings of hemorrhages, cotton wool spots, or congestion of the veins on and around the disc occur in papilledema but usually not in pseudopapilledema. Papilledema must also be distinguished from swelling of the disc due to primary diseases of the optic nerve such as neuritis or optic nerve tumors. Visual acuity is the main feature used in distinguishing between papilledema and disc edema due to optic neuropathies. Patients with optic neuritis or other optic neuropathies have alterations in visual function, whereas acuity remains good in papilledema. Swelling of the optic nerve can also occur in local ocular disorders such as occlusion of the central retinal vein, infarction of the optic nerve, uveitis, and severe ocular hypotony.

Optic Neuritis. Inflammation of the optic nerve may produce edema of the optic disc (papillitis), or the disc may remain normal during the acute phase of the illness (retrobulbar neuritis). Characteristically, there is some impairment of visual acuity and alteration in the visual field. Color perception is often markedly impaired, even in the presence of relatively mild visual loss. In most cases of optic neuritis, vision decreases rapidly, with the deficit becoming maximal within days. Later, the disc becomes atrophic. The prognosis for recovery of vision is good after a single episode, and the patient is usually left with a sector of atrophy of the optic nerve head (temporal pallor). Optic neuritis occurs in individuals who are otherwise healthy and also in individuals with multiple sclerosis. Less commonly, it may be seen in association with collagen vascular disease, sarcoidosis, syphilis, and inflammatory bowel disease. Involvement of the optic nerve probably occurs at some time in most patients with multiple sclerosis, if one can extrapolate from autopsy data and from series of patients investigated by electrophysiologic tests (the visual evoked potential). About 15 per cent of all cases of multiple sclerosis begin with an attack of optic neuritis, but the subsequent signs of multiple sclerosis may not appear for years. Greater than 50 per cent of patients with apparently uncomplicated optic neuritis eventually develop other symptoms and signs of multiple sclerosis if followed long enough. The rate of decline of vision is one of the best means of differentiating optic nerve inflammation, ischemic optic neuropathy, and compressive neuropathy.

Anterior Ischemic Optic Neuropathy. Occlusion of the nutrient vessels of the optic nerve may produce infarction with sudden loss of vision. Anterior ischemic optic neuropathy usually occurs in middle or old age. Swelling of the optic nerve is present at the time of visual loss and most commonly, there is an altitudinal (upper or lower) defect in the visual field. In most cases, the cause is unclear, but there is a high correlation with a history of hypertension. Temporal arteritis should be suspected whenever an individual over the age of 50 develops an acute optic neuropathy. The erythrocyte sedimentation rate is usually but not always elevated, and a biopsy of the temporal artery often shows the characteristic inflammatory lesion. The nonvisual symptoms of temporal arteritis, such as headache, jaw claudication, polymyalgia, malaise, and fever, may be absent or unrecognized. Patients with anterior ischemic optic neuropathy in whom temporal arteritis is suspected should receive daily systemic corticosteroid therapy until the biopsy has been examined. In the case of a positive biopsy, therapy should be continued and the patient's corticosteroid dosage titrated against the erythrocyte sedimentation rate and symptoms. It should be remembered that arteritis affects many blood vessels in the body and a negative biopsy does not rule out the possibility of arteritis elsewhere, including the optic vasonervorum. Recovery of vision in either arteritic or nonarteritic anterior ischemic optic neuropathy is rare.

Compressive Optic Neuropathy. Some patients with a history of slowly progressive visual loss who originally are thought to have optic neuritis are ultimately found to have compression of the optic nerve or chiasm by a neoplasm or aneurysm. Pituitary adenoma, craniopharyngioma, internal carotid aneurysm, glioma, ectopic pinealoma, and meningioma are the most important lesions in this regard. Dysthyroid ophthalmopathy may also cause compressive optic neuropathy, although proptosis and strabismus are more common findings.

Hereditary and Toxic Optic Neuropathies. Dominantly inherited optic atrophy (Kjer's) is associated with mild to moderate visual loss, bilateral central or centrocecal scotomas, and temporal pallor of the optic nerve head. Leber's hereditary optic atrophy typically appears in late adolescent males with sudden visual loss in one eye, followed by involvement of the fellow eye within days to months. The degree of visual loss is usually greater than that seen in dominantly inherited optic atrophy. Occasional cases are reported in females, and inheritance is probably maternal. Tobacco-alcohol amblyopia is an optic neuropathy of moderate severity with central or centrocecal scotomas and temporal pallor. Previously considered secondary to possible toxic effects of ethanol or nicotine, it is likely secondary to chronic nutritional deprivation. There are numerous medications that cause toxic optic neuropathies, such as isoniazid, ethambutol, chlorpropamide, chloramphenicol, penicillamine, and amiodarone. In addition, a number of chemicals may cause optic neuropathy through industrial exposure or environmental contamination, including benzene derivatives, carbon tetrachloride, lead, and methanol.

Disturbances of Pupil Motility and Defects in Accommodation

Accommodation. Accommodation is the process by which the eye refocuses from distant to near objects. Any lesion that damages the third nerve can produce paralysis of accommodation together with pupillary dilatation, ptosis, and ophthalmoplegia. Failure to accommodate results in the sensation of blurred vision. In *Adie's syndrome*, defects in accommodation occur together with a large, sluggish pupil. Paralysis of accommodation may be seen as an isolated finding in diphtheria, and also as part of the characteristic neuro-ophthalmic picture of botulism and iatrogenic effects of anticholinergic medications including antiparkinsonism and antidepressant types.

Pupil Size. With unilateral blindness, patients do not have a direct pupillary response to light but retain an intact consensual reaction. It should be noted that loss of vision in one eye does not produce unequal pupils. The presence of a normal pupillary response to light in a totally blind patient indicates a cortical (or geniculocalcarine) origin for the blindness. Hysteria and malingering must be ruled out in such cases.

Mydriasis. A fixed *dilated pupil* (mydriasis) may accompany any lesion of the third cranial nerve, but it is seen most characteristically with aneurysms and shifts in the cranial contents. In cases of subdural hematoma with pressure on the third nerve, the abnormal pupil is usually on the side of the lesion. In perplexing cases of fixed, dilated pupils without other evidence of disease of the nervous system, one should consider the possibility that the patients are instilling a mydriatic agent into their own eyes or that they have had accidental contact with such a drug. Blunt trauma to the globe may also produce a fixed dilated pupil; often after a period of weeks there is recovery from such traumatic mydriasis, but in some cases it can be permanent. Acute angle closure glaucoma is an important ocular cause of a dilated sluggish pupil.

Miosis. A small pupil (miosis) occurs in Horner's syndrome. Pontine hemorrhages produce bilateral fixed miosis. Iritis is an important ocular cause of a small pupil. Pupils fixed in the midposition are seen in Parinaud's syndrome (see below) and in combined sympathetic and parasympathetic denervation of the globe. The Argyll Robertson pupil is small and does not react to light but does react on near vision. The condition is usually bilateral, but the two pupils may be unequal. Classic Argyll Robertson pupils are usually due to syphilis of the central nervous system, but similar pupillary abnormalities can result from diabetes, trauma, or herpes zoster.

Disorders of Ocular Motility

Diplopia. Diplopia (double vision) generally results from a weakness of the eye muscles supplied by the third, fourth, or sixth cranial nerve. Misalignment of the visual axes produces two images separated horizontally, vertically, or obliquely; the patient can eliminate one of the images by closing either eye. Double (or multiple) vision that is seen with only one eye is rarely of neurologic origin. *Sudden* onset of diplopia is usually due to lesions of the third, fourth, or sixth cranial nerve or nucleus, often associated with other brain stem deficits.

Third nerve palsies (oculomotor) include those with a dilated pupil and those with a normal (spared) pupil. Sudden paralysis of the muscles innervated by the third nerve *with* involvement of the pupil is the characteristic neuro-ophthalmic sign of an aneurysm at or near the junction of the internal carotid artery and posterior communicating artery. Headache is not necessarily present. A patient with a sudden isolated third nerve paralysis with involvement of the pupil should be expeditiously hospitalized. Computerized axial tomographic scanning and arteriography are usually required to appropriately evaluate the problem. Ischemia often associated with diabetes mellitus causes third nerve palsies, but the pupils are characteristically spared. Diabetic oculomotor palsies may also be painful. Patients with diabetes mellitus who develop a pupil-sparing third nerve palsy should not be subjected to invasive studies. The ophthalmoplegia generally resolves within 3 months without specific treatment. Third nerve palsies also occur from herpes zoster, temporal arteritis, migraine syndromes, and sinus mucoceles. Intramedullary lesions of the midbrain may also cause third nerve palsies. Sudden painless third nerve palsy with contralateral hemiplegia or tremor indicates infarction of the midbrain on the side of the ophthalmoplegia. Transtentorial herniation of the brain from brain swelling, expansion of the intracranial masses, or blood clots can produce a third nerve palsy with early involvement of the pupil. Slowly evolving third nerve palsies are seen in basal tumors, granulomas, and infiltrating neoplasms of the midbrain.

Isolated *sixth nerve palsies* (abducens) can occur

from diabetes (ischemic), intracavernous (infraclinoid) aneurysms of the internal carotid artery, basal tumors (especially metastatic lesions, tumors extending from the nasopharynx, cordomas, and meningiomas), herpes zoster, temporal arteritis, spontaneous dural arteriovenous fistulas, and increased intracranial pressure. Abducens neuropathies occurring in patients with increased intracranial pressure are usually due to compression. Sudden lateral rectus muscle paresis with ipsilateral facial paralysis indicates infarction of the pontine tegmentum. Progressive ophthalmoplegia and facial paralysis occur with pontine gliomas.

Fourth nerve palsies (trochlear) are rarer than third or sixth nerve palsies and are most commonly due to trauma. The trauma is either directly to the orbit or to the vertex of the head. The trochlear nerve is then contused by the anterior medullary velum. Other causes are ischemia, tumor (intramedullary or extramedullary), and mesencephalic infarcts.

Combinations of eye muscle palsies may occur with orbital masses, inflammations, or infections; infraclinoid (intracavernous) aneurysms; basal tumors; carotid-cavernous fistulas; cavernous sinus tumors; granulomas of the carotid or inflammations; basilar meningitis; herpes zoster; and brainstem infarcts or tumors. Patients with thiamine deficiency (particularly alcoholics) may develop *Wernicke's encephalopathy,* a disease characterized by the rapid development of ophthalmoplegia in a setting of nystagmus, ataxia, and Korsakoff's psychosis. The ophthalmoplegia generally responds within hours to parenteral thiamine therapy. The nystagmus is apt to be resistant to treatment. It is important to diagnose and treat it with parenteral thiamine without delay. Sudden painful ophthalmoplegia, often with headache and visual loss, can be an indication of infarction of a pituitary adenoma. Painful ophthalmoplegia, associated with periorbital edema, malaise, myalgia, and fever, occurs in some patients with trichinosis. One should be particularly alerted when fever, malaise, and ophthalmoplegia occur in a diabetic. Diabetics are particularly susceptible to orbital cellulitis due to *Mucor* or related fungi; mucormycotic infections of the orbit are almost uniformly fatal if untreated.

It may be difficult or impossible to distinguish on clinical grounds between infections of the orbit and infections of the cavernous sinus. Both produce pain, proptosis, ophthalmoplegia, fever, malaise, and leukocytosis. Obviously, patients presenting with painful ophthalmoplegia with proptosis and fever require immediate in-hospital evaluation. Ophthalmologic consultation should be obtained, since a sterile orbital cellulitis ("orbital pseudotumor"), which is a steroid-responsive, noninfectious inflammatory disorder, may be difficult to distinguish from infections of the orbit or cavernous sinus.

An important orbital cause of painless diplopia is endocrine exophthalmos or the orbitopathy of *Graves' disease*. This disorder occurs in hyperthyroid, euthyroid, or hypothyroid patients and can involve one or both orbits. Manifestations include progressive exophthalmos, retraction of the upper eyelid, injection and congestion of the conjunctiva, and ophthalmoplegia.

Many patients with *myasthenia gravis* have ophthalmoplegia, with or without ptosis. The ophthalmoplegia generally involves more than one muscle and increases as the day wears on. Even if ptosis is not present spontaneously, it can often be induced by having the patient look up for several minutes. This causes the lid gradually to fall. Usually, weakness of eyelid closure is also present. Administration of a short-acting anticholinesterase agent such as edrophonium hydrochloride may reverse the ophthalmoplegia and ptosis, thus establishing the diagnosis. Unfortunately, false-negative reactions may occur. Myasthenia gravis should be considered in the differential diagnosis of all cases of ptosis or ophthalmoplegia in which there is no pupillary involvement.

Lesions of the *medial longitudinal fasciculi,* the small paired tract in the brainstem that integrates the vestibular and ocular motor systems, produce a characteristic disturbance of ocular motility called *internuclear ophthalmoplegia.* Patients with internuclear ophthalmoplegia have midpositioned eyes when they look directly ahead. However, when they gaze to the side opposite the lesion, the ipsilateral eye fails to adduct. The contralateral eye abducts but has coarse, horizontal nystagmus. Both medial rectus muscles contract normally when the patient is asked to converge. Bilateral internuclear ophthalmoplegia is most commonly seen in patients with multiple sclerosis, and it is the most characteristic disturbance of ocular motility in that disease. Unilateral cases are most often due to vascular disease, especially in older patients.

Skew deviation is an acquired vertical deviation in which one eye is higher than the other, usually in all fields of gaze. Sometimes it is difficult to differentiate skew deviation from paralysis of an eye muscle due to a lesion of the lower motor neuron. Skew deviation indicates disease in the cerebellum or brainstem and is the only important *supranuclear* cause of diplopia. Multiple sclerosis, infarctions, and neoplasms of the brainstem or cerebellum are the most common causes.

Gaze Disturbances. The inability of both eyes to look synchronously in a particular direction is termed gaze palsy. The centers for horizontal gaze in the cerebral hemispheres can be damaged by vascular, traumatic, neoplastic, infectious, and inflammatory lesions, and they may discharge as a facet of a focal seizure. In the acute stages of damage to these centers, the eyes remain deviated to the same side as the lesions, and the patient is unable to look in the opposite direction. Gaze palsies due to hemispheric lesions are usually transient, even when the lesion is fixed. Gaze palsies due to pontine lesions impair the patient's ability to look to the side of the lesion, and they tend to be persistent if the lesion is static. Gaze paralysis due to pontine disease is encountered in multiple sclerosis, Wernicke's encephalopathy, tumors, and infarctions.

Vertical gaze is mediated in the pretectum. Lesions of the rostral mesencephalon and the posterior portion of the third ventricle characteristically affect vertical gaze. Impaired *upward gaze* combined with fixed pupils, known as *Parinaud's syndrome*, is often associated with pineal tumors invading adjacent structures but also occurs in vascular and demyelinating lesions of the rostral midbrain. Parkinson's disease and Huntington's chorea are associated with problems of upward gaze. In some cases of postencephalitic parkinsonism and in phenothiazine-induced extrapyramidal syndromes, transient uncontrollable upward deviation of the eyes (oculogyric crises) occurs.

In a disease called *progressive supranuclear palsy*, there is sometimes selective or predominant involvement of *downward gaze* early in the course of the illness. Later, all vertical movements are affected. The impairment of gaze can be overcome by such reflex maneuvers as the doll's eye phenomenon (passively turning the patient's head and inducing an adversive eye movement) or by instilling ice water into the ear canals. Downward gaze paralysis may also be a prominent feature in patients with Huntington's chorea.

Nystagmus. Nystagmus refers to rhythmic alternating movements of the eyes that can occur under both physiologic and pathologic circumstances. It may have either a distinct rapid and a distinct slow component (jerk type) or no distinct rapid and slow phases (pendular type). Nystagmus can be induced in normal individuals by stimulation of the semicircular canals (labyrinths), either by rotation of the patient (as in Bárány's test) or by irrigation of the external auditory canal with cold or hot water (caloric test). Vestibular nystagmus was discussed earlier in the section on dizziness.

Another form of physiologic nystagmus is *opticokinetic nystagmus,* which is induced by having the patient look at a repeating pattern (e.g., stripes) passed in a horizontal or vertical direction in front of his eyes. The patient develops nystagmus with a slow component in the direction toward which the stimulus is being moved, followed by a fast corrective movement back toward the midline. Defects in opticokinetic nystagmus are typically encountered in lesions of the posterior half of the cerebral hemisphere, especially of the parietal lobe. A diminished or absent response is noted when the target is rotated toward the side of the lesion.

Congenital nystagmus may occur as a motor abnormality unaccompanied by any other ocular or neurologic defects. This type of nystagmus may take any form except vertical. Nystagmus develops after the loss of central vision in both eyes when it occurs within the first five years of life. Toxic levels of barbiturates and phenytoin (Dilantin) characteristically produce nystagmus, usually gaze-evoked, with horizontal jerk nystagmus on gaze to the side and upbeating nystagmus on upward gaze. Vertical nystagmus occurs with disease in the pons, medulla, or rostral vermis of the cerebellum. Gaze-evoked nystagmus is common in patients with involvement of the brainstem by multiple sclerosis, tumors, or infarction.

Certain forms of nystagmus have great localizing value. Nystagmus that is downbeating is typical of lesions involving the cervicomedullary junction (e.g., Arnold-Chiari malformation). Nystagmus in which the eyes rhythmically converge or retract into the orbit indicates disease of the mesencephalon. Seesaw nystagmus, in which one eye rotates up and in, while the other eye moves down and out, is associated with *chiasmatic* and *suprasellar lesions* (especially craniopharyngiomas). Acquired discordant nystagmus, in which the two eyes move in different directions or in which the nystagmus is of different amplitude in the two eyes, points to disease of the brainstem (Table 60–9).

Table 60–9. LOCALIZING VALUE OF NONVESTIBULAR NYSTAGMUS

Observed Movement	Probable Site of Lesion
Downbeating	Cervicomedullary junction (Arnold-Chiari malformation)
Convergent or retractory	Mesencephalon
Seesaw	Chiasmatic, suprasellar
Discordant (acquired)	Brainstem

Behavioral Disturbances

Sanford Auerbach

Neurologic disease is often manifested by a disturbance in behavior. At times, these changes in behavior are quite apparent, such as clear alterations in consciousness, language, or personality. These changes may also be quite subtle and apparent only after a close examination. On some occasions, a behavioral disturbance may be recognized but not easily distinguished from a psychiatric disturbance. Therefore, it is critical for the clinician to develop an approach to these problems, to be able to first recognize and then initiate the first steps into an analysis of these problems.

The following approach to the mental status examination may serve as a guide in the identification of symptom complexes and the formulation of specific plans for diagnostic evaluation and therapeutic intervention (Table 60–10). This approach emphasizes an assessment of (1) consciousness and attention; (2) language; (3) spatial organization; (4) memory; (5) general intellectual function; and (6) personality.

One must always keep in mind the great variability in any patient population. Premorbid variability may be due to the influence of educational background, age, and socioeconomic factors. In addition, individual differences in cerebral organization may result in a variable presentation of pathologic states.

Confusional State and Disorders of Consciousness

In clinical terms, *consciousness* refers to the state of the individual's awareness of self and environment. It is best considered in terms of its components, *arousal* and *attention*. Levels of arousal are described by assessing the level of wakefulness and the stimulus required to elicit a response. A comatose patient is totally unarousable; an alert patient responds to normal stimuli. Several terms have been introduced to describe altered states of arousal; but rather than trying to label the level, it is better for the clinician to note the nature of the stimulus required (normal voice, loud voice, pinching, painful stimulation, and so on) and the response elicited (verbalization, groaning, movement, and so on). The anatomic and physiologic correlates of arousal and attention are complex, but a useful simplification is possible. Arousal and attention depend on the integrity of physiologic mechanisms that take their origin in the reticular formation and other structures that lie in the upper brainstem, extending from the middle pons to the hypothalamus. Pharmacologically, this system is largely influenced by central acetylcholine and monoamine systems. It follows that disorders of general attention or arousal can result from structural or metabolic lesions involving the paramedian brainstem tegmentum, diencephalon, or cerebral hemispheres. Table 60–11 lists useful diagnostic procedures for evaluating acute confusional states.

A minimum degree of alertness is necessary for the ability to attend. *Attentional* disorders refer to an inability to maintain concentration. Patients with altered states of alertness are unable to attend fully to the examiner's questions. However, disorders of attention may also be found in patients who are fully alert. These disorders are of three types: (1) general inattention to all stimuli; (2) sensory inattention to stimuli of a specific modality (visual, tactile, auditory); and (3) hemi-inattention or inattention to one side of space.

A *general deficit of attention* can usually be suspected in patients who cannot maintain the usual level of concentration expected during the taking of the medical history. These difficulties result from failure (1) to initiate the focusing of attention, (2) to sustain attention (vigilance), (3) to shift concentration appropriately, (4) to suppress inappropriate distractions (response inhibition), and (5) to manipulate concentration and attention at an appropriate rate. Tests of digit span can be used to quantify parts of

Table 60–10. ESSENTIALS OF NEUROBEHAVIORAL ASSESSMENT

Consciousness
Arousal
Attention
Language
Spatial organization
Memory
General intellectual function
Personality

Table 60–11. DIAGNOSTIC PROCEDURES USED TO STUDY CONFUSIONAL STATES

Correlate data from history and physical examination.
Obtain laboratory screens for toxic-metabolic-infectious disorders.
Obtain electroencephalogram to help document toxic-metabolic disorders, lesions, focal lesions.
Perform cerebrospinal fluid analysis to evaluate for infection.
Perform computerized tomography scan to determine the existence of intracerebral or extracerebral intracranial lesions.

these functions (mostly vigilance), but other tests of mental control function are needed to generate a more complete picture. Asking the patient to spell words backwards, to recite the months of the year in reverse order, or to serially subtract by seven starting from 100 are examples of tests that are considered to be helpful. A general deficit of attention may be mild or severe. When it interferes with daily function, it may be referred to as a *confusional state.*

In *sensory-specific inattention,* certain pathways from thalamus to cortex are usually involved. In the case of inattention for external space in one field (hemispatial), connections to the inferior parietal lobule have been implicated in addition to the frontal lobes. Unlike with the general disorders of attention, the presence of sensory-specific attentional disorders usually suggests a structural lesion, e.g., stroke, tumor, and so on.

Language Syndromes

Aphasia. Aphasia is an acquired disorder of the linguistic aspects of language. Aphasic classification is based on the identification of disorders in language production (speech, writing) and language comprehension (auditory comprehension, reading) (Table 60–12). When this is combined with the assessment of the ability to repeat and name, a classification system emerges that aids in anatomic localization.

The application of this system in anatomic localization can follow certain rules of thumb: (1) Most people have left hemisphere dominance for speech. (2) Nonfluent aphasics have lesions that extend anterior to the central sulcus; fluent aphasics have lesions that extend posterior to the central sulcus. (3) Aphasics with relatively more severe comprehension deficits have lesions posterior to the central sulcus. (4) Aphasics with repetition difficulties have lesions that spare the perisylvian region. (5) All aphasic patients have naming difficulties. When naming is the primary deficit, the term anomic aphasia is used, and the lesion is usually localized in the second temporal gyrus (Table 60–13).

Broca's Aphasia (Expressive Aphasia, Efferent Motor Aphasia, Verbal Aphasia, Motor Aphasia). Patients with Broca's aphasia generally have nonfluent speech output and poor repetition but with relative preservation of comprehension. Nonfluent speech is slow, effortful, agrammatic, and often limited to few content words (telegrammatic). Writing is generally comparable to speech output, and reading comprehension is usually similar to auditory comprehension. A long-lasting Broca's aphasia is invariably associated with a right hemiparesis, affecting the face and right upper extremity most severely.

Wernicke's Aphasia (Receptive Aphasia, Acoustic Aphasia, Syntactic Aphasia). Patients with Wernicke's aphasia have fluent speech output with poor comprehension and poor repetition. Fluent speech is well articulated with phrases of normal length and with normal melody. Output may, however, be contaminated by paraphasic substitutions of words or parts of words. Reading and writing are usually comparable to their other language deficits. Unlike patients with Broca's aphasia, patients with Wernicke's aphasia rarely have a prominent hemiparesis.

Conduction Aphasia (Afferent Motor Aphasia). This type of aphasia is characterized by a prominent deficit in repetition with relatively preserved spontaneous speech and comprehension. Spontaneous speech is fluent, although it is often contaminated by occasional paraphasic substitutions and some word-

Table 60–12. CLASSIFICATION OF APHASIA

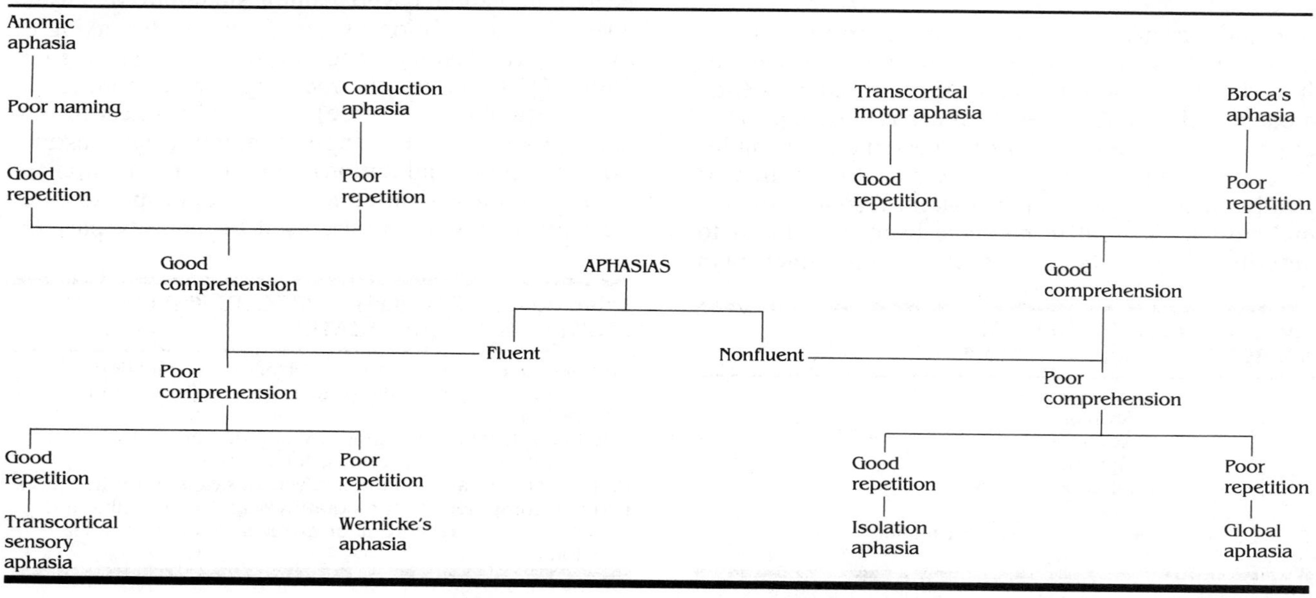

Table 60–13. EXAMINATION OF THE APHASIC PATIENT

Spontaneous speech: Is it fluent (effortless speech with normal melody, rate of production and phrase length)? Or is it nonfluent (slow, labored, hesitant)?
Comprehension: Does the patient understand spoken words? This should be assessed for various categories and at various levels of complexity (objects, body parts, complex ideas).
Repetition: Can the patient repeat words and sentences?
Confrontation Naming: Can the patient name objects when asked?
Reading
Writing

finding difficulty. Comprehension is fairly good in general conversation but may break down on more demanding formal testing. Repetition is markedly impaired. Writing is usually comparable to the level of spontaneous speech. Reading aloud parallels repetition, but reading comprehension parallels auditory comprehension. Significant hemiparesis is rare, but a hemisensory syndrome is not uncommon.

Transcortical Motor Aphasia (Anterior Isolation Syndrome, Dynamic Aphasia). Transcortical aphasia is characterized by a marked reduction in the amount and complexity of spontaneous speech despite retained ability to repeat sentences, to read aloud, and to name objects. Reading comprehension and auditory comprehension are relatively preserved. The relative sparing of repetition abilities distinguishes a transcortical motor aphasia from Broca's aphasia.

Transcortical Sensory Aphasia. This type of aphasia is characterized by impaired auditory comprehension despite preserved repetition and fluent output. Spontaneous speech is fluent but often disrupted by word-finding pauses and occasional paraphasic errors. Reading aloud is possible, but reading comprehension is poor. Writing is usually more affected than spontaneous speech. Hemiparesis or prominent sensory abnormalities are not common.

Anomic Aphasia (Nominal Aphasia, Amnestic Aphasia). Anomia is the inability to generate names in confrontation tasks and in spontaneous speech. As a symptom, it is common to all forms of aphasia. When anomia becomes the predominant feature in an aphasic disorder the term anomic aphasia is used. Auditory and reading comprehension, reading aloud, and repetition are all relatively normal. Spontaneous speech is fluent and marked by a severe word-finding difficulty.

Global Aphasia. In global or total aphasia, all aspects of speech and language are impaired. There is normally an associated hemiparesis and hemisensory deficit. Most patients with a global aphasia secondary to a unilateral lesion retain the ability to communicate nonverbally and to understand a surprising amount of the information contained in conversational language. Unlike patients with more widespread cerebral damage, they usually learn to manage many of the activities of daily living and can become relatively independent.

Isolation Aphasia (Mixed Transcortical Aphasia). In isolation aphasia, meaningful spontaneous speech is scanty or absent and comprehension is severely impaired. The ability to repeat, however, is strikingly spared.

Aphasics often have significant amounts of spontaneous recovery during the first few months after onset. There is also a role for active therapeutic intervention. Current approaches to aphasia therapy emphasize the expansion of preserved abilities and have been shown to be of benefit to many patients.

Aprosodia. Aprosodia is a term used to describe acquired disorders in the nonlinguistic aspects of communication and language. Such patients have difficulties processing the information conveyed in vocal inflections, facial expressions, hand gestures, and the emotional context of speech. Some patients may have difficulties comprehending this information; others have difficulties in producing this information. Aprosodias are associated with lesions of the nondominant hemisphere.

Disorders of Spatial Organization

Patients who have spatial disorganization may not be able to find their way around their home or the hospital; they may present with a particular difficulty in performing common tasks: dressing, eating, using tools, drawing, driving, putting objects together, and so on. These patients may have a disorder in the ability to maintain the appropriate spatial relationship of a set of objects or images—that is to say, a disorder of spatial organization.

The specific presentation depends on the interaction of three factors: (1) The daily activities of the patient: A carpenter, for instance, relies heavily on his ability to arrange objects in an appropriate spatial relationship; a bus driver must keep his bus route in mind. (2) The ability of the patient to recognize the existence of an impairment: Frequently, lesions producing such deficits are associated with the inability to appreciate the existence of a problem or the precise nature of the problem. This combination is not uncommonly seen in patients with lesions of the right hemisphere. The clinician must have a high index of suspicion and, when possible, seek history from friends and family. (3) The specific nature of the disorder: Depending on the acuteness and size of the lesion, disturbances in function vary from patient to patient.

Attentional disorders (general and specific) are of special interest in disorders of spatial organization. Some patients with frontal lobe attentional disorders may seem to fixate on inappropriate stimuli. This results from an inability to maintain attention to the appropriate task and to suppress inappropriate stimuli (see discussion on general attentional disorders). For instance, they may begin a task of drawing a picture of a house, start to draw the roof, and then continue by drawing another roof on top of that, and so on.

Hemi-inattention may often be quite dramatic, and the patient may entirely ignore one side of space. For instance, he may read only one half of a page, copy one half of a figure, eat from one half of his plate. Although this problem occurs with lesions of either hemisphere, it is most common with lesions of the right hemisphere, which result in left-sided hemi-inattention.

Many patients have difficulties referred to as *visuospatial disorders*. They may not be able to organize objects properly in space. For instance, when asked to draw a figure such as a house, the elements (windows, doors, roof, and so on) may be arranged in a haphazard fashion; or when asked to arrange blocks in a simple pattern, they may lose the concept of the overall configuration. These patients usually have right parietal lesions.

We have been discussing components of what could be termed a *right hemisphere syndrome*. It is a syndrome that results from lesions involving right frontal, parietal, and temporal regions. Such patients present with general attentional disorders, hemi-inattention, disorders of topographic memory, and visuospatial disorganization. They are frequently unaware of their disorder, occasionally to the point of denying its very existence. In addition, they frequently display some of the personality changes described.

Management of these disorders is first aimed at identifying the underlying cause and the nature of the specific deficits. It is then important to identify the functional capabilities of the patient and instruct him or her on ways to compensate for deficiencies.

Table 60–14. MEMORY AND AMNESIA

A. Memory
   1. Hypothetical neuropsychologic processes mediating retention
      a. *Short-term memory* refers to immediate retention with rapid decay
      b. *Long-term memory* refers to permanent retention
   2. Clinically derived description relating to time scale of patient's life (relative terms)
      a. *Recent memory*
      b. *Remote memory*
   3. Clinically derived description relating to disorders of memory
      a. *Immediate recall* refers to the ability to recall with total accuracy information that has just been presented
      b. *Ability to learn* refers to new verbal and nonverbal material
      c. *Ability to retrieve* refers to previously learned information

B. Amnesia: An impairment of memory secondary to cerebral malfunction
   1. *Anterograde amnesia* refers to an inability to learn new material after the time of brain injury
   2. *Retrograde amnesia* refers to an inability to recall previously learned material
   3. *Confabulation* is the production of a fabricated statement
      a. Momentary confabulations (embarrassment) usually involve the placing of a past event in the wrong temporal or spatial context in response to a direct question
      b. Fantastic (productive) confabulations refer to the spontaneous production of false memories that the patient believes to be true

Memory Disorders

Memory refers to the effects of previous perceptual experience on present behavior. Several additional phrases such as short-term and long-term memories or recent and remote memories require definition, and these definitions are included in Table 60–14.

Amnesia is a disorder of memory that is independent of confusion or other cognitive impairments. Amnestic disorders have two components: *anterograde* and *retrograde*. These terms are used to describe disorders in learning new material and retaining old information, respectively. These terms are referable to the time of brain injury and are present in all amnestic patients to some extent.

Some amnestic patients *confabulate;* that is, they produce false statements. Usually, these comments represent past personal events that have been mislocalized in time and space. These confabulations are *momentary* and are produced in response to direct questioning, presumably to avoid embarrassment. For instance, when asked about the events of the previous evening, the patient might describe a sequence of events that occurred months or years prior to the present. This momentary type of confabulation is commonly observed in amnestic patients. The other type is called the *fantastic* type and consists of a spontaneous production of a completely false statement believed to be true by the patient. The second type is uncommon and usually implies frontal lobe pathology in addition to a memory disorder.

The examination for memory disorders begins with the medical history. Occasionally, a patient complains of a memory problem, but usually this is omitted in the discussion of the chief complaint. However, the clinician should be alerted by the patient who is considered a "poor historian." There are many reasons why a patient has difficulty in the formulation of an accurate history, and a memory disorder is one of them. The examination should then follow in a logical manner. First, *alertness* and *attention* must be assessed. If these functions are altered, then the examiner should follow the scheme for assessment of confusional syndromes. Second, the examiner should assess *retrieval* of previously acquired information. This should be done for recently acquired information (recent memory) and then for progressively more remote information. The examiner can start with questions related to events of the day (details of meals, schedules, and so on) or current events (political or athletic or in whatever area the patient has some knowledge) and proceed to past personal and past political, athletic, or cultural information. Most of this information is usually assessed in the general medical history; however, questions must be asked for which there is a reliable data base (i.e., questions for which the examiner can be certain of the correct response). Finally, the examiner can assess the ability of the patient to learn new information. This can be done informally by asking the patient to recall information previously discussed. More formally, the physician can ask the patient to recall a list of three unrelated items after 5 to 10 minutes, being assured that the patient is able to recall the objects immediately. The ultimate objective is to distinguish retrograde and anterograde components. This is most easily done in cases in which there is a discrete time of injury (e.g., head trauma).

The pathologic anatomy for amnestic syndromes has usually included medial temporal structures and medial diencephalic structures. The precise interaction of the components of the medial temporal region (hippocampus, parahippocampal structures), medial diencephalic region (dorsal medial nucleus of the thalamus, mamillary bodies), and connecting pathways (fornices) has not been established. The pharmacology of memory is complex but probably involves interaction of acetylcholine, various monoamine neurotransmitters, and neuropeptides.

Post-traumatic amnesia occurs in association with closed head injury, typically in an injury severe enough to cause a *concussion* (transient alteration or loss of consciousness associated with closed head injury). These patients suffer from both retrograde and anterograde components, although post-traumatic amnesia usually refers to the anterograde component. Usually, the length of the anterograde component exceeds that of the retrograde component. In serious injuries, the retrograde component does not allow the patient to recall events immediately preceding the trauma. Even in very mild concussions in which patients are only dazed, they will not recall the seconds preceding the concussive blow. The retrograde component initially may be quite long but then shortens over time (shrinking retrograde amnesia). Unfortunately, the term post-traumatic amnesia is actually a misnomer. During the anterograde component, these patients are usually confused and have generalized disorders of attention. Technically, these patients are suffering from a post-traumatic *confusional* state rather than an amnestic state.

Korsakoff's syndrome is a complex of clinical features associated with (1) anterograde amnesia, (2) a variable and patchy retrograde amnesia with relative preservation of early memories, and in many cases, (3) confabulation. A syndrome may be associated with a variety of pathologic causes, and Korsakoff's syndrome has been associated with metabolic defects or nutritional deficiencies (in particular, of the B-complex vitamins), exogenous toxins, central nervous system infections, trauma, vascular lesions, and surgically induced lesions. Korsakoff's disease or psychosis is the label usually used to describe the alcohol-related syndrome of amnesia.

The term Korsakoff's psychosis is often used to refer to patients with long histories of excessive alcohol use, usually with associated nutritional deficiencies. In many cases, it emerges in patients who initially present with a Wernicke's encephalopathy. *Wernicke's encephalopathy* (note the distinction from Wernicke's aphasia) is associated with thiamine (vitamin B_1) deficiency and indicated by (1) a confusional state, (2) ocular motor dysfunction, and (3) ataxia. A peripheral neuropathy is commonly associated but may be a variable finding. The patient is usually treated with the administration of parenteral thiamine and metabolic correction. As the confusional state begins to clear, the mental status evolves into the confabulatory amnestic state seen in Korsakoff's psychosis. In yet another population of alcoholics, Korsakoff's syndrome seems to develop without apparent episodes of Wernicke's encephalopathy. The clinical features of the memory disorder in the two groups of alcohol-associated Korsakoff's psychosis are identical.

Management of patients with amnestic syndromes involves (1) the *recognition* and *definition* of the memory disorder and any associated disorders, (2) *diagnosis* and *treatment* of the underlying cause, and (3) *direct management* of the amnesia. Therapy usually consists of establishing an environment with appropriate cues available (calendars, clocks, signs, and so on).

Dementia

Dementia has usually been defined by neurologists as a condition representing a deterioration or loss of intellectual function, which includes memory and related cognitive abilities. Unfortunately, variations on this definition are plentiful, and the reader should always take note of which one is being used. Points to be emphasized are the following: (1) dementia refers to a deterioration from a prior state; (2) dementing illnesses may be reversible (e.g., nutritional deficiencies) as well as irreversible; (3) the loss of intellect in dementia is usually poorly defined in most classifications, largely because of the variability across various dementing illnesses; and (4) dementing illnesses may affect patients of all ages.

Dementing illnesses have often been clinically classified on the basis of associated symptoms and underlying causes. This usually results in a long list of disease states that have to be eliminated in a systematic manner. The disease categories cover all possible medical conditions that may affect the brain: degenerative, metabolic, infectious, toxic, endocrinologic, nutritional, traumatic, neoplastic, and vascular. This approach, however, is not always useful to the clinician seeking to assess the symptoms of dementia.

A symptomatic approach considers dementing illness in two main categories: cortical and fronto-limbic (or "subcortical"). A *cortical* dementia implies (1) loss of language function, usually exhibited as a difficulty recalling names and then proceeding to resemble an aphasic syndrome in some ways; (2) a loss of the ability to execute motor tasks on command or spontaneously that can only be explained on the basis of a cognitive deficit (e.g., the patient loses the ability to manipulate utensils for eating despite adequate dexterity and appreciation of what is intended); (3) loss of the ability to grasp the meaning of otherwise well-perceived stimuli; and (4) memory loss. The *fronto-limbic* or subcortical type refers to patients who have the following: (1) slowing of cognitive information; (2) emotional changes; (3) difficulty in manipulating acquired information; and (4) a memory deficit characterized as "forgetting to remember."

The best example of cortical dementia is *Alzheimer's disease.* The onset of this disease can occur anytime from middle age to late life. In patients over 65, the term *senile dementia—Alzheimer type* is in current use. The early symptoms may be mild and are often masked by a relatively preserved personality in a patient who otherwise appears to be free of any neurologic disease. These patients may have difficulties with memory, word finding, and calculation abilities. Slowly they lose the ability to adequately perform their work. The relative preservation of personality and absence of other neurologic stigmata frequently results in the recognition of this disorder only at a more advanced stage. The particular pattern of cognitive deficits may be quite variable and may be dependent on such factors as premorbid functioning, interaction with effects of aging on the brain, interaction with reactive psychiatric changes (particularly depression in earlier stages), and a variability in the disease process, since it may affect different cortical areas at different rates.

Fronto-limbic dementias or subcortical dementias are represented by a wide range of disease states. The most striking feature of this group is slowness in functioning and long latency to respond. This slowness characteristically increases with the increasing difficulty of the task required. The emotional changes can be variable, but as a group these patients frequently appear to be apathetic, having intermittent outbursts of irritability. The difficulty in manipulating acquired information can usually be assessed by noting the patient's ability to handle all of the elements necessary in solving problems. Some patients have difficulties solving problems in arithmetic despite an ability to understand each of the steps required in the solution. Other patients may have particular problems, for example, in organizing the details of how they would change a flat tire. Still others may have particular problems interpreting proverbs in an appropriately abstract manner. These problems are all independent of aphasic difficulties. The memory disorder does not fit the usual pattern of amnestic syndromes described above. With appropriate cues, these patients may indeed demonstrate relatively preserved memory function. The causes of these disorders are diverse and can best be pursued by a search for associated neurologic deficits.

The dementia associated with *normal pressure hydrocephalus* is an example of a reversible form of a subcortical type of dementia. Normal pressure hydrocephalus is the term used by most physicians to refer to patients with large ventricles without apparent obstruction, with normal CSF pressures, and a recognizable clinical syndrome that can be reversed with a shunting procedure. The clinical syndrome consists of a prominent gait disorder, an urgency type of urinary incontinence, and a mild to moderate subcortical type of dementia. Unfortunately, no definitive diagnostic test exists that clearly identifies the shunt-responsive patient. In general, the development of this clinical syndrome over a period of months is sufficient to warrant suspicion. A CT or MRI scan usually shows large ventricles with relatively less cortical atrophy. A cisternogram normally shows ventricular reflux and poor flow over the convexities. Symptoms may improve after the removal of large amounts of cerebrospinal fluid.

Multi-infarct dementia is another form of a subcortical dementia found in patients with multiple subcortical, white and gray matter lacunar infarctions. A history of a step-wise progression of neurologic illnesses together with evidence of multifocal neurologic signs often, but not always, helps distinguish this form of dementia from other types. The MRI scan is most useful in detecting even small infarcts.

Further evaluation of demented patients can include (1) careful medical evaluation for causative factors; (2) a laboratory screen for metabolic disorders; (3) an electroencephalogram to look for evidence of diffuse or focal disease; (4) a cerebrospinal examination for evidence of chronic meningitis, including syphilis in selected cases; and (5) a computed tomography or magnetic resonance imaging scan of the head to document the presence of structural changes. Experimental investigations may include special computerized analyses of the computed tomography or magnetic resonance imaging scan, long latency evoked potentials, and special biochemical analyses. Neuropsychologic evaluation is always useful to document both the degree and the pattern of deficits. Treatment is based on the underlying cause.

Personality Disorders

It is in the realm of personality disorders that the specialties of neurology and psychiatry begin to merge into the field of behavioral neurology. Indeed, as research into the pathophysiology of personality disorders progresses, it seems that brain-behavior relations become ever more important. In general, neurologists are concerned with acquired changes attributable to demonstrable damage to the nervous system.

It is readily accepted that brain damage can influence personality. The task of assessing personality changes and determining the related brain pathology is confounded by three factors:

1. The interaction of premorbid personality and disease. For example, many patients may become depressed as a reaction to physical disease, be it rheumatoid arthritis or a cerebral infarct.

2. Assessment of personality may be impaired by associated neurologic impairments, as in the case of the aphasic who has limited verbal comprehension.

3. Confusion is often generated by the appearance of certain symptom complexes in populations with either psychiatric or neurologic disease. For instance, features of the symptom complex observed in many patients with limbic seizure disorders (temporal lobe epilepsy) are not uncommonly observed in patients with schizophrenia.

There is no standard neurobehavioral approach to the evaluation of personality disorders. There are five major steps, however, that should be considered.

1. The clinician should take notice of the context in which any *change in behavior* has occurred. Psychologically based disorders usually are either chronic or occur within the context of definable situational stresses. One should, therefore, be suspicious of any sudden unexplained changes in personality. In particular, the emergence of a new behavioral disorder in an elderly individual should make the clinician suspicious of an underlying neurologically based cause. Finally, any behavioral change associated with a history of other medical or neurologic disorders should be considered secondary to these medical and neurologic problems until otherwise established.

2. Assessment of the *expression of emotion* requires the differentiation of: (a) A difficulty in emotional control with apparent emotional overflow that is independent of the patient's true mood. Patients with *pseudobulbar palsy* will suddenly begin to cry or laugh with the least amount of provocation. This results from an upper motor neuron lesion of the bulbar musculature and is associated with hyperactive facial and gag reflexes. These patients admit that they have no control over these outbursts of apparent emotion. (b) A difficulty in the translation of emotion into facial expression. These patients cannot adequately produce the expressions associated with happiness, fear, anger, and so on. They will often fail to produce the usual emotional tones in speech. Commonly, this problem is associated with right hemisphere pathology. (c) A difficulty that is reflective of true changes in mood. These changes must be considered independently of the first two elements. For instance, patients with pseudobulbar palsy may also become depressed.

3. The next step is the evaluation of a patient's *ability to comprehend* the information intended in facial expression, vocal intention, or other physical actions. In everyday life, many of our actions and words can carry ambiguous meanings that can be distinguished only by an interpretation of the intended meaning. For instance the statement "I really like this book" can be spoken to convey that the speaker either likes or does not like the book. Similarly, an accurate interpretation of facial expression conveys considerable information in daily communication. Some patients with right hemisphere lesions lose the ability to utilize this information. Not uncommonly they present with behavioral changes related to these difficulties.

4. *Appropriateness of affect* is sometimes difficult to judge and is often confounded by individual reactions to disease. Patients with parietal lobe lesions may initially appear somewhat euphoric or unconcerned about their difficulties. Similarly, patients with frontal lobe lesions may display behavior that is particularly inappropriate when considered in the context of their usual social norms. Patients with frontal lobe disorders may also display considerable emotional variability, with wide swings in mood. Their affect, however, is usually quite shallow. Finally, specific disease states are commonly associated with persistent changes in personality. As described previously, patients with subcortical disease, such as Parkinson's disease, frequently become depressed.

5. The *clinicopathologic correlation* in disorders of emotion and personality can be varied. The preceding discussion has suggested that disease involving the cerebral hemispheres as well as deeper, subcortical structures is involved in these behavioral disorders. Frontal, temporal, and parietal lobes can all be implicated in different changes. Management and treatment of any of these disorders must follow recognition. We urge a high index of suspicion. Once a neurologic disorder is suspected, then appropriate diagnostic evaluations (toxic-metabolic screen, electroencephalogram, cerebrospinal fluid examination, computed tomography or magnetic resonance imaging scan) can be performed.

Cerebral Localization of Specific Syndromes

At this point, it may be useful to look at cerebral localization of function from the point of view of anatomic regions. Each of these points can be discussed within the context of our symptomatic approach. The information here is useful in relationship to the information presented in the section about strokes given later in the chapter.

Frontal Lobes. Lesions of the frontal lobes can result in disorders of attention, of either the generalized or hemi-inattention type. Left frontal lesions are frequently associated with language disorders that vary according to the size and location of the lesion. Elements of Broca's aphasia or a transcortical motor aphasia may be present. A disorder of spatial organization may be present and is usually related to the associated disorder of attention. Disorders of memory are difficult to assess because of attentional disorders, but a subcortical or fronto-limbic type of dementia may develop, marked by slowness, apathy, concreteness, personality changes, and "forgetfulness."

Personality changes are frequently present and may be characterized by disorders in the motor control of emotion (pseudobulbar palsy), especially in bifrontal disease; by difficulty translating emotion into a facial expression, especially in right frontal lesions; by disorders in the comprehension of emotional intention (particularly with right hemisphere disease); and by true disorders of mood. Often, these patients have a shallow affect with elements of euphoria, irritability, and apathy. The precise constellation of signs varies according to lesion size and location.

Parietal Lobes. Unilateral right parietal lobe lesions have been associated with acute confusional syndromes, but lesions of either inferior parietal lobe have been associated with hemi-inattention syndrome. Language disorders are frequently encountered with left parietal lesions. Visuospatial disorders are commonly associated with a right parietal lobe lesion, but the left parietal lobe still plays a role in certain aspects of the details of visuospatial organization. Deficits associated with parietal lobe lesions are frequently encountered in the cortical dementias.

Temporal Lobes. Bilateral temporal lobe lesions, especially those involving medial temporal structures, have been associated with acute confusional syndromes. Left posterior temporal lobe lesions are frequently associated with aphasic difficulties, which vary according to the precise localization. Bilateral lesions of the auditory cortex can result in a deficit in the nonaphasic interpretation of acoustic information (auditory agnosia), which may be most prominent for linguistic information (pure word deafness) or for environmental sounds (auditory sound agnosia or agnosia for environmental sounds). Medial temporal lesions can be associated with an amnestic syndrome, which may be specific for verbal information in left-sided lesions or for spatial organization information in right-sided lesions. Elements of temporal lobe lesions are frequently seen in cortical types of dementias, especially Pick's disease. The relationship of temporal lobe lesions to personality disorders is complex and probably involves limbic connections.

These clinical descriptions are brief and highlight only a few of the commonly observed behavioral disturbances seen with focal hemispheric lesions. However, these descriptions illustrate the value of a symptomatic approach in understanding the importance of brain-behavior relationships in clinical practice.

Epilepsy

Robert G. Feldman
Thomas R. Browne III
David E. Burdette

Epilepsy is a spontaneous, recurrent, stereotypic occurrence. It is a symptom of brain disorders arising from excessive electrical discharging of neurons. In most patients, the cause of epileptic attacks is unknown. In others, after proper observation and tests, a definite explanation may be discovered. A seizure disorder for which no evident cause can be found in the history, in the physical examination, or from special studies is referred to as *primary* or *"idiopathic."* When a seizure appears to be a manifestation of an underlying condition, such as the residua of trauma or the effects of a brain tumor, vascular malformation, intracerebral bleeding, meningitis, encephalitis, hypoglycemia, hypoxia, or withdrawal from drugs or alcohol, it is considered *secondary* or *"symptomatic"* epilepsy. An International Classification System (Table 60–15) of the types of epilepsy encountered clinically is recommended for conventional use. Familiar, older names as well as those from the International Classification are included in this chapter for the purpose of transitional definition from commonly used terms to accepted international nomenclature.

Primary/Idiopathic Epilepsies

GENERALIZED EPILEPSIES

Petit mal "absences," myoclonic seizures, akinetic attacks, and grand mal convulsions are examples of generalized epilepsy, the form of seizure disorder accompanied by loss of consciousness. In *petit mal*

Table 60–15. SUMMARY OF INTERNATIONAL CLASSIFICATION OF EPILEPTIC SEIZURES

I. Partial (Focal, Local) Seizures
  A. Simple partial seizures (consciousness not impaired)
    1. With motor signs
    2. With sensory symptoms
    3. With autonomic symptoms or signs
    4. With psychic symptoms
  B. Complex partial seizures (temporal lobe or psychomotor seizures; consciousness impaired)
    1. Simple partial onset, followed by impairment of consciousness
      a. With simple partial features (A.1–A.4), followed by impaired consciousness
      b. With automatisms
    2. With impairment of consciousness at onset
      a. With impairment of consciousness only
      b. With automatisms
  C. Partial seizures, evolving to secondarily generalized seizures (tonic-clonic, tonic, or clonic)
    1. Simple partial seizures (A), evolving to generalized seizures
    2. Complex partial seizures (B), evolving to generalized seizures
    3. Simple partial seizures, evolving to complex partial seizures, evolving to generalized seizures
II. Generalized Seizures (Convulsive or Nonconvulsive)
  A. Absence (petit mal) seizures
  B. Myoclonic seizures
  C. Clonic seizures
  D. Tonic seizures
  E. Tonic-clonic (grand mal) seizures
  F. Atonic seizures
III. Unclassified Epileptic Seizures (due to incomplete data)

epilepsy, the common feature can be a lapse in attention, an arrest of speech, or only a transitory interruption in thought or comprehension. The attacks consist of absence of awareness lasting 5 to 8 seconds. There are usually no other outward clinical signs or movement. One might easily mistake the blank stare and unresponsiveness in school for "daydreaming" or insolence of a child. Such repeated interruptions interfere with learning unless they are recognized and properly treated. There may simply be sudden head nodding or loss of general muscle tone in atonic and myoclonic seizure types. Loud sounds or bright lights may precipitate myoclonic jerks or akinetic seizures. The electroencephalogram (EEG) in such cases will confirm the diagnosis by revealing bilateral, synchronous, three cycle per second waveforms. This form of generalized, nonfocal seizure disorder usually first appears during childhood and may persist after pubescence. As the patient reaches adolescence, the frequency of absence seizures decreases and EEG shows less active spike and wave discharges during resting interictal recording; provocative tests such as hyperventilation or photic stimulation may be needed to demonstrate the persistence of underlying seizure potentiality.

A *grand mal* convulsion is a form of generalized epilepsy characterized by sudden loss of consciousness and an initial tonic motor phase, in which the patient falls to the ground. There may be vocalizations. The body remains tonic for a few moments with the eyelids and jaws clenched. Trembling of face and limbs follows; increases in amplitude of jerking develop into clonic, irregular shaking of all the extremities. Such tonic-clonic seizures may last for seconds or minutes, accompanied by a loss of sphincter control, hyperventilation, salivation, and sweating. A period of exhaustion follows, lasting from minutes to as long as several hours. The phase of recovery, or *postictal state,* may last for hours with prolonged sleep or stupor.

PARTIAL EPILEPSIES

Simple partial seizures are caused by a local cortical discharge that results in seizure symptoms appropriate to the function of the discharging area of the brain without impairment of consciousness.

Complex partial seizures are caused by a local cortical discharge that does result in impairment of consciousness. Impaired consciousness is defined as the inability to respond normally to exogenous stimuli due to altered awareness or responsiveness.

Simple Partial Seizures. *Focal motor seizures* usually arise in the premotor cortex and cause movements of the contralateral limbs without loss of consciousness. *Jacksonian seizures* are partial seizures consisting of involuntary movements beginning in the hand and spreading to the face, then to the leg; jacksonian seizures may also begin with movements in the foot, and spread up the leg, down the arm, and to the face. This focal type of partial epilepsy may last 20 to 30 seconds without alteration in consciousness. When focal seizures spread to other cortical areas, other movements such as turning of the body are produced, or a generalized convulsion develops. Sometimes following a focal motor seizure, the parts involved may be weakened temporarily in what is known as *postictal paralysis. Focal sensory seizures* are the result of epileptic discharges arising in the sensory cortex. The patient may describe numbness or tingling, coldness, or a sensation of water running over a part of the body. *Special sensory seizures* involving vision, hearing, and equilibrium have been described. Auditory and vertiginous seizures are frequently associated with further spread into temporal lobe structures.

Complex Partial Seizures. The temporal lobe connections with the limbic system, which include the amygdala, hippocampus, thalamus, cingulum, and caudate nucleus, are affected by seizure activity. Seizures affecting these structures lead to disturbed awareness, perception, and memory, as well as impaired interpretation of environmental cues. Seizures that result in semipurposeful behaviors are very difficult to differentiate from behavioral disturbances of psychiatric origin; these have been known as psychomotor or temporal lobe epilepsy. Involvement of deep temporal, pararhinal, and diencephalic structures in psychomotor seizures accounts for both affective disturbance and confusional states with minor alterations in consciousness. There may be additional symptoms that include any combination of cognitive symptoms (deja vu, jamais vu, recall of past events); affective symptoms (fear, anxiety, and occasionally pleasure); psychosensory symptoms (automatisms, i.e., unconscious acts that are "automatic" and for which the patient has no recollection); and spatial disorientation (micropsia, macropsia, and depersonalization). The attack characteristically subsides gradually, with a period of postictal drowsiness or confusion, and often with a distorted memory for the events immediately preceding and following the seizure episode.

Secondary/Symptomatic Epilepsies

Secondary epilepsies are caused by an underlying pathologic condition and are serious symptoms of a process or lesion that must receive primary attention. In the newborn, certain mechanisms that maintain stabilization of the nervous system in the adult are not completely developed. Therefore, immature infants may have seizures associated with structural or metabolic disorders of the brain that would not cause seizures in older children or adults. Some children between the ages of 6 months and 3 years are susceptible to convulsions only at times of fever, but as the threshold for unstable neuronal membrane discharging increases with age, such susceptibility becomes less.

Posttraumatic epilepsy arising from birth trauma results from intracerebral damage from hypoxia of cortical neurons, or it may occur from the effects of intracerebral bleeding and subdural fluid collection. A history of head trauma is obtained in almost one half of all cases of epilepsy, and about 5 to 10 per cent of closed head injuries result in traumatic epilepsy. The initial impact of a severe closed head injury in a child may produce a seizure without serious permanent structural damage or recurrent epilepsy. Injuries that penetrate the skull increase the risk of epilepsy to as high as 50 per cent. Posttraumatic seizures may occur immediately after the injury or even after a lapse of 5 years or more. There is a greater risk of permanent posttraumatic epilepsy in those who have seizures during the first week after injury, suggesting that a cerebral contusion has occurred.

Intracerebral masses, such as tumor or hematoma, produce seizures as a result of changes in the cortical neurons following deprivation of blood supply, distortion of the cortex by the effect of pressure, and edema associated with a mass. As an initial symptom of brain tumor in adults, seizures are reported to occur in 11.3 per cent of patients aged 40 to 49 years, and in 15.4 per cent of those beyond 50 years. Slowly growing tumors, such as meningiomas and oligodendrogliomas, are more likely to cause seizures than more rapidly growing infiltrating ones. Meningiomas, usually located close to the cortex, are associated with seizures in as high as 67 per cent of cases. Tumors located deep in the white matter (gliomas) are likely to produce paralysis or other neurologic symptoms before manifesting themselves as seizures.

Seizures occurring during the first week secondary to a *cerebrovascular infarction* (stroke) are due to acute cerebral ischemic changes and rarely recur following recovery. When they occur months or years after a cerebral infarction they are due to gliosis and tend to recur; therefore, antiepileptic therapy is required indefinitely. Secondary epilepsy results from other primary vascular diseases, including insufficient blood supply to the cerebral cortex due to arteriosclerosis, inflammation of small blood vessels (arteritis), congenital heart disease or cardiac arrhythmias with embolization, or disturbed reflex circulatory control. Epileptic attacks occur during the night in elderly patients, when their blood pressure may fall to a critically low level. Likewise, postural hypotension may induce a seizure associated with syncope. Arteriovenous malformations are often associated with seizures. A cerebral hemorrhage or a cortical infarction due to embolization by thrombi, fat, or air causes acute symptomatic seizures.

Epileptic seizures may also occur as a symptom of *biochemical disturbances* of neuronal function, such as electrolyte imbalances. In such cases, prompt, proper therapy to correct an imbalance will result in full functional recovery. Resolution of the biochemical disturbance should eliminate the cause of the symptomatic seizure. In patients whose epilepsy is caused by other lesions or is idiopathic, electrolyte and other biochemical disturbances may serve as "triggers" of an attack (see under Precipitation of Seizures).

The accumulation of protein breakdown products such as urea, creatinine, and uric acid, and the retention of inorganic and organic acids, including sulfate, result in *renal failure* and acute uremia. The exact mechanism of interference with the function of the nervous system in uremia is not known, but the accumulation of abnormal substances, hypocalcemia, dehydration, acidosis, and hypokalemia may be contributory. Epilepsy that persists after recovery from uremia suggests that irreversible damage to cortical neurons has occurred or that some other underlying lesion exists.

Focal, generalized, or myoclonic seizures may occur in *hepatic encephalopathy*. Stupor and coma are characteristic of the terminal stages of hepatic failure, which is accompanied by an increase in blood ammonia. Cerebral metabolism, either at the level of glutamine synthesis or in the reductive deamination of alpha-ketoglutarate, is affected by increased amounts of blood ammonia. The electroencephalogram reflects increased ammonia by developing generalized slow waves (two to three cycles per second). The cause of the seizures in *hepatic failure* may be an interference of pyridoxal function, the consequent disruption of glutamic acid–gamma-aminobutyric acid pathways, and the resultant decreased cerebral oxygen consumption. Correction of hepatic dysfunction and the fluid-electrolyte imbalance is the best means of treating these seizures; diphenylhydantoin is not effective, and diazepam only masks the problem by depressing the already depressed nervous system.

Endocrine Abnormalities

Adrenal. Adrenal hormone effects on epilepsy and the EEG may be due to a shift of electrolytes or alterations in glucose metabolism. Administration of hydrocortisone to adult epileptics decreased their seizure threshold, in contrast to the antiepileptic effect of ACTH in infants with hypsarrhythmia. Mineralocorticoid effects on seizure frequency result from the attendant electrolyte abnormalities.

Thyroid. Hyperthyroidism and the administration of thyroxine produce acceleration of baseline rhythms on EEG and may produce paroxysmal activity. Epileptics who are in a hyperthyroid state may have a poor response to their anticonvulsant regimen until that imbalance is corrected. Hypothyroidism is associated with seizures as well, but these are usually penultimate to the comatose state in myxedema coma and are not a routine factor to be considered in the poorly controlled epileptic.

Drugs. Drugs that affect the nervous system either as sedatives, tranquilizers, or stimulants can lower seizure threshold. Continued use of relatively high levels of medication for periods of weeks or months followed by abstinence of several days may produce tremulousness, irritability, and often generalized convulsions. Barbiturates, heroin, meperidine, glutethimide, meprobamate, diazepoxide, and alcohol are a few examples of drugs that upon withdrawal may result in seizure. In some individuals, phenothiazines potentiate an underlying seizure tendency but rarely cause seizures of themselves. Stimulants such as amphetamines, pentylenetetrazole (Metrazole), caffeine, and ephedrine also lower the seizure threshold. Common "rum fits" after heavy alcohol intake characteristically begin in individuals who have been chronically intoxicated and then decrease or stop their drinking. The exact mechanism is obscure, but hypomagnesemia and respiratory alkalosis have been suggested as important factors. The EEG pattern is usually normal except in immediate relation to the seizure and often shows heightened sensitivity to photic stimulation (as is true with any drug withdrawal state). Seizures may be precipitated in drinkers unassociated with either alcoholic intoxication or withdrawal from alcohol if there is residual cerebral gliosis produced by previous trauma or hypoxia. Precipitation of seizures in a known epileptic patient by threshold-lowering events is discussed later in this chapter.

Diagnostic Evaluation

It is imperative that an underlying primary cause of a patient's seizures be identified as soon as possible and properly treated, in order that a reversible cerebral disease process not be overlooked and in order to facilitate seizure control. In a patient with a first seizure, the differential diagnosis must include cerebral infection and toxic and metabolic factors. Emergency intervention may be required. Thus, blood for electrolytes, sugar, urea nitrogen, and a toxic chemical and drug screen for sedatives or stimulants must be drawn immediately upon arrival in an emergency room. Examination of cerebrospinal fluid will reveal evidence of subarachnoid hemorrhage, or infection or inflammation such as meningitis or encephalitis. An elevated cerebrospinal fluid protein or xanthochromia will indicate an active process and the possibility of a lesion such as a tumor or subdural hematoma, which would require further neurologic consultation and care.

It is essential that a correct diagnosis be established. If a patient who does not have epilepsy is given the diagnosis label of epilepsy, he or she is unnecessarily subjected to many inconveniences including long-term medication with serious side effects, expensive laboratory tests, loss of driver's license, and possible loss of employment. It is often difficult to stop antiepileptic medication once it has been started for fear of recurrent seizures. Therefore, it is important to be certain before a label is attached.

The best way to diagnose the type of seizure a patient has is to actually observe a seizure. Often the most important differential diagnostic information is history obtained from the patient and/or reliable observers. The physician must elicit the exact details of the aura, ictus, and postictal period of the patient's seizures from observers. The accuracy of such descriptions may be limited by the subjective involvement of a parent, friend, or spouse who is watching the startling event of a convulsion. Videotape monitoring has been used to document clinical seizures. Prolonged observation by videorecording along with ambulatory or telemetered electroencephalographic monitoring may be necessary in some patients in whom the nature of the seizures is unclear. For example, the differential diagnosis of temporal lobe (complex partial) epilepsy from pseudoseizures or hysteria can be greatly aided by video-EEG documentation of the clinical behaviors.

The *electroencephalogram* measures the electrical activity of the brain through the calvarium and scalp by the use of surface electrodes and a very sensitive amplifier system. Artifacts of movement, electrode resistance, and various physiologic phenomena must be recognized and differentiated from the normal brain wave patterns. In a person suspected of having epilepsy, additional waveforms, spikes, and paroxysmal trains of irregular patterns appear intermixed with the background "normal" brain wave pattern. The diagnostic criteria for the various seizure types have been established, and such patterns can be recorded during a seizure or be present during a time of no observable clinical seizures. In fact, the EEG may be abnormal when no seizures are occurring, and may be normal at times even when the patient is known to have epilepsy and may have had abnormal EEG's at other times. Under these circumstances, the EEG study should be repeated in a serial fashion; if necessary, repeat the study after the patient has been kept awake all night. Such sleep deprivation enhances the EEG abnormalities in epilepsy, especially in the complex partial or psychomotor variety. Other special provocative tests may be used in the EEG laboratory, including photic stimulation, hyperventilation, and simultaneous electrocardiographic-electroencephalographic recording.

Radiographic examination of the skull may reveal a fracture line, evidence of long-standing increased intracranial pressure, erosion of the sella turcica, or abnormal calcifications. All these suggest possible conditions that could lead to epilepsy. A small metastatic lesion to the brain may cause a seizure with all neuroradiologic studies normal, but a chest film may reveal the primary neoplasm. Tuberous sclerosis, meningioma, and vascular malformations may show up as calcifications on a skull radiograph. A computerized axial tomogram (CT scan) is indicated in the work-up of a seizure disorder because of its high yield of information about brain tissue content, ventricular size, asymmetries, vascular markings, and possible mass lesions. Arteriograms are useful in documenting abnormal blood vessels (angiomas, arteriovenous malformations) and the blood supply to vascular tremors, which may not be visible on the CT scan. New techniques of imaging using magnetic resonance (MRI) reveal focal, generalized, or vascular processes not visualized on CT scan.

The First Seizure. The occurrence of a generalized convulsion is a frightening experience for the patient's family and for anyone witnessing it. For the patient, loss of consciousness and amnesia for the episode can be devastating to self-image and self-esteem. For this reason, the manner in which the initial attack is handled is important to the future well-being of the patient.

A Single Seizure. An epileptic attack that is symptomatic of high fever, toxic encephalopathy, alcohol withdrawal, or syncope will probably not recur once the primary condition is corrected. In these instances acute circumstances can explain the single seizure. There are otherwise healthy individuals who have a seizure after an all-night party or cramming for exams because of sleep deprivation. The decision to treat or not to treat the initial single seizure is based on (1) detailed information about the circumstances surrounding the event; (2) adequate laboratory data at the time to identify low blood levels of sugar or electrolytes or other toxins; and (3) presence of EEG evidence of epilepsy at least 2 weeks after the seizure. In the absence of confirmatory evidence for a seizure disorder, one would be reluctant to commit a patient to long-term medication, its inconveniences, and potential side effects for prevention of another attack, which might not occur anyway. However, if there is sufficient information to make a diagnosis of epilepsy, adequate therapy must be instituted and continued. Periodic observation and repeat EEG should be done. Often, a single seizure remains as such on medication. In some individuals, medication can be discontinued after a seizure-free period of 5 years or more following a single seizure event. At that time, on no medication and with a normal EEG (best with sleep deprivation stress), the patient may be allowed to go without medication and observed further. Yearly normal EEG's for 3 to 5 more years should help the physician decide that the single seizure was just that and that life-long medication will not be necessary.

The age at which a person has a first seizure may give a clue as to the cause of the condition. A genetic predisposition will reveal itself at any time. During growing years, the underlying tendency for a seizure may be precipitated by threshold-lowering effects of endocrine imbalances and changes associated with pubescence. Likewise, the effects of an early birth trauma, hypoxic event, or infantile febrile illness may not make their appearance as a seizure until adolescence. Vascular malformations are often recognized because of the associated epileptic seizure. Most patients have no clearly identifiable structural abnormality to explain their epileptic tendency, and yet, there may be those in whom a brain tumor must be suspected and may be detected with complete investigation. From 20 to 40 years of age, epilepsy develops most frequently as a result of trauma to the head in which cerebral contusion has occurred. Inflammatory conditions such as vasculitis, meningitis, and neurosyphilis are common causes for seizures that develop in middle age. After cerebrovascular accidents, infarctions may develop a margin of neurons and gliosis that becomes epileptogenic. Prevention of recurrence of seizures is desirable, not only because of its effect on the life style and safety of the patient, but also because there is reason to believe that the longer a person is seizure-free, the better will be the prognosis for future control of seizures. Therefore, identifying the first seizure as a symptom of a primary disorder and institution of appropriate therapy are extremely important.

Therapy

GENERAL APPROACH

Therapy for epilepsy includes certain medications, in appropriate dosages, intended to reduce the frequency and severity of recurrent attacks. To be a successful participant in his or her own therapy program, the epileptic patient must be helped to accept the diagnosis and the various psychological and social ramifications that accompany it. Control of seizures is affected by behavior and attitude of the person with epilepsy as well as the physician directing the therapy.

The willingness of the physician and nurses to be available to answer questions about why a seizure has occurred eventually provides the patient and family with an understanding of the circumstances that can lower seizure threshold—an understanding that can contribute to better control. Managing epilepsy on an expedient or crisis basis is never satisfactory. A continuing patient-doctor relationship must exist in which the physician is committed to help the patient learn ways to reduce, if not eliminate, the frequency and severity of the epileptic attacks. The physician must offer guidance for psychosocial and vocational achievement. An indifference to these matters omits an important aspect of the management of epilepsy. Seizures are controlled by maintaining a balance between those factors that precipitate them and those that prevent them. Avoidance of seizure threshold-lowering events (discussed later) and the addition of medication to raise the threshold make seizures less likely to recur (Fig. 60–2).

DRUG MANAGEMENT

Drug management of the epilepsies requires the selection (Table 60–16) of an effective drug for the particular seizure type; use of the proper dosage to achieve a therapeutic blood level of the specific drug; adjustment of medication to optimal levels for achievement of control with minimal side effects; and choice of alternative or additional drugs if the initial selection fails to stop the seizures or produces untoward effects.

Control of seizures with proper modern prophylactic medication is now almost always assured. It may be necessary to ascertain by gas-liquid chromatography that a therapeutic blood level is achieved by the amount of medicine the patient is taking by mouth. However, the blood level of medication must not be used as the sole criterion for dosages. Both the seizure threshold and the patient's individual susceptibility to particular trigger mechanisms must also be considered.

Prophylactic therapy for generalized seizures requires careful introduction of the proper dose of the appropriate medication. Phenytoin is a very effective drug for preventing recurrent generalized seizures of the generalized (grand mal) type. In recommending an oral dose for an adult, one should take into consideration that different preparations of the same generic drug (e.g., phenytoin) may have different times to peak concentration. Initiation of therapy should be done with *one drug,* preferably phenytoin in doses of 10 to 14 mg. per kg. orally. It is possible to prescribe phenytoin once a day since its half-life is 22 hours. Some patients prefer it twice a day because of gastric irritation when taking 300 mg. or more all at once. A daily intake of 300 to 400 mg. usually provides a therapeutic serum concentration of 15 to 20 micrograms per ml., often reaching steady state after 4 to 5 days. Some patients obtain therapeutic levels with less oral intake than others, and a daily dose of 200 mg. may be sufficient to produce a level of 10 to 20 micrograms per ml. for such patients. There are many epileptic patients who remain completely seizure-free with serum concentrations well below the so-called therapeutic range despite an intake of 300 to 400 mg. per day. In some of these patients, to push the drug dosage higher in order to increase the serum concentration results in toxic side effects. It is absolutely necessary to regulate each patient's medications according to his or her own needs for seizure control and not depend on the serum concentration alone, i.e., to treat the patient, not the blood level.

Absorption from the gastrointestinal system will be affected by the quality of the capsule, changes in pH of the gastric contents, or competition of the drug with other substances for metabolic enzymes. The rates of rise and fall of serum concentration of the drug will be reflected in the quantity distributed to the brain. Because different antiepileptic drugs follow common metabolic pathways, there may be an interference with the eventual serum concentration of the individual drugs when administered together. Enzyme induction is suspected as the mechanism for decreasing serum concentration of the first administered drug, and the inhibition of hepatic metabolism is presumed to be responsible for increases in serum concentration. Therefore, polypharmacy is undesirable. Excretion of drugs is increased when there is renal failure, and in patients with hepatic disease, the rate of inactivation is slowed.

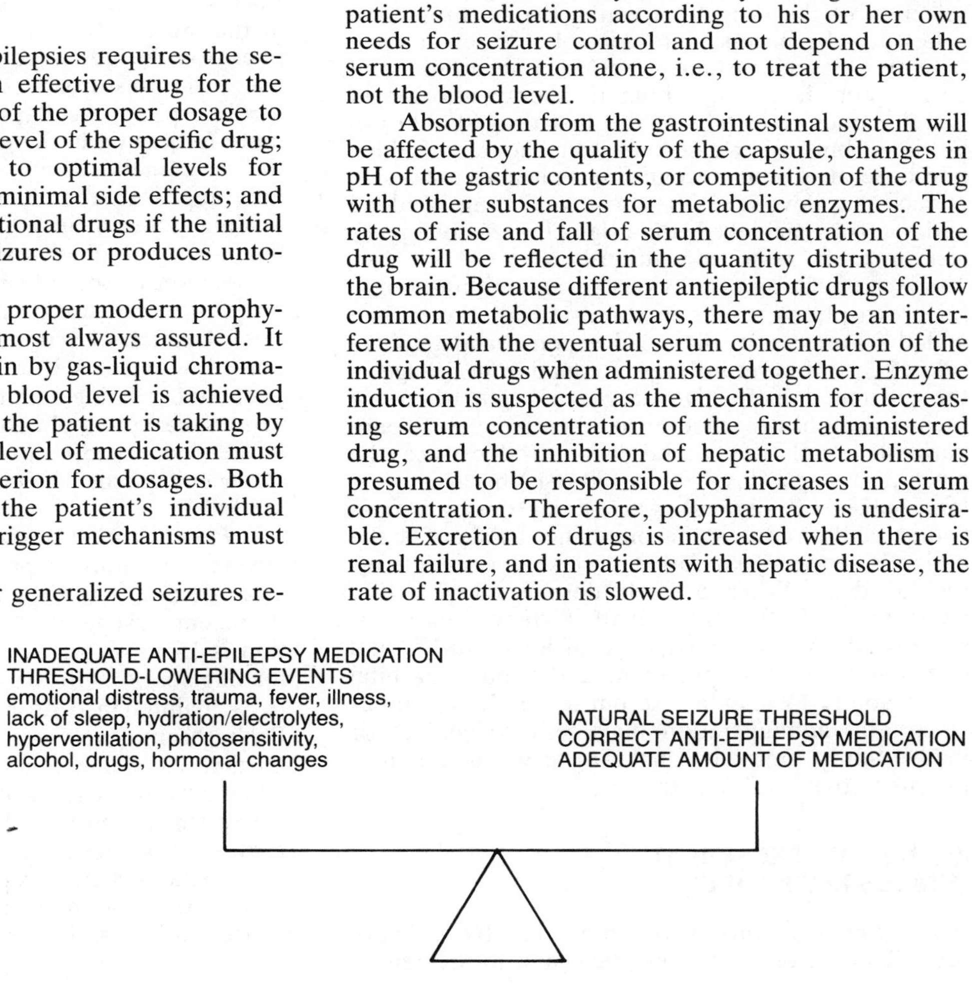

Figure 60–2. Balance between those factors that induce seizures and those that prevent them from occurring.

Table 60–16. ANTIEPILEPTIC DRUGS OF CHOICE

Seizure Type	Drug(s) of First Choice	Alternative Drugs
Simple and complex partial	Phenytoin Carbamazepine	Phenobarbital Primidone
Secondary generalized partial	Phenytoin Carbamazepine Phenobarbital	Primidone
Primary generalized tonic-clonic	Phenytoin Carbamazepine	Phenobarbital* Primidone* Valproic acid*†‡
Absence	Ethosuximide	Valproic acid‡ Clonazepam

*Definitive comparative studies not done; recommended use is based on available non-definitive data.

†Not an FDA-approved indication, unless accompanied by absence seizures.

‡Valproic acid is the drug of choice in patients having both absence and tonic-clonic seizures.

Increases in doses of phenytoin can be made until seizure control and adequate serum concentration are achieved. Toxicity, manifested as nystagmus, ataxia, lethargy, and slurred speech, usually occurs at a level of 18 to 20 micrograms per ml. If the seizures are not controlled despite a therapeutic serum level, reconsideration must be given to the selection of the drug for treating the seizures. Two drugs may be necessary to control seizures in some patients. In such instances, serum concentrations of each agent should be within its therapeutic range. Simultaneous reduction of the first drug should not be done, but rather a second drug should be added one dose at a time, recognizing that additional side effects may develop. When a second drug is added and control is achieved, the original ineffective medication can be removed cautiously.

Accumulation of previously tried and unsuccessful prescriptions results in confusion for the patient and the unnecessary financial expense and additive side effects of several drugs. Reduction in dosage in the presumed ineffective drug can begin when the second drug has reached a therapeutic level. Phenobarbital, usually the second drug introduced, can be given as a single dose (90 to 180 mg.) because of its long half-life (96 hours). Once-a-day dosing is convenient and it reduces noncompliance by avoiding the patient's tendency to forget to take the middle-of-the-day dose. When a single dose is taken before going to sleep, the problem of daytime sedation is eliminated. Another advantage of long half-life and once-a-day dosage of phenytoin and/or phenobarbital is the ability to maintain serum levels despite times when oral administration may be inconvenient or inadvertently omitted. One can "catch up" before the protective level falls too far.

EMERGENCY TREATMENT (STATUS EPILEPTICUS)

Phenytoin (Dilantin) is the most reliable primary drug. To control status epilepticus and to prevent its recurrence, a therapeutic serum concentration must be achieved quickly and maintained effectively. An intravenous loading dose should be given (14 mg. per kg.) followed by maintenance doses of 100 mg. orally or intravenously every 6 to 8 hours to achieve a therapeutic phenytoin serum concentration throughout the first 24 hours after the loading dose. Phenytoin does not depress respiration as much as intravenous doses of diazepam or phenobarbital do, nor does it deeply depress the level of consciousness. When tonic-clonic status epilepticus appears to be refractory, attention must be directed to other possible threshold-lowering factors. Difficulty in achieving control of tonic-clonic status epilepticus should raise concern about the possible presence of a new acute central nervous system process such as meningitis, encephalitis, trauma, or subarachnoid bleeding; metabolic disturbances such as hyponatremia, hypocalcemia, or hypoglycemia; hepatic or renal failure; withdrawal from sedative drugs, including alcohol; or drug intoxication. Sleep deprivation, fever, and noncompliance in taking medications are common precipitants of seizures in people with long-standing epilepsy. Precaution must be taken, when giving phenytoin in emergency situations, to avoid side effects. It should never be given intramuscularly because it is slowly absorbed and precipitates as crystals in the muscle. Serious complications of intravenous phenytoin include hypotension, atrial and ventricular conduction disturbances, ventricular fibrillation, and cardiorespiratory collapse. These complications occur more frequently in the elderly. If the drug is given at the recommended rate of 50 mg. per minute, it will take approximately 20 minutes to administer a full loading dose to an adult. Brain and cerebrospinal fluid levels of phenytoin reach a peak 1 hour after completion of the infusion. Because of this delay of onset of effect, use of an adjunctive drug that has a brief duration of action, such as diazepam, can temporarily control seizures while the loading dose of phenytoin is being administered and absorbed. Intravenous diazepam, phenobarbital, or paraldehyde may be needed to stop an ongoing seizure or to control status epilepticus when a full loading dose of phenytoin fails.

Phenobarbital is given to patients who have had adverse reactions to phenytoin, or who continue to seize despite a full loading dose of phenytoin. The therapeutic range of phenobarbital serum concentration is 15 to 40 micrograms per ml. An intravenous loading dose of 8 to 20 mg. per kg. should be followed by a maintenance dose of 5 mg. per kg. per day. Peak serum levels occur up to 12 hours after an intramuscular injection. Phenobarbital should not be administered intramuscularly for treatment of status epilepticus because of the slow time to peak concentration. In addition, toxic quantities will accumulate if the patient is given repeated injections, and yet the patient will continue to seize until the peak serum concentration and therapeutic level is reached. If seizures do not stop, adjunctive use of diazepam may be necessary, which can cause serious cardiorespiratory depression in the presence of previously administered phenobarbital, since the effects of diazepam and phenobarbital are additive.

Diazepam (Valium) is quickly absorbed and reaches maximal brain concentration 1 minute after the end of an intravenous infusion. The usual adult dosage of intravenous diazepam for status epilepticus is 5 to 10 mg., given over 1 to 2 minutes. Fifty per cent of the serum concentration is metabolized after 20 minutes following intravenous injection, accounting for the failure of diazepam to control serial seizures of status epilepticus when given as the only drug. Intravenous diazepam is most helpful if used when generalized tonic-clonic activity has continued without interruption for 3 to 5 minutes and a patient has received a loading dose of phenytoin that has not yet reached an anticonvulsive effect. The decision to use intravenous diazepam must be given serious consideration because of possible cardiorespiratory depression and hypotension. For this reason other agents, including paraldehyde, may be tried.

Paraldehyde in a dosage of 0.1 to 0.15 mg. per kg. given intravenously or by intramuscular injection deep into the buttocks, 5 ml. at a time in an injection site, may be helpful in controlling status epilepticus. Peak blood levels are reached 20 to 60 minutes after intramuscular injection. The elimination half-life is 3 to 10 hours.

General anesthesia may be necessary in some cases to eliminate seizures. Although the effect wears off after the anesthetic is removed, general anesthesia has value when time to reach peak effect is needed after giving a loading dose of phenytoin. Similarly, total neuromuscular blockade (curarization) can be used to reduce the muscle activity of seizures and reduce the stress of status epilepticus on the heart and the effects of apnea, while waiting for a loading dose to take hold. General anesthesia eliminates the observable movements, making monitoring of seizure activity and recovery difficult.

Antiepileptic Drugs of Choice for Simple Partial, Complex Partial, and Tonic-Clonic Seizures

Simple partial, complex partial, and tonic-clonic seizures are the most common types of seizure disorders in adolescents and adults. Phenytoin (Dilantin), carbamazepine (Tegretol), phenobarbital, and primidone (Mysoline) are the drugs usually employed for treatment (see Table 60–16). Treatment success has been highest with phenytoin and carbamazepine, intermediate with phenobarbital, and lowest with primidone. Double-blind comparisons of phenytoin versus carbamazepine for partial and tonic-clonic seizures have demonstrated no statistically significant difference in efficacy between these two drugs for these seizure types. Thus, phenytoin and carbamazepine are the two most effective drugs for partial and tonic-clonic seizures and have similar efficacy. The choice between phenytoin and carbamazepine for a given patient depends on weighing the advantages and disadvantages of these two drugs other than efficacy (see following).

PHENYTOIN (DILANTIN)

Advantages. (1) Phenytoin is relatively nonsedating; (2) serious toxicity is rare; (3) parenteral administration is possible; (4) a loading dose may be given by the oral or intravenous route; (5) it need be taken only once a day by a majority of adults; and (6) it is relatively inexpensive.

Disadvantages. (1) Phenytoin may cause some sedation and/or impairment of higher intellectual function; (2) there is a relatively high incidence of annoying side effects with chronic administration, including gingival hyperplasia, hirsutism, acne, and coarsening of facial features.

Pharmacokinetics (Table 60–17). Approximately 85 per cent of an orally administered dose of Dilantin, 100 mg. extended-release Kapseals, is absorbed slowly over a period of 24 hours. The rate and extent of absorption for generic phenytoin preparations are highly variable. Intramuscular phenytoin is slowly and erratically absorbed. Phenytoin is 69 to 96 per cent protein-bound and is biotransformed by the liver. Phenytoin has dose-dependent pharmacokinetics with the following consequences: (1) serum concentration increases (or decreases) faster than dosing rate when dosing rate is increased (or decreased); (2) time to reach steady state after change in dosing rate may vary from 5 to 28 days; and (3) serum concentration at one dosing rate does not directly predict serum concentration at another dosing rate.

Usual Dosage. In many adults, 4 to 5 mg. per kg. of Dilantin, 100 mg. Kapseals, may be administered once daily. The daily dose is usually given at bedtime to minimize side effects associated with peak concentration. The following individuals should receive Dilantin Kapseals in at least two divided doses daily: (1) persons who have unacceptable toxic effects associated with peak serum concentration with once-daily administration, (2) children (children have shorter phenytoin elimination half-lives than do adults), and (3) persons who do not obtain complete seizure control with once-daily administration (seizures may occur at time of trough serum concentration). Persons receiving a "prompt release" phenytoin preparation (i.e., not an extended-release preparation) should utilize a dosage regimen of twice daily or three times daily. Phenytoin is available in 30 and 100 mg. capsules and 50 mg. tablets. Note that the only extended-release forms of phenytoin are certain 100 mg. capsules. A syrup for oral dosage and a parenteral form are also available.

Toxicity. Gastric distress occurs with early treat-

Table 60–17. PHARMACOKINETICS OF ANTIEPILEPTIC DRUGS*

Drug	Indications†	Starting Dose (mg. per day)	Maintenance Dose (mg. per day)	Elimination Half-Life (hours)	Time to Steady-State Plasma Concentration (days)	Therapeutic Range of Plasma Concentration (μg. per ml.)
Phenytoin (Dilantin)	T-C, CP	300	300–500	10–34	7–8	10–20
Carbamazepine (Tegretol)	T-C, CP, SP	200	600–1200	14–27	3–4	4–12
Phenobarbital	T-C, CP, SP	90	90–240	46–136	14–21	10–40
Primidone (Mysoline)	T-C, CP, SP	125	750–1500	6–18	4–7	5–12
Ethosuximide (Zarontin)	A	500	500–1500	20–60	7–10	40–120
Valproic acid (Depakene, Depakote)	A	1000	1000–4000	6–15	1–2	40–150
Clonazepam (Clonopin)	A, AT, M	1.5	1.5–20	20–40	—	—

*All values are for adults.
†A, absence; AT, atonic; CP, complex partial; M, myoclonic; SP, simple partial; T-C, tonic-clonic.

ment (can often be alleviated by taking medication with meals).

Dose-related toxic effects include cerebellar signs (ataxia, limb movement, dysarthria, nystagmus); encephalopathy; changes in mental state ranging from dysphoria and mild confusion to coma; choreiform movements; increased seizure frequency.

Idiosyncratic reactions include dermatitis (usually morbilliform and appearing within the first 2 weeks of therapy); agranulocytosis, thrombocytopenia, and aplastic anemia; Stevens-Johnson syndrome; hepatitis; nephritis; lymphoma-like syndrome, thyroiditis; systemic lupus erythematosus; and hyperglycemia.

Other side effects include hirsutism (in an estimated 5 per cent of patients); gingival hyperplasia (can be minimized with careful dental hygiene and avoidance of high serum concentrations); accelerated scar formation; thickening of subcutaneous tissues of face and scalp; Dupuytren's contractures; acne; folic acid, vitamin K, and vitamin D deficiency; low levels of immunoglobulin A; and peripheral neuropathy (usually motor and without clinical manifestations).

Interactions with other antiepileptic drugs are summarized in Table 60–18. The following other drugs may elevate serum phenytoin concentrations: cimetidine, disulfiram, isoniazid, dicumarol, chloramphenicol, methylphenidate, diazepam, sulfamethizole, phenylbutazone, chlorpromazine, chlordiazepoxide, and propoxyphene. Ethanol, phenylbutazone, and salicylates have been reported to lower phenytoin serum concentration. Phenytoin has been reported to lower the levels of the following drugs: digitoxin, dicumarol, metyrapone, dexamethasone, cortisol, contraceptive steroids, 25-hydroxycholecalciferol, and thyroxine.

Intercurrent illnesses affect metabolism of phenytoin. Phenytoin intoxication is not likely in renal disease, but relatively high concentrations of unbound drug are present and may need to be specifically determined at times. There is some risk of phenytoin intoxication in hepatic dysfunction.

CARBAMAZEPINE (TEGRETOL)

Advantages. (1) Carbamazepine definitely causes less sedation and less impairment of higher intellectual function than does phenobarbital or primidone; (2) it probably causes less sedation and impairment of intellectual function than does phenytoin; and (3) it does not have the annoying cosmetic side effects of phenytoin.

Disadvantages. (1) Carbamazepine has been reported to cause serious bone marrow depression and other idiosyncratic reactions in a very small percentage of patients; (2) it may cause diplopia, dizziness, drowsiness, ataxia, or nausea, especially at onset of therapy; (3) parenteral administration is impossible; (4) a loading dose cannot be administered by the oral or intravenous route; (5) it must be given in divided doses; and (6) it is more expensive than alternative drugs.

Pharmacokinetics (see Table 60–17). Approximately 75 to 85 per cent of an orally administered dose of Tegretol 200 mg. tablets is slowly absorbed after oral administration. The bioavailability of generic carbamazepines is usually less than that of Tegretol. Carbamazepine is 70 to 80 per cent protein-bound. Carbamazepine is metabolized by the liver into 32 or more metabolites, some of which (especially epoxide) possess antiepileptic activity. Carbamazepine biotransformation exhibits time-dependent pharmacokinetics (self-induction), which is usually complete within 1 to 2 weeks.

Usual Dosage. Initial adult dosage is 200 mg. twice daily, increased at weekly intervals by adding up to 200 mg. per day, given in three or four daily doses until the best response is obtained. Dosage generally should not exceed 1000 mg. daily in children 12 to 15 years of age, and 1200 mg. daily in patients above 15 years of age. Doses of up to 1600 mg. daily have been used in adults in rare instances. (This exceeds the maximum dose recommended by the manufacturer.) Maintenance dosage is adjusted to the minimum effective level, usually 800 to 1200 mg. daily. Carbamazepine is available as 200 mg. tablets, 100 mg. chewable tablets, and 100 mg. per 5 ml. oral suspension.

Toxicity. Gastric irritability is an effect (usually managed by taking the drug after meals).

Dose-related effects include diplopia or blurred vision; dizziness, drowsiness; ataxia; headache;

Table 60–18. EFFECT OF ADDING A SECOND ANTIEPILEPTIC DRUG ON SERUM CONCENTRATION OF ORIGINAL ANTIEPILEPTIC DRUG

Original Drug	Added Drug	Effect of Added Drug on Serum Concentration of Original Drug
Carbamazepine	Clonazepam	No change
	Phenobarbital	Decrease*
	Phenytoin	Decrease*
	Primidone	Decrease*
Clonazepam	Phenobarbital	Decrease
	Phenytoin	Decrease
	Valproic acid	No change
Ethosuximide	Carbamazepine	Decrease
	Phenobarbital	No change
	Phenytoin	No change
	Primidone	No change
	Valproic acid	Increase or no change
Phenobarbital	Carbamazepine	No change
	Clonazepam	Data uncertain
	Phenytoin	Increase
	Valproic acid	Increase*
Phenytoin	Carbamazepine	Increase*
	Clonazepam	Data uncertain
	Ethosuximide	No change
	Phenobarbital	No change
	Primidone	No change
	Valproic acid	Decrease*
Primidone	Carbamazepine	Increase in derived phenobarbital
	Clonazepam	No change
	Ethosuximide	No change
	Phenytoin	Increase in derived phenobarbital
	Valproic acid	Increase
Valproic acid	Carbamazepine	Decrease*
	Clonazepam	No change
	Ethosuximide	No change
	Phenobarbital	Decrease*
	Phenytoin	Decrease*
	Primidone	Decrease*

*Interactions particularly likely to be encountered in clinical practice.

tremor, dystonia, chorea; depression, irritability; psychosis; convulsions; water retention (inappropriate ADH-like syndrome); congestive heart failure; and cardiac arrhythmias.

Idiosyncratic reactions include anemia, agranulocytosis, leukopenia, thrombocytopenia; hypersensitivity syndrome (dermatitis, eosinophilia, lymphadenopathy, splenomegaly); and cholestatic and hepatocellular jaundice. The rate of fatal idiosyncratic reactions with carbamazepine is estimated currently at 1 in 20,000 to 1 in 1 million patients. Although a matter of concern, this risk is in a range similar to that of other commonly used drugs such as penicillin.

Drug interactions of carbamazepine with other antiepileptic drugs are tabulated in Table 60–18. Propoxyphene, erythromycin, chloramphenicol, and cimetidine may elevate serum carbamazepine concentration. Carbamazepine may accelerate the metabolism of warfarin and tetracycline.

Carbamazepine may precipitate or exacerbate congestive heart failure. Its use should be avoided in this setting or when major arrhythmias are a concern. Serum levels and potential toxicity need to be closely watched if the drug is used in patients with renal or hepatic disease.

GENERIC FORMS OF PHENYTOIN AND CARBAMAZEPINE

In order for a generic antiepileptic drug to be declared "equivalent" to a brandname antiepileptic drug by the FDA, the generic drug must pass certain in vitro dissolution tests and must meet two criteria in comparisons in vivo of brandname drugs versus generic drugs in cross-over studies performed on volunteers. The first in vivo criterion is that mean percentage of difference between brandname and generic drugs should not be more than 20 per cent for values measuring bioavailability (e.g., drug serum concentration, peak drug serum concentration, area under the serum concentration time curve). The second in vivo criterion is that in at least 75 per cent of subjects administered the generic drug, the generic drug has a bioavailability of greater than 75 per cent relative to that of the brandname drug. Note that these two rather loose in vivo criteria would allow a generic antiepileptic drug to be approved as "equivalent" to a brandname drug by the FDA despite its having a bioavailability considerably different from that of the brandname drug in a sizeable percentage of individuals. Switching from a brandname antiepileptic drug to a generic drug of lesser bioavailability may result in a drop in drug serum concentration and a loss of seizure control with resulting loss of driver's license or physical injury. Switching from a brandname antiepileptic drug to a generic drug of greater bioavailability may result in increased drug serum concentration and drug intoxication.

In the authors' opinion, a generic antiepileptic drug should produce a serum concentration that is 90 to 120 per cent of the serum concentration produced by the brandname antiepileptic drug *in all patients* to ensure there will not be problems with breakthrough seizures or antiepileptic drug intoxication at the time of switching from a brandname to a generic drug. None of the generic phenytoin or carbamazepine products currently on the market meet this criterion. Thus, none of the currently marketed generic phenytoin or carbamazepine products can be substituted for a brandname drug without some risk to the patient.

PHENOBARBITAL

Advantages. (1) Serious toxicity is rare; (2) parenteral administration is possible; (3) a loading dose may be given by the oral or intravenous route; (4) phenobarbital is inexpensive; and (5) it need be taken only once a day by a majority of adults.

Disadvantages. (1) It is less effective than phenytoin or carbamazepine, and (2) it causes disabling sedation and/or irritability and/or impairment of higher intellectual function in a high percentage of patients.

Pharmacokinetics (see Table 60–17). Phenobarbital is absorbed slowly (over 6 to 18 hours) but completely from the small intestine. The drug is 40 to 60 per cent protein-bound. Approximately one third of an administered dose of phenobarbital is excreted unchanged in the urine, and two thirds is excreted as metabolites created by hepatic biotransformation. Phenobarbital exhibits linear (non–dose-dependent) pharmacokinetics.

Usual Adult Dosage. The usual dosage is 3 to 5 mg. per kg. per day. Because of phenobarbital's long elimination half-life (approximately 4 days), the drug need be given only once daily (usually at bedtime), unless the toxicity associated with attainment of peak serum concentration causes the patient difficulty. In this case, the drug can be given in two divided doses. The 4-day elimination half-life means that 14 to 21 days are required for attainment of steady-state phenobarbital serum concentration after a change in dosing rate.

Toxicity. Sedation and slowed mentation can occur in relation to dose; ataxia may also occur.

Idiosyncratic reactions include dermatitis; agranulocytosis; aplastic anemia; and hepatitis.

Other side effects include folic acid, vitamin K, and vitamin D deficiency.

Interactions of phenobarbital with other antiepileptic drugs are tabulated in Table 60–18. Folic acid and dicumarol may lower phenobarbital serum concentrations, whereas chloramphenicol may elevate phenobarbital serum concentrations. Phenobarbital may lower serum concentrations of dexamethasone, digitoxin, and chloramphenicol.

The risk of phenobarbital intoxication must be monitored for carefully in patients with renal or hepatic disease.

PRIMIDONE

Advantages. Serious toxicity is rare.

Disadvantages. (1) It is less effective than phenytoin or carbamazepine; (2) there is a very high incidence of toxicity at time of initiation of therapy (nausea, dizziness, ataxia, somnolence); (3) in a high percentage of patients, it causes disabling sedation and/or irritability and/or impairment of higher intellectual function during chronic administration; (4) parenteral administration is impossible; (5) a loading dose cannot be administered by the oral or intravenous route; (6) it is significantly more expensive than phenobarbital; (7) the patient must pay for monitoring of two blood levels (primidone and phenobarbital) each time blood level is checked; and (8) the drug must be given in divided doses.

Pharmacokinetics (see Table 60–17). Primidone is rapidly absorbed from the gastrointestinal tract. Protein binding is minimal. Biotransformation of primidone leads to the formation of two metabolites, phenobarbital and phenylethylmalonamide (PEMA); each has antiepileptic activity, as does primidone per se. The rate of conversion to phenobarbital is enhanced by concurrent use of inducing drugs such as phenytoin. When primidone is given as a monotherapy drug, the derived phenobarbital concentration may be less than the serum concentration of primidone. Concurrent use of inducing drugs will often provide serum concentrations of primidone that are one third those of the metabolically derived phenobarbital. Concurrent use of primidone and phenobarbital should be avoided to prevent phenobarbital toxicity (this is further enhanced if a third drug with metabolic induction qualities is employed).

Usual Adult Dosage. Special care is needed with the initiation of therapy, particularly in patients who are starting drug treatment for the first time. Previous treatment with phenobarbital (which should be discontinued if primidone is to be used) allows a smooth introduction of this drug. The patient should take the initial dose at bedtime, and no more than 125 mg. should be given (50 mg. tablets are available for initiation and it is often best to begin with a dose of this size). Dosage adjustments are made with the goal of attaining serum concentrations no greater than 15 micrograms per ml. (2 hours after ingestion). Primidone is available in 50 mg. and 250 mg. tablets and as a suspension.

Toxicity. Sedation and ataxia are dose-related.

Idiosyncratic reactions include dermatitis, leukopenia and thrombocytopenia, agranulocytosis and aplastic anemia, lymphadenopathy, hepatitis, lupus erythematosus, and personality changes.

The patient should be forewarned about *side effects* such as dizziness, nausea, sedation, and ataxia at the time of initiation of therapy. Rarely, hallucinatory states have also been observed. Thirty per cent of individuals are unable to tolerate this drug and discontinue it during the first three months of administration. Prolonged therapy may be associated with folic acid, vitamin K, and vitamin D deficiency.

Interactions with other antiepileptic drugs are shown in Table 60–18. Isoniazid may inhibit primidone metabolism.

The risk of primidone toxicity is enhanced in instances of renal disease; its effect on hepatic disease is less clear.

VALPROIC ACID (DEPAKENE, DEPAKOTE)

Valproic acid is an expensive and potentially dangerous drug. Valproic acid has not been approved by the FDA for treatment of partial or tonic-clonic seizures unless they are accompanied by absence seizures.

Uncontrolled studies of valproic acid as initial or adjunctive therapy for partial seizures have produced variable results. These studies show that only about 30 per cent of patients with secondary generalized tonic-clonic seizures have good control with valproic acid. Existing medical evidence and medical-legal considerations dictate limited usage of valproic acid for partial seizures or secondary generalized tonic-clonic seizures at the present time. However, uncontrolled studies indicate that valproic acid may possess considerable efficacy for primary generalized tonic-clonic seizures. Valproic acid may be useful as a monotherapy drug for patients with the combination of absence and tonic-clonic seizures. Valproic acid may also be effective monotherapy for myoclonic and tonic-clonic seizures of adolescence.

Other Drugs for Partial and Tonic-Clonic Seizures

Clorazepate dipotassium, phenacemide, mephenytoin, and ethotoin are less consistently effective than are phenytoin, carbamazepine, phenobarbital, and primidone in the treatment of partial or tonic-clonic seizures. However, an occasional patient whose seizures cannot be controlled with the four first-line drugs may respond to clorazepate dipotassium, phenacemide, mephenytoin, or ethotoin. In particular, ethotoin should be considered for patients who have had a good therapeutic response to phenytoin but were forced to discontinue the drug because of toxic effects.

Antiepileptic Drugs of Choice for Absence Seizures

Ethosuximide, valproic acid, and clonazepam are the three drugs used to treat absence seizures (see Table 60–16). These drugs have been shown to have equal efficacy in treatment of absence seizures in definitive, double-blind studies. The selection among these agents is based on weighing advantages and disadvantages, aside from efficacy.

ETHOSUXIMIDE (ZARONTIN)

Advantages and Disadvantages. Ethosuximide is the drug of first choice for patients with only absence seizures because it is extremely effective and most patients experience few or no side effects during chronic administration. Gastrointestinal upset and drowsiness, the common side effects of ethosuximide, tend to occur early in therapy and then diminish as tolerance develops. The drug seldom causes behavioral or cognitive disturbances. About 1 to 7 per cent of patients taking ethosuximide develop leukopenia, which is reversible if detected early.

Pharmacokinetics (see Table 60–17). This drug is readily and almost completely absorbed in the alimentary tract. There is little or no binding to serum proteins. It is transformed in the liver to either a ketone or an alcohol metabolite, which is then excreted with or without glucuronide conjugation.

Usual Adult Dosage. Initial dosage is 500 mg. per day. Dosage thereafter is individualized according to seizure control and serum concentration. Daily dosage may be increased by 250 mg. every 4 to 7 days until seizure control is achieved. Optimal dosage is usually 15 to 30 mg. per kg. per day. Ethosuximide may be administered twice daily unless toxicity associated with peak serum concentration produces unacceptable toxicity, in which case a dosage regimen of three or four times daily should be employed. Ethosuximide is available as a 250 mg. capsule or as a syrup.

Toxicity. Symptoms include gastric irritation; anorexia; nausea and vomiting.

Dose-related signs include drowsiness, dizziness, and headache.

Idiosyncratic occurrences include pancytopenia, agranulocytosis, and aplastic anemia; psychosis; skin rashes; lupus erythematosus; dyskinesia, akinesia, bradykinesia, and parkinsonian changes.

Interactions of ethosuximide with other antiepileptic drugs are summarized in Table 60–18. These interactions rarely cause problems in clinical practice.

Renal and hepatic disorders do not appear to pose major problems for enhanced toxicity of ethosuximide.

VALPROIC ACID (DEPAKENE, DEPAKOTE)

Advantages and Disadvantages. Valproic acid is extremely effective in controlling absence seizures and also has some activity against tonic-clonic seizures. Valproic acid seldom causes leukopenia. Despite the possible advantages of valproic acid, ethosuximide remains the drug of first choice for patients with only absence seizures because (1) the risk of serious fatal hepatotoxic effects as a result of valproic acid administration appears to be greater than the risk of bone marrow depression as a result of ethosuximide administration; (2) the common side effects of valproic acid (gastrointestinal upset, drowsiness, tremor) are more severe and persistent than those of ethosuximide; (3) the longer elimination half-life of ethosuximide allows more constant blood levels with less frequent administration; (4) valproic acid is much more expensive than ethosuximide; (5) valproic acid produces more clinically significant drug interactions with other antiepileptic drugs than does ethosuximide; and (6) the onset of antiabsence effect occurs earlier with ethosuximide than with valproic acid. In patients with both absence and tonic-clonic seizures, valproic acid may be the drug of choice because it has efficacy against tonic-clonic seizures, whereas ethosuximide does not.

Pharmacokinetics (see Table 60–17). Valproic acid is rapidly and completely absorbed after oral administration, with a slight delay in absorption if it is taken after meals. The drug is approximately 90 per cent protein-bound. Protein binding varies with drug serum concentration, and the free fraction increases with increasing serum concentration. Primary metabolism is by hepatic hydroxylation and conjugation with glucuronide; valproate also appears in the bowel and undergoes enterohepatic circulation. Beta and omega oxidation may also take place. Excretion as glucuronide in the urine follows, with minor amounts lost in feces and expired air.

Usual Adult Dosage. Therapy is started at 15 mg. per kg. per day and gradually increased by 5 to 10 mg. per kg. per day every week until therapeutic success is achieved, a maximum dose of 60 mg. per kg. per day is reached, or the serum concentration exceeds 150 micrograms per ml. Valproic acid is available (Depakene) in 250 mg. and 500 mg. tablets and as a syrup; it is also available as enteric-coated divalproex sodium, a stable coordinate compound called Depakote, which is available in 125 mg., 250 mg., and 500 mg. tablets. The absorption of this enteric-coated compound is delayed by about 1 hour, with a peak concentration reached in 3 to 4 hours. Depakene must be administered in three or more divided doses per day; Depakote can usually be administered twice daily and produces fewer gastrointestinal side effects in many patients.

Toxicity. Anorexia, nausea, and indigestion are common early gastrointestinal symptoms, which rarely also include vomiting and diarrhea. These symptoms are reduced with the enteric-coated preparation Depakote.

Dose-related elevations in serum transaminases, tremor, and hyperammonemia are usually transient but could be harbingers of serious hepatic disease.

Hepatic necrosis, thrombocytopenia, pancreatitis, stupor and coma, hair loss, "worsened behaviors," and depression occur in some patients. The risk of hepatic fatality is greatest in children younger than 11 years of age and in persons taking valproic acid in combination with other antiepileptic drugs.

Side effects include weight gain and platelet dysfunction.

Interactions with other antiepileptic drugs are summarized in Table 60–18. Antiepileptic doses of aspirin may displace valproic acid from protein-binding sites and increase valproic acid free fraction threefold. Also, valproic acid metabolism may be inhibited by aspirin.

The use of valproic acid should be avoided in the presence of liver disease. Because of possible effects of valproic acid on hemostasis (thrombocytopenia, platelet dysfunction), persons on valproic acid who are about to undergo surgery should have a thorough hemostatic evaluation.

CLONAZEPAM (CLONOPIN)

Advantages and Disadvantages. Clonazepam is the third drug of choice for absence seizures, because disabling side effects (drowsiness, ataxia, behavior disturbance) and development of tolerance to the antiepileptic effect of the drug are more common with clonazepam than with ethosuximide or valproic acid.

Pharmacokinetics (see Table 60–17). Clonazepam appears to be well absorbed by the alimentary tract. It is 47 per cent protein-bound. Extensive biotransformation takes place, and less than 0.5 per cent is recovered from the urine as clonazepam.

Usual Adult Dosage. The initial dosage is 1.5 mg. per day in three divided doses. An increase of 0.5 to 1 mg. per day is made at 3- to 4-day intervals until seizure control is attained or a maximum dose of 20 mg. per day is reached. A clear correlation between serum clonazepam concentration and seizure control has not been established. Approximately one third of patients receiving clonazepam develop tolerance to the antiepileptic effect of the drug after 1 to 6 months of administration. In some patients the antiepileptic effect of clonazepam can be restored by increasing the dosage. The drug should be withdrawn very slowly to avoid withdrawal seizures. Tablet sizes include 0.5, 1.0, and 2.0 mg.

Toxicity. *Dose-related* symptoms include drowsiness, ataxia, behavioral changes (irritability, depression, psychosis), dysarthria, and diplopia.

Idiosyncratic reactions encountered are skin rash, hair loss, anemia, leukopenia, and thrombocytopenia.

Interactions of clonazepam with other antiepileptic drugs are summarized in Table 60–18. Concurrent use of amphetamines and methylphenidate may cause central nervous system depression and respiratory irregularities. Depressant effects may also be enhanced by alcohol, antianxiety and antipsychotic drugs, antidepressants, and other antiepileptic drugs. In some individuals, concurrent use of valproic acid has been associated with the development of absence seizures.

Renal disease is unlikely to affect the elimination of clonazepam, but the presence of liver disease may require decreased dosage.

Precipitation of Seizures in the Otherwise "Controlled" Patient

Recurrence of seizures in an otherwise "controlled" patient usually follows a reduction in level of anticonvulsant drug in the central nervous system, caused by an inadequate intake of prescribed dosage, by rapid excretion of the drug, or by poor absorption. Whereas the correct amount of an appropriate pharmacologic agent usually serves to prevent recurrence of an attack, in some patients certain other factors have a clear relationship to the clinical precipitation of an epileptic attack. Such "triggers" lower the seizure threshold but are not the primary cause of the epilepsy itself (see Fig. 60–2).

Seizure control can be improved by recognizing the relationship of a number of threshold-lowering events to recurrence of attacks and by using appropriate strategies to reduce their impact on seizure activity. As many as 80 per cent of seizures occur in an apparently fortuitous manner, without evident precipitating cause; the remaining seizures are the result of identifiable threshold-altering and, less commonly, triggering phenomena.

CYCLIC TRIGGERS

Sleep-Wakefulness. The interactions of epilepsy and the sleep-wake cycle are of particular importance. Approximately 25 per cent of persons with epilepsy have seizures predominantly during sleep, whereas 35 to 50 per cent have seizures predominantly while awake. The type of epilepsy determines its occurrence during the sleep-wake cycle. Myoclonic seizures, for example, occur during the early waking period. Grand mal (generalized) and partial seizures are more evenly distributed throughout various states of arousal. Patients with juvenile myoclonic epilepsy are susceptible to seizures when awakened prematurely from sleep, exhibiting a particular sensitivity to sleep deprivation.

Polysomnography in patients having frequent and difficult-to-control seizures may exhibit characteristic changes in sleep architecture. Those with predominantly waking seizures have increased waking after sleep onset (WASO) but normal latencies and amounts of REM and NREM sleep, whereas those with frequent seizures during sleep have a disruption of sleep architecture in a potentially epileptogenic manner. In addition to an increased WASO, seizures cause decreases in the amount of REM and deep NREM sleep and increases in light NREM sleep. Unlike selective REM sleep deprivation, in which a rebound in REM sleep occurs, the decreased REM sleep associated with seizures has no subsequent rebound, thereby implying a more complex relationship. Therapeutic attention to the sleep problem may improve the control of the epilepsy.

Sleep deprivation is a common threshold-lowering event leading to an epileptic attack. The basic mechanisms underlying the effects of sleep deprivation are not known, but roles for relative cortical depolarization, instability of subsequent level of arousal, and impeding of normal reparative functions have been suggested. The use of sleep deprivation in the diagnosis of epilepsy is valuable in bringing out paroxysmal activity in the electroencephalogram. The EEG recording must be made while the patient is awake, but after a full night's sleep deprivation. The avoidance of sleep deprivation is of great importance in seizure control.

Menstruation. Fluctuation in seizure frequency in association with the menstrual cycle occurs in 50 to 80 per cent of women with epilepsy. These women describe a premenstrual exacerbation in seizure frequency. Commonly, this exacerbation is noted at time of ovulation as well as immediately premenstrually and during menstruation; relatively fewer seizures are noted in the midluteal phase. Mechanisms postulated for this cyclic variation include fluid retention, stress, and anticonvulsant concentration variation. Seizure frequency can be related to variations in the ratio of the levels of estrogen to the progesterone level. Animal studies consistently demonstrate an epileptic effect of estrogen and an antiepileptic effect of progesterone. Various pharmacologic treatments, including a trial of acetazolamide administered 5 to 7 days prior to expected menstruation and continued until cessation of menses, have been proposed and used successfully by some. The relative predictability of the seizures should allow modification of activities during times of seizure exacerbation.

Menarche and Menopause. Seizures often appear at menarche. Approximately one third of patients with generalized tonic-clonic or partial seizures had exacerbation of their seizure frequency at menarche, whereas another third remained unchanged, and the final third had fewer seizures. The effects of menopause have not been adequately investigated, although attempts at seizure control by castration were not successful in the past. In general, seizure frequency is reduced after menopause, and control seems easier to achieve on the same drug regimen that was previously less successful.

Pregnancy. Of epileptic women who become pregnant, seizure frequency increases in 25 per cent, decreases in 25 per cent, and remains largely unchanged in 50 per cent. Many potentially exacerbating factors are present, including changes in hormonal balance, fluid balance, and drug metabolism. The most likely cause of seizure exacerbation is the difficulty in maintenance of adequate serum antiepileptic drug levels because of changes in body fluid volume. The potential teratogenicity of anticonvulsant medication must be weighed against the risk of seizure to mother and fetus.

ELECTROLYTE IMBALANCES

Secondary seizures occur as symptoms in pathologic states associated with electrolyte imbalances. Transient changes in electrolyte balance may also serve as triggers of an existing seizure potentiality, which may be secondary to some other cause, or may even be primary or idiopathic. In either situation, correction of the imbalance is necessary.

Sodium. Stability of normal and epileptogenic neurons is based on maintaining ionic equilibrium. Both *hyponatremia* and *hypernatremia* disrupt neuronal membrane stability and lower the epileptic threshold. In animal experiments, a low epileptic threshold is related to a low level of serum sodium and a fall in the ratio of extracellular to intracellular sodium in the brain. *Hyponatremia* may occur as a result of diarrhea, because of excessive sweating, or from increased excretion of sodium in the urine associated with renal disease or diuretics. Loss of sodium may also occur in association with central nervous system diseases such as encephalitis or third ventricle tumors affecting hypothalamic structures. Reduced sodium levels may occur after parenteral administration of hypotonic fluids, acute infections and fever, or acute expansion of extracellular fluid volume from retention of water. Convulsions due to water intoxication and hyponatremia are resistant to anticonvulsant drugs and can be controlled only by correction of the electrolyte imbalance. *Hypernatremic states* may result from central nervous system lesions that cause diabetes insipidus, or from dehydration, sodium retention, or excessive sodium intake. Ironically, too rapid a correction of hypernatremia may lead to seizures as a result of rebound hyponatremia. The risk of seizures due to hyponatremia alone is greatest when the sodium level rapidly falls to less than 120 mEq. per liter.

Hypocalcemia. The calcium ion is integral to normal neuronal function. It functions as a secondary messenger in neurons and plays a critical role in the release of neurotransmitter quanta into the synaptic cleft. When seizures occur in the presence of low serum calcium, they are probably due to the effect of the low concentration of calcium on the permeability of cell membranes to potassium and sodium, with the fall in calcium leading to seizures only indirectly. Conditions resulting in depletion of extracellular calcium cause neuromuscular and neuronal irritability. Low ionic concentration of calcium may occur during treatment of hypernatremic states. Neonatal tetany, hypoparathyroidism, pseudohypoparathyroidism, rickets, steatorrhea, chronic renal disease, and treatment of acidosis with dehydration may all lead to seizures by an initial hypocalcemic effect. Clinical tetany must be differentiated from epileptic phenomena.

Hypomagnesemia. Hypomagnesemia also lowers membrane stability and may be accompanied by secondary seizures. The hypomagnesemic state, like hypocalcemia, is associated with neuromuscular and neuronal irritability. The most common causes include malnutrition, alcoholism, gastrointestinal losses, acute pancreatitis, renal insufficiency, vitamin D intoxication, and hypoparathyroidism.

Hypoglycemia. Hypoglycemia and *hypoxia* cause seizures by depriving the brain of essential materials for oxidative metabolism. In the absence of sufficient glucose, the brain oxidizes other noncarbohydrate substrates, such as lipids and amino acids, but none of these is adequate to maintain normal function for any significant length of time. Hypoglycemia of rapid onset increases risk of seizures. Of the many causes of hypoglycemia that may lead to convulsions, overdoses of drugs such as insulin and tolbutamide are the most common. Excessive alcohol ingestion lowers blood sugar. Hypoglycemia-induced seizures may be associated with hyperinsulinism, with impaired glycogenolysis and glyconeogenesis resulting from hepatic disease, or with lesions of either the anterior lobe of the pituitary or the adrenal cortex. Physiologic hypoglycemia occurring after a large meal may precipitate symptomatic attacks in some individuals who already have a low seizure threshold. Absence seizures (3 hertz spike and wave) are known to be sensitive to hypoglycemia.

Hyperventilation. The direct effect of hyperventilation is to induce hypocapnea, which in turn causes diffuse cerebral vasoconstriction. The mechanism for its epileptogenic effect may involve alkalosis, which causes a reduction in ionic calcium and leads to membrane instability. Some epileptic patients are more sensitive than others to these effects; for example, those with absence seizures are the most susceptible. Hyperventilation produces seizures in almost all untreated absence patients; in those receiving medication there may be seen an enhancement of the 3 hertz spike and wave activity in the EEG without noticeable clinical seizures. When 3 hertz bursts recur for longer than 7 seconds, however, lapses of awareness may be precipitated, or a clinically observable absence attack may be observed. Vigorous hyperventilation causes paroxysmal discharges in 11 per cent of patients with complex partial seizures. Involuntary hyperventilation may occur as the involuntary sequela of sobbing, anxiety, exercise, or sexual activity and may provoke a seizure in those susceptible. Anxiety-induced hyperventilation may require the use of sedative agents. Exercise-induced hyperventilation may occur in the postexercise period. Many reports of exercise-induced epilepsy find that paroxysmal activity on EEG is decreased during exercise and more prevalent immediately following exercise.

HYPERTHERMIA

The effect of hyperthermia to lower the seizure threshold occurs most commonly in infancy and early childhood, although adults may convulse when body temperature is raised quickly to temperatures above 38.8° C (102° F). The pathogenesis of this phenomenon is unclear. Febrile convulsions are seizures that are precipitated by fever alone. It is uncertain whether febrile convulsions predispose individuals toward subsequent seizures or whether they unmask an underlying, pre-existent seizure potentiality.

BEHAVIORAL TRIGGERS

Emotion. Emotional stress is a primary source of exacerbation of seizures in patients with poorly controlled complex partial seizures. The use of behavior modification in such patients is an effective means of decreasing seizure frequency in susceptible patients. The model of stimulus-organism-response (SOR) provides a means of appropriately modifying behavior by providing a conscious awareness of areas of emotional vulnerability that can be triggered by certain cues, changes in the stimulus (S) or the response (R) by a particular person (O). Seizures resulting from a heightened emotional state are a manifestation of dysfunction at the level of the organism (the patient). Behavior modification is directed toward the specific emotional triggers of which the patient may or may not be aware and which predispose that patient to frequent seizures. Modification of the stimulus is required in the treatment of seizures that result from specific triggering mechanisms. The precipitation of an attack by emotional triggers in a patient with epilepsy must be differentiated from a "pseudoseizure" or "hysterical fit" in borderline personality patients who do not actually have epilepsy.

Sensory Precipitants. A subset of seizure disorders exists in which a seizure is the direct sequela of a specific and often well-defined stimulus. These sensory-induced or reflex seizures are believed to occur in at least 5 to 6 per cent of epileptics. They may result from any number of inciting events, most of which may be identified by the sensory type, i.e., visual, auditory, somesthetic, gustatory, or olfactory. Some of the reflex epilepsies appear to be triggered by more complex, associated thought processes, but for simplicity's sake, they will be considered under the sensory stimulus that is primarily involved by that process.

Photosensitive Epilepsy. Those reflex epilepsies in which seizures are the direct result of characteristic retinal stimulation are designated photosensitive. The electroencephalographic correlate of photosensitive epilepsy is the photoconvulsive response. In everyday life, photosensitive epilepsy manifests itself as seizures that occur upon exposure to flickering lights in the environment or upon viewing of characteristic visual patterns such as that of a checkered tablecloth. The most common of these is television epilepsy. The seizures most often described in association with environmental stimuli have been generalized tonic-clonic, with absence, myoclonic, and partial seizures being significantly less common. Much information concerning the epileptogenic characteristics of visual stimuli in photosensitive epilepsy has been obtained through induction of the photoconvulsive response in the EEG laboratory with intermittent photic stimulation and pattern viewing. Characteristics of those patterns most likely to induce seizures include a degree of linearity to the contours within the pattern and its binocular presentation. A patient may self-induce seizures by hand-waving, rapid blinking, or sitting too close to a television set. Attempts to discourage self-induced seizures are difficult because patients often find the seizures pleasurable or relaxing.

Auditory Triggering. Auditory triggering of seizures is exceedingly rare. Seizures precipitated by a simple auditory stimulus are almost exclusively "startle" in nature. The majority are tonic seizures that are induced by a sudden noise; therefore, the term *acousticomotor* is something of a misnomer. The quality of the sound is unimportant; rather, the provocative factor is the "startle."

Musicogenic Epilepsy. Musicogenic epilepsy is more far-reaching than acousticomotor epilepsy, for it is induced both by the hearing of specific musical stimuli and by the inward recalling of the appropriate musical passages. The responsible melodies vary widely in genre, and the seizures tend to be complex partial with the ictal EEG showing paroxysmal discharges over either temporal lobe.

Somatosensory Stimulation. Seizures may be triggered by somatosensory stimulation of a body part. The seizures most often take the form of a tonic, asymmetrical contraction of opposing muscles in the extremity, thereby producing a posturing or athetotic effect. Many of the associated EEG's have minimal or no significant abnormality, but this most likely results from the small size of the focus. As a whole, somatosensory reflex epilepsies respond well to appropriate anticonvulsant therapy, and behavior modification strategies are unneeded.

Gustatory or Eating Epilepsy. Chewing, eating, or drinking may precipitate paroxysmal activity on EEG and clinical myoclonic, absence, and tonic-clonic seizures. Typically, the seizures are complex partial, originating in the temporal lobes, and are characterized by a head drop followed by automatisms and a variable impairment of consciousness. Attempts at isolating a single factor within the act of eating have been largely unsuccessful although occasionally the inciting event is thought to be mastication or gastric distention. It is speculated that the amygdala, the likely focus of masticatory seizures, plays an integral role in the phenomenon of eating epilepsy.

Olfactory Induction. Olfactory induction of seizures is extremely rare. In one study, perfumed air was found to exacerbate temporal lobe spike activity in 16 of 61 patients with temporal lobe epilepsy. These persons may exhibit sudden irritability, mood change, and disturbances in awareness.

Prevention. To minimize the seizure threshold-lowering impact of various conditions, the physician must help the patient identify those endogenous factors and modify them mechanically, and must educate the patient about appropriate behavioral avoidance or manipulation of exogenous factors encountered in daily living.

"Outgrowing" Epilepsy

In a child with epilepsy, the presence of a specific brain lesion, such as congenital cysts, posttraumatic changes, vascular malformations, or tuberous sclerosis, is a definite basis upon which to commit an individual to treatment for a lifetime; when no structural condition is identified, then the prognosis is better. Focal seizures occurring in early life have a more favorable prognosis, but no remissions can be expected when the first seizure occurs after the age of 7 to 9 years. When petit mal type seizures are considered, children may follow one of three courses. One third will have more seizures after puberty; one third continue to have absence seizures of various types; and one third develop grand mal seizures as well.

There are many adults who have what they think is their first seizure but who find when checking with their parents or previous medical records that they had been told that they had outgrown their childhood epilepsy. The prolonged period of being seizure-free may simply be a matter of increasing threshold with increasing age. A person with a history of epilepsy may go through life on no medication whatsoever as long as he or she is not faced with sufficient threshold-lowering factors (see Fig. 60–2) to precipitate an attack at a particular time.

Stopping Medication

Many patients begin to feel confident when their seizures have been controlled for a year or more. Forgetting that it is because of the medication that the seizures are under control, they might miss one dose now and then. If nothing happens, they begin to question the need for as much medicine as they were taking and begin to take one less pill a day. When the serum level falls below the protective level for the patient's personal seizure threshold, an attack will occur. Eighteen months is a frequent time for this to happen, unless the patient is seen and reminded of the need for medication at least every 6 to 10 months. When seizures are well controlled for 5 years or more on medication, the patient must be reminded about the protective nature of the proper dose of the correct medication. The data from a Scandinavian study showed that 30 per cent of such controlled patients will have occurrence of seizures within two years of stopping medication. If no untoward effects develop, prophylactic medication can be relatively inexpensive insurance for maintaining a desired life style.

The expectations of the physician and the patient (and the family) will determine the outcome of the therapy. An optimistic yet realistic attitude has better results than one that accepts recurrent seizures as inevitable. Realistic optimism with a good understanding of seizure threshold and how to keep it elevated is the way to approach treatment of persons with epilepsy.

Understanding by the patient, whether child or adult, and by the patient's family is absolutely essential to the proper management of epilepsy. This requires a clear definition of the patient's capabilities as well as his or her restrictions early in the course of the seizure disorder. The fear that a seizure may come at possibly embarrassing times, such as at a job interview, may itself bring on an attack. In most cases, a child with epilepsy can grow up with a healthy self-image provided the seizures are seriously treated and controlled. The child should not tiptoe through life as a fragile eggshell, but should try to accept the condition, realizing that he or she can be free of seizures if a regimen is strictly maintained that will prevent them.

Admittedly the common emotional reaction to the word "epilepsy" is negative. Epileptic attacks have been a mystery for centuries, and social prejudice and discrimination have long made life difficult for persons with epilepsy. Misconceptions still exist, such as "epileptics have less intelligence than non-epileptics"; "epilepsy is inherited"; "epilepsy is a form of mental illness"; "a common characteristic of epilepsy is a tendency to commit acts of violence"; and so on. Archaic laws applicable to persons with epilepsy remain on the statute books of some states, although improvement has taken place in recent years. Discoveries of effective antiepileptic therapy have brought about some social changes and concomitant increases in job opportunities for persons with epilepsy. In addition, active educational campaigns by organizations concerned with neurology and epilepsy have favorably affected public opinion. However, it is still usually considered a catastrophe when a seizure is experienced by a patient and his or her family. Therefore, careful counseling of both the patient and the family at the earliest opportunity and continuing support are absolutely essential.

Epilepsy and Personality

Evidence suggests that the frequency of emotional disturbance is higher in patients with epilepsy and that increases in stress increase the frequency of seizures. However, the association between a specific personality pattern of disturbance and a specific seizure disorder has yet to be clearly established. A more reasonable view in light of current evidence is that patients with partial complex seizures are more vulnerable to effects of emotional activation because limbic system structures are involved. This involvement has consequences in two ways: (1) control of behavior is more problematic and (2) memory is affected, which in turn influences the way persons cope with the disorder. Because of the retrograde amnesia in these patients, the identification of emotional precipitants is more difficult for them.

Personality patterns in these patients may reflect the role that seizures have played in their lives and the way in which they have been viewed by others, particularly family members. Moreover, patterns within the family may have served to reinforce the patient's status as a "sick" person and such a status perpetuates dependency. The recurrence of seizures reduces self-confidence in a patient whose epilepsy is poorly controlled. He or she is dependent on others during an attack when consciousness is affected. Embarrassment and fear of being rejected by those who witnessed the seizure may follow recovery. Behavior patterns may develop as a result of long-standing, poorly controlled epilepsy. What have been considered unique characteristics of the epileptic personality in cases of temporal lobe epilepsy may simply reflect the person's prolonged accumulation of learned responses to the feeling of having no control over his or her environment.

Parents, teachers, and medical personnel contribute to the patient's view of himself or herself by their behavior and reactions to the patient and the seizures. Parents must be supportive but not overly protective to a point of being suppressive. Teachers and family members must accentuate the abilities of a person with epilepsy rather than the limitations and handicaps. Those who witness seizures often must know how to be helpful both during and after the attack. Through counseling and medical advice, they must be prepared for the possible occurrence of a seizure and must learn to accept the sense of helplessness when it happens. Frustration with failed therapies and interrupted family plans must be met with understanding rather than anger and rejection toward the seizure patient. A thoroughly open program of information and expression of feelings by all members of the family, including the patient, may alleviate behaviors that complicate seizure control and lead to future problems of social and personal adjustment.

Coma and Altered States of Consciousness

Viken Babikian

Consciousness refers to an individual's awareness of inner thoughts, emotions, and surrounding stimuli and is qualified by its content and degree of wakefulness. *Coma* (from the Greek, "deep sleep") denotes a state of deep unconsciousness and markedly reduced physical activity and is characterized by the individual's nonresponsiveness to stimuli. The concept of consciousness, as used in this chapter, is an attribute of human central nervous system functioning. Consciousness and coma are the two extremes of a continuum. *Confusion,* an intermediate state, describes mild disorientation, decreased attention span, lack of thought organization, and difficulty attending to detail and interpreting stimuli. It frequently is associated with decreased alertness. In *stupor,* alertness is severely depressed, mentation is dulled, and physical activity is decreased. Responses to external stimuli are markedly reduced. Confusion and stupor usually indicate diffuse brain dysfunction. *Delirium* is characterized by changes in the content of consciousness, with disorientation, agitation, hallucinations, and illusions dominating the clinical picture. The level of alertness fluctuates. Delirium is observed in the context of metabolic encephalopathy.

Two conditions describing altered states of responsiveness have increasingly been recognized in recent years. The *"locked-in"* syndrome denotes a state of quadriplegia and lower cranial nerve paralysis with preserved consciousness. It is frequently caused by lesions of the basis pontis. Patients in *"alpha-coma"* are unconscious and have electroencephalographic tracings that consist primarily of alpha frequency activity. Alpha-coma has been reported after cardiopulmonary arrest and in patients with brainstem lesions.

Pathophysiology

Our basic understanding of alertness is based to a large extent on the notion of cerebral cortex and brainstem reticular formation interactions. The reticular formation, a diffuse network of glia, neurons, and neural fibers, occupies medial and dorsal areas of the medulla, pons, and midbrain but has indistinct boundaries. Fibers arising from its pontine and mesencephalic components project to the nonspecific reticular and intralaminar nuclei of the thalamus. The latter in turn are thought to project to the cortex either directly or indirectly after further synapsing in specific thalamic nuclei, such as the anterior nucleus ventralis. Cortical areas receiving these projections are incompletely identified but include limbic and orbitofrontal regions. In the cat, high-frequency electrical stimulation of the nonspecific thalamic nuclei, subthalamic area, and pontine or mesencephalic tegmentum can cause widespread desynchronization of the electroencephalogram and arouse the animal. The concept of an ascending reticular activating system (ARAS) has been proposed to describe in a simplified way this alerting effect. It is assumed that the ARAS corresponds to the rostral extension of the reticular formation, the caudal parts of which are located in the pons and medulla and play a role in the induction of sleep. Recent laboratory investigations suggest that acetylcholine and norepinephrine might mediate some of the alerting effect of the ARAS.

Pathologic processes that disrupt the integrity of the reticular formation, its rostral projections, and the cortical mantle and underlying white matter bilaterally alter the individual's level of consciousness. Plum and Posner (1982) have described three basic mechanisms that can affect the organic functioning of this axis:

1. Infratentorial lesions mechanically damage the pontine or mesencephalic paramedian reticular formation (e.g., pontine hemorrhage) or disrupt its functioning by compressing it (e.g., cerebellar tumors with mass effect).

2. Supratentorial space-occupying lesions can depress consciousness by causing transtentorial herniation and by compressing or displacing diencephalic-mesencephalic structures (e.g., large temporal lobe gliomas).

3. Diffuse lesions involving the cortical mantle or subcortical white matter bilaterally (e.g., trauma) and systemic or primarily neurologic metabolic disorders that affect neuronal function (e.g., hypoglycemia, inherited neurologic disorders) also alter consciousness.

Table 60–19 summarizes common clinically recognized causes of coma.

Table 60–19. COMMON CAUSES OF COMA*

I. *Infratentorial lesions*
   A. Vascular disorders
      Brainstem and cerebellar infarction
      Pontine and cerebellar hemorrhage
      Subdural hematoma
      Subarachnoid hemorrhage
   B. Primary or metastatic brain tumors
   C. Infections
      Cerebellar abscess
      Subdural empyema
II. *Supratentorial lesions with mass effect*
   A. Vascular disorders
      Intracerebral hemorrhage
      Subdural hematoma
      Epidural hematoma
      Cerebral infarction
      Subarachnoid hemorrhage
   B. Primary or metastatic brain tumors
   C. Infections
      Intraparenchymal abscess
      Subdural hematoma
      Herpes simplex encephalitis
   D. Head trauma
   E. Pituitary apoplexy
III. *Other etiologies*
   A. Metabolic encephalopathies
      Hypoglycemia
      Hyponatremia and hypernatremia
      Hypocalcemia and hypercalcemia
      Hyperosmolar states
      Hypoxia and ischemia
      Hepatic failure
      Renal failure
      Pulmonary failure
      Myxedema
      Thyroid storm
      Medication and drug overdose
      Ingestion or inhalation of toxins
      Nutritional deficiencies
   B. Head trauma
   C. Infection
      Meningitis
      Encephalitis
      Postinfectious encephalomyelitis
   D. Reye's syndrome
   E. Seizures and postictal states
   F. Disorders of temperature regulation
   G. Advanced degenerative neurologic disorders (acquired or inherited)
      Alzheimer's disease
      Leukodystrophies and demyelinative disorders
   H. Psychiatric "pseudocoma"

*Modified from Plum, F., and Posner, J. B.: The Diagnosis of Stupor and Coma. 3rd edition. Philadelphia, F. A. Davis Company, 1982.

Physical Examination

Review of cardiac rate and rhythm, blood pressure, temperature, respiratory pattern, and general physical findings can provide helpful clues to the cause of coma. The neurologic examination proper is initiated with a period of observation: Are the eyes open? Is the patient vocalizing? yawning? posturing? Is the patient moving all four extremities spontaneously? Is asterixis, myoclonic jerks, or focal twitching observed? An initial impression about the patient's level of alertness and neurologic examination is formulated at this time and verified during the rest of the examination. Presence of nuchal rigidity is checked after cervical fracture has been ruled out.

Although "lethargic," "stuporous," and "obtunded" are commonly used terms to characterize patients with altered consciousness, degree of alertness is best described in terms of patient activity, rather than labeled. Spontaneous activity and response to conversational speech, yelling, shaking, or painful stimuli are recorded. Verbal or nonverbal responses to more than one mode of stimulation are elicited.

Cranial nerve examination includes reviewing the eye positions at rest, testing extraocular movements in response to verbal orders, and oculocephalic (doll's eye phenomenon) and oculovestibular (cold caloric) reflex stimulations. Size, shape, and symmetry of the pupils, direct and consensual pupillary responses to flashed light, and corneal reflexes are recorded. The basic neuroanatomic structures that subserve pupillary responses and extraocular movements are located in the pons and midbrain, and the preceding tests help establish the structural integrity of these pathways and surrounding brain tissue. Pathologic responses on these tests, therefore, have localizing value, whereas normal findings in the unconscious person would suggest a nonstructural cause, since these responses are likely to be affected late in the course of metabolic coma.

Decorticate posturing refers to spontaneous or induced positioning of the extremities, in which an arm is internally rotated and flexed at the elbow, and the ipsilateral leg is extended at the hip, knee, and ankle. In addition, both arm and leg are adducted. *Decerebrate rigidity* is represented by extension of all four extremities, with adduction and internal rotation of both arms and legs proximally. Although bilateral decerebrate posturing is traditionally ascribed to lesions at the mesencephalic level, several well-documented cases suggest that it is also caused by bilateral supratentorial lesions. Unilateral decerebrate posturing can be caused by damage to the motor cortex and its projections to the pons. Decorticate and decerebrate posturing can be present spontaneously following brain damage or can be induced by painful and other stimuli. Rubbing of the sternum and compression of a nailbed provide frequently used painful stimuli. When the response to pain is assessed, stimulus used, areas stimulated, and exact response are recorded. Deep tendon reflex testing can provide further lateralizing or localizing clues.

Laboratory Studies

The importance of a detailed clinical history and physical examination cannot be overemphasized in the evaluation of unconscious patients. Individuals accompanying the patient to the hospital should be questioned in detail before they leave. Information thus gathered will help formulate a tentative diagnosis and orient further diagnostic testing. Laboratory tests can help identify systemic or central nervous system metabolic abnormalities, infection, and central nervous system structural and electroencephalographic changes.

To detect systemic metabolic changes, venous blood is drawn to determine serum glucose, electrolytes, calcium, urea nitrogen, ammonia, and liver transaminase levels. Arterial blood is obtained to determine pH, oxygen and carbon dioxide tensions, and percentage oxygen saturation. Blood and urine are tested for drug levels and the presence of toxins. Most hospitals have the facilities to determine levels of only common medications and drugs, and consult outside toxicology laboratories for more comprehensive testing. Specific requests help accelerate this process. A complete blood count is obtained to detect infection and changes in the hematocrit and platelet count. Computerized tomography indentifies structural brain lesions. With the exception of patients with clearly identified primarily non-neurologic causes of coma, such as hypotension secondary to cardiac arrest, brain computerized tomography scans should be obtained early in all unconscious subjects. In individuals with diencephalic-midbrain junction or posterior fossa nonhemorrhagic lesions, magnetic resonance is the imaging method of choice. Imaging studies should be obtained prior to the lumbar puncture in order to identify and treat herniation, but the puncture should not be delayed when there is a strong clinical suspicion of meningitis. Subarachnoid hemorrhage and central nervous system or meningeal infection are identified by appropriate tests of the cerebrospinal fluid.

Electroencephalography remains the technique of choice to diagnose epilepsy and some metabolic encephalopathies, and to establish functional hemispheric asymmetries. Evoked potentials provide information about the integrity of auditory and sensory pathways. Electroencephalographic and evoked potential testing is frequently repeated to monitor the progression of coma and has been used to predict its outcome.

Therapy

The unconscious patient admitted to the emergency ward might be at risk for further central nervous system damage. Early diagnosis and treatment are therefore critical to prevent progression. The aim of the initial phase of therapy, when a diagnosis has still not been made, is to ensure adequate oxygenation, to stabilize the hemodynamic status, and to treat some readily reversible metabolic disorders. As soon as the cause of unconsciousness is identified, treatment is directed toward the specific cause of coma.

Tracheal intubation and mechanical ventilation may be necessary to maintain adequate oxygenation. Intravenous access is established to administer fluids and medications. The neck is immobilized until cervical radiographs can be obtained to rule out a cervical fracture. To counteract the possibility of hypoglycemia, 50 ml. of a 50 per cent glucose solution is administered intravenously. Chronic alcoholics and patients suspected of malnutrition are given 100 mg. of thiamine as well. Individuals with physical signs of narcotic overdosage receive 0.4 to 0.8 mg. naloxone, injected intravenously, or, if intravenous access is not available, administered intratracheally. In some patients larger doses of naloxone might be needed to reverse the respiratory and central nervous system depressant effects of the narcotic. A 1 or 2 mg. dose of physostigmine is injected intramuscularly or intravenously to carefully monitored subjects with signs of anticholinergic drug overdose; if found effective, this dose is repeated every 60 minutes as necessary.

When increased intracranial pressure and herniation are suspected, mechanical hyperventilation aiming at an arterial P_{CO_2} of 25 to 28 mm Hg is initiated, and 0.25 gram per kg. to 1 gram per kg. of a 20 per cent solution of mannitol is infused intravenously over 20 minutes to achieve a serum osmolarity ranging from 305 to 315 mosm. per liter. Although the use of dexamethasone in the treatment of increased intracranial pressure in trauma and stroke is controversial, dexamethasone (10 mg. followed by 6 mg. every 6 hours) is widely prescribed to treat edema of brain tumors.

Patients with witnessed seizures requiring treatment are bolused with 15 to 18 mg. per kg. phenytoin, injected intravenously at a rate not exceeding 50 mg. per minute. Subjects in status epilepticus can be treated with 5 to 10 mg. intravenous doses of diazepam infused at a rate of no more than 5 mg. per minute, and repeated once when indicated. The anticonvulsive effect of phenytoin is delayed by approximately 20 to 60 minutes after intravenous injection; diazepam has a rapid onset of action but has the disadvantage of depressing the patient's level of alertness and respiratory drive. This could necessitate intubation and mechanical ventilation. If the preceding regimen fails to control the seizures, phenobarbital is administered in 5 mg. per kg. increments intravenously every 30 minutes until the seizures stop, or a total dose of 15 to 20 mg. per kg. is reached. Phenobarbital can also depress the patient's level of consciousness and respiratory drive.

Brain Death

Until the recent past the diagnosis of death was based on the clinical observation of persistent apnea and absence of pulse. With the advent of modern techniques that can maintain cardiovascular and respiratory functions for prolonged periods, this concept has evolved, and brain death is widely accepted today among physicians as a criterion for death. In their *Report on the Diagnosis of Death* to the Presidential Commission for the Study of Ethical Problems in Medicine and Biomedical and Behavioral Research, the Medical Consultants (1982) recognized that "an individual who has sustained either (1) irreversible cessation of circulatory and respiratory functions, or (2) irreversible cessation of all functions of the entire brain, including the brain stem, is dead." They recommended that the determination of death be made in accordance with accepted medical standards, and that at the time of diagnosis hypothermia, drug and metabolic intoxication, neuromuscular blockade, and shock be avoided. Pathologic changes corresponding to clinical brain death consist of extensive necrosis and edema of cerebral tissue.

There is no consensus today with regard to the criteria that help establish the diagnosis of brain death and the laboratory tests that can confirm it unequivocally. Criteria commonly used to establish a clinical diagnosis include cerebral unreceptivity and unresponsivity to painful and other sensory stimuli, apnea, fixed pupils, and absent corneal, oculovestibular, oculocephalic, ciliospinal, cough, gag, and swallowing reflexes. A period of observation varying from 6 to 24 hours is usually recommended to document the persistence of these findings. Laboratory tests used to confirm the clinical impression include electroencephalography showing electrocerebral silence and, in rare cases, cerebral angiography to document the complete absence of cerebral blood flow.

Cerebrovascular Disease

Philip A. Wolf

The abrupt onset of hemiplegia has been known as stroke since the 17th century, denoting a condition of being suddenly rendered unconscious or paralyzed. The unexpected appearance of this frequently devastating illness suggests it is an "accident," as the term "cerebrovascular accident" implies. In recent years it has become clear that stroke, and the atherosclerotic and thrombotic disease underlying it, represents the end-result of a process set in motion many years before.

Stroke is the third leading cause of death in the United States, accounting for approximately 150,000 deaths in 1985, about 7.5 per cent of all deaths. However, mortality statistics understate the importance of stroke as a force in disease and disability; stroke is far more disabling than lethal. Furthermore, stroke is the most common neurologic disease leading to hospitalization of adults and is a significant contributor to long-term disability. It has been estimated that half of stroke survivors are permanently disabled, and a substantial proportion require long-term institutional care. Although stroke incidence increases with age, roughly doubling in successive decades of life, approximately 20 per cent occur below the age of 65 years. Unlike coronary heart disease, which affects men four times as often as women, stroke occurs with nearly equal incidence in women and men. Cerebrovascular disease is responsible for the majority of serious neurologic events in a general hospital. Physicians caring for adults will have to deal with acute stroke patients; those caring for the elderly will encounter stroke patients daily (Table 60–20).

Clinical Features

BRAIN INFARCTION

Two thirds of cases of brain infarction are a consequence of atherosclerosis affecting the carotid, vertebral, or basilar arteries with superimposed thrombus, or of large artery atherothrombosis (Fig. 60–3).

The site and extent of the infarct is determined by the available flow through the obstructed artery and through collaterals. There are three levels of collaterals: (1) the extracranial-intracranial connections between external carotid branches and the internal carotid artery and between the external carotid and other cervical arteries and the vertebral arteries; (2) the circle of Willis; and (3) the pial anastomoses between the major cerebral arteries.

Some brain tissue deprived of oxygen will undergo infarction, whereas adjacent areas will have sufficient flow to sustain tissue viability but not tissue function. Recovery of the physiologic integrity of this ischemic area is responsible in part for the recovery that occurs after stroke, particularly recovery of function in hours or days after the infarct.

Attention is being focused on this marginal area of nonfunctional but still viable brain as a way of limiting the damage from an acute stroke. This ischemic area is called the ischemic penumbra. Intervention to prevent the death of these ischemic cells may be attempted by means such as use of thrombolysins or other agents to restore flow to the ischemic area; use of calcium channel blocking agents to prevent cell death; use of other agents to block excitatory amino acid neurotransmission; use of substances to increase cerebral microcirculatory vasodilation; and preventing local cerebral acidosis.

TRANSIENT ISCHEMIC ATTACKS

The first indication of atherosclerotic arterial narrowing may be the occurrence of transient ischemic attacks (TIA's), episodes of focal cerebral ischemia that precede brain infarction in one half to two thirds of all thrombotic strokes. These episodes are brief, by definition persisting less than 24 hours, usually less than 20 minutes. They may be recurrent, with hundreds of stereotypical episodes over many months preceding the stroke, or there may be a single TIA followed in a day or two by infarction. Episodes of transient brain dysfunction—seizures, syncope, confusional and amnesic episodes—are common in the elderly and may be mistaken for TIA's. Inner ear dysfunction with recurrent dizziness, sometimes with ataxia, is common and in the absence of other clear-cut brainstem signs is rarely an indication of focal brainstem ischemia. Symptoms of carotid and vertebrobasilar artery territory TIA's are given in Table 60–21.

LACUNAR INFARCTION

Nearly 20 per cent of lesions precipitating stroke and about one third of all infarcts are lacunar infarcts.

Table 60–20. DIFFERENTIAL DIAGNOSIS OF STROKE

	Atherothrombotic Infarction	Cerebral Embolism	Intraparenchymatous Hemorrhage	Subarachnoid Hemorrhage
Prior warning	Characteristic	No	No	Uncommon
Onset	Abrupt	Abrupt	Abrupt	Abrupt
Course after onset	Variable—fluctuation, stepwise progression, or maximal at onset	Deficit—maximal at onset, often improvement is rapid	Smooth progression	Maximal deficit at onset
Activity at onset	Usually during sleep	While active, often shortly after rising	While active	Active, often exertion
Initial loss of consciousness	Rare	Rare	Common	Common
Headache	Uncommon	Occasionally	Characteristic	Characteristic
Computed tomography scan—shortly after onset	Normal or decreased density	Normal or decreased density	Hematoma (lesion of increased density)	Blood in subarachnoid space
After 5 to 7 days	Area of decreased density, contrast shows gray matter enhancement	Area or areas of decreased density	Hematoma and surrounding edema mass effect	Bloody CSF under normal or increased pressure
Lumbar puncture	Normal	Normal	Bloody CSF under increased pressure	Bloody CSF under normal pressure
Arteriography—shortly after onset	Occlusion or severe arterial stenosis	Occlusion of intracerebral arteries and multiple branch occlusions	Mass effect	Aneurysm of circle of Willis, arterial spasm

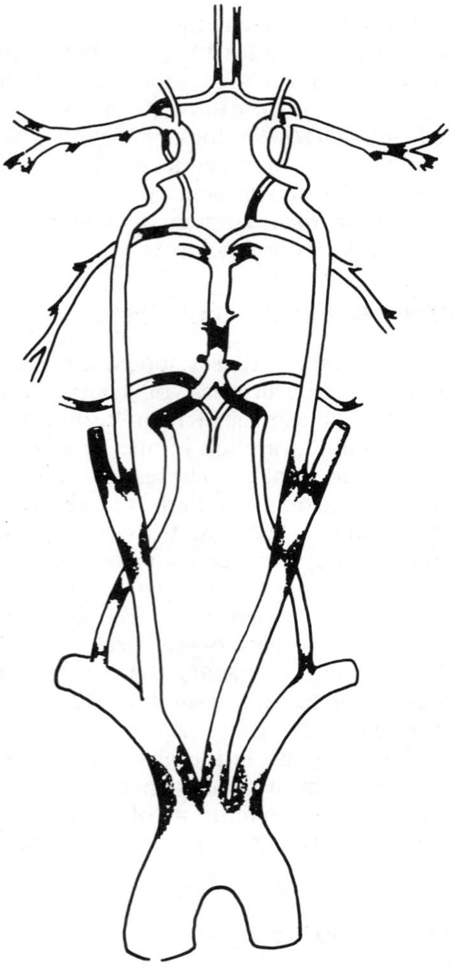

Figure 60–3. Preferred sites for atherosclerotic plaques. (From Toole, J. F.: Diagnosis and Management of Stroke. New York, American Heart Association, 1979.)

Occlusion of small penetrating arteries, 50 to 150 μ in diameter, produces infarcts generally between 0.5 and 1.5 cm. in size. These lacunae occur in the territory of penetrating branches of anterior, middle, and posterior cerebral arteries, and of branches of vertebral and basilar arteries as well. Accordingly, these tend to involve the basal ganglia, internal capsule, and basis points preferentially. The commonest lacunar syndrome is that of *pure motor hemiplegia* from a lacunar infarction in the internal capsule. In this syndrome, pure motor weakness develops without sensory loss, visual field disturbance, or disorder of language or cognitive function. Such deficits tend to have a stuttering onset, so characteristic of thrombotic disease, and evolve in a leisurely fashion over a few days. The pure sensory stroke, the dysarthric "clumsy hand" syndrome, and the syndrome of weakness in the leg and ataxia in the ipsilateral arm are also seen. Lacunar stroke seems to be, as with other stroke syndromes, a consequence of hypertension. In this situation, however, hypertension produces atheroma and thrombosis in some patients and lipohyalin degeneration in others. Multiple lacunar infarcts involving corticospinal and corticobulbar tracts may produce the syndrome of *lacunar state* with dementia and pseudobulbar palsy, including emotional lability.

Table 60–21. CLINICAL FEATURES OF TRANSIENT ISCHEMIC ATTACKS

Carotid Territory (in decreasing frequency)
- Numbness of fingers
- Transient monocular blindness
- Speech disturbance
- Numb and weak hand and arm
- Weak hand
- Numb and weak arm and leg
- Numb face

Vertebrobasilar Territory (in varying combinations)
- Dizziness
- Diplopia
- Dysarthria
- Weakness of part of one or both sides
- Staggering gait
- Veering to one side
- Numbness of part of one or both sides
- Crossed numbness
- Dark or blurred vision
- Partial or total blindness
- Ptosis
- Paralysis of conjugate gaze
- Speechlessness
- Dysphagia

CEREBRAL EMBOLISM

Cerebral embolism is a potentially preventable cause of stroke, and in half the cases a source for embolism can be detected (Table 60–22). The onset is abrupt as the embolus lodges in one of the arteries supplying the brain. The course, after onset, may include a severe neurologic deficit that is only temporary; the symptoms disappear as the embolus fragments and moves distally. In fact, the rapid resolution or clearing

Table 60–22. SOURCES OF CEREBRAL EMBOLI

A. Cardiac sources
  1. Atrial fibrillation with or without rheumatic, congenital, acquired coronary, hypertensive, or luetic heart disease
  2. Myocardial infarction with mural and intraventricular thrombus
  3. Cardiac surgery
  4. Cardiomyopathy and myocarditis
  5. Valvular diseases
     a. Mitral stenosis (rheumatic heart disease)
     b. Prosthetic valve
     c. Bacterial endocarditis, acute and subacute
     d. Prolapsed mitral valve
  6. Marantic endocarditis
  7. Cardiac myxoma

B. Noncardiac sources
  1. Complications of angiography
  2. Paradoxical embolism
  3. Atherosclerotic plaque and ulcers of aorta and major brachiocephalic arteries
  4. Fat, tumor, or air

C. Undetermined source

of the clinical deficit is an important point in the differential diagnosis and one that strongly favors embolism. In such patients, cerebral arteriography within the first 48 hours after onset may disclose embolic material in multiple cerebral branches, thereby confirming the diagnosis. A search for the source of an embolism must be made in each case in which it is suspected. Unfortunately, in many patients documented to have cerebral embolism on arteriography, a source cannot be found; presumably, atherosclerotic lesions of the ascending aorta and brachiocephalic arteries, including the carotid arteries, are the origin of the embolic material.

INTRAPARENCHYMATOUS HEMORRHAGE

The most common site of intraparenchymatous hemorrhage is the putamen, with hemorrhage frequently occurring in the thalamus, pons, cerebellum, and cerebral white matter. Such lesions were previously thought to be uniformly fatal. Recently, CT scanning of large numbers of stroke patients has shown that a proportion of these hemorrhages are restricted in size and that recovery is common. The syndrome of *acute cerebellar hemorrhage* is an important one to recognize, since the hematoma may be evacuated surgically, often with excellent clinical recovery. If the diagnosis is missed, the outcome is frequently fatal. The clinical hallmarks are the sudden onset of dizziness; repeated uncontrollable vomiting; inability to stand and walk after the onset of hemorrhage; and associated ipsilateral facial paresis and gaze palsy. Hemiplegia is not obvious, and the diagnosis of labyrinthitis, viral gastroenteritis, or drug intoxication may be made. The CT scan discloses the hematoma. Cerebellar infarction due to embolism may follow a similar course with progression of signs and symptoms 48 to 72 hours after the ictus as cerebellar edema develops. CT scan discloses the infarct, and the swollen cerebellar hemisphere may be surgically drained with good results.

SUBARACHNOID HEMORRHAGE

Rupture of aneurysm of the circle of Willis produces spontaneous subarachnoid hemorrhage and is responsible for between 5 and 10 per cent of strokes in clinical series. Approximately 90 to 95 per cent of saccular aneurysms lie in the anterior part of the circle of Willis, but determination of the exact vascular site of the aneurysm is difficult to make clinically. Onset is abrupt, with a sudden, violent headache often associated with *transient* loss of consciousness or seizure. Since the bleeding occurs outside of brain substance, there are frequently no lateralizing signs such as hemiparesis, aphasia, or visual field defect. The patient has signs of intracranial bleeding: nuchal rigidity, subhyaloid retinal hemorrhages, and, on lumbar puncture, blood in the cerebrospinal fluid. The outstanding characteristic of subarachnoid hemorrhage is a tendency for the hemorrhage to recur.

Destruction of brain tissue by the initial hemorrhage, infarction of the brain due to arterial spasm, and recurrent hemorrhage constitute the major causes of death and disability following subarachnoid hemorrhage. Overall, the 30-day case fatality rate for subarachnoid hemorrhage is 50 per cent. Patients who have survived the initial hemorrhage with little or no clinical deficit must have their care directed toward the prevention of recurrent hemorrhage.

Disturbance of Motor Function

Jan Kucera
Jeannette Chirico-Post
Marie Saint-Hilaire

Disturbance of motor function may be due to disease of the brain, the spinal cord pathways, the motor nerves and their connections with muscle, or the muscle itself. The first sign of proximal weakness is usually noticed while climbing stairs. Distal weakness is evident when the patient is unable to hold a glass securely or guide a pen without strain. The patient may notice atrophy of muscle, such as wasting of the first dorsal interosseous space or the thenar eminence, appearing insidiously after injury or chronic pressure on a nerve. Sometimes the main complaint is described as progressive weakness following exercise, or as a dysphagia or diplopia, which resolves after rest. A broken leg or other injury may result from an inability to stabilize the hip or may be the effect of previously unrecognized Parkinson's disease or cerebellar ataxia.

In this section, disturbance of movement is discussed from the periphery to the central nervous system, beginning with conditions that affect muscle.

Muscle Weakness

MYASTHENIA GRAVIS

Myasthenia gravis may occur at any age from infancy to old age. The presence of anti-acetylcholine receptor antibodies in patients with myasthenia gravis suggests that an autoimmune mechanism is responsible for the disorder. The commonest symptoms are ptosis, diplopia, dysphagia, dysarthria, marked fatigability, and weakness. Symptoms appear and progress after exercise and are relieved by rest. There is a striking tendency toward involvement of ocular and bulbar muscles, although the axial and appendicular muscles may also be affected, but with normal peripheral sensation, preservation of tendon reflexes, and absence of muscular atrophy.

The degree of severity of myasthenia gravis can be described clinically as follows: group I, ocular involvement only; group II(a), mild, generalized weakness, including ocular involvement; group II(b), moderate severity, including ocular and mild to moderate bulbar involvement; group III, acute severe myasthenia gravis developing over a period of weeks to months, usually requiring tracheostomy and respiratory support because of severe bulbar involvement; group IV, late, severe condition, requiring respiratory support; group V, complete remission, leaving only mild muscle atrophy. Children of myasthenic mothers may show myasthenia at birth.

Although a history of a fluctuant weakness of limb muscles or of increasing difficulty in maintaining the focus of one's eyes as the day progresses is highly suggestive, confirmatory tests using the physiologic principles of neuromuscular transmission are necessary. Repetitive stimulation of a peripheral nerve, such as the ulnar, while the responses of a small muscle in the hand are recorded by electromyograph, may reveal a decrement in amplitude of muscle response as the stimulation is repeated at a constant shock strength. Administration of 10 mg. of edrophonium hydrochloride in 1 ml. of solution will restore the muscle responses. Edrophonium must be administered intravenously in fractional doses, 0.2 ml. (2 mg.) initially, with a lapse of 30 seconds allowed before additional amounts are given, up to the total dose of 10 mg., to avoid arterial hypertension and cardiac irregularities, which otherwise might occur as side effects of the drug. Test administration of edrophonium will help differentiate a cholinergic crisis (i.e., overtreatment) from a myasthenic crisis (insufficient anticholinesterase medication).

Therapy for myasthenia gravis requires the use of two classes of treatment modalities—anticholinesterases and immunosuppression. Initially, neostigmine prostigmine bromide may be given as 15 mg. tablets every 2 to 6 hours, especially at times when fatigue is anticipated, such as before meals, when chewing might become difficult. As few as four or as many as 20 tablets per day may be needed. A longer-acting preparation, pyridostigmine bromide (Mestinon), may be used every 2 to 8 hours. A 60 mg. tablet of pyridostigmine is approximately equivalent to a 15 mg. tablet of neostigmine, and a dose of 60 to 180 mg. may be given at night.

Immunosuppression is usually accomplished alone or in combination with the anticholinesterases. Thymectomy, of benefit to most patients, should be considered early in the course of therapy. Corticosteroid therapy usually takes the form of prednisone given orally either daily or on alternate days in a dose of 25 to 100 mg. The major anticipated problems with the initiation of prednisone therapy are exacerbation of myasthenic symptoms early in the course of therapy and recurrence of symptoms upon reduction of steroids. Plasmapheresis has been used with excellent results in some patients with myasthenia gravis. The role of plasma exchange to assist in the preparation of patients for thymectomy, as well as in symptomatic relief of myasthenic symptoms while awaiting effectiveness of other forms of immunosuppressive therapy, has clearly been established. Azathioprine (Imuran) is usually administered in dosages of 2 to 3 mg. per kg. body weight per day. The effectiveness of azathioprine usually requires some 4 to 6 months of therapy. Serious side effects must be monitored for, including severe hematopoietic depression, infection, and late neoplasm. Patients in myasthenic crisis may require tracheostomy and respiratory support while medications are being readjusted and plasmapheresis is used.

HYPOKALEMIC PERIODIC PARALYSIS

This type of paralysis is a form of recurrent muscle weakness that occurs both sporadically and in families, the usual pattern of inheritance being autosomal dominant. Attacks of muscle paralysis begin in the teenage years, and males are more susceptible. Diffuse muscle weakness or total paralysis may appear after heavy carbohydrate intake, during sleep, or after a day of vigorous exercise. Proximal limb muscles and the trunk are affected more often than the distal muscles. Reflexes are lacking. Recovery ensues after a few hours or in a day. During an attack there is a reduction in serum potassium levels, with the ion presumably moving into the muscle fibers. This causes change in the electrocardiogram. The condition can be alleviated by a diet high in potassium and low in carbohydrate and sodium, and by administration of acetazolamide (Diamox). To abort an attack, 10 gm. of potassium chloride should be given, preferably orally.

In certain families a form of muscle weakness has been described in which the serum potassium is elevated during an attack *(hyperkalemic periodic paralysis)*. The attacks are brief, 30 minutes to 3 hours, and recovery is hastened by exercise. In a severe attack, intravenous calcium gluconate is given. Delayed muscle relaxation after contraction (myotonia) may be demonstrable between the attacks. Maintenance therapy on acetazolamide (Diamox) or chlorothiazide (Diuril) is used.

MUSCULAR DYSTROPHY

Muscular dystrophy includes a group of disorders characterized by weakness and wasting of the striated muscle, a progressive clinical course, and often a hereditary background. Although most patients have their first symptoms early in life, onset may be at any age, depending on the specific form of the disease.

Pseudohypertrophic (Duchenne's) muscular dystrophy appears in the preschool years and affects boys exclusively. The progression is steady, usually necessitating a wheelchair before the end of the patient's first decade, with death in most instances resulting from respiratory or cardiac failure before the late teens. The early symptoms of difficult gait and difficult running or toe-walking are rarely recognized as caused by muscular dystrophy unless the disease has been known in other members of the family. Enlargement of the calves may precede noticeable weakness by many months and actually can be mistaken for unusually good muscular development. The so-called Gowers' sign indicates weakness of proximal muscles. Upon arising from the floor, the patient places hands upon thighs and pushes the trunk up to a standing position. In Duchenne's muscular dystrophy the blood levels of creatine phosphokinase (CPK) are grossly elevated early in the disease, even before clinical symptoms become evident. As the disease progresses, the CPK gradually declines toward normal values. This test is sufficiently specific to cast doubt on a diagnosis of early Duchenne's muscular dystrophy when the CPK values are not elevated.

Muscle biopsy and electromyography can be used together to help confirm the clinical diagnosis. The typical histologic changes are size variation and hyaline degeneration of muscle fibers, with infiltration of fat between muscle bundles. The electromyograph shows short duration, low amplitude, rapidly firing potentials in the presence of a weak muscle contraction. This form of muscular dystrophy is transmitted by a sex-linked recessive mechanism, but the mutation rate is high. Carrier detection is performed by serum CPK determinations. Genetic counseling is an important part of the therapeutic approach to the muscular dystrophies. Treatment is supportive, with attempts to prevent contractures. Sometimes surgical procedures to lengthen the Achilles tendon allow additional months of ambulation before the child is confined to a wheelchair.

Limb-girdle muscular dystrophy has a later onset than Duchenne's dystrophy, affecting the pelvic and shoulder girdle muscles and displaying a benign, slow course. Genetic transmission is by an autosomal recessive mechanism. Symptoms may occur during the first three decades. Muscle biopsy and serum enzyme studies are less valuable in the diagnosis of limb-girdle muscular dystrophy than in pseudohypertrophic muscular dystrophy. The *facioscapulohumeral form of muscular dystrophy* is inherited by an autosomal dominant mechanism, and both sexes are affected with equal frequency. The illness appears early in puberty, and the clinical course is relatively slow and sometimes abortive. It is not unusual for patients to remain ambulatory until an advanced age. The muscles earliest affected are those of the face, shoulder girdle, and upper arms. Involvement of the lower extremities may follow after a decade or two.

Myotonic muscular dystrophy is characterized by symptoms of distal limb muscle weakness and wasting, delayed relaxation of muscles after an initial contraction (myotonia), and certain extramuscular changes consisting of frontal baldness, bilateral lens opacities, and, in males, testicular atrophy. Swallowing difficulties may also be noted. The onset is usually in the second or third decade of life. Inheritance is autosomal dominant. Quinine, procainamide, and phenytoin have been used with variable results to treat the myotonia.

INFLAMMATORY MYOPATHIES

The signs and symptoms of polymyositis, as in certain forms of muscular dystrophy, are predominantly those of proximal muscular weakness of the pelvic and shoulder girdles. Systemic signs and symptoms are rarely present early in the disease. Typically, the onset is insidious, with weakness of the proximal muscles of the upper and lower limbs and a defective swallowing mechanism gradually appearing over weeks to months. Moderate fluctuations in the intensity of the clinical disease are characteristic. Muscular pain and tenderness are more common in the acute form than in subacute or chronic cases. Raising the arms over the head and, especially, maintaining them in an overhead position, as in combing the hair, become difficult. In severe or advanced cases the weakness may be extreme, and the patient is then bedridden. Muscle atrophy is a late occurrence. The link between polymyositis and certain of the connective tissue diseases can be observed in the similarities of the skin manifestations of systemic lupus erythematosus, scleroderma, and dermatomyositis. Furthermore, mild or transitory arthritis occurs in about one third to one half of the cases of polymyositis.

The diagnosis is supported by findings of elevations of serum aldolase and creatine phosphokinase.

These enzymes, which are released as a result of the destructive myopathy, are often, but not always, increased in the acute and subacute stages. *Electromyography* in polymyositis shows abnormal potentials in nearly all stages of the disease. During rest there are small potentials that are indistinguishable from spontaneous fibrillations; upon voluntary movement, a complex, polyphasic pattern of motor unit potentials may be observed. Short bursts of rapidly repeating action potentials that fade away after a brief initial period (pseudomyotonia) have been described. Muscle biopsy will disclose changes if the sample is taken from an affected muscle, the best choice in general being a proximal muscle that is partially but not completely weakened. Histologic features include either primary focal or extensive degeneration of muscle fibers, sometimes with vacuolization; evidence of regeneration, as demonstrated by sarcoplasmic basophilia and the presence of large nuclei and prominent nucleoli; necrosis of a part or the whole of one or more fibers, with phagocytosis; interstitial infiltration of inflammatory cells; and, in long-standing cases, interstitial fibrosis. Treatment for acute polymyositis should include prednisone (50 to 100 mg. per day by mouth). Once recovery begins and the enzyme levels have returned to normal, a lower dosage can be attempted. Maintenance therapy should be continued for months or years with a prednisone dosage ranging from 5 to 20 mg. per day. Some patients will be found to have an underlying malignant disease.

ENDOCRINE AND METABOLIC MYOPATHIES

Chronic thyrotoxic myopathy consists of a progressive weakness and wasting of muscles with or without overt symptoms and signs of thyrotoxicosis. The proximal muscles of the limbs are most severely affected. The bulbar and ocular muscles are usually spared. The serum CPK is normal. The disorder is reversed after correction of the thyroid function. In patients with *hypothyroid myopathy*, weakness of the proximal limb muscles is seen with or without other clinical features of hypothyroidism. The deep tendon reflexes may show a slowness in contraction and relaxation. The serum CPK may be elevated. The weakness disappears after treatment with thyroid hormone.

Patients treated with corticosteroids for months or years sometimes develop *corticosteroid myopathy*, a progressive weakness of the proximal limb muscles. The serum CPK is normal. The muscle biopsy shows decrease in size of the muscle fibers (type II) that normally have high anaerobic glycolytic metabolism. Reduction or discontinuation of corticosteroid administration results in improvement and recovery. A similar myopathy is seen in patients with Cushing's syndrome.

With advancing knowledge of the chemistry of muscle, a number of muscle disorders have been recognized to represent disturbances of carbohydrate or lipid metabolism or the function of mitochondria. *McArdle's disease* (phosphorylase deficiency) is a rare familial disorder caused by an absence of phosphorylase in skeletal muscle. The symptoms start in childhood and consist of painful contracture of vigorously exercised muscles lasting for a few hours. Myoglobinuria may occur. Moderate exercise does not usually lead to symptoms. No abnormalities are present on examination. The usual increase in blood lactic acid following exercise is not present in these patients. The final diagnosis rests on histochemical or biochemical demonstration of absence of phosphorylase in muscle biopsy.

Disorders Involving the Motor Unit

The anterior horn cell, its axon, and its neuromuscular junction together compose a motor unit. A peripheral nerve is made up of the axons of many motor units. Knowledge of the segmental arrangement of nerves is helpful in relating a given muscle paralysis to a lesion of a particular nerve, nerve root, or level of spinal anterior horn cells.

ANTERIOR HORN DISEASES

Primary involvement of the motor neuron occurs in several conditions, of which *amyotrophic lateral sclerosis* (Charcot's or Lou Gehrig's disease) is one. Progressive muscular atrophy and progressive bulbar palsy describe different stages of this disease, in which upper as well as lower motor neurons are affected. When spastic paraparesis is noted, the physician may first think about the possibility of a surgically remediable lesion in the cervical region, such as spondylosis or tumor; then consideration is given to vitamin B_{12} deficiency and demyelinating disease of the spinal cord, such as multiple sclerosis or transverse myelopathy. Bladder function is preserved, but dysarthria, dysphagia, or both may be the earliest symptoms when the process begins in the bulbar nuclei. Weakness of the hands and fingers leads to clumsiness of movement. The process often begins asymmetrically and goes on for 2 to 5 or 7 years, rarely longer without respiratory support and tube feeding. Sudden, large involuntary movements of groups of muscle fibers usually are experienced by the patient before atrophy of muscle is recognized. These spontaneous muscle movements, sometimes accentuated by exercise, are known as fasciculations and can be recorded by electromyography as large, high amplitude, multiphasic potentials of moderate duration occurring at random frequency. Muscle atrophy spreads from areas innervated by one affected spinal nerve segment to another. The shoulder girdle and upper arms are involved early. The palate is affected shortly after the tongue, which shows minute quiverings (fasciculations) on its surface.

Acute anterior poliomyelitis is another disease of motor neurons and produces asymmetrical flaccid paralysis. It is caused by poliovirus infection, with destruction of motor cells in the spinal cord and brainstem. Following systemic infection by the virus, paralysis develops between the second and fifth day, after the appearance of meningeal signs. Progression of motor weakness may continue for another 3 to 5 days; then the clinical picture stabilizes. Respiratory paralysis often results in death when the medullary nuclei are affected in the bulbar form of the illness. Cerebrospinal fluid examination reveals lymphocytosis and normal to moderately elevated protein. The prognosis is poor when the paralysis is extensive. Partially denervated muscles may have some recovery of function, but the degree of residual motor paralysis depends on the total number of ventral horn cells that are permanently destroyed.

Spinal cord tumors involving the cervical region affect anterior horn cells and long tracts. They cause both muscle wasting of the shoulders and upper extremities and local sensory losses. There may also be spasticity in the lower extremities due to corticospinal tract involvement. A neurogenic bladder occurs with spinal cord compression (this is extremely unusual in cases of amyotrophic lateral sclerosis until very late in the illness). *Syringomyelia* may produce muscle atrophy following initial weakness, fasciculations, and sensory deficits, like intramedullary spinal cord tumors but in contrast with amyotrophic lateral sclerosis.

The recognition of treatable motor unit diseases is very important. Sometimes surgical aspiration of a cyst associated with syringomyelia or decompression of the spinal cord by removing a tumor or spondylotic protrusion will ameliorate symptoms.

RADICULOPATHIES

The differential diagnosis of neck-arm pain should include other nerve entrapment syndromes with referral pain, such as thoracic outlet or median nerve compression, ulnar group involvement, or lesions of the radial nerve at the humerus level. Angina pectoris has often been mistaken for cervical radiculopathy and vice versa.

Cervical vertebrae develop degenerative changes at their articulating surfaces as a response to repeated trauma and aging *(spondylosis)*. Incidental radiologic findings of degenerative arthropathic changes with spur formation are found in a high proportion of persons over the age of 50 years without symptoms. These changes involve degeneration of the intervertebral disc (annulus fibrosus) and secondary changes in the vertebral bodies and foramina. Symptoms arise when the nerve roots and/or the spinal cord is impinged upon directly by a spondylotic bar or spur and its blood supply is interfered with. Various symptoms may result from a combination of root and spinal cord involvement. Cervical spondylosis produces impingement on nerve roots, and entrapment syndromes of peripheral nerves simulate motor neuron disease when associated with muscle wasting, fasciculations, and no sensory loss.

Pain associated with cervical radiculopathy is due to traction upon nerve roots and the dural sleeves. Cervical muscle spasm contributes to pain, although it also serves as a "splint" of the cervical spine. Muscle spasm may eliminate the normal curvature (lordosis) of the cervical spine. Straightening is seen on x-ray examination. The location of referred pain and changes in the tendon reflexes are helpful in determining the segmental spinal level involved. Radiculopathy at the fifth and sixth cervical levels often presents as a burning sensation in the ipsilateral suprascapular region, an area supplied by the dorsal scapular nerve; a C7 root impingement may cause an ache in the elbow associated with a pain in the lower neck. When the sensory fibers are affected, pain may radiate from lesions in the middle cervical region (C5–C6) to the middle or index fingers or to the lateral aspect of the arm; with low cervical lesions (C7–C8) the pain may be referred to the hypothenar region and the fourth and fifth fingers. Movement of the neck or percussion of an involved cervical spine may reproduce the discomfort radiating into the arm. Careful muscle testing is useful when weakness is present. The combination of weakness in the biceps muscle and a reduced biceps tendon reflex suggests a C6 involvement.

Lumbosacral radiculopathies result from the same mechanisms as the cervical root syndromes (Table 60–23). Pain in the gluteal region or in the area of the greater trochanter is caused by L5 radiculopathy or intertrochanteric bursitis. Radiation of pain from the sciatic notch down the back of the leg may also occur with L5 root compression. Pain caused by an intrapelvic mass encroaching upon the lumbar plexus or the sciatic nerve must also be kept in mind in the differential diagnosis; therefore, rectal and pelvic examinations should be a part of the work-up for back pain.

Cauda equina tumors produce bilateral leg pain and a perianal burning sensation. As mentioned, intrapelvic masses must be ruled out by rectal examination in every case of low back pain; in some cases sigmoidoscopy and barium enema examinations are necessary. Intravenous pyelography may reveal a pelvic mass such as with endometriosis, which can produce symptoms of lumbar radiculopathy by traction on the lumbar plexus. Sprains of the low back muscles and ligaments may cause pain in the paravertebral regions with radiation down the back of the leg. In such cases the pain is due in part to hamstring muscle spasm. Lateral leg pain may occur with spasm of the tensor fasciae latae. Recurrent back pain associated with menstrual cycles has been attributed by some to psoas muscle spasm.

A burning pain in the knee with reduced knee-

Table 60–23. RADICULAR SYNDROMES*

Nerve Root	Intervertebral Space	Subjective Pain Radiation	Sensory Area	Bladder and Bowel Dysfunction†	Straight Leg Raising‡	Ankle Jerk	Knee Jerk	Motor Signs§
L3	L2–L3	Back to buttocks to posterior thigh to anterior knee region	Hypalgesia in knee region	+/−	Usually −	+	+	Quadriceps weakness
L4	L3–L4	Back to buttocks to posterior thigh to inner calf region	Hypalgesia in inner aspect of lower leg	+/−	Usually − May be +	+	−	Quadriceps and possible anticus weakness
L5	L4–L5	Back to buttocks to dorsum of foot and big toe	Hypalgesia in dorsum of foot and big toe	+/−	+ +	+	+	Weakness of anterior tibialis, big toe extensor, gluteus medius
S1	L5–S1	Back to buttocks to sole of foot and heel	Hypalgesia in heel or lateral foot	+/−	+ + +	−	+	Weakness of gastrocnemius, hamstring, gluteus maximus

+ Present; − absent; +/− may be present or absent.
*Modified from Cailliet: Low Back Pain Syndrome. Philadelphia, F. A. Davis Company, 1968.
†Bladder and bowel dysfunction can occur at any level.
‡Related to extent of nerve root involvement at each level.
§Only the more obvious and functional muscles are listed. (This is not a complete list of muscles innervated.)

jerk and quadriceps reflexes and a weakness of the anterior thigh muscles suggest involvement of lumbar root levels (L3–L4), whereas a reduced Achilles tendon reflex and dysesthesia in the heel indicate S1 root compression. Weakness of the extensor hallucis and the extensor digitorum brevis muscles is usually present with L5 and S1 radiculopathies. Aggravation of low back pain on motion with referred pain down the legs occurs with root syndromes, but these are signs also of intraspinal processes.

Diagnostic Studies. The differential diagnosis of cervical or lumbar radiculopathy may be difficult if considered only on a clinical basis. Pain may be present without objective signs of muscle weakness or reflex changes. Underlying depression reduces a patient's tolerance for discomfort. *Electromyography* (EMG) reveals denervation in some cases of subacute radiculopathy; however, atrophy and weakness are already present by the time the EMG is helpful. Fibrillations, the electrical evidence of denervation in muscle, may be found in the extensor digitorum brevis muscles (S1) or in the triceps (C7) and biceps (C5) muscles. Reduced numbers of discharging motor units are often the only finding. A corresponding change in deep tendon reflexes is the most convincing evidence of a particular nerve root (radicular) injury. *Myelography* has become the best confirmatory test in localizing an impinged nerve root, a spinal cord compression, or other intraspinal abnormality. In some cases, myelography may be negative, but clinical signs and persistent pain may justify an exploration at the appropriate root level. Technical advances in CT scanning have made it possible to visualize a herniated disc, intraspinal masses, or dislocation or fracture in the transverse plane.

Therapeutic Measures. Treatment of radicular syndromes requires both relief of the associated muscle spasms and pain and reduction of the irritation of the nerve root. Excluding cases due to acute protrusions that cause spinal cord or cauda equina compression and require emergency laminectomy, radicular syndromes are managed best by conservative measures in 90 per cent of patients, especially for the first attack. Treatment consists of bed rest on a firm mattress supported by bed boards for 2 to 3 weeks. Hot tub soaks, muscle massage, and analgesics may help. On the other hand, gentle cervical traction (5 to 12 pounds for 20 to 30 minutes, four times a day) with the neck slightly flexed and the patient sitting semiupright is the treatment of choice for acute cervical disc protrusions; this may be followed by physical therapy and the use of a supporting towel or small to medium-sized plastic collar around the neck. For severe spondylosis with or without a ruptured disc, conservative treatment may not suffice. After study of the patient by myelography, appropriate surgical procedures should be considered.

Peripheral Neuropathies

Signs and symptoms of dysfunction of peripheral nerves reflect the location and degree of damage to nerve fibers and their myelin sheaths. The longest peripheral fibers are usually affected earliest; this is the reason for a stocking-glove pattern of sensory loss in polyneuropathy. Motor signs after denervation induce hypotonia and weakness of muscles, hyporeflexia, and atrophy of muscles. In systemic illnesses with polyneuropathy, all nerves are usually affected and will show prolonged conduction velocities, distally more than proximally. The main sensory symptoms of disorders of peripheral nerves include *paresthesias* (numbness, tingling, or other spontaneous sensation in the absence of an actual applied stimulus); *dysesthesias* (painful, unpleasant distortion of actual sensation); *hyperesthesias* (excessive reaction or persistence of sensation to a given stimulus); and *hypoesthesias* (reduced sensibility to a stimulus). In the presence of severe polyneuropathy with dense loss of all sensation in an extremity, the patient may experience curious symptoms during periods of sensory deprivation, especially when the lights are off and no sound is heard. Fingers may show "dancing" movements (pseudoathetosis). This spontaneous movement has been attributed to an attempt by the patient to localize the extremities in space by use of joint sensation.

TRAUMATIC AND ENTRAPMENT NEUROPATHIES

Injuries to several divisions within the cervical plexus or within the lumbar plexus are approached clinically in a manner similar to that for root syndromes, although the signs are usually more obvious. For example, weakness of both the anterior and the posterior muscles of an extremity would be more suggestive of a plexus lesion than of a paresis due to the weakness of the extensor or flexor muscles alone. Therefore, the differentiation of peripheral nerve lesions from plexus lesions requires careful physical examination and thorough knowledge of the anatomy and innervation of the muscles involved (Fig. 60–4). In a region of localized injury and inflammation of a peripheral nerve, delay in conduction caused by damage to the myelin sheath produces weakness in the muscles subserved. Localized pain and distal sensory disturbances appear before weakness and atrophy. Exogenous damage, such as a contusion or a chronic compression of the nerve, produces block of nerve transmission at the point of injury. Repeated trauma from movement of the nerve within an entrapment area usually leads to a reactive inflammatory response, with formation of adhesions, and obstruction of blood supply.

Several examples of mononeuropathies due to entrapment are described in the following.

Occipital Nerve Syndrome. Repeated pressure on the occipital nerve produces a chronic ache, a burning sensation, and tenderness over the mastoid area. Recurrent muscle spasm and headache can also occur. Xylocaine injection of the nerve may give some relief, but occipital neurectomy is often necessary for complete elimination of the symptoms. Occipital neuralgia in elderly patients who rest their head against a high-backed rocking or reclining chair results from compression of the occipital nerve.

Thoracic Outlet Syndromes (Costoclavicular Syndrome, Scalenus Syndrome). The diagnosis of thoracic outlet syndrome is made whenever there is compression of neurovascular elements at any point between the base of the neck and the axilla. The syndrome may be suspected from the history, and suspicion may be strengthened upon hearing an arterial bruit on auscultation over the anterior cervical triangle; this bruit is usually accentuated by abducting and extending the arm. Turning the head in the direction opposite to the side of the lesion may exaggerate the symptoms (Adson's maneuver). The radial pulse will usually disappear as the symptoms are brought out. The neurovascular bundle is composed of the inferior cord of the brachial plexus and the subclavian artery and vein. They have an intimate relationship with the scalenus anterior muscle and tendon and, if any is present, with the cervical rib, an enlarged transverse process, or a fibrous band uniting such a process to the rib.

The mutual relationships of the various structures in the upper thoracic outlet are constantly altered by respiratory movements and movements of the upper extremities. Repeated trauma of the neurovascular bundle from a stretch injury to the arm, from changes in posture due to pregnancy or weight gain, or from the wearing of a heavy pack with shoulder straps may lead to compression entrapment of the nerve, artery, and vein. Nerve conduction studies may be of little help in making this diagnosis except in the presence of prolonged compression of the nerve. Then, a low amplitude median motor response, a low or relatively low amplitude ulnar sensory action potential, relatively low or normal amplitude ulnar motor response, and normal amplitude median sensory action potential are found. Brachial arteriography may be needed to establish convincing criteria for an operation.

Long Thoracic Nerve Syndrome. "Winging of the scapula" due to dorsal scapular nerve entrapment and rhomboid paralysis must be differentiated from entrapment of the long thoracic nerve. This nerve supplies the serratus anterior muscle, which fixes the scapula when forward pressure is exerted with the arm. Winging of the scapula may be greater with serratus anterior than with rhomboid paralysis. Careful surgical release of the scalenus medius muscle is the appropriate treatment, but complete resolution of the winging may not be obtained. Weakness of the serratus anterior may be a late sequela of the Parsonage Turner syndrome or neuralgic amyotrophy.

Radial Nerve Syndrome. The radial nerve (Fig. 60–5) passes posteriorly from the medial to the lateral side of the humerus between the origins of the lateral and medial heads of the triceps muscle. After going through the lateral intramuscular septum, it is located in front of the lateral condyle of the humerus between two other muscles, the brachialis and brachioradialis. It bifurcates, with its deep branch passing under a fibrous edge of the extensor carpi radialis muscle and passing then through a slit in the supinator muscle.

Compression of the fibers may take place at various points of close relationship to muscle edges.

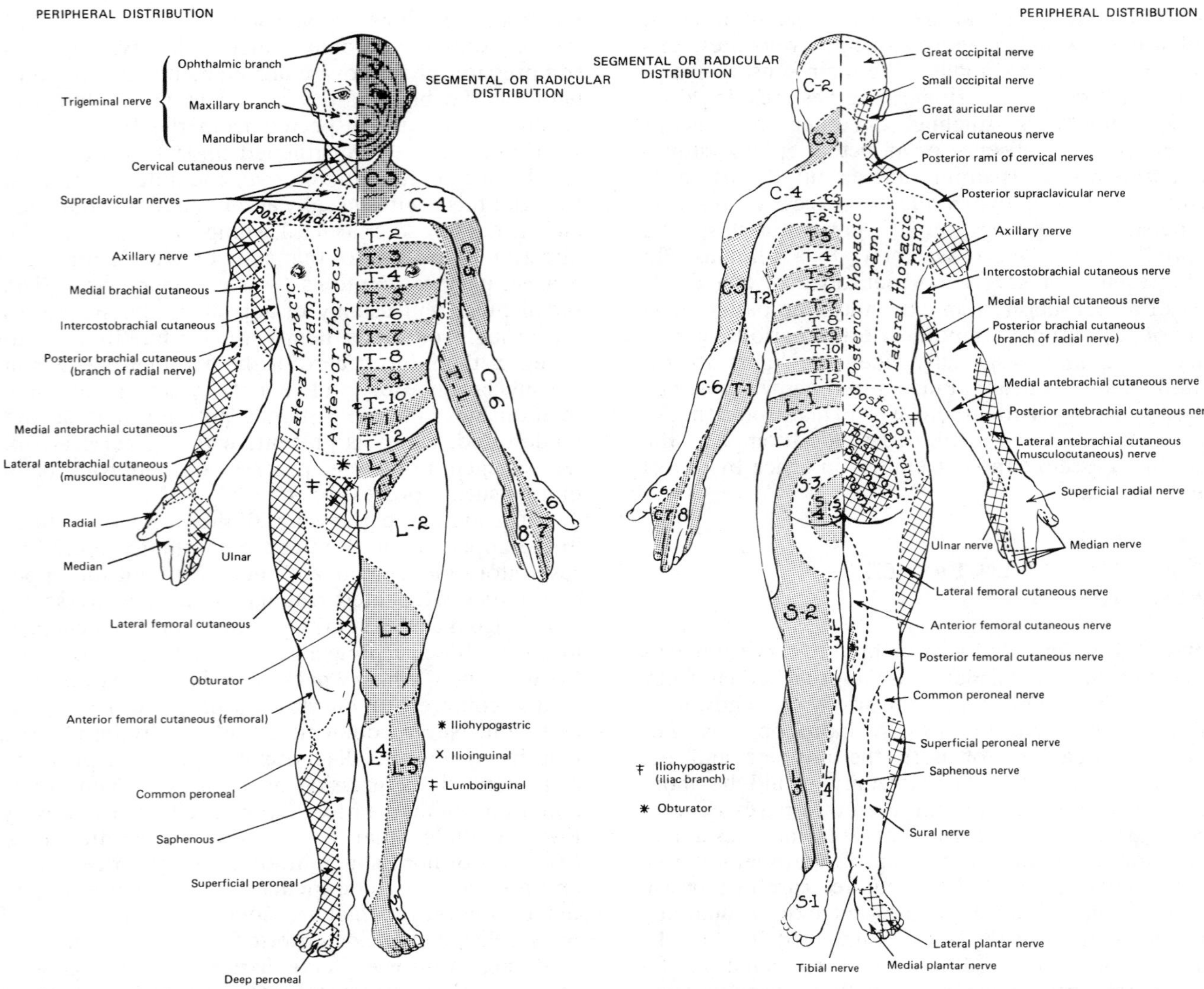

Figure 60–4. Cutaneous innervation. (From Chusid, J. Q.: Correlative Neuroanatomy and Functional Neurology. 19th ed. Los Altos, CA, Lange Medical Publications, 1985.)

The subsequent weakness is then dependent on the site of compression. Compression high in the axilla will result in weakness of extension at the elbow and wrist. Compression of the radial nerve below this level consists of pain in the elbow region with weakness and atrophy in extensor muscles below the elbow. Dorsiflexion or supination of the wrist and extension of the fingers may be especially painful. The superficial branch of the radial nerve courses in the forearm under the brachioradialis muscle, along the extensor carpi radialis longus muscle. Neurologic dysfunction of the superficial branch of the radial nerve occurs in patients when the nerve is entrapped as it penetrates the extensor carpi radialis brevis and before emerging to supply the skin in the region of the metacarpal multiangular joints, just where the strap of a heavy purse may rest. The skin in this area becomes dysesthetic when the superficial branch is compressed or becomes injured, as during removal of a ganglion at the location. The posterior interosseus branch of the radial nerve is a purely muscular branch and can become entrapped as it passes through the interosseus ligament in the forearm. The result of compression of this nerve is paralysis of extensor indicis proprius, leading to an inability to extend the index finger.

Ulnar Nerve Syndrome. The ulnar nerve (Fig. 60–6) passes through the medial intermuscular septum of the upper arm and is located behind the medial epicondyle of the elbow in the "ulnar groove," or cubital tunnel formed by a fibrous expansion of the origin of the common flexor muscle. Trauma, with subsequent scarring, acute or the result of repeated stretching of the nerve within the cubital tunnel, produces symptoms of the ulnar nerve syndrome. The localization of a block in ulnar nerve conduction is reflected in the extent of numbness to pinprick in the sensory distribution of the nerve, and in the amount of weakness and atrophy of the flexor carpi ulnaris and flexor digitorum profundus muscles.

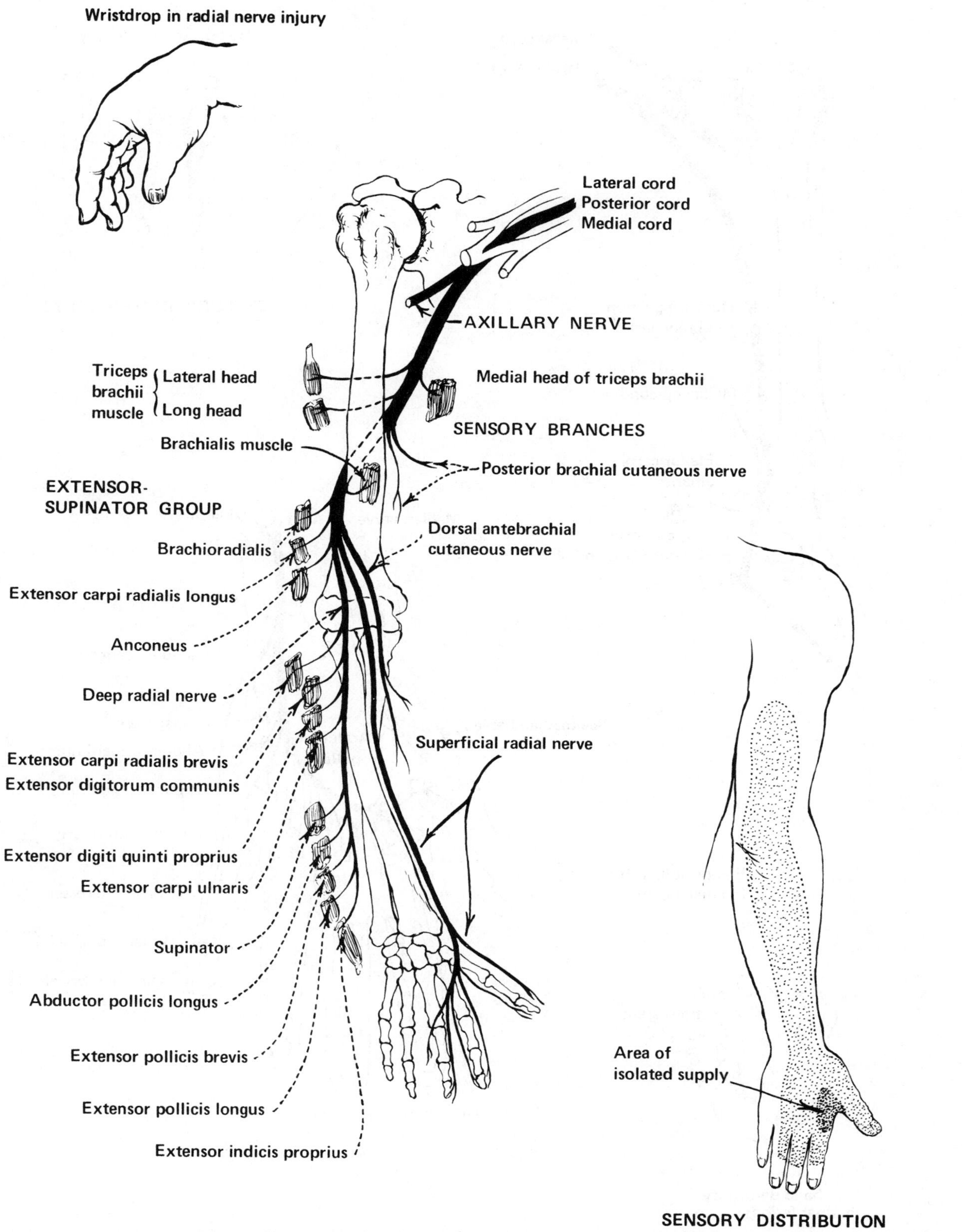

Figure 60–5. The radial (musculospiral) nerve (C6 to C8 and T1). (From Chusid, J. Q.: Correlative Neuroanatomy and Functional Neurology. 19th ed. Los Altos, CA, Lange Publications, 1985.)

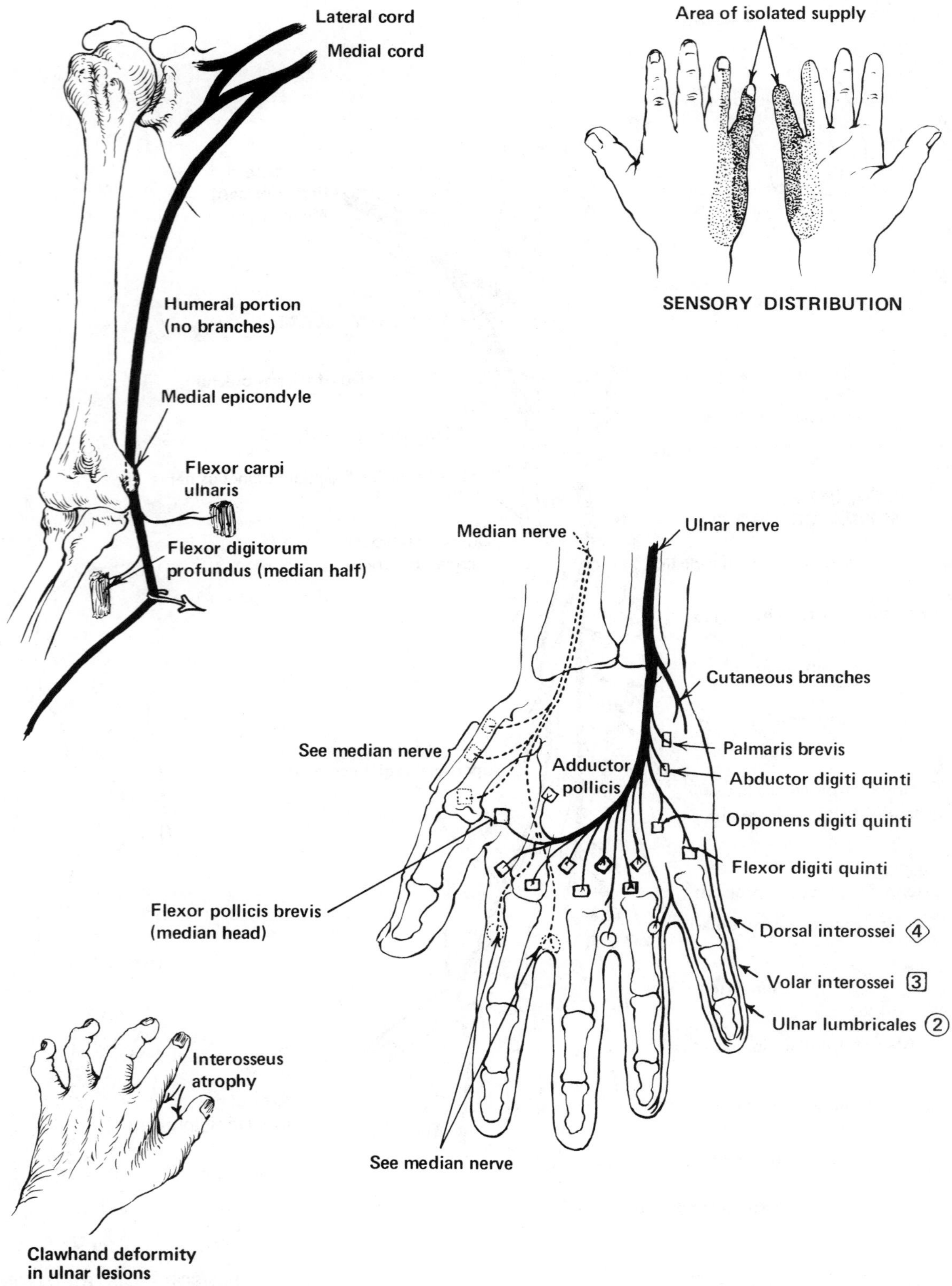

Figure 60–6. The ulnar nerve (C8, T1). (From Chusid, J. Q.: Correlative Neuroanatomy and Functional Neurology. 19th ed. Los Altos, CA, Lange Medical Publications, 1985.)

Nerve conduction velocity studies may reveal prolonged latencies across the elbow, confirming the diagnosis of ulnar neuropathy.

An awkward structural relationship between the tautness of the ulnar nerve and its proximity to the fibrous roof of the tunnel eventually compresses the nerve. *Tardy ulnar nerve palsy* is the term describing a neuropathy arising months or years after an earlier trauma; it is usually unilateral. Occupational hazards may be responsible; for example, a taxi driver who rests his elbow on an armrest, or a traffic policeman or a letter sorter in the post office who makes frequent flexing and extending movements at the elbow, pulling the taut nerve against the wall of the canal, may develop ulnar nerve palsy. A too freely moving ulnar nerve may slide in and out of the groove if the fascial covering over the tunnel is inadequate or if there is a shallow bone groove. Complete dislocation of the nerve may occur with extreme movements of the elbow. The nerve is often palpable as it is moved over the medial epicondyle. Surgical transposition of the nerve anteriorly is the best treatment for a freely moving ulnar nerve.

Injury to the *palmar branch* of the ulnar nerve in the hand may occur. Complaints of burning dysesthsia in the fourth and fifth fingers will accompany the onset of entrapment of the palmar nerve or its superficial branches against the pisiform or hamate bone. Weakness of fine movements of the fingers and atrophy of the interosseus muscles develop later. There are signs of weakness and atrophy without sensory defect when only the *deep branch* is involved. Radiologic examination of the hand may reveal a fracture or dislocation of the pisiform-hamate tunnel.

Median Nerve Syndromes. The median nerve (Fig. 60–7) passes through the pronator teres muscle and then goes under the edge of the flexor digitorum sublimis muscle to the midforearm. It can be traumatized by the fibrous edge of the sublimis bridge or stretched by the ulnar head of the pronator. Constant pressure on the inner aspect of the arm is a common cause of median neuropathy; such occurs as a result of the head of a bed-partner resting on the upper forearm (honeymoon paralysis) or from pressure from the strap of a heavy purse at the susceptible point. Numbness and dysesthesia over the radial side of the palm and the palmar side of the first, second, and third digits and half of the fourth are the main complaints. Motor signs involve the inability to pronate or to flex the wrist and fingers and loss of apposition of the thumb. In the *pronator syndrome*, pressure placed on the median nerve in the proximal portion of the forearm reproduces the symptoms of numbness and tingling. Nerve conduction velocity and electromyographic studies are helpful in differentiating the pronator site of entrapment from the more distal carpal tunnel syndromes. Surgical exploration is often necessary for definitive treatment.

The transverse carpal ligament forms the roof of the carpal tunnel. It is a thick and relatively inelastic structure; it extends from the wrist forward to the medial convexity of the thenar eminence. The motor branch of the median nerve is damaged at the distal edge of the ligament. Both wrists may have aching or pain, but the one used most will show the symptoms first. Carpal tunnel syndrome may be diagnosed when the patient complains of severe pain in the hand, often during sleep, which increases in intensity upon awakening. After several such episodes of nocturnal pain, the patient learns to shake the hand downward, holding it over the side of the bed. Running cold water over the hand and wrist will also give relief. The pain is worse premenstrually. An individual may relate it to dish washing, gardening, crocheting, or any activity requiring exertion of the wrist. Not uncommonly, a young woman in her seventh month of pregnancy may complain of hand pain. Its intensity grows until term and subsides after delivery. It is not necessary to relieve entrapment of the median nerve during pregnancy unless pain becomes very intense. This same person may develop wrist and hand pain later in life after other precipitating circumstances, such as hypothyroidism, rheumatoid arthritis, diabetes, weight gain, or simply wearing a tight bracelet or watch band. Various industrial maneuvers may bring on symptoms of the carpal tunnel syndrome.

The index and middle fingers and sometimes all fingertips are hypersensitive and eventually numb. Weakness of the abductor pollicis brevis muscle develops. Tenderness is present at the wrist. Tapping over the wrist will evoke an electric shock–like sensation in the fingers (Tinel's sign). Electrical studies of the latency of median nerve conduction across the wrist are the best way of making a positive diagnosis of the carpal tunnel syndrome. If the motor latency is greater than 4.0 msec. in the affected hand and less than that in the unaffected one, and if, in addition, the ulnar latencies across the wrist are normal, then the lesion is likely to be in the median nerve at the wrist. The latency time can be prolonged as much as 12 to 17 msec. Motor responses may be completely absent when atrophy becomes significant. An evoked sensory latency, recorded over the nerve at the wrist after an applied stimulus that is sufficient to produce a conducted impulse in the sensory fibers of the index and middle fingers, may show a prolongation when the motor response is either normal or cannot be elicited at all.

Some symptomatic improvement may be afforded by injecting hydrocortisone into the carpal tunnel, but sectioning of the transverse carpal ligament high into the base of the hand is usually necessary to relieve the entrapment.

Lateral Femoral Cutaneous Syndrome. An unpleasant burning sensation in response to touching the lateral aspect of the upper thigh has been called *meralgia paresthetica*. The lateral femoral cutaneous nerve emerges from the lateral border of the psoas major muscle and runs within the lateral wall of the pelvis to reach the iliacus fascia, and goes through an opening in the lateral attachment of the inguinal ligament. Entrapment may occur at the *anterior su-*

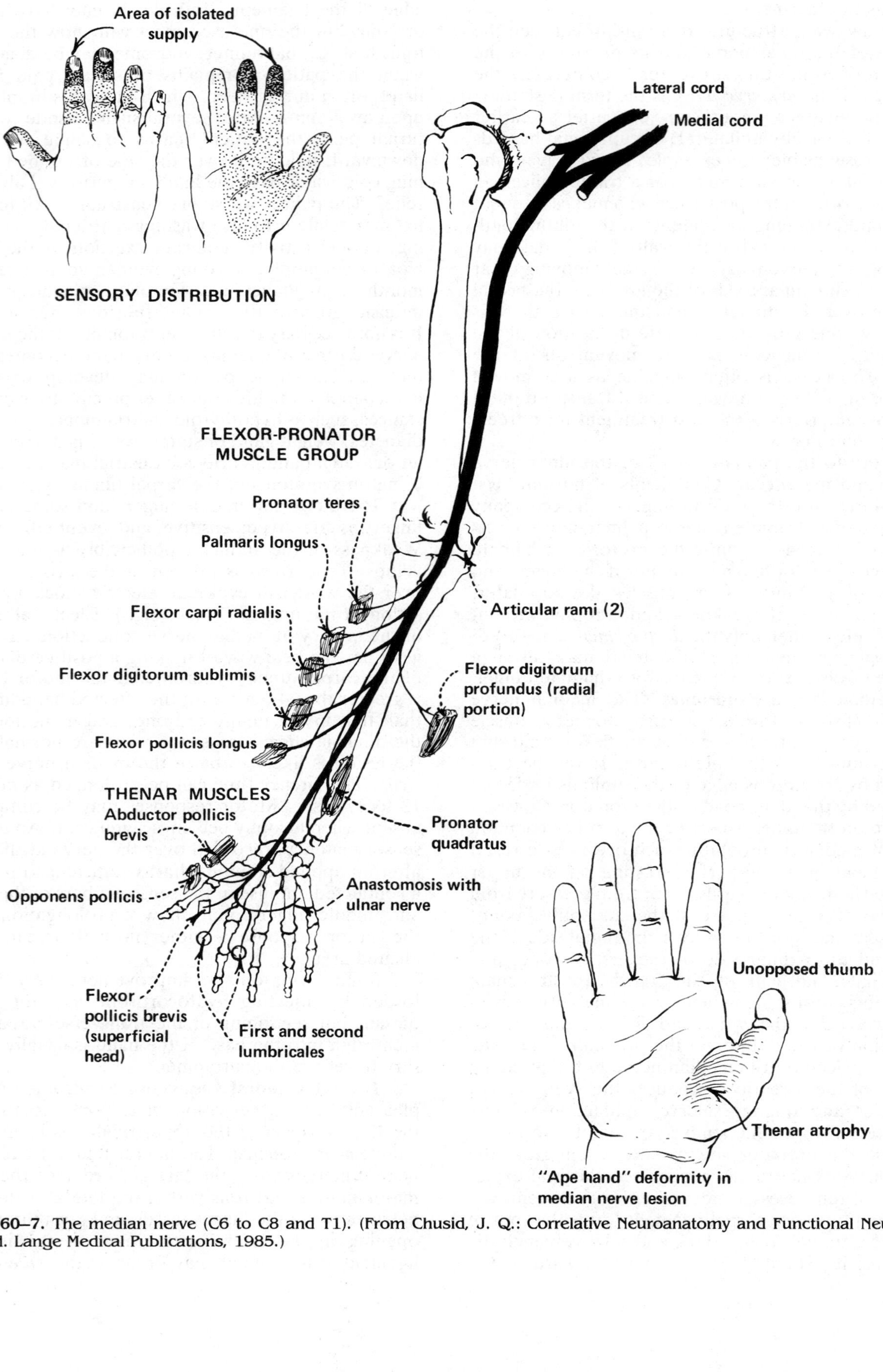

Figure 60–7. The median nerve (C6 to C8 and T1). (From Chusid, J. Q.: Correlative Neuroanatomy and Functional Neurology. 19th ed. Lange Medical Publications, 1985.)

perior spine, where the nerve passes through the lateral end of the inguinal ligament before going to the surface. The nerve may also be tensed against its surrounding muscle and fascia when the leg is abducted, with sudden shifts in trunk posture, following leg or back injuries, or after a marked increase in subcutaneous fat. Direct trauma to the nerve may occur at its site of exit or following a fracture of the anterior portion of the ilium. Rarely, a neuroma may form from repeated trauma on the nerve at the point of exit from the pelvis under the inguinal ligament. An intrapelvic neoplasm occasionally is associated with meralgia paresthetica and must be considered in all cases. In most cases, however, conservative measures are sufficient therapy. Weight reduction, posture correction by shoelifts, or improved walking habits may be sufficient to decrease the traction on the nerve at points of entrapment. Occasionally surgical exploration at the site of entrapment must be performed to give relief.

Ilioinguinal Nerve Syndrome. The ilioinguinal nerve contains fibers from root levels L1 and L2. The nerve is located within the wall of the pelvis and courses through and between the transversalis and internal oblique muscles to reach the round ligament or spermatic cord under the external oblique muscle. Pain may arise at the entrapment point in the region of the anterior spine. Radiation of the pain or dull ache to the groin and genitals from this cause often is attributed to intrapelvic disease or to disturbances in the genitalia.

Obturator Nerve Syndrome. As the obturator nerve passes out of the pelvis, its posterior division goes through the obturator externus muscle, where hip motions may cause pain. Entrapment of the nerve usually occurs in the obturator membrane as it forms a canal against the pubic bone. Adhesions within the pelvis following the rupture of an ovarian cyst have produced obturator nerve entrapment and damage. Numbness may be found on the inner aspect of the thigh, or severe groin pain may radiate down the inner side of the thigh. Adductor weakness may also develop. Intrapelvic exploration of the nerve is the only feasible definitive treatment.

Sciatic Nerve Syndrome. The sciatic nerve is made up of fibers from L4, L5, and S2 roots. After its course within the lumbosacral plexus, it traverses the pelvis and exits via the greater sciatic notch in the floor of the pelvis. External trauma to the sciatic nerve may occur, but traction on the nerve against the rim of the notch, such as may occur with a sudden, severe fall upon the buttocks, usually is the way local damage happens. Ischemia of the sciatic nerve from prolonged sitting, as on a toilet seat, compressing the nerve against the rim of the sciatic notch, may cause local neuropathy. Endometrial cysts may bind down the nerve at the sciatic notch. Mechanical trauma may occur during delivery, from the fetus compressing the nerve against the rim of the sciatic notch. Premonitory signs may be recognized during pregnancy by leg pain and paresthesias in the distribution of the external popliteal and peroneal nerves.

Femoral Nerve Syndrome. Entrapment of the femoral nerve under the inguinal ligament occurs when there is a concomitant femoral triangle hernia. Femoral neuropathy may be produced by wearing a tight panty-girdle or truss for a hernia or as a complication of a hysterectomy. Clinical features include weakness of extension of the knee, absent knee jerk, and hypalgesia over the anterior inferior portion of the thigh. The differential etiologic diagnosis of femoral neuropathy, other than entrapment, includes metabolic causes such as diabetes, uremia, thiamine deficiency, the remote effects of cancer, and vascular infarction of the nerve. Treatment is usually conservative with progressive resistance exercises. Occasionally, to maintain tone and strength of the quadriceps muscle, surgical exploration of the femoral canal may be warranted.

Common Peroneal Nerve Syndrome. The lateral position of the common peroneal nerve as it courses around the fibular neck allows it to be bruised easily (Fig. 60–8). Persons who have thin legs who bump into the corner of a desk drawer or sit with their legs tightly entwined frequently compress the nerve against the bone beneath. The peroneal nerve is the lateral branch of the sciatic nerve that divides anteriorly into superficial, deep peroneal, and recurrent nerves. Entrapment may occur along the fibrous edge of the peroneus longus muscle, over which the deep and superficial branches must pass. The branches of the common peroneal nerve may be damaged in a person wearing an ill-fitting boot or a short leg brace or cast or in a patient whose legs are held in the lithotomy position by improper placement of stirrups. Chronic bed patients whose legs are positioned by pillows may develop foot drop. Weakness of eversion of the foot and sensory changes along the dorsum of the foot and lateral aspect of the lower leg are findings in this syndrome. A complete foot drop with paralysis of dorsiflexion due to peroneal nerve involvement must be differentiated from that due to sciatic nerve or L5–S1 root involvement. Preservation of function of the posterior tibial nerve (i.e., inversion) will be of value in ruling out root involvement, since it too is supplied by those same roots.

OTHER PERIPHERAL NEUROPATHIES

Disturbances of the peripheral nerve may be classified as mononeuropathies, i.e., secondary to trauma and/or entrapment, and polyneuropathies. Generalized polyneuropathies may occur as a result of certain systemic diseases, exposure to toxic substances, as a result of nutritional deficiency, or on a genetic basis. Inflammation of support tissues around the nerves causes secondary effects on the nerves themselves. When the nerves are diseased, there are changes in the nerve cell and its axon or in the Schwann cell and myelin sheath, or both. When the pathologic change is in the perineurium and surrounding connective tissue and blood vessels, it is known as an interstitial

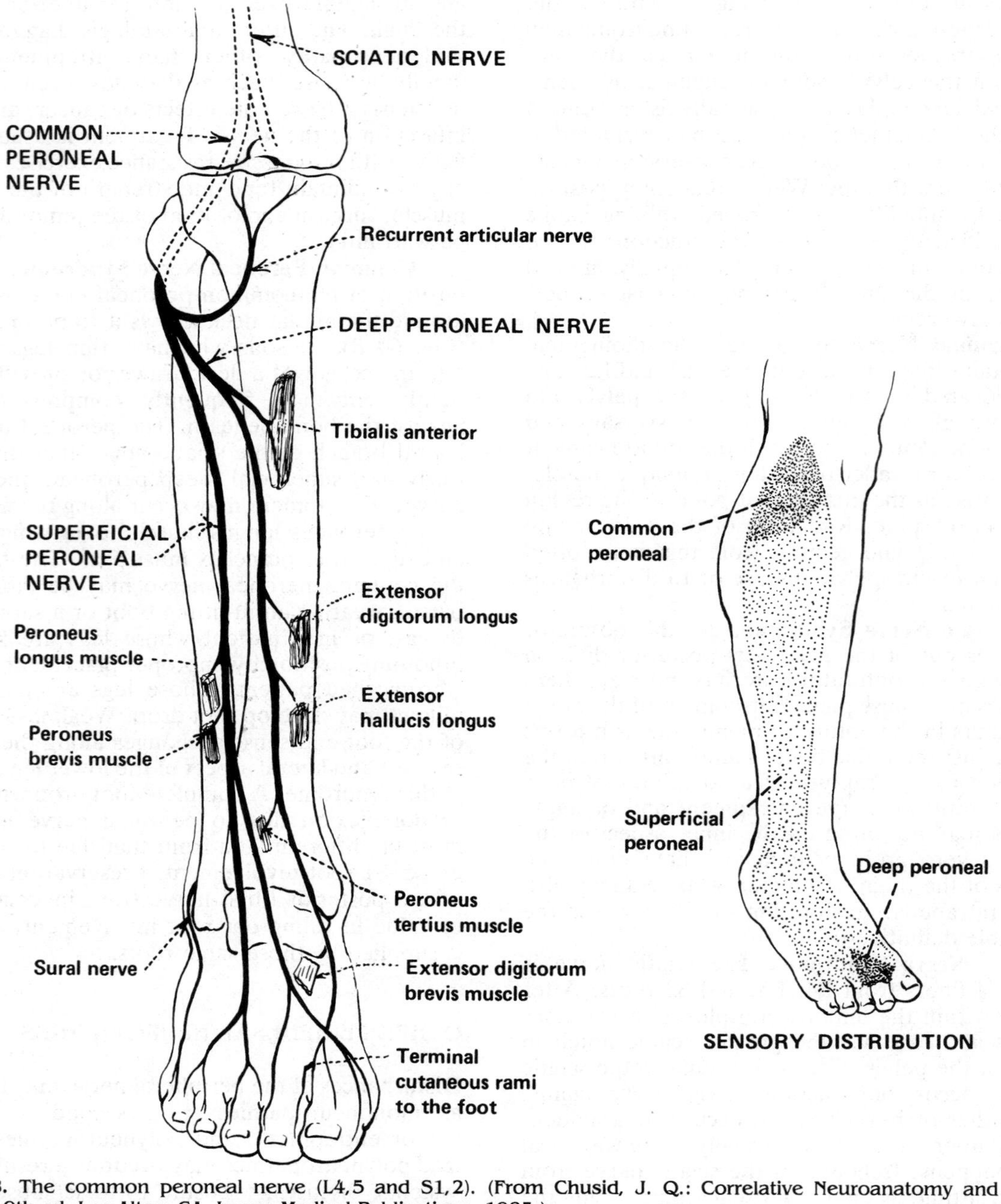

Figure 60–8. The common peroneal nerve (L4,5 and S1,2). (From Chusid, J. Q.: Correlative Neuroanatomy and Functional Neurology. 19th ed. Los Altos, CA, Lange Medical Publications, 1985.)

neuropathy. When the neuron itself is involved, it is called parenchymatous neuropathy. Examples of these neuropathies are described in the following section. Entrapment neuropathies may be concurrent in patients with parenchymatous or interstitial neuropathies, since the underlying condition may serve as a predisposing factor for the effects of compression.

Parenchymatous Neuropathies

NUTRITIONAL AND ALCOHOLIC NEUROPATHIES

Segmental degeneration in the nerve's myelin sheath, swelling of the internodal segments, and droplet formation in the myelin, with subsequent disturbances of nerve conduction, occur in patients with inadequate intake of thiamine and related B-complex vitamins. Although motor and sensory nerves are affected, the sensory fibers show earliest damage. The patient complains of "burning feet" paresthesias. Weakness and atrophy of muscles are common. Hypalgesia and hypoactive reflexes are frequent signs. Treatment includes large doses of thiamine (200 mg.) intramuscularly each day for 10 days, and B-complex vitamins, including vitamin B_{12}, given parenterally to ensure absorption. Mental changes (Korsakoff's syndrome) in the absence of adequate thiamine may develop abruptly in a patient with a chronic nutritional neuropathy. Emergency treatment with replacement vitamins must be used to reverse a Korsakoff's syndrome. Short leg braces and cock-up splints may be needed in patients with motor weaknesses. Physical therapy is usually helpful for muscle strengthening while myelin is replaced by the Schwann cells and nerve conduction is re-established.

TOXIC NEUROPATHIES

Parenchymatous changes in peripheral nerves result from exposure to and absorption of toxic substances, such as certain metals (lead, arsenic, mercury, bismuth), solvents (triorthocresylphosphate, *n*-hexane, trichloroethylene), other substances such as acrylamide, and certain of the compounds used to treat malignancies (vincristine). Histologically, toxic neuropathies are characterized by myelin destruction, paranodal swelling, and damage to axis cylinders, and sometimes neuronal chromatolysis. The symptoms are the same as in the nutritional neuropathies, but the history of exposure should be helpful in making the differential etiologic diagnosis. Chelating agents are useful in the treatment of heavy metal intoxication. Axonal neuropathies caused by toxic solvents are usually irreversible.

CARCINOMATOUS NEUROPATHY

This type of complication of neoplasia may precede any actual signs of cancer. It occurs in about 16 per cent of patients with carcinoma of the lung and 4.4 per cent of those with carcinoma of the breast. Whether the destruction of myelin is related to nutritional factors or to neoplastic toxic substances that interfere with metabolism of the Schwann cells is as yet unknown. Severe polyneuropathies, often sensory more than motor, may herald the presence of cancer long before other evidence is seen.

ACUTE PORPHYRIA NEUROPATHY

Painful paresthesias are often seen in patients who have *acute porphyria* associated with vomiting, constipation, fever, tachycardia, hypertension, and leukocytosis. During the symptoms, the urine contains increased amounts of uroporphyrin. Shortly after the abdominal cramps, a flaccid paralysis may appear involving the arms and legs. Pathologic studies have shown that the spinal cord is spared but that varying degrees of segmental myelin degeneration may occur in the more peripheral parts of the nerves. The actual pathogenesis of porphyric neuropathy is thought to be directly toxic, but this is uncertain. Treatment is symptomatic; barbiturates should be avoided since they exacerbate symptoms; ACTH and cortisone have been used with variable results.

UREMIC NEUROPATHY

Neuropathy of insidious onset, progressively involving sensory and motor functions in a symmetrical distribution in both feet and legs, and, in some instances, hands and forearms, may occur in patients with chronic uremia. Uremic neuropathy has been found to worsen after renal dialysis. The pathogenesis has been attributed to a specific uremic toxic disorder of the nerves rather than to an associated nutritional deficiency.

Interstitial Neuropathies

ALLERGIC AND POSTINFECTIOUS PERIPHERAL NEUROPATHIES

These neuropathies include instances of interstitial infiltration with inflammatory cells following serum therapy, typhoid inoculation, or smallpox vaccination. Sometimes called acute idiopathic polyneuritis, the syndrome of acute infective polyneuritis, or *Guillain-Barré syndrome,* is characterized by ascending motor weakness, areflexia, and distal sensory impairment. The cerebrospinal fluid (CSF) shows a unique change in an albuminocytologic dissociation. That is, at the onset of symptoms, the CSF may have 4 to 5 WBC's and moderately elevated protein, but after 6 to 10 days, the CSF protein may reach remarkably elevated levels (150 to 300 mg. per dl.) with only 2 to 3 WBC's or none. The CSF sugar content is not abnormally high or low. The CSF protein may stay elevated throughout the entire course of illness, returning to normal 4 to 6 months after recovery.

The signs and symptoms usually appear within a week to 10 days following an acute febrile illness, most commonly an upper respiratory infection. Over a period of several days, the weakness may progress to involve the trunk, upper extremities, face, and bulbar muscles. Urinary retention may occur. If the patient survives the initial acute phase and especially the respiratory and vasomotor collapse, which occurs in 30 per cent of cases, the prognosis is very good for complete recovery within 4 to 6 months. Treatment with steroids has no beneficial effect in the course of the illness or the mortality rate. Supportive measures, tracheostomy if necessary, and respiratory assistance are the main methods of management. In uncomplicated cases, the prognosis is usually good. Plasmapheresis instituted in the early stages within the first week of the diagnosis of Guillain-Barré is of benefit. There is a reduction of length of stay in intensive care units and ultimately a shorter length of stay in the hospital secondary to Guillain-Barré syndrome.

VASCULAR AND ISCHEMIC NEUROPATHIES

Thrombosis of a popliteal artery, an interior spinal artery, a femoral artery, or other artery may result in infarction of the area supplied by that particular vessel, and damage to if not destruction of the peripheral nerves subserved. Small nutrient arterial disease such as that in periarteritis nodosa or vasculitis may also cause ischemia in the peripheral nerves. In such conditions, single or multiple nerves may be involved, with secondary necrosis of the myelin and axis cylinders.

DIABETIC NEUROPATHY

In patients with diabetes mellitus, neuropathy is due in part to vascular abnormalities, to some obscure metabolic abnormality in the neuron itself, or to a combination of these. The incidence of neuropathy in patients with diabetes increases with the duration of the disease and the age of the patient. Patients with diabetes have a high incidence of intraneural vascular lesions, consisting of hyalinization, stenosis, and thickening of the small arterial walls. The neuropathy seems to be unrelated to the degree of therapeutic control of the diabetes. Most commonly neuropathy in diabetes involves the lower extremities, often bilaterally, and usually is a predominantly sensory impairment. Isolated cranial nerve palsies, such as third, seventh, and fifth nerve paralyses, are frequently observed in diabetics. In fact, isolated cranial neuropathies may be signs of unsuspected diabetes. There may also be autonomic neuropathy or visceral involvement, leading to vasomotor instability, pilomotor or sudomotor abnormalities, postural hypotension, sexual impotence, and bladder dysfunction. Skin atrophy and pain, paresthesias, absence of deep tendon reflexes, decreased vibration sense, and elevation of spinal fluid protein are common clinical findings.

Disturbances of Tone, Posture, and Movement of Central Origin

The localization of a lesion in the central nervous system is partly based on careful analysis of any disorders of movement. All cortical neurons are organized for special functions. In the frontal areas, anterior to the central gyrus, the neurons are responsible for voluntary movements. The motor cortex has a topographic arrangement in which the knee, trunk, shoulder, and elbow movements are located predominantly on the convexity of the brain. Lower down on the motor strip are the areas dealing with movements of the hand, face, mouth and tongue, swallowing, and speech.

Interruption of the pathway from upper motor neuron to lower motor neuron in the internal capsule or in the corticospinal tract results in a disorder of movements. Other systems are also essential in the control of movement and posture. Sensory feedback is necessary to regulate the accuracy and the amplitude in force of the motor act. Basal ganglia have a complex role, being possibly responsible for the automatic execution of the sequence of motor programs, and for providing a pathway whereby cortical regions involved in certain higher brain functions gain access to motor control mechanisms. The cerebellum is concerned with the coordination of somatic motor activity, the regulation of muscle tone, and mechanisms that influence and maintain equilibrium. Finally, the vestibular system plays a major role in the maintenance of upright posture, antigravity limb responses, muscle tone, and walking. Separation of the spinal reflex mechanisms from the vestibular complex results in decerebrate states.

TONE

Examination of a muscle at rest, whether it is of a limb, the trunk, or the neck, reveals a sense of tension that can be felt when the limb is passively moved. This is called *tone*. *Hypotonia* is a decreased to absent resistance to passive motion, and it is seen in disorders of the cerebellum and posterior columns and early in Huntington's chorea; it is associated with a feeling of flabbiness of the muscle and, on occasion, increased extensibility of muscles and limbs. Hypertonia is an increased resistance to passive motion, which is seen in such disorders as parkinsonism, paraplegia, and hemiplegias of many different kinds. There are several types of hypertonia: spasticity, rigidity, and paratonia. *Spasticity*, which follows lesions of the corticospinal tract, is an increased resistance on passive stretch that suddenly melts or gives way (the lengthening reaction of the muscle); it is often associated with hyperreflexia and clonus. *Rigidity* is an increased resistance through the full range of motion, in both flexion and extension; it is seen in disorders of basal ganglia, in particular putamen and globus pallidus lesions. *Paratonia (gegenhalten)* is a resistance that increases as the limb is passively moved; superficially, the patient seems uncooperative. Although not always present, it is seen in disorders of the parietal lobe and as a nonspecific sign of diffuse encephalopathy.

Paralysis or *plegia* is the inability to perform a movement at all. *Paresis* is a condition of weakness in performing a task. If half the body is involved, as in lesions of the corticospinal or pyramidal tracts above the foramen magnum or high cervical region, a *hemiplegia* or *hemiparesis* results. If only one extremity is involved, it is called a *monoparesis* or *monoplegia*. The anterior horn cell in the spinal cord is the neuron responsible for translating commands from the brain into actions by the muscles. Muscle tone is *flaccid* and weak and atrophy develops when there is damage to the anterior horn cells or the peripheral motor nerves. A paralysis or weakness can also be present as a result of emotional disorders, as, for example, in conversion hysteria.

Disorders of movement are categorized as either *hypokinetic*, with slowness and paucity of voluntary movements, or *hyperkinetic*, manifested by excess involuntary movements. Parkinson's disease is the best example of the hypokinetic disorders.

Parkinsonism is manifested by alterations of muscle tone and posture and the inability to initiate movement, even though there is no weakness. This is called *akinesia*. *Bradykinesia* is very slow movement. During the evolution of bradykinesia to akinesia there can be freezing or halting into a fixed posture in the midst of a muscular movement. The most common hyperkinetic disorder is tremor. Other common hyperkinesias include chorea, athetosis, ballismus, dystonia, tics, and myoclonus. These terms do not imply a specific etiologic agent; rather, they describe symptoms or signs of an underlying disease process. The term "dyskinesia" means abnormal movement. However, it is usually used to refer to "tardive dyskinesia," a choreiform involuntary movement produced by antipsychotic or antiemetic drugs. When patients are asleep, the hyperkinetic movement disorders disappear, but palatal myoclonus and tics may persist.

Chorea refers to quick, continued, fleeting, and unpredictably random movements of the limbs, lips, face, tongue, or body, along with a loss of posture. It must be differentiated from *athetosis*, in which there can be slow, writhing movements and an alternation of hyperextension with pronation and flexion with supination of the arms. Two diseases to be noted here are progressive hereditary chorea (Huntington's disease) and Sydenham's chorea. Huntington's disease is associated with cell loss and atrophy of the caudate nucleus. Sydenham's chorea is an acute disease of childhood associated with rheumatic fever, characterized by emotional lability, hypotonia, and choreiform movements of the muscles of the extremities, face, and trunk. The interval between the initial infection and the onset of neurologic symptoms is usually so long that serologic evidence of the streptococcal infection can be absent. Chorea has also been described with lupus, thyrotoxicosis polycythemia, and Lyme's disease.

Ballismus is an involuntary violent flinging movement of a limb or limbs secondary to a lesion of the subthalamic nucleus. When only one side of the body is involved, it is called *hemiballismus*.

Dystonia is characterized by movements that are of a twisting nature, ranging in speed from rapid to slow, and usually being sustained for a second or longer. When these movements are sustained, the term "dystonic posturing" is used. The great majority of patients have primary torsion dystonia, sporadic or hereditary. Secondary dystonia is caused by a great variety of disorders including Wilson's disease, perinatal cerebral injury, encephalitis, head trauma, stroke, and drugs (L-dopa, neuroleptics, anticonvulsants). Each body part can be affected with dystonic movements in different ways. Spasmodic torticollis and writer's cramp are examples of focal dystonias. *Hemiplegic dystonia* is a posture in which the paralyzed side of the body displays flexion of the upper extremity at the elbow, wrist, and fingers, extension of the leg, and plantar flexion of the foot. *Flexion dystonia* is a persistent attitude of flexion in all the limbs, with the wrists overflexed and pronated, the fingers eventually flexed (although initially extended), the legs flexed on the abdomen, and the feet plantar flexed. It may be seen in the end stage of diffuse cortical disease or trauma. *Akathisia* is a condition in which an individual has "restless legs" and cannot sit still for any period. It is seen as a concomitant of tardive dyskinesia, or following massive doses of phenothiazine, or as a side effect of large doses of L-dopa, which is used in the treatment of parkinsonism.

Tics are stereotypical, sudden, brief movements that recur at irregular intervals in precisely the same manner. They can take any form, such as eye blinking, shrugging, coughing, or twitching of various parts of the body. Tourette's syndrome is a chronic tic disorder with onset in childhood, in which there are both involuntary motor and vocal tics, which are characteristically fluctuating. *Tremor* is a rhythmic alteration in movement, faster than one per second, that tends to be consistent in pattern, amplitude, and frequency; it is usually due to the reciprocal contraction of a muscle group and its antagonist. Tremors take the form of rhythmic flexion-extension, pronation-supination, or abduction-adduction movements that disappear during sleep. Tremor can occur at rest, when a posture is sustained, or with action of the limbs. Rest tremor occurs characteristically with Parkinson's disease. Postural tremor can be "essential," "familial," or "senile." It usually involves the hands, with difficulties writing, but can also involve the head, the voice, and the trunk. Kinetic tremor occurs in cerebellar disease. The amplitude of the tremor increases as the arm is extended or the limb approaches the target.

Apraxia is the failure to perform a given motor act upon request, although the individual retains the ability to make the necessary component movements and understands the request.

In conclusion, the differential diagnosis of disorders of movement must include various processes that destroy the cerebral cortex and its pathways in the hemispheres and cause disturbances of function in the integration of control of postural reflexes. Traumatic lesions to the central nervous system may produce all combinations of pyramidal and extrapyramidal disorders. Multiple sclerosis affects primarily white matter pathways. Degenerative diseases may select either primarily white matter or gray nuclear masses. Cerebrovascular accidents may destroy gray and white matter within specific areas of vascular supply.

CEREBELLAR DISEASE

Cerebellar disease results in abnormalities (1) in the amplitude of individual movements (hypermetria or dysmetria); (2) in combining of elementary movements (asynergia); (3) in speed of alternating movements (adiadochokinesia); (4) in continuity of contractions (akinetic and static tremor); and (5) in speed of initiation and arrest of movement (dyschronometria). Ataxia of gait, with a broad base, is characteristic of cerebellar disease. Truncal ataxia is due to lesions of the vermis; appendicular ataxia, seen as overshoot, and past pointing are associated with lesions of the hemispheres. Use of a walker or cane assists in gait stabilization.

MULTIPLE SCLEROSIS

The cause of multiple sclerosis (MS) is still unknown. Lesions are multiple, with many more plaques existing than can be detected clinically. These silent lesions may become periodically symptomatic or remain dormant. Certain locations in the nervous system appear to be preferentially involved, giving rise to a constellation of symptoms, which in many cases gives a fairly typical clinical picture. The optic nerve and chiasm, the brainstem, the oculomotor system, the cerebellum, and the spinal cord are the most commonly involved sites. Acute loss or diminution of vision in one eye (optic neuropathy), double vision resulting from an internuclear ophthalmoplegia, nystagmus, incoordination and gait ataxia, long tract signs and spasticity, tingling, numbness, signs of posterior column involvement, and urinary frequency and incontinence are among the usual manifestations of the disease.

In making a diagnosis of multiple sclerosis, the differential diagnosis must include all possible remediable conditions. A foramen magnum meningioma or a cerebellar pontine angle tumor (acoustic neuroma) may produce brainstem signs of cranial neural dysfunction, ataxia, and weakness that could be blamed on demyelination in the brainstem. A sudden onset of impotence or sensory and motor signs attributable to the spinal cord may indeed be due to a large demyelinative lesion, but compression by arthritic spondylosis or a tumor within the spinal canal must be considered. Pain syndromes, such as trigeminal neuralgia, or radiculopathic pains may occur as an attack of demyelination, but local entrapment or inflammation of these nerves may produce the same symptoms. Retrobulbar optic neuritis causing visual disturbance in one eye may be associated with subsequent attacks or exacerbations of symptoms affecting other areas of myelin within the central nervous system. Sometimes, MS is a diagnosis of exclusion, but it is one that should be made with the greatest care and suspicion, since the prognosis is so variable from patient to patient and there is no specific therapy yet available.

The list of diagnostic possibilities to be considered is a long and complicated one because MS plaques may occur anywhere in the central nervous system. The symptoms of MS may be bizarre, and their occasionally extremely short duration, measured in hours and even in minutes, not infrequently leads to the diagnosis of hysteria. The first attack of MS may be indistinguishable from a postinfectious encephalomyelitis. In the young adult the suddenness of appearance of symptoms suggests MS rather than cerebrovascular accident. The neurologic complications of the collagenopathies must also be considered, however. Often the inconsistencies of the patient's complaints and findings on examination raise the possibility of psychogenic causes for the disability. This conclusion can be avoided by a careful review of the symptoms, the signs, and the tempo of the illness. If there are a variety of complaints characterized by exacerbations and remissions over a period of months or years and the findings are mainly those of dysfunction within white matter systems, then a suspected diagnosis of multiple sclerosis is justified.

An important feature of the course of the illness is the abrupt onset and occasionally extremely short duration of symptoms. Exacerbations and remissions are common but not completely understood, although the pathophysiologic mechanism of the disease explains certain of its manifestations. Myelin, rather than being destroyed, may simply be edematous, and remission may thus be the result of restoration of function in the myelin sheath. On the other hand, clinical and experimental evidence demonstrates that increases in body temperature and changes in calcium ion concentration, along with other physiologic disturbances, have transient deleterious effects on conductive properties of partially demyelinated fiber tracts, thus accounting for sudden exacerbations of symptoms. Psychological stress and physical trauma may produce similar transient effects on the nervous system of individuals with MS. This pattern of exacerbations and remission is very helpful in the diagnosis of the disease. Clinical evidence can be reinforced by various procedures, ranging from the simple hot bath test to the more sophisticated evoked response studies. In addition to demonstrating previously experienced symptoms, the hot bath test may elicit previously latent neurologic abnormalities. Visual, brainstem, auditory, and somatosensory evoked response studies may also demonstrate the existence of clinically silent lesions.

Magnetic resonance imaging has now become the test of choice to demonstrate plaques in the central nervous system and may be useful to monitor the biologic evolution of plaques and the effects of therapy. The examination of the cerebrospinal fluid for the purpose of demonstrating oligoclonal immunoglobulin G bands can be of value, since in some published series over 90 per cent of patients with definite MS have such bands. Demonstration of immunoglobulin G in CSF in concentrations above 13 to 15 per cent of CSF total protein can be made for up to 60 per cent of MS patients.

The treatment of MS remains controversial. ACTH and oral corticosteroids used for the shortening of acute exacerbations are a tested yet disputed therapy. Baclofen (5 to 30 mg. daily) and diazepam (20 to 30 mg. daily) have been valuable in diminishing spasticity and controlling painful muscle spasm and clonus. In some cases, however, such antispasticity drugs destroy the "spastic crutch" effect, leaving the patient less capable of standing than when previously untreated. Proper nutrition, physiotherapy, prevention and control of bladder infections, and psychological and social support are the mainstays of long-term therapy.

The course of the illness is "predictably unpredictable," and yet may follow several patterns. Prognosis is less discouraging than popularly reported, with one third of patients affected to such a mild degree that interference with normal daily activities is minimal and temporary. One third of patients do eventually become wheelchair-bound, while life expectancy is diminished by only 10 to 15 per cent in the most severe cases.

PARKINSON'S DISEASE

Parkinson's disease is characterized by a tremor of the opposed thumb beating against the first finger (pill rolling) or by a tremor of the roll of the whole hand (dice rolling). Increased tone and plastic rigidity appear first in the flexors of the upper limbs and are associated with delay in initiation of movement. Degrees of bradykinesia and objective rigidity are variable. As the disease progresses, the wrists become flexed and pronated, with fingers extended, and the ankles become plantar flexed. Any attempt to displace any part from this attitude meets with resistance (cog wheeling).

The pathologic process of Parkinson's disease consists principally of loss of pigmented dopaminergic neurons in the substantia nigra. This is associated biochemically with a decreased level of dopamine in the putamen and caudate nucleus.

The most specific treatment in Parkinson's disease is the replacement of brain dopamine by the oral administration of L-dopa. L-Dopa crosses the blood-brain barrier and is transformed into dopamine in the brain. Dopamine itself does not cross the blood-brain barrier. L-Dopa is most often given in combination with carbidopa (as Sinemet) to allow better absorption and higher concentrations of L-dopa in the CNS. The dose of L-dopa must be carefully regulated for each patient, since too-large doses are associated with abnormal involuntary movements, freezing, and confusion. Often the physician mistakes the increased rigidity or akinesia that is due to excess dopamine as a call for more medication; and, as is obvious, increased dosage of L-dopa in such cases causes more trouble. Reduction of dosage leads to improvement.

Long-term use of L-dopa can provide good function for a person with Parkinson's disease as long as care is given to the dosage used. Targets of therapy must be identified, such as ability to get up from a chair, turn over in bed, walk unassisted, or feed and dress oneself. The lowest effective dose should be given on a time schedule that provides sufficient "power" to function, but not enough to produce the signs of excess dopamine effect (Fig. 60–9).

However, chronic administration of L-dopa is associated with complications such as wearing-off effect of the doses or "on-off" phenomenon. The addition of another medication such as bromocriptine is often helpful in these cases. Bromocriptine can also be used de novo in newly diagnosed patients to delay the introduction of L-dopa and its complications, or added early on instead of increasing the dose of L-dopa. Patients who are on a small dose of L-dopa with bromocriptine do better than patients on larger-doses of L-dopa alone. In patients who do not tolerate or respond to bromocriptine, pergolide, a new dopamine agonist, can be effective.

Eldepryl (selegiline hydrochloride, Deprenyl), a monoamine oxidase-B inhibitor, has recently received FDA approval for use as an adjunct to L-dopa (Sinemet) for individuals whose response to L-dopa is less than optimal. In addition, eldepryl is also started at the time of diagnosis, since recent studies have suggested that it may slow the progression of Parkinson's disease.

Besides L-dopa, bromocriptine, pergolide, and

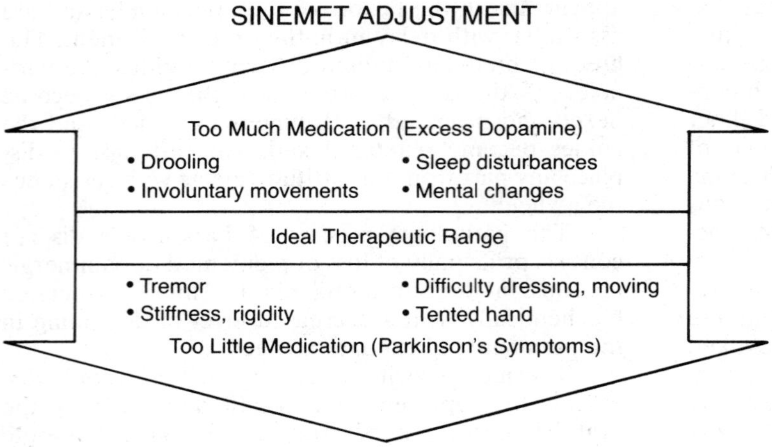

Figure 60–9. Instructional aid for dosage adjustment of carbidopa–levodopa (Sinemet) according to individual need.

eldepryl, a variety of anticholinergic medications are used, principally for the treatment of tremor. These drugs are usually combined with L-dopa. The side effects of trihexyphenidyl (Artane), benztropine mesylate (Cogentin), and amantadine (Symmetrel) are dry mouth, blurred vision, and confusion. In addition to medications, physical therapy and good dietary, fluid, and bowel hygiene must be maintained. The family must be encouraged to include the patient and to be forbearing even though the slowness of movement and speech becomes tedious.

HUNTINGTON'S DISEASE

Huntington's disease is a neurodegenerative disorder resulting from genetic expression at a locus on chromosome 4. This gene is inherited in an autosomal dominant pattern with complete penetrance. The onset of symptoms can vary from childhood to the seventh or eighth decade. Choreiform movements, intellectual decline, and emotional disturbances are cardinal features. Pathologic changes include marked atrophy of the striatum (caudate and putamen), giving the lateral ventricles a characteristically enlarged appearance, demonstrable on CT or MRI scan. Neuronal depletion is also observed in the pallidum, thalamus, cortex, brainstem, and cerebellum. This is reflected by deficiency in gamma-aminobutyric acid (GABA) and acetylcholine in the basal ganglia. Currently available pharmacotherapy for Huntington's disease remains limited to symptomatic relief of movement disorders, depression, and psychotic manifestations, with no alteration of the functional decline of the patients. Disabling chorea and some behavioral outbursts can be reduced by the use of haloperidol. Genetic counseling is important, especially since the marker for the gene has been identified, permitting screening to assess asymptomatic carriers and to make prenatal diagnosis. However, the detection of the gene requires blood samples from affected and unaffected family members, and the accuracy of the test is 95 per cent at best. In addition, subjects undergoing testing for the genetic marker should receive counseling to help them cope with the repercussions of the test findings.

WILSON'S DISEASE (HEPATOLENTICULAR DEGENERATION)

Wilson's disease, a disturbance of copper metabolism with copper overload, is a rare autosomal recessive disorder that may present at any age from 5 to 50 years. Clinical manifestations include severe and progressively disabling tremor of the extremities and eventually difficulties of bulbar function and speech. A constant sign is a circumcorneal brownish discoloration seen with tangential illumination or by slit-lamp examination of the margin of the iris and cornea. Patients show increased urinary excretion of copper (more than 100 micrograms per 24 hours) and depression of serum ceruloplasmin (below 20 mg. per 100 ml.). The neuropathologic changes seen in advanced Wilson's disease are atrophy and cavitation of the putamen, together with a striking hyperplasia of the astrocytes and a loss of nerve cells. Biochemically, copper is present in excess in all regions of the gray matter of the central nervous system. Treatment has been directed toward the use of chelating agents to remove the excess copper. Penicillamine has been preventive in members of certain families with this disease.

References

Adams, R. D. A., and Victor, M.: Principles of Neurology. 4th ed. New York, McGraw-Hill Book Co., 1989.

Barnett, H., et al.: Stroke: Pathophysiology, Diagnosis and Management. London, Churchill Livingstone, 1986.

Browne, T. R., and Feldman, R. G.: Epilepsy: Diagnosis and Management. Boston, Little, Brown & Co., 1983.

Chusid, J. Q.: Correlative Neuroanatomy and Functional Neurology. 19th ed. Los Altos, Lange Medical Publications, 1985. *An easy to use paperback desk reference for signs, symptoms, and anatomical correlations. It provides all necessary information one does not need to memorize.*

Daube, J. R., et al. (Eds): Medical Neurosciences. 2nd ed. Boston, Little, Brown & Co., 1986.

DeJong, R. N.: The Neurologic Examination. 4th ed. London, Harper & Row, 1979. *This book provides the explanations of the various useful techniques of the neurological examination.*

Diamond, S., and Dalessio, D. J.: The Practicing Physician's Approach to Headache. 4th ed. Baltimore, Williams & Wilkins, 1986.

Fisher, C. M.: The neurological examination of the comatose patient. Acta Neurol. Scand., *45* [Suppl 36]:1, 1969.

Fishman, R. A.: Cerebrospinal Fluid in Disease of the Nervous System. Philadelphia, W. B. Saunders Co., 1980.

Guidelines for the Determination of Death: Report of the Medical Consultants of the Diagnosis of Death to the President's Commission for the Study of Ethical Problems in Medicine and Biomedical and Behavioral Research. Neurology, *32*:395, 1982.

Plum, F., and Posner, J. B.: The Diagnosis of Stupor and Coma. 3rd ed. Philadelphia, F. A. Davis Co., 1982. *The best source of information about the anatomy and physiology of disturbance of consciousness. To understand coma and the related neurological phenomena is to overcome one of the most perplexing of clinical challenges in medicine.*

Raskin, N. H.: Headache. 2nd ed. New York, Churchill Livingstone, 1988.

Walsh, F. B., and Hoyt, W. F.: Clinical Neuro-ophthalmology. 4th ed. 5 vols. Baltimore, Williams & Wilkins, 1982–1988.

61

Marriage and Family Counseling

Macaran A. Baird
William J. Doherty

This chapter presents an updated model for understanding the physician-patient-family relationship and for providing primary care marriage and family counseling. Significant progress has been made in clarifying this counseling role for family physicians since the last edition of this text. Previously, the debate within academic and pragmatic family medicine was whether or not family physicians could or should aspire to provide some level of marriage and family counseling to their patients and families. Now it seems realistic to say that many primary care physicians, especially family physicians, are being trained to offer some type of marriage and family counseling. Current questions relate to the depth of counseling skill that is needed by family physicians to competently deliver the appropriate level of counseling.

The increasing integration of marriage and family therapy concepts into the literature of family medicine is one measure of the growing acceptance of such counseling as a legitimate part of family medicine. Over two dozen books from academic and practicing family physicians and family therapists are now available to encourage family physicians and therapists to work together on providing support and therapy to patients and families. *Working With Families in Primary Care* by Janet Christie-Seeley, 1984, proposes a descriptive and teaching concept for a low-key manner in which family physicians may interact with families without raising expectations about intensive therapy. Other studies in recent literature are laying the intellectual foundation that may move family medicine from the provision of good intentions to actual implementation of primary care family counseling for patients and families. The titles of these works indicate the direction family medicine is heading, which is in the direction of a primary care family-centered model based upon a team approach and emphasizing the limits of the physician acting alone as a therapist. Examples of such studies include *Collaborative Health Care: A family-oriented model* (Glenn, 1987); *The Family in Medical Practice: A Family Systems Primer* (Crouch, 1987); *Family Dynamics for Physicians: Guidelines to Assessment and Treatment* (Sawa, 1985); *Principles of Family Systems in Family Medicine* (Henao and Gross, 1985); and Doherty and Baird's two books, *Family Therapy in Family Medicine: Toward the Primary Care of Families* (1983) and *Family-Centered Medical Care: A Clinical Casebook* (1987). Since 1983 a new medical journal, *Family Systems Medicine*,* has provided a forum for ideas "at the interface of family systems and modern medicine."

Family therapy concepts and family systems ideas are becoming part of the language of family medicine. We are moving slowly toward an integrated "biopsychosocial model" of medicine as proposed by Engel (1977) in which the family physician may choose to

**Family Systems Medicine* is published quarterly by FSM, 149 East 78 Street, New York, NY 10021.

function as a primary care marriage and family counselor. However, this model is difficult to implement in practice. We are early in this journey toward integration of biopsychosocial care (Doherty, Baird, and Becker, 1987).

The next section addresses the cornerstone issue—that physicians are involved with the entire family when seeing the individual patient. Both the physician and the patient are part of interacting and overlapping systems. As family therapists such as Minuchin (1974) and Haley (1976) have emphasized, the central unit in family treatment is not the family alone but the therapeutic system, which includes both the family and the helping professional. Family physicians, as physicians of first contact to more than one generation in the family, have repeated contact with families during various predictable and unexpected events and transitions. Therefore, the starting point for a model of the family physician's role in helping families is that the physician is part of a system with patients and families.

The Therapeutic Triangle in Family Practice

The physician-patient relationship is multilateral rather than bilateral. Although most physician-patient encounters are on a one-to-one basis, the therapeutic system operates in units of at least three members—the patient, a member of the patient's family or social support system, and the physician. This therapeutic triangle is outlined in Figure 61–1. Of course, there are other members of the therapeutic system, such as nurses, referring physicians, and other family members and friends, but a three-part system is the most basic building block for viewing multilateral relationships (Haley, 1976).

The Illusion of the Dyad in Medical Practice. Modern medicine has frequently been accused of treating the disease but ignoring the patient as a person. The field of family medicine was created in part to provide an antidote to this problem. Medical schools are now offering limited training in communication skills to increase physicians' sensitivity to patients' emotional needs as well as their physical needs. The holistic medicine movement is attempting to reintegrate the spheres of the body and the mind in health care delivery—in other words, promoting the care of the whole person. These developments represent progress from the impoverished model of the disease-oriented physician. However, much of the writing in this "humanistic" approach to medical care ignores the social context of the physician-patient relationship. This view of the medical relationship as exclusively a one-to-one relationship can be termed "the illusion of the dyad in medical practice." Except in the most extreme form of episodic care, family members are involved in what transpires between the physician and the patient. Therefore, medical practice occurs in the triads rather than dyads. Family members influence the patient's selection of a health care practitioner, expectations for appropriate care, and the evaluation of the diagnosis and the prescribed treatment. Metaphorically, the family is the "ghost in the room" when the physician is interacting with a solitary patient. These influences occur even if the physician has not treated other family members; hence, every physician who deals with patients—whether he or she is a family physician or not—is involved in therapeutic triangles.

Implications of a Triangular Perspective. The clinical potential for viewing the therapeutic system as a triangle is most available to the family physician who has regular access to both the patient and the patient's key social support person(s). (For convenience, this person or persons will be referred to as "family"). Of the three sections in the therapeutic triangle in Figure 61–1, the physician-patient relationship has received the most attention from physicians and researchers alike. Other implications of the triangular perspective that have not received much attention are highlighted in this discussion.

The Family's Support of the Patient. Family physicians who overlook the therapeutic role of the family are failing to recognize a resource group who are probably the greatest full-time physician's assistants. Although physicians typically diagnose and prescribe in the office, medical treatment is usually carried out at home in the family setting. Even when hospital treatment is involved, the current trend is toward brief acute care in the hospital and early release to the home setting for continued care and recuperation. All of physician-prescribed activities, such as hygiene, nutrition, administration of medication, exercise, and rest, are performed with the support of the family. An extensive literature attests to the importance of the family in the patient's recovery from chronic illness (see the review by Pattison and Anderson, 1978; and Doherty and Campbell, 1988). The family's involvement is equally important, moreover, in the treatment of patients' psychosocial problems. Particularly when the patient is not highly motivated to change a behavior pattern, as in alcoholism and obesity, the physician may be powerless to effect an improvement without the involvement of other family members (Harkaway, 1983). In general, outside of the acute care setting of the office and hospital, the physician has relatively limited influence over the patient's cooperation with the treatment plan. The family has potentially the greatest influence. Mobilizing cooperative efforts among all three parts of the therapeutic triangle—patient, family, and physician—should yield the greatest likelihood of success with both medical treatment and changes in life style.

The Physician-Family Relationship. The quality of the physician's relationship with the patient's family may be a crucial influence on the amount of cooperation that occurs between the physician and

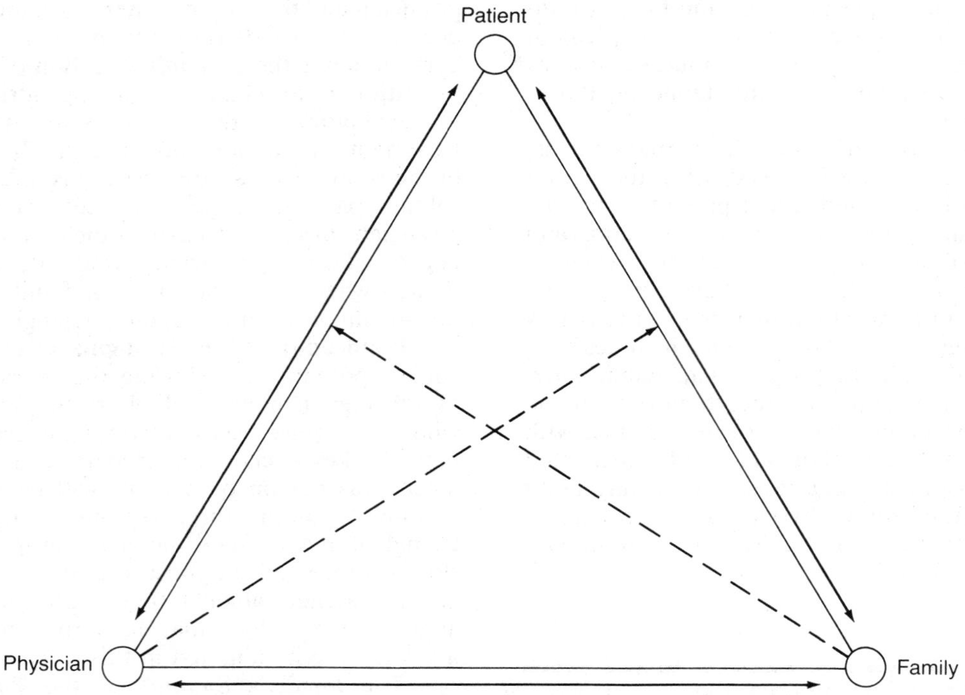

Figure 61–1. The therapeutic triangle in medicine.

the patient. The clearest illustration of this point is the therapeutic triangle consisting of the physician, the child, and the parent. Korsch and Negrette (1972) found that the likelihood of a child receiving proper at-home care after a clinic visit was affected by the mother's feelings about how much interest the physician showed in her as a person. Physicians who related well to the child but not to the mother had poorer cooperation from the family. For adult treatment, it also seems likely that a positive physician-family relationship enables the physician to gain important information about the patient's condition and to enlist the family's support in the treatment program. Generally, one would expect that the more serious or chronic the disease and the more difficult the therapeutic regimen, the more important the physician-family relationship would become.

The Physician's Support of the Patient-Family Relationship. In Figure 61–1, the dotted line connecting the physician to the mid-point between the patient and the family represents the ways in which the physician supports (or undermines) that patient-family relationship. In the field of human development, Urie Bronfenbrenner (1979) has stressed that the quality of primary dyadic relationships (like parent-child or husband-wife) is influenced by the support given to these relationships by significant outsiders. For example, the mother-child relationship depends on the support of the father; marital relationships are strengthened or weakened by the influence of the in-laws. Robert Ryder and colleagues (1971) likewise found evidence for the pivotal influence of family and friends on the development of couples' relationships during courtship and early marriage. As a significant outsider to family relationships, the family physician inevitably has an effect, whether it is for good or ill. For example, by supporting the family in dealing with chronic illness of a member, the physician may help maintain the quality of the family bonds during a period of stress. On the other hand, if a physician actively or passively takes the side of a dissatisfied and anxious wife but does not help her and her husband address their problems, then that physician is unintentionally undermining the marital relationship. There is an irony here: The most positive and intense physician-patient relationships may serve to weaken family relationships if the physician is unaware of being involved in a triangle.

The Family's Support of the Physician-Patient Relationship. Just as the physician is implicated in family relationships, the family is continually either supporting or undermining the physician's relationship with the patient, as suggested by the dotted line in Figure 61–1. In order to protect the interests of its members, the family evaluates the competence and concern of the physician. Circumstances in which the patient's trust in the physician may be tested include a diagnosis of serious illness, an uncertain or mistaken diagnosis, the suggestion by the physician that the symptoms have a nonorganic origin, and a treatment plan that is not working. The triangular model suggests that an important element in the continuation of a trusting and constructive physician-patient relationship is the family's support of the physician's role. Examples of family responses that support the physician-patient relationship are the following: "Dr. Smith usually knows what he is doing. Remember the time he caught Johnny's meningitis?" "Why don't you ask the doctor about whether these pills ought to make you sleepy; I'm sure she'll try to find something else you can take." Examples of undermining responses are the following: "He's not a specialist, you know, so he's probably not up on diabetes." "She probably wouldn't listen to your complaints; she's too busy." On the other hand, when the physician feels like disinvesting from a difficult patient, the family's active support of the physician may help keep the physician-patient relationship therapeutic and keep the patient in the physician's practice.

The concept of therapeutic triangle is a useful first step toward thinking about how a family physician might help families. However, how does a family physician become involved with families in a constructive way without being trained as a full-fledged family therapist? How does this primary care physician gauge the depth of interaction appropriate to the contextual matters we have just reviewed? After several years of struggling with these questions, the authors have proposed a second step toward helping family physicians practice family-centered care within the framework of family medicine. This second step toward implementing family systems concepts focuses upon a physician's progression through several successive "levels of involvement" with families. This concept is explained in the next section.

Five Levels of Counseling Families

As the authors became more experienced in teaching family systems concepts and family-centered care to residents and practicing physicians, we discovered what appears to be a developmental sequence that many physicians seem to go through in reaching sophistication in biopsychosocial and family-centered care (Doherty and Baird, 1986, 1987). These developmental levels of family-centered care help put marriage and family counseling skills in context for family physicians. At each successive level, family physicians can be helpful and therapeutic for patients and families. This concept helps to emphasize that it may not always be necessary or appropriate for family physicians actually to provide intensive marriage and family counseling. But under specific circumstances that relate to the context of the patient, the physician, and the family, some level of this counseling may be entirely appropriate and possible. Each of these levels can be described in terms of the associated knowledge base, personal development, and skills needed by the physician.

There are innumerable ways in which a family physician may provide counseling for patients and families. The degree to which the physician is helpful as a counselor to the couple or family is dependent on many variables such as patient and family needs, physician training, physician energy and time, other available counseling resources, patient preference, and other factors that may be unique to a specific situation. We have chosen to divide this range of physician interactions into five gradients or levels of counseling (Table 61–1). Each level builds upon the previous level of activity and expands to a more complex interaction that requires more training, more time to deliver, and greater commitment from both the physician and the family. Each higher level of counseling assumes competence at all previous levels of involvement. Based upon this framework, we then discuss the role of a family physician in relation to marriage and family counseling (Doherty and Baird, 1987).

At Level One the family physician would focus nearly exclusively on the biomedical aspects of the patient's complaint. The family would be contacted only for legal or perfunctory purposes. Within this framework, even a careful family medical history would be unlikely to reveal family or marital conflicts that might lead to a desire for counseling. Only medical knowledge and skills are necessary. Personal development of the physician is not usually a relevant factor for successful interactions. Level One may be the most comfortable mode of interaction for some family physicians, especially during early training years or the first few years of practice. Occasionally, unmanaged or unmanageable time constraints may cause almost any physician to function at this level. However, with experience and training, most family physicians move beyond Level One and provide some type of support or assistance in response to the patient's family and marital concerns. Once involved, physicians may move on to other levels and offer helpful information, support, specific interventions, or referral for counseling (see Table 61–1).

In this model, Level Two involves a more collaborative interchange between the physician and the patient and family. At this level, the family physician would be aware of the triangular nature of the doctor-patient-family relationship. Through training or practice experience, physicians functioning at this level realize that patients belong to families and that family members are important influences on the patient's health behavior and attitudes. Families are understood as potential allies in the care of an individual patient. The family history may be used to discover not only medical illness patterns but also sources of support or stress for the patient. Conducting a constructive family interview is an achievable skill needed at this level. Patient or family concerns about family relationships would be appropriate to discuss when operating at this level. A collaborative approach to the patient and family would open new sets of data for the physician. The family could be asked for support, for information, or for more resources to assist with the management of the patient's problem. If a major family dysfunction is confounding medical treatment, the physician may be able to identify this problem and refer the patient and the family to a therapist for marriage or family therapy. Collabora-

Table 61–1. LEVELS OF PHYSICIAN INVOLVEMENT WITH FAMILIES

Level One: Minimal Emphasis on the Family	Level Two: Ongoing Medical Information and Advice	Level Three: Feelings and Support	Level Four: Systematic Assessment and Planned Intervention	Level Five: Family Therapy
This baseline level of involvement consists of dealing with families only as necessary for practical and medical-legal reasons but does not include communicating with families as integral to the physician's role or as involving skills for the physician to develop. This level presumably characterizes most types of medical school training in which biomedical issues are the sole conscious focus of patient care	Knowledge base: Primarily medical, plus awareness of the triangular dimension of the physician-patient relationship Personal development: Openness to engage patients and families in a collaborative way Skills 1. Regularly and clearly communicating medical findings and treatment options to family members 2. Asking family members questions that elicit relevant diagnostic and treatment information 3. Attentively listening to family members' questions and concerns 4. Advising families about how to handle the medical and rehabilitation needs of the patient 5. For large or demanding families, knowing how to channel communication through one or two key members 6. Identifying gross family dysfunction that interferes with medical treatment, and referring the family to a therapist	Knowledge base: Normal family development and reactions to stress Personal development: Awareness of one's own feelings in relationship to the patient and family Skills 1. Asking questions that elicit family members' expressions of concerns and feelings related to the patient's condition and its effect on the family 2. Empathically listening to family members' concerns and feelings, and normalizing them where appropriate 3. Forming a preliminary assessment of the family's level of functioning as it relates to the patient's problem 4. Encouraging family members in the efforts to cope as a family with their situation 5. Tailoring medical advice to the unique needs, concerns, and feelings of the family 6. Identifying family dysfunction and fitting a referral recommendation to the unique situation of the family	Knowledge base: Family systems Personal development: Awareness of one's own participation in systems, including the therapeutic triangle, the medical system, one's own family system, and larger community systems Skills 1. Engaging family members, including reluctant ones in a planned family conference or a series of conferences 2. Structuring a conference with even a poorly communicating family in such a way that all members have a chance to express themselves 3. Systematically assessing the family's level of functioning 4. Supporting individual members while avoiding coalitions 5. Reframing the family's definition of their problem in a way that makes problem-solving more achievable 6. Helping the family members view their difficulty as one that requires new forms of collaborative efforts 7. Helping family members generate alternative, mutually acceptable ways to cope with their difficulty 8. Helping the family balance their coping efforts by calibrating their various roles in a way that allows support without sacrificing anyone's autonomy 9. Identifying family dysfunction that lies beyond primary care treatment and orchestrating a referral by educating the family and the therapist about what to expect from one another	Knowledge base: Family systems and patterns whereby dysfunctional families interact with professional and other health care systems Personal development: Ability to handle intense emotions in families and self and to maintain neutrality in the face of strong pressure from family members or other professionals Skills The following is not an exhaustive list of family therapy skills but rather a list of several key skills that distinguish Level Five involvement from primary care involvement with families 1. Interviewing families or family members who are quite difficult to engage 2. Efficiently generating and testing hypotheses about the family's difficulties and interaction patterns 3. Escalating conflict in the family in order to break a family impasse. 4. Temporarily siding with one family member against another 5. Constructively dealing with a family's strong resistance to change 6. Negotiating collaborative relationships with other professionals and other systems who are working with the family, even when these groups are at odds with one another

tion and information exchange are key themes at this level.

At Level Three, the physician would be skilled at collaborative interactions and information exchange but would also be trained to offer supportive counseling to patients and their families to help them deal more successfully with family stress and emotional reactions. Feelings and affectively laden issues are commonly discussed at this level. Family members' reactions to the primary patient's illness may lead to mutual concerns about how the patient or family is coping with the medical problem, with life cycle transitions, work stresses, or any other major life circumstance. At this level, the family physician may become involved in providing supportive counseling while consulting with or referring the patient to a trusted therapist as needed. Hallmarks of this level of counseling by family physicians include a clear grasp of the limitations of the physician's skill, time, and energy, plus a well established network of support for this physician. Such activity presumes that the physician-counselor understands his or her own feelings regarding the patient or family engaged in counseling, a sound knowledge base about normal family development and reactions to stress, and modest skill in assessing how well the family is functioning. (More detail about family assessment is presented later in this chapter.)

Level Four builds upon the previous levels and involves family and marital counseling by the family physician using specific strategies (1) to assess family functioning, (2) to create modest change in family interactions for families trying to cope with a medical issue, (3) to initiate focused interventions for alcohol or drug abuse, (4) to assist families' coping with other crises, and (5) to develop and maintain a supportive network of therapists and community resources to create a therapeutic team. Therefore, much of the information presented in this chapter is most relevant to the physician who strives to interact at Level Four.

Level Five is formal family therapy. This moves beyond the primary care domain into specialized family treatment. The distinguishing feature of family therapy in this model is that the therapist is trained to deal with entrenched family dysfunction, high degrees of family resistance, strongly negative affect, and pressure to draw the therapist into counterproductive coalitions. Few family physicians are prepared for this level of counseling with families without special fellowship experiences. Family therapists usually have at least a master's degree in a mental health field and several years of supervised experience and are certified by national or state organizations. There are a handful of family physician/family therapists in the United States. Most have become full-time medical educators, some have shifted the focus of their practice toward therapy, and others are practicing family-centered care with a team including other family therapists (Doherty and Baird, 1987; Glenn, 1987).

To summarize this concept, we believe that physicians can interact helpfully with families at several different levels. Each of these levels of counseling implies a greater degree of physician involvement, with each having a minimum knowledge base, degree of personal development, and specific skills needed by the physician. Even if a family physician is trained to counsel at all five levels, there are many situations in which the higher levels of counseling are not possible or not appropriate. Just as surgeons do not always operate when consulted for a patient's problem, family physicians who are able to offer marriage and family counseling do not apply these skills unless the situation indicates such an investment for both the physician and the family. Sometimes, the patient and family primarily need their physician to share information in a collaborative manner or simply to inquire how they are feeling about a medical or social crisis. When more involvement with the family is indicated, the family physician may be available and effective at providing primary care level marriage and family counseling. It is appropriate to address the context of the family physician. In the background is the reality of the physician's busy workday and multiple demands upon time, energy, and intellect. Counseling is most meaningful if the physician (1) has established a respectful and caring relationship with the primary patient, (2) has energy and time to offer to the couple or family, (3) has created a supportive network to allow collaboration with therapists or other interested physicians, (4) has structured the work environment to permit extended office or hospital visits, and (5) charges appropriately for the professional counseling efforts. The remainder of this chapter orients the physician to marriage and family counseling at Levels Three and Four. These levels of counseling with families are outlined in Table 61–1.

Assessment and Counseling Techniques at Levels Three and Four

This section discusses specific assessment categories the family physician can use to gain a clearer picture of a family. Generally, a confident assessment of a family's level of functioning requires assessing the whole family, but preliminary hypotheses can be formed from interviewing individual family members.

Unfortunately, the field of family therapy lacks the refined diagnostic categories and procedures available in biomedicine. There are no widely accepted and clinically practical diagnostic tests or instruments that can be used to determine family dysfunction, although quite a large number of instruments have been described in the research literature (Jacob and Tennenbaum, 1988).

Our conviction is that there is no substitute for careful analysis of the family's life situation and interaction patterns and that this analysis can be done only through interacting with the family in the context of the therapeutic triangle. The assessment categories and indicators described here are derived largely from the work of Salvador Minuchin (1974), although almost all family therapists would also use at least our four core dimensions: stress, adaptability, cohesion, and interaction patterns. Olson and associates (1979) have documented the universality among family therapy theories of the concepts of adaptability and cohesion. Interaction patterns, as we have noted, are a more core element in all systems approaches to the family. Finally, stress, which is a trigger for many types of family dysfunction, must be included in a family assessment.

WHAT ARE THE SOURCES OF STRESS ON THIS FAMILY?

Stress occurs when events or situations strain the family's resources. Minuchin divides the sources of family stress (or stressors) into internal and external categories. Prominent among internal sources are family life cycle changes and the illness and disability or death of family members. External sources include stressful contact of one member with extrafamilial forces such as school and work, and stressful contact of the whole family with extrafamilial forces such as the welfare system or a depressed economy. Of course, families often are suffering from both internal and external sources of stress. McCubbin et al. (1980) have discussed how stressors accumulate in families: some families can handle the main stressor such as illness or unemployment but fall apart under added strain, such as of adolescents leaving home or elderly parents becoming more dependent.

The Family Life Cycle as a Stressor. Families move through a common (though not universal) sequence of transitions and transformations, just as the individual human organism goes through predictable changes from infancy to old age. A prominent and universal source of stress for families lies in the challenge of adjusting to a new stage in the family's career (Carter and McGoldrick, 1980). One way to demarcate stages in the family life cycle is as follows: (1) the newly married couple, (2) family with young children, (3) the family with adolescent children, (4) the launching phase, and (5) the older family. An increasingly common variation on this "typical" sequence is a divorce, a period of single parenthood, and remarriage into a "reconstituted family." The main point is that any significant transition can strain the family's resources for reorganizing itself. The presence of stress in a family may suggest "growth pains" more than serious family dysfunction. Minuchin (1974) criticizes some family therapists for being too ready to label a family as dysfunctional when it is merely reacting to a temporary dislocation.

To focus on the family as a social system in transformation, however, highlights the transitional nature of certain family processes. It demands an exploration of the changing situation of the family and its members and of their stresses of accommodation. With this orientation, many more families who enter therapy would be seen and treated as average families in transitional situations, suffering the pains of accommodating to new circumstances (p. 61).

Individual and family problems, then, may stem from the stress of a transitional process in the family's career. A stomach problem may be related to the shakedown process of a new marriage, the burden of a newborn infant, the addition of a second child, the challenge of an emerging adolescent, concern about the physical decline of one's parents, or the fear of being dependent on one's children in old age. Equally or more stressful are the adjustments to being divorced and restarting a family.

Illness and Disability as Stressors. The threat or the reality of the loss of a family member or that member's normal role in the family is tremendously unsettling for the family. In one family we have worked with, the mother was found to have multiple sclerosis. In another family, the husband never resigned himself to his wife's multiple sclerosis and their relationship began a slow decline toward eventual divorce. In neither case did the illness cause the family dysfunction, but it did tax the family system beyond its strength. Both families may have remained functional under less severe stress. In the face of a chronic illness or disability, some families never reorganize and, therefore, suffer severe hardship, whereas other families adjust in such a way that the family needs the individual to remain sick and dependent. It is especially difficult diagnostically to differentiate families who are appropriately supporting their disabled member (such as a retarded child) from families who are oversupporting the member by keeping that person dependent.

Extrafamilial Stressors. The physician may determine that the family is basically healthy but suffering from externally caused stresses affecting either individual family members or the family as a unit. Job-related stress, for example, is reported to be widespread. According to Gunby (1981), the National Center for Health Statistics found that about one in four Americans report that they experience a great deal of emotional stress on the job. In some cases, the physician may want to call upon community resources. In areas where such resources are inadequate, then the physician may want to take the plunge into "community therapy" by trying to bring new resources to the community. In any case, it is important to support the family itself; help it adapt, if necessary; and not imply that the family itself is the focus of the problem.

HOW ADAPTABLE OR RIGID IS THE FAMILY?

In the face of normal and abnormal stress, some families do quite well and other families break apart or develop a dysfunctional stability. According to Minuchin and many other family therapists, the key to family coping is family adaptability. Adaptability is the family's ability to respond flexibly—particularly to modify its interaction patterns if necessary—in the face of stress. Poor adaptability or rigidity is a sure indicator that the family needs specialized therapy instead of primary care counseling.

After Minuchin's (1974) discussion of the misdiagnosis of dysfunction that is ascribed to some families who are experiencing the normal strains of adapting to change, he goes on to discuss the other dimension of family adaptability:

The label of pathology would be reserved for families who in the face of stress increase the rigidity of their transactional patterns and boundaries, and avoid or resist any exploration of alternatives. In average families, the therapist relies on the motivation of family drama, entering into transitional coalitions in order to skew the system and develop a different level of homeostasis (p. 60).

How can family physicians assess the family's level of adaptability? The authors propose two ways: first, through the family's history (as taken verbally from family members and as observed by the family physician), and second, through "nudging" the family in family counseling and observing whether or not it changes. The history approach yields crucial information on precipitating events and on the chronicity of the problems. The longer the family has lived with the problem, the more rigid the family system is apt to be when faced with the task of changing its interaction patterns. For example, alcohol abuse of long duration clearly suggests a family with a low level of adaptability. A more flexible family would have either solved the problem or split apart. The same holds for dependency on prescription drugs, except here physicians may be active participants in the family dysfunction. The authors believe that dependency on prescription drugs generally indicates dysfunction in the therapeutic triangle. In fact, rigid and dependent families frequently draw kindly but unwary physicians into rigid and enmeshed relationships with themselves. This dynamic renders the family more difficult to treat for an outside therapist unless the therapist can change the rigid family/physician interaction pattern (Selvini-Palazzoli et al., 1980).

A second way to assess family adaptability is to engage the family in a counseling relationship and to observe any change that takes place. This approach is similar to the way physicians handle some medical problems of uncertain etiology. Sometimes it is worth beginning treatment with a low-risk medication whose success or failure will yield diagnostic information, such as administering antibiotic therapy for infections of undetermined etiology. In assessing family functioning, the physician may be uncertain from the history about the extent of the family's rigidity. In such cases, primary care family counseling (with an agreed-upon limit of sessions before a referral) gives the physician a much clearer picture of the family's functioning. For example, a Level Four interaction would occur if the physician helps a couple agree to spend a few hours together without the children during the next week. Their success in carrying out the task gives the physician information about their flexibility as well as about the likelihood that they need formal family therapy as opposed to more primary care counseling at Level Four.

HOW COHESIVE IS THE FAMILY?

Some families allow members to support one another emotionally and physically while holding onto an adequate degree of autonomy or separateness. Maintaining the balance between family and self is a continual challenge for all individuals. Too much cohesiveness results in family enmeshment, a situation in which family members are too close to each other; they are overprotective and overreactive to one another's pain (Minuchin, 1974). Diagnostic signs of enmeshment in a family are (1) members speaking for one another; (2) continual interruptions while someone is speaking; (3) high levels of emotionality, such as tears in one member "spreading" quickly to others in the family; (4) overprotective responses; and (5) either an unwillingness to discuss conflicts and negative feelings for fear of hurting someone or reactive conflict in which family members flare up angrily at apparently small provocations.

At the other extreme from an enmeshed family is a disengaged family in which family cohesion is sacrificed in favor of individual autonomy. Family members go their own way, do not respond quickly to emergencies, and are emotionally unreactive to one another. The latter point is crucial to note in the diagnosis of disengagement, since avoidance behavior in a family can also be the temporary result of enmeshed relationships that have become too painful. The key difference is that enmeshed relationships still are highly volatile emotionally, even when members are trying to avoid one another, whereas people in disengaged relationships are generally emotionally shut off from one another, although they engage in conflict if one member provokes the other.

It should be noted that often in dysfunctional families, one subsystem or relationship (for example, mother with adolescent child) may be overly close or enmeshed while another (e.g., father with same adolescent child) may be disengaged. Moreover, terms like enmeshment and disengagement are not precise diagnostic categories with unmistakable behavioral indicators. They are among the best concepts we have in the field, but the dimensions of their boundaries themselves still need to be clarified. A relatively gross assessment of enmeshment or extreme disengagement would be comfortable for physicians functioning at Level Three. To intervene with such families would quickly move to Level Four (planned intervention) and may often require Level Five consultation or referral to initiate family change.

WHICH REPEATED INTERACTION PATTERNS IN THE FAMILY ARE RELATED TO THE PROBLEM?

The answer to this question provides a dynamic quality to family assessment. According to Watzlawick and Weakland (1977), leaders of the interactional school of family therapy, the heart of family assessment is the analysis of the interactional context of dysfunctional behavior, i.e., how the problem can be understood as emerging from the ebb and flow of family behavior within the overall interactional structure. A fine-grained analysis of this interactional context can provide the key to solving the problem by changing its family context. Attempts to change well-established family interaction patterns would involve family counseling at least at Level Four. Frequently, this is the heart of Level Five (formal family therapy). Watzlawick (1977) gives the following example of an interactional diagnosis:

For a relationship to be viable, there has to be a minimum of that kind of mutual understanding which is colloquially referred to as 'knowing where one stands with the partner.' What constitutes that minimum may vary greatly from one individual to another; for whatever reasons in their individual past, some people get along with very little of it, while others need a lot. Assuming now that a husband belongs to the former class of people and his wife the latter, a typical conflict will very probably arise in their marriage. Since the wife does not get enough information from her husband to know 'where she stands' with him, what he thinks and feels about her and their shared life, etc, she is likely to try to get this information by asking him pertinent questions, watching his behavior, searching for further clues, and the like. In all probability he will find these behaviors excessively curious and intrusive. Notice that up to this point there is nothing even remotely 'pathologic' about their relationship. They simply operate with two different ideas about what their degree of understanding and closeness should be, and neither of these ideas is wrong per se—they are simply different. But the situation is unstable and unless they manage to decrease the discrepancy of their views, their interaction is bound to escalate. The more she seeks the missing information, the less likely he is to give it, and the more he withdraws and keeps her at a distance, the harder she will try to establish closeness. Both are thus caught in a 'more of the same' interaction in which, typically, a solution is sought through increased effort that precludes the solution. The rest of this fictitious, yet everyday story is easy to imagine. By the time professional help becomes necessary, her behavior satisfies the established clinical criteria of pathological jealousy (pp. xiii–xiv).

Minuchin (1974) and Haley (1980) emphasize those interaction patterns that maintain clear boundaries (optimal cohesion) across family subsystems so that members can have both the support and the autonomy appropriate to their age and position in the family. Stated simply, Minuchin and Haley believe that parents should cooperate with each other, the couple should give each other more emotional support than either gets from the children, and parents should be in charge of their children. When this family hierarchy is firmly in place, then parents are not likely to either undercontrol or overcontrol their children, and adults are free to work out their problems between themselves. Common dysfunctional interaction patterns that undermine this hierarchical arrangement occur when (1) one parent repeatedly allies with a child against the other parent; (2) the oldest child is thrust into the "parental child" role with inappropriate responsibilities for the other children; (3) one parent develops a closer allegiance with a grandparent than with the co-parent; (4) an unsatisfying marriage leads one parent to derive too much emotional support from a child; (5) the children continually play one parent off against the other; and (6) the family physician or other outside professional gets incorporated into a coalition with one family member against another. Changing these interaction patterns may be accomplished at Level Four if these patterns are recently established and not firmly woven into the fabric of family functioning. However, if initial attempts to confront such patterns are not successful, the physician could recognize that family therapy is indicated (Level Five).

Communication in families can be viewed as an aspect of family interaction patterns. As Watzlawick et al. (1967) maintain, all behavior—both verbal and nonverbal—in an interactional situation has message value, i.e., is communication. Two basic categories for assessing communication in families are (1) the directness of the communication and (2) the congruence of the communication. Directness refers to whether family members communicate through intermediaries (for example, a son tells his mother when he is angry at his father) or can deal in straightforward fashion with one another as individuals. In some families, the members speak for one another; if you ask Sara a question, her mother answers for her. The implicit interactional rule: No one can have a direct relationship (communicate with) Sara except through the mother. Congruence, which is closely linked to directness in communication, refers to whether the verbal and nonverbal channels of communication are sending the same message. When family members are angry with one another, do they laugh or give long speeches or avoid contact? Or do they more congruently express this anger by both words and tone of voice? Families develop implicit rules for what can be communicated about and what cannot: Certain feelings or wants are acceptable and others are negatively sanctioned. Since feelings tend to "leak out" whether they are sanctioned or not, families in which open expression of negative feelings is not permitted will experience high levels of incongruent—and confusing—communication.

Despite the importance of communication in families, however, we do not list it as a separate assessment category because we believe that much "poor communication" stems from larger structural and interactional issues (like ongoing coalitions), which make effective communication nearly impossible. For example, if a father and a daughter are aligned against the mother, then communication between mother and daughter is bound to be skewed. If a husband continues to have an affair against his wife's wishes, their communication will deteriorate severely. The authors note these points because newcomers to family counseling sometimes assume that all family problems stem from "poor communication" and can be solved by getting people to talk more directly with one another. Although it is often helpful to get family members to be more direct and congruent, in our view communication patterns flow inexorably from the underlying dynamics of the family system and, therefore, must be evaluated and dealt with in the context of wider family assessment and treatment issues. In the midst of treating medical problems, a physician may discover such problems in communication. Short-term and well-focused intervention may resolve such difficulties (Level Four). For example, the physician might ask an anxious and constantly intervening mother if the daughter who presented with a medical complaint could answer the pertinent questions directly rather than through the mother: "Mrs. Smith, I have learned a great deal from your description of your daughter's problem. Now, I need to hear more from her."

If several gentle attempts to draw this boundary around the daughter and promote more direct communication fail, then the physician may choose to ask for assistance from a collaborating therapist.

Family Assessment for Family Physicians

The field of family therapy (see ms. p. 61–27) is still searching for reliable, valid, and clinically practical assessment instruments that lead to clear treatment decisions (Jacob and Tennenbaum, 1988). Many of the best assessment instruments are to be used for research purposes only and either are too long for use in family practice offices or require video equipment and trained observers (Cromwell et al., 1976). Brief assessment methods have proved difficult to validate or are poorly related to clinical issues. Academic family physicians have directed some attention to biopsychosocial assessment, including family assessment (Smilkstein, 1978, 1980; Medalie et al., 1981; Henao and Gross, 1985). Although numerous approaches to family assessment are presented in academic centers, the authors have chosen to present only one technique that is especially useful for practicing family physicians—the genogram or family tree.

The Genogram (Family Tree). One way to understand a complex family system, especially a three-generational family or a "reconstituted" family created by the merger of two divorced people, is to diagram the family. The family diagram is used extensively by the Bowen school of family therapy (Bowen, 1978; McGoldrick and Gerson, 1985) and has been used in a limited form by genetic counselors for years. Family medicine has borrowed the approach and expanded it by including both biomedical information and psychosocial information. Depending on the family physician's purposes and available time, the genogram can serve as (1) a quick overview of family members and their interrelationships, (2) a way to visually overlay biomedical and psychosocial information, and (3) a study tool for gaining a comprehensive understanding of multigenerational family systems. See Chapter 74 for instructions and illustrations on how to construct a genogram. Basically, include all members of at least three generations of the family as well as both spouses' families. Ages or birthdates of family members can be added, dead members can be indicated with a slash, and known chronic diseases can be indicated by an appropriate symbol in the box for each member. A key for the symbols should be placed at the bottom of the genogram. Conflict can be symbolized by jagged lines between certain family members. Enmeshment can be marked by extra heavy lines between two or more members, and coalitions by lines separating two members from a third. Divorce can be documented with a disconnected line and the year of the divorce, with the noncustodial parent's new family penciled in. The genogram, then, can be used to store practically any information about the family.

The complexity of the genogram depends on individual needs. Family physicians in busy office practices probably confine themselves to a rapid sketch of the genogram when they are dealing with large family systems. In other cases, when such information can be stored mentally or does not seem especially relevant to the presenting problem, many family physicians do not use a genogram at all. Generally, however, the genogram can be a useful tool for bringing order out of chaos. Its chief limitations are the time spent in construction and the fact that it provides only "static" data and not interactional data about the ebb and flow of the family's interactional structure. It is a useful tool for a more structured interview when family or marital counseling is initiated.

Functions of Level Three Marriage and Family Counseling

Level Three marriage and family counseling assumes that the physician can already function adequately at Level Two. Level Three counseling has four distinct functions or purposes: education, prevention, support, and challenge. Supervision and training assist physicians in understanding their own feelings during these interactions. It is fundamental to this level of counseling for the physician to have insight into his or her emotional responses and appreciate the importance of emotional expression in the family. This moves beyond the "common sense" role of the compassionate physician.

Education. Sometimes families get themselves into trouble because they are faced with unfamiliar situations. New parents argue heatedly over getting up with the baby when he cries at night. The wife of a man depressed over the loss of his job grows progressively more agitated when he does not snap out of his depressive symptoms. A husband is upset over his wife's diminished sexual interest during pregnancy. A recently divorced woman believes that she must be going crazy because of her mood swing, and fears her children will inevitably be damaged by the divorce. If these individuals and families are reasonably well functioning, the above situations lend themselves to a family counseling intervention by the family physician in the role of teacher. Physicians of course have been filling this role for centuries, but generally the teaching has been done mainly with individual patients (usually the wife or mother) rather than with a couple or family. *It is far better to educate all the involved parties as a group.* This way the physician can maintain a relationship with the whole therapeutic triangle. At Level Three counseling, the physician inquires as to the family's feelings about the current crisis or their reaction to the new information presented by the physician.

Many educational efforts are made ineffective, however, when translated by a patient who wants to make a point. Some examples include: "The doctor says to let the kid cry, just like I told you," "The doctor says you're making things worse by nagging me," or in one of our favorites, the mother of three small children told her husband, "The doctor said my stress comes from being cooped up with little kids, so I'm going back to bartending in the evenings." This husband, by the way, tended to be jealous of his wife and she tended to be flirtatious with men.

Educating the couple or whole family gives each member access to the same knowledge and same opportunity to ask questions. With the physician's help, the family can then apply this information or advice to their own situation; for example, clear expectations about the course of an illness can help the family reassign family responsibilities. If education is to lead to action, the commitment of all the involved family members is required; sometimes this means bringing grandparents into family counseling, especially if the doctor's ideas are quite different from the family's traditional notions.

Family sessions also give the physician the opportunity to teach in one of the most effective ways—by modeling. The physician can deal with the depressed, unemployed husband in a way similar to how the wife could deal with her husband, that is, with sympathy for his suffering (address his feelings), with understanding that depression cannot usually be "willed" away (information), but with firm expectations that he will participate in his own recovery and refrain from manipulating others into catering to him unnecessarily. The same kind of modeling can be quite helpful for families trying to cope with the physical illness of a member: The physician can show the family how to combine strong support with clear expectations for the patient's independence. Opportunities for such family life education occur every day in family medicine.

The educational function of family counseling brings to bear the family physician's knowledge in such areas as family dynamics, child development, stress during the life cycle, and mental and physical illness. By assembling the family members to discuss their current difficulty, the physician can more effectively educate, can avoid disturbances in the therapeutic triangle, and can model the behavior being taught. By recognizing and diffusing the affective responses of the patient and family to the information being presented during the educational interaction, the physician may "clear the air" and improve the climate for the sharing of information.

Prevention. Prevention in family counseling may be viewed as a special kind of education concerned with avoiding common problems encountered by families during their life cycles. If education to ameliorate problems is more desirable than waiting until therapy is needed, then preventive family counseling is better still. Since people have routine medical needs throughout their lives, family physicians are uniquely situated to deliver preventive family counseling. Any of the transitional points in the family life cycle is appropriate for such an intervention, but perhaps the most well-documented need is for prophylactic treatment of couples who are expecting their first child. One of the most consistent findings in family sociology is that the average couple experience an enduring decline in marital satisfaction following the birth of the first child, a decline not experienced by couples who do not have children (Rollins and Cannon, 1974). Clinically, the move from a dyad to a triad can be seen as leaving someone feeling outside. The father may feel jealous of his wife's preoccupation with the baby; the wife may feel divided between husband and baby. The husband and father may experience stronger needs to earn money and be successful in his job; thus, at a time when the wife needs him more, the husband may be more preoccupied with the outside world.

The family physician can try to prepare couples for these transitional stresses through preventive marital counseling. Prospective parents tend to be focused on the childbirth to the exclusion of considering their future life as parents. Some ideas can be presented during prenatal visits, and then more intensive preventive counseling can begin after the birth. Issues the physician can bring up include the couple's expectations of each other for child care, their employment plans, their plans to spend time alone as a couple, use of relatives as babysitters for relief from child care burdens, whether and how soon to have another baby, birth control, and child-rearing values and techniques, including those learned in their families origin. To move from Level Two to Level Three with this preventive interaction, the physician would inquire of the husband's and wife's different reactions to these issues. One research finding can be stressed: Couples who maintain a high level of companionship activities may not experience a decline in marital satisfaction after the baby comes.

The transition of the birth of the first child is just one of many examples that could be developed to suggest the place for preventive family counseling. Some other family life cycle stress points are the birth of the second child, the challenges of adolescent children, and the increasing dependency of elderly family members on their adult children. Preparing families for these expectable stresses by presenting information and discussing reactions to it can allow them to cope more successfully.

In addition to preventing problems associated with life-cycle transitions, preventive family counseling can help avoid dysfunctional coping with medical problems. A common illustration is a husband's first myocardial infarction. Here a preventive intervention with the couple should be considered as part of the standard treatment protocol. The danger these couples face, of course, is that their marital roles will quickly resemble a nonsexual nurse-invalid relationship. The preventive counseling should be done with both spouses present, even if one or both appear uncomfortable (and even if the physician is uncomfortable). If the spouses are counseled separately, neither will be certain about what the doctor told the other one. Together they can both hear the good news that the husband is still a man and that she can still be a wife.

Support. Providing support for individuals and families is the foundation of all counseling. Hence, support is involved in the other three functions of family counseling. It is singled out here because sometimes support is all the family physician needs to provide a family. The supportive function of family counseling is aimed at helping the family through a difficult time by being available, by listening attentively, by helping family members express their feelings, by showing one's concern, and by letting the family take responsibility for its own resolution of the difficulty. In a primarily supportive family counseling session, then, the physician would do little in the way of education or problem-solving. This relatively passive counseling role may be quite difficult for physicians who prefer a more active role.

Supportive family counseling is most clearly indicated when a family has suffered the death of one of its members. Since the physician is trained to view the death of a patient as personal failure, he or she may be reluctant to give the family the time and attention required for supportive grief counseling. The emotional force field that families create is nowhere more keenly felt than when a member has died, particularly if the death was unexpected or ill-timed. The death of the family patriarch or matriarch, the death of a spouse/parent during the child-rearing years, and the death of a child are examples of particularly troublesome losses for families. What families need is support through their process of grieving, healing, and recovery. They must learn to accept the loss and to reorganize themselves without the missing member. If not handled carefully, the wound opened by a significant loss may not heal—leading to the impairment of one or more members—or the emotional wound may leave a scar, resulting in a diminished quality of personal and family life.

Challenge. There is an old statement of purpose among pastoral counselors that applies to family physician counselors as well: to comfort the disturbed and to disturb the comfortable. Two goals of challenging the family are comforting the disturbed, which refers to the supportive function of counseling, and shaking up those with an illusory sense of good health or with rigid ways of viewing problems. One of the most effective ways of constructively challenging a family is to offer a family systems perspective on the problem and then stress the urgency of a collaborative solution. The physician can point out a couple's troublesome interactional structure and challenge them gently but firmly to work together at changing it. Also, parents can be challenged to collaborate in disciplining their children instead of arguing about who is responsible for the family troublemaker. A test of the family's adaptability is how it responds and whether or not it changes after the counselor makes a challenging observation about the family's interaction patterns. Some adaptable families have an enlightening experience and begin to change their interaction patterns. Other families reject alternative solutions or are unable to implement them.

Challenging or confronting families about serious problems is a risky but sometimes necessary part of the primary care of families. It is risky because the family may resist, disagree, or verbally attack the physician who is criticizing the family. Why is it sometimes necessary? Since families often become stabilized around the major dysfunctions of their members, a major jolt may be needed to create the possibility of change and healing. Chemical dependency is a classic illustration in primary medical care of the symptom that the family protects in one of its members: Husband: "I have a few beers every evening." Wife: "Yes, he doesn't pass out like he used to. Now my uncle, there was an alcoholic."

Sometimes the family physician may initiate supportive or educational counseling with a family and subsequently discover that the family is more dysfunctional than anticipated. The physician can then switch from an educational supportive/educational mode to a challenging mode. One outcome of a successful challenge concerning a serious family problem can be a referral for therapy. The referral should be made to a known and trusted source, it should be rapid, and it should be followed up to make sure that the family kept the appointment and is progressing in treatment. Successful use of challenge and referral during the process of family counseling can keep the physician out of long-term unproductive counseling relationships and can mobilize the family to accept the more intensive help it needs.

Basic Techniques in Primary Care Family Counseling

Family counseling is more an art than a science, more a fluid series of exchanges than a set of discrete behavioral techniques. Counselors and therapists with widely different styles may arrive at very similar results: Some counselors are more feeling oriented and some more task oriented; some are quite active in the session, others are relatively passive. Despite these differences, the authors believe that there are a number of fundamental guidelines for family counseling by family physicians—guidelines that cut across personality types of the counselor and, to some extent, the kinds of family problems being treated. Eleven basic family counseling techniques are discussed in this section. The first of these are presented within the limits of Level Three counseling techniques.

LEVEL THREE FAMILY COUNSELING TECHNIQUES

Engaging the Family. The first step in any helping effort is to engage the patient, in this case the family. Engaging refers to the process of meeting and establishing the beginning of a trusting relationship with family members. Engaging a couple or family is more difficult than engaging an individual patient. Since they are accustomed to one-to-one relationships, physicians are apt to relate to a couple as "a patient + one," and to a family as "a mother + others." Making personal contact with a family requires making personal contact with each family member. This is the first guideline for engaging a family: Talk to each member separately at the beginning of the session. The conversation can be casual and informative: How old are you? Where do you work? What do you do for fun? How do you like school? You might want to begin with the spouse or parent whom you know the least, for example, the husband whose wife is your primary patient. In other words, it is often useful to begin immediately by building a bridge to the person who is the most distant on the therapeutic triangle. When there is an identified patient like a child who acts out, you should probably not begin by asking that child any questions. A child who is placed under pressure will not communicate if the physician moves in too quickly. Generally, a good rule of thumb is to start interacting with the adult family member whom you may know least well or with the child who seems most removed from the problem.

This warm-up period is intended to put the family at greater ease and to give them a sense of who the physician is. Social time also helps the counselor begin to get a feel for the family, i.e., its mood, activity level, authority structure, language patterns. The counselor is then able to adapt to the family's unique style, a process Minuchin calls "joining the family." Some families are "hot" and some are "cool," some use intellectual language ("We don't communicate"), whereas others talk concretely ("He watches T.V. instead of talking to me"). The counselor can best engage a family initially by employing the language of the family. Similarly, families tend to have a member whose opinion counts most on matters of importance (such as whether to return to family counseling). The family counselor can sense who holds this role and make a special point to honor this member's authority. The underlying goal here is that the counselor communicate to the family an acceptance of them as a family.

In summary, engaging the family involves two steps: (1) social conversation with each family member and (2) adapting the counselor's style to the family's style. If this critical first task has been done well, the next step follows naturally. The question to be addressed is: "Why are we all here?"

Establishing the Agenda

It is often helpful to ask the family about their understanding of the purpose of the family conference. Even if the physician has called the meeting and, therefore, has a particular agenda, individual family members may have different objectives. If the physician begins by announcing *the* agenda, important information may be missed about family members' expectations. For example, at one family conference called by the medical team to summarize the diagnosis and treatment plan for an elderly patient, two family members said that their goal was to find out why grandma kept "worrying herself sick." An unexpectedly useful counseling session followed.

After asking each family member what he or she wants to accomplish in the family conference, the physician can then state his or her goals, and propose a way to try to meet everyone's expectations or to determine what expectations are realistic for this conference and what will require follow-up. By using this procedure to set the agenda, the physician can begin the heart of the family session with all family members in attendance for the discussion.

Switching from Talking About Facts to Talking About Feelings. Perhaps the key skill for a physician in conducting Level Three family counseling is that of moving from discussion about medical facts and treatment plans to family members' emotional responses to the medical problem. Most family conferences begin with a Level Two discussion centering on relevant information. After all, emotional reactions are usually tied to perceptions of the patient's diagnosis and prognosis. During the initial phase of most family conferences, then, the discussion consists of explanations, questions, and answers. Moving to the issue of feelings does not happen automatically, particularly because families have been socialized by medical personnel to "keep to the facts" and not waste valuable professional time with emotional expression.

Here is a useful technique to move the discussion to eliciting an emotional response. After making sure the family has asked all their questions, the physician can say: "Now I'd like to know what this experience has been like for you emotionally," or "How are you folks handling all of this?" If no one responds immediately, the physician can say: "I imagine that this has been upsetting or worrisome for some of you." Most families respond openly to such requests for emotional responses. For those who do not respond, the physician can say in an accepting manner: "Sometimes it's hard to talk about these things." Then the family conference should be brought to a conclusion. The physician's job is to offer emotional support, not to require the family to be open.

Normalizing Feelings. One of the most important contributions a physician can make to a family's emotional well-being during a medical crisis or after a loss is to help family members understand that their emotional responses are understandable and normal. Feelings such as fear, grief, anger, guilt, and relief can accompany a serious medical illness, treatment relapses, death, and life transitions such as divorce. Family members can feel ashamed if they have emotions that do not seem "rational" or "proper." And some families have rules discouraging members from openly sharing their feelings in times of crisis. The presence of an encouraging and gentle physician can help family members open up to each other about painful feelings and accept such feelings as natural. The physician can say things such as: "Many people feel the way you do in this situation." The physician can also normalize a *range* of feelings in the family, indicating that not everyone reacts the same way at the same time. An example is "Right now, John is dealing with this diagnosis by feeling angry at himself for smoking all these years, whereas Linda is feeling a lot of sadness. It's O.K. to feel differently. Both feelings are normal and likely to change as time goes on. There is no "right" way to feel right now, and it would help if you could accept each other's feelings and not argue about who has the right approach."

Avoiding Premature Reassurance. Some physicians equate Level Three counseling with reassurance. When a wife first expresses her fear of her husband dying from a repeated myocardial infarction, the physician who moves too quickly to reassure her cuts off her opportunity to express her feelings more fully and be heard by the physician and her husband. Initially, empathetic responses are better, such as: "I'm sure that's a big worry for right now," or "It's hard living with that fear right now." The physician can then ask the husband if he has the same worry. The result might be the first time the couple has openly expressed their feelings on this subject and can enhance their intimacy as they move through the next phase of recovery. After feelings have been explored to the family's limits or wishes, the physician can offer reassurance about the odds of a repeated myocardial infarction but once again should say that the fear is normal and is something the family will have to live with.

Anticipating Challenges Ahead. Part of the educational task of Level Three family counseling is to help the family anticipate future challenges to their ability to cope with a health problem. An example is a family conference to communicate the diagnosis of Alzheimer's disease. The family physician can gently warn family members about the changes that are likely to occur in the patient's functioning and the increased burdens likely to be felt by the principal caretaker. The physician can say that family members sometimes get into needless conflicts when members disagree about whether to take an optimistic stance ("Dad looked and sounded great today") or a more pessimistic stance ("He may have looked O.K. today, but you don't see him as often as I do"). By counseling in a Level three mode, the physician can help the family deal prospectively with what lies ahead for them, and can encourage them to work together as a family coping unit. The physician can offer to meet again with them to help in this process of family adjustment over time.

A CASE ILLUSTRATION OF LEVEL THREE COUNSELING

The following case example is a case written by Stephen Spann, University of Oklahoma, in *Family-Centered Medical Care: A Clinical Casebook.*

I was called to the rural home of Mrs. M, a 73-year-old widow, mother of 14, who was chronically bedridden. As I drove the 15 winding miles to her hillside home, I remembered her past history.

I had first met Mrs. M some 2 years ago when she was admitted through the emergency room with an acute myocardial infarction. At that time she gave a 5-year history of being confined to bed, secondary to diffuse osteoarthritis and morbid obesity. Her hospital course was stormy; she kept going in and out of multifocal atrial tachycardia and remained on the verge of respiratory failure secondary to restrictive and obstructive lung disease. She was discharged home to the care of a loving extended family. Most of her children lived close by and took turns staying with her, providing her with the best of home care. I made periodic house calls to follow her progress; she did well for some 3 months. She suddenly became acutely ill and was readmitted to the hospital with pneumonia and respiratory failure. Endotracheal intubation and mechanical ventilatory support were required, but the patient survived. During a family meeting prior to discharge, she requested never to be intu-

bated again. The family and I agreed and I sent her back home; she had done well until now, almost 2 years later.

Upon arriving at Mrs. M's home, I found her to be alert but in moderate respiratory distress. My diagnosis was pneumonia with acute respiratory failure. I reviewed our previous contract with Mrs. M and her family, and offered the option of hospital readmission. Mrs. M requested admission for symptomatic relief, insisting that I promise that she would not be intubated for mechanical ventilation. She improved minimally with antibiotics. What initially appeared to be pneumonia proved to be metastatic renal cell carcinoma. The patient was begun on hormonal chemotherapy and sent home on chronic oxygen therapy. In a family meeting prior to discharge, the patient requested to be allowed to die at home and never to return to the hospital. Her family was supportive and continued their usual excellent constant home care.

I sensed that the patient did not have long to live. I visited Mrs. M. and her family as often as I could, although I had little in my curative armamentarium to offer. I directed my efforts toward ensuring her comfort and supporting the family. My visits became longer. Sometimes I stayed long enough for a piece of homemade pie and a cup of tea, taking the time to get to know my patient and the family better. I learned that she had been born nearby, married young, and delivered 10 of her 14 children right there on the side of the hill where she now lay dying. I came to know all of her children who lived in the area and to feel almost like a member of the family myself. Strong, close, and cohesive, the family seemed to be dealing very well with the stress of their mother's terminal illness.

Around 2:00 A.M.*, on a cold winter night, I received a call from one of Mrs. M's daughters who seemed to be in a state of panic. The entire family assembled, and Mrs. M appeared to be dying. "Shouldn't we transfer Mother to the hospital to see if we can do something to save her?" I offered to come to the house immediately. When I arrived I found Mrs. M to be uncomfortable and in moderate respiratory distress. She was lethargic but squeezed my hand in recognition. I increased her oxygen flow and gave her a narcotic injection. She responded quickly and began to rest and breath easier. All of her children were present. I stayed some 2 hours, reassuring them of the correctness of her dying at home, supporting them, and reminiscing with them about her long and full life. Mrs. M died quietly the next afternoon. I attended her wake a few days later and was welcomed by the family as an esteemed friend.*

(DOHERTY AND BAIRD, 1987, pp. 61–63)

Level Four Family Counseling Techniques

There are many situations when more than Level Three counseling is needed. Sometimes the family is trapped in a dysfunctional pattern that needs a specific nudge or intervention to move into a more adaptive pattern. Family physicians can gain a knowledge base, a set of attitudes, and specific skills that are essential to any helper who provides this level of assistance to families. This section presents a brief description of the themes, techniques, and circumstances that are appropriate to this level of counseling families. Fundamental to this discussion is the understanding that this more in-depth counseling is done by a physician who is part of a network of skilled helpers. These techniques are not offered as a manual for family physicians to become independent family therapists but rather as guidelines for those family physicians who wish to become skilled in marriage and family counseling while working as part of an interdisciplinary team. In this discussion, the authors do not presume to present a framework through which family physicians could become autonomous, credentialed family therapists. That degree of expertise (Level Five counseling) is beyond the scope of this chapter. Examples of Level Five family therapy in a family practice setting are found in Doherty and Baird (1987).

Structuring the Session. At this level, initiating a family interview is viewed as the first stage of initiating a planned intervention. Just as a successful artist must be in control of the artistic medium, a successful counselor or therapist must have control over the counseling session. The counselor must be able to decide on the structure of the session and adhere to it within reasonable limits. For example, the time to socialize with each family member may have to be protected from a family member who wants to monopolize the physician's attention. The following is a structuring statement: "Mrs. J., I'd like to come back to that point after I've had a chance to get to know the rest of your family."

Level Four family counseling presents greater control difficulties than does individual counseling. Family members may collude unconsciously with one another to stay away from topics the counselor wants them to discuss. Members may compete for speaking time during the session, or some may withdraw into the background of the conversation. The counselor is apt to be swept away by the family's well-rehearsed interaction patterns. When the family meets the counselor, there is always an underground power struggle; failure to gain control over the counseling sessions after repeated tries indicates that the physician/counselor should seek consultation or refer the family for therapy.

Structuring the session means being able to enforce the physician's rules when they conflict with the family's. The authors suggest several core family counseling rules within the realm of Level Four:

1. Each person has the right to speak without being interrupted. Some families are chronic interrupters; no one finishes an important thought. If the physician permits interruptions, he or she perpetuates this dysfunctional interaction pattern. With an interrupting family, the physician can make the rule explicit: "I would like everyone to get a chance to speak without being interrupted." Then the physician must enforce the rule.

2. When it has been announced what the physician wants to do, the physician should not become sidetracked. If you say the physician wants to ask everyone's opinion, he or she should not let an

argument between two family members prevent every members opinion from being heard. The family will know that the physician did not follow through on his or her intention, and the two combatants unconsciously may have wanted to avoid hearing someone else's response.

3. The physician should steer the family back to the issues at hand when the discussion strays. One of the best ways to avoid confronting a problem is to keep changing the subject, as anyone who has ever served on a committee can attest. An effective counselor has a homing sense for staying with important issues. A common family escape is to complain about people not present in the session, such as in-laws, school teachers, or other physicians. In the presence of one's wife, it may be easier to complain about one's mother than about one's wife. A simple way of getting back on the track is to say "I'd like to return to what you were talking about earlier." After repeated failures to retrack the family, the counselor can confront them about their pattern of moving away from certain issues. This confrontation can be done with a supportive acknowledgment of the family's fear:

Physician: I've noticed that when I ask you to talk about your relationship as a couple, you end up talking about Mr. J's mother. She must be an important person in your marriage. And I think it may be hard for the two of you to just talk about your own relationship. Is that true for you, Mr. J?

4. The physician should resist requests for solutions if he or she thinks the requests are premature or inappropriate. Some patients and families want to jump from a hasty identification of a problem to an immediate solution, preferably one proposed by the physician. In order to spend enough time exploring the problems and getting family members to talk with one another honestly, you may have to sidestep family members' requests for definitive advice. They may be expecting you to write a family prescription after a 20-minute evaluation. The request for a solution can be handed back to the family in a number of ways:

Physician: I think we need to understand more about what's going on first.

Physician: The solution is going to have to come from all of you as a family. I have some ideas to offer, but only you know what kind of family you want to have.

The point here is that the physician/counselor should take responsibility for the timing of the counseling process and, therefore, must resist being pulled into an expert advisor role for a family that has not squarely confronted either its problems or its own resources for change.

5. The physician should take charge of the physical arrangements of the session. The authors prefer to have family members sit in a circle, with the counselor having a favorite chair reserved. It is diagnostically useful to see how family members place themselves within the space you provide; e.g., do the spouses sit far apart? If the physician wants people to change seats during the session so that, for example, a married couple can talk more directly with each other, they should be asked to move.

6. The physician should take charge of who attends the counseling sessions. If the children are asked to be present, insist that they be there. If a child or spouse feels free to show up one time and not the next, the counseling cannot work.

In Carl Whitaker's approach to family therapy, the first significant phase of therapy is the "battle for structure" (Whitaker and Keith, 1981). This issue is just as important for primary care family counseling. It is only when the family perceives the physician as the leader of the session that the family feels secure enough to delve into painful material. Family counseling can begin with an authoritarian flavor and move toward democracy: The counselor controls the sessions at the outset like a parent or teacher, then later, when this leadership role is clearly established, the counselor can let the strings of power return gradually to the family.

Defining the Problem. After each family member has had the opportunity to give an initial statement about the problems that brought the family to counseling, the counselor can move to define these issues more clearly. A common approach used by family therapists is to ask family members to specify the changes they would like to see in the family. This puts the issue in a positive form, i.e., changes they would like to see as opposed to a negative form of complaints about others' behavior. Often this reversal of direction requires coaching from the counselor.

Physician: Mrs. J., what changes would you like to see in your relationship with your husband so you could be happier in your marriage?

Mrs. J.: I just want him to stop avoiding me so much.

Physician: Rather than putting it as what he should stop doing, would you say what you would like him to do more often, or something you would like to see him start doing?

Mrs. J.: I would like him to stay home with me in the evenings and pay some attention to me.

A start has been made toward defining this marital problem. The problem is constructively described as the wife wanting more time and affection than the husband is giving her. "I want to be around you more" is a more positive beginning for problem solving than "You go out too much; you just want to avoid me."

Thus, the first guideline for defining the problem is to specify what changes family members would like to see. Preferably these requests for change should be concrete rather than global.

Mrs. J.: I wish he would be more attentive to me.

Physician: How could he show that he was attentive?

Mrs. J.: By staying home with me once in a while and talking to me instead of watching television.

By asking the wife to specify what sort of specific behavior change she wants from her husband, the counselor has begun the process of helping them find solutions to their problems.

When the physician has helped one person to clarify his or her goals, move on to another. It is very important, especially in marital counseling, that both partners state some change they would like to see occur in the relationship. If Mr. J. feels free of blame by claiming to be perfectly content, then Mrs. J. falls into the role of the complaining shrew. Both partners must accept responsibility for change if change is to occur. An exception is in the area of disciplinary problems of children; sometimes the parents must force a reluctant child to change.

As each problem is clarified, the counselor can summarize the issue for the family. By the end of the first session, the family can be presented with an agenda of changes they have said they want to work on. Further definition of problems continues during subsequent counseling sessions.

History-Taking. Minuchin (1974) recommends taking only a brief history of the presenting problem during the first session. The authors agree with this procedure for family physicians working at Level Four. It is important to learn about the origins of the family problem and how it developed to its present level; however, history-taking need not encompass more than a third of the initial interview. The onset of the problem and previous efforts to cope with the problem are two essential pieces of historical information. Tracing the start of the problem may suggest that the family is suffering a life-cycle adjustment difficulty, as in the case of a couple whose dissatisfaction begins after the birth of a first child or after their last child has left home. Similarly, it is useful to know whether a patient's depression or anxiety began after a particular family event, like an extramarital affair, or has pervaded the patient's life since childhood.

In addition to questions about the origins of the presenting problem, the second important piece of history concerns the family's attempts to solve the problem. The Palo Alto school of family therapy (Weakland et al., 1974) has proposed that families get into trouble not because of the "problem" itself (e.g., depression, acting-out behavior) but because of how the family attempts to solve the problem. Thus the physician/counselor should inquire about the family's coping attempts. How did family members try to help Mr. J. when he got depressed? How did he respond to their gestures? Often people tell a depressed individual to "cheer up," thereby making that person feel worse. Or parents may try to crush their son's incipient rebellion by controlling him more and more closely until the family explodes. The "problem" may have begun as relatively normal behavior on the part of an adolescent or as a normal reaction to situational stress, but the "treatment" made the patient seriously ill.

For family physicians we suggest a problem-focused approach to family counseling (Level Four) that de-emphasizes extensive history-taking and elaborate assessment of all areas of family functioning—activities that would be more appropriate at Level Five. The problem with such comprehensive data gathering is that the physician is left with more information than can be handled. Information overload may result unless the data are matched with advanced therapy skills that more powerfully induce change. Families that can only be helped with the assistance of comprehensive three-generational biopsychosocial family assessment should to be referred to a therapist or seen with a co-therapist who is a professional family therapist. Family physicians, as primary care family counselors, do not have the time or the training for such analysis, and many families do not need this advanced level of care anyway. Minuchin's approach to assessment is taxing and complicating enough for the level of counseling practiced by most family physicians. Furthermore, the authors think the most important outcome in successful interventions is derived from the physician's understanding of the interaction patterns that maintain the problem and that influence the physician/family therapeutic relationship. These dynamics can be assessed only by face-to-face interaction with the family.

Remaining Neutral. The therapeutic triangle is like an electromagnetic field that pulls the counselor in one direction or another. Counseling a family requires an overall stance of neutrality, or stated more positively, an alignment with each member and with the family as a unit. The therapeutic triangle can remain functional in the face of brief coalitions of the counselor with one member against another—as when the counselor supports a wife to confront her husband's drinking behavior—but the counselor's support must be perceived by family members as flowing equally to all members. This is difficult to achieve for a physician who has already formed a bond with a primary patient. In such cases, during the first counseling session with the family, the physician should work especially hard at communicating to other family members that their positions and feelings are understood and appreciated. In other words, the physician can draw on the trust and emotional investment established with the primary patient by temporarily paying more attention to others.

Neutrality flows from an internal state in the counselor rather than from a body of techniques. In other words, the physician must believe that there are no villains and no faultless victims in the family in order to refrain from casting family members in these roles. The husband knows whether or not the physician regards him as an irresponsible person; the wife detects the physician's judgment that she is lucky her husband has stayed with her all these years. If the physician detects these feelings, and often such judgments are involuntary, then he or she should not try to counsel the family. The physician should send them to a therapist or a family physician colleague.

If the physician can avoid taking sides and scapegoating individuals in the family, the following techniques may be helpful in communicating this neutral support to the family:

1. Paraphrase each person's major complaint or proposed solution in terms that sound as reasonable as possible. This communicates to family members that the physician thinks that their feelings are understandable and not stupid or bad.

Mrs. J.: I want him home more in the evening. I can't stand being a single parent. But when I ask him to stay home, he gets mad at me. Am I expecting too much?

Physician: You're saying that he's your husband and you need his support at home with the kids. But when you bring up this problem, you feel like it just leads to a fight. Mr. J., what's your side of this?

Mr. J.: I'd be willing to stay home more in the evenings, but I can't stand it when she nags at me. She doesn't appreciate that I work hard all day.

Physician: If I understand you correctly, the problem for you is not that you don't want to stay home with your wife but that things get so bad between the two of you that you tend to stay away. Is that right?

Mr. J: Yeh, that's right.

The counselor has attempted to communicate to each spouse that each is understood.

2. Juxtapose each person's position on the problem and point out any similarities that are observed. One of the best ways to remain neutral in a conflict is to articulate the positions of both sides in a reciprocal fashion, thereby implicitly saying that neither side has cornered the market on truth and righteousness.

Physician: Both of you are saying that you would like to feel more appreciated by the other. Mrs. J., you feel like your husband doesn't think housework and child care are difficult burdens. Mr. J., you've said that your wife doesn't seem to appreciate your need for relaxation after working outside the home all day. What I hear are two people who very much want support from each other but who are ending up driving each other farther apart. Does that sound like what's going on?

Such interventions serve notice to the couple that the physician sees them as in the same boat, albeit rowing in opposite directions. You are saying that they both have legitimate needs and claims on each other. And you have identified the problem as stemming from their ineffective efforts to give and receive support. Even if one member is an alcoholic, and on this issue the physician may be allying with the other spouse, the physician can openly acknowledge the unhappiness this person feels in the family and the changes he or she wants to see occur. There is a good chance, for example, that the nonalcoholic spouse has denied any personal contribution to family problems by placing all the blame on the partner's drinking. Although the physician does not support an alcoholic husband's self-deceptions about the drinking, he or she can support the husband's effort to escape the scapegoat role in the family.

Encouraging a Collaborative Set. Family members need help discovering that they got into the problem together and must get out together. In Benjamin Franklin's phrase, "If we do not hang together, we will surely hang separately." When family alliances are fragile, the family physician can help by communicating the expectation that the family will work together on the problem.

One way to encourage the family to take a collaborative set is to help them discern the structure they have been working with to create or sustain the problem.

Physician: Mr. and Mrs. J., it's not very surprising to me that you've been having trouble controlling Jimmy's behavior. He's a pretty clever 13 year old who knows how to take advantage of his parents when they're at odds with each other. You each have some pretty good ideas about disciplining him, but you don't have your act together as a parental team.

It is not enough, of course, to point out the mutual participation in the formation of the problem; the physician must also help them change their interactional structure. Generally, resolving family problems requires complementary changes to be made by all participants. A brilliant solution that requires change in only one member is probably doomed to fail. That person will feel unfairly burdened. In the case of the "J." family, it would be a mistake to settle for Mr. J.'s promise to stay home more in the evenings. Unless his wife also behaves differently toward him, he will not stay home long. Setbacks do not contribute to family growth.

Therefore, when helping families negotiate change or when offering suggestions for handling common family problems, the physician should look for tasks or solutions that involve two or more people. When the new parents are arguing over how to handle baby's crying, give them a suggestion that they can implement together rather than one that involves only one partner (typically the mother). A couple whom one of the authors counseled agreed to alternate getting up each night to feed and change their fussy baby. This was their first collaborative parenting venture. They eventually got to the point where they let baby cry and go back to sleep, but at the beginning it was important that they learn to share the nightly burden.

In encouraging a collaborative set in these ways, the family physician is calling on the family's espirit de corps, i.e., their sense of belonging to each other in bad times and good. Fairly well-functioning families respond positively to being approached this way. More debilitated families probably do not get worse but they do not get much better without specialized treatment. The limits of Level Four family counseling and the need for formal family therapy become obvious when the attempt to establish this collaborative set fails.

Facilitating Family Discussion. Generally, it is best for the counselor to begin the first session by talking individually with family members. This procedure helps build rapport with each member and helps establish the counselor's control of the session. At some later point, however, it is often helpful to have family members speak directly with one another. Inducing the family to have such a discussion can be difficult for the novice counselor.

Several moments in family counseling lend themselves to family discussions. When the family is approaching a joint decision, the counselor can step back and ask them to talk with each other about what they want to do. A second appropriate time for family discussion is when a family member tells the counselor something positive about another member, such as:

Husband: I guess I don't tell her very often that I think she is a good wife.

Physician: Why don't you tell her now?

A third case is when someone speaks of poor communication with someone else. If a wife says that her husband does not listen when she tells him something, the counselor can ask her to talk with him in the session. A good rule of thumb for family counseling is that people must first change in the office if they are expected to act differently at home. If they cannot communicate in front of the counselor, then they will not do any better at home.

Sometimes family members are reluctant to speak directly with one another in front of the counselor. Common expressions of this resistance are:

1. "I've already told this to her."
2. "I feel silly."
3. Continuing to speak directly to the counselor instead of the other family member.

If the physician decides to ask the spouse or other family members to talk with each other, the physician must firmly insist that they do so. Gently but persistently repeat your request.

Physician: I know you feel a little strange talking with your husband in front of me, but I'd like you to try it anyway.

Wife: He already knows how I feel about it.

Physician: Tell him again anyway. I'd like to just listen while the two of you talk together.

Sometimes getting two people to interact requires changing the seating arrangement. The spouses can be asked to turn their chairs so they can face each other more directly, and the physician can move his or her chair back to become less central to the family system. One technique the authors have used when spouses continue to look at us instead of at each other is to refrain momentarily from looking at either one of them as they begin talking. Thus they have only each other to look at. Like all counseling techniques, this method has its limits: After one of the authors suggested to a resident that he look away from the couple in order to encourage them to keep talking with each other, the resident proceeded to stare out the window for ten minutes while the couple made befuddled furtive glances in his direction.

When family members engage in serious conversation in the presence of the physician, the physician can learn much about their communication patterns and can coach them in more effective communication and more constructive problem-solving. The trick is for the physician to move into their conversation to make an observation or suggestion, but then to back out again so they can continue talking. This is the essence of coaching as opposed to playing the game oneself.

Wife: When I am depressed, you seem to avoid me all the time.

Husband: No, I don't.

Physician: Would you tell your husband what he does that makes you think he is avoiding you?

Wife: Well, he . . .

Physician: (Pointing to husband) Tell him directly.

Wife: You listen to me for a while and then go putter around your shop or watch baseball or something. You always have something else to do when I'm feeling down.

Husband: (To wife) I don't know how to help you. I just feel awful for you but I don't know what to say after awhile, so I just get up and leave.

Wife: It would help if you stayed and listened to me.

The physician in this vignette was helping this couple deal directly with each other around the issue of how the wife gets support during her depressed moods. Since this couple apparently uses physical distances as a way to handle difficult communication episodes, the physician can help them best by coaching them to talk openly with each other in the counseling sessions. The wife can be helped to tell her husband more directly what she wants from him when she is depressed, and the husband can teach his wife about the limits of his tolerance of her discussions about how badly she feels. If he offers more brief supportive gestures to her, she may feel less inclined to talk about her troubles at great length. At any rate, their best chance of progress lies in their face-to-face interactions in marital counseling.

Dealing with Resistance. Major family resistance to change or to the counseling process should signal the need for a referral to a therapist, but some forms of resistance are inevitable in every counseling relationship. A skilled primary care counselor must know how to deal with at least two forms of resistance: failure to cooperate with the structure of the counseling (missed appointments, lateness, unreasonable time demands), and the tendency to argue with the counselor ("yes, but . . . "). The structuring issue requires an assertive posture from the physician/counselor. Families that miss appointments or come late to sessions should be confronted about the problem. One way to use this resistance therapeutically is to ask what the family is trying to tell the physician by their behavior. If everyone denies any deeper meaning in the uncooperativeness, then the physician can deal with it straightforwardly by telling the family that his or her time is important and that it should be respected. The physician can also confront the family about how high a priority they are placing on the counseling, particularly if other activities become excuses to skip a family session. Unreasonable time demands can be dealt with in a similar straightforward way: "I realize you would like to meet weekly (instead of every two weeks) or in the evenings, but my schedule cannot accommodate that." Two other options are to try to deal directly with the family's doubts about their internal resources for getting through the week by themselves, or refer a particularly demanding family to a therapist who has more time for family sessions.

Arguing with resistive patients and family members is a common pitfall for beginning counselors:

Patient: I don't think I will ever get over this divorce.

Counselor: You will probably be feeling better soon.

Patient: I don't think so. I don't know how you can say that.

Counselor: I've worked with other people in your situation, and I'm sure you'll be feeling better.

Patient: Huh.

It is quite frustrating to have a family member—or a whole family—disagree with one of your most brilliant biopsychosocial observations. The counselor's art generally requires bending with such disagreement rather than meeting it head on. People often need time to assimilate new information about themselves and their families. Two ways to deal with disagreement are (1) to suggest that family members think about what the physician has said, or (2) to encourage them to say more about how they see the issues and how they would like to change things. Their disagreement may not be a sign of resistance at all; they may be closer to the truth and to the best solutions. Therefore, one option is to follow where they lead and see whether or not a common area of agreement can be found. The worst option is to repeatedly try to persuade the family of the wisdom of your position.

Generally, the best approaches to dealing with families' resistance are to be assertive with them when they are uncooperative with the structure of treatment and to follow their thoughts and feelings when they disagree with the physician's assessment of their situation, and then to seek a blending of the physician's view and theirs.

Helping Families Make Behavioral Contracts. Behavioral marital therapists like Jacobson and Margolin (1979) and Stuart (1980) have demonstrated the usefulness of helping couples make clear agreements with each other for changing their interaction patterns. It is often not enough to help couples or families understand their problems better and communicate more honestly with each other; solutions may require agreements or contracts about what each person will do differently in the future. Here, the counselor's role is that of teacher and mediator: the physician should stress the importance of each person making a commitment to change and working out a complementary decision about what behaviors each is willing to change. Some families never move to this stage of decision-making on their problems and other families handle it with unilateral calls for everyone else to change ("If you would pay more attention to me or stop drinking, we wouldn't be having this problem"), or with unilateral confessions of guilt and promises to change ("I know my temper is the problem; I'll try to control it better"). Complementary change offers better promise of success.

Other important ingredients in effective behavioral contracts include:

(1) *A positive emotional environment during the negotiations.* The quality of the outcome depends heavily on the quality of the process. If the family members are speaking angrily or resentfully, then the agreement is unlikely to be implemented successfully: "All right. I'll start cleaning the house more often. You'll be able to eat off the floor by the time I get finished! You'll see!" It is better to wait until negative feelings have subsided and the physician has helped the partners see the benefits of collaboration. Behavioral contracts should be made with calm voices and positive feelings.

(2) *Clear and specific behavior changes agreed to by all parties.* It is not enough for the husband to promise to be "more attentive" and the wife to be "more supportive of his work." They need to nail down the particular behavior that makes each other feel good.

(3) *Good faith commitment by all parties to carry through with the new behaviors.* Jacobson and Margolin (1979) and Stuart (1980) have discussed the value of "good faith" contracts, in which each party is unilaterally committed to following through with change, as opposed to "quid pro quo" contracts, in which each party will change only if the other does. The good faith approach builds positive feelings in problem-solving: "I want to do something that will make you happier, and I will do it because I want to, not just because you will do something for me in return."

(4) *Evaluation to see if the contract is working.* Family members should plan in advance to evaluate the success of their agreement at a later time. There does not have to be a "do or die" quality to the contract; the partners need to learn the importance of renegotiating agreements that are not working.

A CASE ILLUSTRATION OF BEHAVIORAL CONTRACTING

A young woman presented with uncontrolled epilepsy related to marital distress, which she said led her to not taking care of herself. Her biggest complaint about her husband was that he nagged her all the time about not taking care of herself (eating well, getting enough sleep, taking her medicine) and made her feel stupid and incompetent. When the couple was seen together, the underlying interactional power struggle over her health became apparent. He adopted the stern parent role in their relationship and she adopted an admiring but uncooperative child role. The husband felt frustrated and scared by her seizures and continually nagged her about taking better care of herself. She agreed with his criticisms but would get angry at him for putting her down. After they fought, she would apologize for acting irresponsibly, but nothing would change. During the marital counseling session, the counselor pointed out some of these interaction patterns and empathized with the frustration that each partner felt. After these and other issues were explored, the counselor helped them negotiate a behavioral contract. The husband volunteered that one thing he could do would be not to nag her about her health; the wife agreed that she would remind him if she felt his comments sounded like nagging.

By itself, this contract would have been insufficient and negative—an agreement to stop doing something. So the counselor asked the wife what kind of support she would like from her husband. She then asked him to listen to her more when she talked about her frustration at work. He promised to do this as long as he could stop her when she discussed the technical aspects of her job too much; she agreed to this, commenting that such technical talk was probably one way she used to sound smarter than her husband. Thus, the final behavioral contract called for diminishing a negative interaction pattern and enhancing a positive one. The wife could "own" her health behaviors but still ask for support from her husband; he could support her without becoming a frustrated "parent."

Two follow-up sessions over the next 3 months revealed that the couple had followed through on their contract; the wife had experienced no further seizures, marital satisfaction had improved, and the husband was acknowledging that he was more able to work on some of his own career decisions. This brief but planned Level Four intervention was successful. If further intervention were needed to assist this couple, formal family therapy (Level Five) would be indicated.

Assigning Homework. Since families spend at most 1 hour per week in family counseling, most of important changes have to occur at home. An effective way to extend the influence of the family counseling session throughout the week is to assign a task for the family to accomplish before the next session. The task should be designed to provide follow-through on some issue dealt with in the session. For example, a couple who have spent little time alone may be asked to go on a date during the next week. Or an uninvolved father might be assigned the task of supervising his son's homework every night. It is essential that the details of the task be worked out and agreed upon during the counseling session. The couple in the above example should be asked to make specific plans during the counseling session; the father and son should decide what time homework is to be done. Such clarity is particularly important early in the counseling relationship when the family may need a lot of structure from the counselor to change their ways of relating.

The physician should not assign tasks for behavior that the family has not engaged in during the counseling session. A couple who have not communicated effectively about their household responsibilities with the counselor present should not be asked to continue their discussion at home. Save such issues for the next session. However, if they have made a breakthrough on this issue in counseling, then you might ask them to work out the details on their own and report back at the next session. Finally, the homework task should always be followed by the counselor. Failure to do the task suggests either that the family is resisting change or that the task was inappropriate or not agreed upon by the family. In any case, the counselor should see failure to follow through on homework as an important issue for discussion with the family.

A CASE ILLUSTRATION OF LEVEL FOUR COUNSELING

The following case example is a summary of a case written by Dr. William L. Miller, University of Connecticut, in *Family-Centered Medical Care: A Clinical Casebook* (Doherty and Baird, 1987, pp 107–109).

Mrs. B and her new daughter, Glee, had presented no obvious problems to their family physician and nursing team until Glee was 3 months of age. Both had been smiling and charming for the routine visits until Mrs. B returned to work—then everything changed. Over the next 6 months, Mrs. B saw her family physician five times, Glee saw him 13 times, and Mrs. B had called 16 times for assistance. The chief complaint was usually nasal stuffiness.

At a routine visit when the child was 9 months old, the family physician noted edematous turbinates and suspected allergic rhinitis as the cause of most of the problems for the past months. The physician recommended the elimination of dairy products from the child's diet for a trial period, and a few small changes in Glee's bedroom. The excitement of this diagnostic triumph was not shared by the doctor's nurse. "They'll call back. You know, we still haven't seen or talked to Dad."

Following are the words of Dr. Miller:

. . . My exuberance collapsed. We had trained our nurse well; she had seen behind the mask that had so successfully deceived my partner and me. Three hours later, the nurse's words throbbed in my ears as I answered the phone to speak with Mr. B for the first time. He was furious. He demanded to know what was wrong with his daughter and what gave me the right to tell his wife to completely refurbish their house. Evidently, Mrs. B had gone home and taken all the curtains down, thrown out many of Glee's toys, cleaned out Mr. B's closet, and was about to remove the sofa covers when Mr. B arrived home. With the mask removed and the disarming smile no longer mesmerizing me, I remembered all the forgotten clues. Mrs. B suffered nausea for all 9 months of pregnancy; Mr. B was taking Valium chronically before coming to our office; Mr. B never called or appeared in our office; Mr. B remained silent throughout the prenatal consult; and, most obviously, Glee came for frequent office visits for illness though her exams showed her to be healthy. After reassuring Mr. B that I had not prescribed redecorating their home, I began probing into Mr. and Mrs. B's marital relationship. I hit the jackpot! Their marriage had been struggling prior to the pregnancy, but the conflicts were overshadowed by Mrs. B's constant nausea, and then, after birth, by Glee's continuous "need for attention" because of her repeated illnesses that we unwittingly acknowledged by agreeing to see her (and getting paid). Mr. B admitted his anger toward us had been mounting steadily with each new bill from our office because he never thought Glee was sick. I accepted his anger and asked that Mrs. B also join our phone conversation. We all finally agreed that the entire B family would come for the next visit. The family session reinforced the information obtained by telephone. After 20 minutes, Mrs. B agreed to make appointments at our office only at times her husband could also come. She also agreed to argue with her husband instead of immediately going to check on Glee when conflict arose. Mr. B then agreed to listen to his wife when they did argue. In addition to these instructions for improving communication, they were also advised to spend 15 minutes touching each other daily . . .

Subsequently, the B's medical bills decreased, minor health problems with Glee were handled at home and everyone was less frustrated. More intensive marital therapy may become indicated in the future. However, now the physician and family understood the nature of their discomfort. The intervention was initiated indirectly by the nurse when she confronted the physician's optimism over finding a "medical" solution to this complex problem. The physician offered a limited intervention that would be likely to assist a couple who had not spent many years locked into this dysfunctional interaction. A timely Level Four counseling intervention such as this may be unusually effective for a family with a newly developed problem. Very few families would seek formal family therapy at that early stage. Ironically, at a later stage, it is more difficult to resolve, even for a fully trained family therapist.

The Future of Marriage and Family Counseling for Family Physicians. Family counseling skills and a family-centered approach to medical care are becoming familiar to newly trained family physicians. As we have shown in this chapter there is a wide range of counseling activity that is appropriate to the family physician. The academic literature is reflecting that marriage and family counseling by the family physician is realistic if the physician is seen as part of the doctor-patient-family triangle and as one part of an integrated helping team. Major new members of this team for the future will be family therapists, psychiatrists, social workers, nurses, family social scientists, and others who share a systems view of families. Family medicine may lead the other medical specialties toward a biopsychosocial model.

A family systems approach that includes family and marital counseling is an effective vehicle to help achieve this goal. Successful implementation of this model requires not only that family physicians become more skilled in their purposeful interactions with families but that these physicians share their trust and authority with other members of the medical team in order to meet the biopsychosocial needs of patients and families. The challenge for family medicine is to continue to demonstrate the utility of this approach in practice, to develop effective teaching strategies, to develop realistic research relating to these counseling activities, and to keep counseling skills in perspective for the caring, skilled, and busy family physician of tomorrow.

References

Bauman, M. H., and Grace, N. T.: Family process and family practice. J. Fam. Pract., *4*:1135, 1977.

Bowen, M.: Family Therapy in Clinical Practice. New York, Jason Aronson, 1978. *A collection of papers by one of the pioneers of family therapy.*

Bronfenbrenner, U.: The Ecology of Human Development. Cambridge, Mass., Harvard University Press, 1979. *A pioneering book by one of the leading authorities on child development and the family and the social context of child development.*

Carter, E. A., and McGoldrick, M.: The family life cycle and family therapy: An overview. *In* Carter, E. A., and McGoldrick, M. (Eds.): The Family Life Cycle: A Framework for Family Therapy. New York, Gardner Press, 1980. *The best book on the clinical implications of family life cycle changes and transitions.*

Christie-Seeley, J. (Ed.): Working with Families in Primary Care. New York, Praeger, 1984. *One of the first books on this topic written by a family physician.*

Cromwell, R. E., Olson, D. H., and Fournier, D. G.: Diagnosis and evaluation in marital and family counseling. *In* Olson, D. H. (Ed.): Treating Relationships. Lake Mills, IA, Graphic Publishing Company, 1976.

Crouch, M. A., and Roberts, L.: The Family in Medical Practice: A Family Systems Primer. New York, Springer-Verlag, 1987. *An excellent primer that covers basic concepts and includes a valuable appendix of family systems educational programs and resources.*

Doherty, W. J., and Baird, M. A.: Family Therapy in Family Medicine: Toward the Primary Care of Families. New York, Guilford Press, 1983.

Doherty, W. J., and Baird, M. A. (Eds.): Family-Centered Medical Care: A Clinical Casebook. New York, Guilford Press, 1987.

Doherty, W. J., Baird, M. A., and Becker, L. A.: Family Medicine and the Biopsychosocial Model: The Road Toward Integration. *In* Doherty, W. J., Christianson, C. E., and Sussman, M. B. (Eds.): Family Medicine: The Maturing of a Discipline. New York, Haworth Press, 1987.

Engel, G. L.: The Need for a new medical model: A challenge for biomedicine. Science, *198*:129–136, 1977. *The seminal paper from the first proponent of the biopsychosocial model.*

Glenn, M. L.: Collaborative Health Care: A Family-Oriented Model. New York, Praeger, 1987. *An outstanding historical and current statement of our efforts to work as a team toward a biopsychosocial model.*

Gunby, P.: Air controller strike spotlights job stress. J.A.M.A., *246*:1632, 1981.

Haley, J.: Problem Solving Therapy. San Francisco, Jossey-Bass, 1976.

Haley, J.: Leaving Home. New York, McGraw-Hill, 1980.

Harkaway, J. L.: Obesity: Reducing the Larger System. J. Strategic Syst. Fam. Ther., *2*:2–24, 1983. *This paper is a clear explanation of how physicians became part of the problem in chronic obesity.*

Henao, S., and Gross, N. (Eds.): Principles of Family Systems in Family Medicine. New York, Brunner/Mazel, 1985.

House, J. S., Landis, K. R., and Umberson, D.: Social Relationships and Health. Science, *24*:540–545, 1988.

Huygen, F. J. A.: Family Medicine: The Medical Life History of Families. New York, Brunner/Mazel, 1982.

Jacob, T., and Tennebaum, D. L.: Family Assessment: Rationale Methods and Future Directions. New York, Plenum Press, 1988.

Jacobson, N. S., and Margolin, G.: Marital Therapy. New York, Brunner/Mazel, 1979.

Korsch, B. M., and Negrette, V. F.: Doctor-patient communication. Sci. Am., *227*:66, 1972.

McCubbin, H. I., Joy, C. B., Cauble, A. E., et al.: Family stress and coping: A decade review. J. Marriage Fam., *42*:855, 1980. *A review of research in the 1970's on stress and the family.*

McGoldrick, M., and Gerson, R.: Genograms in Family Assessment. New York, W. W. Norton, 1985.

Medalie, J. H., Kitson, G. C., and Zyzanski, S. J.: A family epidemiological model: A practice and research concept for family medicine. J. Fam. Pract., *12*:79, 1981.

Minuchin, S.: Families and Family Therapy. Cambridge, MA, Harvard University Press, 1974. *A classic statement of the structural family therapy approach to family assessment and family treatment.*

Olson, D. H., Sprenkle, D. H., and Russell, C.: Circumplex model of marital and family systems: I. Cohesion and adaptability dimensions, family types, and clinical applications. J. Fam. Pract., *18*:3, 1979.

Pattison, E. M., and Anderson, R. C.: Family health care. Public Health Rev., *7*:83, 1978.

Rakel, R. E.: Principles of Family Medicine. Philadelphia, W. B. Saunders Co., 1978. *This book has useful sections on constructing a family tree and on family-centered record keeping.*

Ransom, D. C., and Massad, R. J.: Family Structure and Function. *In* Rakel, R. E., and Conn, H. F. (Eds.): Family Practice. 2nd ed. Philadelphia, W. B. Saunders Co., 1978.

Rollins, B. C., and Cannon, K. L.: Marital satisfaction over the family life cycle: A re-evaluation. J. Marriage Fam., *36*:271, 1974.

Ryder, R. G., Kafka, J. S., and Olson, D. H.: Separating and joining influences in courtship and early marriage. Am. J. Orthopsychiatry, *41*:450, 1971.

Sawa, R. J.: Family Dynamics for Physicians: Guidelines to Assessment and Treatment. Studies in Health and Human Services. Vol. 4. Lewiston, New York, Edwin Mellen, 1985.

Selvini-Palazzoli, M., Boscolo, L., Cecchin, G., et al.: The problem of the referring person. J. Marital Fam. Ther., *6*:3, 1980. *An interesting article highlighting how physicians can become so close to some families that the referral for therapy is undermined.*

Smilkstein, G.: The family APGAR: A proposal for a family function test and its use by physicians. J. Fam. Pract., *6*:1231, 1978. *The author presents the family APGAR scale, including preliminary evidence for its reliability and validity.*

Smilkstein, G.: Assessment of family function. *In* Rosen, G. M., Geyman, J. P., and Layton, R. H. (Eds.): Behavioral Science in Family Practice. New York, Appleton-Century-Crofts, 1980.

Stuart, R. B.: Helping Couples Change. New York, The Guilford Press, 1980.

Watzlawick, P., and Weakland, J. H. (Eds.): The Interactional View. New York, W. W. Norton and Company, 1977.

Watzlawick, P., Beavin, J. H., and Jackson, D. D.: Pragmatics of Human Communication. New York, W. W. Norton and Company, 1967.

Weakland, J. H., Fisch, R., Watzlawick, P., et al.: Brief therapy: Focused problem resolution. J. Fam. Pract., *13*:141, 1974.

Whitaker, C. A., and Keith, D. V.: Symbolic-experiential family therapy. *In* Gurman, A. S., and Kniskern, D. P. (Eds.): Handbook of Family Therapy. New York, Brunner/Mazel, 1981.

Worby, C., and Gerard, R.: Family dynamics. *In* Rakel, R. E., and Conn, H. F. (Eds.): Family Practice. 2nd ed. Philadelphia, W. B. Saunders Co., 1978.

62

Sexual Health Care: A Life Cycle Approach

Charles E. Driscoll
Georgianna S. Hoffmann

When this material was last revised in 1983 for the third edition of this text, little was yet known of the impact on sexual life styles that would result from the rampant spread of AIDS. Genital herpes infections were causing significant physical and psychologic stigmata and were the focus of concern for sexually active people from 1979 to 1982. Seemingly a product of (and some claimed "punishment" for) the sexual experimentation of the 60's and 70's that was typified by the "free love" and "anything goes" attitude, the herpes epidemic began to modify relationships and sexual behavior. All of that now pales in comparison to the fear and change brought about since 1985 when human immunodeficiency virus (HIV) infection crossed over from being a disease of high-risk groups (homosexuals and I.V. drug users) into the heterosexual population. We are now facing an unparalleled crisis in American health, with 78 per cent or more of cases attributable to the consequences of sexual activity.

Recent data on sex practices (Masters et al., 1988) show that modifications in our expression of sexuality have certainly occurred. Sexual experimentation with multiple sexual partners is declining. Three of four heterosexual singles now say they are more selective of their partners, choosing long-term monogamous relationships. Self-report of oral sex and anal intercourse is somewhat lower in frequency. The condom has become a common word, even for many children, after every household in America received guidelines for safer sex from the U.S. Surgeon General in 1988. The gay community has been very effective in educating its own population about and reduction of high-risk sexual behavior. The alarming fact, however, is that segments of the population (e.g., adolescents and young adults) still refuse to believe they are at risk and engage in sex with many partners in ways that are known to increase HIV transmission. Physicians are obligated to view sexuality as an important component of healthy living and to inquire of and educate their patients in safe and healthy sexual behaviors.

Many people turn first to their family physician for help with sexual concerns. The spontaneous report rate for sexual problems is about 15 per cent, but this is only a very small segment in relation to the rate of report, which is as high as 60 per cent, when sensitive questioning techniques are used. Personal worries over the appropriateness of inquiring about sexuality may have lessened over the past 5 years, but the reluctant patient asks questions in a hesitating, indirect manner or not at all. Routinely assessing for sexual satisfaction allows patients to consider sexuality as an important component of their overall health and to discuss their concerns freely and openly. When sexual concerns are present, skillful recognition and handling of the problem by the physician brings about a positive outcome. Every sexually active person deserves assessment for health risk and education about safe sexual practices.

Talking to Patients About Sexuality

Comfort for the Patient. Sexuality needs to be seen as an acceptable subject for discussion in the medical office. For those patients who initially cannot bring themselves to volunteer information, the permission is implicitly given to open a later discussion. There are several ways to give this permission—permission to think about, talk about, and learn about sex. For example, questions about sex should be included on self-administered intake history questionnaires. Two appropriate questions are, "Sexual difficulties—Yes or No?," or "Sex is entirely satisfactory—Yes or No?." These one-liner questionnaires sometimes open the door for further discussion; follow up the information if they are circled, crossed out, or show any evidence of pencil marks as if there was some hesitation on answering. Verbal history-taking is a more direct approach.

The office setting presents many opportunities for indicating that sex is a permissible topic for discussion. The journal *Medical Aspects of Human Sexuality* may be included among the waiting room magazine selections for patient reading. Medical reference texts about sexuality on the bookshelves allow the patient to see that the doctor has been studying about sex and may presume that sex is an area of his or her knowledge, as are pediatrics, gynecology, and other topics represented in the physician's library. Regularly distributed items for patient education should include pamphlets on self-examination of the breasts or testicles; contraceptive, venereal disease, and safe-sex information; and pamphlets designed for special interest groups such as preventive sexual health care for homosexuals.

To facilitate discussion about specific problems and solutions, the physician may want to have educational aids available in the consulting room. Pipe cleaner figures or wooden artist model dolls with flexible limbs are helpful in illustrating alternatives to traditional sexual positions or habits. Handcrafted cloth dolls complete with genitalia are useful in communicating with children, particularly those who have been sexually abused. In counseling a couple with orgasmic dysfunction, it may be useful to show couples what an electric vibrator looks like to help them decide whether or not they would like to try this aid in their own relationship. Well-illustrated books in a lending library are excellent for those patients who would feel too embarrassed to purchase copies for themselves. There are also a wide variety of films in 16 mm or videocassette format illustrating techniques for improvement of sexual functioning. These are available from companies such as Edcoa, The Center for Marital and Sexual Studies, and MultiMedia Resource Center. Physicians encountering patients with sexual difficulties find that they can accomplish a great deal by having these resources readily available.

Comfort for the Physician. All of these efforts for putting the patient at ease and disseminating information are wasted if physicians cannot deal with or at least conceal their own discomfort with sexual concerns. Verbal and nonverbal cues deliver the true, hidden message that says: "Please don't talk to me about this subject." Comfort with matters of sexual health care does not come automatically; it must be practiced and controlled. Many individuals find sexual topics occasionally embarrassing, distasteful, or sexually arousing. It is permissible for the physician to have these various feelings too, but it is unacceptable to display them before the patient.

To develop a nonjudgmental, caring attitude in a stepwise fashion, the physician can use one or two excellent textbooks on human sexuality, such as the *Textbook of Sexual Medicine* by Kolodny and associates, *Sexual Problems in Medicine* by Lief, and *Human Sexuality* by Masters and associates, to become knowledgeable and to eliminate many myths and incorrect assumptions acquired from previous learning.

Once information has been updated, physicians should assess their personal value system and attitudes toward sexuality. If more knowledge and comfort with sexuality is needed, physicians can participate in a postgraduate continuing education course or a sexual attitude readjustment training session.

Sexual Problems in Family Practice

According to data from the 1985 National Ambulatory Medical Care Survey of the National Center for Health Statistics, the ten most common diagnoses in office practice include six that are directly or indirectly related to issues of sexuality (hypertension, normal pregnancy, health supervision of infant or child, general medical examination, diabetes mellitus, neurotic disorders). Pelvic, breast, and rectal examinations were, respectively, the 5th, 8th, and 10th most commonly specified diagnostic services performed, and symptoms of the genitourinary system account for 5 per cent of the principal reasons for an office visit. There are many areas of health care that exert major influences on sexuality (contraceptive counseling, prenatal care, ischemic heart disease) and others that have a more peripheral or covert effect (hypertension and its drug therapy, medical and post-surgical care, anxiety).

According to one investigation on the scope of sexual health care in medical practice (Burnap and Golden, 1967), the six most frequently occurring sexual problems, listed in descending order of frequency, were "anorgasmia, decreased sexual desire, complaints related to frequency of intercourse, general information seeking, impotence, and dyspareunia (painful intercourse)." Ten and fifteen years later, two studies of physician recall about their patients' consultations (Levenson and Croft, Texas, 1977; and Driscoll et al., Iowa, 1982) essentially agreed on the relative frequency of the problems as shown in Table 62–1. In the Iowa study, all 104 family physicians reported that they delivered some form of medical care that directly involved human sexuality (e.g., contraceptive counseling, obstetric care, Papanicolaou's smears). Surprisingly, the average occurrence of sexual problems presented as either a direct or an important related complaint was only 2 to 10 per cent. Today, if this study was replicated, one might expect incest to move significantly up the list due to more education and greater efforts at detection. It is fair to say that the scope of sexual health care is extremely broad in family practice, being included in as much as 50 to 75 per cent of all the care that family physicians deliver. It may also be fair to note that we as physicians do rather poorly in addressing the subject with our patients.

Recognition and Intervention. Early diagnosis and treatment of sexual dysfunction within the context of the routine examination or treatment for illness can be helpful in preventing the development of more difficult and refractory problems. Early intervention is preventive of needless patient suffering and saves the physician the time that would be spent later in more intensive therapy.

Many factors temporarily affect the level of an individual's sexual desire and of a couple's sexual activity. An extreme but timely example is the phobic reaction to sex experienced by a young woman who learned that a previous sex partner had subsequently contracted HIV infection. Unfortunately, people sometimes have the erroneous belief that everyone else in the world has a perfect sex life and they are the only individuals or couples having difficulties. This myth is especially damaging because it prevents people from seeing that sexual satisfaction is very much tied to knowledge about human sexual response, to communication patterns, and to a willingness to teach the sexual partner about what they like and what is erotically important to them. The myth fails to take into account the fact that a couple's sexual relationship is always subject to the stresses and strains of things outside the relationship—difficulties at work, the advent of children arriving into the family, problems with caring for elderly parents, and so forth. If the family physician can point out the commonality of some of these issues and offer simple education, very often persons respond positively by the alleviation of sexual difficulties. Sometimes simply the opportunity for a couple to air concerns and ventilate feelings can be a very helpful intervention.

Table 62–1. RELATIVE FREQUENCY OF SEXUAL PROBLEMS ENCOUNTERED BY PHYSICIANS

Condition	Per Cent
Erectile dysfunction (2° > 1°)	24.4
Dyspareunia	20.3
Misinformation	15.5
Psychosexual dysfunction	9.4
Premature ejaculation	8.4
Anorgasmia	7.9
Extramarital sex	6.6
Organic sexual dysfunction	2.6
Rape	1.1

The relative frequency of the following sexual problems is less than 1 per cent: homosexuality, masturbation, lesbianism, incest, sexual perversion, zoophilia, and pedophilia.

The classic syndromes of chronic back pain, chronic headache, or chronic fatigue can, of course, be due to many causes. Frequently, they may mask a disorder of sexual desire or satisfaction (Klein, 1984). The physician should understand the syndrome as an unconscious and nondeliberate attempt by the woman or man to avoid sex.

Gender-Specific Symptoms. Symptoms in women that suggest sexual problems include chronic complaints of discomfort during intercourse for which no disease state can be identified, or complaints of chronic congestion, heaviness in the pelvis, and a feeling of discomfort that persists for several days after intercourse. These symptoms indicate that the woman may have reached the plateau stage of arousal but was unable to achieve orgasm and, therefore, had a residual vasocongestion in the pelvic area. She may not have connected the symptoms with lack of orgasmic return, or she may be well aware of the connection but feel embarrassed about raising the question of sexual satisfaction with the physician. A gentle exploration of the woman's sexual history can often help her to begin to allow discussion of her experience and her feelings.

Other indicators that may be connected with sexual problems in women include chronic low level anxiety states and depression. It is common for a woman to feel that if a sexual problem exists within a couple's relationship, it is entirely her fault. The woman may continually assure the doctor that her husband has nothing whatever to do with this problem and that it is entirely her own deficiency. It is important to display a nonjudgmental attitude and explain that the objective is not to assign blame or find fault in either partner but to help the two of them explore their interactions and learn the kinds of things they need to know about each other that will improve their sexual response.

Men may be even more reluctant than women to admit that they have sexual problems. This is probably the result of another damaging sexual myth that men should always desire sexual activity and always be ready to perform; if a man finds his own experience contrary to this myth, he begins to question his masculinity. Vague complaints of urinary difficulties or "chronic prostatitis" that cannot be supported clinically may be the patient's way of directing the doctor's attention to his genitalia in the hope that the physician will discover a correctable condition that could also solve the sexual difficulty. The physician should indicate to the patient that many, if not most, men have occasional episodes of erectile difficulty; usually this occurs when the man is tired, has consumed a heavy meal, or drank too much alcohol. It is also common at times for men to have difficulty delaying ejaculation. If asked in a matter-of-fact way whether or not this has ever happened to him, then the man can feel more comfortable in expressing his own concerns.

Examining the Patient

Once the continuum of sexual health care has been entered, patient counseling begins by taking the sexual history and performing a modified sexologic examination. This assessment examination is an educational tool to inform the patient *and* assure the physician of normal sexual anatomy and physiology. A sexual history and a modified sexologic examination are appropriate in the following situations: premarital examination; annual Papanicolaou's smear and pelvic examination; venereal disease check; obstetric work-up at the prenatal and postpartum examinations; and when the patient presents with contraceptive requests, sexual problems or complaints, bladder or urinary complaints, vaginal infection, and pre-surgical and postsurgical visits (e.g., for vasectomy, tubal ligation, mastectomy, hysterectomy).

The Sexual History. It should come as no surprise that a high correlation exists between routinely taking a sexual history and the identification of sexual problems (Driscoll et al., 1986). From the beginning, the physician should ensure an atmosphere of comfort and confidentiality. Patients who remain clothed during the history-taking are less likely to feel "exposed" when their bodies are covered, even when their private thoughts and activities are brought to the surface. If note-taking is a common practice, do not write the answers to sexual questions. Place the paper and pencil aside and close the record, nonverbally indicating that information about sexual matters does not have to be a part of the patient's chart. Do not artificially segregate questions about sex from the other parts of the history; it is much better to include questions about sex with related areas in the review of the patient's history. Questions about menstrual cycles, bowel movements, or vaginal infections naturally lead to questions about sexual practices, performance, use of contraception, and specific concerns of the patient.

Two important techniques in history-taking are especially useful for the sexual history. First, *unloading* gives the patient a wide range of possibilities for correct answers, so that no matter what the patient replies, it seems to fit the definition of "normal." In this way what the patient considers "right" becomes clear. For example, the physician might say, "Some people have intercourse five times a week, others once a month, and others never at all. How often do you have intercourse?" The second questioning technique is that of *ubiquity*. Inform the patient that the problem that is being asked about is present in many people, perhaps the majority, and the physician would like to know whether or not it is also present in the patient.

There are several general open-ended questions that are to be used routinely. The first is "How satisfactory is your sexual functioning?" This question is appropriate for every sexually active patient. By avoiding the word "intercourse," nothing is assumed about the sexual activities of a patient and, consequently, the patient is more likely to disclose accurate information. The second question (using the technique of *ubiquity*) is: "At some time in their lives most people experience a sexual problem or concern; what type of sexual problems have you had?" A third routine question is particularly important in dealing with adolescents or other people suspected of having a need for sexual information: "Many people have unanswered questions or need information about sexual functioning. What questions do you have about sex?" Add questions for assessing risk factors associated with sexual behavior as follows: "Since beginning regular sexual activity, how many different partners have you had?" "Are your sexual partners male, female or both?" "Have you or your sexual partner ever used I.V. drugs?"

If the answers to all of these questions indicate no problems, record "sexual history negative" in the chart and proceed with history-taking in other areas. If a problem is suspected, pursue the sexual history further by beginning with general questions of a less sensitive nature, such as an inquiry about surgery or infection of the genitals, parity, or contraception, and then proceed to more sensitive areas, such as first sexual encounter and early sexual experiences, fears of sex, self-diagnoses, and sexual behavior patterns. Continue to search for areas of misinformation and supply the necessary facts or a reference when appropriate.

When communication or relationship difficulties are suspected, quantitate the problem by using a rating scale method. Patients may be asked to assess their own sexual functioning and that of their spouse on a scale of 1 to 5; the physician in turn assesses the ratings for congruence.

The Sexologic Examination. This examination includes the primary and secondary sex organs. Traditionally, a pelvic examination takes place in the lithotomy position with over-the-knee draping, presenting a barrier to communication and loss of patient participation in the examination. Changing the table so that the patient can assume a semisitting position and offering a hand-held mirror allows her to observe what is happening during a pelvic examination and permits active participation, learning, and increased patient-physician communication (Fig. 62–1). Warming the vaginal speculum to increase comfort is accomplished by storing it on a heating pad in the examining table drawer or holding it under warm water for a few seconds. A plastic speculum may

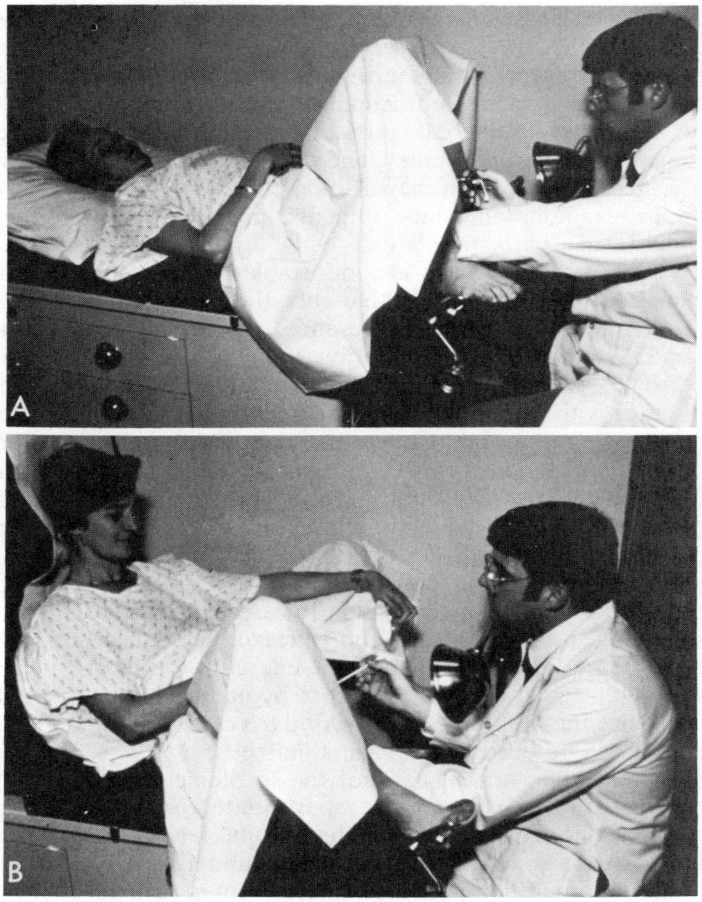

Figure 62–1. *A,* Traditional lithotomy position blocks communication between doctor and patient. *B,* Teaching the patient is facilitated by use of a mirror and a semisitting position.

afford better visibility for the patient. With the patient looking in the mirror, point to anatomic structures, name them, and explain their physiologic function.

Female Sexologic Exam. Begin by examining the vulva for lesions or areas of sensitivity to touch. Check to see that the clitoris is free from the clitoral hood and that no adhesions are present to restrict its movement. If only light touching of the perineum stimulates marked contraction of the bulbocavernosus muscles, the problem of vaginismus may exist. If an organic problem of the sacral nerves (S2,3,4) is suspected, elicit the bulbocavernosus reflex by firmly squeezing the area of the clitoris and observe the anal sphincter for contraction. Inspect the introitus for a Bartholin cyst or previous obstetric trauma to the perineum. Palpate the urethra along the course of the vaginal roof to express exudate and to check for sensitivity of the Gräfenberg spot. The Gräfenberg spot has been described (Addiego et al., 1981; Quadagno, 1988) as a center for physiologic response during orgasm that may be present in a few women. The spot is located beneath the surface of the anterior vaginal wall at the junction of the upper one third and lower two thirds of the vaginal barrel, and is presumed to be the female analogue of the prostate. When the spot is stimulated during sexual activity, or when it is palpated during the normal pelvic examination, the patient may report a sensation of having to urinate followed by a pleasurable sensation. It is unclear whether or not true female ejaculation can occur as a function of this tissue. If historically the Gräfenberg spot is presumed to exist, the patient may be reassured that this is a normal sexual variant.

On speculum examination of the vagina, the physician should search for infections, mucosal lesions, or areas of old obstetric trauma and test any healed lacerations for pain or anesthesia. When performed at the time of examination, Kegel's perineal exercises allow assessment of the tone of the perineal muscles. Ask the patient to push down with a Valsalva maneuver to assess the presence of a cystocele or a rectocele. Examine the tone and integrity of the anus as well. The patient can participate in the bimanual examination by palpating the fundus of the uterus while the physician's examining fingers hold it toward the abdominal wall. Conclude the consultation by performing and teaching a breast self-examination.

Male Sexologic Exam. Begin with inspection of the penis; look for lesions that may be hidden by the uncircumcised foreskin. Compress the meatus between the fingers to assess for stricture that may indicate prior infection. Palpate the shaft of the penis dorsally to rule out the plaquelike lesion of Peyronie's disease. Palpate the testicles and teach self-examination. Check the size of the testicles and follow the vas to the inguinal canal to check for areas of infection, tenderness, or asymmetry. Test the bulbocavernosus reflex (present in 70 per cent of normals) for neurologic disease by squeezing the glans of the penis and looking for anal contraction. Examine the rectum for evidence of venereal warts or poor muscle tone, suggesting penile-anal entry, and do a prostatic exam. The male examination may also be concluded with a breast examination, since reflexive nipple erection should occur with stimulation.

When the physician is comfortable in doing this examination with individual patients, the examination can then be done in the presence of the patient's sexual partner. The examination should always first be done with each partner in private to discuss findings with the patient and obtain consent for the partner to be present. This type of examination gives permission for viewing the sexual organs and often imparts information to both partners that cannot be obtained from self-examination at home. When both partners are present, the squeeze technique for ejaculation control can be taught or the partner's careful digital exploration of the vagina for areas of responsiveness can be included. (The squeeze technique is described later in this chapter.) Generally, the most sensitive vaginal areas for pleasure by manual stimulation are thought to be at 12, 4, and 8 o'clock around the outer one third of the vaginal barrel.

Of course, not all parts of the sexologic examination or sexual history are appropriate for every patient. The physician should have some feeling for the patient's sensitivity and desire to undertake the examination. When patients verbally express the desire not to partake in this line of questioning and when discomfort is noted, the physician should let the topic drop at this office visit. At least the door has been opened for the patient to return at a later time as the need arises.

Predictable Patient and Family Needs for Sexual Health Care

EMERGING SEXUALITY

Sexual development begins at the moment of conception with the determination of chromosomal sex. However, male and female fetuses are initially indistinguishable by their external genitalia and have a bipotential gonadal state until the differentiation into male or female occurs between 8 and 12 weeks of gestation. The presence or absence of circulating levels of testosterone differentiates the external sexual organs regardless of the genetic determinants. A locally acting substance, the müllerian duct inhibitory factor, causes the müllerian duct system to disappear, and circulating testosterone begins to exert its influence on the wolffian duct system. By the 14th week of gestation, internal and external sexual anatomy are clearly different.

Ambiguous Genitalia. Hormonal excess or deficiency, genetic chromosomal accidents, and combinations of these mechanisms have produced sexual anomalies. When a baby is born with a sexual anomaly, the assignment of sex at birth is a particularly delicate situation for the family and medical team. When the genitalia are ambiguous or where there is even the slightest doubt about the true sex of the child, it is best to avoid pronouncing the sexual assignment until further testing can be done. Explain to the parents that, like the condition of cleft palate, a situation in which the baby's lip was not completely finished in utero, the ambiguous genitalia are a condition of unfinished intrauterine development. When thorough attempts at diagnosis have been made, treatment (which may include sex reassignment) is initiated early and subsequent sexual development can be relatively normal despite these genetic mishaps; the loss of fertility is usually the only major consequence (Money and Ehrhardt, 1972).

Sexual Development. This process depends on many factors, and the role of sex education in the home is central. Parental reactions and attitudes need to be examined before the child passes through those stages, and anticipatory guidance should be provided when possible. Advise the parents to use correct names for the genitalia from the start of childhood. Giving answers in a trustworthy and relaxed manner is a skill that needs to be learned and practiced by the parents. The parents should discuss with each other some of the questions and situations they will encounter *before* they arise and reach mutual agreement about their responses. Sex education in childhood is a joint responsibility of parents and should not be allocated to one or the other.

The sexual development most evident in the *newborn and early childhood period* is body exploration and genital fondling by babies. Physiologic manifestations of orgasm, including sweating, rhythmic muscle contractions, and abrupt general relaxation are reported. The child may be subjected to disapproval or discipline by the parents following the occurrence of genital play and may be confused by this message as it contrasts with the pleasing physical sensations. These contradictory messages may provide the early roots for adult sexual problems. Guidance for the parents should include reassurance that this behavior begins at 5 to 6 months of age in almost all infants and nearly always ceases on its own by 10 to 12 months of age without the need for parental intervention.

Later childhood sexual development involves the emergence of *gender identity*, or the internal experience of one's sexual self. The external expression of sexuality is known as the *gender role*. Many traits and behaviors are common to both boys and girls, but the sense of masculinity or femininity characteristically includes the psychosocial tasks of organizing behavior toward peers of the same sex and of the opposite sex and identifying with the sexual anatomy and behavior of the same-sex parent.

By the age of 18 months, gender identity is

developed to the extent that sex reassignment cannot usually be accomplished. By 2 to 2 1/2 years of age, growing children have gained awareness of the difference between boys and girls, so that by age 3 they are able to correctly identify their own sex and the sex of others by their dress. By age 4 to 5 the sex of others is identified by differences in genitalia, primarily the presence or absence of breasts. Most children experiment with their sexuality during childhood and same-sex and opposite-sex play is a normal part of growing up. Sexual curiosity and nudity in young children as they "play doctor" is a normal, anticipated event.

Encourage parents to use the "teachable moment," such as the birth of a new baby into the family, to help explain basic sexual information to their children. When a child becomes old enough to ask questions, answers should be provided when the questions are asked and not put off until later because many times questions lose their importance and are not asked again. Parents should answer only what is asked; they should not supply more information than the child is ready to receive. Some children, however, do not ask questions about sex, and sensitivity to other cues that reveal their need to know is important (for example, the child may make up sexual stories to tell in school about mommy having a baby). It is important for the physician to have references available to suggest for the parents' use so they will give correct information and be able to use appropriate illustrations. Parents should review all information for its content before they place it in front of the child so they can anticipate where questions may arise. Be alert for the child who acts sexually precocious, for example, an 8-year-old child engaging in seductive sexual behavior or acting out sexual intercourse or fellatio with another child. These are signs that the child has been prematurely initiated into adult sexual behaviors and may imply the child is a victim of pedophilia or incest.

Sex education that is begun during early childhood, long before the advent of puberty, prevents some of the misinformation that comes from using peers as the primary informational resource. The arrival of *adolescence* can be less tumultuous when good sex education has already begun. The onset of puberty is accompanied by interest in the opposite sex, yet adolescents do not quite know how to handle their feelings and emotions. Behavior toward the opposite sex is manifested as giggling, teasing, tickling, or kicking—all of which are innocent activities that lead to increased contact. As a result of changing hormone levels, body changes occur, including the development of the primary and secondary sex organs. The first physical sign of pubertile change in girls is typically telarche (breast budding), followed by pubarche (appearance of pubic hair) and, lastly, menarche. Male sexual development usually proceeds through testicular development, the increase in penis size, the appearance of pubic hair, and, finally, attainment of the adult size and shape of the genitalia. The sexual staging of Marshall and Tanner should be performed at each visit to the physician (Tanner, 1962).

Masturbation and fantasy are the principal orgasmic outlets during adolescence. The majority of people *do* masturbate, and *no* physical or psychologic harm results from it. Parents who are aware of this should be advised to avoid eliciting guilt or anxiety in their teenagers. At puberty, sexual desires are heightened, more so in males than in females, and masturbation to orgasm has occurred in 50 to 60 per cent of boys by age 15. Boys begin masturbation earlier than girls, are more likely to masturbate with a friend or in groups, and frequently are taught how to do it by peers. Girls begin later in adolescence (about 40 per cent have tried by age 15), usually do it in private, and tend to learn how on their own. More recent data (Masters et al., 1988) confirm that there is an increasing trend toward more frequent use of masturbation by female teenagers than was reported by Kinsey in the 1950's.

The sexual behavior of later adolescence has become apparent primarily by its outcome—the ever-increasing incidence of teenage pregnancy. Each year, more than one million teenagers become pregnant, about one every 35 seconds, and approximately 40 per cent obtain abortions. Venereal disease is also on the rise among adolescents. Adolescent behavior patterns suggest that as many as 49 per cent of girls may have experienced intercourse by age 15, rising to 69 per cent by age 19. Figures for boys are similar: about 50 per cent experience intercourse by age 15, and approximately 78 per cent or more by age 19 (Masters et al., 1988).

Although peers have much more of an effect and influence on sexual behavior than do parents, parents should continue to provide factual information and be a trustworthy resource for their adolescent. When sexual decision-making is taking place, the child needs help in maintaining self-esteem while resisting peer pressures for early sexual activity. Problems of body image and sexual development should be anticipated and understanding and reassurance given by both parents and physician.

It is important to emphasize the individual nature of the timing of sexual development. Encourage parents to talk with their children about menstruation and wet dreams well in advance of their onset. Fathers may tell their adolescent sons that many boys have wet dreams and that they are normal and expected. Boys should be told that mothers know about wet dreams, too, and will not be angry or surprised by stained bed clothing. Mothers should explain to their adolescent daughters about the menstrual cycle and the use of sanitary napkins or tampons. A relaxed attitude and a demonstration of napkin use, with time allowed for questions and answers, provides not only a basic understanding but also an acceptance of the inconvenience or discomfort of menses. Stressing the specialness of the ability to carry a baby also helps to foster a healthy approach to menstruation. It is, by the way, just as acceptable for mothers to teach boys and for fathers to teach girls if both the parent and the adolescent are comfortable with each other. Advise parents also that other trusted adults (physicians, clergy, and counselors) should be sought when privacy issues make parent-child communication impossible. Excellent references to aid in teaching the adolescent are noted in the references for patient use (Calderone and Ramey, 1982; Hamilton, 1978; Johnson, 1977).

MATURING SEXUALITY

As the individual matures, the sexual value system expands with the accumulation of increasing amounts of material of erotic significance. Body image becomes profoundly important, since the degree to which people accept a person's body as attractive influences the extent to which they are willing to accept their sexuality and to allow intimate bonds to develop. Unfortunately, many people retain the image of themselves as an ugly, acned, and awkward adolescent long after they have become attractive adults in reality. When that sense of adolescent vulnerability is carried over into adult life it can inhibit and restrict the person's ability to relate sexually to a partner. Sexuality and self-esteem are so closely intertwined that when self-esteem is lowered for any reason the individual becomes prone to some degree of sexual dysfunction; and sexual dysfunction, in turn, tends to lower self-esteem. It is important for professionals to avoid using terms such as *frigid* for women and *impotent* for men, since these words carry hurtful connotations that may further damage the patient's self-esteem.

It is unfortunate but true that men and women arrive at sexual maturity with different value systems. For women, the sexual value system contains a great deal of negative content related to being clean, neat, lady-like, and good, together with prohibitions against touching genitalia or being carried away by sexual arousal. For men, the negative content tends to center on a prohibition against experiencing and expressing any type of "unmanly" feelings and the physical demonstration of affection and tenderness is not encouraged. Men have almost always learned to masturbate rapidly to climax during adolescence, whereas many women have not learned how to stimulate their own bodies to reach an orgasmic response. Therefore, the reflex response patterns for a woman have generally not been developed before she attempts to establish a sexual relationship with a partner. On the other hand, men usually have a well-developed sexual response pattern; however, they may not be in touch with their rate of arousal and may have difficulty with ejaculatory control. These differences tend to engender a great deal of disappointment in early sexual encounters as well as feelings that there is something wrong with either the self or the partner.

In most instances, sexual failures derive from the culturally different experiences that men and women have had in growing up. These experiences sometimes prevent people from understanding that sexual activity is not limited to conventional intercourse. It includes a whole continuum of erotic activity from eye contact to talking, listening, holding hands, hugging, self-stimulation, partner stimulation, and perhaps oral-genital contact. Physical touch and skin contact is essential for receiving affirmation, acceptance, and affection. In fact, it may be intimacy rather than sexual activity that is being sought. Sex can serve as a substitute for intimacy or it can be an expression of it.

Whether the young woman reaches orgasm or not during sexual activity depends in part on whether or not she has learned to be orgasmic with self-stimulation. It also requires that she assume responsibility for much of her own sexual arousal and that she participate equally in the initiation of sexual activities. (The person who initiates sexual activity is likely to become aroused more quickly than the person who is the recipient of the advances.) When a woman is willing to play her own part in the sexual dance, she is more likely to be satisfied. For the greatest mutual satisfaction, the man and woman need to be counseled to collaborate and cooperate with each other.

First Pregnancy. The first pregnancy is usually a turning point in early marriage. Couples are generally unaware of the changes in sexual desire and responsiveness that typically occur during a pregnancy, and appropriate counseling is indicated. It is best if the counseling can be done with family-centered maternity care for the couple rather than just with the female partner.

During the first trimester, desire and frequency of intercourse usually decline. This decline may be due to some of the unpleasant physical symptoms of pregnancy or to underlying psychologic factors, such as fear on the part of the couple regarding the potential for harm to the fetus as a result of intercourse. During the second trimester, sexual desire increases again, and some women report their most exquisite period of sexual responsiveness occurred during this period. It has been postulated that increased pelvic congestion may be a factor in increasing sexual desire. In the third trimester, probably as a result of the size of the abdomen and discomfort during intercourse, desire and frequency of intercourse tend to decline. As the woman's body changes, her feelings about her sexual attractiveness may be altered and she needs assurance from her spouse that she is still sexually desirable. Again, fears about the harmful effects of intercourse on the developing fetus usually surface in the couple. There is presently no firm support in the literature for increased risk of infection resulting from sex during pregnancy. Intercourse may be permitted, but alternative forms of sexual pleasuring should also be pointed out. As the abdominal girth increases, a change in coital position will improve comfort. Side-by-side front- or rear-entry positions are often recommended. The physician may suggest the couple use hand or mouth stimulation, but should caution against blowing air into the vagina during oral-genital sex because air embolism may occur. Recommend avoidance of intercourse if there is a history of early miscarriage; if bleeding, spotting, or leaking of amniotic fluid occurs; or if uterine contractions that resemble labor appear before the pregnancy could be viable. Bleeding during pregnancy commonly occurs from trauma to the highly vascular cervix; after confirmation by physical examination, reassure the couple that no harm has been done. Finally, advise the couple that the rates of orgasm with coitus diminish as pregnancy progresses and this should not become a source of deep concern. Changes in location of erogenous zones may occur, but experimentation may solve this problem.

Following pregnancy, sexuality takes another altered course. Predictably, there will be a low level of sexual tension for 4 to 6 weeks postpartum because of low estrogen and high progesterone levels. Advise the couple that as sexual desire begins to return, they may return to sexual activity if contraception has been planned for, if no pain occurs with pressure applied to the episiotomy area, and if the lochia has changed from a reddish to a yellow or brownish color. The use of Kegel's exercises to strengthen the perineal muscles after the stretching caused by childbirth is extremely helpful in the restoration of satisfactory lovemaking (Table 62–2). The interruption in a couple's sexual life by pregnancy requires a slow, gentle return with a new "courting" period to help negotiate the transition. Pregnancy may have caused a decrease in sensitivity of the target organ responses, and more stimulation may be necessary than was needed prior to pregnancy. Women who are lactating need to know that vaginal lubrication is usually insufficient and that some water-soluble lubricant should be used. A lactation response may occur upon achieving orgasm, and the couple needs to be forewarned of this. Likewise, orgasm may result from lactation and breast-feeding, and it is wise to inform the lactating mother of this phenomenon so that she can enjoy it as a normal "side effect" of nursing rather than be embarrassed or disturbed about it.

The reproductive years are encumbered with the raising of children and the intense drive for career success. The fatigue and loss of sleep associated with caring for small children is responsible in large measure for a rather predictable decrease in sexual desire. This decrease may be experienced by the woman more than the man if child rearing is not shared by both. From this problem may result a disparate level of sexual drive expressed by the woman as "he wants sex too much" and by the man as "she doesn't want sex enough." Another common problem is the lack of privacy for intimate behavior. A lock for the bedroom door is a simple solution for inhibited arousal experienced because of fear of discovery by the children.

As the number of dual-career couples increases, so does the pattern of the "workaholic" husband or wife. There is really so much to be done to keep the household going and to keep each person's career afloat that the couple often have very little time and energy left for each other. If this is a choice that both people make and that they are both happy with, the physician need not try to change it. Sometimes, however, an inquiry into the pattern of "busyness" will lead to the discovery that the patient is not really happy with that life style and has used it as a coping mechanism to control sexual anxiety. Use the example of developing a savings account as an analogy for

Table 62–2. KEGEL'S PUBOCOCCYGEUS MUSCLE EXERCISES*

Female

The patient locates the correct muscle by sitting on the toilet with knees as far apart as possible and begins urination; contract perineum only to stop the flow.

Exercises should be practiced 2 to 3 times daily at varying intervals to avoid tenderness and fatigue.

1. Contract the pubococcygeus muscle and hold for a count of 3; relax. Begin with 10, work up to 30, at each practice.
2. Contract and release the pubococcygeus muscle as rapidly as possible in a flicking motion. Begin with 10, work up to 30 or more with each practice.
3. Breathe deeply and imagine drawing air in through the vagina, tightening the muscle as you inhale. Begin with 5, work up to 15, at each practice.
4. Bear down as if having a bowel movement or giving birth, relax, then tighten the pubococcygeus muscle. Begin with 5, work up to 15, at each practice. If done prior to intercourse, vasocongestion and arousal may be enhanced.

Once learned, these exercises may be done at any time, and if associated with things the patient does consistently, it is easier to remember to practice them. Regular practice over a period of months may be necessary before results are noted. Once good muscle tone is established, maintenance exercises of 10 to 30 contractions per day are usually sufficient.

Male

The patient locates the correct muscle by beginning to urinate and then stopping the flow. When the muscle is tightened, the penis will lift slightly.

Exercises 1, 2, and 4 above are recommended to enhance erections and ejaculatory control.

*Adapted from Hartman, W. E., and Fithian, M.: Long Beach, CA, Center for Marital and Sexual Studies, 1972.

developing an improved intimate relationship; as with the bank, when there is no deposit there is no return. Explain that developing an intimate relationship requires spending time together, listening to each other, and touching each other in nonsexual and affectionate ways, which then can lead on into more intimate and sexual activity if the couple is comfortable with this. When sex is attempted separately from this context of intimacy and caring, it tends to be perfunctory and unsatisfactory. Very often, however, the couple has expected themselves and each other to be able to relate sexually without the context of affection and time together. When an authoritative person helps them understand that it simply does not work that way, they can be stimulated to sort out their priorities and to make some changes that may well result in greater satisfaction. If people see intimacy as a legitimate need, they can frequently protect their time together in such a way as to make it quality time and to improve their relationship.

As the marriage relationship develops over time, the partners often begin to communicate with each other more about general issues of daily life—what to do about children, the house, the car, and financial problems—and exhibit less concern for maintaining intimacy. Their sexual development as a couple may fall victim to routinization and boredom.

Midlife. Continuing development of the intimate and erotic aspects of a marital relationship requires that some effort be expended as the marriage matures, yet couples often are afraid, shy, or uninformed about how to introduce variety into their sexual life; old habits are difficult to change. The marriage may continue as a functional unit until the children have grown up and are leaving home, and then the original marriage contract comes up for renegotiation in one way or another.

Unexpected difficulties may arise when, instead of leaving home, the grown children elect to continue to live with their parents or, after having left, return. This "elastic nest" is a development that may coincide with the need to care for elderly parents in the home. In addition to increased stress, the elastic nest syndrome involves a reduction in the privacy that the middle-aged couple may have looked forward to in order to reconstitute their intimate relationship. The physician can encourage careful planning and insistence first upon meeting the needs of the middle-aged couple before offering assistance to the generation on either side.

Predictable developmental crises of midlife have been described, the most important of which involve increasing assertiveness and independence of women and increasing emotionality and sensuousness of men (Sheehy, 1974). Not surprisingly, many people experience a full-blown identity crisis characterized by many of the same features that characterize adolescence—rebelliousness, a desire to be independent, and a wish to be "one's own boss." Unfortunately, this internal upheaval in both the husband and wife usually occurs at the same time that the children are having their first feelings of rebelliousness and confusion, and the couple's intimacy balance almost surely is upset or severely tested. In the marital crises that occur so frequently at this time, the inner restrictions of earlier years tend to be projected onto the partner, and there is often a great deal of blaming. The physician who is aware of this developmental stage can help patients understand that there is great potential for growth in this period if the crisis is handled in a constructive way.

The importance of this struggle for adolescents has come to be respected or, at least, to be recognized. However, in this turbulent period adults face identical tasks that are equally essential for continued growth. Mother and father and adolescents in the family are thus all going through a crisis of identity, with the corresponding role confusion, conflict between dependence and independence, and the desire to form new relationships with people outside the family. It is this last point that often brings the most misfortune to the middle-aged family. In the young, the importance of making friends, forming alliances, and falling in love outside the family is acknowledged as a legitimate part of self-discovery. When this happens in adult life, an extramarital affair results. Various surveys have placed the estimate for extramarital sex by married women and men at between 1 in 4 and 1 in 3. Although an accurate estimate is methodologically difficult to obtain, the incidence of extramarital sexual experiences has increased since the 1950's Kinsey data were recorded, especially for women. A perfectly good marriage may be destroyed because people believe that affairs should not happen if a husband and wife love each other.

In an extramarital relationship, with less at stake emotionally than in their marriage, people allow themselves to experiment more freely with new sexual behaviors—to try them on for size and to see if a new style fits better than an old pattern. The tragedy occurs when husbands and wives fail to see the experimental nature of the affair. Affairs can be very risky and full of potential hurt to all concerned, although increasing numbers of people are having them anyway—sometimes with sexual involvement and sometimes without. This midlife phenomenon should be seen in such a light that irrevocable damage to the person's most important relationships may be avoided.

The reward for managing to survive this period of the family life cycle is the ultimate reorganization of the personality of the partners in the direction of greater autonomy, strength, and commitment. The marriage relationship may be reconstituted and revitalized. The partners involved may emerge with a clearer sense of who they are and, therefore, a greater sense of freedom in the relationship. It is not uncommon for marital partners who are survivors of this kind of struggle to report a sense of remarriage, although to the same spouse.

With greater self-awareness and fewer inhibitions, women often find their interest in and enjoyment of sexual activity increasing and they are willing to take more responsibility for their own and their partner's satisfaction. At the same time, men become more sensual and less genitally oriented. They may begin to experience some changes in response that are perfectly normal but that may make them more cautious in sexual performance and appear to be less interested. The middle-aged man tends to need more time and more direct stimulation to facilitate erection and usually finds that his need to ejaculate is less intense. It is important to understand that orgasm and ejaculation are not the same phenomenon. The two responses nearly always occur together in young men, but in the older man, orgasm may occur without ejaculation if he will let himself experience his sensations instead of trying to force himself to ejaculate. The man's sexual partner should understand this as well to prevent worry about "withholding" of orgasm. Trying to force ejaculation may produce enough anxiety to result in avoidance of sex and, possibly, in erectile dysfunction. (At any age, simultaneous orgasm is at best a happy accident. Too many couples have ruined their sex lives by trying to accomplish this whenever they make love. It often works better to plan tandem orgasms taking turns with who goes first.)

As the natural shifts of midlife occur, there are new delights in store, especially when the couple keep in touch with each other's changes by talking together and sharing feelings with each other. Many people are afraid to share their sexual fears and worries with each other, but when they do, they discover that vulnerability brings intimacy. The family physician can be extremely helpful to such a couple by bringing them together in the office and gently facilitating their discussions about sexual concerns or any other strains that they are experiencing at midlife.

Aging. In both the aging man and woman, the best guarantee of continued function is regular, frequent sexual intercourse or masturbation, or both. Continuing to feel that sensuality and sexuality is an important dimension of life helps improve functioning and enjoyment of sex. Needs of the couple often shift from a primary focus on genital sex to greater needs for intimacy, closeness, and touch. Many older women may have a greater interest in sex than their male partners and need to be given permission to view masturbation as an acceptable alternative.

The menopausal woman may suffer from lack of estrogen, which causes a thin, atrophic vaginal epithelium that does not lubricate well in response to sexual stimulation. Estrogen creams or oral estrogens may be prescribed, and water-soluble lubricants may reduce discomfort. A notable hindrance to the enjoyment of sex in the elderly woman is the occurrence of tetanic uterine contractions that may be noted after the menopause. These tetanic contractions set up a fear of pain and an avoidance cycle that often leads to a precipitous drop in sexual activity. Orally prescribed estrogen therapy alleviates this complication. As the woman ages, the vaginal walls tend to lose some elasticity, and the capability of lengthening the vaginal barrel is reduced. Sudden penile thrusting may injure the vaginal epithelium, and the couple should be slower and more gentle in lovemaking. Orgasm may take longer to occur and may be shorter and less intense. The couple should alter their expectations realistically as they grow older rather than consider these normal changes to be indicative of failure.

Whether or not there is a true male climacteric remains a matter of medical debate; however, it appears that a small percentage of men do suffer from a seriously decreasing testosterone level. If this problem is found in a patient, replacement therapy is indicated. In most men, the decline in circulating testosterone levels appears to be so gradual over a period of time that it is probably only a small factor.

The aging man requires a longer period of direct penile stimulation to achieve full erection, but the erection may last for a longer time. Both the volume of seminal fluid and the force of ejaculation are reduced, and occasionally, retrograde ejaculation may appear. If the aging man does not expect these changes, he may perceive them as the first signs of sexual failure. He may then avoid further attempts at sexual functioning so as not to experience the inevitable disappointment or precipitously seek a new, younger partner in an attempt to rejuvenate himself. Additionally, the loss of elastic tissue in the anterior abdominal wall causes a change in the angle of the erect penis; some males mistake this for a change in the hardness of the erection. The adverse psychologic effect of observing the changes of aging needs to be overcome by counseling so that an occasional normal failure does not lead to serious sexual dysfunction.

After the death of a spouse and after 1 or more years of sexual continence, the reawakening of sexual desire may be difficult to achieve. This problem is described as the "widow's" or the "widower's" syndrome and is often encountered in elderly patients. The man may experience erectile failure as memories of a long-cherished previous spouse block the achievement of intimacy and sexual response with a new partner. The woman who tries to return to sexual activity after a period of continence may find that vaginal atrophy has occurred, making vaginal penetration and coitus very painful. Use of intravaginal estrogen cream, Kegel exercises, and progressively larger sized dilators returns the vaginal barrel to a sexually functioning diameter and length. In both men and women, excellent sexual functioning can be expected to return with adequate professional help and an understanding sexual partner. Sexuality need not die in old age.

Psychosexual Disorders

Disturbances in normal sexual adjustment may be subdivided into three categories: gender identity disorders, paraphilias, and psychosexual dysfunctions.

GENDER IDENTITY DISORDERS

Gender identity disorders involve a discrepancy between the actual anatomic sex of the individual and the sex that is perceived internally by that individual. These disorders may not be discovered until adulthood, but behavioral symptoms and problems with sexual adjustment can usually be traced back into childhood and adolescence. Gender identity disorders are rare and should not be confused diagnostically with the more common feelings of inadequacy about fulfilling expected sexual stereotypes of "maleness" and "femaleness." Most of the time, these disorders can be spotted in an early form during childhood and referral for counseling often fosters normal developmental adjustment. It is improper to tell parents who are concerned about their children's disordered psychosexual development that it is merely a stage that the child is going through and that he or she will probably outgrow the disordered behavior. In adolescence these children are often troubled by severe anxiety, depression, and even suicidal ideation. Failure to identify these psychosexual disorders in their early stages only prolongs the suffering of the child and the family and perhaps endangers the child's life.

Gender Identity Disorder of Childhood. This disorder is marked by a persistent discomfort in a child about his or her own biologic sex and a desire or insistence to be of the other sex (Rekers and Milner, 1979). There is usually a persistent denial of the individual's own anatomic attributes that goes beyond "tomboyishness" or "sissyish" behavior. Girls may insist that they are biologically unable to have children, refuse to urinate in a sitting position, and claim that they will grow up to be men and grow a penis. Boys with this disorder prefer to dress in girls' or women's clothing, regularly prefer girls as playmates, and are judged by cultural standards to exhibit feminine behavior, gestures, and actions. These boys are almost always teased and rejected by their male peers, and attendance at school is usually a problem. The onset of the problem occurs during early childhood, and the majority of boys who cross-dress begin to do so before their 4th birthday; teasing and rejection by male peers with significant social conflict is usually present by age 7 or 8 years of age. During adolescence, one third to two thirds of the male gender–dysphoric patients may develop a homosexual orientation.

Girls with an identity disorder of childhood also express symptoms at an early age, but most begin to give in to social pressures by late childhood or adolescence and only a minority maintain their identity as males. There may be some possibility that boys with this disorder may historically have had extreme and excessive physical or emotional closeness with their mothers and a relative absence of fathering during early formative years. Girls who develop the disorder may have had mothers who were unavailable at an early age, perhaps because of schizophrenia or other psychologic disorders or because of illness, and the girl seems to make a stronger identification with the male role of the father.

When symptoms of gender identity disturbances become apparent, evaluation begins with a medical history and a physical examination. Abnormal or ambiguous genitalia militates against this diagnosis. The parents should be interviewed, and perhaps the child's teacher as well, in order to determine what types of behavior are exhibited. These children are at high risk for developing transsexualism, transvestism, or adult homosexuality; and behavior change, if it is desired, needs to be instituted at an early age. Some symptoms of sexual identity disturbance in girls include chronic rejection of female clothing and appearance; masculine gestures and dress; avoidance of girls as playmates; playing as "one of the boys"; a desire to be given a boy's name; masturbatory behavior while dressed in male clothing; a strong desire to be called a male and to have a penis; and a request for male hormones or sexual reassignment surgery. In boys, the symptoms of sexual identity disturbance include dressing in feminine clothing and the use of cosmetics; feminine gestures and gait; avoidance of boys as playmates; trying to be feminine by joining girls' activities; masturbation with female clothing; an expressed desire to be a female, have children, and breast-feed; and request for removal of the penis or for other sexual reassignment procedures.

Since these problems are complex, detection of a gender identity disorder almost always indicates referral to a child psychiatrist. Family counseling includes encouraging the boy's father or the girl's mother to be as visible and positive a role model as possible. Father-son or mother-daughter activities should be increased in frequency and the disordered behavior actively discouraged. Punishment for cross-gender behavior is not appropriate, however, but the rewarding of appropriate gender behavior is vital. At each regular office visit, progress toward normal sexual identity should be assessed and the family given support.

Transsexualism. This is a later-appearing gender identity disorder, with an estimated prevalence in males of 1:30,000 and 1:100,000 in females; this condition is not merely a variation of homosexuality. It should not be diagnosed until a person has had at least 2 years of persistent and continuous desire to be rid of his or her genitals and live as a member of the opposite sex. If there is a condition of ambiguous genitalia, transsexualism should *not* be diagnosed.

A clear difference between *transsexualism* and *transvestism* exists. The transsexual is very uncomfortable with his or her genitals and finds them repugnant. There is a very intense feeling of inappropriateness about one's anatomic sex, and there are no mental disorders (i.e., schizophrenia). Transvestism, on the other hand, is a paraphilic disorder in which the individual considers himself or herself to be basically of the correct anatomic sex, but who must indulge in recurrent, persistent cross-dressing for the purpose of sexual excitement. Transvestism may be part of a spectrum of behavior that may or may not evolve into transsexualism.

Male transsexualism is more common than the female type, the ratio being perhaps 2 to 1. Because of associated anxiety, depression, and dysfunctional social and occupational adjustment, problems can easily occur as the transsexual attempts to live in the desired gender role. Gender identity problems in childhood often are present before transsexualism develops, but the full syndrome does not usually appear until late adolescence or early adult life. There are probably about 10,000 transsexuals in the United States today, 2000 of whom have changed their sex through surgery.

The role of the physician in the management of transsexualism is first to recognize the gender identity problems of childhood and prevent progression *if possible*. When the behavior pattern has been persistent and chronic, referral to a gender-identity clinic or a sexual reassignment clinic is important so that the patient may receive the concentrated efforts of psychologists, endocrinologists, and sexual reassignment surgeons. The physician needs to remain nonjudgmental and attuned to the family and social problems the patient may experience. Reassurance, kindness, support, a desire to help, and treating the patient as a person have a positive effect. If the family members of the transsexual patient express a need for understanding in this unusual situation, the physician can be helpful by reassuring them that transsexualism is not hereditary and that established family relationships need to be continued and stabilized.

Obviously, transsexualism requires more than just medical treatment. The number of people presenting for sex change operations is increasing at major medical centers in the United States, and concern about how to diagnose and treat these individuals has surfaced. The high costs of elective surgery are a drawback to its widespread use. Family physicians can be of great assistance to the gender identity disorder clinic by providing historical information gained from the prior long-term care of these individuals. Even after referral to such a clinic, the patient certainly needs continuing primary care that is provided in a supportive and understanding manner.

The family physician may also be asked to manage the maintenance of hormone therapy. In the case of the female-to-male change, androgens (testosterone, 250 to 300 mg. intramuscularly each month) are given to redistribute body weight, grow facial hair, lower the pitch of the voice, build muscle mass, and suppress menstruation. Requests for mastectomy are common, followed less often by desire for hysterectomy and oophorectomy. A minority of patients request construction of a phallus. In the male-to-female gender reassignment, estrogen therapy (stilbesterol, 0.05 mg. daily, or conjugated estrogens, 1.25 to 2.5 mg. daily) aids in the development of breasts and in a few cases provides a more feminine appearance to body contours. Estrogens do not raise the pitch of the voice or reduce growth of the beard. Voice training and electrolytic depilation are usually necessary for these problems. Potential risks of hormone therapy, such as vascular thrombosis and malignant breast tumors, should be explained but rarely are patients deterred from proceeding. Penectomy is usually requested, with construction of a vagina using the invaginated scrotal and penile skin. Dilating molds are necessary. As long as the crura (roots of the penis) are kept intact, orgasm may still be possible. Breast augmentation may also be requested.

PARAPHILIAS

The second group of psychosexual disorders, paraphilias, may be defined as the need to perform unusual or bizarre acts in order to obtain sexual excitement. These behaviors are involuntary, repetitive, and usually involve preference of a nonhuman object for sexual arousal, repetitive sexual activity with humans involving real or simulated suffering or humiliation, or repetitive sexual activity with nonconsenting partners. The sexual partner of the paraphiliac may consent to erotic behavior but may end up feeling excluded or superfluous or may possibly be injured in the act. The most common paraphilias are pedophilia (sexual activity with prepubertal children), fetishism (sexual stimulation through nonliving objects), transvestism (cross-dressing), zoophilia (use of animals in sexual activity), exhibitionism (exposing the genitals), voyeurism (looking or "peeping"), sexual masochism (excitement produced through suffering), and sexual sadism (excitement produced by infliction of suffering). Other, atypical paraphilias include coprophilia (with feces), frotteurism (with rubbing), klismaphilia (with enema), mysophilia (with filth), necrophilia (with a corpse), telephone scatologia (lewdness), and urophilia (urine).

Paraphiliacs tend not to regard themselves as ill. They usually come to the physician's attention only after their behavior has brought them into conflict with the law. In these cases, the physician's task is primarily crisis intervention: Some conflict with the law or society needs to be mediated; an often unsuspecting, shocked, and embarrassed family must be counseled and supported; the sexual offender may need support and even physical protection; and referral for psychiatric treatment must be arranged.

Cases of paraphilia are quite complex and the recidivism rate is high, particularly for those who display exhibitionism and pedophilia. The physician should remember that many of these activities carry considerable risk not only to the consenting or nonconsenting partner but also to the paraphiliac. Accidental death has occurred during acts of sexual fetishism and sadomasochism. In the case of patients who exhibit pedophilia, many were themselves victims of sexual abuse. Psychiatric intervention should be undertaken as soon as the problem is discovered.

PSYCHOSEXUAL DYSFUNCTION

The Natural Response Cycle. The complete sexual response cycle can be divided into the following phases (American Psychiatric Association, 1987):

1. Appetitive—fantasies about and a desire for sexual activity.
2. Excitement—a subjective sense of pleasure and the accompanying physiologic changes. The major change in the male consists of penile tumescence, leading to erection and the appearance of Cowper's gland secretion. The major changes in the female consist of generalized vasocongestion in the pelvis, vaginal lubrication, and swelling of the external genitalia. The orgasmic platform is developed—that is, the narrowing of the outer third of the vagina by increased pubococcygeal muscle tension and vasocongestion; vasocongestion of the labia minora, along with breast tumescence; and lengthening and widening of the inner two thirds of the vagina.
3. Orgasm—a peaking of sexual pleasure with release of sexual tension in rhythmic contraction of the perineal muscles and pelvic reproductive organs. In the male, this is preceded by the sensation of ejaculatory inevitability, which is followed by emission of semen caused by contractions of the prostate, seminal vesicles, and urethra. In the female, orgasm is accompanied by contractions of the outer third of the vagina, although these are not always subjectively experienced. Both the male and female experience generalized muscular tension, contractions, and involuntary pelvic thrusting.
4. Resolution—a sense of general well-being and muscular relaxation. Men are physiologically refractory to further erection and orgasm for a period of time. In contrast, women may be able to respond to additional stimulation almost immediately.

The natural sequence typically develops out of desire and proceeds through phases of arousal and plateau (excitement), orgasm, and resolution. The length of time spent in the different phases of the sequence varies greatly from individual to individual, from one sex to the other, and from one occasion to another in the same person (Fig. 62–2).

On a physiologic level, the human sexual response is as natural a function as breathing or digestion. However, the cycle is very sensitive to interference by the critical faculties of the mind as well as the emotions; in other words, what the individual thinks or feels can profoundly affect sexual functioning. Inhibitions of clinical significance may occur at one or more phases in the response cycle.

Psychosexual Dysfunctions. Sex with a partner is the most intimate and vulnerable form of human communication because it involves the sexual value system and self-esteem of two people. It requires the meshing of two sets of expectations, two sets of fears, and two sets of potential problems with communication. Sexual activity is supposed to be pleasurable, but sometimes it seems like a miracle that people ever manage to enjoy themselves. When a patient or couple present with complaints of sexual dysfunction, there is no uninvolved partner. Each person contributes to and is affected by what happens in the sexual relationship. It is not helpful to accept the statement of one partner that it is "all my fault." In fact, the superior stance of the "normal" partner may be part of the problem. The couple's relationship should be the focus of therapy, with collaboration between the partners to determine the desired outcomes. In *either partner*, there may be *physical* factors, *psychologic* factors, and *situational* factors that contribute to the problem. In the *relationship*, there may also be *physical* factors, such as the lack of opportunity because of frequent separation due to illness or travel. When the couple gets back together again, they must go through a period of adjustment. Adverse *emotional* factors include the conspiracy of silence, withdrawal from sexual contact, failure to express feelings, and perhaps a lack of affectionate touch. Interactional factors include power struggles, hurt and hostility, and perhaps a trade off between control over money versus control over sex. This systems approach to the diagnosis of sexual dysfunctions is presented in Figure 62–3.

THE SEXUAL RESPONSE CYCLE

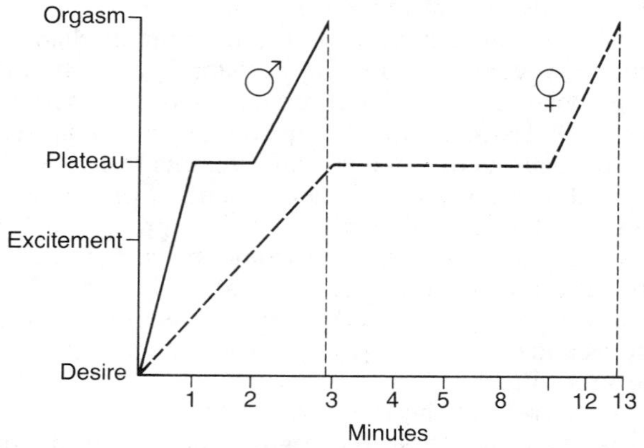

Figure 62–2. The figure illustrates the asynchronous nature of the average male and female response cycles. By prolongation of the plateau phase in the male, the partners may achieve closer proximity of orgasm. For clarity, the gradual tapering of sexual excitement (resolution phase) is not shown in the figure.

Performance anxiety is most commonly responsible for sexual dysfunction. When fears concerning sexual performance dominate a relationship, either or both of the partners sacrifice spontaneity and become careful observers of their own sexual behaviors, sometimes called "spectatoring." As they watch and measure their sexual response and look for physical signs of excitement, the experience ceases to be a naturally occurring, mutually shared expression of need and feeling. The individual becomes unable to focus on pleasurable sensations, and the couple, instead of relating to each other in a warm and spontaneous way, becomes two actors attempting to carry out roles they expect of themselves. Unfortunately, spectatoring usually confirms the worst fears, short-

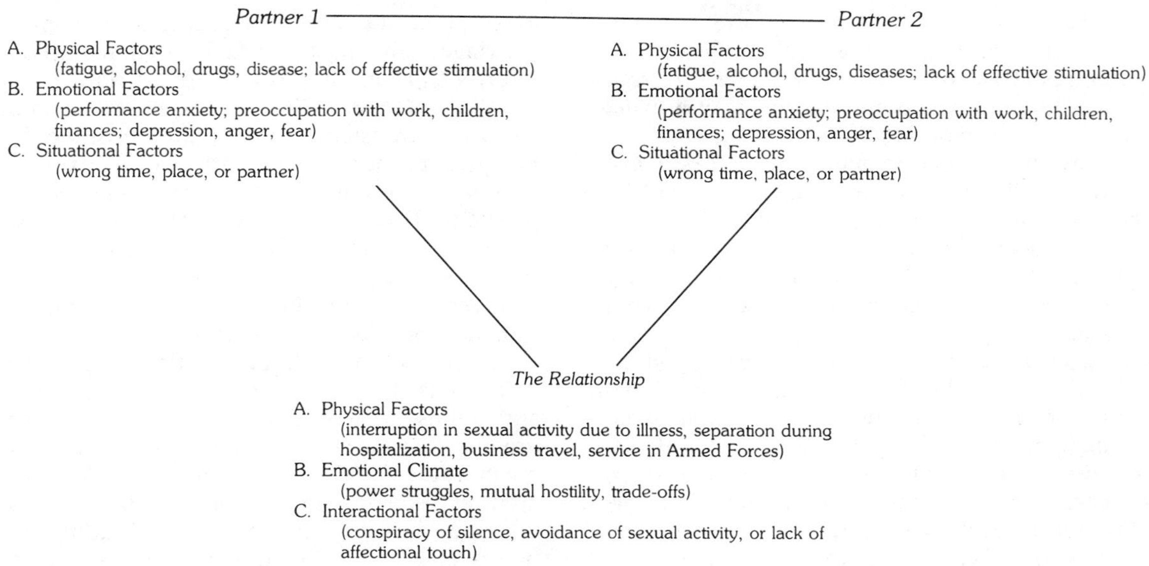

Figure 62–3. A systems approach to the diagnosis of sexual dysfunction.

circuiting the natural response. When both partners have previously been functional and performance anxiety is of short duration, the family physician may help by asking for a ban on intercourse and prescribing *sensate focus exercises* for nondemand pleasuring (Barbach, 1976). Encourage the couple to gently caress and pleasure each other in graduated stages, first by general body caressing and later by genital caressing, but insist on the absence of pressure to move ahead to intercourse so there is time for the natural excitement response to return.

If people are simply told to go home and do these exercises, they often go home and do what they have always done, which produces the end result that they have previously experienced—that is, failure. The physician should break that cycle by having the couple sit down together in the physician's presence, with the physician instructing them to relax, take deep breaths, close their eyes, and gently caress each other's hand. Ask the couple to explore the texture of the skin, the structure, the temperature of each hand slowly, gently, and very carefully. This *guided caress* can be the foundation for change in the way the partners touch each other (Hartman and Fithian, 1972). The presence of the physician can reduce anxiety, help each person focus more intently on what he or she is experiencing, and begin to institute change in the couple's sexual relationship. Instruct the couple to practice this again at home, and then to proceed on to a face caress, then to a foot bath and caress, and finally to an all-over nude body caress but without genital stimulation. The ban on intercourse is maintained throughout the process, even when genital stimulation is added to the body caress. When both partners feel satisfied with the way they have been able to complete these exercises, they are given instruction for the *quiet vagina exercise* (Hartman and Fithian, 1972). If the woman has been having the major difficulty with orgasmic response, she is instructed to insert the man's penis when *she* is ready. If the problem is with the male's erection, the woman is given the authority to initiate penile insertion, which can be accomplished whether or not the penis is fully erect. The couple should simply lie together for 15 or 20 minutes after insertion of the penis with no movement or thrusting and only enough stimulation from the woman's vaginal muscle to maintain the man's erection. Eventually, when both partners feel secure in this exercise, the ban on intercourse is lifted. When one or both members of the couple have long-lasting problems with performance anxiety or deep-seated conflicts about closeness, intimacy, and pleasure, the couple needs more than this level of therapy, and they should be referred to a qualified sex therapist who is able to devote more time to helping them work out their problems.

Disorders of Desire in Both Sexes. Inhibited sexual desire is currently the most common sexual complaint and is expressed as a problem by 30 to 40 per cent of patients seeking help for sexual problems (Kaplan, 1979). It may be a primary condition based on the individual's temperament (some people are simply at the asexual end of the continuum) or upbringing (which might have resulted in a fear of experiencing sexual pleasure). Secondary disorders of desire grow out of repeated disappointment and frustration during sexual encounters, anger towards the partner, or fear of abandonment. Additionally, loss of libido is frequently associated with drugs, fatigue, anxiety, or depression.

Unless they are associated with a treatable condition such as depression, desire disorders are difficult to treat with brief therapy and, therefore, require referral. However, occasionally this problem grows out of distaste related to a partner's poor personal hygiene or style of initiating intimacy. When these factors can be uncovered in the history, the situation can be handled effectively by the family physician.

Excitement Disorders in the Female. In rare instances a woman may report total or partial *sexual anesthesia*, i.e., she experiences no sensation or response to sexual stimulation and may not perceive genital touch at all. This problem may or may not be accompanied by aversion to coitus. The location and extent of the anesthesia is determined by sex history and sexologic examination. Treatment of this disorder is very time consuming and should be referred to a sex therapist.

General sexual dysfunction is a condition in which the woman derives slight or no pleasure from sexual stimulation. Erotic feelings and desire are not experienced; the typical physiologic signs of arousal (lubrication and development of the orgasmic platform) do not occur. These women are frequently anorgasmic but not necessarily so. Lack of pleasure in the experience is the key to diagnosis. These women rarely seek sexual activity of their own accord and may report experiencing irritation rather than pleasurable sensation on being touched. This may be a primary or secondary condition, absolute (with all partners), or situational (under specific conditions and with certain partners but not with others). Occasionally, with a partner of a different race or a different social class or with the use of a specific type of stimulation, the woman might be able to experience arousal.

Objective evidence of this condition in the clinical situation is difficult to obtain. Sexual history can help to differentiate whether the condition is due to psychologic conflict about sexual activity or about the particular partner or whether or not there was inadequate sexual experience necessary to develop a natural response pattern. This condition may also result from repeated frustrating, unsatisfactory, or painful experience with sexual activity, so that the body has simply "given up" trying to respond. Cases in which the woman has been able to become aroused in the past are associated with a better prognosis. The family physician can encourage the couple to place a ban on intercourse and to take part in the sensate focus exercises described previously. If the couple has attempted these exercises without any feeling of progress or if the couple has resisted doing the exercises, it would be wise to refer them to a sex therapist.

Excitement Disorders in the Male. This disorder is characterized by primary or secondary erectile dysfunction. It is estimated that 50 per cent of men have some period of erectile dysfunction during their lifetime (Kaplan, 1979).

Primary erectile dysfunction (never having been able to achieve erection sufficient for intercourse) is rare. In the absence of congenital, acquired physical, or endocrine factors, a psychogenic cause is most likely. Severe sexual anxiety may be related to either religious beliefs, homosexual orientation, or traumatic failure at first coital attempts. It may occur in conjunction with vaginismus in a sexually anxious and inexperienced couple, producing an unconsummated marriage. The problem is of such complexity that referral to a sex therapist is appropriate.

Secondary erectile dysfunction is much more common, and transient episodes are considered normal. Fatigue, preoccupation with work, overeating, or drinking too much can easily cause a temporary problem. Because society puts enormous value on the male's ability to become erect, a single failure can produce performance anxiety that precipitates recurrences, establishing a pattern of dysfunction. If a man experiences erectile problems in 25 per cent or more of coital opportunities, the condition is defined as secondary erectile dysfunction (Masters and Johnson, 1970). It is important to assess for organic factors such as diabetes, circulatory inadequacy (atherosclerosis or venous insufficiency), lowered testosterone production, overuse of alcohol and nicotine, and drug use before concluding that a patient's erectile dysfunction is psychogenic in origin. Ten years ago it was believed that about 15 per cent of cases of erectile failure were organic; however, now that new technologies have improved diagnosis, the organic causes versus psychologic causes are thought to be 50/50. When the sex history suggests an organic cause for the dysfunction (vascular problems, 25 per cent; endocrine problems, 10 per cent; diabetes, 1 to 10 per cent; drugs; neurologic problems; and zinc deficit), treatment for the specific cause should be instituted. All patients with an organic cause have some degree of psychogenic potentiation of the disorder.

When the diagnosis of erectile failure is indeterminate or needs confirmation, erection capability can be tested by measurement of nocturnal penile tumescence with sophisticated electronic equipment in a sleep lab. Two strain gauges on the penis (base of shaft and just below the glans) are used to check for nocturnal erections with an increase in circumference of more than 15 mm. at both gauges. If this occurs, the erectile dysfunction is probably psychogenic (Baum, 1989). The family physician may make this determination using a strip of postage stamps or "plumber's tape" as a substitute for the elaborate electronics. When plumber's tape is placed around a changing cylindrical circumference, it will expand but not contract. Strips of tape are placed circumferentially around the flaccid penis at bedtime and checked the following morning. If the penis is organically unable to erect, the normal pattern of five to seven sleep erections will not occur and the tape or postage stamps will have remained in conformation to the size of the flaccid penis. If erections have occurred, the tape cylinder will have stretched to a larger diameter or the stamp strip will have torn apart. A commercially available product (the Snap Gauge by Dacomed Corporation) measures erections by the breaking of several plastic membranes that snap at different degrees of rigidity. Vasculogenic erectile failure can be documented by measuring the penile systolic blood pressure via a Doppler probe. Penile artery pressure that is 70 per cent or less of brachial artery pressure suggests vascular insufficiency. Performance anxiety and a negative response from the partner may be a part of organic erectile failure, too. Therefore, treatment may need to focus on the psychologic as well as the organic components of the problem.

The treatment plan begins with a ban on intercourse, and the couple is instructed in nondemand pleasuring exercises. A man with erectile failure typically is so concerned with his partner that he does not readily allow himself to share in the pleasurable feelings. When asked how he feels about being caressed, a typical response is, "I don't think she likes doing this." The male needs to focus on himself and to let his partner feel and speak for herself. Many sexually dysfunctional people misread each other's nonverbal communication and tend to define their partner's reaction erroneously as negative, especially if the individual has feelings of rejection about a body part. He fails to understand that the partner could enjoy touching his penis and frequently does not allow the partner to fondle it.

A condition that may be confused with psychogenic impotence is the external iliac "steal syndrome" (Wagner and Green, 1981). The patient may achieve an almost normal erection but is not able to maintain it after coitus is initiated, particularly in the "missionary" position. Some patients may experience gluteal pain soon after their erection disappears. The condition is caused by a restricted blood flow to the lower limbs and pelvic area. Measurement of penile blood pressure is a method frequently used to diagnose this condition. Angiography may be necessary to demonstrate stenosis or occlusion of the penile arteries. Surgical intervention is the treatment of choice for many men with this condition. For others, assurance that their condition has an organic basis, combined with instruction about alternative sexual positions or relief from performance anxiety, may be sufficient.

Many advances have occurred within the past decade in the treatment of organic erectile dysfunction. Mechanical aids include suction devices that draw blood into the penis and sustain erection by a constriction applied to the base of the shaft (Osbon ErecAid), and by external devices that can be worn to enhance rigidity (Synergist Erection System). Yohimbine hydrochloride blocks alpha$_2$-adrenergic receptors and is sometimes able to restore good erectile function in cases of partial failure. Various vasoactive drugs (papaverine, phentolamine, prostaglandin E) have been utilized for intracavernosal injection of the penis. Blood flow into the penis increases by relaxing smooth muscle in the spongy erectile tissue. A caveat about injection therapy is to expect some degree of fibrosis to develop in the shaft of the penis from repeated needle injections. Prolonged erection (priapism) has also been noted as a complication of injection therapy. There are now multiple types of penile implant devices that offer an improvement over the perforated acrylic rods first used in 1960. The device was modernized in 1973 when intermittent erections were accomplished with use of the Scott Inflatable Prosthesis.

The partner of a man with erectile dysfunction tends to be bewildered, blames herself, or attributes the man's erectile problems to problems such as "He doesn't love me anymore"; "I'm not attractive to him"; "He's punishing me"; or "He must have another sexual partner." Although any of those factors may be involved, often they are not. The woman feels disappointed, hurt, angry, frustrated, concerned, or possibly relieved, depending on how she feels about sexual activity. The family physician should determine what factors and feelings are involved, allow their ventilation, and, if appropriate, help the couple begin to get back in touch with each other.

Orgasmic Phase Disorders in the Female. Orgasmic dysfunction refers to the inability to experience orgasm from sexual stimulation. The stages of desire, excitement, and often plateau are experienced, but the woman is unable to break through into orgasm. This condition may be primary, secondary, or situational.

In *primary orgasmic dysfunction* (or primary anorgasmia), the woman has never experienced orgasm by any means including self-stimulation, partner stimulation, fantasy, or dreams. However, when the woman's sex history is explored carefully and some descriptive assistance given, she may realize that she has, in fact, experienced orgasm, though not necessarily involving genital touching. For example, as a little girl, she may have learned to squeeze her thighs together rhythmically and repeatedly while sitting in school and experienced a rising, bubbling sensation in her genital area that was very pleasurable and that induced her to repeat this experience over and over. *Any* experience of orgasm precludes the diagnosis of true primary anorgasmia.

In true primary orgasmic dysfunction, the physiologic response pattern is underdeveloped or inhibited. For whatever reason, the woman has not learned to stimulate herself to orgasm and she has not established her own reflex-response pattern to transfer to her partnership. When repeated arousal to the plateau level has taken place without orgasm, the woman tends to become frustrated at a certain point in the response cycle and arousal is lost. The woman may begin to avoid the disappointment and physical discomfort of unrelieved pelvic congestion by avoiding sexual contact altogether. The woman may not feel free to allow herself to reach orgasm because of negative content in her sexual value system, such as a prohibition against touching genitalia or the strong admonition to keep sexual feelings under control so as to avoid pregnancy or misuse by the man.

Research indicates that one effective treatment for primary anorgasmia is the use of directed masturbation exercises (Barbach, 1976; Heiman et al., 1976). It is not uncommon to encounter considerable firm resistance on the part of the woman who is being encouraged to use this technique. Yet she must, at her own pace, learn how to engage in self-exploration and lower her resistance. It is essential for her to assume responsibility for seeking and utilizing effective sexual stimulation, avoiding the common but erroneous belief that the man is responsible for "giving" her an orgasm. The woman first learns what kinds of stimulation are effective for her and then must be willing to teach her partner.

A negative body image often accompanies primary anorgasmia, and the woman is told to look at herself nude in a mirror in the privacy of her home and carefully assess her feelings about each part of her body. She should note the correctable problems she sees and decide if it is worth the effort to correct them. Those that are uncorrectable must be accepted. Counsel the husband and wife together, suggesting the use of the guided-caress exercises, and a prescription of reading for both partners (Barbach, 1976; Heiman et al., 1976). Their problem can perhaps be overcome by a relatively brief period of office counseling, but if resistances seem too great or the problems too pervasive, referral to a sex therapist is indicated.

In *secondary orgasmic dysfunction*, orgasm has been experienced in the past but not at the present time. This condition may arise from decreased time and attention to courting as a preliminary to intercourse, resulting in "A kiss of the lips, a touch of the breast, and dive for the pelvis disease" (Masters, 1970). Fatigue, the stress of raising young children, preoccupation with careers, and the allocation of too little time for intimacy are the most common contributing factors.

This problem is easiest to treat if it is discovered and dealt with before frustration, anxiety, and negative feelings have grown and before avoidance patterns have developed. Help the couple to discuss the problem openly; transmit information about the human sexual response cycle and the development of the orgasmic platform; teach that sexual interaction does not need to cease with the male's orgasm and ejaculation; give permission to the woman to explore her own sexual sensations and to allow them to come into her partnership; and prescribe guided-caress exercises. If no progress is being made after several follow-up office visits, referral is indicated.

Situational orgasmic dysfunction refers to cases in which orgasm is experienced only occasionally; perhaps with certain kinds of stimulation (for example, with self-stimulation but not with stimulation by the partner). Many authorities believe that this is a normal variation of the female sexual response. However, if the woman wishes to learn how to have orgasm with intercourse, she and her partner are instructed to use the guided-caress exercises to reach a higher state of arousal; then she inserts the penis when she is ready using the female astride position and moves her pelvis so as to receive maximum stimulation for herself.

Alternatively, the couple may be shown the special position that provides the greatest degree of access to the clitoral area while the penis is within the vagina (Fig. 62–4). This is a very restful position for both partners. Intercourse can continue for a long period of time without strain; continued clitoral stimulation can easily be given by the man to his partner, by the woman to herself, or a vibrator may be used. Once the woman has had several successful experiences with orgasm in this fashion, she is usually able to utilize other positions. The man should be informed that a number of women benefit from continued clitoral stimulation during intercourse in order to reach orgasm and that his partner will teach him how she likes to be touched in order to accomplish their mutual goal.

There is a female analogue of premature ejaculation that is rare but can cause difficulty between the couple. The woman usually initiates sexual activity, comes to a very rapid orgasm, and may then turn over and go to sleep, leaving her partner unsatisfied. The physician should explore the dynamics of the couple's interaction, facilitate communication, and accommodate the man's need for effective sexual stimulation. As in the treatment of all dysfunctions, it is important to emphasize the shared responsibility of engaging in sexual activity.

Orgasmic Phase Disorders in the Male. The terms orgasm and ejaculation have traditionally been used interchangeably to describe the male experience of climax. Orgasm, however, can occur without ejaculation (some men in fact learn to have multiple orgasms), and ejaculation can occur with little or no sensation of pleasure or relief. Most notably this occurs when the male ejaculates preceding erection. These patients require referral.

Premature ejaculation is typified by the male becoming erect and ejaculating either just before intercourse or very quickly after insertion. Contemporary society places too much emphasis on the importance of simultaneous orgasms; therefore, this situation becomes a problem for the man's self-esteem and for the woman's sexual satisfaction. In the past, premature ejaculation has been attributed to the presence of psychopathology or hostile feelings toward women. Now it is understood that control of the ejaculatory reflex is largely a matter of conditioning based on learning from early experiences. The adolescent boy who learns to masturbate rapidly to ejaculation develops a rapid response pattern. Early experiences at intercourse in which there is fear of discovery or the man practiced ejaculating in his underwear during heavy petting sessions are precursors for difficulty in ejaculatory control.

The best treatment is a retraining process involving both partners, whereby the man is encouraged to assume a passive role and to focus on his own sensations. After a general body caress, the woman sits facing the man between or astride his legs and begins gentle manual pleasuring of his genitals to bring him erect. As he becomes aroused, he thinks of a scale from 0 (no arousal) to 10 (the point of

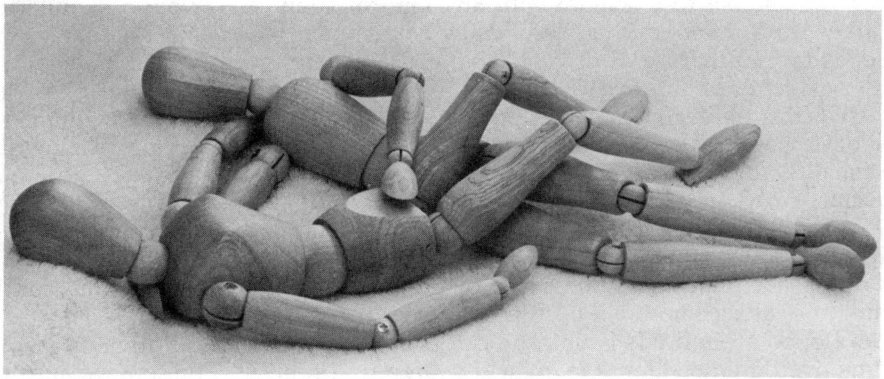

Figure 62–4. In this position, the man lies on his side and the woman lies on her back with both legs over his legs or with one leg over his side and the other leg between his legs. Both partners are supported by the bed, and the woman's breasts, abdomen, and clitoral area are accessible for additional stimulation. This position is useful for sexually dysfunctional couples and during advanced pregnancy or during times of illness or fatigue.

ejaculation). He analyzes his sensations of arousal and signals his partner as he approaches 7 or 8 on that scale (before the point of ejaculatory inevitability). At his signal, the woman performs the *squeeze technique*, placing her thumb on the frenulum of the penis and her first and second fingers just above and below the coronal ridge on the opposite side of the penis. She may use both hands. She firmly grasps the penis for a count of ten so that the man's sense of ejaculatory urgency will diminish. His erection may or may not also diminish. Pleasuring resumes until he signals her again. This procedure is repeated for a total of three times per session. Then he is allowed to go on to ejaculation on the fourth time. The couple is encouraged to repeat this for two more sessions during the first week; during the second week, the use of a lubricant is introduced to approximate the feeling of being inside the vagina. The sessions are repeated as before.

As the man feels more confident with his ejaculatory control, the couple may next use the *stuffing technique*. They use the squeeze only once but sufficiently to allow the penis to lose its erection; then the man's flaccid penis is stuffed inside the vagina with use of the female astride position. The female remains motionless until her partner gets used to being inside the vagina, then she begins to move slowly until he becomes erect. When he reaches the point he has learned to identify, he lets her know, and she disengages and uses the squeeze technique. This procedure of stuffing and squeezing is prescribed for three repetitions with the fourth repetition proceeding to orgasm and done for three sessions.

When vaginal containment can continue for about 5 minutes without ejaculation, the couple can initiate intercourse, use thrusting movements, and allow the man to ejaculate intravaginally. Whenever the man feels a need for assistance with ejaculatory control, he can ask his partner to use the squeeze technique again. If the couple has been separated for awhile, it is sometimes helpful to resume sexual activity by using this learned procedure. A pictorial and clear description of this procedure can be recommended for the patient's reading (Vandervoort and McIlvenna, 1972).

In place of the squeeze technique, other versions of treatment involve the *stop-start maneuver*, in which the couple simply stop moving when the man feels close to ejaculation, focus thoughts on a relaxing scene, breathe deeply, and rest until the man's desire to ejaculate is diminished.

Since the passive role for the man and the active role for the woman may be unfamiliar and anxiety provoking to the couple, support and encouragement from the physician, as well as explicit instruction in procedures, are very important. Make this treatment a playful and pleasurable exercise. When a good relationship exists between the couple, the woman often reports that she obtained considerable sexual arousal and a great deal of pleasure from giving pleasure to the man and assisting him in learning ejaculatory control. Because anorgasmia in the woman and premature ejaculation in the man are a common combination, the treatment is a helpful experience for both partners.

In taking a sex history, it is not uncommon to discover that a man with secondary erectile failure has a previous history of premature ejaculation. The erectile dysfunction is treated first, and the ejaculatory control is dealt with later. The squeeze technique, which includes body caressing and nondemand genital stimulation, may be the best treatment for both conditions.

As men become more willing to discuss their sexual practices, it appears that a number of men may experience retarded ejaculation, or difficulty in ejaculating, particularly as they grow older. This should not be confused with retrograde ejaculation that may result from diabetes, medication, or prior surgery. Anxiety about this normal development may cause even further difficulty and, in some cases, may lead to erectile dysfunction. Some men report that they fake ejaculation on occasion in order to be able to stop the sexual interaction with which they have become tired or bored. If the man continues to pressure himself to ejaculate, performance anxiety tends to interrupt the natural response.

A small percentage of men are unable to ejaculate intravaginally, and this is usually a primary condition. Some of these men can ejaculate with masturbation in private; others can ejaculate with manual or oral partner stimulation, but not during coitus. A few are unable to ejaculate with any kind of stimulation. In a number of cases this may be a condition secondary to the use of drugs (Table 62–3). There is also evidence of the psychogenic origin of the disorder based on rigid religious beliefs, rejection of the spouse, severe hostility and negative feelings, homosexuality, or anxiety in regard to producing pregnancy.

Since the female partner is called upon to participate in the treatment of this disorder, it is important to help her understand the cause of the dysfunction and to deal with her own hostility or distrust that has developed around this issue. The caress activities are employed to heighten the man's awareness of his physical sensations and to improve communication, particularly nonverbal communication patterns, between the couple. The pressure to perform is eliminated. When genital pleasuring takes place, the woman stimulates the man's penis in the way he finds most arousing, with the objective of producing ejaculation manually. The next step is to continue the sex play, keeping the man at a high plateau stage of arousal with the woman in the female astride position. As she excites him to the highest possible level of arousal before ejaculation, she then inserts the penis into the vagina rapidly, continuing penile stimulation with her hands if necessary or with her vaginal muscles. If ejaculation does not occur, the woman dismounts and continues manual stimulation until reinserting the penis at the point of ejaculatory inevitability (Kolodny et al., 1979). Often only one episode of intravaginal ejaculation is needed to reverse the dysfunction. If success is delayed, referral to a sex therapist is the best alternative.

Resolution Phase Disorder in the Male. Priapism in the male may result from systemic disease (sickle

Table 62–3. EFFECTS OF DRUGS ON SEXUALITY

Agent	Desire (Libido)	Excitement (Erection/Lubrication)	Plateau (Delay of Orgasm)	Ejaculation or Orgasm
Hormones				
Androgens	↑	↑	—	↑
Progestins	↓	—	—	↓ M
Estrogens	↓ M ↑ ± F	↓ M	↑ M	↓ M
Corticosteroids	↓	—	—	infertility
Cyproterone acetate	↓	↓ M	↑ M	infertility M
Antihypertensives				
Spironolactone	↓	↓ M	—	—
Prazosin	—	↓	—	—
Diuretics	↓	↓	—	—
Methyldopa	↓	↓	↑	↓
Alpha blockers (clonidine)	↓	↓	—	↓
Beta blockers (propranolol)	↓	↓	—	—
Guanethidine	↓	↓	↑	↓
Enalapril	—	↓	—	—
Reserpine	↓	↓	—	↓
Psychoactives				
Benzodiazepines	↓	—	—	↓
Phenothiazines	↓	↓	—	↓
Monoamine oxidase inhibitors	↓	↓	↑	↓
Tricyclics	↓	↓	↑	↓
Lithium	—	↓	—	—
Alcohol and sedative-hypnotics	↑ Low Doses ↓ High Doses	↑ ↓	↑ ↑	— ↓
Trazodone	—	↑ Priapism	—	—
Stimulants	↑ Low Doses ↓ High Doses	↓ ↓	— —	↑ ↓
Nicotine	—	↓	—	—
Miscellaneous				
Antihistamines	↓	↓	—	—
Cimetidine	↓	↓	—	infertility M
Antiparkinson's medications	↑ M	—	—	↓
Digitalis	↓	↓	—	—
Anticholinergics	—	↓	—	—
Thyroxine	↑	—	—	—
Disulfiram	—	↓	↑	—
Timolol	↓	↓	—	—
L-Tryptophan	↓	↓	—	—
Ephedrine	—	—	—	↑
Naproxen	—	↓	—	—
Clofibrate	↓	↓	—	—
Metoclopramide	↓	↓	—	—

↑ = enhanced/increased/shortened; ↓ = inhibited/decreased/lengthened; — = unknown/uncertain effect; M = male effect only; F = female effect only.

cell disorder, leukemia, metastatic cancer) or drug use (cocaine, papaverine, trazodone and other psychoactive drugs; several antihypertensive agents; tolbutamide). Treatment should be emergent to provide detumesence of the erection, but eventual management is aimed at the underlying medical condition that triggers this abnormal response. Emergent treatment consists of aspiration of the corpora with a large bore needle. Irrigation of the corpora with saline or 10 per cent heparin solution may also be needed.

Vaginismus. The female dysfunction known as *vaginismus* is not easily classified according to the physiologic response cycle model and is considered separately. Vaginismus refers to *involuntary* spastic contraction of the muscles of the outer third of the vagina, occurring reflexively in response to imagined, anticipated, or real attempts at penetration. Vaginismus should be suspected from the sex history if the woman describes difficulty with tampon insertion, profound fears of pelvic examination, or inability to insert a diaphragm, contraceptive foam applicator, or vaginal suppository. This condition can effectively prevent intercourse; however, it does not preclude orgasm for the female. Many women with vaginismus are orgasmic with masturbation or oral stimulation by their partner. The most common presenting complaint is the absence of a sex life. Determine whether or not the couple enjoys mutually pleasurable activities other than intercourse. The couple's self-esteem will rise if they learn that they are, by definition other than intercourse, having sexual activity with each other. Identifying the couple as sexually active with a problem that is usually quite treatable tends to be motivating.

Vaginismus may be a primary condition due to strict religious upbringing, fear of an alcoholic or incestuous parent, or fear of sexual abuse. This condition occurring in combination with primary erectile dysfunction results in an unconsummated marriage; it may be implicated in the development of secondary erectile dysfunction, as the male partner becomes frightened about causing pain for his female partner. Secondary vaginismus may be seen following attempted or completed rape, trauma, or any condition that causes dyspareunia. The most common cause of secondary vaginismus is the "vaginitis-vaginismus syndrome" (Sarrel and Sarrel, 1979). Monilial infections and vaginal herpes are so prevalent that many women are at risk for developing this condition if they continue to have intercourse while the infection is present and thus associate pain with sexual activity. Eventually the woman's vaginal muscles may not permit intercourse as a result of negative conditioning. Prevention requires that both the patient and her partner be given appropriate education and guidance, with a ban on intercourse until the infection is effectively eliminated.

Dyspareunia and vaginismus are distinct forms of female sexual dysfunctions that often occur together, but not always. In addition to infection, causes of dyspareunia are lack of lubrication due to ineffective stimulation, fibrosities in the vaginal wall, traumatic conditions resulting from childbirth, or postmenopausal tetanic uterine contractions.

The physician must be unhurried and gentle in the sexologic examination, allowing the woman to be in control of the examination. A well-lubricated examining finger is held at the introitus without insertion and the woman is asked if she is uncomfortable, avoiding the words "hurt" or "pain." Initial examination is done without the male partner present, but a nurse should be in attendance and she should talk with the woman while the examination is being conducted to allay her anxiety and to help distract her. Proceed very slowly, always assuring the woman that she is in charge of what is going to happen, and attempt to insert one finger into the vaginal orifice to a depth of 1 to 2 inches using posterior pressure on the perineal body. If involuntary contraction of the vaginal muscles occurs, a diagnosis of vaginismus can be made.

This involuntary muscle contraction should be demonstrated to both partners after the woman has been seen alone. The man will then realize that the woman's reaction is not specific to him; it is not a voluntary refusal of intercourse. At this examination, do not proceed with an attempt to insert a speculum. Instruct the woman in the Kegel exercises and prescribe an exercise regimen for her (see Table 62–2). Explain to the patient that doing these exercises will give her voluntary control over her vaginal muscles and that she will eventually be able to relax the muscles to tolerate vaginal containment.

On the second appointment, an examination is repeated to determine progress. If the examining finger can be inserted easily, instruct the woman to go through the Kegel exercises with the examining finger in place to be certain that she is exercising the muscle correctly. After the woman has practiced the exercises with the examining finger in place, then the smallest of a set of well-lubricated plastic dilators may be inserted in the vagina as the examining finger is withdrawn. When this has been accomplished, the woman is given the dilator to insert herself, using lubrication and exercising her muscles before inserting it. It is helpful to have her point the dilator toward her coccyx while it is being inserted. When this has been accomplished fairly easily, she may go on to the next size dilator. She is sent home with the dilators that she has used and is asked to practice inserting them several times a day during the coming week. She should hold them in place for 15 to 20 minutes while she performs the Kegel exercises. She is instructed to do this procedure when she can be comfortably alone and undisturbed; she may choose to stimulate her clitoris simultaneously.

When she has been able to progress to a number 2 dilator comfortably, repeat the pelvic examination using a pediatric speculum or a narrow-bladed "Peterson" speculum. If pelvic pathology is discovered, appropriate treatment is undertaken and the use of the dilators is restricted until recovery occurs. The purchase of an elaborate set of vaginal dilators is unnecessary. It is possible to use the plastic covers from disposable syringes as an inexpensive alternative, using the smallest size and following a progression as the woman is able to tolerate increasing diameters.

As the woman's comfort level increases, her male partner is included: first to watch, then to insert his finger, then the dilator, and finally his penis, with the woman in control in the female astride position. The female may wish to reach orgasm first before attempts at insertion of the penis are made, since the vaginal muscles relax after orgasm. Body caressing and non-demand pleasuring techniques are taught so that treatment is set in the context of related mutual love-play. The treatment is highly successful when the female partner is motivated for intercourse. (If profound concern about pregnancy is one of the causative factors of the condition, reliable birth control must be prescribed and instituted before beginning treatment.) When the couple or the female does not appear to be motivated for intercourse or if both partners have severe and long-standing sexual problems, referral to a sex therapist is indicated.

Alternative Sexual Life Styles

Homosexuality and Bisexuality. Alternate sexual life styles are choices related to sexual preference and not a problem of gender identity. Sexual preferences are usually established in late adolescence and early adulthood. Homosexuality as defined as an aberrant sexual behavior was removed from the *Diagnostic and Statistical Manual* in 1980.

The incidence of homosexuality is estimated at close to 10 to 12 per cent of the total population (Kolodny et al., 1979). Although the changing attitudes of society in the past 25 years have moved toward greater acceptance of homosexuals and a larger number of persons are now willing to identify themselves as homosexual or bisexual, there remains strong negative social pressure against these alternative sexual life styles.

Unfortunately, very few homosexuals initially and spontaneously identify their sexual preference to a physician. This may be because of actual or rumored discrimination in the medical care system. The physician needs to abandon stereotypical ideas about alternative sexual life styles and pay attention to improvement of the quality of primary health care. Bisexual or homosexual patients should be able to expect to be treated with the same sensitivity and dignity as other patients or to have sensitive referral to professionals who are comfortable with their alternative life styles. Primary health care should not vary greatly from those of patients with traditional sexual preferences, and primary emotional needs remain the same. See the following chapter for a discussion of issues important to the health care of homosexuals.

Other Alternative Life Styles. A wide range of alternative life styles may come to the attention of the family physician. Celibacy, practiced by individuals or couples, is increasingly popular. At the same time, the rate of extramarital sexual activities is reported to be increasing, especially among women. Experimentation with consensual extramarital sexual relationships, such as open marriage, swinging, and group marriage in which several individuals live together in a committed relationship, continues to be an alternative to traditional marriage for a segment of the population. Since the partners in such arrangements may be at risk for emotional upheaval and for venereal disease, comprehensive sexual health care requires a careful sex history, a tolerant attitude, and openness to honest discussion.

Sexual Variance and Violence

Rape. Rape is an increasingly common crime of violence in which sex is used as one of the weapons; males as well as females are its victims. The true incidence of rape is unknown, because the vast majority of rapes go unreported. It is estimated that one in four adolescent girls are victims of molestation, forcible rape, or incest, and fewer than 50 per cent of these crimes are reported to law enforcement personnel or physicians (Woodline and Kossoris, 1981). Of those cases that are reported, the assailant goes unapprehended 50 per cent of the time. Males may be more reluctant to report sexual assault than females because of the connotation that since they have not been able to prevent the assault, they are weak or unmasculine.

The age range for victims of rape ranges from infancy to old age. The highest incidence of rape and other types of sexual assault occurs in the adolescent age group, but nearly 10 per cent are less than 10 years of age and approximately 25 per cent are between 10 and 14 years old. These data may be surprising to the physician who has rarely seen a rape victim, since most media dramatizations portray the victim as a young adult or middle-aged woman. Children rarely are portrayed as rape victims although they may account for over 60 per cent of all rape victims. Nearly half of all female rape victims report that they voluntarily agreed to go into a car, house, or apartment with a new male acquaintance, and one quarter of all rape victims report that they voluntarily used alcohol or drugs at the time of assault (Jenny, 1988). There may be some predisposing risk-taking behavior that can be modified by education for prevention of sexual assault.

Helplessness, humiliation, and fear of recurring attacks characterize rape victims and, in fact, a high percentage of victims are raped more than once. Many rapes occur in the victim's own home, resulting in the feeling that "no place is safe." The perpetrator is often known to the victim. The experience of rape produces an acute stress reaction known as the "rape trauma syndrome" that is most severe from 6 weeks to 3 months or more after the attack. The victim's initial feeling after escape is gratitude at being alive. Quickly, however, the survivor's feeling turns to self-blaming and preoccupation with the event, accompanied by a sense of loss of control over his or her life. Depression is a very common sequela, and suicide attempts are fairly frequent. Somatic and sexual problems are also common, since anything that resembles the rape situation is likely to trigger the feelings connected with the initial trauma.

Counseling the victim requires a respectful, accepting, and gentle approach. View the patient as a normal, healthy individual whose current emotional distress results from a serious life crisis, and communicate the conviction that the person will recover. The idea of being a survivor is very important. If the physician is a male, it is reassuring to the female victim to have another woman present during the interview and examination following a rape. Many rape crisis centers can provide advocates who are trained to give both physical and emotional support to the victim during questioning and examination. Assist the victim to regain or maintain control of the situation by ensuring that he or she still has the ability and the opportunity to make choices. Goal-directed counseling, based on a series of graduated steps that delineate the victim's progress toward recovery, conveys an attitude of hopefulness and counteracts depression in rape victims.

The family physician can help the rape victim inform the spouse, partner, or parents about the rape, enlisting empathy and support. The partner or parents may also need help with their own reactions to the rape; rage and a desire for retaliation or revenge are common. Redirecting the focus of attention toward issues of personal safety and the need of the rape victim to retell the story over and over can be useful in the situation. The danger of suicide attempts following a rape, particularly among adolescents, needs to be recognized, and measures must be taken to protect the person during the most stressful period following the attack. It is extremely important to help the person re-establish and maintain a sense of self-esteem, which tends to be badly battered by this kind of experience. If the partner or family is not sympathetic or supportive, put the patient in contact with other individuals who are able to serve in this role.

Sexual Abuse of Children. Physicians in all states are mandatory child abuse reporters; thus it is essential to be aware of the required procedure for the state in which one practices. Authorities agree that sexual abuse is probably the most underdiagnosed, and therefore underreported, type of child abuse. Because it is a criminal offense for any adult to have sexual contact with a child, it is imperative that the physician cooperate in the investigative process.

A random survey from a population of 600 general practitioners and pediatricians in the state of Washington reveals that the majority of the sexual abuse relationships encountered are incestuous intercourse and molestation (Woodline and Kossoris, 1981). Father-daughter incest accounts for approximately 75 per cent of cases of incest; mother-son, father-son, mother-daughter, and brother-sister incest account for the remaining 25 per cent. Nearly 80 per cent of all cases of father-daughter incest involved a stepfather or father substitute such as a live-in boyfriend. This statistic should alert the family physician to children who may be at higher risk. However, incestuous relations can happen in all types of families.

Incest is a symptom of extreme family disorganization; the intergenerational boundaries have been broken and there is confusion over power issues and a betrayal of trust by the caretaking adult. (Alcohol is a major factor in removing the restraints over adult sexual behavior that might otherwise be present.) Sibling or cousin incest may be somewhat less traumatic unless age disparity is present or force is used. When the behavior continues over time, there is always confusion between emotional closeness and sexual intimacy for the child, who is powerless and vulnerable. The child, usually female, who carries the guilty family secret comes to believe that the well-being and continuation of the family is her responsibility. The parental threat aimed at silencing the child enforces this belief. The mother, who may be withdrawn, depressed, or otherwise away from the home, may collaborate consciously or unconsciously in the incestuous father-daughter relationship by absenting herself from sexual relations with her husband and ignoring signs of his inappropriate behavior. She may even insist that the child is lying if the girl comes to her for help—perhaps out of fear that the family will be destroyed economically and emotionally. The situation frequently does not come to light until the daughter is an adolescent and the father begins to excessively control her social activities outside the family. In her anger, the girl may then reveal the secret—her legacy of power over the parent she perceives as unjustly authoritarian and restrictive.

Obviously, a history of sexual abuse may not be offered by either child or parent because of fear or embarrassment. Therefore, the physician must be alert to the possibility of abuse if there are such signs and symptoms as vaginal or penile discharge; genital trauma; lacerations; anal trauma; painful urination or defecation; or the presence of gonorrhea, syphilis, trichomoniasis, or genital warts. When these signs are present, smears obtained from the appropriate orifices should be examined for the presence of spermatozoa. If results are positive, there is strong evidence for the likelihood of sexual abuse. Colposcopic examination of the introitus is a helpful adjunct for detection. Vigorous follow-up should be instituted in such cases. The counseling required in cases of incest is time consuming and more complex than the family physician can be expected to undertake. Preventive counseling might include attention to single-parent families in which the adults may be isolated from a supportive network of other adult relationships. When children are visiting noncustodial parents under conditions of limited sleeping arrangements, encouraging the parents to have the children sleep in their own beds and discussing appropriate intimacy between parents and children could be helpful. Research findings suggest a link between childhood sexual abuse and later drug abuse, juvenile delinquency, and criminal behavior (Burgess et al., 1987). Psychiatric referral assists victims in dealing with their trauma and facilitates breaking the cycle of the abused growing up to become the abuser.

Medical Assessment and Care for the Sexual Abuse Victim. The medical-legal aspects of rape or sexual abuse require a methodical history, a physical examination, and the collection of well-documented laboratory evidence. Evidence collection and examination are best done in a hospital setting according to written protocol. From the moment the victim arrives at the hospital, at least one, and preferably two, of the health care team should remain with him or her at all times. The environment must seem safe to the victim; acceptance of the patient's story, provision of emotional support, and assurance of confidentiality are paramount. A full description of all procedures that will follow should be given, and informed consent should be obtained in writing. Unless the victim of sexual abuse is a minor, reporting the incident and presenting the evidence to the police should only be done after obtaining the patient's permission. When the victim is a minor, the evidence should be collected and the incident reported in accordance with existing state laws regarding child abuse.

A careful history should include the time, place, and circumstances of the rape or sexual abuse incident. The identity of the assailant, if known, should be recorded as well as details of the type and amount of sexual contact. Hand-sewn dolls complete with genitalia and anal and oral openings can be used to help a child explain the details of the occurrence more accurately. Physical force or injury should be documented, including the use or presence of weapons. Any witnesses should be identified. The type and degree of resistance employed by the victim should also be recorded. The occurrences that followed the abusive incident, including behavior that might alter or remove evidence (e.g., changing of clothing, douching, bathing, or urinating) are important. Collection of the victim's past medical and sexual history is also necessary, including date of last menstrual period and information about contraception and last sexual contact prior to the sexual abuse.

A thorough general physical examination used to assess trauma and to treat any injuries requiring immediate attention is performed next. Inspect the skin and clothing by using a Wood's ultraviolet light, since semen has a bright green fluorescence. A genital examination is performed to determine the condition of the hymen and the presence of genital injury, and any secretions noted should be swabbed and examined for the presence of sperm. The pubic hair is inspected and combed into a plain white envelope. Add the comb to the envelope and seal it. Pubic hair plucked from the patient should be collected in a separate envelope and sealed. Fingernail scrapings, which are labeled for each finger, should be obtained in a separate container. Smears should be taken from the vagina, anus, and cervix to be examined later for sperm, gonococci, and detection of prostatic acid phosphatase. Vaginal and rectal specimens may be collected by aspiration after lavage with 10 ml of warmed physiologic sterile saline solution. A wet preparation should be examined immediately for the presence of motile sperm. A urine specimen should be collected for examination for the presence of sperm and for a pregnancy test, and a blood specimen should be obtained for serology. All specimens should be labeled and submitted according to the clinical laboratory recommendations in the hospital with signed receipts collected when specimens are transferred from one individual to the other in order to preserve the chain of evidence. Bimanual examination can be done to detect uterine size and perhaps pre-existent pelvic pathology. After swabbing the anus for secretions to be examined for sperm, a rectal examination is done.

As additional evidence, vegetation and soil from the scene of a rape along with hair, clothing fibers, and blood samples of the suspect may be obtained. It is also customary to keep the victim's clothing that was worn at the time of the assault, particularly the underpants, and to seal them in an envelope for evidence.

Prophylactic treatment against venereal disease can be offered to the patient, since gonorrhea develops in 3 to 4 per cent of rape victims and syphilis develops in 0.1 per cent. The drug of choice for venereal disease prophylaxis is procaine penicillin G, given intramuscularly at a dose of 4.8 million units after 1 gram of probenecid has been taken orally. Oral tetracycline may also be prescribed for prophylaxis of *Chlamydia trachomatis* infection. When antibiotics are given, the patient should be warned that the normal bacterial flora may possibly be altered, causing an overgrowth of *Monilia* with resultant vaginal discharge and itching. It is advisable to repeat venereal disease testing 6 weeks after the acute examination.

Female patients should be advised about the possibility of pregnancy. If an unwanted pregnancy is possible, the patient may be offered 5 days of postcoital estrogen therapy with ethinyl estradiol, 5 mg. per day, or diethylstilbestrol, 50 mg. per day, in divided doses.

The Influence of Illness on Sexuality

Speaking very generally, sexuality may be either enhanced or decreased by any illness or disability;

there may be increased harmony or increased discord. Illness can change sexuality for the better by creating greater closeness, as in cases of terminally ill patients who sense a limitation of time. However, all too often the effect is adverse.

Illness or disability may affect sexual functioning adversely in three ways. First, the illness may affect the somatic part of sexuality by creating pain, immobility, disfigurement, or a change in function. The *psychologic* components of sexual functioning may be altered by fear, anxiety, moods, defensive behavior, or anger—all responses that can be triggered by illness. Finally, a *combination* of effects on the somatic and psychologic systems may be produced when partial sexual dysfunction triggers a psychologic response out of proportion to the event. For example, a partial erectile dysfunction secondary to drugs prescribed for hypertension may lead to a psychologic reaction of anxiety and concern that further worsens the erectile dysfunction. Emotional responses to illness and disability, such as the fear of death, the embarrassment of disability, the need to be dependent, and the denial of illness, commonly alter an individual's feelings about intimacy and sexuality.

The physician who counsels an ill person about sexuality needs to remember that there is usually a change in motivation for sex following illness. Previous motivations may give way to increased needs to secure reassurance and to affirm masculinity or femininity. Sex may also be used to receive nurturing or other secondary gain. For example, a male may use sex as a symbolic test of potency, power, and affirmation of attractiveness. The sexual partner may become overprotective and parental, thereby restricting intimate behavior. (Misguided attempts to protect the partner are more likely to result when not enough information is present to encourage the normal emotional responses.) Anger or feelings of aversion may cause withdrawal of the sexual partner or even abandonment.

RESPONSE CYCLES

Either partner's sexual response cycle may be affected in any one of its phases. Common sexual dysfunctions that result from illness include diminished or abolished desire for sex, incomplete or prolonged excitement, prolongation of the plateau, inhibition or abolishment of orgasm, and prolongation of the resolution phase and refractory period.

Noted sex researcher Domeena Renshaw (Lief and Renshaw, 1981) has categorized eight common sexual difficulties in easy-to-remember fashion: the "Four A's" (anxiety, anger, alcohol, and aging) and the "Four D's" (drugs, depression, deliberate control, and dissociation). Emotions that distress the individual, such as *anxiety* and *anger*, activate the sympathetic system and preclude the occurrence of the normal parasympathetically controlled excitement phase. *Alcohol* has a paradoxical effect: in small amounts, it releases inhibitions and perhaps enhances sexuality; in larger amounts, perhaps as little as two alcoholic beverages, it decreases the ability to perform. *Aging* and illness may interact to significantly alter sexual functioning in ways that may provoke psychologic reactions that intensify the sexual failure.

The three main categories of *drugs* known to alter the sexual cycle are the antihypertensives (exert adverse effects on desire, excitement, and orgasm), the antipsychotics and major tranquilizers (primarily affect orgasm; one well-known response is the retrograde ejaculation caused by Mellaril), and the antihistamines, including anti-Parkinson drugs. (See Table 62–3 for a summary of known drug effects on sexuality.)

Depression, a common sequela of myocardial infarction, often accompanies terminal illness and malignancy, and may occur as a primary endogenous disease. A cardinal symptom of depression is decreased libido. *Deliberate control* of sex may be exerted by the sexual partner of the ill patient, creating a gap in communication and intimacy. Fear of injuring the sexual partner may produce distancing, or at the opposite extreme, fear of loss of the loved one may increase sexual demands. *Dissociation* is the psychotic condition in which there is loss of touch with reality and absent sexual drive.

BASIC RULES

There are six basic rules that physicians should keep in mind when they confront problems of sexuality resulting from illness:

Take a Sex History. All patients deserve inquiry regarding their sexual functioning, but not all patients require counseling or therapy. Illness may provide a legitimate, long-awaited excuse to discontinue sexual activity. When sexual partners are satisfied with the sexual pattern and indicate no desire to change, interference is unwarranted. It is especially important, however, to take a basic sex history of all ill and disabled patients. Patients who may be reluctant to volunteer information on such problems are then given an opportunity to do so. Table 62–4 suggests some areas for questioning.

Give Anticipatory Guidance. Anticipatory guidance may be important in preventing the occurrence of major dysfunction. This is particularly true when surgical procedures are contemplated (Libman and

Table 62–4. ELEMENTS INCLUDED IN THE SEX HISTORY FOR PERSONS WITH ILLNESS

Pre-illness level of functioning
Present level of functioning
Medications being taken
Effects of illness on self-image
Which part of the sexual cycle is affected?
Attitudes, fears, and communication of the *couple*
Desired outcome as a result of intervention

Fichten, 1987). Providing basic information and expectations prior to the procedure usually prevents the sexual dysfunction that is predictable in certain instances. Referral to an expert is not commonly required.

Learn from Other Patients. Learn from the patients themselves what works best for them. Ask people who have suffered some disability or illness about specific sexual problems they have encountered and how they have solved them; pass these useful tips on to other patients. It is often helpful to introduce a patient to someone who has suffered the same illness or disability and who has made a satisfactory adjustment.

Increase the Sexual Repertoire. Always attempt to widen the sexual repertoire of the patient; provide specific alternatives and suggestions for working around the disability.

Perform a Sexologic Examination. Provide an informative and educational examination for the patient. Use a semisitting position, a hand-held mirror, and a good deal of educational information. When this information is provided, the patient will better understand what surgical procedures are about to be performed or how illness has affected the structure and function of the sex organs.

Consultation. The physician should recognize his or her limitations and seek additional consultation when necessary. An understanding and communicative sexual partner is important to the quality of sexual adjustment following illness. If a couple's problems involve more general areas of their relationship, someone better versed in handling sexual problems may be appropriate, or perhaps other types of counseling (e.g., marital, grief) need to be pursued.

COMMON SPECIFIC PROBLEMS

According to Alex Comfort (1978), problems of sexuality created by illness do not often involve major dysfunctions like paraplegia or systemic disease. The three most common problems are interference with the patient's habitual behavior patterns, convalescence from myocardial infarction, and the sequelae of common surgical procedures such as mastectomy and prostatectomy.

Arthritis. To illustrate the alteration of a sexual habit pattern, consider the arthritic patient who has problems with mechanical positioning of the hips. Since it is often painful and contracted with muscular atrophy and weakness, the rheumatoid hip may create difficulties with coital positioning. In most patients, arthritis produces fatigue and pain, both of which depress sexual libido. Often the fingers and hands are severely affected, perhaps to the point of preventing sexual self-stimulation and stimulation of the partner. Stiffness, which presents in the mornings, generally improves toward noon and the patient functions best at midday, tiring at night, with the greatest pain coming at bedtime. Also, some medications used for arthritis can produce depression (cortisone) and depress sexual sensitivity even when they relieve pain (analgesics).

Counseling hints for the patient with arthritis include using a warm room with a warm bed, preferably a warm water bed that will reduce pressure upon joints and decrease the need to expend work because of the self-propelling water wave. Pillows may be used to elevate joints that have contractures. If decreased sexual sensitivity does not result, pain medication should be taken before sexual activity. When a decrease in sexual sensitivity occurs, the pain medication should be taken immediately afterward. The patient may be advised that 2 to 4 hours of pain relief may be the resultant effect of orgasm. Sex is best tried when the patient is well rested; arranging for the couple to be together at midday seems most reasonable. Hot baths and warmup exercises may limber the joints, and at the same time provide sexual stimulation if they are given by the partner. Reduced weight-bearing may be accomplished by the use of side-to-side facing or rear-entry positions. When Sjögren's syndrome is present, additional vaginal lubrication is necessary and may result in a more sensual experience when applied by the partner. There may be a need for surgery in some joints, particularly the hips, to improve sexual functioning.

Diabetes. Approximately 30 per cent of diabetic women have some degree of sexual dysfunction. The problems relate primarily to vaginal dryness, vaginal infections, decreased autonomic function, and atrophy of the vaginal epithelium. These problems lead to delayed arousal, painful or traumatic intercourse, a decline in libido, and anorgasmia. A neurogenic bladder predisposes the woman to dribbling, incomplete emptying, or incontinence; infections are common. Embarrassment about wetness or odor may create an aversion to touch and orogenital contact by the partner.

To help the woman who has sexual difficulties related to diabetes, suggest that the couple regularly use vaginal lubrication to counteract dryness and prescribe topical estrogen therapy to preserve thickness of the vaginal epithelium. When vaginal infection occurs, it should be treated promptly with appropriate agents (usually antimonilials) and advise against intercourse until complete healing of the vaginal lining has occurred (usually 3 weeks). Instruct the couple in alternatives to conventional intercourse for sexual pleasuring. The neurogenic bladder can be more completely emptied prior to intercourse by the Crede maneuver, the Valsalva maneuver, or intermittent self-catheterization. Drugs such as bethanecol, 10 to 25 mg. every 4 to 6 hours, may be used.

Sexual dysfunction may affect as many as 80 per cent of men with Type I diabetes after age 40. Commonly, this is an organic form of erectile failure with a significant secondary psychologic overlay of fear, guilt, or depression. The cause of erectile failure is thought to be secondary to autonomic and sensory neuropathy and perhaps vascular insufficiency. Temporary failure can result from poor diabetic control. Diabetics sometimes have failure of the internal bladder sphincter, leading to retrograde ejaculation. Usually, erectile failure precedes the ejaculation disorder. Most male diabetics with sexual dysfunction related to erectile failure benefit from sex therapy and improved communication for reduction of performance anxiety. Erection may be improved by external suction devices (the VED vacuum erection device or The Synergist Erection System). An empiric trial of therapy with yohimbine, 5 mg. three times per day, may be tried in nonhypertensive diabetics to decrease outflow of blood from the penis. Zinc depletion has been implicated in this problem, and replacement with doses of 220 mg. of zinc sulfate twice daily can be tried.

Intracavernous penile papaverine injections have produced very good results for those motivated patients who respond to its use. Those with neurologic erectile failure will be more responsive than those with vascular impairment. Papaverine is started at a dose of 7 to 8 mg. injected shortly before intercourse, once every 24 hours, and increased as necessary up to a maximum of 30 mg. (1 ml.). Long-term complications include fibrosis of the corpora cavernosa, which may preclude penile prosthesis surgery at a later date. Urologic consultation is warranted before beginning papaverine therapy. The surgical implantation of a rigid or inflatable penile prosthesis is reserved for those patients in whom conservative or medical therapy has failed.

Heart Disease. Papadopoulos (1980) has reported on the sexual concerns and needs of wives of patients who have heart disease. One hundred wives were interviewed, and nearly all wished that they could receive sexual instructions in the presence of their husbands. Many did not. It is wise to remember to include both partners in any sexual counseling in the context of illness.

Depression is nearly always present following myocardial infarction, and many men never return to their previous level of functioning. One third to one half experience a decrease in desire and frequency of sexual activity even up to several years following myocardial infarction. Similar effects are noted in women following the onset of a heart attack. A careful assessment of the patient for the presence of depression may reveal a treatable cause for sexual dysfunction.

The patient with heart disease should know that sexual activity up to and including orgasm requires approximately 5.5 metabolic units of energy expended. If a patient can climb two flights of stairs, he or she has the capacity to perform during sexual intercourse. The average heart rate at orgasm is 115 to 120 beats per minute. Most patients do not experience angina until the heart rate reaches a mean of 145 ($\pm$ 20) beats per minute. These averages would indicate that sexual activity is usually safe. It is wise for the patient to undergo submaximal exercise testing prior to leaving the hospital in order to establish the presence of dysrhythmias or the inability to perform at the required energy level.

Of 5559 sudden deaths in Japan, 18 (0.03 per cent) were related to coitus; however, 14 of the 18 were with extramarital partners (Ueno, 1969). It is advisable that the re-establishment of sexual activity occur with the usual and customary partner, whether within the marriage or without.

In any case, sexual activity should be resumed by pleasuring without intercourse with the introduction of sensate focus and relaxation techniques. These nondemand, nonstress activities allow the patient to resume intimacy immediately without the need for performance that may produce anxiety about angina or a second heart attack. The bedroom should be warm; a warmed water bed may reduce the work output needed for sexual intercourse. Long-acting nitrates may be taken prior to intercourse for prophylaxis of angina. Again, it is wise to avoid sex after meals, smoking, or an argument. When congestive heart failure may be a problem, the avoidance of orthopnea is accomplished through the use of the sitting position. In some cases of chronic heart disease with severe angina, coronary artery bypass surgery may be the only hope to offer for resumption of normal sexual activity.

Cancer. A diagnosis of cancer may be assumed to affect sexuality in a variety of ways because the condition constitutes a crisis that threatens mortality. When the diagnosis is superimposed on pre-existing sexual problems, the impact can be devastating. Even in the case of a couple with an excellent sexual relationship prior to diagnosis, the insult to the patient's body from treatment along with fatigue, emotional turmoil, depression, and pain may severely damage the couple's sexual functioning. In addition to the patient's problems, the partner has his or her own reactions and feelings that require attention. These feelings may include a fear of injuring the patient or being injured themselves by the cancer or its treatment (especially radiation therapy) (Kudsk and Hoffmann, 1987).

Because cancer and its treatment have an impact on body image and therefore on self-esteem with concomitant effects on the patient's partnership, it is essential for the family physician to actively attend to the patient's concerns by introducing the topic of sexual health care even before treatment begins. This may be the most important part of the process of identifying, evaluating, and remedying psychosexual dysfunction following treatment (Schain, 1988). For patients with committed partners, whether they are married or not, heterosexual or homosexual, the *couple* should be considered the unit of care. Attention to the sexual system (see Fig. 62–3) should be a thread woven throughout the patient's diagnostic and treatment experience, staged with sensitivity to the concerns that are uppermost at the time.

The family physician's skill in listening to the patient and his or her partner and individualizing the information given is a vital factor in minimizing the impact of cancer and its treatment on the couple's sexual functioning. For the patient without a partner, the physician's reassurance that the patient is still a valuable person, in fact, the "same" person as before diagnosis, can be greatly therapeutic. In all cases, preserving and enhancing the patient's self-esteem is a critical factor in promoting sexual rehabilitation. It is important for the physician to convey a message of hope; although patience and experimentation may be necessary, sexual healing can occur.

The specific suggestion to resume affectionate and intimate touch as soon as possible after surgery, with a return to intercourse as soon as physical healing has occurred, can help to prevent a conspiracy of silence and a pattern of withdrawal from becoming established. Other sexual activities such as oral or manual techniques can be encouraged when intercourse is medically contraindicated for long periods of time. This can help alleviate discouragement and provide comfort. The healing power of touch and the psychologic effect of uninterrupted intimacy can hasten the patient's recovery and strengthen the relationship. The physician's active support of this process, combined with the invitation to voice concerns, ask questions, and reveal unspoken fears, is an important part of the challenge of caring for the patient with cancer.

Since it is essential to avoid pairing pain with sexual activity, the active involvement of both partners in planning for optimal comfort and pleasure should be facilitated. For some couples, early viewing of the operative area is important for acceptance to occur. For others, "permission" to cover it in an attractive manner is paramount. Cleanliness of both partners is important to reduce the risk of infection. In cases in which vaginal lubrication has been compromised, a water-soluble lubricant such as Lubrin, Personal Lubricant, or Transi-lube should be recommended. Since semen may "burn" friable vaginal tissues (particularly after radiation), the use of a condom can be helpful. A position that is restful for both partners, providing intromission without deep penetration and avoiding pressure on breast or abdominal incisions, is illustrated in Figure 62–4. Putting the patient in touch with people who have successfully recovered from a particular type of cancer can be extremely helpful.

The most important part of counseling the cancer patient about sexuality is to preserve and protect the patient's sense of masculinity or femininity in the face of treatment procedures that may precipitate feelings of mutilation, repulsiveness, and desexualization. It is helpful to present alternatives to the couple's usual and habitual sexual pattern to accommodate their current needs. The information required is usually basic, and there may be simple solutions for what the couple deems an exceedingly difficult problem. The physician's guidance and support for the patient's return to sexual functioning can help to transform a potential tragedy into an experience of growth in communication and intimacy.

References

References for Physician Use

Addiego, F., Belzer, E. G., Comolli, J.: Female ejaculation: A case study. Sex Res. *17*(1):13–21, 1981.

American Psychiatric Association: Diagnostic and Statistical Manual of Mental Disorders. 3rd ed.—Revised. Washington, D.C., American Psychiatric Association, 1987.

Antoniskis, D., Sattler, F. R., and Leedom, J. M.: Importance of assessing risk behavior for AIDS—Why and how to obtain a relevant history. Postgrad. Med., *83*:138–152, 1988.

Baum, N.: Impotence: Organic or psychogenic? Diagnosis *11*(1):37–48, 1989.

Bohlen, J. G., Held, J. P., Sanderson, M.D., et al.: Heart rate, rate-pressure product, and oxygen uptake during four sexual activities. Arch. Intern. Med., *144*:1745–1748, 1984.

Burnap, D., and Golden, J.: Sexual problems in medical practice. J. Med. Educ., *42*:673, 1967.

Burgess, A. W., Hartman, C. R., and McCormack, A.: Abused to abuser: Antecedents of socially deviant behaviors. Am. J. Psychiatry, *144*:1431–1436, 1987.

Butler, R. N., and Lewis, M. I.: Sex After Sixty: A Guide for Men and Women for Their Later Years. New York, Harper and Row, 1976. *For physicians and their patients who wish to understand the normal changes that affect sexual expression in later life. Sensual and sexual options available to choose from are presented. This is a wise and affirming book that contains a great deal of practical guidance.*

Comfort, A. (Ed.): Sexual Consequences of Disability. Philadelphia, George F. Stickley Co., 1978.

DeMoya, D., DeMoya, A., and Lewis, H. R.: RN's Sex Q & A—Candid Advice for You and Your Patients. Oradell, N.J., Medical Economics Books, 1984. *This book is derived from hundreds of questions that nurses and other health professionals have asked editors of a column entitled "Sex Q & A" of the nursing journal "R.N."*

Doherty, W. J., and Baird, M. A.: Family Therapy and Family Medicine: Toward the Primary Care of Families. New York, The Guilford Press, 1983. *Presents a new model for primary care treatment of family problems. Includes excellent section on the treatment of sexual problems in family practice.*

Driscoll, C. E., Coble, R. J., and Caplan, R. M.: The sexual practices, attitudes and knowledge of family physicians. Fam. Pract. Res. J., *1*(4):200–210, 1982.

Driscoll, C. E., Garner, E. G., and House, J. D.: The effect of taking a sexual history on the notation of sexually related diagnoses. Fam. Med., *18*(5):293–295, 1986.

Franger, A. L.: Taking a sexual history and managing common sexual problems. J. Reprod. Med., *33*:639–643, 1988.

Green, R. (Ed.): Human Sexuality: A Health Practitioner's Text. 2nd ed. Baltimore, Williams and Wilkins Company, 1979. *A short, concise reference for practical management of various clinical problems. Particularly good chapters on the homosexual as a patient and the homosexual as a physician. Good reference for topics such as sexual activity in the cardiac patient, marital and sexual counseling after mastectomy, and sexuality in spinal cord–injured patients.*

Hartman, W. E., and Fithian, M. A.: Treatment of Sexual Dysfunction. A Bio-Psycho-Social Approach. Long Beach, CA, Center for Marital and Sexual Studies, 1972. *A complete description of a biopsychosocial approach to the treatment of human sexual dysfunctions, using a dual-sex team approach. The book includes information on body image work, the sexologic examination, guided caress, and use of audiovisual materials in sex therapy.*

Jenny, C.: Adolescent risk-taking behavior and the occurrence of sexual assault. Am. J. Dis. Child., *142*(7):770, 1988.

Johnson, L. E., and Morley, J. E.: Impotence in the elderly. Am. Fam. Physician, *38*:225–240, 1988.

Kaplan, H. S.: Disorders of Sexual Desire. New York, Brunner/Mazel, 1979.

Kentsmith, D. K., and Eaton, M. T.: Treating Sexual Problems in Medical Practice. New York, Arco Publishing, Inc., 1979.

Klein, M.: When talk is not cheap. New Physician, *33*:30–31, 1984.

Kolodny, R. C., Masters, W. H., and Johnson, V. E.: Textbook of Sexual Medicine. Boston, Little, Brown & Co., Inc., 1979. *The best textbook oriented to the needs of clinicians working with patients who have sexual problems. One of the most comprehensive texts available. Since its readibility and illustrations are excellent, this text is a must for the family physician's library.*

Kudsk, E. G., and Hoffmann, G. S.: Rehabilitation of the cancer patient. Primary Care, *14*(2):381–390, 1987.

Levenson, A., and Croft, H.: Patients' sexual problems: Aspects of physicians' qualifications and management. J. Reprod. Med., *18*:27, 1977.

Libman, E., and Fichten, C. S.: Prostatectomy and sexual function. Urology *29*(5):467–478, 1987.

Lief, H. I. (Ed.): Sexual Problems in Medical Practice. Chicago, American Medical Association, 1981. *A guide for the practicing physician in counseling patients with sexual problems. A number of authorities in human sexuality attempt to provide updated information from sexual research in the past decade.*

Lief, H. I., and Renshaw, D. C.: Primary Care of Common Sexual Problems: Diagnostic and Therapeutic Guidelines. American Medical Association Council on Continuing Physician Education, a video clinic with accompanying study guide, 1981. (Approved for two credit hours in Category I.) *A 60-minute videotape that should help to increase the primary care physician's ability to recognize normal and disordered sexual behavior and to understand the physiologic changes of the human sexual response cycle. Appropriate technique of sexual interviewing and history-taking is shown. Explores physicians' attitudes and competence to act in clinical management as educator and counselor. This program may be rented or purchased from the American Medical Association. Council on Continuing Physician Education, 535 North Dearborn Street, Chicago, Illinois 60610.*

Masters, W. H., and Johnson, V. E.: Human Sexual Response. Boston, Little, Brown & Co., Inc., 1966.

Masters, W. H., and Johnson, V. E.: Human Sexual Inadequacy. Boston, Little, Brown & Co., Inc., 1970.

Masters, W. H., Johnson, V. E., and Kolodny, R. C.: Crisis: Heterosexual Behavior in the Age of AIDS. New York, Grove Press, Inc., 1988.

Masters, W. H., Johnson, V. E., and Kolodny, R. C.: Human Sexuality. 3rd ed. Boston, Scott, Foresman and Company, 1988.

Medical Aspects of Human Sexuality. Hospital Publications, Inc., 500 Plaza Drive, Secaucus, NJ 07094. *Published monthly, this journal is an excellent, current source for physicians. Covers diagnosis, therapy and updates on recent literature in the field of sexuality.*

Money, J.: Lovemaps: Clinical Concepts of Sexual/Erotic Health and Pathology, Paraphilia, and Gender Transposition in Childhood, Adolescence, and Maturity. New York, Irvington Publishers, Inc., 1986.

Money, J., and Ehrhardt, A.: Man and Woman, Boy and Girl: The Differentiation and Dimorphism of Gender Identity from Conception to Maturity. Baltimore, MD, Johns Hopkins University Press, 1972.

Ostrow, D. G., and Obermaier, A.: Sexual practices history. *In* Ostrow, D. G., Sandholzer, T. A., and Felman, Y. M.: Sexually Transmitted Diseases in Homosexual Men—Diagnosis, Treatment and Research. New York, Plenum Medical Book Co., 1983.

Papadopoulos: Sexual concerns and needs of the postcoronary patient's wife. Arch. Intern. Med., *140*(1):38, 1980.

Pomeroy, W. B., Flax, C. C., and Wheeler, C. C.: Taking a Sex History: Interviewing and Recording. New York, The Free Press, 1982.

Quadagno, D. M.: Update on the G-Spot. Med. Aspects Hum. Sex., *22*(8):93–94, 1988.

Rekers, G. A., and Milner, G. C.: How to diagnose and manage childhood sexual disorders. Behav. Med., April, 1979, pp. 18–21.

Robinette, M. A., and Moffat, M. J.: Intracorporal injection of papaverine and phentolamine in the management of impotence. Br. J. Urol., *58*:692–695, 1986.

Sarrel, L. J., and Sarrel, P. M.: Sexual Unfolding: Sexual Development and Sex Therapies in Late Adolescence. Boston, Little, Brown & Co., Inc., 1979.

Schain, W. S.: The sexual and intimate consequences of breast cancer treatment. Cancer, *38*(3):154–161, 1988.

Sheehy, G.: Passages: Predictable Crises of Adult Life. New York, E. P. Dutton and Company, Inc., 1974.

Sorensen, R. C.: Adolescent Sexuality in Contemporary America: Personal Values and Sexual Behaviors Ages 13–19. New York, World Publishing, 1973.

Starr, B. D., and Weiner, M. B.: The Starr and Weiner Report on Sex and Sexuality in the Mature Years. New York, Stein and Day, 1981. *Eight hundred senior-citizen respondents reveal that sex is as good for them at this point in their lives as it was when they were younger, and for some it is even better. A comprehensive study that will surely eradicate many of the damaging stereotypes that are prevalent about sex and sexuality in older people. May be recommended to patients.*

Tanner, J. M.: Growth at Adolescence. 2nd ed. Oxford, Blackwell Scientific Publications, 1962.

Trachtenbarg, D. E., Bordeaux, D. R., Guillozet, N., et al.: Monograph No. 26: Sexual Maturation and Genital Problems. Kansas City, MO, American Academy of Family Physicians Home Study Self-Assessment Course, 1981. *Two-booklet self-study review of psychosexual development from neonatal to elderly age groups. Supplemental text on common sexual dysfunction and treatment, sexual abuse and rape, and care of persons with alternate sexual life styles. Reference table regarding drug effects on the sexual response.*

Ueno, M.: The so-called coition death. Nippon Hoigaku Zasshi, *17*:333, 1969.

Vincent, C. E.: Sexual and Marital Health: The Physician As a Consultant. New York, McGraw-Hill, Inc., 1973. *Contains humor as well as clear, practical and detailed information about counseling in sexual and marital health concerns.*

Wagner, G., and Green, R.: Impotence: Physiological, Psychological, Surgical Diagnosis and Treatment. New York, Plenum Press, 1981.

Walz, T. H., and Blum, N. S.: Sexual Health in Later Life. Lexington, MA, D. C. Heath and Company, 1987.

Wolman, B. B., and Money, J.: Handbook of Human Sexuality. Englewood Cliffs, N.J., Prentice-Hall, Inc., 1980. *Part 1 describes developmental and behavioral aspects of sexuality from the onset of human life to its end; Part 2, social, cultural and legal aspects of sexual behavior; and Part 3, sexual aberrations and dysfunctions and their various treatment methods. A blending of medical and psychosocial information with minimal illustration.*

Woodline, B. A., and Kossoris, P. D.: Sexual misuse: Rape, molestation and incest. Symposium on pediatric and adolescent gynecology. Pediatr. Clin. North Am., *28*(2):481, 1981.

References for Patient Use

AIDS: What Young Adults Should Know. Reston, VA, American Alliance for Health, Physical Education, Recreation and Dance, 1987.

An Intimate Parent-Child Talk. What every 8–16 year old MUST know growing up in the 80's and 90's. (A 115-minute videotape.) Sexual information created by Daniel G. Amen, M.D.

Barbach, L. G.: For Each Other: Sharing Sexual Intimacy. Signet, Doubleday & Company, 1984.

Barbach, L. G.: For Yourself: Fulfillment of Female Sexuality—A Guide to Orgasmic Response. New York, Anchor Press, Doubleday, 1976. *A self-help book for women to learn how to become orgasmic. The book includes the feelings and experiences of many women using the group therapy approach to the treatment of sexual problems. It also includes a step-by-step program and is available in paperback.*

Bass, E., and Davis, L.: The Courage to Heal: A Guide for Women Survivors of Child Sexual Abuse. New York, Harper & Row Publishers, 1988.

Calderone, M. S., and Ramey, J. W.: Talking with Your Child About Sex. New York, Balantine Books, 1982. *Helps parents to be less anxious in talking about sex with their children.*

Comfort, A., and Comfort, J.: The Facts of Love. New York, Crown, 1979.

Federation of Feminist Women's Health Center: A New View of a Woman's Body—A Fully Illustrated Guide. New York, Touchstone of Simon & Schuster, 1981. *Self-help and knowledge for the educated, feminist consumer. Illustrations include color plates of variations in the appearance of vulvae and cervices.*

Haeberle, E. J.: The Sex Atlas: A New Illustrated Guide. New York, Seabury Press, 1978.

Hamilton, E.: Sex With Love: A Guide for Young People. Boston, Beacon Press, 1978. *For couples of any age but particularly for young people with an emphasis on tenderness, pleasuring, and expression of feelings.*

Heiman, J., LoPiccolo, L., and LoPiccolo, J.: Becoming Orgasmic: A Sexual Growth Program for Women. Englewood Cliffs, N.J., Prentice-Hall, Inc., 1976. *Self-help book designed for the patient that presents a step-by-step method for the woman herself to learn how to become orgasmic alone and eventually within her partnership. Can be used as an adjunct to counseling for the highly motivated woman or couple.*

Johnson, E. W.: Love and Sex in Plain Language. 3rd ed. Philadelphia, J. B. Lippincott Co., 1977. *Written for preadolescent to adolescent readers and intended to be given by the parents when boys and girls show interest in the subject of sex.*

Lewis, H. R., and Lewis, M. E.: The Parents' Guide to Teenage Sex and Pregnancy. New York, St. Martin's Press, 1980. *Book for parents about adolescent sexuality. It is well researched and medically accurate; an excellent addition to the lending library shelf.*

Masters, W. H., Johnson, V. E., and Kolodny, R. C.: Masters and Johnson on Sex and Human Loving. Boston, Little, Brown & Co., Inc., 1986. *The authors' research applied to a comprehensive discussion aimed at a general audience. Illustrated. Also, it is a useful reference for the physician.*

Money, J., and Tucker, P.: Sexual Signatures: On Being a Man or a Woman. Boston, Little, Brown & Co., Inc., 1975.

Mooney, T. O., Cole, T. M., and Chilgren, R. A.: Sexual Options for Paraplegics and Quadriplegics. Boston, Little, Brown & Co., Inc., 1975. *Includes many photographic illustrations of positions and techniques to enable paraplegics and quadriplegics to engage comfortably and successfully in sexual activity. Important areas of self-esteem and the establishment of good communication in relationships are covered.*

Sex: A Topic of Conversation for Parents of Young Children. Sol Gordon, Mondell Productions, Inc. (A 25 minute videotape.)

Sex: A Topic of Conversation for Parents of Teenagers. Sol Gordon, Mondell Productions, Inc. (A 25 minute videotape.)

Sex: A Topic of Conversation for Teenagers. Sol Gordon, Mondell Productions, Inc. (A 25 minute videotape.)

Task Force on Concerns of Physically Disabled Women. New York, Human Sciences Press, 1978. *Two comprehensive and helpful booklets ("Toward Intimacy" and "Within Reach") discuss different kinds of handicaps as they relate to female sexuality. The book includes reproductive functioning and special considerations for contraceptive measures and discusses modifications necessitated by various physical handicaps.*

Vandervoort, H. E., and McIlvenna, T.: The Yes Book of Sex: You Can Last Longer. San Francisco, Multimedia Resource Center, 1972.

Zilbergeld, B., and Ullman, J.: Male Sexuality: A Guide to Sexual Fulfillment. Boston, Little, Brown & Co., Inc., 1978. *The book is useful in helping a male patient to understand his own particular condition and for facilitating sexual responses. It is also helpful for reducing performance pressure and dispelling myths about male sexuality.*

Other Sources of Information

Center for Marital and Sexual Studies
William E. Hartman and Marilyn A. Fithian, Co-Directors
5199 East Pacific Coast Highway
Long Beach, CA 90804
213–597–4425

Institute for Sex Research
416 Morrison Hall
Indiana University
Bloomington, IN 47401

Masters and Johnson Institute
4910 Forest Park Boulevard
St. Louis, MO 63108
314–361–2377

Sexual Attitude Reassessment Seminar (SAR)
Program in Human Sexuality
Department of Family Practice and Community Health
University of Minnesota Medical School
Minneapolis, MN 55414

Multi-Focus, Inc.
1525 Franklin Street
San Francisco, CA 94109
800–821–0514 (in California 415–673–5100)

Joseph LoPiccolo, Ph.D.
Department of Psychology
University of Missouri—Columbia
210 McAlester
Columbia, MO 65211
314–882–6860

63

Primary Care of the Homosexual Patient

Susan Miller
Donald S. Williamson

Theoretically primary care of the homosexual patient should not differ noticeably from that of a comparable heterosexual patient. However, the nature of the physician-patient relationship has changed in the last 20 years. As a consequence of an increased emphasis on the biomedical and therapeutic needs of patients, sensitivity to psychosocial needs has decreased. This change has led to an increase in adversarial relationships, and nowhere is this potential for conflict more evident than in the care of the homosexual patient. In addition to the increased prevalence of certain physical problems, the physician must face his or her own attitudes, which can have a direct effect on the physician-patient relationship and the quality of care that is rendered. Acknowledgment and acceptance of the *existence* of homosexuality does not necessarily require tacit approval of the behavior.

A successful therapeutic alliance between physician and patient incorporates moral neutrality, collaboration, and confidentiality; it encompasses beliefs concerning illness, death, gender identity, religion, race, and sexuality. Homosexuality is just one of many areas of potential conflict. The successful physician is able to create a therapeutic alliance with patients that separates clinical decisions from moral judgment, while at the same time establishing mutual trust.

This chapter focuses on the primary health care of the homosexual patient and how the patient's sexuality can affect the physician-patient relationship.

Issues in Sexuality

HOMOSEXUALITY

Care of the homosexual patient does not differ fundamentally from care of the heterosexual patient, but the physician's reaction to and understanding of homosexuality may influence the care rendered. Homosexuality elicits competing emotional responses in today's society, based in part on uncertainty regarding the origins of sexual orientation. Authorities disagree on whether sexual orientation is determined genetically or environmentally; probably it is interactional and synergistic. In addition this conflict is exacerbated by religious, social, and political sanctions against homosexual behavior (Richardson, 1987). Homosexuality is a medical term used to describe sexual attraction to a person of the same sex. Current American Psychiatric Association consensus does not consider homosexuality to be an illness or to be associated with increased psychopathology (Richardson, 1987; Council on Scientific Affairs, 1982). Moreover, in contrast to sexual preference, sexual orientation is not generally considered a volitional or learned behavior. If this is true, then sexual orientation is not amenable to change. Although homosexuality is the medical term, *gay* or *lesbian* is the cultural terminology for a specific social identity or life style. Numerous commonly held stereotypes contribute to the confusion surrounding these terms. These negative stereotypes are frequently based on the belief that appearance reliably predicts sexual orientation, i.e., gay men are "effeminate," and lesbian women are "masculine." Other debated theories are that homosexuality can be "cured," occurs secondary to "recruitment," or is a result of "hating members of the opposite sex." The inherent variability in individual behavior discredits generalizations made of all gay or lesbian individuals.

COMING OUT

A process that does not have an explicit counterpart in heterosexual psychosocial development is "coming out." Although all individuals experience a period of psychosexual awareness and development, homosexuality is associated with stigmatization. "Coming out" is defined as the identification, acceptance, and disclosure of one's homosexual orientation. This process is not role-modeled and is frequently disapproved of by society. The perception of being different and in conflict with family expectations may create feelings of guilt, denial, secrecy, or anger. Defense mechanisms include repression, internalized homophobia, promiscuity, or suicide. Frequently, this information is hidden from the biologic family in order to protect them from anticipated grief or despair.

ADOLESCENCE

Adolescent psychosocial development may further complicate the coming out process. During this lifecycle stage, the adolescent often struggles to develop a clear sense of sexual identity, self-confidence, and vocational goals. Adolescents must also balance parental closeness and separation issues. Their fear of parental rejection may result in secrecy to avoid confrontation. In addition, a significant amount of behavioral experimentation occurs. Social isolation and erosion of identity formation may be compounded if a peer support system does not exist. The additional risk of violence (e.g., suicide and accidents), sexually transmitted diseases (Remafedi, 1987), eating disorders, and substance abuse (Martin and Hetrick, 1988) further complicates the care of these patients.

The primary care physician can assist adolescent patients in understanding and effectively managing their sexual development and orientation. Reassurance that the physiologic changes associated with puberty are normal has a positive impact on the development of self-image. Nonjudgmental listening with the protection of confidentiality provides a secure environment for the individual to explore coping strategies.

The most crucial aspect of "coming out" is disclosure to and acceptance by oneself. In this regard the physician should respect the patient's own emotional timetable. Subsequent disclosure to friends often occurs before disclosure to family. In this transitional period, the individual may feign heterosexual behavior in order to maintain biologic familial relationships. The coming out process may be repressed until the individual is in his or her 30's and 40's and has established marital relationships and responsibilities.

Disclosure, whether it occurs in young or middle adulthood, results in a crisis. The physician is frequently a source of information, advice, and support. By offering support and reassurance, the family physician facilitates this discovery process.

SEXUAL HISTORY

The physician does not know that a patient is homosexual unless the individual chooses to reveal this information. Obtaining the medical history is a unique opportunity to establish mutual trust and to develop an appreciation of the patient's own perception of health and disease. Although knowledge of sexual orientation is not essential to the treatment of minor problems, numerous medical conditions associated with sexual activity exist, which may be relevant to a patient's chief complaint. Concealment of this information may delay an accurate diagnosis and the initiation of appropriate therapy.

Discussing sexuality with skill and confidence requires experience. Although obtaining a sexual history often is psychologically intrusive, it need not be. The following technique can be incorporated within a routine review of systems. For example, the physician can begin with any of a series of general questions as shown in Table 63–1. A preliminary question such as "Is there anything about your life style, such as recent travel, sexual practices, diet, or use of drugs, that might help me diagnose your medical condition?" (Owen, 1986) shows a willingness to discuss sensitive issues. The first interview with a patient may not reveal any information, but on follow-up visits, the patient volunteers relevant facts. These questions avoid the use of slang or the assumption of heterosexuality. If an affirmative response to any of these questions is obtained, Table 63–1 also lists examples of direct, follow-up questions that can be asked.

The section on risk factors is especially pertinent if the physician is to decrease the transmission of sexually transmitted diseases. Screening for sexually transmitted diseases will clarify clinical symptoms (i.e., rectal bleeding, sore throat, or anal itching) and focus therapy. Patients are often relieved to have the opportunity to discuss their fears, and the sexual history provides an ideal opportunity to discuss the technical aspects of safe sex. As with any other clinical problem, documentation of onset, severity, frequency, prior therapy, and associated symptoms is essential.

Table 63–1. SEXUAL HISTORY

Screening Questions

Are you sexually active?
Do you have a need for contraception?
(Do you have any children?)
Who is your most important source of emotional support?
Have you ever had a sexual relationship with a man, woman, both, or neither?
Do you have any questions about your sexual function?

Follow-up Questions

Are you having any problems in this relationship?
How would you classify your current sexual behavior?
Is this different from previous sexual practices?
Can you give me an estimate of the number of current or past sexual partners?
Can you describe the duration or intensity of emotional involvement (casual or long-term)?
When and where was your last sexual contact?
Was this behavior typical for you?
Are you satisfied with your ability to perform sexually?

Risk Factors

What is the frequency, type, and last occurrence of sexually transmitted diseases (herpes, gonorrhea, syphilis).
Is the HIV status of you or your significant other known?
What drugs have you used in social situations?
What is your current drug use?
Can you give me an estimate of the number of sexual partners you have had?
Under what circumstances do you practice safe sex?*

*Safe sex is defined as the avoidance of partner's body fluids (semen, vaginal secretions, blood, saliva, urine, and feces) and limitation of the number of sexual partners. Oral sex is not considered to be safe sex.

BIOMEDICAL ISSUES

Such screening questions help develop a working diagnosis. For example, the treatment of viral gastroenteritis differs from the management of giardiasis (Owen, 1986). Although both conditions are associated with the symptom of diarrhea, a knowledge of the individual's sexual orientation guides the evaluation and prompts initiation of appropriate therapy. Owen provides a summary of commonly seen problems (Table 63–2). Ascertainment of potential coexisting sexually transmitted diseases is critically important. In addition, underlying immunosuppression increases the susceptibility to infection and modifies the duration of treatment.

A significant health problem today is undetected chemical abuse. Concomitant use of alcohol and drugs further impairs judgment and increases the risk of transmission. This high-risk behavior is not eradicated by platitudes ("just say no"). Drug users have an increased sense of alienation that makes treatment more difficult. Since relapse is frequent, referral to treatment programs is necessary.

LESBIAN HEALTH CARE ISSUES

Although the prevalence of female homosexuality is estimated at 5 per cent of the general population (Kinsey, 1953), physicians fail to identify most of these women within their clinical practices. Medical problems specific to homosexual women have not been identified (Johnson et al., 1981), although psychosocial issues are pertinent to the management of their care. A major hindrance to physician-patient communication is to assume the patient is heterosexual. This may be as inadvertent as indigent clinics requiring each person to leave with a contraceptive after obtaining a Papanicolaou's smear (Raymond, 1988), or as blatant as projections of homophobia or explicit sexism. The written medical questionnaire may itself project subtle assumptions of heterosexuality.

The commonly perceived social identity for adult women is marriage and motherhood rather than primary provider. If lesbian couples have children through prior marriages, adoption, or artificial insemination, they still seek medical care for their children from either a family physician or pediatrician. Single mothers may not reveal a lesbian sexual identity for fear of child custody suits, loss of child support, or job discrimination. On the average, women earn less money and have less job mobility and security than men (Browning, 1987). These financial consequences of coming out explain a patient's need for reticence and confidentiality.

Additionally, previous violence (rape or abuse) has an impact on a patient's self-esteem. Violence has a tendency to be a recurrent theme in subsequent relationships and, although rare, may occur between women. The difficulties in dealing with violence in heterosexual patients are compounded by secrecy issues of lesbian patients. The patient may conceal this violence because of fear, embarrassment, or guilt.

BISEXUALITY

Bisexuality has been considered an "experimental phase" or a "denial of homosexuality" but may in rare instances be a stable sexual orientation (Lourea, 1985). In contrast, married men who have repressed their sexual orientation until mid-life (before coming out) are not considered to be bisexual.

Bisexual individuals, in addition to facing issues of coming out and parenting, may be more circumspect in their sexual relationships because of the HIV epidemic. Bisexuals provide a potential bidirectional introduction of HIV into both the heterosexual and homosexual populations. Subsequently, these individuals face additional stigmatization, with a further reluctance to reveal their sexual orientation.

The Impact of the HIV Epidemic

The HIV epidemic has forced a re-evaluation of the physician-patient relationship. Physicians may be hesitant to treat patients because of fears of contagion.

Table 63–2. DISEASES ASSOCIATED WITH SEXUAL ACTIVITY*

"Traditional" Sexually Transmitted Diseases	**Enteric Diseases**
Gonorrhea	Shigella
urethral, anal, pharyngeal	*Campylobacter* infection
Chlamydial infections	Amebiasis
nongonococcal urethritis	Giardiasis
nongonococcal proctitis	
lymphogranuloma venereum	**Traumatic Complications of Sexual Intercourse**
Bacterial prostatitis	Rectal injuries
Syphilis	hemorrhoids, anal fissures, lacerations, fistula, abscess, bleeding, sphincter injury
Primary, secondary; early latent, late latent, tertiary stages	Foreign bodies
Chancroid	Genital injuries
	penile bites, edema, penile fracture, perforation (urethra, rectosigmoid), nipple injury, breast abscess, sexual assault
Ectoparasites	
Scabies	**Dermatologic Conditions**
Pediculosis	Allergic reactions to lubricants
	Contact dermatitis
Viral Sexually Transmitted Diseases	Inhaled nitrite burns
Herpes (penile, anal, oropharyngeal)	
Condyloma acuminatum (anal, penile)	
Hepatitis A	
Hepatitis B	
Non-A, non-B hepatitis	
Cytomegalovirus infection	
HIV infection	

*Modified from Owen, W. F.: Diseases in the Homosexual Man Associated with Sexual Activity. Med. Clin. North Am., *70*(3)505, 1986.

Negative attitudes concerning homosexuality can be superimposed on this anxiety. But it is important to remember that sexuality is only one facet of an individual's identity and does not diminish his or her common humanity with all other human beings. The fears and the hopes, the grief and the joys experienced by these individuals are the same.

POLITICAL IDENTITY

The general public, including physicians, is not aware of the extent to which the gay community has created a sense of political and personal identity. Within the gay subculture, individuals exhibit normal productivity, career advancement, and emotional growth. In the late 1970's, sexual freedom was redefined as political liberation and contributed to the spread of the human immunodeficiency virus. The HIV epidemic has curtailed the expression of this sexual freedom by placing a new emphasis on monogamy and celibacy. Current patterns of courtship and marriage are more likely to parallel those behaviors seen in heterosexual couples. Although legal protection of this status does not yet exist, the emotional bonding within the couple remains intense.

EDUCATIONAL ISSUES

Research to date suggests a correlation between HIV-relevant knowledge and alterations in group behavior (Becker, 1988). Although educational strategies have not been limited to celibacy, the emphasis on safe sex or use of sterile equipment has played a critical role in the reduction of sexually transmitted diseases and the transmission of HIV through intravenous drug use. The educational programs developed in San Francisco are an example of an effective approach to behavior modification (Becker, 1988; Reinisch, 1988).

Although lesbians have a low incidence of sexually transmitted diseases, this factor should not lead to a sense of complacency. If a woman or her partner has experienced prior heterosexual behavior or used intravenous drugs, she is at risk for HIV exposure and may unknowingly be seropositive. In addition, female-to-female transmission of the human immunodeficiency virus has been documented (Monzon et al., 1987, Marmor et al., 1986). The role menstruation plays in transmission is unknown.

The issue of parenting further complicates the types of health care that these women seek. Prior to the HIV epidemic, lesbian couples established informal relationships with gay men to facilitate donor insemination. HIV disease has had a direct impact on these relationships and impaired the establishment of parenting opportunities.

HIV TESTING

HIV testing, initiated by a physician, is not benign and, unlike a complete blood count, has legal and emotional ramifications. Legal ramifications may involve confidentiality, public agency reporting, contact tracing, and procedural protection issues (Falk, 1988). Discrimination, insurance cancellation, and loss of employment have occurred secondary to a positive report. Emotional ramifications of a positive HIV antibody test include panic, denial, anger, or hopelessness.

Self-initiated testing may be delayed because individuals do not define their behavior as high risk (e.g., adolescents) or because anonymous testing is unavailable. In addition, patients may refuse testing because of a perceived lack of therapeutic alternatives (Rosner, 1987).

There is a small minority of individuals in all sexual groups who compulsively engage in habitual sexual intercourse with multiple partners. This form of conduct is known as sexually addictive behavior. These individuals are more liable to be exposed to, and to transmit, the HIV infection. Unless the physician is aware of this behavior, he or she will miss the opportunity to detect and counsel high-risk individuals.

PSYCHOSOCIAL ISSUES

Patients with HIV infection often harbor a sense of self-punishment and experience major depression. These reactions accompany changes in body image, guilt, helplessness, loss of significant others, and social isolation. The death of friends is a repetitive and cumulative loss. Suicide is often a considered option (Marzuk et al., 1988). The diagnosis of AIDS often precipitates the "coming out" to biologic family members, which creates an additional crisis situation. The primary physician is vital in facilitating these emotional processes and assisting the patient, his lover, and family in dealing with the anxiety of uncertainty. In addition, the physician needs to face his or her own perceptions of inadequacy and fears of death. Gay men usually are ahead of general society in dealing with the grief and educational issues that are a consequence of this epidemic. They have often served as teachers to health care providers. Perhaps, instead of condemnation, society should recognize the role these men have served as a research source for the natural history of HIV and their altruistic help in the testing of antiviral agents.

TERMINAL CARE

Caring for the terminally ill patient is not necessarily a hopeless process. During this chronic illness, patients and their families often reconsider their values and priorities and become reconciled. The physician can help promote this process by encouraging a sense of self-worth and empowerment and offering nonjudgmental compassion. Through frank communication, tempered by consideration of the patient's desires and beliefs about death and dying, the physician can help the patient and the family prepare for death.

Summary

In summary, homosexuality is a relatively new field for primary care physicians. Much of what is being learned is based on changing societal mores and devastating effects of the HIV epidemic. Future research on the epidemiology, psychosocial issues, and behavioral changes associated with homosexuality will clarify the dilemmas society faces in dealing with the topic.

References

Becker, M. H.: AIDS and behavior change. Public Health Rev., *16*:1–11, 1988. *Summary of behavior changes seen in homosexual men and intravenous drug users in response to the threat of HIV infection.*

Browning, C.: Therapeutic issues and intervention strategies with young adult lesbian clients: A developmental approach. J. Homosex., *14*:45–52, 1987. *An overview of "coming out" processes and developmental issues for lesbian women.*

Council on Scientific Affairs: Health care needs of a homosexual population. J.A.M.A., *248*:736–739, 1982.

Falk, T. C.: AIDS public health law. J. Leg. Med., *9*:529–546, 1988. *Excellent review of the legal issues involved in contact tracing, public health reporting, and civil controls in HIV infection.*

Johnson, S. R., Guenther, S. M., Laube, D. W., et al.: Factors influencing lesbian gynecologic care: A preliminary study. Am. J. Obstet. Gynecol., *140*:20–28, 1981.

Kinsey, A.: Sexual Behavior in the Human Female. Philadelphia, W. B. Saunders, 1953.

Lourea, D. N.: Psychosocial issues related to counseling bisexuals. J. Homosex., *11*:51–62, 1985.

Marmor, M., Weiss, L. R., Lyden, M., et al.: Possible female-to-female transmission of human immunodeficiency virus. Ann. Intern. Med., *105*:969, 1986.

Martin, A. D., and Hetrick, E. S.: The stigmatization of the gay and lesbian adolescent. J. Homosex., *15*:163–183, 1988.

Marzuk, P. M., Tierney, H., Tardiff, K., et al.: Increased rate of suicide in persons with AIDS. J.A.M.A., *259*:1333–1337, 1988.

Monzon, O. T., Capellan, J. M. B.: Female-to-female transmission of HIV. Lancet, *ii*:40–41, 1987.

Owen, W. F.: The clinical approach to the male homosexual patient. Med. Clin. North Am., *70*(3):499–535, 1986. *This is an excellent and comprehensive primer on health care for male homosexual patients.*

Raymond, C. A.: Lesbians call for greater physician awareness, sensitivity to improve patient care. J.A.M.A., *259*:18, 1988. *A commentary describing lesbian health care issues.*

Reinisch, J. M., Sanders, S. A., Ziemba-Davis, M.: The study of sexual behavior in relation to the transmission of human immunodeficiency virus. Am. Psychologist, *43*:921–927, 1988.

Remafedi, G.: Homosexual youth: A challenge to contemporary society. J.A.M.A., *258*:222–225, 1987.

Richardson, D.: Recent challenges to traditional assumptions about homosexuality: Some implications for practice. J. Homosex., *13*:1–2, 1987. *Provides a succinct discussion about the changes in professional attitudes and models of treatment.*

Rosner, F.: Acquired immunodeficiency syndrome: Ethical and psychosocial considerations. Bull. N.Y. Acad. Med., *63*:123–133, 1987.

64

Genetic Problems

James W. Hanson
Andrew M. Barclay

Genetic health care is intended to minimize the burden of genetic disorders and birth defects on individuals, families, and the community. These conditions are common and consume a disproportionate share of our health care resources. Furthermore, such disorders cause substantial anxiety among potentially at-risk persons. Virtually every family that a physician encounters has a personal or a family history of real or potential genetic concerns for which evaluation or counseling may be helpful. For all these reasons, familiarity with a genetic approach to health care is an appropriate and vital component of family medicine.

Principles and Practice of Genetic Counseling

Genetic counseling is a communication process that is intended to help the affected individual and family to:

- comprehend the medical facts (diagnosis, prognosis, and management)
- understand the contribution that heredity makes to the disorder and to its recurrence risk
- understand the alternatives available for dealing with this risk recurrence
- choose that course of action that is most compatible with the individual's goals, values, and religious beliefs
- make the best possible adjustment to the condition and its implications.

There are four components to the genetic counseling process: diagnosis, informative counseling, supportive counseling, and follow-up. An accurate diagnosis is the first prerequisite for genetic counseling, although it is not always possible.

Genetic information may impinge upon reproductive and life-style decisions and chronic aspects of health care. A concerted effort is required if a patient is to have sufficient understanding of his or her condition and is to become an active participant in health care. Furthermore, informative counseling involves communicating with other individuals in the family or community (such as other health care providers, teachers, and social services agents) who have a need to know this information by virtue of their involvement with the management program or because of implications for their own health.

The supportive phase of counseling is intended to help individuals and families cope with the psychologic burdens imposed by the discovery of genetic disorders or birth defect problems. The chronic, handicapping nature of many birth defects and genetic disorders makes the need for supportive care particularly acute for many families. Supportive care must also include a well-thought-out management program to meet the many and often complex needs of individuals and families suffering from one of these conditions.

Finally, careful follow-up is required to assure continuity of care, impart new information, and meet the ever-changing needs of the affected individual and his or her family. Additionally, the family may grow in size, and the next generation also needs guidance and counseling, which must be available as major life decisions are being made. Failure of the follow-up program may be the single most frequent reason for the ultimate failure of the genetic counseling process.

BARRIERS TO EFFECTIVE COUNSELING

In order to be effective, genetic counseling must not only be understood but must also be accepted by families and affected persons. Among the most important barriers to achievement of this understanding and acceptance is the grief reaction. The birth of a child with a birth defect invariably engenders feelings of anger, grief, and guilt similar to those encountered in other crisis situations. The assistance and guidance of a sensitive and concerned physician is of vital importance to families attempting to cope with these feelings while they are trying to make appropriate health care decisions.

A second barrier to effective genetic counseling is inadequate comprehension of information. Many individuals are inadequately informed about health matters in general. When they encounter a problem such as a birth defect in their family, the information may appear complex and frightening. An explanation of the nature of the problem, its prognosis, and other implications in common terms can help the affected individual and family to become more effective participants in their own health care. Furthermore, many of these conditions are unfamiliar to family physicians. Thus, a special attempt by the physician to understand medical aspects of the problem and other related issues is necessary if the family's needs are to be adequately met.

Time is another barrier to the genetic counseling process. Over time, changes may occur in the structure and availability of important services in the community for affected families. Periodic review can help to identify problems engendered by such changes and thereby lead to maintenance of a satisfactory care program.

Various psychosocial factors can also interfere with the genetic counseling process. Many individuals still misconstrue the objectives of genetic counseling and fear that they will be forced to accept blame for the genetic problem or, in the case of a woman with a genetically compromised fetus, have an abortion.

Interpersonal relationships among individuals, families, and health care providers may present an additional barrier to effective counseling. By the nature of his or her ongoing relationship with a family, the family physician has a unique opportunity to build a trusting relationship based on truth telling and a sensitive concern for the welfare of the patients. The physician must be candid and nonjudgmental and must try to build the self-worth of patients and their families.

Finally, the financial considerations engendered by the presence of a genetic problem may influence some family members to inappropriately delay consultation or fail to seek necessary care.

Common situations that indicate a need for genetic consultation are presented in Table 64–1. Referral to genetics consultants can be an invaluable aid to busy family practitioners. However, by the nature of their practice, these genetics specialists are often unable to provide for many ongoing management and psychosocial needs of families. These needs are better handled by the family physician and other community-based resources. Thus it is important for family physicians to become familiar with their role in handling common genetic problems and to develop a comfortable working relationship with regional genetics consultants. This partnership can be highly effective in managing even the most complex genetic health concerns.

Table 64–1. INDICATIONS FOR GENETIC CONSULTATION

Family history of a known genetic disorder or recurrent pathologic condition
Birth defects
Single anomalies
Multiple defect patterns
Mental retardation or developmental delay
Behavioral disorders of genetic origin
Short stature and other growth disorders
Dysmorphic facial features
Infertility, sterility, or fetal wastage
Ambiguous genitalia or abnormal sexual development
Exposure to potentially mutagenic or teratogenic agents
Cancer of genetic origin

THE FAMILY HISTORY

The record on any patient is incomplete until family history information is collected, as such information may be critical to the correct diagnosis. Furthermore, history-taking represents an opportunity to screen for other unrelated, potentially serious health concerns of the patient and his or her family.

The construction of a pedigree as a part of the family history is an appropriate and efficient device for collecting such information. In addition, a pedigree creates a visual representation of family relationships, which are not easily described verbally (see Chapter 74 on the family genogram).

The Genetic Basis of Human Disease

Human disease may be considered as an imbalance between stresses placed upon persons by the environment in which they live and the inborn capacity of each person's body to cope with these stresses. Viewed from this perspective, both the environment and our genetic endowment contribute to nearly all forms of impaired health. Thus, although some problems such as trauma or infection would seem to be predominantly environmental in origin, it is important to recognize that susceptibility to these problems may be controlled by genetic characteristics or that such characteristics may affect aspects of the body's homeostatic coping mechanisms (e.g., wound healing, the inflammatory response).

Three general types of health problems of predominantly genetic origin can be easily identified: chromosomal disorders, monogenic conditions, and multifactorial disorders.

CHROMOSOMAL DISORDERS

Chromosomal disorders are quantitative genetic problems. In such conditions, the body has an incorrect amount of genetic material. The net gain or loss of genes may result in adverse health consequences. Three general types of chromosome problems can be recognized: aneuploidy, structural rearrangements, and mosaicism.

Aneuploidy

Aneuploid conditions are due to the presence of abnormal numbers of chromosomes. They arise through abnormalities in the separation of chromosomes during meiosis (during gametogenesis). As such, they are principally the result of preconceptional factors. Aneuploid embryos are common and probably represent a major cause of first-trimester spontaneous abortion. Aneuploidy is found in only approximately 0.5 per cent of live-born children. Surviving aneuploid children show abnormalities principally of sex chromosomes (XXY, XYY, XXX, XO, and so on) or small autosomes (e.g., trisomy 21, trisomy 18, trisomy 13). Monosomies of autosomal chromosomes are rarely viable.

Polyploidy (the presence of more than two haploid sets of chromosomes) is another nonviable numerical abnormality of chromosomes that may also account for first-trimester miscarriages. Polyploidy accounts for many cases of so-called "blighted ovum" or the "empty gestational sac" syndrome.

Structural Rearrangements

Structural abnormalities of chromosomes are much less frequent than numeric abnormalities. They are the product of chromosomal breakage, followed by rearrangement of chromosomal segments during the repair process. These structural abnormalities may result in loss or gain of chromosomal material, reciprocal exchange of chromosome material between nonhomologous chromosomes, the formation of structurally anomalous chromosomes (e.g., ring chromosomes), or the formation of chromosomes with rearranged segments (e.g., inversions). The presence of structurally abnormal chromosomes within a gamete creates a possibility of formation of a zygote with extra or missing genetic information (the so-called duplication and deficiency syndromes), such as partial monosomy for the short arm of chromosome 5, which is also known as the cri du chat syndrome.

Of particular importance with regard to structural chromosomal rearrangements is the possibility of an asymptomatic carrier state in clinically normal family members. For this reason, recognition of a structural chromosomal abnormality in a child should prompt investigation of both parents to search for the presence of such a carrier state. If such an abnormality is identified, further investigation of the family may be warranted in order to allow identification and counseling of other at-risk family members.

In recent years, the advent of molecular genetic technology has allowed much more detailed analysis of human genetic material. With these techniques, which are discussed further later in this chapter, it is possible to localize genes to specific regions of chromosomes, analyze the structure of genes, and gain insights into their functions. These studies have already revealed that genetically important structural changes in genes and chromosomes, often not visible under the light microscope, are much more common than was believed only a few years ago.

Mosaicism

The third principle category of chromosomal abnormalities is mosaicism. This problem arises because of postzygotic defects in chromosomal separation during somatic cell division (mitosis). Such an abnormality would be expected to produce cell lines (clones) with an abnormal number of chromosomes, some of which could be viable. These viable chromosomally abnormal cells would coexist within the individual in association with other chromosomally normal cell lines, thus creating an individual with a mixture of cell types: a mosaic individual. In general, such mosaic conditions may be associated with slightly less obvious clinical manifestations in an affected individual, although it is important to recognize that individuals identified because of clinical abnormalities most commonly have a sufficiently large population of chromosomally abnormal cells to be of serious consequence. The health care of such individuals is usually similar to that of others affected with the same (but nonmosaic) chromosomal disorder.

The risk of recurrence of a mosaic chromosomal defect in a family is usually low. However, mosaic individuals may themselves be at an increased risk for chromosomally abnormal offspring, should they be able to reproduce.

Gonadal mosaicism (either for aneuploid cell lines or for cell lines with mutant genes of postzygotic origin) may be an important and underappreciated reason for the recurrence of apparently sporadic genetic disorders in families. This factor should be explicitly considered in genetic counseling.

Chromosomal disorders are likely to present in the following ways:

- multiple congenital anomalies; common clinical examples include a child with Down's syndrome (DS), trisomy 13, or trisomy 18

- abnormalities of sexual differentiation and function, including infertility; clinical examples include XO Turner's syndrome, XXY Klinefelter's syndrome, and XO or XY pseudohermaphroditism
- recurrent fetal wastage (especially during the first trimester); occasionally due to balanced parental structural chromosomal rearrangements
- mental retardation, especially when associated with dysmorphic facial features and growth deficiency; such cases are frequently found to be due to chromosomal deletions or additions, especially involving autosomal chromosomes
- certain cancers or cancer syndromes; clinical examples include some cases of retinoblastoma, Wilms' tumor, and the chromosomal breakage syndromes (e.g., Bloom's syndrome, Fanconi's syndrome) associated with lymphoreticular malignancies.

The presence of one or more of these problems in an individual should prompt consideration for chromosome analysis. It is customary to obtain a heparinized blood specimen for leukocyte culture in such cases. However, virtually any tissue can be used, if the tissue is placed into appropriate culture media for the culture of fibroblasts or other similar tissues. If mosaicism is suspected, it is important to sample at least two different cell lines (that is to say, both leukocytes and fibroblasts). Specimens can be collected even postmortem or from aborted material if death occurred less than 2 days previously. In such instances, skin or connective tissue should be obtained for fibroblast culture, and particular efforts should be made to obtain tissue uncontaminated by bacteria.

In the past, the buccal smear has been used to screen for abnormalities of sex chromosomes. The buccal smear should be considered at best a crude screening device, and chromosomal analysis should be carried out if a chromosomal abnormality is truly suspected.

Space does not allow an in-depth discussion of the clinical features or specific diagnostic or therapeutic needs of individuals suffering from one of the wide possible varieties of chromosomal abnormalities. However, this information is available in most standard pediatric texts. Syndromes of particular importance with which clinicians should be familiar are briefly summarized in Table 64–2.

Table 64–2. COMMON CHROMOSOMAL DISORDERS

Condition	Syndrome	Major Manifestations
Autosomal		
Trisomy 21	Down's	Short stature, mental deficiency, cardiac defects, hypotonia
Trisomy 18		Severe growth and mental deficiency, cardiac defects, hypertonicity, renal defects
Trisomy 13		Severe mental deficiency, brain malformations, cleft lip, polydactyly, cardiac defects
Sex chromosomes		
XO	Turner's	Short stature, amenorrhea, infertility, coarctation of aorta, nuchal webbing
XXY	Klinefelter's	Tall stature, hypogonadism, gynecoid habitus

Down's Syndrome. DS is an especially important disorder for family physicians, both as a management model and because of its frequency. Like other major cytogenetic problems, many of these pregnancies end in spontaneous abortion. The incidence of DS births varies from one in 700 to one in 1000 live births, and the incidence increases to one in 100 in offspring of mothers 40 years of age or older. Because of higher birth rates in young women, 75 per cent to 80 per cent of DS infants are born to women under age 35. DS is the most common autosomal cytogenetic disorder that causes mental retardation. Features at birth include hypotonia, a flat occiput, oblique palpebral fissures, epicanthal folds, short ears (less than 6 cm.), short internipple distance, and a wide space between the first and second toe. No effective means to predict the individual's abilities exists in early infancy. DS individuals have an average IQ of 45 (moderate mental retardation range is 40 to 55). There is a large variation in abilities.

The vast majority of infants with DS now survive to adulthood because of more aggressive and more successful care in infancy and childhood. Cardiac defects occur in half of DS infants, and cardiac surgery is successful in DS children. The early use of antibiotics in respiratory and other infections has compensated for the impaired immune response of these children. Otitis media is common; in addition, the DS individual has poor auditory processing so that he or she does not learn well by the auditory route. Cataracts, myopia, and strabismus are also common. After maturation, the male is infertile. Females have a shortened reproductive span but can become pregnant.

Other associated conditions include tracheoesophageal fistula, duodenal stenosis, annular pancreas, and Hirschsprung's disease. Leukemia is more common in those with DS, but is still an unusual occurrence. Both hyperthyroidism and hypothyroidism occur with increased frequency in those with DS. Yearly thyroxine and thyroid-stimulating hormone levels should be measured. Atlantoaxial subluxation occurs in one sixth of those with DS because of laxity of the transverse ligament of the atlas. Those individuals with an anterior dental interval of more than 5 mm. should be followed closely with yearly neurologic examinations to rule out deterioration. Fusion of the upper cervical spine may be needed to prevent atlantoaxial dislocation and paralysis. Lateral cervical spine films of the patient in flexion, neutral, and extension positions should be taken every 3 years. If subluxation is present, activities that stress the neck, such as diving, jumping, and hitting a soccer ball with the head, should be avoided.

Although all DS individuals over the age of 40 demonstrate the neuropathologic features of Alzheimer's disease, only a few of that group of DS individuals appear to show much in the way of cognitive decline before the age of 60. It remains to be seen if younger individuals who received more stimulation in their formative years will demonstrate a measurable cognitive decline by their 5th decade. The use of anticholinergics should be discouraged in those with DS because they may exacerbate memory problems.

MONOGENIC CONDITIONS

A second major category of genetic health problems includes abnormalities of single genes or single gene pairs. These are qualitative abnormalities of gene function and may involve no quantitative abnormality of genetic material, unless a particular gene has been lost or duplicated. Monogenic disorders can be characterized by their pattern of inheritance. These patterns of inheritance are based upon the number of abnormal genes necessary to produce clinical manifestations of the disorder and by the type of chromosome upon which these genes are located. The three principle categories thus defined are autosomal dominant, autosomal recessive, and X-linked recessive. X-linked dominant disorders are relatively infrequent.

Autosomal Dominant

Autosomal dominant disorders are conditions that are clinically manifest when a single dose of abnormal gene is present on one of the autosomes (nonsex chromosomes). Thus, affected individuals usually have one normal and one abnormal copy of the gene in question and have a 50 per cent chance of passing on the abnormal gene each time they reproduce. These genes are often pleiotropic; that is, they may have manifestations in more than one body tissue (e.g., the gene causing neurofibromatosis may produce café au lait spots, tumors, and disturbances of growth). They may vary in the degree to which they cause clinical signs to be manifested in different affected individuals within the same family. This is referred to as variable expression. Some individuals may be so mildly affected as to not be clinically recognizable. In such individuals, the gene is said to be nonpenetrant. It is also important to recognize that not all such conditions are manifest at birth; Huntington's disease, for example, is commonly not clinically manifest until the fourth decade of life.

The pattern of transmission of autosomal dominant disorders within families tends to be vertical. In other words, parent-to-child transmission is common. Both sexes are equally likely to be affected in this situation. It should also be noted that new cases of such disorders may suddenly appear within families. This may be explained either through incomplete penetrance or by mutation in a single egg or sperm cell. In this latter case, the recurrence risk for a couple to have another similarly affected child is low, except for the small possibility of gonadal mosaicism described above. The affected child, however, would have a 50 per cent risk of passing on the condition to his or her own offspring.

Many skeletal dysplasias (e.g., achondroplasia), disorders of connective tissue (e.g., Marfan's syndrome), and neurodegenerative disorders (e.g., Huntington's disease, some cases of bipolar depressive illness) are due to autosomal dominant genes. Some especially frequent dominant monogenic disorders with which the family physician should be generally familiar are presented in Table 64–3.

Autosomal Recessive

Autosomal recessive disorders are those conditions that are manifest only when both members of a gene pair are abnormal. In order for an individual to inherit a double dose of such abnormal autosomal genes, it would ordinarily be necessary for both parents to carry at least a single dose of the abnormal gene. Indeed, it has been estimated that most individuals carry between four and eight recessive deleterious genes. Fortunately, such a carrier state is asymptomatic. Nevertheless, the marriage of two such carrier individuals creates a situation in which there is a 25 per cent risk with each pregnancy for the offspring to inherit a double dose of the abnormal gene, thereby becoming affected.

Inbreeding increases the likelihood of producing

Table 64–3. COMMON AUTOSOMAL DISORDERS

Condition	Major Manifestations
Dominant inheritance	
Neurofibromatosis	Café au lait spots, neurofibromas, growth disturbances
Marfan's syndrome	Tall stature, aortic ectasia, ectopia lentis, scoliosis
Myotonic dystrophy	Muscle wasting, myotonia, behavioral disorders, cognitive defects, arrhythmias, cataracts
Stickler's syndrome	Myopia, joint hypermobility, cleft palate, hearing loss, arthritis
Peroneal muscular atrophy	Distal muscular wasting
Huntington's disease	Dementia, movement disorders
Recessive inheritance	
Phenylketonuria	Mental deficiency, eczema, hypopigmentation
Sickle cell anemia	Anemia, short stature, infections, "crises"
Tay-Sachs disease	Macrocephaly, developmental delay, hyperacusis, seizures, retinal cherry-red spot
Cystic fibrosis	Meconium ileus, bronchiectasis, malabsorption

offspring with autosomal recessive disorders. It is estimated that approximately 1 in 20 whites of Northern European background carries the gene for cystic fibrosis, 1 in 25 Ashkenazi Jews carries the gene for Tay-Sachs disease, and 1 in 10 American blacks carries the gene for sickle cell anemia. For such high-risk populations, screening for the identification of carriers may be a practical consideration in all members of that ethnic group when sensitive, specific, inexpensive carrier tests are available, as is the case for the last-mentioned two conditions.

Autosomal recessive inheritance is characteristic of most enzymatic defects. Thus, disorders that are likely to be recessively inherited include many metabolic errors such as phenylketonuria, galactosemia, maple syrup urine disease, homocystinuria and other aminoacidopathies, some defects of fatty acid metabolism, glycogen storage diseases, most mucopolysaccharidoses, and other storage disorders. In addition, most hemoglobin components and other serum protein variants are also recessively inherited. Several important examples are presented in Table 64–3.

X-linked Recessive

The third major category of monogenic inheritance is X-linked recessive. This pattern of inheritance results from the presence of abnormal recessive genes located upon the X chromosome. Because women have two X chromosomes, they have two copies of each X-linked gene. Recessive abnormal genes located on the X chromosome are usually not manifest in females for this reason. On the other hand, males have a single copy of the X chromosome and thereby have only a single copy of each gene located thereon. The Y chromosome is thought to carry little genetic information other than that relevant to male sexual differentiation. For this reason, the presence of even a single abnormal recessive gene on the X chromosome in the male usually results in a clinical abnormality, whereas females may be asymptomatic carriers of X-linked recessive genes. A carrier female has a 50 per cent risk for each male offspring to be affected and a 50 per cent risk for each female offspring to be a carrier. An affected male has no chance to have an affected son (that is, there is no male-to-male transmission). However, all (100 per cent) of his daughters would be carriers of this condition.

Common examples of X-linked recessive disorders are hemophilias A and B, Duchenne's muscular dystrophy, and androgen insensitivity syndrome (testicular feminization syndrome). Several important X-linked disorders are presented in Table 64–4. X-linked genes probably also account for a substantial proportion of the excess mental retardation found among males.

Fragile X. An especially important disorder causing serious mental deficiency is the fragile X syndrome. This condition is a disorder of the X chromosome in which the lower part of the long arm appears, when visualized through the microscope, to be constricted or broken. Almost all of the affected individuals have serious degrees of mental retardation and may have some or all of the physical and behavioral features presented in Table 64–5. Fragile X syndrome occurs in approximately 1 in 2000 persons and is still underrecognized throughout the world. Females are usually less severely affected, although their communication abilities may be very poor. Fragile X individuals may show autistic behaviors and very poor and repetitive speech.

Genetic testing for fragile X syndrome requires special culture conditions. The proportion of cells demonstrating the abnormality varies; therefore, 50 to 100 cells need to be examined. For these reasons, it is important to specify the suspected diagnosis when ordering chromosomal studies on individuals in whom this diagnosis is being considered.

There appears to be a correlation between the number of affected cells and the degree of retardation in heterozygotes. Prenatal testing of amniocytes is valid if positive (i.e., over 8 per cent of cells affected) but may not be valid if negative, especially in females. Genetic testing should be performed on those with a family history of fragile X or unspecified retardation in a male relative. Testing does not, however, predict perfectly whether or not a couple will give birth to an affected or an unaffected offspring.

Although folic acid levels in those affected are normal, treatment with folic acid in children has been attempted, with equivocal results. The same treatment has shown no benefit in adults. Drugs are generally not helpful in ameliorating autistic behavior, although thioridazine and amphetamine-like drugs have been used with limited success.

Table 64–4. COMMON X-LINKED DISORDERS

Condition	Major Manifestations
Duchenne's muscular dystrophy	Progressive muscular wasting, cardiomyopathy, contractures
Hemophilia A and B	Bleeding
Fragile X syndrome	Mental deficiency, mildly dysmorphic facies, macro-orchidism

Table 64–5. COMMON FEATURES OF FRAGILE X SYNDROME

Feature	Per Cent Occurrence
Macro-orchidism	92
Mitral valve prolapse	81
Hyperextensibility of joints	79
Hand biting	78
Austistic behavior	69
High-arched palate	65
Large or prominent ears	48
Pectus excavatum	32

MULTIFACTORIAL DISORDERS

The third category of genetic human disease is multifactorial disorders, also sometimes referred to as polygenic conditions. This category encompasses many of the more common health problems that show a familial tendency, such as certain common malformations (e.g., cleft lip or palate, congenital heart disease, neural tube defects), coronary artery disease, hypertension, some forms of cancer, diabetes, epilepsy, and possibly schizophrenia. These conditions remain, for the most part, poorly understood in terms of their origin. However, their pattern of occurrence within families can be duplicated through a model that assumes an interaction between multiple factors, some genetic, some environmental. Such a model predicts that the likelihood of recurrence of the same defect within first-degree relatives is higher than in the general population (often within the vicinity of 3 per cent to 5 per cent). Among more distant relatives, the likelihood of sufficient factors aggregating within a particular individual to exceed the threshold of clinical effect is progressively less. As predicted, the incidence of affected individuals among third-degree or more distantly related persons approaches the general population frequency for this group of conditions. Recurrence risk estimates quoted as a part of the genetic counseling process for individuals with multifactorial disorders are derived from empiric risk tables. It is important to be sure that such tables have been derived from data concerning a population similar to the group to which the patient belongs, because there may be significant differences in these figures between populations from different ethnic or geographic groups.

It is vital to distinguish between defects presumed to be multifactorial in origin and defect categories that are etiologically heterogeneous. Multifactorial inheritance can be mimicked by inappropriate lumping together of seemingly similar defects of distinct causes. For instance, facial cleft malformations in children may be associated with certain chromosomal defects (e.g., trisomy 13, partial monosomy of the short arm of chromosome 4), with monogenic disorders (e.g., Van der Woude's syndrome, Stickler's syndrome), or with certain environmental teratogens (e.g. certain anticonvulsants, alcohol), or they may be seen as isolated, single defects in a particular family member. Each of these different causes has distinct genetic and health implications for the affected individual and other family members. Thus, all facial cleft anomalies should not be treated the same way, either medically or in the genetic counseling process. Careful diagnostic evaluation can help to appropriately categorize affected individuals, thereby minimizing this problem.

Genetic Issues in Primary Care

Common genetic concerns can be identified in association with particular phases or events during the life cycle. Presented in the following section are common genetic concerns surrounding the birth of a child, pregnancy, the emerging adult, and the care of the family unit.

GENETIC CONCERNS IN THE NEWBORN PERIOD

Neonatal Screening for Metabolic and Genetic Disorders

Genetic and metabolic screening is a search for persons with genetic and metabolic disorders so that early treatment can lead to the amelioration or avoidance of adverse health consequences such as mental retardation, illness, and death.

Genetic screening is more than a laboratory procedure. It involves a series of steps that logically culminates in the identification and early treatment of affected individuals. Genetic screening should therefore be carried out under controlled conditions and may be considered when the following criteria are met.

1. There is evidence of substantial public benefit and acceptance, including acceptance by the medical community.
2. The feasibility of genetic screening has been investigated and shown to be cost-effective.
3. Appropriate public education can be carried out.
4. Satisfactory test methods and laboratory facilities are available.
5. Resources exist to deal with counseling, follow-up, and other consequences of testing.
6. Means are available to evaluate the effectiveness and success of each step in the process.

Confidentiality should be strictly maintained.

There is general agreement that congenital hypothyroidism and phenylketonuria meet these various requirements to be included in any neonatal metabolic screening program. In addition, many authorities have concluded that galactosemia, branched-chain α-ketoaciduria (maple syrup urine disease), and possibly homocystinuria meet these requirements as well. Furthermore, there are many other metabolic disorders for which appropriate screening methodologies and methods of treatment will undoubtedly become available in the future. Recent National Institutes of Health studies demonstrate that hemoglobin disorders, such as sickle cell anemia, can be effectively included in newborn screening programs. Early identification of such affected infants and early appropriate antibiotic prophylaxis can be life saving.

The family physician should become familiar with the neonatal and metabolic genetic screening program functioning in his or her state and community so that the physician can participate fully and effectively in the appropriate care of newborns. The physician should be familiar with the medical consequences, methods of diagnosis, and treatment of the conditions for which screening is proposed. A good working relationship with medical consultants and referral resources in the area is essential.

It is important to avoid pitfalls in the screening process that act to delay or prevent effective treatment because the failure to diagnose and provide appropriate treatment for affected children may result in a substantial legal liability. For the group of conditions described above, screening not earlier than the 3rd day of life nor later than the 5th day of life is optimal for the efficient detection and early treatment of these conditions. Present-day policies that result in earlier discharges from the hospital have sometimes been used as a justification for not carrying out screening tests on newborns prior to their leaving the hospital. This is an unwise policy, since it results in no screening test being carried out because of the failure of the follow-up process in up to one third of such cases. Furthermore, the screening tests for hypothyroidism and galactosemia are positive for affected individuals, even if carried out on umbilical cord blood.

Whereas it is true that screening before the 3rd day of life may miss some cases of errors of amino acid metabolism, such as phenylketonuria, many cases can be identified even on the 1st day of life because of catabolism of endogenous protein. Thus early screening affords some possibility of detection of affected individuals and avoids the hazards of failure of follow-up or delays in the screening process, which could result in acute illness in children with galactosemia or branched-chain α-ketoaciduria. For these reasons, it is recommended that all children be screened prior to discharge from the hospital and that children who are screened earlier than the 3rd day of life or who otherwise have specimens collected in such a way as to raise concern about the validity of screening results have a repeat screening carried out, generally within 2 weeks.

Birth of a Malformed Child

The birth of a child with congenital anomalies, whether stillborn or live-born, engenders a family crisis. As discussed earlier, parents and other family members may experience an intense grief reaction and can be expected to have many questions about the causes of the child's defects, implications for the child's health (if the child survives), and implications for future reproduction, either for themselves or other family members.

Some parents find it difficult to accept an imperfect child who does not meet their expectations. They should be allowed to express their grief and then move into a problem-solving mode. Despite exemplary prenatal care, most parents feel guilty and blame a particular event in their pregnancy for the problem. Often the parents become hostile and mistrust the medical community. Repeated assurance that they did not cause the problem is necessary; specific advice and support by other new parents of similarly affected children is invaluable.

A common group of needs can be anticipated. Such families need the following:

1. to be informed as soon as a diagnosis is made or a serious problem is suspected
2. to be together when informed, if at all possible
3. to be told the truth, with appropriate terminology that is both sensitive and empathic
4. to have contact with physicians, nurses, and other health care providers with whom they can share feelings and ask questions
5. to have contact with the baby to test their fears and anxieties about their child
6. to receive specific information about the condition, including books, pamphlets, and other written materials when possible
7. to have assistance in preparing to discuss the diagnosis with relatives and friends
8. to meet other parents who have children with similar problems
9. to learn about community resources
10. to have time to grieve and to develop appropriate coping mechanisms.

Even when severe anomalies are present in the infant (living or dead), families should gently be encouraged to see and even hold the baby. If they decline, it is prudent to offer a second opportunity within a few hours if the baby is deceased. If all else fails, photographs may be taken and retained for the medical record should the family wish to see the child or have to cope with associated problems for themselves at a later date. In addition, if the child has died or is likely to die, the family should be encouraged to permit appropriate diagnostic studies so that questions that can be anticipated from the family in the future can be satisfactorily answered.

Appropriate evaluation of the malformed or stillborn neonate can usually be accomplished with facilities available in most hospital settings. Types of studies recommended and information needed for further evaluation of such cases are summarized in Table 64–6. Pictures may be "worth a thousand words," particularly in describing dysmorphic facial features. X-ray studies can be particularly valuable if there is evidence of disproportionate growth of limbs or other body parts. A whole-body, postmortem x-ray can be extremely useful in delineating possible skeletal dysplasias, many of which are genetic in origin. Cultures or serologic studies may help to evaluate the possible role of prenatal fetal infections.

Table 64–6. USEFUL PROCEDURES IN EVALUATING THE MALFORMED OR STILLBORN NEONATE

Photographs	Cultures or titres
X-ray studies	Prenatal history
Autopsy	Family history
Chromosomal analysis	

Table 64–7. PHYSICAL HAZARDS TO THE FETUS

Agent	Congenital Abnormalities
Radiation	
High levels	Microcephaly, possibly ocular defects, mutations, malignancy
Low levels (<10 rads)	Mutations, possibly malignancy, no clear association with birth defects
Heat or fever	Neural tube defects, possibly other central nervous system anomalies, possibly mental retardation
Mechanical factors	
Oligohydramnios Multiple gestation Uterine malformation	Positional deformities, possibly limb reduction defects, possibly mandibular hypoplasia
Amniotic bands	Syndactyly, prenatal limb amputations, atypical facial clefts, exencephaly, encephalocele, thoracogastroschisis, ocular defects

Chromosome analysis is also useful in cases with multiple malformations, and, as described earlier, specimens can be obtained postmortem and shipped to cytogenetics laboratories.

It is important to note that chromosome studies may be relatively expensive procedures. Thus, if they are not carried out on the malformed infant, then the only way to investigate the possibility of a familial chromosomal abnormality at a future point in time would be chromosomal studies on both parents. This approach at best provides only incomplete information about the origin of the child's abnormalities, is twice as expensive for the family, and is less likely to be covered by insurance. Finally, a careful search for internal anomalies and documentation, insofar as is possible, of the nature of suspected defects through a careful autopsy can be extremely useful in the later diagnostic evaluation and counseling of the family of the affected infant. Many families who decline an autopsy will in a matter of a few hours reconsider if the purpose of the study is carefully discussed with them.

A careful history of the prenatal period, searching for possible environmental teratogens to which the mother may have been exposed, can also be informative. This information can be obtained at a later time, as can a careful family history, including a pedigree, which may reveal the presence of suspicious genetic factors in the family.

The choice of which of these procedures to pursue ultimately must remain the responsibility of the attending physician. Likewise, the attending physician may well assume the responsibility for the continuing care of surviving developmentally handicapped children. An adequate diagnosis certainly helps to answer the many questions the family has under these circumstances and facilitates the development of an appropriate treatment and management program.

GENETIC CONCERNS OF PREGNANCY

Exposure to Teratogenic Agents

Teratogens are environmental factors that can cause birth defects in the developing fetus. It has been estimated that from 10 per cent to 20 per cent of birth defects are caused primarily by maternal exposure to such factors at sensitive stages of pregnancy. However, it is becoming increasingly clear

Table 64–8. INFECTIOUS TERATOGENIC AGENTS

Agent*	Fetal Wastage	Growth Deficiency	Mental Deficiency	Congenital Abnormalities
Viruses				
Rubella	+	+	+	Ocular and cardiovascular anomalies, deafness, microcephaly, immune and endocrine disturbances, delayed skeletal development
Cytomegalovirus	+	+	+	Ocular and cardiovascular anomalies, deafness, microcephaly, hydrocephaly, possibly gastrointestinal anomalies
Herpes simplex	+	?	+	Ocular anomalies, microcephaly, patent ductus arteriosus, hypoplastic distal phalanges
Varicella zoster	?	+	+	Ocular anomalies, microcephaly, hypoplastic limbs, neurogenic muscular atrophy, cutaneous defects
AIDS	+	+	+	Fifty per cent or more develop AIDS; no clear association with specific malformations
Bacteria				
Syphilis	+	+	+	Ocular, dental and skeletal anomalies, hydrocephalus, microcephaly, cutaneous lesions, nerve palsies, nephrosis
Mycoplasmas	+	?	?	Possibly neural tube defects, possibly aneuploidy
Parasites				
Toxoplasmosis	+	+	+	Ocular anomalies, microcephaly, hydrocephaly, deafness

*+ = agent causes adverse effect; ? = agent possibly causes adverse effect.

Table 64–9. DRUG AND CHEMICAL HAZARDS TO THE FETUS

Nonprescription Drugs	
Ethyl alcohol	Fetal alcohol syndrome; mental and growth deficiency, fetal wastage; cardiac, ocular, central nervous system, and skeletal malformations; cleft palate; characteristic facies
Tobacco	Growth deficiency, fetal wastage; no clear association with human malformations
Salicylates	Possibly growth deficiency, possibly patent ductus arteriosus
Opiates	Growth deficiency; no clear association with human malformations
Cocaine	Possibly vascular disruption, possibly genitourinary tract anomalies
Caffeine	No clear link to human malformations
Other "street drugs" (e.g., amphetamines, LSD and other hallucinogens, marijuana)	No clear link to human malformations
Prescription Drugs	
Anticancer agents (e.g., folic acid antagonists, alkylating agents)	Fetal wastage; growth and mental deficiency; characteristic facies; central nervous system, ocular, and skeletal malformations; cleft palate; genitourinary tract anomalies; limb malformations
Anticoagulant agents	
Coumarin derivatives	Fetal wastage; growth and mental deficiency; characteristic facies; central nervous system and skeletal anomalies; choanal atresia
Heparin	Possibly fetal wastage
Antibiotics	
Tetracyclines	Dental abnormalities
Streptomycin (and possibly other aminoglycosides)	Hearing loss
Chloroquine	Possibly ocular defects, possibly hearing loss
Others	No consistent association with human malformations
Anticonvulsants	
Oxazolidines (e.g., trimethadione)	Trimethadione syndrome; fetal wastage; growth and mental deficiency; characteristic facies; cardiac, central nervous system, gastrointestinal, genitourinary, and limb malformations; cleft palate
Hydantoins (e.g., phenytoin)	Hydantoin syndrome; growth and mental deficiency; characteristic facies; cardiac, skeletal, and limb malformations; cleft palate; possible association with neuroblastoma
Barbiturates (and primidone)	Possibly barbiturate syndrome; present evidence inconclusive
Valproic acid	Valproate syndrome, spina bifida
Diazepam	Possibly low risk for facial clefts

that genetic factors alone cannot account for the large majority of other congenital anomalies. Thus, it can be expected in the future that more teratogenic agents or combinations of environmental factors in the presence of certain genetically susceptible individuals will be identified as causes of birth defects. It is particularly important to note that such birth defects may be prevented if family physicians can advise their patients as to which hazardous agents to avoid during pregnancy.

An incomplete summary of hazardous infectious, physical, drug, and chemical agents during pregnancy is presented in Tables 64–7, 64–8, and 64–9. Referral of questions regarding this category of agents to teratogen information services is recommended. Often such services are associated with genetics services programs at referral centers. The March of Dimes Birth Defects Foundation publishes a list of such programs. Familiarity with such regional resources can be of great value in dealing with many complex issues raised by exposure to teratogens during pregnancy.

Drug and chemical agents are most prudently avoided during pregnancy whenever possible, and women should be warned before attempting pregnancy. However, should medical therapy for a significant maternal health problem be indicated, potential implications of this therapy for the fetus should be discussed with the family prior to its initiation. Consultation with experts in teratology, prenatal diagnostic studies, and termination of the pregnancy may be considered. In view of the frequency of birth defects, indiscriminate use of therapeutic agents during pregnancy is likely to be associated by chance alone with birth defects in a significant percentage of cases. This can lead to unwarranted parental concerns and even litigation.

It should also be recognized that some maternal metabolic or genetic factors may present hazards to the developing fetus. Poorly controlled juvenile-onset diabetes mellitus, phenylketonuria, and myotonic dystrophy can result in fetal defects.

Finally, it should be mentioned that maternal malnutrition can impair fetal growth. Though mal-

Table 64–10. COMMON EXAMPLES OF PRENATALLY DIAGNOSABLE DISORDERS

Chromosomal disorders
Malformations
Neural tube defects
Limb reduction defects
Body wall defects
Hydrocephaly
Microcephaly
Renal agenesis
Some cardiac malformations
Skeletal dysplasia and other bony anomalies
Congenital infections
Metabolic disorders
Mucopolysaccharidoses and other storage diseases
Aminoacidopathies and other organic acid defects
Urea cycle disorders
Blood dyscrasias
Bleeding disorders
Hemoglobinopathies

nutrition per se has not been associated with an increase in the frequency of congenital anomalies in humans, vitamin deficiency has. Furthermore, it is possible that such problems can potentiate the effects of other more hazardous agents in the developing child.

Preconceptional paternal exposure to most potentially hazardous agents probably presents minimal absolute risks to the fetus and none at all if exposure occurs after conception.

Prenatal Diagnosis of Birth Defects

The development of prenatal diagnosis of birth defects and genetic disorders during the past 2 decades represents a unique and rapidly growing story of medical progress. At present, over 300 such fetal conditions can be identified by one or more of the following prenatal diagnostic techniques: (1) midtrimester transabdominal amniocentesis, (2) ultrasonography and other fetal imaging studies, (3) fetoscopy, (4) aspiration of fetal blood by cordocentesis, (5) chorionic villi sampling, and (6) fetal biopsy. Some of the more common diagnosable conditions are summarized in Table 64–10.

Measurement of maternal serum alphafetoprotein (MSAFP) has been recommended as a routine part of prenatal care. There is an association between elevation of MSAFP levels and neural tube defects and other serious birth defects or medical disorders. Unusually low MSAFP levels are an indicator of increased risk for DS and other severe chromosomal disorders. The family physician should establish a close working relationship with local referral and screening programs and become informed about the availability of testing programs at the local level, protocols for obtaining services, common interpretational issues, and follow-up.

Table 64–11. INDICATIONS FOR PRENATAL DIAGNOSTIC CONSULTATION

Advancing maternal age (>35)
Previous chromosomal abnormality in a child
Previous neural tube defect in a child or parent
Familial chromosomal rearrangement in a parent
High risk for biochemical genetic disorder
High risk for certain malformations or syndromes
Prenatal sex determination for X-linked disorders
High risk for certain skeletal dysplasias
Abnormal maternal serum alphafetoprotein (high or low)
Exposure to teratogenic agents

Presently recognized indications for consideration of prenatal diagnostic studies for the detection of birth defects or genetic disorders are summarized in Table 64–11. The family physician should be familiar with common indications, such as advancing maternal age or the previous birth of a child with a chromosomal abnormality or a neural tube defect, and be able to offer basic counseling.

Benefits of prenatal genetic studies include the following:

- The couple can be reassured that the fetus is normal. This may prevent unnecessary termination.
- Care of the fetus or newborn can be modified.
- The family can be psychologically prepared.
- The option of termination may be presented. A future pregnancy can still offer some couples the opportunity to bear children free from such disorders.

Problems include the following:

- There is a very small risk to the mother or fetus of infection, hemorrhage, or miscarriage (less than 0.5 per cent when expertly done).
- Fetal cell culture failure may result in no diagnosis being made. This does not indicate a serious fetal anomaly, but repeat amniocentesis may be required.
- Normal results from amniocentesis studies or other prenatal diagnostic studies do not eliminate the possibility that the fetus could have other abnormalities or disorders. Many fetal defects are not diagnosable at the present time.

Failure to discuss prenatal diagnostic studies as an option for families at an increased risk for having a child with a birth defect may place the attending physician in serious medicolegal jeopardy. Courts are increasingly holding physicians responsible for the medical and human consequences of such omissions.

GENETIC CONCERNS FOR THE EMERGING ADULT

Growth patterns of other family members are the best predictors of adult height. Likewise, in some families, unusually early or unusually late sexual maturation are normal genetic variants. For this reason, patterns of growth and development can be anticipated, as can the attendant psychologic problems thereby sometimes engendered. In some cases, these problems may be sufficiently serious to warrant medical intervention.

Individuals with connective tissue disorders or skeletal dysplasias should be advised to avoid contact sports and competitive weight-bearing exercises, which might place undue stresses on susceptible joints and tissues. Potential cardiovascular problems can be identified and in many cases appropriately treated to minimize future risks. Supportive counseling can be provided to the individual and family, which may allow better psychologic adaptation to specific conditions or problems.

In a similar vein, occupational choices may be influenced by present or anticipated health considerations, e.g., neuromuscular coordination, visual or auditory impairment, learning difficulties, unusual susceptibility to trauma (e.g., connective tissue disorders, common bleeding problems, certain skeletal dysplasias), and cardiovascular problems. Individuals should understand the prognosis and methods of treatment or management available to them to deal with such health conditions. Individuals with a genetically based susceptibility to environmental factors (allergy, asthma, alpha$_1$-antitrypsin deficiency) may be encouraged to choose occupational environments in which intense exposures to the potential environmental hazard to which they are susceptible may be minimized.

Life-style decisions may be critical. For instance, it is especially important for individuals with alpha$_1$-antitrypsin deficiency to avoid smoking, and those with a familial tendency to the development of maturity-onset diabetes should be counseled to avoid obesity.

Premarital counseling affords another opportunity to the family physician. At this time of life, young adults are concerned about the potential health status of themselves, their spouses, and their future offspring. This is an excellent occasion to review the family history carefully, to search for genetic health concerns, and to discuss the implications of identified problems for both the prospective couple and their offspring. Information can be provided regarding the effects of alcohol, smoking, drugs, and other potentially hazardous environmental agents on the developing fetus.

COMMON GENETIC CONCERNS IN THE CARE OF FAMILIES

Those with a family history of early myocardial infarction may be at an increased risk for genetic reasons. Other risk factors may also be present, including elevated dietary lipids, being overweight, smoking, or consuming too much dietary salt. Some of these factors may have a genetic basis; those that are environmental may be modified. Similar arguments for searching for affected individuals in high-risk families can be advanced for families with an unusual prevalence of cancer, epilepsy, diabetes, certain malformation problems, and certain behavioral disorders. Thus it is clear that a genetic approach to human health problems can contribute much in the case of many common conditions.

Treatment of Genetic Disorders

Effective forms of treatment are available for many genetic conditions, and appropriate medical management can improve the quality of life for the vast majority of affected families. The treatment modalities available are summarized in Table 64–12. In addition, patient education and regular follow-up is essential.

GENETIC ASPECTS OF MEDICAL THERAPEUTICS

Genetic control of the body's response to medical pharmacologic agents is a particular area with which the family physician should become familiar. Drug metabolism is under genetic control. Individuals have different rates of isoniazid acetylation and phenytoin parahydroxylation. Some are prone to malignant hyperthermia when exposed to anesthetic agents. Glucose-6-phosphate dehydrogenase deficiency is a common X-linked recessive metabolic disorder that may predispose the individual to severe hemolytic anemias in the presence of treatment with several common categories of drugs. Many similar examples could be cited.

Table 64–12. MEDICAL AND SURGICAL APPROACHES TO THE TREATMENT OF GENETIC DISORDERS

Medical	
Avoidance of hazardous factors	Halothane in malignant hyperthermia; barbiturates in porphyria
Restriction of dietary components	Galactose in galactosemia; phenylalanine in phenylketonuria
Replacement of physiologic substances	Factor VIII in hemophilia A; thyroxine in cretinism
Supplementation with physiologic substances (pharmacologic amounts)	Calciferol in vitamin D-dependent rickets
Introduction of pharmacologic agents	Cholestyramine for hypercholesterolemia; penicillamine in Wilson's disease
Surgical	
Excision	Colectomy in multiple polyposis of colon
Correction	Repair of cleft lip or palate
Modification	Gastric bypass procedures in Prader-Willi syndrome
Transplantation	Kidneys in polycystic disease, bone marrow in immune deficiency disorders

Such pharmacogenetic differences may explain differences in therapeutic response, re-emphasizing the need for a specific measurement of drug levels when inadequate or toxic responses are obtained to standard therapies. Family members should be informed.

COMPREHENSIVE CARE IN THE COMMUNITY

In order to be effective, genetic health care must be extended into the community setting. As pointed out previously, the family physician may be the team leader in providing a comprehensive management program. However, it is important to recognize that other individuals and professions provide important health, social, and educational services to persons with genetic concerns. The family physician can act as the patient advocate in obtaining important community and regional resources to meet other, nonmedical needs. A listing of organizations and agencies that may be of assistance to families with various members affected with handicapping conditions is available from the National Center for Education in Maternal and Child Health in Washington, D.C. (see reference).

References

General Readings

Bergsma, D.: Birth Defects Compendium. 2nd ed. New York, Alan R. Liss, Inc., March of Dimes Birth Defects Foundation, New York, 1979. *A compendium of brief summaries on a large number of birth defects.*

Bratshaw, M. L., and Perret, Y. M.: Children with Handicaps: A Medical Primer. Baltimore, Paul H. Brookes Publishing Co., 1981. *A superbly organized and logical exposition of the basis of handicapping conditions, with modern, sensible discussions of particular common categorical problems seen in medical practice. Clearly written and thoughtful.*

Garver, K. L., and Marchese, S. G.: Genetic Counseling for Clinicians. Chicago, Year Book Medical Publishers, Inc., 1986. *A synoptic and clinically oriented guide to issues in genetic counseling and related health care services.*

Genetics Support Groups: Volunteers and professionals as partners. *In* Weiss, J. O., et al. (Eds.): Birth Defects: Original Article Series. March of Dimes Birth Defects Foundation, Vol. 22 (2), 1986. *A useful discussion of issues and of roles for volunteers and support groups in the comprehensive care of individuals and families with genetic and birth defect problems.*

Gorlin, R. J., and Cohen, M. M., Jr.: Syndromes of the Head and Neck. 3rd ed. New York, McGraw-Hill Book Co., 1989. *In-depth discussion of defect categories affecting craniofacial structures. Excellent bibliographies.*

Hudis, J.: Teratogen Information Services. New York, March of Dimes Birth Defects Foundation, 1988. *A list of services that provide information on drug and chemical exposures during pregnancy.*

Jackson, L. G., and Schimke, R. N.: Clinical Genetics: A Source Book for Physicians. New York, John Wiley and Sons, 1979. *A detailed discussion of genetic problems encountered in clinical practice. Good sections on multisystemic disorders and genetic aspects of single-system diseases.*

Jones, K. L.: Smith's Recognizable Patterns of Human Malformation. 4th ed. Philadelphia, W. B. Saunders Co., 1988. *The "bible" of syndromology. Concise, easy to read, and eminently usable. Many useful tables and differential guides. Excellent sections on generic issues such as ambiguous genitalia and growth disorders.*

Kelly, T. D.: Clinical Genetics and Genetic Counseling. Chicago, Year Book Medical Publishers, Inc., 1980. *A good general introduction to medical genetics and genetic counseling. Good source of basic information as well as thoughtful discussions of common clinical problems and genetic issues in clinical medicine.*

McKusick, V. A.: Mendelian Inheritance in Man: Catalogs of Autosomal Dominant, Autosomal Recessive, and X-linked Phenotypes. 8th ed. Baltimore, Johns Hopkins University Press, 1988. *A catalogue of all known or suspected single-gene disorders of humans, with synoptic comments and selected bibliographies of relevant medical literature. Easy to use and an excellent reference resource. Updated regularly.*

National Center for Education in Maternal and Child Health: A National List of Voluntary Organizations in Maternal and Child Health. Washington, D.C., 1985. *A comprehensive guide to voluntary organizations and parent support groups that provide services to individuals and families with handicapping conditions and other health problems.*

Sever, J. L., and Brent, R. L.: Teratogen Update: Environmentally Induced Birth Defect Risks. New York, Alan R. Liss, Inc., 1986. *A detailed discussion of several of the most important human teratogens.*

Shepard, T. H.: Catalog of Teratogenic Agents. 5th ed. Baltimore, Johns Hopkins University Press, 1986. *Similar format to that used by McKusick but deals with potentially hazardous environmental agents for fetal development. Easy to use and an excellent resource. Updated regularly.*

Smith, D. W.: Growth and Its Disorders: Basics and Standards, Approach and Classifications, Growth Deficiency Disorders, Growth Excess Disorders, Obesity. Vol. 15 in the series Major Problems in Clinical Pediatrics. Philadelphia, W. B. Saunders Co., 1977. *A practical guide to growth problems. Well organized and straightforward. Penetrating clinical discussions. Very usable.*

Smith, D. W.: Recognizable Patterns of Human Deformation. 2nd ed. Philadelphia, W. B. Saunders Co., 1981. *A companion volume to Smith's Recognizable Patterns of Human Malformation that discusses biomechanical factors contributing to birth defects. Also very usable.*

Standbury, J. B., Wyngaarden, J. B., and Fredrickson, D. S. (Eds.): The Metabolic Basis of Inherited Disease. 5th ed. New York, McGraw-Hill Book Co., 1983. *A basic in-depth reference work on metabolic diseases. Extensive basic science discussion. Some good clinical information.*

Thompson, J. S., and Thompson, M. W.: Genetics in Medicine. Philadelphia, W. B. Saunders Co., 1986. *A clear and concise discussion of basic human genetics and issues in medical practice.*

Williamson, R. A.: Prenatal diagnosis. *In* Pitkin, R. M., and Scott, J. R. (Eds.): Clinical Obstetrics and Gynecology. Vol. 31. Philadelphia, J. B. Lippincott Co., 1988. *A current, comprehensive, and authoritative guide to prenatal diagnosis issues and capabilities. Lists disorders currently diagnosable.*

Zellweger, H., and Simpson, J.: Chromosomes in Man. Spastics International Medical Publications. London, William Heinemann Medical Books, Ltd; Clinics in Developmental Medicine, Nos. 65 and 66. Philadelphia, J. B. Lippincott Co., 1977. *Practical information for clinicians about chromosome problems. Clinical manifestations described in detail. Some social, legal, and psychologic aspects also considered.*

Sources on Specific Genetic Problems

The following references are to comprehensive review-type articles on specific genetic problem categories commonly encountered by the practicing physician. They are up-to-date, clearly written, and well organized. They represent an excellent way of learning more about each of these subjects than is contained in usual texts and would be valuable references in a clinic or hospital library.

Aleck, K. A., and Shapiro, L. J.: Genetic-metabolic considerations in the sick neonate. Pediatr. Clin. North Am., *25*:431, 1978.

Anderson, C. E., Rotter, M. D., and Zonana, J.: Hereditary considerations in common disorders. Pediatr. Clin. North Am., *25*:539–556, 1978.

Fraser, F. C.: The genetics of common birth defects and diseases. *In* Kaback, M. M. (Ed.): Genetic Issues in Pediatric and Obstetric Practice. Chicago, Year Book Medical Publishers, 1981, pp. 45–54.

Golbus, M. S.: The current scope of antenatal diagnosis. Hospital Practice, *17*:179–186, 1982.

Hanson, J. W.: Avoidable hazards in pregnancy: A guide for the primary care physician. Continuing Education, *11*:69–76, 1982.

Hillman, R. E.: Heritable metabolic disorders in the critically ill newborn. *In* Kaback, M. M. (Ed.): Genetic Issues in Pediatric and Obstetric Practice. Chicago, Year Book Medical Publishers, 1981, pp. 185–198.

Holtzman, R. E.: Newborn screening for hereditary metabolic disorders: Desirable characteristics, experience, and issues. *In* Kaback, M. M. (Ed.): Genetic Issues in Pediatric and Obstetric Practice. Chicago, Year Book Medical Publishers, 1981, pp. 455–470.

Neims, A. H., and Manchester, D. K.: Heredity and the response to drugs and environmental chemicals. *In* Kaback, M. M. (Ed.): Genetic Issues in Pediatric and Obstetric Practice. Chicago, Year Book Medical Publishers, 1981, pp. 369–380.

Schimke, R. N.: Genetics and cancer in children: Current concepts. *In* Kaback, M. M. (Ed.): Genetic Issues in Pediatric and Obstetric Practice. Chicago, Year Book Medical Publishers, 1981, pp. 413–441.

Simpson, J. L.: Disorders of sexual differentiation resulting from mutant genes. *In* Kaback, M. M. (Ed.): Genetic Issues in Pediatric and Obstetric Practice. Chicago, Year Book Medical Publishers, 1981, pp. 329–368.

Spranger, J., Benirschke, K., Hall, J. G., et al.: Errors of morphogenesis: Concepts and terms. J. Pediatr., *100*:160, 1982.

65

Anxiety

Wayne Katon
John Geyman

Whether viewed as mental illness, psychiatric problems, stress-related illness, or functional disorders, psychologic dysfunction of individuals in our increasingly complex society may well be more frequent and more incapacitating than any other disease or disorder. Studies sponsored by the National Institute of Mental Health have shown that in the United States, over one half of all patients with mental health disorders are cared for solely by the primary care sector (Regier et al., 1984; Shapiro et al., 1984). Several recent studies have demonstrated that 25 per cent to 33 per cent of primary care patients suffer from a Diagnostic and Statistical Manual of Mental Disorders (DSM-III) mental disorder (Hoeper et al., 1979). Moreover, primary care patients with mental disorders utilize approximately twice as much nonpsychiatric medical care as patients without mental health problems (Hankin and Oktay, 1979). These patients also have a higher incidence of organic illness (Eastwood, 1971). As a result of their long-term contact with all members of the family, family physicians have a special opportunity and responsibility to recognize and manage mental health problems.

Anxiety and depression represent the two most common mental health disorders encountered in everyday medical practice (Marsland et al., 1976). The recent Epidemiologic Catchment Area study that measured the prevalence of mental illness in five major United States cities found that anxiety disorders occurred in 15.4 per cent of the community, second only to disorders of substance abuse, which occurred in 16.7 per cent of the population (Yates, 1986). Two recent studies determined that anxiety represented the fifth and fifteenth most common clinical diagnosis in primary care (Vallbona, 1973; Marsland et al., 1976). Moreover, the 1980–1981 National Ambulatory Medical Care survey (which gathered information on approximately 90,000 visits to a nationally representative sample of private physicians from nine specialty groups) determined that anxiety and nervousness accounted for 11 per cent of all visits to physicians (Schurman et al., 1985). Further evidence of the prevalence of anxiety is provided by a recent survey of 350 primary care physicians, in which anxiety disorders were rated as the most common psychiatric problem seen in their clinics (Orleans et al., 1985). Antianxiety agents in general and benzodiazepines in particular have been consistently the most prescribed medications in the United States over the last 15 to 20 years, and primary care physicians wrote 85 per cent of these prescriptions (Mellinger et al., 1984).

Anxiety is not only caused by social problems but is also frequently precipitated by medical illness. Thus, Zung (1979) has demonstrated that significant anxiety is found in 9 per cent of people in the community, in 32 per cent of people seeking primary care treatment, and in 52 per cent of patients with a known cardiologic illness. Anxiety frequently causes amplification of complaints of chronic medical illness and often worsens a pathophysiologic state in those illnesses (such as angina pectoris, asthma, or peptic ulcer disease) that may be adversely affected by increased sympathetic nervous system arousal (Katon and Roy-Byrne, 1989).

DEFINITION

Anxiety is a fearful emotion accompanied by certain physical symptoms. It may be of acute onset, or it may be a chronic, long-standing problem featuring a variety of physical complaints.

Rickels (1977) describes anxiety in these terms:

Anxiety is perceived as a subjective feeling of heightened tension and diffuse uneasiness defined as the conscious and reportable experience of intense dread and foreboding conceptualized as internally derived and unrelated to external threat. It is not merely fear because it lacks a specific object.

A major change precipitated by the development of the DSM-III in 1980 (American Psychiatric Association, 1980) is that anxiety is no longer thought of as a common unidimensional symptom often necessitating treatment with minor tranquilizers. Instead, advances in psychiatric nosology have developed specific, identifiable diagnostic categories made up of carefully delineated clusters of symptoms (Friedman and Jaffe, 1983). Each of these categories or syndromes has differing etiologic, treatment, and prognostic implications. The DSM-III recognizes the following subclasses of anxiety disorders: phobic, obsessive-compulsive, panic, generalized, posttraumatic stress, and atypical anxiety. This chapter especially focuses on panic disorder and agoraphobia, which are the most common anxiety disorders seen in primary care.

Anxiety disorders must be evaluated in a biopsychosocial framework. Thus, genetic and biologic factors in anxiety need to be evaluated within the social context in which the disorder began, taking into account the psychologic strengths and vulnerabilities of the patient. These disorders occur in a wide variety of patients, ranging from those with strong social support systems and many psychologic strengths to patients who are devoid of social support and have many maladaptive personality traits.

Diagnostic Approaches

SUBTYPES OF ANXIETY

It is especially important to differentiate generalized anxiety disorder or transient states of anxiety associated with life stress from acute panic attacks. There are extremely effective treatments for panic disorder, and accurate diagnosis and early aggressive treatment often decreases potential vocational and social disability.

PANIC DISORDER

The key distinguishing feature of panic disorder is the episodic nature of the panic attacks. Panic attacks are manifest by the sudden onset of intense apprehension, fear, or terror and at least four of the following somatic symptoms: dyspnea (the patient often actually hyperventilates); palpitations; chest pain or discomfort; choking or smothering sensations; dizziness; a feeling of unreality; paresthesia; diaphoresis; faintness; trembling or shaking; hot and cold flashes; nausea or abdominal distress; and fears of dying, going crazy, or losing control during an attack (Table 65–1) (American Psychiatric Association, 1987).

In clinical samples, the onset of panic disorder is generally between the ages of 17 and 30 (mean age 22.5 years) (Sheehan, 1979). In the Epidemiologic Catchment Area study, the highest 6-month prevalence was in those ages 25 to 44 years (Myers et al., 1984). In four recent epidemiologic studies, the prevalence of panic disorder in females was 1.6 per cent to 2.9 per cent and in males was 0.4 per cent to 1.7 per cent (Crowe et al., 1983; Myers et al., 1984; Uhlenhuth et al., 1983; Weissman et al., 1978). Several recent studies have found that patients with panic disorder were overrepresented within the primary care medical system. Katon and colleagues (1986) randomly assessed 195 primary care patients, aged 17 years and older, using a structured psychiatric interview. A total of 6.5 per cent of patients met

Table 65–1. DIAGNOSTIC CRITERIA FOR PANIC DISORDER*

A. At some time during the disturbance, one or more panic attacks (discrete periods of intense fear or discomfort) have occurred that were unexpected, i.e., did not occur immediately before or on exposure to a situation in which the person was the focus of others' attention.

B. Either four attacks, as defined in criterion A, have occurred within a 4-week period, or one or more attacks have been followed by a period of at least a month of persistent fear of having another attack.

C. At least four of the following symptoms developed during at least one of the attacks:
- Shortness of breath (dyspnea) or smothering sensations
- Dizziness, unsteady feelings, or faintness
- Palpitations or accelerated heart rate (tachycardia)
- Trembling or shaking
- Sweating
- Choking
- Nausea or abdominal distress
- Depersonalization or derealization
- Numbness or tingling sensations (paresthesias)
- Flushes (hot flashes) or chills
- Chest pain or discomfort
- Fear of dying
- Fear of going crazy or of doing something uncontrolled

Note: Attacks involving four or more symptoms are panic attacks; attacks involving fewer than four symptoms are limited-symptom attacks.

D. During at least some of the attacks, at least four of the C symptoms developed suddenly and increased in intensity within 10 minutes of the beginning of the first C symptom noticed in the attack.

E. It cannot be established that an organic factor initiated and maintained the disturbance, e.g., amphetamine or caffeine intoxication, hyperthyroidism.

Note: Mitral valve prolapse may be an associated condition, but does not preclude a diagnosis of panic disorder.

*Reprinted with permission from: American Psychiatric Association: Diagnostic and Statistical Manual of Mental Disorders, 3rd ed. revised. Washington, D.C., American Psychiatric Association, 1987, pp. 237–238.

DSM-III criteria for panic disorder alone, and 6.5 per cent met criteria for major depression and panic disorder. Finlay-Jones and Brown (1981), utilizing a structured psychiatric interview, found that 17 per cent of 164 female primary care patients suffered from anxiety neurosis (these patients have panic disorder or generalized anxiety or both), with 8 per cent suffering from anxiety neurosis alone and 9 per cent having anxiety neurosis and major depression.

Three recent controlled studies suggest that panic disorder is often precipitated by stressful life events. These studies found that patients with panic disorder often had a higher frequency than controls of stressful life events that connoted danger and threat (Finlay-Jones and Brown, 1981), events viewed as extremely uncontrollable or undesirable and that caused a severe lowering of self-esteem (Roy-Byrne et al., 1986), and finally events that involved the death or severe illness of a friend or relative (Faravelli, 1985). Panic attacks have also been described after a physical illness, accident or trauma, rape or physical assault, and endocrinologic changes.

Panic disorder is a familial disease, with controlled studies demonstrating that 18 per cent to 40 per cent of first-degree relatives of patients with panic disorder also suffer from this severe anxiety disorder (Noyes et al., 1978; Cohen et al., 1951; Crowe et al., 1983). Moreover, a recent twin study demonstrated a significantly higher concordance for panic disorder in monozygotic twins than in dizygotic twins (Torgerson, 1983). Genetic studies have found that females are affected more frequently than males, with the ratio approaching 2:1. More alcohol abuse is found in the male relatives of panic disorder patients than in the male relatives of controls (Crowe et al., 1983; Noyes et al., 1978; Cohen et al., 1951).

There has been an exponential growth in psychobiologic studies of panic disorder. These studies have demonstrated that patients with panic disorder are more susceptible to developing anxiety attacks than normal controls when challenged with specific provocative agents, including intravenous lactate, air with increased carbon dioxide concentrations, isoproterenol, caffeine, and yohimbine (Roy-Byrne and Cowley, 1988). Whether these tests produce specific, unique biochemical changes in patients with panic disorder or simply produce increased somatic sensations to which patients with panic disorder overreact is still controversial. Recent studies with position emission tomography scanning, magnetic resonance imaging, and brain electrical activity mapping have implicated parahippocampal and temporal lobe abnormalities in panic disorder, and these studies await replication (Roy-Byrne and Cowley, 1988; Katon, 1989). Abnormalities in the benzodiazepine–gamma-aminobutyric acid system and the noradrenergic controls of the sympathetic nervous system have also been recently documented in panic disorder (Katon, 1989), but theories of the primacy of either of these systems in the causation of panic disorder remain controversial.

Table 65–2 shows the usual chronology in the development of panic disorder. Patients often experience the onset of the first panic attack, at times described as the worst experience in their life, after one or a series of life events overwhelm their coping mechanisms. Many patients actually are seen by a family physician after a first or second attack, and early intervention may stop the syndrome at this point. Other patients go on to the second stage, in which panic attacks become more frequent and the patient begins to develop anticipatory anxiety, i.e., anxiety between attacks because of the constant fear another will occur. During this second stage, patients may begin to associate many environmental events with the anxiety and often develop multiple phobias and avoidance behavior. If patients have an attack while driving, they may avoid getting into the car, or if they have an attack while giving a speech, they may avoid public speaking. This pattern may culminate in the third stage, *agoraphobia*, which literally means "a fear of the marketplace" but actually describes the ultimate regressive behavior of being afraid to leave the house because of the association of panic attacks with many environmental stimuli. In DSM-III-R, agoraphobia is defined as a fear of being in places or situations from which escape might be difficult or embarrassing or help might be unavailable in the event of a panic attack. Most patients with agoraphobia actually will leave the house and become involved in activities with a person they see as a protector. Agoraphobic patients often avoid being alone and regressively cling to significant others. Zitrin and coworkers (1978) have shown that almost all agoraphobics have panic attacks. Table 65–3 describes the DSM-III-R criteria for panic disorder with agoraphobia; the DSM-III-R criteria emphasize that agoraphobic avoidance may range from mild to severe (American Psychiatric Association, 1987).

The patient with panic disorder has cognitive, affective, and somatic symptoms and also experiences social consequences to the development of the disorder (Grant et al., 1983) (Table 65–4). The patient often selectively focuses on the somatic components of the panic syndrome and attributes the increased anxiety and tension to the frightening nature of these somatic symptoms. Recent studies have demonstrated that the most common presenting somatic symptoms are cardiologic (chest pain and tachycardia), neurologic (headache, dizziness, faintness, paresthesia), and gastrointestinal (irritable bowel symptoms and epigastric pain) (Katon, 1984). The presentation of cardiologic symptoms may especially lead to costly and potentially dangerous medical tests in patients with panic disorder. Thus, three recent studies have documented that nearly 50 per cent of patients with chest pain and negative angiographic studies suffer from panic disorder (Katon et al., 1988; Beitman et al., 1987; Bass and Wade, 1984). In patients with vague, ill-defined complaints, the physician must be alert to the possibility of panic disorder or major depression as being the underlying etiology and must

Table 65–2. THREE STAGES IN DEVELOPMENT OF PANIC DISORDER

Initial acute panic attack or cluster of attacks ⟶	Panic attacks increase in frequency ⟶ Phobias develop Anticipatory anxiety and avoidance behaviors develop Medical care-seeking dramatically increases for somatic complaints	Agoraphobia Increased dependency Dramatic changes in family system Chronic somatization develops

question the patient specifically about the somatic components of each syndrome.

Panic Disorder and Mitral Valve Prolapse

Patients with panic disorder have been found to have an increased prevalence of mitral valve prolapse (MVP). A recent review of 17 studies found that 18 per cent of patients with panic disorder or agoraphobia met definite criteria for MVP and 27 per cent met probable criteria for MVP versus an average rate of definite MVP of 1 per cent in normal controls and probable or definite MVP in 12 per cent of controls (Margraf et al., 1988). These studies must be understood in the context of recent research on MVP. Wynne (1986) recently suggested that there are really two groups of subjects who carry the diagnosis of MVP. The first consists of persons in whom the disorder is primarily an echocardiographic finding. These people are no more symptomatic than controls, have no more arrhythmias, are often free from the typical auscultatory findings, and have a low risk of complications. The echocardiographic findings in this group are probably anatomic normal variants and reflect the technologic advances in defining valve motion but emphasize the difficulty in differentiating variants of normal valve mobility. The second group consists of patients who typically not only have evidence of prolapse on echocardiography but also have clinical findings of mitral valve regurgitation. These people have symptoms related to valvular insufficiency and appear to have an increased risk of infective endocarditis as well as progressive mitral regurgitation. Two useful markers have been identified to help differentiate between the first group (with trivial) and the second group (with important) MVP: (1) the degree of redundancy of the valve, a finding that can be defined echocardiographically and (2) the presence of mitral regurgitation on physical examination. Nishimura and colleagues (1985) recently found that almost every patient with a complication of MVP had redundant valves as indicated by an increase of mitral valve leaflet thickness of 5 mm. or more.

Evidence from a study by Gorman and colleagues (1988) has determined that the MVP in patients with panic disorder is mild and not associated with thickened mitral valve leaflets (the high-risk group of MVP patients described by Nishimura and colleagues [1985]). Patients with panic disorder and MVP have also been found to respond equally well to treatment with imipramine as patients with panic disorder alone (Gorman et al., 1981). Several cases have been described in which patients with panic disorder and echocardiographically proved MVP had normal echocardiograms after the panic attacks were successfully treated (Gorman et al., 1988). The findings suggest that panic disorder is associated with an increased

Table 65–3. DIAGNOSTIC CRITERIA FOR PANIC DISORDER WITH AGORAPHOBIA*

A. Meets the criteria for panic disorder.
B. Agoraphobia: Fear of being in places or situations from which escape might be difficult (or embarrassing) or in which help might not be available in the event of a panic attack. (Includes cases in which persistent avoidance behavior originated during an active phase of panic disorder, even if the person does not attribute the avoidance behavior to fear of having a panic attack.) As a result of this fear, the person either restricts travel or needs a companion when away from home, or else endures agoraphobic situations despite intense anxiety. Common agoraphobic situations include being outside the home alone; being in a crowd or standing in a line; being on a bridge; and traveling in a bus, train, or car.

Specify current severity of agoraphobic avoidance:
Mild: Some avoidance (or endurance with distress), but relatively normal life style, e.g., travels unaccompanied when necessary, such as to work or to shop; otherwise avoids traveling alone.
Moderate: Avoidance results in constricted life style, e.g., the person is able to leave the house alone but not to go more than a few miles unaccompanied.
Severe: Avoidance results in being nearly or completely housebound or unable to leave the house unaccompanied.
In Partial Remission: No current agoraphobic avoidance, but some agoraphobic avoidance during the past 6 months.
In Full Remission: No current agoraphobic avoidance and none during the past 6 months.

Specify current severity of panic attacks:
Mild: During the past month, either all attacks have been limited-symptom attacks (i.e., fewer than four symptoms), or there has been no more than one panic attack.
Moderate: During the past month, attacks have been intermediate between mild and severe.
Severe: During the past month, there have been at least eight panic attacks.
In Partial Remission: The condition has been intermediate between In Full Remission and Mild.
In Full Remission: During the past 6 months, there have been no panic or limited-symptom attacks.

*Reprinted with permission from: American Psychiatric Association: Diagnostic and Statistical Manual of Mental Disorders, 3rd ed., revised. American Psychiatric Association, 1987, pp. 238–239.

Table 65–4. COMPONENTS OF PANIC DISORDER*

Cognitive	Affective	Somatic	Social
Worry	Anxiety or nervousness	Tachycardia	Dependency
Sense of foreboding	Secondary depression	Hyperventilation (patient complains of shortness of breath)	Vocational limitations
Sense of impending doom or dread	Irritability	Tingling in hands and feet	Isolation
Exaggeration of innocuous situations as dangerous		Diaphoresis	
Exaggeration of probability of harm in specific situations		Dizziness or syncope	
Tendency to be inattentive, distractible		Flushing	
Sense of unreality		Muscle tension	
Rumination		Tremulousness	
Loss of control		Restlessness	
		Chest tightness, pressure on chest (pseudoangina)	
		Headaches, backaches, muscle spasms	

*From Grant B., Katon, W., and Beitman, B.: Panic disorder. J. Fam. Pract., *17*, 909, 1983.

prevalence of MVP, but this seems to be a mild type that is principally an echocardiographic finding of little relevance for treatment and not necessitating prophylactic antibiotic treatment.

PHOBIC DISORDERS

The essential feature of a phobic disorder is the persistent and irrational fear of a specific object, activity, or situation that results in a compelling desire to avoid the dreaded object, activity, or situation. The fear is recognized by the individual as excessive or unreasonable in proportion to the actual danger of the situation, object, or activity (American Psychiatric Association, 1987).

The phobic disorders are classified as agoraphobia (covered in the previous section on panic disorder), the most pervasive and severe form, which almost always occurs secondary to the onset of panic attacks; social phobia; and simple phobia. Simple phobia involves a persistent irrational fear of and compelling desire to avoid an object or a situation in which one is alone or in a public place. Common simple phobias are fears of heights (acrophobia), animals, insects, airplanes, and confined spaces (claustrophobia).

In social phobia, there is a persistent fear of and compelling desire to avoid a situation in which the individual is exposed to public scrutiny by others; the sufferer fears he or she may act in a way that will be humiliating and embarrassing (American Psychiatric Association, 1987).

In simple phobias, psychosocial trauma can often be identified as the original precipitant; for example, being bitten by a dog as a child may lead to a phobia of all dogs. In both simple phobia and social phobia, when the individual is exposed to the phobic stimulus, he or she becomes overwhelmingly fearful and may experience symptoms identical to those of a panic attack. These individuals often have considerable anticipatory anxiety when they know they will be exposed to the phobic stimulus. Patients with simple and social phobias do not have panic attacks when not exposed to the specific phobic stimulus. Their phobias are circumscribed. In terms of patients seeking psychiatric treatment, almost 70 per cent have panic attacks and have developed multiple phobias, and 30 per cent have circumscribed social or simple phobias (Sheehan, 1979).

GENERALIZED ANXIETY DISORDER

Patients with generalized anxiety disorder (GAD) have unrealistic or excessive worry about one or more life circumstances for a period of 6 months or longer during which they are bothered more days than not by these concerns (American Psychiatric Association, 1987). Patients also have at least six of 18 symptoms from three categories: (1) motor tension, (2) autonomic hyperactivity, and (3) vigilance and scanning (Table 65–5). In some patients, symptoms of GAD are life long and persistent, whereas for other patients the symptoms are acute, intermittent, and closely related to environmental stressful events.

In primary care, most patients with symptoms of generalized anxiety disorder develop these symptoms secondary to another major DSM-III disorder such as panic disorder, major depression, alcohol abuse, or an Axis II personality disorder (Katon et al., 1987; Breslau and Davis, 1985). These disorders and organic causes of anxiety must be screened for and ruled out before embarking on treatment of GAD. When these psychiatric and medical causes of GAD are ruled out, only a small subset of patients remains with primary GAD.

Many other patients present with impairment in social relationships (marriage) or occupational functioning and with symptoms of anxiety within 3 months of the onset of a specific stress but do not have enough symptoms to fulfill criteria for GAD. According to the DSM-III-R formulation, these are called adjustment disorders with anxious mood.

Table 65–5. DIAGNOSTIC CRITERIA FOR GENERALIZED ANXIETY DISORDER*

A. Unrealistic or excessive anxiety and worry (apprehensive expectation) about two or more life circumstances, e.g., worry about possible misfortune to one's child (who is in no danger) and worry about finances (for no good reason), for a period of 6 months or longer, during which the person has been bothered more days than not by these concerns. In children and adolescents, this may take the form of anxiety and worry about academic, athletic, and social performance.

B. If another Axis I disorder is present, the focus of the anxiety and worry in A is unrelated to it, e.g., the anxiety or worry is not about having a panic attack (as in panic disorder), being embarrassed in public (as in social phobia), being contaminated (as in obsessive compulsive disorder), or gaining weight (as in anorexia nervosa).

C. The disturbance does not occur only during the course of a mood disorder or a psychotic disorder.

D. At least six of the following 18 symptoms are often present when anxious (do not include symptoms present only during panic attacks):
  Motor tension:
    Trembling, twitching, or feeling shaky
    Muscle tension, aches, or soreness
    Restlessness
    Easy fatigability
  Autonomic hyperactivity
    Shortness of breath or smothering sensations
    Palpitations or accelerated heart rate (tachycardia)
    Sweating or cold clammy hands
    Dry mouth
    Dizziness or lightheadedness
    Nausea, diarrhea, or other abdominal distress
    Flushes (hot flashes) or chills
    Frequent urination
    Trouble swallowing or "lump in throat"
  Vigilance and scanning:
    Feeling keyed up or on edge
    Exaggerated startle response
    Difficulty concentrating or "mind going blank" because of anxiety
    Trouble falling or staying asleep
    Irritability

E. It cannot be established that an organic factor initiated and maintained the disturbance, e.g., hyperthyroidism, caffeine intoxication.

*Reprinted with permission from: American Psychiatric Association: Diagnostic and Statistical Manual of Mental Disorders, 3rd ed., revised. Washington, D.C., American Psychiatric Association, 1987, pp. 252–253.

POSTTRAUMATIC STRESS DISORDER

Patients with posttraumatic stress disorder (PTSD) have experienced a severe catastrophic event that is outside the range of normal human experience and would be distressing to anyone (American Psychiatric Association, 1987). The patient frequently and persistently re-experiences the event by having recurrent, often intrusive images of the trauma and recurrent dreams or nightmares of the event, and by experiencing behavior in which he or she suddenly acts or feels as if the traumatic event were recurring. These behavioral abnormalities include illusions, hallucinations or flashback episodes, and intense psychologic distress when exposed to environmental stimuli that symbolize or resemble an aspect of the traumatic event (Table 65–6). Patients with PTSD persistently avoid stimuli associated with the trauma or experience a numbing of general responsiveness as well as chronic symptoms of increased arousal when exposed to events that symbolize or resemble an aspect of the traumatic event.

In primary care, civilian cases of PTSD are occasionally seen, and these patients may have combinations of symptoms of PTSD, panic disorder, and major depression. Indeed, recent research experience has demonstrated that many PTSD patients have panic attacks during flashback episodes (Mellman and Davis, 1985). Civilian cases are often precipitated by extreme trauma such as a severe automobile accident, industrial accident, or national disaster. Many of these civilian cases become complicated by the legal and disability systems that may unwittingly lead to prolongation of disability. Early intervention with accurate diagnosis and aggressive treatment may prevent occupational and social disability secondary to this disorder.

MEDICAL DIFFERENTIAL DIAGNOSIS

Some studies have shown that in patients referred for mental health problems such as anxiety, depression, and psychosis, from 9 per cent to 42 per cent had medical illnesses that were responsible for their symptoms (Hall et al., 1978; Koranyi, 1979). Anxiety must be differentiated from a host of organic problems, including the various cardiovascular, respiratory, cerebral, metabolic, hormonal, and other disorders listed in Table 65–7. In a patient with a known medical ailment, that illness (including the symptoms, complications, and pharmacologic treatment) should always be suspected as the cause of the psychologic symptoms (Rosenbaum, 1982). For instance, a diabetic patient with hypoglycemic episodes, an asthmatic patient with a toxic aminophylline serum level, and a patient with recent myocardial infarction who is worried and concerned about resuming work and sexual relations may each suffer from symptoms of anxiety. The primary treatment would be adjusting pharmacologic treatment or counseling about the illness and the limitations it imposes on that patient's life (Rosenbaum, 1982).

PSYCHIATRIC DIFFERENTIAL DIAGNOSIS

Patients with anxiety disorders have a high frequency of current depression and frequently a lifetime history of major depression. About 60 per cent of patients with major depression also have a concurrent anxiety disorder (GAD or panic disorder) (Leckman et al., 1983a). Approximately 20 per cent of patients with major depression have panic disorder (Leckman et al., 1983b).

Table 65–6. DIAGNOSTIC CRITERIA FOR POSTTRAUMATIC STRESS DISORDER*

A. The person has experienced an event that is outside the range of usual human experience and that would be markedly distressing to almost anyone, e.g., serious threat to one's life or physical integrity; serious threat or harm to one's children, spouse, or other close relatives and friends; sudden destruction of one's home or community; or seeing another person who has recently been, or is being, seriously injured or killed as the result of an accident or physical violence.

B. The traumatic event is persistently re-experienced in at least one of the following ways:
- Recurrent and intrusive distressing recollections of the event (in young children, repetitive play in which themes or aspects of the trauma are expressed)
- Recurrent distressing dreams of the event
- Sudden acting or feeling as if the traumatic event were recurring (includes a sense of reliving the experience, illusions, hallucinations, and dissociative [flashback] episodes, even those that occur upon awakening or when intoxicated)
- Intense psychologic distress at exposure to events that symbolize or resemble an aspect of the traumatic event, including anniversaries of the trauma

C. Persistent avoidance of stimuli associated with the trauma or numbing of general responsiveness (not present before the trauma), as indicated by at least three of the following:
- Efforts to avoid thoughts or feelings associated with the trauma
- Efforts to avoid activities or situations that arouse recollections of the trauma
- Inability to recall an important aspect of the trauma (psychogenic amnesia)
- Markedly diminished interest in significant activities (in young children, loss of recently acquired developmental skills such as toilet training or language skills)
- Feeling of detachment or estrangement from others
- Restricted range of affect, e.g., unable to have loving feelings
- Sense of a foreshortened future, e.g., does not expect to have a career, marriage, or children, or a long life

D. Persistent symptoms of increased arousal (not present before the trauma), as indicated by at least two of the following:
- Difficulty falling or staying asleep
- Irritability or outbursts of anger
- Difficulty concentrating
- Hypervigilance
- Exaggerated startle response
- Physiologic reactivity upon exposure to events that symbolize or resemble an aspect of the traumatic event (e.g., a woman who was raped in an elevator breaks out in a sweat when entering any elevator)

E. Duration of the disturbance (symptoms in B, C, and D) of at least 1 month.

Specify delayed onset if the onset of symptoms was at least 6 months after the trauma.

*Reprinted with permission from: American Psychiatric Association: Diagnostic and Statistical Manual of Mental Disorders, 3rd ed., revised. Washington, D.C., American Psychiatric Association, 1987, pp. 250–251.

Table 65–7. ORGANIC DISORDERS SIMULATING ANXIETY SYNDROME*

Cardiovascular:	**Metabolic and Hormonal:**
Ischemic heart disease	Thyrotoxicosis
Valvular heart disease	Pheochromocytoma
Cardiomyopathies	Adrenocortical insufficiency
Myocarditis	Hypokalemia
Arrhythmias	Hypoglycemia
Respiratory:	Hyperparathyroidism
Emphysema	Myasthenia gravis
Occult pulmonary embolism	**Nutritional:**
Hamman-Rich syndrome	Thiamine, pyridoxine, or folate deficiency
Scleroderma	Iron deficiency anemia
Cerebral:	**Intoxication:**
Transient cerebrovascular insufficiency	Caffeine
Psychomotor epilepsy	Alcohol
Essential tremor	Sympathomimetics
	Amphetamines

*From Walker, J. I.: The anxious patient. J. Fam. Pract., *12*:4, 733, 1981.

Patients with panic disorder have been demonstrated to have a 50 per cent to 90 per cent risk of having a major depressive episode at some point in their lifetime (Breir et al., 1984; Cloninger et al., 1981; Raskin et al., 1982; Pariser et al., 1979). In a recent primary care study, 50 per cent of patients with panic disorder also suffered from major depression (Katon et al., 1986). Patients with panic disorder or agoraphobia with a history of major depression have been shown to have a more severe anxiety disorder, greater levels of past impairment, and a longer duration of panic disorder or agoraphobia compared with patients with panic disorder or agoraphobia with no history of depression (Breir et al., 1984).

These data suggesting an overlap of panic disorder, agoraphobia, GAD, and depression are supported by the findings of Goldberg (1979) that 67 per cent of patients with mental illness in primary care clinics have mixed symptoms of anxiety and depression. The implication of these data is that a primary care patient with anxiety should be carefully screened for major depression and vice versa. The occurrence of both disorders frequently suggests that antidepressant medication will be needed.

Anxiety is a frequent accompaniment of drug and alcohol abuse and withdrawal, and such abuse must be suspected in patients with persistent requests for antianxiety medications. Moreover, patients with panic disorder, GAD, or social phobias often try to self-medicate with alcohol in order to modulate their anxiety (Quitkin et al, 1972). Although alcohol may temporarily decrease anxiety, the short half-life of this substance frequently leads to worsening anxiety as blood levels of alcohol rapidly decrease. Also, alcohol may have a "kindling" effect on sympathetic nervous system tone, provoking long-lasting increases in arousal after a prolonged period of usage. Alcohol often upsets sleep cycles, a disruption that has also been found to worsen panic disorder (Roy-Byrne and Uhde, 1988).

Recent studies have documented that in approximately one third of alcoholics, panic disorder or severe phobic behavior or both often preceded this substance abuse (Mullaney and Trippett, 1979; Bowen et al., 1984; Smail et al., 1984). Longitudinal chronologic studies have revealed that self-medication with alcohol in these patients temporarily relieves phobic anxiety but actually leads to worsening social phobias; conversely, abstinence from alcohol leads to improvement in phobic behavior (Stockwell et al., 1984).

HISTORY

A systematic approach is required for the accurate diagnosis of the underlying cause of anxiety. As for other clinical problems, this approach should place particular emphasis on the history and physical examination. Further laboratory and x-ray studies should be carefully selected on an individual basis and may often have therapeutic as well as diagnostic value in themselves. These studies often help patients feel that their physicians have taken their complaints seriously.

The history is probably the single best diagnostic tool in the work-up of the anxious patient, whether the anxiety is of an acute or chronic nature. The history-taking process should be sufficiently open-ended and unhurried to elicit the patient's concerns and fears, current life situation, family and other support systems, and concurrent medical problems. Table 65–8 presents a number of symptom cues related to anxiety and depression that are pertinent in the review of symptoms (Goldstein and Brauger, 1971). One particularly useful part of the history, especially in elderly patients with anxiety, is inquiry into the sleep-wake pattern of the patient. A sudden change in this 24-hour pattern frequently represents depression or situational anxiety, which often is related to alterations in a familiar environment (Gadge, 1976).

PHYSICAL EXAMINATION

There are a number of common physical findings of anxiety that are well known to experienced clinicians. The patient looks worried and acts tense. The initial handshake often reveals a moist palm. Increased motor activity is often evident, such as frequent movements, crossing and uncrossing of the legs while sitting, rearranging of clothing, and nervous gestures. The facial muscles may show twitching or tics. Breathing is often rapid and superficial, and in panic disorder, frequent deep, sighing respirations are seen. Associated symptoms include mild tachycardia, muscular tension, and brisk but symmetrical deep tendon reflexes. Other signs suggestive of anxiety include unsteady voice, strained facies, grinding of teeth, dilated pupils, tremor of hands, flushing, and excessive perspiration.

FURTHER DIAGNOSTIC STUDIES

It is important that a complete and adequate diagnostic work-up be carried out in order to elucidate the basis of anxiety, but the extent of this work-up should be individualized. The family physician may have known the patient well over a period of years and may have a good understanding of the patient's life situation, personality structure, concurrent medical problems, and previous laboratory and x-ray studies. Under these circumstances, it may be that no further diagnostic studies are necessary in order to manage the patient's anxiety effectively. However, if the problem is a relatively recent complaint or if the patient is not well known to the physician or has not been fully worked up in the recent past, further diagnostic studies are usually warranted. This work-up should be aimed at detecting previously unrecognized organic disease and assuring the patient that the problem is being taken seriously and will be understood by the physician.

A variety of organic diseases should be considered in assessing the particular constellation of anxiety symptoms experienced by the individual patient. The patient with hyperthyroidism, which is often precipitated by an episode of stress, usually presents with tachycardia, palpitations, moist palms, tremor, weight loss, and subjective apprehension. Heart disease manifested by such events as angina, paroxysmal atrial tachycardia, and paroxysmal nocturnal dyspnea may require differentiation from an anxiety attack. Chronic anxiety may resemble other organic diseases, such as adrenal insufficiency, anemia, hypoglycemia, cerebral arteriosclerosis, and other forms of central nervous system disease.

In view of the sizable differential diagnoses involved with a patient presenting with anxiety, further diagnostic work-up may require such studies as complete blood count, urinalysis, an SMA-12 panel, thyroid function studies, electrocardiogram, chest x-ray examination, and more specific studies if indicated.

It is also helpful to obtain some assessment of the level of function in the patient's family. The Family APGAR score as developed by Smilkstein (1978) provides a valid and convenient diagnostic tool for this purpose. This screening questionnaire can be completed by the patient in less than 10 minutes and yields information that affords assessment of family function in terms of five components: adaptation, partnership, growth, affection, and resolve. An APGAR scoring system, which ranges from a highly functional family (APGAR of 7 to 10) to a severely dysfunctional family (APGAR of 0 to 3), is applied. In addition to the Family APGAR, Smilkstein recommends that the work-up of a severely dysfunctional family also include identification and evaluation of

Table 65–8. MOST FREQUENTLY REPORTED SYMPTOMS OF ANXIETY AND DEPRESSION*

Symptom Categories	Symptom Cues
Intellectual	Difficulty in concentration, poor memory
Anxious mood	Worrying, anticipation of the worst, fearful anticipation, irritability
Tension	Feelings of tension, fatigability, startle response, moved to tears easily, trembling, feelings of restlessness, inability to relax
Fears	Fears of dark, of strangers, of being left alone, of animals, of traffic, of crowds
Depressed mood	Feelings of sadness, hopelessness; the patient expresses pessimism, discouragement, and sadness; facial expression reflects despair or dejection
Feelings of guilt	Self-reproach, feels he or she has let people down, criticizes self to an unrealistic degree
Retardation	Slowness of thought and speech; impaired ability to concentrate, decreased motor activity
Word and activities	Thoughts and feelings of incapacity, fatigue, or weakness related to activities, work, or hobbies; loss of interest in activity, hobbies, or work—either directly reported by patient or indirectly indicated by listlessness, indecision, and vacillation (feels he or she has to push self to work or activities); decrease in actual time spent in activities or decrease in productivity
Hypochondriasis	Patient is absorbed in own physical ailments, preoccupation with health
Insomnia	Difficulty in falling asleep, broken sleep, unsatisfying sleep and fatigue on waking, dreams, nightmares, night terrors, early awakening
Somatic	Pains and aches; twitching; stiffness; myoclonic jerks; grinding of teeth; unsteady voice; increased muscular tone; tinnitus; blurring of vision; hot and cold flushes; feelings of weakness; pricking sensation; easily fatigued; heaviness in limbs, back, or head; backaches; headaches; muscle aches; loss of energy; fatigability
Cardiovascular symptoms	Tachycardia, palpitations, pain in chest, throbbing of vessels, fainting feelings, missing beat
Respiratory symptoms	Pressure or constriction in chest, choking feelings, sighing, dyspnea
Gastrointestinal symptoms	Difficulty in swallowing, breaking wind, abdominal pain, burning sensations, abdominal fullness, nausea, vomiting, borborygmi, loosenss of bowels, loss of weight, constipation
Genitourinary symptoms	Frequency of micturition, urgency of micturition, amenorrhea, menorrhagia, frigidity, premature ejaculation, loss of libido, impotence
Autonomic symptoms	Headache, raising of hair

*From Goldstein, B. F., and Brauger, B.: Pharmacologic considerations in the treatment of anxiety and depression in medical practice. Med. Clin. North Am., 55:487, 1971.

the family's past and present crises as well as assessment of the family's resources.

Management

The family physician has several advantages over other therapists in the management of clinical anxiety. Perhaps most important is the fact that the anxious patient usually perceives the problem as primarily medical rather than psychiatric. The family physician often has a strong physician-patient relationship established with the patient, which facilitates management, and often has seen the patient respond to previous stressful experiences, such as serious illness or death of another family member, divorce, or change of occupation. Knowledge of the patient's past social, medical, and family history is likewise helpful. The family physician is generally the first physician consulted and often sees emotional problems in early stages before fixed patterns of illness have been set.

GENERAL PRINCIPLES

Management of clinical anxiety rests on the following guidelines.

Prerequisites for the Physician. In order to manage the anxious patient effectively, physicians need to understand their own feelings and reactions to patients presenting with this kind of problem. Patience and a nonjudgmental attitude are required of the physician, together with the capacity to identify and encourage the particular interests and goals important to the individual patient.

Adequate Work-up. The importance of an adequate diagnostic work-up has already been stressed as an essential foundation for effective management of the patient with anxiety. The patient must feel that the physician has gathered adequate information and understanding of the problem before any reassurance or counseling can be effective. There is no quicker way to create patient distrust of the physician than for the patient to feel that reassurance or advice is given lightly without sufficient work-up. Equally ineffective is the physician's continued ordering of laboratory tests or x-ray studies after the patient has been assured of the absence of organic disease.

Treatment Based on Etiology. Therapeutic intervention for the anxious patient requires precision in the diagnostic work-up, both in terms of identifying or ruling out organic disease and in terms of understanding the personal concerns of the patient as an individual. Management, to be effective, must be based to the greatest extent possible on the specific organic and psychiatric diagnosis of the patient.

Development of a Therapeutic Plan. A deliberate therapeutic plan must be developed as a joint effort involving the patient as well as the physician. This plan usually involves a series of office visits on a regular basis over a period of time and may require specific kinds of therapeutic intervention, such as the use of counseling or psychotropic drugs or both. Use of such a plan allows the physician an opportunity to periodically reassess the effectiveness and progress of management and to make changes in therapy if indicated.

Avoidance of Common Pitfalls of Management. There are several common pitfalls that may trap the well-intentioned but unwary physician attempting to manage the patient with anxiety. Blazer (1977) has pointed out some of the approaches that should be avoided.

- Do not tell the patient there is really nothing wrong, that "it's all in your head." The difficulty with this approach can be further compounded by cajolery, censure, or an authoritative stance on the part of the physician.
- Do not perform a physical examination, laboratory, or x-ray studies to "prove" that the patient's anxiety is unfounded. This may be part of an ill-advised pretense of sharing the patient's concern as to the cause of anxiety or to confirm a "nothing is wrong with you" approach.
- Do not pretend the patient's complaint is real, then "cure" it with a mock regimen.
- Do not explain in psychiatric terms how the patient's complaint of anxiety can cause somatic symptoms without addressing the patient's real concerns.

Building Support Mechanisms. It is important to identify support mechanisms for the patient, especially for the patient who is divorced, widowed, or elderly. Members of the extended family and friends can frequently be helpful in this respect. Encouraging the development of outside interests may help to reduce the patient's self-absorption with his or her own problems. It is often useful to involve other family members in the development of a therapeutic plan for the patient.

SPECIFIC MANAGEMENT PROBLEMS

It is essential to differentiate the subtype of anxiety the patient is suffering from in order to prescribe specific effective treatment. In the last 10 years, medication has been demonstrated to be effective in double-blind psychopharmacologic treatment trials for many of the subtypes of anxiety. Controlled clinical trials have also demonstrated efficacy of specific psychotherapies, such as cognitive-behavioral therapy.

Panic Disorder

Treatment depends to some extent on the stage of the syndrome. The family physician often sees the patient after the first panic attack, or certainly in the first few months of the syndrome before multiple phobias, anticipatory anxiety, and avoidance behaviors develop (stages 2 and 3). Studies of the general population have revealed that up to one third of the general population have had a panic attack at some point in their lifetime, but most people have never had a cluster of attacks in a short enough period to meet DSM-III-R criteria for panic disorder (Katon et al., 1987; Norton et al., 1985). If the patient has infrequent attacks without the development of phobic behavior or develops a few attacks during severe stress in his or her life, education by the family physician about anxiety and self-relaxation techniques is often quite helpful, together with supportive psychotherapy aimed at helping the patient solve problems and deal with stressful life situations.

Once the panic attacks have begun to increase in frequency and the patient is starting to develop avoidance and phobic behaviors, the following guidelines should be utilized (Katon, 1989; Katon, 1986):

1. Specific pharmacologic therapy should be initiated to completely block panic attacks.
2. Once the panic attacks have ceased, the patient should be encouraged to re-enter situations that he or she may have begun to avoid, such as crowds of people, parties, driving on freeways, or going to the movies. Many of these phobias involve social situations in which the patient commonly had panic attacks.
3. The family physician should take a complete social and psychiatric history to address personality vulnerabilities, current life stresses, and developmental problems that may have provoked the onset of panic attacks or made the person more vulnerable to

life stress. Panic attacks can develop in a broad range of individuals, from those with no prior psychiatric history to patients with severe personality disorders. Patients who develop more severe phobic behavior with panic attacks have been found to have more problems in their family of origin and more maladaptive coping patterns as adults (Joyce et al., 1989; Vitaliano et al., 1987). The family physician may need to refer patients with panic disorder to marital therapy when the patients' attacks develop in the context of marital conflict. In patients experiencing chronic problems with low self-esteem, rejection sensitivity, and poor interpersonal relationships, psychodynamic therapy may be the treatment of choice.

4. Patients should be encouraged to read articles and books about panic disorder, and the family physician should educate the patient about the likely course of the illness. The length of pharmacologic treatment needs to be discussed, as does the possibility of relapse.

Recent double-blind, placebo-controlled studies have documented that there are three pharmacologic classes of medication that are equally effective and significantly more effective than placebo in the treatment of panic disorder:

1. the tricyclic antidepressants
2. the high-potency benzodiazepines
3. the monoamine oxidase inhibitors (Sheehan et al., 1980; Sheehan et al., 1984).

In primary care, the first-line treatment of choice for panic disorder should be the tricyclic antidepressants. These medications are quite safe, and studies of primary care patients have demonstrated that 50 per cent of patients with panic disorder will also have a major depression (Katon et al., 1986). The tricyclic antidepressants are effective therapeutic agents for both disorders. Imipramine is the best-studied drug in the treatment of panic disorder, with at least ten double-blind, placebo-controlled studies demonstrating its efficacy (Roy-Byrne and Katon, 1987). Recent studies have also documented that other tricyclics, such as desipramine, nortriptyline, amitriptyline, clomipramine, and doxepin, are also effective (Lydiard, 1988).

The family physician should begin treatment with 10 to 25 mg. of imipramine (or an alternative antidepressant) and gradually increase the medication by 25 mg. every 4 to 5 days until panic attacks cease. The ultimate dosage of medication needed is quite variable, with some patients responding at a low dosage such as 25 to 50 mg. and others needing up to 300 mg. It is useful for the physician to have a guide to antidepressant side effects, such as that shown in Table 65–9 (Katon and Roy-Byrne, 1988). The physician can then rationally choose alternative antidepressants based on side effects. Thus, if anticholinergic side effects develop when using imipramine, a switch to a medication such as desipramine with lower anticholinergic side effects is helpful. Similarly, if the patient develops orthostatic hypotension when using imipramine, a switch to a medication with decreased orthostatic hypotensive side effects, such as nortriptyline, may be helpful.

A subgroup of patients with panic disorder develop intolerable side effects on all tricyclic antidepressants. Some of these patients can be treated with very low dosages of tricyclics, such as 5 to 10 mg. initially, with a very gradual increase in dosage. Another alternative is to add a low dosage of alprazolam or lorazepam with the tricyclic; this often decreases the initial anxiety and "jitteriness" that can be a transient side effect of tricyclics. However, a small subgroup of patients will not tolerate tricyclic antidepressants at all, and the high-potency benzodiazepines represent an effective second line of treatment. Alprazolam, lorazepam, and clonazepam have all been demonstrated to be more effective than placebo in the treatment of panic disorders (Lydiard, 1988). Patients should be started on 0.5 mg. of alprazolam twice daily, with a gradual increase in 0.5 mg. increments every 2 to 3 days until panic attacks cease. Equivalent dosages of lorazepam and clonazepam to 0.5 mg. of alprazolam are 1.0 mg. of lorazepam and 0.25 mg. of clonazepam (Roy-Byrne et al., in press). One caveat is that patients with prior histories of multiple drug or alcohol abuse, personality disorder, or chronic benign pain probably should not be treated with benzodiazepines because of potential problems with abuse.

Monoamine oxidase inhibitors are potentially the most effective class of medications for panic disorder (Sheehan et al., 1984), but the lack of familiarity of most family physicians with these medications and the potential "hypertensive crisis" that can ensue when the patient does not follow a low-tyramine diet preclude their regular use in primary care. In a patient who has not responded to a tricyclic antidepressant or benzodiazepine, psychiatric consultation may be helpful.

Generalized Anxiety Disorder

In GAD or in less severe transient states of anxiety (adjustment disorder), the following modalities are often helpful.

Psychologic Support. The process of psychologic support by the family physician for patients with anxiety often involves a brief series of office visits to deal with the problem. In selected cases, some kind of family counseling may also be indicated. In one study, for example, it was found that an anxiety state in one or both parents was the most common psychosocial factor found in dysfunctional families with multiple health problems or exaggerated responses to organic illness or both (Schmidt, 1978).

At times, it may be possible for the family physician to provide psychologic support and counseling during a series of follow-up visits linked to other forms of treatment. A patient being treated for duodenal ulcer is a good example of someone well suited to this approach. It takes little time to palpate for epigastric tenderness and evaluate response to

Table 65–9. HETEROCYCLIC PROPERTIES OF ANTIDEPRESSANTS

	Potency of Reuptake Blockade						
	Serotonin	*Norepinephrine*	Dosage (mg.)	H_1	Anticholinergic	Sedation	Orthostatic Hypotension
Tertiary Amines							
Doxepin (Sinequan)	+ + +	+ +	100–300	Highest	Moderate	High	+ + +
Amitriptyline (Elavil)	+ + + +	+ +	100–300	Moderate to high	Highest	High	+ + +
Imipramine (Tofranil)	+ + + +	+ +	100–300	Low	Moderate	Moderate	+ +
Trimipramine (Surmontil)	+	+	100–300	High	Moderate	High	+ + +
Secondary Amines							
Nortriptyline (Pamelor)	+ + +	+ + +	50–125	Low	Low	Moderate	+
Protriptyline (Vivactil)	+ + +	+ + + +	20–60	Low	High	Low	+
Desipramine (Norpramin)	+ +	+ + + +	100–300	Low	Low	Low	+
Amoxapine (Ascendin)	+ +	+ + +	100–300	?	Low	Low	+ +
Tetracyclic							
Maprotiline (Ludiomil)	+	+ + +	100–300	Moderate	Low	Moderate	+ +
Triazolopyridine							
Trazadone (Desyrel)	+ + +	+	150–500	Low	Lowest	High	+ + +
Bicyclic							
Fluoxetine (Prozac)	+ + + +	0	20–80	?	Lowest	Low	0

0 = none, + = slight, + + = moderate, + + + = marked, + + + + = pronounced.

drug and dietary treatment during a series of follow-up visits. The remainder of each visit can be directed to identification of sources of stress and concern in the patient's life that may be subject to treatment through manipulation or counseling. Reassurance can be particularly effective for the anxious patient when combined artfully with treatment of concurrent medical problems.

Under other circumstances, it may be preferable to schedule a brief series of formal sessions for counseling or supportive psychotherapy. Over a span of five or six visits, each as short as 20 to 30 minutes, excellent results can often be obtained. Cathell (1968) suggests that the family physician should not imitate the psychiatrist's technique for treating emotional illness. He believes that the family physician tends to be more directive, authoritative, problem oriented, and pragmatic than psychiatrists are and that the physician's methods should reflect such differences and the particular nature of the practice.

A recent study by Catalan and colleagues (1984) lends support to the effectiveness of brief, effective, problem-focused counseling in the treatment of GAD by primary care physicians. A practice of family physicians that regularly prescribed benzodiazepines for the relief of anxiety was asked to participate in a randomized trial in which new patients with anxiety were treated. The intervention group was scheduled for brief supportive psychotherapy, and the controls were given the physician's usual prescription of a benzodiazepine. The patients were then followed at 3-month intervals. At 3 and 6 months, there were no differences between intervention patients and controls in psychiatric symptoms or distress. Moreover, the brief supportive counseling did not take significantly more physician time, nor did the patients who received psychotherapy tend to self-medicate with drugs or alcohol.

In the just-mentioned study, one subgroup with more severe distress did benefit more from medication. In a second study, patients with this high level of distress were randomized to either benzodiazepine treatment by the family physician or four to five sessions of problem-focused therapy with a psychiatrist (Gath and Catalan, 1988). The psychotherapy patients did equally well compared with the patients treated with benzodiazepines at follow-up. This research team is now entering a third phase of the research in which the brief, problem-focused treatment will be taught to primary care physicians. They will then measure the family physician's efficacy with problem-focused therapy against treatment with benzodiazepines in a controlled clinical trial.

Anstett and Hipskind (1981) have described some useful criteria that assist in predicting successful outcomes of brief office counseling. They observe that successful counseling depends upon agreement of the physician and patient on three issues: the nature of the problem, the goals of counseling, and their respective roles during counseling as well as length and expense of counseling. Table 65–10 lists the patient characteristics found to correlate with successful counseling outcomes. Relaxation techniques can also be quite helpful in decreasing anxiety and are easily taught in two to three half-hour sessions by the family physician. Benson and Klipper, in *The Relaxation Response* (1976), provide a useful relaxation technique that can be mastered by most patients and elucidate a theoretical rationale that may add to patient motivation. A recent study reported excellent

Table 65–10. PATIENT CHARACTERISTICS CORRELATING WITH SUCCESSFUL COUNSELING OUTCOME*

Demographic: relative youth, attractiveness, verbal ability, intelligence, success in other endeavors
Awareness that the problem is psychologic in nature
Presence of "signal anxiety"
Personality traits: persevering, dependable, nonimpulsive, trusting
High motivation for change in self
Faith that the counseling can be helpful
Awareness of how counseling works
Previous successful counseling experience
A personal resource system supportive of the aims of counseling
Absence of debilitating characterologic components in the patient's personality
Previous meaningful interpersonal relationships

*From Anstett, R., and Hipskind, M.: Selecting patients for brief office counseling. J. Fam. Pract., *13*:195, 1981.

results using relaxation training combined with cognitive therapy in the treatment of GAD.

Psychopharmacology of Generalized Anxiety Disorder. The heterogeneous nature of GAD makes evaluation of treatment difficult. GAD is often associated with many other anxiety disorders, such as panic disorder, PTSD, and agoraphobia as well as affective disorders such as major depression (Breslau and Davis, 1985; Katon et al., 1987). In general, benzodiazepines, buspirone, beta-blockers, and antidepressants have all been found to be more effective than placebo in patients with GAD (Roy-Byrne and Katon, 1987).

Multiple studies have demonstrated the efficacy of benzodiazepines in GAD. Recent concerns have centered not on efficacy but on the risks of the chronic use and abuse of benzodiazepines (Roy-Byrne and Katon, 1987). Table 65–11 lists the benzodiazepines available in the United States (Wesson, 1980). The major advantages of the benzodiazepines are (1) their lower potential for dependence and abuse, (2) the lower frequency of side effects and allergic reactions compared with antidepressants or phenothiazines, (3) their low lethality rate, even when taken in overdose, and (4) their believed inability to activate liver microsomal enzymes and therefore not alter the rate of metabolism of other drugs (Wesson, 1980).

In general, abuse of benzodiazepines by primary care patients is infrequent. Almost all abusers of benzodiazepines have had a prior history of substance abuse; therefore patients with a history of substance abuse should probably not be prescribed benzodiazepines, especially long-term (Roy-Byrne and Hummer, 1988). A larger concern for the primary care physician than abuse is the difficulty many anxious patients seem to have in withdrawing from these medications. Both severe rebound anxiety and withdrawal symptoms can be moderate to severe (Pecknold et al., 1988). The benzodiazepines with a short half-life appear especially likely to precipitate rebound anxiety and withdrawal (Roy-Byrne and Katon, 1987). For most patients, the symptoms experienced with drug discontinuation are not enduring and the patient can be supported with brief, regular visits and reassured that the symptoms will subside. Several strategies to decrease rebound symptoms include tapering the medication very slowly, switching from short-acting benzodiazepines to long-acting benzodiazepines prior to tapering, and treating the patient with a tricyclic antidepressant before attempting to taper the benzodiazepine. Because of the problem with discontinuation of these medications, many authorities are recommending shorter-term treatment, i.e., several weeks to 6 months (Roy-Byrne and Hummer, 1988).

One recent important development in the treatment of GAD is the finding demonstrating that tricyclic antidepressants are quite effective in the treatment of GAD (Kahn et al., 1986). This study demonstrated that imipramine was slightly superior in efficacy to chlordiazepoxide, although this increased effectiveness did not become apparent for 3 to 6 weeks. Given the fact that many primary care patients with GAD also suffer from major depression and panic disorder, tricyclic antidepressants may be the safest, most effective treatment of GAD. Also, the antidepressants are much easier to taper, without the rebound anxiety and withdrawal problems seen with benzodiazepines.

A new nonbenzodiazepine alternative anxiolytic medication that appears effective in treating GAD is buspirone (Goa and Ward, 1986). This medication is nonsedating, does not cause any withdrawal symptoms when abruptly discontinued, has no synergistic effects with alcohol or other sedative hypnotic agents, and appears to be as effective as benzodiazepines in the treatment of GAD. Buspirone often takes 2 to 3 weeks to have an effect, and patients who have been treated previously with benzodiazepines tend to report this medication as less effective.

Finally, beta-blockers have been used to treat anxiety, but they generally have a less robust anxiolytic effect than the three classes of medication described earlier and have the added risk of precipitating depression (Roy-Byrne and Katon, 1987).

Phobic Disorders: Simple Phobias, Agoraphobia, and Social Phobias

Simple phobias respond well to the behavior modification techniques of systemic desensitization (Wolpe, 1973) or in vivo exposure (Marks, 1987). In desensitization, the patient learns a relaxation technique and then, through imagery or in vivo, is exposed to a gradual hierarchy of stimuli while in a relaxed state that approaches the phobic object or situation. For instance, if a patient has a fear of dogs, after a relaxation technique is taught and mastered, the patient may sequentially be exposed to a picture of a dog; observe a stuffed animal or a dog in a cage; hold a puppy; and, finally, pet an adult dog. In each step of the hierarchy, if the anxiety of the patient becomes high, the stimulus is withdrawn.

Marks (1987) has demonstrated that in vivo ex-

Table 65–11. BENZODIAZEPINES: GENERIC AND TRADE NAMES AND USUAL ADULT DOSAGES WHEN USED FOR TREATMENT OF ANXIETY*

Name	Range of Adult Dosages (mg. per day)†	Available Tablet or Capsule (mg.)
Alprazolam (Xanax)	0.25–4	0.25, 2.5, 1
Chlordiazepoxide hydrochloride	10–100	5, 10, 25
(Chlordiazachel)	10–100	5, 10, 25
(A-Poxide)	10–100	5, 10, 25
(SK-Lygen)	10–100	5, 10, 25
(Librium)	10–100	5, 10, 25
(Librium injectable)	50–200	50-mg. per ml. ampule
Chlorazepate dipotassium		
(Tranxene)	15–60	3.75, 7.5, 15
(Tranxene SD)‡	11.25–22.5	11.25, 22.5
Diazepam		
(Valium)	4–40	2, 5, 10
(Valium injectable)	5–100§	2-mg. ampules, 5 mg. per ml.
Flurazepam		
(Dalmane)	15–30	15, 30
Halazepam		
(Paxipam)	20–160	20, 40
Lorazepam		
(Ativan)	2–6	1, 2
Oxazepam		
(Serax)	30–120	10, 15, 30
Prazepam		
(Verstran)	20–60	10

*Modified from Wesson, D. R.: Anxiety: Its meaning and psychotropic drug treatment. *In* Buchwald, C., et al. (Eds.): Frequently Prescribed and Abused Drugs. Brooklyn, Career Teacher Center, State University of New York, 1980, p. 25.

†Usually given in divided doses, two to four times daily.

‡Recommended as single daily dose.

§May be given intramuscularly or intravenously; usually not more than 20 mg. in single dose. Intravenous injection rate should not exceed 5 mg. per minute.

posure to the phobic stimulus, either gradually or all at once (flooding), is more effective both in total efficacy and rapidity of cure than desensitization by imagery. Marks (1987) has also shown that in vivo exposure is also an effective technique to treat agoraphobia. The therapist or physician develops a hierarchic list of phobias, placing the weakest fears at one end and the most severe at the other. The patient then decides with the clinician what phobic situations he will "expose" himself or herself to that week. Marks (1987) has demonstrated that exposing the patient rapidly and for long periods to the phobic stimulus maximizes therapeutic efficacy.

In simple phobia, in vivo exposure alone is quite effective. In agoraphobia, evidence from two recent studies shows that imipramine in combination with exposure enhances the effects of exposure (Mavissakalian et al., 1983; Telch et al., 1985). It must be kept in mind that most patients with agoraphobia also have panic disorder and, although exposure therapy may decrease phobic avoidance, the patient may still be left with panic attacks. Thus, the addition of imipramine may ameliorate the panic attacks that often exacerbate phobic behavior. Monoamine oxidase inhibitors and high-potency benzodiazepines have also been shown to be quite effective in the treatment of agoraphobia (Sheehan et al., 1984).

Exposure-based treatments have also been shown to be moderately effective (Alstrom et al., 1984) in social phobias. Recent studies have also reported that monoamine oxidase inhibitors are effective in 70 per cent of the cases of social phobia (Liebowitz, 1987).

Posttraumatic Stress Disorder

Mellman and Davis (1985) have demonstrated that the recurrent intrusive images and feelings of PTSD are often quite similar to those experienced by patients with panic attacks. Indeed, many patients with PTSD have both panic disorder and major depression and try to self-medicate their increased sympathetic nervous system tone with alcohol or sedative hypnotic agents.

Medications with a dampening effect on sympathetic nervous system tone have been found to be quite effective in PTSD. Recent reports have indicated that imipramine and monoamine oxidase inhibitors are quite effective in combat veterans with the disorder (Bleich et al., 1986). Also, clonidine, an alpha$_2$ receptor agonist that diminishes release of norepinephrine (Kolb et al., 1984), and high-dosage propranolol have been found to be moderately effective (Van der Kolk, 1983).

Anecdotal uncontrolled reports have suggested that behavioral, group, and psychodynamic therapy all can be effective in treating PTSD (Fairbank and Nicholson, 1987). These therapies seem to all have in common the reliving and continued exposure to painful thoughts and feelings that may ultimately desensitize the patient to these images and to the autonomic nervous system feelings evoked by them.

References

Alstrom, J. E., Worklund, C. L., Persson, G., et al.: Effects of four treatment methods on agoraphobic women not suitable for insight-oriented psychotherapy. Acta Psychiatr. Scand., *70*:1, 1984.

American Psychiatric Association: Diagnostic and Statistical Manual of Mental Disorders. 3rd ed. Washington, D.C., American Psychiatric Association, 1980.

American Psychiatric Association: Diagnostic and Statistical Manual of Mental Disorders. 3rd ed., revised. Washington, D.C., American Psychiatric Association, 1987.

Anstett, R., and Hipskind, M.: Selecting patients for brief office counseling. J. Fam. Pract., *13*:195, 1981. *This paper presents a useful approach to selecting patients for brief office counseling based upon the characteristics of the patient, the physician, and the physician-patient relationship that are likely to correlate with successful outcomes of counseling.*

Bass, C., and Wade C.: Chest pain with normal coronary arteries: A comparative study of psychiatric and social morbidity. Psychosom. Med., *14*:51, 1984.

Beitman, B. D., Basha, I., Flaker, G., et al.: Atypical or nonanginal chest pain: Panic disorder or coronary artery disease. Arch. Intern. Med., *147*:1548, 1987.

Benson, H., and Klipper, M. Z.: The Relaxation Response. New York, Avon Publishers, 1976.

Blazer, D. G.: Psychopathology of Aging. Kansas City, American Academy of Family Physicians, 1977.

Bleich, A., Siegel, B., Garb, R., et al.: Posttraumatic stress disorder following combat exposure: Clinical features and psychopharmacologic treatment. Br. J. Psychi., *149*:365, 1986.

Bowen, R. C., Cipywny, K. D., D'Aray, C., et al.: Alcoholism, anxiety disorders and agoraphobia. Alcoholism: Clin. Exper. Research, *8*:48, 1984.

Breir, A., Charney, D. S., and Heninger, G. B.: Major depression in patients with agoraphobia and panic disorder. Arch. Gen. Psychi., *41*:1129, 1984.

Breslau, N., and Davis, G. C.: DSM-III generalized anxiety disorder: An empirical investigation of more stringent criteria. Psychi. Research, *14*:231, 1985.

Cahtell, J. L.: Somehow, "GP style" psychotherapy works. Consultant, *8*:12, 1968.

Catalan, J., Gath, D., Edmonds, G., et al.: The effects of nonprescribing of anxiolytics in general practice. I. Controlled evaluation of psychiatric and social outcome. Br. J. Psychi., *144*:593–602, 1984.

Cloninger, C. R., Martin, R. L., Clayton, P., et al.: A blind follow-up and family study of anxiety neurosis. Preliminary analyses of the St. Louis 500. *In*: Klein, D. F., and Rabkin, J. (Eds.): Anxiety: New Research and Changing Concepts. New York, Raven Press, 1981, pp. 137–148.

Cohen, M. E., Badal, D., Kilpatrick, A., et al.: The high familial prevalence of neurocirculatory asthenia (anxiety neurosis, effort syndrome). Am. J. Human Genet., *3*:126, 1951.

Crowe, R. R., Noyes, R., Pauls, D. L., et al.: A family study of panic disorder. Arch. Gen. Psychi., *40*:1065, 1983.

Eastwood, M. R.: Screening for psychiatric disorder. Psychol. Med., *1*:197, 1971.

Fairbank, J. A., and Nicholson, R. A.: Theoretical and empirical issues in the treatment of posttraumatic stress disorder in Vietnam veterans. J. Clin. Psychol., *43*:44, 1987.

Faravelli, D.: Life events preceding the onset of panic disorder. J. Affect. Dis., *9*:103, 1985.

Finlay-Jones, R., and Brown, G. W.: Types of stressful life events and the onset of anxiety and depressive disorders. Psychol. Med., *11*:803, 1981.

Friedman, D., and Jaffe, A.: Anxiety disorders. J. Fam. Pract., *16*:145, 1983.

Gadge, S. W.: Treating the aging patient. *In* Kelly, J. T. (Ed.): Perspectives of Human Aging. Minneapolis, Craftsman Press, 1976, p. 118.

Gath, D., and Catalan, J.: Evaluation of the outcome of brief psychological treatments in primary care. Paper presented at the Treatment of Mental Disorders in General Health Care Settings: A Research Conference. Pittsburgh, June 15–17, 1988.

Goa, K. L., and Ward, A.: Buspirone: A preliminary review of its pharmacological properties and therapeutic efficacy as an anxiolytic drug. Drugs, *32*:114, 1986.

Goldberg, D.: Detection and assessment of emotional disorders in a primary care setting. Int. J. Ment. Health, *8*:30, 1979.

Goldstein, B. F., and Brauger, B.: Pharmacologic considerations in the treatment of anxiety and depression in medical practice. Med. Clin. North Am., *55*:487, 1971.

Gorman, J. M., Fyer, A. F., Gliklick, J., et al.: Effect of imipramine on prolapsed mitral valves of patients with panic disorder. Am. J. Psychi., *138*:977, 1981.

Gorman, J. M., Goetz, R. R., Fyer, M., et al.: The mitral valve prolapse—panic disorder connection. Psychosom. Med., *50*:114, 1988.

Grant, B., Katon, W., and Beitman, B.: Panic disorder. J. Fam. Pract., *17*:907, 1983.

Hall, R. C., et al.: Physical illness presenting as psychiatric disease. Arch. Gen. Psychi., *35*:1315, 1978.

Hankin, J., and Oktay, J. S.: Mental disorder and primary care: An analytic review of the literature. *In* National Institute of Mental Health (Rockville, MD): Series D, No. 7, DHEW Pub. No. (ADM) 78-661. U.S. Government Printing Office, 1979.

Hoeper, E. W., Nyczi, G. R., and Cleary, P. D.: Estimated prevalence of RDC mental disorder in primary care. Int. J. Ment. Health, *8*:6, 1979.

Joyce, P. R., Bushell, J. A., Oakley-Browne, M. A., et al.: The epidemiology of panic symptomatology and agoraphobic avoidance. Comp. Psychi., *30*:303–312, 1989.

Kahn, R. J., McNair, D. M., and Lipman, L. S.: Imipramine and chlordiazepoxide in depressive and anxiety disorders. II. Efficacy in anxious outpatients. Arch. Gen. Psychi., *43*:79, 1986.

Katon, W.: Panic disorder and somatization: A review of 55 cases. Am. J. Med., *77*:101, 1984.

Katon, W.: Panic disorder: Epidemiology, diagnosis and treatment. J. Clin. Psychi., *47*:21, 1986.

Katon, W.: Panic Disorder in the Medical Setting. National Institute of Mental Health, 1989.

Katon, W., Hall, M. L., Russo, J., et al.: Chest pain: Relationship of psychiatric illness to coronary arteriographic results. Am. J. Med., *84*:1, 1988.

Katon, W., and Roy-Byrne, P. P.: Antidepressants in the medically ill: Diagnosis and treatment in primary care. Clin. Chem., *34*:829, 1988.

Katon, W., and Roy-Byrne, P. P.: Panic disorder in the medically ill. J. Clin. Psychi., *50*:299–302, 1989.

Katon, W., Vitaliano, P. P., Russo, J., et al.: Panic disorder: Epidemiology in primary care. J. Fam. Pract., *23*:233, 1986.

Katon, W., Vitaliano, P. P., Anderson, K., et al.: Panic disorder: Residual symptoms after the acute attacks abate. Comp. Psychi., *28*:151, 1987.

Katon, W., Vitaliano, P. P., Russo, J., et al.: Panic disorder: Spectrum of severity and somatization. J. Nerv. Ment. Dis., *175*:12, 1987.

Kolb, L. C., Burris, B. C., and Griffiths, S.: Propranolol and clonidine in the treatment of the chronic post-traumatic stress disorders of war. *In* Van der Kolk, B. A. (Ed.): Post-Traumatic Stress Disorder: Psychological and Biological Sequelae. Washington, D.C., American Psychiatric Press, 1984.

Koranyi, E. K.: Morbidity and rate of undiagnosed physical illness in a psychiatric clinic population. Arch. Gen. Psychi., *36*:414, 1979.

Leckman, J. F., Merikangas, K. P., Pauls, D. L., et al.: Anxiety disorders and depression: Contradictions between family study data and DSM-III convention. Am. J. Psychi., *140*:880, 1983a.

Leckman, J. F., Weissman, M. M., Merikangas, K. R., et al.: Panic disorder and major depression. Arch. Gen. Psychi., *40*:1055, 1983b.

Liebowitz, M. R., Gorman, J. M., Fyer, A. J., et al.: Social phobia: Review of a neglected anxiety disorder. Arch. Gen. Psych., *42*:729–736, 1985.

Lydiard, R. B.: Panic disorder: Pharmacologic treatment. Psychiatric Annuals, *18*:468, 1988.

Margraf, J., Ehlers, A., and Roth, W. T.: Mitral valve prolapse and panic disorder: A review of their relationship. Psychosom. Med., *50*:93, 1988.

Marks, I. M.: Fears, Phobias and Rituals: Panic, Anxiety and Their Disorders. New York, Oxford University Press, 1987.

Marsland, D. W., Wood, M., and Mayo, F.: Content of family practice: A data bank for patient care, curriculum and research in family practice—526,196 patient problems. J. Fam. Pract., *3*:25, 1976.

Mavissakalian, M., Michelson, L., and Dealy, R. S.: Pharmacological treatment of agoraphobia: Imipramine versus imipramine with programmed practice. Br. J. Psychi., *143*:348, 1983.

Mellinger, G. D., Balter, M. B., and Uhlenhuth, E. H.: Prevalence and correlates of long-term regular use of anxiolytics. J.A.M.A., *251*:375, 1984.

Mellman, T. A., and Davis, G. C.: Combat related flashbacks in posttraumatic stress disorder. Phenomenology and similarity to panic attacks. J. Clin. Psychi., *46*:379, 1985.

Mullaney, J. A., and Trippett, C.: Alcohol dependence and phobias: Clinical description and relevance. Br. J. Psychi., *135*:565, 1979.

Myers, J. K., Weissman, M. M., Tischler, G. E., et al.: Six-month prevalence of psychiatric disorders in three communities. Arch. Gen. Psychi., *41*:959, 1984.

Nishimura, R. A., McGoon, M. D., Shub, C., et al.: Echocardiographically documented mitral-valve prolapse: Long-term follow-up of 237 patients. N. Engl. J. Med., *313*:1305, 1985.

Norton, R. G., Harrison, B., Hauch, J., et al.: Characteristics of people with infrequent attacks. Abnorm. Psychi., *94*:216, 1985.

Noyes, R., Clancy, J., Crowe, R., et al.: The familial prevalence of anxiety neurosis. Arch. Gen. Psychi., *35*:1057, 1978.

Orleans, C. T., George, L. K., and Houpt, J. L.: How primary physicians treat psychiatric disorders: A national survey of family practitioners. Arch. Gen. Psychi., *42*:52, 1985.

Pariser, S. F., Jones, B. A., Pinta, E. F., et al.: Panic attacks: Diagnostic evaluations of 17 patients. Am. J. Psychi., *136*:105, 1979.

Pecknold, J., Swinson, R. P., Kuch, K., et al.: Alprazolam in panic disorder and agoraphobia: Results from a multicenter trial. III. Discontinuation effects. Arch. Gen. Psychi., *45*:429, 1988.

Quitkin, F. M., Rifkin, A., Kaplan, J., et al.: Phobic anxiety syndrome complicated by drug dependence and addiction. A treatable form of drug abuse. Arch. Gen. Psychi., *27*:159, 1972.

Raskin, M., Peeke, H. V. S., Dickman, W., et al.: Panic and generalized anxiety disorders: Developmental antecedents and precipitants. Arch. Gen. Psychi., *39*:687, 1982.

Regier, D. A., Myers, K., Kramer, M., et al.: The National Institute of Mental Health Epidemiologic Catchment Area (ECA) program: Historical context, major objectives, and study population characteristics. Arch. Gen. Psychi., *41*:934, 1984.

Rickels, K.: Drug treatment of anxiety. *In* Jarvik, M. E. (Ed.) Psychopharmacology in the Practice of Medicine. New York, Appleton-Century-Crofts, 1977, p. 310.

Rosenbaum, J. F.: The drug treatment of anxiety. N. Engl. J. Med., *7*:401, 1982.

Roy-Byrne, P. P., and Cowley, D.: Panic disorder: Biological aspects. Psychi. Ann., *18*:457, 1988.

Roy-Byrne, P. P., Cowley, D. S., and Katon, W.: Pharmacotherapy of anxiety disorders. *In*: Textbook of Therapeutic Medicine for Practicing Physicians, in press.

Roy-Byrne, P. P., and Hummer, D.: Benzodiazepine withdrawal: Overview and implications for the treatment of anxiety. Am. J. Med., *84*:1041, 1988.

Roy-Byrne, P. P., Geraci, M., and Uhde, T.: Life events and the onset of panic disorder. Am. J. Psychi., *143*:1424, 1986.

Roy-Byrne, P. P., and Katon, W.: An update on treatment of the anxiety disorders. Hosp. Comm. Psychi., *38*:835, 1987.

Roy-Byrne, P. P., and Uhde, T. W.: Exogenous factors in panic disorder: Clinical and research implications. J. Clin. Psychi., *49*:56, 1988.

Schmidt, D. D.: The family as the unit of medical care. J. Fam. Pract., *7*:303, 1978.

Schurman, R. A., Kramer, P. D., and Mitchel, J. B.: The hidden mental health network: Treatment of mental illness by non-psychiatrist physicians. Arch. Gen. Psychi., *42*:89, 1985.

Shapiro, S., Skinner, E. A., Kessler, L. G., et al.: Utilization of health and mental health services: Three epidemiologic catchment area sites. Arch. Gen. Psychi., *41*:971, 1984.

Sheehan, D.: The efficient treatment of phobic disorders. *In* Menschreck, T. (Ed.): Psychiatric Medicine Update. New York, Elsevier, 1979, pp. 189–202.

Sheehan, D. V., Ballenger, J., and Jacobsen, G.: Treatment of endogenous anxiety with phobic, hysterical and hypochondriacal symptoms. Arch. Gen. Psychi., *37*:51, 1980.

Sheehan, D. V., Claycomb, J. B., and Surman, O. S.: Comparison of phenelzine, imipramine, alprazolam and placebo in the treatment of panic attacks and agoraphobia. Paper presented at the American Psychiatric Association Annual Meeting, Los Angeles, 1984.

Smail, P., Stockwell, T., Canter, S., et al.: Alcohol dependence and phobic anxiety states. I. A prevalence study. Br. J. Psychi., *144*:53, 1984.

Smilkstein, G.: The Family APGAR: A proposal for a family function test and its use by physicians. J. Fam. Pract., *6*:1231, 1978.

Stockwell, T., Smail, S., Hodgson, R., et al.: Alcohol dependence and phobic anxiety states. II. A retrospective study. Br. J. Psychi., *144*:58, 1984.

Telch, M. J., Agras, W. S., Taylor, C. B., et al.: Combined pharmacological and behavioral treatment for agoraphobia. Behav. Res. Ther., *23*:325, 1985.

Torgerson, S.: Genetic factors in anxiety disorders. Arch. Gen. Psych., *40*:1085–1092, 1983.

Uhlenhuth, E. H., Bolter, M. D., Mellinger, G. D., et al.: Symptom checklist syndromes in the general population: Corrections with psychotherapeutic drug use. Arch. Gen. Psychi., *40*:1167, 1983.

Vallbona, C.: Monthly Statistical Report. Texas, Casa de Amigo Community Health Clinic, 1973.

Van der Kolk, B. A.: Psychopharmacologic issues in posttraumatic stress disorder. Hosp. Comm. Psychi., *34*:683, 1983.

Vitaliano, P. P., Katon, W., Russo, J., et al.: Coping as an index of illness behavior in panic disorder. J. Nerv. Ment. Dis., *175*:78, 1987.

Weissman, M. M., Myers, J. K., and Harding, P. S.: Psychiatric disorders in a U.S. urban community: 1975–1976. Am. J. Psychi., *135*:459, 1978.

Wesson, D. R.: Anxiety: Its meaning and psychotropic drug treatment. *In* Buchwald, C., et al. (Eds.): Frequently Prescribed and Abused Drugs. Brooklyn, Career Teacher Center, State University of New York, 1980, p. 21–34. *A comprehensive and authoritative perspective on the role of drug therapy in the treatment of anxiety. The indications and risks of specific drugs are presented in detail together with practical guidelines for the drug therapy of the anxious patient.*

Wolpe, J.: The Practice of Behavioral Therapy. 2nd ed. Oxford, Pergammon Press, 1973.

Wynne, J.: Mitral valve prolapse. N. Engl. J. Med., *314*:577, 1986.

Yates, W. R.: The National Institute of Mental Health Epidemiologic Study: Implications for family practice. J. Fam. Pract., *22*:251, 1986.

Zitrin, Z. M., et al.: Behavior therapy, supportive psychotherapy, imipramine and phobias. Arch. Gen. Psychi., *35*:307, 1978.

Zung, W. W. K.: Assessment of anxiety disorder: Qualitative and quantitative approaches. *In* Fann, W. E., Karacan, I., Pokorny, A. D., et al. (Eds.): Phenomenology and Treatment of Anxiety, New York, Spectrum Publications, Inc., 1979, pp. 1–17.

66

Depression

Thomas L. Schwenk
James C. Coyne

Depression is an important concern in family practice for at least three reasons: its prevalence, the key role family physicians have to play in its management as a major public health problem, and its effect on health and medical care, even in its milder forms. Yet, the tasks facing family physicians in detecting and diagnosing depression in their practices and making appropriate treatment decisions are formidable, and the existing psychiatric literature and nosology are not as useful as they first appear.

One review of 60,000 diagnoses from a family practice population found that depression was the tenth most common diagnosis of all conditions and the second most frequent psychiatric problem encountered (Baker, 1974). Although such figures are impressive, it is likely that they underestimate the extent to which family physicians routinely confront depression. The prescription of antidepressants and counseling for depression frequently occur in the absence of a recorded diagnosis (Jencks, 1985), and many cases of depression presented to family physicians may remain undetected. In methodologically rigorous research, prevalence estimates of approximately 6 per cent have been obtained for major depression (Von Korff et al., 1987), and this statistic suggests that it could surpass hypertension as the most frequent illness encountered in family practice.

The efficacy of antidepressants and psychotherapy for depression is well established, but most clinically significant cases of depression go untreated. The costs of untreated depression for the individual, the family, and society as a whole are high. It has been suggested that half of family practice patients with depression have serious difficulties maintaining their normal lives (Johnson and Mellor, 1977), along with an increased risk of suicide. Untreated depression has come to be viewed as a major public health problem, and better detection and treatment of depression by family physicians and other primary care providers has been proposed as its solution (National Institute of Mental Health, 1983). This approach has been advocated because a seriously depressed person is more likely to consult a family physician than a psychiatrist. Indeed, the majority of persons with depression receive treatment for the condition in primary care settings rather than in specialty mental health settings (Sireling et al., 1985). Also, the majority of prescriptions for antidepressants are given in the primary care setting.

Family physicians have been criticized for missing many cases of depression that are presented to them, including perhaps 30 to 50 per cent of all cases of major depression (Von Korff et al., 1987; Freeling et al, 1985). Yet, few family practice patients with significant depressive symptoms complain directly of depression or initially identify depression as their reason for the visit (Duer et al., 1988). Many patients deny that they are depressed even when asked directly. If they volunteer information on depressive symptoms at all, the symptoms often concern somatic complaints or fatigue rather than mood disturbance. The family physician must distinguish these symptoms from the acute and chronic health problems that occur concomitantly with depression in primary care and that serve as patients' stated reasons for the visit. It may require several patient visits and considerable vigilance and probing on the part of the family physician to detect the presence of significant depressive symptoms, distinguish them from other complaints, and make an appropriate diagnosis.

Undoubtedly, there are a large number of depressed family practice patients with relatively unambiguous symptoms or what has been termed "conspicuous psychiatric morbidity." Many of these patients are similar to those seen by psychiatrists, would benefit from treatment, and yet go unrecognized. However, many cases of depression in family practice are more ambiguous, are milder and shorter in duration, and have fewer neurovegetative features than those found in psychiatric settings (Sireling et al., 1985). The advantages of antidepressants over placebo may not extend to such cases, and what constitutes appropriate treatment is unclear. There is a pressing need for diagnostic criteria, treatment guidelines, and medical education that deal with such patients. However, family physicians must routinely make decisions without these aids for the present time.

It should be appreciated that depression, even when not present in the form of a complete syndrome, can have a significant impact on medical care and health outcomes. For instance, patients pejoratively labeled as malingerers on the basis of multiple, recurrent complaints without concurrent physical findings have been found to have significantly higher self-reports of depressive symptoms than controls (Jacobs et al., 1968). It is possible that detection and brief psychotherapeutic treatment of mildly depressed patients could reduce unnecessary outpatient visits, laboratory tests and x-ray studies, and hospitalizations. Furthermore, the patient's depressed mood and accompanying demoralization can also increase the perceived severity and medical intractability of an established chronic illness, as well as increase its impact on a patient's life, and it can decrease the patient's adherence to a long-term or involved regimen. Thus, even when the issue is not one of a formally diagnosable depressive disorder, the suspicion of depressed mood can be important in managing patients who overutilize medical services or who have difficulties adapting to chronic illness.

Classification of Depression and Depressive Syndromes

A major problem in the care of depressed patients by family physicians is the difficulty in classifying and labeling patients with varying degrees of depression and various types of symptom complexes. Ambiguous classification and labeling leads to inadequate treatment. Yet, existing diagnostic criteria are largely derived from work with psychiatric populations in which the spectrum of depressive disorders is narrower than that encountered in family practice. Many family practice patients have chronic or intermittent depressive symptoms and yet are nonclassifiable according to the strict criteria proposed for major depression, dysthymia, adjustment disorder with depressed mood, and other depressive syndromes in the Diagnostic and Statistical Manual of Mental Disorders (DSM III-R; American Psychiatric Association, 1983).

Even so, a careful review of the criteria for major depression (Table 66–1) suggests that this diagnosis fits more family practice patients than is generally appreciated. Misconceptions about these criteria are probably a source of the underdiagnosis of major depression by mental health professionals as well as family physicians. As can be seen, the criteria are based on symptoms and make no reference to precipitating stressors. Regardless of whether patients are facing a recent life change such as divorce or loss of employment that makes their mood state "understandable," if they meet these criteria, they are to be considered depressed and appropriately treated. Mood disturbance is a requirement for diagnosis. The mood disturbance must persist most of the day, nearly every day, for 2 weeks, although a patient can fulfill this criterion and still have periods of a couple of hours at a time in which his or her mood is buoyed up. Sadness and dejection are not requirements, although many depressed patients report these feelings as their principal complaint. A loss of pleasure or interest in all or most usual activities is an alternate way of meeting the mood criteria, and persons having this type of mood disturbance may further complain that all emotional experience, including sadness, has been blunted or inhibited. In severely depressed patients, this inhibition of emotional expression may involve an inability to cry, even though mildly and moderately depressed persons readily cry.

The standard criteria for major depression also have some limitations. The criteria identify an extremely heterogenous group of patients; two patients can be found to be depressed without having a single symptom in common. Further, many patients in a typical family practice have significant depressive symptoms without ever meeting the criteria for this diagnosis. Dysthymia offers a possible diagnostic and therapeutic category for many depressed patients in family practice (see the diagnostic criteria in Table 66–2). Recent epidemiologic studies suggest that dysthymia is more prevalant than previously suspected,

Table 66–1. DSM-III-R CRITERIA FOR MAJOR DEPRESSIVE EPISODE*

At least five of nine of the following symptoms, at least one of which is depressed mood or loss of interest or pleasure

1. Depressed mood
2. Loss of interest or pleasure
3. Significant weight change (> 5 per cent of body weight in 1 month) or appetite change
4. Sleep disturbance
5. Psychomotor agitation or retardation
6. Fatigue or loss of energy
7. Feelings of worthlessness or excessive guilt
8. Cognitive dysfunction
9. Recurrent suicidal ideation

No organic cause or relationship to normal bereavement
No delusions or hallucinations
No associated psychiatric morbidity, such as schizophrenia

*Adapted from American Psychiatric Association: Diagnostic and Statistical Manual of Mental Disorders. 3rd ed. Washington, D.C., American Psychiatric Association, 1983.

Table 66–2. DSM III-R CRITERIA FOR DYSTHYMIA

At least three of the following symptoms present for at least 2 years
1. Decreased effectiveness or productivity at work, school, home
2. Social withdrawal
3. Mood disturbance (irritability or inappropriate anger)
4. Inability to respond with pleasure to rewards
5. Pessimistic, negative, brooding, self-pitying
6. Tearfulness
7. Any of symptoms listed for diagnosis of major depression

*Adapted from American Psychiatric Association: Diagnostic and Statistical Manual of Mental Disorders. 3rd ed. Washington, D.C., American Psychiatric Association, 1983.

yet many patients who have persistent symptoms do not meet the criterion of a duration of 2 full years. Adjustment disorder with depressed mood is another relevant category and refers to symptoms such as depressed mood, tearfulness, and hopelessness that follow a stressful life event and persist no longer than 6 months. Yet, appropriate therapeutic recommendations are not well established for dysthymia or adjustment disorder, and taken together with major depression, they still fail to accommodate the depressive features of many family practice patients. In particular, there is probably a considerable number of patients who suffer intermittent depressive symptoms chronically or episodically but who do not meet the criteria for any of these diagnoses. A recognition that these patients are prone to some mild mood disturbances can reduce the incidence of unnecessary laboratory tests and inappropriate treatment.

Figure 66–1 represents an effort to provide a classification that leads to treatment recommendations, capitalizes on strengths of the DSM III-R criteria, and accommodates the broader range of depressive conditions encountered in family practice. Those diagnoses listed under major depression are more serious and are more deserving of intensive treatment such as combined psychopharmacology and counseling. Patients with diagnoses listed under minor depression generally respond to supportive talk therapy, with vigilance regarding the development of neurovegetative symptoms or more numerous or serious symptoms that signify that the patient has developed major depression, requiring more intensive and usually psychopharmacologic treatment.

MAJOR DEPRESSION

The forms of major depression of greatest importance to family physicians are unipolar primary depressions and depression secondary to a major medical illness or an illness that requires surgery. Bipolar (manic-depressive) illness is considerably less common in primary care and usually requires joint care or care through referral to a psychiatrist, particularly regarding the subtleties of managing lithium administration and blood levels (unless the family physician has experience with these methods). Depressive conditions that are secondary to schizophrenia or substance abuse require attention to the primary disorder, again often requiring psychiatric assistance or significant experience in dealing with patients with those major psychiatric diagnoses.

The diagnosis of unipolar, major depression is based on the DSM III-R criteria listed in Table 66–1. As discussed above, these criteria are relatively clear. However, one source of underdiagnosis is a low index of suspicion in dealing with patients who discount their feelings of apathy, anhedonia, or melancholic mood. Self-administered questionnaires can be used on a screening basis for sensitizing the physician to the need to consider the diagnosis of major depression, although these questionnaires err on the side of greater sensitivity at the expense of specificity.

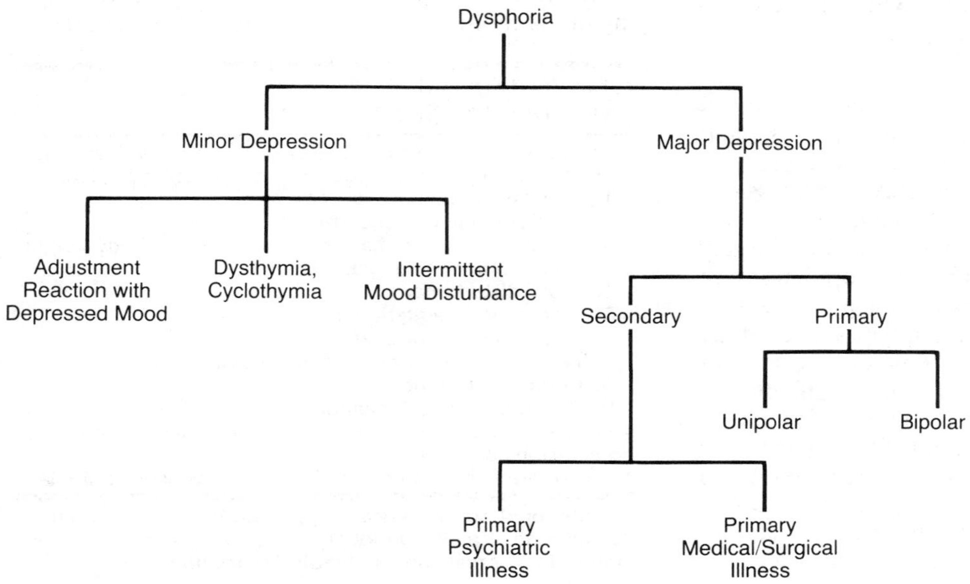

Figure 66–1. Classification of depressive syndromes. (Adapted from Petty, F., Primary Care, *144*:669–683, 1987.)

False-positives that are likely to occur include patients with significant anxiety or neuroticism in the absence of a depressive syndrome. Questionnaires with studied validity in various primary care and medical settings include the Depression Inventory, the Zung Self-Rating Depression Scale, the General Health Questionnaire (GHQ), and the Center for Epidemiologic Studies—Depression Scale (CES-D). A comparison of useful distinguishing features of these self-administered questionnaires is shown in Table 66–3.

Arriving at the diagnosis of major depression secondary to a significant medical illness or an illness that requires surgery is dependent on the physician's awareness of the numerous diseases and syndromes with which depression is associated. Many medical illnesses include symptoms of a psychomotor, cognitive, or neurovegetative type that are identical with those found in depression, making distinction difficult for treatment purposes. (See the later section regarding a more complete discussion of inclusive versus exclusive methods of diagnosing depression in patients with biomedical illness.)

MINOR DEPRESSION

A diagnosis of adjustment disorder with depressed mood can be applied to a patient with up to 6 months of mild mood disturbance, as long as his or her psychomotor and cognitive function continues fairly undisturbed. Dysthymic and cyclothymic patients are those with long-term personality styles including persistent or cyclical dysphoria, self-pity, irrational negativity, and "moodiness," hence the previously used term of "characterologic depression." Patients with this condition exhibit few or none of the neurovegetative symptoms that require psychopharmacologic treatment, nor are they cognitively impaired. These patients rarely respond to antidepressants or intensive psychotherapy but require the use of an interviewing style and a physician-patient relationship that support positive, constructive health behaviors. Some of these patients may have a residual or an impending major depression or an attenuated form of another type of major depression, necessitating careful attention to the longitudinal course of the depressive symptoms, particularly the development of neurovegetative symptoms that would respond to psychopharmacologic therapy.

It should be noted that patients may suffer from an acute episode of major depression superimposed on a dysthymic condition. This phenomenon is more prevalent than once was thought and has been labeled "double depression." The fact that a patient has a history of dysthymia should not distract a physician from the possibility of the emergence of a full syndrome of major depression in the same patient. Antidepressant medication is likely to prove effective in treating the major depression in such patients, in which case they may simply return to their baseline level of dysthymia.

As we have noted earlier, the criteria of the DSM III-R do not accommodate a group of patients who suffer episodic or chronic intermittent depressive conditions or who show recurrent but short-lived periods of lability of mood in the face of everyday life stress. In such states, the patients may be preoccupied with feeling of inadequacy, withdraw from their usual activities, complain, react with resentment and irritability, and otherwise prove demanding and difficult. One alternative to the criteria of the DSM III-R that is widely used in psychiatric and epidemiologic research, the Research Diagnostic Criteria (Spitzer et al., 1978) acknowledges the existence of such persons with the classifications of episodic minor depressive disorder, chronic and intermittent minor depressive disorder, and labile personality. However, such diagnoses have mainly served as exclusion criteria for clinical studies, and so these patients are not well studied. The physician should also be alert to the possibility that what appears to be a minor condition actually may represent the onset of a more serious depressive disorder. A brief review of any history of past depression can be revealing in this regard.

MASKED DEPRESSION

"Masked depression" is a term that is subject to considerable misunderstanding and misuse. It has sometimes been used to broaden the category of

Table 66–3. CHARACTERISTICS OF COMMONLY USED QUESTIONNAIRES FOR DIAGNOSIS OF DEPRESSION

Questionnaire/Instrument	Number of Items	Method of Administration	Characteristics and Use
Minnesota Multiphasis Personality Inventory (MMPI) D-Scale	60 (scale 2)	self-administered	Measures change in severity of depression, outcome of treatment
Beck Depression Inventory (BDI)	21	self-administered	Measures subjective experiences, psychologic components of depression
Zung Self-Rating Depression Scale	20	self-administered or by trained interviewer	Index of depression severity
Center for Epidemiologic Studies—Depression	20	self-administered	Screening general or medical care populations
General Health Questionnaire (GHQ)	28	self-administered	Screening for range of emotional distress in medical care population

depression to include patients who otherwise lack the required symptoms for diagnosis. Formally speaking, the diagnosis of depression requires the presence of mood disturbance. In psychiatric settings, this disturbance generally is the patient's presenting complaint. However, this may not be the case, particularly in family practice, and the physician may have to rely on inference and information from sources other than the patient to decide if mood disturbance is indeed occurring. For instance, the patient may vigorously deny sadness or loss of pleasure, yet a few questions reveal that he or she has largely withdrawn from family and friends and given up exercise and hobbies. In such an instance, a judgment of mood disturbance and, therefore, a diagnosis of depression may be justified.

From this perspective, masked depression refers to a presentation of depression rather than a distinct subtype. The diagnosis involves an often difficult judgment, but one that is frequently required of family physicians. Moreover, since the diagnosis of this presentation of depression largely is based on somatic complaints, particularly chronic pain, this condition represents perhaps the largest reservoir of undiagnosed, treatable depression in the typical family practice.

Patients with masked depression initially present with a nearly inexhaustible list of somatic complaints, with particular emphasis on chronic pain (headache, chest pain, back pain, abdominal pain), gastrointestinal complaints (nausea, diarrhea, constipation, flatulence, bloating, belching, indigestion), neurologic complaints (fainting, fatigue, dizziness, visual blurring), and cardiorespiratory complaints (palpitations, dyspnea, syncope, hyperventilation). These patients appear to have an unexplained selective perception for the somatic manifestations of their psychologic pain, with a corresponding denial of the psychologic and neurovegetative symptoms. The association with panic attacks, hypochondriasis, or common somatoform disorders is unclear (see Chapters 65 and 67), but differentiation from the last two conditions is critical for successful treatment. Depression that is described purely in the form of a list of somatic complaints is eminently more treatable than most somatoform disorders, whereas antidepressant therapy of even moderate dosage is often successful in panic attacks.

Two techniques for differentiating depression from common somatoform disorders are (1) the use of screening questionnaires with relatively higher specificity (see Table 66–3) and (2) the empiric use of antidepressants when the index of suspicion is high. For example, in patients with a past history of major depression or who describe under persistent questioning some component of neurovegetative, psychologic, or cognitive dysfunction, a cautious trial of an antidepressant with a low incidence of serious side effects (see Table 66–4 and Chapter 71) may have both diagnostic and therapeutic value.

Epidemiology and Natural History of Depression

The development of clearer diagnostic criteria, semistructured interview schedules, and rating scales has allowed a marked increase in information available on the epidemiology of depression. Current estimates are that the 6-month prevalence of major depression is 4.4 per cent and the lifetime prevalence is 18 per cent (Weissman and Myers, 1980). Less than half of persons currently experiencing major depression seek professional help. Major depression is 2 to 3 times more common in women than in men, with women 18 to 44 years of age having the highest rate. Depression is most common among persons aged 18 to 44, particularly between the ages of 25 and 34. Although the elderly have high rates of dysphoria, they do not have higher rates of clinical major depression. Apparently, the rate of depression is increasing for persons born after 1935 and the age of onset is decreasing. The mean age of onset of a first episode of depression is now in the 20's. If current trends continue, family physicians can expect to see a greater number of young persons with major depression than in the past.

Although a person's morale or sense of well-being is predictably increased in association with higher income and education, increased rates of major depression apparently are not related to the absence of these benefits. In recent studies, major depression affects equally the rich and poor, the educated and uneducated, blue collar and white collar workers, and blacks and whites. Major depression is related to marital status, with single and formerly married individuals having higher rates than that of married individuals. Yet, the highest rate of depression is found among persons who are married and are not getting along with their spouse. For both men and women, the risk of major depression in an unhappy marriage increases about 25-fold (Weissman, 1987). Major depression is consistently related to recent life events, particularly those involving a loss, with depressed persons having 3 to 6 times as many such events as nondepressed persons. Vulnerability to depression after a life event is substantially increased by having poor social relationships or low social support, particularly for women; for instance, a woman is 3 times more likely to become depressed after a stressful life event if she lacks a confiding relationship (Brown and Harris, 1978). Thus, advances in our understanding of the biomedical aspects of depression should not distract us from its psychosocial dimensions (Coyne, 1987).

The traditional view of major depression has been that it is a relatively benign condition, generally occurring in a single episode in a person's life and remitting without residual problems. However, it now appears that only about half of persons experiencing an episode of major depression suffer only a single episode. The emerging view of depression is that it is

Table 66–4. CHARACTERISTICS OF COMMONLY USED ANTIDEPRESSANTS

Generic Name	Trade Name(s)	Effect on Serotonin Uptake	Effect on Norepinephrine Uptake	Sedating Effect	Anticholinergic Effect	Orthostatic Effect	Usual Dose and Dosage Range (mg./day)
Tricyclic Tertiary Amines							
Amitriptyline	Elavil, Endep	++++	++	++++	++++	++++	150 (75 to 300)
Imipramine	Tofranil, SK-Pramine	++++	++	++	+++	++++	150 (75 to 300)
Doxepin	Sinequan, Adapin	+++	++	+++	++	++	150 (75 to 300)
Tricyclic Secondary Amines							
Desipramine	Norpramin, Pertofrane	+++	++++	+	+	+	150 (75 to 300)
Protriptyline	Vivactil	+++	++++	+	+++	+	30 (15 to 60)
Nortriptyline	Pamelor	+++	+++	++	++	+	75 (50 to 150)
Others							
Amoxapine	Ascendin	++	+++	++	++	++	150 (75 to 300)
Maprotaline	Ludiomil	+	++	++	+	++	150 (75 to 200)
Trazodone	Desyrel	+++	+/−	+++	—	++	300 (200 to 600)
Fluoxetine	Prozac	++++	+/−	+	+	+	20 (20–60)
Monamine Oxidase Inhibitors							
Isocarboxazid		—	—	—	—	—	20 (10 to 50)
Phenelzine		—	—	—	—	—	60 (45 to 90)
Tranylcypromine		—	—	—	—	—	20 (10 to 50)

−, absent; +, slight; ++, moderate; +++, strong; ++++, very strong.

heterogeneous and highly variable in its course, but that it is basically a recurrent, episodic disorder with varying degrees of residual difficulties (Clayton, 1983). Episodes of major depression tend to last between 4 and 8 months, but about 15 per cent of patients with major depression have a chronic course. Relapse after successful treatment is common, with about 50 per cent of patients relapsing within 2 years. This figure decreases with maintenance dosages of antidepressants. On the average, persons who become clinically depressed can expect a mean of between five and six episodes in their lifetimes. For the family physician, this suggests that knowledge of past history can be important in detecting depression, and that inquiries about whether a patient has previously had periods in which he or she felt sad or blue every day for a couple of weeks can be crucial in resolving ambiguous cases.

Recent studies have also shown that obtaining a family history is also important in detecting risk factors for major depression. Although only about 25 per cent of depressed psychiatric patients and possibly fewer family practice patients have a clearly defined family history of depression, persons with a first-degree relative with major depression have a risk of major depression 2 to 3 times that of the general population. Persons who become depressed earlier in life have stronger family histories of depression, and so family physicians should be alert to undetected depression in the parents of adolescents with major depression. Finally, assortative mating is high, with depressed men particularly likely to marry women who are vulnerable to depression.

Studies of dysthymia in the general population have only recently become available. A survey of five communities in the United States found rates from 2.1 to 4.2 per cent (Weissman et al., 1987). It is most prevalent among women under 65 years of age, in the unmarried, and in young persons with low income. It has a surprisingly high co-morbidity with other psychiatric conditions (70 to 75 per cent), particularly major depression, and this raises questions as to whether or not it is a specific disorder. It may often represent the consequence of untreated or only partially remitted episodes of depression that have become chronic, or it may represent a milder manifestation of major depression.

RELATED PSYCHIATRIC CONDITIONS

Major and minor types of depression have many features in common with other psychiatric conditions, and some overlap in diagnostic criteria can occur. The DSM III-R criteria for depression note the need for an absence of hallucinations and delusions and an absence of major psychotic disease. However, early and residual schizophrenia can be exhibited as depression owing to the ill-defined mood alterations and somatic preoccupations often present. The cognitive disturbances can masquerade as dementia, particularly in elderly patients in whom severe cognitive dysfunction is particularly common. In such cases, the symptoms suggesting dementia may disappear with appropriate treatment of the depression.

The DSM III-R criteria allow for the occurrence of major depression in patients who have a pre-existing personality disorder. Diagnosis can be difficult in that such patients' manipulative behavior, poor impulse control, and disordered interpersonal relationships may distract the physician from the presence of their depressive symptoms. Although treatment for depression is still indicated, persons with pre-existing personality disorders do not respond as well as other patients.

The somatic preoccupation of many depressed patients who are seen in primary care can be confused with hypochondriasis and common somatiform disorders. Patients who abuse alcohol, sedatives, or hypnotics can be depressed, as can patients who are withdrawing from cocaine or amphetamines. Accurate diagnosis may require that the patient first complete withdrawal from alcohol or abused drugs. Bereaved patients may pose some diagnostic problems. A patient who otherwise meets the criteria for major depression may still be thought to be experiencing uncomplicated bereavement when his or her condition is judged to be a timely and appropriate reaction to a loss. However, if these symptoms become prolonged or if marked psychomotor retardation or a morbid preoccupation with worthlessness develops, a diagnosis of major depression should be considered. Many depressed patients have significant anxiety symptoms and can be thought to have one of several anxiety disorders (see Chapter 65). Depression and anxiety can best be distinguished by focusing on the neurovegetative and somatic components of depression, since the psychologic symptoms of depression are often similar to those of anxiety.

Biomedical Aspects of Depression

NEUROBIOLOGY OF DEPRESSION

Major depression requiring intensive psychopharmacology and psychotherapy is construed as ultimately being a neuroendocrinologic disorder. Irrespective of the presence of life stresses, major losses, or precipitating events, many patients with major depression have been shown to have major neurobiologic abnormalities. These abnormalities include an excess of 5-hydroxyindoleacetic acid (a serotonin metabolite); abnormalities in the hypothalamopituitary adrenal axis and in the regulation of thyroid-stimulating hormone stimulation by thyrotropin-releasing hormone; and abnormalities in levels of melatonin, luteinizing hormone, growth hormone, and prolactin. For these reasons, previous distinctions between "exogenous" or "reactive" depression due to precipitating events and "endogenous" depression due to biologic abnormalities are considered unhelpful or irrelevent since they neither clarify the etiology of the condition nor predict the success of various therapies. In practical terms, patients can have a neurovegetative form of depression that responds well to antidepressants or requires more serious treatment such as electroconvulsive therapy irrespective of the presence or absence of significant life losses or precipitating events.

However, defined in other ways, the notion of endogenous depression retains some validity. Reactivity to changes in life circumstances *while* patients are depressed has been found to predict the patient's response to biologically oriented treatment, with patients who are less responsive deriving greater benefit. Other predictors include (1) a distinct quality of mood and whether or not there has been a loss of the ability to experience pleasure; (2) psychomotor retardation; (3) feeling worse in the morning than in the evening; and (4) early morning awakening and appetite disturbance. These symptoms are related to measurable abnormalities in the neuroendocrine system and a variety of quantitative measures of sleep disturbance (Clayton and Barrett, 1983). Also, these symptoms have now replaced the absence of precipitating stress as the definitive criteria for endogenous depression. To reduce confusion, the term "reactive" has been abandoned in the United States in favor of "nonendogenous," and "melancholic" has replaced "endogenous." However, some cautions are in order. Most patients in family practice with major depressive disorder are not melancholic, but nonetheless, many are responsive to antidepressants. The distinction is imprecise and its prediction of the patient's response to treatment is relative. Furthermore, many patients with melancholic symptoms face difficult psychosocial circumstances that require adjunctive psychotherapy for the alleviation of these symptoms.

Despite the assumption that major depression is ultimately a neuroendocrinologic disorder, in a carefully selected psychiatric research population only about 60 per cent of severely ill patients demonstrate any such neurohormonal abnormality with the methods that are currently available. The proportion of family practice patients with major depressive disorder may be as low as 20 to 30 per cent. Furthermore, despite initial enthusiasm, efforts to diagnose pharmacologically treatable depression through biologic markers, such as the dexamethasone suppression test, have been relatively unsuccessful in primary care populations, particularly when compared with astute clinical diagnosis that allows recognition of the multiple forms of major depression that can appear in unselected populations.

The dexamethasone suppression test is conducted similarly to that for the diagnosis of Cushing's syndrome, although the method differs somewhat. Despite encouraging results in tertiary populations, the test cannot be recommended in primary care populations because of poor positive predictive value and an unacceptably high rate of false-positive results. It does distinguish between severe and mild depression, but one does not need the dexamethasone suppression test for this purpose, and an exclusive reliance on it would cause many patients who would benefit from antidepressant medication to be missed. The dexamethasone suppression test and other neurohormonal tests, such as the TRH stimulation test, may be useful if done together, but no evidence exists regarding their usefulness in primary care. This is particularly true for differentiating those depressive patients who would benefit from antidepressant therapy, or in distinguishing patients with depression in addition to a chronic illness from depression due to chronic illness. Although it is considered useful as a research tool, dexamethasone suppression test has not proved to be the "gold standard" that it was hoped to be.

DEPRESSION AND BIOMEDICAL ILLNESS

Depression and biomedical illness interact in several complex ways. Major depression may coexist in patients with severe medical illness and may be implicated as an increased risk for certain major illnesses. Chronically ill patients may be more likely to suffer from a secondary depression. Distinguishing depression coexistent with physical illness from depression due to physical illness represents one of the major challenges for the family physician. This distinction is critical for both diagnostic accuracy and treatment efficacy. Chronically ill patients suffer needlessly when major depression is underdiagnosed, usually owing to the physician's ascribing the depressive symptoms to the coexistent illness or dismissing the dysphoric and neurovegetative symptoms as inevitable (therefore, somehow unimportant). Rehabilitation from a major medical illness, such as a myocardial infarction or a cerebrovascular accident, can be slowed tremendously by undiagnosed depression. Less-than-optimal results of rehabilitation can be accepted prematurely if the neurovegetative and psychologic symptoms of depression are undetected, thereby allowing the patient's helpless and hopeless mood to sabotage rehabilitative efforts. Finally, many organic illnesses can have depression as the presenting symptom or include depression as a significant component, and the physician needs to include these organic causes in any differential diagnosis for dysphoria.

Depression can be caused by dozens of organic illnesses (Table 66–5), particularly those of the neurologic, metabolic, and endocrine types. Of particular importance for the family physician are diabetes mellitus, hyperthyroidism or hypothyroidism, postpartum state, cirrhosis, folate and iron deficiencies, infectious mononucleosis, influenza (particularly in the elderly), uremia, occult neoplasm, and the pseudodementia of the elderly with presumed Alzheimer's disease. Some studies suggest that 10 to 20 per cent of patients believed to have a major depression on initial presentation are found eventually to have an undiagnosed organic illness as the actual cause of the depressive symptoms. In addition, at least 200 medications have been implicated in causing depressive symptoms, including several drugs prescribed frequently in primary care (Table 66–6).

Table 66–5. ORGANIC ILLNESSES ASSOCIATED WITH DEPRESSION

Rheumatologic—systemic lupus erythematosus, rheumatoid arthritis
Cardiac—mitral valve prolapse, myocardial infarction, hypertension
Endocrine—hyperthyroidism and hypothyroidism, diabetes mellitus, hypercalcemia, Cushing's syndrome, postpartum state
Gastrointestinal—cirrhosis, inflammatory bowel disease, pancreatitis, intestinal bypass
Hematologic—sickle cell anemia
Nutritional deficiencies—B_{12}, folate, iron, thiamine, niacin
Infectious—encephalitis, hepatitis, influenza, infectious mononucleosis, pneumonia, tuberculosis
Renal—renal transplant, uremia
Neoplastic—intracranial, leukemia, pancreatic, lymphoma
Neurologic—subdural hematoma, multiple sclerosis, CVA, Parkinson's, uncontrolled epilepsy
Miscellaneous—psoriasis, sarcoidosis, drugs (see Table 66–6)

Table 66–6. DRUGS COMMONLY ASSOCIATED WITH DEPRESSION

Amphetamines, other central nervous system stimulants
Barbiturates
Benzodiazepines
Cimetidine
Clonidine
Beta-blockers
Corticosteroids
Indomethacin
Alpha-methyldopa
Oral contraceptives, estrogens
Reserpine, guanethidine
Sulfonamides

In addition to depression being the presenting symptom of severe underlying chronic illness, many common physical illnesses cause (or are associated with) depression. From 20 to 30 per cent of hospitalized patients suffer from major depression, with an additional 20 to 30 per cent suffering moderate depressive symptoms. This prevalence extends across disparate disease categories (e.g., patients with post-myocardial infarction, cerebrovascular accident, renal failure, and terminal cancer), suggesting a possible common neurobiologic pathway modified by psychosocial circumstances or pre-existing psychiatric morbidity. These patients present a diagnostic dilemma. Many of their symptoms satisfy the DSM III-R criteria for diagnosis (e.g., fatigue, loss of pleasure, sleep disturbance, appetite disturbance, and cognitive dysfunction), but it may be unclear whether the symptoms originated from the depression or the biomedical illness.

The family physician can use either an *inclusive* or an *exclusive* approach to the evaluation of these patients. The inclusive approach attributes all symptoms of depression to the diagnostic criteria for depression, irrespective of whether or not the symptoms might actually be due to the associated physical illness. This method is conceptually "clean" because it is based on observable phenomenon but errs on the side of greater sensitivity than specificity, thus causing overdiagnosis of depression. This possibility must be remembered if the patient is exposed to potentially harmful therapies (such as antidepressants or electroconvulsive therapy) for an illness that may not exist.

The exclusive approach eliminates anorexia and fatigue from the list of possible depressive symptoms, since they are so likely to be caused by an organic illness such as cancer. The diagnosis of depression must then be made from four of the remaining six DSM III-R criteria (assuming either depressed mood and loss of interest or pleasure are present). This approach leads to underdiagnosis, especially in patients with certain devastating systemic illnesses, such as cancer, who may benefit most from treatment for major depression. For purposes of greater sensitivity at the expense of specificity, the inclusive approach is recommended, but caution must be used to avoid excessive zeal in the aggressive treatment of every patient diagnosed in this fashion.

Management of the Depressed Patient

EVALUATION OF SUICIDAL RISK

One of the critical objectives for the family physician caring for depressed patients is to assess suicidal risk, both at the initial diagnosis and during subsequent evaluations and continuing care. Studies suggest that most persons who commit suicide consult their family physician during the month prior to their death but do not receive treatment for depression. As many as 70 per cent of patients who commit suicide have one or more active physical illnesses, and these illnesses rather than depression per se may provide the reason for their visit.

The single best indicator of risk for suicide remains a direct or indirect statement of intent. Other correlates of increased suicidal risk are shown in Table 66–7. Of importance is to identify and refer patients at particularly high risk, such as a recently widowed elderly male patient who has coexistent alcoholism and a history of major depression or attempted suicide. Patients who have a major physical illness or a chronic debilitating condition for which there is little hope of improvement and who do not have significant family support are also at high risk. With malignancies and incurable conditions, the critical periods are while the diagnosis and the prognosis have just been presented and when patients are coming to realize the seriousness of their condition.

Table 66–7. CORRELATES OF INCREASED SUICIDE RISK IN DEPRESSED PATIENTS

Increased age (peak risk in men is at 75; in women, between 55 and 65)
Gender (women make more suicide attempts, men are more often successful)
Marital status and social support (in order of decreasing risk: never married, widowed, separated or divorced, married without children, married with children)
Employment (greater in unemployed persons)
Presence of physical illness, especially chronic pain, terminal illness
Coexistent alcoholism or substance abuse
History of prior attempts
Communication to family, friends, or physician of intent, financial plans following death, or specific means of suicide
Positive family history of successful suicide (especially that of parents)

The physician should take seriously any mention of suicide and not be deterred from inquiry by the fear that a frank discussion might lead to suicidal behavior. It is not unusual for even moderately depressed persons to have fleeting thoughts of suicide, and the physician's broaching of the topic may be appreciated by patients as a sign of the physician's recognition of their plight. The assessment of suicidal risk should focus on *intent* and *lethality*. Intent refers to a patient's commitment to an act that is expected to lead to death. Particular concern is warranted when the patient has a definite plan, considers using more than one method at a time, and has made preparations for death or has taken steps not to be discovered. Patients who do not have a well-developed plan but who are extremely impulsive, psychotic, or frequently intoxicated may pose similar risks. Lethality refers to the degree to which particular methods are likely to lead to death. As part of an assessment, the physician may ask outright if the patients are willing to make a commitment or contract not to kill themselves, and if they are, what plans for help they have made if the urge worsens. Patients who cannot credibly make such a commitment should be considered at high risk.

ANTIDEPRESSANTS

Whether major depression begins with precipitating psychosocial stresses or is an intrinsic neurochemical imbalance, the end result in patients with neurovegetative symptoms is a functional depletion of neurotransmitters. Controversy still exists regarding an exclusive and complete description of specific neurotransmitter deficiencies and neural synaptic locations of these deficiencies, but attention has recently shifted from the availability of neurotransmitters to the sensitivity of receptors, primarily histamine H1, muscarinic, and alpha$_1$ adrenoceptor receptor sites. Actions at these receptor sites are also responsible for the usual side effects of tricyclic and similar antidepressants: dry mouth, urinary retention, sedation and orthostatic hypotension.

Drug selection depends upon a number of special clinical situations as well as taking side effects into account (see Table 66–4). For example, patients with a form of depression that has a significant component of anxiety, agitation, or sleep disturbance benefit from the antidepressants with a significant sedative effect, such as amitriptyline, doxepin, or trazodone.

Elderly patients prone to orthostatic hypotension would respond poorly to antidepressants that exacerbate this problem, such as amitriptyline or imipramine. Nortriptyline and desipramine are particularly good for elderly patients with orthostatic problems or prostatic hypertrophy. Patients without dominant neurovegetative symptoms would also benefit from a medication such as desipramine. Predicting the response of patients to one class of antidepressants is difficult, so lack of a response to therapeutic dosages should prompt the physician to check the blood level of the drug (for the purpose of checking patient compliance) or to switch to a different antidepressant. The lethal dose of most cyclic antidepressants may be as low as 1000 to 1500 mg., so no single prescription should exceed this quantity, especially in the early phase of treatment when suicidal risk assessment is difficult and the risk of suicide may fluctuate. The use of fixed combination drug preparations is rarely if ever justified, especially since most combinations include minor or major sedatives that have little role in the treatment of depression.

Antidepressants should be begun at a low dose (typically 25 mg.) and increased to a therapeutic dose in 25- to 50-mg. increments every 3 to 7 days. A convenient routine is to plan to see the patient weekly in the early stages of diagnosis and treatment for medication adjustment and supportive counseling (irrespective of referral for extended mental health care), and adjusting the dosage at each visit. Interim adjustments are useful as well. Compliance is markedly increased by giving the entire dosage in the evening, specifically at dinner time, because peak blood levels are reached in 3 to 4 hours. Side effects should be assessed at each visit, distinguishing the "nuisance" effects such as dry mouth from more serious effects such as hypotension, palpitations, and urinary retention. Once an effective dosage is reached, treatment should continue for 4 to 6 months before withdrawal is even considered. Frequent courses of similar length or continuous treatment for more than a year are not uncommon owing to the relapsing nature of major depression.

Assessing drug interactions is critical in the proper use of antidepressants, particularly because of their potentially widespread use. Important effects occur from the activity of other drugs, such as clonidine (decreased effect), prazosin (increased effect), and anticoagulants (decreased metabolism). Agents that lower the activity of antidepressants include barbiturates, alcohol, oral contraceptives, and cigarette smoking. Increased antidepressant activity is caused by disulfiram (Antabuse), antiseizure medications, and amphetamine derivatives (presumably infrequently used).

The family physician needs to become familiar and comfortable with only a few of the many tricyclics and related antidepressants, choosing those with complementary side effects. Monoamine oxidase inhibitors are used less often by family physicians because severe dietary restriction is necessary with their administration and they can be dangerous without meticulous attention to dietary details. Many family physicians believe that the need for switching from the usual antidepressants to monoamine oxidase inhibitors is an indication for referral of the patient to a psychiatrist.

Some controversy still surrounds the issue of whether to use antidepressants with psychotherapy or each method alone, but most evidence suggests that the two modalities are most effective when they are combined. Patients with major depression have at least a 70 per cent response rate to aggressive psychopharmacologic treatment, with or without psychotherapy. Patients with major depression, as measured by the presence of significant neurovegetative symptoms and standard DSM III-R criteria, are most likely to respond, whereas depression of a characterologic nature, such as cyclothymia or dysthymia, is less responsive. Some studies of family practice patients suggest that even patients with fairly mild depression, as measured by standardized questionnaires or structured interviews, respond well to short courses of antidepressants at less than the usual therapeutic dosage. This is also true for patients with chronic pain syndromes or masked depression. Even some patients with dysthymia who are developing major symptoms suggestive of major depression but do not yet fit the standard criteria may benefit from aggressive antidepressant therapy.

MEDICATION VERSUS PSYCHOTHERAPY

The superiority of antidepressant medication over placebo is well established, but there is still controversy surrounding the relative roles of psychotherapy and antidepressants. Some studies have shown medication to be superior to psychotherapy in the reduction of symptoms and prevention, but the same studies have also shown psychotherapy to be superior in its effect on social functioning. Antidepressant medication has little immediate effect on the interpersonal difficulties that accompany depression, and the effects of antidepressants are markedly reduced when patients are experiencing serious difficulties such as intense marital conflict. Some recent studies have found psychotherapy to be superior to antidepressants, and the most effective types of psychotherapy used have some common features: they are relatively brief, are structured, and emphasize constructive changes in behavior rather than exploration of the past or the achievement of insight. One study in which such therapy was documented as being superior to antidepressants involved general practice patients in England (Blackburn et al., 1981).

Antidepressants are most effective in alleviating sleep disturbance, appetite disturbance, and other neurovegetative symptoms; whereas psychotherapy is most effective in dealing with suicidal feelings and interpersonal problems. However, there is considerable variability in patients' acceptance of treatment.

An all-too-common situation is that of depressed women with marital difficulties being given only antidepressants and then not complying with treatment. If these patients are simply given time to talk about their problems, they are more willing to accept antidepressants.

Contrary to popular belief, there is currently *no* evidence that antidepressant medication interferes with the effectiveness of psychotherapy. For moderate to severe depression, a combined approach is most effective. However, physicians have sometimes allowed psychotherapy to interfere with antidepressant therapy when they underprescribe or inappropriately reduce the dosage because a patient has initiated psychotherapy.

PSYCHOLOGIC MANAGEMENT

Patients suffering from depression benefit from a clear, empathetic, and confident style on the part of the physician. The physician should take care to grasp and acknowledge the nature and focus of the patient's distress. Attempts to minimize or deny this distress will prove self-defeating and threaten the physician's rapport with the patient. However, without denying the reality of the patient's difficulties, it is useful to point out that a hopeless and pessimistic view is frequently a symptom of depression.

Patient Education. Both the patient and his or her family members need information about depression. They should recognize that it is not a matter of personal weakness or failure of will power. It should be pointed out that most episodes of depression resolve within 4 to 8 months. The expected loss of libido associated with depression should be explained to the patient and his or her spouse if there is conflict over sexual dissatisfaction. The patient and the family should be told when to expect the effects of both antidepressant medication and psychotherapy to appear. Specific side effects from antidepressant therapy should be construed as a sign that the drug is beginning to take effect.

Reducing Expectations. Depressed patients and family members should be instructed that depression can prove to be a tremendous drain on one's patience, morale, and energy level, and that all should appreciate that patients are not going to be at their best. Some activities can be put off or responsibilities reduced. Initiating an activity can prove particularly difficult for depressed persons. However, patients should be encouraged to consider whether they would feel better by initiating or deferring the activity, knowing that they have a greater risk of failure in not completing the activity despite their initial efforts.

Antidepressant Activities. Patients should be encouraged to undertake activities that provide some sense of mastery or pleasure. In particular, patients who see themselves as undeserving or self-sacrificing should be encouraged to view such suggestions as a prescription from the physician (Altrocchi et al., 1986). Patients benefit most if they are asked to commit themselves to specific activities and if the physician makes a follow-up inquiry as to whether the activities are actually being undertaken.

Contact with Family Members. The physician should acknowledge that depression is difficult for those who live with the patient. The family members should be encouraged not to take responsibility for the patient's mood but to take responsibility for their own behavior instead. Although family members should be encouraged to be supportive, they should avoid becoming overinvolved in miscarried efforts to prod or coerce patients into activities. "Constructive criticism" from family members is unlikely to be helpful to patients. Sometimes it is helpful for patients and family members to plan special activities or simple protected time together. Family members should also be aware they are at risk for increased infections, complaints of pain, and depression.

ADDITIONAL TREATMENT APPROACHES

Psychotherapy and antidepressants are the mainstay of treatment for depression. In addition to these major approaches, several additional approaches are available. The book *Feeling Good: The New Mood Therapy* (Burns, 1980) is one example of a self-help book that enhances positive thinking and provides a concrete plan for constructive action. Bibliotherapy may also include such books as *A New Guide to Rational Living* (Ellis & Harper, 1975) and *Control Your Depression* (Lewinsohn et al., 1980) or even a number of texts concerning assertion training. A prescription of relaxation exercise or more strenuous aerobic activity such as running, bicycling, swimming, or cross-country skiing may be helpful (Griest et al., 1978). Physical exercise not only may be a useful distraction from negative thinking but may enhance mood directly through poorly understood neurochemical changes. A prescription for exercise similar to that used for cardiac rehabilitation is appropriate.

INDICATIONS FOR REFERRAL

Several events or situations suggest the need for referral of depressed patients by family physicians to psychiatrists or more comprehensive mental health centers. Table 66–8 shows a list of possible indications for referral, none of which are necessarily absolute but all of which bear careful consideration by the family physician who does not have extensive training in caring for complicated depressed patients. The following indications should receive particular consideration: significant suicidal ideation or expressed intent; severe cognitive dysfunction, including self-care and nutritional deficiencies; severe bipolar disorder; or patients' failing multiple courses of antidepressants with documented compliance. Some of these circumstances require hospitalization (e.g., for electrocon-

Table 66–8. INDICATIONS FOR REFERRAL TO A PSYCHIATRIST

Moderate or high suicidal risk (see Table 66–7)
Severe cognitive dysfunction with difficulty in daily living or nutritional deficiencies
Psychotic or delusional symptoms
Lack of family support for observation or care
Significant physical illness complicating antidepressant treatment
Uncertain diagnosis or complicating psychiatric diagnosis such as alcoholism
Bipolar disease
Lack of response to antidepressants (combined with severe neurovegetative symptoms, suggesting need for electroconvulsive treatment)

vulsive therapy), which usually requires referral to a psychiatrist.

Depression in Children and the Elderly

MANAGEMENT OF DEPRESSION IN CHILDREN

The care of depressed children deserves special attention because of the increasing incidence of depression in children and adolescents, the apparently increasing incidence of suicide in adolescents, the devastating effects on families with depressed children, and the superior expertise required of physicians who care for these children. In diagnosing depression, the family physician is in a crucial position to deal with the most common confounding situation, that of distinguishing depression from similar psychologic characteristics that occur in normal development during childhood. The family physician may understand the child's family environment to the extent that any change in behavior is more noticeable, family reaction to the depressed child is more visible, and features suggestive of depression are more detectable than when the case is evaluated by a consultant who has had limited contact with the patient and his or her family.

The incidence of depression, using standard DSM III-R criteria, varies with age, from 1 to 4 per cent in children under 6 years of age to as high as 13 per cent in adolescents and preadolescents. Depression is almost impossible to diagnose in children under 5 years old because of the limited language and cognitive abilities of these patients. In older children, manifestations of low self-esteem, social isolation, sadness, anxiety, school problems, ill-formed suicidal ideation, and failure to make expected weight gains may signal depression. Adolescents show the same manifestations of depression as adults. However, these symptoms may not be apparent at first, and depressed adolescents may come to the attention of the family physician because of parents' complaints of their loss of interest in their appearance, sulkiness, withdrawal from family activites, and retreat to their rooms. Questionnaires and self-report inventories can be used in children older than 6 who have age-appropriate verbal abilities. Children of this age group are thought to be reliable informants. If their report of mood and symptoms differs from that given by the parents, studies show that the children are ultimately more accurate. This fact strongly suggests that a child-centered approach to children with behaviors and mood suggestive of depression is appropriate despite the possible protestations of parents. The use of antidepressants is sufficiently complex, particularly in prepubertal children, that referral is recommended. About 75 per cent of children with major depression respond to antidepressants, and improvement is usually seen first in school behavior and performance. A strong family-centered approach to counseling is best, and the family physician should play a strong role in coordinating and reinforcing such an approach. A comprehensive approach includes a detailed plan for altering the child's family and school environment, individual psychotherapy, psychopharmacologic interventions, attention to family members with associated depression or substance abuse problems, and a commitment to a long-term follow-up plan.

MANAGEMENT OF DEPRESSION IN THE ELDERLY

Depression is a common psychiatric disorder in the elderly, with estimates of prevalence ranging from 5 to 50 per cent. A likely prevalence of dysphoric mood is 15 to 20 per cent and for major depression, 3 to 5 per cent. The suicide rate also increases with age, whether or not it is due to the high incidence of depression. The depressed elderly differ in presentation from other depressed adults by having a higher rate of somatization without mood alteration and by the common problem of depression presenting as dementia, the so-called pseudodementia syndrome. Patients with pseudodementia present with cognitive dysfunction, problems in self-care, and difficulties in concentration and memory. A relentless search for mood disturbance or neurovegetative symptoms is necessary to make the correct diagnosis of depression. The high rate of chronic and terminal illness in the elderly also causes a high rate of secondary depression. Depression associated with polypharmacy is a particular problem, with alcohol, sedatives, antihypertensives, and digitalis being the most common causes.

Treatment follows the recommendations for young adult patients, with a few important modifications. Pharmacokinetics differ considerably in the elderly due to decreased gastrointestinal absorption, altered plasma protein binding, and decreased renal and hepatic clearance, and blood levels are often 50 per cent lower in the elderly for the same dosage given to younger patients. On the other hand, the elderly may be more sensitive to certain side effects of antidepressants, particularly orthostatic hypotension. Also, the elderly already may be taking other classes of medications, which may cause drug interactions. Cardiac effects and organic brain syndrome from the anticholinergic effects are also particular concerns when managing elderly patients. For all of these reasons, an antidepressant with minimal anticholinergic and orthostatic side effects, such as desipramine or trazodone, is frequently used in elderly patients. Severe depression may require electroconvulsive therapy, which is not contraindicated because of age. As in all depressed patients, psychotherapy should include attention to family and living environment and associated illness in family members.

References

Altrocchi, J., Antonuccio, D. O., and Miller, G. D.: Nondrug prescriptions for the depressed adult outpatient. Postgrad. Med. J., *79*:164–181, 1986. *Detailed suggestions for specific assignments to be given to depressed patients, including the scheduling of pleasant activities.*

American Psychiatric Association: Diagnostic and Statistical Manual of Mental Disorders. 3rd ed. (Revised). Washington, D.C., American Psychiatric Association, 1983.

Baker, C.: What's different about family medicine? J. Med. Educ., *49*:229–235, 1974.

Beck, A. T., Ward, C. H., Mendelson, M., et al. An inventory for measuring depression. Arch. Gen. Psychiatry, *4*:561–571, 1961. *The most widely used self-reported measurement of depression. It is useful as a screening instrument.*

Blackburn, I. M., Bishop, S., Glen, A. L., et al. The efficacy of cognitive therapy in depression: A treatment trial using cognitive therapy and pharmacotherapy, each alone and in combination. Br. J. Psychiatry, *139*:181–189, 1984.

Blacker, C. V., and Clare, A. W.: Depressive disorder in primary care. Br. J. Pyschiatry, *150*:737–751, 1987. *A thorough review of depression as it appears to the general and family physician, with particular reference to the relationship of depression to somatic symptoms and physical illness.*

Brown, G. W., and Harris, T. L.: Social Origins of Depression. New York, Free Press, 1978.

Burgin, D.: Depression in children and adolescents. Psychopathology, *19*(suppl. 2):148–155, 1986.

Burns, D.: Feeling Good: The New Mood Therapy. New York, William Morrow, 1980. *Excellent self-help book with specific tasks to provide mastery and pleasure experiences and to counter pessimism and negative thinking. Based on the cognitive approach to psychotherapy, which was shown to be as effective as antidepressant medication with family practice patients. (See Blackburn et al. for the comparative study.)*

Clayton, P. J.: The prevalence and course of the affective disorders. *In* Davis, J. M., and Maas, J. W. (Eds.) The Affective Disorders. Washington, D.C., American Psychiatric Press, 1983.

Clayton, P. D., and Barrett, J. E. (Eds.): Treatment of Depression: Old Controversies and New Approaches. New York, Raven Press, 1983.

Cohen-Cole, S. A., and Stoudemire, A.: Major depression and physical illness. Special considerations in diagnosis and biologic treatment. Psychiatr. Clin. North Am., *10*:1–17, 1987. *In addition to a thorough review of the relationship, a discussion of inclusive and exclusive approaches to diagnosis is included.*

Coyne, J. C.: Depression, biology, marriage and marital therapy. J. Marital Fam. Ther., *13*:393–407, 1987. *Reviews advances in the understanding of both biologic and psychosocial aspects of depression and argues that both perspectives are needed. A special emphasis is placed on the importance of marriage and the family in psychotherapy for depression.*

Duer, S., Schwenk, T. L., and Coyne, J. C.: Medical and psychosocial correlates of depressive symptoms in family practice. J. Fam. Pract., *27* (6): 609–614, 1988.

Ellis, A., and Harper, R. A.: A New Guide to Rational Living. Englewood Cliffs, NJ, Prentice-Hall, 1975. *Self-help book based on the rational-emotive approach to psychotherapy.*

Finlayson, R. E., Martin, L. M.: Recognition and management of depression in the elderly. Mayo Clin. Proc. *57*:115–120, 1982.

Freeling, P., Rao, B. M., Paykel, E. S., et al.: Unrecognized depression in general practice. Br. Med. J., *290*:1880–1883, 1985.

Goldberg, D., and Huxley, P.: Mental Illness in the Community: The Pathways to Psychiatric Care. London, Tavistock Publications, 1980.

Goldberg, I. D.: A scaled version of the General Health Questionnaire. Psychol., Med., 9:139–147, 1979.

Griest, J. H., Klein, M. H., Eischens, R. R., et al.: Running as a treatment for nonpsychotic depression. Behav. Med., *5*: 19–24, 1978.

Hyman, S. E., and Jenike, M. A.: Approach to the patient with depression. *In* Goroll, A. H., May, L. A., and Mulley, A. G. (Eds.) Primary Care Medicine. Philadelphia, J. B. Lippincott, 1987.

Jacobs, T. J., Fogelson, S., and Charles, E.: Depression ratings in hypochondria. N.Y. State J. Med., *25*:3119–3122, 1968.

Jencks, S. F.: Recognition of mental distress and diagnosis of mental disorder in primary care. J.A.M.A., *253*:1903–1907, 1985. *A large-scale study, based on National Ambulatory Medical Care Survey data, describing the lack of relationship between chart diagnoses of mental disorder, the provision of psychotherapeutic and therapeutic listening, and the prescription of psychopharmacologic treatment in primary care practices.*

Johnson, D. A. W., and Mellor, V.: The severity of depression in patients treated in general practice. J. R. Coll. Gen. Pract., *27*:419–22, 1977.

Kamerow, D. B., and Campbell, T. L.: Is screening for mental health problems worthwhile in family practice? An affirmative view and an opposing view. J. Fam. Pract., *25*:181–183, 1987.

Katon, W.: The epidemiology of depression medical care. International J. Psychiatry Med., *17*:93–112, 1987. *A massive review emphasizing that depression is the most common diagnosis in primary care. Underdiagnosis is probably due to the somatizing features of most depression in medical care settings.*

Katon, W., Kleinman, A., and Rosen, G.: Depression and somatization: A review. Am. J. Med., *72*:127–134 (part 1) and 241–247 (part 2), 1982.

Lewinsohn, P. M., Munoz, R. F., Youngren, M. A., et al. Control Your Depression. Englewood Cliffs, NJ, Prentice-Hall, 1979. *Self-help text based on the behavioral approach to psychotherapy.*

National Institute of Mental Health: Mental health services in primary care settings: Report of a conference 1983, April 2–3, 1979. Dept. of Health and Human Services Publication (ADM) 83-995, Series DN No. 2. Rockville, MD, 1983.

Petty, F.: Depression and medical/surgical illness: "Who wouldn't be depressed?" Prim. Care, *14*:669–683, 1987.

Prestidge, R., and Lake, R.: Prevalence and recognition of depression among primary care outpatients. J. Fam. Pract., *25*:67–72, 1987. *The authors note that less than half of all depressed patients in primary care are initially identified and treated. Also, they advocate brief screening interviews and use of depression rating scales.*

Radloff, L. S.: The CES-D scale: A self-report depression scale for research in the general population. Applied. Psychol. Meas., *1*:385, 1977. *Standarized self-report measure developed by the National Institute of Mental Health for epidemiologic studies but now validated as a screening instrument in primary care.*

Richelson, E.: Pharmacology of antidepressants. Psychopathology, *20*(suppl 1):1–12, 1987.

Rodin, G., Voshart, K.: Depression in the medically ill: An overview. Am. J. Psychiatry, *143*:696–705, 1986. *A detailed review of the high incidence of major depression in most major medical and surgical illnesses, with an emphasis on the need for aggressive treatment despite possible interactions between medical and psychiatric treatments.*

Rucker, L., Dietch, J. T.: Depression in primary care: Evolving concepts and approach to therapy. South. Med. J., *79*:215–222, 1986.

Schulberg, H., McClelland, M., and Burns, B. J.: Depression and physical illness: The prevalence, causation, and diagnosis of comorbidity. Clin. Psychology Rev., *7*:145–167, 1987.

Sireling, L. I., Paykel, E. S., Freeling, P., et al.: Depression in general practice: Case thresholds and diagnosis. Br. J. Psychiatry, *147*:113–118, 1985.

Spitzer, R. L., Endicott, J., and Robbins, E.: Research diagnostic criteria: Rationale and reliability. Arch. Gen. Psychiatry, *35*:773–782, 1978.

Von Korff, M., Shapiro, S., Burke, J. D., et al.: Anxiety and depression in a primary care clinic. Arch. Gen. Psychiatry, *44*:152–156, 1987.

Weissman, M. M.: Psychiatric epidemiology: Rates and risks for major depression. Am. J. Public Health, *77*:445–451, 1987.

Weissman, M. M., Leaf, P. L., Bruce, M. L., and Florio, L.: The epidemiology of dysthymia in five communities: Rates, risks, comorbidity, and treatment. Am. J. Psychiatry, *145*:815–819, 1987.

Weissman, M. M., and Myers, J. K.: Psychiatric disorders in a U.S. community: The application of research diagnostic criteria to a resurveyed community sample. Acta. Psychiatr. Scand., *62*:99–111, 1980.

Yates, W. R. (Ed.): Depression. Prim. Care, *14*(4):657–668, 1987. *An excellent review for family physicians, with a particularly functional classification of the many forms of depressions.*

Zung, W. W. K.: A self-rating depression scale. Arch. Gen. Psychiatry, *12*:263–273, 1965.

67

The Somatic Patient

Erich E. Brueschke
Robert E. Zitter

Patients who present to the family physician with complaints for which no organic or physiologic basis can be found tend to be individuals of extremes. On the one hand they are frequently subject to labels such as hypochondriacs or somatizers, but on the other hand they are subjects of extensive tests, procedures, and pharmacologic treatment. Since the symptoms often mimic potentially serious disease but frequently no specific cause is found, this approach represents a failure of the process used in assessing these patients and a lack of appreciation of the characteristics of such patient problems. Most importantly, these patients may receive less than optimal treatment and symptomatic relief, thereby enduring more suffering than is necessary.

This chapter delineates the various psychologic and psychiatric conditions underlying the more common forms of somatization. It is hoped that this discussion will aid the primary care physician in more accurately diagnosing and effectively managing such cases rather than simply ruling out organic disease, an approach that may even prolong somatization and increase the risk of iatrogenesis. The assessment should be aimed at including the most probable causes for the observed problems rather than at an exhaustive attempt to rule out all, frequently unlikely, possibilities first.

Prevalence

Studies consistently document that as many as 50 per cent of patients who consult with their primary care physician have psychosocial problems rather than medical problems (Stoeckle et al., 1964). The majority of these individuals are experiencing depressive or anxiety disorders, or both (Cadoret et al., 1980). Somatoform disorders as well as stress-related physical complaints without accompanying psychiatric diagnoses also account for large numbers of somatic patients.

Many patients suffering from an emotional disorder first present with physical symptoms. Consequently, they consult their primary care physician rather than a mental health professional. Unfortunately, studies indicate that physicians only identify, at best, one-half of the depressed patients who appear for treatment. Cadoret and associates (1980) found that nonspecific functional complaints as well as complaints about pain and anxiety increased in number in the year prior to the diagnosis of depression and decreased to normal levels following the treatment of depression. Based on these and other studies, one can safely conclude that the typical somatic patient is not a malingerer; rather, this individual is likely to be truly in distress and to be experiencing any one of a number of psychiatric disorders or psychologic influences or conditioning. The role of the family physician is to sort out these factors, to determine the presence of anxiety or depression, or both, while using caution in selecting laboratory studies to identify specific problems for treatment.

Somatic Components of Psychiatric Disorders

DEPRESSION

The somatic components of depression may include fatigue; difficulty in sleeping; concentration impairment; poor appetite; increased agitation or anxiety; panic attacks; various pain states; poorly defined, nonspecific physical complaints; and a general sense of not feeling well. Of course, any one of these problems may be the focus of the patient's concern and precipitate a visit to the doctor. Unfortunately, many depressed patients have little or no insight into their depressed state. Older persons, in particular, tend to focus more on somatic concerns than on affective states. A common mistake made by the primary care physician is to treat an individual symptom, e.g., insomnia or chest wall pain, rather than diagnosing the patient's depression and treating this very manageable condition. Thus, it is important to ask about all of the vegetative signs of depression, since the patient may not volunteer this information.

ANXIETY

Anxiety disorders, particularly panic disorders and generalized anxiety, have multiple somatic components. The DSM III-R list of panic disorder symptoms includes dyspnea, palpitations, chest pain, choking sensations, dizziness, unsteady feelings, paresthesias, hot and cold flashes, sweating, faintness, and trembling. Individuals with panic attacks often become progressively more disabled by their frightening symptoms while they move through the traditional medical system, which sometimes takes years. They may become increasingly more hypochondriacal as they focus more and more on their somatic sensations. This heightened somatic concern, in turn, increases the level of anxiety, which is likely to lead to more physical symptoms, thus feeding the patient's hypochondria. All of these factors result in a vicious circle. The traditional medical approach may actually reinforce and strengthen this process rather than break it through the proper education and therapy.

Patients suffering from generalized anxiety disorder usually experience similar autonomic-mediated symptoms along with hypochondriacal tendencies but without the acute panic attacks. It is important for the family physician to question the patient specifically about panic attacks in the usual places, e.g., malls, stores, church, and while driving, since the treatment for panic disorder, which is often antidepressants with supportive counseling, may be inappropriate for generalized anxiety disorder.

SOMATOFORM DISORDERS

Patients diagnosed with any one of the somatoform disorders all share the common feature of presenting with physical symptoms suggestive of organic disease for which there are no demonstrable physical findings. With the exception of malingering or factitious disease, there is no conscious production of symptoms. Therefore, these symptoms are very "real" to the patient. Somatoform disorders include conversion disorder, hypochondriasis, somatization disorder, and somatoform pain disorder. Most of the patients with somatoform disorders have thick medical charts. These patients, who often doctor-shop, face the greatest risk of undergoing needless medical tests and procedures as well as becoming dependent on medication.

Conversion Disorder

Conversion disorder refers to the loss or alteration of physical functioning that suggests physical disorder. The classic conversion symptoms include paralysis, paresthesias, blindness, and seizures. Such symptoms usually start suddenly during a time of acute stress or conflict and disappear quickly. The symptoms are involuntarily produced with no insight into the underlying conflict or secondary gain. Here, the key is for the physician to thoroughly explore the patient's life circumstances without simply concentrating on the medical work-up or prematurely confronting the patient as to the lack of any "real" cause.

Hypochondriasis

Hypochondriasis refers to the fear of having or the belief that one has a serious disease. This is based on the patient's misinterpretation of various normal bodily sensations despite the attempts of others to convince the patient otherwise. AIDS seems to be the most recent fear of hypochondriacal patients. Such individuals often come from alcoholic or dysfunctional families, sometimes with other hypochondriacal family members who are generally anxious and not directly addressing their real issues and anxieties.

Somatization Disorder

Somatization disorder is characterized by recurrent and multiple somatic complaints over many years, usually starting during young adulthood. Individuals with this condition may be the most difficult patients for the primary care physician to manage because of the breadth, number, and frequency of complaints involving so many organ systems. The marked nature of this disorder should "tip off" the physician who should be conservative with medications and diagnostic treatment procedures.

Somatoform Pain Disorder

Somatoform pain disorder simply refers to the preoccupation with pain in the absence of significant or anatomically consistent physical findings. Chronic back pain is probably the most common form of this disorder. This may be the most disabling of the somatoform disorders, often resulting in significant time away from work. Once pain becomes chronic in nature, the prognosis for a successful outcome becomes much poorer due to conditioning factors that will be discussed later in this chapter. Unfortunately, as with many of the problems listed earlier, patients with chronic pain usually move around the medical system for several years before a mental health consultation is considered. Such individuals become clinically depressed at some point due to their increasing limitations. Also, it must be noted that biological relatives of chronic pain patients have a much higher incidence of depression than that found in the general population. A fairly high percentage of the cases of chronic back pain are precipitated by a physical injury or trauma.

ADJUSTMENT DISORDER WITH PHYSICAL SYMPTOMS

In contrast to the somatoform disorders, adjustment disorder with physical symptoms describes individuals who experience stress-related physical symptoms without more global impairment or emotional dysfunction. This type of disorder accounts for a large number of patients, who may be the easiest patients to diagnose and manage. The primary care physician who asks about life stresses should find that most patients with stress-related physical symptoms are reasonably amenable to discussion and education because the relationship between their symptoms and life circumstances can usually be made quite clear.

SUBSTANCE ABUSE

Of course, substance abuse can lead to a host of physical problems, including gastrointestinal disease, liver disease, fatigue, and sleep difficulties. Withdrawal from alcohol and drugs as well as caffeine and nicotine often causes increased anxiety and physical complaints. In very sensitive individuals, excessive caffeine may produce or exacerbate physical symptoms of anxiety such as trembling and anxiety attacks. Periodically, substance abusers or dependent patients may present with physical symptoms for the underlying, sometimes subconscious, purpose of obtaining additional prescriptions such as tranquilizers or pain medications. Thus, a careful evaluation of alcohol, drug, and medication consumption and a medical history is mandatory in the assessment of somatic complaints.

PSYCHOTIC DISORDERS

Psychotic disorders refer to those individuals with an underlying thought disorder, which may be accompanied by intractable physical symptoms, sometimes of a bizarre or unusual nature ("it feels like water rushing through my stomach"). Such patients may be tenuously holding on to a marginal adjustment via somatization. If the physician senses oddities in the patient or finds a family history of more severe mental illness, it would be wise to refer the patient for a more complete psychologic evaluation.

Conditioning Family Factors

Operant conditioning is a powerful way in which physical complaints can develop, strengthen, and be maintained. Behavior that is followed by positive consequences, i.e., positive reinforcement, or by the removal of negative ones, i.e., negative reinforcement, will increase in the future. Those behaviors that are consistently ignored or punished tend to be extinguished. Almost any physical symptom or complaint can inadvertently be reinforced, even by caring persons with good intentions. Examples of reinforcement include attention, affection, and sympathy by family members; financial compensation; time off from work; avoidance of responsibility; addiction to pain medication; attention from health care professionals; and avoidance of focusing on other personal or family problems.

Adult patients who are most likely to have somatic physical symptoms become reinforced are those with poor vocational or interactional skills. For example, a male with chronic back pain with few marketable job skills may not receive much less income on disability than working at a low-paying job. The same patient who also is not assertive in his marriage may get more of his psychologic needs met through complaining of back pain than through his usual marital interactions. Unfortunately, very few patients have any insight into these patterns initially. Thus, it is important for the physician to perform a broad assessment of the patient's functioning in order to formulate workable hypotheses.

Children are very susceptible to inappropriate contingencies operating within a dysfunctional family environment, particularly one with severe marital difficulties. A child may receive subtle or not so subtle reinforcement for sick behavior such as abdominal complaints. This may allow the parents to avoid focusing on their own problems through worrying about the sick child. Such a scenario underlies many school phobias, e.g., the child with gastrointestinal difficulty every weekday morning. We saw a 14-year-old male patient who had "real" diarrhea every morning but not on weekends or vacations. He had missed tremendous amounts of school, and had been hospitalized twice with negative results over a 2-year period. The pattern was obvious to the psychologic consultant. The boy was fine during the rest of the day once it was too late to go to school. He spent much time with his mother during the day, thus clearly receiving attention and reinforcement. The parents, obviously not close emotionally, denied marital problems, but the boy's father worked long hours and the boy's mother appeared quite angry with him. She and her 14-year-old son were close despite her frustration with his "condition." Salvador Minuchin and colleagues (1978) have written extensively about psychosomatic families. Such families tend to be rigid, to be unable to resolve conflict effectively, to lack psychologic language, and to deny psychologic difficulty. A physician must also be concerned about physical, sexual, or emotional abuse in somatic children. Gross and associates (1980) found that 80 per cent of women with pelvic pain of undetermined organic cause came from dysfunctional families in which violence and physical assault occurred frequently.

Another powerful form of conditioning is modeling. A large percentage of somatic patients had a parent or grandparent with chronic, somatic complaints. These patients observe a key family member managing the lives of the rest of the family through somatization. Apley (1975) reported that the incidence of abdominal pain in parents and siblings of children with similar pain was six times higher than in relatives of a control group. In a long-term longitudinal study of abdominal symptoms, Christensen and Mortensen (1975) found that those children with recurrent abdominal pain who continued to experience such problems as adults were much more likely to have their own children develop abdominal difficulties than those adults who did not retain their childhood somatic complaints.

The final conditioning model for physical symptomatology is that of classical conditioning in which symptoms become associated with particular places, people, or situations. One of the best examples is chemotherapy nausea becoming conditioned to the thought or sight of the hospital. Similarly, headaches, chest discomfort, or stomach upset can become associated not only with one's job but even with thinking about work. Avoidance of the aversive situation through these symptoms further reinforces and strengthens them. Additional factors, such as the patient's level of obsessiveness, other sources of reinforcement, and the patient's psychologic status, determine the degree of control the particular symptoms have over a patient's life.

Sociocultural Aspects of Somatic Illness

Rosen and colleagues (1982) discuss the distinction between disease and illness. Disease refers to the malfunctioning of biologic or psychologic processes, or both, whereas illness is defined as perception, evaluation, explanation, and labeling of symptoms by the patient and his family within the context of the social culture. There is significant variability among cultural groups in the way symptoms are perceived and managed. For example, Zborowski (1952) found the response to pain by hospitalized patients differed among ethnic groups, with Italian and Jewish Americans having the greatest emotional response. Somatization appears to be correlated with lower socioeconomic groups, in which it is less acceptable to directly express one's emotions. Of particular interest, there have been several cross-cultural studies of depression recently reviewed by Keeton and Dengerink (1983). It appears that the vegetative signs of depression are the same across cultures and countries. However, the major difference is the perception of affective and cognitive states, e.g., feelings of hopelessness, helplessness, and guilt. This recognition appears to be a more recent phenomenon in American culture, whereas many countries, particularly Middle Eastern and Chinese, express their feelings through somatization. Some languages lack words to describe internal, affective, and feelings states. One interesting study (Racy, 1970) found that as Arabs become more "westernized," their depression becomes more similar to that seen in the American culture. Our own experience confirms these findings; that is, our Middle Eastern patients who have come to the United States in the last few years seem to react to psychosocial stressors through somatization. All in all, due to either the lack of appropriate psychologic language or strong cultural sanctions against talking about emotions as well as the greater legitimacy and acceptability of physical symptoms, many of our patients continue to somaticize. These data emphasize the importance, particularly with depressed patients, of assessing the vegetative signs of depression, the patient's facial expressions, and life circumstances rather than relying solely on the patient's self-report of depression.

Diagnosis

BIOPSYCHOSOCIAL MODEL

A comprehensive, biopsychosocial assessment is the key to developing the diagnosis with the greatest utility for patient management. Obviously, given the many influencing factors discussed earlier as well as the statistical frequency of medical patients with physical findings that are not significant, a narrow biomedical approach is insufficient for a large number of patients. To argue that all possible, organic etiologies should be eliminated *prior* to exploring nonmedical factors is no longer tenable. The preferred approach is to consider the more likely causes of the problem while doing a reasonable *concurrent* investigation into possible biomedical and psychosocial causes. Because the real problem may be neglected, the patient is at greater risk for harm with a more narrow approach to assessment. Most patients accept a multifactorial investigation and welcome a more wholistic inquiry into their health concerns. When the evaluation is conducted within the context of a good doctor-patient relationship, the patient does not feel accused of "being crazy" or "malingering." In fact, the most frustrated patients are those who endure an extensive medical work-up with negative results and no relief of their symptoms only to be dismissed because no "real" cause is found. An uncommon presentation of a common problem (such as an anxiety disorder) is seen more frequently than a common presentation of a rare disorder (such as pheochromocytoma). Therefore, unless some other features of the presentation point to a physical disorder, do not postpone consideration of a likely disorder in order to rule out unlikely problems with time-consuming, costly, and possibly hazardous studies.

THE CLINICAL INTERVIEW

The clinical interview remains the basic assessment tool in the biopsychosocial evaluation. Observational skills are important, particularly for those patients who appear depressed or anxious but have poor insight into these conditions. Occasionally, the doctor identifies inappropriate or bizarre behavior as well as an angry patient. Questioning must include a judicious mixture of open-ended and directed questioning. Open-ended questions are more likely to lead to productive avenues that can be pursued with more specific questions. Starting the interview with mostly directed, leading, or specific questioning is likely to bypass important areas that need to be explored and certainly does not encourage emotional responses.

It is helpful to operationalize the patient's presenting complaints through a functional analysis. A functional analysis consists of three parts: *antecedents, symptomatic behavior*, and *consequences*. Antecedents refer to the triggering stimuli—place, time, day, activity, and people. We have found patients who have physical symptoms that only occur outside of the house, in church, during the week, or at work. Symptomatic behavior can be broken down into physiologic symptoms (e.g., tachycardia, lightheadedness), cognitive behavior (e.g., I am going to die, I am sick, I better lie down), and overt behavior (e.g., leaving the situation, withdrawing, becoming irritable). Finally, as described earlier in this chapter, consequences and benefits of this behavior can include avoidance of stressful situations, attention, nurturance, medications, and financial gain. A functional analysis should provide the clearest and most complete picture that readily leads to intervention.

Particularly in acute cases, it is important to identify life stresses or changes that occurred around the time of onset. It is amazing how many patients cannot make the connection between obvious stressors such as the death of a loved one and the onset of lightheadedness and palpitations. If patients are simply asked "have you been under more stress lately?," the patient may give a negative response. Thus, the physician should make inquiries into specific areas such as the occurrence of a recent death in the family, job change, and relationship difficulties.

We find it clinically useful to distinguish between acute and chronic somatization. Symptoms that have a duration of 6 months or less are usually related to specific environmental stressors or biologically mediated psychiatric disorders such as depression or panic disorder or a combination of these factors. These somatic patients generally have a good prognosis with the proper identification of the disorder, education, and treatment. More chronic cases, particularly in those patients who have somatic symptoms across multiple organ systems for many years, have a poorer prognosis and tend to exhibit more global psychologic impairment. The chronic somatic patient would benefit from the coordinated treatment of both the family physician and a mental health provider.

Research into the patient's family history offers many important clues. A family history of depression, anxiety, alcoholism, and chronic physical problems puts the patient at increased risk for somatic difficulties. Adult children of alcoholics as well as patients who are victims of physical, sexual, and emotional abuse often are hypersensitive to bodily sensations and react to stress somatically.

The patient must be evaluated for the psychiatric disorders described earlier. Again, depression and anxiety disorders account for a large portion of somatic patients. Asking about the vegetative signs of depression often yields a positive response yet is frequently neglected, particularly if the patient denies depression. One can observe atypical depression with only a few vegetative signs and with a more somatic expression, which still responds well to antidepressant or psychologic treatment. Sometimes, patients state that they are depressed because of the physical problems rather than viewing the depression as the causative factor. These patients may still respond well to treatment for the depressive disorder. Of course, a family history of affective illness would place greater weight on treating the depression. Regarding anxiety disorders, the most effective outcome results from inquiring about anxiety attacks in specific places such as stores, church, restaurants, and in the car. One should also ask about phobias and obsessive thoughts.

THE USE OF SELF-MONITORING BY THE PATIENT

Having the patient keep a symptom diary is a cost-effective method of collecting data that helps to educate both the patient and physician. In many cases, these data directly lead to intervention strategies. Other than a constant problem such as fatigue, most symptoms are amenable to this approach. Such diaries serve to actively involve patients in their medical treatment rather than having them simply wait for the physician to solve their problems. Essentially, self-monitoring assists in identifying antecedents of the disorder of which the patient may be unaware.

PSYCHOLOGIC TESTING

In those cases in which the biomedical and psychosocial evaluations are not productive, one may consider a referral for psychologic testing to assist in the decision-making process. The Minnesota Multiphasic Personality Inventory, an extensively used and validated objective personality test, is useful with the somatic patient. It helps to differentiate depressive disorders, anxiety disorders, chronic personality disorders, and psychotic disorders. It is a relatively inexpensive and quick test that can even be scored for use by a computer, producing a computerized summary. Less frequently, projective tests such as the Rorschach and the Thematic Apperception Test (TAT) also can be used for those more ambiguous and complex cases. The main advantage of these tests is that patients do not know what responses are expected; therefore, it is more difficult to influence the test results. These tests are more time consuming and expensive and some psychologists question their validity. Neuropsychologic testing, such as the Halstead-Raitan and Intelligence measures, is desirable when the family physician wants "harder" data on a patient who he suspects may have compromised brain functioning.

Treatment

EDUCATION

Education of the somatic patient is accomplished throughout the biopsychosocial evaluation process. As the family physician gradually puts the pieces of the puzzle together with the patient by identifying antecedents, depressive symptoms, and family dysfunction, the patient is learning to reframe his or her problem in a way that is more conducive to treatment. In many cases, this understanding alleviates the fear of what is wrong medically and allows patients to take more control over their lives. For some patients, education will suffice; for others, additional intervention strategies are necessary to target each problem area. Throughout this assessment and education phase of treatment, the family physician is gaining the confidence of the somatic patient, strengthening the physician-patient relationship.

THERAPY

Of course, therapy should follow directly from the assessment. In acute somatization associated with an environmental stressor, education and supportive counseling may suffice. On the other hand, the family physician may identify long-term, developmental issues, e.g., incest or childhood emotional abuse, which amplify the reaction to environmental stressors and which require formal psychotherapy.

It is best to form a good working relationship with a few mental health professionals to facilitate effective, ongoing communication during the patient's therapy. Mental health providers tend to specialize in different populations and techniques. Some problems such as muscle tension–related physical symptoms or anxiety attacks may respond well to a behavioral approach, including relaxation techniques. On the other hand, family therapy might be more appropriate for a somatic child. In other cases, an expert in medication therapy is indicated.

Patients with chronic somatic complaints are likely to be in need of psychotherapy because of their more global, psychologic impairment. In addition, the more chronic the somatization becomes, the more the individual becomes adjusted to the sick role. This includes a certain amount of reinforcement from significant others. Thus, in long-standing somatic problems such as chronic back pain, the physician and therapist are attempting to modify current factors that are maintaining the physical symptoms as well as the more long-standing, deeper issues. Patients should understand that their symptoms are quite real, that the symptoms are not "in their head," and that they are truly suffering. They should also understand that the family physician, the patient, and the therapist are working together to alleviate the patient's physical difficulties.

Medications, particularly the antidepressants and anxiolytics, can be beneficial in the management of the somatic patient, with or without counseling. Anti-depressants are the treatment of choice for depression-related somatization and panic attacks. Particularly with marked sleep disturbance, sedating antidepressants can offer immediate relief in addition to long-term benefits. Family physicians should become familiar with a few antidepressants, which vary as to the amount of sedation and anticholinergic side effects. Antidepressants offer a major advantage over the anxiolytics in that dependency does not become an issue. With the exception of alprazolam, the anxiolytics do not prevent panic attacks. If one does not question the patient specifically about panic attacks, an anxiolytic may be inappropriately prescribed without much therapeutic benefit. In the case of acute environmental stressors associated with physical symptoms, a short-term trial of an anxiolytic may be helpful as long as the patient clearly understands the rationale. For the *chronically* anxious patient who has associated physical or autonomic symptoms, or both, buspirone may offer significant relief (see chapter 68, Psychotherapeutic Drugs).

With some experience, these medications can be safely and effectively managed by the family physician. Certain patients have side effects to most of the antidepressants, although trazodone and fluoxetine seem to produce fewer side effects. Significant problems due to side effects can be an appropriate basis for referral to a psychiatrist. Also, after a trial of at least 1 to 2 months at a therapeutic dosage of several antidepressants, which can be determined by blood levels, psychiatric consultation is indicated if the patient is not sufficiently responsive.

References

Apley, J.: The Child With Abdominal Pains. Oxford, Blackwell, 1975.

Cadoret, R. J., Widmer, R. B., and North, C.: Depression in family practice: Long-term prognosis and somatic complaints. J. Fam. Pract., *10*:625, 1980. *The relationships between somatic pain, functional complaints, and anxiety were studied in depressed patients over time. Persistence of somatic symptoms after 1 year predicted eventual chronicity of the depression.*

Christensen, M. F., and Mortensen, O.: Long-term prognosis in children with recurrent abdominal pain. Arch. Dis. Child., *50*:110, 1975.

Gross, R., Doerr, H., Caldirola, G., and Ripley, H.: Borderline syndrome and incest in chronic pelvic pain patients. Int. J. Psychiatry Med., *10*:77, 1980.

Keeton, W., and Dengerink, H. A.: Somatization in primary health care. *In* Carr, J. E., and Dengerink, H. A. (Eds.): Behavioral Science in the Practice of Medicine. New York, Elsevier Biomedical, 1983, pp. 105–131. *A discussion of somatization in primary care is presented using literature references and case presentations. The role of reinforcement in sick role behavior and sociocultural factors are both well covered.*

McClynn, T. J., and Metcalf, H. L. (Eds.): Diagnosis and Treatment of Anxiety Disorders—A Physician's Handbook. Washington, D. C.: American Psychiatric Press, 1989. *A practical approach to the anxious patient is presented in two parts. Part One discusses general principles of diagnosis and treatment of anxiety disorders for the primary care physician, and Part Two provides a detailed description of diagnostic criteria and management strategies for each anxiety disorder.*

Minuchin, S., Rosman, B. L., and Baker, L.: Psychosomatic Families. Cambridge, MA, Harvard University Press, 1978. *A description of the family therapy approach to the treatment of psychosomatic families.*

Racy, J.: Psychiatry in the Arab East. Acta Psychiatr. Scand. Supplementum, *21*:1, 1970.

Rosen, G., Kleinman, A., and Katon, W.: Somatization in family practice: A biopsychosocial approach. J. Fam. Pract., *14*:493, 1982. *The authors review the prevalence and consequences of somatization and develop a conceptual model that includes cultural, childhood, psychologic, and environmental factors.*

Stoeckle, J. D., Zola, I. K., and Davidson, G. E.: The quantity and significance of psychological distress in medical patients. J. Chronic Dis., *17*:959, 1964.

Zborowski, M.: Cultural components in responses to pain. J. Soc. Issues, *8*:16, 1952.

68

Substance Abuse

Marc A. Schuckit
Robert E. Rakel
Alan Blum
Kevin M. Sherin
Jan A. Fawcett

Alcohol

Marc A. Schuckit

In most western countries 90 per cent or more of individuals are drinkers of alcoholic beverages at some time during their lives, including almost 70 per cent who currently imbibe alcohol. The percentage of drinkers is higher among men than among women, although the gap between the two sexes may be rapidly closing. Most individuals consume their first drink at approximately age 12 to 14 years, have a maximum quantity and frequency of intake in their late teens to mid-20's, and then decrease the amount of alcohol consumed with each increasing decade.

Unfortunately, during late adolescence and early adulthood temporary alcohol-related problems are highly prevalent. Almost 50 per cent of men and a slightly lower proportion of women experience an alcohol-related blackout (forgetting all or part of what happened during a drinking evening), miss some time from school or work because of drinking, have an alcohol-related accident or a single driving arrest while drinking, and so on. Fortunately, most of these individuals spontaneously moderate their drinking and do not go on to develop the more pervasive and persistent alcohol-related problems that might be labeled alcoholism.

These data underscore the importance of establishing an alcohol intake history in all patients, even those who do not meet alcoholic criteria. Drinking, heavy intake of alcohol, and temporary alcohol-related life problems are so prevalent that it is difficult for us to properly treat any patient without establishing his or her alcohol intake and problem history. Even among nonalcoholics, the usual drinking pattern can contribute to accidents and exacerbate independent medical and psychiatric disorders.

Actual alcoholism fulfilling criteria outlined in the following sections is one of the most prevalent serious disorders in our society. Even utilizing restrictive criteria, the lifetime risk for developing this disorder among men is at least 10 per cent and might

This work was supported by NIAAA grant #05226 and the Veterans Administration Research Service.

be as high as 15 per cent (Robins et al., 1984; Schuckit, 1985a). The rate of similar problems in women is at least 5 per cent.

SOME MYTHS

Most physicians have been trained in central city hospitals where they were inaccurately taught that the average alcoholic lives on skid row, returns to treatment facilities repetitively, and rarely demonstrates long-lasting improvement. If one accepts this stereotype, it is possible to draw the *erroneous* conclusion that alcoholics are exceptionally difficult to treat and that dealing with them is unrewarding. Therefore, it is worthwhile to briefly review two myths that must be set aside if we are to optimize our ability to help our patients.

First, only 5 per cent or so of alcoholics fit the skid row stereotype. The average alcoholic appears in clinical settings in a sober state, looking well groomed, having no smell of alcohol, and lacking many of the other traits we may associate with skid row. This typical patient complains of a variety of medical and emotional problems that must be properly diagnosed if the clinician hopes to avoid unexpected calls in the middle of the night and adverse reactions to ill-advised treatments. In fact, the usual alcoholic man or woman resembles the usual person in society. He or she has a job and financial resources, has close friends and relatives, and is capable of abstaining from alcohol for extended periods of time.

A second important myth is that alcoholics are not likely to improve. To the contrary, numerous studies have documented that the average middle class alcoholic who agrees to enter treatment and completes a rehabilitation program appears to have a 60 to 70 per cent chance of maintaining abstinence for at least 1 year (Neubuerger et al., 1982; Schuckit, 1989). Although few investigations go beyond 12 months of follow-up, there are additional data that once abstinence is achieved for this period of time, the chances of continuing an alcohol-free life style are extremely high. In addition, even without actual treatment there is at least a 20 per cent chance of "spontaneous remission" in which life-long abstinence is achieved even in the absence of formal treatment or participation in self-help groups (Helzer et al., 1985; Ludwig, 1985; Schuckit, 1989).

Pharmacology of Alcohol

Ethanol is a simple molecule that is weakly charged, soluble in both water and fat, and thus widely distributed in the body. The concentration of this substance in blood is loosely predicted by the number of drinks as related to the body weight; that is, in general, the larger the person, the greater amount of alcohol that needs to be consumed for a specific blood alcohol level (BAL). However, there are additional important factors, including the percentage body fat (with increasing age and increasing body fat there is less body water and thus higher BAL's), age (with an increased brain sensitivity and decreased ability of the liver to metabolize alcohol with increasing age), past experiences, concomitant medications, and so on.

The level of alcohol in the blood is expressed as milligrams or grams of ethanol per 100 milliliters (or deciliters) of blood. For example, in most states a person with a BAL of 100 mg. per dl. or 0.100 gram per dl. (the same blood levels using different units) is considered legally drunk. The BAL increases by approximately 20 mg. per dl. for each drink, a level that takes slightly more than an hour to metabolize. This amount of alcohol also contains approximately 10 grams of ethanol, with approximately 100 calories or more—calories "empty" of the usual nutrients such as vitamins.

As a typical central nervous system (CNS) depressant, beverage alcohol decreases the activity of neurons, although some behavioral stimulation can be observed at low blood levels. The clinical effects of the drug are similar to those observed with other brain depressants such as the benzodiazepines (e.g., diazepam or Valium) and barbiturates (in fact, all prescription sleeping pills and most prescription antianxiety drugs). Thus, there is cross-tolerance between all of the brain depressants with the result that simultaneous intake of multiple drugs of this class can (and frequently does) result in a lethal overdose. On the other hand, the repeated intake of any one drug of this class can result in tolerance so that when the first drug is stopped, larger doses of a second brain depressant might be required to achieve the desired clinical effect (e.g., larger doses of a benzodiazepine might be required to induce anesthesia in a sober but recently heavily drinking alcoholic) (Schuckit, 1989).

Tolerance, or the need for larger doses of the drug to achieve the same effects, is a relatively complex phenomenon. First, metabolic or *pharmacokinetic* tolerance is observed when, after 1 to 2 weeks of daily drinking, the liver adapts through induction of enzymes to increase the metabolic rate for ethanol by as much as 30 per cent. Cellular or *pharmacodynamic* tolerance represents the adaptation of the nerve cells to a state of "resistance" to the effects of alcohol. The mechanisms for cellular tolerance are not well understood but probably represent changes in cell membranes and/or neurochemical receptors (perhaps for gamma-aminobutyric acid or serotonin)—changes that contribute to physical dependence. Finally, *behavioral* tolerance represents the learned behavior or practice effects whereby chronic heavy drinkers can perform tasks moderately efficiently even though they are intoxicated. The combination of all three mechanisms contributes to the ability of most relatively healthy alcoholics (i.e., with no severe liver or brain damage) to drink large amounts of alcohol, with cellular tolerance contributing to their ability to be awake and alert at levels of alcohol that might be lethal in others.

The metabolism and excretion of alcohol is relatively straightforward. Low amounts of this substance (between 2 and 10 per cent, depending on the BAL) are excreted directly through sweat, urine, and lungs. The vast majority of ethanol is metabolized in the liver through at least three different mechanisms, each resulting in the same first breakdown product of alcohol, acetaldehyde. The most clinically relevant metabolic pathway occurs through alcohol dehydrogenase in the cell cytosol, after which acetaldehyde is rapidly destroyed by aldehyde dehydrogenase in both the cytosol and mitochondria. Each of these steps requires nicotinamide adenine dinucleotide (NAD) as a cofactor, and it is the lack of availability of this hydrogen receptor that is probably a major rate-limiting step in this metabolic pathway. The second type of oxidation of ethanol, most important at higher BAL's, occurs in the smooth endoplasmic reticulum and is called the microsomal ethanol oxidizing system or MEOS. Third, an unknown percentage of ethanol is also metabolized through the catalase system.

Alcohol is a simple substance that produces effects in almost all body systems. Each drink of alcohol (e.g., 10 ounces of beer, 4 ounces of wine, or 1.5 ounces of 80-proof beverage) results in a BAL of approximately 20 mg. per dl., an amount that takes slightly more than an hour for the body to destroy. With repeated intake of this substance, cellular, metabolic, and behavioral tolerance develops, but the average nontolerant individual is likely to demonstrate behavioral and physical effects with as few as one to two drinks. Ninety per cent or more of alcohol is metabolized in the liver to acetaldehyde, a biologically active substance that is usually rapidly and efficiently destroyed. Reflecting the ability to induce liver enzymes, its position as a "preferred fuel" in the liver where hydrogen receptors are likely to be utilized, and its actions on almost all body systems, it is important to determine the alcohol intake pattern in patients for whom we are prescribing any medication, especially other brain depressant drugs, medications with sedative side effects, and substances metabolized in the liver.

The Diagnosis of Alcoholism

Because 90 per cent of people drink at some time during their lives, and reflecting the fact that moderately heavy intake of alcohol is likely to be observed in the late teens to late 20's, an understanding of the prevalence of drinking and the pharmacology of alcohol can enhance our clinical abilities. The remainder of this chapter focuses on the diagnosis, etiology, usual course, and treatment for severe and pervasive alcohol-related life problems or alcoholism.

Before discussing the actual diagnostic criteria, it is worthwhile to briefly review some biases important in considering any diagnosis (Goodwin and Guze, 1989). Historically, diagnoses in medicine have been used to describe a clinical condition at one point in time, to imply causation, and to predict the most likely course as well as help select the appropriate treatment. Whereas many different diagnostic criteria are available for alcoholism, the most clinically relevant are probably those that meet the last criterion, i.e., those that tell us when to intervene and the treatment approaches with the best asset-to-liability ratio.

From this perspective there are as many as 11 different definitions of alcoholism that have been used in the literature in recent decades (Boyd et al., 1983). However, there is a great amount of overlap in the individuals identified by these diagnostic approaches. Thus, someone who is labeled alcoholic because the quantity and frequency of intake is excessive is also almost certain to demonstrate signs of psychological dependence and is likely to evidence serious life problems related to heavy drinking. If the diagnostic approach is excessively broad, many labeled individuals will probably not go on to develop more severe and pervasive problems; with the very restrictive approaches, diagnosed people will run the expected clinical course, but some men and women who are excluded from the label might also be at risk for severe future problems.

The more formal and official diagnostic criteria for alcoholism are presented in the Revised Third Diagnostic and Statistical Manual of the American Psychiatric Association, the DSM III-R. Here, alcohol abuse, coded as 305.OX, requires evidence of a pattern of "pathologic" alcohol use as evidenced by daily drinking along with efforts to control and some problems including binges, blackouts, and occasional heavy consumption. In addition, to meet criteria for alcohol abuse, some evidence of social and/or occupational functioning impairment over a period of at least 1 month must be evident. Alcohol dependence (coded as 303.9), on the other hand, requires that in addition to such problems there is evidence of tolerance or an abstinence syndrome from alcohol. While the DSM III-R criteria represent a compromise between different schools of thought on diagnostic labeling, unfortunately few research projects have demonstrated the clinical relevance of the distinction between alcohol abuse and alcohol dependence, and it can be difficult (if not impossible) to actually document such concepts as tolerance from a clinical history (Schuckit et al., 1985).

A diagnostic approach of great potential use to the clinician evaluates the occurrence of significant alcohol-related life problems, gathered as part of the usual social history (Schuckit, 1985b; Schuckit, 1986). Once a pattern of problems has been established, the next step is to determine whether the alcohol has contributed to these difficulties. Thus, alcoholism is diagnosed with a history of any of the following: a marital separation or divorce related to alcohol; multiple arrests related to drinking; physical evidence that alcohol has harmed health, including evidence of alcoholic withdrawal; or a job loss or layoff related to drinking. Once patients have fulfilled these criteria, they have demonstrated that they ignored the early warning signs that alcohol was causing a problem and went on to develop major alcohol-related life consequences. In other words, there is evidence that alcohol means more to the person than the problems it has caused. Follow-up studies demonstrate that once these criteria are met, it is possible to predict a high likelihood of continued major life problems from alcohol should drinking continue (Schuckit, 1985b; Schuckit, 1986).

Of course, it is not always possible to obtain all of this information directly from the patient. Although many individuals will admit to major life problems and often agree that it is possible that alcohol contributed to them, an appropriate work-up for any problem in behavioral medicine *requires* that additional information about the patient be obtained. This is usually carried out through an interview with someone who knows about the patient's history, often a relative and usually the spouse.

Finally, it is important at this juncture to briefly review the importance of primary versus secondary alcoholism. Approximately three quarters of alcoholics who present for treatment have no major pre-existent psychiatric disorder. It is these *primary alcoholics* who are the focus of the comments offered in this chapter, and it is usually people in this group who are the subjects in most clinical studies. The natural history and rehabilitation efforts aimed at primary alcoholics are slightly different from those for men and women who developed their alcohol-related life problems only *after* the establishment of another major psychiatric diagnosis (i.e., have secondary alcoholism). Thus, these 20 to 30 per cent of secondary alcoholics often demonstrate pre-existent severe antisocial life problems in all areas of functioning (e.g., have the antisocial personality disorder with secondary alcoholism), or demonstrate severe life problems related to drugs before the onslaught of alcoholism (e.g., have primary drug abuse with secondary alcoholism). It is also probable that the rate of independent and pre-existent major depressive disorders among alcoholics is at least as high as in the general population (perhaps 5 per cent or so), as are the rates of most major anxiety disorders such as panic disorder or agoraphobia (Schuckit, 1986; Schuckit and Monteiro, 1988).

Different diagnostic criteria for alcoholism outline very similar populations. The essential element is documentation of heavy enough and persistent enough intake of alcohol to interfere significantly with health and life functioning, despite which the individual continues to drink. In the 70 to 80 per cent of cases in which alcoholism is the first appearing major psychiatric disorder, the primary alcoholic is likely to run a somewhat predictable clinical course.

Etiology

There is no single cause for alcoholism. It is likely that different individuals develop their pervasive alcohol-related life problems for a variety of reasons. For most it is probable that the interaction of stress, general environment, personality, and biological predisposing factors combine to produce the final alcoholic picture.

It is the last of the influences, biological factors, for which the best data are available. Alcoholism does appear to be a biologically influenced disorder, and there is evidence that genetic factors play an important role. This section places an emphasis on data supporting the importance of genetic factors contributing to the alcoholism risk.

Data from family, twin, and adoption studies all support the importance of genetic influences (Schuckit, 1985c; Goodwin, 1985). First, alcoholism runs strongly in families, with sons and daughters of alcoholics demonstrating a fourfold increased risk for this disorder. The level of risk appears to increase with the number of alcoholic relatives, the severity of alcoholism, and the closeness of the genetic relationship. However, establishing that a disorder is familial does not prove that genetic factors are important because most individuals are raised by their biological parents.

The second approach, twin studies, attempts to separate genetics and environment by comparing the risk for alcoholism in identical twins of alcoholics with the risk for fraternal twins. If the development of alcoholism is related to childhood environment, then the twin of an alcoholic, being born and raised at the same time as the sibling, should be at high risk for the disorder, no matter what kind of twinship is involved. However, if alcoholism is related to genetic factors, the identical twin of an alcoholic (sharing 100 per cent of his or her genes with the affected individual) should have a significantly higher risk for alcoholism than the fraternal twin of an alcoholic (sharing only 50 per cent of the genes, the same as in any full sibling). The majority of twin studies support the conclusion that there is a significantly higher risk for alcoholism in the identical versus the fraternal twin of alcoholics, although not all studies agree (Goodwin, 1985; Gurling et al., 1985).

The third approach, adoption type studies, offers the most compelling evidence that alcoholism is genetically influenced (Goodwin, 1985; Schuckit, 1987). Numerous investigations utilizing the half sibling or formal adoption approaches have demonstrated that sons and daughters of alcoholics have a fourfold increased risk, even when they were adopted close to birth and raised by nonalcoholics. In fact, having an alcoholic rearing parent does not increase the risk any higher than that predicted by severe alcohol-related problems in the biological father or mother.

Recently, a number of laboratories have attempted to identify the biological factors that might be contributing to the risk for alcoholism (Schuckit,

1987). These studies visualize individuals as entering life with a greater or lesser level of biological predisposition, which then interacts with environmental factors to produce the final clinical picture. Most of these investigations have focused on teenage or young adult sons and daughters of alcoholic parents, comparing them in numerous areas with children of nonalcoholics. One such series has repeatedly documented that children of alcoholics demonstrate less intense responses to a three- to five-drink alcohol challenge by showing less subjective feelings of intoxication, less decrement in motor performance measures at a given BAL, less intense or more evanescent changes in hormones after drinking, and/or less post-ethanol change on several electrophysiologic measures (Schuckit, 1987; Schuckit and Gold, 1988). These studies might indicate that some children of alcoholics carry their elevated risk by a relative insensitivity to the effects of beverage alcohol at low BAL's, a time when most people are deciding whether it is appropriate to continue to drink during an evening. Other interesting and potentially important findings in children of alcoholics include the documentation that a significant minority of these offspring may have a lower amplitude of a brain wave (the P300 of the event-related potential) thought to reflect some unique cognitive abilities (Begleiter et al., 1987), might demonstrate different patterns of alpha waves on background cortical electroencephalograms (Ehlers and Schuckit, in press), and might have some specific deficits on neurocognitive and psychomotor test performance (Schuckit et al., 1987).

In summary, although it is not likely that there is any one specific cause for alcoholism, there is ample evidence that genetically influenced biological factors contribute to the predisposition toward this disorder. Several studies are beginning to identify factors that might contribute to the risk, and it is hoped that future follow-ups of higher risk individuals might pinpoint environmental factors that interact with the biological predisposition to produce the disorder. These data might lead to greater understanding of causes, which in turn might contribute to our ability to actually prevent alcoholism before it develops, or might identify more specific or effective treatment approaches. In the interim, the genetic issues underscore the biological rather than moral underpinnings for this highly prevalent and serious disorder.

The Natural History or Usual Clinical Course of Alcoholism

When diagnostic criteria are carefully selected, they can tell us important information about the usual clinical course and help to select among various treatments. Thus, we can be informed about whether the clinical course is likely to be so benign that no interventions are required or if, on the other hand, severe problems are likely to ensue. Of course, even careful diagnoses cannot indicate the exact difficulties a specific patient would have. They can, however, predict the patterns of problems that are likely to ensue.

In this context, the "average" alcoholic is likely to have his or her first drink, first period of intoxication, and first more minor related problems from alcohol during the teenage years, at a time not significantly different from the general population. These generalities apply to primary alcoholics, not the 10 per cent or so of alcoholic males who have major pre-existent antisocial personality disorder or the additional 5 per cent who exhibit severe pre-existent drug-related life difficulties.

By the mid to late 20's, most men and women are beginning to moderate their drinking, probably learning from more minor problems. At the same time, difficulties for alcoholics are likely to escalate, with the first major life problem from drinking appearing in the late 20's to early 40's (Vaillant, 1982; Schuckit, 1989).

Once established, the course of alcoholism is likely to be one of frequent exacerbations and remissions (Ludwig, 1985). In the typical course, alcohol-related problems escalate, precipitating a crisis. In the context of these problems, most individuals will temporarily cease drinking, usually going through mild withdrawal on their own. This period of abstinence lasting days to months for the average middle-class primary alcoholic is usually followed by thoughts that drinking might be "safe" if only carried out at certain times of the day or with certain beverages. The temporary "controlled" drinking is characterized by an ability to go to parties and consume alcohol without problems, and is likely to last for days to months, sometimes longer. The period of "control" is almost inevitably followed by unpredictable times of escalating intake with associated problems, which in turn lead to more problems, more persistent heavy intake, and a crisis that often precipitates another episode of abstinence (Helzer et al., 1985).

Although most alcoholics appear to break into this cycle with active help from clinicians or self-help organizations such as Alcoholics Anonymous (AA), even without formal intervention the course is far from hopeless (Drew, 1968). Several studies have documented that at least 20 per cent or more of alcoholics achieve permanent abstinence without formal intervention (Editorial, 1987; Schuckit, 1989). However, should the alcoholic continue to drink, the life span is shortened by an average of 15 years with the leading causes of death, in decreasing order, being heart disease, cancer, accidents, and suicide.

An important part of the natural history of alcoholism involves the effects of persistent heavy drinking on various body systems. In general, the early stages of alterations in organ functions tend to be reversible, but many body systems deteriorate with permanent levels of damage after repeated alcohol-related insults.

In the *CNS*, temporary problems that can be observed with even one night of heavy drinking include an alcoholic blackout (forgetting all or part of what occurred while drinking) and interference with sleep (falling asleep can be facilitated, but alcohol "fragments" sleep with subsequent bad dreams and a lack of deep sleep) (Schuckit, 1989). With chronic intake of large doses of alcohol, perhaps 5 to 15 per cent of alcoholics develop a deterioration of the nerves to the hands and feet, a peripheral neuropathy. Cerebellar degeneration with accompanying nystagmus and motor incoordination is probably observed in 1 per cent or so of alcoholics (Estrin, 1987). Severe cognitive impairment can take many forms including the thiamine deficiency–related Korsakoff syndrome characterized by profound anterograde and retrograde amnesia, along with possible impairments in visuospatial, abstract, and conceptual reasoning—problems likely to become permanent to greater or lesser degrees in almost two thirds of the individuals meeting diagnostic criteria (Grant, 1987). Less specific forms of cognitive problems, often being reflected by increased size of the brain ventricles, are seen in 20 per cent or more of alcoholics, frequently accompanied by irreversible decreases in intellectual functioning (Harper et al., 1987).

Related to general CNS functioning is the fact that heavy doses of alcohol contribute to severe psychological impairment (Schuckit, 1986). This can include an intense sadness lasting for days to weeks in the midst of heavy drinking, sometimes so severe that it resembles major depressive disorder and probably contributes to the 15 per cent lifetime risk for completed suicide among alcoholics (Brown and Schuckit, 1988). However, when the severe depression is observed only in the context of heavy drinking, it is likely that it will disappear with abstinence alone, and under these circumstances, in primary alcoholics antidepressant medications are rarely required. Similarly, acute alcoholic withdrawal (lasting up to 5 days) and the following protracted period of more mild abstinence symptoms (lasting up to 3 to 6 months) is frequently characterized by severe anxiety that can include panic attacks, phobias, and feelings of generalized anxiety, each of which is likely to decrease spontaneously over a period of months with abstinence alone (Schuckit and Monteiro, 1988). In addition, perhaps 1 to 3 per cent of alcoholics develop auditory hallucinations or paranoid delusions in the absence of any obvious signs of withdrawal—a temporary state of alcohol hallucinosis that is likely to disappear spontaneously within days to weeks (Schuckit, 1989).

Probably reflecting the major role played in alcohol absorption and metabolism, problems in the *gastrointestinal (GI) system* are prevalent among alcoholics (Lieber, 1984; Frank and Raicht, 1985). These include irritation of the esophagus and stomach with resulting esophagitis and gastritis, probably the major causes of upper GI bleeds among alcohol abusers. Problems in the small bowel include the interference one can expect in the absorption of many vitamins and nutrients by ethanol, whereas large bowel difficulties are likely to include periods of diarrhea. Of course, alcohol contributes to pancreatitis (perhaps in 5 per cent of alcoholics). In the liver, the utilization of NAD as the hydrogen receptor with subsequent interference in gluconeogenesis and the accumulation of fatty acids produces numerous systemic effects. Local damage to the liver progresses from reversible stages of fatty infiltration of cells through an actual ballooning and damage of cells (alcoholic hepatitis as well as hyalin sclerosis), on to potentially severe scarring or cirrhosis with subsequent impairment in general functioning of the liver, and alteration in abdominal blood circulation with resulting ascites and a myriad of complications.

The *blood-producing* and *immune systems* are also potentially severely affected. The most common change in red blood cells (RBC's) is an increase in size or mean corpuscular volume (MCV), along with a possible mild anemia. Other forms of anemia, including sideroblastic changes, are more rare and are less likely to occur in the absence of severe malnutrition. Heavy drinking also decreases production of most white blood cells, decreases granulocyte mobility and adherence, and impairs a number of hypersensitivity responses. These changes as well as accompanying alterations in T cell activities might contribute to the very high risk for cancers observed in alcoholics. This is especially true for malignancies involving the head and neck (it is estimated that 70 per cent of cancers in this area above the epiglottis are seen in alcoholics), esophagus, breast, and stomach, factors contributing to the finding that cancers are the second leading causes of death in alcoholics.

Whereas one to two drinks per day in an otherwise healthy individual might be associated with a decreased risk for *cardiovascular* disease, there is evidence that intake over this level might contribute to vascular disease, the leading cause of death among alcoholics (Lang et al., 1985; Criqui, 1986; Saunders, 1987). The greater the alcohol intake, the greater the likelihood of high blood pressure, and it is estimated that heavy drinking is one of the major contributors to mild to moderate hypertension. As a striated muscle toxin, alcohol is also likely to produce heart muscle damage, and ethanol is felt to be the leading cause of idiopathic cardiomyopathy. In addition, higher alcohol levels increase the low density lipoproteins as well as triglycerides and might also contribute to the risk for cerebrovascular accidents (Donahue et al., 1986).

Additional important consequences of heavy drinking include temporary interference with *sexual functioning*, including impotence and testicular atrophy with persistent heavy drinking for men, and menstrual irregularities for women (Irwin et al., 1988). There are also a series of well-documented adverse effects on the developing fetus, which, in its full-blown form of the fetal alcohol syndrome, can include facial changes with epicanthal eye folds, poorly formed concha, small teeth with faulty enamel, cardiac atrial or ventricular septal defects, an aberrant palmar crease, microcephaly, and various levels of mental retardation (Morrow-Tlucak and Ernhart, 1987). Alcohol also contributes to skeletal myopathy characterized by painful and swollen muscles, high levels of muscle enzymes in the blood, and even myoglobinurea. Finally, in this brief review, effects on the *skeletal system* include alterations in calcium metabolism with an increased risk for fractures and osteonecrosis of the femoral head (Bikle et al., 1985).

Once primary alcoholism is diagnosed, the family physician can know a great deal about the potential clinical course. Severe alcohol-related problems alternating with periods of abstinence and short episodes of controlled drinking are likely to continue for many years, although as many as 20 per cent of alcoholics can reach permanent spontaneous remission from drinking. In the course of the heavy intake of alcohol, levels of temporary as well as severe organ impairment can ensue, and many of these factors can also be used in identifying the hidden alcoholic in practice as is outlined in the next section.

Treatment Issues

IDENTIFICATION AND CONFRONTATION OF THE ALCOHOLIC

It should be fairly obvious by this point that the physician should recognize that any patient might have alcoholism. By taking a history of alcohol-related life problems from the patient as well as a resource person, the majority of alcoholic individuals will be identified. However, for those individuals for whom a resource person is not available or when the history is incomplete, there are a number of laboratory tests that can be most helpful in identifying alcohol-abusing individuals (Schuckit and Irwin, 1988).

The first and most sensitive laboratory test is *gamma-glutamyl transferase* (GGT), an enzyme induced in the liver with consumption of five to six or more drinks daily and which has a 70 per cent sensitivity and similar specificity in identifying alcoholics (e.g., GGT blood levels of 40 or more units). Additional tests with slightly less impressive levels of sensitivity and specificity include a high-normal *MCV* (e.g., 90 to 95 cubic microns or higher), as well as an increase in *aspartate transaminase* (SGOT) or *alkaline phosphatase*. Serum *uric acid* levels greater than 7 mg. per dl. as well as *triglycerides* greater than 180 mg. per dl. or high levels of *high density lipoprotein* cholesterol in the absence of exercise are additional clues that a patient might be drinking heavily.

A number of clinical findings should also raise an index of suspicion that a patient might be alcoholic. These include mild and inconsistent levels of hypertension (e.g., 140/90), repeated infections such as pneumonias, and otherwise unexplained cardiac arrhythmias. Additional specific findings that should raise suspicion include cancer of the head and neck, esophagus, or cardia of the stomach as well as, of course, cirrhosis, unexplained hepatitis, pancreatitis, or peripheral neuropathies.

After an alcoholic has been identified, he or she should be confronted with the diagnosis. The presenting complaint can be used as an important entree to an alcohol problem. For instance, the patient complaining of insomnia or hypertension should be told that these are clinically important symptoms and that the laboratory tests and physical findings indicate that alcohol appears to have contributed to the problem. Continued drinking is likely to increase the risk for further medical and psychological difficulties. The physician should then share information about the course of alcoholism and explore possible avenues for attacking the problem.

The first confrontation could be met by the patient with any of several responses. For the patient who absolutely denies that he or she has a drinking problem, it is important to recognize that only rarely does a single confrontation result in important change. Rather, it is necessary to "keep the door open," inviting the patient back for further tests during which additional gentle but firm confrontations are carried out. It is wise to never give up, as many patients think about the confrontation between sessions and after several weeks or months may be willing to consider abstinence, especially after a severe life crisis.

A second potential response is that the patient recognizes that a problem might be present but desires to "cut down" on drinking. As noted previously, almost all alcoholics periodically spontaneously decrease their alcohol intake—the problem is not controlling but staying in control over an extended period of time. Thus, it should be pointed out that the individual has "cut down" many times in the past, but each effort resulted in a subsequent escalation of intake with severe life problems. Thus, controlled drinking does not work over an extended period of time. However, if the patient absolutely insists, a series of guidelines can be established for the patient and *spouse* whereby no more than two drinks (as defined earlier) can be consumed within a 24-hour period. The thought here is that if the individual sticks to the rule (which is very difficult), he or she cannot become intoxicated and problems are not likely to ensue. An additional benefit to this strategy is that the patient then commits himself or herself to controlling and can be urged to agree to try abstinence when the controlled drinking does not work over a long period of time.

The overall goal of all types of confrontation is to get the patient to agree to permanent abstinence. Once this has been acheived, steps are taken to help him or her focus on detoxification (if needed) and rehabilitation, as described in the following.

DETOXIFICATION PROCEDURES

In the presence of alcohol-induced cellular tolerance, any sudden decrease in ethanol can lead to symptoms of withdrawal from its CNS depressant effects. As with most syndromes, patients do not develop every symptom and the usual clinical picture is mild. More common features include a tremor of the hands (shakes or jitters); autonomic nervous system dysfunctions such as increases in pulse, respiratory rate, and body temperature; insomnia, possibly accompanied by bad dreams; feelings of generalized anxiety or panic attacks; and GI upset. Symptoms are likely to begin 5 to 10 hours after decreasing alcohol intake, peak in intensity on day 2 or 3, and improve by day 4 or 5. However, as part of a protracted abstinence picture, anxiety, insomnia, and mild levels of autonomic dysfunction may persist for 6 months or more. These continuing phenomena may contribute to the tendency to return to drinking.

Only about 5 per cent of alcoholics show evidence of severe withdrawal symptoms. These can include grand mal convulsions (usually generalized and rarely focal in nature and most often limited to one or at most two seizures), severe agitation, and intense confusion. Thus, less than 5 per cent of patients develop delirium tremens or DT's, a syndrome characterized by confusion (often with associated delusions and hallucinations), severe agitation, and seizures. It is probable that the likelihood of developing severe withdrawal or DT's is higher with concomitant medical disorders or very high prior levels of alcohol intake.

The treatment of withdrawal is predicted by the clinical picture. The *first* and most important step is to perform a thorough physical examination in all alcoholics. The *second* step is to recognize that even well-nourished middle-class alcoholics are likely to have problems absorbing vitamins from the proximal small intestine and thus require multiple B vitamins, especially 50 to 100 mg. of thiamine daily for a week or more. The *third* step is to recognize that the symptoms are primarily due to cellular adaptation to a CNS depressant followed by a rapid decrease in blood levels. Thus, symptoms can be alleviated by administering any brain depressant, using doses on day 1 that decrease symptoms (usually utilizing pulse and other autonomic symptoms as guidelines), and then decreasing the dose to zero over a 3- to 5-day period. Although any CNS depressant can be effective, the benzodiazepines have the highest margin of safety and are, therefore, the preferred class of drug for the treatment of alcohol withdrawal. Short half-life benzodiazepines (e.g., oxazepam or lorazepam) may be especially useful for patients with liver impairment or pre-existent brain damage, but these drugs must be administered every 4 hours and it is possible that skipping a dose could actually precipitate seizures. Therefore, most clinicians use the longer half-life drugs (e.g., diazepam or chlordiazepoxide), prescribing, for example, 25 mg. of chlordiazepoxide or 10 mg. of diazepam orally every 4 to 6 hours on the first day, decreasing the dose by at least 20 per cent of the original day's dose over each subsequent 24 hours.

The most effective treatment for severe withdrawal such as the DT's remains controversial. It is probable that the state of confusion and agitation will persist for 3 to 5 days regardless of the pharmacologic intervention used, and drugs are given primarily to control behavior rather than to change the course of the syndrome. Many clinicians recommend using benzodiazepines, and doses as large as 300 mg. or more per day of chlordiazepoxide are sometimes required. Other physicians use antipsychotic medications such as thioridazine or haloperidol to control behavior, although these types of drugs have no place in the treatment of mild withdrawal symptoms.

For the usual mild to moderate severity withdrawal, vitamins, general supports, and the judicious use of benzodiazepines are all that is required. Most patients present for treatment in an overhydrated—not dehydrated—state, and, thus, intravenous fluids are rarely needed. Similarly, when seizures or "rum fits" appear, they are usually single and most often respond to benzodiazepine; thus, there is little evidence that anticonvulsants such as phenytoin are effective.

Although alcohol withdrawal is often treated in a hospital, efforts at reducing health care costs have resulted in increasing levels of data about the appropriateness of the outpatient detoxification for alcoholics with mild abstinence syndromes (Hayashida et al., 1989). This is appropriate for patients in good physical condition who demonstrate mild signs of withdrawal despite low BAL's and for those without prior histories of DT's or withdrawal seizures. Such individuals still require a careful physical examination, evaluation of blood tests, vitamin supplementation, and appropriate doses of a benzodiazepine. The drug is given in a *1- to 2-day supply* and should be administered by the patient or spouse four times a day. Patients are asked to *return daily* for evaluation of vital signs, and the patient's family or friends are told to bring him or her to the emergency room if signs and symptoms of severe withdrawal escalate.

Finally, many municipalities have opted to take advantage of the relatively mild intensity of withdrawal symptoms by establishing "social model" detoxification programs. Here, monies are saved by offering a minimal amount of medical care and no prescription medications. Thus, in the optimal setting, patients are screened to rule out severe medical problems, recent seizures, or histories of severe DT's—such more severely impaired individuals are referred to an inpatient medically oriented treatment program. The remainder of patients are given nutrition, vitamins, the opportunity to rest, and a supportive environment in which reassurance and education help them to minimize the levels of discomfort that they experience.

REHABILITATION

Alcoholics who agree to enter treatment can be referred to inpatient or outpatient programs. In general, most rehabilitation efforts follow the general guidelines of increasing the level of motivation for abstinence and helping the patient to re-establish a life style free of alcohol. There is little convincing evidence that one type of program is superior to any other, nor are there well-documented guidelines to help the clinician decide whether to use inpatient or outpatient rehabilitation.

Reflecting the fact that inpatient care is much more expensive, outpatient rehabilitation is attractive. There are common sense guidelines that can help determine those individuals for whom the more intrusive and expensive inpatient care might be more appropriate. These include hospitalization if (1) the patient has medical problems that are difficult to treat outside a hospital; (2) there is enough depression or confusion or other psychiatric symptoms to interfere with outpatient care; (3) the patient has such severe life crises that it is difficult to deal with him or her as an outpatient; (4) outpatient treatment has been attempted but failed; or (5) the patient lives too far from the treatment center to participate in outpatient care. If an inpatient program is required, it would make sense that those with more severe medical problems might be treated in a program associated with a medical facility, those with more severe psychiatric difficulties might be preferentially referred to programs associated with a psychiatric unit, and the remaining patients might be most cost-effectively dealt with in a freestanding facility.

Whether carried out in an inpatient or outpatient setting, efforts aimed at increasing levels of motivation for abstinence include lectures to the patients and families regarding the individual's responsibility for his or her own actions and the course of life problems that can be expected if drinking continues (i.e., the natural history of alcoholism). Motivation is also enhanced through association with AA for the patient and affiliated family groups for the spouse (AlAnon) as well as for the children (Alateen). As part of group counseling or therapy sessions that occur almost daily, patients are repeatedly reminded of the issues of responsibility and problems likely to be experienced in the future.

Patients are also taught how to readjust to a life without alcohol. Important topics for discussion in group counseling include how to occupy free time now that alcohol is no longer an option, how to deal with friends and colleagues who insist that alcohol should not be a problem and the individual should return to drinking, mechanisms for dealing with anger in the spouse and children as well as other relatives, how to deal with job and other environmental stressors that have in the past been dealt with by heavy drinking, and so on. Thus, most groups focus on relatively superficial day-to-day life experiences. This is a process that is begun on a multiple time per week basis during the inpatient or most intensive outpatient mode, but one that must be continued for at least 6 months or longer on at least a once a week basis as part of aftercare. Of course, affiliation with AA offers the individual the model of many people who have been through similar experiences, gives a sober peer group, and for those who so desire, offers a series of steps to be followed in not only staying sober but rebuilding a more fulfilling life.

With the exception of vitamins and short-term use of benzodiazepines during acute withdrawal, the role of medications in alcoholic rehabilitation is extremely limited. As part of a protracted abstinence syndrome, most alcoholics will experience decreasing levels of sleep problems and anxiety symptoms for 3 to 6 months after abstinence is achieved. These can be dealt with through education, reassurance that improvement will occur, and behavior modification through which patients are discouraged from naps, advised to avoid caffeinated beverages in the evening, told to establish a regular retiring and awakening time (behavioral approaches that will improve sleeping patterns), and counseled on how to recognize early signs of escalating anxiety and experiment with alternative behaviors for anxiety release (e.g., exercise, hobbies, meditation, biofeedback). There is *no place* for sleeping pills or antianxiety drugs in the treatment of the average primary alcoholic after acute withdrawal is completed. Similarly, it is likely that no higher a percentage of alcoholics will require antidepressant medications, lithium, or antianxiety drugs than is true in the general population.

One medication that has been used in alcohol rehabilitation is disulfiram (Antabuse), usually prescribed in doses of 250 mg. per day. Unfortunately, this medication has dangers of potential contribution to neuropathies as well as irreversible liver failure, and it is possible that disulfiram contributes to the risk for cardiovascular disease. Recent extensive clinical trials have been unable to document the superiority of disulfiram over placebo (Fuller et al., 1986). Thus, in light of the lack of convincing evidence of efficacy and the documentation of risks for this drug, as well as the possibility of a severe reaction to alcohol while on the medication, it is difficult to recommend this agent for the average patient. It is probable that the use of disulfiram should be reserved for individuals who have shown that it is only on this drug that they have been able to maintain abstinence in the past, or those for whom other treatments have been unsuccessful.

In summary, confrontation, detoxification, and rehabilitation of our alcohol-abusing patients is an important part of the daily practice of family medicine. It is in our own best interests as well as those of our patients to learn how to utilize the past history, pattern of laboratory results, and series of medical problems to identify those individuals who are likely to fulfill criteria for alcoholism. Once a careful history taken from the patient and resource person establishes the presence of this important diagnosis, repeated firm but gentle confrontations are often required to get the individual to admit that intervention is appropriate. The next step in this process is to carry out appropriate detoxification measures, although many alcoholics can be treated as outpatients following a good physical examination and with the judicious use of vitamins and short-term prescription of a benzodiazepine. Rehabilitation follows a series of common sense guidelines and frequently succeeds. The characteristics of the patient are often the best indicators of the outcome, and there are ample data to conclude that for those individuals with families and jobs who are willing to admit their alcoholism and enter a rehabilitation program, between two thirds and three quarters are likely to achieve and maintain long-term abstinence. When clinicians ignore the alcohol-related life problems and do not carry out the procedures necessary for an effective *series* of confrontations, difficulties are likely to continue, the patient is likely to experience deterioration in social functioning and in multiple body systems, and the life span can be significantly shortened.

Nicotine Addiction

Robert E. Rakel
Alan Blum

The power of nicotine addiction became clear when I saw malnourished and hungry people trading food rations for cigarettes.

WILLIAM FOEGE, M.D. (1989), commenting on refugee camps during the Nigerian Civil War.

Tobacco smoking leads to a dependence on nicotine that is indistinguishable from other forms of drug dependence. The diagnostic manual of the American Psychiatric Association (DSM III-R) classifies tobacco dependence as an addiction. In such a dependency, the drug is needed to maintain an optimal state of well-being. Nicotine, the habituating constituent of tobacco, meets the criteria for addiction, since a typical withdrawal syndrome occurs after smoking cessation.

Cigarette smoking is the chief avoidable cause of death in our society. Each year smoking is responsible for 18 per cent of the total deaths in the United States. This is seven times more Americans than were killed in the Vietnam war. "Clearly, smoking has killed more Americans during this century than were killed in battle or died of war-related diseases in all wars ever fought by this nation" (Pollin and Ravenholt, 1984).

Approximately 40 per cent of all deaths from cancer are caused by smoking. In 1985 an estimated 3.6 million years of potential life lost resulted from smoking (MMWR, 1988).

More young women than young men smoke cigarettes and in 1986 lung cancer passed breast cancer as the leading cause of cancer death in women.

Although cigarette smoking among adults declined from 42 per cent to 29 per cent in the United States between 1964 and 1987 (following publication of the Surgeon General's first report on smoking and health in 1964), 32 per cent of men and 27 per cent of women continue to use tobacco daily. Approximately 1.3 million persons per year stop smoking. However, each day approximately 3000 individuals start smoking, most of whom are young (Pierce et al., 1989). Half of high-school seniors who smoke started by age 14 years. Almost half of all smokers born since 1935 started smoking before 18 years of age. Although 80 per cent of those who smoke say they would like to stop, only 20 per cent of those who try actually succeed in stopping for good. The likelihood of success in stopping increases with the number of attempts, and those with a college education are twice as likely to break the habit as are less educated smokers.

In 1964 only a single life insurance company, State Mutual of Massachusetts, offered a reduced price to nonsmokers. Today, virtually all life insurance companies, even those owned by tobacco conglomerates, now offer significant discounts to persons who do not smoke. Actuarial data leave little doubt that the average life expectancy of a 32-year-old man who smokes cigarettes is 72 years, compared with 79 years for someone who does not smoke. Smoking-related chronic obstructive pulmonary disease is the largest cause of disability payments, and lung cancer is no longer a rarity among men and women in their 40's.

Cancer

Forty per cent of all cancer deaths are attributable to cigarette smoking. Besides lung cancer, smoking is the major cause of cancers of the larynx, oral cavity, and esophagus. It is a contributory factor in cancers of the pancreas, bladder, kidney, stomach, and uterine cervix. A dose-response relationship exists between smoking and all of these.

Lung. Male smokers are 22 times more likely to develop lung cancer and female smokers are 12 times more likely when compared with these who never smoked. There is a clear dose-response relationship between lung cancer risk and daily cigarette consumption, and those who smoke more than a pack of cigarettes a day have a risk that is at least 20 times that of nonsmokers.

Unfortunately, early detection does not improve the survival rate for lung cancer. The 5-year survival rate is less than 10 per cent and has not changed since the early 1960's. However, the risk of death from lung cancer is reduced when smoking is discontinued.

Larynx. The risk for laryngeal cancer is 20 to 30 times greater in the smoker. Seventy per cent of oral and 85 per cent of laryngeal cancer deaths are directly attributable to smoking.

Esophagus. Cigarette smoking is a factor in over half of the cases of esophageal cancer, and the 5-year survival is only about 3 per cent. Heavy smokers (more than one pack per day) have 10 times the mortality from esophageal cancer as do nonsmokers.

Pancreas. An equally dismal picture occurs with cancer of the pancreas, for which the 5-year survival rate is only 2 per cent. Because of the nonspecific nature of presenting symptoms and the difficulty of making a diagnosis, the mean survival time after diagnosis is less than 6 months. Smokers have two to three times the risk of pancreatic cancer as do nonsmokers, and the risk is proportional to the amount smoked.

Cervix Uteri and Ovary. Women who smoke cigarettes have four times the risk of nonsmokers of developing cervical cancer. Even women who smoke only 100 cigarettes during their lifetimes more than double their risk of cervical cancer. The risk from smoking is greater in women under 30 years of age than in those older than 30 years (Slattery et al., 1989).

Constituents from cigarette smoke are distributed by the blood throughout the body and have been detected in the cervical mucus of smokers at levels 40 to 50 times those in the serum.

The risk of ovarian cancer is three times greater in women who smoke cigarettes (Qian et al., 1989).

Bladder and Kidney. Forty per cent of bladder cancers are smoking related, and higher rates of kidney cancers are also noted among smokers. Smokers have three to four times the risk of developing bladder cancer than do people who never smoked. The kidneys and bladder are the final common pathway for the concentration of the toxic products of tobacco smoke and provide the longest direct exposure to carcinogens and radioactive substances, such as polonium-210 (^{210}Po), in tobacco smoke.

Leukemia. A greater than 50 per cent increased mortality from leukemia occurs in cigarette smokers (relative risk 1.53) and the response is dose-related. Those smoking more than one pack per day have a twofold increased risk (Kinlen and Rogot, 1988).

Chronic Obstructive Pulmonary Disease (COPD)

Cigarette smoking is the main cause of chronic obstructive pulmonary disea se, which is the leading cause of disability in the United States. Changes in bronchi and the lung parenchyma are proportional to the amount of smoke inhaled. Cigarette smoke inhibits ciliary activity of the bronchial epithelium and the phagocytic activity of macrophages in the alveoli. This results in the decreased clearance of foreign material and bacteria from the lung, which leads to increased infection and tissue destruction (Fig. 68–1).

Cardiovascular Disease

Coronary Heart Disease. Nicotine raises systolic blood pressure, heart rate, and cardiac output and causes vasoconstriction. The relationship between cerebral vasoconstriction and anoxia associated with carbon monoxide due to cigarette smoking could explain the 50 per cent increase in automobile accidents in smokers. The symptoms associated with carbon monoxide intoxication can be a problem, especially for persons with an already compromised coronary circulation. Carbon monoxide has an affinity for hemoglobin (forming carboxyhemoglobin) that is 245 times stronger than that of oxygen. Thus, it reduces oxygen delivery to the myocardium and has a decidedly negative inotropic effect. Carboxyhemoglobin also lowers the threshold for ventricular fibrillation and could explain the higher incidence of sudden death in those who smoke.

The risk of myocardial infarction is proportional to the number of cigarettes smoked. The trend toward the use of filter cigarettes does not appear to have reduced the risk of coronary heart disease. Theoretically, filter cigarettes reduce the amount of tar (the condensate of tobacco smoke that includes over 3000 compounds including more than 40 carcinogens), but they may increase the amount of carbon monoxide, thus contributing to the increased mortality from coronary heart disease. Persons who smoke cigarettes containing low amounts of nicotine have the same degree of risk of myocardial infarction as do those who smoke cigarettes containing larger amounts. Smokers of these low-dose cigarettes still have three times the risk of myocardial infarction as do nonsmokers (Kaufman et al., 1983). The good news is

390,000 Deaths Attributable to Cigarette Smoking

United States, 1985

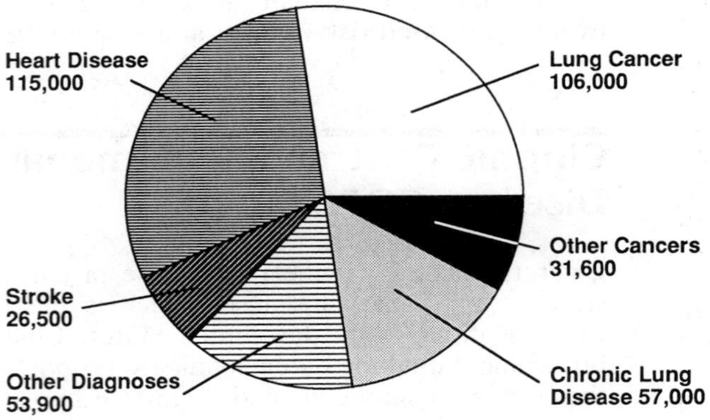

Figure 68–1. Smoking is responsible for more than one of every six deaths in the United States. It remains the single most important preventable cause of death in our society. (From U.S. Dept. of Health and Human Services, Office of Smoking and Health.)

that the risk of sudden death decreases immediately upon stopping and the risk of myocardial infarction decreases within a few years of stopping to a level similar to that in men who have never smoked. This is true even in heavy smokers who have a positive family history of coronary heart disease (Rosenberg et al., 1985).

Three fourths of myocardial infarctions in women below the age of 50 years have been attributed to smoking (Slone et al., 1978). The Chief Medical Examiner of Dade County, Florida, states that a woman between 40 and 50 years of age who dies suddenly is by definition a cigarette smoker until proven otherwise (Davis, 1977). The risk of myocardial infarction increases progressively, to as much as 20-fold in persons smoking 35 or more cigarettes per day. There is no safe level of smoking. Women who smoke only one to four cigarettes a day have 2.5 times greater risk of coronary heart disease. Women who smoke and use oral contraceptives have a risk of heart attack that is 10 times greater than women who do neither.

Silent ischemia probably comprises the majority of all cardiac ischemic events. Patients with coronary heart disease who smoke have three times as many episodes of silent ischemia as do nonsmokers, and the duration of each is 12 times longer (Barry et al., 1989). Frequent episodes of myocardial ischemia, even though asymptomatic, must damage the heart. Since smoking also increases platelet adhesiveness and lowers HDL cholesterol, the association with a higher incidence of myocardial infarction is no surprise.

Benefits from stopping smoking can be demonstrated at all ages. There is no decrease in benefit as one gets older, so it is still worthwhile for someone over age 65 to break the addiction (Hermanson et al., 1988). This benefit can be demonstrated in the cerebral as well as the coronary circulation. Elderly individuals who stop smoking have significantly higher cerebral perfusion levels than do those who continue to smoke. Even those who have smoked for 30 or 40 years have improved cerebral circulation within a relatively short time after stopping smoking (Rogers et al., 1985).

Persons who smoke more than one pack of cigarettes a day are four times more likely to develop Alzheimer's disease than are nonsmokers. As with other smoking-related diseases, this one is also dose-dependent; those smoking less than one pack a day are at 1.6 times the risk.

Stroke. Stroke is the third most common cause of death in the United States. Although hypertension is the greatest risk factor for stroke, cigarette smoking also is a significant factor. The incidence of stroke among smokers is 50 per cent higher than among nonsmokers (40 per cent higher in men and 60 per cent higher among women) (Wolf et al., 1988).

The risk of stroke increases in proportion to the amount of smoking; it is twice as great in those who smoke more than 40 cigarettes per day than in those smoking less than 10 cigarettes per day.

Compared with women who have never smoked, the risk of stroke increases from 2.2-fold in women smoking one to 14 cigarettes per day to 3.7-fold in women smoking 25 or more cigarettes daily (Colditz et al., 1988). A clear dose-response relationship has also been noted by Bonita and associates (1986). They found a threefold increase in the risk of stroke in smokers compared with nonsmokers (Fig. 68–2). The risk is 5.6 times higher in persons smoking more than one pack of cigarettes daily. Cigarette smokers who are also hypertensive have a 20-fold increased risk of stroke.

Smoking may increase the likelihood of thrombosis by increasing the serum fibrinogen, by enhancing platelet aggregation, and by increasing blood viscosity.

The risk of stroke declines rapidly after cessation of smoking and after 5 years is at the level of nonsmokers. This emphasizes that it is never too late to quit no matter how long someone has been smoking.

Subarachnoid Hemorrhage. Habitual smoking increases the risk of subarachnoid hemorrhage 3.9 times for men and 3.7 times for women. The risk

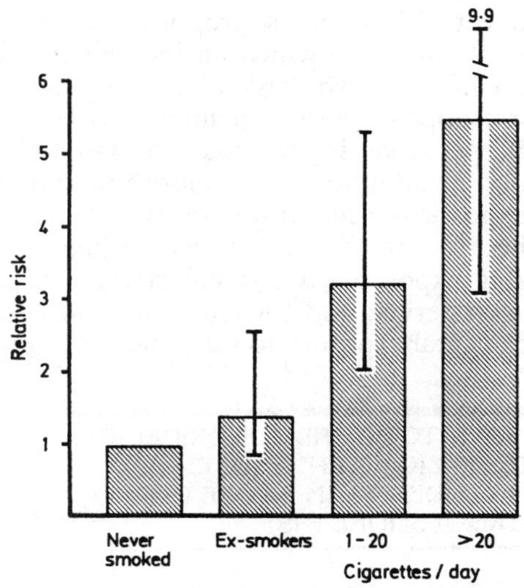

Figure 68–2. Cigarette smoking and risk of stroke, adjusted for age and sex. Bars and 95 per cent confidence limits. (Bonita, R., Scragg, R., and Stewart, A. Br. Med. J., *293*:6–8, 1986.)

increases to 22 times that of nonsmokers in women who both smoke and use oral contraceptives (Bell and Symon, 1979).

One theory is that structural damage occurs in the wall of cerebral vessels, causing aneurysms that are more likely to rupture. In a meta-analysis review of all available data regarding cigarette smoking and stroke, Shinton and Beevers (1989) confirmed the 50 per cent increased risk of stroke associated with cigarette smoking and found that the risk of subarachnoid hemorrhage tripled and was greater in women than in men.

Filter Cigarettes

A mistaken popular belief is that filtered brands of cigarettes (which now comprise more than 97 per cent of those sold in the United States) are safer than nonfiltered cigarettes. Low-tar and low-nicotine filter cigarettes are now advertised widely. Since the addiction is to nicotine, people who smoke low-nicotine cigarettes undergo "compensatory smoking," in which they inhale more frequently and more deeply, in order to maintain their blood nicotine levels. As a result, the tar intake also increases, changing a low-tar cigarette to the high-tar category. Smokers who take 14 puffs per cigarette receive 58 per cent more tar than those taking the standard 8.7 puffs per cigarette. Some manufacturers include perforations in the filter to dilute the smoke with air, advertising these as ultra-low-tar cigarettes. Many smokers, however, block the holes with their lips or their fingers in order to obtain undiluted smoke with a higher concentration of nicotine (Kozlowski et al., 1980).

Cigarettes with reduced yields of nicotine and carbon monoxide are not safer. The fourfold increased risk of myocardial infarction does not vary according to the nicotine content, and the degree of risk is proportionate to the number of cigarettes smoked (Palmer et al., 1989).

Nicotine blood levels are similar for cigarette smokers, pipe smokers, and users of snuff, despite the different methods of absorption. Long-term users of snuff have a 50-fold increased risk for cancer of the cheek and gum (Koop and Luoto, 1982).

Smokeless Tobacco

There are two types of smokeless tobacco: snuff, which is dry or moist, and chewing (spitting) tobacco, which comes as loose-leaf, plug, or twist. Use of these substances increases the frequency of oral-pharyngeal cancers and gum recession. Leukoplakia is found in 18 to 64 per cent of users (Connolly et al., 1986).

A large percentage of the 10 million users of smokeless tobacco in the United States are male adolescents who mistakenly feel this is a relatively safe alternative to smoking. Most users start at 10 to 12 years of age (Evans, 1988) (Fig. 68–3).

Smokeless tobacco contains the same carcinogens as cigarette tobacco but some of them in much greater concentration. Nitrosamines, which are powerful chemical carcinogens, are present at levels up to 14,000 times higher than the federal government allows in bacon and beer (Connolly et al., 1986).

Involuntary (Passive) Smoking

The effects of tobacco on nonsmokers (passive smoking) can be significant. An estimated 15 per cent of the American public is allergic to cigarette smoke. Two thirds of the smoke from a burning cigarette never reaches a smoker's lungs, but instead goes directly into the air. *Sidestream smoke* is that which is emitted into the air from a smoldering cigarette between puffs, whereas *mainstream smoke* is that which the smoker inhales directly during puffing. Although diluted by air prior to being inhaled, sidestream smoke contains greater amounts of toxic substances than does mainstream smoke because of a lower combustion temperature and lack of filtration through the cigarette (Table 68–1).

A nonsmoker who spends one hour in a smoke-filled car on a commuter train inhales as much as if he or she had smoked nine filter cigarettes (Aronow, 1979). It has been estimated that a nonsmoking musician who plays in a smoke-filled club and lives with a chain-smoking roommate inhales the equivalent of 27 cigarettes a day.

Hirayama (1981) demonstrated the increased risk of lung cancer in nonsmoking housewives exposed to the second-hand cigarette smoke of their husbands (Fig. 68–4). The risk from passive smoking was one

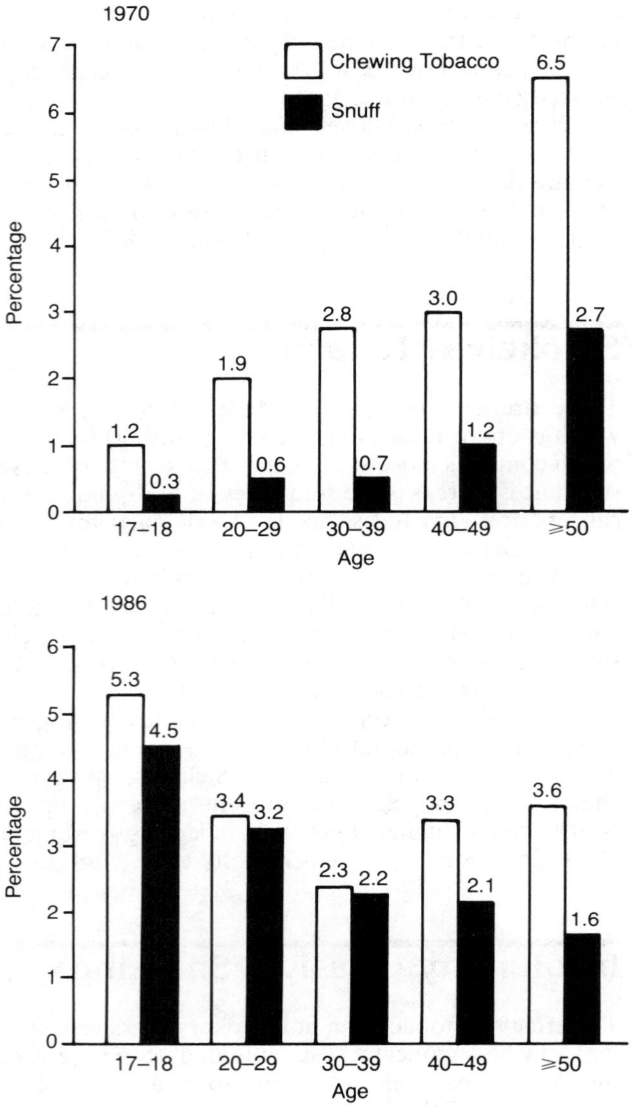

Figure 68–3. Prevalence of chewing tobacco and snuff use among men, 1970 (NHIS) and 1986 (AUTS). (From U.S. Dept. of Health and Human Services.)

half to one third that of direct smoking. A direct dose-response relationship was observed, with the annual mortality from lung cancer being 8.7 per 100,000 for women whose husbands smoked only occasionally and 18.1 per 100,000 for those whose husbands smoked 20 or more cigarettes daily. The wives of heavy smokers had a twofold greater risk of dying from lung cancer than did wives of nonsmoking men. Their risk was half that of women smokers.

A similar study in Sweden found that women with husbands who smoke have three times the risk of developing lung cancer compared with wives of nonsmoking husbands (Pershagen et al., 1987). To date, 14 studies have shown an association between being married to a smoker and having an increased risk of lung cancer. Overall, about one third of lung cancers occur in nonsmokers living with smokers.

Cancer risk appears proportional to the total amount of smoke to which an individual is exposed during a lifetime. The risk of developing cancer of any form appears dose-dependent, increasing by at least 50 per cent in persons exposed only during childhood or adulthood, and more than doubling for those exposed during both periods.

The risk of cancer increases significantly with increasing exposure. It is greatest for cancer of the breast and cervix, and for leukemia and lymphoma. Transplacental exposure to substances absorbed from

Table 68–1. TOXIC AND TUMORIGENIC AGENTS OF CIGARETTE SMOKE; RATIO OF SIDESTREAM SMOKE (SS) TO MAINSTREAM SMOKE (MS)

	Amount per Cigarette		Ratio of Sidestream to Mainstream Smoke
Gas Phase			
Carbon dioxide	10–80	mg	8.1*
Carbon monoxide	0.5–26	mg	2.5*
Nitrogen oxides (NO_x)	16–600	μg	4.7–5.8
Ammonia	10–130	μg	44–73
Hydrogen cyanide	280–550	μg	0.17–0.37
Hydrazine	32	μg	3
Formaldehyde	20–90	μg	51
Acetone	100–940	μg	2.5–3.2
Acrolein	10–140	μg	12
Acetonitrile	60–160	μg	10
Pyridine	32	μg	10
3-Vinylpyridine	23	μg	28
N-Nitrosodimethylamine	4–180	ng	10–830
N-Nitrosoethylmethylamine	1.0–40	ng	5–12
N-Nitrosodiethylamine	0.1–28	ng	4–25
N-Nitrosopyrrolidine	0–110	ng	3–76
Particulate Phase			
Total particulate phase	0.1–40	mg	1.3–1.9*
Nicotine	0.06–2.3	mg	2.6–3.3*
Toluene	108	μg	5.6
Phenol	20–150	μg	2.6
Catechol	40–280	μg	0.7
Stigmasterol	53	μg	0.8
Total phytosterols	130	μg	0.8
Naphthalene	2.8	μg	16
1-Methylnaphthalene	1.2	μg	26
2-Methylnaphthalene	1.0	μg	29
Phenanthrene	2.0–80	μg	2.1
Benz(a)anthracene	10–70	μg	2.7
Pyrene	15–90	ng	1.9–3.6
Benzo(a)pyrene	8–40	ng	2.7–3.4
Quinoline	1.7	μg	11
Methylquinoline	6.7	μg	11
Harmane	1.1–3.1	μg	0.7–2.7
Norharmane	3.2–8.1	μg	1.4–4.3
Aniline	100–1200	ng	30
α-Toluidine	32	ng	19
1-Naphthylamine	1.0–22	ng	39
2-Naphthylamine	4.3–27	ng	39
4-Aminobiphenyl	2.4–4.6	ng	31
N'-Nitrosonornicotine	0.2–3.7	μg	1–5
NNK†	0.12–0.44	μg	1–8
N'-Nitrosoanatabine	0.15–4.6	μg	1–7
N-Nitrosodiethanolamine	0–40	ng	1.2

From The Health Consequences of Smoking: Cancer. A Report of the Surgeon General. DHHS Publication No. (PHS) 82-50179. Rockville, MD, U.S. Department of Health and Human Services, Public Health Service, Office on Smoking and Health, 1982.

*In cigarettes with perforated filter tips, the SS/MS ratio rises with increasing air dilution. In the case of smoke dilution with air to 17 per cent, the SS/MS ratios for TPM rise to 2.14, CO_2 36.5, CO 23.5, and nicotine to 13.1.

†NNK, 4-(methylnitrosamino)-1-(3-pyridyl)-butanone.

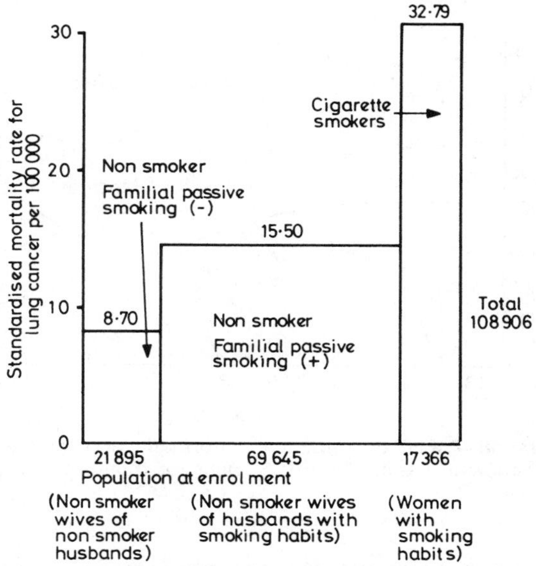

Figure 68–4. Lung cancer mortality in women according to presence or absence of direct and familial indirect smoking. (From Hirayama, T.: Nonsmoking wives of heavy smokers have a higher risk of lung cancer: A study from Japan. Br. Med. J., *282*:1983, 1981.)

the mother's smoking during pregnancy may predispose the infant to cancer later in life (Sandler et al., 1985b).

Passive smoking increases the risk of cervical cancer. Slattery and associates (1989) found that passive exposure to smoke for 3 hours a day increases the risk of a woman's developing cervical cancer 3.43 times. One hour of passive smoking exposes the person to carcinogenic nitrosamines equivalent to smoking one half a pack of filtered cigarettes. Thus, the risk of cancer from passive smoking can be as great as that from personal cigarette smoking.

The risks of passive smoking extend far beyond cancer. It is estimated that tobacco smoke in the home and workplace could be responsible for the deaths of 46,000 nonsmokers annually in the United States. Most of these (32,000) are due to heart disease, making passive smoking the third leading preventable cause of death after alcohol and smoking itself. It is estimated that the risk of myocardial infarction is three times higher for a woman whose husband smokes (Wells, 1988).

Effects on Children. Parents who smoke are more likely to have children who will take up smoking. Indeed, 75 per cent of those who smoke cigarettes had at least one parent who smoked. The risk of a child's taking up smoking doubles with each additional adult family member who smokes. Children of smoking parents are also innocent victims (involuntary smokers) and have been shown to be more likely to suffer from bronchitis and pneumonia during their first year of life and otitis media when older. Numerous studies have shown that they have an increased incidence of cough, bronchitis, and pneumonia that is proportional to the number of cigarettes smoked by the parents, particularly the mother. Asthma is also more prevalent in children whose mothers smoke, and their stature is retarded in proportion to the number of smokers in the home (Rantakallio, 1978). Passive smoking has also been blamed for some instances of sudden infant death syndrome (SIDS).

Small children are victimized more by passive smoking than are adults. Because of more rapid breathing, they inhale larger amounts of harmful substances. Children exposed to their parents' cigarette smoke have six times the average number of respiratory infections. They also have deficits in growth and in intellectual and emotional development, as well as more behavior disorders.

The risk of cancer is increased by 50 per cent in children of men who smoke. The risk of a child developing hematopoietic cancer is 4.6 times greater if both parents smoke (Sandler et al., 1985a).

Pregnancy. A dose-response relationship also exists during pregnancy. The more a pregnant woman smokes, the lower the infant's birth weight is likely to be. On the average, babies born to women who smoke during pregnancy are 200 grams lighter than those of comparable nonsmokers (Fig. 68–5). Heavy smokers have a 130 per cent increased incidence of newborns weighing less than 2500 grams. However, a woman who gives up smoking by her fourth month of gestation will have the same risk as a nonsmoker. The term "fetal tobacco syndrome" provides a label for fetal growth retardation when (1) the mother smoked five or more cigarettes a day throughout the pregnancy; (2) there was no evidence of hypertension in the mother; (3) the newborn has symmetrical growth retardation; and (4) no other cause of intrauterine growth retardation is obvious (Nieburg et al., 1985).

The risk of spontaneous abortion in heavy smokers is 1.7 times that for nonsmokers. Smoking during pregnancy increases the incidence of abruptio placen-

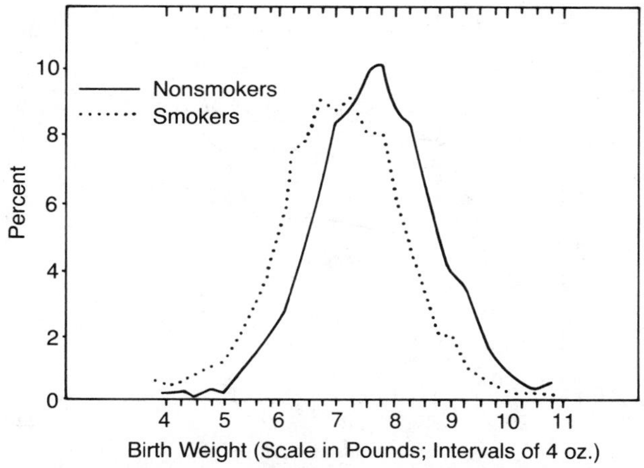

Figure 68–5. Percentage distribution by birth weight of infants of mothers who did not smoke during pregnancy and of those who smoked one pack or more of cigarettes per day. (From U.S. Dept. of Health and Human Services.)

tae, placenta previa, bleeding during pregnancy, and premature rupture of the membranes. It also increases the incidence of premature births and perinatal deaths (Fig. 68–6). Obviously, pregnancy is an opportune time for the family physician to encourage women to discontinue smoking.

About 25 per cent of women who smoke at the beginning of their pregnancy will stop on their own sometime during the nine months. Aggressive intervention programs by physicians could influence another 30 per cent to stop. The greatest effort should be directed toward pregnant unmarried white women, since they are 40 per cent more likely to smoke than are nonpregnant white women (Williamson et al., 1989).

There is strong experimental evidence that maternal smoking causes fetal hypoxia. This could explain the increased incidence of congenital abnormalities noted in babies of smokers (Fig. 68–7). The offspring of mothers who smoke during the three months before or after conception are twice as likely to have a cleft palate compared with those of nonsmokers (Khoury et al., 1989).

Reduced fertility is also a problem in women who smoke cigarettes. Smokers are three to four times more likely to take longer than one year to conceive, and heavy smokers have more difficulty than do light smokers. Spermatozoa from smokers also show more morphologic abnormalities and decreased mobility compared with nonsmokers.

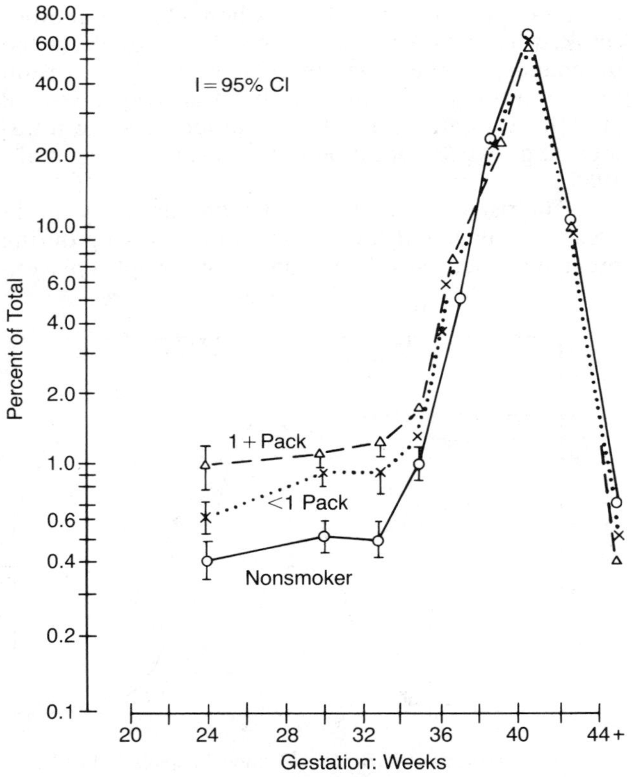

Figure 68–6. Percentage distribution by weeks of gestation of births to nonsmokers, smokers of less than one pack per day, and smokers of one pack per day or more. (From U.S. Dept. of Health and Human Services.)

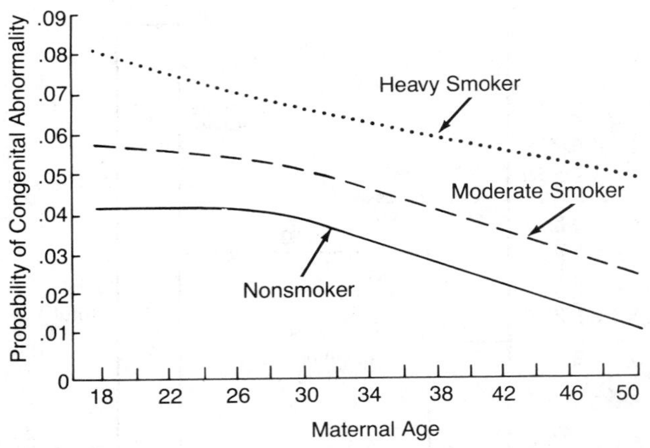

Figure 68–7. Risk of congenital abnormality according to age and smoking habit. (From U.S. Dept. of Health and Human Services.)

The Anti-Smoking Movement

A remarkable grassroots anti-smoking movement that arose in the 1970's has had a major impact on the goal of achieving a smoke-free society and has impelled more traditional health organizations such as the American Medical Association to become more outspoken. The first medical organization to develop office-based and community-wide strategies against tobacco use and promotion was Doctors Ought to Care (DOC), started in 1977 by a family physician at the University of Miami (Blum, 1980).

Other important organizations worthy of the health professional's support include the Coalition on Smoking or Health, a Washington lobbying group composed of the American Cancer Society, American Lung Association, and American Heart Association; Americans for Nonsmokers' Rights, Berkeley, CA;. Action on Smoking and Health (ASH, the oldest and foremost legal resource of the anti-smoking movement located in Washington, DC); the Tobacco Products Liability Project located at Northeastern University School of Law; and local groups of GASP (Group Against Smoking Pollution).

Support comes from a large variety of diverse sources including the comic strip Doonesbury in which a job applicant to a tobacco company blows his chances for employment because he cannot say "Cigarettes do not cause cancer" without laughing.

Smoking Cessation*

Ideally, validity of the abstinence rate for a smoking-cessation method should rest on the performance of

*Method of Alan Blum.

a controlled, double-blind study in which there is a follow-up of at least 6 months' duration of all subjects who started out (Schwartz, 1969, 1979, 1987). Few published outcome evaluations meet such criteria. Despite insufficient evidence to back up their advertised claims of success, expensive commercial aids and clinics for smoking cessation proliferate. The methods include acupuncture, hypnotherapy, biofeedback, rapid smoking, special filters, diets, self-help books and tape cassettes, pocket calculators for keeping track of cigarettes, aversive conditioning with electric shock, and a host of chemical remedies including local anesthetic agents, tranquilizers, nicotine substitutes, and nicotine itself in various forms. Many methods are quite costly, but having to pay a high fee for an alleged smoking cure may be the most motivating aspect of the method's success.

The physician's active involvement in smoking cessation, akin to his or her role in the prevention of smoking among teenagers and children, can be extremely crucial in and of itself. More than a decade ago, at a time when efforts to discourage smoking were much less widespread and accepted, Russell and colleagues (1979) found that 1 to 2 minutes of simple but unequivocal advice on the part of the physician to stop smoking resulted in a cessation rate of over 5 per cent measured at 1 year, as opposed to only 0.3 per cent in the control group. Moreover, when strong advice is given at the time of recovery from a heart attack or other smoking-related disease (combined with a brochure and a promise of follow-up), over 60 per cent stop smoking and stay off cigarettes—measured at 3 years—more than twice the rate of those who receive less definitive advice (Burt et al., 1974).

Although many people are saying they have simply stopped on their own, such individuals may not consciously attribute their success to the increasing social pressures that reinforced their decision. Indeed, efforts to curtail tobacco use have become a cornerstone of nationwide health promotion efforts, in large measure attributable to the outspokenness of former Surgeon General C. Everett Koop. Not only has organized medicine become united in the past few years on the need for more assertive office-based and community-wide strategies to end smoking, but other forces in society including large corporations and governmental agencies have also implemented smoke-free policies.

OBSTACLES TO CHANGE

At the same time, cigarette advertisers, whose livelihoods depend on maintaining the dependence of more than 50 million Americans on tobacco, including 1.25 million teenagers each year who take up smoking, are no shrinking violets. Appeals to freedom, wealth, glamour, manliness, athletic prowess, and sexual attractiveness cannot have failed to undermine public health efforts. This is borne out by the fact that the prevalence of smoking has declined by only 0.5 percentage points per year (Davis, 1989). Moreover, women, blue-collar workers, and minority groups in general are not appreciably reducing their cigarette consumption.

Thus, smoking cessation programs for the individual patient cannot truly succeed in the long run in the absence of both workplace smoking bans and multimedia counteradvertising strategies that weaken the influence of the tobacco industry and reinforce the physician's office-based efforts (Blum, 1980).

Although cigarette smoking becomes an addiction, it is first an entirely learned behavior. The "peer pressure" so often cited by tobacco companies as the reason for adolescent smoking is as much a manufactured product as the cigarettes themselves. The purpose of advertising is not just to sell cigarettes, but also to promote and reinforce the social acceptability of smoking and to encourage complacency toward the enormous social and health toll taken by smoking-caused diseases and fires. Today cigarette manufacturers spend more money annually to promote smoking than is spent to advertise for any other consumer product including automobiles and food.

A variety of factors may inhibit physician involvement in smoking cessation, such as the perceived or real lack of time, the lack of reimbursement by third-party payers for such counseling, and the lack of "peer group" reinforcement in a technologically oriented, tertiary care–centered, highly intellectualized health care system. Nonetheless, physicians might well find that their increased involvement in efforts to promote smoking cessation among patients, regardless of the minimal enhancement in revenue, becomes a practice-building factor as word spreads about the doctors who care.

OFFICE-BASED STRATEGIES

There is much the physician can do to become a better teacher about smoking, in lieu of relegating this role to ancillary personnel, a smoking cessation clinic, or a pamphlet off the shelf. The physician can develop an innovative strategy beginning outside the office or building. A bus bench, billboard, or sign in the parking lot with a straightforward or humorous health promotion message helps establish a thought-provoking and favorable image. In the waiting area, removal of ashtrays and the placement of signs noting that "In the interest of comfort, safety, and health, this is a smoke-free environment" further reinforce the message.

Magazines with cigarette advertisements ought not to appear in the physician's office in the absence of prominent stickers or rubber-stamped messages calling patients' attention to the deceptive, absurd nature of such ads (Table 68–2). Alternatively, felt-tip pens could be made available for patients to contribute their own anti-smoking comments or artwork. A commitment on the part of American phy-

Table 68–2. CIGARETTE ADVERTISING REVENUES AND COVERAGE OF SMOKING AND HEALTH, SELECTED MAGAZINES

	Years Surveyed	Health Articles Discussing Smoking (%)	Cigarette Ad Revenue (% of all)
Reader's Digest	1965–1981	34.4	0
Good Housekeeping	1965–1981	22.1	0
Prevention	1967–1978	15.4	0
Vogue	1965–1981	11.7	5.1
U.S. News and World Report	1965–1981	7.4	14.6
Ladies' Home Journal	1968–1981	7.1	16.3
Time	1965–1981	6.9	17.2
Harper's Bazaar	1968–1981	4.5	7.1
McCall's	1969–1980	4.5	15.1
Newsweek	1969–1981	2.9	15.8
Cosmopolitan	1971–1981	2.3	9.4
Mademoiselle	1966–1981	1.9	7.3
Ms.	1972–1981	0	14.8
Redbook	1970–1981	0	16.1

Note: Magazines listed included a minimum of 60 health-related articles in the years surveyed.
(From Dale, K. C.: American Council on Science and Health Survey: Which magazines report the hazards of smoking? ACSH News and Views, 3:1, 8–10, 1982.

sicians not to let their offices become vehicles for selling cigarettes would make a substantial contribution to health promotion. Although the responsibility for the office-based smoking cessation strategy should rest with the physician, it is invaluable to include all office staff as positive reinforcers for patients. Labeling each chart with a small no-smoking sticker to indicate the need for such reinforcement may be helpful, although care must be taken to avoid stigmatizing the patient as a "smoker." One would do well to reconsider using potentially alienating words such as "smoker" or even "quitter."

The key to successful smoking cessation efforts is a positive approach. A discussion about the diseases caused by smoking and the harmful constituents of tobacco smoke is essential—indeed, the physician must not shrink from imparting, through graphic posters, pamphlets, slides, and other audiovisual aids, the gruesome consequences of smoking—but the benefits of not smoking must be emphasized at least as strongly. Moreover, solely educating patients about the facts of smoking in a single office visit is unlikely to result in behavioral change. On the other hand, the physician can, through the use of creative analogies related to the patient's occupation, hobbies, or romantic interest, succeed in changing the patient's entire attitude toward smoking. For example, naming a partial list of the poisons and irritants in tobacco smoke, such as hydrocyanic acid (cyanide), ammonia, formaldehyde, and carbon monoxide (Table 68–1), may mean little at first. (One pregnant patient proudly stated that she never buys a brand of cigarettes with the warning that mentions harm to the fetus, only those brands that say they contain carbon monoxide.) But by noting that cyanide is the substance used in the gas chamber in executions, that formaldehyde is used to preserve cadavers, or that ammonia is the predominant smell in urine, the physician is likely to cause the patient to think about smoking a bit differently. Similarly, it does little good to talk about carcinogens in tobacco smoke in an age when the public believes "everything causes cancer." Sadly, the concept of relative risk is poorly developed in our society, as all too many people who smoke choose to think their millions-to-one odds of winning the state lottery are better than their one-in-seven chance of actually getting lung cancer.

METAPHORS THAT MOTIVATE

A revocabularization on the part of the physician is essential for making progress in office-based smoking cessation. Instead of "pack-year history," a more relevant term might be the "inhalation count." A pack-a-day smoking patient will breathe in upward of one million doses of cyanide, ammonia, carcinogens, and carbon monoxide in less than 15 years, not including the inhalation of other people's smoke. Another way to emphasize the enormous amount smoked is to state the amount smoked in financial terms: a pack-a-day cigarette buyer will spend in excess of $638 a year (calculated at $1.75 a pack)—or in excess of $8000 in a decade if that money were put into a savings account or bond. Or one can remark about the joyful feeling of finding a $50 bill every few weeks—which is what one would indeed find if the money had not been spent on cigarettes. One patient who began smoking in the Marines at age 18 and who still smoked three packs a day at age 33 remarked ruefully that he had "smoked a Porsche."

Thus, whereas patient education in general and smoking cessation in particular rest on the knowledge on the part of both physician and patient of the deleterious aspects of adverse health behavior, the cognitive component alone is insufficient. Both the physician and the patient must be motivated to succeed. Three keys to office-based smoking cessation are to personalize, individualize, and demythologize.

The physician can learn to *personalize* approaches to smoking cessation by carefully screening the pamphlets and other audiovisual aids available in the office. (Ideally, family physicians should consider producing their own.) It is essential to scrutinize all such material, as one would with a new drug or medical device. Personally handing a brochure to the patient while pointing out and underlining certain passages or illustrations will provide an important reinforcing message. The pamphlets, posters, and signs should be changed or otherwise updated every few weeks or months.

Individualizing the message to the patient is the cornerstone of success in patient education. The same cigarette counseling method cannot be used for a high-school girl, a construction worker, and an executive already showing signs or symptoms of heart disease. In the case of a high-school girl, the physician should not focus on such abstract concepts as emphysema and lung cancer, but rather emphasize the cosmetic unattractiveness of yellow teeth, bad breath, the loss of athletic ability, and the financial drain that results from buying cigarettes. As for the construction worker, the physician might suggest the likelihood of fewer lost paydays, greater physical strength, and even a lengthier sex life were he to stop buying cigarettes.

In talking with the concerned executive, it is especially important to *demythologize* certain beliefs about smoking, such as that the ultra-low-tar cigarettes she is smoking are safer. To the contrary, use of so-called low-tar brands, which should be referred to as "low poison" by the physician, may in fact result in compensatory deeper inhalation of greater concentrations of chemical additives and noxious gases that increase the risk of heart attack. One way to highlight the absurdity of the belief that low-tar cigarettes are safer is to ask rhetorically, Safer than what? Fresh air? or to wonder aloud if it is safer to jump from the 50th story of the Empire State Building instead of the roof. Another analogy is to point out that one would never think of buying a loaf of bread—or any other consumer product—that was advertised as containing "only 2 milligrams of cancer causers." In any event, such dialogue must be practiced over and over again like any medical procedure and individualized to the patient. (Remember that no two construction workers, teenagers, or executives are alike.) The counseling should be designed to call attention not only to the inevitable risks of smoking cigarettes but also to the chemically adulterated tobacco product itself, its inflated price, and the ubiquitous and ludicrous way in which the person's brand is promoted (Blum, 1980b).

COMMON MYTHS

The most important myth surrounding smoking is that it relieves stress. This can be debunked by pointing out that the stress that is relieved is that which resulted from being dependent on cigarettes; this is the essence of addiction. At the same time, it is also important to point out that deep breathing in and of itself has a relaxing effect (Woods, 1988). The second saddest myth, reinforced in advertisements for Virginia Slims, Silva Thins, and a host of new lines of long, thin cigarettes intended for women and girls, is that smoking keeps weight off. Aside from pointing to all the obese women who smoke and attempting to correct the misapprehension that being overweight is a greater health risk than is smoking, one can point out that by damaging the taste buds and other digestive tract cells, smoking does inhibit appetite. But since it also results in more sedentary behavior through loss of lung capacity and cardiovascular fitness, the joke is on the person who smokes. One need not gain weight on stopping smoking if one will relearn to enjoy walking and running as much as one relearns the taste of food. In short, by no means will all persons who stop smoking gain weight. Even among those who do, the average weight gain is less than five pounds (Davis, 1989). Moreover, the slightly lower weight in many who continue to smoke is associated with a higher-risk body fat distribution (Shimokata et al., 1989; Bonithon-Kopp et al., 1989). Because more than 75 per cent of black patients who smoke buy menthol brands, it is important to debunk the myth that this substance in some way "cools" the smoke (U. S. Dept. of Health and Human Services, Surgeon General's Report, 1989). In fact, menthol is an anesthetic that deadens the throat to create the illusion of a less irritating smoke.

Perhaps the biggest myth from the physician's standpoint that has been encouraged in the medical literature is that the patient must be "ready to quit." Although common sense dictates that those who express a greater interest in stopping smoking will have a greater success rate, those patients who do not express an interest in stopping smoking symbolize the overall challenge we face in curbing this pandemic. One of the reasons for lack of motivation of patients may be their sense of inevitability of failure. It is conceivable that by not educating the nonmotivated smoking patient, the physician is in effect reinforcing the notion that it may be too difficult to stop smoking.

Setting a "quit date," the sine qua non of the smoking cessation literature, may rationalize the continuation of an adverse health practice and may strengthen denial. In other words, it is helpful to remind patients that they can stop now. If they do not stop, this does not mean you will not treat them the next time, but it is important to give encouragement and not reinforce excuses. Most authors do feel that a quit date, targeted only one week or a few weeks into the future, is useful for the motivated patient, for whom denial is less of a problem. Its purpose is to let the individual build up resolve or to permit a gradual reduction in daily cigarette consumption. Giving patients a few written reminders (such as lists of the advantages and disadvantages of smoking, the rewards for not smoking and the penalties for lighting up, the situations and environmental influences that encourage one to smoke, and the myths of smoking and smoking cessation) is very helpful (Woods, 1988). A prescription with a no-smoking symbol signed by the physician and included with the other prescriptions is a thoughtful gesture.* The physician should not advise "cutting down," switching to a low-tar cigarette, or changing to a pipe or cigar.

CONSUMER ADVOCACY ROLE

Traditional office-based approaches begin by asking, Do you smoke? How much do you smoke? and When did you start smoking? Although this may provide the physician with relevant data for charting purposes, this approach is all too often a signal for the patient to become defensive and resistant to further discussion, especially if the patient had no intention to stop smoking. There are, however, alternative ways of obtaining information, and at the same time piquing the patient's interest in the subject. By using and identifying with the vocabulary used by the consumer of cigarettes, the physician can adopt (and be perceived in) the role of consumer advocate, as opposed to medical finger-wagger. The most important—and nonthreatening—questions to ask are, What brand do you buy? and How much do you spend on cigarettes? The patient is likely to be surprised and intrigued by these questions, which can be asked at any time in the course of the interview, since they appear to be nonjudgmental. They serve to suggest that the physician is not solely a know-it-all and a preacher on the dangers of the evil weed. In effect, a question about the cost of cigarettes shows concern for the patient's financial well-being. Inquiring as specifically as possible about the brand name—for example, Marlboro/Menthol/Lights/100s/Box—will lead to a greater understanding on the part of the physician of the same vocabulary used by the person who buys cigarettes, and will narrow the communication gap. The patient may even begin to laugh aloud at the foolishness of such a vocabulary, especially as he or she is encouraged to show the physician the package and to appreciate how little information about the product appears beyond the attractive design.

Promotions for various pharmacologic agents, mail order gadgets, and clinics in smoking cessation reinforce the notion that cigarette smoking is primarily a medical problem with a simple, prescribable, nonindividualized solution (Blum, 1984). When a patient requests a "drug that will help me stop smoking," the physician must confront the dilemma of not wishing to dash the patient's expectations while emphasizing that a drug or device is at best an adjunct and not a means of smoking cessation.

It is an unfortunate fact of life that many patients will not stop smoking until they have gotten their money's worth at a special smoking cessation clinic; and it seems that regardless of the method used, the more expensive the better. For the physician and patient who wish to buck this trend, a worthwhile reference is the National Cancer Institute's *Smoking Manual for Physicians*.

APPROACH TO ADOLESCENTS

Children and teenagers who smoke cigarettes pose a special challenge, since they represent the market most carefully nurtured by tobacco advertisers. It is essential to avoid emphasizing the adult and dangerous nature of smoking. Rather, smoking should be referred to as the childish, dumb, and silly-looking practice that it is. The single most important statement the physician can make to an adolescent is, "Come on, you're too old to smoke. That's for the little kids who want to look grown up." Another strategy is for the physician to ask the teenager who smokes to help think of ideas for talking to junior high school and primary school students who are just taking up smoking.

As a general rule in approaching the subject of smoking cessation with a patient, Schwartz and others recommend thinking in terms of a strategy that comprises interventions designed to enhance motivation and those that will help reduce dependence (Schwartz, 1987). Time and commitment on the part of the physician will result in greater success. The biggest obstacle to smoking cessation is complacency on the part of the physician.

*These are available along with a variety of stickers, posters, and newsletters from DOC, 1423 Harper Street, Medical College of Georgia, Augusta, GA 39012.

Controlled Substances

Kevin M. Sherin
Jan A. Fawcett

Development of a working knowledge of the medical issues surrounding drug abuse is a critically important priority for today's family physician. The family physician is in a front-line position for early detection of drug abuse problems and direction of her or his patients toward successful outcomes. This chapter provides an overview of drug abuse disorders beginning with background information, reviewing acute and chronic effects of commonly abused drugs, detailing the clinical approach to recognition of and management of patients, and finally reviewing issues impacting the physician and her or his role in the community. Let us first examine controlled substances from a historical perspective.

Historical Perspective

Drug abuse is considered the number one political problem currently facing the United States. The term "epidemic" is often applied to describe the scope of the problem. Drugs considered abused in epidemic proportions vary with legal status, availability, and cultural relativism. Heroin was a legal drug prior to the turn of the century and was widely prescribed. In 1914, Congress passed the Harrison Narcotic Tax Act, which banned both heroin and cocaine as illegal narcotic drugs (Claussen, 1977). From the 1930's to the 1960's cocaine was viewed as a harmless recreational drug without addictive potential. Yet the powerful psychoactive properties of cocaine have probably been recognized since A.D. 600 (Creger, 1986).

Cocaine abuse is the dominant form of illicit drug use in the United States. In 1963 it was estimated that there were only 10,000 cocaine users domestically. Estimates now place the number of regular users of cocaine at 5 to 10 million (Abelson and Miller, 1985). The advent of the "crack" form in 1985 led to wider availability at low cost, further contributing to increases in consumption. Meanwhile, the last several decades have seen numbers of heroin addicts stabilize at between 500 and 800 thousand nationwide (Kulberg, 1986).

Theories of Addiction

Genetic contributions to chemical dependency have been emphasized (Robins, 1978; Madden, 1979). Children of alcoholics or drug abusers seem to be at higher risk for development of substance abuse disorders (Goodwin et al., 1973). Variations in the biology of metabolism of psychoactive drugs or changes at drug receptor sites in the CNS, e.g., endorphin or dopamine receptors, may play a role here. The significance of social and environmental factors in the development of drug dependence is substantial. Social and cultural factors affecting the acceptability and availability of drugs are important features promoting harmful personal consumption. In the Vietnam experience, wide availability of heroin contributed to high rates of consumption among U.S. servicemen. Motives for drug use include (1) medicinal purposes, (2) symbolic purposes, including peer group acceptance, and (3) pleasurable effects on the mind (Madden, 1979). Constitutional aspects of the individual may provide fertile soil for development of chemical dependency. Some individuals who later abuse drugs possess antisocial personality traits. The individual user even lacking genetic contributions risks development of biological addiction by repeated exposure to psychoactive substances capable of triggering powerful internal reward systems.

Epidemiology

Since 1980 drug abuse patterns in the United States have been relatively stable with the exception of cocaine. It is estimated that 30 million Americans have used cocaine (Abelson and Miller, 1985) and that 5 million use it regularly (Abelson and Miller, 1985). The highest prevalence of cocaine use has been among young white men (ages 18 to 25 years) residing in the west and the northeastern United States (Abelson and Miller, 1985). Use among women is increasing. Recent surveys of United States high-school students' cocaine use showed evidence of a decline (Adams and Kozel, 1985). The present cocaine epidemic is considered to be the fifth and largest stimulant abuse outbreak.

Regular users of cocaine now exceed those of heroin by over fivefold (Fernandez-Pol et al., 1988). Abused drugs showing relative declines since the 1970's include phencyclidine, amphetamines, sedative hypnotics, and hallucinogens. Marijuana use remains relatively stable. Inner city patterns were reflected in a recent study from the Department of Psychiatry at Bronx Lebanon Hospital in New York. These investigators found that 40 per cent of inpatients had used cannabis; 37 per cent alcohol; 20 per cent amphetamines; 12 per cent cocaine; 12 per cent phencyclidine (PCP); 10 per cent barbiturates and other sedative hypnotics; 9 per cent opiates; 1 per cent inhalants; and 1 per cent hallucinogens (Fernandez-Pol et al., 1988).

Pharmacologic Principles

Pharmacologic principles affecting abused drugs include (1) absorption, (2) distribution, (3) metabolism, (4) excretion, (5) tolerance and cross-tolerance, and (6) dependence (Morgan, 1985). Absorption varies with route of intake and may include inhalation (volatile gas or smoke), insufflation (cocaine), oral ingestion, and intravenous (IV) infusion. Peak drug levels occur rapidly with inhalation, intravenous injection, and insufflation; they are more likely to produce fatalities or serious sequelae. Regarding drug distribution, the partition coefficient equals the concentration of oil-dissolved drug versus "water"-dissolved drug, and this ratio reflects lipophilicity and hydrophilicity. Most psychoactive substances readily cross the blood-brain barrier. Nonpolar compounds tend to be lipophilic, have a high partition coefficient, and widely distribute within fat and myelin layers, producing prolonged psychodynamic or physiologic effects.

Psychoactive compounds are metabolized by several pathways (Morgan, 1985). Most are metabolized in hepatocytes via dehydroxylation, deamination, and acetylation. Barbiturates and benzodiazepines induce microsomal enzymes of the P-450 pathway. Tolerance then develops, which promotes cross-tolerance. Alcohol and benzodiazepines have cross-tolerance since they share this common pathway. Psychoactive drug metabolism occurs largely via first-order kinetics; that is, a fixed proportion of metabolite versus substrate is produced, giving the drug a fixed half-life (λ ½). Inert compounds of psychoactive metabolites may be produced. Excretion occurs principally through the kidneys. The Pka of a compound may allow more rapid renal excretion if the urine pH is altered. Alkalinization of urine enhances the excretion of phenobarbital, a weak acid. Emergency medicine physicians indirectly utilize this acid-base principle of enhanced excretion in gastric lavage. Some drugs are recirculated through the acidic environment of the gastric mucosa long after absorption; removal is enhanced by gastric suction, e.g., Doriden (glutethimide). Acidification of urine to enhance excretion is no longer widely used clinically. Phencyclidine toxicity is an exception; clinical outcome is improved with administration of ascorbic acid and Haldol together (Giannini et al., 1987).

Pharmacologic dependence requires a discrete abstinence or physiologic withdrawal syndrome in the drug's absence. Presence of the drug prevents emergence of withdrawal. Stereotyped responses are seen with opiates, sedative hypnotics, depressant drugs, and alcohol. Sedative hypnotic and depressant drug withdrawal mimics delayed alcohol withdrawal. A "low-dose" benzodiazepine withdrawal syndrome includes anxiety and insomnia; it persists for months and responds well to beta blockers (Smith and Wesson, 1983). Opiate withdrawal is characterized by lacrimation, frequent yawning, gastrointestinal disturbance, rhinorrhea, and piloerection.

Acute Effects of Commonly Abused Drugs

COCAINE

Cocaine is an alkaloid extracted from the South American shrub *Erythroxylon coca*. Its pharmacologic properties have been extensively reviewed (Kulberg, 1986) and include powerful stimulant, vasoconstrictive, and anesthetic effects. Cocaine is a powerful euphoric with potent addictive properties. Acute effects include mydriasis, tachycardia, overalertness, talkativeness, flushing, hyperthermia, and emotional lability. Persons with abnormal plasma cholinesterase activity may experience an overdose at lower thresholds. Signs of toxicity include nausea, vomiting, seizures, tachyarrhythmia, hypertensive crisis, strokes, myocardial infarction, extreme anxiety with disorientation, and sudden cardiorespiratory arrest. Abstinence may result in hypersomnia, irritability, dysphoria, and prolonged depression. Smokeable forms (free-basing) have been associated with pneumothorax, pneumomediastinum, and other pulmonary effects (Creger, 1986). Maternal-fetal effects are discussed under chronic effects.

PRESCRIPTION DRUGS

Amphetamines. Amphetamine, phenylpropanolamine, ephedrine, and caffeine have similar central and peripheral toxic effects (Kulberg, 1986). Small doses may produce alertness, lessened fatigue, a sense of well-being, and improved motor skills. Side effects include anxiety, restlessness, insomnia, abdominal cramps, and lassitude. Overdosage results in anxiety, agitation, hallucinations, and seizures. Acute paranoid psychosis is seen with large overdoses. Peripheral effects include elevated blood pressure, diaphoresis, mydriasis, hyperactive bowel sounds, tachycardia, and reflex bradycardia.

Sedative Hypnotics. Benzodiazepines have a high threshold for toxic effects (Kulberg, 1986). Sedation is the hallmark of this class of drugs. An overdose may result in blurring of vision, dysarthria, ataxia, and nystagmus. An acute withdrawal syndrome begins between days 5 and 8 of abstinence. Signs and

Table 68–3. STREET TERMINOLOGY OF ABUSED DRUGS

Class	Example Names
Sedative Hypnotics	Barbs, blues, goofballs, greens and whites, soapers, roaches (Librium)
	Ludes (Quaalude)
	Mean-green (Placidyl)
	Yellow-jackets (phenobarbital)
	Red devils (secobarbital)
Analgesics	
Heroin	Smack, junk, horse, H, brown, skag
Methadone	Dollies, wafers
Darvon	Pinks and grays
Terpin hydrate	Terp
Dilaudid	Fours
Designer Drugs	
MDA	Love drug
MDMA	Ecstasy, Adam
Fentanyl	China white
Stimulants	
Cocaine	Crack, coke, gold dust, flakes, snow, rock
Other stimulants	Speedball (heroin and cocaine)
	Uppers; truck drivers, crank (amphetamines)
	Crossroads, bennies, copilot
Cannabinols	
Marijuana	Reefer, roach, weed, pot, joint, grass, brick, lid
Hashish	Ganja, bhang
Hallucinogens	
LSD	Acid, blue dots, cube, D
Other	Cactus (mescaline)
	Magic mushrooms (psilocybin)
	Pearly gates (morning glory seeds)
PCP	Angel dust, dust, rocket fuel, peacepill, hog, supercoke, super joint, cosmos, goon

Adapted from Appendix C, AMSAODD Review Course Syllabus, Oct. 8–10, 1987. American Medical Society for Alcoholism and other Drug Dependencies, 12 W. 21st St., New York, NY.

symptoms may include insomnia, irritability, seizures, tremulousness, muscle twitching, and delirium. Phenobarbital, glutethimide, and ethchlorvynol withdrawal effects are similar with a difference only in λ ½. Methaqualone is considered a sedative hypnotic.

OPIATES

Opiate overdose produces a clinical triad of respiratory and CNS depression with meiotic pupils (Kulberg, 1986). Muscle flaccidity, hypertension, and hypothermia may also be seen. Euphoria accompanied by brief diaphoresis is a typical dose response in a heroin addict. Noncardiogenic pulmonary edema is a complication of parenteral narcotic overdose (Madden, 1979).

HALLUCINOGENS

Phencyclidine. "Angel dust" or PCP was marketed in the 1950's as a surgical anesthetic and in the 1960's as an animal anesthetic (Kulberg, 1986). This dissociative anesthetic has been associated with violent, bizarre behaviors, radical alterations of sensory stimuli, and supernormal strength often associated with self-injury in the face of anesthesia. Hypertension and bidirectional nystagmus are frequently seen. Hyperthermia may occur in the face of muscle rigidity and rhabdomyolysis. Patients may also appear catatonic.

Lysergic Acid Diethylamide. LSD is an illusionogenic drug (Kulberg, 1986). Actual stimuli are distorted. Sounds, smells, and visual stimuli may be altered or merged. Depersonalization or personality disorganization may lead to panic or a "bad trip." Paresthesias, diaphoresis, ataxia, and tremors may be seen. The sense of passage of time may be slowed (Madden, 1979).

INHALANTS

Volatile Solvent/Propellants. In the 19th century popular agents included ether and chloroform. Toluene and aliphatic chlorinated compounds have replaced these today. Solvent abuse is particularly prevalent among the rural poor in the South (Kulberg, 1986). Acute CNS effects include initial delirium, euphoria, confusion, ataxia, and dysarthria. Bizarre and impulsive behavior can lead to significant morbidity and mortality. Illusions and delusions may follow and the clinical picture may progress to coma. Sudden death can occur and has been attributed to myocardial sensitization (Kulberg, 1986).

Nitrates. These remain popular in homosexual and heterosexual populations for enhanced erection/orgasm. Headache, nausea, palpitations, and dizziness are seen. Giddiness, syncope, and confusion are frequently observed. Sudden death can occur with repeated inhalation. Methemoglobinemia can occur.

Mescaline-Peyote. Toxicity usually occurs 1 to 2 hours following ingestion. The clinical effects are similar to those produced by LSD or PCP. However, there is usually an intact memory for the events, unlike under the influence of PCP (Kulberg, 1986).

Cannabis (Marijuana). Tetrahydrocannabinol is the principal active ingredient. Conjunctival injection and a dreamy state are the principal objective findings in a user (Madden, 1979; Kulberg, 1986). Euphoric enhanced perceptions and altered sense of time are frequent. Toxic doses may alter body image and produce depersonalization, paranoia, and disorientation. Sinus tachycardia occurs frequently.

Chronic Effects of Substance Abuse

COCAINE

Chronic effects of cocaine abuse or dependence are related to the route of intake and have been extensively reviewed (Creger, 1986). Nasal insufflation results in chronic rhinorrhea. Nasal septal atrophy and perforation may also occur (Vilensky, 1982). Chronic sinusitis, sinus osteomyelitis, and brain abscess can accompany insufflation (Shveitzer, 1986). Smokeable forms of cocaine may be associated with pulmonary problems. Intravenous use of cocaine can result in allergic vasculitis, cerebral infarcts, and infectious complications including hepatitis B and AIDS. Oral ingestion has been associated with hepatic damage and intestinal infarcts (Nalbandian et al., 1986). Myocardial fibrosis has been observed in occasional users (Simpson and Edwards, 1986). Maternal use during pregnancy can result in maternal-fetal effects including fetal brain infarcts, intestinal atresia, genitourinary anomalies, prune belly syndrome, intrauterine growth retardation, prematurity, and abruptio placentae (Chasnoff et al., 1985, 1986; Creger, 1986).

STIMULANTS

Stimulant use can result in weight loss and insomnia. Psychiatric sequelae occur with frequent chronic use and may include anxiety, depression, paranoid states, and mood swings. Direct myocardial injury has been described with phenylpropanolamine ingestion (Pentel et al., 1982).

SEDATIVE HYPNOTICS

Prolonged abstinence syndromes associated with sedative hypnotics have already been discussed. Interruption of REM sleep is frequent. Thrombocytopenia, leukopenia, and jaundice clear with abstinence (Stutzman, 1987). Muscle and nervous tissue necrosis can occur with IV use. In the elderly, prescription drug abuse can present with dementia, depression, or both.

OPIATES

Intravenous abusers are at increased risk for endocarditis, brain abscess, pneumonia, lung abscess, viral hepatitis, and HIV-associated diseases. Parkinsonism occurs with one street substitute for heroin. A heroin-associated nephropathy is known to occur. Hemolytic anemia and thrombocytopenia may also occur with chronic opiate abuse (Stutzman, 1987).

HALLUCINOGENS

Chronic use of cannabis and other hallucinogens may result in immunologic suppression. COPD, arrhythmias, rhabdomyolysis, and renal failure also are known to occur (Stutzman, 1987).

INHALANTS

Chronic effects from inhalants include neurotoxicity and pulmonary and renal sequelae. Long-term cerebellar dysfunction in adolescence has been reported. A peripheral neuropathy termed "huffer's neuropathy" has been observed. Pulmonary effects in the form of direct lung injury are suspected. Toluene sniffing can result in muscle weakness, gastroenteritis complaints of pain and hematemesis, neuropsychiatric disorders, and peripheral neuropathy. Renal tubular damage and nonanion gap acidosis are common.

Obtaining the Substance Abuse History

In approaching the substance abuse history, the family physician must be open and friendly yet direct and thorough. An adolescent school physical should include an inquiry that opens the door to this discussion. "It is important for us to be open and honest in discussing health issues, but I want to reassure you that whatever we discuss will be held in strictest confidence. Many young people today are trying out recreational drugs by smoking cigarettes, marijuana, or 'crack.' Have you or your friends tried any of these?" A young adult with rhinorrhea and hypertension could be queried regarding stimulant or cocaine insufflation in the following manner. "I notice that your blood pressure is elevated and your nasal passages are swollen. Are there any over-the-counter nasal sprays or recreational drugs you are currently exposed to that may contribute to this picture?" Finally, the reluctant patient with telltale evidence of substance abuse who persists in denying a problem may undergo a focused physical examination to confirm medical suspicions. The physician may continue obtaining more history of possible adverse effects on school or work performance, social and behavioral change, or breakdown of family and interpersonal relationships. When the individual acknowledges substance abuse, each possible route of intake should be elaborated and recorded in the history. Obtaining data from significant others may be particularly important.

Physical Examination

A focused physical examination should detail target organs that may be affected by commonly abused or suspect drugs. A careful assessment of mental status should be undertaken to exclude overt depression, suicidal ideation, or evidence of thought disorder. A careful neurologic examination should be accomplished with particular attention to tremor, twitching, signs of hyperreflexia, parkinsonism, and pupillary

Table 68–4. PREDICTIVE VALUE OF SCREENING

		Disease Present	Disease Absent	
Test	+	a = 95	b = 990	a + b
	−	c = 5	d = 8910	c + d
	total =	a + c = 100	b + d = 9900	Prevalence 1%

$$\text{Sensitivity} = \frac{a}{a + c} = \frac{95}{95 + 5} = 95\%$$

$$\text{Specificity} = \frac{d}{b + d} = \frac{8910}{990 + 8910} = \frac{8910}{9900} = 90\%$$

$$\text{Positive Predictive Value} = \frac{a}{a + b} = \frac{95}{95 + 990} = 8.7\%$$

$$\text{Negative Predictive Value} = \frac{d}{c + d} = \frac{8910}{8910 + 5} = 99.9\%$$

Adapted from Last, J. M. (Ed.): Public Health and Preventive Medicine. 12th ed. New York, Appleton Century Crofts, 1986, p. 40. Permission granted from publisher and author.

sizes and responses. Blood pressure and pulse should be accurately recorded. Skin findings such as jaundice, diaphoresis, piloerection, skin needle tracks, or abscesses should be noted. EENT examination findings including scleral icterus, nasal mucosal redness, atrophy, ulceration, or pharyngeal erythema are observed. The cardiovascular examination should detect evidence of dysrhythmia, new murmur, or changes in pre-existent heart sounds. Pulmonary findings including increased AP diameter, wheezes, and rhonchi are elicited. Hepatomegaly is noted on the abdominal examination. The maternal-fetal examination seeks to uncover evidence of intrauterine growth retardation or other signs of fetal distress.

Laboratory Findings

A drug abuse or toxicology profile may be obtained to corroborate reportedly abused substances. Clandestine or unindicated testing through the physician's office should be discouraged. Specific drug levels may be assayed when emergency management or detoxification is anticipated. Additional laboratory parameters should be examined based on the findings of the focused history and physical. An IV drug abuser should receive a hepatitis profile. Human immunodeficiency virus (HIV) antibody testing may be offered with appropriate informed consent and pre- and post-test counseling. Cocaine abusers may require sinus radiographs, chest radiographs, or cardiac profiles depending on circumstances. Prescription drug and analgesic abusers require liver and renal function tests. When first-time seizures occur in young persons, an EEG should be done several days following the event. A CT scan of the head is indicated when there is any suspicion of a focal event. Marijuana or "crack" smokers may benefit from pulmonary function screening.

Screening Issues

Screening technologies for drug abuse remain imperfect tools that serve as adjuncts to clinical acumen. The family physician should approach these technologies with caution, particularly with regard to workplace screening. As with any diagnostic test, predictive value is proportionally related to prevalence of the disease in the population (Last, 1986). For example, if 1 per cent of 10,000 railroad workers abused cocaine on the sample day and a sound screening test for benzylecgonine, a cocaine metabolite, is 95 per cent sensitive and 90 per cent specific, the results in Table 68–4 can be anticipated. Therefore, the positive predictive value of a positive test for cocaine where the prevalence is low (1 per cent) is poor (8.7 per cent).

Intervention

DENIAL

Patient denial is a particularly difficult issue for the family physician in approaching chemical dependency intervention. The patient may be frightened or threatened by discussion, detection, or intervention in his or her drug abuse or dependency disorder. Responses vary, including (1) anger, (2) amusement, (3) denial of a problem, or (4) evading the question. The patient's lack of awareness of harmful sequelae of drug abuse may be genuine and related to cognitive or functional impairment; at other times denial is a deliberate ego defense. Regardless of cause, significant disorders must be confronted in a humane, nonjudgmental, and persuasive manner by the concerned physician.

Negotiating patients into chemical dependency treatment involves a process. Social factors help le-

Table 68–5. DETOXIFICATION REGIMENS

Abused Drugs	Toxic Rx	Abstinence Syndrome	Blockade Rx
Cocaine	ABC's/Supportive Benzodiazepines CA blockers Anticonvulsants	Desipramine or Bromocriptine	N/A
Stimulants	Benzodiazepines Charcoal lavage Acidify urine	Minor tranquilizer or Antipsychotic if required	N/A
Sedative hypnotics	Saline diuresis/Supportive	Substitution of short-acting benzodiazepine	N/A
Depressants Phenobarbital	Alkalinize urine Na bicarbonate Respiratory support	*Pentobarbital challenge test + Substitution Rx	N/A
Opiates	Narcan ABC's/Supportive	Clonidine, Darvon, or methadone	Naltrexone
Hallucinogens	Benzodiazepines	N/A	N/A

*Incremental doses of pentobarbital to achieve sedation switch to equivalent total dose of phenobarbital, followed by gradual phenobarbital reduction (30 mg. per day) (Smith and Wesson, 1970).

verage intervention and include (1) spouse or family pressure, (2) legal pressures including DUI charges, and (3) employment issues (absenteeism or threatened job loss). Inpatients can be motivated by economic pressures for failure to follow medical advice resulting in possible loss of reimbursement (option given to sign out against medical advice or enter treatment). Direct referral to chemical dependency facilities is more readily accomplished when family or significant others are actively involved.

DETOXIFICATION

Detoxification is often accomplished on an outpatient basis, although certain drugs may require inpatient treatment. Factors to weigh in assessing outpatient detoxification potential include (1) single or polydrug abuse; (2) presence or absence of social supports; (3) type of abused drug(s); (4) previous failed efforts at outpatient treatment; (5) mental status abnormalities; (6) serious medical complications; and (7) levels of addiction. Often treatment avenues available to patients are determined by reimbursement. Outpatient approaches can be attempted initially. If relapse occurs, inpatient or residential treatment should be pursued. Sedative hypnotic or major depressant detoxification frequently requires inpatient care.

Detoxification regimens are specific to abused agents. Widely accepted protocols (Booker and Benzer, 1987; Salkin, 1987) include those listed in Table 68–5.

Treatment Approaches

Postdetoxification treatment approaches range from self-help groups to highly structured long-term residential programs (Wilford, 1981). Self-help groups are modeled after the 12-step program Alcoholics Anonymous (AA). Drug abuse–specific 12-step programs include Narcotics Anonymous and Cocaine Anonymous. For combined alcohol and drug addictions, Alcoholics Anonymous is a reasonable option. Most chemically dependent patients require specific, directive treatment. Treatments range from inpatient chemical dependency programs to outpatient, partial hospitalization programs. Factors including medical and psychiatric complications, compliance demonstrated by urine drug screens, previous treatment outcomes, reimbursement options, and social supports are evaluated weighing outpatient versus inpatient treatment decisions. Methadone maintenance and naltrexone are viable options for opiate addicted individuals (Schuckit, 1984).

Follow-up Management

Follow-up management is guided by prognosis. Previous failed efforts at rehabilitation do not indicate automatic failure; patients with these disorders often relapse. Patients improve their prognosis if motivated to enter long-term therapeutic communities, e.g., SynAnon. Structured and supportive follow-up care includes monitoring compliance with self-help group attendance, offering supportive psychotherapy, managing aversive or chemotherapeutic regimens, and monitoring urine drug screens. Clinicians may query frequency of attendance at 12-step group meetings, whether patients have obtained a "sponsor," and how they are progressing with "step work." Issues such as changing life style, attending groups, home and job conflicts, personality disorders, and unresolved anger should be evaluated and addressed. Family physicians should familiarize themselves with local resources and consultants in the addictions field (available from the

American Society of Addiction Medicine (ASAM); see Salkin, 1987).

Physician Impairment

Physician impairment is an increasingly recognized issue. Most state medical societies have systems to aid recovering professionals. The Joint Commission on the Accreditation of Healthcare Organizations now requires medical staff bylaws to include impaired physician committees. Physicians seem to have higher rates of chemical dependency than do other populations. This may be related to increased access to pharmaceuticals, higher levels of job stress, or increased awareness and recognition of or lack of alternative outlets for handling illness or anxiety. In at least two recent surveys (Morse et al., 1984; Med World News, 1986), family physicians were found to have higher impairment rates. The American Academy of Family Physicians is developing programs targeting professional awareness and prevention to help combat chemical dependency.

Community and Public Health Issues

Drug abuse prevention research has shown that efforts combining cognitive, behavioral, and social skill learning that increases resistance to pro drug social influences appear to be most effective. The family physician has a responsibility to assist in these community-based prevention efforts. The family physician can further develop knowledge and expertise in this area and serve as a resource in helping to educate community groups. Family practice residency programs and hospitals have developed "speakers bureaus" of physicians willing to speak in schools, churches, and civic and other community groups on various preventive health care issues. Effective approaches include local treatment resources; recovering personalities are particularly helpful in actual presentations. The physician here serves as a resource person knowledgeable about medical sequelae of chemical dependency.

Conclusion

Drug abuse disorders remain an important issue in family practice. Cocaine dependence is currently a major component of this health care burden. Family physicians must acquire skills in recognition of and screening for chemical dependency in their practice. Family practitioners must acquire additional skills in intervention for and/or referral for treatment in order to deliver comprehensive patient care. The family physician should become knowledgeable about physician impairment. The specialty of family practice plays a significant role in enhancing community awareness and in the prevention of these disorders.

References

Abelson, H. I., and Miller, J. D.: A decade of trends in cocaine use in the household population. Natl. Inst. Drug Abuse Res. Monogr. Ser., *61*:35–49, 1985. *A comprehensive monograph series based on Drug Abuse Warning Network (DAWN), which is constantly updated.*

Adams, E. H., and Kozel, N. J.: Cocaine use in America: Introduction and overview. Natl. Inst. Drug Abuse Res. Monogr. Ser., *61*:1–2, 1985.

Adams, E. H., Groerer, J., Rouse, B. A., and Kozel, N. J.: Trends in prevalence and consequences of cocaine use. Adv. Alcohol Subst. Abuse, *6*:49–71, 1986.

American Psychiatric Association: Diagnostic Criteria from the DSM III-R. Washington, DC, American Psychiatric Press, 1987a. *This diagnostic manual represents a compromise between various schools of thought in psychiatry. Some of the diagnoses are carefully studied and substantiated by data, whereas others have little information to guarantee predictive validity.*

American Psychiatric Association: Task Force on Nomenclature and Statistics: Diagnostic and Statistical Manual of Mental Disorders (rev.). 3rd ed. Washington, DC, American Psychiatric Association, 1987b.

Aronow, W. S.: The effect of smoke on the nonsmoker. Fam. Pract. Recertification, *1*:47, 1979.

Barry, J., Mead, K., Nabel, E. G., et al.: Effect of smoking on the activity of ischemic heart disease. J.A.M.A., *261*:398–402, 1989.

Begleiter, H., Porjesz, B., and Bihari, B.: Auditory brainstem potentials in sons of alcoholic fathers. Alcoholism: Clin. Exp. Res., *11*:477–479, 1987. *An interesting study that demonstrates electrophysiological differences between at least a subset of young children of alcoholics and controls.*

Bell, B. A., and Symon, L.: Smoking and subarachnoid haemorrhage. Br. Med. J., *1*:577, 1979.

Bikle, D. D., Genant, H. K., Cann, D., Recker, R. R., et al.: Bone disease in alcohol abuse. Ann. Intern. Med., *103*:42–48, 1985.

Blum, A.: Nicotine chewing gum and the medicalization of smoking. Ann. Intern. Med., *101*:121–123, 1984.

Blum, A.: Medicine vs. Madison Avenue. J.A.M.A., *243*:739–740, 1980.

Blum, A.: Butting in where it counts. Hospital Physician *16*(4):22–35, 1980b.

Bonita, R., Scragg, R., and Stewart, A.: Cigarette smoking and risk of premature stroke in men and women. Br. Med. J., *293*:6–8, 1986.

Bonithon-Kopp, C., Raison, J., Ducimetiere, P., et al.: Smoking wastes a good Parisenne (letters). J.A.M.A. *262*:1185–1186, 1989.

Booker, R., and Benzer, D.: Sub acute care. Chapter VIII, Review Course Syllabus for American Medical Society on Alcoholism and Other Drug Dependencies, 12 W. 21st St., New York, NY 10010, 1987, pp. 189–208. *Excellent overview of follow-up issues for clinicians to consider with chemically dependent patients.*

Boyd, J., Weissman, M., Thompson, W., and Myers, J.: Different definitions of alcoholism. Am. J. Psychiatry, *140*:1309–1313, 1983.

Brown, S. A., and Schuckit, M. A.: Changes in depression among abstinent alcoholics. J. Stud. Alcohol, 49:412–417, 1988.

Burt, A., Thronley, P., Illingworth, D., et al.: Stopping smoking after myocardial infarction. Lancet, *1*:304–306, 1974.

Centers for Disease Control: State-specific estimates of smoking-attributable mortality and years of potential life lost—United States, 1985. MMWR, Vol. 37, November 18, 1988.

Chasnoff, I. J., Burns, W. J., Scholl, S. H., et al.: Cocaine use in pregnancy. N. Engl. J. Med., *313*:666–669, 1985. *A major descriptive work by a pioneer in the field.*

Chasnoff, I. J., Bussey, M. E., Savich, R., et al.: Perinatal cerebral infarction and maternal cocaine use. J. Pediatr., *108*:456–459, 1986.

Cigarette Smoking as a Dependence Process: National Institute on Drug Abuse Research Monograph Series No. 23. Krasnegor, N. A. (Ed.). DHEW Publication No. (ADM) 79-800. Rockville, MD, U.S. Dept. of Health, Education and Welfare, Public Health Service, Alcohol, Drug Abuse, and Mental Health Administration, 1979.

Claussen, J.: Early history of narcotics use and narcotics legislation in the United States. *In* Rock, P. (Ed.): Drugs and Politics. Transaction Books, 1977, pp. 23–24. *A collection of essays examining the social and political aspects of drugs and drug users.*

Colditz, G. A., Bonita, R., Stampfer, M. J., et al.: Cigarette smoking and risk of stroke in middle-aged women. N. Engl. J. Med., *318*:937–941, 1988.

Connolly, G. N., Winn, D. M., Hecht, S. S., et al.: The reemergence of smokeless tobacco. N. Engl. J. Med., *314*:1020–1027, 1986.

Creger, L. L., and Mark, H.: Special report: Medical complications of cocaine abuse. N. Engl. J. Med., *315*:1495–1500, 1986. *A comprehensive review of the acute and chronic medical sequelae of cocaine abuse.*

Criqui, M. H.: Alcohol consumption, blood pressure, lipids, and cardiovascular mortality. Alcoholism: Clin. Exp. Res., *10*:564–569, 1986.

Dale, K. C.: American Council on Science and Health Survey: Which magazines report the hazards of smoking? ACSH News and Views, *3*:1, 8–10, 1982.

Davis, J., Chief Medical Examiner, Dade County, Florida. Personal communication, 1977.

Davis, R., Director, Office on Smoking and Health, U.S. Dept. of Health and Human Services. Personal communication, 1989.

Donahue, R. P., Abbott, R. D., Reed, D. M., and Yano, K.: Alcohol and hemorrhagic stroke. J.A.M.A., *255*:2311–2314, 1986.

Drew, L. R. H.: Alcoholism as a self-limiting disease. Q. J. Stud. Alcohol, *29*:956–967, 1968.

Editorial: Dying for a drink? Lancet, *2*:1249, 1987.

Ehlers, C., and Schuckit, M. A.: EEG changes after ethanol in sons of alcoholics and controls. J. Stud. Alcohol, in press.

Estrin, W. J.: Alcoholic cerebellar degeneration is not a dose-dependent phenomenon. Alcoholism: Clin. Exp. Res., *11*:372–375, 1987.

Evans, R. I.: Smokeless tobacco vs cigarette use among adolescents. Cancer Bull., *40*:355–359, 1988.

Fernandez-Pol, B., Bluestone, H., and Muzruch, M. S.: Inner city substance abuse patterns: A study of psychiatric inpatients. A. J. Drug Alcohol Abuse, *14*:41–50, 1988.

Fishburn, P. M.: National Survey on Drug Abuse: Main Findings: 1979. DHHS Publication No. (ADM) 80-976. Rockville, MD, National Institute of Drug Abuse, 1980.

Frank, D., and Raicht, R. F.: Alcohol-induced liver disease. Alcoholism: Clin. Exp. Res., *9*:66–82, 1985.

Fuller, R. K., Branchey, L., Brightwell, D. R., Derman, R. M., et al.: Disulfiram treatment of alcoholism. A Veterans Administration Cooperative Study. J.A.M.A., *256*:1449–1455, 1986.

Garfinkle, L.: Cancer mortality in nonsmokers: Prospective study by the American Cancer Society. J.N.C.I., *65*:1169, 1980.

Giannini, A. J., et al.: Augmentation of haloperidol by ascorbic acid in phencyclidine intoxication. Am. J. Psychiatry, *144*:1207–1209, 1987.

Goodwin, D. W.: Alcoholism and genetics. Arch. Gen. Psychiatry, *42*:171–174, 1985.

Goodwin, D. W., and Guze, S. B.: Psychiatric Diagnosis. 4th ed. New York, Oxford University Press, 1989. *A classic text introducing the reader to the use of diagnosis for the purpose of establishing prognosis and treatment.*

Goodwin, D. W., Schulsinger, F., Hermansen, L., et al.: Alcohol problems in adoptees raised apart from alcoholic biological parents. Arch. Gen. Psychiatry, *28*:238–243, 1973.

Grant, I.: Alcohol and the brain: Neuropsychological correlates. J. Consult. Clin. Psychol., *55*:310–324, 1987.

Gurling, H. M. D., Phil, M., Grant, S., and Dangl, J.: The genetic and cultural transmission of alcohol use, alcoholism, cigarette smoking and coffee drinking: A review and an example using a log linear cultural transmission model. Br. J. Addict., *80*:269–272, 1985. *Beginning with a twin register in a psychiatric hospital, this study found no strong support for a genetic predisposition. It is highlighted here because it stands out in distinction from many of the other studies.*

Hammond, E. C.: Smoking in relation to the death rates of one million men and women. *In* Haenszel, W. (Ed.): Epidemiological Approaches to the Study of Cancer and Other Chronic Diseases. National Cancer Institute, 1966.

Harper, C., Kril, J., and Daly, J.: Are we drinking our neurones away? Br. Med. J., *294*:534–536, 1987.

Hayashida, M., Alterman, A. I., McLellan, A. T., and O'Brien, C. P.: Comparative effectiveness and costs of inpatient and outpatient detoxification. N. Engl. J. Med., *320*:358–365, 1989.

Health Consequences of Smoking: Cancer. A Report of the Surgeon General. DHHS Publication No. (PHS) 82-50179. Rockville, MD, U.S. Dept. of Health, Education, and Welfare, Public Health Service, Office on Smoking and Health, 1982.

Health Consequences of Smoking for Women. A Report of the Surgeon General. Rockville, MD, U.S. Dept. of Health, Education, and Welfare, Public Health Service, Office on Smoking and Health, 1985.

Helzer, J., Robins, L., Taylor, J., et al.: The extent of long-term moderate drinking among alcoholics. N. Engl. J. Med., *312*:1678–1682, 1985. *While most alcoholics drink in a controlled way for short periods of time, this study demonstrates that only a tiny percentage are able to maintain that control for any extended period of time.*

Hermanson, B., Omenn, G. S., Kronmal, R. A., and Gersh, B. J.: Beneficial six-year outcome of smoking cessation in older men and women with coronary artery disease. N. Engl. J. Med., *319*:1365–1369, 1988.

Herning, R. I., Jones, R. T., Bachman, J., and Mines, A. H.: Puff volume increases when low-nicotine cigarettes are smoked. Br. Med. J., *283*:187, 1981.

Hirayama, T.: Non-smoking wives of heavy smokers have a higher risk of lung cancer: A study from Japan. Br. Med. J., *282*:183, 1981. *Introduces important evidence that those who live with smokers are at increased risk for life-threatening illness.*

Irwin, M., Baird, S., Smith, T. L., et al.: Use of laboratory tests to monitor heavy drinking by alcoholic men discharged from a treatment program. Am. J. Psychiatry, *145*:595–599, 1988.

Kaufman, D. W., Helmrich, S. P., Rosenberg, L., et al.: Nicotine and carbon monoxide content of cigarette smoke and the risk of myocardial infarction in young men. N. Engl. J. Med., *308*:409, 1983.

Khoury, M. J., Govez-Farias, M., and Mulinare, J.: Does maternal cigarette smoking during pregnancy cause cleft lip and palate in offspring? Am. J. Dis. Child., *143*:333–337, 1989.

Kinlen, L. J., and Rogot, E.: Leukemia and smoking habits among United States Veterans. Br. Med. J., *297*:657–659, 1988.

Koop, C. E., and Luoto, J.: The health consequences of smoking: Cancer. Overview of a report of the Surgeon General. Public Health Rep., *97*:318, 1982.

Kozlowski, L. T., Frecker, R. C., Khouw, V., and Pope, M. A.: The misuse of "less-hazardous" cigarettes and its detection: Hole-blocking of ventilation filters. Am. J. Public Health, *70*:1202, 1980.

Kulberg, A.: Substance abuse: Clinical identification and management; pediatric toxicology. Pediatr. Clin. North Am., *33*:331–333, 1986. *A comprehensive review of clinically relevant aspects of substance abuse.*

Lang, R. M., Borow, K. M., Neumann, A., and Feldman, T.: Adverse cardiac effects of acute alcohol ingestion in young adults. Ann. Intern. Med., *102*:742–747, 1985.

Last, J. (Ed.): Public Health and Preventive Medicine. 12th Ed. New York, Appleton Century Crofts, 1986, p. 40.

Law and Medicine/Council Report: Issues in employee drug test-

ing. J.A.M.A., *258*:2095, 1987. *A review of current positions and legal ramifications of employee drug testing.*
Lieber, C. S.: Alcohol and the liver: 1984 update. Hepatology, *4*:1243–1260, 1984. *A broad-based discussion of alcohol-related liver disease written by a renowned expert in the field.*
Ludwig, A. M.: Cognitive processes associated with "spontaneous" recovery from alcoholism. J. Stud. Alcohol., *46*:53–58, 1985. *This paper represents the culmination of a long series of studies on craving and cognitive processes among alcoholics.*
Lundberg, G. (Ed.): Mandatory unindicated urine drug screening: Still chemical McCarthyism. J.A.M.A., *256*:3003–3005, 1986.
Madden, J. S.: A Guide to Alcohol and Drug Dependence. Bristol, UK, John Wright & Sons, Ltd., 1979. *A discussion of basic science and treatment issues of drug dependence.*
Moore, E. C.: Women and health, United States, 1980. Public Health Rep., *95*[Suppl.]: Sept.-Oct., 1980.
Morgan, J. P.: Alcohol and Drug Abuse Curriculum Guide for Pharmacology Faculty. Rockville, MD, National Institute on Drug Abuse, 1985, pp. 3–19.
Morrow-Tlucak, M., and Ernhart, D. B.: Maternal prenatal substance abuse and behavior at age 3 years. Alcoholism: Clin. Exp. Res., *11*:225, 1987.
Morse, R. M., et al.: Prognosis of physicians treated for alcoholism and drug dependence. J.A.M.A., *251*:745, 1984.
Nalbandian, H., et al.: Intestinal ischemia caused by cocaine ingestion. Report of 2 cases. Surgery, *97*:374–376, 1986.
Neubuerger, O. W., Miller, S. I., Schmitz, R. E., et al.: Replicable abstinence rates in an alcoholism treatment program. J.A.M.A., *248*:960–963, 1982. *Based on a sample of middle class alcoholics carefully followed after a private treatment program, the study demonstrates a high rate of continued abstinence.*
New knowledge about nicotine effects. J.A.M.A., *247*:2333, 1982.
Nieburg, P., Marks, J. S., McLaren, N. M., and Remington, P. L.: The fetal tobacco syndrome. J.A.M.A., *253*:2998–2999, 1985.
Novotny, T. Epidemiologist, Office on Smoking and Health, U.S. Dept. of Health and Human Services. Personal communication, 1989.
Palmer, J. R., Rosenberg, L., and Shapiro, S.: "Low-yield" cigarettes and the risk of nonfatal myocardial infarction in women. N. Engl. J. Med., *320*:1569–1573, 1989.
Pentel, P., Mikell, F., and Navoral, S. H.: Myocardial injury after phenylpropanolamine ingestion. Br. Heart J., *47*:51–54, 1982.
Pershagen, G., Svensson, C., Hrubec, Z.: Passive smoking and lung cancer. Am. J. Epidemiol., *125*:17–24, 1987.
Pierce, P., Fiore, M. C., Novotny, T. E., et al.: Trends in cigarette smoking in the United States. J.A.M.A., *261*:61–65, 1989.
Pollin, W., and Ravenholt, R. T.: Tobacco addiction and tobacco mortality. J.A.M.A., *252*:2849–2854, 1984.
Qian, H., Feng, J., Hou, X., et al.: Smoking and reproductive cancer. Female Patient, *14*:42–51, 1989.
Raeburn, P.: Passive smoking may be 10 times deadlier than thought. Houston Post, June 19, 1989.
Rantakallio, P.: Relationship of maternal smoking to morbidity and mortality of the child up to the age of five. Acta Paediatr. Scand., *67*:621, 1978.
Reducing the Health Consequences of Smoking: 25 years of program. A Report of the Surgeon General. DHHS Publication No. (PHS) 89-8411. Rockville, MD, U.S. Dept. of Health, Education and Welfare, Public Health Service. Office of Smoking and Health, 1989. *The definitive summary and analysis of the multifarious problems due to smoking, trends in smoking behavior, and efforts to curb tobacco use.*
Research on Smoking Behavior: National Institute on Drug Abuse Research Monograph Series No. 17. Jarvik, M. E., Cullen, J. W., Gritz, E. R., et al. (Eds.). DHEW Publication No. (ADM) 78-581. Rockville, MD, U.S. Dept. of Health, Education and Welfare, Public Health Service, Alcohol, Drug Abuse, and Mental Health Administration, 1977.
Robins, L. N.: Study childhood predictors of adult outcomes: Replications from longitudinal studies. Psychol. Med., *8*:611–622, 1978.
Robins, L. N., Helzer, J. E., and Guze, S. B.: Lifetime prevalence of specific psychiatric disorders in three sites. Arch. Gen. Psychiatry, *41*:949–958, 1984. *Part of the Epidemiological Catchment Area studies being done worldwide, the paper demonstrates a very high prevalence of alcohol-related problems and alcoholism.*
Rogers, R. L., et al.: Abstention from cigarette smoking improves cerebral perfusion among elderly chronic smokers. J.A.M.A., *253*:2970–2974, 1985.
Rosenberg, L., Kaufman, D. W., Helmrich, S. P., and Shapiro, S.: The risk of myocardial infarction after quitting smoking in men under 55 years of age. N. Engl. J. Med., *313*:1511–1514, 1985.
Russell, M. A. H., Wilson, C., Taylor, C., et al.: Effect of general practitioner's advice against smoking. Br. Med. J., *2*:231–235, 1979. *Discusses the importance of the family physician's involvement in office-based efforts to promote smoking cessation.*
Salkin, M.: Management of emergencies. Chapter VII. Review Course Syllabus for American Medical Society on Alcoholism and Other Drug Dependencies, 12 W. 21st St., New York, NY 10010, 1987.
Sandler, D. P., Everson, R. B., Wilcox, A. J., et al.: Cancer risk in adulthood from early life exposure to parents' smoking. Am. J. Public Health, *75*:487–492, 1985a.
Sandler, D. P., Wilcox, A. J., and Everson, R. B.: Preliminary communication: Cumulative effects of lifetime passive smoking on cancer risk. Lancet, *1*:312–314, 1985b.
Saunders, J. B.: Alcohol: An important cause of hypertension. Br. Med. J., *294*:1045–1046, 1987.
Schuckit, M. A.: Drug and Alcohol Abuse. 3rd ed. New York, Plenum Press, 1989.
Schuckit, M. A.: Biological vulnerability to alcoholism. J. Consult. Clin. Psychol., *55*:301–309, 1987.
Schuckit, M. A.: Genetic and clinical implications of alcoholism and affective disorder. Am. J. Psychiatry, *143*:140–147, 1986. *When alcoholism and depressive disorders are carefully defined, this study demonstrates little convincing evidence of a genetic relationship between the two.*
Schuckit, M. A.: Overview: Epidemiology of alcoholism. *In* Schuckit, M. A. (Ed.): Alcohol Patterns and Problems. Series in Psychosocial Epidemiology, vol. 5. New Brunswick, NJ, Rutgers University Press, 1985a, pp. 1–42.
Schuckit, M. A.: The clinical implications of primary diagnostic groups among alcoholics. Arch. Gen. Psychiatry, *42*:1043–1049, 1985b. *Part of a long series of studies showing that alcoholics with pre-existent psychiatric disorders have prognoses different from those who had no major psychiatric illness before alcoholism.*
Schuckit, M. A.: Genetics and the risk for alcoholism. J.A.M.A., *254*:2614–2617, 1985c.
Schuckit, M. A.: Drug and Alcohol Abuse: A Clinical Guide to Diagnosis and Treatment. New York, Plenum Press, 1984.
Schuckit, M. A., and Gold, E. O.: A simultaneous evaluation of multiple markers of ethanol/placebo challenges in sons of alcoholics and controls. Arch. Gen. Psychiatry, *45*:211–216, 1988. *The culmination of a series of studies demonstrating a decreased reaction to alcohol in children of alcoholics.*
Schuckit, M. A., and Irwin, M.: Diagnosis of alcoholism. Med. Clin. North Am., *72*(5):1133–53, 1988.
Schuckit, M. A., and Monteiro, M. G.: Alcoholism, anxiety, and depression. Brit. J. Addiction, *83*:1373–1380, 1988.
Schuckit, M. A., Butters, N., Lyn, L., and Irwin, M.: Neuropsychologic deficits and the risk of alcoholism. Neuropsychopharmacology, 21:45–53, 1987.
Schuckit, M. A., Zisook, S., and Mortola, J.: Clinical implications of DSM III diagnoses of alcohol abuse and alcohol dependence. Am. J. Psychiatry, *142*:1403–1408, 1985.
Schwartz, J. L.: Review and evaluation of smoking cessation methods: The United States and Canada, 1978–1985. NIH Pub. No. 87-2940. Division of Cancer Prevention and Control, National Cancer Institute, U.S. Dept. of Health and Human Services, 1987. *A unique document, it is the most comprehensive report on the subject of stopping smoking.*
Schwartz, J. L.: Review and evaluation of smoking cessation. Public Health Rep., *94*:558–563, 1979.
Schwartz, J. L.: A critical review and evaluation of smoking control methods. Public Health Rep., *84*:483–506, 1969.

Shimakata, H., Muller, D. C., and Andres, R.: Studies in the distribution of body fat, III: effects of cigarette smoking. J.A.M.A., *261*:1169–1173, 1989.

Shinton, R., and Beevers, G.: Meta-analysis of relation between cigarette smoking and stroke. Br. Med. J., *298*:789–794, 1989.

Shveitzer, V. G.: Osteolytic sinusitis and pneumomediastinum: Deceptive otolaryngologic complications of cocaine abuse. Laryngoscope, *96*:206–210, 1986.

Simpson, R. W., and Edwards, W. D.: Pathogenesis of cocaine induced ischemic heart disease. Arch. Pathol. Lab. Med., *110*:479–484, 1986.

Slattery, M. L., Robison, L. M., Schuman, K., et al.: Cigarette smoking and exposure to passive smoke are risk factors for cervical cancer. J.A.M.A., *261*:1593–1598, 1989.

Slone, D., Shapiro, S., Rosenberg, L., et al.: Relation of cigarette smoking to myocardial infarction in young women. N. Engl. J. Med., *298*:1273, 1978.

Smith, D. E., and Wesson, D. R.: Benzodiazepine dependency syndromes. J. Psychoactive Drugs, *15*:85–95, 1983.

Smith, D. E., and Wesson, D. R.: A new method for treatment of barbiturate dependence. J.A.M.A., *213*:294–295, 1970.

Stutzman, E.: Medical complications. Chapter IX, Review Course Syllabus for American Medical Society on Alcoholism and Other Drug Dependencies, 12 W. 21st St., New York, NY 10010, 1987.

U.S. Dept. of Health and Human Services. *Reducing the Health Consequences of Smoking: 25 Years of Progress. A Report of the Surgeon General.* U.S. Dept. of Health and Human Services, Public Health Service, Centers for Disease Control, Center for Chronic Disease Prevention and Health Promotion, Office on Smoking and Health. DHHS Publication No. (CDC) 89-8411. Prepublication version January 11, 1989. *Also known as the Surgeon General's Report, 1989.*

Vaillant, G. E.: Natural history of male alcoholism. Arch. Gen. Psychiatry, *39*:127–133, 1982. *Part of a series of carefully constructed descriptions of the usual course of alcoholism.*

Vilensky, W.: Illicit and licit drugs causing perforation of the nasal septum. J. Forensic Sci., *27*:958–962, 1982.

Wells, A. J.: An estimate of adult mortality in the United States from passive smoking. Environ. International, *14*:249–265, 1988.

Wilford, B. B.: Drug Abuse: A Guide for the Primary Care Physician. Chicago, American Medical Association, 1981.

Williamson, D. F., Serdula, M. K., Kendrick, J. S., and Binkin, N. J.: Comparing the prevalence of smoking in pregnant and nonpregnant women, 1985 to 1986. J.A.M.A., *261*:70–74, 1989.

Winters, T. H., and Di Franza, J. R.: Radioactivity in cigarette smoke. N. Engl. J. Med., *306*:364, 1982.

Wolf, P. A., D'Aostine, R. B., Sannel, W. B., et al.: Cigarette smoking as a risk factor for stroke. The Framingham Study. J.A.M.A., *259*:1025–1029, 1988.

Woods, P. J.: Smoking and Behavior Control. Roanoke, VA, Hollins College, Dept. of Psychology, 1988.

69

Psychiatric Emergencies

Philip J. Bohnert

It is 5:30 P.M. and you are rushing to finish at the office. You are tired and eager to get home, because you were admitting a patient to the hospital at 1:00 A.M. last night and started making rounds at 7:00 A.M. today, so you would like some rest. Your last patient is Mr. Jones, a successful 52-year-old executive of the Catholic faith, who comes to your office with his wife. She is "very concerned about him" because he has just made his third suicide attempt in the past 3 years. The attempts involved taking 5 to 10 Dalmane capsules; the last time he also got drunk. Each time he managed to let his wife know that he had taken the pills and she summoned paramedical help. She had left him 4 months ago, but returned 1 week ago after his last attempt. They are now working with a psychiatrist on the marriage and his alcoholism. She is encouraged that he has decreased his drinking recently. You have been treating him for multiple sclerosis and he mentions that "My thinking has not been as sharp lately."

Your feelings in response to Mr. Jones' problems are probably very mixed: a sigh of frustration, pressure and responsibility, empathy for Mrs. Jones, uncertainty about the seriousness of the suicidal risk, and simply fatigue and possibly annoyance at having to deal with such a serious problem at this time. You feel confused because of the "mixed signals" that Mr. Jones (and many suicidal patients) may give, and Mr. Jones poses a very demanding challenge.

We physicians are all suffering to some degree from professional stress. Daily we deal with significant pressures: fearful and/or demanding patients, life-threatening illnesses, staff problems and conflicts, not to mention our own internal states of fatigue and other personal stressors. Understandably, much of the time we do not welcome the further strain that comes with psychiatric emergencies, such as Mr. Jones presents. Typically, being overstressed leads either to emotional numbing with avoidance/denial of uncomfortable stimuli, or to hypervigilance. For the physician facing a psychological emergency, these can translate on the one hand into underreacting, e.g., minimizing a patient's comments about "wanting to die," or not pursuing feelings of "falling apart" or being "so furious I feel like killing someone." On the hyperalert side, the family physician can overreact and immediately refer all seriously depressed or angry patients to a hospital or psychotherapist. Our goal in this chapter is to give the family physician reliable, concise information and techniques for assessment and management that can help him or her avoid either "selective inattention" or "hyperreactivity" in three types of emergency situations.

A psychiatric emergency is an acute disturbance in behavior, thinking, or feeling that, if not responded to, will lead to life-threatening or psychologically damaging results. We will focus on the potentially suicidal patient, the decompensating psychotic, and the violent patient.

Practicing medicine is a privilege. The intimacy offered by our patients' sharing of their deepest concerns and feelings can be very gratifying. The opportunity to help heal the body/mind, even a broken spirit, is a special gift. The opportunity to use this gift is greatest when dealing with emergency situations. The chance to help the patient and family resolve a crisis is a remarkable opportunity to "make a difference." For example, suicide is often considered to be the most preventable cause of death next to lung cancer. When we are able to serve someone in a way that saves his or her life or prevents further psychological injury, we are truly fulfilling our Hippocratic ideals.

The Potentially Suicidal Patient

The family physician clearly can be the most potent person in the prevention of suicide. Barraclough (1974) found that two thirds of suicides had seen a family physician in the month before they killed themselves, 40 per cent within a week. Approximately 80 per cent of successful suicides have told someone of their intention (Beskow, 1979). Yet among suicides who were known to have told someone of their intent, only about one of every six of their physicians had known of it (Murphy, 1988). It is well known that the patient considering suicide will usually tell the physician if asked, so apparently many physicians are reluctant to explore this subject. Asking about suicidal thought does not increase the risk; *not* asking can be dangerous. A helpful technique is to use a progressively more open series of questions, such as, "Do you ever feel that life is not worth living? Do you ever *wish* you were dead? Have you ever thought of *hurting* yourself? Have you had any thoughts about *killing* yourself? What have you thought about doing?" This accomplishes two things: It builds trust, and also the gradual build-up makes many patients ready, even impatient, to be asked the more frank questions.

It is important for physicians to be aware of their own feelings, so that evaluation and handling of the potentially suicidal patient is not affected. *Denial* may occur because the physician feels reluctant or inadequate to deal with such a serious problem. This may be because of depression that the physician, or present or past members of the physician's family, had experienced; facing similar feelings in the patient can be an unpleasant reminder. *Anger* can also surface if the physician has a judgmental attitude that "Everyone should be able to handle his own problems," and that thinking about suicide is simply a sign of weakness. *Fear* can complicate management if the physician feels threatened by possible damage to his or her reputation or bad publicity if a patient commits suicide; the best antidote for this is to become confident in the evaluation and management of the suicidal patient.

There are many reasons why the family physician is the most natural person to intercept the potential suicide. First, the most reliable predictor of suicidal risk is a diagnosis of psychiatric illness, particularly depression, alcohol and substance abuse, and schizophrenia. At least two thirds of successful suicides were clinically depressed or abusing alcohol or drugs, conditions that can be picked up by the family physician. Major depression was found to have a prevalence of 6 per cent in a rigorous study (Von Korff et al., 1987); this would make it the most common illness in family practice. It is well known that far more psychiatric patients are initially seen, as well as receive treatment, by their family physician than by psychiatrists or psychologists.

In addition, many medical conditions carry with them a particularly high suicidal risk, most notably AIDS (Marzuk et al., 1988), organic brain syndromes (Black et al., 1985), chronic renal disease with dialysis (Abram et al., 1971; Haenel et al., 1980), multiple sclerosis (Kahana et al., 1971; Barraclough, 1981), Huntington's disease (Schoenfeld et al., 1984; Farrer, 1986), and terminal medical illness, particularly cancer. Peptic ulcer (Knop and Fischer, 1981) and respiratory disease also increase the risk. Table 69–1 lists these high-risk illnesses and also gives a perspective on the approximate distribution of all suicides by diagnosis. The lifetime risk of patients with one of the three most common diagnoses ultimately committing suicide is also indicated, and is surprisingly similar for all three diagnoses (Pitts and Winokur, 1966; Guze and Robins, 1970; Bleuler, 1978).

Although these diseases seem to carry an unusually high risk, many of the less severe illnesses the family physician sees are related to factors that lead to suicidality, such as hopelessness, depression, and a sense of being a burden to others. In fact, there is evidence that an increasing frequency of medical visits without clear need may be a subtle cry for help.

For all these reasons, the family physician has the best opportunity of any health care professional to detect and help prevent suicide.

PREDICTORS OF SUICIDE

Investigators of suicide have collected voluminous data about various parameters related to increased suicidal risk, and most of us are familiar with the usually cited "high-risk factors," such as being male, over 50, living alone, contemplating using a gun or hanging. However, these criteria alone are not nearly adequate when you are faced with a patient and asking yourself, "Is *this patient* sitting in my office now a serious threat to kill himself *at this time?* Is the risk high enough that I should insist on hospitalization?" Table 69–2 prioritizes these risk factors.

Suicide predictors are divided into four categories. *Most reliable* indicates criteria that researchers have shown to be powerful indicators of imminent and/or high risk of suicide. Recent research has been particularly helpful in identifying acute, short-term lethal factors. *Supplemental indicators* refer to information that is also correlated with high suicidal risk, but is less compelling. Nonetheless, these additional criteria can be helpful to the clinician in strengthening or weakening the case for suicidal risk based on the "most reliable" indicators. *Deceptive or equivocal indicators* include issues that often confuse clinicians, especially by falsely reassuring them, e.g., "She only took pills, she's not serious." These are areas that require further questioning to avoid superficial stereotypes and "common wisdom"—actually common

Table 69–1. PATIENTS AT HIGH RISK FOR SUICIDE

	Risk Compared with General Population	Percentage of All Suicides	Lifetime Risk of Successful Suicide
Primary affective disorder	25–487×	50%	15%
Substance abuse, including alcohol	11–20×	25%	15%
Schizophrenia	34×	10%	15%
AIDS	66×		
Diseases affecting the CNS:			
Organic brain syndrome		7%	
Delirium tremens			
Temporal lobe epilepsy	25×		
Huntington's disease	3–23×		
Multiple sclerosis	14×		
Renal disease with dialysis	10–50×		5%
Cancer	2–4×	4%	
Peptic ulcer	2–9×		
Respiratory disease	3×		

misunderstandings—about suicidal risk. Finally, *observations suggesting low risk* give the physician relatively solid evidence that the patient is less seriously suicidal.

The key concept here is to evaluate by the *composite* of factors. The more factors matching those found in suicide "committers," the graver the risk. For example, a *30-year-old woman* (both low-risk factors) who has *recently lost a lover* (moderate risk in a young woman) would usually not be a high risk. However, if she also has a *major depressive disorder,* her risk suddenly rises, since 56 per cent of the suicides in patients with this diagnosis occur by age 30 or younger, within 1 year of the diagnosis (Fawcett, 1988).

Although there may seem to be many factors to consider, the family physician can actually do a well-organized, time-effective assessment by focusing on six areas: *diagnosis, symptoms, demographic/factual data, past history* (including any *precipitating events*), *external resources,* and the *interviewer's own reactions.*

Diagnosis is the first focus. The most powerful risk factor for suicide is the presence of *any serious psychiatric illness*, which is found in over 90 per cent of suicides. Depressive illness is the most common diagnosis, accounting for approximately one half of all suicides, and with a risk 25 times that of the general population (see Table 69–1). This risk increases to a startling 487 times in the severely depressed male (Essen-Moeller et al., 1956). Corroborating this, Fawcett (1988) found patients with major affective disorders killed themselves over 200 times the general population rate in the first year of study. It is imperative that the clinican evaluate any depressed patient closely. Suicidal risk is increased in the presence of either agitation or delusions. The most ominous time is the depressed phase of manic-depressive illness, bipolar type II, since about half these patients commit suicide. The most alarming symptom is hopelessness.

The next largest proportion of suicides are those with alcohol or other substance abuse (25 per cent). The importance of this group is illustrated in the finding of 58 per cent of suicides with this diagnosis by Fowler et al. (1986). Thus, depressives and substance abusers make up approximately three fourths of all suicides. The primary mechanisms in the alcoholic are disinhibition, impaired judgment, and impulsivity. Practically all suicides within this group are precipitated by personal loss, especially if the loss was recent (often within 6 weeks). Two patterns increase the risk, either currently drinking or having been alcoholic for many years. The primary obstacle here is the widespread tendency of physicians to underdiagnose alcoholism (see Chapter 68). The most clear-cut criteria are simply repeated difficulties caused by drinking in a person's work, health, or relationships. Detailed questioning is necessary, rather than accepting such typical responses as "I only drink socially."

Schizophrenics constitute about 10 per cent of the suicide total. They are particularly vulnerable in the depressive, recovery phase. When their course is volatile, with many exacerbations and remissions, risk is particularly high; impulsive acts are typical.

It should be noted that comorbidity of any two of these three diagnoses amplifies the danger.

The family physician should be particularly alert for suicidal potential when treating certain medical illnesses. The patient diagnosed with AIDS is in especially acute peril; in Marzuk's study (1988), *all* of the suicides occurred within 9 months of being diagnosed, all at early stages of the illness, and one fourth of these jumped to their death from the hospital window. There have been several reports of patients with positive HIV antibodies without AIDS, as well as lovers of AIDS patients, who have committed suicide. Patients with diseases affecting the central nervous system may be at higher risk because of neurotransmitter disturbances. Low levels of 5-hydroxyindole acetic acid (5-HIAA), a serotonin metabolite, in the cerebrospinal fluid have been correlated with violent suicide (Brown et al., 1982). Several factors are probably involved with the increased suicide rate in patients with terminal illness, including chronic or severe pain, loss of function, fear of

Table 69–2. PREDICTORS OF SUICIDE: HIGH-RISK INDICATORS

Most Reliable	Supplemental Indicators
Diagnosis Depression, especially: Agitated Delusional Manic-depressive Substance abuse, including alcohol, especially: Disruption/loss Concurrently depressed Concurrently psychotic Drugs *and* alcohol Schizophrenia, especially: Depressive phase Self-destructive voices Dual diagnosis: Depression plus psychosis Substance abuse plus depression Substance abuse plus psychosis AIDS Diseases affecting the CNS Chronic renal disease, dialysis	***Diagnosis*** Organic brain syndrome Terminal illness, especially cancer Chronic respiratory disease Peptic ulcer
Symptoms Hopelessness Anhedonia Severe psychic anxiety Panic attacks Depressive turmoil Moderate alcohol abuse Contemplating hanging or jumping Suicidal impulses Sense of being a burden to others Severe crying, or inability to cry Ideas of reference or persecution Divorced Prior psychiatric hospitalization Threat of financial loss Negative/mixed reaction by interviewer Mood cycling	***Symptoms*** Communication poor Alcoholic: currently drinking Moderate to severe insomnia
Demographic/Factual Data Divorced, widowed, never married, living alone Suicide plans: Lethal method available Recently made or revised will; left note Specific place, time	***Demographic/Factual Data*** Over 65, under 25 Male White, American Indian
Past History Prior psychiatric hospitalization Previous suicidal attempts	***Past History*** Previous suicidal attempts by family Alcoholic: drinking >20 years *No* precipitant
External Resources Personal disruption/loss Financial resources exhausted	***External Resources*** Friends rejecting
Interviewer's Reactions Negative/mixed reaction Uneasy letting patient leave	

disfigurement, loss of family support, depression, and hopelessness.

The *symptoms* listed in Table 69–2 are particularly potent predictors of *acute* suicidal risk; the first six indicators are from Fawcett (1988), the second nine from Motto (1988). (The last four are not symptoms, but are grouped here for convenient identification as indicators of particularly acute risk.) Motto studied 2999 patients hospitalized for a suicidal state or severe depression and found these nine factors to be predictive of patients who committed suicide *within 60 days of discharge*. Four or more of these factors identified 79 per cent of the suicides. Fawcett found hopelessness (focused on by many authors) and anhedonia, "the loss of pleasure or interest," as the two most significant factors. Psychic anxiety was correlated with elevated 24-hour 17-hydroxycorticosteroid levels. He defines depressive turmoil as "the rapid switching of mood from depression to anxiety to anger or vice versa, accompanied by agitation and perturbation." He also found mood cycling ("depression and mania or hypomania") to be important. Patients previously in a psychiatric hospital are at very high risk in the first year after discharge, especially during the first month. Porkorny (1983) found that psychiatrically hospitalized veterans had 10 times the suicide risk of other veterans. The risk correlated with previous suicidal attempts is proportionate to the number of attempts. Finally, an important criterion is the *interviewer's reaction* at the end of the interview. It is useful to ask, "If this were my best friend, would I feel comfortable letting him or her go home?" If the answer is "No," then recommend hospitalization.

Of the *supplemental indicators,* the dramatic two- to threefold increase of suicide in the young in the past 20 years is cause for alarm. Two known factors are increased substance abuse (Marzuk and Mann, 1988) and "cluster" suicides, which occur within 2 weeks of television reporting of a young suicide or a feature movie about adolescent suicide.

The *deceptive or equivocal indicators* merit special elaboration (Table 69–3). The patient most often underestimated for suicidal potential is the one who has made *frequent attempts.* The term "gestures" is falsely minimizing; 50 to 75 per cent of suicide "committers" have tried previously, and 10 per cent of "attempters" are ultimately successful. Tuckman and Youngman (1968) found suicide attempters had a 139-fold increase in eventual suicidal deaths. Of suicide attempters, 1 to 2 per cent will succeed in killing themselves within a year, and 1 to 2 per cent will die each year thereafter, up to a total of about 10 per cent. Therefore, any threat by someone who has attempted suicide previously should be taken seriously. The important question about a person's *religion* is whether he or she is *actively practicing*; if so, this lessens the risk.

Another common myth is that patients who "only" take pills are not serious. This is belied by the fact that one fourth of successful suicides are achieved by taking medication. Helpful clues include whether the patient has overdosed or tried other *"low-lethality" methods* before, whether the patient *thought* the dose was lethal, and whether the patient is upset that he or she was saved.

Table 69–3. FURTHER EVALUATION OF SUICIDAL RISK

Deceptive or Equivocal Indicators, Requiring Further Questioning
Frequent threats, attempts, "gestures"
"Low-lethality" method
Religion stated, especially Catholic
Low-Risk Indicators
Female
25 to 40 years old
Diagnosis of:
Histrionic personality
Obsessive-compulsive
Communication good
Religion, actively practicing
Enjoys work; works regularly
One close relationship

Finally, in this difficult problem, the clinician can sometimes be fortunate enough to notice certain data that can be reassuring that a particular patient is at *lower risk* (see Table 69–3). The "hysterical personality" is more interested in drama than death, and the obsessive-compulsive usually has too much intellectualization and rigid control to do himself in. It is also reassuring if the patient continues talking at length with the physician or mentions future plans, e.g., for an upcoming birthday. Finally, in the author's experience, the most powerful protective factor is having one close relationship.

You now begin to evaluate Mr. Jones, and to sort out the "mixed signals" he is giving. You know that a 52-year-old man is statistically a relatively high risk. However, you know you need more reliable indicators. An external resource that is helpful is the fact that he is a successful, affluent executive, who likes his work. This can provide him some ongoing self-esteem as well as the money to pay for therapy. The fact that he has used a relatively few sedative pills each time and managed to let his wife know each time is mildly reassuring. However, you know that the risk increases in proportion to the number of attempts, so you are concerned. Another possible mitigating factor is the apparent support of his wife; but you find out that she has left him three times and therefore may do it again. This could be especially ominous since Mr. Jones is an alcoholic, which makes him extremely vulnerable to a loss. You are not at all reassured because he reportedly has been drinking less lately; in fact, you know that the alcoholic who is still actively drinking is definitely a greater risk. The fact that he and his wife are working in psychotherapy is positive, although he obviously is not working very hard on his alcoholism if he is still drinking. You were reassured when you heard that he was Catholic, but you prudently questioned him further and discovered that he has not practiced for several years, so that this is not protective. Finally, his multiple sclerosis and impaired mental functioning (declining memory, less clear thinking) definitely put him in the very-high-risk category of diseases affecting the central nervous system. Add to this that his diagnosis of alcoholism has already put him at high risk, and you can confidently decide that Mr. Jones is definitely a serious suicidal threat. This gives you much more confidence and you strongly recommend hospitalization.

Despite the alarming connotations of suicidal ideas, the family physician who develops a diagnostic outline for assessment can feel comfortable that a high level of reliability in evaluating the patient's risk can be reached, and thus move on to management. Principles of immediate and ongoing management are summarized in Table 69–4.

FOLLOW-UP

The benefits of being able to detect and manage the potentially suicidal patient are powerful and very gratifying. When followed 8 years after a suicide attempt, 41 per cent stated that the act had been a turning point in their lives (Retterstol, 1970). After Einstein dealt with serious suicidal impulses as a young adult, he developed a whole new perspective

Table 69–4. MANAGEMENT OF THE SUICIDAL PATIENT

I. **Immediate**
  A. **The doctor as healing agent.** Discussing the patient's suicidal thoughts nonjudgmentally is itself powerfully supportive.
  B. **Get a detailed history, assess the risk.**
  C. **Get help.**
    1. Relatives, friends, clergy ("one close relationship"); to protect and support the patient, supply important information.
    2. Consultation/referral.
    3. Get support for your own emotions.
  D. **Remove lethal methods.** Surprisingly often not insisted upon. Have a relative or friend make sure that this is carried out.
  E. **Get patient to externalize feelings; offer empathy.** Verbalization of the patient's sad, scared, or angry feelings diminishes the likelihood of taking out the feelings on himself.
  F. **Medication.** Lessening the overwhelming discomfort significantly reduces suicidal risk. Prescribe only sublethal amounts. See Chapter 71 for details and dosages.
    1. Sedative for severe insomnia; uninterrupted, around-the-clock depression can become intolerable.
    2. Tranquilizer for agitation. *Not* Valium; may worsen depression.
    3. Antidepressant; some patients respond within a week. "Takes the edge off" the depression for many. Caution: If a listless depressed patient gets mobilized, he may gain enough energy to attempt suicide.
  G. **Electroconvulsive therapy.** Usually only as a "last resort."
  H. **Medicolegal.**
    1. Document level of suicidal risk.
    2. List reasons for deciding this.
    3. Note attempts to manage, e.g., referral to hospital or psychotherapist; if refused, relationships (who) contacted.
    4. Notify relatives.
  I. **Hospitalize.**
    1. If your evaluation of risk factors equates to "high-risk."
    2. All who *attempt* suicide—easier to evaluate the patient and toxicity of an overdose adequately, and enlist the family's help.
    3. Commitment: if patient refuses hospitalization. Know your state's criteria; being "dangerous to himself or others" is most common (Stevenson, 1988). Also be familiar with specific details: where to call, take the patient, etc.
    4. After your best efforts at evaluating the patient, if you still have disturbing feelings about letting the patient leave your office to go home, it is best to hospitalize him. *Pay attention to your intuition!*

II. **Ongoing**
  A. **Psychotherapy, especially for depression, psychosis, alcoholism; referral if needed.** Referral is particularly indicated if the psychodynamics are complicated or the suicidal possibilities warrant close monitoring and/or more intensive psychotherapy. *Frequent* follow-up after discharge is imperative, especially during the first 12 months, when risk is highest. The patient who gets daily contact in a hospital and is then discharged and told to come back in a month is getting a very mixed message.
  B. **Medicate adequately.** At least 50 per cent of suicides are given an inadequate dose of antidepressant medication, receive the medication too briefly, or are seen too infrequently.
  C. **Monitor the initial suicide predictors to track the patient's recovery:** mood, thinking, behavior, and relationships.

that helped lead to his most brilliant and productive years as a theoretician; similar stories by many other major contributors to society are well known. Predicting and preventing a possible suicide is obviously a major service to the patient and can be extremely satisfying to the family physician.

The Decompensating Psychotic

The alarming behavior and thinking of the person who is literally "going crazy" can truly be an emergency situation for the patient's family, the family physician, *and* the physician's office staff. The pathognomonic symptoms of delusion and/or hallucination that characterize full-blown psychosis appear in the later stages of illness—the stage of "psychotic crystallization." However, the clinician can better anticipate/prevent an acute psychotic break, as well as any possible associated violence, by an awareness of the incipient clues of developing psychosis. Table 69–5 shows these "early warning signals" and symptoms of the acute psychotic turmoil, when the patient's mental state is deteriorating but still relatively amenable to intervention. The psychotic depressive or manic will have strong depressive or euphoric affect, in addition to psychomotor retardation or agitation, but the psychotic symptoms evolve as shown in Table 69–5. By detecting early symptoms of decompensation, the family physician can help avert the end-stage of psychotic crystallization, in which the risk of suicide or violence to others is greatest.

The Violent Patient

She was "the love of his life," but as financial and marital problems gradually unravelled his life, retail executive Dan Franklin shot his only child, Terri, with a shotgun, minutes before he killed his wife, her sister, and then himself. Terri's schoolmates and the neighbors were shocked by the killing, although a friend stated that the Franklins had recently begun marital counseling because Dan was battering his wife. A friend of Terri's has spent most of the last two days crying; "I still find myself planning to go to the

Table 69–5. PROGRESSION OF PSYCHOTIC DECOMPENSATION

Early Warning Signals	Acute Psychotic Turmoil	Psychotic Crystallization
Inner (not audible) voice, e.g., conscience	Auditory illusions	Auditory hallucinations
Hyperacuity to sensations	Illusions/ misperceptions	Hallucinations of any type
Feelings of being "different"	Feels "unreal"; "strange" bodily symptoms	Somatic delusions
Blames failures on poor *circumstances*	Blames other *people*	Paranoid "illumination": sees *systematized* plot
Easily slighted, wronged	Feelings of mistreatment, persecution	Delusions of persecution
Excessively, judgmental, righteous	Vengeful against specific people	Urge to kill, possibly on command of delusion

Adapted from Swanson, D., Bohnert, P., and Smith, J.: The Paranoid. Boston, Little, Brown & Co., 1970, p. 41.

football game with her next week and then I realize I can never do that again; I'm going to miss her for a long time."

Indeed she will. Could these deaths have been prevented, by detecting clues that obviously preceded this tragedy, if you had seen any member of this family in your office recently? Also, acts of violence directed toward physicians themselves occur often enough to make us uneasy about the risk to ourselves. Yet most physicians do not develop a systematic approach, using information now available, that would enable them to make a rapid evaluation, leading to management, of the patient who is already or is rapidly becoming violent. We will focus on the principles of instant risk evaluation and short-term management.

INSTANT RISK EVALUATION

The three primary areas on which to focus are present behavior, past history, and diagnosis. Practically all violent behavior comes from patients with the diagnoses listed in Table 69–6; the percentage of total violent acts is indicated in parentheses. Tardiff's excellent, concise approach to management and assessment of violence is shown in Table 69–7. Other high-risk factors include being male, a young adult, and of subnormal intelligence. The same principle of graduated questioning described in the suicidal section is recommended here. The interviewer could begin by asking: "Do you ever lose control of your anger? Have you ever thought about *hurting* someone? Have you ever *hit* anyone?" Follow-up questions could ask about details of previous violence.

MANAGEMENT OF THE VIOLENT PATIENT

Verbal Intervention

The most important skill is the ability to present oneself in a nonthreatening, calming manner (see Table 69–7). Ideally, the physician can be compassionate, yet allow enough physical distance so the patient will not feel "invaded" (Swanson et al., 1970). Do *not* make constant eye contact or stare, or make angry comments, such as "Get hold of yourself." Giving psychological interpretations is also not useful. Avoid "reassuring" touches, especially with the paranoid. The principal underlying motivation for the patient's aggressive behavior is to protect himself or herself against feelings of impotence and fragility. Thus, quick movements toward the patient or aggressive statements should be avoided, since they may provoke a counterattack. The physician should keep at least an arm's length from the patient, to protect himself or herself and give the patient "space." Someone should stay with the patient at all times to maintain the empathic contact. The patient's feelings should be focused upon; the single most effective verbal maneuver is probably the "contact statement." This is simply an acknowledgment of the patient's feelings, e.g., "You really seem angry." This makes the patient feel heard, which usually diminishes the need to act out to have an impact. Attempts to rationalize and talk the patient out of the behavior are generally futile, mostly because they are interpreted by the patient as discounting his or her feelings ("You shouldn't be getting so upset."). At the same time, limit-setting is important so that the patient knows that violence is unacceptable. This is reassuring to the patient, who actually wants to maintain control. The presence of family or friends is often useful to get information and reinforce controls.

The clinician should know his or her feelings, fears, and fantasies about possible violence in advance, as described in dealing with suicidal patients; the physician's own unrecognized anger, denial, and fears can lead to nontherapeutically exaggerated re-

Table 69–6. DIAGNOSES OF VIOLENCE-PRONE PATIENTS

Psychoses	Organic Mental Disorders (20%)	Personality Disorders (20%)	Other
Schizophrenia (30–40%)	Substance abuse	Antisocial	Episodic dyscontrol syndrome
Mania	CNS diseases	Paranoid	Post-traumatic stress disorder
	Systemic diseases	Borderline	
	Seizure disorders		

Table 69–7. VERBAL MANAGEMENT OF VIOLENT PATIENTS

Be concerned for your safety.
Appear calm and in control.
Speak softly in a nonprovocative, nonjudgmental manner.
Both patient and clinician sit, if possible.
Do not tower over patient or stare at the patient.
When the patient begins to talk, listen.
Assess violence potential (following increase risk):
- How well planned is a threat?
- Availability of means for harming others?
- History of previous violence or other impulsive behaviors?
  - If so, what were precipitants, who were the victims, how serious were injuries?
- History of being abused as a child?
- Alcohol or drug abuse?
- Psychosis?
- Know your feelings about violence and reactions to the patient (e.g., denial, anger, fear, projection, bias).

From Tardiff, K.: Violence. *In* Talbott, J. A., et al. (Eds.): American Psychiatric Press Textbook of Psychiatry. Washington, DC, American Psychiatric Press, 1988.

sponses. A very effective strategy is to tell the patient that you feel frightened; this almost always gives the patient a sense of power, which counteracts his primary fear (powerlessness) and obviates the need to prove his potency.

Pharmacologic Treatment

The next step, if verbal methods are not effective, is the use of medication, usually rapid tranquilization. Tardiff (1988) provides an effective regimen (Table 69–8) and states that violent behavior is usually decreased within 20 minutes, with amelioration of psychotic symptoms within 6 hours. Even the act of offering medications often quiets the patient by giving him a feeling that controls are available (Tobias, 1988).

Hospitalization

For some patients, verbal and pharmacologic intervention will not be adequate and hospitalization is necessary. The primary indications for hospitalization in the potentially violent patient are psychosis, intoxication, a recent violent outburst, or an intended victim.

SPECIAL ISSUES

The Patient with a Gun

This is the ultimate fear, and the physician and staff should have a specific, prearranged plan to avoid panic. The ideal reaction is to simply escape. If this is not possible, comply with any requests. Do not ask for the gun immediately, but ask the patient why he feels the need to have it. This introduces mindfulness and, it is hoped, lessens impulsivity. When you do ask for a gun, never accept it directly, but ask the patient to put it on a table or the floor. Since the primary dynamics are impulsivity or a defense against impotence, a calm, respectful attitude is indicated.

Medicolegal Considerations

How is one to prudently "protect intended victims," to conform to the *Tarasoff* decision in California? This duty to warn or protect intended victims is usually necessary only when there are clear indications that the patient is a serious risk to physically harm a specific person (Beck, 1985). It is essential to document factors that led to the evaluation of violence potential, as well as the management decisions whether to hospitalize the patient and/or warn an intended victim.

Table 69–8. USE OF MEDICATIONS WITH VIOLENT PATIENTS

Neuroleptics
- Should be used with caution or not at all in delirious patients and in alcohol or drug toxic or withdrawal states.
- Toxic screen for alcohol and drugs should be done.
- For schizophrenia and mania, use rapid neuroleptization.

Haloperidol
- Low dose: 5 mg. intramuscularly every 4 hours for a maximum of 15–30 mg. a day.
- High dose: 10 mg. every 30 minutes for a maximum of 45–100 mg. a day.

Chlorpromazine
- 10–25 mg. test dose for orthostatic hypotension and observe for 1 hour.
- Low dose: 25 mg. intramuscularly every 4 hours.
- High dose: 75 mg. intramuscularly every 4 hours for a maximum of 400 mg. a day.

Sodium amobarbital (10 per cent solution)
- 200–500 mg. intravenously slowly 0.5–1.0 ml. per minute until sleep.

Diazepam
- 5–10 mg. diluted solution intravenously slowly (with intravenous sodium amobarbital or diazepam, there must be an ability to deal with laryngeal spasm or respiratory depression).

Carbamazepine
- 100–200 mg. twice a day for 1 week and then increase by 100–200 mg. a day until blood levels are from 4–12 ng./ml., usually for a total daily dose of 600 mg. Patients with seizure disorders may need up to 1200 mg. a day.

Propranolol
- 20 mg. three times a day with increases of 60 mg. every 3 to 4 days to a dose not exceeding 640 mg. a day.
- Exclude patients with bronchial asthma, chronic obstructive pulmonary disease, insulin-dependent diabetes, cardiac disease, severe peripheral vascular disease, severe renal disease, and hyperthyroidism.
- Monitor plasma blood levels of concurrent neuroleptics and anticonvulsants.

From Tardiff, K. (Cornell University Medical College): Violence. *In* Talbott, J. A., et al. (Eds.): American Psychiatric Press Textbook of Psychiatry. Washington, DC, American Psychiatric Press, 1988.

References

Abram, H. S., Moore, G. L., and Westervelt, F. B.: Suicidal behavior in chronic dialysis patients. Am. J. Psychiatry, *127*:119–124, 1971.

Barraclough, B. M.: Suicide and epilepsy. *In* Reynolds, E. H., and Trimble, M. R. (Eds.): Epilepsy and Psychiatry. Edinburgh, Churchill Livingstone, 1981.

Barraclough, B., Bunch, J., Nelson, B., et al.: A hundred cases of suicide: Clinical aspects. Br. J. Psychiatry, *125*:355, 1974. *This is particularly pertinent for family physicians, since this study shows that they are the group who have the best chance to detect and prevent suicide in the month and week before the act.*

Beck, J. C. (Ed.): The potentially violent patient and the *Tarasoff* Decision in Psychiatric Practice. Washington, DC, American Psychiatric Press, 1985.

Beskow, J.: Suicide and mental disorder in Swedish men. Acta Psychiatr. Scand. [Suppl.], *277*:1–138, 1979.

Black, D. W., Warrick, G., and Winokur, G.: The Iowa Record Linkage Study: Excess mortality among patients with organic mental disorders. Arch. Gen. Psychiatry, *42*:78–81, 1985.

Bleuler, M.: The Schizophrenic Disorders. New Haven, Yale University Press, 1978.

Brown, L. G., Ebert, M. H., Goger, P. F., et al.: Aggression, suicide and serotonin: Relationships to cerebrospinal fluid amine metabolites. Am. J. Psychiatry, *139*:741–746, 1982.

Essen-Moeller, E., Larsson, H., Uddenberg, C. E., et al.: Individual traits and morbidity in a Swedish rural population. Acta Psychiatr. Neurol. Scand. [Suppl.]:100, 1956.

Farrer, L. A.: Suicide and attempted suicide in Huntington's disease: Implications for preclinical testing of persons at risk. Am. J. Med. Genet., *24*:305–311, 1986.

Fawcett, J.: Predictors of early suicide: Identification and appropriate intervention. J. Clin. Psychiatry [Suppl.], *49*:10, 1988. *A valuable study because it is one of only a handful that focus on short-term predictors of suicide—the most useful for clinicians. A prospective study of 955 patients with major affective disorders begun in 1977, funded by NIMH and involving five academic medical centers.*

Fowler, R. C., Rich, C. L., and Young, D.: San Diego suicide study: II. Substance abuse in young cases. Arch. Gen. Psychiatry, *43*:962, 1986. *One of the most comprehensive studies on suicide. It reveals a tremendous increase in drug abuse (58% frequency) compared with previous studies, a younger than usual suicide age (20 to early 30's), and a typical use of multiple substances.*

Guze, S. B., and Robins, E.: Suicide and primary affective disorders. Br. J. Psychiatry, *117*:437, 1970.

Haenel, T. H., Brunner, F., and Battegay, R.: Renal dialysis and suicide: Occurrence in Switzerland and in Europe. Compr. Psychiatry, *21*:140–145, 1980.

Kahana, E., Leibowitz, U., and Alter, M.: Cerebral multiple sclerosis. Neurology, *21*:1179–1185, 1971.

Knop, J., and Fischer, A.: Duodenal ulcer, suicide, psychopathology and alcoholism. Acta Psychiatr. Scand., *63*:346–355, 1981.

Marzuk, P. M., and Mann, J. J.: Suicide and substance abuse. Psychiat. Ann., *18*:11, 1988. *A survey of substance abusers who committed suicide, and therefore useful to clinicians dealing with this population. Clinical, demographic, and historical characteristics are described, as well as various mechanisms of enhanced suicidal risk. A section on clinical management is also useful.*

Marzuk, P. M., Tierney, H., Tardiff, K., et al.: Increased risk of suicide in persons with AIDS. J.A.M.A., *259*:9, 1988. *This is an excellent study showing the tremendously increased risk of suicide in AIDS patients, disproving previous suggestions that the risk is low. The authors offer very cogent conclusions about clinical management and public health implications, as well as a useful brief survey of increased suicidal risk in other medical illnesses.*

Motto, J. A., and Bostrom, A.: Near-term indicators of suicide risk. Presented at the Regional Symposium of the World Psychiatric Association, Washington, DC, October, 1988. *This is another particularly useful study that discovered nine suicide predictors for the extreme short term (within 60 days of discharge). This and Fawcett's study together are invaluable.*

Murphy, G. E.: Suicide and attempted suicide. *In* Michels, R., et al.: Psychiatry. Philadelphia, J. B. Lippincott, 1988, pp. 9, 17. *This chapter, by one of the most well known researchers of suicide, gives a comprehensive review of the literature. Especially useful are the sections on dealing with suicidal intent (with specific suggestions for interventions) and the physician's role in suicide (reasons for missing the diagnosis; undertreatment).*

Pitts, F. N. Jr., and Winokur, G.: Affective disorder VII: Alcoholism and affective disorder. J. Psychiatr. Res., *4*:37, 1966.

Pokorny, A. D.: Prediction of suicide in psychiatric patients. Arch. Gen. Psychiatry, *40*:249–257, 1983.

Retterstol, N.: Long-Term Prognosis After Attempted Suicide. Springfield, IL, Charles C Thomas, 1970, p. 110.

Schoenfeld, M., Myers, R. H., Cupples, L. H., et al.: Increased rate of suicide among patients with Huntington's disease. J. Neurol. Neurosurg. Psychiatry, *47*:1283–1287, 1984.

Stevenson, J. M.: *In* Suicide. Talbott, J. A., Hales, R. E., and Yudofsky, S. C. (Eds.): American Psychiatric Press Textbook of Psychiatry. Washington, DC, American Psychiatric Press, 1988, pp. 1021–1035. *This is an outstanding survey of the literature, with especially good sections on psychiatric illness and suicide, biological factors, and suicide in the young.*

Swanson, D., Bohnert, P., and Smith, J.: The Paranoid. Boston, Little, Brown & Co., 1970, p. 216.

Tardiff, K.: Violence. *In* Talbott, J. A., Hales, R. E., and Yudofsky, S. C. (Eds.): American Psychiatric Press Textbook of Psychiatry. Washington, DC, American Psychiatric Press, 1988. *The author offers a chapter giving sweeping coverage of the violent patient, including information gathered when he chaired a Task Force of the American Psychiatric Association developing guidelines for the uses of seclusion and restraint. The family physician interested in developing his or her expertise with the violent patient can learn much about responding in an emergency, as well as the extended evaluation of organic mental disorders, psychotic disorders, and nonorganic, nonpsychotic disorders leading to violence. Finally, the management section can help the family physician become well equipped to handle the violent patient.*

Tobias, C. R., Turns, D. M., Lippmann, S., et al.: The violent patient: What to do? South. Med. J., *81*:640, 1988. *This excellent article is "dense" with information about the violent patient, including risk factors, biological and environmental contributors, and verbal and pharmacologic treatment.*

Tuckman, J., and Youngman, W. F.: Assessment of suicide risk in attempted suicides. *In* Resnik, H. L. P. (Ed.): Suicide Behaviors. Boston, Little, Brown & Co., 1968.

Von Korff, M., Shapiro, S., Burke, J. D., et al.: Anxiety and depression in a primary care clinic. Arch. Gen. Psychiatry, *44*:152–156, 1987.

70

Dementia

Richard E. Finlayson

The past century has provided western society with an enviable legacy—increasing longevity. A review of the literature on normal aging by Stein (1988) shows that the percentage of persons in the United States who are over age 65 has increased from 2 per cent to about 12 per cent during the past 100 years. Expectations are that by the middle of the next century this will become a 10-fold increase. This demographic trend is having a notable impact on the prevalence of certain diseases, especially those of a degenerative nature. The dementing disorders, as a group, are problems of late life that cause great personal suffering and economic loss for society.

Recognition that dementia is not an inevitable or direct consequence of growing old (becoming "senile") has been a relatively recent development. The current expansion of interest in this field is gratifying. Butler (1975) recommended that the term "senility" be discarded in favor of "emotional and mental disorders in old age," i.e., a more diagnosis-specific approach to understanding late life intellectual loss. Even as we begin to understand old mysteries, however, we are being confronted with new ones, e.g., the human immunodeficiency virus (HIV). This cause of dementia seems to have the potential for changing at least one way in which we think about dementia, i.e., as a disorder of late life.

In this chapter, the dementia syndrome is described and its causes, epidemiology, diagnosis, and management are discussed.

Definition and Clinical Manifestations

A definition of dementia offered by Maletta (1987) contains several key concepts central to our present understanding of this syndrome:

> A clinical syndrome complex in a patient marked by a gradual, persistent and generalized deterioration of intellectual and emotional function from a previously higher level in an alert individual. This deterioration may be progressive, static or remitting.

Memory loss is the key clinical feature of most cases of early dementia but is difficult to differentiate from "age-associated memory impairment" (Crook et al., 1986). The misplacing of things, forgetting appointments, and the like happens to healthy people so commonly that these lapses hardly can be taken as evidence of illness—*unless* by their frequency and intensity they seriously interfere with that person's life. Families who have taken some note of an older person's failing memory sometimes take comfort in the observation that the loved one can recall a Social Security number, for example. Although such long-term memory may eventually be lost, its preservation is not a reliable finding early in the course of the syndrome. Other impairments in the focal-cognitive process that are sometimes seen include loss of visual-spatial skills and aphasia.

Personality traits that seemed adaptive, or at least were well tolerated by others, may become exaggerated and cause considerable social tension. For example, a retired, previously hard-driving executive may take up a new career at a frenzied pace as a defense against an inner sense of impending psychologic dissolution. Individuals who have been prone to being suspicious may develop paranoid thinking. Sometimes one observes what seems to be a complete reversal of personality. A person who was "independent-minded" (but actually lived denying many dependency needs) may become "clingy" or "under foot" or change from "a tiger into a pussycat."

Because of their diverse characteristics, affective symptoms do not easily lead to or provide a basis for a diagnosis of dementia. Apathy, slowed thinking, depressive moods, restlessness, insomnia, and somatic complaints may be present, however, even before anyone has expressed a serious concern about memory or other cognitive functions.

"Subcortical dementia" (Albert et al., 1974) has been described as a type of dementia in which affective symptoms are prominent. Dementia of the Alzheimer's type (DAT) is a "cortical dementia" according to this schema and is distinguished primarily by memory loss, aphasia, apraxia of speech, and agnosia. In Cummings and Benson's (1984) review of the subject of "subcortical dementia," they record the following features as characteristics: slowness of mental processing, forgetfulness, impaired cognition, apathy, and depression. The syndrome has been linked to various diseases including progressive supranuclear palsy, Huntington's disease, Jakob-Creutzfeldt disease, Parkinson's disease, lacunar state, and depression. HIV dementia has also been described as "subcortical." The validity of the concept—i.e., cortical versus subcortical—remains controversial. We know now, for example, that DAT, the classic "cortical dementia," is not limited to cortical structures but has extensive involvement in subcortical structures, such as the nucleus basalis of Meynert (Whitehouse et al., 1982).

Once a dementia is moderately advanced, it is readily discernible to those living and working in close association with the person that cognition is impaired. He or she may get lost on the way home from work or while at a shopping mall. Self-care diminishes to varying degrees, resulting in poor hygiene and inappropriate dress. Social situations become difficult, even embarrassing. A steady progression of symptoms is characteristic of DAT. Reisberg's (1986) staging of this disorder clearly demonstrates the downhill course. Patients eventually require assistance in being clothed, fed, and bathed and in handling secretions. Language is lost. The person no longer can sit up and finally becomes comatose.

The course of multi-infarct dementia (MID) typically differs from DAT in that the onset is abrupt and the deterioration is stepwise. Personality is relatively spared but emotional lability can be intense. Focal neurologic findings are common. There may be prolonged stable periods, but death can come quickly as a result of an acute cerebrovascular or cardiovascular event. Differentiation of this disorder from DAT can be difficult in the clinical situation—multi-infarct dementia may follow a clinical course similar to that of DAT.

Etiology and Epidemiology

With the exception of HIV dementia, most patients with dementia encountered by the family physician will be elderly. In elderly patients, DAT and MID are responsible for 75 to 85 per cent of reported cases. There are many other causes; some of these can be arrested or reversed. Table 70–1 is based on the Office of Medical Applications of Research, National Institutes of Health (1987) and gives the categories and some examples of reversible and progressive dementia.

Table 70–1. CATEGORIES OF DEMENTIA BASED ON REVERSIBILITY: EXAMPLES OF SOME CAUSES AND DISORDERS

Causes that Can Be Removed or Reversed	Progressive Degenerative Diseases
Intoxications	Without important neurologic findings other than dementia
Prescription drugs	Alzheimer's disease
Illicit drugs	Pick's disease
Carbon monoxide	With important neurologic findings with or without dementia
Heavy metals	Parkinson's disease
Drug combinations	Huntington's disease
Infections	Progressive supranuclear palsy
Any agent capable of affecting brain	Many others
Metabolic disorders	
Endocrinopathies	
Encephalopathy of renal/hepatic failure	
Wilson's disease	
Nutritional disorders	
Thiamine deficiency	
Folate deficiency	
Niacin deficiency	
Vascular	
Hypertension	
Atherosclerosis	
Vasculitis	
Embolic disease	
Cardiac disease	
Space-occupying lesions	
Chronic subdural hematoma	
Brain tumor	
Affective disorders	

Data from Office of Medical Applications of Research, National Institutes of Health (1987).

The category of "intoxication" is particularly important with respect to drug and alcohol use. The vulnerability of older persons to substance misuse, abuse, and dependence has been discussed by Atkinson (1984). Contributing factors that have been suggested in the literature are (1) biologic (e.g., slowed biotransformation and clearance); (2) common medical ailments leading to self-medication with over-the-counter drugs and increased exposure to prescription drugs; and (3) psychosocial stressors (e.g., retirement and loss of spouse).

According to Tarter and Edwards (1985), the dementias associated with alcoholism are due to a wide range of factors, e.g., malnutrition, liver disease, vascular disease, and injury. Empirical data that support the validity of "alcoholic dementia" as a unique syndrome are lacking.

Many infectious agents are capable of causing dementia. There is a "new kid on the block" that may have the potential for changing the age distribution of dementia in a major way. Human immunodeficiency virus (HIV) diseases are capable of producing various neuropsychiatric syndromes including dementia (Holland, 1988; Price et al., 1988). Delirium (which should not be confused with dementia) is common in acquired immune deficiency syndrome (AIDS) as a result of hypoxia secondary to pneumonia and other medical factors. There is strong support from the available evidence that AIDS dementia complex is caused by the direct action of HIV-1. Other treatable causes of encephalopathy (infection and tumor) should be ruled out (Ho, 1989). HIV should be considered in any case of dementia in a patient under age 50 when its well-known risk factors are present. The literature is controversial at this time as to how common dementia is in otherwise asymptomatic carriers or whether the risk of dementia increases as a carrier state persists.

The dementia associated with depression has been described in the literature as a "pseudodementia" (Wells, 1979; Feinberg and Goodman, 1984). The need to differentiate the two disorders arises frequently in community practice because of the problem of overlapping phenomenology. There has been a tendency, however, to dichotomize the issue excessively, based on an assumption that depressed, cognitively impaired persons must have either one or the other disorder. Newer evidence reveals that many patients have both depression and organic dementia. This occurred in 30 per cent of the patients studied by Ron et al. (1979) In a study by Reifler et al. (1982), 23 per cent of a group of 88 cognitively impaired elderly had depression and 85 per cent of these depressed patients had both disorders.

DAT is the most common of all reported causes of dementia (one half to two thirds of cases). Pick's disease, also a progressive dementia, is much less common. A detailed discussion of the pathology and possible causes of DAT is beyond the scope of this chapter. In brief, it is a progressive neuronal degeneration in the cerebral cortex and subcortical nuclei. Loss of cortical neurons and presence of neurofibrillary tangles and senile plaques in the gray matter are characteristics (Perl and Pendlebury, 1986). Various etiologic hypotheses have been advanced—e.g., loss of central cholinergic function, accelerated aging of the brain, genetic factors, aluminum intoxication, infection, and autoimmunity (Kokmen, 1984).

Read and Jarvik (1984) reviewed the topic of cerebrovascular disease in the differential diagnosis of dementia. They noted from the literature that in pathologic studies, the second most common finding in demented patients is the presence of multiple infarctions in brain tissue. The diagnostic entity MID may account for as many as one third of cases of dementia. They listed the following mechanisms: (1) lacunar state; (2) multiple emboli; (3) vasculitis; (4) blood dyscrasias; (5) hypoperfusion; and (6) anoxic episode.

Diagnosis

The clinical history is the single most important source of information. An awareness of the wide range of psychobehavioral disturbances and diverse causes is essential to accurate diagnosis. Once a physician suspects the syndrome from the history, it is important to attempt to document (or rule out) the presence of cognitive impairment. This impairment is easily missed unless specific questions are addressed to the patient and family members. A structured mental status examination such as the "mini-mental state" (Folstein et al., 1975) or the "short test of mental status" (Kokmen et al., 1987) is very useful and much to be preferred over a hit-or-miss attempt at bedside assessment of mental status. It must be emphasized, however, that these simple screening tests are not sufficient in themselves to make a diagnosis of dementia.

Other causes of cognitive disturbance should not be overlooked. Delirium is an acute syndrome characterized by abrupt onset, confusion, fluctuating course (even over minutes), autonomic instability, and visual hallucinations. Although multiple medical factors can contribute to delirium directly, an underlying dementia may predispose the patient to this syndrome. Thus, both may be present. Dementia praecox (schizophrenia) is not a dementia as we now conceptualize it, but it does sometimes lead to progressive deterioration of personality. It is differentiated from dementia by the characteristic thought disorder, auditory hallucinations, and related symptoms.

Physical examination of the older patient should be performed with a knowledge of findings that are related to aging per se. Walshe (1987) discussed neurologic findings that are involutional in origin. These are "generally uniform among the aging population, symmetric and predictable." The clue to abnormality is asymmetrical loss. Various findings that should *not* be attributed to aging include extraocular movement abnormalities, ataxia, absence of deep tendon reflexes, extensor plantar response, and trouble with tandem gait.

Table 70–2 give the recommendations of the Office of Medical Applications of Research, National Institutes of Health (1987) for study of patients with new onset of dementia. An important initial step in diagnosis is the discontinuing of medications that are not absolutely necessary. Those that are known to produce an abstinence syndrome when abruptly

Table 70–2. STANDARD DIAGNOSTIC STUDIES FOR NEW-ONSET DEMENTIA

Complete blood cell count
Electrolyte panel
Screening metabolic panel
Thyroid function tests
Vitamin B_{12} and folate levels
Tests for syphilis and, depending on history, for HIV
Urinalysis
Electrocardiogram
Chest radiograph

Data from Office of Medical Applications of Research, National Institutes of Health (1987).

stopped—e.g., barbiturates, benzodiazepines, and opiates—should be tapered on a standard schedule if dependence is suspected.

When depression is suspected, psychiatric consultation should be considered. The neurologist can be especially helpful in guiding the advanced work-up, i.e., in decisions concerning special diagnostic studies such as electroencephalography, computed tomography of the head, and magnetic resonance imaging. Neuropsychologic assessment is most useful when the history and clinical results of examination are equivocal and for providing a baseline estimation of cognitive performance. The diagnosis of dementia is based on all available evidence but not infrequently it remains tentative. Observation over a period of months may be necessary in order to make a reasonably firm diagnosis. Table 70–3 gives the DSM III-R criteria for diagnosis of dementia. With respect to DAT, it should be emphasized that it is diagnosed not only by exclusion but also by a history that is compatible with the symptoms and course of the illness.

Treatment

The wise physician will keep in mind the possibility of multiple causes of dementia in a given patient. A program that addresses the obvious medical disorders that are treatable and provides psychosocial management from the outset is most desirable.

PSYCHOSOCIAL MANAGEMENT

Family care-givers, themselves usually middle-aged or elderly, constitute the backbone of the informal care of DAT patients. An awareness of their vulnerabilities is very important as the physician begins to talk with them and the patient about this most burdensome and socially disruptive disease.

The initial reaction of the family to the diagnosis commonly involves feelings of anxiety, fear of getting the disease themselves, and guilt. These things should be discussed. A knowledge of the family dynamics, especially the quality of the relationship between the patient and the potential care-givers, is vital. One might anticipate, for example, that an enmeshed family that has had closed boundaries to the community would choose to "handle it" themselves and thus place a greater strain on the care-giver(s), leading perhaps to early breakdown of support.

What do patients and families want and need to know? First and foremost, they must have reliable information about the disease. In the case of DAT, it should be emphasized that the cause is not known at present and a cure is not available. This will help to minimize needless expenditure of time and money in search of miracle cures. The physician will find Reisberg's (1986) Functional Assessment Staging of Alzheimer's Disease (FAST) a useful tool in understanding and interpreting to the family the usual course of this illness. Discussion of the course of the illness is a good format in which to discuss in-home relief services, foster care, and nursing home place-

Table 70–3. DIAGNOSTIC CRITERIA FOR DEMENTIA

A. Demonstrable evidence of impairment in short- and long-term memory. Impairment in short-term memory (inability to learn new information) may be indicated by inability to remember three objects after 5 minutes. Long-term memory impairment (inability to remember information that was known in the past) may be indicated by inability to remember past personal information (e.g., what happened yesterday, birthplace, occupation) or facts of common knowledge (e.g., past presidents, well-known dates).

B. At least one of the following:
  1. impairment in abstract thinking, as indicated by inability to find similarities and differences between related words, difficulty in defining words and concepts, and other similar tasks;
  2. impaired judgment, as indicated by inability to make reasonable plans to deal with interpersonal, family, and job-related problems and issues;
  3. other disturbances of higher cortical function, such as aphasia (disorder of language), apraxia (inability to carry out motor activities despite intact comprehension and motor function), agnosia (failure to recognize or identify objects despite intact sensory function), and "constructional difficulty" (e.g., inability to copy three-dimensional figures, assemble blocks, or arrange sticks in specific designs);
  4. personality change, i.e., alteration or accentuation of premorbid traits.

C. The disturbance in A and B significantly interferes with work or usual social activities or relationships with others.

D. Not occurring exclusively during the course of delirium.

E. Either 1 or 2:
  1. there is evidence from the history, physical examination, or laboratory tests of a specific organic factor (or factors) judged to be etiologically related to the disturbance;
  2. in the absence of such evidence, an etiologic organic factor can be presumed if the disturbance cannot be accounted for by any nonorganic mental disorder, e.g., major depression accounting for cognitive impairment.

Criteria for Severity of Dementia:

Mild: Although work or social activities are significantly impaired, the capacity for independent living remains, with adequate personal hygiene and relatively intact judgment.

Moderate: Independent living is hazardous, and some degree of supervision is necessary.

Severe: Activities of daily living are so impaired that continual supervision is required, e.g., unable to maintain minimal personal hygiene; largely incoherent or mute.

From American Psychiatric Association Committee on Nomenclature and Statistics: Diagnostic and Statistical Manual of Mental Diseases. 3rd ed. (revised). Washington, DC, American Psychiatric Association, 1987, p. 107. By permission of the publisher.

ment. Each type of dementia has features that are of very practical importance to the care-givers and, of course, to the patient.

Recommended reading for families includes (1) *The 36-Hour Day* (Mace and Rabins, 1981); (2) *Alzheimer's Disease and Related Illnesses* (Heston and White, 1983); and (3) *You, Your Parent and the Nursing Home* (Fox, 1986).

The psychosocial perspectives of HIV-related diseases have been discussed by Ostrow et al. (1988). They point out that there is much stress-induced psychopathology with this illness, e.g., anxiety disorders, affective disorders, and psychosis. The medical factors contributing to neuropsychiatric illness are not confined to the action of the virus alone. Thus, management is very complex, requiring multiple medical specialists and supportive personnel. At a very basic level, the patient needs help in dealing with the medical symptoms, the Social Security system, and everyday problems. Listening, lack of fear by the practitioner, and caring are essential elements in the treatment of AIDS patients.

PSYCHOPHARMACOLOGIC TREATMENT

It is important to remember that most patients who are demented have a disorder for which a specific treatment is not available. Behavioral symptoms therefore are the usual target of drug treatment. The medical treatment of the disorders that cause or contribute to dementia and that have established causes and treatment protocols will not be discussed here, with the exception of depression.

There are some general principles of prescribing for the elderly that should be kept in mind. Because of the prevalence of physical disorders in older people, the potential for drug interactions is increased. Discontinue as many unnecessary drugs (including over-the-counter) as possible. Decrease the starting dose of drugs to about half and use divided doses when possible to minimize side effects (e.g., orthostatism, urinary retention). Choose drugs with side effects that are most compatible with the patient's medical problems.

Antipsychotic drugs (neuroleptics) are probably the most widely used for treatment of the restlessness, agitation, and wandering associated with dementia. One advantage of these drugs is the lack of development of tolerance and an abstinence syndrome—common to sedatives and antianxiety drugs. The antipsychotics are hardly a panacea, however. In a controlled study, Risse and Barnes (1986) observed that only about one third of the agitated, demented patients treated with neuroleptics responded to a moderate or marked degree.

The selection of a specific antipsychotic drug usually is based on the side-effect profile. One probably would not use such a drug in a patient with Parkinson's disease. In a patient who is just sensitive to the extrapyramidal side effects, a low-potency drug would be preferable, e.g., thioridazine (Mellaril) or chlorpromazine (Thorazine). The disadvantages of the low-potency group are sedation (if it is not needed), central anticholinergic confusion, and adverse cardiovascular effects.

Consideration of side effects is also important in choosing an antidepressant for the patient who has depression as a primary or an associated problem. This approach can be taken with confidence when using antidepressants because we do not have consistently reliable methods for selecting a specific drug on the basis of efficacy alone. Until we know more about depression in demented patients, the physician should adhere to the same general guidelines for using antidepressants as would be followed in treating a nondemented depressed person.

Barbiturates should be avoided because they are central nervous system depressants. Benzodiazepines, especially those with long half-lives (either parent drug or active metabolites), should be used with caution. Richelson (1984) noted that the half-life of the active metabolite of flurazepam (Dalmane), for example, may be as long as 200 hours in the elderly. Daily administration of this or other long-acting benzodiazepines could be hazardous. Smaller and less-frequent dosing is indicated. Fortunately, we have shorter-acting benzodiazepines available; oxazepam (Serax), alprazolam (Xanax), triazolam (Halcion), lorazepam (Ativan), and temazepam (Restoril) are examples. It should be emphasized, however, that although accumulation problems may be lessened with this latter group, each is capable of producing tolerance, abstinence syndrome, and cognitive and affective problems. Chronic administration should be avoided, when possible, and no drug should be used as a substitute for a sound behavioral management program.

Winograd and Jarvik (1986) have written a very informative and practical article concerning physician management of the demented patient. The reader is referred to this article for further discussion of the topic (see annotated reference).

Acknowledgments

The author thanks Alan J. Wright, M.D., Emre Kokmen, M.D., and Ronald C. Peterson, M.D., for their assistance in preparing this chapter.

References

Albert, M. L., Feldman, R. G., and Willis, A. L.: The "subcortical dementia" of progressive supranuclear palsy. J. Neurol. Neurosurg. Psychiatry, *37*:121, 1974.

Atkinson, R. M.: Substance use and abuse in late life. *In* Atkinson, R. M. (Ed.): Alcohol and Drug Abuse in Old Age. Washington, DC, American Psychiatric Press, 1984, pp. 2–21. *This monograph is a useful guide for diagnosis and management of abuse of alcohol, prescription drugs, and over-the-counter medications by the elderly.*

Butler, R. M.: Psychiatry and the elderly: An overview. Am. J. Psychiatry, *132*:893, 1975. *In this classic article, Butler discusses the psychologic and social factors that have contributed to a form of prejudice called "ageism."*

Crook, T., Bartus, R. T., Ferris, S. H., et al.: Age-associated memory impairment: Proposed diagnostic criteria and measures of clinical change—report of a National Institute of Mental Health work group. Dev. Neuropsychol., 261, 1986.

Cummings, J. L., and Benson, D. F.: Subcortical dementia: Review of an emerging concept. Arch. Neurol., *41*:874, 1984.

Feinberg, T., and Goodman, B.: Affective illness, dementia, and pseudodementia. J. Clin. Psychiatry, *45*:99, 1984. *Four "ideal types" of depression plus dementia syndromes are discussed: (1) depression presenting as dementia; (2) depression with secondary dementia; (3) dementia presenting as depression; and (4) dementia with secondary depression.*

Folstein, M. F., Folstein, S. E., and McHugh, P. R.: "Mini-mental state": A practical method for grading the cognitive state of patients for the clinician. J. Psychiatr. Res., *12*:189, 1975.

Fox, N.: You, Your Parent and the Nursing Home. New York, Prometheus Books, 1986.

Heston, L. L., and White, J. A.: Dementia: A Practical Guide to Alzheimer's Disease and Related Illnesses. New York, W. H. Freeman & Company, 1983. *This book has a very good discussion of the biomedical aspects of dementia.*

Ho, D. D.: The acquired immunodeficiency syndrome (AIDS) dementia complex; UCLA Conference. Ann. Intern. Med., *111*:400–410, 1989.

Holland, J. C. B.: The psychologic and neuropsychologic complications of AIDS. Am. J. Prev. Psychiatry Neurol. (special issue AIDS), *1*:11, 1988.

Kokmen, E.: Dementia—Alzheimer type. Mayo Clin. Proc., *59*:35, 1984.

Kokmen, E., Naessens, J. M., and Offord, K. P.: A short test of mental status: Description and preliminary results. Mayo Clin. Proc., *62*:281, 1987.

Mace, N. L., and Rabins, P. V.: The 36-Hour Day: A Family Guide to Caring for Persons With Alzheimer's Disease, Related Dementing Illnesses, and Memory Loss in Later Life. Baltimore, The Johns Hopkins University Press, 1981. *This is a classic, widely acclaimed guide for families of and other caregivers for demented persons.*

Maletta, G. J.: Diagnosis of dementias. Minn. Med., *70*:378, 1987.

Office of Medical Applications of Research, National Institutes of Health: Differential diagnosis of dementing diseases. J.A.M.A., *258*:3411, 1987. *A wide variety of medical specialists, other scientists, and public organizations involved with the dementias contributed to this excellent document.*

Ostrow, D., Grant, I., and Atkinson, H.: Assessment and management of the AIDS patient with neuropsychiatric disturbances. J. Clin. Psychiatry, *49*:14, 1988.

Perl, D. P., and Pendlebury, W. W.: Neuropathology of dementia. Neurol. Clin., *4*:355, 1986.

Price, R. W., Brew, B., Sidtis, J., et al.: The brain in AIDS: Central nervous system HIV-1 infection and AIDS dementia complex. Science, *239*:586, 1988.

Read, S. L., and Jarvik, L. F.: Cerebrovascular disease in the differential diagnosis of dementia. Psychiatr. Ann., *14*:100, 1984. *The authors emphasize the danger of premature diagnosis of DAT and thereby the possibility of overlooking an opportunity to treat a cardiovascular cause of the dementia. A nice review.*

Reifler, B. V., Larson, E., and Hanley, R.: Coexistence of cognitive impairment and depression in geriatric outpatients. Am. J. Psychiatry, *139*:623, 1982.

Reisberg, B.: Dementia: A systematic approach to identifying reversible causes. Geriatrics, *41*:30, 1986. *This staging of the course of dementia gives the differential diagnostic considerations of each stage.*

Richelson, E.: Psychotropics and the elderly: Interactions to watch for. Geriatrics, *39*:30, 1984.

Risse, S. C., and Barnes, R.: Pharmacologic treatment of agitation associated with dementia. J. Am. Geriatr. Soc., *34*:368, 1986.

Ron, M. A., Toone, B. K., Garralda, M. E., and Lishman, W. A.: Diagnostic accuracy in presenile dementia. Br. J. Psychiatry, *134*:161, 1979.

Stein, E. M.: Normal aging—psychological and sociocultural aspects. *In* Lazarus, L. W. (Ed.): Essentials of Geriatric Psychiatry. New York, Springer Publishing Co., 1988, pp. 1–24.

Tarter, R. E., and Edwards, K. L.: Neuropsychology of alcoholism. *In* Tarter, R. E., and Van Thiel, D. H. (Eds.): Alcohol and the Brain: Chronic Effects. New York, Plenum Publishing, 1985, pp. 217–242.

Walshe, T. M.: Neurologic examination of the elderly patient: Signs of normal aging. Postgrad. Med., *81*:375, 1987.

Wells, C. E.: Pseudodementia. Am. J. Psychiatry, *136*:895, 1979.

Whitehouse, P. J., Price, D. L., Struble, R. G., et al.: Alzheimer's disease and senile dementia: Loss of neurons in the basal forebrain. Science, *215*:1237, 1982.

Winograd, C. H., and Jarvik, L. F.: Physician management of the demented patient. J. Am. Geriatr. Soc., *34*:295, 1986. *The authors provide some very useful aids—e.g., a physician checklist (periodic review), environmental and behavioral management techniques for institutionalized patients, techniques to help cognitive function, management guidelines for insomnia and wandering behavior, and aids for demented patients with instability.*

71

Psychotherapeutic Drugs

Leo E. Hollister

It may be confusing to refer to drugs as psychotherapeutic, for the term has been used traditionally to denote some form of psychologic or social, rather than pharmacologic, treatment. Some persons prefer to use psychotropic, but this epithet is less precise, for it includes any drug with psychic actions, including many, such as hallucinogens, that are not therapeutic.

The original term for these drugs, the modern era of which covers more than three decades, was tranquilizer. This usage was most unfortunate, for it created a great deal of misunderstanding about the nature of these drugs. Their primary action was not merely to make emotionally ill patients more calm or sedated but also to make them better able to cope with their lives. They are not, as they have been derisively called, chemical straightjackets, but rather they may be considered liberating.

A prolific array of names has been used to describe specific classes of psychotherapeutic drugs. Those used to treat anxiety or insomnia have been called sedative-hypnotics (an old term that still has much to commend it), minor tranquilizers (see objections above), and even worse, psychorelaxants, muscle relaxants, or anxiolytics. Drugs used for treating depression are variously known as thymoleptics, psychic energizers (whatever they may be), and psychostimulants (something that they most clearly are not). Drugs used for treating schizophrenia and some other psychoses are called major tranquilizers (a term that permits confusion with the sedative hypnotic group), ataractics, neuroleptics, and psycholeptics. Greatest agreement in terminology is found with lithium carbonate, which is called either an antimanic or mood-stabilizing drug.

The prefix anti has much to recommend it as a label for these drugs. It is based on their predominant clinical use rather than any imputed pharmacologic or therapeutic mode of action. Thus, antianxiety, antidepressant, and antipsychotic leave little doubt about which respective class of drugs is meant. We shall use this nomenclature in this chapter.

General Principles in the Use of Psychotherapeutic Drugs

The physician in family practice will have many occasions for prescribing antianxiety drugs and hypnotics, somewhat fewer occasions to use antidepressants (perhaps fewer than warranted), only infrequent occasions to use antipsychotic drugs, and only rare occasions to use a mood-stabilizing drug. The first two types of drugs will probably be initially prescribed by the family physician. The last two types of drugs are more likely to have been prescribed by another physician, with the family physician being involved in follow-up care and supervision of drug treatment.

When prescribing any kind of drug, we should ideally prefer to make a diagnosis first. This ideal is often not met, particularly when one is dealing with emotional and psychiatric disorders, the etiology of which is uncertain and the diagnosis of which is often controversial. Many times, therefore, the choice of a drug will be determined by the predominant presenting symptom of the patient. Such a symptomatic approach to treatment works only if it is carefully monitored. Because most common symptoms of emotional illness, such as anxiety, insomnia, or the manifold signs of depression, are nonspecific, the symptom may not truly indicate the underlying disorder. When it does not, this deficiency will be made apparent by the patient's course during treatment.

Many psychotherapeutic drugs have nonpsychiatric indications. For instance, phenothiazines are valuable antiemetics. For this indication, the psychiatric effects of the drugs, mainly sedation, are unwanted. On the other hand, some drugs that are used primarily for nonpsychiatric indications, such as the antihistamine diphenhydramine (Benadryl), may possess enough sedative or anticholinergic properties to be useful in psychiatric patients. Thus, the parameters of clinical indications of these drugs are not always clear. When using psychotherapeutic drugs, the physician is faced with two opposing views. On the one hand, we should like to treat with the smallest dose of drug that will do the job and use it for the shortest possible time. On the other hand, we do not want to risk undertreating patients and denying them the benefits that these drugs may offer. No clear guidelines exist for determining how to reconcile these conflicting goals. Each case must be viewed in its entire context and good clinical judgment applied. One simply cannot rely on a cookbook approach, even if one could be found.

Like all other drugs, psychotherapeutic drugs produce unwanted effects and complications that can range from bothersome to serious. As is always the case, the benefits from the drugs must be weighed against the cost of these unwanted effects. If the drugs are being used for proper indications, one can almost always find that the benefits exceed the costs, but the question should be constantly held in mind, as the ratio may shift with the evolution of the disorder.

Sedative-Hypnotic Drugs

This class of drugs includes those used for treating simple anxiety as well as insomnia. Although the drugs used are similar and in many cases overlap, the two indications will be considered separately.

ANXIETY

Anxiety is perceived as a pervasive feeling of apprehension about some unspecified future threat to self-esteem. The somatic manifestations of anxiety are many, affecting virtually all organ systems. In turn, anxiety must be distinguished from other organic illnesses whose symptoms may resemble those of anxiety. Anxiety also accompanies many organic illnesses and psychosomatic complaints. Many more antianxiety drugs are prescribed for such indications than for "psychiatric" anxiety disorders. Although it has been averred that many physicians write prescriptions instead of trying to understand their patients, formal surveys of use of these drugs do not support this idea (Rickels, 1981; Mellinger, Balter and Uhlenhuth, 1984).

Types of Antianxiety Drugs

Seven classes of antianxiety drugs are summarized, with examples of each, in Table 71–1. Three classes, including the benzodiazepines, may be classified as classic *sedative-hypnotics*. Three others have other primary uses, but their ability to sedate can be exploited. They also have a variety of effects on the autonomic nervous system and have been termed *sedative-autonomic*. The seventh class of drugs is represented by buspirone, a drug chemically different from any of the others. This drug is devoid of sedative-hypnotic properties and may be considered a *nonsedative* antianxiety drug. It remains to be seen to what extent this new class of drugs, exemplified by buspirone, will displace benzodiazepines as the most widely used drugs for treating anxiety.

Pharmacology and Pharmacokinetics

The exact mode of action of benzodiazepines in alleviating anxiety and evoking sleep is still unknown. They do not seem to act directly through usual neurotransmitters, such as acetylcholine, norepinephrine, dopamine, or serotonin. The discovery in 1977 of specific receptors in the brain for benzodiazepines triggered a tremendous amount of investigation into the modes of action of these drugs. Benzodiazepine receptors are functionally linked to gamma-aminobutyric acid (GABA) receptors that regulate the opening and closing of chloride ion channels. Both GABA and benzodiazepines enhance the capacity of each other to open these ion channels and to hyperpolarize the postsynaptic cell. The inhibitory neurotransmitter, GABA, is widely distributed in the central nervous system (Paul et al, 1981).

The discovery of an endogenous polypeptide that

Table 71–1. VARIOUS TYPES OF ANTIANXIETY DRUGS

Sedative-Hypnotic
Barbiturates—phenobarbital, butabarbital sodium (Butisol), others
Glycerol derivatives—meprobamate (Miltown and others), tybamate (Solacen)
Benzodiazepines—diazepam (Valium), chlordiazepoxide (Librium), oxazepam (Serax), clorazepate dipotassium (Tranxene), prazepam (Verstran), lorazepam (Ativan), alprazolam (Xanax), others
Sedative-Autonomic
Diphenylmethane antihistamines—diphenhydramine (Benadryl), hydroxyzine (Atarax), others
Tricyclic antidepressants—doxepin (Sinequan)
Phenothiazines or other antipsychotics—trifluoperazine (Stelazine), fluphenazine (Prolixin), haloperidol (Haldol), others
Nonsedative
Azaspirodecanediones—buspirone (Buspar)

binds to these receptors, diazepam-binding inhibitor (DBI), has provided a possible biologic basis for anxiety (Alho et al., 1985). The normal function of the benzodiazepine receptor might be to provide for the development of anxiety or fear, a major defense mechanism. DBI seems to evoke such reactions in animals. This defense mechanism might become disturbed as a result of some inborn abnormality or owing to environmental stimulation early in life that leads to exaggerated responses to stress throughout life. Other sedative-hypnotics, such as barbiturates, bind to other portions of the GABA-benzodiazepine receptor-ion channel, which might explain their similar pharmacologic actions.

Although it seems evident that facilitation of GABA-ergic neurotransmission may account for the anticonvulsant and muscle relaxant actions of benzodiazepines, it is not so evident that they account for the sedative and hypnotic effects. A second, non–GABA-linked benzodiazepine receptor has been postulated for mediating these actions.

Depending on dose, these drugs produce sedation, anticonvulsant and muscle relaxant actions, hypnosis, anesthesia, coma, and death. Therapeutic margins are very large so that death solely as a result of ingestion of benzodiazepines is rare, which is a distinct advantage over the barbiturates. Another advantage is that these drugs do not induce drug-metabolizing enzymes to the same extent that barbiturates do; thus, significant pharmacokinetic interactions with other drugs are uncommon.

Benzodiazepines may not differ much in their modes of action, but they differ considerably in their pharmacokinetic parameters. It is possible, based on plasma half-lives, to classify these agents according to presumed duration of action, even though sometimes the actual duration of action is not entirely predicted by the plasma half-life (Table 71–2). The relative advantages and disadvantages of benzodiazepines with differing half-lives have been the subject of many debates with no resolution (Shader and Greenblatt, 1981).

The mode of action of buspirone (Buspar) is so radically different from that of benzodiazepines that it might provide new leads to the biologic mechanisms of anxiety. Buspirone, which somewhat resembles the antipsychotic butyrophenones chemically, has only weak dopamine-receptor blocking actions. Its major action is mediated through an affinity for 5-HT_{1A} receptors, serotonin receptors of previously unknown function. It does not bind to 5-HT_{1B} receptors, muscarinic cholinergic or calcium channel antagonist receptors. How it may act at the receptor for which it has greatest affinity to relieve anxiety is not known (Peroutka, 1985).

Buspirone is rapidly absorbed, so much so that it has been recommended that it be taken with food to delay absorption and reduce its first-pass metabolism through the liver. First-pass metabolism is large so that systemic bioavailability is low. The elimination half-life is 2.5 to 3.0 hours with less than 1 per cent of the drug excreted unchanged. Despite its extremely short half-life, which might suggest that taken according to usual dosage schedules it would be difficult to attain very high steady-state concentrations of the drug, its antianxiety effect is usually delayed for 2 to 3 weeks (Palmer, 1988).

Indications

The various indications for the benzodiazepines, the most widely used and most versatile group of antianxiety drugs, are shown in Table 71–3. It can be readily appreciated that virtually all of these indications had previously been used for barbiturates. The only indication for buspirone would be treatment of anxiety.

Choice of Drug

Because most of these drugs share a common pattern of pharmacologic actions, except for duration of effect, there is little to choose between them. Diazepam (Valium) has been the most popular of

Table 71–2. PHARMACOKINETIC CLASSIFICATION OF BENZODIAZEPINES

Drug	Active Metabolites	Range T½ (hrs)
Very Long-Acting		
Flurazepam (Dalmane)	Desalkyflurazepam (major activity)	40–100
Long-Acting		
Clorazepate (Tranxene)	Nordiazepam	30–96
Prazepam (Verstran)	Nordiazepam	30–96
Moderately Long-Acting		
Chloridazepoxide (Librium)	Several, including nordiazepam	10–29
Diazepam (Valium)	Nordiazepam	14–61
Halazepam (Praxipam)	Nordiazepam	9–28
Short-Acting		
Alprazolam (Xanax)	None	6–20
Lorazepam (Ativan)	None	9–22
Oxazepam (Serax)	None	6–24
Temazepam (Restoril)	Oxazepam	5–20
Very Short-Acting		
Triazolam (Halcion)	None	2–4

Table 71–3. VARIOUS CLINICAL INDICATIONS FOR BENZODIAZEPINES

Anxiety—with or without physical disorders
Insominia—preferably after proper diagnosis
Muscle relaxation—only in presence of true spasm
Adjunct to analgesics—never used alone for pain
Alcohol withdrawal—intravenous or oral administration, but not intramuscular
Anesthesia—either induction agent or sole anesthesia; intravenous
Anticonvulsant—diazepam intravenously for status epilepticus; clonazepam (Clonepin) for minor seizures

these agents, but recent fears, probably overstated, about dependence on this drug have led to a decline in the total number of prescriptions for all drugs in this class, especially those for diazepam. Lorazepam and alprazolam rival diazepam in popularity. Alprazolam is said to be especially useful in treating acute anxiety attacks (panic states), but other benzodiazepines may also be effective. It is reported to be effective for treating mild depressions, but this indication has not been officially approved.

Short-acting drugs have been recommended for elderly patients or for those with liver disease, both of whom have decreased ability to eliminate drugs. The usual practice, when drug elimination may be impaired, has been simply to decrease the initial dose of a drug that might have a slower elimination rate and to increase dosing intervals. The two main advantages of long-acting drugs have been the need for fewer daily doses, as well as the attenuated withdrawal reaction in cases of abuse. With so little to choose between these drugs, the choice is best determined by the preference of the patient (Hollister, 1984).

The exact role of buspirone remains to be elucidated. It would seem to be most appropriate for patients with mild generalized anxiety who have not been treated previously with a benzodiazepine. It might also be considered for anxious patients with a past history of substance abuse.

Doses and Dosage Schedules

Plasma concentrations obtained from equivalent doses of these drugs in different patients or subjects vary widely. The variability among subjects given single doses of various benzodiazepines may be sixfold. All of these data clearly indicate that using the same dose for all patients is therapeutic nonsense. How can one arrive at a proper dose for a patient clinically, assuming that plasma concentrations as a control are not easily or readily available and may have questionable significance in any case? A reasonable approach would be to establish the minimally effective hypnotic dose of the drug. Such a dose, which could be determined in three or four nights, would provide a guide to the patient's sensitivity to the drug. Daytime doses, perhaps given as needed, might be one third to one half the hypnotic dose.

Drugs with a slow disappearance rate are well suited to single daily dosage. The most appropriate time to give the single dose would be at bedtime so that the hypnotic effects of these drugs could be exploited. A patient with anxiety so severe that drug treatment is required would commonly also have some difficulty sleeping. The "daytime hangover," which is inevitable with those long-acting drugs, may provide precisely the degree of mild sedation compatible with unimpaired daily activities but relief of troublesome symptoms. Fractions of the minimally effective hypnotic dose may be used as needed for particular daytime stresses.

Many patients take benzodiazepines on an as needed basis, either in anticipation of some anxiety-provoking encounter or when symptoms become bothersome. Such practice should be encouraged rather than discouraged. Simply having a supply available for such use is reassuring for some patients. Buspirone, by virtue of its short half-life, should be taken regularly in divided doses.

Duration of Treatment

Anxiety is often episodic, waxing and waning with changes in a person's life. In such cases, treatment might follow the course, drugs being used only when symptoms are discomforting or disabling and not indefinitely.

Diazepam and other benzodiazepines might be assumed to have an average disappearance rate from plasma of 24 hours so that a steady-state plateau of plasma concentration should be attained within a week. A satisfactory result would suggest that an adequate dose had been chosen. If the drug were then discontinued, its disappearance curve would be the obverse of that for its accumulation, so it is likely that a patient would have a residual effect for 2 to 3 days even after such a brief course. By limiting treatment to short courses, problems of tolerance with less loss of efficacy and increased doses with the risk of physical dependence are avoided.

Not all patients who complain of anxiety experience it episodically. Some have anxiety chronically, which may simply represent an unusually high level of "trait" anxiety. These patients often do very well with small doses of some antianxiety drug maintained for longer periods of time. Even so, treatment should be phased out periodically, both to determine whether it is still needed and to reduce the likelihood of "therapeutic-dose dependence." The latter may be a function of the duration of uninterrupted treatment and is unlikely when courses are limited to 4 months or less.

As far as one can tell, buspirone can be used indefinitely, as withdrawal reactions have not been documented with this drug. Still, the basic principle of using the least dose for the shortest possible time applies also with this drug.

Monitoring Treatment

It is especially important to monitor the patient's response to treatment. Failure to respond appreciably to drug therapy within the first week usually augurs a poor later response. The problem may be one of inadequate dose or noncompliance by the patient. If these factors can be eliminated, it is possible that the patient's anxiety may signify a different order of illness, such as depression or schizophrenia. Attempting to treat a nonresponsive patient may lead to a progressive augmentation of dose that may induce dependence on the drug without adequate relief of the original symptoms. On the other hand, a good response to treatment during the first two weeks would be reason to suggest interrupting drug therapy.

Plasma concentrations of these drugs that are "therapeutic" have not been clearly defined, and we cannot recommend any regular laboratory monitoring of drug levels, even if they were widely available. Usually, adequate doses of diazepam produce a combined concentration of diazepam/nordiazepam of 600 ng. per ml. A patient who has responded poorly and who has not attained such levels might be suspected of noncompliance or of having been prescribed an inadequate dose.

Drug Combinations

Benzodiazepines have been combined with most other psychotherapeutic drugs, usually with benefit if the individual patient's needs have been thoroughly considered. An irrational combination occurs when a patient takes one benzodiazepine (e.g., diazepam) for daytime relief of anxiety, and another (e.g., flurazepam) as a hypnotic at night. Most benzodiazepines can be used interchangeably as antianxiety drugs and as hypnotics.

Adverse Effects

Oversedation, the most common side effect, is an extension of desired actions. Patients should be warned about the possibility of sedation from any dose taken during the day. Usually it will be greatest 1 to 2 hours after the drug is taken. Dangerous activities, such as driving an automobile, or making critical judgments should be deferred.

Hostile outbursts are rare and are a function of the patient's personality rather than the drug. Any disinhibiting agent, most notably alcohol but also sedatives, may allow hostile emotions to surface. Depression is also not due to the drug itself, but it may be unmasked by relief of concomitant anxiety. Its emergence might indicate that the antianxiety drug be discontinued and an antidepressant substituted for it.

"Classic" dependence of the alcohol-barbiturate type may ensue when benzodiazepines are misused or abused. Usually chronic doses of 40 mg. per day of diazepam or equivalent doses of other drugs are required. As physicians have control over patients' access to these drugs by prescription, such abuse should be rare in medical practice. Of much greater current concern is development of minor types of withdrawal reactions following prolonged use of therapeutic doses (usually less than 30 mg. per day of diazepam for more than 8 months). Such a long, uninterrupted course of treatment should be avoided whenever possible. Patients with such exposure to these drugs should not be abruptly withdrawn but should be gradually weaned from them (Rickels et al., 1984).

Interactions

Pharmacodynamic interactions with benzodiazepines may involve any number of other drugs with sedative properties, most especially alcohol. Many clinicians routinely urge patients on these drugs to forgo alcohol completely, but that may be self-delusory. Significant interactions tend to occur only when alcohol is present in high concentrations or when large doses of benzodiazepines are taken concurrently.

Pharmacokinetic interactions, in which the presence of one drug alters the absorption, distribution, metabolism, or excretion of another, are rare with the benzodiazepines and of little clinical consequence. The interaction between diazepam and cimetidine, in which the latter drug increases plasma concentrations of the former, has not yet proved to be a problem clinically.

Contraindications

Sedative-hypnotic drugs are best avoided in alcoholics or other patients who abuse social or illicit drugs. Instead, if anxiety needs treatment, one can try buspirone or one of the sedative-autonomic drugs. The latter are rarely abused. Any drug that reduces the level of consciousness may reduce respiratory drive. Thus, these drugs are not indicated in patients with chronic respiratory disease and carbon dioxide retention or in patients with known sleep apnea (see below).

INSOMNIA AND SLEEP DISORDERS

Insomnia, or preferably, hyposomnia, has been defined by patients in many ways: an inability to induce sleep as readily as desired; an inability to stay asleep; an abbreviated period of sleep with premature awakening; a night of sleep interrupted by nightmares and involuntary arousals; or sleep that is not refreshing. Insomnia has many causes. As one gets older, sleep becomes increasingly fragmented and less deep. Whenever possible, this type of physiologic insomnia should be treated with simple reassurance.

Worry or excitement can interfere with sleep. Such causes usually are easily uncovered. Chronic anxiety reactions are almost always accompanied by some degree of sleep disturbance, as are depressive reactions. Psychologic studies of patients referred for sleep laboratory evaluation showed 85 per cent to have at least one scale in the pathologic range on the

Minnesota Multiphasic Personality Inventory. Depression was frequent and more readily recognized as a cause of insomnia in younger rather than older patients. Patients who experience insomnia and also complain of diminished interest and energy, loss of weight, weeping, and anxiety may need treatment for depression.

A careful drug history is imperative when evaluating insomnia. Two commonly taken social drugs may interfere with sleep. Caffeine is generally recognized as having this effect, but it may not do so until the middle years of life. Therefore, persons who were always able to drink their evening cup of coffee without suffering sleep problems may begin to find sleep more difficult and fail to associate the insomnia with its ingestion. Although alcohol is a depressant and often enhances the onset of sleep, heavy drinkers often find that they awaken in the early morning in a stimulated state. It is speculative whether this is a mild withdrawal symptom or the result of secondary release of catecholamines from previous alcoholic intake, but alcohol may interfere with sleep in some persons. Appetite suppressants of the sympathomimetic type can also interfere with sleep (Mellinger, Balter and Uhlenhuth, 1984).

Almost any condition that causes pain will interfere with sleep. The aching joints of a patient with rheumatoid or osteoarthritis should be managed with adequate anti-inflammatory drugs to avoid the need for hypnotics. The nocturnal pain of duodenal ulcer can be prevented from interfering with sleep by a night-time dose of a histamine-2 blocker. Men with enlarged prostates may avoid or reduce their need for trips to the bathroom by decreasing fluid intake and avoiding alcohol before retiring. In short, a search should be made for remediable medical conditions that might interfere with sleep before any hypnotic is prescribed.

Types of Drugs

The distinction between sedative or antianxiety drugs and hypnotics is not clear. Many drugs of the former class serve equally well as hypnotics and enjoy widespread use as such. Drugs commonly labeled hypnotics may often be used in smaller doses as antianxiety agents. Thus, distinctions are often made on the basis of traditional uses, the latter encouraged by promotional claims for a particular drug. Some drugs that are more exclusively promoted as hypnotics are shown in Table 71–4.

The benzodiazepines are now the most widely used hypnotic drugs. Flurazepam (Dalmane), which is promoted for this use in the United States, is the oldest. Virtually any benzodiazepine may be used as a hypnotic. Diazepam is frequently employed as a hypnotic, even though it has never been promoted for this use. Triazolam (Halcion), a newer benzodiazepine, is more potent and has a short half-life. Temazepam (Restoril), which also has a short half-life, has been added to the growing list of benzodiazepine hypnotics.

Many older hypnotics are obsolete and seldom used or have actually been removed from the market, such as methaqualone (Quaalude). Some use of short-acting barbiturates, such as secobarbital sodium, as well as chloral hydrate, remains.

Indications

Reasonable diagnostic efforts should be made before hypnotic drugs are prescribed (Consensus Conference, 1984). It has been suggested that all patients for whom chronic treatment is proposed should first be screened in a sleep disorder clinic, but this hardly seems practical, since one third of the adult population may be troubled with insomnia at times. One should probably consider referring patients who are refractory to the prudent use of hypnotics to a psychiatrist or a sleep laboratory.

Two goals should be kept in mind when prescribing hypnotics: Drugs should be used occasionally and not habitually, and the least amount that will provide symptomatic relief should be used. The patient must be told that insomnia does not seriously damage health; a night of poor sleep will probably be rectified the following night without any pharmacologic intervention. If this premise is accepted, a patient should use a hypnotic drug only after at least two consecutive nights of poor sleep; that should make their use intermittent and relatively infrequent. Patients should be told that after taking a single dose of a drug such as flurazepam, they may still have lingering effects the next night. Thus, taking two consecutive doses of a hypnotic is seldom justified. However, some patients may ignore this advice and use drugs regularly.

Contraindications

Sleep apnea, which is a universal occurrence in young infants and is possibly related to some cases of sudden infant death syndrome, is a definite contraindication to the use of hypnotics. During periods of sleep apnea, respiration ceases totally. This is due to a central mechanism from diminished sensitivity of the respiratory center, a peripheral mechanism of upper airway obstruction, or both. When upper airway obstruction occurs, the patient may resume breathing with marked snorting or gasping sounds, so that the diagnosis may be suggested clinically if such sounds were heard by another who shared the same room or bed with the patient. These episodes cause frequent awakenings that result in poor sleep. Poor nocturnal sleep causes much sleepiness during the day, so that the presenting complaint may be tiredness. Use of hypnotics, which might further depress respiratory drive, would be clearly contraindicated in such cases of sleep apnea.

Choice of Drug

The relative advantages and disadvantages of short- versus long-acting hypnotics are still controver-

Table 71–4. CHARACTERISTICS OF DIFFERENT HYPNOTICS

	Doses (mg.)	Duration of Action	Advantages/Disadvantages
Benzodiazepines			
Flurazepam (Dalmane)	15, 30	Long	Safe; cumulative overdose
Triazolam (Halcion)	1.25, 0.50, 1.0	Short	Safe; amnesic episodes
Temazepam (Restoril)		Short	Safe; bioavailability?
Barbiturates			
Secobarbital (Seconal)	50, 100	Moderate	Genetic; overdose problem; loss of efficiency
Others			
Chloral hydrate	0.5, 2.0	Moderate	Effective; unpleasant

sial. Flurazepam may accumulate and produce a chronic intoxication. Whether triazolam produces rebound anxiety or insomnia is unsettled; a rare complication is anterograde amnesia. The pharmaceutical preparation of temazepam in the U.S. may lead to slow absorption.

With only three benzodiazepines from which to choose as hypnotics, it is probably well to be willing to use all three, depending on the preference of individual patients.

Tricyclic antidepressants may have sedative qualities. A therapeutic trial of a tricyclic antidepressant may be worthwhile if depression is the suspected etiology; occasional treatment with 25-mg. nightly doses is never indicated. Antipsychotics are poor hypnotics. They induce disagreeable reactions in normal patients, and in psychotic patients, they often fail to relieve sleep disturbances. Sedative antihistamines are the active ingredient in many over-the-counter sleep remedies. They would only be considered as prescription drugs were the patient to have some reason not to take benzodiazepines.

Doses and Dosage Schedules

Doses should be the lowest possible. Drugs that are encapsulated do not allow one to try half a dose unit, even though 7.5 mg. of flurazepam might be adequate for some patients. On the other hand, one can crack a 0.25-mg. tablet of triazolam and let the patient try 0.125 mg., which could be effective.

The rule of "one night out of three" for hypnotic use in patients with chronic insomnia should be tried. The fact that virtually all hypnotic drugs distort the normal architecture of sleep, as recorded in sleep laboratories, makes one loath to promote their continual use. Intermittent use may also avoid any tendency for tolerance to the hypnotic effects to develop.

Side Effects

Almost all hypnotic drugs have some type of hangover effects. These effects may be less pronounced with drugs that have short half-lives, such as triazolam and temezapam, as compared with flurazepam, which has a rather long half-life. A long half-life may be desirable for relief of concomitant daytime anxiety. It mitigates against nightly use because of cumulation. Whether rebound anxiety-insomnia is a characteristic of short-lived drugs is questionable (Kales et al, 1983). Anterograde amnesia has been reported in rare instances of triazolam use.

Psychologic dependence may occur frequently with hypnotic drugs, but physical dependence is rare. In the latter instance, daytime doses are almost always taken.

Nondrug Treatment

The relaxation that follows a warm bath, a massage, or the relief of sexual tension can promote sleep. Many insomniacs have developed elaborate rituals for courting sleep, and some seem to work. Boring tasks that do not require close attention, such as watching the many commercials during the late movie on television, often induce sleep. As much of the process of preparing for sleep is a ritual, some conditioned responses may occur naturally. It can be worthwhile to plan some sort of ritual for patients who seek relief from insomnia and link this with drug therapy in order to take advantage of the conditioned reflex aspect of the process of going to sleep. To the extent that drug responses can be "conditioned" by their association with habitual activities, habit alone may substitute for the drug or enhance its effect.

A regular pattern of activities and exercise may facilitate normal sleep. Increasing an insomniac's activity level to the point of moderate fatigue may induce sleep. Sleeping at unusual hours can disrupt the usual pattern. Some insomniacs, especially those troubled by early awakening, may benefit from postponing their bedtime. Pharmacologic doses of the essential amino acid L-tryptophan, such as 2 to 5 grams, have a definite hypnotic effect, but it is doubtful that the amounts contained in the usual glass of warm milk are adequate.

Antidepressants

DEPRESSION

Depression is probably the most frequent emotional disorder. It is a symptom (at one time or another most of us have felt "depressed"); a syndrome (a

Table 71–5. VARIOUS TYPES OF ANTIDEPRESSANT DRUGS AND THEIR USUAL DAILY DOSES

Drugs	Doses (mg.)
Tricyclics	
Imipramine (Tofranil, others)	75–200
Desipramine (Pertofrane, others)	75–200
Amitriptyline (Elavil, others)	75–200
Nortriptyline (Aventyl, others)	75–150
Protriptyline (Vivactil)	20–40
Doxepin (Sinequan)	75–300
Trimipramine (Surmontil)	75–200
"Second-Generation"	
Amoxepine (Asendin)	150–300
Maprotiline (Ludiomil)	75–200
Trazodone (Desyrel)	50–600
Fluoxetine (Prozac)	20–80
Buproprion (Wellbutrin)	100–300
Monoamine Oxidase Inhibitors	
Phenelzine (Nardil)	45–75
Tranylcypromine (Parnate)	10–30
Iscarboxazide (Marplan)	20–50

constellation of nonspecific symptoms from multiple causes); and an illness (one that can be severely disabling or even fatal). Like hypertension, depression may be often a missed diagnosis, yet it is a highly treatable disorder with serious consequences for morbidity and mortality when not recognized and treated.

Diagnostic distinctions are important in prognosis and in planning treatment. Primary affective disorders will have a significant morbidity and mortality. Treatment with drugs is usually basic. Tricyclic antidepressants and monoamine oxidase (MAO) inhibitors are the mainstays for treating unipolar depression. Tricyclics may also be useful in the depressed phase of bipolar depression, and antipsychotics may be required for the manic phase. The role of drug treatment for secondary depressions is smaller, and more emphasis should be placed on psychotherapeutic measures. These depressions seldom become as chronic and disabling as the primary type.

Primary care physicians may prescribe antidepressants without consultation with a psychiatrist if they feel the indications are secure and feel comfortable using these drugs. A sizable portion of antidepressants is prescribed by primary care physicians; the most frequent complaint is that less than optimal doses are used.

Types of Antidepressant Drugs

The large variety of drugs available for treating primary depressions is shown in Table 71–5. Almost all are metabolized in large part by the liver (Hollister, 1981b).

Tricyclic compounds have varying degrees of some of the following pharmacologic actions: blockade of uptake of aminergic neurotransmitters; sedation, possibly related to block of histamine-2 receptors in brain; antimuscarinic action; alpha-adrenergic blocking action; sympathomimetic effects; and quinidinelike actions. Blockade of uptake of aminergic neurotransmitters leads to a decreased number of postsynaptic beta-adrenoreceptors, a change that has been suggested as a common action of all antidepressants (Sulser, 1983).

Monoamine oxidase inhibitors work presynaptically, increasing the amount of aminergic neurotransmitter available for release into the synapse. Whether this difference in mode of action confers special clinical differences is not clear. These drugs may be especially useful for "atypical" depressions characterized by high levels of anxiety, much hypochondriasis, and phobic features; another definition of atypical depression emphasizes reversed vegetative symptoms: hypersomnia, weight gain, agitation, and increased libido. They are useful also in various obsessive-compulsive-phobic syndromes, either alone or combined with antianxiety drugs.

The "second generation" drugs (this term is used because they constitute a variety of chemical structures and modes of action) have been reported to have fewer side effects, relieve depression faster, and cause less problem when taken in overdose. These virtues have been somewhat difficult to prove. Amoxepine and maprotiline work by uptake inhibition, similar to tricyclics. Trazodone seems to work through serotonergic mechanisms, but the precise way is uncertain. Fluoxetine is the first of a coming group of selective uptake inhibitors of serotonin. Buproprion resembles amphetamines chemically but lacks their euphoriant and sympathomimetic effects; side effects have been minor thus far.

Sympathomimetic stimulants have properties that might be expected to make them suitable as antidepressants: blockade of the amine reuptake mechanism, weak inhibition of MAO, increased release of catecholamine neurotransmitters, and possibly direct agonist action of postsynaptic receptors. Clinically, they are not highly regarded, although an occasional patient may do rather well when treated with these agents.

Indications

Indications for tricyclic antidepressants are summarized in Table 71–6. Some are more established

Table 71–6. INDICATIONS FOR VARIOUS ANTIDEPRESSANT DRUGS

Definite Indications	
Depression, mainly endogenous	
Enuresis	
Relief of chronic pain of unknown cause	
Cataplexy in narcoleptics	
Other Indications	
Obsessive-compulsive-phobic states—clomipramine preferred	
School phobia	
Panic disorder	
Attentional deficit syndrome sympathomimetics preferred	

than others, and some involve nonpsychiatric illnesses (Hollister, 1983).

Choice of Drug

Most of these drugs are equally effective for depression, but some patients may respond better to one type than another. It is still reasonable to start treatment with one of the tricyclics. Should that drug fail, some would urge trying another tricyclic that might differ most from the first (such as desipramine, which selectively blocks uptake of norepinephrine, following amitriptyline, which mainly blocks uptake of serotonin). Others would next try either an MAO inhibitor or one of the second generation drugs. Drug therapy may be expected to be effective in 60 to 70 per cent of patients. Electroconvulsive treatment (ECT) is a treatment to be tried when all else fails or when the patient is at immediate risk of suicide.

The sedative, antimuscarinic, and sympathomimetic actions contribute to the most common side effects. Drugs may vary in their proportion of these pharmacologic actions so that patients who refuse treatment or who are noncompliant with one drug may accept another (see Table 71–8). Trazodone has variable, but often considerable, sedative activity but virtually no anticholinergic or sympathomimetic actions. It is also quite safe when overdoses are taken. Fluoxetine lacks sedative, anticholinergic, sympathomimetic actions; its side effects are nausea, headache, jitteriness, and insomnia.

At present, the choice of drug is best made based on the patient's prior response to drugs. Otherwise, it is largely empiric.

Doses and Dosage Schedules

The usual range of daily doses of these drugs is shown in Table 71–5. These ranges apply to patients in the middle years of life who are in good health. Very young or very old patients, ill patients, or patients who are excessively small may require much more conservative doses. The upper range shown is not absolute, but if doses are increased above this level, one might consider concurrent monitoring of plasma concentrations.

Usually, patients are treated with small doses of drug initially with rapid increments to the dose range shown. Therefore, it may take 2 weeks or so until steady-state levels at an effective dose are reached, leading some to ascribe this delay in response purely to this pharmacokinetic phenomenon. When drugs are administered by intravenous infusion, the antidepressant effect occurs more rapidly.

Single daily doses are feasible, although doses are often divided early in treatment. The timing of the daily dose of drug will be determined by the extent of sedation and the effect of the drug on the patient's daytime activities and sleep.

Monitoring Plasma Concentrations

The dose of drug often does not predict the plasma concentration that will be attained in an individual patient. Attempts have been made to define a therapeutic range of plasma concentration for various antidepressants. These are shown in Table 71–7. None of these ranges has been definitely established, but it seems reasonable to believe that exceptionally low concentrations might be associated with an incomplete clinical response and that high concentrations might cause toxicity.

The strongest indication for obtaining a determination of plasma concentration occurs with the patient who responds poorly to what should be an adequate dose. Very low concentrations might suggest noncompliance. Concentrations at the lower end of the presumed therapeutic range might indicate the need for an increased dose. A patient responding adequately to treatment, no matter what the dose, does not need to have plasma concentrations measured (Hollister, 1981a).

Duration of Treatment

Because it is impossible to predict in individual patients how long a depressive episode will last or how long the patient was in an episode prior to being treated, many authorities suggest that treatment be continued for 3 to 4 months following complete remission.

Decision about maintenance treatment must be

Table 71–7. PROPOSED RANGE OF PLASMA CONCENTRATIONS FOR THERAPEUTIC EFFECTS OF VARIOUS TRICYCLIC ANTIDEPRESSANTS

Amitriptyline/Nortriptyline	
	60–200 ng./ml.
	>200 ng./ml.
	80–200 ng./ml.
	>120 ng./ml.
	95–250 ng./ml.
Nortriptyline	
	60–140 ng./ml.
	50–139 ng./ml.
	50–150 ng./ml.
	>100 ng./ml.
	up to 175 ng./ml.
	>200 ng./ml. poorer response
Imipramine/Desipramine	
	>20 ng./ml.
	>180 ng./ml.
	>45 ng./ml. imipramine; >75 ng./ml.
Desipramine	
	>135 ng./ml.
Protriptyline	
	70–170 ng./ml.
Amoxapine	
	200–400 ng./ml.
Maprotiline	
	200–400 ng./ml.

based on many clinical considerations, most important, the natural history of the depressive disorder in a particular patient. The value of maintenance treatment for frequently recurring depression has been well established. Maintenance doses may be only one third of the full therapeutic dose.

Drug Combinations

Antidepressants and lithium are often used together in the depressed phase of bipolar depression. Antipsychotics may have to be added to antidepressants in psychotic or agitated depressions. Antianxiety drugs have been added to antidepressants with some possible benefit. Each clinical situation in which a combination of drugs may be useful must be evaluated separately. Generally, one would prefer to avoid drug combinations, but used judiciously, some have merit.

Side Effects and Interactions

Most side effects of antidepressant drugs stem from unwanted pharmacologic actions. These are summarized in Table 71–8.

The sedative effects of tricyclics may interact pharmacodynamically with other sedative drugs, most commonly alcoholic beverages. The anticholinergic effects may be additive with other drugs that may be given concurrently, such as phenothiazines or antiparkinsonian drugs. Tricyclics impair uptake of some sympatholytic antihypertensive drugs into sympathetic nerve endings, nullifying their therapeutic action. Such interactions have occurred with guanethidine, methyldopa, and clonidine. Often the blood pressure rises acutely, overshooting its original level. The acute hypertensive crisis may be life-threatening.

Monoamine oxidase inhibitors interact with other sympathomimetic drugs or with the indirect sympathomimetic tyramine, resulting in paradoxical hypertension and severe occipital headache. Tyramine is found in a variety of foods and beverages that are likely to be fermented, including ripened cheese and some wines.

Antipsychotics

SCHIZOPHRENIA AND PSYCHOSES

Most family physicians will prefer to have a psychiatrist make the diagnosis of schizophrenia. Many patients are very clearly psychotic, but because craziness comes in many guises, it is well to have a diagnosis made by a specialist. Once the patient is started on drug treatment, the primary responsibility for follow-up may fall on the family physician.

Another situation is that of the patient who has been hospitalized for an acute psychosis but is discharged from the mental hospital on maintenance medication. If a psychiatrist is not available for follow-up or does not wish to undertake it, the responsibility becomes that of the primary care physician. The family physician should insist that an adequate record of the patient's illness be forwarded and that a physician at the hospital be available for consultation or re-referral.

Sometimes the dose of antipsychotics that has been prescribed for the discharged patient may seem monumental. Reduction of dose should be done only in consultation with the referring psychiatrist, as large doses may have been found by long trial and error to be essential for the particular patient. The main goal of the follow-up care of these patients is to ensure that they continue to function adequately and to be alert to the development of any complications of treatment, especially that of tardive dyskinesia, ab-

Table 71–8. PROFILE OF SIDE EFFECTS* OF VARIOUS ANTIDEPRESSANTS

	Sedation	Anticholinergic Action	Orthostatic Hypotension	Sympathomimetic	Quinidinelike Action
Tricyclics					
Amitriptyline (Elavil)	+ + +	+ + +	+ + +	+	+ + +
Imipramine (Tofranil)	+ +	+ + +	+ + +	+ +	+ + +
Doxepin (Sinequan)	+ + +	+ + +	+ +	+	+
Nortriptyline (Aventyl)	+ +	+ +	+	+	+ +
Desipramine (Pertofrane)	+	+	+	+ + +	+ +
Protriptyline (Vivactil)	±	+ +	+	+ +	+
Others					
Amoxapine (Asendin)	+ +	+	+ +	0	?
Maprotiline (Ludiomil)	+ +	+	+ +	0	?
Trazodone (Desyrel)	+ + +	?	0	0	?
Fluoxetine (Prozac)	none of above; see text				
Buproprion (Wellbutrin)	0	0	0	±	?

*Side Effects
Sedation—daytime drowsiness or lethargy, slowed thinking, night-time sedation
Anticholinergic action—dry mouth, blurred vision, constipation, urinary retention, mental confusion in the elderly
Orthostatic hypotension—due to alpha-adrenergic blockage; also includes ejaculatory impotence
Sympathomimetic—tremor, sweating
Quinidinelike action—delayed cardiac conduction times, possible ventricular arrhythmias with fatality

normal movements that resemble Huntington's disease, which appear late in the course of treatment.

Finally, the family physician may be the first to see an aged person whose behavior has been deteriorating. Unless the story is classic for Alzheimer's disease (senile dementia), the patient should be given the benefit of a medical work-up to rule out reversible causes of dementia, delirium, or depression. If these are ruled out and the dreaded diagnosis of Alzheimer's disease must be made, the most effective treatment is judicious use of antipsychotic drugs.

Types of Drugs

The various drugs that have been employed as antipsychotics are listed in Table 71–9. Virtually all are metabolized mainly by the liver. The aliphatic and piperidine phenothiazines are low-potency compounds, the daily therapeutic dose being measured in hundreds of milligrams. The piperazine phenothiazines are high-potency drugs, the usual daily dose being measured in tens of milligrams. Thioxanthenes are generally weaker than their phenothiazine homologs, but some are still considered high-potency drugs. Butyrophenones are also high-potency drugs, although their chemical structure is quite different from that of the phenothiazines or thioxanthenes. The remaining classes of drugs tend to be a mixed group. Potency should never be confused with efficacy, which is roughly the same with equivalent doses of all these drugs (Carlsson, 1978).

Indications

The primary indication for antipsychotics is schizophrenia. Although the drugs are by no means curative and in fact have many deficiencies, they are the best established treatment of this serious disorder. Patients with a diagnosis of schizoaffective disorder may also benefit from the use of these drugs to treat their psychotic symptoms. Acute mania may not respond to lithium alone; the judicious and temporary use of antipsychotics may be extremely helpful. Psychoses of old age are best managed with antipsychotics, although treatment is entirely symptomatic. Some acute brain syndromes, such as the "recovery or intensive-care room syndrome," respond to antipsychotics.

The use of antipsychotics in patients with depression should be limited to those who have psychotic or agitated forms of depression. Minor emotional disorders in which anxiety predominates are best treated with benzodiazepines. Acute brain syndromes associated with illicit drug use or withdrawal from alcohol are best managed with antianxiety drugs; antipsychotic drugs may aggravate the situation.

Table 71–9. VARIOUS TYPES OF ANTIPSYCHOTICS

Class/Drug	Relative Potency	Daily Doses (mg.)
Aliphatic phenothiazine		
Chlorpromazine (Thorazine)	100	100–800
Piperidine phenothiazine		
Thioridazine (Mellaril)	100	100–800
Mesoridazine (Serentil)	50	50–400
Piperazine phenothiazine		
Perphenazine (Trilafon)	10	16–80
Trifluoperazine (Stelazine)	5	5–60
Fluphenazine (Prolixin)	2	4–100
Thioxanthene		
Thiothixene (Navane)	3	5–120
Butyrophenone		
Haloperidol (Haldol)	2	4–150
Dibenzoxazepine		
Loxapine (Loxitane)	10	15–160
Dihydroindolone		
Molindone (Moban)	10	15–225

Choice of Drug

A completely rational choice between antipsychotic drugs currently cannot be made for individual patients. How should we choose one drug from a bewildering array to try in a given patient? The usual dictum has been to learn to use a few drugs well rather than all poorly. One of the most rational ways to narrow the choice of antipsychotics would be to master one of each of the three types of phenothiazines and one of each of the remaining chemical classes of drugs.

A basic assumption in making these choices is that differences within a chemical class are less than differences among classes; this allows the choice of only a single drug for each. The assumption is also made that the puzzling differences between the responses of individual patients to different drugs (a clinical phenomenon that was recognized as soon as more than one drug became available) are largely due to differences in each patient's metabolic handling of the drug, making chemical distinctions important.

Doses and Dosage Schedules

A wide range of doses is used, as therapeutic margins are great for the antipsychotics. Doses shown in Table 71–9 are only rough guides; recent trends are toward using the lowest possible doses except in treatment-resistant patients.

Divided doses are usually given as treatment is started. They minimize the initial impact of many of the unwanted pharmacologic effects (sedation and adrenergic blocking activity) and allow better titration of dose. Doses need not be divided equally, and even at the beginning of treatment, the major daily fraction of dose may be given in the afternoon or evening hours. Unfortunately, this eminently sensible practice in initiating treatment is seldom changed, and patients may stay on divided doses for years. Frequency of dose should be reduced once the full therapeutic dose has been achieved, with the goal of a single daily dose to be given in the evening. Giving the major dose in the evening assists sleep while avoiding excessive daytime sedation.

The majority of patients can be managed with oral medication, but parenteral doses are becoming more popular. The "low-dose" drugs can be given in therapeutic doses parenterally with little difficulty. This procedure would assure that the patient could not be undertreated as a result of some vagary in the drug's absorption or metabolism or the patient's refusal of oral medication. Any patient who does not respond to the orally administered drug should be considered for a trial on parenteral doses before the physician concludes that the drug is ineffective.

Fatty acid esters of drugs with an alcohol moiety are being used increasingly for maintenance therapy in outpatients; decanoate esters of both fluphenazine and haloperidol are currently available. Single intramuscular injections may last for 2 to 4 weeks, thus ensuring drug intake. These preparations have been extremely useful for maintenance therapy, but they have no place in the initial treatment of patients, even though it can be done.

Maintenance Treatment

Maintenance doses should be as low as possible for retaining therapeutic gains. Slow reduction of dose may avoid sudden relapse. Time and again, it has been shown that patients tolerate the reduced drug dose in maintenance very well (Klerman and Tuason, 1980).

"Drug holidays" are another way in which the total exposure of patients to drugs may be reduced. Such an approach is completely empirical because it is impossible to predict in advance who will tolerate interruption of treatment for any substantial period of time, although many patients will. Unless someone is around to watch the patient carefully for signs of relapse so that treatment may be restarted immediately, this approach is neither feasible nor fair to the patient.

Drug Combinations

Little or no rationale exists for combining two antipsychotic drugs. Combinations of the antipsychotic perphenazine and the antidepressant amitriptyline have become extremely popular. Pharmacologically, they do not make much sense, for some of their crucially important actions should oppose each other. Nonetheless, several studies have shown that patients seem to get the best of each drug in the combination. The combination is justified only when the diagnosis is unclear, as in the differential diagnosis between a depressed schizophrenic and a depressed psychotic. Using the combination is a way to cover both possibilities. Extemporaneous combinations of these drugs are preferred because they can be changed as the diagnosis becomes clear, so that eventually a patient may receive one drug or the other. The anticholinergic effect of the tricyclic usually eliminates the need for any antiparkinsonian medication.

Because anxiety in schizophrenics is part of the illness, antipsychotics might be expected to ameliorate it eventually. Antianxiety drugs may be used adjunctively, especially when they do double duty as hypnotics. Mild akathisia may sometimes be mistaken for anxiety. Diphenhydramine or hydroxyzine, both having sedative and anticholinergic actions, may be a better choice than conventional antianxiety drugs.

Antiparkinsonian drugs are used most often in combination with antipsychotics. When antiparkinsonian drugs are used either prophylactically or to treat a drug-induced extrapyramidal syndrome, the drug should be discontinued after several weeks of treatment to determine whether it is still needed. Quite possibly, this well-documented clinical observation that continued antiparkinsonian drugs may not be needed is due to the fact that drug-induced extrapyramidal reactions may be self-limiting.

The basis for using antipsychotic drugs in combination with lithium is established in manic states, and the combination is possibly beneficial in schizoaffective psychoses. Some clinicians find that the addition of lithium provides more control of patients than that obtained by the antipsychotic drug alone.

Side Effects and Complications

The numerous side effects and complications associated with this class of drugs are summarized in Table 71–10. Additional sources provide a more complete discussion of these (Hollister, 1989).

Interactions

Most interactions of antipsychotics are pharmacodynamic, representing the additive sedative, anticholinergic, or alpha-adrenergic blocking effects of

Table 71–10. SIDE EFFECTS AND COMPLICATIONS OF ANTIPSYCHOTICS

Adverse Behavioral Effects
Excitement, akinesia—sedatives or antiparkinsonian drugs
Toxic-confusional state—reduce dose of antipsychotic or antiparkinsonian drug or tricyclic antidepressant
Adverse Central Nervous System Effects
Parkinson syndrome—antiparkinsonian drugs
Dystonic reactions—antiparkinsonian drugs
Akathisia—diphenhydramine
Tardive dyskinesia—reduce or eliminate drug; eliminate antiparkinsonian drugs or tricyclic antidepressants
Adverse Effects on Autonomic Nervous System
Blurred vision, dry mouth, urinary hesitancy, constipation—reduce dose; cholinergic drugs
Orthostatic hypotension—reduce dose; change drug
Metabolic/Endocrine
Amenorrhea, galactorrhea, impotence—reduce dose
Toxic-Allergic
Agranulocytosis—stop drug; another class—rare
Cholestatic jaundice—stop drug; another class—rare
Miscellaneous
Heat stroke, malignant neuroleptic syndrome—stop drug; treat energetically

these drugs when combined with others having similar properties. The quinidinelike effect of thioridazine when combined with similar effects from tricyclic antidepressants may enhance cardiotoxicity. Pharmacokinetic interactions have been described, but most are of no real clinical significance.

Mood-Stabilizing Drugs

MANIC-DEPRESSIVE DISORDERS

Manic-depressive illness is a frequently diagnosed, serious emotional disorder. Patients with cyclic attacks of mania share many attributes with paranoid schizophrenia (grandiosity, bellicosity, paranoid thoughts, and overactivity). The gratifying response of manic-depressive patients to lithium therapy has made such diagnostic distinctions important.

Because of the obvious possible confusion in diagnosis between paranoid schizophrenia on the one hand and manic-depression on the other, most family physicians will refer suspected manic-depressive patients to a psychiatrist for a diagnostic opinion.

Drug Usage

Lithium salts are predominant among drugs of this category. The goal of treatment with such drugs is to avoid the swings in mood that lead to disabling depression or mania.

Carbamazepine (Tegretol) has become an alternative to lithium and may be used when lithium fails or when its side effects preclude adequate treatment. The pharmacologic actions that make both these drugs effective for treating mania is not known. Other anticonvulsants, such as clonazepam (Klonopin) and valproate sodium, have been used experimentally.

When mania is mild, lithium or carbamazepine alone may be an effective treatment. In more severe cases, it is almost always necessary to use some antipsychotic drug concurrently. After mania is controlled, the latter drug may be discontinued and the mood-stabilizer maintained for prophylactic use.

Pharmacology and Pharmacokinetics of Lithium

Unlike antipsychotic or antidepressant drugs, which have a multiplicity of pharmacologic actions on the central or autonomic nervous system, lithium ion produces relatively mild sedation and is devoid of adrenergic blocking or anticholinergic effects. A second attribute of the treatment is that, being an ion, it is easily measured in body fluids such as plasma, urine, or saliva. It is distributed in body water, unlike most of the other lipid-soluble drugs, and is not metabolized, being almost totally excreted by the kidney. Thus, its kinetics can be studied much more easily, and plasma or tissue concentrations can be correlated with clinical effects. A third attribute of considerable interest has been the prophylactic use of the drug in preventing both mania and depression. It is remarkable that a so-called functional psychosis can be controlled so easily by such a simple chemical as lithium carbonate (e.g., Eskalith and others).

Indications for Mood Stabilizers

The manic stage of manic-depressive disorder is the primary indication. Little doubt now exists that these drugs are useful for prevention of recurrent affective episodes. Although cycling of what appear to be endogenous depressions without any mania may be reduced by mood stabilizers, these agents are not treatments for endogenous depression. The addition of mood stabilizers to antipsychotics may be useful in schizoaffective disorders or schizophrenia. Claims that lithium is useful in uncontrollable aggressive behavior or alcoholism are still uncertain.

Doses and Dosage Schedule

One should consider the patient's body weight and age in making an assessment of the appropriate doses of lithium carbonate for starting treatment. The initial volume of distribution of lithium will be the body water, which is approximately 50 per cent of body weight for adult women and 55 per cent for adult men. The proportion of body water may decrease slightly at older age levels. More important in older patients is an inapparent decrease in renal function. Any patient past age 50 is likely to have a decreased creatinine clearance, which may reach 50 per cent or less of the usual normal values without abnormal elevation of serum creatinine. Thus, large patients may require large doses, but older patients will generally require a dose less than predicted for their size.

A dose of 0.5 mEq. per kg. per day will produce serum lithium concentrations in the range of 1.0 mEq. per liter after a week of treatment. A 70-kg. person would require 35 mEq. of lithium per day. With each 300-mg. dosage unit containing approximately 8 mEq., the initial dose would be roughly 1200 mg. per day. If the desired serum lithium concentration is not precisely reached, the dose can be changed in an arithmetic fashion to attain the desired concentration. Usual serum concentrations for treatment of acute mania are 0.8 to 1.2 mEq. per liter; maintenance concentrations range between 0.5 to 0.9 mEq. per liter.

Almost always it is necessary to use divided doses of lithium to avoid gastric distress. Two to four divided doses may be needed, depending on the total daily dose. Medication is best taken with or shortly after meals.

Carbamazepine should be started in doses of 400 to 800 mg. per day and doses adjusted to maintain plasma concentrations similar to those used for treating seizures. Doses should always be divided.

Monitoring Treatment

Serum levels of lithium should be checked at weekly intervals during the first four weeks of treatment but less often (every 4 to 6 weeks) thereafter. As the patient comes under control, doses may be reduced to produce lower plasma concentrations, usually about one half to two thirds the level required to attain remission (Amdisen, 1977). A similar schedule of monitoring plasma concentrations of carbamazepine should be followed.

Maintenance Treatment

The decision to use prophylactic treatment depends on many factors: the frequency and severity of previous episodes, a crescendo pattern of appearance, and the degree to which the patient is willing to follow a program of indefinite maintenance therapy. If the present attack was the patient's first, one might prefer to terminate treatment after it subsided. Anyone with a frequency of one or more episodes of illness a year might be considered to be a prime candidate for maintenance treatment. Even so, if patients are not reliable, efforts might be better spent to alert their families to the initial signs of recurrence and to provide prompt treatment when the disorder recurs. Some patients with mania discontinue treatment voluntarily, for they feel that their spirits and initiative are suppressed by mood stabilizers.

Drug Combinations

Lithium and carbamazepine have been combined when neither has been effective alone. Both drugs may be combined with antipsychotics when mania breaks through a prophylactic treatment program or with antidepressants when depression becomes apparent. Although haloperidol was alleged to be a poor drug to combine with lithium, it seems in retrospect to be no different from other antipsychotics. All antipsychotics may produce more severe extrapyramidal syndromes when combined with mood stabilizers.

Interactions

Because the clearance of lithium is reduced by about 25 per cent by the presence of oral diuretics, doses may have to be reduced by a similar amount. A similar reduction in lithium clearance has been noted with several nonsteroidal anti-inflammatory drugs that block synthesis of prostaglandins. Whether or not this interaction extends to aspirin and acetaminophen is not yet known.

Side Effects and Complications

Many side effects associated with lithium treatment occur at varying times after treatment (Vestergaard, Amdisen, and Schou, 1980). Some are harmless, whereas others may augur the onset of toxicity. It is important to distinguish which side effects may herald toxicity. The more common or important ones are summarized in Table 71–11.

Overdoses

Careful assessment of the state of consciousness and continual monitoring of neurologic signs, vital signs, electrolytes, and arterial blood gases are basic. Blood pressure should be maintained by intravenous fluids, but pressor agents may be required in some cases. Norepinephrine (Levophed) and dopamine (Inotropin) are the preferred agents. Respiration should be assisted when ventilation is impaired. A cuffed endotracheal tube will mitigate against secretions, vomitus, or the return from gavage reaching the lung. Appropriate attempts should be made to rid the body of the drug, using gavage, activated charcoal, and purgatives as first treatments.

SEDATIVE-HYPNOTICS

Benzodiazepines are remarkably safe. Only two cases of successful suicides with overdose of diazepam alone have been documented. Based on observations of 121 cases of poisoning with chlordiazepoxide, it was concluded that when the drug was used alone, symptoms were quite mild, consisting only of drowsiness or stupor. If another drug was also present, its effects usually predominated. Instances of overdose with diazepam have been equally mild, characterized by marked muscle relaxation but little fall in blood pressure or respiratory depression. Oxazepam and clorazepate, being metabolites of diazepam, should prove to have shorter and probably milder courses than the precursor drug. The availability of such safe antianxiety drugs as the benzodiazepines is a distinct advantage. Buspirone appears to be equally safe when taken in overdoses.

ANTIDEPRESSANTS

Paradoxically, drugs used for treating patients at high risk for suicide have a high potential for being used

Table 71–11. SIDE EFFECTS OF LITHIUM

Nausea, loose stools, fine tremor, polyuria—frequently early symptoms—possibly propranolol (Inderal) for tremor
Edema, weight gain—late symptoms; if diuretic is used, reduced lithium dose
Vomiting, coarse tremors, sleepiness, dysarthria—may herald toxicity
Goiter, hypothyroidism—thyroxine
Nephrogenic diabetes insipidus—thiazide diuretics; reduce dose
Contraindications—bradycardia-tachycardia ("sick-sinus") syndrome; pregnancy and lactation

successfully for that purpose. Overdose of tricyclic antidepressants may be quite serious: coma, convulsions, and cardiac abnormalities are the diagnostic triad. Cardiac abnormalities include delayed conduction time and both abnormal atrial and ventricular rhythms. Because the latter may be life threatening, continued monitoring in an intensive care unit is required.

Overdoses of MAO inhibitors are rare. Most toxic effects are attributable to excessive adrenergic stimulation: agitation, delirium, neuromuscular excitability, seizures, and hyperthermia. Coma and shock are late stages. Supportive treatment is usually adequate. Among second-generation drugs, overdoses of amoxapine and maprotiline are every bit as dangerous as those from tricyclics. On the other hand, overdoses of trazodone and fluoxetine appear to cause relatively few problems.

ANTIPSYCHOTICS

General principles of management of overdoses apply to antipsychotics, but some special problems must be met as they arise. Convulsions are best treated by intravenous injections of diazepam or sodium phenytoin. The possibility of increasing central respiratory depression with further doses of a central depressant drug should be balanced against the anticonvulsant effect and only minimally effective doses used. Acute hypotension not responsive to forced fluids may require the use of a pressor agent. Norepinephrine is the logical drug for treatment, being primarily an alpha-adrenergic receptor stimulant. Warm blankets and heat cradles may reverse the trend toward hypothermia, but if one overshoots the mark, fever will ensue. Fever should not be ascribed immediately to some infectious complication in the absence of other evidence.

LITHIUM

Therapeutic overdoses are more common than those due to deliberate or accidental ingestion of the drug. Therapeutic overdoses are usually due to accumulation of lithium as a result of some change in the patient's status, such as diminished electrolytes, use of diuretics, fluctuating renal function, or pregnancy. As tissue levels have already been established, the plasma concentrations of the drug may not be excessively high in proportion to the degree of toxicity; any value over 2 mEq. per liter must be considered as indicating potential toxicity.

A primary consideration is to rid the patient of the drug. Because of the physically large amounts of drug involved (one may be dealing with 30 to 60 grams), absorption is slow. In part this may be due to decreased gastrointestinal motility associated with impaired consciousness. Lavage should be done with a wide-bore tube because the material tends to clump and may be difficult to remove through smaller tubes. Saline cathartics should follow lavage. Charcoal is not an effective adsorbent in this instance. Because lithium is a simple ion, it is dialyzed readily. Both peritoneal dialysis and hemodialysis have been effective, although the latter is preferred. One may wish to use both simultaneously. Dialysis should be sustained until the plasma concentrations fall below the usual therapeutic range.

Supportive measures include assisted respiration and maintained blood pressure, as in most poisonings, and monitoring of the electrocardiograph for the possible development of life-threatening arrhythmias. Special attention must be paid to the bronchial toilet so that if viscous secretions develop, the patient does not asphyxiate. Serum lithium levels should be measured every 4 to 6 hours to assure that effective measures are being taken to eliminate the drug.

Even though a fatal outcome is avoided by excellent management, some patients may develop permanent neurologic sequelae, usually in the form of choreoathetoid disorders, cerebellar signs, and dementia of varying degrees. It is difficult to predict such outcomes, although serious intoxications are more likely to be followed by permanent damage.

Overdoses of carbamazepine have been managed by the supportive measures outlined above.

References

Alho, H., Costa, E., Ferrero, P., et al.: Diazepam-binding inhibitor: A neuropeptide located in selected neural populations of rat brain. Science, *229*:179–181, 1985. *Could this endogenous peptide provide a basis for the biologic mechanism of anxiety?*

Amdisen, A.: Serum lithium monitoring and clinical pharmacokinetics of lithium. Clin. Pharmacokinet., *2*:73, 1977. *Complete review by an authoritative reviewer.*

Carlsson, A.: Antipsychotic drugs, neurotransmitters and schizophrenia. Am. J. Psychiatry, *135*:164, 1978. *The father of the "dopamine hypothesis" of schizophrenia explains the relationships between the actions of antipsychotic drugs and other lines of evidence that led to the formulation of this hypothesis.*

Consensus Conference: Drugs and insomnia. The use of medications to promote sleep. J.A.M.A., *251*:2410–2414, 1984. *Current thinking by a group of experts about the relation of drug treatment to the management of insomnia.*

Hollister, L. E.: Monitoring plasma concentrations of psychotherapeutic drugs. Trends in Pharmacological Sciences, *2*:89, 1981a. *This review covers all psychotherapeutic drugs. With the exception of lithium, most interest in monitoring plasma concentrations of these drugs lies in the tricyclic antidepressants. At the moment, routine monitoring doesn't make sense, but there are some situations in which such a determination may be helpful. The major indication is when a patient who is receiving what should be an adequate dose fails to respond. Noncompliance is frequently the reason.*

Hollister, L. E.: Current antidepressant drugs: Their clinical use. Drugs, *22*:129, 1981b.

Hollister, L. E.: Clinical Pharmacology of Psychotherapeutic Drugs. New York, Churchill-Livingstone, 1989. *More information than most family physicians want or need, but handy as a reference book.*

Hollister, L. E.: Selection of benzodiazepines. J. Drug Ther. Res., *9*:416–422, 1984. *An attempt to sort out the vast number to reduce those a clinician needs to use. Pharmacokinetic differences account for variety of choices. Personal preference of patient and confidence by physician are main criteria.*

Kales, A., Soldatos, C. R., Bixler, E. O., et al.: Early morning insomnia with rapidly eliminated benzodiazepines. Science, *220*:95–97, 1983. *Controversial report of rebound following short-acting drugs. Some see it, others do not. Suggests concept of single-dose withdrawal.*

Klerman, G. L., and Tuason, V. B.: Prevention of relapse of schizophrenia. Arch. Gen. Psychiatry, *37*:16, 1980. *Low-dose maintenance treatment prevents relapse and avoids excessive exposure to antipsychotics.*

Mellinger, G. D., Balter, M. B., and Uhlenhuth, E. H.: Prevalence and correlates of the longterm regular use of anxiolytics. Arch. Gen. Psychiatry, *251*:375–379, 1984.

Mellinger, G. D., Balter, M. B., and Uhlenhuth, E. H.: Insomnia and its treatment. Prevalence and correlates. Arch. Gen. Psychiatry, *42*:225–232, 1985. *Both this paper and the one by the same cited above deal with the prevalence of drug use for treating complaints of anxiety and insomnia. Contrary to some opinion, drugs are not used capriciously for these disorders but rather in an acceptable medical model.*

Palmer, D. P.: Buspirone, a new approach to the treatment of anxiety. FASEB J., *2*:2445–2452, 1988. *If buspirone really works, then we shall have to consider alternative hypotheses to the pathophysiology of anxiety. It would be surprising if such a ubiquitous defense mechanism did not have redundant physiologic mechanisms.*

Paul, S. M., Marangos, P. J., Skolnick, P.: The benzodiazepine-GABA-chloride ionophore receptor complex: Common site of minor tranquilizer action. Biol. Psychiatry, *16*:213, 1981. *Benzodiazepine receptors were clearly not put in the brain awaiting the discovery in the 1950's of this class of drugs. Perhaps a change in receptors or in their endogenous ligands sets the stage for clinical anxiety. Only a minority of people are affected, and they seem to do well on drugs. Could pathologic anxiety be biologically based rather than purely a response to life events?*

Peroutka, S. J.: Selective interaction of novel anxiolytics with 5-hydroxytryptamine 1A receptors. Biol. Psychiatry, *20*:971–979, 1985. *This receptor, looking for a function, may have found one.*

Rickels, K.: Are benzodiazepines overused and abused? Br. J. Pharmacol., *11*:71S, 1981. *Rickels musters the evidence to support the contention that rather than being overused, antianxiety drugs may be underused. Although abuse can occur, with resulting physical dependence, the matter has been greatly exaggerated in regard to the prevalence and severity of the problem.*

Rickels, K., Case, G. W., Winokur, A., et al.: Longterm benzodiazepine therapy: Risks and benefits. Psychopharmacol. Bull., *20*:608–615, 1984. *Short-term treatment, under 4 months, is rarely associated with therapeutic-dose dependence, but this phenomenon becomes more frequent following long-term treatment, over 8 months.*

Shader, R. I., and Greenblatt, J. D.: The use of benzodiazepines in clinical practice. Br. J. Pharmacol., *11*:5S, 1981. *All you want to know about the pharmacokinetics of benzodiazepines, and more. This whole volume, a supplement to the regular issues of the journal, has many articles pertaining to the benzodiazepines.*

Sulser, F.: Mode of action of antidepressant drugs. J. Clin. Psychiatry, *44*:14–20; 1983. *The common mode of action of all antidepressant drugs of different chemical classes is believed to be down-regulation of central beta-adrenergic receptors.*

Vestergaard, P., Amdisen, A., and Schou, M.: Clinically significant side effects of lithium treatment: A survey of 237 patients in long-term treatment. Acta Psychiatr. Scand., *63*:333–345, 1981. *If anyone can speak with authority on the prevalence of side effects from lithium, it is this Danish group. Early side effects are common and may not be of much importance. However, side effects can be the cue to impending toxicity, as this drug has a rather small therapeutic margin. In fact, clinical signs may be a more reliable guide than serum levels that seem to be reasonable.*

72

Interpreting Laboratory Tests

Paul M. Fischer
Lois A. Addison

Since the 1960's, there has been a dramatic shift in the way that clinicians use laboratory tests. The 1960's were marked by the rapid acceptance of "screening panels" which promised the ability to diagnose important conditions while the patient was symptom free. Multichannel chemistry analyzers made it possible to order large numbers of tests and to have the results back within a short period of time. Test ordering became simplified to just deciding which particular "panel" or "profile" was needed.

Since the 1970's, it has become clear that very few of the common tests are useful in screening asymptomatic individuals. This has led to a more rigorous analysis of the clinical role of laboratory tests.

The most widely accepted model for test ordering is based on a test's sensitivity, specificity, and predictive value. These concepts are part of the "decision analysis" description of how clinicians choose diagnostic strategies. Decision analysis is a method of mathematically analyzing the probabilities that are involved in clinical decisions.

Clinicians are often excited to learn about decision analysis. After all, it outlines a "rational" way to view test ordering. These testing concepts have also been endorsed by those who pay for health care and who would therefore like to identify "unnecessary" tests. Toward this end, the American College of Physicians and the Blue Cross and Blue Shield Association have released an entire text on the use and interpretation of common diagnostic tests (Sox, 1987).

We have found these concepts to be theoretically useful but very difficult to translate into day-to-day practice. Our initial enthusiasm has been tempered by realizing that even the very best clinicians do not and cannot function by the narrow rules laid down by the proponents of decision analysis. Tests are used in many ways by clinicians. George Lundberg, M.D. (editor of J.A.M.A.) has identified at least 32 different reasons why physicians order tests, including "nothing else to do" (Lundberg, 1983).

The Problem of a "Gold Standard"

The starting point in decision analysis is to identify a test's sensitivity and specificity. Sensitivity is defined as the percentage of individuals with the disease who have a positive test. Specificity is defined as the percentage of people without the disease who have a negative test. Both concepts depend on a reference, or "gold standard," method to identify whether a person is diseased. Unfortunately, most of the commonly used gold standards are imperfect.

This issue has recently been discussed for tests of ischemic heart disease (Boyko et al., 1988). Coronary angiography is usually used as the gold standard for this illness; however, several studies have now shown that this test frequently misclassifies both the presence and the absence of significant coronary artery stenosis. If a gold standard misclassifies individuals, then both the sensitivity and specificity of a second comparison test will be artificially altered.

The inadequacy of reference tests is a problem for such common diseases as Group A streptococcal pharyngitis and urinary tract infections. In diagnosing patients with sore throats, a throat culture has traditionally been used. More recently, rapid tests which detect group A streptococcal cell wall antigens have become available. Many microbiologists complain that these newer tests are relatively "insensitive," since they have a 10 per cent false negative rate (i.e., in 10 per cent of patients with a negative antigen test, Group A streptococci will grow on a throat culture). However, the colony count in these "false negative" cases is often low. It is therefore not clear whether the patient is a noninfected carrier or an infected patient. The sensitivity of any antigen test can be discredited by employing more sophisticated culture techniques and, therefore, recovering strep from a larger percentage of patients. Group A streptococci can in fact be cultured in up to 60 per cent of "normal" persons if special culture techniques are used (Kellogg and Manzella, 1986).

Some have argued that a rise in streptococcal antibody titers (i.e., ASO titers) should be used as a gold standard in determining who really has group A streptococcal pharyngitis. In one recent study looking at the clinical response to antibiotic therapy in individuals with a positive throat culture, both patients with and without an antibody response showed a dramatic clinical response to antibiotics, compared with individuals with negative throat cultures (Gerber et al., 1988). The authors concluded that the study raised significant questions about the appropriateness of using antibody response to distinguish who has a true streptococcal infection. There is to date no clear agreement on the gold standard for evaluating the common condition of streptococcal pharyngitis.

As another example, consider the diagnosis of urinary tract infections. Until recently, it was not uncommon to tell a woman with urinary frequency, urgency, and dysuria that she "was not infected" because her urine culture grew only 50,000 colonies. This was based on the time-honored level of 100,000 colonies per ml. of urine as a cut-off for "significant bacteriuria." This diagnostic level failed to consider the patient's symptoms, how long the urine had incubated in the bladder, or the specimen's specific gravity. More recent studies have indicated that a colony count as low as 100 may indicate infection in a patient with dysuria. It is therefore impossible to identify a single level of bacteriuria as a "gold standard" for diagnosing UTIs.

These examples illustrate the problem with identifying appropriate gold standards on which to base a test's sensitivity and specificity. Clinicians must be cautious in trusting the published performance characteristics of any test. Unfortunately, there is no precise way to adjust for the errors of an imperfect reference test. Clinicians must rely on common sense.

Problems in Confidence

A second problem is the great variability in reported test sensitivities and specificities. Pronouncements are made that a test has a "95 per cent sensitivity" as if this were for all times and for all patient populations. The next month, an article using the same test reports a "60 per cent sensitivity." No wonder clinicians have a hard time putting these concepts to use!

One reason for this variation is that the accuracy of the reported sensitivity or specificity depends on the size of the population studied. Often the studies have few patients. If the numbers are low, there can be little certainty of the results.

A recommendation has been made that sensitivities and specificities should be reported as a "confidence interval" (Heckerling, 1988). This is the range of values (usually $\pm$ 2 SD) which is supported by the data. For example, if a test is positive in 15 of 20 patients with a disease, the sensitivity is 75 per cent. However, the 95 per cent confidence limits for the sensitivity would be 51 to 91 per cent. This is an extremely wide variation. If the same test is studied with a larger population and 300 of 400 patients with the disease have a positive test, the sensitivity would remain 75 per cent but the 95 per cent confidence limits would be narrowed to between 70 and 79 per cent.

The lesson for the clinician should be to suspect all sensitivity and specificity values. Be especially cautious whenever there is great variation in the values reported for a single test.

Spectrum of Disease

The traditional decision analysis model assumes that either you have a disease or you do not. This simplistic ideal is complicated by the "spectrum" of disease (Ransohoff and Feinstein, 1978). The spectrum of disease is the range of features found in an illness. Every illness is characterized by variation in terms of its chronicity and severity. Test results will similarly vary. The usual pattern is that a test is more likely to be positive when the disease is of a longer duration or greater severity. Many of the reported sensitivities and specificities are optimistically high because of the tendency of researchers to ignore the problem of disease spectrum.

An example is the literature on carcinoembryonic antigen (CEA) testing for colon cancer. The early studies indicated a 90 per cent sensitivity for this test. Most of these studies were done on individuals with very extensive disease. Later studies with more representative samples of colon cancer patients (i.e., some with localized disease and others with extensive disease) showed that the test was sensitive only in patients with extensive cancer.

A test's specificity can be inaccurate because of the variety of nondiseased patients who are studied. (Remember, specificity is defined as the percentage of individuals without the disease who have a negative test.) The early studies on CEA and colon cancer showed specificities of 90 per cent. The nondiseased individuals in these studies were healthy and asymptomatic. Later studies used a more appropriate spectrum of controls (i.e., individuals with other colon diseases or individuals with cancers other than those of the colon). In these later studies, the specificity of CEA testing was greatly reduced.

The Problem of Prevalence

Another concept on which most decision analysis is based is that of disease prevalence. This is the number of individuals with a disease in a population at a given time. There are unfortunately almost no prevalence figures that can be easily "plugged into" a decision analysis formula for real clinical situations. The best that can usually be done in estimating the prevalence of a disease is to state whether it is common, uncommon, or rare.

There are typically two types of prevalence figures in the literature. The first is derived from case series that are seen in referral centers (i.e., What percentage of patients in an endocrinology clinic with the chief complaint of fatigue have hypothyroidism?) These are notoriously inaccurate because of the problem of referral bias.

A second common type of prevalence is from population studies. In this type of research, a sample of individuals in a geographic area is tested (i.e., What percentage of the U.S. population has hypertension?). While this prevalence figure will tell you about the general population, it does not help in deciding what the prevalence of a disease is in the patients who come to your office with a specific complaint (i.e., What is the prevalence of CNS cancer in individuals who present with headache and have a normal neurologic examination?).

Another aspect of prevalence which is usually overlooked is that it varies from one practice site to another and from month to month. Consider for example the differences in the prevalence of HIV disease in San Francisco compared with Omaha. Also consider the prevalence of influenza in February compared with July.

Treatment Assumptions

It is often assumed that understanding a test's predictive value will lead to clear and rational test ordering. However, even when clinicians can agree on the characteristics of a test, they may end up with very different decisions about how to use the test. This has been recently described by DeNeef for the tests used to diagnose group A streptococcal pharyngitis (DeNeef, 1987). DeNeef looked at 21 different strategies for treating adults with pharyngitis. He included a wide range of treatment strategies including the use of empiric antibiotics, culturing, or testing with rapid tests. In the end, it was not principally the characteristics of the test that determined the clinical strategy, but rather the physician's treatment goals, which could be to minimize total cost, minimize adverse outcomes, or minimize the costs of both adverse outcomes and unnecessary antibiotics. It is, to a large extent, the assumptions about therapeutic goals, rather than the characteristics of the test, which determine how a test is used.

Decision Levels

If clinicians cannot easily use sensitivity, specificity, or predictive value in making clinical decisions, what do they use? It is our observation that when interpreting tests, clinicians usually ask two questions:

1. Is it normal or abnormal?
2. If abnormal, is it a little abnormal or very abnormal?

The degree to which the test is abnormal has often been overlooked in discussions about test interpretation (Statland, 1987). It is, however, what clinicians have intuitively used for a long time in deciding whether they should act on a test result. A serum calcium of 10.5 mg. per dl., although outside the usual reference range, will often not catch a clinician's attention. A level of 13 mg. per dl., on the other hand, is impossible to ignore.

Test Interpretation

This chapter reviews many of the common tests that clinicians are called upon to interpret. Each section includes background information about the test, highlighting the most common causes of an "abnormal" test and some of the common pitfalls in the test's interpretation. This information reflects our perspective from work in primary care clinical settings.

Each section includes a table of "normal" values. We have chosen this word, rather than "reference range" or other similar terms, since "normal" is the term which clinicians usually use. "Reference range" is a statistically safe term which meets the laboratory's needs whereas "normal" meets the clinician's needs. ("Mr. Jones, your cholesterol is normal.") When appropriate, differences are indicated between the normal values for adults and children, males and females.

All values are given in both conventional units and Système International (SI) units. Conversion factors (i.e., conventional to SI units) are also given. The adoption of SI units by the U.S. medical literature should be complete by the time the next edition of this text is published.

We have tried to identify the important diagnoses to consider when interpreting an increased or decreased test value. When interpretation is aided by the degree of abnormality, we have indicated the useful diagnostic ranges. These should not be viewed as firm rules, but rather as clinically useful guides.

Finally, we have indicated actions that should be considered in helping to interpret an abnormal test. These actions are sometimes patient history, physical examination findings, or further laboratory testing. The suggested actions are ranked in order to indicate a commonsense plan for further evaluation.

Despite the increasing interest in establishing rules for "appropriate" test ordering, the best that can be said is that there are a few instances when a test is clearly appropriate, a few when it is clearly inappropriate, and many other instances that are open to debate. Clinicians live in a sea of uncertainty.

ALBUMIN

Background

Albumin is produced by the liver and released into the plasma, where it accounts for 90 per cent of the intravascular oncotic pressure. A healthy adult liver is able to produce 12 to 14 grams of albumin per day (Table 72–1). This is reduced with advanced age, poor nutrition, or hepatic disease.

It is unclear how albumin is degraded in the body; however, only very small amounts are normally lost through the urine or the gastrointestinal mucosa. When there is either a reduction in albumin synthesis or an increase in albumin loss, hypoalbuminemia develops. This is often associated with edema.

Serum albumin testing is not recommended for the general screening of healthy individuals. When such routine screening is done, most of the abnormal values are mildly elevated or decreased. These represent the extremes of the normal distribution of values and can usually be ignored. The test is extremely useful in evaluating patients with edema, liver disease, or suspected malnutrition.

An elevated albumin is of no clinical significance. It is most commonly seen in the face of dehydration.

Table 72–1. NORMAL VALUES FOR ALBUMIN

Diagnostic Units: gm./dl. (gm./L.). SI conversion factor = 10

Normal 4.0–6.0 gm./dl. (40–60 gm./L.)

Decreased	Diagnoses to Consider	Actions to Consider
<4.0 (40)	Decreased synthesis Liver insufficiency Malnutrition Malignancy Increased loss Nephrotic syndrome Extensive burns Protein-losing enteropathy Pregnancy Inflammatory illness	1. Dietary history 2. Urinalysis 3. 24-hour urine protein 4. Bilirubin 5. Creatinine 6. Hemoglobin

Values in parentheses are SI units.

Table 72–2. NORMAL VALUES FOR ALKALINE PHOSPHATASE

Diagnostic Units: Units/L.

Normal Adults: 30–120
Children: 50–400
Pregnant women: 30–200

Increased	Diagnoses to Consider	Actions to Consider
120–200	Nonfasting patient specimen Drug effect	1. Repeat test with patient fasting 2. Review patient medications
>200	Increased from bone: Paget's disease Osteomalacia Bony metastasis Hyperparathyroidism Increased from liver: Bile duct stone Biliary cancer Pancreatic cancer Pancreatitis Liver infiltration (sarcoid) Primary biliary cirrhosis Viral hepatitis Severe cirrhosis Other causes: Drug effect Heart failure Hyperthyroidism Lymphoma Leukemia	1. Review patient medications 2. Serum bilirubin, GGT, and aminotransferases 3. RUQ abdominal ultrasound 4. Pelvis or femur x-rays 5. Serum calcium 6. Bone scan

ALKALINE PHOSPHATASE

Background

Alkaline phosphatase (ALP) is a family of enzymes found in nearly all body tissues but which have no known function (Table 72–2). In normal adults, about half of the measured serum ALP is produced by the liver and about half is produced by bone. Children and adolescents have ALP levels two to four times that of a normal adult. This is due to the rapid bone growth in this age group. Women in the third trimester of pregnancy also have an elevated ALP. This is due to production of this enzyme by the placenta. This level returns to normal by one month postpartum.

Liver diseases are usually divided into those which are primarily hepatic and those which are cholestatic. Elevation in aminotransferase is the usual laboratory marker for direct hepatocyte insult. Alkaline phosphatase, on the other hand, is the usual marker for a cholestatic illness. This includes any process that causes an obstruction in the bile ducts (i.e., stone, cancer, pancreatitis, primary biliary cirrhosis). In these illnesses, the ALP and conjugated bilirubin levels are moderately to greatly elevated, while the aminotransferase levels are normal or only mildly elevated (Fischer, 1985). In illnesses that are directly hepatotoxic (i.e., viral hepatitis) the aminotransferase and conjugated bilirubin are greatly elevated, while the ALP may be normal or only mildly elevated. Although alcohol ingestion is often cited as a cause for an elevated ALP, this is rarely the case unless there is advanced cirrhosis or severe alcoholic hepatitis.

The ALP level is elevated in disorders associated with osteoblastic activity (i.e., new bone formation). Paget's disease of bone is the prototypical illness. Ninety per cent of these patients will have an elevated ALP even though most are asymptomatic. Osteoporosis and fractures do not commonly lead to elevated ALP levels.

A gamma glutamyltransferase test (GGT) is useful in differentiating between biliary and bony sources of an elevated ALP. The GGT is usually elevated when the ALP is derived from the liver.

The ALP is not a useful screening test in asymptomatic individuals. Values less than the reference range are of no clinical significance.

Since more than 200 different medications can cause an elevated ALP, a good first step in anyone with an unexplained ALP elevation is a thorough medication review.

AMINOTRANSFERASES

Background

The aminotransferases (or transaminases) are enzymes primarily located within hepatocytes. Alanine aminotransferase (ALAT) used to be referred to as serum glutamic phosphoracetic transaminase (SGPT). Aspartate aminotransferase (ASAT) used to be referred to as serum glutamic oxaloacetic transaminase (SGOT). Increased levels of the two enzymes are due to liver injury and the subsequent leaking of the enzymes from the cells. In general, the level of the aminotransferases reflects the severity of the hepatic injury (Table 72–3).

ALAT is fairly specific for the liver. In contrast, ASAT is also increased in injury to cardiac or skeletal muscle. This fact is useful clinically, since if both enzymes are elevated, a hepatic source is very likely. In most illnesses the ALAT value is greater than the ASAT. The only common exception to this rule is in alcoholic hepatitis, in which the ASAT is higher.

ASAT and ALAT testing are not useful in the screening of healthy individuals. They are, however, extremely useful in diagnosing and monitoring all forms of liver disease. They are also frequently used as screening tests in patients on medications which can produce liver injury (i.e., INH).

Aminotransferase values less than the lower normal limit are infrequently seen and are of little clinical significance. The exceptions to this rule are in advanced cirrhosis and fulminant hepatitis. In these situations a normal or low level can indicate that the disease has progressed so far that few hepatocytes remain.

Table 72–3. NORMAL VALUES FOR AMINOTRANSFERASES

Diagnostic Units: Units/L.

Normal 0–35

Increased	Diagnoses to Consider	Actions to Consider
35–400	Both ALAT and ASAT elevated: Infectious hepatitis Toxic hepatitis Alcoholic hepatitis Shock liver Biliary obstruction Only ASAT elevated: Myocardial infarction Hemolysis (in vivo) Pulmonary infarction Muscular dystrophy	1. Review patient medication 2. Review foreign travel, needle sticks, chemical exposures, and transfusion history 3. Alcohol history 4. Serum bilirubin, alkaline phosphatase 5. Test for viral hepatitis 6. Peripheral smear for hemolysis
>400	Both ALAT and ASAT elevated: Infectious hepatitis Toxic hepatitis Shock liver	

AMYLASE (SERUM)

Background

There are few diseases that are diagnosed with as much certainty, based on a single test, as is pancreatitis from the finding of an elevated amylase (Table 72–4). With very few exceptions, an elevated amylase indicates pancreatitis and a normal amylase rules out this diagnosis. In addition to pancreatitis, patients with abdominal pain and an elevated amylase should be evaluated for a perforated peptic ulcer or mesenteric infarction.

Table 72–4. NORMAL VALUES FOR AMYLASE

Diagnostic Units: Somogyi units/dl. (Units/L.)

Normal 50–150 (0–130)

Increased	Diagnoses to Consider	Actions to Consider
>150 (130)	Pancreatitis: Alcoholic Gallstone Trauma Hyperlipidemia Infectious Drug-induced Familial ERCP Perforating ulcer Mesenteric infarction Salivary gland disease Chronic renal failure Amylase-secreting cancer	1. Alcohol history 2. Abdominal examination 3. Complete drug history 4. RUQ ultrasound 5. Urinary amylase 6. Amylase/creatinine clearance 7. Lipase or amylase isoenzyme

Values in parentheses are SI units.

Table 72–5. NORMAL VALUES FOR BILIRUBIN

Diagnostic Units: mg./dl. (μ mol./L.). SI conversion factor = 17.1
Normal 0.1–1.0 (2–17)

Increased in Newborns	Diagnoses to Consider	Actions to Consider
1.0–10 (17–171)	Direct < 15% of total: Physiologic Breast feeding ABO incompatibility Rh incompatibility Hemorrhage Maternal diabetes Direct > 15% of total: Sepsis TORCH infections Hepatitis Biliary atresia	1. Mother and infant blood type 2. Direct Coombs' tests 3. Hct
10–20 (171–342)	Kernicterus possible	1. Phototherapy or exchange transfusion (base decision on days of age, weight, maturity)
Increased in Adults	**Diagnoses to Consider**	**Actions to Consider**
> 1.0 (17)	Hepatic insufficiency Biliary obstruction Hemolysis Postoperative complications	1. Alcohol history 2. Complete drug history 3. Travel, dietary, and needle stick history 4. Peripheral blood smear 5. Conjugated bilirubin, AST, ALP 6. Reticulocyte count 7. Viral hepatitis tests 8. Direct Coombs' tests 9. RUQ ultrasound

Values in parentheses are SI units.

Amylase is produced by the pancreas, salivary glands, and some tumors (lung). Most of the amylase produced by the pancreas goes directly into the gut. A small fraction is absorbed into the circulation. About one third of the normal serum amylase is pancreatic in origin, while two thirds is from the salivary glands. The amylase in the circulation is excreted primarily by the kidneys. Modest elevations in the serum amylase (i.e., two times normal) can therefore be seen in patients with chronic renal failure.

The degree of amylase elevation does not always correlate with the severity of pancreatic injury. This is particularly true in chronic pancreatitis, in which serum levels may be normal despite ongoing pancreatic injury. In such cases, a urinary amylase or an amylase to creatinine clearance ratio may be helpful.

In unexplained hyperamylasemia, serum lipase or amylase isoenzymes may be helpful tests. Lipase is produced by the pancreas but not by salivary glands.

Low serum amylase levels are rarely of clinical significance.

BILIRUBIN (TOTAL)

Background

Bilirubin is formed from the heme ring as senescent red cells are degraded. It is transported in blood attached to albumin and then delivered to the liver, where it is conjugated and excreted in the bile. The common causes for hyperbilirubinemia are increased red cell destruction, liver diseases, and biliary tract obstruction.

Laboratories measure the total bilirubin and conjugated (i.e., direct) bilirubin (Table 72–5). The unconjugated bilirubin fraction (i.e., indirect) is then obtained by subtraction. For normal serum, less than 15 per cent of the total bilirubin is in the conjugated fraction. The various causes for hyperbilirubinemia have traditionally been divided into those associated with unconjugated bilirubin and those associated with conjugated bilirubin. In practice, many diseases are of a mixed form (i.e., elevation in both conjugated and unconjugated bilirubin).

In hepatic diseases, the bilirubin level is usually proportional to the level of hepatocyte injury. Jaundice is detectable only when the total bilirubin level exceeds 3.0 mg. per dl. Low serum bilirubin levels are of no clinical significance.

BLOOD UREA NITROGEN (BUN)

Background

The BUN is commonly used to measure renal function. The serum creatinine is, however, a much more reliable indicator of the glomerular filtration rate (GFR). This is because in addition to GFR, the

Table 72–6. NORMAL VALUES FOR BLOOD UREA NITROGEN/CREATININE RATIO

Normal 10:1 (BUN to Cr)

Increased Ratio	Diagnoses to Consider	Actions to Consider
>10	High nitrogen load: GI bleeding High-protein diet High catabolism Low urine flow: Dehydration Congestive heart failure	1. Examine for hydration status 2. Examine for CHF 3. Dietary history 4. Drug history (steroids) 5. Stool occult blood
Decreased Ratio	**Diagnoses to Consider**	**Actions to Consider**
<10	High urine flow: Water intoxication SIADH Low-protein diet Protein malnutrition Liver insufficiency	1. Check serum and urine osmolality 2. Check serum sodium 3. Dietary history 4. Bilirubin

BUN is affected by the nitrogen load, the water intake, and the urine flow. If you want to know about the kidney, order a creatinine.

The normal BUN is 8 to 26 mg. per dl. (2.9 to 9.3 mmol. per liter). The SI conversion factor is 0.357 (Table 72–6).

A rise in BUN is seen with renal insufficiency. However, it is not a specific indicator of renal function. A more useful way to use the BUN is to calculate the BUN to creatinine ratio. This ratio can serve as a useful indicator of diseases that result in an abnormal nitrogen load, urine flow, or water intake.

CALCIUM

Background

Calcium is essential for maintenance of the skeleton and for normal neuromuscular function. The

Table 72–7. NORMAL VALUES FOR CALCIUM

Diagnostic Units: mg./dl (mmol/L.). SI conversion factor = 0.2495
Normal 8.8–10.3 (2.20–2.57)

Increased	Diagnoses to Consider	Actions to Consider
10.3–13.0 (2.57–3.24)	Hyperparathyroidism Metastatic cancer Thiazide diuretics Immobilization Vitamin D intoxication Milk-alkali syndrome Multiple myeloma Sarcoidosis Thyrotoxicosis	1. Repeat serum calcium 2. Complete diet and drug history 3. Ionized calcium, albumin, phosphorus, PTH, T_4 4. Chest x-ray 5. Hand x-rays 6. Evaluation for malignancy
>13.0 (3.24)	Hypercalcemic coma	1. Vigorous hydration 2. Furosemide 3. Close monitoring
Decreased	**Diagnoses to Consider**	**Actions to Consider**
7.0–8.8 (1.75–2.20)	Hypoalbuminemia Chronic renal failure Hypoparathyroidism (neck surgery) Malnutrition Vitamin D deficiency: Nutritional Anticonvulsants Malabsorption Liver disease Hypomagnesemia Pancreatitis	1. Serum albumin 2. Complete drug history 3. Alcohol history 4. Serum creatinine, phosphate, magnesium, PTH
<7.0 (1.75)	Hypocalcemic seizures Hypocalcemic arrhythmias	1. IV calcium gluconate 2. Serum ionized calcium 3. Serum magnesium

Values in parentheses are SI units.

usual serum test for calcium measures the total calcium (Table 72–7). About half of the total calcium is bound to albumin. The rest is present in serum in the ionized form. The measurement of ionized calcium can also be specifically ordered.

The serum level of calcium is under the complex control of the parathyroid hormone (PTH) and calcitonin. These hormones and others control the rate at which calcium is absorbed from the gastrointestinal tract, excreted in the urine, and gained or lost to bone.

The most common laboratory abnormality seen is a low total calcium in a patient with a low serum albumin. This is primarily a disorder of serum albumin, not a problem with calcium, since the ionized calcium remains unchanged. In this setting it is possible to mathematically correct the calcium for the decreased albumin (1 gram per dl. reduction in albumin leads to 1 mg. per dl. reduction in calcium).

Hypercalcemia is associated with fatigue, depression, constipation, polydipsia, ulcers, and hypertension. In the outpatient setting, the most common cause for hypercalcemia is hyperparathyroidism (Heath et al., 1980). Many of these patients are asymptomatic. Malignancies are the most common cause for hypercalcemia in the inpatient setting. The most common cancers to produce hypercalcemia are lung, breast, and kidney.

Hypocalcemia produces symptoms that result from neuromuscular excitability. These include carpopedal spasm, seizures, tetany, stiffness, fatigue, memory loss, and confusion.

There is debate about whether serum calcium is an appropriate screening test for asymptomatic individuals. It has frequently been included in screening chemistry panels. The rationale for its use as a screening test has been that hyperparathyroidism is frequently asymptomatic. This argument has recently come into question because of the uncertainty of whether asymptomatic hyperparathyroidism requires any specific therapy.

CHLORIDE

Background

Chloride is the major extracellular anion in the body. Despite this fact, it is a relatively uninteresting analyte and is rarely clinically useful.

Most dietary chloride is absorbed. The level in the body is then controlled by renal excretion (Table 72–8). The primary cause for an abnormal chloride is in response to a shift in the serum CO_2 content. The CO_2 content decreases when there is a metabolic acidosis or metabolic compensation for respiratory alkalosis. In these situations, the chloride increases in response to the reduction in CO_2 content. CO_2 content is increased in cases of metabolic alkalosis or in a metabolic response to respiratory acidosis. In these settings, the chloride is reduced to compensate for the increased CO_2 content.

Chloride can be depleted by either gastrointestinal losses (vomiting) or renal losses (salt-losing renal diseases). In this case, the chloride depletion results in a persistent metabolic alkalosis.

The most frequent use of the chloride test is in calculating the anion gap. This is calculated by subtracting the total measured anions (chloride + bicarbonate) from the total cations (sodium + potassium). The normal range for the anion gap is 16 ± 4 mEq. per liter. Increases in the anion gap indicate the presence of unmeasured anions such as ketoacids, lactic acids, methanol, and so forth.

CHOLESTEROL

Background

The NIH has established a National Cholesterol Education Program. One goal of this program is to have all adults screened for hypercholesterolemia. While there is considerable debate about which cholesterol levels require treatment and the optimal approach to treatment, most people now agree that the screening of adults is probably indicated (Table 72–9). Epidemiologic studies have shown that a 1 per cent decrease in total cholesterol is associated with a 2 per cent decrease in coronary heart disease (CHD) risk.

Considerable variation is often seen in repeated cholesterol values from the same patient. This is due to test accuracy errors (± 3 per cent), test imprecision (± 3 per cent), and day-to-day patient variation (± 7 per cent). In addition, cholesterol has been shown to demonstrate a seasonal variation. Although the studies have been limited, there does *not* appear to be a variation in total cholesterol based on whether the patient is fasting or not. (Fasting is, however, essential in measuring triglycerides and the cholesterol lipoprotein fractions.)

Cholesterol measurements should be used to diagnose hypercholesterolemia much as blood pressure readings are used to diagnose hypertension. Several readings over a period of time are required before a diagnosis can be made (Burke and Fischer, 1988).

If the total cholesterol indicates that the patient is at risk for hypercholesterolemia, the NIH recommends that a fasting lipoprotein analysis be done. The total cholesterol, HDL cholesterol, and triglycerides should be measured. The LDL cholesterol can then be calculated by the formula: LDL cholesterol = total cholesterol − HDL cholesterol − triglycerides divided by 5.

If the LDL cholesterol is between 130 and 160 mg. per dl., then the patient is considered at a borderline high risk for coronary heart disease. If the LDL cholesterol is greater than 160 mg. per dl., then the patient is considered at high risk for CHD. LDL values less than 130 mg. per dl. are desirable (Taylor et al., 1987).

Table 72–8. NORMAL VALUES FOR CHLORIDE

Diagnostic Units: mEq./L. (mmol./L.). SI conversion factor = 1
Normal 95–105 (95–105)

Increased	Diagnoses to Consider	Actions to Consider
>105	Metabolic acidosis: Loss of bicarbonate Production of metabolic acids Respiratory alkalosis with metabolic compensation Dehydration	1. HCO_3, Na, K, pH, BUN, Cl 2. Calculate anion gap
Decreased	**Diagnoses to Consider**	**Actions to Consider**
<95	Metabolic alkalosis: Hydrogen ion loss HCO_3 retention Respiratory acidosis with metabolic compensation Salt-losing renal disease Thiazide diuretics	1. Urinalysis 2. HCO_3, Na, K, pH, BUN, Cl

Values in parentheses are SI units.

The NIH recommends that the decision to treat should be based on a patient's risk factors for CHD and the LDL value. Total cholesterol measurements should be used only for case finding and to follow the response to therapy (NIH, 1985).

CO_2 CONTENT

Background

The CO_2 content of blood is made up of bicarbonate, carbonic acid, and dissolved CO_2. Ninety-five per cent of the total CO_2 content is bicarbonate (HCO_3). Bicarbonate is the second most important anion in serum and is the most available base which is capable of buffering a metabolic acid load. This role in the body's acid-base balance is its principal clinical function. The two mechanisms for control of CO_2 content are respiratory elimination of CO_2 and renal reabsorption of filtered bicarbonate. Bicarbonate can also be lost pathologically through elimination from the gastrointestinal tract (Table 72–10).

The most common CO_2 content abnormality is a

Table 72–9. NORMAL VALUES FOR CHOLESTEROL

Diagnostic Units: mg./dl. (mmol./L.). SI conversion factor = 0.02586
Normal <200 (5.2)

Increased	Diagnoses to Consider	Actions to Consider
200–239 (5.2–6.2)	Borderline risk for CHD: Familial hypercholesterolemia High cholesterol diet Biliary obstruction Nephrotic syndrome Hypothyroidism	1. Repeat cholesterol test 2. Evaluate for CAD risks a. Male sex b. Smoking c. Family history of CHD d. Hypertension e. Diabetes mellitus f. Severe obesity g. History of vascular disease h. LDL less than 35 mg./dl. 3. If patient has known CAD or 2 or more risk factors, order lipoprotein analysis
≥240 (≥6.2)	High risk for CHD: As above	1. Repeat cholesterol 2. Fasting lipoprotein analysis 3. Classify based on LDL a. <130 = desirable b. 130–159 = borderline risk c. ≥160 = high risk
Decreased	**Diagnoses to Consider**	**Actions to Consider**
<140 (<3.6)	Low risk for CHD: Hyperthyroidism Hepatic insufficiency	1. Dietary history 2. Bilirubin 3. T_4, T_3U

Values in parentheses are SI units.

Table 72–10. NORMAL VALUES FOR CO_2

Diagnostic Units: mEq./L. (mmol./L.). SI conversion factor = 1
Normal 22–28 (22–28)

Decreased	Diagnoses to Consider	Actions to Consider
<22	Metabolic acidosis: Bicarbonate loss: Diarrhea Renal tubular acidosis Primary hyperparathyroidism Failure to reabsorb bicarbonate: Triamterene, spironolactone Renal tubular acidosis Production of metabolic acids: Renal failure Diabetic ketoacidosis Lactic acidosis Methanol Ethylene glycol Salicylates Alcoholic ketoacidosis Respiratory alkalosis with compensation: Anxiety Sepsis Salicylates CNS injury	1. Full drug history 2. Serum electrolytes 3. Blood gas 4. Calculate anion gap
Increased	**Diagnoses to Consider**	**Actions to Consider**
>28	Metabolic alkalosis: Volume contraction NG suction Vomiting Potassium depletion Furosemide Cushing's syndrome Chronic respiratory acidosis with compensation	1. Serum electrolytes 2. Blood gas 3. Urine electrolytes

Values in parentheses are SI units.

decreased level due to metabolic acidosis. In this setting, it is useful to calculate the anion gap. This value may provide a clue to the cause of the acidosis.

A metabolic alkalosis may be initiated by the loss of hydrogen ion, as is seen in nasogastric suction. The maintenance of the metabolic alkalosis requires that there be a greater than normal reabsorption of bicarbonate by the kidneys. Therefore, in patients with an elevated CO_2 content, look for diseases that affect the bicarbonate handling by the renal tubules.

CREATININE

Background

Creatinine is released from skeletal muscle and is excreted unchanged in the urine (Beck and Kassirer, 1987). There are few factors other than renal function which affect its serum level. It is therefore the best of the common tests for monitoring renal insufficiency. A rise in creatinine indicates a falling glomerular filtration rate.

The biggest problem with using creatinine as a measure of renal function is that it is a relatively insensitive marker of renal disease. A 50 per cent reduction in renal function from normal leads to a creatinine rise from only 1 mg. per dl. to 2.0 mg. per dl. (Table 72–11). Considerable early renal damage may therefore occur before it becomes apparent by a rising creatinine.

A second problem with interpreting serum creatinine is that it is slow in reacting to sudden changes in renal function. For example, in sudden and severe renal failure (i.e., acute tubular necrosis following shock), the creatinine will rise only 1 mg. per dl. per day. This is despite a creatinine clearance of zero!

Since creatinine is released by skeletal muscle, it is occasionally affected by total muscle mass. Small, elderly women may therefore have a normal creatinine even with a reduced renal function.

A patient's creatinine clearance can be estimated from the formula:

$$\text{CR clearance} = [(140 - \text{age})(\text{weight in kg.})] / (72 \times \text{CR in mg. per dl.}).$$

As a rough guideline, a creatinine of 2 mg. per dl. is equivalent to a creatinine clearance of 50 ml. per minute; a creatinine of 4 mg. per dl. is equal to a creatinine clearance of 20 ml. per minute; and a creatinine of 6 is equivalent to a creatinine clearance of 10 ml. per minute.

A serum creatinine is a useful screening test in

Table 72–11. NORMAL VALUES FOR CREATININE

Diagnostic Units: mg./dl. (μmol./L.). SI conversion factor = 88.4
Normal 0.6–1.2 (50–110)

Increased	Diagnoses to Consider	Actions to Consider
1.2–1.6 (110–141)	Mild renal impairment Muscle injury	1. Repeat test 2. Urinalysis 3. Creatinine clearance
>1.6 (141)	Prerenal failure: Dehydration Blood loss Heart failure Liver failure Intrinsic renal failure: Diabetes mellitus Hypertension SLE Nephrotoxins Glomerulonephritis Acute tubular necrosis Postrenal failure: Urethral obstruction Upper tract obstruction	1. Urinalysis 2. Creatinine clearance 3. Bladder catheterization 4. Renal imaging
>6.0 (530)	Severe renal failure	1. HCO (metabolic acidosis) 2. Serum potassium (hyperkalemia)

Values in parentheses are SI units.

Table 72–12. NORMAL VALUES FOR DIGOXIN

Diagnostic Units: ng./ml. (nmol./L.). SI conversion factor = 1.281
Therapeutic 0.5–2.2 (0.6–2.8)

Decreased	Diagnoses to Consider	Actions to Consider
<0.5 (0.6)	Inadequate dose Noncompliance Poor GI absorption Absorption interference: Kaolin-pectin Antacids Cholestyramine	1. Review medication compliance 2. Review other medications 3. Increase digoxin dose
Increased	**Diagnoses to Consider**	**Actions to Consider**
2.2–3.0 (2.8–3.8)	Excessive digoxin dose Decreased creatinine clearance Level taken prior to 6 hours after a dose Drug interaction: Quinidine Verapamil Antibiotics Nifedipine Amiodarone	1. Evaluate for toxicity 2. Serum K, Ca, Mg, HCO_3 3. Review medication dosing 4. Serum Cr or BUN 5. Review other medications
>3.0 (3.8)	Toxicity very likely	1. Stop digoxin 2. ECG monitoring 3. Correct electrolyte abnormalities

Values in parentheses are SI units.

those patients at risk for renal injury (i.e., patients with hypertension or diabetes). However, it is not a useful test in asymptomatic patients without significant risk factors. This is because of the low prevalence of chronic renal failure in the general population and the low sensitivity of the test. A low serum creatinine is of no clinical significance.

DIGOXIN

Background

The various preparations of digitalis have been used to treat heart failure for more than 200 years. Digoxin is the form that is most commonly prescribed today. In addition to its use in the treatment of heart failure, this drug is frequently used to block the A-V node in atrial tachyarrhythmias. Digoxin has a very narrow therapeutic window. Levels below 0.5 ng. per ml. are generally not therapeutic, while levels over 2.2 ng. per ml. are often associated with toxicity (Table 72–12). The ability to use this medication properly has been enhanced because of the wide availability of serum digoxin levels.

When digoxin is used orally as a tablet, 60 to 85 per cent of the drug is absorbed. The newer gelatin capsules (Lanoxicaps) are associated with a 90 to 100 per cent absorption. The peak effect for the drug ranges from 2 to 6 hours after oral administration. It is impossible to accurately interpret a serum digoxin level drawn within this 6-hour period. During this time, the levels will be high and will not reliably correlate with the steady-state level.

Digoxin is primarily metabolized by the kidney. The half-life of the drug in patients with normal renal function is 1½ days. This is increased to 4 to 5 days in patients who are anuric. The drug's very long half-life means that a steady-state level is not reached until 1 week following a change in dosage of the oral preparation.

Digitalis toxicity is associated with nausea, vomiting, fatigue, confusion, blurred vision, and cardiac disturbances. The most common cardiac problems are ventricular ectopy, A-V block, paroxysmal atrial tachycardia, atrial fibrillation, and ventricular fibrillation. The incidence of digoxin toxicity increases with increasing serum levels. Toxicity is found at lower digoxin levels if accompanied by hypokalemia, alkalosis, hypercalcemia, or hypomagnesemia.

Table 72–13. NORMAL VALUES FOR EOSINOPHILS

Diagnostic Units: percentage of leukocytes (cells × 10^6/L). SI conversion factor = % × WBC
Normal 1–3% (50–350 × 10^6/L.)

Increased	Diagnoses to Consider	Actions to Consider
>3% (350 × 10^6/L.)	Parasite infection Other infections: *Chlamydia* pneumonia Infectious mononucleosis Scarlet fever Chronic active hepatitis Allergic diseases: Asthma Allergic rhinitis Urticaria Drug reaction Autoimmune diseases: Rheumatoid arthritis Ulcerative colitis Regional enteritis Sjögren's Leukemia/lymphoma Eosinophilic syndromes: Hypereosinophilic syndrome Eosinophilic myositis Eosinophilic cystitis Eosinophilic gastritis Pulmonary infiltrates Dermatologic: Atopic dermatitis Eczema Urticaria Pemphigus Scabies Psoriasis Dermatitis herpetiformis	1. Full drug history 2. Travel history 3. Ova and parasites (×2) 4. Sputum for eosinophils 5. Chest x-ray
>10% (1000 × 10^6/L.)	Parasitic infection Drug reaction Eosinophilic syndrome	

Values in parentheses are SI units.

The most common mistake in using serum digoxin levels is "treating the level" instead of "treating the patient." One third of patients with digoxin toxicity have levels that are within the usual therapeutic range. Likewise, levels greater than the normal upper limit may be required in some clinical situations (i.e., to slow the ventricular rate in atrial fibrillation). A wide range of medications can increase or decrease the digoxin level. These are indicated in Table 72–12.

EOSINOPHILS

Background

Eosinophils are granulocytic leukocytes. It is unclear whether their role in the body is to respond to specific antigens (i.e., parasitic infections) or to help in modulating the normal inflammatory reaction. The percentage of eosinophils in a normal differential can be converted to the eosinophil count by multiplying the percentage times the total WBC (i.e., 3 per cent × 10,000 = 300) (Table 72–13).

Slight increases in the number of eosinophils can be seen with many diseases and are rarely clinically significant. On the other hand, it is uncommon to see a marked increase in the number of eosinophils. Drug reactions are the most common cause of high eosinophil counts (i.e., sulfonamides, gold, aspirin, antibiotics, phenytoin, and hydralazine). Parasitic infections, especially tissue-invasive helminths, are the second most common cause of eosinophilia. Noninvasive helminths, encysted parasites, and protozoa do not generally produce eosinophilia.

Low eosinophil counts are sometimes seen in response to an acute viral or bacterial infection. This is due to a suppression of eosinophil production when large numbers of neutrophils are required. Such low eosinophil counts are of no clinical significance.

ERYTHROCYTE SEDIMENTATION RATE (ESR) (WESTERGREN METHOD)

Background

Anticoagulated whole blood is made up of blood cells suspended in plasma. When the blood is allowed to stand for a period of time, the cells settle out. The rate of settling is affected by both red blood cell factors (i.e., shape, size, and hematocrit) and by

Table 72–14. NORMAL VALUES FOR THE WESTERGREN ERYTHROCYTE SEDIMENTATION RATE

Diagnostic Units: (mm./hour)

Normal		Male	Female
	Children	0–10	0–10
	<50 years old	0–15	0–20
	50 to 65 years old	0–20	0–30
	>65 years old	0–38	0–53

Increased	Diagnoses to Consider	Actions to Consider
> 100	Temporal arthritis Polymyalgia rheumatica Multiple myeloma Lymphoma/leukemia Metastatic cancer Sepsis Ulcerative colitis Biliary cirrhosis	1. Serum protein electrophoresis
40–100	Anemia Rheumatoid arthritis Malignancy Viral hepatitis Tuberculosis Ectopic pregnancy Myocardial infarction Rheumatic fever Hyperthyroidism Hypothyroidism Normal pregnancy Oral contraceptives Macrocytosis	1. Evaluate Hb/Hct and RBC morphology 2. Repeat ESR 3. Evaluate thyroid function

Decreased	Diagnoses to Consider	Actions to Consider
	Polycythemia Congestive heart failure Hemoglobinopathy Spherocytosis RBC abnormalities	1. Evaluate Hb/Hct and RBC morphology 2. Ignore isolated low values in asymptomatic patients

Table 72–15. NORMAL VALUES FOR VENOUS GLUCOSE

Diagnostic Units: mg./dl. (mmol./L.). SI conversion factor = 0.05551			
Screening Test: Fasting Glucose			
	Normal	Requires GTT	Diagnostic of Diabetes
Adult	< 115 (6.38)	115–140 (6.38–7.77)	> 140 (7.7) × 2
Child	< 130 (7.22)	130–140 (7.22–7.77)	> 140 (7.77) × 2
Confirmatory Tests: Glucose Tolerance Tests			
Adult: 75 gram oral glucose dose			
	Normal	Impaired Glucose Tolerance	Diabetes
Fasting	< 115 (6.38)	< 140 (7.77)	< 140 (7.77)
30 minutes	< 200 (11.1)	1 of 3 > 200 (11.1)	1 of 3 > 200 (11.1)
60 minutes	< 200 (11.1)		
90 minutes	< 200 (11.1)		
120 minutes	< 140 (7.77)	140–200 (7.77–11.1)	> 200 (11.1)
Child: 1.75 grams glucose per kilogram body weight up to 75 grams			
	Normal	Impaired Glucose Tolerance	Diabetes
Fasting	< 130 (7.22)	< 140 (7.77)	> 140 (7.77)
30 minutes	< 200 (11.1)	< 200 (11.1)	1 of 3 > 200 (11.1)
60 minutes	< 200 (11.1)	< 200 (11.1)	
90 minutes	< 200 (11.1)	< 200 (11.1)	
120 minutes	< 140 (7.77)	140–200 (7.77–11.1)	> 200 (11.1)
Pregnancy			
Screening: O'Sullivan screen 50 grams glucose (patient can be nonfasting) "Positive" if ≥ 140 (7.77) at one hour			
Confirmation: O'Sullivan 3 hour GTT 100 grams oral glucose in a fasting patient The patient is positive for gestational diabetes if two or more of the values are: Fasting: ≥ 105 (5.79) 1 hour: ≥ 190 (10.55) 2 hour: ≥ 165 (9.16) 3 hour: ≥ 145 (8.05)			
Hypoglycemia			
Males: < 55 (3.05) at the same time as patient has symptoms			
Females: < 40 (2.22) at the same time as patient has symptoms			

Values in parentheses are SI units.

plasma factors (fibrinogen and globulins,). The ESR is a measure of the rate of blood cell settling (Table 72–14).

The ESR is a nonspecific test used to diagnose and follow the clinical course of a wide variety of diseases which are characterized by tissue inflammation, infection, or malignancy (Sox and Liang, 1986).

Several methods have been used to perform the ESR. The Westergren or modified Westergren method is preferred. Most of the relevant research on this test has used one of these two methods.

The most common reason for an elevated ESR is anemia. It is therefore essential that a hematocrit or hemoglobin be done on any patient with an elevated ESR. It is impossible to accurately "correct" the ESR value for the degree of anemia.

Any abnormality in red blood cell shape or size can result in a reduced ESR. For this reason, a peripheral smear should be done on all patients. Check that the RBC morphology is normal.

The ESR is not a useful screening test in asymptomatic patients. It is of only limited usefulness in diagnosing patients with vague complaints (i.e., fatigue, abdominal pain). It is, however, extremely useful in evaluating patients who are suspected of having temporal arteritis or polymyalgia rheumatica. It is also useful in following patients who have other connective tissue disorders, such as rheumatoid arthritis. In these patients, the ESR can be a useful indicator of the activity of the disease. The ESR will start to decrease within days of the initiation of steroid therapy. It will then usually fall to a level that is somewhat greater than normal. Treatment with nonsteroidal anti-inflammatory drugs does not lead to a drop in the ESR.

GLUCOSE

Background

Interpreting glucose values can be extremely difficult. The usual reasons for ordering this test are to diagnose diabetes, to follow the course of diabetic treatment, or to diagnose hypoglycemia (Table 72–15).

The American Diabetes Association has defined seven different disorders of glucose metabolism:

1. Type I diabetes mellitus. These patients require insulin to prevent ketoacidosis.

2. Type II diabetes mellitus. These patients are usually obese adults and can be treated with diet or oral hypoglycemic agents (Physicians' Guide to Non–Insulin Dependent [Type II] Diabetes: Diagnosis and Treatment, 1988.)
3. Impaired glucose tolerance. These patients have higher than normal glucose values but less than required to be diagnostic for diabetes.
4. Gestational diabetes mellitus. This represents hyperglycemia only during pregnancy.
5. Previous abnormality of glucose tolerance. This includes patients who have had diabetes when under stress, when obese, or when pregnant but who now have normal glucose tolerance.
6. Potential abnormality of glucose tolerance. This includes patients with close relatives who are diabetic.
7. Other types of diabetes mellitus. These are patients whose diabetes is caused by other conditions such as pancreatic disease, Cushing's syndrome, acromegaly, thyrotoxicosis, or drugs (steroids, estrogen, or thiazide diuretics).

Two common reasons for abnormally elevated glucose testing are drawing specimens after a patient has eaten and drawing the specimen from a vein above an IV infusion.

There are two types of hypoglycemia. The first is postprandial hypoglycemia, also referred to as reactive hypoglycemia. It is most commonly seen in patients with a history of gastric surgery who therefore have very fast stomach emptying times. Their symptoms (i.e., sweating, weakness, anxiety, irritability) occur several hours after eating.

Fasting hypoglycemia is seen primarily in diabetics and alcoholics. Their symptoms (i.e., mental confusion, bizarre behavior, seizures) are more gradual in onset and more persistent. This form of hypoglycemia usually occurs only after a long period of fasting.

Other disorders associated with hypoglycemia are insulinoma, adernal insufficiency, hypopituitarism, and drug-induced hypoglycemia (insulin, sulfonylureas, and salicylates).

It is essential to remember that not all glucose specimens are the same. A random glucose taken 2 hours after lunch should not be treated the same way as a fasting specimen. In addition, there are differences among whole blood, serum, and plasma values. Venous plasma and venous serum glucose values are 15 per cent higher than those present in venous whole blood. Capillary whole blood values are 10 per cent higher than those measured in venous whole blood. Venous plasma and venous serum values are 5 to 7 per cent higher than those found in capillary whole blood. (The values given in Table 72–15 are for venous plasma or venous serum. Specimens other than these should be adjusted accordingly.)

Table 72–15 differentiates screening tests from diagnostic tests. The usual screening test is a fasting glucose. The results of this test may indicate that the patient is normal, may suggest that a diagnostic test (i.e., a glucose tolerance test) be done, or may be diagnostic of diabetes. Note that there are specific screening and diagnostic tests for gestational diabetes (i.e., the O'Sullivan test).

GLYCOSYLATED HEMOGLOBIN (HB A_{1c})

Background

The glycosylation of hemoglobin occurs continuously during a red blood cell's life and is directly related to the average glucose concentration. The measurement of glycosylated HB A_{1c} has therefore become a useful clinical test to assess the "average" glucose control in diabetic patients (Table 72–16). Increased percentages of glycosylated hemoglobin reflect increased hyperglycemia. Once glycosylated, hemoglobin remains as such throughout the red cell's life. The test value can therefore be viewed as a measure of diabetic control for the previous 1 to 3 months. (Physician's Guide to Non–Insulin Dependent [Type II] Diabetes: Diagnosis and Treatment, 1988.)

Hyperglycemia is also associated with the glycosylation of other body proteins. This glycosylation may be the basis for some of the angiopathic and neuropathic changes seen in diabetes. Some clinicians therefore use this test as an assessment of a patient's risk for diabetic complications.

The HB A_{1c} value will not change with rapid hour-to-hour or day-to-day variations in serum glucose. It is therefore not appropriate to use this test in making decisions about insulin dosage in either the acutely ill hospitalized patient or ambulatory diabetics on insulin. Home glucose monitoring is a better source of data for these decisions.

There is wide variation between laboratories on both the "normal" range of values as well as the degree of elevation associated with various levels of hyperglycemia. It is therefore important to know the characteristics of your laboratory's test. The hemoglobin A_{1c} per cent may be falsely elevated with uremia, alcoholism, and aspirin use. The test may be falsely lowered in anemia, hemoglobinopathies, and pregnancy.

HEMOGLOBIN AND HEMATOCRIT

Background

Hemoglobin and hematocrit values are often used interchangeably in clinical practice to measure the oxygen-carrying capacity of a volume of blood (Table 72–17). It is important to remember that they are *not* measures of either the total blood volume or the red blood cell mass.

Most modern hematology instruments directly measure the hemoglobin and calculate the hematocrit from the measured RBC and mean corpuscular vol-

Table 72–16. NORMAL VALUES FOR GLYCOSYLATED HEMOGLOBIN

Diagnostic Units: percentage of total hemoglobin
Normal 5–7% (varies by laboratory)

Increased	Diagnoses to Consider	Actions to Consider
< 9%	Good diabetic control (most glucoses < 200 mg./dl.)	1. No change in therapy
9–14%	Average diabetic control (most glucoses < 300 mg./dl.)	1. Consider home glucose monitoring
> 14%	Poor diabetic control (i.e., persistent hyperglycemia)	1. Evaluate for causes of poor diabetic control

Table 72–17. NORMAL VALUES FOR HEMOGLOBIN

Diagnostic Units: Hemoglobin: gm./dl. (gm./L.). SI conversion factor = 10.0

			Hemoglobin
Normal	Males	Birth	18.5–21.5 (185–215)
		1 month	15.5–18.5 (155–185)
		3 months	13.5–16.5 (135–165)
		6 months	13.0–16.0 (130–160)
		9 months	12.0–14.0 (120–140)
		1 year	10.0–14.0 (100–140)
		2 years	10.5–14.2 (105–142)
		4 years	11.2–14.3 (112–143)
		8 years	12.0–14.8 (120–148)
		14 years	12.5–15.0 (125–150)
		Adult	13.9–16.3 (139–163)
	Females	Birth	18.0–21.0 (180–210)
		1 month	15.8–18.9 (158–189)
		3 months	13.3–16.4 (133–164)
		6 months	12.8–14.8 (128–148)
		9 months	11.7–13.9 (117–139)
		1 year	10.0–14.0 (100–140)
		2 years	10.5–14.2 (105–142)
		4 years	11.3–14.2 (113–142)
		8 years	11.5–14.5 (115–145)
		14 years	11.6–14.8 (116–148)
		Adult	12.0–15.0 (120–150)

Increased	Diagnoses to Consider	Actions to Consider
Hb > 16.5 (165)	Dehydration Diuretic use Polycythemia vera Secondary polycythemia: High altitude Pulmonary disease Cardiac disease Renal tumor	1. Smoking history 2. Check volume status 3. Splenomegaly 4. Urinalysis 5. CBC 6. Platelet count 7. Alkaline phosphatase
Hb > 22 (220)	Severe polycythemia	1. Consider phlebotomy
Decreased	**Diagnoses to Consider**	**Actions to Consider**
Hb < 11 (110)	Blood loss Decreased blood cell survival Decreased marrow production RBC sequestration (spleen)	1. History of chronic disease 2. Menstrual history 3. Stool for occult blood 4. Splenomegaly 5. RBC indices 6. Reticulocyte count 7. Trial on iron therapy 8. Iron, TIBC, ferritin 9. Folate, B_{12}
Hb < 8 (80)	Severe anemia	1. Consider transfusion

Values in parentheses are SI units.

Table 72–18. NORMAL VALUES FOR MEAN CORPUSCULAR VOLUME

Diagnostic Units: cubic microns (fL). SI conversion factor = 1
Normal 76–100

Increased	Diagnoses to Consider	Actions to Consider
100–120	Reticulocytosis Folate deficiency B_{12} deficiency Hypothyroidism Response to chemotherapy	1. Reticulocyte count 2. Serum B_{12} 3. Serum or RBC folate 4. T_4
> 120	Folate deficiency B_{12} deficiency	1. Serum B_{12} 2. Serum or RBC folate
Decreased	**Diagnoses to Consider**	**Actions to Consider**
70–76	Iron deficiency Thalassemia Anemia of chronic disease Hereditary sideroblastic anemia Lead poisoning RBC fragmentation (burns)	1. Reticulocyte count 2. Peripheral smear 3. Serum iron, TIBC, or ferritin 4. Hb electrophoresis
< 70	Severe iron deficiency Thalassemia	1. Reticulocyte count 2. Peripheral smear 3. Serum iron, TIBC, or ferritin 4. Hb electrophoresis

ume (MCV). The hematocrit can also be measured by centrifugation of a microcapillary tube filled with whole blood. When this is done, the hematocrit is defined as the per cent volume of red blood cells after maximal packing has occurred. For most purposes, the hematocrit and hemoglobin are convertible by a factor of 3 (i.e., Hct = 3 × Hb).

It is reasonable to use the hemoglobin and hematocrit interchangeably except for patients with abnormally shaped red blood cells (i.e., sickled cells). In such patients, the measured hematocrit is artificially high because the red blood cells fail to maximally pack. In such individuals, a hemoglobin is a better test to follow.

There is little evidence that the general population benefits from routine hemoglobin or hematocrit screening. Screening, however, may be indicated in groups at high risk for anemia such as infants, pregnant women, the institutionalized elderly, or menstruating females. It is also customary to screen individuals undergoing a procedure which could be associated with blood loss and to screen all hospitalized patients on admission.

The most common abnormal finding is a mild, unsuspected anemia. This condition is usually asymptomatic. The importance of the finding is not based on the need to treat the anemia but rather the need to uncover the anemia's cause. The cause is frequently a clinically important diagnosis (i.e., poor nutrition, menorrhagia, pernicious anemia, colon cancer).

In addition to screening, a hemoglobin or hematocrit is an essential test for any patient in whom anemia is suspected, in whom there is abnormal bleeding, or in whom polycythemia is part of the differential diagnosis.

The most common error in interpreting a hemoglobin or hematocrit value is to rely on it as an indicator of acute blood loss. These are not good measures of total blood volume. Between 12 and 24 hours are required after an acute bleed before fluid equilibration can occur. It is only then that the hemoglobin or hematocrit can be used to indicate the extent of blood loss.

MEAN CORPUSCULAR VOLUME (MCV)

Background

The MCV is the most important of the red blood cell indices. In modern hematology instruments, this value is derived by the degree of impedance disturbance as cells pass between two electrodes. The magnitude of the disturbance indicates the size of the cell.

The primary use of the MCV is to differentiate anemias into macrocytic, normocytic, or microcytic (Table 72–18). This differentiation is useful in theory but is often not helpful in practice. Most anemic patients are normocytic at the time of their diagnosis.

Reticulocytes and other very young RBCs are macrocytic. A rapid marrow release of RBCs will therefore produce an increased MCV. This should not be confused with the other causes of macrocytosis.

It is important to remember that the MCV is an average of all of the cell populations. Mixed populations of macrocytic and microcytic cells may therefore produce a normocytic MCV. This is seen in the early treatment of an iron deficiency anemia (i.e., macrocytic reticulocytes plus microcytic cells) as well as in alcoholic patients who are both iron and folate deficient.

PAP SMEAR

Background

Dr. George Papanicolaou first proposed the use of cytology to detect gynecologic cancers in 1943. The widespread adoption of Pap smear testing in the U.S. has since led to a 70 per cent decrease in mortality from cervical cancer. Despite this fact, there continue to be 50,000 cases per year of cervical carcinoma-in-situ, 13,000 cases of invasive carcinoma, and 7000 cervical cancer deaths.

The Pap classification (i.e., Classes I to V) was used for many years to report Pap smear results. However, this terminology was plagued with variability, inconsistencies, and ambiguity. It has often led to confusion about the clinical implications of a Pap smear report. It is now widely recommended that this older terminology system be replaced by one of the reporting systems outlined in Table 72–19.

Cervical cytology does not represent a clear and continuous spectrum of malignancy (i.e., Classes I to V). Instead, some "abnormal" findings are due to benign conditions. Others are diagnostic of carcinoma. Some indicate dysplastic changes which *may* be a marker for carcinoma. The more severe the dysplasia, the more likely is malignancy. Mild dysplasia may be seen with human papillomavirus (HPV) infection. It is this mild dysplasia (neither normal, nor clearly malignant, nor necessarily benign) which causes the greatest confusion. The current research which associates HPV infections and cervical carcinoma may permit a better understanding of the disease process.

Pap smear reports often say that the "specimen is inadequate." There are multiple reasons for this including scant cellularity, poor fixation, inflammatory cells that obscure the cervical cells, menstrual blood that obscures the cervical cells, or the absence of endocervical cells. Endocervical cells are a marker for specimen collection in the transformation zone of the cervix. The transformation zone is the area from which cervical carcinomas arise. There is debate about whether the absence of endocervical cells is an absolute indication for a repeat specimen.

Pap smear results also indicate other diagnoses. These include infections with *Candida, Gardnerella, Chlamydia, Trichomonas,* cytomegalovirus, and herpes simplex. In some cases, the actual organism is seen (e.g., *Trichomonas*), while in other cases (e.g., herpes simplex) the organism is not seen but cellular changes that are consistent with an infection are seen. The accuracy of diagnosing these various infections by Pap smear is extremely variable. In most cases, further historical and laboratory confirmation is needed to make a specific diagnosis.

A final word of caution: Pap smears are associated with a significant false negative rate (about 30 per cent). There should be little reassurance from a normal follow-up Pap smear after one that shows dysplasia. When in doubt, schedule colposcopy.

Table 72–19. PAP SMEAR CLASSIFICATION SYSTEMS

World Health Organization	Cervical Intraepithelial Neoplasia (CIN)	National Cancer Institute (NCI)	Actions to Consider
Normal	Normal	Normal	1. Routine follow up
Atypical—benign, suggestive of:	Atypical—benign, suggestive of:	Atypical—benign, suggestive of:	1. Clinical correlation 2. Treat specific condition
Mild dysplasia	CIN-1	Low-grade squamous intraepithelial lesion	1. Clinical correlation 2. More frequent follow-up
Moderate dysplasia	CIN-2	High-grade squamous intraepithelial lesion	1. Colposcopy/referral
Severe dysplasia	CIN-3	High-grade squamous intraepithelial lesion	1. Referral
Carcinoma-in-situ	CIN-3	High-grade squamous intraepithelial lesion	1. Referral
Invasive squamous cell carcinoma	Invasive squamous cell carcinoma	Invasive squamous cell carcinoma	1. Referral
Adenocarcinoma	Adenocarcinoma	Adenocarcinoma	1. Referral

Descriptive Terms for Squamous Cell Abnormalities:

Benign reactive changes: This covers a range of conditions that are benign and do not require follow-up, including squamous metaplasia, epithelial response to inflammation, nuclear enlargement, parabasal cells, and hyperplasia of endocervical cells.

Hyperkeratosis: This refers to the presence of keratinized squamous cells without nuclei. It is associated with dysplasia in 10% of patients and may be hard to distinguish from dysplasia. Colposcopy is probably indicated if this finding persists for two consecutive reports.

Parakeratosis: Similar to hyperkeratosis except that the nuclei are retained. Handle in the same manner.

Koilocytosis: This represents vacuolization and enlargement of the epithelial cells. It is pathognomonic for genital warts, even if no warts are seen clinically.

Dyskeratosis: This refers to a mismatch between the nuclear and cytoplasmic maturation. It is commonly seen with condyloma but may also represent malignant changes.

PLATELET COUNT

Background

The normal adult platelet count ranges from 140 to 400 × 10^9 per liter. Counts below 140 × 10^9 per liter indicate thrombocytopenia. Counts greater than 400 × 10^9 per liter indicate thrombocytosis (Table 72–20).

Platelet counts are routinely reported on specimens sent for complete blood counts. This is because most modern cell counters do an automated platelet count as a part of their routine testing. Because of this fact, the most common platelet count abnormality is a small increase or decrease from normal in an otherwise asymptomatic individual. There is usually no benefit from further evaluating or even repeating the platelet count in these cases.

There is little justification for ordering screening platelet counts on asymptomatic outpatients or as a part of the admission testing on hospitalized patients. The one exception to this would be an individual who is admitted for a major surgical procedure. The platelet count is, however, useful in the evaluation of patients with abnormal bleeding, bruising, purpura, petechiae, or splenomegaly.

Thrombocytopenia can be caused by a reduction in the marrow's production of platelets (either from marrow suppression or infiltration), increased destruction of platelets, or sequestration of platelets in the spleen. A platelet count is also a very useful indicator of marrow sensitivity to cytotoxic medications in the treatment of cancer.

It should be remembered that platelets may be adequate in number but defective in function. Medications are the most common cause of abnormal platelet function (i.e., aspirin, other nonsteroidal anti-inflammatory drugs, alcohol, and penicillins).

POTASSIUM

Background

Potassium is the major cation in the intracellular fluid. Ninety-eight per cent of the total body potassium is contained within the cells. The kidneys are responsible for regulation of the extracellular potassium. Hypokalemia and hyperkalemia are principally due either to renal disorders or to abnormalities in the intake of potassium.

It is not useful to test healthy outpatients for this electrolyte. However, the test is very useful for patients with renal disease, those on diuretics, and patients who complain of weakness (Table 72–21). It is also customary to obtain a serum potassium on all acutely ill hospitalized patients. Disorders of potassium are common in hospitalized patients because of the frequent use of IVs and nasogastric suction.

Table 72–20. NORMAL VALUES FOR PLATELET COUNT

Diagnostic Units: platelets × 10^9/L.
First week of life: 84–478
After first week of life: 140–400

Decreased	Diagnoses to Consider	Actions to Consider
100–400	Response to viral illness Response to bacterial illness	1. Repeat test
50–100 (may have bleeding with major surgery)	Thrombocytopenia purpura Post transfusion Spleen sequestration Marrow infiltration (i.e., leukemia) Response to cytotoxic drugs	1. History of all medications 2. Alcohol history 3. Examine for splenomegaly 4. CBC 5. Trial off all medications 6. Bone marrow biopsy
20–50 (may have bleeding with minor procedure)	Thrombocytopenia Marrow infiltration DIC	1. Platelet transfusion for any procedure
< 20 (may have spontaneous GI or CNS hemorrhage)	Severe thrombocytopenia	1. Platelet transfusion
Increased	**Diagnoses to Consider**	**Actions to Consider**
400–600	Splenectomy Infection Blood loss Inflammatory bowel disease Collagen vascular disease	1. Repeat test
600–1000	Malignancy Polycythemia vera	1. Evaluate for malignancy
> 1000 (may have spontaneous thrombosis and bleeding)	Severe thrombocytosis	1. Administer antiplatelet drugs

Table 72–21. NORMAL VALUES FOR POTASSIUM

Diagnostic Units: mEq./L. (mmol./L.). SI conversion factor = 1
Normal 3.5–5.0 (3.5–5.0)

Increased	Diagnoses to Consider	Actions to Consider
5.0–7.5	Hemolyzed specimen Drugs: Potassium-sparing diuretics NSAID ACE inhibitors Potassium supplementation Decreased renal excretion: Acute renal failure Chronic renal failure Addison's disease Acidosis Tissue destruction	1. Repeat K on new specimen 2. Drug and diet history 3. Check ECG for peaked T 4. Creatinine 5. Serum electrolytes 6. Urine electrolytes
>7.5	Hyperkalemic arrhythmias Hyperkalemic paralysis	1. ECG for peaked T, wide QRS, absent P 2. Calcium gluconate 3. Glucose/insulin infusion 4. Bicarbonte 5. Ion exchange resins
Decreased	**Diagnoses to Consider**	**Actions to Consider**
3.5–2.5	Renal loss: Thiazide or loop diuretics Renal tubular acidosis Hyperaldosteronism Gastrointestinal loss: Vomiting Diarrhea Inadequate dietary potassium Inadequate IV potassium Insulin therapy Metabolic alkalosis	1. Drug and diet history 2. Serum electrolytes 3. Urine electrolytes 4. ECG for ST sagging, T depression, and U waves 5. Monitor for digoxin toxicity 6. Administer oral potassium
< 2.5	Hypokalemic arrhythmias	1. Monitor closely for arrhythmias and paralysis 2. Administer IV and oral potassium

Values in parentheses are SI units.

The most commonly seen potassium disorder is a mild hypokalemia in patients on a thiazide or loop diuretic. These patients are often asymptomatic, and it is unclear whether such patients benefit from treatment. Mild hypokalemia can also be associated with vague complaints such as weakness, muscle cramps, and paresthesias. More severe hypokalemia may cause arrhythmias, a paralytic ileus, or paralysis. All hypokalemic patients on digoxin require treatment because of the increased risk for digoxin toxicity with even mild hypokalemia.

The most common reason for hyperkalemia is hemolysis of red blood cells during blood collection or processing. In some cases, these specimens have red serum. If in doubt, retest the patient prior to undergoing a long work-up for real hyperkalemia.

Hyperkalemia is associated with patient complaints of weakness or paralysis. Severe hyperkalemia (potassium greater than 8) is associated with bradycardia, hypotension, ventricular fibrillation, and cardiac arrest.

When there is suspicion of a laboratory error, a quick and useful maneuver is to do an ECG. Clinically significant hyperkalemia or hypokalemia is usually associated with the ECG findings indicated in Table 72–21.

PROTEIN (TOTAL)

Background

The total protein measured by the laboratory includes albumin plus the various globulins (Table 72–22). Fibrinogen, another blood protein, is not measured since it is depleted when serum clots.

Decreased levels of total protein are seen in a wide variety of illnesses. In most cases, these diseases are better followed by the albumin since it is the albumin fraction which is usually reduced. A reduction in albumin is also a better guide to edematous states since it is responsible for 90 per cent of the oncotic pressure.

Increased levels of total protein are occasionally seen and usually lead to an evaluation for multiple myeloma. In fact, myeloma can be associated with increased, normal, or decreased total protein levels.

When there is a question about the interpretation of any abnormal total protein, it is useful to obtain a protein electrophoresis. This test separates the albumin from the various globulins. The electrophoretic pattern may be diagnostically helpful. Immunologic typing should be done for any electrophoretic "spike" to further test for myeloma.

Table 72–22. NORMAL VALUES FOR PROTEIN

Diagnostic Units: gm./dl. (gm./L.). SI conversion factor = 10.0
Normal 6–8 (60–80)

Decreased	Diagnoses to Consider	Actions to Consider
< 6 (60)	Decreased synthesis: Liver insufficiency Malnutrition Malignancy Increased loss: Nephrotic syndrome Extensive burns Protein-losing enteropathy Inflammatory illness Myeloma Overhydration	1. Dietary history 2. Urinalysis 3. 24-hour urine protein 4. Bilirubin 5. Creatinine 6. Protein electrophoresis
Increased	**Diagnoses to Consider**	**Actions to Consider**
> 8 (80)	Dehydration Multiple myeloma Sarcoidosis Monoclonal gammopathy Chronic inflammation	1. Creatinine, BUN 2. Protein electrophoresis 3. Chest x-ray

Values in parentheses are SI units.

PROTHROMBIN TIME

Background

The prothrombin time (PT) is the only coagulation test commonly used in the outpatient setting (Table 72–23). It is the time required to initiate clotting when tissue thromboplastin is mixed with blood. The PT is a measure of both the extrinsic clotting system (i.e., Factor VII) as well as those factors common to both the intrinsic and extrinsic system (i.e., Factor X, Factor V, prothrombin, and fibrinogen) (Hirsh and Levine, 1987).

A prothrombin time is not considered a useful screening test for asymptomatic patients, even those undergoing a surgical procedure. It is most commonly used in monitoring the anticoagulation effects of patients on warfarin (Coumadin). It is also a useful test for evaluating any patient with abnormal bleeding. It is important to note that the PT is normal in patients with classic hemophilia (i.e., Factor VIII deficiency) and those with von Willebrand's disease.

There has been a great deal of confusion about PT testing. A broad range of values have been called "normal" by different laboratories. In addition, there has been disagreement about appropriate therapeutic PT levels in patients on warfarin.

Many of these problems are due to the fact that the test relies on thromboplastin reagents which vary considerably in their clotting activity. Those used today are less responsive than those that were used in the early studies on therapeutic anticoagulation. This has led to some clinicians unknowingly over-anticoagulating their patients.

PT results may be reported in seconds, as a ratio compared with normal controls, or as an internationalized normalized ratio (INR). The international normalized ratio is standardized to the World Health Organization's reference thromboplastin. It is essential that the clinician know which of these reporting

Table 72–23. NORMAL VALUES FOR PROTHROMBIN TIME

Normal	Seconds	Patient/Control Ratio (rabbit brain thromboplastin)	INR*
	11–13	0.9–1.1	0.8–1.3
Anticoagulation Therapy	**Seconds**	**Patient/Control Ratio (rabbit brain thromboplastin)**	**INR***
Treatment of deep vein thrombosis	15–18.5	1.3–1.6	2.0–3.0
Treatment of pulmonary embolism	15–18.5	1.3–1.6	2.0–3.0
Prevention of embolism in atrial fibrillation or tissue heart valves	15–18.5	1.3–1.6	2.0–3.0
Prevention of embolism in patients with prosthetic heart valves	18.5–21	1.6–1.8	3.0–4.5
Prevention of embolism in patients with recurrent emboli	18.5–21	1.6–1.8	3.0–4.5

Increased	Diagnoses to Consider	Actions to Consider
	Liver disease Malabsorption DIC Warfarin therapy Factor II, V, VII, X deficiency Vitamin K deficiency	1. Liver enzymes, bilirubin 2. PTT 3. Clotting factor assays 4. Serum carotene 5. 72-hour stool fat 6. Administer vitamin K

*INR: International Normalization Ratio

systems is being used to assure adequate anticoagulation without risking unnecessary bleeding.

RETICULOCYTE COUNT

Background

Reticulocytes are immature red blood cells which have extruded their nucleus but contain residual basophilic staining material. They are released from the marrow into the peripheral blood and then take one to two days to change into mature red blood cells.

A reticulocyte count is the ratio of reticulocytes compared with the total number of red blood cells (Table 72–24). Since normal red blood cells have a 120-day life span, about 1 per cent of red blood cells are destroyed and replaced each day. Since the newly released cells are reticulocytes, a normal reticulocyte count is about 1 per cent.

The reticulocyte count serves as a measure of the marrow's responsiveness to an anemia. In an anemia caused by the marrow's underproduction of red cells, the reticulocyte count will be low. In anemia caused by a short red cell life (i.e., as with hemolysis or blood loss), a healthy marrow will respond with an increase in red blood cell production and, therefore, an elevated reticulocyte count.

There are two corrections usually done on the reticulocyte count. The first is the correction for the anemia. Since the reticulocyte count is a function of both the number of reticulocytes and the number of mature red blood cells, a decrease in the number of red blood cells could result in an increase in the uncorrected reticulocyte count, even if the number of reticulocytes remains the same. This would give the false impression of an active marrow response, even though the marrow had not actually responded. The corrected reticulocyte count is equal to the uncorrected reticulocyte count times the patient's hematocrit divided by 45.

A second correction factor should be made whenever there are nucleated red blood cells seen on the peripheral smear. This is an indication that the marrow is very active in releasing blood cells. The reticulocytes are therefore released earlier in their development, and they therefore spend a longer period in the peripheral circulation before developing into mature cells. This correction involves dividing the corrected reticulocyte count (as calculated above) by the number of days that are required for maturation of the reticulocyte:

Hematocrit level	Maturity in days
40–45	1.0
35	1.5
25	2.0
15	2.5

SODIUM

Background

Sodium is the major cation in the extracellular fluid. To interpret this test properly it is necessary to think about it not as a measure of total body sodium but rather as a measure of both the total body water and the effective circulatory volume (Table 72–25). In normal situations the serum osmolality is used by the body to adjust the serum sodium. When the osmolality increases, thirst increases so more water is taken in and antidiuretic hormone (ADH) is secreted, so less free water is lost by the kidneys. When

Table 72–24. NORMAL VALUES FOR RETICULOCYTE COUNT RANGES

Diagnostic Units: percentage reticulocytes (corrected)
Normal: Newborn to two weeks of age: 2.5 to 6.5
Males older than two weeks: 0.8 to 2.5
Females older than two weeks: 0.8 to 4.1

Increased	Diagnoses to Consider	Actions to Consider
> 2.5 in males > 4.1 in females	Hemorrhage Hemolytic anemia Response to treatment for a nutritional anemia Marrow recovery after reversible suppression	1. CBC 2. Menstrual history 3. Stool for occult blood 4. Peripheral smear for hemolysis 5. Complete drug history 6. Coombs' test 7. Hb electrophoresis
Decreased	**Diagnoses to Consider**	**Actions to Consider**
< 0.8	Nutritional anemia Anemia of chronic disease Aplastic anemia Marrow infiltration Septicemia	1. CBC 2. History of chronic malignant, inflammatory, or infectious disease 3. Complete drug history 4. Iron, ferritin, TIBC 5. Folate, B_{12} 6. Bone marrow biopsy
< 0.2	Aplastic anemia	

Table 72–25. NORMAL VALUES FOR SODIUM

Diagnostic Units: mEq./L. (mmol./L.). SI conversion factor = 1
Normal: 135–147 (135–147)

Increased	Diagoses to Consider	Actions to Consider
> 147	Fluid loss in excess of salt: Sweating Diarrhea Diabetes mellitus (osmotic diuresis) Diabetes insipidus Hyperaldosteronism Reduced fluid intake: Altered mental status (unable to drink) Vomiting Excessive salt intake: Infant formula Hypertonic NG feeding Salt poisoning	1. Clinical ssessment of fluid status 2. Serum electrolytes 3. Serum BUN/creatinine 4. Serum glucose 5. Urine specific gravity 6. Give PO fluids
> 160	CNS symptoms if an acute change	1. Slow hydration with isotonic saline (reduce serum sodium no faster than 10 mEq./L. each day)
Decreased	**Diagnoses to Consider**	**Actions to Consider**
< 135	Excess water: Psychogenic polydipsia Excessive IV hydration Decreased effective circulatory volume: Diuretic therapy Congestive heart failure Cirrhosis Nephrotic syndrome Dehydration with free water access Inability to excrete water: Renal failure (Cr Cl < 15) SIADH Sodium depletion: Gastrointestinal loss Excessive sweating Adrenal insufficiency Pseudohyponatremia	1. Clinical assessment of fluid status 2. Urine/serum osmolality 3. Urine protein 4. BUN, creatinine 5. Urine specific gravity 6. Serum albumin 7. Serum electrolyte 8. Water restriction
< 120	CNS symptoms are likely due to brain swelling	1. Administer hypertonic saline (3%) until sodium is 125 mEq./L.

Values in parentheses are SI units.

osmolality decreases, thirst is turned off and ADH secretion is suppressed. In situations where the effective circulatory volume is reduced (i.e., heart failure), the body may sacrifice a normal osmolality in an effort to maintain the circulatory volume. In this setting, the sodium falls as fluid is retained in an effort to maintain the circulation.

A serum sodium cannot be properly interpreted without a physical examination of the patient's volume status. In hypovolemic states there will be an orthostatic blood pressure drop, decreased skin turgor, dry mucous membranes, and weight loss. Hypovolemia may be associated with either a normal, an increased, or a decreased serum sodium. To a large extent this depends on the patient's access to free water. Hypovolemia leads to thirst. If this results in drinking fluids that are low in sodium, hyponatremia follows.

Heart failure, cirrhosis, and nephrotic syndrome are frequent causes of hypervolemia (i.e., edematous states). In each case, the total body water is increased but the effective circulating volume is decreased. Therefore, ADH is stimulated and free water is retained. This leads to hyponatremia.

Pseudohyponatremia is seen with hyperglycemia, severe hyperlipidemia, or hyperproteinemia. In these situations, the presence of other solutes in the serum results in artificially low serum sodium values (if measured by flame photometry).

Testing for serum sodium is not useful in the routine screening of healthy individuals. However, it is very useful in patients with heart failure, liver disease, chronic renal failure, and other edematous states. All acutely ill hospitalized patients should be tested, since serum sodium is often altered by intravenous therapy or nasogastric suction. In addition, patients on lithium therapy should have their sodium evaluated because this drug can lead to nephrogenic diabetes insipidus.

THEOPHYLLINE

Background

Drug level monitoring is extremely important when using medications that have serious toxic effects

Table 72–26. VALUES FOR THEOPHYLLINE

Diagnostic Units: μg./ml. (μmol./L.). SI conversion factor = 5.55

Therapeutic
10–20 (56–111)

Decreased	**Diagnoses to Consider**	**Actions to Consider**
<10 (56)	Noncompliance Inadequate dosage Change in drug metabolism Trough level Use of short ½ life theophylline	1. Review drug compliance 2. Check time of last dose 3. Is patient a new smoker? 4. Is drug being absorbed? 5. Increase dose or frequency by 100% if level is < 5 by 50% if level is 5–8 by 20% if level is 8–10
Increased	**Diagnoses to Consider**	**Actions to Consider**
20–35 (111–194)	Excessive dose Excessive dosing frequency Erythromycin alters drug metabolism Cimetidine alters drug metabolism Liver disease Heart failure	1. Complete drug history 2. Examine for side effects 3. Decrease dose
> 35 (194)	Dosing error Intentional overdose	1. Examine for side effects 2. Hospitalize to monitor 3. Administer activated charcoal
> 50	Seizures or arrhythmias very likely	1. Consider charcoal hemoperfusion

Values in parentheses are SI units.

and that display wide variations in absorption or metabolism (Taylor, 1986). Theophylline is such a drug, and measurement of theophylline levels has therefore become a common practice (Table 72–26).

The bioavailability of theophylline is the fraction of drug absorbed. Following absorption, the level in the blood reaches a peak, which is the highest drug concentration. For currently available theophylline preparations, the dose-to-peak time varies from 2 to 12 hours. Theophylline is then metabolized by the liver and excreted by the kidneys. The time required to decrease the drug concentration in the blood by 50 per cent is referred to as its half-life. The half-life for theophylline is 8 to 9 hours and does not vary with the type of theophylline preparation. After 4 to 5 consecutive doses of theophylline have been taken, the drug reaches a steady state. A drug level drawn just before the next dose is the lowest steady-state level and is referred to as a trough level.

The theophylline level is affected by a variety of factors including the type of theophylline preparation, the frequency of dosing, the patient's size, and the patient's age. The metabolism of theophylline can be decreased (and therefore the serum level increased) by liver disease, pulmonary disease, heart failure, and the concomitant use of erythromycin or cimetadine. Smoking, on the other hand, increases theophylline metabolism and therefore decreases the theophylline level.

There is often debate about whether a peak or a trough level is better in managing a patient on theophylline. The answer depends on what information is needed. In general, the peak level is used to assess toxicity, while the trough is a useful measure of the dosing adequacy.

High levels of theophylline are associated with nausea, vomiting, diarrhea, headache, insomnia, agitation, tachycardia, seizures, tremor, and fever. The occurrence of toxic side effects tends to be very individual. Some patients will have seizures, tachyarrhythmias, or circulatory collapse at a theophylline level of 50. Others remain asymptomatic at this level.

It is essential that a complete dosing history be taken whenever a theophylline level is drawn. It is impossible to interpret the value without knowing which preparation of theophylline is being taken, whether the person has been compliant with the medication, and the timing of the last dose.

THYROXIN (T_4)

Background

Thyroxin is the principal hormone secreted by the thyroid gland. It is almost completely bound to proteins in the circulation. Most of the binding is to thyroxin-binding globulin (TBG), but a small amount is also bound to albumin. The active form of the hormone is free thyroxin (i.e., thyroxin not bound to protein). Thyroxin is used in the body to regulate tissue metabolism.

The most common screening thyroid test is the serum thyroxin. Unfortunately, this test measures total thyroxin rather than just the active hormone (i.e., free T_4). Many of the test abnormalities that are therefore seen are due to abnormal levels of

Table 72–27. NORMAL VALUES FOR THYROXIN

Diagnostic Units: µg./dl. (nmol./L.). SI conversion factor = 13.0
Normal: 5.5–12.5 (72–163)

Increased	Diagnoses to Consider	Actions to Consider
> 12.5 (163)	Hyperthyroidism Elevated TBG: Birth control pills Pregnancy Estrogens Liver disease Drugs: Propranolol Amphetamines Contrast media Amiodarone Heparin	1. Complete drug history 2. T_4 index 3. Sensitive TSH 4. Free T_3 5. Thyroid uptake scan
Decreased	**Diagnoses to Consider**	**Actions to Consider**
< 5.5 (72)	Hypothyroidism Decreased TBG: Malnutrition Liver diseases Nephrotic syndrome Androgens Glucocorticoids Sick thyroid syndrome	1. T_4 index 2. TSH 3. Albumin 4. Urinary protein

Values in parentheses are SI units.

thyroid-bonding globulin instead of the active hormone.

The free T_4 level can be approximated by ordering a T_3 uptake test and calculating the free T_4 index (Table 72–27). This index approximates the free T_4. If it is increased, it suggests hyperthyroidism. If it is decreased, it suggests hypothyroidism.

When using the T_4 or the T_4 index as screening tests, there frequently remain cases in which the diagnosis is uncertain. If there is concern about hypothyroidism, a thyroid-stimulating hormone (TSH) test is usually helpful. If there is concern about hyperthyroidism, the free T_3 is useful. Low level TSH tests have been introduced which are low in hyperthyroidism.

Thyroxin-binding globulin levels and free T_4 levels are available but are rarely used diagnostically. In difficult cases, the response to thyrotropin-releasing hormone (TRH) can be used to sort out both hyperthyroid and hypothyroid diagnoses.

URIC ACID

Background

The serum level of uric acid is based on the balance between the rate at which purines are absorbed or produced by the body compared with their metabolism and excretion (Table 72–28). Increased levels can be due to increased purine absorption (i.e., a high protein diet), increased production (i.e., leukemia), or reduced purine excretion (i.e., chronic renal failure).

There is no evidence that uric acid in solution causes any disease. All of the diseases associated with hyperuricemia are due to deposition of uric acid crystals. These illnesses include acute gouty arthritis, gouty tophi, gouty nephropathy, and urolithiasis. Low uric acid levels are occasionally seen in patients with renal tubular defects and are of no clinical significance.

The most common test abnormality is hyperuricemia in an asymptomatic patient. The frequency of this finding is due to the addition of uric acid as an analyte on many screening panels. There is wide agreement that in the absence of acute gouty arthritis, tophi, renal disease, or renal stones, these patients require no treatment. Most patients with chronic renal failure will have hyperuricemia owing to the kidney's reduced ability to excrete uric acid. These patients' uric acid levels are usually less than 10 and do not require treatment if the patient is asymptomatic.

A uric acid less than 7 is sometimes seen in a patient with acute gout. This is believed to be due to a urate diuresis that occurs in response to the joint inflammation. The diagnosis of acute gouty arthritis must be based on the microscopic identification of urate crystals in synovial fluid. Many patients have been misdiagnosed as having gout when they in fact had another form of arthritis (i.e., osteoarthritis) but also had incidental, asymptomatic hyperuricemia.

WHITE BLOOD CELL COUNT (WBC)

Background

Changes in the white blood cell count (WBC) are seen with many infectious, hematologic, inflammatory, and neoplastic diseases. This variety of diseases makes the WBC a nonspecific test. It can, however, be a sensitive indicator of disease in some clinical situations (Shapiro, 1987). Its degree of increase or decrease often correlates with the severity of the disease process. Following changes in the WBC

Table 72–28. NORMAL VALUES FOR URIC ACID

Diagnostic Units: mg./dl. (µmol./L.). SI conversion factor = 60
Normal: 2.5–7.0 (150–420)

Increased	Diagnoses to Consider	Actions to Consider
> 7.0 (420)	Gout Diuretics Chronic renal failure High protein diet Leukemia, lymphoma	1. Tap inflamed joint 2. Complete dietary history 3. Complete drug history 4. Serum creatinine 5. 24-hour urinary uric acid 6. Colchicine trial 7. CBC

Values in parentheses are SI units.

Table 72–29. NORMAL RANGES FOR WHITE BLOOD CELL COUNT

Diagnostic Units: cells/cu. mm. (cells × 10^9/L.). SI conversion factor = 0.001

Age	Average	95% Range
Birth	18,100	9,000–30,000
12 hours	22,800	13,000–38,000
24 hours	18,900	9,400–34,000
1 week	12,200	5,000–21,000
2 months	11,000	5,500–18,000
1 year	11,400	6,000–17,500
2 years	10,600	6,000–17,000
6 years	8,500	5,000–14,500
10 years	8,100	4,500–13,500
20 years	7,500	4,500–11,500
Adult	6,500	3,200–9,800

Decreased	Diagnoses to Consider	Actions to Consider
500–3200 (0.5–32) in adults	Infections: Severe bacterial infection Influenza Infectious mononucleosis Typhoid fever Drugs: Cytotoxic Idiosyncratic Congestive splenomegaly Felty's syndrome SLE Megaloblastic anemia Aplastic anemia Congenital neutropenia	1. Complete drug history 2. Peripheral smear 3. Platelet count 4. CBC 5. Mono test 6. ANA 7. Folate, B_{12} levels 8. Bone marrow biopsy
< 500 (0.5)	At risk for severe bacterial infections	1. Frequent examinations 2. Antibiotics for fever

Increased	Diagnoses to Consider	Actions to Consider
9800–30,000 (9.8–30) in adults	Physiologic reaction to stress Infection Tissue destruction Leukemia Cancer Hemorrhage Splenectomy	1. Symptom-directed physical examination 2. Peripheral smear
> 30,000 (30)	Leukemia Leukemoid reaction	1. Peripheral smear 2. Examine for hepatomegaly and splenomegaly

Values in parentheses are SI units.

over time can therefore provide useful information about the course of an illness (Table 72–29).

Five types of white blood cells are commonly counted in the WBC differential; the neutrophil, lymphocyte, monocyte, eosinophil, and basophil (Table 72–30). Changes in the relative percentages of these cells are recognized as useful patterns by clinicians in many common illnesses (i.e., leukocytosis and a shift to the left in bacterial diseases).

Leukopenia usually indicates neutropenia. This is defined as less than 2 × 10^9 per liter neutrophils in whites or 1.5 × 10^9 per liter in blacks. In patients receiving chemotherapy, neutropenia of less than 0.5 × 10^9 per liter is often associated with severe infec-

Table 72–30. NORMAL VALUES FOR WHITE BLOOD CELL DIFFERENTIAL COUNT BY AGE

Age	Segmented Neutrophils %	Band Neutrophils %	Eosinophils %	Basophils %	Lymphocytes %	Monocytes %
Birth	47	14	2.2	0.6	31	5.8
1 week	34	11.8	4.1	0.4	41	9.1
1 year	23	8.1	2.6	0.4	61	4.8
4 years	3447	8.0	2.8	0.6	50	5.0
12 years	51	8.0	2.5	0.5	38	4.4
20 years		8.0	2.7	0.5	33	5.0

tions. In patients with congenital neutropenia, at the same reduced neutrophil level, there is usually no infection. This indicates that the former patients have both a quantitative and a qualitative neutrophil defect.

Lymphopenia is defined as less than 1.5×10^9 per liter. It is frequently seen in association with a wide variety of physiologic stresses and is of no clinical significance. Reductions in monocytes, eosinophils, and basophils are occasionally seen and are not clinically useful.

An increased WBC count can be seen with a wide variety of diseases. The average WBC count tends to be higher in children than adults (see Tables 72–29 and 72–30). Most elevated WBC counts are below 30,000 cells per cu. mm. Counts greater than 30,000 are usually due to leukemia or a leukemoid reaction. It is obviously important to differentiate between these two diagnoses.

References

Beck, L. H., and Kassirer, J. P.: Serum electrolytes, serum osmolality, blood urea nitrogen, and serum creatinine. *In* Sox, H. C. (Ed.): Common Diagnostic Tests: Use and Interpretation. Philadelphia, American College of Physicians, 1987, pp. 317–329.

Boyko, E. J., Alderman, B. W., and Barron, A. E.: Reference test errors bias the evaluation of diagnostic tests for ischemic heart disease. J. Gen. Intern. Med., *3*:476–481, 1988.

Burke, J. J., Fischer, P. M.: A Clinician's Guide to the Office Management of Cholesterol. J.A.M.A., *259*:3444–3448, 1988. *This article reviews some of the analytic factors that should be considered in interpreting a cholesterol value.*

DeNeef, P.: Selective testing for streptococcal pharyngitis in adults. J. Fam. Pract., *25*:347–351, 1987.

Fischer, P. M.: Alkaline phosphatase value, elevated. *In* Taylor, R. B. (Ed.): *Difficult Diagnosis.* Philadelphia, W. B. Saunders, 1985, pp. 6–13. This short chapter reviews the biochemistry of ALP and presents a clinical decision flow chart for the investigation of an elevated value.

Gerber, M. A., Randolph, M. F., and Mayo, D. R.: The group A streptococcal carrier state, a reexamination. Am. J. Dis. Child., *142*:562–565, 1988.

Heath, H., Hodgson, S. F., and Kennedy, M. A.: Primary hyperparathyroidism: Incidence, morbidity, and potential economic impact in a community. N. Engl. J. Med., *302*:189–193, 1980. *This classic article reviews the cases of hyperparathyroidism that were detected in the Mayo Clinic following the widespread adoption of periodic chemistry testing. The authors raise the issue of whether this is a disease that merits detection in the asymptomatic state.*

Heckerling, P. S.: Confidence in diagnostic testing. J. Gen. Intern., Med. *3*:604–606, 1988.

Hirsh, J., and Levine, M. N.: The optimal intensity of oral anticoagulant therapy. J.A.M.A., *258*:2723–2726, 1987. *This is an excellent review of the use of PT testing including the therapeutic ranges recommended by the NIH and American College of Chest Physicians, National Conference on Antithrombotic Therapy.*

Kellogg, J. A., and Manzella, J. P.: Detection of Group A streptococci in the laboratory or physician's office. J.A.M.A., *255*:2638–2642, 1986.

Lundberg, G. D.: Using the Clinical Laboratory in Medical Decision Making. Chicago, American Society of Clinical Pathologists Press, 1983.

National Institutes of Health: Lowering blood cholesterol to prevent heart disease, consensus conference. J.A.M.A., *253*:2080–2086, 1985. *This is the report that outlines the NIH's recommendations for treatment of hypercholesterolemia.*

Physician's Guide to Non-Insulin Dependent (Type II) Diabetes: Diagnosis and Treatment. American Diabetes Association, Alexandria, Virginia, 1988. *This inexpensive and short monograph reviews the current classifications of all types of diabetes, describes how diagnosis should be made, and discusses the treatment of Type II diabetic patients. It is appropriately conservative in its assessment of the HBA_{1c} test. The text is clear and brief. The diabetic field changes very quickly. This short reference provides the current information directly from the ADA.*

Ransohoff, D. F., and Feinstein, A. R.: Problems of spectrum and bias in evaluating the efficacy of diagnostic tests. N. Engl. J. Med., *299*:926–929, 1978.

Shapiro, M. F., and Greenfield, S.: The complete blood count and leukocyte differential count: an approach to their rational application. Ann. Intern. Med., *106*:65–74, 1987. *This is a very harsh but scholarly review of the CBC and its indications. It was one of several papers that were commissioned by Blue Cross/Blue Shield in collaboration with the American College of Physicians. Its recommendations are likely to be used in future algorithims relating to diagnosis.*

Sox, H. J. (Ed.): Common Diagnostic Tests, Use and Interpretation. Philadelphia, American College of Physicians, 1987.

Sox, H. C., and Liang, M. H.: The erythrocyte sedimentation rate: guidelines for rational use. Ann. Intern. Med. *104*:515–523, 1986. *This critical review of the literature attempts to define appropriate clinical use for the test. The manuscript was one of several commissioned by the Blue Cross and Blue Shield Association and prepared in cooperation with the American College of Physicians. It is likely that its very conservative recommendations will serve as the basis for future reimbursement policies.*

Statland, B. E.: Clinical Decision Levels for Lab Tests. Oradell, N.J., Medical Economics Books, 1987.

Taylor, A. T.: Office Therapeutic Drug Monitoring. Prim. Care, *13*:743–760, 1986. *This is a very nice summary of drug metabolism, therapeutic drug monitoring, and how these measurements can be made in the office laboratory. Several case examples are given.*

Taylor, W. C., Pas, T. M., Shepard, D. S., et al.: Cholesterol reduction and life expectancy: A model incorporating multiple risk factors. Ann. Intern. Med. *106*:605–614, 1987. *This article looks at the treatment of hypercholesterolemia and analyzes the benefit from cholesterol reduction. For persons between 20 and 60 years of age who are at risk for coronary heart disease, a gained life expectancy of 3 days to 3 months is determined for a life-long program of cholesterol reduction.*

Part V

Management of the Practice

73

The Problem-Oriented Medical Record

Robert E. Rakel

A well-prepared medical record is among the most useful tools available to a family physician. When functioning effectively, it communicates the relevant facts regarding patient care to all health personnel involved and allows for the easy documentation and retrieval of information vital to the patient's ongoing care. The information should be organized in a systematic, logical, and consistent manner and should accurately reflect the patient's state of health. Orderly recording of data is vital to efficient care, and although the information should be simplified as much as possible, it must likewise be both complete and accurate. Information placed in the office record should not be gathered and stored just because it is available and may someday be useful; it should be accumulated on the basis that it is needed at present or will at some future time be needed for providing good patient care. We must avoid merely accumulating data and allowing the record to be "untouched by human thought" (Murnaghan, 1973). Family medicine involves the care of patients over a prolonged period of time. Acute illnesses cannot be treated as totally isolated events but must be viewed in the total perspective of a person's or a family's long-term care. A pregnant woman, for example, may have a slightly elevated blood pressure, which should be compared with readings prior to and following pregnancy to assess its true importance. (Similarly, her smoking habits, alcohol intake, caffeine intake, weight, and other physiologic and psychologic functions should be noted and followed.)

An office record system will maintain its usefulness and efficiency over time only if it is individually designed to match the objectives and the personality of the physician using it. The chart should be developed and organized based upon the individual physician's preferences and needs. Some will enjoy using flow sheets frequently; others will be turned off by them. Some will prefer, and will be able to maintain, an adequate medication list; others may find it impossible to keep such a list current. The ideal record must also be kept simple and must not handicap or confine the busy physician's productivity by requiring unnecessary paper work. Merely accumulating a large amount of data is not productive; however, a well-organized record may actually require fewer data and yet be more informative than many present systems. The lengthy, illegible, and poorly organized office record of the past has developed into a logical, well-structured account that lends itself to quick and easy retrieval of information and ready assessment of the patient's present health care needs and potential health hazards. It also assists the physician in predicting the patient's potential future state of health by identifying significant risk factors.

The Source-Oriented Medical Record

The traditional office record of the past was structured according to the source of material contained in the record; thus, it is called the source-oriented medical record (SOMR). In such a record, laboratory data, electrocardiographic reports, consultants' reports, physicians' notes, consultants' notes, nurses' notes, and x-ray reports are all filed independently in separate areas. Material organized in this way becomes primarily a diary of past events and is of relatively limited value in ongoing patient care, although it was probably adequate for the crisis-oriented, episodic care of patients with acute illness, which has too often constituted the bulk of primary medical care.

Although the SOMR is relatively easy to maintain, its disadvantages are that support for action taken is frequently lacking and it takes considerable time for those unfamiliar with the patient to get a complete review of the problems, especially to trace the history of any particular problem. According to Weed (1971), "The record is not a static repository of medical observations structured in the meaningless order of source, but a precise instrument of communication."

The Problem-Oriented, or Patient-Oriented, Medical Record (POMR)

The stimulus for change in record-keeping came in 1969, when Weed developed the problem-oriented medical record (POMR). Although this innovative concept was originally applied to the hospital record, its principles have served as the nucleus for major changes in outpatient records as well. The "pure" form proposed by Weed has required some modification to be adapted to family practice, but its basic concepts serve as an excellent foundation for an efficient office medical record. The POMR has also been called the "patient-oriented medical record," since it helps to avoid depersonalization and emphasizes individuality of the patient by listing the specific problems unique to that person. Hence, the patient is not just another person with gallbladder disease but an individual with a unique combination of associated problems that identify him as different from other patients with gallbladder disease.

The POMR achieves its maximum potential in the hands of a family physician. It works especially well in the continuing care of patients with chronic illness and in complex cases involving multiple problems. Since these are areas in which family physicians are especially effective, it is no wonder that they are the greatest promoters of the POMR. Now that many patients who suffer from previously fatal illnesses are surviving, the family physician is involved in the continuing care of ever increasing numbers of the chronically ill. Management of patients with these chronic illnesses requires a dynamic record that accurately reflects at all times the patient's present and past medical problems and assists the physician in remaining aware of other potential problems that can become significant at any time.

Improved Communication

As our society becomes more mobile and medical technology becomes increasingly complex, we need a well-organized medical record system that permits easy communication and transfer of information among health professionals, both within the same office and at separate sites. No longer can the record be a document understood only by the physician who places data in it. It must permit other physicians, as well as an increasing number of other health personnel, who also depend on the record, to readily assess the patient's condition, understand the plan of management, and recognize all elements important to the patient's ongoing care. As long as the record is able to communicate information in this manner, it will serve as an effective tool for all members of the health care team.

The maintenance of a complete and well-organized medical record over a prolonged period of time contributes to high-quality care by permitting attention to be focused on preventive measures. The need for a uniform, organized collection of information in the office record will increase as more physicians practice in groups and a larger portion of costs is paid by third parties. Increased emphasis is being placed on the assessment of the quality of care, and outpatient records need to be organized in a manner that permits review, just as hospital records are reviewed. Terminology is also being influenced by third-party payers. The physician and other health professionals, such as the dentist, nurse, and therapist, are now called providers, and the office visit is an encounter. It is hoped that in family practice an encounter will remain a friendly interaction between physician and patient, rather than follow Webster's definition of "a meeting of adversaries or hostile persons to engage in conflict." It is no wonder that many physicians bristle at the use of this term to refer to their relationships with patients.

Improved patient care must remain the primary objective of any newly structured record system. As Murnaghan (1973) stated: "Data collection and information systems cannot be justified if they subvert the process of patient care and fail to benefit the patient and provider either directly or indirectly. The growth of public, as opposed to private, responsibility for personal health services means that more and more data requirements will be placed upon the providers of care." Data collection must not be allowed to become threatening to either the patient or the physician but must be an obvious asset to the care and management of all problems related to patients.

Patient Access to Medical Records

Use of the computer in medical recordkeeping has focused more attention on confidentiality of the medical record. Access to medical records for management purposes is being given to more and more nonhealth professionals who are neither sensitive to patients' concerns about confidentiality nor bound by strong ethical or professional codes of conduct regarding the use of such information. A fine balance between confidentiality and access will have to be struck.

The Federal Privacy Act of 1974 (Public Law 93–579) establishes the patient's right to obtain the medical record in federal institutions. A number of states also have statutes as well as precedent court decisions permitting direct access of patients to their medical records. Controversy still exists about the effect this will have on clinical care. Although there is no proof that sharing the record with the patient improves the quality of care, there is general agreement that it improves patient understanding and compliance. Schade, a family physician in Los Gatos, California, allows patients to keep their own complete medical record, and he maintains only a brief office record in note form. Patients thus have the record available if they are seen in an emergency room or by a consultant or when moving to a new area. He believes that making the records available to the patients not only enables them to develop a keen understanding of their medical problems and treatment but actually discourages rather than encourages the incidence of filing malpractice suits (Schade, 1976).

One survey of patients (Michael and Bordley, 1982) found that 80 per cent felt they should be permitted to see their medical record, but they were not convinced that possessing a copy was as important as reading it. Regardless of local law, the best policy is to allow patients to examine and copy their records upon request unless there is valid medical reason for refusing to do so. Tufo and colleagues (1977) gave patients copies of their medical records in an attempt "to provide a clear statement of problems and plans to emphasize self-help and patient responsibility." They feel that the patient's audit of the record provides feedback concerning the accuracy of the information and the level of patient understanding.

Fischbach and associates (1980) promote the involvement of the patient; in developing their problem list and progress notes, they state: "The attitude that 'what you don't know won't hurt you' is proving unrealistic; it is what patients do not know, but vaguely suspect, that causes them corrosive worry."

Sharing the medical record with the patient certainly has its place and can be of value, yet discretion is called for since it can also be harmful. For example, some elderly patients may become depressed or confused by seeing a problem list containing 10 to 12 items and multiple medications. Patients with emotional problems may have difficulty understanding or coping with the content of progress notes.

Information Retrieval

The medical record is rapidly becoming less the private property and sole responsibility of the physician and more the joint responsibility and common property of the physician, other health providers, and the patient. Information in the medical record should be highly visible, clear, and concise so that it can be retrieved easily to allow for effective and efficient use of time by the physician and other health professionals.

The use of facsimile (fax) transmission greatly facilitates the transfer of medical information including the electrocardiogram. In many ways, fax transmission is superior to telephone voice communication, express mail, and electronic mail. It can be especially useful in emergency care (Yamamoto and Wiebe, 1989).

Medical Information Cards

Medical identification cards are becoming increasingly popular in our mobile society. Such a card contains microfilm of selected portions of an individual's medical record and is carried as a wallet card. This document serves as a "medical passport" and identifies the nature of the patient's medical problems, such as a recent myocardial infarction, diabetes mellitus, drug allergies, anticoagulant medication, and immunization status. These data give an accurate composite picture of the patient's health status to physicians other than the patient's personal physician during an emergency or when the patient is traveling outside the community.

Laser optic technology has made possible the use of credit card size plastic cards that can store up to 800 pages of data. These cards record x-rays, CT and MRI scans, as well as electrocardiograms. A special read-write unit and an IBM compatible computer are needed to use the card. A special software package ensures confidentiality of the medical record. The patient's picture and signature can be invisibly imbedded in the card making forgery or transfer impossible.

Conversion to a New System

A well-organized and clearly developed medical record will make the provision of excellent medical care readily apparent. It will, however, just as readily expose poor or inadequate care. Physicians who have converted their office record systems to the problem-oriented format undergo a humbling experience as numerous weaknesses in their previous system are uncovered. Problems are frequently identified that had been lost in the record, and laboratory abnormalities are uncovered that were not investigated further. One physician discovered that blood pressure readings had been taken for only a third to a half of all patients in his practice. Another noted that he had been paying too little attention to preventive measures or to the follow-up of potentially serious problems. The most valuable detection is the uncovering of a considerable amount of buried and almost forgotten clinical data. The conversion of an SOMR to any new form of record system, whether it be the POMR or others, will involve a reassessment and reorganization of the record system that will be of value to the physician and the patient by uncovering these problems and placing all facts into a refreshing new perspective.

When records are converted to a problem-oriented format, it is best to begin conversion with the most active records and leave less active ones until later. It is most helpful to start all new patients in the POMR format and to convert established patients with chronic diseases who are seen frequently. High school students, or other temporary help, can be hired to work in the evening to type index cards and transfer record contents to new jackets. The physician should prepare the problem list. Although this is a time-consuming activity, the review it requires will be worth the trouble by reacquainting the physician with previously forgotten aspects of the patient's care.

Transfer of Information

It is important that the family physician incorporate the patient's entire medical background into the record so that the total comprehensive picture is constantly available to the physician and to other health personnel who have need of it. Valuable medical information is often scattered in a variety of locations and thus becomes relatively inaccessible or unavailable when needed.

When new patients are seen, a strong effort should be made to acquire all medical information from other physicians, government services, hospitals, and other health agencies previously involved in the patient's care. A great deal of unnecessary effort and expense results when each physician, in turn, must establish full medical data for every patient, since a variety of diagnostic tests and therapeutic trials must be needlessly repeated. When the transferred record is in the form of the POMR or some similarly concise system, putting it to use is a simple matter for the new physician and sending it on is a painless experience for the former physician because he knows that it can be interpreted readily and will be of benefit to his former patient's care. Central computerization of the medical record in the future may obviate much of this problem. In countries with a national health service, such as Great Britain, the medical record is considered state property and is automatically transferred with patients when they move to a new community.

A study by Birtwhistle and Anderson (1989) showed that only half (52 per cent) of family physicians regularly request previous records on their patients. When information was obtained, there was a preference for short summaries of the patient's problems and copies of previous consultation reports as well as hospital discharge summaries. Somewhat of a surprise was the opinion that office progress notes were seldom useful.

A well-organized record system, such as the POMR, also allows the referring family physician to communicate the patient's total health status more effectively to consulting physicians by submitting the problem list with the consultation request. This prevents the specialist from merely "treating his own disease" and ensures awareness of all of the patient's medical, social, and psychiatric problems, as well as the problems for which the consultation is being requested. When a cardiologist is asked to consult about a seriously ill patient in the coronary care unit, the problem list clearly illustrates other problems to be considered and managed and makes the need for continuing involvement by the family physician readily apparent. Subspecialists are prevented from concentrating on a single part to the detriment of the whole patient.

Legibility

Legibility is necessary if any data, no matter how systematically organized, are to be retrieved and collated in a rapid, accurate, and useful manner that will permit the quick review of a patient's total health status. The well-known illegibility of physicians' handwriting is an understandable product of conditioning during many years of rapid note taking. This handicap, the greatest barrier to effective communication and good records, is now being removed as a rapidly increasing number of physicians turn to dictating their records and using secretarial services for transcription to obtain clearly typed progress notes. This improved legibility is an obvious advantage in group practices, in which more than one physician and several nurses or other health professionals are likely to depend upon the same chart. The POMR, because of its structure, lends itself well to dictation with a minimum of confusion.

Minimum Requirements for the Office Records

The American Board of Family Practice has incorporated a review of office records into its recertification procedure. Table 73–1 lists those items considered by the Board to be essential to a good office record.

Organization of a Record System

FILING

A record-keeping system, no matter how well organized, is of little value if the medical record cannot be

Table 73–1. OFFICE RECORD CONTENT RECOMMENDATIONS
(American Board of Family Practice*)

Recognizing the importance of the medical record in the provision of continuing, comprehensive, family-oriented health care, the American Board of Family Practice recommends that at least the following information should be available in the patient's office chart. The Board does not advocate any particular record-keeping system but recognizes that there are certain principles of record-keeping which enable information to be used effectively in patient care.

A. Records must be legible.

B. In order for records to allow an efficient and rapid review of the patient's total health picture, or a particular health problem, by family physicians and associates, consultants, and allied health personnel, the clinical record should contain the following:

1. The patient's profile
   * Age (birth date)
   * Sex
   * Occupation
   * Education
   * Economic status
   * Family structure
   * Activity pattern
   * Height
   * Weight
   * Habitus
   * Blood pressure
2. Information about possible risk factors
   * History of familial or hereditary disease
   * Alcohol or drinking habits
   * Smoking habits
   * Environmental risks
   * Life style
   * Stress factors
3. A notation which clearly indicates the presence or absence of specific
   * Allergies
   * Drug idiosyncrasies or intolerances
4. Adequate information about the past history, such as
   * Previous illness
   * Previous surgery
   * Recurrent minor problems
5. Adequate information to clearly and easily identify
   * The primary problem
   * Associated or other problems
   * Medications the patient is taking
   * Current immunization status
   * Results of pertinent laboratory and/or X-ray examinations
6. Well-organized and clinically informative progress notes which clearly provide adequate current information about
   * The patient's health status
   * Observations about the patient's problems
   * Conclusions
   * Tests
7. Adequate information to clearly and easily provide information about the
   * Therapeutic or management plan for each element of the patient's health care
   * Patient education for each problem

*From Recertification Handbook for Diplomates, American Board of Family Practice, Lexington, Kentucky, 1988.

found. Much time can be saved by using an efficient filing system.

Alphabetic Filing Systems

This is a popular method of record storage, especially for small practices. Records are filed alphabetically according to surname. Because of the similarity of many names, however, misfiling is common. Strong ethnic backgrounds in a community may lead to heavy concentrations of similar names. Family filing is also difficult with the alphabetic system, particularly when there are different surnames in the family.

Color coding of alphabetical filing systems will limit misfiling and ease retrieval. Each letter has a distinctive color. Colored labels representing the first two letters of the patient's last name are fixed to the tab on each file.

Numeric Systems

Terminal digit filing appears to be the more efficient system for family practice. Fewer charts are misfiled using this system, and it allows for a more rapid and accurate placement and retrieval of records. The only significant disadvantage is the need to maintain an alphabetic and numeric cross-reference index.

Color Coding

Color-coded terminal digit filing largely eliminates the possibility of misfiling or at least limits it to a narrow area. Ten colors are used, one for each of the 10 Arabic numerals 0 (zero) to 9, as opposed to the large number of colors needed in alphabetic systems. This permits ready recognition of visually distinct categories, especially when open shelving is used. Records are arranged according to the last two digits. Each number is keyed to a color on the record jacket edge. The two colors representing the two digits are easily recognized if the record is misfiled. Records with the same two terminal digits are then arranged in sequence according to the numbers preceding the two terminal digits. Thus, chart 00–00–13 will be followed by 00–01–13, 00–02–13, and so on (Fig. 73–1). Color coding can also be an advantage when added to alphabetic systems, but misfiling is common when there are many charts filed under common family names such as Smith, Jones, and Young.

Open Shelving

Color-coded terminal digit filing works best with open-shelf filing, although it can be adapted to drawer files as well. Shelves are better than drawers, however, since they can be stacked higher and it is easier for more than one person to have access to them at a time.

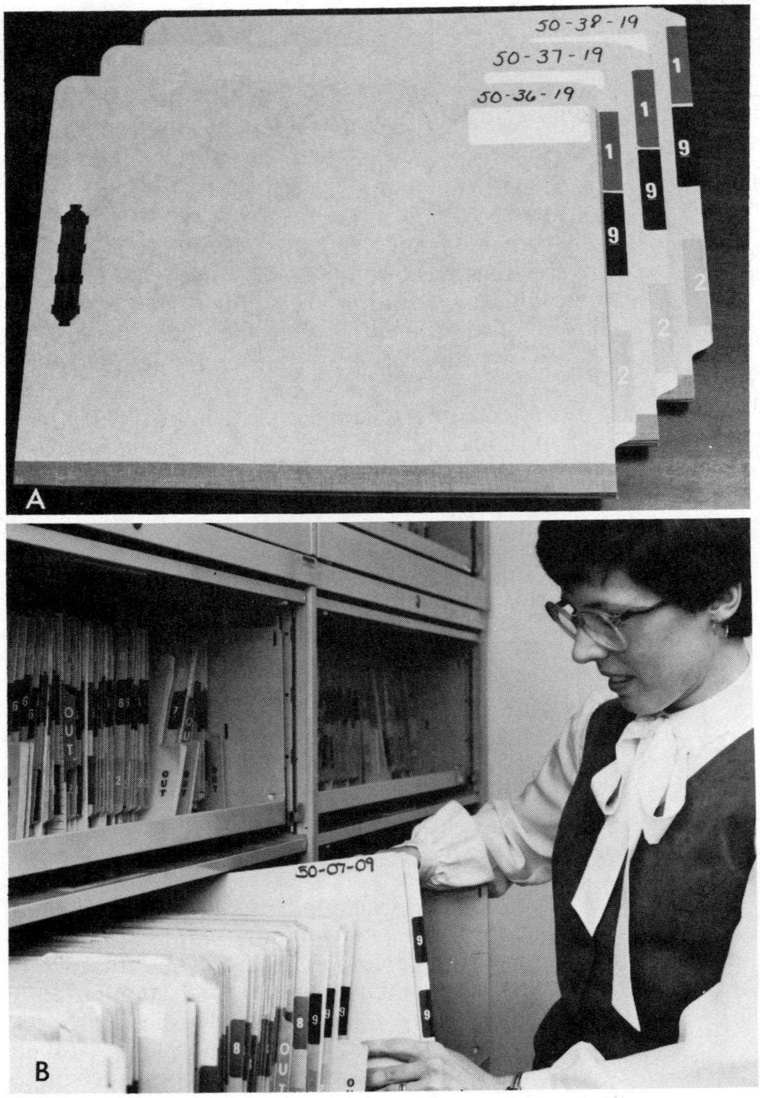

Figure 73–1. Color-coded terminal digit charts.

Inactive Records

Purging of inactive records avoids burdening the record system with unused charts. To keep the unnecessary volume to a minimum, records of patients who have not been seen for 2 or 3 years should be considered inactive and removed from the active file. This weeding out can be a relatively simple process. A color-coded tab or mark corresponding to the year can be added to the margin of each chart (Figs. 73–1 and 73–2). Each year the color is changed when a member of the family is seen so that the color represents the most recent year in which the patient or family was seen. If yellow was the color 3 years ago, it is an easy task to pull all charts with yellow tabs. For the system to work, however, the receptionist or nurse must check this tab each time the chart is pulled to make sure the color corresponds to the current year. A list of preprinted dates can also be stamped on the chart with check marks indicating the most recent year of chart use (Fig. 73–2).

Family Charts

The physician's care of families is facilitated by a record system that focuses on the family. Family folders are filed under the name of the head of the household or the person responsible for the account. This is especially important when family members have different names. Sometimes the family is filed according to all persons living together in the same residence regardless of who is paying for the care. With the numeric filing system, there is only one possible shelf location for the family folder regardless of the variety of surnames involved. Even if surnames vary within a family because of children from previous marriages or because the wife's parents live with the

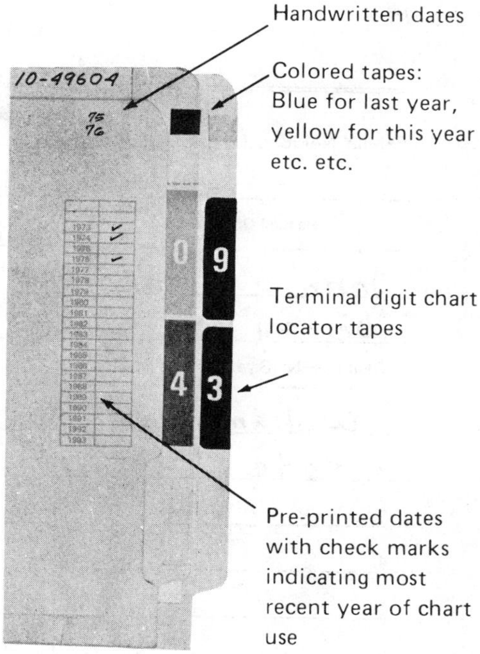

Figure 73–2. Designating year of most recent chart use for purging inactive records. (From Sullivan, R. J., Jr.: Medical Record and Index Systems for Community Practice. Cambridge, MA, Ballinger Publishing Co., 1979.)

family, each individual is identified by a one- or two-digit modifier within the family number.

The family folder usually consists of an outer file jacket containing selected family information as well as the individual charts of each family member (Fig. 73–3). The first item in the family folder is the *family registration form* (Fig. 73–4) containing family demographic data that are usually obtained at the first office visit. It maintains a prominent location in the chart because it is a ready source of reference for the names and ages of all family members and includes occupational and insurance information. The purpose of the family chart is to provide the physician with as much information as possible relating to factors involving the entire family that could have an impact on the health of any individual member. It is important for the physician to note when the problems involving one family member influence the health of another.

Family Member Visit Register. Family stress may become evident by a clustering of problems in many family members. The *family member visit register* can assist the family physician in identifying these problems early. Widmer, Cadoret, and North (1980) have shown that early signs of depression include an increased number of visits by all family members and

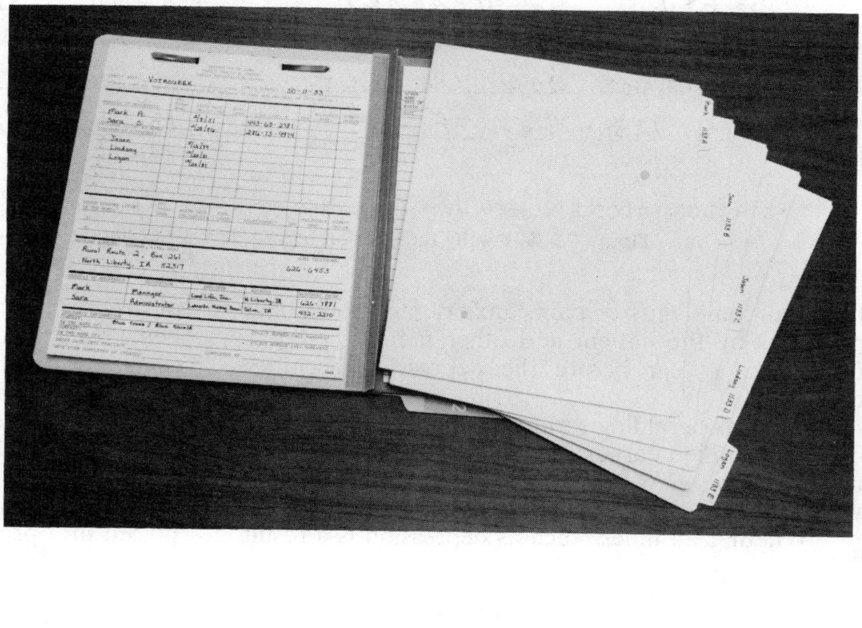

Figure 73–3. Family folder containing individual patient records.

MR-3 11/88

DEPARTMENT OF FAMILY MEDICINE
FAMILY REGISTRATION RECORD

FAMILY NAME: Wagner PATIENT NUMBER: 10-25-68

Head(s) Of Household:	Sex M/F	Check If Lives At Home	Birth Date (Mo/Day/Yr)	Soc. Sec. #	Highest School Level Completed	Ethnic Origin (W,B,H,E,O)*
John	m	✓	01/03/49	416-01-3241	2yrs col.	W
Betty	F	✓	09/06/50	513-60-5214	college	W
CHILDREN: (Give last name if different)			/ /			
1. William	m	✓	12/14/70	- -		
2. Kate	F	✓	10/10/74	- -		
3.			/ /	- -		
4.			/ /	- -		
5.			/ /	- -		
6.			/ /	- -		

Other Persons Living In The Home:	Birth Date (Mo/Day/Yr)	Highest School Level Completed	Relationship	Ethnic Origin (W,B,H,E,O)*
1. Tom Johnson	09/22/20	high school	wife's father	W
2.	/ /			
3.	/ /			

MAILING ADDRESS: (Street, City, Zip) HOME TELEPHONE

8834 Elm Deer Park, Texas 432-7641

HEAD(S) OF HOUSEHOLD	OCCUPATION(S)	EMPLOYER(S)	BUSINESS PHONE(S)
John	salesman	self-employed	481-3289
Betty	teacher	Houston ISD	521-2800

NEAREST RELATIVE: Joe Wagner RELATIONSHIP: father

ADDRESS: 12304 Fern Forest, Houston, TX 77044 459-6092 932-1626
(Street, City, State, Zip, Home Phone, Business Phone)

* ETHNIC ORIGIN CODES (optional): W = White or Caucasian; B = Black or Afro-American; H = Hispanic or Mexican-American; E = East Asian; O = Other

Figure 73–4. Family registration record. (Baylor College of Medicine, Houston, Texas.)

frequent complaints of pain, anxiety, and functional problems by the patient and other family members for up to a year before the depression becomes obvious.

Patterns heralding serious diseases of this nature can be identified earlier if the family physician maintains an overview of the interpersonal dynamics within a family.

Whether an illness such as depression is a result of stress that affects the entire family, with one person being the "weak link," or whether the symptoms of the ill person affect the others is currently undecided. Experiments with techniques similar to the family member visit register will help the family physician monitor these factors and discover new clues to the early diagnosis of significant problems.

The family member visit register (Fig. 73–5) is placed in a prominent area of the family folder and

FAMILY MEMBER VISIT REGISTER

NAME DALY

NUMBER 50-00-03

Given Name	LLOYD	DAWN	PEGGY	KEVIN	MICHELLE	MRS. VAN	
Date of Birth	3/18/39	5/12/41	11/29/60	8/20/64	5/5/71	4/20/02	
DATE	PROBLEM	PROBLEM	PROBLEM	PROBLEM	PROBLEM	PROBLEM	PROBLEM
3/17/75	ulcer						
4/3/75		Headache			well child exam	BP check	
4/7/75				sore throat			
5/12/75			school prob.				
5/30/75	Alcoholism						
7/8/75		Fatigue					
7/23/75		Depression					
8/19/75				Cough			
9/4/75	Ulcer check						
9/22/75						BP check	
10/1/75					Otitis media		
10/10/75					FU-OM		
11/12/75			Drug Prob.				
12/6/75		Depression					
1/17/76				Laceration			
2/10/76		Marital Prob.					

Figure 73–5. Family member visit register, University of Iowa.

records the dates, names, and major reasons for visits by all family members. A glance at this form shows whether other recent problems prominent within the family have a bearing on the present complaint. It may also serve as a reminder to the physician to ask about the progress of another family member who was recently ill. In this way the physician can assess the degree of recovery or the likelihood of a continuing disability and can be constantly prepared to deal with family problems in addition to serving as the personal physician for individual family members.

Family Genogram. Also contained within the outside family folder is the *family genogram* (see Chapter 74). By noting shared family problems, the physician can be alerted to problems that could be related to the present symptoms or to other disorders that should be considered and evaluated in addition to the presenting problem.

It is useful to have a corner or prominent area in the chart to record events that are important occurrences in the patient's life so that these can be recalled and mentioned during subsequent visits. Reference to or questions about events such as the birth of a grandchild, move into a new home, or trip abroad will be appreciated by the patient.

CHART ORGANIZATION

The organization of material within the chart will vary with the type of chart selected, but in all cases the material should be organized in a consistent and predefined manner. If a folder is used, the problem list is usually the top sheet on the left, with the family registration record beneath it. The top sheet on the right contains the most recent progress notes, with previous progress notes beneath it, followed by the data base, electrocardiograms, and correspondence. If possible, each of these sections should be divided by tabs or by some other method to allow easy identification, perhaps by using different colors for each section. A more economical method than purchasing chart dividers is to cut away the edge of progress note pages to make the underlying data base accessible (Fig. 73–6).

USING THE POMR

Although the POMR, as developed by Weed, was originally directed toward organization of the hospital record, it was rapidly adapted to the outpatient setting. Its usefulness in family practice was first demonstrated by Bjorn and Cross (1970). Numerous publications and articles appearing since 1969 have developed the basic concepts further and have suggested many variations, which provide myriad choices for the individual physician. Physicians are encouraged to review the literature and then to select those components with which they feel most comfortable and which appear most useful in their particular practice. The design of any component should be varied when necessary to match individual preference.

Weed describes four basic elements as the nucleus of the POMR: the data base, problem list, initial plan, and progress notes. Although his initial plan applies primarily to the complete work-up of a new office patient or the admission work-up of a hospitalized patient, most physicians prefer to incorporate it into ongoing patient care as a feature of the progress note (Fig. 73–7). The logical approach to record-keeping, then, calls first for the establishment of a data base, after which a problem list is developed, initial plans are identified, and the patient's progress is monitored with continual updating of the data base and problem list.

PROBLEM LIST

Although the problem list is developed largely from information accumulated in the data base, it is the most important single ingredient of the POMR. If there is limited enthusiasm for using all components of the POMR, development of a problem list alone will be of significant benefit. Addition of a data base will enhance its usefulness, but full benefits can be realized only when structured progress notes are also incorporated.

A problem is anything that requires diagnosis or management or that interferes with quality of life as perceived by the patient. It can be either a firm diagnosis, a physical symptom, or a social or economic problem. It is any physiologic, pathologic, psychologic, or social item of concern to either the patient or the physician. A problem is any item that physicians believe they cannot afford to miss or that requires ongoing concern or attention.

The problem list serves as a comprehensive over-

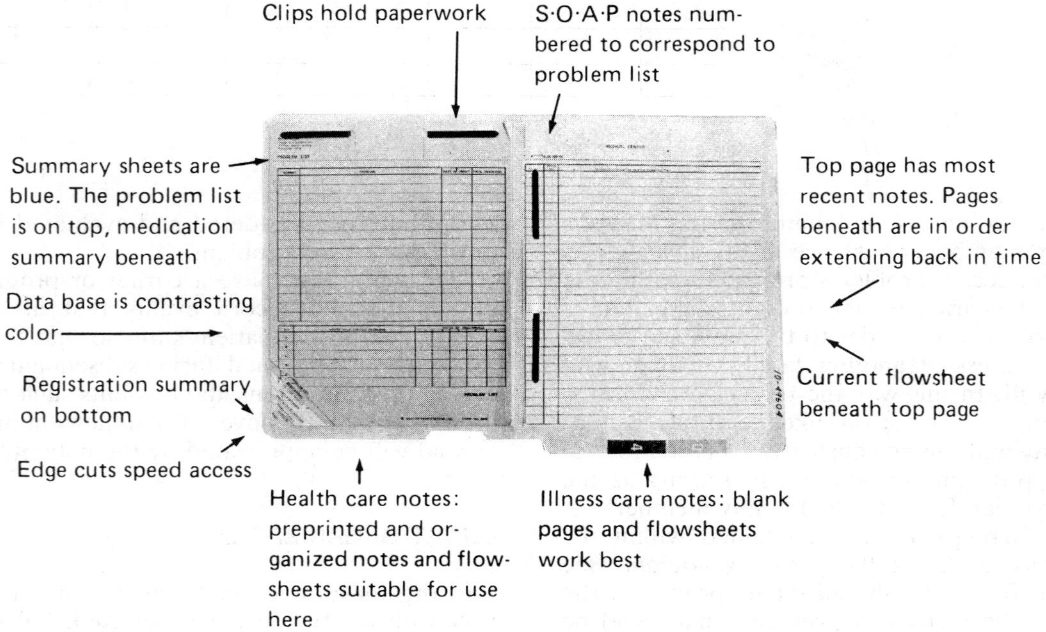
Clips hold paperwork
S·O·A·P notes numbered to correspond to problem list
Summary sheets are blue. The problem list is on top, medication summary beneath
Data base is contrasting color
Registration summary on bottom
Edge cuts speed access
Top page has most recent notes. Pages beneath are in order extending back in time
Current flowsheet beneath top page
Health care notes: preprinted and organized notes and flowsheets suitable for use here
Illness care notes: blank pages and flowsheets work best

Figure 73–6. One method of arranging the chart using the problem-oriented format. (From Sullivan, R. J., Jr.: Medical Record and Index Systems for Community Practice. Cambridge, Massachusetts, Ballinger Publishing Co., 1979.)

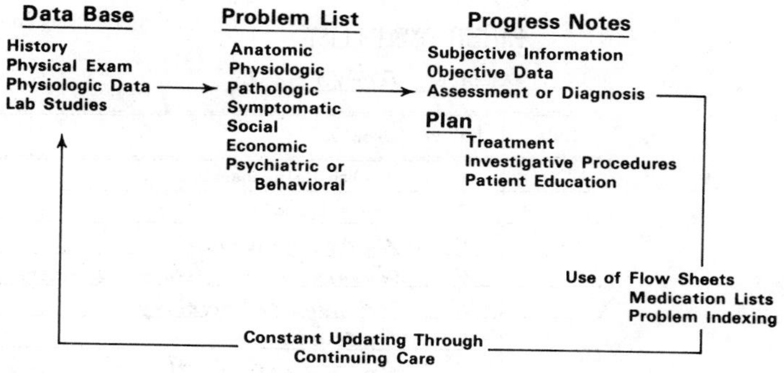

Figure 73–7. Basic elements of the problem-oriented medical record.

view of the patient's present and past state of health. It indicates whether the problems are active or have occurred in the past but are at present inactive. The problem list is a reminder of what has occurred so that the physician can be helped to remember that the patient had a cholecystectomy or hysterectomy and thus does not continue to ask about the function of these organs while obtaining a history.

Problems can be any of the following:

1. Anatomic (hernia)
2. Physiologic (jaundice of unknown etiology)
3. A sign (hepatomegaly)
4. A symptom (dyspnea, fatigue)
5. Economic (financial difficulty)
6. Social (marital discord, spouse alcoholic)
7. Psychiatric (depression)
8. Physical handicap (paralysis, amputation)
9. Specific diagnosis (acute rheumatic fever)
10. Abnormal laboratory test (elevated blood urea nitrogen, elevated sedimentation rate)
11. Risk factor (family history of diabetes mellitus or of cancer)

Risk factors can either be included in the major problem list or listed separately, as in Figure 73–8.

Each problem is numbered, and the progress notes are keyed by number to the appropriate problem on the list, thereby reflecting its present state of resolution. The management of each problem is consistently identified throughout the text by this same number.

The types of illness seen by a family physician are often more appropriately described as symptoms or undifferentiated problems than as diseases. *Disease* implies a full understanding of the pathology and etiology of the illness, whereas many of the illnesses encountered by the family physician involve a varying degree of insight into the underlying etiology and a varying severity of the illness, which occasionally resolves while still in the undifferentiated state.

The problem list is a dynamic picture of the patient's health problems and is continually changed by updating, as new problems are added or old problems are carried to a greater degree of resolution. It should contain all of the patient's continuing problems and should have a prominent position in the record, so as to constantly remind the physician to care for the whole patient and not to limit attention to the problem that may be temporarily outstanding. One value of the problem list is that it continually "stares back at you" and prevents the physician from focusing on too limited an area to the exclusion of the patient's total health picture. With such a format, it is possible to rapidly orient oneself to the most important current problem without forgetting the others.

All problems can be kept in proper perspective. One physician on call for another can rapidly grasp the essential nature of a case by scanning the problem list and thereby can make a more rational decision regarding the acute presenting problem. To do this however, the problems should be *printed* for ease of reading and rapid scanning. The POMR also allows for more efficient use of allied health personnel, by permitting the physician to effectively communicate an assessment of the patient's problems and their management.

In the traditional SOMR, it is difficult to retrieve and correlate information about one particular problem. In the POMR, this information is arranged according to the problem for which it is intended. The basic concept of the POMR is that the problem is the functional unit. All activities relating to the care of the patient, including progress notes, history, physical findings, and therapy, refer to the specific problem for which treatment was initiated. The constant surveillance of the patient's state of health by the physician and allied health personnel and their efforts toward establishing effective health maintenance require constant monitoring of health hazards and risk factors. These risk factors should be identified on the problem list and should serve constantly to alert all health personnel to their presence.

It has been appropriately said that the main value of the POMR is not its structure but its honesty. The POMR demands that all problems be described straightforwardly and at their present stage of development and resolution, no matter how elementary the terms used to describe them may be. It insists that physicians list only what they *know* to be present, not what they *think* to be present. The principle to be followed is "record what is known, not what is supposed." The POMR discourages guesswork and

PATIENT PROBLEM LIST

NAME *Wanda Smith*
DATE OF BIRTH *8-25-21*
FAMILY # *50-13-62*
HOSPITAL # *70-59438*

Code	No.	Problem	Date Onset	Date Recorded	Comments:
	1	Health Maintenance			
	2	Acute Episode			
	3.	*Hypertension*	*1970*	*1/14/82*	
	4.	*Degenerative Joint Disease*	*1976*	*1/14/82*	
	5.	*S/P Hysterectomy*	*1976*		*Fibroid*
	6.	*Depression*	*1980*		
	7.	*Rt. Carotid Bruit, Asymptomatic*	*1981*		

ALLERGIES:

Code	RISK FACTORS	Date	Comments:
	Strong Family History of Diabetes		
	Carcinoma of Breast in Mother		

IMMUNIZATIONS	DATE	DATE	DATE	DATE	DATE	IMMUNIZATIONS	DATE	DATE	DATE
DTP						Influenza			
TOPV						Pneumovax	*1/14/82*		
Indicate one: DT, Td, Tet Tox									
Tuberculin Test									
MMR									

3/82

Figure 73–8. Problem list, University of Iowa.

insists on an accurate listing of actual problems and observed facts. As Weed (1971) has said, "The problem list should not contain diagnostic guesses; it should simply state the problems at a level of refinement consistent with the physician's understanding, running the gamut from the precise diagnosis to the isolated, unexplained finding."

The POMR does not demand excessive compulsiveness but does require that all significant factors be displayed so that they cannot be ignored. Abnormal data should be placed on the problem list and accounted for. The logic behind clinical decisions will be apparent in the POMR, and caution should be taken to avoid drawing conclusions prematurely; for example, a combination of a low hemoglobin level and an elevated reticulocyte count does not equal iron deficiency anemia. More information is necessary to reach that conclusion.

Design of the Problem List

The problem list can be structured in a variety of ways. Physicians should select those components considered most desirable and arrange them in the manner most appropriate to their practice. Most practices design their own problem list, but a large variety of formats are available commercially. The University of Iowa problem list (see Fig. 73–8) has separate columns for coding, problem number, problem, date of onset of problem, date problem recorded, and comments. Another format is that used at Baylor College of Medicine listing acute and chronic problems on the same page (Fig. 73–9).

Acute, Self-Limited Problems. Some programs use a separate problem list for acute, self-limited problems, since only chronic problems should be placed on the master problem list. These temporary problems can be listed separately, as shown in Figure 73–9, or on a separate page entirely. The frequency of recurrence is indicated by dates of occurrence. In this manner, recurring acute problems, such as otitis media or acute bronchitis that can be potentially threatening to the patient's future health, can be identified and transferred to the major problem list.

An alternative method for identifying acute prob-

MR-1-11/88

BAYLOR FAMILY PRACTICE CENTER
PROBLEM LIST
Please Print

Name Smith, Sandra   Date of Birth 7-13-32

NO.	DATE	CHRONIC PROBLEMS AND RISK FACTORS	COMMENTS
1.	2/86	HEALTH MAINTENANCE	
2.	2/86	Hypertension	
3.	2/86	FH Colon CA	
4.	7/89	CA Breast	(L) Mastectomy - 2 pos. nodes
5.	9/89	Depression	
		ALLERGIES	PCN

		ACUTE PROBLEMS	RECURRENCES											
	3/20/86	Bronchitis												
	5/30/87	Low back pain												
	6/21/87	Contact dermatitis												
	6/88	Vaginitis												
	3/89	UTI												

Figure 73–9. Problem list, Baylor College of Medicine, Houston, Texas.

lems is to list them as "Problem No. 2," as in Figure 73–8. When this method is used, all acute, self-limited problems are labeled Problem No. 2 in the progress notes, with the name of the problem also listed next to the heading of No. 2. In a similar manner, the label "Problem No. 1" is permanently assigned to health maintenance activities and stresses the emphasis on preventive measures in family practice.

Some systems prefer to use letters for the acute problems, assigning the next letter in the alphabet to each new acute problem whether or not a separate acute problem list is used. Others believe that temporary problems can be handled in the progress notes only and need not be identified on the problem list. This simplifies the record system but runs the risk of failing to recognize recurring acute problems that deserve greater visibility and continuous monitoring. Most acute and temporary problems that are encountered, however, are self-limiting and usually do not recur with a frequency that requires their being placed on the master problem list.

Components of the Problem List. Legibility is an important component of the problem list. Problems should be either typed or printed in large letters to support the major function of the list: that the problems be "visible at a glance."

A variety of methods can be used to illustrate the active or inactive status of each problem. Those problems that have been resolved but may have an impact upon the patient's future health must be retained on the problem list for continued visibility. A resolved problem can be transferred to a separate inactive column, or it can be identified by indicating the date of resolution under "comments" or in a separate column. It can also be identified by drawing a line or arrow through the problem.

When a higher level of understanding or sophistication is reached for any active problem or combination of problems, these should be changed to a single, new problem. This resolution to a higher level can be indicated by listing the date of resolution of the earlier problem and adding the newer problem at the bottom of the list. Another method is to draw an arrow from the previous problem to the newer designation while maintaining the same problem number and position on the problem list, space permitting. If a comment column is used, the reason for this change can be noted. Otherwise, future information can be identified by placing over the arrow the date of the office visit at which information leading to the increased resolution was obtained. An example of such a change in problem status is the listing of "dyspnea on exertion" and "peripheral edema" as separate problems that are then resolved to "congestive heart failure," once the presence of renal disease has been ruled out. Another example would be the change of the problem of "pain, right knee" to "degenerative joint disease" when x-ray exams identify the specific cause.

Family Problem List. Family problem lists are a method of depicting the problems of each family member on the same page, along with problems that involve the entire family unit (Fig. 73–10). Many family physicians prefer to include this information as part of the family genogram instead of using a family problem list.

Whatever the method of organization, this comprehensive, visible, and concise overview of problems enables the physician to provide family-oriented care while keeping the ongoing problems of individual members in proper perspective. The only real disadvantage of a family problem list is the limited amount of space available and, thus, the limited amount of information that can be documented. If a family problem list is used, it should be prominently displayed in the family folder and should be the only place that master problems are listed. This should force the physician to look at the family as a whole. Unfortunately, there is some risk that the physician may focus on the individual's record to the exclusion of information in the family folder.

The family problem list emphasizes the fact that no one in the family can have a problem without affecting other members in some manner; in fact, the problems of greatest importance are those that by their very nature affect each family member (Grace et al., 1977). The family problem list gives the physician an awareness of the entire family's health problems. It serves as a reminder of the problems of other members who are not being seen but may need attention or follow-up.

DATA BASE

The data base is the first step toward developing the problem list. It is the platform upon which the structure of the POMR depends for stability. The data base consists of the history (chief complaint, present illness, past history, systems review, and social history), physical examination, physiologic data, and baseline laboratory studies. The data base on each patient varies depending upon age, sex, and race. Each physician should define the minimum amount of data that will be collected on all patients in the practice so that office personnel can assist in assuring that this minimum is accomplished. The collection of most elements of the data base can be assigned to allied health professionals who can obtain the information prior to the physician's involvement.

The data base serves as the groundwork for each patient's future care and should include those tests that are effective screening procedures for significant disease or are likely to be good reference points for future problems; for example, elevations of blood pressure can have a significant long-term detrimental effect, and a mild elevation may go undetected if an earlier baseline determination is not available for comparison. The data base should concentrate on the problem that cannot afford to be missed and should include those tests that are of greatest value in detecting these problems. Active debate will continue

FAMILY PROBLEM LIST

NAME	ADDRESS	PHONE
Simpson	1842 Eastwood	337-2104

Problem No.	Date	PROBLEM DESCRIPTION	Problem No.	Date	PROBLEM DESCRIPTION
		William DOB 2/6/39			Margaret DOB 6/6/41
1	1969	Alcoholism	1	1964	Obesity
2	1969	Chronic underemployment	2	1969	Recurrent tension headaches
3	7/70	Allergic rhinitis	3	1974	Depression
4	2/72	Hypertension, essential	4	1974	Contraception
5			5	1976	Cholecystectomy
6			6		
7			7		
8			8		
9			9		
10			10		
11			11		
12			12		
		Ann DOB 10/29/60			James DOB 8/21/64
1	1970	Allergic rhinitis	1	4/70	Asthma
2	11/73	School problem	2	2/75	Behavior problem
3	6/76	Recurrent abdominal pain	3		
4			4		
5			5		
6			6		
		Gary DOB 4/4/71			DOB
1	6/74	Allergic rhinitis	1		
2	10/74	Recurrent otitis media	2		
3	2/75	Penicillin allergy	3		
4			4		
5			5		
6			6		

PROBLEMS OF FAMILY AS A WHOLE

1. Economic problems
2. Marital discord
3. Parent - child conflict
4. Allergies

Figure 73–10. Family problem list. (From Grace, N. T., Neal, E. M., Wellock, C. E., and Pile, D. D.: The family-oriented medical record. J. Fam. Prac., 4:91–98, 1977.)

regarding the need for various routine tests; the issue of which test is the most reliable indicator of potentially significant disease will be settled only by further research. Tests to be emphasized in the data base are those that detect disease at its earliest, presymptomatic phase so that the normal course of the disease can be interrupted and its impact minimized.

A complete data base is so essential to the success of the POMR that many physicians place "incomplete data base" as "Problem No. 1" on the list, where it remains until all required data have been obtained. A commitment should be made to obtain all of the data within a given period of time. If a complete history and physical examination cannot be obtained at one visit, information can still be collected bit by bit during a series of visits over a period of time. The visibility of an incomplete data base as Problem No. 1 serves as a constant reminder to continue accumulating the data, regardless of the nature of the episodic visit.

Health Maintenance Forms

A variety of forms have been developed to help monitor routine screening activities. These usually indicate the tests that should be performed at different ages to detect potentially serious disease in its earliest stage. Figure 73–11 *A* and *B* illustrates the elements identified by faculty and residents at Baylor College of Medicine as those that should be monitored periodically from 20 to 79 years of age. Clear blocks indicate that the examination or test should be done at that age; shaded blocks indicate the test is not recommended but information can still be added at that age if the test was not performed when indicated earlier.

History

A variety of new methods for obtaining the medical history have been developed to save the physician time and still allow for an in-depth accumulation of valuable historical information. These health history questionnaires are available as printed forms for the patient to complete, either in the office waiting room or at home prior to the visit. A questionnaire can be either self-designed (see Fig. 74–1) or purchased commercially. If a significant number of positive findings appear on the general health history questionnaire, more detailed preprinted questionnaires are also available in cardiovascular, gas-

A

BAYLOR FAMILY PRACTICE CENTER
HEALTH MAINTENANCE PROFILE

PATIENT______________________ DATE __________

AGE	20	21	22	23	24	25	26	27	28	29	30	31	32	33	34	35	36	37	38	39	40	41	42	43	44	45	46	47	48	49
BLOOD PRESSURE																														
INTERIM H & P																														
HEARING EXAM																														
VISION CHECK																														
TONOMETRY																														
BREAST EXAM																														
MAMMOGRAPHY																														
PAP SMEAR																														
LIPOPROTEIN PROFILE																														
URINALYSIS																														
HEMATOCRIT																														
PPD																														
Td																														
STOOL GUAIAC																														
DIGITAL RECTAL EXAM																														
SIGMOIDOSCOPY																														
EKG (as indicated)																														
CXR (as indicated)																														

RUBELLA TITER/VACCINE	BASELINE EVALUATION DATE:	IF GIVEN, CHECK AND INDICATE DATE. VACCINE	CHECK IF TITER INDICATES IMMUNITY. TITER

ADDITIONAL RECOMMENDED SCREENING

Key: N = Normal/Performed A = Abnormal R= Refused

These are general recommendations for the population at large. They should be modified as needed on a case by case basis. Please consult your personal physician regarding the specific tests and schedule recommended for you.

Figure 73–11. *A* and *B*, Health maintenance profile, Baylor College of Medicine, Houston, Texas.

B

BAYLOR FAMILY PRACTICE CENTER
HEALTH MAINTENANCE PROFILE

PATIENT Dorothy Sanford DATE

AGE	50	51	52	53	54	55	56	57	58	59	60	61	62	63	64	65	66	67	68	69	70	71	72	73	74	75	76	77	78	79
BLOOD PRESSURE						N																								
INTERIM H & P						N																								
HEARING EXAM						N																								
VISION CHECK						N																								
TONOMETRY						N																								
BREAST EXAM						N																								
MAMMOGRAPHY						N																								
PAP SMEAR						N																								
LIPOPROTEIN PROFILE						A																								
URINALYSIS						N																								
HEMATOCRIT						N																								
PPD																														
Td																														
STOOL GUAIAC						N																								
DIGITAL RECTAL EXAM						N																								
SIGMOIDOSCOPY						N																								
EKG (as indicated)						N																								
CXR (as indicated)																														
FLU VACCINE						✓																								
PNEUMOVAX																														

ADDITIONAL RECOMMENDED SCREENING

Key: N= Normal/Performed A= Abnormal R= Refused

These are general recommendations for the population at large. They should be modified as needed on a case by case basis. Please consult your personal physician regarding the specific tests and schedule recommended for you. MR-4, 3-23-88

Figure 73–11 *Continued*

trointestinal, respiratory, or obstetric/gynecologic systems.

When a complete history is being obtained, it is important to have available the records from the patient's previous physicians because the patient may have an unrealistic impression of the pathologic findings present, and accurate assessment of past problems is possible only by reviewing the actual records or a summary from the physicians involved. This information should become a permanent part of the data base and should serve as a reference point for all present and future difficulties in the same areas.

Physical Examination and Physiologic Data

One advantage of using a printed physical examination sheet is the ability to easily identify information that has been obtained in part but has yet to be completed. A highly structured "check-off" format is sometimes used. This makes it possible to set a goal for completeness and to know when that goal has been reached or what remains to be done. With a nonstructured, open-ended format, it is difficult to tell how much remains incomplete. The structured method, as developed by the Promis Clinic in Hampden Highlands, Maine, permits the easy identification of items to be obtained by allied health professionals prior to the physician's examination. It also allows for the comparison of data on four successive complete evaluations. Illustrations of body parts can be used in addition to the written report to depict abnormalities detected during a physical examination.

Some practices insist upon a comprehensive data base for all new patients and will not accept patients for treatment beyond the second visit for an episodic illness until the standard comprehensive examination is completed. Following the completion of this examination, the patient is sent a summary of the findings, including a problem list and the plans for following each problem. The patient is asked to review the material for accuracy and to keep it for a permanent record.

Laboratory Data

A valuable time-saving practice is to transfer all laboratory report slips to a standard laboratory data sheet (Fig. 73–12). This method avoids the bulk and confusion that a mass of laboratory slips in a variety of colors and sizes contributes to the medical record. Fears that mistakes can be made when transferring the data have been shown to be mostly unfounded, and the significant amount of time saved in retrieving and comparing a sequence of laboratory information arranged side by side chronologically is well worth the time and effort involved. This ability to follow the variations of a single or multiple tests over time on a single page is of significant benefit in maintaining an accurate overview of the patient's laboratory data, especially when compared with the system of "shingling" laboratory slips that requires a variety of slips to be found and lifted if one is to follow a sequence of tests such as serum potassium, T_4, glucose, or cholesterol.

Standard computer printouts of laboratory tests performed outside the office are popular and are reported in a variety of formats. Some of these can be designed to allow placement in the chart so that chronologic documentation of single tests is possible.

It is also useful to document chronologically the dates and results of Papanicolaou smears, electrocardiograms, x-ray exams, and other selected items. The actual report forms (if they contain a more detailed description of an abnormality) can be filed to the rear of the chart. Once complete information is transferred to the appropriate section of the data base form, the slip can be discarded.

The data base should also identify all allergies and should include a summary of all immunizations, hospitalizations, and consultations. In this manner, the physician can note at a glance whether a patient has any allergies, has ever been hospitalized, or has ever required consultation by other physicians. Organizing data in this manner may take slightly longer, but the time saved in retrieval more than compensates for the effort. The chronologic order of information in both the progress notes and the laboratory data is particularly useful in family practice because changes over time and frequency of involvement can be visualized and coordinated. When there is an abnormal laboratory or physiologic finding that cannot be explained by a problem already on the problem list, it is included as a new problem and maintains that visibility until it is resolved by further diagnosis or treatment.

Progress Notes

Well-organized and logically structured progress notes in combination with the problem list are the secret of the POMR's effectiveness in promoting continuing patient care. Progress notes are divided into four main components: subjective information, objective data, assessment, and plan (Fig. 73–13). These components correspond to the history, physical examination, diagnosis, and treatment sections of the traditional record. The acronym SOAP is used to describe the POMR format of a progress note and is a more descriptive and more easily pronounced term than would be the acronym HPEDT. An essential feature of any useful record is the organization of major components of the progress notes, placing the most important features in a consistent and readily identifiable position. The historical or subjective data should consistently occupy one specific position and the plan of management, or therapeutic data, another. The actual location is insignificant, as long as each maintains a separate, easily located, and readily visible identity.

Each progress note is keyed by number to its problem on the problem list, and the problem number and title serve as headings for each progress note. In

PATIENT NAME Jones, Betty

BLOOD CHEMISTRY

PROFILES

	NORMAL RANGE			
DATE		11-1-74	10-16-75	8-18-76
TOT PROTEIN	5.9-8.0	7.1	6.8	7.3
ALBUMIN	3.2-5.0	3.8	4.0	3.7
Ca	8.8-11.0	9.7	10.0	10.2
IN. PO_4	2.2-4.8	2.9	2.7	3.0
CHOL	150-220	228	244	215
GLUCOSE	71-117	85	95	83
BUN	5-24	10	13	12
URIC ACID	2.3-6	3.2	3.3	3.7
ALK PHOS	0.6-2.5	1.1	1.0	1.3
LDH	280-770	538	544	575
TOT BIL	0.2-1.0	0.5	0.4	0.5
SGOT	10-49	20	24	26
Na	135-150	141	136	142
K	3.0-5.0	5.4	5.0	4.8
Cl	94-110	102	98	99
CO_2				
BUN				
CREATININE	0.2-1.7	0.8	1.0	1.2

INDIVIDUAL TESTS

DATE		11-1-74	10-16-75	8-18-76	9-13-76
VDRL		Neg			
T3	.80-1.20	.99			
T4	4.0-11.0	9.3			
Free Thyroxine index	3.2-13.2	9.2			
Cholesterol	150-220	228	244	215	220

Figure 73–12. Laboratory data form, University of Iowa.

this manner, all information pertaining to a particular problem and the ongoing plan for managing that problem are easily identified throughout the record. This system allows for rapid assessment of a problem and its stage of resolution by all health personnel. It prevents the POMR from being a disorganized "flight of ideas," as is so frequently the case with the SOMR. Progress notes in the SOMR format are usually long and the information is randomly arranged. Progress notes in the POMR format are in outline form and frequently contain more data, although fewer words (Fig. 73–14).

Every problem need not be described in a progress note at each visit. Comments need be made regarding only those problems that are pertinent to that visit and for which some change of status or new information is noted. Likewise, every item or component of the progress note need not be commented upon at each visit. If there is no change in status or no new information available, that section, whether it be the subjective, objective, assessment, or plan, should be omitted or a dash inserted to indicate "no need for comment." Meaningless terms such as "doing well" or "status quo" are of little value and should be avoided. All progress information is documented chronologically, and health professionals other than the physician insert their comments or observations in the same manner as the physician.

As new information is accumulated during each visit, the progress notes are used to provide feedback to continually update and modify the problem list. It is also possible to describe more than one problem per visit.

Subjective Information. This includes the history of the problem and all descriptive information perceived as important by the patient, including symptoms and feelings. This is an interpretation of the problem from the patient's point of view.

Objective Data. This term refers to those items noted on examination by the physician or allied health personnel. These data include all measurements and factual information obtained by independent observers, and they represent the facts undistorted by bias. Information within this section should also be arranged consistently in the same order; e.g., data concerning blood pressure, temperature, pulse, and respiration. There is, by the way, no firm rule that objective data follow the subjective. Some physicians

POMR
Progress Note

Date ____ Pt. Name __________ Age ____
Prob. No. ____ Title ______________

S	Subjective Information	Present Complaint Symptoms Family and Social History Past History
O	Objective Information	Physical Findings Physiological Data Laboratory Data
A	Assessment	Diagnosis Present Status of Problem
P	Plan	Therapy Medication Procedures Investigations Laboratory Tests Identify "Rule-outs" Patient Education

Figure 73–13. Major components of the POMR progress note.

prefer to have the objective first so that it can be located more easily.

Assessment. This refers to either the diagnosis or a description of the problem at its present stage of resolution. Guesswork is not permitted, and only the degree of resolution that can be supported by data is described.

Problem-solving techniques are a fundamental component of traditional medical education. Problem recognition, however, is too often modified by a haste to play the academic game of one-upmanship and to establish a diagnosis rapidly and with the least amount of data. The POMR lays bare any attempt to short cut the establishment of a sound diagnosis based on the logical acquisition of adequate data. This does not mean, however, that a differential diagnosis is to be avoided, since all "rule-outs" and potential causes for the problem should be reflected accurately in the record so that the problem can be pursued to a definite conclusion. This conclusion may be either the complete disappearance of the sign or symptoms without a final diagnosis ever being reached or the combining of a variety of symptoms and signs into a definite diagnosis.

Plan. This refers to the diagnostic and therapeutic modalities used in the management of the problem. This section should include all present medications, laboratory tests, procedures (such as exercise or inhalation therapy), further diagnostic plans (such as x-ray studies), patient education (such as informative literature and diet instruction), counseling methods, and the use of consultants. The entire plan (or treatment) section is the most important portion of the progress notes and should be prominently located so that it can be easily found, since future evaluation requires the comparison of outcome with previous treatment plans to determine whether the results obtained match previous expectations. In this manner, the success or failure of earlier plans can be measured. The use of a green or red pen to write the plan will make this section stand out and be easily identified.

A well-thought-out plan helps to maintain continuity of care and allows the physician to communicate to an associate on call the plans for the patient's management. Three major subdivisions constitute the execution of the plan:

1. *Diagnostic studies* should contain the "rule-outs" and the tests to be used in this process of differential diagnosis, e.g., to rule out peptic ulcer,

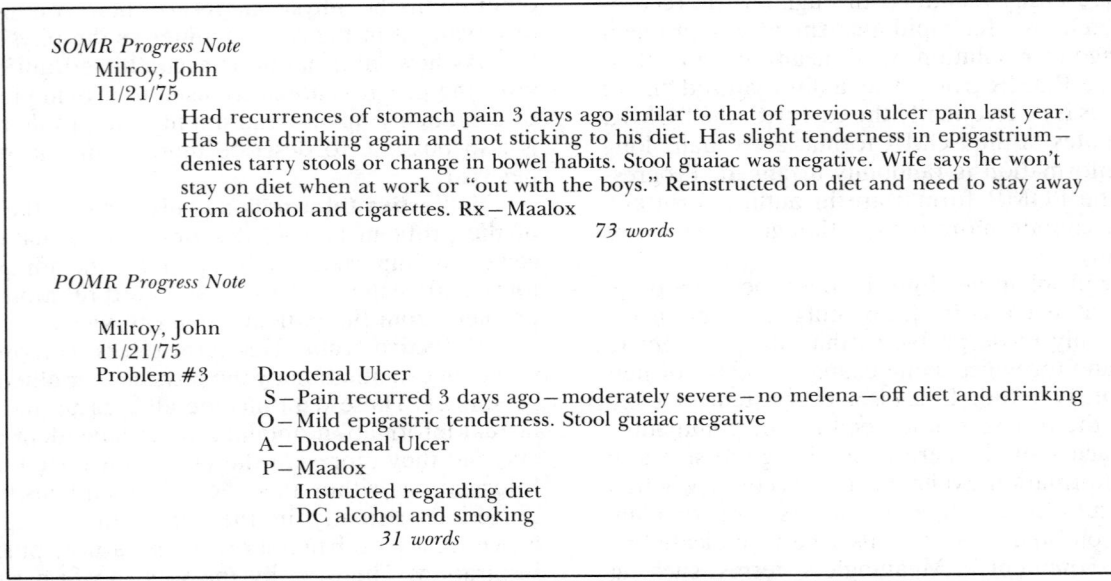

SOMR Progress Note
Milroy, John
11/21/75

Had recurrences of stomach pain 3 days ago similar to that of previous ulcer pain last year. Has been drinking again and not sticking to his diet. Has slight tenderness in epigastrium—denies tarry stools or change in bowel habits. Stool guaiac was negative. Wife says he won't stay on diet when at work or "out with the boys." Reinstructed on diet and need to stay away from alcohol and cigarettes. Rx—Maalox

73 words

POMR Progress Note

Milroy, John
11/21/75
Problem #3 Duodenal Ulcer
S—Pain recurred 3 days ago—moderately severe—no melena—off diet and drinking
O—Mild epigastric tenderness. Stool guaiac negative
A—Duodenal Ulcer
P—Maalox
Instructed regarding diet
DC alcohol and smoking

31 words

Figure 73–14. Comparison of volume and organization of SOMR and POMR progress notes.

obtain an upper gastrointestinal tract series, stool guaiac determination, and so forth. Under the heading of diagnostic studies would also be included the laboratory tests to be done at the next visit. The nurse or laboratory technician will then be alerted to obtain these prior to the physician's involvement. The diagnostic studies category means that more information is needed, and it lists the tests to be conducted to assist in the future evaluation of a problem.

2. *Therapeutic measures* include medications and other treatment modalities.

3. *Patient education* consists of the factors necessary for patient understanding and compliance. This, too, is often a neglected area and therefore warrants visibility by including it as a regular item in the progress notes. The patient education section is of greatest importance for patients with chronic problems, since treatment of one form or another will be a constant feature throughout their lives. The patient should know what to expect from treatment, what side effects are possible, and how a specific medication might react with other drugs or foods. Unexpected events should be avoided as much as possible so that maximum compliance will be maintained. The patient also needs adequate insight into the problem to know when to seek help without further delay. When patient instruction is given, whether this be the distribution of an American Heart Association booklet on hypertension or information about the hazards of smoking, it should be documented in the record so that other health personnel who share responsibility for continuing education of the patient will remain informed.

Hospital Discharge Summaries

These summaries should also be organized in the POMR format, with each problem being identified and numbered and the pertinent information "SOAPed." This record (the discharge summary) is then incorporated into the office record at the appropriate chronologic point to assist in the continuing care of the patient during future office visits.

Avoiding Legal Pitfalls

Juries have a tendency to believe that if an event is not recorded it never occurred, so a complete and accurate medical record is the physician's best defense in a malpractice suit. Often there is a 2- or 3-year delay before a case reaches court and recall from memory will be difficult. Therefore, an accurate and legible record is essential.

Every page of the medical record should bear the patient's name. Progress notes should be signed, dated, arranged chronologically, and typed or written in ink, never pencil.

Derogatory, trivial, or loose comments about patients or colleagues should not be recorded; they could prove embarrassing if publicized during a legal review. Similarly, vague and ambiguous statements, such as "the patient is feeling better," should be avoided.

ALTERING A RECORD

Adding or changing a statement is no problem if done correctly and if no suit is pending. However, altering the record after a suit has been filed is the kiss of death. This is considered tampering and arouses suspicions that are difficult to dispel. If it is necessary to change an entry in the chart because of an error, the inaccurate material should be crossed out with a single line so that the words remain legible. The change should be initialed and the date and time noted in the margin with a note explaining why the change was made.

DOCUMENTING PHONE CALLS

It is wise to document every telephone call received in the office. Requests for prescription refills should be documented in the medical record as should any call involving medical advice or treatment.

WORDS TO AVOID

Medical records are not privileged and confidential; the information belongs to the patient. Maligning or deprecatory remarks are certainly inappropriate. Words that should be avoided are "simple," "routine," and "uncomplicated," since they suggest a guarantee or predict a good outcome. If the patient is described as uncooperative, the reasons should be documented. Similarly, if patients refuse certain diagnostic tests or procedures this should be documented along with the reason for recommending the test. The fact that the patient was informed of the need for the test is also important. A suit has never been successfully brought because the physician gave the patient too much information.

Flow Sheets

Flow sheets are a useful adjunct to any medical record system, particularly when the POMR is used in conjunction with continuing patient care and the management of chronic illnesses. It is sometimes difficult to review the course of a single problem over time using progress notes because a great deal of page turning is required to pick out that problem on successive visits. Placing the prolonged course of a single problem, or even selected multiple problems, on one flow sheet greatly facilitates comprehension and management. Flow sheets are also useful in any clinical situation requiring the monitoring of multiple laboratory and therapeutic data over a long period of time. They present an overview of the illness, compressing events over time onto one page, and allow the physician to identify current values as well as observe trends in the course of a disease. Flow sheets permit speedy retrieval of data and facilitate the ongoing analysis of the stage of chronic illness by indicating changing trends in response to therapy.

Once the parameters to be monitored have been identified, the flow sheet serves as a constant reminder to review these items and acts as an early warning system for potential problems by indicating variations from the previous pattern or baseline. Such sheets allow for a large amount of physiologic and management data to be accumulated in a compact area and observed at a glance.

When laboratory data have been entered on the flow sheet, they can be, but do not need to be, entered on the data base form as well. Just as with the data base form, the laboratory slip is filed elsewhere or discarded and is not retained in the chart. Avoid double entry whenever possible because one or the other will frequently be omitted, resulting in confusion or extra time spent searching. The flow sheet permits ready comparison of all determinations of a single test. It also permits physiologic and laboratory data to be monitored on the same time scale as therapeutic management. When material is categorized in this manner, physicians tend to write more concise and clearer notes, including fewer irrelevant details.

The time required to enter data on a flow sheet is much less than the time that is lost in sorting out disorganized information in the traditional record. A partially used flow sheet, however, can be more inefficient than none at all, since the physician is then required to search back and forth among the flow sheet, progress notes, and data base for the complete information.

The flow sheet can be a simple piece of graph paper, a self-designed form (Fig. 73–15), or a preprinted form. In each instance, the left-hand column should contain the elements considered essential to the ongoing management of the problems being followed. Just as the data base must be individually designed for each practice, the flow sheet must be suited to the preferences of the physician and must be designed to measure those items considered most important in the management of the illnesses for which it is used.

Items to be monitored on a flow sheet usually include:

1. Frequency of symptoms
2. Physiologic data, such as weight, edema, and blood pressure
3. Laboratory data, such as fasting blood glucose levels, urine cultures, and serum potassium and serum cholesterol levels
4. Medications
5. Nondrug therapy, such as diet and physical therapy
6. Patient compliance
7. Patient education

Flow sheets serve as memory aids and guard against the possibility of important aspects of a patient's continuing care being overlooked by the physician. For example, when monitoring the course of a diabetic patient, the physician may forget to regularly check the fundi or peripheral pulses for potential vascular change. Listing these as areas to be evaluated at prescribed intervals, along with the blood glucose level and other specifics, will serve as a reminder to all office personnel. The data-gathering activities of allied health personnel can easily be incorporated into the structure of the flow sheet by identifying those parameters to be measured at the next visit prior to the physician's examination. The flow sheet should monitor problems at intervals that will reflect the degree of stability of the illness; the more acute and unstable the problem, the more frequently measurements will be required. Items should be monitored often enough to ensure good care without undue expense. In an intensive care unit, the intervals between items are minutes or hours, whereas in the outpatient setting, they are days, weeks, or months.

The chart format of a flow sheet also minimizes problems caused by illegible handwriting. Effective use of flow sheets may obviate the need for progress notes when repeated visits relate only to the ongoing management of the chronic illnesses followed on the flow sheet. When progress notes are necessary, "see flow sheet" will frequently suffice in lieu of entries in the objective and plan categories.

Well-Child Care Forms

A variety of methods for documenting well-child care has been developed. These provide reminders of the normal developmental milestones during early development, immunizations and laboratory tests, patient education, and physical examination. The form shown in Figure 73–16 not only permits the documentation of well-child care up to school entry but also serves as a reminder of those features that should be checked periodically on physical examinations, such as hips (for dysplasia), vision, and hearing. Standard patient education handouts are developed for each age group, and brief developmental milestones are documented. If there is any question as to whether these have been reached, a complete Denver Development Test is done. Since this form is accompanied by a growth chart, the appropriate box is checked when the measurement is plotted on the growth chart, including head circumference until 12 months and adding blood pressure at age 4 years. If significant abnormalities are found during the physical examination, they are more thoroughly documented in the standard progress note format, as are intercurrent acute illnesses (see also Eggertsen et al., 1980, and Margolis, 1977). A similar form continues this format for ages 5

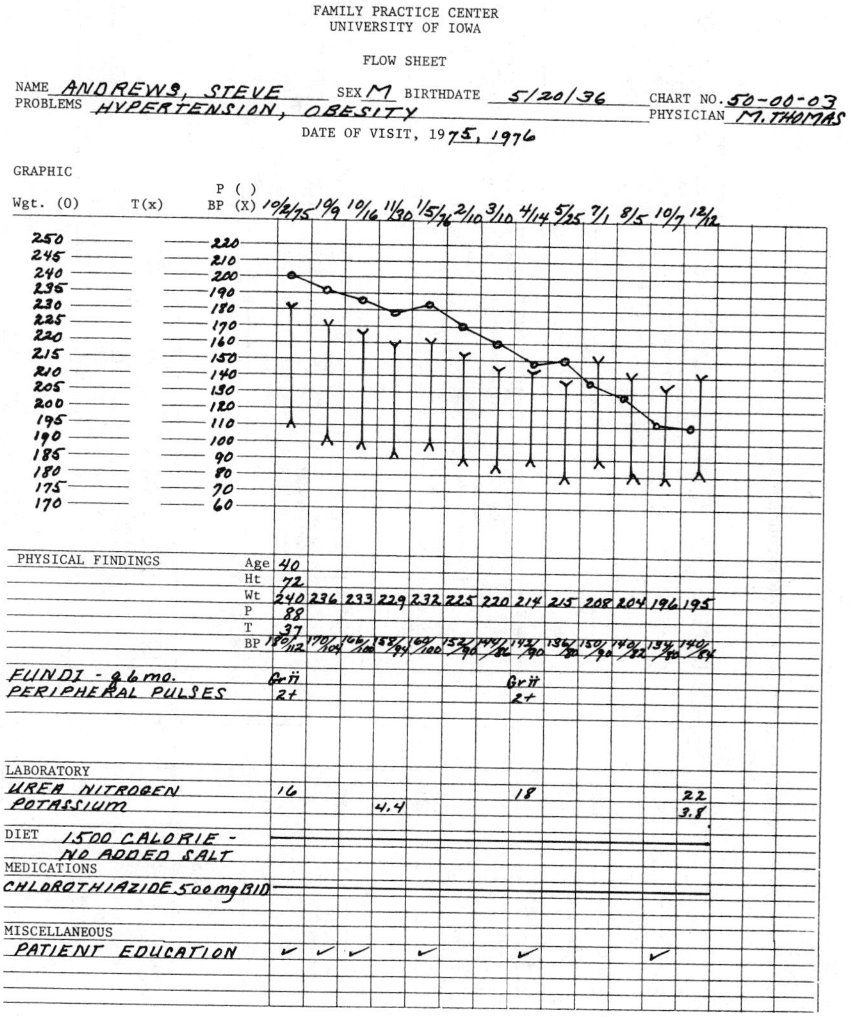

Figure 73–15. Flow sheet for a patient with hypertension and obesity, University of Iowa, Family Practice Center. (From Rakel, RE.: Principles of Family Medicine. Philadelphia, W. B. Saunders Co., 1977.)

through 18 years, so that on two pages well-child care from birth to age 18 can be succinctly documented.

Medication Lists

Almost from the beginning, medication lists have been a component of the problem-oriented medical record as it is used in family practice. Chronic medications are frequently documented below the problem list or in a similar prominent location. It is difficult, however, to keep these lists current, for as soon as omissions occur, the list becomes more trouble than it is worth since it must be checked against the progress notes for accuracy. A variety of other methods are in use, the most accurate involving a direct copy of all prescriptions written. Figure 73–17 is an illustration of the medication list used at the University of Iowa, where pressure-sensitive paper, upon which the prescription is placed when written, is used. Although redundancy occurs, the usefulness of this list lies in its accuracy. Problems arise only if prescriptions are written without being placed over the appropriate area on this sheet.

One way to avoid this problem is to use a medication list such as that developed in the Department of Family Medicine at Baylor College of Medicine (Fig. 73–18). Prescriptions are fixed along the left side of the page by a perforation. An actual copy of the medication prescribed is left on the underlying pressure sensitive sheet. Two medications can be written (one on each line) and the prescription form removed from the page after which the patient's name and physician's signature are entered. If these names are entered before the prescription form is removed, the names will appear on the pressure sensitive sheet on top of the next prescription since the forms are shingled to save space. No loose prescription pads are used so this almost ensures an accurate record of all medications prescribed, plus their strength, quantity, instructions, and number of refills. Space is also allotted for recording the date and reason for discontinuing a drug.

THE UNIVERSITY OF IOWA
DEPARTMENT OF FAMILY PRACTICE
CHILD HEALTH CARE FORM

Name ______________________

Date of Birth ______________________

☑ NORMAL ☒ = ABNORMAL

Birth History ______________ Labor and delivery record in chart ☐

Newborn Exam ______________ Newborn exam record in chart ☐

Birth Weight ______ Gms. ______ Lbs. Breastfeeding ☐ Formula ☐

AGE	ACTUAL AGE	DATE	HT. WT. HC.	DEVELOPMENT	PHYSICAL EXAM		IMMUNIZATIONS/ LABORATORY	EDUCATION
2 WKS.			☐ ☐ ☐	Moro Reflex Symmetrical motor activity	HENT Eyes Lungs Heart Abd.	G.U. Skel. Neuro Skin	PKU (or at 4 wks.)	Hand Out No. 1 Fluoride Iron Vitamins Auto Seat
			ASSESSMENT:				________ M.D. (signed)	
1 MO.			☐ ☐ ☐	Smiles in response to Mother	Blink Red reflex HENT Eyes Lungs Heart	Abd. G.U. Skel. Neuro. Skin		Hand Out No. 2 Nutrition
			ASSESSMENT:				________ M.D. (signed)	
2 MOS.			☐ ☐ ☐	Briefly follows object Vocalizes Head up to 45°	Check hips Femoral pulse Hernia HENT Eyes Lungs	Heart Abd. G.U. Skel. Neuro. Skin	DPT-1 TOPV-1	Hand Out No. 3 Nutrition Recheck fluoride iron vitamins
			ASSESSMENT:				________ M.D. (signed)	
4 MOS.			☐ ☐ ☐	Rolls over Follows object 180° Grasps Sits w/head steady Squeals	Turns toward sound HENT Eyes Lungs Heart	Abd. G.U. Skel. Neuro. Skin	DPT-2 TOPV-2	Hand Out No. 4 Nutrition
			ASSESSMENT:				________ M.D. (signed)	
6 MOS.			☐ ☐ ☐	Feeds self crackers Sits without support Passes cube hand to hand Reaches for objects	Symmetrical light reflection HENT Eyes Lungs Heart	Abd. G.U. Skel. Neuro. Skin	DPT-3 TOPV-3	Hand Out No. 5 Nutrition Discuss solid foods Ipecac Fear of strangers
			ASSESSMENT:				________ M.D. (signed)	

CHILD HEALTH CARE FORM (continued)

AGE	ACTUAL AGE	DATE	HT. WT. HC.	DEVELOPMENT	PHYSICAL EXAM		IMMUNIZATIONS/ LABORATORY	EDUCATION
9 MOS.			☐ ☐ ☐	Peek-a-boo, bye-bye Pulls self to standing Thumb-finger grasp Imitates sounds	Vision-follows dropped object HENT Eyes Lungs Heart	Abd. G.U. Skel. Neuro. Skin	Hct. Sickle cell test if appropriate TBN	Hand Out No. 6 Nutrition Check Amt. of Milk Wean from bottle Discuss discipline
			ASSESSMENT:				________ M.D. (signed)	
12 MOS.			☐ ☐ ☐	Walks holding on Mama, Dada Drinks from cup Plays pat-a-cake	Check hips Cover-uncover test Test hearing HENT Eyes Lungs Heart	Abd. G.U. Skel. Neuro. Skin	(MMR at 15 mos.)	Hand Out No. 7 Nutrition Appetite normal Household safety
			ASSESSMENT:				________ M.D. (signed)	
18 MOS.			☐ ☐	Feeds self w/spoon Walks backward Removes garment Knows simple anatomy	HENT Eyes Lungs Heart Abd.	G.U. Skel. Neuro. Skin	MMR (at 15 mos.) DPT Booster TOPV Booster	Hand Out No. 8 Nutrition Toilet training Discipline
			ASSESSMENT:				________ M.D. (signed)	
2 YRS.			☐ ☐	Puts on clothing Combines 2-3 words Runs well; Stairs one step at a time Draws 1; circular scribbling	HENT Eyes Lungs Heart Abd.	G.U. Skel. Neuro. Skin		Hand Out No. 9 Dental visit Need for peer companionship but unable to share Matches TV supervision
			ASSESSMENT:				________ M.D. (signed)	
3 YRS.			☐ ☐	Dresses w/help Knows full name and age Stand on 1 foot for 1 second Speaks in sentences Draws 0 Toilet trained	Vision Hearing Blood pressure HENT Eyes Lungs	Heart Abd. G.U. Skel. Neuro. Skin		Hand Out No. 10 Knives & electricity TV supervision Dental hygiene
			ASSESSMENT:				________ M.D. (signed)	
4 YRS.			☐ ☐ B. P. /	Dresses self Hops on one foot Draws man w/head and 2-4 parts Knows 3 of 4 colors	Blood pressure HENT Eyes Lungs Heart	Abd. G.U. Skel. Neuro. Skin		Hand Out No. 11 Water safety Traffic safety
			ASSESSMENT:				________ M.D. (signed)	

Figure 73–16. Child Health Care Form, University of Iowa.

Name: Jones, Robert

DRUG ALLERGIES Penicillin — Date of Birth: 7-13-32 — Chart No.: 50-16-32 — Date:

Date	Prescription	Strng.	Quant.	Sig.	# Refills	Problem	Subsequent Refill Information	
5/4/82	Hydrochlorothiazide	50mg	100	i twice daily to lower blood pressure	0		7/1/82 #100	
5/4/82	Tetracycline	250mg	40	i four times daily until gone	0			
9/14/82	Theodur	200mg	120	ii tabs P.O. b.i.d.	4			
9/14/82	Hydrochlorothiazide	50mg	120	i tab P.O. b.i.d	2			
10/19/82	Tetracycline	250mg	40	i tab qid	0			

Figure 73–17. Medication list, University of Iowa, Family Practice Center.

Evaluating Quality of Care

Many physicians perceive "audit" as a threatening term, whereas to others it serves as a source of intellectual stimulation. The challenge is to assess clinical performance and improve professional competence. Bjorn and Cross (1970) have designed their practice to include an ongoing audit system, both internal and external, accomplished by review by office staff and visiting consultants. Their enthusiasm for such auditing procedures indicates that such methods can serve as a source of professional stimulation and improved patient care. They conclude that the practicing physician who does not develop an efficient audit system will "suffer from apathy, bitterness and the general dissatisfaction of conducting a practice devoid of basic intellectual gratifications integral to continued professional growth." A willingness to be reviewed by peers can certainly result in professional stimulation. To be successful, however, audit must be viewed as an experience in learning and as an exciting, intellectually rewarding exercise.

Weed (1971) emphasizes that to be effective and fair, record audit must relate to defined criteria. Everyone must know what is to be measured and how this is to be done. He equates this process with defining the length and width of a football field and the rules of play before the game has begun, rather than after it is under way. Unfortunately, too many audit procedures used in hospitals and clinics today avoid defining specific criteria for audit or do so after the fact. Both the physician and the reviewer should understand what standards are to be used in the review. This involves developing criteria of excellence that all agree to in advance and against which performance can be measured.

Since each patient is unique, it is difficult to design criteria of excellence that apply to all patients with a given problem, such as peptic ulcer. An extensive list of 40 criteria will include many inappropriate items, resulting in a "poor score" that is inaccurate. A brief or limited list of criteria that apply to most patients will give better scores but poor discrimination. Greenfield and colleagues (1978) describe a method of "criteria mapping" that applies branching logic to an extensive list of criteria, result-

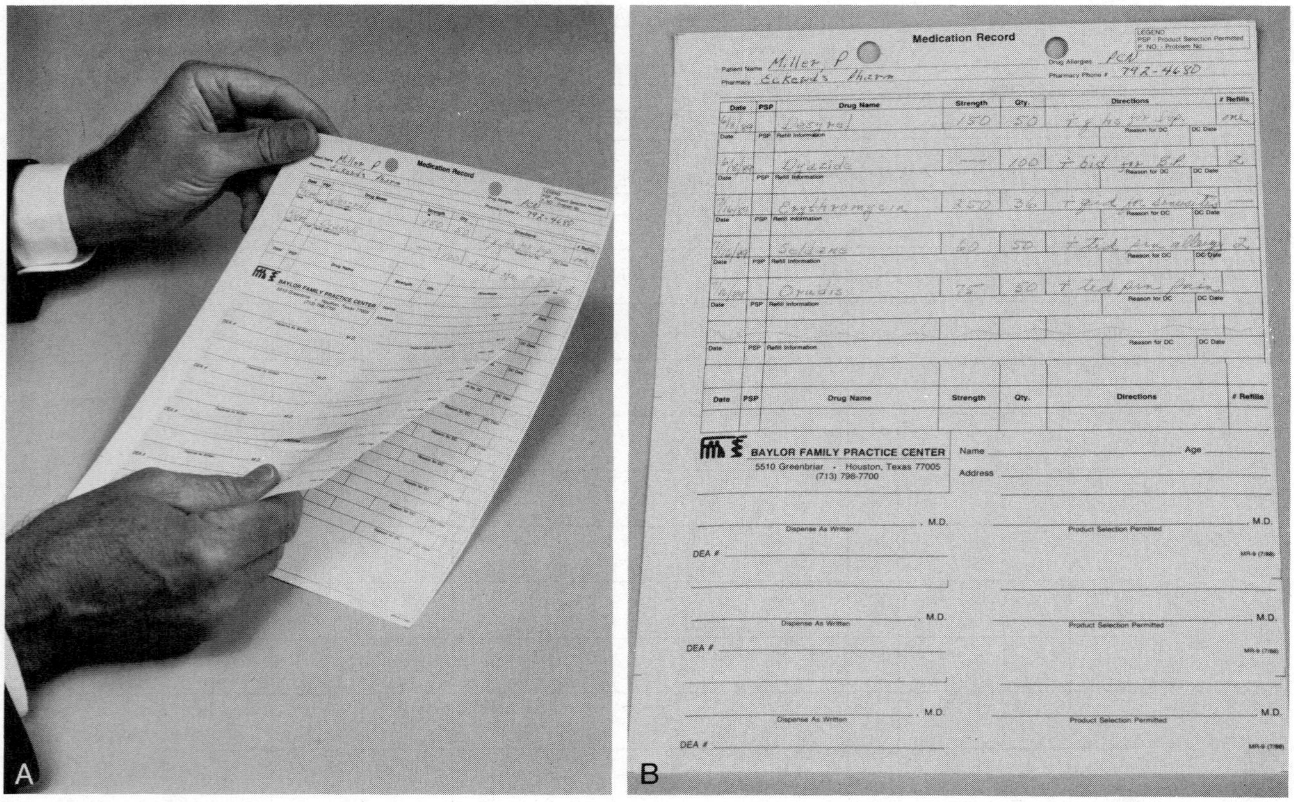

Figure 73–18. Medication record, Baylor College of Medicine, Houston, Texas. *A*, Shingled prescription forms attached along left margin overlying pressure-sensitive copy. *B*, Three of the six forms, containing up to two prescriptions each, have been used.

ing in a patient-specific approach and a more valid assessment of medical care than either the extensive or the limited list of criteria.

Many audits are primarily a content review, involving an analysis of whether or not desired components of the record are properly documented and in place. Evaluating the process of care increases the value of the audit, but a thorough and proper analysis requires the establishing of criteria of excellence so that performance can be measured against these criteria. After standards have been set, the audit determines whether the standards have been met and then assesses the effect of these standards on patient care. The knowledge gained by the audit process should be used to bring about required change, and reaudit should be performed to see if this change did in fact occur and whether or not it was effective. Thus, audit is an ongoing process that continually evaluates quality of care and the ability to improve that quality based upon knowledge gained.

Measurements of outcome of care are the most useful, yet the most difficult, measurements of physician performance. In addition to actual outcome, other components of quality of care include patient expectations, patient satisfaction, and physician satisfaction with outcomes.

The POMR lends itself well to record audit because it encourages the accumulation of data with a minimum of ambiguity. Since there is a defined location for all data relating to a particular problem, it is easy to determine the presence or absence of those data. The data base defines the measurements to be obtained for each patient. The plan category relating to each problem clearly indicates the physician's logic and intended course of action. In this manner, the auditor is not required to guess whether the prednisone was intended for asthma, arthritis, or some other problem. Such an organized office record system documents the logic of the physician's approach to a problem and preserves it for review by peers, whether the purpose be education, recertification, relicensure, or reimbursement.

The Computerized Medical Record

Attempts to develop a computerized ambulatory record have so far met with limited enthusiasm. Two such systems are the computer-stored ambulatory record (COSTAR) developed at Massachusetts General Hospital and the problem-oriented medical information system (PROMIS) developed by the University of Vermont. Many commercial systems are available for scheduling appointments, billing, and insurance processing, but computerization of the medical record has not been universally accepted. An effective computerized system should promote better patient care by stabilizing costs, improving accessibility of information, and facilitating the quality of care.

Problem Indexing in Practice

Now that the computer is available for billing and for other office functions, problem indexing in family practice can be an especially useful tool. It permits easy retrieval of charts required for audit as part of the recertification process of the American Board of Family Practice (ABFP). The ABFP has identified 20 problems for which charts may need to be retrieved and reviewed for self-audit (Table 73–2). Computerization allows for easy expansion of these 20 items to include all 371 items in the World Organization of National Colleges and Academies of Family Practice (now called WONCA) classification or the 4000 or more items in the Hospital International Classification of Disease Adapted for Use in the United States (HICDA).

The advantages of problem indexing include:

1. Easy retrieval of records of patients with common problems or of those receiving similar medications.

2. Recall of patients when discoveries indicate new treatments that are likely to be more effective than the one currently being used.

3. Identification of patients for whom medications must be changed because new hazards of therapy have been identified; e.g., the sudden recall of the drug ticrynafen (Selacryn).

4. Recall of patients with chronic problems requiring periodic evaluation; e.g., recurrent urinary tract infections or chronic lung disease.

Table 73–2. 20 PROBLEM CATEGORIES USED IN THE OFFICE RECORD REVIEW OF THE AMERICAN BOARD OF FAMILY PRACTICE*

Coronary Artery Disease
Hypertension
Urinary Tract Infection
Allergy
Duodenal Ulcer
Diabetes Mellitus
Chronic Heart Failure
Arthritis (Osteo, Rheumatoid, Gouty)
Urethral Discharge
Chronic Obstructive Pulmonary Disease
Carcinoma of the Breast
Depressive Disorders
Menstrual Disorders
Well-Child Care
Irritable Bowel Syndrome
Geriatric Patient
Alcoholism & Alcohol Abuse
Acute Appendicitis
Low Back Pain
Normal Pregnancy (Delivered)

*From the American Board of Family Practice Recertification Application, American Board of Family Practice, Lexington, Kentucky, 1989.

5. Self-audit of physician performance to evaluate effectiveness in selected areas.

6. Audit of the problems encountered in the practice to identify areas of prominence when designing a continuing education program.

7. Analysis of the content of the practice to assist in the design of appropriate curricular objectives for undergraduate and graduate teaching programs.

8. Collection of data for clinical investigation and other research efforts.

9. Retrieval of cases for recertification.

References

Ambulatory Medical Care Records: Uniform Minimum Basic Data Set. A report of the United States National Committee on Vital and Health Statistics. Lilienfield, A. M., chairman. U.S. Department of Health, Education and Welfare, National Center of Health Statistics. Vital and Health Statistics Documents and Committee Reports, Series 4, No. 16, D.H.E.W. Publication No. (HRA) 75–1453.

Birtwhistle, R. V., and Anderson, J. E.: Transferring records when patients change family doctors. Can. Fam. Physician, *35*:51–55, 1989.

Bjorn, J. C., and Cross, H. D.: Problem Oriented Practice. Chicago, Modern Hospital Press, 1970. *The is a pragmatic text, written by two family physicians. It describes their practices, which incorporated Weed's principles of the problem-oriented medical record (POMR), and covers the specific forms and techniques used. Emphasis is placed on the value of self-audit and consultant audits in private practice, and they explain the manner in which the POMR contributes to the process of evaluation of care. This text and Weed's book are the first two classics relating to the POMR.*

Easton, R. C.: Problem-Oriented Medical Record Concepts. New York, Appleton-Century-Crofts, 1974. *This text is presented in a workbook format which will be of value to students. It describes the basic concepts of the POMR and a variety of methods for its implementation. Working questions and review questions are included in each chapter. Content is aimed at both the inpatient and outpatient application of POMR.*

Eggertsen, S. C., Schneeweiss, R., and Bergman, J. J.: An updated protocol for pediatric health screening. J. Fam. Pract., *10*:25–37, 1980.

Feldman, W. S.: Pitfalls in documenting medical records. Med. Aspects Human Sexuality, pp. 49–57, June 1987.

Fischbach, R. L., Sionelo-Bayog, A., Needle, A., et al.: The patient and practitioner as co-authors of the medical record. Patient Counseling and Health Education, First Quarter, pp. 1–5, 1980.

Froom, J., et al.: An integrated medical record and data system for primary care (in eight parts). J. Fam. Pract., *4*:951 to *5*:1007, 1977. *Each article emanates from the Family Medicine Program at the University of Rochester, Highland Hospital. There are various authors for each of the eight parts, but Froom has written most of them.*

Grace, N. T., Neal, E. M., Wellock, C. E., et al.: The family-oriented medical record. J. Fam. Pract., *4*:91–98, 1977. *Includes an example of the single-page family problem list developed in practice.*

Hiller, M. D., and Seidel, L. F.: Patient care management systems, medical records, and privacy: A balancing act. Public Health Rep., *97*:332–345, 1982.

Hurst, J. W., and Walker, H. K.: The Problem Oriented System. New York, Medcom, Inc., 1972.

Margolis, C. Z.: The Pediatric Problem-Oriented Record. Pleasantville, N.Y., Docent Corp., 1977.

Michael, M., and Bordley, C.: Do patients want access to their medical records? Med. Care, *20*:432–435, 1982.

Murnaghan, J. G.: Ambulatory medical care data. Review of the conference proceedings. Report of a conference on ambulatory care records, Chicago, April 1972. Med. Care, *11*(Suppl):13, 1973.

Recertification Handbook of Diplomates. American Board of Family Practice, Lexington, Kentucky, 1988.

Recertification Instruction Handbook. Application and Office Record Review, 1989 Recertification Examination. American Board of Family Practice, Lexington, Kentucky, 1989.

Ruth, D. H., Rigden, S., and Brunworth, D.: An integrated family-oriented problem-oriented medical record. J. Fam. Pract. *8*:1179–1184, 1979.

Schade, H. I.: My patients take their medical records with them. Med. Econ., pp. 75–81, May 6, 1976.

Schade, H. I.: Office Policies Statement of the Schade Medical Clinic, Los Gatos, California, 1980.

Shapiro, D. M.: A family data base for the family oriented medical record. J. Fam. Pract., *13*:881–887, 1981.

Sullivan, R. J., Jr.: Medical Record and Index Systems for Community Practice. Cambridge, Mass., Ballinger Publishing Co., 1979. *This is one of a series of six manuals on rural health center development produced by the Health Services Research Center of the University of North Carolina at Chapel Hill. It focuses on record filing and indexing as well as design of a problem-oriented record.*

Tufo, H. M., Bouchard, R. E., Rubin, A. S., et al.: Problem-oriented approach to practice: II. Development of the system through audit and implication. J.A.M.A., *238*:502–505, 1977.

Walker, H. K., Hurst, J. W., and Woody, M. F.: Applying the Problem Oriented System. New York, Medcom Press, 1973. *An excellent reference emphasizing the practical application of principles illustrated in Weed's and in Cross and Bjorn's original works. Of special value is the description of the role of allied health professionals in the utilization of the POMR. Experiences at the Promis Clinic of Cross, Bjorn, and Burger at Hampden Highlands, Maine, and in other practices are also of great interest.*

Weed, L. L.: Medical Records, Medical Education and Patient Care. Chicago, The Press of Case Western Reserve University, distributed by Year Book Medical Publishers, Inc., 1971. *This text describing the POMR is a classic. Unfortunately, it is directed toward the hospital application rather than the outpatient or office use. Weed's basic principles are well presented, however.*

Widmer, R. B., Cadoret, R. J., and North, C. S.: Depression in family practice: some effects on spouses and children. J. Fam. Pract. *10*:45, 1980.

Yamamoto, L. G., and Wiebe, R. A.: Improving medical communication with facsimile (fax) transmission. Am. J. Emerg. Med., *7*:203–208, 1989.

74

The Family Genogram

Standard Genogram Structure

Robert E. Rakel

The family genogram is a tool used by physicians to summarize on one page a large amount of information relating to the family. It includes a family's hereditary background and the risk this places on current members, along with other major medical, social, and interactional influences. The genogram is also referred to as the family pedigree, family tree, or genealogic chart.

The genogram should indicate those conditions in the family that have hereditary significance, but it can also be used to depict problems of a less well-defined hereditary nature that appear to have a high incidence in a family. Even if these problems are not purely genetic, they may be related to social or environmental factors or to family traits or habits that predispose future family members to the likelihood of that problem developing. The genogram can also demonstrate problems of unknown etiology that are common in a family. Regardless of the cause of the problem, demonstrating its trend throughout succeeding generations of a family is valuable, because it gives offspring some idea of whether they might develop the condition. Thus, charting the incidence of cancer, heart disease, or asthma in a family alerts the individual patient to factors that should be watched for closely.

The genogram supplements the problem list, giving the physician an overview of the main problems affecting the family over three or more generations.

Genograms make it easier for a clinician to keep in mind family members, patterns, and events that may have recurring significance in a family's ongoing care.

(McGoldrick and Gerson, 1985)

The greatest barrier to the universal adoption of the genogram by practicing physicians is the time required to develop one. The search for methods that require minimal physician and office staff time continues. Jolly and colleagues (1980) found that the average time required to complete a genogram (using pretrained patients) was 16 minutes, with a range of 9 to 30 minutes.

Family History

Family background and family influences are not merely incidental items to be considered briefly during the care of an individual; they are essential to the continuing and comprehensive care of that individual and family. The family history has long been a major component of the medical record, since information concerning family background is a potential source of valuable diagnostic information. Too often, however, family data are treated superficially when the physician asks questions regarding the frequency of hereditary or transmissible problems within the family. This ritualistic inquiry is often no more than a recitation by the physician of diseases, such as tuberculosis and diabetes, for which a yes or no answer is requested and that yields data of only limited usefulness. The astute diagnostician delves into the patient's background more thoroughly, attempting to uncover subtle trends or relationships between significant past events and the present problem. The family physician usually accumulates a complete family history over a period of time, gradually adding items to the picture during a series of patient visits. In this way the patient, by asking other family members for additional data and clarification, is able to add more information at subsequent visits. Families usually enjoy developing a family genogram and cooperate in constructing one that not only reflects their lineage but also remains a dynamic picture that can be of medical value to future generations.

The family history can be obtained on a standard questionnaire that becomes a permanent part of the record, such as the Baylor Health History Questionnaire (Fig. 74–1). A primary objective is to search for problems in the family's background that are possible threats to the health of present family members and their future offspring. The degree of susceptibility of any individual can be identified by noting the frequency of occurrence in previous family members. The amount of family data that can be collected in this manner is limited, however, and much more information is available when history forms of this type are supplemented by a genogram.

One example of an important hereditary influence is inborn errors of metabolism. Although these are rare and normally occur at a rate of only one in every 10,000 births, the carriers of these diseases experience a rate of one per every 100 births or less. The probability of one carrier marrying another is sufficiently high to cause concern, and since many of these disorders can be prevented or managed if diagnosed early, the identification of these affected individuals, or carriers, assumes greater importance. Over a thousand genetic abnormalities caused by single mutant genes in humans have been identified.

Studies in Northern Ireland and British Columbia show that up to 6 per cent of persons born in those areas are affected by a serious genetic disease at some time in their lives. Someone born in those regions and relocating to another area may not be identified as potentially transmitting a problem inherent in the previous region unless a complete family history and genogram are obtained.

Basic Design of the Genogram

The purpose of the family genogram is to develop a realistic overview of the family's background and potential health problems. The techniques and symbols used should be those that physicians consider most meaningful in their practice and with which they feel most comfortable. Because the objective is to provide this information at a glance, the chart should be kept simple and brief. The more complicated the symbols and the more cluttered the design, the more time and effort it takes to construct the chart and to retrieve the information. (In a few instances, however, such increased detail may be worth the time.) Symbols requiring the least possible amount of explanation should be selected to represent specific problems.

The standard family genogram chart consists of three or more generations, representing all members of both spouses' families. The generations can be identified by roman numerals (Fig. 74–2). The first-born members of each generation are the farthest to the left, with siblings following to the right in order of birth. A single generation is represented on the same line, and symbols should all be the same size. In generation I, it is traditional to place the husband's symbol on the left. The children of that marriage are indicated on the next generation line. In later generations, the first pregnancy (or first-born child) is placed to the left. The family name is placed above each major family unit, and the given names are placed below each symbol (Fig. 74–3*A*). An indication of either the patient's age or birthdate with each symbol is also useful. When ages are shown, it is important to indicate the date on which the chart was developed so that these ages can be adjusted over time. The other method is to show the dates of birth as in Figure 74–3*B*.

There is often one member of the family who is of greater medical significance because of a chronic disease or an overwhelming problem. If such an individual is the major reason for developing a genogram, this person is called the *index person* (similar to the *proband*) and is identified by an arrow, double square, or double circle (Fig. 74–4).

The components of a genogram include the following:

1. Three or more generations
2. The names of all family members
3. Age or year of birth of all family members
4. Any deaths, including age at or date of death and cause
5. Significant diseases or problems of family members
6. Indication of members living together in the same household
7. Dates of marriages and divorces
8. A listing of first-born of each family to the left, with siblings listed sequentially to the right
9. A key depicting all symbols used

Baylor Family Practice Center
Health History Questionnaire

Today's Date ____________

Single ______
Married ______
Divorced ______
Widowed ______
Separated ______

Name ____________ Occupation ____________

All previous occupations ____________

Education: Years in high school ______ Years college ______ Degrees ______

Birthplace ____________ Date of Birth ____________

NOTE: This is a confidential record of your medical history and will be kept in this office. Information contained here will not be released to any person except when you have authorized us to do so.

Family History	If Living: Age	Health	If Deceased: Age at Death	Cause
Father				
Mother				
(Circle) 1. Brother/Sister				
2. Brother/Sister				
3. Brother/Sister				
4. Brother/Sister				
Spouse				
(Circle) 1. Son/Daughter				
2. Son/Daughter				
3. Son/Daughter				
4. Son/Daughter				

Has any blood relative or husband or wife ever had:	Check if Yes	Relationship if Yes
Allergies		
Asthma		
Arthritis		
Glaucoma		
Cancer		
Tuberculosis		
Diabetes		
Heart Trouble		
High Blood Pressure		
Stroke		
Epilepsy/Seizures		
Substance Abuse		
Depression/Emotional Prob.		
Suicide		
Kidney Trouble		
Birth Defects		
Sickle Cell Anemia		
Mental Retardation		

PERSONAL HISTORY: Please complete blanks in sections below

Date of last physical examination: ____________ Physician ____________

HOSPITALIZATIONS: List all, for illness or surgery, beginning with the most recent:

Date	Reason	Hospital	Physician

CURRENT MEDICATIONS: Circle those you use.

Laxatives
Aspirin
Vitamins
Tranquilizers
Hormones
Antacids
Birth Control Pills
Decongestants
Nasal Sprays
Cortisone
Diet Pills
Diuretics/Water Pills
Cold/Allergy Pills

LIST ANY ADDITIONAL MEDICATIONS YOU TAKE:

DATE OF LAST:

Pap Smear ______
Mammogram ______
Cholesterol ______
EKG (or treadmill) ______
Stool test (blood) ______
Sigmoidoscopy ______

HAVE YOU HAD X-RAYS OF: **Date** **Result**

Chest
Stomach (Upper GI)
Colon (Barium Enema)
Others: ____________

WEIGHT: Now ______
1 yr. ago ______
Desired ______

ALCOHOLIC BEVERAGES:
Never ______ Less than
6 drinks/week ______
7-24 drinks/week ______
Over 24/week ______
Ever treated for alcoholism? ______

RECREATIONAL DRUGS:
Marijuana ______
Cocaine ______
Heroin ______
Other ______
Ever treated for drug dependency? ______

HABITS: Use seat belts? ______

TOBACCO: Never ______
Cigarettes ______ (______ packs/day)
Cigars ______ Pipe ______
Age started smoking ______
Age stopped smoking ______
Snuff ______ Chewing tobacco ______

ANY SPECIAL DIET? ______
Type: ______

EXERCISE? Type: ______

Frequency, distance or amount: ______

PLEASE TURN OVER

MR-2,4-88

Figure 74–1. Baylor College of Medicine Health History Questionnaire.

Illustration continued on following page

PERSONAL HISTORY - Circle any of the items listed below that apply to you (past or present):

Measles (10 day)
German Measles (3 day)
Mumps
Chicken pox
Whooping Cough
Scarlet fever/Scarlatina
Diphtheria
Pneumonia
Influenza
Pleurisy
Any eye disease, injury, impaired sight
Any ear disease, injury, impaired hearing
Any troubles with nose, sinuses, mouth, throat
Problems with your teeth
Rheumatic fever
Rheumatism
Any bone or joint disease
Neuritis or neuralgia
Bursitis, sciatica or lumbago
Stiff, swollen or painful joints
Polio or meningitis
Bladder or kidney infection or stones
Gonorrhea, syphilis, or herpes
Chlamydia, Venereal warts
Anemia
Yellow jaundice or hepatitis
Tuberculosis
Mononucleosis
Diabetes
Hypoglycemia

High blood pressure
Low blood pressure
Cancer
Food, chemical or drug poisoning
Received blood or plasma transfusions
Broken or cracked bones
Concussion or head injury
Knocked unconscious
Dislocations
Severe lacerations
Recent sprains
Frequent infections or boils
Hay fever or asthma
Hives
Eczema
Fainting spells
Convulsions or seizures
Frequent or severe headaches
Dizziness
Anxiety/tension
Difficulty remembering or concentrating
Difficulty sleeping
Frequent crying spells
Work or family problems
Thoughts about committing suicide
Nervous breakdown
Paralysis or numbness
Enlarged thyroid or goiter
Enlarged glands
Skin problems

Recent change in appetite or eating habits
Chest pain or angina pectoris
Spitting up of blood
Night sweats
Shortness of breath
Palpitation or fluttering heart
Heart murmur
Swelling of hands, feet or ankles
Extreme tiredness or weakness
Varicose veins
Albumin, sugar, blood or pus in urine
Difficulty urinating
Get up at night to urinate
Abnormal thirst
Stomach trouble or ulcer
Colitis or other bowel disease
Liver or gall bladder disease
Hemorrhoids
Rectal bleeding
Constipation or diarrhea
Black bowel movements
Change in bowel or bladder habits
Indigestion or difficulty swallowing
Change in a wart or mole
Hoarseness or cough
Non-healing sores
Lumps in breasts or elsewhere
Unusual bleeding or discharge
Tubal infections
Sex is not satisfactory

MEN ONLY: Have you ever had swellings of or lumps on testicles?
Yes No
Do you do regular testicular self-exam? Yes No

WOMEN ONLY: Do you do regular breast self-exam? Yes No

Menstrual History
Age at onset_____________ Date of last period_____________
Cycle (from start to start) _____________ days
Usual duration of flow _____________ days.
Flow is _________ Heavy _________ Medium _________ Light
Pain or cramps _____________ Periods irregular _____________
Have had vaginal infections or frequent discharge _____________
Have taken birth control pills or used an IUD _____________
Have had abnormal PAP _________ Date of last PAP _________

Pregnancies: Total number _____________
How many children born alive _____________
How many stillbirths _____________
How many premature _____________
How many Cesarean sections _____________
How many miscarriages _____________
How many abortions _____________

IMMUNIZATIONS: List year of most recent immunization
Rubella _____________
Measles and mumps_____________
Tetanus_____________
Polio _____________
Diphtheria _____________
Influenza _____________
Hemophilus influenza _____________
Pneumonia (Pneumovax) _____________
Hepatitis _____________

EXPOSURES: Have you been exposed to
Lead_____________
DES _____________
Asbestos_____________
Others (Chemicals, Noise, etc.) _____________

ALLERGIES: Are you allergic to
Penicillin, sulfa, other antibiotics _____________
Aspirin, codeine or morphine _____________
Any other medicines? _____________
Insect bites or stings _____________
Any foods? _____________

____
Physician's Signature Date Reviewed

Figure 74–1 *Continued*

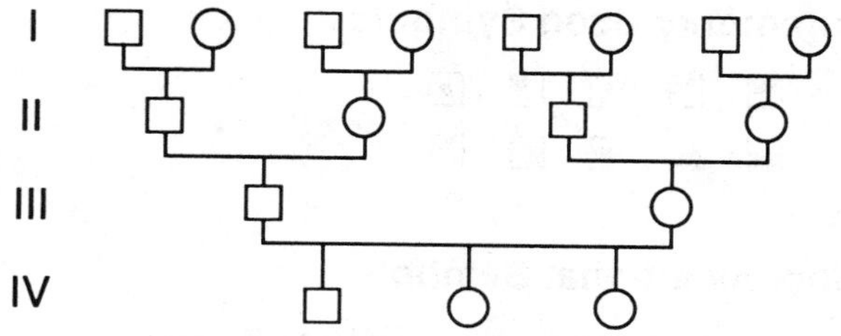

Figure 74–2. Basic genogram structure.

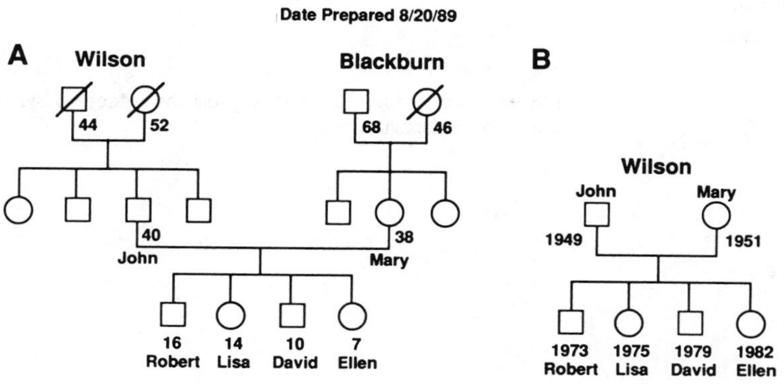

Figure 74–3. Basic genogram containing family names, first names, and ages or birthdates.

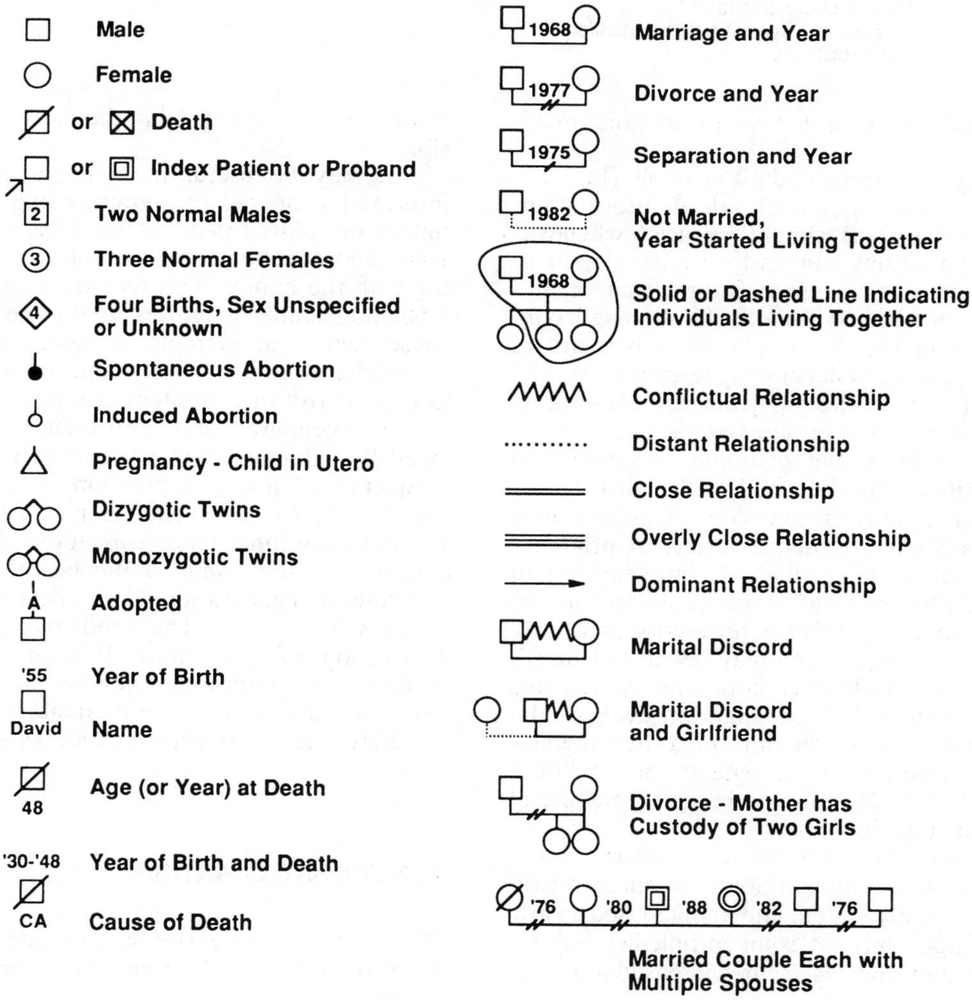

Figure 74–4. Standard genogram symbols.

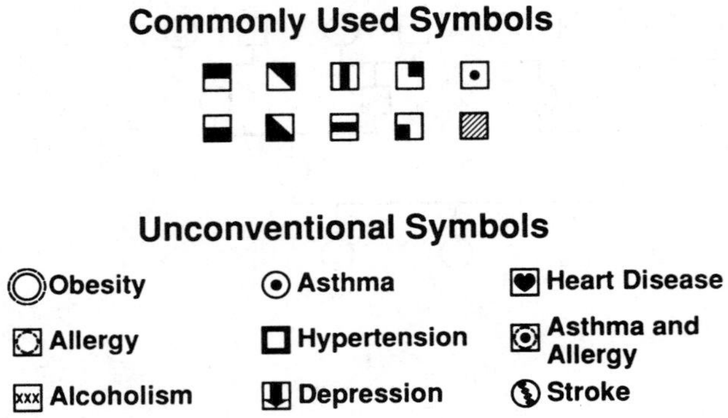

Commonly Used Abbreviations

ALC	Alcoholic
ALL	Allergy
ARTH	Arthritis
CA	Cancer
CAD	Coronary Artery Disease
CVA	Cerebrovascular Accident
DEP	Depression
DM	Diabetes Mellitus
GI	GI Tract Disease
HBP or HT	Hypertension
MI	Myocardial Infarction
MVP	Mitral Valve Prolapse
PUD	Peptic Ulcer Disease
SLE	Systemic Lupus Erythematosis
TB	Tuberculosis

Figure 74–5. Individually designed (or selected) symbols and common abbreviations.

10. Symbols selected for simplicity and maximum visibility.

Familiarity with the standard symbols (Fig. 74–4) allows for more rapid retrieval of information. These standard symbols should be used whenever possible, but variations can easily be developed to provide more accurate or useful information. Examples of unconventional or individually designed symbols are shown in Fig. 74–5. These symbols are of greatest value to the physician who designs them, and the symbols chosen by the physician depend entirely upon his or her personal preference.

Standard symbols that maintain simplicity and avoid competition can be used with most family genograms, since only a few conditions normally require representation. When a variety of problems are represented in one genogram, the selection of symbols should be made with special care to assure that they are noncompetitive. Cluttered symbols are more difficult to interpret and may defeat the chart's primary purpose. Additional notations on selected individuals regarding their occupation, level of education, general state of health, or other medical problems can usually be listed beneath the symbol or beneath the chart to give a more complete picture of that individual (Fig. 74–6).

When family members assist in constructing a genogram, they may gain additional insight into risks inherent in the family system and an increased awareness of the importance of some problems. For example, if repeated suicides occur, increased attention can be given to recognizing the early signs of depression.

It may be useful to highlight critical medical information on the genogram, using a yellow highlighter or colored pen. In this way, significant problems can be immediately recognized by anyone working with the family. This technique may be useful in educating family members about the importance of these items. For example, if cancer or heart disease is highlighted, the family can be told about the particular risk of continuing cigarette smoking.

The genogram shown in Figure 74–7 was developed by a family practice resident investigating the frequency of manic depression in a family and its relationship to alcoholism (Geron, 1976). An apparent X-linked inheritance was noted. Of medical significance to the family is the fact that the affected individuals in generation III first developed symptoms at ages 22 and 32. The predictive significance for generation IV is obvious. Prompt recognition and treatment of symptoms will be possible when the problems first occur rather than later, after significant hardship has been experienced, as is so often the case.

FUNCTIONAL CHARTING

An additional dimension can be added to the genogram by including the functional components shown

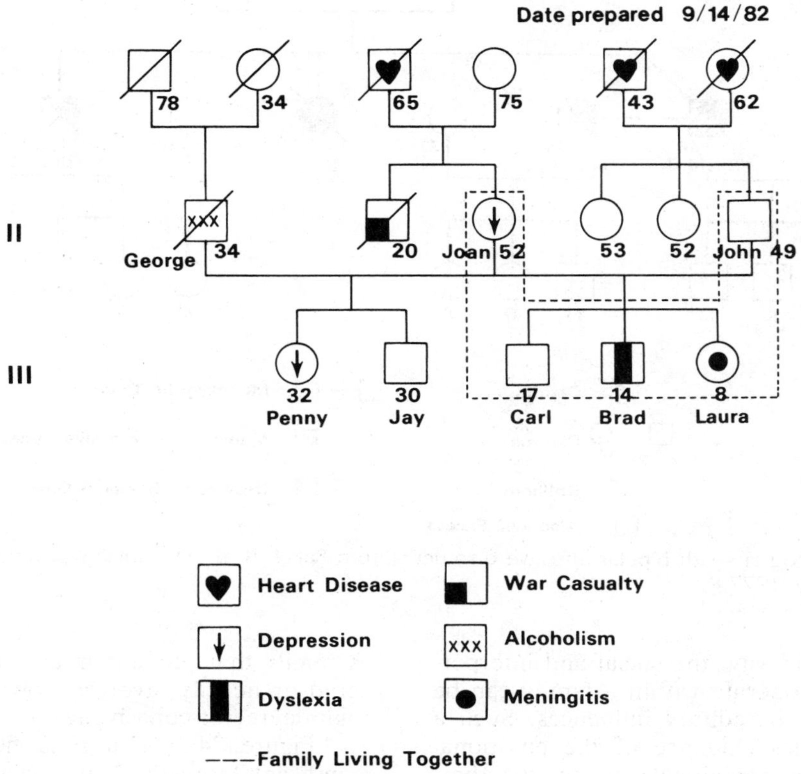

Joan (52)
Back Injury
Rectal fissure

Penny (32)
Schoolteacher
Migraine headaches

Jay (30)
Sailor
2 children
Divorced
Abdominal pain after father's death

Carl (17)
Hives
Allergy to dust
Undescended testicle

Brad (14)
Premature birth
Hyperkinetic—on Ritalin
Inferiority complex

Laura (8)
Meningococcal meningitis
Wears corrective shoes

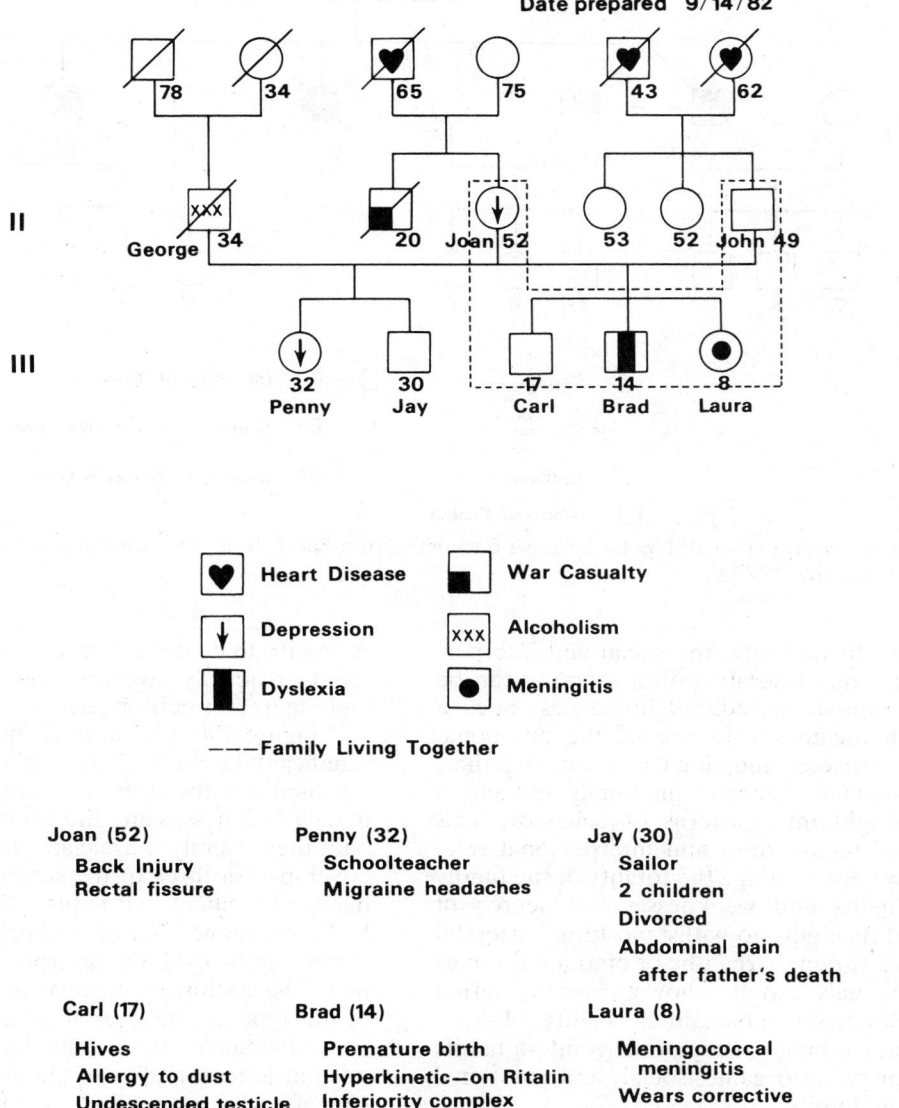

Figure 74–6. Family genogram with additional information on each individual at bottom of chart.

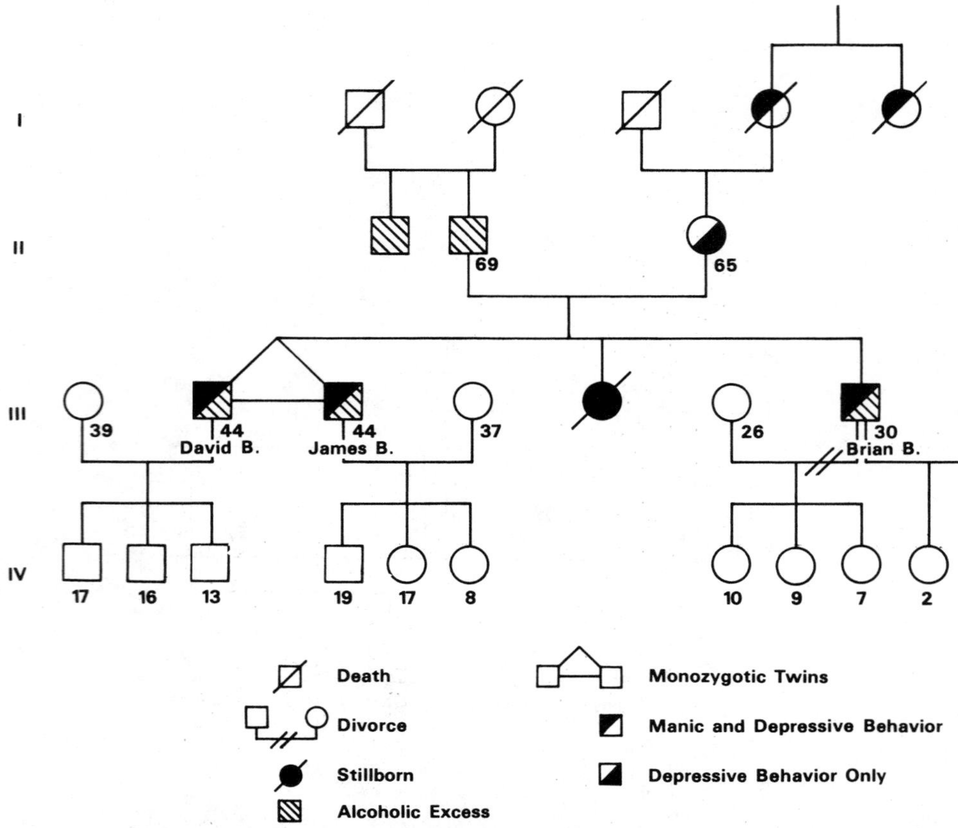

Figure 74–7. Family genogram with bipolar affective disorder. (From Rakel, R. E.: Principles of Family Medicine. Philadelphia, W. B. Saunders Company, 1977.)

in Figure 74–4. In this way, the social and interpersonal influences that operate within a family can be shown in addition to hereditary influences. Such a picture, which includes evidence of the emotional relationships between individuals living together, gives a more dynamic image of the family and allows for greater insight into patterns of behavior. This visualization of family roles and interpersonal relationships allows one to judge the totality of the family unit—its strengths and weaknesses, its degree of solidarity, and its ability to withstand future stressful situations. The varying strengths of emotional bonds between individuals can be shown, as can marital discord and dominant personalities. Figure 74–8 incorporates many functional components into a family chart and depicts the organic, social, and emotional problems of the family.

CHARTS SHOWING CHANGES OVER TIME

An individual's or family's significant medical events over a period of time can be condensed into a single composite picture, using a variety of charting techniques. These methods conceptualize significant stresses that occur in an individual or family over time and involve the sequencing of noteworthy events within the family that may have a causal relationship. A family that remains intact in spite of a very cluttered or heavily involved flow chart demonstrates a high degree of cohesiveness.

Figure 74–9 is a time flow chart that shows significant biomedical and sociomedical events in a troubled family over 7½ years. It illustrates the impact of illnesses and life events on family members and their family physician. In this family, cancer developed in three of the seven children, the mother made five suicide attempts, and the only daughter had a pregnancy out of wedlock. The two periods of severe family dysfunction from 1973 to 1974 and 1978 to 1979 are shown with vertical shading. A flow chart of this type not only provides a sequential analysis of an individual's life events but, when the vertical portion is reviewed, also shows how the same event can affect various family members. Chronic crisis-ridden families such as this need to be recognized early by the family physician.

In the Netherlands, Huygen (1978) collected data for 30 years on the families in his practice. Figure 74–10 depicts the care of a family over a 23-year period. An X marks visits for skin problems. Prenatal care is depicted on a separate line from the wife's other medical visits. This family is similar to many American families in which the husband seeks medical care much less frequently than do the wife and children.

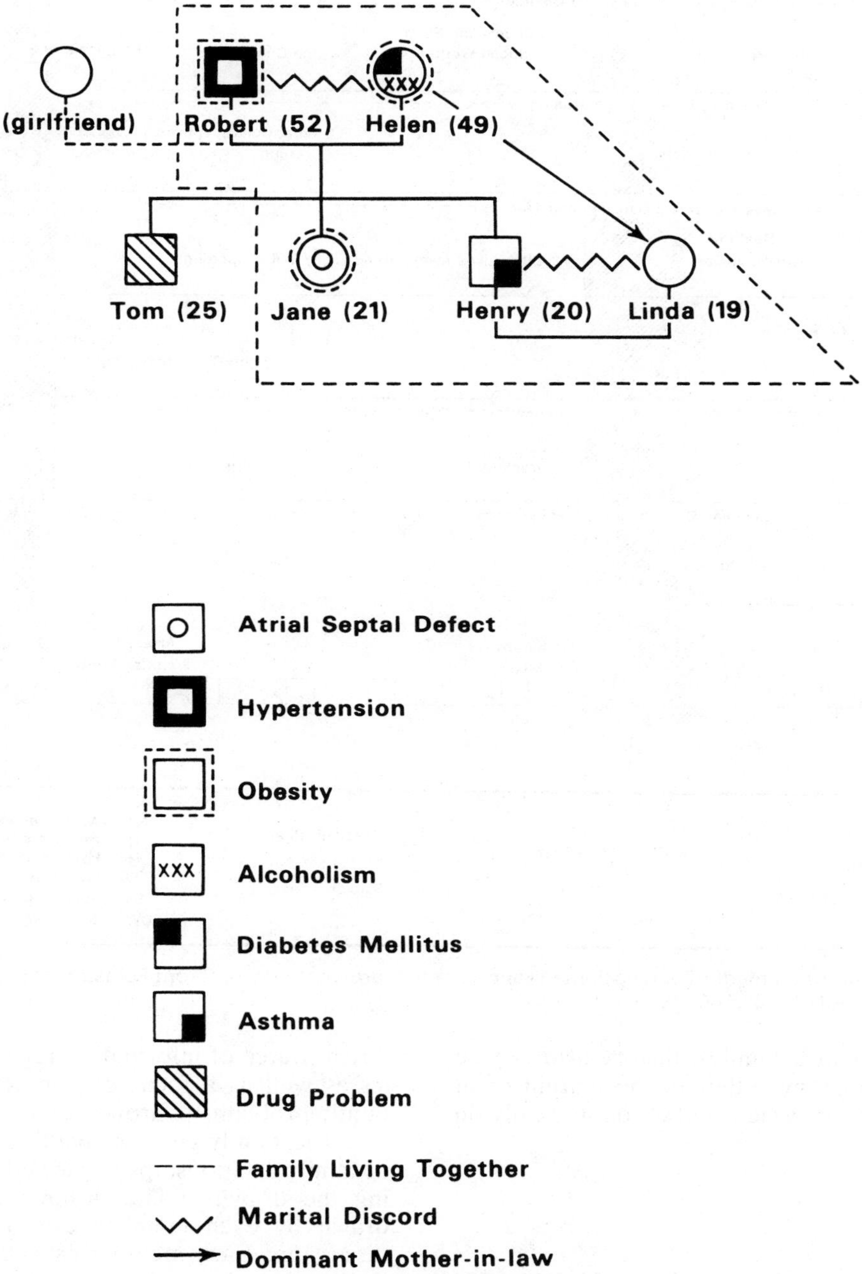

The Dobson family chart, 3/6/76.

Figure 74–8. Family genogram incorporating functional components. (From Rakel, R. E.: Principles of Family Medicine. Philadelphia, W. B. Saunders Company, 1977.)

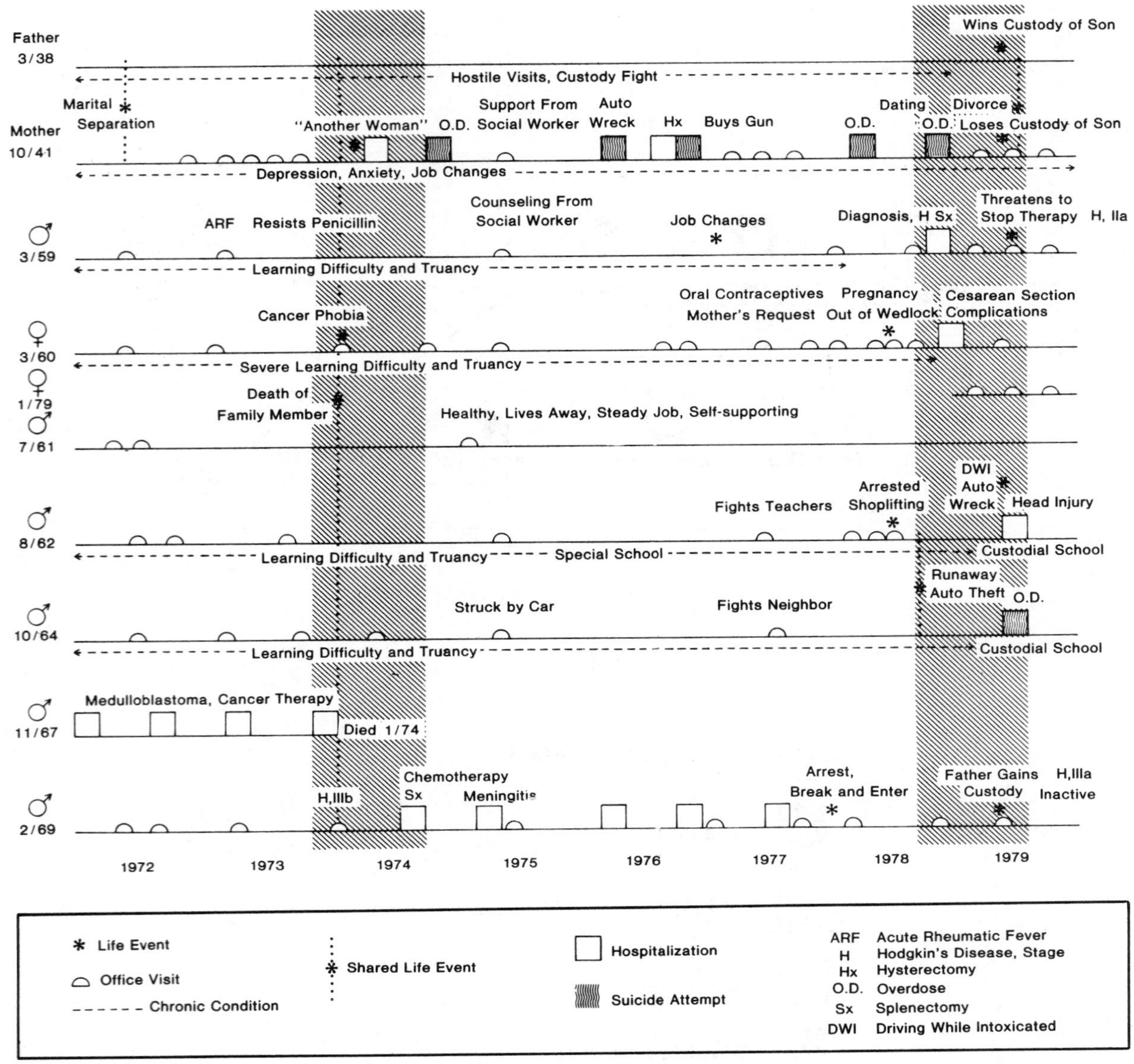

Figure 74–9. Flow chart of biomedical and sociomedical events that are interrelated. (From Rainsford, G. L., and Schuman, S. H.: The family in crises. J.A.M.A., *246*:60, 1981.)

Critical events in a family's history also can be shown on the genogram, either in the margin or at the bottom, or they may be listed chronologically on a separate page.

FAMILY CIRCLE

The family circle (Fig. 74–11) is a way to depict the emotional relationships of a family as depicted by one member (arrow). The size of the circle indicates importance; the distance from others reflects the degree of emotional attachment or closeness. Significant others, including friends and pets, may also be included if the person feels they are part of "family." The date is very important because these relationships will almost always change over time. The family circle requires only 2 or 3 minutes to complete and can be a rich source of information regarding family dynamics as well as a focus of opportunity for discussing family problems (Thrower et al., 1982).

The family circle provides at a glance a picture of family relationships as viewed by the person making the drawing. The differences in family circles drawn by each member can serve as a focus for discussion. Each member can also be asked to draw the family as he or she would like it to be. The family circle "is among the most value-free, nonjudgmental methods for discussing emotional and relationship problems without focusing on individual pathology" (Thrower et al., 1982). It can complement the genogram and add useful information about family dynamics.

Some family physicians prefer to use the genogram to show functional relationships, but in some families this can lead to a complicated diagram that

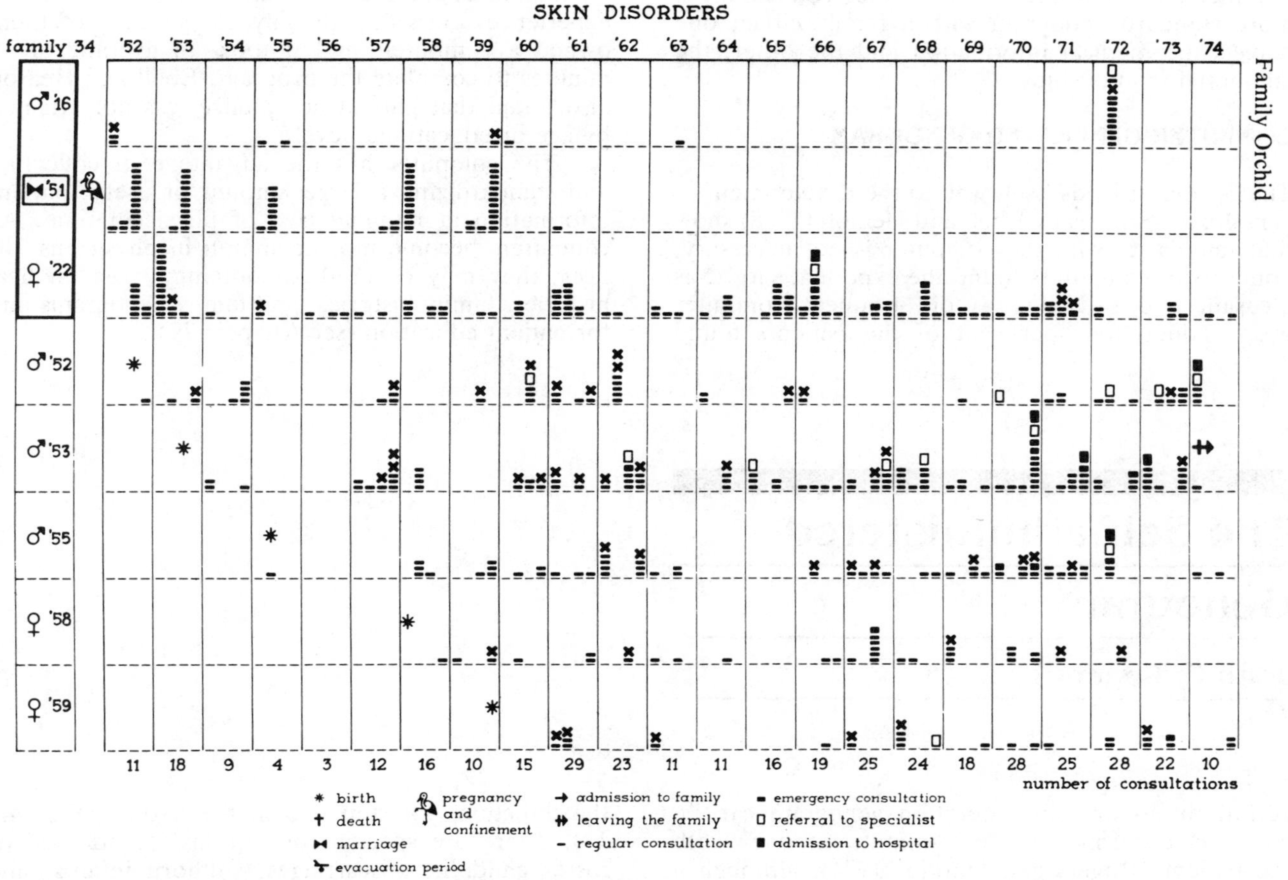

Figure 74–10. Family chart with visits for skin disorders indicated by an X. (From Huygen, F. J. A.: Family Medicine: The Medical Life History of Families. Nijmegen, The Netherlands, Dekker and Van de Vegt, 1978.)

Figure 74–11. Family circle chart. (From Birrer, R. B.: Urban Family Medicine. New York, Springer-Verlag, 1987.)

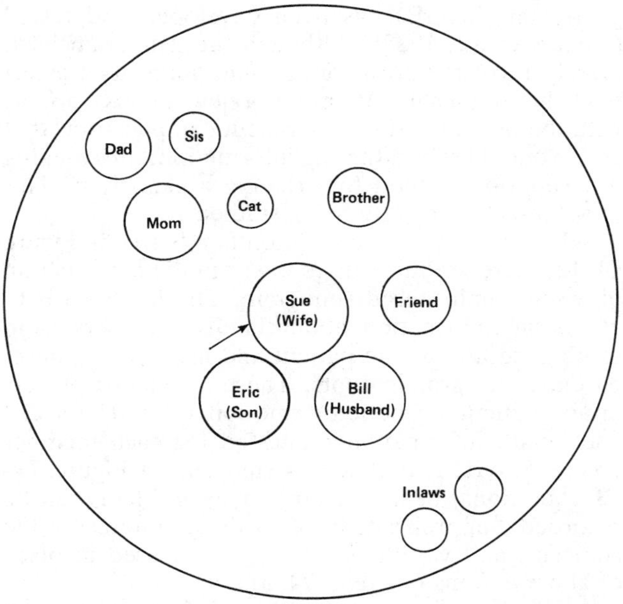

"My husband, son and I are the most important to me. My mom is also very important, but I don't feel as close to her as I feel to my friend. I feel very distant from my dad."

is difficult to interpret. Others prefer to combine a more standard genogram with a family circle; one depicts the medical information and the other, the emotional relationships.

COMPUTER-GENERATED GENOGRAM

The computer lends itself well to the development of genograms. Studies by Ebell and Heaton (1988) show that familiarity with the computer is not necessary; nonusers of computers found the experience to be as pleasant and satisfying as did frequent computer users. Ninety-four per cent of the patients found creation of a computerized genogram to be a pleasant experience, even though only 15 per cent of them owned a computer, and it took an average of 19 minutes to complete the program. Ebell and Heaton also noted that patient acceptance was not affected by age or educational level.

The computer has the advantage of collecting and standardizing a large amount of useful patient information at minimal cost of physician time. As computers become more common in physicians' offices, they may be used for obtaining past medical histories, family histories, and family genograms and for patient education (see Chapter 79).

The Self-administered Genogram

John C. Rogers

A full three- or four-generation genogram can be constructed during a 15- to 20-minute interview with the patient (Rogers and Durkin, 1984), although a sketchy two-generation genogram can be obtained in about 5 minutes. In consideration of the time constraints of a busy office practice, a self-administered genogram (SAGE) has been developed and tested (Rogers et al., 1985). Although the genogram itself merely records information, some authorities assert that the physician-patient interview builds rapport with the patient and has therapeutic implications that go beyond merely gathering information, thus making it a superior method for creating a genogram. This hypothesis is currently being studied.

Beginning with the skeleton family tree in Figure 74–12, there are three major steps in the construction of a self-administered genogram. The first step is to get basic information about family members from three generations: the patient and his or her spouse, parents, and grandparents. These are major players in any patient's genetic or emotional life. The social and health information requested for each member on the SAGE is outlined as step one in Figure 74–13. Additional health or emotional problems can be recorded if appropriate or of particular interest to the clinician, and various symbols can be used in place of abbreviations (see Fig. 74–5).

The second step is to gather information about other members in the family who do not appear on the skeleton tree, i.e., the patient's children and brothers and sisters. Aunts and uncles of the patient can be included as well, but they are not included in the directions for step two of the SAGE (Fig. 74–14). There are specific conventions for adopted or foster children, miscarriages, stillborn infants, and any current pregnancy of unknown sex (see Fig. 74–4). For these individuals, name, date of birth (and date of death, if appropriate), and social or health problems are the only information requested.

The third step is to get information about other marriages or long-term, intimate relationships of the patient and his or her spouses, parents, or grandparents. The convention for diagraming these relationships on the SAGE is described in Figure 74–15. Children from these relationships can be added using the same conventions as in step two. Clinicians sometimes use other conventions or develop their own idiosyncratic symbols or abbreviations, especially for particularly sensitive issues such as sexual affairs (see Figs. 74–4 and 74–8).

Once the few conventions for the use of genogram symbols have been mastered, many patients are able to complete SAGE skeleton family trees, as in Figure 74–16.

Reading Genograms

Experienced family physicians and family therapists can scan and interpret genograms within moments. On the other hand, inexperienced learners, such as students or residents, must be taught a step-by-step, systematic approach to reading this diagnostic tool.

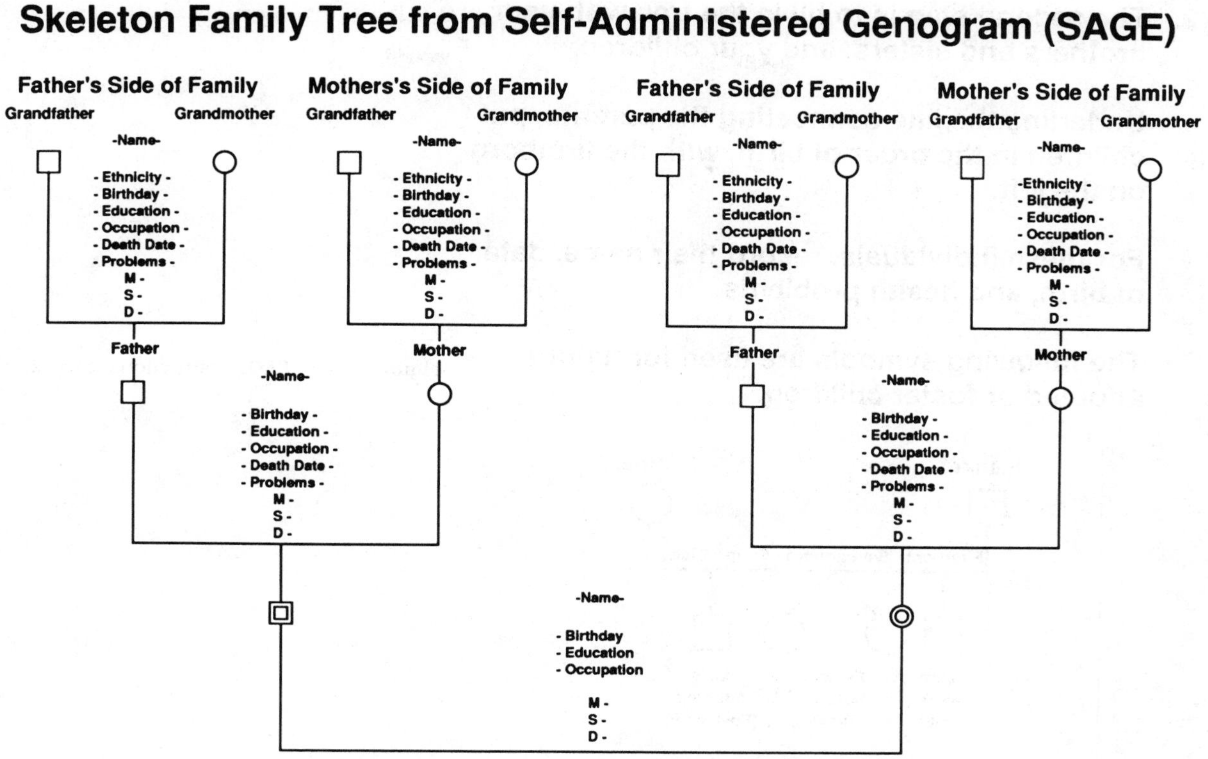

Figure 74–12. Skeleton family tree for SAGE.

Throughout the tree, women are ○'s and men are □'s.

Step 1. The first step is to get information about you, your spouse, parents, and grandparents.

Please fill in the social and health information for each person on the <u>Skeleton Family Tree</u>.

For dates of birth, death, marriages, or divorces, please record Month-Day-Year whenever possible.

For problems, please note any problems with health or daily living. If any members of your family have or have had any of the following conditions you may use the shorthand titles in parentheses.

• High Blood Pressure	(HBP)
• Heart Disease	(HRT DIS)
• Stroke	(CVA)
• Alcohol Problems	(ALC)
• Depression	(DEP)
• Nerve problems	(NERVES)
• Diabetes	(DM)
• Cancer	(CA)
• Drug problems	(DRUG PROB)
• Anxiety	(ANX)
• Emotional problems	(EMO PROB)
• Chronic symptoms	(HEADACHES, BACK PAIN, STOMACH PAIN, ETC.)

Figure 74–13. SAGE instructions, Step 1.

Step 2. The second step is to fill in the tree with your brothers and sisters, and your children.

Underline the line connecting the parents, put children in the order of birth, with the firstborn on the left.

For these individuals, record their name, date of birth, and health problems.

The following symbols are used for natural, adopted or foster children.

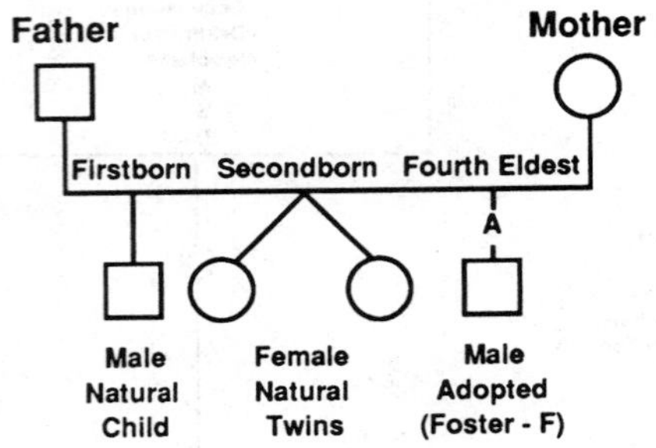

Figure 74–14. SAGE instructions, Step 2.

The four components of the family genogram are structure, demographics, events, and problems.

Structure. This refers to the composition of the index patient's current family unit and is a function of marital status (single, married, separated, divorced, widowed) and parental status (no children or natural, foster, or adopted children or stepchildren). The genogram in Figure 74–16 displays a number of different types of structure: single adult, single parent, childless couple, nuclear family, and blended family. These are the most frequent family structures recorded on genograms, but others may be encoun-

Step 3. The third step is to get information about any other marriages for you, your spouse, or your parents.

Put these marriages to the outside of the marriages already on the Skeleton Tree.

Please specify Month-Day-Year for marriages, separations, and divorces.

Use slash marks to show relationships that have ended.

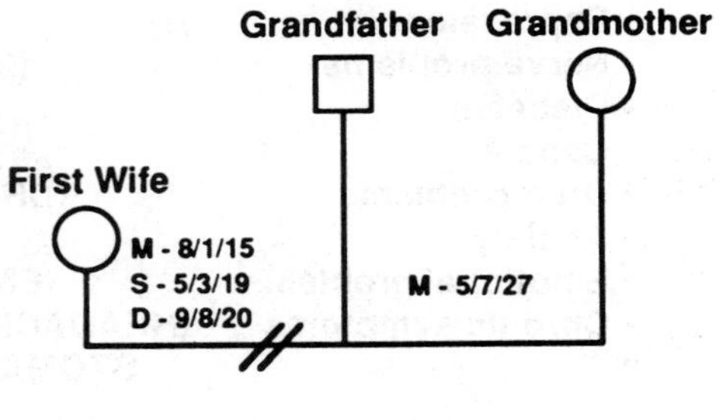

Figure 74–15. SAGE instructions, Step 3.

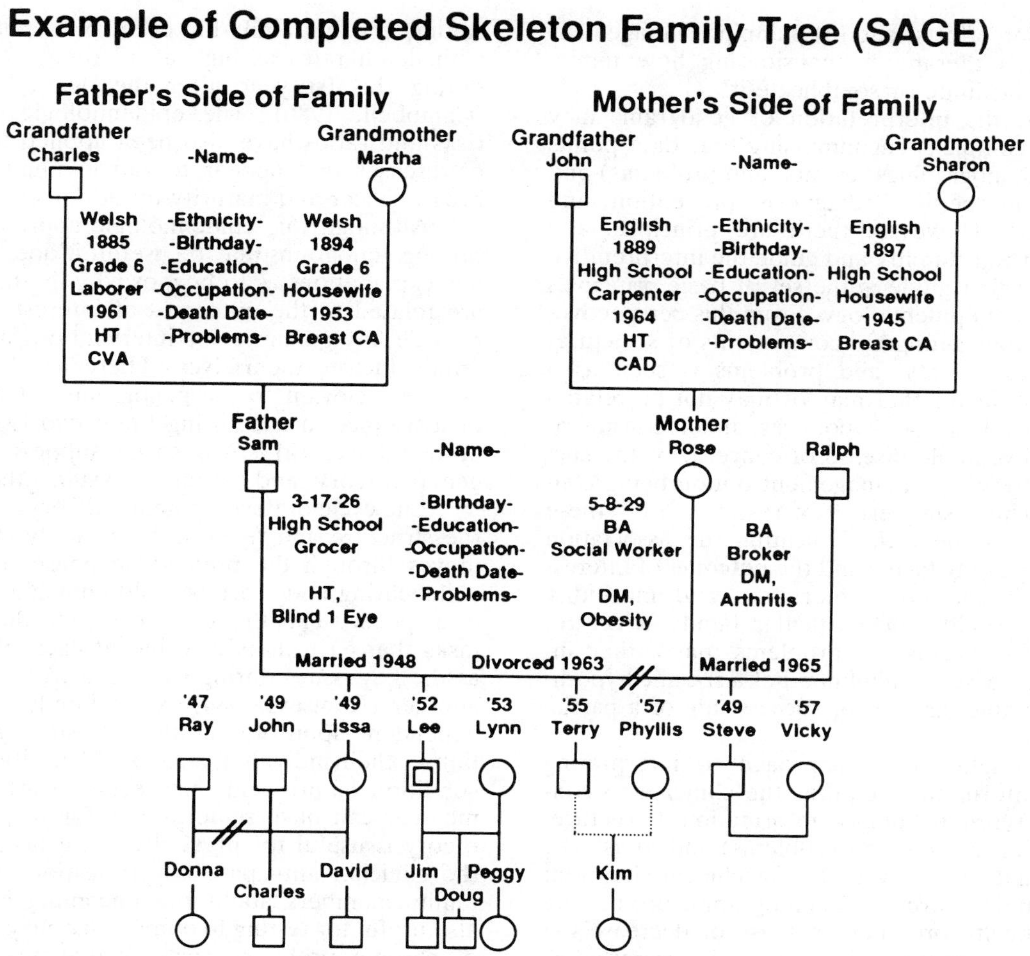

Figure 74–16. Example of completed SAGE.

tered, especially if there are more than two generations living together, other long-term relationships, or individuals living together without legal bonds.

Family Demographic Information. This includes ethnicity, education, and occupation. Specific information about each of these three factors may be important, as well as the consistency or lack of consistency for the items among the family members. Hence, the clinician reading this part of the genogram notes the ethnicity, education, and occupation of the index patient and how those compare with the demographics of other members of the family.

Family Life Events. A number of major life events are recorded on genograms, including marriage, separation, and divorce; birth and death; and major social or health problems. Life events related to beginning or ending education, changes in occupational status, or leaving home can often be inferred from information on the genogram. The clinician reading the genogram notes what events have occurred, the time sequence, and whether there has been a confluence or pileup of events.

Social and Health Problems. Here the genogram reader notes the type and number of problems and their consistency among family members.

Interpretation

The four-step protocol for reading the genogram extracts relevant information but does not deal with the meaning or implications of the family information—that requires interpretation. The full interpretation of the information depends upon the type of clinical decisions that need to be made. There is no such thing as a "normal genogram," so the interpretation of the reading is clearly dependent upon the clinical situation to which the family information is being applied.

Family information is used predominantly in three types of situations: (1) evaluating a somatic complaint by testing biopsychosocial hypotheses about what caused the condition, (2) assessing a patient's risk for biomedical and mental disorders in order to implement appropriate primary and secondary prevention efforts, and (3) planning management of a patient's therapy by considering how family factors may facilitate or complicate it.

At first, the interpretation of genograms may seem to be complex, encompassing four data points (structure, demographics, events, and problems) and three possible decisions (diagnosis, prevention, and management). However, there are principles and theories that can simplify and guide the interpretative process. The first guide is the set of basic principles and methods of epidemiology. From this perspective, each of the four genogram components of structure, demographics, events, and problems is seen as a potential risk factor that may or may not be related to the biopsychosocial hypothesis under consideration, the preventable disease of concern, or the success or failure of the management option being considered. The simplest expression of these relationships is the ratio indicating the association between the family factor and the outcome of interest (relative risk and odds, mortality, and morbidity ratios). Specifically, the particular family structure, demographics, events, or problems may either increase or decrease the likelihood of a specific hypothesis, preventable disease, or success rate of a particular therapy.

This straightforward approach to interpreting genogram information requires the clinician to consider four types of family information (structure, demographics, events, and problems) and to ask the questions that are relevant to the clinical situation: Does the family's structure, demographic profile, life events, or health problems increase or decrease the likelihood of a specific biopsychosocial hypothesis? Do they increase or decrease the patient's risk of developing a specific preventable condition? Do they increase or decrease the success rate of a particular management option? From the answers to the four questions about each type of genogram information, the clinician can interpret how family information is related to the hypothesis, preventable condition, or management option.

For example, the family structure variable of marital status has been studied in relation to a number of health outcomes. It is well documented th t nonmarried persons have increased death rates for all major causes of death: cardiovascular diseases, infectious diseases, malignancies, accidents, homicides, and suicides. The age-specific death rates for widowed or divorced individuals is from two to four times higher than those of their married peers (Lynch, 1977). The demographic variable of education has also been related to mortality ratios; individuals with the lowest levels of education have the highest death rates for malignant neoplasms, cardiovascular and renal diseases, diabetes, tuberculosis, influenza, cirrhosis of the liver, accidents, and suicides. Breast cancer is the exception to this trend; in this situation, women with higher education have a higher death rate than those with lower education (Syme and Berkman, 1976). Mortality ratios have also been studied for the family life event of a spouse's death, with death rates as high as 12 times normal noted during the 1st year after the death of a spouse (Campbell, 1986). The epidemiologic concepts of risks and ratios have also been applied to a number of diseases that appear to run in families, such as breast cancer and maturity-onset diabetes mellitus.

Although this epidemiologic approach to interpreting genograms may be useful, it does not provide any explanations as to how or why the family factors are related to the outcomes of interest, nor does it provide any guidance for interventions aimed at the family factors themselves. There are four theories that are relevant to the genogram that may also be of assistance in addressing these two issues: (1) life cycle theory, (2) stress–social support theory, (3) genetic theory, and (4) family systems theory.

Life cycle or developmental theory describes how the structure and function of a family changes as it moves through the predictable phases of marriage: childbearing and rearing, child launching, and death of a spouse. This theory specifies the developmental tasks that each individual has at each phase as well as the key issues during transition from one stage to another (Ramsey, 1984). Since family members are dependent upon one another for successful completion of their individual stage and transitional tasks, a condition or problem that seems to affect only one member can have ramifications for the family. This theory is useful for preventive care because it helps the clinician anticipate key transitions and educate family members about the upcoming change. It is also useful for testing hypotheses about exacerbations of chronic problems such as diabetes or asthma; frequency of acute illnesses; or onset of apparently psychosomatic problems such as headache, backache, fatigue, or abdominal pain.

Whereas family life cycle theory uses both family structure and some information about family events for interpreting the genogram, the stress–social support theory uses all four categories of genogram information: structure, demographics, events, and problems. This theory asserts that stressful life events can cause illness unless buffered by social support. In addition, social support itself may have an independent beneficial effect on health, regardless of the presence or absence of stressful events (Smilkstein, 1978; Medalie, 1978). The four categories of genogram information provide the data by which the stress and support can be determined. Clearly the genogram does not include all things that may be stressors or all sources of support, and these other areas may need to be explored by the clinician using this theoretic framework to interpret the genogram.

Genetic theory dominates most attempts to understand how health problems are transmitted from one family generation to another. This theory includes Mendelian transmission of autosomal dominant, autosomal recessive, sex-linked recessive, and intermediate inheritance as well as the issue of genetic susceptibility. The last requires information about environmental factors as well as familial tendencies (Warrell, 1987). This theory is relevant to the diagnosis and prevention of specific biologic diseases as well as some mental disorders and can be used to generate risk predictions for first- and second-degree relatives of those afflicted with particular conditions (Warrell, 1987; Smeraldi et al., 1981; Pauls et al., 1979).

Family systems theory is a rubric that includes several family function constructs and theories developed by a number of experts. Bowen's Intergenerational Family Systems Theory is the framework most closely associated with the use of the genogram by family therapists in their clinical work. A discussion of that theory is beyond the scope of this chapter because it requires a level of abstraction about family processes that is not pertinent to the practices of most family physicians. See Chapter 4 and Bray et al. (1987) for a further discussion.

Once the clinician has completed the four-step protocol for reading the genogram, epidemiologic principles and life cycle, stress–social support, and genetic theories can be used to guide the interpretation. Following this two-part procedure ensures a systematic reading and interpretation of the genogram and allows for effective use of routine family information in clinical decision-making. The theoretic principles used for the interpretation of the genogram can also guide the clinician as additional family information is gathered or therapeutic interventions are designed and implemented.

This chapter attempts to show that the family genogram, when accurately derived and correctly interpreted, can help family physicians make more efficient use of basic family information as they make their daily decisions. The assumption is that knowing more about the entire family allows the clinician to be more effective. The genogram can guide the physician into more in-depth psychologic assessments of the family and help him or her explore subtle problems that may have originated from the family situation.

Clinical Examples

CASE I: KATHRYN

Kathryn is a 2-year-old child who is seen 2 days after her second birthday complaining that her stomach burns. Functional abdominal pain may be one of the biopsychosocial hypotheses to be considered. The genogram in Figure 74–17 may be useful in testing this hypothesis. The genogram is read as follows:

Family structure:	Single-parent family with one child at home
Family demographics:	High school–educated parents, mother employed; status consistent with that of other family members

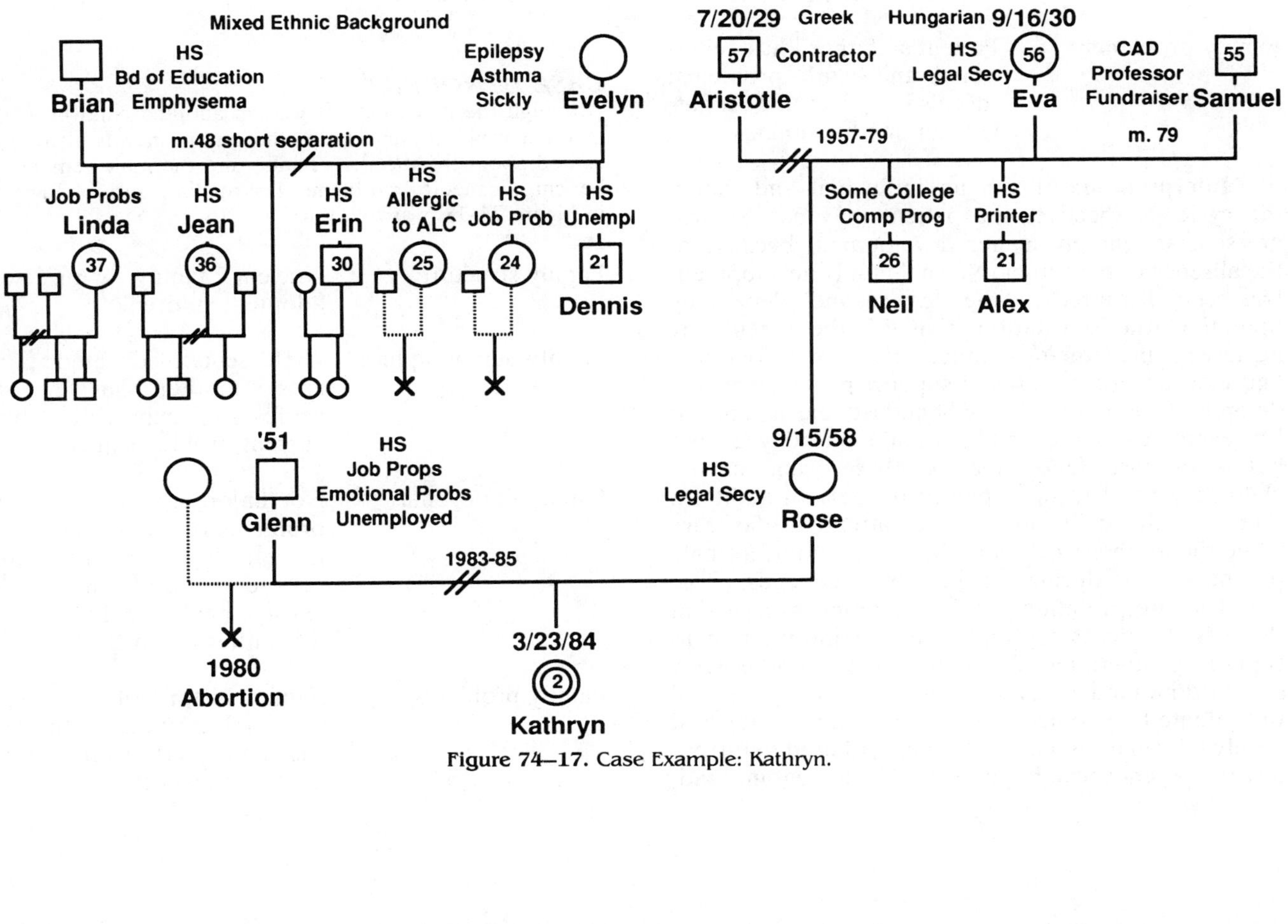

Figure 74–17. Case Example: Kathryn.

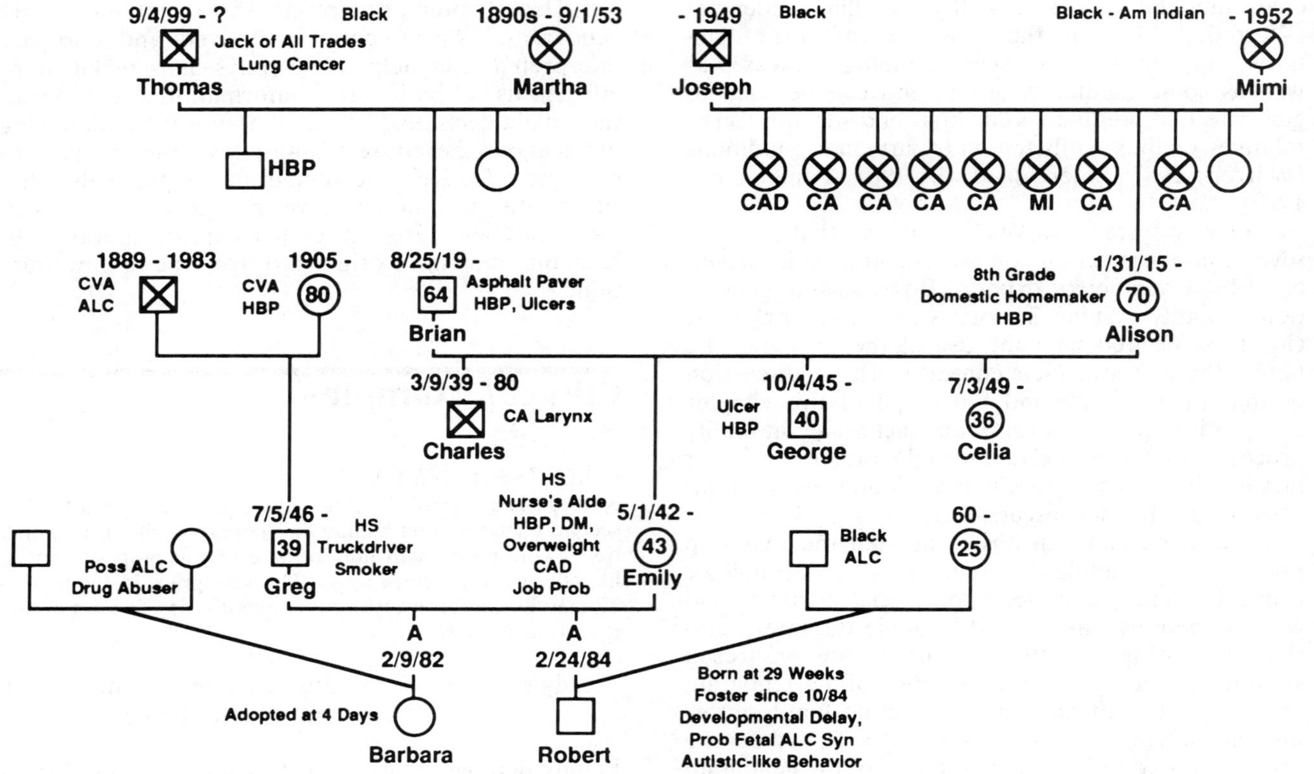

Figure 74–18. Case Example: Robert.

Family life events:	Divorce of patient's parents 1 year prior to visit; patient's birthday 2 days prior to visit
Family problems:	Patient's father has emotional and work problems; this also appears to be a pattern among his siblings.

Interpretation. From an individual and family life cycle perspective, the patient may not be progressing adequately in her development because of the absence of her father. Normal family development has been disrupted by the divorce and, depending upon the father's visitation privileges, the patient may be having inadequate contact with a male parental figure. From a stress–social support perspective, the divorce of the parents within the last year is a major life event, as is the child's second birthday 2 days before the visit. The impact of these events on the child may need to be explored further. In addition, there are the daily problems of attending day care while the mother works and the fact that only a single parent is home during evenings and weekends.

The interpretation of this genogram suggests that there is the necessary and sufficient information to support a functional abdominal pain hypothesis. A standard biomedical evaluation is of course indicated to evaluate that clinical hypothesis, and more focused family information may need to be gathered to further test the psychosocial hypothesis. The genogram reading and interpretation provide a guide to help the clinician efficiently gather the most relevant additional family data.

CASE II: ROBERT

Although the index patient was an adopted child brought in for a well-baby check-up, the physician was also concerned about the mother's health and the management of her chronic medical problems. The reading of the genogram in Figure 74–18 is as follows:

Family structure:	Nuclear family with two adopted children
Family demographics:	High school–educated parents; mother has health profession experience but current problems at work
Family life events:	No major life events; daily problems of child's developmental delay and behavior problems and mother's chronic health problems and difficulties at work
Family problems:	Family history of hypertension and cardiovascular disease and a very strong family history of cancer.

Interpretation. From the epidemiologic and genetic points of view, the mother's risk for cardiovascular disease has interacted with her current risk factors of high blood pressure, diabetes, and obesity to cause heart disease. She is also at risk for malignancy, so the status of her cancer-screening efforts as well as primary cancer-prevention efforts are of concern. From the stress–social support perspective, the stresses of young, adopted children along with the mother's own health problems may not be adequately buffered by the support of the husband, who is a truck driver and is out of town a great deal. The presence of a confidant to support the mother is a very important area to explore. The mother's ability to care for her own health needs may be compromised by the demands of her children and the apparent lack of support.

In this situation, the family information may be central to the preventive health activities of the family physician as well as to the management of chronic medical problems. Again, the genogram reading and interpretation provide the clinician with guidance as to fruitful areas to explore during brief office visits.

References

Arbogast, R. C., Scratton, J. M., and Krick, J. P.: The family as patient: Preliminary experience with a recorded assessment of schema. J. Fam. Pract., *7*:1151, 1978. *Looks at the family diagrammatically and descriptively, using a family interview questionnaire that includes phases of the family life cycle, the psychosocial interior of the family, and the social milieu.*

Birrer, R. B.: Urban Family Medicine. New York, Springer-Verlag, 1987.

Bray, J. H., Harvey, D. M., and Williamson, D. S.: Intergenerational family relationships: An evaluation of theory and measurement. Psychotherapy, *24*:516, 1987.

Campbell, T. L.: Family's Impact on Health: A Critical Review and Annotated Bibliography. National Institute of Mental Health. Series on No. 6, Department of Health and Human Services Pub. No. (adm) 86–1461. Washington, D.C.: Supt. of Docs., United States Govt. Print. Off., 1986. *This comprehensive review summarizes the current knowledge about the impact of family on both the mental and physical health of its members.*

Duhl, F. J.: The use of the chronologic chart in general systems family therapy. J. Marital. Fam. Ther., *7*:361, 1981. *Describes a method for documenting family events and their impact on each family member using a chronologic chart.*

Ebell, M. H., and Heaton, C. J.: Development and evaluation of a computer genogram. J. Fam. Pract., *27*:536, 1988.

Friedman, H., Rohrbaugh, M., and Krakauer, S.: The time-line genogram: Highlighting temporal aspects of family relationships. Fam. Proc., *27*:293, 1988.

Geron, M.: Genetics of Bipolar Affective Disorder and Its Application in Family Practice. Paper presented at the Annual Research Symposium, Department of Family Practice, Iowa City, University of Iowa, June 26, 1976.

Gordon, H.: The family history and the pedigree chart. Postgrad. Med., *52*:123, 1972. *An excellent brief outline of the major components of a pedigree chart.*

Huygen, F. J. A.: Family Medicine: The Medical Life History of Families. Nijmegen, The Netherlands, Dekker and Van de Vegt, 1978. *A thorough documentation of continuing medical care and the complexities of family health over a period of 30 years by a family physician in Holland. His observations of the medical problems of the families he treated are supplemented by 25 family charts.*

Jolly, W., Froom, J., and Rosen, M.: The genogram. J. Fam. Pract., *10*:251, 1980.

Kertesz, J.: Urban family mapping. *In* Bierrer, R. B. (Ed.): Urban Family Medicine. New York, Springer-Verlag, 1987, pp. 72–81.

Like, R. C., Rogers, J., and McGoldrick, M.: Reading and interpreting genograms: A systematic approach. J. Fam. Pract., *26*:407, 1988.

Lynch, J. J.: The Broken Heart: The Medical Consequences of Loneliness. New York, Basic Books, Inc., Publishers, 1977. *This book explores in depth the medical consequences of marital status and the availability of support and companionship.*

McGoldrick, M., and Gerson, R.: Genogram in Family Assessment. New York, W. W. Norton & Co., 1985. *This is an excellent book on genograms written by a psychiatric social worker and a family therapist. Genograms of famous families such as those of Freud, Fonda, Kennedy, and Roosevelt are used to illustrate structure and interpretation.*

Medalie, J. H.: Family Medicine Principles and Applications. Baltimore, Waverly Press, Inc., 1978.

Pauls, D. L., Noyes, R, and Crowe, R. R.: The familial prevalence in second-degree relatives of patients with anxiety neurosis (panic disorder). J. Affect. Dis., *1*:279, 1979.

Prince-Embury, S.: The family health tree: A form for identifying physical symptom patterns within the family. J. Fam. Pract., *18*:75, 1984.

Rainsford, G. L., and Schuman, S. H.: The family in crisis. J.A.M.A., *246*:60, 1981.

Ramsey, C. N.: Developmental Theory of Families: The Family Life Cycle. *In* Rakel, R. E. (Ed.): Textbook of Family Practice. Philadelphia, W. B. Saunders Co., 1984, pp. 41–49.

Rogers, J., and Durkin, M.: The semi-structure genogram interview. I, Protocol. II, Evaluation. Fam. Sys. Med., *2*:176, 1984.

Rogers, J., Durkin, M., and Kelly, K.: The family genogram: An underutilized clinical tool. New Jers. Med., *82*:887, 1985.

Rogers, J., and Cohn, P.: Impact of a screening family genogram on first encounters in primary care. Fam. Pract. *4*:291, 1987.

Smeraldi, E., Negri, F., Hembuch, R. C., and Kidd, K. K.: Familial patterns and possible modes of inheritance of primary affective disorders. J. Affect. Dis., *3*:173, 1981.

Shapiro, D. M.: A family data base for the family oriented medical record. J. Fam. Pract. *13*:881, 1981. *Provides an outline for a written summary of a family data base that is analogous to the traditional history and physical for an individual.*

Smilkstein, G.: The cycle of family function: A conceptual model for family medicine. J. Fam. Pract., *6*:1231, 1978.

Stevenson, I.: The Diagnostic Interview. 2nd ed. New York, Harper & Row, 1971. *The chapter "Variations in Interviews" contains a variety of charts correlating changes to life stresses over time. There is a good presentation on the correlations between emotions and symptoms over time and ways of detecting these in the interview as well as depicting them graphically.*

Syme, S. L., and Berkman, L.: Social class, susceptibility, and sickness. Am. J. Epidemiol., *104*:1, 1976.

Thompson, J. S., and Thompson, M. W.: Genetics in Medicine. 2nd ed. Philadelphia, W. B. Saunders Co., 1973. *Although the book deals primarily with the chromosomal and clinical aspects of genetics, the chapter "Patterns of Transmission of Genes and Traits" presents the fundamentals of inheritance and includes the symbols commonly used in pedigree charts.*

Thrower, S. M., Bruce, W. E., and Walton, R. F.: The family circle method for integrating family systems concepts in family medicine. J. Fam. Pract., *15*:451, 1982. *Using circles to represent themselves within a larger circle that represents the family, members illustrate in graphic form their interpretation of relationships within the family. The drawings provide, at a glance, patterns of closeness, of alliances, and of power that can be of help to the physician caring for the family.*

Warrell, D. A. (Ed.): Oxford Textbook of Medicine. 2nd ed. Oxford, Oxford University Press, 1987, pp. 4.10–4.36. *This comprehensive text gives a thorough overview of genetic mechanisms and disorders.*

Zander, L. I.: Recording family and social history. J. Coll. Gen. Pract., *27*:518, 1977.

75

The Economics of Family Practice

E. Lee Taylor

The highest use of capital is not to make more money, but to make money do more for the betterment of life.

HENRY FORD

Economics is the science of the production and distribution of goods and services. Medical economics is that part of the national economy that focuses on the production and distribution of health care goods and services. It is imperative that family physicians in this modern, complex, and rapidly changing medical economics system have an understanding of the basic national economic system and the role that medical economics plays within the system. Without that understanding, it would be difficult for any physician to maintain a practice that meets the growing demand for delivery of high-quality health care services in the most cost-effective manner.

The Law of Economics: Supply and Demand

One basic law of economics—the law of supply and demand—states that *when demand for a product or service is high, price will rise, and when the demand for a product or service decreases, the price will fall, provided all external forces remain stable.* The external forces that affect supply and demand in the health care system are numerous. The effects each force may have on the supply or demand side of the economic scale would require volumes to explain. One can see from Figure 75–1 that it is an almost impossible task to perfectly balance the economic elements of medical care. Many of these forces may affect either side of the scale—supply or demand for health care service.

A perspective of the present-day medical economy can be gained by a review of its historical development. Knowledge of the rapid changes in our health care system will provide some understanding of the many external forces that have produced the present medical economic environment.

The Evolution of Modern Medical Economics

Before 1940, there was really little interest in medicine, especially by the federal government. Most people, except the indigent, paid their own medical bills. The indigent were cared for by physicians who agreed to provide services to the poor in exchange for hospital privileges. A small number of group health insurance plans existed, but relatively few people belonged or subscribed to them. Medical care, in comparison with other costs, was not considered to be terribly expensive. The government financed only 20 per cent of the total national health care costs at that time. Today, the government's share of health care has more than doubled to over 40 per cent of total national health care expenditures (Campion, 1984). Many events have led to today's high health care costs and large expenditures for health care. Most have occurred since 1940.

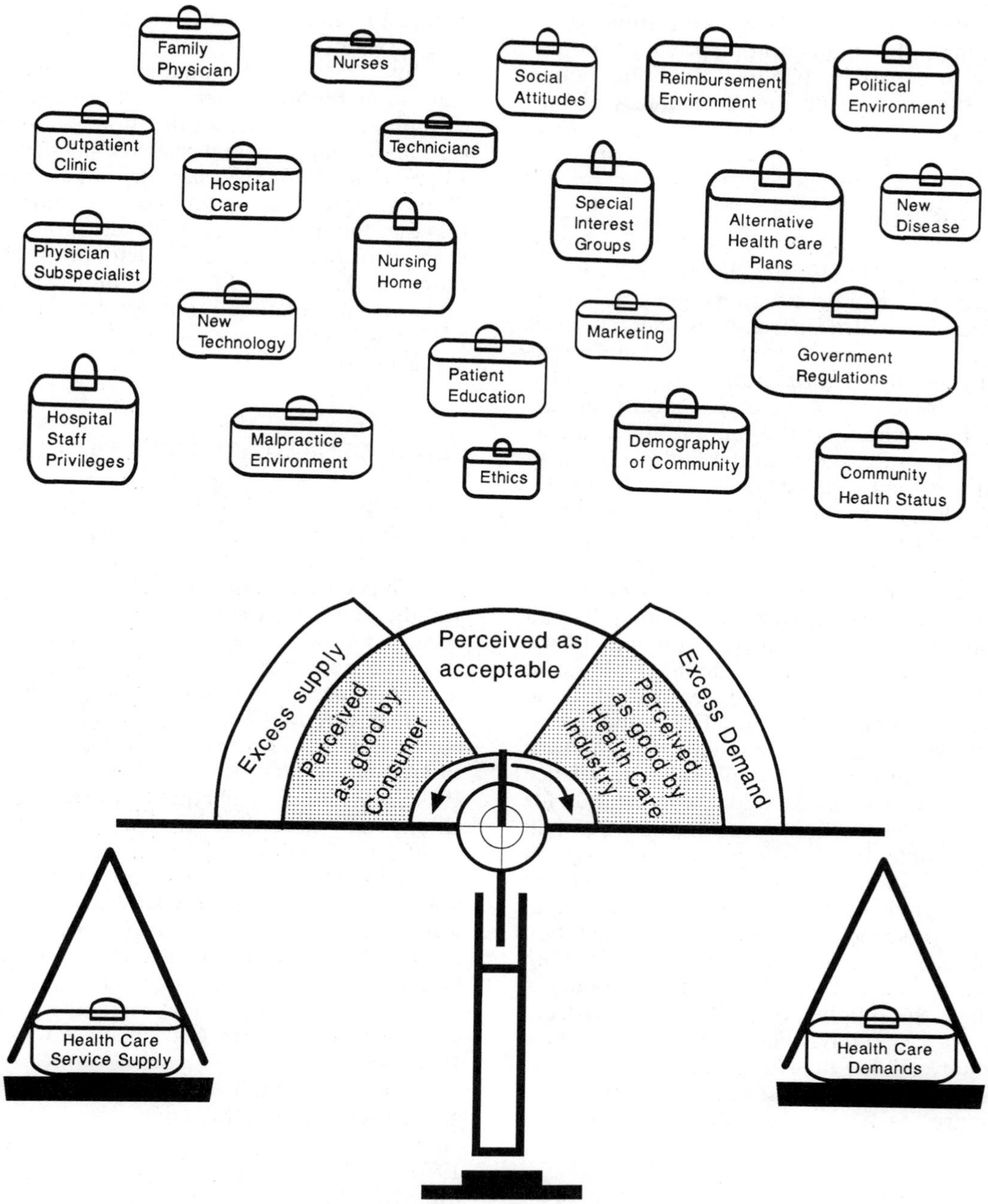

Figure 75–1. Health care economic scale and additional economic weights.

THE MOVE TO SPECIALIZATION

World War II brought about rapid changes in the health care system. During this time, antibiotics, anesthesia, and many medical and surgical techniques were developed and improved at a rapid pace. Before the war, most physicians were general practitioners; only 5256 physicians, or fewer than 25 per cent of physicians in the United States, were in specialty training. By 1946, the physicians in specialty training had increased by 70 per cent. Most physicians leaving the military after the war went back to specialty training because of increased technology and the new G.I. Bill of Rights, which provided educational stipends for veterans. These stipends supplemented these physicians' residency incomes and made additional training affordable. The federal government also started programs that subsidized medical schools and hospitals with large amounts of research funds. Consequently, the age of specialization was inevitable. By the 1950's, almost 20,000 physicians were in specialty training (Campion, 1984).

By 1946, the general practitioners were feeling a drastic reduction in both their numbers and their influence. Within the medical profession, some were losing hospital privileges because specialized hospital staffs were often requiring board certification or residency training rather than granting privileges on the basis of proven capability (Council on Long Range Planning, 1988). As a result, the American Academy of General Practice was formed in 1947.

PHYSICIAN SHORTAGE

As specialization continued, the shortage of primary care physicians (general practitioners, general internists, and general pediatricians) grew worse. The lack of primary care physicians, especially family physicians, and a general shortage and geographic maldistribution of physicians became a concern of the profession, the public, and the federal government. In 1948, the Ewing Report from the Federal Security Agency and a bill introduced by Senator Claude D. Pepper (D., Fla.) proposed a 5-year program of support for medical schools to address the predicted shortage of 42,000 physicians by 1960. The amount of federal funds to subsidize medical schools for research, training, and construction grew rapidly, and increasing specialization continued (Campion, 1984).

The 1950's saw the concern about a physician shortage continuing, and a series of reports led to the passage of the Health Professions Education Assistance Act of 1963. This act was intended to increase enrollment in medical and other allied health science schools. It provided loans to students and funds for renovating and constructing new facilities. Around the early to middle 1960's, the perception was that more economic stimulus was needed to increase health manpower. Federal legislation to fund operational support for schools was provided contingent on each school increasing its enrollment (Council on Medical Education, 1982). This funding stimulated the increase in the number of medical schools from 85 in 1957 to 127 today. The number of medical school graduates more than doubled, from 7264 in 1963, at the time the legislation was passed, to 15,667 by 1981 (Figure 75–2).

PRIMARY CARE DEVELOPMENT

Until the 1960's, real efforts were not made to control specialization. Even when efforts were made, there were no limits or restrictions, just more encouragement for medical school graduates to choose primary care specialties. The 1960's produced several reports indicating the need for primary care physicians. The Ad Hoc Committee on Education for Family Practice (The Willard Report) recommended that family practice be designated a specialty and that board certification be provided (Council on Medical Education, 1982). By 1969, The American Board of Family Practice was established; family practice became the 20th specialty and formal residency programs began. In 1971, the American Academy of General Practice changed its name to the American Academy of Family Physicians.

In 1975, the Coordinating Council on Medical Education reported that the percentage of primary care physicians (general practitioners, general internists, and general pediatricians) had decreased from 43 per cent of all physicians in 1965 to 34 per cent in 1972. Congress had attempted to stimulate interest for the family practice specialty with the Family Practice of Medicine Act in October of 1970. At that time, the American Boards of Internal Medicine and Pediatrics were advised to make primary care careers in their specialties more attractive (Council on Medical Education, 1982).

PUBLIC DEMAND AND EXPECTATIONS

Before 1940, medical care was not considered an important issue because medicine was frequently considered ineffective. During and after the war, with the advent of antibiotics, new surgical procedures, and the therapeutic success of medicine, medical care became a desired and demanded service of our society. The new demand for medical services created the rapid spread of health insurance. The number of people covered by health insurance grew from a very few in 1940, to 72.3 per cent of the population in the 1960's, and to 86.4 per cent of the population by the 1970's. With the enactment of Medicare for the elderly and Medicaid for the indigent in 1965, a significant additional demand was placed upon the profession for medical care and health care services. Many of the health care services being purchased were no longer personal, out-of-pocket expenses paid for by the individual consumer. Not only did the number of patients per physicians increase, but the number of visits per patient increased also. Physician visits per patient per year increased from three in 1940 to five in 1984.

Society's greater expectations from medical care also produced a malpractice crisis. The number of claims increased from 2.9 per 100 physicians before 1976 to 6.2 per 100 physicians by 1981. The size of awards to patients also increased, as did the premiums for professional liability insurance, at a rate of 14 per cent annually after 1976 (Campion, 1984).

EVOLUTION OF HOSPITAL AND SERVICES CARE

Many factors contributed to the growth of hospitals. Some of these were increased medical technology, new surgical procedures, federal grants for research, the Hill-Burton Act of 1946, private health insurance, and specialty training for physicians. As public demand for the quality of care being provided in hospitals rose, annual admissions increased from 13.6 million in 1940 to 36.2 million in 1980. Outpatient

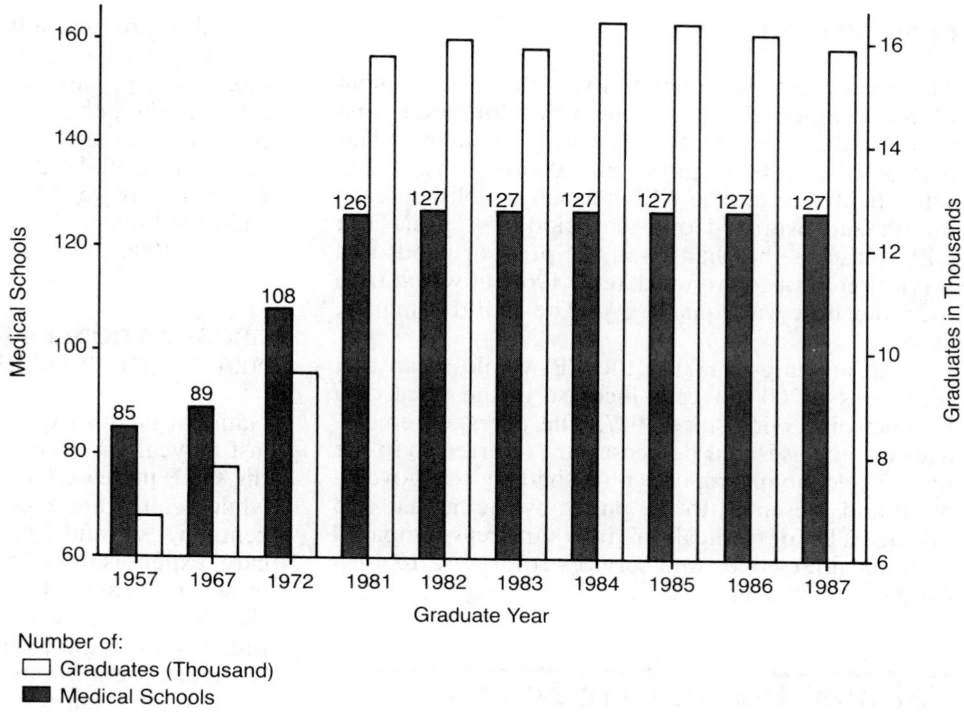

Figure 75–2. Medical school growth and graduates, 1957–1987. (From Crowley, A., Etzel, S., and Shaw, H. JAMA, *258*(8)[1957 after Campion, 1984].)

visits to hospitals increased by 44 per cent between 1970 and 1979 (Campion, 1984).

As accessibility to health care grew, so did cost. This was logical, but it was the degree of growth in expense that caused concern. In 1970, the Nixon administration recognized that the Medicare hospital program would cost $2.7 billion more than anticipated 5 years earlier. At this time, the focus of the federal government began to shift from the previous concern for access to health care to cost containment. As the cost of hospital care increased, many programs were instituted by the federal government to review hospital utilization and to limit the number of hospitals days and services provided during an admission (Campion, 1984).

The prospective payment system was enacted in 1983, a system of hospital reimbursement based on over 400 Diagnosis-Related Groups (DRGs). Under DRGs, hospitals are reimbursed at a fixed rate for diagnosis and treatment of the DRG, regardless of the length of stay or service provided. The prospective payment system has encouraged hospitals to provide only required services and to reduce the length of stay in the hospital.

As of 1986, the average length of stay in hospitals had decreased and was at a 16-year low for patients under 65 years of age and at a 5-year low for patients 65 years of age and older. These shorter lengths of stay are due to the prospective payment system implemented by the federal government in 1983 and the response of the health care profession to pressure from private businesses and health care insurance companies to reduce health care costs (Arnett and Freeland, 1987).

Understanding General Economics

As evidenced by the historical events since 1940, we have seen the effects of technology, public attitudes, demand for services, politics, and the massive federal economic stimulus that has brought us to today's complex system of medical economics.

To gain an understanding of today's medical economic environment, it is necessary to understand how the national economy is measured and evaluated. This will give physicians a better understanding of why there is so much private, public, and political interest in health care costs. Some important terms often used in describing the medical economic environment are described below.

GROSS NATIONAL PRODUCT

The gross national product (GNP) is the total market value of final goods and services produced by a national economy over a specific period of time. This is usually reported on an annual basis and is frequently used to measure the standard of living and the rate of economic growth. The rate of growth of a specific product or service is expressed as a percentage of the total GNP.

CONSUMER PRICE INDEX

The consumer price index (CPI) is the measurement of the average change in the price for goods and services that are bought for everyday living. This includes the costs for physicians, dentists, drugs, and other health care. The CPI is usually published each month and averaged over a period of 1 year. The CPI measures the changes in the price of goods and services from a reference date of 1967, at which time the index base was equal to 100 (The World Almanac, 1988).

An increase of 300 in the CPI would mean that there was a 200 per cent increase in the price of a product or service since 1967. The average percentages of increases and decreases are referred to in the medical economic reports published by the government and presented to the public by the media. The average CPI for medical care in urban areas compared with all other goods and services from 1982 to 1985 can be seen in Figure 75–3.

National Health Care Economics Today

From 1940 to 1986, the percentage allocation of national health expenditures between private and public sources almost reversed. In 1940, 80 per cent of health care expenditures came from private sources and 20 per cent from the public. By 1986, expenditures from private sources had decreased to 59 per cent and the public allocation had increased to 41 per cent. Twenty-nine per cent of the public allocation came from federal government sources (Reuter, 1988). Figure 75–4*A* and *B* demonstrates the source and distribution of the national health care expenditures in 1986.

GROSS NATIONAL PRODUCT MEASUREMENT OF HEALTH CARE COSTS

National health expenditures have increased for the last 50 years as a per cent of the GNP. In the 1970's the GNP increased at a rate of 2 to 6 per cent a year while health care expenses grew at a rate of 12.7 per cent. In 1980 and 1981 the growth of national health care expenses was 15 per cent, whereas the GNP grew at an annual rate of only 8.3 per cent. The slowdown in growth is probably due to increasing pressure from the federal government and the public to reduce health care costs, especially the costs of hospital inpatient services.

The highest health care expenditures on a national basis are for hospital care and physician services. Before 1965 and the enactment of Medicare and Medicaid programs, national expenditures for hospital care were $13.9 billion. This had increased to

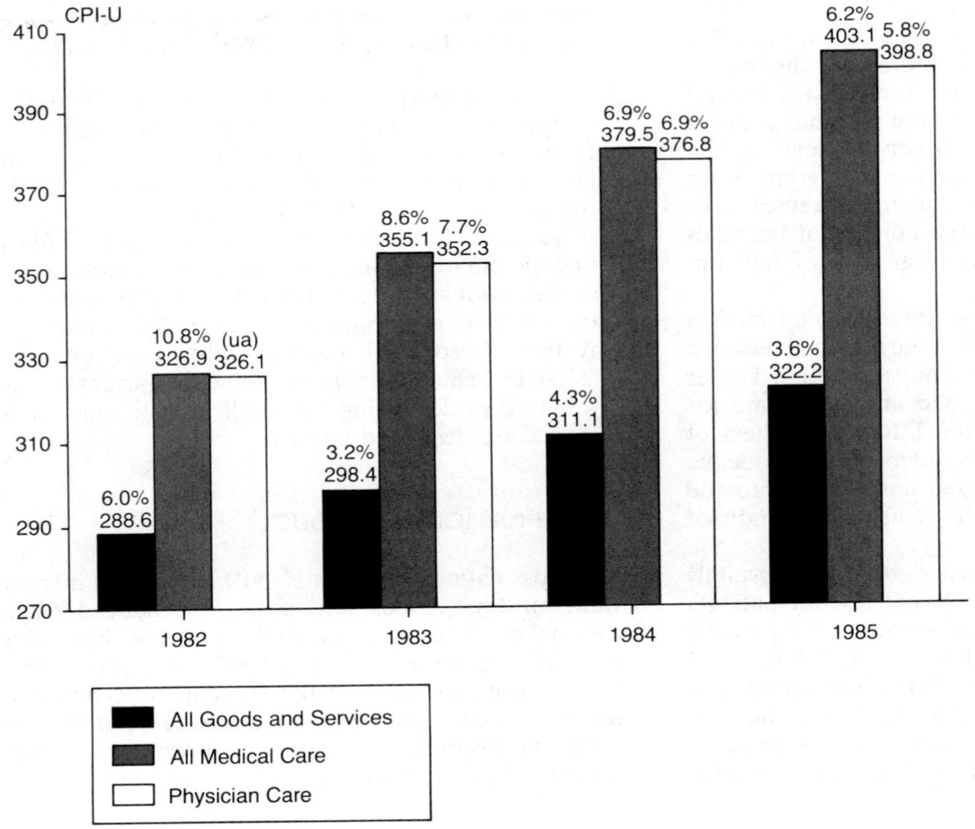

Figure 75–3. Average consumer price index—urban (CPI-U), 1982–1985. (Medical care versus all goods and services.) (From The World Almanac and Book of Facts. 1988, pp. 109–110; Bureau of Labor Statistics, U.S. Labor Dept.)

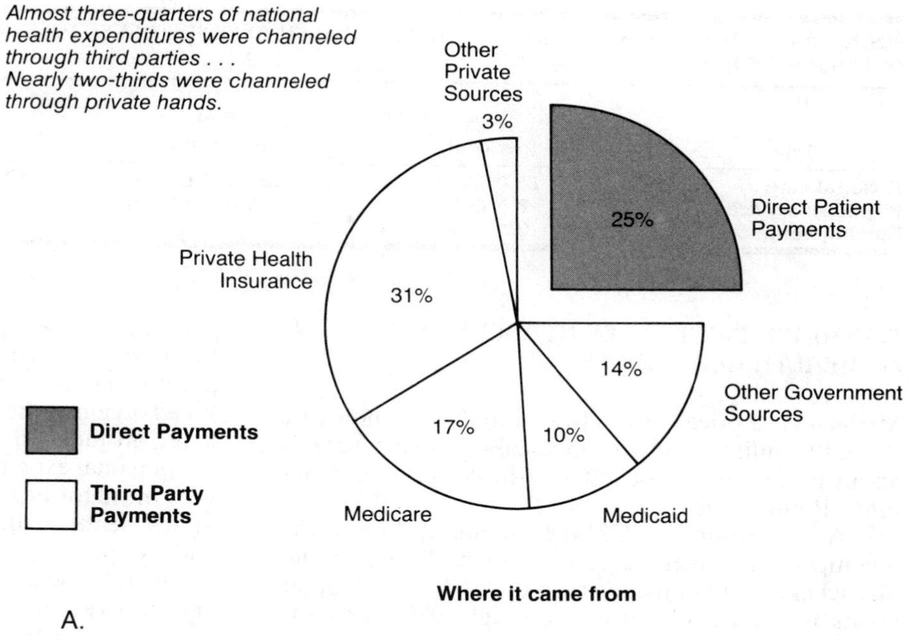

Figure 75–4. The nation's health dollar, 1986. (From Arnett, R., Freedland, M., et al.: National health care expenditures: 1986–2000. Health Care Financing Review, 8(4):3, 1987.)

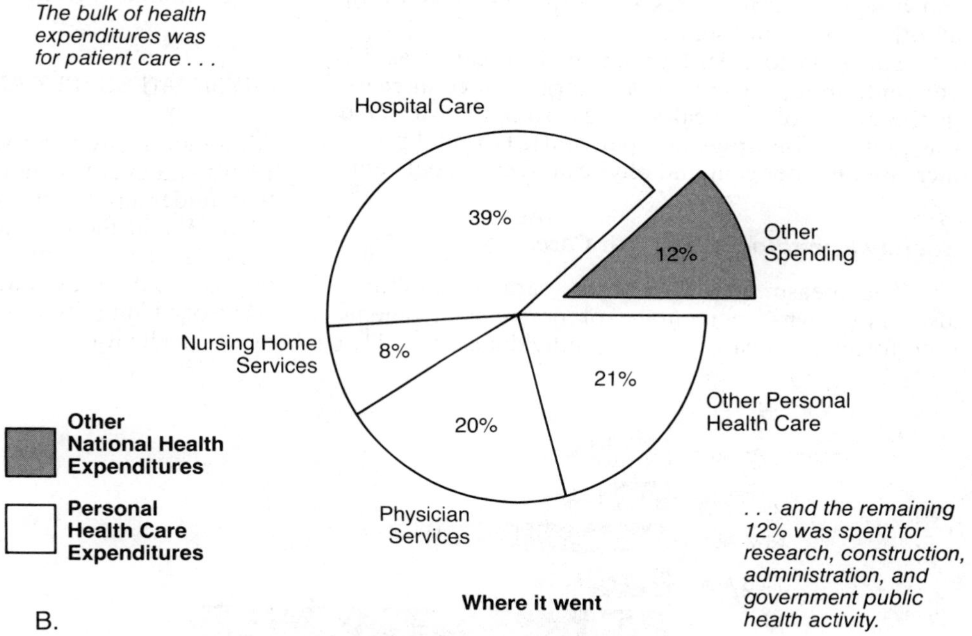

$176.6 billion by 1986. By 1986, physician service payments, which account for 20 per cent of the national health care dollar, had increased to 10 times the total 1965 charges (Reuter, 1988). One should note, however, that the percentage of the health care dollar that was spent for physician services ranged from 18.9 per cent to 20.5 per cent of total health care expenditures over the 21-year period (Table 75–1).

It is important to remember that after passage of the Medicare and Medicaid legislation in 1965, financial access to health care was provided for many who previously had had no health care coverage. Hospital admission rates increased 25 per cent, surgical procedures increased by 40 per cent, and the number of hospital days per person over 65 years of age rose 50 per cent. Since the group of these aged 65 or older accounts for 10 to 12 per cent of the population and needs more medical care than the younger segment of our society, it is not surprising that they account for over one fourth of the total medical expenditures (Campion, 1984). It was during this time of Medicaid and Medicare implementation, as discussed previously, that the number of medical school graduates was doubled to meet the demand for services.

Table 75–1. PARTIAL LIST OF UNITED STATES HEALTH EXPENDITURES, 1965–1990 (BILLIONS OF DOLLARS)

Type	1965 (per cent)	1980 (per cent)	1986 (per cent)	1990 (Projected in per cent)
Hospital care	$ 14.0 (33.4)	$101.6 (41.0)	$179.6 (39.2)	$250.4 (38.7)
Physician service	8.5 (20.3)	46.8 (18.9)	92.0 (20.1)	132.6 (20.5)
Nursing home care	2.1 (5.0)	20.4 (8.2)	38.1 (8.3)	129.0 (19.9)

CONSUMER PRICE INDEX MEASUREMENTS OF HEALTH CARE COSTS

Medical care prices have grown rapidly, as shown by the CPI. Inflation in the medical economic area is about twice the rate of inflation in the general economy (Reuter, 1988).

As an example of CPI measurement, Figure 75–3 compares the average CPI for all medical care and physician care with the average total CPI for all other goods and services from 1982 through 1985. The costs for medical services and total medical care have shown significant increases above the average CPI for all other goods and services.

The 1985 to 1986 CPI for medical care was 7.7 per cent, another increase. The largest price increase in the group of medical services from 1985 to 1986 was prescription drugs (8.6 per cent). Hospital prices increased 6.0 per cent and physician fees 7.2 per cent.

Society Spending on Health Care

The measurement of health care expenditures also shows what percentage of personal income is used for medical care. In 1986, individuals spent 11.6 per cent of their personal or household income for health care expenses. This amounted to about $1837 per person (Arnett et al., 1987).

To gain some perspective about the standard of living attitudes of our society, one needs to compare the personal expenditures for all products and services with those for health care. Table 75–1 lists the United States health expenditures from 1965 through 1986 and the projected expenditures for 1990. Figure 75–5 illustrates what consumers spend for many goods and services in their daily living. A comparison of these two documents brings closer some concept of the economic attitude of our society.

PHYSICIAN SUPPLY AND DEMAND

Although a physician shortage was predicted in the 1950's and every economic effort was made to correct that undersupply, the nation faced a new issue in 1978: Would there be too many physicians in 1990 if the present rate of production continued? To address that issue, the Graduate Medical Education National Advisory Committee was established by the Department of Health and Human Services. After 2 years

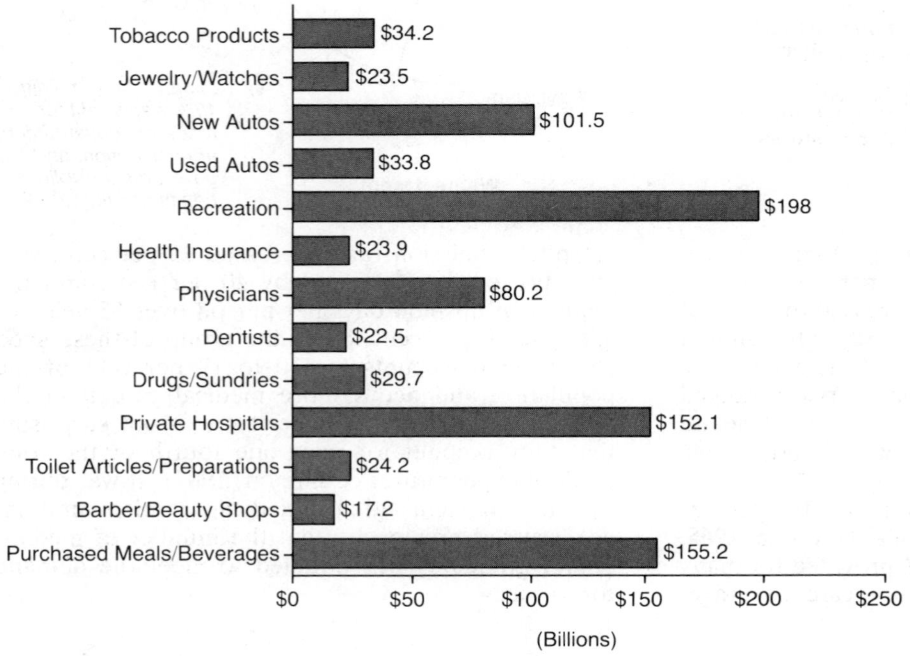

Figure 75–5. Personal consumption expenditures in the United States. (From The World Almanac and Book of Facts, 1988, p. 113; and Bureau of Economic Analysis, U.S. Commerce Dept.)

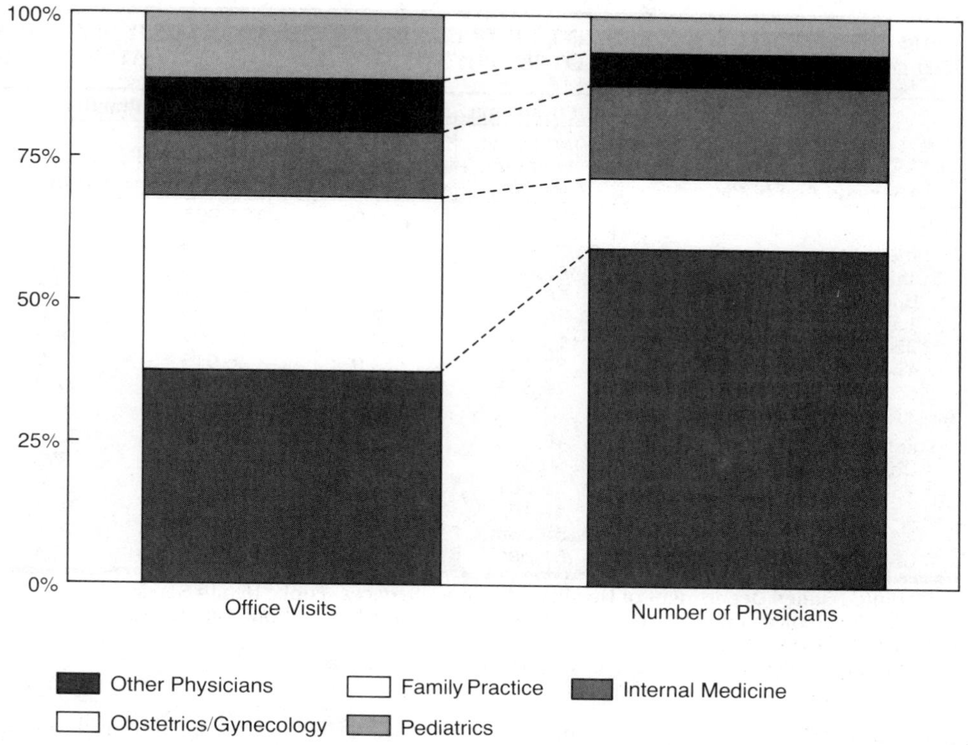

Figure 75–6. Ambulatory office visits to primary care specialists in the United States, 1985. (From American Medical Association, December 31, 1985 [physician numbers]; National Center for Health Statistics, 1985 Summary [office visits]; National Ambulatory Medical Care Survey, January 23, 1987, No. 128, p. 3; and American Academy of Family Physicians, 1987, p.22 [family practice].)

of study, the committee reported in 1980 that there would be an oversupply of 75,000 physicians by 1990 if the present rate of graduation from medical schools continued. As a result of this report, Congress decreased and eliminated much of the funding to medical schools that had begun in 1963 (Council on Medical Education, 1982).

In July 1988, a council appointed to advise congress on federal policies regarding physician supply and demand for services, The Council on Graduate Medical Education, reported the following (Residency Assistance Program Newsletter, 1988):

- There is an undersupply of family physicians.
- There is a geographic maldistribution of physicians, with few physicians in many rural and inner-city areas.
- There is an adequate supply of pediatricians.
- There may be an impending undersupply of general internists.
- More minorities should be represented in medicine.
- The present health care financing system decreases the attractiveness of certain disciplines to students and presents incentives that tend to produce a concentration of physicians in what may be oversupplied specialties.

By 1988, it appeared that the physician supply of medical school graduates was remaining stable or decreasing slightly. The trend has been a decrease of approximately 200 graduates per year since 1986 (Jonas and Etzel, 1988).

Future changes in reimbursement policy may play a greater role in increasing the number of primary care physicians, including family physicians. There have been discrimination patterns in the reimbursement system in the following ways:

- Physicians in rural areas have not been reimbursed at the same rate as those in urban areas. This includes reimbursements from Medicare.
- Primary care physicians, including family physicians in some cases, have received lower reimbursement than other specialists or subspecialists for performing the same procedures.

In 1988, The Harvard Resource Based Relative Value Scale study, directed by William S. Hsiao, was submitted to the Health Care Financing Administration for review. The reimbursement design, if accepted by Congress, will compensate more for cognitive skills and reduce the rate for some procedural and surgical treatments. It must first go through a series of hearings, including hearings held by Congress and organized medicine. The Health Care Financing Administration will also submit its own recommendations to Congress. It is expected that primary care physicians will receive more equitable reimbursements for the time they spend with patients (Director's Newsletter, 1988). A long, drawn out debate is expected, with the largest opposition coming from the surgical and internal medicine subspecialists

Table 75–2. NUMBER AND PER CENT DISTRIBUTION OF OFFICE VISITS BY SEX AND AGE OF PATIENT AND BY FAMILY PHYSICIANS AND OTHER PHYSICIANS IN THE UNITED STATES FOR 1985*

Sex and Age of Patient	All Physicians		Family Practice		Other Physicians†	
	Number of Visits in Thousands	*Per cent Distribution*	*Number of Visits in Thousands*	*Per cent Distribution*	*Number of Visits in Thousands*	*Per cent Distribution*
Total	636,386	100.0	193,995	100.0	442,391	100.0
Female						
Total female	387,480	60.9	117,685	60.7	269,795	61.0
Under 15 years	58,175	9.1	14,699	7.6	43,475	9.8
15–24 years	48,883	7.7	16,679	8.6	32,204	7.3
25–44 years	118,557	18.6	35,797	18.5	82,760	18.7
45–64 years	82,331	12.9	26,915	13.9	55,416	12.5
65 years and over	79,535	12.5	23,595	12.2	55,940	12.6
Male						
Total male	248,906	39.1	76,310	39.3	172,593	39.0
Under 15 years	60,594	9.5	14,960	7.7	45,633	10.3
15–24 years	25,081	3.9	9,672	5.0	15,408	3.5
25–44 years	57,167	9.0	20,251	10.4	36,917	8.3
45–64 years	55,060	8.7	17,081	8.8	37,978	8.6
65 years and over	51,004	8.0	14,346	7.4	36,657	8.3

*United States Department of Health and Human Services, Public Health Service, National Center for Health Statistics, National Ambulatory Medical Care Survey: Unpublished Data, and Facts About Family Practice. Kansas City, MO. American Academy of Family Physicians, p. 23.

†Excludes physicians in anesthesiology, pathology, and radiology.

because of the possibility of a reduction in some of their fees.

Family Practice Physician Supply and Demand

In 1975, family physicians accounted for 13.8 per cent of the total physician population. As of 1989, they account for about 11.9 per cent of the total (Council on Long Range Planning and Development, 1988). Part of this decreased percentage is a result of the increased number of graduates from medical schools and the overall increase in physicians.

Although composing only 11.9 per cent of the physician population, family physicians handle 30.5 per cent of the more than 636 million office-based outpatient visits per year in the United States. (Internists handle 11.6 per cent and pediatricians 11.4 per cent. [Council on Long Range Planning and Development, 1988].) Representing only 11.9 per cent of the physician supply, this country's family physicians handle approximately one third of the nation's total office visits (Figure 75–6).

The 1985 demographic analysis of family practice office visits compared with visits to other physicians can be seen in Table 75–2. It should be noted that about 20 per cent of office visits to family physicians were made by patients 65 years of age or older. Visits to family physicians accounted for 30 per cent of the total geriatric office visits to all physicians. With the rapidly growing geriatric population now approaching 12 per cent of the United States population, this is economically significant since all patients over 65 years of age are covered under the Medicare program. The aging population will continue to place an increasing demand on the specialty of family practice as well as on the entire health care system.

Distribution of Family Physicians

The geographic distribution of family practice graduates as of 1987 can be seen in Figure 75–7. Of the 1987 family practice graduates, 42.9 per cent practice in geographic areas with a population less than 25,000 and 27.6 per cent practice in areas more than 25 miles from a large city.

This geographic trend appears to be more common for family physicians than for the other primary care specialists. From 1970 to 1983, the overall physician supply increased in metropolitan and in rural areas, but the percentage slightly decreased in rural areas (Mead and Seidman, 1986). Although the Graduate Medical Education National Advisory Committee in its 1980 report predicted physician oversupply in many specialty areas (including pediatrics, obstetrics and gynecology, and certain internal medicine subspecialties), the trend toward specialization has continued. The recent Report of the Council on Graduate Medical Education has confirmed that the trend toward specialization continues, increasing further the undersupply of family physicians. From 1970 to 1983, internal medicine showed an increase of physicians of 95.6 per cent; pediatrics, 80.6 per cent; obstetrics and gynecology, 55.3 per cent; surgical specialists, 51.3 per cent; and family practice, 10.7 per cent (Mead and Seidman, 1986).

The annual report for 1987 of the American Board of Medical Specialties indicates that 51.2 per cent of those completing internal medicine residencies subspecialize and do not enter primary care. About 9.1 per cent of the obstetrics and gynecology residents

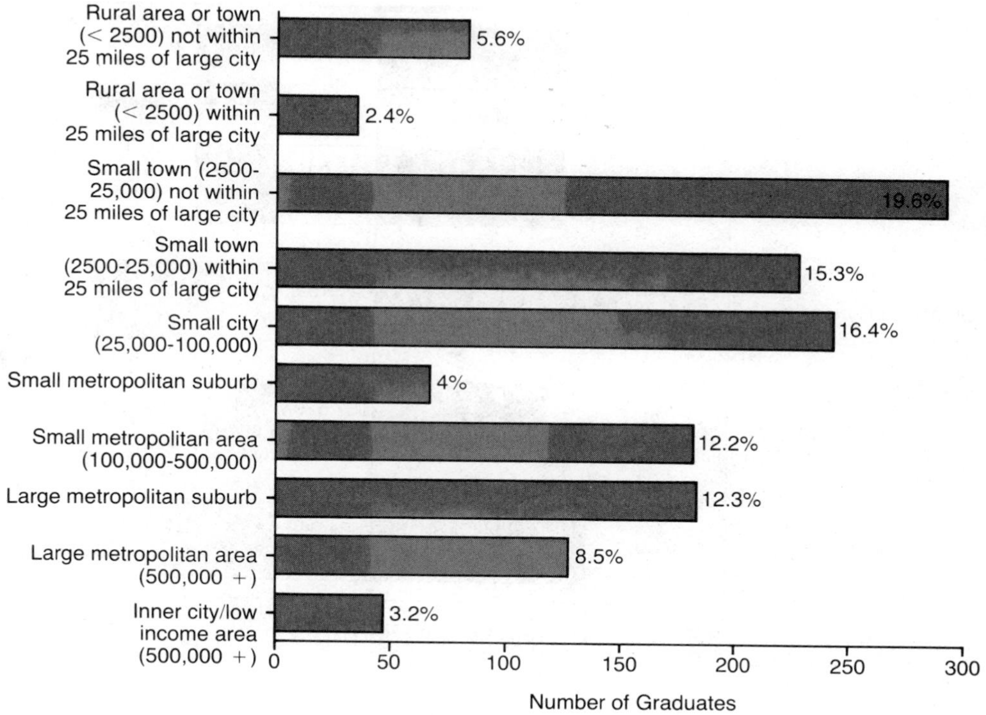

Figure 75–7. Distribution of residents graduating in 1987 by community size. (From American Academy of Family Physicians, Reprint No. 155N, 1988.)

and 19.7 per cent of pediatricians also subspecialize (Table 75–3). This means that 26,727 of those specialists do not enter primary care and must remain in larger metropolitan areas in and around large hospitals or medical centers in order to be provided with the consultations and high-technology equipment necessary to practice their subspecialties.

Family Practice Income

Family physicians, although not the most financially rewarded physicians in the medical profession, do very well economically. There are many factors that affect an individual's income. The economics of the community and the nation; the number of years one is in practice; the practice type; and, of course, the time and dedication one places in patient care and practice management all have an impact on personal economics.

Figure 75–8 compares the incomes and expenses of the primary care specialties with 1987 receipts. This information is provided by an ongoing survey that is conducted periodically by the journal *Medical Economics*. This survey is representative of specialty, geographic area, and age of physician. Overall, there are some general trends that can be seen from the *Medical Economics* continuing survey.

One trend is that all physicians' incomes tend to peak when physicians are between 40 and 49 years of age and reach their highest levels when physicians have been in practice between 10 and 20 years. In addition, the survey shows that 37 per cent of the family physicians surveyed had median practice earnings of $100,000 or more after expenses and before taxes. Approximately 62 per cent of physicians of all specialties surveyed had net incomes of more than $100,000 (Owens, A. 1988).

Figure 75–9 shows the number of patient encounters necessary for primary care specialties to generate the expenses and income illustrated in Fig-

Table 75–3. GENERAL AND SUBSPECIALTY CERTIFICATES ISSUED FROM 1977 THROUGH 1986 TO PRIMARY CARE SPECIALTIES*

Specialty	General Certificates Issued	Subspecialty Certificates Issued	Subspecialty Certificates as a Percentage of General Certificates
Family practice	26,506	—	—
Internal medicine	45,068	23,055	51.2
Obstetrics and gynecology	8,542	776	9.1
Pediatrics	14,664	2,896	19.7

*American Board of Medical Specialties: Annual Report. Evanston, IL, 1987, pp. 64–65.

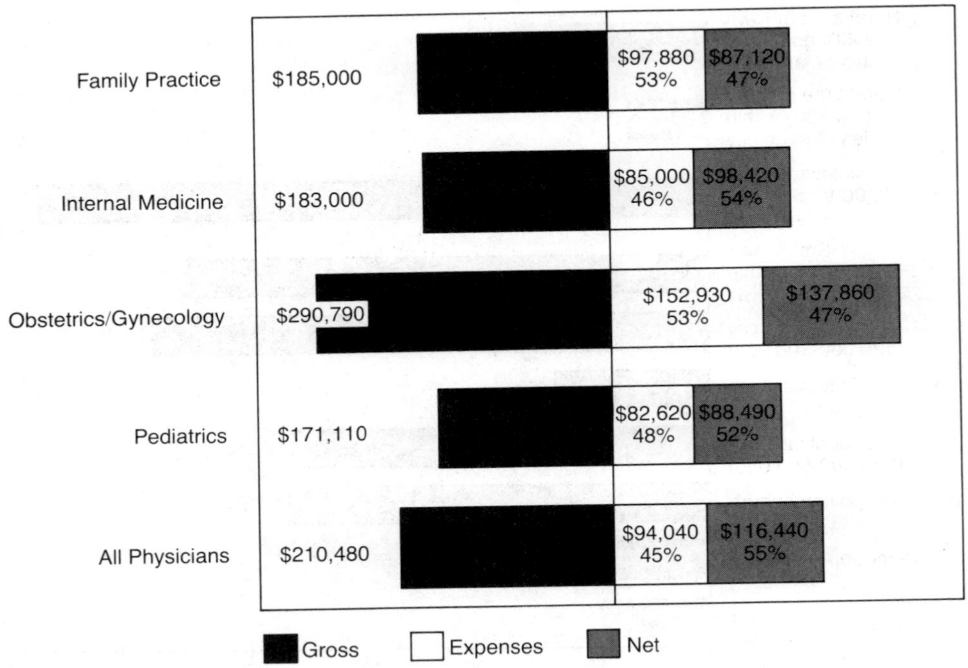

Figure 75–8. Median incomes and expenses of primary specialties from 1987 practice receipts (gross – expenses = net). (From Owens, A.: How much did your earnings grow last year? Copyright by Med. Econ., September 5, 1988, p. 161.)

ure 75–8. This includes all patient encounters, including office visits, home visits, nursing home visits, and hospital visits.

Alternative Health Care Plans

The alternative health care plans, such as Health Maintenance Organizations (HMOs) and Preferred Provider Organizations (PPOs) are heavily recruiting family physicians because of their broad base of expertise in providing health care to all ages and both sexes. It is imperative that family physicians understand these health care systems very thoroughly in order to avoid economic pitfalls (see Chapter 76).

HEALTH MAINTENANCE ORGANIZATIONS

HMOs experienced rapid growth as a result of the federal law enacted in 1973 to provide federal grants to private HMOs. This law was a result of pressure from private industry to cut health care costs. As of

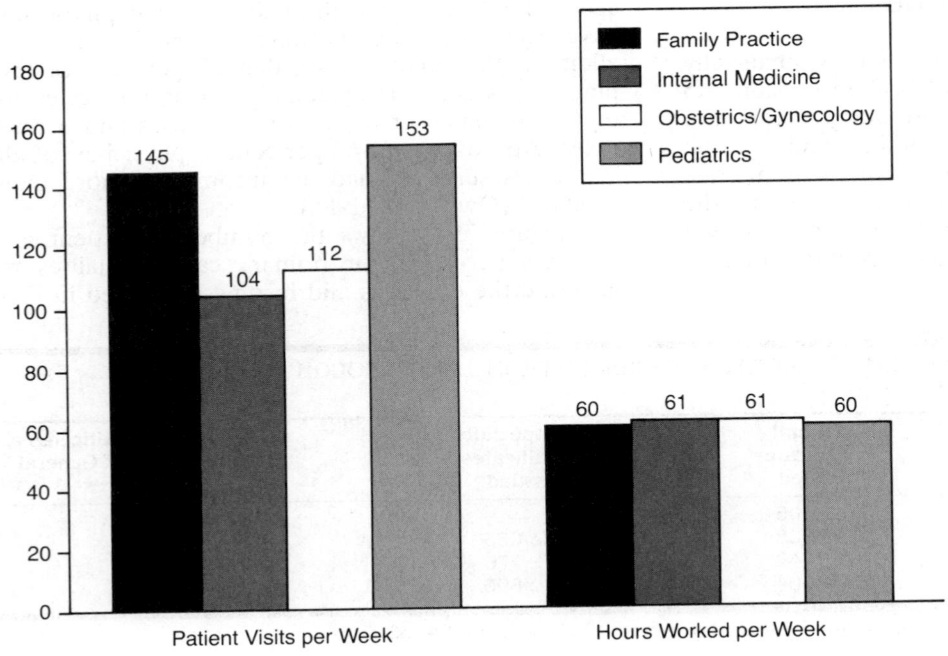

Figure 75–9. Median number of patient encounters and hours worked per week by primary care specialists, 1987. (From Owens, A.: How low can productivity go? Medical Econ., December 7, 1987, pp. 174, 190.)

1985, over 21 million Americans were enrolled in prepaid plans such as HMOs. This number is expected to increase to approximately 50 per cent of the population by the year 2000 (Aluise, 1988).

HMOs have several unique characteristics that differ from traditional health insurance. A fixed number of patients enroll in a plan with a physician or group practice. A contract is entered into in order to provide comprehensive health care services to patients enrolled in the plan. The physician receives a fixed amount of money to provide specifically defined care and services. This fixed payment per enrollee is received regardless of use by the enrollee. Some patients use more than the allocation; some use less. Few patients use none of this allocation.

The physician is at risk financially and can experience an economic loss if costs for excessive visits, health services, or serious illnesses exceed the fixed allocations per patient or enrollee. The process of providing care to an HMO community must be monitored very closely, and the family physician must be very careful to assess the amount of administrative time that the HMO places upon his present practice and office staff. In addition to financial and administrative burdens, the family physician must be aware of the possibility of being placed in an adversarial relationship with a patient when he or she denies a patient's requests for laboratory and x-ray procedures or consultation services that may be unnecessary but that the patient perceives as otherwise. As a so-called gatekeeper in this system, the family physician may often find that he or she is in another adversarial role with consultants regarding the number of visits or health care services the consultant perceives as necessary (Aluise, 1988).

PREFERRED PROVIDER ORGANIZATIONS

The PPOs combine the philosophy of fee for service with an HMO type of health care plan. PPOs operate within a system that comprises a panel of health care providers and includes physicians, hospitals, diagnostic centers, and other entities to form a contractual team concept. A fee schedule for each service is negotiated and agreed upon before the service is provided. Patients are given a choice of services within that health care system. The fee schedule is usually 10 per cent to 20 per cent less than the area's prevailing charges. In PPOs, cost-effective health care is encouraged through incentives for patients to use more outpatient services such as surgery and health care and rehabilitation services. They are also required to have preadmission certification and second opinions. They closely monitor costs and productivity patterns of the physicians and other providers of health care services. Some malpractice policies may not cover a physician while participating in a PPO contract (Aluise, 1988).

As of July 1986, 650 plans enrolling 24 million people were in business. Membership growth has been over 25 per cent annually. Many concerns have been expressed regarding the possible conflict of prepaid arrangements and the potential for lowering the quality of care and placing the patient at risk by limiting services. Consequently, physicians must continue to maintain high ethical standards and be patients' advocates. Third-party payers can be held liable if they are considered to have unreasonable cost-containment provisions that may adversely influence medical decisions (Cook and Rodnick, 1988).

Future Directions

The present medical economy has evolved at a rapid pace, primarily since 1940. The influence upon the medical economic environment has come from numerous sources: the government, the public, special-interest groups, professional societies, and the explosion of scientific knowledge and technology. The federal government has played a significant role in the advancement of health care access and quality of care in this country; however, it must also accept and share the responsibility for the increased costs that have been created by social medical programs. Although political leaders are focusing upon the cost-effective side of health care costs in the face of a large national budget deficit, they will find it difficult to place any of the burden on private citizens. Health care is now viewed as a basic right and not an economic commodity, as other goods and services are considered to be.

The federal government must address several issues. Physician supply and reimbursement policies affect medical students' selections of specialties and often influence physicians to choose geographic locations away from needy rural or urban areas. Little has been done to provide incentives for students to enter family practice or to practice in rural areas. The number of students who have chosen family practice as a specialty has fallen far below the level that had been expected. The national goal had been for 50 per cent of all graduates to enter primary care specialties, with half of that number entering family practice (Rakel and Pisacano, 1984). The number of students entering family practice each year has ranged from 10 to 15 per cent and has never reached that goal. Overall, rural and inner-city areas have had little gain in overall physician supply, although 42.9 per cent of family practice graduates go to these areas.

The federal government, medical schools, and state legislatures must provide visible and positive encouragement as well as economic stimulus in order to increase student interest in family practice. Family physicians as well as all other physicians must practice more management and understand the political and economic facets of health care delivery.

In 1978, Rogers recognized problems we still have a decade later:

- Academic medical center faculties do a poor job of preparing physicians for a generalist role.
- Family physicians and general internists in rural areas receive less remuneration than specialists who practice fewer hours in major hospitals. This needs to be corrected.
- Physicians do not have a sufficient understanding of the financial aspects of health care.
- A geographic maldistribution of physicians creates problems of access to health care for many patients.
- Health care is not being adequately delivered on an ambulatory basis.

Efforts to correct the situation have been slow because of the misdirection of medical education, economic stimuli, and political attitudes within our medical schools and the medical profession. Family physicians will determine their destiny by their participation in and response to these challenges, but appropriate stimuli from medical schools and the political and professional environment will be mandatory to reach any type of medical economic balance in our society.

Acknowledgment

I would like to express my appreciation to the following individuals who have contributed their patience and unswerving efforts to this chapter.

Mrs. Jamie Wise for her secretarial skills and patience.

Ms. Priscilla Roberts for her editorial assistance.

Mr. Terry Stone for his illustration and graphic assistance.

The Honorable Ronnie G. Flippo, U.S. Congressman, 8th District, Alabama, and his staff for providing U.S. Government health care analysis information through the Library of Congress.

References

A Report of the Council on Medical Education, American Medical Association, Future Directions for Medical Education. Chicago, Illinois, American Medical Association 1982, pp. 77–86. *This paperback, available for the AMA, provides a total history of medical education in a concise format. The book is divided into two sections; the first half is the actual report and the second half is a historical survey of the major factors and events that influenced medical education to the early 1980's.*

Aluise, J. J.: Essentials of Family Medicine. Baltimore, Williams and Wilkins, 1988.

American Academy of Family Physicians (AAFP) Directors Newsletter Kansas City, Missouri, Oct. 14, 1988.

American Board of Medical Specialties Annual Report and Reference Handbook. Evanston, Ill., American Board of Medical Specialties, 1987.

Arnett, R., Freeland, M., McKusick, D., et al.: National health expenditures: 1986–2000. Health Care Financing Review, Health Care Financ. Admin., *8*:1, 1987. *This government publication is a thorough analytic survey that analyzes all facets of health care, its history, and its present and future projections.*

Braude, J. M.: Complete Speakers and Toastmaster's Library: Remarks of Famous People. Englewood, N.J., Prentice Hall, 1965.

Campion, F. D.: The AMA and U.S. Health Policy Since 1940. Chicago, Chicago Review Press, 1984. *Campion provides a detailed history of the total evolution of American medicine from 1940 through the early 1980's, with detailed events of a political, social, and economic nature. This book should be a reference for any student or physician who desires an in-depth understanding of how medicine has reached such exponential growth and public attention.*

Cook, J. V., and Rodnick, J. E.: Evaluating HMO/IPA contracts for family physicians: One group's exposures. J. Fam. Pract., *26*:325, 1988.

Council on Long Range Planning and Development, American Medical Association: The future of family practice. J.A.M.A., *260*:1272, 1988. *This report of the American Medical Association was developed in cooperation with the American Academy of Family Physicians. It reviews the history and development of family practice, discusses some of its strengths and weaknesses, and identifies the new challenges and opportunities that face the 20-year-old specialty.*

Council on Medical Education: Future Directions for Medical Education. Chicago, American Medical Association, 1982. *This paperback, available from the American Medical Association, provides a total history of medical education in a concise format. The book is divided into two sections: The first half is the actual report, and the second half is a historical survey of the major factors and events that influenced medical education through the early 1980's.*

Director's Newsletter. Kansas City, Mo., American Academy of Family Physicians, Oct. 14, 1988.

Facts About Family Practice. Kansas City, Mo., American Academy of Family Physicians, 1987. *This 135-page paperback of factual material and statistics regarding the specialty of family practice covers supply and distribution of physicians and demographic, economic, and educational statistics taken from the American Medical Association's data file, the Department of Health and Human Services, and the American Academy of Family Physicians. It is a good reference for family physicians seeking a data base for entering practice or comparing an established practice with survey results and other statistics about family practices.*

Jonas, H. S., and Etzel, S. I.: Undergraduate medical education. J.A.M.A., *260*:1067, 1988.

Mead, D., and Seidman, B.: National Physician Trends from 1970–1983. Chicago, American Medical Association, Department of Data Release Services, 1986.

Owens, A.: How low can productivity go? Med. Econ., *64*:174, 1987.

Owens, A.: How much did your earnings grow last year? Med. Econ., *65*:159, 1988. *This article is an extensive analysis of a* Medical Economics *continuing survey of physicians of different specialities, geographic locations, and age groups. It is well done, and the graphics simplify the many economic areas. Usually different issues of* Medical Economics *will concentrate on a specific economic area, i.e., expenses, income, and other appropriate areas of practice economics.*

Rakel, R. E.: Textbook of Family Practice. 3rd ed. Philadelphia, W. B. Saunders Co., 1984, p. 3.

Residency Assistance Program Newsletter, American Academy of Family Physicians. Kansas City, MO, *2*:2–3, 1988.

Reuter, J. A.: Health Care Expenditures and Prices. Major Issues System Brief. The Library of Congress, Washington, D.C., Congressional Research Service, 1988, pp. 1–12.

Rogers, D. E.: American Medicine Challenge for the 1980's. Cambridge, MA, Ballinger Publishing Co., 1978, pp. 77–86. *Rogers describes, predicts and makes recommendations for medicine to meet the challenges we are facing today from the education system to actual health care delivery.*

The World Almanac and Book of Facts 1988, published for Birmingham Post Herald, New York, New York, Newspaper Enterprise Association, Inc., 1987, p. 109.

76

Managed Health Care

Robert Eidus
Michael A. Stocker

Managed health care is a system of reimbursement for health care services that is designed to control costs while preserving quality of care. The system of controls is generally a combination of incentives to providers of health care and rules whose adherence to by both providers and patients is necessary to guarantee reimbursement. The emergence of managed health care is a result of the desire of individuals to ensure access to health care in the 1920's and 1930's, combined with the recognition in the 1960's and 1970's that cost containment is an issue for the country as a whole. Manifestations of these concerns were the Medicare Act of 1965, which addressed individual issues of access and affordability, and the Health Maintenance Organization (HMO) Act of 1973, which addressed the national concern for cost containment.

Health care costs, which grew at a linear and affordable rate through the first three quarters of the century, have escalated dramatically in the last 15 years. Adding to the pressure for reform is the fact that health care spending seems to be highly inefficient and without commensurate value for the dollars expended. Current United States health care expenditures exceed 11 per cent of its gross national product. This is double the amount spent by many other industrialized nations. Despite this expenditure, our longevity and perinatal mortality rate, as measures of the overall health of our society, are worse than those of many other industrialized nations. Attempts to control costs have met with varying success. Medicare has had great difficulty in controlling costs and is moving toward increased regulatory control. The demand for health care services has outstripped American society's willingness to pay for them. HMOs, which control cost through a combination of rules and incentives, have met with mixed success to date. Traditional indemnity health insurance also now recognizes the need for reform.

Health Care and Cost

Victor Fuchs (1972) has developed a model (Fig. 76–1) for assessing the value of health care expenditures. Point C maximizes the value of gain in health care benefit per dollar input. Typically, developing countries that have recently made rapid gains in the areas of public health and hygiene find their cost-benefit ratio to be on this slope of the curve. Point A on the curve indicates that at some point no additional expenditure of health care dollars will result in any appreciable improvement in the overall health of the population. At point B, a dollar input into the health care system results in a dollar value output in terms of health care benefits. Beyond that point, for every dollar input, there is less than a dollar value to the general population. Few people will argue that the United States currently is closer to point A than point B—hence, the mandate for more cost-effective management of the health care dollar.

The main causes for escalation of health care costs are the proliferation of medical technology, the rapid increase in the number of health care providers, an increase in public demand for health care services,

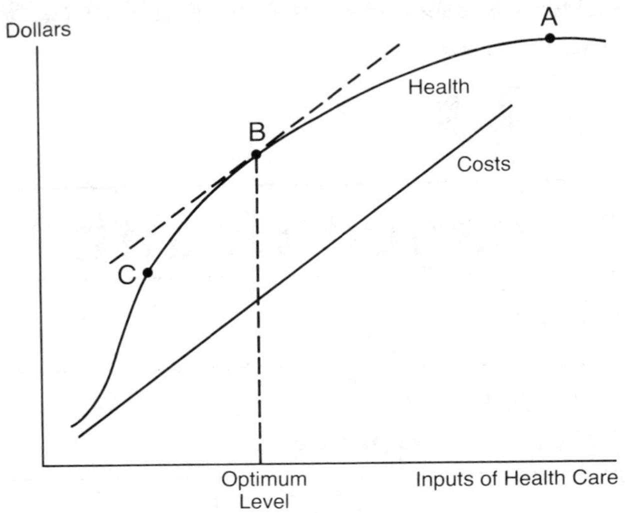

Figure 76–1. Determination of optimum level of health care utilization.

and the removal of direct payment from the patient to the health care provider with the advent of third-party payers. Most of the new health care technologies have been what is referred to as secondary or halfway technologies (Thomas, 1974). Secondary technologies tend to deal with disease once the illness becomes manifest. These technologies can halt the progression of but not reverse, cure, or prevent further pathophysiology. Examples of such technologies are coronary artery bypass grafting and respirators. Secondary technologies tend to be very expensive. This is in contrast to primary (complete) technologies, which are designed to attack and prevent the cause of pathology. Primary technologies reflect a full understanding of causation and pathophysiology. Examples are polio and smallpox immunization programs. These programs are quite inexpensive and tend to fall at point A on Fuchs' curve. Unfortunately, the number of secondary technologies far exceeds primary technologies at present.

The proliferation of health care providers has caused a secondary increase in demand for health care services as well as costs per procedure. Many of these services have a marginal cost-benefit ratio. The utilization of procedures such as tonsillectomy, hysterectomy, coronary angiography, and carotid endarterectomy varies greatly from community to community, and the variation cannot be explained by differences in the overall health of the populations leading to the actual need for such services (Chassin et al., 1986). In an affluent, highly educated society, the demand for health care services is often in excess of the need. These expectations are accentuated by the removal of direct payment from the patient to the provider of health care services.

Health Insurance

For the first half of the 20th century, there was only a small market for health care insurance. Most middle- and upper-class economic groups were able to pay directly for their health care services. Lower-class economic groups were treated as charity cases by both hospitals and doctors. Health care providers were therefore limited in what they could charge by what the patient could afford to pay. Gradually, however, a larger segment of society found that they were unable to pay for health care services. The Great Depression of the 1930's increased the number of individuals exposed to this problem. From this developed, in the late 1930's, the widespread availability of nonprofit (Blue Cross and Blue Shield) and commercial insurance for both hospital care and physician services. Historically, these plans did not cover preventive health care services and emphasized reimbursement of surgical procedures. In 1965 and 1966, with the creation of Medicare and Medicaid, millions of additional people were afforded health care insurance coverage. Therefore, by the late 1960's, most health care was reimbursed by a third-party payer. The provider (physician) and recipient (patient) then no longer were directly accountable to each other for the costs of health care services rendered. This lack of mutual financial accountability has been a potent stimulus for the increased demand by both physicians and patients for the provision of health care services. Commercial and nonprofit insurers have not recently been able to predict their costs reliably. Their revenues generated have often been insufficient to cover costs. In 1987, nongovernmental health insurers had a net loss of over 3 billion dollars with Blue Cross/Blue Shield absorbing approximately half of the losses. Adding significantly to the problem is the overall federal budget deficit. Thus, the societal imperative for managed health care has been set in motion.

Until recently, most physicians have felt that the payment for health care services is solely a relationship between the patient and the insurers and the physician is not and should not be involved. Managed health care attempts to establish a relationship of mutual accountability between the patient, the insurer, and the provider of health care services. Thus, the third party is no longer merely a payer of health care services but now is an active participant in the process. It is predicted that, by the year 2000, virtually all health care will be managed to some degree. Traditional indemnity insurance plans are putting managerial controls on their payment of benefits. Governmental health insurance is regulating care aggressively and is studying the implementation of new types of fee structures. Perhaps the most aggressive attempt at control, although not necessarily the most effective, is mandatory assignment. Under mandatory assignment, physicians are not permitted to bill for the balance of payment, with the exception of copayments and deductibles, for fees in excess of "allowable charges." This regulatory control has been implemented in some states and considered by others as well as by the United States Congress.

GENERAL FEATURES OF MANAGED HEALTH CARE

There are certain general features that are common to almost all forms of managed health care. These features include utilization review, mandatory second opinions, case management, same-day surgery, defined limitations of coverage, and variations in benefits. When utilized collectively, they have a modest effect on controlling costs.

Utilization Review. This is the review of health care services before, during, and after the services are being rendered. Concurrent review is performed by nurses and physicians during the actual use of services. The reviewer looks specifically at whether or not the patient's illness meets the severity of illness criteria, both for admission and for continued hospitalization. In addition, there is a determination of whether or not services provided are clinically indicated. Insurers who actively utilize this form of management must have the ability to receive accurate information about the current status of the patient and must be able to intercede to prevent utilization or deny payment for unnecessary services. Preadmission notification is utilized to identify some of the problems addressed in concurrent or retroactive review before they occur. Typically, hospitals and physicians are required to notify the insurer in advance for elective admissions. Preadmission notification offers the opportunity for education and direction to more cost-effective ways of providing care. Utilization review is becoming commonplace with all insurance companies and HMOs, and it is expected that they will become more aggressive by not paying for nonauthorized services.

Mandatory Second Opinions. Many common procedures are overutilized. These include hysterectomy, tonsillectomy, coronary angiography, coronary artery bypass surgery, carotid endarterectomy, cataract surgery, cesarean section, and septoplasty. These procedures, which are among the most frequently performed, tend to lack clearly defined, objective clinical indications and require a high degree of physician judgment. Nevertheless, when panels of experts in a given field have retroactively reviewed the indications for performing these procedures, there is a consensus that a large percentage of these procedures were not clinically indicated. Insurance companies often designate certain procedures as requiring a second opinion prior to the performance of surgery. The effectiveness of traditional second opinion programs has been limited, although one hospital achieved a 34 per cent reduction in the number of cesarean sections performed (Myers and Gleicher, 1988). As a result, managed care organizations are moving toward the development of independent panels of regional consultants or computerized decision-making algorithms to objectively assess indications for procedures. Application of predetermined criteria could call into question as much as 17 per cent of coronary angiography procedures and 32 per cent of carotid endarterectomies, with larger numbers being equivocal in terms of clinical indicators (Merrick et al., 1986; Chassin, et al., 1987).

Case Management. This is distinct from the role of the primary care physician as case manager. Traditionally, case management has referred to the coordination of the delivery of health care services to patients who have complex medical illnesses that require the overlapping of primary, secondary, tertiary, and long-term care and rehabilitative services. Typically, these services are coordinated by an experienced nurse clinician who has expertise in utilization review, rehabilitation, or the provision of home care services. The case manager's role is to coordinate care after clinical decisions have been made by the physician (e.g., the use of a respirator at home). The case manager is also responsible for the orderly transfer of medical information from one health care provider to another.

Same-Day Surgery. Although the charges for health care services provided in hospitals are highly regulated, outpatient care fees are not. Therefore, charges for these services often vary significantly from actual costs, and opportunities for negotiation of fees exist. Changing the site does not always decrease the cost. Some hospitals, in an effort to maximize reimbursement, have made some outpatient surgical procedures more expensive than if they were performed as inpatient procedures. Over the past decade, many procedures thought only to be appropriate in a hospital setting are now provided safely in the outpatient setting. These include cataract surgery, herniorrhaphy, dilatation and curettage, vasectomy, and endoscopy. Typically, these short-procedure units develop their own indications for utilization as well as their own quality assurance mechanisms. Third-party payers can independently develop their own clinical indications for utilization and require that certain procedures only be done on an outpatient basis.

Defined Provider Panels. Although these are most commonly associated with alternative delivery systems, they may also be associated with traditional forms of insurance. In traditional insurance plans, defined provider panels are usually associated with reduced copayments or the elimination of balance billing. Usually, these provider panels are defined as "participating physicians and hospitals." Defined provider panels may be composed of primary physicians, consultants, diagnostic facilities, and hospitals. By limiting provider panels, there is an increased ability to monitor quality and cost-effectiveness. In addition to fee restrictions, participating physicians and facilities agree to participate in preadmission authorization, second opinion, utilization review, and quality assurance activities.

Benefits Management. Increasingly, insurance companies and alternative delivery systems are placing limitations on the breadth of coverage. Traditionally, most plans exclude experimental procedures and cosmetic surgery. These are usually defined within the benefits policy. In addition to this, managed health care is now looking at specific procedures. Procedures are increasingly scrutinized in terms of medical efficacy and necessity. Procedures that are not medically efficacious—those that offer no benefits over other, less costly procedures—may not be paid for. Examples of such procedures could include radial keratotomy and use of gastric balloons. In addition, diagnostic or therapeutic modalities that are deemed not medically necessary may be excluded from coverage.

Benefits Variation (Cost Sharing). By putting some of the responsibility for payment on the patient, it is possible to modify utilization patterns. Three common benefits variations are copayments, deductibles, and coinsurance. They are defined as follows:

- Copayment is a fixed payment per encounter, regardless of the amount of the bill. For example, $5.00 may be charged for an office visit to a physician.
- A deductible is a first dollar payment by the insured up to a set threshold. For example, the first $500.00 of hospital claims in a given year may be paid by the patient.
- Coinsurance is payment by the patient of a fixed percentage of the total bill. For example, 20 per cent of outpatient costs may be charged to the patient.

Copayments, deductibles, and coinsurance act not only to decrease the cost of services to the insurer but also to actually decrease utilization and, hence, total costs of medical care. In addition, the level of cost shifting may be modified to influence patients to utilize the most cost-effective facilities. For example, copayments are usually much higher for the use of an emergency room than for a primary care physician's office. These reimbursement mechanisms are commonly used to provide options to enrollees about their choice of services. For example, patients have the opportunity to select and utilize a defined provider panel in exchange for reduced out-of-pocket expenses. In some systems, patients must select this option in advance, with the opportunity to change provided on a yearly basis. In other systems, they have the option to make the decision whenever they utilize services (point of service).

The impact of benefits variation on the utilization of services is, in part, based on disposable income. Patients in lower socioeconomic groups are more likely to use fewer services when cost-sharing mechanisms are used. This is especially true for the utilization of services such as periodic health maintenance and check-ups for chronic illness such as hypertension, diabetes, and mental health. In order to distribute the change in utilization of services equally throughout income ranges, some insurers make the total out-of-pocket expenses a percentage of total income. For example, out-of-pocket payments for services for an individual may be limited to 1 per cent of annual income.

Benefits variation balances the desire for patient satisfaction with the need to control costs. In general, unrestricted access to physicians and hospitals with no out-of-pocket expenses is associated with a high level of member satisfaction and increased costs of health care. Restrictions on the use of hospitals and providers result in a decrease in the number of choices for the patient and also decrease the cost of medical services. As the cost of care becomes a greater problem, restrictions will continue to be placed on access to physicians and hospitals. In this setting, insurers and physicians have an obligation to make sure that the restrictions on the use of care or the financial burdens to the patient do not compromise quality of care (Relman, 1983).

PREFERRED PROVIDER ORGANIZATIONS

Preferred Provider Organizations (PPOs) are an intermediate step between HMOs and indemnity insurance. PPOs may be developed by insurance companies, group practices, medical staffs, hospitals, or medical societies as a method of preserving market share. Large employers may develop their own PPOs to control costs.

Typically, a PPO is a system in which, if a subscriber chooses a preferred provider, there is a reduced deductible or reduced copayment or both. In turn, employers or insurance companies negotiate discounted fees with preferred providers. Thus, a subscriber has the choice of seeing a preferred provider or any other health care provider who is not a member of the PPO. When a subscriber goes out of the system, he or she incurs additional responsibility for the medical costs.

Fee discounting, which is a major feature of PPOs, is a weak method of cost containment, especially when not supported by utilization controls. Providers, whether they be physicians, hospitals, or others, who have their fees discounted may compensate for this, either by increasing the frequency of utilization or by increasing the complexity of the billed services. Since total cost is a combination of cost per service, frequency of services, and intensity of services provided, using only fee discounting is not as effective as taking all three factors into account. The overall effectiveness of a PPO is largely a function of the insurer's ability to identify and recruit quality and cost-effective providers. PPOs that do not use a great deal of selectivity in defining their provider panels will not be successful.

HEALTH MAINTENANCE ORGANIZATIONS

HMOs have their origin in the United States in the late 1920's and early 1930's. The origin of the modern-day HMO can be traced to the provision of care for employees of the Los Angeles Department of Water and Power by Ross and Loos, provision of medical and worker's compensation care by Henry Garfield for employees of Henry Kaiser who were working on the Grand Coulee Dam, and care for New York City employees promoted by Mayor La Guardia. These experiments have evolved into the Ross-Loos Clinic (now the CIGNA Health Plan of California), the Kaiser-Permanente Plan, and the Health Insurance Plan of Greater New York (Starr, 1982).

HMOs, which as late as the 1970's enrolled only 2 per cent of the nation in their health plans, now occupy 12 per cent of the market. In some states, market penetration is as high as 40 per cent. It is estimated that by the year 2000, 25 per cent of the nation's population will be enrolled in HMOs. In addition, Medicare and many Medicaid programs have entered into contractual agreements with HMOs. HMOs differ from other forms of health care delivery in the following ways:

- HMOs are financially at risk for the costs of health care administered to enrollees and are responsible for the access, availability, and quality of care rendered.
- The breadth of medical coverage, including ambulatory care, health promotion, and disease prevention, is comprehensive, with patients bearing only minimal out-of-pocket expenses beyond payment of the premium.
- There is a defined panel of providers, usually including physicians and hospitals. To receive benefits, enrollees are required to use this defined provider panel unless there is prior authorization by the HMO.
- When paying physicians, especially primary care physicians, fee-for-service is the exception. Most HMOs reimburse for physician services at the primary care level either by salary or by capitation. Specialists and ancillary services may be paid for by methods other than fee-for-service, including a discounted fee-for-service with a holdback.
- Most HMOs employ a gatekeeper physician system that supervises access to health care resources. Although many organizations, including the American Academy of Family Physicians, do not like the term "gatekeeper" to describe the sole or major function of the primary care physician case manager, it is an important aspect of case management and a potent method of cost containment. Proponents of such systems feel that the use of a physician in this manner is an effective alternative to other, more oppressive regulatory controls. As the term implies, in order to receive specialist or hospital services, enrollees must first go through the primary care physician who is typically a pediatrician, internist, or family physician. By controlling access in this manner, coordination of care and cost containment become centered around the primary care physician. Gatekeeping works by reducing duplication of services through the coordination of care, preventing an enrollee from selecting the wrong type of specialist for his or her needs, and reducing unnecessary consultations when necessary services are required but can be provided by the primary care physician.
- Physicians have incentives for cost-effective care. This, along with the use of limited provider panels and gatekeepers, is one of the more controversial aspects of HMOs. Although there is a potential for overzealous behavior on the part of providers to maximize these incentives, HMOs realize that part of the reason for the proliferation in health care costs in traditional fee-for-service reimbursement is that providers have incentives for overutilization. HMOs further realize that, although physician fees only make up a fraction of total health care costs, physician-directed decisions to order consultations, diagnostic tests, medication, and hospitalization account for the vast majority of health care expenditures. Hence, physicians must assume their proper share of responsibility for health care costs. Incentives are used to influence behavior toward a desired goal.

Structure of Health Maintenance Organizations

There are 700 HMOs currently operating in the United States, and they assume several forms. Major categories are staff model, group model, and independent practice association (IPA). Staff model HMOs generally own the facilities from which they render care, and there is no separate contracted physician organization. Group model HMOs are similar to staff model HMOs except that the HMO contracts directly with a group of physicians for health care services. Group and staff models may or may not own their own hospitals. Physicians are generally on salary, with some type of additional incentive system. Because of the large capital expense, these HMOs need a high concentration of enrollees in a specific geographic area. They have the advantage of centralized access to utilization and quality assurance data and records. However, they have the most restricted provider panels. In an IPA model, the HMO contracts with individual practitioners. Typically, family physicians contract only for primary care services. These services usually include preventive, diagnostic, and treatment services; injections; immunizations; patient education; and hospital care. Other services may also be included. In some situations, the IPA can act as an intermediary for the individual practitioner. Some IPAs accept risk by receiving a fixed amount for health care services and then subcontracting with individual physicians within their IPA. In others, the HMO contracts directly with individual physicians. This model is referred to as a direct contract model. IPAs are the fastest-growing segment of HMOs in terms of enrollee membership, principally because of the expanded provider panel, which offers a greater choice to prospective members. This may, however, reduce an IPA's ability to control costs.

Provider Reimbursement and Incentives

HMOs have a responsibility to contain costs and at the same time provide quality medical services. In containing costs, two of the most powerful tools that an HMO has are the gatekeeper system and capitation. Utilization can vary depending on the reimbursement incentives regardless of the medical necessity for the procedure. Physicians, hospitals, and other health care providers are usually paid for their services by one of four methods: (1) unit of service rendered (fee-for-service), (2) diagnosis (diagnosis-related groups, (3) salary, and (4) membership (capitation). In fee-for-service payment, health care providers have a financial incentive to maximize income by increasing the frequency of services and increasing the intensity of services. Therefore, providers have incentives to do more costly and invasive procedures and provide services more frequently. In order to maximize reimbursement when being paid by diagnosis, providers have an incentive to maximize the frequency of utilization and minimize intensity. Therefore, providers (usually hospitals) have an incentive to see enrollees more often but provide less intensive services. Physicians who are salaried and who have no other incentive programs attached to their performance are relatively incentive neutral. Typically in an HMO setting, salaried physicians do have other incentives, either in the form of a salary withholding or a bonus. Usually these incentives are related to individual productivity, cost-effectiveness, satisfaction, or a combination thereof.

Reimbursement by membership, whether at a fixed rate or adjusted for age and sex, is referred to as capitation. In this reimbursement method, physicians have an incentive to minimize intensity and minimize frequency of services. In this setting, it is incumbent on the HMO to have appropriate quality assurance activities. Without sacrificing quality, however, good physicians can also alter utilization, depending on reimbursement incentives. For example, one study showed that the ordering of chest x-rays and ECGs, usually highly profitable procedures, was less in a group of internists paid by capitation than it was in a group of internists paid on a fee-for-service basis (Epstein et al., 1986).

Assessment of Individual Health Maintenance Organizations

Primary care physicians will come into contact with some manner of managed health care. There are several points to consider when deciding whether or not to participate. For physicians in private practice, a determination should be made about whether or not the HMO can supply a sufficient number of patients to justify the changes in office procedures that each HMO requires. This can best be determined by looking at similar offices that have joined the HMO and the growth of new offices in other service areas.

Reimbursement should be adequate. Basic to the assessment of reimbursement adequacy is an understanding of income and the risk the primary care physician assumes for the delivery of services. In general, the greater the responsibility required of the primary care physician and the greater the risk, the greater should be the compensation. There should also be some sharing of risk for the primary care physician for difficult and expensive cases. A convenient way to assess income potential and risk is to determine the amount of reimbursement per encounter. This is accomplished by totaling all revenues (fees-for-service, capitation, copayments, withholdings, and incentive distributions) and dividing by the number of encounters. Withholdings and incentive distributions are the portions at risk.

In addition, it is useful to know whether risk is pooled and then borne by many or all physicians who participate in the HMO or only by individual physicians. If the portion of the income at risk is determined by the activities of all physicians in the HMO, then there is less variation in income return; however, income will also not be as closely related to each physician's ability to control costs.

A well-managed HMO should have a full time medical director. This person should be available, understand the physician practice setting, and have the ability to effect financial reimbursement in situations in which the system clearly does not provide adequate compensation.

The HMO should make available its method of tracking the performance of the primary care office. This usually includes information about the number of units of service and the cost per unit of services. This information should be reported at least every 6 months, and the HMO should have an assessment mechanism to help those offices that are doing poorly under the reimbursement system.

The HMO should have a system for measuring the quality of care and detecting significant variations in care. Because of the restricted nature of the network of physicians in an HMO and the fact that they are organized into a single delivery system, the HMO is able to provide quality-of-care information not available in an unmanaged system. The adequacy of the quality assurance system is an important issue in determining the quality of the HMO itself.

The HMO should be financially solvent. In most states, the quickest way to determine financial solvency is to call the state department that regulates HMOs, usually the state's department of insurance or department of health. Determining the strength of an HMO's backers (e.g., a hospital and an insurance company) and reviewing an annual report is another way of determining an HMO's fiscal health.

Finally, the physician should analyze, from a personal point of view, his or her own practice style and the HMO's reimbursement system. Physicians should realize that all reimbursement incentives can be abused. Therefore, it is reasonable for the HMO to monitor physician practice patterns. The practicing physicians in the plan should, however, have significant input into the monitoring process.

Ethical Issues

Many ethical questions have arisen with the growth and popularity of HMOs. Among them are the following: What is the role of for-profit corporations in the delivery of health care? What is the role of the family physician as rationer of health care? Is it ethical to have incentives to control health care cost?

Critics of HMOs argue that, given the limited resources available for health care, there is no room for corporate profit in the equation. It is also argued that physicians should not be rationers of health care with individual patients. Furthermore, many critics of managed health care feel strongly that incentives to withhold or reduce the intensity of health care to patients are unethical (Hilman, 1987).

Advocates of managed health care believe there is enough waste and inefficiency in the health care system so that if any HMO, be it for-profit or nonprofit, is able to control costs of health care, preserve quality, and make health care insurance more affordable and available, then there is a great societal benefit. They point to the current 37 million people in the United States who do not have health insurance, over half of whom are members of families with at least one person employed. They feel that HMOs breed competition, which is beneficial. Furthermore, they argue that the attempts of for-profit and nonprofit institutions to control the bottom line are virtually identical.

With respect to rationing, most medical directors of HMOs feel that the primary care physician should provide medical services for the individual patient up to the level at which the maximum medical benefit is achieved. In addition, they argue that the incentives for overutilization in the fee-for-service method of reimbursement are just as harmful as the incentives for underutilization in capitation. Both require utilization and quality assurance controls and the participation of ethical physicians.

Family Physicians and Health Maintenance Organizations

Family physicians and HMOs have areas of mutual interest and benefit. Family physicians can look to HMOs to reimburse them more equitably for cognitive and preventive health care services. In addition, HMOs recognize the central role of the primary care physician. In most HMOs, the relative importance of the primary care physician with respect to specialists is augmented and the discrepancies in reimbursement are reduced. HMOs, on the other hand, are looking for proof from family medicine that family physicians are well trained not only in a wide breadth of primary care services but also in preventive health care, cost-effective health care, clinical decision making, and the role of the physician case manager (Jacobs and Mott, 1987).

In addition, to the extent that family physicians are trained and comfortable working within an organizational framework and have a firm understanding of medical ethics and health care economics, they gain a strong competitive advantage over other primary care specialties. Since employers and employees as well as HMOs are looking for these skills, their acquisition by a large body of family physicians will enhance the position of family practice.

Quality Assurance

Society, although desiring cost containment, is not willing to see this achieved at the expense of quality. Therefore HMOs must demonstrate that their quality of care is equal to or better than that of unmanaged systems. To date, there have also been very few good studies comparing quality of care between various systems. Principally, studies have looked at patient satisfaction as an index of quality. There have also been few studies that measure medical outcomes. What data currently exist suggest that care rendered within HMOs is comparable to or better than care given in unmanaged systems. Nevertheless, significant problems do exist in making these comparisons. HMOs vary in their delivery of care and ability to internally monitor quality. Also, staff model HMOs, on which most of the research has been concentrated, measure quality very differently than do IPA models. Finally, the migratory status of the American population makes long-term studies very difficult. HMOs will increasingly need to devote a significant amount of their budgets to quality assurance activities.

Management information systems need to become increasingly sophisticated so that retroactive, concurrent, and prospective quality assurance activities can be carried out. As health care becomes more aggressively managed in all spheres, there will be a commensurate need for effective quality assurance activities.

Future Issues and Challenges for Health Maintenance Organizations

With the vast array of health care benefits and the highly mobile nature of the American population, there is a rapid movement of people from one type of health care plan to another. The transient nature of enrollees' participation in a particular HMO or type of health care system impedes the ability of a population to receive continuity of care and the benefits of preventive health care. HMOs need to develop a method of attracting those people who are more likely to stay within a managed health care system over time. In addition, other innovative ways to ensure continuity of care, even when enrollees transfer into and out of various HMOs, need to be developed. All types of health care delivery systems, including HMOs, need to develop increasingly sophisticated ways of measuring quality, so that the cost of these services will be incorporated into health care premiums. In addition, HMOs need to work with employees, enrollees, and providers in order to achieve a relationship of trust and mutual dependence. IPA model HMOs need to concentrate more on their medical delivery systems than on marketing. To achieve this, many of these HMOs need to develop a more restricted provider panel as their ability to measure cost-effectiveness and quality parameters for physicians improves.

HMOs, like family practice, have grown out of a societal mandate. For HMOs, this mandate is to control costs and preserve quality. HMOs, both collectively and individually, will be increasingly under pressure to demonstrate that they are achieving these goals. If they succeed, their position in the health care system will be maintained and enhanced. If they are unable to succeed in either of these areas, HMOs will be replaced by another system, most likely involving increased regulation and centralization.

References

Bertakis, K., and Robbins, J.: Gatekeeping in primary care: A comparison of internal medicine and family practice. J. Fam. Pract., *24*:305, 1987. *A controlled study comparing continuity of care and referral patterns between internal medicine and family practice ambulatory training sites. Laboratory costs were higher and measures of continuity of care were lower for the group receiving care from the internal medicine clinic.*

Brook, R. H., Ware, J. E., Rodgers, W. H., et al.: Does free care improve adults health? N. Engl. J. Med., *309*:1426. *Follow-up of the classic Rand health care experiment. Subjects were randomly assigned to free care or insurance with cost sharing. Those in the free care group had significantly higher utilization. Persons with poor vision and those with low income and hypertension had better outcomes when provided with free care.*

Chassin, M., Brook, R., Park, R. E., et al.: Variations in the use of medical and surgical services by the Medicare population. N. Engl. J. Med., *314*:285, 1986.

Chassin, M. R., Kosecoff, J., Park, R. E., et al.: Does inappropriate use explain geographic variations in the use of health care services? J.A.M.A., *258*:2533, 1987.

Cherkin, D. C., Rosenblatt, R. A., Schneeweiss, R., et al.: The use of medical resources by residency-trained family physicians and general internists: Is there a difference? Med. Care, *25*:455, 1987. *A comparison of 132 family physicians and 102 general internists. All were practicing, residency trained, and were postresidency for the same length of time. Family physicians spent less time with hypertensive patients and ordered fewer tests. They were less likely to order consultations or hospitalizations across their entire practice.*

Ellsbury, K. E., and Schneeweiss, R.: Physician knowledge and attitudes about health insurance after the introduction of capitated health plans. J. Fam. Pract., *26*:57, 1988.

Epstein, A., Begg, C., and McNeil, B.: The use of ambulatory testing in prepaid and fee-for-service group practices. N. Engl. J. Med., *314*:1089, 1986. *A comparison of utilization of ECGs and chest x-rays in two internal medicine group practices. The group receiving payment by fee-for-service had significantly higher usage than the group being paid by capitation.*

Fuchs, V.: Health care and the United States economic system. Milbank Memor. Fund Quarter., *50*:211, 1972.

Fuchs, V. R.: The rationing of medical care. N. Engl. J. Med., *311*:1572, 1984.

Ginzberg, E.: U.S. health policy. J.A.M.A., *260*:3647, 1988.

Harris, J. M., Jr.: The Role of the Medical Director in the Fee for Service/Prepaid Medical Group. Denver, Center for Research in Ambulatory Health Care Administration, 1983.

Herman, J. M.: Utilization review and the family physician. Fam. Med., *20*:215, 1988.

Hillman, A. L.: Financial incentives for physicians in HMOs. N. Engl. J. Med., *317*:1743, 1987. *Describes various incentive systems used in 302 HMOs and categorizes them. It concludes that certain incentives, if used in conjunction with each other, might adversely affect quality of care.*

Jacobs, O., and Mott, P.: Physician characteristics and training emphasis considered desirable by leaders of HMOs. J. Med. Ed., *62*:725, 1987.

Kosecoff, J., Chassin, M. R., Fink, A., et al.: Obtaining clinical data on the appropriateness of medical care in community practice. J.A.M.A., *258*:2538, 1987.

Merrick, N., Brook, R., Fink, A., et al.: Use of carotid endarterectomy in five California Veterans Administration Medical Centers. J.A.M.A., *256*:2531, 1986.

Myers, A. A., and Gleicher, N.: A successful program to lower caesarean-section rates. N. Engl. J. Med., *319*:1511, 1988.

Newhouse, J. P., Manning, W. G., and Morris, C. N.: Some interim results from a controlled trial of cost sharing in health insurance. N. Engl. J. Med., *305*:1501, 1981.

Relman, A. S.: The Rand health insurance study: Is cost sharing dangerous to your health? N. Engl. J. Med., *309*:1453, 1983.

Siu, A. L., Leibowitz, A., Brook, R., et al.: Use of the hospital in a randomized trial of prepaid care. J.A.M.A., *259*:1343, 1988. *Longitudinal study of patients randomly assigned to a large staff model HMO or a fee-for-service plan without cost sharing. They were studied for 3 or 5 years. A reduction in hospitalization rates was achieved by the HMO, largely through the avoidance of "discretionary surgery." No outcome differences were detected.*

Starr, P.: The Social Transformation of American Medicine. New York, Basic Books, 1982. *Classic, prize-winning book on the evolution of medicine in the United States from a trade to a profession and its current status. Good explanations of the origin and evolution of health care insurance and HMOs, including the 1973 federal legislation.*

Thomas, L.: The Lives of a Cell: Notes of a Biology Watcher. New York, Viking Press, 1974.

77

Accounting Systems

Jack Valancy

Accounting is the language of business. A working knowledge of accounting systems enables the family physician to understand his or her professional finances. Even if financial gain is not the physician's prime motivation, the practice should be operated in a businesslike manner.

General Accounting

ACCOUNTANT AND BOOKKEEPER

The family physician should match his or her needs to the variety of accounting services available. Most physicians, especially those just starting in practice, need only basic accounting services:

- Setting up and auditing the practice's bookkeeping system
- Preparing the practice's financial reports
- Preparing professional and personal tax returns.

A good accountant is more than a technician who manipulates figures. The accountant should explain practice finances, answer the physician's questions, and may advise the physician in matters such as minimizing tax burden, leasing equipment, obtaining credit, and setting up a retirement plan. The accountant should anticipate problems by staying abreast of changes in tax laws and rulings that could affect the physician.

Although anyone can represent himself or herself as an accountant, the family physician should retain a *certified public accountant (CPA)* who is licensed to practice within the state. The accountant should have experience serving physicians with similar needs. To find an accountant, the physician can ask colleagues and check with the local society of CPAs. The physician should ask several prospective accountants to outline the services they propose to provide and to estimate their annual cost. In addition, the physician should ask for and check client references.

It is important that the accountant understand and support the physician's financial objectives. The family physician should ask each prospective accountant about his or her approach to specific situations. An aggressive accountant who engages in "creative" approaches to reduce the physician's tax burden increases the risk of triggering an Internal Revenue Service audit and incurring financial penalties. Conversely, the physician with an overly conservative accountant who "plays it safe" might pay more taxes than necessary.

A bookkeeper does routine accounting tasks such as paying bills and posting transactions. The practice's accountant and bookkeeper should coordinate their efforts. Smaller medical practices usually do not have enough bookkeeping work to keep a full-time bookkeeper busy. In some practices, the employee who does the bookkeeping has other responsibilities as well. Other practices hire a part-time bookkeeper to work a few days a month. Some accounting firms employ bookkeepers who are available to their clients as needed.

FINANCIAL STATEMENTS

An effective accounting system provides precise, current information about where the practice's money comes from *(revenues)*, where it goes *(expenses)*, what it owns *(assets)*, what it owes *(liabilities)*, and what it is worth *(capital)*.

The fundamental relationships between these elements is expressed in the following accounting equations:

$$\text{Assets} = \text{Liabilities} + \text{Capital}$$

$$\text{Income} = \text{Revenues} - \text{Expenses}$$

The information in the accounting equations appears in two basic financial statements: the *balance sheet* and the *income statement*. The balance sheet shows the practice's financial position on a specific date (Table 77–1). The income statement shows revenues and expenses over a period of time (Table 77–2). The practice's accountant prepares financial statements at the end of each accounting period, typically a month, a quarter, and a year.

GENERAL LEDGER: THE ACCOUNTING CYCLE

The *general ledger process*, or the *accounting cycle*, begins when transactions are recorded on *source documents*, such as patient encounter forms, invoices, and receipts. The information is posted to a *journal*, which is a chronologic list of all transactions. Examples of journals in a medical practice are the *daysheets* used to record patient account charges, payments, and adjustments and checking account *registers*, which list checks as they are prepared.

Transaction information is transcribed from the journal to the appropriate *account ledgers* for assets, liabilities, capital, revenues, and expenses. The account ledgers are organized according to a *chart of accounts*, which groups together similar accounts. For example, asset accounts may be numbered 100 to 199; liability accounts, 200 to 299; and so on.

Transactions are recorded following either the *cash* or *accrual* method of accounting. With the cash method, all money that is actually spent or received during an accounting period is included in that period. Under the accrual method, however, expenses and revenues are charged to the period in which they are incurred or earned, even if the money is actually spent or received at a different time. The cash method of accounting is simpler and is used by most taxpayers, including physicians.

Double entry bookkeeping assures that the accounting equations remain in balance. As the name implies, each transaction generates offsetting entries, *debits* and *credits*, to two or more accounts. Each transaction's total debits must equal its total credits. An account's balance is the difference between the sums of its debit and credit entries.

The preparation of a *trial balance* assures that all accounts are in balance before the financial statements are prepared. The sum of all debit entries in all accounts is compared with the sum of all credit entries. If these totals are not equal, there are errors in the accounting system.

An *audit trail* is a technique of cross-referencing transactions through the accounting cycle, from source documents to financial statements. By following the audit trail, the history of each transaction may be traced and errors detected and corrected.

Table 77–1. BALANCE SHEET

Jay Mitchell, M.D.
Balance Sheet
December 31, 1989

Assets	
Cash	$ 7,215
Accounts receivable	10,285
Furniture, equipment, and office improvements	26,200
Less: accumulated depreciation	(6,457)
Total assets:	37,243
Liabilities	
Loan #1 (fixed loan)	$10,350
Loan #2 (line of credit)	9,702
Total liabilities	$20,052
Capital	
Owner's equity	$15,000
Retained earnings	2,191
Total capital (net worth):	$17,191
Total liabilities and capital:	$37,243

Table 77–2. INCOME STATEMENT

Jay Mitchell, M.D.
Income Statement
for the year ended December 31, 1989

Revenues from professional services	$167,240
Expenses	
Auto	$2,255
Books and subscriptions	654
Contributions	250
Depreciation	1,207
Drugs and medical supplies	6,672
Dues	865
Employee benefits	2,390
Insurance	5,650
Office cleaning and maintenance	782
Office payroll	34,854
Pension plan contributions	6,200
Continuing medical education	1,465
Rent	10,200
Taxes	4,817
Telephone	2,176
Utilities	559
Total expenses	$80,996
Practice income	$86,244

PAYROLL

Federal regulations require that employers maintain accurate records of hours worked and earnings for each employee not exempt from the *Fair Labor*

Standards Act (see the following for information about exempt employees). These records should include the time the worker begins and ends each shift and the time taken for unpaid meal and break periods. Employees should complete their own time record. Time clocks are not necessary, but they may be helpful if accurate timekeeping is difficult.

The Fair Labor Standards Act mandates that employers pay nonexempt employees 1½ times their hourly wage for every hour over 40 they work in 1 week. Some states have stricter overtime laws. Overtime pay must be computed on a weekly basis—that is, seven consecutive 24-hour periods. Thus, it is most convenient to pay employees every 1 or 2 weeks, rather than once or twice a month.

Several tests can be used to determine if an employee is exempt from the record keeping and overtime pay requirements of the Fair Labor Standards Act. In general, employees whose work requires the exercise of discretion and independent judgment and who earn more than a certain amount may qualify as exempt. In a medical practice, the office manager, head nurse, and laboratory technicians might qualify as exempt employees.

Employers are obligated to pay taxes based on their employees' compensation. These include:

- Federal, state, and local income taxes
- Social security (Federal Insurance Contributions Act [FICA])
- Unemployment compensation
- Worker's compensation.

Some of these taxes are withheld from the employees' pay; others are contributed by the employer. At the end of each year, employers must provide employees and federal, state, and local governments with records of employee compensation and taxes withheld. Penalties for failing to pay payroll taxes on a timely basis are severe. In order to become known to various government agencies, an employer must have a *Federal employer identification number*, analogous to an individual's social security number.

ACCOUNTS PAYABLE

A medical practice deals with many different suppliers of goods and services. Although some require cash on delivery (COD) or in advance, most vendors establish *trade accounts* for their customers. This arrangement is convenient for ordering goods and services by telephone. Payment usually is due upon the receipt of an invoice.

A *purchase order* is a formal, detailed written order to a vendor for specific goods and services. Purchase orders should be prepared for major purchases, items that are available in different styles or colors, and items that are made to order.

Many practices find it convenient to pay bills twice a month, when the payroll is prepared. Payments are classified according to type of expense (e.g., rent, supplies, insurance), as determined by the practice's chart of accounts.

A *one-write* or *pegboard system* may be used to prepare checks and simultaneously record the amounts in various expense categories on a *check register (daysheet):* Each check has a carbon stripe on its back that transfers data to the daysheet. Each daysheet can accommodate data from roughly 25 to 30 checks. The checks and daysheets have holes in their left margins. A board with protruding pegs is used to align the checks over the daysheet. The daysheet has several columns to the right of the check that are used for classifying expenses.

Some pegboard check-writing systems are designed to be used for payroll preparation as well. The checks have spaces across their tops for recording gross pay, deductions, and net pay. A carbon stripe behind this area transfers data to the employee's payroll record card, which is inserted between the check and daysheet. (Pegboard systems for maintaining patient accounts are described in the Patient Accounting section, which follows.)

Another method for preparing checks and classifying expenses is to use two-part voucher checks, which have a large stub for recording payment information. The original check, which is negotiable, is forwarded to the payee with the stub attached. The duplicate copy, which is nonnegotiable, remains in the practice.

A *petty cash fund* is used to pay minor practice expenses without writing a check. A specific total amount, such as $50, is set for the fund. A check written to "cash" is used to obtain bills and coins for the fund. As cash is withdrawn, receipts or *petty cash vouchers* for the purchases are filed. The cash remaining, plus the total of the receipts and vouchers, should always equal the total amount of the fund. Additional checks are written to replenish the fund as needed.

A *change fund* is a set amount of bills and coins used to make change for patients as necessary at the front desk. A check written to "cash" funds the change fund. The total amount of the change fund does not vary from day to day.

ACCOUNTING CONTROL

There are three good reasons for maintaining accounting control:

1. *Preventing and detecting errors.* Without good accounting control, it is virtually impossible to detect and correct errors in the practice's accounting system. Maintaining daily controls helps reveal minor errors before they become major problems.

2. *Reducing embezzlement.* Although it is impossible to entirely prevent embezzlement, good accounting controls reduce the risk.

3. *Establishing a valid base for comparison.* Keeping complete and accurate records establishes a

valid data base for measuring the financial performance of the practice.

Some specific techniques for maintaining accounting control follow:

- Use prenumbered source documents in sequence.
- Reconcile transactions as often as practical: daily, weekly, or monthly.
- Correct errors immediately. Document corrections.
- Separate accounting tasks among employees. For example, one employee could open the mail and endorse checks; another could post the payments to patient accounts.
- Deposit all cash, checks, and credit card documents daily.
- *Proof* the practice's accounts receivable monthly. That is, compare the daysheet's running total with the sum of individual account balances.
- Follow all control procedures designed for the specific accounting and bookkeeping systems used.
- Review bills as they are paid. Only partners in the practice should be authorized to sign checks.
- Monitor the petty cash and change funds.
- Make unannounced spot checks of various aspects of financial operations.
- Have the practice's accountant audit the accounting systems regularly, at least every 2 years.
- Have staff members covered under a fidelity bond, which reimburses the practice for losses resulting from employee theft. This form of insurance is often part of the physician's business owner's insurance policy. Prosecution of the offender might be required in order to collect damages.

For further information, see Figure 77–1.

Patient Accounting

An effective patient accounting system is crucial to the financial well-being of a family practice. Fair financial policies and sound procedures applied in a consistent manner can minimize difficulties for the physician, patients, and staff.

FINANCIAL POLICIES

Established financial policies guide the business relationships between family physicians and their patients. Without explicit guidelines, physicians, patients, and staff are likely to have different expectations; and routine matters can become sensitive issues. Financial policies include, but are not limited to, the following issues:

- When payment for services is expected
- The conditions for granting professional courtesy, discounts, or charity care
- Whether the practice participates in health insurance programs such as Medicare, Blue Shield, and managed care plans (e.g., Health Maintenance Organizations, Preferred Provider Organizations)
- The conditions for accepting assignment of insurance benefits
- The conditions for preparing and submitting insurance claims for patients
- How the practice pursues delinquent accounts
- Whether patients are discharged from the practice for nonpayment of fees

Information about the practice's financial policies should be presented to patients in a clear, matter-of-fact manner. Some physicians prefer their staff to inform patients when the initial appointment is scheduled. Other physicians are more comfortable if the patient is informed at the end of the initial visit. If a patient is about to incur an unusually large fee, it is good to confirm the financial arrangements before the services are rendered.

Reinforcing an oral explanation of the practice's financial policies with written information is very helpful. This information may be contained in a *practice information brochure* that explains all pertinent policies and procedures, or in a separate *patient accounting brochure.* A statement inviting the patient to discuss financial matters with the staff should be included to solicit questions before problems arise.

FEES

For the most part, patients complain about physicians' fees because they perceive inconsistencies. Family physicians should carefully evaluate the services they provide and the corresponding fees they charge. Complete explanations to patients of services and fees can minimize complaints.

Professional fees should reflect the time, effort, training, skill, and resources required to render the service. A fair guideline for establishing fees is to observe the going rates in the area. To estimate these rates, the family physician may:

- Request copies of the *prevailing charge report* for family physicians in the geographic area from the local Medicare intermediary. The prevailing charge includes the *customary (median) charges* for 75 per cent of the claims submitted to Medicare during the preceding 12-month base period, adjusted by an economic factor index.
- Contact the local Blue Shield plan to determine reimbursement rates under their *usual, customary,* and *reasonable (UCR) guidelines.*
- Check *Physician Marketplace Statistics*, published by the American Medical Association (AMA), for data on physicians' average fees for selected services and procedures, office visits, and hospital visits.
- Check *Medical Economics* magazine for their survey of fees by specialty and region.

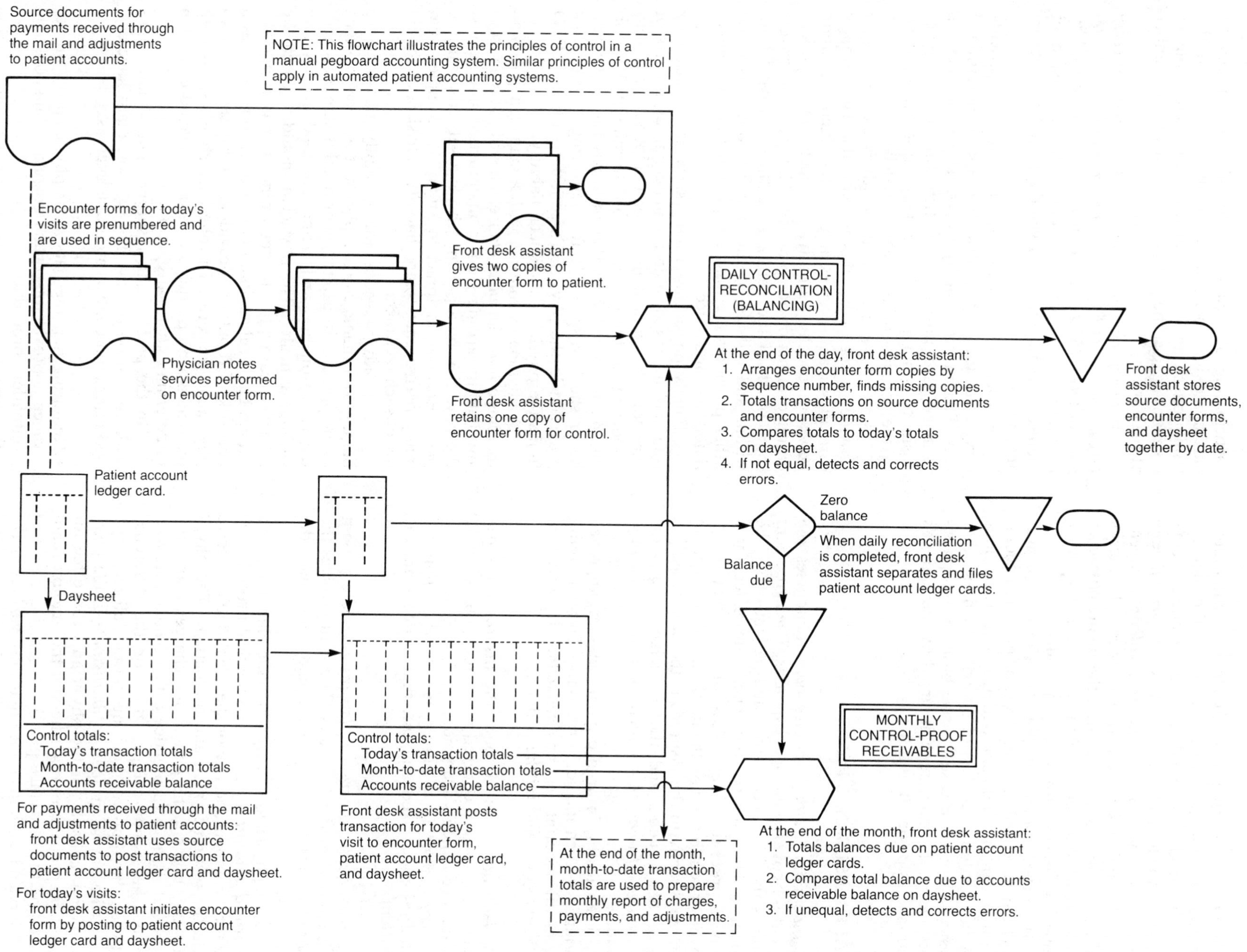

Source documents for payments received through the mail and adjustments to patient accounts.
NOTE: This flowchart illustrates the principles of control in a manual pegboard accounting system. Similar principles of control apply in automated patient accounting systems.
Encounter forms for today's visits are prenumbered and are used in sequence.
Physician notes services performed on encounter form.
Front desk assistant gives two copies of encounter form to patient.
Front desk assistant retains one copy of encounter form for control.
DAILY CONTROL-RECONCILIATION (BALANCING)
At the end of the day, front desk assistant:
1. Arranges encounter form copies by sequence number, finds missing copies.
2. Totals transactions on source documents and encounter forms.
3. Compares totals to today's totals on daysheet.
4. If not equal, detects and corrects errors.
Front desk assistant stores source documents, encounter forms, and daysheet together by date.
Patient account ledger card.
Zero balance
Balance due
When daily reconciliation is completed, front desk assistant separates and files patient account ledger cards.
Daysheet
Control totals:
Today's transaction totals
Month-to-date transaction totals
Accounts receivable balance
Control totals:
Today's transaction totals
Month-to-date transaction totals
Accounts receivable balance
MONTHLY CONTROL-PROOF RECEIVABLES
For payments received through the mail and adjustments to patient accounts:
front desk assistant uses source documents to post transactions to patient account ledger card and daysheet.
For today's visits:
front desk assistant initiates encounter form by posting to patient account ledger card and daysheet.
Front desk assistant posts transaction for today's visit to encounter form, patient account ledger card, and daysheet.
At the end of the month, month-to-date transaction totals are used to prepare monthly report of charges, payments, and adjustments.
At the end of the month, front desk assistant:
1. Totals balances due on patient account ledger cards.
2. Compares total balance due to accounts receivable balance on daysheet.
3. If unequal, detects and corrects errors.

Figure 77–1. Daily and monthly patient accounting system controls.

Restraint of trade—that is, acting alone or with others to hinder a competitor's free actions in the marketplace—is illegal. Prohibited activities include agreeing how much to charge for specific services *(price fixing)* and agreeing not to compete *(controlling competition)*. Although it is unlikely that a few casual remarks will trigger *antitrust* proceedings, the family physician should avoid detailed discussions of fees and other competitive issues with other physicians.

Almost all practicing physicians extend professional courtesy, reduce their fees, or provide uncompensated care to indigent patients. Fee reductions may be granted to a class of patients (such as other physicians) or on a case-by-case basis. Some physicians accept the amount reimbursed by the patient's insurance as payment in full.

HEALTH INSURANCE PLANS

An *indemnity health insurance plan* reimburses the patient for covered medical expenses. The agreement involves the insurance carrier and patient only. The patient is liable for the physician's entire fee for a medical procedure, regardless of the amount approved or reimbursed by the insurance plan. Payment is made directly to the insured. If the patient assigns his or her benefits and the physician accepts the *assignment of benefits*, payment is made to the physician.

The health insurance plan sets an approved amount for each medical procedure. The plan reimburses this amount, less any *deductible* or *copayment* amounts to be paid by the patient.

- A *deductible* is an amount the insured must pay each year toward covered medical expenses before insurance benefits are paid.
- A *copayment* is a percentage of the approved charges, or a fixed amount, that is due from the patient.

A *service health insurance plan* provides the patient with covered medical services. The plan involves the insurance carrier, the patient, and sometimes the physician.

If the physician *participates* in the plan, the plan's *approved amount* for a covered medical procedure is the total compensation he or she is entitled to receive from the insurance plan and the patient. The physician may not bill the patient for charges above the approved amount (a practice called *balance billing*). He or she is not compensated for the difference between the approved amount and the full fee.

If the physician *does not participate* in the plan, the patient is liable for the physician's entire fee for a medical procedure, regardless of the amount reimbursed by the insurance plan.

Service health insurance plans use various incentives to encourage their subscribers to see participating physicians and discourage them from seeing nonparticipating physicians. In considering whether to participate in a service health insurance plan, the family physician should weigh possible reductions in revenues against the prospect of an increased number of patients.

Managed care plans include *Preferred Provider Organizations (PPOs)* and *Health Maintenance Organizations (HMOs)*. Such plans are characterized by a greater degree of control over the provision of medical care than indemnity and service health insurance plans.

Physicians who belong to PPOs agree to provide services to the plan's subscribers for predetermined fees. Patients are usually free to choose among the primary care physicians participating in the plan. Visits to other providers usually must be approved by the patient's primary care physician.

An HMO is a system of health care delivery that provides a set of benefits to patients. The primary care physician receives a predetermined *capitation payment*, usually monthly, for each HMO patient enrolled in his or her practice. This payment covers some or all of the patient's health care costs, both within and outside of the practice. Specialists and other providers are paid a capitated rate or a negotiated fee-for-service.

Family physicians usually serve in a *gatekeeper* role and are responsible for managing all aspects of care for each patient in his or her panel. It is very important for the physician to determine if the capitation amount will be sufficient to pay for all the care he or she is responsible for delivering. A *stop loss* provision in the physician's contract with the HMO limits the physician's financial liability.

A physician's contract with a managed care plan that has a *hold harmless* clause relieves the plan from any liability arising from a malpractice suit against the physician by a patient who is a subscriber in the plan. Because malpractice suits are complex and many parties may share liability, physicians should avoid such contracts.

It is advantageous for a family physician to belong to a managed care plan if it attracts patients to the practice, its capitation or reimbursement schedule is reasonable, and claims are paid quickly and without difficulty. The physician should research the managed care plan to determine if it is financially stable, has a substantial number of subscribers, has a network of reputable providers, and is responsive to physicians' concerns. The physician should speak with physicians who participate in the managed care plan to determine their satisfaction.

In the past, health insurance plans paid claims with little or no review. Today, most plans have cost and utilization control programs such as:

- Requiring that the patient or physician obtain advance approval for certain hospital admissions and outpatient procedures
- Requiring that the patient obtain a second opinion for certain procedures

- Requiring discharge planning for hospitalized patients
- Reviewing the physician's treatment plan for the patient

BASIC FUNCTIONS OF A PATIENT ACCOUNTING SYSTEM

All patient accounting systems, whether manual or automated, perform the following seven basic functions. Different types of patient accounting systems are described later in this section.

Storing of Patient Demographic and Insurance Information

This information includes the patient's name, address, telephone number, date of birth, sex, person responsible for paying the account, alternative address, specific types of insurance coverages and insurance contract numbers, and notations for any courtesies or discounts to be extended. This information usually is obtained at or before the patient's first visit by having the patient complete a *patient information form*. This form may also include a statement authorizing the practice to release information to obtain reimbursement from insurance carriers and a statement authorizing payment of benefits directly to the practice. Having these signed statements on file eliminates the need for the patient to sign individual insurance forms. Filing a photocopy of the patient's insurance identification card reduces the risk of errors in transcribing policy information.

Posting and Storing Transactions

All transactions (charges, payments, and adjustments) should be recorded on source documents:

- *Encounter forms* (also called *superbills, charge tickets*, and *routing* slips) are used to record charges, payments, and adjustments made at the time of service (see the section on Processing Insurance Claims, which follows, for more information about superbills).
- Payment or adjustment *vouchers* (forms) and *registers* (lists) are created as these transactions are processed.
- A *remittance advice* is a document attached to a bill that is returned with a payment in order to identify the patient's account.

In order to maintain a valid statistical base of charges, payments, and adjustments, the full charge for the service provided and the amount of any adjustment should be recorded. Recording the net value of the charge less adjustments distorts statistics of practice operations.

Computer Systems. Computer systems can process payments and adjustments in several ways.

In a *balance forward* system, payments and adjustments are posted against the patient's undifferentiated balance due. Balance forward processing is less complicated than other systems, but it is also less precise. It is suited to practices in which patients are responsible for the full amount of fees, regardless of insurance reimbursement. (This is the way payments and adjustments are posted to patient account ledger cards in a manual system. Notations are used to relate payments and adjustments to charges.)

In an *open item* system, payments and adjustments are posted against individual charges. Open item processing is appropriate in practices in which the amount owed by patients for specific procedures depends on the amount of insurance reimbursement received. Here, the additional precision of knowing the balance remaining on specific charges is worth the extra effort required to maintain an open item system.

An *open claim* system is similar to an open item system, except that payments and adjustments are posted against the balance remaining on an insurance claim, which may contain several individual charges.

Controlling System Operations

It is important to maintain system control in order to detect and correct errors before they cause problems. The *daily reconciliation* (or *balancing*) process compares transaction totals derived from source documents with the totals on the daysheet. When reconciliation is completed, the source documents, calculator tapes, and daysheets should be bundled together and stored for at least a year. Additional system control procedures are described in the previous section on Accounting Control.

Producing Patient Bills

A copy of the encounter form can be the first bill a patient receives. If the family physician's policy is to obtain payment at the time of service, the front desk assistant should request payment. Signs alone are not effective for collecting payments.

Bills are customarily mailed to patients on a monthly basis, at the same time each month. They must be accurate, detailed, clear, and professional looking. Bills should show the outstanding balance of the account at the beginning of the billing period; all charges, payments, and adjustments posted during the period; and the account balance at the end of the period. Some family physicians have the policy that payment is not expected from the patient until after insurance reimbursement has been received or denied. In this situation, all charges submitted for reimbursement should be identified and the amount currently due from the patient should be clearly shown.

Processing Insurance Claims

According to AMA guidelines, physicians are obligated to help their patients obtain reimbursement of their medical costs from insurance carriers. At the very least, this means providing patients with a *superbill:* an encounter form that identifies the practice and contains information about the services rendered, fees, and diagnosis. Patients may submit a copy of the superbill along with a claim form to their insurance carrier.

Many family physicians prepare and submit insurance claims for their patients, particularly if reimbursement is likely. Insurance claim processing can be complex, and it is important that the practice's procedures are efficient. Virtually every insurance carrier publishes a provider manual and has representatives to advise practices how to submit insurance claims properly. Educational programs that train staff to process insurance claims are widely available.

Most insurance carriers accept claims submitted on the standard *HCFA 1500* (or *universal*) *claim form*. As a courtesy, the family physician should provide these to patients who prepare and submit their own insurance claims.

It is important that correct procedure and diagnosis codes be used on insurance claims. Incorrect or missing codes could cause a claim to be underpaid or rejected. The *Current Procedural Terminology* (CPT) coding system is generally accepted for coding procedures, although some carriers require other codes. Current procedural terminology code books are updated annually and are available from the AMA. The *International Classification of Diseases, 9th edition, Clinical Modification* (ICD.9.CM) coding system generally is used for diagnoses. Code books are available from the United States Government Printing Office and other sources, including the AMA.

The family physician should ensure that his or her staff prepares insurance forms promptly, neatly, and completely. A duplicate copy should be kept on file in the event that a claim must be researched or resubmitted. The staff should follow up with the insurance company if reimbursement is lower than expected or if the claim has been outstanding for longer than usual or rejected in error.

Electronic media claim submission (also called *paperless processing*) eliminates the need to prepare and submit insurance claims on paper forms. A computer system with the appropriate capabilities can prepare claims on magnetic tape or disk or transmit them directly to the insurance carrier's or a claims processing clearing-house's computer over ordinary telephone lines. The advantages of electronic submission of insurance claims include faster payment, lower risk of underpayment or rejection, and time and money saved in forms preparation.

Identifying and Pursuing Delinquent Accounts

The best way to manage delinquent accounts is to prevent them from becoming delinquent in the first place. The process begins when the patient is informed of the practice's financial policies. It continues with the consistent performance of patient accounting procedures.

An *aged trial balance* is a list of unpaid accounts with the outstanding balances classified by the time elapsed since the date of service in columns labeled current, 31–60, 61–90, 91–120, and 120+. Although a computer system can produce this report easily, compiling this information by hand is a tedious process. Alternatively, in a manual system delinquent accounts can be identified by manually reviewing patient ledger cards.

If a charge for which the patient is responsible remains unpaid for more than a month, the second bill mailed to the patient should carry a brief reminder, or *dunning message*. If payment is not received, messages of increasing severity should appear on the next several bills. More active techniques for requesting payment are recommended if the account is more than 60 or 90 days past due.

Telephone calls are much more effective than written communications in collecting past due amounts. The purpose of the call is to ask the responsible party what he or she plans to do about the outstanding amount. It is not intended to threaten or harass. Rather, the practice is attempting to maintain communications with the responsible party throughout the collection process. To protect confidentiality, the caller should not leave messages that suggest the nature of the call. Calls should not be made at odd hours or at the individual's place of work. The staff member who places the call should be friendly but firm and, above all, remain in control. If the responsible party claims that an error has been made, the caller should offer to investigate and get back to him or her. Appropriate consideration should be given to patients experiencing legitimate financial hardship.

Every call should end with an agreement that the responsible party will pay a specific amount by a specific date. The staff member who obtains this commitment should follow up on unfulfilled promises to pay.

Collection letters can be useful when other attempts to collect have been ignored. A *final notice* letter tells the responsible party that further action will be taken if the entire amount is not paid by a specific date or if the practice is not contacted to make other arrangements. Further action could mean taking the patient to small-claims court or referring the matter to a collection agency or an attorney.

If the family physician takes a patient to small-claims court or retains the services of a collection agency or attorney, consideration should be given to discharging the patient from the practice. Unless the patient is being treated for an acute, serious condition, the physician is not obligated to continue providing medical care without compensation. The family physician should send the patient a letter via registered or certified mail with receipt of delivery. The letter should state that, effective on a specific date 2 weeks to a month hence, the physician is discharging the patient from his or her care and that, with the patient's signed approval, medical records will be forwarded to the physician of the patient's choice.

Producing Reports

Each month, the family physician should keep track of:

- gross charges (*productivity*, or the full value of services provided)
- payments received
- adjustments.

Many group practices use this information to calculate a portion of each physician's compensation.

The physician should also be aware of:

- accounts receivable balance
- accounts receivable aging.

This information helps to determine the success of the practice's financial policies and the performance of the patient accounting system.

ACCOUNTS RECEIVABLE MANAGEMENT

Collection Ratio

The *collection ratio* measures the general effectiveness of a practice's patient accounting system. It is expressed as a percentage of gross charges collected. The formula is:

$$\text{Collection ratio} = \frac{\text{Total payments}}{\text{Gross charges}}$$

Because the amount of charges, payments, and adjustments varies from month to month, it is best to calculate the collection ratio based on an average of the previous 3, 6, or 12 months.

A practice's collection ratio should be as high as possible considering the practice's unique circumstances. For example, the collection ratio might be low because the practice serves poor people or because it participates heavily in health insurance plans. The collection ratio is one of several bench marks against which the performance of the practice's patient accounting system may be measured. Other factors include the practice's accounts receivable ratio, the practice's rate of growth, and complaints and compliments received from patients.

Accounts Receivable Ratio

The *accounts receivable ratio* measures how fast patient accounts are being paid. It is expressed as the equivalent number of months of gross charges contained in the practice's accounts receivable. The formula is:

$$\text{Accounts receivable ratio} = \frac{\text{Total accounts receivable}}{\text{Average monthly gross charges}}$$

As with the collection ratio, the appropriate level of a practice's accounts receivable ratio depends on the practice's unique circumstances. A low collection ratio (less than 2:1) is desirable. However, it might be high (above 3:1) because few patients pay at the time of service or because the practice participates heavily in many insurance plans.

Bad debts are amounts owed to the practice that are considered uncollectible. They should be removed from the accounts receivable (written off) on a regular basis. If these amounts remain, the practice's total accounts receivable will grow indefinitely and the accounts receivable ratio will be distorted.

PATIENT ACCOUNTING SYSTEMS

Pegboard System

The *pegboard system*, also called the *one-write system*, is simple, reliable, and not very expensive to install and operate. It is suited to practices with a small number of unpaid accounts (less than 250). The basic components of a pegboard system are:

- encounter form (superbill)
- patient ledger card
- daysheet.

These three items are arranged on a pegboard, a piece of wood or metal with a line of pegs down the left edge. Each day, a daysheet, which has holes on its left edge, is placed on the pegboard. The daysheet is ruled in columns: date; patient name; description of service; and amount of charges, payments, and adjustments. The encounter forms and patient ledger cards have identical columns.

An encounter form, which also has holes on its left edge, is placed on the pegboard before the patient is treated. It is aligned on the pegboard over the next available line on the daysheet. Individual patient ledger cards are slipped between the encounter form and daysheet. Carbon paper or carbonless forms transfer all entries to all forms simultaneously. This saves time and virtually eliminates transcription errors.

The encounter form is then clipped to the patient's medical chart, which is routed to the physician. At the conclusion of the visit, the physician notes the services rendered and the patient's diagnosis. To save time, the most common procedures and diagnoses and their corresponding CPT and ICD.9.CM codes are preprinted on the encounter form. The encounter form is forwarded to the assistant at the front desk. He or she replaces it and the ledger card on the pegboard and records the patient's charges, payments, and adjustments.

If the encounter form is a single sheet perforated vertically, the patient is given the right side and the left side remains in the practice as a control copy. If the encounter form has two pages, one is the patient's receipt and one remains in the practice as a control copy. Encounter forms with a third page may be used to prepare the insurance claims. It is either given to the patient or forwarded to the practice's insurance clerk. Payments received through the mail and adjustments are recorded on the patient ledger cards and daysheet as well.

At the end of the day, the practice's front desk assistant totals the charges, payments, and adjustments recorded on the encounter forms and other source documents. These totals are compared with the corresponding totals on the daysheet. If they are equal, the daysheet is in balance. If not, the assistant attempts to find and correct the error(s).

Patient bills are prepared by photocopying the ledger cards. Insurance claims are prepared from information on copies of encounter forms. Delinquent accounts are identified by manually reviewing the ledger cards. Reports are prepared by compiling the information on the daysheet. As the number of active accounts in the practice grows, these tasks can become very tedious, and using an automated system might be more efficient.

Batch-processing Service Bureau

Practices that use a *batch-processing service bureau* forward all patient information forms and transaction source documents to an outside firm for processing by a computer system. The documents are grouped into batches for control purposes. Manual patient ledger cards and daysheets are not used. Instead, *patient account activity lists* are produced. Daily *transaction journals*, which are the equivalent of daysheets, are produced as batches of source documents are processed. For control purposes, totals of transactions derived from source documents are compared with totals calculated by the computer system from the same data. The computer system automatically creates patient bills and insurance claims (on paper or electronically), identifies and produces collection tools for delinquent accounts, and produces reports.

The advantage of using a batch-processing service bureau is that a computer is used to perform what would otherwise be tedious manual tasks. Some tasks, such as creating reports, cost too much in labor and time to do manually. The disadvantage of a batch-processing service bureau is that patient account information available in the practice is not up-to-date: The results of processing usually are not returned to the practice for a week or more.

Time-sharing Service Bureau

With a *time-sharing service bureau*, computer terminals, and sometimes printers, are located in the practice. They communicate with a computer system in another location. Rather than send documents to the service bureau, the practice's staff members enter information through the computer terminals. As with the batch-processing service bureau, the computer system automatically creates patient bills and insurance claims, identifies delinquent accounts, and produces reports. Printing of patient bills and insurance claims is usually done on high-speed printers at the service bureau.

Using a time-sharing service bureau has all the advantages of using a batch-processing service bureau plus up-to-the-minute information about patient accounts. The disadvantage is that labor costs may be somewhat higher because the practice's staff is responsible for data entry. In addition, continuing operating costs of this type of system could be higher than others.

In-house Computer System

As the name implies, all computer equipment is located in the practice with an *in-house computer system*. The practice's staff uses the computer system to perform all billing, insurance, and collection functions. The family physician should have an agreement with the vendor to support both the hardware and software. The advantages of an in-house system are that the practice has a great degree of control over billing, insurance, and collection functions and that continuing costs of operation, including labor costs, might be lower than other alternatives. The disadvantages, which are not unique to in-house systems, are that the computer hardware or software may be deficient in some way or that the vendor will fail to provide adequate support. A good precaution against problems with this or any other type of patient accounting system is to request and check references of other users of the specific systems under consideration.

References

American Medical Association Medical Collections Study Course (OP-134), Insurance Coding Study Course (OP-411), and Insurance Processing Study Course (OP-426). Chicago, American Medical Association. *Good training materials for employees who perform patient accounting functions. Each course includes a workbook and audio tape. Workbooks are also available separately.*

CPT—1989:Physicians Current Procedural Terminology 1989. 4th ed. Chicago, American Medical Association, 1989. *This is a compilation of descriptive terms and identifying codes for reporting medical procedures performed by physicians. Order item number OP–341/9a to receive the minibook for medical specialties, including family practice, at no additional charge. AMA publications may be ordered by writing to Book and Pamphlet Fulfillment, American Medical Association, P.O. Box 10946, Chicago, Ill. 60610–0946 or by calling 800–621–8335.*

Farber, L. (Ed.): Medical Economics Encyclopedia of Practice and Financial Management. Oradell, N.J., Medical Economics Co., 1985. *A comprehensive, clearly written reference. Medical Economics Co. publishes* Medical Economics *magazine and many books on practice management. One can write for their current catalog at the following: Medical Economics Books, Oradell, N.J. 07649.*

Health Insurance Claim Form. Chicago, American Medical Association. *HCFA-1500 claim forms are available in pads, snap-apart format, and continuous-feed.*

The International Classification of Diseases, 9th ed., Clinical Modification. Washington, D.C., United States Department of Health and Human Services, 1980. Publication number (PHS) 80–1260. *The ICD.9.CM is the generally accepted system of coding diseases and injuries. It is also available from the AMA.*

McCue, J. D.: Private Practice: Surviving the First Year. Lexington, Mass., Collamore Press, 1981. *Good advice on all facets of setting up a medical practice, beginning with whether to enter private practice at all.*

Medical Practice Finance: A Guide for Physicians. Chicago, American Medical Association, 1985.

Physician Marketplace Statistics. Chicago, American Medical Association, 1988. *Includes data on physician's average fees for selected services and procedures and office and hospital visits.*

Soukhanov, A. H., and Haverty, J. R. (Eds.): Webster's Medical Office Handbook. Springfield, Mass., G. & C. Merriam Co., 1975. *This well-written book covers every important aspect of medical office management. It is highly recommended as a reference for office staff.*

Valancy, J.: Microcomputers and Your Practice: A Guide for Physicians. Chicago, Pluribus Press, 1985. *Covers the basics of computer hardware and software, selection and implementation of a computer system, and common applications in medical practices. Pluribus Press, 160 East Illinois Street, Chicago, Ill. 60611, 800–225–3775.*

78

Personnel and Time Management

Duane M. Johnson

In the past, a family physician who practiced compassionate, quality medical care could usually be assured a financially and professionally rewarding career. No longer is that the case.

In today's ever-changing health care market, physicians face many complexities in practice. Strategic practice planning, marketing, competition, cost containment, and computerization are but a few of the foreign concepts that now regularly permeate private practice activities.

Yet historically, the two most important elements of family medicine practice management still remain at the top of the list: personnel and time management.

Why personnel management? Because the nature of medical service revolves around people relationships. Family medicine is a "people business"— people (physicians and staff) serving people (patients).

For example, patients judge a family physician not just on clinical skills but also on how staff relate to them and how efficient they seem. Patients view personnel as direct extensions of the physician, making no differentiations, especially if an outcome is negative.

One must remember that patients have not been to medical school and cannot measure medical expertise. They measure everything that they can measure—what surrounds the actual clinical service, such as the physician's staff representatives. A patient's confidence in a family physician's skills frequently rides not on the physician's brief intervention but on staff interactions.

Physicians discover that personnel management is vital when reading a practice's financial statement. Most family physicians will note quickly that payroll is the single largest expense in their professional lives. Payroll typically runs between 16 and 18 per cent of gross revenue. It never goes away during practice years; instead it usually becomes larger. Carefully selected, well-trained, and effectively managed employees are an asset that will return significant dividends for a family physician.

But what about time management? Why is it important?

Time is the most precious commodity in the practice. It is the life's blood of the practice.

If I were asked to describe in one sentence the business of a family physician, I would put it as follows: A family physician sells clinical skill time units to people. These clinical skill time units are called patient appointments.

If the scheduling and time management of both the family physician and staff are not well controlled and managed, then that physician will suffer significant loss of monetary potential and could even go bankrupt.

Then, too, when a physician's time is mismanaged, many patients, especially in physician-deficient geographic areas, are deprived of professional health care services.

Personnel Organization and Management

Most family physicians find it exciting to be in family medicine. They enjoy the challenge of creating and providing diverse services that help people with their health care needs as well as accumulating monetary benefits from the business of private practice. But effective personnel and time management are required to be successful.

As difficult as it may be to accept, a private family practice is indeed a business. Moreover, it must be perceived and organized with personnel and time managerial principles similar to those of other businesses to produce positive results for patients, physicians, and staff.

Fortunately, nothing in personnel organizational design or the daily execution of practice time activities as a professional business has to detract from the delivery of high-quality patient care. Organizational and other business guidelines are not unethical, unprofessional, or illegal. In fact, the opposite is true. The more carefully a family physician implements organizational business, personnel, and time management principles in the practice, the greater will be the quality, ethics, professionalism, and legal compliance of patient service.

The cornerstone of personnel management is organization. Organizational problems interfere with the practice's overall efficiency and result in lost dollars.

PRACTICE GOALS

To develop a productive organizational structure, the first step is to clearly and explicitly define practice goals. The physician needs to determine specifically and measurably what the organization of people is to accomplish and at what quality level.

Defining goals is the only way to make the best possible use of available resources. In family medicine, those resources include not only the physician's but also the staff's time and skills.

How a family practice is organized (including how many people are needed) is certainly affected by time frames and time limits. Although in family medicine the ratio of assistants to physicians generally runs two and a half to three assistants per physician, the actual number of staff members needed should be determined by empiric means.

Factors such as whether it is a solo or a group practice, where the practice is located, how much the physician delegates, whether it is a fast-paced or slow-paced office, and whether or not x-ray and laboratory equipment are in the office determine the number of assistants needed at the practice.

Once practice goals and standards are targeted, actions and tasks required to accomplish them can be listed and the organization can take shape. Goals themselves are not performable; only the actions or tasks that lead to their fulfillment are do-able. Therefore, goals and standards lay the foundation upon which the organizational structure is built.

It is important to review annually the practice tasks, policies and procedures regarding telephone handling, scheduling, record keeping, patient relations, collections and insurance, marketing, and overall management structure to ensure that present actions are guiding the practice in the desired direction.

Job Descriptions

When goal-oriented actions and tasks are detailed and written, they can be placed together into logical task groups, each of which is then called a job or job description (Fig. 78–1).

To be useful, job descriptions must be carefully thought out and developed. In addition, the number of tasks placed in a job description must be "time calculated" to determine how long they take to accomplish on the average. Then the logical number of tasks that can be done in the time available for that job can be assigned. Also, tasks that logically go with one another should be placed in the same job list; this will maximize efficiency. For instance, if completing one task involves doing half of another, the two should be assigned to the same job (Fig. 78–2).

Formal written job descriptions also serve the total personnel schemata (Fig. 78–3). For example, a written job description provides guidelines for training new employees since the job description spells out the tasks that new staff person must do. It is also a key management tool in reviewing the performance of established personnel.

A job description is a vital communication tool for both management and staff. It defines clearly for each employee what is expected of him or her. It allows management a baseline from which to measure performance and salary levels.

When all tasks necessary to accomplish the practice's objectives are placed in job descriptions, the practice's organization has been focused and the number of personnel needed has been defined (Fig. 78–4).

Practices that are successful tend to be people oriented. Most physicians realize the importance of the patient as a person. Staff members, no less important as people, are a family physician's largest professional investment. When properly selected, trained, and managed, they rapidly become the practice's second greatest asset after the physician.

SUCCESSFUL FUNCTIONING

There are a few cardinal rules essential to the successful functioning of any family practice organization. First, someone on the practice team must be *accountable* for every task that needs to be performed in the organization. In other words, every practice physician and staff member should have a list of tasks that the team depends on them to accomplish. This raises the consistent level of excellence in the practice.

A second cardinal rule is that every position in the practice must be doubly covered. Each member of the practice team should know how to perform

JOB DESCRIPTION

Job Description For:

Reports To:

Responsibilities:

Duties of the Job:

Job Requirements:

Job Relationships:

Authority Boundaries:

Figure 78–1. Sample job description form. (©1989 Practice Productivity, Inc., Atlantic, GA—Personnel Policies and Procedures Manual.)

JOB DESCRIPTION: Medical Receptionist
REPORTS TO: Office Manager

RESPONSIBILITIES: Responsible for receiving patients and visitors, determining their needs and directing them accordingly. Answers telephone, makes appointments, receives payments, and issues receipts. Performs other clerical and administrative tasks as required.

DUTIES OF THE POSITION:

- Greets visitors and patients, determines their needs, and directs them accordingly.
- Answers questions and gives information directly or on the telephone within the limits of his or her knowledge and medical practice policies.
- Makes and checks off appointments, giving routine nonmedical instructions in preparation for the patient's visit to the practice.
- Retrieves medical records from files and prepares charge slips and attaches them to the medical record for use in conjunction with the patient's visit.
- Retrieves and files medical records, letters, reports, and miscellaneous items as requested. Purges medical records monthly.
- Collects fees, issues receipts, and counsels patients concerning their accounts when necessary. Counts and balances money at the end of the day.
- Types hospital lists. Types hospital orders for physicians. Schedules hospital admissions. Schedules surgery. Secures information from hospitals concerning consultations.
- Researches files to determine whether or not patient has visited the practice before. Makes up medical records for new patients.
- Opens practice, does housekeeping chores, runs errands, and closes practice, as required.
- Handles refills for prescriptions according to medical practice policy.
- Performs other duties as required.

JOB REQUIREMENTS:

- Graduation from high school with courses in English and typing. Completion of a medical assistant course at the junior college level is desirable. Previous patient contact work in a medical practice is an advantage. If the applicant does not have experience, 3 months on-the-job training will be provided.
- Be able to operate a sound-recording device and operate an electric typewriter and type 60 words per minute with accuracy.
- Possess the tact required for work situations that involve dealing with patients to secure payment of delinquent accounts.
- Possess the tact to deal effectively with patients, physicians, and other employees in the environment.
- Possess a preference for dealing with people who are ill and need help.
- Possess the verbal ability to discuss medical and financial problems with patients and be clearly understood.

JOB RELATIONSHIPS:

Does not supervise any other employees. Receives supervision from the Office Manager.

AUTHORITY BOUNDARIES:

Reports to the Office Manager in all matters.

Figure 78–2. Job description for a medical receptionist. (©1989 Practice Productivity, Inc., Atlantic, GA—How to Establish or Join a Successful Medical Practice, pp. 17–18.)

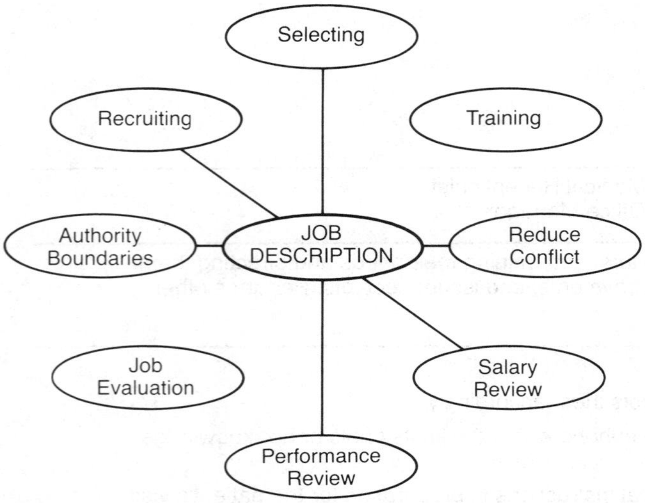

Figure 78–3. Hub and Spokes design job description. (©1989 Practice Productivity, Inc., Atlanta, GA—Personnel Policies and Procedures Manual, p. 5.)

another job or series of tasks so that no one person is indispensable (except the physicians). This cross-training allows the practice to function acceptably when there is illness, vacation, overload, or termination.

Third, salary ranges, based on community supply and demand for the particular job skills required in each position, should be determined prior to hiring. A physician should pay for the job that is being done, not the person doing it.

The final cardinal rule is that communication structures between physicians, physicians and manager, and manager and employees should be clearly defined. Communication is the tool that reduces misunderstandings, which underlie many practice failures. Therefore, great effort should be made to assure that regular communication occurs between various practice team members. Without effective communication, there can be little team relationship, and an organization of any type, especially one that focuses on service to people, must have good relationships among its members to function well.

Office Manager

Another organizational necessity when a practice has three or more employees is an office manager. This position is analogous to that of an orchestra leader. A manager coordinates the physicians and directs day-to-day practice activities in accordance with the physicians' policies and procedures.

The office manager is the administrative head of the practice. That person has responsibility for implementing policies and facilitating communication between physicians and staff and even between the physicians themselves. The manager relieves the physicians of the pressure and time requirements of daily management, enabling them to focus on clinical services and income production. The physicians' only management obligation is to manage the manager.

It is critical that family physicians never abdicate total control of the practice to the manager. If that is done, the practice will not become the type of organization the physicians want it to be. Instead, it will be formed in the image of the manager.

OTHER FACTORS IN PERSONNEL MANAGEMENT

A brief review of a few other personnel management items follows:

Recruiting. This is the search of the community to create the largest possible pool of *qualified* candidates. The physician should use every available service: newspaper advertisements, private employment agencies, schools and colleges, other health care

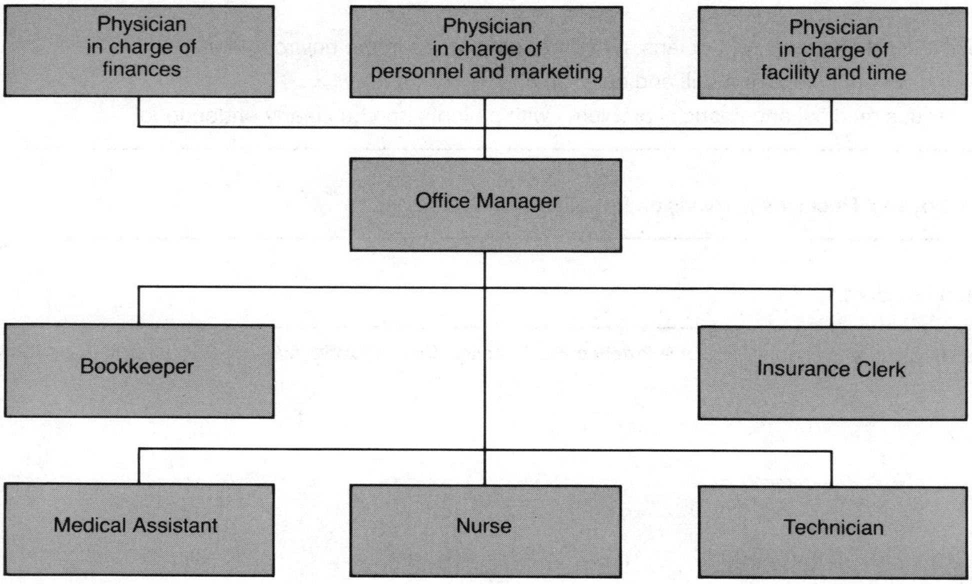

Figure 78–4. Organization chart for a typical three-physician medical office. (©1989 Practice Productivity, Inc., Atlanta, GA—Personnel Policies and Procedures Manual, p.10.)

providers, medical associations, placement listings, and medical assistant staff society services.

Selecting. This is the process of elimination, utilizing interviews, tests of performance of actual job tasks, and checking of job references.

Training. Training never ends, but it should be organized. Performance of the job description duties or list of accountable tasks is the training objective. The trainer should have the new employee watch the task being performed, perform it, and teach it back to the trainer. The trainer should then establish and maintain monitors of quality control on what the employee does. Training also includes orienting a new employee to general practice activities and circumstances of the practice.

Performance Review. This communication approach should be utilized formally once a year. This vital tool can effect positive reinforcement, correct deficiencies, examine problems, say thank you, and provide stimulation and motivation for improving performance. All reviews should be documented in writing in the individual employee's file folder.

Salary Review. Appropriate salaries attract good employees. Salaries for various practice jobs should be researched and evaluated once a year. Raises should be given based on improved performance, not tenure.

Termination. If problems with an employee persist after a documented performance review explaining dissatisfactions, then that employee should be terminated. A cardinal rule when terminating an employee is always to preserve the dignity of the individual, even though he or she typically is unhappy with the outcome. Another reminder is always to be careful not to mishandle the procedure to ensure that legal repercussions do not occur. In particular, one should be sure to document everything.

Personnel Policies and Procedures. Every family practice needs to establish the rules. These should be a set of straightforward communications about a myriad of items that could cause team misunderstandings if not clarified. Some examples are rules about working hours, vacation, sick leave, holidays, smoking, health benefits, and personal use of telephones. These also involve legal obligations of employers to employees. Advisers should assist physicians in developing this important communication tool.

Because a family physician spends more money for payroll than any other expense, from a business sense, it is in a physician's best interest to maximize the use of personnel through effective management.

Time Management

One of the wisest reminders a family physician can ever be given is that he or she is a person first and a physician second. Physicians should be careful to not allow their practices to swallow their whole lives—all their time.

VALUING TIME

The first principle of time management is to value time. If a person does not value time, why expend energy to manage it?

Time is the most valuable asset any human being has: physician, staff, and patient. It should not be squandered.

How a physician uses each 24 hours will not only affect practice outcomes but also have a dramatic impact on a doctor's personal health and relationships with others. The key is the balance between practice and personal time.

Physicians are notorious for letting life get out of balance by mismanaging their time. Some never experience the joy of knowing their children while they are growing up. Others have ruined their health; still others have neglected their marriages and are now divorced. Those family physicians who seem to be in control have obviously established their personal, professional, and practice goals in that order.

PLANNING TIME USAGE

Since time does move onward and since a physician cannot control time, the only thing he or she can control is how to spend that time. A brief investment of time to review and plan time usage should be scheduled every day, with a greater amount of time scheduled once a week to summarize.

Planning is the key to effective time management. A physician should clarify personal, professional, and practice goals once a quarter; keep a time log and analyze time habits once every 6 months; document daily and weekly "to do" lists; stay aware, organized, and on target; and cultivate time management habits.

Time management habits that physicians typically need to cultivate are controlling their telephone usage; delegating responsibility and authority; keeping meeting times to a minimum; managing patients and not allowing patients to manage them; doing as much as possible correctly the first time; and focusing time on pursuing targeted goals.

When all other things have been put into proper perspective, one of the most critical decisions a physician must make is how much time to devote to the medical profession. Proper allocations to family and self will typically be of utmost importance.

Once determined, the professional time allocation must be properly used. Time management in a family practice is money management.

Delegating

The family physician needs to ask the following time management questions: Am I doing things that are better left to my staff? Am I really performing tasks a physician needs to perform and leaving the other tasks to the staff? If not, those tasks should be delegated. The family physician should continually think about what tasks can be given away.

Practice managers should alleviate most physicians of writing performance reviews; scheduling work hours; screening, hiring, training, and terminating employees; ordering supplies; and check writing.

Clinical personnel can handle many routine clinical tasks. When a physician delegates clinical tasks to the staff in front of the patient, the patient usually finds it very acceptable. Of course, clinical personnel must be carefully trained so malpractice risks will not dramatically increase.

Many times, the physician's delegating to a staff member enhances that employee's morale and sense of importance. Much of patient education should be either delegated to the staff or supplied by the physician on videotape or audiotape or in printed form.

All delegated tasks should be carefully reviewed for legal ramifications, and quality control monitoring should be consistently performed.

Scheduling

Scheduling appointments is the most difficult area for a family physician to control, but it can be done reasonably well. At the heart of scheduling is the recognition that a scheduling plan is very individualized.

Common types of scheduling difficulties need to be identified and data gathered about them, and then predictions about the physician's practice based on those data need to be implemented in the schedule itself.

Following are a few other suggestions of data to be researched and predicted:

- The average number of patients seen per physician per day and the type of visit
- The average number of new patients seen per physician per day
- The average amount of time spent with each type of patient by all people involved in service (i.e., physician, medical assistants, clerical assistants to process incoming patients)
- The number of emergency patients seen by day of week
- The patterns of visitation (e.g., Mondays are regularly busy)
- The number of procedures and time needed for each procedure per day
- The average patient waiting time

After the data have been gathered and analyzed, an individual schedule for each doctor is designed. Designated time slots to work in emergency patients; to perform quick check-ups and routine follow-ups; to examine new patients; and to handle other long, time-consuming visits are planned. In other words, a predictable, integrated schedule allowing for each type of patient is mapped out in advance before patient names are scheduled.

The scheduling plan must be realistic about the amount of time the physician has available. It must be followed with vigorous discipline in order not to violate it.

In other words, the schedule must be customized for the way each physician functions based on what has normally happened in previous days, weeks, and months.

An appointment schedule is individually designed, not purchased from a local supplier or stationery store. Many practices, for example, use colored pencils to shade or identify the various time slots, such as red for emergencies, blue for short visits, yellow for long visits, and so on.

An appointment-scheduling procedure manual should be written so that all scheduling staff can be trained to handle this crucial function of the practice and can refresh their memory on scheduling.

Physician Extenders

A number of family physicians have increased their time by using a physician's assistant or nurse practitioner. These physician extenders can see primary care patients with minor problems under a physician's supervision. This allows a physician to focus on the significantly more serious patient health problems.

Time management and scheduling are critical to a family physician, both personally and professionally. When one handles segments of time that cannot be recaptured, discipline is required. An intelligent structure plus the discipline to make it work will contain and maximize this critical control tool.

Time management and scheduling will never be perfect, but they must be empirically worked with to create positive results. That means periodic re-evaluations must be done because, as in life, you are never adjusted, but always adjusting.

79

The Use of Personal Computers in Medicine

Abdulla M. Abdulla
Cathi Chambley Miller
John S. Henke

Since its introduction a little more than 10 years ago, the personal computer has become a part of virtually every segment of the business world, including the medical profession. For many years, physicians have been accustomed to using computerized laboratory equipment for performing intricate tasks, making complex calculations, and printing detailed reports. This equipment, including laboratory instruments such as chromatographs and spectrophotometers, and diagnostic tools such as computerized tomographic and single-photon emission tomography thallium scanners have taken advantage of the size, speed, and precision of microprocessor chips similar to those found in personal computers. Due to the complexity of many diagnostic tools and the vast amount of paperwork involved in maintaining patient records for a hospital or private practice, the use of computers in the health-care profession has seen dramatic growth. As computer systems become more widely utilized, and as the ease of use and the overall familiarity of the health-care worker with computerized equipment increases, there will continue to be growth in the number of computer users as well as in the number of applications available.

Computers have been in use in hospitals and medical schools for many years; however, those computers were generally the large mainframes or minicomputers that took up a great deal of floor space. Additionally, the operations of those computer systems were usually too complex for the novice to understand. An inexperienced user was not able to tap into the power of these computers because there was no interface between the user and the computer that was easily understood, and because there were few applications that would be pertinent to the daily business of a medical practice. The introduction of personal computers, which were originally conceived as a product for the home, brought a sudden demand for packages that could be used by any person in any profession.

Standardization of Hardware and Disk Operating Systems

Initially, there was little uniformity between computer systems, with each company designing a proprietary computer and operating system software or disk operating system. Systems were developed using the

CP-M, Apple DOS, IBM PC-DOS, and other operating systems, each being basically incompatible with the other. This disparity between systems generated a good deal of initial confusion among most medical practitioners, who were concerned with issues such as cost-efficiency and investment protection. This led to many physicians and other health care workers consciously to decide to wait before purchasing a specific computer system for their practice. Within the last few years, however, there has been a move toward standardization within the computer industry so that the number of choices of operating systems has been reduced and unified while the number of personal computer manufacturers has increased. This means that a health care professional can now select a computer system that meets his or her needs in terms of software performance while having a large selection of computers from which to select the model having the desired features at the right price. Within this large computer industry, the leading operating systems that are currently available are Unix, Xenix and DOS, which run on IBM or compatible types of personal computers as well as Apple's Macintosh computers and Unix or Xenix specific systems made by AT&T, Burroughs, Unisys and others. ProDOS, which is used by the Apple II systems, and Macintosh, a system unique to the Macintosh computers, are both popular systems. The Apple II has seen little growth for medical software mostly due to the memory demands of complex software. However, the newer Macintosh system is quickly achieving a foothold in a great many areas of the medical profession. Each operating system has features that distinguish it from the others, and each offers something unique to medical practice.

Spread Sheet and Data Base Systems

The move to personal computers in the medical office was ensured with the introduction of software such as Lotus 1-2-3 (spread sheet) and dBASE (data base). With these powerful software packages, a skilled and determined user could create programs that would fully computerize routine paperwork tasks such as accounting and record keeping. As the development of these applications shifted from the end-user to full-time developers, more job-specific packages became available. In other words, because these developers had the time and resources to create full-featured, complex applications, the particular needs of many businesses were met. Medical professionals, including physicians, hospital administrators, and records managers, began to see the possibilities of integrating computer systems into their workplace. The functions and abilities that appealed to these potential computer users were not developed with a specific market in mind; rather, the packages were designed to have enough features to appeal to persons in every business in which information processing and accounting procedures take a high priority. The medical professional has been able to take advantage of many of these programs, particularly those that allow the physician to automate patient accounting, patient records, word processing, and scheduling.

The Role of Computers

The reasons for using computer systems in the health care field are the same as those for any other business. Computers speed up the retrieval of information and produce accurate financial or statistical information. Because a computer system can store and retrieve information at a high rate of speed, reports detailing financial, medical, scheduling, or other information can be generated on a timely basis. This allows the organization to know the status of any record almost immediately. In this way, an administrator can review the financial status of a hospital and a physician can review the status of any patient's treatment. By utilizing systems for using data base and accounting procedures, the volume of paper that must be stored by any office or hospital can be reduced to a fraction, because all records are stored electronically.

Use of Computers in the Medical Office

Word Processors. Initially, personal computers were introduced into the medical office to address only a few basic needs. The first of those needs, word processing, was met by programs that introduced simplicity and speed into the creation of any document, from correspondence to patient notes. Word processing programs were especially important to the physician who spent a great deal of time documenting research for publication because the turn-around time for editing changes was greatly decreased with this system. The editing of documents that were created on a computer was much faster than editing those documents that were created manually and the productivity of both the physician and the typist was increased. As word processing programs gained more features, the quality of the documents that could be produced improved.

Patient Scheduling. One of the greatest problems facing most medical practices is patient scheduling. Patient scheduling must allow a reasonable time between appointments, but this allowance is difficult to incorporate into the schedule because the practitioner has a responsibility to generate income while best serving the needs of his or her patients. Scheduling programs have been designed that divide the physician's time into increments of any size, and a patient is placed in the earliest available time slot. If that appointment time is not convenient, the scheduling clerk can continue to search the schedule to find a more convenient appointment time. Other programs allow the scheduling clerk to enter the best day and time and place the patient in the first slot which fits those criteria.

Staff Scheduling. Staff scheduling is always difficult, especially when the medical office must juggle conflicting schedules of several busy doctors with the needs of a large office staff. Scheduling becomes vital to hospital staff, which needs an adequate number of nurses and other staff members available to provide acceptable levels of patient care without a large outlay in overtime pay for overstaffing. Most offices and many hospital wards and departments continue to schedule manually, although the time involved can be prohibitive when patient load and staff requests fluctuate. Programs that automate the scheduling of staff can be of significant benefit, especially if those programs allow input pertaining to patient load and staff requests. One such program is What'sBest, by General Optimization, which allows the scheduler to enter information about staff requirements and individual scheduling requests into a Lotus 1-2-3 template. The information is then used in a mathematical model that determines the schedule. Other programs have been developed using other methods, however the basic premise behind staff scheduling remains the same: Utilize the staff most efficiently to meet needs without incurring large overtime expenses.

Bookkeeping. In addition to word processing and scheduling, another application of computers that immediately caught on in the medical industry was automated bookkeeping. The health care profession requires an accounting system that keeps general ledger, accounts receivable and accounts payable records. These tasks can be performed by a variety of accounting programs, ranging from straightforward and simple systems to complex systems. Larger practices and most hospitals require systems that also maintain records of cash disbursements and create and print checks. The system must also be complex enough to allow the entry of fixed assets, such as buildings, large equipment, and instruments; depreciation of assets; and inventory control. Of course, all health care practices require a system that performs payroll tasks, figures earnings for salaried and hourly employees, and maintains state and Federal income tax and FICA deduction records, as well as other deductions for medical insurance, 401K, or other employee programs.

Patient Accounting. Patient accounting is perhaps the most commonly computerized task in the medical office and in hospitals. The ability to quickly and efficiently provide patients and billing officers with up-to-date records of patient charges and payments allows the hospital and office to track the income from patient accounts, perform aging on past-due accounts, and provide the physician and accountant with a concise report on the financial well-being of the business. A well-designed medical billing program allows the bookkeeper to create a file on each patient, showing dates of service, service performed, charge, payment amount, and payment date. Many packages are available that are generally sophisticated enough for use by many types of businesses and can easily automate any medical practice. Accounting packages also are available that were created specifically for the medical office. These packages track items that are most useful to the physician, so that he or she can determine what procedures are most cost effective for the practice. In a group practice, it is highly desirable to use a program that allows tracking of the income and expenses of each producer, including nursing and therapist staff members.

Many medical billing programs also allow the billing officers to generate insurance forms so that the process of filing for insurance payment can be performed routinely with each visit rather than monthly or bi-monthly for all patients in the system. Electronic claims generation makes filing insurance claims faster and easier for the office worker and relieves the burden of insurance filing from the patient. Electronic claims allow the physician or other administrator to be assured that insurance payment will not be delayed because of improperly filed forms or other patient delays. This is especially important for practices or hospitals having a large number of Medicare and Medicaid patients, since the policies concerning the filing and payment of claims can be confusing and stringent. Electronic claims generation applications are included in some medical office systems, and are also available as single packages that can be added to existing systems. Some programs, such as MediMac by HealthCare Communications, allows the physician to enter information necessary to file insurance claims, including demographics, diagnoses, treatment plans, and charges. Many of these programs trade information with other programs; for example MediMac can share information with the Great Plains accounting packages and Microsoft File data bases.

Record Keeping of Patients' Files. One of the most important data base needs of a medical practice is to place the records of patients on the computer system. Data base programs that allow the physician to enter demographic information on each patient as well as the diagnoses, treatments, and insurance information have been designed for many medical specialties. These specialty-specific programs allow, for example, the cardiologist to enter only information that is normally obtained from cardiac patients, whereas a neurologist would need another specific set of information. No matter what specialty the system is used for, the patient records should contain a place for handwritten notes, which would be entered into the database at the end of the day. Some programs offer the ability to add almost unlimited note lengths, whereas others offer various options that allow the physician to select options from predetermined entries.

With a patient data base, each patient has a record in the system. As with most manual systems, the initial information set contains the demographic information and the patient medical history. Programs have been developed that allow these entries to be made by a receptionist or admitting clerk or by the patient or a family member. Patient history systems can follow an item-by-item entry process. However, more sophisticated programs, such as Historymaker 4 by Medical Logic International, have menus containing the most common choices and allow for entry of unusual items. However, other programs let the patient or clerk enter information based on yes or no questions.

Patient records that contain information detailing the results of laboratory and other diagnostic tests help the physician diagnose an illness and follow the treatment and response of any patient. Any program that can immediately print reports based on this information becomes more and more important, especially in growing practices or practices in which patients are seen less frequently. Having the information at hand allows the physician or therapist to concentrate on current symptoms or improvements rather than on reviewing the patient's history. Physician's orders for a patient can be entered into a patient record system so that those orders become part of the patient's records. This entry system also reduces any errors or delays in treatment due to the illegibility of a physician's handwriting. By using a data base system, the physician is able to review previous treatment programs and determine any changes that should be made immediately upon examining a patient rather than after locating and reviewing the handwritten notes or locating a patient chart. The addition of a modem and a computer at the physician's home could allow remote access of such information while he or she took a call at home. Obviously, an access security system would be of paramount importance in maintaining the confidentiality of the patients and the practice.

Storage of Digitized Diagnostic Tests. One of the newest uses for data base systems is to maintain records of patient diagnostic images such as x-ray studies, CT scans, and magnetic resonance studies. With the use of sophisticated scanning equipment, these film images can be digitized and stored on media such as WORM drives (Write Once, Read Many times). By storing these images electronically, an x-ray study archive need no longer maintain vast storerooms of film. Another advantage of disk storage is the speed of accessibility of the data; a search of computer-archived images is much faster than a manual search through rows of shelves. Electronic images cannot be misfiled, and these images can be transferred electronically to other computers quickly so that there is no delay through mailing. Another advantage of digitized images is the number of software products that allow the physician to view the image at a variety of intensities and shades while providing the ability to manipulate the image by zooming in on a specific point of interest. By giving the physician or technician the ability to more accurately identify images, the computer becomes a tool that enhances the diagnostic ability of the physician. Finally, the addition of a relatively inexpensive Fax card and printer to the physician's computer at home and the availability of a Fax machine in the hospital emergency room or the coronary care unit allows the transmission of electrocardiograms to the cardiologist's home. The cardiologist can then provide the interpretation and emergency orders prior to leaving for the hospital. This system can be particularly valuable in expediting the use of thrombolytic therapy in acute myocardial infarction, particularly if the emergency room physician has doubts about the interpretation of the electrocardiogram.

Customized Data Base Systems. Data bases can also be constructed to provide immediate access to other information needed to provide an efficient and high level of patient care. There are several programs available that provide information about a patient's disease or treatments based on information in a previously created data base. For example, SOAP, a drug interaction program by Patient Medical Records Inc., allows the health care provider to enter the patient information into a data base and relate the information about the patient's illness and drug therapy to another data base that contains information on a vast number of drugs, the possible drug to drug and drug to disease interactions. This data base also contains information about the dosage and side effects of a specific drug treatment.

As medical technology has made tremendous strides within the past 25 years, especially within the field of transplantation, the need has arisen for a data base containing information on organ donors and patients in need of transplants. One such data base, the United Network for Organ Sharing, is available to virtually all transplant programs through modem link-up. These organ-donor matching programs store information about the vast number of patients in need and is updated and searched each time an organ becomes available. Matches are made on the basis of best match of blood and tissue type. When a match is found, the hospital and physician as well as the organ recipient are immediately notified of the availability of an organ, its location, and pertinent tissue information. If the organ is accepted and the transplant performed successfully, the patient is removed from the data base listing. Unfortunately, because of the vast numbers of patients needing transplants and the limited supply of suitable donor organs, patients are often removed from the data base because of their death.

Another use for a data base has already been applied by hospitals, like the Georgia Baptist Medical Center. At that hospital, each surgical resident adds information to a data base of surgical procedures in which he or she has participated. This information allows the resident to examine the completeness of his or her experience while aiding the attending staff, especially the department chairman, to evaluate the performance of each member of the surgical staff. This type of data base can also be used to collect more general information on the types and frequency of surgical procedures used, giving the hospital administration a tool for evaluating the effectiveness of the surgical staff as a whole or individually. With the expected advent of mandatory quality assurance demands by federal and private medical insurance companies, this mode of record keeping will become commonplace.

Networking of Computers. Information about patients and treatment procedures can be shared between several personal computers in the same office, between two or more offices, and with a hospital computer. For example, the medical office could enter patient demographic information into a hospital computer and expedite remote hospital admissions, saving time and paperwork for the hospital and the patient. Information can also be shared between two offices so that upon making a referral, a physician need not mail copies of the patient's record. This increase in speed of data sharing can allow the physician more time to review information and gather any additional data that could be vital to the care of the patient, thereby improving patient care and facilitating the productivity of the physician and the staff. Information is exchanged between computers by the use of communications packages and the appropriate mechanical link-up system. This system consists of a modem and telephone lines between two computer sites, or in an office situation, can be a Local Area Network, or LAN. An LAN is composed of computers, wiring, and additional communications equipment that allows computers to share programs or data. LANs allow each computer in the network to continue to do its own processing while adding the ability to share information between users. This means that a medical office can have one station in which the patient histories are routinely recorded, but that those histories are available to the physician while he is working with the computer in his office.

Electronic Mail. Electronic (E-) mail systems in which each user has an address and can write memos that are made available to a particular user takes advantage of LAN technology. Physicians have been able to use E-mail to enhance the quick exchange of information.

On-Line Data Base Services. Physicians are also finding that on-line database services are available as aids in diagnosing and planning treatments of diseases and injury. These services are usually compilations of the latest literature on any variety of medical topics. By using these on-line services, a physician can have immediate access to the latest information on treatments that he or she may not be familiar with or on disease states that may be outside his or her area of experience. With this information, a physician can immediately decide on a treatment or can consult with the appropriate specialists. In an emergency situation, these services can be used to review the best treatment or technique for trauma or other acute conditions that require immediate and appropriate intervention. Other on-line services consist of airline schedules and reservation capabilities, stock-market information, the Associated Press News Wire service (in which the information is grouped into special medical categories such as AIDS, Disease and Medical Alerts, New Drugs and Medical Research, and Malpractice/Insurance/Legal), Literature Specialty search of the EMPIRES biomedical literature data base, AMA Washington Report, AIDS information service, USA Today News Service, Medicom Drug Interaction Database, Continuing Medical Education Courses, AMA/Net Professional Group Services, and AMA/Net Public Information Services. Many of these services are accessible through the AMA/Net which is an on-line medical information network of the American Medical Association.

Expert Systems and Artificial Intelligence. Developments in the field of artificial intelligence has generated a great deal of excitement among members of the medical community. Creating computer systems that appear to think, or artificial intelligence, has been a goal of many computer developers and users for decades. By developing a system that is artificially intelligent, a developer creates a system that can solve problems based on certain rule-based knowledge that the computer has within its memory and information about a particular situation that is entered by a user. The use of computerized data bases of knowledge and the ability of a personal computer to quickly search for responses in answer to data base queries has lead to the creation of expert systems for many complex business problems. For the medical community, these expert systems can be highly useful in aiding the physician in determining the diagnosis and treatment plan for any patient. One of the most widely used expert systems for diagnosis is DXplain, developed by physicians at Massachusetts General Hospital and available through AMA/NET. Like others developed for use by medical professionals, this expert system is meant to be used as a tool for the diagnosis made by the physician. An expert system is not able to replace a physician, since it cannot make judgments based on knowledge of the patient's unique personality, perception of pain, or other traits that all physician's must consider in making diagnoses. An expert system does give the physician some guidelines to use in evaluating a potential diagnosis and may present diagnoses not being considered by the physician, perhaps because of the rarity of the problem or because there were hidden problems that were not presented. The system must constantly be updated to include the latest medical findings on new diseases and new treatments or it will quickly lose its relevance and importance as a diagnostic tool.

Education. Education is one area in which the personal computer has made an early and important impact, and this impact is felt as much in the field of medical education as in any other. Since medical education encompasses the education of nurses, physicians, technologists, therapists, and other health care workers as well as continuing education of these professionals and counselling of patients, the programs that are produced for creating medical education software generally require a great deal of flexibility in their design. As a general rule, these "authoring systems" are actually a shell in which the educator designs the specific questions, answers, graphics, and educational information that he or she wishes to present to the student. A complete medical education system normally consists of a computer, a monitor, and appropriate software. However, a printer, a videotape or videodisc player, or a CD-ROM or WORM drive may also be part of such systems. Most good authoring systems, such as Precept by C.M.E. Systems, Inc., and CourseBuilder by TeleRobotics International, allow the instructor to create lessons or examinations that integrate graphics, animation, video, sound, and text to simulate real-life situations or fully explain complex medical concepts. The use of computer-based patient education is another exciting application. From time to time, patient education programs have been offered through Physicians and Computers (a magazine edited by two of the authors) and have covered such areas as Diet and Nutrition, Breast Cancer, Hypertension, and Sexual Dysfunction Following Myocardial Infarction.

Desktop Publishing. The introduction of desktop publishing and desktop presentation software packages has had an impact on the area of education. These types of programs give the medical educator and office staff the ability to integrate text and graphics into a visually pleasing format so that the information can be more easily read and understood by the target audience. Presentations are also a valuable aid for the researcher who spends a great deal of time and money in preparing visual aids. The medical field has been highly receptive of these programs because of the obvious need to create materials that adequately explain difficult concepts to a variety of target audiences.

Computer-Aided Design. Researchers find that the ability of personal computers to store and analyze data can make numerous contributions to their productivity. For example, personal computers are being used by medical researchers in the field of biomedical engineering. These researchers use programs such as VersaCAD to perform Computer-Aided Design (CAD) of prosthetics, including artificial limbs. The Jarvik-7 artificial heart and its predecessors were designed, in part, by using personal computers. Computers also played another role in the development of the artificial heart; as the instruments delivering air pressure and testing blood gases and blood flow perform their calculation, this information is fed to a personal computer that displays to the physician and the assistants the status of the artificial heart and, therefore, the status of the patient. Uses such as this are expected to increase as technology plays a greater role in the development of alternative therapy for disease states. As we stated earlier, computerized tomography scanners and other instruments work through the use of microprocessors. Like the artificial heart, these instruments can make this information compatible with a personal computer so that the information can be used immediately, or can be stored as part of the patient record so that the data can be reviewed at any time.

Statistical Analysis. Another important ability of the personal computer is statistical analysis, which is used most extensively by researchers. In the past, the compilation of data into statistics was a time-consuming task, with the generation of considerable anxiety over the accuracy of the final figures. Mainframe and minicomputers reduced the anxiety, but entering the data was still a painstaking task. Personal computers and statistical packages have introduced a new ease into compiling statistics for the researcher, who can enter the data as it is gathered and evaluate that data using a variety of statistical methods quickly and cost effectively. The speed of this process often decreases the amount of time it takes a researcher to introduce his or her findings as part of a published work, allowing the researchers to spend more time in the clinic or lab and less time interacting with data entry workers.

Transportion Planning. With the emphasis on speed of intervention as a factor in the survival of many critically ill or injured patients, the importance of emergency transportation becomes increasingly apparent. Transplantation teams have also focused attention on the speed at which donor organs must be recovered and delivered to the recipient. Computers can be used to schedule flight personnel and to log flight plans for medical transport units, including helicopters and airplanes. The dispatching unit can alert the staff through modem and beepers, then it can locate the best flight plan and file that flight plan with a computer controlling flights from a nearby airport. All these tasks are routinely performed by people, who must search maps, then verbally file a flight plan. Using the computer can drastically reduce the time it takes to get the emergency transport team in the air. Transportation planning software can also be used by dispatchers of regular ground ambulances, allowing the transportation unit to track mileage, time in route, vehicle upkeep, and other information that would help maintain an efficient means of transporting ill or injured patients quickly and safely.

The applications of personal computers in the medical field increase almost daily as more and more health care professionals find programs that allow them to automate one or more of their tasks. As the power and speed of computers increase, the number of practitioners who find them indispensable in their practice will also increase. The applications introduced here do not begin to cover the number of specific uses of medical software, and of course, like desktop publishing, new applications are being introduced that soon will become integrated into many levels of the medical community.

References

Argento, J.: DXplain: Diagnoses at your Fingertips. Physicians and Computers, *5*(11):8–10, 1988. *Explains a computer service in which the user of a personal computer can link, via modem, with a large data base and seek aid in diagnosing difficult medical problems.*

Dejean, D.: This WORM can help your practice turn. Physicians and Computers, *6*(6):9–12, 1988. *Discusses optical imaging software and hardware. An application is also described in which surgical procedures are explained to the patient.*

Dejean, D.: Hope and glory: Men, medicine, and PCs. PC Computing, *1*(2):64–79, 1988. *Describes the way in which computers have helped scientists develop the artificial heart and limbs.*

Illa, R. How to make your history taking easier. Physicians and Computers *4*(8):8–13, 1987. *Describes a software package that allows the patient to enter his own medical history.*

Lant, J.: PaperChase: Medical information at your fingertips. Physicians and Computers, February *5*(10):16–22, 1988. *Describes an online information retrieval system.*

Rasmus, D.: Expert input. *MacUser* *4*(1):136–150, 1988. *Gives information about artificial intelligence, and compares two programs that are available for creating your own artificial intelligence system on the Macintosh.*

80

Risk Management

Richard G. Roberts

Few topics inflame the passions of physicians as much as medical malpractice. Professional liability issues touch every physician. In the 1986 American Medical Association (AMA) Survey of Physician and Public Opinion on Health Care Issues, physicians identified malpractice as the number one problem facing medicine (Harvey, 1986). The 1988 AMA survey revealed that two thirds of physicians expect that the professional liability problem will worsen. Malpractice concerns shape the practice of medicine and, in turn, affect the access to and cost of medical care. Recognizing the public import of malpractice, the United States Congress, three major federal agency reports, and the legislatures of all 50 states have addressed the issue of medical liability over the past 15 years. Despite the attention and resources that have been devoted to the study of medical malpractice, the problem looms more complex, controversial, and costly than ever.

Physicians are frustrated by their collective inability to remedy the professional liability problem. When confronted by clinical challenges, physicians collect and analyze patient data and then formulate and implement an action plan. When confounded by courthouse condemnations, physicians suffer significant physical and emotional symptoms and alter their practices (Charles et al., 1984). For physicians, the medical malpractice drama is played out on an unfamiliar stage before judges, juries, and legislatures. Forced to read from a script which they had no hand in drafting, in an alien (legal) language they do not comprehend, physicians feel a loss of control and respond with indignation. In this way, however, physicians are similar to patients who believe they were unfairly or incompetently treated by the equally mysterious medical care system. Not surprisingly, "physician expectations about the professional liability system are often as unrealistic as their patients' expectations about medicine" (United States Department of Health and Human Services, 1987).

To regain control of the malpractice colossus, physicians must better inform themselves of the nature and dimensions of the problem and be willing to take a fresh look at its complexities. Adlai Stevenson once said, "If we value the pursuit of knowledge, we must be free to follow wherever that search may lead us." This chapter is dedicated to that search. The dimensions and history of the malpractice crisis will be examined, along with a discussion of possible solutions. The chapter will then focus on risk management as the means by which the individual family physician can have the greatest impact on malpractice prevention. Risk management issues will be viewed from a general perspective, a systems (treatment setting and payment) perspective, and a focused perspective by analyzing those areas of practice that pose the greatest liability risks for the family physician.

The Medical Malpractice Crisis

DIMENSIONS OF THE CRISIS

When engaged in a debate on professional liability, physicians find it disconcerting that not everyone agrees with the premise that there is a medical malpractice crisis. The Association of Trial Lawyers of America (ATLA) has argued that the "crisis" is really a malpractice **insurance** crisis, not a malpractice **litigation** crisis (Association of Trial Lawyers of America, 1984). ATLA also has contended that the crisis is the result of "a few bad doctors." Support for this contention is found in a 4-year study of Los Angeles County physicians in the 1970's in which 46 doctors (0.6 per cent of the 8000) were named in 10 per cent of the suits and were responsible for 30 per cent of all payments made (Phelps, 1977).

There is good evidence to suggest that there is more negligence committed than is ever recognized, litigated, or compensated. A frequently cited study is the Medical Insurance Feasibility Study (MIFS) conducted in 1974 by the California Medical Association and California Hospital Association. The MIFS involved the review of 20,864 California hospital admissions in 1974. That study found that 4.65 per cent of admissions involved potentially compensable events (PCEs). A PCE was defined as a disability caused by health care management. The authors concluded that only 0.79 per cent of all hospital admissions represented PCEs that were accompanied by evidence sufficient to establish claims of legal liability (i.e., negligence), as there were many PCEs that were felt to be nonpreventable. Nevertheless, these 0.79 per cent legally viable PCEs, when extrapolated to the 3,011,000 California hospital admissions in 1974, could have resulted in 23,000 lawsuits. It was estimated, however, that only 1 in 10 of the patients with a legally meritorious PCE ever filed a claim and only 1 in 25 ever received any compensation. The results of this landmark study are used to support the contention that there is more malpractice committed than is compensated and that a no-fault approach to medical negligence might be prohibitively more expensive than the current fault-based tort system.

Other appraisals of the number of negligently injured patients who pursue a malpractice action range from 1 in 6 (Schwartz and Komesar, 1978) to 1 in 15 (Pocincki et al., 1973). Trial attorneys are estimated to turn away approximately three out of four possible malpractice cases because the basis for liability was felt to be too difficult to prove or the award potential was too small (Somers, 1977).

Increased Frequency of Suits

The number of malpractice suits against physicians has been on the rise. In 1956, 1 out of 65 American doctors was sued; in 1983, about 1 out of 5 physicians insured by doctor-owned companies was named in a suit (American Medical Association, 1984). Since the mid-1970's, the number of claims filed each year has increased 10 to 20 per cent.

Increased Size of Awards

The largest malpractice award paid out in the U.S. through 1956 was $230,000, which equated to about $1 million in 1984 dollars when inflation was factored in. By 1984, there were several birth injury claims with ultimate payouts in excess of $100 million. Average paid losses increased 70 per cent from 1981 ($42,000) to 1983 ($72,000) (Reynolds et al., 1987). Over the past decade, the annual growth in the size of malpractice awards has averaged 20 to 30 per cent.

Increased Liability Insurance Premiums

Given the increasing frequency of suits and the increasing size of awards, it is not surprising that malpractice insurance premiums have continued their rapid rise. From 1982 to 1984, average premiums for physicians rose 41 per cent, from $5800 to $8400. Annual malpractice premiums now exceed $200,000 for some practitioners. A survey by the American Academy of Family Physicians in 1986 reported that family physicians paid an average premium of approximately $3000, or $6000 if obstetrics was included. Physicians paid an estimated $3.0 billion in premiums in 1984. However, some contend that these numbers are misleading in that physicians continue to spend only about 4 per cent of their gross revenues on liability insurance premiums, the same as for the past decade (Bovbjerg and Havighurst, 1985). Moreover, it is argued, while the physician is the one who initially shoulders the burden of the premium rise, it is ultimately the public that pays for the rise in the form of higher medical care costs.

Costs of Medical Malpractice

In addition to the premiums that doctors pay, malpractice generates other costs. For example, defensive medicine costs health care consumers an extra $15 billion per year. Defensive medicine practices are those changes in physician behavior (e.g., additional time spent with the patient, extra recordkeeping, more laboratory or diagnostic procedures) that are medically unwarranted but are intended to reduce the probability of a malpractice suit. Another malpractice cost is the loss of physician time spent in litigation activities (e.g., attorney meetings, depositions, at trial).

There are additional medical liability costs that are not as directly apparent. Many feel that physicians have become increasingly wary of their patients, viewing patients as potential plaintiffs who must be kept at arm's length. This wariness may not serve the patient's best interest in that it can hinder the sense of mutual commitment and trust that the therapeutic alliance demands.

The writings of psychiatrist Sara Charles, a leading authority on the response of physicians to the malpractice crisis, have alerted the public to another less obvious cost: As a result of being named in a malpractice suit, 96 per cent of physicians suffer physical or emotional symptoms, 62 per cent order extra tests for "protection," 42 per cent stop seeing certain types of patients, 28 per cent stop performing certain procedures, and 57 per cent feel their families suffer (Charles et al., 1984). Dr. Charles has concluded "that malpractice litigation, the chronic character of involvement with the legal process, and the resultant stress on both sued and nonsued physicians may in the long run not serve the public interest or the quality of medicine. It may diminish rather than enhance the integrity and availability of medical care"

(Charles et al., 1985). Other writers have noted that the threat or fear of a malpractice claim may be more stressful than an actual claim (Connelly, 1988).

The indirect malpractice costs that seem to most interest the public and lawmakers relate to the affordability and availability of medical care. The detrimental impact of malpractice issues on the cost of and access to medical care is most evident in obstetrics. The American College of Obstetricians and Gynecologists (ACOG) has calculated that obstetricians who completed training in 1986 will be named in an average of eight suits during their careers. In 1986, ACOG estimated that liability insurance costs added between $40 and $873 to the cost of each delivery, depending on the state. A 1985 survey of ACOG members revealed that one out of eight had recently quit obstetrics because of malpractice concerns; about one in four had decreased their level of high-risk obstetrics. A similar survey by the American Academy of Family Physicians in 1986 reported that nearly 25 per cent of family physicians had given up obstetrics because of malpractice fears. One study reports that 50 per cent of family physicians will discontinue obstetrics if their malpractice premiums rise to $12,000 (Rosenblatt and Wright, 1987). These changes in physician practices have an impact on access to obstetrical care: In 1986, 17 Alabama counties were without obstetric care, California obstetricians admitted to two thirds more cesarean deliveries because of a fear of suits, and islanders on Molokai, Hawaii, were forced to travel to Oahu for obstetric care (American College of Obstetricians and Gynecologists, 1986a).

HISTORY OF THE CRISIS

To clarify the reasons for the current medical malpractice system, a brief review of the history of malpractice is in order. Malpractice issues have shadowed physicians for millennia. Physicians were originally held to a standard of strict liability: If the results were less than desired, the physician was held liable. No matter that the physician put forward a best effort or that the patient was so ill that no physician could have effected a cure, the physician was liable and the penalties could be severe. The Code of Hammurabi, promulgated in Babylonia around 2000 B.C., mandated that if a physician treated a patient "and caused him to die, one shall cut off the doctor's hands" (Ghitelman, 1987). Roman law later distinguished between acts involving dolus (malice) and culpa (negligence).

The first malpractice case recorded in the English courts occurred in 1329. *Cross v. Guthrey*, 2 Root 90 (Conn., 1794), was the first medical liability claim heard by an American appeals court. By the mid-1800's, malpractice suits had become so frequent that many physicians were no longer performing surgery. The crisis abated during the Reconstruction Era but began to resurface at the turn of the century. State medical societies became very active in the defense of malpractice claims and had an enviable record of successful defenses during the early 1900's. After World War II, the number of suits began to rise sharply, and the trend upward continues today. The common thread appears to be that when times are more prosperous, more people can afford medical care, resulting in more potential exposures to iatrogenic injury and more malpractice litigation.

The watershed year of 1975 saw a number of insurance carriers refusing to underwrite doctors. Up until that time, medical malpractice was not even reported separately, with companies treating it as any other line of property and casualty insurance. The 1975 crisis stimulated a number of state legislatures to pass medical malpractice tort reform packages. In addition, physicians responded to the exit of the commercial carriers by forming doctor-owned professional liability companies, which now insure the majority of U.S. physicians. The tort reforms of 1975 provided only a temporary respite as malpractice claims became more frequent and costly by the early 1980's, triggering steep increases in malpractice insurance premiums.

ELEMENTS OF MALPRACTICE

Most malpractice suits against doctors involve claims of negligence, rather than breach of contract, battery, product liability, or other legal theories. For defendant physicians, malpractice litigation appears to be a dark abyss into which they are about to fall. To plaintiff attorneys, a malpractice suit seems an insurmountable mountain to be climbed. The plaintiff has the burden of proving, with evidence, the following four elements in order to prevail in a malpractice case: **duty, injury, negligence,** and **proximate cause**.

Duty

A physician has a duty to exercise reasonable care when undertaking the treatment of a patient. That duty is said to exist only when there is a doctor-patient relationship. A physician is not obliged to enter into a doctor-patient relationship with any person simply because that person desires to become that doctor's patient. Physicians, like everyone else, have the right to decide to whom they will provide professional services.

There are, however, limits placed on the doctor's right to decide. For example, a physician may not abandon an established patient nor may a physician refuse treatment to a patient who has reasonably relied on the doctor's apparent willingness to treat all comers (e.g., the emergency department physician in a general hospital that advertises its emergency services). When a doctor wishes to terminate an established relationship with a patient, he or she must make available alternative and equivalent medical coverage until the patient has had a reasonable opportunity to establish a new doctor-patient relationship (2 weeks is customarily considered reasonable). Similarly, when an on-duty emergency department physician seeks to avoid entering into a professional relationship with a particular patient, he or she is obliged to make arrangements for another physician to attend to that patient's emergency needs. When it is not reasonable for a patient to assume or rely on the services of a particular physician (e.g., when the doctor is a passerby at the scene of an accident on a roadway), the physician has no duty to offer assistance and the patient has no right to demand treatment. While codes of medical ethics may denounce the physician's driving past the accident victim, the law does not require that the doctor stop and help the victim.

The physician must use caution when offering medical advice. For example, a California doctor was successfully sued by a patient he had never met. The patient called the physician one evening and requested advice regarding the atypical chest pain that he was suffering. The doctor advised the patient that his symptoms could probably wait until the young man's personal physician became available the next morning. The patient was later found to be in the midst of an anterior wall myocardial infarction and suffered complications that he alleged were due to the falsely reassuring advice given to him over the telephone. Despite the fact that the doctor had never met nor sent a bill to the patient, the physician was adjudged negligent and assessed damages for failing to perform an adequate evaluation (i.e., a sufficient history and physical examination) before providing telephone advice that the patient *relied* on. The crucial issue was whether a reasonable patient was in a position to rely on the doctor's advice. If the patient was reasonable in relying on the doctor, a doctor-patient relationship was said to exist and the physician owed the patient a duty to provide reasonable care—to provide the same level of expertise and care that he would for any of his usual patients, regardless of whether a fee was charged or paid.

Injury

The plaintiff must prove an injury resulted from the doctor's negligence. Most plaintiffs have obvious injuries; frivolous claims for trivial injuries are uncommon. A federal study of over 73,000 closed claims reported that only 15.7 per cent of claimants had solely emotional or insignificant injuries—all other patients had disability or death (United States General Accounting Office, 1987).

Negligence

Doctors are not guarantors of perfect results. They are only required to perform at a level equivalent to that of a similar practitioner. The difficulty is over how to decide the adequacy of the physician's performance, given the inability of the jury to decide such issues. Aristotle recommended that physicians should be the ones to decide cases of malpractice (Amundson, 1977). In 15th century London, when guilds held authority over the various trades, physicians were obliged to present all serious cases to guild leaders within a few days after initiating treatment. If guild leaders felt that the physician's treatment was acceptable, the doctor was provided a solid defense against any malpractice claims (Walton, 1985). The concept that it must be other physicians who determine the appropriateness of a particular physician's treatment is crucial to an understanding of malpractice. A patient cannot successfully sue a doctor unless another physician, an expert witness, is willing to testify for the plaintiff that the defendant doctor failed to meet the standard of care.

The standard of care is "that degree of care and skill which is exercised by the average practitioner in the same or similiar circumstances" (*Shier v. Freedman*, 58 Wis.2d 269, 206 N.W.2d 166, 1973). It is important to note that the physician is expected to perform at a level similar to that of the *average*, not *best*, practitioner. Physician-experts and juries are often confused by this point and attempt to impose the highest standard of care. Early on, physicians were held to the standard of care that was exhibited in their own communities. However, as professional isolation became less of a problem, physicians were increasingly held to a specialty or national, rather than local, standard of care. One particularly vexing problem for family physicians is that the physician-experts testifying against them may be of a different specialty (e.g., an orthopedist testifying against a family physician's management of a Colles' fracture). While some will argue that only a family physician can testify against another family physician, others will contend that any physician with experience managing the condition in question should be able to testify as to the standard of care. Finally, there have been cases where the court has imposed its own standard of care, believing the profession's standard to be inadequate. "Custom is relevant in determining the standard of care because it illustrates what is feasible, it suggests a body of knowledge of which the defendant should be aware and it warns of the possibility of far-reaching consequences if a higher standard is required. . . . But custom should never be conclusive." (*Darling v. Charleston Community Memorial Hospital*, 33 Ill.2d 326, 211 N.W.2d 253, 1965).

Proximate Cause

The final element that the plaintiff must prove is that the negligent performance of the physician was the proximate cause of the patient's injury. The plaintiff must first show that the doctor's negligence was the cause in fact of the alleged injury. Two formulas can be used to demonstrate cause in fact: "but for"—the injury would not have occurred but for the negligence; or "substantial factor"—when several possible causes exist (e.g., the patient failed to keep the appointment and the doctor misread the x-ray), the doctor's error was a substantial factor in the resultant injury. Once cause in fact has been proven, the plaintiff must prove that the defendant's mistake was so closely connected in time and space and of such significance that legal liability should be imposed (i.e., proximate cause).

For example, if a surgeon amputates the wrong limb, the patient would be able to show that the injury (the amputation) would not have occurred but for the doctor's mistake and that the error was of such significance that liability should be imposed. Proximate cause becomes a more elusive concept, however, when the patient's original prognosis was poor. As an example, a smoker presents with an abnormal chest x-ray and hip pain that 2 months later are diagnosed as metastatic bronchogenic carcinoma. The physician's failure to diagnose the cancer for 2 months could be said to have reduced the patient's chance for survival, but the chance for survival was poor even at the first visit. Traditionally, the patient could not prevail on the causation question unless the prenegligence odds for survival were more likely than not (i.e., greater than 50 per cent probability). In the bronchogenic carcinoma example, the patient's chance for survival was less than 50 per cent, even at the first visit. Therefore, under traditional doctrine, the doctor would not be held liable for failure to diagnose the cancer at the first visit. However, some jurisdictions have begun to recognize that no matter how poor the patient's chances of survival were at the first visit, they were reduced by some amount because of the doctor's delayed diagnosis. This "loss of a chance" doctrine further complicates the causation question (Shoenberger, 1985). The proof of causation usually requires expert testimony. There are certain acts, however, whereby the negligence and causation are so obvious that a lay jury is deemed able to make that determination (e.g., a hemostat unintentionally left behind in the abdomen). In such cases, the doctrine of res ipsa loquitur ("the thing speaks for itself") is invoked, and no expert testimony is required. The burden of proof then shifts to the defendant to show mitigating circumstances in order to avoid liability.

POSSIBLE SOLUTIONS TO THE CRISIS

It is not surprising, given the complexity of medical malpractice, that there are no simple solutions. Each malpractice crisis has stimulated change which temporized events until the next crisis arose. The better physicians do, the better patients expect them to do. A smarter defense bar is matched by a more shrewd plaintiffs' bar. Tort reforms are diluted by constitutional challenges, mercurial legislatures, sympathetic juries, and judges persuaded by new theories of legal liability. Advances in medical science empower physicians to do more, exposing patients to greater risks of iatrogenesis, and to do better, inspiring patients to expect better. The multifactorial nature of medical malpractice demands a multifaceted approach.

Public Education

Rising and unrealistic patient expectations engender patient dissatisfaction. All members of society (physicians, media, public) share a responsibility to equilibrate patients' hopes with medicine's realities.

Improved Legal Defense

Doctors must actively participate in their own defense. There are several excellent references that guide the defendant-doctor through the litigation process (American College of Obstetricians and Gynecologists, 1986b, and Gass, 1984). Physicians must help their defense counsel to stay current with advances in medical knowledge. The defense bar needs to better update its members on innovative defenses and changing medical theory and practice.

Change the Dispute Resolution (Tort) System

Most appealing to physicians is the proposal to change the tort system. Many believe that the current litigation system is too destructive, expensive, inefficient, and unfair. For example, only 20 to 30 cents out of every malpractice premium dollar goes to the successful plaintiff-patient, the other 70 to 80 cents is consumed by administrative fees, court costs, expert witness fees, and defense and plaintiff attorney charges. The experience in California following passage of its Medical Injury Compensation Reform Act (MICRA) legislation in 1975 suggests that certain tort reforms will help to moderate premium increases—from 1975 to 1986, California went from one of the ten most expensive to one of the ten least expensive states for malpractice premiums. On average, states can expect that capping awards will decrease the severity of malpractice claims by 23 per cent; allowing the offset of collateral benefits will reduce claim frequency by 14 per cent and severity by 11 to 18 per cent; and trimming statutes of limitation by one year will cut claim frequency by 8 per cent (Danzon, 1986). Professor Danzon's studies, however, disprove several commonly held beliefs: Limits on attorney contingency fees, per capita income, and the number of attorneys per capita have no statistically significant effect on the frequency and severity of malpractice claims. The degree of urbanization and the number of doctors, not lawyers, are the most powerful predictors of malpractice litigation for an area. Tort system changes that intuitively seem prudent may not produce their desired results. Moreover, while tort reforms may provide some stabilization of premiums, their effect is temporary. As demonstrated over the past 60 years, increasing medical care utilization, improving technology with its additional risk for iatrogenesis, and rising patient expectations drive up malpractice premiums at a 20 per cent per annum rate, regardless of tort reform. Therefore, physicians should be clear in their understanding of the implications of tort reform proposals before advocating focused or wholesale changes (Abraham, 1988).

Improve the Quality of Medical Practice

It may seem self-evident, but the individual physician is best able to reduce the risk of malpractice litigation by practicing personable and high-quality medicine. Public education, improved legal defense, and tort reform are best accomplished by medical and other organizations. While the profession can enhance the quality of medical practice through the development of scientifically validated standards of care, it is the individual practitioner who must apply those standards. The best protection against a malpractice suit is a conscientious physician who practices reflective medicine, a style of practice that continuously recognizes medicine's ability to do harm, reflects on the patient's progress, and strives to keep the patient satisfied. For example, more than one third of general medicine admissions may suffer iatrogenic illnesses (Steel et al., 1981); the cost of surgical misadventures can also be high (Couch et al., 1981). High-quality medicine is reflective medicine; reflective medicine is the cornerstone of risk management.

Risk Management

GENERAL PERSPECTIVE

As traditionally defined, risk management is an administrative undertaking designed to protect the financial assets of an organization. As applied to the health care system, risk management is the systematic process of identifying, evaluating, and addressing potential and actual risks. The health care industry spends more on risk management, as a percentage of assets, than any other industry (Monagle, 1985). A more practical definition for the clinician is that risk management is a style of practice that attempts to prevent and control patient injuries, malpractice claims, and malpractice claim losses (Sanders, 1987). Quality assurance and risk management are often used interchangeably, although quality assurance more typically involves actual problems (rather than risks), and it is less concerned with financial or legal consequences. More than 75 years ago, Codman urged the profession to reflect on the quality of medical practice (Codman, 1914). Since that time, several methods for evaluating the process and outcome of medical care have been developed: incident reporting systems (where an incident is any happening, with or without injury, involving a patient mishap or a patient's serious expression of dissatisfaction), generic outcome screens (where certain outcomes, such as maternal deaths, are always reviewed), and clinical indicators (where indicators, such as postoperative infection rates, can be used to highlight potential problem areas). Others outside the profession have become increasingly interested in the quality of care provided, including third-party payors such as the federal government and private insurers.

There are at least three elements to consider when evaluating quality of care—the process that the physician used (e.g., tests ordered, procedures performed), the outcome achieved (e.g., cure, improvement, death), and the patient's satisfaction with the care provided. The first two elements are addressed by the remainder of this, or any other, medical textbook; the third element, along with other general issues, will be examined below. Every malpractice suit requires an unhappy patient. It is difficult, although not impossible, for patients to sue doctors whom they like. Physicians at the highest risk of suit have the following attributes: They are male, 40 to 45 years old, surgical specialists, uncomfortable with emotions, less likely to seek consultation, disparaging of others, and poor recordkeepers. Doctors who spend more time with their patients per visit have fewer claims (Adams and Zuckerman, 1984). Most patients willingly wait 15 minutes for the doctor. When the waiting time is expected to exceed 30 minutes, the patient should be informed of the reason for the delay and should be offered an opportunity to reschedule.

Rapport must go beyond the physician. All members of the office staff (receptionist, nurse, business manager, bill collector) are crucial to the creation and maintenance of good patient relationships. The patient's expectation of privacy and confidentiality must be respected by all members of the health care team. As a primary care specialist, the family physician should be available, or make arrangements to have a competent colleague available, to handle any after-hours emergencies. The telephone can be both helpful and harmful for the physician. It can build patient rapport and enhance physician availability. Making a follow-up phone call shortly after a patient's hospital discharge speaks volumes, returning calls in a prompt and reliable fashion fosters trust, and calling test results promotes patient awareness. Telephone conversations should be documented, and the physician should not hesitate to insist on seeing the patient if advice cannot be safely given without examining the patient (Roberts, 1988).

SYSTEMS PERSPECTIVE

The setting in which medical care is provided has an impact on malpractice risk. Four out of five malpractice suits arise out of hospital care; the remaining 20 per cent arise in the outpatient setting. Serious illness, high-risk procedures, multiple caregivers with the potential for miscommunication, loss of patient autonomy in a regimented routine—all of these factors increase the risk of an unhappy outcome for the hospitalized patient. The family physician is often able to enhance patient outcome and satisfaction through long-standing knowledge of the patient, coordination of care, and communication of the patient's progress to the family. In this way, the family physician can reduce the risk of an unsatisfactory result and subsequent litigation.

While committees and other review entities have long safeguarded hospital quality, the assessment of ambulatory care adequacy is a nascent science (Kelly and Mamlin, 1974). Patients perceive the doctor's office as an extension of the physician, from the decor to the currency of the waiting room periodicals to the friendliness of the staff. It is up to the physician to develop a system of practice in the office that promotes high quality care. Checklists (e.g., for health maintenance or for routine follow-up of common conditions) can serve as useful memory joggers. A requirement that no report (lab, x-ray, consultant) is filed in the chart without the doctor's initials can minimize the likelihood of an overlooked abnormality. Tickler files to remind staff to contact a patient for an important recheck at a particular time can militate against a delayed diagnosis. Computerization of the medical office holds great promise for relieving the physician and office staff of much of this tedium (McDonald, 1976). A review process should be developed to ascertain whether unplanned hospitalizations were the result of suboptimal outpatient management. Patient cancellation of or failure to keep an appointment should be documented; when several have not been kept, it would be wise to consider contacting the patient. The patient's progress should be monitored and diagnostic caution should be exercised—if a specific complaint has not been diagnosed after several visits, consultation may be a prudent next step.

Additional liability risks are posed by the evolving mechanisms of paying for health care. In *Wickline v. California* (No. B010156, 2nd Dist.), the plaintiff suffered from Leriche's syndrome and underwent vascular surgery on her leg, after prior approval by Medi-Cal. Postoperative complications caused the surgeon to request an additional 8 days of hospitalization, but Medi-Cal granted only 4 extra days. The patient was discharged within the 4 days and then suffered further complications at home, with the ultimate result being an above-knee amputation. The patient sued Medi-Cal (but not her doctors) for limiting her days of hospitalization. The Court of Appeals found in favor of Medi-Cal, but stated: ". . . the physician who complies without protest with the limitations imposed by a third-party payor, when his medical judgment dictates otherwise, cannot avoid his ultimate responsibility for his patient's care. He cannot point to the health care payor as the liability scapegoat when the consequences of his own determinative medical decisions go sour." How vigorously a physician must protest a third-party payor's utilization review decision is unclear. Before entering into any contractual arrangement where a physician's usual referral or hospitalization practices may be affected, the physician should have an attorney review the contract for potential liability risk (Robinson, 1988).

FOCUSED PERSPECTIVE

It is difficult to extract general recommendations from an analysis of malpractice cases because each case represents unique individuals and facts. Moreover, claims information is usually organized in a manner that best serves the business interests of the insurance carrier and not necessarily in a form that can help to educate physicians as to behaviors that affect liability. Finally, there is no clearinghouse that collects malpractice data, as that information is considered proprietary and therefore a "trade secret" for many carriers. It is nevertheless possible, by reviewing available claims data and case law, to describe certain conditions and practices that are most likely to result in a malpractice suit. This section will discuss the seven leading allegations made against family physicians, and it will highlight the management errors on which the issue of liability most commonly appears to turn.

Failure to Diagnose

About one third of cases against family physicians involve an allegation of failure to diagnose, or to timely diagnose, certain conditions. In over one half of the failure-to-diagnose cases, the condition in question is cancer, especially cancer of the breast, lung, colon, or testes. Every breast mass in a woman must be taken to diagnosis, either by following it to resolution (e.g., after the next menses) or by definitive studies (e.g., needle or open biopsy). Physicians should not be falsely reassured by negative mammogram studies, as mammography has a false negative rate of 20 per cent. Physicians should also be familiar with the various guidelines for screening for breast cancer and with the controversies that surround them (Roberts, 1986a). Pneumonia in an at-risk patient (smoker, asbestos worker, etc.) should be considered lung cancer until subsequent chest x-rays document clearing. Rectal bleeding in an adult over 40 years should not be attributed to hemorrhoids unless endoscopy or radiologic studies have ruled out bowel cancer. A testicular mass or swelling should not be written off as epididymitis unless careful follow-up demonstrates resolution or a tissue diagnosis is made. Failure to diagnose has also been a problem in myocardial infarction, where excessive reliance is placed on falsely negative electrocardiograms or cardiac enzymes; in pulmonary embolus, where an arterial blood gas can help sort out the adult with confusing chest pain or dyspnea; and in appendicitis, where abdominal pain must first be considered a surgical condition until proven otherwise. Physicians are not necessarily expected to diagnose all these conditions at the first visit; rather, they are expected to document a careful patient assessment and vigilant management plan with clearly understood patient instructions (Sanders, 1986).

Negligent Obstetrical Practices

Birth-related injuries represent the second most frequent and the most expensive claims against family physicians. While most suits allege negligence around the time of delivery, it is becoming increasingly clear that the birth process is much less important than prenatal factors in causing cerebral palsy, mental retardation, or neonatal seizures (Perkins, 1987). It is therefore vitally important that the pregnancy be accurately dated, that risk factors be appropriately screened and managed, that the labor be properly attended and followed, and that complications be recognized and treated or, as necessary, referred (Roberts, 1986b). Physicians must be familiar with published standards that may be used against them in court (American College of Obstetricians and Gynecologists, 1989). Despite such vigilance and optimal care, unhappy outcomes can result. When confronted by a neurologically impaired child with tremendous needs, it has been difficult for juries and judges to deny compensation, even where the physician was not at fault. Therefore, obstetrical claims have been put forward as an example of the inadequacies of the tort system, which depends on fault, and of the need for a new approach.

Negligent Management of Fractures/Trauma

Carpal navicular (scaphoid), cervical spine, and femoral head fractures have been troublesome. A "sprained wrist" should be immobilized in a thumb spica cast if there is anatomic snuff box tenderness and a question of a navicular fracture, regardless of the initial x-ray—repeat films 1 or 2 weeks later can finally rule out a fracture. Any significant head or neck trauma should be treated with spinal immobilization until x-rays exclude a cervical spine fracture. Certain femoral head fractures can remain elusive until subsequent films or tomography demonstrates their presence. Careful neurologic examination can ascertain the presence of subtle injury to nerve or tendon. Soft tissue injuries must be evaluated for the possibility of foreign bodies, infection, or compartment syndrome (Dunn, 1987). Injuries around the popliteal fossa warrant a careful examination of the distal circulation.

Failure to Obtain Timely Consultation

The broad scope of family practice leaves the family physician vulnerable to charges of practicing in another specialty area. Training, experience, and demonstrated competence, and not only a physician's specialty status, are the criteria used by the courts to determine whether a doctor was reasonable in taking on a patient with a certain condition. When inexperienced or uncomfortable with a particular problem, the prudent physician will obtain consultation from a local colleague, telephone another specialist, or transfer the patient to a referral center. Failure to do so, when combined with an untoward result, can increase the physician's liability risk.

Negligent Treatment with Drugs

Certain medications, particularly coumadin, psychoactive drugs, and cardiovascular medicines, frequently cause undesired or dangerous side effects. The use of these agents must be monitored (prothrombin times, medication checks, electrolytes), and the patient must be advised on signs of drug-related problems. Drug information handouts are readily obtained and can serve to document that the patient was apprised of potential drug toxicity. One other frequent medication error involves the prescribing of a compound to which the patient was allergic. Many times the prescription is given despite an overlooked notation in the record of the patient's allergy! Routinely asking each patient about drug allergies before each prescription can reduce the risk of such an oversight (Robertson, 1985).

Negligent Performance of a Procedure

It is difficult to prove that a procedure was negligently performed, given that it is usually years later when a malpractice case goes to trial and given that there will be little evidence to prove exactly what was done. Consequently, this is a less common allegation. However, physicians must be careful to undertake only those procedures that they are trained and competent to do.

Failure to Obtain Informed Consent

Many defense lawyers contend that plaintiffs allege failure to obtain informed consent when the case is otherwise weak. About 1 in 10 malpractice cases involves an informed consent issue. Physicians are especially troubled by this allegation, believing that they must do the impossible: inform patients of all possible risks. This is not necessarily the case (Curran, 1986). Informed consent is not a signed form drafted by a hospital lawyer. It is a relationship between doctor and patient that allows a discussion about the nature of the illness; the various treatment options and their respective outcomes, risks, and benefits; and the consequences of undertaking or forgoing the available treatments. Serious or frequent risks should be discussed. Informed consent is a dialogue, not a monologue, and the physician can strengthen the doctor-patient relationship by empathizing with the patient's magical thinking ("I wish this were a risk-free procedure") and by sharing the uncertainty that lies ahead (Gutheil et al., 1984).

THE FOUR Cs OF RISK MANAGEMENT

The only guarantee for avoiding a medical malpractice suit is to avoid medical practice. The best physicians have and will be named as defendants, sometimes correctly, sometimes not. The diligent and reflective practitioner can reduce the risks of malpractice by adhering to the four Cs of risk management: compassion, communication, competence, and charting.

Compassion. Physicians must show compassion toward their patients and also toward their colleagues and themselves. It is tempting, as one listens to a patient's woeful tale, to condemn a prior physician's "suboptimal care." Caution should be exercised before commenting on another caregiver, however, until all the facts have been reviewed (i.e., the prior medical record and not just the patient's version of the events). Hasty statements may unfairly impugn another and may expose the maker of the statements to a slander suit. Disagreements over patient care, or "jousting," should not be gratuitously aired in the medical record. Similarly, physicians should not draw guilt-stricken conclusions about their own performances until all the facts are in (Rasinski, 1982).

Communication. Besides informing patients and their families, doctors should endeavor to inform fellow physicians (e.g., sign-out rounds to covering colleagues), nurses, and other providers (e.g., treatment plan discussions). Nurses and allied health personnel can foster good doctor-patient rapport if they enjoy good rapport with and respect from the doctor. Nurses' notes should be read, and, where disagreements arise, they should be addressed. The physician should ask the nurse to read back telephone orders to minimize misinterpretation.

Competence. When confronted by an emergency, physicians should perform to the best of their abilities and, if necessary, consult with or transfer the patient to another physician as soon as it is feasible.

Charting. Physician sentiment regarding the medical record range from viewing it as a minor irritation to a major nemesis. Nevertheless, approximately one third of malpractice cases are lost because of an inadequate record. Long after memories have faded, the record can serve as a doctor's friend or foe when asked to serve as a witness to the physician's actions. The record must be legible, accurate, consistent, timely, objective, and complete as to significant issues. Entries should be dated and timed (some now note the time spent with patients even in the office setting). Changes to the record must be obvious, without any attempt at concealment. For example, an incorrect phrase should have a single line drawn through it, and the correction should be dated and initialed.

The practitioner has no absolute protection against a medical malpractice suit. Compassionate, competent, and conscientious physicians can diminish, but not eliminate, the risk of suit. Practicing reflective medicine can reduce patient injury and dissatisfaction, and it can represent the best prophylaxis against malpractice litigation. "An ounce of malpractice prevention is worth a ton of money" (Massanari, 1987).

References

Abraham, K. S.: Medical liability reform: a conceptual framework. J.A.M.A., *260*(1):68–72, 1988. *An excellent overview of tort reform and the various elements that must be considered.*

Adams, E. K., and Zuckerman, S.: Variation in the growth and incidence of medical malpractice claims. J. Health Polit. Policy Law, *9*(3):475–488, 1984.

American Academy of Family Physicians: The Family Physician and Obstetrics: A Professional Liability Study. Kansas City, Mo, 1986.

American College of Obstetricians and Gynecologists: Malpractice at a Glance. ACOG, Washington, D.C., 1986a.

American College of Obstetricians and Gynecologists: Litigation Assistant: A Guide for the Defendant Physician. ACOG, Washington, D.C., 1986b. *A very readable monograph that helps the defendant doctor to better understand the preparation and conduct of a malpractice trial.*

American College of Obstetrician and Gynecologists: Standards for Obstetric-Gynecologic Services. 7th ed. ACOG, Washington, D.C., 1989.

American Medical Association Special Task Force on Professional Liability and Insurance: Reports 1, 2 & 3. A.M.A., Chicago, 1984 and 1985.

Amundson, R.: Liability in the physician in classical Greek legal theory and practice. J. Hist. Med., *32*:172–203, 1977.

Association of Trial Lawyers of America: Statement on the Subject of Medical Malpractice before the Committee on Labor and Human Resources, 98th Congress, 2nd Session, July 10, 1984.

Bovbjerg, R. R., and Havighurst, C. C.: Medical malpractice: an update for noncombatants. Business and Health, pp. 38–42, September 1985.

California Medical Association, California Hospital Association: Report on the Medical Insurance Feasibility Study. San Francisco, Sutter Publications, 1977. *Over 20,000 California hospital admissions were reviewed to assess the incidence of patient injury due to physician error.*

Charles, S. C., Wilbert, J. R., and Kennedy, E. C.: Physicians' self-reports of reactions to malpractice litigation. Am. J. Psychiatry, *141*(4):563–556, 1984. *A study of 154 Cook County physicians who had been sued, this article was the first to focus on the impact of malpractice litigation on physician well-being.*

Charles, S. C., Wilbert, J. R., and Franke, K. J.: Sued and nonsued physicians' self-reported reactions to malpractice litigation. Am. J. Psychiatry, *142*(4):437–440, 1985.

Codman, E. A.: The product of a hospital. Surg. Gynecol. Obstet., *18*:491–496, 1914.

Connelly, J. E.: Malpractice: living with the threat. Pharos, pp. 26–29, Summer 1988.

Couch, N. P., Tilney, N. L., Rayner, A. A., et al.: The high cost of low-frequency events: the anatomy and economics of surgical mishaps. N. Engl. J. Med., *304*(11):634–637, 1981.

Curran, W. J.: Informed consent in malpractice cases: a turn toward reality. N. Engl. J. Med., *314*(7):429–31, 1986.

Danzon, P. M.: The frequency and severity of medical malpractice claims: new evidence. Law Contemp. Prob., *49*(2):59–84, 1986. *This scholarly article, by an economist, evaluates the impact that various factors have on medical malpractice claims.*

Dunn, J. D.: Risk management in emergency medicine. Emerg. Med. Clin. North Am., *5*(1):51–69, 1987.

Gass, H. H.: A Guide for the Defendant Doctor. Physician Guide, Southfield, MI, 1984.

Ghitelman, D.: The natural history of malpractice. MD, pp. 59–

81, April 1987. *An entertaining and informative review of the history of medical malpractice litigation over the past 4000 years.*

Gutheil, T. G., Bursztajn, H., and Brodsky, A.: Malpractice prevention through the sharing of uncertainty. N. Engl. J. Med., *311*(1):49–51, 1984. *This article analyzes the patient's perspective on medical decision-making and offers a fresh approach to the doctrine of informed consent and doctor-patient relationships.*

Harvey, L. K.: American Medical Association Survey of Physician and Public Opinion on Health Care Issues, A.M.A., Chicago, 1986 and 1988.

Kelly, C. R., and Mamlin, J. J.: Ambulatory medical care quality-determination by diagnostic outcome. J.A.M.A., *227*(10): 1155–1157, 1974.

Massanari, M.: Risk management: an epidemiologic approach. Infect. Control, *8*(1):3–6, 1987.

McDonald, C. J.: Protocol-based computer reminders, the quality of care and the nonperfectability of man. N. Engl. J. Med., *295*(24):1351–1355, 1976.

Monagle, J. F.: Risk Management: A Guide for Health Care Professionals. Aspen, Rockville, MD, 1985. *A comprehensive introduction to the science of risk management as applied to the health care industry.*

Perkins, R. P.: Perspectives on perinatal brain damage. Obstet. Gynecol., *69*(5):807–819, 1987. *A good review of recent studies on birth-related brain damage. The author concludes that the cause for neurologic deficit in neonates is prenatal rather than perinatal.*

Phelps, C. E.: Experience Rating in Medical Malpractice Insurance. Rand Corp., Santa Monica, CA, 1977.

Pocincki, L. S., Dogger, S. J., and Schwartz, B. P.: The incidence of iatrogenic injuries. Appendix, Report of the Secretary's Commission on Medical Malpractice (DHEW Pub. No. [OS] 73-89). U.S. Government Printing Office, Washington, D.C., 1973.

Rasinski, D.: Risk Management in Practice. American Society of Internal Medicine (Pub. No. 353R4M), Washington, D.C., 1982. *A succinct discussion of the nine Rs of malpractice prevention.*

Reynolds, J. A. (Ed.): Malpractice. Med. Econ., pp. 38–41, April 18, 1988.

Reynolds, R. A., Rizzo, J. A., and Gonzalez, M. L.: The cost of medical professional liability. J.A.M.A. *257*(20):2776–2781, 1987.

Robinson, R.: A primer on how to analyze contracts and avoid the traps. Consultant, *28*(7):74–75, July 1988. *An excellent introduction to the contractual pitfalls of HMOs and PPOs.*

Roberts, R. G.: The telephone. Wis. Med. J., pp. 9–10, 1988.

Roberts, R. G.: Breast cancer and malpractice: how to protect your patient and yourself. Fem. Pat., *11*:81–94, 1986a. *An in-depth review of the current controversies in the diagnosis and treatment of breast cancer, along with a discussion of legal strategies to reduce liability risk.*

Roberts, R. G.: Family Physicians and Obstetrical Malpractice. American Academy of Family Physicians, Kansas City, MO, 1986b. *Liability issues in and recommendations regarding obstetrical malpractice are detailed.*

Robertson, W. O.: Medical Malpractice: A Preventive Approach. Univ. of Washington, Seattle, 1985. *A ground-breaking treatise that demonstrates principles of medical malpractice law through the use of case studies.*

Rosenblatt, R. A., and Wright, C. L.: Rising malpractice premiums and obstetric practice patterns—the impact on family physicians in Washington state. West. J. Med., *146*:746–748, 1987.

Sanders, P. S.: Confronting professional liability: a roundtable discussion of medical risk management. Minn. Med., *70*:142–148, 1987.

Sanders, P. S.: Risk Management and the Family Physician. American Academy of Family Physicians, Kansas City, MO, 1986.

Schwartz, W. B., and Komesar, N. K.: Doctors, damages and deterrence—an economic view of medical malpractice. N. Engl. J. Med. *298*(23):1282–1289, 1978. *A provocative analysis of the strengths and failings of the current malpractice system.*

Shoenberger, A. E.: Medical malpractice injury—causation and valuation of the loss of a chance to survive. J. Leg. Med., *6*(1):51–83, 1985.

Somers, H. M.: The malpractice controversy and the quality of patient care. Mil. Mem. Fund Q., pp. 193–231, Spring 1977. *An insightful presentation on the sociology and politics of medical malpractice.*

Steel, K., Gertman, P. M., Crescenzi, C., et al.: Iatrogenic illness on a general medical service at a university hospital. N. Engl. J. Med., *304*(11):638–642, 1981.

United States Department of Health and Human Services: Report of the Task Force on Medical Liability and Malpractice. U.S DHHS, Washington, D.C., August 1987.

United States General Accounting Office. Medical Malpractice: Characteristics of Claims Closed in 1984. U.S. GAO (HRO-87-55). Washington, D.C., 1987. *This federal study analyzes 73,472 medical malpractice claims closed in 1984.*

Walton, M. T.: The advisory jury and malpractice in 15th century London: the case of William Forest. J. Hist. Med., *40*:478–482, 1985.

Part VI

Research in Family Medicine

81

Statistical Methods

Peter C. O'Brien
Marc A. Shampo
John W. Bachman

Advances in medicine depend on numeric data. Statistics deals with the collection, presentation, and interpretation of numeric data.

Family physicians trying to understand this field may find themselves confused. Its terms seem obscure, for example, standard deviation, standard error, or paired *t*, two-sample *t*, Student *t*. Moreover, the statistical section of a paper is often presented in small print, tempting readers to skip over it without questioning the judgment of the author. Finally, statistics may be misused and thus misleading.

This chapter provides a basic view of medical statistics to clarify the family physician's understanding of this important, pervasive subject. The chapter is divided into three sections: (1) presentation of numeric data; (2) interpretation of numeric data; and (3) working with a statistician on a research project.

Presentation of Numeric Data

Family physicians often need to review or present numeric data. This section discusses some methods. A well-chosen method may reveal relationships not readily understood from looking at a large set of numbers and convey to the reader a clear impression of the data.

RAW DATA

The Tally

For few data, a simple listing of numbers suffices. Each number is important. A good example of a tally is a list of the serum creatinine values of five patients.

GRAPHIC DISPLAYS

As one deals with large amounts of numbers, each number may become less important and trends or relationships become more important. Graphs provide a quick visual impression of data.

Scatter Diagram

For small sets of data, individual points may be plotted in a scatter diagram. Each point in the scatter diagram is determined by two values. For example, in Figure 81–1, each point represents a single patient, and its location is determined by the patient's age (on the horizontal scale) and IgE value (on the vertical scale).

The first step in preparing a scatter diagram is to determine the range for each variable so that the axes may be properly labeled. The graph should be approximately square, with no values plotted on the axes themselves. For a scatter diagram it is not necessary to start either axis at 0.

A scatter diagram should be one of the first steps

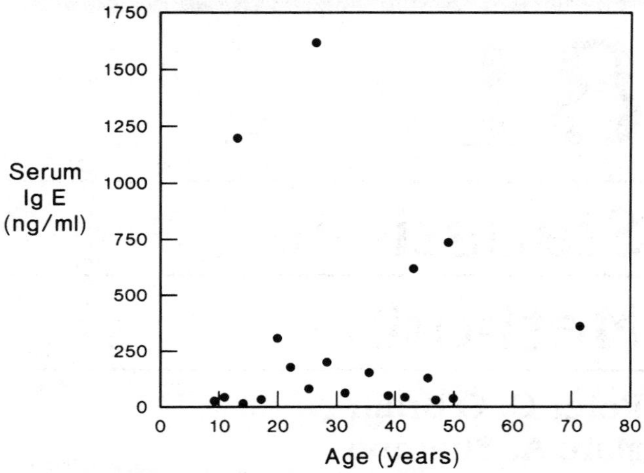

Figure 81–1. Scatter diagram showing fictitious data relating IgE value with age. (From O'Brien, P. C., and Shampo, M. A.: Statistics for clinicians. 3. Graphic displays—scatter diagrams. Mayo Clin. Proc. *56*:196, 1981. By permission of Mayo Foundation.)

in data analysis. Data features that otherwise might go undetected may become obvious on the scatter diagram.

Histogram

A very useful graph for the presentation of numeric data is the histogram, in which frequency is represented by area. For example, Figure 81–2 shows the distribution of serum triglyceride values from 96 6-year-old boys. By examining this graph, one readily sees that there are more values in the interval 41 to 50 mg. per dl. than in any other interval and that most of the values are less than 71 mg. per dl. To provide an understanding of histograms, we will work through the steps that produced Figure 81–2 (see Table 81–1).

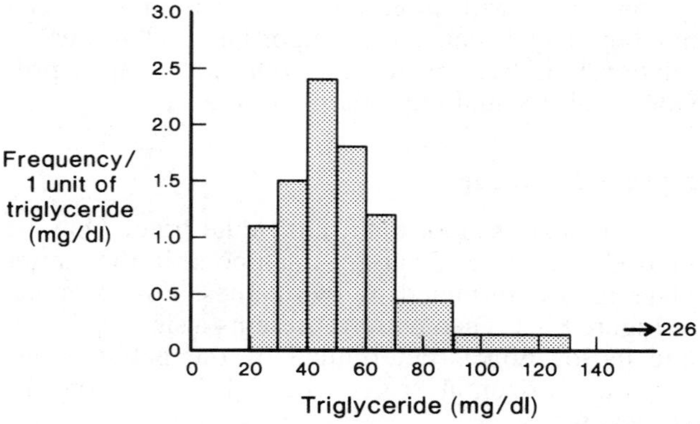

Figure 81–2. Histogram of triglyceride values from 96 6-year-old boys corresponding to data in Table 81–1. Abscissa (x-axis) has unequal intervals corresponding to column B in Table 81–1. Ordinate (y-axis) has values corresponding to column D in Table 81–1. (From O'Brien, P. C., and Shampo, M. A.: Statistics for clinicians. 2. Graphic displays—histograms, frequency polygons, and cumulative distribution polygons. Mayo Clin. Proc., *56*:126, 1981. By permission of Mayo Foundation.)

Step 1. List the observations in order of size, indicating the frequency with which each observation occurs.

Step 2. Form *class intervals*. Group the data items according to intervals of interest or in such a way as to ensure that each interval contains some minimal number of observations. The intervals can be unequal (columns A and B, Table 81–1).

When forming these class intervals—except in the case of very large data sets—one should keep in mind the twin objectives of accurate detail and reliable overall description of the distribution. These considerations are shown in Figure 81–3. Apparently, many of the peaks that appear with the use of 0.1 as the interval width are artifacts—notice that they disappear when an interval width of 0.3 is used. Conversely, with intervals of 1.0, virtually all detail is lost. However, no recommendation will be made for choosing between the two histograms in the middle (class intervals of 0.3 or 0.5) other than to point out that, as will often be the case, the informed judgment of the investigator will likely serve better than any rule of thumb.

Step 3. Determine *frequencies*. In column C of Table 81–1 are the frequencies, or the number of observations that fall within each interval (the number of subjects whose triglyceride values fall within each interval). If all of the intervals were of equal width, these frequencies would suffice to determine the relative heights of the bars to be plotted in the histogram. Since the widths of the intervals are unequal and the frequency is to be represented by area (width × height), one must solve: frequency = width × height.

Thus, $\text{height} = \dfrac{\text{frequency}}{\text{width}} = \text{frequency per}$ unit of measurement (frequency per 1 mg. per dl. of triglyceride), as recorded in column D.

Step 4. Plot the graph, using the widths and heights determined.

Frequency Polygon

To draw a frequency polygon, one simply connects the midpoints of the tops of successive bars of the histogram, as shown in Figure 81–4*A*.

Frequency polygons provide a useful method for comparing two data sets on the same graph. If the sets are not of the same size, their distributions first are made proportional, usually by conversion to a percentage basis. A frequency polygon comparison of triglyceride values from the 96 6-year-old boys in our previous example with the corresponding values from 64 6-year-old girls is shown in Figure 81–4*B*.

Cumulative Distribution Polygon

Another useful method for displaying the distribution of a data set is the cumulative distribution polygon (Fig. 81–5). This graph is constructed by

Table 81–1. DISTRIBUTION OF SERUM TRIGLYCERIDE CONCENTRATIONS IN 96 6-YEAR OLD BOYS*

Serum Triglycerides, mg./dl. *(A)*	Width of Interval *(B)*	Frequency *(C)*	Height [C/B] *(D)*	Cumulative Per Cent of Subjects *(E)*
21–30	10	11	1.1	11.4
31–40	10	15	1.5	27.0
41–50	10	24	2.4	52.0
51–60	10	18	1.8	70.8
61–70	10	12	1.2	83.3
71–90	20	9	0.45	92.7
91–130	40	6	0.15	99.0
226	1	1	1.0	100.0

*From O'Brien, P. C., and Shampo, M. A.: Statistics for clinicians. 2. Graphic displays—histograms, frequency polygons, and cumulative distribution polygons. Mayo Clin. Proc., *56*:126, 1981. By permission of Mayo Foundation.

connecting consecutive points from the cumulative distribution column E of Table 81–1 with straight-line segments. The result shows the percentage of observations less than any given value. Any desired percentile can be obtained from it as well. For example, Figure 81–5 indicates that among the set of 96 triglyceride observations in our familiar example, 80 mg. per dl. corresponds to the 88th percentile (88 per cent of the observations were less than 80 mg. per dl.).

Cumulative distribution polygons can be plotted together just as frequency polygons can, and this provides another way to compare sets of data.

Box-Plot

Occasionally, one wants to compare more than two groups. One approach is to plot the mean and standard deviation, as shown in Figure 81–6. Although this is the most common way of graphing this type of data, a relatively newer approach, which is becoming increasingly popular, is called the box-plot, as shown in Figure 81–7. This type of graph is especially informative because it displays the mean and median, the 25th and 75th percentiles, and the largest and smallest values (see data for obese fe-

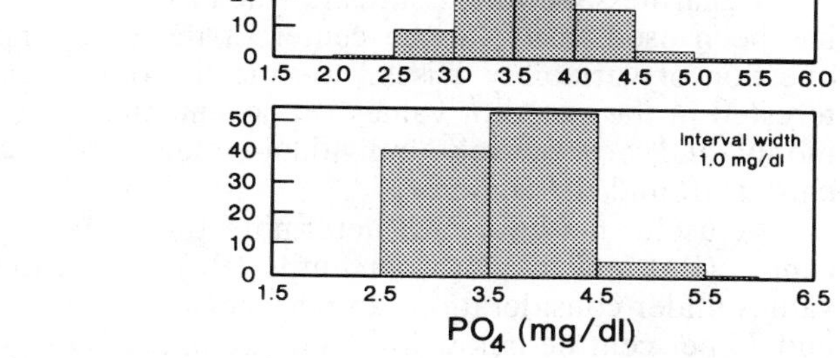

Figure 81–3. Histograms of PO_4 levels in 329 females plotted with interval width of 0.1, 0.3, 0.5, and 1.0 mg./dl. (From O'Brien, P. C., and Shampo, M. A.: Statistics for clinicians. 2. Graphic displays—histograms, frequency polygons, and cumulative distribution polygons. Mayo Clin. Proc. *56*:126, 1981. By permission of Mayo Foundation.)

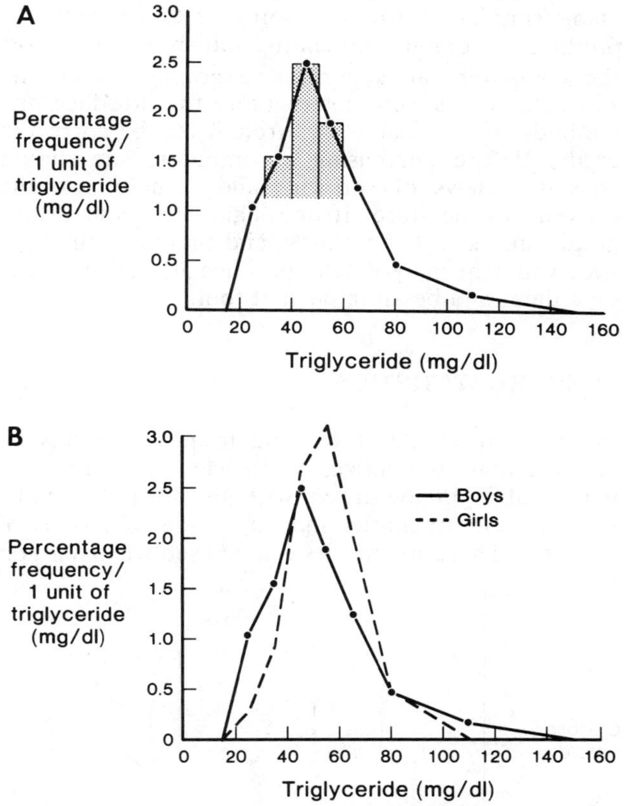

Figure 81–4. Frequency polygons representing serum triglyceride values. Frequencies are expressed as percentages within data sets. *A,* Data from 96 boys (from Fig. 81–2 and Table 81–1). *B,* Data from 96 boys and 64 girls. (From O'Brien, P. C. and Shampo, M. A.: Statistics for clinicians. 2. Graphic displays—histograms, frequency polygons, and cumulative distribution polygons. Mayo Clin. Proc. *56*:126, 1981. By permission of Mayo Foundation.)

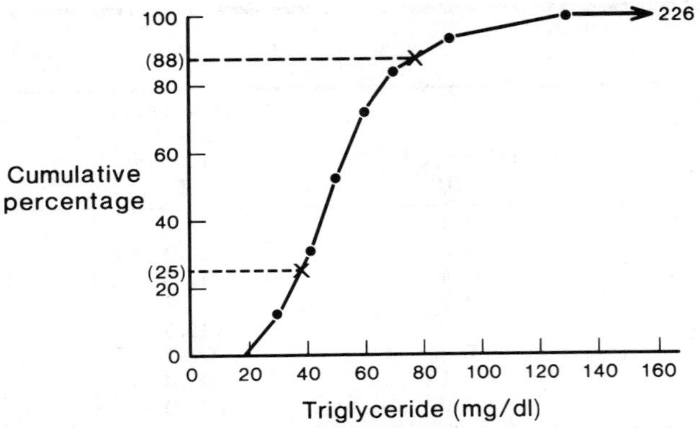

Figure 81–5. Cumulative distribution polygon of triglyceride values from 96 boys (from column E in Table 81–1). (From O'Brien, P. C., and Shampo, M. A.: Statistics for clinicians. 2. Graphic displays—histograms, frequency polygons, and cumulative distribution polygons. Mayo Clin. Proc. 56:126, 1981. By permission of Mayo Foundation.)

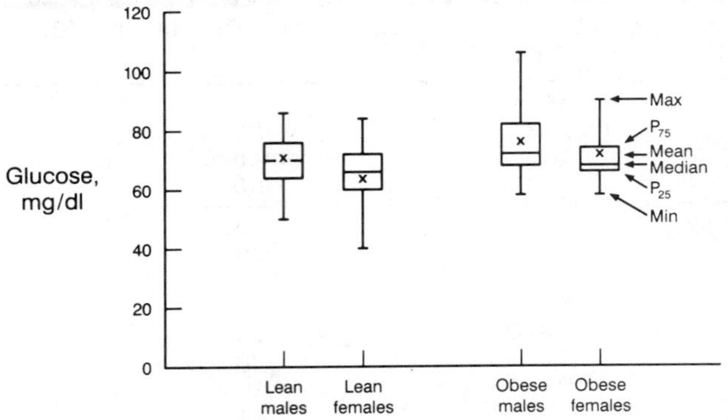

Figure 81–7. Box-plots showing the mean and median, the 25th and 75th percentiles, and the largest and smallest values for serum glucose in four groups of patients. (Both Fig. 81–6 and Fig. 81–7 were derived from the same data.)

males). Modifications of this graph are available to provide even more information.

Computer Assistance in Graphing

If one has a small computer, graphing can be made simpler. Currently, software is available to produce line graphs, bar charts, and area charts. Also the computer can superimpose graphs. Often the software comes with instructions to introduce the methods. If one makes an error, it can be corrected easily. Before purchasing a computer, one should consult reviews of software and actually use the software in the store. If one makes frequent use of graphs in his or her business and practice, this software will help analyze data, produce attractive charts, save time, and be an important tool.

SUMMARY STATISTICS

In the medical literature, one frequently reads an abstract that summarizes an article, presenting the main feature of the article without all of its details. In statistics, summaries may be made of groups of numbers. These summaries can be used when a graph is cumbersome and the data set too large for presentation of all the values in a table.

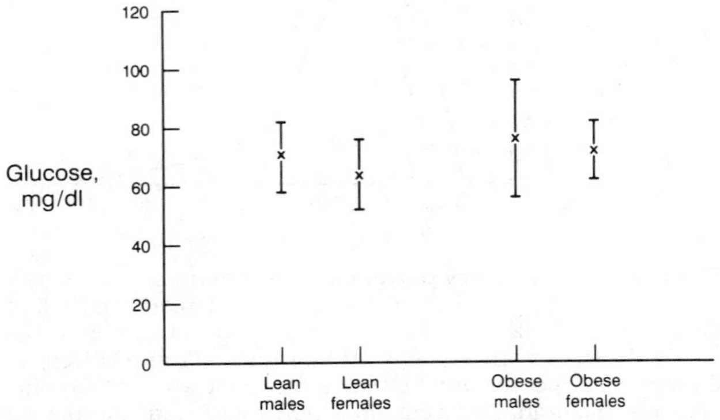

Figure 81–6. Graph of means and standard deviations, comparing serum glucose values in four groups of patients.

Typical Values

The two most important statistics for representing the typical value (that is, the center of a set of data) are the mean and the median.

Mean (Average Number). The mean is computed by summing the individual data points, then dividing this sum by the number of observations *(n)* in the data set. We illustrate with the following hypothetical data: −2, 0, 2, 4, 6 ($n = 5$). The mean ($\bar{x}$) is:

$$\frac{-2 + 0 + 2 + 4 + 6}{5} = \frac{10}{5} = 2.$$

Median (Middle Number). If n is odd, the median is defined as the middle value: half the other observations are equal to it or smaller and half are equal to it or larger. For the data set (−2, 0, 2, 4, 6), the median is 2. If n is even, one takes the midpoint between the two inner values: the median of (1, 5, 6, 7) is 5.5, and the median of (4, 10, 18, 36) is 14.

Variability

Regardless of which statistic (mean or median) has been used to locate the center of the data, the question of variability arises. Specifically, one is interested in the range of values that occur most commonly and how closely individual values tend to cluster around the center.

A useful method is to determine the 25th percentile (P_{25}) and the 75th percentile (P_{75}). Of all the values under consideration, 25 per cent lie below P_{25} and 75 per cent lie below P_{75}. The *interquartile range* extends from the value at P_{25} to the value at P_{75}, and this range includes 50 per cent of the data points. In some instances, an investigator may find other percentiles more appropriate.

In very small data sets, an informative statement

regarding variability is given by the *range*—the smallest value and the largest. However, a disadvantage of the range is that it depends heavily on the size of n: as more observations are included (as n becomes larger), the range usually gets larger (though it may remain unchanged). The range also may be greatly influenced by an occasional observation differing widely from the rest.

Another statistic that is commonly used to describe the variability in a set of data is the *standard deviation*. This usage of the standard deviation appears to derive largely from the mistaken belief that 95 per cent of the observations can be expected to lie within two standard deviations from the mean. The falsity of this proposition is easily demonstrated, for it is true only under special, infrequently occurring conditions. Thus, the appropriateness of the standard deviation for descriptive purposes is somewhat limited. However, it is useful in other contexts (relating to the sample mean), which will be discussed later. The computations required for calculating the standard deviation are illustrated below.

Consider the data set $-2, 0, +2, +4, +6$ ($n = 5$ and $\bar{x} = +2$).

Step 1. Square the deviation of each individual value from the mean.

Step 2. Sum the squared deviations.

Step 3. Divide the sum by $n - 1$. The result is called the *variance* (s^2).

Step 4. Obtain the standard deviation (s) by taking the square root of the variance ($\sqrt{s^2}$).

Example:

Step 1.

Original data	Deviation from mean of +2	Deviation squared
−2	4	16
0	2	4
+2	0	0
+4	2	4
+6	4	16

Step 2. Sum of squared deviations $= 40$

Step 3. ($n = 5$)

$$s^2 = \frac{\text{Sum of squared deviations}}{n - 1} = \frac{40}{4} = 10$$

Step 4. $s = \sqrt{10} = 3.16$.

Limitations of the mean and the standard deviation are illustrated in Figure 81–8, which shows several diverse distributions having the same mean and standard deviation. Let the clinician beware.

Outliers and Skewness

An evaluation of serum urea values in a series of seven patients showed values of 36, 38, 39, 41, 44, 46, and 103. The value of 103, clearly dissimilar to the other six observations, is termed an "outlier." When it is included, the mean is 49.6, which is larger

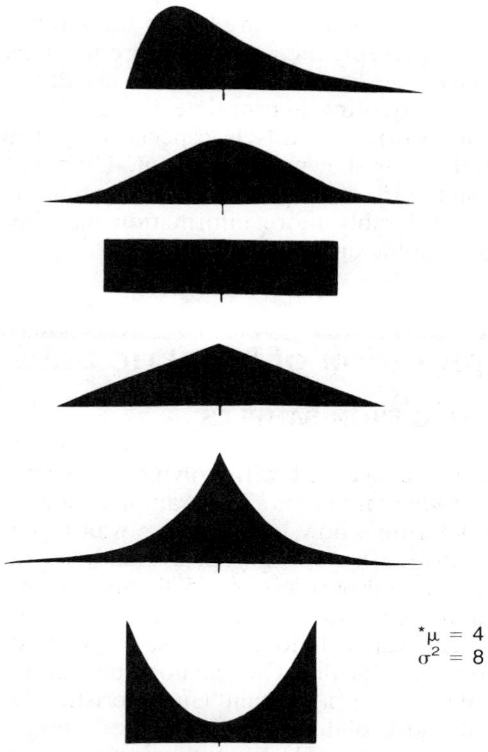

Figure 81–8. Six data sets with the same mean ($\bar{x}$ = 4) and the same standard deviation (s = 2.83). (From Elveback, L.: A discussion of some estimation problems encountered in establishing "normal values." *In* Gabrieli, E. R. (ed.): Clinically Oriented Documentation of Laboratory Data. New York, Academic Press, 1972, p. 117. By permission of the publisher.)

than six of the seven data points. The standard deviation, 23.8, is more than twice the range of the remaining six points when the outlier is omitted. Clearly, in this instance, the mean and standard deviation do not provide an accurate description of the set of data. In this case, the data would be described more accurately by a statement that the median value is 41, six values range from 36 to 46, and one value is 103.

As an example of skewness, consider seven measurements of serum triglycerides: 90, 93, 97, 103, 111, 126, 153 mg. per dl. The mean and standard deviation are 110.4 and 22.4, respectively. Note that the span from the smallest value to the median is only 13 units, 90 to 103, while the span from the median to the largest value is 50 units, 103 to 153. (When the values are arranged in order of increasing size and those greater than the median are more spread out than those less than the median, we say the data are skewed to the right, as appears in Figure 81–8, *top*. This is a common occurrence, particularly with data that cannot be negative, such as the usual laboratory measurements. Less frequently, one encounters data that are skewed to the left.) Again the mean and standard deviation fail to represent accurately the typical values and dispersion. The median (103) and range (90 to 153) would convey this information better.

Generally, when data are highly skewed or when outliers are present, the center is more meaningfully measured by the median. Variability usually is best described by quoting appropriate percentiles or the range (or both), and this is especially appropriate when outliers or skewness is present. Ultimately, of course, summary descriptive statistics remain a summary. Considerably more information may be conveyed by graphic displays.

Interpretation of Numeric Data

ESTIMATING FROM SAMPLES

Often when concerned with solving problems, one deals with *many* numbers. For example, suppose you wish to determine how long patients wait to be seen in your offices. In starting your evaluation, you find that you and your partners see 2500 patients a month. It would be a monumental task to measure how long each patient waited before being seen. Most studies have a similar difficulty. One cannot study all patients with a disease or a certain characteristic. One is forced, because of limitations of time, energy, and cost, to select a sample from the larger group, for example, 100 patients visiting your practice. By studying such samples, one hopes to obtain insight into the larger population, that is, the 2500 patients who visit the offices of your group each month.

Consequently, one must consider the sample very carefully. Does the sample of patients that you select represent the patients in your practice? From that sample, can you make reliable inferences about the patients in your practice?

How does one obtain a representative sample? Ideally, a sample should be selected randomly (although this ideal is seldom possible in medical research, and equivalence to a random sample is often all that can be hoped for). In the example involving waiting time, 100 consecutive patients may not be representative. Waiting times on Monday may be longer than waiting times on Wednesday because of increased rechecks from the previous weekend. A random selection from the population should eliminate any bias in your study.

Suppose you obtained a random sample of 100 patients and found that the mean waiting time was 20 minutes, the standard deviation was 5 minutes, and the range was 2 to 35 minutes. This gives you a fair idea of what is happening in your practice. Of course, if you studied the entire population (all 2500 patients), there probably would be some differences. Your intuition tells you that such differences would not be great. A statistic called the *standard error of the mean* ($SE_{\bar{x}}$) can help you determine how closely you can expect the sample estimate to approximate the true (population) value.

One of the major determinants of the standard error is the sample size. Again using our example, how confident would you be in generalizing if your data were obtained from only five patients? Or if your sample amounted to 25, 100, or 200 patients? As the numbers in the sample increase, one should feel more confident about inferences concerning the population. And since the standard error measures the reliability of a sample mean, one would expect the standard error to decrease as the sample size increases. This it does, because the standard error is determined by dividing the standard deviation *(s)* by the square root of the sample size *(n)*. In our example concerned with waiting time, where n was 100 and the standard deviation 5,

$$SE_{\bar{x}} = \frac{s}{\sqrt{n}} = \frac{5}{\sqrt{100}} = \frac{5}{10} = 0.5$$

Having the standard error, one can calculate the *95 per cent confidence interval (95% CI)*. For samples comprising 60 or more items, without skewness or outliers, this is done with the formula:

$$95\%\ CI = \bar{x} \pm 2 \cdot SE_{\bar{x}}$$

In our example, where the mean waiting time was 20 minutes and the standard error of the mean 0.5,

$$\begin{aligned} 95\%\ CI &= 20 \pm 2 \cdot 0.5 \\ &= 20 \pm 1 \\ &= 19 \text{ to } 21 \text{ minutes} \end{aligned}$$

The definition of 95 per cent confidence interval is frequently abused. The tendency is to say that 95 per cent of the time the value in the population lies between the calculated limits. In our example, one might say 95 per cent of the time the population mean is between 19 and 21 minutes. This is totally false. Our population mean either is present in the interval or not. The correct statement is that the method used to calculate the interval works 95 per cent of the time (in providing limits that bracket the population mean). Thus, the range between 19 and 21 minutes has been determined with a method that produces an interval which includes the mean waiting period 95 times out of 100. Although it is possible that the interval 19 to 21 minutes may not contain the true mean for the population of 2500 patients, it has been constructed by a method that works with 95 per cent of samples like ours (same n, drawn similarly from the population).

COMPARING DATA

Student t *Test*

Progress in medicine depends on experimentation. By taking a sample, one obtains an idea of how things are. By changing the environment (experimenting), one may try to change the outcome. How can one assess whether the change makes a difference? The Student *t* test provides information that helps in this decision.

Paired *t* Test. This technique is used with paired observations. The study design begins with observations from a sample. The experimental changes are applied and then the same group of subjects is restudied. Graphically, this is demonstrated in Figure 81–9. The first question we address in the data analysis is: Do the experimental conditions have any effect on outcome?

To decide whether there is a "statistically significant difference" in the data (that is, a difference, however small, that would not occur by chance), one uses probability.

To test the null hypothesis (no difference), one should recognize that if a characteristic is measured and is remeasured later, there will be differences. Sometimes the observed difference may be large and misleading, even though no real difference exists. An example may be seen in gambling. A slot machine is adjusted to return $1.00 for every $1.20 inserted. Someone develops a "new technique" and wins a jackpot. As he repeats the technique, he encounters

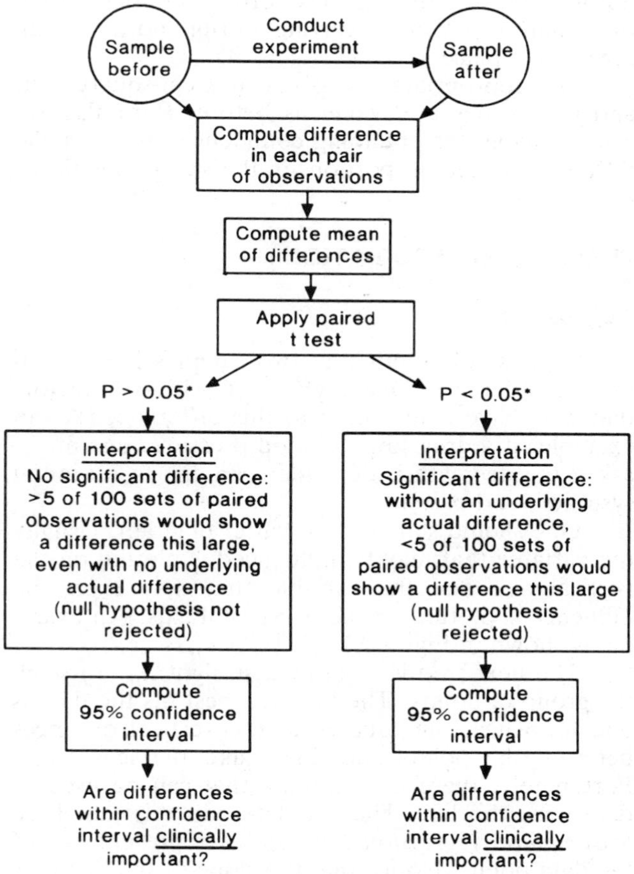

Figure 81–9. Schema of analysis for difference in paired data. Asterisks indicate that limits other than 0.05 could be used. (Modified from O'Brien, P. C., Shampo, M. A., and Bachman, J. W.: Statistics for family physicians. In Rakel, R. E. (ed.): Textbook of Family Practice. 3rd Ed. Philadelphia, WB Saunders Co., 1984, p. 295.)

losses; and eventually he finds that he is losing more than winning. For a while, however, he was misled by a large difference from normal.

By using appropriate statistical methods, one can determine the probability that a difference as large as the one observed in the sample will occur solely by chance (that is, in the absence of any real effect from the experimentally imposed condition). For example, when application of the Student *t* test to the paired data sets gives a probability of 0.10 ($P = 0.10$), one knows that the chance of obtaining this outcome if no real difference exists is only 10 per cent.

Besides wondering whether there is a real treatment effect, one would like to know how large it is likely to be. Once again, by using formulas and tables, the 95 per cent confidence limits of the difference can be found. For example, if a difference of 20 mm. Hg in blood pressure was calculated to have a 95% CI of 20 ± 10 mm. Hg, one could reasonably expect this interval to include the average reduction to be achieved with the drug in the population.

The size of the difference may be as crucial as its existence. For example, if a drug produces a "statistically significant" lowering of blood pressure, that difference is almost certainly real (the null hypothesis of no change is rejected), and yet it may be too small to have clinical importance. (In medical literature, the term "significant" should be reserved for the type of statistical significance described here.) It is essential to remember that a difference may be statistically significant but not important.

Two-Sample *t* Test. In studies that may be affected by unintentional biases—psychologic influences, for example, in tests of antihypertensive drugs—definitive evaluation requires data from two samples: *experimental* and *control.*

The *control sample* consists of patients who are like the others, but they are given only a *placebo,* that is, a preparation that resembles the experimental drug in all outward respects but has no biologic capability of affecting blood pressure. The result obtained in the experimental group will be compared with that obtained in the control group.

Notice that although both samples have been obtained from the same population, they are distinct and independent of each other. Also, we are dealing with the mean and standard deviation of each sample: There is no matching of individual observations from one sample with individual observations in the other sample (Fig. 81–10). By logic similar to that applied with the paired *t* test (but different formulas and tables), one can again obtain a *P* value, indicating the probability of obtaining a difference as large as we observed in our study if in fact there is no treatment effect. As before, the *P* value provides a basis for deciding whether or not to reject the null hypothesis of no difference. Confidence intervals may also be constructed to measure the magnitude of any effect.

Limitations of *t* Tests. A family physician does

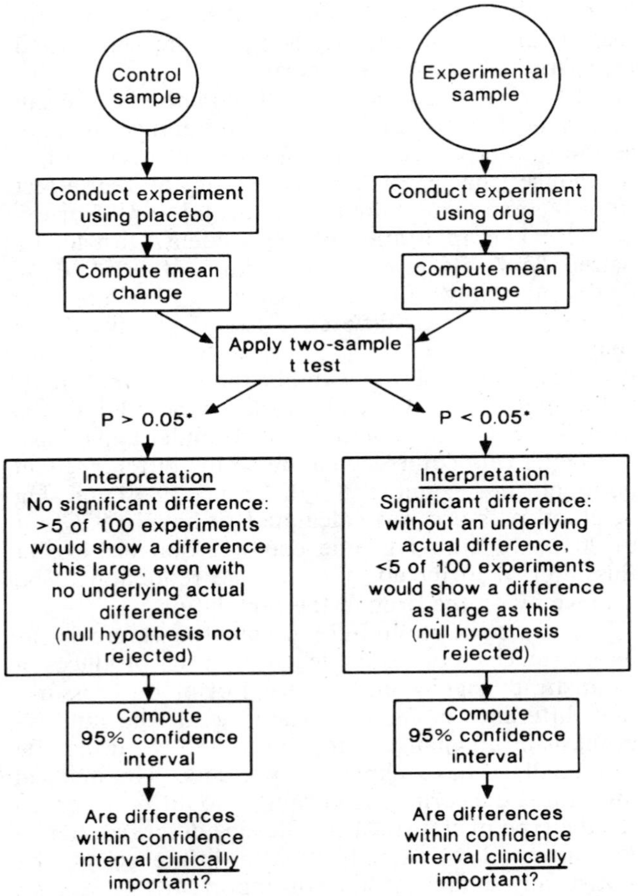

Figure 81–10. Schema of analysis for difference between two independent samples. Asterisks indicate that limits other than 0.05 could be used. (Modified from O'Brien, P. C., Shampo, M. A., and Bachman, J. W.: Statistics for family physicians. *In* Rakel, R. E. (ed.): Textbook of Family Practice. 3rd Ed. Philadelphia, WB Saunders Co., 1984, p. 295.)

not need to know how *t* tests are done. What he or she needs to know is that they are based on probability and sampling.

First, in reviewing study results, the physician should ask, Was the sample similar to the patients in his or her own practice? Is the *P* value small enough to be convincing? Regardless of statistical significance, is the potential difference large enough to be of interest? The answers to these questions will depend on clinical considerations.

As an example, if an antihypertensive drug has toxic effects, you may want to be assured about the magnitude of the reduction. How large is the average reduction and what percentage of patients achieve a clinically important reduction? Remember, your ultimate concern will be clinical significance, not statistical significance. Do not be misled to think that statistics can answer this question for you (although it can help). Ultimately, the decision is yours.

The second point is that the *t* test does not detect small differences with small samples as well as it does with large samples. The size of the 95 per cent confidence interval is helpful in evaluating this capability: the smaller the sample, the wider the interval.

Third, the *t* test depends on summary statistics such as the mean and is not applicable to samples with skewness or outliers.

The fourth point is the need for a well-designed and carefully followed study plan. To avoid any possibility of bias (intentional or unintentional) on the part of the patient, physician, or other study personnel, the choice of treatment (drug or placebo) should be determined randomly and in such a way that only the statistician or the drug manufacturer (or both) knows which patients have received which agent.

Chi-Square Test

The previous examples dealt with observations of variables that are called "continuous," because they have a continuum of values (blood pressures, IgE values). Different tests must be used when variables are discrete, or "dichotomous." Such variables are observed as yes-no or normal-abnormal. In this circumstance, interest centers on the *proportion* of normals and whether this proportion differs between the group of patients receiving a drug and the group receiving a placebo.

The appropriate test is called a chi-square test, and it provides a *P* value as before. Formulas are also available for obtaining confidence limits for the difference in the proportions in the two populations.

EVALUATING ASSOCIATIONS

Regression

Suppose one finds that two samples have a significant difference. One might want to look for factors that may have contributed to this difference. As an example, if a drug lowers blood pressure, one might ask if the decrease is dependent on age or on initial systolic blood pressure.

One should start with a scatter diagram. Usually the variable that may be influenced is plotted on the vertical axis and the variable that may exert the influence is plotted on the horizontal axis. An example is shown in Figure 81–11.

The next step is to draw a straight line through the group of points. The line that best fits the data is one for which the squares of the vertical distances between the points and line make the least sum. Fortunately, there is a formula that can be used to determine this line. The line determined is called the *least-squares regression line,* and it represents all of the data points. Notice that the slope of the line (the amount by which it rises or falls per unit change along the horizontal axis) measures the strength of the association, as does the closeness of the points to the regression line.

The third step involves the familiar question:

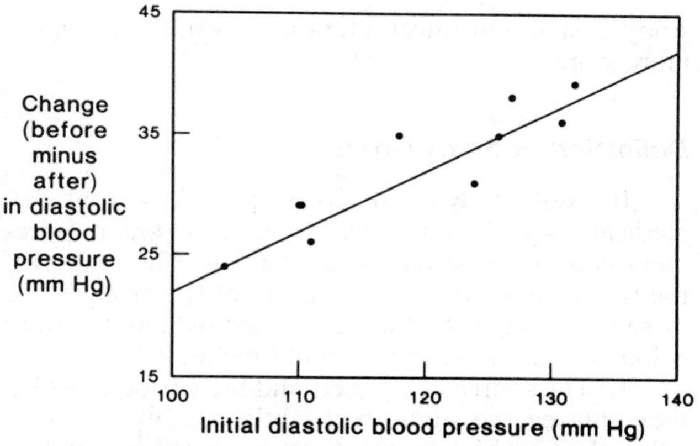

Figure 81–11. Scatter diagram (with regression line): initial diastolic blood pressure and change in diastolic pressure. (Modified from O'Brien, P. C., and Shampo, M. A.: Statistics for clinicians. 7. Regression. Mayo Clin. Proc. *56*:452, 1981.)

What is the probability of observing a slope as large as the one in our study if in fact no association exists? This probability (*P* value) can be computed and so can the 95 per cent confidence limits for the slope.

We have shown how the association between two variables may be quantified by fitting a straight line to the data. In doing so we have considered only the simplest of situations. In practice, other factors may require attention: for example, how to modify the analysis if the scatter diagram reveals outliers or skewness or associations that are nonlinear, or how to evaluate additional variables (such as sex or obesity).

Two other considerations regarding the regression line should be remembered. First, in graphing the regression line the steepness of the line depends on how the axes are scaled (whether large or small units are used). Second, extension of the regression line beyond the plotted data may give rise to absurd implications.

EVALUATING A NEW DIAGNOSTIC PROCEDURE

When a new medical procedure has been developed, such as computer-assisted scanning, it is necessary to evaluate the contribution to patient care that will result from its use. In this situation, the subjective opinion of the physician responsible for patient care will be essential, and perhaps it will determine the ultimate decision as to the procedure's usefulness. However, it is desirable also to perform studies that will provide objective, quantitative data. Three aspects that should be considered are (1) the reliability of the procedure; (2) its accuracy; and (3) how it compares with conventional methods.

Reliability

The reliability of a method is its ability to provide the same answer in repeated observations of the same phenomenon.

A simple example would be a new method of hitting a target in archery. One would call the method reliable if the arrows clustered in the same area. To determine the reliability of a method, several techniques may be used, each evaluating a different aspect of reliability: (1) have different people or institutions apply the method and find if their results are consistent and (2) have the same person or institution repeat the observations and find if results are consistent.

Accuracy

The accuracy of a procedure is measured by its ability to give the right answer. In archery, it would be how often the archer hits a bull's-eye. In medicine, an example would be how often results from a new method to identify urinary tract infection agree with results obtained by the method accepted as definitive—urine culture. Often accuracy is expressed by the error rates, that is, the proportion of false-positive results and the proportion of false-negative results. A test result is false positive if it is positive but the actual status of the patient is negative (patient does not have the disease). Similarly, a false negative means that the test result is negative but the patient's actual status is positive (patient has the disease). The possibilities for classification of the study results are indicated in Table 81–2. With the notation in Table 81–2, the proportions of false positives and false negatives are b/(b + d) and c/(a + c), respectively.

A parallel set of terms is also often used in describing the accuracy of a test. Rather than focusing on the error rates, it focuses on the proportion of patients whose conditions are classified correctly. Thus, the *sensitivity* of a test is defined as the proportion of patients with the disease who are correctly classified by the test. Similarly, the *specificity* of a test is defined as the proportion of patients without the disease who are correctly classified by the test as being disease-free. In terms of the notation in Table 81–2,

$$\text{sensitivity} = a/(a + c)$$
$$\text{specificity} = d/(b + d).$$

Another pair of useful numbers that can be derived

Table 81–2. ACCURACY OF TEST RESULTS

	Disease Status		
Test Result	***Positive (patient has disease)***	***Negative (patient does not have disease)***	***Total***
Positive	a	b	a + b
Negative	c	d	c + d
Total	a + c	b + d	a + b + c + d

The two-by-two table clarifies relationships between test characteristics (sensitivity and specificity) and predictive values of positive and negative test results.

from Table 81–2 is the positive and negative predictive values, which give the probability that the patient has the disease when the test is positive or does not have the disease when the test is negative. These probabilities are a/(a + b) and d/(c + d), respectively.

Comparative Studies

The usual objective of a comparative study is to compare the accuracy of the experimental method (for example, computed tomography) with the accuracy of one or more other methods (such as conventional roentgenography), which, although perhaps more accepted, are not regarded as definitive. An important first step is to define the patient group to be studied. It is essential in this type of study that eligibility for the study should not depend in any way on the outcome of either the experimental or the conventional method. For this reason, the patient's entry into the study should be determined before he or she is examined by either method. Once a patient is admitted to the study, examination by each method should be done without knowledge of the results of the competing method. Additional knowledge (certain clinical information, for example) should not be available with either method (unless such information is considered an integral part of that method).

For ascertaining the relative accuracy of the two methods, the true status of the patients must be known. For example, if method A indicates the presence of a tumor when method B does not, resolution of this difference may be obtained from subsequent surgery. In this situation, the willingness to do surgery should be the same when A is positive and B is negative as when A is negative and B is positive. If it is known beforehand that the rate of false positives for each method is near zero, this difficulty does not arise.

In the absence of a definitive diagnosis, the best that can be done is to measure *agreement* between methods A and B without attempting to measure relative accuracy.

Decision

After studies such as those described above (and perhaps others), the ultimate question, *Is this innovation a worthwhile improvement*? remains to be answered by physicians, who will consider also its safety, convenience, cost, and probably many more factors.

SURVIVORSHIP STUDIES

Although survivorship studies present some unique problems, which we will consider in detail, this example of a research study will also be useful to illustrate some important considerations involving study design and interpretation of results that apply more generally.

Definition of Study Group

In every study of survivorship, as in virtually all medical research on human subjects, the first requirement is to describe the group studied. The reader of the report must be told the nature of the group so he or she can judge whether his or her patient or group is like it. The description should include:

1. The source of subjects and the period in which they entered the study, with notice of any considerable selection bias (practice in a general hospital or a specialty clinic, and so forth).
2. The medical problem of interest: what it was and how its presence was determined.
3. The treatment, if any.
4. All exclusions of subjects from the study and the reasons for them.
5. Characteristics of the study group: their age and sex distributions and, if pertinent, their area of residence, occupation, economic status, race, and so on.
6. Complicating features (associated diseases and so forth) if it seems they may affect survival.

Data Collection and Accounting

Completeness of Follow-Up. The problem in follow-up is the practical difficulty of making it complete enough. Much effort and many stratagems may be justified, because a case "lost to follow-up" cannot be ignored and must be reported. No amount of sophisticated mathematical manipulation can overcome failure of follow-up in a sizable number of instances.

Initial Event. In survivorship studies, each case must have an initial event from whose date the period of observation is counted. This may be birth for congenital disease; but usually it is diagnosis, surgery, or beginning of treatment. Although the onset of disease might be very meaningful, dating of onset is often difficult.

Accounting of Follow-Up Period. Usually the initial event does not occur simultaneously in all cases, and consequently the lengths of follow-up are not equal at any given date. Thus it is necessary that survival rates be specific for a fixed interval of time after the initial event in each case (for example, 5-year survival). Simply providing the number of subjects alive at latest follow-up divided by the number in the study is useless, because the meaning of such a statistic depends on how long each patient is known to have survived, which typically varies considerably from case to case. The appropriate computations are often complex. However, an outline is presented by O'Brien and Shampo (1981) and a more detailed but nontechnical discussion is provided by Berkson and Gage (1950). Also, this is a relatively new area in statistics, and new methods of analysis are continually being developed.

Presentation of Results

Generally the most effective method for describing the survival experience of a group of patients is to graph survival rates against time, as shown in Figure 81–12.

To provide perspective on the outcome of an analysis, a comparison with normal survivorship may be shown. The appropriate norm is experience in a segment of the general population, adjusted (from published tables) to match the study group with respect to age, sex, and perhaps other features that seem pertinent. These rates will indicate the survivorship that would have been expected in the study group if it had been representative of the general population. In addition, expected 5-year or 10-year rates might be presented in the text.

Comment

The principal concern is to point out the need to take varying lengths of follow-up into account in studying survivorship.

Two other ideas remain for presentation here. First, interpretation of results of survivorship studies is often difficult. Because such studies generally are *observational* rather than experimental, questions arise regarding what has caused the differences that are found.

To illustrate: suppose that two different surgical techniques were used to treat patients having the same disease and that 10-year follow-up was obtained on all patients treated with each method. It would be tempting to attribute any difference in survivorship to the difference in surgical techniques. Such a conclusion might not be valid, however, because the disparity could be a result of other factors. For

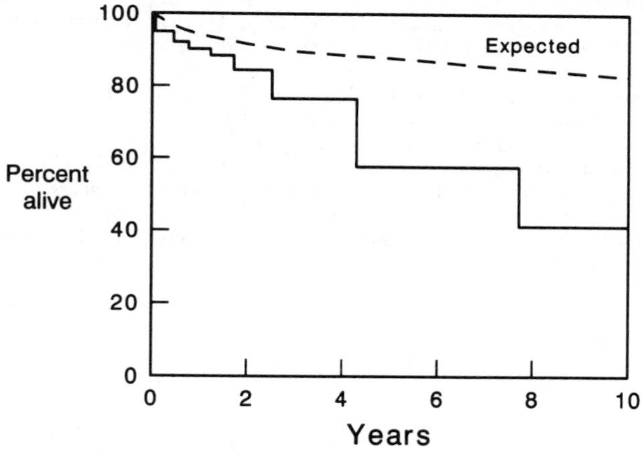

Figure 81–12. Survivorship (actuarial analysis): as observed in study group *(solid line)* and as derived from population segment similar in regard to age, sex, and date of birth *(broken line)*. (From O'Brien, P. C., and Shampo, M. A.: Statistics for clinicians. 11. Survivorship studies. Mayo Clin. Proc. *56*:709, 1981. By permission of Mayo Foundation.)

example, the two groups of patients may have been dissimilar with respect to factors that influence the choice of surgical technique (possibly severity of the illness or age of the patient). Unfortunately, sophisticated statistical algorithms are of only limited usefulness in attempts to distinguish effects due to the factor of interest (surgery) from effects due to other causes.

In order to establish the relative merits of the two surgical techniques, it would be best to design an experiment specifically with this purpose in mind. Ideally, patients would be assigned randomly to either method, enabling a statistician to make a valid probability statement in comparing the two procedures.

Notice that this was the approach in the *experimental* studies described previously. For example, the experimental study comparing two samples (control and experimental groups) was designed carefully, in advance of data collection, so that a direct comparison could be made of the reduction of blood pressure by each of the two drugs used. When a difference between drug effects is observed in a properly designed experimental study, one can make a valid probability statement regarding the hypothesis that it was caused entirely by other factors instead.

Thus, although an observational study is often considerably more convenient and less expensive than a carefully designed experiment, one must also consider the quality and interpretability of the results ultimately to be obtained.

A second important principle is that, for any study design, statistics can only establish an association and cannot define the cause and the effect. For example, statistics may establish an association between having a yellow-stained index finger and the occurrence of lung cancer. However, it is obvious that although the association is strong, "yellow finger" does not cause cancer. In this case, the observed association between yellow finger and lung cancer is merely an artifact resulting from the association between smoking and lung cancer.

Working with a Statistician on a Research Project

In a review of five medical journals, Altman (1980) found statistical errors or errors of omission in 44 to 72 per cent of the articles. In addition, 20 per cent of the statistical procedures were unidentified.

Although journals are increasingly using statisticians to help review articles, the family physician has a responsibility to be critical of articles and to keep an eye on letters to the editor.

If you choose to do research in family practice, the first step is to formulate clearly the question your study is intended to answer. The next step is to talk with a statistician. The statistician will assist you in designing the study (to ensure that the answers ob-

Table 81–3. STATISTICAL DISPLAY AND ANALYSIS*

Methods for Display of Data	
Graphs	***Summary Statistics***
Scatter diagram	Mean (average)
Histogram	Median (middle number)
Frequency polygon	Range
Cumulative distribution polygon	Percentile (interquartile range)
	Standard deviation
Survival curve	
Statistical Procedures	
Procedure	***Example of Use***
Paired *t* test	Before treatment vs. after
Two-sample *t* test	Placebo-treated vs. experimentally treated
Chi-square	Association between discrete variables: smoking (yes-no) vs. lung cancer (yes-no)
Regression	Association between two continuous variables: blood pressure and weight

*From O'Brien, P. C., Shampo, M. A., Bachman, J. W.: Statistics for family physicians. *In* Rakel, R. E. (Ed.): Textbook of Family Practice. 3rd ed. Philadelphia, W.B. Saunders Company, 1984, p. 295. By permission of the publisher.

tained are valid and that the sample size is sufficient to detect the effects that you are interested in), setting up data collection procedures, planning and implementing data analysis, interpreting and presenting the results, and preparing the manuscript.

As mentioned at the outset, the purpose of this chapter is to help you read the medical literature, recognize situations that require statistical expertise, and communicate effectively with a statistician when those situations arise. How does one go about locating a statistician?

Although there are a number of private consulting firms available, probably the simplest and most cost-effective strategy is to seek help from a large university. Most such institutions have a statistics department. A brief telephone call to the department chairman usually will suffice for referral to a statistician suitable for your needs. (Statisticians tend to specialize in different areas, much as physicians do.)

If you feel nervous as you approach your first meeting with the statistician, recognize this as a normal and quite common reaction. Remember that it is the statistician's responsibility to cut through the technical jargon and address your specific needs. You, on the other hand, should be prepared to explain those needs, remembering that the statistician lacks your medical background. Make sure you can state very specifically which questions your study is intended to answer, as this will be the starting point for the collaborative effort. From this point, the process should move quite naturally to considerations of study design, data collection, data analysis, and interpretation of results. Expect to meet with the statistician on a continuing basis as the study moves through these stages. If at any time the statistician's recommendations seem to violate "common sense," insist on a satisfactory, comprehensible explanation. The problem may well lie in the mathematical formulation rather than in your lack of mathematical sophistication.

A summary of some of the information discussed earlier in the chapter is presented in Table 81–3.

References

Altman, D. G.: Statistics and ethics in medical research: misuse of statistics is unethical. Br. Med. J., *281*:1182, 1980.

Berkson, J., and Gage, R. P.: Calculation of survival rates for cancer. Proc. Staff Meet. Mayo Clin., *25*:270, 1950. *A nontechnical discussion of the actuarial method.*

Boardman, T. J.: The future of statistical computing on desktop computers. Am. Stat., *36*:49, 1982.

Breslow, N. E., and Day, N. E.: Statistical Methods in Cancer Research. Vol. 1. The Analysis of Case-Control Studies. Lyon, International Agency for Research on Cancer, 1980.

Dixon, W. J., and Massey, F. J., Jr.: Introduction to Statistical Analysis. New York, McGraw-Hill, 1969.

Elveback, L. R.: How high is high? A proposed alternative to the normal range. Mayo Clin. Proc., *47*:93, 1972.

Elveback, L. R.: The population of healthy persons as a source of reference information. Hum. Pathol., *4*:9, 1973.

Fleiss, J. L.: Statistical Methods for Rates and Proportions. New York, John Wiley & Sons, 1973.

Kalbfleisch, J. D., and Prentice, R. L.: The Statistical Analysis of Failure Time Data. New York, John Wiley & Sons, 1980. *An extensive review of methods for studying survivorship data. The mathematics is more sophisticated.*

Kleinbaum, D. G., and Kupper, L. L.: Applied Regression Analysis and Other Multivariable Methods. North Scituate, Massachusetts, Duxbury Press, 1978.

Lehmann, E. L.: Nonparametrics: Statistical Methods Based on Ranks. San Francisco, Holden-Day, 1975. *A comprehensive review of statistical methods that avoid mathematical assumptions.*

Miller, R. G., Jr., Efron, B., Brown, B. W., Jr., et al.: Biostatistics Casebook. New York, John Wiley & Sons, 1980. *An excellent view of statistics as it is actually practiced.*

O'Brien, P. C., and Shampo, M. A.: Statistics for clinicians. Mayo Clin. Proc., *56*:45, 1981. *A 45-page collection of papers from which this chapter was derived.*

Ostle, B.: Statistics in Research. Ames, The Iowa State University Press, 1963.

82

Research Methodology

Richard L. Holloway
John C. Rogers

The clinician contemplating involvement in the research process has five primary considerations: (1) area of interest, (2) questions, (3) research thinking, (4) the research team, and (5) research techniques. Every researcher works within an area of interest and becomes knowledgeable about other scholars, appropriate journals, pertinent academic meetings or societies, the reputed centers of excellence, and the cutting edges in that area. Choosing one area of focus is one of the most difficult steps in the transition from generalist-clinician to clinician-researcher. Research questions are specific inquiries within the broader area of interest and must be even more narrowly focused than is often comfortable for the comprehensive care-oriented family physician.

In the transition to researcher, the clinician's thinking also must take on new dimensions. Differential diagnosis, rapid hypothesis testing, therapeutic trials, intuitive clinical judgment, and efficient problem-solving must be supplemented by detached inquiry, prolonged planning, repeated refinement, precise logic, and other thought processes not confined to allotted research time. Just as clinical work is often discussed socially with colleagues, research also becomes a social activity. Colleagues in the research enterprise are just as skilled and essential as the diverse members of the clinical care "team."

Research techniques often pose the most threatening domain to clinicians considering a "sampling" of research. The domain encompasses new and specialized knowledge that can appear threatening to professionals accustomed to being masters of complex information. A basic familiarity with this new knowledge is important, but mastery is not essential since consultants in specialized areas are available and represent important members of the clinician's new "team."

The final domain of the research world is an acknowledgment of the limits of what one person can accomplish, what one project can address, and what research itself can offer. Inadequate respect for limits can lead to disillusionment and failure.

Area of Interest

Many beginning researchers draw a firm boundary between their clinical and research lives, as if one has nothing to do with the other. The tasks of the clinic and the tasks of research are quite different, but the passions that drive us and that create curiosity and a desire to solve problems are essentially the same. Thus, research should involve an area that evokes passion, curiosity, and desire. Although this concept may seem elementary, it cannot be underestimated. Researchers need to care about a project enough to see it through to completion. In fact, a reasonable guideline for generating a research question is that it must be important enough to warrant consideration and narrow enough to make the answer feasible. Otherwise, the world of investigation is wide open.

Involvement in research often begins with a deliberate, systematic effort. This is a familiar method used by many funding agencies that support research activities, including the federal government. The war on cancer, begun in the 1960's, and research on geriatrics and AIDS are examples of deliberate, systematic efforts to find solutions to specific problems.

Investigators also may enter research and produce relatively spontaneous or unintended outcomes. For example, a researcher might attempt to resolve one problem and find the answer to another problem. Another individual may bring together several unrelated elements and make a single new discovery. Thomas Edison probably is the best known example of a person who made a discovery in this way. He tested thousands of potential filament materials for an electric light bulb, but using results from previous experimentation led to his success. In the medical world, Alfred Vogel provides an excellent example of someone who sought the answer to one problem and found something else. While testing mercuric salicylide as a treatment for syphilis treatment, he produced the first potent diuretic.

In addition to the systematic search and fortuitous discovery, other factors can have an impact on the selection of an interest area. The issue of AIDS is probably the most current prominent example of how social and cultural forces can affect what we choose to investigate. Physical and climatic changes also offer opportunities for new areas of investigation. Recently, research into the greenhouse effect has demonstrated the enormous impact of physical and climatic changes on our approach to research problems or on the character they might acquire.

The best way to enter research is to think in terms of recent concerns or unresolved problems. This may provide clues to important areas of research. When an idea occurs, jot it down; collect groups of research ideas and look for the emergence of a common thread or theme, which may reveal a fundamental topic area to be addressed by the investigator. Motivation delivered from this "core of doubt" is invaluable to the research process. At every step of the process, the researcher returns to that core and is reminded of what he or she was really trying to find.

THE LITERATURE SEARCH

Drawing from an established body of knowledge can enrich the researcher's understanding of the study area. The literature search can determine if a particular study has already been done, but its usefulness does not end there. Chances are the study has been done before but perhaps not in just the same way or with a different emphasis or context. A review of the literature can give important support to the choice of topic as well as ensure the study has not been done before.

Secondary Sources. Begin reviewing the literature by conducting a general reading program in the area of interest. Typically, this involves a review of secondary sources, usually textbooks or review articles, in which authors present the works of others rather than their own research. The goal is to get an overview that provides clues to definitions, historical data, classic studies, and perhaps even a bibliography or list of references. In addition, a secondary review can give information about key investigators and important centers or institutions where the seminal work has been conducted.

However, a secondary review is only a beginning and has significant limitations. In secondary sources, authors present the work of others and, as such, incorporate their own biases into the array of literature chosen for review. Furthermore, the information rarely is as current as that found in primary sources. Secondary sources can generate and help determine the scope and usefulness of various works. References in secondary sources should be used to develop a starting point from which to begin a literature search.

Primary Sources. Primary literature sources are usually journal articles, although they can be book chapters, technical reports, dissertations, or government documents. Primary sources contain the author's report on his or her original work. Once an area of interest has been identified, one should concentrate more and more on a narrow band of primary sources, which usually are not part of a general reading program because they tend to be more specific. Concentrating on a particular area helps to identify primary sources that focus on a specific aspect of the research.

When reviewing the literature, do not forget the human element. One of the true joys of the research process is the development of colleagues. People who research a given area usually are accessible and delighted to talk with others interested in that particular area. The researchers should not be intimidated by the thought of calling a world-renowned expert to discuss a particular research area. People who have spent a long time researching a given area have valuable insights and advice on how to proceed.

Research Questions

In the process of identifying and declaring an area of interest, a number of potential research questions come to mind. Many will be dismissed as the literature leads to greater familiarity with the field. New questions are stimulated and others are refined as the reading reveals what questions have been asked and how they have been addressed. Through the iterative process of reading and questioning, the researcher's questions become more specific and the procedures necessary for addressing the questions become more apparent.

A persistent issue in family medicine research has been the link between the clinical and research worlds. A barrier to understanding the research process has arisen from the assumption that research questions and findings must have immediate clinical applicability to be useful in family medicine. Because the purpose of research is to build a knowledge base, that assumption simply is not true. Clinical applicability usually follows the research process by a period of time. Sometimes research questions and their associated findings never result in clinical applicability. Clinical practice has a natural independence from the research process, a point that needs underscoring. To be sure, research questions are expected to be useful at some level in clinical reasoning and to clinical practice. But to limit research only to questions with immediate applicability to clinical practice is to unduly restrict the researcher's creativity and may undermine the ultimate utility of the research and development process.

A researcher begins by asking a question driven by the "core of doubt" and suggested by the existing research, then sets out purposefully and systematically to answer that research question. The researcher does not try to prove a point, support a set of beliefs, or find reasons for a specific predetermined course of action. Instead, the researcher tests a range of plausible hypotheses about factors that may or may not be related to a particular outcome. Often, research is best done in teams because team members can share differing perspectives on hypothesized connections.

Research Thinking

Physicians are socialized throughout medical school, residency training, and practice to the types of thinking expected within clinical medicine. Unstated presumptions and rules govern how to gather and evaluate evidence, how to develop diagnostic formulations from incomplete and conflicting information, how to test clinical hypotheses, and how to choose among therapeutic options. This type of thinking is not formalized, usually occurs unconsciously, and continues after the clinical encounters are over, such as during lunch, dinner, recreation, and social events. Researchers' thinking differs in some respects, but experienced investigators' thinking also may become subconscious, occurring at all times (even in dreams) and evolving through an extended socialization process.

Although various authors disagree about the nature of research reasoning, a point of consensus is that the purpose of research is to build knowledge. The researcher uses a combination of methods aimed at building a fundamental understanding of a phenomenon. Researchers use data collection and deduction to develop answers to these questions. Deduction comes in the formulation of a question and the development of logical reasoning around the topic. The process requires nothing but the researcher's brain and can occur at any time of the day or night, irrespective of allotted research time.

Research questions arise, in part, from some theoretical understanding of a phenomenon. Whether this theoretical understanding has been formalized into a structured body of work or merely exists as a common understanding among clinicians, theories produce questions through the logic of deductive reasoning. Questions also may evolve through inductive reasoning such as from a well-established line of empirical research that has suggested future study. Every physician has seen the last paragraph of a research article suggesting that because of the observed findings, future investigators should examine questions X, Y, and Z. Research questions arising from theoretical understanding and induction are part of the process Thomas Kuhn characterized as "normal science."

HYPOTHETICAL REASONING

To aid in the formulation of sound research questions, researchers have developed a reasoning process that begins with the assumption that an experimental intervention does not differ from a control group (the way the things typically are done under normal circumstances). This reasoning, called the null hypothesis, presupposes that the results will be the same for the experimental intervention and the control group. Although this may seem peculiar, it stands to reason that the researcher would begin with an assumption supporting the way "things are" rather than with an assumption favoring a successful intervention.

The task of the researcher then is to see whether or not the experimental intervention produces a result that differs from the normal condition. This assumption, which underlies the entire research process, is critical to understanding the rest of research methodology. Understanding of statistical significance, biases in research design, selection biases, sampling, and other forms of research reasoning are rooted in the fundamental principle of assuming no difference between the experimental intervention and normal conditions.

The researcher begins by asking what is the probability that results of an experimental intervention would have occurred by chance? The answer comes in the form of a probability statement, such as the probability of the results, occurring by chance is less than 5 per cent ($P < 0.05$).

Answers to research questions rely on a delicate linkage between the conceptual understanding of a question and the testing of that question under normal conditions. If the results of an experimental intervention are sufficiently improbable by chance, the researcher concludes the research hypothesis is tenable. Notice that we use the term "tenable" rather than true. If we err on the side of caution, it is because the research process has a level of credibility that may carry an overrated force of truth. Research reasoning is probabalistic and relies on a linkage between the researcher's brain and the data he or she collects.

The Research Team

With few exceptions, clinicians work on a one-to-one basis with patients. Other members of the health care team are called in to assist in increasing the efficiency of the physician and to perform services the physician does not provide. The family physician feels a sense of responsibility to the patient and assumes the role of case manager and primary provider. In a research project, the principal investigator assumes a similar role. The principal investigator drives the project. Also, the principal investigator energizes the process through the "core of doubt," dictates the specific techniques necessary through his or her questions, and determines what coworkers (co-investigators) or consultants are needed through his or her limitations. Other members of the team (research assistants, programmers, and secretaries) carry out tasks that may increase the efficiency of the investigators; whereas, co-investigators and consultants lend expertise the principle investigator does not personally possess. Colleagues who are not directly involved in a project become invaluable as the principle investigator strives to be at the cutting edge of research in the area, refines questions and designs, revises grants and manuscripts, and advances his or her thinking. The more people who know about and have discussed a project, the stronger is the foundation of the project. But with few exceptions, research cannot be completed successfully by a committee but only by a principal investigator who has the motivation to complete a project. From this leadership, the other players in the process conduct their roles and perform their tasks.

Research Techniques

The research process requires some general techniques and some highly specialized techniques. Through reading, a researcher becomes familiar with the design, measurement, and analytic procedures frequently employed in the field. Specialization is inevitable if a researcher wants to develop a program of research and contribute substantially to a body of knowledge. Resisting this aspect of research socialization is futile; accepting it as a natural part of the research role is extremely rewarding and beneficial.

A few general research techniques provide a necessary foundation for specialization. They include (1) developing hypotheses, (2) selecting subjects, (3) choosing designs, and (4) assessing internal validity.

DEVELOPING HYPOTHESES

Once a question has been developed, a researcher probably has some expectation of the results. Since any expectation may bias the results, a researcher can impose many controls to reduce the amount of bias inherent in the research process. Research expectations are called *hypotheses*, since they are speculations about the relationship between and among the variables within the question.

Defining Variables. Simply stated, a variable is anything that varies. Variables are implicit in the research question itself and give it meaning. For example, "Is patient compliance enhanced by patient education?" represents a question that has been researched and discussed frequently in family medicine. Within that question, two variables emerge: patient compliance and patient education. One need not look beyond the research question to find the variables of interest. Certainly, other variables might emerge that have an impact on the outcome of the question, but the first step is to look at the question itself and to determine the central variables of interest to the researcher. Additional variables will come later, including confounding variables that interfere with the researcher's ability to draw conclusions about the relationships among the basic variables of a study.

With a question like the one involving patient compliance and patient education, a researcher might hypothesize that systemic patient education would improve compliance. This hypothetical relationship suggests that the use of patient education in a prescribed number of patient encounters will produce greater levels of compliance than would be seen with no patient education. This is just one interpretation of how the question might be investigated.

Operational Definitions. For each variable of compliance and patient education, the researcher has a conceptual understanding. At this point the researcher is still working on the level of abstract thinking, and the understanding of compliance and patient education need not come from any source other than experience. The next step in defining variables produces a level of information that most researchers do not have readily available. To measure a variable such as compliance or patient education, the researcher needs to develop specific definitions. These definitions, called operational definitions, provide an understanding of the operations the researcher will use to define each variable. Compliance might be defined as a specific formula or outcome measurement, such as blood tests, self-reports, urine samples, or pill counts.

Patient education might be defined in terms of a specific activity within parameters defined by the researcher. In this example, patient education is the independent variable because the researcher can manipulate the variable as a purposeful intervention. Independent variables are manipulated to have an effect on an outcome (or dependent variable), in this case compliance.

After operationally defining variables, the researcher develops working hypotheses, which suggest how variables might relate to one another. At this point, the hypotheses become more specific. For example, in a study of patient education and compliance, the researcher might hypothesize that compliance will be enhanced by a systematic application of patient education, as predicted by a specific set of findings in previous literature. After refining the research question with well-defined variables that can be manipulated (independent) or measured as an outcome (dependent), the researcher invokes the null hypothesis to help remove bias from the study.

SELECTING A REPRESENTATIVE SAMPLE

Researchers frequently ask statistical consultants what sample size is needed to ensure the validity of results. The answer is two-fold, but perhaps it is simpler than one might imagine. The basic principles of subject selection are sample size and sample representativeness, each of which warrants significant and independent attention.

The first and perhaps most important job of the researcher is to determine the representativeness of the sample. Under ideal circumstances, subjects should be selected randomly from a defined population and randomly assigned to treatment or control conditions under experimentally controlled circumstances. Though conditions are rarely ideal, the sample always should be selected in a purposeful, systematic manner that should provide a truly representative group of individuals from a defined population. Before considering sample size, the researcher must ensure that each member of the sample is as representative as possible of a defined population. A population is a theoretically infinite set of individuals with some shared characteristics. These characteristics may be as few or as numerous as is reasonable for the purposes of research. For example, a study often focuses on a population of individuals who have a particular disease. The researcher begins by defining the characteristics of the disease, then seeks to sample individuals who have those characteristics.

Sample size becomes a consideration only after the population has been defined. Numerous guidelines and texts give excellent direction for selecting research samples. Each formula for calculating sample size considers at least some of the following elements:

- The relative homogeneity or heterogeneity of the individuals within the population. The more individuals differ, the larger the sample size needed.
- The number of planned comparisons the researcher will make. The more planned comparisons, the larger the sample size.
- Meaningful differences. As a general rule, larger sample sizes allow detection of smaller differences. From a practical standpoint, however, a researcher must ask whether or not a difference is worth detecting. A blood pressure drop of a single point, for example, may not be clinically useful, even though it may be "significant." The researcher must anticipate a useful or meaningful change in scores and choose the sample size accordingly.

Other aspects of choosing a sample size include practical considerations such as resources available and the kind of precision the researcher wishes to have with regard to results. A consulting statistician can calculate a precise sample size that is tailored to the research question.

CHOOSING EXPERIMENTAL STUDIES

There are many ways to characterize research designs because disciplines use many different names for designs and categorizations. Family medicine researchers have used approaches from a variety of disciplines across a number of topics. For the purposes of this chapter, the epidemiologist's approach to research designs is used. Figure 82–1 shows that research designs initially can be categorized by the way subjects are assigned to research studies. When the investigator has control over the assignment of subjects, a study is an experiment, as described in Table 82–1. When the investigator does not have control over subject assignment and must rely on observation of subjects in their natural setting, the investigation is an observational study, which is discussed later.

Experimental studies come in two basic forms. Community trials, so named because they often involve intact communities or groups, entail controlled assignment of subjects but are not necessarily randomized. In other words, the experimenter uses the groupings as they exist in a clinic, community, classroom, or other natural grouping. A true randomized experiment, sometimes referred to as a randomized clinical trial, involves both random selection of subjects from a defined population and random assignment of those subjects either to an experimental or control group. Simultaneous assignment of subjects to experimental and control groups affords the experimenter an opportunity to observe the effect of the independent variable on the dependent variable in the absence of any extraneous effects. Investigators use before-and-after measurement of subjects as a way of determining the impact of the experimental treatment. A control group is desirable and can be used in conjunction with before-and-after measurements for a complete set of controls.

The beauty of an experiment rests in its simplicity and control. No other study type can truly claim to assess causal relationships, and none can be conducted with the flexibility the experiment affords. There are many experimental designs, but each shares the fundamental principles of randomization and control. Multiple variables may be explored, and a great deal of precision may be obtained.

CHOOSING OBSERVATIONAL STUDIES

When assignment of subjects to experimental and control groups is not possible, observational studies

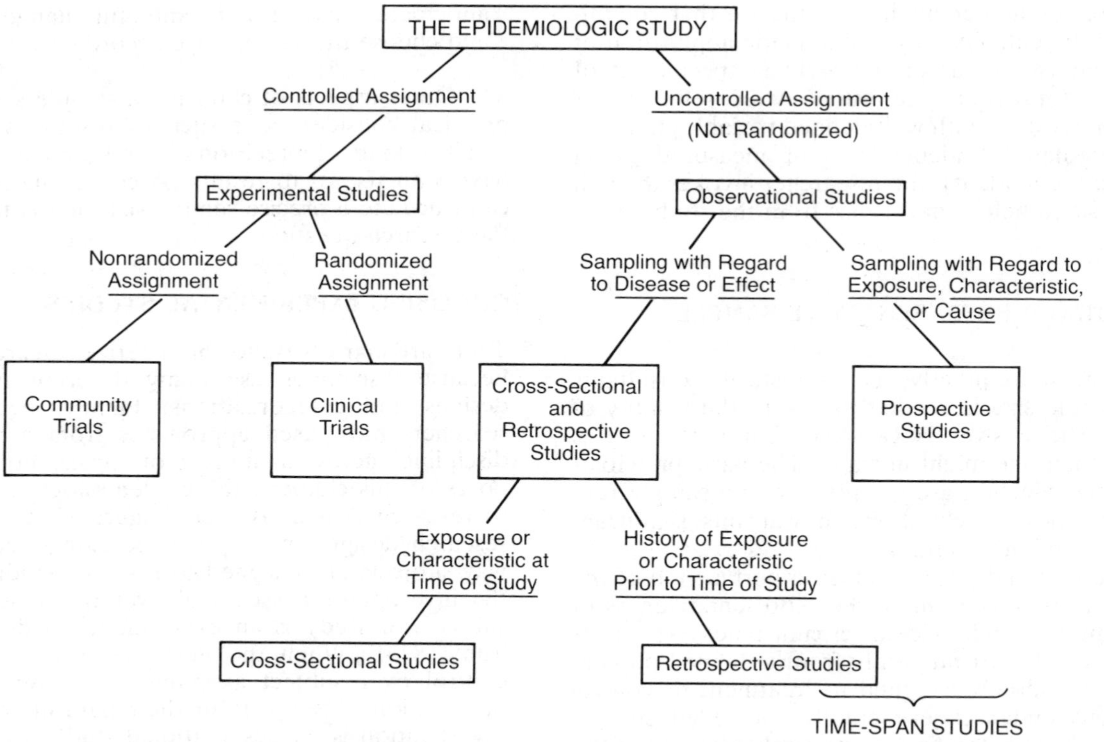

Figure 82–1. The anatomy of an epidemiologic study. (From Lilienfeld, A. M., and Lilienfeld, D. E.: Foundations of Epidemiology. 2nd ed. New York, Oxford University Press, 1980.)

are conducted. Examining individuals in their natural setting is an extremely useful approach to determining the strength of relationships among variables as one would encounter them in a clinic or community. As a tradeoff, observational designs tend to sacrifice control for generalizability. Although experiments are well controlled, they tend to be somewhat limited in their generalizability to applied settings. Observational studies cannot control for the many variables encountered in the natural setting, but their generalizability is greater because they are conducted in the very setting to which their results will be applied. The following brief descriptions provide an overview of observational study types.

Case Report and Case Series. These reports are well known to most medical readers and are extremely useful for describing symptomatology and potential underlying causes of new diseases. In particular, unusual or rare diseases have often been described first in case reports or cases series. Although they are the most basic of studies, they have great value for reporting new information and potential relationships between variables.

Population Studies. These studies seek to de-

Table 82–1. STRENGTHS AND WEAKNESSES OF EXPERIMENTS

Methodology	Strengths	Weaknesses	Interpretation
Sources of Control:	High control	Independent variables rarely have the strength of variables in natural setting	Attribute causation by control over subject selection and comparison
Comparative administration of treatment and controls	Variables manipulated	Limited generalizability	
Random assignment and selection of subjects	Can be replicated	Expensive	
Baseline period of observation before intervention, another measurement after			

scribe the characteristics of a broad population of individuals of interest to the investigator. For example, a variety of studies has focused on the diagnostic patterns of family physicians, beginning with the "Virginia Study" by Marsland and his colleagues. Population studies provide a wealth of information on an entire population of interest, such as doctors, patients with a certain diagnosis, or other defined groups.

Longitudinal Studies. These are population studies conducted over time to discover patterns in characteristics or diseases. Useful fluctuations and trends that do not appear immediately can be observed over time.

Although Table 82–2 lists no particular strengths for the first four types of observational studies, this does not mean they have none. They merely fall into a relatively special category of studies that seek only to describe and not to draw any speculations about relationships between variables. They have little control over any of the facets of the subject under study, and adhere fairly precisely to a description of what happened. In fact, studies that exceed these boundaries should be viewed with some skepticism, since they probably have overstepped the capabilities of a purely descriptive study. The next group of study types in the table can provide some explanation of relationships.

Cross-Sectional Studies. The relationship between a disease and other characteristics of interest may be examined using a single data base covering a single period in time. Cross-sectional studies often involve existing chart data bases, census data, or other data bases collected on a broad population of interest by federal agencies or other organizations. The purpose of such a study is to establish correlations that may be studied further. Even though quickness is listed as a strength, this means quickness relative to other types of studies. A cross-sectional study is not easy to do, as anyone who has attempted one will testify.

An inherent problem of cross-sectional studies relates to irregularities in data bases and the difficulty of getting complete data sets for each individual in the sample. However, given that these problems have been overcome, a cross-sectional study can be accomplished relatively rapidly but requires a keen eye for observations and relationships. A cross-sectional approach has inherent weaknesses, however. Because data may have been collected over periods of time for many different reasons, a cross-sectional study has no specific time frame. Typically, a researcher needs large numbers to support any conclusions about the speculative nature of relationships within a cross-sectional data base. Sample sizes must be calculated on the basis of all potentially planned comparisons within the data base. Finally, existing cases in a data base may not necessarily represent all the cases in a population of interest.

A good cross-sectional study is not paralyzed by these weaknesses but acknowledges them and allows the reader to draw conclusions from the data presented. A well-done cross-sectional study may give an investigator a good estimate of disease prevalence.

Case-Control Studies. These well-known studies, which account for studies found in a large proportion

Table 82–2. STRENGTHS AND WEAKNESSES OF OBSERVATIONAL STUDIES

Study Types	Methodology	Strengths	Weakness	Interpretation
Case report study Case series study Population study Longitudinal study	General observation of the relationship of the disease (variable) and basic characteristics (person, place, time)	(See text)	Limits generalization from results—empirically not as much control as more sophisticated methods	Description of what happened
Cross-sectional studies	Examines the relationship between disease and other characteristics of interest as they exist in a defined population at one time	Quick	No time frame Need large numbers of subjects Existing cases may not be representative of all cases	Prevalence of disease
Case-control studies (retrospective)	Compares persons with disease and persons without disease with regard to how frequently the attribute was present	Easy (time and money) Fewer subjects Tests multiple exposure hypothesis No attrition	Cannot measure risk Information collected for other reasons Existent disease only	Comparative frequencies of risk factors of those with and without disease
Cohort studies (incidence prospective)	Study population is free of disease; attributes of interest are measured and followed over a period of time; development of the disease is measured	Measures relative risk Less biased information on exposed persons	Money and time Attrition Single (few) exposure categories End-points difficult to define	Measures the relative attributable risk of disease development

of the medical literature, compare a "diseased" group to a "nondiseased" group and trace back potential antecedent conditions that may have led to the disease. A well-done case-control study can offer important information to the clinician and the experimenter without the need to wait for years for results to appear, as is the case with a prospective study. Their proliferation probably results from the fact they are relatively easy to conduct when compared with the more expensive and demanding cohort study. Case-control studies require fewer subjects than many other types of studies, and they can test multiple exposure hypotheses that are constructed in a systematic fashion.

Over the years, case-control studies have been the subject of many disagreements among epidemiologists, and clinicians should be aware of the studies' weaknesses. Case-control studies depend upon accurate exposure information. Typically, an investigator first determines who has a disease and who does not and then asks parallel questions of each group. This seemingly simple strategy has many potential pitfalls. Subjects recall exposure information with varying degrees of accuracy, so the information they give may be biased by extraneous influences that cannot be controlled by design alone. Controlling for these weaknesses requires a well-designed questionnaire that is handled by capable questioners.

Though case-control studies theoretically have no attrition, as noted in the "strengths" column, subjects often must be excluded for reasons other than the study's purposes. For example, some people are too sick to respond, some die during the study, some have complicating disease factors that would alter the results of the study if included, and others simply refuse to participate.

The outcome of a case-control study is a comparison of risk factors of people with or without the disease, sometimes called a relative risk ratio. Relative risk ratios have become an extremely important component of modern epidemiology. They give the clinician an opportunity first to determine the relative risk of those who do and do not have the exposure categories investigated and then to offer sound clinical advice.

Prospective Studies. The prospective study has a tremendous amount of strength because it is conducted over a long period of time, studies a population that is "free of disease," and observes the development of various disease conditions of interest. It has the power of watching exposure characteristics before a disease develops and therefore can make attributional claims.

These strengths do not come without their costs, however. Prospective studies tend to be expensive, take a lot of time, and have problems because of loss of subjects due to attrition. Furthermore, the investigators need to decide early on what they will evaluate; therefore, only a few exposure characteristics can be observed simultaneously. As new ones develop, additional studies must begin.

True end-points are difficult to define in a prospective study. As an end-point, the determination of mortality has been deemed relatively simple by the experts (although points of disagreement still exist) but morbidity is an ongoing problem with multiple interpretations that must be agreed upon by the investigators. However, the payoffs of such a study seem worth the additional work. A well-done cohort study measures the relative risk of disease development between exposed and unexposed groups. The strengths of conclusions that can be drawn are extremely compelling and usually are heeded seriously.

ASSESSING INTERNAL VALIDITY

The purpose of research design is to control for unintended influences that might interfere with the understanding of the relationship between the independent and dependent variables. As a result, the design must cover a range of potential unintended influences. These unintended influences have a number of different names, but they commonly are called *threats to internal validity*. A study's internal validity may be defined by its freedom from unintended influences. Therefore, the more a study can control threats, the more likely it will be to support conclusions about the causal relationship between the independent and dependent variables.

A refined organization of threats to internal validity was introduced by Campbell and Stanley (1963). Since the introduction of their terminology, threats to internal validity have been discussed at length and authors differ on the specific interpretation of different kinds of threats to internal validity. For the purposes of this discussion, we have categorized threats to internal validity into four basic areas:

- *Time and history*. Effects due to historical events or the maturation of subjects.
- *Experimentation and observation*. Effects resulting from the performance of the experiment itself.
- *Selection*. Biases due to assignment or attrition of subjects.
- *Regression to the mean*. An effect due to the selection of subjects from extreme groups.

Time and History. A caption underneath a picture of a particularly disheveled W. C. Fields states, "Things happened." Things happen during the performance of a research project, too, and a good design controls for the impact of unintended historical events. Two major sources account for the majority of time and history effects. *History* refers to events that occur outside the study but that have an impact on the outcome of the study. For example, a dissertation student at the University of Minnesota was interested in studying the effects of Tylenol marketing on the drug-consuming public. He scheduled his study for 1982. His timing was particularly poor since that was the year that a number of cases of "Tylenol tampering" were reported in Chicago. Could these effects have been avoided? Perhaps, but only if one were to select a particularly insulated sample that was protected from any knowledge of the events surrounding the tampering incidents.

Maturation can exert an effect as subjects grow older during a study. Sometimes observed effects are only due to the fact that subjects aged not that they grew smarter, learned patient education materials any better, or responded very well to treatment. "Tincture of time" is a common clinical term for the self-resolution of an illness. Maturation also can be effectively controlled by the use of a control group. At the very least, a control group can reveal the effect maturation had on subjects, as compared with the effect of an intervention.

Experimentation and Observation. The numerous effects of experimentation and observation have inspired texts, articles, journals, books, pamphlets, and probably a few leaflets. Some of the most prominent effects follow.

Repeated measurement occurs when the investigator uses a number of measurements over a period of time to observe profiles within patients. This is particularly evident in studies of issues such as blood pressure, serum levels, and liver functions. Subjects may respond differently at the beginning of the study and can become used to the measurement. The researcher must determine how much variation is due to true observed differences as opposed to how much variation involves acclimation to the measurement.

Experimental effects parade under a number of fairly colorful names, such as the Hawthorne effect, the halo effect, the John Henry effect, and others. Each of these effects refers to subjects' responses to the process of being studied. The Hawthorne effect, for instance, refers to a subject's response to the novelty of participating in an experiment. (This effect is so named because of its association with an electrical company's Hawthorne plant, where a study of worker productivity was conducted in the early 20th century.) The halo effect reflects the tendency of raters, observers, or any tool of measurement used to generalize across a number of categorizations when the effects in only a single categorization is known. This type of effect can be observed in clinical ratings, educational studies, and a number of other ratings-based experiments.

The John Henry effect is named for its association with the legendary John Henry of the 19th century, who beat the steam-powered railroad spike–driving machine in a contest. John Henry was the control group in this experiment, and he beat out the experimental group (the steam-powered machine). This happens in real experiments, too. If the control group learns of its status, the members attempt to outperform the experimental group. This has been observed in a number of community trials involving health promotion and emphasizes the need to protect the control group from knowledge of the experimental materials.

Observer bias may occur in any kind of study that uses observers as a primary source of measurement. The best way to overcome this bias is to train observers carefully and make sure they are not tempted to rely on their own internal criteria for measurement but use the criteria set by the study.

A final effect of experimentation and observation, which demands much more discussion than is possible here, is that of recall biases (selective recall). As mentioned above, many studies, particularly those using retrospective methodologies such as case-control studies, require subjects to recall something about their past behaviors. Although this may seem like a simple task, everyone has a tendency to recall some things better than others. When asked to recall particulars of health or specific exposure characteristics, many people have difficulty because of being biased by their current state of health. Many studies involve people who are seriously ill. They tend to recall vividly some parts of their behavior and suppress others. It is only human nature to do so. As might be expected, case-control studies are particularly vulnerable to this type of bias. The best case-control studies are those that control recall bias as thoroughly as possible. They employ highly structured questionnaires, present questions in several different ways to check the validity of responses, and make use of trained raters and observers who consistently follow a rigorous course.

Having collected data, a rigorous investigator calculates the reliability of any questionnaires used and determines the reliability of the observers who conducted the interviews. The researcher can then be assured that data were collected in a consistent and correct fashion.

Selection. Selection effects arise any time subjects have not been selected and assigned randomly to experimental and control conditions. Any time nonrandom methods are used, individuals can be assigned to experimental conditions in a way that might bias the sample. This bias may become evident through unbalanced responses to questions, one study group containing people who have more of a certain characteristic, or in more healthy people being contained in one group than another. Randomization is the only way to control completely for such unintended influences, but as a secondary measure, investigators often measure as many important characteristics as possible as to account for potential differences. The problem with such a strategy is the impossibility of measuring all characteristics of interest. However, given a selective list of important characteristics, an investigator may support the case that bias has been reduced.

One of the primary sources of control in an experiment is the control group. An ideal control group would consist of members who are identical in every respect to the experimental group but who have not received the experimental treatment or intervention. A control group typically is selected at the same time as the experimental group by random selection from a defined population. Only through randomization can the experimenter be relatively sure that any extraneous characteristics have been equally distributed between groups.

Other forms of control include crossover designs, in which members of the control and experimental groups literally cross from one to the other after a period of time. This assures the experimenter that nothing inherent to the control or experimental groups might have caused some differences. Double-blind studies control for the effect of the expectations of the experimenter on the study. In double-blind study, a physician who does not know the identity of experimental and control groups administers treatments to reduce the potential for bias.

Attrition is particularly problematic in long-term investigations, such as cohort studies. Attrition is also a factor in questionnaire-based studies that depend upon high response rates for accurate results. The only universal rule of thumb is to make sure that as many people as possible from the beginning of the study are represented in the sample at the end of the study. Many investigators who conduct long-term studies have employed relatively elaborate strategies to keep people in their studies to ensure the validity of their results. For example, investigators conducting a hypertension reduction program in Minnesota sought advice from clinical psychologists to determine why individuals were leaving the study and to devise strategies to keep them in. Any time a study subject is lost to follow-up, a potentially important piece of information is lost.

Regression to the Mean. The final threat to internal validity is regression to the mean, a peculiar phenomenon that occurs when subjects have been selected on the basis of extreme scores of one form or another. When individuals have been selected because of an extreme characteristic (high blood pressure, for example), the categorization of "extremeness" is a relatively arbitrary one. If everyone with a diastolic pressure of greater than 100, for example, was categorized as high, one might argue that 100 is an inappropriate figure. Ninety-nine might be better, or even 101. The point is that the choice is arbitrary and thus is subject to error. The cutoff point depends on precision measurement to classify individuals as above or below 100. Individuals who are erroneously classified for whatever reason are not "true members" of the extreme group. Statistically, the more one diverges from the average score, the more likely it is that an error will occur from the measurement to the "true" score.

Extreme scores have a natural tendency to rebound slightly on repeated measurement. This is not due to any inaccuracy on the part of the investigator or anything else. It is merely a statistical phenomenon reflecting the fact that the more extreme the score, the less probable it is! In studies that depend on extreme scores, erroneously classified individuals sometimes may represent true scores that are somewhat lower or higher. This may interfere with a treatment intended to raise or lower scores, so the investigator may not know whether a change in those scores reflects treatment efficacy or a statistical phenomenon. A control group provides a good remedy for this kind of problem, as does careful attention to the statistical significance assigned to the study.

As clearly indicated, research designs have plenty of potential for error. Words like "bias" and "control" have loaded meanings in their everyday usage and can scare even the most hardy clinician away from research. Honest research depends upon the researcher's disclosing as much information as possible so other people might replicate the study and determine whether or not the results fit their own setting and circumstances. Eliminating bias and controlling for unintended influences are challenges in every study.

References

Berg, A. O., Gordon, M. J., and Cherkin, D. C.: Practice Based Research in Family Medicine. Kansas City, MO, American Academy of Family Physicians, 1986.

Campbell, D. T., and Stanley, J. C.: Experimental and Quasi-experimental Designs for Research. Chicago, IL, Rand McNally & Co., 1963.

Feinstein, A. R.: Clinical Biostatistics. St. Louis, MO, C. V. Mosby Co., 1977.

Friedman, G. L.: Primer of Epidemiology. New York, McGraw-Hill, 1980.

Gehlbach, S. H.: Interpreting the Medical Literature: A Clinician's Guide. Lexington, MA, D.C. Health & Co., 1982.

Geyman, J. P. (Ed.): Special issue on research in family practice. J. Fam. Pract., 7:1, 1978.

Kerlinger, F. N.: Foundations of Behavioral Research. New York, Holt Rinehart & Winston, Inc., 1973. *For the serious researcher who will explore behavioral or educational topics, this book is the most thorough overview available. This text is an excellent reference for the beginner as well as the advanced researcher, since it covers a staggering array of topics from building a research knowledge base through various analytic techniques.*

Krathwohl, D. R.: How to Prepare a Research Proposal. Syracuse, NY, Syracuse University Bookstore, 1966.

Kuhn, T.: The Structure of Scientific Revolutions. Chicago, IL, University of Chicago Press, 1964. *A scientific revolution is a displacement of the conceptual network through which scientists view the world and results in significant shifts in the criteria determining the legitimacy of both problems and proposed solutions. This notion is believed to be relevant to family medicine research, especially that dealing with the biopsychosocial model. This essay on the history and philosophy of science provides investigators with an understanding of how their work fits on the "normal to extraordinary research" continuum.*

Leaverton, P. E.: A Review of Biostatistics: A Program for Self-Instruction. Boston, MA, Little Brown & Co., Inc. 1986.

Lilienfeld, A. M., and Lilienfeld, D. E.: Foundations of Epidemiology. 2nd ed. New York, Oxford University Press, 1980. *The title of this book is most appropriate. The authors are clear, concise, and complete in their treatment of the basic research design and technique information. The flow diagram in this chapter is reproduced from this book. An excellent starting place for the clinical or epidemiologic researcher.*

Marks, R. G.: Designing a Research Project and Analyzing Research Data: The Basics of Biomedical Research Methodology. Belmont, CA, Wadsworth, 1982.

Marsland, D. W., Wood, M., and Mayo, F.: Content of Family Practice. *In* Geyman, J. P. (ed.): A Statewide Study in Virginia with Its Clinical, Educational, and Research Implications. New York, Appleton-Century-Crofts, 1976.

Riegelman, R. K.: Studying a Study and Testing a Test: How to Read the Medical Literature. Boston, MA, Little Brown & Co., Inc., 1981. *This is a very appropriate text for the busy physician who wants a no-nonsense introduction to reading the medical literature. It provides succinct descriptions of study designs, epidemiologic rates, and statistical tests. Its greatest strength is the "uniform framework" it provides for each major task: studying a study, testing a test, rating a rate, and selecting a statistic. At the end of each of these sections, the summary provides a series of questions that serve as a handy checklist for the appropriate task. The flow-catching exercises allow the reader to try out his or her newfound skills. This is a superb text for residency journal clubs.*

Sackett, D. L., Haynes, R. B., and Tugwell, P.: Clinical Epidemiology: A Basic Science for Clinical Medicine. Boston, MA, Little Brown & Co., Inc., 1985. *This book is just as valuable to the clinicians who never do research as it is to the few who do. The three major sections on diagnosis, management, and keeping up to date are filled with practical illustrations, questions, and suggestions that reveal the logic of clinical medicine. By reading this book, clinicians do gain knowledge, but more importantly, physicians receive instruction in how to critically analyze their daily clinical problems and dilemmas. This is not a dry textbook on epidemiology but rather a fascinating and practical guide for the intelligent practice of medicine.*

83

Interpreting the Medical Journal Literature

John W. McCall, III
Larry Culpepper

"There are only a handful of ways to do a study properly, but one thousand ways to do it wrong"

(McMaster University, #V, 1981)

Problem of Keeping up

The number of scientific journals has increased an estimated four-fold over the last decade, with the medical sciences representing the most explosive field. The total number of medical journal publications increased seven and one-half times (Bowker, 1988). Today there are well over 20,000 biomedical journals (McMaster University, 1981A); new articles appear at a rate of at least one every 26 seconds (Krogh, 1985). Therefore, even a speed reader who reads 24 hours a day, could not keep up with all the medical literature. "If practitioners were to attempt to keep up with the literature by reading two articles per day, in 1 year they would fall 55 centuries behind. Put another way, if physicians were to read everything of possible biomedical relevance, they would need to read 5,500 articles per day" (Haynes et al., 1986*A*). Given this information, why should one even attempt to keep up—is it necessary?

First Principle: Understand Why It Is Important to Keep Up With The Medical Literature

Several studies have documented journal reading to be the most important continuing education activity in terms of physician preference, frequency with which it is used, amount of time devoted to it, and frequency with which it leads to changes in practice. "The use of medical journals consistently ranks above the use of other sources of literature such as newsletters, textbooks, and monographs, as well as above the use of other means of continuing education such as personal contact with colleagues, making of clinical rounds, continuing education courses, and contact with pharmaceutical representatives" (Haynes et al., 1986*A*).

Reasons for keeping up with the medical journal literature in clinical practice include: (1) to stay current with medical trends and maintain competence; (2) to seek solutions to specific patient care problems; and (3) to nourish a personal sense of curiosity and interest about medical conditions. Regular journal reading yields insights into the clinical course and prognosis of human illness, new diagnostic procedures, new treatments, and dangerous drug interactions and side effects. The ultimate application of keeping up is to make rational decisions about changing one's practice of medicine. Good reading habits and skills should contribute to the appropriate and timely adoption of new knowledge into practice.

Before one can read competently, minimal skills and a basic strategy on "how to read" must be developed. "Even the most diligent readers will be little better for their efforts if they lack the ability to sort the valuable contributions from trivial or misleading articles" (Gehlbach et al., 1980). Many physicians lack the skills, or if they have the skills, they may have low confidence in their ability to read critically. These skills are seldom taught formally during medical school or residency training. Almost 60 per cent of all graduating medical students responding to a 1988 questionnaire reported that the time devoted to the teaching of literature analysis skills was inadequate (AAMC, 1988). A result of regular reading is the development of competence and confidence in distinguishing new findings that are reliable and valid from those that are not and deciding when new information should lead to a change in clinical practice (Table 83–1).

Second Principle: Determine What to Read

Once the need is recognized and the commitment is made, the next step is to decide on what to read. For this step, it is important to have a working knowledge of the types of journals and types of articles in those journals.

Journals, like people, have unique personalities that reflect their mission or special focus. Two methods for classifying journals are by topic, i.e., general purpose to highly specialized; or by the type of articles most often published, i.e., original research, review, established protocols for treating their patients, and so on. Under the first method, there are three categories: (1) general, e.g., *New England Journal of Medicine, JAMA*, and *Lancet*; (2) medical speciality, e.g., *Journal of Family Practice, Annals of Internal Medicine*, and *Pediatrics*; and, (3) subspecialties, e.g., *Circulation* and *Archives of Dermatology*. In addition to the *Journal of Family Practice*, major family medicine journals include the *American Family Physician*, the *Journal of the American Board of Family Practice*, and *Family Medicine* (a joint publication of the Society of Teachers of Family Medicine and the North American Primary Care Research Group). International journals of note include *Family Practice: An International Journal* and the *Journal of the Royal College of General Practice*.

The typical family physician should read at least 6 to 8 journals. These journals should represent a mix from the two methods weighted toward the patient composition of the physician's practice. A physician's list of regularly read journals should fit his or her reading style and provide a mix of original research and review articles. In addition, Reinharth advocates that some journals and articles be selected

Table 83–1. A GRAMMAR FOR INTERPRETING THE MEDICAL LITERATURE

First Principle:	Understand *why* it is important to keep up with the medical literature		
Second Principle:	Determine *what* to read		
Third Principle:	Determine *whether or not* to read an article		
	Rule One:	Look at the title to determine general interest	
	Rule Two:	Verify the article's relevance by reading the summary or abstract	
	Rule Three:	Scan the article to determine technical complexity	
Fourth Principle:	Determine *how* to read medical journals		
	Rule One:	Understand the general concepts	
		Step 1:	Know the standard article format for most clinical studies
		Step 2:	Be skeptical
		Step 3:	Do not judge an article by the journal in which it is published
		Step 4:	There is more to an article than the abstract
		Step 5:	Recognize that there is no such thing as a perfect study
		Step 6:	Judge the author's treatment of contradictory studies
		Step 7:	Recognize that validity and reliability are crucial
	Rule Two:	Determine *what* is being studied	
		Step 1:	Determine the study questions or hypothesis
		Step 2:	Identify the specific study variables under study
		Step 3:	Determine how the variables are defined and measured
	Rule Three:	Determine *who* is being studied	
		Step 1:	Determine the characteristics of the study subjects
		Step 2:	Determine how subjects were selected
		Step 3:	Determine whether or not the sample size is adequate
	Rule Four:	Determine the type of study and assess validity	
	Rule Five:	Determine how the data have been statistically analyzed	
		Step 1:	Recognize the fundamental importance of good descriptive statistics
		Step 2:	Determine the types of inferential statistics used
	Rule Six:	Understand that statistical tests do not determine causation by themselves	
	Rule Seven:	Decide whether or not the results and recommendations warrant any change in your clinical practice	

outside of the physician's specialty and include some basic science articles (Reinharth, 1986).

Regarding the mix of original articles versus review articles or other nonoriginal contributions, Haynes and associates (1986A) strongly condemn the reading of any article that is not original and peer reviewed. However, Patrick (1988) describes this approach for the family physician as narrow-minded. Our view is that the mixture of reading material should reflect the purpose for reading. Physicians often encounter a patient with an unusual disease or combination of diseases about which they need specific information. For this purpose, scanning a textbook, followed by reading a quality review article is an excellent initial approach. This process may be followed by scanning articles from "how to" journals such as *Patient Care* to identify practical insights. Finally, scanning original research articles helps identify recent advances. In contrast, reading generally should include a few good review articles as they appear and scanning reports of original research.

Good clinical review articles often include enough basic science background to allow physicians who regularly read them to stay attuned to current findings. We recommend that the reading of basic science articles for the typical family physician be limited, unless one simply finds pleasure in such reading. Original articles regarding new drugs should be limited primarily to clinical trials and postmarketing (FDA release) reports. Studies investigating drugs that are close to being licensed by the FDA for general use are referred to as Phase III studies. Of very limited interest for clinical application are reports of animal studies (Phase I) or preliminary human trials (Phase II). Parts II and III of the articles by Haynes and associates (1986 B and C) provide further information about deciding which journals to read.

Third Principle: Determine Whether or Not to Read an Article

Once one decides on a general game plan of what to read, the next step is to determine the rules related to whether to read a particular article. Gehlbach (1988) describes this process as learning how to "taste" an article; it also has been described as separating the "wheat from the chaff" (McMaster University, 1981A).

RULE ONE: LOOK AT THE TITLE TO DETERMINE GENERAL INTEREST

The reader should have a vested interest in the article to be read. Look at the title. If the article is not interesting or appears not to be relevant to the reader's practice, move on.

RULE TWO: VERIFY THE ARTICLE'S RELEVANCE BY READING THE SUMMARY OR ABSTRACT

"At issue here is not whether the article's results are true, but whether the results, if true, are useful" (McMaster University, 1981A). The question to ask is whether the new clinical information would be of practical use for the reader, given his or her particular practice setting and patients. Would the differences lead to different results?

RULE THREE: SCAN THE ARTICLE TO DETERMINE TECHNICAL COMPLEXITY

If the technical complexity of the article far exceeds the ability of the reader to comprehend it, the effort would be inefficient and frustrating.

Fourth Principle: Determine How to Read Medical Journals

RULE ONE: UNDERSTAND THE GENERAL CONCEPTS

Step 1: Know the Standard Article Format for Most Clinical Studies

This format usually consists of the abstract or summary; the introduction (definition of the problem and review of the literature); the methods (design of the study, description of the sample, data collecting procedures, any treatment administered, and data analysis); the results (of data analysis); the discussion (of results and study limitations, relationship of results to previous studies); the summary or conclusions, or both; and the bibliography. A quick scanning of the abstract, introduction, and conclusions usually lets the reader identify whether or not articles with interesting titles are truly of interest. If so, more time can be spent on the results, discussion, and methods sections.

Step 2: Be Skeptical

The reader should be skeptical of all articles. One should not accept a study's results and conclusions as "truths" unless one understands the general techniques of critical reading and has reviewed the study and understood its limitations. These involve the ability to understand the format of an article, analyze the process by which the study was done, recognize the limitations of the work, and critique the results and interpretation. The critical reader should ask the following seven questions (Crocker, 1977): What is the purpose of the study? How does this research relate to the current body of knowledge in the professional discipline? What measures are used? Do the sample size and sampling procedures permit results to be generalized to a larger population? What is the design of the study and what are its inherent limitations? What is the outcome of the data analysis? What (if any) are the implications for practice?

Step 3: Do Not Judge an Article by the Journal in Which It Is Published

A naive view is that one does not have to worry about the credibility of an article (validity and reliability) if it appears in a peer-reviewed journal, particularly a prestigious one. Although some journals do have more rigorous standards than others, to use this factor to judge the merits of a particular article is dangerous. "The review and editorial policies of even the best and most highly respected journals provide incomplete protection from error . . ." (McMaster University, 1981A).

It also is dangerous to judge the validity of an article by its packaging; i.e., the right jargon and inclusion of complicated tables generated by sophisticated computer statistical packages does not ensure quality. An outstanding parody on this line of thinking is the article "The Teething Virus" (Bennett and Brudno, 1986). The tragic side to this humorous article, according to the authors, is that they get requests for additional copies from physicians who think it is legitimate. Only after a critical review can the physician derive valid and useful conclusions from an article and appropriately apply its findings to practice (Cuddy et al., 1983).

Step 4: There Is More to an Article Than the Abstract

The good abstract is informative and should be able to stand apart from the article, but it cannot be the sole basis for a critical opinion of the study's validity. A complete abstract should include information that identifies the purpose of the study, research design, methods, results, conclusions, and recommendations. Sometimes, the author's abstract of the article contains more wishing than reality and presents a distorted view of the work that follows.

Step 5: Recognize That There Is No Such Thing as a Perfect Study

At the opposite extreme, there are those who are overly critical of everything published and only consider the weaknesses of a study. To operate at this extreme is a folly equal to overlooking all weaknesses of an article. There is a big difference between the ideal study design (as in any blueprint) and the final product. The critical questions are (1) do the strengths outweigh the weaknesses and (2) is there something in the study that adds new knowledge that improves patient care. Every research publication is likely to have a flaw; occasionally, some flaws invalidate the entire study. However, even when overt investigator bias or a design flaw is in evidence, it is incorrect to immediately reject the author's conclusion or substitute the opposite view. "The only conclusion that a reader should make from a poorly designed study is that no conclusion can be made" (Elenbaas et al., 1983B).

As discussed later, different study designs are particularly susceptible to different problems. An informed reader should be aware of these when evaluating an article. When a design flaw or other bias is identified, the reader should consider whether it is likely to make the findings more or less extreme than those actually reported. Often, a study design problem may be such that a perfect study would have found an even more extreme finding than that reported. In such cases, the existence of the finding can be accepted from the flawed study even though the estimate of the strength of a reported finding might be subject to question.

Step 6: Judge the Author's Treatment of Contradictory Studies

It is the responsibility of the investigator to include both sides of an issue in the literature review, usually presented in the introduction. A literature review should relate the current study to previous studies and show how this study attempts to answer questions not resolved by preceding studies. An important indicator of author bias is the treatment of contradictory studies. The critical reader should assess whether or not the author has emphasized only particular previous results that favor his or her objective and ignored those that disagree or discount his or her findings. A related serious error that occasionally is committed is that an author selects a previously published study and draws conclusions regarding efficacy by comparing its results with the results of the current study (Elenbaas et al., 1983B).

Step 7: Recognize That Validity and Reliability Are Crucial

The core issues for how to read the medical journal literature are summarized in two words: validity and reliability. Reliability is the degree of consistency between repeated measures of the same thing, i.e., if I repeated the study would I get the same data? Validity is the degree to which a study achieves the aim for which it was designed. For example, does it represent the truth? Is it unbiased? Is it applicable to practice? Will the patients we see and treat respond in the same way as those described in the study? Does the paper really support its claims? Of the two concepts, validity is the most important, but it is also the most difficult to assess and the more subjective of the two (although the two are not mutually exclusive). A study's findings may be very reliable yet invalid.

There are two types of validity: internal and

external. Internal validity usually refers to the ability of the study design to measure what it was intended to measure within the confines of the study. External validity is more commonly referred to by physicians as "generalizability." Generalizability has to do with whether or not conclusions can be applied to a setting different from that used for the study, including the reader's practice. "The reader should be wary of statements of invalid extrapolation to clinical situations that were not within the study scope" (Elenbaas et al., 1983B). Different types of studies are prone to different internal validity problems. These will be discussed after we have identified the various types of studies. Generalizability is discussed further under Rule Three.

RULE TWO: DETERMINE WHAT IS BEING STUDIED

Step 1: Determine the Study Questions or Hypothesis

What is the subject of the investigation? Is it hypertension, pregnancy outcome, patient compliance, or treatment efficacy? More specifically, what is at issue, e.g., a relationship, an effect, or a cause? In short, what is the hypothesis? The research question or hypothesis usually is included in the introduction as part of the statement of the problem, although it is usually implied rather than formally stated. A hypothesis is a statement of the predicted outcome of the study design, and results are compared to it.

Step 2: Identify the Specific Variables under Study

These can usually be identified in the abstract, introduction, or methods sections. Variables are so named because they may vary according to the circumstances surrounding them at any given time. Descriptive studies report information about variables of interest and the relationships among them.

In analytic studies, there are two types of variables: independent variables and dependent variables (e.g., smoking and cancer, monosaturated fats and cholesterol, family well-being and diabetic control). The independent variables can be described simply as the variables under study, which are presumed to influence the dependent variable. A dependent variable is exactly that. It is defined as being dependent on other variables for its outcome, shape, or existence. Therefore, a study that has a title such as, "The effect of passive smoking on lung cancer mortality rates of non-smoking female airline attendants," is saying that passive smoking has been identified as the independent variable and lung cancer mortality as the dependent variable.

A special group of independent variables are referred to as "confounding" variables. Confounding variables are ones that are associated with the independent variables of interest in the study and also are independent risk factors for the disease of interest (the outcome). Differences in outcomes between groups in a study actually may be due to the confounding variable rather than to the independent variable under study. For example, if various occupations are being investigated for the risk of lung cancer, and it also is known that smoking varies between occupations, unless the frequency of smoking in the various groups is taken into account in the analysis, associations between the occupational risk of interest and lung cancer will not be valid. Confounding variables are particularly important to analytic studies that seek to draw cause-and-effect conclusions. Although authors might not specifically label variables as confounding variables, the readers should observe whether or not other risk factors known to affect the outcomes in question in the study have been taken into consideration, particularly if they also are likely to be related to the potential cause under study.

Step 3: Determine How the Variables Are Defined and Measured

These elements are referred to as "operational definitions." The specific definitions and measures greatly influence the results and are directly related to the issue of validity considered later. For example, how does the investigator actually define and measure passive smoking, family well-being, diabetic control, or monosaturated fats? In many articles, the variable definitions and measures are not reported and the reader is asked to assume that they were adequate, valid, and reliable. Sometimes they are reported in fine print or as footnotes to save space. Find them and do not assume that print size is related to level of importance.

RULE THREE: DETERMINE WHO IS BEING STUDIED

Rule Three is critical when it comes to making a decision about the applicability of study findings to clinical practice. A study's methods and procedures may be very reliable, but the results still may not be applicable to patients in a different practice. The characteristics of the sample have a great deal to do with this question of external validity or generalizability—the appropriateness of applying the findings from a study setting to a specific practice. In determining who is being studied, several steps must be followed.

Step 1: Determine the Characteristics of the Study Subjects

This factor includes such characteristics as the subjects' age, sex, occupation, education, and medical condition. What were the "inclusion and exclusion criteria?" Investigators sometimes restrict their study to a very homogeneous group of subjects. For example, studies of aspirin in the prevention of cardiac or stroke events might be restricted to white males between the ages of 45 and 65. One view is that such a restriction limits the application of the study findings. However, it greatly reduces the likelihood of erroneous conclusions due to age, sex, or race differences between intervention and control groups. Thus, a reader is left with greater confidence of the validity of the study but is also left with the sometimes difficult decision of deciding the biologic plausability of applying the results to individuals who were not represented in the study.

For family physicians, the generalizability of studies conducted on hospitalized patients and patients from subspecialty referral practices, clinics, and emergency rooms is often questionable. Such studies may involve patients who are different enough from those of family physicians that the results of a similar study done with the family physician's practice would be different. These differences may be of a demographic nature (e.g., age, race, sex, education, inner city-rural population, and married-single parent). They may be subtle; duration and severity of illness, time differences in diagnostic assessment, compliance, practice staffing, and physician continuity are a few such areas of difference that might affect the results of a study. For example, in studies investigating treatment of urinary tract infections, few women at initial presentation in private practice had antibody-coated bacteria in their urine (which possibly indicates the duration and the severity of infection), whereas such was commonly found in hospital clinic patients and in a majority of emergency room patients.

Step 2: Determine How Subjects Were Selected

This information goes beyond simple inclusion and exclusion criteria. This question actually refers to the type of sample—random (or probability) sample versus a nonrandom (or availability) sample. It is the method used to obtain a "representative" sample, i.e., a sample that is typical of the entire population from which the sample was drawn. Most clinical studies are based on "availability" samples, which include all subjects (up to a certain number) that meet the inclusion and exclusion criteria.

A false assumption is to equate "randomized" with a "random sample." A randomized study often uses an availability sample and assigns the patient or subject to one group or another based on the principle of "randomness," i.e., giving each subject equal chance of being put in one group or another. On the other hand, a true "random" sample gives an equal chance of being in the study to every subject meeting inclusion criteria in the population. Theoretically, a nonrandom or availability sample could be just as representative of some population as a random sample if the investigator knows all the important characteristics of the population to be studied and carefully selects subjects based on them. However, most investigators are not willing to make such an assumption (nor should the reader) and opt for a random sample whenever feasible.

Step 3: Determine Whether or Not the Sample Size Is Adequate

Sample size is a very important question, since it directly affects statistical significance and, therefore, error type (see Rule Five). Unfortunately, the answer to this question is usually much more elusive than we like to think and often is more an art than a science. Mathematical formulas for determining sample size do exist, but they are highly dependent on the validity of specific information used in the calculations about the condition in the population to be studied. Consequently, the number produced by a sample size formula is no more reliable than the assumptions used. Accurate data for such use often is not available. In reality, the critical reader cannot do much more than determine whether or not the sample size appears reasonable within the context of the practical limitations of the study, i.e., time, resources, complexity of the exclusion and inclusion criteria, and rarity of the disease or variables under study. One advantage of studies that report results using confidence intervals is that the breadth of such intervals provides a good indication of sample size adequacy (see the statistical section discussed later).

RULE FOUR: DETERMINE THE TYPE OF STUDY AND ASSESS VALIDITY

With the general concepts covered, it is time to construct a specific framework for dissecting journal articles that report clinical or epidemiologic findings. To start, determine the type of study from the title, abstract, or introduction. This imposes a logical structure to the article, guides the reader in assessing critical issues, and narrows the possible conclusions. For example, one would approach a descriptive article (e.g., prevalence or cross-sectional study) differently than an analytic study (e.g., case-control or cohort study).

We recommend that the inexperienced reader not memorize a complicated taxonomy of research designs. In fact, certain types of studies are sometimes referred to in different ways, e.g., cross-sectional or prevalence, retrospective or case-control, or prospective or cohort study. Very often, a study may be a combination of two or more classical types. A quick test of the reader's level of ability to comprehend types of studies may be found in the response to the question, "Does a clear mental image emerge when one reads the following: a multicenter, prospective, randomized, double-blind, crossover clinical trial?" Until a reader gains confidence with his or her own classification system and set of definitions, we recommend that a practical approach is to keep one or more glossary of terms close by. A glossary of terms can be found in most epidemiologic textbooks or textbooks on clinical research methods.

In a very broad sense, there are only two types of studies: descriptive and analytic. Types of descriptive studies include case reports and series, correlational studies, and cross-sectional (also termed prevalence) studies. Case reports and their expansion into case series are the most basic types of studies and often serve to alert the medical community of new medical phenomena. In cross-sectional studies, all information is gathered at the same time from participants available at that time. Because of this they are sometimes called prevalence surveys.

Cross-Sectional Studies. This type of study has two major problems. First, since study focuses on one point in time, the relative contribution of frequency of occurrence, severity of a disease, and effectiveness of any treatment cannot be separated. For example, a frequent but rapid fatal disease is underrepresented in the study population, whereas an infrequent but chronic disease is overrepresented. Second, since information about both diseases and their potential causes are collected at the same time, it may be very difficult to decide whether or not the potential cause really preceded the disease.

In correlational studies, information on entire populations rather than individuals is used. The major limitation of such studies is the inability to link data at the individual level. For instance the frequency of cigarette smoking in various countries has been correlated with the frequency of cardiac deaths. It is assumed that smokers are the ones dying more frequently of cardiac disease. A related concern is the lack of ability to control for the effects of confounding variables. For instance, diet actually may lead to cardiac deaths rather than cigarette smoking, with diet varying across countries in a pattern related to cigarette smoking.

A major disadvantage of all descriptive study types is that no cause-and-effect relationship can be established. The advantages, however, are that they can be done simply and economically and are useful for identifying potential relationships for investigation using analytic study designs. For example, case reports provided the first evidence of the existence of AIDS. These were followed by cross-sectional studies that began to identify how prevalent the condition was and the characteristics of patients affected. This information could not prove cause-effect relationships but provided an informed basis for the design of case-control and cohort studies of hypotheses regarding blood, sexual, and other transmission vectors.

In analytic studies, the investigator exercises direct or indirect control over the variables of interest so that cause-and-effect conclusions can be drawn from comparisons between groups of subjects. Variables of interest may be exposures to potential causes of disease (e.g., smoking), preventive measures, diagnostic tests, treatments, or other medically related events. These types of studies often involve observations that span a significant period of time. Analytic studies may be divided into intervention studies, including clinical trials and quasiexperimental designs, and observational studies, including case control studies and cohort studies. Each of these designs has particular advantages and is prone to specific validity problems. These elements are discussed in more detail in sections that follow.

Intervention Studies. In these studies, the investigator intervenes to control the treatment, diagnostic test, preventive measure, or the exposure (potential cause of a disease) under investigation. The outcomes of interest are subsequently measured, and the experience of those individuals receiving the intervention is compared with that of those who did not. Sometimes the comparison is between two or more "active" agents, between an active agent and a placebo, or between an active agent and a control group in which no intervention is made. At times, ethical considerations preclude the use of a control group, and the study compares the results of the currently accepted treatment with those of an experimental treatment. The comparison group may be the same patients as those receiving the intervention with measurements taken at an earlier point in time (self-controls), or a different group of patients who measured at the same time or at an earlier time (the latter are often referred to as "historical" controls) may be used.

The key questions for assessing the validity of an intervention study include: How comparable were the intervention and comparison populations? What was done with information about patients who either did not agree to take part in the study or who left the study (including those who died) before final outcome measurements were obtained? How comparable were the effects of being in the study for the two groups other than the specific intervention under investigation? How adequate were the measurements in measuring the changes of interest? Was compliance measured and how was information about patients who were not compliant managed?

With regard to the first and second questions, the double-blind randomized clinical trial is the gold standard. In this design, subjects are enrolled and informed consent is obtained prior to randomly assigning the patients to receive the intervention under investigation or a placebo (or alternative treatment). For large samples, this design, if properly carried out, has a very high likelihood of revealing that the control and intervention groups are similar in all characteristics other than the intervention. Most other intervention designs also seek to obtain groups that are equal with regard to all characteristics other than the intervention under study. In articles reporting such studies, the first table should be a presentation of the characteristics of the controlled and intervention groups. Did the investigators' randomization or other selection process really result in equal comparison and intervention groups? If not, how likely is it that the differences have affected the results? Were differences in socioeconomic factors or geographic location likely to lead to different outcomes? Was the morbidity of the two groups and the severity of illness equivalent? For studies using historical controls, were other changes in medical care or society during the intervening time likely to alter the outcome?

In addition, the reader must determine the difference between the beginning sample and the sample the investigator finally used. The reader must determine the characteristics of the patients who withdrew from the study or who were lost to follow-up. For studies in which this is an issue, a second table in the article should contrast the baseline characteristics of those who completed the study with those who withdrew before completion and any differences between the comparison and intervention groups. This information may be used to evaluate the likely effects of those dropping out on the reported study outcome. In most situations, the most valid approach to analyzing data is to leave information on patients who dropped out in the group to which they were originally randomized. Were the dropout rate and the reasons for dropping out similar in the two groups? Did patients who dropped out actually represent an adverse outcome such as death? Did patients with the most severe disease or patients with a specific comorbidity leave the intervention group more frequently? Did patients drop out due to side effects or poor compliance (possibly indicating the occurrence of side effects)? When more than 10 to 20 per cent of subjects drop out of a study, the validity of the results becomes increasingly tenuous. Similarly, measurement of compliance is crucial to knowing whether or not the intervention group actually received the intervention. This is particularly important in studies with negative results.

Investigators routinely present t-tests or other tests that judge the statistical significance of differences in groups or between groups and those lost to follow-up. However, such tests are of little value in deciding the larger questions of the effects of group differences or of those patients who are lost to follow-up on the study results. This is a matter of judgment. If certain outcomes primarily occurred in certain groups of patients or in those lost to follow-up, would the conclusions be different?

The nature and adequacy of the measurement tools used must be understood for the reader to know what an intervention has actually achieved. For such instruments, knowing whether or not they have undergone a standardization and validation process is important. In assessing measurement tools, the reader should ask not only whether or not the measurement instrument was appropriate to the change of interest, but whether or not it adequately reflected changes in the range of interest. Functional assessment tools may be used as an example. Although several tools can adequately measure the functional status of patients, the maximum discriminating ability of these tools is among patients who have significant existing disability (e.g., cane- or wheelchair-dependent) as opposed to those with less severe disability.

Traditionally, the best measures have been considered to be those reflecting direct biologic information such as blood pressure, weight, or morbidity outcomes (new heart attacks, deaths). Reports of symptoms and other questionnaire data are thought to be "softer" and more open to differing interpretations by respondents. In this area, one dilemma of interest to family physicians is that while "hard" biologic data may be the most important in deciding whether an intervention works, "soft" life information, which is only obtainable through questionnaires, may be important in deciding the overall value of the new intervention.

Cohort Studies. Cohort studies are used primarily to investigate the effects of exposure to some condition on the subsequent development of an outcome (usually a disease). Cohort studies are particularly suited to the study of possible causes, including rare causes, in common diseases. They must be very large and, consequently, costly and inefficient if the outcome occurs infrequently or requires a long follow-up interval. These studies also can help determine time relationships between being exposed and the development of the outcome.

In cohort studies, two or more groups are set up, with subjects allocated based on exposure status. These studies generally are done prospectively; that is, the groups are constructed at a time when all subjects are free of the outcome (usually a disease). The groups should be similar in all characteristics known to be related to the outcomes of interest. One group is the exposed group, the other group is the unexposed comparison group. The groups are then followed for an interval of time, and the rates of developing the outcome for the exposed and unexposed groups are compared. Two issues are critical to the validity of the results of cohort studies.

First, the exposed and unexposed groups must indeed be similar in all other characteristics related to the outcome(s), except for the exposure of interest. For some cohort studies, particularly those focusing on occupational exposure, data from the general population often is used since the general population is rarely exposed. However, such studies may be subject to a "health worker" bias, since the comparison group taken from the general population may include individuals with chronic illness and life-style habits that prevent them from working.

Crucial to the validity of the study is that whatever procedures are used to identify outcomes must be applied equally to both exposed and unexposed individuals. To ensure that the groups being compared are similar with respect to characteristics that might affect the disease outcome, except for the determinant understudy, it is important to check that the information obtained from the two groups is adequate and of comparable quality. Thus, for example, the validity of a study should be questioned if the cause of death for the comparison group was determined from death certificates, and the cause of death for the exposed group was determined from hospital records. The adequacy and nature of measurement tools, as was discussed in relation to intervention studies, is equally important for cohort studies.

A second major problem in cohort studies is the information on subjects lost to follow-up. If the number of patients lost to follow-up is related to the exposure of interest or to the outcomes, the validity of the results will be in jeopardy. Concerns regarding those patients lost to follow-up discussed for intervention studies apply to cohort studies as well.

Case-Control Studies. Although cohort studies are particularly useful for investigating the possible effects of exposures, case-control studies are used for identifying one or more causes of a single disease, particularly a rare disease. Since both the exposure and the development of the disease have occurred at the time of the study, the case-control study can be conducted far more rapidly and less expensively than cohort studies, which require a follow-up period. Thus, case-control studies are of great value in studying rare diseases and particularly those with long latent periods. However, case-control studies are not very useful in investigating rare exposures, unless study groups can be identified for which the exposure is not uncommon (such as special occupational groups).

In case-control studies, subjects are identified by whether they have the disease (cases) or do not have the disease (controls). Cases are usually identified from an available population, such as patients attending a practice or admitted to a set of hospitals who have the disease. In reading a case-control report, one should look for a very specific set of criteria by which patients were judged to have the disease. Whenever possible, cases should be represented by individuals identified at the time of diagnosis (incident cases) rather than all those existing at a point in time (prevalent cases). Otherwise, the prevalent cases will reflect determinants not only of the development of the disease but of disease chronicity.

The selection of the control group is the most critical issue in designing a valid case-control study. In general, controls should be individuals who, if they had developed the disease, would have been counted as cases in the study. Thus, controls represent nondiseased members of the larger theoretical population of which the cases represent all the diseased individuals. If cases and controls have been adequately selected, differences in exposure rates in the two groups may be considered to be associated with the frequency of developing the disease. (Such association does not necessarily imply a cause-and-effect relationship.) Of note, the control group in most studies should not be the general population for the same reasons that were discussed under the section on cohort studies.

As with previously discussed study designs, the sources of information should be ones that give comparable quality information for both cases and controls. The results of probing for exposure information may be different in different settings, e.g., smoking or drug abuse history may be probed in greater detail at the time of hospitalization than at the time of initial office work-up. If office records are used to obtain the information on controls, office records also should be used to obtain information on cases. Otherwise, the results may represent differences in how the information was obtained rather than in true patient status.

Case-control studies have the potential of developing more problems than clinical trials or cohort studies. Sometimes in ways that are not immediately obvious, the selection of cases or controls depends on the exposure being investigated. This factor will invalidate a case-control study. For example, in a recent study of the relationship of pancreatic cancer to caffeine intake, controls were selected from the practices of gastroenterologists who were the physicians for the cases. However, patients seeing gastroenterologists for reasons other than pancreatic cancer are likely to have been instructed in the past or to have decreased their coffee intake spontaneously. In this particular example, the finding of an increased rate of caffeine intake among those with pancreatic cancer was invalid. A second major problem for case-control studies is the role of recall on the part of study subjects giving information. Individuals with the disease are likely to ponder potential causes and recall exposures that have been forgotten by the nondiseased controls.

Retrospective and Prospective Studies. The reader will frequently encounter these two terms, which refer to the temporal sequencing of study events rather than the basic design. A retrospective study is one in which all the events have occurred (both exposure and outcome) prior to data collection. Retrospective studies are usually those in which subjects are examined for some common factor in their history, and the studies are often descriptive in design. Case-control studies are also retrospective. Prospective studies are ones in which subjects are followed from identification of the characteristic of interest to the time of outcome, e.g., disease. In many instances, a prospective approach is used simply to observe the effects of a treatment or other event over time. Most intervention studies and cohort studies are conducted prospectively.

RULE FIVE: DETERMINE HOW THE DATA HAVE BEEN STATISTICALLY ANALYZED

The overall objective of the statistical analyses reported in an article is to reduce the data into simple groupings with numerical values that can be interpreted in unbiased ways. In reality, this part of the article may leave many readers confused. Consequently, many readers skim data analysis information.

This makes the reader almost totally dependent on the investigator to make judgments about the appropriateness of the analyses and limits the reader in making an informed decision about changing clinical practice based on the results. The following steps may be helpful in evaluating the statistical sections of articles.

Step 1: Recognize the Fundamental Importance of Good Descriptive Statistics

The reader may not understand all the nuances of statistics, but all readers should be able to make some judgment about the results and recommendations of an article based on good frequency tables, e.g., numbers, percentages, and means. A good article, even one constrained by space, should have good descriptive statistics as a foundation to the results section.

Step 2: Determine The Types of Inferential Statistics Used

There are three basic types of inferential statistics: (1) tests of statistical significance, (2) tests of association or strength, and (3) tests or techniques that have predictive capability.

Tests of Statistical Significance. Frequently used tests of significance are the chi-square test and the t-test (see pp. 1805–1806.) Analyses of variance or covariance are basically t-tests for assessing the difference in means for more than two groups. They also allow for statistically taking into account the effects of other variables, including potential confounding variables. A test of significance is reported in terms of the "P" value. Most studies that use inferential statistical techniques begin with a test of significance to determine the P value. The P value is the probability that a finding involving grouped data could have occurred by chance. Simply interpreted, $P < .05$ means that there is at least a 95 per cent probability that the finding did not occur by chance alone and a less than 5 per cent probability that the finding occurred by chance.

Conclusions using P values are subject to error in two directions. An alpha or type I error is the error of deciding that a finding is not due to chance alone when in fact it is. On the other hand, a beta or type II error is the error of concluding that the finding is due to chance when in fact it is not. A small sample greatly increases the chance of making a beta or type II error. Although there is nothing magical about a finding of $P < .05$, this has become a benchmark for statistical significance. However, the reader should always keep the concepts of statistical error (alpha and beta) in mind in making his or her own interpretation. If the results are "negative" (P value $> .05$), then a report of the "power" of an analysis is useful. It is the chance that a type II error did not occur.

Tests of Association. A test of association, such as a relative risk ratio (RR) or odds ratio (OR), is a test of the strength of the relationship between two or more variables or outcomes. The relative risk is the ratio of the likelihood of an event occurring in one group in comparison to its occurring in a second group (often called the comparison or reference group). For example, a value of 1 indicates an equal chance, a value of 1.3 equals a 30 per cent increase in the likelihood of the event occurring, a value of 2 equals a doubling in likelihood, and a value of 0.7 would indicate a 30 per cent decrease in likelihood. Confidence intervals are often reported for relative risk measures or other statistics. They indicate the range within which the true value is likely to be at a given level of certainty. For example, RR = 1.5 (90% C.I. 1.3–1.8) indicates that the best estimate is a 50-per cent increase in the risk of the event occurring, with a 90-per cent chance that the true value lies between a 30- and 80-per cent increase in risk. Larger samples give narrower confidence intervals, indicating more precision in the result obtained. Relative risks give information about the magnitude of the findings as well as the certainty of the estimate. They are related to P values in that if $P < .05$, the 95-per cent confidence interval does not include 1.0. If the P value exactly equals .05, one extreme of the 95-per cent confidence interval would be 1.0 (e.g., 95% C.I. 1.0–1.8).

An R value or correlation coefficient is another statistic indicating an association between variables. It has a range of -1 to $+1$. If there is no linear relationship between two variables, the value of the coefficient is 0. If there is a perfect positive linear relationship the value is $+1$, and if there is a perfect negative linear relationship the value is -1. However, two variables can have a correlation coefficient close to zero and still have a strong nonlinear relationship (Norusis, 1986). A correlation coefficient measures the strength of the relationship but relays no information about statistical significance, nor can causation or prediction be assumed.

Tests of Prediction. Common statistical techniques employed for this purpose include some types of analysis of variance and covariance, multiple regression, and logistic regression. These last two elements often report results in terms of relative risks adjusted for the effects of other variables.

Determining the appropriateness of a test or a set of tests is often difficult and requires a level of expertise that is beyond the scope of this chapter. There are a number of assumptions that must be considered in determining statistical test appropriateness, such as sample size, level of measurement of the data, type of sample distribution or shape (normal or otherwise), and power. If the reader is concerned about the appropriateness of a test, it may be necessary to consult an introductory statistics textbook.

RULE SIX: UNDERSTAND THAT STATISTICAL TESTS DO NOT DETERMINE CAUSATION BY THEMSELVES

A cause-and-effect relationship can never be established by a statistical test alone. Statistical significance only indicates that the association between two variables is not likely to be due to chance alone. For example, a comparison of mortality and morbidity between hospitals and steel mills would find a stronger association or correlation between hospitals and the incidence of mortality and morbidity than that found in steel mills. However, this does not mean that hospitals are a major cause of mortality. In addition, if one was interested in studying the cause of fires, one would find a very high correlation between fires and fire trucks; however, it would be foolish to assume that fire trucks cause fires.

The decision to consider a relationship to be one of cause and effect requires considertion of several issues other than statistical results. First, one must determine whether or not the design of the research reported was of an analytic nature (i.e., case-control, cohort, or interventional design) and whether or not the results can be considered valid based on issues already discussed. Descriptive studies cannot prove a cause-and-effect relationship.

Additional criteria that can help in assessing an article on a cause-and-effect relationship include information about the temporal sequence of events reported, the strength of the association reported, the presence of a dose-response relationship, the biologic credibility of the proposed association, and the consistency of the findings with other published work. The first three of these issues can be evaluated using information presented in the article. An absolute criteria for a cause-and-effect relationship is that the cause preceeded the effect. This is easily confirmed in clinical trials and cohort studies. However, it is a critical issue to confirm in assessing a case-control report. The greater the magnitude of the observed association, the less likelihood that it is due to factors not considered by the investigators, including undiscovered causes. Similarly, the presence of a dose-response relationship can be considered somewhat supportive of a cause-and-effect relationship if other criteria are met. However, by itself, it is a weak criteria since such a dose-response relationship may be due to the influence of extraneous variables. The lack of a dose-response relationship may simply indicate the existence of an all-or-nothing type of phenomena.

If the study is judged to be indicative of a cause-and-effect relationship based upon the above criteria, further support for the relationship might be inferred from the investigator's reporting of other supportive articles in the review of the literature (introductory and discussion sections). Further support can be derived from general knowledge about the logical plausability of the relationship. This is not an absolute requirement, since cause-and-effect associations often are identified years prior to development of an understanding of the specific biologic pathways involved. Once again, this can be judged, in part, based on the author's discussion and introductory sections.

RULE SEVEN: DECIDE WHETHER OR NOT THE RESULTS AND RECOMMENDATIONS WARRANT ANY CHANGE IN CLINICAL PRACTICE

A considerable percentage of the medical literature provides support for the use of new diagnostic studies, medications, and the changing of history-taking and patient education efforts about new potential causes of diseases. Over time, many initial reports are questioned or disproven by subsequent studies. For example, it is not uncommon for drugs to be removed from the market within 1 or 2 years of release because of newly discovered side effects. Two thirds of the studies appearing in medical journals have been judged to contain some unwarranted conclusions (Sheehan, 1980). Therefore, it is important for the physician to be aware of the pitfalls discussed in this chapter—when to reject, when to delay in making changes, or when to institute actual changes in clinical practice. The clinician-reader needs to develop an approach for deciding when to put new findings into practice.

We propose the following steps for the physician to take in making such decisions. First, articles that report completely new causes of disease or first-time reports of the effectiveness of a diagnostic test or treatment should be viewed as preliminary only. A reader should identify whether the results, if supported in the future, would be applicable to his or her practice. If so, the reader can keep an eye out for further supportive literature. Another practical reason to develop an understanding of major new reports is that if they also are reported by the news media, patients may question the physician about the findings.

If other articles subsequently report the same findings, the reader may seriously consider incorporating the findings into practice. The validity of such articles must first be verified by critical reading: "Before accepting the conclusions of such studies, clinicians should be satisfied that the improved patient outcomes following therapy are so great that they cannot be explained by one or more biases in the assembly of the study patients or in the assessment or interpretation of their responses to therapy" (McMaster University, 1981B).

As a second step, the opinion of clinical experts should be obtained prior to clinical application. Editorials accompanying articles may serve this purpose. In addition, the physician may want to discuss them with colleagues in appropriate specialties. Consultants frequently have additional information available to them from subspecialty meetings and discussions with university-based investigators. Generally, one should not consider using a new medication or procedure prior to its use by the local consultants. Because of the increased frequency with which subspecialty consultants see patients with diseases in their area, they are likely to be more aware of practical issues and potential complications in the treatment of these patients. For a new medication, once the conditions mentioned earlier have been satisfied, the physician may decide to begin its use in his or her practice. To start, we recommend use with particularly reliable patients who are likely to recognize and report side effects early. As the physician gains experience, it is reasonable to use new clinical tools that have demonstrated advantage on a routine basis.

A final activity in keeping up with the literature is keeping up with changes in medical literature itself: "In the next decade, I believe academics and publisher will have to increase their efforts to make medical publications more relevant and to keep practitioners up-to-date. The general medical journal will have to change. Though it will still be the first to report important results, it will become less a multispecialty showcase, less an archive for curiosities, and more a forum for critical analysis and rapid exchange of comment. Its ultimate task will be to firmly integrate new results into the existing body of knowledge. This means the journals will have to link academics, medical educators, professional writers, and learned societies more closely—a big job, but medical journals will have to respond to the increasingly complex challenge of keeping up" (Morgan et al., 1985). However, the responsibility and the challenge to keep up and to do so correctly has and primarily will remain with the physician.

References

Alguire, P. C., Massa, M. O., Lienhart, K. W., et al: A package workshop for teaching critical reading of the medical literature. Med. Teach., *10*:85, 1988.

Association of American Medical Colleges: Graduation Questionnaire Results. Washington, DC, 1988.

Bennett, H. J., and Brudno, D. S.: The teething virus. Pediatr. Infect. Dis. J., *5*:399–401, 1986.

Bowker, R. R.: Ulrich's news: serials trends: scientific publishing boom. R. R. Bowker's International Serials Database, *1*:2, 1988.

Crocker, L. M.: Linking research to practice: suggestions for reading a research article. Am. J. Occup. Ther., *31*:34–39, 1977. *The general format for reporting research results is described. In addition, seven major questions to be asked by critical readers are presented. The article is concise and easy to follow.*

Cuddy, P. G., Elenbaas, R. M., and Elenbaas, J. K.: Evaluating the medical literature, part I: abstract, introduction methods. Ann. Emerg. Med., *12*:549–555, 1983. *A thorough three-part series on evaluating the medical literature (see the next two references). The series begins with information on how to evaluate article abstracts in part I and concludes with suggestions on how to critically evaluate the results and discussion section of a journal article in part III. The series is based on the premise that there is probably no such thing as a perfect study.*

Elenbaas, R. M., Elenbaas, J. K. and Cuddy, P. G.: Evaluating the medical literature, part II: statistical analysis. Ann. Emerg. Med., *12*:610–620, 1983A.

Elenbaas, J. K., Cuddy, P. G. and Elenbaas, R. M.: Evaluating the medical literature, part III: results and discussion. Ann. Emerg. Med., *12*:679–686, 1983B.

Gehlbach, S. H.: Tasting an article. *In* Gahlbach, S. H.: Interpreting The Medical Literature. New York, Macmillan Pub. Co. Second edition, 1988. *This is the first chapter of a 14-chapter 218-page book on interpreting the medical literature. The chapter covers the issue of validity, reasons to read, the bones of an article, and approaching an article and serves as an introduction to the more detailed chapters that follow.*

Gehlbach, S. H., et al.: Teaching residents to read the medical literature. J. Med. Educ., *55*:362–365, 1980.

Geyman, J. P.: Critical reading habits and the maturation of family medicine. J. Fam. Pract., *25*:115, 1987.

Gonnella, J. S.: Selecting and reading research articles. J. Med. Educ., *55*:883–884, 1980.

Haynes, R. B., McKibbon, K. A., Fitzgerald, P., et al: How to keep up with the medical literature: I. Why try to keep up and how to get started. Ann. Intern. Med., *105*:149–153, 1986A. *In this first of six articles on keeping up with the medical literature, three strategies are described to enhance the efficiency and effectiveness of journal reading. This extensive series of articles gives a comprehensive treatment to a number of important issues.*

Haynes, R. B., McKibbon, K. A., Figzgerald, P., et al.: How to keep up with the medical literature: II. Deciding which journals to read regularly. Ann. Intern. Med., *105*:309–312, 1986B.

Haynes, R. B., McKibbon, K. A., Fitzgerald, P., et al.: How to keep up with the medical literature: III. Expanding the number of journals you read regularly. Ann. Intern. Med., *105*:474–478, 1986C.

Inui, T. S.: Critical reading seminars for medical residents: Report of a teaching technique. Med. Care, *19*:122–124, 1981.

Kantor, S. M., and Griner, P. F.: Educational needs in general internal medicine as perceived by prior residents. J. Med. Educ., *56*:748–756, 1981.

Kern, D. C., Parrino, T. A., Corst, D. R., et al.: The lasting value of clinical skills. J.A.M.A., *254*:70–76, 1985.

Krogh, C. L.: A checklist system for critical review of medical literature. Med. Educ., *10*:392–395, 1985. *A short, easy to read article covering eleven helpful suggestions for critical reading. The approach was devised in a family practice setting for teaching physicians to review medical literature quickly while remaining critical of what is read.*

LeFevre, M.: Statistical analysis in family medicine research. J. Fam. Med., *20*(5):359–363, 1988. *A clearly written introductory article on statistical analysis for the nonstatistician. The article reviews concepts fundamental to any statistical analysis, the primary reasons to submit data to analysis, and selection of the appropriate statistical test.*

McMaster University: How to read clinical journals: I. Why to read them and how to start reading them critically. Can. Med. J., *124*:555–558, 1981. *In this first of a comprehensive five-part series on how to read clinical journals, ten reasons to read clincal journals and five steps in how to read them are presented and discussed. The series is designed for busy clinicians who are striving to keep abreast of important advances in clinical diagnosis, of new insights into the clinical course and prognosis of human illness, of breakthroughs in our understanding of etiology of disease, and of clinically significant improvements in therapeutics.*

McMaster University: How to read clinical journals: III. To learn the clinical course and prognosis of disease. Can. Med. J., *124*:869–872, 1981A.

McMaster University: How to read clinical journals: V. To distinguish useful from useless or even harmful therapy. Can. Med. J., *124*:1156–1162, 1981B.

Morgan, P.: Are physicians learning from what they read in journals? Can. Med. J., *133*:263, 1985.

Norusis, M. J.: The SPSS guide to data analysis. Chicago, IL, SPSS Inc., 1986.

Patrick, J. K.: Controlling the medical magazine monster. J. Arkansas Med. Soc., *84*:480–482, 1988.

Reinharth, D.: Keeping up with the medical literature. Ann. Intern. Med., *105*:807–808, 1986.

Riegelman, R. K.: Studying a study and testing a test: How to read the medical literature. Boston, MA, Little Brown & Co., Inc., 1981.

Sheehan, T. J.: The medical literature: Let the reader beware. Arch. Intern. Med., *140*:472, 1980.

Woods, J. R., and Winkle, C. E.: Journal club format emphasizing techniques of critical reading. Med. Teach., *10*:85, 1988.

Woods, J. R., and Winkle, C. E.: Journal club format emphasizing techniques of critical reading. J. Med. Educ., *57*:799–801, 1982.

Appendix I Laboratory Values of Clinical Importance

Rex B. Conn

Introduction

The quantitative procedures carried out in a clinical laboratory represent measurements of substances normally present within rather narrow ranges of concentration. In order to use such data, we must know the values to be expected in a normal individual and what is considered a significant deviation from normal. Actually, there can be no sharp dividing line between abnormal and normal values, since there is a gradual transition during any pathologic process from what is clearly normal to what is clearly a pathologic condition.

In medicine, it is a logical impossibility to define normality, and the term "reference values" has replaced the earlier term "normal values." Reference values are derived from statistical studies on subjects believed to have no condition that might affect the measurements under consideration. The traditional and most widely used statistical approach is to carry out the measurement on a large group of subjects and to set the reference limits at the mean value plus or minus two standard deviations. Since values obtained for many measurements are not Gaussian in distribution, additional steps are frequently used in calculation of the reference ranges. The important consideration is that the reference ranges derived by these statistical methods contain only 95 per cent of the reference population. Thus, a value slightly outside the reference range might be due either to chance distribution or to an underlying pathologic process.

A single reference range for all individuals may be inadequate for some clinical measurements. Values obtained on presumably normal persons may vary because of age, sex, body build, race, environment, and state of gastrointestinal absorption. A universal caveat in the use of reference values is that for many procedures the reference range will vary with the method used. This is particularly true for enzyme measurements and measurements based upon immunochemical principles.

The International System of Units for Laboratory Measurements (Le Système International D'Unités)

An extensive modification of the metric system has been adopted by clinical laboratories in many countries. This adaptation is the International System of Units (Le Système International d'Unités), usually abbreviated S.I. units. Whereas the metric system utilizes the centimeter, the gram, and the second as basic units, the International System uses the meter, the kilogram, and the second as well as four other basic units.

The International System is a coherent approach to all types of measurement that utilizes seven dimensionally independent basic quantities: mass, length, time, thermodynamic temperature, electric current, luminous intensity, and amount of substance. Each of these quantities is expressed in a clearly defined *base unit* (Table 1).

Two or more base units may be combined to provide *derived units* (Table 2) for expressing other measurements such as mass concentration (kilograms per cubic meter) and velocity (meters per second). Standardized prefixes (Table 3) for base and derived units are used to express fractions or multiples of the base units so that any measurement can be expressed in a value between 0.001 and 1000.

MEDICAL APPLICATIONS

The most profound change in laboratory reports will result from expressing concentration as amount per volume (moles per liter) rather than mass per volume (milligrams per 100 milliliters). The advantages of the former expression can be seen in the following:

Conventional Units

1.0 gram of hemoglobin
Combines with 1.37 ml of oxygen
Contains 3.4 mg of iron
Forms 34.9 mg of bilirubin

S.I. Units

1.0 mmol of hemoglobin
Combines with 4.0 mmol of oxygen
Contains 4.0 mmol of iron
Forms 4.0 mmol of bilirubin

Chemical relationships between lactic acid and pyruvic acid and the glucose from which both are derived, as well as the relationship between bilirubin and the binding capacity of albumin, are other examples of chemical relationships that will be clarified by using the new system.

There are a number of laboratory and other medical measurements for which the S.I. units appear to offer little advantage, and some that are disadvantageous because the change would require replacement or revision of instruments such as the sphygmomanometer. The cubic meter is the derived unit for volume; however, it is inappropriately large for medical measurements, and the liter has been retained. Thermodynamic temperature expressed in kelvins is not more informative for medical measurements. Since the Celsius degree is the same as the kelvin degree, the Celsius scale is used. Celsius rather than centigrade is the preferred term.

Selection of units for expressing enzyme activity presents certain difficulties. Literally dozens of different units have been used in expressing enzyme activity, and interlaboratory comparison of enzyme results is impossible unless the assay system is precisely defined. In 1964, the International Union of Biochemistry attempted to remedy the situation by proposing the International Unit for enzymes. This unit was defined as the amount of enzyme that will catalyze the conversion of 1 micromole of substrate per minute under standard conditions. Difficulties remain, however, as enzyme activity is affected by temperature, pH, the type and amount of substrate, the presence of inhibitors, and other factors. Enzyme activity can be expressed in S.I. units, and the katal has been proposed to express activities of all catalysts, including enzymes. The katal is that amount of enzyme that catalyzes a reaction rate of 1 mole per second. Thus,

Table 1. BASE UNITS

Property	Base Unit	Symbol
Length	metre	m
Mass	kilogram	kg
Amount of substance	mole	mol
Time	second	s
Thermodynamic temperature	kelvin	K
Electric current	ampere	A
Luminous intensity	candela	cd

Table 2. DERIVED UNITS

Derived Property	Derived Unit	Symbol
Area	square metre	m^2
Volume	cubic metre	m^3
	litre	l
Mass concentration	kilogram/cubic metre	kg/m^3
	gram/litre	g/l
Substance concentration	mole/cubic metre	mol/m^3
	mole/litre	mol/l
Temperature	degree Celsius	C = K − 273.15

Table 3. STANDARD PREFIXES

Prefix	Multiplication Factor	Symbol
atto	10^{-18}	a
femto	10^{-15}	f
pico	10^{-12}	p
nano	10^{-9}	n
micro	10^{-6}	μ
milli	10^{-3}	m
centi	10^{-2}	c
deci	10^{-1}	d
deca	10^{1}	da
hecto	10^{2}	h
kilo	10^{3}	k
mega	10^{6}	M
giga	10^{9}	G
tera	10^{12}	T

adoption of the katal as the unit of enzyme activity would provide no more information than is obtained when results are expressed in International Units.

Hydrogen ion concentration in blood is customarily expressed as pH, but in S.I. units it would be expressed in nanomoles per liter. It appears unlikely that the very useful pH scale will be discarded.

Pressure measures, such as blood pressure and partial pressures of blood gases, would be expressed in S.I. units using the pascal, a unit that can be derived from the base units for mass, length, and time. This change probably will not be adopted in the early phases of the conversion to S.I. units. Similarly, a proposed change in expressing osmolality in terms of the depression of freezing point is inappropriate, because osmolality may be calculated from vapor pressure as well as freezing point measurement.

CONVENTIONS

A number of conventions have been adopted to standardize usage of S.I. units:

1. No periods are used after the symbol for a unit (kg not kg.), and it remains unchanged when used in the plural (70 kg not 70 kgs).
2. A half space rather than a comma is used to divide large numbers into groups of three (e.g., 5 400 000 not 5,400,000).
3. Compound prefixes should be avoided (nanometer not millimicrometer).
4. Multiples and submultiples are used in steps of 10^3 or 10^{-3}.
5. The degree sign for the temperature scales is omitted (38 C not 38°C).
6. The preferred spelling is metre not meter, litre not liter.
7. Report of a measurement should include information on the system, the component, the kind of quantity, the numerical value, and the unit. For example: *System,* serum. *Component,* glucose. *Kind of quantity,* substance concentration. *Value,* 5.10. *Unit,* mmol/l.
8. The name of the component should be unambiguous; for example, "serum bilirubin" might refer to unconjugated bilirubin or to total bilirubin. For acids and bases, the maximally ionized form is used in naming the component; for example, lactate or urate rather than lactic acid or uric acid.

TABLES OF REFERENCE VALUES

Tables accompanying this article indicate "normal values" for most of the commonly performed laboratory tests. The title of the tables has been changed from the "normal values" of previous years to "reference values" to conform to current usage. The reference value is given in conventional units, and the value in S.I. units is calculated from these figures. Notes (page 1848) provide additional information.

REFERENCE VALUES IN HEMATOLOGY

	Conventional Units		S.I. Units		Notes
Acid hemolysis test (Ham)	No hemolysis		No hemolysis		
Alkaline phosphatase, leukocyte	Total score 14–100		Total score 14–100		
Carboxyhemoglobin	Up to 5% of total		0.05 of total		a
Cell counts					
Erythrocytes					
Males	4.6–6.2 million/cu mm		4.6–6.2 × 10^{12}/l		
Females	4.2–5.4 million/cu mm		4.2–5.4 × 10^{12}/l		
Children (varies with age)	4.5–5.1 million/cu mm		4.5–5.1 × 10^{12}/l		
Leukocytes					
Total	4500–11,000/cu mm		4.5–11.0 × 10^{9}/l		
Differential	*Percentage*	*Absolute*			
Myelocytes	0	0/cu mm	0/1		b
Band neutrophils	3–5	150–400/cu mm	150–400 × 10^{6}/l		
Segmented neutrophils	54–62	3000–5800/cu mm	3000–5800 × 10^{6}/l		
Lymphocytes	25–33	1500–3000/cu mm	1500–3000 × 10^{6}/l		
Monocytes	3–7	300–500/cu mm	300–500 × 10^{6}/l		
Eosinophils	1–3	50–250/cu mm	50–250 × 10^{6}/l		
Basophils	0–0.75	15–50/cu mm	15–50 × 10^{6}/l		
Platelets	150,000–350,000/cu mm		150–350 × 10^{9}/l		
Reticulocytes	25,000–75,000/cu mm 0.5–1.5% of erythrocytes		25–75 × 10^{9}/l		b
Bone marrow, differential cell count					
	Range	*Average*	*Range*	*Average*	
Myeloblasts	0.3–5.0%	2.0%	0.003–0.05	0.02	a
Promyelocytes	1.0–8.0%	5.0%	0.01–0.08	0.05	
Myelocytes: Neutrophilic	5.0–19.0%	12.0%	0.05–0.19	0.12	
Eosinophilic	0.5–3.0%	1.5%	0.005–0.03	0.015	
Basophilic	0.0–0.5%	0.3%	0.00–0.005	0.003	
Metamyelocytes	13.0–32.0%	22.0%	0.13–0.32	0.22	
Polymorphonuclear neutrophils	7.0–30.0%	20.0%	0.07–0.30	0.20	
Polymorphonuclear eosinophils	0.5–4.0%	2.0%	0.005–0.04	0.02	
Polymorphonuclear basophils	0.0–0.7%	0.2%	0.00–0.007	0.002	
Lymphocytes	3.0–17.0%	10.0%	0.03–0.17	0.10	
Plasma cells	0.0–2.0%	0.4%	0.00–0.02	0.004	
Monocytes	0.5–5.0%	2.0%	0.005–0.05	0.02	
Reticulum cells	0.1–2.0%	0.2%	0.001–0.02	0.002	
Megakaryocytes	0.3–3.0%	0.4%	0.003–0.03	0.004	
Pronormoblasts	1.0–8.0%	4.0%	0.01–0.08	0.04	
Normoblasts	7.0–32.0%	18.0%	0.07–0.32	0.18	
Coagulation tests					
Antithrombin III (synthetic substrate)	80–120% of normal		8–1.2 of normal		
Bleeding time (Duke)	1–5 min		1–5 min		
Bleeding time (Ivy)	Less than 5 min		Less than 5 min		
Bleeding time (template)	2.5–9.5 min		2.5–9.5 min		
Clot retraction, qualitative	Begins in 30–60 min Complete in 24 hrs		Begins in 30–60 min Complete in 24 h		
Coagulation time (Lee-White)	5–15 min (glass tubes) 19–60 min (siliconized tubes)		5–15 min (glass tubes) 19–60 min (siliconized tubes)		

REFERENCE VALUES IN HEMATOLOGY *Continued*

	Conventional Units	S.I. Units	Notes
Euglobulin lysis time	2–6 hrs at 37°	2–6 h at 37 C	
Factor VIII and other coagulation factors	50–150% of normal	0.50–1.5 of normal	a
Fibrin split products (Thrombo-Wellco test)	Less than 10 mcg/ml	Less than 10 mg/l	
Fibrinogen	200–400 mg/dl	5.9–11.7 μmol/l	c
Fibrinolysins	0	0	
Partial thromboplastin time, activated (APTT)	20–35 sec	20–35 sec	
Prothrombin consumption	Over 80% consumed in 1 hr	Over 0.80 consumed in 1 h	a
Prothrombin content	100% (calculated from prothrombin time)	1.0 (calculated from prothrombin time)	a
Prothrombin time (one stage)	12.0–14.0 sec	12.0–14.0 sec	
Tourniquet test	Ten or fewer petechiae in a 2.5 cm circle after 5 min	Ten or fewer petechiae in a 2.5 cm circle after 5 min	
Cold hemolysin test (Donath-Landsteiner)	No hemolysis	No hemolysis	
Coombs' test			
Direct	Negative	Negative	
Indirect	Negative	Negative	
Corpuscular values of erythrocytes (values are for adults; in children, values vary with age)			
MCH (mean corpuscular hemoglobin)	27–31 picogm	0.42–0.48 fmol	d
MCV (mean corpuscular volume)	80–96 cu micra	80–96 fl	
MCHC (mean corpuscular hemoglobin concentration)	32–36%	0.32–0.36	a
Haptoglobin (as hemoglobin binding capacity)	100–200 mg/dl	16–31 μmol/l	d
Hematocrit			
Males	40–54 ml/dl	0.40–0.54	a
Females	37–47 ml/dl	0.37–0.47	
Newborn	49–54 ml/dl	0.49–0.54	
Children (varies with age)	35–49 ml/dl	0.35–0.49	
Hemoglobin			
Males	14.0–18.0 grams/dl	2.17–2.79 mmol/l	d
Females	12.0–16.0 grams/dl	1.86–2.48 mmol/l	
Newborn	16.5–19.5 grams/dl	2.56–3.02 mmol/l	
Children (varies with age)	11.2–16.5 grams/dl	1.74–2.56 mmol/l	
Hemoglobin, fetal	Less than 1% of total	Less than 0.01 of total	a
Hemoglobin A_{1c}	3–5% of total	0.03–0.05 of total	a
Hemoglobin A_2	1.5–3.0% of total	0.015–0.03 of total	a
Hemoglobin, plasma	0–5.0 mg/dl	0–0.8 μmol/l	d
Methemoglobin	0–130 mg/dl	4.7–20 μmol/l	e
Osmotic fragility of erythrocytes	Begins in 0.45–0.39% NaCl Complete in 0.33–0.30% NaCl	Begins in 77–67 mmol/NaCl Complete in 56–51 mmol/l NaCl	
Sedimentation rate			
Wintrobe: Males	0–5 mm in 1 hr	0–5 mm/h	
Females	0–15 mm in 1 hr	0–15 mm/h	
Westergren: Male	0–15 mm in 1 hr	0–15 mm/h	
Females	0–20 mm in 1 hr	0–20 mm/h	
(May be slightly higher in children and during pregnancy)			

REFERENCE VALUES FOR BLOOD, PLASMA, AND SERUM
(For some procedures the reference values may vary depending upon the method used)

	Conventional Units	S.I. Units	Notes
Acetoacetate plus acetone, serum			
Qualitative	Negative	Negative	
Quantitative	0.3–2.0 mg/dl	3–20 mg/l	
Adrenocorticotropin (ACTH), plasma			
6 AM	10–80 picogm/ml	10–80 ng/l	
6 PM	Less than 50 picogm/ml	Less than 50 ng/l	
Alanine aminotransferase, *see* Transaminase			
Aldolase, serum	0–11 milliunits/ml (30°)	0–11 units/l (30 C)	f
Aldosterone			
Adult, supine	3–10 nanogm/dl	0.08–0.3 nmol/l	
standing			
male	6–22 nanogm/dl	0.17–0.61 nmol/l	
female	5–30 nanogm/dl	0.14–0.8 nmol/l	
Alpha amino nitrogen, serum	3.0–5.5 mg/dl	2.1–3.9 mmol/l	
Ammonia (nitrogen), plasma	15–49 mcg/dl	11–35 μmol/l	
Amylase, serum	25–125 milliunits/ml	25–125 units/l	
Anion gap	8–16 mEq/liter	8–16 mmol/l	
Ascorbic acid, blood	0.4–1.5 mg/dl	23–85 μmol/l	
Aspartate aminotransferase, *see* Transaminase			
Base excess, blood	0 ± 2 mEq/liter	0 ± 2 mmol/l	
Bicarbonate, serum	23–29 mEq/liter	23–29 mmol/l	
Bile acids, serum	0.3–3.0 mg/dl	3.0–30.0 mg/l	
Bilirubin, serum			
Direct	0.1–0.4 mg/dl	1.7–6.8 μmol/l	
Indirect	0.2–0.7 mg/dl (Total minus direct)	3.4–12 μmol/l (Total minus direct)	
Total	0.3–1.1 mg/dl	5.1–19 μmol/l	
Calcium, serum	4.5–5.5 mEq/liter 9.0–11.0 mg/dl (Slightly higher in children) (Varies with protein concentration)	2.25–2.75 mmol/l (Slightly higher in children) (Varies with protein concentration)	
Calcium, ionized, serum	2.1–2.6 mEq/liter 4.25–5.25 mg/dl	1.05–1.30 mmol/l	
Carbon dioxide content, serum			
Adults	24–30 mEq/liter	24–30 mmol/l	
Infants	20–28 mEq/liter	20–28 mmol/l	
Carbon dioxide tension (P_{CO_2}), blood	35–45 mm Hg	35–45 mm Hg	g
Carotene, serum	40–200 mcg/dl	0.74–3.72 μmol/l	
Ceruloplasmin, serum	23–44 mg/dl	230–440 mg/l	h
Chloride, serum	96–106 mEq/liter	96–106 mmol/l	
Cholesterol, serum			
Total	150–250 mg/dl	3.9–6.5 mmol/l	
Esters	68–76% of total cholesterol	0.68–0.76 of total cholesterol	a
Cholinesterase			
Serum	0.5–1.3 pH units	0.5–1.3 pH units	f
Erythrocytes	0.5–1.0 pH unit	0.5–1.0 pH unit	f
Copper, serum			
Males	70–140 mcg/dl	11–22 μmol/l	
Females	85–155 mcg/dl	13–24 μmol/l	
Cortisol, plasma			
8 AM	6–23 mcg/dl	170–635 nmol/l	
4 PM	3–15 mcg/dl	82–413 nmol/l	
10 PM	Less than 50% of 8 AM value	Less than 0.5 of 8 AM value	
Creatine, serum	0.2–0.8 mg/dl	15–61 μmol/l	
Creatine kinase, serum (CK, CPK)			
Males	12–80 milliunits/ml (30°)	12–80 units/l (30 C)	f
	55–170 milliunits/ml (37°)	55–170 units/l (37 C)	f
Females	10–55 milliunits/ml (30°)	10–55 units/l (30 C)	f
	30–135 milliunits/ml (37°)	30–135 units/l (37 C)	f
Creatine kinase isoenzymes, serum			
CK-MM	Present	Present	
CK-MB	Absent	Absent	
CK-BB	Absent	Absent	
Creatinine, serum	0.6–1.2 mg/dl	53–106 μmol/l	
Cryoglobulins, serum	0	0	
Fatty acids, total, serum	190–420 mg/dl	7–15 mmol/l	i
nonesterified, serum	8–25 mg/dl	0.30–0.90 mmol/l	
Ferritin, serum	20–200 nanogm/ml	20–200 μg/l	

REFERENCE VALUES FOR BLOOD, PLASMA, AND SERUM *Continued*
(For some procedures the reference values may vary depending upon the method used)

	Conventional Units	S.I. Units	Notes
Fibrinogen, plasma	200–400 mg/100 ml	5.9–11.7 μmol/l	c
Folate, serum	1.8–9.0 nanogm/ml	4.1–20.4 nmol/l	
Erythrocytes	150–450 nanogm/ml	340–1020 nmol/l	
Follicle-stimulating hormone (FSH), plasma			
Males	4–25 milliunits/ml (I.U.)	4–25 IU/l	
Females	4–30 milliunits/ml (I.U.)	4–30 IU/l	
Postmenopausal	40–250 milliunits/ml (I.U.)	40–250 IU/l	
Gamma glutamyltransferase			
Males	6–32 milliunits/ml (30°)	6–32 units/l (30 C)	f
Females	4–18 milliunits/ml (30°)	4–18 units/l (30 C)	f
Gastrin, serum	0–200 picogm/ml	0–200 ng/l	
Glucose (fasting)			
Blood	60–100 mg/dl	3.33–5.55 mmol/l	
Plasma or serum	70–115 mg/dl	3.89–6.38 mmol/l	
Growth hormone, serum	0–10 nanogm/ml	0–10 μg/l	
Haptoglobin, serum	100–200 mg/dl (As hemoglobin binding capacity)	16–31 μmol/l (As hemoglobin binding capacity)	d
Hydroxybutyric dehydrogenase, serum (HBD)	0–180 milliunits/ml (30°)	0–180 units/l (30 C)	f
17-Hydroxycorticosteroids, plasma	8–18 mcg/dl	0.22–0.50 μmol/l	j
Immunoglobulins, serum			
IgG	550–1900 mg/dl	5.5–19.0 g/l	
IgA	60–333 mg/dl	0.60–3.3 g/l	
IgM	45–145 mg/dl	0.45–1.5 g/l	
IgD	0.5–3.0 mg/dl	5–30 mg/l	
IgE	<500 nanogm/ml (Varies with age in children)	<500 μg/l (Varies with age in children)	
Insulin, plasma (fasting)	5–25 microunits/ml	36–179 pmol/l	
Iodine, protein bound, serum	3.5–8.0 mcg/dl	0.28–0.63 μmol/l	k
Iron, serum	75–175 mcg/dl	13–31 μmol/l	
Iron binding capacity, serum			
Total	250–410 mcg/dl	45–73 μmol/l	
Saturation	20–55%	0.20–0.55	a
Lactate, blood, venous	4.5–19.8 mg/dl	0.5–2.2 mmol/l	
arterial	4.5–14.4 mg/dl	0.5–1.6 mmol/l	
Lactate dehydrogenase, serum (LD, LDH)	45–90 milliunits/ml (I.U.) (30°) 100–190 milliunits/ml (37°)	45–90 units/l (30 C) 100–190 units/l (37 C)	f
LDH_1	22–37% of total	0.22–0.37 of total	
LDH_2	30–46% of total	0.30–0.46 of total	a
LDH_3	14–29% of total	0.14–0.29 of total	
LDH_4	5–11% of total	0.05–0.11 of total	
LDH_5	2–11% of total	0.02–0.11 of total	
Leucine aminopeptidase, serum	14–40 milliunits/ml (30°)	14–40 units/l (30 C)	f
Lipase, serum	0–1.5 units (Cherry-Crandall)	0–1.5 units (Cherry-Crandall)	f
Lipids, total, serum	450–850 mg/dl	4.5–8.5 g/l	m
Lipoprotein cholesterol, serum			
LDL cholesterol	60–180 mg/dl	600–1800 mg/l	
HDL cholesterol	30–80 mg/dl	300–800 mg/l	
Luteinizing hormone (LH), serum			
Males	6–18 milliunits/ml (I.U.)	6–18 IU/l	
Females, premenopausal	5–22 milliunits/ml (I.U.)	5–22 IU/l	
midcycle	3 times baseline	3 times baseline	
postmenopausal	Greater than 30 milliunits/ml (I.U.)	Greater than 30 IU/l	
Magnesium, serum	1.5–2.5 mEq/liter 1.8–3.0 mg/dl	0.75–1.25 mmol/l	
5′-Nucleotidase, serum	3.5–12.7 milliunits/ml (37°)	3.5–12.5 units/l (37 C)	f
Nitrogen, nonprotein, serum	15–35 mg/dl	10.7–25.0 mmol/l	
Osmolality, serum	285–295 mOsm/kg serum water	285–295 mmol/kg serum water	n
Oxygen, blood			
Capacity	16–24 vol % (varies with hemoglobin)	7.14–10.7 mmol/l (varies with hemoglobin)	o
Content Arterial	15–23 vol %	6.69–10.3 mmol/l	o
Venous	10–16 vol %	4.46–7.14 mmol/l	o
Saturation Arterial	94–100% of capacity	0.94–1.00 of capacity	a
Venous	60–85% of capacity	0.60–0.85 of capacity	a
Tension, Po_2 Arterial	75–100 mm Hg	75–100 mm Hg	g
P_{50}, blood	26–27 mm Hg	26–27 mm Hg	g

Table continued on following page

REFERENCE VALUES FOR BLOOD, PLASMA, AND SERUM *Continued*
(For some procedures the reference values may vary depending upon the method used)

	Conventional Units	S.I. Units	Notes
pH, arterial, blood	7.35–7.45	7.35–7.45	p
Phenylalanine, serum	Less than 3 mg/dl	Less than 0.18 mmol/l	
Phosphatase, acid serum	0.11–0.60 milliunit/ml (37°) (Roy, Brower, Hayden)	0.11–0.60 units/l	f
Phosphatase, alkaline, serum (ALP)	20–90 milliunits/ml (30°) (Values are higher in children)	20–90 units/l (30 C) (Values are higher in children)	f
Phosphate, inorganic, serum			
Adults	3.0–4.5 mg/dl	1.0–1.5 mmol/l	
Children	4.0–7.0 mg/dl	1.3–2.3 mmol/l	
Phospholipids, serum	6–12 mg/dl (As lipid phosphorus)	1.9–3.9 mmol/l (As lipid phosphorus)	
Potassium, serum	3.5–5.0 mEq/liter	3.5–5.0 mmol/l	
Prolactin, serum			
Males	1–20 nanogm/ml	1–20 μg/l	
Females	1–25 nanogm/ml	1–25 μg/l	
Protein, serum			
Total	6.0–8.0 grams/dl	60–80 g/l	m
Albumin	3.5–5.5 grams/dl	35–55 g/l	q
	52–68% of total	0.52–0.68 of total	a
Globulin			
$Alpha_1$	0.2–0.4 gram/dl	2–4 g/l	m
	2–5% of total	0.02–0.05 of total	a
$Alpha_2$	0.5–0.9 gram/dl	5–9 g/l	m
	7–14% of total	0.07–0.14 of total	a
Beta	0.6–1.1 grams/dl	6–11 g/l	m
	9–15% of total	0.09–0.15 of total	a
Gamma	0.7–1.7 grams/dl	7–17 g/l	m
	11–21% of total	0.11–0.21 of total	a
Protoporphyrin, erythrocyte	27–61 mcg/dl packed RBC	0.48–1.09 μmol/l packed RBC	
Pyruvate, blood	0.3–0.9 mg/dl	0.03–0.10 mmol/l	
Sodium, serum	136–145 mEq/liter	136–145 mmol/l	
Sulfates, inorganic, serum	0.8–1.2 mg/dl	83–125 μmol/l	
Testosterone, plasma			
Males	275–875 nanogm/dl	9.5–30 nmol/l	
Females	23–75 nanogm/dl	0.8–2.6 nmol/l	
Pregnant	38–190 nanogm/dl	1.3–6.6 nmol/l	
Thyroid-stimulating hormone (TSH), serum	0–7 microunits/ml	0–7 milliunits/l	
Thyroxine, free, serum	1.0–2.1 nanogm/dl	13–27 pmol/l	
Thyroxine (T_4), serum	4.4–9.9 mcg/dl	57–128 nmol/l	
Thyroxine binding globulin (TBG), serum (as thyroxine)	10–26 mcg/dl	129–335 nmol/l	
Thyroxine iodine, serum	2.9–6.4 mcg/dl	229–504 nmol/l	k
Triiodothyronine (T_3), serum	150–250 nanogm/dl	2.3–3.9 nmol/l	
Triiodothyronine (T_3) uptake, resin (T_3RU)	25–38% uptake	0.25–0.38 uptake	a
Transaminase, serum			
SGOT (aspartate aminotransferase, AST)	8–20 milliunits/ml (30°) 7–40 milliunits/ml (37°)	8–20 units/l (30 C) 7–40 units/l (37 C)	
SGPT (alanine aminotransferase, ALT)	8–20 milliunits/ml (30°) 5–35 milliunits/ml (37°)	8–20 units/l (30 C) 5–35 units/l (37 C)	f f
Triglycerides, serum	40–150 mg/dl	0.4–1.5 g/l 0.45–1.71 mmol/l	r
Urate, serum			
Males	2.5–8.0 mg/dl	0.15–0.48 mmol/l	
Females	1.5–7.0 mg/dl	0.09–0.42 mmol/l	
Urea			
Blood	21–43 mg/dl	3.5–7.3 mmol/l	
Plasma or serum	24–49 mg/dl	4.0–8.3 mmol/l	
Urea nitrogen			
Blood	10–20 mg/dl	7.1–14.3 mmol/l	k
Plasma or serum	11–23 mg/dl	7.9–16.4 mmol/l	
Viscosity, serum	1.4–1.8 times water	1.4–1.8 times water	
Vitamin A, serum	20–80 mcg/dl	0.70–2.8 μmol/l	
Vitamin B_{12}, serum	180–900 picogm/ml	133–664 pmol/l	

REFERENCE VALUES FOR URINE
(For some procedures the reference values may vary depending upon the method used)

	Conventional Units	S.I. Units	Notes
Acetone and acetoacetate, qualitative	Negative	Negative	
Albumin			
Qualitative	Negative	Negative	
Quantitative	10–100 mg/24 hrs	10–100 mg/24 h 0.15–1.5 μmol/24 h	q
Aldosterone	3–20 mcg/24 hrs	8.3–55 nmol/24 h	
Alpha amino nitrogen	50–200 mg/24 hrs	3.6–14.3 mmol/24 h	
Ammonia nitrogen	20–70 mEq/24 hrs	20–70 mmol/24 h	
Amylase	1–17 units/hr	1–17 units/h	f
Amylase/creatinine clearance ratio	1–4%	0.01–0.04	
Bilirubin, qualitative	Negative	Negative	
Calcium			
Low Ca diet	Less than 150 mg/24 hrs	Less than 3.8 mmol/24 h	
Usual diet	Less than 250 mg/24 hrs	Less than 6.3 mmol/24 h	
Catecholamines			
Epinephrine	Less than 10 mcg/24 hrs	Less than 55 nmol/24 h	
Norepinephrine	Less than 100 mcg/24 hrs	Less than 590 nmol/24 h	
Total free catecholamines	4–126 mcg/24 hrs	24–745 nmol/24 h	s
Total metanephrines	0.1–1.6 mg/24 hrs	0.5–8.1 μmol/24 h	t
Chloride	110–250 mEq/24 hrs (Varies with intake)	110–250 mmol/24 h (Varies with intake)	
Chorionic gonadotropin	0	0	
Copper	0–50 mcg/24 hrs	0–0.80 μmol/24 h	
Cortisol, free	10–100 mcg/24 hrs	27.6–276 nmol/24 h	
Creatine			
Males	0–40 mg/24 hrs	0–0.30 mmol/24 h	
Females	0–100 mg/24 hrs (Higher in children and during pregnancy)	0–0.76 mmol/24 h (Higher in children and during pregnancy)	
Creatinine	15–25 mg/kg body weight/24 hrs	0.13–0.22 mmol•kg^{-1}body weight/24 h	
Creatinine clearance			
Males	110–150 ml/min	110–150 ml/min	
Females	105–132 ml/min (1.73 sq meter surface area)	105–132 ml/min (1.73 m^2 surface area)	
Cystine or cysteine, qualitative	Negative	Negative	
Dehydroepiandrosterone	Less than 15% of total 17-ketosteroids	Less than 0.15 of total 17-ketosteroids	a
Males	0.2–2.0 mg/24 hrs	0.7–6.9 μmol/24 h	
Females	0.2–1.8 mg/24 hrs	0.7–6.2 μmol/24 h	
Delta aminolevulinic acid	1.3–7.0 mg/24 hrs	10–53 μmol/24 h	
Estrogens			
Males			
Estrone	3–8 μg/24 hrs	11–30 nmol/24 h	
Estradiol	0–6 μg/24 hrs	0–22 nmol/24 h	
Estriol	1–11 μg/24 hrs	3–38 nmol/24 h	
Total	4–25 μg/24 hrs	14–90 nmol/24 h	u
Females			
Estrone	4–31 μg/24 hrs	15–115 nmol/24 h	
Estradiol	0–14 μg/24 hrs	0–51 nmol/24 h	
Estriol	0–72 μg/24 hrs	0–250 nmol/24 h	
Total	5–100 μg/24 hrs (Markedly increased during pregnancy)	18–360 nmol/24 h (Markedly increased during pregnancy)	u
Glucose (as reducing substance)	Less than 250 mg/24 hrs	Less than 250 mg/24 h	
Hemoglobin and myoglobin, qualitative	Negative	Negative	

Table continued on following page

REFERENCE VALUES FOR URINE *Continued*
(For some procedures the reference values may vary depending upon the method used)

	Conventional Units	S.I. Units	Notes
Homogentisic acid, qualitative	Negative	Negative	
17-Hydroxycorticosteroids			
Males	3–9 mg/24 hrs	8.3–25 μmol/24 h	j
Females	2–8 mg/24 hrs	5.5–22 μmol/24 h	
5-Hydroxyindoleacetic acid			
Qualitative	Negative	Negative	
Quantitative	Less than 9 mg/24 hrs	Less than 47 μmol/24 h	
17-Ketosteroids			
Males	6–18 mg/24 hrs	21–62 μmol/24 h	l
Females	4–13 mg/24 hrs (Varies with age)	14–45 μmol/24 h (Varies with age)	
Magnesium	6.0–8.5 mEq/24 hrs	3.0–4.3 mmol/24 h	
Metanephrines (see Catecholamines)			
Osmolality	38–1400 mOsm/kg water	38–1400 mmol/kg water	n
pH	4.6–8.0, average 6.0 (Depends on diet)	4.6–8.0, average 6.0 (Depends on diet)	p
Phenolsulfonphthalein excretion (PSP)	25% or more in 15 min 40% or more in 30 min 55% or more in 2 hrs (After injection of 1 ml PSP intravenously)	0.25 or more in 15 min 0.40 or more in 30 min 0.55 or more in 2 h (After injection of 1 ml PSP intravenously)	a
Phenylpyruvic acid, qualitative	Negative	Negative	
Phosphorus	0.9–1.3 gram/24 hrs	29–42 mmol/24 h	
Porphobilinogen			
Qualitative	Negative	Negative	
Quantitative	0–0.2 mg/dl Less than 2.0 mg/24 hrs	0–0.9 μmol/l Less than 9 μmol/24 h	
Porphyrins			
Coproporphyrin	50–250 mcg/24 hrs	77–380 nmol/24 h	
Uroporphyrin	10–30 mcg/24 hrs	12–36 nmol/24 h	
Potassium	25–100 mEq/24 hrs (Varies with intake)	25–100 mmol/24 h (Varies with intake)	
Pregnanediol			
Males	0.4–1.4 mg/24 hrs	1.2–4.4 μmol/24 h	
Females			
Proliferative phase	0.5–1.5 mg/24 hrs	1.6–4.7 μmol/24 h	
Luteal phase	2.0–7.0 mg/24 hrs	6.2–22 μmol/24 h	
Postmenopausal phase	0.2–1.0 mg/24 hrs	0.6–3.1 μmol/24 h	
Pregnanetriol	Less than 2.5 mg/24 hrs in adults	Less than 7.4 μmol/24 h in adults	
Protein			
Qualitative	Negative	Negative	
Quantitative	10–150 mg/24 hrs	10–150 mg/24 h	m
Sodium	130–260 mEq/24 hrs (Varies with intake)	130–260 mmol/24 h (Varies with intake)	
Specific gravity	1.003–1.030	1.003–1.030	
Titratable acidity	20–40 mEq/24 hrs	20–40 mmol/24 h	
Urate	200–500 mg/24 hrs (With normal diet)	1.2–3.0 mmol/24 h (With normal diet)	
Urobilinogen	Up to 1.0 Ehrlich unit/2 hrs (1–3 PM) 0–4.0 mg/24 hrs	Up to 1.0 Ehrlich unit/2 h (1–3 PM) 0–6.8 μmol/24 h	
Vanillylmandelic acid (VMA) (4-hydroxy-3-methoxymandelic acid)	1–8 mg/24 hrs	5–40 μmol/24 h	

REFERENCE VALUES FOR THERAPEUTIC DRUG MONITORING

Drug	Therapeutic Range	Toxic Levels	Proprietary Names
Antibiotics			
Amikacin, serum	15–25 mcg/ml	Peak: >35 mcg/ml Trough: >5–8 mcg/ml	Amikin
Chloramphenicol, serum	10–20 mcg/ml	>25 mcg/ml	Chloromycetin
Gentamicin, serum	5–10 mcg/ml	Peak: >12 mcg/ml Trough: >2 mcg/ml	Garamycin
Tobramycin, serum	5–10 mcg/ml	Peak: >12 mcg/ml Trough: >2 mcg/ml	Nebcin
Anticonvulsants			
Carbamazepine, serum	5–12 mcg/ml	>12 mcg/ml	Tegretol
Ethosuximide, serum	40–100 mcg/ml	>100 mcg/ml	Zarontin
Phenobarbital, serum	10–30 mcg/ml	Vary widely because of developed tolerance	
Phenytoin, serum (diphenylhydantoin)	10–20 mcg/ml	>20 mcg/ml	Dilantin
Primidone, serum	5–12 mcg/ml	>15 mcg/ml	Mysoline
Valproic acid, serum	50–100 mcg/ml	>100 mcg/ml	Depakene
Analgesics			
Acetaminophen, serum	10–20 mcg/ml	>250 mcg/ml	Tylenol Datril
Salicylate, serum	100–250 mcg/ml	>300 mcg/ml	
Bronchodilator			
Theophylline (aminophylline)	10–20 mcg/ml	>20 mcg/ml	
Cardiovascular drugs			
Digitoxin, serum	15–25 nanogm/ml (Specimen obtained 12–24 hrs after last dose)	>25 nanogm/ml	Crystodigin
Digoxin, serum	0.8–2 nanogm/ml (Specimen obtained 12–24 hrs after last dose)	>2.4 nanogm/ml	Lanoxin
Disopyramide, serum	2–5 mcg/ml	>5 mcg/ml	Norpace
Lidocaine, serum	1.5–5 mcg/ml	>5 mcg/ml	Anestacon Xylocaine
Procainamide, serum	4–10 mcg/ml *10–30 mcg/ml (*Procainamide + *N*-Acetyl Procainamide)	>16 mcg/ml *>30 mcg/ml	Pronestyl
Propranolol, serum	50–100 nanogm/ml	Variable	Inderal
Quinidine, serum	2–5 mcg/ml	>10 mcg/ml	Cardioquin Quinaglute Quinidex Quinora
Psychopharmacologic drugs			
Amitriptyline, serum	*120–150 nanogm/ml (*Amitriptyline + Nortriptyline)	*>500 nanogm/ml	Amitril Elavil Endep Etrafon Limbitrol Triavil
Bupropion	25–100 nanogm/ml	N/A	Wellbutrin
Desipramine, serum	*150–300 nanogm/ml (*Desipramine + Imipramine)	*>500 nanogm/ml	Norpramin Pertofrane
Fluoxitine	100–800 nanogm/ml (Lower levels may provide adequate clinical response)	N/A	Prozac
Haloperidol	3–20 nanogm/ml	N/A	Haldol
Imipramine, serum	*150–300 nanogm/ml (*Imipramine + Desipramine)	*>500 nanogm/ml	Antipress Imavate Janimine Presamine Tofranil
Lithium, serum	0.8–1.2 mEq/liter (Specimen obtained 12 hrs after last dose)	>2.0 mEq/liter	Lithobid Lithotabs
Nortriptyline, serum	50–150 nanogm/ml	>500 nanogm/ml	Aventyl Pamelor
Trazodone	900–2100 nanogm/ml	N/A	Desyrel

REFERENCE VALUES IN TOXICOLOGY

	Conventional Units	S.I. Units	Notes
Arsenic, blood	3.5–7.2 mcg/dl	0.47–0.96 μmol/l	
Arsenic, urine	Less than 100 mcg/24 hrs	Less than 1.3 μmol/24 h	
Bromides, serum	0	0	
	Toxic levels: Above 17 mmol/l	Toxic levels: Above 17 mmol/l	
Carbon monoxide, blood	Up to 5% saturation	Up to 0.5 saturation	
	Symptoms occur with 20% saturation	Symptoms occur with 0.20 saturation	a
Ethanol, blood	Less than 0.005%	Less than 1 mmol/l	
Marked intoxication	0.3–0.4%	65–87 mmol/l	
Alcoholic stupor	0.4–0.5%	87–109 mmol/l	
Coma	Above 0.5%	Above 109 mmol/l	
Lead, blood	0–40 mcg/dl	0–2 μmol/l	
Lead, urine	Less than 100 mcg/24 hrs	Less than 0.48 μmol/24 h	
Mercury, urine	Less than 100 mcg/24 hrs	Less than 50 nmol/24 h	

REFERENCE VALUES FOR CEREBROSPINAL FLUID

	Conventional Units	S.I. Units	Notes
Cells	Fewer than 5/cu mm; all mononuclear	Fewer than 5/μl; all mononuclear	
Chloride	120–130 mEq/liter	120–130 mmol/l	
	(20 mEq/liter higher than serum)	(20 mmol/l higher than serum)	
Electrophoresis	Predominantly albumin	Predominantly albumin	
Glucose	50–75 mg/dl	2.8–4.2 mmol/l	
	(20 mg/dl less than serum)	(1.1 mmol/less than serum)	
IgG			
Children under 14	Less than 8% of total protein	Less than 0.08 of total protein	a,m
Adults	Less than 14% of total protein	Less than 0.14 of total protein	
Pressure	70–180 mm water	70–180 mm water	g
Protein, total	15–45 mg/dl	0.150–0.450 g/l	m
	(Higher, up to 70 mg/dl, in elderly adults and children)	(Higher, up to 0.70 g/l, in elderly adults and children)	

REFERENCE VALUES FOR GASTRIC ANALYSIS

	Conventional Units	S.I. Units	Notes
Basal gastric secretion (1 hour)			
Concentration	(Mean ± 1 S.D.)	(Mean ± 1 S.D.)	
Males	25.8 ± 1.8 mEq/liter	25.8 ± 1.8 mmol/l	
Females	20.3 ± 3.0 mEq/liter	20.3 ± 3.0 mmol/l	
Output	(Mean ± 1 S.D.)	(Mean ± 1 S.D.)	
Males	2.57 ± 0.16 mEq/hr	2.57 ± 0.16 mmol/h	
Females	1.61 ± 0.18 mEq/hr	1.61 ± 0.18 mmol/h	
After histamine stimulation			
Normal	Mean output 11.8 mEq/hr	Mean output 11.8 mmol/h	
Duodenal ulcer	Mean output 15.2 mEq/hr	Mean output 15.2 mmol/h	
After maximal histamine stimulation			
Normal	Mean output 22.6 mEq/hr	Mean output 22.6 mmol/h	
Duodenal ulcer	Mean output 44.6 mEq/hr	Mean output 44.6 mmol/h	
Volume, fasting stomach content	50–100 ml	50–100 ml	
Emptying time	3–6 hrs	3–6 h	
Color	Opalescent or colorless	Opalescent or colorless	
Specific gravity	1.006–1.009	1.006–1.009	
pH (adults)	0.9–1.5	0.9–1.5	p

GASTROINTESTINAL ABSORPTION TESTS

	Conventional Units	S.I. Units
D-Xylose absorption test	After an 8 hour fast, 10 ml/kg body weight of a 0.05 solution of D-xylose is given by mouth. Nothing further by mouth is given until the test has been completed. All urine voided during the following 5 hours is pooled, and blood samples are taken at 0, 60, and 120 minutes. Normally 0.26 (range 0.16–0.33) of ingested xylose is excreted within 5 hours, and the serum xylose reaches a level between 25 and 40 mg/100 dl after 1 hour and is maintained at this level for another 60 minutes.	No change
Vitamin A absorption	A fasting blood specimen is obtained and 200,000 units of vitamin A in oil is given by mouth. Serum vitamin A level should rise to twice fasting level in 3 to 5 hours.	No change

REFERENCE VALUES FOR FECES

	Conventional Units	S.I. Units	Notes
Bulk	100–200 grams/24 hrs	100–200 g/24 h	
Dry matter	23–32 grams/24 hrs	23–32 g/24 h	
Fat, total	Less than 6.0 grams/24 hrs	Less than 6.0 g/24 h	
Nitrogen, total	Less than 2.0 grams/24 hrs	Less than 2.0 g/24 h	
Urobilinogen	40–280 mg/24 hrs	40–280 mg/24 h	
Water	Approximately 65%	Approximately 0.65	a

REFERENCE VALUES FOR IMMUNOLOGIC PROCEDURES

	Conventional Units
Lymphocyte subsets	
T cells	60–85%
B cells	1–20%
T-helper cells	35–60%
T-suppressor cells	15–30%
T-H/S ratio	1.5–2.5
Complement	
C3	85–175 mg/dl
C4	15–45 mg/dl
CH_{50}	25–55 H_{50} units/ml
Tumor markers	
Carcinoembryonic antigen (CEA)	
(Roche)	Less than 5 nanogm/ml
(Abbott)	Less than 4.1 nanogm/ml
Alpha-fetoprotein (AFP)	Less than 10–30 nanogm/ml (depends on method)

REFERENCE VALUES FOR SEMEN ANALYSIS

	Conventional Units	S.I. Units	Notes
Volume	2–5 ml; usually 3–4 ml	2–5 ml; usually 3–4 ml	
Liquefaction	Complete in 15 min	Complete in 15 min	
pH	7.2–8.0; average 7.8	7.2–8.0; average 7.8	p
Leukocytes	Occasional or absent	Occasional or absent	
Count	60–150 million/ml Below 60 million/ml is abnormal	60–150 million/ml Below 60 million/ml is abnormal	
Motility	80% or more motile	0.80 or more motile	a
Morphology	80–90% normal forms	0.80–0.90 normal forms	a

ORAL GLUCOSE TOLERANCE TEST

The oral glucose tolerance test (OGTT) may be unnecessary if the fasting plasma glucose concentration is elevated (venous plasma ≥140 mg/dl or 7.8 mmol/l) on two occasions. The OGTT should be carried out only on patients who are ambulatory and otherwise healthy and who are known not to be taking agents that elevate the plasma glucose (see reference 10). The test should be conducted in the morning after at least 3 days of unrestricted diet (≥150 grams of carbohydrate) and physical activity. The subject should have fasted for at least 10 hours but no more than 16 hours. Water is permitted during the test period; however, the subject should remain seated and should not smoke throughout the test.

The dose of glucose administered should be 75 grams (1.75 grams per kg of ideal body weight, up to a maximum of 75 grams for children). Commercial preparations containing a suitable carbohydrate load are acceptable. If criteria for gestational diabetes are used, a dose of 100 grams of glucose is required.

A fasting blood sample should be collected, after which the glucose dose is taken within 5 minutes. Blood samples should be collected at 30 minute intervals for 2 hours (for gestational diabetes, fasting 1, 2, and 3 hours). The following diagnostic criteria have been recommended by the National Diabetes Data Group:

Normal OGTT in Nonpregnant Adults	Fasting venous plasma glucose <115 mg/dl (6.4 mmol/l); ½ h, 1 h, and 1½ h OGTT venous plasma glucose <200 mg/dl (11.1 mmol/l); 2 h OGTT venous plasma glucose <140 mg/dl (7.8 mmol/l)
Diabetes Mellitus in Nonpregnant Adults	Both the 2 hour sample *and* some other sample taken between administration of the 75 gram glucose dose and 2 hours later must show a venous plasma glucose ≥200 mg/dl (11.1 mmol/l)
Impaired Glucose Tolerance in Nonpregnant Adults	Three criteria must be met: Fasting venous plasma glucose <140 mg/dl (7.8 mmol/l); ½ h, 1 h, or 1½ h OGTT value ≥200 mg/dl (11.1 mmol/l); 2 h OGTT venous plasma glucose between 140 and 200 mg/dl (7.8 and 11.1 mmol/l)
Gestational Diabetes	Two or more of the following values after a 100 gram oral glucose challenge must be met or exceeded: (values are for venous plasma glucose)

Fasting	105 mg/dl	5.8 mmol/l
1h	190 mg/dl	10.6 mmol/l
2h	165 mg/dl	9.2 mmol/l
3h	145 mg/dl	8.1 mmol/l

Notes

a. Percentage is expressed as a decimal fraction.
b. Percentage may be expressed as a decimal fraction; however, when the result expressed is itself a variable fraction of another variable, the absolute value is more meaningful. There is no reason, other than custom, for expressing reticulocyte counts and differential leukocyte counts in percentages or decimal fractions rather than in absolute numbers.
c. Molecular weight of fibrinogen = 341,000 daltons.
d. Molecular weight of hemoglobin = 64,500 daltons. Because of disagreement as to whether the monomer or tetramer of hemoglobin should be used in the conversion, it has been recommended that the conventional grams per deciliter be retained. The tetramer is used in the table; values given should be multiplied by 4 to obtain concentration of the monomer.
e. Molecular weight of methemoglobin = 64,500 daltons. See note d above.
f. Enzyme units have not been changed in these tables because the proposed enzyme unit, the katal, has not been universally adopted (1 International Unit = 16.7 nkat).
g. It has been proposed that pressure be expressed in the pascal (1 mm Hg = 0.133 kPa); however, this convention has not been universally accepted.
h. Molecular weight of ceruloplasmin = 151,000 daltons.
i. "Fatty acids" includes a mixture of different aliphatic acids of varying molecular weight. A mean molecular weight of 284 daltons has been assumed in calculating the conversion factor.
j. Based upon molecular weight of cortisol 362.47 daltons.
k. The practice of expressing concentration of an organic molecule in terms of one of its constituent elements originated when measurements included a heterogeneous class of compounds (nonprotein nitrogenous compounds, iodine-containing compounds bound to serum proteins). It was carried over to expressing measurements of specific substances (urea, thyroxine), but the practice should be discarded. For iodine and nitrogen 1 mole is taken as the monoatomic form, although they occur as diatomic molecules.
l. Based upon molecular weight of dehydroepiandrosterone 288.41 daltons.
m. Weight per volume is retained as the unit because of the heterogeneous nature of the material measured.
n. The proposal that osmolality be reported as freezing point depression using the millikel-vin as the unit has not been received with universal enthusiasm. The milliosmole is not an S.I. unit, and the unit used here is the millimole.
o. Volumes per cent might be converted to a decimal fraction; however, this would not permit direct correlation with hemoglobin content, which is possible when oxygen content and capacity are expressed in molar quantities. One millimole of

hemoglobin combines with 4 millimoles of oxygen.

p. Hydrogen ion concentration in S.I. units would be expressed in nanomoles per liter; however, this change has not received general approval. Conversion can be calculated as antilog (−pH).

q. Albumin is expressed in grams per liter to be consistent with units used for other proteins. Concentration of albumin may be expressed in mmol/l also, an expression that permits assessment of binding capacity of albumin for substances such as bilirubin. Molecular weight of albumin is 65,000 daltons.

r. Most techniques for quantitating triglycerides measure the glycerol moiety, and the total mass is calculated using an average molecular weight. The factor given assumes a mean molecular weight of 875 daltons for triglycerides.

s. Calculated as norepinephrine, molecular weight 169.18 daltons.

t. Calculated as metanephrine, molecular weight 197.23 daltons.

u. Conversion factor calculated from molecular weights of estrone, estradiol, and estriol in proportions of 2:1:2 daltons.

References

1. AMA Drug Evaluations, 6th ed. Chicago, American Medical Association, 1986.
2. AMA Council on Scientific Affairs: J.A.M.A. *253*:2552, 1985.
3. Goodman, A. G., Gilman, L. S., Rall, T. W., and Murad, F.: Goodman and Gilman's The Pharmacological Basis of Therapeutics, 7th ed. New York, Macmillan, 1985.
4. Henry, J. B.: Clinical Diagnosis and Management by Laboratory Methods, 17th ed. Philadelphia, W. B. Saunders Company, 1984.
5. Henry, R. J., Cannon, D. C., and Winkleman, J. W.: Clinical Chemistry—Principles and Techniques, 2nd ed. New York, Harper & Row, 1974.
6. International Committee for Standardization in Hematology, International Federation of Clinical Chemistry and World Association of Pathology Societies: Clin. Chem. *19*:135, 1973.
7. Lundberg, G. D., Iverson, C., and Radulescu, G.: J.A.M.A. *255*:2247, 1986.
8. Miale, J. B.: Laboratory Medicine—Hematology, 6th ed. St. Louis, C. V. Mosby, 1982.
9. National Diabetes Data Group: Diabetes *28*:1039, 1979.
10. Page, C. H., and Vigourex, P.: The International System of Units (S.I.). U.S. Department of Commerce, National Bureau of Standards, Special Publication 330, 1974.
11. Physicians' Desk Reference, 43rd ed. Oradell, N.J., Medical Economics Company, 1989.
12. Scully, R. E., McNeely, B. U., and Mark, E. J.: N. Engl. J. Med. *314*:39, 1986.
13. Tietz, N. W.: Clinical Guide to Laboratory Tests. Philadelphia, W. B. Saunders Company, 1983.
14. Tietz, N. W.: Textbook of Clinical Chemistry. Philadelphia, W. B. Saunders Company, 1986.
15. Williams, W. J., Beutler, E., Erslev, A. J., and Lichtman, M. A.: Hematology, 3rd ed. New York, McGraw-Hill Book Company, 1983.

Some of the values have been established by the Clinical Pathology Laboratories, Emory University Hospital, Atlanta, Georgia, or by the Clinical Laboratories, Thomas Jefferson University Hospital, Philadelphia, Pennsylvania, and have not been published elsewhere.

Appendix II

NOMOGRAM FOR THE DETERMINATION OF BODY SURFACE AREA OF CHILDREN AND ADULTS

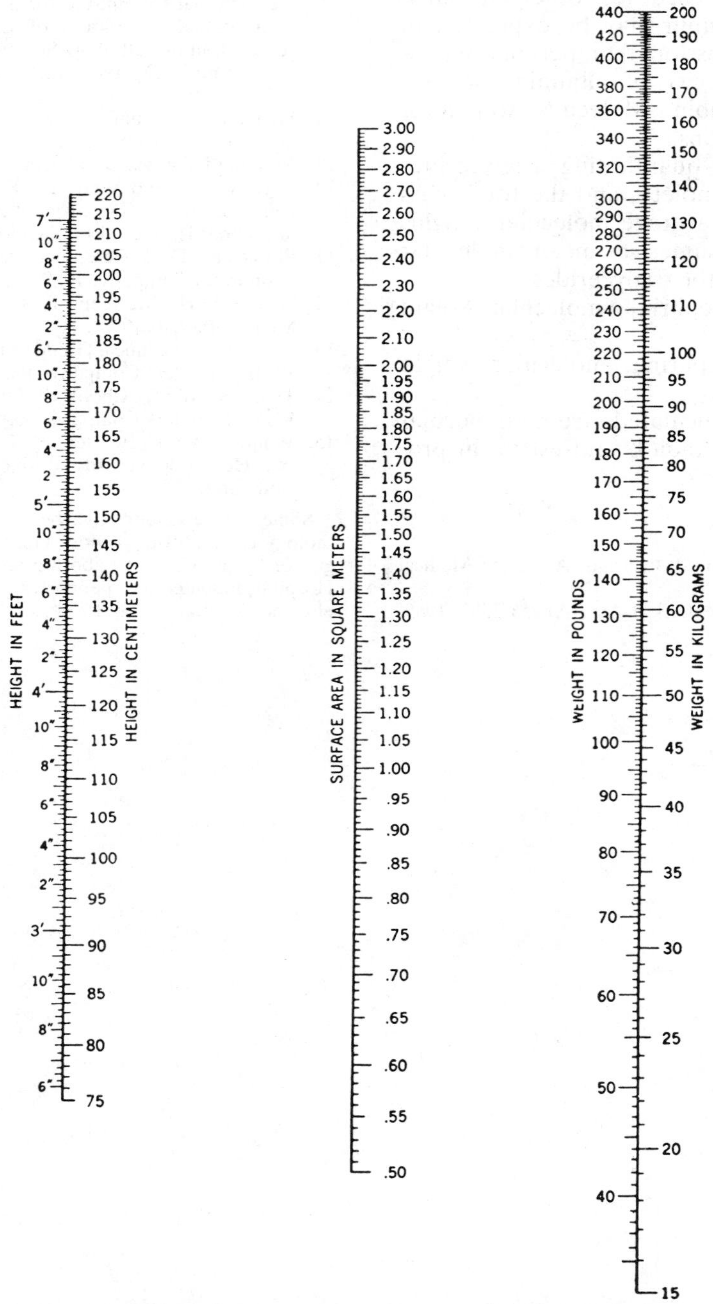

*From Boothby, W. M., and Sandiford, R. B.: Boston Med. Surg. J., *185*:337, 1921.

Appendix III

CONVERSION OF APOTHECARY'S MEASURES TO METRIC EQUIVALENTS

Weights

Apothecary	*Metric* Approximate		More Nearly Accurate
1 grain	60 mg	0.06 gm	0.06479 gm
2 grains	120 mg	0.12 gm	
3 grains	180 mg	0.2 gm	
5 grains	300 mg	0.3 gm	
15 grains	1000 mg	1.0 gm	
60 grains or 1 dram		4.0 gm	3.88 gm
240 grains or 4 drams, 1/2 oz		15.0 gm	
480 grains or 8 drams, 1 oz.		30.0 gm	31.103 gm
			31.103 gm (Troy)
			28.350 gm (Avoir.)
12 oz or 1 pound		360.0 gm	373.24177 gm
12 oz or 1 pound		260.0 gm	373.24177 gm (Troy)
16 oz or 1 pound		480.0 gm	453.592 gm (Avoir.)
3/4 grain		45 mg	
1/2 grain		30 mg	
3/8 grain		23 mg	
1/4 grain		15 mg	
1/6 grain		10 mg	
1/8 grain		8 mg	
1/10 grain		6 mg	
1/16 grain		4 mg	
1/32 grain		2 mg	
1/64 grain		1 mg	
1/100 grain		0.6 mg	
1/250 grain		0.25 mg	
1/300 grain		0.2 mg	
1/1000 grain		0.06 mg	

Liquid Measures

Apothecary	Approximate	More Nearly Accurate
1 minim	0.06 ml	0.06161 ml
3 minims	0.2 ml	
15 minims	1.0 ml	0.92415 ml*
60 minims, 1 fl. dram	4.0 ml	3.6967 ml
480 minims 1 fl oz.	30.0 ml	29.5737 ml
16 fl oz or 1 pt	500.0 ml	473.179 ml
32 fl oz or 1 qt	1000.0 ml	946.358 ml

*1 ml is equal to 16.23 minims.
Quantity of drug prescribed in grams per 2 ounces (60 ml) gives dose in grains per dram.

Appendix IV

CONVERSION OF POUNDS TO KILOGRAMS

Pounds → ↓	0	1	2	3	4	5	6	7	8	9
0	0.00	0.45	0.90	1.36	1.81	2.26	2.72	3.17	3.62	4.08
10	4.53	4.98	5.44	5.89	6.35	6.80	7.25	7.71	8.16	8.61
20	9.07	9.52	9.97	10.43	10.88	11.34	11.79	12.24	12.70	13.15
30	13.60	14.06	14.51	14.96	15.42	15.87	16.32	16.78	17.23	17.69
40	18.14	18.59	19.05	19.50	19.95	20.41	20.86	21.31	21.77	22.22
50	22.68	23.13	23.58	24.04	24.49	24.94	25.40	25.85	26.30	26.76
60	27.21	27.66	28.12	28.57	29.03	29.48	29.93	30.39	30.84	31.29
70	31.75	32.20	32.65	33.11	33.56	34.02	34.47	34.92	35.38	35.83
80	36.28	36.74	37.19	37.64	38.10	38.55	39.00	39.46	39.91	40.37
90	40.82	41.27	41.73	42.18	42.63	43.09	43.54	43.99	44.45	44.90
100	45.36	45.81	46.26	46.72	47.17	47.62	48.08	48.53	48.98	49.44
110	49.89	50.34	50.80	51.25	51.71	52.16	52.61	53.07	53.52	53.97
120	54.43	54.88	55.33	55.79	56.24	56.70	57.15	57.60	58.06	58.51
130	58.96	59.42	59.87	60.32	60.78	61.23	61.68	62.14	62.59	63.05
140	63.50	63.95	64.41	64.86	65.31	65.77	66.22	66.67	67.13	67.58
150	68.04	68.49	68.94	69.40	69.85	70.30	70.76	71.21	71.66	72.12
160	72.57	73.02	73.48	73.93	74.39	74.84	75.29	75.75	76.20	76.65
170	77.11	77.56	78.01	78.47	78.92	79.38	79.83	80.28	80.74	81.19
180	81.64	82.10	82.55	83.00	83.46	83.91	84.36	84.82	85.27	85.73
190	86.18	86.68	87.09	87.54	87.99	88.45	88.90	89.35	89.81	90.26
200	90.72	91.17	91.62	92.08	92.53	92.98	93.44	93.89	94.34	94.80

Appendix V

TABLE OF TEMPERATURE EQUIVALENTS CELSIUS (CENTIGRADE): FAHRENHEIT SCALE

Celsius: Fahrenheit $°F = (°C \times 9/5) + 32$				Fahrenheit: Celsius $C = (°F - 32) \times 5/9$					
C°	F°	C°	F°	F°	C°	F°	C°	F°	C°
−50	−58.0	49	120.2	−50	−46.7	99	37.2	157	69.4
−40	−40.0	50	122.0	−40	−40.0	100	37.7	158	70.0
−35	−31.0	51	123.8	−35	−37.2	101	38.3	159	70.5
−30	−22.0	52	125.6	−30	−34.4	102	38.8	160	71.1
−25	−13.0	53	127.4	−25	−31.7	103	39.4	161	71.6
−20	−4.0	54	129.2	−20	−28.9	104	40.0	162	72.2
−15	+5.0	55	131.0	−15	−26.6	105	40.5	163	72.7
−10	14.0	56	132.8	−10	−23.3	106	41.1	164	73.3
−5	23.0	57	134.6	−5	20.6	107	41.6	165	73.8
0	32.0	58	136.4	0	−17.7	108	42.2	166	74.4
+1	33.8	59	138.2	+1	−17.2	109	42.7	167	75.0
2	35.6	60	140.0	5	−15.0	110	43.3	168	75.5
3	37.4	61	141.8	10	−12.2	111	43.8	169	76.1
4	39.2	62	143.6	15	−9.4	112	44.4	170	76.6
5	41.0	63	145.4	20	−6.6	113	45.0	171	77.2
6	42.8	64	147.2	25	−3.8	114	45.5	172	77.7
7	44.6	65	149.0	30	−1.1	115	46.1	173	78.3
8	46.4	66	150.8	31	−0.5	116	46.6	174	78.8
9	48.2	67	152.6	32	0	117	47.2	175	79.4
10	50.0	68	154.4	33	+0.5	118	47.7	176	80.0
11	51.8	69	156.2	34	1.1	119	48.3	177	80.5
12	53.6	70	158.0	35	1.6	120	48.8	178	81.1
13	55.4	71	159.8	36	2.2	121	49.4	179	81.6
14	57.2	72	161.6	37	2.7	122	50.0	180	82.2
15	59.0	73	163.4	38	3.3	123	50.5	181	82.7
16	60.8	74	165.2	39	3.8	124	51.1	182	83.3
17	62.6	75	167.0	40	4.4	125	51.6	183	83.8
18	64.4	76	168.8	41	5.0	126	52.2	184	84.4
19	66.2	77	170.6	42	5.5	127	52.7	185	85.0
20	68.0	78	172.4	43	6.1	128	53.3	186	85.5
21	69.8	79	174.2	44	6.6	129	53.8	187	86.1
22	71.6	80	176.0	45	7.2	130	54.4	188	86.6
23	73.4	81	177.8	46	7.7	131	55.0	189	87.2
24	75.2	82	179.6	47	8.3	132	55.5	190	87.7
25	77.0	83	181.4	48	8.8	133	56.1	191	88.3
26	78.8	84	183.2	49	9.4	134	56.6	192	88.8
27	80.6	85	185.0	50	10.0	135	57.2	193	89.4
28	82.4	86	186.8	55	12.7	136	57.7	194	90.0
29	84.2	87	188.6	60	15.5	137	53.3	195	90.5
30	86.0	88	190.4	65	18.3	138	58.8	196	91.1
31	87.8	89	192.2	70	21.1	139	59.4	197	91.6
32	89.6	90	194.0	75	23.8	140	60.0	198	92.2
33	91.4	91	195.8	80	26.6	141	60.5	199	92.7
34	93.2	92	197.6	85	29.4	142	61.1	200	93.3
35	95.0	93	199.4	86	30.0	143	61.6	201	93.8
36	96.8	94	201.2	87	30.5	144	62.2	202	94.4
37	98.6	95	203.0	88	31.0	145	62.7	203	95.0
38	100.4	96	204.8	89	31.6	146	63.3	204	95.5
39	102.2	97	206.6	90	32.2	147	63.8	205	96.1
40	104.0	98	208.4	91	32.7	148	64.4	206	96.6
41	105.8	99	210.2	92	33.3	149	65.0	207	97.2
42	107.6	100	212.0	93	33.8	150	65.5	208	97.7
43	109.4	101	213.8	94	34.4	151	66.1	209	98.3
44	111.2	102	215.6	95	35.0	152	66.6	210	98.8
45	113.0	103	217.4	96	35.5	153	67.2	211	99.4
46	114.8	104	219.2	97	36.1	154	67.7	212	100.0
47	116.6	105	221.0	98	36.6	155	68.3	213	100.5
48	118.4	106	222.8	98.6	37.0	156	68.8	214	101.1

Appendix VI Recommendations of the U.S. Preventive Services Task Force, 1989

The U. S. Department of Health and Human Services convened the U.S. Preventive Services Task Force in 1984. The mandate of this expert panel was to evaluate the effectiveness of clinical preventive services—screening tests, counseling interventions, immunizations, and chemoprophylactic regimens—based on a systematic review of scientific evidence in published clinical research. Over a period of 5 years, the task force studied the evidence for 169 preventive interventions, reviewing about 2500 relevant clinical trials and other epidemiologic studies. The 481-page report of the task force, the *Guide to Clinical Preventive Services,* was published in 1989.[1] It is the most extensive work to date in the field of preventive services. This appendix presents an overview of the task force methodology and a brief summary of the recommendations in the *Guide*.

Methodology

The U.S. Preventive Services Task Force adopted a structured methodology for reviewing the evidence and developing clinical practice recommendations. In developing their methodology, the U.S. task force drew on the experience and prior example of a similar effort undertaken by the Canadian Task Force on the Periodic Health Examination.[2] The reader is referred to the *Guide to Clinical Preventive Services* for details about this methodology. Recommendations were based almost entirely on the quality of the scientific evidence. Criteria were used to select 60 conditions that represented the leading causes of death and disability in the United States and to select preventive services to be evaluated for each of these conditions.

Preventive services selected were then required to satisfy predetermined criteria of effectiveness before being recommended for inclusion in periodic health examination. The determination of whether a preventive service met these criteria was based on a systematic review of the literature. Supporting evidence was graded on the basis of the quality of relevant studies; greater emphasis was given to well-conducted studies and to those studies whose designs provided more persuasive evidence of effectiveness. The final recommendations reflect the quality of the supporting evidence. Preventive services were generally not recommended for routine use if the science indicated that they were ineffective.

The recommendations summarized in this appendix apply only to *asymptomatic* persons who have no clinical evidence of the target condition. Thus, recommendations against the routine performance of a screening test would not necessarily apply to patients with suspicious signs or symptoms, a history of the target condition, or known risk factors for the disease. Also, the recommendations apply only to activities in the clinical setting. They should not be extrapolated for use in other activities, such as in shopping center health screening booths, public education campaigns, or legislative or regulatory actions. Finally, the term clinician also is used to include nonphysician primary care providers (e.g., nurses, nurse practitioners, physicians' assistants). These other providers often play an important role in the delivery of preventive services and may perform them more effectively than physicians.

Recommendations

Only short excerpts from the *Guide to Clinical Preventive Services* are included in this appendix, and the reader is referred to the original document for further details. The task force recommendations and the individual chapters in the report itself are organized around the 60 target conditions evaluated by the panel. Condensed versions of the task force recommendations begin each chapter; they are reprinted in this appendix. The remainder of each chapter, not included here, provides a complete review of the scientific evidence for the preventive service, a summary of relevant official recommendations from other groups, and detailed instructions for the practitioner that include information on dosages, recommended frequency, and other specifics.

Tables

The preventive services recommended by the task force for inclusion in the periodic health examination are then summarized in this appendix in eight tables, organized by age group. The reader should refer to appropriate chapters in the *Guide to Clinical Preventive Services* to obtain more detailed information about the proper indications for specific preventive services than can be provided in these tables. The preventive services listed reflect only those topics evaluated by the task force.

The tables are provided for general guidance. Clinicians should use individual judgment to determine what is most appropriate for each patient, and they may wish to add other preventive services to this list. The patient's medical history, risk factors, and other individual circumstances must be considered in designing an appropriate periodic health examination for each patient. Since the evaluations were defined by specific preventive services, general procedures such as the medical history and the physical examination were not examined in their entirety.

A frequency schedule for periodic health visits is recommended in each table. These intervals are considered clinically prudent; however, scientific data are lacking to determine the optimal frequency for such visits. Clinicians should exercise discretion in selecting an appropriate schedule, especially for patients with abnormal signs or symptoms and those with chronic illnesses. The preventive services listed in each table are not necessarily recommended at every periodic visit. For example, although thyroid function tests may be clinically prudent in elderly women, they are not recommended annually even though periodic visits in this age group are recommended once a year.

Many of the preventive services in the tables are recommended only for members of high-risk groups and are not considered appropriate in the routine examination of all persons in the age group. This is due to differences in disease risk among individuals in different risk categories and the effectiveness of some preventive services in only certain populations. The specific risk groups for which the maneuver is considered appropriate are identified by an annotated high-risk code accompanying each table. The reader should refer to appropriate chapters in the *Guide to Clinical Preventive Services* for more detailed criteria to help identify individuals at increased risk.

Risk factors that are especially important for clinicans to identify at an early stage but that are not considered appropriate for routine screening are listed under the heading *Remain Alert For*. Many of the disorders appearing under this heading are often overlooked by clinicians owing to failure to recognize suggestive signs or symptoms or the importance of early identification.

Although the preventive services listed in the tables can serve as the basis for designing periodic health examinations devoted entirely to disease prevention, they may also be performed during visits for other reasons (e.g., illness visits, chronic disease checkups) when indicated. For patients with limited access to care, the illness visit may provide the only realistic opportunity for the clinician to discuss prevention. In addition, certain illness visits provide excellent opportunities for related preventive interventions (e.g., smoking cessation counseling for the smoker presenting with acute bronchitis).

Busy clinicians may not be able to perform all recommended preventive services during a single clinical encounter. The clinician should use discretion in selecting appropriate preventive services from these lists and may wish to give special emphasis to preventive services aimed at the leading causes of illness and disability in the age group. Age-specific leading causes of death are listed in each table to aid the clinician in making this assessment. Recommended preventive services that cannot be performed by the clinician can then be scheduled for a later visit.

Immunizations appearing in the tables are those recommended on a routine basis and do not apply to persons with special exposures to infected individuals. The reader is referred to the *Guide to Clinical Preventive Services* for detailed guidelines on immunization in such circumstances.

Acknowledgment

The authors wish to acknowledge the assistance of Douglas B. Kamerow, M.D., M.P.H. and Steven H. Woolf, M.D., M.P.H., Office of Disease Prevention and Health Promotion, U.S. Public Health Service.

References

1. U.S. Preventive Services Task Force: Guide to Clinical Preventive Services. Baltimore, MD, Williams & Wilkins, 1989.
2. Canadian Task Force on the Periodic Health Examination: The periodic health examination. Can. Med. Assoc. J. *121*:1194–1254, 1979.

1. Screening for Asymptomatic Coronary Artery Disease

Recommendation. Clinicians should emphasize the primary prevention of coronary artery disease by periodically screening for high blood pressure and high serum cholesterol and by routinely investigating behavioral risk factors for coronary artery disease such as tobacco use, dietary fat and cholesterol intake, and inadequate physical activity. Secondary prevention of coronary artery disease (screening) by performing routine electrocardiography to screen asymptomatic persons is not recommended. It may be clinically prudent to perform screening electrocardiograms (ECGs) in certain high-risk groups. Routine resting or exercise ECG screening before entering athletic programs is not recommended for asymptomatic children, adolescents, or young adults.

2. Screening for High Blood Cholesterol

Recommendation. Periodic measurement of total serum cholesterol is most important for middle-aged men, and it may also be clinically prudent in young men, women, and the elderly. All patients should receive periodic counseling regarding dietary intake of fat (especially saturated fat) and cholesterol.

3. Screening for Hypertension

Recommendation. Blood pressure should be measured regularly in all persons 3 years of age and above.

4. Screening for Cerebrovascular Disease

Recommendation. There is currently insufficient evidence to recommend for or against auscultation for carotid bruits or noninvasive testing for carotid stenosis as effective screening strategies to prevent cerebrovascular disease in asymptomatic persons. It may be clinically prudent to include cervical auscultation in the physical examination of patients with established risk factors for cerebrovascular or cardiovascular disease. All persons should be screened for hypertension, and some should be tested for high blood cholesterol. Clinicians should also provide counseling about smoking, exercise, and dietary fat consumption.

5. Screening for Peripheral Arterial Disease

Recommendation. Routine screening for peripheral arterial disease in asymptomatic persons is not recommended. Clinicians should be alert for signs of peripheral arterial disease in persons at increased risk and should thoroughly evaluate those patients with clinical evidence of vascular disease.

6. Screening for Breast Cancer

Recommendation. All women over age 40 should receive an annual clinical breast examination. Mammography every 1 to 2 years is recommended for all women beginning at age 50 and concluding at approximately age 75 unless pathology has been detected. It may be prudent to begin mammography at an earlier age for women at high risk for breast cancer. Although the teaching of breast self-examination is not specifically recommended at this time, there is insufficient evidence to recommended any change in current breast self-examination practices.

7. Screening for Colorectal Cancer

Recommendation. There is insufficient evidence to recommend for or against fecal occult blood testing or sigmoidoscopy as effective screening tests for colorectal cancer in asymptomatic persons. There are also inadequate grounds for discontinuing this form of screening where it is currently practiced or for withholding it from persons who request it. It may be clinically prudent to offer screening to persons aged 50 and older with known risk factors for colorectal cancer.

8. Screening for Cervical Cancer

Recommendation. Regular Papanicolaou (Pap) testing is recommended for all women who are or who have been sexually active. Pap smears should begin with the onset of sexual activity and should be repeated every 1 to 3 years at the physician's discretion. They may be discontinued at age 65 if previous smears have been consistently normal.

9. Screening for Prostate Cancer

Recommendation. There is insufficient evidence to recommend for or against routine digital rectal examinations as an effective screening test for prostate cancer in asymptomatic men. Transrectal ultrasound and serum tumor markers are not recommended for routine screening in asymptomatic men.

10. Screening for Lung Cancer

Recommendation. Screening asymptomatic persons for lung cancer by performing routine chest radiography or sputum cytology is not recommended.

11. Screening for Skin Cancer

Recommendation. Routine screening for skin cancer is recommended for persons at high risk. Clinicians should advise all patients with increased outdoor exposure to use sunscreen preparations and other measures to protect their skin from ultraviolet rays. Currently, there is no evidence for or against counseling patients to perform skin self-examination.

12. Screening for Testicular Cancer

Recommendation. Periodic screening for testicular cancer by testicular examination is recommended for men with a history of cryptorchidism, orchiopexy, or testicular atrophy. There is insufficient evidence of clinical benefit or harm to recommend for or against routine screening of other asymptomatic men for testicular cancer. Clinicians should advise adolescent and young adult males to seek prompt medical attention for testicular symptoms such as pain, swelling, or heaviness. Currently, there is insufficient evidence for or against counseling patients to perform periodic self-examination of the testicles.

13. Screening for Ovarian Cancer

Recommendation. Screening for asymptomatic women for ovarian cancer is not recommended. It is prudent to examine the uterine adnexa when performing a gynecologic examination for other reasons.

14. Screening for Pancreatic Cancer

Recommendation. Routine screening for pancreatic cancer in asymptomatic persons is not recommended.

15. Screening for Oral Cancer

Recommendation. Routine screening of asymptomatic persons for oral cancer by primary care clinicians is not recommended. It may be prudent for clinicians to perform careful examinations for cancerous lesions of the oral cavity in patients who use tobacco or excessive amounts of alcohol as well as in those with suspicious symptoms or lesions detected through self-examination. All patients should be counseled to receive regular dental examinations, to discontinue the use of all forms of tobacco, and to limit consumption of alcohol. Persons with increased exposure to sunlight should be advised to take protective measures to protect their lips and skin from the harmful effects of ultraviolet rays.

16. Screening for Diabetes Mellitus

Recommendation. An oral glucose tolerance test for gestational diabetes mellitus is recommended for all pregnant women between 24 and 28 weeks of gestation. Routine screening for diabetes in asymptomatic nonpregnant adult patients, using plasma glucose measurement or urinalysis, is not recommended for the general population, but it may be appropriate in selected high-risk groups.

17. Screening for Thyroid Disease

Recommendation. Screening for congenital hypothyroidism is recommended for all neonates during the first week of life. Routine screening for thyroid disorders is otherwise not warranted in asymptomatic adults or children. Persons with a history of irradiation to the upper body may benefit from regular physical examination of the thyroid.

18. Screening for Obesity

Recommendation. All children and adults should receive periodic height and weight measurements.

19. Screening for Phenylketonuria

Recommendation. Screening for phenylketonuria (PKU) is recommended for all newborns prior to discharge from the nursery. Infants who are tested before 24 hours of age should receive a repeat screening test before the third week of life. Routine prenatal screening for maternal PKU is not recommended.

20. Screening for Hepatitis B

Recommendation. All pregnant women should be tested for hepatitis B surface antigen at their first prenatal visit. The test may be repeated in the third trimester in women at increased risk of exposure during pregnancy.

21. Screening for Tuberculosis

Recommendation. Tuberculin skin testing of asymptomatic persons should be performed on those at high risk of acquiring tuberculosis.

22. Screening for Syphilis

Recommendation. Routine screening for syphilis in asymptomatic persons is recommended for those in high-risk groups and for pregnant women.

23. Screening for Gonorrhea

Recommendation. Routine testing for gonorrhea in asymptomatic persons is recommended for persons at high risk and for pregnant women. An ophthalmic antibiotic should be applied topically to the eyes of all newborns immediately after birth to prevent ophthalmia neonatorum.

24. Screening for Infection with Human Immunodeficiency Virus

Recommendation. Screening for infection with human immunodeficiency virus (HIV) should be offered periodically to persons seeking treatment for sexually transmitted diseases, intravenous drug users, homosexual and bisexual men, and others at increased risk of infection. Testing should also be offered to pregnant women (or women contemplating pregnancy) who are at increased risk for HIV infection. Testing should not be performed in the absence of informed consent and adequate pretest and post-test counseling. Clinicians should be careful to use proper tests and qualified laboratories. Seropositive persons require adequate post-test counseling, and partners should be properly notified. Persons with negative tests results also require counseling and repeat testing when appropriate.

25. Screening for Chlamydial Infection

Recommendation. Routine testing for *Chlamydia trachomatis* infection is recommended for asymptomatic persons at high risk of infection. Pregnant women in high-risk categories should be tested at the first prenatal visit. Ophthalmic antibiotics should be applied topically to the eyes of all newborns immediately after birth to help prevent ophthalmia neonatorum.

26. Screening for Genital Herpes Simplex

Recommendations. Screening for genital herpes simplex virus (HSV) infection is recommended for pregnant women with active lesions.

27. Screening for Asymptomatic Bacterium Hematuria and Proteinuria

Recommendation. Period urine testing of asymptomatic persons is recommended for those with diabetes mellitus and for pregnant women. In addition, it may also be clinically prudent to screen preschool children and persons aged 60 and older.

28. Screening for Anemia

Recommendation. All infants and pregnant women should be tested for anemia. Routine screening of other asymptomatic persons for anemia is not recommended in the absence of clinical indications.

29. Screening for Hemoglobinopathies

Recommendation. Hemoglobin analysis is recommended for all newborns at risk for hemoglobin disorders. Hemoglobin analysis should also be discussed and offered to adolescents and young adults at risk for hemoglobinopathies and should be performed routinely at the first prenatal visit on all pregnant black women. All screening efforts should be accompanied by comprehensive counseling and treatment services.

30. Screening for Lead Toxicity

Recommendation. Annual lead screening is recommended for all children aged 9 months to 6 years who are at high risk for the development of lead toxicity, especially those who live in or frequently visit older housing that is dilapidated or undergoing renovation.

31. Screening for Diminished Visual Acuity

Recommendation. Vision screening is recommended for all children once before entering school, preferably at age 3 or 4. Routine vision testing is not recommended as a component of the periodic health examination of asymptomatic school children. Clinicians should be alert for signs of ocular misalignment when examining all infants and children. Vision screening of adolescents and adults is not recommended, but it may be appropriate in the elderly.

32. Screening for Glaucoma

Recommendation. There is insufficient evidence to recommend routine performance of tonometry by primary care physicians as an effective screening test for glaucoma. It may be clinically prudent, however, to advise patients aged 65 and older to be tested periodically for glaucoma by an eye specialist.

33. Screening for Hearing Impairment

Recommendation. Screening should be performed on all neonates at high risk for hearing impairment. High-risk children who have not been tested at birth should be screened before age 3, but there is insufficient evidence of accuracy to recommend routine audiologic testing of all children in this age group. There is also insufficient evidence of benefit to recommend for or against hearing screening of asymptomatic children beyond age 3. Screening is not recommended for asymptomatic adolescents or adults not exposed routinely to excessive noise. Elderly patients should be evaluated regarding their hearing, counseled regarding the availability and use of hearing aids, and referred appropriately for any abnormalities.

34. Screening for Intrauterine Growth Retardation

Recommendation. Women at increased risk for delivering a growth-retarded infant should receive ultrasound examination early in the second trimester to determine gestational age and in the third trimester to measure the size of critical fetal structures. Routine ultrasound screening is otherwise not recommended in normal pregnancies, although physicians may wish to consider ultrasound dating in pregnant women with uncertain menstrual histories. All pregnant women should receive appropriate counseling regarding smoking, alcohol and other drug abuse, and nutrition.

35. Screening for Preeclampsia

Recommendation. All pregnant women should receive systolic and diastolic blood pressure measurements at the first prenatal visit and periodically throughout the third trimester.

36. Screening for Rubella

Recommendation. Serologic testing for rubella antibodies should be performed at the first clinical encounter with all pregnant and nonpregnant women of childbearing age who lack evidence of immunity. Susceptible nonpregnant women who agree not to become pregnant for 3 months should be vaccinated. Susceptible pregnant women should not be vaccinated until immediately after delivery.

37. Screening for Rh Incompatibility

Recommendation. All pregnant women should receive ABO/Rh blood typing and testing for anti-Rh(D) antibody at their first prenatal visit. Unsensitized Rh-negative women should receive Rh(D) immune globulin at 28-30 weeks' gestation and within 72 hours after delivery, as well as after spontaneous or therapeutic abortion, ectopic pregnancy, amniocentesis, antepartum placental hemorrhage, or a transfusion of Rh-positive blood products.

38. Screening for Congenital Birth Defects

Recommendation. Amniocentesis for karyotyping should be offered to pregnant women aged 35 and older. Maternal serum alpha-fetoprotein should be measured on all pregnant women during weeks 16 to 18 in locations that have adequate counseling and follow-up services. Ultrasound examination is not recommended as a routine screening test for congenital defects.

39. Screening for Fetal Distress

Recommendation. Fetal heart rate should be measured by auscultation on all women in labor to detect signs of fetal distress. Electronic fetal monitoring should not be performed routinely on all women in labor. It should be reserved for pregnancies at increased risk of fetal distress.

40. Screening for Postmenopausal Osteoporosis

Recommendation. Routine radiologic screening to detect low bone mineral content is not recommended.

41. Screening for Risk of Low Back Injury

Recommendation. Screening asymptomatic persons for risk of low back injury is not recommended. Routine spinal radiographs of asymptomatic persons are also not recommended.

42. Screening for Dementia

Recommendation. Screening for cognitive impairment among asymptomatic persons is not recommended.

43. Screening for Abnormal Bereavement

Recommendation. Clinicians aware of the impending or recent death of a patient's loved one should assess potential risk factors for abnormal grieving and should provide emotional support for mourning. Clinicians should also remain alert for the signs and symptoms of pathologic bereavement.

44. Screening for Depression

Recommendation. The performance of routine screening tests for depression in asymptomatic persons is not recommended. Clinicians should maintain an especially high index of suspicion for depressive symptoms in those persons at increased risk for depression.

45. Screening for Suicidal Intent

Recommendation. Routine screening for suicidal intent is not recommended. Clinicians should be alert to signs of suicidal ideation in persons with established risk factors. Persons suspected of suicidal intent should be questioned regarding the extent of preparatory actions and referred for further evaluations if evidence of suicidal behavior is detected. Clinicians should be alert to symptoms of depression and should routinely ask patients about their use of alcohol and other drugs.

46. Screening for Violent Injuries

Recommendation. Routine screening interviews or examinations for evidence of violent injuries are not recommended. Children and adults presenting with unusual injuries should be examined with attention to possible abuse or neglect, and efforts should be made to prevent subsequent violent injury. Counseling and referral should be offered to those persons at high risk of becoming victims or perpetrators of violence.

47. Screening for Alcohol and Other Drug Abuse

Recommendation. All adolescents and adults should be asked to describe their use of alcohol and other drugs. Routine measurement of biochemical markers and drug testing are not recommended as the primary method of detecting alcohol and other drug abuse in asymptomatic persons. Persons in whom alcohol or other drug abuse or dependence is confirmed should receive appropriate counseling, treatment, and referrals. All persons who use alcohol, especially pregnant women, should be encouraged to limit their consumption, and all persons who use alcohol or other intoxicating drugs should be counseled about the dangers of operating a motor vehicle or performing other potentially dangerous activities while intoxicated.

48. Counseling to Prevent Tobacco Use

Recommendation. Tobacco cessation counseling should be offered on a regular basis to all patients who smoke cigarettes, pipes, or cigars and to those who use smokeless tobacco. The prescription of nicotine gum may be an appropriate adjunct for some patients. Adolescents and young adults who do not currently use tobacco products should be advised not to start.

49. Exercise Counseling

Recommendation. Clinicians should counsel all patients to engage in a program of regular physical activity, tailored to their health status and personal lifestyle.

50. Nutritional Counseling

Recommendation. Clinicians should provide periodic counseling regarding dietary intake of calories, fat (especially saturated fat), cholesterol, complex carbohydrates (starches), fiber, and sodium. Women and adolescent girls should receive counseling on calcium and iron intake, and pregnant women should receive specific information on nutritional guidelines during pregnancy. Parents should also be counseled about the nutritional requirements in infancy and early childhood.

51. Counseling to Prevent Motor Vehicle Injuries

Recommendation. All patients should be urged to use occupant restraints (safety belts and child safety seats) for themselves and others, to wear safety helmets when riding motorcycles, and to refrain from driving while under the influence of alcohol or other drugs.

52. Counseling to Prevent Household and Environmental Injuries

Recommendation. Patients who use alcohol or other drugs should be warned against engaging in potentially dangerous activities while intoxicated. It may also be clinically prudent to provide counseling on other measures to reduce the risk of unintentional household or environmental injuries from falls, drownings, fires or burns, poisoning, and firearms.

53. Counseling to Prevent Human Immunodeficiency Virus Infection and Other Sexually Transmitted Diseases

Recommendation. Clinicians should take a complete sexual and drug use history on all adolescent and adult patients. Sexually active patients should be advised that abstaining from sex or maintaining a mutually faithful monogamous sexual relationship with a partner known to be uninfected are the most effective strategies to prevent infection with human immunodeficiency virus or other sexually transmitted diseases. Patients should also receive counseling about the indications and proper methods for using condoms and spermicides in sexual intercourse and about the health risks associated with anal intercourse. Intravenous drug users should be encouraged to enroll in a drug treatment program and should be warned against sharing drug equipment or using unsterilized needles and syringes. All patients should be offered testing in accordance with recommendations on screening for syphilis, gonorrhea, chlamydia, genital herpes, hepatitis B, and infection with human immunodeficiency virus.

54. Counseling to Prevent Unintended Pregnancy

Recommendation. Clinicians should obtain a complete sexual history from all adolescent and adult patients. Sexually active women who do not want to become pregnant and men who do not want to have a child should receive detailed counseling on methods to prevent unintended pregnancy. Sexually active patients should also receive information on measures to prevent sexually transmitted diseases.

55. Counseling to Prevent Dental Disease

Recommendation. All patients should be encouraged to visit a dental care provider on a regular basis. Primary care clinicians should counsel patients regarding daily tooth brushing, dental flossing, the appropriate use of fluoride for caries prevention, avoiding sugary foods, and risk factors for developing baby bottle tooth decay. Children living in communities with inadequate water fluoridation should receive appropriate dietary fluoride supplements. While examining the mouth, clinicians should be alert for obvious signs of oral diseases.

56. Childhood Immunizations

Recommendation. All children without established contraindications should receive diphtheria-tetanus-pertusis (DTP), oral poliovirus (OPV), measles-mumps-rubella (MMR), and conjugate *Haemophilus influenzae* type b vaccines in accordance with recommended schedules. A tetanus-diphtheria (Td) booster should be administered between the ages of 14 and 16 years and every 10 years thereafter.

57. Adult Immunizations

Recommendation. Pneumococcal vaccine should be administered at least once and influenza vaccine should be administered annually to all persons aged 65 and older and to persons in selected high-risk groups. Hepatitis B vaccine should be offered to homosexually active men, intravenous drug users, and others at high risk for infection. All adults should receive tetanus-diphtheria toxoid boosters at least once every 10 years. Vaccination against measles and mumps should be provided to all adults who lack evidence of immunity.

58. Postexposure Prophylaxis

Recommendation. Postexposure prophylaxis should be provided to selected persons with exposures to *Haemophilus influenza* type b disease, meningococcal infection, hepatitis A, hepatitis B, tuberculosis, and rabies.

59. Estrogen Prophylaxis

Recommendation. Although routine postmenopausal estrogen replacement is not recommended, estrogen therapy should be considered for asymptomatic women who are at increased risk for osteoporosis, who lack known contraindications, and who have received adequate counseling about potential benefits and risks.

60. Aspirin Prophylaxis

Recommendation. Low-dose aspirin therapy should be considered for men aged 40 and over who are at significantly increased risk for myocardial infarction and who lack containdications to the drug. Patients should understand the potential benefits and risks of aspirin therapy before beginning treatment.

Table 1. BIRTH TO 18 MONTHS
Schedule: 2, 4, 6, 15, 18 Months*

Leading Causes of Death: Conditions originating in perinatal period
Congenital anomalies
Heart disease
Injuries (nonmotor vehicle)
Pneumonia/influenza

First Week: Ophthalmic antibiotics[1]
Hemoglobin electrophoresis (HR4)[1]
T4/TSH[2]
Phenylalanine[2]
Hearing (HR1)

Screening	Parent Counseling	Immunizations and Chemoprophylaxis
Height and weight Hemoglobin and hematocrit[3] HIGH-RISK GROUPS Hearing[4] (HR1) Erythrocyte protoporphyrin (HR2)	***Diet*** Breast-feeding Nutrient intake, especially iron-rich foods ***Injury Prevention*** Child safety seats Smoke detector Hot water heater temperature Stairway gates, window guards, pool fence Storage of drugs and toxic chemicals Syrup of ipecac, poison control telephone number ***Dental Health*** Baby bottle tooth decay ***Other Primary Preventive Measures*** Effects of passive smoking	Diphtheria-tetanus-pertussis (DTP) vaccine[5] Oral poliovirus vaccine (OPV)[6] Measles-mumps-rubella (MMR) vaccine[7] *Haemophilus influenzae* type b (Hib) conjugate vaccine[8] HIGH-RISK GROUPS Fluoride supplements (HR3)

Remain Alert For: Ocular misalignment
Tooth decay
Signs of child abuse or neglect

This list of preventive services is not exhaustive. It reflects only those topics reviewed by the U.S. Preventive Services Task Force. Clinicians may wish to add other preventive services on a routine basis, and after considering the patient's medical history and other individual circumstances. Examples of target conditions not specifically examined by the Task Force include:

Developmental disorders	Metabolic disorders
Musculoskeletal malformations	Speech problems
Cardiac anomalies	Behavioral disorders
Genitourinary disorders	Parent family dysfunction

*Five visits are required for immunizations. Because of lack of data and differing patient risk profiles, the scheduling of additional visits and the frequency of the individual preventive services listed in this table are left to clinical discretion (except as indicated in other footnotes).

1. At birth. 2. Days 3 to 6 preferred for testing. 3. Once during infancy. 4. At age 18-month visit, if not tested earlier. 5. At ages 2, 4, 6, and 15 months. 6. At ages 2, 4, and 15 months. 7. At age 15 months. 8. At age 18 months.

High-Risk Categories

HR1 Infants with a family history of childhood hearing impairment or a personal history of congenital perinatal infection with herpes, syphilis, rubella, cytomegalovirus, or toxoplasmosis; malformations involving the head or neck (e.g., dysmorphic and syndromal abnormalities, cleft palate, abnormal pinna); birthweight below 1500 g; bacterial meningitis; hyperbilirubinemia requiring exchange transfusion; or severe perinatal asphyxia (Apgar scores of 0 to 3, absence of spontaneous respirations for 10 minutes, or hypotonia at 2 hours of age).

HR2 Infants who live or frequently visit housing built before 1950 that is dilapidated or undergoing renovation; who come in contact with other children with known lead toxicity; who live near lead processing plants or whose parents or household members work in a lead-related occupation; or who live near busy highways or hazardous waste sites.

HR3 Infants living in areas with inadequate water fluoridation (less than 0.7 parts per million).

HR4 Newborns of Caribbean, Latin American, Asian, Mediterranean, or African descent.

Table 2. AGES 2–6
Schedule: See Footnote*

Leading Causes of Death: Injuries (nonmotor vehicle)
Motor vehicle crashes
Congenital anomalies
Homicide
Heart disease

Screening	Patient and Parent Counseling	Immunization and Chemoprophylaxis
Height and weight Blood pressure Eye examination for amblyopia and strabismus[1] Urinalysis for bacteriuria HIGH-RISK GROUPS Erythrocyte protoporphyrin[2] (HR1) Tuberculin skin test (PPD) (HR2) Hearing[3] (HR3)	***Diet and Exercise*** Sweets and between-meal snacks, iron-enriched foods, sodium Caloric balance Selection of exercise program ***Injury Prevention*** Safety belts Smoke detector Hot water heater temperature Window guards and pool fence Bicycle safety helmets Storage of drugs, toxic chemicals, matches, and firearms Syrup of ipecac, poison control telephone number ***Dental Health*** Tooth brushing and dental visits ***Other Primary Preventive Measures*** Effects of passive smoking HIGH-RISK GROUPS Skin protection from ultraviolet light (HR4)	Diphtheria-tetanus-pertussis (DTP) vaccine[4] Oral poliovirus vaccine (OPV)[4] HIGH-RISK GROUPS Fluoride supplements (HR5)

Remain Alert For: Vision disorders
Dental decay, malignment, premature loss of teeth, mouth breathing
Signs of child abuse or neglect
Abnormal bereavement

This list of preventive services is not exhaustive. It reflects only those topics reviewed by the U.S. Preventive Services Task Force. Clinicians may wish to add other preventive services on a routine basis, and after considering the patient's medical history and other individual circumstances. Examples of target conditions not specifically examined by the Task Force include:

Developmental disorders	Behavioral and learning disorders
Speech problems	Parent/family dysfunction

*One visit is required for immunizations. Because of lack of data and differing patient risk profiles, the scheduling of additional visits and the frequency of the individual preventive services listed in this table are left to clinical discretion (except as indicated in other footnotes).

1. Ages 3–4. 2. Annually. 3. Before age 3, if not tested earlier. 4. Once between ages 4 and 6.

High-Risk Categories

HR1 Children who live in or frequently visit housing built before 1950 that is dilapidated or undergoing renovation; who come in contact with other children with known lead toxicity; who live near lead processing plants or whose parents or household members work in a lead-related occupation; or who live near busy highways or hazardous waste sites.

HR2 Household members of persons with tuberculosis or others at risk for close contact with the disease; recent immigrants or refugees from countries in which tuberculosis is common (e.g., Asia, Africa, Central and South America, Pacific Islands); family members of migrant workers; residents of homeless shelters; or persons with certain underlying medical disorders.

HR3 Children with a family history of childhood hearing impairment or a personal history of congenital perinatal infection with herpes, syphilis, rubella, cytomegalovirus, or toxoplasmosis; malformations involving the head or neck (e.g., dysmorphic and syndromal abnormalities, cleft palate, abnormal pinna); birthweight below 1500 g; bacterial meningitis; hyperbilirubinemia requiring exchange transfusion; or severe perinatal asphyxia (Apgar scores of 0–3, absence of spontaneous respirations for 10 minutes, or hypotonia at 2 hours of age).

HR4 Children with increased exposure to sunlight.

HR5 Children living in areas with inadequate water fluoridation (less than 0.7 parts per million).

Table 3. AGES 7–12
Schedule: See Footnote*

Leading Causes of Death: Motor vehicle crashes
Injuries (nonmotor vehicle)
Congenital anomalies
Leukemia
Homicide
Heart disease

Screening	Patient and Parent Counseling	Chemoprophylaxis
Height and weight Blood pressure HIGH-RISK GROUPS Tuberculin skin test (PPD) (HR1)	***Diet and Exercise*** Fat (especially saturated fat), cholesterol, sweets and between-meal snacks, sodium Caloric balance Selection of exercise program ***Injury Prevention*** Safety belts Smoke detector Storage of firearms, drugs, toxic chemicals, matches Bicycle safety helmets ***Dental Health*** Regular tooth brushing and dental visits ***Other Primary Preventive Measures*** HIGH-RISK GROUPS Skin protection from ultraviolet light (HR2)	HIGH-RISK GROUPS Fluoride supplements (HR3)

Remain Alert For: Vision disorders
Diminished hearing
Dental decay, malalignment, mouth breathing
Signs of child abuse or neglect
Abnormal bereavement

This list of preventive services is not exhaustive. It reflects only those topics reviewed by the U.S. Preventive Services Task Force. Clinicians may wish to add other preventive services on a routine basis, and after considering the patient's medical history and other individual circumstances. Examples of target conditions not specifically examined by the Task Force include:

Developmental disorders	Behavioral and learning disorders
Scoliosis	Parent/family dysfunction

*Because of lack of data and differing patient risk profiles, the scheduling of visits and the frequency of the individual preventive services listed in this table are left to clinical discretion.

High-Risk Categories

HR1 Household members of persons with tuberculosis or others at risk for close contact with the disease; recent immigrants of refugees from countries in which tuberculosis is common (e.g., Asia, Africa, Central and South America, Pacific Islands); family members of migrant workers; residents of homeless shelters; or persons with certain underlying medical disorders.

HR2 Children with increased exposure to sunlight.

HR3 Children living in areas with inadequate water fluoridation (less than 0.7 parts per million).

Table 4. AGES 13–18
Schedule: See Footnote*

Leading Causes of Death: Motor vehicle crashes
Homicide
Suicide
Injuries (nonmotor vehicle)
Heart disease

Screening

History
Dietary intake
Physical activity
Tobacco/alcohol/drug use
Sexual practices

Physical Examination
Height and weight
Blood pressure
HIGH-RISK GROUPS
Complete skin examination (HR1)
Clinical testicular examination (HR2)

Laboratory/Diagnostic Procedures
HIGH-RISK GROUPS
Rubella antibodies (HR3)
VDRL/RPR (HR4)
Chlamydial testing (HR5)
Gonorrhea culture (HR6)
Counseling and testing for HIV (HR7)
Tuberculin skin test (PPD) (HR8)
Hearing (HR9)
Papanicolaou smear (HR10)[1]

Counseling

Diet and Exercise
Fat (especially saturated fat), cholesterol, sodium, iron,[2] calcium[2]
Caloric balance
Selection of exercise program

Substance Use
Tobacco: cessation/primary prevention
Alcohol and other drugs: cessation/primary prevention
Driving/other dangerous activities while under the influence
Treatment for abuse
HIGH-RISK GROUPS
Sharing/using unsterilized needles and syringes (HR12)

Sexual Practices
Sexual development and behavior[3]
Sexually transmitted disease: partner selection, condoms
Unintended pregnancy and contraceptive options

Injury Prevention
Safety belts
Safety helmets
Violent behavior[4]
Firearms[4]
Smoke detector

Dental Health
Regular tooth brushing, flossing, dental visits

Other Primary Preventive Measures
HIGH-RISK GROUPS
Discussion of hemoglobin testing (HR13)
Skin protection from ultraviolet light (HR14)

Immunizations and Chemoprophylaxis

Tetanus diphtheria (Td) booster[5]
HIGH-RISK GROUPS
Fluoride supplements (HR15)

Table 4. AGES 13–18 *Continued*
Schedule: See Footnote*

Remain Alert For:	Depressive symptoms Suicide risk factors (HR11) Abnormal bereavement Tooth decay, malalignment, gingivitis Signs of child abuse and neglect

This list of preventive services is not exhaustive. It reflects only those topics reviewed by the U.S. Preventive Services Task Force. Clinicians may wish to add other preventive services on a routine basis, and after considering the patient's medical history and other individual circumstances. Examples of target conditions not specifically examined by the Task Force include:

Developmental disorders	Behavioral and learning disorders
Scoliosis	Parent / family dysfunction

*One visit is required for immunizations. Because of lack of data and differing patient risk profiles, the scheduling of additional visits and the frequency of the individual preventive services listed in this table are left to clinical discretion (except as indicated in other footnotes).

1. Every 1–3 years. 2. For females. 3. Often best performed early in adolescence and with the involvement of parents. 4. Especially for males. 5. Once between ages 14 and 16.

High-Risk Categories

HR1 Persons with increased recreational or occupational exposure to sunlight, a family or personal history of skin cancer, or clinical evidence of precursor lesions (e.g., dysplastic nevi, certain congenital nevi).

HR2 Males with a history of cryptorchidism, orchiopexy, or testicular atrophy.

HR3 Females of childbearing age lacking evidence of immunity.

HR4 Persons who engage in sex with multiple partners in areas in which syphilis is prevalent, prostitutes, or contacts of persons with active syphilis.

HR5 Persons who attend clinics for sexually transmitted diseases; attend other high-risk health care facilities (e.g., adolescent and family planning clinics); or have other risk factors for chlamydial infection (e.g., multiple sexual partners or a sexual partner with multiple sexual contacts).

HR6 Persons with multiple sexual partners or a sexual partner with multiple contacts, sexual contacts of persons with culture-proven gonorrhea, or persons with a history of repeated episodes of gonorrhea.

HR7 Persons seeking treatment for sexually transmitted diseases; homosexual and bisexual men; past or present intravenous (IV) drug users; persons with a history of prostitution or multiple sexual partners; women whose past or present sexual partners were HIV-infected, bisexual, or IV drug users; persons with long-term residence or birth in an area with high prevalence of HIV infection; or persons with a history of transfusion between 1978 and 1985.

HR8 Household members of persons with tuberculosis or others at risk for close contact with the disease; recent immigrants or refugees from countries in which tuberculosis is common (e.g., Asia, Africa, Central and South America, Pacific Islands); migrant workers; residents of correctional institutions or homeless shelters; or persons with certain underlying medical disorders.

HR9 Persons exposed regularly to excessive noise in recreational or other settings.

HR10 Females who are sexually active or (if the sexual history is thought to be unreliable) aged 18 or older.

HR11 Recent divorce, separation, unemployment, depression, alcohol or other drug abuse, serious medical illnesses, living alone, or recent bereavement.

HR12 Intravenous drug users.

HR13 Persons of Caribbean, Latin American, Asian, Mediterranean, or African descent.

HR14 Persons with increased exposure to sunlight.

HR15 Persons living in areas with inadequate water fluoridation (less than 0.7 parts per million).

Table 5. AGES 19–39
Schedule: Every 1–3 Years*

Leading Causes of Death:	
	Motor vehicle crashes Homicide Suicide Injuries (nonmotor vehicle) Heart disease

Screening

History
- Dietary intake
- Physical activity
- Tobacco/alcohol/drug use
- Sexual practices

Physical Examination
- Height and weight
- Blood pressure
- HIGH-RISK GROUPS
  - Complete oral cavity examination (HR1)
  - Palpation for thyroid nodules (HR2)
  - Clinical breast examination (HR3)
  - Clinical testicular examination (HR4)
  - Complete skin examination(HR5)

Laboratory/Diagnostic Procedures
- Nonfasting total blood cholesterol
- Papanicolaou smear[1]
- HIGH-RISK GROUPS
  - Fasting plasma glucose (HR6)
  - Rubella antibodies (HR7)
  - VDRL/RPR (HR8)
  - Urinalysis for bacteriuria (HR9)
  - Chlamydial testing (HR10)
  - Gonorrhea culture (HR11)
  - Counseling and testing for HIV (HR12)
  - Hearing (HR13)
  - Tuberculin skin test (PPD) (HR14)
  - Electrocardiogram (HR15)
  - Mammogram (HR3)
  - Colonoscopy (HR16)

Counseling

Diet and Exercise
- Fat (especially saturated fat), cholesterol, complex carbohydrates, fiber, sodium, iron[2], calcium[2]
- Caloric balance
- Selection of exercise program

Substance Use
- Tobacco: cessation/primary prevention
- Alcohol and other drugs:
  - Limiting alcohol consumption
  - Driving/other dangerous activities while under the influence
  - Treatment for abuse
- HIGH-RISK GROUPS
  - Sharing/using unsterilized needles and syringes (HR18)

Sexual Practices
- Sexually transmitted diseases: partner selection, condoms, anal intercourse
- Unintended pregnancy and contraceptive options

Injury Prevention
- Safety belts
- Safety helmets
- Violent behavior[3]
- Firearms[3]
- Smoke detector
- Smoking near bedding or upholstery
- HIGH-RISK GROUPS
  - Back-conditioning exercises (HR19)
  - Prevention of childhood injuries (HR20)
  - Falls in the elderly (HR21)

Dental Health
- Regular tooth brushing, flossing, dental visits

Other Primary Preventive Measures
- HIGH-RISK GROUPS
  - Discussion of hemoglobin testing (HR22)
  - Skin protection from ultraviolet light (HR23)

Immunizations

- Tetanus-diphtheria (Td) booster[4]
- HIGH-RISK GROUPS
  - Hepatitis B vaccine (HR24)
  - Pneumococcal vaccine (HR25)
  - Influenza vaccine[5] (HR26)
  - Measles-mumps-rubella vaccine (HR27)

Table 5. AGES 19–39 *Continued*
Schedule: Every 1–3 Years*

Remain Alert For:	Depressive symptoms Suicide risk factor (HR17) Abnormal bereavement Malignant skin lesions Tooth decay, gingivits Signs of physical abuse

This list of preventive services is not exhaustive. It reflects only those topics reviewed by the U.S. Preventive Services Task Force. Clinicians may wish to add other preventive services on a routine basis, and after considering the patient's medical history and other individual circumstances. Examples of target conditions not specifically examined by the Task Force include:

- Chronic obstructive pulmonary disease
- Hepatobiliary disease
- Bladder cancer
- Endometrial disease
- Travel-related illness
- Prescription drug abuse
- Occupational illness and injuries

*The recommended schedule applies only to the periodic visit itself. The frequency of the individual preventive services listed in this table is left to clinical discretion, except as indicated in other footnotes.

1. Every 1–3 years. 2. For women. 3. Especially for young males. 4. Every 10 years. 5. Annually.

High-Risk Categories

HR1 Persons with exposure to tobacco or excessive amounts of alcohol, or those with suspicious symptoms or lesions detected through self-examination.

HR2 Persons with a history of upper-body irradiation.

HR3 Women aged 35 and older with a family history of premenopausally diagnosed breast cancer in a first-degree relative.

HR4 Men with a history of cryptorchidism, orchiopexy, or testicular atrophy.

HR5 Persons with family or personal history of skin cancer, increased occupational or recreational exposure to sunlight, or clinical evidence of precursor lesions (e.g., dysplastic nevi, certain congenital nevi).

HR6 Markedly obese, persons with a family history of diabetes, or women with a history of gestational diabetes.

HR7 Women lacking evidence of immunity.

HR8 Prostitutes, persons who engage in sex with multiple partners in areas in which syphilis is prevalent, or contacts of persons with active syphilis.

HR9 Persons with diabetes.

HR10 Persons who attend clinics for sexually transmitted diseases; attend other high-risk health care facilities (e.g., adolescent and family planning clinics); or have other risk factors for chlamydial infection (e.g., multiple sexual partners or a sexual partner with multiple sexual contacts, age less than 20).

HR11 Prostitutes, persons with multiple sexual partners or a sexual partner with multiple contacts, sexual contacts of persons with culture-proven gonorrhea, or persons with a history of repeated episodes of gonorrhea.

HR12 Persons seeking treatment for sexually transmitted diseases; homosexual and bisexual men; past or present intravenous (IV) drug users; persons with a history of prostitution or multiple sexual partners; women whose past or present sexual partners were HIV-infected, bisexual, or IV drug users; persons with long-term residence or birth in an area with high prevalence of HIV infection; or persons with a history of transfusion between 1978 and 1985.

HR13 Persons exposed regularly to excessive noise.

HR14 Household members of persons with tuberculosis or others at risk for close contact with the disease (e.g., staff of tuberculosis clinics, shelters for the homeless, nursing homes, substance abuse treatment facilities, dialysis units, correctional institutions); recent immigrants or refugees from countries in which tuberculosis is common; migrant workers; residents of nursing homes, correctional institutions, or homeless shelters; or persons with certain underlying medical disorders (e.g., HIV infection).

HR15 Men who would endanger public safety were they to experience sudden cardiac events (e.g., commercial airline pilots).

HR16 Persons with a family history of familial polyposis coli or cancer family syndrome.

HR17 Recent divorce, separation, unemployment, depression, alcohol or other drug abuse, serious medical illnesses, living alone, or recent bereavement.

HR18 Intravenous drug users.

HR19 Persons at increased risk for low back injury because of past history, body configuration, or type of activities.

HR20 Persons with children in the home or automobile.

HR21 Persons with older adults in the home.

HR22 Young adults of Caribbean, Latin American, Asian, Mediterranean, or African descent.

HR23 Persons with increased exposure to sunlight.

HR24 Homosexually active men, intravenous drug users, recipients of some blood products, or persons in health-related jobs with frequent exposure to blood or blood products.

HR25 Persons with medical conditions that increase the risk of pneumococcal infection (e.g., chronic cardiac or pulmonary disease, sickle cell disease, nephrotic syndrome, Hodgkin's disease, asplenia, diabetes mellitus, alcoholism, cirrhosis, multiple myeloma, renal disease, or conditions associated with immunosuppression).

HR26 Residents of chronic care facilities or persons suffering from chronic cardiopulmonary disorders, metabolic diseases (including diabetes mellitus), hemoglobinopathies, immunosuppression, or renal dysfunction.

HR27 Persons born after 1956 who lack evidence of immunity to measles (receipt of live vaccine on or after birthday, laboratory evidence of immunity, or a history of physician-diagnosed measles).

Table 6. AGES 40–64
Schedule: Every 1–3 Years*

Leading Causes of Death: Heart disease
Lung cancer
Cerebrovascular disease
Breast cancer
Colorectal cancer
Obstructive lung disease

Screening

History
Dietary intake
Physical activity
Tobacco/alcohol/drug use
Sexual practices

Physical Examination
Height and weight
Blood pressure
Clinical breast examination[1]
HIGH-RISK GROUPS
- Complete skin examination (HR1)
- Complete oral cavity examination (HR2)
- Palpation for thyroid nodules (HR3)
- Auscultation for carotid bruits (HR4)

Laboratory/Diagnostic Procedures
Nonfasting total blood cholesterol
Papanicolaou smear[2]
Mammogram[3]
HIGH-RISK GROUPS
- Fasting plasma glucose (HR5)
- VDRL/RPR (HR6)
- Urinalysis for bacteriuria (HR7)
- Chlamydial testing (HR8)
- Gonorrhea culture (HR9)
- Counseling and testing for HIV (HR10)
- tuberculin skin test (PPD) (HR11)
- Hearing (HR12)
- Electrocardiogram (HR13)
- Fecal occult blood/sigmoidoscopy (HR14)
- Fecal occult blood/colonoscopy (HR15)
- Bone mineral content (HR16)

Counseling

Diet and Exercise
Fat (especially saturated fat), cholesterol, complex carbohydrates, fiber, sodium calcium[4]
Caloric balance
Selection of exercise program

Substance Use
Tobacco cessation
Alcohol and other drugs:
- Limiting alcohol consumption
- Driving/other dangerous activities while under the influence
- Treatment for abuse

HIGH-RISK GROUPS
- Sharing/using unsterilized needles and syringes (HR19)

Sexual Practices
Sexually transmitted diseases; partner selection, condoms, anal intercourse
Unintended pregnancy and contraceptive options

Injury Prevention
Safety belts
Safety helmets
Smoke detector
Smoking near bedding or upholstery
HIGH-RISK GROUPS
- Back-conditioning exercises (HR20)
- Prevention of childhood injuries (HR21)
- Falls in the elderly (HR22)

Dental Health
Regular tooth brushing, flossing, and dental visits

Other Primary Preventive Measures
HIGH-RISK GROUPS
- Skin protection from ultraviolet light (HR23)
- Discussion of aspirin therapy (HR24)
- Discussion of estrogen replacement therapy (HR25)

Immunizations

Tetanus-diphtheria (Td) booster[5]
HIGH-RISK GROUPS
- Hepatitis B vaccine (HR26)
- Pneumococcal vaccine (HR27)
- Influenza vaccine (HR28)[6]

Remain Alert For: Depressive symptoms
Suicide risk factors (HR17)
Abnormal bereavement
Signs of physical abuse or neglect
Malignant skin lesions
Peripheral arterial disease (HR18)
Tooth decay, gingivitis, loose teeth

Table 6. AGES 40–64 *Continued*
Schedule: Every 1–3 Years*

This list of preventive services is not exhaustive. It reflects only those topics reviewed by the U.S. Preventive Services Task Force. Clinicians may wish to add other preventive services on a routine basis, and after considering the patient's medical history and other individual circumstances. Examples of target conditions not specifically examined by the Task Force include:

Chronic obstructive pulmonary disease	Travel-related illness
Hepatobiliary disease	Prescription drug abuse
Bladder cancer	Occupational illness and injuries
Endometrial disease	

*The recommended schedule applies only to the periodic visit itself. The frequency of the individual preventive services listed in this table is left to clinical discretion, except as indicated in other footnotes.

1. Annually for women. 2. Every 1 to 3 years for women. 3. Every 1–2 years for women beginning at age 50 (age 35 for those at increased risk). 4. For women. 5. Every 10 years. 6. Annually.

High-Risk Categories

HR1 Persons with a family or personal history of skin cancer, increased occupational or recreational exposure to sunlight, or clinical evidence of precursor lesions (e.g., dysplastic nevi, certain congenital nevi).

HR2 Persons with exposure to tobacco or excessive amounts of alcohol, or those with suspicious symptoms or lesions detected through self-examination.

HR3 Persons with a history of upper-body irradiation.

HR4 Persons with risk factors for cerebrovascular or cardiovascular disease (e.g., hypertension, smoking, CAD, atrial fibrillation, diabetes) or those with neurologic symptoms (e.g., transient ischemic attacks) or a history of cerebrovascular disease.

HR5 Markedly obese persons with a family history of diabetes, or women with a history of gestational diabetes.

HR6 Prostitutes, persons who engage in sex with multiple partners in areas in which syphilis is prevalent, or contacts of persons with active syphilis.

HR7 Persons with diabetes.

HR8 Persons who attend clinics for sexually transmitted diseases, attend other high-risk health care facilities (e.g., adolescent and family planning clinics), or have other risk factors for chlamydial infection (e.g., multiple sexual partners or a sexual partner with multiple sexual contacts).

HR9 Prostitutes, persons with multiple sexual partners or a sexual partner with multiple contacts, sexual contacts of persons with culture-proven gonorrhea, or persons with a history of repeated episodes of gonorrhea.

HR10 Persons seeking treatment for sexually transmitted diseases; homosexual and bisexual men; past or present intravenous (IV) drug users; persons with a history of prostitution or multiple sexual partners; women whose past or present sexual partners were HIV-infected, bisexual, or IV drug users; persons with long-term residence or birth in an area with high prevalence of HIV infection; or persons with a history of transfusion between 1978 and 1985.

HR11 Household members of persons with tuberculosis or others at risk for close contact with the disease (e.g., staff of tuberculosis clinics, shelters for the homeless, nursing homes, substance abuse treatment facilities, dialysis units, correctional institutions); recent immigrants or refugees from countries in which tuberculosis is common (e.g., Asia, Africa, Central and South America, Pacific Islands); migrant workers; residents of nursing homes, correctional institutions, or homeless shelters; or persons with certain underlying medical disorders (e.g., HIV infection).

HR12 Persons exposed regularly to excessive noise.

HR13 Men with two or more cardiac risk factors (high blood cholesterol, hypertension, cigarette smoking, diabetes mellitus, family history of CAD); men who would endanger public safety were they to experience sudden cardiac events (e.g., commercial airline pilots); or sedentary or high-risk males planning to begin a vigorous exercise program.

HR14 Persons aged 50 and older who have first-degree relatives with colorectal cancer; a personal history of endometrial, ovarian, or breast cancer; or a previous diagnosis of inflammatory bowel disease, adenomatous polyps, or colorectal cancer.

HR15 Persons with a family history of familial polyposis coli or cancer family syndrome.

HR16 Perimenopausal women at increased risk for osteoporosis (e.g., Caucasian race, bilateral oophorectomy before menopause, slender build) and for whom estrogen replacement therapy would otherwise not be recommended.

HR17 Recent divorce, separation, unemployment, depression, alcohol or other drug abuse, serious medical illnesses, living alone, or recent bereavement.

HR18 Persons over age 50, smokers, or persons with diabetes mellitus.

HR19 Intravenous drug users.

HR20 Persons at increased risk for low back injury because of past history, body configuration, or type of activities.

HR21 Persons with children in the home or automobile.

HR22 Persons with older adults in the home.

HR23 Persons with increased exposure to sunlight.

HR24 Men who have risk factors for myocardial infarction (e.g., high blood cholesterol, smoking, diabetes mellitus, family history of early-onset CAD) and who lack a history of gastrointestinal or other bleeding problems, and other risk factors for bleeding or cerebral hemorrhage.

HR25 Perimenopausal women at increased risk for osteoporosis (e.g., Caucasian, low bone mineral content, bilateral oopherectomy before menopause or early menopause, slender build) and who are without known contraindications (e.g., history of undiagnosed vaginal bleeding, active liver disease, thromboembolic disorders, hormone-dependent cancer).

HR26 Homosexually active men, intravenous drug users, recipients of some blood products, or persons in health-related jobs with frequent exposure to blood or blood products.

HR27 Persons with medical conditions that increase the risk of pneumococcal infection (e.g., chronic cardiac or pulmonary disease, sickle cell disease, nephrotic syndrome, Hodgkin's disease, asplenia, diabetes mellitus, alcoholism, cirrhosis, multiple myeloma, renal disease or conditions associated with immunosuppression).

HR28 Residents of chronic care facilities and persons suffering from chronic cardiopulmonary disorders, metabolic diseases (including diabetes mellitus), hemoglobinopathies, immunosuppression, or renal dysfunction.

Table 7. AGES 65 and Over
Schedule: Every Year*

Leading Causes of Death: Heart disease
Cerebrovascular disease
Obstructive lung disease
Pneumonia/influenza
Lung cancer
Colorectal cancer

Screening

History
Prior symptoms of transient ischemic attack
Dietary intake
Physical activity
Tobacco/alcohol/drug use
Functional status at home

Physical Examination
Height and weight
Blood pressure
Visual acuity
Hearing and hearing aids
Clinical breast examination[1]
HIGH-RISK GROUPS
- Auscultation for carotid bruits (HR1)
- Complete skin examination (HR2)
- Complete oral cavity examination (HR3)
- Palpation of thyroid nodules (HR4)

Laboratory/Diagnostic Procedures
Nonfasting total blood cholesterol
Dipstick urinalysis
Mammogram[2]
Thyroid function tests[3]
HIGH-RISK GROUPS
- Fasting plasma glucose (HR5)
- Tuberculin skin test (PPD) (HR6)
- Electrocardiogram (HR7)
- Papanicolaou smear[4] (HR8)
- Fecal occult blood/Sigmoidoscopy (HR9)
- Fecal occult blood/Colonoscopy (HR10)

Counseling

Diet and Exercise
Fat (especially saturated fat), cholesterol, complex carbohydrates, fiber, sodium, calcium[3]
Caloric balance
Selection of exercise program

Substance Use
Tobacco cessation
Alcohol and other drugs:
- Limiting alcohol consumption
- Driving/other dangerous activities while under the influence
- Treatment for abuse

Injury Prevention
Prevention of falls
Safety belts
Smoke detector
Smoking near bedding or upholstery
Hot water heater temperature
Safety helmets
HIGH-RISK GROUPS
- Prevention of childhood injuries (HR12)

Dental Health
Regular dental visits, tooth brushing, flossing

Other Primary Preventive Measures
Glaucoma testing by eye specialist
HIGH-RISK GROUPS
- Discussion of estrogen replacement therapy (HR13)
- Discussion of aspirin therapy (HR14)
- Skin protection from ultraviolet light (HR15)

Immunizations

Tetanus-diphtheria (Td) booster[5]
Influenza vaccine[1]
Pneumococcal vaccine
HIGH-RISK GROUPS
- Hepatitis B vaccine (HR16)

Table 7. AGES 65 and Over
Schedule: Every Year*

Remain Alert For:	Depression symptoms Suicide risk factors (HR11) Abnormal bereavement Changes in cognitive function Medications that increase risk of falls Signs of physical abuse or neglect Malignant skin lesions Peripheral arterial disease Tooth decay, gingivitis, loose teeth

This list of preventive services is not exhaustive. It reflects only those topics reviewed by the U.S. Preventive Services Task Force. Clinicians may wish to add other preventive services on a routine basis, and after considering the patient's medical history and other individual circumstances. Examples of target conditions not specifically examined by the Task Force include:

- Chronic obstructive pulmonary disease
- Hepatobiliary disease
- Bladder cancer
- Endometrial disease
- Travel-related illness
- Prescription drug abuse
- Occupational illness and injuries

*The recommended schedule applies only to the periodic visit itself. The frequency of the individual preventive services listed in this table is left to clinical discretion, except as indicated in other footnotes.

1. Annually. 2. Every 1 to 2 years for women until age 75, unless pathology detected. 3. For women. 4. Every 1 to 3 years. 5. Every 10 years.

High-Risk Categories

HR1 Persons with risk factors for cerebrovascular or cardiovascular disease (e.g., hypertension, smoking, CAD, atrial fibrillation, diabetes) or those with neurologic symptoms (e.g., transient ischemic attacks) or a history of cerebrovascular disease.

HR2 Persons with a family or personal history of skin cancer, or clinical evidence of precursor lesions (e.g., dysplastic nevi, certain congenital nevi), or those with increased occupational or recreational exposure to sunlight.

HR3 Persons with exposure to tobacco or excessive amounts of alcohol, or those with suspicious symptoms or lesions detected through self-examination.

HR4 Persons with a history of upper-body irradiation.

HR5 Markedly obese persons with a family history of diabetes, or women with a history of gestational diabetes.

HR6 Household members of persons with tuberculosis or others at risk for close contact with the disease (e.g., staff of tuberculosis clinics, shelters for the homeless, nursing homes, substance abuse treatment facilities, dialysis units, correctional institutions); recent immigrants or refugees from countries in which tuberculosis is common (e.g., Asia, Africa, Central and South America, Pacific Islands); migrant workers; residents of nursing homes, correctional institutions, or homeless shelters; or persons with certain underlying medical disorders (e.g., HIV infection).

HR7 Men with two or more cardiac risk factors (high blood cholesterol, hypertension, cigarette smoking, diabetes mellitus, family history of CAD); men who would endanger public safety were they to experience sudden cardiac events (e.g., commercial airline pilots); or sedentary or high-risk males planning to begin a vigorous exercise program.

HR8 Women who have not had previous documented screening in which smears have been consistently negative.

HR9 Persons who have first-degree relatives with colorectal cancer; a personal history of endometrial, ovarian, or breast cancer; or a previous diagnosis of inflammatory bowel disease, adenomatous polyps, or colorectal cancer.

HR10 Persons with a family history of familial polyposis coli or cancer family syndrome.

HR11 Recent divorce, separation, unemployment, depression, alcohol or other drug abuse, serious medical illnesses, living alone, or recent bereavement.

HR12 Persons with children in the home or automobile.

HR13 Women at increased risk for osteoporosis (e.g., Caucasian, low bone mineral content, bilateral oopherectomy before menopause or early menopause, slender build) and who are without known contraindications (e.g., history of undiagnosed vaginal bleeding, active liver disease, thromboembolic disorders, hormone-dependent cancer).

HR14 Men who have risk factors for myocardial infarction (e.g., high blood cholesterol, smoking, diabetes mellitus, family history of early-onset CAD) and who lack a history of gastrointestinal or other bleeding problems, or other risk factors for bleeding or cerebral hemorrhage.

HR15 Persons with increased exposure to sunlight.

HR16 Homosexually active men, intravenous drug users, recipients of some blood products, or persons in health-related jobs with frequent exposure to blood or blood products.

Table 8. PREGNANT WOMEN[1]

First Prenatal Visit

Screening

History
Genetic and obstetric history
Dietary intake
Tobacco/alcohol/drug use
Risk factors for intrauterine growth retardation and low birth-weight
Prior genital herpetic lesions

Laboratory/Diagnostic Procedures
Blood pressure
Hemoglobin and hematocrit
ABO/Rh typing
Rh(D) and other antibody screen
VDRL/RPR
Hepatitis B surface antigen (HBsAg)
Urinalysis for bacteriuria
Gonorrhea culture
HIGH-RISK GROUPS
- Hemoglobin electrophoresis (HR1)
- Rubella antibodies (HR2)
- Chlamydial testing (HR3)
- Counseling and testing for HIV (HR4)

Counseling

Nutrition
Tobacco use
Alcohol and other drug use
Safety belts
HIGH-RISK GROUPS
- Discuss amniocentesis (HR5)
- Discuss risks of HIV infection (HR4)

Remain Alert for: Signs of physical abuse

This list of preventive services is not exhaustive. It reflects only those topics reviewed by the U.S. Preventive Services Task Force. Clinicians may wish to add other preventive services on a routine basis, and after considering the patient's medical history and other individual circumstances. Examples of target conditions not specifically examined by the Task Force include:
- Counseling on warning signs and symptoms
- Physical findings of abdominal and cervical examination
- Tay-Sachs disease
- Childbirth education
- Teratogenic and fetotoxic exposures

Table 8. PREGNANT WOMEN[1] *Continued*

Follow-Up Visits
Schedule: See Footnote*

Screening
Blood pressure
Urinalysis for bacteriuria

Screening Tests at Specific Gestational Ages

14–16 Weeks:
Maternal serum alpha-fetoprotein (MSAFP)[2]
Ultrasound cephalometry (HR8)

24–28 Weeks:
50 g oral glucose tolerance test
Rh(d) antibody (HR9)
Gonorrhea culture (HR10)
VDRL/RPR (HR11)
Hepatitis B surface antigen (HBsAg) (HR12)
Counseling and testing for HIV (HR13)

36 Weeks:
Ultrasound examination (HR14)

Counseling

Nutrition
Safety belts
Discuss meaning of upcoming tests
HIGH-RISK GROUPS
Tobacco use (HR6)
Alcohol and other drug use (HR7)

*Because of lack of data and differing patient risk profiles, the scheduling of visits and the frequency of the individual preventive services listed in this table are left to clinical discretion, except for those indicated at specific gestational ages.

1. See also Tables 4 to 6 for other preventive services for women. 2. Women with access to counseling and follow-up services, skilled high-resolution ultrasound and amniocentesis capabilities, and reliable, standardized laboratories.

High-Risk Categories

HR1 Black women.

HR2 Women lacking evidence of immunity (proof of vaccination after the first birthday or laboratory evidence of immunity.)

HR3 Women who attend clinics for sexually transmitted diseases, attend other high-risk health care facilities (e.g., adolescent and family planning clinics), or have other risk factors for chlamydial infection (e.g., multiple sexual partners or a sexual partner with multiple sexual contacts).

HR4 Women seeking treatment for sexually transmitted diseases; past or present intravenous (IV) drug users; women with a history of prostitution or multiple sexual partners; women whose past or present sexual partners were HIV-infected, bisexual, or IV drug users; women with long-term residence or birth in an area with high prevalence of HIV infection in women; or women with a history of transfusion between 1978 and 1985.

HR5 Women aged 35 and older.

HR6 Women who continue to smoke during pregnancy.

HR7 Women with excessive alcohol consumption during pregnancy.

HR8 Women with uncertain menstrual histories or risk factors for intrauterine growth retardation (e.g., hypertension, renal disease; short maternal stature; low prepregnancy weight; failure to gain weight during pregnancy; smoking, alcohol and other drug abuse; and history of a previous fetal death or growth-retarded baby).

HR9 Unsensitized Rh-negative women.

HR10 Women with multiple sexual partners or a sexual partner with multiple contacts, or sexual contacts of persons with culture-proven gonorrhea.

HR11 Women who engage in sex with multiple partners in areas in which syphilis is prevalent, or contacts of persons with active syphilis.

HR12 Women who engage in high-risk behavior (e.g., intravenous drug use) or in whom exposure to hepatitis B during pregnancy is suspected.

HR13 Women at high risk (see HR4) who have a nonreactive HIV test at the first prenatal visit.

HR14 Women with risk factors for intrauterine growth retardation (see HRB).

Index

Note: Page numbers in *italics* refer to illustrations; page numbers followed by t refer to tables.